Mucosal Immunology

Mucosal Immunology

Third Edition

Edited by

Jiri Mestecky
Professor of Microbiology and Medicine
Department of Microbiology
The University of Alabama at Birmingham
Birmingham, Alabama

John Bienenstock
University Professor
McMaster University
Hamilton, Ontario
Canada

Michael E. Lamm
Joseph R. Kahn Professor of Pathology
Case Western Reserve University
School of Medicine
Cleveland, Ohio

Lloyd Mayer
Professor and Chairman
Immunology Center
Dorothy and David Merksamer Professor
    of Medicine
Mount Sinai Medical Center
New York, New York

Jerry R. McGhee
Professor of Microbiology
Department of Microbiology
The University of Alabama at Birmingham
Birmingham, Alabama

Warren Strober
Chief, Mucosal Immunity Section
Laboratory of Clinical Investigation
National Institute of Allergy and Infectious
    Diseases
National Institutes of Health
Bethesda, Maryland

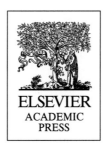

ELSEVIER
ACADEMIC
PRESS

Amsterdam • Boston • Heidelberg • London
New York • Oxford • Paris • San Diego
San Francisco • Singapore • Sydney • Tokyo

ELSEVIER
ACADEMIC
PRESS

30 Corporate Drive, Suite 400, Burlington, MA 01803, USA
525 B Street, Suite 1900, San Diego, CA 92101-4495, USA
84 Theobald's Road, London WC1X 8RR, UK

This book is printed on acid-free paper.

Library of Congress Cataloging-in-Publication Data

Mucosal immunology / edited by Jiri Mestecky ... [et al.].–3rd ed.
   p. ; cm.
  Includes bibliographical references and index.
  ISBN 0-12-491543-4 (set) – ISBN 0-12-491544-2 (v. 1)–ISBN 0-12-491545-0 (v. 2)
  1. Mucous membrane–Immunology. I. Mestecky, Jiri, 1941-
  [DNLM: 1. Mucous Membrane–immunology. 2. Immunity, Mucosal–physiology. QS
  532.5.M8 H236 2004]
  QR185.9.M83M84 2004
  616.07′9–dc22

                                                      2004059493

British Library Cataloguing in Publication Data
A catalogue record for this book is available from the British Library
ISBN: 0-12-491543-4

For all information on all Academic Press publications
visit our website at www.academicpress.com

Printed in the United States of America

04 05 06 07 08 09 9 8 7 6 5 4 3 2 1

In Memoriam

Malcolm Artenstein
Merrill W. Chase
Anne Ferguson
Robert Good
Joseph Heremans
Graham Jackson
Otakar Koldovsky
Frederick Kraus
Henry Kunkel
Goro Mogi
Eva Orlans
Richard Rothberg
Roberta Shahin
Masaharu Tsuchiya
Robert Waldman

For their lasting contributions
to the field of Mucosal Immunology

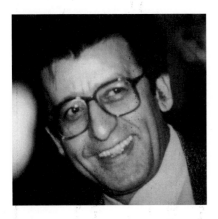

We dedicate the third edition of *Mucosal Immunology* to its founding editor, Pearay L. Ogra, our friend and colleague, in appreciation of his many contributions to our discipline

The Editors

Preface to the First Edition

Only 25 years ago, a multidisciplinary group of some three dozen individuals met for the first time in Vero Beach, Florida, under the auspices of the National Institute of Child Health and Human Development (NICHHD) to discuss a recently identified immunoglobulin, secretory IgA. Since that historic workshop, seven international congresses have been held to discuss secretory immunoglobulins and mucosal immunology, and there have been a number of scientific meetings on immunological mechanisms in such mucosal sites as respiratory tract, gut, genital tract, mammary glands, and periodontal tissues. The last International Congress of Mucosal Immunology, held in 1992 in Prague, Czechoslovakia, was attended by nearly 1000 participants.

The recognition that defenses are mediated via mucosal barriers dates back several thousand years. Ingestion of *Rhus* leaves to modify the severity of reactions to poison ivy is a centuries old practice among native North Americans. The modern concepts of local immunity, however, were developed by Besredka in the early 1900s, followed by the discovery of IgA in 1953 and its isolation and characterization in 1959. Studies in the early 1960s demonstrated the presence of IgA in a unique form in milk and, shortly thereafter, in other external secretions. These studies were followed by the discovery of the secretory component and the identification of the J chain. These remarkable observations were soon complemented by the characterization of the bronchus-associated lymphoid tissue (BALT) and the gut-associated lymphoid tissue (GALT), the observation of circulation of antigen-sensitized or reactive IgA B cells from BALT and GALT to other mucosal surfaces such as the genital tract and the mammary glands, and the definition of mucosal T cells. In the past decade, our concept of the mucosal immune system has been expanded to include M cells and mechanisms of mucosal antigen processing, regulatory T lymphocytes and other effector cell mechanisms, neuropeptides, and the network of interleukins and other cytokines. Finally, the biological significance of the mucosal immune system increasingly is being realized in the context of human infections acquired via mucosal portals of entry, including conventional infections as well as new syndromes such as acquired immune deficiency associated with infection by HIV.

Despite the tremendous progress made in the acquisition of new knowledge concerning the common mucosal immune system, mucosal infections, and oral immunization, no single text covering the entire spectrum of mucosal immunity was available. Therefore, this handbook was organized to develop a perspective of the basic biology of the components that constitute the framework of the common mucosal immune system, as well as of the infectious and immunologically mediated disease processes of the mucosae. Virtually all chapters have been authored by original investigators responsible for key observations on which current concepts are based.

Part I, Cellular Basis of Mucosal Immunity, provides an introductory overview and a historical perspective of the mucosal immune system (Chapter 1), followed by 10 comprehensive chapters (Section A) on development and physiology of mucosal defense (Chapters 2–11). These chapters address structure and function of mucosal epithelium, cellular basis of antigen transport, mucosal barrier, innate humoral factors, bacterial adherence, development and function of mucosal immunoglobulin, and epithelial and hepatobiliary transport. Section B (Chapters 12–19) focuses on cells, regulation, and specificity in inductive and effector sites. The inductive site chapters discuss characteristics of mucosa-associated lymphoid tissue (MALT), Peyer's patches, regulation of IgA B cell development, diversity and function of mucosal antigen-presenting cells, oral tolerance, peptidergic circuits, role of B-1 cells, and lymphocyte homing. The chapters on effector sites (Section C) present information about cytokines, mucosal Ig-producing cells, regulatory T cells, intraepithelial cells, mucosal IgE, inflammation and mast cells, cytokines in liver, cytotoxic T cells in mucosal effector sites, and immunity to viruses (Chapters 20–29). Section D addresses mucosal immunization and the concepts of mucosal vaccines. These chapters discuss passive immunization, vaccine development for mucosal surfaces, antigen delivery systems, mucosal adjuvants, and approaches for generating specific secretory IgA antibodies (Chapters 30–34).

Part II, Mucosal Diseases, addresses the secretory immune system with special reference to mucosal diseases. Section E consists of chapters on the stomach, intestine, and liver, and includes diseases of GALT and intestinal tract, α chain and related lymphoproliferative disorders, gastritis and peptic ulcer, malabsorption syndrome, food allergy, intestinal infections, and diseases of the liver and biliary tract (Chapters 35–42). Section F covers selected areas of lung and lower airway and includes chapters on BALT and pulmonary diseases, mucosal immunity in asthma, respiratory infections, and inhalant allergy (Chapters 43–46). Section G presents information on the oral cavity, upper airway, and mucosal regions in the head and neck (Chapters 47–50), as well as ocular immunity, tonsils and adenoids, and middle ear. Sections H and I are devoted to mammary glands and genitourinary tract, respectively. These sections consist of chapters on milk, immunological effects of breast feeding (Chapters 51 and 52), IgA nephropathy, immunology of female and male reproductive tracts, endocrine regulation of genital immunity, mucosal immunopathophysiology of HIV infection, and genital infections relative to maternal and infant disease (Chapters 53–58).

The information reviewed in the different chapters in this handbook will be of considerable interest to diverse groups of clinicians, basic and clinical immunologists, biologists, veterinarians, and public health workers interested in understanding the application of basic biology to virtually all immunological or infection-mediated disease processes of external mucosal surfaces. This handbook will be of particular importance to students of medicine and pediatrics, including individuals studying gastroenterology and pulmonology, ophthalmology, gynecology, infectious disease, otolaryngology, periodontal disease, sexually transmitted disease, and especially mucosal immunology.

Pearay L. Ogra
Jiri Mestecky
Michael E. Lamm
Warren Strober
Jerry R. McGhee
John Bienenstock

Preface to the Second Edition

Since the publication of the First Edition of *Mucosal Immunology* (then called *Handbook of Mucosal Immunology*) in 1994, an enormous amount of new information has become available concerning the structure and function of the mucosal immune system. The Editors therefore decided to update and expand the original text to encompass this new information and to maintain the volume as the primary reference work of the field. The broadened content of the second edition, and therefore its increased size, reflects the rapid expansion of new information and interest, and hence the impact our discipline is having on immunology and biology in general. It is becoming obvious that the phylogenetic development of the entire immune system is inseparable from that of its mucosal compartment. Indeed, one can provide many convincing arguments that stimulation with environmental antigens, which are encountered in everyday life primarily at mucosal surfaces, results in a strategic distribution of cells involved in the initiation of humoral and cellular immune responses at such sites. Notable advances have been made in our knowledge of the regulation of mucosal immune responses. This involves a better understanding of how immune responses are generated and thus how the mucosal immune system maintains host defense at mucosal surfaces. In addition, it involves deeper insights recently acquired into the nature of negative or tolerogenic responses (mucosal tolerance) in the mucosal immune system and how the mucosal immune system avoids untoward responses to ubiquitous antigens and the possible induction of self-reactive responses.

The implications of these advances have been applied in several clinical areas. These include the development of several new mucosal vaccine preparations consisting of either live attenuated organisms or nonreplicating antigens that provide protection for several mucosal viral infections such as rotavirus and influenza virus infection, and for mucosal bacterial infections such as infection with *S. typhi* and *V. cholerae*. These vaccines are the harbinger of others to come based on recent increases in the understanding of mucosal adjuvants. On the other side of the coin, the induction of oral tolerance is now being tested as an approach to the treatment of autoimmune diseases such as juvenile diabetes mellitus, rheumatoid arthritis, and multiple sclerosis.

Finally, the balance between mucosal responsiveness and unresponsiveness is being explored within the context of a series of newly developed models of chronic mucosal inflammation. These models are providing a wealth of new information not only concerning immune response in general, but also concerning the pathogenesis of various types of mucosal inflammation such as inflammatory bowel disease and gluten-sensitive enteropathy. These advances in our understanding of mucosal immune system function, of course, are based on numerous new studies of the way individual components of the system operate. This edition of *Mucosal Immunology* addresses these issues with new discussions and analyses such as mucosal B cell function and the development of IgA-producing plasma cells; the function of epithelial cells as antigen-presenting cells and secretors of cytokines and chemokines; and the function of mucosal T cells both in the lamina propria and in the epithelial cell compartments.

The Second Edition is a considerably larger volume with nearly 100 chapters. Several important changes have been made in this edition. The sections on the development and physiology of mucosal defense, inductive and effector tissues and cells of the mucosal immune system, functional characteristics of mucosal cells and tissues, mucosal immunity and infections, antigen delivery systems, mucosal adjuvants, and the male genital tract have either been enlarged or newly added. As a result of these changes, as well as the dedicated work of our many contributors, we hope *Mucosal Immunology* will continue to be the starting place for the knowledge and study of the mucosal immune system.

Publication of this rather large volume would not have been possible without the dedication and collaboration of the authors of the individual chapters. We recognize with gratitude the contributions of a most helpful staff at Academic Press, especially Dr. Kerry Willis and Mr. Aaron Johnson. We also recognize the contributions of Ms. Diane Zimmerman (University of Texas Medical Branch), Ms. Ruby Zuppert (Case Western Reserve University), Ms. Wendy Abbott and Ms. Sheila D. Turner (University of Alabama at Birmingham), Ms. Sarah Kaul (National Institutes of Health), Ms. Linda Builder (McMaster University), and Ms. Maria Bethune (University of Alabama at Birmingham).

It is our pleasure to submit this volume to interested readers. We sincerely hope that this second edition will provide new stimuli for research not only in mucosal immunology but in the related fields of theoretical and practical immunology.

Pearay L. Ogra
Jiri Mestecky
Michael E. Lamm
Warren Strober
John Bienenstock
Jerry R. McGhee

Preface to the Third Edition

Mucosal immunology has grown in the last decade from a discipline of perhaps peripheral interest to the mainstream immunologist into a major subspecialty with implications for the physiology of the entire immune system. An enormous and highly variable load of foreign substances, which includes indigenous mucosal microbiota as well as environmental and food antigens encountered mainly at the vast surface areas of mucosal membranes, has resulted during evolution in a strategic distribution of specialized cells involved in the uptake, processing, and presentation of antigens, the production of antibodies, and cell-mediated immunity at the front line of host defense. Furthermore, the great majority of infectious diseases and potential agents of bioterrorism directly afflicts or is acquired through the mucosal surfaces of the respiratory, gastrointestinal, and genitourinary tracts. In addition to the induction of protective responses to infectious agents, the unique immunoregulatory mechanisms involved in the parallel induction of mucosal tolerance efficiently prevent the overstimulation of the systemic compartment of the immune system. Exploitation of the principles of mucosal immunology has not only had a profound impact on theoretical immunology, but has also captured the attention of investigators working in applied fields including autoimmunity, allergy, infectious diseases of gastrointestinal and respiratory tract, sexually transmitted diseases, human immunodeficiency virus infections, and the development of vaccines for human and veterinary medicine. The publication of three editions of *Mucosal Immunology* within 10 years reflects the impressive expansion of new information and the impact the discipline has had on basic immunologic principles and their practical implications. Thus, the third updated and expanded edition of *Mucosal Immunology* will provide essential information and an invaluable source of inspiration for investigators in this field as well as related research endeavors.

The foundations of modern mucosal immunology were laid in the early 1960s. The authors of the chapters in this volume have been important contributors and witnesses of the remarkable progress in mucosal immunology. We hope that their unique insights, together with the enthusiasm of younger colleagues of the next generation, have resulted in a volume that provides inspiration and broadens the application of the principles of mucosal immunology to other biomedical disciplines.

The assembly of a volume of this size and scope required dedicated effort of many individuals who provided invaluable contributions at various stages of production. The editors of the third edition of *Mucosal Immunology* would like to thank the founding editor, Dr. Pearay L. Ogra, for his leadership in the first and second editions; therefore, we dedicate this book to him. We also thank the authors of the individual chapters for their excellent contributions and cooperation. We gratefully acknowledge the efforts of our administrative co-workers, namely, Maria D. Crenshaw, Lydia Lopez, Sandra Martinez, Sheila D. Turner, Kelly R. Stinson, and Susan Brill, for their contributions in the completion and assembly of this book. Finally, we thank Margaret MacDonald and Victoria Lebedeva of *Elsevier* for their exemplary dedication, invaluable help, and deeply appreciated patience.

Jiri Mestecky
John Bienenstock
Michael E. Lamm
Lloyd Mayer
Jerry R. McGhee
Warren Strober

Contributors

Mohammed D. Abd-Alla
Department of Medicine, University of Minnesota, Minneapolis, Minnesota

Soman N. Abraham
Departments of Pathology and Molecular Genetics and Microbiology, Duke University Medical Center, Durham, North Carolina

David Adams
Liver Research Laboratories, University of Birmingham Institute of Clinical Science, MRC Centre for Immune Regulation, Queen Elizabeth Hospital, Edgbaston, Birmingham, United Kingdom

Deborah J. Anderson
Fearing Research Laboratory, Department of Obstetrics, Gynecology, and Reproductive Biology, Brigham and Women's Hospital, Harvard Medical School, Boston, Massachusetts

Charles J. Arntzen
Arizona State University Biodesign Institute and School of Life Sciences, Tempe, Arizona

T. Prescott Atkinson
Department of Pediatrics, Division of Pediatric Allergy, University of Alabama at Birmingham, Birmingham, Alabama

Espen S. Baekkevold
Laboratory for Immunohistochemistry and Immunopathology (LIIPAT), Institute of Pathology, University of Oslo, The National Hospital, Rikshospitalet, Oslo, Norway

A. Dean Befus
Pulmonary Research Group, Department of Medicine, Faculty of Medicine, University of Alberta, Edmonton, Alberta, Canada

Lesley Ann Bergmeier
Guy's, Kings, and St. Thomas' Medical and Dental Schools, London, United Kingdom

Göran Bergsten
Department of Medical Microbiology, University of Lund, Lund, Sweden

M. Cecilia Berin
Department of Pediatrics, Mount Sinai School of Medicine, New York, New York

Joel M. Bernstein
Department of Otolaryngology and Pediatrics, State University of New York at Buffalo, School of Biomedical Sciences, Buffalo, New York

Charles L. Bevins
Departments of Immunology, Gastroenterology, and Colorectal Surgery, The Cleveland Clinic Foundation Research Institute, Cleveland, Ohio

John Bienenstock
Departments of Medicine & Pathology and Molecular Medicine, McMaster University, Hamilton, Ontario, Canada

Brian L. Bishop
Department of Molecular Genetics and Microbiology, Duke University Medical Center, Durham, North Carolina

Jan Bjersing
Department of Rheumatology and Inflammation Research, Göteborg University, Göteborg, Sweden

Richard S. Blumberg
Division of Gastroenterology, Harvard Medical School, Brigham and Women's Hospital, Boston, Massachusetts

Libuse A. Bobek
Department of Oral Biology, University at Buffalo, Buffalo, New York

Nadiya Boiko
Department of Biology, University of Pennsylvania, Philadelphia, Pennsylvania, and Department of Genetics and Plant Physiology, Uzhhorod National University, Uzhhorod, Ukraine

Nicolaas A. Bos
Department of Cell Biology, Immunology Section, University of Groningen, Groningen, The Netherlands

Kenneth L. Bost
Department of Biology, University of North Carolina at Charlotte, Charlotte, North Carolina

Prosper N. Boyaka
Department of Microbiology, University of Alabama at Birmingham, Birmingham, Alabama

Per Brandtzaeg
Laboratory for Immunohistochemistry and Immunopathology (LIIPAT), Institute of Pathololgy, University of Oslo, The National Hospital, Rikshospitalet, Oslo, Norway

David E. Briles
Department of Microbiology, University of Alabama at Birmingham, Birmingham, Alabama

Jeremy H. Brock
Department of Immunology, University of Glasgow, Glasgow, Scotland

Richard A. Bronson
Department of Obstetrics and Gynecology, Stony Brook Health Science Center, Stony Brook, New York

William R. Brown
Department of Gastroenterology, University of Colorado School of Medicine, Denver, Colorado

Mark G. Buckley
Allergy and Inflammation Research, Division of Infection, Inflammation, and Repair, School of Medicine, University of Southampton, Southampton, United Kingdom

Eugene C. Butcher
Laboratory of Immunology and Vascular Biology, Department of Pathology, Stanford University School of Medicine, Stanford, California; and The Center for Molecular Biology and Medicine, The Veterans Affairs Palo Alto Health Care System, Palo Alto, California

John E. Butler
Department of Microbiology and Interdisciplinary Immunology Program, The University of Iowa, Iowa City, Iowa

Hege S. Carlsen
Laboratory for Immunohistochemistry and Immunopathology (LIIPAT), Institute of Pathololgy, University of Oslo, The National Hospital, Rikshospitalet, Oslo, Norway

Gail H. Cassell
Infectious Disease Drug Discovery Research and Clinical Investigation, Lilly Research Laboratories, Indianapolis, Indiana

Sabina Cauci
Department of Biomedical Sciences and Technologies, University of Udine, Udine, Italy

John J. Cebra
Department of Biology, University of Pennsylvania, Philadelphia, Pennsylvania

Stephen J. Challacombe
Department of Oral Medicine and Pathology, Guy's Hospital, London, United Kingdom

Hilde Cheroutre
La Jolla Institute for Allergy & Immunology, San Diego, California

Rachel Chikwamba
Arizona State University Biodesign Institute and School of Life Sciences, Tempe, Arizona

Noel K. Childers
Department of Oral Biology, University of Alabama at Birmingham, Birmingham, Alabama

Robert L. Clancy
Department of Pathology, University of Newcastle, Newcastle, New South Wales, Australia

Richard W. Compans
Department of Microbiology and Immunology, Emory University School of Medicine, Atlanta, Georgia

Richard A. Cone
Jenkins Department of Biophysics, Johns Hopkins University, Baltimore, Maryland

Lynette B. Corbeil
Department of Pathology, UCSD Medical Center, University of California at San Diego, San Diego, California

Mardi A. Crane-Godreau
Department of Physiology, Dartmouth Medical School, Lebanon, New Hampshire

Allan W. Cripps
School of Medicine, Griffith University, Queensland, Australia

Charlotte Cunningham-Rundles
Division of Clinical Immunobiology, Mount Sinai School of Medicine, New York, New York

Roy Curtiss, III
Biodesign Institute and School of Life Sciences, Arizona State University, Tempe, Arizona

Cecil Czerkinsky
Faculte de Medecine-Pasteur, Universite de Nice, Nice, France

Steven J. Czinn
Department of Pediatrics, Case Western Reserve University, Cleveland, Ohio

Ype de Jong
Division of Immunology, Beth Israel Hospital, Boston, Massachusetts

Gordon Dent
Centre for Molecular Biomedicine, School of Life Sciences, Keele University, Keele, United Kingdom

Mark T. Dertzbaugh
United States Army Medical Research Institute of Infectious Disease, Fort Detrick, Maryland

Victor J. DiRita
Department of Microbiology and Immunology, University of Michigan Medical School, Ann Arbor, Michigan

Rainer Duchmann
Medical Department, Charité Universitätsmedizin Berlin, Campus Benjamin Franklin, Free University of Berlin, Berlin, Germany

Charles O. Elson
Division of Gastroenterology and Hepatology, Department of Medicine, University of Alabama at Birmingham, Birmingham, Alabama

Steven N. Emancipator
Department of Pathology, Case Western Reserve University, Cleveland, Ohio

Mary K. Estes
Department of Molecular Virology and Microbiology, Baylor College of Medicine, Houston, Texas

Sidonia Fargarasan
Laboratory of Mucosal Immunology, RIKEN Research Centre for Allergy and Immunology, Yokohama City, Japan

Ana M. C. Faria
Departamento de Bioquímica e Imunologia, Instituto de Ciências Biológicas, Universidade Federal de Minas Gerais, Belo Horizonte, Brazil

Inger Nina Farstad
Laboratory for Immunohistochemistry and Immunopathology (LIIPAT), Institute of Pathololgy, University of Oslo, The National Hospital, Rikshospitalet, Oslo, Norway

Paul L. Fidel, Jr.
Department of Microbiology, Louisiana State University Health Science Center, New Orleans, Louisiana

Hans Fischer
Department of Medical Microbiology, University of Lund, Lund, Sweden

George Fogg
Department of Pediatrics and Communicable Diseases, University of Michigan Medical School, Ann Arbor, Michigan

Kohtaro Fujihashi
Departments of Oral Biology and Microbiology, and
The Immunobiology Vaccine Center, University of
Alabama at Birmingham, Birmingham, Alabama

Francesco M. Fusi
Department of Obstetrics and Gynecology, University of
Milano, Instituto Scientifico, Ospedale San Raffaele,
Milan, Italy

Ivan J. Fuss
Laboratory of Clinical Investigation, National Institute
of Allergy and Infectious Disease, National Institutes of
Health, Bethesda, Maryland

Thomas Ganz
Departments of Medicine and Pathology, UCLA School
of Medicine, Los Angeles, California

Roberto P. Garofalo
Department of Pediatric Immunology, Allergy, and
Rheumatology, University of Texas Medical Branch,
Galveston, Texas

Robert J. Genco
State University of New York, University at Buffalo,
Buffalo, New York

Andrew T. Gewirtz
Epithelial Pathobiology Division, Department of
Pathology and Laboratory Medicine, Emory University,
Atlanta, Georgia

Maree Gleeson
Hunter Area Pathology Services, Newcastle, New South
Wales, Australia

Gabriela Godaly
Department of Medical Microbiology, University of
Lund, Lund, Sweden

Randall M. Goldblum
Pediatric Child Health Research Center, University
of Texas Medical Branch, Galveston, Texas

Katherine S. Grant
Department of Physiology, Dartmouth Medical School,
Lebanon, New Hampshire

Harry B. Greenberg
Department of Microbiology and Immunology, Veterans
Affairs Hospital, Stanford University, Palo Alto,
California

Hans Michael Haitchi
Allergy and Inflammation Research, Division of
Infection, Inflammation, and Repair, School of
Medicine, University of Southampton, Southampton,
United Kingdom

George Hajishengallis
Department of Microbiology, Immunology, and
Parasitology, Louisiana State University, New Orleans,
Louisiana

Hiromasa Hamada
Department of Microbiology and Immunology, Keio
University School of Medicine, Tokyo, Japan

Lars Åke Hanson
Department of Clinical Immunology, Göteborg
University, Göteborg, Sweden

R. Doug Hardy
Division of Infectious Diseases, University of Texas
Southwestern Medical Center, Dallas, Texas

M. Veronica Herias
Department of Public Health and Food Safety, Faculty
of Veterinary Medicine, Utrecht University,
The Netherlands

Georg Herrler
Institut für Virologie, Tierärztliche Hochschule
Hannover, Hannover, Germany

John E. Herrmann
Division of Infectious Diseases and Immunology,
University of Massachusetts Medical School, Worcester,
Massachusetts

Douglas C. Hodgins
Department of Pathobiology, Ontario Veterinary
College, University of Guelph, Guelph, Ontario, Canada

Frank Hoentjen
Postdoctoral Research Fellow, University of North
Carolina, Chapel Hill, North Carolina; and Free

University Medical Center, Amsterdam,
The Netherlands

Stephen T. Holgate
Allergy and Inflammation Research, Division of
Infection, Inflammation, and Repair, School of
Medicine, University of Southampton, Southampton,
United Kingdom

Judith H. Holloway
Tissue Infection and Repair, Division of Infection,
Inflammation, and Repair, School of Medicine,
University of Southampton, Southampton, United
Kingdom

Jan Holmgren
Department of Medical Microbiology and Immunology,
and Göteborg University Vaccine Research Institute,
Göteborg University, Göteborg, Sweden

Edward W. Hook III
Department of Medicine, Division of Infectious
Diseases, University of Alabama at Birmingham,
Birmingham, Alabama

Joan S. Hunt
Department of Anatomy and Cell Biology, University of
Kansas Medical Center, Kansas City, Kansas

Mark D. Inman
Firestone Institute for Respiratory Health, St. Joseph's
Healthcare, and Department of Medicine, McMaster
University, Hamilton, Ontario, Canada

Heikki Irjala
Department of Medical Microbiology, University of
Lund, Lund, Sweden

Hiromichi Ishikawa
Department of Microbiology and Immunology, Keio
University School of Medicine, Tokyo, Japan

Takeru Ishikawa
Department of Otorhinolaryngology, Kumamoto
University School of Medicine, Kumamoto, Japan

Juraj Ivanyi
Department of Oral Medicine & Pathology, Guy's
Campus, Medical and Dental Schools of Kings College,
London, United Kingdom

Susan Jackson
Department of Microbiology, University of Alabama at
Birmingham, Birmingham, Alabama

Sirpa Jalkanen
Medicity Research Laboratory and Department of Medical
Microbiology, University of Turku, Turku, Finland

Edward N. Janoff
Mucosal and Vaccine Research Center and Infectious
Disease Section, Veterans Affairs Medical Center,
University of Minnesota School of Medicine,
Minneapolis, Minnesota

Han-Qing Jiang
Department of Biology, University of Pennsylvania,
Philadelphia, Pennsylvania

Charlotte S. Kaetzel
Department of Microbiology, Immunology, & Molecular
Genetics, and Department of Pathology & Laboratory
Medicine, University of Kentucky, Lexington,
Kentucky

Yutaka Kanamori
Department of Microbiology and Immunology, Keio
University School of Medicine, Tokyo, Japan;
Department of Pediatric Surgery, Graduate School of
Medicine, The University of Tokyo, Tokyo, Japan

Loren C. Karp
Inflammatory Bowel Disease Center, Cedars–Sinai
Medical Center, Los Angeles, California

Tomohiro Kato
Department of Endoscopy, Jikei University School of
Medicine, Tokyo, Japan

Marcus E. Kehrli, Jr.
Agricultural Research Service, National Animal Disease
Center, Ames, Iowa

Brian L. Kelsall
Laboratory of Clinical Investigation, National Institute
of Allergy and Infectious Disease, National Institutes of
Health, Bethesda, Maryland

Michael A. Kerr
Department of Clinical Biochemistry and Immunology,
General Infirmary at Leeds, Leeds, United Kingdom

Mogens Kilian
Department of Medical Microbiology and Immunology, University of Aarhus, Aarhus, Denmark

Hiroshi Kiyono
Division of Mucosal Immunology, Department of Microbiology and Immunology, Institute of Medical Science, The University of Tokyo, Tokyo, Japan; Departments of Microbiology and Oral Biology, The Immunobiology Vaccine Center, University of Alabama at Birmingham, Birmingham, Alabama

Katherine L. Knight
Department of Microbiology and Immunology, Stritch School of Medicine, Loyola University of Chicago, Maywood, Illinois

Marina Korotkova
Department of Clinical Immunology, Göteborg University, Göteborg, Sweden

George Kraal
Department of Molecular Cell Biology, VU University Medical Center, Amsterdam, The Netherlands

Jean-Pierre Kraehenbuhl
Swiss Institute for Experimental Cancer Research and Institute of Biochemistry, University of Lausanne, Epalinges, Switzerland

Arthur M. Krieg
Coley Pharmaceutical Group, Wellesley, Massachusetts

Mamidipudi T. Krishna
Allergy and Inflammation Research, Division of Infection, Inflammation, and Repair, School of Medicine, University of Southampton, Southampton, United Kingdom

Frans G. M. Kroese
Department of Cell Biology, Immunology Section, University of Groningen, Groningen, The Netherlands

Mitchell Kronenberg
La Jolla Institute for Allergy & Immunology, San Diego, California

Yuichi Kurono
Department of Otolaryngology, Faculty of Medicine, Kagoshima University, Kagoshima, Japan

William H. Kutteh
Division of Reproductive Endocrinology, Department of Obstetrics and Gynecology, University of Tennessee, Memphis, Tennessee

Mi-Na Kweon
Mucosal Immunology Section, International Vaccine Institute, Seoul, Korea; and Division of Mucosal Immunology, Institute of Medical Science, The University of Tokyo, Tokyo, Japan

Michael E. Lamm
Department of Pathology, Case Western Reserve University, Cleveland, Ohio

Nicole Lazarus
Laboratory of Immunology and Vascular Biology, Department of Pathology, Stanford University School of Medicine, Stanford, California; and the Center for Molecular Biology and Medicine, The Veterans Affairs Palo Alto Health Care System, Palo Alto, California

Leo LeFrançois
Division of Immunology, Department of Internal Medicine, University of Connecticut Health Center, Farmington, Connecticut

Thomas Lehner
Guy's, Kings, and St. Thomas' Medical and Dental Schools, London, United Kingdom

Robert I. Lehrer
Department of Medicine and Molecular Biology Institute, UCLA School of Medicine, Los Angeles, California

Francisco Leon
Laboratory of Clinical Investigation, National Institute of Allergy and Infectious Disease, National Institutes of Health, Bethesda, Maryland

Myron M. Levine
Center for Vaccine Development, University of Maryland School of Medicine, Baltimore, Maryland

David Lim
House Ear Institute, Los Angeles, California

Tong-Jun Lin
Department of Microbiology and Immunology and Department of Pediatrics, Dalhousie University, Halifax, Nova Scotia, Canada

George P. Lomonossoff
John Innes Centre, Norwich, United Kingdom

Knut E. A. Lundin
Department of Medicine and Institute of Immunology, Rikshospitalet University Hospital, Oslo, Norway

Ann-Charlotte Lundstedt
Department of Medical Microbiology, University of Lund, Lund, Sweden

Nils Lycke
Department of Medical Microbiology and Immunology, Göteborg University, Göteborg, Sweden

Thomas T. MacDonald
Division of Infection, Inflammation, and Repair, University of Southampton School of Medicine, Southampton, United Kingdom

Richard T. Mahoney
Arizona State University Biodesign Institute and School of Life Sciences, Tempe, Arizona

Denis Martin
Unité de Recherche en Vaccinologie, Centre Hospitalier, Universitaire de Québec, Québec, Canada

Hugh S. Mason
Arizona State University Biodesign Institute and School of Life Sciences, Tempe, Arizona

Keisuke Masuyama
Department of Otorhinolaryngology, Yamanashi University School of Medicine, Yamanashi, Japan.

Lloyd Mayer
Immunology Center, Mount Sinai Medical Center, New York, New York

Donald M. McDonald
Cardiovascular Research Institute, Comprehensive Cancer Care Center, and Department of Anatomy, University of California at San Francisco, San Francisco, California

M. Juliana McElrath
Program in Infectious Diseases, Clinical Research Division, Fred Hutchinson Cancer Research Center, and Department of Medicine, University of Washington, Seattle, Washington

Jerry R. McGhee
Department of Microbiology, University of Alabama at Birmingham, Birmingham, Alabama

Jiri Mestecky
Departments of Microbiology and Medicine, University of Alabama at Birmingham, Birmingham, Alabama

Suzanne M. Michalek
Department of Microbiology, University of Alabama at Birmingham, Birmingham, Alabama

Christopher J. Miller
Center for Comparative Medicine and Department of Veterinary Pathology, Microbiology, and Immunology, School of Veterinary Medicine, and California National Primate Research Center, University of California at Davis, Davis, California

Robert D. Miller
Department of Biology, University of New Mexico, Albuquerque, New Mexico

Goro Mogi
Department of Otolaryngology, Oita Medical University, Oita, Japan

Øyvind Molberg
Department of Rheumatology and Institute of Immunology, Rikshospitalet University Hospital, Oslo, Norway

Zina Moldoveanu
Department of Microbiology, University of Alabama at Birmingham, Birmingham, Alabama

Giovanni Monteleone
Cattedra di Gastroenterologia, Department Medicina Interna, Università Tor Vergata, Rome, Italy

Paul C. Montgomery
Department of Immunology and Microbiology, Wayne State University School of Medicine, Detroit, Michigan

Itaru Moro
Department of Pathology, Nihon University School of Dentistry, Tokyo, Japan

Richard P. Morrison
Department of Medicine, University of Alabama at Birmingham, Birmingham, Alabama

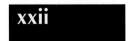

Keith Mostov
Department of Anatomy, Department of Biochemistry and Biophysics, and Cardiovascular Research Institute, University of California, San Francisco, California

Allan McI. Mowat
Department of Immunology and Bacteriology, Division of Immunology, Infection, and Inflammation, University of Glasgow, and Western Infirmary, Glasgow, Scotland, United Kingdom

Brian R. Murphy
Respiratory Viruses Section, Laboratory of Infectious Diseases, National Institute of Allergy and Infectious Disease, National Institutes of Health, Bethesda, Maryland

James P. Nataro
Center for Vaccine Development, University of Maryland School of Medicine, Baltimore, Maryland

John G. Nedrud
Department of Pediatrics and Institute of Pathology, Case Western Reserve University, Cleveland, Ohio

Marian R. Neutra
Department of Pediatrics, Harvard Medical School, and Gastrointestinal Cell Biology Laboratory, Children's Hospital, Boston, Massachusetts

Stella Nowicki
Department of Obstetrics and Gynecology and Department of Microbiology and Immunology, University of Texas Medical Branch, Galveston, Texas

Paul M. O'Byrne
Firestone Institute for Respiratory Health, St. Joseph's Healthcare, and Department of Medicine, McMaster University, Hamilton, Ontario, Canada

Itzhak Ofek
Department of Human Microbiology, Sackler Faculty of Medicine, Tel-Aviv University, Tel-Aviv, Israel

Pearay L. Ogra
Division of Infectious Diseases, Children's Hospital, Buffalo, New York

Derek T. O'Hagan
Chiron Corporation, Emeryville, California

Yoshitaka Okamoto
Department of Otorhinolaryngology, Chiba University School of Medicine, Chiba, Japan

Carlos J. Orihuela
Department of Infectious Diseases, St. Jude Children's Research Hospital, Memphis, Tennessee

Albert D. M. E. Osterhaus
Department of Virology, Erasmus University, Rotterdam, The Netherlands

Nancy L. O'Sullivan
Department of Anatomy and Cell Biology, and of Immunology and Microbiology, Wayne State University School of Medicine, Detroit, Michigan

Robert L. Owen
Department of Medicine, University of California San Francisco; Gastroenterology Section, Veterans Affairs Medical Center, San Francisco, California

Roy C. Page
Regional Clinical Dental Research Center, University of Washington, Seattle, Washington

Margaret B. Parr
Department of Anatomy, School of Medicine, Southern Illinois University, Carbondale, Illinois

Earl L. Parr
Department of Anatomy, School of Medicine, Southern Illinois University, Carbondale, Illinois

Viviana Parreño
Institute of Virology, Center of Research in Veterinary Science, National Institute of Agricultural Technology, Buenos Aires, Argentina

David W. Pascual
Veterinary Molecular Biology, Montana State University, Bozeman, Montana

Jane V. Peppard
Aventis Pharmaceuticals, Bridgewater, New Jersey

Margaret G. Petroff
Department of Anatomy and Cell Biology, University of Kansas Medical Center, Kansas City, Kansas

Jeffrey Pudney
Fearing Research Laboratory, Department of Obstetrics, Gynecology, and Reproductive Biology, Brigham and Women's Hospital, Harvard Medical School, Boston, Massachusetts

Jonathan I. Ravdin
Department of Medicine, University of Minnesota, Minneapolis, Minnesota

Kathryn B. Renegar
Department of Pediatric Infectious Diseases, Vanderbilt University, Nashville, Tennessee

Ki-Jong Rhee
Department of Microbiology and Immunology, Stritch School of Medicine, Loyola University of Chicago, Maywood, Illinois

Guus F. Rimmelzwaan
Department of Virology, Erasmus University, Rotterdam, The Netherlands

Anna-Karin Robertson
Center for Molecular Medicine, Karolinska Institute, Stockholm, Sweden

Harriett L. Robinson
Division of Microbiology and Immunology, Yerkes Primate Research Center of Emory University, Atlanta, Georgia

Kenneth L. Rosenthal
Centre for Gene Therapeutics, Department of Pathology & Molecular Medicine, McMaster University Health Sciences Centre, Hamilton, Ontario, Canada

Marc E. Rothenberg
Division of Allergy and Immunology, Department of Pediatrics, Cincinnati Children's Hospital Medical Center, Cincinnati, Ohio

Barry T. Rouse
Department of Microbiology, The University of Tennessee at Knoxville, Knoxville, Tennessee

Jeffrey B. Rubins
Mucosal and Vaccine Research Center and Pulmonary Section, Veterans Affairs Medical Center, University of Minnesota School of Medicine, Minneapolis, Minnesota

Michael W. Russell
Department of Microbiology and Immunology, and of Oral Biology, University at Buffalo, Buffalo, New York

Linda J. Saif
Food Animal Health Research Program, Ohio Agricultural Research and Development Center, The Ohio State University, Wooster, Ohio

Marko Salmi
Medicity Research Laboratory, University of Turku; and National Public Health Institute, Turku, Finland

Hugh A. Sampson
Department of Pediatrics, Mount Sinai School of Medicine, New York, New York

Patrick Samuelsson
Department of Medical Microbiology, University of Lund, Lund, Sweden

Luca Santi
Arizona State University Biodesign Institute and School of Life Sciences, Tempe, Arizona

R. Balfour Sartor
Departments of Medicine and Microbiology & Immunology and Multidisciplinary Center for IBD Research and Treatment, University of North Carolina, Chapel Hill, North Carolina

Dwayne C. Savage
Department of Microbiology, University of Tennessee at Knoxville, Knoxville, Tennessee

D. Scott Schmid
Viral Immunology Section, Centers for Disease Control and Prevention, Atlanta, Georgia

Nathan Sharon
Department of Membrane Research and Biophysics, Weizmann Institute of Science, Rehovot, Israel

Penelope J. Shirlaw
Department of Oral Medicine and Pathology, Guy's and St. Thomas' Medical School, London, United Kingdom

Phillip D. Smith
Division of Gastroenterology and Hepatology, Department of Medicine, University of Alabama at

Birmingham, and The Research Service, Veterans Administration Medical Center, Birmingham, Alabama

Leslie E. Smythies
Division of Gastroenterology and Hepatology, Department of Medicine, University of Alabama at Birmingham, Birmingham, Alabama

Ludvig Sollid
Institute of Immunology, Rikshospitalet University Hospital, Oslo, Norway

P. Frederick Sparling
Department of Microbiology and Immunology, University of North Carolina, Chapel Hill, North Carolina

Paul W. Spearman
Department of Pediatric Infectious Diseases, Vanderbilt University, Nashville, Tennessee

Jo Spencer
Department of Histopathology, United Medical and Dental Schools of Guy's and St. Thomas' Hospitals, St. Thomas Campus, London, United Kingdom

Warren Strober
Mucosal Immunity Section, Laboratory of Host Defense, National Institute of Allergy and Infectious Disease, National Institutes of Health, Bethesda, Maryland

Wen Su
Department of Histopathology, United Medical and Dental Schools of Guy's and St. Thomas' Hospitals, St. Thomas Campus, London, United Kingdom

David A. Sullivan
Schepens Eye Research Institute and Department of Ophthalmology, Harvard Medical School, Boston, Massachusetts

Catharina Svanborg
Department of Medical Microbiology, University of Lund, Lund, Sweden

Ann-Mari Svennerholm
Department of Medical Microbiology and Immunology, and Göteborg University Vaccine Research Institute, Göteborg, Sweden

Maj-Lis Svensson
Department of Medical Microbiology, University of Lund, Lund, Sweden

Stephan R. Targan
Division of Gastroenterology, Inflammatory Bowel Disease Center, and Immunobiology Institute, Cedars–Sinai Medical Center; and UCLA School of Medicine, Los Angeles, California

Martin A. Taubman
Department of Immunology, The Forsyth Institute, Boston, Massachusetts

Esbjörn Telemo
Department of Rheumatology and Inflammation Research, Göteborg University, Göteborg, Sweden

Jorma Tenovuo
Institute of Dentistry, University of Turku, Turku, Finland

Cox Terhorst
Division of Immunology, Beth Israel Hospital, Boston, Massachusetts

Helena Tlaskalova-Hogenova
Department of Gnotobiology and Immunology, Institute of Microbiology, Czech Academy of Sciences, Prague, Czech Republic

Debra A. Tristram
Department of Pediatrics, East Carolina University, Greenville, North Carolina

Elaine Tuomanen
Department of Infectious Diseases, St. Jude Children's Research Hospital, Memphis, Tennessee

Brian J. Underdown
Department of Pathology, Faculty of Health Sciences, McMaster University, Hamilton, Ontario, Canada

Marjolein van Egmond
Departments of Molecular Cell Biology and Surgical Oncology, VU University Medical Center, Amsterdam, The Netherlands

Matam Vijay-Kumar
Epithelial Pathobiology Division, Department of Pathology and Laboratory Medicine, Emory University, Atlanta, Georgia

Sharon W. Wahl
Oral Infection and Immunity Branch, National Institute of Dental and Craniofacial Research, National Institutes of Health, Bethesda, Maryland

W. Allan Walker
Departments of Nutrition and Pediatrics, Massachusetts General Hospital, Boston, Massachusetts

Richard L. Ward
Division of Infectious Diseases, Children's Hospital Medical Center, University of Cincinnati, Cincinnati, Ohio

Casey T. Weaver
Department of Pathology, University of Alabama at Birmingham, Birmingham, Alabama

Howard L. Weiner
Center for Neurologic Diseases, Brigham and Women's Hospital, Harvard Medical School, Boston, Massachusetts

Robert C. Welliver
Division of Infectious Diseases, Children's Hospital, Buffalo, New York

Charles R. Wira
Department of Physiology, Dartmouth Medical School, Lebabon, New Hampshire

Jenny M. Woof
Division of Pathology and Neuroscience, University of Dundee Medical School, Dundee, United Kingdom

Andrew C. Wotherspoon
Department of Histopathology, The Royal Marsden NHS Trust, London, United Kingdom

Kenneth R. Youngman
Laboratory of Immunology and Vascular Biology, Department of Pathology, Stanford University School of Medicine, Stanford, California; and the Center for Molecular Biology and Medicine, The Veterans Affairs Palo Alto Health Care System, Palo Alto, California

Lijuan Yuan
Food Animal Health Research Program, Ohio Agricultural Research and Development Center, The Ohio State University, Wooster, Ohio

Martin Zeitz
Medical Department, Charité Universitätsmedizin Berlin, Campus Benjamin Franklin, Free University of Berlin, Berlin, Germany

Contents

Historical Aspects of Mucosal Immunology

Jiri Mestecky

Departments of Microbiology and Medicine, University of Alabama at Birmingham, Birmingham, Alabama

John Bienenstock

Departments of Medicine, Pathology, and Molecular Medicine, McMaster University, Hamilton, Ontario, Canada

Jerry R. McGhee

Department of Microbiology, University of Alabama at Birmingham, Birmingham, Alabama

Michael E. Lamm

Department of Pathology, Case Western Reserve University, Cleveland, Ohio

Warren Strober

Mucosal Immunology Section, National Institute of Allergy and Infectious Disease, National Institutes of Health, Bethesda, Maryland

John J. Cebra

Department of Biology, University of Pennsylvania, Philadelphia, Pennsylvania

Lloyd Mayer

Immunology Center, Mount Sinai Medical Center, New York, New York

Pearay L. Ogra

Division of Infectious Diseases, Children's Hospital, University of Buffalo, Buffalo, New York

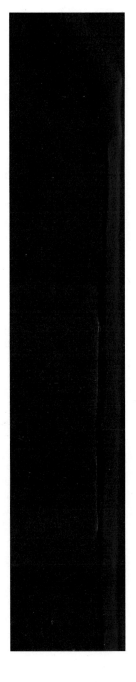

"Historia est testis temporum, lux veritatis, vita memoriae, magistra vitae, nuntia vetustatis" (History is the witness of time, the light of truth, the essence of remembrance, the teacher of life, the messenger from times past).

Marcus Tullius Cicero (106–43 BC)

"Who controls the past controls the future . . ."

George Orwell (1903–1950) From 1984

For millennia, the empirical experience of past generations suggested that those who survived certain diseases became resistant to repeated attacks. For example, plague survivors could attend to the needs of the sick and deceased without becoming sick again (Thucydides, 5th century BC). The earliest recorded and surprisingly successful attempt to enhance resistance to a harmful substance—in this case a plant poison—was described in great detail by the king of Pontus (a territory on the Black Sea Coast of Turkey), Mithridates VI-Eupator (about 132–63 BC) (Reinach, 1890). To protect himself against a highly probable attempt on his life by numerous adversaries to his rather despotic rule, Mithridates invented a universal antidote to the then commonly used plant-derived poisons. The formula found in his archives in his own handwriting consisted of two dried nuts, two figs, and 20 leaves of rue (an aromatic Eurasian plant, the "herb-of-grace" from which volatile oil used in ancient medicine can be expressed), which were crushed and mixed with salt. More importantly, the blood of ducks fed unspecified poisonous weeds was added before ritual ingestion of this mixture every morning. In fear of being captured by his enemies, the King always carried in the hilt of his scimitar a lethal dose of poison extracted from the plants given to the ducks. The protective effect of everyday ingestion of trace amounts of plant poisons apparently present in the ducks' blood was soon to be demonstrated under most dramatic circumstances. Mithridates had successively added to his kingdom of Pontus other provinces (Cappadocia and lands extending as far as the Crimea); his territorial conquest brought him into conflict with Rome. After his last and fateful battle of the third Mithridatian War with the Romans, and betrayal by his own son Farnaces II, who instigated an army revolt against his father, the desperate Mithridates attempted suicide by ingesting the poison hidden in his sword. Although the poison from the same vial was lethal for his daughters Mithridatis and Nysa, the king survived. Whether the dose was insufficient (he shared it with two additional persons) or Mithridates was "immune" to the poison remains disputable. In desperation, the unlucky king ordered his Gallic mercenary Bituit to stab him shortly before being captured by mutinous soldiers. These dramatic events captured the attention of the prolific French playwright Jean Racine (1639–1699) and inspired him to write the famous tragedy *Mithridate* (1673). A century later, Wolfgang Amadeus Mozart (1756–1791) composed at the age of 14 his highly successful youthful opera seria *Mitridate, Re di Ponto*, which premiered in December 1770, in Milan. Thus, the story of Mithridates, understandably devoid of its immunologic undertones, survives for posterity.

In the 5th century AD, wise men highly venerated for their experience, judgment, and wisdom, called sages, recommended in the Babylonian Talmud for the treatment of rabies that: "If one is bitten by a mad dog, he may eat his liver and be cured" (section Moed, tractat Yoma, chapter 8, segment 84). According to other sources, the diaphragm of a rabid dog should also have been ingested. Although there are no reports suggesting the success of such treatment, based on the current knowledge, it is not surprising that this recommended practice was not widely accepted and remained of historical interest.

The roots of mucosal immunity also can be traced to documents dated in 900 AD. The Chinese developed a secret ritual to ward off the dreaded scourge of their time, smallpox, which we now know was caused by the variola virus. As part of this Chinese ritual, the scabs of healed pustules were ground up and used as an inhalant. In many instances, this earliest form of nasal immunization worked so well that the practice made its way into India. However, in some instances this risky practice actually resulted in a fatal infection. Nevertheless, modifications of the practice spread from India to Turkey, where in 1717 Lady Mary Wortley Montagu (1689–1762) learned of it and brought the practice of variolation back to England. Her adaptation, although still risky, worked in many instances. Later in that century, Dr. Edward Jenner (1749–1823), who knew of and practiced this method

of treatment, worried about the inherent risks of spread of the disease. He astutely recognized that milkmaids often developed handsores closely resembling smallpox pustules; however, the lesions healed and in all cases they were immune to smallpox. As we now appreciate, the cowpox lesions were caused by *Vaccinia* virus, which, although related to the smallpox virus, was much less virulent for humans. The infection, however, did induce an immunity to smallpox (Jenner, 1798). The actual practice of using *Vaccinia* (from the Latin *Vacca*, cow) was adapted to describe use of attenuated bacteria or viruses, or inactivated bacterial toxins or recombinant proteins as *vaccines*, which of course is the accepted terminology today. Interestingly, 1996 was proclaimed the year of the vaccine in recognition of Jenner's contributions 200 years earlier. A complete worldwide vaccination program by the World Health Organization and other health agencies resulted in eradication of smallpox in 1979.

MUCOSAL MICROBIOTA

Based on Pasteur's work on the microbial nature of fermentation, it was widely believed that the presence of bacteria in the intestine was essential for the life of the host (Leidy, 1849). However, Metchnikoff (1903, 1908) tended to regard the intestinal flora as hostile, inducing toxemia in the host, and proposed that the process of premature aging could be prevented by altering the intestinal microbiota. Surprisingly, this doctrine found a fertile ground in the early 20th century and drastic forms of treatment, including high enemas or even therapeutic colectomies, were used to prevent intestinal autointoxication (Lane, 1926). On the other hand, many workers devoted themselves to determining whether life could be maintained with a sterile intestinal tract. One of the first was Schottelius (1899), who was able to rear chicks under sterile conditions. Nuttal and Thierfelder (1895) achieved some success with mammals: they removed embryonic guinea pigs by cesarean section and maintained them uncontaminated for several weeks. The conclusion was that bacteria in the intestinal tract were not necessary for mammalian life, when an appropriate diet was provided. Cohendy (1912) finally showed that "prolonged" life was possible in the absence of gut bacteria by rearing chicks for up to 40 days under germfree (GF) conditions.

Contemporary approaches were motivated by the belief that GF animals were invaluable tools for discrimination of genetically determined immune mechanisms, spontaneously available, from those induced by environmental antigens, especially intestinal microflora (for review see Sterzl *et al.*, 1987). This belief was supported by experiments done in many countries using guinea pigs: Glimstedt in Sweden (1932); Reyniers (1932) at the Lobund Institute, United States; and Miyakawa *et al.* (1958) in Japan. It was found that the wasting syndrome, which developed in thymectomized newborns, could be ameliorated by raising the altered animals under conditions that prevented intestinal colonization.

It has also been known for decades that gut commensal microbes colonizing the neonatal mammal effect the activation and development of the *systemic* immune system, especially to increase circulating specific and "natural" antimicrobial antibodies (Tlaskalová *et al.*, 1970; Carter and Pollard, 1971; Berg and Savage, 1975; Kim, 1979; Tlaskalová-Hogenová and Stepánková, 1980). Piglets were chosen because they displayed considerable fetal insulation, provided by a six-layered epithelial-chorial placenta. This barrier is impermeable not only to cells but also to larger protein molecules such as immunoglobulins (Ig) (Sterzl and Silverstein, 1967), and passive maternal antibodies are obtained after birth with early suckling of colostrum. Newborns were delivered into sterile bags and transferred into a laminar flow room containing sterilized cages (Trávnícek *et al.*, 1975). Similar approaches have proved effective for obtaining and maintaining GF rats, mice, and rabbits (Gustafsson, 1948; Carter and Pollard, 1971; Berg and Savage, 1975; Tlaskalová-Hogenová and Stepánková, 1980). Of these GF mammalian models, only piglets can be deprived of colostrums and milk and denied any passive immunity *via* maternal antibodies. Without the passive protection provided by the colostrum, piglets exposed to normal environmental microbes or artificially colonized with a "nonpathogenic" *Escherichia coli* die in 48 to 72 hours of bacterial septicemia (Trnka *et al.*, 1959). However, such colostrum-deprived, sterile piglets can be maintained under GF conditions with an appropriate diet.

Professor Joseph Leidy (1849) wrote that "from the opinion so frequently expressed that contagious diseases and some others might have their origin and reproductive character through the agency of cryptogamic spores . . . I was led to reflect upon the possibility of plants of this description existing in healthy animals, as a natural condition; or at least, apparently so, as in the case of *Entozoa*." Leidy reasoned that the wet epithelial surfaces of the body could provide a rich culture medium for commensal microbes. Perhaps the first systematic analyses of these commensal microbes were provided by Schaedler, Dubos, and their coworkers (Schaedler *et al.*, 1965a,b; Dubos *et al.*, 1965). They stated that "mice and other mammals normally harbor an extensive bacterial flora, not only in the large intestine, but also in the stomach and small intestine. Although this flora plays an essential role in the development and well being of its host, its exact composition is not known" (Schaedler *et al.*, 1965a). Unfortunately, their final lament is still true. However, the three seminal papers of Schaedler, Dubos, and coworkers offered the first comprehensive characterization of a portion of the gut microflora (using both aerobic and anaerobic *in vitro* culture) and employing the very models we still depend on today to assess the interactions of gut microbes with the gut-associated lymphoid tissue (GALT)—the natural colonization of neonates and the deliberate colonization of axenic (GF) mice with particular gut commensal bacteria.

Shortly after the gut lamina propria of several mammalian species (humans, rabbits, rats, and mice) was found to contain an abundance of secretory plasma cells (Crabbé *et al.*, 1965; Crandall *et al.*, 1967; Pierce and Gowans, 1975; Cebra

et al., 1977), most of which made IgA, it was noted that both GF adult mice (Crabbé *et al.*, 1970) and neonatal mice (for review see Parrott and MacDonald, 1990) had a paucity of such cells. Thus, the absence of gut microbes seemed to forestall the natural development of the abundant population of IgA plasma cells normally present in gut lamina propria. As early as 1968, Crabbé *et al.* (1968) were able to demonstrate that colonization of formerly GF mice with normal intestinal flora could stimulate the development of IgA plasma cells to normal levels within 4 weeks; furthermore, they showed that oral administration of the protein antigen ferritin to GF mice led to the appearance of antigen-specific IgA plasma cells in gut lamina propria (Crabbé *et al.*, 1969). Pollard made the significant observations that Peyer's patches of GF mice contained mainly "primary" (quiescent) B-lymphoid follicles, but that some enteric bacteria could activate germinal center (GC) reactions, whereas others were less effective (Pollard and Sharon, 1970; Carter and Pollard, 1971). Pollard and Sharon (1970), Foo and Lee (1972), and Berg and Savage (1975) all agreed that some enteric bacteria were more effective than others in stimulating the development of specific circulating antibodies. Thus, they tend to support the notion of autochthonous versus normal gut microbiota.

Coincident with these observations, in 1971, Peyer's patches were found to be sites for the preferred generation and accumulation of *precursors* for IgA plasma cells (Craig and Cebra, 1971), which could immigrate to and selectively populate all mucosal tissues (Cebra *et al.*, 1977). Thus, it became relevant to link the development of specific, IgA-committed B cells in Peyer's patches to the appearance and accumulation of specific IgA plasmablasts in the gut lamina propria or elsewhere in mucosal tissues and to try to implicate particular gut microbes as effective stimuli of these perturbations.

HEALING POWERS OF SECRETIONS: HISTORY OF BREASTFEEDING

Injured animals lick their wounds to clean them and also to hasten their healing. In many ancient cultures, squirting milk in the nose or conjunctiva of sick children and the application of urine or saliva to skin injuries were common medical practices. Lactational products of human and other mammalian species have long been associated with unique healing powers. Human milk, especially mother's own milk, has been considered a complete food for infants of all mammals in many ancient scriptures. More than 2500 years ago, with the evolution of agricultural civilization and domestication of mammals, it was proposed by Charak Sutrasthana that milk obtained from buffalo, cow, sheep, camel, donkey, horse, elephant, and goat, when fed to humans, can improve insomnia, appetite, and sexual drive, help ascites, piles, infestations by worms, skin disorders, muscle weakness, and a variety of other ailments (Athavale, 1977). As investigations by Koch began to establish research methods to study the etiology and pathogenesis of infectious disease in the 1800s, classic observations by Escherich (1888) provided, for the first time, evidence that intestinal flora of the human neonate is exquisitely sensitive to human milk. In studies carried out with coliform bacteria, he observed that bacteria isolated from the feces of persons on a meat diet possess a very intense ability to solubilize and split complex nitrogen compounds (egg albumin, casein), whereas bacteria from the feces of milk-fed babies utilize only small amounts of such compounds. Escherich stated: "It is noteworthy in connection with this latter property that it must be more than coincidence that if one spreads the feces of milk-fed babies on gelatin plates, not a single colony capable of liquefying the gelatin is found. However, most of the types from the feces of meat-fed persons will liquefy gelatin to a glue-like peptone. Further, both types show a particular effect on different types of sugar that are fermented with the production of acid. They give extensive growth on potato and finally in animal experiments demonstrate pathogenic properties" (Escherich, 1888).

Empirical experience supporting the notion that breast milk may protect against diarrheal diseases of children was reviewed by Hanson et al. (1988): "Analyses of infant mortality in diarrhoea from Sweden and Finland in the early 19th century showed that there was a peak during the summer. This increased mortality was related to the frequent 'summer diarrhoea' during the warm months of July and August. But this peak of mortality was primarily seen in areas where mothers did not breast-feed. In nearby areas where breast-feeding was the rule, there was no increase, or only a minor increase, in the infant mortality in diarrhoea during the summer. The difference did not relate primarily to socioeconomic factors since breast-feeding could be seen in very poor populations, whereas in the same area the farmers' wives had to leave their babies at home to be fed cow's milk through an unhygienic cow horn while working in the fields during the harvest."

The earliest scientifically documented contribution to our knowledge of milk as an important source of mucosal immunity and its functions in *in vivo* settings is based on studies by Paul Ehrlich (1854–1915) who, in 1892, demonstrated that maternal immunization and subsequent breastfeeding induced protection against the toxic substances ricin and abrin in suckling mice (Ehrlich, 1892). Based on his studies on transfer of immunity through milk, he clearly emphasized the natural breastfeeding of children and raised his voice against artificial feeding. His studies attempted to document the benefit of breastfeeding in mumps, typhus, and measles. Furthermore, he discussed the possible protective role of breastfeeding on congenital syphilis.

It is now well established that bifidobacteria predominate in the feces of the breast-milk-fed infant. Human, but not cow's, milk contains factors that stimulate colonization with bifidobacteria. This observation was largely possible because of the discovery in 1953 of *Bifidobacterium bifidum*, a subspecies of bifidobacteria that requires human milk for its growth. Over the years, bifidobacterium has been used anecdotally and more recently under controlled conditions as a therapeutic modality to prevent and treat diarrheal disease, induce immunomodulation, detoxify the gastrointestinal tract, and restore normal intestinal flora (for review see Bezkorovainy and Miller-Catchpole, 1989). Clinical experience in many countries over the past 2 centuries has suggested a strong link between breastfeeding and protection against diarrheal diseases and against fertility and childbearing (Jelliffe and Jelliffe, 1977).

Biologic linkage of the milk and mammary glands to the mucosal immune system was recognized initially by identification of immunoglobulins in milk by Gugler and von Muralt (1959) and Hanson (1961). Subsequent studies led to the identification of secretory IgA (S-IgA) in human milk (Hanson and Johansson, 1961). As these studies were being carried out in Europe, the presence of IgA was demonstrated in other external mucosal secretions by Tomasi and his coworkers (Chodirker and Tomasi, 1963; Tomasi and Zeigelbaum, 1963; Bienenstock and Tomasi, 1968) in the United States. These observations were followed by the definition of antiviral, antibacterial, and antiparasitic activity in S-IgA and other milk immunoglobulins; demonstration of a diverse spectrum of cellular elements and antigen-specific, cell-mediated immune responses; recovery of cytokines; and identification of other nonimmunologic defense factors in mammalian products of lactation.

Finally, several studies have identified intestinal and respiratory tract axes in homing of IgA-committed, antibody-forming cells from the intestinal Peyer's patches and bronchus-associated lymphoid tissues to the mammary glands (Montgomery et al., 1974, 1978; Goldblum et al., 1975; Roux et al., 1977; Fishaut et al., 1981; also see subsequent discussion). During the past 20 years it has become clear that many of the observations made by our ancestors have been proved to be accurate. These include the effects of breastfeeding on mucosal infections, childhood allergy, birth spacing, childhood survival, as well as effects on modulation of immune response and its regulation in autoimmune diseases.

ANTIBODIES OF EXTERNAL SECRETIONS

This discovery of antibodies in external secretions, or more specifically in gastrointestinal tract secretions, should be credited to a Russian pathologist, Alexandre Besredka (1870–1940), who initiated studies at the Pasteur Institute (which he headed) with two species of bacteria (Besredka, 1919). He used toxin-producing *Shigella dysenteriae* for work on enteric infections, and *Bacillus anthracis*, which Pasteur himself had used earlier in studies to develop an anthrax vaccine. Besredka clearly showed that oral immunization of rabbits with *S. dysenteriae* led to a solid immunity in the gastrointestinal tract that was unrelated to titers of serum antibodies. He also showed that cutaneous immunization with anthrax toxoid resulted in serum antibodies associated with resistance to challenge. Besredka (1919, 1927) deduced that both types of bacteria caused disease in part by production of exotoxins, and in the case of dysentery a local antibody response was protective.

The first direct demonstration of antibodies in stool was provided by A. Davies (1922), who studied fecal extracts from patients recovering from *S. dysenteriae* infection. Agglutinin titers as high as 1:80 were noted; however, peak titers occurred in bloody mucus, and he failed to see antibodies in normal, immunized subjects. Even so, he correctly deduced that most of the antibody activity present was derived by local synthesis and secretion into the gastrointestinal tract.

Studies of local antibody responses in the gastrointestinal tract and their role in protection from infection require a more appropriate infection agent and animal disease model than the dysentery-induced fatal infection of rabbits used by Besredka (1919). One can trace the first successful model, the guinea pig, to Robert Koch (1843–1910), who showed that the disease cholera could be reproduced by direct injection of *Vibrio cholerae* into the duodenum or by oral dosing with vibrios in 5% carbonate to neutralize stomach acidity, a method still in use for oral immunization to the present time. Nevertheless, opium was required to reduce intestinal peristalsis and to allow growth of *V. cholerae* in the small intestine, with subsequent diarrhea and death from dehydration (Koch, 1885). The model for cholera was more suitable for definitive demonstration that antibodies were produced locally in the gastrointestinal tract, because the diarrhea results from an intoxication (by cholera toxin), which is produced by noninvasive *V. cholerae*, as opposed to the dysentery model of Besredka (1919), in which *S. dysenteriae* actually invades the epithelium and causes a bloody diarrhea with sloughing of intestinal mucosa with possible plasma antibody transudates. Nevertheless, both Besredka (1919) and Davies (1922) reached the correct conclusion that gut mucosal antibodies were locally produced and not serum derived using the dysentery model in rabbits or convalescing humans, respectively.

The studies of Burrows, Havens, Koshland, and their coworkers were the first definitive evidence that antibodies to cholera in feces, termed *coproantibodies*, were indeed induced in guinea pigs after deliberate vaccination or oral infection with *V. cholerae*. In fact, in an elegant series of studies it was clearly established that either intraperitoneal vaccination or suboptimal oral infection led to the presence of coproantibodies, which preceded the development of serum antibodies (Burrows *et al.*, 1947; Burrows and Ware, 1953; Burrows and Havens, 1948). Furthermore, the presence of these coproantibodies correlated with protection from oral challenge with live vibrios. Additional work using prior irradiation and intraperitoneal immunization led to the induction of fecal antibodies in the absence of serum antibody responses, and again protection from challenge was achieved (Koshland and Burrows, 1950).

The essential protective role of intestinal antibodies in survival was demonstrated 35 years ago in a unique model of GF, colostrum-deprived newborn piglets (Rejnek *et al.*, 1968). Because of the absent transplacental transport of antibodies, these animals deprived of milk die of septicemia with environmental bacteria, as described earlier. However,

after ~2–3 days, the intestinal absorption of antibodies from milk into the circulation ceases and they remain in the gut lumen. Although all control animals given *E. coli* orally succumbed to infection, piglets that also orally received immune milk or serum (or isolated antibodies) survived irrespective of the source of Ig isotype. These experiments convincingly demonstrated that antibodies function locally within the intestinal lumen and prevent otherwise fatal infection with commensal microbiota.

Studies on experimental infection of mice with influenza virus were also providing evidence for a local protection. For example, immunity to influenza correlated directly with the presence of antibodies in tracheal–bronchial washes, and not in serum. Furthermore, the presence of antibodies in the murine respiratory tract actually prevented experimental influenza infection (Fazekas de St. Groth and Donnelly, 1950a,b). Thus, studies performed in animals provided strong evidence that secretory antibodies were not mere transudates of antibodies from plasma and that resistance to mucosal infections correlated better with the titers of antibodies in the relevant secretion than in serum. However, the importance of secretory antibodies and their accumulation, as a response to the influenza virus infection, was predicted by Francis and Brightman (1941) and Francis *et al.* (1943). Although the original publications are unavailable, Shvartsman and Zykov (1976) reviewed a large number of papers from 1938 to 1972, generated by Russian and East European investigators (Soloviev, Parnes, Zakstelskaya, Smorodintsev, Zhdanov, Sokolov, Slepushkin, Ikic, Sarateanu, Cajal, and their coworkers). These studies concerned the immunobiologic properties of secretory antibodies induced in animals by systemic and mucosal immunizations, immunologic memory, designs of live vaccines, and differences in immune responses induced by various influenza virus vaccines (live or inactivated) given to tens of thousands of vaccinees by the oral, nasal, or systemic routes. Retrospectively, we must regret that results of these studies were either not published or printed in journals unavailable (or not read) in other countries.

When IgA was shown to be the major isotype in the secretions (see subsequent discussion), it was logical to infer that such protection was mediated by IgA antibodies. In the ensuing years, a number of laboratories went on to demonstrate, both clinically and experimentally, the ability of IgA antibodies to confer protection against a variety of infectious agents that affect mucosal membranes. In some studies, protection was shown directly; in others, resistance to infection best correlated with specific IgA antibody content in the particular secretion. Some of the key observations were made by Smith *et al.* (1967), Ogra *et al.* (1968), and Fubara and Freter (1973). From such studies, together with the knowledge that IgA antibodies in milk are not absorbed from the gut of the suckling infant (Ammann and Stiehm, 1966), it could be concluded that IgA antibodies in mucosal secretions can act as a luminal barrier to inhibit the attachment and penetration of antigens, including intact microbes. A consistent observation was that IgA-deficient individuals have increased serum antibodies to food antigens (Buckley and Dees, 1969), indicative of a deficient intestinal barrier. Further support for the immune barrier concept came from work by Williams and Gibbons (1972), who showed that S-IgA antibodies can prevent bacteria from adhering to epithelial cells, and Walker *et al.* (1972), who showed that oral immunization can reduce the subsequent absorption of the same antigen. Moreover, the barrier function of S-IgA could be aided by its relative resistance to degradation by proteases (Brown *et al.*, 1970).

The discovery of IgA with its unique properties and predominance in almost all external secretions deserves a closer examination. In the early 1950s, many investigators studying the properties of human myeloma proteins noted that not all "γ-globulins" fulfilled the criteria as then defined by low–molecular-weight and carbohydrate-poor (7S), or high-molecular-weight and carbohydrate-rich (19S) antibodies (for review, see Heremans, 1974). It appeared that some proteins with an electrophoretic mobility in the β-region differed from both 7S and 19S antibodies in their precipitability with inorganic salts (*e.g.*, $ZnSO_4$) and displayed antigenic properties distinct from both 7S and 19S antibodies (Slater *et al.*, 1955). Although some of these myeloma proteins with β electrophoretic mobility shared the same molecular weight with 7S antibodies, their carbohydrate content was remarkably higher. These findings prompted Slater *et al.* (1955) to postulate the existence of an additional class of antibodies.

Drawing on this knowledge and exploiting novel immunochemical techniques, Heremans and his coworkers demonstrated in a series of papers (Heremans, 1959; Heremans *et al.*, 1959, 1963; Carbonara and Heremans, 1963) that the carbohydrate-rich, serologically peculiar β-globulin constituted a type of antibody that was distinct from 7S and 19S globulins and was also present in normal human serum. The designation as IgA was accepted in 1964, and all previous synonyms, such as βx, $β_{2A}$-globulin, $γ_{1A}$, and γA, were abandoned.

Antibodies were found in milk by Gugler and von Muralt (1959), as mentioned earlier. In parotid saliva, immunoglobulins were identified by Ellison *et al.* (1960) and by Kraus and Sirisinha (1962). The presence of additional antigenic determinants on milk compared with serum antibodies was noted by Hanson (1961) and Hanson and Johansson (1962). In several outstanding papers, Tomasi and coworkers (Chodirker and Tomasi, 1963; Tomasi and Ziegelbaum, 1963; Tomasi *et al.*, 1965) demonstrated the predominance of IgA in a polymeric (p) form (11S) in many external secretions of human origin and provided a structural explanation for additional antigenic determinants on S-IgA by the discovery of a novel, IgA-associated polypeptide—secretory piece—later renamed secretory component (SC). The independent identification of a previously observed polypeptide, thought to be an aberrant L chain, as a novel component, joining (J) chain, in pIgA from the serum of myeloma patients (Halpern and Koshland, 1970) and in polymeric serum IgM and S-IgA from human colostrum (Mestecky *et al.*, 1971), resulted in the proposal of a molecular formula

for rabbit (O'Daly and Cebra, 1971) and human (Mestecky *et al.*, 1972) dimeric S-IgA as $(α_2L_2)_2 \cdot SC_1 \cdot J_1$. By then, the well-established preponderance of IgA in external secretions had prompted numerous studies that resulted in several models of selectivity of IgA transport (for review, see Brandtzaeg, 1981). Some investigators speculated that monomeric IgA was assembled into polymers within epithelial cells through incorporation of SC (Tomasi *et al.*, 1965; South *et al.*, 1966). Infusion of IgA-containing plasma to children with low serum levels of IgA led to the appearance of IgA in the saliva. Contrary to the SC-dependent polymerization of IgA, Lawton and Mage (1969) and Bienenstock and Strauss (1970) convincingly demonstrated by immunochemical studies of rabbit and human S-IgA that the polymerization is SC independent and must occur within IgA-secreting plasma cells *before* their product is taken up by epithelial cells. The importance of the polymeric configuration and the presence of J chain for efficient SC binding was predicted by Mach (1970, addendum) and documented by Radl *et al.* (1971, 1974). Based on previous extensive histochemical studies of the distribution of component chains of S-IgA in tissue sections performed in several laboratories (*e.g.*, Tomasi *et al.*, 1965; Tourville *et al.*, 1969; Poger and Lamm, 1974), but mainly his own, Brandtzaeg (1974) proposed that SC on epithelial cells functions as a receptor for J chain–containing pIgA, which is transported into external secretions. Further evidence to support this contention was provided by *in vitro* studies of pIgA- or IgM-binding *live* human adenocarcinoma epithelial cell lines of intestinal origin (Crago *et al.*, 1978; Nagura *et al.*, 1979; Brandtzaeg and Prydz, 1984) and costaining for SC and IgA on isolated intestinal epithelial cells (Brandtzaeg, 1978).

The structural–cellular interactions responsible for an extremely effective transport of pIgA from the circulation into the bile of mice and rats, the so-called "liver pump" (Jackson *et al.*, 1977; Lemaitre-Coelho *et al.*, 1977), were explored in the late 1970s and early 1980s in several laboratories. Immunohistochemical and functional studies of liver cells from many vertebrate species convincingly demonstrated that the murine, rat, and rabbit but not human hepatocytes express SC (see Chapter 12) responsible for the binding and selective transport of pIgA present in a free form as well as in the form of low-molecular-weight immune complexes.

Extensive studies concerning the interaction of Igs with various cell populations resulted in the discovery of cellular receptors specific for the Fc fragment of Igs of some but not all isotypes. The binding of radiolabeled IgA of various molecular forms, including S-IgA, to human neutrophils (Spiegelberg *et al.*, 1974) and monocytes (Fanger *et al.*, 1980) led to the discovery of Fcα receptors and their participation in cell activation and promotion of phagocytosis. Importantly for many subsequent studies of biologic functions of IgA (*e.g.*, activation of complement and opsonization), aggregated myeloma IgA proteins of both subclasses and polyclonal S-IgA bound better than free IgA and the Fcα receptors differed remarkably in their specificities from the Fcγ receptors (Spiegelberg *et al.*, 1974; Lawrence *et al.*, 1975).

Antigenic differences among various human IgA myeloma proteins resulted in the discovery, in 1966, of IgA subgroups, later reclassified as subclasses, by four independent groups of investigators (Feinstein and Franklin, 1966; Kunkel and Prendergast, 1966; Vaerman and Heremans, 1966; Terry and Roberts, 1966). Their structural uniqueness, including differences in heavy–light chain covalent bonding (Grey *et al.*, 1968), carbohydrate structures, existence of genetic variants (allotypes) that are restricted to the IgA2 subclass (Kunkel *et al.*, 1969), characteristic distribution in systemic and mucosal compartments, and medical importance such as sensitivity to proteases produced by bacterial pathogens, and their association with diseases (*e.g.*, IgA nephropathy), are described in pertinent chapters of this book.

Although an increased resistance of S-IgA compared with serum immunoglobulins to proteolytic enzymes was observed by Brown *et al.* (1970), the presence of an Fc fragment of IgA in stools indicated that at least a fraction of intestinal IgA is cleaved *in vivo* by enzyme(s) of enteric microbial origin (Mehta *et al.*, 1973). This finding resulted in the discovery of bacterial proteases that cleave IgA1 into Fab and Fc fragments: *Streptococcus sanguis, Neisseria gonorrhoeae, Neisseria meningitidis* (Plaut *et al.*, 1974, 1975), *Streptococcus pneumoniae*, and *Haemophilus influenzae* (Kilian *et al.*, 1979; Male, 1979) were initially identified as producers of unique IgA1 proteases.

ANATOMIC STUDIES OF MUCOSAL ORGANS AND THEIR FUNCTIONAL IMPLICATIONS

Current extensive studies of lymphoid cell trafficking as related to the induction of mucosal immune responses or tolerance have emphasized the role of unique lymphoepithelial structures associated with the intestinal and respiratory tract. These structures were described in the intestine by Johannes Conrad Peyer (1653–1712), a Swiss anatomist and naturalist who lived most of his life in what is now known as Schaffhausen in the vicinity of Lake Constance. It was here that he first noted in 1673 the structures that subsequently bear his name: *Peyer's patches*. He published his observations in 1677 in a treatise entitled *Exercitatio anatomico—medica de glandulis intestinorum, earumque usu et affectionibus. Cui subjungitur anatome ventriculi galliinacei* (Peyer, 1677). It is noteworthy that Peyer's original treatise of 1677 was published in exactly the same form for a second time in 1681 by H. Wetstenium in Amsterdam. This accounts for the confusion as to when Peyer originally published his work. At that time it was common to publish the same work in more than one place. In *Garrison and Morton's Medical Bibliography*, it is stated that these same structures were first described by Johannes Nicolau Pechlin (1672) in his treatise titled *De purgantium medicamentorum facultatibus exercitatio nova* (Pechlin, 1672; Norman, 1991). Additionally, it has been suggested

that the same structures had already been noted in 1645 by Marco Aurelio Severino (1580–1656), who was a professor of anatomy and surgery in Naples (Schmidt, 1959).

As indicated in his title, Peyer actually described these structures as glands, because when he squeezed them, he saw a milky fluid (chyle) emerging from what he thought were these structures. It was only with the advent of microscopes and histology that it became clear that these structures contained mononuclear cells (lymphocytes) and were lymphoid nodules, not secretory glands.

Peyer was a physician who studied medicine in Basel and subsequently Paris and Montpellier. After his studies he returned to his birthplace, where he became the pupil of Johannes Jakob Wepfer, whose son-in-law was Johannes Conrad Brunner, who first described the duodenal glands that now carry his name. Considering Peyer's close association with Wepfer and Brunner, it is not surprising that Peyer thought that the lymphatic nodules were secreting glands.

The role and function of Peyer's patches remained obscure for 160 years when William Wood Gerhard published a classic study of patients dying from typhus (Gerhard, 1837). Louis, the great Parisian clinician under whom Gerhard studied, had originally described a triad that involved enlargement of Peyer's patches, mesenteric glands, and spleen in what was at that time termed *dothinenteritis* or typhoid fever, which also included typhus, these two diseases not having yet been differentiated. Gerhard differentiated them and pointed out the lack of involvement of Peyer's patches in typhus, quoted in *A Bibliographical History of Medicine* (Talbott, 1970).

It was widely thought that the lymphatic glands or nodules were involved in some way in defense mechanisms of the intestinal tract, especially because they were clearly enlarged in various intestinal infections such as typhoid fever. However, relatively little new significant information on these structures became available until the 20th century. Jolly (1913) coined the name *lympho-epithelial organs* and applied it to Peyer's patches and the bursa of Fabricius because of the close relationship between lymphatic tissue and the mucosal epithelium. Aschoff (1926), quoted by Ehrich (1929), classified them with lymphatic tissue of the mucous membranes of the digestive, respiratory, reproductive, and urinary systems, in a group distinct from lymph glands and nodes. However, it was not until 1935 that Hummel stated that Peyer's patches "are located at the beginnings of lymph channels rather than in their course" (Hummel, 1935). She did a careful study of intestinal lymphoid tissue and classified it according to the presence or absence of well-formed germinal centers, which were dependent on age and exposure to intestinal contents. Sanders and Florey (1940) published a paper on the effects of the removal of lymphatic tissue. They coined the name *peyerectomy* and successfully carried out the surgical removal of visible Peyer's patches and other lymphoid tissue including the spleen to study the effect on the hypertrophy of residual lymphoid tissue and numbers of circulating lymphocytes. Clearly, peyerectomy caused a decrease in the number of circulating lymphocytes and interestingly, hypertrophy of intrahepatic lymphoid tissue. Jacobson *et al.* (1961) showed that mice could be protected from otherwise fatal total body irradiation by the shielding of a single Peyer's patch.

In a light and dissecting microscopic study of human Peyer's patches, Cornes (1965) showed that the number of patches increase with age to about 12 years and then decline rapidly to age 20, followed by a slower but steady decrease in number of visible lymphoid aggregates up to old age. All these observations led eventually to the experiments of Cooper *et al.* (1966), who showed in rabbits that the surgical removal of the sacculus rotundus, appendix, and Peyer's patches followed by x-irradiation, led to a selective deficiency of antibody-producing capacity to a range of antigens while leaving delayed hypersensitivity and rejection of skin allografts intact.

Joel *et al.* (1970) observed that the lymphoid epithelium of mouse Peyer's patches had the capacity to take up and retain India ink particles selectively. The first description of *follicle-associated epithelium* overlying gut-associated lymphoid tissue (GALT) was provided by Bockman and Cooper (1973). As they clearly state in their review (Bockman and Cooper, 1973; Bockman and Stevens, 1977) of the previous literature, others had described micropinocytotic activity in such lymphoepithelium before them as well as the unusual nature of this epithelium (Faulk *et al.*, 1970). However, Bockman and Cooper showed selective pinocytosis by this epithelium in the chicken bursa, rabbit appendix, and mouse Peyer's patches. This work was expanded by Owen and Jones (1974) in an ultrastructural study of human Peyer's patch tissue. It was in this last paper that these authors first used the term *M* for microfold cell, a name that appears to have been retained and is now in general use. Experiments by Schaffner *et al.* (1974) and Sorvari *et al.* (1975) clearly showed the selective pinocytotic capacity of chicken bursal lymphoepithelium in regard to environmental and luminal antigens. In 1977, Owen, as well as Bockman and Stevens, published their separate papers describing a specific and selective uptake of tracer molecules.

Because of similarities in appearance between rabbit intestinal lymphoid tissue in the appendix and sacculus rotundus, Archer *et al.* (1963) suggested that the lymphoid tissue in the intestine might be analogous to the avian bursa of Fabricius. The differentiation of the role of the bursa of Fabricius in its regulation of B-cell development from that of the thymus and its role in T-cell development had occurred as a result of the pioneering work of Glick *et al.* (1956), in a now classic paper on the role of the bursa in antibody production. A series of papers by Cooper, Percy, Good, and associates supported this view of gut-associated lymphoid tissue (GALT), which was subsequently overtaken by the concept that in mammals the bone marrow may serve as the actual bursal equivalent (for review, see Waksman and Ozer, 1976).

In their paper on "The route of re-circulation of lymphocytes in the rat," Gowans and Knight (1964) clearly showed for the first time that lymphocytes circulated from blood to lymph and back again, and that this migration from blood to lymph occurred as a result of a special affinity by lymphocytes for the endothelium of postcapillary venules. The same paper showed that thoracic duct lymphoblasts were retained primarily in the bowel and that Peyer's patches were a major site for localization of recirculating small lymphocytes obtained from rat thoracic duct lymph. Griscelli *et al.* (1969), Hall and Smith (1970), and Hall *et al.* (1972) showed that lymphoblasts from the thoracic duct were localized or homed primarily to the intestine. The latter authors postulated that they might be "particularly concerned with furnishing the IgA antibodies that protect mucous surfaces in general and the gut in particular." Coincident with these publications from Hall's group, Craig and Cebra (1971) directly demonstrated that Peyer's patches were enriched in lymphoid precursors for IgA plasmablasts, by cell transfer into sublethally, x-irradiated allogeneic rabbits or congenic, IgA-allotype distinct mice (see Cebra *et al.*, 1977). Copious, predominantly IgA plasmablasts were observed in the spleens of recipient allogeneic rabbits and in the intestinal lamina propria of recipient congenic mice following such cell transfers. These studies were closely followed by findings that Peyer's patches were required for efficient uptake of antigen from the gut lumen and dissemination of specifically stimulated IgA antibody-forming cells throughout the gut lamina propria, using pairs of Thiry-Vella intestinal loops (Robertson and Cebra, 1976; Cebra *et al.*, 1977). Further relevant studies showed that the enhanced potential of Peyer's patch B cells to generate specific IgA plasmablasts *in vitro* and *in vivo* was correlated with their markedly higher content of IgA memory B cells compared with systemic lymphoid organs (Cebra *et al.*, 1977; Gearhart and Cebra, 1979; Fuhrman and Cebra, 1981). It was subsequently shown (Rudzik *et al.*, 1975) that the localization of IgA-containing cells in the spleen was due to an allogeneic effect.

Bienenstock *et al.* (1973a,b) published definitive papers on what they termed *bronchus-associated lymphoid tissue* (BALT) and deemed it analogous to the GALT described originally by Good, Cooper, and coworkers (see previous discussion). It may be pertinent that Klein (1875) had noted morphologic similarities between the bronchial and intestinal lymphoid follicles and stated remarkably that "these lymphoid follicles in the bronchial walls are therefore in every respect analogous to the lymph follicles found in other mucous membranes, e.g. tonsils and in the intestine...." Bienenstock (1974) concluded that "this lymphoid tissue might be part of a more universal mucosal lymphoid system" and in 1974 coined the term *common mucosal immunological system* in the Proceedings of the Second International Congress of Immunology.

Studies of the origin, migration, and homing of lymphoid cells from GALT and BALT to other mucosal sites were of basic importance for parallel attempts to induce specific immune responses in external secretions. Montgomery *et al.* (1974, 1978) found that specific IgA antibody could be induced in the mammary secretions of rabbits by oral and bronchial immunization. This observation was confirmed and extended by the experiments of Goldblum *et al.* (1975)

in the human. In the same year, Rudzik *et al.* (1975) and McWilliams *et al.* (1975, 1977) offered further data suggesting a common mucosal immunologic system when they showed that cells derived from GALT, BALT, or mesenteric lymph nodes repopulated bronchial and intestinal lamina propria with IgA-containing cells. This general concept that cells migrate from one mucosal site to another and there provide protection against the immunizing antigen received considerable support and development as a result of the experiments of many investigators. Thus, Michalek *et al.* (1976) demonstrated that oral immunization with *Streptococcus mutans* induces salivary IgA antibodies that protected rats from the development of dental caries. Roux *et al.* (1977) and Weisz-Carrington *et al.* (1978, 1979) showed that mesenteric lymph node blasts homed to the murine lactating mammary gland and that this homing was under hormonal influence. The parallel induction of specific IgA antibodies in saliva and tears of orally immunized individuals extended the commonness of the mucosal immune system to the oral cavity and ocular system in humans (Mestecky *et al.*, 1978). Finally, this work was extended to the female reproductive tract of experimental animals (McDermott and Bienenstock, 1979; McDermott *et al.*, 1980).

Many investigators have contributed to the development of the concept of the common mucosal immune system from its first proposal. It is now thought that the mucosal immune system may be more generalized even than originally thought. Although mucosal-associated lymphoid tissue (MALT) has been used to describe this concept (Bienenstock *et al.*, 1979), it is widely assumed that the solitary lymphoid follicles or nodules often found in mucosal tissues may be part of this generalized system. Indeed, Ham (1969), in his classic textbook of histology, suggested that these isolated mucosal lymphoid follicles were "a characteristic of wet epithelial surfaces." Thus, the concept of a common mucosal immune system may well comprise all mucosal surfaces including the nasal, lacrimal, mammary, and salivary glands, the mucosal part of the bronchial tract, intestine, and both female and male reproductive tracts. The extent to which the skin is involved in this system remains to be determined.

In addition to lymphocytes in Peyer's patches and lamina propria, the epithelial lining of some mucosal surfaces, intestines in particular, contains large numbers of unique cells—intraepithelial lymphocytes (IEL) (see Chapter 30). The discovery and initial characterization of the "round cells" (runde Zellen) as leukocytes were made by Weber (1847) and Eberth (1864) and were followed by numerous papers from other German investigators (for reviews see Wolf-Heidegger, 1939; Ferguson, 1977). Considering the rather limited repertoire of available methodologies to study the function of IEL, several researchers predicted with an admirable foresight that IEL may rejuvenate the aging epithelial cells. For example, Guieysse-Pellissier (1912), Goldner (1929), and Bunting and Huston (1921) proposed that the gut was the graveyard of lymphocytes. Based on extensive studies concerning the presence of lymphocytes within the intestinal epithelium of many species, Fichtelius

(1967, 1970) speculated that these cells, called theliolymphocytes, represented a mammalian analog of avian bursa of Fabricius (a "bursa-equivalent") that influences the maturation of B cells. Extensive studies carried out from the early 1960s to the late 1970s (for review see Ferguson, 1977) provided detailed morphologic description and characterization of IEL at the light and electron microscopic levels, their distribution throughout the gut, precise localization and relationship to the villous epithelium, initial quantitative data, and their proliferative potential. Furthermore, it was demonstrated that the numbers and phenotypes of IEL display marked variations in patients with celiac disease, dermatitis herpetiformis, tropical sprue, giardiasis, and other gastrointestinal disorders, but not in Crohn's disease or ulcerative colitis (Ferguson, 1977).

MUCOSAL VACCINATION

The seminal contributions of Paul Ehrlich to the field of mucosal immunity are rarely appreciated in modern literature, yet his outstanding studies performed more than 100 years ago must impress current researchers with their simplicity, perfection of execution, and impact on the future development of mucosal immunology. The protective effect of oral immunization with highly toxic substances of plant origin (ricin, abrin, and robin) was demonstrated in three animal species (mainly mice, but also guinea pigs and rabbits) (Ehrlich, 1891a, 1891b). After having determined the precise lethal dose (for both systemic and oral administration) of abrin and ricin, Ehrlich immunized these animals by the oral route with initially minute but subsequently increasing doses given for up to 40 consecutive days. After such treatment, animals became immune to a subcutaneous challenge with ricin at doses that were 400- to 800-fold greater than the normally lethal amount. Furthermore, the blood from immunized animals contained protective antiricin "matter" (*ein antitoxischer Körper*) transferable to unimmunized animals. For historical precision we should remind ourselves that the terms *Antikörper* in German and *antibody* in English were used for the first time by an Austrian-born American pathologist, Karl Landsteiner (1868–1943), in 1900. The discoverers of these "matters," Emil von Behring (1854–1917) and Shibasaburo Kitasato (1852–1931), did not use such terminology in their landmark paper (Behring and Kitasato, 1890) on the passive protection of animals with sera from tetanus toxin-immunized animals, published in 1890, only 1 year before Ehrlich's studies. In contrast to systemic immunization with ricin or abrin, which may cause severe local reactions even at small doses, oral immunization was much safer, although higher doses were required to achieve immunity. However, the most astounding finding of Ehrlich's studies concerned the immunity induced in the *eyes of orally* immunized animals. Ricin and especially abrin are extremely toxic when given in the conjunctival sac: panophthalmia with subsequent necrosis of the eye follows. Surprisingly, orally immunized animals tolerated intraconjunctival application of concentrated ricin or abrin ointments or solutions without any ill effects! The exquisite specificity of the protective "matters" was convincingly demonstrated by the lack of immunity to ricin in abrin-immunized animals and vice versa. Therefore, without knowledge of the existence of antibodies in external secretions or the migratory patterns of antibody-secreting cells, Paul Ehrlich inadvertently demonstrated in 1891 the concept of the common mucosal immune system! Only 1 year later, in 1892, Ehrlich documented the protective property of milk taken from immunized dams and given to suckling pups (see earlier discussion).

The first attempts at vaccination against bacterial diseases through the intestinal tract were carried out in Pasteur's laboratory before 1880 (for reviews, see Calmette, 1923; Gay, 1924). Pasteur (1880), Roux, and Chamberland protected chickens against chicken cholera by ingestion of food containing *Bacillus avisepticus* (now *Yersinia multocida*), although the feeding of anthrax spores to sheep was less effective than the subcutaneous injection of attenuated vaccines **(Table 1)**.

A series of attempts followed between 1892 and 1903, when many scientists (e.g., Klemperer, 1892) induced immunity to *V. cholerae* and *Salmonella typhi* by the ingestion of killed or living bacteria by animals and even humans (see in Calmette, 1923). Interestingly, *serum* agglutinins were considered the indicators of protection. This contention met with considerable criticism from Besredka, Calmette, and Gay. The last author wrote in 1924: "It is particularly true that a general reaction as evidenced by serum antibodies is no indication of a superior local protection, for example in the intestine, if we admit that this exists." (!) Various other bacteria such as *Mycobacterium tuberculosis*, *Yersinia pestis*, and *Corynebacterium diphtheriae* were also given orally with some degree of success (Calmette, 1923). However, bacteria that infect through the intestinal tract, where their pathogenic effects are manifest, remained in focus . . . "to protect certain areas of increased susceptibility by the process of local immunization or to close certain 'portals of entry' by the same process" (Gay, 1924). The efficacy of oral immuniza-

Table 1 Selected List of Bacterial and Food Antigens Used in Mucosal Immunization Studies in Humans and Animals

Antigen	Results and Comments	Author
Yersinia multocida (chicken cholera)	Oral immunization; protection induced	Pasteur, 1880
Vibrio cholerae	Oral immunization, moderate protection	Klemperer, 1892; Metchnikoff, 1903[a]
Mycobacterium tuberculosis	Serum antibodies induced by oral immunization	Calmette and Guérin 1906–1923[a]
Yersinia pestis		
Corynebacterium diphtheriae		
Shigella dysenteriae	Limited protection	Besredka, 1919, 1927
Salmonella typhi	Oral immunization preferable to systemic	Vaillant, 1922[a]
Streptococcus pneumoniae	Protection achieved by nasal immunization	Bull and McKee, 1922
	Protection achieved by oral immunization	Ross, 1930
Abrin, ricin, robin	Oral immunization results in systemic and mucosal protection	Ehrlich, 1891a, 1981b
Cow's milk and whey	Prevention of anaphylaxis by feeding	Besredka, 1909
Cow's milk, ox blood, egg white, zein, oats	Decrease in systemic reactivity after prolonged but not short ingestion of these antigens	Wells and Osborne, 1911
Dinitrochlorobenzene	Inhibition of systemic (skin) reactivity after hapten feeding; inability to suppress skin sensitivity by oral immunization in previously sensitized animals[b]	Chase, 1946
Poison ivy	Oral ingestion results in decreased skin reactivity in a few studies; discouraged for lack of efficacy	Stevens, 1945
Horse serum and meat	Sensitization for anaphylaxis	Rosenaw and Anderson, 1907[a]
Proteins from rice, corn, and oat flour	Precipitins in serum	Magus, 1908[a]

[a] Data from Bull and McKee (1929); Chase (1946); Gay (1924); Stevens (1945); Klingman (1958); Wells and Osborne (1911); Calmette (1923).
[b] See Table 3.

tion in the protection against intraperitoneal challenge with *Streptococcus pneumoniae* in a rat model was demonstrated in a series of papers by Ross (1930). A single or even better, repeated ingestion of heat-killed, desiccated, mechanically disrupted, or bile acids–dissolved pneumococci induced a high degree of protection against 10^3–10^4 lethal doses, curiously, as short as 48 hours after immunization. Feeding of rats' tissues of animals killed by pneumococci or living or acid-killed pneumococci was also protective. Sera of orally immunized animals did not contain any agglutinins or precipitins; external secretions were not examined.

As described in the previous section on Antibodies of External Secretions, the concept of oral or intestinal immunization was brought to prominence by Besredka (1919, 1927). Although his immunization studies with *S. typhi* in a rabbit model met with considerable skepticism (Gay, 1924), his later reports using *S. dysenteriae*, again in a rabbit model, demonstrated that when killed cultures were given *per os*, protection was local in that antibodies were found first locally in the intestine rather than in the general circulation (Besredka, 1919). Similar results were obtained by Masaki (1922) with *V. cholerae* in a rabbit model. In several studies, Besredka stressed the importance of giving bile before or with the administration of oral vaccines.

The validity of results obtained in animal models was soon tested in humans. Vaillant (1922) used Besredka's vaccine during an outbreak of typhoid fever: among 1236 subjects immunized orally, there were only 2 cases of typhoid (0.17%); in 173 who received subcutaneous vaccine, 4 cases were recorded (2.3%); and among 600 unvaccinated individuals, 50 cases were observed (8.3%)! Later, Besredka (1927) reported the results of immunization of students in a military academy: among 253 students immunized subcutaneously, 10 cases of typhoid occurred (4%), whereas in those who received the oral vaccine with bile (268 subjects), 5 cases of infection were recorded (1.9%).

The current revival of interest in intranasal immunization initialized by Waldman *et al.* (1968) should also be viewed from a historical perspective. Bull and McKee (1929) immunized rabbits intranasally with a suspension of killed pneumococci before challenge with the live pathogen. A single intranasal immunization performed 11 days before challenge protected all animals from death (**Table 2**), whereas 83% of rabbits immunized once 8 days before challenge, and 57% of unimmunized controls, succumbed. To detect antibody responses, the authors used the complement-fixation test performed with *sera* from these animals. In the absence of such antibodies, the authors concluded that the protection was independent of serum antibodies. In light of our current knowledge, it is likely that IgA-mediated protective responses were induced but were not detectable in serum because of the extremely rapid elimination of IgA from the circulation of rabbits. Moreover, complement fixation is inappropriate to test for the presence of IgA antibodies. Antibodies in nasal secretions were not examined. In the authors' defense, antibody isotypes and their different complement-binding properties were unknown, and the discovery of antibodies in nasal secretions was 40 years away.

The seminal role of inductive sites of MALT in the generation of immune responses at the site of vaccination as well as in secretions and tissues of anatomically remote mucosae and glands has been exploited with increasing frequency in the design of vaccines that can be administered by mucosal routes. Although many such vaccines and unique delivery systems are currently being explored, it may be useful to illustrate the "mucosal" history of a vaccine against poliomyelitis—a dreadful disease that is likely to be eliminated from the world.

Efforts to develop immunoprophylaxis against polioviruses began immediately after the first isolation of the virus. Both killed and live virus vaccine candidates were developed as early as 1910, although at that time information on the existence of three distinct poliovirus types was not available. During the early 1930s, studies were undertaken to vaccinate humans with infected monkey spinal cord suspensions inactivated with formalin or sodium ricinoleate (Kolmer *et al.*, 1935; Brodie and Park, 1936). However, these trials failed for lack of adequate controls, failure or inability to standardize vaccine preparations, and lack of reproducible quantitative methodologies for virus titration. The battle against polio began seriously at the national level in the United States with the establishment of the National Foundation for Infantile Paralysis—March of Dimes organization in 1938 with the first Franklin D. Roosevelt Birthday Ball to support clinical

Table 2 Protection Achieved by Intranasal Immunization of Rabbits with *Streptococcus pneumoniae*

No. of Treatments	Died (%)	Infected but Recovered (%)	Escaped Infection (%)
4	7.7	7.7	84.6
2	14.3	14.3	71.4
1 (11 days before infection)	0	83.4	16.6
1 (8 days before infection)	83.4	0	16.6
Normal rabbits (10 series of 6)	57	27.0	16.0

Modified from Bull and McKee (1929).

research aid, at Georgia Warm Springs Foundation in 1939 (Smith, 1991). Furthermore, during World War II, information became available regarding the distinct antigenic types of the virus, their ability to induce specific antibody responses after inactivation, the ability of inactivated virus to induce protection against intracerebral challenge (Morgan, 1948; Bodian, 1949), and the capacity of polioviruses to replicate *in vitro* in human and primate tissue culture cells (Enders *et al.*, 1949; Enders, 1952). Other wartime efforts directed toward the control of epidemics of influenza with an inactivated vaccine resulted in a renewed interest in the development of formalin-inactivated poliovaccines (Salk, 1953). The introduction of tissue culture techniques and the characterization of the poliovirus passage in tissue culture is a landmark and represents the cornerstone of our current knowledge of cell–virus interaction. These observations significantly facilitated the development of other live attenuated or inactivated vaccine candidates (Koprowski *et al.*, 1952, Jervis *et al.*, 1956; Sabin, 1955). The inactivated type of polio vaccine (Salk IPV) was licensed in 1955 and the Sabin oral live attenuated polio vaccine (Sabin OPV) was licensed in 1961 to 1962 (Report of the Commission on the Cost of Medical Care, 1964). The concept of *alimentary resistance* induced following naturally acquired wild poliovirus infection was proposed by Koprowski *et al.* (1956). However, the development of S-IgA antibody responses following oral immunization with Sabin polio vaccine was first demonstrated in the late 1960s (Ogra *et al.*, 1968). In additional investigations, it was observed that Salk IPV in general did not induce a consistent level of mucosal immunity to reinfection, although the induced circulating antibodies were found to be highly effective in the prevention of viremia and systemic infection (Ogra and Karzon, 1969, 1971).

Following licensing of the Salk vaccine, a mass vaccination campaign was initiated under the auspices of the March of Dimes. The incidence of poliomyelitis fell precipitously as more and more children were immunized.

By 1965, the incidence of paralytic disease displayed a low incidence not recorded in the previous 6 decades. From 1950 to 1954, the average number of poliomyelitis cases reported per year was 38,727. On the other hand, in 1961 the total number of poliomyelitis cases had declined to 1312; of these, 988 cases were reported to be paralytic. This represented a more than 95% decline in the incidence of disease from the previous 5-year period (Berkovich *et al.*, 1961). It is estimated that almost a 90% reduction in the number of poliomyelitis cases was attained with Salk IPV alone before the introduction of OPV. The death rate from poliomyelitis had declined to 0.1 in 100,000 in 1961 compared with an annual death rate of 1.9 in 1915 to 1924, and 1.2 in 1945 to 1954. The 1961 figures represent the lowest death rate observed for any reporting period in the United States during the previous 5 decades (Report of the Commission on the Cost of Medical Care, 1964). However, a relative increase in the incidence of type 3 virus outbreaks was observed in 1959 and 1960. In these clusters, more than 50% of the subjects had received three or more doses of IPV

(Berkovich *et al.*, 1961; Gresham, 1962). Other investigations carried out during that time also suggested that the reduction in the incidence of paralytic polio could not be entirely accounted for by the known efficacy of the IPV or the number of persons immunized with IPV (Bodian, 1961). From a historical perspective, it is gratifying to note that poliomyelitis has been eradicated in most of the Americas and Europe and will be virtually eliminated in the rest of the world. This success is largely the result of orally administered vaccines associated with the development of effective serum and secretory antibody responses to the virus. However, as late as the 1950s, experts in infectious diseases stated that "neither passive immunization by human immune or animal serum nor active immunization by vaccines can be advised" against poliovirus infection (Harries and Mitman, 1951).

ORAL TOLERANCE

The precise origin of the frequently claimed beneficial effect of eating plants in the prevention and treatment of skin rashes caused by repeated exposure to certain plants is shrouded in mystery. Although Dakin (1829) states, "Some good meaning, mystical, marvelous physicians, or favored ladies with knowledge inherent, say the bane will prove the best antidote, and hence advise the forbidden leaves to be eaten, both as a preventive and cure to the external disease," we have no information as to the historical basis for this traditional treatment. Gilmore (1911) refers to a practice of chewing plant leaves used by some tribes of American Indians. The "bane" or leaves consumed belong to representatives of some 50 species of plants called "poison vine, ivy, or oak" of the genus *Rhus*, later reclassified as *Toxicodendron*, with species *toxicodendron*, *radicans*, *diversilobum*, and *vernix*, which are native to North America. In Japan, the sap of the lac tree (*Rhus vernicifera*), called *kiurushi*, displays a skin-sensitizing ability, as well as chemical structures and physical properties, analogous to its American counterpart (for reviews, see Stevens, 1945; Klingman, 1958). The effectiveness of inducing systemic tolerance, in this case to skin delayed-type hypersensitivity reactions, by feeding fresh or dried plants (or their ether, alcohol, or oil extracts) was controversial despite extensive studies performed in hypersensitive patients and experimental animals (Kligman, 1958). Oral therapy with ether extracts of fresh leaves, sometimes combined with systemic hyposensitization, was successful in the hands of several investigators (*e.g.*, Duncan, 1916; Shelmire, 1941), whereas others reported no improvement, as summarized in detail by Stevens (1945) and Klingman (1958). Although the skin, anal orifice, and oral mucosa are in that order excellent sensitizing sites that become inflamed on reexposure to poisoning, the intestinal mucosa is apparently refractory (Silvers, 1941).

Extensive systematic studies of immune responses, and anaphylaxis in particular, to plant and animal proteins were carried out at the beginning of this century in many laboratories, but the experiments reported by A. Besredka and

H.G. Wells (1875–1943) should attract the attention of mucosal immunologists. It appears that Besredka (1909) was the first investigator to make several observations that were relevant to the concept of anaphylaxis and its prevention by ingestion or rectal administration of protein antigens, in this case milk and milk whey. In an extensive series of experiments, Besredka demonstrated that the injection of milk to previously systemically sensitized animals resulted in fatal anaphylaxis within a few minutes. However, no sensitization occurred when milk was administered rectally or orally. Most importantly, the administration of whole milk or milk whey by the oral or rectal route prevented "sensitization" to the subsequent injection of milk and thus provided a safe and good way for "anti-anaphylactic vaccination." These studies were shortly followed by those of Wells and Osborne (1911), who contributed enormously in this now classical paper to our comprehension of oral tolerance: (1) guinea pigs fed on animal (cow's milk, egg white, ox blood) or plant (corn or oats) proteins are at first *rendered sensitive* to these proteins, as demonstrated by anaphylactic reactions when the proteins are injected systemically; (2) feeding of plant proteins extended to a few weeks or months makes experimental animals *refractory to anaphylaxis*; (3) this refractory condition seems to be reached more easily with vegetable proteins of *natural food* than with animal proteins, perhaps because of their presence in the diet from the time of weaning; and (4) *young animals* fed vegetable proteins immediately after weaning became completely refractory to any reaction against injected proteins. Analogous studies of cutaneous hypersensitivity and the induction of serum precipitins in marasmic and normal infants fed cow's milk proteins, egg white, sheep serum, or almond flower were performed by Du Bois *et al.* (1925). The authors concluded that the ingestion of these antigens leads to the appearance of specific "precipitins" in blood and, in many cases, to cutaneous hypersensitiveness in both marasmic and normal infants. Because the results of the intracutaneous test were obtained within 1 hour after the injection, it is likely that they reflect the presence of IgE antibodies, whereas the serum "precipitins" were represented mainly by IgG antibodies.

Inhibition of skin manifestations of delayed-type hypersensitivity to a hapten, 2,4-dinitrochlorobenzene, by prior feeding was reported by Chase (1946). A cursory look at one simple table in this rather brief paper of such basic importance tells the story without need for involved statistical analysis **(Table 3)**. Guinea pigs given, by the oral route, 1% solution of the hapten in olive oil for 6 consecutive days and again two to three times after an 8-day rest displayed "... a very considerable diminution [of skin reactions upon challenge] in groups that had received prior feeding of the chemical." To demonstrate the specificity of unresponsiveness induced by feeding hapten (2,4-dinitrochlorobenzene), tolerized animals were systemically sensitized with a second, unrelated hapten (o-chlorobenzoyl chloride). When such animals received a simultaneous series of intracutaneous injections with both haptens, they reacted only to the second hapten. Other findings in this landmark paper concern the

Table 3 Inhibition of Hypersensitivity Reactions by Hapten Feeding

Hypersensitivity Rated as	Prior Feeding of Allergen (%) (93 Animals)	Controls (%) (77 Animals)
High	3.2	74.0
Good	0.0	16.9
Moderate	8.6	5.2
Weak	20.4	3.9
Low	46.2	0.0
Very faint, or entirely negative	21.5	0.0

Modified from Chase (1946).

longevity of tolerance (at least 31 weeks) induced by feeding, and the *failure of oral treatment* to diminish the degree of hypersensitivity in animals *with established sensitivity* to the hapten induced by the systemic route! The potential for inhibiting the development of skin sensitization by giving antigens through oral (Chase, 1946) or systemic (Sulzberger, 1930) routes is sometimes referred to as the Chase-Sulzberger phenomenon. Detailed examination of Sulzberger's and Chase's papers, however, leads to the conclusion that the single feature common to both studies is that inhibition of *skin* sensitization can be achieved when the hapten is first given by another route. To inhibit skin sensitization, in contrast to Chase's oral route, Sulzberger *injected* the hapten (arsphenamine) into the heart, muscles, tongue, peritoneal cavity, lungs, or testes of experimental animals. Therefore, it is likely that different mechanisms of prevention of subsequent skin sensitization were involved.

Attempts to induce systemic unresponsiveness by prior feeding of hapten or antigen in humans had been reported infrequently until the recent revival of interest in oral tolerance. Poison ivy or oak extracts were used with variable results, as summarized in admirable completeness by Stevens (1945). In more recent literature, oral desensitization with the same allergen was largely unsuccessful and therefore discouraged (Klingman, 1958). Sulfonamides, introduced into medicine before World War II, are known inducers of allergic reactions when given *per os* or applied to the skin: eczematous dermatitis ensues in some patients. In a limited study, Park (1944) administered small doses of sulfanilamide orally to desensitize allergic patients with success. Grolnick (1951) used another known skin sensitizer—krameria—by the oral route in an attempt to achieve inhibition of subsequent skin sensitization, although unsuccessfully. These experiments were of considerable medical importance because krameria, an extract of the roots of Brazilian or Peruvian rhatany (shrubs or herbs of the family *Leguminosae*) was used frequently as an astringent and listed as an official tincture in the U.S. Pharmacopoeia. Grolnick administered large doses three times daily for 2 weeks, followed by a double dose for up to 8 weeks) of the diluted tincture before the skin sensitization regimen. However, no difference in the frequency or intensity of skin reactions was observed between orally "desensitized" subjects and controls (no oral ingestion) when skin sensitization with krameria was induced. Using the same hapten, 2,4-dinitrochlorobenzene, as Chase (1946), Lowney (1968, 1973) observed reduced incidence and intensity of cutaneous sensitization in individuals given this hapten orally by application of a 2% solution in acetone on the buccal mucosa: 8 of 17 (47%) individuals were tolerant in the experimental group, compared with 1 of 26 (4%) subjects in the control group. The efficacy of feeding this hapten in capsules on the suppression of subsequent contact sensitization was dose dependent: small amounts (< 20 mg) had no effect, whereas higher doses (> 20 mg) induced a significant decrease in reactivity.

Induction of systemic unresponsiveness to an ingested antigen—bovine serum albumin (BSA)—was studied in adults by Korenblat et al. (1968). Observing that the sera from more than 80% of normal children but only 7% of adults older than 40 years of age contained anti-BSA or anti-α-lactalbumin antibodies, the authors tested for possible oral tolerance by systemic immunization with BSA. Indeed, those individuals who had no anti-BSA antibodies did not respond to a systemic or oral challenge. By contrast, serum anti-BSA titers were increased by systemic immunization in individuals with preexisting antibodies. In retrospect, these results are reminiscent of the previously mentioned studies of Wells and Osborne (1911), indicating that ingestion of proteins led first to the induction of responses that decreased on prolonged feeding of the antigen.

IMMUNOPATHOLOGY

IgA deficiency

Selective deficiency of IgA (or β_2A or γ1A according to previous terminology) was described by Giedion and Scheidegger (1957), Fudenberg et al. (1962), and West et al. (1962). Interestingly, these initial reports contained descriptions of patients whose symptoms presaged the clinical profiles of patients with IgA deficiency as defined in later, more extensive studies of the condition. Some of the patients, for instance, had respiratory infections and thus predicted the major clinical manifestation of IgA deficiency, that is, chronic upper and lower respiratory infections leading in the untreated state to bronchiectasis and respiratory failure. In addition, one patient had steatorrhea and malabsorption and was therefore representative of another symptom complex in IgA deficiency, a non-gluten-sensitive sprue-like syndrome marked by villous atrophy, malabsorption, and at times, intestinal nodular lymphoid hyperplasia. The origin of this symptom complex, initially described in depth by Crabbé and Heremans (1966), is still poorly understood, although most students of IgA deficiency consider it to be an autoimmune manifestation of the disease (McCarthy et al., 1978). On this basis, it must be differentiated from gastrointestinal

problems due to infections of the gastrointestinal tract such as giardia or salmonella infection, which have been shown to occur more frequently in IgA deficiency than in normals by Ammann and Hong (1971). Finally, one patient in the West series had a lupus-like syndrome and was thus indicative of the rather strong association of IgA deficiency with autoimmunity, as later shown by the increased incidence of "silent" IgA deficiency in autoimmune diseases and the increased incidence of antibodies against self-proteins or food proteins and frank autoimmunity in IgA-deficient patients themselves (Buckley and Dees, 1969; Ammann and Hong, 1971; Cassidy et al., 1973). The basis of this association was later investigated by Cunningham-Rundles et al. (1978), who showed that IgA-deficient patients absorb an increased amount of intact macromolecules from the food into the bloodstream and, in addition, manifest high levels of circulating antigen–antibody complexes following food ingestion that presumably arise as a result of prior antibody responses to the absorbed food protein. In addition, these investigators showed that the presence of absorbed food molecules and antigen–antibody complexes in the circulation correlated with the presence of autoantibodies or autoimmune disease. Thus, they postulated that in the absence of IgA, the gastrointestinal tract manifests reduced barrier function and permits entry of macromolecules, some of which cross-react with self-antigen and give rise to autoantibody responses (Cunningham-Rundles et al., 1981).

Another early milestone in the history of IgA deficiency was the discovery in 1964 by Rockey et al. (1964) that IgA deficiency can occur in ostensibly healthy individuals. This finding was later expanded by epidemiologic studies of blood bank donors, which established that IgA deficiency is mainly a "submerged" immunodeficiency occurring in 1/300–1/2000 individuals in various Caucasian populations (Hanson et al., 1983). The existence of such seemingly silent IgA deficiency has prompted studies to determine the factors that result in increased susceptibility to infection. One factor, first identified by Oxelius et al. (1981), relates to the finding that a subset of patients with IgA deficiency also have IgG subclass deficiency, and thus are at further risk for infection. Indeed, as subsequently shown by Björkander et al. (1985), many, but not all, patients with associated IgG subclass deficiency had a greater frequency of infections than patients with IgA deficiency alone. Another factor, identified by Mellander et al. (1986), relates to the ability of IgA-deficient patients to manifest compensatory IgM or IgG antibody responses that then presumably provide sufficient protection at mucosal surfaces to prevent infections; it should be noted here that in humans, IgM like IgA can be transported to the mucosal surface via the polymeric Ig receptor. Finally, the level of IgA produced in patients may be a factor in the occurrence of infection. Thus, patients whose immune systems produce virtually no IgA may be at greater risk than those that produce reduced amounts of IgA. Two caveats concerning silent IgA deficiency are in order. First, as emphasized by Cunningham-Rundles et al. (1980), such unidentified immunodeficiency may in fact be a risk factor for gastrointestinal neoplasia or, as mentioned earlier, autoimmunity. Second, although silent IgA deficiency may be silent in the relatively clean environments of Western, industrialized countries, it may lead to disease in less developed countries that have environments more closely approximating those that led to the evolution of the immune system.

The finding that some patients with IgA deficiency do produce some IgA and thus have what might be called a partial IgA deficiency relates to the important studies of Savilahti and Pelkonen (1979) showing that a sizable group of IgA-deficient patients, mostly those who have partial IgA deficiency, exhibit transient IgA deficiency that eventually reverts to normal. The causes of such transient deficiency are presently unclear. Among the possibilities that have been suggested is exposure to certain viruses and drugs (particularly anticonvulsants) as well as certain insults to the immune system such as graft-versus host disease, all of which have been associated with IgA deficiency in one way or another (Savilahti and Pelkonen, 1979; Elfenbein et al., 1976). Whether such transient IgA deficiency is qualitatively different from complete IgA deficiency remains to be explored, as does the question of whether all forms of IgA deficiency require an environmental trigger.

Yet another observation concerning IgA deficiency that was made in the early years following its discovery was that of LaPlane et al. (1962) showing that the deficiency occurs in relatives of patients with common variable immunodeficiency (CVI). This observation was the first to suggest that IgA deficiency and CVI are related diseases and to suggest that these immunodeficiencies have a common genetic basis. These possibilities were later put on a firmer footing by the discovery that the two diseases share a common set of HLA haplotypes and that IgA deficiency occasionally evolves into frank panhypogammaglobulinemia (see Chapter 64). In addition, it eventually became apparent that the immunologic abnormalities found in IgA deficiency and CVI were fundamentally similar and thus the two deficiencies represented two ends of the same disease spectrum. As for genetic studies of IgA deficiency (and CVI), these begin with the studies of Koistinen (1975), who noted familial clustering of IgA deficiency and the studies of Van Thiel et al. (1977) showing the occurrence of kindreds with IgA deficiency and various autoimmune diseases. Ambrus et al. (1977) showed that IgA deficiency was associated with HLA-B8 and thus ushered in a series of studies of MHC genes in IgA deficiency and CVI.

The previous considerations bring us to studies of the immunopathogenesis of IgA deficiency (and CVI). In the late 1970s and throughout the 1980s, evidence was accumulated that established that although IgA deficiency (and CVI) may sometimes be associated with class-specific suppressor T cells, the more constant and more basic deficit resides in the B cells. In particular, it was shown by Mitsuya et al. (1981) and Pereira et al. (1982) that IgA B cells in IgA deficiency (and all B cells in CVI) manifest defective class switching and terminal differentiation. Interestingly, this defect in patients with CVI appears to be hierarchical in the sense that upon *in vitro* stimulation, IgA differentiation is most affected, IgG differentiation is next most affected, and IgM differentiation is least affected.

Renal diseases

Mucosal infections of the respiratory tract and diseases of the gastrointestinal tract or liver may result in the alteration of IgA metabolism and the deposition of IgA1 in the glomerular mesangium and skin. Berger and Hinglais (1968) and Berger (1969) described a new form of glomerulonephritis characterized by prominent codeposits of IgA and IgG in the glomerular mesangium. The disease, now termed *IgA nephropathy*, or according to its discoverer, *Berger's disease*, is the most common cause of glomerulonephritis in the world.

Subsequent studies indicated that the mesangial deposition of IgA1 also may be present in other diseases including Henoch-Schönlein purpura (HSP), systemic lupus erythematosus, dermatitis herpetiformis, alcoholic liver cirrhosis, and inflammatory bowel disease. Although HSP in children was first described by Heberden (1801), and then by Schönlein (1837), and Henoch (1874), its relationship to IgA nephropathy was elucidated relatively recently. Interestingly, based on the careful review of historical records of the symptoms and duration of the disease, Davies (1991) speculated that the kidney failure and ultimate death of W. A. Mozart was due to HSP.

Gluten-sensitive enteropathy (GSE)-celiac disease and celiac sprue

The discovery of GSE is credited to W. K. Dicke, a Dutch pediatrician, who noted during the mid-1930s that one of his patients repeatedly developed diarrhea and rash soon after the ingestion of bread (Dicke, 1941). Notwithstanding the fact that, in retrospect, the clinical syndrome in this patient is better classified as allergy to wheat protein rather than GSE (which is a nonallergic immunologic hypersensitivity and does not result in immediate symptoms), Dicke generalized this observation to a larger group of children with chronic diarrhea and wasting who probably did have GSE. On this basis, in a 1940 meeting of the Dutch Pediatric Society, he proposed a wheat-free diet for children with GSE (then called Gee-Herter syndrome). There is a persistent anecdote that Dicke subsequently became convinced of his theory in the early 1940s during the German occupation of Holland when he noted that the children with GSE actually improved in spite of the general food shortage (which of course included a wheat shortage) and suffered relapses at one point when wheat was air-lifted into Holland by the Allies (Smits, 1989). Finally, in the late 1940s, Dicke teamed up with several Dutch scientists, particularly J. H. Van de Kamer, who had devised a method of measuring fat excretion in the stool to formally show that feeding of certain cereal grains to patients with GSE led to increased fat excretion (*i.e.*, fat malabsorption) (Van de Kamer et al., 1953). This result, published as a Ph.D. thesis by Dicke in 1950, was rapidly reproduced in other parts of Europe and GSE was thus uniquely defined as a diarrheal syndrome due to cereal grain protein hypersensitivity (Dicke, 1950).

In the approximately 50 years that have elapsed since this singular discovery, there have been many important additional landmarks in the study of GSE. In the 1950s, it was shown that GSE is characterized by the presence of villous atrophy and that the loss of absorptive surface that results from such atrophy is responsible for the main clinical manifestation of the disease—malabsorption and nutrient deficiency (Paulley, 1954; Shiner, 1960). This discovery also enabled clinicians in the 1960s to link the skin disease, dermatitis herpetiformis, to GSE because patients with dermatitis herpetiformis could also be shown to have various degrees of villous atrophy and to have amelioration of disease with a gluten-free diet (Shuster et al., 1968). The existence of two clinical forms of gluten sensitivity led to the increasing use of the term *gluten-sensitive enteropathy* rather than celiac disease as the more inclusive name for the disease. Finally, during this early period of the study of GSE, it was also established that the offending protein in gluten causing GSE was the wheat prolamin known as gliadin; as shown later, similar components of rye and oat grains also cause GSE (Dicke et al., 1950).

In the 1960s and early 1970s, the first evidence that GSE was associated with gluten-specific immune dysfunction appeared in studies showing that patient mucosal tissue displayed evidence of increased immunologic activity, including increased numbers of plasma cells in lamina propria and increased intraepithelial cells (Eidelman et al., 1966; Ferguson and Murray 1971). In addition, it was shown that high serum IgA levels prevalent in GSE tend to fall after the institution of a gluten-free diet (Asquith et al., 1969), and feeding of gluten to patients with quiescent disease leads to a prompt increase in IgA and IgM synthesis, some of which is gluten specific (Loeb et al., 1971). Finally, the first evidence that T-cell immunity might be involved in GSE appeared with a report from Ferguson et al. (1975) showing that lymphocytes from patients produce a cytokine upon exposure to gluten (migration-inhibition factor). At this point, strong evidence that the disease was in fact due to an immunologic abnormality was then provided by Falchuk et al. (1974) and Katz et al. (1976), who used organ culture techniques to show that gliadin was not directly toxic to patient tissue, but instead required the stimulation of an "endogenous mechanism," which results in the secretion of soluble mediators of villous atrophy and which is inhibitable by steroids. The "endogenous mechanism" was at that time assumed to be and was later proven to be an immunologic reaction resulting in the production of IFN-γ (Przemioslo et al., 1995).

These developments were now expanded, beginning in the early 1970s and extending into the 1980s, by the discovery that GSE is strongly associated with a particular set of MHC genes. The initial finding here was made by Falchuk et al. (1972), who showed that GSE is associated with the MHC class I gene encoding HLA-B8. This observation was later followed by those of Keuning et al. (1976) and Tosi et al. (1983), who demonstrated that GSE was associated with the MHC class II genes encoding HLA-DR3, HLA-DR7, and most importantly, HLA-DQ2.

Inflammatory bowel disease

The inflammatory bowel diseases (IBDs), Crohn's disease and ulcerative colitis, are commonly thought to have been "discovered" relatively recently, that is, in the last 100 years. Review of the historical record, however, quickly discloses that although the prevalence of these diseases may have vastly increased during this period, the first cases were recognized hundreds of years ago and numerous cases were described in the British medical literature in the last half of the 19th century. Thus, as far as ulcerative colitis is concerned, the first clearly reported case can be traced back to Wilks and Moxon (1875), who described a young woman with ulcerations involving the entire colon and who ultimately died of the complications of bloody diarrhea. Over the next 25–40 years hundreds of cases of ulcerative diseases of the colon were reported, not only in Britain, but also in other European countries and ulcerative colitis was a major gastrointestinal disease at the time of the Congress of Medicine held in Paris in 1913. Similarly, with respect to Crohn's disease, the first case was reported by Wilks (1859) who described a 42-year-old woman with inflammation of both the colon and terminal ileum who died after several months with diarrhea and fever; this patient was initially said to have ulcerative colitis, but on reevaluation of the findings much later was found to have had Crohn's disease. Similar cases were reported by Fenwick (1889) and Dalziel (1913) on 13 patients with more or less classic findings of Crohn's disease, which were attributed to a mycobacterial agent other than *Mycobacterium tuberculosis* (Tietze, 1920; Moschcowitz and Wilensky, 1923). In the ensuing 20 years, numerous instances of gastrointestinal disease resembling Crohn's disease were reported that finally crystallized the idea that Crohn's disease is a separate and unique disease entity. In 1932, two young physicians, an internist and a surgeon, presented findings related to what they proposed was a new clinical and pathologic entity: terminal ileitis with granulomatous inflammation. Ginzburg and Oppenheimer (1932) reported on 51 cases of granulomatous inflammation of the bowel that were not tuberculous, amebic, or syphilitic. They proposed six categories, including one with isolated terminal ileitis characterized by fissuring, longitudinal ulcers, granulomatous inflammation, stenotic bowel, and the propensity to fistulize. This series was published in 1932 in the *Transactions of the American Gastroenterological Association* with only Ginzburg and Oppenheimer as authors. One month later, Burrill B. Crohn presented 14 cases of pure ileitis and published a landmark paper describing the clinical, pathologic, radiographic, and therapeutic features of the disease. Cases from both studies were from the service of Dr. A. A. Berg, a noted Mount Sinai surgeon (Chief of Service). Dr. Crohn's paper, published in the *Journal of the American Medical Association*, received the critical acclaim and notice, hence the disease designation Crohn's disease. The initial presentation by Dr. Ginzburg did not include Crohn's name and this has led to some debate regarding the appropriate naming of the disease. The Scots refer to terminal ileitis as Dalziel's disease, the world as Crohn's disease, and Ginzburg, until his death in the 1990s, as Ginzburg's disease. The Crohn et al. (1932) publication was able to establish a new disease entity and ultimately to provide its eponymous name, not because it contained a more extensive series of cases of chronic intestinal inflammation than earlier reports, but rather because it provided specific evidence that the inflammation was not due to a known infectious agent, particularly M. tuberculosis, and was therefore a new type of inflammatory bowel disease. Thus, it justifiably stands as a landmark in the history of gastrointestinal disease and mucosal immunopathology.

More complete clinical and pathologic characterization of ulcerative colitis and Crohn's disease followed the initial definition of these diseases as outlined previously. Ulcerative colitis was characterized as a relatively superficial disease usually beginning in the rectum and then extending proximally to involve the descending colon in some patients and the entire colon in others; in addition, the characteristic microscopic findings of the disease were identified including epithelial cell hyperplasia and goblet cell depletion, the presence of crypt abscesses, and a mixed lamina propria infiltrate of lymphocytes and eosinophils (Warren and Sommers, 1954). In contrast, Crohn's disease was defined by the presence of focal lesions of the small intestine, most commonly involving the terminal ileum but also frequently involving the ascending colon; furthermore, the lesions themselves were shown to be characterized by transmural thickening, luminal narrowing, fistula formation, and fibrosis (Warren and Sommers, 1948). Finally, Crohn's disease, on microscopic examination, was shown to be a granulomatous inflammation sometimes associated with the presence of giant cells, and although crypt abscesses were also present in Crohn's inflammation, overall granulocytic infiltration was far less prominent than in ulcerative colitis (Warren and Sommers, 1948; Rappaport et al., 1951). On the basis of these distinctive morphologic features, ulcerative colitis and Crohn's disease could clearly be defined as different pathologic entities. Nevertheless, they remained grouped as members of the inflammatory bowel disease spectrum because they both were idiopathic inflammations of the intestine without an obvious infectious etiology. In addition, they were found to be genetically related diseases in that patients with one of the forms of inflammatory bowel disease frequently had family members with the other form (Jackman and Bargen, 1942).

For many years, the cause of both ulcerative colitis and Crohn's disease was assumed to be infectious in nature and one after another candidate organism was championed as the causative agent. In the 1920s, for instance, diplostreptococci, organisms ordinarily found in the oral cavity, were considered the cause of ulcerative colitis, and in the ensuing decades, Pseudomonas aeruginosa, E. coli, Entamoeba histolyt-

ica, and Chlamydiae were likewise considered. Later in the 1950s and 1960s, these bacterial and parasitic candidate organisms lost favor—instead, various viruses were believed to be the etiologic agent. A similar pattern emerged for Crohn's disease beginning in the era before Crohn's report with the assumption that the disease was due to a mycobacterial infection; it was in fact the exclusion of mycobacterial infection by animal inoculation, syphilis by serologic testing, and actinomycosis by histologic findings, that allowed Crohn's disease to emerge as a separate entity (Crohn et al., 1932). This initial exclusion of an infectious etiology, however, did not stop the search for an infectious agent and in the period extending from 1952 to 1985, numerous organisms were proposed as causes of Crohn's disease including various bacterial, chlamydial, and viral organisms. The last enjoyed a particular vogue throughout the 1970s and into the 1980s, but was all but eliminated as a possibility by the inability to culture viral organisms from lesions (Phillpots et al., 1980). Of note, interest in the mycobacterial etiology of Crohn's disease resurfaced in the late 1970s and 1980s with the emergence of evidence that the disease was caused by an atypical cell wall–deficient mycobacterial species (Chiodini et al., 1984). Ultimately, however, this idea also failed because the putative organism could not be found in lesional tissues by sophisticated immunologic and culture techniques and because there was no evidence that the putative organism caused an immune response. The latter fact was particularly influential in light of the emerging belief among many students of the disease that IBD is basically an immunologic dysfunction.

The concept that IBD might be due to a nonallergic immunologic dysfunction was first seriously considered by Kirsner et al. (1961), who conducted the first series of studies of a possible immunologic dysfunction in IBD, taking the approach of creating animal models of bowel inflammation that resembled IBD. One such model was created in rabbits and was based on the "Auer" procedure, which consisted of stimulating antibody responses to a given antigen and then inducing mucosal deposition of antigen–antibody complexes by subsequently applying the antigen to the colon that had been preexposed to formalin (Kraft et al., 1963). An inflammation was thereby achieved that resembled ulcerative colitis histologically, but which differed from ulcerative colitis in that it was self-limited. In later studies by Mee et al. (1979), a similar rabbit model was created, except for the fact that investigators preimmunized the animals with E. coli, a member of the normal mucosal microflora (Mee et al., 1979), and the ulcerative colitis-like disease obtained was persistent. Taken together, these experiments suggested that IBD may result from an initial insult, followed by an inappropriate and sustained immunologic response to normal flora. A similar conclusion can be drawn from the almost forgotten studies of Halpern et al. (1967), who induced chronic ulcerative colitis-like lesions in rats by injecting the latter with strains of live or dead E. coli in Freund's adjuvant. Interestingly, in this case, the colitis could be prevented by prefeeding with E. coli, which in retrospect suggests that induction of tolerance with

the inducing antigen (by feeding) affected colitis production and that colitis was a result of a failure of mucosal immunoregulation.

Later studies of animal models, conducted in the 1970s, enlarged on the previous themes. In one model studied during this period, the contactant dinitrochlorobenzene was used to induce colitis, providing an early suggestion that T cells rather than B cells might be the key elements in the inflammatory response of IBD (Onderdonk et al., 1978). In another model, it was shown that in mice and other animals wherein colitis had been induced by carrageenan, the coadministration of metronidazol prevented colitis induction (Broberger and Perelman, 1959). This again suggested a role of intestinal microflora. Overall, these early animal studies presaged current concepts of IBD that hold that both ulcerative colitis and Crohn's disease are due to an abnormality of immunoregulation and an inappropriate response to antigens in the mucosa environment.

The 1950s and 1960s, in addition to the above described animal model work, saw the advent of the first studies of human IBD from an immunologic point of view. The pioneering work that was conducted by Broberger and Perlmann (1959) and their various colleagues provided evidence that patients with IBD, particularly those with ulcerative colitis, developed antibodies to gut constituents, either bacterial antigens or cross-reactive self-antigens present in epithelial cells. Later it became apparent that these "autoantibodies" were most likely not disease specific and probably occurred secondary to tissue injury; nevertheless, they paved the way to future studies showing that ulcerative colitis is associated with the production of particular autoantibodies such as antineutrophil cytoplasmic antibody (ANCA) and antitropomyosin.

Perlmann and Broberger (1963) and their colleagues also introduced the idea that IBD was characterized by the development of cytotoxic cells, which were ultimately shown by Shorter et al. (1970) to be natural killer (NK) cells capable of mediating antibody-dependent cell-mediated cytotoxic reactions against epithelial cells, perhaps in conjunction with the antiepithelial cell antibodies alluded to earlier (Perlmann and Broberger, 1963; Shorter et al., 1970). This cytotoxicity phenomenon also proved to be disease nonspecific, but was nevertheless important because it focused attention on cell-mediated immunologic processes as a cause of IBD. With these studies, the stage was now set for studies of T cells, first at the cellular level and later at the cytokine level (Hodgson et al., 1978; Elson et al., 1981). These, together with the newer animal models that have come along in the past 5 years, strongly suggest that ulcerative colitis and Crohn's disease represent different kinds of dysregulated mucosal immune responses induced by antigens in the normal microflora.

CODA

As authors of this treatise, we are well aware of dangers inherent in writing historical reviews: inadvertent omission of some important articles, overemphasis of some but underappreciation of other contributions, and subjective differences in the perception or interpretation of published data. Nevertheless, we hope that ultimately this review, which covers relevant topics from ancient past to the late 1970s and early 1980s, will provide interesting and stimulating background information. We sincerely hope that the outstanding accomplishments of our predecessors and still active contemporaries who initiated research in this area and published their work more than 30 years ago will find appreciative readers.

REFERENCES

Ambrus, M., Hernádi, E., and Bajtai, G. (1977). Prevalence of HLA-A1 and HLA-B8 antigens in selective IgA deficiency. Clin. Immunol. Immunopathol. 7, 311–314.

Ammann, A. J., and Hong, R. (1971). Selective IgA deficiency: Presentation of 30 cases and a review of the literature. Medicine 50, 223–236.

Ammann, A. J. and Stiehm, E. R. (1966). Immune globulin levels in colostrum and breast milk, and serum from formula- and breast-fed newborns. Proc. Soc. Exp. Biol. Med. 122, 1098–1100.

Archer, O. K., Sutherland, D. E. R., and Good, R. A. (1963). Appendix of the rabbit: A homologue of the bursa in the chicken. Nature 200, 337–339.

Aschoff, L. (1926). Die lymphatischen Organe. Beiheft Med. Klin.

Asquith, P., Thompson, R. A., and Cooke, W. T. (1969). Serum-immunoglobulins in adult coeliac disease. Lancet 2, 129–131.

Athavale, B. (1977). Bala-Veda Pediatrics and Ayurveda Proceedings of the XV International Congress of Pediatrics, pp. 1–190. New Delhi. Shilp Associates, Bombay.

Behring, von E. and Kitasato, S. (1890). Ueber das Zustandekommen der Diphtheric Immunität und der Tetanus-Immunität bei Thieren. Deutsch. Med. Wochenschr. 16, 1113–1114.

Berg, R. D. and Savage, D. C. (1975). Immune responses of specific pathogen-free and gnotobiotic mice to antigens of indigenous and nonindigenous microorganisms. Infect. Immun. 11, 320–329.

Berger, J. (1969). IgA glomerular deposits in renal disease. Transplant. Proc. 1, 939–944.

Berger, J. and Hinglais, N. (1968). Les dépôts intercapillaires d'IgA-IgG. J. Urol. Néphrol. 74, 694–695.

Berkovich, S., Picketing, J. E., and Kibrick, S. (1961). Paralytic poliomyelitis in Massachusetts, 1959. A study of the disease in a well vaccinated population. N. Engl. J. Med. 264, 1323–1326.

Besredka, A. (1909). De l'anaphylaxie. De l'anaphylaxie lactique. Ann. Inst. Pasteur 23, 166–176.

Besredka, A. (1919). De la vaccination contre les états typhoides par la voie buccale. Ann. Inst. Pasteur. 33, 882–903.

Besredka, A. (1927). Local Immunization. Baltimore: Williams & Wilkins.

Bezkorovainy, A. and Miller-Catchpole, R. (1989). Biochemistry and Physiology of Bifidobacteria, 1–192. Boca Raton, FL: CRC Press.

Bienenstock, J. (1974). The physiology of the local immune response and the gastrointestinal tract. In Progress in Immunology, Vol. 4. Clinical Aspects I (eds. L. Brent and J. Holborow), 197–207. Amsterdam: North Holland American Elsevier.

Bienenstock, J., Johnston, N., and Perey, D. Y. E. (1973a). Bronchial lymphoid tissue. I. Morphologic characteristics. Lab. Invest. 28, 686–692.

Bienenstock, J., Johnston, N., and Perey, D. Y. E. (1973b). Bronchial lymphoid tissue. II. Functional characteristics. Lab. Invest. 28, 693–698.

Bienenstock, J., McDermott, M., and Befus, D. (1979). A common mucosal immune system. In Immunology of Breast Milk (eds. P. L. Ogra and D. L. Dayton), 91–104. New York: Raven Press.

Bienenstock, J. and Strauss, H. (1970). Evidence for synthesis of human colostral γA as 11S dimer. J. Immunol. 105, 274–277.

Bienenstock, J. and Tomasi, T. B., Jr. (1968). Secretory γA in normal urine. J. Clin. Invest. 47, 1162–1171.

Björkander, J., Bake, B., Oxelius, V. A., and Hanson, L. Å. (1985). Impaired lung function in patients with IgA deficiency and low levels of IgG2 or IgG3. N. Engl. J. Med. 313, 720–724.

Bockman, D. E. and Cooper, M. D. (1973). Pinocytosis by epithelium associated with lymphoid follicles in the bursa of Fabricius, appendix, and Peyer's patches. An electron microscopic study. Am. J. Anat. 136, 455–477.

Bockman, D. E. and Stevens, W. (1977). Gut-associated lymphoepithelial tissue: Bidirectional transport of tracer by specialized epithelial cells associated with lymphoid follicles. J. Reticuloendothel. Soc. 21, 245–254.

Bodian, D. (1949). Differentiation of types of poliomyelitis viruses. I. Reinfection experiments in monkeys (second attacks). Am. J. Hyg. 49, 200–224.

Bodian, D. (1961). Poliomyelitis immunization. Mass use of oral vaccine in the United States might prevent definitive evaluation of either vaccine. Science 134, 819–822.

Brandtzaeg, P. (1974). Mucosal and glandular distribution of immunoglobulin components: Differential localization of free and bound SC in secretory epithelial cells. J. Immunol. 112, 1553–1559.

Brandtzaeg, P. (1978). Polymeric IgA is complexed with secretory component (SC) on the surface of human intestinal epithelial cells. Scand. J. Immunol. 8, 39–52.

Brandtzaeg, P. (1981). Transport models for secretory IgA and secretory IgM. Clin. Exp. Immunol. 44, 221–232.

Brandtzaeg, P. and Prydz, H. (1984). Direct evidence for an integrated function of J chain and secretory component in epithelial transport of immunoglobulins. Nature 311, 71–73.

Broberger, O. and Perlmann, P. (1959). Autoantibodies in human ulcerative colitis. J. Exp. Med. 110, 657–674.

Brodie, M. and Park, W. H. (1936). Active immunization against poliomyelitis. Am. J. Public Health 26, 119–125.

Brown, W. R., Newcomb, R. W., and Ishizaka, K. (1970). Proteolytic degradation of exocrine and serum immunoglobulins. J. Clin. Invest. 49, 1374–1380.

Buckley, R. H. and Dees, S. C. (1969). Correlation of milk precipitins with IgA deficiency. N. Engl. J. Med. 281, 465–469.

Bull, C. G. and McKee, C. M. (1929). Respiratory immunity in rabbits. VII. Resistance to intranasal infection in the absence of demonstrable antibodies. Am. J. Hyg. 9, 490–499.

Bunting, C. H. and Huston, J. (1921). Fate of the lymphocyte. J. Exp. Med. 33, 593–600.

Burrows, W., Elliott, M., and Havens, I. (1947). Studies on immunity in Asiatic cholera. The excretion of coproantibody in experimental enteric cholera in the guinea pig. J. Infect. Dis. 81, 261–281.

Burrows, W. and Havens, I. (1948). Studies on immunity to Asiatic cholera. V. The absorption of immune globulin from the bowel and its excretion in the urine and feces of experimental animals and human volunteers. J. Infect. Dis. 82, 231–250.

Burrows, W. and Ware, L. L. (1953). Studies on immunity to Asiatic cholera. VII. Prophylactic immunity to experimental enteric cholera. J. Infect. Dis. 92, 164–174.

Calmette, A. (1923). Les vaccinations microbiennes par voie buccale. Ann. Inst. Pasteur 37, 900–920.

Calmette, A. and Guérin, C. (1901). Recherches sur la vaccine experimentale. Ann. Inst. Pasteur 15, 161–168.

Carbonara, A. O. and Heremans, J. F. (1963). Subunits of normal and pathological γ1A-globulins β2A-globulins. Arch. Biochem. Biophys. 102, 137–143.

Carter, P. B. and Pollard, M. (1971). Host responses to "normal" microbial flora in germ-free mice. J. Reticuloendothelial. Soc. 9, 580–587.

Cassidy, J. T., Petty, R. E., and Sullivan, D. B. (1973). Abnormalities in the distribution of serum immunoglobulin concentrations in juvenile rheumatoid arthritis. J. Clin. Invest. 52, 1931–1936.

Cebra, J. J., Gearhart, P. J., Kamat, R., Robertson, S. M., and Tseng, J. (1977). Origin and differentiation of lymphocytes involved in the secretory IgA response. In Origins of Lymphocyte Diversity, Cold Spring Harbor Symp. Quant. Biol. 41, 201–215.

Chase, M. V. (1946). Inhibition of experimental drug allergy by prior feeding of the sensitizing agent. Proc. Soc. Exp. Biol. Med. 61, 257–259.

Chiodini, R. J., Van Kruiningen, H. J., Thayer, W. R., Merkal, R. S., and Coutu, J. A. (1984). Possible role of mycobacteria in inflammatory bowel disease. I. An unclassified Mycobacterium species isolated from patients with Crohn's disease. Dig. Dis. Sci. 29, 1073–1079.

Chodirker, W. B., and Tomasi, T. B., Jr. (1963). Gamma-globulins: Quantitative relationships in human serum and nonvascular fluids. Science 142, 1080–1081.

Cohendy, M. (1912). Expériences sur la vie sans microbes. Compt. Rend. Acad. Sci. 154, 533–536.

Combiesco, D. and Calab, G. (1924). De l'immunisation contre Staphylocoque pyogéne par la voie buccale, chez le lapin. Comp. Rend. Seanc. Soc. Biol. Filial. 91, 734–735.

Combiesco, D., Magheru, A., and Calab, G. (1923). Vaccination preventive contre la dysentérie par la voie digestive, chez le lapin. Compt. Rend. Seanc. Soc. Biol. Filial. 88, 904–906.

Cooper, M. D., Perey, D. Y., McKneally, M. F., Gabrielsen, A. E., Sutherland, D. E. R., and Good, R. A. (1966). A mammalian equivalent of the avian bursa of Fabricius. Lancet 1, 1388–1391.

Cornes, J. S. (1965). Number, size, and distribution of Peyer's patches in the human small intestine. Part I. The development of Peyer's patches. Gut 6, 225–233.

Crabbé, P. A., Bazin, H., Eyssen, H., and Heremans, J. F. (1968). The normal microbial flora as a major stimulus for proliferation of plasma cells synthesizing IgA in the gut. Int. Arch. Allergy 34, 362–375.

Crabbé, P. A., Carbonara, A. O., and Heremans, J. E. (1965). The normal human intestinal mucosa as a major source of plasma cells containing γA-immunoglobulin. Lab. Invest. 14, 235–248.

Crabbé, P. A. and Heremans, J. F. (1966). Lack of gamma A-immunoglobulin in serum of patients with steatorrhoea. Gut 7, 119–127.

Crabbé, P. A., Nash, D. R., Bazin, H., Eyssen, H., and Heremans, J. F. (1969). Antibodies of the IgA type in intestinal plasma cells of germfree mice after oral or parenteral immunization with ferritin. J. Exp. Med. 130, 723–744.

Crabbé, P. A., Nash, D. R., Bazin, H., Eyssen, H., and Heremans, J. F. (1970). Immunohistochemical observations on lymphoid tissues from conventional and germ-free mice. Lab. Invest. 22, 448–457.

Crago, S. S., Kulhavy, R., Prince, S. J., and Mestecky, J. (1978). Secretory component on epithelial cells is a surface receptor for polymeric immunoglobulins. J. Exp. Med. 147, 1832–1837.

Craig, S. W. and Cebra, J. J. (1971). Peyer's patches: An enriched source of precursors for IgA-producing immunocytes in the rabbit. J. Exp. Med. 134, 188–200.

Crandall, R. B., Cebra, J. J., and Crandall, C. A. (1967). The relative proportions of IgG-, IgA-, and IgM-containing cells in rabbit tissues during experimental trichinosis. Immunology 12, 147–158.

Crohn, B. B., Ginzburg, L., and Oppenheimer, G. D. (1932). Regional ileitis: A pathologic and clinical entity. J. Am. Med. Assoc. 99, 1323–1329.

Cunningham-Rundles, C., Brandeis, W. E., Good, R. A., and Day, N. K. (1978). Milk precipitins, circulating immune complexes, and IgA deficiency. Proc. Natl. Acad. Sci. U.S.A. 75, 3387–3389.

Cunningham-Rundles, C., Brandeis, W. E., Pudifin, D. J., Day, N. K., and Good, R. A. (1981). Autoimmunity in selective IgA deficiency: Relationship to anti-bovine protein antibodies, circulating immune complexes and clinical diseases. Clin. Exp. Immunol 45, 299–304.

Cunningham-Rundles, C., Pudifin, D. J., Armstrong, D., and Good, R. A. (1980). Selective IgA deficiency and neoplasia. Vox Sang. 38, 61–67.

Dakin, R. (1829). Remarks on a cutaneous affliction, produced by certain poisonous vegetables. Am. J. Med. Sci. 4, 98–100.

Dalziel, T. K. (1913). Chronic interstitial enteritis. Br. Med. J. 2, 1068–1070.

Davies, A. (1922). An investigation into the serological properties of dysentery stools. Lancet 2, 1009–1012.

Davies, P. J. (1991). Mozart's death: A rebuttal of Karhausen. Further evidence for Schönlein-Henoch syndrome. J. R. Soc. Med. 84, 737–740.

Dicke, W. K. (1941). Eenvoudig dieet bij het syndroom van Gee-Herter. NT Geneesk 85, 1715–1721.

Dicke, W. K. (1950). Coeliac disease. Investigation of the harmful effects of certain types of cereal on patients with coeliac disease. Thesis, Utrecht, The Netherlands.

Dserzgowdky, S. K. (1910). Ueber die aktive Immunisierung des Menschen gegen Diphtherie. *Zeitschr. Immunitätsforsch. Exp. Therap.* 3, 602.

Du Bois, R. O., Schloss, O. M., and Anderson, A. F. (1925). The development of cutaneous hypersensitivities following the intestinal absorption of antigenic protein. *Proc. Soc. Exp. Biol. Med.* 23, 176–180.

Dubos, R., Schaedler, R. W., Costello, R., and Hoet, P. (1965). Indigenous, normal, and autochthonous flora of the gastrointestinal tract. *J. Exp. Med.* 12, 67–75.

Duncan, C. H. (1916). Autotherapy in ivy poisoning. *N. Y. Med. J.* 104, 901.

Eberth, C. J. (1864). Ueber den feineren Bau der Darmschteinhaut. *Würzburger Natur. Wissenschaft. Zeitschr.* 5, 22–33.

Ehrich, W. (1929). Studies of the lymphatic tissue. *Am. J. Anat.* 43, 347–371.

Ehrlich, P. (1891a). Experimentelle Untersuchungen über Immunität. I. Ueber Ricin. *Deutsch Med. Wochenschr.* 17, 976–979.

Ehrlich, P. (1891b). Experimentelle Untersuchungen über Immunität. II. Ueber Abrin. *Deutsch Med. Wochenschr.* 17, 1218–1219.

Ehrlich, P. (1892). Ueber Immunität durch Vererbung und Säugung. *Zeitschr. Hyg. Infekt. Krankh.* 12, 183–203.

Eidelman, S., Davis, S. D., Lagunoff, D., and Rubin, C. E. (1966). The relationship between intestinal plasma cells and serum immunoglobulin A (IgA) in man. *J. Clin. Invest.* 45, 1003.

Elfenbein, G. J., Anderson, P. N., Humphrey, R. L., Mullins, G. M., Sensenbrenner, L. L., Wands, J. R., and Santos, G. W. (1976). Immune system reconstitution following allogeneic bone marrow transplantation in man: A multiparameter analysis. *Transplant. Proc.* 8, 641–646.

Ellison, S. A., Mashimo, P. A., and Mandel, I. D. (1960). Immunochemical studies of human saliva. I. The demonstration of serum proteins in whole and parotid saliva. *J. Dent. Res.* 39, 892–898.

Elson, C. O., Graeff, A. S., James, S. P., and Strober, W. (1981). Covert suppressor T cells in Crohn's disease. *Gastroenterology* 80, 1513–1521.

Enders, J. F. (1952). General preface to studies on the cultivation of poliomyelitis viruses in tissue culture. *J. Immunol.* 69, 639–643.

Enders, J. F., Weller, T. H., and Robbins, F. C. (1949). Cultivation of the Lansing strain of poliomyelitis virus in cultures of various human embryonic tissues. *Science* 109, 85–87.

Enlows, E. M. A. (1925). Vaccination by mouth against bacillary dysentery. *Publ. Health Report* 40, 639–649.

Escherich, T. (1888). The intestinal bacteria of the neonate and breast-fed infant. *Rev. Infect. Dis.* 10, 1220–1225.

Falchuk, Z. M., Gebhard, R. L., Sessoms, C., and Strober, W. (1974). An in vitro model of gluten sensitive enteropathy: Effect of gliadin on intestinal epithelial cells of patients with gluten sensitive enteropathy in organ culture. *J. Clin. Invest.* 53, 487–500.

Falchuk, Z. M., Rogentine, G. N., and Strober, W. (1972). Predominance of histocompatibility antigen HLA-A8 in patients with gluten-sensitive enteropathy. *J. Clin. Invest.* 51, 1602–1606.

Fanger, M. W., Shen, L., Pugh, J., and Bernier, G. M. (1980). Subpopulations of human peripheral granulocytes and monocytes express receptors for IgA. *Proc. Natl. Acad. Sci. U.S.A.* 77, 3640–3644.

Faulk, W. P., McCormick, J. N., Goodman, J. R., Yoffey, J. M., and Fudenberg. H. H. (1970). Peyer's patches: Morphologic studies. *Cell. Immunol.* 1, 500–520.

Fazekas de St. Groth, S. and Donelley, M. (1950a). Studies in experimental immunology of influenza. III. Antibody response. *Aust. J. Exp. Biol. Med. Sci.* 28, 45–60.

Fazekas de St. Groth, S. and Donelley, M. (1950b). Studies in experimental immunology of influenza IV. The protective value of active immunization. *Aust. J. Exp. Biol. Med. Sci.* 28, 61–75.

Feinstein, D. and Franklin, E. C. (1966). Two antigenically distinguishable subclasses of human γA myeloma proteins differing in their heavy chains. *Nature* 212, 1496–1498.

Fenwick, S. (1889) Clinical Lectures on Some Obscure Disease of the Abdomen. London: T & A Churchill.

Ferguson, A. (1977). Intraepithelial lymphocytes of the small intestine. *Gut* 18, 921–937.

Ferguson, A., MacDonald, T. T., McClure, J. P., and Holden, R. J. (1975). Cell-mediated immunity to gliadin within the small-intestinal mucosa in coeliac disease. *Lancet* 1, 895–897.

Ferguson, A. and Murray, D. (1971). Quantitation of intraepithelial lymphocytes in human jejunum. *Gut* 12, 988–994.

Fichtelius, K.-E. (1967). The mammalian equivalent to bursa Fabricii of birds. *Exp. Cell Res.* 46, 231–234.

Fichtelius, K.-E. (1970). Cellular aspects on the phylogeny of immunity. *Lymphology* 3, 50–59.

Fishaut, M., Murphy, D., Neifert, M., McIntosh, K., and Ogra, P. L. (1981). Bronchomammary axis in the immune response to respiratory syncytial virus. *J. Pediatr.* 99, 186–191.

Foo, M. C. and Lee, A. (1972). Immunological response of mice to members of the autochthonous intestinal microflora. *Infect. Immun.* 6, 525–532.

Francis, T., Jr. and Brightman, I. J. (1941). Virus-inactivating capacity of nasal secretions in the acute and convalescent stages of influenza. *Proc. Soc. Exp. Boil. Med.* 48, 116–117.

Francis, T., Jr., Pearson, H. E., Sullivan, E. R., and Brown, P. M. (1943). The effect of subcutaneous vaccination with influenza virus upon the virus-inactivating capacity of nasal secretions. *Amer. J. Hyg.* 37, 294–300.

Fubara, E. S. and Freter, R. (1973). Protection against enteric bacterial infection by secretory IgA antibodies. *J. Immunol.* 111, 395–403.

Fudenberg, H., German, J. L., III, and Kunkel, H. G. (1962). The occurrence of rheumatoid factor and other abnormalities in families of patients with agammaglobulinemia. *Arthr. Rheumat.* 5, 565–588.

Fuhrman, J. A. and Cebra, J. J. (1981). Special features of the priming process for a secretory IgA response: B cell priming with cholera toxin. *J. Exp. Med.* 153, 534–544.

Gay, F. P. (1924). Local resistance and local immunity to bacteria. *Physiol. Rev.* 4, 191–214.

Gerhard, W. W. (1837). On the typhus fever which occurred in Philadelphia in the Spring and Summer of 1836. *Am. J. Med. Sci.* 18, 289–322.

Gearhart, P. J. and Cebra, J. J. (1979). Differentiated B lymphocytes: Potential to express particular antibody variable and constant regions depends on site of lymphoid tissue and antigen load. *J. Exp. Med.* 149, 216–227.

Giedion, A. and Scheidegger, J. J. (1957). Kongenitale Immunparese bei Fehlen spezifischer β_2- Globuline und quantitativ normalen γ-Globulinen. *Helvet. Paediatr. Acta* 12, 241–259.

Gilmore, R. M. (1911). Uses of plants by Indians. In *Thirty-third Annual Report. Department of Agriculture, Entomology and Plant Quarantine Review*, 100.

Ginzburg, L. and Oppenheimer, G. D. (1932). Non-specific granulomata of the intestine (Inflammatory tumors and structures of bowel). *Transact. Am. Gastroenterol. Assoc.* 35, 241–283.

Glick, B., Chang, T. S., and Jaap, R. G. (1956). The bursa of Fabricius and antibody production. *Poultry Sci.* 35, 224–225.

Glimstedt, G. (1932). Das Leben ohne Bakterien. Sterile Aufziehung von Meerschweinchen. *Vehandl. Anat. Ges. Anat. Anz.* 75, 78–89.

Goldblum, R. M., Ahlstedt, S., Carlsson, B., Hanson, L. Å., Jodal, U., Lidin-Janson, G., and Sohl-Åkerlund, A. (1975). Antibody-forming cells in human colostrum after oral immunization. *Nature* 257, 797–799.

Goldner, J. (1929). Le probléme de la régénération de l'epithélium intestinal. *Bull. Histol. Appliq. Physiol.* 6, 79–95.

Gowans, J. L. and Knight, E. J. (1964). The route of re-circulation of lymphocytes in the rat. *Proc. R. Soc. Lond. [Biol.]* 159, 257–282.

Gresham, G. E., Joseph, J. M., Farber, R. E., and Silverman, C. (1962). Epidemic of type 3 paralytic poliomyelitis in Baltimore, Maryland, 1960. *Public Health Rep.* 77, 349–355.

Grey, H. M., Abel, C. A., Yount, W. J., and Kunkel, H. G. (1968). A subclass of human γA-globulins (γA2) which lacks the disulfide bonds linking heavy and light chains. *J. Exp. Med.* 128, 1223–1236.

Griscelli, C., Vassalli, P, and McCluskey, R. T. (1969). The distribution of large dividing lymph node cells in syngeneic recipient rats after intravenous injection. *J. Exp. Med.* 130, 1427–1451.

Grolnick, M. (1951). Studies on contact-dermatitis. VIII. The effect of feeding of antigen on the subsequent development of skin sensitization. *J. Allergy* 22, 170–174.

Gugler, E. and von Muralt, G. (1959). Ueber immuno-elektrophoretische Untersuchungen an Frauenmilch-Proteinen. 2. *Mitt. Schweiz. Med. Wochenschr.* 89, 925–929.

Guieysse-Pellissier, A. (1912). Caryanabiose et greffe nucleaire. *Arch. Anat. Microscop.* 13, 1–94.

Gustafsson, B. (1948). Germfree rearing of rats. *Acta Pathol. Microbiol. Scand.* 22, 1–132.

Hall, J. G., Parry, D. M., and Smith, M. E. (1972). The distribution and differentiation of lymph-borne immunoblasts after intravenous injection into syngeneic recipients. *Cell Tissue Kinet.* 5, 269–281.

Hall, J. G. and Smith, M. E. (1970). Homing of lymph-borne immunoblasts to the gut. *Nature* 226, 262–263.

Halpern, B., Zweibaum, A., Oriol Palau, R., and Morard, J. C. (1967). Experimental immune ulcerative colitis. In *Immunopathology. International Symposium* eds. P. Miescher and P. Grabar, 161–178. Basel, Switzerland: Schwabe and Co.

Halpern, M. S. and Koshland, M. E. (1970). Novel subunit in secretory IgA. *Nature* 228, 1276–1278.

Ham, A. W. (1969). *Histology*, 313. Philadelphia: JP Lippincott.

Hanson, L. Å. (1961). Comparative immunological studies of the immune globulins of human milk and of blood serum. *Int. Arch. Allergy Appl. Immunol.* 18, 241–267.

Hanson, L. Å., Adlerberth, I., Carlsson, B., Coffman, K., Dahlgren, U., Nilsson, K., Jalil, F., and Roberton, D. (1988). Mucosal immunity—from past to present. *Monogr. Allergy* 24, 1–8.

Hanson, L. Å., Björkander, J., and Oxelius, V. A. (1983). Selective IgA deficiency. In *Primary and Secondary Immunodeficiency Disorders* (R. Chandra, ed.), pp. 62–84. Churchill-Livingston, Edinburgh, Scotland.

Hanson, L. Å. and Johansson, B. (1961). Immunological characterization of chromatographically separated protein fractions from human colostrum. *Int. Arch. Allergy Appl. Immunol.* 20, 65–79.

Harries, E. H. R., Mitman, M., with collaboration of Taylor, I. (1951). *Clinical Practice in Infectious Diseases*, 448. Baltimore: Williams & Wilkins.

Heberden, W. (1801). *Commertarii di Marlbaun. Historia et Curatione.* London: Payne.

Henoch, E. H. H. (1874). Ueber eine eigenthümliche Form von Purpura. *Berliner Klin. Wochenschr.* 51, 641–643.

Heremans, J. F. (1959). Immunochemical studies on protein pathology. The immunoglobulin concept. *Clin. Chim. Acta* 4, 639–646.

Heremans, J. F. (1974). Immunoglobulin A. In *The Antigens* (ed. M. Sela), vol. 2, 365–522. New York: Academic Press.

Heremans, J. F., Heremans, M. T., and Schultze, H. E. (1959). Isolation and description of a few properties of the β_2A-globulin of human serum. *Clin. Chim. Acta* 4, 96–102.

Heremans, J. F., Vaerman, J. -P., and Vaerman, C. (1963). Studies on the immune globulins of human serum. II. A study of the distribution of anti-*Brucella* and anti-diphtheria antibody activities among γ_{ss-} γ_{1M-} and γ_{1A}-globulin fractions. *J. Immunol.* 91, 11–17.

Hodgson, H. J., Wands, J. R., and Isselbacher, K. J. (1978). Decreased suppressor cell activity in inflammatory bowel disease. *Clin. Exp. Immunol.* 32, 451–458.

Hummel, K. P. (1935). The structure and development of the lymphatic tissue in the intestine of the albino rat. *Am. J. Anat.* 57, 351–383.

Jackman, R. J. and Bargen, J. A. (1942). Familial occurrence of chronic ulcerative colitis (thrombo ulcerative colitis). *Am. J. Dig. Dis. Nutr.* 9, 147–149.

Jackson, G. D. F., Lemaitre-Coelho, I., and Vaerman, J. -P. (1977). Transfer of MOPC-315 IgA to secretions in MOPC-315 tumor-bearing and normal BALB/c mice. *Protides Biol. Fluids* 25, 919–922.

Jacobson, L. O., Marks, E. K., Simmons, E. L., and Gaston, E. O. (1961). Immune response in irradiated mice with Peyer's patch shielding. *Proc. Soc. Exp. Biol. Med.* 108, 487–493.

Jelliffe, D. B. and Jelliffe, E. F. P. (1977). Current concepts in nutrition. "Breast is best": Modern meanings. *N. Engl. J. Med.* 297, 912–915.

Jenner, E. (1798). *An Inquiry into the Causes and Effects of the Variolae Vaccinae, a Disease Discovered in Some of the Western Counties of England, particularly Gloucestershire, and Known by the Name of the Cow Pox.* London: Sampson Low.

Jervis, G. A., Koprowski, H., McGee, E. L., Nelsen, D. J., Norton, T. W., and Stokes, J., Jr. (1956). Immunization of children by the feeding of living attentuated Type I and Type II poliomyelitis virus and the intramuscular injection of immune serum globulin. *Am. J. Med. Sci.* 232, 378–388.

Joel, D. D., Sordat, B., Hess, M. W., and Cottier, H. (1970). Uptake and retention of particles from the intestine by Peyer's patches in mice. *Experientia* 26, 694.

Jolly, J. (1913). Sur les organes lymphoepitheliaux. *Comp. Rend. Soc. Biol. T.* 74, 540–543.

Katz, A. J., Falchuk, Z. M., Strober, W., and Shwachman, H. (1976). Gluten-sensitive enteropathy. Inhibition by cortisol of the effect of gluten protein in vitro. *N. Engl. J. Med.* 295, 131–135.

Keuning, J. J., Pena, A. S., van Leeuwen, A., van Hooff, J. P., and van Rood, J. J. (1976). HLA-DW3 associated with coeliac disease. *Lancet* 1, 506–508.

Kilian, M., Mestecky, J., and Schrohenloher, R. E. (1979). Pathogenic species of the genus *Haemophilus* and *Streptococcus pneumoniae* produce immunoglobulin A1 protease. *Infect. Immun.* 26, 143–149.

Kim, Y. B. (1979). Role of antigen in ontogeny of the immune response. In *Microbiology 1979* (ed. D. Schlessinger) pp. 343–348. American Society for Microbiology, Washington, D.C.

Kirsner, J. B. (1961). Experimental "colitis" with particular reference to hypersensitivity reactions in the colon. *Gastroenterology* 40, 307–312.

Klein, E. (1875). *The Anatomy of the Lymphatic System. II. The Lung.* London: Smith and Elder.

Klemperer, G. (1892). Untersuchungen über künstlichen Impfschutz gegen Choleraintoxication. *Berliner Klin. Wochenschr.* 29, 789–793.

Klingman, A. M. (1958). Poison ivy (*Rhus*) dermatitis. *Arch. Dermatol.* 77, 149–180.

Koch, R. (1885). Zweiter Konferenz zur Erörterung der Cholerafrage. *Deutsch. Med. Wochenschr.* 37A, 1–60.

Koistinen, J. (1975). Selective IgA deficiency in blood donors. *Vox Sang.* 29, 192–202.

Kolmer, J. A., Klugh, G., Jr., and Rule, A. M. (1935). A successful method for vaccination against acute anterior poliomyelitis. *J. Am. Med. Assoc.* 104, 456–460.

Koprowski, H., Jervis, G. A., and Norton, T. W. (1952). Immune responses in human volunteers upon oral administration of a rodent-adapted strain of poliomyelitis virus. *Am. J. Hyg.* 55, 108–126.

Korenblat, P. E., Rothberg, R. M., Minden, P., and Farr, R. S. (1968). Immune responses of human adults after oral and parenteral exposure to bovine serum albumin. *J. Allergy* 41, 226–235.

Koshland, M. E. and Burrows, W. (1950). Quantitative studies of the relationship between fecal and serum antibody. *J. Immunol.* 65, 93–103.

Kraft, S. C., Fitch, F. W., and Kirsner, J. B. (1963). Histologic and immunohistochemical features of the Auer "colitis" in rabbits. *Am. J. Pathol.* 43, 913–927.

Kraus, F. W. and Sirisinha, S. (1962). Gamma globulin in saliva. *Arch. Oral. Biol.* 7, 221–233.

Kunkel, H. G. and Prendergast, R. A. (1966). Subgroups of γA immune globulins. *Proc. Soc. Exp. Biol. Med.* 122, 910–913.

Kunkel, H. G., Smith, W. K., Joslin, F. G., Natvig, J. B., and Litwin, S. D. (1969). Genetic marker of the γA2 subgroup of γA immunoglobulins. *Nature* 223, 1247–1248.

LaPlane, R., Burtin, P., Curioni, S., Houet, C., Graveleau, D., and LeBalle, J. C. (1962). Sur un cas d'agammaglobulinemie atypique. Etude biologique et génétique. *Ann. Pediat.* 38, 281–290.

Lane, W. A. (1926). The prevention of the disease. *Surg. Gynecol. Obstet.* 42, 196–208.

Lawrence, D. A., Weigle, W. O., and Spiegelberg, H. L. (1975). Immunoglobulins cytophilic for human lymphocytes, monocytes, and neutrophils. *J. Clin. Invest.* 55, 368–376.

Lawton, A. R., 3rd and Mage, R. G. (1969). The synthesis of secretory IgA in the rabbit. I. Evidence for synthesis as an 11S dimer. *J. Immunol.* 102, 693–697.

Leidy, J. (1849). On the existence of entophyta in healthy animals as a natural condition. *Proc. Acad. Natl. Sci. Phila.* 4, 225–233.

Lemaitre-Coelho, I., Jackson, G. D. F., and Vaerman, J. -P. (1977). Rat bile as a convenient source of secretory IgA and free secretory component. *Eur. J. Immunol.* 7, 588–590.

Lipton, M. M. and Steigman, A. J. (1963). Human coproantibodies against polio viruses. *J. Infect. Dis.* 112, 57–66.

Loeb, P. M., Strober, W., Falchuk, Z. M., and Laster, L. (1971). Incorporation of L-leucine-^{14}C into immunoglobulins by jejunal biopsies of patients with celiac sprue and other gastrointestinal diseases. *J. Clin. Invest.* 50, 559–569.

Lowney, E. D. (1968). Immunologic unresponsiveness to a contact sensitizer in man. *J. Invest. Dermatol.* 51, 411–417.

Lowney, E. D. (1973). Suppression of contact sensitization in man by prior feeding of antigen. *J. Invest. Dermatol.* 61, 90–93.

Mach, J. P. (1970). *In vitro* combination of human and bovine free secretory component with IgA of various species. *Nature* 228, 1278–1282.

Male, C. (1979). Immunoglobulin A1 protease production by *Haemophilus influenzae* and *Streptococcus pneumoniae*. *Infect. Immun.* 26, 254–261.

Masaki, S. (1922). Du mécanisme de l'infection cholérique et de la vaccination contré le choléra par voie buccale. *Compt. Rend. Seanc. Soc. Biol. Filial.* 86, 532–534.

McCarthy, D. M., Katz, S. I., Gazze, L., Waldmann, T. A., Nelson, D. L., and Strober, W. (1978). Selective IgA deficiency associated with total villous atrophy of the small intestine and an organ-specific anti-epithelial cell antibody. *J. Immunol.* 120, 932–938.

McDermott, M. R. and Bienenstock, J. (1979). Evidence for a common mucosal immunologic system. I. Migration of B immunoblasts into intestinal, respiratory, and genital tissues. *J. Immunol.* 122, 1892–1898.

McDermott, M. R., Clark, D. A., and Bienenstock, J. (1980). Evidence for a common mucosal immunologic system. II. Influence of the estrous cycle on B immunoblast migration into genital and intestinal tissues. *J. Immunol.* 124, 2536–2539.

McWilliams, M., Phillips-Quagliata, J. M., and Lamm, M. E. (1975). Characteristics of mesenteric lymph node cells homing to gut-associated lymphoid tissue in syngeneic mice. *J. Immunol.* 115, 54–58.

McWilliams, M., Phillips-Quagliata, J. M., and Lamm, M. E. (1977). Mesenteric lymph node B lymphoblasts which home to the small intestine are precommitted to IgA synthesis. *J. Exp. Med.* 145, 866–875.

Mee, A. S., McLaughlin, J. E., Hodgson, H. J. F., and Jewell, D. P. (1979). Chronic immune colitis in rabbits. *Gut* 20, 1–5.

Mehta, S. K., Plaut, A. G., Calvanico, N. J., and Tomasi, T. B., Jr. (1973). Human immunoglobulin A: Production of an Fc fragment by an enteric microbial proteolytic enzyme. *J. Immunol.* 111, 1274–1276.

Mellander, L., Björkander, J., Carlsson, B., and Hanson, L. Å. (1986). Secretory antibodies in IgA deficient and immunosuppressed individuals. *J. Clin. Immunol.* 6, 284–291.

Mestecky, J., Kulhavy, R., and Kraus, F. W. (1972). Studies on human secretory immunoglobulin A. II. Subunit structure. *J. Immunol.* 108, 738–747.

Mestecky, J., McGhee, J. R., Arnold, R. R., Michalek, S. M., Prince, S. J., and Babb, J. L. (1978). Selective induction of an immune response in human external secretions by ingestion of bacterial antigen. *J. Clin. Invest.* 61, 731–737.

Mestecky, J., Zikan, J., and Butler, W. T. (1971). Immunoglobulin M and secretory immunoglobulin A: Presence of a common polypeptide chain different from light chains. *Science* 171, 1163–1165.

Metchnikoff, E. (1903). In *The Nature of Man* (ed. P. C. Mitchell), 72–73, New York: G. P. Putman.

Metchnikoff, E. (1908). In *The Prolongation of Life* (ed. P. C. Mitchell), 58–83, 150–183. New York: G. P. Putman.

Michalek, S. M., McGhee, J. R., Mestecky, J., Arnold, R. R., and Bozzo, L. (1976). Ingestion of *Streptococcus mutans* induces secretory IgA and caries immunity. *Science* 192, 1238–1240.

Mitsuya, H., Osaki, K., Tomino, S., Katsuki, T., and Kishimoto, S. (1981). Pathophysiologic analysis of peripheral blood lymphocytes from patients with primary immunodeficiency. I. Ig synthesis by peripheral blood lymphocytes stimulated with either pokeweed mitogen or Epstein-Barr virus *in vitro*. *J. Immunol.* 127, 311–315.

Miyakawa, M., Iijima, S., Kishimoto, H., Kobayashi, R., Tajima, M., Isomura, N., Asano, M., and Hong, C. (1958). Rearing germfree guinea pigs. *Acta Pathol. Jpn.* 8, 55.

Montgomery, P. C., Connelly, K. M., Cohn, J., and Skandera, C. A. (1978). Remote-site stimulation of secretory IgA antibodies following bronchial and gastric stimulation. *Adv. Exp. Med. Biol.* 107, 113–122.

Montgomery, P. C., Rosner, B. R., and Cohn, J. (1974). The secretory antibody response. Anti-DNP antibodies induced by dinitrophenylated type 3 pneumococcus. *Immunol. Commun.* 3, 143–156.

Morgan, I. M. (1948). Immunization of monkeys with formalin-inactivated poliomyelitis viruses. *Am. J. Hyg.* 48, 394–406.

Moschcowitz, E. and Wilensky, A. D. (1923). Non-specific granulomata of the intestine. *Am. J. Med. Sci.* 166, 48–66.

Mowat, A. M. and Ferguson, A. (1981). Hypersensitivity in the small intestinal mucosa. V. Induction of cell-mediated immunity to a dietary antigen. *Clin. Exp. Immunol.* 43, 574–582.

Nagura, H., Nakane, P. K., and Brown, W. R. (1979). Translocation of dimeric IgA through neoplastic colon cells in vitro. *J. Immunol.* 123, 2359–2368.

Norman, J. M. (1991). *Garrison and Morton's Medical Bibliography*. Menston, England: Scolar Press.

Nuttall, G. H. F. and Thierfelder, H. (1895). Thierisches Leben ohne Bakterien im Verdauungskanal. *Z. Physiol. Chem.* 21, 109–121.

O'Daly, J. A. and Cebra, J. J. (1971). Chemical and physicochemical studies of the component polypeptide chains of rabbit secretory immunoglobulin A. *Biochemistry* 10, 3843–3850.

Ogra, P. L. and Karzon, D. T. (1969). Poliovirus antibody response in serum and nasal secretions following intranasal inoculation with inactivated poliovaccine. *J. Immunol.* 102, 15–23.

Ogra, P. and Karzon, D. (1971). Formation and function of poliovirus antibody in different tissues. *Prog. Med. Virol.* 13, 156–193.

Ogra, P. L., Karzon, D. T., Righthand, F., and MacGillivray, M. (1968). Immunoglobulin response in serum and secretions after immunization with live and inactivated poliovaccine and natural infection. *N. Engl. J. Med.* 279, 893–900.

Onderdonk, A. B., Hermos, J. A., Dzink, J. L., and Bartlett, J. G. (1978). Protective effect of metronidazole in experimental ulcerative colitis. *Gastroenterology* 74, 521–526.

Owen, R. L. (1977). Sequential uptake of horseradish peroxidase by lymphoid follicle epithelium of Peyer's patches in the normal unobstructed mouse intestine: an ultrastructural study. *Gastroenterology* 72, 440–451.

Owen, R. L. and Jones, A. L. (1974). Epithelial cell specialization within human Peyer's patches: An ultrastructural study of intestinal lymphoid follicles. *Gastroenterology* 66, 189–203.

Oxelius, V. A., Laurell, A. B., Lindquist, B., Golebiowska, H., Axelsson, U., Bjorkander, J., and Hanson, L. Å. (1981). IgG subclasses in selective IgA deficiency: Importance of IgG2-IgA deficiency *N. Engl. J. Med.* 304, 1476–1477.

Park, R. G. (1944). Sulphonamide allergy. The persistence and desensitization. *BMJ* 2, 816–817.

Parrott, D. and MacDonald, T. T. (1990). The ontogeny of the mucosal immune system in rodents. In *Ontogeny of the Immune System of the Gut* (ed. T. T. MacDonald), 51–67. Boca Raton, FL: CRC Press.

Pasteur, L. (1880). De l'attenuation du virus du choléra des poules. *Compt. Rend. Acad. Sci.* 91, 673–680.

Paulley, L. W. (1954). Observation on the aetiology of idiopathic steatorrhoea jejunal and lymph-node biopsies. *Brit. Med. J.* 2, 1318–1321.

Pechlin, J. N. (1672). De purgantium medicamentorum facultatibus exercitatio nova *treatise*.

Pereira, S., Webster, D., and Platts-Mills, T. (1982). Immature B cells in fetal development and immunodeficiency: Studies of IgM, IgG, IgA, and IgD production *in vitro* using Epstein-Barr virus activation. *Eur. J. Immunol.* 12, 540–546.

Perlmann, P. and Broberger, O. (1963). In vitro studies in ulcerative colitis. II. Cytotoxic action of white blood cells from patients on human fetal colon cells. *J. Exp. Med.* 117, 717–733.

Peyer, J. C. (1677). *Exercitatio Anatomico-Medica de Usu et Affectionibus. Cui Subjungitur Anatome Ventriculi Galliinacei.* Onophrius et Waldkirch, Schaffhausen.

Peyer, J. C. (1681). Exercitatio Anatomico-Medica de Glandulis Intestinorum, Earumque Usu et Affectionibus. Cui Subjungitur Anatome Ventriculi Gallinacei. Amsterdam: H. Wetstenium.

Phillpots, R. J., Hermon-Taylor, J., Teich, N. M., and Brooke, B. N. (1980). A search for persistent virus infection in Crohn's disease. *Gut* 21, 202–207.

Pierce, N. F. and Gowans, J. L. (1975). Cellular kinetics of the intestinal immune response to cholera toxoid in rats. *J. Exp. Med.* 142, 1550–1563.

Plaut, A. G., Gilbert, J. V., Artenstein, M. S., and Capra, J. D. (1975). *Neisseria gonorrhoeae* and *Neisseria meningitidis:* Extracellular enzyme cleaves human immunoglobulin A. *Science* 190, 1103–1105.

Plaut, A. G., Wistar, R., Jr., and Capra, J. D. (1974). Differential susceptibility of human IgA immunoglobulins to streptococcal IgA protease. *J. Clin. Invest.* 54, 1295–1300.

Poger, M. E. and Lamm, M. E. (1974). Localization of free and bound secretory component in human intestinal epithelial cells. A model for the assembly of secretory IgA. *J. Exp. Med.* 139, 629–642.

Pollard, M. and Sharon, S. (1970). Responses of the Peyer's patches in germ-free mice to antigenic stimulation. *Infect. Immun.* 2, 96–100.

Przemioslo, R. T., Lundin, K. E., Sollid, L. M., Nelufer, J., and Ciclitira, P. J. (1995). Histological changes in small bowel mucosa induced by gliadin sensitive T lymphocytes can be blocked by anti-interferon gamma antibody. *Gut* 36, 874–879.

Radl, J., Klein, F., van den Berg, P., de Bruyn, A. M., and Hijmans, W. (1971). Binding of secretory piece to polymeric IgA and IgM paraproteins *in vitro. Immunology* 20, 843–852.

Radl, J., Schuit, H. R. E., Mestecky, J., and Hijmans, W. (1974). The origin of monomeric and polymeric forms of IgA in man. *Adv. Exp. Med. Biol.* 45, 57–65.

Rappaport, H., Burgoyne, F. H., and Smetana, H. F. (1951). The pathology of regional enteritis. *Milit. Surg.* 109, 463–488.

Reinach, T. (1890). Mithridate Eupator. Roi de Pont, pp. 283–285, 409–410. Paris: Firmin-Didot.

Rejnek, J., Travnicek, J., Kostka, J., Sterzl, J., and Lanc A. (1968). Study of the effect of antibodies in the intestinal tract of germ-free baby pigs. *Folia Microbiol.* 13, 36–42.

Report of the Commission on the Cost of Medical Care. (1964). The economic significance of the prevention of paralytic poliomyelitis 1955–1961. *J. Am. Med. Assoc.* 29–46.

Reyniers, J. A. (1932). The use of germfree guinea pigs in bacteriology. *Proc. Indiana Acad. Sci.* 42, 35–37.

Robertson, S. M. and Cebra, J. J. (1976). A model for local immunity. *Ricerca Clin. Lab.* 6, 105–119.

Rockey, J. H., Hanson, L. Å., Heremans, J. F., and Kunkel, H. G. (1964). Beta-2A-aglobulinemia in two healthy men. *J. Lab. Clin. Med.* 63, 205–212.

Ross, V. (1930). Oral immunization against pneumococcus. Use of bile salt dissolved organisms, etc., time of appearance of immunity and dosage. *J. Exp. Med.* 51, 585–607.

Roux, M. E., McWilliams, M., Phillips-Quagliata, J. M., Weisz-Carrington, P., and Lamm, M. E. (1977). Origin of IgA-secreting plasma cells in the mammary gland. *J. Exp. Med.* 146, 1311–1322.

Rudzik, O., Clancy, R. L., Perey, D. Y. E., Day, R. P., and Bienenstock, J. (1975). Repopulation with IgA-containing cells of bronchial and intestinal lamina propria after transfer of homologous Peyer's patch and bronchial lymphocytes. *J. Immunol.* 114, 1599–1604.

Sabin, A. B. (1955). Characteristics and genetic potentialities of experimentally produced and naturally occurring variants of poliomyelitis virus. *Ann. N.Y. Acad. Sci.* 61, 924–938.

Salk, J. E. (1953). Principles of immunization as applied to poliomyelitis and influenza. *Am. J. Public Health* 43, 1384–1398.

Sanders, A. G. and Florey, H. W. (1940). The effects of the removal of lymphoid tissue. *Br. J. Exp. Pathol.* 21, 275–287.

Savilahti, E. and Pelkonen, P. (1979). Clinical findings and intestinal immunoglobulins in children with partial IgA deficiency. *Acta Paediatr. Scand.* 68, 513–519.

Schaedler, R. W., Dubos, R., and Costello, R. (1965a). The development of the bacterial flora in the gastrointestinal tract of mice. *J. Exp. Med.* 122, 59–66.

Schaedler, R. W., Dubos, R., and Costello, R. (1965b). Association of germ-free mice with bacteria isolated from normal mice. *J. Exp. Med.* 122, 77–83.

Schaffner, T., Mueller, J., Hess, M. W., Cottier, H., Sordat, B., and Ropke, C. (1974). The bursa of Fabricius: A central organ providing for contact between the lymphoid system and intestinal content. *Cell. Immunol.* 13, 304–312.

Schmidt, J. E. (1959). *Medical Discoveries: Who and When.* Springfield, IL: Charles C. Thomas.

Schönlein, J. L. (1837). Allgemeine und specielle Pathologie und Therapie. Würzburg, Germany: Herisan.

Schottelius, M. (1899). Die Bedeutung der Darmbakterien für die Ernahrung. *Arch. Hyg.* 34, 210–243.

Shelmire, B. (1941). Hyposensitization of poison ivy. *Arch. Dermatol. Syphil.* 44, 983–998.

Shiner, M. and Doniach, I. (1960). Histopathologic studies in steatorrhea. *Gastroenterology* 38, 419–440.

Shorter, R. G., Huizenga, K. A., ReMine, S. G., and Spencer, R. J. (1970). Effects of preliminary incubation of lymphocytes with serum on their cytotoxicity for colonic epithelial cells. *Gastroenterology* 58, 843–850.

Shuster, S., Watson, A. J., and Marks, J. (1968). Coeliac syndrome in dermatitis herpetiformis. *Lancet* 2, 1101–1106.

Shvartsman, Ya. S. and Zykov, M. P. (1976). Secretory anti-influenza immunity. *Adv. Immunol.* 22, 291–330.

Silvers, S. H. (1941). Stomatitis venenata and dermitis of anal orifice from chewing poison leaves (*Rhus toxicodendron*). *J. Am. Med. Assoc.* 116, 2257.

Slater, R. J., Ward, S. M., and Kunkel, H. G. (1955). Immunological relationships among the myeloma proteins. *J. Exp. Med.* 101, 85–108.

Smith, C. B., Bellanti, J. A., and Chanock, R. M. (1967). Immunoglobulins in serum and nasal secretions following infection with type 1 parainfluenza virus and injection of inactivated vaccines. *J. Immunol.* 99, 133–141.

Smith, J. S. (1991). *Patenting the Sun: Polio and Salk Vaccine.* New York: Anchor Books Doubleday.

Smits, B. J. (1989). History of coeliac disease. *Br. Med. J.* 298, 387.

Sorvari, T., Sorvari, R., Ruotsalainen, P., Toivanen, A., and Toivanen, P. (1975). Uptake of environmental antigens by the bursa of Fabricius. *Nature* 253, 217–219.

South, M. A., Cooper, M. D., Wollheim, F. A., Hong, R., and Good, R. A. (1966). The IgA system. I. Studies of the transport and immunochemistry of IgA in the saliva. *J. Exp. Med.* 123, 615–627.

Spiegelberg, H. L., Lawrence, D. A., and Henson, P. (1974). Cytophilic properties of IgA to human neutrophils. *Adv. Exp. Med. Biol.* 45, 67–74.

Sterzl, J., Mandel, L., and Stepankova, R. (1987). The use of gnotobiological models for the studies of immune mechanisms. *Nahrung* 31, 599–608.

Sterzl, J. and Silverstein, A. M. (1967). Developmental aspects of immunity. *Adv. Immunol.* 6, 337–459.

Stevens, F. A. (1945). Council on pharmacy and chemistry. Report of the council: Status of poison ivy extracts. *J. Am. Med. Assoc.* 127, 912–921.

Sulzberger, M. B. (1930). Arsphenamine hypersensitivity in guinea-pigs. II. Experiments demonstrating the role of the skin, both as originator and as site of hypersensitiveness. *Arch. Dermatol. Syphil.* 22, 839–849.

Talbott, J. H. (1970). A Biographical History of Medicine, 734–736. New York: Grune & Stratton.

Terry, W. D. and Roberts, M. S. (1966). Antigenic heterogeneity of human immunoglobulin A proteins. *Science* 153, 1007–1008.

Thucydides. (1951). *The Complete Writings of Thucydides: The Peloponnesian War.* (transl. J. H. Finley, Jr.), 112. New York: The Modern Library.

Tietze, A. (1920). Ueber entzundliche Dickdarmgeschwulste. *Ergeb. Chir. Orthop.* 12, 211–273.

Tlaskalová, H. and Stepánková, R. (1980). Development of antibody formation in germ-free and conventionally reared rabbits: the role of intestinal lymphoid tissue in antibody formation to *E. coli* antigens. *Folia Biol.* 26, 81–93.

Tlaskalová, H., Sterzl, J., Hájek, P., Pospísil, M., Ríha, I., Marvanová, H., Kamarytová, V., Mandel, L., Kruml, J., and Kováru, F. (1970). The development of antibody formation during embryonal and postnatal periods. In *Developmental Aspects of Antibody Formation and Structure* (eds. J. Sterzl and I. Ríha), 767–790. Prague: Academia Publishing House.

Tomasi, T. B., Jr., Tan, E. M., Solomon, A., and Prendergast, R. A. (1965). Characteristics of an immune system common to certain external secretions. *J. Exp. Med.* 121, 101–124.

Tomasi, T. B., Jr. and Zigelbaum, S. O. (1963). The selective occurrence of γ1A globulins in certain body fluids. *J. Clin. Invest.* 42, 1552–1560.

Tosi, R., Vismara, D., Tanigaki, N., Ferrara, G. B., Cicimarra, F., Buffolano, W., Follo, D., and Auricchio, S. (1983). Evidence that celiac disease is primarily associated with a DC locus allelic specificity. *Clin. Immunol. Immunopathol.* 28, 395–404.

Tourville, D. R., Adler, R. H., Bienenstock, J., and Tomasi, T. B., Jr. (1969). The human secretory immunoglobulin system: Immunohistological localization of γA, secretory "piece," and lactoferrin in normal human tissues. *J. Exp. Med.* 129, 411–429.

Trávnícek, J., Kovaru, F., Mandel, L., Stozicky, V., and Kruml, J. (1975). The delivery of piglets for germfree rearing by caesarean section in a closed system. *Acta Vet.* 33, 297.

Trnka, Z., Sterzl, J., Lanc, A., and Mandel, L. (1959). Natural and experimental infections in agammaglobulinemic piglets. *Giorn. Malattie Infet. Parasitarie* 11, 330.

Vaerman, J. P. and Heremans, J. F. (1966). Subclasses of human immunoglobulin A based on differences in the alpha polypeptide chains. *Science* 153, 647–649.

Vaillant, L. (1922). Note sur l'emploi du vaccine bilié de Besredka par la voie buccale dans quelques foyers épidémiques de fiévre typhoïde. *Ann. Inst. Pasteur* 36, 149–156.

Van de Kamer, J. H., Weijers, H. A., and Dicke, W. K. (1953). Coeliac disease. IV. An investigation into the injurious constituents of wheats in connection with their action on patients with coeliac disease. *Acta Paediatr.* 42, 223–230.

Van Thiel, D. H., Smith, W. I., Jr., Rabin, B. S., Fisher, S. E., and Lester, R. (1977). A syndrome of immunoglobulin A deficiency, diabetes mellitus, malabsorption, a common HLA haplotype. Immunologic and genetic studies of forty-three family members. *Ann. Intern. Med.* 86, 10–19.

Waksman, B. H. and Ozer, H. (1976). Specialized amplification elements in the immune system. The role of nodular lymphoid organs in the mucosal membranes. *Prog. Allergy* 21, 1–113.

Waldman, R. H., Kasel, J. A., Fulk, R. V., Mann, J. J., Togo, Y., Hornick, R. B., Heiner, G. T., and Dawkins, A. T. (1968). Influenza antibody in human respiratory secretions after subcutaneous or respiratory immunization with inactivated virus. *Nature* 218, 594–595.

Walker, W. A., Isselbacher, K. J., and Bloch, K. J. (1972). Intestinal uptake of macromolecules: Effect of oral immunization, *Science* 177, 608–610.

Warren, S. and Sommers, S. C. (1948). Cicatrizing enteritis (regional ileitis) as a pathologic entity: Analysis of 120 cases. *Am. J. Pathol.* 24, 475–497.

Warren, S. and Sommers, S. C. (1954). Pathology of regional ileitis and ulcerative colitis. *J. Am. Med. Assoc.* 154, 189–193.

Weber, E. H. (1847). Ueber den Mechanismus der Einsaugung des Speisesaftes beim Menschen und bei einigen Tieren. *Arch. Anat. Physiol. Wissensch. Med.* 7, 400–402.

Weisz-Carrington, P., Roux, M. E., McWilliams, M., Phillips-Quagliata, J. M., and Lamm, M. E. (1978). Hormonal induction of the secretory immune system in the mammary gland. *Proc. Natl. Acad. Sci. U.S.A.* 75, 2928–2932.

Weisz-Carrington, P., Roux, M. E., McWilliams, M., Phillips-Quagliata, J. M., and Lamm, M. E. (1979). Organ and isotype distribution of plasma cells producing specific antibody after oral immunization: Evidence for a generalized secretory immune system. *J. Immunol.* 123, 1705–1708.

Wells, H. G. and Osborne, T. B. (1911). The biological reactions of the vegetable proteins. I. Anaphylaxis. *J. Infect. Dis.* 8, 66–124.

West, C. D., Hong, R., and Holland, N. H. (1962). Immunoglobulin levels from the newborn period to adulthood and in immunoglobulin deficiency states. *J. Clin. Invest.* 41, 2054–2064.

Wilks, S. (1859). Morbid appearances in the intestine of Miss Bankes. *London Med. Gazzette* 2, 264.

Wilks, S. and Moxon, W. (1875). *Lectures on Pathological Anatomy.* Lindsay & Blakiston.

Williams, R. C. and Gibbons, R. J. (1972). Inhibition of bacterial adherence by secretory immunoglobulin A: A mechanism of antigen disposal. *Science* 177, 697–699.

Wolf-Heidegger, G. (1939). Zur Frage der Lymphocytenwanderung durch das Darmepithel. *Zeitschr. Mikrosc. Anat. Forsch.* 45, 90–103.

Part I

Mucosal Immune System

Section A

Mucosal Barrier:
Development and Physiology
of Mucosal Defense

Development and Physiology of Mucosal Defense: An Introduction

Chapter

1

Lloyd Mayer

Immunology Center, Mount Sinai Medical Center, New York, New York

W. Allan Walker

Mucosal Immunology Laboratory, Massachusetts General Hospital, Boston, Massachusetts

The primary function of the small intestine is to absorb nutrients into the circulation (Field and Frizzell, 1991). During the course of this activity, the intestine is exposed to a wide variety of antigens derived from foods, resident bacteria, and invading microorganisms. These need to be limited by a barrier that will allow absorption of nutrient molecules. In addition, the intestine transports macromolecules that are important in growth and development, for example, epidermal growth factor (EGF) (Weaver and Walker, 1988; Weaver et al., 1990; Carpenter and Wahl, 1991) and maternal IgG (Simister and Rees, 1985; Rodewald and Kraehenbuhl, 1984). Thus any mechanism that acts as a barrier must also allow entry of physiologically important molecules whose size is comparable to that of many antigens.

The lumen of the intestine is capable of harboring harmful microorganisms (Snyder, 1991); to mount an immune response against these potential pathogens, the mucosal immune system must survey antigens in the lumen. There is good evidence that immunosurveillance by the small intestine depends on transport of antigens across the gut (Mowat, 1987). However, such transport must occur in a controlled manner to avoid harmful immune responses. Nevertheless, there are times when the control of antigen entry breaks down, and this may lead to an excessive influx of antigens, which may ultimately cause disease (Sanderson and Walker, 1993). Both Crohn's disease (Malin et al., 1996) and necrotizing enterocolitis (Israel, 1994) are associated with increased uptake of macromolecules. These two diseases remain among the most important problems facing those investigating diseases of the intestine in children.

MACROMOLECULAR ABSORPTION

To maintain immunosurveillance, antigens are transported across the intestine in physiologic amounts, but pathologic transport may occur when the mucosal barrier is breached. This barrier consists of two main components **(Fig. 1.1)**. Extrinsic mechanisms will limit the amount of antigen reaching the surface of the intestine; the intrinsic barrier consists of the structural and functional properties of the intestine itself.

There is both clinical and experimental evidence that antigens traverse the epithelium and enter the circulation (Warshaw and Walker, 1974; Paganelli et al., 1979), but for the most part, this transport is not harmful and may at times be beneficial.

Production of immunoglobulins directed toward luminal antigen depends on immunologically intact antigen interacting with membrane-bound immunoglobulins on the surface of B cells that are located beyond the intestinal epithelium (Kagnoff, 1989; Elson et al., 1986). Mechanisms that allow passage of antigen through the intestinal epithelium in controlled amounts are therefore an essential prelude to B-cell activation.

T-cell responses, on the other hand, are initiated by presentation of short peptides bound to major histocompatibility complexes (MHCs) (Unanue, 1984). As luminal antigen can activate mucosal T cells [as occurs, for example, in celiac disease (Marsh, 1992)], the intestine must process luminal antigen to peptides of the size that can bind to MHC molecules and in turn interact with T-cell receptors. Antigens can be processed in three ways by the intestine. First, peptide

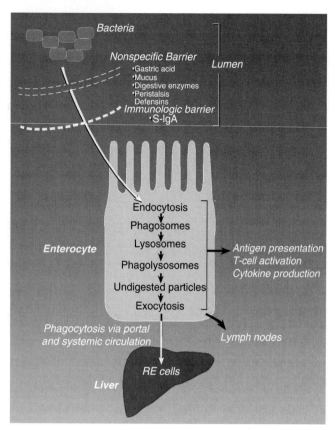

Fig. 1.1. Barriers to macromolecular absorption. Antigen entry is prevented by physiologic and immunologic mechanisms in the gastrointestinal tract as well as by the physical structure of the epithelium itself. Reticuloendothelial (RE) cells consist of Kupffer's cells lining the bile ducts in the liver. Reproduced with permission from Sanderson and Walker (1993).

Table 1.1. Physiologic Transport of Macromolecules across the Intestinal Epithelium

1. Receptor-bound transport across enterocytes
2. Passage across M cells
3. Uptake, processing, and presentation in association with class II MHC molecules

reactions are beneficial and are described in other chapters of this book. There will be times, however, when excessive antigen crosses the intestine, causing more widespread immune reactions. These reactions could result in gastrointestinal disease (Sanderson and Walker, 1993) or even systemic illness such as eczema (Majamaa and Isolauri, 1996).

Macromolecules cross intestinal epithelial cells (IECs) in two ways of which we can be certain. They can be shuttled through absorptive cells using specific receptors—in which case only those macromolecules that bind to a receptor will pass—or they can pass through specialized epithelial cells termed microfold cells (M cells; see Chapter 7). A further possibility is that antigenic fragments cross epithelial cells for presentation by class II MHC molecules at the basolateral surface (Table 1.1). Hershberg and colleagues (1998) have documented that this can occur in an *in vitro* model of IEC antigen presentation. They transfected T84 cells with MHC class II molecules and showed that processing of tetanus toxoid can occur (by the presence of cathepsins B and D) and that processed peptides can be presented to DR-restricted T-cell hybridomas. *In vivo* it is well documented that in the neonate there is immaturity of tight junctions (see the following text) and that in this situation paracellular transport of macromolecules occurs (Strobel *et al.*, 1984; Strobel and Ferguson, 1986; Beach *et al.*, 1982).

Receptor-bound transport

Most of the macromolecules that are required can be made *de novo;* however, this is not always the case. For example, certain growth factors including EGF, transforming growth factor-α, and nerve growth factor are all polypeptides that are transported across the intestine (Chu and Walker, 1991). IgG can also be transported across the intestine at times (Simister and Rees, 1985). The newborn makes very little immunoglobulin, and most circulating antibody is IgG derived passively from the mother. For the most part, in humans IgG is transferred by the placenta during late gestation, whereas in many animals the transfer occurs from maternal milk through the proximal small intestine. The transfer of IgG across the gut is mediated by receptors similar to those present in human placenta (Sedmark *et al.*, 1991). They bind to the Fc portion of the immunoglobulin molecule.

Macromolecules are transferred by a mechanism that is altogether different from those that transport nutrients such as glucose and amino acids. Nutrient molecules enter the intestinal cell cytoplasm at the apical membrane and exit the basolateral membrane. Macromolecules, on the other hand, transverse the cell **(Fig. 1.2)** in membrane-bound compartments that invaginate from the apical membrane. The first

fragments could be generated during transit in the lumen with proteins acted on by luminal proteases (*e.g.*, pepsin, trypsin, chymotrypsin—luminal pre-processing); second, antigen can be processed during epithelial transport (intracellular epithelial processing); and third, antigen could be processed from whole antigen that has traversed the epithelium and reached antigen-presenting cells in the mucosal immune system (macrophages and dendritic cells in the lamina propria). In any case, uptake of antigen by the epithelium is essential. Moreover, the pathway by which the antigen or its products reach the immune system of the gut may critically affect the type of immune response generated. Thus an understanding of the mechanisms whereby antigen is handled is central to the study of the mucosal immune response.

PHYSIOLOGIC TRANSPORT

Sampling of luminal antigen by the mucosa is likely to be a physiologic phenomenon, which will result in appropriate immune responses by the gut. These will include the local production of secretory IgA (S-IgA) and mechanisms that lead to oral tolerance (Thompson and Staines, 1991). Such

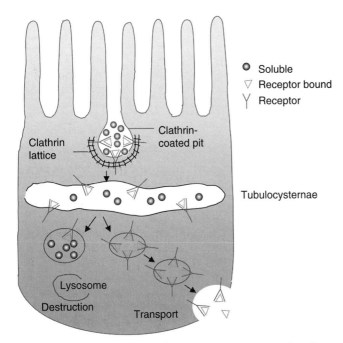

Soluble
Receptor bound
Receptor

Clathrin
lattice

Clathrin-
coated pit

Tubulocysternae

Lysosome
Destruction   Transport

Fig. 1.2. Macromolecular endocytosis in enterocytes. The plasma membrane between microvilli invaginates to form vesicles. Clathrin, a protein that forms a membrane lattice, controls the curvature of the membrane. Macromolecules can enter the vesicle bound to surrounding membrane by its own receptor or by nonspecific attraction; they can also enter free in solution. After entry they move to the tubulocysternae, where they are sorted and pass either to vesicles that travel toward the lysosome or to vesicles that traverse the cell to the basolateral pole. Membrane-bound molecules are more likely than those in solution to traverse the cells. Reprinted with permission from Sanderson and Walker (1993).

step in this process is attachment to receptors on the apical surface of enterocytes.

In young mice maternal IgG absorption shows features characteristic of a membrane receptor transport: IgG is selectively absorbed (Jones and Waldmann, 1972; Guyer *et al.*, 1976), and its absorption shows saturation kinetics (Brambell, 1966). Binding is pH dependent, occurring at pH 6, not at pH 7.4 (Rodewald, 1976).

As the contents of the upper jejunum are at low pH, the conditions are ideal for binding (Jones and Waldmann, 1983). Moreover, intracellular membrane compartments are acidic, and so binding would be maintained after invagination of surface membrane and formation of vesicles (Abrahamson and Rodewald, 1981). The IgG receptor has now been isolated, its gene cloned, and the nucleic acid sequencing determined. From this, the amino acid sequence has been deduced (Simister and Mostov, 1989; Mikulska *et al*, 2000). It is a molecule homologous to class I MHCs. It is bound in its active form to β2 macroglobulin. Despite the homology, the two molecules have very different functions, and their assembly is different. Recent studies have suggested that this molecule is expressed in adult bowel as well, both in rodents and in man. Bidirectional transepithelial transport of IgG has been noted both *in vitro* and *in vivo* (intestine and lung) (McCarthy *et al.*, 2000; Yoshida *et al.*, 2004; Bitonti *et al.*, 2004).

The Fc receptor is able to move across the epithelial cell. The transcytosis occurs in both directions. The receptor is carried with the membrane trafficking from lumen to serosa and returns by another membrane transport mechanism. Some membrane proteins contain specific amino acid sequences that direct the protein within the cell, for instance, the polymeric IgA receptor (Casanova *et al.*, 1991), which transports the IgA from the basolateral membrane to the apical membrane (Chapter 12). However, the amino acid sequences that determine the movement of the Fc receptor have not been elucidated.

Transfer of maternal IgG in the neonatal rodent falls markedly at weaning (after 21 days of age, a phenomenon known as closure). This is now known to be caused by the decrease in expression of the Fc receptor gene (Simister and Mostov, 1989). Thus factors in breast milk may affect Fc receptor gene expression. The Fc receptor has been detected in humans (Mikulska *et al.*, 2000; Yoshida *et al.*, 2004). It is present in the placenta and transfers maternal immunoglobulin *in utero* during the later stages of gestation. Israel *et al.* (1993) have shown that the Fc receptor may be present on small intestinal epithelium in the first trimester and may possibly function early in the transfer of maternal IgG from amniotic fluid to the fetus. As alluded to previously above, this receptor is expressed on adult epithelium *(in vivo)* and may play a role in the transport of IgG or IgG immune complexes from the lumen to the lamina propria.

The mechanisms involved in the transit of membrane-bound ligands to the basolateral pole of the enterocyte are still poorly understood. In electron microscopic studies, the apical membrane of absorptive cells can be seen invaginating to form endosomes (Fig. 1.2). On the inner aspect of these developing membrane compartments, there appear to be regular arrays of clathrin (Knutton *et al.*, 1974; Gonnella and Neutra, 1984; Shibata *et al.*, 1983), a protein designed to form lattices around membrane vesicles. It has a central role in the budding and fusion of membrane vesicles (Brodsky, 1984). In particular, clathrin assembly at the surface membrane of cells promotes the endocytosis of external receptors (Steinman *et al.*, 1983).

Further transit into the cell may occur by the movement of separated vesicles (Fig. 1.2). Hopkins *et al.* (1990) have challenged this concept and favor a single transport compartment called the endosomal reticulum that extends from the cell surface. The shape and movement of these intracellular compartments will depend on the structural proteins that make up the cytoskeleton of the cell.

Cells specialized for macromolecular transport (M cells)

Generation of secretory immune responses by the intestinal mucosa depends on transfer of antigens across the epithelium. Any loss of the molecular structure of the antibody recognition sites, the epitopes, during transport would render them unrecognizable by B cells. The passage of intact macromolecules across the gut is at variance with the role of the gut as a macromolecular barrier. For macromolecules to cross the gut in a controlled manner, specialized epithelial cells have evolved that overlie lymphoid follicles (Bockman and Cooper, 1973; Owen, 1977). These M cells, discussed in detail in Chapter 7, have features that facilitate controlled entry of antigens and larger particles through the intestinal epithelium. Recent data have shed light on the development of these cells. Elegant studies by Kerneis *et al.* (1997) defined the differentiation of normal absorptive epithelium into M cells by the presence of subepithelial Peyer's patch (PP) lymphocytes. This was shown to be dependent upon cell contact (migration into the overlying epithelium) and in fact was found to depend upon the presence of B cells in the epithelial monolayer. Notch, expressed by B cells, interacts with its ligand on epithelial cells (Sander and Powell, 2004), triggering their differentiation into M cells. In support of this concept, mice deficient in B cells (e.g., μ heavy chain knock-out mice) are deficient in PPs and lack M cells (Golovkina *et al.*, 1999).

More recently non-PP lymphoid follicles have been reported to exist in the distal small intestine (Lorenz *et al.*, 2003) and cells sharing phenotypic similarity to M cells have been reported to overlie these structures. Whether they function in a manner comparable to M cells has not been reported.

Enterocytes as antigen-presenting cells

Effective immune responses to antigenic proteins require the help of T lymphocytes. Stimulation of T cells in turn depends on exogenous antigen being presented by antigen-presenting cells (APCs) (Unanue, 1984). The APC must internalize, digest, and link a small fragment of the antigen to a surface glycoprotein (the major histocompatibility complex class II or HLA-D in humans) that interacts with a T-cell receptor (TCR). A number of cells of the immune system can act as APC, including B cells, macrophages, and dendritic cells. The ability of these cells to present antigen depends on the expression of class II MHC on their surface (Unanue, 1984). Class II MHC are also present in epithelia of the normal small intestine, particularly on villous cells, of the small intestine in both humans (Wiman *et al.*, 1978) and rodents (Kirby and Parr, 1979; Mason *et al.*, 1981). *In vitro* studies (Bland and Warren, 1986; Mayer and Shlien, 1987; Kaiserlian *et al.*, 1989) have demonstrated that isolated enterocytes from rat and human small intestine can present antigens to appropriately primed T cells (Chapter 25). This raises the possibility that in the intestine class II MHC might present peptides from cellular membrane compartments to cells of the immune system that are localized below the epithelium. In support of this concept, class II MHC molecules have been detected in adult rat jejunum villi in association with intracellular organelles (Mayrhofer and Spargo, 1990). Class II molecules were never detected in the microvillus brush border or vesicles at the base of microvilli. However, organelles below the terminal web and throughout the apical cytoplasm were stained specifically. Basolateral membranes clearly showed class II MHC molecules. These molecules are therefore in an ideal position for binding with polypeptides that may have been taken up and processed within the epithelial cell **(Fig. 1.3)**. Interestingly, the expression of class II MHC in the gastrointestinal epithelium is increased in a number of

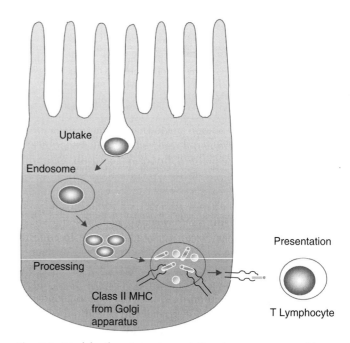

Fig. 1.3. Model of antigen presentation by enterocytes. Macromolecules can enter the membrane-bound organelle of the enterocyte. Instead of binding to the surrounding membrane or being destroyed in lysosomes, antigen is processed within the endosomal component into fragments that can bind to class II MHC on the inner membrane of the components. From there they are presented on the basolateral surface of the cell. (Drawing prepared with the help of Dr. L. Mayer.) Reprinted with permission from Sanderson and Walker (1993).

diseases. In Crohn's disease (Selby *et al.*, 1983; Mayer *et al.*, 1991), there is enhanced expression on enterocytes from inflamed areas. Moreover, the effect of enterocytes from inflamed tissue is to stimulate helper T lymphocytes (Mayer and Eisenhardt, 1990). Increased expression of class II MHC is also evident in the small intestine in patients with autoimmune enteropathy (Hill *et al.*, 1991) and in graft-versus-host disease (Mason *et al.*, 1981). Certain gastrointestinal infections increase class II MHC expression, for example, in the stomach infected with *Helicobacter pylori* (Engstrand *et al.*, 1989) and in the intestine infested with nematode parasites (Masson and Perdue, 1990).

If class II MHC molecules transport peptides derived from luminal macromolecules, then these diseases will lead to an increase in the presentation of these peptides to the gastrointestinal immune systems. This may cause further inflammation and further presentation of luminal antigens, leading to a vicious cycle. Some drugs used to treat inflammatory bowel disease reduce class II expression in epithelial cells. The drug 5-ASA, for example, reduces the class II MHC expression that occurs in cultured cells expressing class II MHC in response to interferon-γ (Crotty *et al.*, 1992). T-cell activation depends not only on presentation of antigen by class II MHC but also on the attachment of separate surface molecules to molecules on the APC. The molecules on the surface of APC include intercellular adhesion molecule 1 (ICAM-1) [which binds to leukocyte function–associated antigen 1 (LFA-l)] on the T cell and the costimulatory molecules B7-l (CD80) and B7-2 (CD86) which both bind to CD28 and CTLA-4 (Freeman *et al.*, 1989, 1991, 1993; Linsley *et al.*, 1991; Azuma *et al.*, 1993; Hathcock *et al.*, 1993). A functional distinction probably exists between the ICAM-1/LFA-1 bond and the other two bonds (Liu *et al.*, 1992). ICAM-1 is thought to provide support for the weak (Matsui *et al.*, 1991) class II MHC/TCR bond, whereas CD80/CD86 transmit specific stimulatory signals through their ligands to T cells (Damle *et al.*, 1992). Lack of binding by CD80/CD86 to CD28 may result in T-cell tolerance (Schwartz *et al.*, 1990) because blocking of CD28 during antigen presentation leads to clonal anergy in T cells (Harding *et al.*, 1992) with absence of T-cell proliferation and interleukin-2 (lL-2) production.

Cells of the small intestinal epithelium do not express CD80 **(Fig. 1.4)** (Bloom *et al.*, 1995). It is tempting to speculate that epithelial cell antigen presentation may therefore downregulate primary T-cell responses under normal circumstances. Under these circumstances, the epithelial cell's role as a barrier to antigen absorption would not only be passive. The epithelium could actively inhibit the immune responses initiated by the passage of antigen that has leaked through to professional APC in the lamina propria (which do express costimulatory molecules). In disease states, however, such an inhibition of T cell activation may be inappropriate. *H. pylori* induces expression of costimulatory molecules on gastric epithelium (Ye *et al.*, 1997), and CD86 is expressed by epithelial cells isolated from patients with ulcerative colitis (Nakazawa *et al.*, 1999). It is important to note however that the majority of lymphocytes in the lamina propria are memory cells. Such cells are less dependent upon co-stimulatory signals.

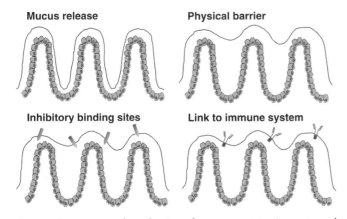

Fig. 1.4. Four proposed mechanisms for mucus protection; rate and quantity of mucus release, viscous blanket (physical barrier), competitive binding sites, and link to the intestinal immune system. Reprinted with permission from Snyder and Walker (1987).

BARRIERS PREVENTING PATHOLOGIC TRANSPORT

Physiologic passage of macromolecules is essential for the development of immune responses by the intestine; uncontrolled penetration of antigens, however, could initiate pathologic processes that lead to gastrointestinal disease states. For antigen transport to be controlled, nonspecific entry into the circulation must be limited. This is done in two ways: first, by restricting the amount of antigen reaching the surface of the intestine (extrinsic barrier) and second, by the physical characteristics of the intestine itself (intrinsic barrier) (Fig. 1.1).

Many barrier mechanisms are not fully developed at birth, and there is good evidence that antigen transport in the neonatal period is less restricted than in adults. In animals the changes in antigen absorption from newborn to adult are particularly evident (closure). Initially, the phenomenon was applied to the transport of immunoglobulins (Brambell, 1966), but significant changes in absorption have been documented for antigens that do not have specific transport receptors. Radiolabeled bovine serum albumin (BSA) (Udall *et al.*, 1981b) was fed in physiologic amounts to rabbits at birth, 1 week, 2 weeks, 6 weeks, and 1 year of age, and the plasma radioactivity was measured. The study was designed to ensure that the radioactivity measured corresponded to protein absorption. From 1 week of age, there was a marked fall in the transport of BSA across the intestine. Moreover, in a later study (Udall *et al.*, 1981a), it was found that the development of the mucosal barrier depended on the type of feeding during the neonatal period. Naturally breast-fed rabbits had lower plasma BSA levels than did formula-fed rabbits, suggesting that breast milk affects the development of the mucosal barrier. This chapter reviews how different components of the barrier develop, particularly as a fall in antigen absorption has been demonstrated in humans also. Milk proteins penetrate more readily in infancy than in adults. In one study α-lactalbumin absorption decreased with age (Axelsson *et al.*, 1989). In a second study, formula-fed neonates had greater levels of β-lactoglobulin than older infants (Roberton *et al.*, 1982).

Extrinsic barrier
Proteolysis and gastrointestinal acidity
There are many ways by which antigen access to the epithelium will be limited (Fig. 1.1). Proteolysis will destroy the structure of antigens and thus destroy epitopes for immunologic recognition. Altering the proteolytic capacity of the gastrointestinal tract affects macromolecular uptake. In everted gut sacs (Walker *et al.*, 1975) taken from rats who had previously undergone ligation of the pancreatic duct, transport of horseradish peroxidase (HRP) was greater than in sacs made in sham-operated animals. Furthermore prior feeding of pancreatic extract decreased the uptake of HRP. The effects of digestion on macromolecular uptake have been elegantly confirmed by feeding rats aprotinin (a trypsin inhibitor) together with lysine vasopressin (Saffron *et al.*, 1979). This

peptide hormone is absorbed through the intestine in sufficient quantities to have a noticeable affect on fluid retention when fed orally. When given together with aprotinin, however, the effects of vasopressin are more marked, implying that more has reached the surface of the intestine because of reduced proteolysis.

Neutralizing gastric acidity (which reduces the activity of gastric enzymes) also increases antigen transport. When oral feeds of sodium bicarbonate were given to rats at the same time as BSA, increased BSA was found in the gut (Walker *et al.*, 1975). These findings have important consequences because deficiencies of pancreatic enzymes occur in various diseases. Patients with cystic fibrosis, in which pancreatic activity is severely affected, have an increased incidence of cow's milk allergy, presumably because of increased antigen uptake. Also, gastric acidity (Hyman *et al.*, 1985) and pancreatic activity (Lebenthal and Lee, 1982) may be less in the newborn, and this may have consequences on the development of the mucosal barrier.

In addition to the acid secreted into the stomach, the epithelial cells of the IEC create an acid microclimate. Mucus and the outer glycocalyx of the intestinal epithelium are composed of negatively charged carbohydrate side chains. This negative charge reduces the diffusibility of hydrogen ions within the surface layer of the cell. Any pH at the apical surface of the epithelium will therefore be maintained in the region. Studies on the absorption of salicylic acid (Lucas, 1984), a weak electrolyte, indicated that its uptake was much greater than expected when the bulk phase of the intestine was alkaline. In fact, the absorption of salicylate in experiments was equivalent to that expected had the bulk phase been at a pH of 2 lower than in fact it was. Absorption of weak bases was altered in the opposite direction to weak acids in rat small intestine (Winne, 1977). In a relationship of absorption against pH, the uptake of a weak electrolyte should be at 50% of its maximum when the pH of the absorptive surface is equal to the electrolyte's pK. These data resulted in the proposal that the microclimate of the small intestinal surface is acidic. Direct experiments measuring the pH of the surface with microelectrodes have confirmed this prediction in both human and rodents (Rechkemmer *et al.*, 1986; Lucas, 1983; Daniel *et al.*, 1985; Rechkemmer, 1992).

The microclimate changes during ontogeny. In the suckling rat the microclimate is even more acidic than that of the adult. Weak acids (such as short-chain fatty acids) will be particularly well absorbed under these conditions. Said *et al.* (1987) showed not only that age differences resulted in differences in the acid microclimate but also that the microclimate was maintained by mucus. The addition of a mucolytic agent (*N*-acetyl cysteine) reduced the acidity of the apical surface.

Although mucus impedes the free diffusion of hydrogen ions into the bulk phase, it does not generate acidity. Hydrogen ions are secreted by the epithelial cells in exchange for sodium ions by a Na^+/H^+ antiporter in the intestinal apical membrane. Sodium passes readily into epithelial cells down its concentration gradient, causing

hydrogen ions to be pumped into the apical space, where they are trapped by the negatively charged mucopolysaccharide side chains, as discussed previously. Removal of sodium from the bulk phase causes a reduction in the microclimate (Shimada, 1987). An investigation of how the microclimate might alter the uptake of antigens or invading organisms has never been undertaken. However, the acidity has a marked effect on the absorption of smaller molecules. For weak electrolytes (such as short-chain fatty acids), sodium removal would indirectly alter absorption by increasing the pH, which maintains the weak acid in its more soluble form. The acid microclimate has a direct effect on transport of dipeptides (Lister *et al.*, 1995), which, unlike amino acids, are transported into the cell in association with hydrogen ions. Based on the work in rodents (Said *et al.*, 1987), it appears that neonates would produce a microclimate sufficient for these absorptive functions. However, little is known about the microclimate in the preterm neonate, and this remains an interesting area for further study.

Peristalsis

The time available for absorption will depend on the speed of luminal contents down the bowel. It is a common experience in clinical gastroenterology that uptake of nutrients in patients with limited absorptive capacity (such as short bowel syndrome) is improved by reduced intestinal motility with agents such as loperamide (Remington *et al.*, 1983). There is good reason to believe that antigen absorption will also be limited by peristaltic action. An association between motility and antigen absorption has important implications. First, motility patterns change with development (Bisset *et al.*, 1986; Milla 1996), and this may contribute to alterations in antigen uptake with age. Second, gastrointestinal disease can affect the motility of the intestine (Mayer *et al.*, 1988) and may result in changes in antigen absorption, although such changes may be small relative to the effect that a disease has on the physical barrier created by the intestine itself. Nevertheless, antibody-antigen complex formation in the mucus coat, coupled with peristalsis, causes rapid expulsion of antigens from the small intestine (Snyder and Walker, 1987).

Mucus coat

Structure. The mucus coat lining the intestine is composed of a solution of glycoproteins (mucin) of molecular weights ranging from one to several million daltons (Chapter 4). Intestinal mucin molecules are made up of carbohydrate side chains (70% to 80%) bound to a protein skeleton. This protein core has a high proportion of serine, threonine, and proline residues (Allan, 1981; Forstner, 1978), and the carbohydrate moieties are attached to it by means of *N*-acetyl galactosamine. Five carbohydrates moieties (*N*-acetyl galactosamine, *N*-acetyl glucosamine, fucose, galactose, and sialic acid) are arranged in side chains of 2 to 22 sugars in length. The exact composition of the molecules of mucin can vary greatly. There are clear differences between animal species. Even within localized regions of the intestinal tract, mucus molecules appear to be a heterogeneous group. At least six different mucin species have been identified following separation on diethylaminoethyl-cellulose chromatography in both rats and humans (Podolsky, 1985). Each species had distinct carbohydrate and amino acid composition. Marked changes in the composition of mucin occur with development. The mucin from the small intestine of newborn rats contains more protein than does adult rat mucin (Shub *et al.*, 1983). The carbohydrate content also changes as the animals grow. Not only does the total carbohydrate ratio increase with age, but the types of sugar moieties change also: newborn rat mucin has less fucose and *N*-acetyl galactosamine than does mucin from adult rats.

Function. Viscous coat. There are a number of ways by which mucus offers protection to the intestinal wall (Fig. 1.4). First, it provides a mucus blanket. The physical characteristics of this blanket are determined by the chemical structure of the glycoprotein molecules themselves. The sticky quality of the mucus is an important mechanism for preventing penetration of organisms. The motility of *Entamoeba histolytica* trophozoites (Leitch *et al.*, 1985), for example, is significantly decreased by mucus. The increased viscosity that mucus provides to the luminal solution will enhance the depth of the unstirred layer overlying the surface of the intestine. This will reduce the diffusion of molecules toward the intestinal surface (Strocchi and Levitt, 1991). The effect will be most marked for larger molecules, and this will limit absorption of antigens rather than nutrient molecules, which are smaller.

Competitive binding
The carbohydrate moieties that make up most of the mucus structure are analogous to the glycoprotein and glycolipid receptors that exist on the enterocyte membrane (Gibbons, 1981). They could therefore act as competitors to the binding of proteins and microorganisms at the enterocyte surface. Many infectious agents adhere to epithelial cells through cell surface molecules (fimbria, pili, and flagella) (Freter, 1981; Chapter 3), which have carbohydrate-binding properties. Indeed, competition between salivary mucus glycoproteins and receptors on buccal epithelium has already been shown for binding of pathogenic streptococci (Williams and Gibbons, 1975). Furthermore, it is possible that the invasiveness of *Shigella flexneri* in primates depends in part on the lack of barrier function of mucus (Denari *et al.*, 1986). Guinea pig colonic mucus inhibits invasion of HeLa cells by *Shigella*, whereas monkey colonic mucus (and by implication, human mucus) does not.

Mucin release
Release of mucus into the gastrointestinal tract will act as a barrier by generating a stream that draws luminal contents away from epithelial cells. Both nonspecific and immunologic agents can initiate mucus release. The role of nonimmunologic agents and their relationship to endogenous agents that alter mucus secretion is not well understood (Snyder and Walker, 1987). Cholinergic agents (Specian and Neutra, 1980) and mustard oil (Neutra *et al.*, 1982) cause goblet cell release, but a number of regulatory peptides (including histamine, serotonin, and α-adrenergic and β-adrenergic agents) have no effect. Nevertheless, immunologic phenomena cause goblet cells to release mucus (see the following text).

Immunologic barrier
The adequacy of immune function in the gastrointestinal tract affects the attachment and penetration of bacteria and toxins (Chapter 3). This has been elegantly shown (Winner *et al.*, 1991) by implantation of IgA-secreting hybridomas under the skin of infant mice, who are then inoculated with cholera. IgA appears in large amounts in the small intestine as S-IgA (see Chapter 14). When the hybridomas are implanted that secrete IgA interacting with the antigen on the surface of *Vibrio cholerae*, mortality from cholera is dramatically reduced (Winner *et al.*, 1991).

It is also likely that IgA prevents the transfer of antigens across the gut. This hypothesis is supported by studies of patients with selective IgA deficiency. These patients have increased circulating immune complexes and precipitating antibodies to absorbed bovine milk proteins (Cunningham-Rundles *et al.*, 1978), with peak concentrations occurring between 1 and 2 hours after milk ingestion (Cunningham-Rundles *et al.*, 1979).

Innate immunity encompasses appropriate defense responses that are not adaptive (Medzhitov and Janeway, 1997). This definition excludes the involvement of lymphocytes but includes other cell types that respond to molecular patterns. This concept is well developed in macrophages, but enterocytes also recognize specific patterns, especially those derived from bacteria. For example, chemotactic cytokines are released from epithelial cells following invasion by *Salmonella* (Eckmann *et al.*, 1993) or attachment of *H. pylori* (Crowe *et al.*, 1995). In addition, the metabolite of resident bacteria (butyrate) enhances chemokine secretion by epithelial cells stimulated by proinflammatory agents. Innate immunity has an older phylogeny than adaptive immunity. The epithelial cell's early evolution, compared with the lymphocyte's, is consistent with its role in innate immunity. More recently several groups have defined the presence of pattern recognition receptors (PRRs) recognizing moieties expressing common molecular patterns (pathogen-associated molecular patterns or PAMPs) by microorganisms on epithelial cells (Cario *et al.*, 2000). These PRRs or toll-like receptors (TLRs) recognize distinct bacterial or viral products and trigger an inflammatory response. Although they were originally defined on classical APCs, their presence on epithelial cells raises questions regarding the ability of the absorptive epithelium to sense luminal pathogens. Ligation of TLRs on classical APCs results in the activation of nuclear factor kappa B (NFκB), an event that would be poorly tolerated in the gut. Epithelial cells however fail to express many of the associated molecules required for optimal signaling through the TLR (e.g., MD2, CD14), and this observation may account for the nonresponsiveness of the epithelium to bacterial products such as LPS (Abreu *et al.*, 2001, 2003).

Interestingly, intracellular PRRs exist as well. NOD2 recognizes muramyl dipeptide (a component of peptidoglycan) and is expressed by monocytes and epithelium (Ogura *et al.*, 2001). Mutations in NOD2 occur in a subpopulation of patients with Crohn's disease (Ogura *et al.*, 2001; Hugot *et al.*, 2001). Such defects might account for the failure of intestinal epithelium to clear intracellular bacteria (Bonen *et al.*, 2003).

Combined effects of immunologic and nonimmunologic barriers

Both oral and parenteral immunization with specific antigens can reduce their uptake by the intestine (Walker *et al.*, 1972, 1973). These observations may well be a combined effect of immunologic and nonimmunologic components of the mucosal barrier. Proteolysis of intestinal antigens was considerably greater in immunized animal than in nonimmunized controls (Walker *et al.*, 1975). It is likely that this enhanced proteolysis is the result of interaction of immune complexes in the mucus coat. This augmented protective process is illustrated in **Figure 1.5.**

Another example of combined protection is the increased discharge of goblet cell mucus occurring in intestinal anaphylaxis. Lake and colleagues (1980) have shown, using radiolabeled goblet cell mucus to quantitate release, that IgE-mediated mast cell discharge of histamine results in enhanced mucus release into the intestinal tract. This may explain why parasites are eventually expelled from the intestine, together with mucus (Miller and Nawa, 1979). Figure 1.2 illustrates possible mechanisms of immune complex-mediated goblet cell mucus release on the intestinal surface.

Yang *et al.* (2000) defined another function for luminal IgE. She showed that normal epithelial cells express the low affinity Fc receptor for IgE (CD23) and that this molecule transports IgE immune complexes rapidly across the epithelium resulting in the activation of mucosal mast cells and consequent chloride secretion by epithelial cells.

Intrinsic barrier
Once antigens have negotiated the many components of the extrinsic barrier mechanism, there is a considerable physical barrier to further penetration. This barrier results from the surfaces of the enterocytes and the tight junctions formed among them. However, this barrier is not impervious to the passage of antigens, as was once thought. The integrity of this barrier is often reduced in diseases of the gastrointestinal tract.

Microvillous structure
Microvilli could constitute a significant barrier because of their size and charge. In the intestinal epithelium of children (Phillips *et al.*, 1979), there are 40 microvilli of 100-nm diameter every 5 μm. Thus, if microvilli beat in unison, the distance between them is only 25 nm, which is the same order of magnitude as the same macromolecules—the dimensions of albumin, for example, are 3 × 13 nm. Microvilli are also negatively charged and therefore stain easily with ruthenium red (Jacobs, 1983); thus a charged molecule may be significantly inhibited even if its diameter is well below 25 nm.

The site of invagination of apical plasma membrane has been demonstrated to be between microvilli (Knutton *et al.*,

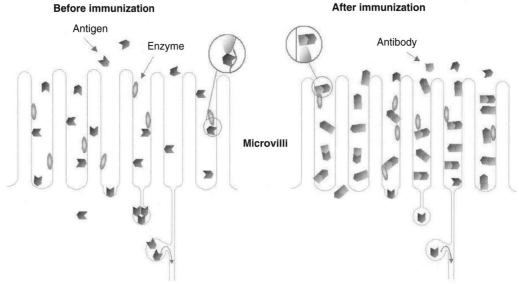

Before immunization   **After immunization**

Antigen   Enzyme   Antibody

Microvilli

Fig. 1.5. Schematic representation of the processing of protein antigen at the surface of the gut. Prior to immunization, a small portion of ingested protein escapes intraluminal digestion and is taken up by the enterocyte and transported to the intercellular spaces. After immunization, antibodies present on the gut surface interact with antigen to form complexes, thereby preventing or decreasing the binding of antigen to, and subsequent pinocytosis of antigen by, intestinal epithelial cells. Antigens complexed with antibodies in the mucus coat (glycocalyx) may be degraded by pancreatic enzymes absorbed by the gut surface; consequently, there is less antigen available by intestinal epithelial cells. Reprinted with permission from Walker *et al.* (1975).

1974; Gonnella and Neutra, 1984; Shibata *et al.*, 1983). Thus it is likely that antigens have to pass the microvillus "barrier" to enter the cell. This has direct relevance to disease processes, for any agent that strips of microvilli or affects their formation will alter the barrier function of the intestine. The microvillus structure is greatly altered by infections of cryptosporidia or enteropathogenic *Escherichia coli* (Ulshen and Rollo, 1980).

Further support for the concept of a microvillous barrier comes from morphologic studies of M cells. The function of these cells is macromolecular transport. Unlike absorptive cells, they do not have well-developed microvilli. As every morphologic feature of these cells is in keeping with their function, this would suggest that microvilli do constitute a significant barrier.

Enterocyte surface membrane. At the base of the microvilli, the surface of the enterocyte consists of plasma membrane. As in other cells, this is composed of a lipid bilayer in which membrane-bound proteins are situated. This bilayer presents a considerable barrier to antigen transport because of its physical structure. In fact it is highly unlikely that antigens can cross this lipid bilayer into the enterocyte cytosol. However, invagination of apical membranes occurs regularly, allowing macromolecules to be carried into the cell within membrane-bound compartments (Fig. 1.2). Indeed, a large number of compartments exist beneath the apical surface of the enterocyte into which antigens can be transferred. Some of this activity is physiologic and has been described in an earlier section; however, bystander molecules can be carried into the cell by this process. This was clearly demonstrated in electron micrographs, which showed HRP inside membrane-bound compartments (Cornell *et al.*, 1971). Stern and Walker (1984) have shown that binding to the surface of the enterocyte is an important determinant as to whether macromolecules are transported across the cell. For both BSA and β-lactoglobulin, absorption was nonsaturable and correlated with binding to the intestinal surface. Membrane-bound macromolecular transport can be distinguished from molecules moving freely in the lumen of compartments of the enterocyte (Gonnella and Neutra, 1984) in newborn rat ileum.

Binding to the surface of the cell depends on the structure of the antigen and the chemical composition of the microvillous membrane. Both these factors can vary. The structure of the antigen depends on the actual antigen itself. BSA binds less efficiently to the surface of the intestine than β-lactoglobulin and in consequence is transported less readily (Stern and Walker, 1984). In addition, structural alterations in antigen caused by proteolysis might also affect its binding, as this will change the physicochemical characteristics of the molecule. For example, the gliadin fraction B3 (Stern *et al.*, 1988) binds less well to microvillous membrane protein than the pure gliadin peptide B3142.

Intracellular organelles and enzymes
Antigens that enter enterocytes from the lumen are affected by a number of different factors that will influence transport

to the basolateral surface. Of primary importance is the rate of vesicular passage to the basolateral membrane. This will depend on the rate of endocytosis, the proportion of vesicles being divided toward the lysosome, and the speed of travel of membrane-bound compartments. The rate of breakdown of products held in membrane compartments is determined by lysosomally derived enzymes. These include proteases such as cathepsin B and D and those that catalyze carbohydrate breakdown such as acid phosphatase and mannosidase. It is the degree to which the organellar contents encounter such enzymes that determines the rate of intracellular destruction of macromolecules. This encounter can be in the lysosome or in endocytic vesicles (Dinsdale and Healy, 1982). We know that such enzymes are present in IEC and at levels of activity that can influence macromolecular transport. In the rat (Davies and Messer, 1984), cathepsin B and D activity can be found throughout the length of the intestine, particularly in the middle and distal thirds. Interestingly, this activity peaks in the second week of age and then progressively falls. The ontogeny of macromolecular transport (Udall *et al.*, 1981b) in no way reflects this pattern, emphasizing that it is the importance of interaction between membrane-bound compartment flow and enzyme activity that is of prime importance. This is more clearly seen in the piglet, in which intestinal cathepsin B and D levels do not alter with age (Ekstrom and Westrom, 1991), yet closure can be clearly demonstrated in the same animals in the second day of life.

Although cathepsins are capable of destroying macromolecular biological activity, they may not completely digest the protein molecule, and the final steps in digestion of peptides may be by peptidases (Vaeth and Henning, 1982) in the cytoplasm.

Junctions between cells
The physical barrier that prevents penetration of antigen across the intestinal epithelium consists of two main components: the epithelial cells (the transcellular route) and the spaces between cells (the paracellular route). The pathophysiology of this latter pathway has been well reviewed (Madara, 1989, 1990a, b; Gumbiner, 1987; Powell, 1981). The pathway consists of the tight junctions (or zonulae occludens) and the subjunctional space.

The subjunctional space is not a significant barrier as molecules as large as HRP can diffuse freely between the serosa and this space. However, the tight junctions (TJs) offer a substantial barrier to diffusion of large molecules, although it is permeable to water and small ions (Frizzell and Schultz, 1972). Claude and Goodenough (1973) demonstrated a correlation between the structure of the TJs as seen in freeze fracture preparations and passive electrical permeability in a number of epithelial preparations. The preparations, when viewed under the electron microscope, show a network of characteristic anastomosing strands. The composition of these strands is under investigation, but it is likely that they are proteins of high tensile strength. In tight epithelia (such as the gallbladder), there are many such strands, whereas in more permeable epithelia (such as mammalian proximal small intestine), there are few. The relationship between density and epithelial resistance has been confirmed in IEC (Madara and Dharmasathaphorn, 1985). T84 cells grow as confluent monolayers in culture. In the first 10 days after passage, the junctions become increasingly tight, as judged by transepithelial resistance. This resistance was found to correlate with the number of strands formed between cells.

The barrier formed by the TJs is preserved even when epithelial cells themselves are extruded at the villous tip. The band from the tight junction moves away from the apex down the lateral aspect of the cell as the cell is extruded (Madara, 1990b). Eventually younger cells beneath the extruding cell form TJs at the very moment that the old cell is lost. Thus preservation of a TJ network is a function whose importance overrides that of epithelial cell viability.

Cell-cell adhesion depends on a family of molecules, the cadherins, which bind either to catenins or to plakoglobin, which in turn binds to catenins (Hinck *et al.*, 1994; Nathke *et al.*, 1994). These interactions not only preserve the epithelial cell barrier but also prevent epithelial cells from breaking away from their monolayers, as is seen in intestinal neoplasia. Interestingly, suppressing the normally expressed E-cadherin in the epithelia with a dominant-negative N-cadherin (NCAD) disrupts cell-cell interactions (Hermiston and Gordon, 1995a). Transgenic mice, in which distinct areas of the intestinal epithelium expressed NCAD, exhibited changes in the lamina propria only in those areas that expressed the NCAD gene (Hermiston and Gordon, 1995b). The changes in the lamina propria included infiltration with lymphocytes and histiocytes, IgA- or IgG-secreting plasma cells, and increased expression of class II MHC. By 3 months of age, crypt distortion and crypt abscesses appeared. Chimeras expressing NCAD along the entire crypt-villous axis had greater disease than those with NCAD expression confined to the villous epithelium. This animal model exemplifies the importance of the epithelial barrier in the prevention of inflammatory bowel disease.

The TJ is a dynamic structure whose resistance varies with events taking place in the epithelium and intestinal lumen. Changes in paracellular absorption occur during active transport of nutrients by epithelial cells, particularly in relation to smaller molecules. Pappenheimer and colleagues (Pappenheimer and Reiss, 1987; Pappenheimer, 1987; Madara and Pappenheimer, 1987) have calculated that the rate of uptake from the lumen of molecules smaller than 5500 Da was proportional to the rate of fluid absorption, a concept known as solvent drag. The application of an alternating current across isolated intestine, with and without mucosa, gave an estimate of the impedance of the intestinal mucosa. The impedance falls with the stimulation of sodium-coupled solute transport across the enterocyte. It is, therefore, possible that sodium-coupled solute transport triggers contraction of cytoskeletal elements of the enterocyte, which in turn pull open TJ. These predictions have been confirmed by electron microscopy (Madara and Pappenheimer, 1987). Sodium-dependent solutes such as

glucose and amino acids induce expansion of intercellular spaces associated with condensation of microfilaments of the actin-myosin ring associated with the TJ. Although these observations have enormous importance for the physiology of absorption of nutrients, their impact on our understanding of macromolecular transport has yet to be fully assessed. The calculated pore radius of the open TJ (5 nm) is similar to that of small macromolecules: glucose/sodium transport will in fact allow the passage of a polypeptide 11 amino acids long (MP-l) (Atisook and Madara, 1991), but larger immunogenic proteins may not pass through this route under physiologic conditions. HRP, for example, does not pass TJ (Atisook and Madara, 1991) even when it has been rendered permeable to MP-l.

On the other hand, *pathologic* insults to the intestine may open these pores sufficiently to allow passage of antigens. The macromolecular permeability of the gut in disease models needs to be reexamined using Pappenheimer's methodology. Macromolecular markers of different sizes, change, and hydrophilicity have all been used independently *in vivo* in both animals and humans, but the physical characteristics of these molecules have not been used to predict pore size in disease. An important model of increased permeability caused by intestinal inflammation is the effect of mast cell–dependent reactions in the rat intestine following *Nippostrongylus brasiliensis* infection. Increased amounts of BSA can be detected immunologically in the circulation following infection with the organism after mild systemic anaphylaxis (Bloch *et al.*, 1979). Similarly, transfer of ^{51}Cr-labeled ethylenediamine tetraacetic acid (EDTA) and ovalbumin is enhanced (Ramage *et al.*, 1988). It should be possible to make an estimate of the physical characteristics of the paracellular pathway during inflammation.

The permeability of the TJ can be examined *in vitro*. This enables workers to study the effects of epithelial events that are seen *in vivo*. Monolayers of epithelial cells (T84) have effective TJs, producing a resistance of around 1500 Ω/cm^2. Application of interferon-γ (Madara and Stafford, 1989) reduces the resistance and allows easier permeation of large sugars; Interferon-γ levels are increased in the mucosa of patients with Crohn's disease because of T-cell activation (Chapter 71). Bowel inflammation is characterized by the transepithelial passage of polymorphonuclear neutrophils (PMN). This phenomenon has been produced *in vitro* by putting chemotactic agents and PMN on different sides of the monolayer (Nash *et al.*, 1987). The passage of neutrophils opens TJs, reducing monolayer resistance and allowing transfer of large sugars.

CONCLUSIONS

The mucosal barrier, like the skin, defines the boundary between the host and its environment. Unlike the skin, the mucosae of the gut and respiratory tract must absorb substances that are essential for life. To be selective, the intestinal mucosa has developed a complex network composed of elements that are extrinsic to the intestine itself, as well as those defined by intestinal structure.

The challenges for the future lie in defining the role of this barrier in the establishment of gastrointestinal disease. It will also be interesting to examine whether cellular elements in the mucosal immune system can recognize antigens without their needing to penetrate the intestinal epithelium. The observations that members of the immunoglobulin super-family are found on the surface of the epithelium and that lymphocytes can pass into the intestinal lumen make this a tantalizing possibility.

REFERENCES

Abrahamson, D.R. and Rodewald, R. (1981). Evidence for the sorting of endocytic vesicle contents during the receptor-mediated transport of 19G across the newborn rat intestine. *J. Cell. Biol.* 91, 270–280.

Abreu, M.T., Vora, P., Faure, E., Thomas, L.S., Arnold, E.T., and Arditi, M. (2001). Decreased expression of Toll-like receptor-4 and MD-2 correlates with intestinal epithelial cell protection against dysregulated proinflammatory gene expression in response to bacterial lipopolysaccharide. *J. Immunol.* 167, 1609–1616.

Abreu, M.T., Thomas, L.S., Arnold, E.T., Lukasek, K., Michelsen, K.S., and Arditi, M. (2003). TLR signaling at the intestinal epithelial interface. *J. Endotoxin Res.* 9, 322–330.

Allan, A. (1981). Structure and function of gastrointestinal mucus. In *Physiology of the Gastrointestinal Tract*, vol. 7, pp. 617–639, Raven, New York.

Atisook, K. and Madara, J.L. (1991). An oligopeptide permeates intestinal tight junctions at glucose-elicited dilatations. Implication for oligopeptide absorption. *Gastroenterology* 100, 719–724.

Axelsson, L., Jakobsson, L., Lindberg, T., Poleberger, S., Benediktsson, B., and Raiha N. (1989). Macromolecular absorption in preterm and term infants. *Acta Paediatr. Scand.* 78, 532–537.

Azuma, M., lto, D., Yagita, H., Okumura, K., Phillips, J.H., Lanier, L.L., and Somoza, C. (1993). B70 antigen is a second ligand for CTLA-4 and CD28. *Nature* 366, 76–79.

Beach, R.C., Menzies, I.S., Clayden, G.S., and Scopes, J.W. (1982). Gastrointestinal permeability changes in the preterm neonate. *Arch. Dis. Child.* 57, 141–145.

Bissett, W.M., Watt, J.B., Rivers, R.P.A., and Milla, P.J. (1986). The ontogeny of small intestinal motor activity. *Pediatr. Res.* 20, 692.

Bitonti, A.J., Dumont, J.A., Low, S.C., Peters, R.T., Kropp, K.E., Palmobella, V.J., Stattel, J.M., Lu, Y., Tan, C.A., Song, J.J., Garcia, A.M., Simister, N.E., Spiekermann, G.M., Lencer, W.I., and Blumberg, R.S. (2004). Pulmonary delivery of an erythropoietin Fc fusion protein in nonhuman primates through an immunoglobulin transport pathway. *Proc. Natl. Acad. Sci. USA* 101, 9763–9768.

Bland, P.W. and Warren L.G. (1986). Antigen presentation by epithelial cells of the rat small intestine. I. Kinetics, antigen specificity and blocking by anti-Ia antisera. *Immunology* 58, 1–8.

Bloch, K.J., Bloch, D.B., Stems, M., and Walker, W.A. (1979). Intestinal uptake of macromolecules. VI. Uptake of protein antigen in vivo in normal rats and rats infected with *Nippostrongylus brasiliensis* or subjected to mild systemic anaphylaxis. *Gastroenterology* 77, 1038–1044.

Bloom, S., Simmons, D., and Jewell, D.P. (1995). Adhesion molecules intercellular adhesion molecule (ICAM-1), ICAM-3 and B7 are not expressed by epithelium in normal or inflamed colon. *Clin. Exp. Immunol.* 101, 157–163.

Bockman, D.E. and Cooper, M.D. (1973). Pinocytosis by epithelium associated with lymphoid follicles in the bursa of Fabricius, appendix and Peyer's patches. An electron microscopic study. *Am. J. Anat.* 136, 455–478.

Bonen, D.K., Ogura, Y., Nicolae, D.L., Inohara, N., Saab, L., Tanabe, T., Chen, F.F., Foster, S.J., Duerr, R.H., Brant, S.R., Cho, J.H., and

Nunez, G. (2003). Crohn's disease-associated NOD2 variants share a signaling defect in response to lipopolysaccharide and peptidoglycan. *Gastroenterology* 124, 140–146.

Brambell, F.W. (1966). The transmission of immunity from mother to young and the catabolism of immunoglobulins. *Lancet* 2, 1087–1093.

Brodsky, F.M. (1984). Living with clathrin: its role in intracellular membrane traffic. *Science* 242, 1396–1402.

Cario, E., Rosenberg, I.M., Brandwein, S.L., Beck, P.L., Reinecker, H.C., and Podolsky, D.K. (2000). Lipopolysaccharide activates distinct signaling pathways in intestinal epithelial cell lines expressing Toll-like receptors. *J. Immunol.* 164, 966–972.

Carpenter, G. and Wahl, M.I. (1991). The epidermal growth factor family. In *Peptide Growth Factors and Their Receptors 1* (M.B. Spom and A.B. Roberts, eds.), pp. 69–171. Springer-Verlag, New York.

Casanova, J.E., Apodaca, G., and Mostov, K.E. (1991). An autonomous signal for basolateral sorting in the cytoplasmic domain of the polymeric immunoglobulin receptor. *Cell* 66, 65–75.

Chu, S.H. and Walker, W.A. (1988). Development of the gastrointestinal mucosal barrier: changes in phospholipid head groups and fatty acid composition of intestinal microvillas membranes from newborn and adult rats. *Pediatr. Res.* 23, 439–442.

Chu, S.H. and Walker, W.A. (1991). Growth factor signal transduction in human intestinal cells. *Adv. Exp. Med. Biol.* 310, 107–112.

Claude, P. and Goodenough, D.A. (1973). Fracture faces of zonulae occludentes from "tight" and "leaky" epithelia. *J. Cell Biol.* 58, 390–440.

Cornell, R., Walker, W.A., and Isselbacher, K.J. (1971). Small intestinal absorption of horseradish peroxidase. A cytochemical study. *Lab. Invest.* 25, 42–48.

Crotty, B., Hoang, P., Dalton, H.R., and Jewell, D.P. (1992). Salicylates used in inflammatory bowel disease and colchicine impair interferon-γ-induced HLA-DR expression. *Gut* 33, 59–64.

Crowe, S.E., Alvarez, L., Dytoc, M., Hunt, R.H., Muller, M., Sherman, P., Patel, J., Jin, Y., and Ernst, P.B. (1995) Expression of interleukin 8 and CD54 by human gastric epithelium after *Helicobacter pylori* infection *in vitro*. *Gastroenterology* 108, 65–74.

Cunningham-Rundles, C., Brandeis, W.E., Good, R.A., and Day, N.K. (1978). Milk preciptins, circulating immune complexes, and IgA deficiency. *Proc. Natl. Acad. Sci. USA* 75, 3387–3389.

Cunningham-Rundles, C., Brandeis, W.E., Good, R.A., and Day, N.K. (1979). Bovine antigens and the formation of circulating immune complexes in selective immunoglobulin A deficiency. *J. Clin. Invest.* 64, 272–279.

Damle, N.K., Klussman, K., Linsley, P.S., and Aruffo, A. (1992). Differential costimulatory effects of adhesion molecules B7, ICAM-l, LFA-3, and VCAM-1 on resting and antigen-primed CD4+ T lymphocytes. *J. Immunol.* 148, 1985–1982.

Daniel, H., Neugebauer, B., Kratz, A., and Rehner, G. (1985). Localization of acid microclimate along intestinal villi of rat jejunum. *Am. J. Physiol.* 248, G293-G298.

Davies, P.H. and Messer, M. (1984). Intestinal cathepsin B and D activities of suckling rats. *Biol. Neonate* 45, 197–202.

Denari, G., Hale, T.L., and Washington, O. (1986). Effect of guinea pig or monkey colonic mucus on Shigella aggregation and invasion of HeLa cells by *Shigella flexneri* 1b and 2a. *Infect. Immun.* 51, 975–978.

de Santa Barbara, P., van den Brink, G.R., Roberts, D.J. (2003). Development and differentiation of the intestinal epithelium. *Cell. Mol. Life Sci.* 60, 1322–1332.

Dinsdale, D. and Healy, P.I. (1982). Enzymes involved in protein transmission by the intestine of the newborn lamb. *Histochem. J.* 14, 811–821.

Eckmann, L., Huang, G.T., Smith, J.R., Morzycka-Wroblewska, E., Kagnoff, M.F. (1994). Increased transcription and coordinate stabilization of mRNAs for secreted immunoglobulin alpha heavy chain and kappa light chain following stimulation of immunoglobulin A expressing B cells. *J. Biol. Chem.* 269, 33102–33108.

Ekstrom, G.M. and Westrom, B.R. (1991). Cathepsin B and D activities in intestinal mucosa during postnatal development in pigs. Relation to intestinal uptake and transmission of macromolecules. *Biol. Neonate* 59, 314–321.

Elson, C.O., Kagnoff, M.F., Fiocchi, C., Befus, A.D., and Targan, S. (1986). Intestinal immunity and inflammation: recent progress. *Gastroenterology* 91, 746,–768.

Engstrand, L., Scheyliius, A., Pahlson, C., Grimelius, L., Schwan, A., and Gustavsson, S. (1989). Association of *Campylobacter pylori* with induced expression of class II transplantation antigen on gastric epithelial cells. *Infect. Immun.* 57, 827–832.

Field, M. and Frizell, RA. (1991). Intestinal absorption and secretion. In *The Gastrointestinal System* (S. G. Schultz, ed.), vol. IV. American Physiology Society, Bethesda, Maryland.

Forstner, I. (1978). Intestinal mucins in health and disease. *Digestion* 17, 234–263.

Freeman, G.J., Freedman, A.S., Segil, J.M., Lee, G., Whitman, I.F., and Nadler, L.M. (1989). B7, a new member of the Ig superfamily with unique expression on activation and neoplastic B cells. *J. Immunol.* 143, 2714–2722.

Freeman, G.J., Gray, G.S., Gimmi, C.D., Lombard, D.B., Zhou, T.J., White, M., Fingeroth, I.D., Gribben, J.G., and Nadler, L.M. (1991). Structure, expression, and T cell costimulatory activity of the murine homologue of the human B lymphocyte antigen B7. *J. Exp. Med.* 174, 625–631.

Freeman, G.J., Gribben, I.G., Boussiotis, V.A., Ng, I.W., Restivo, V.A., Lombard, L.A., Gray, G.S., and Nadler L.M. (1993). Cloning of B7-2: a CTLA-4 counter-receptor that costimulates human T cell proliferation. *Science* 262, 909–911.

Freter, R. (1981). Mechanisms of association of bacteria with mucosal surfaces. In: Elliot, O'Connor, Whelen, 80th CIBA Foundation Symposium, pp. 36–47. Pitman Medical, London.

Frizze1, R.A. and Schultz, S.G. (1982). Ionic conductance of extracellular shunt pathway in rabbit ileum. *J. Gen. Physiol.* 59, 318–346.

Gibbons, R.A. (1981). Mucus of the mammalian genital tract. *Br. Med. Bull.* 34, 34–38.

Golovkina, T.V., Shlomchik, M., Hannum, L., and Chervonsky, A. (1999). Organogenic role of B lymphocytes in mucosal immunity. *Science* 286, 1965–1968.

Gonnella, P.A. and Neutra, M.R. (1984). Membrane-bound and fluid-phase macromolecules enter separate prelysosomal compartments in absorptive cells of suckling rat ileum. *J. Cell Biol.* 99, 909–917.

Gumbiner, B. (1987). The structure, biochemistry, and assembly of epithelial TIs. *Am. J. Physiol.* 253, C749–C758.

Guyer, R.L., Koshland, M.E., and Knopf, P.M. (1976). Immunoglobulin binding by mouse intestinal epithelial cell receptors. *J. Immunol.* 117, 587–593.

Harding, F.A., McArthur, I.G., Gorss, J.A., Raulet, D.H., and Allison, I.P. (1992). CD28-mediated signalling co-stimulates murine T cells and prevents induction of anergy in T cell clones. *Nature* 365, 607–609.

Hathcock, K.S., Laszlo, G., Dickler, H.B., Bradshaw, I., Linsley, P., and Hodes, R.J. (1993). Identification of an alternative CTLA-4 ligand costimulatory for T cell activation. *Science* 262, 905–907.

Hermiston, M.L. and Gordon, J.L. (1995a). In vivo analysis of cadherin function in the mouse intestinal epithelium. Essential roles in adhesion, maintenance of differentiation, regulation of programmed cell death. *J. Cell Biol.* 129, 489–506.

Hermiston, M.L. and Gordon, J.L. (1995b) Inflammatory bowel disease and adenomas in mice expressing a dominant mutant negative N-cadherin. *Science* 270, 1203–1207.

Hershberg, R.M., Cho, D.H., Youakim, A., Bradley, M.B., Lee, J.S., Framson, P.E., and Nepom, G.T. (1998). Highly polarized HLA class II antigen processing and presentation by human intestinal epithelial cells. *J. Clin. Invest* 102, 792–803.

Hill, S.M., Milla, P.J., Bottazzo, G.F., Mirakian, R. (1991). Autoimmune enteropathy and colitis: is there a generalised autoimmune gut disorder? *Gut* 32, 36–42.

Hinck, L., Nathke, I.S., Papkoff, J., and Nelson, W.J. (1994). Dynamics of cadherin/catenin complex formation: novel protein interactions and pathways of complex assembly. *J. Cell Biol.* 125, 1327–1340.

Hopkins, C.R., Gibson, A., Shipman, M., and Miller, K. (1990). Movement of internalized ligand-receptor complexes along a continuous endosomal reticulum. *Nature* 346, 335–339.

Hugot, J.P., Chamaillard, M., Zouali, H., Lesage, S., Cezard, J.P., Belaiche, J., Almer, S., Tysk, C., O'Morain, C.A., Gassull, M., Binder, V., Finkel, Y., Cortot, A., Modigliani, R., Laurent-Puig, P., Gower-Rousseau, C., Macry, J., Colombel, J.F., Sahbatou, M., Thomas, G. (2001). Association of NOD2 leucine-rich repeat variants with susceptibility to Crohn's disease. *Nature* 411, 599–603.

Hyman, P.E., Clarke, D.D., Everett, S.L., Sonne, B., Steward, D., Harada, T., Walsh, J.H., and Taylor, I.L. (1985). Gastric acid secretory function in preterm infants. *J. Pediatr.* 106, 467–471.

Israel, E.J. (1994). Neonatal necrotizing enterocolitis, a disease of the immature intestinal mucosal barrier. *Acta Paediatr. Scand. Suppl.* 396, 27–32.

Israel, E.J., Pang, K.Y., Harmatz, P.R., and Walker, W.A. (1987). Structural and functional maturation of rat gastrointestinal barrier with thyroxine. *Am J. Physiol.* 252, 762–767.

Israel, E.J., Simister, N., Freiberg, E., Caplan, A., and Walker W.A. (1993). Immunoglobulin G binding sites on the human foetal intestine: a possible mechanism for the passive transfer of immunity from mother to infant. *Immunology* 79, 77–81.

Ingkaran, N. and Abidin, Z. (1981). Intolerance to food proteins. In *Pediatric Nutrition* (Lifshitz, F. ed.), p. 453. Marcel Decker, New York.

Jacobs, L.R. (1983). Biochemical and ultrastructural characterization of the molecular topography of the rat intestinal microvillous membrane. Asymmetric distribution of hydrophilic groups and anionic binding sites. *Gastroenterology* 85, 46–54.

Jones, E.A. and Waldmann, T.A. (1972). The mechanism of intestinal uptake and transcellular transport of IgG in the newborn rat. *J. Clin. Invest.* 51, 2916–2927.

Kagnoff, M.F. (1989). General characteristics and development of the immune system. In *Immunology and Disease of the Gastrointestinal Tract* (M.H. Sleisenger and J.S. Fordtran, eds.), 4th. ed., pp. 114–143. Saunders, Philadelphia, PA.

Kaiserlian, D., Vidal, K., and Revillard, J-P. (1989). Murine enterocytes can present soluble antigen to specific class ll-restricted CD4+ T cells. *Eur. J. Immunol.* 19, 1513–1516.

Kerneis, S., Bogdanova, A., Kraehenbuhl, J.P., and Pringault, E. (1997). Conversion by Peyer's patch lymphocytes of human enterocytes into M cells that transport bacteria. *Science* 277, 949–952.

Kirby, W.N. and Parr, E.L. (1979). The occurrence and distribution of H-2 antigens on mouse intestinal epithelial cells. *J. Histochem. Cytochem.* 27, 746–750.

Knutton, S., Limbrick, A.R., and Robertson, J.D. (1974). Regular structures in membranes: membranes in the endocytic complex of ileal epithelial cells. *J. Cell Biol.* 62, 679–694.

Kraehenbuhl, J.P., Pringault, E., and Neutra, M.R. (1997). Review article: Intestinal epithelia and barrier functions. *Aliment. Pharmacol. Ther.* 11 Suppl 3, 3–8; discussion 8–9.

Lake, A.M., Bloch, K.J., Sinclair, K.J., and Walker, W.A. (1980). Anaphylactic release of intestinal goblet cell mucus. *Immunology* 39, 173–178.

Lebenthal, E. and Lee, P.C. (1982). Altemate pathways of digestion and absorption in early infancy. *J. Pediatr. Gastroenterol. Nutr.* 3, 1–3.

Leitch, G.J., Dickey, A.D., Udezuler, I.A., and Bailey, G.B. (1985). *Entamoeba histolytica* trophozoites in the lumen and mucus blanket of rat colons studied in vivo. *Infect. Immun.* 47, 68–73.

Linsley, P.S., Brady, W., Grosmire, L., Aruffo, A., Damle, N.K., and Ledbetter, J.A. (1991). Binding of the B cell activation antigen B7 to CD28 costimulates T cell proliferation and interleukin 2 mRNA accumulation. *J. Exp. Med.* 173, 721–730.

Lister, N., Sykes, A.P., Bailey, P.D., Boyd, C.A., and Bronk, J.R. (1995). Dipeptide transport and hydrolysis in isolated loops of rat small intestine: effects of stereospecificity. *J. Physiol.* 484, 173–182.

Liu, Y., Jones, B., Aruffo, A., Sullivan, K.M., Linsley, P.S., and Janeway, C.A. (1992). Heat-stable antigen is a costimulatory molecule for CD4 T cell growth. *J. Exp. Med.* 175, 437–445.

Lorenz, R.G., Chaplin, D.D., McDonald, K.G., McDonough, J.S., and Newberry, R.D. (2003). Isolated lymphoid follicle formation is inducible and dependent upon lymphotoxin-sufficient B lymphocytes, lymphotoxin beta receptor, and TNF receptor I function. J. Immunol. 170, 5475–5482.

Lucas, M.L. (1983). Determination of acid surface pH in vivo in rat proximal jejunum. Gut 24, 734–739.

Lucas, M.L. (1984). Weak electrolyte absorption and the acid microclimate. In Intestinal Absorption and Secretion (E. Skadhauge and K. Heintze, eds.), pp. 39–54. MTP, Lancaster.

MacDonald, T.T., Hutchings, P., Choy, M.Y., Murch, S., and Cooke, A. (1990). Tumor necrosis factor-alpha and interferon- gamma production measured at the single cell level in normal and inflamed human intestine. Clin. Exp. Immunol. 81, 301–305.

Madara, J.L. (1989). Loosening TJs. Lessons from the intestine. J. Clin. Invest. 83, 1089–1094.

Madara, J.L. (1990a). Maintenance of the macromolecular barrier at cell extrusion sites in intestinal epithelium: physiological rearrangement of tight junctions. J. Membr. Biol. 116, 177–184.

Madara, J.L. (1990b). Pathobiology of the intestinal epithelial barrier. Am. J. Pathol. 137, 1273–1281.

Madara, J.L. and Dharmsathaphorn, K. (1985). Occluding junction structure-function relationships in a cultured epithelial monolayer. J. Cell. Biol. 101, 2124–2133.

Madara, J.L. and Pappenheimer, J.R. (1987). Structural basis for physiological regulation of paracellular pathways in intestinal epithelia. J. Membr. Biol. 100, 149–164.

Madara, J.L. and Stafford, J. (1989). Interferon-γ directly affects barrier function of cultured intestinal epithelial monolayers. J. Clin. Invest. 83, 724–727.

Malin, M., Isolauri, E., Pikkarainen, P., Karikoski, R., and Isolauri J. (1996). Enhanced absorption of macromolecules: a secondary factor in Crohn's disease. Dig. Dis. Sci. 41, 1423–1428.

Marsh, M.N. (1992). Gluten, major histcompatibility complex, and the small intestine. A molecular and immunobiologic approach to the spectrum of gluten sensitivity (celiac sprue). Gastroenterology 102, 330–354.

Mason, D.W., Dallman, M., and Barclay, A.N. (1981). Graft-versus-host disease induces expression of Ia antigen in rat epidermal cells and gut epithelium. Nature 293, 150–151.

Masson, S.D. and Perdue, M.H. (1990). Changes in distribution of Ia antigen on epithelium of the jejunum and ileum in rats infected with Nippostrongylus brasiliensis. Clin. Immunol. Immunopathol. 57, 83–95.

Matsui, K., Boniface, J.J., Reay, P.A., Schlid, H., Frazekas-de-St Groth, B., and Davis, M.M. (1991). Low affinity interaction of peptide-MHC complexes with T cell receptors. Science 254, 1788–1791.

Mayer, E.A., Raybould, H., and Koelbel, C. (1988). Neuropeptides, inflammation and motility. Dig. Dis. Sci. 33, 71S–77S.

Mayer, L. and Shlien, R. (1987). Evidence for function of Ia molecules on gut epithelial cells in man. J. Exp. Med. 166, 1471–1483.

Mayer, L. and Eisenhardt, D. (1990). Lack of induction of suppressor T cells by intestinal epithelial cells from patients with inflammatory bowel disease. J. Clin. Invest. 86, 1255–1260.

Mayer, L., Eisenhardt, D., Salomon, P., Bauer, W., Pious, R., and Piccinini, L. (1991). Expression of class II molecules on intestinal epithelial cells in humans. Differences between normal and inflammatory bowel disease. Gastroenterology 100, 3–12.

Mayrhofer, G. and Spargo, L.D.J. (1990). Distribution of class II major histocompatibility antigens in enterocytes of the rat jejunum and their association with organelles of the endocytic pathway. Immunology 70, 11–19.

McCarthy, K.M., Yoong, Y., and Simister, N.E. (2000). Bidirectional transcytosis of IgG by the rat neonatal Fc receptor expressed in a rat kidney cell line: a system to study protein transport across epithelia. J. Cell Sci. 113, 1277–1285.

Medzhitov, R. and Janeway, C.A. (1997). Innate immunity: impact on the adaptive immune response. Curr. Opin. Immunol. 9, 4–9.

Mikulska, J.E., Pablo, L., Canel, J., and Simister, N.E. (2000). Cloning and analysis of the gene encoding the human neonatal Fc receptor. Eur. J. Immunogenet. 27, 231–240.

Milla, P.J. (1996). Intestinal motility during ontogeny and intestinal pseudoobstruction in children. Pediatr. Clin. North Am. 43, 511–532.

Miller, H.R.P. and Nawa, Y. (1979). Immune regulation of intestinal goblet cell differentiation. Nouv. Rev. Fr. Hematol. 21, 31–45.

Mostov, K.E. and Simister, N.E. (1985). Transcytosis. Cell 42, 389–390.

Nakazawa, A., Watanabe, M., Kanai, T., Yajima, T., Yamazaki, M., Ogata, H., Ishii, H., Azuma, M., and Hibi, T. (1999). Functional expression of costimulatory molecule CD86 on epithelial cells in the inflamed colonic mucosa. Gastroenterology 117, 536–545.

Nash, S., Stafford, J., and Madara, J.L. (1987). Effects of polymorphonuclear leukocyte transmigration on the barrier function of cultured intestinal epithelial monolayers. J. Clin. Invest. 80, 1104–1113.

Nathke, I.S., Hinck, L., Swedlow, J.R., Papkoff, J. and Nelson, W.J. (1994). Defining interactions and distribution of cadherin and catenin complexes in polarized epithelial cells. J. Cell Biol. 125, 1341–1352.

Neutra, M.R., O'Malley, L.J. and Specian, R.D. (1982). Regulation of intestinal goblet cell secretion. II. A survey of potential secretagogue. Am. J. Physiol. 242, G380–G387.

Ogura, Y., Bonen, D.K., Inohara, N., Nicolae, D.L., Chen, F.F., Ramos, R., Britton, H., Moran, T., Karaliuskas, R., Duerr, R.H., Achkar, J.P., Brant, S.R., Bayless, T.M., Kirschner, B.S., Hanauer, S.B., Nunez, G., and Cho, J.H. (2001). A frameshift mutation in NOD2 associated with susceptibility to Crohn's disease. Nature 411, 603–606.

Ogura, Y., Inohara, N., Benito, A., Chen, F.F., Yamaoka, S., and Nunez, G. (2001). Nod2, a Nod1/Apaf-1 family member that is restricted to monocytes and activates NFκB. J. Biol. Chem. 276, 4812–4818.

Owen, R.L. (1977). Sequential uptake of horseradish peroxidase by lymphoid follicle epithelium of Peyer's patches in the normal unobstructed mouse intestine: an ultrastructural study. Gastroenterology 72, 440–451.

Paganelli, R., Levinsky, R.J., Brostoff, J. and Wraith, D.G. (1979). Immune complexes containing food proteins in normal and atopic subjects after oral challenge and effect of sodium cromoglycate on antigen absorption. Lancet. 1, 1270–1272.

Pappenheimer, J.R. (1987). Physiological regulation of transepithelial impedance in the intestinal mucosal of rat and hamster. J. Membr. Biol. 100, 137–148.

Pappenheimer, J.R. and Reiss, K.Z. (1987). Contribution of solvent drag through intercellular junctions to absorption of nutrient by the small intestine of the rat. J. Membr. Biol. 100, 123–136.

Phillips, A.D., France, N.E. and Walker-Smith, J.A. (1979). The structure of the enterocyte in relation to its position on the villus in childhood: an electron microscopical study. Histopathology 3, 117–130.

Podolsky, D.K. (1985). Oligosaccharide structure of isolated human colonic mucin species. J. Biol. Chem. 260, 15510–15515.

Powell, D.W. (1981). Barrier function of epithelia. Am. J. Physiol. 241, G275–G288.

Ramage, J.K., Stanisz, A., Scicchitano, R., Hunt, R.H. and Perdue, M.H. (1988). Effect of immunologic reactions on rat intestinal epithelium. Correlation of increased permeability to chromium 51-labeled ethylene diaminetetraacic acid and ovalbumin during acute inflammation and anaphylaxis. Gastroenterology 94, 1368–1375.

Rechkemmer, G. (1992). Transport of weak electrolytes. In: Gastrointestinal System IV. Handbook of Physiology, Pp. 371–388 American Physiologic Association, Washington, DC.

Rechkemmer, G., Wahl, M., Kuschinsky, W. and von Engelhardt, W. (1986). pH-microclimate at the luminal surface of the intestinal mucosa of guinea pig and rat. Pfluegers Arch. 407, 33–40.

Remington, M., Malagelada, J.R., Zinsmeiste, A. and Fleming, C.R. (1983). Abnormalities in gastrointestinal motor activity in patients with short bowels: effect of a synthetic opiate. Gastroenterology 85, 629–636.

Roberton, D.M., Paganelli, R., Dinwiddie, R. and Levinsky, R.J. (1982). Milk antigen absorption in the preterm and term neonate. Arch. Dis. Child. 57, 369–372.

Rodewald, R. (1976). pH-dependent binding of immunoglobulins to intestinal cells of the neonatal rat. J. Cell Biol. 71, 666–669.

Rodewald, R. and Kraehenbuhl, J.P. (1984). Receptor-mediated transport of IgG. *J. Cell Biol.* 99, 159s–164s.

Saffron, M., Franco-Saenz, R., Kong, A., Pepthadjopoulos, D., and Szoka, F. (1979). A model for the study of oral administration of peptide hormones. *Can. J. Biochem.* 57, 548–553.

Said, H.M., Smith, R., and Redha, R. (1987). Studies on the intestinal surface acid microclimate: developmental aspects. *Pediatr. Res.* 22, 497–499.

Sander, G.R., Powell, B.C. (2004). Expression of notch receptors and ligands in the adult gut. *J. Histochem. Cytochem.* 52, 509–516.

Sanderson, I.R. and Walker, W.A. (1993). Uptake and transport of macromolecules by the intestine: possible role in clinical disorders (An update). *Gastroenterology* 104, 622–629.

Schwartz, R.H., Bogema, S. and Thorne, M.M. (1990). A cell culture model for T lymphocyte clonal anergy. *Science* 248, 1349–1356.

Sedmak, D.D., Davis, D.H., Singh, U., and van de Winkel, J.G. (1991). Expression of IgG Fc receptor antigens in placenta and on endothelial cells in humans. An immunohistochemical study. *Am. J. Pathol.* 138, 175–181.

Selby, W.S., Janossy, G., Mason, D.Y., and Jewell, D.P. (1983). Expression of HLA-DR antigens by colonic epithelium in inflammatory bowel disease. *Clin. Exp. Immunol.* 53, 614–618.

Shibata, Y., Arima, T., and Yamamoto, T. (1983). Regular structures on the microvillar surface membrane of ileal cells in suckling at intestine. *J. Ultrastruct. Res.* 85, 70–81.

Shimada, T. (1987). Factors affecting the microclimate pH in rat jejunum. *J. Physiol.* 392, 113–127.

Shub, M.D., Pang, K.Y., Swann, D.A., and Walker, W.A. (1983). Age-related changes in chemical composition and physical properties of mucus glycoproteins from rat small intestine. *Biochem. J.* 215, 405–411.

Simister, N.E. and Mostov, K.E. (1989). An Fc receptor structurally related to MHC class I antigens. *Nature* 337, 184–187.

Simister, N.E. and Rees, A.R. (1985). Isolation and characterization of an Fc receptor from neonatal rat small intestine. *Eur. J. Immunol.* 15, 733–738.

Snyder, J.D. (1991). Bacterial infections. In: *Pediatric Gastrointestinal Disease: Pathophysiology, Diagnosis, Management* (Walker, W.A., Goulet, O., Kleinman, R.E., Sherman, P.M., Schneider, B.L., Sanderson, I.R., eds.), pp. 527–537. B.C. Decker, Toronto.

Snyder, J.D. and Walker, W.A. (1987). Structure and function of intestinal mucin: developmental aspects. *Int. Arch. Allergy Appl. Immunol.* 82, 351–356.

Specian, R.D. and Neutra, M.R. (1980). Mechanism of rapid mucus secretion in goblet cells stimulated by acetylcholine. *J. Cell Biol.* 85, 626–640.

Steinman, R.M., Mellman, I.S., Mueller, W.A., and Cohn, Z.A. (1983). Endocytosis and the recycling of plasma membrane. *J. Cell Biol.* 96, 1–27.

Stern, M. and Walker, W.A. (1984). Food proteins and the gut mucosal barrier. I. Binding and uptake of cow's milk proteins by rat jejunum in vivo. *Am. J. Physiol.* 246, G556–G562.

Stern, M. and Gellermann, B. (1988). Food proteins and maturation of small intestinal microvillus membranes (MVM). I. Binding characteristics of cow's milk proteins and concanavalin A to MVM from newborn and adult rats. *J. Pediatr. Gastroenterol. Nutr.* 7, 115–121.

Stern, M., Gellermann, B., Belitz, H.D., and Wieser, H. (1988). Food proteins and maturation of small intestinal microvillus membranes (MVM). II. Binding of gliadin hydrolysate fractions and of the gliadin peptide B3142. *J. Pediatr. Gastroenterol. Nutr.* 7, 122–127.

Strobel, S. and Ferguson, A. (1984). Immune responses to fed protein antigens in mice. 3. Systemic tolerance or priming is related to age at which antigen is first encountered. *Pediatr. Res.* 18, 588–594.

Strobel, S. and Ferguson, A. (1986). Modulation of intestinal and systemic immune responses to a fed protein antigen, in mice. *Gut* 27, 829–837.

Strocchi, A. and Levitt, M.D. (1991). A reappraisal of the magnitude and implications of the intestinal unstirred layer. *Gastroenterology* 101, 843–847.

Thompson, H.S.G. and Staines, N.A. (1991). Could specific oral tolerance be a therapy for autoimmune disease? *Immunol. Today* 12, 396–399.

Udall, J.N., Colony, P., Fritze, L., Pang, K., Trier, J.S., and Walker, W.A. (1981a). Development of gastrointestinal mucosal barrier. II. The effect of natural versus artificial feeding on intestinal permeability to macromolecules. *Pediatr. Res.* 15, 245–249.

Udall, J.N., Pang, K., Fritze, L., Kleinman, R., and Walker, W.A. (1981b). Development of gastrointestinal mucosal barrier. II. The effect of age on intestinal permeability to macromolecules. *Pediatr. Res.* 15, 241–244.

Ulshen, M.H. and Rollo, J.L. (1980). Pathogenesis of *Escherichia coli* gastroenteritis in man—another mechanism. *N. Engl. J. Med.* 302, 99–101.

Unanue, E.R. (1984). Antigen presenting function of the macrophage. *Annu. Rev. Immunol* 2, 395–428.

Vaeth, G.F. and Henning, S.J. (1982). Postnatal development of peptidase enzymes in rat small intestine. *J. Pediatr. Gastroenterol. Nutr.* 1, 111–117.

Walker, W.A., Isselbacher, K.J., and Bloch, K.J. (1972). Intestinal uptake of macromolecules: effect of oral immunization. *Science* 177, 608–610.

Walker, W.A., Isselbacher, K.J., and Bloch, K.J. (1973). Intestinal uptake of macromolecules. II. Effect of parenteral immunization. *J. Immunol* 111, 221–226.

Walker, W.A., Wu, M., Isselbacher, J.K., and Bloch, K.J. (1975). Intestinal uptake of macromolecules IV. The effect of duct ligation on the breakdown of antigen and antigen-antibody complexes on the intestinal surface. *Gastroenterology* 69, 1123–1229.

Warshaw, A.L. and Walker, W.A. (1974). Intestinal absorption of intact antigenic protein. *Surgery* 76, 495–499.

Weaver, L.T., Gonnella, P.A., Israel, E.J., and Walker, W.A. (1990). Uptake and transport of epidermal growth factor by the small intestinal epithelium of the fetal rat. *Gastroenterology* 98, 828–837.

Weaver, L.T. and Walker, W.A. (1988). Epidermal growth factor and the developing human gut. *Gastroenterology* 94, 845–847.

Williams, R.C. and Gibbons, R.J. (1975). Inhibition of streptococcal attachment of receptors on human buccal epithelial cells by antigenically similar salivary glycoproteins. *Infect. Immun.* 11, 711–715.

Wiman, K., Curman, B., Forsum, U., Klareskog, L., Malmnas-Tjernlund, I.U., Rask, L., Tragardhl, L., and Person, P.A. (1978). Occurrence of Ia antigens on tissues on non-lymphoid origin. *Nature* 276, 711–713.

Winne, D. (1977). Shift of pH-absorption curves *J. Pharmatokinet. Biopharm.* 5, 53–94.

Winner, L.S., Mack, J., Weltzin, R.A., Mekalanos, J.J., Kraehenbuhl, J.P., and Neutra, M.R. (1991). New model for analysis of mucosal immunity: intestinal secretion of specific monoclonal immunoglobulin A from hybridoma tumors protects against *Vibrio cholerae* infection. *Infect. Immun.* 59, 977–982.

Yang, P.C., Berin, M.C., Yu, L.C., Conrad, D.H., and Perdue, M.H. (2000). Enhanced intestinal transepithelial antigen transport in allergic rats is mediated by IgE and CD23 (Fc epsilon RII). *J. Clin. Invest.* 106, 879–886.

Ye, G., Barrera, C., Fan, X., Gourley, W.K., Crowe, S.E., Ernst, P.B., and Reyes, V.E. (1997). Expression of B7-1 and B7-2 costimulatory molecules by human gastric epithelial cells: potential role in CD4 + T cell activation during *Helicobacter pylori* infection. *J. Clin. Invest.* 99, 1628–1636.

Yoshida, M., Claypool, S.M., Wagner, J.S., Mizoguchi, E., Mizoguchi, A., Roopenian, D.C., Lencer, W.I., and Blumberg, R.S. (2004). Human neonatal Fc receptor mediates transport of IgG into luminal secretions for delivery of antigens to mucosal dendritic cells. *Immunity* 20, 769–783.

Mucosal Microbiota

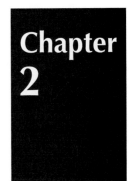

Dwayne C. Savage

Department of Microbiology, University of Tennessee at Knoxville, Knoxville, Tennessee

INTRODUCTION

The normal skin, the mucosal surfaces, and the lumen of the alimentary canal of adult humans harbor microbial cells in numbers that in aggregate can be estimated to outnumber animal cells in the body. The population of animal cells has been estimated at about 10^{13}. The population of microbial cells has been estimated at over 10^{14} (Savage 1977). With its number of microorganisms exceeding by at least tenfold its number of animal cells, the human can be regarded as an elaborate vessel in which microorganisms can survive and propagate. Alternatively, the human can be regarded as a biologic organism composed of both eukaryotic animal cells and eukaryotic and prokaryotic microbial cells (Savage 1986). A large body of evidence supports that latter concept.

Adult mammals, including humans, depend for their nutrition to a greater or lesser extent upon microbial processes in the alimentary canal (Savage 1986). Adult humans gain as much as 10% of their carbon and energy from microbial processes in their large bowel (Roberfroid *et al.* 1995). The epithelial cells of the cecum and colon are dependent for their carbon and energy on butyric acid, a fermentation end product of intestinal microorganisms (Roberfroid *et al.* 1995). The microbial and animal components of the body interact in many other physiologic and biochemical ways (Bry *et al.* 1996; Grubb *et al.* 1989). Such evidence supports a concept that the animal and microbial cells of man have coevolved in symbiosis to a high degree of interdependency (Savage 1977, 1986, 2002; Stevens and Hume 1995). One result of that coevolution involves certain immunologic functions (Cebra 1999; Henderson *et al.* 1996). This chapter presents information on the microbial populations on normal mucosal surfaces in humans (the indigenous microbiota) and then evaluates some evidence on how those populations interact with immunologic functions.

Until recently, the microbial species in the indigenous microbiota of human body surfaces have been identified by investigators using conventional techniques and laboratory culture media. During recent years, however, efforts to detect and identify members of the biota have been impacted by the techniques of molecular biology and genetics (Tannock 2002; Savage 2002). Use of such techniques has yielded new evidence on the genera and species of organisms in the biota, and is expanding and changing knowledge gained from conventional technology. In describing the microbiota, therefore, the chapter presents information gained from conventional technology and then discusses some findings gained from use of molecular methods. The methods used are not described in detail. Readers are referred to cited publications for those details.

MICROORGANISMS INDIGENOUS TO MUCOSAL SURFACES

Indigenous microorganisms colonize in adult humans the skin and the mucosal surface of the oral cavity, the upper respiratory tract, the urogenital tract, and much of the gastrointestinal (GI) canal (Hentges 1993; Tannock 1995). The organisms interact with the host's immunologic system in complex ways. The interactions begin when the microbiota develops during succession in the neonate and continue throughout life (Berg 1983). As is amplified in the following text, however, the biota during succession differs from the adult biota ("climax biota"). In addition, the populations of various bacterial species in the biota differ in elderly adults from those in young and middle-aged adults (Mitsuoka 1992). Therefore, the biota of neonates and the aged may interact with the immunologic system in ways differing from those of the biota of young and middle-aged adults (Percival *et al.* 1996). Such differences may complicate understanding of how the mucosal microbiota interacts with the immunologic system.

The climax mucosal microbiota in the normal adult, its succession in neonates, and its changes in advanced age

Skin

The microbiota of the skin is not obviously a subject for a chapter devoted to mucosal microorganisms. Microbial components of that biota are often found on mucosal surfaces, however, such as those of the nasopharynx and external sex organs, and are therefore addressed here.

The keratinizing integument of the adult human body, and especially the hair follicles and various glands in that epithelium, are colonized by a microbial biota (Tannock 1995). Prominent in that biota, as assessed by conventional methods, are certain species of the bacterial genera: *Acinetobacter* (Seifert *et al.* 1997), *Corynebacterium* (Chiller *et al.* 2001), *Micrococcus* (Chiller *et al.* 2001), *Propionibacterium* (Till *et al.* 2000), and *Staphylococcus* (Chiller *et al.* 2001). Species of the lipophilic yeast *Malassezia* (Till *et al.* 2000) and fungi of certain genera, for example, *Pityrosporum* (Tannock 1995), may also be considered members of the biota. These organisms vary in number from site to site on the skin. Their populations are influenced, both in level and makeup, by numerous endogenous factors, including secretions predominating in given areas and the density and type of glands and hair follicles (Tannock 1995). They are influenced as well by exogenous factors such as antibacterial drugs and cosmetics (Holland and Bojar 2002). Their succession (development) in neonates and condition in the elderly have apparently not been systematically studied.

Molecular approaches have been applied in studies in which microorganisms on the skin have been identified (Davies *et al.* 2001). Seifert *et al.* (1997) used polymerase chain reaction (PCR) to amplify 16S rDNA from *Acinetobacter* species isolated from skin on various areas of the adult body and identified the isolates by restriction endonuclease analysis. They also used sodium dodecyl-page electrophoresis (SDS-PAGE), ribotyping, and DNA-DNA hybridization technology to identify some of the isolates. The cultures were also identified by conventional methods. The molecular methods proved to be as effective as the conventional ones in identifying the bacteria. Using a similar approach, Gaitanis *et al.* (2002) used molecular methods to identify isolates of *Malassezia* species cultured from pathologic skin scales and identified by conventional methods.

However, these investigators also compared findings from that approach with findings from experiments in which they extracted DNA from the scale samples and used restriction fragment length polymorphism-PCR technology (RFLP-PCR) to identify the yeasts to species. The molecular analysis proved to be as useful as culture technology for identifying species of the yeasts in the skin specimens and to be faster and possibly more sensitive (Gaitanis *et al.* 2002).

Nasopharynx/oropharynx

The indigenous biota of the anterior nares of the normal adult human generally reflects the bacterial biota of the skin (Hentges 1993). As determined with conventional methods, predominating species in the skin biota are of the gram-positive, aerobic genera *Staphylococcus* and *Corynebacterium* and of the anaerobic, gram-positive genus *Propionibacterium* (**Table 2.1**). Similar genera and species can occur in the nasopharynx. In this site, however, bacteria of certain aerobic gram-negative species can also be found (Table 2.1).

The biota of the surface of the mucous membranes of the oropharynx in normal adults also consists only of bacterial species. Some of these derive from the nasopharynx; and some derive from the mouth. Those are outnumbered many times over, however, by numerically dominant aerobes of the gram-positive genus *Streptococcus*. *Mycoplasma* and members of the aerobic, gram-negative genus *Haemophilus* are reported also to be members of the indigenous oropharyngeal biota (Table 2.1).

Numerous studies have been published in which the focus has been on culturing and identifying with conventional methods bacteria from the nasopharynx and oropharynx in neonates (Tannock 1995). Likewise, several reports exist in the literature of findings from culturing of bacteria from the throats of children of various ages (Hokama *et al.* 1996). Most of these investigations have not involved systematic study of the succession of the oropharyngeal biota. Rather, they have been focused on recovery of organisms of particular species, especially beta-hemolytic streptococci,

Table 2.1. Indigenous Microbiota of the Human Upper Respiratory Tract[a]

Gram Characteristic	Genus	Location[b]
Not applicable	*Mycoplasma*	OP
Positive	*Staphylococcus*	AN
	Corynebacterium	AN
	Propionibacterium[c]	AN
	Streptococcus[d]	OP
Negative	*Moraxella*	NP
	Haemophilus	OR and NP
	Neisseria	OR and NP

[a]From Tannock (1995) and Hentges (1993).
[b]OP, oropharynx; AN, anterior nares; NP, nasopharynx.
[c]Strict anaerobe.
[d]Seventeen species, some of which are strict anaerobes.

Staphylococcus aureus, or *Escherichia coli.* Typical of such studies was a recent analysis of the succession of various streptococcal species in the infant nasopharynx (Kononen *et al.* 2002). In spite of the limitations of such studies, evidence from them supports a conclusion that neonates delivered in natural birth acquire within hours to days in their nasopharynx and oropharynx a pioneer biota consisting mainly of streptococci and staphylococci (Tannock 1995). These bacteria rapidly establish populations that may contain in the infant higher numbers of *S. aureus* than are found in adults. That biota appears to reach climax (adult condition) early in childhood and, except during periods of respiratory illness and treatment with antibacterial drugs, persists throughout life. Molecular methods have apparently not yet been applied to systematic analysis of the respiratory biota.

Oral cavity

The indigenous microbiota of the adult mouth, as assessed by conventional methods, involves bacterial species of numerous genera **(Table 2.2)**. A few of the species are facultative in their energy-generating metabolism and can grow in atmospheres either free of or containing oxygen. Most of them, however, are strictly anaerobic and must be cultured in atmospheres free of oxygen (Loesche 1994). The various species preferentially colonize certain sites in different parts of the buccal cavity with strict anaerobes predominating in subgingival plaque. The populations of the various species, especially in subgingival areas, tend to vary in size with the quality of the dental hygiene of the individuals being sampled.

The first systematic study of the oral microbiota in succession was probably that published by McCarthy *et al.* (1965). These investigators sampled for microbial culturing the mouths of 51 newborn and 44 1-month-old infants. They repeated samples on the latter group at ages 8 and 12 months. Streptococci were dominant in the mouth throughout the first year of life, comprising 98% of the cultivable bacteria within 2 days of birth and 70% after 12 months. *Streptococcus salivarius* was isolated from half of the neonates; staphylococci, and species of *Lactobacillus, Neisseria,* and *Veillonella* were occasionally isolated (McCarthy *et al.* 1965). These findings were confirmed and expanded by Pearce *et al.* (1995), who focused on succession of streptococcal species, and by Kononen *et al.* (1999), who focused on succession of anaerobic components of the biota.

In the latter study, Kononen *et al.* (1999) took saliva samples at 2, 6, and 12 months of age from 44 healthy Caucasian infants, cultured strictly anaerobic bacteria from the samples, and using conventional methods, identified the isolates to genus and species. *Veillonella* species were most frequently cultured from the 2-month-old infants. *Prevotella, Fusobacterium,* and *Porphyromonas* species were only occasionally isolated from the 2-month-olds but were often recovered from salivas from older babies. *Capnocytophaga* and *Actinomyces* species were often recovered from 1-year-old children. Organisms appearing in early months in the infant mouth tended to persist into adulthood (Kononen *et al.* 1999). These findings and those from the earlier studies suggest that oral mucosal tissues and mucosa distal to the mouth are exposed within days after birth to a bacterial biota consisting largely of streptococcal species. Within about 2 months thereafter, however, other components of the biota, especially strictly anaerobic ones, appear and thereafter increase in population. The oral biota of elderly individuals reflects their states of dental hygiene (Tannock 1995).

Table 2.2. Indigenous Members of the Microbiota of the Mouth[a]

Gram Characteristic	Genus	In Saliva and on Tongue	In Plaque[b]
Not applicable	*Treponema*[c]	+	+
Positive	*Streptococcus*[d]	+	+
	Lactobacillus[e]	+	+
	Actinomyces[e]	+	+
Negative	*Fusobacterium*[e]		+
	Capnocytophaga[e]		+
	Prevotella[e]		+
	Porphyromonas[e]		+
	Actinobacillus[e]		+
	Veillonella[e]		+
	Desulfovibrio[e]		+

[a]From Loesche (1994).
[b]Supragingival, subgingival, or both.
[c]Microaerophilic.
[d]Both facultative and anaerobic species.
[e]Strict anaerobes.

Molecular technologies have been used in studies of the oral microbiota. They have been applied in identifying to species bacterial isolates obtained by conventional culture and used to identify bacterial species from their DNAs in aspirates of oral secretions. One approach in which isolates of the organisms were cultured by conventional methods and identified by 16S rRNA PCR-RFLP analysis and 16S rRNA gene sequencing yielded evidence that *Capnocytophaga granulosa* and *Capnocytophaga haemolytica* occur in subgingival plaque in adults with chronic periodontitis (Ciantar *et al.* 2001). A similar study in which strains of *Fusobacterium nucleatum* were cultured from 19 individuals in four families (8 parents and 11 children, all with healthy mouths) revealed that the children shared with one or the other of their parents at least one strain and also had at least one unique strain of the anaerobe. Those bacterial isolates had been identified by ribotyping (Suchett-Kay *et al.* 1999).

In a study of the second type, Munson *et al.* (2002) extracted DNA and cultured isolates from aspirates of infected root canals. 16S rDNA sequences from 624 DNA clones and 261 cultured isolates were identified by comparison with database sequences. Sixty-five taxa were identified, of which 26 were found by the molecular methods alone. The investigators concluded that the direct molecular analysis of genes in the aspirates revealed a more diverse microflora associated with endodontic infections than was revealed by culture methods alone (Munson *et al.* 2002). As discussed in the following text, similar findings have been made when molecular tools were applied to identifying bacterial species in body sites other than the mouth.

The urogenital tract

The male. The periurethral biota of the penis generally reflects that of the skin with staphylococci and corynebacteria predominating. An aerobic organism unique to the area, *Mycobacterium smegmatis*, may occasionally be cultured.

Molecular technology has apparently yet to be used for identifying members of the biota of the penis.

The female. Studies in which conventional microbiologic techniques were used have revealed that the periurethral biota of premenarcheal girls and menarcheal women generally reflects that of the skin and cervix with species of *Lactobacillus*, *Staphylococcus*, and *Corynebacterium* predominating (Marrie *et al.* 1980). The microbiota of the mucosal epithelium of the cervix and vagina of premenarcheal females is similar to that of menarcheal women and is composed of species of the periurethral biota and other gram-positive and gram-negative genera **(Table 2.3)**. Populations of species of gram-positive, metabolic anaerobes of the genus *Lactobacillus* predominate in both cases but are much higher in menarcheal than premenarcheal women. The bacterial populations undergo cyclical shifts in size that are related to the menstrual cycle (Redondo-Lopez *et al.* 1990). They also vary depending upon behavioral factors including use of vaginal, but not oral, contraceptives (Eschenbach *et al.* 2000; Gupta *et al.* 2000) and frequency of sexual intercourse (Schwebke *et al.* 1999).

The populations of lactobacilli are higher on the vaginal epithelium of menarcheal than premenarcheal females because estrogen in menarcheal women stimulates deposits of glycogen in the vaginal mucosa (Hentges 1993). The lactobacilli ferment and produce organic acids from the glycogen and form populations of substantial size on the mucosal epithelium. The fermentation end products of those populations lower the vaginal pH to 4.4–4.6. In postmenarcheal women with declining levels of estrogen, the lactobacilli populations and those of staphylococci and corynebacteria decline, the vaginal pH rises, and populations of some gram-positive and gram-negative anaerobes (e.g., coliforms) increase (Marrie *et al.* 1980).

The neonate's vagina is sterile at birth. Within 24 hours, however, it is colonized with corynebacteria, staphylococci,

Table 2.3. Indigenous Members of the Vaginal Mucosal Microbiota During the Reproductive Years[a]

Gram Characteristic	Genus	Average Population[b]	Isolation Frequency[c]
Not applicable	*Candida*	2.1	25
Positive	*Corynebacterium*	8.8	25
	Lactobacillus	8.9	90
	Micrococcus	2.0	5
	Peptococcus[d]	8.0	10
	Streptococcus	8.5	15
	Staphylococcus	7.1	35
Negative	*Escherichia*	4.6	5
	Gardnerella	9.3	15

[a]Adapted from Sobel and Chaim (1996).
[b]CFU/ml washing.
[c]Percentage of cultured microorganisms.
[d]Strict anaerobe.

and nonhemolytic streptococci, primarily deriving from the mother's vaginal biota (Mandar and Mikelsaar 1996). After a few days, lactobacilli appear as glycogen is deposited in the vaginal mucosa resulting from maternal estrogen in the neonatal blood. A biota then develops resembling that of the adult. After the passively transferred estrogen is excreted and the glycogen disappears; the *Lactobacillus* populations decline. At menarche, as glycogen is again deposited in the mucosa, the characteristic climax biota dominated by lactobacilli again develops (Hentges 1993; Hillier and Lau 1997; Marrie *et al.* 1980; Samsioe 1998).

Molecular technology has been applied in studies of the vaginal microbiota, especially in studies in which the aim has been to amplify information on strains and species of lactobacilli. These lactic acid bacteria produce compounds that inhibit growth of vaginal pathogens and are important components of the biota of women during their reproductive years. Antonio *et al.* (1999) used whole chromosomal DNA hybridization probes for known *Lactobacillus* species to identify isolates cultured from sexually active women. They found that strains of *Lactobacillus crispatus* and *Lactobacillus jensenii* are the most frequently isolated members of the vaginal biota (Antonio *et al.* 1999).

Ventura *et al.* (2000) demonstrated that amplified ribosomal DNA restriction analysis (ARDRA) is a reliable and rapid method for identifying to species and subspecies level *Lactobacillus* isolates from the vagina. Similarly, Vasquez *et al.* (2002) have demonstrated that such isolates can be typed by randomly amplified polymorphic DNA (RAPD) analysis and identified to species by temporal temperature gradient gel electrophoresis, mutiplex PCR, and 16S ribosomal DNA sequencing. Their study not only confirmed the findings of Antonio *et al.* (1999) but also revealed for the first time that *Lactobacillus iners* is one of the predominating species of the vaginal biota (Vasquez *et al.* 2000).

Burton *et al.* (2003) recently reported findings from use of PCR-denaturing gradient gel electrophoresis and sequencing of the V2-V3 region of the 16S rRNA gene (PCR-DGGE) to identify *Lactobacillus* species in samples of vaginal secretions from premenopausal women. This technology eliminated the need for culturing the bacteria and revealed that nearly 80% of the individuals possessed DNA sequences with high levels of similarity to *Lactobacillus* sequences. Sequences homologous to *L. iners* were the most commonly found and were detected in 42% of the women studied (Burton *et al.* 2003), confirming the findings of Vasquez *et al.* (2002). As in studies of the oral biota, use of molecular technology has proved to be a rapid and accurate approach for identifying bacteria and is expanding and extending knowledge of the vaginal microbiota.

Gastrointestinal canal

Molecular technologies have been used since the mid-1990s to identify indigenous bacteria in the GI tract (Millar *et al.* 1996; Vaughan *et al.* 2000; Wang *et al.* 1996). Findings in numerous papers published since 1996 have attested to the utility of a variety of molecular approaches for rapidly iden-

tifying cultured isolates and for detecting and identifying bacteria from DNA in intestinal specimens (Savage 2002; Tannock 2002). The technologies have proved so successful that seven European laboratories have cooperated in a joint project to develop, refine, and apply molecular methods "towards facilitating elucidation of the complex composition of the human intestinal microflora and to devise robust methodologies for monitoring the gut flora in response to diet" (Blaut *et al.* 2002, p. 2203). The activities of those laboratories and of others around the world have begun to advance and alter understanding of the intestinal microbiota gained in earlier years by culturing technologies. The following paragraphs continue the paradigm of presenting information on the biota as has been developed with the latter technologies. Rather than presenting molecular findings at the end of this section on the GI microbiota, however, I give those findings where they seem to me best to illustrate how our understanding of the biota is being altered by molecular technologies.

Stomach. Gastric acidity creates in the human stomach an environment that is inimical to microbial survival (Hentges 1993). Therefore, the stomach is, in general, free of an indigenous microbiota. One bacterial species, *Helicobacter pylori*, has the capacity, however, to overcome the acidity and to colonize gastric mucosal epithelium (Lee *et al.* 1993). This organism can be found on the mucosal epithelium of the antrum and occasionally the fundus of the stomach in a large proportion of individuals tested (Lee *et al.* 1993; Elitsur *et al.* 2002). It is recognized to be the etiologic agent of acute and chronic gastritis and to be involved in the etiology of peptic ulcers and gastric neoplasia (Guillemin *et al.* 2002; Lee *et al.* 1993). In spite of evidence supporting such etiologic roles, it can be cultured from many adults (Lee *et al.* 1993) and even some children (Elitsur *et al.* 2002) who are free of symptoms of gastric disease. These findings support the opinion of some investigators that populations of *H. pylori* on the stomach mucosa constitute an indigenous gastric microbiota. Molecular methods involving a variety of approaches have been developed for rapidly identifying *H. pylori* in cultured specimens and in situ in the stomach (Tham *et al.* 2001). These approaches have confirmed histologic findings that the bacterium associates intimately with the gastric mucosal epithelium (Tham *et al.* 2001).

Small intestine. As has the stomach, the upper two-thirds of the small bowel—the duodenum, jejunum and proximal ileum—has been thought to be free of a microbiota (Hentges 1993). The distal one-third of the small bowel (ileum) has a microbiota reflecting that of the large intestine. The upper small bowel has yielded in cultures of luminal content and biopsies of the mucosa bacteria of genera and species found in areas proximal to it (Savage 1983a). The bacteria are mainly species of streptococci and staphylococci presumably passing from the mouth and oropharynx into the stomach during eating of a meal. Those organisms have been considered to be transients in the area and to pass through the small bowel with the digesta. In some cases, however, bacterial species in high numbers can be cultured from the mucosa in that area.

Children with irritable bowel syndrome or celiac disease have bacteria of various species in substantial populations on the mucosal epithelium of the jejunum for prolonged periods after food has passed through (Ciampolini *et al.* 1996). These findings, made in a developed Western country, are reminiscent of earlier findings that a complex, largely gram-negative biota colonizes the small bowel epithelium in many if not most clinically normal individuals in certain areas of India (Savage 1986). Taken together, such pieces of evidence suggest that the mucosal epithelium of the upper small bowel can harbor a microbiota under certain circumstances. In addition, they suggest that, even though the surface is not permanently colonized with bacteria, microorganisms may persist on it in substantial numbers for prolonged periods. These findings may have implications for understanding how the intestinal microorganisms interact with the immunologic system.

Large intestine. The indigenous microbiota of the normal adult human colon has been extensively studied with culture methods for isolating, identifying, and enumerating bacteria. The biota has proved to be enormous. The aggregate bacterial populations can exceed 100 trillion (10^{14}) cells. Indeed, the mucosal surface and the lumen of the large bowel harbor 99.9% of the human indigenous microbiota (Finegold *et al.* 1983; Holdeman *et al.* 1976; Savage 1977, 1986, 1989). Estimates vary on the number of genera and species involved. However, hundreds of species in 40 to 50 bacterial genera have been cultured and identified from feces and bowel content (Finegold *et al.* 1983; Holdeman *et al.* 1976). Both gram-negative and gram-positive, facultative, microaerophilic, and strictly anaerobic species have been identified. The populations of anaerobes outnumber those of the microaerophiles and facultatives by as much as 1000 to 1. The bacteria colonize both the digesta in the lumen and the mucosal epithelium.

Particular bacterial genera and species in huge populations predominate in the biotas of most individuals (Finegold *et al.* 1983; Holdeman *et al.* 1976). Each individual may have stable populations of certain species, however, that are characteristic of their biota (Holdeman *et al.* 1976). The lists of the known genera and species occupy many pages in books. For reasons of space, those lists are not reproduced here. **Table 2.4** contains a list of the predominating bacterial genera. The interested reader should consult Finegold *et al.* (1983), Hentges (1993), Holdeman *et al.* (1976), and Tannock (1995) for listings of the genera and species of bacteria found in feces and colonic content. In addition to the bacterial biota, many individuals also harbor members of archael genera (particularly methanogenic prokaryotes) in their colonic biota (Table 2.4). The reader is referred to Miller and Wolin (1986) for information on those microorganisms.

Methods for culturing from natural specimens (e.g., feces or colonic content) and identifying strictly anaerobic bacteria to genus and species are cumbersome, time consuming, labor intensive, and expensive. As a result, efforts to culture and identify isolates of the hundreds of bacterial species in the colonic biota have been accomplished in only a few lab-

oratories in the world (Finegold *et al.* 1983; Holdeman *et al.* 1976; Mitsuoka 1992). Results from those studies have generally agreed on the major components of the biota but have differed in details. Methods (e.g., sampling, diluents, culture media, incubation of media) tend to vary from laboratory to laboratory. The differing approaches tend to yield differing results, especially in describing minor elements of the biota. More important, no culture methods used are adequate for culturing bacteria in the numbers that can be estimated from microscopic counts of smears of either feces or colonic content (Matsuki *et al.* 2002). These observations have stimulated aggressive efforts to bring molecular technologies to bear on identifying bacterial isolates cultured from feces and for identifying bacterial species from their genes in samples of those materials **(Table 2.5)**.

Studies involving molecular technology have confirmed findings from conventional studies on the size and diversity of prokaryotic populations in the colon (Matsuki *et al.* 2002). In addition, they have revealed that the molecular methods are more rapid than, and as reliable as, methods based on cultural technologies for identifying members of the biota isolated from feces. They have also led, in direct analysis of DNAs in feces, to discovery of species that have never been cultured and identified with conventional tools. Findings from such molecular studies will undoubtedly be important for analyses of how the biota and immunologic system interact.

Whatever the technologies used, most studies of the colonic microbiota involve sampling of feces. Such samples are probably representative of the biota in the lumen but give little or no information on the mucosal biota. The biota specific to the mucosal epithelium has been difficult to assess (Savage 1983a). Investigators have usually relied on specimens taken at biopsy in living subjects or on samples of mucosal tissue taken at autopsy of individuals killed in accidents. Biopsies often derive from patients suffering some disease of the small bowel, colon, or rectum. Samples taken at autopsy are rarely obtained immediately following death of the individual. Results from biopsies must be regarded with caution because nothing is known about how the patient's disease and its treatment influence the outcome of the microbiologic analysis of the specimens. The results of cultures taken at autopsy may be influenced by postmortem changes in the mucosa (Savage 1983a). Several such studies involving cultural technologies have suggested, nevertheless, that the mucosal microbiota probably reflects in content of bacterial species the biota culturable from feces (Table 2.4; Savage 1983a). Moreover, estimates of number of bacteria on mucosal surfaces able to grow aerobically compared with the numbers able to grow only anaerobically reflect estimates of aerobic and anaerobic populations in feces (Finegold *et al.* 1983). These and other experimental findings have suggested a hypothesis that the mucosal biota is a reservoir for inoculating the luminal content (Freter *et al.* 1983; Savage *et al.* 1995).

That concept has been challenged, however, by findings from a study of the colonic mucosal microbiota involving molecular technologies (Zoetendal *et al.* 2002a). Using

Table 2.4. Indigenous Microbiota in Human Feces[a]

Gram Characteristic	Genus[b]	Frequency[c]	Population[d]
Not applicable	*Methanococcus* and other methane-producing Archeae	50	Unknown
Positive	*Clostridium*	100	10
	Bifidobacterium	74	10
	Eubacterium	94	11
	Lactobacillus	78	10
	Streptococcus	≥99	10
	Peptococcus	≥33	10
	Peptostreptococcus	≥45	10
	Propionibacterium	≥9	9
Negative	*Bacteroides*	≥99	11
	Fusobacterium	≥18	8
	Butyrivibrio	≤1	8
	Actinomyces	≤8	9
	Acidaminococcus	20	9
	Coprococcus	≤6	9
	Gaffkya	≤1	12
	Megasphaera		9
	Ruminococcus	5	10
	Sarcina	45	6
	Veillonella	≥6	8
	"Facultatives"	34	9
		98	

[a]From Finegold *et al.* (1983), Tannock (1995), and Hentges (1993).
[b]All are anaerobic bacteria except "facultatives," which grow either aerobically or anaerobically.
[c]Percentage of individuals sampled.
[d]Estimated average $\log_{10}$.

denaturing-gradient gel electrophoresis analysis (DGGE) of 16S rDNA PCR amplicons, these investigators tested whether or not the bacterial species detectable in biopsies are the same as those in the fecal biota of normal human adults. They found that the predominating mucosal biota is host specific and differed significantly in composition from the fecal biota. This important finding is provocative and should stimulate more research on bacterial populations present on the mucosa and in feces.

Based upon use of conventional methods for identifying isolates from feces, indigenous bacteria have been demonstrated to colonize the neonatal colon in a pattern resembling ecologic succession (Cooperstock and Zedd 1983; Hentges 1993; Savage 1977). This pattern begins at birth and can be influenced by many factors, not the least of which are the circumstances of the birth (whether natural or cesarean), the neonatal diet, and possibly even birth weight (Sakata *et al.* 1985). The bacterial species culturable from feces, especially in the early stages of succession, can differ

in infants born in vaginal delivery from those delivered by cesarean section, especially when the latter infants are delivered into controlled environments (Wharton *et al.* 1994). Likewise, the predominating bacterial species can differ in infants fed at the breast as compared with those fed formula (Benno *et al.* 1985; Wharton *et al.* 1994). Those fed at the breast have predominating populations of bifidobacterial species, and those fed formula tend to have high populations of gram-negative anaerobes and lactobacilli. Whether born by cesarean section or by natural birth, however, and whether or not they consumed mothers' milk or formula, by the time they consume solid food, most infants have a fecal biota similar to that of the adult (Cooperstock and Zedd 1983). No reports are available about microorganisms colonizing colonic mucosal surfaces in healthy neonates, infants, and young children.

Molecular tools have recently been applied to identifying bacteria in the feces of infants. Millar *et al.* (1996) used PCR to amplify the V3 region of 16S rDNA in DNA extracted

Table 2.5. Application of Molecular Technologies for Detecting in Feces and Identifying Bacterial Species in the Human Fecal Microbiota[a]

Publication	Subjects	Sampling	Methods[b]	Major Findings	Major Conclusions
Wang *et al.* (1996)	Adults/infants	Feces; anaerobic bacteria of certain species	Quantitive 16S rRNA PCR	PCR titers highest for anaerobic bacteria of certain species	Method simple, rapid; eliminates DNA isolation
Franks *et al.* (1998)	Adults	Feces; anaerobic bacteria of certain species	16S rRNA-FISH	Probes detected anaerobes in feces at numbers comparable	Fecal anaerobe populations normally vary over time
Suau *et al.* (1999)	Adult	DNA extracted from feces	PCR amplification of clones of 16S	95% of clones in three major anaerobic groups	Majority of clones from hitherto unknown bacterial species
Matsuki *et al.* (1999)	Adults/infants	DNA extracted from feces	PCR amplification of bifidobacterial 16S rDNAs from isolates	Species of *Bifidobacterium* identified and detected in feces	Method allows *Bifidobacterium* species to be rapidly and accurately identified in feces
Walter *et al.* (2001)	Adults	DNA extracted from feces	PCR-DDGE of clones of 16S bacterial rDNAs	Genera of lactic acid bacteria (LAB) identified in feces	Approach more effective than culture in identifying LAB
Matsuki *et al.* (2002)	Adults	DNA extracted from feces and bacterial isolates from feces	PCR amplification and sequencing of 16S rDNA from isolates and feces	Genera of anaerobic bacteria identified and detected in feces	Approaches used should contribute to study of composition and dynamics of fecal microbiota
Satokari *et al.* (2001)	Adults	DNA extracted from feces and *Bifidobacterium* isolates from feces	PCR-DGGE detection of 520bp fragment of 16S ribosomal DNA	Subjects had stable host-specific fecal populations of bifidobacteria; *B. adolescentis* most common species	Methods used validated for qualitative analysis of complex bifidobacterial communities
Requena *et al.* (2002)	Adults/infants	DNA extracted from feces and *Bifidobacterium* isolates from feces	PCR-DGGE detection of 301bp transaldolase gene of *Bifidobacterium* and real-time quantitative PCR targeting of 101bp transaldolase gene	Subtypes of bifidobacterial isolates detected with 301bp probe; bifidobacterial species detected and quantitated in feces with 101bp probe	Quantitative PCR effective for estimating bifidobacterial populations in adults, but not as effective as using 16S rDNR-targeting PCR in infants
Zoetendal *et al.* (2002b)	Adults	Feces; *Ruminococcus obeum*-like anaerobic bacteria	16S rRNA-targeted probes for *R. obeum* and FISH	Probes detected that *R. obeum*-like bacteria comprise from 2.2% to 16% of bacterial community in feces	*R. obeum*-like bacteria are numerically important in human fecal microbiota

[a]Listing not exhaustive.
[b]PCR, polymerase chain reaction; FISH, quantitative-fluorescence-*in situ* hybridization; DGGE, denaturing-gradient gel electrophoresis.

from feces and from cultured isolates from preterm infants. Their goal was to assess the extent to which bacterial species not detected by culture contribute to the fecal microbiota of those infants. The amplicons from the fecal DNA and DNA extracted from cultured isolates were compared by PCR-DGGE (Table 2.5). A substantial number of amplicons found in most of the infants were not found in cultured isolates. However, most of the amplicons of uncultured genetic types had 90% sequence identity with sequences from known intestinal bacteria cultured from adult human feces. As with term infants, therefore, preterm infants born in vaginal deliveries are exposed at birth to fecal bacteria that colonize their colons.

Harmsen *et al.* (2000) used novel molecular technologies to examine the bacterial species in the feces of term infants. These investigators cultured isolates from feces and used fluorescence in situ hybridization (FISH) with 16S rRNA targeted oligonucleotide probes to assess the bacterial species present in feces from infants consuming either breast milk or formula during the first 20 days after normal birth. The media used for culturing isolates from feces proved to be insufficiently selective and unsuitable for quantitative analysis of fecal biota. Nevertheless, both the cultural methods and use of the FISH technique demonstrated that the infants were colonized soon after birth by a complex biota similar to that of adults. Shortly thereafter, a succession began that led to a biota in breast-fed infants with species of *Bifidobacterium* predominating and to a biota in formula-fed infants with *Bacteroides* and bifidobacterial species predominating. These findings generally confirmed others made with conventional tools on the succession of the fecal biota in infants. They have added as well the novel observation that babies fed on formula have high populations of *Bacteroides* and bifidobacteria as well as of lactobacilli. Species of the latter bacteria have been reported to dominate in feces of formula-fed infants in numerous studies in which conventional technologies have been used (Benno *et al.* 1985; Wharton *et al.* 1994).

In a study focused on *Lactobacillus* strains, Matsumiya *et al.* (2002) tested whether or not *Lactobacillus* strains are transmitted from mother to infant during birth. They used arbitrarily primed PCR (AP-PCR) with enterobacterial repetitive intergenic sequences (ERIC1R and ERIC2) primers to identify strains isolated from the feces of newborns and from the vaginas of their mothers. Only about one-fourth of infants were found to acquire vaginal lactobacilli from their mothers. The strains did not long persist in the infant gut but were replaced after birth by lactobacilli from milk and unknown sources (Matsumiya *et al.* 2002).

Findings on succession of the mucosal microbiota suggest that indigenous microorganisms interact with the immunologic system of neonates and infants up to 2 or more years old in ways that may differ from such interactions in young and middle-aged adults (see the following text). As noted, the populations of the various bacterial genera increase and decrease during succession. The child's immunologic system, therefore, presumably is exposed to microbial antigens that vary over time in quantity and quality. That antigenic

exposure occurs during the time maternal antibodies are circulating in the neonates' blood and thereafter as those antibodies clear from the system and the infants' own immunologic systems assume full responsibility for resistance to disease. These phenomena make for considerable complexity for investigators interested in the immunologic responses to the indigenous mucosal microbiota.

The colonic microbiota of individuals in advanced age, as evaluated with conventional technologies, differs qualitatively and quantitatively from that of young and middle-aged adults (Benno *et al.* 1985; Hebuterne 2003; Mitsuoka 1992). Compared to the biota of younger adults, the biota of the aged contains larger populations of clostridia of various species and smaller populations of bifidobacteria and lactobacilli (Hebuterne 2003; Mitsuoka 1992). Diversity in the various bacterial species present also changes with aging. For example, diversity in *Bacteroides* species increases and that of *Bifidobacterium* species decreases (Hopkins and Macfarlane 2002; Saunier and Dore 2002). Likewise, the capacity of species of bifidobacteria to adhere to intestinal mucus also decreases in the elderly (He *et al.* 2001).

Since the data mentioned previously were derived from analyses of feces, little can be said about the mucosal microbiota of the colon in elderly individuals. The findings suggest, nevertheless, that as with infants, the mucosal immunologic system of persons of advanced age may experience net contact with indigenous bacteria differing from that experienced by young and middle-aged persons. The findings also suggest that, as is known for neonates and infants, "colonization resistance" in the aged differs from that in the young and the middle-aged.

THE MUCOSAL MICROBIOTA AND "COLONIZATION RESISTANCE" (NATURAL DEFENSE)

The mucosal microbiota in various areas of the body has been known for many years to have the capacity either to limit the growth of, or to kill, certain transient microbial pathogens entering their habitats. Some strains of *S. aureus* in the nasopharynx can prevent pathogenic strains of the same bacterium from colonizing the mucosal surface (Tannock 1995). The biota of the normal vagina can prevent *Candida albicans* and certain other microbial pathogens from colonizing the mucosal epithelium of that area of the body (Redondo-Lopez *et al.* 1990). The biota of the GI canal is known to prevent *Clostridium difficile* from proliferating on the cecal and colonic epithelium (Tannock 1995; van der Waaij 1989). The GI microbiota also restricts to relatively low levels the indigenous populations of *E. coli* and other coliform bacteria (Freter *et al.* 1983). These phenomena have been called "colonization resistance" (Gaya and Verhoef 1988).

The mechanisms of colonization resistance are far from understood. Nutritional competition is, however, established as an important mechanism (Roberfroid *et al.* 1995). Indigenous coliform populations are suppressed in the cecum of adult mice, at least partially, by nutritional competition with anaerobic elements of the indigenous microbiota (Freter *et al.* 1983). Similarly, populations of *C. difficile* may be suppressed by nutritional competition with the murine cecal microbiota (Wilson and Perini 1988). Some evidence suggests, however, that the populations of that pathogen may also be suppressed by volatile short-chain fatty acids that are end products of anaerobic bacterial metabolism in the colon and cecum (Su *et al.* 1987). That finding is echoed in observations that lactic acid and hydrogen peroxide produced by lactobacilli may be involved in suppression by the indigenous biota of microbial pathogens in the vagina (Hillier *et al.* 1993; Redondo-Lopez *et al.* 1990).

In addition to nutritional competition and toxicity of metabolic end products, factors such as bacteriocins and competition for mucosal adhesion sites may also be involved in the capacity of indigenous biota to suppress pathogens (Savage 1983b). That capacity, then, is likely to entail multiple mechanisms. One fact is established, however: The mechanisms involve net processes exerted by the microbiota as a whole. Colonization resistance to a particular microbial pathogen is rarely reproducibly demonstrated in ex-GF animals colonized with one, two, or several indigenous microbial species (Freter *et al.* 1983; Savage 1983b). Even when a single bacterial species can be shown to inhibit a pathogen, that inhibition takes place against a background of a full biota (Alak *et al.* 1997). Therefore, to function optimally, colonization resistance requires the entire indigenous microbiota operating as a kind of organ. A similar circumstance may be involved in the interactions of the indigenous mucosal microbiota and the immunologic system.

THE MUCOSAL MICROBIOTA AND IMMUNOLOGIC SYSTEM

The capacity of humans to mount immunologic responses develops and functions in an environment that includes the indigenous microbiota of mucosal surfaces (Ouwehand *et al.* 2002). That biota interacts with cells that mediate those responses and influences those cells as they mature in infants and children and as they function in adults. The mechanisms mediating the ways in which the biota interacts with immunologic systems have been under study for many years (Gaskins 1997; Henderson *et al.* 1996; Tannock 1995). The studies began with observations made with germfree (GF) animals.

GF animals have been available for experimental use for over 80 years (Gustafsson 1984). From the earliest days, investigators realized that such animals differed in many ways from their conventional counterparts with a microbiota. Most of the differences were physiologic; some were anatomic. One of the most striking anatomic differences was observed in the gut-associated lymphoid tissue (GALT) in the Peyer's patches and lamina propria of the intestines. Those tissues in conventional animals were prominent and stocked with monocytic cells in large numbers. By contrast,

in GF animals, they tended to be hypocellular, containing few monocytic elements (Bealmear *et al.* 1984).

These early observations led to intense experimental interest in the immunologic systems of GF animals of many species including mice, rats, guinea pigs, rabbits, swine, chickens, and monkeys. Findings from those early experiments have been reviewed (Bealmear *et al.* 1984; Berg 1983). This text summarizes only some of the most important observations.

By comparison with conventional animals, the blood of GF animals contains IgG in only small amounts and IgM in low to undetectable amounts. In addition, GF animals produce no detectable IgA. In spite of these humoral deficits, the animals are able to mount both cellular and humoral responses to antigenic challenge. Delayed hypersensitivity responses (DTH) generally develop at rates comparable to the rates at which they develop in conventionals. Humoral and secretory responses develop at somewhat slower rates than those of animals with a microbiota, but eventually reach similar quantitative levels. These findings have been interpreted to mean that GF animals are fully competent immunologically but are not challenged by environmental and microbial antigens that impact on the conventional animal (Bealmear *et al.* 1984; Berg 1983). They have also been interpreted to mean that the immunologic system in a "normal" conventional animal is the product of interacting immunologic processes and molecules from indigenous microorganisms.

Studies of the mechanisms by which the indigenous biota on mucosal surfaces interacts with the body's immunologic system have been focused on two interrelated phenomena: (1) The system is tolerant of the indigenous microbiota, and (2) the microbiota communicates with the intestinal cytokine network. The following text summarizes some findings that illustrate recent approaches to study of the mechanisms underlying those phenomena. The summary is not exhaustive and includes only findings from studies that indicate the focus and direction of current research in the area.

The immunologic system is tolerant of the indigenous microbiota

In 1983, Berg reviewed information available at the time on antibody responses to antigens of bacteria in the intestinal microbiota. He discussed "natural antibodies" and concluded that serum and secretions of healthy adult human subjects contain in low titers IgA, IgG, and IgM antibodies reactive with antigens of indigenous intestinal bacteria. Berg cautioned that such antibodies could be induced by dietary as well as microbial antigens, but highlighted evidence concerning antibodies induced by antigens of indigenous bacteria (Berg 1983). In particular, he compared antibody responses to indigenous and nonindigenous bacteria either injected into or given orally to GF rodents. He concluded that the results supported a hypothesis that certain bacteria indigenous to the gastrointestinal tract do not elicit as great a host immune response as do various nonindigenous bacteria (Berg 1983).

The evidence for tolerance to antigens of indigenous bacteria was discussed in some detail by Gaskins (1997), who concluded his review, "The complex and paradoxical relationship between the animal host and the autochthonous microbiota residing in its gastrointestinal tract provide a consummate model system to investigate mechanisms underlying oral tolerance." That tolerance has been under study by Cebra and his colleagues (Cebra 1999, p. 585).

In one study, Shroff et al. (1995) associated GF mice with various gram-negative and gram-positive bacteria and found that not all organisms able to colonize the gut induced an efficient humoral immune response in the mucosa. In another effort, Shroff et al. associated GF mice with the facultative anaerobic bacterium *Morganella morganii* and observed that the organism rapidly colonized the guts of the gnotobiotes and stimulated in them hypertrophy of Peyer's patches, including germinal center reactions (GCR), and development of specific IgA (Shroff et al. 1995). The GCR peaked 14 days after the animals were colonized and thereafter began to wane. The bacteria translocated to mesenteric lymph nodes until the onset of the specific IgA response. Shroff et al. (1995) suggested that a secretory IgA (S-IgA) response to the facultative anaerobe attenuates chronic stimulation of GCR even though the bacteria persist in the gut.

S-IgA is known to clear transient intestinal pathogens such as *Salmonella typhimurium* and *Vibrio cholerae* from the guts of mice (Apter et al. 1993; Michetti et al. 1992). S-IgA does not, however, clear indigenous anaerobic bacteria from the intestine even though such bacteria in feces may be coated with them (van der Waaij et al. 1994). Such findings confirm that the mucosal immunologic system is tolerant of bacterial components of the intestinal biota (Berg 1983). The mechanisms of that tolerance may come from research on how the microbiota interacts with the cytokine network.

The indigenous microbiota communicates with the cytokine network

In a comprehensive and important review of information available at the time on how the microbiota and immunologic systems interact, Henderson et al. (1996, p. 1) wrote, "We propose that the ability of the multicellular organism to live harmoniously with its commensal microflora must depend on mutual signaling involving eukaryotic cytokines and prokaryotic cytokine-like molecules." They referred to the latter molecules as "bacteriokines" and described them as diverse bacterial molecules that can "selectively induce the synthesis of both pro-inflammatory and immunomodulatory/anti-inflammatory cytokines." Henderson et al. listed such bacterial molecules, including protein toxins, cell-surface polysaccharides, endotoxin-associated proteins, lipoproteins, peptidoglycan, and many others. They emphasized that certain of the molecules can downregulate proinflammatory cytokine networks and that cytokines can bind to bacteria and influence their behavior. They stated their view that the indigenous biota and the eukaryotic animal cells of man are in constant communication (Henderson et al. 1996). Henderson and Wilson (1998) recently reaffirmed the view.

Recent evidence for the "bacteriokine" hypothesis has come from the interest of numerous investigators in certain properties of butyric acid. As noted earlier, this compound is an end product of bacterial metabolism in the colon and is the energy source for colonocytes (Saemann et al. 2002). It has recently been discovered to have antiinflammatory activity and may mediate that activity by interfering in intestinal epithelial and lamina propria cells with transcription factors critical for synthesis of proinflammatory cytokines (Saemann et al. 2002). These findings may have important implications for treatment of inflammatory bowel disease (IBD) (Segain et al. 2000).

The etiology of IBD may involve antigens of the indigenous biota. For example, in diseases such as Crohn's disease and ulcerative colitis, the intestinal mucosa is infiltrated with T lymphocytes responsive to microbial antigens (Duchmann et al. 1995). These authors tested a hypothesis that IBD results when normal immunologic tolerance to antigens of the indigenous biota is broken in the human intestine. They used an *in vitro* system to assay for the capacity of sonicates of bacteria from the intestine to induce proliferation of mononuclear cells from inflamed and normal intestinal mucosa and blood from patients with IBD, and from normal mucosa and blood from individuals free of the disease. The sonicates were able to induce proliferation in the mononuclear cells from inflamed but not from normal intestine. They were unable, however, to induce proliferation in cells from the blood of either the patients or normal individuals. Only sonicates from bacteria derived from an individual other than the person whose cells were being tested were able to induce intestinal mononuclear cells (Duchmann et al. 1995).

Kuhn et al. (1993) have also been interested in IBD and have been studying immune cell functions in chronic enterocolitis generated by gene targeting in interleukin-10–deficient (IL-10–deficient) mice. They suggested that the bowel inflammation in their animals originates from uncontrolled immune responses stimulated by enteric antigens, and that IL-10 is an essential immunoregulator controlling such responses in genetically intact mice. More recently, they have demonstrated that the colitis in their IL-10–deficient animals is mediated by aberrant cytokine production (Berg et al. 1996) and T helper cell 1–type CD4(+) cells (Davidson et al. 1996).

Duchmann et al. (1999) tested T-lymphocyte specificity and cross-reactivity toward antigens from various species of facultative and anaerobic bacteria from the intestinal biota. T-cell clones were isolated with phytohemagglutinin from peripheral blood and biopsy specimens of inflamed and non-inflamed colon from patients with IBD and from normal controls. The clones were restimulated with various isolates of intestinal bacteria. *Bifidobacterium* and *Bacteroides* isolates specifically stimulated CD4+TCRαβ lymphocytes from both blood and biopsies from patients with IBD. Clones isolated from the patients and the normal subjects were reactive with facultative bacteria from a person other than themselves. Clones from patients with IBD were stimulated also, however, by facultative bacteria from their own biota.

The investigators concluded from the findings that immune responses to antigens from the intestinal biota involve a complex network of T-cell specificities (Duchmann *et al.* 1999).

Those findings provide support for the hypothesis that the systemic and intestinal immune systems are normally tolerant of the intestinal biota and that the tolerance is broken in IBD. They also suggested that each individual may be unique in tolerance to indigenous biota (Duchmann *et al.* 1995, 1999). Such findings hold important implications for future research on the mechanisms by which mucosal microbiota communicates with the cytokine network.

Such communication may require the entire indigenous microbiota. The entire biota, engaging in "cross-talk" (Bry *et al.* 1996) with the cytokine network, may inhibit inflammation in the mucosa. It may also prevent secretory immunoglobulins reactive with bacterial members of the biota from removing the biota from the mucosal surface. Therefore, an intact intestinal microbiota may be necessary not only for effective colonization resistance, but also for effective communication with the cytokine network. In other words, the indigenous microbiota may function as an accessory "organ" in the human body (Savage 1989).

One function of that accessory organ is to cooperate with the immunologic system in the most important game of preventing disease. This game goes on throughout life, but may proceed by different rules in neonates, young children, and the aged from the way it is played in young and middle-aged adults. Such differences may be illustrated by interesting findings of several research groups who are testing a postulate that atopic allergy in young children is caused by exposure to intestinal biotas of abnormal composition in infancy (Kalliomaki *et al.* 2001). Such findings should inspire experimental work for many years to come.

CONCLUSION

Microorganisms, principally bacteria, colonize the skin and mucosal surfaces in most areas of the adult human body. Gram-positive, aerobic bacteria predominate on the skin and the mucosa of the nasopharynx and oropharynx. Over 200 species of gram-positive and gram-negative bacteria of several facultative and strictly anaerobic genera colonize the surface of the teeth and mucosal surfaces of the mouth (oral cavity). Gram-positive and gram-negative facultative and anaerobic bacteria also colonize the mucosal surface and lumen of major portions of the GI tract. In this case, however, over 400 to 500 species of as many as 40 to 50 genera are involved. The anaerobic bacteria predominate by manyfold in both the buccal cavity, the distal one-third of the small intestine, and large intestine. Functional anaerobes also predominate on vaginal surfaces. In this case, however, most of the organisms are members of the genus *Lactobacillus*. In aggregate, the microbial populations on all mucosal surfaces exceed 100 trillion (1×10^{14}) cells. This enormous population, over 99% of which is found in the large intestine, constitutes an indigenous microbiota. This biota establishes on the various mucosal surfaces after birth in patterns that can be recognized as ecologic successions. The indigenous microbiota functions in "colonization resistance" to inhibit nonindigenous microorganisms and certain indigenous microbial pathogens from proliferating in the mucosal habitats. In addition, this biota interacts with the immunologic system throughout life. Secretory antibodies develop to antigens of some bacterial species in the biota, and "bacteriokines" produced by bacterial members of the biota communicate with the cytokine network. This communication ("cross-talk") results in immunologic nonreactivity (tolerance) to the microbiota. When this tolerance is broken, inflammation can result that damages the mucosae.

REFERENCES

Alak, J. I. B., Wolf, B. W., Mdurvwa, E. G., Pimentil-Smith, G. E., and Adeyemo, O. (1997). Effect of *Lactobacillus reuteri* on intestinal resistance to *Cryptosporidium parvum* infection in a murine model of acquired immunodeficiency syndrome. *J. Infect. Dis.* 175, 218–221.

Antonio, M. A. D., Hawes, S. E., and Hillier, S. L. (1999). The identification of vaginal *Lactobacillus* species and the demographic and microbiologic characteristics of women colonized by these species. *J. Infect. Dis.* 180, 1950–1956.

Apter, F. M., Michetti, P., Winner, L. S., III, Mack, J. A., Mekalanos, J. J., and Neutra, M. R. (1993). Analysis of the roles of anti-lipolysaccharide and anti-cholera toxin immunoglobulin A (IgA) antibodies in protection against *Vibrio cholerae* and cholera toxin by use of monoclonal IgA antibodies in vivo. *Infect. Immun.* 61, 5279–5285.

Bealmear, P. M., Holtermann, O. A., and Mirand, E. A. (1984). Influence of the microflora on the immune response. Part 1. General characteristics of the germ-free animal. Part 2. Gnotobiotic animals in immunological research. In *The Germ-Free Animal in Biomedical Research* (eds. M. E. Coates and B. E. Gustafsson), 335–386. London: Laboratory Animals Ltd.

Benno, Y., Sawada, K, and Mitsuoka, T. (1985). The intestinal microflora of infants: Composition of fecal flora in breast-fed and bottle-fed infants. *Microbiol. Immunol.* 28, 975–986.

Berg, R. (1983). Host immune response to antigens of the indigenous intestinal flora. In *Human Intestinal Microflora in Health and Disease*, (ed. D. J. Hentges), 101–128. New York: Academic Press.

Berg, D. J., Davidson, N., Kuhn, R., Muller, W., Menon, S., Holland G., Thompson-Snipes, L., Leach, M. W., and Rennick, D. (1996). Enterocolitis and colon cancer in interleukin-10 deficient mice are associated with aberrant cytokine production and CD4+ TH1-like responses. *J. Clin. Invest.* 98, 1010–1020.

Blaut, M., Collins, M. D., Welling, G. W., Dore, J., van Loo, J., and de Vos, W. (2002). Molecular biological methods for studying the gut microbiota: The EU human gut flora project. *Brit. J. Nutr.* 87, S203–S211.

Bry, L., Falk, P. G., Midtvedt, T., and Gordon, J. I. (1996). A model of host-microbial interactions in an open mammalian ecosystem. *Science* 273, 1380–1383.

Burton, J. P., Cadieux, P. A., and Reid, G. (2003). Improved understanding of the bacterial vaginal microbiota of women before and after probiotic instillation. *Appl. Environ. Microbiol.* 69, 97–101.

Cebra, J. J. (1999). Influences of microbiota on intestinal immune system development. *Am. J. Clin. Nutr.* 69, 1046S–1051S.

Chiller, K., Selkin, B. A., and Murakawa, G. J. (2001). Skin microflora and bacterial infections of the skin. *J. Invest. Dermatol. Symp. Proc.* 6, 170–174.

Ciampolini, M., Bini, S., and Orsi, A. (1996). Microflora persistence on duodenojejunal flat or normal mucosa in time after a meal in children. *Physiol. Behavior* 60, 1551–1556.

Ciantar, M., Spratt, D. A., Newman, H. N., and Wilson, M. (2001). *Capnocytophaga granulose* and *Capnocytophaga haemolytica*: Novel species in subgingival plaque. *J. Clin. Periodontol.* 28, 701–705.

Cooperstock, M. S., and Zedd, A. J. (1983). Intestinal flora of infants. In *Human Intestinal Microflora in Health and Disease* (ed. D. J. Hentges), 79–100. New York: Academic Press.

Davidson, N. J., Leach, M. W., Fort, M. M., Thompson-Snipes, L., Kuhn, R., Muller, W., Berg, D. J., and Rennick, D. M. (1996). T helper cell 1-type CD4+ T cells, but not B cells, mediate colitis in interleukin 10-deficient mice. *J. Exp. Med.* 184, 241–251.

Davies, C. E., Wilson, J. J., Hill, K. E., Stephens, P., Hill, C. M., Harding, K. G., and Thomas, D. W. (2001). Use of molecular techniques to study microbial diversity in the skin: Chronic wound repair reevaluated. *Wound Repair Regen.* 9, 332–340.

Duchmann, R., Kaiser, I., Hermann, E., Mayet, W., Ewe, K., and Zumbuschenfelde, K. H. M. (1995). Tolerance exists towards resident intestinal flora but is broken in active inflammatory bowel-disease (IBD). *Clin. Exp. Immunol.* 102, 448–455.

Duchmann, R., May, E., Heike, M., Knolle, P., Neurath, M., and Meyer zum Buschenfelde, K. H. (1999). T cell specificity and cross reactivity towards enterobacteria, bacteroides, bifidobacterium and antigens from resident intestinal flora in humans. *Gut* 44, 812–818.

Elitsur, Y., Lawrence, Z., and Triest, W. E. (2002). Distribution of *Helicobacter pylori* organisms in the stomachs of children with *H. pylori* infection. *Human Pathol.* 33, 1133–1135.

Eschenbach, D. A., Patton, D. L., Meier, A., Thwin, S. S., Aura, J., Stapleton, A., and Hooton, T. M. (2000). Effects of oral contraceptive pill use on vaginal flora and vaginal epithelium. *Contraception* 62, 107–112.

Finegold, S. M., Sutter, V. L., and Mathisen, G. E. (1983). Normal indigenous intestinal flora. In *Human Intestinal Microflora in Health and Disease* (ed. D. J. Hentges), 3–32. New York: Academic Press.

Franks, A. H., Harmsen, H. J. M., Raangs, G. C., Jansen, G. J., Schut, F., and Welling, G. W. (1998). Variations of bacterial populations in human feces measured by fluorescent in situ hybridization with group-specific 16S rRNA-targeted oligonucleotide probes. *Appl. Environ. Microbiol.* 64, 3336–3345.

Freter, R., Brickner, H., Botney, M., Cleven, D., and Aranki, A. (1983). Mechanisms that control bacterial populations in continuous-flow culture models of mouse large intestinal flora. *Infect. Immun.* 39, 676–685.

Gaitanis, G., Velegraki, A., Frangoulis, E. I., Mitroussia, A., Tsigonia, A., Tzimogianni, A., Katsambas, A., and Legakin, J. J. (2002). Identification of *Malassezia* species from patient skin scales by PCR-RFLP. *Clin. Microbiol. Infect.* 8, 162–173.

Gaskins, H. R. (1997). Immunological aspects of host/microbiota interactions at the intestinal epithelium. In *Gastrointestinal Microbiology* (eds. R. I. Mackie, B. A. White, and R. E. Isaacson), Vol. 2, 537–587. New York: Chapman and Hall.

Gaya, H., and Verhoef, J., eds. (1988). Current topic: colonization resistance. *Eur. J. Clin. Microbiol. Infect. Dis.* 7, 91–113.

Grubb, R., Midtvedt, T., and Norin, E., eds. (1989). *The Regulatory and Protective Role of the Normal Microflora*, 1–416. New York: Stockton.

Guillemin, K., Salama, N. R., Tompkins, L. S., and Falkow, S. (2002). Cag pathogenicity island-specific responses of gastric epithelial cells to *Helicobacter pylori* infection. *Proc. Natl. Acad. Sci. U.S.A.* 99, 15136–15141.

Gupta, K., Hillier, S. L., Hooton, T. M., Roberts, P. L., and Stamm, W. E. (2000). Effects of contraceptive method on the vaginal microbial flora: A prospective evaluation. *J. Infect. Dis.* 181, 595–601.

Gustafsson, B. E. (1984). The germ-free animal: Its potential and its problems. In *The Germ-Free Animal in Biomedical Research* (eds. M. E. Coates and B. E. Gustafsson), 1–10. London: Laboratory Animals Ltd., Litho Service.

Harmsen, H. J., Wildeboer-Velco, A. C., Raangs, G. C., Wagendorp, A. A., Klijn, N., Bindels, J. G., and Welling, G. W. (2000). Analysis of intestinal flora development in breast-fed and formula-fed infants by using molecular identification and detection methods. *J. Pediatr. Gastroenterol. Nutr.* 30, 61–67.

He, F., Ouwehand, A. C., Isolauri, E., Hosoda, M., Benno, Y., and Salminen, S. (2001). Differences in composition and mucosal adhesion of bifidobacteria isolated from healthy adults and healthy seniors. *Curr. Microbiol.* 43, 351–354.

Hebuterne, X. (2003). Gut changes attributed to ageing: Effects on intestinal microflora. *Curr. Opin. Clin. Nutr. Metab. Care* 6, 49–54.

Henderson, B., and Wilson, M. (1998). Commensal communism and the oral cavity. *J. Dent. Res.* 77, 1674–1683.

Henderson, B., Poole, S., and Wilson, M. (1996). Microbial/host interactions in health and disease: Who controls the cytokine network? *Immunopharmacology* 35, 1–21.

Hentges, D. J. (1993). The anaerobic microflora of the human body. *Clin. Infect. Dis.* 16, S175–S180.

Hillier, S. L., and Lau, R. J. (1997). Vaginal microflora in postmenopausal women who have not received estrogen replacement therapy. *Clin. Infect. Dis.* 25, S123–S126.

Hillier, S. L., Krohn, M. A., Rabe, L. K., Klebanoff, S. J., and Eschenbach, D. A. (1993). The normal vaginal flora, H_2O_2-producing lactobacilli, and bacterial vaginosis in pregnant women. *Clin. Infect. Dis.* 16, S273–S281.

Hokama, T., Hamamoto, I., Takenaka, S., Hirayama, K., Yara, A., and Adjei, A. (1996). Throat microflora in breastfed and formula-fed infants. *J. Trop. Pediatr.* 42, 324–326.

Holdeman, L. V., Good, I. J., and Moore, W. E. C. (1976). Human fecal flora: Ariation in bacterial composition within individuals and a possible effect of emotional stress. *Appl. Environ. Microbiol.* 31, 359–375.

Holland, K. T., and Bojar, R. A. (2002). Cosmetics: What is their influence on the skin microflora? *Am. J. Clin. Dermatol.* 3, 445–449.

Hopkins, J. J., and Macfarlane, G. T. (2002). Changes in predominant bacterial populations in human faeces with age and with *Clostridium difficile* infection. *J. Med. Microbiol.* 51, 448–454.

Kalliomaki, M., Kirjavainen, P., Erola, E., Kero, P., Salminen, S., and Isolauri, E. (2001). Distinct patterns of neonatal gut microflora in infants in whom atopy was and was not developing. *J. Allergy Clin. Immunol.* 107, 129–131.

Kononen, E., Jousimies-Somer, H., Bryk, A., Kilp, T., and Kilian, M. (2002). Establishment of streptococci in the upper respiratory tract: Longitudinal changes in the mouth and nasopharynx up to 2 years of age. *J. Med. Microbiol.* 51, 723–730.

Kononen, E., Kanervo, A., Takala, A., Asikainen, S., and Jousimies-Somer, H. (1999). Establishment of oral anaerobes during the first year of life. *J. Dent. Res.* 78, 1634–1639.

Kuhn, R., Lohler, J., Rennick, D., Rajewsky, K., and Muller, W. (1993). Interleukin-10-deficient mice develop chronic enterocolitis. *Cell* 75, 263–274.

Lee, A., Fox, J., and Hazell, S. (1993). Pathogenicity of *Helicobacter pylori*: A perspective. *Infect. Immun.* 61, 1601–1610.

Loesche, W. J. (1994). Ecology of the oral flora. In *Oral Microbiology and Immunology* (eds. R. J. Nisengard and M. G. Newman), 307–319. Philadelphia: Saunders.

Mandar, R., and Mikelsaar, M. (1996). Transmission of mothers' microflora to the newborn at birth. *Biol. Neonate* 69, 30–35.

Marrie, T. J., Swantee, C. A., and Hartlen, M. (1980). Aerobic and anaerobic urethral flora of healthy females in various physiological age groups and of females with urinary tract infections. *J. Clin. Microbiol.* 11, 654–659.

Matsuki, T., Watanabe, K., Tanaka, R., Fukuda, M., and Oyaizu, H. (1999). Distribution of bifidobacterial species in human intestinal microflora examined with 16S rRNA-gene-targeted species-specific primers. *Appl. Environ. Microbiol.* 65, 4506–4512.

Matsuki, T., Watanabe, K., Fujimoto, J., Miyamoto, Y., Takada, T., Matsumoto, K., Oyaizu, H., and Tanaka, R. (2002). Development of 16S rRNA-gene-targeted group-specific primers for the detection and identification of predominant bacteria in human feces. *Appl. Environ. Microbiol.* 68, 5445–5451.

Matsumiya, Y., Kato, N., Watanabe, K., and Kato, H. (2002). Molecular epidemiological study of vertical transmission of vaginal

Lactobacillus species from mothers to newborn infants in Japanese, by arbitrarily primed polymerase chain reaction. *J. Infect. Chemother.* 8, 43–49.

McCarthy, C., Snyder, M. L., and Parker, R. B. (1965). The indigenous oral flora of man. I. The newborn to the 1-year-old infant. *Arch. Oral. Biol.* 10, 61–70.

Michetti, P., Mahan, M. J., Slauch, J. M., Mekalanos, J. J., and Neutra, M. R. (1992). Monoclonal secretory immunoglobulin A protects mice against oral challenge with the invasive pathogen *Salmonella typhimurium*. *Infect. Immun.* 60, 1786–1792.

Millar, M. R., Linton, C. J., Cade, A., Glancy, D., Hall, M., and Jalal, H. (1996). Application of 16S rRNA gene PCR to study of bowel flora of preterm infants with and without necrotizing enterocolitis. *J. Clin. Microbiol.* 34, 2506–2510.

Miller, T. L., and Wolin, M. J. (1986). Methanogens in human and animal intestinal tract. *Syst. Appl. Microbiol.* 7, 223–229.

Mitsuoka, T. (1992). Intestinal flora and aging. *Nutr. Rev.* 50, 438–446.

Munson, M. A., Pitt-Ford, T., Chong, B., Weightman, A., and Wade, W. G. (2002). Molecular and cultural analysis of the microflora associated with endodontic infections. *J. Dent. Res.* 81, 761–766.

Ouwehand, A., Isolauri, E., and Salminen, S. (2002). The role of the intestinal microflora for the development of the immune system in early childhood. *Eur. J. Nutr.* 41, 132–137.

Pearce, C., Bowden, G. H., Evans, M., Fitzsimmons, S. P., Johnson, J., Sheridan, M. J., Wientzen, R., and Cole, M. F. (1995). Identification of pioneer viridans streptococci in the oral cavity of human neonates. *J. Med. Microbiol.* 42, 67–72.

Percival, R. S., Marsh, P. D., and Challacombe, S. J. (1996). Serum antibodies to commensal oral and gut bacteria vary with age. *FEMS Immunol. Med. Microbiol.* 15, 35–42.

Redondo-Lopez, V., Cook, R. L., and Sobel, J. D. (1990). Emerging role of lactobacilli in the control and maintenance of the vaginal bacterial microflora. *Rev. Infect. Dis.* 12, 856–872.

Requena, T., Burton, J., Matsuki, T., Munro, K., Simon, M. A., Tanaka, R., Watanabe, K., and Tannock, G. W. (2002). Identification, detection, and enumeration of human *Bifidobacterium* species by PCR targeting the transaldolase gene. *Appl. Environ. Microbiol.* 68, 2420–2427.

Roberfroid, M. B., Fornet, F., Bouley, C., and Cummings, J. H. (1995). Colonic microflora: Nutrition and health. Summary and conclusions of an International Life Sciences Institute (ILSI) [Europe] workshop held in Barcelona, Spain. *Nutr. Rev.* 53, 127–130.

Saemann, M. D., Bohmig, G. A., and Zlabinger, G. J. (2002). Short-chain fatty acids: Bacterial mediators of a balanced host-microbial relationship in the human gut. *Wien. Klin. Wochenschr.* 114, 289–300.

Sakata, H., Yoshioka, H., and Fujita, K. (1985). Development of the intestinal flora in very low birth weight infants compared to normal full-term newborns. *Pediatrics* 144, 186–190.

Samsioe, G. (1998). Urogenital aging: A hidden problem. *Am. J. Obstet. Gynecol.* 178, S245–S249.

Satokari, R. M., Vaughan, E. E., Akkermans, A. D., Saarela, M., and de Vos, W. M. (2001). Bifidobacterial diversity in human feces detected by genus-specific PCR and denaturing gradient gel electrophoresis. *Appl. Environ. Microbiol.* 67, 504–513.

Saunier, K., and Dore, J. (2002). Gastrointestinal tract and the elderly: Functional foods, gut microflora and healthy ageing. *Digest. Liver Dis.* 34, S19–S24.

Savage, D. C. (1977). Microbial ecology of the gastrointestinal tract. *Annu. Rev. Microbiol.* 31, 107–133.

Savage, D. C. (1983a). Associations of indigenous microorganisms with gastrointestinal epithelial surfaces. In *Human Intestinal Microflora in Health and Disease* (ed. D. J. Hentges), 55–78. New York: Academic Press.

Savage, D. C. (1983b). Factors influencing biocontrol of bacterial pathogens in the intestine. *Food Technol.* 41, 82–87.

Savage, D. C. (1986). Role of the gastrointestinal microflora in mammalian nutrition. *Annu. Rev. Nutr.* 6, 155–178.

Savage, D. C. (1989). The normal human microflora composition. In *The Regulatory and Protective Role of the Normal Microflora* (eds. R. Grubb, T. Midvedt, and E. Norin), 3–18. London: Stockton.

Savage, D. C. (2002). Intestinal bacteriology for the 21st century. *Biosci. Microflora* 20, 107–114.

Savage, D. C., Lundeen, S. G., and O'Connor, L. T. (1995). Mechanisms by which indigenous microorganisms colonize epithelial surfaces as a reservoir of the luminal microflora in the gastrointestinal tract. *Microecol. Therapy* 21, 27–36.

Schwebke, J. R., Richey, C. M., and Weiss, H. L. (1999). Correlation of behaviors with microbiological changes in vaginal flora. *J. Infect. Dis.* 180, 1632–1636.

Segain, J. P., Raingeard de la Bletiere, D., Bourrielle, A., Leray, V., Gervois, N., Rosales, C., Ferrier, L., Gonnet, C., Blottiere, H. M., and Galmiche, J. P. (2000). Butyrate inhibits inflammatory responses through NfkapaB inhibition: Implications for Crohn's disease. *Gut* 47, 397–403.

Seifert, H., Dijkshoorn, L., Gerner-Smidt, P., Pelzer, N., Tjernberg, I., and Vaneechoutte, M. (1997). Distribution of *Acinetobacter* species on human skin: Comparison of phenotypic and genotypic identification methods. *J. Clin. Microbiol.* 35, 2819–2825.

Shroff, K. E., Meslin, K., and Cebra, J. J. (1995). Comensal enteric bacteria engender a self-limiting humoral mucosal immune response while permanently colonizing the gut. *Infect. Immun.* 63, 3904–3913.

Sobel, J. D., and Chain, W. (1996). Vaginal microbiology of women with acute recurrent vulvovaginal candidiasis. *J. Clin. Microbiol.* 34, 2497–2499.

Stevens, C. E., and Hume, I. D. (1995). *Comparative Physiology of the Vertebrate Digestive System.* Cambridge: Cambridge University Press.

Su, W. J., Waechter, M. J., Bourlioux, P., Dolegeal, M., Fourniat, J., and Mahuzier, G. (1987). Role of volatile fatty acids in colonization resistance to *Clostridium difficile* in gnotobiotic mice. *Infect. Immun.* 55, 1686–1691.

Suau, A., Bonnet, R., Sutren, M., Godon, J.-J., Bibsio, G. R., Collins, M. D., and Dore, J. (1999). Direct analysis of genes encoding 16S rRNA from complex communities reveals many novel molecular species within the human gut. *Appl. Environ. Microbiol.* 65, 4799–4807.

Suchett-Kay, G., Decoret, D., and Barsotti, O. (1999). Intra-familial distribution of *Fusobacterium nucleatum* strains in healthy families with optimal plaque control. *J. Clin. Periodontol.* 26, 401–404.

Tannock, G. W. (1995). *Normal Microflora: An Introduction to Microbes Inhabiting the Human Body*, 1–115. London: Chapman and Hall.

Tannock, G. W. (2002). Analysis of the intestinal microflora using molecular methods. *Eur. J. Clin. Nutr.* 56, S44–S49.

Tham, K. T., Peek, R. M., Jr., Atherton, J. C., Cover, T. L., Perez-Perez, G. I., Shyr, Y., and Blaser, M. J. (2001). *Helicobacter pylori* genotypes, host factors, and gastric mucosal histopathology in peptic ulcer disease. *Human Pathol.* 32, 264–273.

Till, A. E., Goulden, V., Cunliffe, W. J., and Holland, K. T. (2000). The cutaneous microflora of adolescent, persistent and late-onset acne patient does not differ. *Brit. J. Dermatol.* 142, 885–892.

Van der Waaij, D. (1989). The ecology of the human intestine and its consequences for overgrowth by pathogens such as *Clostridium difficile*. *Annu. Rev. Microbiol.* 43, 69–87.

Van der Waaij, L. A., Mesander, G., Limburg, P. C., and van der Waaij, D. (1994). Direct flow cytometry of anaerobic bacteria in human feces. *Cytometry* 16, 270–279.

Vasquez, A., Jakobsson, T., Ahrne, S., Forsum, U., and Molin, G. (2002). Vaginal *Lactobacillus* flora of healthy Swedish women. *J. Clin. Microbiol.* 40, 2746–2749.

Vaughan, E. E., Schut, F., Heilig, H. G., Zoetendal, E. G., de Vos, W. M., and Akkerman, A. D. (2000). A molecular view of the intestinal ecosytem. *Curr. Issues Intest. Microbiol.* 1, 1–12.

Ventura, M., Casas, I. A., Morelli, L., and Callegari, M. L. (2000). Rapid amplified ribosomal DNA restriction analysis (ARDRA) identification of *Lactobacillus* spp. Isolated from fecal and vaginal samples. *Syst. Appl. Microbiol.* 23, 504–509.

Walter, J., Hertel, C., Tannock, G. W., Lis, C. M., Munro, K., and Hannes, W. P. (2001). Detection of *Lactobacillus*, *Pediococcus*, *Leuconostoc*, and *Weissella* species in human feces by using group-specific PCR primers and denaturing gradient gel electrophoresis. *Appl. Environ. Microbiol.* 67, 2578–2585.

Wang, R. F., Cao, W. W., and Cerniglia, C. E. (1996). PCR detection and quantitation of predominant anaerobic-bacteria in human and animal fecal samples. *Appl. Environ. Microbiol.* 62, 1242–1247.

Wharton, B. A., Balmer, S. E., and Scott, P. H. (1994). Sorrento studies of diet and fecal flora in the newborn. *Acta Paediatr. Japonica* 38, 579–584.

Wilson, K. H., and Perini, F. (1988). Role of competition for nutrients in suppression of *Clostridium difficile* by the colonic microflora. *Infect. Immun.* 56, 2610–2614.

Zoetendal, E. G., von Wright, A., Vilpponen-Salmela, T., Ben-Amor, K., Akkermans, A. D. L., and de Vos, W. M. (2002a). Mucosa-associated bacteria in the human gastrointestinal tract are uniformly distributed along the colon and differ from the community recovered from feces. *Appl. Environ. Microbiol.* 68, 3401–3407.

Zoetendal, E. G., Ben-Amor, K., Harmsen, H. J. M., Schut, F., Akkermans, A. D. L., and de Vos, W. M. (2002b). Quantification of uncultured *Ruminococcus obeum*-like bacteria in human fecal samples by fluorescent in situ hybridization and flow cytometry using 16S rRNA-targeted probes. *Appl. Environ. Microbiol.* 68, 4225–4232.

Adhesion of Bacteria to Mucosal Surfaces

Chapter 3

Soman N. Abraham

Departments of Pathology and Molecular Genetics and Microbiology, Duke University Medical Center, Durham, North Carolina

Brian L. Bishop

Department of Molecular Genetics and Microbiology, Duke University Medical Center, Durham, North Carolina

Nathan Sharon

Department of Membrane Research and Biophysics, Weizmann Institute of Science, Rehovot, Israel

Itzhak Ofek

Department of Human Microbiology, Sackler Faculty of Medicine, Tel-Aviv, University, Tel-Aviv, Israel

INTRODUCTION

An overwhelming number of infectious diseases are initiated by bacterial colonization of the mucosal surfaces of the genitourinary, gastrointestinal, or respiratory tracts. Since mucosal colonization by bacteria is preceded by bacterial attachment to epithelial cells or to mucins coating these mucosal cells, intensive studies have focused on the cellular and molecular aspects underlying the adhesion of bacteria. These studies have revealed that many bacteria express on their surfaces, frequently in the form of specialized organelles, adhesins that seek and bind to cognate receptors on the surface of mucosal cells. The specific binding interaction between the bacterial adhesins and host receptors allows the bacteria to firmly attach to particular sites on the mucosal surfaces and thereby resist dislocation by the hydrokinetic forces that typically act on these surfaces.

Although adhesion of bacteria to mucosal surfaces is an important determinant of mucosal colonization, especially in determining its site and density, it is becoming increasingly clear that this is not the complete story. Several critical postadhesion events are necessary for the bacteria to successfully establish themselves on the mucosal surfaces and to initiate infection. These events, triggered by the adhesion of the bacteria to their complementary receptor on the mucosal cells, include alterations to the expression of virulence factors by the bacteria on one hand and induction of physiologic changes on the mucosal surface. The latter include proliferation of epithelial cells, increased mucus secretion, endocytosis of adherent bacteria, and release of proinflammatory and antiinflammatory

mediators by mucosal and submucosal cells. This chapter briefly reviews the current state of knowledge of bacterial adhesins and their mucosal cell receptors. It then discusses selected postadhesion events and describes how they influence mucosal colonization. Finally, it shows how the knowledge gained provides a basis for the development of antiadhesion agents that can block and even reverse bacterial colonization of mucosal surfaces and their harmful postadhesive events.

BACTERIAL ADHESION CHARACTERISTICS

Classification

The adhesion interactions of more than 100 bacterial pathogens of human and farm animals have been investigated (Ofek 1994). Based on these studies, three main types of adhesin–receptor interactions have been described (**Table 3.1**). The first type, probably shared by the majority of bacterial pathogens studied, is based on lectin–carbohydrate recognition in which the lectin is either on the bacteria or on the mucosal surface. The second type, of which a significant number of cases are known, involves protein–protein recognition between a protein on the bacteria and a complementary protein on the mucosal surface. The third type, and perhaps the least well characterized, involves binding interactions between hydrophobic moieties of proteins and lipids in which the lipid is either on the host cell or on the bacterial surface. The contribution of hydrophobicity to bacterial adhesion to mucosal surfaces is often underestimated because it is responsible for the initial, weak, and reversible interaction that precedes the other, more obvious, binding interactions between microorganisms and their target cells (Doyle 2000; Ofek 1994). The formation of bacterial biofilms on inert and abiotic surfaces of various medical devices has resulted in many infections (Donlan 2002). Bacterial hydrophobicity has been shown to play a dominant role in the formation of such biofilms (Di Martino *et al.* 2003; Faille *et al.* 2002).

Lectins as adhesins

A large number of adhesins are carbohydrate specific and therefore considered as lectins, which bind the bacteria to the carbohydrate moieties of glycoproteins or glycolipids present on epithelial and other cells of the host. Examples of lectin-adhesins and their sugar specificities are shown in **Table 3.2**. The lectins can be either in the form of fimbrial structure, capsule, or as an outer membrane component in gram-negative bacteria. The adhesin-lectin binds to complementary sugars presented in glycoproteins and/or glycolipids on animal cell surface. Methods have been developed for the detection of new lectin/adhesins and their complementary receptors (Goldhar 1994; Hatakeyama *et al.* 1996). A more comprehensive list of lectin-adhesins may be found in a number of reviews (Cassels and Wolf 1995; Karlsson 1995; Ofek 1994; Sakarya and Oncu 2003).

The adhesion mediated by lectin–sugar interaction can be inhibited by either a simple or complex carbohydrate structure, which competes with the host cell glycoprotein or glycolipids on the carbohydrate binding domain of the bacterial adhesin-lectin (reviewed in Schengrund 2003; Sharon and Ofek, 2000). In general, the affinity of sugars to the adhesin-lectin is low, in the millimolar range. An increase of several orders of magnitude in the inhibitory potency of monovalent carbohydrates can be achieved by suitable chemical derivatization (Firon *et al.* 1987; Sorme *et al.* 2002). It can also be obtained by their attachment to polymeric carriers to form multivalent ligands (Ofek *et al.* 1996).

Some bacterial lectins may recognize internal sequences as well. For example, the crystal structure has confirmed that the tip adhesin PapG of P fimbriae recognizes internal Galα(1–4)-Gal sequences on cell surface glycolipids (Table 3.2). Another interesting feature of the carbohydrate–lectin interaction is that at least in some cases (e.g., *Helicobacter pylori*), the binding of the bacterial lectin-adhesin to glycolipids is dependent on the linkage of fatty acids to the sugar moieties **(Table 3.3)**. For example, molecular modeling shows that the preferred conformation for *Helicobacter* lectin in glycolipids is the hydrogen bonding between the O_2 of the fatty acid and glucose (Karlsson 1995).

The study of bacterial lectin-adhesins, especially when these molecules are associated with fimbrial structures, has been hampered because it was difficult to separate the lectins in pure soluble form that exhibits the carbohydrate binding specificity of the whole bacteria. A major breakthrough was achieved by preparing a fusion protein involving ZZ protein of staphylococcal protein A and the amino terminal region of PapG, the adhesin molecule associated with P fimbriae of uropathogenic *Escherichia coli* (Hansson *et al.* 1995). Three fusion proteins, each derived from three distinct clones of *E. coli* and exhibiting different fine receptor specificity, were constructed and purified by using IgG affinity columns. The three fusion proteins derived from PapGI, PapGII, and PapGIII exhibited identical fine sugar specificity to that of the native fimbriae-associated proteins. In a similar manner,

Table 3.1. Types of Adhesin–Receptor Interactions in Bacterial Adhesion to Mucosal Surfaces

Type of Interaction	Bacterial Ligand (and Example)	Receptor on Epithelial Cell (and Example)	References
Lectin–carbohydrate	Lectin (type 1 fimbriae) Polysaccharide (LPS of gram-negative bacteria)	Glycoprotein (uroplakin 1a on bladder cells) Lectin (lectin on corneal epithelial cells)	Wu *et al.* 1996 Zhou *et al.* 2001 Zaidi *et al.* 1996
Protein–protein	Fibronectin-binding proteins (F protein of *Streptococcus pyogenes*)	Fibronectin (fibronectin on respiratory cells)	Ensenberger *et al.* 2001 Hanski and Caparon 1992 Hanski *et al.* 1996
Hydrophobin–protein	Glycolipid (lipoteichoic acid of *S. pyogenes*)	Lipid receptors (lipid-binding region fibronectin on epithelial cells)	Courtney 1990 Hasty and Courtney 1996
	Lipid-binding proteins (surface protein of *Campylobacter* species)	Membrane lipid (phospholipids and sphingolipids of cells)	Guerry *et al.* 2002 Sylvester *et al.* 1996 Szymanski and Armstrong 1996

Table 3.2. Examples of Various Types of Receptor–Adhesin Relationships in Bacterial Adhesion to Animal Cells[a,b]

Type	Bacteria and Clone	Host Cell	Adhesin	Receptor	Attachment Site of Receptor
A.	*Escherichia coli*, UTI	RBC	Dr fimbriae	Dr-BG	Dr specific
	E. coli, ETEC	RBC	AFA II	Dr-BG	AFA II specific
	E. coli, pigs	RBC	F 1845 fimbriae	Dr-BG	F 1845 specific
B.	*Streptococcus pyogenes*	Mucosal	LTA	FN	NH2 terminal
	Staphylococcus aureus	Mucosal	FBP	FN	NH2 terminal
C.	*E. coli*	Uroepithelial	P fimbriae, Fso	P-BG	Gal(1-4)Gal
		Pyelonephritis	P fimbriae, Fso F/H	FN	ND
D.	*E. coli*	RBC	Type 1 fimbriae	66-kDa Gp	OligoMan
		PMN	Type 1 fimbriae	CD11/18 Gp	OligoMan
		Macrophages	Type 1 fimbriae	CD48 Gp[c]	OligoMan
		Mast cells	Type 1 fimbriae	CD48 Gp[d]	OligoMan
		Uroepithelial		Uroplakin 1a	OligoMan[e]

[a]Adapted from Ofek and Doyle 1994.
[b]Gp, Glycoprotein; RBC, red blood cells; PMN, polymorphonuclear leukocytes; LTA, lipoteichoic acid; FBP, fibronectin-binding protein; NH2 terminal, amino terminal region; ND, not defined; OligoMan, oligomannoside; FN, fibronectin; BG, blood group.
[c]Baorto *et al.* 1997.
[d]Malaviya *et al.* 1999.
[e]Wu *et al.* 1996; Zhou, *et al.* 2001.

Table 3.3. Examples of Carbohydrates as Attachment Sites for Bacteria Colonizing Mucosal Surfaces[a]

Organism	Target Tissue	Carbohydrate Structure	Form[b]
Escherichia type 1	Urinary tract	Manα3[Manα3(Manα6)]	GP
P	Urinary tract	Galα1-4Gal	GSL
S	Neural	NeuAc(α23)Galβ3GalNAc	GSL
CFA/1	Intestine	NeuAc(α2-8)	GP
CS3	Intestine	GalNAcβ1-4Gal	GP
K1	Endothelial cells	GlcNAcβ1-4GlcNAc	GP
K99	Intestine	NeuGc(α2-3)Galβ4Glc	GSL
Helicobacter pylori	Stomach	NeuAc(α2-3)Gal	GSL
	Lewis-b blood group	Lactosyl ceramide	GP
		Glucose-fatty acid	GSL
Neisseria gonorrhoeae	Genital	Galβ1-4Glcβ	GSL
		NeuAc(α2-3)Galβ1-4GlcNAc	GP
Pseudomonas aeruginosa	Intestine	Galβ3GlcNAc	GP
		Fucose	GP
		Mannose	GP
	Respiratory	GalNAcβ1-4Gal	GSL
Haemophilus influenza	Respiratory	GalNAcβ1-4Gal	GSL
Streptococcus pneumoniae	Respiratory	GlcNAcβ3Gal	GP
Mycoplasma pneumoniae	Respiratory	NeuAc(α2-3)-GalβGlcNAc	GP
Streptococcus suis	Respiratory	Galα1-4Gal	GP
Klebsiella pneumoniae	Respiratory	Galα1-4Gal	GP
	Enteropathogenic	Galα1-4Gal	GP

[a]Based on Sharon and Lis 1997; Ofek and Doyle, 1994; and Karlsson, 1995.
[b]Predominant form: GP, glycoproteins; GSL, glycolipids.

the adhesin tip of type 1 fimbriae (FimH) was purified by producing both FimH/His-tag and FimH/MalE fusion proteins (Schembri *et al.* 2000; Thankavel *et al.* 1997). In many cases, purified fimbrial adhesins are stable only when complexed with their chaperones in the periplasmic space or in association with the fimbrial structures. Fimbrial purification of the adhesin alongside its chaperone stabilizes the purified adhesin while also maintaining its receptor specificity, as has been shown with FimH and its chaperone FimC (Choudhury *et al.* 1999). It is anticipated that many fimbrial lectins will be purified and their combining sites identified through fusion proteins or adhesin/chaperone pairs. Both methods will stabilize the proteins and retain their carbohydrate binding activity.

Bacterial oligosaccharides and lipopolysaccharides as adhesins

Mammalian macrophages express lectins that recognize complementary carbohydrate structures on bacterial surfaces and mediate nonopsonic phagocytosis of bacteria (Ofek *et al.* 1995). In all these cases, the carbohydrate structures recognized by the macrophage lectins were either contained in the capsular polysaccharides or in the lipopolysaccharides of the outer membrane of gram-negative bacteria. A more comprehensive review on the role of macrophage lectin–bacteria polysaccharide interaction in the infectious process may be found elsewhere (Keisari *et al.* 1997; Ofek *et al.* 1995; Ofek and Sharon 1988; Palaniyar *et al.* 2002). Evidence has been accumulated to suggest that the lipooligosaccharide/lipopolysaccharide (LOS/LPS) of the outer membrane of gram-negative bacteria participate in mediating adhesion of the microorganisms to nonprofessional phagocytes, including mucosal cells, as well as to mucus constituents (Jacques 1996). For example, it has been shown that LOS of *Haemophilus ducreyi* contributes to adherence to human keratinocytes, and LOS biosynthesis mutants have reduced adherence to bronchial epithelium (Gibson *et al.* 1997; Swords *et al.* 2000). Additional evidence for this notion is based either on comparing the adhesion of LPS mutants to

their parent strains or on showing that extracted LPS inhibit adhesion of the bacteria. Because the lipid A moiety of LPS is inserted into the outer membrane, most studies were aimed at defining the residues contained in the polysaccharide moiety of LPS, which is exposed. A compelling evidence for adhesin activity of LPS was obtained in a study showing that isolated *Vibrio mimicus* LPS and, especially its polysaccharide moiety, caused direct hemagglutination of rabbit erythrocytes (Alam *et al.* 1996). In another study, it was found that the heptose-3-deoxy-D-manno-2-octulosonic residue contained in the inner core region of LPS is recognized by a lectinlike receptor on the plasma membrane of rat hepatocytes (Parent 1990). The inner core LPS with a terminal glucose residue of *Pseudomonas aeruginosa* was also found to be necessary for the bacteria to bind to and be internalized by corneal epithelial cells (Zaidi *et al.* 1996). In many cases the lectinlike receptor on the mammalian cells involved in binding the bacterial LOS/LPS has been identified (Blake *et al.* 1995; Jeannotte *et al.* 2003; Mey *et al.* 1996; Nassif and So 1995; Swords *et al.* 2000). These receptors, which function in normal host biology, have been coopted by the bacteria as the bacterial adhesins purposely mimic the glycolipid structure of the natural host ligands (Harvey *et al.* 2001).

Common themes

A number of common themes have emerged regarding the interactions between bacteria and mucosal cells. The most notable is the concept that pathogenic bacteria attach to mucosal cells typically through multiple adhesive interactions. Thus a bacterium may express several adhesin moieties, each with a specificity for a distinct receptor molecule on the epithelial cell surface (for examples, see **Table 3.4**). These multiple bacterial adhesins may be structurally similar but may exhibit different binding specificities such as the type 1 and P fimbriae of uropathogenic *E .coli*. Alternatively, they may be composed of structurally and chemically dissimilar adhesins such as the lipoteichoic acid (LTA) and proteinaceous adhesins of *Streptococcus sanguis*. Some pathogens (e.g., *Neisseria gonorrhoeae*) produce two lectin-adhesins,

Table 3.4. Selected Bacterial Clones Expressing Multiple Adhesins[a]

Bacterial Clone	Source of Isolation	Adhesion	Characteristics
Escherichia coli	Pyelonephritis	Type P Type 1	Fimbrial lectin
Staphylococcus saprophyticus	Urinary	Gal-GlcNAc	Peripheral lectin
		Lipoteichoic acid	Fibrillar hydrophobin
Neisseria gonorrhoeae	Urogenital	Pilus	Pilin adhesin
		Opa	Outer membrane protein
Streptococcus sanguis	Dental plaque	Protein	Peripheral hydrophobin
		Protein	Fimbriae
		Protein	Peripheral lectin
		Lipoteichoic acid	Fibrillar hydrophobin

[a]Adapted from Ofek and Doyle 1994.

each exhibiting specificity for distinct carbohydrate structures, one of which is found in glycolipids and the other on glycoproteins. In many instances, these distinct adhesins are expressed by different subpopulations of a bacterial clone. By generating several phenotypic variants expressing adhesins of distinct specificities, a given bacterial clone will increase the repertoire of tissues that it can colonize and also introduce an antigenic variability that enhances its ability to withstand the multifaceted defenses of the host. In those instances in which multiple adhesins are expressed simultaneously on the same organism, each adhesin appears to complement the other functionally. For example, the cell surface LTA and the M protein that are coexpressed on the surface of *S. pyogenes* have both been implicated in mediating bacterial binding to Hep-2 cells (reviewed in Courtney *et al.* 2002). Adhesion of *S. pyogenes* to the cells appears to involve a two-step process, the first of which is mediated by the interaction of LTA with fibronectin molecules on the host cells (Hasty and Courtney 1996) and the second of which is mediated by binding of M protein to sialic acid modification of different receptors and glycosaminoglycans (Frick *et al.* 2003; Ryan *et al.* 2001).

Now that the identity of many bacterial adhesins and their cognate receptors on the host cells have been characterized, a number of general features can be noticed (Table 3.2). A particular receptor may contain more than one attachment site specific for two or more adhesins. This is illustrated by the three different clones of *E. coli*, each of which produces distinct adhesin that binds to a different region of the same receptor molecules of Dr blood group. Another general feature is that two different pathogens each expressing structurally distinct adhesins can exhibit the same receptor specificity on host cells. This is the case with *Staphylococcus aureus* and *S. pyogenes*, both of which bind the amino terminal region of fibronectin found on mucosal cells. The adhesin on *S. aureus* is a fibronectin-binding protein, whereas the adhesin on *S. pyogenes* is lipoteichoic acid (Table 3.2). The finding that several different respiratory tract pathogens seem to be able to recognize the carbohydrate sequence GalNAcβ4Gal is yet another example in which distinct adhesins on different bacteria appear to be recognizing the same receptor (Table 3.3). It has been suggested that the GalNAcβ4Gal carbohydrate sequence is preferentially accessible in the glycolipid of the respiratory epithelium and this allows firm binding of a diverse group of respiratory pathogens bearing adhesins specific for this sequence. In some cases, however, recognition of a specific carbohydrate sequence is not enough to mediate bacterial tropism. This becomes apparent when comparing the different tissues and animal species that are colonized as the result of a Galα(1–4)Gal–specific adhesin. Uropathogenic P-fimbriated *E. coli* (Dodson *et al.* 2001), the pig pathogen *Streptococcus suis* (Tikkanen *et al.* 1995), and the respiratory/enteropathogenic P-like fimbriated *Klebsiella pneumoniae* (Przondo-Mordarska *et al.* 1996) all recognize this carbohydrate sequence, yet have different tropisms.

Conversely, the same bacterial adhesin can bind to several distinct receptors on different cell types. Such receptors are called isoreceptors. Cases in point are the different receptors identified for the type 1 fimbriae for *E. coli*. Several molecules ranging in size from 110–145 kDa have been described as receptors for type 1 fimbriae on different cell types (Table 3.2). It is believed that all these glycoprotein receptors share a common oligomannose-containing attachment site for FimH, the adhesin moiety of type 1 fimbriae. In view of the fact that the critical factor determining FimH binding is a specific carbohydrate structure and not the protein, it is not surprising that the type 1 fimbrial receptor on different cell types is not the same protein molecule because the level of glycosylation of proteins in different cell types varies widely. An adhesin molecule may contain multiple domains, each with distinct receptor specificity as is the case of the filamentous hemagglutinin adhesin of *Bordetella pertussis* (reviewed in Locht *et al.* 2001). The hemagglutinin has been cloned and sequenced and contains at least three domains. One domain is arginin-glycin-aspartic (RGD) sequence, which mediates binding of *Bordetella* to a CR3 integrin present on pulmonary macrophages (Relman *et al.* 1989); the hemagglutinin also contains two carbohydrate-binding domains, one of which is specific for galactose (Tuomanen *et al.* 1988) and the other for sulfated sugars (Menozzi *et al.* 1994).

A feature of bacterial adhesins is that they are commonly associated with surface structures (Mulvey 2002; Ofek 1994). Typical examples are the fimbrial adhesins of *E. coli*, consisting of an assembly of several hundred proteins, usually different kinds (Gaastra and Svennerholm 1996). In many cases only one protein carries the receptor-binding site. However, in at least one case, it was found that two proteins associated with same type of fimbriae function as adhesins with distinct receptor specificity. For example, two subunits on *E. coli* P fimbriae have been implicated in adhesion (reviewed in Mulvey 2002; Wullt *et al.* 2001). The first is PapG, which mediates the characteristic Galα(1–4)Gal binding properties of P fimbriae, and the second subunit is PapE, which is responsible for promoting bacterial binding to fibronectin. Interestingly, both PapG and PapE subunits are located at the distal ends of the peritrichously arranged fimbrial filaments and make up the unique fibrillum tip structure.

Bacterial adhesins have been directly implicated in tissue tropism because they mediate bacterial adherence to particular cell types and receptors. It has been shown that slight allelic variations in the adhesin binding pocket can target bacteria to different mucosal surfaces. Crystal structures of FimH have detailed the mannose-binding pocket for over 200 uropathogenic strains of *E. coli*, and it has been shown that these strains that colonize the bladder have a highly conserved FimH structure as opposed to intestinal colonizing strains (Hung *et al.* 2002). Therefore bacterial tissue tropism can be directly influenced by allelic alterations in the adhesin structure itself. Additionally, the adhesin-binding pocket specificity can be modulated by the fimbrial structure on which it is presented. For example, the fine sugar-binding specificity of *E. coli* FimH has been shown to be altered when expressed on the type 1 fimbrial shaft of *K. pneumoniae* (Madison *et al.* 1994). The magnitude of adhesion also is influenced by the physical state of the adhesin structure as shown for *Neisseria meningitidis*, which exhibits high-adhesiveness to tissue culture cells when the organisms express fimbriae in bundles as compared with variants expressing long and distinct fimbriae (Marceau *et al.* 1995). Even variations in the location of the adhesin-genes may affect the receptor specificity as shown for the MrkD fimbrial adhesin encoded by an *mrk* gene cluster in *K. pneumoniae* (Hornick *et al.* 1995). The organisms contain multiple copies of the *mrk* genes, which may be present on both plasmid and chromosome. The chromosomal genes encode for adhesin with a receptor specificity distinct from that encoded by plasmid *mrk* genes.

INTERACTION WITH THE EXTRACELLULAR MATRIX

As indicated previously, mucosal cells are often covered by a layer of mucus (sometimes referred to as the extracellular matrix [ECM]), which is composed of a heterogeneous mixture of proteins exhibiting various degrees of glycosylation. ECM components are found underlying epithelial tissues or surrounding cells. They consist of several different structural glycoproteins, including mucins, collagens, elastin, fibronectin, fibrinogen, laminin, and proteoglycans; for example, chondroitin sulfate proteoglycan and heparin

sulfate proteoglycan. Many mucosal colonizers express adhesins that specifically recognize one or more constituents in the extracellular matrix. The same three categories of recognition depicted in Table 3.1 exist between bacteria and the extracellular matrix; for example, the interaction may result from either protein–protein, lipid–protein, or lectin–sugar interactions. A number of bacterial lectins were found to recognize the oligosaccharide side chains of ECM molecules, including binding of type 1 fimbriae, G fimbriae, and S fimbriae to laminin, among others (Kukkonen *et al.* 1998; Valkonen *et al.* 1994). Of particular interest is the family of respiratory mucins, which contain carbohydrate structures recognized by bacteria that colonize the upper respiratory tract (Scharfman *et al.* 1996). For example, the attachment of *P. aeruginosa* to respiratory mucin is mediated by flagellin (Lillehoj *et al.* 2002). A more thorough discussion on ECM–bacteria interactions may be found in excellent reviews (Hasty *et al.* 1994; Menozzi *et al.* 2002; Patti *et al.* 1994; *et al.* Patti and Hook 1994). Among the various ECM components, interactions with fibronectin have been studied the most at both the molecular and cellular levels. This is probably because it is found on the surface of many types of host cells including mucosal cells, and as such, it may act as a receptor for bacterial adhesion and colonization. Nevertheless, the adhesion of bacteria to extracellular matrix components other than fibronectin is increasingly becoming recognized. Examples of recent studies describing specific structures that mediate binding of bacteria to such ECM components are shown in **Table 3.5**. A remarkable feature is

Table 3.5. Examples of Bacterial Adhesins Mediating Binding of the Bacteria to ECM Glycoproteins

Bacteria	Bacterial Adhesin	ECM Component	References
Borrelia burgdorferi	DbpA and DbpB	Proteoglycan decorin	Fischer *et al.* 2003
	Protein A (Osp A) and 70-kDa protein	Plasminogen	Hu *et al.* 1995
	Fn-BA		
Haemophilus influenzae	P2 and P5 outer membrane protein	Repiratory mucin	Devies *et al.* 1995 Kubiet and Ramphal 1995 Reddy *et al.* 1996
Neisseria, gonorrhoeae	Opa protein	Proteoglycan	van Putten and Paul 1995
Pseudomonas aeruginosa	57-kDa and 59-kDa outer membrane proteins and proteins 42–48-kDa and 77–85-kDa flagellar 65.9-kDa FliF (MS ring)	Laminin Respiratory mucins	Plotkowski *et al.* 1996 Arora *et al.* 1996 Scharfman *et al.* 1996
Mycobacterium bovis	28-kDa protein	Heparin	
Escherichia coli	GafD protein of G fimbriae	Laminin	Saarela *et al.* 1996
Bordetella pertussis	Filamentous hemagglutinin	Heparin	Hannah *et al.* 1994
Helicobacter pylori	Lipopolysaccharide and 25-kDA protein	Laminin	Valkonen *et al.* 1997
Listeria monocytogenes	ActA outer membrane protein	Heparin	Alvarez-Dominguez *et al.* 1997

that many bacterial species studied express on their surfaces at least two proteins that bind specific ECM components. In the case of *Helicobacter pylori,* the laminin specific adhesin may be either a 25-kDa sialic acid–binding lectin, which recognizes sialyl residues of laminin, or lipopolysaccharide, which recognizes yet unidentified regions in laminin. Many studies have established fibronectin as an important receptor for *S. pyogenes* and other bacteria on mucosal surfaces (Courtney *et al.* 1990; Joh *et al.* 1999; Ofek 1994). At least six different molecules on *S. pyogenes* surfaces were found to recognize fibronectin, including lipoteichoic acid, protein F/Sfb, a 28-kDa fibronectin-binding protein, glyceraldehyde-3-phosphate dehydrogenase, serum opacity factor, a 54-kDa fibronectin-binding protein, and FBP54 (reviewed in Cunningham 2000; Hasty and Courtney 1996). Why a bacterial pathogen should have evolved multiple adhesins for the same ECM is unclear.

ADHESION-DEPENDENT EVENTS

Although the contribution of bacterial adherence to colonization of mucosal surfaces has been well recognized for several decades (reviewed in Ofek and Beachey 1980), its involvement in subsequent steps of the infectious process was largely unclear until the last decade. Several activities that are intimately related to the infectious process have emerged that are so-called adhesion-dependent or are immediate consequences of adhesion (reviewed in Finlay and Cossart 1997; Wullt *et al.* 2002). Apparently, the specific interaction between bacterial adhesins and their complementary receptors on mucosal cells elicits a variety of distinct responses in the host cells as well as in the bacteria, which can markedly affect the course of the infectious process. These findings point to some intriguing and novel functions for bacterial adhesins on mucosal surfaces as well as in deeper tissue. This section reviews evidence of selected examples of bacterial adhesin-mediated responses in the bacteria and in various host cells and their contribution to the infectious process. Since many of these observations involve uropathogenic *E. coli,* we will examine the implications of these findings in the context of the urinary tract wherever pertinent.

Induction of bacterial virulence genes
The urinary tract is relatively inhospitable to bacterial colonization. To establish an infection, bacteria must be able to sense this hostile environment and to modulate its protein expression profile to ensure their survival. There is now evidence that the bacteria can do so by using their adhesins as sensory organelles. It has been shown that host cell contact by the P fimbriae of *E. coli* can induce the CPX two-component signal transduction system, which has been shown to alter virulence gene transcription such as the *Pap* gene cluster (Hung *et al.* 2001; reviewed in Raivio and Silhavy 1999). These findings point to an intriguing new function for bacterial P fimbriae, namely, that of a sensory organelle. The

strategic location of PapG at the distal tips of the peritrichously arranged fimbriae probably facilitates this purported role. This finding is one of an increasing number of cases that show that bacterial pathogens are intrinsically capable of responding to important cues from host cells following interactions between complementary cell surface molecules (Abraham *et al.* 1998; Cotter and Miller 1996; Finlay and Cossart 1997). In addition, these observations provide a molecular basis for previous findings that various bacteria obtain a growth advantage following attachment to host cells. This has been demonstrated for type 1–fimbriated *E. coli* as well as for *N. gonorrhoeae,* which exhibit shorter lag period times when adhering to tissue culture cells (Bessen and Gotschlich 1986; Zafriri *et al.* 1987). Microarray data have confirmed that *Neisseria* attachment to host cells can alter the expression of a panoply of virulence genes including various adhesins, transporters, and capsule proteins (Dietrich *et al.* 2003; Grifantini *et al.* 2002).

Induction of cytokine responses from mucosal cells
In addition to evoking responses among adherent bacteria, the specific coupling of bacterial adhesins with their receptors on the mucosal cells also elicits a range of cellular responses. For example, the specific coupling of the P fimbrial adhesin to its complementary Galα(1–4)Gal-containing receptor epitopes on uroepithelial cells elicits the release of several immunoregulatory cytokines, including interleukin (IL)-1a, IL-b, IL-6, and IL-8 (Svanborg *et al.* 1996; Wullt *et al.* 2001). Some intriguing clues to the underlying intracellular molecular links between fimbriae-mediated attachment to the cell surface and cellular cytokine production have emerged. The specific attachment of PapG adhesin of P fimbriae to the Galα(1–4)Gal oligosaccharides on globoseries glycolipids, which are localized to the outer leaflet of the lipid bilayer of the epithelial cell membrane, triggers intracellular release of ceramides (Hedlund *et al.* 1996; Wullt *et al.* 2002). These PapG-elicited ceramides may be derived from the globoseries receptor itself or from neighboring sphingomyelin molecules by the generation of endogenous sphingomyelinases (Hedlund *et al.* 1996; Svanborg *et al.* 1996; Wullt *et al.* 2001; Wullt *et al.* 2002). Ceramide is known to be a critical second messenger in signal transduction processes in the cell and can activate the Ser/Thr family of protein kinases and phosphatases with Ser/Thr specificity, leading eventually to cytokine production. Interestingly, this bacterial adhesin-mediated mechanism of signaling is not unlike pathways known to be utilized by immunoregulatory cytokines such as tumor necrosis factor alpha (TNFα) and IL-1 when evoking cellular responses (Svanborg *et al.* 1996; Wullt *et al.* 2001; Wullt *et al.* 2002). Thus, in this instance, the bacterial adhesin appears to be functionally mimicking the host's immunoregulatory molecules. Type 1 fimbriae of uropathogenic *E. coli* also stimulate a cytokine response from uroepithelial cells that is distinct from that evoked by P fimbriae (Connel *et al.* 1996). This difference may be caused by host toll-like receptor 4 activation, which is dependent on type 1 fimbrial adhesion (Mysorekar 2002; Schilling, 2003).

Induction of cytokine responses from inflammatory cells

The capacity of bacterial adhesins to elicit cytokine response is not confined to mucosal cells. Indeed, type 1 fimbriae of uropathogenic *E. coli* are capable of binding to and eliciting immunoregulatory products from activating a wide range of inflammatory cells, including macrophages, neutrophils, mast cells, and B and T lymphocytes *in vitro* (reviewed in Connel *et al.*, 1996b). Evidence that these interactions may occur *in vivo* with significant physiologic effects comes from intraperitoneal injection of *E. coli* expressing type 1 fimbriae into mice, which resulted in the generation of a large spike in extracellular TNFα and leukotriene B4 (LTB4) in the peritoneal fluid (Malaviya *et al.* 1996; Malaviya 2000). The role of the fimbrial adhesin, FimH, is evidenced by the finding that intraperitoneal challenge with a FimH minus isogenic mutant exhibited only a limited TNFα/LTB4 response (Malaviya *et al.* 1996). The cellular source of both the TNFα and LTB4 in the mouse peritoneum was determined to be mast cells because mice genetically deficient in mast cells exhibited a limited response following intraperitoneal injection of type 1 fimbriae. Notably, the TNFα and LTB4 response of mast cells was accompanied by a large influx of neutrophils into the peritoneum, which is consistent with the fact that both mediators are potent neutrophil chemoattractants (Malaviya *et al.* 1996; Malaviya 2000). Thus one of the immediate outcomes of type 1 fimbriae–mediated activation of mast cells is recruitment of neutrophils to sites of bacterial challenge. More recently, mast cell–dependent neutrophil recruitment has been shown to elicit macrophage influx into the skin, another important site of bacterial invasion (von Stebut 2003). Because mast cells are found preferentially in mucosal surfaces, including the urinary tract, the interaction of type 1 fimbriae of *E. coli* with mast cells proximal to the uroepithelium could contribute to the influx of neutrophils and macrophages from surrounding blood vessels, leading to their translocation through the epithelial barrier and subsequent entry into the lumen of the urinary tract. Indeed, the presence of neutrophils in the urine is an early and often diagnostic indication of urinary tract infection. The excessive transepithelial migration of neutrophils during infections may predispose this barrier to increased bacterial penetration, as suggested for other mucosal surfaces (Finlay and Cossart 1997), and raises the possibility that facets of the host's immune response may be co-opted by pathogenic bacteria to facilitate their virulence.

Impact of bacteria-elicited inflammatory responses

Evaluating the physiologic effects of adhesin-elicited cytokines at sites of bacterial infection is generally difficult because of their numerous and complex effects (Henderson *et al.* 1996; Malaviya *et al.* 1996). Using microarray to analyze host cell responses, it is possible to determine the variety and range of cytokines produced upon bacterial attachment, even though it does little to detail their immune effects. For example, microarray analysis of mouse bladders infected with uropathogenic *E. coli* has confirmed that proteins essential to epithelial proliferation, secretion of proinflammatory mediators, and epithelial barrier function are upregulated (Mysorekar *et al.* 2002). Even though these proteins are upregulated, their effects on bacterial pathogenesis have yet to be determined. Some of the various responses evoked in the urinary tract following the adherence of uropathogenic *E. coli* to the urinary mucosae are illustrated in **Figure 3.1**. In general, proinflammatory cytokines serve to initiate and regulate the innate and specific immune responses of the host to an infectious agent. These responses include increased mucus secretion and the recruitment and activation of a variety of phagocytic cells, all of which could potentially affect the early elimination of the pathogen (Henderson *et al.* 1996; Malaviya *et al.* 1996; Uehling *et al.* 1999). However, not all these responses have their intended effects. Indeed, some of the adhesin-triggered secreted products of host cells may have severe pathophysiologic effects on the surrounding tissue, particularly when released in excess or at inopportune times (Malaviya *et al.* 1996). Although direct evidence for this is still lacking, there is considerable circumstantial evidence supporting the notion that the many proteases, oxygen radicals, and cytotoxic cytokines secreted by inflammatory cells following activation by type 1–fimbriated *E. coli* (Malaviya *et al.* 1996; Malaviya *et al.* 1994; Tewari *et al.* 1994) are detrimental to the host and foster bacterial pathogenesis. For example, the neutrophil elastases, oxygen radicals, and other cytotoxic agents stimulated from neutrophils following their interaction with type 1 fimbriae of *E. coli* in the kidney are major contributors to renal scarring (Brown *et al.* 1998; Steadman *et al.* 1988; Topley *et al.* 1989). In several instances, the critical determinant of whether an inflammatory response favors the host or pathogen is dependent on other prevailing factors, including the host's immune status and the intrinsic virulent capabilities of the pathogen. The number of bacteria at the site of infection is potentially another critical factor in light of the findings that certain bacteria have the capacity of "quorum sensing" (de Kievit and Iglewski 2000; Passador *et al.* 1993), that is, they possess the capability of measuring their population density at a given site and to coordinately turn on the expression of a battery of new virulence factors upon reaching a critical density, presumably to mount an effective challenge to the host's immune response.

Induction of bacterial phagocytosis

In addition to eliciting a variety of pharmacologically active mediators from various host cells, bacterial adhesins also elicit uptake of bacteria by phagocytic cells of the host under serum-free conditions. The process has been coined "lectinophagocytosis," in analogy to opsonophagocytosis, in which recognition between the microorganisms and the phagocytic cells is mediated by serum constituents termed opsonins (mainly IgG antibodies and the C3b and C3bi fragments of the C3 component of complement) (Ofek *et al.* 1995; Ofek and Sharon 1988). The best characterized system of lectinophagocytosis is that of bacteria carrying mannose-specific type 1 fimbrial lectins capped by the FimH adhesin.

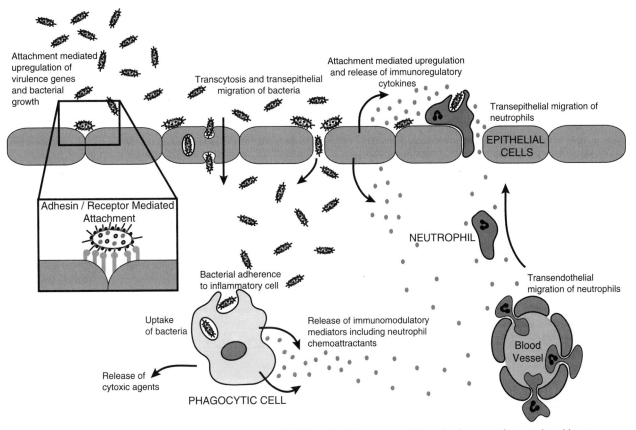

Fig. 3.1. Diagrammatic depiction of bacterial adherence to epithelial and inflammatory cells and subsequent bacterial and host responses.

That a bacterial adhesin that promotes bacterial colonization and infection would also promote ingestion by phagocytic cells is somewhat of a paradox. However, new evidence has emerged that suggests that the type 1 fimbriae-elicited bacterial phagocytosis by macrophages was actually advantageous to the bacterial population (Baorto *et al.* 1997). *In vitro* survival assays revealed that unlike *E. coli* phagocytosed via opsonin-mediated processes, *E. coli* internalized via type 1 fimbriae survived much of the intracellular killing process of macrophages. By associating with CD48, a glycosylphosphoinisitol-linked moiety on the surface of macrophages, the bacteria gain access to a host membrane domain called lipid rafts that facilitates endocytosis, which bypasses the normal phagocytic killing mechanisms of the macrophages (Baorto *et al.* 1997). Entry of many different gram-positive and gram-negative bacteria into host cells has been shown to be mediated by lipid raft endocytosis (Duncan *et al.* 2002). This finding provides a molecular basis for earlier observations showing that, compared with bacteria ingested via opsonophagocytosis, bacteria subjected to lectinophagocytosis are markedly less sensitive to killing by phagocytes (reviewed in Ofek *et al.* 1995). It is noteworthy that lectinophagocytosis comes into play only at body sites with poor opsonizing capacity, such as the urinary mucosa, which

may help explain why type 1–fimbriated *E. coli* is the singular most frequent pathogen at this site (Hagberg *et al.* 1981).

Lipid raft–mediated lectinophagocytosis also mediates invasion of nonphagocytic cells such as epithelial and endothelial cells. The ability of uropathogenic *E. coli* to enter bladder epithelium and safely replicate has been suggested as an effective bacterial counterbalance to host defensive immunity (Schilling *et al.* 2003). This invasive ability is also adhesin specific, as *E. coli* uptake by bladder epithelium is mediated through FimH attachment but not through PapG (Martinez *et al.* 2000). As a host defensive measure, soluble mannosylated proteins with bacterial FimH specificity have been shown to be produced that can inhibit bacterial attachment and entry into phagocytic and nonphagocytic cells alike (Pak *et al.* 2001).

In summary, the coupling of the bacterial adhesin with the host receptor is not an inanimate event but rather a very active process that signals a myriad of responses in the host cells and in the bacteria itself. In the urinary tract, adherent *E. coli* appear capable of inducing the expression of bacterial genes that would favor their growth in the urine and elicit a range of immune responses from host cells, facets of which could be coopted by the bacteria to favor their survival (Fig. 3.1).

CONCLUDING REMARKS

Experiments in animals have proved that it is possible to prevent infections by blocking the adhesion of the pathogen to target tissue. These findings have provided an impetus for the development of antiadhesion drugs for the prevention and therapy of microbial infections in humans (reviewed in Ofek *et al.* 1996; Sharon and Ofek 2002). New classes of drugs such as these are in great need because of the increased occurrence of pathogenic organisms that are resistant to conventional antibiotics. The advantages of inhibiting adhesion to prevent bacterial colonization of mucosal surfaces rely on the assumption that the spread of strains with genotypic resistance to the method applied would be much slower than in the case of employing approaches aimed at killing the organisms.

Because lectin-mediated adhesion is a mechanism shared by many pathogens (see the preceding text), most investigators have focused their efforts on preventing bacterial infections by blocking the pathogen's lectins. A number of strategies have been suggested, including mucosal immunity to induce S-IgA antiadhesin antibodies, metabolic inhibitors of the expression of adhesion (e.g., sublethal concentration of antibiotics), dietary inhibitors, and receptor analogues (reviewed in Ofek 1994; Sharon and Ofek 2002). In the latter strategy, the lectin-adhesin is inhibited by sugars specific for the lectin and is probably the most attractive approach today for the synthesis of antiadhesive drugs **(Table 3.6)**. This was originally demonstrated in the late 1970s, when it was shown that methyl α-mannoside can protect mice against urinary tract infection by type 1–fimbriated *E. coli*; methyl α-glucoside, which is not recognized by the bacteria, was not effective (Aronson *et al.* 1979). Subsequent studies

by many other groups with *E. coli*, both type 1 and P fimbriated, with type 1–fimbriated *K. pneumoniae*, as well as with other pathogenic microorganisms, have confirmed and extended the initial results and have proven beyond any doubt the drug potential of antiadhesive compounds (Table 3.6) (Beuth *et al.* 1995; Sharon and Ofek 2000; Zopf *et al.* 1996). Thus, 11 derivatives of galabiose that inhibit the adhesion of P-fimbriated *E. coli* to animal cells *in vitro* prevented urinary tract infections in mice and monkeys by the bacteria (Ohlsson *et al.* 2002). Antibodies against mannose-containing compounds present on epithelial cells prevented urinary tract infection in mice by type 1–fimbriated *E. coli*. Sialylated glycoproteins, administered orally, protected colostrum-deprived newborn calves against lethal doses of enterotoxigenic *E. coli* K99. In a clinical trial in humans, patients with otitis externa (a painful swelling with secretion from the external auditory canal) caused by *P. aeruginosa* were treated with a solution of galactose, mannose, and N-acetylneuraminic acid (Beuth *et al.* 1996). The results were fully comparable with those obtained with conventional antibiotic treatment. Attractive candidates are oligosaccharides, such as those found in human milk and other body fluids that have been shown to inhibit the adhesion to cells and tissues of strains of *H. pylori* or certain streptococci (Sharon and Ofek 2000; Zopf *et al.* 1996). Use of dietary inhibitors, especially milk, which is rich in carbohydrates, is another attractive strategy to block adhesion and prevent infections (Sharon and Ofek 2000). However, other dietary produce may also contain adhesion inhibitory activity and may be used to prevent bacterial infections. For example, cranberry juice contains at least two inhibitors of urinary pathogenic *E. coli* and has been successfully used to prevent urinary tract infections in elderly women (Ofek *et al.* 1991). Another attractive strategy is probiotic prevention urinary tract

Table 3.6. Inhibitors of Bacterial Lectin/Adhesin as Antiadhesion Drugs for Preventing Infection in Experimental Animals[a,b]

Bacteria	Animal, Site	Inhibitor
Escherichia coli type 1	Mice, UT	MeαMan
	Mice, GIT	Mannose
	Mice, UT	Anti-Man antibodies
Klebsiella pneumoniae type 1	Rats, UT	MeαMan
Shigella flexneri type 1	Guinea pigs, eye	Mannose
Escherichia coli type P	Mice	Globotetraose
	Monkeys	Galα4GalβOMe
Escherichia coli K99 glycoproteins	Calves, GIT	Glycopeptides of serum
Pseudomonas aeruginosa	Human ear	Gal+ Man+NeuAc
Helicobacter pylori	Piglet stomach	Oligosaccharide NE0080
Streptococcus pneumoniae	Rabbit lungs	Oligosaccharide NE1530
Streptococcus pneumoniae	Mouse lungs	GlcNAc

[a]Adapted from Sharon 1996; Sharon and Ofek 2000.
[b]UT, urinary tract; GIT, gastrointestinal tract; Me, methyl; Gal, glactose; NeuAc, Neuraminic acid; Man, mannoside; GlcNAc, N-acetylglucosamine.

infections that utilize nonvirulent *Lactobacillus* to deplete the vaginal surface of receptors for more virulent bacteria such as *Pseudomonas* and *Klebsiella* (Osset *et al.* 2001; Reid 2002). By coupling antibacterial drugs to either lectins or antisaccharide antibodies, it is possible to target antibiotics to the lipid raft endocytic pathway and directly to the intracellular bacterial niche (McIntosh *et al.* 2002).

These findings illustrate the great potential of simple carbohydrates in the prevention of infections caused by bacteria that express surface lectins. Moreover, they raise hopes for the development of antiadhesive drugs for human use. The development of antiadhesion therapy targeted at the microbial lectins has been hampered by the great difficulty in large-scale synthesis of the required inhibitory saccharides. Alternatives are glycomimetics, compounds that structurally mimic the inhibitory carbohydrates, but which may be more readily obtainable. Eventually, a cocktail of inhibitors, or a polyvalent one, will have to be used, since many infectious agents express multiple specificities. The emerging collection of microbial lectin crystal structures and the elucidation of the essential atomic structure needed for binding specificity will definitely benefit the design of such drugs in the future.

REFERENCES

Abraham, S. N., Jonsson, A. B., and Normark, S. (1998). Fimbriae-mediated host-pathogen cross-talk. *Curr. Opin. Microbiol.* 1, 75–81.

Alam, M., Miyoshi, S. I., Tomochika, K. I., and Shinoda, S. (1996). Purification and characterization of novel hemagglutinins from *Vibrio mimicus*: A 39-kilodalton major outer membrane protein and lipopolysaccharide. *Infect. Immun.* 64, 4035–4041.

Alvarez-Dominguez, C., Vazquez-Boland, J. A., Carrasco-Marin, E., Lopez-Mato, P., and Leyva-Cobian, F. (1997). Host cell heparan sulfate proteoglycans mediate attachment and entry of *Listeria monocytogenes*, and the listerial surface protein ActA is involved in heparan sulfate receptor recognition. *Infect. Immun.* 65, 78–88.

Aronson, M., Medalia, O., Schori, L., Mirelman, D., Sharon, N., and Ofek, I. (1979). Prevention of colonization of the urinary tract of mice with *Escherichia coli* by blocking of bacterial adherence with methyl alpha-D-mannopyranoside. *J. Infect. Dis.* 139, 329–332.

Arora, S. K., Ritchings, B. W., Almira, E. C., Lory, S., and Ramphal, R. (1996). Cloning and characterization of *Pseudomonas aeruginosa fliF*, necessary for flagellar assembly and bacterial adherence to mucin. *Infect. Immun.* 64, 2130–2136.

Baorto, D. M., Gao, Z., Malaviya, R., Dustin, M. L., van der Merwe, A., Lublin, D. M., and Abraham, S. N. (1997). Survival of FimH-expressing enterobacteria in macrophages relies on glycolipid traffic. *Nature* 389, 636–639.

Bessen, D., and Gotschlich, E. C. (1986). Interactions of gonococci with *HeLa* cells: Attachment, detachment, replication, penetration, and the role of protein II. *Infect. Immun.* 54, 154–160.

Beuth, J., Ko, H. L., Pulverer, G., Uhlenbruck, G., and Pichlmaier, H. (1995). Importance of lectins for the prevention of bacterial infections and cancer metastases. *Glycoconj. J.* 12, 1–6.

Beuth, J., Stoffel, B., and Pulverer, G. (1996). Inhibition of bacterial adhesion and infections by lectin blocking. *Adv. Exp. Med. Biol.* 408, 51–56.

Blake, M. S., Blake, C. M., Apicella, M. A., and Mandrell, R. E. (1995). Gonococcal opacity: Lectin-like interactions between Opa proteins and lipooligosaccharide. *Infect. Immun.* 63, 1434–1439.

Brown, J. F., Chafee, K. A., and Tepperman, B. L. (1998). Role of mast cells, neutrophils and nitric oxide in endotoxin-induced damage to the neonatal rat colon. *Br. J. Pharmacol.* 123, 31–38.

Cassels, F. J., and Wolf, M. K. (1995). Colonization factors of diarrheagenic *E. coli* and their intestinal receptors. *J. Ind. Microbiol.* 15, 214–226.

Choudhury, D., Thompson, A., Stojanoff, V., Langermann, S., Pinkner, J., Hultgren, S. J., and Knight, S. D. (1999). X-ray structure of the FimC-FimH chaperone–adhesin complex from uropathogenic *Escherichia coli*. *Science* 285, 1061–1066.

Connel, I., Agace, W., Klemm, P., Schembri, M., Marild, S., and Svanborg, C. (1996). Type 1 fimbrial expression enhances *Escherichia coli* virulence for the urinary tract. *Proc. Natl. Acad. Sci. USA* 93, 9827–9832.

Cotter, P. A., and Miller, J. F. (1996). Triggering bacterial virulence. *Science* 273, 1183–1184.

Courtney, H., Hasty, D., and Ofek I. (1990). Hydrophobic characteristic of pyogenic streptococci. In *Microbial Cell Surface Hydrophobicity* (eds. Doyle, R. J., and Rosenburg, M.), 361-386. Washington: American Society of Microbiology Publication.

Courtney, H. S., Hasty, D. L., and Dale, J. B. (2002). Molecular mechanisms of adhesion, colonization, and invasion of group A streptococci. *Ann. Med.* 34, 77–87.

Cunningham, M. W. (2000) Pathogenesis of group A streptococcal infections. *Clin. Microbiol. Rev.* 13, 470–511.

Davies, J., Carlstedt, I., Nilsson, A. K., Hakansson, A., Sabharwal, H., van Alphen, L., van Ham, M., and Svanborg, C. (1995). Binding of *Haemophilus influenzae* to purified mucins from the human respiratory tract. *Infect. Immun.* 63, 2485–2492.

de Kievit, T. R., and Iglewski, B. H. (2000). Bacterial quorum sensing in pathogenic relationships. *Infect. Immun.* 68, 4839–4849.

Dietrich, G., Kurz, S., Hubner, C., Aepinus, C., Theiss, S., Guckenberger, M., Panzner, U., Weber, J., and Frosch, M. (2003). Transcriptome analysis of *Neisseria meningitidis* during infection. *J. Bacteriol.* 185, 155–164.

Di Martino, P., Cafferini, N., Joly, B., and Darfeuille-Michaud, A. (2003). *Klebsiella pneumoniae* type 3 pili facilitate adherence and biofilm formation on abiotic surfaces. *Res. Microbiol.* 154, 9–16.

Dodson, K. W., Pinkner, J. S., Rose, T., Magnusson, G., Hultgren, S. J., and Waksman, G. (2001). Structural basis of the interaction of the pyelonephritic *E. coli* adhesin to its human kidney receptor. *Cell* 105, 733–743.

Donlan, R. M. (2002). Biofilms: Microbial life on surfaces. *Emerg. Infect. Dis.* 8, 881–890.

Doyle, R. J. (2000). Contribution of the hydrophobic effect to microbial infection. *Microbes Infect.* 2, 391–400.

Duncan, M. J., Shin, J. S. and Abraham, S. N. (2002). Microbial entry through caveolae: variations on a theme. *Cell Microbiol.* 4, 783–791.

Ensenberger, M. G., Tomasini-Johansson, B. R., Sottile, J., Ozeri, V., Hanski, E., and Mosher, D. F. (2001). Specific interactions between F1 adhesin of *Streptococcus pyogenes* and N-terminal modules of fibronectin. *J. Biol. Chem.* 276, 35606–35613.

Faille, C., Jullien, C., Fontaine, F., Bellon-Fontaine, M. N., Slomianny, C., and Benezech, T. (2002). Adhesion of *Bacillus* spores and *Escherichia coli* cells to inert surfaces: Role of surface hydrophobicity. *Can. J. Microbiol.* 48, 728–738.

Finlay, B. B., and Cossart, P. (1997). Exploitation of mammalian host cell functions by bacterial pathogens. *Science* 276, 718–725.

Firon, N., Ashkenazi, S., Mirelman, D., Ofek, I., and Sharon, N. (1987). Aromatic alpha-glycosides of mannose are powerful inhibitors of the adherence of type 1 fimbriated *Escherichia coli* to yeast and intestinal epithelial cells. *Infect. Immun.* 55, 472–476.

Fischer, J. R., Parveen, N., Magoun, L., and Leong, J. M. (2003). Decorin-binding proteins A and B confer distinct mammalian cell type-specific attachment by *Borrelia burgdorferi*, the Lyme disease spirochete. *Proc. Natl. Acad. Sci. USA* 100, 7307–7312.

Frick, I. M., Schmidtchen, A., and Sjobring, U. (2003). Interactions between M proteins of *Streptococcus pyogenes* and glycosaminoglycans promote bacterial adhesion to host cells. *Eur. J. Biochem.* 270, 2303–2311.

Gaastra, W., and Svennerholm, A. M. (1996). Colonization factors of human enterotoxigenic *Escherichia coli* (ETEC). *Trends Microbiol.* 4, 444–452.

Gibson, B. W., Campagnari, A. A., Melaugh, W., Phillips, N. J., Apicella, M. A., Grass, S., Wang, J., Palmer, K. L., and Munson, R. S., Jr.

(1997). Characterization of a transposon Tn916-generated mutant of *Haemophilus ducreyi* 35000 defective in lipooligosaccharide biosynthesis. *J. Bacteriol.* 179, 5062–5071.

Goldhar, J. (1994). Bacterial lectinlike adhesins: Determination and specificity. *Methods Enzymol.* 236, 211–231.

Grab, D. J., Givens, C., and Kennedy, R. (1998). Fibronectin-binding activity in *Borrelia burgdorferi1. Biochim. Biophys. Acta* 1407, 135–145.

Grifantini, R., Bartolini, E., Muzzi, A., Draghi, M., Frigimelica, E., Berger, J., Randazzo, F., and Grandi, G. (2002). Gene expression profile in *Neisseria meningitidis* and *Neisseria lactamica* upon host-cell contact: From basic research to vaccine development. *Ann. N.Y. Acad. Sci.* 975, 202–216.

Guerry, P., Szymanski, C. M., Prendergast, M. M., Hickey, T. E., Ewing, C. P., Pattarini, D. L., and Moran, A. P. (2002). Phase variation of *Campylobacter jejuni* 81-176 lipooligosaccharide affects ganglioside mimicry and invasiveness *in vitro. Infect. Immun.* 70, 787–793.

Hagberg, L., Jodal, U., Korhonen, T. K., Lidin-Janson, G., Lindberg, U., and Svanborg Eden, C. (1981). Adhesion, hemagglutination, and virulence of *Escherichia coli* causing urinary tract infections. *Infect. Immun.* 31, 564–570.

Hannah, J. H., Menozzi, F. D., Renauld, G., Locht, C., and Brennan, M. J. (1994). Sulfated glycoconjugate receptors for the *Bordetella pertussis* adhesin filamentous hemagglutinin (FHA) and mapping of the heparin-binding domain on FHA. *Infect. Immun.* 62, 5010–5019.

Hanski, E., and Caparon, M. (1992). Protein F, a fibronectin-binding protein, is an adhesin of the group A streptococcus *Streptococcus pyogenes. Proc. Natl. Acad. Sci. USA* 89, 6172–6176.

Hanski, E., Jaffe, J., and Ozeri, V. (1996). Proteins F1 and F2 of *Streptococcus pyogenes:* Properties of fibronectin binding. *Adv. Exp. Med. Biol.* 408, 141–150.

Hansson, L., Wallbrandt, P., Andersson, J. O., Bystrom, M., Backman, A., Carlstein, A., Enquist, K., Lonn, H., Otter, C., and Stromqvist, M. (1995). Carbohydrate specificity of the *Escherichia coli* P-pilus papG protein is mediated by its N-terminal part. *Biochim. Biophys. Acta* 1244, 377–383.

Harvey, H. A., Swords, W. E., and Apicella, M. A. (2001). The mimicry of human glycolipids and glycosphingolipids by the lipooligosaccharides of pathogenic *Neisseria* and *Haemophilus. J. Autoimmun.* 16, 257–262.

Hasty, D. L., and Courtney, H. S. (1996). Group A streptococcal adhesion: All of the theories are correct. *Adv. Exp. Med. Biol.* 408, 81–94.

Hasty, D. L., Courtney H., Sokurenko E., and Ofek I. (1994). Bacteria–extracellular matrix interactions. In *Fimbriae, Adhesion, Genetics, Biogenesis, and Vaccines* (ed. Klem, P.). Boca Raton, FL: CRC Press.

Hatakeyama, T., Murakami, K., Miyamoto, Y., and Yamasaki, N. (1996). An assay for lectin activity using microtiter plate with chemically immobilized carbohydrates. *Anal. Biochem.* 237, 188–192.

Hedlund, M., Svensson, M., Nilsson, A., Duan, R. D., and Svanborg, C. (1996). Role of the ceramide-signaling pathway in cytokine responses to P-fimbriated *Escherichia coli. J. Exp. Med.* 183, 1037–1044.

Henderson, B., Poole, S., and Wilson, M. (1996). Bacterial modulins: A novel class of virulence factors which cause host tissue pathology by inducing cytokine synthesis. *Microbiol. Rev.* 60, 316–341.

Hornick, D. B., Thommandru, J., Smits, W., and Clegg, S. (1995). Adherence properties of an *mrkD*-negative mutant of *Klebsiella pneumoniae. Infect. Immun.* 63, 2026–2032.

Hu, L. T., Perides, G., Noring, R., and Klempner, M. S. (1995). Binding of human plasminogen to *Borrelia burgdorferi. Infect. Immun.* 63, 3491–3496.

Hung, D. L., Raivio, T. L., Jones, C. H., Silhavy, T. J., and Hultgren, S. J. (2001). Cpx signaling pathway monitors biogenesis and affects assembly and expression of P pili. *EMBO J,* 20, 1508–1518.

Hung, C. S., Bouckaert, J., Hung, D., Pinkner, J., Widberg, C., DeFusco, A., Auguste, C. G., Strouse, R., Langermann, S., Waksman, G., and Hultgren, S. J. (2002). Structural basis of tropism of *Escherichia coli* to the bladder during urinary tract infection. *Mol. Microbiol.* 44, 903–915.

Jacques, M. (1996). Role of lipo-oligosaccharides and lipopolysaccharides in bacterial adherence. *Trends. Microbiol.* 4, 408–409.

Jeannotte, M. E., Abul-Milh, M., Dubreuil, J. D., and Jacques, M. (2003). Binding of *Actinobacillus pleuropneumoniae* to phosphatidylethanolamine. *Infect. Immun.* 71, 4657–4663.

Joh, D., Wann, E. R., Kreikemeyer, B., Speziale, P., and Hook, M. (1999). Role of fibronectin-binding MSCRAMMs in bacterial adherence and entry into mammalian cells. *Matrix Biol.* 18, 211–223.

Karlsson, K. A. (1995). Microbial recognition of target-cell glycoconjugates. *Curr. Opin. Struct. Biol.* 5, 622–635.

Keisari, Y., Kabha, K., Nissimov, L., Schlepper-Schafer, J., and Ofek, I. (1997). Phagocyte–bacteria interactions. *Adv. Dent. Res.* 11, 43–49.

Kubiet, M., and Ramphal, R. (1995). Adhesion of nontypeable *Haemophilus influenzae* from blood and sputum to human tracheobronchial mucins and lactoferrin. *Infect. Immun.* 63, 899–902.

Kukkonen, M., Saarela, S., Lahteenmaki, K., Hynonen, U., Westerlund-Wikstrom, B., Rhen, M., and Korhonen, T. K. (1998). Identification of two laminin-binding fimbriae, the type 1 fimbria of *Salmonella enterica* serovar typhimurium and the G fimbria of *Escherichia coli,* as plasminogen receptors. *Infect. Immun.* 66, 4965–4970.

Lillehoj, E. P., Kim, B. T., and Kim, K. C. (2002). Identification of *Pseudomonas aeruginosa* flagellin as an adhesin for Muc1 mucin. *Am. J. Physiol. Lung Cell. Mol. Physiol.* 282, L751–756.

Locht, C., Antoine, R., and Jacob-Dubuisson, F. (2001). *Bordetella pertussis,* molecular pathogenesis under multiple aspects. *Curr. Opin. Microbiol.* 4, 82–89.

Madison, B., Ofek, I., Clegg, S., and Abraham, S. N. (1994). Type 1 fimbrial shafts of *Escherichia coli* and *Klebsiella pneumoniae* influence sugar-binding specificities of their FimH adhesins. *Infect. Immun.* 62, 843–848.

Malaviya, R., Ross, E. A., MacGregor, J. I., Ikeda, T., Little, J. R., Jakschik, B. A., and Abraham, S. N. (1994). Mast cell phagocytosis of FimH-expressing enterobacteria. *J. Immunol.* 152, 1907–1914.

Malaviya, R., Ikeda, T., Ross, E., and Abraham, S. N. (1996). Mast cell modulation of neutrophil influx and bacterial clearance at sites of infection through TNF-alpha. *Nature* 381, 77–80.

Malaviya, R., Gao, Z., Thankavel, K., Vander Merwe, P. A., and Abraham, S. N. (1999). The mast cell tumor necrosis factor alpha response to FimH-expressing *Escherichia coli* is mediated by the glycosylphosphatidylinositol-anchored molecule CD48. *Proc. Natl. Acad. Sci. USA* 96, 8110–8115.

Malaviya, R., Abraham, S. N. (2000). Role of mast cell leukotrienes in neutrophil recruitment and bacterial clearance in infectious peritonitis. *J. Leukoc. Biol.* 67, 841–846.

Marceau, J. J., Beretti, J. L., and Nassif, X. (1995). High adhesiveness of encapsulated *Neisseria meningitidis* to epithelial cells is associated with the formation of bundles of pili. *Mol. Microbiol,* 17, 855–863.

Martinez, J. J., Mulvey, M. A., Schilling, J. D., Pinkner, J. S., and Hultgren, S. J. (2000). Type 1 pilus-mediated bacterial invasion of bladder epithelial cells. *EMBO J.* 19, 2803–2812.

McIntosh, D. P., Tan, X. Y., Oh, P., and Schnitzer, J. E. (2002). Targeting endothelium and its dynamic caveolae for tissue-specific transcytosis *in vivo:* A pathway to overcome cell barriers to drug and gene delivery. *Proc. Natl. Acad. Sci. USA* 99, 1996–2001.

Menozzi, F. D., Mutombo, R., Renauld, G., Gantiez, C., Hannah, J. H., Leininger, E., Brennan, M. J., and Locht, C. (1994). Heparin-inhibitable lectin activity of the filamentous hemagglutinin adhesin of *Bordetella pertussis. Infect. Immun.* 62, 769–778.

Menozzi, F. D., Pethe, K., Bifani, P., Soncin, F., Brennan, M. J., and Locht, C. (2002). Enhanced bacterial virulence through exploitation of host glycosaminoglycans. *Mol. Microbiol.* 43, 1379–1386.

Mey, A., Leffler, H., Hmama, Z., Normier, G., and Revillard, J. P. (1996). The animal lectin galectin-3 interacts with bacterial lipopolysaccharides via two independent sites. *J. Immunol.* 156, 1572–1577.

Mulvey, M. A. (2002). Adhesion and entry of uropathogenic *Escherichia coli*. *Cell. Microbiol.* 4, 257–271.

Mysorekar, I. U., Mulvey, M. A., Hultgren, S. J., and Gordon, J. I. (2002). Molecular regulation of urothelial renewal and host defenses during infection with uropathogenic *Escherichia coli*. *J. Biol. Chem.* 277, 7412–7419.

Nassif, X., and So, M. (1995). Interaction of pathogenic neisseriae with nonphagocytic cells. *Clin. Microbiol. Rev.* 8, 376–388.

Ofek, I., and Doyle, R. (1994). *Bacterial Adhesion to Cells and Tissues.* London/New York: Chapman and Hall.

Ofek, I., and Beachey, E. H. (1980). Bacterial adherence. *Adv. Intern. Med.* 25, 503–532.

Ofek, I., and Sharon, N. (1988). Lectinophagocytosis: A molecular mechanism of recognition between cell surface sugars and lectins in the phagocytosis of bacteria. *Infect. Immun.* 56, 539–547.

Ofek, I., Goldhar, J., Zafriri, D., Lis, H., Adar, R., and Sharon, N. (1991). Anti-*Escherichia coli* adhesin activity of cranberry and blueberry juices. *N. Engl. J. Med.* 324, 1599.

Ofek, I., Goldhar, J., Keisari, Y., and Sharon, N. (1995). Nonopsonic phagocytosis of microorganisms. *Annu. Rev. Microbiol.* 49, 239–276.

Ofek, I., Kahane, I., and Sharon, N. (1996). Toward anti-adhesion therapy for microbial diseases. *Trends Microbiol.* 4, 297–299.

Ohlsson, J., Jass, J., Uhlin, B. E., Kihlberg, J., and Nilsson, U. J. (2002). Discovery of potent inhibitors of PapG adhesins from uropathogenic *Escherichia coli* through synthesis and evaluation of galabiose derivatives. *Chembiochem* 3, 772–779.

Osset, J., Bartolome, R. M., Garcia, E., and Andreu, A. (2001). Assessment of the capacity of *Lactobacillus* to inhibit the growth of uropathogens and block their adhesion to vaginal epithelial cells. *J. Infect. Dis.* 183, 485–491.

Pak, J., Pu, Y., Zhang, Z. T., Hasty, D. L., and Wu, X. R. (2001). Tamm-Horsfall protein binds to type 1 fimbriated *Escherichia coli* and prevents *E. coli* from binding to uroplakin Ia and Ib receptors. *J. Biol. Chem.* 276, 9924–9930.

Palaniyar, N., Nadesalingam, J., and Reid, K. B. (2002). Pulmonary innate immune proteins and receptors that interact with gram-positive bacterial ligands. *Immunobiology* 205, 575–594.

Parent, J. B. (1990). Membrane receptors on rat hepatocytes for the inner core region of bacterial lipopolysaccharides. *J. Biol. Chem.* 265, 3455–3461.

Passador, L., Cook, J. M., Gambello, M. J., Rust, L., and Iglewski, B. H. (1993). Expression of *Pseudomonas aeruginosa* virulence genes requires cell-to-cell communication. *Science* 260, 1127–1130.

Patti, J. M., and Hook, M. (1994). Microbial adhesins recognizing extracellular matrix macromolecules. *Curr. Opin. Cell. Biol.* 6, 752–758.

Patti, J. M., Allen, B. L., McGavin, M. J., and Hook, M. (1994). MSCRAMM-mediated adherence of microorganisms to host tissues. *Annu. Rev. Microbiol.* 48, 585–617.

Plotkowski, M. C., Tournier, J. M., and Puchelle, E. (1996). *Pseudomonas aeruginosa* strains possess specific adhesins for laminin. *Infect. Immun.* 64, 600–605.

Przondo-Mordarska, A., Smutnicka, D., Ko, H. L., Beuth, J., and Pulverer, G. (1996). Adhesive properties of P-like fimbriae in *Klebsiella*-species. *Zentralbl. Bakteriol.* 284, 372–377.

Raivio, T. L., and Silhavy, T. J. (1999). The sigmaE and Cpx regulatory pathways: Overlapping but distinct envelope stress responses. *Curr. Opin. Microbiol.* 2, 159–165.

Reddy, M. S., Bernstein, J. M., Murphy, T. F., and Faden, H. S. (1996). Binding between outer membrane proteins of nontypeable *Haemophilus influenzae* and human nasopharyngeal mucin. *Infect. Immun.* 64, 1477–1479.

Reid, G. (2002). The potential role of probiotics in pediatric urology. *J. Urol.* 168, 1512–1517.

Relman, D. A., Domenighini, M., Tuomanen, E., Rappuoli, R., and Falkow, S. (1989). Filamentous hemagglutinin of *Bordetella pertussis*: Nucleotide sequence and crucial role in adherence. *Proc. Natl. Acad. Sci. USA* 86, 2637–2641.

Ryan, P. A., Pancholi, V., and Fischetti, V. A. (2001). Group A streptococci bind to mucin and human pharyngeal cells through sialic acid–containing receptors. Infect. Immun., 69, 7402–7412.

Saarela, S., Westerlund-Wikstrom, B., Rhen, M., and Korhonen, T. K. (1996). The GafD protein of the G (F17) fimbrial complex confers adhesiveness of *Escherichia coli* to laminin. *Infect. Immun.* 64, 2857–2860.

Sakarya, S., and Oncu, S. (2003). Bacterial adhesins and the role of sialic acid in bacterial adhesion. *Med. Sci. Monit.* 9, RA76–82.

Scharfman, A., Kroczynski, H., Carnoy, C., Van Brussel, E., Lamblin, G., Ramphal, R., and Roussel, P. (1996). Adhesion of *Pseudomonas aeruginosa* to respiratory mucins and expression of mucin-binding proteins are increased by limiting iron during growth. *Infect. Immun.* 64, 5417–5420.

Schembri, M. A., Hasman, H., and Klemm, P. (2000). Expression and purification of the mannose recognition domain of the FimH adhesin. *FEMS Microbiol. Lett.* 188, 147–151.

Schengrund, C. L. (2003). "Multivalent" saccharides: Development of new approaches for inhibiting the effects of glycosphingolipid-binding pathogens. *Biochem. Pharmacol.* 65, 699–707.

Schilling, J. D., Martin, S. M., Hunstad, D. A., Patel, K. P., Mulvey, M. A., Justice, S. S., Lorenz, R. G., and Hultgren, S. J. (2003). CD14- and toll-like receptor–dependent activation of bladder epithelial cells by lipopolysaccharide and type 1 piliated *Escherichia coli*. *Infect. Immun.* 71, 1470–1480.

Sharon, N. (1996). Carbohydrate-lectin interactions in infectious diseases. *Adv. Exp. Med. Biol.* 408, 1–8.

Sharon, N. and Lis, H. (1997). Microbial lectins and their glycoprotein receptors. In *Glycoproteins II* (Montreuil, J., Vliegenthart, J. F. G., and Schachter, H., eds.), 475–506. Amsterdam, Elsevier.

Sharon, N., and Ofek, I. (2000). Safe as mother's milk: Carbohydrates as future anti-adhesion drugs for bacterial diseases. *Glycoconj. J.* 17, 659–664.

Sharon, N., and Ofek, I. (2002). Fighting infectious diseases with inhibitors of microbial adhesion to host tissues. *Crit. Rev. Food. Sci. Nutr.* 42, 267–272.

Sorme, P., Qian, Y., Nyholm, P. G., Leffler, H., and Nilsson, U. J. (2002). Low micromolar inhibitors of galectin-3 based on 3'-derivatization of N-acetyllactosamine. *Chembiochem* 3, 183–189.

Steadman, R., Topley, N., Jenner, D. E., Davies, M., and Williams, J. D. (1988). Type 1 fimbriate *Escherichia coli* stimulates a unique pattern of degranulation by human polymorphonuclear leukocytes. *Infect. Immun.* 56, 815–822.

Svanborg, C., Hedlund, M., Connell, H., Agace, W., Duan, R. D., Nilsson, A., and Wullt, B. (1996). Bacterial adherence and mucosal cytokine responses: Receptors and transmembrane signaling. *Ann. N.Y. Acad. Sci.* 797, 177–190.

Swords, W. E., Buscher, B. A., Ver Steeg Ii, K., Preston, A., Nichols, W. A., Weiser, J. N., Gibson, B. W., and Apicella, M. A. (2000). Nontypeable *Haemophilus influenzae* adhere to and invade human bronchial epithelial cells via an interaction of lipooligosaccharide with the PAF receptor. *Mol. Microbiol.* 37, 13–27.

Sylvester, F. A., Philpott, D., Gold, B., Lastovica, A., and Forstner, J. F. (1996). Adherence to lipids and intestinal mucin by a recently recognized human pathogen, *Campylobacter upsaliensis*. *Infect. Immun.* 64, 4060–4066.

Szymanski, C. M. and Armstrong, G. D. (1996). Interactions between *Campylobacter jejuni* and lipids. *Infect. Immun.* 64, 3467–3474.

Tewari, R., Ikeda, T., Malaviya, R., MacGregor, J. I., Little, J. R., Hultgren, S. J., and Abraham, S. N. (1994). The PapG tip adhesin of P fimbriae protects *Escherichia coli* from neutrophil bactericidal activity. *Infect. Immun.* 62, 5296–5304.

Thankavel, K., Madison, B., Ikeda, T., Malaviya, R., Shah, A. H., Arumugam, P.M., and Abraham, S.N. (1997). Localization of a domain in the FimH adhesin of *Escherichia coli* type 1 fimbriae capable of receptor recognition and use of a domain-specific antibody to confer protection against experimental urinary tract infection. *J. Clin. Invest.* 100, 1123–1136.

Tikkanen, K., Haataja, S., Francois-Gerard, C., and Finne, J. (1995). Purification of a galactosyl-alpha 1-4-galactose-binding adhesin from the gram-positive meningitis-associated bacterium *Streptococcus suis*. *J. Biol. Chem.* 270, 28874–28878.

Topley, N., Steadman, R., Mackenzie, R., Knowlden, J. M., and Williams, J. D. (1989). Type 1 fimbriate strains of *Escherichia coli* initiate renal parenchymal scarring. *Kidney Int.* 36, 609–616.

Tuomanen, E., Towbin, H., Rosenfelder, G., Braun, D., Larson, G., Hansson, G. C., and Hill, R. (1988). Receptor analogs and monoclonal antibodies that inhibit adherence of *Bordetella pertussis* to human ciliated respiratory epithelial cells. *J. Exp. Med.* 168, 267–277.

Uehling, D. T., Johnson, D. B., and Hopkins, W. J. (1999). The urinary tract response to entry of pathogens. *World. J. Urol.* 17, 351–358.

Valkonen, K. H., Wadstrom, T., and Moran, A. P. (1994). Interaction of lipopolysaccharides of *Helicobacter pylori* with basement membrane protein laminin. *Infect. Immun.* 62, 3640–3648.

Valkonen, K. H., Wadstrom, T., and Moran, A. P. (1997). Identification of the N-acetylneuraminyllactose-specific laminin-binding protein of *Helicobacter pylori*. *Infect. Immun.* 65, 916–923.

van Putten, J. P., and Paul, S. M. (1995). Binding of syndecan-like cell surface proteoglycan receptors is required for *Neisseria gonorrhoeae* entry into human mucosal cells. *EMBO J.* 14, 2144–2154.

Von Stebut, E., Metz, M., Milon, G., Knop, J., and Mauer, M. (2003). Early macrophage influx to sites of cutaneous granuloma formation is dependent on MIP-1 alpha/beta released from neutrophils recruited by mast cell derived TNF alpha. *Blood* 101, 210–215.

Wu, X. R., Sun, T. T., and Medina, J. J. (1996). *In vitro* binding of type 1-fimbriated *Escherichia coli* to uroplakins Ia and Ib: Relation to urinary tract infections. *Proc. Natl. Acad. Sci. USA* 93, 9630–9635.

Wullt, B., Bergsten, G., Connell, H., Rollano, P., Gebratsedik, N., Hang, L., and Svanborg, C. (2001). P-fimbriae trigger mucosal responses to *Escherichia coli* in the human urinary tract. *Cell. Microbiol.* 3, 255–264.

Wullt, B., Bergsten, G., Samuelsson, M., and Svanborg, C. (2002). The role of P fimbriae for *Escherichia coli* establishment and mucosal inflammation in the human urinary tract. *Int J. Antimicrob. Agents* 19, 522–538.

Zafriri, D., Oron, Y., Eisenstein, B. I., and Ofek, I. (1987). Growth advantage and enhanced toxicity of *Escherichia coli* adherent to tissue culture cells due to restricted diffusion of products secreted by the cells. *J. Clin. Invest.* 79, 1210–1216.

Zaidi, T. S., Fleiszig, S. M., Preston, M. J., Goldberg, J. B., and Pier, G. B. (1996). Lipopolysaccharide outer core is a ligand for corneal cell binding and ingestion of *Pseudomonas aeruginosa*. *Invest. Ophthalmol. Vis. Sci.* 37, 976–986.

Zhou, G., Mo, W. J., Sebbel, P., Min, G., Neubert, T. A., Glockshuber, R., Wu, X. R., Sun, T. T., and Kong, X. P. (2001). Uroplakin Ia is the urothelial receptor for uropathogenic *Escherichia coli*: Evidence from *in vitro* FimH binding. *J. Cell. Sci.* 114, 4095–4103.

Zopf, D., Simon, P., Barthelson, R., Cundell, D., Idanpaan-Heikkila, I., and Tuomanen, E. (1996). Development of anti-adhesion carbohydrate drugs for clinical use. *Adv. Exp. Med. Biol.* 408, 35–38.

Mucus

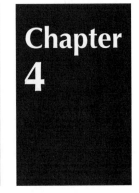

Chapter 4

Richard A. Cone

Jenkins Department of Biophysics, Johns Hopkins University, Baltimore, Maryland

The slimy is docile. Only at the very moment when I believe that I possess it, behold by a curious reversal, it possesses me. Here appears its essential character: its softness is leech-like. . . . It is a soft, yielding action, a moist and feminine sucking, it lives obscurely under my fingers. . . . (Sartre, 1981)

INTRODUCTION

This slimy and somewhat repellant substance is often ignored, but mucus serves a multitude of immune functions. Some are not readily apparent, and others are not easy to investigate. Many functions of mucus can only be studied *in vivo* or in fresh, unmanipulated samples that are often difficult to obtain. Our current level of ignorance of mucus is caused in part by a certain lack of glamour that tends to repel rather than attract interest. Indeed, in textbooks, lecture slides, and papers on mucosal immunology, the cartoons of the mucosal surface usually focus on the cells of the mucosal immune system, B cells, T cells, M cells, Langerhans cells, with the blanket of mucus often completely missing—out of sight, out of mind. Only after 20 years of intensive research to develop an acquired immune deficiency syndrome (AIDS) vaccine has research interest finally shifted to create *mucosal* vaccines for human immunodeficiency virus (HIV) that might exclude infectious entry. This shift helped reveal a lack of research interest in the mechanisms by which this virus is transmitted in mucus: We still do not know whether HIV first enters the sexual partner as a cell-free virus or whether HIV is more likely to be actively transported into the partner by infected "Trojan horse leukocytes," ameboid cells in cervical mucus or semen that can migrate through epithelia to reach lymph nodes. It is in mucus, the watery gel on the surface of the epithelium, that immune functions usually prevent the infectious entry of pathogens and the injurious entry of toxins. With further research on the protective functions that occur in mucus, we may learn how to augment mucosal immune defenses to prevent the initial entry of pathogens and toxins, how to "exclude" them before they infect.

This chapter discusses some of the physical and chemical properties of mucus that help protect epithelial surfaces.

More extensive discussion of the synthesis, secretion, and biochemistry of mucus can be found in excellent reviews by Taylor *et al.* (2003), Davies *et al.* (2002), Forstner *et al.* (1995), Neutra and Forstner (1987), Lichtman *et al.* (1996), and Forstner (1995). For recent reviews of mucin peptide structure and evolution, see Dekker *et al.* (2002), Desseyn *et al.* (2000), van Klinken *et al.* (1995), Gendler and Spicer (1995), and Gum (1995). For mucins in gastrointestinal (GI) disease, see Corfield *et al.* (2000).

THE MUCOSAL SURFACE IS A PROTECTIVE "ECOSYSTEM"

Mucus secretions sustain complex, thriving, and local ecosystems. Mucus gels, formed by secreted mucins, are loaded with cells, bacteria, nutrients, protective factors, and wastes. Many of the constituents, including the secreted mucins, are specific to the particular mucosal surface, an environmental niche that supports each microecosystem. It is the complexity and marked diversity of mucins (Roussel *et al.* 1988) that help make each ecosystem unique.

Secreted mucins are long fibrous peptides coated with a complex array of glycans. Currently, 14 mucin-type glycoproteins have been assigned to the *MUC* gene family (see Dekker *et al.* 2002). Each mucin gene is highly polymorphic, several different mucin genes are expressed at each type of mucosal surface, and some epithelial cells express more than one mucin gene (Dekker *et al.* 2002; Dessyn *et al.* 2000; Gendler and Spicer 1995). In addition, the diversity of oligosaccharides attached to mucins is remarkable; the respiratory mucins of a single person probably contain several hundred different glycans, and there are considerable variations between individuals (Roussel *et al.* 1988; Lamblin *et al.* 1991; Tabak 1995). However, the distribution of O-glycans attached to mucins does not differ significantly between the right and left glands in the same individual. Certain mucosal microbiota, both commensals and pathogens, have been shown to bind specifically to mucins secreted at the sites they inhabit, or infect, including *Pseudomonas aeruginosa*, which binds tracheobronchial mucins and infects the lungs (Vishwanath and Ramphal 1985), as well as several other bacteria and viruses that bind specifically to different glycan structures (Tabak 1995; Cohen and Laux 1995). Most commensal bacteria do not degrade mucins, but a few symbiotic bacteria are well adapted to "graze" on the mucins secreted by the intestine, enabling the host to recycle some of the mucin components it sheds (see the following text). These symbiotes adapt specifically to the host's mucins; for example, microorganisms in the gut have been shown to produce blood group–degrading enzymes specific to the blood group glycans of the host mucins (Hoskins *et al.* 1985). Moreover, the composition of mucins and their glycosylation vary not only during development but also depending on the host's diet and the presence and activity of specific commensals and pathogens. Thus the mucins help create local ecosystems at different epithelial sites, helping select and support specific arrays of commensals and helping define and defend against the specific pathogens to which each epithelium is susceptible.

Mucus not only helps support and define these mucosal ecosystems, but it helps regulate them in concert with the rest of the mucosal immune system. Mucus acts as the outermost sensory "organ" of the mucosal immune system because the mucus blanket, similar to a cell membrane, is a selectively permeable barrier. Mucus must enable rapid entry and exit of nutrients, gases, and wastes, while excluding pathogens and toxins. Thus mucus helps select and regulate what the cellular immune system will encounter. In addition, the mucus blanket selectively nurtures and helps

regulate commensal microbes, the abundant "microbiota" that colonize most mucosal surfaces (see Chapter 2). Commensals are often friendly and protective organisms that help reduce or prevent colonization by pathogens. However, commensals remain friendly only if the mucosal immune system, by regulating the secretion rates and composition of mucus as well as the array of secreted antibodies and other protective factors, maintains adequate control of commensal populations—many commensals, merely by overgrowing or by migrating to another mucosal ecosystem, become pathogenic. In helping maintain this control, mucus also acts as the outermost effector organ of the mucosal immune system.

In performing its numerous functions, mucus is continuously secreted, then shed and discarded, or digested and recycled. Its lifetime is short, often measured in minutes to hours, and both the sensory and effector functions mediated in mucus are rapid; mucus secretion and shedding rates can change within seconds and can increase dramatically to wash away toxic substances. Characteristic thicknesses, secretion rates, and mucociliary transport rates are shown in **Figure 4.1** along with some structural features of the mucus coat.

The composition of mucus is also continuously regulated by varying secretion rates of different mucin types, ions, proteins, lipids, and water. The array of secreted antibodies in mucus changes continuously to deal with the ever-changing flux of antigens and pathogens arriving on the epithelial surface and the continual activities of commensal populations. Thus the protective functions of mucus are dynamic

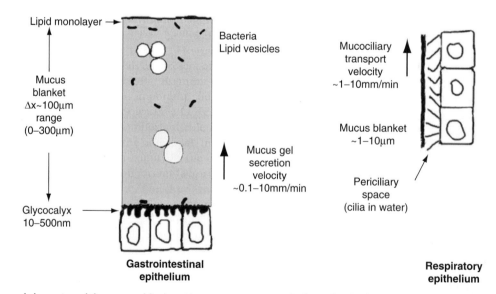

Fig. 4.1. Structure and dynamics of the mucus blanket. Humans secrete a total of ~10 liters of mucus per day (Moore 1976). Most bacteria populate the outermost surfaces of the mucus blanket (Sherman *et al.* 1987), although a few adhere directly to the epithelial cells (Poulsen 1994). The thickness, Δx, of the mucus blanket varies with mucosal activity and anatomic site, as do the transport rates indicated by the range of velocities with which the mucus coat moves outward and the rates of lateral transport by mucociliary transport. The ranges in these rates reflect in part the difficulties in measuring mucus transport rates (see Forstner 1995). Diffusional transit times through a mucus blanket, Δt, increase exponentially with the thickness of the blanket, as Δx^2, requiring that the thickness of the blanket be regulated not only to ensure rapid diffusional exchange rates but also to provide adequate time for secreted antibodies and other protectants to be maximally effective against incoming toxins and pathogens.

processes, depending on relative rates of outward secretion and inward diffusion, and on the relative rates of mucus shedding and microbial growth. Unlike the systemic immune system, the mucosal immune system continuously encounters, monitors, and regulates a thriving array of microbes and toxins that are ever present and ever changing. Continuous regulation of mucus secretions helps keep these microbes and toxins at bay, on the outer mucosal surfaces, most of the time.

GEL PROPERTIES OF MUCUS THAT HELP PROTECT MUCOSA

Mucus is a viscoelastic gel

Mucus is a sticky (viscid) slippery gel with viscoelastic properties that are regulated to ensure efficient transport and shedding of the mucus blanket. Viscoelasticity is regulated primarily by regulating the mucin to water secretion ratio and also by regulating lipid, protein, and ion content, especially Ca^{++} content (Raynal et al. 2003). Mucus has sufficient adhesive and elastic strength to be retained on the epithelial surface despite the shearing forces of swallowing, peristalsis, eyelid blinking, and copulation. In the lungs, mucus elasticity must be sufficient to resist the force of gravity; if it becomes too thin and watery, mucus can run downward and clog the alveoli. Crucial for mucus transport and shedding is the shear dependence of its viscosity. Motions that create large changes in velocity over short distances, that is, high shear rates, cause the viscosity of mucus to fall precipitously. Thus mucus is a "non-Newtonian" fluid that is unlike water, honey, and oils, all of which are Newtonian fluids whose viscosities have little if any shear dependence. When mucus is rapidly sheared, a slippage plane forms between layers of mucus, and within this slippage plane, the viscosity becomes waterlike. As this occurs, the sliding force is said to overcome the "yield strength," and as long as the mucus continues to slip, the viscosity in the slippage plane remains low, making mucus an excellent lubricant. **Figure 4.2** illustrates the location of the slippage plane and emphasizes that unstirred layers of mucus adhere to, and move with, both of the sliding surfaces. These unstirred layers are crucial for creating the selective permeability of the mucus blanket. Also, the unstirred layer can help mechanically stabilize the surface; the "pellicle" of unstirred mucus that adheres to teeth slows

the rate at which the enamel demineralizes (Nieuw Amerongen et al. 1987).

Figure 4.3 is a summary of viscosity measurements performed on a variety of mucus secretions. It illustrates that despite variations in the biochemical structure of mucins and differences in mucus composition, the viscoelasticity of many mucus secretions is quite similar. In particular, the viscous drag exerted by mucus is very large at low shear rates, some 10^4–10^6 times greater than the viscous drag of water. However, with the maximum shear rates that occur physiologically, the viscous drag of mucus, as shown by the extrapolated lines in Figure 4.3, decreases so much it begins to approach the minimal viscous drag of water.

What Figure 4.3 does not show is that, when the steady shear rate stops, the viscoelasticity of mucus recovers, or heals, restoring much of its elasticity and viscosity within seconds and fully recovering more slowly over minutes to hours (Taylor et al. 2003; Bell et al. 1985). Without this healing action, mucus once sheared by coughing would drip back into the lungs, cilia could not move mucus efficiently out of the sinuses, inner ears, lungs, or reproductive tracts, and snails, slugs, and other gastropods would be unable to move. Gastropods produce local contractile waves that travel along the surface of their feet, rapidly shearing mucus locally, allowing the local contraction to slip forward easily while the rest of the foot remains still, gripping firmly with mucus that is not being sheared and hence has high viscosity (Denny 1980; Silberberg 1990). If the viscoelasticity of mucus did not heal after slipping, the noncontracting parts of the foot would slip backward while the contracting parts were slipping forward. The healing process reveals that mucus is not a covalently cross-linked gel, since cross-linked gels, such as polyacrylamide gels used for electrophoresis, tear irreparably when sheared. Mucus is a gel formed not only by the entangling of mucin fibers, but also by multiple but well-spaced low-affinity bonds between the long, thin, and flexible fibers of mucin. The thermal diffusional motions of these fibers cause them to reentangle and to reassociate rapidly after being pulled apart sideways at a slippage plane. Thus it is the diffusional reentanglement and rebonding of the fibers that "heals" the mucus, a healing process that can be repeated indefinitely. Only if mucus is subjected to large and rapid shear motions sufficient to break the longer mucin fibers does its viscoelasticity begin to degrade.

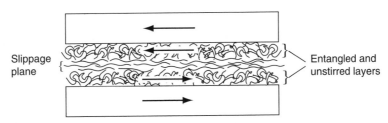

Fig. 4.2. Mucus forms a slippage plane that leaves intact an unstirred layer adhering to each surface. Although stirring actions, such as swallowing and peristalsis, can deliver substances close to epithelial surfaces, molecules and viruses, and nonmotile bacteria must diffuse through an unstirred layer before they can contact epithelial cells.

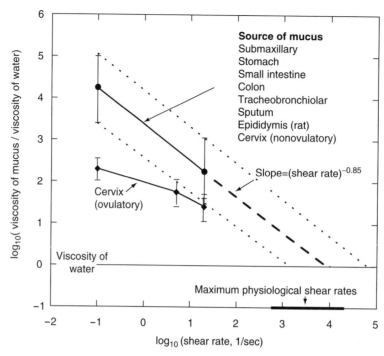

Fig. 4.3. Mucus viscosity decreases as the shear rate increases, making mucus an excellent lubricant that both clings and slips. Log_{10} [mucus viscosity] is shown as a function of log_{10} [shear rate] in units of 1/sec. Mucus viscosity at constant shear is given in relative units with respect to the viscosity of water, 0.01 mPas. Shear rate is the velocity gradient, dv/dx, between two surfaces sliding past each other. High shear rates occur at mucosal surfaces during eye blinks, coughing, vomiting, bowel movements, copulation, and ejaculation, and at the cellular level, comparably high shear rates are created by cilia, sperm flagella, and bacterial flagella. (An object of radius r moving through a fluid with velocity v, creates a shear rate of approximately v/r.) In all these physiologic cases, maximum shear rates occur in the range of $\sim 10^3 – 10^4$ per second. The data summarized in this figure were derived from several different rheologic techniques applied to mucus obtained from many different mucosal sites: Pig submaxillary gland (Sellers *et al.* 1988a), pig stomach, small intestine, and colon (Sellers *et al.* 1987, 1988b, 1991); human lung (Yeates *et al.* 1996; Jeanneret-Grosjean *et al.* 1988; Rubin *et al.* 1992); human sputum (Yeates *et al.* 1996), rat epididymis (Usselman and Cone 1983); human nonovulatory cervix (unpublished observations, Zeitlin and Cone 1997); human and bovine cervix (Wolf *et al.* 1977a,b). Viscosity at steady shear rate, η', was derived from oscillating ball and oscillating cone-and-plate rheometric observations using $\eta' = (G^* \sin\delta)/\eta = G''/\omega$ where $\tan\delta$ = viscous strain/elastic strain and ω = rad/sec. For an excellent review, see Yeates *et al.* (1996). Given the differences in measuring techniques and temperatures ($\sim 20°$C to $37°$C), and the different epithelial sources and mucin concentrations ($\sim 2\%$ to 9%) in the various mucus samples, the range of results, shown by the vertical bars, is remarkably small. However, other mucus secretions have significantly lower mucin concentrations, such as tear film, saliva ($\sim 0.1\%$ to 0.5%), and ovulatory cervical mucus ($\sim 0.5\%$ to 1.5%) and hence have significantly lower viscosities, as illustrated by ovulatory cervical mucus.

Mucus transport requires well-regulated viscoelasticity

When a mucus gel is displaced only a short distance (small strain), mucin fibers stretch rather than disentangle or pull apart and hence tend to spring back when the displacing force is released. This elastic property of mucus is critical for mucociliary transport. Cilia on the epithelial surfaces of the respiratory tract continuously sweep mucus shed from the eyes, sinuses, middle ears, nose, and lungs into the pharynx. The particles and pathogens trapped within these mucus secretions are thereby delivered to the stomach where they are rapidly inactivated by acid. Tear film is cleansed and replaced in this way every ~ 10 seconds, nasal mucus is cleansed and replaced within ~ 10 minutes (Schuhl 1995), and respiratory mucus is transported up and out of the lungs at rates of $\sim 5–10$ cm/min. When the tip of a cilium sweeps the surface of a mucus blanket, it sweeps with a shearing motion

that is small and fast enough that the mucus gel acts primarily by elastic rather than by viscous forces, greatly enhancing the efficiency of this transport mechanism (Silberberg 1990). Also, the beating cilia apparently push the mucus blanket away from the cell surface, forming a water layer next to the epithelial cell surface, the periciliary layer (see Figure 4.1). Thus most ciliary motions occur within the low viscosity of water, and only the tips of the cilia sweep against the viscoelastic mucus gel.

Cilia can only transport mucus if it has appropriate viscoelasticity. If respiratory mucus becomes too runny, gravity overcomes ciliary transport, and mucus runs out of the nose as well as sliding down into the lungs. On the other hand, if mucus becomes too firm, as in cystic fibrosis, it becomes too viscous to be transported by cilia. Thus the viscoelasticity of mucus must be closely regulated to obtain the best compromise between the elasticity needed to prevent gravitational flow, and provide efficient ciliary transport, and the low viscosity needed to allow rapid transport and clearance (Silberberg 1990). Indeed, the viscoelasticity of respiratory mucus appears to be "tuned" to the small, rapid sweeping motions of cilia. Under normal conditions, respiratory mucus is relatively thicker, somewhat slowing mucus transport, but when irritants, such as cigarette smoke (Rubin *et al.* 1992), or allergens (Hattori *et al.* 1993) are encountered, more dilute mucin is secreted, decreasing viscoelasticity into the optimal range for maximizing mucociliary clearance (Hattori *et al.* 1993).

During a cough, the explosive blast of air creates large displacements at high shear rates that overcome the yield strength of mucus; the mucin fibers begin to pull apart and disentangle at the slippage plane and the outer layer of mucus is driven rapidly along by the flow of air. The blast of air can also create waves in the mucus coat that grow in size and shear rates until blebs of mucus are flung from their crests and expelled (King 1987; Tomkiewicz *et al.* 1994). In pursuing observations of mucus clearance by coughing, mayonnaise was found to be a readily available substitute that reasonably simulates the non-Newtonian viscoelasticity of mucus. As with ciliary transport, mucus that is too thick cannot readily be cleared by coughing.

Swallowing and peristaltic transport also require close regulation of the viscoelasticity of mucus. The sensation of oral dryness (xerostomia), a significant problem for many elderly people, appears to be caused by saliva with inadequate viscoelasticity because people can have this problem even when their salivary flow rates are normal (Fox *et al.* 1987; Narhi 1994). Infertility occurs in males with cystic fibrosis from the atrophy of the epididymis and vas deferens (Dean and Santis 1994; Dumur *et al.* 1996), apparently because epididymal mucus becomes too viscoelastic to be transported by peristalsis, leading to blockage and atrophy. Similarly, overly thick mucus in the ducts leading from the liver, gallbladder, and pancreas can block transport of bile salts and digestive enzymes, disabling the digestive actions of the gut, especially for fats, which end up undigested in the feces.

Viscoelasticity of mucus can block motility of sperm and bacteria

Only during the time of ovulation, when cervical mucus becomes less viscoelastic, can human sperm swim through this mucus, increasing their abilities to reach the upper reproductive tract. Ovulatory mucus contains a relatively large amount of MUC5B mucin (Gipson *et al.* 2001) and is capable of being stretched between two fingers into a thread several centimeters in length ("*spinnbarkeit*"). During most of the rest of the menstrual cycle and throughout pregnancy, nonovulatory mucus is thicker and breaks apart when stretched between the fingers. The concentration of mucins in nonovulatory mucus is only moderately increased (twofold to fourfold), but this markedly increases its viscoelasticity, making nonovulatory cervical mucus virtually impenetrable to sperm (Moghissi and Syner 1970; Wolf *et al.* 1977a,b). In small rodents, the viscoelasticity of mucus is

also used in the male reproductive tract to immobilize sperm during the time they are stored in the caput epididymis of the testis (Usselman and Cone 1983; Usselman *et al.* 1985). This storage mucus protects rat sperm from being killed by the high shear rates that occur during ejaculation of these relatively large sperm through relatively small epididymal ducts: the rat sperm stored within a bolus of mucus are subjected to much less shear since the slippage plane occurs between the bolus and the epithelial surface (Baltz *et al.* 1990). The viscous drag of rat epididymal mucus is comparable with that of mucus samples from many other mucosal surfaces, as indicated in Figure 4.3; this viscoelasticity is just thick enough to block *Escherichia coli* as well as sperm from swimming (Usselman and Cone 1983). Thus it is likely that many mucus secretions are sufficiently viscoelastic to block the motility of many types of bacteria. Indeed, most intestinal bacteria populate the outer, lumenal surface of the mucus blanket. Nevertheless, some types of bacteria seem especially well designed to penetrate normal mucus, notably *Helicobacter pylori* and *Vibrio cholerae*, both of which are capable of swimming through intestinal mucus (Schrank and Verwey 1976). Leukocytes (Parkhurst and Saltzman 1994), and probably other ameboid cells, can also migrate through relatively thick mucus. In response to infections with *H. pylori*, the viscoelasticity of gastric mucus *increases* (Markesich *et al.* 1995), suggesting that, as with nonovulatory cervical mucus, thicker mucus may help prevent entry by motile pathogens.

Saliva and tear fluid have markedly lower viscoelasticity and are readily penetrable by motile bacteria. Thus, on some mucosal surfaces, the viscoelasticity of the gel is not, by itself, sufficient to trap or prevent entry by motile bacteria. However, the high rate at which tear film and saliva are secreted and replaced creates a potent defense against bacterial colonization and overgrowth. Decreased secretion rates of these fluids lead to increased infection rates; diminished flow of saliva increases susceptibility to dental cavity formation (caries) and to opportunistic yeast infections (thrush mouth) (Tabak 1995). During sleep, saliva is secreted more slowly, and the reduced flow rate leads to an increase in bacterial colonization causing "morning breath" on waking.

Thickness and secretion rates of the mucus blanket vary greatly with epithelial site, and status

As Ivan P. Pavlov (1849–1936) demonstrated, simply the anticipation of eating food stimulates the secretion of saliva and gastric mucus. Fear has the opposite effect, slowing salivary secretion, thinning the mucus layers and reducing their lubricant ability, an effect that is well known to public speakers, hence, the traditional glass of water. In addition to neural control, mucus secretion rates are also regulated by many different types of local stimuli that have yet to be identified or fully elucidated (Dartt 2002; McNamara and Basbaum 2002; Deplancke and Gaskins 2001; Forstner 1995; Forstner *et al.* 1995; Neutra and Forstner 1987). The thickness of the mucus blanket is determined by the balance between the rate of secretion and rate of degradation and shedding. Toxic and irritating substances can greatly stimulate mucus secretion, increasing the thickness of the mucus blanket "shield" while efficiently and rapidly moving the irritants away from the epithelium. Secreting new mucus is markedly more efficient than simply washing the surface, because rinsing the surface fails to refresh the unstirred layer adhering to the epithelium. In contrast, by continuously secreting new mucus, the unstirred layer is continuously and rapidly replaced. Thus pathogens and irritants must continuously migrate or diffuse "upstream" to reach the epithelium. Even in an absorptive epithelium such as the small intestine, where water is flowing inward through and being filtered through the mucus coat, irritants and pathogens must advance through a blanket of mucus gel that is moving *outward* if they are to reach the epithelial surface.

In the human GI tract, the mucus blanket is thickest in the stomach (180 μm; range 50–450 μm) and colon (110–160 μm) (Kerss *et al.* 1982; Sandzen 1988; Copeman *et al.* 1994). In the small intestine, the thickness varies greatly depending on digestive activity. For instance, with a fibrous diet, the outer "sloppy" layer of mucus in the rat intestine can be wiped away by the movement of the chyme, but a firmly adherent inner layer of mucus still covers the epithelial surface (Strugala *et al.* 2003; Szentkuti and Lorenz 1995). In addition, a thin mucus coat is likely to adhere to the chyme. As reported by Florey (1962), intestinal mucus is "tenacious" and wraps up particles so they do not come in direct contact with epithelial cells: "particles of India ink injected into the stomach of a cat became wrapped up in little balls of mucin ... [that] were gradually bound together, and they appeared in the feces as small masses firmly held together by mucin." Gruber *et al.* (1987) observed what happened to a variety of test particles and found that irrespective of the size, density, or composition, GI mucus formed them into mucus-covered "slugs." Even the unusually thin mucus secreted in tear film wraps particles in a mucus coat, as can be noticed on removing an irritating particle from the eyelid. In the intestine, the cells least protected by mucus and most exposed to the chyme are the M cells on the domes of the Peyer's patches. No mucus is secreted in the region surrounding these cells, which protrude relatively unprotected into the lumen (Neutra and Forstner 1987). Thus M cells are positioned as sensory outposts for cellular immune functions, transcytosing the particles that impinge on their surface into the interior of the patch. Since these are likely to be particles that mucus has failed to trap and "wrap," mucus thereby helps select those antigens most likely to require the production of specific antibodies to help exclude them.

Lipid layer and mucin-bound lipids help provide selective permeability

Figure 4.1 illustrates two additional barrier structures of the mucus blanket, the glycocalyx on the lumenal surface of the epithelial cells (Ito 1974) and the lipid layer that forms on the surfaces of many types of mucus blankets (Rubin 2002; Davenport 1972; Lichtenberger 1995). Both these structures contribute significantly to the selective permeability of the mucus blanket. The lipids in and on the surfaces of mucus blanket, together with saccharides on mucins, also serve as scavengers against free radical attack (Lamont 1992; Lichtenberger 1995).

A lipid layer significantly impedes the evaporation of water from the tear film covering the eyes, a major problem for birds in flight, and enhances its lubricant properties needed for cleansing and blinking. The lipid layer is formed in part by cationic surfactants, including dipalmitoyl-phosphatidylcholine (DPPC), whose positively charged head groups bind to the highly negatively charged mucins that form the mucus gel, while the aliphatic chains form a continuous hydrophobic monolayer facing the outer surface of the gel. The surfactants secreted in the lungs not only prevent alveolar collapse by reducing the surface tension but also probably increase the ability of respiratory mucus to trap hydrophobic airborne particles. In the GI tract, the lipid layer significantly impedes the diffusion of gastric acid (see the following text). The presence of this hydrophobic surface layer can be observed by placing a drop of water on the surface of the mucus blanket and observing the angle with which the drop contacts the surface. The contact angle is largest (implying the most hydrophobic surface) when the drop of water is placed on gastric mucus and on colon mucus. The angle is usually smaller (implying a less hydrophobic surface) in the small intestine, but there are considerable variations with different species (Lichtenberger 1995).

The glycocalyx is the most concentrated glycoprotein layer in the mucosal surface. It is composed, in part, with short nonsecreted mucin fibers anchored in the cell membrane and forms a dense glycoprotein coat ranging from 10–500 nm in thickness in which the mucin fibers are packed more closely than in secreted mucus gel (Ito 1974; Frey *et al.* 1996; Maury 1995). The role of the glycocalyx in regulating access of microparticles to the apical membranes of epithelial cells in the gut has been examined in a recent elegant study in which the membrane-binding subunit of cholera toxin (CTB) was used as a binding ligand for probe particles about 6, 30, and 1000 nm in diameter (Frey *et al.* 1996). CTB binds tightly and specifically to a ganglioside (GM1) that protrudes only about 2.5 nm above the membrane lipid bilayer (McDaniel *et al.* 1986). Hence the CTB on the probes had to approach within this distance to bind to the cell membrane surface. All three probes stuck to the mucus blanket, but in regions where the mucus blanket had been adequately removed or washed away, the 6-nm probe, which was comparable in size to many nutrient molecules and toxins, adhered to all cell types facing the lumen of the gut; the 30-nm probe, which was comparable in size to a small virus, failed to bind to enterocytes, which were covered with a glycocalyx about 500-nm thick; but these viral-sized particles did bind to the M cells, which were covered with a much thinner 20–30 nm glycocalyx. The 1000-nm "bacterial size" probe failed to bind to any cell surface. Although not the intended aim of the study, the results also revealed the extent to which all three probes were trapped in the mucus blanket and could only approach or penetrate the glycocalyx in areas where the mucus blanket had been adequately removed. In places where intestinal chyme wipes away the mucus blanket, the glycocalyx thus forms the final filter that can prevent pathogens from adhering to epithelial cells.

Protective roles of the unstirred mucus layer

Most epithelial surfaces are covered by a continuous blanket of mucus despite the vigorous stirring actions of blinking eyelids, coughing, chewing, and swallowing. The shear-dependent viscosity of mucus helps maintain an unstirred layer of gel through which particles must diffuse before they can contact epithelial cells. Even the mucus that wraps particles of chyme forms an unstirred layer around the particle. These unstirred layers of mucus form a diffusional barrier that helps create much of the selective permeability of the mucus blanket:

- The viscidity of the mucus gel traps most large particles, whatever their surface properties. Regardless of stirring and slipping actions occurring within the mucus, particles that stick to the mucus will not penetrate an unstirred layer.
- Even molecules that are so small they could readily diffuse between the mucin fibers cannot penetrate the unstirred layer if they stick tightly to mucins or to the glycocalyx.
- As the thickness of the unstirred layer, Δx, increases, it takes more time for a particle to diffuse through the unstirred layer. Since the diffusional transit time, Δt, increases exponentially, $\Delta t \propto \Delta x^2$, even a small increase in the thickness of the unstirred layer can markedly increase the transit time, and this can significantly enhance protective actions by:
  - Increasing duration of exposure to acid inactivation, digestive enzymes, free radical scavengers (Lichtenberger 1995), and other protective actions before the pathogen or toxin can contact the epithelium.
  - Increasing the number of antibodies that can accumulate on the surface of a pathogen before it can contact the epithelium.
  - Increasing the effective concentration of secreted antibodies and other protective constituents in the unstirred layer. Secreted protective factors diffuse outward through the mucus coat and become diluted or otherwise dispersed in the layers of mucus being stirred and shed by the epithelium; thus the thicker the unstirred layer, the higher the concentration of protectants near the epithelium. Indeed, the adherent unstirred layer of mucus acts as a "matrix" that stores and deploys numerous protectants near the epithelium (Davies *et al.* 2002; Taylor *et al.* 2003).

Although an intact unstirred layer offers significant protection, if an unstirred layer becomes too thick, it will slow the exchange of gases, nutrients, and wastes, and a thick unstirred layer may become too viscoelastic to shed. Stasis, or blocked flow, of a mucus secretion can lead to bacterial overgrowth and infections. Thus, to function well, the thickness of the unstirred layer, like the viscoelasticity of mucus, must be regulated to achieve a balance; thick enough to protect, but not so thick that exchange rates, and shedding or secretion, are compromised.

Gastric protection requires continuous secretion

As Louis Pasteur (1822–1895) demonstrated, germs abound in our environment, and the greatest influx arrives in food, drink, and the mucus secretions of others. A major role of the stomach is to sterilize pathogens delivered to it in mucus secretions from the eyes, nose, lungs, and mouth. Gastric acidity plays a major role in this sterilization process, but its broad-spectrum action is also cytotoxic for host cells. Gastric mucus thus plays a crucial role in preventing gastric injury.

How the stomach digests meat, but not itself, is a question actively investigated for centuries; Réaumur (1683–1757) showed gastric juice can liquefy meat *in vitro*, Spallanzani (1729–1799) showed that meat enclosed in a wire cage he swallowed (attached to a string) was digested in his stomach, as he could see by pulling the cage back out, and Prout (1785–1850) showed that the stomach does indeed begin to digest itself soon after death. It has been known for some time that continuous secretion of mucus helps prevent self-digestion of the stomach, but the details of the protective mechanisms are still under investigation.

In the stomachs of rats, rabbits, frogs, guinea pigs, and humans (Schreiber and Scheid 1997, and references therein), a large pH gradient is maintained across the mucus blanket with pH values at the epithelial surface near pH 7 even when the luminal pH is 2, a 10^5-fold concentration gradient across a watery gel only ~200 μm thick. Some of the leading ideas for explaining how this can occur are the following.

Can mucus itself block the rapid diffusion of acid? Observations of hydrochloric acid (HCl) diffusing through isolated samples of gastric mucus reveal that it retards the rate of diffusion of acid, but only modestly: $D_{HCl \text{ in mucus}}/D_{HCl \text{ in water}} \approx 1/4$ (Livingston and Engel 1995; Nicholas *et al.* 1991; Williams and Turnberg 1980). In fact, water itself can have a larger effect on the rate at which acid diffuses; D_{HCl} slows 10-fold as the pH rises from 3.5 to 7.7 (Nicholas *et al.* 1991). Is mucus secreted outward faster than acid diffuses inward? The velocity with which gastric mucus is secreted outward, v, is about 3 μm/min in guinea pig (and histamine stimulation can increase v to about 8 μm/min; Schreiber and Scheid 1997). The thickness of the mucus blanket, Δx, is ~200 μm, so the blanket is refreshed (replaced) within $\Delta x/\Delta v$ ~1 hour. The diffusion constant for HCl in gastric mucus falls from ~30×10^{-7} to ~1×10^{-7} cm²/sec as the pH rises from the luminal pH of ~1–2 to the epithelial pH of ~7 (Nicholas *et al.* 1991). Using these values to estimate the diffusional transit time, Δt, given by the Einstein relation, $\Delta t = \Delta x^2/2D$, suggests HCl will diffuse through the mucus blanket within ~10 min, much less than the hour it takes to replace the mucus blanket. This indicates that outward secretion of mucus significantly reduces the arrival of acid at the epithelial surface, but is not adequate by itself to account for the entire pH gradient.

Can bicarbonate secretion by the epithelium neutralize HCl before it reaches the epithelium? This "mucus-bicarbonate" barrier hypothesis (Heatley 1959) proposes that the bicarbonate secreted by the epithelium counteracts acidic influx. The mucus/bicarbonate pH gradient can be rapidly dissipated when the pH falls below ~2.5 (Lichtenberger 1995), and it now appears that the primary effect of bicarbonate secretion may be to raise the pH sufficiently to slow the diffusion of acid in water since bicarbonate alone is insufficient to neutralize the HCl above pH 3–5 (Vadgama and Alberti 1983; Nicholas et al. 1991).

Can the layer of lipid on the surface of gastric mucus slow the inward flux of acid? A lipid layer, if continuous, can be nearly impermeant to ions and protons, since they are nearly insoluble in lipids. Cell membranes are based on this fundamental property of the lipid bilayers. The amount of surface-active lipids in gastric mucus is comparable to that in respiratory mucus (Slomiany et al. 1989; for reviews, see Lichtenberger 1995; Slomiany and Slomiany 1991). The presence of a lipid layer on the surface of the mucus blanket can be observed not only by placing a drop of water on the surface, but also by electron microscopy. The microscopic images reveal that the lipid (monolayer) on the mucus gel surface is often discontinuous; hence this layer is not likely to confer the impermeability to protons and ions of a cell membrane. However, in gastric mucus there are additional membranous vesicles below the surface that may also reduce permeability of the mucus blanket to ions, and these seem well positioned to replace rapidly any breaks in the outermost monolayer. In addition, the gastric mucosa can rapidly incorporate both luminally and systemically administered precursors of neutral and phospholipids, and both their biosynthesis and secretion appear to be tightly regulated (Lichtenberger 1995). Agents that disrupt the hydrophobic surface of gastric mucus, such as aspirin and other nonsteroidal antiinflammatory drugs (NSAIDs), can cause gastric inflammation. H. pylori, the bacteria now known to colonize the stomach and cause ulcers, decrease surface hydrophobicity and can do so both enzymatically and by generating large amounts of ammonium within the mucus blanket (Lichtenberger 1995). Finally, milk, as well as the lipids extracted from milk, can provide effective protection against acid, ethanol, and stress-induced ulcerogenesis (Dial and Lichtenberger 1987). Taken together, there is convincing evidence that lipid layers provide significant protection against gastric acid, but again, acting alone, they are probably insufficient to create the entire pH gradient. In particular, the pH gradient does not change sharply at the surface of the blanket but extends through most of its thickness.

In summary, it appears that all of the preceding mechanisms contribute to maintaining the large pH gradient across gastric mucus: the lipid layers probably reduce the permeability of the mucus blanket to gastric acid more than the mucus gel itself, but without continuous secretion of bicarbonate and mucus, lumenal acid would soon accumulate at the epithelial surface.

How is acid delivered to the gastric lumen? The details of the outward transport of acid are less well understood. HCl is known to be secreted by parietal cells in the crypts, but how it traverses the mucus blanket to reach the gastric lumen is unknown. Holm and Flemstrom (1990), using a pH-sensitive dye to observe gastric acid secretion in vivo in the rat, observed discrete blue (acidic) spots directly above the crypts during active HCl secretion. Since the HCl is actively secreted (pumped) and is probably much less viscous than the mucus blanket, Fabry (1990) suggested that it may push through the mucus blanket by a process of viscous fingering. When a low viscosity fluid is injected into a high viscosity fluid, it forms channels through which the low viscosity fluid flows without mixing. (Anyone who has kneaded dough or clay has experienced, upon adding a small amount of additional water, that the water initially "squirts" out of the high-viscosity fluid and only slowly mixes after repeated kneading.) Bhaskar et al. (1991, 1992) demonstrated that viscous fingering occurred when HCl was injected into solutions of gastric mucin when the solution was above pH 4, but not when the solution was more acidic than pH 4. Viscous fingering in mucus should depend significantly on mucin concentration, lipid and protein content, and ionic strength, as well as pH, and Schreiber and Schied (1997) attempted to create viscous fingering by microinjecting acid with a pH-sensitive dye directly into gastric mucus layers in gastric explants from guinea pigs. The dye never expanded or flowed as would be expected from viscous fingering, and thus whether viscous fingering actually occurs during the transport of gastric HCl remains in question.

Schreiber and Scheid (1997) raise the interesting possibility that protons secreted by the gastric mucosa are buffered by the continuously secreted mucus. Mucins are stored in a highly condensed form in vesicles that accumulate high concentrations of Ca^{++}. The Ca^{++} can form crosslinks between the numerous anionic sites (carboxyls and sulfates) on the tips of the mucin glycans. Calcium may also help condense mucins by calcium-mediated protein cross-links (Raynal et al. 2003). During the process of secretion, Ca^{++} ions diffuse away from the granule and are rapidly exchanged with extracellular Na^+ and K^+ ions as well as protons. Thus in the process of being secreted, mucins can accumulate protons and transport them toward the lumen as the mucus gel moves toward the lumen. Schreiber and Scheid (1997) further report that pepsinogen becomes converted to pepsin within the more acidic outer layers of mucus, and pepsin in turn enzymatically decreases the buffer capacity of the mucus, thereby releasing protons near the lumenal surface of the mucus blanket. Key evidence that supports this concept is their finding that mucus incubated with pepsinogen and acidified to pH 1 released significant amounts of additional acid, 50 mM. If no pepsinogen was added, the mucus did not release this additional acid. Thus continuous secretion of gastric mucus may not only help protect the stomach from acid, it may also be instrumental in delivering acid to the lumen. However, the biochemical mechanism by which pepsin causes the release of acid from mucins is not known.

"Viscidity": What makes mucus sticky?

Mucus sticks to most surfaces and most small particles—it is a universal, though weak, adhesive. All but the largest filter-feeding animals gather food by using mucus to trap water-borne particles. Many fish coat their mouths with mucus which, together with any particles of food adhering to it, is periodically expelled from the mouth with a gulp, rather like a cough, then swallowed, digested, and recycled (Sanderson, *et al.* 1996). Similarly, mucus is used to protect lungs from airborne particles, nearly all of which stick to respiratory mucus before they reach the alveoli. Like filter-feeding fish, we swallow, digest, and recycle this mucus after sterilizing it with gastric acid. The universal adhesive character of mucus also enables gastropods to cling and crawl along all types of surfaces, including slippery surfaces coated with algae.

What makes mucus so sticky—and what does *not* stick to mucus? The answers to these questions help explain the selective permeability of the mucus blanket. How is it that metabolites, gases, and wastes that must be exchanged through the mucosal surface readily diffuse through the mucus blanket without sticking to it? Detailed answers to these questions are just beginning to emerge. In broad outline, the mucin fibers that form mucus gel are like long flexible strings densely coated with short glycans, most of which are tipped with a negative charge (carboxyl or sulfate groups). These glycosylated and highly hydrophilic regions are separated by "naked," relatively hydrophobic regions of the protein that probably fold into somewhat hydrophobic globules or "beads" that are often stabilized by multiple internal disulfide bonds. Since each mucin fiber consists of a flexible array of alternating hydrophilic and hydrophobic regions, by conforming to the surface of an incoming particle, an array of low-affinity hydrophilic and/or hydrophobic bonds can develop between the flexible fibers of the gel and the particle. Thus, in addition to bonds that commensal bacteria form with specific glycans on mucins, a mucus gel can stick to any surface with which it can form multiple low-affinity bonds. Low-affinity bonds, of course, have very short half-lives, typically being broken by thermal energy within fractions of a second, but if the mucus gel makes numerous low-affinity bonds with the particle, at any given time one or more low-affinity bonds will keep the particle linked to mucin fibers, and the particle will remain stuck, held in place by the elasticity of the linked and entangled gel. Just as polyvalent antibodies, such as IgM, can bind to a pathogen with essentially permanent high "avidity" by making multiple low-affinity bonds, the mucus gel can trap a particle with permanent high "viscidity" when the flexible, but elastically linked and entangled, fibers of mucins that form the gel make numerous low-affinity bonds to the particle.

The term "viscidity" may help emphasize not only the importance of the multiple low-affinity bonds that can be made by mucin fibers but also that to create "viscidity" the mucin fibers must form an elastic gel; if the gel had no elasticity, it would not exert an elastic recoil to a particle adhering to it, and the particle would migrate or diffuse as in a purely viscous fluid. The instant the elasticity of a mucus gel is lost by dilution, or by breaking the bonds that link mucin fibers together, a fiber that had been continually detaching and reattaching to a trapped particle would begin instead to diffuse away, allowing the particle to migrate. Thus only when the mucin fibers form an *elastic* gel can they create the viscidity that keeps the particle trapped in the gel while the low-affinity bonds "flicker" on and off.

MUCUS GEL STRUCTURE

Mucins are long, thin, and flexible "wormlike chains" with negatively charged glycosylated regions interspersed with globular hydrophobic peptide "beads"

Figure 4.4 depicts several structural features of a generalized mucin fiber of the type secreted to form mucus gels. A cell-associated mucin is shown for comparison. In solution, each secreted mucin acquires the entropically most favored configuration of a random coil. If the ends of the fiber are pulled apart or if the coil is compressed or flattened, it will react elastically with a force that resists these deformations because the thermal motions of every "link" in the chain will act to pull back against an elongating force and push against a compressing force: elongations and compressions both reduce the number of possible configurations and the entropy of the coil.

Progress in characterizing the structures of secreted and cell-associated mucins has greatly accelerated recently with the use of monoclonal antimucin antibodies that have enabled sequencing of the genes for several mucins (*MUC1* to *MUC13*); for excellent reviews of this progress see Dekker *et al.* 2002; Desseyn *et al.* 2000; van Klinken *et al.* 1995; Gendler and Spicer 1995; Strous and Dekker 1992. Sequence analysis shows mucins to be a heterogeneous group of molecules that appear to form two distinct families (Dekker *et al.* 2002). One family is "cell-associated": MUC1, MUC3A, MUC3B, MUC4, MUC12, and MUC13 all contain a transmembrane domain. They range from 100–500 nm in length, and though much shorter than secreted mucins, are long enough to reach outward well beyond the glycocalyx where they help make the initial specific interactions between cells (Springer 1990) and play many roles in cell signaling. Significant alterations in cell-attached mucins occur in cellular development, infections, and tumors. The second family is "secreted" mucins: MUC2, MUC5AC, MUC5B, MUC6, and MUC7 (Dekker *et al.* 2002; Van Klinken *et al.* 1995; Thornton *et al.* 1996, 1997). As illustrated in Figure 4.4, all of these secreted mucins except MUC7 are extremely long molecules, up to several microns in length, longer than the diameters of many types of cells.

All mucins have high amounts of proline (P), threonine (T), and/or serine (S) residues, constituting 20% to 55% of the amino acid composition and concentrated in one or several major "PTS" regions of the peptide. These PTS regions are highly glycosylated with oligosaccharides *O*-linked to most of the threonine and serines, resulting in 40% to 80%

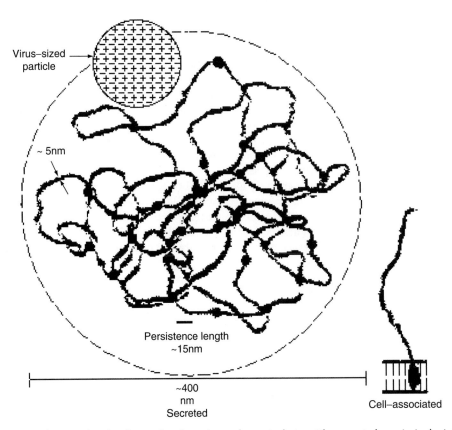

Fig. 4.4. Relative dimensions of secreted and cell-associated mucins and a typical virus. The secreted mucin is depicted as a random coil of about 5 mucin monomers linked end-to-end to have an overall length of ~2 μm. The fuzzy surface of the fiber suggests the "bottle brush" array of negatively charged glycans that make the fiber ~5–10 nm in diameter, and the curvatures in the random coil approximate a persistence length of 15 nm. In a mucus gel, 10–100 of these random coils overlap and entangle. The "beads" distributed along the fiber represent the Cys-subdomains, naked protein regions rich in cysteines that fold into globular structures with some hydrophobic surfaces. The hydrophobic surfaces of the beads adsorb lipid molecules and also likely form numerous weak low-affinity hydrophobic bonds between mucin fibers, increasing the viscosity of the mucus gel. The virus particle (100-nm diameter) is shown densely covered with + and − charges at one tenth of the actual charge density of a poliovirus.

O-linked glycans by weight in the mature secreted mucins. In addition to the "bottle brush" regions of *O*-linked glycans, there are many *N*-linked sulfate–bearing glycans located near both ends of mucin monomers, comprising 2% to 3% by weight. The "bottle brush" heavily glycosylated regions are separated by "naked" protein regions with a peptide composition comparable to globular proteins. These naked protein regions are thus sufficiently hydrophobic that they may fold into globular "beads" that are stabilized by multiple disulfide bonds (Sheehan *et al.* 1986). Purified mucins contain little α helix or β pleated sheet secondary structure (Shogren *et al.* 1989; Gerken *et al.* 1989). The naked protein "beads" are the most hydrophobic regions of mucins, binding fluorescent lipid probes with a K_D ~10^{-5} M; pronase digestion, which eliminates most of the naked regions, almost completely eliminates lipid probe binding (Shankar *et al.* 1990, 1991). The naked regions are also the most antigenic sites on mucins, and disulfide reduction reduces their reactivity with antimucin antibodies (Mantle *et al.* 1984). The epitope revealed by disulfide reduction is shared by a variety of human mucins (Sheehan *et al.* 1991a).

In Figure 4.4, the thick fuzzy lines depict the glycosylated and negatively charged "bottle brush" regions, and the interspersed "beads" depict the folded naked and hydrophobic protein regions. In mucus gels, which typically have mucin concentrations of 2% to 5%, each mucin overlaps/entangles with on the order of 10 to 100 other mucins. In addition to mucins entangling with each other, the hydrophobic bead regions of each mucin probably adsorb significant amounts of lipids, and these in turn may form numerous low-affinity bonds between overlapping mucins that increase the viscoelasticity of the gel. Delipidating mucins and treating mucus with lysolecithin significantly decrease gel viscoelasticity (Murty *et al.* 1984; Slomiany *et al.* 1986).

Structure and dimensions of the glycan "bottle brush"

The glycosylated PTS regions of epithelial mucins contain large and variable numbers of tandem repeats of a peptide sequence. For example, in MUC1, a cell-associated mucin present on most mucosal epithelia, there are 30 to 90 tandem repeats of a 20 amino acid sequence, a genetic polymorphism that yields mucin monomers ranging from about 150–450 nm in length. MUC2, a mucin secreted by many mucosal surfaces, has 51 to 115 tandem repeats, yielding glycosylated PTS regions about 50–200 nm in length (Lancaster *et al.* 1990; Toribara *et al.* 1991; see van Klinken *et al.* 1995). The glycans are attached to these PTS regions by the *O*-linked *N*-acetylgalactosamine (GalNAc) to which 1 to 20 additional sugars are attached, many of which terminate with sialic acid or sulfate groups. The peripheral sugars of these glycans form the ABH and Lewis blood group specificities of mucins (Neutra and Forstner 1987). As with cell-associated mucins, alterations in the peripheral sugars of secreted mucins occur during certain immune responses, infections, and in tumors (Forstner *et al.* 1995). The glycans extend about 0.5–5 nm from the peptide core, so the total diameter of the glycosylated region, as inferred biochemically, is about 3–10 nm. The dense packing of the saccharides linked directly to the peptide stiffen it to become a chain that extends axially about 2.5 Å per peptide (compared with 1.5 Å for an α helix). The negatively charged carboxyls on the outer tips of the glycans repel each other, helping create the "bottle brush" array that somewhat further increases the stiffness of the glycosylated region; the addition of the initial *O*-linked GalNAc increases the persistence length of the random coil peptide almost six-fold, from 1 nm to about 6 nm, while the charged carboxyls cause an additional doubling of the persistence length to about 15 nm (Shogren *et al.* 1989). It is this partial stiffening of the peptide chain that creates a "wormlike," rather than a fully flexible, chain. Thus each glycosylated region is a flexible, negatively charged fiber about 3–10 nm in diameter and 50–200 nm in length.

Each monomer of secreted mucin contains one or more glycosylated regions. In Figure 4.4, a secreted mucin fiber ~2 µm in length is shown with 20 glycosylated regions separated by naked protein "beads." The glycosylated regions are depicted as ~7-nm wide, ~100-nm long, and with curvatures suggestive of the observed persistence length.

Mucin monomers are linked end-to-end in long chains

The molecular mass of secreted mucins ranges between 0.5 and 40 MDa (Sheehan *et al.* 1995; Carlstedt and Sheehan 1988). These huge molecules, typically several µm long, are formed by linking numerous mucin monomers, each about 0.2–0.6 µm in length, end to end (Sheehan *et al.* 1991b; Carlstedt and Sheehan 1984). Sulfhydryl reagents such as dithiothreitol (DTT) that break disulfide bonds quickly "dissolve" most mucus gels by dissociating mucin fibers into their monomeric subunits. This chain-breaking process nearly abolishes the viscoelastic gel properties of mucus. The separated monomers do not aggregate and remain as individual random coils. Thus, after reducing the disulfides, interactions between the glycosylated and naked protein regions of individual monomers are insufficient to cause monomers to gel, unless the monomer concentration is greatly increased, in which case the gel that forms is mostly viscous, with relatively little elasticity.

The mechanisms that link mucin monomers together are being actively investigated. It is likely that in many cases disulfide bonds between the globular domains near the ends of the monomers link monomers together (Carlstedt and Sheehan 1984). As shown in **Figure 4.5**, there are disulfide-rich domains (D-domains) arrayed near both ends of mucin monomers. Sequence analysis of mucin genes also suggest that a "cystine knot" at the amino terminal and one of several cysteine-rich domains (D-domains) near the carboxyl terminal may be involved in oligomerization via noncovalent affinity bonds (van Klinken *et al.* 1995). Reduction-insensitive bonds form some links between MUC2 monomers (Herrmann *et al.* 1999). In addition, calcium-dependent protein interactions provide reversible cross-links between MUC5B monomers in salivary mucus (Raynal *et al.* 2003). Finally, recent observations show that three MUC2 monomers can be linked by their N termini to form trimers (Godl *et al.* 2002), thus producing a branched network of mucins. The D-domains that form the trefoil-like bonds are highly resistant to protease digestion, perhaps because of their multiple internal disulfide bonds. Just as glycosylation protects the extended fibrous regions from proteolysis, multiple disulfide bonds may do the same for the unglycosylated globular domains in mucins, a property of major importance in the digestive tract.

Mucin monomers are linked together before being secreted (Godl *et al.* 2002; Dekker *et al.* 1991; McCool *et al.* 1994; Tytgat *et al.* 1995), and ~90% of SH groups in secreted mucins are involved in S-S bonds (Mantle *et al.* 1990). When a mucin-filled vesicle is secreted, the mucin fibers swell explosively to form an entangled ball of mucus gel (Verdugo 1984). This tendency for stored mucins to swell is apparently a source of artifact that causes mucus-secreting cells to swell into "goblet"-shaped cells during fixation for microscopy. When epithelia are prepared by fast-freezing followed by freeze substitution, mucus-secreting cells are not goblet-shaped but have straight lateral sides, like their neighboring epithelial cells (Sandoz *et al.* 1985; Verdugo 1990).

Ionic control of mucus swelling, and viscoelasticity

Mucin granules can increase some 500-fold in volume within 50 milliseconds of being secreted (Verdugo 1984, 1990). This explosive swelling of mucin fibers is driven not only by the diffusional (thermal) expansion of the flexible mucin fibers but also by the repulsion between the negatively charged glycosylated regions that emerges as divalent ions diffuse out of the gel and are exchanged by monovalent ions. Mucins stored in a secretory vesicle are copackaged with Ca^{++} that condenses the mucins by shielding and cross-linking the negatively charged glycans. Two monovalent counterions diffuse inward to replace the efflux of each Ca^{++}, approximating a Donnan equilibrium, and this increase in osmotic pressure contributes to the speed of swelling (Tam and Verdugo 1981; Verdugo 1991).

Changes in ionic strength cause mucus gels to shrink or swell, and this can markedly alter the viscoelasticity since gel

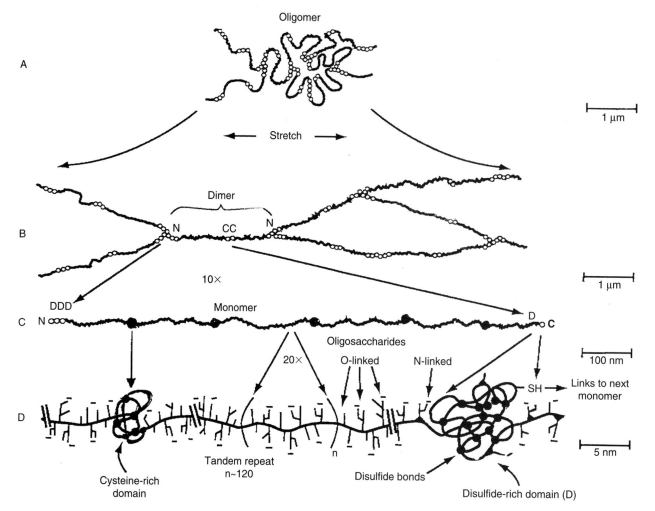

Fig. 4.5. Major biochemical features of gel-forming mucins. The genes for all the major gel-forming secreted mucins characterized to date, *MUC2, MUC5AC, MUC5B, MUC6* (Dekker *et al.* 2002; van Klinken *et al.* 1995; Thornton *et al.* 1996, 1997), are all located on chromosome locus 11p15. They are very large, have considerable overall homology in their nonglycosylated regions, and may have evolved through gene duplication of one ancestral gene (Dessyn *et al.* 1998). Their large RNAs (14–24 kilobases) all exhibit variable-length polymorphism (Debailleul *et al.* 1998). **A,** Several mucin monomers are shown linked together in an oligomeric gel. **B,** "Stretching" the gel helps clarify the linkages between monomers. Mucins first form dimers linked by a disulfide bond between disulfide-rich (D) domains near the carboxyl terminals (Perez-Vilar and Hill 1998a). Dimers then form oligomers linked by disulfide bonds between D-domains near their amino terminals (Perez-Vilar *et al.* 1998b; van Klinken *et al.* 1998). In addition, the amino terminals of MUC2 form trimers between trypsin-resistant globular domains that likely create branched networks, not just linear polymers. Both the glycosylated and the globular domains of these branched networks are likely to resist being digested in the GI tract (Godl *et al.* 2002). In saliva, MUC5B monomers are linked together with Ca^{++}-dependent protein interactions that may also create branched networks (Raynal *et al.* 2003). **C,** The number and distribution of D-domains vary significantly between mucins (see Desseyn *et al.* 1997; 2000); D-domains are homologous to those in the von Willebrand clotting factor where they also form oligomeric disulfide bonds between fibrous monomers (Keates *et al.* 1997). In addition to a D-domain, there is a cystine knot (11 Cys, 85 aa) at the carboxyl terminal end of *MUC2, MUC5AC,* and *MUC5B.* Almost the entire length of these gel-forming mucins are PTS tandem-repeat regions that are highly glycosylated. The number of repeats can be very large with n = 135 in pig submaxillary mucin (Eckhard *et al.* 1997). Also, the number of amino acids per tandem repeat varies greatly between mucins; from eight amino acids in *MUC5AC* to 169 in *MUC6.* **D,** Glycans are attached to most of the threonine and serine residues in the PTS regions. N-linked glycans are attached to relatively sparse but specific peptide sequences NX(S or T), mostly near the ends of the monomers. In contrast, *O*-linked glycans attach densely to the S and T residues apparently without requiring specific peptide sequences. Similarly, the size, structure, and composition of glycans depend on the epithelial site at which the mucin is synthesized rather than the peptide sequence (see Karlsson *et al.* 1997). The glycans form a "bottle brush" array with most glycan tips being negatively charged with a sialic acid (carboxyl group) or a sulphate group. The D-domains (351–375 aa in length) form globular folded structures (β strands devoid of α helix) stabilized by numerous disulfide bonds (●). Arrayed along the glycosylated PTS domains of *MUC2, MUC5AC,* and *MUCB* (but not *MUC6*), are several Cys-subdomains (10 Cys, 108 aa in length) that are well conserved and appear to be unique to these gel-forming mucins (Dekker *et al.* 2002). The PTS regions between the globular Cys-subdomains are about 100-400 aa in length (see Desseyn *et al.* 2000; Dekker *et al.* 2002), suggesting specific functional roles. These domains, by adhering weakly to each other, might contribute to zigzag "accordion" folding during storage prior to secretion and also to the lipid-dependent viscoelasticity of the secreted gel. In addition, they are appropriately spaced to provide low-affinity linkage sites for antibodies that have accumulated on the surfaces of pathogens (see Padgett 1995).

viscosity at constant shear rates increases exponentially, approximately as [mucin]$^{2-3}$ (Wolf et al. 1977a). Increasing the concentration of monovalent cations, such as Na$^+$, causes mucus to shrink, and high concentrations of multivalent cations, such as Ca^{++}, collapse the gel. Acidity can also collapse mucus gels, but by a different mechanism; as the pH becomes more acidic, the carboxyl groups (sialic acid) on the glycans become protonated, reducing the negative charge on the glycosylated regions. Gastric mucins condense when exposed to high acidity, greatly increasing their viscoelasticity (Lamont 1992). Perhaps to help counteract this acid-induced shrinking and condensation, the O-linked glycans of gastric mucins have fewer sialic acid groups, and the less glycosylated regions have more N-linked glycans with "acid-resistant" sulfate groups (sulfates remain negatively charged even when exposed to pH 1). Gastric mucus is exposed to a wide range of pH, and switching from carboxyl to sulphate groups helps reduce the extent to which gastric mucus swells and shrinks, and this probably helps keep the viscoelasticity of gastric mucus in the appropriate range.

It is likely that many epithelia regulate the ionic environment as a means to regulate the viscoelasticity of mucus (Forstner 1995). An outstanding example is cystic fibrosis, a condition caused by malfunction of ion transport, perhaps by nonfunctional chloride$^-$ channels. In this disease, mucus secretions throughout the body become too viscoelastic to be cleared efficiently, causing stasis, greatly increasing the incidence of bacterial infections. In addition, even the normal shedding of epithelial cells, whose debris is normally swept away, begins to collect, and the dispersal of fibers of DNA, which can be even longer than mucin fibers, further increases the viscoelasticity of mucus. Indeed, enzymatic cleavage of DNA markedly reduces the viscosity of cystic fibrotic mucus (Shak et al. 1990; Yeates 1996), and recombinant human DNase is now being used to help loosen and clear respiratory mucus of patients with cystic fibrosis (Shak 1995; Ulmer et al. 1996).

The structural arrangement of mucin fibers in mucus gels is not yet known

The molecular structure of a mucus gel is difficult to observe and numerous attempts have been made to prepare mucus for electron microscopy with methods designed to cause minimal distortion to the actual structural array of mucin fibers. When fresh mucus is prepared for electron microscopy, most fixation methods yield a random mesh of thick individual fibers about 30–100 nm in diameter (Yudin et al. 1989; Poon and McCoshen 1985; Chretien et al. 1975), or about 10-fold thicker than the 3–10 nm diameter of a mucin fiber determined biochemically. In contrast, when individual purified mucin fibers are flowed onto a grid and then lightly shadowed with heavy metal, electron microscope images reveal smooth, curvilinear fibers with a diameter of about 5–7 nm (Sheehan et al. 1986; Slayter et al. 1991), which is reasonably consistent with the diameter expected from the biochemical structure. Moreover, if individual fibers are not flowed onto the grid, but simply allowed to settle, they appear "kinky" and flexible with curvatures that appear reasonably consistent with the ~15-nm persistence length inferred from the behavior of mucin fibers as random coils in solution (Shogren et al. 1989). The much thicker (and straighter) fibers typically seen in images of mucus gels are probably thickened in part from the tendency of other constituents of a mucus gel (antibodies, lysozyme, lactoferrin, albumin, etc.) to adsorb to, and hence thicken, the mucin fibers during preparation of the gel for electron microscopy. The metals used to increase electron contrast also increase the apparent fiber diameter. However, these two effects can at most double the apparent thickness of mucin fibers because mucins typically comprise a major fraction of the nondialyzable dry weight of mucus. Thus the published evidence to date suggests that conventional fixation methods and even fast freezing followed by freeze substitution somehow cause mucin fibers to become 3–10 times thicker than an individual mucin fiber. Perhaps fixation causes multiple fibers to clump together, but another possibility is suggested by the somewhat ribbonlike images obtained in fast-frozen preparations fixed by freeze substitution (Yudin et al. 1989) as well as by the "kinky" shapes seen when isolated mucin fibers are deposited with minimal flow onto the electron microscope grid. Mucin fibers fixed within a mucus gel might thicken by condensing *longitudinally* with zigzag folds. In this case successive hydrophobic beads might tend to cluster together with the interspersed glycosylated regions, folding into hairpin loops. Such a folding mechanism might reduce the tendency for mucin fibers to become overly entangled in the process of being deposited in the storage granule or during the explosive swelling process upon secretion. Recently, a new method for fixing mucus has been developed by A. I. Yudin in which glutaraldehyde is delivered to fresh mucus in dimethyl sulfoxide (DMSO) (Olmsted et al. 2001). With this procedure, fixation neither shrinks nor expands the gel, and there is no tendency, as with other methods, for the outer surface of the gel to become fixed leaving the inner regions unfixed. Apparently DMSO enables glutaraldehyde to diffuse well into the gel before reacting. Examples of ovulatory cervical mucus and sperm flagella fixed by this method are shown in **Figure 4.6**. The individual mucin fibers appear to be kinked and folded, with individual fibers appearing to be ~10–15 nm in diameter, reasonably consistent with their biochemical structure and unlike the much too thick fibers seen in all previous electron microscope images of mucins. In addition, DMSO/glutaraldehyde fixation provides images suggestive of fibers clustered together by small beadlike structures consistent with the hypothesis that hydrophobic globular protein domains, but not the glycosylated PTS regions, tend to adhere to each other (Olmsted et al. 2001).

When vigorously motile sperm are present in cervical mucus while it is being fixed with the DMSO/glutaraldehyde method or by freeze substitution after fast freezing (Yudin et al. 1989), the mucin fibers on one side of motile sperm

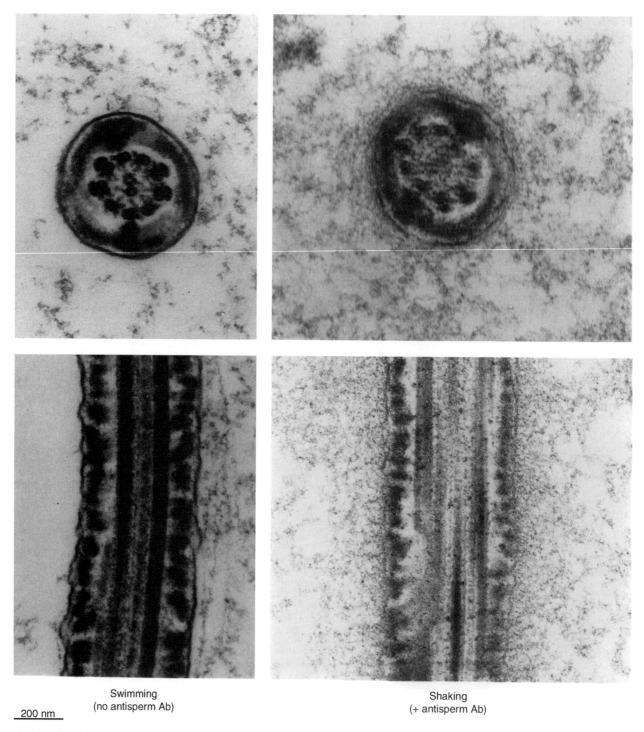

Swimming
(no antisperm Ab)

Shaking
(+ antisperm Ab)

200 nm

Fig. 4.6. Flagella of motile human sperm in ovulatory cervical mucus prepared for electron microscopy by fixation with glutaraldehyde delivered in DMSO. The mucin fibers appear thin and kinked. In the absence of antisperm antibodies, sperm swim rapidly through ovulatory mucus, and the sideways movements of the flagella compress the mucin fibers on one side and rarify them on the other. In contrast, if antisperm antibodies are present, sperm remain motile but simply shake in place, and in this case mucin fibers can be seen condensed uniformly on all sides of the flagella, consistent with the hypothesis that antibodies can trap pathogens by making them adhere to mucin fibers. Scale: 200 nm. (Micrographs provided by A. I. Yudin and D. F. Katz.)

flagella are compressed while those on the other side are rarified, as can be seen in both longitudinal and transverse sections of the flagella of sperm that were swimming at the time of fixation or fast freezing. This motility-induced displacement of mucin fibers, together with the apparent diameter of individual mucin fibers, suggests that the DMSO/glutaraldehyde fixation method gives a reasonably accurate image of mucin fibers as they occur in a mucus gel. However, further observations with other techniques will be needed before a more detailed structure of mucin fibers in a mucus gel can be developed.

SELECTIVE PERMEABILITY AND TRAPPING IN MUCUS

Viruses are small enough to diffuse through mucus

Early investigations of diffusion through mucus gels demonstrated that small molecules can readily diffuse through mucus, but a few early observations suggested that larger molecules, such as globular proteins, were too large to penetrate intestinal mucus. This seemed reasonable, since the end products of digestion, such as monosaccharides and disaccharides, or small peptides, could penetrate the mucus coat to reach the enterocytes, but the mucus coat would prevent the (larger) digestive enzymes from attacking these cells. However, more recent work clearly demonstrates that particles much larger than digestive enzymes, even virus-sized

particles, can readily diffuse through mucus gels. **Figure 4.7** shows the speed with which particles of various sizes diffuse through fresh samples of human cervical mucus compared with the speed with which they diffuse in water. The ratio of the diffusion constant in mucus, D_{mucus}, divided by the diffusion constant in water, D_{water}, is shown as a function of particle size (Stokes diameter) for several proteins and antibodies and for two virus-sized particles. These observations were made with fluorescently labeled probes using fluorescence recovery after photobleaching (FRAP) to quantify diffusion rates. This method minimally perturbs the mucus gel and is not subject to many of the errors that plagued earlier observations (i.e., unstirred layers, clogged filters, and uncontrolled perturbations of mucus gel structure and thickness).

As can be seen in Figure 4.7, virus-sized particles can readily diffuse through mucus. These observations were made in ovulatory cervical mucus, which is less concentrated than most mucus secretions. However, human papilloma virus freely diffused through even the thickest nonovulatory cervical mucus samples studied. Thus papilloma virus must be much smaller than the cut-off size for particles diffusing in cervical mucus.

The cut-off size for a filter is determined in part by the fiber spacing, and an analysis of diffusion rates similar to those shown in Figure 4.7 indicates that the effective fiber spacing in ovulatory mucus is ~100 nm (Olmsted *et al.* 2001). Mucin fiber spacing is likely to change only slowly

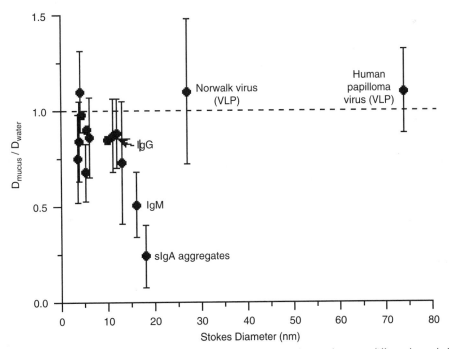

Fig. 4.7. Diffusion in midcycle cervical mucus. Proteins, antibodies, and virus-sized particles can diffuse through human cervical mucus almost as rapidly as they diffuse through water. D_{mucus}/D_{water} is plotted as a function of the diameter of the diffusing particles. $D_{mucus}/D_{water} = 1$ indicates particles that diffuse equally rapidly in mucus as in water. These include lysozyme, lactoferrin, and pepsin, and two virus-sized particles (capsids), Norwalk virus and human papilloma virus. Note that antibodies can also diffuse through mucus, but IgM and small aggregates of S-IgA diffuse significantly more slowly in mucus than in water even though they are much smaller than human papilloma virus. (Padgett 1995; Saltzman *et al.* 1994; and Henry *et al.* 1992; see Olmsted *et al.* 2001 for additional details.)

with mucin concentration, decreasing approximately as the square root of concentration. Because mucin concentrations range from ~1% in ovulatory mucus to <5% in thick, colonic mucus, the cut-off size in GI tract mucus is probably at least $1/\sqrt{5} \approx 1/2$ the cut-off size for ovulatory cervical mucus; hence particles ~50–100 nm should be small enough to penetrate most mucus gels. Virus particles that infect mucosal surfaces are ~100 nm or less in diameter (polio, 28 nm; hepatitis B, 43 nm; adenoviruses, 60–90 nm; rotavirus, 75 nm; HIV, 120 nm). This suggests that viruses, by shedding virtually all metabolic machinery, may have evolved to become small enough to penetrate the mucus gels that cover their target cells.

Multiple low-affinity bonds can trap particles in mucus

If virus-sized spheres of latex are mixed into mucus, unlike virus particles, they stick so firmly and polyvalently to mucin fibers that the gel wraps around them, forming thick cables and sheets of mucin fibers, wrapping them in mucus much as Florey (1962) described for India ink particles in the intestine. This wrapping effect is a strikingly easy observation to make with fluorescently labeled latex microspheres (Olmsted *et al.* 2001). Such particles, although small enough to diffuse readily between mucin fibers, most assuredly do not penetrate mucus gels—they are trapped by mucus viscidity. Even when latex microspheres are heavily carboxylated to cover them with negative charge, or coated with covalently bound bovine serum albumin or casein (excellent proteins for blocking enzyme-linked immunosorbent assay [ELISA] plates), they still adhere to mucus, and if they diffuse at all, they diffuse significantly slower than in water.

Mucus viscidity can trap particles by forming low-affinity polyvalent hydrophobic and ionic bonds, but not molecules that are too small to make polyvalent bonds

The surface of latex beads is hydrophobic, and hence detergents are typically used to keep such beads in suspension. That mucus still binds these detergent-coated beads with such viscidity reveals how well mucus gels can trap hydrophobic surfaces, even when coated with detergents. This also helps explain why some small molecules diffuse more slowly through mucus than other molecules of similar size: molecules that partition into oil, or other nonpolar solvents, diffuse more slowly through mucus than through water, and their diffusion constants in mucus decrease in proportion to their nonpolar/polar partition coefficient as would be expected if their diffusion rate is retarded in proportion to the fraction of time they are bound or partition into hydrophobic surfaces in the mucus gel (Matthes *et al.* 1992; Larhed *et al.* 1997). Small relatively hydrophobic molecules, like testosterone, or molecules with small hydrophobic patches, such as serum albumin, although retarded by mucus, can still diffuse through the gel because small molecules, unlike virus-sized latex beads, do not make multiple bonds with different fibers of gel; they bind to a fiber monovalently, with a low-affinity bond that

persists for only a short time. Thus they are not trapped polyvalently, with viscidity.

Because the glycosylated regions of mucin fibers are densely coated with negatively charged carboxyl groups, and numerous sulphate groups are present toward the ends of many mucin fibers, mucus can also bind positively charged particles with high viscidity; indeed, polyvalent cations collapse the gel around them.

How do viruses avoid sticking to mucus?

As revealed by virus-sized latex microspheres, virus particles are large enough to make highly polyvalent bonds with a mucus gel. How do viruses avoid sticking to mucus? How do they avoid making any low-affinity bonds? This question has yet to be investigated directly, but the surfaces of many viruses, such as poliovirus, are densely coated equally with both positive and negative charges, as are most monomeric soluble proteins (see Wada and Nakamura 1981). This creates a densely charged, yet neutral, surface. The virus depicted in Figure 4.4 is shown densely coated with positive and negative charges, yet the actual surface density of these charges on a poliovirus is tenfold greater than shown because the average distance between charges is 5 Å. Such a densely charged but neutral surface will neither be repelled nor attracted to the negatively charged regions of mucins. If viruses were highly negatively charged, although less likely to stick to mucin fibers, they would also be less likely to enter (partition into) the negatively charged mucus gel or glycocalyx. Conversely, if viruses were positively charged they would become tightly wrapped in mucus. Equally important, by being densely coated with charged groups, viruses will not bind the hydrophobic surfaces of mucin fibers. Thus viruses appear well designed to penetrate mucus by being small enough, neutral in net surface charge, and coated densely with charged groups that prevent hydrophobic bonding.

Nanoparticles are being actively investigated not only to create better mucosal vaccines but also to increase the efficiency of orally delivered drugs (Florence 1997). These investigations make clear that nanoparticles are absorbed primarily by the M cells. They also reveal that most such particles stick to mucus (Behrens *et al.* 2002). It is likely that nanoparticles, modeled not only on the size but also the surface charge properties of virus particles, may be delivered more efficiently to the M cells because fewer may be lost in feces or wrapped in mucus, like India ink, as described by Florey (1962).

Secreted antibodies collaborate with mucin fibers to trap pathogens in mucus

As is well known, at least to mucosal immunologists, more antibodies are secreted into external secretions than into blood (Mestecky *et al.* 1986; Conley and Delacroix 1987). What are the roles of all these secreted antibodies? How do they protect mucosal surfaces? (For a recent review, see Corthesy and Kraenhenbuhl, 1999.) Some mechanisms are well established. For example, secreted antibodies, like mucins, can exclude pathogens (Stokes *et al.* 1975) by blocking the adhesins or other receptor sites used by pathogens to adhere to epithelial target cells as well as tooth surfaces (Williams and Gibbons 1972; Tramont 1977; Svanborg-Edén and Svennerholm 1978; Hajishengallis *et al.* 1992; Chapter 3), and secreted antibodies, especially polyvalent IgA and IgM, can agglutinate pathogens into clusters too large to diffuse through mucus. Also, after being agglutinated by antibodies, motile pathogens and commensals make little or no forward progress. In addition, not only IgA, but also IgA-antigen immune complexes are transported from the basolateral to the apical surface by transcytosis through epithelial cells, and thus even when pathogens or toxins gain access to mucosal tissues, the IgA secretion process may help eliminate them from the tissue by delivering them into mucus (Lamm *et al.* 1995; Kaetzel *et al.*1994; Chapter 15). Finally, it is noteworthy that in early childhood, as the mucosal immune system matures, an increasing fraction of both pathogens and commensals observed in fresh samples of nasopharyngeal mucus become coated with secreted antibodies until by adolescence, the majority of pathogens, and commensals, are coated with secreted antibodies (Stenfors and Räisänen 1991). There is another mechanism by which secreted antibodies exclude pathogens, a potent protective mechanism that has been little recognized outside the field of immunocontraception.

The "shaking phenomenon"
The presence of antisperm antibodies in cervical mucus, or in semen, correlates with infertility in humans. Such antibodies usually do not kill sperm, there being little if any active complement present in these mucus secretions. Instead they simply agglutinate sperm, which remain motile for hours without making forward progress. In addition, if individual sperm enter cervical mucus, they soon start to shake in place, progress no further, and finally die hours later. This is called "the shaking phenomenon." How do secreted antibodies trap these highly motile cells in mucus?

Kremer and Jager (1976, 1992), who first described the shaking phenomenon, proposed that antibodies secreted into cervical mucus would bind to the mucus fibers and trap sperm as they swim into the mucus; similarly, sperm coated with antibodies secreted in semen would also be trapped as antibodies on the sperm surface contact fibers of cervical mucus. This hypothesis is supported by the finding that antibodies from which the Fc domains have been enzymatically removed no longer cause sperm to shake in place in mucus (Jager *et al.* 1981; Bronson *et al.* 1987). One function of the Fc domain of a secreted antibody may thus be to bind to mucus fibers, thereby forming an adhesive cross-link between an antigen bound to the Fab moieties and a mucin fiber.

Antisperm antibodies that cause sperm to shake in place in ovulatory cervical mucus also cause mucin fibers to adhere to the surface of the flagella, as can be seen in Figure 4.6. As mentioned previously, in the absence of antisperm antibodies, when sperm swim through mucus, they compress mucin fibers on one side of the flagellum, while rarifying the mucin fibers on the other. Note that no mucins appear to adhere to the flagellar surface facing the rarified region of mucus gel. In contrast, if antisperm antibodies are present, mucus fibers condense uniformly on all sides of the flagella, as can be seen in both longitudinal and transverse sections of the flagella of sperm shaking in place. Thus electron microscopic evidence also supports the hypothesis that antibodies cross-link antigens to mucin fibers. (The antibodies do not otherwise hinder the motility of sperm. This can be demonstrated simply by thinning the mucus to lower its viscoelasticity, in which case the sperm again swim vigorously forward. This reveals the crucial role of the viscoelasticity of the gel in trapping pathogens by the shaking phenomenon.)

That secreted antibodies can trap pathogens and antigens in mucus, making them "mucophilic," has been observed in many settings: (1) As in cervical mucus, antisperm antibodies added to nasal and salivary mucus also cause sperm to shake in place (Olmsted 2000); (2) *Salmonella typhimurium* coated with S-IgA adhere to the mucus blanket in rat intestines and to a column of pig gastric mucin (Magnusson and Stjernstrom 1982); (3) *Campylobacter jejuni* are trapped in the mucosal blanket of the rabbit intestine only if specific S-IgA is present (McSweegan *et al.* 1987); (4) *Staphylococcus aureus* and *P. aeruginosa* are agglutinated by purified fractions of the low-molecular-weight salivary mucin MG2 only if S-IgA specific for these pathogens is present (Biesbrock *et al.* 1991a,b); and (5) *Trichinella spiralis* larvae are trapped in rat intestinal mucus if antibodies specific for this parasite are delivered to this mucus by any of several routes; adding monoclonal antibodies directly to samples of the mucus, passively immunizing rat pups with milk by nursing *T. spiralis*–infected dams, and by passively immunizing pups with milk from uninfected dams that were themselves passively immunized intravenously with monoclonal antibodies (Carlisle *et al.* 1991). In all four settings, it did not matter how the antibodies were delivered to the mucus; if and only if specific antibodies were present did the pathogens and parasites become trapped in mucus. In these tests, nonimmune mucus did not trap or agglutinate the bacteria or parasites. The results of these studies help demonstrate that topically and orally applied antibodies can be highly effective at trapping pathogens in mucus. Even antibodies that fail to aggregate bacteria, or sperm, in the absence of mucus can be highly effective at trapping them in a mucus gel.

How do secreted antibodies bind to mucus fibers?
If antibodies can diffuse through mucus, how can they form adhesive cross-links to mucin fibers that will trap a motile pathogen? As was shown above in Figure 4.7, antibodies diffuse through mucus more slowly than in water even though larger virus-sized particles diffuse just as rapidly in mucus as in water. This suggests that antibodies are retarded by repeatedly making short-lived low-affinity bonds with mucin fibers. Similar diffusion measurements were performed in human salivary mucus (Padgett 1995); when water was withdrawn to concentrate salivary mucus, D_{mucus}/D_{water} for antibodies decreased with increasing mucin concentration as expected

for equilibrium binding between antibodies and mucins: $D_{mucus}/D_{water} \propto 1/[1 + (\text{mucin})]$. Assuming D_{mucus}/D_{water} is the fraction of time the antibodies are free to diffuse, and $1 - D_{mucus}/D_{water}$ is the fraction of time they spend bound to mucin fibers, then, in cervical mucus gels with dry weights ranging 1% to 5% as well as in salivary mucus gels with dry weights ranging 1% to 10%, IgG was bound between ~10% to 60% of the time, and IgM was bound between 30% to 80% of the time. Thus, throughout the physiologic range of mucin concentrations, antibodies are free to diffuse through mucus about half of the time, enabling them to accumulate rapidly on antigenic particles, and yet antibodies also spend about half of the time bound to mucin fibers. This low but significant antibody–mucus affinity appears appropriate if a role of secreted antibodies is to trap antigenic particles in mucus. Even though the low-affinity bond each antibody makes with a mucin fiber is weak and short lived, at any given time a subset of the antibodies bound to the surface of an antigenic particle will bind polyvalently to the elastic mucus gel.

Are weak low-affinity bonds strong enough to trap vigorously motile sperm and bacteria? The forward thrust of a human sperm is about 20 pN, significantly smaller than the measured strength of single-affinity bonds (Baltz et al. 1988; Baltz and Cone 1990; Kishino and Yanagida 1988; Florin et al. 1994). Thus multiple low-affinity bonds are more than strong enough to trap sperm and bacteria in mucus gels.

The nature of the low-affinity bonds formed between antibodies and mucus gels is unknown. That the Fab moiety does not bind to mucins was clearly demonstrated by observing the diffusion rates in mucus of IgM and IgM-Fc$_5\mu$, the pentameric Fc core that remains after all 10 Fab groups have been removed. Both IgM and IgM-Fc$_5\mu$ are equally retarded by mucus, indicating that it is the Fc core, not the Fab groups, that mediate affinity bonding to mucins (Olmsted et al. 2001).

Antibodies must function well in many types of mucus secretions throughout the body; thus the antibody–mucin affinity must be well controlled. Given the marked differences in glycosylation of different mucins in different sites in the body, and the differences in pH, ionic strength, and nonmucin components of mucus, antibodies probably bind to conserved protein domains, such as the cysteine rich domains that are well spaced along most secreted mucin fibers rather than to the highly variable glycosylated regions.

Several investigators have tried and failed to detect direct binding between antibodies and purified mucins (Crowther et al. 1985; Iontcheva et al. 1997; Olmsted 2000; and see Clamp 1977). This suggests that another component in mucus may be needed to form low-affinity links between antibodies and mucins. One such candidate is the IgG Fc binding protein identified by Kobayashi et al. (1989, 1991). This protein is stored and secreted from mucin granules in goblet cells present in many mucosal epithelia (except the conjunctiva). The mRNA for this mucinlike protein indicates it has 12 tandem repeats of a 400–amino acid cysteine-rich domain that resembles similar domains in secreted mucins (Harada et al. 1997). The 12 domains appear to bind up to three IgG molecules, and they bind aggregated IgG more tightly than monomeric IgG. Thus this IgG Fc binding protein could link antibodies to mucins if these cysteine-rich domains bind with low affinity to similar conserved domains on the gel-forming mucins.

Recently, secretory component (SC) has been shown to have a new role in immune exclusion (Phalipon et al. 2002). Nasally delivered dimeric/polymeric IgA is markedly more effective when bound to SC (to form S-IgA) than without SC in protecting mice against bacterial infection of the respiratory tract. SC helps retain S-IgA in the mucus lining of the respiratory tract, where it traps bacteria in mucus, thereby excluding them from the epithelial surface, and transporting them away with the mucus. Unlike IgG Fc binding protein, SC appears to adhere to the mucus gel via its carbohydrate residues. Human mucus retards the diffusion of aggregates of human S-IgA, but only slightly more than it retards IgM (Olmsted et al. 2001). Hence the bonds SC makes with the mucus gel are low enough in affinity to allow S-IgA to diffuse through mucus to accumulate on the surfaces of the bacteria, but high enough to help retain (or partition) S-IgA in mucus.

MUCUS–COMMENSAL RELATIONSHIPS

The mucus "rainforest"

At least 500 different types of bacteria, yeast, protozoa, and worms live in the mucus ecosystem of the human gut (Neutra and Forstner 1987; see Chapter 2). Most of the time most of these organisms cause little trouble to their host. However, many of them can switch from being commensals to pathogens if they overgrow their welcome, especially if they penetrate the mucus blanket and cling to the surfaces and/or penetrate the epithelial cells. Enterotoxigenic E. coli (ETEC) become pathogenic only when they adhere to the enterocytes (Gaastra and de Graaf 1982); similarly V. cholerae must attach to the villus to produce diarrhea (Schrank and Verwey 1976), and mucus has been shown to bind cholera toxin (Strombeck and Harrold 1974). Thus microbes that release toxins are likely to be most irritating when they attach to epithelial cells and thereby deliver toxins directly to the cell surface. Commensals can also become pathogenic simply by entering some "new territory," disrupting the normal commensal population at some other epithelial site, or colonizing an otherwise unpopulated site, as when E. coli from the GI tract initiate a urinary tract infection simply by colonizing a new epithelial site, the bladder.

Many commensals have specific receptors, or adhesins, with which they bind to secreted as well as cell-associated mucins (Cohen and Laux 1995; Lichtman et al. 1996). By clinging to the unstirred layer, they will slow the rate at which they are swept away and shed by the host. At any given mucosal surface, the secreted mucins and the cell-attached mucins can have many of the same protein and glycosylated surfaces. Thus bacterial adhesins that adhere to the mucus gel may also adhere to the epithelial cell surface; indeed, uropathogenic *E. coli* that do not stick to mucus do not adhere to urethral epithelial cells, although those that stick to mucus can also adhere to the epithelial cells (Fujita *et al.* 1989). This reveals a major protective function of secreted mucins: By secreting mucins that are closely similar to the cell-associated mucins, pathogens can be kept from attaching to the epithelial cell surface—the pathogen will stick to the mucus gel before it can reach the target cell. Mucins, as well as specific glycans present on mucins, have been shown to block bacterial attachment to epithelial cell surfaces. Also, in saliva, a small monomeric secreted mucin is an especially effective agglutinator of streptococci (Tabak 1995). This defense mechanism of secreting and shedding "false targets," the same molecular structures to which pathogens and commensals might adhere to epithelial target cells, helps keep both pathogens and commensals at bay in mucus. This strategy may be augmented by secreting mucin monomers more rapidly than the larger gel-forming oligomeric mucins (Davies *et al.* 2002).

Grazing on mucus

Most commensals do not degrade mucins. For example, *E. coli* appears to feed entirely on phosphatidylserine (Krivan *et al.* 1992). The commensals and pathogens that do degrade mucus slowly begin to colonize the human gut over the first several months to 2 years of human life (Midtvedt *et al.* 1994). The small subset of bacteria that "graze" on mucus cling to specific glycans and nibble (cleave) specific sugars from the tips of the glycans (Neutra and Forstner 1987). Moreover, this subset of grazing microbes act cooperatively, each supplying glycosidases other strains lack. As long as the host secretes mucus fast enough, this arrangement is completely symbiotic. Mucins can only be slowly digested by host enzymes, and most mucins would be shed in feces relatively undigested were it not for the small subset of commensals that specialize in eating mucins. This is made evident by germfree animals that produce less mucus, yet their cecums become engorged with mucus. Soon after germfree animals are provided with commensal bacteria, the excess mucus in the cecum is digested, and yet the rate of mucus secretion increases (Szentkuti *et al.* 1990; Enss *et al.* 1992).

Some non–mucin-degrading commensals, such as lactobacilli (Ruseler-van Embden *et al.* 1995), can adhere directly to epithelial cell surfaces without causing irritation. Indeed, lactobacilli are the dominant microbiota in the healthy human vagina. These commensals are the predominant source of the lactic acid that acidifies the vaginal fluid to approximately pH 4 (Boskey *et al.* 2001), and other microbial inhibitors such as peroxide, that suppress the growth of many other commensals that might otherwise become pathogenic. The most common vaginal disorder, bacterial vaginosis, is an overgrowth of commensal bacteria that can occur when lactobacilli are suppressed (see Chapters 99–101).

Regulating mucosal microbiota with secreted antibodies and mucus

Secreted antibodies participate in a simple negative-feedback regulatory process that can keep commensals and pathogens from overpopulating or invading an epithelial surface. In the intestine, as is now well established (Neutra and Forstner 1987), antigen particles impinging on M cells are transcytosed into Peyer's patches, delivered to B and T lymphocytes which, if stimulated, initiate the clonal expansion of B cells. These B cells migrate to nearby mucosal surfaces (and more slowly to other mucosal surfaces) where they secrete antibodies, typically pIgA, that can specifically bind the antigen. The antigen-specific antibodies are then secreted into the mucus as S-IgA where they are free to diffuse and will accumulate on the surface of antigen particles to which they bind specifically. Thus these secreted antibodies are likely to trap in mucus any antigen-bearing particle on which they accumulate, and thereby decrease the amount of this antigen that will impinge on the M cells. This simple negative feedback loop will automatically arrive at an appropriate average rate of production of S-IgA. If more than enough antigen-specific antibody is being secreted, little if any antigen will arrive at the M cell, and few if any B cells will be stimulated to make antibody against this antigen. On the other hand, if too little antigen-specific antibody is being secreted, more antigen will impinge on the M cell. In this feedback loop, mucus participates both as a sensory and effector organ, helping select what reaches the M cell, helping the secreted antibodies to trap, and thereby exclude the antigen.

The specificity of secreted antibodies can play another major role in regulating mucosal microbiota. Unlike broad-spectrum protective factors or therapeutic drugs, specific antibodies can completely eliminate and prevent recolonization by a specific microbe from an epithelial region while leaving the remaining microbiota intact. This has been strikingly demonstrated with topical oral applications of monoclonal antibodies against *Streptococcus mutans*, the acid-producing bacterium that, by adhering to tooth enamel, is usually responsible for dental caries (Ma *et al.* 1990). After a 9-day oral treatment with monoclonal antibody, the oral microbiota of the subjects remained free of *S. mutans* more than 2 years; in contrast, *S. mutans* recolonized within days of oral treatment with a broad-spectrum microbicide, chlorhexidine. Apparently, once *S. mutans* is specifically eliminated, other commensals occupy its environmental niche and thereby help prevent its recolonization (Lehner *et al.* 1992a).

CONCLUDING PERSPECTIVES

Mucus helps protect epithelial surfaces in many different ways, as a lubricant that protects against mechanical damage while enabling rapid cleansing and shedding of mucosal surfaces, as a regulated nutrient medium in which whole ecosystems thrive, usually symbiotically, and as a filter whose permeability is regulated by mucins, antibodies, lipids, and other nonmucin factors. Although major features of some of these functions are now emerging, many of the molecular mechanisms are unknown, and most of the regulatory mechanisms are completely unknown. What is the actual structure of a mucus gel? How are antibodies lightly bound to mucins? What cellular and tissue mechanisms regulate the viscoelasticity of mucus? What regulates the secretion rates of specific mucins and their glycosylation? Not only are mucins biochemically complex, but their interactions with mucosal microbiota must be even more complex.

Despite our present level of ignorance of mucus and its functions, we are approaching the ability to create safer and more effective agents for augmenting the protective functions of mucus, such as the development of nanoparticles for improved mucosal delivery of drugs and vaccines (see Florence 1997; Lehner *et al.* 1992b; Mestecky and McGhee 1992), hyperimmune milk for preventing GI infections (Tacket *et al.* 1988, 1992), and the development of monoclonal antibodies that can be delivered topically (for reviews, see Zeitlin *et al.* 2000; Cone and Whaley 1994) as well as systemically to provide passive immune protection of mucosal surfaces against commensal bacteria such as *S. mutans* (Ma *et al.* 1990), motile pathogens such as *V. cholerae* (Winner *et al.* 1991), and sexually transmitted disease (STD) pathogens, including HIV (Parren *et al.* 2001; Veazey *et al.* 2003; Mascola *et al.* 2003; Ruprecht *et al.* 2003; Kozlowski and Neutra 2003).

ACKNOWLEDGMENTS

Thanks to Thomas R. Moench, Kevin J. Whaley, Sharon Achilles, Elizabeth Boskey, Larry Zeitlin, and Denis Wirtz for help with the manuscript, Ashley I. Yudin and David F. Katz for providing unpublished micrographs for Figure 4.5, and Emily Martin for introducing me to Sartre's discourse on the repulsiveness of the slimy in human consciousness.

REFERENCES

Baltz, J. M., and Cone, R. A. (1990). The strength of non-covalent biological bonds and adhesions by multiple independent bonds. *J. Theor. Biol.* 142, 163–178.

Baltz, J. M., Katz, D. F., and Cone, R. A. (1988). Mechanics of sperm-egg interaction at the zona pellucida. *Biophys. J.* 54, 643–654.

Baltz, J. M., Williams, P. O., and Cone, R. A. (1990). Dense fibers protect mammalian sperm against damage. *Biol. Reprod.* 43, 485–491.

Behrens, I., Pena, A. I., Alonso, M. J., and Kissel, T. (2002). Comparative uptake studies of bioadhesive and non-bioadhesive nanoparticles in human intestinal cell lines and rats: The effect of mucus on particle adsorption and transport. *Pharm. Res.* 19, 1185–1193.

Bell, A. E., Sellers, L. A., Allen, A., Cunliffe, W. J., Morris, E. R., and Ross-Murphy, S. B. (1985). Properties of gastric and duodenal mucus. *Gastroenterology* 88, 269–280.

Bhaskar, K. R., Gong, D. H., Bansil, R., Pajevic, S., Hamilton, J. A., Turner, B. S., and LaMont, J. T. (1991). Profound increase in viscosity and aggregation of pig gastric mucin at low pH. *Am. J. Physiol.* 261, G827–G832.

Bhaskar, K. R., Garik, P., Turner, B. S., Bradley, J. D., Bansil, R., Stanley, H. E., and LaMont, J. T. (1992). Viscous fingering of HCl through gastric mucin. *Nature* 360, 458–461.

Biesbrock, A. R., Reddy, M. S., and Levine, M. J. (1991). Interaction of a salivary mucin-secretory immunoglobulin A complex with mucosal pathogens. *Infect. Immun.* 59, 3492–3497.

Boskey, E. R., Cone, R. A., Whaley, K. J., and Moench, T. R. (2001). Origins of vaginal acidity: High D/L lactate ratio is consistent with bacteria being the primary source. *Hum. Reprod.* 16, 1809–1813.

Bronson, R. A., Cooper, G. W., Rosenfeld, D. L., Gilbert, J. V., and Plaut, A. G. (1987). The effect of an IgA1 protease on immunoglobulins bound to the sperm surface and sperm cervical mucus penetrating ability. *Fertil. Steril.* 47, 985–991.

Carlisle, M. S., McGregor, D. D., and Appleton, J. A. (1991a). The role of the antibody Fc region in rapid expulsion of Trichinella spiralis in suckling rats. *Immunology.* 74, 552–558.

Carlisle, M. S., McGregor, D. D., and Appleton, J. A. (1991b). Intestinal mucus entrapment of *Trichinella spiralis* larvae induced by specific antibodies. *Immunology* 74, 546–551.

Carlstedt, I., and Sheehan, J. K. (1984). Macromolecular properties and polymeric structure of mucus glycoproteins. *Ciba Found. Symp.* 109, 157–172.

Carlstedt, I., and Sheehan, J. K. (1988). Structure and macromolecular properties of mucus glycoproteins. *Monogr. Allergy* 24, 16–24.

Chretien, F. C., Cohen, L., Borg, V., and Psychoyos, A. (1975). Human cervical mucus during the menstrual cycle and pregnancy in normal and pathological conditions. *J. Reprod. Med.* 14, 192–196.

Clamp, J. R. (1977). The relationship between secretory immunoglobulin A and mucus. *Biochem. Soc. Trans.* 5, 1579–1581.

Cohen, P. S., and Laux, D. C. (1995). Bacterial adhesion to and penetration of intestinal mucus *in vitro*. *Methods Enzymol.* 253, 309–314.

Cone, R. A., and Whaley, K. J. (1994). Monoclonal antibodies for reproductive health: Part I. Preventing sexual transmission of disease and pregnancy with topically applied antibodies. *Am. J. Reprod. Immunol.* 32, 114–131.

Conley, M. E., and Delacroix, D. L. (1987). Intravascular and mucosal immunoglobulin A: Two separate but related systems of immune defense? *Ann. Int. Med.* 106, 892–899.

Copeman, M., Matuz, J., Leonard, A. J., Pearson, J. P., Dettmar, P. W., and Allen, A. (1994). The gastroduodenal mucus barrier and its role in protection against luminal pepsins: The effect of 16,16 dimethyl prostaglandin E2, carbopol-polyacrylate, sucralfate and bismuth subsalicylate. *J. Gastroenterol. Hepatol.* 9, S55–S59.

Corfield, A. P., Myerscough, N., Longman, R., Sylvester, P., Arul, S., and Pignatelli, M. (2000). Mucins and mucosal protection in the gastrointestinal tract: New prospects for mucins in the pathology of gastrointestinal disease. *Gut* 47, 589–594.

Corthesy, B., and Kraehenbuhl, J. P. (1999). Antibody-mediated protection of mucosal surfaces. *Curr. Top. Microbiol. Immunol.* 236, 93–111.

Crowther, R., Lichtman, S., Forstner, J., and Forstner, G. (1985). Failure to show secretory IgA binding by rat intestinal mucin. *Fed. Proc.* 44, 691. (Abstr.).

Dartt, D. A. (2002). Regulation of mucin and fluid secretion by conjunctival epithelial cells. *Progr. Retin. Eye Res.* 21, 555–576.

Davenport, H. W. (1972). Why the stomach does not digest itself. *Sci. Am.* 226, 87–93.

Davies, J. R., Herrmann, A., Russell, W., Svitacheva, N., Wickstrom, C., and Carlstedt, I. (2002). Respiratory tract mucins: Structure and expression patterns. *Novartis Found. Symp.* 248, 76–88; discussion 88–93, 277–282.

Dean, M., and Santis, G. (1994). Heterogenicity in the severity of cystic fibrosis and the role of CFTR gene mutations. *Hum. Genet.* 93, 364–368.

Debailleul, V., Laine, A., Huet, G., Mathon, P., d'Hooghe, M. C., Aubert, J. P., and Porchet, N. (1998). Human mucin genes MUC2, MUC3, MUC4, MUC5AC, MUC5B, and MUC6 express stable and extremely large mRNAs and exhibit a variable length polymorphism. An improved method to analyze large mRNAs. *J. Biol. Chem.* 273, 881–890.

Dekker, J., van der Ende, A., Aelmans, P. H., and Strous, G. J. (1991). Rat gastric mucin is synthesized and secreted exclusively as filamentous oligomers. *Biochem. J.* 279, 251–256.

Dekker J., Rossen, J.W., Buller, H.A., and Einerhand, A.W. (2002). The *MUC* family: An obituary. *Trends Biochem. Sci.* 27, 126–31.

Denny, M. (1980). The role of gastropod pedal mucus in locomotion. *Nature* 285, 160.

Deplancke, B., and Gaskins, H.R. (2001). Microbial modulation of innate defense: Goblet cells and the intestinal mucus layer. *Am. J. Clin. Nutr.* 73, 1131S–1141S.

Desseyn, J.L., Aubert, J.P., Porchet, N., and Laine A. (2000). Evolution of the large secreted gel-forming mucins. *Mol. Biol Evol* 17, 1175–1184.

Desseyn, J. L., Guyonnet-Duperat, V., Porchet, N., Aubert, J. P., and Laine, A. (1997). Human mucin gene *MUC5B*, the 10.7-kb large central exon encodes various alternate subdomains resulting in a super-repeat: Structural evidence for a 11p15.5 gene family. *J. Biol. Chem.* 272, 3168–3178.

Dial, E. J., and Lichtenberger, L. M. (1987). Milk protection against experimental ulcerogenesis in rats. *Digest. Dis. Sci.* 32, 1145–1150.

Dumur, V., Gervais, R., Rigot, J. M., Delomel-Vinner, E., Decaestecker, B., Lafitte, J. J., and Roussel, P. (1996). Congenital bilateral absence of the vas deferens (CBAVD) and cystic fibrosis transmembrane regulator (CFTR): correlation between genotype and phenotype. *Hum. Genet.* 97, 7–10.

Enss, M. L., Grosse-Siestrupp, H., Schmidt-Wittig, U., and Gartner, K. (1992). Changes in colonic mucins of germfree rats in response to the introduction of a 'normal' rat microbial flora. Rat colonic mucin. *J. Exp. Anim. Sci.* 35, 110–119.

Fabry, T. L. (1990). How the parietal secretion crosses the gastric mucus without being neutralized. *Gastroenterology* 98, A42.

Florence, A. T. (1997). The oral absorption of micro- and nanoparticulates: Neither exceptional nor unusual. *Pharmaceut. Res.* 14, 259–266.

Florey, H. W. (1962). The secretion and function of intestinal mucus. *Gastroenterology* 43, 326–329.

Florin, E. L., Moy, V. T., and Gaub, H. E. (1994). Adhesion forces between individual ligand-receptor pairs. *Science* 264, 415–417.

Forstner, G. (1995). Signal transduction, packaging and secretion of mucins. *Annu. Rev. Physiol.* 57, 585–605.

Forstner, J. F., Oliver, M. G., and Sylvester, F. A. (1995). Production, structure, and biologic relevance of gastrointestinal mucins. In *Infections of the Gastrointestinal Tract* (eds. M. J. Blaser, P. D. Smith, J. I. Ravdin, H. B. Greenberg, and R. I. Guerrant), pp.71–88. New York: Raven Press, Ltd.

Fox, P. C., Busch, K. A., and Baum, B. J. (1987). Subjective reports of xerostomia and objective measures of salivary gland performance. *J. Am. Dent. Assoc.* 115, 581–584.

Frey, A., Giannasca, K. T., Weltzin, R., Giannasca, P. J., Reggio, H., Lencer, W. I., and Neutra, M. R. (1996). Role of the glycocalyx in regulating access of microparticles to apical plasma membranes of intestinal epithelial cells: Implications for microbial attachment and oral vaccine targeting. *J. Exp. Med.* 184, 1045–1059.

Fujita, K., Yamamoto, T., Yokota, T., and Kitagawa, R. (1989). *In vitro* adherence of type 1-fimbriated uropathogenic *Escherichia coli* to human ureteral mucosa [published erratum appears in *Infect. Immun.* 58, 579 (1990)]. *Infect. Immun.* 57, 2574–2579.

Gaastra, W., and de Graaf, F. K. (1982). Host-specific fimbrial adhesins of noninvasive enterotoxigenic *Escherichia coli* strains. *Microbiol. Rev.* 46, 129–161.

Gendler, S. J., and Spicer, A. P. (1995). Epithelial mucin genes. *Annu. Rev. Physiol.* 57, 607–634.

Gerken, T. A., Butenhof, K. J., and Shogren, R. (1989). Effects of glycosylation on the conformation and dynamics of O-linked glycoproteins: Carbon-13 NMR studies of ovine submaxillary mucin. *Biochemistry* 28, 5536–5543.

Gipson, I. K., Moccia, R., Spurr-Michaud, S., Argueso, P., Gargiulo, A. R., Hill, J. A. 3rd, Offner, G. D., and Keutmann, H. T. (2001). The amount of MUC5B mucin in cervical mucus peaks at midcycle. *J. Clin. Endocrinol. Metab.* 86, 594–600.

Godl, K., Johansson, M. E., Lidell, M. E., Morgelin, M., Karlsson, H., Olson, F. J., Gum, J. R., Jr., Kim, Y. S., and Hansson, G. C. (2002). The N terminus of the MUC2 mucin forms trimers that are held together within a trypsin-resistant core fragment. *J. Biol. Chem.* 277, 47248–47256.

Gruber, P., Longer, M. A., and Robinson, J. R. (1987). Some biological issues in oral, controlled drug delivery. *Adv. Drug Deliv. Rev.* 1, 1–18.

Gum, J. R., Jr. (1995). Human mucin glycoproteins: Varied structures predict diverse properties and specific functions. *Biochem. Soc. Transact.* 23, 795–799.

Hajishengallis, G., Nikolova, E., and Russell, M.W. (1992). Inhibition of *Streptococcus mutans* adherence to saliva-coated hydroxyapatite by human secretory immunoglobulin A (S-IgA) antibodies to cell surface protein antigen I/II: reversal by IgA1 protease cleavage. *Infect. Immun.* 60, 5057–5064.

Harada, N., Iijima, S., Kobayashi, K., Yoshida, T., Brown, W. R., Hibi, T., Oshima, A., and Morikawa M. (1997). Human IgG Fc binding protein (FcgammaBP) in colonic epithelial cells exhibits mucin-like structure. *J. Biol. Chem.* 272, 15232–15241.

Hattori, M., Majima, Y., Ukai, K., and Sakakura, Y. (1993). Effects of nasal allergen challenge on dynamic viscoelasticity of nasal mucus. *Ann. Otol. Rhinol. Laryngol.* 102, 314–317.

Heatley, N. G. (1959). Mucusubstance as a barrier to diffusion. *Gastroenterology* 37, 304–314.

Henry, B. T., Adler, J., Hibberd, S., Cheema, M. S., Davis, S. S., and Rogers, T. G. (1992). Epi-fluorescence microscopy and image analysis used to measure diffusion coefficients in gel systems. *J. Pharm. Pharmacol.* 44, 543–549.

Herrmann, A., Davies, J. R., Lindell, G., Martensson, S., Packer, N. H., Swallow, D. M., and Carlstedt I. (1999). Studies on the "insoluble" glycoprotein complex from human colon: Identification of reduction-insensitive MUC2 oligomers and C-terminal cleavage. *J. Biol. Chem.* 274, 15828–15836.

Holm, L., and Flemstrom, G. (1990). Microscopy of acid transport at the gastric surface *in vivo*. *J. Intern. Med.* 732, 91–95.

Hoskins, L. C., Agustines, M., McKee, W. B., Boulding, E. T., Kriaris, M., and Niedermeyer, G. (1985). Mucin degradation in human colon ecosystems: Isolation and properties of fecal strains that degrade ABH blood group antigens and oligosaccharides from mucin glycoproteins. *J. Clin. Investig.* 75, 944–953.

Iontcheva, I., Oppenheim, F. G., and Troxler, R. F. (1997). Human salivary mucin MG1 selectively forms heterotypic complexes with amylase, proline-rich proteins, statherin, and histatins. *J. Dent. Res.* 76, 734–743.

Ito, S. (1974). Form and function of the glycocalyx on free cell surfaces. *Philosoph. Trans. R. Soc. Lond, B,: Biol. Sci.* 268, 55–66.

Jager, S., Kremer, J., Kuiken, J., and Mulder, I. (1981). The significance of the Fc part of antispermatozoal antibodies for the shaking phenomenon in the sperm-cervical mucus contact test. *Fertil. Steril.* 36, 792–797.

Jeanneret-Grosjean, A., King, M., Michoud, M. C., Liote, H., and Amyot, R. (1988). Sampling technique and rheology of human tracheobronchial mucus. *Am. Rev. Respir. Dis.* 137, 707–710.

Kaetzel, C. S., Robinson, J. K., and Lamm, M. E. (1994). Epithelial transcytosis of monomeric IgA and IgG cross-linked through antigen to polymeric IgA: A role for monomeric antibodies in the mucosal immune system. *J. Immunol.* 152, 72–76.

Karlsson, N. G., Herrmann, A., Karlsson, H., Johansson, M. E., Carlstedt, I., and Hansson, G. C. (1997). The glycosylation of rat intestinal Muc2 mucin varies between rat strains and the small and large intestine: A study of O-linked oligosaccharides by a mass spectrometric approach. *J. Biol. Chem.* 272, 27025–27034.

Keates, A. C., Nunes, D. P., Afdhal, N. H., Troxler, R. F., and Offner, G. D. (1997). Molecular cloning of a major human gall bladder mucin: Complete C-terminal sequence and genomic organization of MUC5B. *Biochem. J.* 324, 295–303.

Kerss, S., Allen, A., and Garner, A. (1982). A simple method for measuring thickness of the mucus gel layer adherent to rat, frog and human gastric mucosa: Influence of feeding, prostaglandin, N-acetylcysteine and other agents. *Clin. Sci.* 63, 187–195.

King, M. (1987). The role of mucus viscoelasticity in cough clearance. *Biorheology* 24, 589–597.

Kishino, A., and Yanagida, T. (1988). Force measurements by micromanipulation of a single actin filament by glass needles. *Nature* 334, 74–76.

Kobayashi, K., Blaser, M. J., and Brown, W.R. (1989). Identification of a unique IgG Fc binding site in human intestinal epithelium. *J. Immunol.* 143, 2567–2574.

Kobayashi, K., Hamada, Y., Blaser, M. J., and Brown, W.R. (1991). The molecular configuration and ultrastructural locations of an IgG Fc binding site in human colonic epithelium. *J. Immunol.* 146, 68–74.

Kozlowski, P. A., and Neutra, M. R. (2003). The role of mucosal immunity in prevention of HIV transmission. *Curr. Mol. Med.* 3, 217–228.

Kremer, J., and Jager, S. (1976). The sperm cervical mucus contact test: A preliminary report. *Fertil. Steril.* 27, 335–340.

Kremer, J., and Jager, S. (1992). The significance of antisperm antibodies for sperm–cervical mucus interaction. *Hum. Reprod.* 7, 781–784.

Krivan, H. C., Franklin, D. P., Wang, W., Laux, D. A., and Cohen, P. S. (1992). Phosphatidylserine found in intestinal mucus serves as a sole source of carbon and nitrogen for salmonellae and *Escherichia coli. Infect. Immun.* 69, 3943–3946.

Lamblin, G., Lhermitte, M., Klein, A., Houdret, N., Scharfman, A., Ramphal, R., and Roussel, P. (1991). The carbohydrate diversity of human respiratory mucins: A protection of the underlying mucosa? *Am. Rev. Respir. Dis.* 144, S19–S24.

Lamm, M. E., Nedrud, J. G., Kaetzel, C. S., and Mazanec, M. B. (1995). IgA and mucosal defense. *Acta Pathol. Microbiol. Immunol. Scand.* 103, 241–246.

Lamont, J. T. (1992). Mucus: The front line of intestinal mucosal defense. *Ann. N.Y. Acad. Sci.* 664, 190–201.

Lancaster, C. A., Peat, N., Duhig, T., Wilson, D., Taylor-Papadimtriou, J., and Gendler, S. J. (1990). Structure and expression of the human polymorphic epithelial mucin gene: an expressed VTNR unit. *Biochem. Biophys. Res. Commun.* 173, 1019–1029.

Larhed, A. W., Artursson, P., Grasjo, J., and Bjork, E. (1997). Diffusion of drugs in native and purified gastrointestinal mucus. *J. Pharm. Sci.* 86, 660–665.

Lehner, T., Ma, J. K., and Kelly, C. G. (1992a). A mechanism of passive immunization with monoclonal antibodies to a 185,000 M(r) streptococcal antigen. *Adv. Exp. Med. Biol.* 327, 151–163.

Lehner, T., Bergmeier, L. A., Panagiotidi, C., Tao, R., Brookes, R., Klavinskis, L. S., Walker, P., Walker, J., Ward, R. G., Hussain, L., Gearing, A. J. H., and Adams, S.E. (1992b). Induction of mucosal and systemic immunity to a recombinant simian immunodeficiency viral protein. *Science* 258, 1365–1369.

Lichtenberger, L. M. (1995). The hydrophobic barrier properties of gastrointestinal mucus. *Annu. Rev. Physiol.* 57, 565–583.

Lichtman, S. N., Sherman, P., and Mack, D. R. (1996). The role of mucus in gut protection. *Curr. Opin. Gastroenterol.* 12, 584–590.

Livingston, E. H., and Engel, E. (1995). Modeling of the gastric gel mucus layer: Application to the measured pH gradient. *J. Clin. Gastroenterol.* 21 (Suppl. 1):S120–S124.

Ma, J. K., Hunjan, M., Smith, R., Kelly, C., and Lehner, T. (1990). An investigation into the mechanism of protection by local passive immunization with monoclonal antibodies against *Streptococcus mutans. Infect. Immun.* 58, 3407–3414.

Magnusson, K. E., and Stjernstrom, I. (1982). Mucosal barrier mechanisms: Interplay between secretory IgA (S-IgA), IgG and mucins on the surface properties and association of salmonellae with intestine and granulocytes. *Immunology* 45, 239–248.

Mantle, M., Forstner, G. G., and Forstner, J. F. (1984). Antigenic and structural features of goblet-cell mucin of human small intestine. *Biochem. J.* 217, 159–167.

Mantle, M., Stewart, G., Zayas, G., and King, M. (1990). The disulfide-bond content and rheological properties of intestinal mucins from normal subjects and patients with cystic fibrosis. *Biochem. J.* 266, 597–604.

Markesich, D. C., Anand, B. S., Lew, G. M., and Graham, D.Y. (1995). *Helicobacter pylori* infection does not reduce the viscosity of human gastric mucus gel. *Gut* 36, 327–329.

Mascola, J. R., Lewis, M. G., VanCott, T. C., Stiegler, G., Katinger, H., Seaman, M., Beaudry, K., Barouch, D. H., Korioth-Schmitz, B., Krivulka, G., Sambor, A., Welcher, B., Douek, D. C., Montefiori, D. C., Shiver, J. W., Poignard, P., Burton, D. R., and Letvin, N. L. (2003). Cellular immunity elicited by human immunodeficiency virus type 1/simian immunodeficiency virus DNA vaccination does not augment the sterile protection afforded by passive infusion of neutralizing antibodies. *J. Virol.* 77, 10348–10356.

Matthes, I., Nimmerfall, F., Vonderscher, J., and Sucker, H. (1992). Mucus models for investigation of intestinal absorption mechanisms. 4. Comparison of mucus models with absorption models *in vivo* and *in situ* for prediction of intestinal drug absorption. (in German). *Pharmazie* 47, 787–791.

Maury, J., Bernadec, A., Rigal, A., and Maroux, S. (1995). Expression and glycosylation of the filamentous brush border glycocalyx (FBBG) during rabbit enterocute differentiation along the crypt-villus axis. *J. Cell Science* 108, 2705–2713.

McCool, D. J., Forstner, J. F., and Forstner, G. G. (1994). Synthesis and secretion of mucin by the human colonic tumor cell line LS180. *Biochem. J.* 302, 111–118.

McDaniel, R. V., Sharp, K., Brooks, D., McLaughlin, A. C., Winiski, A. P., Cafiso, D., and McLaughlin, S. (1986). Electrokinetic and electrostatic properties of bilayers containing gangliosides GM1, GD1a, or GT1: Comparison with a nonlinear theory. *Biophys. J.* 49, 741–752.

McNamara, N., and Basbaum, C. (2002). Signaling networks controlling mucin production in response to Gram-positive and Gram-negative bacteria. *Glycoconj. J.* 18, 715–722.

McSweegan, E., Burr, D. H., and Walker, R. I. (1987). Intestinal mucus gel and secretory antibody are barriers to *Campylobacter jejuni* adherence to INT 407 cells. *Infect. Immun.* 55, 1431–1435.

Mestecky, J., and McGhee, J. R. (1992). Prospects for human mucosal vaccines. *Adv. Exp. Med. Biol.* 327, 13–23.

Mestecky, J., Russell, M. W., Jackson, S., and Brown, T. A. (1986). The human IgA system: A reassessment. *Clin. Immunol. Immunopathol.* 40, 105–114.

Midtvedt, A. C., Carlstedt-Duke, B., and Midtvedt, T. (1994). Establishment of a mucin-degrading intestinal microflora during the first two years of human life. *J. Pediatr. Gastroenterol. Nutr.* 18, 321–326.

Moghissi, K. S., and Syner, F. N. (1970). Studies on human cervical mucus: Mucoids and their relation to sperm penetration. *Fertil. Steril.* 21, 234–239.

Moore, E. W. (1976). *Physiology of Intestinal and Electrolyte Absorption.* American Gastroenterological Society. Baltimore: Milner-Fenwick.

Murty, V. L. N., Sarosiek, J., Slomiany, A., and Slomiany, B. L. (1984). Effect of lipids and proteins on the viscosity of gastric mucus glycoprotein. *Biochem. Biophys. Res. Comm.* 121, 521–529.

Narhi, T. O. (1994). Prevalence of subjective feelings of dry mouth in the elderly. *J. Dent. Res.* 73, 20–25.

Neutra, M. R., and Forstner, J. F. (1987). Gastrointestinal mucus: Synthesis, secretion, and function. In *Physiology of the Gastrointestinal Tract* (ed. L. R. Johnson), 975–2008, New York: Raven Press.

Nicholas, C. V., Desai, M., Vadgama, P., McDonnell, M. B., and Lucas, S. (1991). pH dependence of hydrochloric acid diffusion through gastric mucus: Correlation with diffusion through a water layer using a membrane-mounted glass pH electrode. *Analyst* 116, 463–467.

Nieuw Amerongen, A. V., Oderkerk, C. H., and Driessen, A. A. (1987). Role of mucins from human whole saliva in the protection of tooth enamel against demineralization *in vitro. Caries Res.* 21, 297–309.

Olmsted, S. S. (2000). Three mechanisms of mucus that protect epithelial surfaces. Ph.D. thesis, Johns Hopkins University.

Olmsted, S. S., Padgett, J. L., Yudin, A. I., Whaley, K. J., Moench, T. R., and Cone, R. A. (2001). Diffusion of macromolecules and virus-like particles in human cervical mucus. *Biophys. J.* 81, 1930–1937.

Padgett, J. L. (1995). Macromolecules and virus-like particles diffuse through human mucus. Ph.D. thesis, Johns Hopkins University.

Parkhurst, M. R., and Saltzman, W. M. (1994). Leukocytes migrate through three-dimensional gels of midcycle cervical mucus. *Cell Immunol* . 156, 77–94.

Parren, P. W., Marx, P. A., Hessell, A. J., Luckay, A., Harouse, J., Cheng-Mayer, C., Moore, J. P., and Burton, D. R. (2001). Antibody protects macaques against vaginal challenge with a pathogenic R5 simian/human immunodeficiency virus at serum levels giving complete neutralization *in vitro. J. Virol.* 75, 8340–8347.

Perez-Vilar, J., and Hill, R. L. (1998a). The carboxyl-terminal 90 residues of porcine submaxillary mucin are sufficient for forming disulfide-bonded dimers. *J. Biol. Chem.* 273, 6982–6988.

Perez-Vilar, J., Eckhardt, A. E., DeLuca, A., and Hill, R. L. (1998b). Porcine submaxillary mucin forms disulfide-linked multimers through its amino-terminal D-domains. *J. Biol. Chem.* 273, 14442–14449.

Phalipon, A., Cardona, A., Kraehenbuhl, J. P., Edelman, L., Sansonetti, P. J., and Corthesy, B. (2002). Secretory component: A new role in secretory IgA-mediated immune exclusion *in vivo. Immunity* 17, 107–115.

Poon, W. W., and McCoshen, J. A. (1985). Variances in mucus architecture as a cause of cervical factor infertility. *Fertil. Steril.* 44, 361–365.

Poulsen, L. K., Lan, F., Kristensen, C. S., Hobolth, P., Molin, S., and Krogfelt, K. A. (1994). Spatial distribution of *Escherichia coli* in the mouse large intestine inferred from rRNA in situ hybridization. *Infect. Immun.* 62, 5191–5194.

Raynal, B. D., Hardingham, T. E., Sheehan, J. K., and Thornton, D. J. (2003). Calcium-dependent protein interactions in MUC5B provide reversible cross-links in salivary mucus. *J. Biol. Chem.* 278, 28703–28710.

Roussel, P., Lamblin, G., Lhermitte, M., Houdret, N., Lafitte, J. J., Perini, J. M., Klein, A., and Scharfman, A. (1988). The complexity of mucins. *Biochimie* 70, 1471–1482.

Rubin, B.K. (2002). Physiology of airway mucus clearance. *Respir. Care* 47, 761–768.

Rubin, B. K., Ramirez, O., Zayas, J. G., Finegan, B., and King, M. (1992). Respiratory mucus from asymptomatic smokers is better hydrated and more easily cleared by mucociliary action. *Am. Rev. Respir. Dis.* 145, 545–547.

Ruprecht, R. M., Ferrantelli, F., Kitabwalla, M., Xu, W., and McClure, H. M. (2003). Antibody protection: Passive immunization of neonates against oral AIDS virus challenge. *Vaccine* 21, 3370–3373.

Ruseler-van Embden, J. G., van Lieshout, L. M., Gosselink, M. J. and Marteau, P. (1995). Inability of *Lactobacillus casei* strain GG, *L. acidophilus*, and *Bifidobacterium bifidum* to degrade intestinal mucus glycoproteins. *Scand. J. Gastroenterol.* 30, 675–680.

Saltzman, W. M., Radomsky, M. L., Whaley, K. J., and Cone, R. A. (1994). Antibody diffusion in human cervical mucus. *Biophys J.* 66, 508–515.

Sanderson, S. L., Stebar, M. C., Ackermann, K. L., Jones, S. H., Batjakas, I. E., and Kaufman, L. (1996). Mucus entrapment of particles by a suspension-feeding Tilapia (Pisces: Cichlidae). *J. Exp. Biol.* 199, 1743–1756.

Sandoz, D., Nicolas, G., and Laine, M. C. (1985). Two mucous cell types revisited after quick-freezing and cryosubstitution. *Biol. Cell* 54, 79–88.

Sandzen, B., Blom, H., and Dahlgren, S. (1988). Gastric mucus gel layer thickness measured by direct light microscopy: An experimental study in the rat. *Scand. J. Gastroenterol.* 23, 1160–1164.

Sartre, J-P. (1981). *Existential Psychoanalysis.* Washington, DC: Regnery Gateway.

Schrank, G. D., and Verwey, W. F. (1976). Distribution of cholera organisms in experimental *Vibrio cholerae* infections: Proposed mechanisms of pathogenesis and antibacterial immunity. *Infect. Immun.* 13, 195–203.

Schreiber, S., and Scheid, P. (1997). Gastric mucus of the guinea pig: Proton carrier and diffusion barrier. *Am. J. Physiol.* 272, G63–G70.

Schuhl, J. F. (1995). Nasal mucociliary clearance in perennial rhinitis. *J. Invest. Allergol. Clin. Immunol.* 5, 333–336.

Sellers, L. A., Allen, A., Morris, E. R., and Ross-Murphy, S. B. (1987). Mechanical characterization and properties of gastrointestinal mucus gel. *Biorheology* 24, 615–623.

Sellers, L. A., Allen, A., Morris, E. R., and Ross-Murphy, S. B. (1988a). Submaxillary mucins: Intermolecular interactions and gel-forming potential of concentrated solutions. *Biochem. J.* 256, 599–607.

Sellers, L. A., Allen, A., Morris, E. R., and Ross-Murphy, S. B. (1988b). Mucus glycoprotein gels: Role of glycoprotein polymeric structure and carbohydrate side-chains in gel-formation. *Carbohydr. Res.* 178, 93–110.

Sellers, L. A., Allen, A., Morris, E. R., and Ross-Murphy, S. B. (1991). The rheology of pig small intestinal and colonic mucus: Weakening of gel structure by non-mucin components. *Biochim. Biophys. Acta* 1115, 174–179.

Shak, S. (1995). Aerosolized recombinant human DNase I for the treatment of cystic fibrosis. *Chest* 107, 65S–70S.

Shak, S., Capon, D. J., Hellmiss, R., Marsters, S. A., and Baker, C. L. (1990). Recombinant human DNase I reduces the viscosity of cystic fibrosis sputum. *Proc. Natl. Acad. Sci. U.S.A.* 87, 9188–9192.

Shankar, V., Naziruddin, B., Reyes de la Rocha, S., and Sachdev, G. P. (1990). Evidence of hydrophobic domains in human respiratory mucins: Effect of sodium chloride on hydrophobic binding properties. *Biochemistry* 29, 5856–5864.

Shankar, V., Virmani, A.K., Naziruddin, B., and Sachdev, G. P. (1991). Macromolecular properties and polymeric structure of canine tracheal mucins. *Biochem. J.* 276, 525–532.

Sheehan, J. K., Oates, K., and Carlstedt, I. (1986). Electron microscopy of cervical, gastric, and bronchial mucus glycoproteins. *Biochem. J.* 239, 147–153.

Sheehan, J. K., Richardson, P. S., Fung, D. C., Howard, M., and Thornton, D. J. (1995). Analysis of respiratory mucus glycoproteins in asthma: A detailed study from a patient who died in status asthmaticus. *Am. J. Respir. Cell Mol. Biol.* 13, 748–756.

Sheehan, J. K., Boot-Handford, R. P., Chantler, E., Carlstedt, I., and Thornton, D. J. (1991a). Evidence for shared epitopes within the 'naked' protein domains of human mucus glycoproteins. *Biochem. J.* 274, 293–296.

Sheehan, J. K., Thornton, D. J., Somerville, M., and Carlstedt, I. (1991b). Mucin structure: The structure and heterogenicity of respiratory mucus glycoproteins. *Am. Rev. Respir. Dis.* 144, S4–S9.

Sherman, P., Fleming, N., Forstner, J., Roomi, N., and Forstner, G. (1987). Bacteria and the mucus blanket in experimental small bowel bacterial overgrowth. *Am. J. Pathol.* 126, 527–534.

Shogren, R., Gerken, T. A., and Jentoft, N. (1989). Role of glycosylation on the conformation and chain dimensions of O-linked glycoproteins: Light-scattering studies of ovine submaxillary mucin. *Biochemistry* 28, 5525–5536.

Silberberg, A. (1990). On mucociliary transport. *Biorheology* 27, 295–307.

Slayter, H. S., Wold, J. K., and Midtvedt, T. (1991). Intestinal mucin of germ-free rats: Electron-microscopic characterization. *Carbohydr. Res.* 222, 1–9.

Slomiany, B. L., Sarosiek, J., Liau, Y. H., Laszewicz, W., and Slomiany, A. (1986). Lysolecithin affects the viscosity, permeability, and peptic susceptibility of gastric mucin. *Scand. J. Gastroenterol.* 21, 1073–1079.

Slomiany, B. L., Murty, V. L., Mandel, I. D., Zalesna, G., and Slomiany, A. (1989). Physico-chemical characteristics of mucus glycoproteins and lipids of the human oral mucosal mucus coat in relation to caries susceptibility. *Arch. Oral Biol.* 34, 229–237.

Slomiany, B. L., and Slomiany, A. (1991). Role of mucus in gastric mucosal protection. *J. Physiol. Pharmacol.* 42, 147–161.

Springer, T. A. (1990). Adhesion receptors of the immune system. *Nature* 346, 425–434.

Stenfors, L. E., and Räisänen, S. (1991). Secretory IgA- and IgG-coated bacteria in the nasopharynx of children: An immunofluorescence study. *Acta Oto-Laryngol.* 111, 1139–1145.

Stokes, C. R., Soothill, J. F., and Turner, M. W. (1975). Immune exclusion is a function of IgA. *Nature* 255, 745–746.

Strombeck, D. R., and Harrold, D. (1974). Binding of cholera toxin to mucins and inhibition by gastric mucin. *Infect. Immun.* 10, 1266–1272.

Strous, G. J., and Dekker, J. (1992). Mucin-type glycoproteins. *Crit. Rev. Biochem. Mol. Biol.* 27, 57–92.

Strugala ,V., Allen, A., Dettmar, P. W., and Pearson, J. P. (2003). Colonic mucin: Methods of measuring mucus thickness. *Proc. Nutr. Soc.* 62, 237–243.

Svanborg-Eden, C., and Svennerholm, A. M. (1978). Secretory immunoglobulin A and G antibodies prevent adhesion of *Escherichia coli* to human urinary tract epithelial cells. *Infect. Immun.* 22, 790–797.

Szentkuti, L., and Lorenz, K. (1995). The thickness of the mucus layer in different segments of the rat intestine. *Histochem. J.* 27, 466–472.

Szentkuti, L., Riedesel, H., Enss, M. L., Gaertner, K., and VonEngelhardt, W. (1990). Pre-epithelial mucus layer in the colon of conventional and germ-free rats. *Histochem. J.* 22, 491–497.

Tabak, L. A. (1995). In defense of the oral cavity: structure, biosynthesis, and function of salivary mucins. *Annu. Rev. Physiol.* 57:547–564.

Tacket, C. O., Losonsky, G., Link, H., Hoang, Y., Guesry, P., Hilpert, H., and Levine, M. M. (1988). Protection by milk immunoglobulin concentrate against oral challenge with enterotoxigenic *Escherichia coli. N. Engl. J. Med.* 318, 1240–1243.

Tacket, C. O., Binion, S. B., Bostwick, E., Losonsky, G., Roy, M. J., and Edelman, R. (1992). Efficacy of bovine milk immunoglobulin concentrate in preventing illness after *Shigella flexneri* challenge. *Am. Trop. Med. Hyg.* 47, 276–283.

Tam, P. Y., and Verdugo, P. (1981). Control of mucus hydration as a Donnan equilibrium process. *Nature.* 292, 340–342.

Taylor, C., Allen, A., Dettmar, P. W., and Pearson, J. P. (2003). The gel matrix of gastric mucus is maintained by a complex interplay of transient and nontransient associations. *Biomacromolecules* 4, 922–927.

Thornton, D. J., Carlstedt, I., Howard, M., Devine, P. L., Price, M. R., and Sheehan, J. K. (1996). Respiratory mucins: Identification of core proteins and glycoforms. *Biochem. J.* 316, 967–975.

Thornton, D. J., Howard, M., Khan, N., and Sheehan, J. K. (1997). Identification of two glycoforms of the MUC5B mucin in human respiratory mucus: Evidence for a cysteine-rich sequence repeated with the molecule. *J. Biol. Chem.* 272, 9561–9566.

Tomkiewicz, R. P., Biviji, A., and King, M. (1994). Effects of oscillating air flow on the rheological properties and clearability of mucous gel simulants. *Biorheology* 31, 511–520.

Toribara, N. W., Gum, J., Culhane, P. J., Legace, R. E., Hicks, J. W., Petersen, G. M., and Kim, Y. S. (1991). *MUC-2* human small intestinal mucin gene structure: Repeated arrays and polymorphism. *J. Clin. Invest.* 88, 1005–1013.

Tramont, E. C. (1977). Inhibition of adherence of *Neisseria gonorrhoeae* by human genital secretions. *J. Clin. Invest.* 59, 117–124.

Tytgat, K. M., Bovelander, F. J., Opdam, F. J., Einerhand, A. W., Buller, H. A., and Dekker, J. (1995). Biosynthesis of rat MUC2 in colon and its analogy with human MUC2. *Biochem. J.* 309, 221–229.

Ulmer, J. S., Herzka, A., Toy, K. J., Baker, D. L., Dodge, A. H., Sinicropi, D., Shak, S., and Lazarus, R. A. (1996). Engineering actin-resistant human DNase I for treatment of cystic fibrosis. *Proc. Natl. Acad. Sci. USA* 93, 8225–8229.

Usselman, M. C., and Cone, R. A. (1983). Rat sperm are mechanically immobilized in the caudal epididymis by "immobilin," a high molecular weight glycoprotein. *Biol. Reprod.* 29, 1241–1253.

Usselman, M. C., Cone, R. A., and Rossignol, D. P. (1985). Rat cauda epididymal fluid is a mucus. *J. Androl.* 6, 315–320.

Vadgama, P., and Alberti, K. G. (1983). The possible role of bicarbonate in mucosal protection and peptic ulceration. *Digestion* 27, 203–213.

van Klinken, B. J., Dekker, J., Buller, H. A., and Einerhand, A. W. (1995). Mucin gene structure and expression: Protection vs. adhesion. *Am. J. Physiol.* 269, G613–G627.

van Klinken, B. J. W., Einerhand, A. W. C., Buller, H. A., and Dekker, J. (1998). The oligomerization of a family of four genetically clustered human gastrointestinal mucins. *Glycobiology* 8, 67–75.

Veazey, R. S., Shattock, R. J., Pope, M., Kirijan, J. C., Jones, J., Hu, Q., Ketas, T., Marx, P. A., Klasse, P. J., Burton, D. R., and Moore, J. P. (2003). Prevention of virus transmission to macaque monkeys by a vaginally applied monoclonal antibody to HIV-1 gp120. *Nat. Med.* 9, 343–346.

Verdugo, P. (1984). Hydration kinetics of exocytosed mucins in cultured secretory cells of the rabbit trachea: A new model. *Ciba Found. Symp.* 109, 212–225.

Verdugo, P. (1990). Goblet cells secretion and mucogenesis. *Ann. Rev. Physiol.* 52, 157–176.

Verdugo, P. (1991). Mucin exocytosis. *Am. Rev. Respir. Dis.* 144, S33–S37.

Vishwanath, S., and Ramphal, R. (1985). Tracheobronchial mucin receptor for *Pseudomonas aeruginosa*: predominance of amino sugars in binding sites. *Infect. Immun.* 48, 331–335.

Wada, A., and Nakamura, H. (1981). Nature of the charge distribution in proteins. *Nature* 293, 757–758.

Williams, R. C., and Gibbons, R. J. (1972). Inhibition of bacterial adherence by secretory immunoglobulin A: A mechanism of antigen disposal. *Science* 177, 697–699.

Williams, S. E., and Turnberg, L. A. (1980). Retardation of acid diffusion by pig gastric mucosa: A potential role in mucosal protection. *Gastroenterology* 79, 299–304.

Winner, L. 3rd, Mack, J., Weltzin, R., Mekalanos, J. J., Kraehenbuhl, J. P., and Neutra, M. R. (1991). New model for analysis of mucosal immunity: Intestinal secretion of specific monoclonal immunoglobulin A from hybridoma tumors protects against *Vibrio cholerae* infection. *Infect. Immun.* 59, 977–982.

Wolf, D. P., Blasco, L., Khan, M. A., and Litt, M. (1977a). Human cervical mucus. I. Rheologic characteristics. *Fertil. Steril.* 28, 41–46.

Wolf, D. P., Blasco, L., Khan, M. A., and Litt, M. (1977b). Human cervical mucus. II. Changes in viscoelasticity during the ovulatory menstrual cycle. *Fertil. Steril.* 28, 47–52.

Yeates, D. B., Besseris, G. J., and Wong, L. B. (1996). Physicochemical properties of mucus and its propulsion. In *The Lung: Scientific Foundations* (eds. R. G. Crystal, J. B. West, P. J. Barnes, and E. R. Weibel). Philadelphia: Raven Publishers.

Yudin, A. I., Hanson, F. W., and Katz, D. W. (1989). Human cervical mucus and its interaction with sperm: A fine-structured view. *Biol. Reprod.* 40, 661–671.

Zeitlin, L., Cone, R. A., Moench, T. R., and Whaley, K. J. (2000). Preventing infectious disease with passive immunization. *Microbes Infect.* 2, 701–708.

Innate Humoral Defense Factors

Chapter 5

Michael W. Russell

Department of Microbiology and Immunology, and of Oral Biology, University at Buffalo, Buffalo, New York

Libuse A. Bobek

Department of Oral Biology, University at Buffalo, Buffalo, New York

Jeremy H. Brock

Department of Immunology, University of Glasgow, Glasgow, Scotland

George Hajishengallis

Department of Microbiology, Immunology, and Parasitology, Louisiana State University, New Orleans, Louisiana

Jorma Tenovuo

Institute of Dentistry, University of Turku, Turku, Finland

INTRODUCTION

During the past decade, the field of Innate Immunity has assumed greater importance because of its role in the early phase of the immune response to pathogens. As a result, the term has become somewhat restricted in its meaning to refer to the events associated with the initial recognition of and response to pathogens by the antigenically nonspecific cells and molecules of the immune system. However, innate or nonspecific defense against infectious agents has a much older history, and the exocrine secretions of the body contain many, highly diverse humoral (i.e., soluble) factors that protect the body from the majority of potential pathogens that enter along with food and air, or by intimate contact between individuals. These are the principal subjects of this chapter.

The contribution of innate defense factors to the protection of mucosal surfaces against microbial colonization and aggression is probably greatly underestimated. Evidence for this is seen in IgA-deficient subjects who lack S-IgA antibodies in their secretions and yet are not severely compromised, even though the deficiency may be partially compensated by secretory IgM or small amounts of IgG in secretions (see Chapter 64). Furthermore, innate defense mechanisms help to define the minimal requirements for successful colonization by commensal and pathogenic organisms: those that cannot adapt to these conditions will be incapable of maintaining themselves within the host. Much of the earlier work on innate defense systems in mucosal secretions was performed in saliva or milk, which are readily accessible in large quantities. However, it has

become apparent that similar mechanisms operate in most secretions, although with significant differences of detail. Increased attention to the antimicrobial factors present in the genital tract occasioned by the acquired immune deficiency syndrome (AIDS) epidemic, for example, has revealed that this tract has multiple non–immunoglobulin-based defense mechanisms (Quayle 2002).

It is important to note that the mucosal surfaces first present a mechanical barrier, consisting of the epithelium itself, which varies from a single columnar cell layer in the gastrointestinal and respiratory tracts to a stratified and sometimes keratinized epithelium in the mouth and lower female genital tract (vagina). Most such surfaces are reinforced by the copious secretion of mucus, which is propelled by peristaltic or ciliary action and is thought to physically entrap microparticles including microorganisms; however, specific interactions between mucins and bacterial receptors may also be involved (Lichtman *et al.* 1996; see also Chapter 4). Furthermore, mucosal surfaces desquamate, and there is a considerable turnover of epithelial cells (estimated at 10^{11} per day from the human small intestine alone; Potten and Morris 1988), which, on shedding, carry with them a burden of attached microorganisms.

Sensitive immunochemical assays can usually reveal the presence of complement proteins, especially the major components such as C3, in various secretions. Furthermore, epithelial cells have been found to synthesize complement components C3, C4, and factor B (Strunk *et al.* 1988). However, the concentrations of complement components present are usually well below those found in serum, and consequently it is uncertain whether the classical or alternate complement pathway operates as a fully functional system in secretions.

Phagocytes represent a major component of innate defense at the cellular level, and all classes of phagocytes, including macrophages, neutrophils, eosinophils, and mast cells, occur within mucosal tissues. Some of them develop special characteristics in accordance with their location, for example, mucosal mast cells (Chapter 36) and lamina propria macrophages (Chapter 26). Although the activities of phagocytes may be largely confined to the tissues themselves, at least under normal healthy circumstances, rather than taking place within the lumen, the microenvironment close to the mucosal surface may permit phagocytic activity, as in the case of alveolar macrophages. As most secretions are hypotonic, phagocytes probably do not survive with functional activity for long in the bulk fluid phase. However, their contents may be released upon lysis or through surface degranulation and thereby contribute to the soluble antimicrobial factors in the secretions. Part of the lactoferrin and lysozyme, as well as myeloperoxidase (as distinct from salivary peroxidase) found in whole saliva or milk, for example, originates from neutrophils emigrating in the gingival crevice or in the lactating mammary gland (Moldoveanu et al. 1982). Milk, however, is isotonic, and contains variable numbers of both macrophages and neutrophils, depending upon the stage of lactation and both exogenous and endogenous stimuli. Huge numbers of neutrophils accumulate rapidly in milk in response to infection (mastitis), but their phagocytic activities are compromised by constituents of milk, particularly casein, which they ingest in competition with the microorganisms. This results in premature activation, diversion, and attenuation of the neutrophil intracellular killing mechanisms (Grazioso and Buescher 1996).

PATTERN-RECOGNITION RECEPTORS

Innate immune recognition is mediated by a series of germline–encoded receptors, known as pattern-recognition receptors (PRRs), which detect virulent microorganisms through recognition of invariant pathogen-associated molecular patterns (PAMPs) (Akira 2001). Of particular importance are PRRs involved in lipopolysaccharide (LPS) recognition and subsequent activation of signaling events. Such molecules include LPS-binding protein (LBP), CD14, β_2 integrins, and toll-like receptors (TLRs) (Akira 2001). Studies in wild-type and PRR-deficient mice as well as human macrophages activated by LPS, taxol, or bacterial fimbriae suggest that TLRs, CD14, and β_2 integrins form a functional multireceptor complex that coordinates induction of intracellular signals (Perera et al. 2001; Hajishengallis et al. 2002). TLRs constitute an evolutionarily conserved PRR family, which serves as central signal-transducing elements for induction of immunoregulatory genes that trigger innate immunity and instruct the development of adaptive immunity, and the induced regulatory and proinflammatory molecules include cytokines, chemokines, cellular adhesion molecules, and costimulatory molecules. Not surprisingly, TLRs are expressed mainly in cells that mediate first-line defense, such as neutrophils, monocytes/macrophages, dendritic cells, and mucosal epithelial cells (Cario and Podolsky 2000; Zarember and Godowski 2002).

PRRs are likely to play an important role in mucosal defense, not only as cell surface receptors, but also as humoral factors. Indeed, at least some PRRs are naturally found in soluble form, which may have a contributory or regulatory effect on the function of the cell-associated version. A classic example is CD14, a 55-kDa glycoprotein that can be attached to the cell membrane by means of a glycosylphosphatidyl-inositol (GPI) anchor and is therefore devoid of a cytoplasmic domain (Haziot et al. 1988). In addition to the membrane form of CD14 (mCD14), the molecule can also be found in two soluble forms (sCD14), one of which is proteolytically liberated from its GPI anchor (48-kDa sCD14), and a second that escapes from the cell membrane (55-kDa sCD14) (Bufler et al. 1995; Haziot et al. 1988). sCD14 can be found in serum at 2–3 μg/ml and in other biologic fluids such as milk, cerebrospinal fluid, and urine (Bussolati et al. 2002; Labéta et al. 2000; Landmann et al. 2000).

Like mCD14, sCD14 also binds LPS, and the resulting complexes can activate mucosal epithelial and other cells that do not express mCD14 (Pugin et al. 1993). The activating signals are transduced by TLRs (Akira 2001). Milk-derived sCD14 may facilitate neonatal intestinal epithelial cell responses to LPS (Labéta et al. 2000), but conversely, injury may be induced by LPS in renal tubular epithelial cells leading to proteinuria (Bussolati et al. 2002). In contrast to the agonistic activity of sCD14 in mCD14-negative cells, high levels of sCD14 may inhibit LPS-induced TNF-α release in monocytes/macrophages by competing with mCD14 for LPS (Haziot et al. 1994). sCD14 levels are upregulated in sepsis (Landmann et al. 2000), possibly mitigating the severity of disease, since LPS lethality in mice was diminished by recombinant sCD14 (Haziot et al. 1995).

The LPS-binding protein, which is an acute-phase protein, transfers LPS monomers from micelles to CD14, resulting in cell activation, or from aggregates or sCD14-LPS complexes to high-density lipoprotein (HDL), resulting in LPS neutralization (Akira 2001). Thus low LBP concentrations may enhance the biologic activity of LPS, whereas during the acute phase high concentrations may be inhibitory, as suggested by the protective effect of LBP against endotoxin shock in mice (Lamping et al. 1998).

Although soluble forms of human TLRs have not been reported, an alternatively spliced murine TLR4 mRNA has been described, which results in expression of a secretory form of TLR4 (sTLR4) devoid of transmembrane and intracellular domains (Iwami et al. 2000). Functionally, sTLR4 inhibits LPS-induced NF-κB activation and TNF-α release.

Other humoral PRRs have also been reported to suppress the inflammatory function of membrane PRRs. Pulmonary surfactant protein A (SP-A) inhibits TLR2-dependent, Staphylococcus aureus peptidoglycan-induced TNF-α release in human monocytic cells and rat alveolar macrophages by binding directly to TLR2 (Murakami et al. 2002a). SP-A can also engage CD14 and prevent cellular activation in response to certain serotypes of LPS (Sano et al. 1999).

Soluble PRRs therefore allow the innate immune system to regulate cellular activation positively or negatively. The property of soluble PRRs to mediate agonistic or antagonistic effects renders them attractive tools for manipulating the innate immune system and its instructive role in the development of adaptive immunity. For example, the identification and application of PRR recognition domains that can act as decoy receptors may help develop novel strategies aiming at downregulating the immune response in various chronic inflammatory diseases.

LYSOZYME

Since the initial discovery of lysozyme in 1922 in tears and nasal secretions by Alexander Fleming, a huge literature has accumulated on its structure, function, genetics, biosynthesis, regulation, enzyme activity, and properties, and the reader is referred to a definitive monograph that summarizes much of this information (Jollès 1996). Enzymatically, lysozyme (muramidase; EC 3.2.1.17) hydrolyzes the β(1-4) glycosidic bond between N-acetylmuramic acid and N-acetyl-D-glucosamine in bacterial peptidoglycan (Chipman and Sharon 1969).

Conventional or type c lysozyme has been identified widely in mammals, birds, reptiles, and even in insects. Some forms of lysozyme c bind calcium. A different enzyme, designated lysozyme g, is found only in birds, and enzymes with similar activity occur in plants and bacteriophages. Lysozyme c was the first enzyme to be sequenced and resolved by X-ray crystallography and to have its mechanism of action proposed. Identical forms of lysozyme c occur in various human body fluids and tissues, and it is abundant in the specific granules of neutrophils. The concentrations of lysozyme in different secretions vary widely **(Table 5.1)**. Concentrations can also differ markedly between species: for example, human milk contains approximately 3000 times higher levels of lysozyme than does

cow's milk (Chandan *et al.* 1964). Lysozyme within a given fluid may originate from different sources: for example, in human saliva, lysozyme is produced by the salivary glands and by oral phagocytes derived from the gingival crevices (Korsrud and Brandtzaeg 1982; Moro *et al.* 1984).

Lysozyme consists of a single polypeptide chain of 119–130 amino acid residues; the human enzyme contains 129 residues, M_r 14,600, pI 10.5. There are four disulfide bridges that stabilize the molecule in a compact ellipsoidal shape (for review, see Jollès and Jollès 1984). The crystallographic structure **(Fig. 5.1)** reveals two domains: one α-helical domain comprising the N-terminal and C-terminal segments, and a smaller β-sheet domain (for review, see Strynadka and James 1996). Glu35 and Asp52 are highly conserved in the active site. Genetically, type c lysozyme is encoded by a relatively small 10-kb gene of four exons with three introns (Irwin *et al.* 1996).

Although lysozymes isolated from different species or even from different tissues of the same species show similar biologic activity, they differ biochemically and in specific activity. Human lysozyme has a higher specific activity and more potent antibacterial effect against oral microorganisms than hen egg-white lysozyme (Iacono *et al.* 1980). However, few species of bacteria are directly lysed by lysozyme, and other modes of action independent of its enzymatic activity have been described, including the activation of bacterial autolysins, bacterial aggregation, blocking bacterial adherence, and the inhibition of acid production by oral microorganisms (Iacono *et al.* 1985; Laible and Germaine 1985; Twetman *et al.* 1986; Wang and Germaine 1991). Moreover, cell walls of oral streptococci weakened by cleavage of peptidoglycan become susceptible to lysis by the addition of detergents or monovalent anions such as bicarbonate, fluoride, thiocyanate, and chloride, which predominate in saliva (Pollock *et al.* 1987). When treated with high concentrations of lysozyme in the absence of salt or detergent, *Streptococcus*

Table 5.1. Concentrations of Some Major Innate Humoral Factors in Human Secretions

Factor	Saliva[a,b]	Milk	Tears	Intestinal	Genital	Respiratory
Lysozyme	10–80 µg/ml (unst. parotid) 10–200 µg/ml (unst. whole)	55–75 µg/ml	1.2–1.3 mg/ml	43–106 µg/ml		
Lactoferrin	7–20 µg/ml (unst. parotid) 8.5–24 µg/ml (stim. whole)	1–3 mg/ml, 4–15 mg/ml (colostrum)	1.7 mg/ml	1–26 µg/ml (pancreatic juice)	1.2 mg/ml (semen)	~50–150 µg/ml (BAL)
Peroxidase	2–13 µg/ml (stim. whole) 1–7 µg/ml (unst. whole)	10–15 µg/ml (colostrum), less in late milk	30–40 µg/ml			

[a]Other factors in saliva (whole): Histatins, 14–47 µg/ml; Cystatin S, 7.3–8.2 µM; Cystatin SN, 2.8 µM; *MUC7*, 133 µg/ml; Secretory leukocyte protease inhibitor, 1–10 µg/ml
[b]Stim., stimulated; unst., unstimulated; BAL, bronchoalveolar lavage.

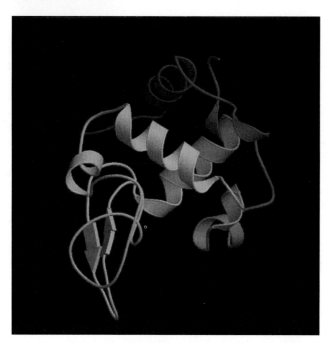

Fig. 5.1. Ribbon diagram showing the molecular structure of human lysozyme (Protein Data Bank ID#1JWR; Higo and Nakasako 2002).

c after the divergence of birds and mammals, as it retains the conserved calcium-binding residues found in lysozyme c (McKenzie and White 1991). Although normally devoid of muramidase or antibacterial activity, a variant form of α-lactalbumin has been reported to induce apoptosis in tumor cells (Svensson *et al.* 2000). This variant, designated HAM-LET (human α-lactalbumin made lethal to tumor cells), was found to be in oligomeric "molten globule" conformation and could be induced by the release of calcium at low pH in the presence of oleic acid (Svensson *et al.* 2000). As these conditions may occur in the nursing infant stomach, the authors speculated that HAMLET could serve to protect the infant gut. This form of α-lactalbumin has also been reported to be bactericidal against *Streptococcus pneumoniae* (Håkansson *et al.* 2000).

LACTOFERRIN

Lactoferrin is a member of the transferrin family of iron-binding proteins. Like plasma transferrin, lactoferrin can reversibly bind two ferric ions, but unlike transferrin it is primarily a protein of exocrine secretions (Table 5.1) and neutrophil granules and has no clearly defined role in iron transport or metabolism. Nevertheless, a plethora of functions have been proposed for lactoferrin, but despite much research there is still no consensus as to which, if any, are important *in vivo*.

Many of the proposed functions of lactoferrin relate to antimicrobial, antiinflammatory, and immunomodulatory activities, and these will be discussed in this chapter. Others, such as its possible role in iron absorption and neonatal development, fall outside the scope of this book and will not be dealt with here. For a comprehensive review of all aspects of lactoferrin structure and function, see Schryvers and Vogel (2002).

Biosynthesis and structure

Lactoferrin is synthesized by a variety of mucosal tissues, major sites being the mammary gland and the genital tract (reviewed by Teng 2002). Concentrations vary in different tissues and between different species, and indeed some mammals (e.g., rats and rabbits) contain no lactoferrin in their milk (Masson and Heremans 1971). The other major source of lactoferrin is the secondary granules of neutrophils. Lactoferrin is synthesized by myeloid precursors, rather than the mature neutrophil itself (Rado *et al.* 1987). Significant synthesis also occurs in the kidney, but only minimal synthesis occurs in liver and spleen (Teng 2002).

Lactoferrins from a number of species have been identified and characterized structurally. Like all members of the transferrin family, they are single-chain glycoproteins with a molecular weight of about 80 kDa, and lactoferrins typically show a 60% sequence homology with serum transferrin (Baker 1994). The polypeptide chain is folded into two lobes, which show ~40% sequence homology, indicative of an ancestral gene duplication (**Fig. 5.2**). Each lobe is in turn

mutans exhibits areas of cell wall dissolution without cell lysis (Cho *et al.* 1982). Its cationic property (pI 10.5) may allow lysozyme to exert bactericidal activity analogous to other cationic proteins, and although binding to oral bacteria is strongly dependent on pH and ionic strength, bacteriolysis caused by lysozyme may be physiologically significant in the oral environment where these parameters can fluctuate markedly. However, there is no clear evidence that salivary levels of lysozyme are related to the occurrence of dental caries or periodontal disease (Tenovuo 1989). Remarkably, lysozyme is reported to display inhibitory activity against human immunodeficiency virus–1 (HIV-1) (Lee-Huang *et al.* 1999).

Several synergistic effects between lysozyme and other nonimmunoglobulin or immunoglobulin defense factors have been reported. These include a bactericidal effect on *S. mutans* exerted by lysozyme and iron-depleted lactoferrin (Soukka *et al.* 1991), and the inhibition of glucose uptake in oral streptococci by lysozyme and components of the salivary peroxidase/H_2O_2/SCN^- system, including the oxidation product, hypothiocyanite (Lenander-Lumikari *et al.* 1992). Possibly the membrane damage caused by the cationic nature of lysozyme facilitates the diffusion of thiocyanate oxidation products into the cell. Lysozyme was reported to synergize also with secretory IgA (S-IgA) antibody and complement to cause lysis of *Escherichia coli*, but these reports were not confirmed by other studies. It is possible that other contaminating factors contributed to the effects observed.

Lysozyme displays sequence homology with α-lactalbumin, an abundant protein in milk, which together with galactosyltransferase forms lactose synthase. It is thought that α-lactalbumin evolved from calcium-binding lysozyme

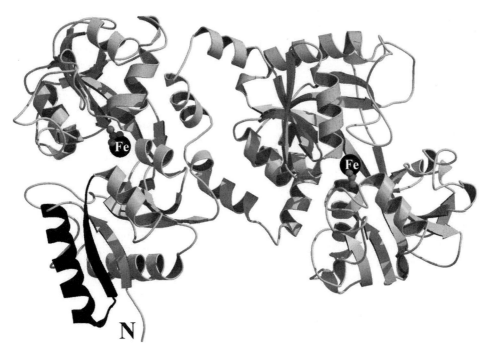

Fig. 5.2. Ribbon diagram showing the structural organization of the lactoferrin molecule. The N-lobe is on the left, the C-lobe on the right. In each lobe the bound iron atom is shown as a black sphere in the center, with its associated carbonate ion. The antibacterial domain on the surface of the N-lobe is highlighted in black, and the N-terminus, where a cluster of positively charged residues is found, is labeled N. Figure courtesy of Heather Baker.

folded into two domains, separated by a cleft in which each iron-binding site is located. In all cases the ferric iron is liganded to an aspartic acid, two tyrosines, and a histidine, together with two oxygen atoms from a synergistically bound carbonate ion, without which lactoferrin cannot bind iron (Baker 1994).

Iron binding and release are associated with conformational changes in the protein. When lactoferrin is in the iron-free (apo) form, the interdomain cleft adopts an "open" configuration, but binding of iron (and carbonate) causes the cleft to close and become locked in this configuration (Anderson *et al.* 1990). One consequence of this is that the open apo form is more susceptible to denaturation and proteolytic digestion than is the Fe-bound (holo) form. Iron is released by lowering the pH, but in lactoferrin the degree of stabilization of the lobe structure is greater than in transferrin, and consequently iron release does not occur until pH ~3 is reached, whereas in transferrin iron release occurs at pH ~5.5 (Mazurier and Spik 1980). This probably explains why transferrin but not lactoferrin can donate iron to cells via receptor-mediated endocytosis.

Interaction of lactoferrin with other molecules and cell surfaces

Another important structural difference between lactoferrin and transferrin is that, whereas transferrin has a pI of around 5.5–6.0 (Hovanessian and Awdeh 1976), lactoferrin is a highly basic protein with a pI of about 9 (Moguilevsky *et al.* 1985). This is because of the presence of several surface regions with high positive charge, most notably near the

N-terminus of the molecule, which in the case of human lactoferrin has four consecutive arginines at positions 2–5. The high pI of lactoferrin makes it an extremely "sticky" protein, and as a result it binds readily to other macromolecules (Lampreave *et al.* 1990), which probably enables it to adhere to mucosal surfaces. The "stickiness" of lactoferrin has also hampered attempts to characterize true lactoferrin receptors. Lactoferrin-binding sites with affinities comparable with those exhibited by specific receptors have been identified on hepatocytes (McAbee and Esbensen 1991), monocytes/macrophages (Birgens *et al.* 1993), activated T lymphocytes (Mazurier *et al.* 1989), mammary epithelial cells (Rochard *et al.* 1992), and intestinal brush border cells. However, only the enterocyte brush border receptor has so far been cloned and functionally expressed (Suzuki *et al.* 2001). This, and probably many other receptors, interacts with the basic N-terminal region of lactoferrin (El Yazidi-Belkoura *et al.* 2001). Of particular interest is a report that activated γδ T cells express lactoferrin receptors and show enhanced *in vitro* proliferation in the presence of lactoferrin (Mincheva-Nilsson *et al.* 1997).

The consequences of lactoferrin–cell interactions are generally poorly understood. Interaction with hepatocytes leads to internalization and degradation of lactoferrin (McAbee *et al.* 1993), and internalization by T lymphocytes has also been reported (Bi *et al.* 1996). However, monocytes show no appreciable internalization of bound lactoferrin (Ismail and Brock 1993). Interaction of lactoferrin with T lymphocytes results in mitogen-activated protein (MAP) kinase activation (Dennin-Duthille *et al.* 2000), but otherwise little is known about what if any cell signaling events are triggered by lacto-ferrin–receptor interactions.

Function

Despite a very large number of studies of lactoferrin function, a clearly defined role for lactoferrin has yet to emerge. Unlike transferrin, there is no good evidence that it plays a major role in iron transport. Lactoferrin does not enhance iron absorption from the gut (Hernell and Lonnerdal 2002), and indeed lactoferrin knockout mice show no abnormalities of iron status (Ward *et al.* 2003). Most of the proposed functions are based predominantly on *in vitro* studies, and in many cases the mechanisms involved are unknown. In those cases where more is known, the activity is usually attributable either to lactoferrin's iron-binding properties or to its basicity. In particular, peptides containing the basic N-terminal region of lactoferrin ("lactoferricins") have been isolated and shown to be more active than the intact protein.

Antimicrobial activity

Lactoferrin has been reported to inhibit the growth or reduce the infectivity of a wide range of infectious agents, including bacteria, viruses, and various parasites. Many different organisms and mechanisms have been implicated, and in the following discussion, particular attention will be given to potential mucosal pathogens.

Antibacterial activity

One of the first functions attributed to lactoferrin was bacteriostatic activity, following the demonstration that lactoferrin could inhibit the growth of various bacteria *in vitro*. The activity was only shown by apo-lactoferrin, and addition of iron abolished activity, indicating that inhibition of microbial iron uptake was involved. A large range of microorganisms is susceptible to this activity, including mucosal pathogens such as enteropathogenic *E. coli*, *Salmonella* spp., and *Vibrio cholerae*. This field has been extensively reviewed by Weinberg (2001). However, many bacteria can overcome the bacteriostatic effect of iron-withholding by lactoferrin; some secrete low–molecular-weight high-affinity iron chelators (siderophores), which can remove iron from lactoferrin or possibly scavenge iron from other host sources (Brock *et al.* 1991), and others, notably *Haemophilus* spp. and meningococci, express specific lactoferrin receptors, regulated by bacterial iron levels, which allow the organism to acquire lactoferrin-bound iron (Gray-Owen and Schryvers 1996). Inhibition of growth may not be the only consequence of iron withholding by lactoferrin; in the case of *Pseudomonas aeruginosa*, lack of iron prevents the organisms from forming a biofilm and thus making them more susceptible to other host defense mechanisms (Singh *et al.* 2002). In contrast, Fe-lactoferrin could inhibit binding of *Actinobacillus actinomycetemcomitans* to buccal epithelial cells, whereas apo-lactoferrin was ineffective (Fine and Furgang 2002), suggesting that low iron levels might actually aid colonization.

However, iron withholding may not be the only mechanism by which lactoferrin inhibits bacteria. A bactericidal effect, independent of iron-binding activity, was first demonstrated by Arnold *et al.* (1977), and subsequent investigation showed that this involved increased membrane permeability (Ellison and Giehl 1991) and was mediated by the basic N-terminal region of lactoferrin, the isolated lactoferricin peptides being more active than intact lactoferrin (Bellamy *et al.* 1992). The effect can in some cases be abrogated by bacterial proteases, which presumably digest the lactoferricin peptide (Ulvatne *et al.* 2002). The bacterial molecules to which lactoferrin or its peptide binds vary. In *S. aureus* binding is to the cell wall teichoic acid (Vorland *et al.* 1999), whereas in *E. coli* it is to lipopolysaccharide (Vorland *et al.* 1999) and porins (Sallmann *et al.* 1999). In *S. pneumoniae* lactoferrin binds to pneumococcal surface protein A (Hammerschmidt *et al.* 1999), and in *Gardnerella vaginalis* a 120-kDa surface protein is responsible (Jarosik and Land 2000), though this may be more analogous to the iron-regulated receptors mentioned previously.

A novel antibacterial activity of lactoferrin has been demonstrated in which it inactivates two colonization factors, the IgA1 protease and the Hap adhesin, on *Haemophilus influenzae*, as the result of an intrinsic serine protease activity (Hendrixson *et al.* 2003), suggesting that lactoferrin is a truly bifunctional protein. The possibility that this activity might be caused by a contaminating milk protease bound to lactoferrin seems to be ruled out as both milk and recombinant human lactoferrin were active. In a rather similar model, lactoferrin bound to and caused proteolytic cleavage of the hemoglobin receptor of *Porphyromonas gingivalis*, thus preventing the organism from obtaining hemoglobin-bound iron (Shi *et al.* 2000). However, in this case the proteolytic activity may have originated in the bacterium as the lactoferricin peptide was also active, yet does not contain the region thought to be responsible for the serine protease activity of lactoferrin itself (Hendrixson *et al.* 2003).

Although the antibacterial effect of lactoferrin has been amply confirmed *in vitro*, evidence for its *in vivo* activity, especially clinical data, is less convincing. The facts that lactoferrin occurs in high concentration (~1mg/ml) in human milk, and that breastfed babies are less susceptible than bottle-fed babies to gastrointestinal infection, suggest that lactoferrin might be an important protective factor in breast milk, but attempts to modify the gastrointestinal flora of newborn bottle-fed infants by supplementing formula milks with lactoferrin have failed to demonstrate such a role (Roberts *et al.* 1992). However, there is some evidence that lactoferrin can protect against bacterial infection in animal models. Experimental *Helicobacter* infections were ameliorated by oral administration of lactoferrin (Wang *et al.* 2001). This appears to be the result of the glycan moiety of lactoferrin interfering with bacterial adherence, rather than of iron deprivation. Colonization of the kidney in murine *S. aureus* infection was reduced by either systemic or oral administration of lactoferrin (Bhimani *et al.* 1999), and joint inflammation in experimental murine *S. aureus* infectious arthritis was reduced by local administration of lactoferrin (Guillen *et al.* 2000). Oral administration of lactoferrin or the lactoferricin peptide also reduced the overgrowth and translocation of enterobacteria that occurred in mice fed bovine milk (Teraguchi *et al.* 1995), and oral recombinant human lactoferrin reduced the severity of systemic *E. coli* infection in neonatal rats infected by the oral route (Edde *et al.* 2001). It has also been shown that lactoferrin could protect rabbits against experimental *Shigella flexneri* infection, through a mechanism involving inhibition by the basic N-terminal region of lactoferrin of bacterial uptake by host cells (Gomez *et al.* 2003). An interesting antibacterial effect of lactoferrin that clearly depends upon its iron-binding properties was reported by Schaible *et al.* (2002), who showed that β_2-microglobulin-knockout mice, which suffer from an iron overload condition similar to human hemochromatosis, became less susceptible to tuberculosis following treatment with lactoferrin. These studies in experimental animals suggest that lactoferrin might have a therapeutic effect on certain types of bacterial infection in man, and it is to be hoped that appropriate clinical studies can be devised.

Antiviral activity

Lactoferrin has been reported to prevent infection by a variety of viruses (for review, see van der Strate *et al.* 2001). Both DNA and RNA viruses are susceptible, including cytomegalovirus, HIV, herpesvirus, hepatitis B and C viruses, rotavirus, respiratory syncytial virus, and enterovirus 71. Lactoferrin appears to be most effective at the early stages of infection and can act either by blocking viral receptors on host cells or by binding directly to the virus itself. The molecular mechanisms involved vary. In the case of rotavirus, lactoferrin blocks entry into enterocytes by a mechanism that is independent of iron saturation but is enhanced by desialylation of the protein and can be mimicked by two tryptic peptides that do not, however, involve the lactoferricin region of the molecule (Superti *et al.* 2001). This also seems to be the case for anti–hepatitis C activity, in which a peptide from the C-terminal region of lactoferrin binds to hepatitis C virus E2 protein and prevents interaction with the host cell (Nozaki *et al.* 2003). In contrast, the ability of lactoferrin to inhibit *in vitro* hepatitis B virus infection is dependent upon interaction with the hepatocyte rather than the virus (Hara *et al.* 2002). The lactoferricin region is partly, but not entirely, responsible for the ability of lactoferrin to inhibit binding of HIV to CXCR4 or CCR5 receptors (Berkhout *et al.* 2002).

The vast majority of studies refer to *in vitro* antiviral activity, and there is much less evidence for an antiviral role for lactoferrin *in vivo*. However, lactoferrin administered to suckling mice improved survival rates in experimental hantavirus infection (Murphy *et al.* 2001). Protection against cytomegalovirus infection in mice has also been reported, though this appeared to result from enhanced natural killer (NK) cell activity rather than to direct antiviral activity (Shimizu *et al.* 1996). Finally, a clinical trial of bovine lactoferrin in hepatitis C virus infection caused a temporary improvement in 6 out of 45 patients (Okada *et al.* 2002).

Antiparasitic activity

A number of antiparasitic effects of lactoferrin have been reported, though the role of lactoferrin as an antiparasitic molecule remains ill defined, and mechanisms, when elucidated, tend to be parasite specific. For example, the basic properties of lactoferrin are responsible for its ability to prevent *Plasmodium bergei* from invading fibroblasts (Shakibaei and Frevert 1996) and inhibited CD36-mediated and thrombospondin-mediated binding of *Plasmodium falciparum*–infected erythrocytes to epithelia (Eda *et al.* 1999). Lactoferrin can inhibit *in vitro* growth of *P. falciparum* (Kassim *et al.* 2000) and *Pneumocystis carinii* (Cirioni *et al.* 2000), in the latter case resulting from an iron-withholding mechanism. Other parasites such as *Tritrichomonas foetus* (Grab *et al.* 2001), *Treponema pallidum* (Alderete *et al.* 1988), and *Leishmania chagasi* (Wilson *et al.* 2002) possess mechanisms by which they can remove iron from lactoferrin, which might therefore be expected to enhance rather than inhibit growth.

Modulation of immune and inflammatory responses

While the antimicrobial effects of lactoferrin have been known for decades, it has more recently become apparent that lactoferrin can influence immune and inflammatory responses. In some cases, antimicrobial activity has been found to result from immunomodulatory activity, rather than a direct antimicrobial effect.

One mechanism by which lactoferrin may exert an antiinflammatory effect is via the binding of non–transferrin bound iron at inflammatory foci and thus rendering it unable to catalyze potentially harmful free-radical reactions (Guillen *et al.* 2000). Another mechanism depends upon the previously mentioned ability of lactoferrin to bind to bacterial LPS (reviewed by Baveye *et al.* 1999). This results in impairment of LPS binding to soluble or surface CD14 on monocytes (Baveye *et al.* 2000b) and the subsequent production of interleukin-6 (IL-6)(Mattsby-Baltzer *et al.* 1996), TNFα, and nitric oxide (Choe and Lee 1999). In neutrophils, lactoferrin inhibits binding of LPS to L-selectin and subsequent production of reactive oxygen species (Baveye *et al.* 2000a). It also inhibits LPS-mediated IL-8 production by endothelial cells (Elass *et al.* 2002). This activity is mediated by the basic N-terminal region of lactoferrin (Zhang *et al.* 1999). In a murine model of endotoxemia, lactoferrin was found to be most effective at reducing parameters of endotoxic shock when administered 1 hour before LPS; administration of lactoferrin either 18 hours before LPS, or following the development of endotoxemia, was less effective (Kruzel *et al.* 2002).

Orally administered lactoferrin, or its basic N-terminal peptides, can also reduce the severity of dextran sulfate–induced colitis in mice (Haversen *et al.* 2003). The mechanism is unknown, but could involve interference of binding of dextran to mucosal cells as the result of charge neutralization.

Although most reports have shown lactoferrin to have an antiinflammatory and immunosuppressive effect, there are some studies showing contrary results. Immobilized, but not soluble, lactoferrin stimulates eosinophil activation (Thomas *et al.* 2002), suggesting that lactoferrin bound to airway epithelial cells might exacerbate asthma (though a similar scenario in the gut might result in enhanced antiparasitic activity). Induction of collagen-induced arthritis in mice constitutively expressing human lactoferrin was found to develop more severely than in congenic controls (Guillen *et al.* 2002). It was suggested that this may be the result of lactoferrin skewing the immune response toward a proinflammatory type 1 rather than an antiinflammatory type 2 response. Lactoferrin has also been reported to act as a transactivator by upregulating transcription of the *IL-1β* gene (Son *et al.* 2002), an activity that may relate to the proposal that lactoferrin can act as a transcription factor (He and Furmanski 1995).

In summary, despite extensive research, much remains to be learned about lactoferrin. Thanks largely to the crystallographic studies of Baker *et al.* (1998), we now have a fairly complete knowledge of the structure of lactoferrin and its iron-binding properties. There is increasing evidence that lactoferrin may be a genuinely multifunctional protein, with iron-binding, release of basic peptides, and perhaps proteolytic activity being required in different functional scenarios. However, it must be remembered that many proposed functions of lactoferrin are based entirely on *in vitro* studies, and *in vivo* data supporting many of these are lacking. Even with extensively studied areas such as the role of the basic N-terminal lactoferricin peptides, we still do not know if such peptides are actually produced *in vivo* in functionally significant quantities, if at all. It is to be hoped that future research will focus on the *in vivo* relevance of functions based on *in vitro* studies, and eventually lead to clinical evaluation of lactoferrin as a useful prophylactic or therapeutic agent.

PEROXIDASES

Peroxidase activity is found in exocrine secretions including milk, tears, and saliva as well as in vaginal fluid (Table 5.1). Most of the activity is derived from enzymes synthesized in the glands that produce the secretions. Contributions also come from polymorphonuclear leukocytes (myeloperoxidase; MPO) and possibly from eosinophils (eosinophil peroxidase; EPO). As comprehensive discussion of the various members of the peroxidase family is beyond the scope of this chapter, attention will focus on human salivary peroxidase (hSPO), human lactoperoxidase (hLPO), and, for comparative purposes, bovine lactoperoxidase (bLPO). The latter enzyme has been studied extensively because of its ready availability in high purity and because it has many properties in common with hSPO and hLPO.

Structure of peroxidases

Human SPO is a ~75-kDa protein that is secreted by the parotid glands. The gene for hSPO has been cloned and sequenced (Kiser *et al.* 1996), and its sequence is similar (except for two nucleotides) to hLPO, which suggests that these two enzymes are in fact products of the same gene expressed in different tissues (salivary and mammary glands). The amino acid sequence of hSPO displays 99.4% identity to the C-terminal fragment of hLPO (Dull *et al.* 1990). Additionally, hSPO shares high amino acid identity to other mammalian peroxidases **(Table 5.2)**.

A high degree of homology exists between hSPO and bLPO, and their C-terminal 324 amino acids show 84% homology (Dull *et al.* 1990). However, hSPO has fewer cysteine, methionine, and isoleucine residues and more alanine, glycine, proline, and serine residues than bLPO. Their carbohydrate compositions differ, and hSPO is also more sensitive to inactivation by azide (Månsson-Rahemtulla *et al.* 1988). The bLPO molecule consists of a single polypeptide chain with one heme group, which is covalently attached to the protein via two ester linkages. The sequence of bLPO can be aligned with human peroxidases to reveal the following similarities: MPO, 55.4%; EPO, 54%; and thyroid peroxidase, 44.6%.

bLPO probably has an ellipsoidal structure in solution (Paul and Ohlsson 1985) and has properties that are similar to those of other small globular proteins. Inferences about the higher order structure of hSPO can be made based on amino acid composition and solution properties. The mosaic of hydrophobic and charged groups on the surface of hSPO is responsible for its strong affinity for many different kinds of surfaces (Pruitt and Adamson 1977; Pruitt *et al.* 1979). Since absorbed hSPO retains its enzyme activity, attachment to surfaces does not block donor access to the heme group; thus the surface-binding sites and the heme group are not in immediate proximity.

Preparations of bLPO from bovine milk are heterogeneous (Paul and Ohlsson 1985). A major fraction of bLPO consists of a single polypeptide chain of 78.5 kDa. Subfractions of

Table 5.2. Identity of hSPO cDNA Polypeptide Sequence with Those of Other Peroxidases

Peroxidase Polypeptide[a]	Percent Similarity to hSPO[b]	Percent Identity with hSPO[c]
bLPO	90.7	83.0
hLPO	99.4	99.7
hMPO	70.6	52.2
hEPO	67.1	50.4
hTPO	62.1	42.4

[a]bLPO, bovine lactoperoxidase; hLPO, human lactoperoxidase; hMPO, human myeloperoxidase; hEPO, human eosinophil peroxidase; hTPO, human thyroid peroxidase; hSPO, human salivary peroxidase.
[b]Similarity reports both identical and conservatively substituted shared amino acids; polypeptide sequences analyzed using GenBank BESTFIT.
[c]Identity reports only identical amino acids shared between two polypeptide sequences analyzed using GenBank BESTFIT.

lower molecular mass are derived by loss of carbohydrate groups and by deamidation of asparagine or glutamine residues. hSPO from human saliva is also heterogeneous (Månsson-Rahemtulla *et al.* 1988), and at least three major forms of 78, 80, and 280 kDa have been reported. Human milk contains at least two peroxidases (Pruitt *et al.* 1991), hLPO and MPO (derived from milk leukocytes), the relative amounts of which vary widely from sample to sample and depend on the stage of lactation. The properties of hLPO are similar to those of hSPO.

Peroxidase-mediated defense mechanisms

Peroxidases protect mucosal surfaces from microorganisms by catalyzing the peroxidation of halides (Cl^-, Br^-, I^-, and the pseudohalide, thiocyanate ion SCN^-) to generate reactive products that have potent antimicrobial properties. MPO and EPO catalyze the peroxidation of Cl^-, Br^-, I^-, and SCN^-, but bLPO, hLPO, and hSPO do not catalyze the peroxidation of Cl^-. In the absence of halides and SCN^-, peroxidases behave as catalases and degrade H_2O_2 to water and oxygen. The catalase and peroxidase activities of these enzymes also protect mucosal surfaces by preventing the accumulation of toxic products of oxygen reduction.

Peroxidase kinetics and reaction mechanisms are very complex (for review, see Pruitt and Kamau 1991). The products of the reactions and mechanisms depend on the particular enzyme, the particular donor, the relative concentrations of enzyme, H_2O_2, and donors, the pH, and temperature. For mucosal defense mechanisms, the most significant peroxidase reactions are those related to catalase activity and to thiocyanate oxidation by hSPO, MPO, and hLPO. Although the actual reactions are complex and include multiple intermediates, the net reactions of the peroxidation of thiocyanate at physiologic concentrations are:

$$SCN^- + H_2O_2 \rightarrow OSCN^- + H_2O$$
$$OSCN^- + H^+ \rightarrow HOSCN$$

Peroxidation of SCN^- occurs via compound I, in which both oxidizing equivalents of peroxide have been transferred to the heme group. The hypothiocyanite ion $OSCN^-$ is in equilibrium with its conjugate acid (HOSCN, pK_a = 5.3). The net peroxidation reaction may be in an apparent state of dynamic equilibrium *in vivo* (Pruitt *et al.* 1986), which minimizes the concentration of H_2O_2 and maximizes the concentrations of HOSCN and $OSCN^-$. Both sets of reactions consume toxic H_2O_2 and generate products that are harmless to the host. These same reactions can protect some bacteria from H_2O_2 toxicity (Adamson and Carlsson 1982). However, HOSCN and $OSCN^-$ inhibit the growth and metabolism of many species of bacteria (for review, see Pruitt and Reiter 1985).

The major limiting factor for SCN^- peroxidation in human saliva is the availability of H_2O_2, as shown by experiments in which the addition of H_2O_2 to human saliva *in vivo* (Månsson-Rahemtulla *et al.* 1983) or *in vitro* (Tenovuo *et al.* 1981) resulted in increased concentrations of HOSCN and $OSCN^-$. However, concentrations of SCN^- below 0.6 mM

may also be limiting (Pruitt *et al.* 1982), and in human milk, the concentrations of SCN^- are usually below this level. The low peroxidase concentration in human milk also may be a limiting factor (Pruitt and Kamau 1991; Pruitt *et al.* 1991).

The thiocyanate ion is a critical component of the hSPO system; it is secreted by salivary, mammary, lacrimal, and gastric glands, and can originate from several sources. Salivary SCN^- concentration varies considerably and depends, for example, on diet and smoking habits. However, the major source of SCN^- is the detoxification of CN^- primarily in the liver by the enzyme, thiosulfate-cyanide sulfurtransferase, which catalyzes the transfer of a sulfur atom from thiosulfate to CN^-, to yield nontoxic SCN^-. Normal plasma levels of SCN^- are 20–120 µM, but in secreted fluids containing hSPO, hLPO or bLPO, the levels are much higher. Thiocyanate is found in parotid, submandibular, and whole saliva as well as in gingival crevicular and dental plaque fluids (Tenovuo 1985) and milk (Pruitt and Kamau 1991). Average concentrations of SCN^- in saliva of non-smokers have been reported to range from 0.35 mM to 1.24 mM, whereas the reported range for smokers varies from 1.38 mM to 2.74 mM (Tenovuo 1985). In human milk, mean values of 0.021 mM to 0.122 mM have been reported with large variations from sample to sample (Pruitt and Kamau 1991).

Thus SCN^- is concentrated 10-fold to 20-fold from plasma into the salivary glands in humans and animals, apparently by active transport. Tenovuo *et al.* (1982b) showed that the concentration of SCN^- in whole saliva rises on initial stimulation and then gradually declines. However, in no instance does the secretion rate of SCN^- (concentration of $SCN^- \times$ secretion flow rate) in whole stimulated saliva drop below that of unstimulated saliva, indicating that the SCN^- transport system is able to maintain SCN^- levels despite the increased dilution resulting from stimulation. Thus, active transport of SCN^- may be increased by stimulation. Active transport of SCN^- into saliva may also provide a recycling mechanism for this important ion: as saliva is swallowed continuously, SCN^- would be reabsorbed into the blood by the gastrointestinal uptake and concentrated again in the salivary glands.

MPO catalyzes the oxidation of Cl^- by H_2O_2 to form water and a highly reactive oxidizing agent, the hypochlorite ion (OCl^-), which activates latent collagenase, elastase, gelatinase, and cathepsin that are present in leukocytes and inactivates circulating protease inhibitors, causing tissue injury (Weiss 1989). The cytocidal hypohalous acid oxidants can also be produced by EPO through oxidation of halides (Br^-, Cl^-, and I^-) in the absence of SCN^-. Although the hypohalous acid oxidants mediate the killing of bacteria and the extracellular destruction of invading helminthic parasites (Gleich and Adolphson 1986), these oxidants are also extremely tissue destructive (Slungaard and Mahoney 1991). However, SCN^- has been shown to be the preferred substrate for both MPO and EPO, although it is present in serum in significantly lower concentrations than the other halides (Thomas and Fishman 1986; Slungaard and

Mahoney 1991). This preference for SCN⁻ results in generation of HOSCN and OSCN⁻, which are nontoxic to human cells and tissues (Hänström *et al.* 1983; Slungaard and Mahoney 1991; Tenovuo and Larjava 1984; Thomas and Fishman 1986). Thus SCN⁻ protects a variety of tissues from damage that could occur as a result of peroxidase-catalyzed oxidation of Cl⁻ and Br⁻. For example, in the reaction that accompanies the respiratory burst of leukocytes, the oxidation of the Cl⁻ ion by MPO may generate toxic products (Weiss 1989).

Antimicrobial spectrum of mucosal peroxidase systems

The peroxidase–SCN⁻ system has antibacterial effects against many *Streptococcus* species (Pruitt and Reiter 1985), some periodontitis-associated bacteria (Tenovuo 1985; Courtois *et al.* 1992, Ihalin *et al.* 1998), and anaerobic mucosal pathogens **(Table 5.3)**. In streptococci the system inhibits glucose incorporation, glycolysis, and acid production by cariogenic bacteria (Pruitt and Reiter 1985; Lenander-Lumikari and Loimaranta 2000); it also affects the cytoplasmic membrane and inhibits various membrane oxidases and reductases in the respiratory chain and formation of the electrochemical proton gradient in *E. coli*. The reduction of bacterial acid production by the peroxidase system is enhanced in the presence of S-IgA (Tenovuo *et al.* 1982a), but this effect does not depend on specific antibodies.

Table 5.3. Selected Mucosal and Oral Pathogens that Are Susceptible to Inhibition by the hSPO or bLPO System[a]

Gram-positive bacteria
  Mutans streptococci (capable of initiating dental caries)
  Lactobacilli
Gram-negative bacteria
  Actinobacillus actinomycetemcomitans
  Porphyromonas gingivalis
  Helicobacter pylori
  Listeria monocytogenes
  Salmonella typhimurium
  Escherichia coli
Viruses
  Human immunodeficiency virus (HIV)
  Herpes simplex type 1
  Respiratory syncytial virus (RSV)
Yeasts
  Candida albicans
  Candida krusei

[a]Many observations are only from *in vitro* studies and depend on the concentration of the inhibitory agent. See reviews by Pruitt and Reiter (1985), Tenovuo (1998), and Lenander-Lumikari and Loimaranta (2000).

Although the peroxidase-mediated effects on gram-positive bacteria are merely bacteriostatic at neutral pH, gram-negative bacteria such as *E. coli* and *P. gingivalis* are killed (Fadel and Courtois 1999; Shin *et al.* 2001). In addition to bacterial species, yeasts and many viruses (Table 5.3) are sensitive to the peroxidase–SCN⁻ systems (Pourtois *et al.* 1990; Mikola *et al.* 1995).

Enhancement of salivary peroxidase systems

Mimicking salivary antibacterial capacity has been achieved in commercial products by adding the bLPO system, lactoferrin, or lysozyme into various oral health care products targeted to patients with hyposalivation or xerostomia. In these products bLPO is supplemented with KSCN, and the necessary H_2O_2 is generated in the mouth by a glucose–glucose oxidase system. The original rationale was to elevate *in vivo* concentrations of HOSCN/OSCN⁻ to bactericidal levels, and although they indeed appear to increase salivary OSCN⁻ concentrations, there is no clinical evidence that they enhance the antimicrobial activity of human saliva *in vivo* (Tenovuo 2002). Interestingly, recent observations indicate that antimicrobial activity against mucosal pathogens can greatly be enhanced if bLPO is replaced by horseradish peroxidase (which does not oxidize SCN⁻ at pH > 6), and iodide is used as the oxidizable agent instead of SCN⁻ (Ihalin *et al.* 2003).

OTHER FACTORS

In addition to the major and better known innate factors described previously, there are numerous other antimicrobial agents of a wide variety found in different secretions. Some of these, especially those present in saliva, have been the subject of intensive investigation at the molecular level in recent years.

Low–molecular-weight inhibitors

Inorganic and organic acids present in many secretions are known to have antimicrobial properties. For example, neutralization of stomach hydrochloric acid results in a 1000-fold reduction in the infectious dose of *Salmonella typhi* (Mims *et al.*, 1995). Lactic acid (largely produced by lactobacilli) is believed to be of substantial importance in the maintenance of vaginal health and to inhibit the growth of organisms involved in bacterial vaginosis as well as HIV (see Chapter 99). Human milk contains a large number of oligosaccharides (apart from lactose), some of which are present in concentrations of up to 1–2 g/L, but because they are excreted intact in infants' urine, they are thought not to have significant nutritive value. Several have been found to resemble carbohydrate structures present in bacterial cell walls, for example, those of group B streptococci (Pritchard *et al*, 1992), giving rise to speculation that they might be able to interfere with bacterial adherence to host cells, as has been reported in the case of the adherence of *E. coli* to uroepithelial cells (Coppa *et al.* 1990). Sialyllactose and fucosylated milk oligosaccharides have also been found to inhibit cholera toxin and the heat-stable enterotoxin of *E. coli* (Idota *et al.* 1995; Newburg *et al.* 1990), presumably by interfering with the binding of these toxins to the carbohydrates on their receptors.

High–molecular weight glycoprotein agglutinins

Salivary mucins are reported to form heterotypic complexes with various other proteins, including lysozyme and α-amylase, as well as S-IgA, and thereby enhance their binding and agglutinating properties (Biesbrock *et al.* 1991; Iontcheva *et al.* 1997). The salivary agglutinin, a 300–400-kDa glycoprotein that occurs in parotid secretion and binds various oral streptococci (Rundegren 1986), has been found to be identical to the scavenger receptor gp-340, which is present in bronchoalveolar fluid and also binds to lung surfactant protein D (Ligtenberg *et al.* 2001).

Collectins

The collectins constitute a family of lectins that possess triple-helical collagenlike domains as well as C-terminal Ca^2—dependent lectin domains (Holmskov *et al.* 1994). The best known are serum mannose-binding lectin (MBL-A), which can initiate complement activation by binding to IgA (Roos *et al.* 2001), and bovine conglutinin, which interacts with the complement breakdown product, iC3b, and is able to neutralize influenza A virus (Hartshorn *et al.* 1993). Liver-type mannose-binding lectin (MBL-C) has recently been identified not only in liver but also in the small intestine, where it is presumed to play a role in mucosal defense (Uemura *et al.* 2002). SP-A and SP-D (which is closely related to conglutinin) occur in the lung surfactant and are synthesized by type II alveolar cells (Hoppe and Reid 1994). SP-A and possibly SP-D can bind to bacteria and viruses via carbohydrate groups and promote their phagocytosis by alveolar macrophages, possibly through interaction with the C1q or related receptors (Nepomuceno *et al.* 1997).

Cationic antimicrobial peptides

A large number of peptides or small proteins having antimicrobial activity and sharing the general characteristic of a high content of arginine and lysine residues, which confer a high isoelectric point, have been described in a wide variety of secretions and tissues. These include defensins, cathelicidins, and intestinal cryptdins, as well as magainins from amphibian skin and insect cecropins and are discussed in Chapter 6. It was noted previously that some of the antibacterial effects of lysozyme are probably because of its cationic nature. Nuclear histones have bactericidal properties *in vitro*, but whether this is of any significance *in vivo* is debatable.

Angiogenins

Angiogenin was originally discovered as a protein from human carcinoma cells having the ability to stimulate vasculogenesis in the chorioallantoic membrane of chicks and is now known to comprise a family of up to four proteins in various mammalian species. However, several observations have suggested that angiogenins, which are released by the liver into the circulation in the acute-phase response, may be involved in defense against infection. Angiogenin-4 has now been found to be expressed by intestinal Paneth cells in mice, especially when stimulated by gut commensal bacteria such as *Bacteroides thetaiotaomicron* (Hooper *et al.* 2003). It is a 144-residue protein and member of the ribonuclease family, secreted along with lysozyme from Paneth cell granules, giving rise to crypt concentrations exceeding 1 mM. It displays potent bactericidal activity against gram-positives such as *Enterococcus faecalis*, *Listeria monocytogenes*, *S. pneumoniae*, and the yeast *Candida albicans* at concentrations as low as 1 μM. Other angiogenins demonstrate different antimicrobial activities *in vitro*. Thus it is proposed that angiogenins constitute a new family of peptides involved in innate defense.

Proline-rich proteins

The proline-rich proteins (PRPs) are a large family of salivary proteins produced by parotid and submandibular glands. PRPs constitute nearly 70% of the total protein of human saliva and proline accounts for about 25% to 40% of the amino acids (Bennick 1982). PRPs are further subdivided into three groups, acidic, basic, and glycosylated, encoded by six genes, characterized by a variable number of tandem repeats of about 60 base-pairs (Azen and Maeda 1988). The basic and glycosylated PRPs are encoded by four genes, *PRB1* to *PRB4*; the acidic by two genes, *PRH1* and *PRH2*. PRPs are synthesized as precursor proteins (~150 amino acids), many of which are cleaved before secretion giving rise to a large number of PRPs in saliva (more than 20 have been identified). Further variability in PRPs arises by differential RNA processing, and some acidic PRP phenotypes are products of an allelic gene. Interestingly, the submandibular gland expresses only the acidic types.

Functional roles of acidic PRPs include binding to hydroxyapatite (thus becoming a part of the acquired enamel pellicle of teeth), binding of calcium ions and inhibition of crystal growth of calcium phosphate in supersaturated solutions, thereby helping to maintain tooth integrity (reviewed by Lamkin and Oppenheim 1993). All these functions are accomplished through the amino-terminal region of the molecule, which is highly acidic. The carboxyl-terminal domain of acidic PRPs was implicated in bacterial binding, especially for type 1 fimbriae of *Actinomyces viscosus*. This binding, which may facilitate the formation of dental plaque, happens only when PRPs are adsorbed to hydroxyapatite, not with the free soluble protein. The bound protein undergoes a conformational change in the carboxy-terminal of the molecule, exposing receptors for bacterial attachment, so-called "cryptitopes" (hidden epitopes; Gibbons 1990). This provides an efficient means for *A. viscosus* to bind to teeth without being cleared from the oral cavity. Hydroxyapatite-bound acidic PRPs also bind *S. mutans* and *Streptococcus gordonii*. *S. mutans* binds more strongly to the larger PRPs, and in the case of *S. gordonii*, the binding is localized to the two carboxyl-terminal residues (reviewed by Lamkin and Oppenheim 1993). The acidic PRPs on the tooth surface are degraded into peptides having potential defense properties by dental plaque proteolysis (Madapallimattan and Bennick 1990). A recent study showed the possible release of a pentapeptide (Arg106-Gly107-Arg108-Pro109-Gln110) having antimicrobial properties from acidic PRPs by the proteolytic activity of commensal *Streptococcus* and *Actinomyces* spp. The synthetic pentapeptide desorbed bound bacteria and counteracted sucrose-induced decrease of dental plaque pH *in vitro* (Li *et al.* 2000). PRPs from submandibular-sublingual saliva were also found to inhibit herpes simplex virus 1 replication (Gu *et al.* 1995) and were identified as receptors for *C. albicans* (O'Sullivan *et al.* 1997).

Another acidic PRP is expressed in human lacrimal glands (Dickinson and Thiesse 1995). It shares 45.5% homology with salivary PRP-1 and appears to be expressed also in salivary glands, but its function is unknown, although it is thought to interact with ocular microbes.

In contrast, the functions of the basic PRPs, which are expressed only in parotid saliva, have not been well characterized, but they effectively form insoluble complexes with both condensed tannin and tannic acid, which do not bind to acidic or glycosylated PRPs (Baxter *et al.* 1997; Lu and Bennick 1998). These findings suggest that PRPs play a role in protection against harmful dietary tannins (reviewed by Bennick 2002). Parotid salivary basic proline-rich proteins have been shown to inhibit HIV-1 infectivity, independent of secretory leukocyte protease inhibitor or thrombospondin (Robinowitch *et al.* 2001). It was postulated that the mechanism involves virus–host cell interaction, possibly the binding of the basic proline-rich proteins to the gp120 coat of HIV-1.

Glycosylated PRP also binds to microorganisms, and depending on its presence in the tooth pellicle or saliva, it facilitates the adherence of bacteria to oral surfaces or their clearance from the mouth, respectively (reviewed by Bennick 2002).

Mucins

Before the genes encoding the human salivary mucins were cloned, there was evidence for at least two types of structurally and functionally distinct salivary mucins, MG1 and MG2, the high–molecular-weight (>1000 kDa) and the low–molecular weight (125 kDa) mucin glycoproteins, respectively (Levine *et al.* 1987). These heavily O-glycosylated molecules (85% and 68% for MG1 and MG2, respectively) with tandem repeats in the apo-protein core, are produced by submandibular/sublingual as well as minor salivary glands. MG2 is assumed to exist as a monomer, although it can form dimers and tetramers *in vitro* (Mehrotra *et al.* 1998), whereas MG1 is an oligomer composed of multiple disulfide-linked subunits.

Salivary mucins, as part of viscoelastic mucus, contribute to formation of a protective film on both soft and hard tissues of the oral cavity. MG1 plays a bigger role in mucosal and enamel surface coating, while MG2 is involved in modulation of the microbial flora (reviewed by Levine 1993; Tabak 1995, 1998). As "amphifunctional" molecules (Levine 1993), they regulate the oral microbiota by facilitating the

attachment and proliferation of some microorganisms, and the binding and clearance of others, depending upon their intraoral location. Salivary mucins interact with respiratory (e.g., *P. aeruginosa*), cariogenic (e.g., *S. mutans*), and periodontal pathogens (e.g., *P. gingivalis*), the opportunistic yeast *C. albicans*, and even with HSV-1 and HIV-1 viruses (reviewed by Schenkels *et al.* 1996). A high–molecular-weight glycoprotein (most probably mucin) complexed with α-amylase in human saliva inhibits *S. mutans* glucosyltransferase and may thereby contribute to the control of *S. mutans* colonization in the oral cavity (Jespersgaard *et al.* 2002).

Molecular cloning of the genes encoding the salivary mucins revealed that MG2 is encoded by *MUC7* gene (Bobek *et al.* 1993). *MUC7* protein core is composed of 357 amino acid residues and contains six tandem repeats of 23 amino acids. MG1 is a mixture of at least two mucins, encoded by *MUC5B* and *MUC4* (respiratory mucins). *MUC5B*, the major component, codes for a protein of 3570 amino acids, containing tandem repeats consisting of four superrepeats of 528 residues each (Desseyn *et al.* 1997), and is classified as a gel-forming mucin. *MUC4* is a membrane-bound mucin and is the largest mucin identified to date. Protection of oral epithelial surfaces is likely to involve both gel-forming and membrane-bound mucins, which are expressed by salivary glands and epithelia (Offner and Troxler 2000). The membrane-bound *MUC1* and *MUC4* mucins constitute a protective mucin barrier layer, preventing access by bacteria, fungi, and viruses, and both may form a scaffold upon which *MUC5B* assembles to form multimers.

Recently it was demonstrated that *MUC7*-derived peptides (possibly generated *in vivo* by proteolytic enzymes) can directly kill bacteria and fungi *in vitro*, making *MUC7* a multifaceted, critical component of the oral defense system (Satyanarayana *et al.* 2000; Liu *et al.* 2000; Bobek and Situ, 2003). *MUC7* D1, a 51-residue peptide derived from its N-terminus, and *MUC7* 20-mer, spanning residues 32–51 of *MUC7* **(Fig. 5.3)**, possess antifungal activities that are comparable with or exceed the antifungal activity of histatin 5 (Satyanarayana *et al.* 2000; Bobek and Situ 2003). These peptides are effective against the wild-type, azole-resistant, and amphotericin B–resistant *C. albicans* and *Cryptococcus neoformans*, respectively, and against *Candida glabrata*, *Candida krusei*, and *Saccharomyces cerevisiae*. In comparison with histatin 5, the fungicidal activity of *MUC7* 20-mer against *C. albicans* seems to be independent of fungal metabolic activity. Although it crosses the fungal cell membrane and accumulates inside the cells, mitochondria are not the targets of *MUC7* 20-mer in either *C. albicans* and *C. neoformans*. The 20-mer also showed potent bactericidal activity against *S. mutans*, *S. gordonii*, *P. gingivalis*, *A. actinomycetemcomitans*, *P. aeruginosa*, and *E. coli* (Bobek and Situ 2003). Other *MUC7* peptides were shown to bind or to kill oral streptococci and *A. actinomycetemcomitans* (Liu *et al.* 2000, 2002). Although the *MUC7* peptides are potent against a broad range of microorganisms *in vitro*, it remains to be determined if they are effective *in vivo*. Thus far, the results of two preliminary studies indicated that these peptides, as

Peptide	Amino acid sequence	Net charge
	```1 10 20 30 40 50```	
51-mer	EGRERDHELRHRRHHHQSPKSHFELPHYPGLLAHQKPFIRKSYKCLHKRCR	+8
15-mer	RERDHELRHRRHHHQ	+5
20-mer	LAHQKPFIRKSYKCLHKRCR	+7
12-mer	FIRKSYKCLHKRCR	+6

Fig. 5.3. *MUC7*-derived peptides exhibiting antimicrobial activity. Numbers above the sequences correspond to the actual amino acid position numbers of the native *MUC7*. Data from Bobek and Situ (2003).

well as histatin 5, were not effective against *C. albicans* in animal models of candidiasis (Intini *et al.* 2003, and unpublished results).

Histatins

Histatins are a family of at least 12 small, histidine-rich, cationic peptides secreted into human saliva by salivary glands with significant *in vitro* antimicrobial activity, especially against fungi such as *Candida* (Pollock *et al.* 1984; Oppenheim *et al.* 1988). Histatins 1, 3, and 5 **(Fig. 5.4)** are the most abundant, and they have been credited with most of the anticandidal activity, histatin 5 being the most effective (Xu *et al.* 1991). Histatins 1 and 3 are encoded by *HIS1* and *HIS2* genes, respectively (Sabatini *et al.* 1993); histatin 5 is a proteolytic product of histatin 3, and all the other histatins are believed to arise from histatins 1 and 3 by proteolytic processing. Besides killing the wild-type *C. albicans*, histatins have been found to be effective in the *in vitro* killing of *Candida* species resistant to the commonly used antimycotics, fluconazole, and amphotericin B (Tsai and Bobek 1997a; Helmerhorst *et al.* 1999a), as well as of *C. neoformans* (Tsai and Bobek 1997b) and *Aspergillus fumigatus* (Helmerhorst *et al.* 1999a). Histatin 5 and its analogues exhibit synergestic effects with amphotericin B against *Aspergillus*, *Candida*, and *Cryptococcus* strains, and against an amphotericin B-resistant *C. albicans* laboratory mutant (van't Hof *et al.* 2000).

Despite numerous studies, the mechanism of histatin antifungal action remains unclear. Earlier studies showed that histatins, unlike other cationic, more amphipathic antimicrobial peptides, do not exert their antifungal action through pore

formation (by altering membrane permeability leading to cell lysis). Rather, they act through a multistep mechanism, in which histatin is internalized by *C. albicans*, possibly through a histatin-binding protein (Edgerton *et al.* 1998), and targeted to energized mitochondria (Helmerhorst *et al.* 1999b). The killing of *C. albicans* is accompanied by the release of intracellular potassium ions (Pollock *et al.* 1984; Xu *et al.* 1999) and intracellular ATP (Koshlukova *et al.* 1999). Histatins inhibit respiration and induce the formation of reactive oxygen species in *C. albicans* cells as well as isolated mitochondria, which leads to cell death (Helmerhorst *et al.* 2001). Histatin 5 toxicity to *C. albicans* is concomitant with a decrease in cellular volume, closely coupled with loss of intracellular ATP, and with cell cycle arrest (Baev *et al.* 2002).

Growth-inhibitory activity and the bactericidal effects of histatins were first shown against *S. mutans* (MacKay *et al.* 1984). Histatins inhibit hemagglutination of *P. gingivalis* (Murakami *et al.* 1990), thereby inhibiting colonization by these bacteria, and inhibit coaggregation between *P. gingivalis* and *Streptococcus mitis* (Murakami *et al.* 1991). Histatins also inhibit proteases from *P. gingivalis* (Nishikata *et al.* 1991), both Arg-gingipain and Lys-gingipain, as well as host matrix metalloproteinases (Gusman *et al.* 2001). A histatin 5–derived peptide, P-113 (spanning amino acids 4–15), previously identified as the smallest fragment that retains anticandidal activity comparable with that of the parent compound (Rothstein *et al.* 2001), also shows antibacterial activity against *P. aeruginosa*, *E. coli*, and *S. aureus*, the prominent pathogens of cystic fibrosis (CF) patients (Sajjan *et al.* 2001). This peptide was not active in the presence of purulent sputum from CF patients, but the mirror-image peptide, P-113D (with amino acids in the D configuration) retained significant activity in the presence of sputum and thus shows potential as an inhalant in chronic suppressive therapy for CF patients. The inhibitory effect of histatin 5 on the leukotoxic activity of *A. actinomycetemcomitans*, which is strongly implicated in the pathogenesis of juvenile periodontitis, suggests a new biologic function of histatins in the oral cavity (Murakami *et al.* 2002b).

Histatins as natural antimicrobial peptides show little or no toxicity toward mammalian cells and a low tendency to elicit resistance and thus have great potential to be developed into a novel class of antimicrobials, although few *in vivo* studies

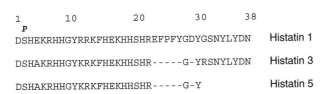

```
1        10        20        30        38
P
DSHEKRHHGYRRKFHEKHHSHREFPFYGDYGSNYLYDN      Histatin 1

DSHAKRHHGYKRKFHEKHHSHR-----G-YRSNYLYDN      Histatin 3

DSHAKRHHGYKRKFHEKHHSHR-----G-Y              Histatin 5
```

Fig. 5.4. Histatin sequences. There are two primary gene products, histatin 1 and histatin 3; histatin 5 is generated by proteolytic cleavage of histatin 3. Histatin 1 is phosphorylated on serine 2. Gaps (–) are shown in the sequences of histatin 3 and 5 to reveal the homology within histatins. Data from Troxler *et al.* (1990).

have been published. Histatin derivatives have some efficacy against experimental gingivitis in beagle dogs (Paquette *et al.* 1997) and in human clinical trials (Mickels *et al.* 2001; Van Dyke *et al.* 2002). A mouth rinse formulation of P-113 has been evaluated in a phase II multicenter clinical trial (Van Dyke *et al.*2002), which suggested that it is safe and reduces the development of gingival bleeding, gingivitis, and plaque in human experimental gingivitis. Histatin 5 has also been examined for efficacy against *C. albicans* infection in a murine model of vulvo-vaginal candidiasis and a rat model of oral candidiasis in comparison with clotrimazole, the "gold standard" in candidiasis treatment (Intini *et al.* 2003; and unpublished data), but the results showed that histatin 5 delivered in Pluronic F127 gel was not effective in either model.

Cystatins

Human salivary cystatins belong to family 2 of the cystatin superfamily, all being derived from a common ancestor (reviewed by Bobek and Levine 1992). Most (but not all) members of this superfamily are potent inhibitors of cysteine proteinases. Salivary cystatins are encoded by four related genes: *CST1, 2, 4,* and *5,* encoding cystatins SN, SA, S, and D, respectively. Cystatins SN, SA, and S are 121–amino acid proteins with about 88% identity; cystatin D contains 122 residues and shows about 55% sequence homology with the other salivary cystatins. *CST1* and *4* are expressed also in a few other tissues in the body, primarily in exocrine epithelia (Dickinson *et al.* 2002), but little is known about the functions of cystatins in other secretions. It is proposed that salivary cystatins evolved from an ancestral housekeeping gene, *CST3,* encoding the ubiquitously expressed cystatin C. Potential functions of type 2 cystatins are direct inhibition of endogenous and exogenous cysteine proteinases, control of mineralization at the tooth surface, antibacterial and antiviral activities, and modulation of the immune system (reviewed by Dickinson 2002). The results of studies concerning salivary cystatin levels with respect to increased oral inflammation and periodontal disease are controversial: cystatin levels have been reported to decline, to increase, or not to change (reviewed by Dickinson 2002).

In vitro, salivary cystatin SN inhibits human lysosomal cathepsins B, H, and L, and cystatin SA inhibits cathepsin L, which is involved in periodontal tissue destruction (Baron *et al.* 1999a), suggesting that salivary cystatins SA and SN are involved in the control of proteolytic events *in vivo*. Cystatin S did not inhibit these proteases, but was able to bind more calcium and bind more rapidly to carbonated apatite than SA or SN, suggesting that its primary role in the oral environment is likely involvement with the mineral balance of the teeth; previous findings showed cystatin S to bind hydroxyapatite and to be a major component of enamel pellicle (reviewed by Bobek and Levine 1992). Cystatins SN and SA, but not S, are also good inhibitors of papain and related enzymes from plants, suggesting that they may block the noxious effects of dietary cysteine proteinases and protect other salivary proteins from degradation.

Cystatins have been shown to be taken up by cells and to interfere with viral replication dependent on host or viral cysteine proteinases. Thus cystatin SN inhibits replication of herpes simplex virus-1 (Gu *et al.* 1995; Weaver-Hiltke and Bobek 1998) but not as effectively as cystatin C, and cystatin D inhibits replication of coronavirus (Collins and Grubb 1998). The cystatins present in tears and saliva only weakly inhibit adenain, a cysteine proteinase of adenovirus, and thus are unlikely to play a significant role in inhibiting adenovirus infections *in vivo* (Ruzindana-Umunyana and Weber 2001).

Many types of cystatins have a wide range of effects on immune cells (reviewed by Dickinson 2002). The list now includes SD-type cystatins, SA1 and SA2, which have been found to adhere to human fibroblasts through cell surface molecules, mainly CD58, leading to expression and release of IL-6 (Kato *et al.* 2002). Salivary cystatins thus may regulate the cytokine network in gingival connective tissues. It would also be interesting to determine whether SD-type cystatins have a role in suppressing oral cancer.

Secretory leukocyte protease inhibitor

Secretory leukocyte protease inhibitor (SLPI), found in the highest concentrations in saliva but present also in breast milk and genital secretions, is an 11.7-kDa protein that exhibits antimicrobial activities and is thought to play a critical role in mucosal defense. SLPI is a potent inhibitor of serine proteinase (such as human leukocyte elastase) and is also capable of inhibiting HIV-1 infectivity *in vitro* (McNeely *et al.* 1995). In salivary glands, SLPI was shown to be produced by acinar epithelial cells of both parotid and submandibular glands, to traverse the ductal system, and accumulate in the mouth. As the virus is localized to interstitial mononuclear cells within the salivary gland, it meets SLPI in the oral cavity, where the inhibitor may impede infection of additional target cells (Wahl *et al.* 1997). These findings suggest that SLPI may be partially responsible for the low rate of oral transmission of HIV-1. SLPI blocks HIV-1 infection of macrophages and primary T cells at concentrations (1–10 μg/ml) that occur naturally in saliva (Shugars and Wahl 1998), and the mechanism appears to involve blocking of uptake of HIV-1 into CD4-positive target cells through interaction with cell surface molecules other than the primary HIV-1 receptor (CD4), rather than through a direct effect on the virus replication.

Although numerous studies report that SLPI protects cultured mononuclear cells against infection, the inhibition of HIV-1 infection of human macrophages is highly variable (Konopka *et al.* 1999), and one study even showed that HIV-1 replication is unaffected by human SLPI (Turpin *et al.* 1996). These discrepancies have been attributed to factors such as variability of macrophage susceptibility to HIV infection and to the quality of SLPI preparations. Purified and refolded SLPI protein expressed from a newly cloned synthetic gene reduced HIV-1 (Ba-L) infection in differentiated human monocytic THP-1 cells, although the commercially available preparations of SLPI did not (Shine *et al.* 2002). This finding warrants a thorough reinvestigation of the molecular and structural basis for the anti-HIV activity of SLPI.

Since elderly individuals are particularly susceptible to mucosal infections, Shugars *et al.* (2001) have assessed salivary production of SLPI in an aged cohort. Their findings indicated that SLPI production (and also production of lysozyme, but not of lactoferrin and total protein) is diminished among healthy community-dwelling older adults, particularly elderly males, but the impact of this on the increased risk of oral disease with advanced age remains to be determined. In infant saliva SLPI has been shown to play an important role in reducing HIV-1 transmission from mother to child through breast milk of HIV-1–infected mothers (Farquhar *et al.* 2002).

Besides SLPI, however, there are other nonimmune endogenous inhibitors of HIV-1 in oral secretions, including thrombospondin, lactoferrin, mucins, cystatins, and PRPs. Thrombospondin, which aggregates the virus and blocks virus–CD4 interaction during viral entry, is also effective at physiologic concentration (Crombie *et al.* 1998), whereas the others inhibit HIV only at supraphysiologic concentrations. In addition, Baron *et al.* (1999b) presented evidence that saliva disrupts HIV-infected mononuclear leukocytes, thus preventing virus multiplication and cell-to-cell transmission through its hypotonicity.

ACKNOWLEDGMENTS

We would like to acknowledge the inspiration of Drs. Bruno Reiter (MWR and JHB), Michael J. Levine (LAB), and Kenneth M. Pruitt, senior author of this chapter in previous editions (JT), who introduced us to the subject and launched us on our scientific careers. We also dedicate this chapter in memoriam to Dr. Britta Månsson-Rahemtulla, who contributed greatly to our understanding of salivary peroxidase and who coauthored this chapter in previous editions.

REFERENCES

Adamson, M., and Carlsson, J. (1982). Lactoperoxidase and thiocyanate protect bacteria from hydrogen peroxide. *Infect. Immun.* 35, 20–24.

Akira, S. (2001). Toll-like receptors and innate immunity. *Adv. Immunol.* 78, 1–56.

Alderete, J. F., Peterson, K. M., and Baseman, J. B. (1988). Affinities of *Treponema pallidum* for human lactoferrin and transferrin. *Genitourin. Med.* 64, 359–363.

Anderson, B. F., Baker, H. M., Norris, G. E., Rumball, S. V., and Baker, E. N. (1990). Apolactoferrin demonstrates ligand-induced conformational change in transferrins. *Nature* 344, 784–787.

Arnold, R. R., Cole, M. F., and McGhee, J. R. (1977). A bactericidal effect for human lactoferrin. *Science* 197, 263–265.

Azen, E. A., and Maeda, N. (1998). Molecular genetics of human salivary proteins and their polymorphisms. *Adv. Hum. Genet.* 17, 141–199.

Baev, D., Li, X. S., Dong, J., Keng, P., and Edgerton, M. (2002). Human salivary histatin 5 causes disordered volume regulation and cell cycle arrest in *Candida albicans*. *Infect. Immun.* 70, 4777–4784.

Baker, E. N. (1994). Structure and reactivity of transferrins. *Adv. Inorg. Chem.* 41, 389–463.

Baker, E. N., Anderson, B. F., Baker, H. M., MacGillivray, R. T. A., Moore, S. A., Peterson, N. A., Shewry, S. C., and Tweedie, J. W. (1998). Three-dimensional structure of lactoferrin. Implications for function, including comparisons with transferrin. *Adv. Exp. Med. Biol.* 443, 1–14.

Baron, A., DeCarlo, A., and Featherstone, J. (1999a). Functional aspects of the human salivary cystatins in the oral environment. *Oral Dis.* 5, 234–240.

Baron, S., Poast, J., and Cloyd, M. W. (1999b). Why is HIV rarely transmitted by oral secretions? Saliva can disrupt orally shed, infected leukocytes. *Arch. Intern. Med.* 159, 303–310.

Baveye, S., Elass, E., Mazurier, J., Spik, G., and Legrand, D. (1999). Lactoferrin: A multifunctional glycoprotein involved in the modulation of the inflammatory process. *Clin. Chem. Lab. Med.* 37, 281–286.

Baveye, S., Elass, E., Fernig, D. G., Blanquart, C., Mazurier, J., and Legrand, D. (2000a). Human lactoferrin interacts with soluble CD14 and inhibits expression of endothelial adhesion molecules, E-selectin and ICAM-1, induced by the CD14-lipopolysaccharide complex. *Infect. Immun.* 68, 6519–6525.

Baveye, S., Elass, E., Mazurier, J., and Legrand, D. (2000b). Lactoferrin inhibits the binding of lipopolysaccharides to L-selectin and subsequent production of reactive oxygen species by neutrophils. *FEBS Lett.* 469, 5–8.

Baxter, N. J., Lilley, T. H., Haslam, E., and Williamson, M. P. (1997). Multiple interactions between polyphenols and a salivary proline-rich protein repeat result in complexation and precipitation. *Biochemistry* 36, 5566–5577.

Bellamy, W., Takase, M., Yamauchi, K., Wakabayashi, H., Kawase, K., and Tomita, M. (1992). Identification of a bactericidal domain of lactoferrin. *Biochim. Biophys. Acta* 1121, 130–136.

Bennick, A. Salivary proline-rich proteins. (1982). *Mol. Cell. Biochem.* 45, 83–99.

Bennick, A. (2002). Interaction of plant polyphenols with salivary proteins. *Crit. Rev. Oral Biol. Med.* 13, 184–196.

Berkhout, B., van Wamel, J. L., Beljaars, L., Meijer, D. K., Visser, S., and Floris, R. (2002). Characterization of the anti-HIV effects of native lactoferrin and other milk proteins and protein-derived peptides. *Antiviral Res.* 55, 341–355.

Bhimani, R. S., Vendrov, Y., and Furmanski, P. (1999). Influence of lactoferrin feeding and injection against systemic staphylococcal infections in mice. *J. Appl. Microbiol.* 86, 135–144.

Bi, B. Y., Liu, J. L., Legrand, D., Roche, A. C., Capron, M., Spik, G., and Mazurier, J. (1996). Internalization of human lactoferrin by the Jurkat human lymphoblastic T-cell line. *Eur. J. Cell. Biol.* 69, 288–296.

Biesbrock, A. R., Reddy, M. S., and Levine, M. J. (1991). Interaction of a salivary mucin-secretory immunoglobulin A complex with mucosal pathogens. *Infect. Immun.* 59, 3492–3497.

Birgens, H. S., Hansen, N. E., Karle, H., and Kristensen, L. O. (1993). Receptor binding of lactoferrin by human monocytes. *Br. J. Haematol.* 54, 383–391.

Bobek, L. A., and Levine, M. J. (1992). Cystatins: Inhibitors of cysteine proteinases. *Crit. Rev. Oral Biol. Med.* 3, 307–332.

Bobek, L. A., and Situ, H. (2003). MUC7 20-mer: Investigation of antimicrobial activity, secondary structure and possible mechanism of antifungal action. *Antimicrob. Agents Chemother.* 47, 643–652.

Bobek, L. A., Tsai, H., Biesbrock, A. R., and Levine, M. J. (1993). Molecular cloning, sequence, and specificity of expression of the gene encoding the low molecular weight human salivary mucin (MUC7). *J. Biol. Chem.* 268, 20563–20569.

Brock, J. H., Williams, P. H., Licéaga, J., and Wooldridge, K. G. (1991). Relative availability of transferrin-bound iron and cell-derived iron to aerobactin-producing and enterochelin-producing strains of *Escherichia coli* and to other microorganisms. *Infect. Immun.* 58, 3185–3190.

Bufler, P., Stiegler, G., Schuchmann, M., Hess, S., Kruger, C., Stelter, F., Eckerskorn, C., Schutt, C., and Engelmann, H. (1995). Soluble lipopolysaccharide receptor (CD14) is released via two different mechanisms from human monocytes and CD14 transfectants. *Eur. J. Immunol.* 25, 604–610.

Bussolati, B., David, S., Cambi, V., Tobias, P. S., and Camussi, G. (2002). Urinary soluble CD14 mediates human proximal tubular epithelial cell injury induced by LPS. *Intl. J. Mol. Med.* 10, 441–449.

Cario, E., and Podolsky, D.K. (2000). Differential alteration in intestinal epithelial cell expression of toll-like receptor 3 (TLR3) and TLR4 in inflammatory bowel disease. *Infect. Immun.* 68, 7010–7017.

Chandan, R. C., Shahani, K. M., and Holly, R. G. (1964). Lysozyme content of human milk. *Nature* 204, 76–77.

Chipman, D. M., and Sharon, N. (1969). Mechanism of lysozyme action. *Science* 165, 454–465.

Cho, M. I., Holt, S. C., Iacono, V. J., and Pollock, J. J. (1982). Effects of lysozyme and inorganic anions on the morphology of *Streptococcus mutans* BHT: Electron microscopic examination. *J. Bacteriol.* 151, 1498–1507.

Choe, Y-H., and Lee, S-W. (1999). Effect of lactoferrin on the production of tumor necrosis factor-α and nitric oxide. *J. Cell. Biochem.* 76, 30–36.

Cirioni, O., Giacometti, A., Barchiesi, F., and Scalise, G. (2000). Inhibition of growth of *Pneumocystis carinii* by lactoferrins alone and in combination with pyrimethamine, clarithromycin and minocycline. *J. Antimicrob. Chemother.* 46, 577–582.

Collins, A. R., and Grubb, A. (1998). Cystatin D, a natural salivary cysteine protease inhibitor, inhibits coronavirus replication at its physiologic concentration. *Oral Microbiol. Immunol.* 13, 59–61.

Coppa, G. V., Gabrielli, O., Giorgi, P., Catassi, C., Montanari, M. P., Varaldo, P. E., and Nichols, B. L. (1990). Preliminary study of breastfeeding and bacterial adhesion to uroepithelial cells. *Lancet* 335, 569–571.

Courtois, P., Majerus, P., Labbé, M., Vanden Abbeele, A., Yourassowsky, E., and Pourtois, M. (1992). Susceptibility of anaerobic microorganisms to hypothiocyanite produced by lactoperoxidase. *Acta Stomatol. Belg.* 89, 155–162.

Crombie, R., Silverstein, R. L., MacLow, C., Pearce, S. F., Nachman, R. L., and Laurence, J. (1998). Identification of a CD36-related thrombospondin 1-binding domain in HIV-1 envelope glycoprotein gp120: relationship to HIV-1-specific inhibitory factors in human saliva. *J. Exp. Med.* 187, 25–35.

Desseyn, J. L., Guyonnet-Duperat, V., Porchet, N., Aubert, J. P., and Laine, A. (1997). Human mucin gene *MUC5B*, the 10.7-kb large central exon encodes various alternate subdomains resulting in a super-repeat: Structural evidence for a 11p15.5 gene family. *J. Biol. Chem.* 272, 3168–3178.

Dhennin-Duthille, I., Masson, M., Damiens, E., Fillebeen, C., Spik, G., and Mazurier, J. (2000). Lactoferrin upregulates the expression of CD4 antigen through the stimulation of the mitogen-activated protein kinase in the human lymphoblastic T Jurkat cell line. *J. Cell. Biochem.* 79, 583–593.

Dickinson, D. P. (2002). Salivary (sd-type) cystatins: over one billion years in the making-but to what purpose? *Crit. Rev. Oral Biol. Med.* 13, 485–508.

Dickinson, D. P., and Thiesse, M. (1995). A major human lacrimal gland mRNA encodes a new proline-rich protein family member. *Invest. Ophthalmol. Vis. Sci.* 36, 2020–2031.

Dickinson, D. P., Thiesse, M., and Hicks, M. J. (2002). Expression of type 2 cystatin genes CST1-CST5 in adult human tissues and the developing submandibular gland. *DNA Cell Biol.* 21, 47–65.

Dull, T. J., Uyeda, C., Strosberg, A. D., Nedwin, G., and Seilhamer, J. J. (1990). Molecular cloning of cDNAs encoding bovine and human lactoperoxidase. *DNA Cell Biol.* 9, 499–509.

Eda, S., Eda, K., Prudhomme, J. G., and Sherman, I. W. (1999). Inhibitory activity of human lactoferrin and its peptide on chondroitin sulfate A-, CD36-, and thrombospondin-mediated cytoadherence of *Plasmodium falciparum*-infected erythrocytes. *Blood* 94, 326–332.

Edde, L., Hipolito, R. B., Hwang, F. F., Headon, D. R., Shalwitz, R. A., and Sherman, M. P. (2001). Lactoferrin protects neonatal rats from gut-related systemic infection. *Am. J. Physiol.* 281, G1140–G1150.

Edgerton, M., Koshlukova, S. E., Lo, T. E., Chrzan, B. G., Straubinger, R. M., and Raj, P. A. (1998). Candidacidal activity of salivary histatins: Identification of a histatin 5-binding protein on *Candida albicans*. *J. Biol. Chem.* 273, 20438–20447.

El Yazidi-Belkoura, I., Legrand, D., Nuijens, J., Slomianny, M. C., van Berkel, P., and Spik, G. (2001). The binding of lactoferrin to glycosaminoglycans on enterocyte-like HT29-18-C1 cells is mediated through basic residues located in the N-terminus. *Biochim. Biophys Acta* 1568, 197–204.

Elass, E., Masson, M., Mazurier, J., and Legrand, D. (2002). Lactoferrin inhibits the lipopolysaccharide-induced expression and proteoglycan-binding ability of interleukin-8 in human endothelial cells. *Infect. Immun.* 70, 1860–1866.

Ellison, R. T. and Giehl, T. J. (1991). Killing of Gram-negative bacteria by lactoferrin and lysozyme. *J. Clin. Invest.* 88, 1080–1091.

Fadel, M., and Courtois, P. (1999). Effect of peroxidase-generated hypothiocyanite on the survival rate of *Porphyromonas gingivalis* NCTC 11834. *Med. Sci. Res.* 27, 667–669.

Farquhar, C., VanCott, T. C., Mbori-Ngacha, D. A., Horani, L., Bosire, R. K., Kreiss, J. K., Richardson, B. A., and John-Stewart, G. C. (2002). Salivary secretory leukocyte protease inhibitor is associated with reduced transmission of human immunodeficiency virus type 1 through breast milk. *J. Infect. Dis.* 186, 1173–1176.

Fine, D. H., and Furgang, D. (2002). Lactoferrin iron levels affect attachment of *Actinobacillus actinomycetemcomitans* to buccal epithelial cells. *J. Periodontol.* 73, 616–623.

Gibbons, R. J., Hay, D. I., Childs, W. C., and Davis, G. (1990). Role of cryptic receptors (cryptitopes) in bacterial adhesion to oral surfaces. *Arch. Oral Biol.* 35 (Suppl.), 107s–114s.

Gleich, G. J., and Adolphson, C. R. (1986). The eosinophilic leukocyte: Structure and function. *Adv. Immunol.* 39, 177–253.

Gomez, H. F., Ochoa, T. J., Carlin, L. G., and Cleary, T. G. (2003). Human lactoferrin impairs virulence of *Shigella flexneri*. *J Infect. Dis.* 187, 87–95.

Grab, D. J., Lonsdale-Eccles, J. D., Oli, M. W., and Corbeil, L. B. (2001). Lactoferrin-binding proteins of *Tritrichomonas foetus*. *J. Parasitol.* 87, 1064–1070.

Gray-Owen, S. D., and Schryvers, A. B. (1996). Bacterial transferrin and lactoferrin receptors. *Trends Microbiol.* 4, 185–191.

Grazioso, C. F., and Buescher, E. S. (1996). Inhibition of neutrophil function by human milk. *Cell. Immunol.* 168, 125–132.

Gu, M., Haraszthy, G. G., Collins, A. R., and Bergey, E. J. (1995). Identification of salivary proteins inhibiting herpes simplex virus 1 replication. *Oral Microbiol. Immunol.* 10, 54–59.

Guillen, C., McInnes, I. B., Vaughan, D., Speekenbrink, A. B., and Brock, J. H. (2000). The effects of local administration of lactoferrin on inflammation in murine autoimmune and infectious arthritis. *Arthritis Rheum.* 43, 2073–2080.

Guillen, C., McInnes, I. B., Vaughan, D. M., Kommajosyula, S., Van Berkel, P. H., Leung, B. P., Aguila, A., and Brock, J. H. (2002). Enhanced Th1 response to *Staphylococcus aureus* infection in human lactoferrin-transgenic mice. *J. Immunol.* 168, 3950–3957.

Gusman, H., Travis, J., Helmerhorst, E. J., Potempa, J., Troxler, R. F., and Oppenheim, F. G. (2001). Salivary histatin 5 is an inhibitor of both host and bacterial enzymes implicated in periodontal disease. *Infect. Immun.* 69, 1402–1408.

Hajishengallis, G., Martin, M., Sojar, H. T., Sharma, A., Schifferle, R. E., DeNardin, E., Russell, M. W., and Genco, R. J. (2002). Dependence of bacterial protein adhesins on toll-like receptors for proinflammatory cytokine induction. *Clin. Diag. Lab. Immunol.* 9, 403–411.

Håkansson, A., Svensson, M., Mossberg, A.K., Sabharwal, H., Linse, S., Lazou, I., Lönnerdal, B., and Svanborg, C. (2000). A folding variant of α-lactalbumin with bactericidal activity against *Streptococcus pneumoniae*. *Mol. Microbiol.* 35, 589–600.

Hammerschmidt, S., Bethe, G., Remane, P.H., and Chhatwal, G.S. (1999). Identification of pneumococcal surface protein A as a lactoferrin-binding protein of *Streptococcus pneumoniae*. *Infect. Immun.* 67, 1683–1687.

Hänström, L., Johansson, A., and Carlsson, J. (1983). Lactoperoxidase and thiocyanate protect cultured mammalian cells against hydrogen peroxide toxicity. *Med. Biol.* 61, 268–274.

Hara, K., Ikeda, M., Saito, S., Matsumoto, S., Numata, K., Kato, N., Tanaka, K., and Sekihara, H. (2002) Lactoferrin inhibits hepatitis B virus infection in cultured human hepatocytes. *Hepatol. Res.* 24, 228–235.

Hartshorn, K. L., Sastry, K., Brown, D., White, M. R., Okarma, T. B., Lee, Y. M., and Tauber, A. I. (1993). Conglutinin acts as an opsonin for influenza A viruses. *J. Immunol.* 151, 6265–6273.

Haversen, L. A., Baltzer, L., Dolphin, G., Hanson, L. A., and Mattsby-Baltzer, I. (2003). Anti-inflammatory activities of human lactoferrin in acute dextran sulphate-induced colitis in mice. *Scand. J. Immunol.* 57, 2–10.

Haziot, A., Chen, S., Ferrero, E., Low, M. G., Silber, R., and Goyert, S. M. (1988). The monocyte differentiation marker, CD14, is anchored to the cell membrane by a phosphatidylinositol linkage. *J. Immunol.* 141, 547–552.

Haziot, A., Rong, G. W., Bazil, V., Silver, J., and Goyert, S. M. (1994). Recombinant soluble CD14 inhibits LPS-induced tumor necrosis factor-a production by cells in whole blood. *J. Immunol.* 152, 5868–5876.

Haziot, A., Rong, G. W., Lin, X. Y., Silver, J., and Goyert, S. M. (1995). Recombinant soluble CD14 prevents mortality in mice treated with endotoxin (lipopolysaccharide). *J. Immunol.* 154, 6529–6532.

He, J., and Furmanski, P. (1995). Sequence specificity and transcriptional activation in the binding of lactoferrin to DNA. *Nature* 373, 721–724.

Helmerhorst, E. J., Reijnders, I. M., van't Hof, W., Simoons-Smit, I., Veerman, E. C., and Amerongen, A. V. (1999a). Amphotericin B- and fluconazole-resistant *Candida* spp., *Aspergillus fumigatus*, and other newly emerging pathogenic fungi are susceptible to basic antifungal peptides. *Antimicrob. Agents Chemother.* 43, 702–704.

Helmerhorst, E. J., Breeuwer, P., van't Hof, W, Walgreen-Weterings, E., Oomen, L. C., Veerman, E. C., Amerongen, A. V., and Abee, T. (1999b). The cellular target of histatin 5 on *Candida albicans* is the energized mitochondrion. *J. Biol. Chem.* 274, 7286–7891.

Helmerhorst, E. J., Troxler, R. F., and Oppenheim, F. G. (2001). The human salivary peptide histatin 5 exerts its antifungal activity through the formation of reactive oxygen species. *Proc. Natl. Acad. Sci. USA* 98, 14637–14642.

Hendrixson, D. R., Qiu, J., Shewry, S. C., Fink, D. L., Petty, S., Baker, E. N., Plaut, A. G., and St. Geme, J. W. (2003). Human milk lactoferrin is a serine protease that cleaves *Haemophilus* surface proteins at arginine-rich sites. *Mol. Microbiol.* 47, 607–617.

Hernell, O., and Lonnerdal, B. (2002). Iron status of infants fed low-iron formula: No effect of added bovine lactoferrin or nucleotides. *Am. J. Clin Nutr.* 76, 858–864.

Higo, J., and Nakasako, M. (2002). Hydration structure of human lysozyme investigated by molecular dynamics simulation and cryogenic X-ray crystal structure analyses: On the correlation between crystal water sites, solvent density, and solvent dipole. *J. Comput. Chem.* 23, 1323–1336.

Holmskov, U., Malhotra, R., Sim, R. B., and Jensenius, J. C. (1994). Collectins: collagenous C-type lectins of the innate immune defense system. *Immunol. Today* 15, 67–74.

Hooper, L. V., Stappenbeck, T. S., Hong, C. V., and Gordon, J. I. (2003). Angiogenins: A new class of microbicidal proteins involved in innate immunity. *Nat. Immunol.* 4, 269–273.

Hoppe, H.-J., and Reid, K. B. M. (1994). Collectins—soluble proteins containing collagenous regions and lectin domains—and their roles in innate immunity. *Protein Sci.* 3, 1143–1158.

Hovanessian, A. G., and Awdeh, Z. L. (1976). Gel isoelectric focussing of human-serum transferrin. *Eur. J. Biochem.* 68, 333–338.

Iacono, V. J., MacKay, B. J., DiRienzo, S., and Pollock, J. J. (1980). Selective antibacterial properties of lysozyme for oral microorganisms. *Infect. Immun.* 29, 623–632.

Iacono, V. J., Zove, S. M., Grossbard, B. L., Pollock, J. J., Fine, D. H., and Greene, L. S. (1985). Lysozyme-mediated aggregation and lysis of the periodontal microorganism *Capnocytophaga gingivalis* 2010. *Infect. Immun.* 47, 457–464.

Idota, T., Kawakami, H., Murakami, Y., and Sugawar, M. (1995). Inhibition of cholera toxin by human milk fractions and sialyllactose. *Biosci. Biotechnol. Biochem.* 59, 417–419.

Ihalin, R., Loimaranta, V., Lenander-Lumikari, M., and Tenovuo, J. (1998). The effects of different (pseudo)halide substrates on peroxidase-mediated killing of *Actinobacillus actinomycetemcomitans*. *J. Period. Res.* 33, 421–427.

Ihalin, R., Pienihäkkinen, K., Lenander, M., Tenovuo, J., and Jousimies-Somer, H. (2003). Susceptibilities of different *Actinobacillus actinomycetemcomitans* strains to lactoperoxidase-iodide-hydrogen peroxide combination and different antibiotics. *Int. J. Antimicrob. Agents,* 21, 434–440.

Intini, G., Aguirre, A., and Bobek, L. A. (2003). Efficacy of human salivary mucin *MUC7*-derived peptide and of histatin 5 in murine model vulvo-vaginal candidiasis. *Int. J. Antimicrob. Agents,* 22, 594–600.

Iontcheva, I., Oppenheim, F. G., and Troxler, R. F. (1997). Human salivary mucin MG1 selectively forms heterotypic complexes with amylase, proline-rich proteins, statherin, and histatins. *J. Dent. Res.* 76, 734–743.

Irwin, D. M., Yu, M., and Wen, Y. (1996). Isolation and characterization of vertebrate lysozyme genes. *EXS* 75, 225–241.

Ismail, M., and Brock, J. H. (1993). Binding of lactoferrin and transferrin to the human promonocytic cell line U937: Effect on iron uptake and release. *J. Biol. Chem.* 268, 21618–21625.

Iwami, K. I., Matsuguchi, T., Masuda, A., Kikuchi, T., Musikacharoen, T., and Yoshikai, Y. (2000). Naturally occurring soluble form of mouse toll-like receptor 4 inhibits lipopolysaccharide signaling. *J. Immunol.* 165, 6682–6686.

Jarosik, G. P., and Land, C. B. (2000). Identification of a human lactoferrin-binding protein in *Gardnerella vaginalis*. *Infect. Immun.* 68, 3443–3447.

Jespersgaard, C., Hajishengallis, G., Russell, M. W., and Michalek, S. M. (2002). Identification and characterization of a nonimmunoglobulin factor in human saliva that inhibits *Streptococcus mutans* glucosyltransferase. *Infect. Immun.* 70, 1136–1142.

Jollès, P. (ed.) Lysozymes: Model enzymes in biochemistry and biology, *EXS*, vol. 75. Basel, Switzerland: Birkhäuser Verlag.

Jollès, P., and Jollès, J. (1984). What's new in lysozyme research? *Mol. Cell. Biochem.* 63, 165–189.

Kassim, O. O., Ako-Anai, K. A., Torimiro, S. E., Hollowell, G. P., Okoye, V. C., and Martin, S. K. (2000). Inhibitory factors in breastmilk, maternal and infant sera against in vitro growth of *Plasmodium falciparum* malaria parasite. *J. Trop. Pediatr.* 46, 92–96.

Kato, T., Imatani, T., Minaguchi, K., Saitoh, E., Okuda, K. (2002). Salivary cystatins induce IL-6 expression via cell surface molecules in human gingival fibroblasts. *Mol. Immunol.* 39, 423–430.

Kiser, C. S., Caterina, J., Engler, J. A., Rahemtulla, B., and Rahemtulla, F. (1996). Cloning and sequence analysis of the human salivary peroxidase-encoding cDNA. *Gene* 173, 261–264.

Konopka, K., Shine, N., Pretzer, E., and Duzgunes, N. (1999). Secretory leukocyte protease inhibitor (SLPI): oxidation of SLPI does not explain its variable anti-HIV activity. *J. Dent. Res.* 78, 1773–1776.

Korsrud, F. R., and Brandtzaeg, P. (1982). Characterization of epithelial elements in human major salivary glands by functional markers: Localization of amylase, lactoferrin, lysozyme, secretory component, and secretory immunoglobulins by paired immunofluorescence staining. *J. Histochem. Cytochem.* 30, 567–666.

Koshlukova, S. E., Lloyd, T. L., Araujo, M. W., and Edgerton, M. (1999). Salivary histatin 5 induces non-lytic release of ATP from *Candida albicans* leading to cell death. *J. Biol. Chem.* 274, 18872–18879.

Kruzel, M. L., Harari, Y., Mailman, D., Actor, J. K., and Zimecki, M. (2002). Differential effects of prophylactic, concurrent and therapeutic lactoferrin treatment on LPS-induced inflammatory responses in mice. *Clin. Exp. Immunol.* 130, 25–31.

Labéta, M. O., Vidal, K., Nores, J. E., Arias, M., Vita, N., Morgan, B. P., Guillemot, J. C., Loyaux, D., Ferrara, P., Schmid, D., Affolter, M., Borysiewicz, L.K., Donnet-Hughes, A., and Schiffrin, E. J. (2000). Innate recognition of bacteria in human milk is mediated by a milk-derived highly expressed pattern recognition receptor, soluble CD14. *J. Exp. Med.* 191, 1807–1812.

Laible, N. J., and Germaine, G. R. (1985). Bactericidal activity of human lysozyme, muramidase-inactive lysozyme, and cationic polypeptides against *Streptococcus sanguis* and *Streptococcus faecalis:* Inhibition by chitin oligosaccharides. *Infect. Immun.* 48, 720–728.

Lamkin, M. S., and Oppenheim, F. G. (1993). Structural features of salivary function. *Crit. Rev. Oral Biol. Med.* 4, 251–259.

Lamping, N., Dettmer, R., Schroder, N. W., Pfeil, D., Hallatschek, W., Burger, R., and Schumann, R. R. (1998). LPS-binding protein protects mice from septic shock caused by LPS or gram-negative bacteria. *J. Clin. Invest.* 101, 2065–2071.

Lampreave, F., Piñeiro, A., Brock, J. H., Castillo, H., Sánchez, L., and Calvo, M. (1990). Interaction of bovine lactoferrin with other proteins of milk whey. *Int. J. Biol. Macromol.* 12, 2–5.

Landmann, R., Müller, B., and Zimmerli, W. (2000). CD14, new aspects of ligand and signal diversity. *Microb. Infect.* 2, 295–304.

Lee-Huang, S., Huang, P. L., Sun, Y., Kung, H. F., Blithe, D. L., and Chen, H. C. (1999). Lysozyme and RNases as anti-HIV components in β-core preparations of human chorionic gonadotropin. *Proc. Natl. Acad. Sci. USA* 96, 2678–2681.

Lenander-Lumikari, M., and Loimaranta, V. (2000). Saliva and dental caries. *Adv. Dent. Res.* 14, 40–47.

Lenander-Lumikari, M., Månsson-Rahemtulla, B., and Rahemtulla, F. (1992). Lysozyme enhances the inhibitory effects of the peroxidase system on glucose metabolism of *Streptococcus mutans. J. Dent. Res.* 71, 484–490.

Levine, M. J. (1993). Salivary macromolecules. A structure/function synopsis. *Ann. N.Y. Acad. Sci.* 694, 111–116.

Levine, M. J., Reddy, M. S., Tabak, L. A., Loomis, R. E., Bergey, E. J., Jones, P. C., Cohen, R. E., Stinson, M. W., and Al-Hashimi, I. (1987). Structural aspects of salivary glycoproteins. *J. Dent. Res.* 66, 436–441.

Li, T., Bratt, P., Jonsson, A. P., Ryberg, M., Johansson, I., Griffiths, W. J., Bergman, T., and Stromberg, N. (2000). Possible release of an ArgGlyArgProGln pentapeptide with innate immunity properties from acidic proline-rich proteins by proteolytic activity in commensal streptococcus and actinomyces species. *Infect. Immun.* 68, 5425–5429.

Lichtman, S. N., Sherman, P., and Mack, D. R. (1996). The role of mucus in gut protection. *Curr. Opin. Gastroenterol.* 12, 584–590.

Ligtenberg, T. J. M., Bikker, F. J., Groenink, J., Tornoe, I., Leth-Larsen, R., Veerman, E. C. I., Amerongen, A. V. N., and Holmskov, U. (2001). Human salivary agglutinin binds to lung surfactant protein-D and is identical with scavenger receptor protein gp-340. *Biochem. J.* 359, 243–248.

Liu, B., Rayment, S. A., Gyurko, C., Oppenheim, F. G., Offner, G. D., and Troxler, R. F. (2000). The recombinant N-terminal region of human salivary mucin MG2 *(MUC7)* contains a binding domain for oral streptococci and exhibits candidacidal activity. *Biochem. J.* 345, 557–564.

Liu, B., Rayment, S. A., Soares, R. V., Oppenheim, F. G., Offner, G. D., Fives-Taylor, P., and Troxler, R. F. (2002). Interaction of human salivary mucin MG2, its recombinant N-terminal region and a synthetic peptide with *Actinobacillus actinomycetemcomitans. J. Periodontal. Res.* 37, 416–424.

Lu, Y., and Bennick, A. (1998). Interaction of tannin with human salivary proline-rich proteins. *Arch. Oral Biol.* 43, 717–728.

Lee-Huang, S., Huang, P. L., Sun, Y., Kung, H. F., Blithe, D. L., and Chen, H. C. (1999). Lysozyme and RNases as anti-HIV components in β-core preparations of human chorionic gonadotropin. *Proc. Natl. Acad. Sci. USA* 96, 2678–2681.

MacKay, B. J., Denepitiya, L., Iacono, V. J., Krost, S. B., and Pollock J. J. (1984). Growth-inhibitory and bactericidal effects of human parotid salivary histidine-rich polypeptides on *Streptococcus mutans. Infect. Immun.* 44, 695–701.

Madapallimattam, G., and Bennick, A. (1990). Phosphopeptides derived from human salivary acidic proline-rich proteins: Biological activities and concentration in saliva. *Biochem J.* 270, 297–304.

Månsson-Rahemtulla, B., Pruitt, K. M., Tenovuo, J., and Le, T. M. (1983). A mouth rinse which optimizes *in vivo* generation of hypothiocyanite. *J. Dent. Res.* 62, 1062–1066.

Månsson-Rahemtulla, B., Rahemtulla, F., Baldone, D. C., Pruitt, K. M., and Hjerpe, A. (1988). Purification and characterization of human salivary peroxidase. *Biochemistry* 27, 233–239.

Masson, P. L., and Heremans, J. F. (1971). Lactoferrin in milk from different species. *Comp. Biochem. Physiol. B* 39, 119–129.

Mattsby-Baltzer, I., Roseanu, A., Motas, C., Elverfors, J., Engberg, I., and Hanson, L.Å. (1996). Lactoferrin or a fragment thereof inhibits the endotoxin-induced interleukin-6 response in human monocytic cells. *Pediatr. Res.* 40, 257–262.

Mazurier, J., and Spik, G. (1980). Comparative study of the iron-binding properties of human transferrins. I. Complete and sequential iron saturation and desaturation of the lactotransferrin. *Biochim. Biophys. Acta* 629, 399–408.

Mazurier, J., Legrand, D., Hu, W.-L., and Spik, G. (1989). Expression of human lactotransferrin receptors in phytohaemagglutinin-stimulated human peripheral blood lymphocytes: Isolation of the receptors by antiligand-affinity chromatography. *Eur. J. Biochem.* 179, 481–487.

McAbee, D. D., and Esbensen, K. (1991). Binding and endocytosis of apo- and holo-lactoferrin by isolated rat hepatocytes. *J. Biol. Chem.* 266, 23624–23631.

McAbee, D. D., Nowatzke, W., Oehler, C., Sitaram, M., Sbaschnig, E., Opferman, J. T., Carr, J., and Esbensen, K. (1993). Endocytosis and degradation of apo- and holo-lactoferrin by isolated rat hepatocytes are mediated by recycling calcium-dependent binding sites. *Biochemistry* 32, 13749–13760.

McKenzie, H. A., and White, F. H. (1991). Lysozyme and alpha-lactalbumin: structure, function, and interrelationships. *Adv. Protein Chem.* 41, 173–315.

McNeely, T. B., Dealy, M., Dripps, D. J., Orenstein, J. M., Eisenberg, S. P., and Wahl, S. M. (1995). Secretory leukocyte protease inhibitor: A human saliva protein exhibiting anti-human immunodeficiency virus 1 activity *in vitro. J. Clin. Invest.* 96, 456–464.

Mehrotra, R., Thornton, D. J., and Sheehan, J. K. (1998). Isolation and physical characterization of the *MUC7* (MG2) mucin from saliva: Evidence for self-association. *Biochem. J.* 334, 415–422.

Mickels, N., McManus, C., Massaro, J., Friden, P., Braman, V., D'Agostino, R., Oppenheim, F., Warbington, M., Dibart, S., and Van Dyke, T. (2001). Clinical and microbial evaluation of a histatin-containing mouthrinse in humans with experimental gingivitis. *J. Clin. Periodontol.* 28, 404–410.

Mikola, H., Waris, M., and Tenovuo, J. (1995). Inhibition of herpes simplex virus type 1, respiratory syncytial virus and echovirus type 11 by peroxidase-generated hypothiocyanite. *Antiviral Res.* 26, 161–171.

Mims C. A., Dimmock N. J., Nash A. and Stephen J. (1995) Mims' Pathogenesis of Infectious Disease. Academic Press, San Diego.

Mincheva-Nilsson, L., Hammarstrom, S., and Hammarstrom, M-L. (1997). Activated human γδ T lymphocytes express functional lactoferrin receptors. *Scand. J. Immunol.* 46, 609–618.

Moguilevsky, N., Retegui, L.A., and Masson, P.L. (1985). Comparison of human lactoferrins from milk and neutrophilic leucocytes. *Biochem. J.* 229, 353–359.

Moldoveanu, Z., Tenovuo, J., Mestecky, J., and Pruitt, K. M. (1982). Human milk peroxidase is derived from milk leukocytes. *Biochim. Biophys. Acta* 718, 103–108.

Moro, I., Umemura, S., Crago, S. S., and Mestecky, J. (1984). Immunohistochemical distribution of immunoglobulins, lactoferrin, and lysozyme in human minor salivary glands. *J. Oral Pathol.* 13, 97–104.

Murakami, Y., Amano, A., Takagaki, M., Shizukuishi, S., Tsunemitsu, A., and Aimoto, S. (1990). Purification and characterization from human parotid secretion of a peptide which inhibits hemagglutination of *Bacteroides gingivalis* 381. *FEMS Microbiol. Lett.* 60, 275–279.

Murakami, Y., Nagata, H., Amano, A., Takagaki, M., Shizukuishi, S., Tsunemitsu, A., and Aimoto, S. (1991). Inhibitory effects of human salivary histatins and lysozyme on coaggregation between *Porphyromonas gingivalis* and *Streptococcus mitis. Infect. Immun.* 59, 3284–3286.

Murakami, S., Iwaki, D., Mitsuzawa, H., Sano, H., Takahashi, H., Voelker, D. R., Akino, T., and Kuroki, Y. (2002a). Surfactant protein A inhibits peptidoglycan-induced tumor necrosis factor-alpha secretion in U937 cells and alveolar macrophages by direct interaction with toll-like receptor 2. *J. Biol. Chem.* 277, 6830–6837.

Murakami, Y., Xu, T., Helmerhorst, E. J., Ori, G., Troxler, R. F., Lally, E. T., and Oppenheim, F. G. (2002b). Inhibitory effect of synthetic histatin 5 on leukotoxin from *Actinobacillus actinomycetemcomitans*. *Oral Microbiol. Immunol.* 17, 143–149.

Murphy, M. E., Kariwa, H., Mizutani, T., Tanabe, H., Yoshimatsu, K., Arikawa, J., and Takashima, I. (2001). Characterization of *in vitro* and *in vivo* antiviral activity of lactoferrin and ribavirin upon hantavirus. *J. Vet. Med. Sci.* 63, 637–645.

Nepomuceno, R. R., Henschen-Edman, A. H., Burgess, W. H., and Tenner, A. J. (1997). cDNA cloning and primary structure analysis of C1qR(P), the human C1q/MBL/SPA receptor that mediates enhanced phagocytosis *in vitro*. *Immunity* 6, 119–129.

Newburg, D. S., Pickering, L. K., McCluer, R. H., and Cleary, T. G. (1990). Fucosylated oligosaccharides of human milk protect suckling mice from heat-stable enterotoxin of *Escherichia coli*. *J. Infect. Dis.* 162, 1075–1080.

Nishikata, M., Kanehira, T., Oh, H., Tani, H., Tazaki, M., and Kuboki, Y. (1991). Salivary histatin as an inhibitor of a protease produced by the oral bacterium *Bacteroides gingivalis*. *Biochem. Biophys. Res. Commun.* 174, 625–630.

Nozaki, A., Ikeda, M., Naganuma, A., Nakamura, T., Inudoh, M., Tanaka, K., and Kato, N. (2003). Identification of a lactoferrin-derived peptide possessing binding activity to hepatitis C virus E2. *J. Biol. Chem.*, 278, 10162–10173.

Offner, G. D., and Troxler, R. F. (2000). Heterogeneity of high-molecular-weight human salivary mucins. *Adv. Dent. Res.* 14, 69–75.

Okada, S., Tanaka, K., Sato, T., Ueno, H., Saito, S., Okusaka, T., Sato, K., Yamamoto, S., and Kakizoe, T. (2002). Dose-response trial of lactoferrin in patients with chronic hepatitis C. *Jpn. J. Cancer Res.* 93, 1063–1069.

Oppenheim, F. G., Xu, T., McMillian, F. M., Levitz, S. M., Diamond, R. D., Offner, G. D., and Troxler, R. F. (1988). Histatins, a novel family of histidine-rich proteins in human parotid secretion. Isolation, characterization, primary structure, and fungistatic effects on *Candida albicans*. *J. Biol. Chem.* 263, 7472–7477.

O'Sullivan, J. M., Cannon, R. D., Sullivan, P. A., and Jenkinson, H. F. (1997). Identification of salivary basic proline-rich proteins as receptors for *Candida albicans* adhesion. *Microbiology* 143, 341–348.

Paquette, D. W., Waters, G. S., Stefanidou, V. L., Lawrence, H. P., Friden, P. M., O'Connor, S. M., Sperati, J. D., Oppenheim, F. G., Hutchens, L. H., and Williams, R. C. (1997). Inhibition of experimental gingivitis in beagle dogs with topical salivary histatins. *J. Clin. Periodontol.* 24, 216–222.

Paul, K.-G., and Ohlsson, P.-I. (1985). The chemical structure of lactoperoxidase. In *The Lactoperoxidase System: Chemistry and Biological Significance* (eds. K. M. Pruitt and J. O. Tenovuo), 15–29. New York: Marcel Dekker.

Perera, P.-Y., Mayadas, T. N., Takeuchi, O., Akira, S., Zaks-Zilberman, M., Goyert, S. M., and Vogel, S. N. (2001). CD11b/CD18 acts in concert with CD14 and toll-like receptor (TLR) 4 to elicit full lipopolysaccharide and taxol-inducible gene expression. *J. Immunol.* 166, 574–581.

Pollock, J. J., Denepitiya, L., MacKay, B. J., and Iacono, V. J. (1984). Fungistatic and fungicidal activity of human parotid salivary histidine-rich polypeptides on *Candida albicans*. *Infect. Immun.* 44, 702–707.

Pollock, J. J., Lotardo, S., Gavai, R., and Grossbard, B. L. (1987). Lysozyme-protease-inorganic monovalent anion lysis of oral bacterial strains in buffers and stimulated whole saliva. *J. Dent. Res.* 66, 467–474.

Potten, C. S., and Morris, R. J. (1988). Epithelial stem cells *in vivo*. *J. Cell Sci.* Suppl. 10, 45–62.

Pourtois, M., Binet, C. Van Tieghem, N., Courtois, P. Vandenabbeele, A., and Thiry, L. (1990). Inhibition of HIV infectivity by lactoperoxidase-produced hypothiocyanite. *J. Biol. Buccale* 18, 251–253.

Pritchard, D. G., Gray, B. M., and Egan, M. L. (1992). Murine monoclonal antibodies to type Ib polysaccharide of group B streptococci bind to human milk oligosaccharides. *Infect. Immun.* 60, 1598–1602.

Pruitt, K. M., and Adamson, M. (1977). Enzyme activity of salivary lactoperoxidase adsorbed to human enamel. *Infect. Immun.* 17, 112–116.

Pruitt, K. M., and Kamau, D. N. (1991). The lactoperoxidase systems of bovine and human milk. In *Oxidative Enzymes in Foods* (eds. D. S. Robinson and N. A. M. Eskin), 133–174. London: Elsevier Applied Science.

Pruitt, K. M., and Reiter, B. (1985). Biochemistry of peroxidase system: antimicrobial effects. In *The Lactoperoxidase System. Chemistry and Biological Significance* (eds. K. M. Pruitt and J. O. Tenovuo), 143–178. New York: Marcel Dekker.

Pruitt, K. M., Adamson, M., and Arnold, R. (1979). Lactoperoxidase binding to streptococci. *Infect. Immun.* 25, 304–309.

Pruitt, K. M., Tenovuo, J., Fleming, W., and Adamson, M. (1982). Limiting factors for the generation of hypothiocyanite ion, an antimicrobial agent, in human saliva. *Caries Res.* 16, 315–323.

Pruitt, K. M., Tenovuo, J., Månsson-Rahemtulla, B., Harrington, P., and Baldone, D. C. (1986). Is thiocyanate peroxidation at equilibrium *in vivo*? *Biochim. Biophys. Acta* 870, 385–391.

Pruitt, K. M., Rahemtulla, F., Månsson-Rahemtulla, B., Baldone, D. C., and Laven, G. T. (1991). Peroxidases in human milk. *Adv. Exp. Biol. Med.* 310, 137–144.

Pugin, J., Schurer-Maly, C. C., Leturcq, D., Moriarty, A., Ulevitch, R. J., and Tobias, P. S. (1993). Lipopolysaccharide activation of human endothelial and epithelial cells is mediated by lipopolysaccharide-binding protein and soluble CD14. *Proc. Natl. Acad. Sci. USA* 90, 2744–2748.

Quayle, A. J. (2002). The innate and early immune response to pathogen challenge in the female genital tract and the pivotal role of epithelial cells. *J. Reprod. Immunol.* 57, 61–79.

Rado, T. A., Wei, X., and Benz, E. J. (1987). Isolation of lactoferrin cDNA from a human myeloid library and expression of mRNA during normal and leukemic myelopoiesis. *Blood* 70, 989–993.

Roberts, A. K., Chierici, R., Sawatzki, G., Hill, M. J., Volpatos, S., and Vigi, V. (1992). Supplementation of an adapted formula with bovine lactoferrin: 1. Effect on the infant faecal flora. *Acta Paediatr.* 81, 119–124.

Robinovitch, M. R., Ashley, R. L., Iversen, J. M., Vigoren, E. M., Oppenheim, F. G., and Lamkin, M. (2001). Parotid salivary basic proline-rich proteins inhibit HIV-I infectivity. *Oral Dis.* 7, 69–70.

Rochard, E., Legrand, D., Lecocq, M., Hamelin, R., Crepin, M., Montreuil, J., and Spik, G. (1992). Characterization lf lactotransferrin receptor in epithelial cell lines from non-malignant human breast, benign mastopathies and breast carcinoma. *Anticanc. Res.* 12, 2047–2052.

Roos, A., Bouwman, L. H., van Gijlswijk-Janssen, D. J., Faber-Krol, M. C., Stahl, G. L., and Daha, M. R. (2001). Human IgA activates the complement system via the mannan-binding lectin pathway. *J. Immunol.* 167, 2861–2868.

Rothstein, D. M., Spacciapoli, P., Tran, L. T., Xu, T., Roberts, F. D., Dalla Serra, M., Buxton, D. K., Oppenheim, F. G., and Friden, P. (2001). Anticandida activity is retained in P-113, a 12-amino-acid fragment of histatin 5. *Antimicrob. Agents Chemother.* 45, 1367–1373.

Rundegren, J. (1986). Calcium-dependent salivary agglutinin with reactivity to various oral streptococcal species. *Infect. Immun.* 53, 173–178.

Ruzindana-Umunyana, A., and Weber, J. M. (2001). Interactions of human lacrimal and salivary cystatins with adenovirus endopeptidase. *Antiviral Res.* 51, 203–214.

Sabatini, L. M., Ota, T., and Azen, E. A. (1993). Nucleotide sequence analysis of the human salivary protein genes *HIS1* and *HIS2*, and evolution of the STATH/HIS gene family. *Mol. Biol. Evol.* 10, 497–511.

Sajjan, U. S., Tran, L. T., Sole, N., Rovaldi, C., Akiyama, A., Friden, P. M., Forstner, J. F., and Rothstein, D. M. (2001). P-113D, an antimicrobial peptide active against *Pseudomonas aeruginosa*, retains activity in the presence of sputum from cystic fibrosis patients. *Antimicrob. Agents Chemother.* 45, 3437–4344.

Sallmann, F. R., Baveye-Descamps, S., Pattus, F., Salmon, V., Branza, N., Spik, G., and Legrand, D. (1999). Porins OmpC and PhoE of *Escherichia coli* as specific cell-surface targets of human lactoferrin. *J. Biol. Chem.* 274, 16107–16114.

Sano, H., Sohma, H., Muta, T., Nomura, S., Voelker, D. R., and Kuroki, Y. (1999). Pulmonary surfactant protein A modulates the cellular response to smooth and rough lipopolysaccharides by interaction with CD14. *J. Immunol.* 163, 387–395.

Satyanarayana, J., Situ, H., Narasimhamurthy, S., Bhayani, N., Bobek, L. A., and Levine, M. J. (2000). Divergent solid-phase synthesis and candidacidal activity of *MUC7* D1, a 51-residue histidine-rich N-terminal domain of human salivary mucin *MUC7*. *J. Pept. Res.* 56, 275–282.

Schaible, U. E., Collins, H. L., Priem, F., and Kaufmann, S. H. (2002). Correction of the iron overload defect in beta-2-microglobulin knockout mice by lactoferrin abolishes their increased susceptibility to tuberculosis. *J. Exp. Med.* 196, 1507–1513.

Schenkels, L. C. P. M., Gururaja, T. L., and Levine, M. J. (1996). Salivary mucins: Their role in oral mucosal barrier function and drug delivery. In *Oral Mucosal Drug Delivery* (ed. M. J. Rathbone), 191–220. New York: Marcel Dekker.

Schryvers, A. B., and Vogel, H. J. (2002). Lactoferrin: Structure, function, and applications. *Biochem. Cell. Biol.* 80, 1–168.

Shakibaei, M., and Frevert, U. (1996). Dual interaction of the malaria circumsporozoite protein with the low density lipoprotein receptor-related protein (LRP) and heparan sulfate proteoglycans. *J. Exp. Med.* 184, 1699–1711.

Shi, Y., Kong, W., and Nakayama, K. (2000). Human lactoferrin binds and removes the hemoglobin receptor protein of the periodontopathogen *Porphyromonas gingivalis*. *J. Biol. Chem.* 275, 30002–30008.

Shimizu, K., Matsuzawa, H., Okada, K., Tazume, S., Dosako, S., Kawasaki, Y., Hashimoto, K., and Koga, Y. (1996). Lactoferrin-mediated protection of the host from murine cytomegalovirus infection by a T-cell-dependent augmentation of natural killer cell activity. *Arch. Virol.* 141, 1875–1889.

Shin, K., Hayasawa, H., and Lönnerdal, B. (2001). Inhibition of *Escherichia coli* respiratory enzymes by the lactoperoxidase-hydrogen peroxide-thiocyanate antimicrobial system. *J. Appl. Microbiol.* 90, 489–493.

Shine, N. R., Wang, S. C., Konopka, K., Burks, E. A., Duzgunes, N., and Whitman, C. P. (2002). Secretory leukocyte protease inhibitor: inhibition of human immunodeficiency virus-1 infection of monocytic THP-1 cells by a newly cloned protein. *Bioorg. Chem.* 30, 249.

Shugars, D. C., and Wahl, S.M. (1998). The role of the oral environment in HIV transmission. *J. Am. Dent. Assoc.* 129, 851–858.

Shugars, D. C., Watkins, C. A., and Cowen, H. J. (2001). Salivary concentration of secretory leukocyte protease inhibitor, an antimicrobial protein, is decreased with advanced age. *Gerontology* 47, 246–253.

Singh, P. K., Paresek, M. R., Greenberg, E. P., and Welsh, M. J. (2002). A component of innate immunity prevents bacterial biofilm development. *Nature* 417, 552–555.

Slungaard, A., and Mahoney, J. R. Jr. (1991). Thiocyanate is the major substrate for eosinophil peroxidase in physiologic fluids. Implications for cytotoxicity. *J. Biol. Chem.* 266, 4903–4910.

Son, K. N., Park, J., Chung, C. K., Chung, D. K., Yu, D. Y., Lee, K. K., and Kim, J. (2002). Human lactoferrin activates transcription of *IL-1beta* gene in mammalian cells. *Biochem. Biophys. Res. Comm.* 290, 236–241.

Soukka, T., Lumikari, M., and Tenovuo, J. (1991). Combined inhibitory effect of human lactoferrin and lysozyme against *Streptococcus mutans* serotype c. *Microbial Ecol. Health Dis.* 4, 259–264.

Strunk, R. C., Eidlin, D. M., and Mason, R. J. (1988). Pulmonary alveolar type II epithelial cells synthesize and secrete proteins of the classical and alternative complement pathways. *J. Clin. Invest.* 81, 1419–1426.

Strynadka, N. C., and James, M. N. (1996). Lysozyme: A model enzyme in protein crystallography. *EXS* 75, 185–222.

Superti, F., Siciliano, R., Rega, B., Giansanti, F., Valenti, P., and Antonini, G. (2001). Involvement of bovine lactoferrin metal saturation, sialic acid and protein fragments in the inhibition of rotavirus infection. *Biochim. Biophys. Acta* 1528, 107–115.

Suzuki, Y. A., Shin, K., and Lonnerdal, B. (2001). Molecular cloning and functional expression of a human intestinal lactoferrin receptor. *Biochemistry* 40, 15771–15779.

Svensson, M., Sabharwal, H., Hakansson, A., Mossberg, A. K., Lipniunas, P., Leffler, H., Svanborg, C., and Linse, S. (1999). Molecular characterization of alpha-lactalbumin folding variants

that induce apoptosis in tumor cells. *J. Biol. Chem.* 274, 6388–6396.

Svensson, M., Hakansson, A., Mossberg, A. K., Linse, S., and Svanborg, C. (2000). Conversion of alpha-lactalbumin to a protein inducing apoptosis. *Proc. Natl. Acad. Sci. USA* 97, 4221–4226.

Tabak, L. A. (1995). In defense of the oral cavity: structure, biosynthesis, and function of salivary mucins. *Annu. Rev. Physiol.* 57, 547–564.

Tabak, L. A. (1998). Protein structure and function relationships: Mucins. In *Oral Biology at the Turn of the Century* (eds. B. Guggenheim and S. Shapiro), 189–197. Basel, Switzerland: S. Karger.

Teng, C. T. (2002). Lactoferrin gene expression and regulation: An overview. *Biochem. Cell Biol.* 80, 7–16.

Tenovuo, J. (1985). The peroxidase system in human secretions. In *The Lactoperoxidase System. Chemistry and Biological Significance* (eds. K. M. Pruitt and J. Tenovuo), 101–122. New York: Marcel Dekker.

Tenovuo, J. (1989). Nonimmunoglobulin defense factors in human saliva. In *Human Saliva: Clinical Chemistry and Microbiology* (ed. J. O. Tenovuo), vol. 2, 55–91. Boca Raton, FL: CRC Press.

Tenovuo, J. (1998). Antimicrobial function of human saliva: How important is it for oral health? *Acta Odontol. Scand.* 56, 250–256.

Tenovuo, J. (2002). Clinical applications of antimicrobial host proteins lactoperoxidase, lysozyme and lactoferrin in xerostomia: Efficacy and safety. *Oral Dis.* 8, 23–29.

Tenovuo, J., and Larjava, H. (1984). The protective effect of peroxidase and thiocyanate against hydrogen peroxide toxicity assessed by the uptake of [³H]-thymidine by human gingival fibroblasts cultured *in vitro*. *Arch. Oral Biol.* 29, 445–451.

Tenovuo, J., Månsson-Rahemtulla, B., Pruitt, K. M., and Arnold, R. (1981). Inhibition of dental plaque acid production by the salivary lactoperoxidase antimicrobial system. *Infect. Immun.* 34, 208–214.

Tenovuo, J., Moldoveanu, Z., Mestecky, J., Pruitt, K. M., and Månsson-Rahemtulla, B. (1982a). Interaction of specific and innate factors of immunity: IgA enhances the antimicrobial effect of the lactoperoxidase system against *Streptococcus mutans*. *J. Immunol.* 128, 726–731.

Tenovuo, J., Pruitt, K. M., and Thomas, E. L. (1982b). Peroxidase antimicrobial system of human saliva: hypothiocyanite levels in resting and stimulated saliva. *J. Dent. Res.* 61, 982–985.

Teraguchi, S., Shin, K., Ogata, T., Kingaku, M., Kaino, A., Miyauchi, H., Fukuwatari, Y., and Shimamura, S. (1995). Orally administered bovine lactoferrin inhibits bacterial translocation in mice fed bovine milk. *Appl. Environ. Microbiol.* 61, 4131–4134.

Thomas, E. L., and Fishman, M. (1986). Oxidation of chloride and thiocyanate by isolated leukocytes. *J. Biol. Chem.* 261, 9694–9702.

Thomas, L. L., Xu, W., and Ardon, T. T. (2002). Immobilised lactoferrin is a stimulus for eosinophil activation. *J. Immunol.* 169, 993–999.

Troxler, R. F., Offner, G. D., Xu, T., vanderSpek, J. C., and Oppenheim, F. G. (1990). Structural relationship between human salivary histatins. *J. Dent. Res.* 69, 2–6.

Tsai, H., and Bobek, L. A. (1997a). Studies of the mechanism of human salivary histatin-5 candidacidal activity with histatin-5 variants and azole-sensitive and -resistant *Candida* species. *Antimicrob. Agents Chemother.* 41, 2224–2228.

Tsai, H., and Bobek, L. A. (1997b). Human salivary histatin-5 exerts potent fungicidal activity against *Cryptococcus neoformans*. *Biochim. Biophys. Acta.* 1336, 367–369.

Turpin, J. A., Schaeffer, C. A., Bu, M., Graham, L., Buckheit, R. W. Jr., Clanton, D., and Rice, W. G. (1996). Human immunodeficiency virus type-1 (HIV-1) replication is unaffected by human secretory leukocyte protease inhibitor. *Antiviral Res.* 29, 269–277.

Twetman, S., Lindqvist, L., and Sund, M. L. (1986). Effect of human lysozyme on 2-deoxyglucose uptake by *Streptococcus mutans* and other oral microorganisms. *Caries Res.* 20, 223–229.

Uemura, K., Saka, M., Nakagawa, T., Kawasaki, N., Thiel, S., Jensenius, J. C., and Kawasaki, T. (2002). L-MBP is expressed in epithelial cells of mouse small intestine. *J. Immunol.* 169, 6945–6950.

Ulvatne, H., Haukland, H. H., Samuelsen, O., Kramer, M., and Vorland, L. H. (2002). Proteases in *Escherichia coli* and *Staphylococcus aureus* confer reduced susceptibility to lacto-ferricin B. *J. Antimicrob. Chemother.* 50, 461–467.

Van der Strate, B.W., Beljaars, L., Molema, G., Harmsen, M. C., and Meijer, D. K. (2001). Antiviral activities of lactoferrin. *Antiviral Res.* 52, 225–239.

Van Dyke, T., Paquette, D., Grossi, S., Braman, V., Massaro, J., D'Agostino, R., Dibart, S., and Friden, P. (2002). Clinical and microbial evaluation of a histatin-containing mouthrinse in humans with experimental gingivitis: A phase-2 multi-center study. *J. Clin. Periodontol.* 29, 168–176.

Van't Hof, W., Reijnders, I. M., Helmerhorst, E. J., Walgreen-Weterings, E., Simoons-Smit, I. M., Veerman, E. C., and Amerongen, A. V. (2000). Synergistic effects of low doses of histatin 5 and its ana-logues on amphotericin B anti-mycotic activity. *Antonie Van Leeuwenhoek* 78, 163–169.

Vorland, L. H., Ulvatne, H., Rekdal, O., and Svendsen, J. S. (1999). Initial binding sites of antimicrobial peptides in *Staphylococcus aureus* and *Escherichia coli. Scand. J. Infect. Dis.* 31, 467–473.

Wahl, S. M., Worley, P., Jin, W., McNeely, T. B., Eisenberg, S., Fasching, C., Orenstein, J. M., and Janoff, E. N. (1997). Anatomic dissoci-ation between HIV-1 and its endogenous inhibitor in mucosal tissues. *Am. J. Pathol.* 150, 1275–1284.

Wang, Y.-B., and Germaine, G. R. (1991). Effect of lysozyme on glucose fermentation, cytoplasmic pH, and intracellular potassium con-centrations in *Streptococcus mutans* 10449. *Infect. Immun.* 59, 638–644.

Wang, X., Hirmo, S., Willen, R., and Wadstrom, T. (2001). Inhibition of *Helicobacter pylori* infection by bovine milk glycoconjugates in a Balb/cA mouse model. *J. Med. Microbiol.* 50, 430–435.

Ward, P. P., Mendoza-Meneses, M., Cunningham, G. A., and Conneely, O. M. (2003). Iron status in mice carrying a targeted disruption of lactoferrin. *Mol. Cell. Biol.* 23, 178–185.

Weaver-Hiltke, T. R., and Bobek, L. A. (1998). Transfection of COS cells with human cystatin cDNA and its effect on HSV-1 replication. *Ann. N.Y. Acad. Sci.* 842, 204–208.

Weinberg, E. D. (2001). Human lactoferrin: A novel therapeutic with broad spectrum potential. *J. Pharm. Pharmacol.* 53, 1303–1310.

Weiss, S. J. (1989). Tissue destruction by neutrophils. *N. Engl. J. Med.* 320, 365–376.

Wilson, M. E., Lewis, T. S., Miller, M. A., McCormick, M. L., and Britigan, B. E. (2002). *Leishmania chagasi:* Uptake of iron bound to lactoferrin and transferrin requires an iron reductase. *Exp. Parasitol.* 100, 196–207.

Xu, T., Levitz, S. M., Diamond, R. D., and Oppenheim, F. G. (1991). Anticandidal activity of major human salivary histatins. *Infect. Immun.* 59, 2549–2554.

Xu, Y., Ambudkar, I., Yamagishi, H., Swaim, W., Walsh, T. J., and O'Connell, B. C. (1999). Histatin 3-mediated killing of *Candida albicans:* Effect of extracellular salt concentration on binding and internalization. *Antimicrob. Agents Chemother.* 43, 2256–2262.

Zarember, K. A., and Godowski, P. J. (2002). Tissue expression of human toll-like receptors and differential regulation of toll-like receptor mRNAs in leukocytes in response to microbes, their products, and cytokines. *J. Immunol.* 168, 554–561.

Zhang, G-H., Mann, D. M., and Tsai, C-M. (1999). Neutralization of endotoxin *in vitro* and *in vivo* by a human lactoferrin-derived peptide. *Infect. Immun.* 67, 1353–1358.

Defensins and Other Antimicrobial Peptides and Proteins

Robert I. Lehrer

Department of Medicine and Molecular Biology Institute, UCLA School of Medicine, Los Angeles, California

Charles L. Bevins

Departments of Immunology, Gastroenterology, and Colorectal Surgery, The Cleveland Clinic Foundation Research Institute, Cleveland, Ohio

Tomas Ganz

Departments of Medicine and Pathology, UCLA School of Medicine, Los Angeles, California

INTRODUCTION

Endogenous antimicrobial peptides are widely distributed among vertebrates. Most are amphiphilic, polycationic molecules with an α-helical, cystine-stabilized β-sheet, or proline-rich structure. They represent elements of a robust, ancestral animal immune system that predates the advent of lymphocytes and immunoglobulins. Secreted and cell-associated antimicrobial peptides enable their hosts to resist incursions by potential pathogens. From a pathogen's perspective, these peptides present a series of barriers to evade or overcome. In humans (and other mammals), defensins and cathelicidins are the principal antimicrobial peptides of neutrophils and epithelial cells. Many mucosal surfaces are bathed by antimicrobial proteins, including lysozyme, lactoferrin, secretory leukoprotease inhibitor (SLPI), and secretory phospholipase A2.

Defensins

All defensins have a largely β-sheet structure and contain three intramolecular cystine disulfide bonds. The smallest, θ-defensins, are circular peptides that contain 18 residues, α-defensins have between 29 and 35 residues, and β-defensins have up to 45 **(Fig. 6.1)**. To date, more than 100 α-defensin, β-defensin, and θ-defensin molecules have been reported, and humans express six different α-defensins and *at least* four β-defensins. Additional human defensin/defensinlike genes exist in five different chromosomal loci, but their expression and

properties remain to be characterized. α-Defensins occur in the neutrophils of humans, rats, rabbits, guinea pigs, and hamsters, but not in those of mice, horses, pigs, and sheep. Although the small intestinal Paneth cells of mice express at least 6 (Ouellette *et al.* 2000; Selsted *et al.* 1992) and possibly as many as 20 α-defensins (Ouellette and Selsted 1996), only two very dissimilar defensin species are found in human Paneth cells (Mallow *et al.* 1996). Two atypical α-defensins exist in rabbit kidney, but their functions remain uncertain (Bateman *et al.* 1996; Wu *et al.* 1998). Thus far, with the exception of rabbit alveolar macrophages, mononuclear phagocytes are not known to produce appreciable amounts of α-defensins.

Although many human epithelial cells constitutively express human β-defensins *(HBD-1)*, this peptide is particularly abundant in the distal renal tubules and in other parts of the genitourinary tract. *HBD-2*, originally recovered from psoriatic skin (Harder *et al.* 1997), is induced in various epithelia by inflammatory signals. In the epidermis, it is present in very low amounts unless induced by interleukin-1 (IL-1) (Liu *et al.* 2003). The *HBD-3* gene was found by genomic searching (Jia *et al.* 2001) and the corresponding peptide was isolated from psoriatic skin (Harder *et al.* 2001). *HBD-4* is highly expressed in the testis (epididymis) and less abundantly in the gastric antrum (Garcia *et al.* 2001b). Since about 50 different β-defensin genes have been identified in the mouse (Scheetz *et al.* 2002), sorting out their functions and relationships to human biology is unlikely to be a simple task.

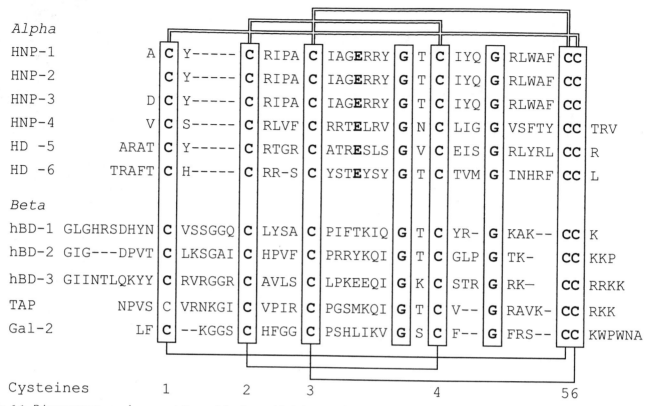

Fig. 6.1. Primary structures of representative α-defensins and β-defensins. The α-defensins (and the cells that contain them) include HNP 1–4 (human neutrophils), HD 5 and 6 (human Paneth cells), RabNP-1 (rabbit granulocytes and alveolar macrophages), and RatNP-1 (rat neutrophils). The β-defensins (and the cells that contain them) include Gal-2 (gallinacin-2, chicken granulocytes), TAP (tracheal antimicrobial peptide, bovine respiratory tract epithelia), BNBD-12 (bovine granulocytes), and hBD-1, -2, and -3 (human epithelial cells). The generally conserved or invariant residues found in both subfamilies have been boxed. The respective cysteine connectivity of α-defensins and β-defensins is shown above and below the sequences.

GENERAL PROPERTIES OF DEFENSINS

Structure of mature defensins

Figure 6.1 shows the primary amino acid sequences of eleven defensins. The six α-defensins are of human origin: HNP 1–4 from leukocytes, and HD-5 and 6 from intestinal cells. The five α-defensins include human hBDs 1–3, bovine "tracheal antimicrobial peptide" (TAP), and gallinacin-2 from chicken leukocytes. Highly conserved residues are boxed and/or bolded. Cysteines 5 and 6 are contiguous and near the carboxy-terminus in both α-defensins and β-defensins, and one of them is covalently linked to the cysteine nearest the amino terminus. Consequently, defensins are complexly folded, macrocyclic molecules.

By x-ray crystallography, human defensin HNP-3 is an elongated ellipsoid, 26 × 15 × 15 Å, dominated by a three-stranded, cystine-stabilized antiparallel β-sheet (Hill *et al.* 1991). The highly conserved Arg[6] and Glu[14] residues form a salt bridge spanning the only non–β-sheet portion of the molecule and the invariant glycine[24] occupies the third position of a Type I turn. HNP-3 crystallizes as a dimer that configures a six-stranded β-sheet stabilized by hydrophobic interactions and hydrogen bonds. That the invariant

glycine[18] is located at the dimer interface suggests that dimer formation may be an essential element of defensin-mediated activity. A dimer of the human α-defensin HNP-3 is illustrated in **Figure 6.2**.

Crystallographic analyses of *HBD-1* (Hoover *et al.* 2001) and *HBD-2* (Hoover *et al.* 2000) found very similar structures for the monomers, including the presence of a short, N-terminal, α-helical segment not present in α-defensins. It is noteworthy that a similarly positioned helical region exists in the defensinlike antimicrobial peptides of insects and plants (*e.g.*, wheat purothionine). The solution structures reported for HBDs 1, 2, and 3 show them to have similar tertiary structures, with a short helical segment preceding a three-stranded antiparallel beta-sheet (Schibli *et al.* 2002). Whereas *HBD-1* and *HBD-2* were monomeric in solution, *HBD-3* was a dimer.

Structural studies on *HBD-2* also revealed some structural similarities with MIP-3α/CCL20, a chemokine showing high affinity for CCR-6 (Perez-Canadillas *et al.* 2001). Both molecules have a rigid conformation of the N-terminal CC motif, as well as the narrow groove between the N-loop and the β2-β3 hairpin. Interestingly, *HBD-2* also binds to CCR-6 and exhibits chemoattractant activity for dendritic cells

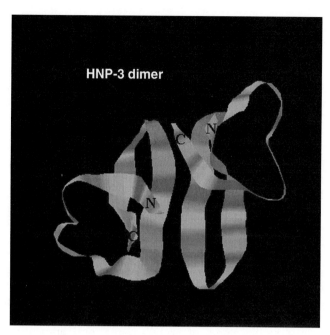

Fig. 6.2. A dimer of human α-defensin HNP-3. The figure is based on coordinates obtained from X-ray crystallography (Hill *et al.* 1991).

through its interaction with this chemokine receptor (Yang *et al.* 1999).

The θ-defensins, initially discovered in rhesus macaque neutrophils, have a remarkable structure, so far unique among mammalian peptides. These 18–amino acid (aa) peptides with three intramolecular disulfide bonds have a cyclic amide backbone (Tang *et al.* 1999; Leonova *et al.* 2001), formed from two nonapeptides by a novel posttranslational ligation reaction. The nonapeptides are encoded by two θ-defensin genes very similar to conventional α-defensins except that they are shortened by a "premature" stop codon, and contain only three cysteines. Either homodimers or heterodimers can be joined to form a mature θ-defensin peptide.

Structure and location of defensin genes
Many different defensin genes have been sequenced. The myeloid α-defensin (DEFA) genes have similar layouts, with three exons that correspond approximately to the 5′-untranslated region, signal sequence/propiece, and mature defensin region (Linzmeier *et al.* 1993). The genes for HD-5 and 6, α-defensins expressed predominantly within the human intestine, have only two exons as do the DEFB genes that encode β-defensins, suggesting that the evolution of α-defensins involved both deletional and insertional events. Although dissimilar in their genomic sequence, the genes for HD-5 and HD-6 show considerable sequence similarity in their proximal 5′-flanking regions, which presumably contain elements involved in their tissue-specific expression (Mallow *et al.* 1996; Salzman *et al.* 2003). The DEFA genes encoding human myeloid and enteric α-defensins are clustered on human chromosome 8 (Linzmeier *et al.* 1999). The human

DEFB genes that encode *HBD-1*, HDB-2, and HDB-3 contain two exons and are all within a few hundred kilobases from the myeloid α-defensin locus on chromosome 8p23 (Liu *et al.* 1997; Peng *et al.* 2001). This region is also home to a DEFT pseudogene that is highly homologous to the genes encoding the α-defensins of rhesus monkeys. θ-defensin (DEFT) genes evidently arose in an Old World monkey when the mutation of a preexisting α-defensin gene placed a premature stop codon within Exon 3 of a DEFA gene. Additional defensin and defensinlike genes have been identified in four other chromosomal loci, but their tissue expression and biology remain to be characterized (Schutte *et al.* 2002).

Activities of defensins
Gram-positive and gram-negative bacteria
A review of the antimicrobial activity of defensins against gram-positive and gram-negative bacteria is available (Lehrer *et al.* 1993). Briefly, defensins are effective broad-spectrum microbicides, especially when present in high local concentrations or acting in low–ionic strength media. High local concentrations occur within phagolysosomes, in the capillary-like lumen of small intestinal crypts, and at interfaces between effector and target cells.

Rabbit defensins NP-1 and NP-2 bind with high affinity to *Pseudomonas aeruginosa* PAO1, forming small surface blebs and permeabilizing its outer membrane. This process, sometimes called "self-promoted uptake" (Sawyer *et al.* 1988), allows the polycationic peptide molecules to displace divalent cations that link adjacent lipopolysaccharide (LPS) molecules. The consequent permeability changes allow otherwise excluded molecules, such as lysozyme, to enter the periplasmic space and attack the bacterium further. Viljanen and coworkers (Viljanen *et al.* 1988) noted that human defensins increased the outer membrane's permeability to hydrophobic probes (e.g., rifampin) in *P. aeruginosa*, *Escherichia coli*, and *Salmonella typhimurium*. Bactericidal concentrations of HNP-1 permeabilized the outer and inner membranes of *E. coli*, causing immediate and simultaneous cessation of macromolecular synthesis and respiration (Lehrer *et al.* 1989a).

Permeabilization of microbial cell membranes is a hallmark of defensin-mediated antimicrobial activity. Especially with human defensins, such permeabilization is prevented by treatments that inhibit the target cell's metabolism, growth, or transmembrane protonmotive force (Lehrer *et al.* 1989a). Defensins permeabilize artificial phospholipid membranes only when a transmembrane electronmotive force of sufficient magnitude and correct polarity is applied (Kagan *et al.* 1990). Membrane conductance increases as the second to fourth power of the defensin concentration, suggesting that two to four defensin molecules interact to form a channel in this system. Wimley and associates (Wimley *et al.* 1994) examined interactions between human defensins and lipid bilayers. They found that HNP-2 (net charge, +3) bound to and permeabilized unilamellar vesicles composed of anionic phospholipids, but not those formed of electroneutral phospholipids. Data from experiments with entrapped markers of different sizes suggested that multimeric HNP-2 formed aqueous pores with a maximum diameter of ~25 Å. If such pores formed in bacterial membranes, they should allow passage of defensin monomers and even dimers (~26 × 15 × 15 Å) to more interior sites.

Certain bacteria are intrinsically resistant to defensins, including *Neisseria gonorrhoeae* (Qu *et al.* 1996a), *Burkholderia cepacia*, *Burkholderia pseudomallei* (Jones *et al.* 1996), and *Brucella spp.* (Martinez de Tejada *et al.* 1995). What can make bacteria resistant has been partially explained by identifying mutations that *increase* bacterial susceptibility to antimicrobial peptides. Studies on the intracellular enteric pathogen *S. typhimurium* revealed the importance of the two-component regulatory system, PhoP/PhoQ. PhoQ is a magnesium-binding sensor kinase that responds to ionic and other environmental changes by phosphorylating PhoP, a DNA-binding protein that can activate numerous genes, including some needed for resistance to antimicrobial peptides and intracellular survival (Miller *et al.* 1990; Chamnongpol *et al.* 2003). These include important aspects of LPS structure (Ernst *et al.* 2001), and expression of an outer membrane protease that cleaves, and presumably inactivates, certain antimicrobial peptides (Guina *et al.* 2000).

Studies with *Staphylococcus aureus* associated its relative resistance to defensins and other cationic antimicrobial peptides to the modification of its membrane phospholipids with L-lysine (Kristian *et al.* 2003) and of its lipoteichoic acids with D-alanine (Collins *et al.* 2002). Both modifications reduce electrostatic binding of the peptides to the staphylococcal surface. *N. gonorrhoeae* may owe its defensin-resistance to an energy-dependent "mtr" efflux pump (Shafer *et al.* 1998). These findings suggest that interactions with cationic antimicrobial peptides may have profoundly influenced bacterial evolution.

In summary, the effect of defensins on microbes can be envisioned to occur in stages. Electrostatic adsorption to anionic sites on or near the target cell's membrane or (for certain defensins) to sugars in microbial glycoproteins or LPS result in locally high concentrations that promote defensin aggregation and multimer formation. Insertion of defensins into microbial membranes is assisted by their positive charge and by the target cell's transmembrane potential. The ensuing membrane disruption and channel formation permit intracytoplasmic entry of defensins and allow essential microbial components to leak out. Unless repaired, these events lead to irreversible target cell injury.

Fungi

Mammalian defensins can kill various fungal pathogens, including *Candida* spp., *Cryptococcus neoformans*, and hyphae and germinating spores of *Rhizopus oryzae* and *Aspergillus fumigatus* (reviewed in Lehrer *et al.* 1993). In recent years, the antifungal properties of defensins have been studied more by botanists and agriculturists than by immunologists. This reflects the importance of fungi as plant pathogens (Thomma *et al.* 2002) and the likely utility of transgenic plants. Plant defensins, like those of mammalian origin,

probably owe their antifungal properties to an ability to induce membrane permeabilization (Thevissen *et al.* 1999).

Mycobacteria, spirochetes, and protozoa

Both human and rabbit defensins show activity against mycobacteria, including *M. tuberculosis* (Miyakawa *et al.* 1996; Sharma *et al.* 2000) and *M. avium-intracellulare* (Ogata *et al.* 1992), even in the presence of divalent cations or physiologic salt concentrations. Although the plasma membrane of *M. tuberculosis* is the principal target for HNP-1 action, its DNA may be a secondary target (Sharma and Khuller 2001). Human neutrophils can ingest and kill both *M. avium* (Hartmann *et al.* 2001) and *M. tuberculosis*, and the latter is apparently subdued by nonoxidative mechanisms (Kisich *et al.* 2002). *In vivo*, mycobacteria that evaded or survived the attentions of neutrophils would likely find a defensin-free sanctuary once resident within a macrophage, because the only mammalian macrophages known to contain significant quantities of defensins are alveolar macrophages of the rabbit.

In a rabbit model of syphilis, large local amounts of defensins were seen during the first 24 hours. This subsided, but reappeared on days 10 to 16, when healing began (Borenstein *et al.* 1991). The Nichols strain of *Treponema pallidum* was neutralized by rabbit defensins *in vitro* and *in vivo*. *Borrelia burgdorferi*, the causative agent of Lyme disease, is also susceptible to defensins (Lusitani *et al.* 2002).

The effect of defensins on protozoans has received little study, at least in vertebrates. Human α-defensin HNP-1, mouse Paneth cell defensin-2 and defensin-3 (cryptdins), and rabbit α-Defensin NP-2 killed trophozoites of *Giardia lamblia*, especially when the concentrations of sodium chloride and divalent cations were low (Aley *et al.* 1994).

Antiviral properties

Both α-defensins (Zhang *et al.* 2002) and θ-defensins (Cole *et al.* 2002) can protect cells from infection by HIV-1 *in vitro*. Persons infected with human immunodeficiency virus–1 (HIV-1) whose α,β CD8 T cells maintain the ability to produce and release α-defensins may exhibit relative resistance to developing acquired immune deficiency syndrome-defining (AIDS-defining) symptoms, compared with HIV-infected subjects whose T cells are defective in this regard (Zhang *et al.* 2002). θ-Defensins act by blocking an early step in the uptake process, and their ability to do so correlates with their ability to bind gp120 with high affinity (Cole *et al.* 2002). α-defensins also bind gp120 with high affinity, but their mechanisms of action against HIV-1 has not yet been defined.

α-Defensins also protect cells from infection by herpes simplex virus (HSV) types 1 and 2 in tissue culture media (Daher *et al.* 1986), by interfering with an early step in the infection process (Sinha *et al.* 2003). Human and rabbit α-defensins also neutralized vesicular stomatitis and influenza A/WSN virus, but lacked significant activity against cytomegalovirus, reovirus, and echovirus (Daher *et al.* 1986). Among the nonenveloped viruses, only adenoviruses have so far been reported to be susceptible to defensins (Gropp *et al.* 1999; Bastian and Schafer 2001).

Cytotoxic activity

Purified human defensins kill various normal and tumor cell targets in a concentration and time-dependent fashion (reviewed in Lehrer *et al.* 1993) and show synergistic activity when combined with sublytic concentrations of hydrogen peroxide. Defensin molecules bound to mammalian target cells with biphasic kinetics, similar to those with *Candida albicans*. K562 cells exposed to 20 µg/ml of radiolabeled HNP-1 bound approximately 4.3×10^9 defensin molecules per cell. This initial binding did not cause cytolysis and was comparable in defensin-resistant and defensin-sensitive targets cells. After 5 to 10 minutes, sensitive targets became permeable to trypan blue (molecular weight = 960 Da) and manifested enhanced transmembrane ion flux. Membrane-bound defensin molecules became progressively more difficult to dislodge by adding serum, and after 3 to 4 hours, the cells began releasing ^{51}Cr-labeled cytoplasmic components. Strand breaks and adenosine triphosphate–ribosylation (ADP-ribosylation) were first detected in K562 and Raji targets 6–8 hours after incubation with HNP, and these increased to maximal levels by 18 hours. DNA was not degraded into nucleosome-sized fragments. Other experiments suggested that the initial defensin-induced pores were voltage dependent and that defensin-mediated injury to mammalian cells depended on an energized target cell membrane. Since defensins are bound by α2-macroglobulin and other normal serum components, it is not surprising that defensins were minimally, if at all, cytotoxic in the presence of serum. Whether and where defensins are cytotoxic *in vivo* is not known.

Other properties of defensins

Although most studies of defensins have examined their antimicrobial properties, considerable evidence suggests that some defensins also play other roles, including immunomodulation, hormonal regulation, opsonization, and stimulating wound repair. Human neutrophil defensins are chemotactic for human monocytes (Territo *et al.* 1989), T-cells (Chertov *et al.* 1996), and immature dendritic cells (Yang *et al.* 2000) *in vitro*, so that their release from neutrophils could provide a signal to mobilize immunocompetent mononuclear cells. Defensins also induce the synthesis of interleukin-8 (IL-8), a C-X-C cytokine, by human airway epithelial cells, possibly providing a mechanism to recruit additional neutrophils to sites of inflammation (Van Wetering *et al.* 1997). The α-defensins of human neutrophils were shown to act as adjuvants to enhance systemic IgG antibody response (Lillard *et al.* 1999). Murine β-defensin MBD-2 acted as an adjuvant for tumor immunization, by providing a costimulatory signal via the toll-like receptor 4 (Biragyn *et al.* 2002). It is not yet clear whether these activities are shared by other defensins.

Rabbit NP-3a ("corticostatin") and certain other α-defensins bound reversibly to the adrenocorticotropic hormone (ACTH) receptor of rat adrenal cells *in vitro* and inhibited ACTH-stimulated steroidogenesis (Zhu and Solomon 1992). Rabbit defensins NP-1 and NP-2 greatly enhanced the ability of rabbit alveolar macrophages to ingest bacteria and fungi under serum-free conditions (Fleischmann *et al.* 1985). Defensins were mitogenic for fibroblasts (Murphy *et al.* 1993), and small daily injections of rabbit defensins accelerated wound healing in rats (Kudriashov *et al.* 1990). Guinea pig defensins were reported to release histamine from rat mast cells *in vitro* (Yamashita and Saito 1989).

DEFENSINS IN MYELOID CELLS

Role in mucosal host defense

Most normal mucosal surfaces contain considerably more epithelial cells than neutrophils or macrophages. Notable exceptions include the gingival crevices that surround teeth, which are bathed in high concentrations of neutrophils and their components. Neutrophil defensin concentrations as high as 1 mg/ml have been detected in such fluids (T. Ganz and K. Miyasaki, unpublished) and could play an important role in controlling local microbial proliferation.

In other locations, neutrophils and macrophages are rapidly recruited to epithelial surfaces when the primary mucosal defenses are overwhelmed by microbial invaders. The important function of these secondary defenses is illustrated by the particularly severe impact of neutropenia on the integrity of oral and gastrointestinal mucosae and the characteristic involvement of periodontal tissues in congenital or acquired neutrophil disorders.

Cellular localization of myeloid defensins

Each human neutrophil contains several thousand cytoplasmic granules that are divided into three principal subtypes, called primary (or azurophil), secondary (or specific), and tertiary. These subtypes can be distinguished by buoyant density, when they are made during the neutrophil's maturation, their response to secretagogues, and their composition. About 30% to 50% of the protein content of the azurophil granules consists of defensins. Relatively small amounts of defensins are released extracellularly after phagocytosis or secretagogue exposure, as the peptides are preferentially delivered phagosomes that contain opsonized bacteria (Joiner *et al.* 1989). This targeted delivery of defensins not only places them where they are most needed, but it also helps minimize any potential cytotoxicity to host tissues. The high concentrations of defensins in human neutrophils are not unique: α-defensins are similarly plentiful in the granules of rabbit neutrophils (~10–15 µg/million cells) and rabbit alveolar macrophages (~2 µg/million cells). Although myeloid defensins (HNPs) 1–4 are most abundant in neutrophils, HNP-1 is also highly expressed by natural killer (NK) cells (Obata-Onai *et al.* 2002; Agerberth *et al.* 2000) and can be produced by other lymphocytes (Agerberth *et al.* 2000).

Structure and production of myeloid defensin precursors

Although human blood neutrophils contain about 5 µg of defensins per million cells, defensin mRNA is not detectable in Northern blots of mature neutrophils, indicating that defensin synthesis is restricted to the neutrophil's bone marrow precursors. Myeloid α-defensins are synthesized as 90–95-aa prepropeptides with a generally well-conserved signal sequence, followed by an anionic propiece and the C-terminally placed defensin domain. Nevertheless, nearly all of the defensin in neutrophil azurophil granules is found to be completely processed to 29–30-aa mature peptides (Harwig *et al.* 1992).

Posttranslational defensin processing has been studied in metabolically labeled HL-60 and CML cells (Valore and Ganz 1992). Their earliest defensin intermediate contained 75 aa and arose by cotranslational removal of the 19-residue signal sequence. Considerable quantities of this 75-aa form were secreted into the medium, and the remainder was proteolytically processed over 20 hours via a 56-aa intermediate into the mature 29-aa and 30-aa defensins. Mature human neutrophils also contained minor amounts (0.25% of total defensins) of incompletely processed 39-aa, 34-aa, and 32-aa defensins (Harwig and Ganz 1992).

This pattern of synthesis and posttranslational processing was substantially reproduced when the HNP-1 defensin cDNA was transduced into defensinless murine 32D and 32D cl3 cells (Liu and Ganz 1995). These transgenic lines accumulated mature defensin in acidified vacuoles corresponding to lysosomes or immature granules. In contrast, two transgenic, defensin-producing nonmyeloid cell lines (an embryonic NIH 3T3 cell line and the pituitary adenoma cell line AtT-20) failed to process the 75-aa prodefensin, indicating that the requisite processing pathway may be tissue specific.

To study the role of the propiece in preproHNP-1, a series of in-frame deletions between the signal peptidase site and the aminoterminus of the mature defensin region (aa 21–64) was constructed, packaged, and transduced into the 32D cl3 granulocytic cell line. Deletions in the amino-terminal two-fifths of the propiece had only minor effects on defensin biosynthesis and did not interfere with accumulation of mature defensin in the granules of 32D cl3 cells. Deletions in the carboxyterminal three-fifths of the propiece diminished net defensin synthesis, blocked constitutive secretion of prodefensin, and interfered with defensin accumulation in cytoplasmic granules. These effects were reproduced by the smaller deletion Δ_{40-51}, which contains a highly conserved secondary structure. Therefore, propiece residues 40–51 appear to be essential for subcellular trafficking and sorting of human neutrophil α-defensins (Liu and Ganz 1995).

β-defensins in animal leukocytes

Instead of containing α-defensins like those found in human, rabbit, rat, hamster, and guinea pig neutrophils, bovine neutrophils contain an impressive array of β-defensin peptides (Selsted *et al.* 1993). Whereas myeloid α-defensins have free amino termini, about half of the β-defensins isolated from bovine neutrophils had a pyroglutamate residue at their amino terminus. This moiety characteristically results from enzymatic modification of an amino-terminal glutamine residue and could confer resistance to proteolytic cleavage by local proteases or alter other biologic properties. The β-defensin peptides from neutrophils manifest antibacterial activity against gram-positive and gram-negative bacteria, but because different *in vitro* assay conditions were used, direct comparison of the relative activity of bovine epithelial and neutrophil β-defensins is not yet possible.

β-defensins ("gallinacins") were also isolated from the leukocytes of chickens (Harwig *et al.* 1994) and turkeys (Evans *et al.* 1994). Two of the three chicken gallinacins differed at only three amino-acid residues and had comparable antibacterial and antifungal activities. The third gallinacin differed at over half of the amino acids and exerted antibacterial activity, but lacked the antifungal activity seen with the other two (Harwig *et al.* 1994). The β-defensins of turkeys showed good activity against *C. albicans*, *Salmonella enteriditis*, and *Campylobacter jejuni*, but were relatively ineffective against *Pasteurella multocida* at 16 µg/ml, the highest peptide concentration tested. They did not neutralize infectious bronchitis virus, an enveloped coronavirus (Evans *et al.* 1995). In normal chickens, the expression of gallinacin-3 was especially prominent in the tongue, bursa of Fabricius, and trachea. It also occurred in other organs, including skin, esophagus, air sacs, large intestine, and kidney. The tracheal expression of gallinacin-3 increased significantly in chickens experimentally infected with *Haemophilus paragallinarum* (Zhao *et al.* 2001).

α-DEFENSINS IN ENTERIC PANETH CELLS

Role of endogenous intestinal antibiotics

Despite continual entry of microorganisms from swallowed food and oral secretions, the normal small intestine contains only a sparse resident flora. Why? Although multiple factors contribute, the ability of intestinal enterocytes and Paneth cells to secrete antimicrobial molecules is likely to play a significant role. Through their differential antimicrobial activities, these molecules could contribute to selecting the normal intestinal flora, which may afford protection from pathogenic bacteria that enter the intestine. Since the intestinal epithelium stem cells reside in the intestinal crypts, secretion of Paneth cell defensins into the crypt lumen **(Figure 6.3)** could provide a protective barrier for this vital proliferative compartment.

Identification of enteric α-defensins in Paneth cells

Paneth cells, first described over 100 years ago, are located at the base of the crypts of Lieberkühn. They are more abundant in the region of the ileum and jejunum and less so in the duodenum. The high density of Paneth cells in the distal

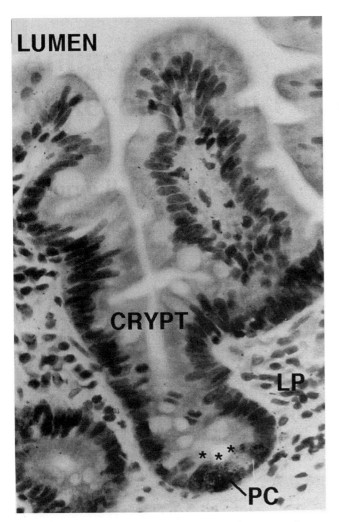

Fig. 6.3. Human small intestine, immunostained for HD-5. A longitudinally cut tubular crypt is prominent and contains several Paneth cells (PC) that contain numerous large, immunoreactive granules (asterisks). The intestinal lumen and the lamina propria (LP) have been labeled. Reproduced from Porter *et al.* (1997a) with permission.

small intestine might signify a role in preventing adverse consequences from reflux of colonic flora into the ileum. Paneth cells contain an extensive endoplasmic reticulum and Golgi network and are filled with numerous, apically located eosinophilic secretory granules whose secretion is stimulated by cholinergic agonists or the entry of bacteria or lipopolysaccharide into the intestinal lumen (Satoh 1988; Qu *et al.* 1996b).

Ouellette and colleagues (Ouellette *et al.* 1989) identified an α-defensin among several prominently expressed RNA messages in the postnatal mouse small intestine. Because this mRNA was expressed in Paneth cells at the base of small intestinal crypts, the corresponding peptides were named "cryptdins." Cryptdin mRNA levels were normal in germfree and nude mice, suggesting that expression was independent of T-cell signals or acquisition of the intestinal flora. Independently, two α-defensin genes (*HD-5* and

HD-6) expressed in human Paneth cells were detected (Jones and Bevins 1992, 1993). In contrast to the six characterized murine enteric defensin genes, which had very high (85%) nucleotide similarity, *HD-5* and *HD-6* were not as closely related, presumably having duplicated and diverged before their murine counterparts (Bevins *et al.* 1996). The striking difference in murine and human enteric defensin gene numbers remains enigmatic. Paneth cells also secrete larger antimicrobial polypeptides, including lysozyme and secretory phospholipase A2 (see sections on "Identification of enteric α-defensins in Paneth cells" and "Developmental regulation of enteric α-defensin expression" in this chapter).

Antimicrobial activity of enteric α-defensins

Native mature defensins (cryptdins) have antibacterial and activity comparable with myeloid defensins (Selsted *et al.* 1992; Eisenhauer *et al.* 1992) and can kill the protozoan parasite *Giardia lamblia* (Aley *et al.* 1994). Recombinant human small intestinal defensin HD-5 was effective against *Listeria monocytogenes*, *S. typhimurium*, and *C. albicans* (Porter *et al.* 1997b; Ghosh *et al.* 2002). It showed minimal cytotoxic activity against human intestinal cell lines (Porter *et al.* 1997a).

Developmental regulation of enteric α-defensin expression

Morphologically identifiable Paneth cells appear in the mouse intestine immediately before birth. Thereafter, murine α-defensin mRNA levels and defensin immunoreactivity increase gradually and reach adult levels by the fourth postnatal week, paralleling expansion of the Paneth cell population. Mice reared in a germfree environment express comparable levels of enteric α-defensins (Ouellette *et al.* 1989; Putsep *et al.* 2000). In humans, a sensitive RT-PCR assay can detect mRNA encoding human enteric defensins HD-5 and HD-6 at 13.5 weeks' gestation, close to the time that morphologically distinguishable Paneth cells can be identified by electron microscopy. At approximately 24 weeks' gestation, HD-5 and HD-6 mRNA was detected in Paneth cells of the small intestinal crypt by *in situ* hybridization. By Northern blot analysis, the levels were approximately 100-fold lower than in adults. The ability to detect human enteric defensin mRNA prenatally indicates that its expression is at least partially constitutive and governed by a developmental program that operates without direct stimulation by microbes or their products.

Like their hematopoietic counterparts, intestinal α-defensins are initially synthesized as prepropeptides. However, unlike the myeloid defensins, Paneth cell defensins are stored as propeptides, exclusively so in humans (Porter *et al.* 1998; Ouellette *et al.* 2000; Ghosh *et al.* 2002). The posttranslational processing of these epithelial α-defensins appears to be an important regulatory step in the generation of bioactive peptides in the small intestine. However, the pathways of processing appear to be quite different in mice and humans. In mice, the matrix metalloprotease matrilysin (matrix metalloproteinase 7) has been identified as an essential enzyme in the processing of small intestinal α-defensins (Wilson *et al.* 1999). In humans, the orthologous small intestine α-defensins are processed to mature peptides during or after secretion into the small intestinal lumen by the serine protease trypsin (Ghosh *et al.* 2002). In both species, the proteases mediating this α-defensin processing are expressed by Paneth cells.

The role of Paneth cell defensins

The hypothesis that intestinal defensins contribute to the regulation of microbial flora in the small intestine received support from studies in matrilysin-deficient mice. Matrilysin (matrix metalloproteinase 7) is expressed specifically in Paneth cells. In mice with a targeted disruption of the intestinal prodefensin-processing protease, matrilysin, Paneth cell defensin precursors were not processed to active mature peptides. The mice had increased susceptibility to intestinal infections with gram-negative organisms (Wilson *et al.* 1999). Detailed analysis of secretions from the isolated crypts of normal and matrilysin-deficient mice indicated that the antimicrobial activity of crypt secretions was largely the result of defensins and that it was greatly impaired in matrilysin-deficient mice (Ayabe *et al.* 2000).

In another model, the transgenic expression of human defensin-5 in the Paneth cells of mice increased their resistance to orally administered *S. typhimurium* but, as might be expected, did not protect against infection by the peritoneal route (Saltzman *et al.*, 2003). In the aggregate, these models point to a central role for Paneth cell defensins as regulators of small intestinal flora and as enteroprotective molecules.

EPITHELIAL β-DEFENSINS

Bovine "tracheal antimicrobial peptide" (TAP) and other animal β-defensins

Bovine tracheal extracts contain an abundant peptide called "TAP," or tracheal antimicrobial peptide, that exhibited antimicrobial activity *in vitro* against *Klebsiella pneumoniae*, *S. aureus,* and *C. albicans* (Diamond *et al.* 1991). Sequence analysis revealed similarity of this molecule to defensins expressed in leukocytes and to its designation as the first epithelial β-defensin. TAP expression was found in the pseudostratified columnar epithelial cells of conducting airway and nasal mucosa (Diamond *et al.* 1993). A hallmark of TAP expression, like several more recently described epithelial β-defensins of humans and mice, is inducible expression in response to bacterial LPS and some inflammatory cytokines (Diamond *et al.* 1996; Russell *et al.* 1996; Diamond *et al.* 2000). A canonical NF-kB recognition site in the 5′-flanking region of the *TAP* gene was important in the transcriptional regulation of this gene by bacterial products (Diamond *et al.* 2000). *In vivo* inoculation of pathogenic bacteria into the bovine lung caused a rapid and dramatic increase in β-defensin expression in the conducting airway epithelium, which was not seen in the adjacent control lobe (Stolzenberg *et al.* 1997).

In bovine tracheal epithelial cells, β-defensin induction by LPS appears to be dependent on epithelium-derived CD14, a well-characterized LPS-binding protein (Diamond *et al.* 1996). This suggests that local expression of CD-14 might provide epithelial cells with the capacity to recognize bacterial products at mucosal surfaces and initiate local defense responses such as antimicrobial peptide production.

Several additional sites of β-defensin expression were identified in cattle, including squamous epithelial cells of the tongue (Schonwetter *et al.* 1995) and epithelial cells of the small intestine and colon (Tarver *et al.* 1998). mRNA encoding a bovine lingual β-defensin ("LAP") was markedly increased in epithelia surrounding naturally occurring tongue lesions, suggesting an integral role for antimicrobial peptides in local inflammatory responses. The antimicrobial activity of LAP and TAP was very similar, and LAP expression was enhanced in bovine trachea after LPS or TNF-α application (Russell *et al.* 1996). In mice, epithelial expression of β-defensins is also observed in the mucosal epithelium of the respiratory and digestive tracts (Morrison *et al.* 1999; Bals *et al.* 1999; Jia *et al.* 2000).

Similar to humans, mice express a noninducible β-defensin in kidney tubule cells and mucosal epithelia of several organ systems (Huttner *et al.* 1997). Recent studies of mice rendered deficient in this epithelial β-defensin through targeted homologous recombination have shown a minimal phenotype (Moser *et al.* 2002; Morrison *et al.* 2002). Further studies of these mice may be necessary to elucidate the functional role of this β-defensin.

Human epithelial β-defensins

A systematic characterization of the peptides present in human blood ultrafiltrates provided the first evidence for the existence of *HBD-1*, the first characterized human β-defensin (Bensch *et al.* 1995). *HBD-1* shared the nine invariantly conserved amino acids present in β-defensins from bovine and avian cells. Although free *HBD-1* was present in nanomolar concentrations in human plasma, an abundant *HBD-1* message occurred in the kidney and vagina (Bensch *et al.* 1995). Several *HBD-1* peptides, generated by differential posttranslational proteolysis at the N-terminus, were the predominant cationic peptides in urine. When tested, using urine as a growth medium, they displayed antibacterial activity against *E. coli*. *In situ* hybridization and immunostaining localized their site of production to the distal tubules of the kidney as well as the various epithelia of the female genital tract (Valore *et al.* 1998).

HBD-1 is also present in human conducting-airway epithelia (McCray and Bentley 1997) as well as in epithelia of many other tissues and in certain glands (Zhao *et al.* 1996). Expression of *HBD-1* by lung epithelia is developmentally regulated, in a manner reminiscent of the α-defensins found in rabbit lung macrophages (McCray and Bentley 1997). Circumstantial evidence implicates the impaired function of *HBD-1*, consequent to high bronchial fluid salinity (Smith *et al.* 1996), as a contributing factor in respiratory tract colonization by *P. aeruginosa* in cystic fibrosis patients (Goldman *et al.* 1997).

HBD-2 was first detected as an abundant cationic peptide and an antimicrobial component in the flaking epidermis of patients with psoriasis (Harder *et al.* 1997). It is produced by differentiated keratinocytes in the epidermis under the influence of inflammatory signals, principally IL-1 (Liu *et al.* 1998, 2002, 2003) and secreted in lamellar bodies into the space between keratinocytes, along with the lipids that make the epidermis impermeable to water (Oren *et al.*, 2003). There, *HBD-2* reaches concentrations sufficient for antimicrobial activity (Liu *et al.* 2002). *HBD-2* is active against a broad range of microbes, with the significant exception of the skin pathogen *S. aureus* (Harder *et al.* 1997; Liu *et al.* 2002).

HBD-3 was detected more or less simultaneously by genomic methodologies (Jia *et al.* 2001; Garcia *et al.* 2001a) and by direct extraction of the peptide from psoriatic skin (Harder *et al.* 2001). *HBD-3* is one of the most cationic defensins known, with a charge of +11 at neutral pH. Unlike *HBD-2*, *HBD-3* is active against *S. aureus* and even *B. cepacia*, at least under low ionic strength conditions. The skin and the tonsils appear to have the highest levels of expression, but *HBD-3* is detectable in other epithelial and nonepithelial tissues as well. The mechanisms of its regulation have not yet been reported.

Genomic analysis indicates that many additional human β-defensin genes and related genes exist, but they remain to be characterized at the peptide level (Schutte *et al.* 2002).

EVOLUTIONARY CONSIDERATIONS

The α-defensin and β-defensin families almost certainly arose by divergence from an ancestral premammalian defensin and not by convergent evolution. This conclusion is supported by the proximity of human α-defensin and β-defensin genes within 150 kb on chromosome 8p23 (Liu *et al.* 1997). Defensinlike molecules not assignable to either defensin family have been identified in invertebrates. Hemocytes of the horseshoe crab, *Tachypleus tridentatus*, contain an antibacterial peptide ("big defensin") whose C-terminal 37 residues have a cysteine structure resembling that of mammalian β-defensins and a primary sequence similar to rat myeloid α-defensins (Saito *et al.* 1995). When the unusually long, 35-residue amino-terminal extension of

big-defensin was cleaved by tryptic digestion, both the defensinlike domain and the amino-terminal extension had antimicrobial properties. An extremely defensinlike antiviral peptide was also identified in the sea anemone, *Anemonia sulcata* (Driscoll *et al.* 1989).

The primary structural resemblance between avian β-defensins (gallinacins) and certain cytostatic (Marquardt *et al.* 1988) and myotoxic peptides in snake venoms (**Fig. 6.4**) also suggests that the progenitors of β-defensins had potential to become weapons of offense, as well as of host defense. The same can be said about the antimicrobial insect defensins, which show striking structural similarity to certain toxic peptides found in scorpion venom (Cociancich *et al.* 1993).

Given such findings, it is reasonable to postulate the antiquity of defensins as host-defense molecules. An evolutionary relationship between vertebrate defensins and the structurally more distant defensins of insects and plants is possible, but lacks convincing supporting data.

OTHER MUCOSAL DEFENSE MOLECULES

Calprotectin

Calprotectin, a member of the widespread calcium-binding S-100 protein family, is present in remarkably high concentration in the cytoplasm of human neutrophils (Brandtzaeg *et al.* 1995). The calprotectin molecule is composed of light (MRP8) and heavy (MRP14) subunits. Although not secreted from intact neutrophils, calprotectin release from dead and dying neutrophils creates high concentrations of the protein in inflammatory or abscess fluids and in the intestinal tract lumen of patients with inflammatory bowel disease. Calprotectin is also found in reactive tissue macrophages, in nonkeratinizing squamous epithelia, and in reactive epidermal cells. The C-terminal portion of calprotectin's heavy chain, MRP14, is identical to a peptide called neutrophil immobilizing factor, "NIF." Calprotectin concentrations of 50–250 µg/ml inhibit growth by *S. aureus*, *S. epidermidis*, and *E. coli*. Even lower concentrations (4–32 µg/ml) inhibit growth by *C. albicans*, possibly by depriving the *Candida* cells of zinc. Calprotectin purified from rat inflammatory peritoneal cells was markedly cytotoxic for mitogen-stimulated lymphocytes and for various tumor cell lines, in

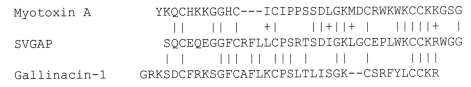

Fig. 6.4. From serpent's tooth to chicken soup. Myotoxin A is a myotoxic peptide from the venom of *Crotalus viridis viridis,* the prairie rattlesnake (Fox *et al.* 1979). SVGAP stands for snake venom growth arresting peptide (Marquardt 1988), and is described in U.S. patent 4774318. Gal-1 is the chicken β-defensin gallinacin-1, originally isolated from chicken heterophils (Harwig *et al.* 1994) and later found in chicken soup (Lehrer unpublished). The disulfide pairing patterns (1:5, 2:4, 3:6) of myotoxin A (Fox *et al.* 1979) and avian β-defensins (Harwig, unpublished) are identical.

which it induced apoptosis. Epithelial cell calprotectin might protect host cells from microbes that invade the cytoplasm directly or by lysing phagosomal membranes.

The murine MRP8 protein (also called CP10 or S100A8) is chemotactic for myeloid cells but this property is not shared by human calprotectin. Homozygous disruption of *MRP8* (*S100A8*) gene in mice causes embryonic death by day 9.5 but *MRP14* (*S100A9*)-deficient mice are viable and healthy (Manitz *et al.* 2003) even though their neutrophils lack both *MRP8/14* partners. Initial studies of these mice detected only very mild defects in neutrophil cytoskeletal organization and migration, but the activity of these neutrophils in microbicidal assays has not been reported.

Lysozyme (muramidase)

Lysozyme was discovered over 75 years ago by Fleming, who called it a "remarkable bacteriolytic ferment" and did not patent it—or penicillin, which he discovered a few years later. This very cationic 14.3-kDa protein enzymatically attacks the β1-4 glycosidic bonds between N-acetylglucosamine and N-acetylmuramic acid, which stabilize bacterial peptidoglycans. Gram-positive bacteria susceptible to the lytic action of lysozyme include *Bacillus subtilis*, *Bacillus megaterium*, and *Micrococcus luteus* (*nee lysodeicticus*). Lysozyme also exerts bactericidal activity by nonenzymatic, nonbacteriolytic mechanisms. It is a remarkably abundant component of phagocytic leukocytes, and also of tears, saliva, and many other secretions. The detection of abundant lysozyme in Paneth cell granules yielded the first clue that these intestinal epithelial cells were important in host defense (Peeters and Vantrappen 1975). Most gram-negative bacteria are resistant to lysozyme, except under very low ionic strength conditions. This is caused largely by the protective effects of their outer membrane, which covers and masks their peptidoglycan layer. Lysozyme may function most effectively in conjunction with other antimicrobial factors, especially those capable of permeabilizing the outer membrane.

Recent experiments in mice deficient in lysozyme-M (Ganz *et al.*, 2003) showed delayed killing of the lysozyme-sensitive *M. luteus*, but the major abnormality in these mice was the highly exaggerated inflammatory response to these bacteria and to peptidoglycan. Peptidoglycan is a potent inflammatory stimulus, in part through its binding to TLR-2 and by peptidoglycan recognition proteins. Whatever lysozyme may contribute to antibacterial activity, it appears to be critically important for eliminating bacterial peptidoglycan, thus extinguishing the strong signal to innate immunity and inflammation generated by this characteristic bacterial macromolecule.

Lactoferrin

Lactoferrin is a 78-kDa single-chain glycoprotein that can bind one or two molecules of ferric iron. It is found in various secretions, including tears, milk, and semen, and also in the secretory granules of neutrophils. Intestinal cells and mononuclear phagocytes have surface receptors for lactoferrin, but do not synthesize it. Certain bacteria (e.g., *N. gonorrhoeae*, *Neisseria meningitidis*, and *Moraxella catarrhalis*) also possess lactoferrin receptors and use them to acquire iron. Lactoferrin or lactoferricin-treated gram-negative bacteria release LPS, develop electron-dense "membrane blisters," and become sensitized to lysozyme—all consistent with outer membrane damage. Lactoferrin binds bacterial lipopolysaccharide with high affinity and also binds various other proteins. Exposure of lactoferrin to pepsin (its normal fate when ingested in milk) releases an antimicrobial polypeptide, "lactoferricin" comprising the amino-terminal lactoferrin residues (Tomita *et al.* 1994). Lactoferricin kills many bacteria and *C. albicans*, but is ineffective against *Proteus* and *Serratia* species and *P. cepacia*. Lactoferrin also inhibits microbial adherence to and invasion of epithelial cells.

Lactoferrin has a higher affinity for iron than its plasma homolog transferrin, and its iron binding is less affected by acid pH. These characteristics may allow it to function as an iron-sequestering substance in mucosal secretions and inflammatory fluids. Because iron is an essential metal for all living organisms, sequestration of iron is an effective means of inhibiting microbial growth. Iron starvation also interferes with bacterial biofilm formation. Even under conditions that otherwise promote biofilm formation, lactoferrin-exposed bacteria remain in the planktonic form, presumably allowing the more mobile bacterial population to disperse and reach iron sources (Singh *et al.* 2002).

Secretory phospholipase A$_2$ (PLA$_2$)

Phospholipase A$_2$ enzymes remove fatty acids from the middle (*sn*-2) carbon atom of phosphoglycerides. Several phospholipase A$_2$ enzymes occur in mammalian cells, but only the 14-kDa secretory PLA$_2$ (sPLA$_2$) has potent microbicidal properties, principally against gram-positive bacteria (Harwig *et al.* 1995; Weinrauch *et al.* 1996). sPLA$_2$ differs from pancreatic PLA$_2$ structurally and in preferring phospholipids prominent in bacterial membranes [e.g., phosphatidylglycerol (PG) and phosphatidylethanolamine (PE)] over phosphatidylcholine as substrates. PLA$_2$ is present in granules of human neutrophils and small intestinal Paneth cells. sPLA$_2$ is released from neutrophils exposed to secretagogues, such as phorbol esters or calcium ionophores, and by Paneth cells exposed to cholinergic agonists, bacteria, or LPS. Serum sPLA$_2$ levels are greatly elevated in patients with sepsis and rise sharply within 3 hours after the experimental administration of lipopolysaccharide to uninfected patients. High concentrations of sPLA are also present in human tears. The antimicrobial specialization of this phospholipase is probably a result of its unusually high net positive charge and a cluster of positively charged residues near its N-terminus that facilitate its interaction with bacteria and access to its phospholipid target (Weiss *et al.* 1991).

Proteinase inhibitors

SLPI is a 107-aa (12.7-kDa) nonglycosylated peptide with a bipartite structure. It is very abundant in many human secretions, including seminal plasma, cervical mucus, nasal secretions, and tears. SLPI has received many alternative names, including human seminal plasma inhibitor-I (HUSI-I), cervix uteri secretion inhibitor (CUSI), bronchial secretory inhibitor (BSI), and bronchial mucus inhibitor (MPI). Mice deficient in SLPI show impaired wound healing (Ashcroft *et al.* 2000; Zhu *et al.* 2002), but their response to infection has not been reported yet. *In vitro*, SLPI shows low-level activity against bacteria and fungi (Hiemstra 2002) and may also have anti-HIV activity. If the high concentrations of SLPI in many epithelial secretions compensate for its low intrinsic potency, its antimicrobial activity could be biologically important.

SLPI is synthesized as a 132-aa prepropeptide with a 25-aa signal peptide. Each of its two structurally similar domains contains four intradomain disulfide bonds in the "four-disulfide-core" pattern also present in wheat germ agglutinin and neurophysin. The C-terminal domain of SLPI (residues 55–107) shows homology to the second domain of chelonianin, a basic protease inhibitor from Red Sea turtle, and is responsible for the molecule's prominent antiprotease activity (Masuda *et al.* 1995). SLPI holoprotein and its N-terminal domain (residues 1–54) have microbicidal properties (Hiemstra *et al.* 1996). Other protease inhibitors with antimicrobial properties include aprotinin, a 58-aa protease inhibitor in bovine mast cells (Pellegrini *et al.* 1996), and ENAP-2, a four-disulfide core protein found in equine granulocytes (Couto *et al.* 1992). Multifunctionality may be a common attribute of other proteins involved in host defense.

Antimicrobial ribonucleases

Eosinophils, as well as other myeloid and epithelial cells, contain cationic antimicrobial proteins belonging to the ribonuclease family (Rosenberg and Domachowske 2001). In humans, eosinophil cationic protein (ECP) and eosinophil-derived neurotoxin (EDN) are among the principal components of eosinophil granules. ECP is broadly antimicrobial (Lehrer, 1989b) and toxic to helminths (Hamann *et al.* 1987, 1990), but EDN is nearly inactive in these assays. Both ECP and EDN show antiviral activity (Rosenberg and Domachowske 2001) against respiratory RNA viruses: respiratory syncytial virus (RSV) and a related murine virus. New members of the antimicrobial ribonuclease family likely to be important in defending body surfaces include RNase 7, an abundant component of human epidermis (Harder and Schroder 2002) and angiogenin 4, an antimicrobial protein of murine Paneth cell granules (Hooper *et al.* 2003). The specific role of these proteins in host defense remains to be defined.

BPI

Bactericidal permeability-increasing protein (BPI) (Elsbach and Weiss 1998) is found in the azurophil (primary) granules of human and rabbit neutrophils, but like defensins, may be absent from mouse neutrophils. It is a 55-kDa cationic protein and a member of a family of lipid-binding proteins, two of which, BPI and lipopolysaccharide-binding protein (LBP) avidly bind to bacterial lipopolysaccharide. *In vitro*, BPI is specifically active against selected gram-negative bacteria at concentrations as low as nanomolar, and this activity is wholly contained in a 25-kDa amino terminal fragment. The mechanism of activity of BPI against bacteria depends on the initial high-affinity interaction with LPS in the outer membrane. The resulting rapid permeabilization of the outer membrane is followed by a slower process that culminates in the disruption of the inner membrane of gram-negative bacteria with attendant loss of viability (Wiese *et al.* 1997). More recently, BPI was also identified as a component of human eosinophil granules and as a lipoxin-inducible protein in mucosal epithelia (Canny *et al.* 2002). *In vitro* studies suggest that BPI contributes to the killing of gram-negative bacteria in isolated epithelia and neutrophils.

Cathelin-associated peptides ("cathelicidins")

The neutrophils of humans, pigs, cattle, sheep, mice, and other mammals contain a variety of structurally diverse antimicrobial peptides collectively called "cathelicidins." These peptides were grouped together because they are synthesized at the carboxy-terminal portion of a precursor containing a highly conserved domain, approximately 100 amino acids long, called "cathelin" (Zanetti *et al.* 1995; Ganz and Weiss 1997). Some of these peptides have amphipathic α-helical structures, others form compact, defensin-like β-sheets stabilized by intramolecular cystine disulfide bonds, and still others are remarkably rich in proline, arginine, or tryptophan residues. The genes for cathelicidins contain four exons, the first three of which encode most of the conserved cathelin domain. Exon 4 specifies the last few cathelin residues, including the cleavage site and the mature peptide. The 5′ flanking sequences of this gene family contain motifs for binding NF-κB, IL-6, GM-CSF, and NF-1, suggesting that synthesis responds to mediators generated early during infection.

The sole known human cathelicidin is named hCAP18 or FALL39/LL37 (Agerberth *et al.* 1995; Cowland *et al.* 1995; Larrick *et al.* 1995). Unlike defensins, which are fully processed before they are stored in the azurophil granules of the neutrophil, the human cathelicidin peptide is stored in the specific (secretory) granules as hCAP18, a cathelin-containing, 140-residue, 17-kD propeptide. During or after secretion, hCAP18 undergoes proteolytic processing by proteinase 3 (Sorensen *et al.* 2001) to liberate LL-37, the 37-residue, α-helical antimicrobial peptide at its C-terminus (Gudmundsson *et al.* 1996). The analogous proteolytic processing of bovine cathelicidins (proBac5 and proBac7) and porcine cathelicidins (proprotegrins 1–3) is mediated by trace amounts of neutrophil elastase (Panyutich *et al.* 1997; Scocchi *et al.* 1992).

mRNA for hCAP18 is found in testis (Malm *et al.* 2000), inflamed keratinocytes (Frohm *et al.* 1997; Agerberth *et al.* 1995), and airway epithelia (Bals *et al.* 1998). *In vitro*, LL-37 displayed both LPS binding (Hirata *et al.* 1995) and microbicidal activities (Agerberth *et al.* 1995) against *E. coli*. The abundance of LL-37 in neutrophil specific granules is about a third that of lactoferrin or lysozyme, the principal proteins of specific granules (Borregaard *et al.* 1995).

In addition to microbicidal activity, certain cathelicidins also have chemoattractant activity. For example, the human cathelicidin LL-37 is chemotactic for neutrophils, monocytes, and T cells, but not for dendritic cells. This activity is likely mediated through binding to the formyl-peptide receptorlike 1 receptor (De *et al.* 2000). The proline-rich porcine cathelicidin PR-39 can induce upregulation of syndecans, heparan sulfate proteoglycans involved in the repair process at the site of skin wounds (Gallo *et al.* 1994).

Although the pig has a large number of cathelicidin genes, the most active antimicrobial peptides in porcine skin wounds are protegrins, secreted from neutrophils as proprotegrins and activated by proteolytic cleavage by neutrophil elastase (Panyutich *et al.* 1997). *In vitro*, inhibition of neutrophil elastase by specific inhibitors blocked the conversion of proprotegrins to protegrins and largely ablated the stable antimicrobial activity secreted by porcine neutrophils (Shi and Ganz 1998). The application of neutrophil elastase inhibitor to porcine wounds decreased the concentration of mature protegrin in wound fluid and impaired the clearance of bacteria from wounds. The deficit could be restored by supplementing the wound fluid with synthetic protegrin *in vitro* or *in vivo* (Cole *et al.* 2001). Thus protegrins act as natural antibiotics that contribute to the clearance of microbes from wounds.

Strong evidence for the antibacterial function of cathelicidins in the skin comes from studies of dermal infections in mice with an ablated gene for CRAMP (cathelin-related antimicrobial peptide). CRAMP, normally the main murine cathelicidin (Nizet *et al.* 2001), is the murine homolog of human hCAP18. In CRAMP-knockout mice, the skin lesions caused by experimental Group A *Streptococcus* inoculation were larger lesions and had higher numbers of viable bacteria than those seen in control mice. As in pigs, infiltrating neutrophils appeared to be the chief source of cathelicidins in inflamed skin. Epithelial cells also produced cathelicidins, but it is not clear if their production was quantitatively significant. How or if epithelial cathelicidins undergo proteolytic processing remains to be defined.

ACKNOWLEDGMENTS

Many of our previous and ongoing studies have been supported by grants from the National Institutes of Health, including: AI 32234, 32738, and 50843 to C. B.; AI 37945 and 22837 to R. I. L.; and HL46809, AI46514, and AI48167 to T. G. The continuing support of the Will Rogers Institute is gratefully acknowledged. We thank Ken Miyasaki for his artistic rendering of the human defensin dimer, all our past and present collaborators for putting up with us, and antimicrobial peptides for being there.

REFERENCES

Agerberth, B., Gunne, H., Odeberg, J., Kogner, P., Boman, H. G., and Gudmundsson, G. H. (1995). FALL-39, a putative human peptide antibiotic, is cysteine-free and expressed in bone marrow and testis. *Proc. Natl. Acad. Sci. USA* 92, 195–199.

Agerberth, B., Charo, J., Werr, J., Olsson, B., Idali, F., Lindbom, L., Kiessling, R., Jornvall, H., Wigzell, H., and Gudmundsson, G. H.

(2000). The human antimicrobial and chemotactic peptides LL-37 and alpha-defensins are expressed by specific lymphocyte and monocyte populations. *Blood* 96: 3086–3093.

Aley, S. B., Zimmerman, M., Hetsko, M., Selsted, M. E., and Gillin, F. D. (1994). Killing of *Giardia lamblia* by cryptdins and cationic neutrophil peptides. *Infect. Immun.* 62, 5397–5403.

Ashcroft, G. S., Lei, K., Jin, W., Longenecker, G., Kulkarni, A. B., Greenwell-Wild, T., Hale-Donze, H., McGrady, G., Song, X. Y., and Wahl, S. M. (2000). Secretory leukocyte protease inhibitor mediates non-redundant functions necessary for normal wound healing. *Nat. Med.* 6, 1147–1153.

Ayabe, T., Satchell, D. P., Wilson, C. L., Parks, W. C., Selsted, M. E., and Ouellette, A. J. (2000). Secretion of microbicidal α-defensins by intestinal Paneth cells in response to bacteria. *Nat. Immunol.* 1, 113–118.

Bals, R., Wang, X., Zasloff, M., and Wilson, J. M. (1998). The peptide antibiotic LL-37/hCAP-18 is expressed in epithelia of the human lung where it has broad antimicrobial activity at the airway surface. *Proc. Natl. Acad. Sci. USA* 95, 9541–9546.

Bals, R., Wang, X., Meegalla, R. L., Wattler, S., Weiner, D. J., Nehls, M. C., and Wilson, J. M. (1999). Mouse beta-defensin 3 is an inducible antimicrobial peptide expressed in the epithelia of multiple organs. *Infect. Immun.* 67, 3542–3547.

Bastian, A. and Schafer, H. (2001). Human alpha-defensin 1 (HNP-1) inhibits adenoviral infection *in vitro*. *Regul. Pept.* 101, 157–161.

Bateman, A., MacLeod, R. J., Lembessis, P., Hu, J., Esch, F., and Solomon, S. (1996). The isolation and characterization of a novel corticostatin/defensin-like peptide from the kidney. *J. Biol. Chem.* 271, 10654–10659.

Bensch, K. W., Raida, M., Magert, H. J., Schulz-Knappe, P., and Forssmann, W. G. (1995). hBD-1: A novel beta-defensin from human plasma. *FEBS Lett.* 368, 331–335.

Bevins, C. L., Jones, D. E., Dutra, A., Schaffzin, J., and Muenke, M. (1996). Human enteric defensin genes: Chromosomal map position and a model for possible evolutionary relationships. *Genomics* 31, 95–106.

Biragyn, A., Ruffini, P. A., Leifer, C. A., Klyushnenkova, E., Shakhov, A., Chertov, O., Shirakawa, A. K., Farber, J. M., Segal, D. M., Oppenheim, J. J., and Kwak, L. W. (2002). Toll-like receptor 4-dependent activation of dendritic cells by beta-defensin 2. *Science* 298, 1025–1029.

Borenstein, L. A., Ganz, T., Sell, S., Lehrer, R. I., and Miller, J. N. (1991). Contribution of rabbit leukocyte defensins to the host response in experimental syphilis. *Infect. Immun.* 59, 1368–1377.

Borregaard, N., Sehested, M., Nielsen, B. S., Sengelov, H., and Kjeldsen, L. (1995). Biosynthesis of granule proteins in normal human bone marrow cells: Gelatinase is a marker of terminal neutrophil differentiation. *Blood* 85, 812–817.

Brandtzaeg, P., Gabrielsen, T. O., Dale, I., Muller, F., Steinbakk, M., and Fagerhol, M. K. (1995). The leucocyte protein L1 (calprotectin): A putative nonspecific defence factor at epithelial surfaces. *Adv. Exp. Med. Biol.* 371A, 201–206.

Canny, G., Levy, O., Furuta, G. T., Narravula-Alipati, S., Sisson, R. B., Serhan, C. N., and Colgan, S. P. (2002). Lipid mediator-induced expression of bactericidal/ permeability-increasing protein (BPI) in human mucosal epithelia. *Proc. Natl. Acad. Sci. USA* 99, 3902–3907.

Chamnongpol, S., Cromie, M., and Groisman, E. A. (2003). Mg2+ Sensing by the Mg2+ Sensor PhoQ of *Salmonella enterica*. *J. Mol. Biol.* 325, 795–807.

Chertov, O., Michiel, D. F., Xu, L., Wang, J. M., Tani, K., Murphy, W. J., Longo, D. L., Taub, D. D., and Oppenheim, J. J. (1996). Identification of defensin-1, defensin-2, and CAP37/azurocidin as T-cell chemoattractant proteins released from interleukin-8-stimulated neutrophils. *J. Biol. Chem.* 271, 2935–2940.

Cociancich, S., Goyffon, M., Bontems, F., Bulet, P., Bouet, F., Menez, A., and Hoffmann, J. (1993). Purification and characterization of a scorpion defensin, a 4kDa antibacterial peptide presenting structural similarities with insect defensins and scorpion toxins. *Biochem. Biophys. Res. Commun.* 194, 17–22.

Cole, A. M., Shi, J., Ceccarelli, A., Kim, Y. H., Park, A., and Ganz, T. (2001). Inhibition of neutrophil elastase prevents cathelicidin activation and impairs clearance of bacteria from wounds. *Blood* 97, 297–304.

Cole, A. M., Hong, T., Boo, L. M., Nguyen, T., Zhao, C., Bristol, G., Zack, J. A., Waring, A. J., Yang, O. O., and Lehrer, R. I. (2002). Retrocyclin: A primate peptide that protects cells from infection by T- and M-tropic strains of HIV-1. *Proc. Natl. Acad. Sci. USA* 99, 1813–1818.

Collins, L. V., Kristian, S. A., Weidenmaier, C., Faigle, M., van Kessel, K. P., van Strijp, J. A., Gotz, F., Neumeister, B., and Peschel, A. (2002). *Staphylococcus aureus* strains lacking D-alanine modifications of teichoic acids are highly susceptible to human neutrophil killing and are virulence attenuated in mice. *J. Infect. Dis.* 186, 214–219.

Couto, M. A., Harwig, S. S., Cullor, J. S., Hughes, J. P., and Lehrer, R. I. (1992). eNAP-2, a novel cysteine-rich bactericidal peptide from equine leukocytes. *Infect. Immun.* 60, 5042–5047.

Cowland, J. B., Johnsen, A. H., and Borregaard, N. (1995). hCAP-18, a cathelin/pro-bactenecin-like protein of human neutrophil specific granules. *FEBS Lett.* 368, 173–176.

Daher, K. A., Selsted, M. E., and Lehrer, R. I. (1986). Direct inactivation of viruses by human granulocyte defensins. *J. Virol.* 60, 1068–1074.

De, Y., Chen, Q., Schmidt, A. P., Anderson, G. M., Wang, J. M., Wooters, J., Oppenheim, J. J., and Chertov, O. (2000). LL-37, the neutrophil granule- and epithelial cell-derived cathelicidin, utilizes formyl peptide receptor-like 1 (FPRL1) as a receptor to chemoattract human peripheral blood neutrophils, monocytes, and T cells. *J. Exp. Med.* 192, 1069–1074.

Diamond, G., Zasloff, M., Eck, H., Brasseur, M., Maloy, W. L., and Bevins, C. L. (1991). Tracheal antimicrobial peptide, a cysteine-rich peptide from mammalian tracheal mucosa: Peptide isolation and cloning of a cDNA. *Proc. Natl. Acad. Sci. USA* 88, 3952–3956.

Diamond, G., Jones, D. E., and Bevins, C. L. (1993). Airway epithelial cells are the site of expression of a mammalian antimicrobial peptide gene. *Proc. Natl. Acad. Sci. USA* 90, 4596–4600.

Diamond, G., Russell, J. P., and Bevins, C. L. (1996). Inducible expression of an antibiotic peptide gene in lipopolysaccharide-challenged tracheal epithelial cells. *Proc. Natl. Acad. Sci. USA* 93, 5156–5160.

Diamond, G., Kaiser, V., Rhodes, J., Russell, J. P., and Bevins, C. L. (2000). Transcriptional regulation of beta-defensin gene expression in tracheal epithelial cells. *Infect. Immun.* 68, 113–119.

Driscoll, P. C., Gronenborn, A. M., Beress, L., and Clore, G. M. (1989). Determination of the three-dimensional solution structure of the antihypertensive and antiviral protein BDS-I from the sea anemone *Anemonia sulcata*: A study using nuclear magnetic resonance and hybrid distance geometry-dynamical simulated annealing. *Biochemistry* 28, 2188–2198.

Eisenhauer, P. B., Harwig, S. S., and Lehrer, R. I. (1992). Cryptdins: Antimicrobial defensins of the murine small intestine. *Infect. Immun.* 60, 3556–3565.

Elsbach, P., and Weiss, J. (1998). Role of the bactericidal/permeability-increasing protein in host defence. *Curr. Opin. Immunol.* 10, 45–49.

Ernst, R. K., Guina, T., and Miller, S. I. (2001). *Salmonella typhimurium* outer membrane remodeling: Role in resistance to host innate immunity. *Microbes Infect.* 3, 1327–1334.

Evans, E. W., Beach, G. G., Wunderlich, J., and Harmon, B. G. (1994). Isolation of antimicrobial peptides from avian heterophils. *J. Leukoc. Biol.* 56, 661–665.

Evans, E. W., Beach, F. G., Moore, K. M., Jackwood, M. W., Glisson, J. R., and Harmon, B. G. (1995). Antimicrobial activity of chicken and turkey heterophil peptides CHP1, CHP2, THP1, and THP3. *Vet. Microbiol.* 47, 295–303.

Fleischmann, J., Selsted, M. E., and Lehrer, R. I. (1985). Opsonic activity of MCP-1 and MCP-2, cationic peptides from rabbit alveolar macrophages. *Diagn. Microbiol. Infect. Dis.* 3, 233–242.

Fox, J. W., Elzinga, M., and Tu, A. T. (1979). Amino acid sequence and disulfide bond assignment of myotoxin a isolated from the venom of Prairie rattlesnake *(Crotalus viridis viridis)*. *Biochemistry* 18, 678–684.

Frohm, M., Agerberth, B., Ahangari, G., Stahle-Backdahl, M., Liden, S., Wigzell, H., and Gudmundsson, G. H. (1997). The expression of the gene coding for the antibacterial peptide LL-37 is induced in human keratinocytes during inflammatory disorders. *J. Biol. Chem.* 272, 15258–15263.

Gallo, R. L., Ono, M., Povsic, T., Page, C., Eriksson, E., Klagsbrun, M., and Bernfield, M. (1994). Syndecans, cell surface heparan sulfate proteoglycans, are induced by a proline-rich antimicrobial peptide from wounds. *Proc. Natl. Acad. Sci USA* 91, 11035–11039.

Ganz, T., and Weiss, J. (1997). Antimicrobial peptides of phagocytes and epithelia. *Semin. Hematol.* 34, 343–354.

Ganz, T., Gabayan, V., Liao, H. I., Liu, L., Oren, A., Graf, T., and Cole, A. M. (2003). Increased inflammation in lysozyme M-deficient mice in response to *Micrococcus luteus* and its peptidoglycan. *Blood* 101, 2388–2392.

Garcia, J. R., Jaumann, F., Schulz, S., Krause, A., Rodriguez-Jimenez, J., Forssmann, U., Adermann, K., Kluver, E., Vogelmeier, C., Becker, D., Hedrich, R., Forssmann, W. G., and Bals, R. (2001a). Identification of a novel, multifunctional beta-defensin (human beta-defensin 3) with specific antimicrobial activity: Its interaction with plasma membranes of *Xenopus oocytes* and the induction of macrophage chemoattraction. *Cell Tissue Res.* 306, 257–264.

Garcia, J. R., Krause, A., Schulz, S., Rodriguez-Jimenez, F. J., Kluver, E., Adermann, K., Forssmann, U., Frimpong-Boateng, A., Bals, R., and Forssmann, W. G. (2001b). Human beta-defensin 4: A novel inducible peptide with a specific salt-sensitive spectrum of antimicrobial activity. *FASEB J.* 15, 1819–1821.

Ghosh, D., Porter, E., Shen, B., Lee, S. K., Wilk, D., Drazba, J., Yadav, S. P., Crabb, J. W., Ganz, T., and Bevins, C. L. (2002). Paneth cell trypsin is the processing enzyme for human defensin-5. *Nat. Immunol.* 3, 583–590.

Goldman, M., Anderson, G., Stolzenberg, E. D., Kari, U. P., Zasloff, M., and Wilson, J. M. (1997). Human beta-defensin-1 is a salt-sensitive antibiotic in lung that is inactivated in cystic fibrosis. *Cell* 88, 553–560.

Gropp, R., Frye, M., Wagner, T. O., and Bargon, J. (1999). Epithelial defensins impair adenoviral infection: Implication for adenovirus-mediated gene therapy. *Hum. Gene Ther.* 10, 957–964.

Gudmundsson, G. H., Agerberth, B., Odeberg, J., Bergman, T., Olsson, B., and Salcedo, R. (1996). The human gene *FALL39* and processing of the cathelin precursor to the antibacterial peptide LL-37 in granulocytes. *Eur. J. Biochem* 238, 325–332.

Guina, T., Yi, E. C., Wang, H., Hackett, M., and Miller, S. I. (2000). A PhoP-regulated outer membrane protease of *Salmonella enterica* serovar typhimurium promotes resistance to alpha-helical antimicrobial peptides. *J. Bacteriol.* 182, 4077–4086.

Hamann, K. J., Barker, R. L., Loegering, D. A., and Gleich, G. J. (1987). Comparative toxicity of purified human eosinophil granule proteins for newborn larvae of *Trichinella spiralis*. *J. Parasitol.* 73, 523–529.

Hamann, K. J., Gleich, G. J., Checkel, J. L., Loegering, D. A., McCall, J. W., and Barker, R. L. (1990). *In vitro* killing of microfilariae of *Brugia pahangi* and *Brugia malayi* by eosinophil granule proteins. *J. Immunol.* 144, 3166–3173.

Harder, J., Bartels, J., Christophers, E., and Schroeder, J.-M. (1997). A peptide antibiotic from human skin. *Nature* 387, 861–862.

Harder, J., Bartels, J., Christophers, E., and Schroder, J. M. (2001). Isolation and characterization of human beta-defensin-3, a novel human inducible peptide antibiotic. *J. Biol. Chem.* 276, 5707–5713.

Harder, J. and Schroder, J. M. (2002). RNase 7, a novel innate immune defense antimicrobial protein of healthy human skin. *J. Biol. Chem.* 277, 46779–46784.

Hartmann, P., Becker, R., Franzen, C., Schell-Frederick, E., Romer, J., Jacobs, M., Fatkenheuer, G., and Plum, G. (2001). Phagocytosis and killing of *Mycobacterium avium* complex by human neutrophils. *J. Leukoc. Biol.* 69, 397–404.

Harwig, S. S., Park, A. S., and Lehrer, R. I. (1992). Characterization of defensin precursors in mature human neutrophils. *Blood* 79, 1532–1537.

Harwig, S. S., Swiderek, K. M., Kokryakov, V. N., Tan, L., Lee, T. D., Panyutich, E. A., Aleshina, G. M., Shamova, O. V., and Lehrer, R. I. (1994). Gallinacins: Cysteine-rich antimicrobial peptides of chicken leukocytes. *FEBS Lett.* 342, 281–285.

Harwig, S. S., Tan, L., Qu, X. D., Cho, Y., Eisenhauer, P. B., and Lehrer, R. I. (1995). Bactericidal properties of murine intestinal phospholipase A2. *J. Clin. Invest.* 95, 603–610.

Hiemstra, P. S., Maassen, R. J., Stolk, J., Heinzel-Wieland, R., Steffens, G. J., and Dijkman, J. H. (1996). Antibacterial activity of antileukoprotease. *Infect. Immun.* 64, 4520–4524.

Hiemstra, P. S. (2002). Novel roles of protease inhibitors in infection and inflammation. *Biochem. Soc. Trans.* 30, 116–120.

Hill, C. P., Yee, J., Selsted, M. E., and Eisenberg, D. (1991). Crystal structure of defensin HNP-3, an amphiphilic dimer: Mechanisms of membrane permeabilization. *Science* 251, 1481–1485.

Hirata, M., Zhong, J., Wright, S. C., and Larrick, J. W. (1995). Structure and functions of endotoxin-binding peptides derived from CAP18. *Prog. Clin. Biol. Res.* 392, 317–326.

Hooper, L. V., Stappenbeck, T. S., Hong, C. V., and Gordon, J. I. (2003) Angiogenins: A new class of microbicidal proteins involved in innate immunity. *Nat. Immunol.* 4, 269–273.

Hoover, D. M., Rajashankar, K. R., Blumenthal, R., Puri, A., Oppenheim, J. J., Chertov, O., and Lubkowski, J. (2000). The structure of human beta-defensin-2 shows evidence of higher-order oligomerization. *J. Biol. Chem.* 275, 32911–32918.

Hoover, D. M., Chertov, O., and Lubkowski, J. (2001). The structure of human beta-defensin-1. New insights into structural properties of beta-defensins. *J. Biol. Chem.* 276, 39021–39026.

Huttner, K. M., Kozak, C. A., and Bevins, C. L. (1997). The mouse genome encodes a single homolog of the antimicrobial peptide human beta-defensin 1. *FEBS Lett* 413, 45–49.

Jia, H. P., Wowk, S. A., Schutte, B. C., Lee, S. K., Vivado, A., Tack, B. F., Bevins, C. L., and McCray, P. B., Jr. (2000). A novel murine beta-defensin expressed in tongue, esophagus, and trachea. *J. Biol. Chem.* 275, 33314–33320.

Jia, H. P., Schutte, B. C., Schudy, A., Linzmeier, R., Guthmiller, J. M., Johnson, G. K., Tack, B. F., Mitros, J. P., Rosenthal, A., Ganz, T., and McCray, P. B., Jr. (2001). Discovery of new human beta-defensins using a genomics-based approach. *Gene* 263, 211–218.

Joiner, K. A., Ganz, T., Albert, J., and Rotrosen, D. (1989). The opsonizing ligand on *Salmonella typhimurium* influences incorporation of specific, but not azurophil, granule constituents into neutrophil phagosomes. *J. Cell Biol.* 109, 2771–2782.

Jones, D. E. and Bevins, C. L. (1992). Paneth cells of the human small intestine express an antimicrobial peptide gene. *J. Biol. Chem.* 267, 23216–23225.

Jones, D. E. and Bevins, C. L. (1993). Defensin-6 mRNA in human Paneth cells: Implications for antimicrobial peptides in host defense of the human bowel. *FEBS Lett.* 315, 187–192.

Jones, A. L., Beveridge, T. J., and Woods, D. E. (1996). Intracellular survival of *Burkholderia pseudomallei. Infect. Immun.* 64, 782–790.

Kagan, B. L., Selsted, M. E., Ganz, T., and Lehrer, R. I. (1990). Antimicrobial defensin peptides form voltage-dependent ion-permeable channels in planar lipid bilayer membranes. *Proc. Natl. Acad. Sci. USA* 87, 210–214.

Kisich, K. O., Higgins, M., Diamond, G., and Heifets, L. (2002). Tumor necrosis factor alpha stimulates killing of *Mycobacterium tuberculosis* by human neutrophils. *Infect. Immun.* 70, 4591–4599.

Kristian, S. A., Durr, M., van Strijp, J. A., Neumeister, B., and Peschel, A. (2003). MprF-mediated lysinylation of phospholipids in *Staphylococcus aureus* leads to protection against oxygen-independent neutrophil killing. *Infect. Immun.* 71, 546–549.

Kudriashov, B. A., Kondashevskaia, M. V., Liapina, L. A., Kokriakov, V. N., Mazing IuA., and Shamova, O. V. (1990). (Effect of defensin on the process of healing of aseptic skin wound and on the permeability of blood vessels). *Biull. Eksp. Biol. Med.* 109, 391–393.

Larrick, J. W., Hirata, M., Balint, R. F., Lee, J., Zhong, J., and Wright, S. C. (1995). Human CAP18: A novel antimicrobial lipopolysaccharide-binding protein. *Infect. Immun.* 63, 1291–1297.

Lehrer, R. I., Barton, A., Daher, K. A., Harwig, S. S., Ganz, T., and Selsted, M. E. (1989a). Interaction of human defensins with *Escherichia coli*: Mechanism of bactericidal activity. *J. Clin. Invest.* 84, 553–561.

Lehrer, R. I., Szklarek, D., Barton, A., Ganz, T., Hamann, K. J., and Gleich, G. J. (1989b). Antibacterial properties of eosinophil major basic protein and eosinophil cationic protein. *J. Immunol.* 142, 4428–4434.

Lehrer, R. I., Lichtenstein, A. K., and Ganz, T. (1993). Defensins: Antimicrobial and cytotoxic peptides of mammalian cells. *Annu. Rev. Immunol.* 11, 105–128.

Leonova, L., Kokryakov, V. N., Aleshina, G., Hong, T., Nguyen, T., Zhao, C., Waring, A. J., and Lehrer, R. I. (2001). Circular minidefensins and posttranslational generation of molecular diversity. *J. Leukoc. Biol.* 70, 461–464.

Lillard, J. W., Jr., Boyaka, P. N., Chertov, O., Oppenheim, J. J., and McGhee, J. R. (1999). Mechanisms for induction of acquired host immunity by neutrophil peptide defensins. *Proc. Natl. Acad. Sci. USA* 96, 651–656.

Linzmeier, R., Michaelson, D., Liu, L., and Ganz, T. (1993). The structure of neutrophil defensin genes. *FEBS Lett.* 321, 267–273.

Linzmeier, R., Ho, C. H., Hoang, B. V., and Ganz, T. (1999). A 450-kb contig of defensin genes on human chromosome 8p23. *Gene* 233, 205–211.

Liu, L., and Ganz, T. (1995). The pro region of human neutrophil defensin contains a motif that is essential for normal subcellular sorting. *Blood* 85, 1095–1103.

Liu, L., Zhao, C., Heng, H. H. Q., and Ganz, T. (1997). The human β-defensin-1 and α-defensins are encoded by adjacent genes: Two peptide families with differing disulfide topology share a common ancestry. *Genomics* 43, 316–320.

Liu, L., Wang, L., Jia, H. P., Zhao, C., Heng, H. H. Q., Schutte, B. C., McCray, P. B. J., and Ganz, T. (1998). Structure and mapping of the human β-defensin *HBD-2* gene and its expression at sites of inflammation. *Gene* 222, 237–244.

Liu, A. Y., Destoumieux, D., Wong, A. V., Park, C. H., Valore, E. V., Liu, L., and Ganz, T. (2002). Human beta-defensin-2 production in keratinocytes is regulated by IL-1, bacteria, and the state of differentiation. *J. Invest. Dermatol.* 118, 275–281.

Liu, L., Roberts, A. A., and Ganz, T. (2003). By IL-1 signaling, monocyte-derived cells dramatically enhance the epidermal antimicrobial response to lipopolysaccharide. *J. Immunol.* 170, 575–580.

Lusitani, D., Malawista, S. E., and Montgomery, R. R. (2002). *Borrelia burgdorferi* are susceptible to killing by a variety of human polymorphonuclear leukocyte components. *J. Infect. Dis.* 185, 797–804.

Mallow, E. B., Harris, A., Salzman, N., Russell, J. P., DeBerardinis, R. J., Ruchelli, E., and Bevins, C. L. (1996). Human enteric defensins: Gene structure and developmental expression. *J. Biol. Chem.* 271, 4038–4045.

Malm, J., Sorensen, O., Persson, T., Frohm-Nilsson, M., Johansson, B., Bjartell, A., Lilja, H., Stahle-Backdahl, M., Borregaard, N., and Egesten, A. (2000). The human cationic antimicrobial protein (hCAP-18) is expressed in the epithelium of human epididymis, is present in seminal plasma at high concentrations, and is attached to spermatozoa. *Infect. Immun.* 68, 4297–4302.

Manitz, M. P., Horst, B., Seeliger, S., Strey, A., Skryabin, B. V., Gunzer, M., Frings, W., Schonlau, F., Roth, J., Sorg, C., and Nacken, W. (2003). Loss of S100A9 (MRP14) results in reduced interleukin-8-induced CD11b surface expression, a polarized microfilament system, and diminished responsiveness to chemoattractants *in vitro. Mol. Cell. Biol.* 23, 1034–1043.

Marquardt, H., Todaro, G. J., and Twardzik, D. R. Snake venom growth arresting peptide. Oncogen and Seattle, WA. (US 4774318-A 3). 9-27-1988. (U.S. Patent Office Register).

Martinez de Tejada, G., Pizarro-Cerda, J., Moreno, E., and Moriyon, I. (1995). The outer membranes of *Brucella* spp. are resistant to bactericidal cationic peptides. *Infect. Immun.* 63, 3054–3061.

Masuda, K., Kamimura, T., Watanabe, K., Suga, T., Kanesaki, M., Takeuchi, A., Imaizumi, A., and Suzuki, Y. (1995). Pharmacological activity of the C-terminal and N-terminal domains of secretory leukoprotease inhibitor in vitro. *Br. J. Pharmacol.* 115, 883–888.

McCray, P. B. J., and Bentley, L. (1997). Human airway epithelia express a beta-defensin. *Am. J. Respir. Cell Mol. Biol.* 16, 343–349.

Miller, S. I., Pulkkinen, W. S., Selsted, M. E., and Mekalanos, J. J. (1990). Characterization of defensin resistance phenotypes associated with mutations in the phoP virulence regulon of *Salmonella typhimurium. Infect. Immun.* 58, 3706–3710.

Miyakawa, Y., Ratnakar, P., Rao, A. G., Costello, M. L., Mathieu-Costello, O., Lehrer, R. I., and Catanzaro, A. (1996). *In vitro* activity of the antimicrobial peptides human and rabbit defensins and porcine leukocyte protegrin against *Mycobacterium tuberculosis*. *Infect. Immun.* 64, 926–932.

Morrison, G. M., Davidson, D. J., and Dorin, J. R. (1999). A novel mouse beta defensin, Defb2, which is upregulated in the airways by lipopolysaccharide. *FEBS Lett.* 442, 112–116.

Morrison, G., Kilanowski, F., Davidson, D., and Dorin, J. (2002). Characterization of the mouse beta defensin 1, Defb1, mutant mouse model. *Infect. Immun.* 70, 3053–3060.

Moser, C., Weiner, D. J., Lysenko, E., Bals, R., Weiser, J. N., and Wilson, J. M. (2002). beta-Defensin 1 contributes to pulmonary innate immunity in mice. *Infect. Immun.* 70, 3068–3072.

Murphy, C. J., Foster, B. A., Mannis, M. J., Selsted, M. E., and Reid, T. W. (1993). Defensins are mitogenic for epithelial cells and fibroblasts. *J. Cell Physiol.* 155, 408–413.

Nizet, V., Ohtake, T., Lauth, X., Trowbridge, J., Rudisill, J., Dorschner, R. A., Pestonjamasp, V., Piraino, J., Huttner, K., and Gallo, R. L. (2001). Innate antimicrobial peptide protects the skin from invasive bacterial infection. *Nature* 414, 454–457.

Obata-Onai, A., Hashimoto, S., Onai, N., Kurachi, M., Nagai, S., Shizuno, K., Nagahata, T., and Mathushima, K. (2002). Comprehensive gene expression analysis of human NK cells and CD8(+) T lymphocytes. *Int. Immunol.* 14, 1085–1098.

Ogata, K., Linzer, B. A., Zuberi, R. I., Ganz, T., Lehrer, R. I., and Catanzaro, A. (1992). Activity of defensins from human neutrophilic granulocytes against *Mycobacterium avium-Mycobacterium intracellulare*. *Infect. Immun.* 60, 4720–4725.

Oren, A., Ganz, T., Liu, L., and Meerloo, T. (2003). In human epidermis, beta defensin-2 is packaged in lamellar bodies. *Exp. Mol. Path.* 74, 180–182.

Ouellette, A. J., Greco, R. M., James, M., Frederick, D., Naftilan, J., and Fallon, J. T. (1989). Developmental regulation of cryptdin, a corticostatin/defensin precursor mRNA in mouse small intestinal crypt epithelium. *J. Cell Biol.* 108, 1687–1695.

Ouellette, A. J., and Selsted, M. E. (1996). Paneth cell defensins: Endogenous peptide components of intestinal host defense. *FASEB Journal* 10, 1280–1289.

Ouellette, A. J., Satchell, D. P., Hsieh, M. M., Hagen, S. J., and Selsted, M. E. (2000). Characterization of luminal Paneth cell alpha-defensins in mouse small intestine. Attenuated antimicrobial activities of peptides with truncated amino termini. *J. Biol. Chem.* 275, 33969–33973.

Panyutich, A., Shi, J., Boutz, P. L., Zhao, C., and Ganz, T. (1997). Porcine polymorphonuclear leukocytes generate extracellular microbicidal activity by elastase-mediated activation of secreted proprotegrins. *Infect. Immun.* 65, 978–985.

Peeters, T. and Vantrappen, G. (1975). The Paneth cell: A source of intestinal lysozyme. *Gut* 16, 553–558.

Pellegrini, A., Thomas, U., Bramaz, N., Klauser, S., Hunziker, P., and von Fellenberg, R. (1996). Identification and isolation of the bactericidal domains in the proteinase inhibitor aprotinin. *Biochem. Biophys. Res. Commun.* 222, 559–565.

Peng, J. H., Schutte, B. C., Schudy, A., Linzmeier, R., Guthmiller, J. M., Johnson, G. K., Tack, B. F., Mitros, J. P., Rosenthal, A., Ganz, T., and McCray, P. B. (2001). Discovery of new human beta-defensins using a genomics-based approach. *Gene* 263, 211–218.

Perez-Canadillas, J. M., Zaballos, A., Gutierrez, J., Varona, R., Roncal, F., Albar, J. P., Marquez, G., and Bruix, M. (2001). NMR solution structure of murine CCL20/MIP-3 alpha, a chemokine that specifically chemoattracts immature dendritic cells and lymphocytes through its highly specific interaction with the beta-chemokine receptor CCR6. *J. Biol. Chem.* 276, 28372–28379.

Porter, E. M., Liu, L., Oren, A., Anton, P. A., and Ganz, T. (1997a). Localization of human intestinal defensin 5 in Paneth cell granules. *Infect. Immun.* 65, 2389–2395.

Porter, E. M., vanDam, E., Valore, E. V., and Ganz, T. (1997b). Broad-spectrum antimicrobial activity of human intestinal defensin 5. *Infect. Immun.* 65, 2396–2401.

Porter, E. M., Poles, M. A., Lee, J. S., Naitoh, J., Bevins, C. L., and Ganz, T. (1998). Isolation of human intestinal defensins from ileal neobladder urine. *FEBS Lett.* 434, 272–276.

Putsep, K., Axelsson, L. G., Boman, A., Midtvedt, T., Normark, S., Boman, H. G., and Andersson, M. (2000). Germ-free and colonized mice generate the same products from enteric prodefensins. *J. Biol. Chem.* 275, 40478–40482.

Qu, X. D., Harwig, S. S., Oren, A. M., Shafer, W. M., and Lehrer, R. I. (1996a). Susceptibility of *Neisseria gonorrhoeae* to protegrins. *Infect. Immun.* 64, 1240–1245.

Qu, X. D., Lloyd, K. C., Walsh, J. H., and Lehrer, R. I. (1996b). Secretion of type II phospholipase A2 and cryptdin by rat small intestinal Paneth cells. *Infect. Immun.* 64, 5161–5165.

Rosenberg, H. F. and Domachowske, J. B. (2001). Eosinophils, eosinophil ribonucleases, and their role in host defense against respiratory virus pathogens. *J. Leukoc. Biol.* 70, 691–698.

Russell, J. P., Diamond, G., Tarver, A. P., Scanlin, T. F., and Bevins, C. L. (1996). Coordinate induction of two antibiotic genes in tracheal epithelial cells exposed to the inflammatory mediators lipopolysaccharide and tumor necrosis factor alpha. *Infect. Immun.* 64, 1565–1568.

Saito, T., Kawabata, S., Shigenaga, T., Takayenoki, Y., Cho, J., Nakajima, H., Hirata, M., and Iwanaga, S. (1995). A novel big defensin identified in horseshoe crab hemocytes: Isolation, amino acid sequence, and antibacterial activity. *J. Biochem. (Tokyo)* 117, 1131–1137.

Salzman, N., Ghosh, D., Huttner, K. M., Paterson, Y., and Bevins, C. L. 2003. Protection against enteric salmonellosis in transgenic mice expressing a human intestinal defensin. *Nature* 422, 522–526.

Satoh, Y. (1988). Effect of live and heat-killed bacteria on the secretory activity of Paneth cells in germ-free mice. *Cell Tissue Res.* 251, 87–93.

Sawyer, J. G., Martin, N. L., and Hancock, R. E. (1988). Interaction of macrophage cationic proteins with the outer membrane of *Pseudomonas aeruginosa*. *Infect. Immun.* 56, 693–698.

Scheetz, T., Bartlett, J. A., Walters, J. D., Schutte, B. C., Casavant, T. L., and PB Jr, B. M. (2002). Genomics-based approaches to gene discovery in innate immunity. *Immunol. Rev.* 190, 137–145.

Schibli, D. J., Hunter, H. N., Aseyev, V., Starner, T. D., Wiencek, J. M., McCray, P. B., Jr., Tack, B. F., and Vogel, H. J. (2002). The solution structures of the human beta-defensins lead to a better understanding of the potent bactericidal activity of HBD3 against *Staphylococcus aureus*. *J. Biol. Chem.* 277, 8279–8289.

Schonwetter, B. S., Stolzenberg, E. D., and Zasloff, M. A. (1995). Epithelial antibiotics induced at sites of inflammation. *Science* 267, 1645–1648.

Schutte, B. C., Mitros, J. P., Bartlett, J. A., Walters, J. D., Jia, H. P., Welsh, M. J., Casavant, T. L., and McCray, P. B., Jr. (2002). Discovery of five conserved beta-defensin gene clusters using a computational search strategy. *Proc. Natl. Acad. Sci. USA* 99, 2129–2133.

Scocchi, M., Skerlavaj, B., Romeo, D., and Gennaro, R. (1992). Proteolytic cleavage by neutrophil elastase converts inactive storage proforms to antibacterial bactenecins. *Eur. J. Biochem.* 209, 589–595.

Selsted, M. E., Miller, S. I., Henschen, A. H., and Ouellette, A. J. (1992). Enteric defensins: Antibiotic peptide components of intestinal host defense. *J. Cell Biol.* 118, 929–936.

Selsted, M. E., Tang, Y. Q., Morris, W. L., McGuire, P. A., Novotny, M. J., Smith, W., Henschen, A. H., and Cullor, J. S. (1993). Purification, primary structures, and antibacterial activities of beta-defensins, a new family of antimicrobial peptides from bovine neutrophils. *J. Biol. Chem.* 268, 6641–6648.

Shafer, W. M., Qu, X., Waring, A. J., and Lehrer, R. I. (1998). Modulation of *Neisseria gonorrhoeae* susceptibility to vertebrate antibacterial peptides due to a member of the resistance/nodulation/division efflux pump family. *Proc. Natl. Acad. Sci. USA* 95, 1829–1833.

Sharma, S., and Khuller, G. (2001). DNA as the intracellular secondary target for antibacterial action of human neutrophil peptide-I against *Mycobacterium tuberculosis* H37Ra. *Curr. Microbiol.* 43, 74–76.

Sharma, S., Verma, I., and Khuller, G. K. (2000). Antibacterial activity of human neutrophil peptide-1 against *Mycobacterium tuberculosis* H37Rv: In vitro and ex vivo study. *Eur. Respir. J.* 16, 112–117.

Shi, J., and Ganz, T. (1998). The role of protegrins and other elastase-activated polypeptides in the bactericidal properties of porcine inflammatory fluids. *Infect. Immun.* 66, 3611–3617.

Singh, P. K., Parsek, M. R., Greenberg, E. P., and Welsh, M. J. (2002). A component of innate immunity prevents bacterial biofilm development. *Nature* 417, 552–555.

Sinha, S., Cheshenko, N., Lehrer, R. I., and Herold, B. C. (2003). NP-1, a rabbit alpha-defensin, prevents the entry and intercellular spread of herpes simplex virus type 2. *Antimicrob. Agents Chemother.* 47, 494–500.

Smith, J. J., Travis, S. M., Greenberg, E. P., and Welsh, M. J. (1996). Cystic fibrosis airway epithelia fail to kill bacteria because of abnormal airway surface fluid. *Cell* 85, 229–236.

Sorensen, O. E., Follin, P., Johnsen, A. H., Calafat, J., Tjabringa, G. S., Hiemstra, P. S., and Borregaard, N. (2001). Human cathelicidin, hCAP-18, is processed to the antimicrobial peptide LL-37 by extracellular cleavage with proteinase 3. *Blood* 97, 3951–3959.

Stolzenberg, E. D., Anderson, G. M., Ackermann, M. R., Whitlock, R. H., and Zasloff, M. (1997). Epithelial antibiotic induced in states of disease. *Proc. Natl. Acad. Sci. USA* 94, 8686–8690.

Tang, Y. Q., Yuan, J., Osapay, G., Osapay, K., Tran, D., Miller, C. J., Ouellette, A. J., and Selsted, M. E. (1999). A cyclic antimicrobial peptide produced in primate leukocytes by the ligation of two truncated alpha-defensins. *Science* 286, 498–502.

Tarver, A. P., Clark, D. P., Diamond, G., Russell, J. P., Erdjument-Bromage, H., Tempst, P., Cohen, K. S., Jones, D. E., Sweeney, R. W., Wines, M., Hwang, S., and Bevins, C. L. (1998). Enteric beta-defensin: Molecular cloning and characterization of a gene with inducible intestinal epithelial cell expression associated with *Cryptosporidium parvum* infection. *Infect. Immun.* 66, 1045–1056.

Territo, M. C., Ganz, T., Selsted, M. E., and Lehrer, R. (1989). Monocyte-chemotactic activity of defensins from human neutrophils. *J. Clin. Invest.* 84, 2017–2020.

Thevissen, K., Terras, F. R., and Broekaert, W. F. (1999). Permeabilization of fungal membranes by plant defensins inhibits fungal growth. *Appl. Environ. Microbiol.* 65, 5451–5458.

Thomma, B. P., Cammue, B. P., and Thevissen, K. (2002). Plant defensins. *Planta* 216, 193–202.

Tomita, M., Takase, M., Wakabayashi, H., and Bellamy, W. (1994). Antimicrobial peptides of lactoferrin. *Adv. Exp. Med. Biol.* 357, 209–218.

Valore, E. V., and Ganz, T. (1992). Posttranslational processing of defensins in immature human myeloid cells. *Blood* 79, 1538–1544.

Valore, E. V., Park, C. H., Quayle, A. J., Wiles, K. R., McCray, P. B., and Ganz, T. (1998). Human beta-defensin-1: An antimicrobial peptide of urogenital tissues. *J. Clin. Invest.* 101, 1633–1642.

Van Wetering, S., Mannesse-Lazeroms, S. P., van Sterkenburg, M. A., Daha, M. R., Dijkman, J. H., and Hiemstra, P. S. (1997). Effect of defensins on interleukin-8 synthesis in airway epithelial cells. *Am. J. Physiol.* 272, L888–L896.

Viljanen, P., Koski, P., and Vaara, M. (1988). Effect of small cationic leukocyte peptides (defensins) on the permeability barrier of the outer membrane. *Infect. Immun.* 56, 2324–2329.

Weinrauch, Y., Elsbach, P., Madsen, L. M., Foreman, A., and Weiss, J. (1996). The potent anti-*Staphylococcus aureus* activity of a sterile rabbit inflammatory fluid is due to a 14-kD phospholipase A2. *J. Clin. Invest.* 97, 250–257.

Weiss, J., Wright, G., Bekkers, A. C., van den Bergh, C. J., and Verheij, H. M. (1991). Conversion of pig pancreas phospholipase A2 by protein engineering into enzyme active against *Escherichia coli* treated with the bactericidal/permeability-increasing protein. *J. Biol. Chem.* 266, 4162–4167.

Wiese, A., Brandenburg, K., Lindner, B., Schromm, A. B., Carroll, S. F., Rietschel, E. T., and Seydel, U. (1997). Mechanisms of action of the bactericidal/permeability-increasing protein BPI on endotoxin and phospholipid monolayers and aggregates. *Biochemistry* 36, 10301–10310.

Wilson, C. L., Ouellette, A. J., Satchell, D. P., Ayabe, T., Lopez-Boado, Y. S., Stratman, J. L., Hultgren, S. J., Matrisian, L. M., and Parks, W. C. (1999). Regulation of intestinal alpha-defensin activation by the metalloproteinase matrilysin in innate host defense. *Science* 286, 113–117.

Wimley, W. C., Selsted, M. E., and White, S. H. (1994). Interactions between human defensins and lipid bilayers: Evidence for formation of multimeric pores. *Protein Sci.* 3, 1362–1373.

Wu, E. R., Daniel, R., and Bateman, A. (1998). RK-2: A novel rabbit kidney defensin and its implications for renal host defense. *Peptides* 19, 793–799.

Yamashita, T., and Saito, K. (1989). Purification, primary structure, and biological activity of guinea pig neutrophil cationic peptides. *Infect. Immun.* 57, 2405–2409.

Yang, D., Chertov, O., Bykovskaia, S. N., Chen, Q., Buffo, M. J., Shogan, J., Anderson, M., Schroder, J. M., Wang, J. M., Howard, O. M., and Oppenheim, J. J. (1999). Beta-defensins: Linking innate and adaptive immunity through dendritic and T cell CCR6. *Science* 286, 525–528.

Yang, D., Chen, Q., Chertov, O., and Oppenheim, J. J. (2000). Human neutrophil defensins selectively chemoattract naive T and immature dendritic cells. *J. Leukoc. Biol* 68, 9–14.

Zanetti, M., Gennaro, R., and Romeo, D. (1995). Cathelicidins: A novel protein family with a common proregion and a variable C-terminal antimicrobial domain. *FEBS Lett.* 374, 1–5.

Zhang, L., Yu, W., He, T., Yu, J., Caffrey, R. E., Dalmasso, E. A., Fu, S., Pham, T., Mei, J., Ho, J. J., Zhang, W., Lopez, P., and Ho, D. D. (2002). Contribution of human alpha-defensin 1, 2, and 3 to the anti-HIV-1 activity of CD8 antiviral factor. *Science* 298, 995–1000.

Zhao, C. Q., Wang, I., and Lehrer, R. I. (1996). Widespread expression of beta-defensin HBD-1 in human secretory glands and epithelial cells. *FEBS Lett.* 396, 319–322.

Zhao, C. Q., Nguyen, T., Liu, L., Sacco, R. E. , Brogden, K. A. and Lehrer, R. I. (2001). Gallinacin-3, an inducible epithelial beta-defensin in the chicken. *Infect. Immun.* 69, 2684–2691.

Zhu, Q. and Solomon, S. (1992). Isolation and mode of action of rabbit corticostatic (antiadrenocorticotropin) peptides. *Endocrinology* 130, 1413–1423.

Zhu, J., Nathan, C., Jin, W., Sim, D., Ashcroft, G. S., Wahl, S. M., Lacomis, L., Erdjument-Bromage, H., Tempst, P., Wright, C. D., and Ding, A. (2002). Conversion of proepithelin to rpithelins. Roles of SLPI and elastase in host defense and wound repair. *Cell* 111, 867–878.

Cellular and Molecular Basis for Antigen Transport Across Epithelial Barriers

Chapter 7

Marian R. Neutra

Department of Pediatrics, Harvard Medical School, and Gastrointestinal Cell Biology Laboratory, Children's Hospital, Boston, Massachusetts

Jean-Pierre Kraehenbuhl

Swiss Institute for Experimental Cancer Research and Institute of Biochemistry, University of Lausanne, Epalinges, Switzerland

INTRODUCTION

Foreign antigens and microorganisms on mucosal surfaces of the oral and nasal cavities and the gastrointestinal, respiratory, and genital tracts are separated from cells of the mucosal immune system by epithelial barriers. To obtain samples of the external environment on mucosal surfaces, the immune system relies on the close collaboration of epithelial cells with antigen-presenting and lymphoid cells. The challenge faced by epithelial tissues is to transport antigen samples across these barriers without compromising the integrity and protective functions of the epithelium. Antigen-sampling strategies at diverse mucosal sites differ dramatically because they are adapted to the cellular organization of the local epithelial barrier, but in all cases, these strategies involve collaboration between epithelial cells and dendritic cells (DCs). For example, in both stratified and simple epithelia, the mucosal immune system sends motile DCs into the narrow intraepithelial spaces and even to the outer limit of the epithelium, where they may obtain samples of foreign material. In simple epithelia where intercellular spaces are sealed by tight junctions, specialized epithelial M cells deliver samples of foreign material by vesicular transport from the lumen directly to DCs and lymphoid cells on the basolateral side of the epithelium.

The fates of antigens and pathogens that cross epithelial barriers differ depending on the mucosal site: for example, they may be released at M-cell basolateral surfaces and taken up by intraepithelial or subepithelial DCs associated with organized mucosal lymphoid tissues, or they may be carried by DCs to distant inductive sites (Masurier *et al.* 1998; MacPherson and Liu, 1999) **(Fig. 7.1)**. In both cases, the phenotype of the DC that captures antigen in or under the epithelium may influence the immunologic outcome of antigen uptake. There is evidence that different subpopulations of DCs play distinct roles in determining the nature of immune responses *in vivo* (Pulendran *et al.* 1999; Maldonado-Lopez *et al.* 1999). These early events at mucosal surfaces may determine the immunologic outcomes of antigen transport and the efficacy of mucosal vaccine strategies.

ANTIGEN TRANSPORT ACROSS STRATIFIED EPITHELIA

Barrier function of stratified squamous epithelia

Stratified squamous epithelia form barriers to antigens in the oral cavity and oral pharynx including the palatine and lingual tonsils, the anal canal, the male foreskin, and the female vagina and ectocervix. These mucosal surfaces are covered by nonkeratinized or parakeratinized epithelia that consist of multilayered cells joined by desmosomes. Although small molecules and proteins can diffuse into the uppermost cell layers, these epithelia provide a permeability barrier to macromolecules by secretion of a glycolipoprotein substance into the narrow intercellular spaces of the lower stratified layers (Farbman 1988). There are many regional variations in the thickness, surface cell phenotypes, and protein expression in stratified squamous epithelia that are determined both by genetic factors and by the local environment. In the vagina and exocervix of some species, for example, fluctuations in hormonal signals over the course of the female cycle have dramatic effects on epithelial thickness, endocytic activity of epithelial cells, and turnover of Langerhans cells (Young and Hosking 1986; Yeaman *et al.* 1998). Proteins administered to the luminal surface of the vagina in mice can be taken up

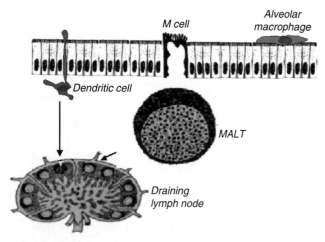

Fig. 7.1. Antigen sampling across simple epithelia. **(See page 1 of the color plates.)** Dendritic cells (DCs) migrate into stratified epithelia in the skin and the vagina (Langerhans cells) or into simple epithelia in the airways and intestine. Some DCs *(shown at left)* may open tight junctions, sample antigens and microorganisms, and then migrate to local organized lymphoid tissues or draining lymph nodes. In the epithelium associated with mucosal lymphoid follicles, specialized M cells *(center)* take up and transport antigens to intraepithelial and subepithelial lymphocytes and DCs. In the lung, macrophages located on the surface of the alveolar epithelium *(right)* can phagocytose antigens, particles, and microorganisms.

by stratified epithelial cells, but such epithelia have no mechanism for directional transcytosis. In addition, there is no evidence for vectorial transport across these barriers. It is unlikely that proteins, other macromolecules, or microbes can passively diffuse through stratified epithelia. Thus the immune system obtains samples of intact foreign antigens from these mucosal surfaces through the activities of motile DCs.

Role of dendritic cells in stratified epithelia

Intraepithelial DCs are present in the stratified epithelia of the oral cavity (Weinberg *et al.* 1987; Okato *et al.* 1989) and vagina (Miller *et al.* 1992a; Yeaman *et al.* 1998; Parr and Parr 1999). These DCs express gp40, a cell surface marker also found on Langerhans cells of the epidermis, and are assumed to be functionally equivalent to Langerhans cells. DCs insinuate themselves between epithelial cells and may even extend processes to the outer limit of the epithelium, apparently to obtain samples of antigens or pathogens from the mucosal surface or from intercellular spaces of the epithelium (Miller *et al.* 1994; Spira *et al.* 1996; Zhang *et al.* 1999; Perry 1994; Anderson 1996). In the oropharynx, high concentrations of intraepithelial DCs occur in the tonsils (Weinberg *et al.* 1987), and these could present antigens either locally in the organized lymphoid tissue of the tonsillar mucosa or after migration to draining lymph nodes (Okato *et al.* 1989). Whether the immunologic outcome of antigen sampling by DCs and macrophages in organized tonsillar lymphoid tissue differs from the outcome of DC sampling in the general buccal epithelium is unknown. DCs also migrate into pseudostratified and simple epithelia of the airways, as described in the following text.

A separate population of DCs that expresses major histocompatibility complex (MHC) II but does not express the gp40 antigen marker of Langerhans cells is found in the connective tissues under stratified mucosal epithelia. Relatively little is known about the function of these submucosal DCs. In the mouse vagina, submucosal DCs were shown to capture viral antigens, migrate to draining lymph nodes, and induce antiviral immune responses independently of the intraepithelial DCs (King *et al.* 1998; Zhao *et al.* 2003). Submucosal DCs of the vagina also differ from intraepithelial DCs in their expression of adhesion molecules and receptors for mucosally transmitted pathogens (Jameson *et al.* 2002). Both intraepithelial and submucosal DC populations may be infected by simian immunodeficiency virus (SIV) or human immunodeficiency virus (HIV) during sexual transmission. Early after oral exposure to SIV or chimeric simian–human immunodeficiency virus (SHIV), infected mononuclear cells were detected by *in situ* hybridization in the lingual and palatine tonsils (Stahl-Hennig *et al.* 1999). During SIV infection of monkey cervicovaginal mucosa, intraepithelial and subepithelial DCs were the first detectable sites of viral replication (Miller *et al.* 1993; Spira *et al.* 1996).

ANTIGEN SAMPLING ACROSS SIMPLE EPITHELIA

A large proportion of the body's mucosal surface area is covered by simple epithelia consisting of a single layer of epithelial cells. Antigen sampling across simple epithelia of the intestines, airways, and genital tract can involve multiple cell types, including epithelial cells and bone marrow–derived leukocytes such as alveolar macrophages and DCs that migrate into the epithelial layer and position themselves on the epithelial surface or between epithelial cells. The subsequent immune response depends in part on which cell type first takes up the antigen.

Polarity of simple epithelia

Simple epithelia consist of polarized cells that can internalize macromolecules from either their apical, lateral, or basal cell surfaces. Polarity is established and maintained through the extrinsic signals provided by homotypic interaction of adhesion molecules such as E-cadherin at the lateral surface and heterotypic interaction of integrins with extracellular matrix components at the basal surface (Knust 2002; Sheppard 1996). These interactions transmit signals internally, resulting in polarized cytoskeletal and signaling networks. The tight junctions that seal the apical poles of epithelial cells provide efficient diffusion barriers and prevent lateral diffusion of membrane glycolipids and proteins between apical and basolateral domains of the plasma membrane. The apical domain of epithelial cells, including intestinal cells, contains specialized components such as microvilli, clathrin coats pits, caveolae, and adhesion sites stabilized by submembrane cytoskeleton not present in nonpolarized cell types. Maintenance of the apical and basolateral domains involves sorting of membrane components vesicles in the trans-Golgi network (TGN) and budding of vesicles enriched in components destined for either the apical or basolateral domain (Matter and Mellman 1994). In addition, specific components "incorrectly" inserted into one domain either from the biosynthetic pathway or from transcytotic vesicles can be resorted to the opposite side by selective endocytosis and transcytosis.

Interactions of simple epithelia with environmental antigens

In order to interact with cells of the immune system, antigens have to cross the barriers formed by epithelia of mucosal tissues. They may follow either a transcellular or a paracellular pathway. The transcellular pathway is mediated by vesicular transport, and the paracellular route occurs through the tight junctions, the tightness of which can be modulated by soluble environmental factors such as bacterial products or host mediators such as hormones and cytokines. Some factors including TNF-α, interferon-$\gamma\gamma$, interleukin-4 (IL-4), and IL-13 increase epithelial permeability (Colgan et al. 1994; Obiso et al. 1997), and others including TGF-$\beta\beta$ and IL-15 enhance barrier function (Planchon et al. 1994; Stevens et al. 1997). Regulation of paracellular and transcellular pathways plays a crucial role in preventing undesirable immune responses against food antigens and the microflora and in triggering responses that contribute to the elimination of invading pathogens.

Uptake of macromolecules, particulate antigens, and microorganisms across intact simple epithelia can occur by active transepithelial vesicular transport, but in vivo, access to epithelial surfaces and transport is restricted by multiple mechanisms (Kraehenbuhl and Neutra 2000). These include local secretions containing mucins and secretory IgA antibodies and cell surface specializations such as cilia, closely packed microvilli, and the glycocalyx, a thick (400–500 nm) layer of membrane-anchored glycoproteins (Maury et al. 1995). The glycocalyx of enterocytes is an effective diffusion barrier that contains large, negatively charged integral membrane mucin-like molecules, adsorbed pancreatic enzymes, and stalked intramembrane glycoprotein enzymes responsible for terminal digestion. Thus the glycocalyx appears to be designed to prevent the uptake of antigens and pathogens by enterocytes, while providing a highly degradative microenvironment that promotes the digestion and absorption of nutrients. This thick, highly glycosylated layer is impermeable to most macromolecular aggregates, particles, viruses, and bacteria and prevents their direct contact with the microvillus membrane (Apter et al. 1993; Frey et al. 1996; Mantis et al. 2000). However, many proteins and microbial products do gain access to intestinal epithelial cell surfaces, and these cells express potential scavenger receptors such as the mannose-6-phosphate–binding protein (Murayama 1990) or ganglioside GM1.

There is considerable evidence that epithelial cells, in particular enterocytes, can endocytose small amounts of intact proteins and peptides (Rubas and Grass 1991). The fate of the molecules varies, but most proteins that are taken up are transported to lysosomes and degraded. Nevertheless, enterocytes have been shown to transport small amounts of intact proteins and peptides across the epithelium. The ability of epithelial cells to internalize and transport luminal antigens from one cell surface to the other involves the directed movement of membrane vesicles. The nature and function of the compartments that comprise endocytic pathways directed either toward the degradative lysosomal compartment or to other destinations and the common molecular mechanisms that mediate sorting of membrane components were first elucidated in cultured cell lines (Courtoy 1991). It is likely that these apply to most polarized epithelial cells in mucosal tissues. Luminal antigens, whether transcytosed or directed into antigen-processing compartments, must be taken up either by fluid phase or receptor-mediated endocytosis via clathrin-coated or noncoated pits and vesicles. In epithelial cells the internalized vesicles fuse to form an "early endosome." Certain proteases are delivered into early endosomal compartments and the endosomal lumen acidifies to pH 6.0–6.2, a milieu in which certain ligands are released from their receptors (Maxfield and Yamashiru 1991). Membrane proteins, lipids, and content may be sorted in the early endosomes or in the TGN for rapid return to the same cell surface (recycling), transport along the degradative pathway (including antigen processing), or transport to the opposite membrane domain (transcytosis). In intestinal cell lines and enterocytes in vivo, there are distinct sets of apical and basolateral early endosomes that are functionally and compositionally different (Fujita et al. 1990; Gruenberg 2001). Apical and basolateral early endosomes cannot fuse with each other, but both can fuse with common "late endosomes." Transport of antigens from one side of an epithelium to the other is not accomplished by simple movement of a vesicle derived from one plasma membrane and fusion with the opposite side. Transcytosis requires a complex series of events including formation and fusion of endosomes, polarized recycling of membrane vesicles, and directional information provided by G proteins and by the highly polarized cytoskeleton of epithelial cells (Mostor and Cardone 1995).

Epithelial signaling in response to environmental antigens

Epithelial cells of mucosal tissues are able to recognize microbe-associated molecular patterns (MAMPs) on environmental microorganisms via pattern-recognition receptors, a heterogeneous family of proteins that include the toll-like receptors (TLRs). Human epithelial intestinal cells express TLR2, TLR3, TLR4, and TLR5. In the human gut, TLR3 and TLR5 are more abundant than TLR2 and TLR4 on colonocytes and villi enterocytes (Cairo and Podolsky 2000; Cairo et al. 2000). This distribution reflects the ability of the epithelium to sense flagellated enteropathogenic bacteria, including Salmonella typhimurium, Escherichia coli, Vibrio cholerae, and dsRNA enteroviruses such as reovirus and rotavirus. TLRs provide a link between recognition of MAMPs and signal transduction resulting in activation of the NFκB pathway. The NFκB transcription factor is essential for innate defenses because it regulates the expression of antimicrobial agents, cytokines, and chemokines (Dwinnell et al. 1999; Eckmann et al. 1995). Flagellin, the subunit of *Salmonella* flagella, is the major factor that triggers the proinflammatory gut epithelial cell response via TLR5. In human intestinal epithelial cell lines, flagellin also induces the NFκB-dependent upregulation of the chemokine CCL20, also known as macrophage inhibitory protein-3α (MIP-3α), or liver and activation-regulated chemokine (LARC). CCL20 attracts immature DCs as well as B and T cells that express CCR6. Thus, through MAMPs and TLRs, epithelial cells are able to link innate to adaptive immunity by attracting DCs that activate naive T lymphocytes. In addition, these signaling pathways can modulate the function of the epithelium itself.

ANTIGEN SAMPLING IN THE AIRWAYS

The lining of the airways, including nasopharynx, trachea, bronchi, and bronchioles varies from pseudostratified to simple epithelium. Although all of these epithelia are sealed by tight junctions, they have an extensive immune surveillance system (Zuercher et al. 2002) and at least two distinct antigen-sampling mechanisms. One of these mechanisms is widespread: in both upper and lower respiratory tract, intraepithelial DCs form a contiguous network, with up to 700 DCs per mm². These MHC class II–positive cells appear to sample inhaled antigens and migrate rapidly to draining lymph nodes. They are migratory cells, spending a short (average 2-day) time in the respiratory mucosa, and in this respect, they are comparable with the subepithelial DCs in the intestinal mucosa.

The nasal cavities and bronchi also have an alternative sampling system in the form of mucosal lymphoid follicles with overlying follicle-associated epithelium containing M cells (Bienenstock and Clancy 1994). In mice, organized lymphoid tissues with M cells form a strip along the floor of the nasal cavity, whereas in humans such tissue is concentrated in the nasopharyngeal tonsils or adenoids. Nasopharyngeal and bronchial M cells are structurally similar to their counterparts in intestine. Nasopharyngeal M cells of humans can take up antigens (Fujimura 2000), and bronchial M cells in mice have been shown to take up viral particles (Morin et al. 1994). However, the relative roles of the intraepithelial dendritic cell network and the organized lymphoid follicles in immune responses to antigens and pathogens are not clear. In the lung, macrophages migrate into alveolar spaces and patrol the surface of the delicate alveolar epithelium. It has been proposed that sampling of antigens by alveolar macrophages allows T-cell activation and expression of T-cell effector function, while selectively inhibiting T-cell proliferation (Upham et al. 1995).

ANTIGEN SAMPLING IN THE INTESTINAL EPITHELIUM

The role of intestinal epithelial cells

Soluble antigens that diffuse through the glycocalyx at the luminal surfaces of intestinal epithelial cells may be taken up and enter the early endosomal compartment. As discussed previously and reviewed elsewhere in this volume, such antigens can either go on to intracellular digestion in lysosomes, be transported across the cells by transcytosis, or enter antigen-processing compartments (**Fig. 7.2**). Evidence from *in vitro* systems suggests that some antigens can be transported across human enterocytes by receptor-mediated endocytosis in the form of antigen–antibody complexes. Murine and human enterocytes express MHC class I and II molecules as well as certain cathepsins required for antigen processing (Kaisetlain 1999). The role of endosomal compartments and vesicular traffic in antigen processing and MHC class II presentation has been investigated in intestinal cell lines (Zimmer et al., 2000; Hershberg et al. 1997, 1998). Antigens taken up apically or basolaterally are presented on the basolateral cell surface, and presentation is much more efficient when antigen internalization is mediated by receptors, as shown for antigens coupled to the B subunit of cholera toxin (Sun et al. 1994).

In response to inflammatory cytokines such as interferon-γ (IFN-γ) and TNF-α, enterocytes (especially in the crypts) upregulate expression of conventional class I molecules associated with β2–microglobulin. In addition, class I related CD1d molecules that are not associated with β2–microglobulin are expressed at the surfaces of intestinal epithelial cells and appear to function as antigen-presenting molecules for specific lipids rather than conventional peptide antigens (Burden and Kronenberg 1999; Porcelli and Modlin 1999; see also Chapter 25). CD1 proteins interact with several specialized populations of T cells, but the precise biologic functions mediated through these interactions remain to be determined. The possible role of antigen uptake by enterocytes in induction of immune responses or immune tolerance has been reviewed (Shao et al. 2001) and is discussed in detail elsewhere in this volume.

The role of dendritic cells

DCs, the only professional cells able to present antigens to naïve T lymphocytes, are derived from circulating monocytes (Banchereau and Steinman 1998) and migrate into mucosal tissues and epithelia following chemokine gradients. In the intestine, DCs are concentrated in great numbers under the follicle-associated epithelium (Ruedl et al. 1996; Kelsall and Strober 1996), but DCs also occur in the lamina propria and within the villus epithelium (MacPherson and Liu 1999). *In vitro*, immature DCs have been shown to be capable of migrating between epithelial cells, opening tight junctions, and capturing antigens via their dendrites. This phenomenon was associated with the upregulation of DC genes encoding epithelial adhesion and tight junction proteins including E-cadherin, occludin, and ZO-1 (Rescigno 2002; Rescigno et al. 2001). *In vivo*, *S. typhimurium* and nonpathogenic *E. coli* were found to stimulate the recruitment of DCs into the villus epithelium, and this was followed by uptake of bacteria by the recruited cells. CCL20 expression was found to be upregulated in the epithelium on villi of the small intestine in response to challenge with *Salmonella*, and this would be expected to attract DCs expressing CCR6. The epithelial CCL20 response is also elicited by *Salmonella* flagellin, a lig-

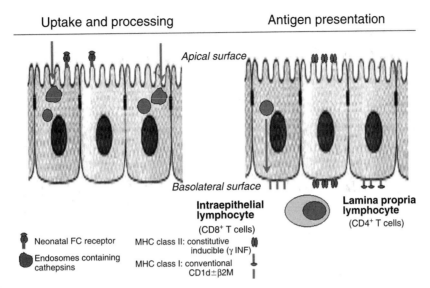

Fig. 7.2. Antigen uptake, processing, and presentation by intestinal epithelial cells. **(See page 1 of the color plates.)** Antigen uptake and processing: In the small intestine, villus enterocytes can endocytose antigens from the lumen and direct them into endosomes where they may be processed and loaded onto presentation molecules. Membrane components such as neonatal Fc receptors may enhance internalization of antigens (Spiekerman *et al.* 2002). Antigens are transported from early apical endosomes to a late endosomal compartment common to incoming apical and basolateral endocytic pathways. The late endosomes contain proteolytic enzymes, for example, cathepsins, that process antigens. Antigen presentation: Intestinal enterocytes express both class I and class II MHC molecules. These include conventional MHC 1 and CD1d, a nonclassical member of the MHC gene family, which may or may not be associated with β2 microglobulin (β2M). Conventional MHC II is synthesized with invariant chain in response to inflammatory signals such as γ-interferon (γ-IFN). Unconventional MHC II not associated with invariant chain is constitutively expressed on enterocytes.

and for TLR5 (Sierro *et al.* 2001). Flagellin appears to act via TLR5 to induce secretion of CCL20 by epithelial cells, and CCL20 may recruit immature DCs to the gut epithelium. Flagellin also triggers production of Th2 cytokines in bone marrow–derived and mesenteric lymph node DCs, and flagellin is a potent stimulator of antigen-specific IL-4 secretion by CD4$^+$ T cells as well as IgG1 antibody responses. As with TLR4 and TLR9 ligands, TLR5-mediated DC activation by flagellin requires MyD88 and induces NFκB-dependent transcription and IL-12p40 secretion. However, flagellin does not trigger secretion of the Th1 cytokine IL-12 p70 or high levels of proinflammatory cytokines. Thus the epithelial CCL20 response in the gut epithelium and recruitment of DCs provides an important link between innate and adaptive immune responses (Izadpanah *et al.* 2001).

Once intraepithelial DCs have taken up antigens or microorganisms, they are thought to leave the villus epithelium and migrate into the lamina propria and/or to draining lymph nodes (Huang *et al.* 2000; MacPherson *et al.* 1995). When an attenuated *S. typhimurium* strain defective in M-cell uptake was administered to mice by the oral route, the bacteria appeared very rapidly in CD18$^+$ cells, both DCs and macrophages, circulating in peripheral blood. The fact that no systemic infection occurred after oral *Salmonella* inoculation into CD18-deficient mice confirmed the importance of CD18$^+$ phagocytic cells in transport of bacteria from the intestine to other organs such as spleen.

Antigen sampling by DCs in the epithelium and lamina propria of the intestine may have both immune suppressive and stimulatory functions. It has been suggested that these

DCs may play a role in generating T cell–independent IgA antibody responses that are directed against commensal bacteria of the intestinal flora, perhaps by presenting native antigens to local naïve B cells (Fagarson *et al.* 2001). Such T cell–independent immune responses are thought to be an evolutionarily primitive form of specific immune defense designed to prevent the normal gut flora from invading the host. In addition, commensals that have crossed the mucosal barrier could be coated by commensal-specific IgA and either be transported back into the lumen by polymeric Ig receptor–mediated (pIgR-mediated) transcytosis or taken up locally and degraded by macrophages expressing Fc μ/α receptors.

SPECIALIZED ANTIGEN-TRANSPORTING EPITHELIA: THE FAE AND M CELLS

Special features of the follicle-associated epithelium

In contrast to the villus and surface epithelium of the intestine, the epithelium overlying mucosal lymphoid follicles (follicle-associated epithelium or FAE) appears to be designed to allow access of macromolecules, particles, and microorganisms to the local epithelial surface and to promote their uptake by transepithelial transport (Neutra *et al.* 1999, 2001). Apical surfaces of cells throughout the FAE are distinct from those of the surrounding villi. Although follicle-associated enterocytes, like their counterparts on villi, are coated with a thick glycoprotein coat or "glycocalyx" (Frey *et al.* 1996), they are not identical to villus cells. FAE enterocytes express lower levels of digestive enzymes (Owen and Bhalla 1983; Savidge and Smith

1995), and mucus-secreting goblet cells are scarce (Owen 1999). Numbers of defensin-producing and lysozyme-producing Paneth cells are reduced in follicle-associated crypts (Giannasca *et al.* 1994). Cells of the entire FAE do not express pIgR and therefore are unable to transport protective secretory IgA (S-IgA) into the intestinal lumen (Pappo and Owen 1988). All of these features tend to reduce antimicrobial defenses and promote local contact of intact antigens and pathogens with the FAE surface. In addition, glycosylation patterns of epithelial cells in the entire FAE differ from those on villi, indicating that glycosyltransferase activities in the FAE are distinct (Gebert and Hach 1993; Giannasca *et al.* 1999; Sharma *et al.* 1996). This may facilitate the recognition and adherence of microorganisms to the FAE.

FAE enterocytes constitutively express the chemokine CCL20. Under normal conditions, CCL20 is produced by intestinal FAE epithelial cells but not villus cells of both humans and mice (Tanaka *et al.* 1999; Iwasaki and Kelsall 2000; Cook *et al.* 2000). The fact that CCL20 has selective chemotactic activity for naive B and T lymphocytes and DCs that express CCR6 receptors suggests that it may be involved in constitutive formation and/or maintenance of organized mucosal lymphoid tissues, as discussed in the following text. CCL20 expression was transiently induced in epithelial cells *in vitro* by flagellin and by the cytokines TNF-α and IL-1 (Sierro *et al.*, 2001). Thus CCL20 could play a key role in the induction of new lymphoid follicles that has been observed in response to gram-negative enterobacteria. In mice lacking the chemokine receptor CCR6, DCs expressing CD11c and CD11b are absent from the subepithelial dome regions of Peyer's patches, and these mice have an impaired humoral immune response to orally administered antigen and to enteropathogenic rotavirus (Cook *et al.* 2000). DCs are present in the normal mouse FAE (Iwasaki *et al.* 2001), and additional DCs may be recruited into the FAE after oral administration of lipopolysaccharide (LPS) or cholera toxin (Anosova, N., Shreedher, V., and Neutra, M. R., unpublished).

The distinct nature of the FAE suggests that tissue-specific transcription factors may control the expression of multiple FAE-specific genes. In support of this idea, transgenic mice carrying a reporter gene under the control of a modified L-pyruvate kinase promoter (SVPK) exhibited strong transgene expression in Peyer's patch FAE, but not in adjacent villus cells (El Bahi *et al.* 2002). The interaction of the FAE with underlying connective tissue cells is also distinct. The FAE lacks the subepithelial myofibroblasts that form a sheath under the epithelium of villi, and the basal lamina of the FAE differs from that of villi: it lacks laminin-2 subunits (Sierro *et al.* 2000) and is highly porous, containing holes that presumably reflect frequent migration of cells into and out of the epithelium (McClugage *et al.*, 1986). However, the cardinal feature of the FAE is the presence of M cells.

Interaction of antigens with M cells

M cells are highly specialized epithelial cells that are joined to their neighbors by tight junctions that restrict the paracellular pathway, but M cells provide functional openings in the epithelial barrier through transepithelial vesicular transport activity. The fact that M-cell differentiation is largely restricted to the FAE reduces the inherent risk of transporting foreign material and microbes across the epithelial barrier by ensuring immediate uptake by DCs and exposure to the organized inductive machinery of the mucosal immune system. M-cell tight junctions define two major plasma membrane domains, apical and basolateral. The basolateral domain includes a large, invaginated subdomain that forms an intraepithelial "pocket" **(Figs. 7.3 and 7.4)** (Neutra *et al.* 2000). The pocket contains specific subpopulations of lymphocytes (Brandtzaeg *et al.* 1999), and this domain presumably displays adhesion molecules that promote docking of the intraepithelial lymphocytes that occupy this unique site in the FAE.

The apical membranes of M cells seem designed to promote adherence and uptake of foreign materials from the lumen (Neutra *et al.* 1999). They generally lack regular brush borders and instead have variable microvilli or microfolds interspersed with large plasma membrane subdomains that function in endocytosis. M cells conduct clathrin-mediated endocytosis of ligand-coated particles (Frey *et al.* 1996), adherent macromolecules (Bye *et al.* 1984; Neutra *et al.* 1987), and viruses (Sicinski *et al.* 1990) **(Fig. 7.5)**. M cells also conduct fluid-phase pinocytosis (Bockman and Cooper 1973; Owen 1977), actin-dependent phagocytosis (Neutra *et al.* 2003), and macropinocytotic engulfment involving dis-

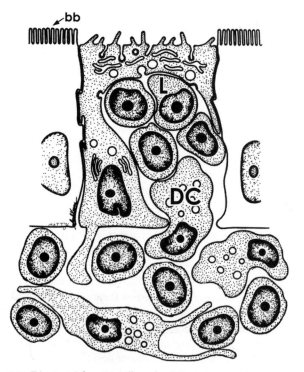

Fig. 7.3. Diagram of an M cell in the follicle-associated epithelium of the intestine. The basolateral surface of the M cell forms an intraepithelial pocket that contains B and T lymphocytes (L) and the occasional dendritic cell (DC). M cells may send cytoplasmic extensions into the subepithelial tissue. Many lymphocytes and a network of dendritic cells (D) are present under the follicle-associated epithelium. (Reproduced from Neutra *et al.* 1996.)

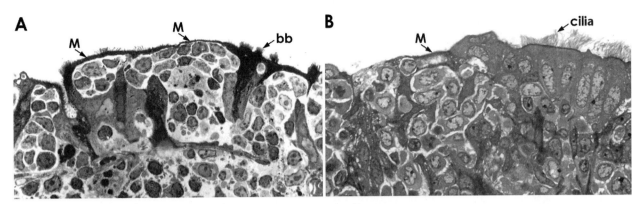

Fig. 7.4. Light micrographs of M cells. **A,** M cells in the follicle-associated epithelium of rabbit Peyer's patch. The epithelium contains numerous M cells that have relatively flat apical surfaces, lack brush borders (bb), and have pale nuclei in their basal cytoplasm. Lymphocytes with small, dense nuclei are present in very large intraepithelial M-cell pockets. Phagocytic cells and lymphocytes are congregated under the epithelium. **B,** M cells in human nasopharyngeal tonsils (adenoids). M cells are present in the pseudostratified, ciliated epithelium lining the deep crypts of the adenoids. They are recognized by their flat apical surfaces that have no cilia and by the clusters of lymphocytes in their large, complex intraepithelial pockets.

ruption of the apical cytoskeletal organization (Jones *et al.* 1994). M-cell membranes are particularly accessible to luminal particles because they lack a thick brush border glycocalyx (Frey *et al.* 1996; Mantis *et al.* 2000) (Fig. 7.5), and integral membrane hydrolytic enzymes (Owen and Bhalla 1983; Savidge and Smith 1995). Rapid binding and uptake of polystyrene or latex beads that adhere to M cells (Pappo and Ermak 1989; Shreedhar *et al.* 2003) and transport of other microparticles (Ermak *et al.* 1995) and liposomes (Childers *et al.* 1990; F. Zhou *et al.* 1995; Chen *et al.* 1996) suggest that particles or microorganisms with hydrophobic surfaces can adhere nonspecifically to M-cell surfaces.

Much remains to be learned about the specific adhesion molecules that may be present on M-cell apical surfaces. Human colonic (but not Peyer's patch) M cells express intercellular adhesion molecule 1 (ICAM-1) (Ueki *et al.* 1995), a molecule that is upregulated on apical membranes of intestinal enterocytes under conditions of inflammation and microbial infection (Huang *et al.* 2000; Kagnoff and Eckmann 1997). This suggests that the presence of this molecule on M cells may be a response to contact with pathogens or their products. In mice, α4/β1 integrin expression is detected in the apical membranes of M cells, and it has been suggested that this integrin may be exploited by pathogenic *Yersinia* to attach and invade (Marra and Isberg 1997; Clark *et al.* 1998; Schulte *et al.* 2000). In several species including humans, M-cell apical membranes display oligosaccharide structures that distinguish them from other epithelial cells (Giannasca *et al.* 1994, 1999; Clark *et al.* 1993; Neutra *et al.* 1999; Lelouard *et al.* 1999). It is tempting to think that certain pathogens can exploit M cell–specific carbohydrate structures to attach to M cells and invade the mucosa. Lectin and antibody probes also revealed variations in the glycosylation patterns of individual M cells within a single FAE (Giannasca *et al.* 1994, 1999). This diversity might expand the possible microbial lectin–M cell surface carbohydrate interactions of the local M-cell population and allow the M cells to "sample" a wider

variety of microorganisms. The M cell–specific carbohydrates in other intestinal regions (cecum, appendix, colon, and rectum) and in other species, including monkeys and humans, are distinct from those in BALB/c mouse Peyer's patches (Gebert and Hach 1993; Falk *et al.* 1994; Giannasca *et al.* 1994, 1999; Jepson *et al.* 1993; Lelouard *et al.* 1999), and there is no single, universal carbohydrate epitope that can serve to identify all M cells in all species.

Although the FAE does not secrete polymeric immunoglobulins, S-IgA that has been transported into the lumen adheres selectively to the apical membranes of M cells in mice, rabbits, and humans (Roy and Varvayanis 1987; Weltzin *et al.* 1989; Mantis *et al.* 2002). In rabbits and mice, exogenous mouse monoclonal IgA, mouse monoclonal IgA-antigen complexes, and human polyclonal S-IgA adhere to apical membranes of M cells and are transported into the intraepithelial pocket. Neither IgM nor IgG binds to mouse M cells. IgA binding is not dependent on secretory component (SC) and is not mediated by asialoglycoprotein receptors, pIgR, or CD89 (Mantis *et al.* 2002). M cells appear to express a novel IgA receptor that recognizes an epitope spanning the first and second constant domains of IgA (Mantis *et al.* 2002). Although the function of the IgA–M-cell interaction is unknown, there is some evidence that uptake of specific IgA-antigen complexes by M cells can induce a secretory immune response (Corthesy *et al.* 1996; F. Zhou *et al.* 1995). One possibility is that the IgA–M cell interaction may promote uptake of IgA-opsonized commensal microorganisms, promoting the maintenance of anticommensal immune responses that could control the luminal microflora and clear microorganisms from the mucosa (MacPherson *et al.* 2000). IgA-antigen complexes might also interact with leukocytes in the M-cell pocket or in underlying lymphoid tissue. IgA receptors in this microenvironment have not been defined, but the novel Fc α/μ receptor identified on macrophages, B cells, and DCs might play a role (Sakamoto *et al.* 2000; Shibuya *et al.* 2000). Alternatively, immature DCs, which are abundant in the subepithelial dome region of

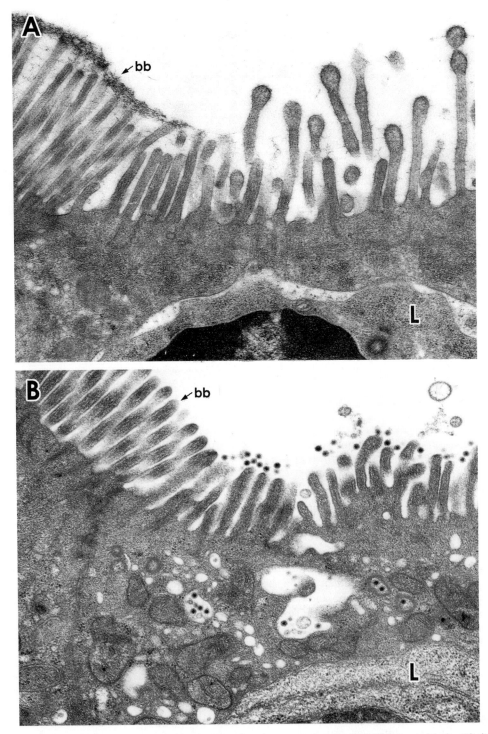

Fig. 7.5. Electron micrographs showing the apical surfaces of an M cell and an enterocyte in the follicle-associated epithelium. **A,** Glycocalyx. The M cell *(at right)* has irregular microvilli with a thin glycoprotein coat. In contrast, the enterocyte *(at left)* has closely-packed microvilli covered by a thick glycocalyx (arrowheads). A lymphocyte (L) is seen in the intraepithelial pocket of the M cell. (Micrograph by Dr. Paul Giannasca.) **B,** Uptake of reovirus. Reovirus (Type 1 Lang) was injected into the ileum of an adult mouse, and Peyer's patch tissue was collected 1 hour later. Reovirus particles are associated with the apical surface of an M cell but not with the microvilli of the neighboring enterocyte. Viral particles are present in M-cell apical endosomes, some of which are clathrin coated. (Micrograph by Dr. Richard Weltzin.)

organized mucosal lymphoid tissues (Iwasaki and Kelsall 2000), might bind S-IgA via the carbohydrate residues on SC. Carbohydrate-mediated binding of S-IgA to immature DCs was demonstrated *in vitro,* and was shown not to induce DC maturation (Heystek *et al.* 2002).

Transepithelial transport across M cells

Macromolecules, particles, and microorganisms taken up at the M-cell apical surface are internalized into endosomal tubules and vesicles and large multivesicular bodies that lie between the apical membrane and the intraepithelial pocket (Figs. 7.3, 7.5). The large vesicles contain the late endosome/lysosome membrane marker lgp120 and generate an acidic internal milieu (Allan *et al.* 1993). Immunocytochemical analysis revealed the presence of an endosomal protease, cathepsin E in rabbit M cells (Finzi *et al.* 1993), but the possible presence of other endosomal hydrolases in M-cell transport vesicles has not yet been examined. MHC class II antigens on M-cell membranes have been documented in subpopulations of M cells of some species (Allan *et al.* 1993). It is not yet known to what extent endocytosed materials are degraded during transepithelial transport, or whether M cells participate in the processing and presentation of antigens. In any case, transepithelial vesicular transport is the major vesicular pathway in M cells, and macromolecules and particles can be released at the pocket membrane as rapidly as 10–15 minutes later.

The pocket and its content of immigrant cells allows M cells to be identified in tissue sections, and the phenotypes of the cells in the M-cell pocket have been described in rodents (Jarry *et al.* 1989; Ermak and Owen 1994), rabbits (Ermak *et al.* 1990), and humans (Brandtzaeg *et al.* 1999) and are discussed elsewhere in this volume. Antigens and pathogens released into the M-cell pocket would first contact these cellular inhabitants, but almost nothing is known about the interactions that occur in this intraepithelial space. It is likely that most antigens and pathogens transported across the FAE by M cells are captured by immature DCs in the subepithelial dome (SED) region (Kelsall and Strober 1996; 1999). Live attenuated *S. typhimurium* and *Listeria monocytogenes* were detected in SED DCs after oral feeding (Hopkins *et al.* 2000; Pron *et al.* 2001). In organized mucosal lymphoid tissues such as the Peyer's patches, the site of initial antigen entry via M cells and capture by DCs occurs in close proximity to organized T-cell and B-cell zones. There is evidence that antigens or pathogens endocytosed by immature DCs in the SED region are ferried by DCs to the adjacent interfollicular T-cell zones where antigen presentation would be expected to occur (Iwasaki and Kelsall 2000). Indeed, subepithelial DCs of Peyer's patches were recently shown to migrate to adjacent T-cell areas in response to an injected parasite antigen and to express maturation markers in the T-cell zones (Iwasaki and Kelsall 2000). Subepithelial DCs did not migrate after ingesting inert fluorescent particles, but particle-containing cells moved to adjacent T-cell areas in response to CT or live

Salmonella (Shreedhar *et al.* 2003). The behavior of antigen-containing or pathogen-containing DCs and their patterns of migration into and out of the dome region are in need of further investigation. Although DC movements and accompanying cellular interactions are likely to be important determinants of mucosal immune responses, they may also facilitate dissemination of infectious agents that exploit the M-cell transport pathway (Pron *et al.* 2001).

EXPLOITATION OF ANTIGEN TRANSPORT PATHWAYS BY MUCOSAL PATHOGENS

Sampling of microorganisms by the mucosal immune system, whether it occurs by DC capture or M-cell transport, carries the risk that pathogens may exploit these mechanisms to cross epithelial barriers and invade the body. In stratified epithelia the antigen uptake and migratory activities of intraepithelial DCs, coupled with their ability to form close associations with T cells, are particularly well suited for rapid dissemination of pathogens that infect lymphoid tissues (Banchereau and Steinman 1998). For example, DCs derived from the epidermis were readily infected after exposure to HIV *in vitro* (Ayehunie *et al.* 1994; Pope *et al.* 1994), and conjugates of DCs and memory T cells showed efficient infection and viral production by the T cells (Ayehunie *et al.* 1994). Available evidence indicates that transmission of SIV across intact vaginal epithelium of monkeys may be mediated by $CD4^+$ DCs (Miller *et al.* 1989, 1992b; Spira *et al.* 1996). Thinning of the epithelium during the menstrual cycle or after progesterone treatment was associated with an increase in the efficiency of vaginal transmission (Marx *et al.* 1996).

The M-cell transport system provides a rapid entry route into the mucosa and thus plays a key role in the pathogenesis of certain bacterial and viral diseases. Since M cells of the intestine are continuously exposed to the lumen of the gut and are relatively accessible to pathogens, the risk of pathogen invasion at these sites is high. Viral and bacterial pathogens successfully exploit M-cell transport, as has been extensively reviewed (Siebers and Finlay 1996; Phalipon and Sansonetti 1999; Neutra *et al.* 2003). Uptake of microorganisms by M cells may also be crucial for maintenance of a normal bacterial flora in the intestine. M cells can transport commensal, noninvasive bacteria into Peyer's patches, and this may play a role in regulating endogenous microbial populations in the lumen or in eliminating and inactivating bacteria that have crossed the mucosal epithelium. Little is known about the processing of commensal bacteria in Peyer's patches or the mechanisms whereby the normal flora is maintained, but there is evidence that it involves T cell–independent IgA antibody responses (MacPherson *et al.* 2000). Uptake of nonpathogenic bacteria in neonates may be crucial for maturation of the mucosal immune system and for development of tolerance to food antigens (Cebra 1999; Cebra *et al.* 1999).

Transport of bacteria by M cells

Diverse gram-negative bacteria bind selectively to M cells, including *V. cholerae* (Owen *et al.* 1986; Winner *et al.* 1991), some strains of *E. coli* (Inman and Cantey 1983; Uchida 1987), *Salmonella typhi* (Kohbata *et al.* 1986), *S. typhimurium* (Jones *et al.* 1994), *Shigella flexneri* (Wassef *et al.* 1989), *Yersinia enterocolitica* (Grutzkau *et al.* 1990), *Yersinia pseudotuberculosis* (Fujimura *et al.* 1992), and *Campylobacter jejuni* (Walker *et al.* 1988). Rabbit M cells can efficiently transport bacillus Calmette-Guerin (Fujimura 1986), and *Mycobacterium paratuberculosis*, inoculated into ligated ileal loops of calves, entered organized mucosal lymphoid tissues presumably via M-cell transport (Momotani *et al.* 1988). Certain gram-positive bacteria such as *L. monocytogenes* can also adhere to and are transported by M cells. The molecular mechanisms involved in M-cell adherence and uptake of bacteria are largely unknown. It is likely that they involve a sequence of molecular interactions, including initial recognition (perhaps via a lectin–carbohydrate interaction), followed by more intimate associations that could require expression of additional bacterial genes, processing of M-cell surface molecules, activation of intracellular signaling pathways, and recruitment of integral or submembrane M-cell proteins to the interaction site. Some salient examples are briefly described here.

The vast majority of the many types of *E. coli* found in the intestine do not selectively adhere to epithelial cells. Certain pathogenic strains that do adhere and colonize and/or invade the mucosa also interact with M cells, but with dramatic differences. In ligated rabbit appendix, *E. coli* strain O:124 were taken up into phagosomelike vesicles and then released into the intraepithelial pocket (Uchida 1987). In contrast, the rabbit pathogen *E. coli* RDEC-1, a strain analogous to enteropathogenic *E. coli* (EPEC) in humans, rapidly induced "pedestals" on M cells identical to those later seen on enterocytes (Inman and Cantey 1983). Initial attachment to M cells is mediated by a plasmid-encoded AF/R1 pilus that is known to recognize a sialoglycoprotein complex in rabbit brush border preparations (Rafiee *et al.* 1991). Induction of the pedestals involves a complex sequence of events orchestrated by the bacterium from a chromosomal pathogenicity island. The bacterium uses a type III secretion system to insert a bacterial product (translocated intimin receptor, Tir) into the host cell membrane, which, when phosphorylated, serves as receptor for the bacterial ligand, intimin. This interaction results in a cascade of cell signal transduction events that culminate in formation of an actin-supported pedestal that supports the bacterium (DeVinney *et al.* 1999). Although pedestal formation is thought to prevent transcytosis by M cells, some uptake nevertheless occurs and infection of humans with EPEC evokes a vigorous immune response (Karch *et al.* 1987).

The earliest stage of infection by invasive bacterial pathogens such as *Salmonella* and *Shigella* involves bacterial translocation through M cells. Differences in the diseases caused by these organisms reflects their diverse effects on host cells after M-cell transport (Neutra *et al.* 2003). For example, *Shigella* infections are limited to the mucosa, while *Salmonella* spreads systemically (Sansonetti and Phalipon 1999). *In vitro* assays have shown that invasion of enterocytes by *Shigella* occurs at the basolateral (but not the apical) cell surface (Mounier *et al.* 1992). *In vivo*, *Shigella* apparently uses M-cell transport to gain access to the basolateral side of the FAE and adjacent epithelium (Wassef *et al.* 1989; Mathan and Mathan 1991; Sansonetti 1991; Sansonetti *et al.* 1996). Uptake into cells occurs through a macropinocytic process that is induced by secretion of bacterial proteins (Ipa) through a type III secretory apparatus. Shigellae then lyse the phagosome membrane, escape into the cytoplasm, and initiate a complex actin-based motility process (Bourdet-Sicard *et al.* 2000) that facilitates their spread from cell to cell (Sansonetti *et al.* 1994). Intracellular shigellae induce activation of NFκB that results in production of IL-8 by epithelial cells (Philpott *et al.* 2000), influx of polymorphonuclear leukocytes into the lamina propria, and mucosal destruction (Wassef *et al.* 1989; Sansonetti 1991; Sansonetti *et al.* 1996). The inflammatory process leads to rapid disruption of the epithelial barrier, thereby facilitating further *Shigella* invasion (Sansonetti and Phalipon 1999).

After oral administration in mice, *S. typhimurium* cross the intestinal barrier and cause a lethal septicemia that closely mimics typhoid fever caused by *S. typhi* in humans. Following injection into ligated intestinal loops in mice, *S. typhimurium* preferentially adheres to M cells of the FAE (Jones *et al.* 1994; Clark *et al.* 1994). A carbohydrate epitope containing galactose linked β(1-3) to galactosamine serves as receptor for *S. typhimurium* on Caco-2 cells (Giannasca *et al.* 1996), but the structure that mediates attachment to M cells *in vivo* is not known. M cells are sites of rapid entry, but *Salmonella* can also enter via the villus epithelium (Takeuchi 1967; Vasquez-Torres *et al.* 1999). The long Lpf fimbriae of *S. typhimurium* seem to mediate adherence to M cells of the murine FAE (Baumler *et al.* 1996). Other adherence mechanisms probably exist, however, since *lpf* mutants show reduced but still significant colonization of murine Peyer's patches. Uptake of the bacteria by M cells occurs by macropinocytosis, and during this process, the bacterium has cytotoxic effects that eventually result in destruction of M cells and the FAE as well as severe inflammatory lesions in Peyer's patches (Kohbata *et al.* 1986; Jones *et al.* 1994, Jones and Falkow 1996). The type III secretion system encoded in the SPI1 pathogenicity island, which allows delivery of *Salmonella* invasion proteins (Sip) into host cells, is likely to be important for invasion and cytotoxicity in M cells, because SPI1 mutants do not destroy the FAE or M cells (Jones *et al.* 1994; Penheiter *et al.* 1997). After crossing of the FAE, *Salmonella* are captured by DCs (Hopkins *et al.* 2000). There is also evidence that small numbers of *Salmonella* can enter the lamina propria mouse of intestinal villi via an M cell–independent pathway that involves capture by intraepithelial DCs, as described previously (Vazques-Torres *et al.* 1999).

Transport of viruses by M cells

Viruses are relatively simple structures that generally depend on adherence to enter endocytic pathways of host epithelial cells. Adherence to M-cell surfaces may be sufficient to ensure entry into Peyer's patch mucosa, because adherent particles and macromolecules are efficiently transcytosed by these cells. Some viral surface proteins have enzymatic activity (Colman et al. 1983; Bisaillon et al. 1999), but there is no evidence that such activity is required for adherence to M cells. Two closely related viral pathogens, reovirus in mice and poliovirus in humans, have been shown to use selective adherence to M cells as an invasion strategy (Wolf et al. 1981; Sicinski et al. 1990), and M-cell transport of several other animal viruses has also been documented (reviewed by Siebers and Finlay 1996).

The mouse pathogen reovirus adheres selectively to M cells and uses this pathway to enter the intestinal mucosa (J. L. Wolf et al. 1981). Reovirus binds to M cells in the Peyer's patches, colon (Owen et al. 1990), and airways of mice and in Peyer's patches of rabbits (Helander et al. 2003). Proteolytic processing of the outer capsid of reovirus in the mouse intestinal lumen increases viral infectivity (Bodkin et al. 1989; Bass et al. 1990) and is required for M-cell adherence (Amerongen et al. 1994). Intestinal proteases remove the outermost capsid protein (sigma 3) and induce a conformational change in the sigma 1 protein that results in its extension up to 45 nm from the viral surface (Nibert et al. 1991; Lee and Gilmore 1998). Recent studies in one of our laboratories have shown that reovirus type 1 binding to M cells is mediated by interaction of the extended Σ 1 protein with a specific sialic acid–containing trisaccharide on the M-cell apical surface (Helander et al. 2003). This determinant is present on all epithelial cells, but appears to be more accessible on M cells (Mantis et al. 2000; Helander et al. 2003). Adherent reovirus is endocytosed by M cells in clathrin-coated pits (Figure 7.5B) and is released into the intraepithelial pocket and subepithelial dome region where it infects phagocytes that are most likely DCs (Kelsall and Strober 1996). Reovirus is unable to adhere to the apical membranes of enterocytes but can infect the entire epithelium from the basolateral side. This underscores the importance of the brush border glycocalyx in protection of enterocytes against luminal pathogens.

Poliovirus enters the body by the oral route and has been shown to proliferate in Peyer's patches before spreading systemically (Racaniello and Ren 1996). Live, attenuated poliovirus was known to evoke a protective mucosal immune response (Ogra and Karzon 1969) long before the ultrastructure and antigen-transporting activity of M cells was first described (Bockman and Cooper 1973). When explants of human Peyer's patch mucosa were exposed in vitro to wild poliovirus type 1 or to the attenuated Sabin strain, and were then examined by electron microscopy, the virus adhered selectively to M cells and was endocytosed (Sicinski et al. 1990). The receptor for poliovirus on neuronal target cell membranes is a member of the immunoglobulin superfamily, and transgenic mice expressing the receptor can be infected by injection of virus (Mendelsohn et al.. 1989). When these mice were challenged orally, viral replication was not detected in the intestinal mucosa, but the nasal mucosa was infected. The mice developed paralytic disease (Racaniello and Ren 1996). It is not known whether the

binding site that poliovirus uses to adhere to M cells is the same or different from that used on target neurons. Nevertheless, the ability of poliovirus to exploit M-cell transport for penetration of the epithelial barrier have led to testing of poliovirus-based oral vaccine vectors for delivery of foreign antigens, either as recombinant viral particles (Crotty et al. 2001) or as pseudovirus particles (Choi et al. 1991; Morrow et al. 1999).

Rectal or vaginal exposure to infected semen can result in HIV transmission (Milman and Sharma 1994), and studies of SIV transmission in monkeys have shown that free SIV can infect via intact rectal or vaginal mucosa (Pauza et al. 1993; Clerici et al. 1994; Lehner et al. 1996; Miller et al. 1989). Evidence to date indicates that HIV and SIV can exploit multiple antigen uptake mechanisms, including M cells, intraepithelial DCs, and vesicular transepithelial transport pathways, to cross epithelial barriers (Amerongen et al. 1991; Kraehenbuhl and Wain-Hobson 1996; Miller et al. 1994; Spira et al. 1996; Bomsel 1997). Normal epithelial cells in vivo do not become infected (Fox et al. 1989), but in vitro studies have shown that isolated epithelial cells can internalize and release virus directly onto target cells (Meng et al. 2002; Dezutti et al. 2001). Whether this occurs in vivo is not known.

In the rectum and recto-anal junction, organized lymphoid tissues and M cells are numerous (O'Leary and Sweeney 1986), and entry of HIV is relatively efficient (Milman and Sharma 1994). There is indirect evidence that M cells may be involved in HIV entry. Using mouse and rabbit mucosal explants in organ culture, we showed that HIV-1 can adhere to M cells and that these cells can transport HIV across the epithelial barrier (Amerongen et al. 1991). If HIV transport occurs via M cells, the virus would have rapid access to organized mucosal lymphoid tissues rich in target T cells, macrophages, and DCs. Intestinal enterocytes are also a potential entry site. Intestinal epithelial cells of humans and monkeys in vivo do not express CD4, but their membranes do contain an alternate receptor, galactosylceramide (Holgersson et al. 1988; Butor et al. 1996), a glycosphingolipid that can mediate HIV infection of neoplastic intestinal epithelial cell lines such as HT29 and Caco-2 cells in culture (Yahi et al. 1992; Fantini et al. 1993; Furuta et al. 1994). When HIV-infected cells were applied to epithelial monolayers in culture, virus crossed the epithelium, presumably by a transcytotic vesicular pathway (Bomsel 1997). Recently one of our laboratories has confirmed that free or cell-associated HIV-1 can infect poorly differentiated Caco-2 cell monolayers and cross the monolayer by transcytosis and that transcytosis results in infection of mononuclear target cells on the serosal side of the epithelium. We further demonstrated that CCR5 or CXCR4 chemokine receptors, together with galactosylceramide, are required for infection of these epithelial cells by non–syncytium-inducing (NSI) or syncytium-inducing (SI) HIV-1, respectively, and for transcytosis to occur (Fotopoulos et al. 2002). M-like cells obtained by coculture of Caco-2 cells and B cells in vitro also transmitted the virus when the cells expressed galactosylceramide and the appropriate chemokine receptor. These results suggest that transcytosis of HIV-1 across M cells *in vivo* may be receptor mediated. It is not clear how HIV particles or HIV-infected cells would gain access to glycolipids in enterocyte membranes *in vivo*, however, because enterocytes throughout the human intestine have brush borders coated with a continuous, 400–500 nm–thick glycocalyx.

PLASTICITY OF ANTIGEN SAMPLING MECHANISMS AT EPITHELIAL SURFACES

Both resident (FAE and M cell) and migratory (Langerhans cells and DCs) antigen-sampling systems associated with simple or stratified epithelia can be modulated by environmental and host factors. The interplay of exogenous microorganisms with epithelial cells and underlying mucosal cells has complex and poorly understood effects on epithelial antigen-uptake systems. On the other side, endogenous hormonal influences can modulate both the behavior of migratory antigen-presenting cells and the structure and function of the epithelia barrier.

Role of commensal microflora
Microorganisms play a crucial role in development of organized mucosal lymphoid tissues. In the gut, colonization by nonpathogenic organisms results in establishment of complex stable societies that maintain their composition despite exposure to an ever-changing luminal environment. The microflora is able to influence the differentiation program of mucosal epithelial cells, thereby creating favorable niches (Bry *et al.* 1996) while shaping the host's adaptive mucosal defense system (Bos *et al.* 2001; Cebra 1999; Cebra *et al.* 1999; Chapter 18, this volume). Germfree mice have a reduced number of Peyer's patches, even though they are fully immunocompetent, but lymphoid follicles and M cells increase in number after exposure to a single bacterial species (Savidge *et al.* 1991) or after transfer to a normal animal house environment (Smith *et al.* 1987). Repopulating germfree mice with a single nonpathogenic microorganism (*Clostridium indolis*) was sufficient to restore the normal number of Peyer's patches (S. Kerneis, unpublished data). Microorganisms also modulate the migration of professional antigen-presenting cells and lymphocytes into simple or stratified epithelia (Holt *et al.* 1994; Eriksson *et al.* 1996).

Role of microbial pathogens
When certain pathogenic microorganisms bind to host epithelial cells, they activate signal transduction pathways that result in the activation of membrane-associated enzymes such as tyrosine protein kinases that modulate the expression of epithelial cell transcription factors (Rosenshine *et al.* 1992; Bliska *et al.* 1993; Eckmann *et al.* 1995; Jones and Falkow 1996). These factors control the expression of chemokines and cytokines (Savkovic *et al.* 1996). For instance, respiratory syncytial virus in the lung (Jamaluddin *et al.* 1996) and *Helicobacter pylori* in the stomach (Segal *et al.*

1996) have been shown to trigger the release of CXCL-8 (IL-8), IL-6, and CCL5 (Rantes). Such signaling molecules may directly or indirectly upregulate endothelial addressins on mucosal small venules, thus facilitating polynuclear and mononuclear cell extravasation (Butcher 1999; Wagner *et al.* 1996). As a result, these factors may cause recruitment of antigen-presenting cells into the mucosa (Eckmann *et al.* 1995, Hsu *et al.* 1995; Jung *et al.* 1995). For example, the release of epithelial chemokines mediates the recruitment of monocytes into the lung (Holt 1994, 2000; McWilliam *et al.* 1994; Sozzani *et al.* 1995), and these can differentiate into immature DCs. *In vitro*, granulocyte-macrophage colony-stimulating factor (GM-CSF) has been found to play a major role in inducing monocytes to differentiate into immature DCs, and TNF-α stimulates the switch of DCs from the sampling to the antigen-presentation mode (Banchereau and Steinman 1998). Some chemokines form gradients by binding to extracellular matrix components, thus supporting the directional migration of leukocytes toward the epithelium (Madara 1994). These signaling mechanisms could play an indirect role in FAE differentiation by promoting the assembly of lymphoid follicles. On the other hand, viral and bacterial pathogens that infect M cells can cause selective loss of this cell type (Bass *et al.* 1988; Jones *et al.* 1994), and this could compromise the ability of the FAE to transport antigens in a selective, controlled manner.

Role of endogenous host factors
In the female genital tract, sexual steroids may modulate the antigen-sampling capacity of the cervical and vaginal epithelia. During the luteal phase of the sexual cycle in rodents, nonhuman primates, and humans, the thickness of the epithelium decreases (Miller *et al.* 1989, 1992b; Young and Hosking 1986; Yeaman *et al.* 1998). This phenomenon, which can be mimicked in monkeys by administration of progesterone (Marx *et al.* 1996), increases the access of DC processes to the epithelial surface and thus may facilitate sampling of antigens, microorganisms (Miller *et al.* 1989), and vaccines (Hopkins *et al.* 1995). In rodents (but not in monkeys), the number of DCs in the vagina is upregulated during the luteal phase (Miller *et al.* 1992a). On the other hand, a study testing the effectiveness of vaginal administration in humans showed that immunization during the follicular phase of the menstrual cycle resulted in stronger antibody responses than immunization during the luteal phase (Kozlowski *et al.* 2002). Thus the effects of hormones show significant species differences.

Plasticity of FAE and M cells
Differentiation of the FAE and M cells is subject to exogenous influences from the lumen and endogenous influences from mucosal cells (for review, see Finke and Kraehenbuhl 2002). The cells of the FAE in the intestine, like all intestinal epithelial cells, are derived from stem cells in the crypts. In adult small intestine, each crypt is a clonal unit harboring a ring of anchored stem cells near the crypt base that gives rise to multiple cell types that migrate upward in columns onto

several adjacent villi (Schmidt *et al.* 1985; Potten and Morris 1988; Gordon and Hermiston 1994). The molecular mechanisms that regulate proliferation and differentiation as the cells migrate from the crypt to the villus are beginning to be understood. The epithelium of the FAE is derived from the crypts surrounding the mucosal lymphoid follicles. The follicle-associated crypts are unusual in that they contain two distinct axes of migration from the same ring of crypt stem cells: cells on one wall of the crypt differentiate into absorptive enterocytes, goblet and enteroendocrine cells that migrate onto the villi, and cells on the opposite wall of the same crypt acquire features of M cells and distinct follicle-associated enterocytes (Bye *et al.* 1984; Gebert *et al.* 1992, 1999; Giannasca *et al.* 1994; Savidge and Smith 1995). As they emerge from the crypt, differentiating M cells begin endocytic activity, fail to assemble brush borders, and acquire immune cells in their characteristic intraepithelial pocket.

There is indirect evidence that cell contacts and/or soluble factors from mucosal lymphoid follicles play an important role in the induction of FAE and M cells (Debard *et al.* 2001). The fact that the follicle-facing side of follicle-associated crypts shows distinct features, including immature M cells and a lack of pIgR expression (Pappo and Owen 1988; Giannasca *et al.* 1994; Gebert *et al.* 1999) indicates that factors produced by mucosa-associated lymphoid tissues (MALT) may act very early in the differentiation pathway, inducing crypt cells to commit to FAE phenotypes. On the other hand, factors or cells from the follicle or the lumen may also act later, to convert some of the FAE enterocyte-like cells to antigen-transporting M cells. The possibility of enterocyte–M cell conversion is supported by the observation that cells with both enterocyte and M-cell features are present in FAE (Gebert *et al.* 1992; Kernéis *et al.* 1996) and that M-cell numbers have been observed to increase after *Salmonella* infection (Savidge *et al.* 1991) and within hours after challenge with a nonintestinal bacterium (Borghesi *et al.* 1996, 1999).

The importance of lymphoid cells in the induction of the FAE is supported by the fact that injection of Peyer's patch lymphocytes into the submucosa of syngeneic mice resulted in local assembly of a new lymphoid follicle and the *de novo* appearance of FAE with typical M cells (Kernéis *et al.* 1997). Immunodeficient SCID mice lack mucosal follicles and identifiable M cells, but follicles with FAE appeared after injection of Peyer's patch cells and fractions enriched in B cells were most effective in reconstituting these structures (Savidge and Smith 1995). Other lines of evidence indicate that B cells play a crucial role. In B cell–deficient mice, the size of the mucosal follicles and the number of M cells are dramatically reduced, but some identifiable M cells are still present (Debard *et al.* 2001; Sierro *et al.* 2000). In contrast, T cell–deficient nude mice have small Peyer's patches with FAE and M cells (Ermak and Owen 1987). Induction of new lymphoid follicles is accompanied by induction of FAE and M cells, as documented in inflamed ileal mucosa (Cuvelier *et al.* 1993). Cytokines are likely to play a role in this phenomenon.

The three-way interaction of epithelium, lymphoid cells, and microorganisms seen in the FAE provides a dramatic demonstration of the phenotypic plasticity of the intestinal epithelium and probably of all simple epithelia.

The role of endogenous factors in development of organized MALT (Finke and Kraehenbuhl 2002) is evidenced by the fact that rudimentary Peyer's patches appear at predictable locations in the small intestine before birth. The fact that Peyer's patches do not form in lymphotoxin (LT) single-knockout and TNF-α/LT double-knockout mice suggests that LT is involved in the induction of organized mucosal lymphoid tissues (De Togni *et al.* 1994; Eugster *et al.* 1995; Futterer *et al.* 1998). A role for LT was supported by experiments in which soluble LTαβ trimers expressed in transgenic mice altered the development of Peyer's patches but not of peripheral lymph nodes (Ettinger *et al.* 1996). The interruption of a B cell–specific chemokine receptor gene impaired the formation of Peyer's patches and inguinal lymph nodes, but not other peripheral lymph nodes (Forster *et al.* 1996). More recently, lymphocytes expressing CD4 but lacking CD3 were shown to play a key role in development of Peyer's patches: adoptive transfer of CD4+CD3− hematopoietic progenitor cells restored Peyer's patch formation and resulted in a higher than normal number of patches (Finke *et al.* 2002).

The requirement for lymphocytes and their products for induction of mucosal follicles and FAE *in vivo* have guided the development of an *in vitro* system that mimics some of the features of the FAE. Murine Peyer's patch lymphocytes cocultured with monolayers of a well-differentiated human enterocyte (Caco-2 cell) line induced disorganization of the enterocyte brush borders and the loss of cell surface sucrase-isomaltase. This was paralleled by a gain of transcytotic activity, as evidenced by temperature-dependent translocation of inert latex particles and *V. cholerae* from the apical to the basolateral compartment. Human B (Raji) but not T (Jurkat) lymphoid cells were able to induce the same changes: again, the Caco-2 cells lost the brush borders typical of villus-type absorptive enterocytes and acquired apical surface features and transcytotic activity typical of M cells (Kernéis *et al.* 1997). This supports the hypothesis that the differentiation pathways of intestinal epithelial cells and the capacity for transepithelial antigen transport can be modulated by lymphocyte–epithelial interactions.

CONCLUSIONS

Although epithelia of all mucosal surfaces maintain a selective barrier, they have mechanisms for providing samples of the external environment to the immune system. Several distinct strategies are used to accomplish this: some epithelia allow transepithelial traffic of professional antigen-presenting DCs, and others produce a specialized antigen-transporting epithelial phenotype, the M cell. The specific molecular recognition systems and nonspecific adherence mechanisms that determine the efficiency of these transport pathways are poorly understood, and much remains to be learned about the fates of transported antigens and the factors that determine the nature and magnitude of the resulting immune responses.

ACKNOWLEDGMENTS

We are grateful to the current and former members of our laboratories who have contributed to the work summarized in this review. The authors are supported by NIH Research Grants HD17557, AI33384, and NIH Center Grant DK34854 to the Harvard Digestive Diseases Center (MRN) and by the Swiss National Science Foundation Grant 31.37155.93 and Swiss League Against Cancer Grant 373.89.2 (JPK).

REFERENCES

Allan, C. H., Mendrick, D. L., and Trier, J. S. (1993). Rat intestinal M cells contain acidic endosomal-lysosomal compartments and express Class II major histocompatibility complex determinants. *Gastroenterology* 104, 698–708.

Amerongen, H. M., Weltzin, R. A., Farnet, C. M., Michetti, P., Haseltine, W. A., and Neutra, M. R. (1991). Transepithelial transport of HIV-1 by intestinal M cells: A mechanism for transmission of AIDS. *J. Acquir. Immune Defic. Syndr.* 4, 760–765.

Amerongen, H. M., Wilson, G. A. R., Fields, B. N., and Neutra M. R. (1994). Proteolytic processing of reovirus is required for adherence to intestinal M cells. *J. Virol.* 68, 8428–8432.

Anderson, D. J. (1996). The importance of mucosal immunology to problems in human reproduction. *J. Reprod. Immunol.* 31, 3–19.

Apodaca, G. (2001). Endocytic traffic in polarized epithelial cells: Role of the actin and microtubule cytoskeleton. *Traffic* 2, 149–159.

Apter, F. M., Michetti, P., Winner, L. S., III, Mack, J. A., Mekalanos, J. J., and Neutra, M. R. (1993). Analysis of the roles of antilipopolysaccharide and anti-cholera toxin IgA antibodies in protection against *Vibrio cholerae* and cholera toxin using monoclonal IgA antibodies *in vivo*. *Infect. Immun.* 61, 5279–5285.

Ayehunie, S., Bruzzese, A. M., Groves, R. W., Kupper, T. S., and Langhoff, E. (1994). HIV-1 transmission by mucosal Langerhans cells, blood dendritic cells, and monocytes *in vitro*. *Reg. Immunol.* 6, 105–111.

Balk, S. P., Burke, S., Polischuk, J. E., Frantz, M. E., Yang, L., Porcelli, S., Colgan, S. P., and Blumberg, R. S. (1994). β2-microglobulin-independent MHC class Ib molecule expressed by human intestinal epithelium. *Science* 265, 259–262.

Banchereau, J., and Steinman, R. M. (1998). Dendritic cells and the control of immunity. *Nature* 392, 245–252.

Bass, D. M., Trier, J. S., Dambrauskas, R., and Wolf, J. L. (1988). Reovirus type 1 infection of small intestinal epithelium in suckling mice and its effect on M cells. *Lab. Invest.* 55, 226–235.

Bass, D. M., Bodkin, D., Dambrauskas, R., Trier, J. S., Fields, B. N., and Wolf, J. L. (1990). Intraluminal proteolytic activation plays an important role in replication of type 1 reovirus in the intestines of neonatal mice. *J. Virol.* 64, 1830–1833.

Batlle, E., Henderson, J. T., Beghtel, H., van den Born, M. M. W., Sancho, E., Huis, G., Meeldijk, J., Robertson, J., van de Wetering, M., Pawson, T., and Clevers, H. (2002). Beta-catenin and TCF mediate cell positioning in the intestinal epithelium by controlling the expression of EphB/EphrinB. *Cell* 111, 251–263.

Baumler, A. J., Tsolis, R. M., and Heffron, F. (1996). The *lpf* fimbrial operon mediates adhesion of *Salmonella typhimurium* to murine Peyer's patch. *Proc. Natl. Acad. Sci. USA* 93, 279–283.

Bienenstock, J., and Clancy, R. (1994). Bronchial mucosal lymphoid tissue. In *Handbook of Mucosal Immunology* (eds. P. L. Ogra, J.

Mestecky, M. E. Lamm, J. R. McGhee, W. Strober, J. Bienenstock), 529–538. New York, Academic Press.

Bisaillon, M., Bernier, L., Sénéchal, S., and Lemay, G. (1999). A glycosyl hydrolase activity of mammalian reovirus sigma1 protein can contribute to viral infection through a mucus layer. *J. Mol. Biol.* 286, 759–773.

Bliska, J. B., Galan, J. E., and Falkow, S. (1993). Signal transduction in the mammalian cell during bacterial attachment and entry. *Cell* 73, 903–920.

Bockman, D. E., and Cooper, M. D. (1973). Pinocytosis by epithelium associated with lymphoid follicles in the bursa of Fabricius, appendix, and Peyer's patches. An electron microscopic study. *Am. J. Anat.* 136, 455–478.

Bodkin, D. K., Nibert, M. L., and Fields, B. N. (1989). Proteolytic digestion of reovirus in the intestinal lumen of neonatal mice. *J. Virol.* 63, 4676–4681.

Bomsel, M. (1997). Transcytosis of infectious human immunodeficiency virus across a tight epithelial cell line barrier. *Nat. Med.* 3, 42–47.

Borghesi, C., Regoli, M., Bertelli, E., and Nicoletti, C. (1996). Modifications of the follicle-associated epithelium by short-term exposure to a non-intestinal bacterium. *J. Pathol.* 180, 326–332.

Borghesi, C., Taussig, M. J., and Nicoletti, C. (1999). Rapid appearance of M cells after microbial challenge is restricted at the periphery of the follicle-associated epithelium of Peyer's patch. *Lab. Invest.* 79, 1393–1401.

Bos, N. A., Jiang, H. Q., and Cebra, J. J. (2001). T cell control of the gut IgA response against commensal bacteria. *Gut* 48, 762–764.

Bourdet-Sicard, R., Egile, C., Sansonetti, P. J., and Tran Van Nhieu, G. (2000). Diversion of cytoskeletal processes by *Shigella* during invasion of epithelial cells. *Microb. Infect.* 2, 813–819.

Brandtzaeg, P., Baekkevold, E. S., Farstad, I. N., Jahnsen, F. L., Johansen, F. E., Nilsen, E. M., and Yamanaka, T. (1999). Regional specialization in the mucosal immune system: What happens in the microcompartments? *Immunol. Today* 20, 141–151.

Bry, L., Falk, P. G., Midtvedt, T., and Gordon, J. I. (1996). A model of host-microbial interactions in an open mammalian ecosystem. *Science* 273, 1380–1383.

Burden, N., and Kronenberg, M. (1999). CD1-mediated immune responses to glycolipids. *Curr. Opin. Immunol.* 11, 326–331.

Butcher, E. C., Williams, M., Youngman, K., Rott, L., and Briskin, M. (1999). Lymphocyte trafficking and regional immunity. *Adv. Immunol.* 72, 209–253.

Butor, C., Couedel-Courteille, A., Guilet, J. G., and Venet, A. (1996). Differential distribution of galactosylceramide, H antigen, and carcinoembryonic antigen in rhesus macaque digestive mucosa. *J. Histochem. Cytochem.* 44, 1021–1031.

Bye, W. A., Allan, C. H., and Trier, J. S. (1984). Structure, distribution and origin of M cells in Peyer's patches of mouse ileum. *Gastroenterology* 86, 789–801.

Cario, E., and Podolsky, D. K. (2000). Differential alteration in intestinal epithelial cell expression of toll-like receptor 3 (TLR3) and TLR4 in inflammatory bowel disease. *Infect. Immun.* 68, 7010–7017.

Cario, E., Rosenberg, I. M., Brandwein, S. L., Beck, P. L., Reinecker, H. C., and Podolsky, D. K. (2000). Lipopolysaccharide activates distinct signaling pathways in intestinal epithelial cell lines expressing toll-like receptors. *J. Immunol.* 164, 966–972.

Cebra, J. J. (1999). Influences of microbiota on intestinal immune system development. (1999). *Am. J. Clin. Nutr.* 69, 1046S–1051S.

Cebra, J. J., Jiang, H-Q., Sterzl, J., and Tlasalova-Hogenova, H. (1999). The role of mucosal microbiota in the development and maintenance of the mucosal immune system. In *Mucosal Immunology* (eds. R. Ogra, J. Mestecky, J. McGhee, J. Bienenstock, M. Lamm, and W. Strober), 267–280. San Diego: Academic Press.

Chen, H., Torchilin, V., and Langer, R. (1996). Lectin-bearing polymerized liposomes as potential oral vaccine carriers. *Pharm. Res.* 13, 1378–1383.

Childers, N. K., Denys, F. R., McGhee, J. F., and Michalek, S. M. (1990). Ultrastructural study of liposome uptake by M cells of rat Peyer's patches: An oral vaccine system for delivery of purified antigen. *Regional Immunol.* 3, 8–16.

Choi, W. S., Pal-Ghosh, R., and Morrow, C. D. (1991). Expression of human immunodeficiency virus type 1 (HIV-1) gag, pol, and env proteins from chimeric HIV-1-poliovirus minireplicons. *J. Virol.* 65, 2875–2883.

Clark, M. A., Jepson, M. A., Simmons, N. L., Booth, T. A., and Hirst, B. H. (1993). Differential expression of lectin-binding sites defines mouse intestinal M-cells. *J. Histochem. Cytochem.* 41, 1679–1687.

Clark, M. A., Jepson, M. A., Simmons, N. L., and Hirst, B. H. (1994). Preferential interaction of *Salmonella typhimurium* with mouse Peyer's patch M cells. *Res. Microbiol.* 145, 543–552.

Clark, M. A., Hirst, B. H., and Jepson, M. A. (1998). M-cell surface β1 integrin expression and invasin-mediated targeting of *Yersinia pseudotuberculosis* to mouse Peyer's patch M cells. *Infect. Immun.* 66, 1237–1244.

Clerici, M., Clark, E. A., Polacino, P., Axberg, I., Kuller, L., Casey, N. I,. Morton, W. R., Shearer, G. M., and Benveniste, R. E. (1994). T-cell proliferation to subinfectious SIV correlates with lack of infection after challenge of macaques. *AIDS* 8, 1391–1395.

Colgan, S. P., Parkos, C. A., Matthews, J. B., Dandrea, L., Awtrey, C. S., Lichtman, A. H., Delparcher, C., and Madara, J. L. (1994). Interferon-gamma induces a cell-surface phenotype switch on T84 intestinal epithelial cells. *Am. J. Physiol.* 267, C402–C410.

Colman, P. M., Varghese, J. N., and Laver, W. G. (1983). Structure of the catalytic and antigenic sites in influenza virus neuraminidase. *Nature (Lond.)* 303, 41–47.

Cook, D. N., Prosser, D. M., Forster, R., Zhang, J., Kuklin, N. A., Abbondanzo, S. J., Niu, X. D., Chen, S. C., Manfra, D. J., Wiekowski, M. T., Sullivan, L. M., Smith, S. R., Greenberg, H. B., Narula, S. K., Lipp, M., and Lira, S. A. (2000). CCR6 mediates dendritic cell localization, lymphocyte homeostasis, and immune responses in mucosal tissue. *Immunity* 12, 495–503.

Corthesy, B., Kaufmann, M., Phalipon, A., Peitsch, M., Neutra, M. R., and Kraehenbuhl, J. P. (1996). A pathogen-specific epitope inserted into recombinant secretory immunoglobulin is immunogenic by the oral route. *J. Biol. Chem.* 52, 33670–33677.

Courtoy, P. J. (1991). Dissection of endosomes. In *Intracellular Trafficking of Proteins* (eds. C. J. Steer and J. A. Hanover), 103–156. Cambridge: Cambridge University Press.

Crotty, S., Miller, C. J., Lohman, B. L., Neagu, M. R, Compton, L., Lu, D., Lu, F. X., Fritts, L, Lifson, J. D., and Andino, R. (2001). Protection against simian immunodeficiency virus vaginal challenge by using Sabin poliovirus vectors. *J. Virol.* 75, 7435–7452.

Cuvelier, C. A., Quatacker, J., Mielants, H., de Vos, M., Veys, E., and Roels, H. (1993). M cells are damaged and increased in number in inflamed human ileal mucosa. *Eur. J. Morphol.* 31, 87–91.

De Togni, P., Goellner, J., Ruddle, N. H., Streeter, P. R., Fick, A., Mariathasan, S., Smith, S. C., Carlson, R., Shornick, L. P., Strauss-Schoenberger, J., Russell, J. H., Karr, R., and Chaplin, D. D. (1994). Abnormal development of peripheral lymphoid organs in mice deficient in lymphotoxin. *Science* 264, 703–706.

Debard, N., Sierro, F., Browning, J., and Kraehenbuhl, J. P. (2001). Effect of mature lymphocytes and lymphotoxin on the development of the follicle-associated epithelium and M cells in mouse Peyer's patches. *Gastroenterology* 120, 1173–1182.

DeVinney, R., Knoechel, D. G., and Finlay, B. B. (1999). Enteropathogenic *Escherichia coli*: cellular harassment. *Curr. Opin. Microbiol.* 2, 83–88.

Dezzutti, C. S., Guenthner, P. C., Cummins, Jr. J. E., Cabrera, T., Marshall, J. H., Dillberger, A., and Lal, R. B. (2001). Cervical and prostate primary epithelial cells are not productively infected but sequester human immunodeficiency virus type 1. *J. Infect. Dis.* 183, 1204–1213.

Donnenberg, M. S., Kaper, J. B., and Finlay, B. B. (1997). Interactions between enteropathogenic *Escherichia coli* and host epithelial cells. *Trends Microbiol.* 5, 109–114.

Druben, D. G., and Nelson, W. J. (1996). Origins of cell polarity. *Cell* 84, 335–344.

Dwinell, M. B., Eckmann, L., Leopard, J. D., Varki, N. M., and Kagnoff, M. F. (1999). Chemokine receptor expression by human intestinal epithelial cells. *Gastroenterology* 117, 359–367.

Eckmann, L., Kagnoff, M. F., and Fierer, J. (1995). Intestinal epithelial cells as watchdogs for the natural immune system. *Trends Microbiol.* 3, 118–120.

El Bahi, S., Caliot, E., Bens, M., Bogdanova, A., Kerneis, S., Kahn, A., Vandewalle, A., and Pringault, E. (2002). Lymphoepithelial interactions trigger specific regulation of gene expression in the M cell-containing follicle-associated epithelium of Peyer's patches. *J. Immunol.* 168, 3713–3720.

Eriksson, K., Ahlfors, E., George-Chandy, A., Kaiserlian, D., and Czerkinsky, C. (1996). Antigen presentation in the murine oral epithelium. *Immunology* 88, 147–152.

Ermak, T. H., and Owen, R. L. (1987). Phenotype and distribution of T lymphocytes in Peyer's patches of athymic mice. *Histochemistry* 87, 321–325.

Ermak, T. H., and Owen, R. L. (1994). Differential distribution of lymphocytes and accessory cells in mouse Peyer's patches. *Am. J. Trop. Med. Hyg.* 50, 14–28.

Ermak, T. H., Steger, H. J., and Pappo, J. (1990). Phenotypically distinct subpopulations of T cells in domes and M-cell pockets of rabbit gut-associated lymphoid tissues. *Immunology* 71, 530–537.

Ermak, T. H., Dougherty, E. P., Bhagat, H. R., Kabok, Z., and Pappo, J. (1995). Uptake and transport of copolymer biodegradable microspheres by rabbit Peyer's patch M cells. *Cell Tissue Res.* 279, 433–436.

Ettinger, R., Browning, J. L., Michie, S. A., van Ewijk, W., and McDevitt, H. O. (1996). Disrupted splenic architecture, but normal lymph node development in mice expressing a soluble lymphotoxin-beta receptor-IgG1 fusion protein. *Proc. Natl. Acad. Sci. USA* 93, 13102–13107.

Eugster, H. P., Müller, M., Karrer, U., Car, B. D., Schnyder, B., Eng, V. M., Woerly, G., Le Hir, M., di Padova, F., Aguet, M., Zinkernagel, R. M., Bluethmann, H., and Ryffel, B. (1995). Multiple immune abnormalities in tumor necrosis factor and lymphotoxin-alpha double-deficient mice. *Int. Immunol.* 8, 23–36.

Fagarasan, S., Kinoshita, K., Muramatsu, M., Ikuta, K., and Honjo, T. (2001). *In situ* class switching and differentiation to IgA-producing cells in the gut lamina propria. *Nature* 413, 639–643.

Falk, P., Roth., K. A., and Gordon, J. I. (1994). Lectins are sensitive tools for defining the differentiation programs of epithelial cell lineages in the developing and adult mouse gastrointestinal tract. *Am. J. Physiol.* 266, G987–G1003.

Fantini, J., Cook, D. G., Nathanson, N., Spitalnik, S. L., and Gonzalez-Scarano, F. (1993). Infection of colonic epithelial cell lines by type 1 human immunodeficiency virus (HIV-1) is associated with cell surface expression of galactosyl ceramide, a potential alternative gp120 receptor. *Proc. Natl. Acad. Sci. USA* 90, 2700–2704.

Farbman, A. I. (1988). The oral cavity. In *Cell and Tissue Biology* (ed. L. Weiss), 573–594. Baltimore: Urban and Schwartzenberg.

Finke, D., and Kraehenbuhl, J.P. (2002). Formation of Peyer's patches. *Curr. Opin. Gen. Dev.* 11, 562–569.

Finke, D., Acha-Orbea, H., Mattis, A., Lipp, M., and Kraehenbuhl, J.-P. (2002). CD4+ CD3– cells induce Peyer's patch development: Role of alpha4beta1-integrin-activation by CXCR5. *Immunity* 17, 363–373.

Finzi, G., Cornaggia, M., Capella, C., Fiocca, R., Bosi, F., and Solcia, E. (1993). Cathepsin E in follicle associated epithelium of intestine and tonsils: Localization to M cells and possible role in antigen processing. *Histochemistry* 99, 201–211.

Forster, R., Mattis, A. E., Kremmer, E., Wolf, E., Brem, G., and Lipp, M. (1996). A putative chemokine receptor, blr1, directs B cell migration to defined lymphoid organs and specific anatomic compartments of the spleen. *Cell* 87, 1037–1047.

Fotopoulos, G., Harari, A., Michetti, P., Trono, D., Pantaleo, G., and Kraehenbuhl, J. P. (2002). Transepithelial transport of HIV-1 by M cells is receptor mediated. *Proc. Natl. Acad. Sci. USA* 99, 9410–9414.

Fox, C. H., Kotler, D., Tierney, A., Wilson, C. S., and Fauci, A. S. (1989). Detection of HIV-1 RNA in the lamina propria of patients with AIDS and gastrointestinal disease. *J. Infect. Dis.* 159, 467–471.

Frey, A., Lencer, W. I., Weltzin, R., Giannasca, K. T., Giannasca, P. J., and Neutra, M. R. (1996). Role of the glycocalyx in regulating access of microparticles to apical plasma membranes of intestinal epithelial cells: Implications for microbial attachment and oral vaccine targeting. *J. Exp. Med.* 184, 1045–1060.

Fujimura, Y. (1986). Functional morphology of microfold cells (M cells) in Peyer's patches. Phagocytosis and transport of BCG by M cells into rabbit Peyer's patches. *Gastroenterol. Jpn.* 21, 325–335.

Fujimura, Y. (2000). Evidence of M cells as portals of entry for antigens in the nasopharyngeal lymphoid tissue of humans. *Virchows Arch.* 436, 560.

Fujimura, Y., Kihara, T., and Mine, H. (1992). Membranous cells as a portal of *Yersinia pseudotuberculosis* entry into rabbit ileum. *J. Clin. Electron Microsc.* 25, 35–45.

Fujita, M., Reinhart, F., and Neutra, M. (1990). Convergence of apical and basolateral endocytic pathways at apical late endosomes in absorptive cells of suckling rat ileum. *J. Cell Sci.* 97, 385–394.

Furuta, Y., Erikkson, K,. Svennerholm, B., Fredman, P., Horal, P., Jeansson, S., Vahlne, A., Holmgren, J., and Czerkinsky, C. (1994). Infection of vaginal and colonic epithelial cells by the human immunodeficiency virus type 1 is neutralized by antibodies raised against conserved epitopes in the envelope glycoprotein gp120. *Proc. Natl. Acad. Sci. USA* 91, 12559–12563.

Fütterer, A., Mink, K., Luz, A., Koscovilbois, M. H., and Pfeffer, K. (1998). The lymphotoxin beta receptor controls organogenesis and affinity maturation in peripheral lymphoid tissues. *Immunity* 9, 59–70.

Gebert, A., and Hach, G. (1993). Differential binding of lectins to M cells and enterocytes in the rabbit cecum. *Gastroenterology* 105, 1350–1361.

Gebert, A., Hach, G., and Bartels, H. (1992). Co-localization of vimentin and cytokeratins in M-cells of rabbit gut-associated lymphoid tissue (GALT). *Cell Tiss. Res.* 269, 331–340.

Gebert A., Fassbender, S., Werner, K., and Weissferdt, A. (1999). The development of M cells in Peyer's patches is restricted to specialized dome-associated crypts. *Am. J. Pathol.* 154, 1573–1582.

Gewirtz, A. T., Navas, T. A., Lyons, L., Godowski, P. J., and Madara, J. L. (2001). Bacterial flagellin activates basolaterally expressed TLR5 to induce epithelial proinflammatory gene expression. *J. Immunol.* 167, 1882–1885.

Giannasca, K. T., Giannasca, P. J., and Neutra, M. R. (1996). Adherence of *Salmonella typhimurium* to Caco-2 cells: Identification of a glycoconjugate receptor. *Infect. Immun.* 64, 135–145.

Giannasca, P. J., Giannasca, K. T., Falk, P., Gordon, J. I., and Neutra, M. R. (1994). Regional differences in glycoconjugates of intestinal M cells in mice: Potential targets for mucosal vaccines. *Am. J. Physiol.* 267, G1108–G1121.

Giannasca, P. J., Giannasca, K. T., Leichtner, A. M., and Neutra, M. R. (1999). Human intestinal M cells display the sialyl Lewis A antigen. *Infect. Immun.* 67, 946–953.

Gordon, J. I., and Hermiston, M. L. (1994). Differentiation and self-renewal in the mouse gastrointestinal epithelium. *Curr. Opin. Cell. Biol.* 6, 795–803.

Gruenberg, L. (2001). The endocytic pathway: A mosaic of domains. *Nat. Rev. Mol. Cell Biol.* 2, 721–730.

Grutzkau, A., Hanski, C., Hahn, H., and Riecken, E. O. (1990). Involvement of M cells in the bacterial invasion of Peyer's patches: A common mechanism shared by *Yersinia enterocolitica* and other enteroinvasive bacteria. *Gut* 3, 1011–1015.

Helander, A., Silvey, K. J., Mantis, N. J., Hutchings, A. B., Chandran, K., Lucas, W. T., Nibert, M. L., and Neutra, M. R. (2003). The viral sigma 1 protein and glycoconjugates containing alpha 2-3-linked sialic acid are involved in type 1 reovirus adherence to M cell apical surfaces. *J. Virol.* 77, 7964–7977.

Hershberg, R. M., Framson, P. E., Cho, D. H., Lee, L. Y., Kovats, S., Beitz, J., Blum, J. S., and Nepom, G. T. (1997). Intestinal epithelial cells use two distinct pathways for HLA class II antigen processing. *J. Clin. Invest.* 100, 204–215.

Hershberg, R. M., Cho, D. H., Youakim, A., Bradley, M. B., Lee, J. S., Framson, P. E., and Nepom, G. T. (1998). Highly polarized Hla class II antigen processing and presentation by human intestinal epithelial cells. *J. Clin. Invest.* 102, 792–803.

Heystek, H. C., Moulon, C., Woltman, A. M., Garonne, P., and van Kooten, C. (2002). Human immature dendritic cells efficiently bind and take up secretory IgA without the induction of maturation. *J. Immunol.* 168, 102–107.

Hoffmann, J. A., Kafatos, F. C., Janeway, C. A., and Ezekowitz, R. A. (1999). Phylogenetic perspectives in innate immunity. *Science* 284, 1313–1318.

Holgersson, J., Stromberg, N., and Breimer, M. E. (1988). Glycolipids of human large intestine: Differences in glycolipid expression related to anatomical localization, epithelial/non-epithelial tissue and the ABO, Le, and Se phenotypes of the donors. *Biochemie* 70, 1565–1574.

Holt, P. G. (2000). Antigen presentation in the lung. *Am. J. Respir. Crit. Care Med.* 162, S151–S156.

Holt, P. G., Schon-Hegrad, M. A., and McMenamin, P. G. (1990). Dendritic cells in the respiratory tract. *Int. Rev. Immunol.* 6, 139–149.

Holt, P. G., Haining, S., Nelson, D. J., and Sedgwick, J. D. (1994). Origin and steady-state turnover of class II MHC-bearing dendritic cells in the epithelium of the conducting airways. *J. Immunol.* 153, 256–261.

Hopkins, S., Kraehenbuhl, J. P., Schoedel, F., Potts, A., Peterson, D., De Grandi, P., and Nardelli-Haefliger, D. (1995). A recombinant *Salmonella typhimurium* vaccine induces local immunity by four different routes of immunization. *Infect. Immun.* 63, 3279–3286.

Hopkins, S., Niedergang, F., Courthésy-Theulaz, I.E., and Kraehenbuhl, J. P. (2000). A recombinant *Salmonella typhimurium* vaccine stain is taken up and survives within murine Peyer's patch dendritic cells. *Cell Microbiol.* 2, 56–68.

Hsu, N., Young, L. S., and Bermudez, L. E. (1995). Response to stimulation with recombinant cytokines and synthesis of cytokines by murine intestinal macrophages infected with the *Mycobacterium avium* complex. *Infect. Immun.* 63, 528–533.

Huang, F. P., Platt, N., Wykes, M., Major, J. R., Powell, T. J., Jenkins, C. D., and MacPherson, G. G. (2000). A discrete subpopulation of dendritic cells transports apoptotic intestinal epithelial cells to T cell areas of mesenteric lymph nodes. *J. Exp. Med.* 191, 435–443.

Inman, L. R., and Cantey, J. R. (1983). Specific adherence of *Escherichia coli* (strain RDEC-1) to membranous (M) cells of the Peyer's patch in *Escherichia coli* diarrhea in the rabbit. *J. Clin. Invest.* 71, 1–8.

Inman, L. R., and Cantey, J. R. (1984). Peyer's patch lymphoid follicle epithelial adherence of a rabbit enteropathogenic *Escherichia coli* (strain RDEC-1): Role of plasmid-mediated pili in initial adherence. *J. Clin. Invest.* 74, 90–95.

Iwasaki, A., and Kelsall, B. L. (2000). Localization of distinct Peyer's patch dendritic cell subsets and their recruitment by chemokines macrophage inflammatory protein (MIP)-3 alpha, MIP-3 beta, and secondary lymphoid organ chemokine. *J. Exp. Med.* 191, 1381–1393.

Iwasaki, A., and B. L. Kelsall. (2001). Unique functions of CD11b+, CD8a+ and double-negative Peyer's patch dendritic cells. *J. Immunol.* 166, 4884–4890.

Izadpanah, A., Dwinell, M. B., Eckmann, L., Varki, N. M., and Kagnoff, M. F. (2001). Regulated MIP-3alpha/CCL20 production by human intestinal epithelium: Mechanism for modulating mucosal immunity. *Am. J. Physiol.* 280, G710–G719.

Jamaluddin, M., Garofalo, R., Ogra, P. L., and Brasier, A. R. (1996). Inducible translational regulation of the nf-il6 transcription factor by respiratory syncytial virus infection in pulmonary epithelial cells. *J. Virol.* 70, 1554–1563.

Jameson, B., Baribaud, F., Pohlmann, S., Ghavimi, D., Mortari, F., Doms, R. W., and Iwasaki, A. (2002). Expression of DC-SIGN by dendritic cells of intestinal and genital mucosae in humans and rhesus macaques. *J. Virol.* 76, 1866–1875.

Jarry, A., Robaszkiewicz, M., Brousse, N., and Potet, F. (1989). Immune cells associated with M cells in the follicle-associated epithelium of Peyer's patches in the rat. *Cell Tissue Res.* 225, 293–298.

Jepson, M. A., Clark, M. A., Simmons, N. L., and Hirst, B. H. (1993). Epithelial M cells in the rabbit caecal lymphoid patch display distinctive surface characteristics. *Histochemistry* 100, 441–447.

Jones, B. D., and Falkow, S. (1996). Salmonellosis: Host immune responses and bacterial virulence determinants. *Annu. Rev. Immunol.* 14, 533–561.

Jones, B. D., Ghori, N., and Falkow, S. (1994). *Salmonella typhimurium* initiates murine infection by penetrating and destroying the specialized epithelial M cells of the Peyer's patches. *J. Exp. Med.* 180, 15–23.

Jung, H. C., Eckmann, L., Yang, S. K., Panja, A., Fierer, J., Morzycka-Wroblewska, E., and Kagnoff, M. F. (1995). A distinct array of proinflammatory cytokines is expressed in human colon epithelial cells in response to bacterial invasion. *J. Clin. Invest.* 95, 55–65.

Kagnoff, M. F., and Eckmann, L. (1997). Epithelial cells as sensors for microbial infection. *J. Clin. Invest.* 100, S51–S55.

Kaiserlian, D. (1999). Antigen sampling and presentation by epithelial cells in mucosal tissues. *Curr. Top. Microbiol. Immunol.* 236, 55–78.

Karch, H., Heesemann, J., Laufs, R., Kroll, H. P., Kaper, J. B., and Levine, M. M. (1987). Serological response to type 1-like somatic fimbriae in diarrheal infection due to classical enteropathogenic *Escherichia coli. Microb. Pathog.* 2, 425–434.

Kelsall, B. L., and Strober, W. (1996). Distinct populations of dendritic cells are present in the subepithelial dome and T cell regions of murine Peyer's patches. *J. Exp. Med.* 183, 237–247.

Kelsall, B. L., and Strober, W. (1999). Gut-associated lymphoid tissue: Antigen handling and T cell responses. In *Mucosal Immunology* (eds. R. Ogra, J. Mestecky, J. R. McGhee, J. Bienenstock, M. E. Lamm, and W. Strober), 293–318. San Diego: Academic Press.

Kernéis, S., Bogdanova, A., Colucci-Guyon, E., Kraehenbuhl, J. P., and Pringault, E. (1996). Cytosolic distribution of villin in M cells from mouse Peyer's patches correlates with the absence of a brush border. *Gastroenterology* 110, 515–521.

Kernéis, S., Bogdanova, A., Kraehenbuhl, J. P., and Pringault, E. (1997). Conversion by Peyer's patch lymphocytes of human enterocytes into M cells that transport bacteria. *Science* 277, 948–952.

King, N. J. C., Parr, E. L., and Parr, M. B. (1998). Migration of lymphoid cells from vaginal epithelium to iliac lymph nodes in relation to vaginal infection by herpes simplex virus type 2. *J. Immunol.* 160, 1173–1180.

Knust, E. (2002). Regulation of epithelial cell shape and polarity by cell–cell adhesion. *Mol. Membr. Biol.* 19, 113–120.

Kohbata, S., Yokobata, H., and Yabuuchi, E. (1986). Cytopathogenic effect of *Salmonella typhi* GIFU 10007 on M cells of murine ileal Peyer's patches in ligated ileal loops: An ultrastructural study. *Microbiol. Immunol.* 30, 1225–1237.

Kozlowski, P. A., Williams, S. B., Lynch, R. L., Flanigan, T. P., Patterson, R. R., Cu-Uvin, S., and Neutra, M. R. (2002). Differential induction of mucosal and systemic antibody responses in women after nasal, rectal, or vaginal immunization: Influence of the menstrual cycle. *J. Immunol.* 169, 566–574.

Kraehenbuhl, J.-P., and Neutra, M. R. (2000). Epithelial M cells: Differentiation and function. *Annu. Rev. Cell Dev. Biol.* 16, 301–332.

Kraehenbuhl, J.-P., and Wain-Hobson, S. (1996). Breaching barriers. *Nat. Med.* 2, 1080–1082.

Lee, P. W. K., and Gilmore, R. (1998). Reovirus cell attachment protein sigma 1: Structure–function relationships and biogenesis. In *Reoviruses. I: Structure, Proteins, and Genetics* (eds. K. L. Tyler and M. B. A. Oldstone), 137–153. Berlin: Springer-Verlaag.

Lehner, T., Bergmeier, L., Tao, L., Brookes, R., Hussain, L., Klavinskis, L., and Mitchell, E. (1996). Mucosal receptors and T- and B-cell immunity. In *Development and Applications of Vaccines and Gene Therapy in AIDS, vol. 4.* (eds. G. Giraldo, D. P. Bolognesi, M. Salvatore, and E. Beth-Giraldo), 21–29. Basel: Karger.

Lelouard, H., Reggio, H., Mangeat, P., Neutra, M. R., and Montcourrier, P. (1999). Mucin related epitopes distinguish M cells and enterocytes in rabbit appendix and Peyer's patches. *Infect. Immun.* 67, 357–367.

Macpherson, A. J., Gatto, D., Sainsbury, E., Harriman, G. R., Hengartner, H., and Zinkernagel, R. M. (2000). A primitive T cell-independent mechanism of intestinal mucosal IgA responses to commensal bacteria. *Science* 288, 2222–2226.

MacPherson, G. G., and L. M. Liu. (1999). Dendritic cells and Langerhans cells in the uptake of mucosal antigens. *Curr. Top. Microbiol. Immunol.* 256, 33–54.

MacPherson, G. G., Jenkins, C. D., Stein, M. J., and Edwards, C. (1995). Endotoxin-mediated dendritic cell release from the intestine: Characterization of released dendritic cells and TNF dependence. *J. Immunol.* 154, 1317–1322.

Madara, J. L. (1994). Migration of neutrophils through epithelial monolayers. *Trends Cell Biol.* 4, 4–7.

Madara, J. L., Nash, S., Moore, R., and Atisook, K. (1990). Structure and function of the intestinal epithelial barrier in health and disease. *Monogr. Pathol.* 31, 306–324.

Maldonado-Lopez, R., De Smedt, T., Michel, P., Godfroid, J., Pajak, B., Heirman, C., Thielemans, K., Leo, O., Urbain, J., and Moser, M. (1999). CD8 alpha(+) and CD8 alpha(−) subclasses of dendritic cells direct the development of distinct T helper cells *in vivo. J. Exp. Med.* 189, 587–592.

Mantis, N. J., Frey, A., and Neutra, M. R. (2000). Accessibility of glycolipid and oligosaccharide epitopes on rabbit villus and follicle-associated epithelium. *Am. J. Physiol.* 278, G915–G923.

Mantis, N. J., Cheung, M. C., Chintalacharuvu, K. R., Rey, J., Corthesy, B., and Neutra, M. R. (2002). Selective adherence of immunoglobulin A to murine Peyer's patch M cells: Evidence for a novel IgA receptor. *J. Immunol.* 169, 1844–1851.

Marra, A., and Isberg, R. R. (1997). Invasin-dependent and invasin-independent pathways for translocation of *Yersinia pseudotuberculosis* across the Peyer's patch intestinal epithelium. *Infect. Immun.* 65, 3412–3421.

Marx, P. A., Spira, A. I., Gettie, A., Dailey, P. J., Veazey, R. S., Lackner, A. A., Mahoney, C. J., Miller, C. J., Claypool, L. E., Ho, D. D., and Alexander, N. J. (1996). Progesterone implants enhance SIV vaginal transmission and early virus load. *Nat. Med.* 2, 1084–1089.

Masurier, C., Salomon, B., Guettari, N., Pioche, N., Lachapelle, F., Guigon, M., and Klatzmann, D. (1998). Dendritic cells route human immunodeficiency virus to lymph nodes after vaginal or intravenous administration to mice. *J. Virol.* 72, 7822–7829.

Mathan, M. M., and Mathan, V. I. (1991). Morphology of rectal mucosa of patients with shigellosis. *Rev. Infect. Dis.* 13 (suppl. 4), S314–S318.

Matter, K., and Mellman, I. (1994). Mechanisms of cell polarity: sorting and transport in epithelial cells. *Curr. Opin. Cell Biol.* 6, 545–554.

Maury, J., Nicoletti, C., Guzzo-Chambraud, L., and Maroux, S. (1995). The filamentous brush border glycocalyx: A mucin-like marker of enterocyte hyper-polarization. *Eur. J. Biochem.* 228, 323–331.

Maxfield, F. R., and Yamashiro, D. J. (1991). Acidification of organelles and the intracellular sorting of proteins during endocytosis. In *Intracellular Trafficking of Proteins* (eds. C. J. Steer and J. A. Hanover), 157–182. Cambridge: Cambridge University Press.

McClugage, S. G., Low, F. N., and Zimmy, M. L. (1986). Porosity of the basement membrane overlying Peyer's patches in rats and monkeys. *Gastroenterology* 91, 1128–1133.

McWilliam, A. S., Nelson, D., Thomas, J. A., and Holt, P. G. (1994). Rapid dendritic cell recruitment is a hallmark of the acute inflammatory response at mucosal surfaces. *J. Exp. Med.* 179, 1331–1336.

Mendelsohn, C. L., Wimmer, E., and Racaniello, V. R. (1989). Cellular receptor for poliovirus: Molecular cloning, nucleotide sequence, and expression of a new member of the immunoglobulin superfamily. *Cell* 56, 855–865.

Meng, G., Wei, X., Wu, X., Sellers, M. T., Decker, J. M., Moldoveanu, Z., Orenstein, J. M., Graham, M. F., Kappes, J. C., Mestecky, J., Shaw, G. M., and Smith, P. D. (2002). Primary intestinal epithelial cells selectively transfer R5 HIV-1 to CCR5+ cells. *Nat. Med.* 8, 150–156.

Miller, C. J., Alexander, N. J., Sutjipto, S., Lackner, A. A., Gettie, A., Hendrickx, A. G., Lowenstine, L. J., Jennings, M., and Marx, P. A. (1989). Genital mucosal transmission of simian immunodeficiency virus: Animal model for heterosexual transmission of human immunodeficiency virus. *J. Virol.* 63, 4277–4284.

Miller, C. J., McChesney, M., and Moore, P. F. (1992a). Langerhans cells, macrophages, and lymphocyte subsets in the cervix and vagina of rhesus macaques. *Lab. Invest.* 67, 628–634.

Miller, C. J., Vogel, P., Alexander, N. J., Sutjipto, S., Hendrickx, A. G., and Marx, P. A. (1992b). Localization of SIV in the genital tract of chronically infected female rhesus macaques. *Am. J. Pathol.* 141, 655–660.

Miller, C. J., McGhee, J. R., and Gardner, M. B. (1993). Mucosal immunity, HIV transmission, and AIDS. *Lab. Invest.* 68, 129–145.

Miller, C. J., Vogel, P., Alexander, N. J., Dandekar, S., Hendrickx, A. G., and Marx, P. A. (1994). Pathology and localization of simian immunodeficiency virus in the reproductive tract of chronically infected male rhesus macaques. *Lab. Invest.* 70, 255–262.

Milman, G., and Sharma, O. (1994). Mechanisms of HIV/SIV mucosal transmission. *AIDS Res. Human Retrovir.* 10, 1305–1312.

Momotani, E., Whipple, D. L., Thiermann, A. B., and Cheville, N. F. (1988). Role of M cells and macrophages in the entrance of *Mycobacterium paratuberculosis* into domes of ileal Peyer's patches in calves. *Vet. Pathol.* 25, 131–137.

Morin, M. J., Warner, A., and Fields, B. N. (1994). A pathway for entry of reoviruses into the host through M cells of the respiratory tract. *J. Exp. Med.* 180, 1523–1527.

Morrow, C. D., Novak, M. J., Ansardi, D. C., Porter, D. C., and Moldoveanu, Z. (1999). Recombinant viruses as vectors for mucosal immunity. *Curr. Top. Microbiol. Immunol.* 236, 255–274.

Mostov, K. E., and Cardone, M. H. (1995). Regulation of protein traffic in polarized epithelial cells. *Bioessays* 17, 129–138.

Mounier, J., Vasselon, T., Hellio, R., Lesourd, M., and Sansonetti, P. J. (1992). *Shigella flexneri* enters human colonic Caco-2 cells through the basolateral pole. *Infect. Immun.* 60, 237–248.

Murayama, Y., Okamoto, T., Ogata, E., Asano, T., Iiri, T., Katada, T., Ui, M., Grubb, J. H., Sly, W. S., and Nishimoto, I. (1990). Distinctive regulation of the functional linkage between the human cation-independent mannose 6-phosphate receptor and GTP-binding proteins by insulin-like growth factor-II and mannose 6-phosphate. *J. Biol. Chem.* 265, 17456–17462.

Neutra, M. R., Phillips, T. L., Mayer, E. L., and Fishkind, D. J. (1987). Transport of membrane-bound macromolecules by M cells in follicle-associated epithelium of rabbit Peyer's patch. *Cell Tiss. Res.* 247, 537–546.

Neutra, M. R., Frey, A., and Kraehenbuhl, J.-P. (1996). Epithelial M cells: Gateways for mucosal infection and immunization. *Cell* 86, 345–348.

Neutra, M. R., Mantis, N. J., Frey, A., and Giannasca, P. J. (1999). The composition and function of M cell apical membranes: Implications for microbial pathogenesis. *Semin. Immunol.* 11, 171–181.

Neutra, M. R., Mantis, N. J., and Kraehenbuhl, J.-P. (2001). Collaboration of epithelial cells with organized mucosal lymphoid tissues. *Nat. Immunol.* 2, 1004–1009.

Neutra, M. R., Sansonetti, P. J., and Kraehenbuhl, J. P. (2003). M cells and microbial pathogens. In *Infections of the GI Tract* (eds. M. J. Blaser, P. D. Smith, J. I. Ravdin, H. B. Greenberg, and L. Guerrant), 163–178. New York: Raven Press.

Nibert, M. L., Furlong, D. B., and Fields, B. N. (1991). Mechanisms of viral pathogenesis: Distinct forms of reoviruses and their roles during replication in cells and host. *J. Clin. Invest.* 88, 727–734.

Obiso, R. J., Azghani, A. O., and Wilkins, T. D. (1997). The *Bacteroides fragilis* toxin fragilysin disrupts the paracellular barrier of epithelial cells. *Infect. Immun.* 65, 1431–1439.

Ogra, P. L., and Karzon D. T. (1969). Distribution of poliovirus antibody in serum, nasopharynx, and alimentary tract following segmental immunization of lower alimentary tract with poliovaccine. *J. Immunol.* 102, 1423–1430.

Okato, S., Magari, S., Yamamoto, Y., Sakanaka, M., and Takahashi, H. (1989). An immuno-electron microscopic study on interactions among dendritic cells, macrophages, and lymphocytes in the human palatine tonsil. *Arch. Histol. Cytol.* 52, 231–240.

O'Leary, A. D., and Sweeney, E. C. (1986). Lymphoglandular complexes of the colon: Structure and distribution. *Histopathology* 10, 267–283.

Owen, R. L. (1977). Sequential uptake of horseradish peroxidase by lymphoid follicle epithelium of Peyer's patches in the normal unobstructed mouse intestine: An ultrastructural study. *Gastroenterology* 72, 440–451.

Owen, R. (1999). Uptake and transport of intestinal macromolecules and microorganisms by M cells in Peyer's patches: A personal and historic perspective. *Semin. Immunol.* 11, 1–7.

Owen, R. L., and Bhalla, D. K. (1983). Cytochemical analysis of alkaline phosphatase and esterase activities and of lectin-binding and anionic sites in rat and mouse Peyer's patch M cells. *Am. J. Anat.* 168, 199–212.

Owen, R. L., Pierce, N. F., Apple, R. T., and Cray, W. C. J. (1986). M cell transport of *Vibrio cholerae* from the intestinal lumen into Peyer's patches: A mechanism for antigen sampling and for microbial transepithelial migration. *J. Infect. Dis.* 153, 1108–1118.

Owen, R. L., Bass, D. M., and Piazza, A. J. (1990) Colonic lymphoid patches. A portal of entry in mice for type I reovirus administered anally. *Gastroenterology* 98, A468.

Pappo, J., and Ermak, T. H. (1989). Uptake and translocation of fluorescent latex particles by rabbit Peyer's patch follicle epithelium: A quantitative model for M cell uptake. *Clin. Exp. Immunol.* 76, 144–148.

Pappo, J., and Owen, R. L. (1988). Absence of secretory component expression by epithelial cells overlying rabbit gut-associated lymphoid tissue. *Gastroenterology* 95, 1173–1177.

Parr, M. E., and Parr, E. L. (1999). Female genital tract immunity in animal models. In *Mucosal Immunology* (eds. P. L. Ogra, J. Mestecky, M. E. Lamm, W. Strober, J. Bienenstock, and J. R. McGhee), 1395–1410. San Diego: Academic Press.

Pauza, C. D., Emau, P., Salvato, M. S., Trivedi, P., MacKensie, D., Malkovsky, M., Uno, H., and Schultz, K. T. (1993). Pathogenesis of SIV mac51 after atraumatic inoculation of the rectal mucosa in rhesus monkeys. *J. Med. Primatol.* 22, 154–161.

Penheiter, K. L., Mathur, N., Giles, D., Fahlen, T., and Jones, B. D. (1997). Non-invasive *Salmonella typhimurium* mutants are avirulent because of an inability to enter and destroy M cells of ileal Peyer's patches. *Mol. Microbiol.* 24, 697–709.

Perry, M. E. (1994). The specialized structure of crypt epithelium in the human palatine tonsil and its functional significance. *J. Anat.* 185, 111–127.

Phalipon, A., and Sansonetti, P. J. (1999). Microbial-host interactions at mucosal sites: Host response to pathogenic bacteria at mucosal sites. *Curr. Top. Microbiol. Immunol.* 236, 163–190.

Philpott, D. J., Yamaoka, S., Israël, A., and Sansonetti, P. J. (2000). Invasive *Shigella flexneri* activates NFkB through an LPS-dependant innate intracellular response and leads to IL-8 expression in epithelial cells. *J. Immunol.* 165, 903–914.

Planchon, S. M., Martins, C. A. P., Guerrant, R. L., and Roche, J. K. (1994). Regulation of intestinal epithelial barrier function by TGF-beta-1: Evidence for its role in abrogating the effect of a T-cell cytokine. *J. Immunol.* 153, 5730–5739.

Pope, M., Betjes, M. G., Romani, N., Hirmand, H., Cameron, P. U., Hoffman, L., Gezelter, S., Schuler, G., and Steinman, R. M. (1994). Conjugates of dendritic cells and memory T lymphocytes from skin facilitate productive infection with HIV-1. *Cell* 78, 389–398.

Porcelli, S., and Modlin, R. (1999). The CD1 system: Antigen-presenting molecules for T cell recognition of lipids and glycolipids. *Annu. Rev. Immunol.* 17, 297–329.

Potten, C. S., and Morris, R. J. (1988). Epithelial stem cells *in vivo*. *J. Cell Sci.* 12, 495–503.

Pron, B., Boumalia, C., Jaubert, F., Berche, P., Milon, G., Geissman, F., and Gaillard, J. L. (2001). Dendritic cells are early cellular targets of *Listeria monocytogenes* after intestinal delivery and are involved in bacterial spread in the host. *Cell. Microbiol.* 3, 331–340.

Pulendran, B., Smith, J. L., Caspary, G., Brasel, K., Pettit, E., Maraskovsky, E., and Malizcewski, C. R. (1999). Distinct dendritic cell subsets differentially regulate the class of immune responses *in vivo*. *Proc. Natl. Acad. Sci. USA.* 96, 1036–1041.

Racaniello, V. R., and Ren, R. (1996). Poliovirus biology and pathogenesis. *Curr. Top. Microbiol. Immunol.* 206, 305–325.

Rafiee, P., Leffler, H., Byrd, J. C., Cassels, F. J., Boedeker, E. C., and Kim, Y. S. (1991). A sialoglycoprotein complex linked to the microvillus cytoskeleton acts as a receptor for pilus (AF/R1) mediated adhesion of enteropathogenic *Escherichia coli* (RDEC-1) in rabbit small intestine. *J. Cell. Biol.* 115, 1021–1029.

Rescigno, M. (2002). Dendritic cells and the complexity of microbial infection. *Trends Microbiol.* 10, 425–431.

Rescigno, M., Urbano, M., Valzasinam, B., Francolini, M., Bonasio, R., Rotta, G., Kraehenbuhl, J. P., Granucci, F., and Ricciardi-Castagnoli, P. (2001). Dendritic cells express tight junction proteins and penetrate gut epithelial monolayers to sample bacteria. *Nat. Immunol.* 2, 361–367.

Rosenshine, I., Donnenberg, M. S., Kaper, J. B., and Finlay, B. B. (1992). Signal transduction between enteropathogenic *Escherichia coli* (EPEC) and epithelial cells: EPEC induces tyrosine phosphorylation of host cell proteins to initiate cytoskeletal rearrangement and bacterial uptake. *EMBO J.* 11, 3551–3560.

Roy, M. J., and Varvayanis, M. (1987). Development of dome epithelium in gut-associated lymphoid tissues: Association of IgA with M cells. *Cell Tissue Res.* 248, 645–651.

Rubas, W. and Grass, G. M. (1991). Gastrointestinal lymphatic absorption of peptides and proteins. *Advanced Drug Delivery Reviews* 7, 15–69.

Ruedl, C., Reiser, C., Bock, G., Wick, G., and Wolf, G. (1996). Phenotypic and functional characterization of CD11c+ dendritic cell population in mouse Peyer's patches. *Eur. J. Immunol.* 26, 1801–1806.

Sakamoto, N., Shibuya, K., Shimizu, Y., Yotsumoto, K., Miyabayashi, T., Sakano, S., Tsuji, T., Nakayama, E., Nakauchi, H., and Shibuya, A. (2001). A novel Fc receptor for IgA and IgM is expressed on both hematopoietic and non-hematopoietic tissues. *Eur. J. Immunol.* 31, 1310–1316.

Sansonetti, P. J. (1991). Genetic and molecular basis of epithelial cell invasion by *Shigella* species. *Rev. Infect. Dis.* 13, 285–292.

Sansonetti, P. J., and Phalipon, A. (1999). M cells as ports of entry for enteroinvasive pathogens: Mechanisms of interaction, consequences for the disease process. *Sem. Immunol.* 11, 193–203.

Sansonetti, P. J., Mounier, J., Prevost, M. C., and Mege, R. M. (1994). Cadherin expression is required for the spread of *Shigella flexneri* between epithelial cells. *Cell* 76, 829–839.

Sansonetti, P. J., Arondel, J., Cantey, J. R., Prévost, M. C., and Huerre, M. (1996). Infection of rabbit Peyer's patches by *Shigella flexneri*: Effect of adhesive or invasive bacterial phenotypes on follicle-associated epithelium. *Infect. Immun.* 64, 2752–2764.

Savidge, T. C., and Smith, M. W. (1995). Evidence that membranous (M) cell genesis is immunoregulated. *Adv. Exp. Med. Biol.* 371A, 239–241.

Savidge, T. C., Smith, M. W., James, P. S., and Aldred, P. (1991). Salmonella-induced M-cell formation in germ-free mouse Peyer's patch tissue. *Am. J. Pathol.* 139, 177–184.

Savkovic, S. D., Koutsouris, A., and Hecht, G. (1996). Attachment of a noninvasive enteric pathogen, enteropathogenic *Escherichia coli*, to cultured human intestinal epithelial monolayers induces transmigration of neutrophils. *Infect. Immun.* 64, 4480–4487.

Schmidt, G. H., Wilkinson, M. M., and Ponder, B. A. J. (1985). Cell migration pathway in the intestinal epithelium: an *in situ* marker system using mouse aggregation chimeras. *Cell* 40, 425–429.

Schulte, R., Kernéis, S., Klinke, S., Bartels, H., Preger, S., Kraehenbuhl, J.-P., Pringault, E., and Autenrieth, I. B. (2000). Translocation of *Yersinia enterocolitica* across reconstituted intestinal epithelial monolayers is triggered by *Yersinia* invasin binding to beta 1 integrins apically expressed on M-like cells. *Cell. Microbiol.* 2, 173–185.

Segal, E. D., Falkow, S., and Tompkins, L. S. (1996). *Helicobacter pylori* attachment to gastric cells induces cytoskeletal rearrangements and tyrosine phosphorylation of host cell proteins. *Proc. Natl. Acad. Sci. USA* 93, 1259–1264.

Shao, L., Serrano, D., and Mayer, L. (2001). The role of epithelial cells in immune regulation in the gut. *Semin. Immunol.* 3, 163–176.

Sharma, R., van Damme, E. J. M., Peumans, W. J., Sarsfield, P., and Schumacher, U. (1996). Lectin binding reveals divergent carbohydrate expression in human and mouse Peyer's patches. *Histochem. Cell Biol.* 105, 459–465.

Sheppard, D. (1996). Epithelial integrins. *Bioessays* 18, 655–660.

Shibuya, A., Sakamoto, N., Shimizu, Y., Shibuya, K., Osawa, M., Hiroyama, T., Eyre, H. J., Sutherland, G. R., Endo, Y., Fujita, T., Miyabayashi, T., Sakano, S., Tsuji, T., Nakayama, E., Phillips, J. H., Lanier, L. L., and Nakauchi, H. (2000). Fc alpha/mu receptor mediates endocytosis of IgM-coated microbes. *Nat. Immunol.* 1, 441–446.

Shreedhar, V. K., Kelsall, B. L., and Neutra, M. R. (2003). Cholera toxin induces migration of dendritic cells from the subepithelial dome region to T- and B-cell areas of Peyer's Patches. *Infect. Immun.* 71, 504–509.

Sicinski, P., Rowinski, J., Warchol, J. B., Jarzcabek, Z., Gut, W., Szczygiel, B., Bielecki, K., and Koch, G. (1990). Poliovirus type 1 enters the human host through intestinal M cells. *Gastroenterology* 98, 56–58.

Siebers, A., and Finlay, B. B. (1996). M cells and the pathogenesis of mucosal and systemic infections. *Trends Microbiol.* 4, 22–29.

Sierro, F., Pringault, E., Simon Assman, P., Kraehenbuhl, J. P., and Debard, N. (2000). Transient expression of M cell phenotype by enterocyte-like cells of the follicle-associated epithelium of mouse Peyer's patches. *Gastroenterology* 119, 734–743.

Sierro, F., Dubois, B., Coste, A., Kaiserlian, D., Kraehenbuhl, J. P., and Sirard, J. C. (2001). Flagellin stimulation of intestinal epithelial cells triggers CCL20-mediated migration of dendritic cells. *Proc. Natl. Acad. Sci. USA* 98, 13722–13727.

Smith, M. W., James, P. S., and Tivey, D. R. (1987). M cell numbers increase after transfer of SPF mice to a normal animal house environment. *Am. J. Pathol.* 128, 385–389.

Sozzani, S., Sallusto, F., Luini, W., Zhou, D., Piemonti, L., Allavena, P., Vandamme, J., Valitutti, S., Lanzavecchia, A., and Mantovani, A. (1995). Migration of dendritic cells in response to formyl peptides, c5a, and a distinct set of chemokines. *J. Immunol.* 155, 3292–3295.

Spiekermann, G. M., Finn, P. W., Ward, E. S., Dumont, J., Dickinson, B. L., Blumberg, R. S., and Lencer, W. I. (2002). Receptor-mediated immunoglobulin G transport across mucosal barriers in adult life: Functional expression of FcRn in the mammalian lung. *J. Exp. Med.* 196, 303–310.

Spira, A. I., Marx, P. A., Patterson, B. K., Mahoney, J., Koup, R. A., Wolinsky, S. M., and Ho, D. D. (1996). Cellular targets of infection and route of viral dissemination after an intravaginal inoculation of simian immunodeficiency virus into rhesus macaques. *J. Exp. Med.* 183, 215–225.

Stahl-Hennig, C., Steinman, R. M., Tenner-Racz, K., Pope, M., Stolte, N., Matz-Rensing, K., Grobschupff, G., Raschdorff, B., Hunsmann, G., and Racz, P. (1999). Rapid infection of oral mucosal-associated lymphoid tissue with simian immunodeficiency virus. *Science* 285, 1261–1265.

Stevens, A. C., Matthews, J., Andres, P., Baffis, V., Zheng, X. X., Chae, D. W., Smith, J., Strom, T. B., and Maslinski, W. (1997). Interleukin-15 signals T84 colonic epithelial cells in the absence of the interleukin-2 receptor beta-chain. *Am. J. Physiol* 35, G1201–G1208.

Sun, J. B., Holmgren, J., and Czerkinsky, C. (1994). Cholera toxin B subunit: An efficient transmucosal carrier-delivery system for induction of peripheral immunological tolerance. *Proc. Natl. Acad. Sci. USA* 91, 10795–10799.

Takeuchi, A. (1967). Electron microscope studies of experimental *Salmonella* infection. I. Penetration into the intestinal epithelium by *Salmonella typhimurium*. *Am. J. Pathol.* 50, 109–136.

Tanaka, Y., Imai, T., Baba, M., Ishikawa, I., Uehira, M., Nomiyama, H., and Yoshie, O. (1999). Selective expression of liver and activation-regulated chemokine (LARC) in intestinal epithelium in mice and humans. *Eur. J. Immunol.* 29, 633–642.

Uchida, J. (1987). An ultrastructural study on active uptake and transport of bacteria by microfold cells (M cells) to the lymphoid follicles in the rabbit appendix. *J. Clin. Electron Microsc.* 20, 379–394.

Ueki, T., Mizuno, M., Uesu, T., Kiso, T., and Tsuji, T. (1995). Expression of ICAM-1 on M cells covering isolated lymphoid follicles of the human colon. *Acta Med. Okayama* 49, 145–151.

Upham, J. W., Strickland, D. H., Bilyk, N., Robinson, B. W., and Holt, P. G. (1995). Alveolar macrophages from humans and rodents selectively inhibit T-cell proliferation but permit T-cell activation and cytokine secretion. *Immunology* 84, 142–147.

Vazquez-Torres, A., Jones-Carson, J., Baumler, A. J., Falkow, S., Valdivia, R., Brown, W., Le, M., Berggren, R., Parks, W. T., and Fang, F. C. (1999). Extraintestinal dissemination of Salmonella by CD18-expressing phagocytes. *Nature* 401, 804–808.

Wagner, N., Lohler, J., Kunkel, E. J., Ley, K., Leung, E., Krissansen, G., Rajewsky, K., and Muller, W. (1996). Critical role for beta-7 integrins in formation of the gut-associated lymphoid tissue. *Nature* 382, 366–370.

Walker, R. I., Schauder-Chock, E. A., and Parker, J. L. (1988). Selective association and transport of *Campylobacter jejuni* through M cells of rabbit Peyer's patches. *Can. J. Microbiol.* 34, 1142–1147.

Wassef, J. S., Keren, D. F., and Mailloux, J. L. (1989). Role of M cells in initial antigen uptake and in ulcer formation in the rabbit intestinal loop model of Shigellosis. *Infect. Immun.* 57, 858–863.

Weinberg, D. S., Pinkus, G. S., and Murphy, G. F. (1987). Tonsillar epithelial dendritic cells: Demonstration by lectin binding, immunohistochemical characterization, and ultrastructure. *Lab. Invest.* 56, 622–628.

Weltzin, R. A., Lucia Jandris, P., Michetti, P., Fields, B. N., Kraehenbuhl, J.-P., and Neutra, M. R. (1989). Binding and transepithelial transport of immunoglobulins by intestinal M cells: Demonstration using monoclonal IgA antibodies against enteric viral proteins. *J. Cell Biol.* 108, 1673–1685.

Winner, L. S. III., Mack, J., Weltzin, R. A., Mekalanos, J. J., Kraehenbuhl, J.-P., and Neutra, M. R. (1991). New model for analysis of mucosal immunity: Intestinal secretion of specific monoclonal immunoglobulin A from hybridoma tumors protects against *Vibrio cholerae* infection. *Infect. Immun.* 59, 977–982.

Wolf, J. L., Rubin, D. H., Finberg, R., Kauffman, R. S., Sharpe, A. H., Trier, J. S., and Fields, B. N. (1981). Intestinal M cells: A pathway for entry of reovirus into the host. *Science* 212, 471–472.

Yahi, N., Baghdiguian, S., Moreau, H., and Fantini, J. (1992). Galactosyl ceramide (or a closely related molecule) is the receptor for human immunodeficiency virus type 1 on human colon epithelial HT29 cells. *J. Virol.* 66, 4848–4854.

Yeaman, G. R., White, H. D., Howell, A., Prabhala, R., and Wira, C. R. (1998). The mucosal immune system in the human female reproductive tract: Potential insights into the heterosexual transmission of HIV. *AIDS Res. Hum. Retrovir.* Suppl 1, S57–S62.

Young, W. G., and Hosking, A. R. (1986). Langerhans cells in murine vaginal epithelium affected by oestrogen and topical vitamin A. *Acta Anat.* 125, 59–64.

Zhang, Z. Q., Schuler, T., Zupancic, M., Wietgrefe, S., Staskus, K. A., Reimann, K. A., Reinhart, T. A., Rogan, M., Cavert, W., Miller, C. J., Veazey, R. S., Notermans, D., Little, S., Danner, S. A., Richman, D. D., Havlir, D., Wong, J., Jordan, H. L., Schacker, T. W., Racz P., Tenner-Racz, K., Letvin, N. L., Wolinsky, S., and Haase, A. T. (1999). Sexual transmission and propagation of SIV and HIV in resting and activated CD4+ T cells. *Science* 286, 1353–1357.

Zhou, F., Kraehenbuhl, J.-P., and Neutra, M. R. (1995). Mucosal IgA response to rectally administered antigen formulated in IgA-coated liposomes. *Vaccine* 13, 637–644.

Zhao, X., Deak, E., Soderberg, K., Linehan, M., Spezzano, Zhu, J., Knipe, D. M., and Iwasaki, A. (2003). Vaginal submucosal dendritic cells, but not Langerhans cells, induce protective Th1 responses to herpes simplex virus-2. *J. Exp. Med.* 197, 153–162.

Zimmer, K. P., Buning, J., Weber, P., Kaiserlian, D., and Strobel, S. (2000). Modulation of antigen trafficking to MHC class II-positive late endosomes of enterocytes. *Gastroenterology* 118, 128–137.

Zuercher, A. W., Coffin, S. E., Thurnheer, M. C., Fundova, P., and Cebra, J. J. (2002). Nasal-associated lymphoid tissue is a mucosal inductive site for virus-specific humoral and cellular immune responses. *J. Immunol.* 168, 1796–1803.

Structure and Function of Intestinal Mucosal Epithelium

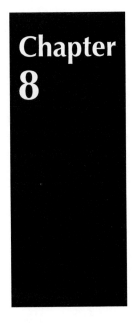

Chapter 8

Tomohiro Kato

Department of Endoscopy, Jikei University School of Medicine, Tokyo, Japan

Robert L. Owen

Department of Medicine, University of California San Francisco; Gastroenterology Section, Veterans Affairs Medical Center, San Francisco, California

INTRODUCTION

The mucosal epithelial layer forms the interface between the luminal contents of the intestines and the tissue compartments of the gastrointestinal tract. This area is the site for digestion and absorption of various essential nutrients, yet it also must function as a barrier against various harmful agents and infectious pathogens. Protecting against such agents are many nonimmunologic factors including gastric acid, pancreatic juice, bile, motility, mucus, glycocalyx, and cell turnover. In addition to these physiologic barriers, an immunologic barrier is created and maintained by the immune defense system, which includes the gut-associated lymphoid tissue-immunoreactive (GALT-immunoreactive) cells distributed throughout the intestinal tract and the systemic immune system. Much has been learned about GALT, but many questions about its structure and function remain unanswered. The mucosal epithelium in GALT, which functions as the leading edge of the immunologic barrier, differs in many ways from the absorptive epithelium elsewhere in the intestinal tract **(Fig. 8.1)**. This chapter first describes the absorptive mucosa and then the GALT mucosa.

INTESTINAL ABSORPTIVE EPITHELIUM

The total mucosal surface in the adult human gastrointestinal tract extends to 200–300 m², the largest area of the body in contact with the external environment. This mucosal surface is covered with a one-cell–thick layer, the mucosal epithelium, which is composed of columnar absorptive cells, goblet cells, undifferentiated crypt epithelial cells, Paneth cells, enteroendocrine cells, tuft cells, cup cells, and intraepithelial lymphocytes (IELs). Although not part of the epithelium, mucus on the surface of the mucosa shields the mucosal epithelial cells from direct contact with the intestinal luminal environment. Beneath the mucosal epithelium is the connective and supportive tissue called the lamina propria. In this tissue are various immunocompetent cells including dendritic cells, macrophages, and lymphocytes, which form a functional unit with the mucosal epithelial cells.

Structure of the absorptive epithelium
Mucosal epithelial cells

Absorptive epithelial cells (enterocytes), which are about 25 μm in height, 8 μm in width, and columnar in shape, constitute the majority of the mucosal epithelium. Their surface has numerous tightly packed microvilli, which are covered with glycocalyx and a thick mucus layer. The regular longitudinal cores of microvilli are interconnected by a terminal web, which is composed of bundles of 20–30 interlacing actin filaments. At their apices, the enterocytes are connected with adjacent epithelial cells mainly by junctional complexes consisting of three major components: tight junctions (zonula occludens), adhesion junctions (zonula adherens), and desmosomes (macula adherens). In addition to the junctional complexes, the lateral membranes interact by means of cell adhesion molecules (CAMs), gap junctions, and interdigitations (Boyer and Thiery 1989). The tight junction, which completely encircles the apical end of absorptive cells as a beltlike band, plays a role in separating the external and internal environments and functions as a selective barrier. The adhesion junction, located in the apical region of absorptive cells just below the tight junction, is connected to actin filaments in the cytoplasm and is thought to anchor each cell to adjacent cells. The desmosome functions like the adhesion junction, connected to intermediate filaments in the cytoplasm. Gap junctions, which are located in the basolateral membrane in other epithelial cells and directly mediate cell-to-cell communication, also have been identified provisionally in intestinal absorptive cells (Suzuki *et al.* 1977; Kataoka *et al.* 1989).

The glycocalyx, which is the surface layer just above the luminal membrane of the absorptive cell, contains various

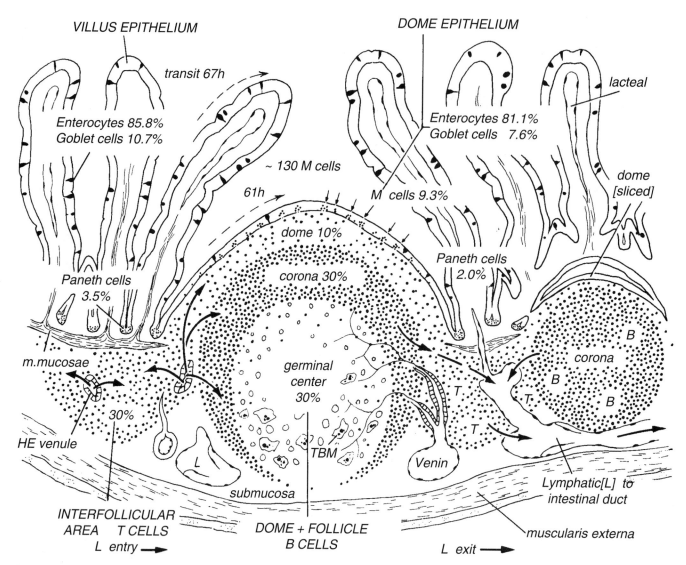

Fig. 8.1. Diagram of an ileal Peyer's patch in the mouse. Peyer's patch lymphoid nodules are composed of three major parts: follicular area (germinal center, corona, and dome), interfollicular (parafollicular) area beneath villi, and dome epithelium. The right follicle beneath villi is sliced tangentially, through the lower slopes of the dome and the lymphocyte corona only. Curved arrows on the left show the influx of lymphocytes across postcapillary high endothelial venules (HEV), which mediate selective immigration of lymphocytes. Arrows on the right show the exit pathway of stimulated lymphocytes into submucosal lymphatics. M cells are difficult to distinguish by light microscopy and are inferred from the location of groups of lymphoid cells (small arrows) in the follicle epithelium. (Migration rates in hours [h] and cell distribution numbers in this figure are from Smith and Peacock 1980 and Abe and Ito 1977. T, T lymphocyte; B, B lymphocyte; TBM, tingible body macrophage; m, muscularis. Diagram courtesy of E. Hamish Batten.)

enzymes and nonenzymatic proteins including disacchari-dases, peptidases, receptors, and transport proteins, all of which are necessary for digestion and absorption of nutrients. The major component of the glycocalyx is carbohydrate anchored into the surface of microvilli.

The smooth endoplasmic reticulum and mitochondria are more abundant in the apical than in the basal cytoplasm. The nucleus normally is located in the basal cytoplasm below the rough endoplasmic reticulum, so enterocytes maintain a characteristic polarity. The basolateral membrane, which begins below the junctional complex, contains abundant Na^+, K^+-ATPase and adenylate cyclase and differs from the

apical membrane in function. Interlocking folds are produced by adjacent cells, interdigitating their lateral membranes, which are separated by a 30-nm–wide intercellular space.

The basal membrane also is separated by a 30-nm space from the basal lamina. Junctional structures called hemidesmosomes anchor basal membrane to basal lamina. Hemidesmosomes are thought to connect with intermediate filaments of the cytoplasm, as do desmosomes. The basal lamina has numerous round or oval pores and is composed of collagen, laminin, fibronectin, and glycosaminoglycans (Hay 1981; Ohtsuka *et al.* 1992). Ultrastructurally, basal lamina consists of a lamina densa 20–50 nm thick that lies between two thin electron lucent layers: the lamina rata externa below and the lamina rata interna above (Dobbins 1990). Although the function of the basal lamina is unclear, researchers believe it gives polarity to the absorptive cells and guides migration of enterocytes from their crypts of origin to their eventual desquamation sites.

Goblet cells, present in both small and large intestine, increase in number from the proximal to the distal portion of the intestine and are located on villi and in crypts. The goblet cell microvilli are irregular in shape and sparse in number but contain actin filaments. The terminal web is poorly developed in goblet cells, facilitating release of mucus granules from the apical cytoplasm. Mucus granules are synthesized above the nucleus in endoplasmic reticulum and Golgi apparatus and are supported by a goblet-shaped sheath that is composed of inner and outer layers of microtubules and intermediate filaments and keeps its shape before and after release of granules (Specian and Neutra 1984). Mucus granules are released in response to acetylcholine stimulation, but regulation of release is unclear.

Undifferentiated epithelial stem cells are located in the midcrypts and produce daughter cells that continuously migrate upward to the crypt mouth and downward to the crypt base. These cells differentiate into absorptive cells and goblet cells above and into Paneth cells and enteroendocrine cells below. The microvilli of crypt cells are shorter and sparser than are microvilli of mature absorptive cells. The terminal web and the junctional complex of crypt cells are undeveloped, and the tight junction of these cells is structurally irregular. However, its density is very high (Marcial et al. 1984). In crypt cells, smooth and rough endoplasmic reticulum is sparse, whereas ribosomes, mitochondria, and Golgi apparatus are relatively abundant. Small granules (0.1–1.5 μm), the functions of which are unknown, are released from crypt cells into the lumen in response to cholinergic stimuli. The undifferentiated crypt epithelial cells mature as they migrate to the summit of the villi, commonly in 3–5 days. From the crypt, cells migrate in a direct line toward the desquamation zone on the villus tip and, similarly, to the apex of the dome in GALT (Schmidt et al. 1985). The migration rate is thought to depend on extraluminal and luminal factors: extraluminal factors consist of hormones, growth factors such as epidermal growth factor (EGF) and transforming growth factor (TGF), cytokines, and neural and vascular factors; luminal factors consist of nutrition, motility, and microflora (Levine 1991). The crypt is recognized to be a major site of secretion of water and minerals into the lumen (Madara and Trier 1987).

Paneth cells commonly are located in the crypts of the small intestine, but occasionally appear in the stomach and large intestine in some disease states. Their characteristic features are their pyramidal shape and, in the apical cytoplasm, various secretory granules that contain proteins including lysozyme, tumor necrosis factor (TNF) (Keshav et al. 1990), and cryptdin (Ouellette et al. 1989). These secretory granules are thought to prevent proliferation of crypt microorganisms by their strong antimicrobial action. Paneth cells also contain IgA and IgG, possibly from phagocytosis of immunoglobulin-coated microorganisms (Rodning et al. 1976).

Enteroendocrine cells are distributed throughout the gastrointestinal tract. The main function of these cells is to release hormones into capillaries in the connective tissue in response to changes in the external environment. These cells contain various distinctive kinds of secretory granules and are classified structurally into closed and open types. Both commonly are located in the epithelium adjacent to the lamina propria, surrounded by other mucosal epithelial cells. Open type cells have a narrow apical surface in direct contact with the lumen and are presumed to react to stimuli from the tissue environment and from the lumen. Closed type cells have no contact with the luminal environment (Dobbins 1990).

Tuft cells, also called *caveolated cells* or *fibrovesicular cells*, have been discovered in the stomach, intestine, and colon of humans, dogs, mice, and rats (Nabeyama and Leblond 1974; Owen 1977; Blom and Helander 1981). These cells are attached to surrounding absorptive cells by regular junctional complexes. On the surface, they have very long microvilli with filaments that are ~5 μm in length, sometimes reaching deep into the cytoplasm. Tuft cells have many caveolae or pits between the bases of microvilli that extend down to the level of the nucleus. The function of these pits is not known, but they are suspected to act as chemical sensors for the luminal milieu.

Cup cells, discovered by Madara (1982) in guinea pig, rabbit, and monkey intestine, have not yet been reported in humans. These cells stain more lightly than adjacent absorptive cells with toluidine blue stain, have abundant intermediate filaments, and have lower alkaline phosphatase activity on their surfaces than adjacent absorptive cells. Cup cells have shorter microvilli with a cuplike concavity, small mitochondria, and few vesicular bodies. The function of these cells is unknown.

IELs have special characteristics that are distinct from those of other lymphocytes. The average number of IELs per 100 absorptive cells is 20 in normal adult human jejunum and decreases distally in the gut (Dobbins 1986). These cells are located above the basal lamina in the epithelial layer and are separated from adjacent enterocytes by a 10-nm to 20-nm space. These lymphocyte–epithelial cell contacts have no junctional structure. Histochemically, almost all IELs are recognized to be $CD3^+$ (pan T cell). Among these cells, 5% to 15% express CD4 (helper/inducer phenotype), and the remaining cells express CD8 (cytotoxic/suppressor phenotype). These distributions contrast with other areas such as peripheral blood and lamina propria, where the $CD4^+$ phenotype is overwhelmingly predominant. Although the T-cell receptors that mediate antigen recognition are composed predominantly of αβ chains on lymphocytes, in the intestinal epithelium the proportion of γδ-positive lymphocytes is much larger than in the peripheral blood and lamina propria (Jarry et al. 1990). Thus, γδ-positive lymphocytes are thought to have a special role in the intestine. The microenvironment within the intestinal epithelium may influence the differentiation of IELs (Guy-Grand *et al.* 1991). Although the functions of IELs are unclear, some possibilities are cytotoxicity, lymphokine secretion, regulation of renewal of mucosal epithelium, and tolerance (Cerf-Bensussan and Guy-Grand 1991; see Chapter 30).

Mucus layer and glycocalyx

Mucus is composed of 1% mucin, 1% free protein, 1% dialyzable salts, and >95% water. Mucus contains albumin, immunoglobulin (mainly secretory IgA; S-IgA), α1-antitrypsin, lysozyme, lactoferrin, and EGF. In the mucus, the characteristic highly viscous and elastic substance is mucin, which is produced mainly in goblet cells as heavily glycosylated glycoprotein (Rhodes 1990). Mucus is not digested because of its resistance to various enzymes and is thought to protect epithelial cells from digestion by enzymes produced by intestinal flora and by pancreatic and biliary juice. The release of mucus from goblet cells is stimulated by neurogenic factors and by alterations in environmental factors, including bacterial infection, parasitic infestation, and the resident intestinal flora. Mucus secretion from goblet cells is triggered by two mechanisms: direct stimulation by immune complexes and chemical agents and indirect stimulation by mediators released by histamine and lymphokines (Snyder and Walker 1987). Mucus can protect epithelium against the adherence of such organisms as *Entamoeba histolytica, Yersinia enterocolitica,* and enteropathogenic *Escherichia coli* by trapping microorganisms and by covering binding sites with mucin and with S-IgA (Magnusson and Stjernström 1982; Chadee *et al.* 1987; Mantle *et al.* 1989; Sajjan and Forstner 1990). Mucin also inhibits the epithelial attachment of such parasites as *Nippostrongylus brasiliensis* and *Trichinella spiralis* (Miller 1987), whereas other components in mucus, including lysozyme, S-IgA, and lactoferrin, have antibacterial activity (see Chapters 4 and 11). The glycocalyx on microvilli forms a zone for digestion and absorption. The mucus layer and rapid turnover of absorptive cells are useful for the protection and regeneration of glycocalyx, because some bacteria can digest important proteins in it by direct contact (Jonas *et al.* 1978; see Chapter 4).

Resident microflora

The resident microflora is composed of at least 400 species of bacteria, of which major components are streptococci, lactobacilli, *Bacteroides,* and enterobacteria. The upper intestinal bacterial count is low in number (<10^5 cfu/ml) and increases distally (terminal ileum, 10^6 per ml; colon, 10^{11} per ml). Intestinal bacterial numbers are regulated by the flow rate of luminal contents (intestinal motility) and by mucus and the antibacterial effects of gastric, pancreatic, and biliary juice. Some of the bacteria produce enzymes that degrade mucin, which is thought to be one of their mechanisms of survival (Rhodes 1989). Resident microflora are known to coexist within the intestinal tract and maintain a stable environment by precluding attachment of enteropathogens (see

Chapter 2). The flora can eliminate foreign pathogens by producing antimicrobial substances (colicins, short-chain fatty acids; Iglewski and Gerhardt 1978; Byrne and Dankert 1979) and by stimulating the growth of mucosal epithelium (Thompson and Trexler 1971). Interestingly, bacteria such as *Lactobacillus, Bacteroides,* and *Clostridium* have been reported also to exist within the intestinal mucosa. Ultrastructurally, these organisms adhere firmly to the mucus layer in crypts of the distal small intestine (Savage 1970; see Chapter 2).

Intestinal epithelial functions

Uptake and transport of nutrients, minerals, water, and nonnutrient materials

Digestion and absorption of nutrients are the primary functions of the gastrointestinal tract. Mucosal absorptive cells, also called enterocytes, have primary digestive and absorptive functions. The apical surface of absorptive cells consists of the glycocalyx and plasma membrane, which contains various enzymes and carriers for digestion and absorption. Sodium is important for the absorption of nutrients and other minerals because its electrical gradient regulates their movement into absorptive cells. Na$^+$, K$^+$-ATPase mainly regulates the gradient of Na$^+$ by secretion and absorption on basolateral membranes; Na$^+$ goes in and out with other minerals and nutrients through the brush border membrane. Water and ions are thought to pass through tight junctions (paracellular pathway) in addition to the route across epithelial cells (transcellular pathway).

Barrier to entrance of microorganisms, particles, and macromolecules

In the intestinal lumen, pancreatic and biliary juice, mucus, glycocalyx, intestinal motility, and resident microflora interact to limit colonization by enteropathogens. Pancreatic and biliary juices, along with S-IgA and lysozyme, have antibacterial activities in some species (Williams *et al.* 1975; Rubinstein *et al.* 1985; Bassi *et al.* 1991). Even if pathogens begin to invade the epithelium, the process may be restricted by local mechanisms and terminated as tiny lesions. Protection is provided by the epithelial cell and by the environment surrounding epithelial cells. Turnover of crypt cells increases the rate of epithelial renewal in response to the invasion of harmful pathogens that damage surface cells. Lesions will be washed by mucus and other secretions in conjunction with intestinal motility and will be repaired by cell migration. Evidence suggests that IELs can kill virus-infected target cells and bacteria in experimental animals (London *et al.* 1989; Tagliabue *et al.* 1984), but no information about such a role for IELs in humans is available (see Chapter 30).

Chemical messengers including neuropeptides, gastrointestinal hormones, and lymphokines affect barrier factors. Substance P, somatostatin, and cholecystokinin (CCK) influence the production of mucin and IgA (Stanisz *et al.* 1986; Freier *et al.* 1987); interferon-γ (IFN-γ) modulates the barrier function of absorptive cells (Madara and Stafford

1989). Although the roles of these mediators are not elucidated completely, they are thought to contribute to the multifactorial network of nonimmunologic mucosal defense mechanisms described earlier and to immunologic mechanisms described in subsequent chapters (see Chapters 34, 35, and 38).

Antigen presentation and immunologic functions of intestinal epithelium

Pathogens and other harmful agents including bacteria, viruses, parasites, and allergenic macromolecules are mixed with nutrient materials in the intestine. Despite protective mechanisms, these harmful agents can cross the mucosal barrier via three major routes: the transcellular route, the paracellular route across cell-to-cell junctions, including tight junctions, and via M cells, which are specially differentiated epithelial cells in Peyer's patches (see subsequent discussion). Uptake mechanisms are separated into receptor-mediated and non–receptor-mediated pathways. The route of uptake of nonnutrients is believed to be primarily paracellular. In fact the tight (occluding) junctions can change configuration in response to luminal contents, with formation of intrajunctional dilatations, permitting relatively large nutrients up to 5500 in molecular weight to pass through (Madara and Trier, 1987). However, the transcellular route through absorptive cells has been recognized to play a special role in initiation of mucosal and systemic infection and, possibly, in antigen presentation, because absorptive cells are the first point of contact for many luminal constituents.

For absorptive cells to function as antigen-presenting cells (APCs), uptake, endosomal degradation, processing, and presentation of antigen to immunocompetent cells (such as T cells and macrophages) restricted by major histocompatibility complex (MHC) class II proteins would be required. This process of delivery of coherent and recognizable antigenic information also requires cytokines and, possibly, control by hormones and the nervous system. APCs must express MHC class II proteins on their surfaces to initiate the process of presentation. Normal absorptive cells in humans and rats do, in fact, express on their apical surfaces MHC class I molecules, which present peptides derived from degradation of intracellular proteins, as well as MHC class II molecules, which present peptides derived from degradation of extracellular proteins (Hirata et al. 1986; Mayer et al. 1991; see Chapter 25). MHC class II expression of HLA-DR is absent in esophagus and stomach, reaches detectable levels in the duodenum, then is more highly expressed in distal small intestine, with maximal expression in the ileum. Passing down the large intestine, expression decreases again and is barely detectable in the rectum (Mayer et al. 1991; Qin et al. 1988). Expression of this antigen presentation molecule for extracellular proteins thus corresponds to the increasing concentration of intraluminal microorganisms in the small intestine and decreases in the colon where a protective coat of mucus separates the intestinal microbial load from the surface of intestinal epithelial cells. CD8[+] IELs are reported to secrete IFN-γ (Cerf-Bensussan et al. 1984), which can stimulate absorptive cells further to express MHC

class II proteins (Hirayama et al. 1987) and protect against infection by viruses. Beside these classical MHC I/II molecules, additional factors contribute to maintenance of the intestinal luminal environment. Absorptive cells are local sites of complement biosynthesis upregulated by proinflammatory cytokines and downregulated by IL-4. (Bamba and Andoh 1998). CD1d, a nonclassical MHC class I–like molecule, expressed first as mRNA in intestinal crypts, then as CD1 protein in villi, appears to function as a novel antigen-presenting molecule for nonpeptide (lipid) bacterial antigens. (Kim and Blumberg 1998; Bleicher et al. 1990). Colonic epithelial cells produce a variety of interleukins, including IL-1, IL-8, IL-10, TNF-α, and TGF-β, which increase following bacterial invasion, providing signals to underlying mucosal cells that the mucosal barrier has been breached (Eckmann et al. 1993). These observations indicate that epithelial absorptive cells function not only in electrolyte transport and nutrient absorption but also in immune surveillance as first responders to intraluminal events, communicating with inflammatory cells and as APCs, at least under special circumstances (Chapters 24 and 25).

Cryptopatches, located in the lamina propria near intestinal crypts, were described and named by Kanamori and colleagues in 1996. They were able to identify approximately 1500 such cryptopatches, each containing about 1000 closely packed lymphocytes, distributed throughout the murine small and large intestine. Cryptopatches are present and continue to produce IEL precursor cells in germfree and athymic nude mice. Most of these cryptopatch lymphocytes express c-kit, IL-7R, Thy1, and lymphocyte function–associated antigen (LFA-1), but not CD3, TCR-αβ, TCR-γδ, sIgM, and B220. IELs are now thought to be derived in large part from these cryptopatches, independent of the thymus or other lymphoid tissues (Oida et al. 2000; Saito et al. 1998).

MUCOSAL EPITHELIUM IN GUT-ASSOCIATED LYMPHOID TISSUE

GALT is a general term for lymphoid tissues distributed in intestine, including aggregated lymphoid nodules in Peyer's patches, the appendix vermiformis (Uchida 1988), colonic patches (Owen et al. 1991), and solitary lymphoid nodules. In its entirety, GALT is the largest lymphoid organ in the body.

The typical GALT structures can be observed most easily in Peyer's patches (Heel et al. 1997). Peyer's patches are groups of lymphoid follicles in the small intestinal mucosa (**Figs. 8.1** and **8.2**). Although their numbers and distribution differ among individuals and in different species, some features are characteristic: Peyer's patches are located along the antimesenteric side of the small intestine and are most prominent in the terminal ileum. The number and size of Peyer's patch follicles decrease with age.

Structure of the follicle epithelium

Morphologically, Peyer's patch nodules are separated into three major domains: the follicular area, the parafollicular

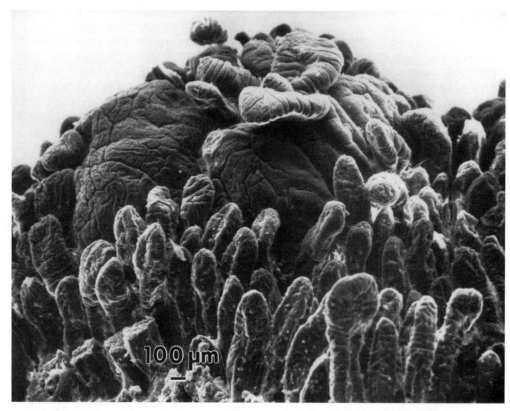

Fig. 8.2. Scanning electron micrograph of a dome-shaped lymphoid nodule surrounded by numerous finger-shaped villi in human Peyer's patch. Note that surfaces of villi are covered with whitish-colored mucus drops that are absent over the surfaces or the lymphoid nodule. (Reprinted with permission from Owen and Jones 1974. Epithelial cell specialization within human Peyer's patches: An ultrastructural study of intestinal lymphoid follicles. *Gastroenterology* 66, 189–203. Baltimore: Williams and Wilkins.)

area, and the follicle-associated epithelium (FAE). Histologically, intestinal lymphoid nodules differ from lymph nodes because they have no capsule, no medulla, no afferent lymphatic ducts, and no clear border. The FAE is a one-cell–thick lining layer that forms the interface between the intestinal lymphoid apparatus and the intestinal luminal environment, and its constituent epithelial cells are generated within surrounding crypts that also supply enterocytes to villi adjacent to lymphoid nodules. FAE is composed of specially differentiated M cells, columnar epithelial cells, IELs, infrequent mucus-secreting goblet cells, and occasional tuft cells. GALT is further described in Chapters 21 and 22.

M cells

By dissecting microscopy, small protruding domes can be distinguished among the villi in Peyer's patches. By scanning electron microscopy (SEM), M cells are found scattered over the dome, surrounded by absorptive cells **(Fig. 8.3)**.

Since Schmedtje described M cells (which he termed lymphoepithelial cells) covering dome-shaped lymphoid follicles in the rabbit appendix (Schmedtje 1965, 1966), similar cells have been discovered in many organs and species. Such cells were identified by Owen and Jones (1974) in human small intestine and termed M cells. M cells also have been found

in nonintestinal lymphoid aggregates, including tonsils (Owen and Nemanic 1978) and bronchi (Bienenstock and Befus 1984; see Chapter 20). M cells occupy ~50% of FAE surface area in rabbits and 10% of intestinal lymphoid follicle surface area in humans and mice.

M cells play an important role in antigen sampling, taking up particles from the intestinal lumen and transporting them to lymphocytes and macrophages enfolded in pockets in the basolateral surfaces of M cells (Gebert *et al.* 1996). **Figure 8.4** shows M cells typical of the lymphoid follicles in human ileum.

M cells have shared and unique structural features in comparison with other mucosal epithelial cells in the intestine **(Fig. 8.5)**. M cells have tight junctions and desmosomes in contact with adjacent columnar epithelial cells and interdigitating lateral membranes **(Fig. 8.6)**. The processes on their luminal surfaces are spaced more widely and often are shorter and more irregular in shape than the microvilli of absorptive cells: these processes consist of "microfolds" in humans (hence, the name "M" cell; Fig. 8.3). Sometimes longer microfolds reach out to surround microorganisms in the intestinal lumen. M cells in other species were found to have specialized microvilli rather than microfolds. Consequently, the term *M cell* now denotes "membranous"

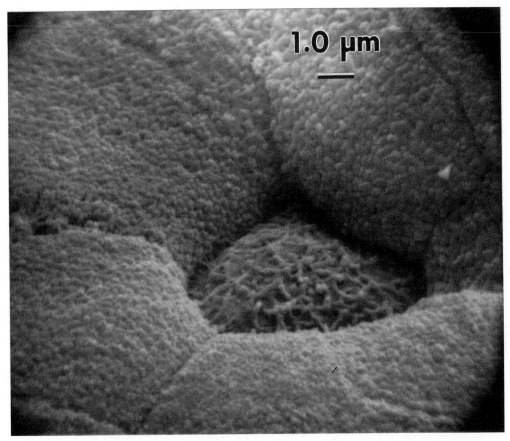

Fig. 8.3. Scanning electron micrograph of the surface of a human Peyer's patch lymphoid nodule. The M cell in the center is surrounded by polygonal absorptive cells that possess numerous tall, closely packed, regular microvilli on their apices. Note the irregular and short microfolds of the M cell.

or "membranelike," reflecting the role of M cells in separating the luminal and intercellular domains, yet facilitating movement from one to the other. Ultrastructurally, microfolds in human M cells and comparable M-cell microvilli in other species have fewer microfilaments such as actin and a less highly developed apical terminal web than do adjacent absorptive cells. The apical cytoplasm of M cells has closely packed mitochondria and numerous rounded, tubular, or oval microvesicles but few lysosomes (Owen *et al.* 1988a; **Fig. 8.7**).

The M cell typically has an extracellular space called the central hollow or pocket, which invaginates its basolateral membrane and surrounds enfolded lymphoid cells **(Fig. 8.8)**. Within these pockets lie one or more lymphocytes, macrophages, plasma cells, or, rarely, polymorphonuclear leukocytes. Immunohistochemical studies of human M-cell pockets from ileal Peyer's patches of patients undergoing colonoscopy found, on average, equal numbers of phenotypically heterogeneous B (CD19+/20+) cells and T (CD3+) cells, mostly of the CD45RO+ memory phenotype, predominantly of the CD4+ subset. There were occasional IgA or IgM plasma cells but few macrophages (CD68+) (Farstrad *et al.*, 1994). Often the apical portion of the M cell is com-

pressed into a thin membranelike band of cytoplasm by the lymphocyte-filled pocket, which also displaces the nucleus of the M cell basally. Three-dimensional reconstruction of M cells in rabbit Peyer's patches reveals a labyrinth formed by large openings joining adjacent hollows, allowing free passage of lymphocytes from M cell to M cell (Regoli *et al.* 1995a). Golgi apparatus and endoplasmic reticulum are located just above the nucleus in M cells (Fig. 8.4). The well-developed microvesicular system, sparse lysosomes, and enfolded lymphocytes are morphologic correlates of the transport function of M cells (see subsequent discussion). No connective junctions are ultrastructurally demonstrable between M cells and enfolded cells, but adhesion molecules, cytokines, and complementary cytoskeletal structures form a complex relationship. Enfolded cells intrude into the M cell from its basal or lateral surface, presumably in response to homing signals and come in contact with surveillance information in the form of macromolecules, particles, and microorganisms transported from the intestinal lumen by M cells. This lymphoid cell traffic in and out of M-cell pockets is facilitated by the numerous holes that can be observed in the basal lamina after removal of mucosal epithelium.

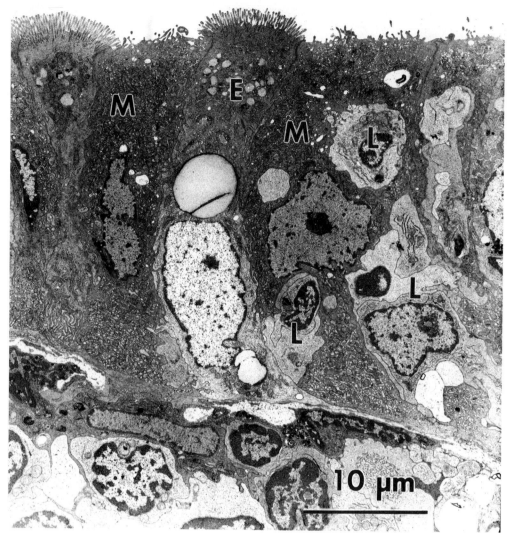

Fig. 8.4. Transmission electron micrograph of human Peyer's patch follicle epithelium. M cells (M) are shorter than enterocytes (E), which are covered by tightly packed microvilli. The M cells on the right enfold lymphocytes (L) in their pockets, whereas the M cell on the left contains no lymphocyte.

M cells in rabbits express an unusual pattern of intermediate filaments in their cytoplasm, that is, predominantly vimentin (Gaidar 1989) with lesser amounts of cytokeratin (Jepson *et al.* 1992), compared with other epithelial cells, in which vimentin is absent and cytokeratin predominates. This M-cell expression of intermediate filaments, which is more typical of cells of mesenchymal origin than of epithelial cells, their phagocytic activity, and their accommodation in shape to enfolded cells, give M cells a superficial resemblance to macrophages. Increased vimentin has not been found in M cells of other species, but porcine M cells contain cytokeratin 18, which is absent from enterocytes and is thus a useful M-cell marker (Gebert *et al.* 1994). In rats cytokeratin 8 is found in higher concentration in M cells, which also fail to stain for alkaline phosphatase, compared with surrounding enterocytes (Rautenberg *et al.* 1996). In humans no distinctive pattern of intermediate filaments has yet been identified.

The layer of glycocalyx and mucus on M cells is quite sparse, compared with that on adjacent columnar cells. Consequently, the microvilli on the surface of M cells can be observed easily by SEM (Fig. 8.3). Human, rabbit, and mouse apical M-cell membranes are rich in sialyl Lewis A antigen, specific mucin-related antigens, and $\beta1$ integrin, compared with adjacent enterocytes (Giannasca *et al.* 1999; Lelouard *et al.* 1999; Clark *et al.* 1998b).

No universal markers for M cells that are useful across species lines have been identified. However, in various species, a variety of different types of markers for M cells are available, including mesenchymal intermediate filaments, mucin-related epitopes, and lectin-binding sites. Even receptors, such as ganglioside G_{M1}, which are present on the surfaces of both enterocytes and M cells, can be utilized for identification when the enhanced accessibility of such receptors, because of the thinner surface glycocalyx, produces a

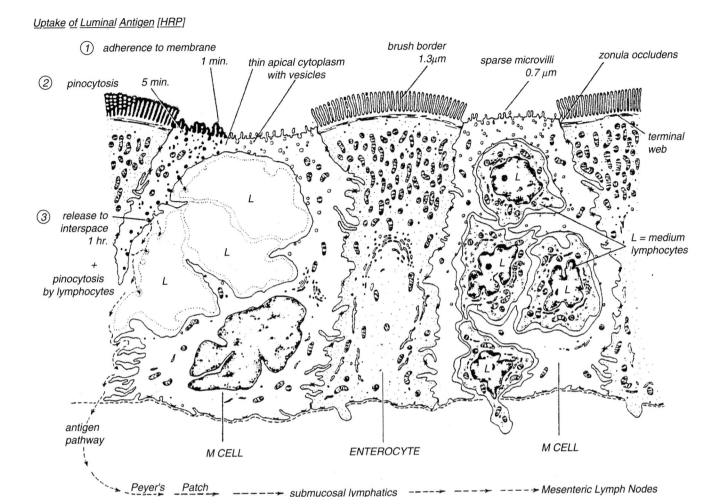

Uptake of Luminal Antigen [HRP]

Fig. 8.5. A diagram of the ultrastructural arrangement of enterocytes (stippled), M cells, and intraepithelial lymphocytes in follicle epithelium of Peyer's patch. On the right, four lymphocytes (L) are enfolded in the central hollow of an M cell. On the left, note the thin apical cytoplasm of the M cell, its lateral interdigitations, and three enfolded lymphocytes (L) shown only in dotted outline. Over the luminal surface, black lines show horseradish peroxidase (HRP) adhering to follicle epithelium 1 minute after being injected into mouse ileum. The time sequence (1–3) shows pinocytotic transfer through the M cell into its central hollow, with some uptake by enfolded lymphoid cells (Owen 1977). Antigens transported by M cells also pass downward through the basal lamina into the lymphoid follicles and are carried into mesenteric lymph nodes for induction of local or systemic immune responses. (Diagram courtesy of E. Hamish Batten.)

relative adherence specificity for M cells (Frey *et al*. 1996). Whether the differential characteristics of M-cell apical membranes that investigators exploit for M-cell localization play roles in their luminal antigen sampling function is not yet clear. The surface of M-cell microvilli has more esterase activity and much less alkaline phosphatase and sucrase-iso-maltase activity than the surface of microvilli of adjacent absorptive cells (Owen and Bhalla 1983). The functional significance of this enzymatic pattern remains uncertain, but has been used to advantage by Smith and colleagues (1987) in examining changes in patterns of M-cell distribution over follicle domes in mice when luminal microbial populations increase. In rabbits there is also a differential distribution of alkaline phosphatase in enterocytes and M cells, but vimentin remains a better M-cell marker (Jepson *et al*.

1993). The low lysosome content of M cells is one morphologic feature, which clearly correlates with M-cell ability to transport antigens from the intestinal lumen with little enzymatic degradation (Owen *et al*. 1986a).

The surface of M cells has been found to interact with S-IgA in uptake of intestinal particles. The surface of the M cell has binding sites for S-IgA (Roy and Varvayanis 1987; Weltzin *et al*. 1989; Kato 1990; **Fig. 8.9**), but lacks secretory component (Pappo and Owen 1988). Immunohistochemically, the human M cell expresses MHC class II HLA-DR antigen on its apical and basolateral membrane, analogous to the dendritic cell and macrophage, which are known to be APCs (Nagura *et al*. 1991). This feature of M cells, in conjunction with the fact that M cells take up complexes containing S-IgA (Zhou *et al*. 1995), suggests that these cells may function as APCs as well

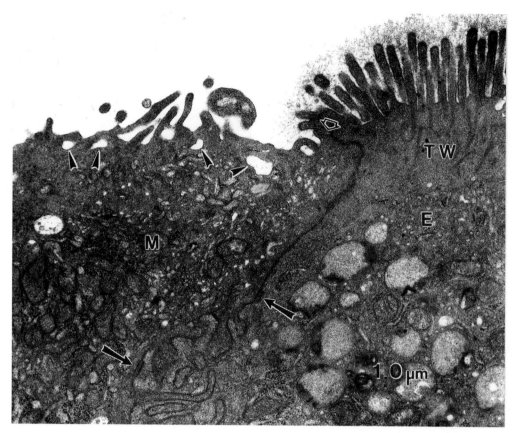

Fig. 8.6. Transmission electron micrograph showing the junction between a columnar enterocyte (E) and an M cell (M) in human Peyer's patch. The M cell has characteristic microfolds, absent terminal web, sparse glycocalyx, and numerous pinocytotic vesicles (arrowheads) in its apical cytoplasm compared with the adjacent enterocyte, which has thick glycocalyx, regular microvilli, and microvillus cores extending down into the terminal web (TW). The interface is composed of a tight junction (open arrowhead), several desmosomes (arrows), and lateral interdigitations.

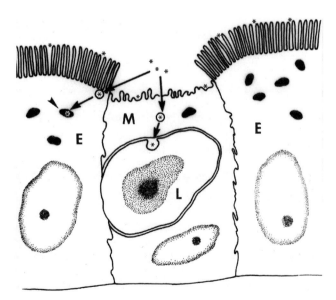

Fig. 8.7. Diagrammatic model of uptake and transport of luminal antigens by M cells (M). The M cell has only a rare lysosome, compared with numerous lysosomes (arrowhead) in adjacent enterocytes (E). When particulate antigens (asterisks) are taken up by enterocytes, they are diverted into lysosomes and digested. In M cells, antigens escape lysosomal degradation and either are taken up by lymphoid cells (L) in the central hollow or pass into the intercellular space. (Reprinted with permission from Owen *et al.* 1986a and Wiley-Liss.)

as antigen-transporting cells. M cells from jejunal Peyer's patches contain acidic endosomal and prelysosomal structures but few lysosomelike structures (Fig. 8.7) and express IL-1 and MHC class II determinants, indicating that they have at least some capacity to present endocytosed antigens directly to lymphocytes (Nagura *et al.* 1991; Allan *et al.* 1993). In humans M cells in Peyer's patches stain for HLA-DR but not for intercellular adhesion molecule-1 (ICAM-1). In contrast, colonic M cells express ICAM-1 but do not display HLA class II antigens, suggesting that in the colon M cells may transport but not present antigen (Ueki *et al.* 1995).

Putative M cells have been recognized morphologically in human fetuses by week 17 of gestation (Moxey and Trier 1978). Although M cells clearly derive from intestinal epithelial cells, their differentiation pathways remain controversial. Three pathways have been proposed. One is M-cell development from mature columnar epithelial cells that overlie domes in intestinal lymphoid structures. Another is M-cell development directly from undifferentiated stem cells in crypts that lie between lymphoid domes and adjacent villi (Bhalla and Owen 1982). A third possible pathway is generation from stem cells of undifferentiated cells capable of becoming either M cells or enterocytes on the dome surface. Some evidence supports each of these pathways. Bye *et al.* (1984) observed morphologically immature M cells, with rapid induction of cells with the M-cell phenotype over follicle domes thus suggests that M cells can derive from differentiated absorptive enterocytes. This hypothesis is further supported by M-cell development in a differentiated absorptive enterocyte cell line after the monolayer is infiltrated by Peyer's patch lymphocytes (Kernéis *et al.* 1997) and by M-cell appearance in neonatal rabbit lymphoid domes more rapidly after influx of lymphocytes into FAE than can be accounted for by migration from crypts (reviewed by Savidge 1996). Not only do intraluminal lymphocytes and luminal microorganisms seem to drive full expression of the M-cell phenotype over domes, but also dedifferentiation back to the enterocyte phenotype is suggested by restriction of apoptosis to the top of domes where few M cells are found (Sierro *et al.* 2000).

The extracellular matrix (ECM) under the FAE may be a factor in proliferation, differentiation, migration, and apoptosis of dome epithelial cells. Sierro *et al.* (2000) found differences between crypts of domes and villi in laminins (Ln) that are major components of ECM. They found absence of the α2 subunit of laminins 2 and 4 in the crypts of follicle domes, which correlated with an absence of smooth muscle actin-positive myofibroblasts under the FAE. Based on these observations, they speculate that ECM may affect FAE-specific differentiation.

Caco-2 cells, derived from a human colonic cell adenocarcinoma, display properties of fetal ileal epithelial cells with multipotent phenotypes (Engle *et al.* 1998); that is, they behave as intestinal crypt cells with differentiation depending on local environment. Utilizing this cell line, Kernéis *et al.* (1997) demonstrated that clones of differentiated enterocytes from the human Caco-2 cell line, when cocultured with mouse Peyer's patch lymphocytes, take on characteristics of M cells. They enfold lymphocytes, develop disorganized apical microvilli, and lose both sucrase-isomaltase, a brush border hydrolase characteristic of differentiated enterocytes, and villin, an actin-associated protein involved in assembly of the apical cytoskeleton. Mouse Peyer's patch lymphocytes induce similar changes in the mouse ICcl-2 cell line, indicating that the inductive factors and their receptors must be conserved across species. Induced M cells from both lines are able to transcytose latex beads, replicating an M-cell function not otherwise present in Caco-2 cells. These investigators were also able to induce formation of M cells *in vivo* by injecting Peyer's patch lymphocytes beneath the duodenal mucosa of mice at sites lacking organized lymphoid tissue. Peyer's patch–like structures developed with well-organized lymphoid follicles and follicle-associated epithelium containing epithelial cells with disorganized microvilli, pockets filled with lymphocytes, lack of polymeric Ig receptors, and binding sites for *Ulex europaeus* agglutinin 1 (UEA), which are characteristic for M cells in mice. This suggests that Peyer's patch formation may be controlled by the distribution of high endothelial venules, which induce extravasation of cells that form lymphoid aggregates rather than by distribution of specialized stem cells, uniquely capable of differentiating into M cells. From their *in vivo* experiments, this group of investigators was unable to determine whether M-cell

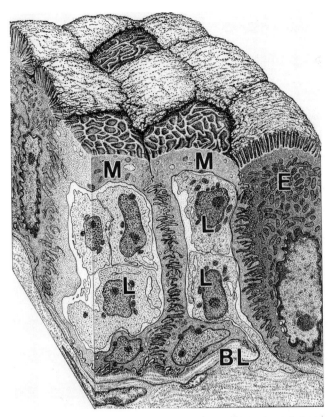

Fig. 8.8. Three-dimensional illustration of M cells (M) interdigitating with adjacent enterocytes (E). In their central hollows, M cells enfold several lymphocytes (L), one of which is migrating through a pore in the basal lamina (BL). (Reprinted with permission from Owen and Nemanic 1978.)

features shared by mature M cells and crypt cells, in all regions of the follicle dome. After intraperitoneal injection of [3H]-thymidine into mice, only crypt cells are labeled for the first 12 hours. Radiolabeled nuclei of immature M cells are first observed near crypt mouths in mice after 24 hours, and mature M cells are labeled after 48 hours. In the mouse, model immature M cells, seen first in upper parts of specialized oval-mouthed dome-associated crypts, can be recognized not only by their morphology but also by binding to UEA1 lectin (Gebert *et al.* 1999). Furthermore, in rabbits many vimentin-labeled M-cell precursors are observed deeper in crypts, down to the zone of rapidly dividing cells (Lelouard *et al.* 2001). These observations indicate that M-cell precursors derive from crypt stem cells deep in crypts. Regardless of their final differentiation steps, M cells ultimately derive from undifferentiated stem cells in the crypts surrounding domes.

Whether they also develop from already differentiated absorptive enterocytes remains controversial. Introduction of *Streptococcus pneumoniae* into rabbit ileal loops for 1 hour induced heightened infiltration of the follicle epithelium with lymphocytes and a marked increase of the proportion of M cells in the follicle epithelium, even though migration of cells from intestinal crypts to the dome apex takes 60 hours (Borghesi *et al.* 1996; Meynell *et al.* 1999). This apparent

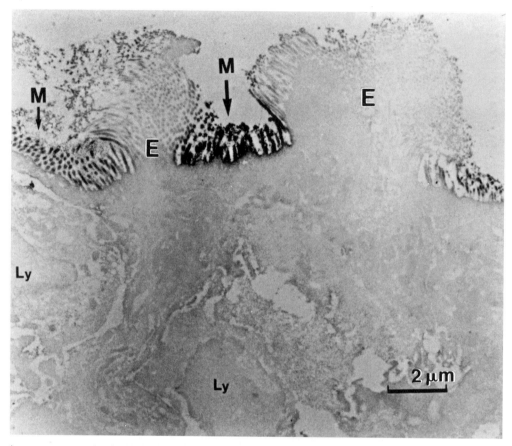

Fig. 8.9. Immunoelectron micrograph of rabbit Peyer's patch follicle epithelium treated with antisecretory IgA antibody and horseradish peroxidase–conjugated secondary antibody. Electron-dense areas of enzyme reaction product are prominent over the short irregular microvilli of the M cells (M) with enfolded lymphocytes (Ly), compared with the adjacent enterocytes (E). Reaction product is presumed to show binding sites of S-IgA on M cells, which may take up IgA-antigen complexes. (Reprinted with permission from Kato 1990.)

induction took place in crypts or by conversion of differentiated absorptive enterocytes. This model may be useful for investigating cytoskeletal rearrangement and signaling when M cells take up various luminal pathogens. Immunodeficient severe combined immunodeficiency (SCID) mice and B-cell–deficient mice lack mucosal follicles and identifiable M cells (Savidge et al. 1994; Loffert et al. 1994), whereas T-cell–deficient nude mice have small Peyer's patches and FAE with M cells (Ermak and Owen 1987). These data suggest that B cells and their regulating cytokines may play a role in formation of FAE including M cells (Hamzaoui and Pringault 1998).

Where M cells go is unclear, since more M cells are present on the edges of domes than on the apices, where desquamation and death of enterocytes generally occur. The life span of M cells is also uncertain. According to the study of Bye et al. (1984), they migrate from the crypt to the dome base within 24 hours and to the summit of the dome within 72 hours. This life span is essentially identical to that of villus epithelial cells. Numbers of cells with labeled nuclei over domes gradually decrease between days 5 and 14, and no labeled cells are present by day 14 (Bye et al. 1984). Sierro et al. (2000), investigating apoptosis in mouse Peyer's patches,

reported that apoptosis was not present on the sides of domes where M cells disappear, whereas apoptotic enterocytes were numerous at the top of the domes in Peyer's patches.

GALT in specific pathogen-free (SPF) animals is poorly developed, although its basic structure is present. Exposure to the intestinal flora is essential for the complete development of GALT. M cells also need microbial exposure to proliferate. The total number of M cells increases in mice after transfer from an SPF to a conventional environment (Smith et al. 1987), whereas the ratio of M cells to FAE is reported not to be changed by such transfer (Sicinski et al. 1986). The invagination by lymphocytes had been considered essential to M-cell development, but lymphocytes do not seem to be necessary for morphologic maturation, since mature M cells can be recognized even in mice depleted of lymphocytes by total lymphoid irradiation (Ermak et al. 1989).

Other follicle epithelial cells

In addition to M cells, columnar absorptive cells, IELs, and tuft cells are present in FAE. The structure of absorptive cells in FAE resembles that of enterocytes on villi, but these two populations of enterocytes may differ in surface characteristics and function (Figure 8.5). In rabbits, secretory component is absent not only from M cells but also from absorptive cells in FAE (Pappo and Owen 1988). The majority of IELs in FAE are CD8[+] T cells, as in villus epithelium (see Chapter 30), but the ratio of CD4[+] to CD8[+] lymphocytes in FAE (4 : 10) is greater than among IELs of villi (0.6 : 10). Lymphocytes in FAE are often large lymphoblast forms, which are thought to be immature and immunologically uncommitted, compared with the mature effector IELs found among enterocytes that cover villi. Ermak *et al.* (1994) found that in rabbit Peyer's patch epithelium, one third of lymphocytes are B cells and the rest are CD4[−], CD8[−], and MHC II[+], and macrophages, B cells, and CD4[+] cells are concentrated in the dome just beneath the FAE. This suggests that the activation of the CD4[+] cells involved in IgA–B cell differentiation takes place in the dome and not in the M-cell pockets. FAE is involved in induction of helper T-cell functions, possibly as a consequence of M-cell uptake and transport of antigens from the intestinal lumen (Bjerke *et al.* 1988). Intraluminal bacterial antigens can stimulate migration of lymphocytes from pockets through channels in the apices of M cells (Regoli *et al.* 1994). Whether these lymphocytes play a role in surveillance or in cellular immune defense remains conjectural.

M-cell function

Several important immunologic and pathophysiologic functions are recognized for M cells. M cells capture antigens from the intestinal lumen and transport them to enfolded lymphocytes and macrophages. Some of these lymphoid cells are presumed to influence IgA production directly in the germinal centers of lymphoid follicles, but this concept has been difficult to prove. Kabok *et al.* (1995) were able to induce production of antiferritin antibody by incubating isolated rabbit Peyer's patch lymphoid follicles with ferritin in organ culture for 7 days. Other stimulated lymphoid cells migrate through lymphatics to mesenteric lymph nodes and via the thoracic duct to the general circulation, then ultimately return by migration and homing receptors to mucosal tissues as IgA-producing plasma cells (Fig. 8.1).

Mucosal surveillance

Antigen uptake. M cells take up and transport a wide variety of sizes and types of intestinal antigens and microorganisms. This unique process may depend in part on factors that include mediators released by immunocompetent cells, hormonal factors, and nervous control. To study M-cell function, investigators have focused on M cells of Peyer's patches, often using ligated intestinal segments and high concentrations of organisms to facilitate detection of uptake that, under physiologic conditions, would occur less frequently yet would be sufficient for induction of immunologic responses. Some of the macromolecules and microorganisms for which uptake and transport by M cells has been confirmed are discussed in the following sections (see also **Table 8.1**).

Particles and macromolecules. Native ferritin (rat; Bockman and Cooper 1973), cationized ferritin (rabbit; Bye *et al.* 1984), horseradish peroxidase (rabbit; Owen 1977; von

Table 8.1. Substances and Microorganisms Taken Up by M Cells

Particles and Macromolecules
Native ferritin
Cationized ferritin
Horseradish peroxidase
Ricinus communis agglutinins I and II
Wheat germ agglutinin
Cholera toxin
Picibanil (OK-432)
600-nm to 750-nm diameter latex particles
Liposomes and IgA-coated liposomes

Viruses
Reovirus type 1 and type 3
Poliovirus type 1
Human immunodeficiency virus type 1 (HIV-1)
Mouse mammary tumor virus (MMTV)

Bacteria
Vibrio cholerae
Salmonella typhi
Salmonella typhimurium
Bacillus Calmette-Guérin (BCG)
Mycobacterium paratuberculosis
Brucella abortus
Streptococcus pyogenes
Streptococcus pneumoniae
Campylobacter jejuni
Yersinia enterocolitica
Yersinia pseudotuberculosis
Shigella flexneri
Salmonella enteriditis
Escherichia coli RDEC-1 strain
Escherichia coli O:124 K:72 strain
Streptococcus pneumoniae R36a
Mycobacterium avium subsp. *Paratuberculosis*
Listeria monocytogenes

Parasites
Cryptosporidium
Eimeria coecicola

Rosen 1981), *Ricinus communis* agglutinins I and II (rabbit; Neutra *et al.* 1987), wheat germ agglutinin (rabbit; Neutra *et al.* 1987), cholera toxin (guinea pig; Shakhlamov *et al.*, 1981), Picibanil (OK-432, a streptococcal biologic response modifier; rabbit; Nagasaki *et al.* 1988), 600-nm to 750-nm diameter latex particles (rabbit; Pappo and Ermak 1989), and IgA-coated and uncoated liposomes (mice; Zhou *et al.* 1995) have been shown to be transported by M cells. There is great interest in characteristics that influence M-cell uptake of particles because M cells may be a useful delivery route for vaccines and pharmaceutical agents (Florence 1997).

Particle size affects uptake. Polylactic polyglycolic acid copolymer (PLGA), a biodegradable carrier particle in a 100-nm size, is taken up at a 15-fold to 250-fold higher rate compared with 500-nm, 1-μm, or 10-μm particles (Desai *et al.* 1996). Protein coating can also greatly influence particle binding and uptake by M cells. In mice, binding and uptake is less enhanced by bovine growth hormone than by bovine serum albumin and more enhanced by human IgG than by bovine growth hormone or bovine serum albumin (Smith *et al.* 1995).

Viruses. Reovirus type 1 and type 3 (mouse; Wolf *et al.* 1983), poliovirus type 1 (human; Sicinski *et al.* 1990), human immunodeficiency virus type 1 (HIV-1; mouse and rabbit; Amerongen *et al.* 1991), and mouse mammary tumor virus (MMTV; mouse; Bevilacqua *et al.* 1989) have been shown to be transported by M cells. Within the intestine, enzymatic digestion of native reovirus particles to intermediate subviral particles is necessary for uptake by M cells, presumably by revealing adherence sites (Amerongen *et al.* 1994).

Bacteria. Vibrio cholerae (rabbit; Owen *et al.* 1986b), *Salmonella typhi* (mouse; Kohbata *et al.* 1986), *Salmonella typhimurium* (mouse; Jones *et al.* 1994), BCG *(Bacillus* Calmette-Guérin; rabbit; Fujimura 1986), *Mycobacterium paratuberculosis* (calf; Momotani *et al.* 1988), *Brucella abortus* (calf; Ackermann *et al.* 1988), *Streptococcus pyogenes* (rabbit; Nagasaki *et al.* 1988) *Streptococcus pneumoniae* (rabbit; Regnoli *et al.* 1995b), *Campylobacter jejuni* (rabbit; Walker *et al.* 1988), *Yersinia enterocolitica* (mouse; Grützkau *et al.* 1990; Autenrieth and Firsching 1996), *Yersinia pseudotuberculosis* (rabbit; Fujimura *et al.* 1989), *Shigella flexneri* (rabbit; Wassef *et al.* 1989; mouse; Jensen *et al.* 1998), *Salmonella enteriditis* (rabbit; Kamoi 1991), RDEC-1 strain of *Escherichia coli* (rabbit; Inman and Cantey 1984), O:124 K:72 strain of *E. coli* (rabbit; Uchida 1987) , *S. pneumoniae* R36a (rabbit; Borghesi *et al.* 1996), *Mycobacterium avium* subsp. *paratuberculosis* (goat; Sigurdardottir *et al.* 2001), and *Listeria monocytogenes* (mouse; Jensen *et al.* 1998) have been shown to be transported by M cells.

Parasites. Cryptosporidium (guinea pig; Marcial and Madara 1986) has been shown to be taken up. In rabbits, the coccidian parasite, *Eimeria coecicola*, is taken up by both M cells and lymphocytes in Peyer's patches, sacculus rotundus, and appendix (Pakandl *et al.* 1996). Even under optimizing conditions, observation of uptake of *Giardia muris* trophozoites has not been possible, although they were found in the pocket within mouse M cells (Owen *et al.* 1981).

Information about M-cell function in absorption of nutrients is limited; however, no absorption of lipid by M cells of mice was observed (Bye *et al.* 1984). M cells are also capable of reverse transport of some substances into the intestinal lumen, as demonstrated by the fact that injected horseradish peroxidase can be seen to move from the tissue into the lumen through M cells (Bockman and Stevens 1977).

The mechanism by which M-cell uptake of various antigens from the intestinal lumen is regulated remains unclear.

One factor may be glycoproteins on the M-cell surface. IgA antibodies in the lumen can selectively adhere to M cells in mice and rabbits, regardless of their antigen specificities (Roy *et al.* 1987). The mechanism of IgA binding to M cells is not known, but monoclonal IgA was shown to mediate uptake of antigen (Weltzin *et al.* 1989). The fate of IgA-antigen complexes after uptake into Peyer's patches is not known.

Although the range of microorganisms and other particles taken up by M cells is wide, these cells also exhibit selectivity of uptake, and specific characteristics impede or facilitate attachment, uptake, and transport. M cells take up viable and killed *M. paratuberculosis*. M cells take up, transport, and present living *V. cholerae* **(Fig. 8.10)**, but killed *Vibrio* are scarcely taken up by M cells. When suspensions of 10^9 *Vibrio* killed by acidification, formalin treatment, ultraviolet irradiation, or heating were injected into ligated intestinal segments of rabbit intestine containing Peyer's patches, none were taken up after 180 minutes. Motile noninvasive but colonizing living *Vibrio* of the same strain were taken up readily by M cells when administered in the same concentration (Owen *et al.* 1988b). Because cholera toxin stimulates a variety of cellular processes, mutant *Vibrio* that produce neither the A nor the B subunit of cholera toxin were administered and found to be taken up by M cells as efficiently as toxigenic strains. In contrast, a toxin-producing but nonmotile strain, CVD 49, was not taken up, indicating that one of the most important determinants of bacterial uptake is whether organisms can reach the M-cell surface, either by motility or by lateral spread across the colonized mucosal surface (Owen *et al.* 1988a).

Even different strains of the same microorganism have very different interactions with M cells. Among *E. coli*, the O:124 K:72 strain is taken up and presented but the O:124 RDEC-1 strain can adhere to the M-cell surface without being transported.

For *S. typhimurium*, the M cell is an important entry portal. This entry requires ruffling and cytoskeletal remodeling of the M-cell apical surface, which depends on a type III protein secretion system encoded by genetic components clustered on pathogenicity island 1 (Penheiter *et al.* 1997; Clark *et al.* 1998a; Galan 1999). Mutants of *S. typhimurium* that no longer secrete proteins involved in invasion of tissue culture cells also fail to induce ruffling of M cells, uptake of *S. typhimurium*, and invasion of intact Peyer's patches (Penheiter *et al.* 1997).

Reovirus type 1 is taken up by M cells only, but type 3 is taken up by M cells and columnar cells in FAE (Wolf *et al.* 1983). Further, after passage through M cells, reovirus type 1 passes through the basolateral membrane of these cells to adjacent columnar epithelial cells and proliferates there, finally producing an inflammatory lesion (Weiner *et al.* 1988). The entry of reovirus type 1 requires reovirus-1 attachment protein, which interacts with receptors such as lectin on M-cell apical membranes (Silvey *et al.* 2001).

Whether the relatively weak alkaline phosphatase activity on the apical surface of the M cell has functional significance

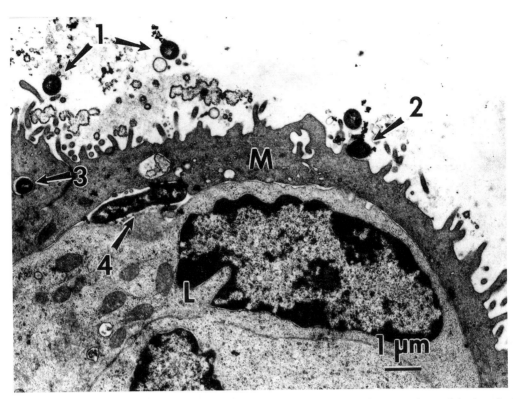

Fig. 8.10. Transport of tritium-labeled *Vibrio cholerae* by rabbit M cells (M). Vibrios (1) lie in the mucus layer of the intestinal lumen. Vibrio 2 is adherent to M-cell microvilli. After uptake, vibrio 3 is transported within a vesicle through the cytoplasm. Finally, vibrio 4 lies within the central hollow, adjacent to an enfolded lymphocyte (L). (Reprinted with permission from Owen *et al*. 1988b.)

is unclear. The very few lysosomes and the well-developed vesicular transport system in its apical cytoplasm contribute to the function of the M cell as the gateway to the immune defense system (Fig. 8.7). This function as a gatekeeper seems to depend on the equilibrium between the motility, colonizing potential, and invasiveness of pathogens and the defensive competence of M cells and associated macrophages and dendritic cells. The efficiency and vigor with which M cells function as the gateway for antigen sampling contribute to a pathophysiologic role of M cells as entry points for invasion by virulent pathogens (Fujimura and Owen 1996; Siebers and Finlay 1996). Some types of intestinal infection, particularly typhoid fever and intestinal tuberculosis, occur initially in Peyer's patches. Virulent pathogens such as *S. typhi* and *S. flexneri* invade M cells and subsequently precipitate the destruction of Peyer's patches. Thus the M cell seems to be a target cell as well as a conduit for some virulent pathogens that cause enteritis in clinical settings (Vazquez-Torres and Fang 2000).

In M cells, whether initiation of an immune response or systemic invasion occurs may depend on binding to the M-cell apical membrane and on the ability of M cells and associated phagocytic cells to digest and inactivate microorganisms. The apical membrane of M cells has been shown to have an enhanced capacity to bind S-IgA, possibly because of its thin glycocalyx compared with adjacent columnar cells (Fig. 8.9). This ability of M cells to bind S-IgA may protect them against the luminal environment and may accelerate M-cell uptake of luminal antigens that are complexed with IgA to boost an existing immune response. The former possibility is supported by the fact that the mouse intestinal mucosa can be protected against virulent *V. cholerae and S. typhimurium* infection by secretion of hybridoma-derived IgA specific to each bacterium (Winner *et al*. 1991; Michetti *et al*. 1992). The latter suggestion is supported by the fact that transport of some viruses by M cells is accelerated by monoclonal IgA antibodies directed against proteins of these viruses (Weltzin *et al*. 1989; see Chapter 7).

The range of mechanisms for capture and uptake of various antigens from the intestinal lumen, and for antigen processing and presentation to enfolded cells, is complex and incompletely understood. Gebert and Hach (1993) have shown that M cells of the rabbit cecum selectively bind lectins specific for fucose and *N*-acetylgalactosamine. These lectins bind to the apical membrane and to the membranes of vesicles in the cytoplasm of M cells. In contrast, rabbit enterocytes selectively bind galactose-specific lectins. In rabbit jejunal Peyer's patches, M cells and enterocytes do not show differences in surface glycoconjugates. UEA selectively binds to α–L-fucose targets on mouse Peyer's patch M cells *in vivo* and is rapidly endocytosed and transported to M-cell basolateral membranes (Clark *et al*. 1995b), but UEA is absent over mouse cecal patch M cells (Clark *et al.* 1994). *Euonymus europaeus* lectin, a lectin with complex carbohydrate specificity, binds to both mouse Peyer's patch and cecal patch M cells (Clark *et al.* 1995a). No lectin has yet been identified that binds to rabbit Peyer's patch M cells, but *E. europaeus* binds differentially to M cells in the periphery of rabbit cecal patches (Clark *et al.* 1995a). Although UEA and other lectins stain M cells in mice, no lectin has yet been found that can distinguish M cells in humans (Sharma *et al.* 1996). Adherence of microorganisms to glycoconjugates on M-cell surfaces may be a critical determinant of variations in microbial uptake and colonization at different levels in the gastrointestinal tract. Even binding sites that are shared by M cells and enterocytes are more accessible for microbial adherence on M cells, which lack mucus and the thick glycocalyx coat present over microvilli of enterocytes. Characterization of M-cell receptor sites that bind microorganisms and antigenic molecules may be critical for the logical development of oral immunizing agents; see Chapters 7 and 55).

Antigen processing. Using immunohistochemical techniques, investigators have shown that M cells express IL-1 and MHC class II molecules (Ia antigen in mice, HLA-DR in humans; Nagura *et al.*, 1991). Previously researchers believed that no digestive mechanism was involved in transport through the M cell. However, Allan and associates (1993) showed that M cells possess acidic endosomal, prelysosomal, and lysosomal compartments and express MHC class II determinants in their prelysosomal and lysosomal structures. These data show that M cells have some potential for processing endocytosed agents and presenting them to the enfolded immunocompetent cells. In mice, IgM plasma cells, macrophages, and T cells that express the CD8 molecule are located in close proximity to M cells and could receive such processed antigen (Jarry *et al.* 1989). Other APCs such as dendritic cells and macrophages exist beneath the FAE (Mowat and Viney 1997).

Dendritic cells in Peyer's patches are divided into three types by their cell surface markers and distribution: myeloid dendritic cells with CD11b+/CD11c+/DEC205−, lymphoid dendritic cells with CD8α+/CD11c+/DEC205+, and double-negative dendritic cells with CD11c+/CD8α−CD11b−. Myeloid dendritic cells are mainly located in dome, and lymphoid cells are mainly in interfollicular areas of Peyer's patches (Iwasaki *et al.* 2000). Dendritic cells in the dome express MHC-I/II, costimulatory molecule (B7-1, CD80, B7-2, CD86), intercellular adhesion molecule-1 (ICAM-1), and mucosal addressin cell adhesion molecule-1 (MAdCAM 1), strongly suggesting that they function as APCs (Ruedl *et al.* 1996). Double-negative dendritic cells are observed only in mucosa-associated lymphoid tissues such as GALT, including Peyer's patches. They locate in not only dome and interfollicular areas but also FAE (Iwasaki *et al.* 2001). These cells extend processes into the FAE and are thought to communicate with M cells in information processing, but their interactions and division of functions remain unclear.

Although the fact that all necessary elements for initiation of intestinal immune responses are present in Peyer's patch

follicles has been clearly demonstrated, proving that M-cell uptake is an essential step in this process has not been possible. Isolation and culture of M cells, which would be helpful in elucidating their various features, have not yet been accomplished.

Target for migration and homing of lymphoblasts
Before lymphoblasts can reach FAE to be enfolded within M cells and brought in contact with various antigens in Peyer's patches, they must leave the systemic circulation via postcapillary venules (PCV) (Fig. 8.1). This directed migration is mediated by high endothelial venules (HEV) in Peyer's patches. In homing, naive T lymphocytes are controlled by surface markers peculiar to each mucosal site; the HEVs have receptors recognized by lymphocyte adhesion molecules. Naive T cells express L-selectin and integrin $\alpha_4\beta_7$ on their surface, which can recognize MAdCAM-1 on HEV in Peyer's patches (Butcher *et al.* 1999). After naive T lymphocytes contact HEV, they are stimulated to cross the walls of the HEV and migrate into the interfollicular tissue and marginal zones of follicles by CC-chemokines such as secondary lymphoid-tissue chemokine (SLC) (Willimann *et al.* 1998; Pachynski *et al.* 1998; Warnock *et al.* 2000; see Chapter 34).

Factors that guide the next step of migration, that is, from HEVs in the parafollicular domain to FAE, remain under investigation. Extracellular matrix components, arrayed along the migration pathway from HEVs to the apices of follicle domes, may provide the physical basis for this directional cell traffic (Ohtsuka *et al.* 1992). The migratory stimulus for lymphoid cells to move from follicle domes into and out of M-cell pockets is unknown.

Lymphocytes of B-cell lineage finally return to the gut mucosa as mature IgA-producing plasma cells. The migration process of these cells from GALT back to the gut is reported to require 4–6 days (Hall 1979). B lymphocytes from GALT also can go to other mucosal sites, including mammary glands, salivary glands, bronchial tissues, and the genitourinary tract, and there become stationary plasma cells that produce IgA (Bienenstock and Befus 1980; see Chapter 20).

Other mucosal associated lymphoid tissues (MALT). Lymphoid tissues comprising MALT are distributed in various locations. Bronchus-associated and nasal-associated lymphoid tissues (BALT, NALT) are of special importance because of their rapid and continual exposure to airborne particulate antigens and microorganisms from the external environment. Both BALT and NALT are very similar in structure to Peyer's patches, also consisting of lymphoid follicles, domes, interfollicular areas, and follicle-associated epithelium. Whether they function as inductive sites for initiating immune responses to airborne agents is still under investigation.

The surface epithelium covering NALT consists of numerous ciliated epithelial cells, a few mucus goblet cells, and numerous M cells. M cells take up various antigens from the mucosal lumen and transport them to underlying immunocompetent cells. They are thus similar to M cells in Peyer's patches in structure and particulate transport. However, whether M cells function as APCs is still unclear. Although NALT has some similarities to Peyer's patches, it differs in tissue morphology, lymphoid migration patterns, and HEV-binding properties and is not MHC class II–positive under normal conditions (Kuper *et al.* 1992).

BALT aggregates are concentrated mainly around bifurcations of major bronchus divisions (Plesch 1982). Compared with Peyer's patches, BALT structure is less specialized and not so extensively infiltrated with lymphocytes, but does contain attenuated surface epithelial cells in close contact with lymphocytes that are similar to M cells in Peyer's patches. The relatively sparse lymphoid tissue in BALT may reflect its more limited microbial exposure compared with Peyer's patches in the intestine.

REFERENCES

Abe, K., and Ito, T. (1977). A qualitative and quantitative morphologic study of Peyer's patches of the mouse. *Arch. Histol. Jpn.* 40, 407–420.

Ackermann, M. R., Cheville, N. F., and Deyoe, B. L. (1988). Bovine ileal dome lymphoepithelial cells: Endocytosis and transport of *Brucella abortus* strain 19. *Vet. Pathol.* 25, 28–35.

Allan, C. H., Mendrick, D. L., and Trier, J. S. (1993). Rat intestinal M cells contain acidic endosomal-lysosomal compartments and express class II major histocompatibility complex determinants. *Gastroenterology* 104, 698–708.

Amerongen, H. M., Weltzin, R., Farnet, C. M., Michetti, P., Haseltine, W. A., and Neutra, M. R. (1991). Transepithelial transport of HIV-1 by intestinal M cells: A mechanism for transmission of AIDS. *J. AIDS* 4, 760–765.

Amerongen, H. M., Wilson, G. A., Fields, B. N., and Neutra, M. R. (1994). Proteolytic processing of reovirus is required for adherence to intestinal M cells. *J. Virol.* 68, 8428–8432.

Autenrieth, I. B., and Firsching, R. (1996). Penetration of M cells and destruction of Peyer's patches by *Yersinia enterocolitica*: An ultrastructural and histological study. *J. Med. Microbiol.* 44, 285–294.

Bamba, T., and Andoh, A. (1998). Regulation of mucosal inflammation and clinical outcome in inflammatory bowel disease. In *Bioregulation and Its Disorders in the Gastrointestinal Tract* (eds. T. Yoshikawa and T. Arakawa), 243–252. Tokyo: Blackwell Science.

Bassi, C., Fontana, R., Vesentini, S., Cavallini, G., Marchiori, L., Falconi, M., Corrà, S., and Pederzoli, P. (1991). Antibacterial and mezlocillin-enhancing activity of pure human pancreatic fluid. *Int. J. Pancreatol.* 10, 293–297.

Bevilacqua, G. Marchetti, A. and Biondi, R. (1989). Ultrastructural features of the intestinal absorption of mouse mammary tumor virus in newborn BALB/cfRIII mice. *Gastroenterology* 96, 139–145.

Bhalla, D. K., and Owen, R. L. (1982). Cell renewal and migration in lymphoid follicles of Peyer's patches and cecum: An autoradiographic study in mice. *Gastroenterology* 82, 232–242.

Bienenstock, J., and Befus, A. D. (1980). Mucosal immunology. A review. *Immunology* 41, 249–270.

Bienenstock, J., and Befus, D. (1984). Gut- and bronchus-associated lymphoid tissue. *Am. J. Anat.* 170, 437–445.

Bjerke, K., Brandtzaeg, P., and Fausa, O. (1988). T cell distribution is different in follicle-associated epithelium of human Peyer's patches and villous epithelium. *Clin. Exp. Immunol.* 74, 270–275.

Bleicher, P. A., Balk, S. P., Hagen, S. J., Blumberg, R. S., Flotte, T. J., and Terhorst, C. (1990). Expression of murine CD1 on gastrointestinal epithelium. *Science* 250, 679–682.

Blom, H., and Helander, H. F. (1981). Quantitative ultrastructural studies on parietal cell regeneration in experimental ulcers in rat gastric mucosa. *Gastroenterology* 80, 334–343.

Bockman, D. E., and Cooper, M. D. (1973). Pinocytosis by epithelium associated with lymphoid follicles in the bursa of Fabricius, appendix, and Peyer's patches. An electron microscopic study. *Am. J. Anat.* 136, 455–478.

Bockman, D. E., and Stevens, W. (1977). Gut-associated lymphoepithelial tissue: Bi-directional transport of tracer by specialized epithelial cells associated with lymphoid follicles. *J. Reticuloendothel. Soc.* 21, 245–254.

Borghesi, C., Regoli, M., Bertelli, E., and Nicoletti, C. (1996). Modifications of the follicle-associated epithelium by short-term exposure to a non-intestinal bacterium. *J. Pathol.* 180, 326–332.

Boyer, B., and Thiery, J. P. (1989). Epithelial cell adhesion mechanisms. *J. Membrane Biol.* 112, 97–108.

Butcher, E. C., Williams, M., Youngman, K., Rott, L., and Briskin, M. (1999). Lymphocyte trafficking and regional immunity. *Adv. Immunol.* 72, 209–253.

Bye, W. A., Allan, C. H., and Trier, J. S. (1984). Structure, distribution, and origin of M cells in Peyer's patches of mouse ileum. *Gastroenterology* 86, 789–801.

Byrne, B. M., and Dankert, J. (1979). Volatile fatty acids and aerobic flora in the gastrointestinal tract of mice under various conditions. *Infect. Immun.* 23, 559–563.

Cerf-Bensussan, N., and Guy-Grand, D. (1991). Intestinal intraepithelial lymphocytes. *Gastroenterol. Clin. North Am.* 20, 549–576.

Cerf-Bensussan, N., Quaroni, A., Kurnick, J. T., and Bhan, A. K. (1984). Intraepithelial lymphocytes modulate Ia expression by intestinal epithelial cells. *J. Immunol.* 132, 2244–2252.

Chadee, K., Petri, W. A., Jr., Innes, D. J., and Ravdin, J. I. (1987). Rat and human colonic mucins bind to and inhibit adherence lectin of *Entamoeba histolytica*. *J. Clin. Invest.* 80, 1245–1254,

Clark, M. A., Jepson, M. A., Simmons, N. L., and Hirst, B. H. (1994). Differential surface characteristics of M cells from mouse intestinal Peyer's and caecal patches. *Histochem. J.* 26, 271–280.

Clark, M. A., Jepson, M. A., and Hirst, B. H. (1995a). Lectin binding defines and differentiates M-cells in mouse small intestine and caecum. *Histochem. Cell Biol.* 104, 161–168.

Clark, M. A., Jepson, M. A., Simmons, N. L., and Hirst, B. H. (1995b). Selective binding and transcytosis of *Ulex europaeus* 1 lectin by mouse Peyer's patch M-cells *in vivo*. *Cell Tissue Res.* 282, 455–461.

Clark, M. A., Hirst, B. H., and Jepson, M. A. (1998a). Inoculum composition and *Salmonella* pathogenicity island 1 regulate M-cell invasion and epithelial destruction by *Salmonella typhimurium*. *Infect. Immun.* 66, 724–731.

Clark, M. A., Hirst, B. H., and Jepson, M. A. (1998b). M-cell surface β1 integrin expression and invasin-mediated targeting of *Yersinia pseudotuberculosis* to mouse Peyer's patch M cell. *Infect. Immun.* 66, 1237–1243.

Desai, M. P., Labhasetwar, V., Amidon, G. L., and Levy, R. J. (1996). Gastrointestinal uptake of biodegradable microparticles: effect of particle size. *Pharm. Res.* 13, 1838–1845.

Dobbins, W. O., III (1986). Human intestinal intraepithelial lymphocytes. *Gut* 27, 972–985.

Dobbins, W. O., III (1990). Biopsy interpretation-electron microscopy. In *Diagnostic Pathology of the Intestinal Mucosa: An Atlas and Review of Biopsy Interpretation*, 23–94. New York, Springer Verlag.

Eckmann, L., Jung, H. C., Schurer-Maly, C., Panjam, A., Morzycka-Wroblewska, E., and Kagnoff, M. F. (1993). Differential cytokine expression by human intestinal epithelial cell lines: Regulated expression of interleukin 8. *Gastroenterology* 105, 1689–1697.

Engle, M. J., Goetz, G. S., and Alpers, D. H. (1998). Caco-2 cells express a combination of colonocyte and enterocyte phenotypes. *J. Cell. Physiol.* 174, 362–369.

Ermak, T. H., and Owen, R. L. (1987). Phenotype and distribution of T lymphocytes in Peyer's patches of athymic mice. *Histochemistry* 87, 321–325.

Ermak, T. H., Steger, H. J., Strober, S., and Owen, R. L. (1989). M cells and granular mononuclear cells in Peyer's patch domes of mice depleted of their lymphocytes by total lymphoid irradiation. *Am. J. Pathol.* 134, 529–537.

Ermak, T. H., Bhagat, H. R., and Pappo, J. (1994). Lymphocyte compartments in antigen-sampling regions of rabbit mucosal lymphoid organs. *Am. J. Trop. Med. Hyg.* 50 Suppl., 14–28.

Farstad, I. N., Halstensen, T. S., Fausa, O., and Brandtzaeg, P. (1994). Heterogeneity of M-cell-associated B and T cells in human Peyer's patches. *Immunology.* 83, 457–464.

Florence, A. T. (1997). The oral absorption of micro- and nanoparticulates: Neither exceptional nor unusual. *Pharmaceut. Res.* 14, 259–266.

Freier, S., Eran, M., and Faber, J. (1987). Effect of cholecystokinin and of its antagonist, of atropine, and of food on the release of Immunoglobulin A and Immunoglobulin G specific antibodies in the rat intestine. *Gastroenterology* 93, 1242–1246.

Frey, A., Giannasca, K. T., Weltzin, R., Giannasca, P. J., Reggio, H., Lencer, W. I., and Neutra, M. R. (1996). Role of the glycocalyx in regulating access of microparticles to apical plasma membranes of intestinal epithelial cells: Implications for microbial attachment and oral vaccine targeting. *J. Exp. Med.* 184, 1045–1059.

Fujimura, Y. (1986). Functional morphology of microfold cells (M cells) in Peyer's patches: Phagocytosis and transport of *BCG* by M cells into rabbit Peyer's patches. *Gastroenterol. Jpn.* 21, 325–335.

Fujimura, Y., and Owen, R. L. (1996). M cells as portals of infection: Clinical and pathophysiological aspects. *Infect. Agents Dis.* 5, 144–156.

Fujimura, Y., Ohtani, K., Kamoi, R., Kato, T., Kozuka, K., Miyashima, N., Uchida, J., Kihara, T., and Mine, H. (1989). An ultrastructural study of ileal invasion process of *Yersinia pseudotuberculosis* in rabbits. *J. Clin. Electron Microscopy* 22, 712–713.

Gaidar, Y. A. (1989). Vimentin-positive epithelial cells in the cupolas of the aggregated lymphoid noduli (Peyer's patches) of the rabbit. *Arkh. Anat. Gistol. Embr.* 97, 84–88.

Galan, J. E. (1999). Interaction of *Salmonella* with host cells through the centisome 63 type III secretion system. *Curr. Opin. Microbiol.* 2, 46–50.

Gebert, A., and Hach, G. (1993). Differential binding of lectins to M-cells and enterocytes in the rabbit cecum. *Gastroenterology* 105, 1350–1361.

Gebert, A., Rothkotter, H. J., and Pabst, R. (1994). Cytokeratin 18 is an M-cell marker in porcine Peyer's patches. *Cell Tissue Res.* 276, 213–221.

Gebert, A., Rothkotter, H. J., and Pabst, R. (1996). M cells in Peyer's patches of the intestine. *International Rev. Cytol.* 167, 91–159.

Gebert, A., Fassbender, S., Werner, K., and Weissferdt, A. (1999). The development of M cells in Peyer's patches is restricted to specialized dome-associated crypts. *Am. J. Pathol.* 154, 1573–1582.

Giannasca, P. J., Giannasca, K. T., Leichtner, A. M., and Neutra, M. R. (1999). Human intestinal M cells display the sialyl Lewis A antigen. *Infect. Immun.* 67, 946–953.

Grützkau, A., Hanski, C., Hahn, H., and Riecken, E. O. (1990). Involvement of M cells in the bacterial invasion of Peyer's patches: A common mechanism shared by *Yersinia enterocolitica* and other enteroinvasive bacteria. *Gut* 31, 1011–1015.

Guy-Grand, D., Cerf-Bensussan, N., Malissen, B., Malassis-Seris, M., Briottet, C., and Vassalli, P. (1991). Two gut intraepithelial CD8+ lymphocyte populations with different T cell receptors: A role for the gut epithelium in T cell differentiation. *J. Exp. Med.* 173, 471–481.

Hall, J. (1979). Lymphocyte recirculation and the gut: The cellular basis of humoral immunity in the intestine. *Blood Cells* 5, 479–492.

Hamann, A., Jablonski-Westrich, D., Jonas, P., and Thiele, H.-G. (1991). Homing receptors reexamined: Mouse LECAM-1 (MEL-14 antigen) is involved in lymphocyte migration into gut-associated lymphoid tissue. *Eur. J. Immunol.* 21, 2925–2929.

Hamzaoui, N., and Pringault, E. (1998). Interaction of microorganisms, epithelium, and lymphoid cells of the mucosa-associated lymphoid tissue. *Ann. N.Y. Acad. Sci.* 859, 65–74.

Hay, E. D. (1981). Extracellular matrix. *J. Cell Biol.* 91, 205s–223s.

Heel, K. A., McCauley, R. D., Papadimitriou, J. M., and Hall, J. C. (1997). Review: Peyer's patches. *J. Gastroenterol. Hepatol.* 12, 122–136.

Hirata, I., Austin, L. L., Blackwell, W. H., Weber, J. R., and Dobbins, W. O., III (1986). Immunoelectron microscopic localization of HLA-DR antigen in control small intestine and colon and in inflammatory bowel disease. *Dig. Dis. Sci.* 31, 1317–1330.

Hirayama, K., Matsushita, S., Kikuchi, I., Iuchi, M., Ohta, N., and Sasazuki, T. (1987). HLA-DQ is epistatic to HLA-DR in controlling the immune response to schistosomal antigen in humans. *Nature* 327, 426–430.

Iglewski, W. J., and Gerhardt, N. B. (1978). Identification of an antibiotic-producing bacterium from the human intestinal tract and characterization of its antimicrobial product. *Antimicrob. Agents Chemother.* 13, 81–89.

Inman, L. R., and Cantey, J. R. (1984). Peyer's patch lymphoid follicle epithelial adherence of a rabbit enteropathogenic *Escherichia coli* (strain RDEC-I)-Role of plasmid-mediated pili in initial adherence. *J. Clin. Invest.* 74, 90–95.

Iwasaki, A., and Kelsall, B. L. (2000). Localization of distinct Peyer's patch dendritic cell subsets and their recruitment by chemokines, macrophage inflammatory protein (MIP)-3α, MIP-3β, and secondary lymphoid organ chemokine. *J. Exp. Med.* 191, 1381–1394.

Iwasaki, A., and Kelsall, B. L. (2001). Unique functions of CD11b+, CD8α+, and double-negative Peyer's patch dendritic cells. *J. Immunol.* 166, 4884–4890.

Jarry, A., Robaszkiewicz, M., Brousse, N., and Potet, F. (1989). Immune cells associated with M cells in the follicle-associated epithelium of Peyer's patches in the rat. *Cell Tissue Res.* 255, 293–298.

Jarry, A., Cerf-Bensussan, N., Brousse, N., Selz, F., and Guy-Grand, D. (1990). Subsets of CD3+ (T cell receptor αβ or γδ) and CD3+ lymphocytes isolated from normal human gut epithelium display phenotypical features different from their counterparts in peripheral blood. *Eur. J. Immunol.* 20, 1097–1103.

Jensen, V. B., Harty, J. T., and Jones, B. D. (1998). Interactions of the invasive pathogens *Salmonella typhimurium, Listeria monocytogenes,* and *Shigella flexneri* with M cells and murine Peyer's patches. *Infect. Immun.* 66, 3758–3766.

Jepson, M. A., Mason, C. M., Bennett, M. K., Simmons, N. L., and Hirst, B. H. (1992). Co-expression of vimentin and cytokeratins in M cells of rabbit intestinal lymphoid follicle-associated epithelium. *Histochem. J.* 24, 33–39.

Jepson, M. A., Simmons, N. L., Hirst, G. L., and Hirst, B. H. (1993). Identification of M cells and their distribution in rabbit intestinal Peyer's patches and appendix. *Cell Tissue Res.* 273, 127–136.

Jonas, A., Krishnan, C., and Forstner, G. (1978). Pathogenesis of mucosal injury in the blind loop syndrome: Release of disaccharidases from brush border membranes by extracts of bacteria obtained from intestinal blind loops in rats. *Gastroenterology* 75, 791–795.

Jones, B. D., Ghori, N., and Falkow, S. (1994). *Salmonella typhimurium* initiates murine infection by penetrating and destroying the specialized epithelial M cells of the Peyer's patches. *J. Exp. Med.* 180, 15–23.

Kabok, Z., Ermak, T. H., and Pappo, J. (1995). Microdissected domes from gut-associated lymphoid tissues: A model for M cell transepithelial transport *in vitro. Adv. Exp. Med. Biol.* 371A, 235–238.

Kamoi, R. (1991). Morphological studies of *Salmonella enteriditis* uptake by microfold cells (M cells) of the Peyer's patch. *Kawasaki Igakkaishi* 17, 225–235. (in Japanese).

Kanamori, Y., Ishimaru, K., Nanno M., Maki K., Ikuta, K., Nariuchi H., and Ishikawa, H. (1996). Identification of novel lymphoid tissues in murine intestinal mucosa where clusters of c-kit+ IL-7R+ Thy1+ lympho-hemopoietic progenitors develop. *J. Exp. Med.* 184, 1449–1459.

Kataoka, K., Tabata, J., Yamamoto, M., and Toyota, T. (1989). The association of gap junctions with large particles in the crypt epithelium of the rat small intestine. *Arch. Histol. Cytol.* 52, 81–86.

Kato, T. (1990). A study of secretory immunoglobulin A on membranous epithelial cells (M cells) and adjacent absorptive cells of rabbit Peyer's patches. *Gastroenterol. Jpn.* 75, 15–23.

Kerneis, S., Bogdanova, A., Kraehenbuhl, J. P., and Pringault, E. (1997). Conversion by Peyer's patch lymphocytes of human enterocytes into M cells that transport bacteria. *Science* 277, 949–952.

Keshav, S., Lawson, L., Chung, L. P., Stein, M., Perry, V. H., and Gordon, S. (1990). Tumor necrosis factor mRNA localized to

Paneth cells of normal murine intestinal epithelium by *in situ* hybridization. *J. Exp. Med.* 171, 327–332.

Kim, H. S., and Blumberg, R. S. (1998). A nonclassical major histocompatibility complex molecule: CD1d expression by epithelial cells. In *Bioregulation and Its Disorders in the Gastrointestinal Tract* (ed. T. Yoshikawa and T. Arakawa), 291–301. Tokyo: Blackwell Science.

Kohbata, S., Yokoyama, H., and Yabuuchi, E. (1986). Cytopathogenic effect of *Salmonella typhi* GIFU 10007 on M cells of murine ileal Peyer's patches in ligated ileal loops. An ultrastructural study. *Microbial. Immunol.* 30, 1225–1237.

Kuper, C. F., Koornstra, P. J., Hameleers, D. M., Biewenga, J., Spit, B. J., Duijvestijn, A. M., van Breda Vriesman, P. J., and Sminia, T. (1992). The role of nasopharyngeal lymphoid tissue. *Immunol. Today.* 13, 219–224.

Lelouard, H., Reggio, H., Mangeat, P., Neutra, M., and Montcourrier, P. (1999). Mucin related epitopes distinguish M cells and enterocytes in rabbit appendix and Peyer's patches. *Infect. Immun.* 67, 357–367.

Lelouard, H., Sahuquet, A., Reggio, H., and Montcourrier, P. (2001). Rabbit M cells and dome enterocytes are distinct cell lineages. *J. Cell Sci.* 114, 2077–2083.

Levine, G. M. (1991). Regulation of intestinal mucosal growth. In *Growth of the Gastrointestinal Tract: Gastrointestinal Hormones and Growth Factors* (eds. J. Morisset and T. E. Solomon), 175–189. Boca Raton, Florida: CRC Press.

Löffert, D., Schaal, S., Ehlich, A., Hardy, R. R., Zou, Y. R., Müller, W., and Rajewsky, K. (1994). Early B-cell development in the mouse: Insights from mutations introduced by gene targeting. *Immunol. Rev.* 137, 135–153.

London, S. D., Cebra, J. J., and Rubin, D. H. (1989). Intraepithelial lymphocytes contain virus-specific, MHC-restricted cytotoxic cell precursors after gut mucosal immunization with Reovirus serotype 1/Lang. *Reg. Immunol.* 2, 98–102.

Madara, J. L. (1982). Cup cells: Structure and distribution of a unique class of epithelial cells in guinea pig, rabbit, and monkey small intestine. *Gastroenterology* 83, 981–994.

Madara, J. L., and Pappenheimer, J. R. (1987). Structural basis for physiological regulation of paracellular pathways in intestinal epithelia. *J. Membr. Biol.* 100, 149–164.

Madara, J. L., and Stafford, J. (1989). Interferon-γ directly affects barrier function of cultured intestinal epithelial monolayers. *J. Clin. Invest.* 83, 724–727.

Madara, J. L., and Trier, J. S. (1987). Functional morphology of the mucosa of the small intestine. In *Physiology of the Gastrointestinal Tract* (ed. L. R. Johnson), 1209–1249. Raven Press, New York.

Magnusson, K.-E., and Stjernström, 1. (1982). Mucosal barrier mechanisms. Interplay between secretory IgA (S-IgA), IgG and mucins on the surface properties and association of *Salmonellae* with intestine and granulocytes. *Immunology* 45, 239–248.

Mantle, M., Basaraba, L., Peacock, S. C., and Gall, D. G. (1989). Binding of *Yersinia enterocolitica* to rabbit intestinal brush border membranes, mucus, and mucin. *Infect. Immun.* 57, 3292–3299.

Marcial, M. A., and Madara, J. L. (1986). *Cryptosporidium*: Cellular localization, structural analysis of absorptive cell-parasite membrane–membrane interactions in guinea pigs, and suggestion of protozoan transport by M cells. *Gastroenterology* 90, 583–594.

Marcial, M. A., Carlson, S. L., and Madara, J. L. (1984). Partitioning of paracellular conductance along the ileal crypt-villus axis: A hypothesis based on structural analysis with detailed consideration of tight junction structure–function relationship. *J. Membrane Biol.* 80, 59–70.

Mayer, L., Eisenhardt, D., Salomon, P., Bauer, W., Plous, R., and Piccinini, L. (1991). Expression of class II molecules on intestinal epithelial cells in humans: Differences between normal and inflammatory bowel disease. *Gastroenterology* 100, 3–12.

Meynell, H. M., Thomas, N. W., James, P. S., Holland, J., Taussig, M. J., and Nicoletti, C. (1999). Up-regulation of microsphere transport across the follicle-associated epithelium of Peyer's patch by exposure to *Streptococcus pneumoniae* R36a. *FASEB J.* 13, 611–619.

Michetti, P., Mahan, M. J., Slauch, J. M., Mekalanos, J. J., and Neutra, M. R. (1992). Monoclonal secretary immunoglobulin A protects

mice against oral challenge with the invasive pathogen *Salmonella typhimurium*. *Infect. Immun.* 60, 1786–1792.

Miller, H. R. P. (1987). Gastrointestinal mucus: A medium for survival and for elimination of parasitic nematodes and protozoa. *Parasitology* 94, S77–S100.

Momotani, E., Whipple, D. L., Thiermann, A. B., and Cheville, N. F. (1988). Role of M cells and macrophages in the entrance of *Mycobacterium paratuberculosis* into domes of ileal Peyer's patches in calves. *Vet. Pathol.* 25, 131–137.

Mowat, A. McI., and Viney, J. L. (1997). The anatomical basis of intestinal immunity. *Immunol. Rev.* 156, 145–166.

Moxey, P. C., and Trier, J. S. (1978). Specialized cell types in the human fetal small intestine. *Anat. Rec.* 191, 269–286.

Nabeyama, A., and Leblond, C. P. (1974). "Caveolated cells" characterized by deep surface invaginations and abundant filaments in mouse gastrointestinal epithelia. *Am. J. Anat.* 140, 147–166.

Nagasaki, S., Kamoi, R., Kato, T., Kozuka, K., Miyashima, N., Fujimura, Y., Uchida, J., and Kihara, T. (1988). M cell transport of *Streptococcus pyogenes*, Su strain, ATCC 2106 and OK-432 from the intestinal lumen into rabbit Peyer's patches. *J. Clin. Electron Microsc.* 21, 588–589.

Nagura, H., Ohtani, H., Masuda, T., Kimura, M., and Nakamura, S. (1991). HLA-DR expression on M cells overlying Peyer's patches is a common feature of human small intestine. *Acta Pathol. Jpn.* 41, 818–823.

Neutra, M. R., and Kraehenbuhl, J.-P. (1992). Transepithelial transport and mucosal defense I: the role of M cells. *Trends Cell Biol.* 2, 134–138.

Neutra, M. R., Phillips, T. L., Mayer, E. L., and Fishkind, D. J. (1987). Transport of membrane-bound macromolecules by M cells in follicle-associated epithelium of rabbit Peyer's patch. *Cell Tissue Res.* 247, 537–546.

Ohtsuka, A., Piazza, A. J., Ermak, T. H., and Owen, R. L. (1992). Correlation of extracellular matrix components with the cytoarchitecture of mouse Peyer's patches. *Cell Tissue Res.* 269, 403–410.

Oida, T., Suzuki, K., Nanno, M., Kanamori, Y., Saito, H., Kubota, E., Kato, S., Itoh, M., Kaminogawa, S., and Ishikawa, H. (2000). Role of gut cryptopatches in early extrathymic maturation of intestinal intraepithelial T cells. *J. Immunol.* 164, 3616–3626.

Ouellette, A. J., Greco, R. M., James, M., Frederick, D., Naftilan, J., and Fallon, J. T. (1989). Developmental regulation of cryptdin, a corticostatin/defensin precursor mRNA in mouse small intestinal crypt epithelium. *J. Cell Biol.* 108, 1687–1695.

Owen, R. L. (1977). Sequential uptake of horseradish peroxidase by lymphoid follicle epithelium of Peyer's patches in the normal unobstructed mouse intestine: An ultrastructural study. *Gastroenterology* 72, 440–451.

Owen, R. L., and Bhalla, D. K. (1983). Cytochemical analysis of alkaline phosphatase and esterase activities and of lectin-binding and anionic sites in rat and mouse Peyer's patch M cells. *Am. J. Anat.* 168, 199–212.

Owen, R. L., and Jones, A. L. (1974). Epithelial cell specialization within human Peyer's patches: An ultrastructural study of intestinal lymphoid follicles. *Gastroenterology* 66, 189–203.

Owen, R. L., and Nemanic, P. (1978). Antigen processing structures of the mammalian intestinal tract: An SEM study of lymphoepithelial organs. *Scanning Electron Microsc.* 2, 367–378.

Owen, R. L., Allen, C. L., and Stevens, D. P. (1981). Phagocytosis of *Giardia muris* by macrophages in Peyer's patch epithelium in mice. *Infect. Immun.* 33, 591–601.

Owen, R. L., Apple, R. T., and Bhalla, D. K. (1986a). Morphometric and cytochemical analysis of lysosomes in rat Peyer's patch follicle epithelium: Their reduction in volume fraction and acid phosphatase content in M cells compared to adjacent enterocytes. *Anat. Rec.* 216, 521–527.

Owen, R. L., Pierce, N. F., Apple, R. T., and Cray, W. C., Jr. (1986b). M cell transport of *Vibrio cholerae* from the intestinal lumen into Peyer's patches: A mechanism for antigen sampling and for microbial transepithelial migration. *J. Infect. Dis.* 153, 1108–1118.

Owen, R. L., Cray, W. C., Jr., Ermak, T. H., and Pierce, N. F. (1988a). Bacterial characteristics and follicle surface structure: Their roles in Peyer's patch uptake and transport of *Vibrio cholerae. Adv. Exp. Med. Biol.* 237, 705–715.

Owen, R. L., Pierce, N. F., and Cray, W. C., Jr. (1988b). Effects of bacterial inactivation methods, toxin production, and oral immunization on uptake of *Vibrio cholerae* by Peyer's patch lymphoid follicles. In *Advances in Research on Cholera and Related Diarrheas* (eds. S. Kuwahara and N. F. Pierce), 189–197. Tokyo: KTK Scientific Publishers.

Owen, R. L., Piazza, A. J., and Ermak, T. H. (1991). Ultrastructural and cytoarchitectural features of lymphoreticular organs in the colon and rectum of adult BALB/c mice. *Am. J. Anat.* 190, 10–18.

Pachynski, R. K., Wu, S. W., Gunn, M. D., and Erle, D. J. (1998). Secondary lymphoid-tissue chemokine (SLC) stimulates integrin $\alpha_4\beta_7$-mediated adhesion of lymphocytes to mucosal addressin cell adhesion molecule-1 (MAdCAM-1) under flow. *J. Immunol.* 161, 952–956.

Pakandl, M., Gaca, K., Drouet-Viard, F., and Coudert, P. (1996). *Eimeria coecicola Cheissin* 1947: Endogenous development in gut-associated lymphoid tissue. *Parasitol. Res.* 82, 347–351.

Pappo, J., and Ermak, T. H. (1989). Uptake and translocation of fluorescent latex particles by rabbit Peyer's patch follicle epithelium: A quantitative model for M cell uptake. *Clin. Exp. Immunol.* 76, 144–148.

Pappo, J., and Owen, R. L. (1988). Absence of secretary component expression by epithelial cells overlying rabbit gut-associated lymphoid tissue. *Gastroenterology* 95, 1173–1177.

Penheiter, K. L., Mathur, N., Giles, D., Fahlen, T., and Jones, B. D. (1997). Non-invasive *Salmonella typhimurium* mutants are avirulent because of an inability to enter and destroy M cells of ileal Peyer's patches. *Molec. Microbiol.* 24, 697–709.

Plesch, B. E. (1982). Histology and immunohistochemistry of bronchus associated lymphoid tissue (BALT) in the rat. *Adv. Exp. Med. Biol.* 149, 491–497.

Qin, O. Y., el-Youssef, M., Yen-Lieberman, B., Sapatnekar, W., Youngman, K. R., Kusugami, K., and Fiocchi, C. (1988). Expression of HLA-DR antigens in inflammatory bowel disease mucosa: Role of intestinal lamina propria mononuclear cell-derived interferon gamma. *Dig. Dis. Sci.* 33, 1528–1536.

Rautenberg, K., Cichon, C., Heyer, G., Demel, M., and Schmidt, M. (1996) Immunocytochemical characterization of the follicle-associated epithelium of Peyer's patches: Anti-cytokeratin 8 antibody (clone 4.1.18) as a molecular marker for rat M cells. *European J. Cell Biol.* 71, 363–370.

Regoli, M., Borghesi, C., Bertelli, E., and Nicoletti, C. (1994). A morphological study of the lymphocyte traffic in Peyer's patches after an *in vivo* antigenic stimulation. *Anat. Rec.* 239, 47–54.

Regoli, M., Bertelli, E., Borghesi, C., and Nicoletti, C. (1995a). Three-dimensional (3D) reconstruction of M cells in rabbit Peyer's patches: Definition of the intraepithelial compartment of the follicle-associated epithelium. *Anat. Rec.* 243, 19–26.

Regoli, M., Borghesi, C., Bertelli, E., and Nicoletti, C. (1995b). Uptake of a gram-positive bacterium (*Streptococcus pneumoniae* R36a) by the M cells of rabbit Peyer's patches. *Anatomischer Anzeiger* 177, 119–124.

Rhodes, J. M. (1989). Colonic mucus and mucosal glycoproteins: The key to colitis and cancer? *Gut* 30, 1660–1666.

Rhodes, J. M. (1990). Mucus and inflammatory bowel disease. In *Inflammatory Bowel Diseases*, ed. 2 (eds. R. N. Allan, M. R. B. Keighley, J. Alexander-Williams, and C. F. Hawkins), 171–179. London: Churchill Livingstone.

Rodning, C. B., Wilson, I. D., and Erlandsen, S. L. (1976). Immunoglobulins within human small-intestinal Paneth cells. *Lancet* 1, 984–987.

Roy, M. J., and Varvayanis, M. (1987). Development of dome epithelium in gut-associated lymphoid tissues: association of IgA with M cells. *Cell Tissue Res.* 248, 645–651.

Rubinstein, E., Mark, Z., Haspel, J., Ben-Ari, G., Dreznik, Z., Mirelman, D., and Tadmor, A. (1985). Antibacterial activity of pancreatic fluid. *Gastroenterology* 88, 927–932.

Ruedl, C., Rieser, C., Böck, G., Wick, G., and Wolf, H. (1996). Phenotypic and functional characterization of CD11c+ dendritic cell population in mouse Peyer's patches. *Eur. J. Immunol.* 26, 1801–1806.

Saito, H., Kanamori, Y., Takemori, T., Nariuchi, H., Kubota, E., Takahashi-Iwanaga H., Iwanaga, T., and Ishikawa, H. (1998). Generation of intestinal T cells from progenitors residing in gut cryptopatches. *Science.* 280, 275–278.

Sajjan, S. U., and Forstner, J. F. (1990). Role of the putative "link" glycopeptide of intestinal mucin in binding of piliated *Escherichia coli* serotype O:157 H:7 strain CL-49. *Infect. Immun.* 58, 868–873.

Santos, L. M. B., Lider, O., Audette, J., Khoury, S. J., and Weiner, H. L. (1990). Characterization of immunomodulatory properties and accessory cell function of small intestine epithelial cells. *Cell. Immunol.* 127, 26–34.

Savage, D. C. (1970). Association of indigenous microorganisms with gastrointestinal mucosal epithelia. *Am. J. Clin. Nutr.* 23, 1495–1501.

Savidge, T. C. (1996). The life and times of an intestinal M cell. *Trends Microbiol.* 4, 301–306.

Savidge, T. C., Smith, M. W., Mayel-Afshar, S., Collins, A. J., and Freeman, T. C. (1994). Selective regulation of epithelial gene expression in rabbit Peyer's patch tissue. *Arch. Eur. J. Physiol.* 428, 391–399.

Schmedtje, J. F. (1965). Some histochemical characteristics of lymphoepithelial cells of the rabbit appendix. *Anat. Rec.* 151, 412–413 (Abstract).

Schmedtje, J. F. (1966). Fine structure of intercellular lymphocyte clusters in the rabbit appendix epithelium. *Anat. Rec.* 154, 417 (Abstract).

Schmidt, G. H., Wilkinson, M. M., and Ponder, B. A. J. (1985). Cell migration pathway in the intestinal epithelium: An *in situ* marker system using mouse aggregation chimeras. *Cell* 40, 425–429.

Shakhlamov, V. A., Gaidar, Y. A., and Baranov, V. N. (1981). Electron-cytochemical investigation of cholera toxin absorption by epithelium of Peyer's patches in guinea pigs. *Bull. Exp. Biol. Med.* 90, 1159–1161.

Sharma, R., van Damme, E. J., Peumans, W. J., Sarsfield, P., and Schumacher, U. (1996). Lectin binding reveals divergent carbohydrate expression in human and mouse Peyer's patches. *Histochem. Cell Biol.* 105, 459–465.

Sicinski, P., Rowinski, J., Warchol, J. B., and Bem, W. (1986). Morphometric evidence against lymphocyte-induced differentiation of M cells from absorptive cells in mouse Peyer's patches. *Gastroenterology* 90, 609–616.

Sicinski, P., Rowinski, J., Warchol, J. B., Jarzabek, Z., Gut, W., Szczygiel, B., Bielecki, K., and Koch, G. (1990). Poliovirus type I enters the human host through intestinal M cells. *Gastroenterology* 98, 56–58.

Siebers, A. and Finlay, B. B. (1996). M cells and the pathogenesis of mucosal and systemic infections. *Trends Microbiol.* 4, 22–29.

Sierro, F., Pringault, E., Assman, P. S., Kraehenbuhl, J. P., and Debard, N. (2000). Transient expression of M-cell phenotype by enterocyte-like cells of the follicle-associated epithelium of mouse Peyer's patches. *Gastroenterology* 119, 734–743.

Sigurdardottir, O. G., Press, C. M., and Evensen, Ø. (2001). Uptake of *Mycobacterium avium* subsp. *Paratuberculosis* through the distal small intestinal mucosa in goats: An ultrastructural study. *Vet. Pathol.* 38, 184–189.

Silvey, K. J., Hutchings, A. B., Vajdy, M., Petzke, M. M., and Neutra, M. R. (2001). Role of immunoglobulin A in protection against reovirus entry into murine Peyer's patches. *J. Virol.* 75, 10870–10879.

Smith, M. W., and Peacock, M. A. (1980). "M" cell distribution in follicle-associated epithelium of mouse Peyer's patch. *Am. J. Anat.* 159, 167–175.

Smith, M. W., James, P. S., and Tivey, D. R. (1987). M cell numbers increase after transfer of SPF mice to a normal animal house environment. *Am. J. Pathol.* 128, 385–389.

Smith, M. W., Thomas, N. W., Jenkins, P. G., Miller, N. G., Cremaschi, D., and Porta, C. (1995). Selective transport of microparticles across Peyer's patch follicle-associated M cells from mice and rats. *Exp. Physiol.* 80, 735–743.

Snyder, J. D., and Walker, W. A. (1987). Structure and function of intestinal mucin: Development aspects. *Int. Arch. Allergy Appl. Immunol.* 92, 351–356.

Specian, R. D., and Neutra, M. R. (1994). Cytoskeleton of intestinal goblet cells in rabbit and monkey: The theca. *Gastroenterology* 97, 1313–1325.

Stanisz, A. M., Befus, D., and Bienenstock, J. (1986). Differential effects of vasoactive intestinal peptide, substance P, and somatostatin on immunoglobulin synthesis and proliferations by lymphocytes from Peyer's patches, mesenteric lymph nodes, and spleen. *J. Immunol.* 136, 152–156.

Suzuki, H., Konno, T., Igarashi, Y., and Yamamoto, T. (1977). The occurrence of electron dense intercellular materials and gap junctions in the human intestinal epithelium. *Tohoku J. Exp. Med.* 121, 301–313.

Tagliabue, A., Boraschi, D., Villa, L., Keren, D. F., Lowell, G. H., Rappuoli, R., and Nencioni, L. (1984). IgA-dependent cell-mediated activity against enteropathogenic bacteria: Distribution, specificity, and characterization of the effector cells. *J. Immunol.* 133, 988–992.

Thompson, G. R., and Trexler, P. C. (1971). Gastrointestinal structure and function in germ-free gnotobiotic animals. *Gut* 12, 230–235.

Uchida, J. (1987). An ultrastructural study on active uptake and transport of bacteria by microfold cells (M cells) to the lymphoid follicles in the rabbit appendix. *J. Clin. Electron Microscopy* 20, 379–394.

Uchida, J. (1988). Electron microscopic study of microfold cells (M cells) in normal and inflamed human appendix. *Gastroenterol. Jpn.* 23, 251–262.

Ueki, T., Mizuno, M., Uesu, T., Kiso, T., and Tsuji, T. (1995). Expression of ICAM-1 on M cells covering isolated lymphoid follicles of the human colon. *Acta Med. Okayama* 49, 145–151.

Vazquez-Torres, A., and Fang, F. C. (2000). Cellular routes of invasion by enteropathogens. *Curr. Opin. Microbiol.* 3, 54–59.

von Rosen, L., Podjaski, B., Bettmann, I., and Otto, H. F. (1981). Observations on the ultrastructure and function of the so-called "Microfold" or "Membranous" cells (M cells) by means of peroxidase as a tracer. *Virchow's Arch. Pathol. Anat.* 390, 289–312.

Walker, R. I., Schmauder-Chock, E. A., Parker, J. L., and Burr, D. (1988). Selective association and transport of *Campylobacter jejuni* through M cells of rabbit Peyer's patches. *Can. J. Microbiol.* 34, 1142–1147.

Warnock, R. A., Campbell, J. J., Dorf, M. E., Matsuzawa, A., McEvoy, L. M., and Butcher, E. C. (2000). The role of chemokines in the microenvironmental control of T versus B cell arrest in Peyer's patch high endothelial venules. *J. Exp. Med.* 191, 77–88.

Wassef, J. S., Keren, D. F., and Mailloux, J. L. (1989). Role of M cells in initial antigen uptake and in ulcer formation in the rabbit intestinal loop model of shigellosis. *Infect. Immun.* 57, 858–863.

Weiner, D. B., Girard, K., Williams, W. V., McPhillips, T., and Rubin, D. H. (1988). Reovirus type 1 and type 3 differ in their binding to isolated intestinal epithelial cells. *Microb. Pathogen.* 5, 29–40.

Weltzin, R., Lucia-Jandris, P., Michetti, P., Fields, B. N., Kraehenbuhl, J. P., and Neutra, M. R. (1989). Binding and transepithelial transport of immunoglobulins by intestinal M cells: Demonstration using monoclonal IgA antibodies against enteric viral proteins. *J. Cell Biol.* 108, 1673–1685.

Williams, R. C., Showalter, R., and Kern, F., Jr. (1975). *In vivo* effect of bile salts and cholestyramine on intestinal anaerobic bacteria. *Gastroenterology* 69, 483–491.

Willimann, K., Legler, D. F., Loetscher, M., Roos, R. S., Delgado, M. B., Clark-Lewis, I., Baggiolini, M., and Moser, B. (1998). The chemokine SLC is expressed in T cell areas of lymph nodes and mucosal lymphoid tissues and attracts activated T cells via CCR7. *Eur. J. Immunol.* 28, 2025–2034.

Winner, L., III, Mack, J., Weltzin, R., Mekalanos, J. J., Kraehenbuhl, J.-P., and Neutra, M. R. (1991). New model for analysis of mucosal immunity: Intestinal secretion of specific monoclonal immunoglobulin A from hybridoma tumors protects against *Vibrio cholerae* infection. *Infect. Immun.* 59, 977–982.

Wolf, J. L., Kauffman, R. S., Finberg, R., Dambrauskas, R., Fields, B. N., and Trier, J. S. (1983). Determinants of reovirus interaction with the intestinal M cells and absorptive cells of murine intestine. *Gastroenterology* 85, 291–300.

Zhou, F., Kraehenbuhl, J. P., and Neutra, M. R. (1995). Mucosal IgA response to rectally administered antigen formulated in IgA-coated liposomes. *Vaccine* 13, 637–644.

Mucosal Immunoglobulins

Chapter 9

Jiri Mestecky

Departments of Microbiology and Medicine, University of Alabama at Birmingham, Birmingham, Alabama

Itaru Moro

Department of Pathology, Nihon University School of Dentistry, Tokyo, Japan

Michael A. Kerr

Department of Clinical Biochemistry and Immunology, General Infirmary at Leeds, Leeds, United Kingdom

Jenny M. Woof

Division of Pathology and Neuroscience, University of Dundee Medical School, Dundee, United Kingdom

INTRODUCTION

Although immunoglobulins (Ig) of all isotypes are present in various external secretions, their absolute levels and relative distributions are characteristically different from those of plasma. Furthermore, there are marked variations in both Ig levels and isotypes among various secretions and even in the same secretion collected at different times or using a different method of collection. Realization of these facts is of paramount importance in studies of the normal physiology of the entire mucosal immune system because the results concerning the isotype distribution, molecular forms of Igs, duration of humoral responses, and so forth, generated in one compartment of the mucosal immune system, for example, intestine, may not be valid for other compartments (e.g., the genitourinary tract). These explicit and intrinsic characteristics of individual compartments of the mucosal immune system reflect marked differences in the dominant source of Ig (local production of Ig in mucosal tissues vs. the bone marrow, lymph nodes, and spleen), expression of epithelial receptors responsible for transport of locally produced or plasma-derived Ig, and regulation of the Ig transport by hormones, cytokines, and other environmentally derived substances of cellular receptors that participate in the distribution of Ig into external secretions.

IMMUNOGLOBULINS OF THE EXTERNAL SECRETIONS

The predominance of IgA over Ig of other isotypes in most external secretions is considered as the characteristic hallmark (Tomasi and Bienenstock 1968; Heremans 1974). However, comparative studies of the Ig levels and isotypes in individual external secretions collected from humans, common experimental animals, and livestock reveal that in some secretions the relative level of IgG may be quite high or even exceed that of IgA. Compilation of data generated in many laboratories reflects a high degree of heterogeneity in the absolute as well as relative levels of Ig in various human external secretions, because of differences in the collection procedures and processing of samples and assays used for measurements (**Table 9.1**). It is quite obvious that the levels of IgA and IgG in human external secretions are well below serum levels (with the exception of colostrum) and that IgA is dominant in most secretions.

Secretory IgA (S-IgA)

Human IgA is heterogenous with respect to its molecular form and subclasses. Plasma or serum IgA is primarily represented by monomeric (m) IgA with two heavy (H) and two light (L-κ or L-λ) chains (**Fig. 9.1A**). A small proportion (<1–20%) of serum IgA occurs in polymeric (p) forms, chiefly as dimers (**Fig. 9.1B**), with some trimers and tetramers. In contrast, the typical and dominant form of IgA in external secretions is represented by polymeric molecules composed of two to four mIgA molecules covalently linked through their Fc region and associated with one molecule of the joining (J) chain and one molecule of secretory component (SC) which is the extracellular segment of the epithelial polymeric Ig receptor (pIgR) (**Fig. 9.1C**) (for details see the following text and Chapter 12). There are two IgA subclasses—IgA1 and IgA2—that display a characteristic distribution in serum (~84% IgA1 and ~16% IgA2) and various external secretions (Conley and Delacroix 1987;

Table 9.1. Levels (in μg/ml) of Ig in Selected Human Body Fluids[a]

Fluid	IgA	IgG	IgM
Serum	500–3,500	7,000–12,000	500–1,500
Tears	80–400	trace–16	0–18
Parotid saliva	15–319	0.4–5	0.4
Colostrum and milk	470–12,340	40–168	50–610
Intestinal fluid	166	4	8
Urine	0.1–1.0	0.06–0.6	
Ejaculate	12–23	16–33	0–8
Uterine cervical fluid	3–333	1–285	5–118

[a]Abbreviated from Table 1 of Appendix I of this volume.

Mestecky and Russel 1986). This structural uniqueness of S-IgA, as compared with its serum counterpart, was documented by early comparative studies of physicochemical properties and antigenic determinants. The difference in the sedimentation constant of serum versus S-IgA (7 S vs. 11 S) was consistent with the dimeric form of S-IgA (for reviews, see Heremans 1974; Tomasi and Bienenstock 1968). The antigenic unique-ness of S-IgA was revealed by Hanson (1961) and Tomasi *et al.* (1965), who determined that the presence of additional anti-genic determinants on S-IgA was caused by the additional polypeptide chain—secretory "piece," later renamed SC—which is acquired during the transepithelial transport of pIgA (see Chapter 12). In the early seventies, an additional polypep-tide—J chain—was identified as a component of pIgA, S-IgA,

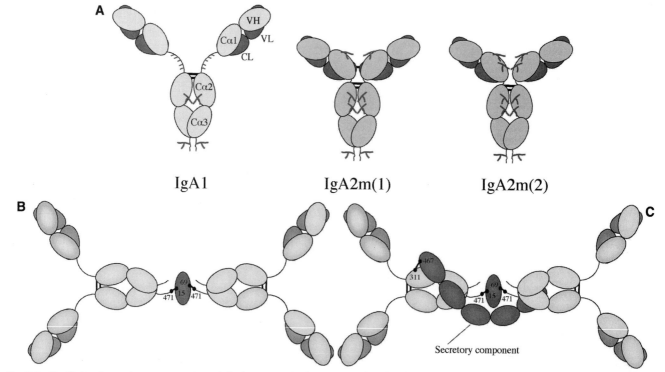

Fig. 9.1. (A–C) A schematic representation of the human IgA of various molecular forms. **(See page 2 of the color plates)** Light chains are shown in dark orange, with the different heavy chains in shades of yellow/gold. Carbohydrates are shown in blue; *N*-linked glycans are branched, and *O*-glycans on the IgA1 hinge are shorter unbranched structures. In IgA2m(1) the usual heavy–light chain disulfide bonds are missing, and instead a disulfide bridge forms between the two light chains. **A,** mIgA. **B,** A schematic representation of human dIgA (J chain in red). For clarity, the distance separating the IgA monomers and J chain has been purposefully increased. Disulfide bridges between α-chain tailpieces and J chain are highlighted with the position of the cysteine residues involved labeled. Cys 471 in the tailpiece of one IgA monomer binds Cys 15 of J chain, while Cys 471 in the tailpiece of the other monomer binds Cys 69 of J chain. The Cys 471 residues of the remaining tailpieces, shown unbound, may interact with other free Cys residues such as Cys 311 (Prahl *et al.*, 1971). **C,** Schematic representation of human S-IgA (SC in blue). J chain–IgA disulfide bridges are highlighted as in **B.** In addition, the disulfide bridge between Cys 311 of a heavy chain of one IgA monomer and Cys 467 in domain V of SC is indicated.

and IgM (Halpern and Koshland 1970; Mestecky *et al.* 1971). The role of J chain in the formation of pIg and the interactions with SC will be described later and also in Chapters 12 and 32.

A variable proportion of IgA in human external secretions is present in the form of mIgA and pIgA devoid of SC. For example, almost one-half of pIgA in the hepatic bile (Kutteh *et al.* 1982b; Delacroix and Vaerman 1983) and 10% of pIgA in colostrum (Mestecky *et al.* 1970) lack SC. The proportion of pIgA forms relative to mIgA also differs in various secretions (Table 1 in Appendix I).

In addition to the monomeric and polymeric forms, IgA in humans, hominoid primates (e.g., gorilla and chimpanzee), and lagomorphs (e.g., rabbits and hares) occurs in the form of subclasses encoded for by two (primates) to thirteen (lagomorphs) constant region genes; other species display only one constant region gene (see Chapters 10 and 11). Subclass-specific structural differences in the constant regions of heavy chains are of importance in their biologic properties, including the differential sensitivities to bacterial proteases (see Chapter 15).

Most S-IgA in humans is derived from local synthesis and not from the circulation (for reviews, see Conley and Delacroix 1987; Mestecky *et al.* 1986, 1991). A relatively high proportion of Ig-producing cells in the mucosal lymphoid tissue is committed to the IgA isotype. This fact, in conjunction with the presence of the specific pIgR expressed on mucosal epithelial cells (see Chapter 12), accounts for the high relative concentration of IgA in mucosal secretions.

S-IgA and S-IgM can also be detected at low levels (about 10 μg/ml) in serum (Iscaki *et al.* 1979; Delacroix and Vaerman 1981; Kvale and Brandtzaeg 1986), and these levels are elevated in patients with liver diseases and in lactating women (Delacroix and Vaerman 1983). The reasons for the elevation of S-IgA in liver disease are not entirely known, but could result from the release of SC from damaged biliary epithelial cells, which would complex with pIgA in blood, or defective clearance of S-IgA and S-IgM, which might enter the blood after retrograde transport from mucosal tissue.

Other immunoglobulins in human external secretions

Although an initial study (Brandtzaeg *et al.* 1968) suggested that the presence of IgM in human external secretions is not dependent on SC-mediated transport, subsequently it was documented that IgM in the external secretions is also associated with SC, as a result of its transport into the secretions by the pIgR (Brandtzaeg 1981, 1985). However, the concentration of S-IgM is substantially lower than that of S-IgA because of the lower proportion of IgM-producing cells in mucosal tissues (Chapter 32). IgM also may not be transported as well as pIgA because of a molecular weight restriction in SC-dependent transport and slower diffusion kinetics in reaching the pIgR (Natvig *et al.* 1997). In some species such as rodents and rabbits, pIgR-dependent transport of IgM may not occur (Underdown *et al.* 1992). On the other hand, a compensatory increase of IgM is observed in mucosal tissues and secretions of IgA-deficient individuals (Plebani *et al.* 1983; Arnold *et al.* 1977; Brandtzaeg *et al.*

1968, 1999; Chapter 64), and IgG may also play a compensatory role (Brandtzaeg *et al.* 1986). However, in cases of IgA-subclass and IgG-subclass deficiencies, the compensatory effects of IgG may not be manifested (Brandtzaeg *et al.* 1986; Chapter 64).

In most species, the concentration of IgG in mucosal secretions is approximately the same as or somewhat greater than that of IgM. The proportion of IgA to IgG in external secretions not only varies from site to site (e.g., saliva vs. genital tract fluids) but also depends on the method and time of collection. This is particularly evident in the case of female genital tract secretions: IgA and IgG levels vary with the menstrual cycle (see Chapter 95), and invasive methods of collection favor increased IgG levels (see Appendix I). Nevertheless, certain human external secretions such as uterine cervical fluid (Kutteh *et al.* 1996), urine (Svanborg Eden *et al.* 1985), vaginal washes, and seminal plasma (unpublished data) contain, relative to IgA, a high proportion of IgG, and this isotype may actually be dominant. IgG is thought to enter the mucosal secretions nonspecifically via paracellular transport, fluid-phase endocytosis, or through receptor-mediated transport (e.g., FcγRn) (Spiekermann *et al.* 2002; Chapter 13).

IgE has been detected in extremely low concentrations in the respiratory and gastrointestinal secretions and is often associated with allergic responses at the mucosae (Brown *et al.* 1975; Mygind *et al.* 1975; Jonard *et al.* 1984). There is little evidence that IgE is transported specifically into mucosal secretions. Increases in permeability of mucosal tissue as a result of allergic reactions may perhaps increase the concentration of IgE in mucosal secretions.

Low concentrations of IgD are found in milk and saliva: this may reflect selective synthesis of IgD in some mucosal tissues but not facilitated transport to the mucosal secretions (Leslie and Teramura 1977).

Species-dependent variability of Ig isotypes in external secretions

There are significant differences in levels and distribution of Ig in external secretions and in serum among various species. Therefore, such marked differences should always be considered in the interpretation of experimental data and their relevance to the mucosal immune system of humans. Specifically, in most species of common experimental animals (e.g., mice, rats, and rabbits), both serum and S-IgA are present predominantly in the form of J chain–containing polymers. In addition to epithelial cells, hepatocytes of these species also express pIgR, which is involved in an extremely effective transport of pIgA from the circulation into the bile and eventually into the gut lumen (see Chapters 11 and 12). Consequently, the main source of S-IgA in the gut lumen of these species is the bile. Furthermore, immunohistochemical studies demonstrated that biliary IgA also may originate from plasma cells locally dispersed in the liver of some species (Nagura *et al.* 1983; Manning *et al.* 1984; Jackson *et al.* 1978; Altorfer *et al.* 1987).

In contrast to humans and hominoid primates, who display two IgA subclasses, other species examined have only one IgA isotype, which is structurally similar to human IgA2 (see the following text). However, lagomorphs, such as rabbits and hares express thirteen IgA subclasses but only one IgG (see Chapter 10).

Further differences have been noted in the dominance of Ig isotypes in the milk from humans and various species of animals (see Chapter 103). Mammary gland epithelial cells of cows, horses, sheep, and goats express in addition to pIgR, a receptor for IgG, the dominant isotype in milk of these species. The functional importance of milk IgG became obvious in studies of colostrum-deprived and milk-deprived animals. In the absence of the transplacental transport of IgG, ingestion of colostrum and milk is absolutely essential for the survival of newborn animals. IgG in colostrum and milk is actively transported from the gut lumen into the circulation during approximately the first 36 hours of life and thus provides life-saving passive immunity to the offspring.

IgA STRUCTURE AND ARRANGEMENT OF COMPONENT CHAINS

In contrast to Ig isotypes that occur exclusively in a monomeric form (IgG, IgD, and IgE) or predominantly polymeric form (IgM), IgA is found in both forms with a characteristic distribution in various body fluids. Depending on the methodology used, 80% to 99% of serum IgA in healthy individuals consists of mIgA. In liver diseases, the proportion of pIgA in serum is increased, and in IgA multiple myelomatosis, pIgA is usually dominant.

By contrast, IgA in almost all external secretions is represented by S-IgA with a dominance of dimers (sedimentation constant 11 S) (Fig. 9.1C) over tetramers (15.5 S). In saliva and milk, the proportion of dimeric and tetrameric S-IgA is approximately 3 : 2 (Brandtzaeg et al. 1970; Zikan et al. 1972; Halpern and Koshland 1973). The proportion of mIgA varies in individual external secretions; in saliva, intestinal washings, tears, and milk mIgA represents 5% to 10% of total IgA; in urine, cervical fluid, and bile, about 20% to 60% is mIgA (Kutteh et al. 1982b, 1993; Delacroix and Vaerman 1983; Svanborg Eden et al. 1985).

Physical properties of IgA

Early investigations into the shape and dimensions of mIgA, dimeric IgA (dIgA), and S-IgA relied on electron microscopy of various IgA preparations. In 1970, Svehag and Bloth examined S-IgA from human and rabbit colostrums, which displayed flexible Y-shaped molecules with two arms of length 65–75 Å, and a third of 50–55 Å. On the basis of these images, a model in which two mIgA were superimposed on each other was proposed. However, the purification process used involved mild reduction in 0.1 M β-mercaptoethanol, which may have been sufficient to break disulfide bonds between monomers (Mestecky et al. 1974a) while leaving inter-H and L-H bonds intact. The images therefore possibly represent mIgA. This interpretation is in keeping with later observations from this group (Bloth and Svehag 1971) and

those of two other groups (Munn et al. 1971; Dourmashkin et al. 1971). Using electron microscopy images, they reported dIgA molecules to have a double Y-shaped appearance. Munn et al. (1971) found that both human myeloma dIgA1 and mouse myeloma dIgA (MOPC 315) had very similar double Y-shaped appearances, with two mIgA molecules interacting via the tips of their Fc regions. The length of the Fab arms was estimated at 70 Å, with the length of the joined Fc regions (Fc–Fc) measuring 125 Å. Dourmashkin et al. (1971) also imaged human myeloma dIgA and the MOPC 315 mouse myeloma proteins and found both to have double Y shapes, with apparent flexibility. For human dIgA, they estimated Fab length to be 70 ± 9 Å, and Fc–Fc length to be 138 ± 26 Å. Bloth and Svehag (1971) found both human colostral and myeloma dIgA contained double Y-shaped structures of dimensions Fab length, 70 Å; Fc–Fc length, 140 Å (dIgA) and 145–155 Å (S-IgA). If it is assumed that the Fc regions are arranged end to end, then the Fc–Fc length should represent around twice the length of a single Fc. These studies therefore would give average approximate values for Fc length of 63 Å (Feinstein et al. 1971), 69 Å (Dourmashkin et al. 1971), and 70 Å (Bloth and Svehag 1971), which fit very well with available estimates of other Fc regions. For example, from x-ray crystal data an IgG1 Fc was reported to be 65 Å long (Guddat et al. 1993). Thus the Fc–Fc length estimates are compatible with an end-to-end arrangement of the Fc regions. Interestingly, hydrodynamic data from sedimentation and viscosity experiments are compatible with this same extended arrangement of the two Fc regions (Björk and Lindh 1974).

Electron microscopy experiments have also been informative regarding the flexibility of IgA molecules. A wide variation in the angle between the Fab arms was noted (Feinstein et al. 1971; Munn et al. 1971) along with some limited degree of flexibility between the two Fc regions (Munn et al. 1971). Although early work had questioned the level of flexibility in IgA (Weltman and Davis 1970), fluorescence polarization and spin-label techniques later revealed that the segmental flexibility in IgA is comparable to that seen in IgG (Zagyansky and Gavrilova 1974; Dudich et al. 1980; Liu et al. 1981).

Recent work has utilized solution structural techniques such as X-ray and neutron scattering to provide information on the structure of human mIgA (Boehm et al. 1999; Furtado et al. 2004). Essentially, the IgA Fab and Fc regions are modeled using the known crystal structures for the corresponding IgG fragments. A molecular dynamics curve fit search method is used to generate several thousand random hinge structures connecting the Fab and Fc regions in any orientation. Scattering curves are calculated for these models and tested against the experimental scattering data collected for human IgA samples allowing the best-fit models to be selected. This process has predicted that human IgA1 and IgA2 adopt average T-shaped structures **(Fig. 9.2)**. Given the apparent flexibility of IgA, the T shape presumably reflects a mean of the many possible conformations in which the Fab arms flex in relation to the Fc. Possibly the most important

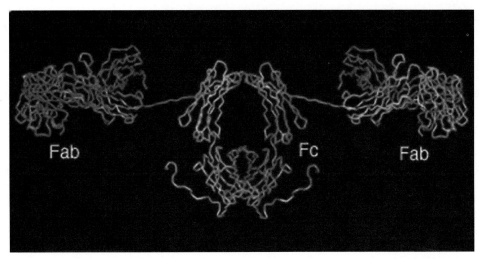

Fig. 9.2. Molecular model of human IgA1 (PDB accession Iiga). The light chains are shown in red, one heavy chain in blue and the other in orange.

Table 9.2. Physicochemical and Biologic Properties of IgA and Component Chains

	IgA1	IgA2	J chain	SC	S-IgA
Molecular mass			15.6 kDa	~76 kDa	
Monomer	~150 kDa	~150 kDa			
Polymer	~320 kDa (dimer)	~320 kDa (dimer)			~390 kDa (dimer)
	~620 kDa (tetramer)	~620 kDa			~690 kDa (tetramer)
Molecular formular					$(\alpha_2 L_2)_{2-4} \cdot J \cdot SC$
Monomer	$\alpha 1_2 L_2$	$\alpha 2_2 L_2$			
Polymer	$(\alpha 1_2 L_2)_{2-4} \cdot J$	$(\alpha 2_2 L_2)_{2-4} \cdot J$			
Sedimentation coefficient			1.28 S	4.7 S	11 S (dimer)
					15.5 S (tetramer)
Monomer	7 S	7 S			
Dimer	~9.5 S	~9.5 S			
Extinction coefficient					
(E 280 nm, 1%, 1 cm)	13.4	13.4	6.53 (275 nm, max)	12.7	13.4
Glycans					
Number of chains	See Fig. 9.4 and Table 9.3		1 *N*-linked	6-7 *N*-linked	
Biologic properties[a]					
Total body pool (mg/kg)	185 ± 49	24.5 ± 7.6			Small amount
Total circulating pool (mg/kg)	101 ± 26	14 ± 4.4			present in plasma
Intravascular (%)	55	57			
Synthetic rate (mg/kg per day)	24 ± 5	4.3 ± 1			
Circulation half-life (days)	6	4.5			

[a]Data valid for systemic IgA but not S-IgA.

revelation from these studies was the predicted extended reach of the Fab arms of human IgA1, compared with those of human IgG1 and IgA2. This may afford IgA advantages in terms of enhanced avidity for antigens spaced at greater distances apart. This may be particularly relevant at the mucosal surface, for example, in the recognition of pathogenic bacteria, many of which have repeated antigenic structures along their surfaces.

Polypeptide chain structure of mIgA, pIgA, and S-IgA

The physicochemical properties of individual chains in IgA of various molecular forms are summarized in **Table 9.2**. Molecules of mIgA contain two α1 or two α2 chains, mutually linked by inter-α chain disulfide bridges, and two κ or two λ chains (Fig. 9.1A). Although in IgA1 α and λ chains are linked by disulfides, in IgA2 molecules inter-α–L chains bonds may be absent, depending on the α2 chain allotype (see the following text). A distinguishing feature of pIgA (Fig. 9.1B), as well as pentameric IgM, is the presence of J chain, a polypeptide incorporated into pIg molecules within antibody-producing cells (Parkhouse and Della Corte 1973; Brandtzaeg 1983, 1985; Koshland 1985; Mestecky and McGhee 1987; Brewer and Corley 1997). Though controversial, the majority of stoichiometric studies indicate that each molecule of pIg, whether dimer, tetramer, or pentamer, contains only one molecule of J chain (Halpern and Koshland 1973; Zikan et al. 1986). However, it appears that different pIgA myeloma proteins display a highly variable content of J chain (Brandtzaeg and Prydz 1984; Vaerman et al. 1998b). Furthermore, J chain is highly susceptible to proteolysis (Koshland et al. 1977); this finding may explain the failure to detect J chain in some pIgA molecules. In native pIgA, some antigenic determinants of J chain are poorly exposed, suggesting that this polypeptide may be at least partially obscured by the Fc region of pIgA. However, in the absence of relevant crystallographic analyses, the precise nature of α-chain and J-chain interactions remains enigmatic. Cleavage of interchain disulfide bonds is usually sufficient to release J chain from pIgA and S-IgA, suggesting that only weak noncovalent interactions exist between J chain and the Fc region of pIgA and S-IgA (Mestecky et al. 1972).

Studies on the structure of dIgA undertaken by chemical and mutational analysis, respectively, indicate that dIgA consists of two mIgA molecules linked end to end with J chain attaching or bonding both mIgA subunits at cysteine (Cys) 471 of one α chain belonging to each monomer subunit (Bastian et al. 1992; Krugmann et al. 1997). The two remaining Cys 471 residues of each α chain may link to each other (Fig. 1B).

The single most important distinguishing feature of S-IgA with respect to serum IgA is the presence of a single molecule of SC per one molecule of S-IgA (Mestecky et al. 1972) (Fig. 9.1C). In addition to its crucial role in the transport of pIgA to mucosal secretions, SC has been shown to increase the stability of S-IgA when compared with mIgA and pIgA molecules and enhance the resistance to proteolysis. Thus the cleavage of disulfide bonds under mildly reducing conditions and in the absence of dissociating agents (e.g., urea, guanidine HCl, acetic acid, etc.) results in a prompt depolymerization of pIgA into the component mIgA units while the same treatment applied to S-IgA has a much less pronounced depolymerizing effect (Mestecky et al. 1974a). Intrinsically high resistance of IgA to common proteolytic enzymes (e.g., pepsin, trypsin, and chymotrypsin) can be further enhanced by SC (Brown et al. 1970; Underdown and Dorrington 1974; Lindh 1975; Crottet and Corthesy 1998). Presumably, this increased resistance to proteolysis confers on S-IgA molecules a significant functional advantage in the gastrointestinal milieu. Nevertheless, tryptic fragments of S-IgA can be generated by cleavage at increased (50° to 60°C) temperatures (Zikan et al. 1972). However, the presence of SC does not appear to influence the sensitivity of S-IgA1 to bacterial IgA1 proteases when compared with pIgA1 (see Chapter 15).

In vitro experiments convincingly demonstrated that SC binds only to pIgA or IgM (Mach 1981; Radl et al. 1971; Weiker and Underdown 1975; Brandtzaeg 1981, 1985). The discovery of J chain in these immunoglobulins led to the postulation that this small polypeptide is instrumental in SC binding (Mach 1970; Appendix to his paper). Brandtzaeg (1985) has maintained that SC binding by pIgA and IgM is dependent on the presence of J chain: pentameric IgM that lacks J chain did not bind SC efficiently, and the ability of pIgA to bind SC in solution or on the surface of SC-bearing epithelial cells was related to the J-chain content (Brandtzaeg 1978, 1983, 1985; Brandtzaeg and Prydz 1984; Vaerman et al. 1998a). However, the means by which the presence of J chain leads to such remarkable enhancement of SC binding is not clear. Previous structural studies of human S-IgA cleaved by cyanogen bromide indicated that J chain and SC are bound to different fragments of the α chain and are not connected by disulfide bridges (Mestecky et al. 1974c). This result suggests that the incorporation of J chain is required to create a conformational change in pIgA and IgM that ultimately generates the SC-binding site.

Results concerning the structure of IgA, SC, and J chain indicate that both SC and J-chain display Ig-domain–like folding of their polypeptide chains (Mostov et al. 1984; Zikan et al. 1985; Pumphrey 1986). Therefore, the mutual interactions between the Fc portion of dIgA, J chain, and SC are likely to be based on the complementarities of their domain-like structures. Although crystallographic analyses of the Fc regions of IgA with J chain and SC have not been generated, chemical and immunochemical studies indicate that the binding of J chain–containing pIgA with SC is initiated by noncovalent interactions between the first domain of SC and Cα3 domain followed by the formation of disulfide bridges with one of the component mIgA molecules (Frutiger et al. 1986; Bakos et al. 1991; Hexham et al. 1999; Underdown et al. 1977; Garcia-Pardo et al. 1979; Fallgren-Gebauer et al. 1995). It appears that both H chains of pIgA (Geneste et al. 1986) and J chain contribute to the binding site for pIgR *in vivo* and SC *in vitro* as evidenced by studies of J chain–knockout mice, J chain–deficient pIgA molecules, and inhibitions of pIgA–pIgR or SC interactions by anti–J-chain reagents

(Johansen *et al.* 2000; Vaerman *et al.* 1998a; Hendrickson *et al.* 1996). Furthermore, details of pIgA–pIgR interactions that occur on the surfaces and during the epithelial cell transcytosis are described in Chapter 12.

α *chains*

Human α1 and α2 chains comprise one variable (V) and three constant (C) region domains, the same as γ chains of IgG and δ chains of IgD (**Table 9.3**, Figs. 9.1 and 9.2). However, IgA as compared with IgG and IgD displays several important structural differences: the presence of a unique hinge region between the Cα2 and Cα3 domains and the extension of the α-chain C terminus by some 18 amino acid residues over the C terminus of γ chains, δ chains, and ε chains (Table 9.3). In this respect, the α chains are analogous to the μ chain (Putnam 1989).

Molecular modelers had based earlier proposals of structures of the Cα domains on the equivalent domains in IgG, which have been generated by X-ray crystallographic techniques (Mattu *et al.* 1998; Boehm *et al.* 1999; Royle *et al.* 2003). Although these predictions served as useful working models, the precise details of domain pairing within the Fc of IgA are now revealed in the crystal structure of the complex of human IgA1 Fc with the extracellular portion of human FcαRI (Herr *et al.* 2003). Overall, Fcα resembles the Fc regions of IgG and IgE but with notable differences in the arrangement of interchain disulphides and the position of *N*-linked glycans. The IgA Fc possesses two-fold symmetry stabilized by extensive interactions between the Cα3 domains, reminiscent of those seen between the equivalent domains in IgG and IgE. The two α chains are anchored to each other at the top of the Cα2 domains by a disulphide bridge between Cys 241 on each chain (Cys 241 is lacking in the truncated Fc present in the crystal, but the bridge is assumed to exist), and two further ones between Cys 299 and Cys 242 on opposite chains. This arrangement gives a compact, planar configuration to the Cα2 pair when viewed from the side. The *N*-linked sugar moieties attached to Asn 263 are externally located, lying on the outer surface of the Cα2 domains with considerable additional contacts with the Cα3 domains. This contrasts markedly with the equivalent glycans in IgG and IgE, which are positioned between the CH2 domains and contact only these domains.

The primary amino acid structures of α chains of human (both subclasses and allotypes), gorilla, chimpanzee, orang-utan, gibbon, macaque, dog, pig, rabbit, mouse, rat, cow, horse, possum, echnida, chicken, and duck IgA have been obtained by amino acid and/or DNA sequence analyses (**Fig. 9.3**) (Abel and Grey 1968; Burnett *et al.* 1989; Kawamura *et al.* 1991, 1992; Patel *et al.* 1995; Brown and Butler 1994; Knight *et al.* 1984; Kratzin *et al.* 1975; Mansikka 1992; Putnam *et al.* 1979; Torano and Putnam 1978; Tsuzukida *et al.* 1979; Tucker *et al.* 1981; Yang *et al.* 1979; Brown *et al.* 1997; Belov *et al.* 2002; Lundquist *et al.* 2001; Wagner *et al.* 2003).

Studies of the V_H genes expressed by the intestinal plasma cells revealed that such genes used by IgA-producing or IgG-producing cells are significantly more highly mutated than those used by IgM (Boursier *et al.* 1999). Furthermore, the tendency to lose or gain potential *N*-glycosylation sites from the higher frequency of somatic hypermutation within the V_H region of IgA produced in mucosal tissues, such as the intestine, may greatly increase the diversity and thus specificity of IgA antibodies (Dunn-Walters *et al.* 2000).

Comparative studies of H chains of all isotypes have indicated a considerable degree of general structural homology between individual domains; however, the number of domains within the C region and the presence and structure of the hinge region are typical of each isotype (Table 9.3). Of all C_H region domains of all five isotypes, the C_H1 domains are most alike in their primary structures. Similarities in primary structures of domains comprising the Fc region of various isotypes display a striking homology when aligned

Table 9.3. Comparative Properties of Human Ig H Chains[a]

Isotype	Amino Acid Residues			Glycans	
	C_H Domains	C Region	Hinge Region	*N*-linked	*O*-linked
γ1	3	330	15	1	0
γ2	3	326	12	1	0
γ3	3	375	62	2	0
γ4	3	326	12	1	0
α1	3	353	26	2–5[b]	3–5
α2	3	340	13	4–12[b]	0
μ	4	451	0	5	0
δ	3	384	64	3	4–5
ε	4	428	0	6	0

[a]Based on Putnam (1989).
[b]Based on analyses of IgA myeloma proteins (Endo *et al.* 1994). The numbers include both complex and high-mannose type *N*-linked chains within the entire (V and C region) α chains.

Cα1 Domain

A

```
              120                    140                    160
               |                      |                      |
HU  1    .ASPTSPKVFPLSLC...STQPDGNVVIACLVQGFFPQEPLSVTWSESGQGVTARNFPPS
HU  2-1  .------------D...--PQ-----V----------------------N--------
HU  2-2  .------------D...--PQ-----V----------------------N--------
CHI 1    ..-----------D...-NPQ-----V-----------------------------T----
CHI 2    ..-----------D...-NPQ-----V----------------N---T-----
GOR 1    .-------------.-------D--V------------------------------
GOR 2    .------------D...-------D--V--------------------N--V-------
ORA      ..---------NF-...-I-------V-----------------------------
GIB 1    ..-----------.---------V--------------------------T----
GIB 2    ..-----------D...---------V-----------------N--------N---T----
CYN      ..---R--------E...G--S-.---V-----------------N----K--A---VI----
BOV      .E-E---SI-----G...NND-A-Q---G---------SA------NQN-DS-SV----..
DOG      .E-K---S--------..HQESE-Y---G---------P--VN---NAGKDSTSVK----M
PIG      .V-E----I---T-G...-SE-A-Y-------RD---S---T----P-RE--IV----..
MOU      .E-ARN-TIY--T-P...PALSSDP-I-G--IHDY--SGTMN---GK--KDI-TV----.
RAT      .E-AKD-TIY--RPP...PSPSSDP-T-G--I-NY--SGTMN---GK--KDISVI----.
RAB 1    .DPA-T-IL-----P.CPLSGQ..P--VG--I-----LG--N-K-TI--EN-...T---V
RAB 2    DLENS--DLI--PCP...ILE-GEPM--G--IR----RG--T---NV--ES-...I---V
RAB 4    .VPA-P-II---TCPGCVLKDTSATI-AG--IR----RG--G---NDNRANL...T---V
RAB 5    .-TAA--RL---IHPRCALKDTSAT-IAG--IR----LG----S-NA--KN-...T---V
RAB 6    DPVN-R-ILI--PSP...ILG-GEP---G--IR----LG------NT--ENL...T---V
RAB 7    .EPAAT-DI---N-PLRV-DGNSQT--VG--IR----PS--R-S-NV-RENMSVY----A
RAB 9    .DPA-T-SL-----P.CPECAH..P--VG--IR----LG--N-S-NG-EG--...I---V
RAB 10   .EAA-NLEL--MTCPR...PR-EQT--VG--IR-.--LD----S-DV--EN-RVY----A
RAB 11   .EPA-T-GIY----PLRV-DGNSQT--VG--IR----LG--R-S-NV-REN-SIY----A
RAB 12   .--A-T-SL---I-P.GPVSGE..T--VG--IR----LG--N-S-NG-EGD-...I---V
RAB 13   ....................NSQY--VG--IR----PG----S-TVN-EN-S-Y----A
ECH      S-TK-T-T-----AYQ.SNSED..P-S-G---T-Y--.--VE---NNQNKDGSTARTF-A
POS      .NPKV--RL----SF...YSETSDSI-LG--AYR---.--VDM--DY--S-G-V--Y-..
HEN      .--ASR-TLYQ-LPLP.SDCPD.P--T-G---TS-L-.P-VT---TTG-AADATAVTSLP
DUC      ..--A-R-TAY--VPV..TDCKDGS--T-G---TD---.--VT---VSG..VTGDQLTF-A
```

Fig. 9.3. Alignment of amino acid sequence of the α-chain constant regions from various species generated using the clustalW program. (See http://www.ebi.ac.uk/clustalw/index.html). In the Cα1, Cα2, and Cα3 domains dashes indicate identity with the prototype sequence (human IgA1), and dots indicate deletions at that position, and for the hinge region, the full sequence is given for each antibody. Numbering is according to the commonly adopted scheme used for IgA1 Bur (Putnam *et al.* 1979a). The isotypes shown are human IgA1 (HU 1), human IgA2 of IgA2m(1) allotype (HU 2-1), human IgA2 of IgA2m(2) allotype (HU 2-2), chimpanzee IgA1 (CHI 1), chimpanzee IgA2 (CHI 2), gorilla IgA1 (GOR 1), gorilla IgA2 (GOR 2), orangutan IgA (ORA), gibbon IgA1 (GIB 1), gibbon IgA2 (GIB 2), cynomolgus monkey (crab-eating macaque, *Macaca fascicularis*) IgA (CYN), bovine IgA (BOV), canine IgA (DOG), porcine IgA (PIG), murine IgA (MOU), Norway rat IgA (RAT), rabbit IgA1 (RAB 1), rabbit IgA2 (RAB 2), rabbit IgA4 (RAB 4), rabbit IgA5 (RAB 5), rabbit IgA6 (RAB 6), rabbit IgA7 (RAB 7), rabbit IgA9 (RAB 9), rabbit IgA10 (RAB 10), rabbit IgA 11 (RAB 11), rabbit IgA12 (RAB 12), rabbit IgA13 (RAB 13), echnida IgA (ECH), possum IgA (POS), chicken IgA (HEN), and duck IgA (DUC). Only the rabbit subclasses known to be expressed are shown (Spieker-Polet *et al.* 1993). Sequences are taken from the translations of nucleic acid sequences using the following accession numbers: J00220 (HU 1), J00221 (HU 2-1 and HU 2-2), X53702 (CHI 1), X53706 (CHI 2), X15045 (GOR 1), X53707 (GOR 2), X53704 (ORA), X53708 (GIB 1), X53709 (GIB 2), X53705 (CYN), AF109167 (BOV), L36871 (DOG), U12594 (PIG), V00785 (MOU), AJ510151 (RAT), X51647 (RAB 1), X82108 (RAB 2), X82110 (RAB 4), X82111 (RAB 5), X82112 (RAB 6), X82113 (RAB 7), X82115 (RAB 9), X82116 (RAB 10), X82117 (RAB 11), X82118 (RAB 12), X82119 (RAB 13), AF416951 (ECH), AF027382 (POS), S40610 (HEN), AJ314754 (DUC). Domain boundaries (Cα1-hinge, Cα2-Cα3) comply with exon–intron boundaries. Where these are not available (PIG, RAT, ECH, POS, HEN), boundaries were estimated by comparison with the most closely homologous IgA sequences. Since the hinge and Cα2 domains are encoded in a single exon, the beginning of the Cα2 was taken as the first Cys residue encoded by this exon in human IgA1. Other sequences were then aligned to give maximum identity. The mouse IgA hinge sequence is that of the BALB/c (Igh-2ᵃ) allotype (Phillips-Quagliata 2002). In chicken and duck IgA, there is no hinge, but an extra domain exists between those domains aligned as Cα1 and Cα2 here. The potential *O*-glycosylation sites in the hinge of human serum IgA1 are residues 225, 228, 230, 232 and 236, although residues 225 and 236 are not always occupied (Mattu *et al.* 1998). **A** and **B,** Cα1 domain; **C,** hinge region; **D** and **E,** Cα2 domain; **F** and **G,** Cα3 domain; **H,** tailpiece.

B

```
                     180                 200                 220
                      |                   |                   |
HU  1    QDASGDLYTTSSQLTLPATQCLAGKSVTCHVKHYTNPSQDVTVPCP..
HU  2-1  -----------------------PD----------------------..
HU  2-2  -----------------------PD--------------S-------R..
CHI 1    ---------------------------------------------R..
CHI 2    --------------------------------T------------R..
GOR 1    -----------------------PD---------N-----------R..
GOR 2    ---------M-------------PDC-------N----S------R..
ORA      --PT-G---------------QD-----------------------R..
GIB 1    -----G---------------E----------E-------------R..
GIB 2    -----G---------------E----------E-------------R..
CYN      -----G--------------A--P-RE------E--------A---V..
BOV      AVLA-S---M--------SL-PK-Q----Q-Q-LSKA-KT-A---IIQ
DOG      KA-T-S---M--------A--PDDS--K-Q-Q-ASS--KA-S---K..
PIG      PAQA-G---M-------VE--P-DQILK-Q-Q-LSKS--S-N---K..
MOU      AL---GR--M-------VE-PE-E--K-S-Q-DS--V-ELD-N-S..
RAT      AP---.P--MC------AE-PK-T--KYY-QYN-S-VRELS-E--GP
RAB 1    -LDTSG------L-N-TDEE-PT..C-A---E-N.EVDRYLIL---..
RAB 2    PSPPSS----Y-L-R---E--PEEN--A-R-E-N.-KG------S-P.
RAB 4    -S-TSS----C-V-S---E--P--N--A-R-E-N.-KR--L----L..
RAB 5    PSGTSGP---C-L-S-TPE--PEDDN-V---E-NYDKG-NL--LY-..
RAB 6    -S-TSS----C-L-R-L-E--PEEN--A---E-NYDKG-H----S-P.
RAB 7    PTGTSGP--AC-E-I--V----EYD-AA---EYNSVINESLP--F-..
RAB 9    PSP-SS------L-S-TDD--PRDGN-----E-NYDEG--L----Q..
RAB 10   -SGTSG-N-AC-L-S--SD--P-DDN-----V-NNE.G--LP---HP.
RAB 11   PTGTSGP--AC-E-I--D----EYD-AA---EYNSVINESLP--F-..
RAB 12   PSPPSS------L-N-TIEE-PK..C-I---E-N.EVHR-LIL---..
RAB 13   -SGTSGP--AC-E-I--V----GQ--AA---EYNSVINESLP--F-..
ECH      VLE-SGY-VL--L-V---D--PES-AYQ-K-N--GS.-RTAN-D-K..
POS      AMLI--A--QA-V-D---D--SNTQAYE-Q-Q--.DT-ANL----K..
HEN      VATT-GT-SLTTA--V-RE-L.Q-NEFV-RAQ-AAT.GA--KETIG..
DUC      VQNG-SY--V-----V--SSY.D-QNFQ-K-T-APT.-TSLSEDIT..
```

Fig. 9.3, Continued

according to the invariant Cys and tryptophan (Trp) residues (Putnam 1989). In particular, the highly homologous position of Cys residues that participate in the formation of intradomain disulfide bridges is critical in maintaining the common structural features of all domains, irrespective of their Ig isotypes.

IgA and IgM display the highest degree of sequence homologies in their Fc regions that comprise Cα2 and Cα3 domains and the tailpiece of IgA and Cμ3 and Cμ4 domains and the tailpiece of IgM (Low et al. 1976). This high degree of primary structure homologies between IgA and IgM appears to reflect their close evolutionary origin (see Chapters 10 and 11). Furthermore, IgA and IgM molecules share important structure–function similarities such as the ability to form polymers, bind J chain through their penultimate Cys residues in a structurally analogous tailpiece (Mestecky et al. 1974b; Mestecky and Schrohenloher 1974),

and interact with epithelial pIgR essential for the selective transepithelial transport of pIg (Brandtzaeg et al. 1981, 1985). Moreover, S-IgM functionally replaces S-IgA in the majority of the IgA-deficient individuals (Plebani et al. 1983; Arnold et al. 1977; Brandtzaeg et al. 1968, 1999).

In humans, hominoid primates (e.g., gorilla and chimpanzee), and in lagomorphs (e.g., rabbits and hares), multiple gene segments encoding C_H region are responsible for the existence of IgA subclasses in these species (see Chapters 10 and 11). However, structural homologies of IgA subclasses within one species are very high. For example, the percentage homology between C domains in human IgA1 and IgA2 are 90% for C_H1, 93% for C_H2, and 98% for C_H3 (Putnam 1989). In other words, with the exception of the hinge region, the primary structures of the α1 and α2 constant regions differ by some 14 out of 340 residues (van Loghem and Biewenga 1983).

Hinge

C

```
                        222                      240
                         |                        |
         HU   1         VPSTPPTPSPSTPPTPSPS
         HU   2-1                      VPPPPP
         HU   2-2                      VPPPPP
         CHI  1         GPSTPCPPTPSTPPTPSPS
         CHI  2                       VPPPPP
         GOR  1         VPSTPPTPSPSTPPTPSPP
         GOR  2                       VPPSPP
         ORA           VPRPTPTPSTPPCPPPS
         GIB  1                     VPLPTPPHP
         GIB  2                      APPPHP
         CYN                        SETKPCL
         BOV                        DSSSCCVPN
         DOG                        DNSHPCHPCPS
         PIG                        VLPSDPCPQ
         MOU                        GPTPPPPITIPS
         RAT                         KPSLV
         RAB  1                     DTHSSCPPTS
         RAB  2        ACNESTIEPPTTPTCPCPCPSPS
         RAB  4        ACNKPTIEPPTKPTCPCPCPSPS
         RAB  5        ECQPPTPSPTTPTTCPCPCPLPS
         RAB  6        ECQPPTPGPSDTTTCPCPCPSPS
         RAB  7                    DPCEQCHCPS
         RAB  9                    DCHCYCPPTS
         RAB  10       ECREPIIDPTPCPTT
         RAB  11                   DPCEQCHCPS
         RAB  12                   DCSIPPIT
         RAB  13       DCCPANSCCTCPSSSSRNLISG
         ECH                       RKNPGVCPDP
         POS                       AVQDPSQ
```

Fig. 9.3, Continued

The major difference between human IgA1 and IgA2 subclasses occurs in the hinge region, which consists of 26 amino acids in IgA1 and 13 in IgA2 molecules (Fig. 9.3 and Table 9.3). The amino acid sequence of the hinge region in IgA1 is reminiscent of that of mucins with multiple serine (Ser), threonine (Thr), and Proline (Pro) residues. Furthermore, three to five O-linked glycan side chains are present **(Fig. 9.4)**. The hinge region of the α1 chain is one of a very limited number of natural substrates for bacterial IgA1 proteases that cleave IgA1 molecules into Fab and Fc fragments with functionally important biologic consequences (see Chapter 15). It has been postulated that the presence of the extended hinge region of IgA1 molecules confers greater segmental flexibility of Fab regions and a more extended reach between Fab tips in IgA1 than IgA2 (Pumphrey 1986; Boehm et al. 1999; Furtado et al. 2004).

When the primary structures of the C_H regions of α chains from various species are compared, the degree of similarity increases from the C_H1 to the C_H3 domain. For example, the percentage homology between human IgA1 and mouse IgA is: 51% in C_H1, 55% in C_H2, 69% in C_H3, and 61% in the C-terminal tailpiece (Putnam 1989). The most outstanding difference was seen in the hinge region (only 18% homology).

The α1 and α2 chains contain an unusually high number (17) of Cys residues involved in the formation of disulfide bridges within a single α chain (intrachain) and between component chains of mIgA, pIgA, and S-IgA. These linkages

Cα2 Domain

D

```
               241                    260                    280
                |                      |                      |
HU  1    CC..HPRLSLHRPALEDLLLGSEANLTCTLTGLRDASGVTFTWT....PSSGKSAVQGPP
HU  2-1  --.------------------------------------A-----...-----------
HU  2-2  --.------------------------------------A-----...-----------
CHI 1    --.----L-------------------------------A---S....-----------
CHI 2    --.------------------------------------A-----...-----------
GOR 1    --.--------------------------------------------...------E---
GOR 2    --.------------------------------------A-----...-------I----
ORA      -G..Q-Q-----------------------------TN---A------...-----N---R--
GIB 1    --..Q-----------------------------------------...-----N-----S
GIB 2    --..Q-----Q-------F---------------------A-----...-----N----L-
CYN      -D..K-----R-----------------------NP--A------...-----N---QS-
BOV      .-..E-S--VQP----------N-S-----S--KS-E-AS---N....-TG--T----S-
DOG      -N..E-----QK----------N-S-----S--K-PK-A----N....--K--EPI-KN-
PIG      --..K-S--QP---A-----N-S-----S--KKSE--S---Q....-G--D---AS-
MOU      .-..Q-S--Q----------D-SI----N---NPE-AV---E....--T--D---KKA
RAT      .-..R-----Q-----------S-----R--KEPT-AV---Q....-TT--D---KEA
RAB 1    -G..E-S---Q--D-R------D-S-----R--K-PKDAV---E...-TN-NEP--QS-
RAB 2    -G..K-S---Q--D-G----N-N-S-----R--LNPE-AV---E...-TF--EP--QS-
RAB 4    -G..K-S---Q--D-G----D-N-S-----R--LNPE-AV---N....-TN--EP--QSA
RAB 5    -G..E-S---Q--D-G----N-N-S-----R--L-PE-AV---E....-TF--EP--LS-
RAB 6    -G..E-S---Q--F-R----N-N-S-----R--KNPE-AV---E....-TN-NKP--QSV
RAB 7    -E..E-S---Q--D-R------D-S-----R--KYPEDAV---E....-TN-NEP--QS-
RAB 9    -G..E-S---Q--DIG----E-K-S-----S--K-PE-AV---E....-TN-NEP--QSV
RAB 10   -G..E-S---Q--DIG----E-K-S-----S--K-PE-AV---E....-TN-NEP--QST
RAB 11   -E..E-S---Q--D-R------D-S-----R--K-PE-AV---E....-TN-NEP--QS-
RAB 12   -G..E-S---Q--DIG----E-K-S-----S--K-PE-AV---E....-TN-NEP--QSV
RAB 13   -...Q-S---Q--D-G-----RD-S-----S--KNPEDAV---E....-TN-NEP--QRA
ECH      -P..TVSV--LP-S-DS-F-DKG-----E---VANVQ-AN-S-SAP..--VTAKP-R--A
POS      --SKTAYV--SP-S--S----TG-------S--KSST--E---ARTPA-A-TL-PI--TA
HEN      .ATPQLQV--LP-T--E--VSHN-TV--VVSNAAA-D--SVS-SRS..SGG-LDVS-TE.
DUC      SPESKLEVT-LP-S----YISQN-SV--VATN..APQDLK-S-SRS..EGTALDV-T-E-
```

Fig. 9.3, Continued

include inter α-α chain bonds within mIgA, α-L–chain bonds, α-α chain disulfides connecting two mIgA in pIgA, α-J chain bonds in pIgA, and α chain–SC bonds in S-IgA. A probable assignment of individual Cys residues to various intra-α–chain or inter-α–chain disulfides has been proposed (Fallgren-Gebauer et al. 1995). The structural significance of some of these Cys residues has been revealed by site-directed mutagenesis studies. For example Cys residue 133 is essential for the formation of the inter-L-α1–chain disulfide bridge. In IgA2, this residue is deleted, and Cys 220 is probably involved in L-α–chain disulfides. However, in IgA2 of A2m(1) allotype (see the following text), most of the molecules lack these L-α chain bridges; instead, dimerized L chains are present (Jerry and Kunkel 1974). The lack of for-mation of L-α2 chain disulfides is caused by the presence of Pro in position 221, which interferes with the formation of the disulfide bridge between L chain and Cys 220 (Chintalacharuvu and Morrison 1996).

Several investigators addressed the question concerning the structural features of the α (and also μ) chain that facilitate the formation of pIgA and IgM (Atkin et al. 1996; Wiersma et al. 1997; Wiersma and Shulman 1995; Sørensen et al. 1996, 1999; Smith et al. 1995; Braathen et al. 2002). The ability of IgA and IgM to form polymers has been associated with the presence of the 18–amino acid C-terminal tailpieces on α chains and μ chains, which include the penultimate Cys residue to which J chain is attached (Mestecky et al. 1974b; Mestecky and Schrohenloher 1974). Indeed, the addition of

```
E
                     300                     320                     340
                      |                       |                       |
HU  1      ERDLCGCYSVSSVLPGCAEPWNHGKTFTCTAAYPESKT.PLTATLSKS..
HU  2-1    ------------------Q-----E-------H--L--.----NIT--..
HU  2-2    ------------------Q-----E-------H--L--.----NIT--..
CHI 1      ------------------------E---------------.----NIT--..
CHI 2      ------------------Q-----E-------H--L-N.----NIT--..
GOR 1      ----------------------------------------.---------..
GOR 2      ---------------------KN---------H-----.----NIT--..
ORA        -----------------D-----Q------EH--L--.Q---------..
GIB 1      -----------I------------------Q---E-.Q---------..
GIB 2      -----------I----Q---NRE-----EH--L--.----NIT--..
CYN        K--P-----------------NRV------EH--LE-.Q----I--P..
BOV        K--S-------------D---S-Q--S-SVTH----S.S----IK-DL.
DOG        ---S-------------D-----D--S---TH----S.-I-VSIT-TT.
PIG        T--S--------I----D---K-E--S----HS-L-S.A----IT-PK.
MOU        VQNS----------R--S-AS-K--VTH---G-..--G-IA-VT.
RAT        VQ-S----T---------R--N-E------TH--FE-P.--GEIA-VT.
RAB 1      Q--P-----------T-TA-TE----VTH--IEGSS----IR-DTG
RAB 2      QL-H-----------VL--A-TE----VTH--IEGDS--G-I--DT.
RAB 4      Q--H-----------A-TV----VTH--IDSGS----I--DT.
RAB 5      RL-H-----------AA--A-TK-N--VTH--I-GVS--DII--DT.
RAB 6      QSYP-----------A-TE----VTH--IEGG----KI--DT.
RAB 7      Q--P-----------A-TE----VTH--IEGGS----I--DT.
RAB 9      QSYP-----------A-TE----VTH--IEGGS----I-I-R.
RAB 10     QSYP-----------A-TE----VTH--IEGGS----I-R...
RAB 11     Q--P-----------A-TE----VTH--IEGSS----I--DT.
RAB 12     QSYP-----------A-TE----VTH--IEGGS---KI-R...
RAB 13     Q---S---------SS--T-KARTE----VTH--IDSGS----I-R...
ECH        V--GQ-K-TIT-T-EV-TDE-MQ-HS-S--VTH--LRE.-I-K-IA-TS.
POS        -Q-SS-K-------EI-T-E-IR-DV-S--VSH--IE-..T-K-IY-PKV
HEN        D-QAD-R-T-R-F-RV---E--G-E--G-SVR.E-GVV.VAEESIR-ET.
DUC        QKQEN-L-RLT---KI---E--S-ES---GV-G--IQG.SV-KSVQ-DL.
```

Fig. 9.3, Continued

this tailpiece to IgG results in the formation of pIgG with interesting functional consequences (Sørensen *et al.* 1996; Smith *et al.* 1995). On the other hand, the deletion of the α-chain tailpiece completely prevented formation of pIgA (Atkin *et al.* 1996). Domain swapping experiments between IgA and IgM have suggested a role for the Cα3 and Cμ4 domains in determining polymer size and J-chain incorporation (Braathen *et al.* 2002). Furthermore, substitution of penultimate Cys 471 with Ser (Atkin *et al.* 1996) or normally *N*-glycosylated asparagine (Asn) 459 with alanine (Ala) in the α chain (Atkin *et al.* 1996) or Asn 563 with Tyr- in the μ chain (Wiersma *et al.* 1997) diminished J-chain incorporation and reduced the assembly of polymers. The linkage of Cys 471 in mIgA remains controversial. According to Prahl *et al.* (1971), Cys 471 forms a disulfide bridge with Cys located elsewhere on the α chain

(possibly Cys 311) but not to a homologous Cys 471 on the second α chain in mIgA or pIgA (Fallgren-Gabauer *et al.* 1995). Molecular modeling based on X-ray and neutron scattering suggested that Cys 311–Cys 471 represented a possible linkage conformation, although it should be borne in mind that the scattering analyses were not sensitive to the presence of the tailpiece (Boehm *et al.* 1999).

The human IgA2 subclass exists in two allotypic forms termed IgA2m(1) and IgA2m(2) (Wang and Fudenberg 1974; van Loghem and Biewenga 1983). The third variant, IgA2(n) so far described in a single individual may represent another allotype that arose through recombination or gene conversion between the two IgA2 alleles (Chintalacharuvu *et al.* 1994). A major structural difference between the IgA2m(1) and IgA2m(2) allotypes concerns the arrange-

Cα3 Domain

F

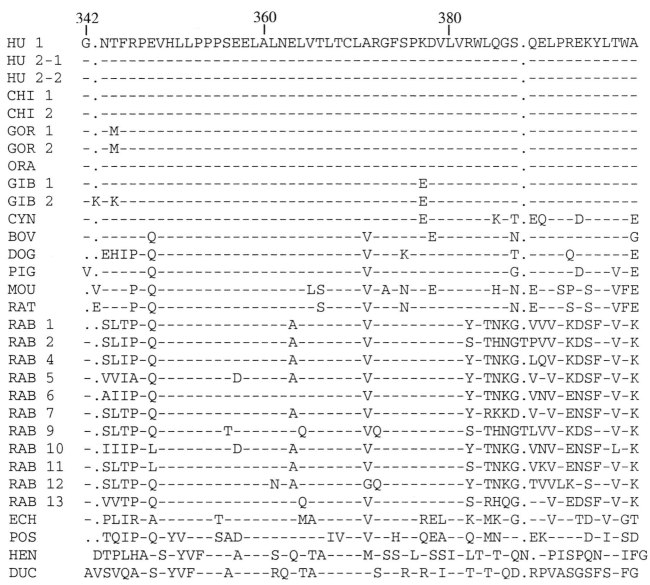

```
               342                  360                    380
                |                    |                      |
HU  1      G.NTFRPEVHLLPPPSEELALNELVTLTCLARGFSPKDVLVRWLQGS.QELPREKYLTWA
HU  2-1    -.---------------------------------------------.------------
HU  2-2    -.---------------------------------------------.------------
CHI 1      -.---------------------------------------------.------------
CHI 2      -.---------------------------------------------.------------
GOR 1      -.-M------------------------------------------.------------
GOR 2      -.-M------------------------------------------.------------
ORA        -.---------------------------------------------.------------
GIB 1      -.------------------------------------E--------.------------
GIB 2      -K-K---------------------------------E--------.------------
CYN        -.-----------------------------------E-------K-T.EQ---D-----E
BOV        -.-----Q-----------------------V-------E-------N.----------G
DOG        ..EHIP-Q----------------------V---K-----------T.---Q-----E
PIG        V.-----Q----------------------V-----------------G.-----D---V-E
MOU        .V---P-Q---------------------LS----V-A-N--E------H-N.E--SP-S--VFE
RAT        .E---P-Q--------------------S----V---N------N.E---S-S--VFE
RAB 1      ..SLTP-Q---------------A-------V---------Y-TNKG.VVV-KDSF-V-K
RAB 2      -.SLIP-Q---------------A-------V---------S-THNGTPVV-KDS--V-K
RAB 4      -.SLIP-Q---------------A-------V---------Y-TNKG.LQV-KDSF-V-K
RAB 5      -.VVIA-Q----------D----A-------V---------Y-TNKG.V-V-KDSF-V-K
RAB 6      -.AIIP-Q----------------------V---------Y-TNKG.VNV-ENSF-V-K
RAB 7      -.SLTP-Q---------------A-------V---------Y-RKKD.V-V-ENSF-V-K
RAB 9      -.SLTP-Q-------T-------Q-----VQ---------S-THNGTLVV-KDS--V-K
RAB 10     -.IIIP-L----------D----A-------V---------Y-TNKG.VNV-ENSF-L-K
RAB 11     -.SLTP-L---------------A-------V---------S-TNKG.VKV-ENSF-V-K
RAB 12     -.SLTP-Q------------N-A-------GQ---------Y-TNKG.TVVLK-S--V-K
RAB 13     -.VVTP-Q---------------Q-----V---------S-RHQG.--V-EDSF-V-K
ECH        -.PLIR-A------T--------MA-----V-----REL--K-MK-G.--V--TD-V-GT
POS        ..TQIP-Q-YV---SAD---------IV--V--H--QEA--Q-MN--.EK----D-I-SD
HEN        DTPLHA-S-YVF---A---S-Q-TA----M-SS-L-SSI-LT-T-QN.-PISPQN--IFG
DUC        AVSVQA-S-YVF---A----RQ-TA------S--R-R-I--T-T-QD.RPVASGSFS-FG
```

Fig. 9.3, Continued

ment of inter-α–L-chain disulfide bridges (Grey et al. 1968). The A2m(2) allotype differs from the A2m(1) allotype and the IgA1 isotype in six positions, two of which are in the Cα1 domain (residues 212 and 221) and four of which are located in the Cα3 domain (residues 411, 428, 458, and 467). The A2m(1) allotype is a hybrid of IgA1 and A2m(2) and may have arisen by a gene conversion event (Tsuzukida et al. 1979; Tucker et al. 1981).

Population studies of the IgA2 allotypes revealed a characteristic racial and ethnic distribution. In Caucasians, the overwhelming proportion of IgA2 is of the A2m(1) allotype, whereas in Africans and in African-Americans, the A2m(2) allotype dominates (Wang and Fudenberg 1974; Van Loghem and Biewenga 1983). Interestingly, American Indians, Australian Aborigines, and Eskimos resemble Caucasians in this respect.

Glycan moiety

Glycans contribute 6% to 7% of total molecular mass in human IgA1 and 8% to 10% in human IgA2 myeloma proteins (Tomana et al. 1976). The higher carbohydrate content in IgA2 proteins is the result of additional N-linked oligosaccharide side chains (Torano et al. 1977; Endo et al. 1994). Although the primary structures of carbohydrate side chains

G

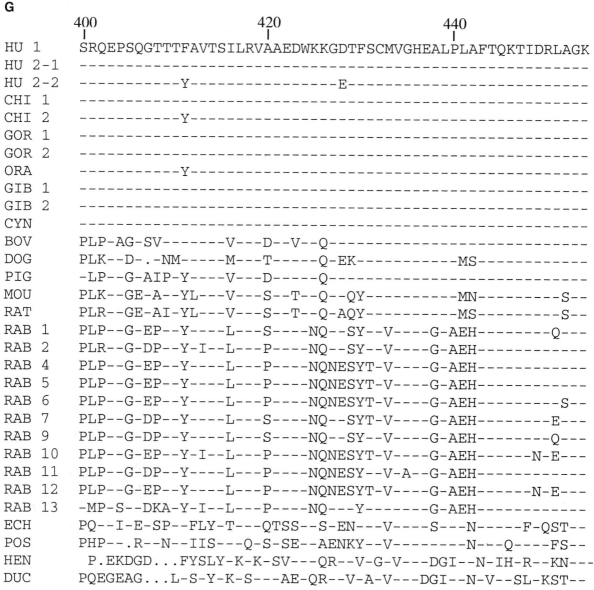

```
               400                   420                   440
                |                     |                     |
HU  1   SRQEPSQGTTTFAVTSILRVAAEDWKKGDTFSCMVGHEALPLAFTQKTIDRLAGK
HU  2-1 ------------------------------------------------------
HU  2-2 -----------Y---------------------E--------------------
CHI 1   ------------------------------------------------------
CHI 2   -----------Y------------------------------------------
GOR 1   ------------------------------------------------------
GOR 2   ------------------------------------------------------
ORA     -----------Y------------------------------------------
GIB 1   ------------------------------------------------------
GIB 2   ------------------------------------------------------
CYN     ------------------------------------------------------
BOV     PLP-AG-SV-------V---D--V--Q---------------------------
DOG     PLK--D-.-NM-----M---T-----Q-EK-----------MS-----------
PIG     -LP--G-AIP-Y----V---D-----Q---------------------------
MOU     PLK--GE-A--YL---V---S--T--Q--QY----------MN---------S--
RAT     PLR--GE-AI-YL---V---S--T--Q-AQY----------MS---------S--
RAB 1   PLP--G-EP--Y----L---S----NQ--SY--V----G-AEH-------Q---
RAB 2   PLR--G-DP--Y-I--L---P----NQ--SY--V----G-AEH-----------
RAB 4   PLP--G-EP--Y----L---P----NQNESYT-V----G-AEH-----------
RAB 5   PLP--G-EP--Y----L---P----NQNESYT-V----G-AEH-----------
RAB 6   PLP--G-EP--Y----L---P----NQNESYT-V----G-AEH---------S--
RAB 7   PLP--G-DP--Y----L---S----NQ--SYT-V----G-AEH-------E---
RAB 9   PLP--G-DP--Y----L---S----NQ--SY--V----G-AEH-------Q---
RAB 10  PLP--G-EP--Y-I--L---P----NQNESYT-V----G-AEH------N-E---
RAB 11  PLP--G-DP--Y----L---P----NQNESY--V-A--G-AEH-----------
RAB 12  PLP--G-EP--Y----L---P----NQNESYT-V----G-AEH------N-E---
RAB 13  -MP-S--DKA-Y-I--L---P----NQ---Y-------G-AEH-----------
ECH     PQ--I-E-SP--FLY-T---QTSS--S-EN---V----S---N-----F-QST--
POS     PHP--.R--N--IIS---Q-S-SE--AENKY--V--------N---Q----FS--
HEN      P.EKDGD...FYSLY-K-K-SV---QR--V-G-V---DGI--N-IH-R--KN---
DUC     PQEGEAG...L-S-Y-K-S---AE-QR--V-A-V---DGI--N-V--SL-KST--
```

Fig. 9.3, Continued

have been determined for a few myeloma and polyclonal IgA proteins, remarkable variability in the content, composition, and number of oligosaccharide side chains was noted (Baenziger and Kornfeld 1974a; Tomana *et al.* 1976; Wold *et al.* 1990; Endo *et al.* 1994; Mattu *et al.* 1998; Royle *et al.* 2003). Statistically significant differences in the content of fucose (Fuc), mannose (Man), and *N*-acetyl glucosamine (GlcNAc) were determined on α1 and α2 chains; the most striking difference was the presence of *N*-acetyl galactosamine (GalNAc) in IgA1 and its absence in IgA2 (Tomana *et al.* 1976). The prototype structures of Asn-linked (*N*-linked) carbohydrate side chains detected in IgA1 and IgA2 myeloma proteins are shown in Fig. 9.4. It should be emphasized that

the number, the type, and the terminal sugar residues vary between proteins of IgA subclasses as well as among individual myeloma proteins within a single subclass. Although the *N*-linked side chains shown in Fig. 9.4A are present in all IgA molecules (Baenziger and Kornfeld 1974a), high-Man type chains (Fig. 9.4B) are not; some IgA molecules, irrespective of the subclass, lack such chains (Endo *et al.* 1994). Interestingly, the high-Man type side chain containing IgA molecules interact through their terminal Man residues with corresponding receptors expressed on gram-negative (Enterobacteriaceae) and gram-positive (lactobacilli) bacteria and inhibit their adherence to epithelial cells (Wold *et al.* 1990; Adlerberth *et al.* 1996; see also Chapter 14).

```
H
                      460
                       |
HU   1     PTHVNVSVVMAEVDGTCY
HU   2-1   -----------------
HU   2-2   ---I--------A-----
CHI  1     -----------------
CHI  2     ---I-------------
GOR  1     -----------------
GOR  2     -----------------
ORA        -----------------
GIB  1     -----------------
GIB  2     -----------------
CYN        -----------------
BOV        ----------S----V--
DOG        --------------I--
PIG        -----------AE-I--
MOU        --N-S---I-S-G--I--
RAT        --N-----I-S-G--I--
RAB  1     ---------V-D-E-V--
RAB  2     ---------V-D-E-V--
RAB  4     ---------V-D-E-V--
RAB  5     ---------V-D-E-V--
RAB  6     ---------V-D-E-V--
RAB  7     ---------V-D-EAV--
RAB  9     ---------V-D-EAV--
RAB  10    ---------V-D-E-V--
RAB  11    ---------V-D-EAV--
RAB  12    --Q------V-D-EAV--
RAB  13    ---------V-D-EAV--
ECH        -ST--LT---SDAA----
POS        --N-----I-SD-S----
HEN        AS-------LSDA-V---
DUC        --Q------LSDA-S---
```

Fig. 9.3, Continued

The hinge region of IgA1 contains three to five short chains linked to Ser and Thr residues by *O*-linked glycosidic bonds (Baenziger and Kornfeld 1974b; Field *et al.* 1989, 1994; Hiki *et al.* 1995; Mattu *et al.* 1998). These side chains are composed of GalNAc, galactose (Gal), *N*-acetyl neuraminic acid (NeuNAc), and, in some proteins, GlcNAc (Fig. 9.4D) (Pierce-Cretel *et al.* 1981, 1989; Royle *et al.* 2003). The prototype structures of *O*-linked glycans described in human IgA1 proteins are shown in Fig. 9.4C. By analogy with *N*-linked side chains, a considerable degree of heterogeneity in the composition of *O*-linked carbohydrates has been described with respect to the content of Gal and NeuNAc (Field *et al.* 1989, 1994; Royle *et al.* 2003). Many different glycan epitopes, including Galβ1,4 and β1,3 linked, sialic acid α2-3 and α2-6 linked, and Fuc α1-4, 3 and 2 linked, suggest that these glycans represent bacterial adhesin-binding sites (Royle *et al.* 2003). Because only a few serum proteins contain *O*-linked carbohydrates (e.g., IgD, C1 inhibitor, fetuin, interleukin-6 [IL-6], and IL-2), which are recognized by the lectin jacalin (Hortin 1990; Kabir 1998), affinity chromatography employing this lectin can be used for purification of IgA1 from various body fluids (Roque-Barreira and Campos-Neto 1985). Although early work questioned the specificity of jacalin for IgA1 (Aucouturier *et al.* 1988, 1989), it is now established as a useful means to purify IgA1 selectively (Skea *et al.* 1988; Biewenga *et al.* 1989).

The total carbohydrate content of S-IgA is considerably higher than that of serum IgA because both J chain and SC are rich in carbohydrates (Tomana *et al.* 1972, 1978; Mizoguchi *et al.* 1982; Neidermeier *et al.* 1972; Baenziger 1979; Hughes *et al.* 1999; Royle *et al.* 2003), as described in

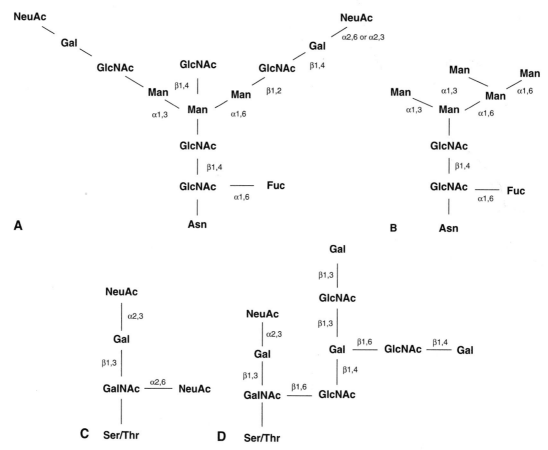

Fig. 9.4. Prototype structures of *N*-linked (**A** and **B**) and *O*-linked (**C** and **D**) glycan side chains of human IgA proteins. Structures **A** and **B** occur in IgA proteins of both subclasses; structures **C** and **D** are present only in the hinge region of IgA1. NeuNAc, *N*-acetyl neuraminic (sialic) acid; Gal, galactose; GlcNAc, *N*-acetyl glucosamine; Man, mannose; Fuc, fucose; and GalNAc, *N*-acetyl galactosamine. ±Gal or ±NeuNAc indicates that some chains terminate at the site of the preceding sugar. For example, structure **C** may occur as GalNAc→Ser, Galβ1→3GalNAc→Ser or NeuNAcα2→3Galβ1→3GalNAc→Ser.

detail subsequently. Serum IgA1 Fc *N*-glycans are reported to be fully galactosylated, suggesting that they occupy positions on the protein surface exposed to sugar modification enzymes (Mattu *et al.* 1998). This is in keeping with the highly accessible position on the surface of the Cα2 and Cα3 domains that they are revealed to occupy by X-ray crystallography. Interestingly, the equivalent sugars on S-IgA appear more truncated (Royle *et al.* 2003).

IgA subclasses

Immunochemical, protein sequencing, and molecular biology studies revealed the existence of IgA subclasses in several species. Two IgA subclasses have been described in humans (for reviews, see Mestecky and Russell 1986; Mestecky *et al.* 1989) as well as in hominoid primates (Kawamura *et al.* 1990, 1992; Ueda *et al.* 1988); thirteen IgA isotypes have been reported in lagomorphs (e.g., rabbits) but not in other mammalian species (Burnett *et al.* 1989, and see Chapters 10 and 11).

Ueda *et al.* (1988) and Kawamura *et al.* (1990, 1992) reported genomic sequences of α-chain genes from several

hominoid species. Their data show clearly the presence of IgA1 and IgA2 molecules in some species, although all features (e.g., the extended hinge in IgA1) were not always present (Sumiyama *et al.* 2002). These authors suggest that gene conversion was a major avenue to creating the IgA subclasses in humans and their immediate predecessors (**Fig. 9.5**).

Using polyclonal and monoclonal antibodies specific for human IgA1 and IgA2, several groups of investigators determined that serum IgA is represented primarily by the IgA1 subclass (about 85% of total serum IgA; for reviews, see Mestecky and Russell 1986; Conley and Delacroix 1987). This value mirrors the proportion of IgA1-secreting and IgA2-secreting cells in the bone marrow (Skvaril and Morell 1974; Crago *et al.* 1984), and in conjunction with additional data (Alley *et al.* 1982; Hijmans 1987), indicates that almost all serum IgA originates from this source.

The proportion of IgA1 to IgA2 varies in individual secretions. Currently available results obtained using polyclonal (Delacroix *et al.* 1982) or monoclonal anti-IgA1 and anti-IgA2 reagents (Ladjeva *et al.* 1989; Kutteh *et al.* 1996) do not include all external secretions. Because most S-IgA in

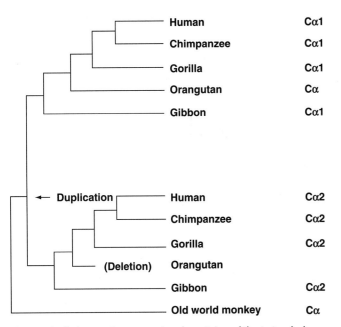

Fig. 9.5. A phylogenetic tree tracing the origins of the IgA subclasses in hominoid primates and humans. (Adapted with permission from that of Kawamura *et al.* 1992.)

humans is of local origin, this IgA1 to IgA2 ratio apparently reflects the characteristic distribution of IgA1-secreting and IgA2-secreting cells in various tissues (Crago *et al.* 1984; Kett *et al.* 1986; Kutteh *et al.* 1988; Burnett *et al.* 1987). Although IgA1-producing cells predominate in most mucosal tissues and glands, in the large intestine, and in the female genital tract, the IgA2 cells equal or outnumber IgA1-positive cells. Lymph nodes contain a mixed proportion of IgA1 and IgA2 cells, depending on the source.

Despite the high degree of identity in the primary structures of human IgA1 and IgA2 molecules, an understanding of the functional differences among the IgA subclasses is related to the structural differences between the two isotypes. The extended hinge region in IgA1 renders it highly susceptible to unique IgA1-specific proteases produced by several bacterial species, including many important human pathogens (see Chapter 15). Furthermore, this extended hinge theoretically confers added segmental flexibility and increased antigen-binding ability on IgA1 molecules compared with IgA2 molecules, although this hypothesis has not been demonstrated experimentally (Pumphrey 1986). IgA1 molecules are predicted, on the basis of scattering studies, to have much greater reach between their Fab arms than IgG (Boehm *et al.* 1999) or IgA2m(1) molecules (Furtado *et al.* 2004) which may confer improved antigen binding of distantly spaced antigens.

Differences in the glycans of human IgA1 and IgA2 antibodies (Tomana *et al.* 1972, 1976; Baenziger and Kornfeld 1974a, b; Torano *et al.* 1977; Putnam 1989; Wold *et al.* 1990; Endo *et al.* 1994) would be expected to influence a number of important properties of these molecules, some of which have been demonstrated experimentally. For example, the

removal of terminal NeuNAc substantially shortens the half-life of IgA molecules in the circulation because of the exposure of Gal and GalNAc residues that are recognized by the asialoglycoprotein receptor (ASGP-R) on hepatocytes (Ashwell and Harford 1982; Stockert *et al.* 1982; Tomana *et al.* 1988). Because of the availability of terminal Gal and GalNAc residues, IgA1 proteins bind better than IgA2 to the ASGP-R expressed on hepatocytes or on the human hepatoma cell line HepG2 (Tomana *et al.* 1988; Rifai *et al.* 2000). Functional differences between IgA1 and IgA2 proteins, including the inhibition of bacterial adherence to epithelial cells, and interactions with the complement system, fibronectin, and cellular receptors, are discussed in detail in Chapter 15.

Studies of the IgA subclass association of naturally or artificially induced serum and secretory antibodies specific for different types of antigens revealed several potentially important findings (for reviews, see Mestecky and Russell 1986; Mestecky *et al.* 1989). In colostrum (Ladjeva *et al.* 1989) or saliva (Brown and Mestecky 1985), antibodies specific for protein antigens were found predominantly to be of the IgA1 subclass. By contrast, antibodies to bacterial lipopolysaccharide and lipoteichoic acid in these fluids were of the IgA2 subclass. However, in serum, such antibodies were present as IgA1 (Russell *et al.* 1986; Moldoveanu *et al.* 1987), suggesting that they were derived from another tissue, probably bone marrow, and were induced by a different stimulatory pathway. The differences in the IgA subclass distribution of specific antibodies were even more accentuated in response to local or systemic infection or immunization. Although low levels of IgA1 and IgA2 antibodies to influenza A virus were detected before infection, IgA1 accounted for most of the rise in antihemagglutinin levels seen after infection (Brown *et al.* 1985). However, in serum, almost all IgA antibodies were of the IgA1 subclass before and after the infection. Systemic immunization with pneumococcal polysaccharide vaccine induced a vigorous serum response in IgG and IgA isotypes. However, when analyzed by an enzyme-linked immunospot (ELISPOT) assay for specific antibody-secreting cells, IgA-producing cells predominated in the peripheral blood (Lue *et al.* 1988). Furthermore, examination with monoclonal anti-IgA1 and anti-IgA2 reagents revealed the predominance of IgA2 cells producing specific antipolysaccharide antibodies. Comparable results were obtained in another concurrent, although independent, study (Heilman *et al.* 1988). Subsequent immunizations of another group of young adult volunteers with tetanus toxoid or with polysaccharides from *Haemophilus influenzae* or *Neisseria meningitidis* induced low numbers of IgA-secreting cells, predominantly of subclass IgA1 against tetanus toxoid, but a high frequency of IgA antipolysaccharide-producing cells (Tarkowski *et al.* 1990).

Collectively, these results indicate that the character of an antigen apparently influences the outcome of the immune response with respect to the IgA subclass. Similar conclusions were reached in studies of the distribution of specific IgG subclass antibodies induced by systemic immunizations with protein or polysaccharide antigens (Hammerström and Smith 1986). The mechanisms that regulate the isotype responses to various types of antigens remain speculative. Processing of different antigens and the involvement of different types of T-helper cells and lymphokines (McGhee *et al.* 1989) represent attractive avenues for future investigations.

J chain

In the early 1970s, comparative studies of the polypeptide chain composition of pIg (S-IgA, pIgA, and IgM) with that of IgG revealed an additional polypeptide chain in polymeric immunoglobulin with a fast electrophoretic mobility (for reviews, see Inman and Mestecky 1974; Koshland 1985). Subsequent studies revealed that this chain was glycosylated, with a molecular mass of 15 to 16 kDa, and was linked by disulfide bridges to the Fc fragment of polymeric IgM or IgA of secretory and serum (myeloma) origin (Mestecky and Schrohenloher 1974; Mestecky *et al.* 1974b; Garcia-Pardo *et al.* 1981). Based on the given criteria (molecular mass, fast electrophoretic mobility, characteristic amino acid composition, and immunochemical cross-reactivity), the presence of J chain has been established, with varying degrees of confidence, in pIg from many vertebrate species including mammals (human, monkey, rabbit, mouse, pig, dog, goat, cat, cow, horse, rat, guinea pig, and sheep), birds (chicken and pheasant), reptiles (turtle), amphibians (frog and toad), and fishes (catfish and sharks) (Kobayashi *et al.* 1973; Inman and Mestecky 1974; Koshland 1985; Mikoryak *et al.* 1988; Kulseth and Rogne 1994; Takahashi *et al.* 2000; Hohman *et al.* 1997, 2003). Molecular biologic approaches combined with immunochemical techniques revealed that J chain is also expressed in some invertebrates (Takahashi *et al.* 1996).

Sequence analyses of mouse genomic DNA revealed that J chain–encoding information is contained in four exons of a single gene located on chromosome 5; in humans, the J-chain gene is on chromosome 4 (Max and Korsmeyer 1985; Koshland 1985; Matsuuchi *et al.* 1986). A pseudogene for human J chain is present on chromosome 8 (Max *et al.* 1994). A comparative analysis of mouse, human, cow, possum, turtle, frog, and nurse shark J-chain genes showed that J-chain DNA is highly conserved among various animal species (Koshland 1985; Max and Korsmeyer 1985; Kulseth and Rogne 1994; Hohman *et al.* 1997; 2003).

Domain structure

Despite the low degree of sequence homology with H and L chains, studies of the secondary structure of J chain have been interpreted to suggest that it folds into an eight-stranded antiparallel β-barrel (with 35% β-sheet and the remainder in random coil) (Zikan *et al.* 1985; Pumphrey 1986). An alternative model suggests a two-domain model in which the first domain has a high propensity for forming β-sheets and the second domain displays a mixture of α-helical and β-strand propensities (Frutiger *et al.* 1992; Koshland 1985).

Primary structure

The primary structures of vertebrate J chains have been determined in mouse, human, rabbit, bullfrog, South African

clawed frog (*Xenopus laevis*), possum, chicken, turtle, and nurse shark and cow, as well as partially in earthworm **(Fig. 9.6)**. J chain consists of ~137 amino acid residues and displays a high degree of sequence homology (approximately 70%) among species (Koshland 1985; Max and Korsmeyer 1985; Mikoryak *et al.* 1988; Kulseth and Rogne 1994; Hohman *et al.* 1997). These findings (summarized in Figure 9.6), in conjunction with remarkable similarity in physicochemical properties and interspecies cross-reactivities (Kobayashi *et al.* 1973), suggest that many of the features of J chain are conserved through evolution. With the exception of nurse shark (Hohman *et al.* 2003), J chains are rich in acidic (aspartic acid [Asp], glutamic acid [Glu]) amino acid residues and low in glycine (Gly), Ser, and phenylalanine (Phe); Trp is absent (Inman and Mestecky 1974). Six of the eight cysteine residues form three intrachain disulfide bridges (Cys 12–Cys 100, Cys 17–Cys 91, and Cys 108–Cys 133); the other two residues (Cys 14 and Cys 68) are involved in disulfide bonds that link J chain to the penultimate cysteine residues of α and μ chains (Mestecky *et al.* 1974b; Mestecky and Schrohenloher 1974; Frutiger *et al.* 1992; Bastian *et al.* 1992; Atkin *et al.* 1996). Studies of the nurse shark J chain revealed several unexpected findings. Unlike all other J chains analyzed so far, nurse shark J chain is not acidic and, therefore, displays unusual electrophoretic mobility in alkaline-urea gels. Of eight Cys residues found in J chains of other species, Cys 7 and 8 are absent. On the other hand, highly conserved Cys 1, 4, 5, and 6 residues and the *N*-glycosylation site (Asn 50-52) are also present in the nurse shark J chain. Examination of various tissues for the presence of J chain transcripts revealed unusual distribution: relative abundance in the spleen, gills, esophagus, and muscle (the μ-chain transcript is not found in this tissue) and surprising absence in the gut (spiral valve) (Hohman *et al.* 2003). The authors speculate that in the nurse shark the J chain may not play a role in Ig assembly.

Carbohydrate of J chain

Approximately 8% of the molecular mass of J chain is contributed by a single carbohydrate side chain linked to Asn residue 48 by an *N*-glycosidic bond. This chain consists of Fuc, Man, Gal, GlcNAc, and NeuNAc (Niedermeier *et al.* 1972; Baenziger 1979). A detailed analysis of the *N*-glycan structures on J chain from S-IgA has recently been reported (Royle *et al.* 2003). The presence of the carbohydrate side chain at Asn 48 appears to be critical to polymer formation between J chain and the mIgA subunits (Krugmann *et al.* 1997).

Secretory component

Identification of SC as part of the transport receptor for pIgA began with immunohistochemical studies in which specific antisera to the (secretion-specific) "secretory piece" established its presence not only within the S-IgA molecule (Hanson 1961) but as a component of mucosal epithelial cells (Tomasi *et al.* 1965; South *et al.* 1986; Brandtzaeg 1978; Crago *et al.* 1978; Nagura *et al.* 1979). Subsequently, SC was isolated free in mucosal secretions as well as associated with

```
                                                          α/μ
                                                          ☆ ▽
human         1 --------MKNHLLFWGV-LAVFIKAVHVKAQE-DE-R----IVLVDNKCKCARITSRII   45
cow           1 --------MKNCLLFWGV-LAIFVMAVLVTAQD-ENER----IVV-DNKCKCARITSRII   45
mouse         1 --------MKTHLLLWGV-LAIFVKVVLVTGDD-EATI----LADN--KCMCTRVTSKII   44
rabbit        1 ----------------------------EDESTV----LVDN--KCQCVRITSRII       22
possum        1 --------MKRSLLFCGL-LAGLCGALLVTAQDYDEDEGRI-LVDNKCK--CVRVTSRLV   48
chicken       1 --------MKSSLP-WVA-LAVSLGFVLVAGYQWD-DGEERVLVNN--KCKCVTVTSKFV   47
turtle        1 --------MKTSLLLWGV-LAVFLGAALVTGYE-DEEAEEHVLVDN--KCKCARVTSKFV   48
bullfrog      1 -MDKC-SVLSAALLLLFA-VYVTGQT-------YREQEYI--LANNKCK--CVKISSRFV   46
Xenopus levis 1 ML-KHVA-LQAAVLLLLS-GSISTQLYETGT-YYDEDAENHVLVENKCK--CIKVTSKFV   54
nurse shark   1 ------------MMKSKDML-GVLAAILFYTALSAAKSERNLLVSSKCKLLE--VSSKMI   45
```

```
                                           α/μ
                                           ▽          ●
human         46 RSSEDPNEDIVE--RNIRIIVPLNNRE▓ISDPTSPLRTRFVYHLSDLCKKCDPTEVELDN  103
cow           46 PSAEDPSQDIVE--RNVRIIVPLNSRE▓ISDPTSPMRTKFVYHLSDLCKKCDTTEVELED  103
mouse         45 PSTEDPNEDIVE--RNIRIVVPLNNRE▓ISDPTSPLRRNFVYHLSDVCKKCDPVEVELED  102
rabbit        23 RDPDNPSEDIVE--RNIRIIVPLNTRE▓ISDPTSPLRTEFKYNLANLCKKCDPTEIELDN   80
possum        49 PSPDNPDEKIVE--RNIRLIVPLKNRE▓ISDPTSPVRTTFVYRLSELCNKCDPVEVEVGN  106
chicken       48 PSKDNPEEEVLE--RNIRIIVPLKSRE▓ISDPTSPLRTTFVYRMTELCKKCDPVEIELGG  105
turtle        49 PSKDNPQEEVLV--RNIRVIVPLLSRK▓ISDPTSPVRTTFVYRLSELCKKCDPTEVELGD  106
bullfrog      47 PSTERPGEEILE--RNIQITIPTSSRM▓ISDPYSPLRTQFVYNLWDICQKCDPVQLEIGG  104
Xenopus levis 55 PSKENPNEKILE--RDIEIRIPLKARE▓ISDPTSPLRTNFVYKLSDLSKKCDPVEVELGG  112
nurse shark   46 VTELPNGEKVEQLVRDIKIIVPLRSRE▓ISDPTSPIRTKFVYKISDFCKNCGRQESPQEP  105
```

```
                      ●              ☆          ¥
human         104 QIVTATQS--NICDEDSATE-TCYTYDRNKCYRAVVP----------------------  137
cow           104 QVVTASQS--NICDSDAE---TCYTYDRNKCYTNRVK--------------------    135
mouse         103 QVVTATQS--NICNEDDGVPETCYMYDRNKCYTTMVP----------------------  137
rabbit         81 QVFTASQS--NICPDDDYSE-TCYTYDRNKCYTTLVP----------------------  114
possum        107 EVVLATQS--NRCDEEN--ET-CYTYDRNKCYTSTAS--------------------    138
chicken       106 ETYQAQQS--NSCNEPET----CYTYNRDKCYTTTFP--------------------    136
turtle        107 RVITAEQS--N▓CSSSDT----CYTYDRNKCYTTTFP--------------------    137
bullfrog      105 IPVLASQP--S-CSKPDD--E-CYTYDRNKCYTTEVN--------------------    135
Xenopus levis 113 ETVLVSQA--N-CHKSDD--T-CYTYDRNKCYTRDIP--------------------    143
nurse shark   106 QCKPKPPPTDE-CYAHDDQS-CR-DYQR---YLGTAKYSKHQEEHLIQKPTVRPFETTVD  159
```

```
                  ¥
human         138 ------LVYGGE-TKMVETALTPDACYPD                    159
cow           136 ------LSYRGQ-TKMVETALTPDSCYPD                    157
mouse         138 ------LRYHGE-TKMVQAALTPDSCYPD                    159
rabbit        115 ------ITHRGG-TRMVKATLTPDSCYPD                    136
possum        139 ------L-YLGGETRTVTTALTPESCYSD                    160
chicken       137 ------FVYHGE-TKHIQAALTPTSCYAE                    158
turtle        138 ------FFYGGK-INTVQAALTPESCYAD                    159
bullfrog      136 ------FKYNDQIIKKKV-PLTPDSCYE-                    156
Xenopus levis 144 ------FTIGGKIEMRKA-ALNPESCYE-                    164
nurse shark   160 PNSFSDAP--------------------                    167
```

Fig. 9.6. Amino acid sequence of human, cow, mouse, rabbit, brushtail possum, chicken, turtle, bullfrog (*Rana catesbeiana*), *Xenopus laevis*, and nurse shark J chains. *N*-glycosylation site is marked by an arrow. The conserved Cys (C) residues are indicated by bold symbols above the sequences. (Data are from Hughes *et al.* 1990; Frutiger *et al.* 1992; Max and Korsmeyer 1985; Matsuuchi *et al.* 1986; Kulseth and Rogne 1994; Mikoryak *et al.* 1988; Hohman *et al.* 1997, 2003.)

S-IgA. The exquisite binding specificity for polymeric but not monomeric immunoglobulin was established (Mach 1970; Radl *et al.* 1971; Brandtzaeg 1984, 1985; Weiker and Underdown 1975). For a more complete discussion of the structure, genetics, and function of pIgR, see Chapter 12.

Domain structure

In most species, SC (molecular mass about 70–83 kDa) consists of five immunoglobulin-like domains with definite but relatively low homology to the γ-chain variable region (Mostov *et al.* 1984). In addition to the five-domain form, rabbits synthesize a truncated three-domain form (Frutiger et al. 1987). Within the basolateral membrane of mucosal epithelial cells, SC consists of five extracellular domains, a transmembrane segment, and a cytoplasmic domain. The term "pIgR" was proposed to differentiate between the membrane form of the transport receptor and the cleaved soluble form known as SC (Mostov et al. 1984).

Primary amino acid sequence

The amino acid sequences of pIgR have been determined completely for eight species and partially for four others and are shown in Chapter 12 (Eiffert et al. 1984, 1991; Mostov et al. 1984; Banting et al. 1989; Kulseth et al. 1995; Verbeet et al. 1995; Piskurich et al. 1995; Adamski and Demmer 1999; Taylor et al. 2002; Peters et al. 2003). In addition to the intrachain disulfide bonds that are thought to be buried within each domain, several of the domains have "extra" disulfide bonds. One of these, located in the fifth domain, is susceptible to disulfide interchange. Data from Fallgren-Gebauer et al. (1995) suggest that only one Cys residue from this labile disulfide bond is linked to one Cys 311 in the $C\alpha 2$ domain.

Carbohydrate

Approximately 22% of the total molecular mass of SC is contributed by carbohydrates (Tomana et al. 1978). The five to seven oligosaccharide side chains contain GlcNAc, Fuc, Man, Gal, and NeuNAc attached by N-glycosidic bonds (Mizoguchi et al. 1982; Hughes et al. 1999). Studies of rabbit SC indicate one common glycosylation site at the Asn residue at position 400 and a second site in the N-terminal domain that varies among different allotypes (Frutiger et al. 1988). In a recent study of the glycans present in human S-IgA (Royle et al., 2003), the majority of structures on human SC were found to be fully galactosylated, nonbisected biantennary structures, but there was a much greater range of structures present than on IgA heavy chain or J chain. Some triantennary structures and a small proportion of tetraantennary structures were also noted. The majority of N-glycans were sialylated, and over 65% of the structures contained core Fuc, with some structures having outer-arm Fuc. The range of glycans present on SC was found to include all the different Lewis and sialyl-Lewis epitopes, indicating that these glycans may bind lectins and bacterial adhesins. Together with the N-linked and O-linked glycans on the α chain of S-IgA, these SC-associated glycans may therefore act as a means by which S-IgA can bind to bacteria, in addition to antigenic recognition via the Fab arms (Wold et al. 1990; Schroten et al. 1998; Phalipon et al. 2002). Further, the finding that serum pIgA but not S-IgA can bind Man-binding lectin, an important activator of the complement system, could be accounted for by masking of terminal GlcNac and Man residues on the IgA heavy chains by SC in S-IgA.

BIOSYNTHESIS AND ASSEMBLY OF IgA

Monomeric IgA

The L chains and α chains that become assembled intracellularly into mIgA molecules are synthesized on separate sets of polyribosomes and are assembled into the monomeric unit through several pathways (Heremans 1974). Depending on the cell type studied, various types of pairings of H and L chains occur early on polyribosomes, but the glycosylated (attachment of GlcNAc, Man, and Fuc on N-linked and GalNAc in O-linked glycan) molecule of mIgA is assembled in the Golgi apparatus. Additional carbohydrate residues (Gal and NeuNAc) are attached during the intracellular passage of mIgA from the Golgi apparatus to the cell surface and ultimate secretion into the medium.

Polymeric IgA

Early investigations of the biosynthetic pathways of mouse IgA suggested that, in cells secreting pIgA, most of the intracellular IgA was present as monomers and that polymerization occurred shortly before or at the time of secretion (Parkhouse 1971). This hypothesis is supported by subsequent comparative and quantitative biochemical studies of the molecular forms of intracellular versus secreted IgA in cell lysates and tissue culture supernatants of normal peripheral blood mononuclear cells stimulated *in vitro* with pokeweed mitogen or transformed with Epstein-Barr virus (EBV) and lymphoblastoid cell lines, which indicated that, although small amounts of pIgA were detected in some cell lysates, most intracellular IgA occurred in a monomeric form (even when the predominant form of secreted IgA was polymeric) (Buxbaum et al. 1974; Kutteh et al. 1982a, 1983; Moldoveanu et al. 1984). Nevertheless, intracellular IgA in human intestinal plasma cells occurs in both pIgA and mIgA forms in approximately equal proportions (Kutteh et al. 1982a). Furthermore, the presence of intracellular polymers can easily be demonstrated by an SC-binding test performed on fixed IgA-producing cells (Radl et al. 1974; Brandtzaeg 1973, 1983; Moro et al. 1990). However, it must be emphasized that the intracellular affinity of pIgA for free SC is a qualitative but not quantitative immunofluorescence test. When IgA from cell lysates of pIgA-producing cells were examined, after molecular-sieve chromatography, for SC binding and presence of J chain, only a small proportion of true intracellular pIgA was present (Moldoveanu et al. 1984).

Distribution of cells synthesizing monomeric and polymeric IgA

Analyses of molecular forms of IgA in perfusates and supernatants of *in vitro* cultured tissue explants as well as immunohistochemical studies of mucosal tissues and glands clearly demonstrated that separate populations of pIgA-secreting and mIgA-secreting cells exist that display a characteristic tissue distribution (for reviews, see Brandtzaeg 1983; Mestecky and McGhee 1987; Mestecky et al. 1991; Brandtzaeg et al. 1999). Typically, most of the IgA cells in the normal human bone marrow produce mIgA (they do not express J chain and do not bind SC) (Crago et al. 1984; Alley et al. 1982; Kutteh et al. 1982a; Radl et al. 1974), whereas the majority of such cells in the intestinal lamina propria produce pIgA, express J chain, and bind SC. The spleen and lymph nodes from different locations display a variable proportion of pIgA-secreting and mIgA-secreting cells. Under pathologic conditions (e.g., IgA multiple myelomatosis), the bone marrow may contain predominantly J chain–positive cells, which produce pIgA (Radl *et al.* 1974; Mestecky *et al.* 1980).

Role of glycosylation in IgA assembly and secretion

There is evidence of species differences in the role played by carbohydrates in IgA secretion. Murine IgA was not secreted when the *N*-linked glycosylation sites were removed by site directed mutagenesis (Taylor and Wall 1988). By contrast, the assembly and secretion of human mIgA1 was relatively unaffected by mutation of one or both *N*-linked glycan-attachment sites (Chuang and Morrison 1997; Mattu *et al.* 1998). In addition, coexpression of the CH2 domain glycosylation mutant with J chain produced dimers. However, while the tailpiece glycosylation mutant was found to be secreted in dimeric forms on coexpression with J chain, the incorporation of J chain into the dimers was reduced (Atkin *et al.* 1996), and there was evidence of secretion of higher molecular weight polymers (Chuang and Morrison 1997). Mutant J chain engineered to lack its one *N*-linked glycan chain caused markedly reduced dimer assembly, suggesting a requirement for the glycan moiety in J-chain function (Krugmann *et al.* 1997).

Benzyl 2-acetamido-2-deoxy-α-D-galactopyranoside (BADG), an inhibitor that blocks synthesis of *O*-linked hinge region glycans beyond the first GalNAc, did not significantly affect intracellular assembly and secretion of IgA1 (Gala and Morrison 2002), suggesting that *O*-linked sugars probably have little influence on Ig assembly.

Role of J chain in the polymerization of immunoglobulins

The role of J chain in polymerization of IgA, particularly in the assembly of dimeric and tetrameric molecules of IgA in human cells, has not been studied as much as the J-chain participation in the assembly of IgM. The association of J chain with pIg but not mIg in serum and secretions raised the possibility that J chain either initiated or regulated the formation of intracellular polymers. The following observations seem consistent with this hypothesis: (1) Ig-producing cells in the subepithelium of the gastrointestinal and respiratory tracts, as well as in the interstitium of mammary, salivary, and lacrimal glands, prominently display the presence of intracellular J chain and primarily produce pIgA (Brandtzaeg *et al.* 1999; Johansen *et al.* 2000); and (2) by contrast, IgG-containing or IgA-containing plasma cells from the normal bone marrow that secrete mIgA are uniformly J-chain negative (Radl *et al.* 1974; Crago *et al.* 1984; Kutteh *et al.* 1982a; Brandtzaeg 1985; Mestecky and McGhee 1987; Brandtzaeg *et al.* 1999).

Since a small proportion of intracellular Ig is linked to J chain, this chain has been proposed to initiate polymerization by binding first to intracellular mIgA or mIgM that subsequently is linked to another monomer, forming a dimeric molecule (for reviews, see Brandtzaeg 1983, 1985; Koshland 1985; Mestecky and McGhee 1987).

However, Stott (1976) observed that pIgM could be detected in lysates of certain mouse cell lines in a tetrameric form lacking J chain. This polypeptide, linked to mIgM, was added as a last step in the process of polymerization. This view is further supported by Brewer and Corley (1997): in a few hybridoma cell lines studied, the J chain was incorporated into pentamers at the late stage of polymer assembly and did not appear to serve as a nucleus of polymerization as originally proposed (Koshland 1985). These data suggest that J chain may not initiate polymerization but may regulate the degree and form of pIg. Site-directed mutagenesis of Cys residues of α or μ chains involved in J-chain binding, and transfection of μ-chain and L-chain genes into J-chain-negative cells, show further that J chain may not be necessary for polymerization (Cattaneo and Neuberger 1987; Davies *et al.* 1989). *In vitro* studies concerning the role of J chain in IgM polymerization reported that covalently linked IgM polymers were synthesized *in vitro* in good yield in the absence of J chain (Bouvet *et al.* 1987). By contrast, Niles *et al.* (1995) claimed that, at least for IgM, J chain was required for pentamer IgM synthesis in transfection experiments. However, in murine cell lines secreting IgM, J chain was not necessary for polymerization or secretion of assembled molecules from IgM-producing cells (Fazel *et al.* 1997; Brewer and Corley 1997). Other experiments revealed that the proper assembly of IgM into pentamers requires the presence of J chain whereas hexameric forms of IgM are always devoid of J chain (Randall *et al.* 1990, 1992a,b; Brewer *et al.* 1994; Hughey *et al.* 1998). Thus it appears that the J chain plays a regulatory role in the IgM pentamer–hexamer biosynthesis. Interestingly, hexameric IgM displays important biologic advantages over pentamers in activation of complement (Brewer *et al.* 1994; Wiersma *et al.* 1998).

Studies of structural requirements for assembly of pIgA and pIgM revealed several important points: (1) tailpieces of the μ chain and α chain are necessary for polymerization of IgA and IgM (Wiersma *et al.* 1997; Atkin *et al.* 1996; Yoo *et al.* 1999; Sørensen *et al.* 2000); (2) penultimate Cys residue of the α-chain and μ-chain tailpieces are necessary for polymerization (Sitia *et al.* 1990; Wiersma and Shulman 1995; Atkin *et al.* 1996); (3) both Cys 14 and Cys 68 and the presence of glycans on Asn 48 of the J chain are necessary for pIgA formation (Krugmann *et al.* 1997); and (4) the presence of Cα2 and Cα3 domains of the α chain, and corresponding Cμ3 and Cμ4 domains of the μ chain plays an important role in efficient formation of polymers and incorporation of J chain (Sørensen *et al.* 2000; Yoo *et al.* 1999). Taken together, available data suggest that complex noncovalent and covalent interactions between α chain (or μ chain) Fc region domains and tailpieces and J chain are most likely required for the formation of pIgA or pIgM. However, in the absence of crystallographic data, we still lack essential information concerning the precise arrangement and intermolecular interactions of these component polypeptides in the assembled pIgA or pIgM molecules. However, at the present time, it could be argued that the weight of evidence favors an end-to-end arrangement of the mIgA in dIgA and S-IgA. As summarized in the preceding text, electron microscopic measurements of the two Fc regions are consistent with such a configuration. Hydrodynamic analyses further support this arrangement (Björk and Lindh 1974). Moreover, the effects of mutagenesis of Cys residues of both the tailpiece of IgA and J chain lend themselves to an interpretation that the most likely arrangement in dIgA places the mIgA in the end-to-end configuration (Krugmann *et al.* 1997).

The role of J chain in Ig polymerization and pIgR-mediated transepithelial transport was elucidated in J chain–deficient mice (Hendrickson *et al.* 1995, 1996; Lycke *et al.* 1999; Erlandsson *et al.* 1998, 2001). In comparison to wild-type mice, markedly increased levels of serum mIgA and decreased levels of biliary and fecal IgA were observed, suggesting an impaired transport of IgA by pIgR-dependent hepatobiliary transport. Interestingly, levels of IgA in milk, intestinal surface, and nasal wash were similar or even higher than in wild-type mice. The authors speculated that J chain was not necessary for IgA transport and an alternative mechanism might be involved (Hendrickson *et al.* 1996). Contrary to these conclusions, Lycke *et al.* (1999) reported some 90% reduction in the level of intestinal IgA with functional impairment of intestinal immunity.

The role of J chain in the generation of pIgR-binding site interactions of IgA and SC domains are described in detail in Chapter 12.

J-chain expression in B cells not producing polymeric immunoglobulins

In the bone marrow of patients with multiple myeloma, J chain is frequently detected by immunofluorescent staining of plasma cells synthesizing monomeric Ig such as IgG, IgD, or only L and H chains or no Ig-related chains at all (Mestecky *et al.* 1980, 1990, 1997). Similarly, J chain has been detected in IgG plasma cells from normal human mucosal tissues and systemic inflammatory sites, and in mitogen-stimulated peripheral blood lymphocytes (Mestecky *et al.* 1977, 1980; Brandtzaeg 1983, 1985; Moro *et al.* 1990; Brandtzaeg *et al.* 1999). The expression of J chain in cells that are not engaged in the synthesis of polymers has been interpreted as a sign of clonal immaturity (Brandtzaeg 1985). Extensive studies of human cells from leukemic patients, established lymphoid cell lines, and EBV-transformed fetal bone marrow cells (depleted of surface Ig-positive cells) revealed that J chain may be expressed in the cytoplasm of human lymphocytes from the earliest stages of their differentiation along the B-cell axis (McCune *et al.* 1981; Kutteh *et al.* 1983; Hajdu *et al.* 1983; Max and Korsmeyer 1985; Kubagawa *et al.* 1988; Mestecky *et al.* 1977, 1997). Thus cells phenotypically characterized as null, pro-B, or pre-B cells contain J chain, frequently in the absence of μ chain. EBV-transformed fetal bone marrow cells or cells from a few patients with a clinically established diagnosis of multiple myeloma display the morphologic features of plasma cells but contain no intracellular Ig; in the former, the cells exhibit a germline configuration or abortive VDJ rearrangement of H-chain gene segments (Kubagawa *et al.* 1988). Surprisingly, J-chain mRNA has also been detected in human thymic but not in peripheral T cells (Bertrand *et al.* 1996). Earlier reports indicating that in murine lymphocytes of B-cell lineage J chain is expressed

only in Ig-secreting cells (Koshland 1985; Wallin *et al.* 1999) were recently challenged by Erlandsson *et al.* (2001), who demonstrated the presence of J-chain message in murine B-cell lymphoma and transformed pre-B–cell lines. Studies performed on murine and human lymphoid cell lines suggest that the intracellular synthesis of J chain and Ig is mutually independent and is differentially regulated (Randall *et al.* 1992; Emilie *et al.* 1988; Matsui *et al.* 1989; Rao *et al.* 1998).

IgA METABOLISM

IgA production

Considering the distribution in various body fluids of the major Ig isotypes and their catabolic rates, clearly IgA is synthesized in humans in quantities (about 66 mg/kg of body weight per day) that exceed by far the combined daily synthesis of all other Ig isotypes (for reviews, see Mestecky *et al.* 1986; Conley and Delacroix 1987). In humans, mIgA present in the circulation is produced mainly in the bone marrow (Hijmans 1987; Alley *et al.* 1982; Kutteh *et al.* 1982a); pIgA for external secretions is produced mostly locally in mucosal tissues **(Fig. 9.7)**. The lower concentration of IgA than IgG in human serum is the result of the more rapid catabolism of IgA (the half-life of IgA is ~6 days versus ~20 to 25 days for IgG) (for review, see Mestecky and Russell 1986), in conjunction with the fact that cells engaged in the production of IgA for the mucosal compartment (e.g., gastrointestinal tract, salivary gland) do not contribute significantly to the circulatory pool (Conley and Delacroix 1987).

Liver as a major site of IgA catabolism

The importance of the liver in IgA metabolism was established by a series of studies performed in animals and in humans with liver diseases. Experiments by Jackson *et al.* (1978) pointed out that the liver transported pIgA from

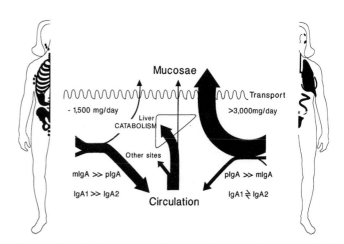

Fig. 9.7. Quantitative aspects of IgA production in humans, including various molecular forms (mIgA and pIgA, IgA1, and IgA2) and their distribution in the systemic and mucosal compartments. (Based on the studies summarized in Conley and Delacroix 1987; Mestecky *et al.* 1986; and Mestecky and McGhee 1987.)

blood to bile in rats. Vaerman and Delacroix (1984) proposed that, in rodents, the liver functions as an "IgA pump" that regulates serum levels of IgA by transporting circulating pIgA into the bile. By this mechanism, significant quantities of IgA are delivered into the intestinal tract of rodents; pIgR present on the surface of rat hepatocytes was identified as the most important receptor responsible for its selective and efficient transport of pIgA into bile in several species in which pIgA is the primary form of circulating IgA (see Chapters 11 and 12).

Interactions between pIgA and hepatocytes are strongly species dependent: pIgR has been found on hepatocytes of many species (rat, rabbit, and mouse), but not on human hepatocytes (for reviews, see Delacroix and Vaerman 1983; Delacroix et al. 1982; Rose et al. 1981; Vaerman and Delacroix 1984; Mestecky et al. 1991; Mestecky and McGhee 1987; Brown and Kloppel 1989; and Chapters 11 and 12). Consequently, the extent to which pIgR-mediated clearance of pIgA occurs is highly species dependent (see Chapter 11).

Role of other receptors in hepatic catabolism of IgA
In addition to pIgR, IgA interactions with hepatocytes can also be mediated through the hepatic ASGP-R or hepatic binding protein (Stockert et al. 1982; Tomana et al. 1988). The presence and properties of ASGP-R have been described for hepatocytes from several species (Ashwell and Harford 1982). ASGP-R, which recognizes terminal Gal and GalNAc residues of desialylated glycoproteins, has been proposed, in addition to pIgR, to play an important role in the endocytosis of IgA by hepatocytes (for reviews, see Brown and Kloppel 1989; Mestecky et al. 1991). The binding of glycoproteins, including IgA, to ASGP-R depends on Ca^{++} and is therefore inhibitable by chelating agents (e.g., EDTA). Bound IgA is internalized and the IgA-containing vesicles fuse with lysosomes, resulting in intracellular degradation.

The site of catabolism of IgA was studied in animal models (Moldoveanu et al. 1988, 1990; Rifai et al. 2000). Mice and monkeys (*Macaca fuscata*) were used as representatives of species with pIgR-positive and pIgR-negative hepatocytes, respectively; however, both species display ASGP-R on hepatocytes. In both species, the liver was identified as the organ with the highest uptake of mIgA and pIgs. Although both parenchymal (hepatocytes) and nonparenchymal cells were involved in the catabolism, the hepatocytes were more active. Other tissues and organs, including muscles, kidneys, skin, and spleen, also catabolized IgA, although to a much lower degree than the liver. However, there appear to be some differences with respect to the catabolism of human IgA in monkeys and mice related to the IgA1 or IgA2 subclass. Moldoveanu et al. (1988, 1990) demonstrated that irrespective of the subclass, pIgA with a well-characterized glycan composition (Tomana et al. 1976; Endoh et al. 1994) is cleared from plasma at the same rate, and the liver was by far the most important organ in the IgA uptake. Furthermore, the uptake of human IgA1 and IgA2 myeloma proteins by human hepatoma cell line HepG2, which expresses ASGP-R, indicated a binding preference of pIgA1 > SC > mIgA1 >

pIgA2 (Tomana et al. 1988). Recently, Rifai et al. (2000) demonstrated that the clearance of *human* IgA proteins from *murine* circulation depends on their subclass. Although IgA2 was cleared by the liver and hepatic ASGP-R, only a small percentage of IgA1 was cleared through this pathway; apparently an alternative, ASGP-R-independent pathway may be involved. However, it is conceivable that the remarkable heterogeneity in the glycosylation patterns (with respect to the number of *N*-linked and *O*-linked chains, presence of truncated forms, glycosylation of V_H or even V_L domains) of IgA proteins of the same subclass and even of a single myeloma protein, as well as species-specific differences (mice vs. monkeys and human Hep G2 cells) may account for this variance.

Thus the liver is involved in catabolism of circulatory Ig, including pIgA and mIgA (Stockert et al. 1982; Moldoveanu et al. 1988, 1990; Tomana et al. 1988). In humans only negligible amounts (about 1 mg/kg per day) of the total IgA produced in the bone marrow, spleen, and lymph nodes (about 20 mg/kg per day) reach the external secretions and are not catabolized (Delacroix and Vaerman 1983; Conley and Delacroix 1987).

REFERENCES

Abel, C. A., and Grey, H. M. (1968). Studies on the structure of mouse γA myeloma proteins. *Biochemistry* 1, 2682–2688.

Adamski, F. M., and Demmer, J. (1999). Two stages of increased IgA transfer during lactation in the marsupial, *Trichosurus vulpecula* (Brushtail possum). *J. Immunol.* 162, 6009–6015.

Adlerberth, I., Ahrne, S., Johansson, M. L., Molin, G., Hanson, L. A., and Wold, A. E. (1996). A mannose-specific adherence mechanism in *Lactobacillus plantarum* conferring binding to the human colonic cell line HT-29. *Appl. Environ. Microbiol.* 62, 2244–2251.

Alley, C. D., Nash, G. S., and MacDermott, R. P. (1982). Marked *in vitro* spontaneous secretion of IgA by human rib bone marrow mononuclear cells. *J. Immunol.* 128, 2604–2608.

Altorfer, J., Hardesty, S. J., Scott, J. H., and Jones, A. L. (1987). Specific antibody synthesis and biliary secretion by the rat liver and intestinal immunization with cholera toxin. *Gastroenterology* 93, 539–549.

Arnold, R. R., Cole, M. F., Prince, S., and McGhee, J. R. (1977). Secretory IgM antibodies to *Streptococcus mutans* in subjects with selective IgA deficiency. *Clin. Immunol. Immunopathol.* 8, 475–486.

Ashwell, G., and Harford, J. (1982). Carbohydrate-specific receptor of the liver. *Annu. Rev. Biochem.* 52, 531–554.

Atkin, J. D., Pleass, R. J., Owens, R. J., and Woof, J. M. (1996). Mutagenesis of the human IgA1 heavy chain tailpiece that prevents dimer assembly. *J. Immunol.* 157, 156–159.

Aucouturier, P., Duarte, F., Mihaesco, E., Pineau, N., and Preud'homme, J. L. (1988). Jacalin, the human IgA1 and IgD precipitating lectin, also binds IgA2 of both allotypes. *J. Immunol. Methods* 113, 185–191.

Aucouturier, P., Pineau, N., Kobayashi, K., and Preud'homme, J. L. (1989). Methodological pitfalls in immunoglobulin subclass assays: An investigation of anti-Ig subclass monoclonal antibody and jacalin reactivity. *Protides Biol. Fluids* 36, 61–69.

Baenziger, J. (1979). Structure of the oligosaccharide of human J chain. *J. Biol. Chem.* 254, 4063–4071.

Baenziger, J., and Kornfeld, S. (1974a). Structure of the carbohydrate units of IgA1 immunoglobulin. I. Composition, glycopeptide isolation, and structure of the asparagine-linked oligosaccharide units. *J. Biol. Chem.* 249, 7260–7269.

Baenziger, J., and Kornfeld, S. (1974b). Structure of the carbohydrate units of IgA1 immunoglobulin. II. Structure of the O-glycosidically linked oligosaccharide units. *J. Biol. Chem.* 249, 7270–7281.

Bakos, M. A., Kurosky, A., and Goldblum, R. M. (1991). Characterization of a critical binding site for human polymeric Ig on secretory component. *J. Immunol.* 147, 3419–3426.

Banting, G., Brake, B., Braghetta, P., Luzio, J. P., and Stanley, K. K. (1989). Intracellular targetting signals of polymeric immunoglobulin receptors are highly conserved between species. *FEBS Lett.* 254, 177–183.

Bastian, A., Kratzin, H., Eckart, K., and Hilschmann, N. (1992). Intra- and interchain disulfide bridges of the human J chain in secretory immunoglobulin A. *Hoppe-Seyler's Z. Biol. Chem.* 373, 1255–1263.

Belov, K., Zenger, K. R., Hellman, L., and Cooper, D. W. (2002). Echidna IgA supports mammalian unity and traditional Therian relationship. *Mamm. Genome* 13, 656–663.

Bertrand, F. E. 3rd, Billips, L. G., Gartland, G. L., Kubagawa, H., and Schroeder, H. W., Jr. (1996). The J chain gene is transcribed during B and T lymphopoiesis in humans. *J. Immunol.* 156, 4240–4244.

Biewenga, J., Hiemstra, P. S., Steneker, I., and Daha, M. R. (1989). Binding of human IgA1 and IgA1 fragments to jacalin. *Mol. Immunol.* 26, 275–281.

Björk, I., and Lindh, E. (1974). Gross conformation of human secretory immunoglobulin A and its component parts. *Eur. J. Biochem.* 45, 135–145.

Bloth, B., and Svehag, S. E. (1971). Further studies on the ultrastructure of dimeric IgA of human origin. *J. Exp. Med.* 133, 1035–1042.

Boehm, M. K., Woof, J. M., Kerr, M. A., and Perkins, S. J. (1999). The Fab and Fc fragments of IgA1 exhibit a different arrangement from that in IgG: A study by X-ray and neutron solution scattering and homology modelling. *J. Mol. Biol.* 286, 1421–1447.

Boursier, L., Dunn-Walters, D. K., and Spencer, J. (1999). Characteristics of IgVH genes used by human intestinal plasma cells from childhood. *Immunology* 97, 558–564.

Bouvet, J.-P., Pieres, R., Iscaki, S., and Pillot, J. (1987). IgM reassociation in the absence of J chain. *Immunol. Lett.* 15, 27–31.

Braathen, R., Sørensen, V., Brandtzaeg, P., Sandlie, I., and Johansen, F. E. (2002). The carboxyl-terminal domains of IgA and IgM direct isotype-specific polymerization and interaction with the polymeric immunoglobulin receptor. *J. Biol. Chem.* 277, 42755–42762.

Brandtzaeg, P. (1973). Two types of IgA immunocytes in man. *Nature New Biol.* 243, 142–143.

Brandtzaeg, P. (1978). Polymeric IgA is complexed with secretory component (SC) on the surface of human intestinal epithelial cells. *Scand. J. Immunol.* 8, 39–52.

Brandtzaeg, P. (1981). Transport models for secretory IgA and secretory IgM. *Clin. Exp. Immunol.* 44, 221–232.

Brandtzaeg, P. (1983). Immunohistochemical characterization of intracellular J-chain and binding site for secretory component (SC) in human immunoglobulin (Ig)-producing cells. *Mol. Immunol.* 20, 941–966.

Brandtzaeg, P. (1985). The role of J chain and secretory component in receptor-mediated glandular and hepatic transport of immunoglobulins in man. *Scand. J. Immunol.* 22, 111–146.

Brandtzaeg, P., and Prydz, H. (1984). Direct evidence for an integrated function of J chain and secretory component in epithelial transport of immunoglobulins. *Nature* 311, 71–73.

Brandtzaeg, P., Fjellanger, I., and Gjeruldsen, S. T. (1968). Immunoglobulin M: Local synthesis and selective secretion in patients with immunoglobulin A deficiency. *Science* 160, 789–791.

Brandtzaeg, P., Fjellanger, I., and Gjeruldsen, S. T. (1970). Human secretory immunoglobulins. I. Salivary secretions from individuals with normal or low levels of serum immunoglobulins. *Scand. J. Immunol.* S12, 3–83.

Brandtzaeg, P., Kelt, K., Rognum, T. O., Söderström, R., Björkander, J., Söderström, T., Petrusson, B., and Hanson, L. A. (1986). Distribution of mucosal IgA and IgG subclass-producing immunocytes and alterations in various disorders. *Monogr. Allergy* 20, 179–194.

Brandtzaeg, P., Farstad, I. N., Johansen, F. E., Morton, H. C., Norderhaug, I. N., and Yamanaka, T. (1999). The B-cell system of human mucosae and exocrine glands. *Immunol. Rev.* 171, 45–87.

Brewer, J. W., and Corley, R. B. (1997). Late events in assembly determine the polymeric structure and biological activity of secretory IgM. *Mol. Immunol.* 34, 323–331.

Brewer, J. W., Randall, T. D., Parkhouse, R. M. E., and Corley, R. B. (1994). IgM hexamers? *Immunol. Today* 15, 165–168.

Brown, T. A., and Mestecky, J. (1985). Immunoglobulin A subclass distribution of naturally occurring salivary antibodies to microbial antigens. *Infect. Immun.* 49, 459–462.

Brown, T. A., Murphy, B. R., Radl, J., Haaijman, J. J., and Mestecky, J. (1985). Subclass distribution and molecular form of immunoglobulin A hemagglutinin antibodies in sera and nasal secretions after experimental secondary infection with influenza A virus in humans. *J. Clin. Microbiol.* 22, 259–264.

Brown, W. R., and Butler, J. E. (1994). Characterization of a Cα gene of swine. *Mol. Immunol.* 31, 633–642.

Brown, W. R., and Kloppel, T. M. (1989). The liver and IgA: Immunological, cell biological and clinical implications. *Hepatology* 9, 763–784.

Brown, W. R., Borthisle, B. K., and Chen, S. T. (1975). Immunoglobulin E (IgE) and IgE-containing cells in human gastrointestinal fluids and tissues. *Clin. Exp. Immunol.* 20, 227–237.

Brown, W. R., Newcomb, R. W., and Ishizaka, K. (1970). Proteolytic degradation of exocrine and serum immunoglobulins. *J. Clin. Invest.* 49, 1374–1380.

Brown, W. R., Rabbani, H., Butler, J. E., and Hammarström, L. (1997). Characterization of the bovine Cα gene. *Immunology* 91, 1–6.

Burnett, D., Crocker, J., and Stockley, R. A. (1987). Cells containing IgA subclasses in bronchi of subjects with and without chronic obstructive lung disease. *J. Clin. Pathol.* 40, 1217–1220.

Burnett, R. C., Hanley, W. C., Zhai, S. K., and Knight, K. L. (1989). The IgA heavy-chain gene family in rabbit: Cloning and sequence analysis of 13 Cα genes. *EMBO J.* 8, 4041–4047.

Butler, J. E. (1983). Bovine immunoglobulins: An augmented review. *Vet. Immunol. Immunopathol.* 4, 43–152.

Buxbaum, J. N., Zolla, S., Scharff, M. D., and Franklin, E. C. (1974). The synthesis and assembly of immunoglobulins by malignant human plasmocytes. III. Heterogeneity of IgA polymer assembly. *Eur. J. Immunol.* 4, 367–369.

Cattaneo, A., and Neuberger, M. S. (1987). Polymeric immunoglobulin M is secreted by transfectants of non-lymphoid cells in the absence of immunoglobulin J chain. *EMBO J.* 112, 1401–1406.

Chintalacharuvu, K. R., and Morrison, S. L. (1996). Residues critical for H-L disulfide bond formation in human IgA1 and IgA2. *J. Immunol.* 157, 3443–3449.

Chintalacharuvu, K. R., Raines, M., and Morrison, S. L. (1994). Divergence of human α-chain constant region gene sequences: A novel recombinant α2 gene. *J. Immunol.* 152, 5299–5304.

Chuang, P. D., and Morrison, S. L. (1997). Elimination of N-linked glycosylation sites from the human IgA1 constant region: Effects on structure and function. *J. Immunol.* 158, 724–732.

Conley, M. E., and Delacroix, D. L. (1987). Intravascular and mucosal immunoglobulin A: Two separate but related systems of immune defense? *Ann. Intern. Med.* 106, 892–899.

Crago, S. S., Kulhavy, R., Prince, S. J., and Mestecky, J. (1978). Secretory component of epithelial cells is a surface receptor for polymeric immunoglobulins. *J. Exp. Med.* 147, 1832–1837.

Crago, S. S., Kutteh, W. H., Moro, I., Allansmith, M. R., Radl, J., Haaijman, J. J., and Mestecky, J. (1984). Distribution of IgA1-, IgA2- and J chain-containing cells in human tissues. *J. Immunol.* 132, 16–18.

Crottet, P., and Corthesy, B. (1998). Secretory component delays the conversion of secretory IgA into antigen-binding competent F(ab')₂: A possible implication for mucosal defense. *J. Immunol.* 161, 5445–5453.

Davies, A. C., Roux, K. H., Pursey, J., and Shulman, M. J. (1989). Intermolecular disulfide bonding in IgM: Effect of replacing cysteine residues in the μ heavy chain. *EMBO J.* 8, 2519–2526.

Delacroix, D. L., and Vaerman, J.-P. (1981). A solid phase, direct competition, radioimmunoassay for quantitation of secretory IgA in human serum. *J. Immunol. Methods* 40, 345–358.

Delacroix, D. L., and Vaerman, J.-P. (1983). Function of the human liver in IgA homeostasis in plasma. *Ann. N.Y. Acad. Sci.* 409, 383–401.

Delacroix, D. L., Dive, C., Rambaud, J. C., and Vaerman, J. P. (1982). IgA subclasses in various secretions and in serum. *Immunology* 47, 383–385.

Delacroix, D. L., Furtado-Barreira, G., de Hemptinne, B., Goudswaard, J., Dive, C., and Vaerman, J.-P. (1983). The liver in the IgA secretory immune system: Dogs, but not rats and rabbits, are suitable models for human studies. *Hepatology* 3, 980–988.

Dourmashkin, R. R., Virella, G., and Parkhouse, R. M. (1971). Electron microscopy of human and mouse myeloma serum IgA. *J. Mol. Biol.* 56, 207–208.

Dudich, E. I., Dudich, I. V., and Timofeev, V. P. (1980). Fluorescence polarization and spin-label study of human myeloma immunoglobulins A and M: Presence of segmental flexibility. *Mol. Immunol.* 17, 1335–1339.

Dunn-Walters, D., Boursier, L., and Spencer, J. (2000). Effect of somatic hypermutation on potential *N*-glycosylation sites in human immunoglobulin heavy chain variable regions. *Mol. Immunol.* 37, 107–113.

Eiffert, H., Quentin, E., Decker, J., Hillmeir, S., Hufschmidt, M., Klingmuller, D., Weber, M. H., and Hilschmann, N. (1984). The primary structure of the human free secretory component and the arrangement of the disulfide bonds. *Hoppe-Seyler's Z. Physiol. Chem.* 365, 1489–1495.

Eiffert, H., Quentin, E., Wiederhold, M., Hillemeir, S., Decker, J., Weber, M., and Hilschmann, N. (1991). Determination of the molecular structure of the human free secretory component. *Hoppe-Seyler's Z. Biol. Chem.* 372, 119–128.

Emilie, D., Karray, S., Merle-Beral, H., Debre, P., and Galanaud, P. (1988). Induction of differentiation in human leukemic B cells by interleukin 2 alone: Differential effect on the expression of μ and J chain genes. *Eur. J. Immunol.* 18, 1479–1483.

Endo, T., Mestecky, J., Kulhavy, R., and Kobata, A. (1994). Carbohydrate heterogeneity of human myeloma proteins of the IgA1 and IgA2 subclasses. *Mol. Immunol.* 31, 1415–1422.

Erlandsson, L., Andersson, K., Sigvardsson, M., Lycke, N., and Leanderson, T. (1998). Mice with an inactivated joining chain locus have perturbed IgM secretion. *Eur. J. Immunol.* 28, 2355–2365.

Erlandsson, L., Akerblad, P., Vingsbo-Lundberg, C., Kallberg, E., Lycke, N., and Leanderson, T. (2001). Joining chain-expressing and -nonexpressing B cell populations in the mouse. *J. Exp. Med.* 194, 557–570.

Fallgren-Gebauer, E., Gebauer, W., Bastian, A., Kratzin, H., Eiffert, H., Zimmerman, B., Karas, M., and Hilschmann, N. (1995). The covalent linkage of the secretory component to IgA. *Adv. Exp. Med. Biol.* 371A, 625–628.

Fazel, S., Wiersma, E. J., and Shulman, M. J. (1997). Interplay of J chain and disulfide bonding in assembly of polymeric IgM. *Int. Immunol.* 9, 1149–1158.

Feinstein, A., Munn, E., and Richardson, N. (1971). The three-dimensional conformation of γM and γA globulin molecules. *Ann. N.Y. Acad. Sci.* 190, 104–121.

Field, M. C., Dwek, R. A., Edge, C. J., and Rademacher, T. W. (1989). *O*-linked oligosaccharides from human serum immunoglobulin A1. *Biochem. Soc. Trans.* 17, 1034–1035.

Field, M. C., Amatayakul-Chantler, S., Rademacher, T. W., Rudd, P. M., and Dwek, R. A. (1994). Structural analysis of the *N*-glycans from human serum immunoglobulin A1: Comparison of normal human serum immunoglobulin A1 with that isolated from patients with rheumatoid arthritis. *Biochem. J.* 299, 261–275.

Frutiger, S., Hughes, G. J., Hanly, W. C., and Kingzette, M., and Jaton, J.-C. (1986). The amino-terminal domain of rabbit secretory component is responsible for noncovalent binding to immunoglobulin A dimers. *J. Biol. Chem.* 261, 16,673–16,681.

Frutiger, S., Hughes, G. J., Fonck, C., and Jaton, J.-C. (1987). High and low molecular weight rabbit secretory components. *J. Biol. Chem.* 262, 1712–1715.

Frutiger, S., Hughes, G. J., Hanly, W. C., and Jaton, J.-C. (1988). Rabbit secretory components of different allotypes vary in their carbohydrate content and their sites of N-linked glycosylation. *J. Biol. Chem.* 263, 812–8125.

Frutiger, S., Hughes, G. I., Paquet, N., Luthy, R., and Jaton, J.-C. (1992). Disulfide bond assignment in human J chain and its covalent pairing with immunoglobulin M. *Biochemistry* 31, 12,643–12,647.

Furtado, P. B., Whitty, P. W., Robertson, A., Eaton, J. T., Almogren, A., Kerr, M. A., Woof, J. M., and Perkins, S. J. (2004). Solution structure determination of monomeric human IgA2 by x-ray and neutron scattering, analytical ultracentrifugation and constrained modeling: a comparison with monomeric human IgA1. *J. Mol. Biol.* 338, 921–941.

Gala, F. A., and Morrison, S. L. (2002). The role of constant region carbohydrate in the assembly and secretion of human IgD and IgA1. *J. Biol. Chem.* 277, 29005–29011.

Garcia-Pardo, A., Lamm, M. E., Plaut, A. G., and Frangione, B. (1979). Secretory component is covalently bound to a single subunit in human secretory IgA. *Mol. Immunol.* 16, 477–482.

Garcia-Pardo, A., Lamm, M. E., Plaut, A. G., and Frangione, B. (1981). J chain is covalently bound to both monomer subunits in human secretory IgA. *J. Biol. Chem.* 256, 11,734–11,738.

Geneste, C., Iscaki, S., Mangalo, R., and Pillot, J. (1986). Both Fcα domains of human IgA are involved in *in vitro* interaction between secretory component and dimeric IgA. *Immunol. Lett.* 13, 221–226.

Grey, H. M., Abel, C. A., Yount, W. J., and Kunkel, H. G. (1968). A subclass of human γA-globulins (γA2) which lacks the disulfide bonds linking heavy and light chains. *J. Exp. Med.* 128, 1223–1236.

Guddat, L. W., Herron, J. N., and Edmundson, A. B. (1993). Three-dimensional structure of a human immunoglobulin with a hinge deletion. *Proc. Natl. Acad. Sci. USA* 90, 4271–4275.

Hajdu, I., Moldoveanu, Z., Cooper, M. D., and Mestecky, J. (1983). Ultrastructural studies of human lymphoid cells. μ and J chain expression as a function of B cell differentiation. *J. Exp. Med.* 158, 1993–2006.

Halpren, M. S., and Koshland, M. E. (1970). Novel subunit of secretory IgA. *Nature* 228, 1276–1278.

Halpern, M. S., and Koshland, M. E. (1973). The stoichiometry of J chain in human secretory IgA. *J. Immunol.* 111, 1653–1660.

Hammerström, L., and Smith, C. I. E. (1986). IgG subclass changes in response to vaccination. *Monogr. Allergy* 19, 241–252.

Hanson, L. A. (1961). Comparative immunological studies of the immune globulins of human milk and of blood serum. *Int. Arch. Allergy Appl. Immunol.* 18, 241–267.

Heilman, C., Barington, T., and Sigsgaard, T. (1988). Subclass of individual IgA-secreting human lymphocytes: Investigation of *in vivo* pneumococcal polysaccharide-induced and *in vitro* mitogen-induced blood B cells by monolayer plaque-forming cell assay. *J. Immunol.* 140, 1496–1499.

Hendrickson, B. A., Conner, D. A., Ladd, D. J., Kendall, D., Casanova, J. E., Corthesy, B., Max, E. E., Neutra, M. R., Seidman, C. E., and Seidman, J. G. (1995). Altered hepatic transport of immunoglobulin A in mice lacking the J chain. *J. Exp. Med.* 182, 1905–1911.

Hendrickson, B. A., Rindisbacher, L., Corthesy, B., Kendall, D., Waltz, D. A., Neutra, M. R., and Seidman, J. G. (1996). Lack of association of secretory component with IgA in J chain-deficient mice. *J. Immunol.* 157, 750–754.

Heremans, J. F. (1974). Immunoglobulin A. In *The Antigens*, vol. 2 (ed. M. Sela), 365–522. New York: Academic Press.

Herr, A. B., Ballister, E. R., and Bjorkman, P. J. (2003). Insights into IgA-mediated immune responses from the crystal structures of human FcαRI and its complex with IgA1-Fc. *Nature* 423, 614–620.

Hexham, J. M., White, K. D., Carayannopoulos, L. N., Mandecki, W., Brisette, R., Yang, Y.-S., and Capra, J. D. A human immunoglobulin (Ig) A Cα3 domain motif directs polymeric Ig receptor-mediated secretion. *J. Exp. Med.* 189, 747–751.

Hijmans, W. (1987). Circulating IgA in humans. *Adv. Exp. Med. Biol.* 216B, 1169–1174.

Hiki, Y., Horii, A., Iwase, H., Tanaka, A., Toda, Y., Hotta, K., and Kobayashi, Y. (1995). O-linked oligosaccharide on IgA1 hinge region in IgA nephropathy: Fundamental study for precise structure and possible roles. *Contrib. Nephrol.* 111, 73–84.

Hohman, V. S., Stewart, S. E., Willett, C. E., and Steiner, L. A. (1997). Sequence and expression pattern of J chain in the amphibian *Xenopus laevis. Mol. Immunol.* 34, 995–1002.

Hohman, V. S., Stewart, S. E., Rumfelt, L. L., Greenberg, A. S., Avila, D. W., Flajnik, M. F., and Steiner, L. A. (2003). J chain in the nurse shark: Implications for function in a lower vertebrate. *J. Immunol.* 170, 6016–6023.

Hortin, G. L. (1990). Isolation of glycopeptides containing O-linked oligosaccharides by lectin affinity chromatography on jacalin-agarose. *Analyt. Biochem.* 191, 262–267.

Hughes, G. J., Frutiger, S., Paquet, N., and Jaton, J.-C. (1990). The amino acid sequence of rabbit J chain in secretory immunoglobulin A. *Biochem. J.* 271, 641–647.

Hughes, G. J., Reason, A. J., Savoy, L., Jaton, J., and Frutiger-Hughes, S. (1999). Carbohydrate moieties in human secretory component. *Biochim. Biophys. Acta* 1434, 86–93.

Hughey, C. T., Brewer, J. W., Colosia, A. D., Rosse, W. F., and Corley, R. B. (1998). Production of IgM hexamers by normal and autoimmune B cells: Implications for the physiologic role of hexameric IgM. *J. Immunol.* 161, 4091–4097.

Inman, F. P., and Mestecky, J. (1974). The J chain of polymeric immunoglobulins. *Contemp. Top. Mol. Immunol.* 3, 111–141.

Iscaki, S., Geneste, C., d'Azambuja, S., and Pillot, J. (1979). Human secretory component. II. Easy detection of abnormal amounts of combined secretory component in human sera. *J. Immunol. Methods* 28, 331–339.

Iwata, A., Iwase, T., Ogura, Y., Takahashi, T., Matsumoto, N., Yoshida, T., Kamei, N., Kobayashi, K., Mestecky, J., and Moro, I. (2002). Cloning and expression of the turtle (*Trachemys scripta*) immunoglobulin joining (J)-chain cDNA. *Immunogenetics* 54, 513–519.

Jackson, G. D. F., Lemaitre-Coelho, I., Vaerman, J. P., Bazin, H., and Beckers, A. (1978). Rapid disappearance from serum of intravenously injected rat myeloma IgA and its secretion into bile. *Eur. J. Immunol.* 8, 123–126.

Jerry, L. M., and Kunkel, H. G. (1974). Special characteristics of the IgA2 subclass. *Adv. Exp. Med. Biol.* 45, 151–160.

Johansen, F. E., Braathen, R., and Brandtzaeg, P. (2000). Role of J chain in secretory immunoglobulin formation. *Scand. J. Immunol.* 52, 240–248.

Johansen, F. E., Braathen, R., and Brandtzaeg, P. (2001). The J chain is essential for polymeric Ig receptor-mediated epithelial transport of IgA. *J. Immunol.* 167, 5185–5192.

Jonard, P. P., Rambaud, J. C., Dive, C., Vaerman, J. P., Galian, A., and Delacroix, D. L. (1984). Secretion of immunoglobulins and plasma proteins from jejunal mucosa. *J. Clin. Invest.* 74, 525–535.

Kaartinen, M., Imir, T., Klockars, M., Sandholm, M., and Mäkela, O. (1978). IgA in blood and thoracic duct lymph: Concentration and degree of polymerization. *Scand. J. Immunol.* 7, 229–232.

Kabir, S. (1998). Jacalin: A jackfruit (*Artocarpus heterophyllus*) seed-derived lectin of versatile applications in immunobiological research. *J. Immunol. Methods* 212, 193–211.

Kaetzel, C. S., Robinson, J. K., Chintalacharuvu, K. R., Vaerman, J. P., and Lamm, M. E. (1991). The polymeric immunoglobulin receptor (secretory component) mediates transport of immune complexes across epithelial cells: A local defense function for IgA. *Proc. Natl. Acad. Sci. USA* 88, 8796–8800.

Kawamura, S., Omoto, K., and Ueda, S. (1990). Evolutionary hypervariability in the hinge region of the immunoglobulin α gene. *J. Mol. Biol.* 215, 201–206.

Kawamura, S., Tanabe, H., Watanabe, Y., Kurosaki, K., Saitou, N., and Ueda, S. (1991). Evolutionary rate of immunoglobulin α noncoding region is greater in hominoids than in Old World monkeys. *Mol. Biol. Evol.* 8, 743–752.

Kawamura, S., Saitou, N., and Ueda, S. (1992). Concerted evolution of the primate immunoglobulin α-gene through gene conversion. *J. Biol. Chem.* 267, 7359–7367.

Kett, K., Brandtzaeg, P., Radl, J., and Haaijman, J. J. (1986). Different subclass distribution of IgA-producing cells in human lymphoid organs and various secretory tissues. *J. Immunol.* 136, 3631–3635.

Knight, K. L., Martens, C. L., Stoklosa, C., and Schneiderman, R. D. (1984). Genes encoding α-heavy chains of rabbit IgA: Characterization of cDNA encoding IgA-γ subclass α-chains. *Nucleic Acids Res.* 12, 1657–1670.

Kobayashi, K., Vaerman, J.-P., Bazin, H., Lebacq-Verheyden, A.-M., and Heremans, J. F. (1973). Identification of J-chain in polymeric immunoglobulins from a variety of species by crossreaction with rabbit antisera to human J-chain. *J. Immunol.* 111, 1590–1594.

Koshland, M. E., Chapuis, R. M., Recht, B., and Brown, J. C. (1977). Selective proteolysis of the J chain component in human polymeric immunoglobulin. *J. Immunol.* 118, 775–781.

Koshland, M. E. (1985). The coming of age of the immunoglobulin J chain. *Annu. Rev. Immunol.* 3, 425–453.

Kratzin, H., Altevogt, P., Ruban, E., Kortt, A., Staroscik, K., and Hilschmann, N. (1975). The primary structure of a monoclonal IgA-immunoglobulin (IgA Tro.). II. The amino acid sequence of the H-chain, α-type, subgroup III; structure of the complete IgA-molecule. *Hoppe-Seyler's Z. Physiol. Chem.* 356, 1337–1342.

Krugmann, S., Pleass, R. J., Atkin, J. D., and Woof, J. M. (1997). Structural requirements for assembly of dimeric IgA probed by site-directed mutagenesis of J chain and a cysteine residue of the α chain CH2 domain. *J. Immunol.* 159, 244–249.

Kubagawa, H., Burrows, P. D., Grossi, C. E., Mestecky, J., and Cooper, M. D. (1988). Precursor B cells transformed by Epstein-Barr virus undergo sterile plasma-cell differentiation: J chain expression without immunoglobulin. *Proc. Natl. Acad. Sci. USA* 85, 875–879.

Kulseth, M. A., and Rogne, S. (1994). Cloning and characterization of the bovine immunoglobulin J chain cDNA and its promoter region. *DNA Cell Biol.* 13, 37–42.

Kulseth, M. A., Krajci, P., Myklebost, O., and Rogne, S. (1995). Cloning and characterization of two forms of bovine polymeric immunoglobulin receptor cDNA. *DNA Cell. Biol.* 14, 251–256.

Kutteh, W. H., Prince, S. J., and Mestecky, J. (1982a). Tissue origins of human polymeric and monomeric IgA. *J. Immunol.* 128, 990–995.

Kutteh, W. H., Prince, S. J., Phillips, J. O., Spenny, J. G., and Mestecky, J. (1982b). Properties of immunoglobulin A in serum of individuals with liver diseases and in hepatic bile. *Gastroenterology* 82, 184–193.

Kutteh, W. H., Moldoveanu, Z., Prince, S. J., Kulhavy, R., Alonso, F., and Mestecky, J. (1983). Biosynthesis of J-chain in human lymphoid cells producing immunoglobulins of various isotypes. *Mol. Immunol.* 20, 967–976.

Kutteh, W. H., Hatch, K. D., Blackwell, R. E., and Mestecky, J. (1988). Secretory immune system of the female reproductive tract: I. Immunoglobulin and secretory component-containing cells. *Obstet. Gynecol.* 71, 56–60.

Kutteh, W., Hammond, K., Prince, S., Wester, R., and Mestecky, J. (1993). Production of immunoglobulin A by the cerix of the human female genital tract. In *Reproductive Immunology* (eds. F. Dondero and P.M. Johnson), vol. 97:151–158. New York: Raven Press.

Kutteh, W. H., Prince, S. J., Hammonds, K. R., Kutteh, C. C., and Mestecky, J. (1996). Variations in immunoglobulins and IgA subclasses of human uterine cervical secretions around the time of ovulation. *Clin. Exp. Immunol.* 104, 538–542.

Kvale, D., and Brandtzaeg, D. (1986). An enzyme-linked immunosorbent assay for differential quantitation of secretory immunoglobulins of the A and M isotypes in human serum. *J. Immunol. Methods.* 86, 107–114.

Ladjeva, I., Peterman, J. H., and Mestecky, J. (1989). IgA subclasses of human colostral antibodies specific for microbial and food antigens. *Clin. Exp. Immunol.* 78, 85–90.

Leslie, G. A., and Teramura, G. (1977). Structure and biological functions of human IgD. XIV. The development of a solid-phase radioimmunoassay for the quantitation of IgD in human sera and secretions. *Int. Arch. Allergy Appl. Immunol.* 54, 451–456.

Lindh, E. (1975). Increased resistance of immunoglobulin A dimers to proteolytic degradation after binding of secretory component. *J. Immunol.* 114, 284–286.

Liu, B. M., Cheung, H. C., and Mestecky, J. (1981). Nanosecond fluorescence spectroscopy of human immunoglobulin A. *Biochemistry* 20, 1997–2003.

Low, T. L. K., Liu, Y.-S. V., and Putnam, F. W. (1976). Structure, function, and evolutionary relationships of Fc domains of human immunoglobulins A, G, M, and E. *Science* 191, 390–392.

Lue, C., Tarkowski, A., and Mestecky, J. (1988). Systemic immunization with pneumococcal polysaccharide vaccine induces predominant IgA2 response of peripheral blood lymphocytes and increases of both serum and secretory anti-pneumococcal antibodies. *J. Immunol.* 140, 3793–3800.

Lundqvist, M. L., Middleton, D. L., Hazard, S., and Warr, G. W. (2001). The immunoglobulin heavy chain locus of the duck: Genomic organization and expression of D, J, and C region genes. *J. Biol. Chem.* 276, 46729–46736.

Lycke, N., Erlandsson, L., Ekman, L., Schon, K., and Leanderson, T. (1999). Lack of J chain inhibits the transport of gut IgA and abrogates the development of intestinal antitoxic protection. *J. Immunol.* 163, 913–919.

Mach, J. P. (1970). *In vitro* combination of human and bovine secretory component with IgA of various species. *Nature* 228, 1278–1282.

Manning, R. J., Walker, P. G., Carter. L., Barrington, P. J., and Jackson, G. D. F. (1984). Studies on the origins of biliary immunoglobulins in rats. *Gastroenterology* 87, 173–179.

Mansikka, A. (1992). Chicken IgA H chains. *J. Immunol.* 149, 855–861.

Matsui, K., Nakanishi, K., Cohen, D. I., Hada, T., Furuyama, J., Hamaoka, T., and Higashino, K. (1989). B cell response pathways regulated by IL-5 and IL-2. Secretory μH chain-mRNA and J chain mRNA expression are separately controlled events. *J. Immunol.* 142, 2918–2923.

Matsunuchi, L., Cann, G. M., and Koshland, M. E. (1986). Immunoglobulin J chain gene from the mouse. *Proc. Natl. Acad. Sci. USA* 83, 456–460.

Mattu, T. S., Pleass, R. J., Willis, A. C., Kilian, M., Wormald, M. R., Lellouch, A. C., Rudd, P. M., Woof, J. M., and Dwek, R. A. (1998). The glycosylation and structure of human serum IgA1, Fab and Fc regions and the role of *N*-glycosylation on Fcα receptor interactions. *J. Biol. Chem.* 273, 2260–2272.

Max, E. E., and Korsmeyer, J. S. (1985). Human J chain gene: Structure and expression in B lymphoid cells. *J. Exp. Med.* 161, 832–849.

Max, E. E., Jakan, N., Yi, H., and McBride, W. O. (1994). A processed J chain pseudogene on human chromosome 8 that is shared by several primate species. *Mol. Immunol.* 31, 1029–1036.

McCune, J. M., Fu, S. M., and Kunkel, H. G. (1981). J chain biosynthesis in pre-B cells and other possible precursors of B cells. *J. Exp. Med.* 154, 138–145.

McGhee, J. R., Mestecky, J., Elson, C. O., and Kiyono, H. (1989). Regulation of IgA synthesis and immune responses by T cells and interleukins. *J. Clin. Immunol.* 9, 175–199.

Mestecky, J., and McGhee, J. R. (1987). Immunoglobulin A (IgA): Molecular and cellular interactions involved in IgA biosynthesis and immune response. *Adv. Immunol.* 40, 153–245.

Mestecky, J., and Russell, M. W. (1986). IgA subclasses. *Monogr. Allergy* 19, 277–301.

Mestecky, J., and Schrohenloher, R. E. (1974). Site of attachment of J chain to human immunoglobulin M. *Nature* 249, 650–652.

Mestecky, J., Kraus, F. W., and Voight, S. A. (1970). Proportion of human colostral immunoglobulin-A molecules containing the secretory determinant. *Immunology* 18, 237–243.

Mestecky, J., Zikan, J., and Butler, W. T. (1971). Immunoglobulin M and secretory immunoglobulin A: Presence of a common polypeptide chain different from light chains. *Science* 171, 1163–1165.

Mestecky, J., Kulhavy, R., and Kraus, F. W. (1972). Studies on human secretory immunoglobulin A. II. Subunit structure. *J. Immunol.* 108, 738–747.

Mestecky, J., Schrohenloher, R. E., Kulhavy, R., Wright, G. P., and Tomana, M. (1974a). Association of S-IgA subunits. *Adv. Exp. Med. Biol.* 45, 99–109.

Mestecky, J., Schrohenloher, R. E., Kulhavy, R., Wright, G. P., and Tomana, M. (1974b). Site of J chain attachment to human polymeric IgA. *Proc. Natl. Acad. Sci. USA* 71, 544–548.

Mestecky, J., Kulhavy, R., Wright, G. P., and Tomana, M. (1974c). Studies on human secretory immunoglobulin A. VI. Cyanogen bromide cleavage. *J. Immunol.* 113, 404–412.

Mestecky, J., Winchester, R. J., Hoffman, T., and Kunkel, H. G. (1977). Parallel synthesis of immunoglobulins and J chain in pokeweed mitogen-stimulated normal cells and in lymphoblastoid cell lines. *J. Exp. Med.* 145, 760–765.

Mestecky, J., Preud'homme, J.-L., Crago, S. S., Mihaesco, E., Prchal, J. T., and Okos, A. J. (1980). Presence of J chain in human lymphoid cells. *Clin. Exp. Immunol.* 39, 371–385.

Mestecky, J., Russell, M. W., Jackson, S., and Brown, T. A. (1986). The human IgA system: A reassessment. *Clin. Immunol. Immunopathol.* 40, 105–114.

Mestecky, J., Lue, C., Tarkowski, A., Ladjeva, I., Peterman, J. H., Moldoveanu, Z., Russell, M. W., Brown, T. A., Radl, J., Haaijman, J. J., Kiyono, H., and McGhee, J. R. (1989). Comparative studies of the biological properties of human IgA subclasses. *Protides Biol. Fluids* 36, 173–182.

Mestecky, J., Moldoveanu, Z., Julian, B. A., and Prchal, J. T. (1990). J chain disease: A novel form of plasma cell dyscrasia. *Am. J. Med.* 88, 411–416.

Mestecky, J., Lue, C., and Russell, M. W. (1991). Selective transport of IgA: Cellular and molecular aspects. *Gastroenterol. Clin. North Am.* 20, 441–471.

Mestecky, J., Moro, I., Moldoveanu, Z., Takahashi, T., Iwase, T., Kubagawa, H., and Cooper, M. D. (1997). Immunoglobulin J chain: Early differentiation marker of human B cells. *Ann. N.Y. Acad. Sci.* 815, 111–113.

Mikoryak, C. A., Morgolies, M. N., and Steiner, L. A. (1988). J chain in *Rana catesbeiana* high molecular weight Ig. *J. Immunol.* 140, 4279–4285.

Mizoguchi, A., Mizuochi, T., and Kobata, A. (1982). Structures of the carbohydrate moieties of secretory component purified from human milk. *J. Biol. Chem.* 257, 9612–9621.

Moldoveanu, Z., Egan, M. L., and Mestecky, J. (1984). Cellular origins of human polymeric and monomeric IgA: Intracellular and secreted forms of IgA. *J. Immunol.* 133, 3156–3162.

Moldoveanu, Z., Brown, T. A., Ventura, M. T., Michalek, S. M., McGhee, J. R., and Mestecky, J. (1987). IgA subclass responses to lipopolysaccharide in humans. *Adv. Exp. Med. Biol.* 216B, 1199–1205.

Moldoveanu, Z., Epps, J. M., Thorpe, S. R., and Mestecky, J. (1988). The sites of catabolism of murine monomeric IgA. *J. Immunol.* 141, 208–213.

Moldoveanu, Z, Moro, I., Radl, J., Thorpe, S. R., Komiyama, K., and Mestecky, J. (1990). Catabolism of autologous and heterologous IgA in non-human primates. *Scand. J. Immunol.* 32, 577–583.

Moro, I., Iwase, T., Komiyama, K., Moldoveanu, Z., and Mestecky, J. (1990). Immunoglobulin A (IgA) polymerization sites in human immunocytes: Immunoelectron microscopic study. *Cell Struct. Funct.* 15, 85–91.

Mostov, K. E., Friedlander, M., and Blobel, G. (1984). The receptor for transepithelial transport of IgA and IgM contains multiple immunoglobulin-like domains. *Nature* 308, 37–43.

Munn, E. A., Feinstein, A., and Munro, A. J. (1971). Electron microscope examination of free IgA molecules and of their complexes with antigen. *Nature* 231, 527–529.

Mygind, N., Weeke, B., and Ullman, S. (1975). Quantitative determination of immunoglobulins in nasal secretion. *Int. Arch. Allergy Appl. Immunol.* 49, 99–107.

Nagura, H., Nakane, P. K., and Brown, W. R. (1979). Translocation of dimeric IgA through neoplastic colon cells *in vitro. J. Immunol.* 123, 2359–2368.

Nagura, H., Tsutsumi, Y., Hasegawa, H., Watanabe, K., Nakane, P. K., and Brown, W. R. (1983). IgA plasma cells in biliary mucosa: A likely source of locally synthesized IgA in human hepatic bile. *Clin. Exp. Immunol.* 54, 671–680.

Natvig, I. B., Johansen, F. E., Nordeng, T. W., Haraldsen, G., and Brandtzaeg, P. (1997). Mechanism for enhanced external transfer of dimeric IgA over pentameric IgM: Studies of diffusion, binding to the human polymeric Ig receptor, and epithelial transcytosis. *J. Immunol.* 159, 4330–4340.

Niedermeier, W., Tomana, M., and Mestecky, J. (1972). The carbohydrate composition of J chain from human serum and secretory IgA. *Biochim. Biophys. Acta* 257, 527–530.

Niles, M. J., Matsuuchi, L., and Koshland, M. E. (1995). Polymer IgM assembly and secretion in lymphoid and nonlymphoid cell lines: Evidence that J chain is required for pentamer synthesis. *Proc. Natl. Acad. Sci. USA* 92, 2884–2888.

Parkhouse, R. M. E. (1971). Immunoglobulin A biosynthesis. Intracellular accumulation of 7S subunits. *FEBS Lett.* 16, 71–73.

Parkhouse, R. M. E., and Della Corte, E. (1973). Biosynthesis of immunoglobulin A (IgA) and immunoglobulin M (IgM). *Biochem. J.* 136, 607–609.

Patel, M., Selinger, D., Mark, G. E., Hickey, G. J., and Hollis, G. F. (1995). Sequence of the dog immunoglobulin α and ε constant region genes. *Immunogenetics* 41, 282–286.

Peters, I. R., Helps, C. R., Batt, R. M., Day, M. J., and Hall, E. J. (2003). Quantitative real-time RT-PCR measurement of mRNA encoding α-chain, pIgR and J-chain from canine duodenal mucosa. *J. Immunol. Methods* 275, 213–222.

Phalipon, A., Cardona, A., Kraehenbuhl, J. P., Edelman, L., Sansonetti, P. J., and Corthesy, B. (2002). Secretory component: A new role in secretory IgA-mediated immune exclusion *in vivo*. *Immunity* 17, 107–115.

Phillips-Quagliata, J. M. (2002). Mouse IgA allotypes have major differences in their hinge regions. *Immunogenetics* 53, 1033–1038.

Pierce-Cretel, A., Decottignies, J. P., Wieruszeski, J. M., Strecker, G., Montreuil, J., and Spik, G. (1989). Primary structure of twenty three neutral and monosialylated oligosaccharides O-glycosidically linked to the human secretory immunoglobulin A hinge region determined by a combination of permethylation analysis and 400-MHz 1H-NMR spectroscopy. *Eur. J. Biochem.* 182, 457–476.

Pierce-Cretel, A., Pamblanco, M., Strecker, G., Montreuil, J., and Spik, G. (1981). Heterogeneity of the glycans O-glycosidically linked to the hinge region of secretory immunoglobulins from human milk. *Eur. J. Biochem.* 114, 169–178.

Piskurich, J. F., Blanchard, M. H., Youngman, K. R., France, J. A., and Kaetzel, C. S. (1995). Molecular cloning of the mouse polymeric Ig receptor: Functional regions of the molecule are conserved among five mammalian species. *J. Immunol.* 154, 1735–1747.

Plebani, A., Mira, E., Mevio, E., Monafo, V., Notarangelo, L. D., Avanzini, A., and Ugazio, A. C. (1983). IgM and IgD concentrations in the serum and secretions of children with selective IgA deficiency. *Clin. Exp. Immunol.* 53, 689–696.

Prahl, J. W., Abel, C. A., and Grey, H. M. (1971). Carboxy-terminal structure of the α chain of human IgA myeloma proteins. *Biochemistry* 10, 1808–1812.

Pumphrey, R. S. H. (1986). Computer models of the human immunoglobulins: Binding sites and molecular interactions. *Immunol. Today* 7, 206–211.

Putnam, F. W. (1989). Structure of the human IgA subclasses and allotypes. *Protides Biol. Fluids* 36, 27–37.

Putnam, F. W., Yu-Sheng, V. L., and Low, T. L. K. (1979). Primary structure of a human IgA1 immunoglobulin. IV. Streptococcal IgA1 protease digestion, Fab and Fc fragment and the complete amino acid sequence of the α1 heavy chain. *J. Biol. Chem.* 254, 2865–2874.

Radl, J. F., Klein, M. H., van den Berg, P., de Bruyn, A. M., and Hijmans, W. (1971). Binding of secretory piece to polymeric IgA and IgA para-proteins *in vitro*. *Immunology* 20, 843–852.

Radl, J., Schuit, H. R. E., Mestecky, J., and Hijmans, W. (1974). The origin of monomeric and polymeric forms of IgA in man. *Adv. Exp. Med. Biol.* 45, 57–65.

Randall, T. D., King, L. B., and Corley, R. B. (1990). The biological effects of IgM hexamer formation. *Eur. J. Immunol.* 20, 1971–1979.

Randall, T. D., Parkhouse, R. M., and Corley, R. B. (1992a). J chain synthesis and secretion of hexameric IgM is differentially regulated by lipopolysaccharide and interleukin 5. *Proc. Natl. Acad. Sci. USA* 89, 962–966.

Randall, T. D, Brewer, J. W., and Corley, R. B. (1992b). Direct evidence that J chain regulates the polymeric structure of IgM in antibody-secreting B cells. *J. Biol. Chem.* 267, 18002–18007.

Rao, S., Karray, S., Gackstetter, E. R., and Koshland, M. E. (1998). Myocyte enhancer factor-related B-MEF2 is developmentally expressed in B cells and regulates the immunoglobulin J chain promoter. *J. Biol. Chem.* 273, 26123–26129.

Rifai, A., Fadden, K., Morrison, S. L., and Chintalacharuvu, K. R. (2000). The N-glycans determine the differential blood clearance and hepatic uptake of human immunoglobulin (Ig)A1 and IgA2 isotypes. *J. Exp. Med.* 191, 2171–2182.

Roque-Barreira, M. C., and Campos-Neto, A. (1985). Jacalin: An IgA-binding lectin. *J. Immunol.* 134, 1740–1743.

Rose, M. E., Orlans, E., Payne, A. W. R., and Hesketh, P. (1981). The origin of IgA in chicken bile: Its rapid active transport from blood. *Eur. J. Immunol.* 11, 561–564.

Royle, L., Roos, A., Harvey, D. J., Wormald, M. R., Van Gijlswijk-Janssen, D., Redwan El-R. M., Wilson, I. A., Daha, M. R., Dwek, R. A., and Rudd, P. M. (2003). Secretory IgA N- and O-glycans provide a link between the innate and adaptive immune systems. *J. Biol. Chem.* 278, 20140–20153.

Russell, M. W., Mestecky, J., Julian, B. A., and Galla, J. H. (1986). IgA-associated renal diseases: Antibodies to environmental antigens in sera and deposition in immunoglobulins and antigens in glomeruli. *J. Clin. Immunol.* 6, 74–86.

Schroten, H., Stapper, C., Plogmann, R., Kohler, H., Hacker, J., and Hanisch, F. G. (1998). Fab-independent antiadhesion effects of secretory immunoglobulin A on S-fimbriated *Escherichia coli* are mediated by sialyloligosaccharides. *Infect. Immun.* 66, 3971–3973.

Sitia, R., Neuberger, M., Alberini, C., Bet, P., Fra, A., Valetti, C., Williams, G., and Milstein, C. (1990). Developmental regulation of IgM secretion: The role of the carboxy-terminal cysteine. *Cell* 60, 781–790.

Skea, D. L., Christopoulous, P., Plaut, A. G., and Underdown, B. J. (1988). Studies on the specificity of the IgA-binding lectin, jacalin. *Mol. Immunol.* 25, 1–6.

Skvaril, F., and Morell, A. (1974). Distribution of IgA subclasses in sera and bone marrow plasma cells of 21 normal individuals. *Adv. Exp. Med. Biol.* 45, 433–435.

Smith, R. I., Coloma, M. J., and Morrison, S. L. (1995). Addition of a μ-tailpiece to IgG results in polymeric antibodies with enhanced effector functions including complement-mediated cytolysis by IgG4. *J. Immunol.* 154, 2226–2236.

Sørensen, V., Rasmussen, I. B., Norderhaug, L., Natvig, I., Michaelsen, T. E., and Sandlie, I. (1996). Effect of the IgM and IgA secretory tailpieces on polymerization and secretion of IgM and IgG. *J. Immunol.* 156, 2858–2865.

Sørensen, V., Sundvold, V., Michaelsen, T. E., and Sandlie, I. (1999). Polymerization of IgA and IgM: Roles of Cys309/Cys414 and the secretory tailpiece. *J. Immunol.* 162, 3448–3455.

Sørensen, V., Rasmussen, I. B., Sundvold, V., Michaelsen, T. E., and Sandlie, I. (2000). Structural requirements for incorporation of J chain into human IgM and IgA. *Int. Immunol.* 12, 19–27.

South, M. A., Cooper, M. D., Wolheim, F. A., Hong, R., and Good, R. A. (1986). The IgA system. I. Studies of the transport and immunochemistry of IgA in the saliva. *J. Exp. Med.* 123, 615–627.

Spiekermann, G. M., Finn, P. W., Ward, E. S., Dumont, J., Dickinson, B. L., Blumberg, R. S., and Lencer, W. I. (2002). Receptor-mediated immunoglobulin G transport across mucosal barriers in adult life: Functional expression of FcRn in the mammalian lung. *J. Exp. Med.* 196, 303–310.

Spieker-Polet, H., Yam, P. C., and Knight, K. L. (1993). Differential expression of 13 IgA-heavy chain genes in rabbit lymphoid tissues. *J. Immunol.* 150, 5457–5465.

Stockert, R. J., Kressner, M. S., Collins, J. C., Sternlieb, I., and Morell, A. G. (1982). IgA interactions with the asialoglycoprotein receptor. *Proc. Natl. Acad. Sci. USA* 79, 6229–6231.

Stott, D. I. (1976). Biosynthesis and assembly of IgM. Addition of J chain to intracellular pools of 8S and 19S IgM. *Immunochemistry* 13, 157–163.

Sumiyama, K., Saitou, N., and Ueda, S. (2002). Adaptive evolution of the IgA hinge region in primates. *Mol. Biol. Evol.* 19, 1093–1099.

Svanborg Edén, C., Kulhavy, R., Mårild, S., Prince, S. J., and Mestecky, J. (1985). Urinary immunoglobulins in healthy individuals and children with acute pyelonephritis. *Scand. J. Immunol.* 21, 305–313.

Svehag, S. E., and Bloth, B. (1970). Ultrastructure of secretory and high-polymer serum immunoglobulin A of human and rabbit origin. *Science* 168, 847–849.

Takahashi, T., Iwase, T., Takenouchi, N., Saito, M., Kobayashi, K., Moldoveanu, Z., Mestecky, J., and Moro, I. (1996). The joining (J) chain is present in invertebrates that do not express immunoglobulins. *Proc. Natl. Acad. Sci. USA* 93, 1886–1891.

Takahashi, T., Iwase, T., Tachibana, T., Komiyama, K., Kobayashi, K., Chen, C. L., Mestecky, J., and Moro, I. (2000). Cloning and expression of the chicken immunoglobulin joining (J)-chain cDNA. *Immunogenetics* 51, 85–91.

Tarkowski, A., Lue, C., Moldoveanu, Z., Kiyono, H., McGhee, J. R., and Mestecky, J. (1990). Immunization of humans with polysaccharide vaccines induces systemic, predominantly polymeric IgA2-subclass antibody responses. *J. Immunol.* 144, 3770–3778.

Taylor, A. K., and Wall, R. (1988). Selective removal of α heavy-chain glycosylation sites causes immunoglobulin A degradation and reduced secretion. *Mol. Cell. Biol.* 8, 4197–4203.

Taylor, C. L., Harrison, G. A., Watson, C. M., and Deane, E. M. (2002). cDNA cloning of the polymeric immunoglobulin receptor of the marsupial *Macropus eugenii* (tammar wallaby). *Eur. J. Immunogenet.* 29, 87–93.

Tomana, M., Mestecky, J., and Niedermeier, W. (1972). Studies on human secretory immunoglobulin A. IV. Carbohydrate composition. *J. Immunol.* 108, 1631–1636.

Tomana, M., Niedermeier, W., Mestecky, J., and Skvaril, F. (1976). The differences in carbohydrate composition between the subclasses of IgA immunoglobulins. *Immunochemistry* 13, 325–328.

Tomana, M., Niedermeier, W., and Spivey, C. (1978). Microdetermination of monosaccharides in glycoproteins by gas-liquid chromatography. *Analyt. Biochem.* 89, 110–118.

Tomana, M., Kulhavy, R., and Mestecky, J. (1988). Receptor-mediated binding and uptake of immunoglobulin A by human liver. *Gastroenterology* 94, 762–770.

Tomasi, T. B., and Bienenstock, J. (1968). Secretory immunoglobulins. *Adv. Immunol.* 9, 1–96.

Tomasi, T. B., Jr., Tan, E., Solomon, A., and Prendergast, R. A. (1965). Characteristics of an immune system common to certain external secretions. *J. Exp. Med.* 121, 101–124.

Torano, A., and Putnam, F. W. (1978). Complete amino acid sequence of the α2 heavy chain of a human IgA2 immunoglobulin of the A2m(2) allotype. *Proc. Natl. Acad. Sci. USA* 75, 966–969.

Torano, A., Tsuzukida, Y., Liu, Y.-S. V., and Putnam, F. W. (1977). Location and structural significance of the oligosaccharides in human IgA1 and IgA2 immunoglobulins. *Proc. Natl. Acad. Sci. USA* 74, 2301–2305.

Tsuzukida, Y., Wang, C. C., and Putnam, F. W. (1979). Structure of the A2m(1) allotype of human IgA: A recombinant molecule. *Proc. Natl. Acad. Sci. USA* 76, 1104–1108.

Tucker, P. W., Slightom, J. L., and Blattner, F. R. (1981). Mouse IgA heavy chain gene sequence: Implications for evolution of immunoglobulin hinge exons. *Proc. Natl. Acad. Sci. USA* 78, 7684–7688.

Ueda, S., Matsuda, F., and Honjo, T. (1988). Multiple recombinational events in primate immunoglobulin ε and α genes suggest closer relationship of human to chimpanzees than to gorillas. *J. Mol. Evol.* 27, 77–83.

Underdown, B. J., and Dorrington, K. J. (1974). Studies on the structural and conformational basis for the relative resistance of serum and secretory immunoglobulin A to proteolysis. *J. Immunol.* 112, 949–959.

Underdown, B. J., DeRose, J., and Plaut, A. (1977). Disulfide bonding of secretory component to a single monomer subunit in human secretory IgA. *J. Immunol.* 118, 1816–1821.

Underdown, B. L, Switzer, I. C., and Jackson, G. D. F. (1992). Rat secretory component binds poorly to rodent IgM. *J. Immunol.* 149, 487–491.

Vaerman, J.-P., and Delacroix, D. L. (1984). Role of the liver in the immunobiology of IgA in animals and humans. *Contrib. Nephrol.* 40, 17–31.

Vaerman, J.-P., Langendries, A., Giffroy, D., Brandtzaeg, P., and Kobayashi, K. (1998a). Lack of SC/pIgR-mediated epithelial transport of a human polymeric IgA devoid of J chain: *In vitro* and *in vivo* studies. *Immunology* 95, 90–96.

Vaerman, J.-P., Langendries, A. E., Giffroy, D. A., Kaetzel, C. S., Fiani, C. M., Moro, I., Brandtzaeg, P., and Kobayashi, K. (1998b). Antibody against the human J chain inhibits polymeric Ig receptor-mediated biliary and epithelial transport of human polymeric IgA. *Eur. J. Immunol.* 28, 171–182.

van Loghem, E., and Biewenga, J. (1983). Allotypic and isotypic aspects of human immunoglobulin A. *Mol. Immunol.* 20, 1001–1007.

Verbeet, M. P., Vermeer, H., Warmerdam, G. C., de Boer, H. A., and Lee, S. H. (1995). Cloning and characterization of the bovine polymeric immunoglobulin receptor-encoding cDNA. *Gene* 164, 329–333.

Wagner, B., Greiser-Wilke, I., and Antczak, D. F. (2003). Characterization of the horse (Equus caballus) IGHA gene. *Immunogenetics* 55, 552–560.

Wallin, J. J., Rinkenberger, J. L., Rao, S., Gackstetter, E. R., Koshland, M. E., and Zwollo, P. (1999). B cell-specific activator protein prevents two activator factors from binding to the immunoglobulin J chain promoter until the antigen-driven stages of B cell development. *J. Biol. Chem.* 274, 15959–15965.

Wang, A. C., and Fundenberg, H. H. (1974). IgA and evolution of immunoglobulins. *J. Immunogenet.* 1, 3–31.

Weiker, J., and Underdown, B. J. (1975). A study of the association of human secretory component with IgA and IgM proteins. *J. Immunol.* 114, 1337–1344.

Weltman, J. K., and Davis, R. P. (1970). Fluorescence polarization study of a human IgA myeloma protein: Absence of segmental flexibility. *J. Mol. Biol.* 54, 177–185.

Wiersma, E. J., and Shulman, M. J. (1995). Assembly of IgM: Role of disulfide bonding and noncovalent interactions. *J. Immunol.* 154, 5265–5272.

Wiersma, E. J., Chen, F., Bazin, R., Collins, C., Painter, R. H., Lemieux, R., and Shulman, M. J. (1997). Analysis of IgM structures involved in J chain incorporation. *J. Immunol.* 158, 1719–1726.

Wiersma, E. J., Collins, C., Fazel, S., and Shulman, M. J. (1998). Structural and functional analysis of J chain-deficient IgM. *J. Immunol.* 160, 5979–5989.

Williams, A. F. (1986). A year in the life of the immunoglobulin superfamily. *Immunol. Today* 8, 298–303.

Wold, A. E., Mestecky, J., Tomana, M., Kobata, A., Ohbayashi, H., Endo, T., and Svanborg-Eden, C. (1990). Secretory immunoglobulin A carries oligosaccharide receptors for *Escherichia coli* type I fimbrial lectin. *Infect. Immun.* 58, 3073–3077.

Yang, C. Y., Kratzin, H., Götz, H., and Hilschmann, N. (1979). Die Primärstruktur eines monoklonalen IgA1 Immunoglobulins (Myelomprotein Tro). VII. Darstellung, Reinigung und Charakterisierung der Disulfidbrücken. *Hoppe-Seyler's Z. Physiol. Chem.* 360, 1919–1940.

Yoo, E. M., Coloma, M. J., Trinh, K. R., Nguyen, T. Q., Vuong, L. U., Morrison, S. L., and Chintalacharuvu, K. R. (1999). Structural requirements for polymeric immunoglobulin assembly and association with J chain. *J. Biol. Chem.* 274, 33771–33777.

Zagyansky, Y. A., and Gavrilova, E. M. (1974). Segmental flexibility of human myeloma immunoglobulins A. *Immunochemistry* 11, 681–682.

Zikan, J., Mestecky, J., Schrohenloher, R. E., Tomana, M., and Kulhavy, R. (1972). Studies on human secretory immunoglobulin A. V. Trypsin hydrolysis at elevated temperatures. *Immunochemistry* 9, 1185–1193.

Zikan, J., Novotny, J., Trapane, T. L., Koshland, M. E., Urry, D. W., Bennett, J. C., and Mestecky, J. (1985). Secondary structure of the immunoglobulin J chain. *Proc. Natl. Acad. Sci. USA* 82, 5905–5909.

Zikan, J., Mestecky, J., Kulhavy, R., and Bennett, J. C. (1986). The stoichiometry of J chain in human secretory dimeric IgA. *Mol. Immunol.* 23, 541–544.

Organization and Expression of Genes Encoding IgA Heavy Chain, Polymeric Ig Receptor, and J Chain

Katherine L. Knight and Ki-Jong Rhee

Department of Microbiology and Immunology, Stritch School of Medicine, Loyola University Chicago, Maywood, Illinois

Genes encoding IgA heavy chains, polymeric Ig receptors, and J chains have been cloned from several species. The aim of this chapter is to discuss the structure and expression of these genes as well as to compare and contrast the IgA genes of various species.

IgA HEAVY CHAIN GENES

Basic structure

Genes encoding the Cα regions of IgA heavy chains have been cloned from the genomes of man (Flanagan *et al.*, 1984), mouse (Tucker *et al.*, 1981), cattle (Knight *et al.*, 1988), sheep (White *et al.*, 1998), rat (Brüggemann *et al.*, 1986), rabbit (Burnett *et al.*, 1989), pig (Brown and Butler, 1994), dog (Patel *et al.*, 1995), horse (Wagner *et al.*, 1997), marsupial (Aveskogh and Hellman, 1998), chicken (Mansikka, 1992), duck (Magor *et al.*, 1998), and several nonhuman primates, including gorilla, chimpanzee, orangutan, gibbon, and Old World monkey (Kawamura *et al.*, 1989; Ueda *et al.*, 1988; Kawamura *et al.*, 1990). Except for primates and rabbits, all mammals studied have a single IgA subclass and, accordingly, a single Cα gene in their germline. Two IgA subclasses and two Cα germline genes are found in humans, whereas rabbits have 13 nonallelic Cα germline genes and 11 IgA subclasses.

Domain structure

As with other C_H genes, the Cα genes of each mammalian species studied have a separate exon that encodes each domain—Cα1, Cα2, and Cα3—as diagrammed in **Figure 10.1**. The hinge region is not encoded as a separate exon but instead is encoded at the 5′ end of the Cα2 exon. The hinge

regions vary in size from 3 codons in the pig Cα gene (Brown and Butler, 1994) to as many as 19 codons in four of the rabbit Cα genes (Burnett *et al.*, 1989). Kawamura *et al.* (1990) showed that the Cα1 and Cα2 genes of chimpanzee, gorilla, and gibbon have hinge structures similar to those of the human Cα1 and Cα2 genes, respectively. In contrast, the hinge region of the Cα gene of Old World monkeys was markedly different from that of any hominoid Cα gene examined. It appears that the hinge region is the least evolutionarily conserved region of the α chain (Scinicariello and Attanasio, 2001).

In contrast to mammalian Cα genes, which encode three domains, the chicken Cα gene encodes a heavy chain with four domains. Mansikka (1992) showed that of the four domains, Cα2 was the least similar to mammalian Cα genes, suggesting that the Cα2 domain was deleted in mammals during evolution. Such deletions throughout evolution may explain the diversity of the sizes of hinge regions in mammals.

Comparison of the proteins encoded by Cα genes of various species showed that the Cα3 domain was the most highly conserved (Brown and Butler, 1994; Burnett *et al.*, 1989). Also, the 19 amino acid extension at the C-terminal end of the secreted form of α heavy chains, encoded at the 3′ end of the Cα3 exon, is highly conserved among species. Especially conserved are the codons for the terminal amino acids Cys and Tyr. Further, the transmembrane (TM) and cytoplasmic tail (CT) sequences found at the C-terminal end of the membrane form of α heavy chains are highly conserved among species. Both the TM and CT are encoded by one small exon, αM, located approximately 2 to 4 kb 3′ of Cα3 (Word *et al.*, 1983; Zhai, S.-K., and Knight, K. L., unpublished data).

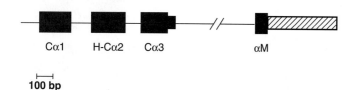

Fig. 10.1. Intron-exon structure of Cα genes. The boxes represent the exons that encode the Cα1 domain; hinge (H) and Cα2 domain; Cα3 domain and secreted tail; and membrane/cytoplasmic domain (αM). The open box with slanted lines represents 3′-untranslated regions of the RNA.

Location of Cα genes in the IgH locus

In all mammalian species studied, including mouse, rat, cattle, horse, human, and rabbit, the Cα genes appear to reside as the 3′-most IgH gene and usually reside 10 kb to 12 kb 3′ of a Cε gene (Shimizu *et al.*, 1982; Brüggemann *et al.*, 1986; Knight *et al.*, 1988; Burnett *et al.*, 1989; Flanagan and Rabbits, 1982; Hofker *et al.*, 1989; Wagner *et al.*, 1997). In mouse, the C_H gene order is $5′-J_H-C_\mu-C_\delta-C_{\gamma3}-C_{\gamma1}-C_{\gamma2b}-C_{\gamma2a}-C_\epsilon-C_\alpha-3′$ (Shimizu *et al.*, 1982). Similarly in rat, the order is $5′-J_H-C_\mu-C_\delta-(C_{\gamma2c}-C_{\gamma2a})-C_{\gamma1}-C_{\gamma2b}-C_\epsilon-C_\alpha-3′$ (Brüggemann *et al.*, 1986). The cattle and horse Cα genes are known to reside 3′ of Cε, but they have not yet been linked by overlapping phage or cosmid clones to Cμ or Cγ genes (Knight *et al.*, 1988; Wagner *et al.*, 1997). In humans, the C_H gene order differs from that in rodents, presumably because of a duplication of a cluster of two Cγ genes, one Cε and one Cα gene (**Fig. 10.2**). The gene order in humans is $5′-J_H-C_\mu-C_\delta-C_{\gamma3}-C_{\gamma1}-\psi C_\epsilon-C_\alpha1-\psi C_\gamma-C_{\gamma2}-C_{\gamma4}-C_\epsilon-C_\alpha2-3′$ (Flanagan and Rabbits, 1982; Hofker *et al.*, 1989). In chickens and ducks, however, the Cα gene is located in between the Cμ and Cυ genes; the C_H gene order is $5′-J_H-C_\mu-C_\alpha-C_\upsilon-3′$ (Lundqvist *et al.*, 2001; Zhao *et al.*, 2000). More surprising is that the Cα gene is in an inverted transcriptional orientation, and thus class switch to IgA expression requires inversion of the ~27-kb region that includes both Cμ and Cα genes (Lundqvist *et al.*, 2001; Magor *et al.*, 1999). The presence of an inverted Cα gene raises questions as to the evolution of immunoglobulin gene loci in vertebrates.

Allelic polymorphism

Allelic polymorphisms of Cα genes have been identified by restriction fragment length polymorphism (RFLP) studies in human (Hendriks *et al.*, 1988; Bottaro *et al.*, 1989), horse (Wagner *et al.*, 1997), cattle (Knight *et al.*, 1987; Brown *et al.*, 1997), pig (Brown *et al.*, 1995), and rabbit (Knight,

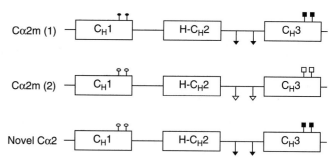

Fig. 10.3. Three allelic forms of human Cα2 genes. The novel α2 gene may have derived from recombination or gene conversion between the two Cα2 alleles, Cα2m(1) and Cα2m(2). Adapted from Chintalacharuvu *et al.* (1994).

unpublished data). Chintalacharuvu *et al.* (1994) identified and characterized a novel human Cα2 gene, presumably an allelic form of Cα2. This gene appears to have developed by recombination or gene conversion between the two Cα2 alleles, α2m(1) and α2m(2) (**Fig. 10.3**). Recently, two alleles of the Cα gene in rhesus macaques have been described (Scinicariello and Attanasio, 2001). The functional significance of these allelic variants remains to be elucidated; however, the IgA variants could differ in resistance to proteolytic enzymes or in the ability to protect mucosal surfaces.

Cα genes of human, rabbit, and other lagomorphs

The Cα gene found in most mammals appears to have undergone duplication in humans, rabbits, and other lagomorphs. In humans, a second Cα gene most likely resulted from duplication of approximately 60 kb of DNA, $5′-C_\gamma-C_\gamma-C_\epsilon-C_\alpha-3′$, containing one Cα gene. In rabbits, the 13 nonallelic Cα genes all reside 3′ of Cε and presumably are the result of multiple duplications of the Cα genes. The 13 Cα genes span a minimum of 160 kb of DNA (Burnett *et al.*, 1989), and nine of the genes have been linked to the $5′-C_\mu-C_\gamma-C_\epsilon-3′$ gene cluster by overlapping cosmid and fosmid clones (**Fig. 10.4**) (Burnett *et al.*, 1989; Volgina *et al.*, 2000). The remaining four Cα genes are in separate or overlapping phage or fosmid clones. It has been difficult to isolate genomic clones that link these genes to the large cluster, even though multiple genomic libraries were screened.

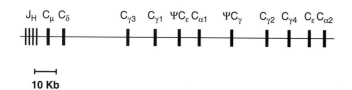

Fig. 10.2. Organization of the human J_H and C_H Ig locus.

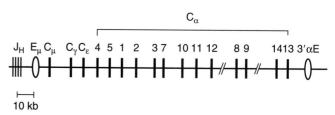

Fig. 10.4. Organization of 13 rabbit germline Cα genes. Cα genes are indicated by solid boxes (Burnett *et al.*, 1989). $C_\alpha13$ and $C_\alpha14$ are positioned 3′ of $C_\alpha8$ and $C_\alpha9$ because of the presence of 3αE 3′ of $C_\alpha13$. Adapted from Volgina *et al.* (2000).

Because of the large number of Cα genes in rabbit as compared with other mammals, Burnett *et al.* (1989) investigated whether multiple copies of Cα genes were also found in other lagomorphs. Southern blots of DNA from members of the two families of lagomorphs, Leporidae and Ochotonidae, hybridized with rabbit C_α probes revealed multiple hybridizing fragments in each sample of DNA **(Fig. 10.5)**. These data indicate that multiple Cα genes are found in animals throughout the order Lagomorpha and that the expansion of Cα genes occurred in a common ancestor. Similar attempts to identify mammals belonging to an order other than Lagomorpha that have multiple Cα genes have so far been unsuccessful. However, among humans, more than 40% of the Mongoloid population are heterozygous for the α1 gene duplication and may provide a basis for further alterations of the human Cα1 gene, resulting in a new subclass of IgA (Rabbani *et al.*, 1996). Thus, we do not yet know, in evolutionary terms, when the expansion of the Cα genes occurred and whether it is continuing.

Expression of Cα genes

In rabbits, the 13 germline Cα genes appear expressible by nucleotide sequence analysis (Burnett *et al.*, 1989). By using probes specific to each of the 13 Cα genes, Spieker-Polet *et al.* (1993) performed RNase protection studies of mRNA from mucosal tissues, including Peyer's patches, mammary tissue, appendix, gut, salivary gland, and mesenteric lymph nodes, and they identified mRNA representing each of the Cα genes except Cα3 and Cα8. Presumably, then, at least 11 IgA isotypes should be found in rabbit mucosal secretions. Surprisingly, Spieker-Polet *et al.* (1993) found that in lung and tonsil, one Cα gene, $C_\alpha 4$, was expressed predominantly. Further, $C_\alpha 4$ is highly expressed in the duodenum-jejunum but not in the lower part of the ileum (Spieker-Polet *et al.*, 1999). It is not clear whether the differential expression of $C_\alpha 4$ is because of differences in the presence or concentration of factors that promote or inhibit switching to specific Cα genes or whether IgA4 B cells specifically home to these

tissues. In the latter case, we could expect IgA4 to be functionally distinct from the other IgA isotypes and to serve a specific function in lung, tonsil, and small intestine.

The differential expression of IgA isotypes in various tissues is also found in humans (Crago *et al.*, 1984; Brandtzaeg *et al.*, 1986; Mestecky and Russell, 1986; Kett *et al.*, 1986). For example, IgA1 represents 80% to 95% of the IgA in serum, whereas in external secretions, IgA1 generally represents only 30% to 50% of the IgA. The factors responsible for the differential expression are not known. Because IgA1 and IgA2 are differentially susceptible to IgA proteases, the differential expression may result from different distribution of IgA proteases in various tissues (Plaut *et al.*, 1975; see chapter on IgA proteases by Kilicus, M., and Russell, M.W.). Other possibilities for the differential expression include local factors that promote isotype switching to either $C_\alpha 1$ or $C_\alpha 2$ or preferential homing of IgA1 or IgA2 B cells to different tissues. The functional significance of the multiple IgA isotypes in both rabbit and human remains to be elucidated.

Control of expression by IgH enhancers

Ig gene expression is regulated by *cis*-acting elements, including the intronic enhancer Eμ (Banerji *et al.*, 1983; Gillies *et al.*, 1983; Grosschedl and Baltimore, 1985) and enhancers 3′ of Cα genes (Dariavach *et al.*, 1991; Lieberson *et al.*, 1991; Matthias and Baltimore, 1993; Michaelson *et al.*, 1995; Pettersson *et al.*, 1990). The Eμ enhancer is located in the intronic region between J_H gene segments and the μ chain gene, and it controls events of early B cell development, including rearrangement of V, D, and J gene segments (Chen *et al.*, 1993; Serwe and Sablitzky, 1993). Enhancers 3′ of Cα genes include HS1,2; HS3A; HS3B; and HS4 in the murine *Igh* complex and HS1,2, HS3, and HS4 in the human *Igh* complex (Chen and Birshtein, 1997; Michaelson *et al.*, 1995; Mills *et al.*, 1997). Whereas these enhancers are associated with both human Cα genes, *Cα1* and *Cα2*, only a single HS1,2 enhancer is found in the rabbit *Igh* locus, even though it contains 13 Cα genes (Volgina *et al.*, 2000).

The HS1,2 and HS3 enhancers appear to be active primarily in plasma cells (Arulampalam *et al.*, 1994; Singh and Birshtein, 1993), whereas HS4 is active throughout B cell development (Michaelson *et al.*, 1995). These enhancers are known to control isotype switching via germline transcription (Pinaud *et al.*, 2001), regulate heavy chain expression in plasma cells (Shi and Eckhardt, 2001), and may stimulate somatic hypermutation of Ig genes (Terauchi *et al.*, 2001). The mechanism by which the enhancers in the 3′ *Igh* region contribute to Ig gene expression and whether some activities are specific for Cα genes remain to be elucidated.

CLASS SWITCHING

For a B cell to express Ig of the IgA isotype, class switching must occur. Class switching occurs in IgM-bearing lymphocytes by a DNA rearrangement of the Cα gene to a region

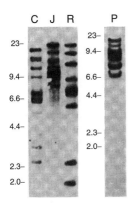

Fig. 10.5. Southern analysis of lagomorph genomic DNA with the rabbit Cα probe. DNA samples, from cottontail rabbit (C), jackrabbit (J), domestic rabbit (R), and pika (P), were restricted with BamHI. Reprinted with permission from Burnett *et al.* (1989) and Oxford University Press.

downstream of the rearranged VDJ gene (reviewed by Jessberger *et al.*, 1996). During switch rearrangement, all C_H genes 5′ of the $C\alpha$ gene are deleted from the germline (Yaoita and Honjo, 1980; Kataoka *et al.*, 1981; von Schwedler *et al.*, 1990; Rabbits *et al.*, 1990; Irsch *et al.*, 1994). The rearrangement generally occurs by recombination between GC-rich tandem direct repeat sequences, termed switch regions (Nikai *et al.*, 1981), which are found 5′ of each C_H gene except C_δ (Davis *et al.*, 1980; Obata *et al.*, 1981). By isolating IgA+ cells from normal human donors and hybridizing for DNA deleted during the switch from IgM to IgA, Irsch *et al.* (1994) showed that switch recombination can occur on both alleles. Although most switch recombination events occur in *cis*, there have been descriptions of switch recombination occurring in *trans*, with the VDJ gene of one chromosome recombining with the C_H region of the other (Kipps and Herzenberg, 1986; Kingzette *et al.*, 1998). In rabbit, a relatively high percentage (3%–7%) of *trans*-associated serum IgA is found, as determined in rabbits heterozygous for allotypic markers present on the V_H and C_H regions (Pernis *et al.*, 1973; Knight *et al.*, 1974). Kingzette *et al.* (1998) developed rabbit hybridomas that produced *trans*-IgA molecules, and by analyzing the IgH chromosomal region of these hybridomas they found that the hybridomas had undergone a *trans*-chromosomal DNA recombination within the Ig switch region.

Role of TGF-β in IgA class switching

Of several factors shown to direct or enhance class switching to IgA, TGF-β is the most potent. When TGF-β is added to LPS- or pokeweed mitogen-stimulated IgA− B cells, IgA expression is induced (Coffman *et al.*, 1989; Lebman *et al.*, 1990a; Kim and Kagnoff, 1990; van Vlasselaer *et al.*, 1992; Ehrhardt *et al.*, 1992). Similarly, retinoic acid plus TGF-β can induce IgA switch in murine B cells (Tokuyama and Tokuyama, 1997). Fagarasan *et al.* (2001) identified IgA switch recombination circle DNA in lamina propria lymphocytes, suggesting that IgA switch can occur in the gut lamina propria, regulated by the local environment. A critical role of TGF-β for IgA switch in vivo was demonstrated by Cazac and Roes (2000), who by using the Cre/loxP system generated mice in which the TGF-β type II receptor was inactivated by cell type–specific mutagenesis and found no IgA-expressing cells.

We do not yet know the exact mechanism by which class switching to IgA is induced. Just prior to switching, the chromatin structure of the switch region is altered, as evidenced by DNase I hypersensitivity, hypomethylation, and germline transcription (Stavnezer–Nordgren and Sirlin, 1986; Stavenzer *et al.*, 1988; Schmitz and Radbruch, 1989; Lebman *et al.*, 1990b; Severinson *et al.*, 1990). The germline transcripts originate in the I region, which is approximately 2 kb 5′ of the switch region and includes a TATA-less promoter and a small I exon (Lebman *et al.*, 1990b; Radcliffe *et al.*, 1990). The germline transcripts themselves include the I exon spliced to the unrearranged C_H1 exon, and they do not generally appear to code for a functional protein and thus are termed sterile transcripts. Regulation of germline transcrip-

tion is through the I-region promoter, in which several *cis* elements have been described as important for both general and cytokine-directed transcription.

The necessity of germline transcripts for class switching was demonstrated in mice lacking the I-region promoter for the $C\gamma1$ gene. In these mice, there are no germline transcripts for IgG1, and switching to IgG1 is abolished (Jung *et al.*, 1993). Harriman *et al.* (1996) showed that the I exon sequence itself is not required for switching, as long as the locus remains transcriptionally active. They knocked out the $I\alpha$ exon in mice and replaced it with another transcriptionally active gene. In these mice, levels of serum and secreted IgA were normal. Furthermore, B cells from these mice were able to undergo isotype switching *in vitro* as efficiently as control B cells (Harriman *et al.*, 1996). Therefore, the $I\alpha$ exon can be replaced with an unrelated but transcribed gene, and switching to IgA is not affected. Presumably, if transcription of the unrelated gene did not occur, switching would also not occur. Even though germline transcription is critical for class switching, transcription of the sterile RNA alone does not regulate the IgA isotype switch. Using single-cell PCR analysis, Spieker-Polet *et al.* (1999) found sterile IgA transcripts of multiple $C\alpha$ genes in single rabbit B cells when cultured with TGF-β and IL-2. Furthermore, with the exception of $C\alpha3$ and $C\alpha8$, functional analysis of the $I\alpha$ promoter regions of the rabbit $C\alpha$ genes did not show a strong correlation between promoter activity and *in vivo* expression of the various IgA isotypes (Spieker-Polet *et al.*, 2002). Therefore, differential expression of IgA isotypes is further regulated subsequent to expression of germline transcripts.

The $I\alpha$ promoter region contains several recognition elements for transcription factors, including a TGF-β response element (TGF-βRE), a cAMP response element (CRE), and a site that binds proteins of the ETS family (Xie *et al.*, 1999). Several authors showed that TGF-βRE, CRE, and ETS are required for optimal promoter activity in human and mouse B cell lines (Nilsson *et al.*, 1995; Lin and Stavnezer, 1992; Zan *et al.*, 1998). TGF-β signaling occurs through the Smad protein family (Heldin *et al.*, 1997; Massagué and Chen, 2000; Yang *et al.*, 1999). Upon TGF-β receptor stimulation, Smad proteins are phosphorylated and translocate to the nucleus, where they cooperatively regulate the transcription of genes with other transcription factors (Chen *et al.*, 1996; Zhang *et al.*, 1998). Shi and Stavnezer (1998) identified several binding sites for Smad proteins and core binding factors (CBP) within the TGF-βRE. Smads bind directly to the TGF-βRE and cooperate with CBP to stimulate germline transcription (Hanai *et al.*, 1999; Pardali *et al.*, 2000). Furthermore, Zhang and Derynck (2000) showed that TGF-β-induced germline transcription requires DNA binding of CREB to the CRE site and of Smads to TGF-βRE sites. Disruption of either binding site abolishes TGF-β-induced transcription.

Requirement for AID in isotype switching

The protein activation-induced cytidine deaminase (AID) was discovered in a mouse B cell line undergoing class switching (Muramatsu *et al.*, 1999). Mice deficient in AID are unable to undergo somatic hypermutation of the Ig genes and to undergo class switch to other isotypes, including to IgA (Muramatsu *et al.*, 2000). Similarly, patients with hyper-IgM syndrome in which the B cells cannot switch to other isotypes all had mutations in the AID gene (Revy *et al.*, 2000). AID belongs to a family of RNA editing enzymes, changing the base cytosine to uridine by deamination (Muramatsu *et al.*, 1999). APOBEC-1 is another member of this family that edits the RNA transcript encoding apolipoprotein B (Teng *et al.*, 1993). It has been suggested that AID might function similarly to APOBEC-1 or, alternatively, AID might function independent of its deaminase activity and act directly in DNA recombination. Tian and Alt (2000) transcribed switch regions *in vitro* and demonstrated that they form RNA-DNA complexes that can recruit DNA-repair enzymes. The discovery of AID as a molecule required for switch recombination has generated considerable excitement among scientists, and the next step is to determine how it functions in switch recombination in combination with other molecules that regulate switch recombination, such as proteins of the SWAP complex (Borggrefe *et al.*, 1998).

POLYMERIC IG RECEPTOR/SECRETORY COMPONENT GENES

Polymeric Ig receptor (pIgR) mediates the transport of polymeric Ig across the epithelium into secretions (see chapter by Mostov, K., and Kaetzel, C. S.). The polymeric Ig binds to the receptor at the basolateral cell surface and is internalized via receptor-mediated endocytosis. The complex is then transcytosed to the apical cell surface where the polymeric Ig is secreted along with a portion of the pIgR, known as secretory component (SC) (Brandtzaeg, 1974; Mostov and Blobel, 1982; Solari and Kraehenbuhl, 1984). Mostov *et al.* (1984) first cloned the pIgR gene from a rabbit cDNA library, and subsequently Deitcher and Mostov (1986) isolated the genomic pIgR gene from a rabbit genomic DNA library. By analyzing the deduced amino acid sequence, Deitcher and Mostov (1986) identified five extracellular domains that are structurally similar to Ig domains, suggesting that pIgR is a member of the Ig superfamily (Mostov *et al.*, 1984; Hunkapiller and Hood, 1989). The sixth domain is highly hydrophobic and spans the cell membrane. The seventh, or cytoplasmic, domain is unusually large: it is composed of 103 amino acids.

The pIgR genes have also been cloned as cDNAs from human (Eiffert *et al.*, 1984; Davidson *et al.*, 1988; Krajci *et al.*, 1989, 1992), mouse (Piskurich *et al.*, 1995), cattle (Kulseth *et al.*, 1995; Verbeet *et al.*, 1995a), rat (Banting *et al.*, 1989), and possum (Adamski and Demmer, 1999). When the amino acid sequences encoded by the pIgR genes cloned from all six mammalian species were compared, most of the regions identified with specific functions were found to be highly conserved. For example, the 23–amino acid sequence in domain 1 that is required for the noncovalent interaction with polymeric Ig is conserved (Frutiger *et al.*,

1986; Bakos *et al.*, 1991 and 1994), as is the extra disulfide bond in domain 5 that forms a covalent bond with dimeric IgA (Cunningham-Rundles and Lamm, 1975; Fallgreen-Gebauer *et al.*, 1993). The cytoplasmic domain encoding 103 amino acids and containing several sorting signals is the most highly conserved portion of the pIgR gene. These signals are required for basolateral sorting, transcytosis, and endocytosis of pIgR (Mostov, 1994) and include crucial Tyr and Ser residues.

The human pIgR gene was localized to the q31–q41 region of chromosome 1 by analyzing human x rodent somatic cell hybrids (Davidson *et al.*, 1988; Krajci *et al.*, 1991 and 1992). The bovine pIgR gene maps to region q13 on chromosome 16, and two allelic RFLP were identified (Kulseth *et al.*, 1994). The mouse pIgR gene is localized to the long arm of chromosome 1 (Kushiro and Sato, 1997). Genomic clones of pIgR from rabbit (Deitcher and Mostov, 1986) and human (Krajci *et al.*, 1992) showed that the pIgR gene contains 11 exons and spans approximately 18 kb **(Fig. 10.6)**. Human pIgR gene has a large intron between exons 1 and 2, and the rat and mouse pIgR genes have a large intron between exons 2 and 3 (Fodor *et al.*, 1997; Verbeet *et al.*, 1995b). Exons 1 and 2, which encode the large 5'-untranslated region of pIgR mRNA, and transcriptional regulation of the pIgR gene are discussed by Mostov and Kaetzel (see Chapter 12).

The regions of pIgR responsible for targeting it to the basolateral surface, for endocytosis and for transcytosis, have been elucidated and serve as an excellent model for understanding intracellular protein traffic (for example, see Mostov *et al.*, 1986; Breitfeld *et al.*, 1989; Schrader *et al.*, 1990; Apodaca *et al.*, 1991; Casanova *et al.*, 1991; Mostov, 1994; Lipschutz *et al.*, 2003; van IJzendoorn *et al.*, 2002; Wang *et al.*, 2000).

J CHAIN GENES

J chain is a 15-kD (137 amino acid) protein found covalently associated with dimeric secretory IgA (SIgA) and polymeric IgM (reviewed by Koshland, 1985). J chain has been cloned in several species, including mouse (Mather *et al.*, 1981; Cann

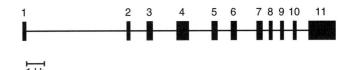

Fig. 10.6. Human pIgR gene. Human pIgR comprises 11 exons spanning 18 kb on chromosome 1q. Exon 2 encodes the initiator AUG codon and most of the leader peptide; exon 3 encodes the N-terminal amino acid of mature, transmembrane pIgR; exons 3, 5, and 6 encode the extracellular domains 1, 4, and 5, respectively; and exon 4 encodes domains 2 and 3, which are deleted by alternate splicing in one form of rabbit pIgR (Deitcher and Mostov, 1986). Data are from Krajci *et al.* (1992) and Piskurich *et al.* (1997). Adapted from Mostov and Kaetzel (1999).

et al., 1982), human (Max and Korsmeyer, 1985; Matsuuchi *et al.*, 1986), cattle (Kulseth and Rogne, 1994), chicken (Takahashi *et al.*, 2000, 2002); possum (Adamski and Demmer, 1999), bullfrog (Mikoryak *et al.*, 1988; Hohman and Steiner, 2000), clawed toad (Hohman *et al.*, 1997), turtle (Iwata *et al.*, 2002), shark (Hohman *et al.*, 2003), and even earthworm (Takahashi *et al.*, 1996). Amino acid sequences of purified J chain have been determined in the rabbit (Hughes, 1990). The chromosomal location of the J chain gene has been determined for mouse and human; in mouse it resides on chromosome 5 (Yagi *et al.*, 1982) and in human, on the long arm of chromosome 4 (Max *et al.*, 1986). The genomic organization of murine J chain consists of four exons distributed over 7.3 kb **(Fig. 10.7)** (Matsuuchi *et al.*, 1986). Unlike Ig genes, J chain genes do not undergo rearrangement during B cell differentiation (Yagi and Koshland, 1981; Matsuuchi *et al.*, 1986).

The J chain protein has been highly conserved evolutionarily and is approximately 73% identical among mammals (Kulseth and Rogne, 1994). Furthermore, the predicted amino acid sequence of earthworm J chain is between 56% and 69% homologous to those of the mammalian J chains (Takahashi *et al.*, 1996). When J chain interacts with IgA, it forms a disulfide bond with the penultimate cysteine residue of IgA and links IgA monomers together in an end-to-end configuration, with J chain in the middle (Atkin *et al.*, 1996; Krugmann *et al.*, 1997). Several groups have proposed 3-D structures for the J chain protein, either that of an Ig-like molecule with a single domain (Zikan *et al.*, 1985) or that of a non-Ig-like molecule with two domains (Cann *et al.*, 1982; Frutiger *et al.*, 1992). Resolution of the 3-D structure of J chain awaits x-ray crystallographic or nuclear resonance imaging data.

The function of J chain has yet to be fully understood. It is known to be involved in but not required for polymeric IgM and dimeric IgA assembly, as well as transport of sIgA across the mucosal epithelium. J chain–deficient mice have elevated serum monomeric IgA levels, but dimeric IgA is also present. Thus J chain is not required for assembly of the dimers (Hendrickson *et al.*, 1995). J chain knockout mice also have lower bile and fecal IgA levels than do wild-type mice, a circumstance suggesting that J chain is required for efficient transport of sIgA into the bile (Hendrickson *et al.*, 1995).

Additional studies of IgA transport with J chain knockout mice showed that breast milk, nasal wash, and intestinal mucosal surface all had normal levels of IgA in comparison with levels in wild-type mice (Hendrickson *et al.*, 1996). However, the S-IgA found at these locations in J chain–deficient mice was mostly monomeric and was not associated with SC (Hendrickson *et al.*, 1996). Thus, J chain is not essential for transport of monomeric IgA but rather functions in forming a stable association between dimeric IgA and SC. It is not known whether J chain knockout mice respond normally to mucosal challenge. Because J chain is expressed in invertebrates (Takahashi *et al.*, 1996), which have no adaptive immune response, J chain may have functions other than polymeric Ig transport and assembly.

In mouse and human, expression of J chain is not restricted only to cells that produce polymeric IgM and IgA. In mouse, J chain expression is found in plasma cells and activated B cells, regardless of isotype (Koshland *et al.*, 1985). Kimura *et al.* (2001) examined expression of murine J chain and μ heavy chain in fetal tissues and found that μ heavy chain expression preceded that of J chain. However, in humans, J chain is expressed in precursor B cells, prior to the expression of Ig (McCune *et al.*, 1981; Iwase *et al.*, 1993; Mestecky *et al.*, 1997). Iwase *et al.* (1993) performed *in situ* PCR for J chain expression on human fetal liver sections and found that the expression of J chain preceded that of μ by at least 1 week. Furthermore, FACS separation of different stages of phenotypically defined B lineage cells from fetal and adult bone marrow, followed by RT-PCR for J chain, showed that J chain was expressed at all stages of B cell development, even the earliest stage prior to expression and rearrangement of the Ig heavy chain (Bertrand *et al.*, 1996; Mestecky *et al.*, 1997). In addition, J chain is expressed during all stages of fetal thymocyte development (Bertrand *et al.*, 1996). Together, these data suggest that J chain expression is regulated differently than Ig expression.

Analysis of the promoter region of J chain in mice showed that it contains two tissue-specific elements, a decanucleotide and pentadecanucleotide, as well as an octamer element (Sigvardsson *et al.*, 1993). These elements are also found in the human and mouse V_κ genes, mouse V_λ genes, and heavy chain enhancers (Mills *et al.*, 1983; Falkner *et al.*, 1984; Parslow *et al.*, 1984; Mage *et al.*, 1989). Their presence in both Ig and J chain genes suggests that expression of Ig and J chain genes are, to some extent, coordinately regulated. Elements that regulate the expression of J chain prior to Ig expression have not yet been defined.

Koshland and colleagues studied the regulation of J chain expression by IL-2. IL-2 is produced by T cells during an immune response and can bind to the IL-2R present on activated B cells. This interaction has been shown to upregulate J chain expression, presumably in B cells differentiating into plasma cells. Using a cloned murine B cell line (BCL1) stimulated by IL-2, Minie and Koshland (1986) demonstrated that IL-2 induces a DNase hypersensitivity region in the J chain promoter and enhancer regions (Kang *et al.*, 1998), suggesting that expression of the J chain gene is regulated by

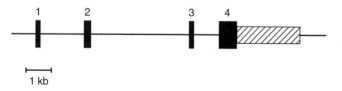

Fig. 10.7. Mouse J chain gene. The murine J chain gene comprises 4 exons spanning 7.3 kb. Exon 1 encodes the 5′ UTR and the leader peptide. Exons 2 and 3 encode the N-terminal half of the protein (amino acids 1–67), whereas exon 4 encodes the C-terminal half of the protein (amino acids 68–137) as well as the 3′ UTR. Adapted from Matsuuchi *et al.* (1986).

chromatin accessibility (Kang *et al.*, 2000). Further mutation and deletion analysis using this region in reporter-gene transfection assays identified two positive regulatory elements, JA and JB, within this region (Lansford *et al.*, 1992; Shin and Koshland, 1993). The JB region was shown to be activated by the transcription factor PU.1 (Shin and Koshland, 1993), whereas the JA region is activated by B-MEF2 (Rao *et al.*, 1998). In addition, promoter deletion analysis revealed a negative regulatory region (JC) upstream of the JA and JB elements. The protein responsible for binding the JC region and repressing J chain expression is called B cell lineage–specific activator protein (BSAP) (Rinkenberger *et al.*, 1996). IL-2 binding relieves this repression by downregulating BSAP and by increasing the amount of the positive regulators (Rinkenberger *et al.*, 1996). In addition, a fourth regulatory protein, the upstream stimulatory factor (USF), binds to an E-box motif immediately upstream from the BSAP binding site (Wallin *et al.*, 1999). Binding of BSAP to the JC region prevents binding of USF and prevents B-MEF2 from interacting with the J chain promoter. Only after BSAP levels decrease are USF and B-MEF2 able to bind to their respective promoter elements and activate J chain transcription. Thus, the tight transcriptional regulation of J chain makes an excellent model system to study activation-induced B cell differentiation.

PRODUCTION OF RECOMBINANT SECRETORY IgA (S-IgA)

S-IgA is the most abundant form of Ig in mucosal secretions, and the production of recombinant S-IgA would be valuable for passive immunizations against various mucosal infections. However, the synthesis of S-IgA requires the production of Ig heavy chain, Ig light chain, and J chain by plasma cells and secretory component, which is synthesized in epithelial cells and becomes associated with dimeric IgA during pIgR-mediated transcytosis. Several attempts have been made to generate intact S-IgA *in vitro* by associating dimeric IgA with recombinant SC produced in cell lines (Cottet and Corthésy, 1997; Crottet *et al.*, 1999; Lipschutz *et al.*, 2003). S-IgA obtained by this method exhibits properties similar to those of natural S-IgA (Crottet and Corthésy, 1999; Lüllau *et al.*, 1996). A more ideal process for production of S-IgA *in vitro* would be to have the S-IgA heavy chains, light chains, J chains, and SC all expressed in the same cell. Such recombinant S-IgA molecules have been successfully obtained by several investigators in CHO cells (Berdoz *et al.*, 1999; Johansen *et al.*, 1999), BHK-21 cells (Vidarsson *et al.*, 2001), and hybridomas (Chintalacharuvu and Morrison, 1997). In addition, Ma *et al.* (1995) developed a transgenic plant that expressed the recombinant S-IgA through successive crosses of plants expressing each of the S-IgA components individually. For clinical applications, post-translational modification of products of these "single cell" expression systems will need to be evaluated (Bakker *et al.*, 2001; Schweikart *et al.*, 1999). Even so, these expression systems lead to the exciting possibility that recombinant S-IgA of desired specificity may be produced in large quantities for therapeutic purposes (Ma *et al.*, 1998).

CONCLUSIONS

A secretory immune system is present in most if not all mammals, including primitive mammals such as insectivores, monotremes, and marsupials. Genes encoding IgA heavy chains have been cloned from several mammals, including man, mouse, rat, rabbit, pig, horse, and cattle; these Cα genes are highly similar to each other and easily can be used as probes to clone Cα genes of other mammals. Of nonmammalian species, IgA-like molecules in chicken and duck have been described. Most mammalian species seem to have one or two IgA isotypes expressed in secretions, but rabbits have at least 11 IgA isotypes. The presence of 11 IgA isotypes in rabbits is intriguing, and it will be important to evaluate their individual roles in secretory immunity.

Genes encoding pIgR are cloned from rabbit, human, mouse, cattle, rat, and possum, whereas J chain genes have been cloned from mouse, human, cattle, chicken, possum, bullfrog, clawed toad, turtle, shark, and earthworm. Experiments with the J chain gene will help elucidate the role of J chain in polymeric Ig, including S-IgA, as well as roles independent of Ig polymers. Experiments with the pIgR gene will elucidate the means by which IgA is transcytosed across the epithelium.

REFERENCES

Adamski, F. M., and Demmer, J. (1999). Two stages of increased IgA transfer during lactation in the marsupial, *Trichosurus vulpecula* (Brushtail possum). *J. Immunol.* 162, 6009–6015.

Apodaca, G., Bomsel, M., Arden, J., Breitfeld, P. P., Tang, K., and Mostov, K. E. (1991). The polymeric immunoglobulin receptor. A model protein to study transcytosis. *J. Clin. Invest.* 87, 1877–1882.

Arulampalam, V., Grant, P. A., Samuelsson, A., Lendahl, U., and Pettersson, S. (1994). Lipopolysaccharide-dependent transactivation of the temporally regulated immunoglobulin heavy chain 3′ enhancer. *Eur. J. Immunol.* 24, 1671–1677.

Atkin, J. D., Pleass, R. J., Owens, R. J., and Woof, J. M. (1996). Mutagenesis of the human IgA1 heavy chain tailpiece that prevents dimer assembly. *J. Immunol.* 157, 156–159.

Aveskogh, M., and Hellman, L. (1998). Evidence for an early appearance of modern post-switch isotypes in mammalian evolution; cloning of IgE, IgG and IgA from the marsupial *Monodelphis domestica. Eur. J. Immunol.* 28, 2738–2750.

Bakker, H., Bardor, M., Molthoff, J. W., Gomord, V., Elbers, I., Stevens, L. H., Jordi, W., Lommen, A., Faye, L., Lerouge, P., and Bosch, D. (2001). Galactose-extended glycans of antibodies produced by transgenic plants. *Proc. Natl. Acad. Sci. USA* 98, 2899–2904.

Bakos, M. A., Kurosky, A., and Goldblum, R. M. (1991). Characterization of a critical binding site for human polymeric Ig on secretory component. *J. Immunol.* 147, 3419–3426.

Bakos, M. A., Widen, S. G., and Goldblum, R. M. (1994). Expression and purification of biologically active domain I of the human polymeric immunoglobulin receptor. *Mol. Immunol.* 31, 165–168.

Banerji, J., Olson, L., and Schaffner, W. (1983). A lymphocyte-specific cellular enhancer is located downstream of the joining region in immunoglobulin heavy chain genes. *Cell* 33, 729–740.

Banting, G., Brake, B., Braghetta, P., Luzio, J. P., and Stanley, K. K. (1989). Intracellular targetting signals of polymeric immunoglobulin receptors are highly conserved between species. *FEBS Lett.* 254, 177–183.

Berdoz, J., Blanc, C. T., Reinhardt, M., Kraehenbuhl, J.-P., and Corthésy, B. (1999). *In vitro* comparison of the antigen-binding and stability properties of the various molecular forms of IgA antibodies assembled and produced in CHO cells. *Proc. Natl. Acad. Sci. USA* 96, 3029–3034.

Bertrand, F. E., Billips, L. G., Gartland, G. L., Kubagawa, H., and Schroeder, J., H. W. (1996). The J chain gene is transcribed during B and T lymphopoiesis in humans. *J. Immunol.* 96, 4240–4244.

Borggrefe, T., Wabl, M., Akhmedov, A. T., and Jessberger, R. (1998). A B-cell-specific DNA recombination complex. *J. Biol. Chem.* 273, 17025–17035.

Bottaro, A., Gallina, R., DeMarchi, M., and Carbonara, A. O. (1989). Genetic analysis of new restriction fragment length polymorphisms (RFLP) in the human IgH constant gene locus. *Eur. J. Immunol.* 19, 2151–2157.

Brandtzaeg, P. (1974). Mucosal and glandular distribution of immunoglobulin components: Differential localization of free and bound SC in secretory epithelial cells. *J. Immunol.* 112, 1553–1559.

Brandtzaeg, P., Kett, K., Rognum, T. O., Soderstrom, R., Bjorkander, J., Soderstrom, T., Petrusson, B., and Hanson, L. A. (1986). Distribution of mucosal IgA and IgG subclass-producing immunocytes and alterations in various disorders. *Monogr. Allergy* 20, 179–194.

Breitfeld, P. P., Harris, J. M., and Mostov, K. E. (1989). Postendocytotic sorting of the ligand for the polymeric immunoglobulin receptor in Madin-Darby canine kidney cells. *J. Cell Biol.* 109, 475–486.

Brown, W. R., and Butler, J. E. (1994). Characterization of a Cα gene of swine. *Mol. Immunol.* 31, 633–642.

Brown, W. R., Kacskovics, I., Amendt, B. A., Blackmore, N. B., Rothchild, M., Shinde, R. and Butler, J. E. (1995). The hinge deletion allelic variant of porcine IgA results from a mutation at the splice acceptor site in the first Cα intron. *J. Immunol.* 154, 3836–3842.

Brown, W. R., Rabbani, H., Butler, J. E., and Hammarström, L. (1997). Characterization of the bovine Cα gene. *Immunology* 91, 1–6.

Brüggemann, M., Free, J., Diamond, A., Howard, J., Cobbold, S., and Waldmann, H. (1986). Immunoglobulin heavy chain locus of the rat: Striking homology to mouse antibody genes. *Proc. Natl. Acad. Sci. USA* 83, 6075–6079.

Burnett, R. C., Hanly, W. C., Zhai, S.-K., and Knight, K. L. (1989). The IgA heavy-chain gene family in rabbit: cloning and sequence analysis of 13 Cα genes. *EMBO J.* 8, 4041–4047.

Cann, G. M., Zaritsky, A., and Koshland, M. E. (1982). Primary structure of the immunoglobulin J chain from the mouse. *Proc. Natl. Acad. Sci. USA* 79, 6656–6660.

Casanova, J. E., Apodaca, G., and Mostov, K. E. (1991). An autonomous signal for basolateral sorting in the cytoplasmic domain of the polymeric immunoglobulin receptor. *Cell* 66, 65–75.

Cazac, B. B., and Roes, J. (2000). TGF-β receptor controls B cell responsiveness and induction of IgA in vivo. *Immunity* 13, 443–451.

Chen, J., Young, F., Bottaro, A., Stewart, V., Smith, R. K., and Alt, F. W. (1993). Mutations of the intronic IgH enhancer and its flanking sequences differentially affect accessibility of the J$_H$ locus. *EMBO J.* 12, 4635–4645.

Chen, X., Rubock, M. J., and Whitman, M. (1996). A transcriptional partner for MAD proteins in TGF-β signalling. *Nature* 383, 691–696.

Chen, C., and Birshtein, B. K. (1997). Virtually identical enhancers containing a segment of homology to murine 3′IgH-E(hs1,2) lie downstream of human Ig Cα1 and Cα2 genes. *J. Immunol.* 159, 1310–1318.

Chintalacharuvu, K. R., Raines, M., and Morrison, S. L. (1994). Divergence of human alpha-chain constant region gene sequences. A novel recombinant alpha2 gene. *J. Immunol.* 152, 5299–5304.

Chintalacharuvu, K. R., and Morrison, S. L. (1997). Production of secretory immunoglobulin A by a single mammalian cell. *Proc. Natl. Acad. Sci. USA* 94, 6364–6368.

Coffman, R. L., Lebman, D. A., and Shrader, B. (1989). Transforming growth factor β specifically enhances IgA production by lipopolysaccharide-stimulated murine β lymphocytes. *J. Exp. Med.* 170, 1039–1044.

Cottet, S., and Corthésy, B. (1997). Cellular processing limits the heterologous expression of secretory component in mammalian cells. *Eur. J. Biochem.* 246, 23–31.

Crago, S. S., Kutteh, W. H., Moro, I., Allansmith, M. R., Radl, J., Haaijman, J. J., and Mestecky, J. (1984). Distribution of IgA1-, and IgA2- and J chain-containing cells in human tissues. *J. Immunol.* 132, 16–18.

Crottet, P., and Corthésy, B. (1999). Mapping the interaction between murine IgA and murine secretory component carrying epitope substitutions reveals a role of domains II and III in covalent binding to IgA. *J. Biol. Chem.* 274, 31456–31462.

Crottet, P., Cottet, S., and Corthésy, B. (1999). Expression, purification and biochemical characterization of recombinant murine secretory component: a novel tool in mucosal immunology. *Biochem. J.* 341, 299–306.

Cunningham-Rundles, C., and Lamm, M. E. (1975). Reactive half-cystine peptides of the secretory component of human exocrine immunoglobulin A. *J. Biol. Chem.* 250, 1987–1991.

Dariavach, P., Williams, G. T., Campbell, K., Pettersson, S., and Neuberger, M. (1991). The mouse IgH 3′-enhancer. *Eur. J. Immunol.* 21, 1499–1504.

Davidson, M. K., Le Beau, M. M., Eddy, R. L., Shows, T. B., DiPietro, L. A., Kingzette, M., and Hanly, W. C. (1988). Genetic mapping of the human polymeric immunoglobulin receptor gene to chromosome region 1q31–q41. *Cytogenet. Cell Genet.* 48, 107–111.

Davis, M. M., Kim, S. K., and Hood, L. E. (1980). DNA sequences mediating class switching in α-immunoglobulins. *Science* 209, 1360–1365.

Deitcher, D. L., and Mostov, K. E. (1986). Alternative splicing of rabbit polymeric immunoglobulin receptor. *Mol. Cell. Biol.* 6, 2712–2715.

Ehrhardt, R. O., Strober, W., and Harriman, G. R. (1992). Effect of transforming growth factor (TGF)-beta 1 on IgA isotype expression. TGF-beta 1 induces a small increase in sIgA+ B cells regardless of the method of B cell activation. *J. Immunol.* 148, 3830–3836.

Eiffert, H., Quentin, E., Decker, J., Hillemeir, S., Hufschmidt, M., Klingmuller, D., and Weber, M. H. (1984). The primary structure of human free secretory component and the arrangement of disulfide bonds. *Hoppe Seylers Z. Physiol. Chem.* 365, 1489–1495.

Fagarasan, S., Kinoshita, K., Muramatsu, M., Ikuta, K., and Honjo, T. (2001). In situ class switching and differentiation to IgA-producing cells in the gut lamina propria. *Nature* 413, 639–643.

Falkner, F. G., and Zachau, H. G. (1984). Correct transcription of an immunoglobulin κ gene requires an upstream fragment containing conserved sequence elements. *Nature* 310, 71–74.

Fallgreen-Gebauer, E., Gebauer, W., Bastian, A., Kratzin, H. D., Eiffert, H., Zimmerman, B., Karas, M., and Hilschmann, N. (1993). The covalent linkage of secretory component to IgA. Structure of sIgA. *Biol. Chem. Hoppe Seyler* 374, 1023–1028.

Flanagan, J. G., and Rabbitts, T. H. (1982). Arrangement of human immunoglobulin heavy chain constant region genes implies evolutionary duplication of a segment containing γ, ε, and α genes. *Nature* 300, 709–713.

Flanagan, J. G., Lefranc, M.-P., and Rabbitts, T. H. (1984). Mechanisms of divergence and convergence of the human immunoglobulin α1 and α2 constant region gene sequences. *Cell* 36, 681–688.

Fodor, E., Feren, A., and Jones, A. (1997). Isolation and genomic analysis of the rat polymeric immunoglobulin receptor gene terminal domain and transcriptional control region. *DNA Cell Biol.* 16, 215–225.

Frutiger, S., Hughes, G. J., Hanly, W. C., Kingzette, M., and Jaton, J. (1986). The amino-terminal domain of rabbit secretory component is responsible for noncovalent binding to immunoglobulin A dimers. *J. Biol. Chem.* 261, 16673–16681.

Frutiger, S., Hughes, G. J., Paquet, N., Luthy, R., and Jaton, J. C. (1992). Disulfide bond assignment in human J chain and its covalent pairing with IgM. *Biochemistry.* 31, 12643–12647.

Gillies, S. D., Morrison, S. L., Oi, V. T., and Tonegawa, S. (1983). A tissue-specific transcription enhancer element is located in the major intron of a rearranged immunoglobulin heavy chain gene. *Cell* 33, 717–728.

Grosschedl, R., and Baltimore, D. (1985). Cell-type specificity of immunoglobulin gene expression is regulated by at least three DNA sequence elements. *Cell* 41, 885–897.

Hanai, J., Chen, L. F., Kanno, T., Ohtani-Fujita, N., Kim, W. Y., Guo, W.-H., Imamura, T., Ishidou, Y., Fukuchi, M., Shi, M.-J., Stavnezer, J., Kawabata, M., Miyazono, K., and Ito, Y. (1999). Interaction and functional cooperation of PEBP2/CBF with Smads. Synergistic induction of the immunoglobulin germline Cα promoter. *J. Biol. Chem.* 274, 31577–31582.

Harriman, G. R., Bradley, A., Das, S., Rogers-Fani, P., and Davis, A. C. (1996). IgA class switch in Iα exon-deficient mice. *J. Clin. Invest.* 97, 477–485.

Heldin, C.-H., Miyazono, K., and ten Dijke, P. (1997). TGF-β signaling from cell membrane to nucleus through SMAD proteins. *Nature* 390, 465–471.

Hendrickson, B. A., Conner, D. A., Ladd, D. J., Kendall, D., Casanova, J. E., Corthésy, B., Max, E. E., Neutra, M. R., Seidman, C. E., and Seidman, J. G. (1995). Altered hepatic transport of immunoglobulin A in mice lacking the J chain. *J. Exp. Med.* 182, 1905–1911.

Hendrickson, B. A., Rindisbacher, L., Corthésy, B., Kendall, D., Waltz, D. A., Neutra, M. R., and Seidman, J. G. (1996). Lack of association of secretory component with IgA in J chain–deficient mice. *J. Immunol.* 157, 750–754.

Hendriks, R. W., Mensink, E. J. B. M., de Lange, G., and Schuurman, R. K. B. (1988). Two PvuII RFLPs recognized by a human immunoglobulin alpha heavy chain probe (IgHA1). *Nucleic Acids Res.* 16, 2365.

Hofker, M. H., Walter, M. A., and Cox, D. W. (1989). Complete physical map of the human immunoglobulin heavy chain constant region gene complex. *Proc. Natl. Acad. Sci. USA* 86, 5567–5571.

Hohman, V. S., Stewart, S. E., Willett, C. E., and Steiner, L. A. (1997). Sequence and expression pattern of J chain in the amphibian, *Xenopus laevis. Mol. Immunol.* 34, 995–1002.

Hohman, V. S., and Steiner, L. A. (2000). The sequence of J chain in an amphibian, *Rana catesbeiana. Immunogenetics* 51, 587–590.

Hohman, V. S., Stewart, S. E., Rumfelt, L. L., Greenberg, A. S., Avila, D. W., Flajnik, M. F., and Steiner, L. A. (2003). J chain in the nurse shark: implications for function in a lower vertebrate. *J. Immunol.* 170, 6016–6023.

Hughes, G. J., Frutiger, S., Paquet, N., and Jaton, J. (1990). The amino acid sequence of rabbit J chain in secretory immunoglobulin A. *Biochem. J.* 271, 641–647.

Hunkapiller, T., and Hood, L. (1989). Diversity of the immunoglobulin gene superfamily. *Adv. Immunol.* 44, 1–63.

Irsch, J., Irlenbusch, S., Radl, J., Burrows, P. D., Cooper, M. D., and Radbruch, A. H. (1994). Switch recombination in normal IgA1+ B lymphocytes. *Immunology* 91, 1323–1327.

Iwase, T., Saito, I., Takahashi, T., Chu, L., Usami, T., Mestecky, J., and Moro, I. (1993). Early expression of human J chain and mu chain gene in the fetal liver. *Cell Struct. Funct.* 18, 297–302.

Iwata, A., Iwase, T., Ogura, Y., Takahashi, T., Matsumoto, N., Yoshida, T., Kamei, N., Kobayashi, K., Mestecky, J., and Moro, I. (2002). Cloning and expression of the turtle (*Trachemys scripta*) immunoglobulin joining (J)-chain cDNA. *Immunogenetics* 54, 513–519.

Jessberger, R., Wabl, M., and Borggrefe, T. (1996). Biochemical studies of class switch recombination. *Curr. Top. Microbiol. Immunol.* 217, 191–202.

Johansen, F.-E., Natvig Norderhaug, I., Røe, M., Sandlie, I., and Brandtzaeg, P. (1999). Recombinant expression of polymeric IgA: incorporation of J chain and secretory component of human origin. *Eur. J. Immunol.* 29, 1701–1708.

Jung, S., Rajewsky, K., and Radbruch, A. (1993). Shutdown of class switch recombination by deletion of a switch region control element. *Science* 259, 984–987.

Kang, C. J., Sheridan, C., and Koshland, M. E. (1998). A stage-specific enhancer of immunoglobulin J chain gene is induced by interleukin-2 in a presecretor B cell stage. *Immunity* 8, 285–295.

Kang, C. J., Oh, U., and Koshland, M. E. (2000). Dynamic chromatin remodeling in the vicinity of J chain gene for the regulation of two stage-specific genes during B cell differentiation. *Mol. Cells* 10, 32–37.

Kataoka, T., Miyata, T., and Honjo, T. (1981). Repetitive sequences in class-switch recombination regions of immunoglobulin heavy chain genes. *Cell* 23, 357–368.

Kawamura, S., Omoto, K., and Ueda, S. (1989). Nucleotide sequence of the gorilla immunoglobulin alpha 1 gene. *Nucleic Acids Res.* 17, 6732.

Kawamura, S., Omoto, K., and Ueda, S. (1990). Evolutionary hypervariability in the hinge region of the immunoglobulin alpha gene. *J. Mol. Biol.* 215, 201–206.

Kett, K., Brandtzaeg, P., Radl, J., and Haaijman, J. J. (1986). Different subclass distribution of IgA-producing cells in human lymphoid organs and various secretory tissues. *J. Immunol.* 136, 3631–3635.

Kim, P. H., and Kagnoff, M. F. (1990). Transforming growth factor beta 1 increases IgA isotype switching at the clonal level. *J. Immunol.* 145, 3773–3778.

Kimura, M., Takahashi, T., Iwata, A., Matsumoto, N., Ogura, Y., Akagi, T., Akima, S., Kobayashi, K., and Moro, I. (2001). Ontogeny of the murine Ig joining chain gene and protein. *Scand. J. Immunol.* 54, 613–618.

Kingzette, M., Spieker-Polet, H., Yam, P.-C., Zhai, S.-K., and Knight, K. L. (1998). Trans-chromosomal recombination within the Ig heavy chain switch region in B lymphocytes. *Proc. Natl. Acad. Sci. USA* 95, 11840–11845.

Kipps, T. J., and Herzenberg, L. A. (1986). Homologous chromosome recombination generating immunoglobulin allotype and isotype switch variants. *EMBO J.* 5, 263–268.

Knight, K. L., Malek, T., and Hanly, W. C. (1974). Recombinant rabbit secretory immunoglobulin molecules: Alpha chains with maternal (paternal) variable-region allotypes and paternal (maternal) constant-region allotypes. *Proc. Natl. Acad. Sci. USA* 71, 1169–1173.

Knight, K. L., Suter, M., and Becker, R. S. (1988). Genetic engineering of bovine Ig: Construction and characterization of hapten-binding bovine/murine chimeric IgE, IgA, IgG1, IgG2 and IgG3 molecules. *J. Immunol.* 140, 3654–3659.

Koshland, M. E. (1985). The coming of age of the immunoglobulin J chain. *Annu. Rev. Immunol.* 3, 425–453.

Krajci, P., Solberg, R., Sandberg, M., Oyen, O., Jahnsen, T., and Brandtzaeg, P. (1989). Molecular cloning of the human transmembrane secretory component (poly-Ig receptor) and its mRNA expression in human tissues. *Biochem. Biophys. Res. Commun.* 158, 783–789.

Krajci, P., Grzeschik, K. H., Geurts van Kessle, A. H. M., Olaisen, B., and Brandtzaeg, P. (1991). The human transmembrane secretory component (poly-Ig receptor); molecular cloning, restriction fragment length polymorphism and chromosomal sublocalization. *Hum. Genet.* 87, 642–648.

Krajci, P., Kvale, D., Tasken, K., and Brandtzaeg, P. (1992). Molecular cloning and exon-intron mapping of the gene encoding human transmembrane secretory component (the poly-Ig receptor). *Eur. J. Immunol.* 22, 2309–2315.

Krugmann, S., Pleass, R. J., Atkin, J. D., and Woof, J. M. (1997). Structural requirements for assembly of dimeric IgA probed by site-directed mutagenesis of J chain and a cysteine residue of the α-chain CH2 domain. *J. Immunol.* 159, 244–249.

Kulseth, M. A., and Rogne, S. (1994). Cloning and characterization of the bovine immunoglobulin J chain cDNA and its promoter region. *DNA Cell Biol.* 13, 37–42.

Kulseth, M. A., Toldo, S. S., Fries, R., Womack, J., Lien, S., and Rogne, S. (1994). Chromosomal localization and detection of DNA polymorphisms in the bovine polymeric immunoglobulin receptor gene. *Anim. Genet.* 25, 113–117.

Kulseth, M. A., Krajci, P., Myklebost, O., and Rogne, S. (1995). Cloning and characterization of two forms of bovine polymeric immunoglobulin receptor cDNA. *DNA Cell Biol.* 14, 251–256.

Kushiro, A., and Sato, T. (1997). Polymeric immunoglobulin receptor gene of mouse: sequence, structure and chromosomal location. *Gene* 204, 277–282.

Lansford, R. D., McFadden, H. J., Siu, S. T., Cox, J. S., Cann, G. M., and Koshland, M. E. (1992). A promoter element that exerts positive and negative control of the interleukin 2-responsive J-chain gene. *Proc. Natl. Acad. Sci. USA* 89, 5966–5970.

Lebman, D. A., Lee, F. D., and Coffman, R. L. (1990a). Mechanism for transforming growth factor β and IL-2 enhancement of IgA expression in lipopolysaccharide-stimulated B cell cultures. *J. Immunol.* 144, 952–959.

Lebman, D. A., Nomura, D. Y., Coffman, R. L., and Lee, F. D. (1990b). Molecular characterization of germ-line immunoglobulin A transcripts produced during transforming growth factor type β-induced isotype switching. *Proc. Natl. Acad. Sci. USA* 87, 3962–3966.

Lieberson, R., Giannini, S., Birshtein, B., and Eckhardt, L. (1991). An enhancer at the 3′ of the mouse immunoglobulin heavy chain locus. *Nucleic Acids Res.* 19, 933–937.

Lin, Y. A., and Stavnezer, J. (1992). Regulation of transcription of the germ-line Igα constant region gene by an ATF element and by novel transforming growth factor-β1-responsive elements. *J. Immunol.* 149, 2914–2925.

Lipschutz, J. H., Lingappa, V. R., and Mostov, K. E. (2003). The exocyst affects protein synthesis by acting on the translocation machinery of the endoplasmic reticulum. *J. Biol. Chem.* 278, 20954–20960.

Lüllau, E., Heyse, S., Vogel, H., Marison, I., von Stockar, U., Kraehenbuhl, J.-P., and Corthésy, B. (1996). Antigen binding properties of purified immunoglobulin A and reconstituted secretory immunoglobulin A antibodies. *J. Biol. Chem.* 271, 16300–16309.

Lundqvist, M. L., Middleton, D. L., Hazard, S., and Warr, G. W. (2001). The immunoglobulin heavy chain locus of the duck. Genomic organization and expression of D, J, and C region genes. *J. Biol. Chem.* 276, 46729–46736.

Ma, J. K.-C., Hiatt, A., Hein, M., Vine, N. D., Wang, F., Stabila, P., van Dolleweerd, C., Mostov, K., and Lehner, T. (1995). Generation and assembly of secretory antibodies in plants. *Science* 268, 716–719.

Ma, J. K.-C., Hikmat, B. Y., Wycoff, K., Vine, N. D., Chargelegue, D., Yu, L., Hein, M. B., and Lehner, T. (1998). Characterization of a recombinant plant monoclonal secretory antibody and preventive immunotherapy in humans. *Nat. Med.* 4, 601–606.

Mage, R. G., Newman, B. A., Harindranath, N., Bernstein, K. E., Becker, R. S., and Knight, K. L. (1989). Evolutionary conservation of splice sites in sterile Cμ transcripts and of immunoglobulin heavy chain (IgH) enhancer region sequences. *Mol. Immunol.* 26, 1007–1010.

Magor, K. E., Warr, G. W., Bando, Y., Middleton, D. L., and Higgins, D. A. (1998). Secretory immune system of the duck (*Anas platyrhynchos*). Identification and expression of the genes encoding IgA and IgM heavy chains. *Eur. J. Immunol.* 28, 1063–1068.

Magor, K. E., Higgins, D. A., Middleton, D. L., and Warr, G. W. (1999). Opposite orientation of the α- and υ-chain constant region genes in the immunoglobulin heavy chain locus of the duck. *Immunogenetics* 49, 692–695.

Mansikka, A. (1992). The chicken IgA heavy chains: implications concerning the evolution of H chain genes. *J. Immunol.* 149, 855–861.

Massagué, J., and Chen, Y.-G. (2000). Controlling TGF-β signaling. *Genes Dev.* 14, 627–644.

Mather, E. L., Alt, F. W., Bothwell, A. L. M., Baltimore, D., and Koshland, M. E. (1981). Expression of J chain RNA in cell lines representing different stages of B lymphocyte differentiation. *Cell* 23, 369–378.

Matsuuchi, L., Cann, G. M., and Koshland, M. E. (1986). Immunoglobulin J chain gene from the mouse. *Proc. Natl. Acad. Sci. USA* 83, 456–460.

Matthias, P., and Baltimore, D. (1993). The immunoglobulin heavy chain locus contains another B-cell-specific 3′ enhancer close to the α constant gene. *Mol. Biol.* 13, 1547–1553.

Max, E. E., and Korsmeyer, S. J. (1985). Human J chain gene. Structure and expression in B lymphoid cells. *J. Exp. Med.* 161, 832–849.

Max, E. E., McBride, O. W., Morton, C. C., and Robinson, M. A. (1986). Human J chain gene: chromosomal localization and associated restriction fragment length polymorphisms. *Proc. Natl. Acad. Sci. USA* 83, 5592–5596.

McCune, J. M., Fu, S. M., and Kunkel, H. G. (1981). J chain biosynthesis in pre–B cells and other possible precursors of B cells. *J. Exp. Med.* 154, 138–145.

Mestecky, J., and McGhee, J. R. (1987). Immunoglobulin A (IgA): molecular and cellular interactions involved in IgA biosynthesis and immune response. *Adv. Immunol.* 40, 153–245.

Mestecky, J., Moro, I., Moldovveanu, Z., Takahaski, T., Iwase, T., Kubagawa, H., and Cooper, M. D. (1997). Immunoglobulin J chain: An early differentiation marker of human B cells. *Ann. N.Y. Acad. Sci.* 815, 111–113.

Michaelson, J. S., Giannini, S. L., and Birshtein, B. K. (1995). Identification of 3′ alpha-hs4, a novel Ig heavy chain enhancer element regulated at multiple stages of B cell differentiation. *Nucleic Acids Res.* 23, 975–981.

Mikoryak, C. A., Margolies, M. N., and Steiner, L. A. (1988). J chain in *Rana catesbeiana* high molecular weight Ig. *J. Immunol.* 140, 4279–4285.

Mills, F. C., Fisher, L. M., Kuroda, R., Ford, A. M., and Gould, H. J. (1983). DNase I hypersensitive sites in the chromatin of human μ immunoglobulin heavy-chain genes. *Nature* 306, 809–812.

Mills, F. C., Harindranath, N., Mitchell, M., and Max, E. E. (1997). Enhancer complexes located downstream of both human immunoglobulin Cα genes. *J. Exp. Med.* 186, 845–858.

Minie, M. E., and Koshland, M. E. (1986). Accessibility of the promoter sequence in the J-chain gene is regulated by chromatin changes during B-cell differentiation. *Mol. Cell. Biol.* 6, 4031–4038.

Mostov, K. E., and Blobel, G. (1982). A transmembrane precursor of secretory component. *J. Biol. Chem.* 257, 11816–11821.

Mostov, K. E., Friedlander, M., and Blobel, G. (1984). The receptor for transepithelial transport of IgA and IgM contains multiple immunoglobulin-like domains. *Nature* 308, 37–43.

Mostov, K. E., de Bruyn Kops, A., and Deitcher, D. L. (1986). Deletion of the cytoplasmic domain of the polymeric immunoglobulin receptor prevents basolateral localization and endocytosis. *Cell* 47, 359–364.

Mostov, K. E. (1994). Transepithelial transport of immunoglobulins. *Annu. Rev. Immunol.* 12, 63–84.

Mostov, K. E., and Kaetzel, C. S. (1999). Immunoglobulin transport and the polymeric immunoglobulin receptor. In *Mucosal Immunology* (eds. Ogra et al.), 2nd ed., 181–212. San Diego: Academic Press.

Muramatsu, M., Sankaranand, V. S., Anant, S., Sugai, M., Kinoshita, K., Davidson, N. O. and Honjo, T. (1999). Specific expression of activation-induced cytidine deaminase (AID), a novel member of the RNA-editing deaminase family in germinal center B cells. *J. Biol. Chem.* 274, 18470–18476.

Muramatsu, M., Kinoshita, K., Fagarasan, S., Yamada, S., Shinkai, Y., and Honjo, T. (2000). Class switch recombination and hypermutation require activation-induced cytidine deaminase (AID), a potential RNA editing enzyme. *Cell* 102, 553–563.

Nikaido, T., Nakai, S., and Honjo, T. (1981). Switch region of immunoglobulin Cmu gene is composed of simple tandem repetitive sequences. *Nature* 292, 845–848.

Nilsson, L., Grant, P., Larsson, I., Pettersson, S., and Sideras, P. (1995). The human Iα1 region contains a TGF-β1 responsive enhancer and a putative recombination hotspot. *Int. Immunol.* 7, 1191–1204.

Obata, M., Kataoka, T., Nakai, S., Yamagishi, H., Takahashik N., Yamakami-Kataoka, Y., Nikaido, T., Shimizu, A., and Honjo, T. (1981). Structure of a rearranged γ1 chain gene and its implication to immunoglobulin class-switch mechanism. *Proc. Natl. Acad. Sci. USA* 78, 2437–2441.

Pardali, E., Xie, X.-Q., Tsapogas, P., Itoh, S., Arvanitidis, K., Heldin, C.-H., ten Dijke, P., Grundström, T., and Sideras, P. (2000).

Smad and AML proteins synergistically confer transforming growth factor β1 responsiveness to human germ-line IgA genes. *J. Biol. Chem.* 275, 3552–3560.

Parslow, T. G., Blair, D. L., Murphy, W. J., and Granner, D. K. (1984). Structure of the 5′ ends of immunoglobulin genes: a novel conserved sequence. *Proc. Natl. Acad. Sci. USA* 81, 2650–2654.

Patel, M., Selinger, D., Mark, G. E., Hickey, G. J., and Hollis, G. F. (1995). Sequence of the dog immunoglobulin alpha and epsilon constant region genes. *Immunogenetics* 41, 282–286.

Pernis, B., Pernis, B., Forni, L., Dubiski, S., Kelus, A. S., Mandy, W. J., and Todd, C. W. (1973). Heavy chain variable and constant region allotypes in single rabbit plasma cells. *Immunochemistry* 10, 281–285.

Pettersson, S., Cook, G., Bruggemann, M., Williams, G., and Neuberger, M. (1990). A second B cell–specific enhancer 3′ of the immunoglobulin heavy-chain locus. *Nature* 344, 165–168.

Pinaud, E., Khamlichi, A. A., Le Morvan, C., Drouet, M., Nalesso, V., Le Bert, M., and Cogné, M. (2001). Localization of the 3′ IgH locus elements that effect long-distance regulation of class switch recombination. *Immunity* 15, 187–199.

Piskurich, J. F., Blanchard, M. H., Youngman, K. R., France, J. A., and Kaetzel, C. S. (1995). Molecular cloning of the mouse polymeric Ig receptor. Functional regions of the molecule are conserved among five mammalian species. *J. Immunol.* 154, 1735–1747.

Piskurich, J. F., Youngman, K. R., Phillips, K. M., Hempen, P. M., Blanchard, M. H., France, J. A., and Kaetzel, C. S. (1997). Transcriptional regulation of the human polymeric immunoglobulin receptor gene by interferon-γ. *Mol. Immunol.* 34, 75–91.

Plaut, A. G., Gilbert, J. V., Artenstein, M. S., and Capra, J. D. (1975). *Neisseria gonorrhoeae* and *Neisseria meningitidis*: extracellular enzyme cleaves human immunoglobulin A. *Science* 190, 1103–1105.

Rabbani, H., Pan, Q., Kondo, N., Smith, C. I., and Hammarström, L. (1996). Duplications and deletions of the human IGHC locus: evolutionary implications. *Immunogenetics* 45, 136–141.

Rabbits, T. H., Forster, A., Dunnick, W., and Bentley, D. L. (1980). The role of gene deletion in the immunoglobulin heavy chain switch. *Nature* 283, 351–356.

Radcliffe, G., Lin, Y.-C., Julius, M., Marcu, K. B., and Stavnezer, J. (1990). Structure of germline immunoglobulin α heavy-chain RNA and its location on polysomes. *Mol. Cell. Biol.* 10, 382–386.

Rao, S., Karray, S., Gackstetter, E. R., and Koshland, M. E. (1998). Myocyte enhancer factor-related B-MEF2 is developmentally expressed in B cells and regulates the immunoglobulin J chain promoter. *J. Biol. Chem.* 273, 26123–26129.

Revy, P., Muto, T., Levy, Y., Geissmann, F., Plebani, A., Sanal, O., Catalan, N., Forveille, M., Dufourcq-Labelouse, R., Gennery, A., Tezcan, I., Ersoy, F., Kayserili, H., Ugazio, A. G., Brousse, N., Muramatsu, M., Notarangelo, L. D., Kinoshita, K., Honjo, T., Fischer, A., and Durandy, A. (2000). Activation-induced cytidine deaminase (AID) deficiency causes the autosomal recessive form of the hyper-IgM syndrome (HIGM2). *Cell* 102, 565–575.

Rinkenberger, J. L., Wallin, J. J., Johnson, K. W., and Koshland, M. E. (1996). An interleukin-2 signal relieves BSAP (Pax5)–mediated repression of the immunoglobulin J chain gene. *Immunity* 5, 377–386.

Schmitz, J., and Radbruch, A. (1989). An interleukin 4–induced DNase I hypersensitive site indicates opening of the gamma 1 switch region prior to switch recombination. *Int. Immunol.* 1, 570–575.

Schrader, C. E., George, A., Kerlin, R. L., and Cebra, J. J. (1990). Dendritic cells support production of IgA and other non-IgM isotypes in clonal microculture. *Int. Immunol.* 2, 563–570.

Schweikart, F., Jones, R., Jaton, J. C., and Hughes, G. J. (1999). Rapid structural characterisation of a murine monoclonal IgA alpha chain: heterogeneity in the oligosaccharide structures at a specific site in samples produced in different bioreactor systems. *J. Biotechnol.* 69, 191–201.

Scinicariello, F., and Attanasio, R. (2001). Intraspecies heterogeneity of immunoglobulin α-chain constant region genes in rhesus macaques. *Immunology* 103, 441–448.

Serwe, M., and Sablitzky, F. (1993). V(D)J recombination in B cells is impaired but not blocked by targeted deletion of the immunoglobulin heavy chain intron enhancer. *EMBO J.* 12, 2321–2327.

Severinson, E., Fernandez, C., and Stavnezer, J. (1990). Induction of germ-line immunoglobulin heavy chain transcripts by mitogens and interleukins prior to switch recombination. *Eur J. Immunol.* 20, 1079–1084.

Shi, M.-J., and Stavnezer, J. (1998). CBFα3 (AML2) is induced by TGF-β1 to bind and activate the mouse germline Igα promoter. *J. Immunol.* 161, 6751–6760.

Shi, X., and Eckhardt, L. A. (2001). Deletional analyses reveal an essential role for the hs3b/hs4 IgH 3′ enhancer pair in an Ig-secreting but not an earlier-stage B cell line. *Int. Immunol.* 13, 1003–1012.

Shimizu, A., Takahashi, N., Yaoita, Y., and Honjo, T. (1982). Organization of the constant-region gene family of the mouse immunoglobulin heavy chain. *Cell* 28, 499–506.

Shin, M. K., and Koshland, M. E. (1993). Ets-related protein PU.1 regulates expression of the immunoglobulin J-chain gene through a novel Ets-binding element. *Genes Dev.* 7, 2006–2015.

Sigvardsson, M., Olsson, L., Hogbom, E., and Leanderson, T. (1993). Characterization of the joining chain (J-chain) promoter. *Scand. J. Immunol.* 38, 411–416.

Singh, M., and Birshtein, B. K. (1993). NF-HB (BSAP) is a repressor of the murine immunoglobulin heavy-chain 3′ alpha enhancer at early stages of B-cell differentiation. *Mol. Cell. Biol.* 13, 3611–3622.

Solari, R., and Kraehenbuhl, J.-P. (1984). Biosynthesis of the IgA antibody receptor: a model for the transepithelial sorting of a membrane glycoprotein. *Cell* 36, 61–71.

Spieker-Polet, H., Yam, P.-C., and Knight, K. L. (1993). Differential expression of 13 IgA-heavy chain genes in rabbit lymphoid tissues. *J. Immunol.* 150, 5457–5465.

Spieker-Polet, H., Yam, P.-C., Arbieva, Z., Zhai, S.-K., and Knight, K. L. (1999). In vitro induction of the expression of multiple IgA isotype genes in rabbit B cells by TGF-β and IL-2. *J. Immunol.* 162, 5380–5388.

Spieker-Polet, H., Yam, P.-C., and Knight, K. L. (2002). Functional analysis of Iα promoter regions of multiple IgA heavy chain genes. *J. Immunol.* 168, 3360–3368.

Stavenzer, J., Radcliffe, G., Lin, Y.-C., Nietupski, J., Berggren, L., Sitia, R., and Severinson, E. (1988). Immunoglobulin heavy-chain switching may be directed by prior induction of transcripts from constant-region genes. *Proc. Natl. Acad. Sci. USA* 85, 7704–7708.

Stavnezer-Nordgren, J., and Sirlin, S. (1986). Specificity of immunoglobulin heavy chain switch correlates with activity of germline heavy chain genes prior to switching. *EMBO J.* 5, 95–102.

Takahashi, T., Iwase, T., Takenouchi, N., Saito, M., Kobayashi, K., Moldoveanu, Z., Mestecky, J., and Moro, I. (1996). The joining (J) chain is present in invertebrates that do not express immunoglobulins. *Proc. Natl. Acad. Sci. USA* 93, 1886–1891.

Takahashi, T., Iwase, T., Tachibana, T., Komiyama, K., Kobayashi, K., Chen, C. L., Mestecky, J., and Moro, I. (2000). Cloning and expression of the chicken immunoglobulin joining (J)-chain cDNA. *Immunogenetics* 51, 85–91.

Takahashi, T., Kimura, M., Matsumoto, N., Iwata, A., Ogura, Y., Yoshida, T., Kamei, N., Komiyama, K., Mestecky, J., and Moro, I. (2002). Cloning of the chicken immunoglobulin joining (J)-chain gene and characterization of its promoter region. *DNA Cell Biol.* 21, 81–90.

Teng, B., Burant, C. F., and Davidson, N. O. (1993). Molecular cloning of an apolipoprotein B messenger RNA editing protein. *Science* 260, 1816–1819.

Terauchi, A., Hayashi, K., Kitamura, D., Kozono, Y., Motoyama, N., and Azuma, T. (2001). A pivotal role for DNase I-sensitive regions 3b and/or 4 in the induction of somatic hypermutation of IgH genes. *J. Immunol.* 167, 811–820.

Tian, M., and Alt, F. W. (2000). Transcription-induced cleavage of immunoglobulin switch regions by nucleotide excision repair nucleases *in vitro*. *J. Biol. Chem.* 275, 24163–24172.

Tokuyama, H., and Tokuyama, Y. (1997). Retinoic acid induces the expression of germ-line Cα transcript mainly by a TGF-β-independent mechanism. *Cell. Immunol.* 176, 14–21.

Tucker, P. W., Slightom, J. L., and Blattner, F. R. (1981). Mouse IgA heavy chain gene sequence: Implications for evolution of immunoglobulin hinge exons. *Proc. Natl. Acad. Sci. USA* 78, 7684–7688.

Ueda, S., Matsuda, F., and Honjo, T. (1988). Multiple recombinational events in primate immunoglobulin epsilon and alpha genes suggest closer relationship of human to chimpanzees than to gorillas. *J. Mol. Evol.* 27, 77–83.

van IJzendoorn, S. C., Tuvim, M. J., Weimbs, T., Dickey, B. F., and Mostov, K. E. (2002). Direct interaction between Rab3b and the polymeric immunoglobulin receptor controls ligand-stimulated transcytosis in epithelial cells. *Dev. Cell* 2, 219–228.

van Vlasselaer, P., Punnonen, J., and de Vries, J. E. (1992). Transforming growth factor-β directs IgA switching in human B cells. *J. Immunol.* 148, 2062–2067.

Verbeet, M. P., Vermeer, H., Warmerdam, G. C., de Boer, H. A., and Lee, S. H. (1995a). Cloning and characterization of the bovine polymeric immunoglobulin receptor-encoding cDNA. *Gene* 164, 329–333.

Verbeet, M. P., Vollebregt, E., van Amersfoorth, S., Kaetzel, C., He Lee, S., and de Boer, H.A. (1995b). Cloning and genome structure of the murine polymeric immunoglobulin receptor gene. *J. Cell. Biochem. Suppl.* 19A, 252.

Vidarsson, G., van der Pol, W. L., van den Elsen, J. M., Vilé, H., Jansen, M., Duijs, J., Morton, H. C., Boel, E., Daha, M. R., Corthésy, B., and van de Winkel, J. G. (2001). Activity of human IgG and IgA subclasses in immune defense against *Neisseria meningitidis* serogroup B. *J. Immunol.* 166, 6250–6256.

Volgina, V. V., Kingzette, M., Zhai, S.-K., and Knight, K. L. (2000). A single 3′α has1,2 enhancer in the rabbit IgH locus. *J. Immunol.* 165, 6400–6405.

von Schwedler, U., Jack, H. M., and Wabl, M. (1990). Circular DNA is a product of the immunoglobulin class switch rearrangement. *Nature* 345, 452–456.

Wagner, B., Siebenkotten, G., Leibold, W., and Radbruch, A. (1997). Organization of the equine immunoglobulin constant heavy chain genes: I. Cε and Cα genes. *Vet. Immunol. Immunopathol.* 12, 1–13.

Wallin, J. J., Rinkenberger, J. L., Rao, S., Gackstetter, E. R., Koshland, M. E., and Zwollo, P. (1999). B cell–specific activator protein prevents two activator factors from binding to the immunoglobulin *J* chain promoter until the antigen-driven stages of B cell development. *J. Biol. Chem.* 274, 15959–15965.

Wang, E., Brown, P. S., Aroeti, B., Chapin, S. J., Mostov, K. E., and Dunn, K. W. (2000). Apical and basolateral endocytic pathways of MDCK cells meet in acidic common endosomes distinct from a nearly-neutral apical recycling endosome. *Traffic* 1, 480–493.

White, G. P., Roche, P., Brandon, M. R., Newton, S. E., and Meeusen, E. N. T. (1998). Cloning and characterization of sheep (*Ovis aries*) immunoglobulin α chain. *Immunogenetics* 48, 359–362.

Word, C. J., Mushinski, J. F., and Tucker, P.W. (1983). The murine immunoglobulin α gene expresses multiple transcripts from a unique membrane exon. *EMBO J.* 2, 887–898.

Xie, X.-Q., Pardali, E., Holm, M., Sideras, P., and Grundström, T. (1999). AML and Ets proteins regulate the Iα1 germ-line promoter. *Eur. J. Immunol.* 29, 488–498.

Yagi, M., and Koshland, M. E. (1981). Expression of the J chain gene during B cell differentiation is inversely correlated with DNA methylation. *Proc. Natl. Acad. Sci. USA* 78, 4907–4911.

Yagi, M., D'Eustachio, P., Ruddle, F. H., and Koshland, M. E. (1982). J chain is encoded by a single gene unlinked to other immunoglobulin structural genes. *J. Exp. Med.* 155, 647–654.

Yang, X., Letterio, J. J., Lechleider, R. J., Chen, L., Hayman, R., Gu, H., Roberts, A. B. and Deng, C. (1999). Targeted disruption of SMAD3 results in impaired mucosal immunity and diminished T cell responsiveness to TGF-β. *EMBO J.* 18, 1280–1291.

Yaoita, Y., and Honjo, T. (1980). Deletion of immunoglobulin heavy chain genes from expressed allelic chromosome. *Nature* 286, 850–853.

Zan, H., Cerutti, A., Dramitinos, P., Schaffer, A., and Casali, P. (1998). CD40 engagement triggers switching to IgA1 and IgA2 in human B cells through induction of endogenous TGF-β: evidence for TGF-β but not IL-10-dependent direct Sμ → Sα and sequential Sμ→ Sγ, Sγ→ Sα DNA recombination. *J. Immunol.* 161, 5217–5225.

Zhang, Y., Feng, X. H., and Derynck, R. (1998). Smad3 and Smad4 cooperate with c-Jun/c-Fos to mediate TGF-β-induced transcription. *Nature* 394, 909–913.

Zhang, Y., and Derynck, R. (2000). Transcriptional regulation of the transforming growth factor-β-inducible mouse germ line Igα constant region gene by functional cooperation of Smad, CREB, and AML family members. *J. Biol. Chem.* 275, 16979–16985.

Zhao, Y., Rabbani, H., Shimizu, A., and Hammarström, L. (2000). Mapping of the chicken immunoglobulin heavy-chain constant region gene locus reveals an inverted α gene upstream of a condensed υ gene. *Immunology* 101, 348–353.

Zikan, J., Novotny, J., Trapane, T. L., Koshland, M. E., Urry, D. W., Bennett, J. C., and Mestecky, J. (1985). Secondary structure of the immunoglobulin J chain. *Proc. Natl. Acad. Sci. USA* 82, 5905–5909.

Phylogeny and Comparative Physiology of IgA

Chapter
11

Jane V. Peppard
Aventis Pharmaceuticals, Bridgewater, New Jersey

Charlotte S. Kaetzel
Department of Microbiology, Immunology, & Molecular Genetics, and Department of Pathology & Laboratory Medicine, University of Kentucky, Lexington, Kentucky

Michael W. Russell
Department of Microbiology and Immunology, and of Oral Biology, University at Buffalo, Buffalo, New York

ORIGINS OF MUCOSAL IMMUNITY

Proteins of the immunoglobulin (Ig) superfamily in several invertebrate phyla, including Annelida, Arthropoda, Echinodermata, and Mollusca, and in Holothuroidea, which are related to the chordate ancestors of the vertebrates, have been recorded (Du Pasquier, 1993). Ig variable region–like domains, some with chitin-binding properties, have been identified in the protochordate amphioxus (*Branchiostoma floridae*) (Cannon *et al.*, 2002), and Ig-like molecules occur in the Agnatha (lamprey and hagfish), but these are very different from those of jawed fish (Varner *et al.*, 1991). Cells of lymphocyte morphology expressing immune function–associated proteins have been found in the lamprey (*Petromyzon marinus*) (Uinuk-ool *et al.*, 2002). True immune systems with antibodies are generally considered to have evolved with the Gnathostomata (jawed vertebrates), and it has been suggested that the development of jaws and predatory feeding habits in the early Placoderms led also to the evolution of immune systems, complete with gut-associated lymphoid tissues (GALT), as protection against the higher rates of microbial and parasitic infection that resulted (Matsunaga and Rahman, 1998). Although there has been considerable effort devoted to the study of the molecular origins and evolution of Ig genes among different classes of fish as well as Amphibia (Schluter *et al.*, 1997), there are large gaps in understanding, particularly concerning the origins of IgA and its physiological functions as we know it in mammals. The origins of J chain and secretory component (SC), as necessary adjuncts to IgA in mammalian systems, are also obscure.

Equally uncertain is when a fully functional mucosal immune system, again as we understand it in mammals, evolved. Primitive GALT occurs in the Agnatha, which lack a true spleen and thymus, and the typhlosole and Leydig's organ represent lymphoid tissues in the anterior intestine of the ammocoete larva of the lamprey and elasmobranchs, respectively (Zapata and Amemiya, 2000). Teleost fish such as carp (*Cyprinus carpio*), channel catfish (*Ictalurus punctatus*), rainbow trout (*Salmo gairdneri*), plaice (*Pleuronectes platessa*), and seabream (*Sparus aurata*) can be immunized orally, anally, or even by immersion in antigens, which induce antibody responses in skin, intestinal mucus, bile, and to a lesser degree, serum (Fletcher and White, 1973; Georgopoulou and Vernier, 1986; Lobb, 1987; Rombout *et al.*, 1986; Ortuño *et al.*, 2002), implying the existence of a mucosal immune system (Hart *et al.*, 1988; St. Louis-Cormier *et al.*, 1984). Although fish do not have organized lymphoid follicles resembling Peyer's patches, uptake of antigens has been demonstrated by epithelial cells, especially in the hind gut (Rombout *et al.*, 1985). It is interesting, too, that gill cells of rainbow trout can trap and take up microparticulate antigen (Torroba *et al.*, 1993). Catfish eggs also contain Ig (Hayman and Lobb, 1993), and the transfer of antibody from immunized females into their eggs has been demonstrated in the plaice (Bly *et al.*, 1986).

COMPARISON OF IgA FROM EXTANT SPECIES

The mammalian mucosal immune system is the best characterized, and IgA has been found to be the major Ig of most (but not all) human secretions (Heremans, 1974). Vaerman (1970) identified IgA in several other mammalian species by means of "first-order criteria" such as antigenic cross-reactivity with human IgA, as well as by "second-order criteria," including association with SC, transport into secretions, and the presence of corresponding plasma cells in submucosal connective tissue, all of which define a secretory Ig system. Thus IgA was demonstrated in the serum and secretions (particularly milk), and IgA-containing intestinal plasma cells were found in the dog, cat, cow, goat, sheep, pig, horse, and hedgehog (Vaerman, 1970, 1973; Vaerman *et al.*, 1969). In addition, Vaerman (1970) summarized previous work describing IgA in various primates, rabbit, mouse, and rat, as well as in other species where the evidence was suggestive but not definitive. However, the functional characteristics of secretory Igs, such as those defined by "second-order criteria," are also found in IgM and other Ig isotypes. For example, IgX fulfills the role of a mucosal Ig in amphibians (Mussman *et al.*, 1996a), but this isotype does not appear to be ancestral to the IgA, which assumes this function in birds and mammals, and may have evolved from IgY. Although the anatomical structures typical of the mucosal immune system in mammals are not developed in ectothermic vertebrates (Zapata and Amemiya, 2000), marsupials such as the opossum, *Didelphis albiventris*, have well-developed Peyer's patches and IgA-containing plasma cells in the intestinal lamina propria (Coutinho *et al.*, 1993).

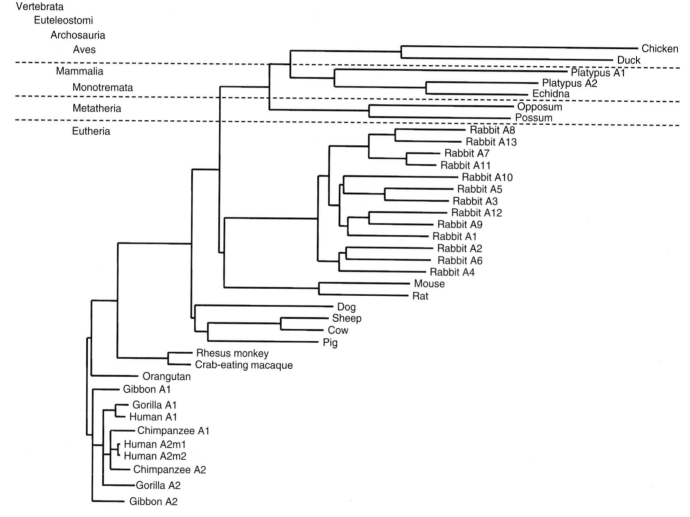

Fig. 11.1. Phylogenetic relationships among vertebrate IgA heavy chain amino acid sequences. The phylogenetic tree was built using the neighbor joining method (Saitou and Nei, 1987); horizontal distances are related to the degree of divergence among the sequences following a multiple sequence alignment. GenBank accession numbers: chicken (*Gallus gallus*), S40610; duck (*Anas platyrhynchos*), U27222; platypus (*Ornithorhynchus anatinus*) A1, Y055778; A2, AY055779; echidna (*Tachyglossus aculeatus*), AF416951; opossum (*Monodelphis domestica*), AF108225; possum (*Trichosurus vulpecula*), AF027382; rabbit (*Oryctolagus cuniculus*) A1, X51647; A2, X82108; A3, X82109; A4, X82110; A5, X82111; A6, X82112; A7, X82113; A8, X82114; A9, X82115; A10, X82116; A11, X82117; A12, X82118; A13, X82119; mouse (*Mus musculus*), D11468; rat (*Rattus norvegicus*), AJ510151; dog (*Canis familiaris*), L36871; sheep (*Ovis aries*), AF024645; cow (*Bos taurus*), AF109167; pig (*Sus scrofa*), U12594; rhesus monkey (*Macaca mulatta*), AY039245; crab-eating macaque (*Macaca fascicularis*), X53705; orangutan (*Pongo pygmaeus*), X53704; gibbon (*Hylobates lar*) A1, X53708; A2, X53709; gorilla (*Gorilla gorilla*) A1, X53703; A2, X53707; chimpanzee (*Pan troglodytes*) A1, X53702; A2, X53706; human (*Homo sapiens*), A1, J00220; A2m1, J00221; A2m2, S71043.

The cloning and sequencing of α-chain genes have now confirmed the presence of IgA in several orders of eutherians and in marsupials and monotremes, as well as birds. In the following sections, some salient features of the structure of IgA from those species for which sequence data are available are discussed (see also Chapter 9). Analysis of Cα sequences allows the construction of a phylogram expressing their relationships **(Fig. 11.1)**. The Comparative Immunoglobulin Workshop Web site (http://www.medicine.uiowa.edu/CIgW/) has information about Igs, including IgA, in species of veterinary importance.

Mammalia

Primates

The α heavy chains of several primate species have been sequenced (Kawamura et al., 1992), revealing interesting evolutionary developments. One of the most remarkable structural aspects of human IgA relates to the occurrence of two subclasses, IgA1 and IgA2, of which the former has an elongated hinge region that is rich in proline residues. Furthermore, the IgA1 hinge has an exact repeat of eight residues and contains O-linked oligosaccharides, which are unusual among Igs. IgA2 lacks this elongated hinge, having only five contiguous proline residues. Among anthropoid apes, the chimpanzee (Pan troglodytes) and gorilla (Gorilla gorilla) also have two IgA subclasses whose hinge regions are very similar to those of the respective human proteins. The orangutan (Pongo pygmaeus) has only one IgA that resembles human IgA1 and has apparently lost its IgA2 (Cole et al., 1992; Kawamura et al., 1990), whereas the gibbon (Hylobates lar) has two IgA subclasses similar to those of other apes. Monkeys appear to have only one IgA isotype, but considerable heterogeneity exists in the hinge region (Sumiyama et al., 2002), which is quite different from that of the apes. Evidence has been presented for the existence of two allotypes of IgA in rhesus macaques (Macaca mulatta), with further allelic polymorphism in the hinge region (Scinicariello and Attanasio, 2001). The recognition of baboon (Papio anubis) IgA by monoclonal antibodies specific for human IgA1 and IgA2 (Shearer et al., 1997) suggested the possibility of two subclasses in these animals, but this has not been confirmed by molecular studies.

The predicted secondary structures of primate IgA (Kawamura et al., 1990) suggest that the IgA1 hinges are largely random coils and that the IgA2 hinges comprise coil and β-turns, whereas the macaque IgA hinge assumes a β-sheet. It is interesting that the hinge regions of gorilla and chimpanzee IgA1, like that of human IgA1, have the sequences that render them susceptible to cleavage by bacterial IgA1 proteases (Cole and Hale, 1991; Qiu et al., 1996) (see also Chapter 15). Indeed, IgA hinge-region heterogeneity has been interpreted as evidence of evolution in response to the diversity of bacterial IgA proteases (Sumiyama et al., 2002). Genetic analysis of the entire H chain locus of primates indicates that the whole primordial Cγ-Cγ-Cε-Cα region has been duplicated in the common ancestor of the apes after its divergence from the monkeys to give rise to the multiple subclasses, although some of the duplicated genes have since become deleted or rendered silent in certain extant species (Kawamura and Ueda, 1992).

Rodents

Six allotypes of mouse IgA have been identified serologically in inbred strains of laboratory mice, and the Cα chains have been sequenced in comparison with that of a wild mouse (Mus pahari), revealing differences that may account for the antigenic epitopes (Phillips-Quagliata, 2002). Considerable variation occurs in the hinge region, which in the Igh-2^a allotype present in BALB/c contains a potential O-glycosylation site. Further similarity with human IgA2 allotypes arises from the disposition of Cys residues such that IgA from BALB/c mice seems to lack disulfide bonds between the H and L chains, whereas in C57Bl/6 and NZB strains IgA has the usual H-L disulfide bonds.

The rat α chain has been sequenced (S. Hobbs, personal communication; EMBL accession number: AJ510151). Two IgA allotypes have been described (Bazin et al., 1974), and the hinge region is quite different from that of the mouse.

Rabbits

The remarkable aspect of IgA in rabbits and their allies (Lagomorpha) is that there are 13 distinct subclasses (Burnett et al., 1989), of which most are expressible and all are potentially functional (Schneiderman et al., 1989). The C_H2 and C_H3 domains are the most conserved, whereas the C_H1 and hinge regions are quite variable. The level of expression, however, differs in various tissues: for example, 10 Cα genes are variously expressed in small intestine, appendix, mesenteric lymph node, and mammary gland, seven Cα genes are significantly expressed in the submandibular salivary gland, and only IgA4 is expressed in tonsil and lung (Spieker-Polet et al., 1993). Moreover, expression in Peyer's patches varies both within and between animals. IgA3 and IgA8, however, are not normally expressed at all (Spieker-Polet et al., 1999). Although the most frequently expressed subclass, IgA4, is the most 5' in the α-chain locus and some evidence suggests sequential switching, the ontogeny of expression does not appear to follow the order of the isotypes on the genome. However, what regulates this expression remains unclear, because all 13 Cα genes have similar Iα promoter sequences, although recent findings reveal that the promoters for unexpressed Cα3 and Cα8 are defective (Spieker-Polet et al., 2002). However, the relative expression levels for the other subclasses do not appear to be related to their respective promoter activities or to their response to TGF-β in vitro. It has been proposed that local microenvironments dependent on the intestinal microbiota influence isotype expression (Spieker-Polet et al., 1999). Moreover, the functional significance of multiple IgA subclasses remains a mystery, especially because rabbits have only one IgG isotype.

Pigs

The α-chain of pig IgA has been sequenced (Brown and Butler, 1994). Only one isotype is present, and the constant region shows a remarkable degree of homology (72%–73% overall) with human IgA1 and IgA2. However, the hinge region is quite different; two allotypes (a and b) exist, having six or two hinge residues, and were thought to have arisen from alternative splicing of the Cα1 exon to the hinge-Cα2 exon (Brown *et al.*, 1995). The expression of the two allotypes is regulated in heterozygotes by mechanisms that may involve endogenous and exogenous factors (Navarro *et al.*, 2000). Cleavage of pig IgA by the swine pathogen *Actinobacillus pleuropneumoniae* is thought to be due to the action of a nonspecific protease (Negrete-Abascal *et al.*, 1994; and see Chapter 15).

Ruminants

Early misunderstandings led to confusion of bovine IgA with its IgG1, which also has fast electrophoretic mobility, and the misperception that IgG1 was the predominant mucosal Ig. Large quantities of IgG1 are indeed transferred from the circulation into the mammary gland prior to parturition, so that the colostrum and milk contain more IgG1 than IgA (Butler *et al.*, 1972). This provides vital passive immune protection for the newborn calf, which receives no transplacental Ig *in utero* and must absorb colostral IgG through the intestinal epithelium during its first 24 hours *post partum*. Nevertheless, bovine milk and other secretions contain significant levels of S-IgA (Mach and Pahud, 1971), and IgA is abundantly synthesized in the mucosae of the gut and respiratory tract, as well as in salivary and lacrimal glands (Butler *et al.*, 1972). The bovine Cα gene has now been sequenced (Brown *et al.*, 1997). There is only one isotype, but evidence exists for allotypic polymorphism (De Benedictis *et al.*, 1984; Knight *et al.*, 1988). The hinge region is short and consists only of serine and cysteine residues. Bovine IgA displays 75% homology with pig IgA.

Sheep Cα chain gene has also been cloned and sequenced (White *et al.*, 1998). Not surprisingly, it shows closest homology with bovine Cα (89% identity) and progressively less homology with pig, hominoid, mouse, rabbit, and possum sequences. The hinge region is short but quite different from the bovine IgA hinge. Restriction analysis suggests that there is only one gene locus, but with the possibility of allelic variation.

Horses

The horse Cα gene has been cloned (Wagner *et al.*, 1997); there is only one gene copy, but restriction fragment length polymorphism among different animals suggests the possibility of four allotypes. Equine Cα has now been sequenced (Wagner *et al.*, 2003).

Carnivores

The sequence of the dog Cα chain (Patel *et al.*, 1995) reveals 65% and 70% overall homology with the corresponding chains of mouse and human, respectively, with the C_H3 domain being the most highly conserved. The hinge region of 10 amino acid residues is quite different from that of other species. Feline secretory IgA has been purified (Yamada *et al.*, 1992), and although IgA myelomas have occasionally been reported, the Cα gene has not been sequenced.

Marsupials and monotremes

An immunoglobulin resembling eutherian IgA was first reported from the marsupial *Setonix brachyuris* (quokka) by Bell *et al.* (1974), and α-chains have now been cloned and sequenced from the marsupials *Monodelphis domestica* (short-tailed opossum) and *Trichosurus vulpecula* (common brushtail possum) and the monotremes *Ornithorhynchus anatinus* (duck-billed platypus) and *Tachyglossus aculeatus* (short-billed echidna) (Aveskogh and Hellman, 1998; Belov *et al.*, 1998; Vernersson *et al.*, 2002; Belov *et al.*, 2002). Marsupial IgA (α-chains) closely resemble their eutherian counterparts in that they have three constant domains plus a short hinge region. Some minor nucleotide differences between clones suggest allotypic variation, although isotypic differences cannot be ruled out on the basis of the small number of clones sequenced so far. In contrast, 13 clones of monotreme α-chain segregate into 3 α1 and 10 α2 forms (Vernersson *et al.*, 2002). Together with comparative data on mammalian γ-chain and ε-chain sequences, α-chain sequence data support the theory that all the post-switch isotypes in mammals arose before the evolutionary separation of monotremes from marsupials and eutherians about 150–170 million years ago (Belov *et al.*, 2002).

Studies on lactation in the brushtail possum have indicated a biphasic pattern of S-IgA transport into the mammary glands that accords with the unique breeding biology of marsupials (Adamski and Demmer, 1999). The first phase of increased expression of the components of S-IgA (Cα chain, J chain, and pIgR) occurs briefly after the birth of the young when they transfer to the pouch to complete their development. A second phase of increased S-IgA expression, representing a second colostrum-like phase, takes place later, just before the young exit the pouch after completing their "external gestation."

Aves

Information on IgA (as well as most aspects of immunology) in birds is confined to a few species of commercial or agricultural interest in three orders, the Galliformes (chicken, turkey), Anseriformes (duck, goose), and Columbiformes (pigeon), leaving the great majority of nearly 10,000 extant species unexamined in this respect.

Work in the early 1970s from several laboratories demonstrated a homolog of mammalian IgA in the chicken (*Gallus domesticus*), antigenically distinct from IgM and IgY (formerly designated IgG; Warr *et al.*, 1995) and present as a minor component in serum but abundant in various secretions such as egg white (Lebaq-Verhayden *et al.*, 1974; Orlans and Rose, 1972; Leslie and Martin, 1973; Bienenstock *et al.*, 1973). Like IgY, chicken IgA lacks a hinge region and has four C_H domains similar to mammalian IgM and IgE, rather than the three found in mammalian IgA or IgG (Warr *et al.*, 1995). It has been suggested that Cυ2 (of IgY) may have contracted to become the hinge region of the mammalian α chain (Mansikka, 1992), although the hinge region of IgA is encoded at the 5′ end of the Cα2 exon rather than by a separate exon, as is the case for other Ig hinge regions (Tucker *et al.*, 1981). Mansikka (1992) also noted that chicken IgA bears a closer resemblance to IgM of the African clawed frog (*Xenopus laevis*) than to amphibian IgY or IgX (see Amphibia section). At the DNA level, 35%–37% overall homology of the deduced amino acid sequence of chicken Cα with human, mouse, and rabbit Cα has been demonstrated, with 41% homology between Cα3 of human and Cα4 of chicken. This homology is consistent with the evolution of IgA before the divergence of birds and mammals (Mansikka, 1992). Although antigenic similarity between human and chicken IgA is weak, nevertheless both chicken IgA and human dimeric (but not monomeric) IgA bind to the chicken pIgR (see later section), such that human IgA is transported into bile *in vivo* (Rose *et al.*, 1981). This confirms the existence of structural homology between these molecules in the region (Cα2 and Cα3 for human IgA) where SC binds. IgA has also been demonstrated in the turkey (*Meleagris gallopavo*; Galliformes) and the pigeon (*Columba livia*; Columbiformes) (Goudswaard *et al.*, 1977), and strong antigenic cross-reactivity has been demonstrated between the bile Igs of turkey and chicken (Hädge and Ambrosius, 1988).

It initially appeared that ducks and geese (Anseriformes) lacked a distinct secretory Ig resembling mammalian IgA and that IgM fulfilled this function (reviewed in Higgins and Warr, 1993), as happens in IgA-deficient humans. Chicken bile contains IgM as well as IgA (Bienenstock *et al.* 1973). However, as in other vertebrates, duck (*Anas platyrhynchos*) IgM is polymeric, possibly tetrameric rather than pentameric, and it occurs at low concentrations in serum (Ng and Higgins, 1986). Biliary Ig was demonstrated to resemble serum IgM but with additional antigenic determinants, and its 10-fold higher concentration suggested an active transport process. Biliary Ig of the goose (*Anser anser*) is strongly cross-reactive with that of the duck but not with that of the chicken or turkey (Hädge and Ambrosius, 1988). However, the deduced amino acid sequence of duck bile Ig most closely resembles the α chain of chickens (51% homology at the Cα4 domain) and can thus be considered an IgA homolog (Magor *et al.*, 1998). As in the chicken, duck IgA contains four Cα domains with no hinge region. Expression of the α chain is strongest in respiratory, alimentary, and reproductive tracts and is stronger than μ chain in these locations. Furthermore, whereas μ chain is present in 1-day-old ducklings, α chain mRNA does not appear until 14–20 days after hatching, consistent with the delayed development of IgA-dependent mucosal immune responsiveness in these birds. So far, no homolog of pIgR has been identified in ducks, but the molecular weight of intact bile Ig is consistent with a tetrameric molecule that would include an 85-kDa SC and a 15-kDa J chain. In functional terms, heterologous polymeric Igs (human IgA and IgM), but not IgG, injected intravenously appear in duck bile, although they appear to be degraded in the process (D. Higgins, personal communication). Furthermore, the antibody activity (e.g., induced by oral or intranasal influenza virus) of biliary Ig appears to be distinct from serum Ig responses (Higgins *et al.*, 1988). Thus, in birds, as in mammals, physiological compartmentalization and specialization of secretory and circulatory immunity have evolved.

The Ig H-chain locus in chickens and ducks is organized differently from the mammalian counterpart. The constant region genes are located in order: μ, α, υ (there is no δ gene) (Zhao *et al.*, 2000; Lundqvist *et al.*, 2001). Moreover, the α gene is in inverse transcriptional orientation, implying that switching to IgA must involve a gene inversion event.

Comparison of functions as well as structure of avian and mammalian IgA also supports the notion that they are similar. Evidence has accumulated confirming the existence of specific mucosal IgA antibody responses that are important in host defense against intestinal pathogens, for example, in fowl coccidiosis caused by *Eimeria* spp. (Davis *et al.*, 1978; Rose *et al.*, 1984). Responses to *E. tenella* include specific biliary IgA antibodies (Mockett and Rose, 1986) whose primary and secondary response kinetics are fully reminiscent of IgA responses to *E. nieschulzi* infection in rats (Rose *et al.*, 1984). In the development of vaccines for poultry, mucosal immune responses have been studied against infectious agents such as rotavirus (Myers *et al.*, 1989) and *Campylobacter jejuni* (Cawthraw *et al.*, 1994), where specific IgA antibodies were detected in bile and intestinal contents. Ocular challenge of chickens with infectious bronchitis virus induces specific IgA in lacrimal secretions (Toro *et al.*, 1996). Furthermore, in a remarkable example of convergent evolution, pigeons produce in their crop a secretion called "crop milk" with which they feed their young, and this milk contains Igs, predominantly IgA, transported from the circulation (Goudswaard *et al.*, 1979). However, this IgA is monomeric and not associated with SC.

SECRETORY IMMUNOGLOBULINS IN ECTOTHERMIC VERTEBRATES

No homolog of IgA has been identified in the earlier classes of vertebrates, yet it is clear that these animals have mucosal immune systems with secretory Igs, although they differ from those found in mammals (Bengten *et al.*, 2000).

Reptilia

The garter snake (*Thamnophis ordinides*) has three antigenically distinct serum Ig classes: a macroglobulin isotype classified as IgM and two ~9S Igs called Ig-1 and Ig-2 (Coe *et al.*, 1976). The 20.5S Ig was also found in bile and intestinal fluid (Portis and Coe, 1975). Although no antigenic distinction could be detected between the IgM found in serum and secretions, quantification relative to Ig-1 suggested that biliary and intestinal IgM is preferentially secreted. The same study showed that turtle (*Chrysemys picta*) bile also contains IgM. Tortoise (*Testudo hermanni*) bile and gut secretions contain predominantly IgM over 8.5S IgY and another 5.7S Ig, and the plasmacytes of the intestinal mucosae produce largely IgM (Vaerman *et al.*, 1975c). Hädge and Ambrosius (1983) were unable to detect in reptiles (or amphibians) an Ig that cross-reacted well with chicken IgA, but they concluded that reptilian (and amphibian) IgY might be a precursor of mammalian IgA (Hädge and Ambrosius, 1986).

These modern reptiles, however, are far removed from the extinct common ancestors of birds and mammals. If avian IgA is indeed a true homolog of mammalian IgA, then it might be hypothesized to have arisen during early reptilian evolution prior to the divergence of both bird and mammal precursors. Perhaps a search for IgA homologs among other reptilian orders, e.g., Crocodylia, or the relic species *Sphenodon punctata* (New Zealand tuatara; Rhynchocephalia) would be revealing.

Amphibia

Several species of clawed toad *(Xenopus)* have been shown to have three Ig classes, termed IgM, IgY, and IgX (Hsu *et al.*, 1985; Amemiya *et al.*, 1989; Mussman *et al.*, 1996b, Hadj-Azimi, 1979). IgX is quite similar to IgM at the cDNA level and in its physicochemical properties, but it is antigenically distinct and is detectable in serum at only low levels. IgM- and IgX-positive B cells, but not IgY cells, are found abundantly in the intestinal epithelium, whereas IgX-positive cells are virtually absent from the spleen (Mussmann *et al.*, 1996a), suggesting that IgX might be functionally analogous to IgA in these animals. Systemic immunization against dinitrophenyl (DNP)–keyhole limpet hemocyanin or trinitrophenyl-Ficoll results in good titers of specific IgM and IgY in serum but elicits very slight increases in IgX. Again, therefore, a separation between mucosal and humoral responses seems established in this species.

It has been reported that the neotenous salamander, the axolotl *(Ambystoma mexicanum)*, synthesizes only two classes of Igs, termed IgM and IgY (Fellah and Charlemagne, 1988). IgM, present in serum early in development, is the major specific antibody synthesized after parenteral antigenic challenge (Fellah *et al.*, 1992). The IgY H (υ) chain is most closely related to *Xenopus* υ chain, with 40% identical amino acid residues (Fellah *et al.*, 1993). However, in the axolotl, IgY occurs in the serum later during development than IgM and is relatively insensitive to immunization. Immunofluorescence detects IgY in the stomach and intestinal mucosae of animals between 1 and 7 months of age. It is intriguing that some anti-mammalian SC antibodies are reported to recognize a protein in the same tissues and to detect an ~80-kDa molecule in western blots of tissue extracts, giving rise to the suggestion that axolotl IgY might be analogous to IgA (Fellah *et al.*, 1992).

Fish

Although no secretory Ig homologous to IgA has been demonstrated in any taxon of fish, some interesting variations on the theme of secretory Igs exist. Several observations have suggested the existence of a mucosal immune system in Teleostei (bony fish). The serum of the sheepshead *(Archosargus probatocephalus)* contains two Ig forms, one ~16S (HMW Ig) and the other ~6S (LMW Ig). Serum HMW Ig is composed of two antigenically indistinct species, a tetrameric covalently linked 700-kDa form and a second subpopulation where the molecule is assembled as two noncovalent subunits, of ~350kDa each. J chain has been found in Ig of sheepshead and in the catfish (Lobb and Clem, 1981a), implying the existence of polymeric forms. In cutaneous mucus of the sheepshead, an Ig antigenically indistinguishable from the serum HMW Ig has been demonstrated; a second dimeric Ig has also been found, a subset of which is covalently linked and associated with a 95-kDa polypeptide

suggested to be an analogue of SC (Lobb and Clem, 1981b). Biliary Ig appears to be related to the HMW Ig of serum, but its H chain is slightly smaller (55kDa), and it occurs exclusively as a non–covalently linked dimer; however, no SC-like chain has been detected (Lobb and Clem, 1981c). Active transport of either serum Ig form to cutaneous mucus or to bile could not be demonstrated, suggesting that the Igs found in these secretions are locally produced (Lobb and Clem, 1981d). Multiple arrangements of a tetrameric Ig have been found in the catfish (Ghaffari and Lobb, 1989). In carp the serum Ig and that of skin mucus are physicochemically similar, containing predominantly tetrameric but also dimeric and monomeric forms; however, monoclonal antibodies distinguish between the two. One antibody, specific for mucus Ig, also reacted with many lymphoid cells in the gut and with the skin epithelium, liver sinusoids, and bile ducts, suggesting uptake of this Ig for secretion (Rombout *et al.*, 1993).

The lack of affinity maturation seen in the antibodies of fish (Warr, 1995) makes it difficult to follow specific immune responses, especially in scant mucosal secretions. However, numerous studies have shown that antigens delivered into the gut are taken up by the tissue and that the production of specific antibodies in the bile and mucosae ensues, sometimes with the development of protective immunity (reviewed in Hart *et al.*, 1988). In addition, some studies have indicated that the separation of circulatory and secretory antibody responses, well-known in mammals, exists also in fish. For example, oral administration of killed *Vibrio anguillarum* to carp induces specific antibody in skin mucus and bile, whereas none is detected in serum (Rombout *et al.*, 1986). Immersion of catfish in DNP-albumin can elicit anti-DNP activity in cutaneous mucus more than in serum (Lobb, 1987). With the need for successful vaccination strategies for commercially reared fish, where mass oral vaccination makes economic and practical sense (Hart *et al.*, 1988), further information in this area should be forthcoming.

The complexities of the tetrameric IgM-like proteins, which are the major form of Ig in various types of fish, have cast doubt on whether they represent the primordial Ig isotype. The Elasmobranchi (sharks and rays) have additional classes of large multidomain Igs, designated IgX(R), IgW, NAR, and NARC, that may be more ancestral (Greenberg *et al.*, 1996; Schluter *et al.*, 1997). The lungfish, *Protopterus aethiopicus* (Dipnoi, which are the most closely related fish to tetrapods), has been found to have, in addition to high- and low-molecular-weight IgM and IgN resembling the teleost Igs, another Ig that is considered orthologous to elasmobranch IgW (Ota *et al.*, 2003). This IgW heavy chain has a C-terminal secretory tailpiece with a subterminal Cys residue, as found in IgM and also in IgA, but no homology with IgA is suggested. Analysis of a homolog of IgD in the catfish suggests that it may be closely related to the ancestral Ig (Wilson *et al.*, 1997), but a phylogram of the relationships between Ig constant regions places the α heavy chain genes in a large cluster that also contains the μ, γ, υ, and ε heavy chain genes separate from the δ genes.

Exactly when in vertebrate evolution IgA first appeared is uncertain. Because mammals and birds have recognizable

IgA, including S-IgA, presumably IgA or its immediate precursor must have evolved with or before the appearance of reptiles (**Fig. 11.2**), and if that is true, then it seems likely that an Ig akin to IgA, or its relic, should exist in reptiles. Indeed, it has been suggested (Hädge and Ambrosius, 1984) that IgY, which first appears in amphibians and is the predominant serum Ig also in reptiles and birds, is a homolog of IgA. This interpretation, however, is based on antigenic cross-reactivity data; alignment of amino acid sequences from diverse species suggests that the relationship of the υ, γ, and ε clusters to each other is much closer than any of these to μ or α (Warr et al., 1995). In either case, however, IgA would appear to predate IgG in phylogeny.

ORIGINS OF J CHAIN

J chain was originally discovered as a component polypeptide associated with mouse and human polymeric Igs, both IgA and IgM (see Chapter 9), although its exact role in Ig polymerization has still not been fully clarified. Nevertheless, J chain appears to be important in maintaining the correct conformation of assembled chains and in interacting *in vivo* with pIgR on epithelial cell and hepatocytes, as well as *in vitro* with SC to form S-IgA or S-IgM. For example, J chain knockout mice have increased plasma and decreased bile and fecal levels of IgA, although serum IgM levels are normal (Hendrickson et al., 1995). J chain has been sequenced in the human, mouse, cow, rabbit, brushtail possum, chicken, turtle (*Trachemys scripta*), bullfrog (*Rana catesbiana*), *Xenopus*, and nurse shark (*Ginglymostoma cirratum*) (Hughes et al., 1990; Kulseth and Rogne, 1994; Matsuuchi et al., 1986;

Max and Korsmeyer, 1985; Adamski and Demmer, 1999; Mikoryak et al., 1988; Takahashi et al., 2000; Iwata et al., 2002; Hohman et al., 1997, 2000, 2003) and also identified in several other mammals and in both teleost and cartilaginous fish (Hadji-Azimi and Michea-Hamzehpour, 1976; Hagiwara et al., 1985; Klaus et al., 1971; Kobayashi et al., 1973; Lobb and Clem, 1981c; Mestecky et al., 1975; Moriya and Ichikawa, 1991; Trebichavsky et al., 1985). The high degree of serological cross-reactivity found between different species' J chains (Kobayashi et al., 1973) is reflected in a high degree of homology in the sequences that have been determined, implying conservation of this polypeptide across eons of evolution. However, although not secreted independently of polymeric Ig, J chain is synthesized early in B cell development, prior to the expression of Ig chains (McCune et al., 1981; Mestecky et al., 1997), and is found also in some B cells that express IgG; these findings point to a role, at present unknown, in some other aspect of B cell development or Ig expression. J chain is also expressed early in human development (in fetal liver beginning at the 6th gestational week) (Iwase et al., 1993). Perhaps consistent with such another function, J chain precedes Ig in phylogeny, as well as in ontogeny.

These considerations led to an examination of the occurrence of J chain homologs in invertebrates (Takahashi et al., 1996). Reverse-transcription-polymerase-chain-reaction analysis using oligonucleotide primers based on consensus gene sequences of mammalian J chains revealed the presence of J chain mRNA in coelomate invertebrates, including slug (*Incilaria bilineata*), oyster (*Crassostrea gigas*), clam (*Meretrix lusoria*), sea cucumber (*Stichopus japonica*), earthworm (*Eisenia foetida*), shrimp (*Penaeus japonicus*), crab (*Portunus trituberculatus*), silkworm (*Bombyx mori*), butterfly (*Artogenia rapae-crucivora*), spider (*Nepila clavata*), and sea squirt (*Ascidea japonica*) but not in much more primitive invertebrates such as sea anemone (*Metridium senile*) and amoeba (*Acanthamoeba castellani*). In addition, J chain transcripts were found in lamprey (*Lampetra japonica*) and lizard (*Eumeces latiscutatus*). The earthworm J chain gene sequence was reported to be 70% homologous with those of mammals, and extracts of whole earthworms revealed immunoreactive protein in western blot analysis with antihuman J chain antiserum. Immunohistochemical staining for J chain was demonstrated in skin mucous cells, intestinal epithelial cells, and macrophage-like cells of earthworm and slug, suggesting its possible involvement in defense, but otherwise its function in invertebrates remains a mystery because they do not produce Igs. Comparison of the earthworm J chain sequence with that of all vertebrates so far sequenced (Hohman et al., 2003), however, has raised questions concerning the identification of J chain in invertebrates.

ORIGINS OF SECRETORY COMPONENT

Although the molecular and cell biology of SC and its function as the pIgR that transports polymeric Ig across epithelia

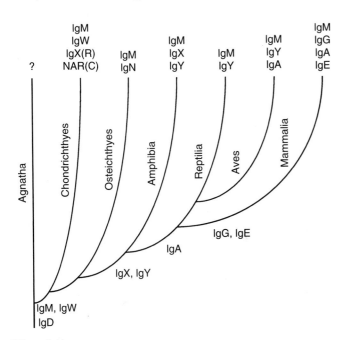

Fig. 11.2. Simplified phylogram of immunoglobulins in relation to vertebrate evolution.

have been comprehensively elucidated in recent years (see Chapter 12), its phylogenetic origins have not been as well examined as those of J chain. Because SC is a member of the Ig superfamily (Mostov et al., 1984), although its homologies are more with V domains rather than C domains, it presumably has ancient roots even if its proximal antecedents are uncertain. Expression of pIgR by mucosal epithelia and association of SC with polymeric Ig has been identified in the usual cast of eutherian mammals, including humans, pigs, cows, dogs, sheep, goats, rabbits, horses, guinea pigs, rats, and mice (Bourne, 1969; Mach et al., 1969; Mach, 1970; Pahud and Mach, 1970; Tourville et al., 1970; Reynolds and Johnson, 1971; O'Daly and Cebra, 1971; Pahud and Mach, 1972; Allen and Porter, 1973; Vaerman et al., 1975a,b; Piskurich et al., 1995; Pierre et al., 1995). Expression of pIgR mRNA and protein has recently been characterized for two marsupial species, the brushtail possum (*Trichosurus vulpecula*) (Adamski and Demmer, 1999) and the tammar wallaby (*Macropus eugenii*) (Taylor et al., 2002). Elevated expression of pIgR and transfer of IgA has been shown to occur in two stages in the mammary gland of marsupials (Adamski and Demmer, 1999; 2000). The first colostral-like stage occurs for a brief period after birth of the pouch young, and the second stage, unique to marsupials, occurs just before the young leave the pouch. Elucidation of the complete amino acid sequences for pIgR from eight mammalian species (six eutherian and two marsupial) has revealed considerable evolutionary divergence **(Fig. 11.3)**. The similarity in amino acid sequence among pIgR homologs in humans, cows, pigs, and rodents is on the order of 65%–70%, whereas the more distantly related rabbit pIgR is only 46%–53% homologous to other eutherians (Kaetzel et al., 2003). Although the overall homology among pIgR proteins is surprisingly low, the sequence of the Ig-binding motif near the N-terminus of pIgR is highly conserved (see Chapter 12). The selective conservation of this functional motif may explain the observation that SC/pIgR from humans, rodents, and rabbits can efficiently bind and transport polymeric (p) IgA from most

mammalian species (Mach, 1970; Underdown and Socken, 1978; Tamer et al., 1995). This conservation of function and the parallels between the phylograms for IgA and pIgR (Figs. 11.1 and 11.3) suggest the possibility that these proteins may have coevolved. DNA and protein parsimony analyses have placed the possum and wallaby pIgR sequences, which are 82% identical at the protein level, in a clade sister to the eutherian species (Taylor et al., 2002). The marsupial pIgR proteins are about 50% homologous to eutherian pIgR proteins, but it has not been determined whether marsupial pIgR can bind or transport eutherian pIgA.

As described above, there is clear evidence for a homolog of mammalian IgA in the external secretions of avian species. Furthermore, SC-like proteins have been found in association with pIgA in the chicken (Peppard et al., 1983; Peppard et al., 1986). Partial nucleotide and amino acid sequences have recently been reported for the extracellular Ig-like domains of chicken pIgR (GenBank accession numbers BM426916 and BG712734), where homology between chicken and mammalian pIgRs ranges from 40% to 50% (Kaetzel et al., 2003). However, the homology between chicken and mammalian sequences is considerably higher in the Ig-binding motif (see Chapter 12). There has not been a systematic search among the lower vertebrates for pIgR or its homologs, or for proteins that might fulfill an analogous function of transporting Igs into secretions. Evidence that amphibians may express an SC-like protein comes from the report that secretory IgY in the gut of the axolotl is associated with a 78-kDa molecule that reacts with antisera to mammalian SC (Fellah et al., 1992). In *Xenopus*, 11 pseudogenes (GenBank accession number AL645786) have been shown to bear some sequence similarity to mammalian pIgR cDNAs, but no protein homolog of pIgR has been identified in this species. There is some evidence that SC-like proteins may also be expressed in mucosal tissues of fish. The dimeric Ig found in skin mucus of the sheepshead is associated with a 95-kDa protein that may be an equivalent of SC (Lobb and Clem, 1981b), but this protein has not been further charac-

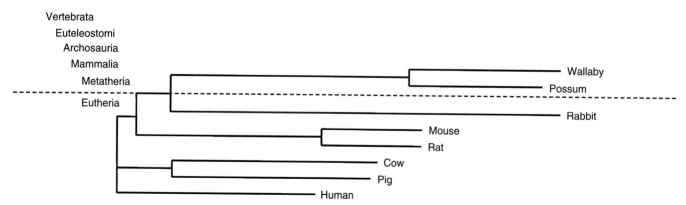

Fig. 11.3. Phylogenetic relationships among mammalian pIgR amino acid sequences. The phylogenetic tree was built as described for Figure 11.1. GenBank accession numbers: wallaby (*Macropus eugenii*), AF317205; possum (*Trichosurus vulpecula*), AF091137; rabbit (*Oryctolagus cuniculus*), X00412; mouse (*Mus musculus*), U06431; rat (*Rattus norvegicus*), X15741; cow (*Bos taurus*), X81371; pig (*Sus scrofa*), AB032195; human (*Homo sapiens*), X73079.

terized. The Ig found in sheepshead bile appears to be different from that found in either serum or skin mucus and is not associated with an SC-like molecule (Lobb and Clem, 1981c,d). More recently, screening of EST libraries from various fish species, including the zebrafish (*Danio rerio*) (GenBank accession number BF717724), the Japanese flounder (*Paralichthys olivaceus*) (GenBank accession number AU050700), and the Atlantic salmon (*Salmo salar*) (GenBank accession number BG936477), has led to the identification of short cDNA fragments encoding putative proteins with 26%–34% amino acid sequence similarity to mammalian pIgRs. These low-level sequence similarities must be interpreted with caution until the pIgR-like proteins are further characterized, especially considering the sequence homology between pIgR and Ig V domains. Clearly, further work needs to be done to elucidate the mechanism by which Ig is secreted in fish skin mucus and other discharges.

It therefore remains an intriguing speculation, subject to investigation, that pIgR may have evolved with the function of transporting polymeric Ig across epithelia to form secretory Ig in fish and amphibians, long before the appearance of IgA. In that connection, it appears that high-molecular-weight Igs from the bullfrog and nurse shark have the ability to bind human SC (Underdown and Socken, 1978). Furthermore, pIgR binds to IgM, which, together with J chain (which is essential for pIgR recognition of polymeric Ig), is phylogenetically older than IgA. If this is true, then when pIgA evolved at some later period in tetrapod phylogeny, there may have already existed a molecule for transporting it across epithelia, although this does not necessarily mean that the mechanism of transepithelial transport was as fully developed as that which now operates in extant mammals and birds. Furthermore, other mechanisms appear to exist for the transport of IgA, including monomeric and secretory forms, through the mammalian liver into bile. These include uptake through the asialoglycoprotein receptor (ASGP-R), which normally leads to intracellular lysosomal degradation of the bound protein. It is known that the ASGP-R and the pIgR start out on the same intracellular pathway but are segregated during transition through the endosomal compartment (Geuze *et al.*, 1984), and switching of human pIgA from ASGP-R to pIgR has been demonstrated in rat liver (Schiff *et al.*, 1984). Membrane-bound galactosyltransferase has also been implicated in the binding of IgA by cells *in vitro* (Tomana *et al.*, 1993a,b). Whether these pathways represent evolutionary hangovers from more primitive Ig transepithelial transport mechanisms is unknown.

COMPARATIVE PHYSIOLOGY OF IgA

Circulating IgA

IgA is synthesized in a variety of different sizes, including monomers, dimers, tetramers, and even higher polymeric forms. A single clone of cells can synthesize different forms of IgA (Moldoveanu *et al.*, 1984; Peppard and Jackson,

1987), and it has been suggested that IgA-secreting cells lodged in different organs can produce IgA with different size profiles (Kutteh *et al.*, 1982a; Brandtzaeg, 1983; Crago *et al.*, 1984). However, the proportions of circulating monomeric (m)IgA and pIgA, as well as total plasma IgA concentrations, vary significantly between different species of mammals and, in particular, between primates and other orders (Vaerman, 1970, 1973). Whereas in human plasma, IgA is usually present at 2 to 3 mg/ml and is predominantly (85% to 95%) monomeric, other nonprimate animals have much lower concentrations of circulating IgA, typically 0.3 mg/ml or less, which corresponds to the approximate concentration of pIgA in human serum. Moreover, the predominant form of plasma IgA in most animals is polymeric, although (as discussed below) in certain species, pIgA is actively and rapidly transported from the plasma to the bile by the liver. In rats, much of this plasma pIgA appears to come from the intestine and is delivered into the circulation from the lymph drainage of the gut through the thoracic duct, which contributes 10 mg of IgA to the plasma pool each day (Kaartinen *et al.*, 1978; Gyure *et al.*, 1990). Molecular size differences of IgA in different species have also led to discrepancies in the measurement of IgA concentration and of its molecular forms, especially when methods dependent on diffusion (e.g., single radial immunodiffusion) are used, because pIgA is underestimated relative to mIgA (Delacroix *et al.*, 1982c).

Circulating half-lives have been estimated for IgA in some species. However, as pIgA binds to pIgR, the rates of clearance of mIgA and pIgA differ considerably in species in which rapid hepatobiliary transport of pIgA occurs (see subsequent discussion). In rats, for example, pIgA is cleared too fast to obtain a relevant measurement of half-life, whereas the clearance of mIgA is similar to that of IgM, with a half-life of about 27 hours (Peppard and Orlans, 1979). In mice, mIgA has been reported to have a final (equilibrium) circulating half-life of about 24 hours, compared with about 10 hours for pIgA (Rifai and Mannik, 1983). In humans and rhesus monkeys, which have similar plasma levels of predominantly mIgA, the circulating half-lives of IgA are given as follows: human IgA1, 5.9 days; IgA2, 4.5 days (Morell *et al.*, 1973); monkey IgA, 4.5 days (Challacombe and Russell, 1979). These rates are also comparable with the corresponding half-lives of circulating IgM. Studies with a residualizing label have shown that the principal site of catabolism of mIgA is the liver in both mice and macaques (Moldoveanu *et al.*, 1988, 1990).

In those species in which it has been directly measured, the contribution of plasma pIgA to secretions (other than bile, as discussed below) is minimal, and the ample supply of pIgA in secretions is predominantly of local origin (rats: Dahlgren *et al.*, 1981; Lemaitre-Coelho *et al.*, 1982; Sullivan and Allansmith, 1984; Peppard and Montgomery, 1987; mice: Russell *et al.*, 1982; Koertge and Butler, 1986b; Mazanec *et al.*, 1989; sheep: Scicchitano *et al.*, 1984a, 1986; Sheldrake *et al.*, 1984; canine saliva: Montgomery *et al.*, 1977; human saliva: Delacroix *et al.*, 1982b; Kubagawa *et al.*, 1987). Milk in early lactation may be an exception: a higher proportion of IgA may be delivered from plasma, at least in mice and sheep (Halsey *et al.*, 1982; Sheldrake *et al.*, 1985).

It therefore seems that the physiology of IgA in humans (and probably other primates) is significantly different from that of the commonly used experimental animals, particularly because of the exceptionally high additional amount of circulating mIgA. Moreover, in humans and the anthropoid apes, this "extra" mIgA is predominantly also of the IgA1 subclass, which is distinctly different from most other forms of IgA (as discussed in the preceding section, Mammalia). As the biological functions of circulating IgA are poorly understood (see Chapter 14), the consequences of these differences are correspondingly obscure.

Hepatobiliary transport of polymeric IgA

In the higher vertebrates, a distinctive feature of pIgA is its ability to be transported across epithelia into secretions by means of the pIgR. From the mid-1960s, a transcytotic pathway involving SC was already known in principle to exist in the gut and secretory sites such as salivary, lacrimal, and mammary glands, but the mechanism was uncertain; as later reviewed by Brandtzaeg (1985), about eight different schemes had been proposed. However, in the late 1970s, the demonstration by several groups that the hepatocytes, which are also cells of epithelial origin, are capable of efficiently picking up and swiftly transporting pIgA across the liver and into bile in mice (Jackson *et al.*, 1977) and rats (Orlans *et al.*, 1978; Jackson *et al.*, 1978) permitted unequivocal demonstration

that SC acted as a cell surface receptor for pIgA on hepatocytes (Orlans *et al.*, 1979; Mullock *et al.*, 1980) in the same way as it did on epithelial cells (Crago *et al.*, 1978; Kühn and Kraehenbuhl, 1979). The subsequent elucidation of SC-mediated transcytosis of pIgA brought it to the attention of cell biologists, who found it to be an accessible model for a unique pathway of intracellular vesicular transport (Sztul *et al.*, 1983; Geuze *et al.*, 1984; Mullock *et al.*, 1987; Hubbard, 1991).

Using hepatobiliary transport as a model system to examine cross-species molecular interactions, experiments *in vivo*, in which rodent or human pIgA was injected intravenously into different experimental animals and its appearance in bile monitored, revealed major differences between species **(Table 11.1)**. Whereas rat, rabbit, and chicken liver transports rat and human pIgA into bile very efficiently, the livers of sheep, dog, cat, pig, and guinea pig are incapable of doing so, with mouse and hamster falling in an intermediate category. In sheep, however, homologous pIgA is transported, and mouse pIgA is more efficiently transported in rats than in mice. Examination of bile for pIgA content in various species in which transport is poor revealed that dog and cat bile, and some human and guinea pig biles, contain several pIgA forms (Orlans *et al.*, 1983). Collectively, these observations suggest that multiple factors influence the extent of pIgA transhepatic transport in different species. The degree of structural homology between the receptor binding site of the injected and endogenous IgA influences the ability of the injected IgA to compete with endogenous IgA for pIgR binding and also to complete the transport pathway intact. In

Table 11.1. Cross-Species Comparison of Hepatobiliary Transport of pIgA

% of injected ^{125}I-pIgA recovered in bile by 3–6 hours (IgA source species)					
Recipient species	**Human**	**Rat**	**Mouse**	**Sheep**	**Dog**
Rat	30[a, b]	30[c]	15[a], 60[d]	20[a]	
Mouse			28[d,e]		
Rabbit	35[a], 52[f]	35[a]			
Human	<3[g]				
Chicken	40[h]				
Sheep	<1[i]	<1[i]		5[a], 20[i]	
Guinea pig	<1[j]	<1[j]			
Dog	<3[k]				<1[k]
Hamster	20[l]				

[a]Orlans *et al.*, 1983.
[b]Vaerman and Lemaitre-Coelho, 1979.
[c]Orlans *et al.*, 1978.
[d]Koertge and Butler, 1986a.
[e]Delacroix *et al.*, 1985.
[f]Delacroix *et al.*, 1982a.
[g]Delacroix *et al.*, 1982b.
[h]Rose *et al.*, 1981.
[i]Scicchitano *et al.*, 1984b.
[j]Hall *et al.*, 1980.
[k]Delacroix *et al.*, 1983.
[l]Vaerman and Langendries, 1997.

addition, the concentration of endogenous IgA in comparison with injected heterologous IgA and the cell surface availability of the pIgR must be important factors.

The question of whether this transport mechanism exists in humans has been debated because although many investigators have demonstrated the presence of pIgA, S-IgA, and free SC in human bile samples (Nagura *et al.*, 1981; Delacroix *et al.*, 1982b; Kutteh *et al.*, 1982b; Orlans *et al.*, 1983; Mullock *et al.*, 1985; Vuiton *et al.*, 1985; Perez *et al.*, 1991), intravenous injection of radiolabeled pIgA into humans revealed little evidence of transhepatic transport (Dooley *et al.*, 1981; Delacroix *et al.*, 1982b), and there is contradictory evidence concerning the presence of the pIgR in human hepatocytes (Hsu and Hsu, 1980; Perez *et al.*, 1989; Nagura *et al.*, 1981; Krajci *et al.*, 1991). Similar to humans, macaques neither show consistent hepatocyte staining for pIgR nor transport pIgA from the circulation into bile (Daniels and Schmucker, 1987). It also has been suggested that dogs, in which hepatic staining for pIgR similar to that in human liver and little evidence of pIgA transport have been observed, are similar to humans (Delacroix *et al.*, 1983). In normal conditions, the pIgA that is transported into most secretions using pIgR is produced predominantly locally by plasma cells underlying the mucosae. The evolutionary origins and functional significance of the removal of pIgA from the plasma through active hepatobiliary transport as it exists in certain rodents are unclear. Because some of the species in which this transport is most active are coprophagous (rats, rabbits, mice), perhaps it serves as a mechanism for delivering large quantities of S-IgA antibodies into the top of the intestinal tract to control the load of fecal microorganisms. Some estimates indicate that in rats, 90% of intestinal S-IgA is delivered by this mechanism (Lemaitre-Coelho *et al.*, 1978). In addition, hepatobiliary clearance of antigen bound to IgA antibody has been demonstrated in rats and mice *in vivo* (Peppard *et al.*, 1981, 1982; Russell *et al.*, 1981; Socken *et al.*, 1981), and it has been suggested that this pathway provides the added functionality of eliminating undegradable bacterial antigens or food antigens inadvertently absorbed by the intestine (Russell *et al.*, 1983; Brown *et al.*, 1984).

CONCLUSIONS

Of all the isotypes of Ig in humans, IgA is the most heterogeneous on account of its multiple molecular forms as well as subclasses (Russell *et al.*, 1992); other species share the heterogeneity of molecular forms, which undoubtedly reflect the variety of physiological functions performed by IgA and the different physiological niches in which these are carried out. Even among the few species and orders of mammals that have been studied, it is clear that there are significant differences in the mucosal immune system and its best known effector molecule, S-IgA, by which these species protect themselves against the daily onslaught of environmental antigens and potential pathogens and regulate their com-

mensal microbiota. Although it is beyond the scope of this discussion, the most ancient lineages of extant vertebrates also reveal a remarkable heterogeneity of Ig structure, despite having an apparently more limited range of Ig isotypes. Though lacking an isotype that is clearly homologous to mammalian or avian IgA, ectothermic vertebrates nevertheless have anatomical structures and mechanisms (albeit poorly understood) for delivering specialized forms of Ig to their mucosal surfaces. Investigation of some of these "missing links" in the evolution of the immune system may well cast light on the remaining mysteries of human mucosal immunity and the origins and functions of IgA in particular.

REFERENCES

Adamski, F.M., and Demmer, J. (1999). Two stages of increased IgA transfer during lactation in the marsupial, *Trichosurus vulpecula* (brushtail possum). *J. Immunol.* 162, 6009–6015.

Adamski, F.M., and Demmer, J. (2000). Immunological protection of the vulnerable marsupial pouch young: two periods of immune transfer during lactation in *Trichosurus vulpecula* (brushtail possum). *Dev. Comp. Immunol.* 24, 491–502.

Allen, W.D., and Porter, P. (1973). Localization by immunofluorescence of secretory component and IgA in the intestinal mucosa of the young pig. *Immunology* 24, 365–374.

Amemiya, C.T., Haire, R.N., and Litman, G.W. (1989) Nucleotide sequence of a cDNA encoding a third distinct *Xenopus* immunoglobulin heavy chain isotype. *Nucleic Acids Res.* 17, 5388–5395.

Ardavín, C.F., and Zapata, A. (1987). Ultrastructure and changes during metamorphosis of the lympho-hemopoietic tissue of the larval anadromous sea lamprey *Petromyzon marinus*. *Dev. Comp. Immunol.* 11, 79–93.

Aveskogh, M., and Hellman, L. (1998). Evidence for an early appearance of modern post-switch isotypes in mammalian evolution; cloning of IgE, IgG and IgA from the marsupial *Monodelphis domestica*. *Eur. J. Immunol.* 28, 2738–2750.

Bazin, H., Beckers, A., Vaerman, J.-P., and Heremans, J.F. (1974). Allotypes of rat immunoglobulins I. An allotype at the α-chain locus. *J. Immunol.* 112, 1035–1041.

Bell, R.B., Stephens, C.J., and Turner, K.J. (1974). Marsupial immunoglobulins: an immunoglobulin molecule resembling eutherian IgA in serum and secretions. *J. Immunol.* 113, 371–378.

Belov, K., Harrison, G.A., and Cooper, D.W. (1998). Molecular cloning of the cDNA encoding the constant region of the immunoglobulin A heavy chain (Cα) from a marsupial: *Trichosurus vulpecula* (common brushtail possum). *Immunol. Lett.* 60, 165–170.

Belov, K., Zenger, K.R., Hellman, L., and Cooper, D.W. (2002). Echidna IgA supports mammalian unity and traditional Therian relationship. *Mamm. Genome* 13, 656–663.

Bengten, E., Wilson, M., Miller, N., Clem, L.W., Pilström, L., and Warr, G.W. (2000). Immunoglobulin isotypes: structure, function, and genetics. *Curr. Topics Microbiol. Immunol.* 248, 189–219.

Bienenstock, J., Perey, D.Y.E., Gauldie, J., and Underdown, B.J. (1973). Chicken γA: physicochemical and immunochemical characteristics. *J. Immunol.* 110, 524–533.

Bly, J.E., Grimm, A.S., and Morris, I.G. (1986). Transfer of passive immunity from mother to young in a teleost fish: haemagglutinating activity in the serum and eggs of plaice, *Pleuronectes platessa* L. *Comp. Biochem. Physiol.* 84A, 309–313.

Bourne, F.J. (1969). IgA immunoglobulin from porcine milk. *Biochim. Biophys. Acta* 181, 485–487.

Brandtzaeg, P. (1983). Immunohistochemical characterization of intracellular J-chain and binding site for secretory component (SC) in human immunoglobulin (Ig)-producing cells. *Mol. Immunol.* 20, 941–966.

Brandtzaeg, P. (1985). Role of J chain and secretory component in receptor-mediated glandular and hepatic transport of immunoglobulins in man. *Scand. J. Immunol.* 22, 111–146.

Brown, T.A., Russell, M.W., and Mestecky, J. (1984). Elimination of intestinally absorbed antigen into the bile by IgA. *J. Immunol.* 132, 780–782.

Brown, W.R., and Butler, J.E. (1994). Characterization of a Cα gene of swine. *Mol. Immunol.* 31, 633–642.

Brown, W.R., Kacskovics, I., Amendt, B.A., Blackmore, N.B., Rothschild, M., Shinde, R., and Butler, J.E. (1995). The hinge deletion allelic variant of porcine IgA results from a mutation at the splice acceptor site in the first Cα intron. *J. Immunol.* 154, 3836–3842.

Brown, W.R., Rabbani, H., Butler, J.E., and Hammarström, L. (1997). Characterization of the bovine Cα gene. *Immunology* 91, 1–6.

Burnett, R.C., Hanly, W.C., Zhai, S.K., and Knight, K.L. (1989). The IgA heavy-chain gene family in rabbit: cloning and sequence analysis of 13 Cα genes. *EMBO J.* 8, 4041–4047.

Butler, J.E., Maxwell, C.F., Pierce, C.S., Hylton, M.B., Asofsky, R., and Kiddy, C.A. (1972). Studies on the relative synthesis and distribution of IgA and IgG1 in various tissues and body fluids of the cow. *J. Immunol.* 109, 38–46.

Cannon, J.P., Haire, R.N., and Litman, G.W. (2002). Identification of diversified genes that contain immunoglobulin-like variable regions in a protochordate. *Nature Immunol.* 3, 1200–1207.

Cawthraw, S., Ayling, R., Nuijten, P., Wassenaar, T., and Newell, D. G. (1994). Isotype, specificity and kinetics of systemic and mucosal antibodies to *Campylobacter jejuni* antigens, including flagellin, during experimental oral infections of chickens. *Avian Dis.* 38, 341–349.

Challacombe, S.J., and Russell, M.W. (1979). Estimation of the intravascular half-lives of normal rhesus monkey IgG, IgA and IgM. *Immunology* 36, 331–338.

Coe, J.E., Portis, J.L., and Thomas, L.A. (1976). Immune response in the garter snake (*Thamnophis ordinoides*). *Immunology* 31, 417–424.

Cole, M.F., and Hale, C.A. (1991). Cleavage of chimpanzee secretory immunoglobulin A by *Haemophilus influenzae* IgA1 protease. *Microb. Pathog.* 11, 39–46.

Cole, M.F., Hale, C.A., and Sturzenegger, S. (1992). Identification of two subclasses of IgA in the chimpanzee (*Pan troglodytes*). *J. Med. Primatol.* 21, 275–278.

Coutinho, H.B., King, G., Sewell, H.F., Tighe, P., Coutinho, V.B., Robalinho, T.I., and Carvalho, A.B. (1993). Immuno-cytochemical study of Peyer's patches follicular-associated epithelium in the marsupial, *Didelphis albiventris. Dev. Comp. Immunol.* 17, 537–548.

Crago, S.S., Kulhavy, R., Prince, S.J., and Mestecky, J. (1978). Secretory component on epithelial cells is a surface receptor for polymeric immunoglobulins. *J. Exp. Med.* 147, 1832–1837.

Crago, S.S., Kutteh, W.H., Moro, I., Allansmith, M.R., Radl, J., Haaijman, J.J., and Mestecky, J. (1984). Distribution of IgA1-, IgA2- and J chain–containing cells in human tissues. *J. Immunol.* 132, 16–18.

Dahlgren, U., Ahlstedt, S., Hedman, L., Wadsworth, C., and Hanson, L.Å. (1981). Dimeric IgA in the rat is transferred from serum into bile but not into milk. *Scand. J. Immunol.* 14, 95–98.

Daniels, C.K., and Schmucker, D.L. (1987). Secretory component–dependent binding of immunoglobulin A in the rat, monkey and human: a comparison of intestine and liver. *Hepatology* 7, 517–521.

Davis, P.J., Parry, S.H., and Porter, P. (1978). The role of secretory IgA in anticoccidial immunity in the chicken. *Immunology* 34, 879–888.

De Benedictis, G., Capalbo, P., and Dragone, A. (1984). Identification of an allotypic IgA in cattle serum. *Comp. Immunol. Microbiol. Infect. Dis.* 7, 35–42.

Delacroix, D.L., Denef, A.M., Acosta, G.A., Montgomery, P.C., and Vaerman, J.P (1982a). Immunoglobulin in rabbit hepatic bile: selective secretion of IgA and IgM and active plasma-to-bile transfer of polymeric IgA. *Scand. J. Immunol.* 16, 343–350.

Delacroix, D.L., Hodgson, H.J.F., McPherson, A., Dive, C., and Vaerman, J.P. (1982b). Selective transport of polymeric immunoglobulin A in bile. Quantitative relationships of monomeric and polymeric immunoglobulin A, immunoglobulin M and other proteins in serum, bile and saliva. *J. Clin. Invest.* 70, 230–241.

Delacroix, D.L., Meykens, R., and Vaerman, J.P. (1982c). Influence of molecular size of IgA on its immunoassay by various techniques. I. Direct and reversed single radial immunodiffusion. *Mol. Immunol.* 19, 297–305.

Delacroix, D.L., Furtado-Barreira, G., de Hemtinne, B., Goudswaard, J., Dive, C., and Vaerman, J.P. (1983). The liver in the IgA secretory immune system. Dogs, but not rats and rabbits, are suitable models for human studies. *Hepatology* 3, 980–988.

Delacroix, D.L, Malburny, G.N., and Vaerman, J.P. (1985). Hepatobiliary transport of plasma IgA in the mouse: contribution to clearance of intravascular IgA. *Eur. J. Immunol.* 15, 893–899.

Dooley, J.S., Potter, B.J., Thomas, H.C., and Sherlock, S. (1982). A comparative study of the biliary secretion of human dimeric and monomeric IgA in the rat and in man. *Hepatology* 2, 323–327.

Du Pasquier, L. (1993). Evolution of the immune system. In *Fundamental Immunology*, 3rd ed. (ed. W.E. Paul), 199–233. New York: Raven Press, Ltd.

Fellah, J.S., and Charlemagne, J. (1988) Characterization of an IgY-like low molecular weight immunoglobulin class in the Mexican axolotl. *Mol. Immunol.* 25, 1377–1386.

Fellah, J.S., Iscaki, S., Vaerman, J.P., and Charlemagne, J. (1992). Transient developmental expression of IgY and secretory component like protein in the gut of the axolotl (*Ambystoma mexicanum*). *Dev. Immunol.* 2, 181–190.

Fellah J.S., Kerfourn, F., Wiles, M.V., Schwager, J., and Charlemagne, J. (1993). Phylogeny of immunoglobulin heavy chain isotypes: structure of the constant region *of Ambystoma mexicanum* upsilon chain deduced from cDNA sequence. *Immunogenetics* 38, 311–317.

Fletcher, T.C., and White, A. (1973). Antibody production in the plaice (*Pleuronectes platessa* L.) after oral and parenteral immunization with *Vibrillo anguillarum* antigens. *Aquaculture* 1, 417–428.

Georgopoulou, U., and Vernier, J.M. (1986). Local immunological response in the posterior intestinal segment of the rainbow trout after oral administration of macromolecules. *Dev. Comp. Immunol.* 10, 529–537.

Geuze, H.J., Slot, J.W., Strous, G.J.A M., Peppard, J., von Figura, K., Hasilik, A., and Schwartz, A.L. (1984). Intracellular receptor sorting during endocytosis: Comparative immunoelectron microscopy of multiple receptors in rat liver. *Cell* 37, 195–204.

Ghaffari, S.H., and Lobb, C.J. (1989). Cloning and sequence analysis of channel catfish heavy chain cDNA indicate phylogenetic diversity within the IgM immunoglobulin family. *J. Immunol.* 142, 1356–1365.

Goudswaard, J., Noordzij, A., van Dam, R.H. van der Donk, J.A., and Vaerman, J.-P. (1977). The immunoglobulins of turkey (*Meleagris gallopavo*). Isolation and characterisation of IgG, IgM and IgA in body fluids, eggs and intraocular tissue. *Poultry Sci.* 56, 1847–1856.

Goudswaard, J., van der Donk, J.A, van der Gaag, I., and Noordzij, A. (1979). Peculiar IgA transfer in the pigeon from mother to squab. *Dev. Comp. Immunol.* 3, 307–319.

Greenberg, A.S., Hughes, A.L., Guo, J., Avila, D., McKinney, E.C., and Flajnik, M.F. (1996). A novel "chimeric" antibody class in cartilaginous fish: IgM may not be the primordial immunoglobulin. *Eur. J. Immunol.* 26, 1123–1129.

Gyure, L.A., Hall, J.G., Hobbs, S.M., Jackson, L.E., and Sinnett, H. (1990). The concentration of IgA in hepatic lymph. In *Advances in Mucosal Immunology*, (eds. T. T. MacDonald, S. J. Challacombe, P. W. Bland, C. R. Stokes, R. V. Heatley, and A. McI. Mowat), 570–573. Dordrecht, The Netherlands: Kluwer Academic Publishers.

Hädge, D., and Ambrosius, H. (1983). Evolution of low molecular weight immunoglobulins. III. The immunoglobulin of chicken bile: not an IgA. *Mol. Immunol.* 20, 597–606.

Hädge, D., and Ambrosius, H. (1984). Evolution of low molecular weight immunoglobulins. IV. IgY-like immunoglobulins of birds, reptiles and amphibians, precursors of mammalian IgA. *Mol. Immunol.* 21, 699–707.

Hädge, D., and Ambrosius, H. (1986). Evolution of low molecular weight immunoglobulins V. Degree of antigenic relationship between the 7S immunoglobulins of mammals, birds, and lower vertebrates to the turkey IgY. *Dev. Comp. Immunol.* 10, 377–385.

Hädge, D., and Ambrosius, H. (1988). Comparative studies on the structure of biliary immunoglobulins of some avian species. II. Antigenic properties of the biliary immunoglobulins of chicken, turkey, duck and goose. *Dev. Comp. Immunol.* 12, 319–329.

Hadji-Azimi, I. (1979). Anuran immunoglobulins. A review. *Dev. Comp. Immunol.* 3, 223–243.

Hadji-Azimi, I., and Michea-Hamzehpour, M. (1976). *Xenopus laevis* 19S immunoglobulin: ultrastructure and J chain isolation. *Immunology* 30, 587–591.

Hagiwara, K., Kobayashi, K., Kajii, T., and Tomonaga, S. (1985). J chain–like component in 18S immunoglobulin of the skate *Raja kenojei*, a cartilaginous fish. *Mol. Immunol.* 22, 775–778.

Hall, J.G., Gyure, L.A., and Payne, A.W.R. (1980). Comparative aspects of the transport of immunoglobulin A from blood to bile. *Immunology* 41, 899–902.

Halsey, J.F., Mitchell, C., Meyer, R., and Cebra, J.J. (1982). Metabolism of immunoglobulin A in lactating mice: origins of immunoglobulin A in milk. *Eur. J. Immunol.* 12, 107–112.

Hart, S., Wrathmell, A.B., Harris, J.E., and Grayson, T.H. (1988). Gut immunology in fish: a review. *Dev. Comp. Immunol.* 12, 453–480; see also erratum (1989) published in *Dev. Comp. Immunol.* 13, 93–100.

Hayman, J.R., and Lobb, C.J. (1993). Immunoglobulin in the eggs of the channel catfish (*Ictalurus punctatus*). *Dev. Comp. Immunol.* 17, 241–248.

Hendrickson, B.A., Conner, D.A., Ladd, D.J., Kendall, D., Casanova, J.E., Corthesy, B., Max, E. E., Neutra, M.R., Seidman, C.E., and Seidman, J.G. (1995). Altered hepatic transport of immunoglobulin A in mice lacking the J chain. *J. Exp. Med.* 182, 1905–1911.

Heremans, J.F. (1974). Immunoglobulin A. In *The Antigens* (ed. M. Sela), vol. 2, 365–522. New York: Academic Press Inc.

Higgins, D.A., and Warr, G.W. (1993). Duck immunoglobulins: structure, functions and molecular genetics. *Avian Pathol.* 22, 211–236.

Higgins, D., Shortridge, K.F., and Ng, P.L.K. (1988). Bile immunoglobulin of the duck (*Anas platyrhynchos*). II. Antibody responses in influenza A virus infection. *Immunology* 62, 499–504.

Hohman, V.S., Stewart, S.E., Willett, C.E., and Steiner, L.A. (1997). Sequence and expression pattern of J chain in the amphibian, *Xenopus laevis*. *Mol. Immunol.* 34, 995–1002.

Hohman, V.S., and Steiner, L.A. (2000). The sequence of J chain in an amphibian, *Rana catesbeiana*. *Immunogenetics* 51, 587–590.

Hohman, V.S., Stewart, S.E., Rumfelt, L.L., Greenberg, A.S., Avila, D.W., Flajnik, M.F., and Steiner, L.A. (2003). J chain in the nurse shark: implications for function in a lower vertebrate. *J. Immunol.* 170, 6016–6023.

Hsu, E., Flajnik, M.F., and Du Pasquier, L. (1985). A third immunoglobulin class in amphibians. *J. Immunol.* 135, 1998–2004.

Hsu, S.M., and Hsu, P.L. (1980). Demonstration of IgA and secretory component in human hepatocytes. *Gut* 21, 985–989.

Hubbard, A.L. (1991). Targeting of membrane and secretory proteins to the apical domain in epithelial cells. *Semin. Cell Biol.* 2, 365–374.

Hughes, G.J., Frutiger, S., Paquet, N., and Jaton, J.-C. (1990). The amino acid sequence of rabbit J chain in secretory immunoglobulin A. *Biochem. J.* 271, 641–647.

Iwase, T., Saito, I., Takahashi, T., Chu, L., Usami, T., Mestecky, J., and Moro, I. (1993). Early expression of human J chain and μ chain gene in the fetal liver. *Cell Struct. Funct.* 18, 297–302.

Iwata, A., Iwase, T., Ogura, Y., Takahashi, T., Matsumoto, N., Yoshida, T., Kamei, N., Kobayashi, K., Mestecky, J., and Moro, I. (2002). Cloning and expression of the turtle (*Trachemys scripta*) immunoglobulin joining (J)–chain cDNA. *Immunogenetics* 54, 513–519.

Jackson, G.D.F., Lemaitre-Coelho, I., and Vaerman, J. P. (1977). Transfer of MOPC-315 IgA to secretions in MOPC-315 tumour-bearing and normal BALB/c mice. *Prot. Biol. Fluids* 25, 919–922.

Jackson, G.D.F., Lemaitre-Coelho, I., and Vaerman, J.P. (1978). Rapid disappearance from serum of intravenously injected rat myeloma IgA and its secretion into bile. *Eur. J. Immunol.* 8, 123–126.

Junghans, R.P., and Anderson, C.L. (1996). The protection receptor for IgG catabolism is the β2-microglobulin-containing neonatal intestinal transport receptor. *Proc. Natl. Acad. Sci. USA* 93, 5512–5516.

Kaartinen, M. (1978). Liver damage in mice and rats causes tenfold increase of blood immunoglobulin A. *Scand. J. Immunol.* 7, 519–522.

Kaartinen, M., Imir, T., Klockaars, M., Sandholm, M., and Mäkelä, O. (1978). IgA in blood and thoracic duct lymph: concentration and degree of polymerization. *Scand. J. Immunol.* 7, 229–232.

Kaetzel, C.S., Traicoff, J.L., and Huddleston, C. (2003). Evolution of the PIGR gene. *Manuscript in preparation.*

Kawamura, S., and Ueda, S. (1992). Immunoglobulin C_H gene family in hominoids and its evolutionary history. *Genomics* 13, 194–200.

Kawamura, S., Omoto, K., and Ueda, S. (1990). Evolutionary hypervariability in the hinge region of the immunoglobulin alpha gene. *J. Mol. Biol.* 215, 201–206.

Kawamura, S., Saitou, N., and Ueda, S. (1992). Concerted evolution of the primate immunoglobulin α-gene through gene conversion. *J. Biol. Chem.* 267, 7359–7367.

Klaus, G.G.B., Halpern, M.S., Koshland, M.E., and Goodman, J.W. (1971). A polypeptide chain from leopard shark 19S immunoglobulin analogous to mammalian J chain. *J. Immunol.* 107, 1785–1787.

Knight, K.L., Suter, M., and Becker, R.S. (1988). Genetic engineering of bovine Ig. Construction and characterization of hapten-binding bovine/murine chimeric IgE, IgA, IgG1, IgG2, and IgG3 molecules. *J. Immunol.* 140, 3654–3659.

Kobayashi, K., Vaerman, J.-P., Bazin, H., Lebacq-Verheyden, A.-M., and Heremans, J.F. (1973). Identification of J-chain in polymeric immunoglobulins from a variety of species by cross-reaction with rabbit antisera to human J-chain. *J. Immunol.* 111, 1590–1594.

Koertge, T.E., and Butler, J.E. (1986a). Dimeric mouse IgA is transported into rat bile five times more rapidly than into mouse bile. *Scand. J. Immunol.* 24, 567–574.

Koertge, T.E., and Butler, J.E. (1986b). Dimeric M315 is transported into mouse and rat milk in degraded form. *Molec. Immunol.* 23, 839–845.

Krajci, P., Meling, G.I., Tasken, K., Rognum, T., and Brandtzaeg, P. (1991). Studies on tissue-specific expression of messenger RNA for the human transmembrane secretory component and its regulation by cytokines in a colonic carcinoma cell line. In *Frontiers of Mucosal Immunology* (eds. M. Tsuchiya, H. Nagura, T. Hibi, and I. Moro), vol. 1, 307–310. Amsterdam: Excerpta Medica.

Kubagawa, H., Bertoli, L.F., Barton, J.C., Koopman, W.J., Mestecky, J., and Cooper, M.D. (1987). Analysis of paraprotein transport into saliva by using anti-idiotype antibodies. *J. Immunol.* 138, 435–439.

Kühn, L.C., and Kraehenbuhl, J.P. (1979). Role of secretory component, a secreted glycoprotein, in the specific uptake of IgA dimer by epithelial cells. *J. Biol. Chem.* 254, 11072–11081.

Kulseth, M.A., and Rogne, S. (1994). Cloning and characterization of the bovine immunoglobulin J chain cDNA and its promoter region. *DNA Cell Biol.* 13, 37–42.

Kutteh, W.H., Prince, S.J., and Mestecky, J. (1982a). Tissue origins of human polymeric and monomeric IgA. *J. Immunol.* 128, 990–995.

Kutteh, W.H., Prince, S.J., Phillips, J.O., Spenney, J.G., and Mestecky, J. (1982b). Properties of immunoglobulin A in serum of individuals with liver disease and in hepatic bile. *Gastroenterology* 82, 184–193.

Lebacq-Verhayden, A.M., Vaerman, J.P and Heremans, J.F. (1974). Quantification and distribution of chicken immunoglobulins IgA, IgM and IgG in serum and secretions. *Immunology* 27, 683–692.

Lemaitre-Coelho, I., Jackson, G.D.F., and Vaerman, J.-P. (1978). Relevance of biliary IgA antibodies in rat intestinal immunity. *Scand. J. Immunol.* 8, 459–463.

Lemaitre-Coelho, I., Yamakido, M., Montgomery, P.C., Langendries, A.E., and Vaerman, J.P. (1982). Selective excretion of IgA in rat bronchial secretions: lack of significant contribution from plasma IgA. *Immunol. Comm.* 11, 441–453.

Leslie, G.A., and Martin, L.N. (1973). Studies on the secretory immunologic system of fowl. III. Serum and secretory IgA of the chicken. *J. Immunol.* 110, 1–9.

Lobb, C.J. (1987). Secretory immunity induced in catfish, *Ictalurus punctatus*, following bath immunization. *Dev. Comp. Immunol.* 11, 727–738.

Lobb, C.J., and Clem, L.W. (1981a). Phylogeny of immunoglobulin structure and function-X. Humoral immunoglobulins of the sheepshead, *Archosargus probatocephalus. Dev. Comp. Immunol.* 5, 271–282.

Lobb, C.J., and Clem, L.W. (1981b). Phylogeny of immunoglobulin structure and function XI. Secretory immunoglobulins in the cutaneous mucus of the sheepshead, *Archosargus probatocephalus. Dev. Comp. Immunol.* 5, 587–596.

Lobb, C.J., and Clem, L.W. (1981c). Phylogeny of immunoglobulin structure and function-XII Secretory immunoglobulins in the bile of the murine teleost *Archosargus probatocephalus. Molec. Immunol.* 18, 615–619.

Lobb, C.J., and Clem, L.W. (1981d). The metabolic relationships of the immunoglobulins in fish serum, cutaneous mucus, and bile. *J. Immunol.* 127, 1525–1529.

Lundqvist, M.L., Middleton, D.L., Hazard, S., and Warr, G.W. (2001). The immunoglobulin heavy chain locus of the duck: Genomic organization and expression of D, J, and C region genes. *J. Biol. Chem.* 276, 46729–46736.

Mach, J.P., Pahud, J.J., and Isliker, H. (1969). IgA with "secretory piece" in bovine colostrum and saliva. *Nature* 223, 952–955.

Mach, J.P. (1970). *In vitro* combination of human and bovine free secretory component with IgA of various species. *Nature* 228, 1278–1282.

Mach, J.-P., and Pahud, J.J. (1971). Secretory IgA, a major immunoglobulin in most bovine external secretions. *J. Immunol.* 106, 552–563.

Magor, K.E., Warr, G.W., Bando, Y., Middleton, D.L., and Higgins, D.A. (1998). Secretory immune system of the duck (*Anas platyrhynchos*). Identification and expression of the genes encoding IgA and IgM heavy chains. *Eur. J. Immunol.* 28, 1063–1068.

Mansikka, A. (1992). Chicken IgA H chains. Implications concerning the evolution of H chain genes. *J. Immunol.* 149, 855–861.

Matsunaga, T, and Rahman, A. (1998). What brought the adaptive immune system to vertebrates? The jaw hypothesis and the seahorse. *Immunol. Rev.* 166, 177–186.

Matsuuchi, L., Cann, G.M., and Koshland, M.E. (1986). Immunoglobulin J chain gene from the mouse. *Proc. Natl. Acad. Sci. USA* 83, 456–460.

Max, E.E., and Korsmeyer, S.J. (1985). Human J chain gene. Structure and expression in lymphoid cells. *J. Exp. Med.* 161, 832–849.

Mazanec, M.B., Nedrud, J.G., Liang, X., and Lamm, M.E. (1989). Transport of serum IgA into murine respiratory secretions and its implications for immunization strategies. *J. Immunol.* 142, 4275–4281.

McCune, J.M., Fu, S.M., and Kunkel, H. G. (1981). J chain biosynthesis in pre-B cells and other possible precursor B cells. *J. Exp. Med.* 154, 138–145.

Mestecky, J., Kulhavy, R., Schrohenloher, R.E., Tomana, M., and Wright, G.P. (1975). Identification and properties of J chain isolated from catfish macroglobulin. *J. Immunol.* 115, 993–997.

Mestecky, J., Moro, I., Moldoveanu, Z., Takahashi, T., Iwase, T., Kubagawa, H., and Cooper, M.D. (1997). Immunoglobulin J chain, an early differentiation marker of human B cells. *Ann. N.Y. Acad. Sci.* 815, 111–113.

Mikoryak, C.A., Margolies, M.N., and Steiner, L.A. (1988). J chain in *Rana catesbiana* high molecular weight Ig. *J. Immunol.* 140, 4279–4285.

Mockett, A.P., and Rose, M.E. (1986). Immune responses to eimeria: quantification of antibody isotypes to *Eimeria tenella* in chicken serum and bile by means of the ELISA. *Parasite Immunol.* 8, 481–489.

Moldoveanu, Z., Egan, M.L., and Mestecky, J. (1984). Cellular origins of human polymeric and monomeric IgA: intracellular and secreted forms of IgA. *J. Immunol.* 133, 3156–3162.

Moldoveanu, Z., Epps, J.M., Thorpe, S.R., and Mestecky, J. (1988). The sites of catabolism of murine monomeric IgA. *J. Immunol.* 141, 208–213.

Moldoveanu, Z., Moro, I., Radl, J., Thorpe, S.R., Komiyama, K., and Mestecky, J. (1990). Site of catabolism of autologous and heterologous IgA in non-human primates. *Scand. J. Immunol.* 32, 577–583.

Montgomery, P.C., Khaleel, S.A., Goudswaard, J., and Virella, G. (1977). Selective transport of an oligomeric IgA into canine saliva. *Immunol. Comm.* 6, 633–642.

Morell, A., Skvaril, F., Noseda, G., and Barandun, S. (1973). Metabolic properties of human IgA subclasses. *Clin. Exp. Immunol.* 13, 521–528.

Moriya, O., and Ichikawa, Y. (1991). Detection of J chain in chicken polymeric immunoglobulins in their native conformation. *Med. Sci. Res.* 19, 83–85.

Mostov, K.E., Friedlander, M., and Blobel, G. (1984). The receptor for transepithelial transport of IgA and IgM contains multiple immunoglobulin-like domains. *Nature* 308, 37–43.

Mullock. B.M., Hinton, R.H., Dobrota, M., Peppard, J., and Orlans, E. (1980). Distribution of secretory component in hepatocytes and its mode of transfer into bile. *Biochem. J.* 190, 819–826.

Mullock, B.M., Shaw, L.J., Fitzharris, B.M., Peppard, J.V., Hamilton, M.J.R., Simpson, M.T., Hunt, T. M., and Hinton, R. H. (1985). Sources of protein in human bile. *Gut* 26, 500–509.

Mullock, B.M., Hinton, R.H., Peppard, J.V., Slot, J.W., and Luzio, J.P. (1987) The preparative isolation of endosome fractions: a review. *Cell Biochem. Funct.* 5, 235–243.

Mussmann, R., Du Pasquier, L., and Hsu, E. (1996a). Is *Xenopus* IgX an analog of IgA? *Eur. J. Immunol.*, 26, 2823–2830.

Mussmann, R., Wilson, M., Marcuz, A., Courtet, M., and Du Pasquier, L., (1996b). Membrane exon sequences of the three *Xenopus* Ig classes explain the evolutionary origin of mammalian isotypes *Eur. J. Immunol.* 26, 409–14.

Myers, T.J., Schat, K.A., and Mockett, A.P. (1989). Development of immunoglobulin class–specific enzyme-linked immunosorbent assays for measuring antibodies against avian rotavirus. *Avian Dis.* 33, 53–59.

Nagura, H., Smith, P.D., Nakane, P.K., and Brown, W.R. (1981). IgA in human bile and liver. *J. Immunol.* 126, 587–595.

Navarro, P., Christensen, R.K., Weber, P., Rothschild, M., Ekhardt, G., and Butler, J.E. (2000). Porcine IgA allotypes are not equally transcribed or expressed in heterozygous swine. *Mol. Immunol.* 37, 653–664.

Negrete-Abascal, E., Tenorio, V. R., Serrano, J.J., Garvia, C., and de la Garza, M. (1994). Secreted proteases from *Actinobacillus pleuropneumoniae* serotype 1 degrade porcine gelatin, hemoglobin and immunoglobulin A. *Can. J. Vet. Res.* 5, 83–86.

Ng, P.L.K., and Higgins, D.A. (1986). Bile immunoglobulins of the duck (*Anas platyrhynchos*). 1. Preliminary characterization and ontogeny. *Immunology* 58, 323–327.

O'Daly, J.A., and Cebra, J.J. (1971). Chemical and physicochemical studies of the component polypeptide chains of rabbit secretory immunoglobulin A. *Biochemistry* 10, 3843–3850.

Orlans, E., and Rose, M.E. (1972). An IgA-like immunoglobulin in the fowl. *Immunochemistry* 9, 833–838.

Orlans, E., Peppard, J.V., Reynolds, J.R., and Hall, J.G. (1978). Rapid active transport of immunoglobulin A from blood to bile. *J. Exp. Med.* 147, 588–592.

Orlans, E., Peppard, J., Fry, J.F., Hinton, R.H., and Mullock, B.M. (1979). Secretory component as the receptor for polymeric IgA on rat hepatocytes. *J. Exp. Med.* 150, 1577–1581.

Orlans, E., Peppard, J.V., Payne, A.W.R., Fitzharris, B.M., Mullock, B.M., Hinton, R.H., and Hall, J.G. (1983). Comparative aspects of the hepatobiliary transport of IgA. *Ann. N.Y. Acad. Sci.*, 409, 411–427.

Ortuño, J., Cuesta, A., Rodríguez, A., Esteban, M.A., and Meseguer, J. (2002). Oral administration of yeast, *Saccharomyces cerevisiae*, enhances the cellular innate immune response of gilthead seabream (*Sparus aurata* L.). *Vet. Immunol. Immunopathol.* 85, 41–50.

Ota, T., Rast, J.P., Litman, G.W., and Amemiya, C.T. (2003). Lineage-restricted retention of a primitive immunoglobulin heavy chain isotype within the Dipnoi reveals an evolutionary paradox. *Proc. Natl. Acad. Sci. USA* 100, 2501–2506.

Pahud, J.J., and Mach, J.P. (1970). Identification of secretory IgA, free secretory piece and serum IgA in the ovine and caprine species. *Immunochemistry* 7, 679–686.

Pahud, J.J., and Mach, J.P. (1972). Equine IgA and secretory component. *Int. Arch. Allergy Appl. Immunol.* 42, 175–186.

Patel, M., Selinger, D., Mark, G.E., Hickey, G.J., and Hollis, G.F. (1995). Sequence of dog immunoglobulin alpha and epsilon constant region genes. *Immunogenetics* 41, 282–286.

Peppard, J.V., and Jackson, L.E. (1987). Variability in the molecular sizes of IgA secreted by individual hybridoma cell lines. *Adv. Exp. Med. Biol.* 216B, 1207–1213.

Peppard, J.V., and Montgomery, P.C. (1987). Studies on the origin and composition of IgA in rat tears. *Immunology* 62, 193–198.

Peppard, J.V., and Orlans, E. (1979). The biological half-lives of four rat immunoglobulin isotypes. *Immunology* 40, 683–686.

Peppard, J., Orlans, E., Payne, A., and Andrew, E. (1981). The elimination of circulating complexes containing polymeric IgA by excretion in the bile. *Immunology* 42, 83–89.

Peppard, J.V., Orlans, E., Andrew, E., and Payne, A.W.R. (1982). Elimination into bile of circulating antigen by endogenous IgA antibody in rats. *Immunology* 45, 467–472.

Peppard, J.V., Rose, M.E., and Hesketh, P. (1983). A functional homologue of mammalian secretory component exists in chickens. *Eur. J. Immunol.* 13, 566–570.

Peppard, J.V., Hobbs, S.M., Jackson, L.E., Rose, M.E., and Mockett, A.P.A. (1986). Biochemical characterisation of chicken secretory component. *Eur. J. Immunol.* 16, 225–229.

Perez, J.H., Van Schaik, M., Mullock, B.M., Bailyes, E.M., Price C.P., and Luzio, J.P. (1991). The presence and measurement of secretory component in human bile and blood. *Clin. Chim. Acta* 197, 171–187.

Perez, J.H., Wight, D.G.D., Wyatt, J.I., Van Schaik, M., Mullock, B.M., and Luzio, J.P. (1989). The polymeric immunoglobulin A receptor is present on hepatocytes in human liver. *Immunology* 68, 474–478.

Phillips-Quagliata, J.M. (2002). Mouse IgA allotypes have major differences in their hinge regions. *Immunogenetics* 53, 1033–1038.

Pierre, P.G., Havaux, X.B., Langendries, A., Courtoy, P.J., Goto, K., Maldague, P., and Vaerman, J.-P. (1995). Mouse secretory component. *Adv. Exp. Med. Biol.* 371A, 629–632.

Piskurich, J.F., Blanchard, M.H., Youngman, K.R., France, J.A., and Kaetzel, C.S. (1995). Molecular cloning of the mouse polymeric Ig receptor. Functional regions of the molecule are conserved among five mammalian species. *J. Immunol.* 154, 1735–1747.

Portis, J.L and Coe, J.E. (1975). IgM: the secretory immunoglobulin of reptiles and amphibians. *Nature* 258, 547–548.

Qiu, J., Brackee, G.P., and Plaut, A.G. (1996). Analysis of the specificity of bacterial immunoglobulin A (IgA) proteases by a comparative study of ape serum IgAs as substrates. *Infect. Immun.* 64, 933–937.

Reynolds, H.Y., and Johnson, J.S. (1971). Structural units of canine serum and secretory immunoglobulin A. *Biochemistry* 10, 2821–2827.

Rifai, A., and Mannik, M. (1983). Clearance kinetics and fate of mouse IgA immune complexes prepared with monomeric or polymeric IgA. *J. Immunol.* 130, 1826–1832.

Rombout, J.H.W.M., Lamers, C.H.J., Helfrich, M.H., Dekker, A., and Taverne-Thiele, J.J. (1985). Uptake and transport of intact macromolecules in the intestinal epithelium of carp (*Cyprinus carpio* L.) and the possible immunological implications. *Cell Tissue Res.* 239, 519–530.

Rombout, J.W., Blok, L.J., Lamers, C.H., and Egberts, E. (1986). Immunization of carp (*Cyprinus carpio*) with a *Vibrio anguillarum* bacterin: indications for a common mucosal system. *Dev. Comp. Immunol.* 10, 341–351.

Rombout, J.H.W.M., Taverne, N., van de Kamp, M., and Taverne-Thiele, A.J. (1993). Differences in mucus and serum immunoglobulins of Carp (*Cyprinus carpio* L.). *Dev. Comp. Immunol.* 17, 309–317.

Rose, M.E., Orlans, E., Payne, A.W.R., and Hesketh, P. (1981). The origin of IgA in chicken bile: its rapid active transport from blood. *Eur. J. Immunol.* 11, 561–564.

Rose, M.E., Peppard, J.V., and Hobbs, S.M. (1984). Coccidiosis: characterization of antibody responses to infection with *Eimeria nieschulzi*. *Parasite Immunol.* 6, 1–12.

Russell, M.W., Brown, T.A., and Mestecky, J. (1981). Role of serum IgA. Hepatobiliary transport of circulating antigen. *J. Exp. Med.* 153, 968–977.

Russell, M.W., Brown, T.A., and Mestecky, J. (1982). Preferential transport of IgA and IgA immune complexes to bile compared with other secretions. *Molec. Immunol.* 19, 677–682.

Russell, M.W., Brown, T.A., Claflin, J.L., Schroer, K., and Mestecky, J. (1983). IgA-mediated hepatobiliary transport constitutes a natural pathway for disposing of bacterial antigens. *Infect. Immun.* 42, 1041–1048.

Russell, M.W., Lue, C., van den Wall Bake, A.W.L., Moldoveanu, Z., and Mestecky, J. (1992). Molecular heterogeneity of human IgA antibodies during an immune response. *Clin. Exp. Immunol.* 87, 1–6.

Saitou, N., and Nei, M. (1987). The neighbor-joining method: a new method for reconstructing phylogenetic trees. *Mol. Biol. Evol.* 4, 406–425.

Schiff, J.M., Fisher, M.M., and Underdown, B.J. (1984). Receptor-mediated biliary transport of immunoglobulin A and asialoglycoprotein: sorting and missorting of ligands revealed by two radiolabeling methods. *J. Cell. Biol.* 98, 79–89.

Schiff, J.M., Fisher, M.M., Jones, A.L., and Underdown, B.J. (1986). Human IgA as a heterovalent ligand: switching from asialoglycoprotein receptor to secretory component during transport across the rat hepatocyte. *J. Cell Biol.* 102, 920–931.

Schluter, S.F., Bernstein, R.M., and Marchalonis, J.J. (1997). Molecular origins and evolution of immunoglobulin heavy-chain genes of jawed vertebrates. *Immunol. Today* 18, 543–549.

Schneiderman, R.D., Hanly, W.C., and Knight, K.L. (1989). Expression of 12 rabbit IgA Cα genes as chimeric rabbit-mouse IgA antibodies. *Proc. Natl. Acad. Sci. USA* 86, 7561–7565.

Scicchitano, R. Husband, A.J., and Cripps, A.W. (1984a). Immunoglobulin-containing cells and the origin of immunoglobulins in the respiratory tract of sheep. *Immunology* 52, 529–537.

Scicchitano, R. Husband, A.J., and Cripps, A.W. (1984b). Biliary transport of serum IgA in sheep. *Immunology* 53, 121–129.

Scicchitano, R., Sheldrake, R.F., and Husband, A.J (1986). Origin of immunoglobulins in respiratory tract secretion and saliva of sheep. *Immunology* 58, 315–321.

Scinicariello, F., and Attanasio, R. (2001). Intraspecies heterogeneity of immunoglobulin α-chain constant region genes in rhesus macaques. *Immunology* 103, 441–448.

Shearer, M.H., Corbitt, S.D., Stanley, J.R., White, G.L., Chodosh, J., Chanh, T.C., and Kennedy, R.C. (1997). Purification and characterization of secretory IgA from baboon colostrum. *J. Immunol. Methods* 204, 67–75.

Sheldrake, R.F., Husband, A.J., Watson, D.L., and Cripps, A.W. (1984). Selective transport of serum-derived IgA into mucosal secretions. *J. Immunol.* 132, 363–368.

Sheldrake, R.F., Scicchitano, R., and Husband, A.J. (1985). The effect of lactation on the transport of serum-derived IgA into bile of sheep. *Immunology* 54, 471–477.

Socken, D.J., Simms, E.S., Nagy, B., Fisher, M.M., and Underdown, B.J. (1981). Transport of IgA antibody-antigen complexes by the rat liver. *Mol. Immunol.* 18, 345–348.

Spieker-Polet, H., Yam, P.-C., and Knight, K.L. (1993). Differential expression of 13 IgA-heavy chain genes in rabbit lymphoid tissues. *J. Immunol.* 61, 5457–5465.

Spieker-Polet, H., Yam, P.C., Arbieva, Z., Zhai, S.K., and Knight, K.L. (1999). *In vitro* induction of the expression of multiple IgA isotype genes in rabbit B cells by TGF-β and IL-2. *J. Immunol.* 162, 5380–5388.

Spieker-Polet, H., Yam, P.C., and Knight, K.L. (2002). Functional analysis of Iα promoter regions of multiple IgA heavy chain genes. *J. Immunol.* 168, 3360–3368.

St. Louis-Cormier, E.A., Osterland, C.K., and Anderson, P.D. (1984). Evidence for a cutaneous secretory immune system in a rainbow trout (*Salmo gairdneri*). *Dev. Comp. Immunol.* 8, 71–80.

Stockert, R.J., Kressner, M.S., Collins, J.C., Sternlieb, I., and Morell, A.G. (1982). IgA interaction with the asialoglycoprotein receptor. *Proc. Natl. Acad. Sci. USA* 79, 6229–6231

Sullivan, D.A., and Allansmith, M.R. (1984). Source of IgA in tears of rats. *Immunology* 53, 791–798.

Sumiyama, K., Saitou, N., and Ueda, S. (2002). Adaptive evolution of the IgA hinge region in primates. *Mol. Biol. Evol.* 19, 1093–1099.

Sztul, E.S., Howell, K.E., and Palade, G.E (1983). Intracellular and transcellular transport of secretory component and albumin in rat hepatocytes *J. Cell Biol.* 97, 1582–1591.

Takahashi, T., Iwase, T., Takenouchi, N., Saito, M., Kobayashi, K., Moldoveanu, Z., Mestecky, J., and Moro, I. (1996). The joining (J) chain is present in invertebrates that do not express immunoglobulins. *Proc. Natl. Acad. Sci. USA* 93, 1886–1891.

Takahashi, T., Iwase, T., Tachibana, T., Komiyama, K., Kobayashi, K., Chen, C.L.H., Mestecky, J., and Moro, I. (2000). Cloning and expression of the chicken immunoglobulin joining (J)-chain cDNA. *Immunogenetics* 51, 85–91.

Tamer, C.M., Lamm, M.E., Robinson, J.K., Piskurich, J.F., and Kaetzel, C.S. (1995). Comparative studies of transcytosis and assembly of secretory IgA in Madin-Darby canine kidney cells expressing human polymeric Ig receptor. *J. Immunol.* 155, 707–714.

Taylor, C.L., Harrison, G.A., Watson, C.M., and Deane, E.M. (2002). cDNA cloning of the polymeric immunoglobulin receptor of the marsupial *Macropus eugenii* (tammar wallaby). *Eur. J. Immunogenet.* 29, 87–93.

Tomana, M., Zikan, J., Kulhavy, R., Bennett, J.C., and Mestecky, J. (1993a). Interactions of galactosyltransferase with serum and secretory immunoglobulins and their component chains. *Mol. Immunol.* 30, 277–286.

Tomana, M., Zikan, J., Moldoveanu, Z., Kulhavy, R., Bennett, J. C., and Mestecky, J. (1993b). Interactions of cell-surface galactosyltransferase with immunoglobulins. *Mol. Immunol.* 30, 265–275.

Toro, H., Reyes, E., Redmann, T., and Kaleta, E.F. (1996). Local and systemic specific antibody response of different chicken lines after ocular vaccination against infectious bronchitis. *Zbl. Veterinärmed. B* 43, 449–454.

Torroba, M., Anderson, D.P., Dixon, O.W., Casares, F., Varas, A., Alonso, L., Gomez del Moral, M., and Zapata, A. G. (1993). *In vitro* antigen trapping by gill cells of the rainbow trout: an immunohistochemical study. *Histol. Histopathol.* 8, 363–367.

Tourville, D.R., Ogra, S.S., Lippes, J., and Tomasi, T.B. (1970). The human female reproductive tract: Immunohistological localization of γA, γG, γM, secretory "piece," and lactoferrin. *Am. J. Obstet. Gynecol.* 108, 1102–1108.

Trebichavsky, I., Zikan, J., Mestecky, J., and Mandel, L. (1985). Ontogeny of J chain expression in pig lymphocytes. *Immunol. Lett.* 10, 287–291.

Tucker, P.W., Slightom, J.L., and Blattner, F.R. (1981). Mouse IgA heavy chain gene sequence: implications for evolution of immunoglobulin hinge exons. *Proc. Natl. Acad. Sci. USA* 78, 7684–7688.

Uinuk-ool, T., Mayer, W.E., Sato, A., Dongak, R., Cooper, M.D., and Klein, J. (2002). Lamprey lymphocyte-like cells express homologs of genes involved in immunologically relevant activities of mammalian lymphocytes. *Proc. Natl. Acad. Sci. USA* 99, 14356–14361.

Underdown, B.J., and Socken, D.J. (1978). A comparison of secretory component–immunoglobulin interactions amongst different species. *Adv. Exp. Med. Biol.* 107, 503–511.

Vaerman, J.P. (1970). *Studies on IgA Immunoglobulins in Man and Animal*, 1–292. Thesis. Louvain, Belgium: Sintal.

Vaerman, J.-P. (1973). Comparative immunochemistry of IgA. *Res. Immunochem. Immunobiol.* 3, 91–161.

Vaerman, J.P., and Langendries, A. (1997). Hepatobiliary transport of IgA in the golden Syrian hamster (*Mesocricetus auratus*). *Immunol. Lett.* 55, 19–26.

Vaerman, J.P., and Lemaitre-Coelho, I. (1979). Transfer of circulating human IgA across the rat liver into the bile. In *Protein Transmission through Living Membranes* (ed. W. A. Hemmings), 383–397. Amsterdam: Elsevier.

Vaerman, J.P., Heremans, J.F., and Van Kerckhoven, G. (1969). Identification of IgA in several mammalian species. *J. Immunol.* 103, 1421–1423.

Vaerman, J.-P., Heremans, J.F., Bazin, H., and Beckers, A. (1975a). Identification and some properties of rat secretory component. *J. Immunol.* 114, 265–269.

Vaerman, J.P., Naccache-Corbic, M.C., and Heremans, J.F. (1975b). Secretory component of the guinea-pig. *Immunology* 29, 933–944.

Vaerman, J.P., Picard, J., and Heremans, J.F. (1975c). Structural data on chicken IgA and failure to find IgA in the tortoise. *Adv. Exp. Med. Biol.* 64, 185–195.

Varner, J., Neame, P., and Litman, G.W. (1991). A serum heterodimer from hagfish (*Eptatretus stoutii*) exhibits structural similarity and partial sequence identity with immunoglobulin. *Proc. Natl. Acad. Sci. USA* 88, 1746–1750.

Vernersson, M., Aveskogh, M., Munday, B., and Hellman, L. (2002). Evidence for an early appearance of modern post-switch immunoglobulin isotypes in mammalian evolution (II); cloning of IgE, IgG1 and IgG2 from a monotreme, the duck-billed platypus, *Ornithorhynchus anatinus*. *Eur. J. Immunol.* 32, 2145–2155.

Vuiton, D.A., Seilles, E., Claude, P., Sava, P., and Delacroix, D.L. (1985). Gall bladder: the predominant source of bile IgA in man? *Clin. Exp. Immunol.* 62, 185–192.

Wagner, B., Siebenkotten, G., Leibold, W., and Radbruch, A. (1997) Organization of the equine immunoglobulin constant heavy chain genes I. Cε and Cα genes. *Vet. Immunol. Immunopathol.* 60, 1–13.

Wagner, B., Greiser-Wilke, I., and Antczak, D.F. (2003). Characterization of the horse (*Equus caballus*) IGHA gene. *Immunogenetics* 55, 552–560.

Warr, G.W., Magor, K.E., and Higgins, D.A. (1995). IgY: clues to the origin of modern antibodies. *Immunol. Today* 16, 392–398.

Warr, G.W. (1995). The immunoglobulin genes of fish. *Dev. Comp. Immunol.* 19, 1–12.

White, G.P., Roche, P., Brandon, M.R., Newton, S.E., and Meeusen, E.N.T. (1998). Cloning and characterization of sheep (*Ovis aries*) immunoglobulin α chain. *Immunogenetics* 48, 359–362.

Wilson, M., Bengtén, E., Miller, N.W., Clem, L.W., Du Pasquier, L., and Warr, G.W. (1997). A novel chimeric Ig heavy chain from a teleost fish shares similarities to IgD. *Proc. Natl. Acad. Sci. USA* 94, 4593–4597.

Yamada, T., Matsuda, M., Ashida, Y., Tsuchiya, R., Wada, Y., Matsubara, T., and Kobayashi, K. (1992). Isolation of secretory IgA from feline bile and bile IgA levels in growing cats. *J. Vet. Med. Sci.* 54, 717–721.

Zapata, A., and Amemiya, C.T. (2000). Phylogeny of lower vertebrates and their immunological structures. *Curr. Topics Microbiol. Immunol.* 248, 67–107.

Zhao, Y., Rabbani, H., Shimizu, A., and Hammarstrom, L. (2000). Mapping of the chicken immunoglobulin heavy-chain constant region gene locus reveals an inverted α gene upstream of a condensed υ gene. *Immunology* 101, 348–353.

Immunoglobulin Transport and the Polymeric Immunoglobulin Receptor

Charlotte S. Kaetzel

Department of Microbiology, Immunology, & Molecular Genetics, and Department of Pathology & Laboratory Medicine, University of Kentucky, Lexington, Kentucky

Keith Mostov

Department of Anatomy, Department of Biochemistry and Biophysics, and Cardiovascular Research Institute, University of California, San Francisco, California

Mucosal surfaces are protected by a physically vulnerable monolayered epithelium covering an enormous surface area, perhaps 300 to 400 m^2 in adult humans. These surfaces are continuously bombarded by potentially infectious agents such as bacteria, viruses, fungi, and parasites, in addition to soluble dietary and environmental substances. The first line of specific immunological defense against these environmental antigens is provided by antibodies in external secretions. In humans, the predominant type of antibody in most external secretions is secretory IgA (S-IgA), resulting from selective transport of polymeric IgA across epithelial cells lining mucosal surfaces (reviewed in Mestecky *et al.*, 1991; Norderhaug *et al.*, 1999b). The magnitude of this transport process is impressive: it has been estimated that approximately 3 g of S-IgA are transported daily into the intestines of the average adult (Mestecky *et al.*, 1986; Conley and Delacroix, 1987) (see subsequent section, Tissue-Specific Expression of pIgR). Transport of polymeric Ig (IgA and to a lesser extent IgM) across mucosal epithelial cells is mediated by the polymeric immunoglobulin receptor (pIgR). Smaller amounts of other isotypes of antibodies, as well as monomeric IgA, can also enter external secretions by transudation from serum or by other receptor-mediated processes.

Nearly 40 years ago Tomasi *et al.* (1965) isolated S-IgA and demonstrated that it was an IgA dimer linked to a glycoprotein of about 80 kDa (originally designated the "secretory piece" and now called secretory component [SC]). Because most of the serum IgA is monomeric, the question arose of whether IgA dimers in S-IgA were assembled from serum-derived monomeric IgA or derived from locally synthesized dimeric IgA. Two landmark experiments demonstrated that the IgA in colostrum is synthesized by local plasma cells as an 11S dimer. Lawton and Mage (1969) examined the distribution of *b* locus light chain allotypic markers in colostral IgA from heterozygous rabbits. If the S-IgA were assembled from serum-derived monomeric IgA, one would expect to find random assortment of the light chain markers. However, immunoprecipitation with antiallotypic antibodies revealed that individual S-IgA molecules contained either the *b4* or *b5* marker, but not both, suggesting that the IgA dimers were assembled within local plasma cells. Similar results were obtained by Bienenstock and Strauss (1970), who demonstrated that individual S-IgA molecules from human colostrum contained either κ or λ light chains but not both. The concept of local origin of S-IgA was upheld by later studies in which transport of locally synthesized pIg into jejunal secretions (Jonard *et al.*, 1984) and saliva (Kubagawa *et al.*, 1987) was found to be significantly greater than transport of serum-derived pIg.

Further support of the model of local synthesis of pIgA came with the discovery of the "joining" (J) chain, a peptide of about 15 kDa that was found to be a subunit of pIgA and pentameric IgM isolated from colostrum (Halpern and Koshland, 1970; Mestecky *et al.*, 1971). Subsequent studies demonstrated that J chain was expressed by a high percentage of IgA- and IgM-secreting plasma cells in mucosal tissues and exocrine glands (Brandtzaeg, 1974c; Nagura *et al.*, 1979a; Korsrud and Brandtzaeg, 1980; Kutteh *et al.*, 1982; Brandtzaeg, 1983a; Crago *et al.*, 1984; Brandtzaeg and Korsrud, 1984), and that expression of J chain was correlated with *in vitro* binding of SC to immunocytes in tissue sections (Brandtzaeg, 1974c, 1983a; Brandtzaeg and Korsrud, 1984). Current evidence suggests that J chain is not essential for polymerization of IgA and IgM, but the presence of J chain is required for binding of pIg to SC (see subsequent section, Binding of pIg to pIgR).

Immunohistochemical studies with specific antibodies to SC demonstrated that this subunit of S-Ig is synthesized not by plasma cells but by epithelial cells lining mucous membranes and exocrine glands (Tourville *et al.*, 1969; O'Daly *et al.*, 1971; Poger and Lamm, 1974; Brandtzaeg, 1974a; Brown *et al.*, 1976; Crago *et al.*, 1978) (see subsequent section, Regulation of pIgR Expression). Thus production of S-IgA and S-IgM was shown to require cooperation between local plasma cells producing pIg and the overlying epithelial cells. By the mid-1970s it was clear that SC was somehow involved in transport of pIg through the epithelial cell, and various models were proposed for this process (Poger and Lamm, 1974; Brandtzaeg, 1974a,b; Crago *et al.*, 1978; Hopf *et al.*, 1978; Brandtzaeg, 1978; Nagura *et al.*, 1979b; Orlans *et al.*, 1979). These investigators localized SC to the basolateral surface of mucosal epithelial cells and (in rodents but not humans) the sinusoidal surface of hepatocytes (see subsequent section, Hepatobiliary Transport of IgA). It was further shown that pIgA could bind to the surface of SC-expressing cells and that binding could be blocked by antibodies to SC. These observations strongly suggested that SC was acting as the receptor for endocytosis of pIgA by the epithelial cell. Furthermore, pIgA and SC were detected in intracellular vesicles that were presumably involved in transcytosis of pIgA across the cell (O'Daly *et al.*, 1971; Brandtzaeg, 1974a; Brown *et al.*, 1976; Poger and Lamm, 1974). The paradox was that SC was a soluble secretory protein, whereas one would expect that a receptor for endocytosis of IgA would be an integral membrane protein. This paradox was resolved with the discovery that SC is a proteolytic fragment of an integral membrane protein, known as the polymeric immunoglobulin receptor (pIgR) (Mostov *et al.*, 1980).

The concept that the transmembrane precursor for SC is a receptor for pIg led to proposal of the model for the transepithelial transport of IgA by pIgR, shown in **Figure 12.1**. pIgR is synthesized as an integral membrane protein in the rough endoplasmic reticulum and then travels to the Golgi apparatus. In the last station of the Golgi, known as the trans-Golgi network (TGN), pIgR is sorted into vesicles that deliver it to the basolateral surface of the epithelial cell. At that surface pIgR can bind to pIgA that is produced by plasma cells, most commonly found in the lamina propria underlying the epithelium. pIgR and bound pIgA are then endocytosed and delivered to endosomes. The receptor and ligand move through a series of endocytotic and transcytotic vesicles and are ultimately delivered to the apical plasma membrane. There the extracellular, ligand-binding portion of pIgR is cleaved off and released together with the IgA into external secretions. This cleaved fragment is the SC. (See subsequent section, pIgR Trafficking and Signals, for a more detailed description of the pathway of pIgR transcytosis.) Most exocrine fluids contain both bound SC (i.e., present in

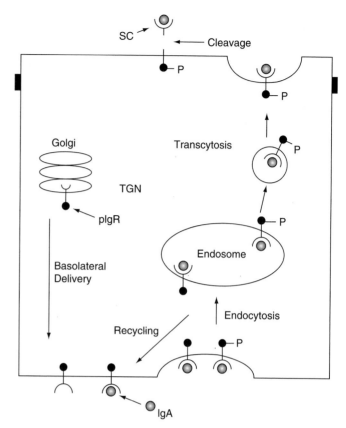

Fig. 12.1. Pathway of pIgR through an epithelial cell. A simplified epithelial cell is illustrated, with the apical surface at the top and the basolateral surface at the bottom.

S-IgA), and free SC (i.e., not bound to S-IgA) (Brandtzaeg, 1973), implying that transcytosis and cleavage of pIgR occur in both the presence and absence of pIg ligand. Mice with two disrupted alleles at the *Pigr* locus have markedly reduced IgA in external secretions, accompanied by elevated serum IgA (Johansen *et al.*, 1999; Shimada *et al.*, 1999), indicating that pIgR is required for transcytosis of pIg across mucosal epithelia *in vivo*.

STRUCTURE AND FUNCTION OF pIgR

Conserved structural features

The complete amino acid sequence of pIgR has been determined for eight mammalian species, six eutherian and two metatherian (see Chapter 11). In addition, partial amino acid sequences have been reported for pIgR from sheep (GenBank AJ313189), dog (GenBank AY081057), and chicken (GenBank BM426916, BG712734). Alignment of these sequences revealed a number of structural features that are highly conserved. The basic structure of pIgR comprises an N-terminal extracellular region of approximately 620 amino acids, a 23 amino acid membrane–spanning region, and a 103 amino acid C-terminal cytoplasmic region **(Figs. 12.2 and 12.3)**. The extracellular region of pIgR is the

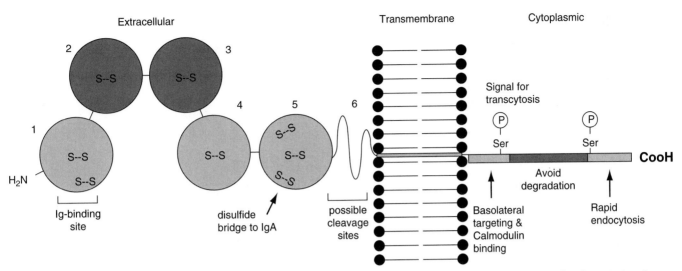

Fig. 12.2. Model of pIgR structure. **(See page 3 of the color plates.)** The extracellular region of pIgR (which is cleaved at the apical surface to form SC) comprises five immunoglobulinlike domains and a sixth domain of unrelated structure. Domains 1, 4, and 5 (yellow) are encoded by single exons that are always included in pIgR mRNA. Domains 2 and 3 (blue) are encoded by a single exon that is sometimes deleted by alternative splicing of rabbit pIgR mRNA. Intradomain disulfide bonds that are conserved in all known pIgR sequences are noted. Multiple sites of SC cleavage in domain 6 have been proposed. The cytoplasmic domain of pIgR contains highly conserved signals for intracellular sorting, endocytosis, and transcytosis.

ligand-binding portion of the molecule conferring specificity for pIg. This region contains five domains with homology to immunoglobulin variable domains and a sixth nonimmunoglobulinlike domain connecting to the transmembrane region (Mostov *et al.*, 1984; Eiffert *et al.*, 1984). Interspecies homology is greatest in domain 1, especially within segments that have been shown to be critical for immunoglobulin binding (Fig. 12.3) (see next section). Domains 2 and 3 are encoded by a single exon, which is frequently spliced out in rabbit pIgR mRNA (Deitcher and Mostov, 1986) but not in other species, suggesting that the functional role of domains 2 and 3 may be species-specific. Each of the five immunoglobulinlike extracellular domains contains an internal disulfide bond, characteristic of immunoglobulin homology units, that is conserved in all known species of pIgR (Eiffert *et al.*, 1984; Piskurich *et al.*, 1995) (Figs. 12.2 and 12.3). A second internal disulfide bond is found in all species in domains 1 and 5 and in some species in domains 2, 3, and 4. A third, highly conserved disulfide bond is found in domain 5. In human secretory IgA, the "extra" disulfide bond in domain 5 has been shown to rearrange to form a disulfide bond with cysteine residues in one of the α heavy chains of S-IgA (Fallgren-Gebauer *et al.*, 1993) (see next section).

The sixth extracellular domain of pIgR has a more random structure than the five immunoglobulin homology domains and is poorly conserved across species (Fig. 12.3). Proteolytic cleavage of pIgR within this domain leads to the release of SC from the apical surface of epithelial cells, either free or bound to pIg. In normal rat hepatocytes and in Madin–Darby canine kidney (MDCK) epithelial cells transfected with rabbit pIgR cDNA, cleavage has been shown to be catalyzed by a leupeptin-sensitive endopeptidase that is restricted to the bile

canalicular membrane of hepatocytes and the apical membrane of epithelial cells (Musil and Baenziger, 1987a, 1988; Solari *et al.*, 1989; Breitfeld *et al.*, 1989; Sztul *et al.*, 1993). However, determination of the precise cleavage site has been complicated by ambiguous results regarding the C terminus of SC. In one study, SC purified from human colostrum (pooled from multiple women) was found to have a ragged C terminus, varying from Ala550 to Lys559, with Ser552 as the dominant C-terminal residue (noted with an arrow, Fig. 12.3) (Eiffert *et al.*, 1984). The Ser at this position is conserved in all known pIgR sequences except rabbit, which diverged significantly from other pIgR sequences in this region. In another study, in which colostrum from one woman was used, a single C terminus of human SC at Arg585 was found (also noted by an arrow in Fig. 12.3) (Hughes *et al.*, 1997). The Arg at this position is poorly conserved across species but is preceded by an invariant proline residue. This proline may cause a bend in the protein chain, exposing nearby residues to proteolytic attack. Multiple C termini in human SC could result from trypsinlike cleavage of pIgR at Lys559 or Arg585, followed by additional exopeptidase cleavage. In contrast to human SC, a C terminus of Ala-Glu was reported for purified rabbit SC (Kuhn *et al.*, 1983). Since three instances of the dipeptide Ala-Glu are present in domain 6 of rabbit pIgR (underlined in Fig. 12.3), these data do not permit precise localization of the cleavage site. Alignment of pIgR sequences revealed significant interspecies homologies at two of the three potential Ala-Glu termini of rabbit SC (noted by arrows at residues Glu577 and Glu589 of human pIgR in Fig. 12.3). The Glu at position 577 of human pIgR is conserved in all known species except cow, which contains a Glu→Gln substitution. The Ala at position 588 of human pIgR is conserved in all eutherian (but not metatherian) species, although the adjacent Glu residue is

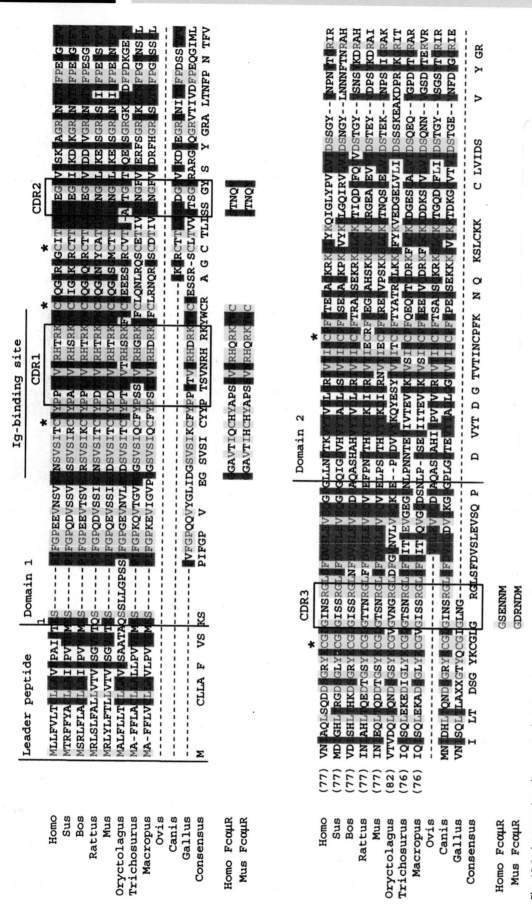

Fig. 12.3. Interspecies alignment of pIgR protein sequences. **(See pages 4–6 of the color plates.)** Full-length sequences were aligned for *Homo sapiens* (X73079), *Sus scrofa* (AB032195), *Bos taurus* (X81371), *Rattus norvegicus* (X15741), *Mus musculus* (U06431), *Oryctolagus cuniculus* (X00412), *Trichosurus vulpecula* (AF091137), and *Macropus eugenii* (AF317205). Partial sequences were aligned for *Ovis aries* (AJ313189), *Canis familiaris* (AY081057), and *Gallus gallus* (BM426916 and BG712734). Numbering of amino acids begins with the first residue of the mature protein (domain 1). Yellow shading indicates sequence identity among all species (excluding those species with no overlapping sequence at that position). Blue shading indicates sequence identity among six or more species. Sequences of the three complementarity-determining regions (CDRs) in domain 1 are boxed. Also shown are homologous sequences within the Ig-binding site and CDRs for the Fcαμ receptor (FcαμR) from *Homo sapiens* (AY063125) and *Mus musculus* (AB048834). Asterisks denote conserved cysteine residues involved in intrachain and interchain disulfide bonding. The arrows in domain 6 indicate potential sites of SC cleavage. Plus signs denote conserved residues in the cytoplasmic domain that have been shown to be required for basolateral targeting and rapid endocytosis. Residues known to be phosphorylated are denoted "P." See text for explanation of domain structure and conserved motifs.

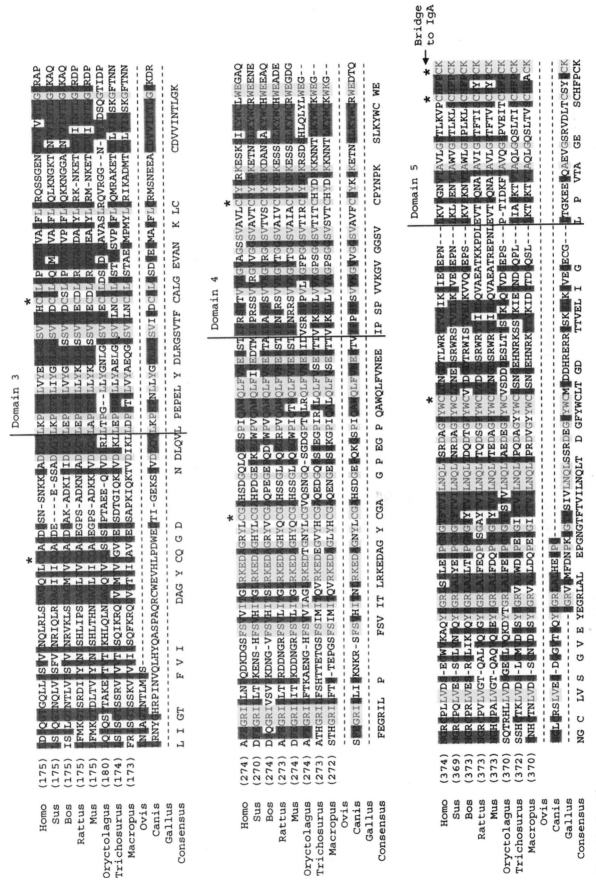

Fig. 12.3. Cont'd

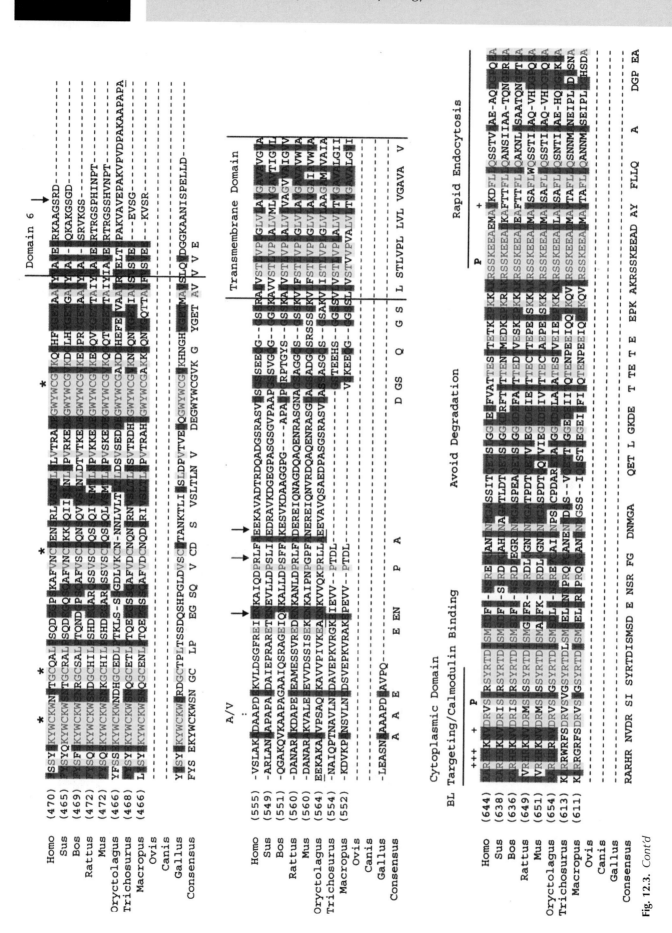

Fig. 12.3. *Cont'd*

found only in human, pig, and rabbit pIgR. A single nucleotide polymorphism has recently been discovered that causes a change in amino acid 560 of human pIgR from alanine to valine (Hirunsatit et al., 2003; Obara et al., 2003) (noted in Fig. 12.3). This polymorphism is associated with increased risk for nasopharyngeal cancer in certain Asian populations, and it has been suggested that reduced cleavage of pIgR may increase the risk of Epstein-Barr virus entry into nasopharyngeal epithelial cells (see subsequent section, Unique Functions of pIg and pIgR in Mucosal Epithelia). In this regard it is noteworthy that possum and wallaby pIgR have a valine residue at the homologous position (Fig. 12.3); it would be interesting to determine whether this naturally occurring sequence difference affects the rate of cleavage of pIgR.

Given the multiplicity of observed C termini for SC, the differing amino acid residues at potential cleavage sites, and the random structure of domain 6, it is likely that multiple proteases can cleave pIgR to SC. Furthermore, the extracellular orientation of pIgR at the apical surface may allow access to both cell-associated and secreted proteases. It has recently been reported that carbohydrate residues of pIgR anchor S-IgA to mucus lining the epithelial surface (Phalipon et al., 2002), raising the possibility that mucus-associated proteases may participate in SC cleavage. Another mechanism for SC cleavage is suggested by the finding that serine proteases released by activated neutrophils cleaved pIgR from the surface of human bronchial epithelial cells (Pilette et al., 2003).

The transmembrane region of pIgR is the most highly conserved domain of the protein, with interspecies differences involving only conservative substitutions of one hydrophobic amino acid for another (Fig. 12.3). The perfectly conserved Pro residue in the center of this core sequence may participate in signal transduction following ligand binding, by causing a bend in the α-helical structure of the membrane-spanning domain (Mostov et al., 1984) (see subsequent section, Regulation of pIgR Traffic). Finally, the cytoplasmic domain of pIgR contains a number of highly conserved intracellular sorting signals that interact with cytoplasmic proteins to direct pIgR through the transcytotic pathway (see subsequent sections, pIgR Trafficking and Signals, Regulation of pIgR Traffic).

Binding of pIg to pIgR

The extracellular region of pIgR, which after proteolytic cleavage is known as SC, is the ligand-binding portion of the molecule. The association of pIgR with pIg involves multiple structural elements that participate in both noncovalent and covalent bonds. The apparent association constants (K_a) for binding of human and rabbit SC to pIgA in solution are on the order of 10^8 M^{-1} (Brandtzaeg, 1985; Kuhn and Kraehenbuhl, 1979a), similar to those observed for antigen-antibody reactions. Estimates of the K_a for binding of dimeric IgA to rabbit pIgR on the surface of epithelial cells have ranged from 10^8 to 10^9 M^{-1} (Kuhn and Kraehenbuhl, 1979b). The K_a for the binding of human pIgR to pen-

tameric IgM is 8–30 times higher than that for pIgA (Brandtzaeg, 1977; Socken and Underdown, 1978; Roe et al., 1999). In vivo, however, the external transfer of pIgA appears to be considerably more efficient than that of IgM on a molar basis (reviewed in Natvig et al., 1997). In carefully controlled studies, human pIgA and pIgM were found to be transported at similar rates across monolayers of MDCK cells transfected with human pIgR (Natvig et al., 1997). However, pIgM was found to diffuse more slowly than pIgA across semipermeable membranes in vitro and was selectively retained in mucosal basement membrane zones in vivo. It has been suggested that the smaller pIgA molecule may be transferred to external secretions more effectively than pentameric IgM because of its preferential diffusion through the extracellular matrix and basement membrane (Natvig et al., 1997). Unlike its human homolog, pIgR from rabbits and rodents binds poorly to IgM (Socken and Underdown, 1978; Underdown et al., 1992; Roe et al., 1999), thus explaining the observation that IgM is not transported from blood to bile in rats (Orlans et al., 1979) (see subsequent section, Hepatobiliary Transport of IgA).

Binding of pIgR to pIgA or pentameric IgM requires the presence of J chain connecting the Ig subunits (reviewed in Johansen et al., 2000). The requirement for J chain was established by comparing the binding of human monomeric IgA, polymeric IgA, and pentameric IgM, with and without J chain, to the surface of human intestinal epithelial cells expressing pIgR (Brandtzaeg and Prydz, 1984). It was subsequently shown that human polymeric IgA lacking J chain was neither transported from blood to bile and rats nor transported across monolayers of MDCK cells expressing human pIgR (Vaerman et al., 1998a). In vivo studies in J chain–deficient mice demonstrated that the presence of J chain was obligatory for pIgR-mediated hepatic transport of IgA and intestinal transport of both IgA and IgM (Hendrickson et al., 1995, 1996; Lycke et al., 1999). Furthermore, IgA derived from J chain–deficient mice was not transported across monolayers of MDCK cells expressing pIgR (Hendrickson et al., 1995). These data suggested an important structural role for J chain in pIgR binding, which could involve either direct contact with pIgR or maintenance of pIg in a conformation that supports binding of pIgR. Antibodies to J chain and (to a lesser extent) soluble J chain dimers were found to inhibit binding of SC to pIgA and pentameric IgM, suggesting that pIgR may bind to the J chain moiety of pIg (Brandtzaeg, 1975a). Antibodies to J chain also inhibited hepatobiliary transport of human pIgA injected intravenously into rats and transport of human pIgA across monolayers of MDCK cells expressing human pIgR (Vaerman et al., 1998b). Recent studies in which mutant forms of human J chain were used have led to the identification of structural features of J chain that are required for pIgR binding (Johansen et al., 2001). Both the C terminus of J chain and two intrachain disulfide bridges (Cys13:Cys101 and Cys109:Cys134) were found to be required for binding of pIgA to pIgR but were not required for polymerization of IgA. Non–covalently stabilized IgA polymers with mutant J chain bound free SC with high affinity but were transcytosed by pIgR-expressing MDCK cells with reduced efficiency. Thus, J chain appears to bind directly to pIgR and to maintain pIg in a conformation optimal for pIgR binding and transcytosis.

Recent experiments with chimeric "domain swap" immunoglobulins revealed that the C-terminal domains of human IgA ($C\alpha3$) and IgM ($C\mu4$) are required for J-chain binding, polymerization, and association with pIgR (Hexham *et al.*, 1999; Chintalacharuvu *et al.*, 2001; Braathen *et al.*, 2002). Mutation of amino acids 402–410 in an exposed external loop of the $C\alpha3$ domain of IgA1 abrogated binding of dimeric IgA to rabbit and human pIgR, suggesting that this region contributes directly to pIgR binding (Hexham *et al.*, 1999). This $C\alpha3$ motif, when fused to green fluorescent protein or present in phage peptides, was sufficient to direct epithelial transcytosis via pIgR (White and Capra, 2002). Chimeric immunoglobulins in which the $C\alpha3$ domain of IgA2m(2) was substituted for the $C\gamma3$ domain of IgG1 formed polymers with J chain and were transported across monolayers of MDCK cells expressing human pIgR (Chintalacharuvu *et al.*, 2001). However, transport of the chimeric immunoglobulins was significantly less efficient than that of native IgA2m(2), suggesting that the native conformation of dimeric IgA, in addition to specific sequences in the $C\alpha3$ domain, is necessary for optimal pIgR binding and transcytosis. Chimeric IgM molecules in which the $C\alpha3$ domain of IgA was substituted for the $C\mu4$ domain of IgM were able to bind both rabbit and human pIgR, while native IgM bound only human pIgR (Braathen *et al.*, 2002). Thus the species specificity of pIgR binding maps to the C-terminal domain of IgM. For all the chimeric immunoglobulins described above, polymerization in the presence of J chain was an absolute requirement for pIgR binding. The complex interaction between pIg and pIgR therefore requires native polymeric conformation and sequence elements with the J chain and the C-terminal domains of IgA and IgM.

Multiple elements in the extracellular immunoglobulinlike domains of pIgR appear to participate in its noncovalent association with pIg. Several independent observations support a pIg-binding role for domain 1. Isolated domain 1 from rabbit, cow, and human pIgR, prepared by digestion of SC (Frutiger *et al.*, 1986; Beale, 1988; Bakos *et al.*, 1991a) or molecular cloning (Bakos *et al.*, 1994), was shown to bind pIg with high affinity. Furthermore, a monoclonal antibody directed against an epitope in domain 1 of human pIgR was found to inhibit binding of free SC to pIgA (Bakos *et al.*, 1991b). To localize further the pIg-binding site within domain 1, Bakos *et al.* (1991a) used peptide mapping to identify a 23–amino acid sequence with immunoglobulin binding activity, albeit with ninefold lower affinity for pIgA than that of isolated domain 1 for pIgA. Whereas binding of intact domain 1 was specific for pIg, the synthetic peptide bound monomeric IgA and IgG just as well as polymeric IgA and IgM, suggesting that the overall structure of domain 1 may contribute to both the affinity and the specificity of pIg-binding. Molecular modeling of the three-dimensional struc-

ture of rabbit pIgR, on the basis of its homology to immunoglobulin variable domains, indicated that the conserved immunoglobulin-binding site spanned an exposed loop analogous to the CDR1 loop of Ig V domains (Coyne *et al.*, 1994). The "CDR1-like" loop is flanked by Cys residues, which are conserved in all known pIgR sequences (including chicken), as well as in the related Ig-binding site of the $Fc\alpha/\mu$ receptor in humans and mice (Fig. 12.3). In human SC, these Cys residues have been shown to form an intrachain disulfide bond, which may stabilize the structure of the "CDR1-like" loop (Fallgreen-Gebauer *et al.*, 1993). In the context of full-length rabbit pIgR, point mutations within CDR1 significantly diminished pIgA binding (Coyne *et al.*, 1994). pIgA binding was also abrogated by mutation of exposed loops analogous to CDR2 and CDR3, suggesting that all three CDRs may contribute to affinity and specificity of pIg binding. These observations suggest that interactions between pIgR and pIg may be similar to interactions between the variable regions of antibodies and their cognate antigens. To determine whether elements in domain 1 contribute to the species specificity of pIgR binding to pentameric IgM, Roe *et al.* (1999) transfected MDCK cells with human/rabbit chimeric pIgR molecules in which the entire domain 1 or the individual CDR-like loops were interchanged. Whereas all the chimeric pIgR molecules mediated binding and transcytosis of pIgA, only those containing domain 1 from human pIgR mediated binding and transcytosis of pentameric IgM. Within domain 1, the CDR2-like loop of human pIgR was the most essential for pentameric IgM binding. The CDR1-like loop but not the CDR3-like loop further contributed to the specificity of IgM binding.

Whereas domain 1 of pIgR is essential for pIg binding, the other extracellular immunoglobulinlike domains contribute to binding affinity. Tryptic fragments of human SC containing either domains 1 and 2 or domains 1, 2, and 3 were shown to bind pIgA with 15-fold lower affinity than did full-length SC (i.e., domains 1–5 of pIgR) (Bakos *et al.*, 1991a). The affinity of isolated domain 1 relative to full-length SC was found to be 33-fold lower for pIgA and 79-fold lower for pIgM (Bakos *et al.*, 1994). Effects of domain deletions in the context of cell-associated human pIgR have been studied by molecular cloning (Norderhaug *et al.*, 1999a). Combined deletion of domains 2 and 3 of pIgR eliminated binding and transcytosis of pIgA across transfected MDCK cells but did not affect binding and transcytosis of pentameric IgM. By contrast, combined deletion of domains 4 and 5 caused a twofold decrease in affinity of pIgR for pIgA and a fourfold decrease in affinity of pIgR for IgM. Crottet and coworkers (Crottet *et al.*, 1999; Crottet and Corthesy, 1999) studied the pIg-binding function of mouse SC by epitope substitutions within the CDR-like loops of domains 1, 2, and 3. As was seen with human pIgR/SC, mutation of the domain 1 CDR3 of domain 1 abrogated pIgA binding. Mutations within domains 2 and 3 did not appreciably affect pIgA-binding affinity but prevented covalent binding between SC and dimeric IgA. Because the critical Cys residue for covalent binding is in domain 5 of SC (see below), these authors suggested that domains 2 and 3 may be necessary for maintaining the correct orientation of domain 5 to allow disulfide bonding with the Cα3 domain of IgA. A role for domains 2 and 3 in pIg binding has also been reported for bovine SC (Beale, 1988). A fragment containing domains 1, 2, and 3 bound pIgM with equivalent affinity, as did full-length SC, whereas a fragment containing domain 1 and part of domain 2 bound pIgM with threefold lower affinity. By contrast, domain 1 of rabbit pIgR was found to bind pIgA with equivalent affinity, as did full-length SC (Frutiger et al., 1986). Furthermore, deletion of domains 2 and 3 in the context of full-length SC (Frutiger et al., 1986) or pIgR (Coyne et al., 1994) did not diminish binding to pIgA. These species-specific differences in pIgA-pIgR interactions may provide a functional explanation for species-specific differences in alternative splicing of the exon encoding domains 2 and 3 in pIgR mRNA (see subsequent section, Expression and Processing of pIgR mRNA).

A unique feature of the S-IgA molecule is the presence of a highly conserved disulfide bond between Cys residues in domain 5 of SC and the Cα2 domain of one of the α-heavy chains in pIgA (Figs. 12.2 and 12.3). Peptide mapping of human S-IgA has identified the participating residues as Cys468 in domain 5 of SC and Cys311 of the α-heavy chain (Fallgreen-Gebauer et al., 1993). Similar disulfide bonds have been identified in S-IgA from other species, and the orthologous Cys residue is perfectly conserved in all known species of pIgR, including chicken (see arrow in Fig. 12.2 denoting "disulfide bridge to IgA"). Disulfide bonding between pIgR and pIgA has been shown to occur late in the transcytotic pathway (Chintalacharuvu et al., 1994), and normal transcytosis of the pIgR-pIgA complex can occur under conditions in which disulfide bonding is prevented (Chintalacharuvu et al., 1994; Tamer et al., 1995). Therefore, the significance of disulfide bonding between pIgR and pIgA may not be to facilitate transcytosis but rather to prevent dissociation of the S-IgA complex in the harsh milieu of external secretions. Unlike pIgA, pentameric IgM does not form a covalent bond with pIgR during epithelial transcytosis (Brandtzaeg, 1975b, 1977).

Unique functions of pIg and pIgR in mucosal epithelia

With each round of pIg transport, epithelial cells "sacrifice" the extracellular domain of pIgR as cleaved SC, either free or complexed to pIg (Fig. 12.1). It is reasonable to assume that the metabolic cost of synthesizing a new molecule of pIgR for each round of pIg transport is compensated for by immune functions contributed by SC. Surface plasmon resonance–based binding experiments indicated that purified S-IgA and pIgA antibodies had identical binding affinities for immobilized antigen (Lullau et al., 1996). Similarly, S-IgA was found to be no more effective than pIgA in its ability to neutralize influenza virus in vitro (Renegar et al., 1998). A surprising finding was that mice with two disrupted *Pigr* alleles had significantly higher numbers of IgA-secreting cells in the intestinal lamina propria than did wild-type mice (Uren et al., 2003). Thus pIgR does not appear to enhance

the production or antigen-binding properties of S-IgA. However, the presence of SC has been shown to enhance both the stability and effector functions of pIg. It has long been appreciated that bound SC protects the S-IgA molecule from proteolytic degradation in vitro (Lindh, 1975; Mestecky et al., 1991; Renegar et al., 1998), and this protective mechanism has subsequently been demonstrated in vivo in the gastrointestinal tract (Chintalacharuvu and Morrison, 1997; Crottet and Corthesy, 1998) and the oral cavity (Ma et al., 1998). The presence of bound SC has also been shown to inhibit degradation of pIgA by neutrophil elastase, thus enhancing the effectiveness of humoral immunity in the respiratory tract (Pilette et al., 2003).

In addition to its role in protecting mucosal IgA from proteolytic degradation, pIgR and SC have been shown to confer novel effector functions on mucosal pIg. One such novel pIgR-dependent function of pIgA is to neutralize intracellular pathogens, such as viruses, directly within epithelial cells. Intracellular neutralization of viruses by pIgA demonstrates that the humoral immune response can effect an immune function previously ascribed only to the cellular immune response. This phenomenon was originally observed in pIgR-expressing MDCK cells infected with either Sendai or influenza virus, using antibodies directed against membrane glycoproteins (hemagglutinin-neuraminidase) found on the surface of virions (Mazanec et al., 1992, 1995). HIV and measles virus have also been shown to be neutralized inside epithelial cells by pIgA antibodies to envelope glycoproteins (Bomsel et al., 1998; Yan et al., 2002). A likely explanation for these results is that the newly synthesized viral glycoproteins that move from the TGN to the cell surface pass through an endosomal compartment that contains transcytosing pIgA. The most likely location would be the apical recycling compartment, because this has already been shown to be a key polarized sorting location (Bomsel et al., 1998). It has recently been reported that mice with two disrupted *Pigr* alleles had reduced protection against influenza virus infection following intranasal immunization (Asahi et al., 2002). This reduced protection could be attributed to a lack of intracellular neutralization as well as reduced immune exclusion by S-IgA in nasal secretions. In another study, no differences in induction of influenza virus–specific CD8+ T cells were found in pIgR$^{-/-}$ mice compared with controls (Uren et al., 2003).

Rotaviral diarrhea causes approximately 500,000 deaths annually worldwide and is responsible for significant morbidity among children in the United States, especially in lower income groups (Miller and McCann, 2000). Development of a rotavirus vaccine has been hampered by the high level of antigenic diversity in its envelope glycoproteins (Laird et al., 2003). Intracellular neutralization of virus by pIgA to internal viral antigens has been found to be a major mechanism for protection against rotavirus infection in mice (Burns et al., 1996). Mice bearing tumors secreting nonneutralizing pIgA specific for the inner-capsid protein VP6 were protected, whereas mice bearing tumors secreting neutralizing pIgA specific for the outer-membrane hemagglutinin VP4 were not protected. Similar results were observed following vaccination with DNA plasmids encoding VP6 (Chen *et al.*, 1997), which caused the production of nonneutralizing mucosal IgA antibodies, or intraperitoneal injection of a nonneutralizing IgA monoclonal antibody to VP6 (Feng *et al.*, 2002). In this case the mechanism is less clear, because the pIgA is directed against an internal antigen of the virion, which would be exposed only after virus uncoating in the cytoplasm. Transcytosis of pIgA is clearly involved, because mice lacking J chain, which are deficient in pIgR-mediated transcytosis, were not protected by intranasal vaccination with VP6 (Schwartz-Cornil *et al.*, 2002). Feng *et al.* (2002) demonstrated intracellular neutralization of rotavirus *in vitro* by delivering anti-VP6 pIgA to the cytoplasm of infected epithelial cells by lipofection. Significantly, the neutralization titers were similar against a variety of rotavirus serotypes and subgroups. The anti-VP6 antibodies appeared to inhibit viral transcription at the start of the intracellular phase of the viral replication cycle. By contrast, other investigators did not observe intracellular neutralization *in vitro* when anti-VP6 IgA was administered to the basolateral surface of polarized epithelial cells expressing pIgR, which would target pIgA to the transcytotic pathway (Ruggeri *et al.*, 1998). It remains to be determined how pIgA antibodies may be delivered to the cytoplasm of rotavirus-infected enterocytes *in vivo*.

A rather different type of interaction of pIgA and viruses is illustrated by the finding that pIgA antibodies to Epstein-Barr virus (EBV) can actually facilitate entry of virus into epithelial cells by pIgR-mediated endocytosis (Sixbey and Yao, 1992; Gan *et al.*, 1997; Lin *et al.*, 1997, 2000). The fate of internalized EBV appears to depend on the degree of epithelial cell polarization. In rat liver *in vivo* and in polarized monolayers of MDCK cells *in vitro*, pIgA-EBV complexes were transcytosed rapidly across the epithelial cell without establishing infection. In contrast, entry of pIgA-EBV complexes into unpolarized cells led to productive infection and expression of EBV antigens. On the basis of these findings, it was suggested that pIgR-mediated transcytosis of pIgA-EBV complexes through the nasopharyngeal epithelium could facilitate endogenous spread of EBV in long-term virus carriers, with infection being confined to cells with altered polarity from prior cytopathology. Significantly, it has been reported that a single nucleotide polymorphism that may affect pIgR cleavage is associated with increased risk of nasopharyngeal cancer in certain Asian populations (Hirunsatit *et al.*, 2003) (see previous section, Conserved Structural Features).

A second novel pIgR-mediated function is transcytosis of locally formed immune complexes (IC) from the lamina propria to the lumenal surface of mucosal epithelial cells. Thus, in addition to the role of S-IgA in immune exclusion, locally produced pIg antibodies within the mucosa may serve to trap antigens derived from the environment, diet, and luminal microbiota or synthesized in the mucosal tissue during infections. Such pIgA-mediated trapping would by itself be an anti-inflammatory mechanism in competition with the

formation of potentially harmful IC containing IgM or IgG antibodies. Moreover, external transport of pIgA IC by mucosal epithelia could be an efficient and potentially less harmful clearance mechanism than their systemic elimination after they reach the circulation. It has been demonstrated *in vitro* that epithelial cells expressing pIgR can vectorially transport IC containing pIgA from the basolateral surface to release at the apical face; the antigen remains undegraded and bound to the pIgA antibody throughout transcytosis (Kaetzel *et al.*, 1991). Monomeric IgA and IgG antibodies, when cross-linked via antigen to pIgA, were also shown to participate in pIgR-mediated epithelial trancystosis (Kaetzel *et al.*, 1994). In addition to IC comprising soluble protein antigens, pIgR has been shown to mediate transcytosis of whole viruses and bacteria complexed to pIgA across polarized monolayers of epithelial cells (Gan *et al.*, 1997; Yan *et al.*, 2002; Zhang *et al.*, 2000). A mucosal IgA-mediated excretory immune system has been demonstrated *in vivo* in mice immunized mucosally with ovalbumin antigen (Robinson *et al.*, 2001). Uptake of antigen into intestinal epithelial cells occurred only from the basolateral aspect, and only when antigen complexed to IgA antibody was present in the lamina propria. Secretory epithelia might therefore participate in the clearance of IgA IC *in vivo* directly at sites where they are most likely to be formed.

Streptococcus pneumoniae is a major human pathogen, causing diseases ranging from relatively mild otitis media to potentially fatal sepsis, pneumonia, and meningitis (Alonso de Velasco *et al.*, 1995). Several novel interactions between pIgR and *S. pneumoniae* have recently been characterized (reviewed in Kaetzel, 2001). Human pIgR/SC has been shown to bind specifically to a polymorphic surface protein of *S. pneumoniae*, variously named SpsA, CbpA, and PspC (Hammerschmidt *et al.*, 1997, 2000; Zhang *et al.*, 2000). Studies with deletional mutants of human pIgR demonstrated that CbpA binds via the immunoglobulinlike domains 3 and 4 (Lu *et al.*, 2003; Elm *et al.*, 2004). In a cell culture model of bacterial invasion, free SC was found to block invasion of epithelial cells by *S. pneumoniae* (Zhang *et al.*, 2000b). However, in the absence of free SC or S-IgA antibody, expression of human pIgR in human nasopharyngeal cells and MDCK cells facilitated pneumococcal adherence and invasion. A subsequent study suggested that the ability of *S. pneumoniae* to co-opt the pIgR transcytosis machinery may be strain-specific (Brock *et al.*, 2002). Thus the role of pIgR in preventing or facilitating invasion of respiratory epithelial cells by *S. pneumoniae* is likely to depend on both host and bacterial factors, especially the levels of S-IgA antibodies and free SC in mucosal secretions.

Recent studies have revealed novel functions for SC following secretion, either as free SC or bound to S-IgA (reviewed in Phalipon and Corthesy, 2003). Free SC has been shown to limit infection or reduce morbidity by binding to bacterial components such as *Clostridium difficile* toxin A (Dallas and Rolfe, 1998), fimbriae of enterotoxigenic *Escherichia coli* (de Oliveira *et al.*, 2001), and (as described above) choline-binding proteins from some strains of *S. pneumoniae*. S-IgA was shown to be more protective than pIgA in a mouse model of respiratory tract infection by *Shigella flexneri*, due to carbohydrate-dependent adherence of S-IgA to the mucus lining of the epithelium of the upper airway (Phalipon *et al.*, 2002).

In addition to its roles in exclusion, neutralization, and excretion of pathogens, pIgR/SC may protect epithelial surfaces by reducing inflammation associated with host immune responses. Free SC has been shown to form a high-molecular-weight complex with IL-8 secreted by primary cultures of human bronchial epithelial cells, inhibiting its activity as a neutrophil chemoattractant (Marshall *et al.*, 2001). Other investigators reported that monomeric and polymeric IgA triggered efficient phagocytosis of heat-killed *Neisseria meningitidis* by human neutrophils, but S-IgA did not (Vidarsson *et al.*, 2001). By contrast, S-IgA was found to be more potent than serum IgA in stimulating degranulation and superoxide production by human eosinophils (Motegi and Kita, 1998; Motegi *et al.*, 2000). Thus the presence of SC in mucosal secretions, free or complexed as S-IgA, may differentially modulate the host immune response to inflammatory stimuli. A novel anti-inflammatory role for for pIgR-pIgA has recently been suggested by the demonstration that intracellular pIgA can neutralize lipopolysaccharide (LPS) of *S. flexneri* in a murine intestinal epithelial cell line that expresses pIgR (Fernandez *et al.*, 2003). LPS-specific pIgA antibodies were found to colocalize with LPS in an apical recycling compartment, preventing LPS-induced NF-κB activation and induction of a proinflammatory response. Given that S-IgA antibodies to LPS constitute a major component of the protective immune response to shigella infection (Phalipon and Sansonetti, 1999), pIgR-mediated intracellular delivery of anti-LPS pIgA may be important for minimizing inflammatory damage to the epithelium. This mechanism could also minimize inflammatory responses to LPS derived from commensal bacteria in the gut. In this regard it is significant that LPS has been shown to upregulate pIgR expression in intestinal epithelial cells (Schneeman and Kaetzel, 2003) (see subsequent section, Regulation of pIgR Expression).

pIgR as a marker for targeting of mucosal epithelial cells

Receptor-mediated endocytosis of foreign DNA has been explored as a mechanism for selective gene delivery, and the localization of pIgR on the surface of mucosal epithelial cells makes it an attractive target. The utility of pIgR as a targeting molecule was first demonstrated with use of an Fab fragment of anti-pIgR antibody, complexed via polylysine to an expression plasmid, to induce expression of a reporter gene in a human intestinal epithelial cell line (Ferkol *et al.*, 1993). Intravenous delivery of a similar targeting vector in rats caused tissue-specific expression of the reporter gene in liver and lung, demonstrating the feasibility of this approach *in vivo* (Ferkol *et al.*, 1995). Complications arising from immune responses to the Fab portion of the targeting vector (Ferkol *et al.*, 1996) were largely overcome by development

of bifunctional proteins in which a single chain Fv with specificity for the extracellular domain of pIgR was fused to a functional protein (Gupta *et al.*, 2001). This approach has now been used to target active α1-antitrypsin to the surface of respiratory epithelia in cultures of polarized cells (Eckman *et al.*, 1999; Ferkol *et al.*, 2000) and in human tracheal xenografts (Ferkol *et al.*, 2003). As described above, short peptides comprising the Cα3 motif of IgA may be sufficient for targeting pIgR and directing epithelial transcytosis (White and Capra, 2002). Thus, in addition to its natural roles in mucosal immunity, pIgR may prove to be an important target molecule for delivery of novel therapeutic agents.

REGULATION OF pIgR EXPRESSION

Tissue-specific expression of pIgR

Shortly after the initial discovery of S-IgA, an immunohistological survey of normal human tissues demonstrated the presence of pIgR in bronchial epithelial cells, salivary glands, gallbladder, renal tubules, pancreatic glandular and ductular epithelial cells, the ductular epithelium of sweat glands, and the epithelial lining of the small and large bowel (Tourville *et al.*, 1969). Subsequent studies confirmed the widespread epithelial distribution of pIgR, although the magnitude of expression varies considerably among anatomic sites and is influenced in a tissue-specific manner by cytokines and hormones (see subsequent section, Regulation of pIgR Expression by Cytokines and Hormones).

The gut mucosa contains most of the immunoglobulin-producing cells in the body and is therefore quantitatively the major effector organ of humoral immunity. The selectivity and capacity of the pIgR-mediated transport mechanism *in vivo* has been studied in normal adult volunteers by jejunal perfusion (Jonard *et al.*, 1984). The average jejunal secretion rate for 11 individuals was 217 μg/40 cm/min for pIgA, 132 μg for albumin, 35 μg for IgG, and 15 μg for mIgA. To determine the contribution of serum versus local origin of these proteins, a relative coefficient of excretion was calculated as the jejunum-to-serum concentration ratio expressed relative to that of albumin. The relative coefficient of excretion was about 218 for pIgA, compared with 0.83 for IgG and 1.98 for mIgA, consistent with local synthesis and/or selective transepithelial transport of pIgA. Measurement of transport of intravenously injected ^{125}IpIgA into jejunal secretions of two volunteers demonstrated that only 2% of total jejunal pIgA was derived from plasma; thus approximately 98% of the pIgA was derived from local synthesis. Conley and Delacroix (1987) later extrapolated the data of Jonard *et al.* (1984) to the length of the entire intestine and compared the total estimated concentration of IgA in intestinal secretions to their own data on intravascular pools of IgA. From these calculations they concluded that the average adult human secretes into the intestine approximately 42.4 mg of IgA/kg body weight/day, of which approximately 39.5 mg represents pIgR-mediated transport of locally synthesized pIgA. Prigent-Delecourt *et al.* (1995) adapted this approach to measuring IgA secretion from colonic mucosa, using pancolonic perfusion in 10 normal volunteers. The secretion rate of pIgA was 153 µg/min (220 mg/day), compared with 8.5 µg for mIgA, 33.5 µg for IgG, 17 µg for IgM, and 104 µg for albumin. The relative coefficient of excretion was 277 for pIgA, 6 for IgM, and 2.2 for mIgA, In addition, all the pIgA in the colonic perfusates was linked to SC, and 12% of the total SC was present in free form. As was the case for the small intestine, these data from the colon are consistent with local synthesis and pIgR-mediated transport of pIgA (and probably also IgM).

There are distinct regional and microtopographical variations in the level of pIgR expression along the GI tract. The importance of pIgR-mediated transcytosis of IgA in gastric mucosa has been questioned on the basis of reports that IgA isolated from gastric mucus did not appear to be associated with SC (Spohn and McColl, 1979a, 1979b). Two groups of investigators reported that immunohistochemical staining of normal gastric mucosa was negative for pIgR in the foveolae, gastric body glands, and pyloric glands of antral and body epithelium (Isaacson, 1982a; Valnes et al., 1984). However, pIgR expression was observed in the isthmus zone of the antral epithelium, which contains actively proliferating epithelium from which more specialized cells are replaced.

Measurement of pIgR protein and mRNA in normal intestinal tissues in humans and animals has demonstrated that expression of pIgR is high along the length of the small and large bowel and rectum, especially in the gland crypts (Tourville et al., 1969; O'Daly et al., 1971; Poger and Lamm, 1974; Brandtzaeg, 1974a, 1974b; Brown et al., 1976; Brandtzaeg and Baklien, 1976; Brown et al., 1977; Brandtzaeg and Baklien, 1976; Brandtzaeg, 1978; Momotani et al., 1986; Ha and Woodward, 1998; Hansen et al., 1999; Blanch et al., 1999; Sun et al., 2003; Peters et al., 2003). High pIgR expression has also been observed in duodenal Brunner's glands, which are formed by cellular division from the bottom of the duodenal crypts (Coutinho et al., 1996b). Expression of pIgR in regenerating cells in the intestinal crypts parallels that seen in the isthmus zone of the gastric antral epithelium and suggests that pIgR synthesis may be associated with immature, rapidly dividing cells in the gastrointestinal (GI) tract. An early study had suggested that pIgR is also produced by intestinal goblet cells (Tourville et al., 1969), but subsequent studies with improved fixation techniques showed unequivocally that pIgR expression is restricted to columnar epithelial cells and is not found in Paneth, goblet, or enteroendocrine cells (Brandtzaeg, 1974b; Brown et al., 1976, 1977; Brandtzaeg, 1978). In the Peyer's patches, the specialized follicle-associated epithelium (including M cells) has been shown to lack pIgR expression and does not appear to participate in pIgR-mediated transport of IgA (Bjerke and Brandtzaeg, 1988; Pappo and Owen, 1988).

In addition to direct transport of IgA across intestinal epithelial cells, other sources of IgA in GI fluids include saliva (approximately 2.9 mg/kg body weight/day) and hepatic bile (approximately 1.2 mg/kg body weight/day) (Conley and Delacroix, 1987). pIgR is expressed abundantly in the glandular acinar and ductular epithelium of parotid and submandibular salivary glands (Tomasi et al., 1965; Rossen et al., 1968; Tourville et al., 1969; Brandtzaeg, 1974a; Korsrud and Brandtzaeg, 1982), where it transports primarily locally synthesized pIgA (Kubagawa et al., 1987). Chewing has been shown to stimulate secretion of S-IgA by human parotid glands (Proctor and Carpenter, 2001), and studies with experimental animals have demonstrated the importance of sympathetic nerve stimulation in this process (Carpenter et al., 1998; Proctor et al., 2000). In the human hepatobiliary system, pIgR has generally been reported to be expressed only by the gallbladder and portal bile duct epithelia (Brandtzaeg, 1985; Nagura et al., 1981; Tomana et al., 1988), although some investigators have reported low but detectable staining of human hepatocytes with one of several monoclonal antibodies to SC (Foss-Bowman et al., 1983; Hsu and Hsu, 1980; Perez et al., 1989). By contrast, rodents, rabbits, and some other species exhibit abundant expression of pIgR by hepatocytes, thus allowing transport of pIgA from blood to bile (see subsequent section, Hepatobiliary Transport of IgA).

Transport of pIgA by pIgR in the upper respiratory tract is an important component of the specific defense of airway mucosae (reviewed in Brandtzaeg et al., 1996; Kim and Malik, 2003). Immunohistochemical studies have demonstrated that pIgR is expressed by epithelial cells in the nasal mucosa, palatine and pharyngeal tonsils, trachea, tracheobronchial glands, and bronchi (Rossen et al., 1968; Tourville et al., 1969; Brandtzaeg, 1974a, 1984; Fiedler et al., 1991; Finkbeiner et al., 1993; Rossel et al., 1993; Perry, 1994; Ferkol et al., 1995). As in the GI tract, pIgR expression is highest in columnar epithelial cells of the crypts and submucosal glands and is lacking in the follicle-associated epithelium of the bronchus-associated lymphoid tissue (Gehrke and Pabst, 1990).

By contrast to the epithelium of the upper respiratory tract, pIgR expression is low in pulmonary alveolar cells (Rossen et al., 1968; Rossel et al., 1993). Only trace amounts of pIgR mRNA have been detected in RNA extracted from whole lungs (Krajci et al., 1989; Piskurich et al., 1995), indicating that pIgR synthesis in the lower airway is minimal. The decreasing gradient of pIgR expression proceeding from the upper to lower respiratory tract is reflected by corresponding decreases in the ratio of IgA to IgG in salivary secretions, tracheal washes, and bronchoalveolar lavage (Daniele, 1990). The contrast of pIgR expression in the upper versus lower airway was illustrated by studies of gene transfer in vivo by targeting pIgR (Ferkol et al., 1995) (see previous section, pIgR as a Marker for Targeting of Mucosal Epithelial Cells). A DNA carrier consisting of Fab anti-SC linked to poly-L-lysine was used to introduce plasmids containing reporter genes into airway epithelial cells in rats. Significant levels of reporter gene activity were observed in the lung, but immunocytochemistry revealed that expression of these genes was localized to the surface epithelium of the airways and the submucosal glands and not the bronchioles and alveoli.

The female genital tract is an important component of the common mucosal immune system, and significant levels of S-IgA and free SC are found in uterine and vaginal secretions (Sullivan and Wira, 1983; Sullivan et al., 1984b; Wira and Sullivan, 1985; Stern and Wira, 1986; Kutteh and Mestecky, 1994; Kutteh et al., 1996; Quesnel et al., 1997; Johansson and Lycke, 2003). Two lines of evidence suggested that the IgA in human cervical mucus was predominantly derived from the local immune system: first, the IgA was predominantly polymeric; second, the IgA1:IgA2 ratio in cervical mucus paralleled the proportions of IgA1 to IgA2 plasma cells in the lamina propria of the uterine cervix (Kutteh et al., 1996). However, the amount of IgG in cervical mucus was found to exceed that of IgA. The IgG:albumin ratio was similar in cervical mucus and serum, suggesting that the IgG was derived from transudation of serum immunoglobulin. Thus both the local and systemic immune systems appear to contribute to humoral immunity in the female reproductive tract.

Immunohistochemical studies of humans and rats demonstrated that expression of pIgR is compartmentalized within female reproductive tissues (Tourville et al., 1970; Kutteh et al., 1988; Parr and Parr, 1989a; Kutteh et al., 1990; Bjercke and Brandtzaeg, 1993; Kutteh and Mestecky, 1994; Kaushic et al., 1995; Fichorova and Anderson, 1999) and is profoundly influenced by hormonal changes in the menstrual or estrus cycle (see subsequent section, Regulation of pIgR Expression by Cytokines and Hormones). Staining for pIgR was strongest in the columnar epithelial cells of the fallopian tubes, endometrial glands, and endocervix, was weak but detectable in the squamous epithelium of the ectocervix and vagina, and was absent in the ovaries and myometrium. The functional significance of pIgR expression in the uterus was confirmed by demonstrating that ex vivo cultures of polarized cells from the endometrium, endocervix, and ectocervix (but not the vagina) specifically bound and transported pIgA (Ball et al., 1995; Richardson et al., 1995; Fahey et al., 1998). Papillomavirus-immortalized cell lines from human ectocervical, endocervical, and vaginal epithelium were found to express pIgR at low levels, but the functional significance of this observation was not investigated (Fichorova et al., 1997; Fichorova and Anderson, 1999).

The presence of S-IgA in seminal fluid suggests that the male urogenital tract may also participate in the common mucosal immune system (Uehling, 1971; Rümke, 1974; Witkin et al., 1981). In one study of 75 men, the average concentration of S-IgA (134 mg/100 ml) exceeded that of IgG by 27-fold, suggesting that the S-IgA was derived predominantly from local synthesis and not transudation from serum. An extensive immunofluorescence study of pIgR distribution in the male rat demonstrated highest expression in the excretory ducts of the coagulating gland, the excretory ducts of the ventral and dorsolateral prostate gland, the ejaculatory duct, and the acini and ducts of the urethral gland (Parr and Parr, 1989b). Weak staining was observed in the parenchyma of the ventral prostate gland, and all other tissues were negative, including testis, epididymis, ductus deferens, ampullary gland, seminal vesicle, coagulating gland, dorsolateral prostate gland, bulbourethral gland, preputial gland, penis, and urinary bladder. Bright staining for SC was seen along the entire length of the urethral epithelium at the apical border of cells, but no intracellular staining was observed, suggesting that free SC or S-IgA may have been adherent to the surface of the cells and not actually synthesized at that location. It is interesting to note, however, that IgA-containing plasma cells were detected only in the urethral gland in the bulbous part of the urethra and not at other sites where pIgR was present. In another study, total levels of IgA and pIgR were measured by radioimmunoassay in reproductive tissues of the male rat (Stern et al., 1992). High levels of pIgR were detected in the prostate, presumably reflecting expression in the epithelium of the excretory ducts. Expression of pIgR was 20-fold lower in the seminal vesicles than in the prostate and was barely detectable in the testes, vas deferens, and epididymis. Significant levels of IgA were observed in the prostate, seminal vesicles, epididymis, testes, and vas deferens, but the source of the IgA was not determined. Few data are available on the distribution of pIgR in the human male reproductive tract. One immunohistochemical study of penile urethrae from 15 male patients at autopsy demonstrated positive expression of pIgR in the urethral epithelium and scattered IgA-positive plasma cells along the length of the urethral mucosa (Pudney and Anderson, 1995).

S-IgA is a major protein of normal human urine, with an estimated average daily excretion of 1.1 mg (Bienenstock and Tomasi, 1968). The presence in urine of SC, both free and bound to IgA, suggests that one or more tissues in the urinary system produce pIgR and actively transport pIgA (Bienenstock and Tomasi, 1968; Remington and Schafer, 1968; Svanborg Edén et al., 1985). An early study of sections of apparently unaffected tissue from six surgically removed kidneys showed positive staining for SC in renal tubular epithelium but not glomeruli (Tourville et al., 1969). In a later study of 17 biopsy specimens from normal renal allograft donors, SC was not found in renal tubular cells (Dobrin et al., 1975). An absence of SC staining was also noted in kidneys of normal male rats (Parr and Parr, 1989b). However, significant levels of SC were seen in tubular epithelial cells, but not glomeruli, from 51 patients with various forms of renal damage (Dobrin et al., 1975), and levels of urinary S-IgA and free SC were found to be elevated in acute pyelonephritis (Svanborg Edén et al., 1985; Greenwell et al., 1995). In subsequent studies in which more sensitive methods were used, pIgR mRNA and protein were detected in normal rat kidney, and levels were elevated following water deprivation, treatment with vasopressin, or ischemia (Rice et al., 1998, 1999). Taken together, these data suggest that pIgR is normally expressed at low levels in the kidney, but expression levels may be elevated in renal disease. However, epithelial cells in the lower urinary tract may normally express pIgR and transport pIgA into urine. Expression of pIgR has been observed in urethral epithelium and urethral glands of normal humans and rats (Parr and Parr, 1989a,b; Pudney and Anderson, 1995).

Expression of pIgR by a number of exocrine glands allows an additional route for locally synthesized pIgA to be transported into external secretions. Most prominent among these is the lactating mammary gland. S-IgA is the major immunoglobulin of colostrum and milk from many mammalian species, whereby it contributes to passive immunity of the suckling young (Bienenstock and Strauss, 1970; Lamm and Greenberg, 1972; Pahud and Mach, 1972; Nagura *et al.*, 1978; Hanson, 1982; Brandtzaeg, 1983b; Sheldrake *et al.*, 1984; Hahn-Zoric *et al.*, 1989; Hayani *et al.*, 1991; Cruz *et al.*, 1991; Goldblum and Goldman, 1994; Giugliano *et al.*, 1995; Rosato *et al.*, 1995; Adamski and Demmer, 1999, 2000; Kumura *et al.*, 2000; van der Feltz *et al.*, 2001; Rincheval-Arnold *et al.*, 2002b; Taylor *et al.*, 2002). As described previously (in the first section), an early study of allotype markers in colostral IgA of rabbits provided direct evidence of local assembly of S-IgA in the mammary gland (Lawton and Mage, 1969). Expression of pIgR by the mammary gland epithelium was subsequently confirmed by immunoelectron microscopy (Kraehenbuhl *et al.*, 1975). An immunofluorescence study of normal breast tissue from 10 women indicated that expression of pIgR in the nonlactating mammary gland is confined to ductal epithelial cells (Harris *et al.*, 1975). A later study of breast tissue from one woman in the eighth month of pregnancy and a second woman in the eighth month of lactation demonstrated variable levels of pIgR expression in alveolar epithelial cells and high levels in ductal epithelial cells (Brandtzaeg, 1983b). The subepithelial connective tissue contained large numbers of IgA-producing plasma cells, suggesting that most of the S-IgA in lacteal secretions was derived from local synthesis and transport. Studies involving experimental animals indicate that expression of pIgR is upregulated by hormones during pregnancy and lactation (see subsequent section, Regulation of pIgR Expressin by Cytokines and Hormones), thus accommodating the increased demand for secretion of S-IgA.

Other glandular epithelial tissues that have been reported to express pIgR include the lacrimal gland (Franklin *et al.*, 1973; Allansmith and Gillette, 1980; Sullivan *et al.*, 1984a; Kelleher *et al.*, 1991; Lambert *et al.*, 1994; Gao *et al.*, 1995; Hunt *et al.*, 1996), the sweat glands of the skin (Tourville *et al.*, 1969; Imayama *et al.*, 1995; Imayama *et al.*, 1994), the pancreas (Tourville *et al.*, 1969), and the thymus (Tomasi and Yurchak, 1972). The subepithelial interstitia of the lacrimal glands (Franklin *et al.*, 1973; Allansmith *et al.*, 1976) and sweat glands (Okada *et al.*, 1988) contain large numbers of IgA-producing plasma cells, indicative of local synthesis and transport of pIgA. By contrast, few if any IgA-producing plasma cells were observed in pancreas (Tourville *et al.*, 1969). Significant concentrations of SC and S-IgA have been detected in pure pancreatic juice (Saito *et al.*, 1985; Hayakawa *et al.*, 1993), but the source of the IgA is unclear.

In the thymus, significant expression of pIgR was observed in Hassall's corpuscles in the relative absence of immunoglobulins (Tomasi and Yurchak, 1972). *In vitro* culture of tissue explants from seven thymuses demonstrated that pIgR was synthesized locally and not transported from extrathymic sites. It has recently been demonstrated that the transcription factor AIRE promotes ectopic expression of peripheral tissue–restricted antigens in medullary epithelial cells of the thymus (Anderson *et al.*, 2002). Expression of pIgR in thymic epithelium may therefore represent a mechanism for achieving central tolerance for this tissue-specific antigen. By contrast, pIgR mRNA was not detected in extracts of spleens from humans (Krajci *et al.*, 1989), cows (Verbeet *et al.*, 1995a), or mice (Blanch *et al.*, 1999). There has been one report of pIgR expression by a murine B cell lymphoma derived from gut-associated lymphoid tissue (Phillips-Quagliata *et al.*, 2000). It is not known whether pIgR expression occurs naturally on a small cohort of normal B cells or whether its expression in T560 cells resulted from the transformation process. It has recently been reported that levels of IgA⁺B220⁻ B cells are elevated in the intestinal lamina propria of pIgR-deficient mice, suggesting that pIgR may play a role in mucosal B cell homeostasis (Uren *et al.*, 2003).

Ontogeny of pIgR expression

Although IgA-producing immunocytes do not appear in significant numbers until after birth, expression of pIgR has been observed in various secretory tissues during human fetal development. In one study, pIgR expression was observed in bronchial epithelium as early as 8 to 12 weeks of gestation and in kidney tubules, gastric epithelium, and the amnion by 13 to 17 weeks (Ogra *et al.*, 1972). In another study of the developing lung, pIgR expression was observed in the serous bronchial epithelium near the duct openings at 16 weeks, in goblet cells at 20 weeks, and in bronchiolar epithelium at 22 weeks (Takemura and Eishi, 1985). Evidence of cleavage of pIgR to SC during fetal development was provided by detection of free SC in amniotic fluid at 16 weeks of gestation, which then increased with gestational age from 26 to 40 weeks (Cleveland *et al.*, 1991). Expression of pIgR in intestinal and salivary gland epithelium was seen somewhat later (16–29 weeks), coinciding with a loss of expression in gastric epithelium (Brandtzaeg *et al.*, 1991; Crago *et al.*, 1978; Ogra *et al.*, 1972; Moro *et al.*, 1991). Recently, a comprehensive series of studies examined expression of various components of the secretory immune system throughout the first and second trimesters of pregnancy (reviewed in Gurevich *et al.*, 2003). Expression of pIgR was widely distributed among epithelial tissues of embryos and fetuses during the first trimester. Detectable as early as week 4 of pregnancy, pIgR represented one of the earliest appearing markers for ectoderm- and endoderm-derived structures. As organogenesis progressed, pIgR expression became restricted to epithelial cells lining mucous membranes, exocrine glands, and other sites of tissue barriers, such as the chorion, amnion, epidermis, mesothelium, and choroid plexus epithelium of the brain ventricles. At no time was pIgR expression seen in tissues of mesodermal origin, such as adrenal glands, the myocardium and endocardium, and the endothelium of capillaries. By contrast, IgA- and IgM-secreting immunocytes did not appear in significant numbers until the second trimester of preganancy and were distributed throughout epithelial and lymphoid tissues. Thus, the earlier expression of pIgR appears to prepare the epithelia of mucosal, glandular, and other barriers for the eventual role of pIg transport.

From a developmental point of view, expression of pIgR can be contrasted in tissues of endodermal, ectodermal, and mesodermal origin (see previous section). In humans, expression of pIgR is widespread in tissues of endodermal origin, including the epithelial linings of the GI and respiratory tracts, the submandibular salivary glands, the palatine tonsils, and the endoderm-derived structures of the genitourinary tract (i.e., the female vagina, the male prostate, and the male and female urethral epithelium). This general pattern of endodermal expression may also explain the presence of pIgR in the pancreas and thymus. However, regional influences may overrule the general pattern of pIgR expression in the developing endoderm. For example, the liver and biliary apparatus are all derived from the endoderm, but in humans pIgR expression appears to be suppressed in hepatocytes while maintained in the gallbladder and bile ducts. Likewise, there is a decreasing gradient of pIgR expression in the endoderm-derived tissues of the upper versus lower respiratory tract. Expression of pIgR is clearly not limited to tissues of endodermal origin, however. Ectoderm-derived tissues that express pIgR include the mammary glands, the sweat glands of the skin, the nasal cavities and olfactory epithelium, the parotid salivary glands, and the lacrimal glands. Certain mesodermal tissues in the female genital tract also express pIgR, i.e., the fallopian tubes, the uterus, and the cervix, but not the ovaries. In summary, expression of pIgR is strictly limited to epithelial cells, is widespread in tissues of endodermal origin, and is also seen in certain glandular epithelia of ectodermal and mesodermal origin.

In humans, expression of pIgR in salivary gland epithelium increases dramatically after the second postnatal week but decreases to the perinatal level around the sixth month (Burgio *et al.*, 1980; Hayashi *et al.*, 1989; Thrane *et al.*, 1991). In the intestinal crypts, mature levels of pIgR expression and signs of external IgA and IgM transport are seen at 1–2 weeks after birth (Brandtzaeg *et al.*, 1991). Postnatal increases in pIgR expression suggest that the secretory epithelium is exposed to stimulatory factors that enhance pIgR expression, perhaps associated with dietary changes and microbial colonization (see subsesquent section, Regulation of pIgR Expression by Microbial Products).

In rodents, the onset of pIgR expression in all tissues appears to be delayed until the postnatal period, coincident with the appearance of IgA-producing plasma cells in the lamina propria (Nagura *et al.*, 1978; Huling *et al.*, 1992). Increases in dietary amines at the time of weaning (associated with the transition from milk to solid food) have been shown to upregulate pIgR expression in the small intestine (Buts *et al.*, 1993). A recent study examined the role of passive and adaptive immunity in regulating pIgR expression in developing murine enterocytes by cross-fostering pups of normal and recombination-activating gene (RAG)–deficient dams (Jenkins *et al.*, 2003). In the absence of milk-derived pIgA (RAG-deficient dams), wild-type pups had significantly higher expression of pIgR mRNA. By contrast, mice lacking adaptive immunity (RAG-deficient pups) had significantly reduced pIgR expression, regardless of whether they were suckled by wild-type or RAG-deficient dams. Thus both passive and adaptive immunity were found to influence the development of enterocyte pIgR expression, suggesting that coordinated mechanisms may regulate antibody production and transport in the gut.

Regulation of pIgR expression by cytokines and hormones

A unique feature of pIgR is that it makes only one trip across epithelial cells before being cleaved and released at the apical surface. Because there is a 1:1 stoichiometry between SC and dimeric IgA in S-IgA, it follows that there must be one molecule of pIgR produced by the epithelial cell for every molecule of dimeric IgA that is transported. Upregulation of pIgR expression would thus increase the capacity of mucosal epithelial cells to transport dimeric IgA. Regulation of pIgR expression in mucous membranes involves complex interactions among multiple cell types, including lamina propria mononuclear cells (lymphocytes and macrophages), intraepithelial lymphocytes, and epithelial cells. A key role for proinflammatory cytokines in pIgR regulation has been demonstrated. Treatment with recombinant interferon-γ (IFN-γ), tumor necrosis factor (TNF), and/or interleukin (IL)-1 has been shown to upregulate pIgR protein and mRNA levels in a variety of cell types, including HT-29 human colon carcinoma cells (Sollid *et al.*, 1987; Kvale *et al.*, 1988; Phillips *et al.*, 1990; Youngman *et al.*, 1994; Denning, 1996; Blanch *et al.*, 1999; Nilsen *et al.*, 1999; Bruno *et al.*, 2003), CaLu-3 human lung carcinoma cells (Loman *et al.*, 1997; Ackermann *et al.*, 1999), human endometrial cells (Menge and Mestecky, 1993), human keratinocytes (Nihei *et al.*, 1996), rat uterus (Wira *et al.*, 1991; Prabhala and Wira, 1991), rat lacrimal gland (Kelleher *et al.*, 1991), and sheep mammary gland (Rincheval-Arnold *et al.*, 2002a). Although the effects of the Th1-type cytokine IFN-γ and the Th2-type cytokine IL-4 are often antagonistic, with respect to pIgR regulation these cytokines are synergistic (Phillips *et al.*, 1990; Youngman *et al.*, 1994; Denning, 1996; Ackermann *et al.*, 1999; Loman *et al.*, 1999). In one study with HT-29 cells, vitamin A was found to be required for pIgR regulation by IFN-γ and IL-4, suggesting that retinoic acid signaling pathways may enhance the cytokine signaling pathways. Recent studies have shed light on the signaling pathways and transcription factors that mediate the regulation of *PIGR* gene transcription by IFN-γ, TNF, and IL-4 (see subsequent section, Transcriptional Regulation).

Several studies have demonstrated a role for endogenous proinflammatory cytokines in pIgR regulation. Supernatants from human intestinal lamina propria mononuclear cells, activated *in vitro* with phorbol ester and calcium ionophore, induced expression of pIgR in HT-29 cells to levels far exceeding those achieved with recombinant cytokines (Youngman *et al.*, 1994). Antibody-mediated neutralization of cytokines in the culture supernatants suggested roles for both IFN-γ and TNF, with IFN-γ acting as the central regulator. By contrast, no effect of endogenous IL-4 was demonstrated. In another study, supernatants from human neutrophils activated with IL-8 and formylmethionylleucylphenylalanine were shown to upregulate pIgR expression in CaLu-3 cells (Pilette *et al.*, 2003). The increase in pIgR expression was correlated with phosphorylation of IκB-α and p38 MAPK, hallmarks of signaling by proinflammatory cytokines. In an *in vivo* study with autoimmune prone (NZB × NZW)F$_1$ mice, calorie restriction was found to decrease expression of IFN-γ, IL-10, and IL-12 as well as pIgR in submandibular salivary glands (Muthukumar *et al.*, 2000). In humans, increased production of IFN-γ (and to a lesser extent TNF) by intraepithelial and lamina propria lymphocytes was shown to correlate with increased expression of pIgR by gastric epithelial cells in *Helicobacter pylori* infection (Ahlstedt *et al.*, 1999). No correlation was seen between IL-4 levels and pIgR expression.

Expression of pIgR is also regulated by hormones, in a cell-type-specific manner. In human uterus, pIgR levels vary significantly during the menstrual cycle, with the highest expression seen during the luteal phase (Sullivan *et al.*, 1984b; Bjercke and Brandtzaeg, 1993). In rat uterine and vaginal tissues and in uterine secretions, pIgR and SC levels were found to be highest at proestrus, intermediate at estrus, and lowest during diestrus (Sullivan and Wira, 1983; Parr and Parr, 1989a; Kaushic *et al.*, 1995). However, SC and S-IgA levels in vaginal secretions were maximal at estrus and reduced at all other stages of the cycle (Sullivan and Wira, 1983), perhaps reflecting differences in the rate of secretion or stability of SC.

Estradiol has been shown to upregulate pIgR expression in human endometrium and endometrial cell lines (Menge and Mestecky, 1993), and in rat uterus pIgR expression is elevated by estrogen and antagonized by progesterone (Sullivan *et al.*, 1983; Wira *et al.*, 1984; Stern and Wira, 1988; Wira *et al.*, 1991; Richardson *et al.*, 1993; Kaushic *et al.*, 1995). By contrast, pIgR expression in rabbit mammary gland is upregulated by prolactin and antagonized by estrogen and progesterone (Rosato *et al.*, 1995). In the male reproductive tract, including the prostate and seminal vesicles, pIgR expression is upregulated by androgens (Stern *et al.*, 1992). An interesting finding is that androgens also upregulate pIgR expression in the lacrimal gland of male rats, where SC output in tears is significantly higher than in female rats (Sullivan *et al.*, 1984a; Vanaken *et al.*, 1998). The discovery of androgen-responsive elements in the human *PIGR* gene has shed light on the mechanisms of hormone-dependent regulation of pIgR expression (see subsequent section, Transcriptional Regulation).

Glucocorticoids have been reported to upregulate pIgR expression *in vivo* in rat serum, saliva, and bile (Wira and Rossoll, 1991) and *ex vivo* in primary cultures of rat hepatocytes (Wira and Colby, 1985). By contrast, glucocorticoids were found to downregulate pIgR mRNA levels in organ cultures of rabbit mammary gland. Little is known about glucocorticoid regulation of pIgR expression in humans, although no effect was seen on SC levels in tracheal aspirates of human infants treated with dexamethasone (Watts and Bruce, 1995). Species-specific regulation of pIgR expression by glucocorticoids may be related to the presence or absence of glucocorticoid-responsive DNA elements that regulate *PIGR* gene transcription (see subsequent section, Transcriptional Regulation).

Regulation of pIgR expression by microbial products

In addition to being regulated by host-derived factors, pIgR expression can be modulated directly by microbes and their metabolic products. Butyrate, a bacterial fermentation product and important energy source in the colon, has been reported to upregulate pIgR expression and to enhance the response to certain cytokines in the human colonic epithelial cell line HT-29 (Kvale and Brandtzaeg, 1995). A role for commensal bacteria in pIgR regulation was suggested by the observation that pIgR expression was increased when germ-free mice were colonized with *Bacteroides thetaiotaomicron*, a prominent organism of the normal mouse and human intestinal microflora (Hooper *et al.*, 2001). Changes in composition of the intestinal microflora may explain the recently reported roles for passive and adaptive immunity in the ontogeny of pIgR expression in mice (Jenkins *et al.*, 2003) (see previous section, Ontogeny of pIgR Expression). Viruses have been shown to upregulate pIgR expression directly in epithelial cells, independent of the production of cytokines by lymphoid and myeloid cells. Infection of primary cultures of rat lacrimal and salivary gland epithelial cells with cytomegalovirus or sialodacryoadenitis induced an acute increase in pIgR production (Huang *et al.*, 1996; Wickham *et al.*, 1997). Infection with reovirus has been shown to upregulate pIgR protein and mRNA levels in the human HT-29 cells (Pal *et al.*, 2003).

A direct role for bacteria and viruses in pIgR regulation suggests that the innate immune system may "prime" epithelial cells for transport of pIg produced during the adaptive immune response. Host cells mediate innate immune responses to microbial components through Toll-like receptor (TLR) signaling (reviewed in Barton and Medzhitov, 2003; Takeda and Akira, 2003). Intestinal epithelial cells have been shown to express a wide variety of TLRs, the expression of which is upregulated during intestinal inflammation (Cario and Podolsky, 2000; Hausmann *et al.*, 2002; Abreu *et al.*, 2003). We have recently discovered that pIgR expression is upregulated in HT-29 cells by bacterial LPS, a ligand for TLR4, and double-stranded RNA, a ligand for TLR3 (Schneeman and Kaetzel, 2003). Upregulation of pIgR levels by LPS may be very significant in light of the recent discovery that pIgR can participate in intracellular neutralization of LPS by epithelial cells (Fernandez *et al.*, 2003) (see previous section, Unique Functions of pIg and pIgR in Mucosal Epithelia). Enhanced uptake and neutralization of LPS by pIgR-pIgA may be an important mechanism by which intestinal inflammation is controlled in the presence of commensal bacteria. Similarly, upregulation of pIgR expression by double-stranded RNA may enhance antiviral immunity, given the important role of pIgR-pIgA in intracellular neutralization of viruses, including rotavirus, which has a double-stranded RNA genome (see previous section, Unique Functions of pIg and pIgR in Mucosal Epithelia). The closely related reovirus, which also has a double-stranded RNA genome, has been shown to upregulate pIgR expression in HT-29 cells (Pal *et al.*, 2003). Significantly, ultraviolet light–inactivated reovirus induced a stronger increase in pIgR expression than did live virus, suggesting that viral components but not viral replication is required for induction of pIgR production. It is possible that viruses with single-stranded RNA or double-stranded DNA genomes may transiently produce double-stranded RNA species at sufficient levels to upregulate pIgR through the TLR3 pathway. Alternatively, these viruses may utilize other innate immune pathways to upregulate pIgR levels in epithelial cells. Signaling through various TLRs could also enhance pIgR expression by other classes of microorganisms, perhaps explaining the observation that pIgR expression was enhanced in the small intestine of rats treated with *Saccharomyces boulardii* (Buts *et al.*, 1990). Increased expression of pIgR in response to a variety of probiotic organisms could contribute to increased secretion of anti-inflammatory S-IgA in the intestine, thus providing broad-spectrum protection against enteral pathogen infection and enteritis.

Dysregulation of pIgR expression in disease states

It has generally been observed that pIgR is upregulated in disease states characterized by widespread tissue inflammation, including gastritis (Chen and Tobe, 1974; Isaacson, 1982a; Valnes *et al.*, 1984), celiac disease (Baklien *et al.*, 1977; Scott *et al.*, 1981), dermatitis herpetiformis (Scott *et al.*, 1981), ankylosing spondylitis (Feltelius *et al.*, 1994), strongyloidiasis (Coutinho *et al.*, 1996a), pancreatitis (Hayakawa *et al.*, 1993), Sjögren's syndrome (Thrane *et al.*, 1992; El Kaissouni *et al.*, 1996), obstructive sialadenitis (Brandtzaeg *et al.*, 1992), tonsillitis (Brandtzaeg, 1988), nephritis (Dobrin *et al.*, 1975; Svanborg Edén *et al.*, 1985; Greenwell *et al.*, 1995), urinary tract infection (Uehling and Steihm, 1971), and bronchopneumonia (Thrane *et al.*, 1994), as well as in victims of sudden infant death syndrome (Thrane *et al.*, 1994). Upregulation of pIgR expression in these diverse conditions can most likely be explained by stimulatory effects of local cytokines (see previous section, Regulation by Cytokines and Hormones). By contrast, reduced pIgR expression in atopic dermatitis, perhaps secondary to an imbalance of Th2 versus Th1 cytokine production, has been reported (Imayama *et al.*, 1994). Levels of SC

and S-IgA in external secretions are also reduced in Behçet's disease, leading to the suggestion that dysregulation of the secretory immune system is involved in the etiology of this chronic inflammatory disease (Abdou *et al.*, 1978; Hamza *et al.*, 1991; Hamza and Makni, 1995).

In untreated celiac disease, enhanced pIg transport associated with upregulation of pIgR expression probably explains why the serum levels of pIgA and IgM generally are only marginally increased, despite the markedly expanded jejunal IgA- and IgM-producing cell populations (Brandtzaeg, 1991). However, the transport capacity of pIgR may be insufficient in certain patients, with unusual proliferation of intestinal IgA immunocytes, resulting in excessive levels of pIgA in serum (Colombel *et al.*, 1988).

Reduced pIgR expression has been noted in regenerating and dysplastic colonic epithelium in inflammatory bowel disease (Rognum *et al.*, 1987); the investigators suggested that butyrate deficiency, secondary to inflammatory bowel disease, could influence pIgR expression along with other aspects of mucosal immune responses. Other dietary deficiencies also have been shown to impact pIgR expression and transport of pIgA. In rats and mice, severe protein malnutrition has been shown to result in reduced pIgR expression in various epithelia and decreased S-IgA levels in tears, saliva, bile, and intestinal secretions (Sullivan *et al.*, 1993; Ha and Woodward, 1997). By contrast, experimental vitamin A deficiency was reported to cause significant increases in total salivary pIgR and S-IgA secretion, although the IgA response to specific infectious agents was depressed (Gangopadhyay *et al.*, 1996). In the HT-29 human colon carcinoma cell-line, vitamin A was shown to be required for upregulation of pIgR expression by IL-4 and IFN-γ (Sarkar *et al.*, 1998).

Expression of pIgR has been widely studied as a potential prognostic variable for colon carcinoma. In eight independent investigations involving a large number of colorectal carcinomas and adenomas, the mode of pIgR expression was found to be correlated with tumor progression (Poger *et al.*, 1976; Rognum *et al.*, 1980, 1982; Isaacson, 1982b; Arends *et al.*, 1984; Wiggers *et al.*, 1988; Koretz *et al.*, 1994; Krajci *et al.*, 1996). In normal intestinal mucosa, pIgR expression was found to be high but to be regulated with respect to both cell type and microtopographical site. By contrast, pIgR expression in most intestinal adenomas was found to be somewhat reduced but homogeneous in pattern, perhaps reflecting a loss of regulatory potential. Finally, pIgR expression was found to be markedly lower and quite heterogeneous in colorectal adenocarcinoma, and tumor-related death was more frequent when primary tumors exhibited an absence or low levels of pIgR. To study the possible mechanism of loss of pIgR expression during progression of colon cancer, Krajci *et al.* (1996) measured pIgR mRNA and protein expression in 33 colorectal adenomas and 19 colorectal carcinomas. In the adenomas, pIgR mRNA levels were positively correlated with pIgR protein levels, and both were negatively related to histological grade. By contrast, the correlation between pIgR mRNA and protein tended to break down in the carcinomas, with frequent instances of positive pIgR mRNA but loss of pIgR protein expression. These investigators concluded that reduced pIgR expression in colorectal adenomas may be a transcriptional defect reflecting the degree of cellular dysplasia, whereas reduced or absent pIgR expression in colorectal adenomas may reflect a combination of transcriptional and post-transcriptional defects, with occasional diallelic gene deletions. We have recently described a cell culture model of colonic adenoma to carcinoma progression, where loss of pIgR expression occurs in late-stage adenomas at the time of acquisition of a tumorigenic phenotype (Traicoff et al., 2003). Elucidation of mechanisms of transcriptional and post-transcriptional regulation of the *PIGR* gene (see subsequent sections, Transcriptional Regulation and Expression and Processing of pIgR RNA) may shed light on the dysregulation of pIgR expression in colorectal cancer.

Reduced expression of pIgR has been associated with airflow obstruction in chronic obstructive pulmonary disease (Pilette et al., 2001) and with cellular dysplasia in lung cancer (Harris and South, 1981; Brooks and Ernst, 1984; Espinoza et al., 1984; Loosli and Hurlimann, 1984; Kodama et al., 1985; Kondi-Paphitis and Addis, 1986; Popper et al., 1987; Kawai et al., 1988; Ordonez, 1989; Ishida et al., 1990a,b; Hirata et al., 1990; Brown et al., 1993). Small cell and squamous cell carcinomas were consistently negative for pIgR, whereas expression of pIgR in other histologic lung tumor types was positively correlated with degree of differentiation and/or cell of origin. We have recently demonstrated that decreased pIgR expression in non–small cell lung cancer is correlated with decreased expression of the upstream stimulatory factor family of transcription factors (Khattar and Kaetzel, unpublished data), which have been shown to be required for basal transcription of the *PIGR* gene (see subsequent section, Transcriptional Regulation).

Two recent studies have identified a number of single-nucleotide polymorphisms (SNPs) in the human *PIGR* gene that are associated with increased risk of nasopharyngeal cancer (Hirunsatit et al., 2003) and IgA nephropathy (Obara et al., 2003). Significantly, both of these groups identified the same SNP, a C-to-T transition at codon 580 that causes an amino acid substitution of alanine to valine. This amino acid is found in the sixth extracellular domain of pIgR (Fig. 12.3), leading to the suggestion that the valine polymorphism may render pIgR less susceptible to proteolytic cleavage and release from the apical cell surface (see previous section, Conserved Structural Features). In nasopharyngeal cancer, increased uptake of Epstein-Barr virus and loss of cell polarity may result from accumulation of pIgR on the cell surface. In IgA nephropathy, dysfunction of the transport pathway for excretion of IgA immune complexes may lead to elevated levels of immune complexes in the systemic circulation and accumulation in renal glomeruli. The association of this polymorphism with two disparate disease states highlights the fundamental homeostatic role of pIgR-mediated transcytosis of polymeric IgA.

ORGANIZATION AND REGULATION OF THE *PIGR* GENE

Chromosomal localization and exon-intron structure of the *PIGR* gene

It has been demonstrated that pIgR is encoded by a single copy gene in the human, bovine, rat, and mouse (Davidson et al., 1988; Krajci et al., 1991; Kulseth et al., 1994; Koch et al., 1995; Kushiro and Sato, 1997; Martín et al., 1997). In situ hybridization on metaphase chromosomes and discordancy analysis of interspecies somatic hybrids have assigned the human pIgR gene (locus *PIGR*) to region q31–q41 on chromosome 1 (Davidson et al., 1988; Krajci et al., 1991), the bovine *PIGR* gene to region q13 on chromosome 16 (Kulseth et al., 1994), and the mouse *Pigr* gene to the long arm of chromosome 1 (Kushiro and Sato, 1997; Sato, 1998). Genetic linkage was demonstrated between the human *PIGR* gene and the polymorphic DNA marker pYNZ23 (locus D1S58), which is linked to other markers residing in 1q32 (Krajci et al., 1992a). This suggested a close relation of *PIGR* to loci encoding three complement regulatory factors, decay accelerating factor, and the complement receptors CR1 and CR2. The mapping of chromosome 1 in the human genome project (National Center for Biotechnology Information, USA) led to the precise localization of the *PIGR* gene on band 1q32.1 within a cluster of immunologically relevant genes (**Fig. 12.4A**). Significantly, the *PIGR* gene is immediately flanked by the gene encoding the Fcα/μ receptor, which contains a highly homologous immunoglobulin-binding site (Fig. 12.3; see previous section, Binding of pIg to pIgR). The chromosomal localization of the mouse *Pigr* gene is very similar to that of its human counterpart, including linkage to the Fcα/μR gene (National Center for Biotechnology Information, Mouse Genome Project).

The human *PIGR* gene comprises 11 exons and 10 introns spanning 17,944 base pairs (Krajci et al., 1992b; Piskurich et al., 1997; Verbeet et al., 1995b; Traicoff et al., 2003) (see Chapter 10). Exons 1 and 2 encode the large 5′-untranslated region (UTR) of pIgR mRNA (see subsequent section, Expression and Processing of pIgR mRNA). The initiator AUG codon and most of the leader peptide are also encoded by exon 2, whereas the N-terminal amino acid of mature, transmembrane pIgR is encoded within exon 3. Extracellular domains 1, 4, and 5 are encoded by exons 3, 5, and 6, respectively. Domains 2 and 3 are encoded by exon 4, which is sometimes deleted by alternate splicing of rabbit pIgR mRNA (see subsequent section, Expression and Processing of pIgR mRNA). Therefore, with the exception of exon 4, the portion of the *PIGR* gene encoding the extracellular Ig-like domains is organized according to the "one domain/one exon" rule characteristic of the Ig superfamily (Williams and Barclay, 1988). Exons 7–11 encode domain 6, the transmembrane region and the cytoplasmic tail. The complete sequence of exon 11 has recently been determined, revealing the presence of an unusually long 3′-UTR (Traicoff et al., 2003) (see subsequent section, Expression and Processing of pIgR mRNA).

A

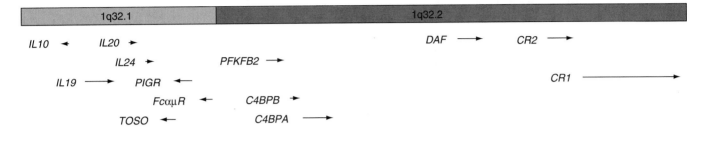

B

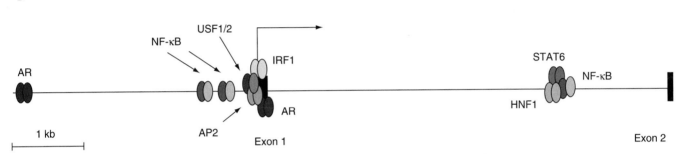

Fig. 12.4. Chromosomal localization of the human *PIGR* gene and binding sites for transcription factors. **(See page 3 of the color plates.)** **A,** Localization of the *PIGR* gene in band q32.1 of chromosome 1, in a cluster of immunologically relevant genes (National Center for Biotechnology Information, USA). Other genes in this region include interleukin (*IL*) *10, 19, 20,* and *24*; regulator of Fas-induced apoptosis (*TOSO*); Fcαμ receptor (*Fcαμr*); 6-phosphofructo-2-kinase/fructose-2,6-bisphosphatase 2 (*PFKFB2*); complement component 4 binding proteins (*C4BP*) *A* and *B*; decay-accelerating factor (*DAF*), and complement receptors (*CR*) *1* and *2*. Arrows indicate relative size and direction of transcription of individual genes. **B,** Binding sites for regulatory transcription factors in the 5'-flanking, promoter, exon 1, and intron 1 regions of the human *PIGR* gene. Abbreviations: AR, androgen receptor; NF-κB, nuclear factor κB; USF, upstream stimulatory factor; AP, activator protein; IRF, interferon regulatory factor; HNF, hepatocyte nuclear factor; STAT, signal transducer and activator of transcription.

Analyses of genomic databases have recently identified 21 SNPs within and flanking the human *PIGR* gene (Hirunsatit *et al.*, 2003; Obara *et al.*, 2003; Traicoff *et al.*, 2003). Three of these SNPs are located within exons, one of which results in an amino acid change from alanine to valine at amino acid 563 in domain 6 (Fig. 12.3; see previous section, Conserved Structural Features). The frequency of alanine at this position was found to be about 75% in one study of normal Chinese and Thai populations (Hirunsatit *et al.*, 2003) and 85% in another study of normal Japanese (Obara *et al.*, 2003). Significantly, homozygosity for valine at this position was associated with increased risk for nasopharyngeal cancer and IgA nephropathy (see previous section, Dysregulation of pIgR Expression in Disease States).

Transcriptional regulation of the *PIGR* gene
Analysis of the human and rodent *PIGR* genes has led to the identification of a number of transcriptional regulatory elements in the 5'-flanking region, exon 1 and intron 1

(Fig. 12.4B). A single start site for transcription of pIgR mRNA was detected with use of RNA from normal human intestine (Piskurich *et al.*, 1997; Johansen *et al.*, 1998) and benign prostate hypertrophy (Verrijdt *et al.*, 1997) (see bent arrow in Fig. 12.4B). The sequences of the human, rat, and mouse *PIGR* genes are significantly homologous in the region spanning 206 base pairs (bp) upstream of the transcription start site and the end of exon 1 (Martín *et al.*, 1997; Fodor *et al.*, 1997; Hempen *et al.*, 2002). The region 5' to position –206 is completely different for the rodent *Pigr* genes, suggesting an evolutionary divergence with possible regulatory significance.

The human, rat, and mouse *PIGR* promoters have the identical sequence "TTTAA" approximately 30 bp upstream of the transcription start site. Whereas the consensus sequence for the TATA box, a regulatory motif that helps to define the position of initiation of mRNA position (Sharp, 1992), is "TATAA," a statistical analysis of promoter elements from eukaryotic genes found the nucleotide

"T" in the second position of the TATA box in 10% of the genes surveyed (Bucher, 1990). It is therefore likely that the "TTTAA" elements in the promoter of the human, rat, and mouse *PIGR* genes interact with ubiquitous TATA-binding proteins to regulate initiation of transcription of pIgR mRNA. The region between approximately 100 bp upstream and 30 bp downstream of the transcription start site has been found to be sufficient for basal transcription of the human *PIGR* (Piskurich et al., 1997; Verrijdt et al., 1997; Johansen et al., 1998) rat *Pigr* (Fodor et al., 1997), and mouse *Pigr* (Martín et al., 1998a) genes linked to heterologous reporter genes. Mutational analyses have demonstrated that an "E-Box" motif at position −71 of the human *PIGR* gene and −74 of the mouse *Pigr* gene is essential for basal promoter activity (Martín et al., 1998b; Johansen et al., 1998; Hempen et al., 2002; Solorzano-Vargas et al., 2002). E-Box motifs with the sequence "$CAC^G/_ATG$" bind to transcription factors of the basic helix-loop-helix/leucine zipper family, including the Myc, upstream stimulatory factor (USF), and TFE subfamilies (Beckmann et al., 1990; Fisher et al., 1991; Meier et al., 1994; Sirito et al., 1998; Kiermaier et al., 1999; Lüscher and Larsson, 1999). We have recently demonstrated that USF-1 and -2 but not c-Myc binds to the *PIGR* E-Box *in vitro* and *in vivo* and enhances promoter activity (Bruno et al., 2004) (Fig. 12.4B). We also found that activator protein-2 (AP2) binds to a site adjacent to the USF site and may regulate *PIGR* promoter activity (Hempen et al., 2002) (Fig. 12.4B).

Investigations into the molecular mechanisms of pIgR regulation in HT-29 human intestinal epithelial cells demonstrated that Fcα/μ and TNF upregulate pIgR mRNA levels by a mechanism involving *de novo* protein synthesis (Piskurich et al., 1993; Piskurich et al., 1997; Krajci et al., 1993; Kaetzel et al., 1997). These observations suggest that Fcα/μ and TNF may induce synthesis of one or more factors that enhance transcription of the *PIGR* gene. Analyses of regulatory regions within and flanking the human *PIGR* gene have identified several transcription factor binding sites that mediate transcriptional responses to proinflammatory cytokines. An element in exon 1 binds members of the interferon regulatory factor (IRF) family of cytokine-inducible transcription factors (Piskurich et al., 1997; Haelens et al., 1999) (Fig. 12.4B). The sequence of this IRF1 binding site is perfectly conserved in the mouse and rat *Pigr* genes (Blanch et al., 1999). Treatment of HT-29 cells with IFN-γ or TNF leads to the appearance of activated Signal Transducer and Activator of Transcription (STAT)1 in the nucleus and increased transcription of the IRF1 gene (Piskurich et al., 1997; Kaetzel et al., 1997b; Blanch et al., 1999). Inhibitors of tyrosine phosphorylation (which would inhibit activation of STAT1) potently inhibit the ability of IFN-γ to increase cellular pIgR levels in HT-29 cells (Denning, 1996). Treatment of primary cultures of sheep mammary gland epithelial cells has been shown to activate STAT1 and STAT5 and to induce coordinate expression of

IRF1 and pIgR mRNA (Rincheval-Arnold et al., 2002a). An *in vivo* role for IRF1 was demonstrated by the observation that mice with two disrupted *Irf1* alleles had significantly lower expression of pIgR mRNA in liver and intestine than did wild-type mice (Blanch et al., 1999).

Binding of TNF and IL-1 to cell surface receptors initiates a signal transduction pathway leading to the activation and nuclear translocation of the transcription factor NF-κB (Hehlgans and Mannel, 2002; Dunne and O'Neill, 2003). Two NF-kB binding sites have been identified in the 5′-flanking region of the human *PIGR* gene (Takenouchi-Ohkubo et al., 2000) (Fig. 12.4B). Mutation of these sites caused a modest decrease in *PIGR* promoter activity in response to TNF. It has recently been demonstrated that a novel NF-κB site in intron 1 cooperates with the IRF-1 site in exon 1 to mediate TNF-induced transcription of the human *PIGR* gene (Schjerven et al., 2001) (Fig. 12.4B). This element is also found in intron 1 of the mouse *Pigr* gene (Kushiro and Sato, 1997). Thus activation of NF-κB by TNF and likely by IL-1) can enhance *PIGR* gene transcription directly (by binding of the NF-κB to cognate response elements) and indirectly (by inducing IRF-1 expression). We have demonstrated that treatment of a number of human epithelial cell lines with IL-1 causes coordinate increases in IRF1 and pIgR mRNA (Blanch et al., 1999; Khattar et al., 2003).

Recent studies have also demonstrated mechanisms by which the Th2 cytokine IL-4 enhances transcription of the human *PIGR* gene. Binding of IL-4 to cell surface receptors was shown to induce activation and nuclear translocation of STAT6, which binds to an IL-4 responsive enhancer region in intron 1 of the *PIGR* gene (Schjerven et al., 2000) (Fig. 12.4B). Inhibitors of tyrosine phosphorylation (which would inhibit activation of STAT6) had previously been shown to block IL-4 induction of pIgR mRNA (Denning, 1996). STAT6 activation also was found to mediate a delayed transcriptional activation of the *PIGR* gene by induction of a *de novo* synthesized protein that cooperates with STAT6 bound to its cognate element in intron 1. This result was consistent with earlier observations that induction of pIgR mRNA by IL-4 can be blocked by inhibitors of protein synthesis (Nilsen et al., 1999; Ackermann et al., 1999). It was subsequently demonstrated that hepatocyte nuclear factor (HNF)-1 and STAT6 cooperate with other as-yet-unidentified transcription factors to enhance *PIGR* gene transcription (Schjerven et al., 2003) (Fig. 12.4B). Both the HNF-1 and STAT6 sites are also found in intron 1 of the mouse *Pigr* gene (Kushiro and Sato, 1997), suggesting that the mechanism of IL-4 regulation may be conserved across species.

Significant advances have also been made in our understanding of transcriptional regulation of the *PIGR* gene by hormones. Androgen-responsive elements have been identified in the 5′-flanking region and exon 1 of the human *PIGR* gene (Verrijdt et al., 1999; Haelens et al., 1999; Verrijdt et al.,

2000; Haelens *et al.*, 2001) (Fig. 12.4B). These elements bound the glucocorticoid receptor as well, albeit more weakly than the androgen receptor. In transient transfection assays, these elements were found to confer higher responsiveness to androgens than to glucocorticoids. A unique glucocorticoid-responsive element has been identified in the 5′-flanking region of the mouse *Pigr* gene, within a region that is not homologous to the human *PIGR* gene (Li *et al.*, 1999).

Expression and processing of pIgR mRNA

Northern blot analysis demonstrated a single pIgR mRNA transcript in human, bovine, sheep, rat, mouse, possum, and wallaby tissues (Krajci *et al.*, 1989; Traicoff *et al.*, 2003; Kulseth *et al.*, 1995; Verbeet *et al.*, 1995a; Rincheval-Arnold *et al.*, 2002b; Banting *et al.*, 1989; Piskurich *et al.*, 1995; Kushiro and Sato, 1997; Adamski and Demmer, 1999; Taylor *et al.*, 2002). By contrast, two prominent pIgR mRNA transcripts were detected in rabbit tissues (about 3.6 and 2.9 kb) (Mostov *et al.*, 1984). In each species, the tissue distribution of pIgR mRNA closely paralleled the tissue distribution of pIgR protein (see previous section, Tissue-Specific Expression of pIgR). This correlation suggests that tissue-specific expression is regulated primarily by the level of pIgR mRNA. Further characterization of the two rabbit pIgR mRNA products and the proteins they encoded revealed that exon 4 (encoding extracellular domains 2 and 3) had been spliced out of the shorter transcript (Deitcher and Mostov, 1986). Analysis of bovine pIgR mRNA by a sensitive RT-PCR technique revealed a rare, shorter mRNA transcript analogous to the rabbit pIgR 2.9-kb mRNA (Kulseth *et al.*, 1995). Although species other than rabbit may occasionally produce the shorter form of pIgR mRNA, it is clear that there is a strong selective pressure to produce the longer form. As discussed above, the selective retention or loss of domains 2 and 3, encoded by exon 4, could impact on the affinity of the pIg-pIgR interaction in species other than rabbit (see previous section, Binding of pIg to pIgR). In this context it is noteworthy that the size of exon 4 of pIgR mRNA (657 nucleotides [nt] in the human) is larger than 99% of vertebrate internal exons (Berget, 1995). The "exon definition" model of mRNA splice site recognition predicts that the size of internal exons must be sufficiently small to allow interactions between splicing structures associated with the 5′ and 3′ ends of each exon (Berget, 1995). The preferential retention of exon 4 of pIgR mRNA in most species may therefore represent a novel mechanism that has evolved in the presence of functional selection. A detailed analysis of exon 4 from the mouse *Pigr* gene revealed the presence of a cryptic RNA splice site corresponding to the boundary of domains 3 and 4 in pIgR protein (Bruce *et al.*, 1999). Multiple exonic and intronic features were found to suppress usage of this cryptic splice site and to promote constitutive inclusion of exon 4 in pIgR mRNA (Bruce and Peterson, 2001).

The unusually long 5′ and 3′ UTRs of pIgR mRNA offer the potential for regulation at the level of mRNA processing, stability, and/or translation. The lengths of the 5′ UTRs of pIgR mRNA are 185, 179, and 181 nt for human, rat, and mouse, respectively (Piskurich *et al.*, 1997; Fodor *et al.*, 1997; Martín *et al.*, 1997) (the complete sequence of the pIgR 5′ UTRs has not been reported for other species). This places the 5′ UTR of pIgR mRNA in the upper 25% in size for typical vertebrate mRNAs, a feature generally associated with regulation of translation efficiency (Kozak, 1987). Although no studies have directly measured efficiency of pIgR mRNA translation, the observation that many colorectal cancers produce pIgR mRNA but not pIgR protein (Krajci *et al.*, 1996) suggests the possibility of dysregulation of pIgR translation (see previous section, Dysregulation of pIgR Expression in Disease States).

The 3′ UTRs of pIgR mRNA are also extremely long, and interspecies homology is quite low except in selected sites such as the cleavage/polyadenylation signal (Koch *et al.*, 1995; Traicoff *et al.*, 2003). The complete 1793-nt sequence of the 3′ UTR of human pIgR mRNA has recently been determined, revealing the presence of two tandem *Alu* repeats, as well as elements that could affect mRNA processing and stability (Traicoff *et al.*, 2003). The 1416-nt 3′ UTR of rat pIgR mRNA is exceptional in that at least six unique sequences have been identified for this region in RNA from rat liver (Koch *et al.*, 1995). All of the pIgR mRNA transcripts contained unusual S1-nuclease sensitive microsatellite elements consisting of multiple tandem d[GGA] and d[GAA] repeats, which are also found in mouse pIgR mRNA (Kushiro and Sato, 1997) but not in any other species yet studied. The microsatellite repeats in the 3′ UTRs of rodent pIgR mRNAs are located in approximately the same position as the *Alu* repeats in human pIgR mRNA, suggesting that this location may represent a genomic "hotspot" for insertion of repetitive elements. Attenuation of gene expression was observed when a 359-bp fragment containing the microsatellite elements from rat pIgR mRNA was inserted into the 3′ UTR of a luciferase reporter gene, suggesting that it may act as a negative regulatory element (Aoki *et al.*, 1997). Biochemical analysis of this negative regulatory region revealed the presence of intramolecular triplexes stabilized by supercoiling, which appeared to inhibit transcription of pIgR mRNA. By contrast, the 1183-nt 3′ UTR of bovine pIgR mRNA (Kulseth *et al.*, 1995; Verbeet *et al.*, 1995a) and the 1068-nt 3′ UTR of rabbit pIgR mRNA do not contain long stretches of repetitive elements, and their regulatory functions have not been investigated. It is interesting to note that the 3′ UTR is considerably shorter in pIgR mRNA from two marsupial species, 480 nt for the common brushtail possum (Adamski and Demmer, 1999) and 485 nt for the tammar wallaby (Taylor *et al.*, 2002). The long pIgR 3′ UTR characteristic of eutherian mammals may therefore represent an evolutionarily recent acquisition of novel mechanisms for regulating the transcription and/or stability of pIgR mRNA.

pIgR TRAFFICKING AND SIGNALS

Experimental systems for analyzing transcytosis of pIgR

pIgR has an unusually complex pathway in the cell, moving first to the basolateral surface and then to the apical surface (Fig. 12.1). Transcytosis of pIgR has, in fact, been an extremely useful model system to elucidate the pathways and mechanisms of polarized membrane traffic in epithelial cells (reviewed in Mostov et al., 2000; O'Brien et al., 2002; Mostov et al., 2003). Epithelial cells form sheets that line cavities or cover an organism externally. A circumferential tight junction divides the plasma membrane of each cell into two domains: the apical plasma membrane faces the lumen of the cavity, whereas the basolateral plasma membrane faces adjoining cells and the underlying basement membrane and connective tissue. These two domains of the plasma membrane differ in their protein and lipid compositions, reflecting the different functions served by the two surfaces in a polarized cell.

Most of our understanding of pIgR trafficking has come from two experimental systems. The first is rat liver, where expression of pIgR by hepatocytes allows transcytosis of pIgA from blood to bile (see subsequent section, Hepatobiliary Transport of IgA). In rat hepatocytes pIgR is directed first to the sinusoidal surface, which is equivalent to the basolateral surface. Transcytosis is to the bile canalicular surface, equivalent to the apical surface, where free SC and S-IgA are released into bile (reviewed in Brown and Kloppel, 1989) (see subsequent section, The Pathway of Transcytosis of pIgR in Rat Hepatocytes). A great advantage of rat liver is that highly purified subcellular fractions can be isolated that are enriched in vesicles involved in the transcytosis of pIgR (Sztul et al., 1991, 1993; Vergés et al., 1999). As a second experimental system, the cloned cDNA for pIgR has been expressed in MDCK cells, which form a tight, well-polarized monolayer when cultured on permeable supports (Mostov and Deitcher, 1986; Tamer et al., 1995). The transfected pIgR behaves in the MDCK cells as it does in vivo and serves as a useful model to study protein trafficking.

Basolateral sorting signal of pIgR

Integral proteins of the plasma membrane are synthesized in the rough endoplasmic reticulum and sent to the Golgi apparatus. As the proteins move through the last compartment of the Golgi, the trans-Golgi network (TGN), they are sorted into vesicles that can deliver them to either the apical or basolateral surface of polarized epithelial cells (Mostov et al., 2000; Nelson and Yeaman, 2001). Although it was originally thought that sorting to the basolateral surface was by default (i.e., did not require a specific sorting signal), studies with pIgR have shown that basolateral sorting requires a sorting signal in the cytoplasmic domain of the membrane

protein (Casanova et al., 1991). pIgR spans the membrane once and contains a carboxyl-terminal, cytoplasmic domain of 103 amino acids. An extensive series of deletions and point mutations have been made in the pIgR cytoplasmic domain, which have uncovered several distinct sorting signals that control trafficking of the pIgR (Figs. 12.2 and 12.3). The 17 amino acids of this cytoplasmic domain that lie closest to the membrane comprise a signal that is necessary and sufficient for targeting from the TGN to the basolateral surface (Fig. 12.3). This 17-residue segment can be transplanted to a heterologous reporter molecule and directs the delivery of this molecule to the basolateral surface (Casanova et al., 1991). Studies on other basolaterally targeted proteins have demonstrated that mutations in their cytoplasmic domains can cause mistargeting to the apical surface, presumably by inactivation of a basolateral signal (reviewed in Mostov et al., 2000). Analysis of the 17-residue basolateral sorting signal of pIgR by alanine scanning mutagenesis suggests that three residues are crucial for basolateral sorting (Aroeti et al., 1993). Individual point mutations of His656, Arg657, or Val660 to Ala largely blocked basolateral targeting. Detailed analysis of this signal suggest that it contains two distinct portions (Reich et al., 1996). Two clathrin adaptor proteins, AP1-B and AP-4, have been implicated in sorting of proteins to the basolateral surface, although it is not known if either of these is specifically involved in trafficking of the pIgR (Folsch et al., 1999; Simmen et al., 2002; Gan et al., 2002).

After reaching the basolateral surface, proteins can be endocytosed and delivered to endosomes. From the endocytic pathway, proteins can be recycled to the basolateral surface, sent to late endosomes and lysosomes for degradation, or transcytosed to the opposite, apical surface. The endocytotic pathway is therefore like the biosynthetic (TGN) pathway, capable of polarized sorting for delivery of proteins to the apical or basolateral surfaces. We found that the 17-residue basolateral sorting signal controls basolateral sorting in both pathways (Aroeti and Mostov, 1994). Ala point mutations that decrease TGN-to-basolateral sorting and correspondingly increase TGN-to-apical sorting have the same effect on sorting that occurs after endocytosis. In other words, these point mutations decrease recycling in the endocytotic pathway back to the basolateral surface and correspondingly increase transcytosis to the apical surface. These data suggest that polarized sorting in both the biosynthetic and endocytotic pathways might occur in the same location and/or use similar molecules. One hypothesis is that molecules are first delivered from the TGN to a compartment of the endosomal system and are then sorted to the basolateral surface (Orzech et al., 2000).

Pathway of pIgR transcytosis

The pathway for transcytosis of pIgR has been analyzed in detail and found to involve at least two and most likely three distinct endosomal compartments (Apodaca et al., 1994; Brown et al., 2000; Wang et al., 2000; Futter et al., 1998; Gibson et al., 1998; Leung et al., 2000; Casanova et al., 1999) (reviewed in Rojas *et al.*, 2002; Mostov *et al.*, 2003) **(Fig. 12.5)**. The pIgR and bound pIgA first undergo clathrin-mediated endocytosis from the basolateral plasma mem-

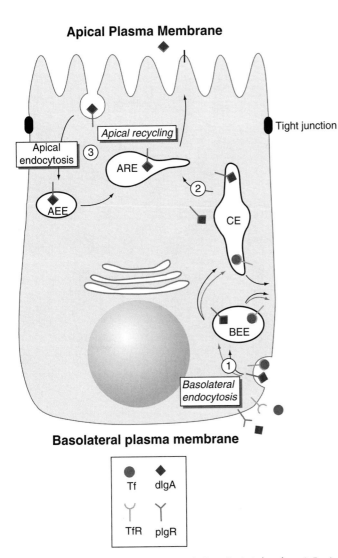

Apical Plasma Membrane

Apical recycling

Apical endocytosis

③

ARE

②

Tight junction

AEE

CE

BEE

①

Basolateral endocytosis

Basolateral plasma membrane

Tf   dIgA

TfR   pIgR

Fig. 12.5. Pathway of transcytosis of dimeric IgA by the pIgR. An epithelial cell is shown, with the basolateral plasma membrane depicted as a blue line and the apical plasma membrane as a red line. Dimeric IgA (dIgA) binds to the pIgR at the basolateral plasma membrane and is endocytosed (step 1). The dIgA and pIgR are delivered to basolateral early endosomes (BEE) and then to common endosomes (CE). Transferrin (Tf) also binds to the transferrin receptor (TfR) at the basolateral surface and is also endocytosed and delivered to BEE and CE. A small portion of the dIgA and pIgR is recycled from BEE and CE to the basolateral surface, while the majority of Tf and TfR is recycled from BEE and CE to the basolateral surface. Much of the pIgR and dIgA are then transferred from CE to apical recycling endosomes (ARE) (step 3). From there, the pIgR and dIgA are exocytosed to the apical plasma membrane. At the apical plasma membrane, the extracellular, ligand-binding portion of pIgR is proteolytically cleaved off to yield SC, which is released together with the dIgA in external secretions. Cleavage of pIgR to SC is not instantaneous; therefore, uncleaved pIgR bound to dIgA can also be endocytosed (step 3) and delivered to apical early endosomes (AEE). This dIgA and pIgR can be recycled via ARE back to the apical plasma membrane.

brane and delivery to basolateral early endosomes (BEE). BEE contain all of the diverse molecules endocytosed from the basolateral surface. Some molecules, including some of the transferrin and its receptor and even probably some pIgR, can be recycled from BEE back to the basolateral surface. Other molecules are sorted from BEE to late endosomes and lysosomes for degradation. Much of the pIgR and pIgA are next sent via a microtubule-dependent process to a predominantly tubular compartment. We refer to this compartment as the common endosome (CE) because it also receives membrane-bound molecules endocytosed from the apical surface. Some transferrin and its receptor reach the CE and are recycled from there to the basolateral surface. The pIgR and pIgA, however, are next transferred to a third compartment, known as the apical recycling endosome (ARE), which is a tubulovesicular compartment clustered just beneath the center of the apical surface. There is some controversy as to whether or not the ARE is truly a distinct compartment from the CE (Sheff *et al.*, 2002). However, the ARE has a significant enrichment of pIgR and pIgA relative to transferrin, in comparison with the CE. Most important, the BEE and CE have a more acidic pH (approximately 5.5), whereas the ARE has a more neutral pH (6.8), which in our opinion is good evidence that the ARE is a distinct compartment. Transport through the endocytotic pathway to the apical surface depends on both microtubules and actin microfilaments and is controlled by small GTPases of the Rho family (reviewed in Apodaca, 2001).

REGULATION OF pIgR TRAFFIC

Virtually all membrane traffic events appear to be tightly regulated (Bomsel and Mostov, 1992; Mostov *et al.*, 2000). Transcytosis of pIgR is regulated at multiple levels and provides an excellent model to study the regulation of membrane traffic (reviewed in Rojas *et al.*, 2002; Mostov *et al.*, 2003. The internalization of pIgR from the basolateral plasma membrane is regulated by phosphorylation (Okamoto *et al.*, 1994). pIgR contains two tyrosine-based internalization signals, which resemble internalization signals found in other rapidly endocytosed receptors (Okamoto *et al.*, 1992) (Fig. 12.3). However, phosphorylation of Ser726, which is distantly located from both of these tyrosine-based signals, is required for rapid endocytosis of pIgR. It is possible that phosphorylation of Ser726 alters the folding of the cytoplasmic domain of pIgR, thereby exposing one of the tyrosine-based internalization signals to the endocytotic machinery.

From both the biosynthetic and endocytotic pathways, the pIgR basolateral sorting signal helps direct pIgR to the basolateral surface. This sorting signal can be thought of as a "basolateral retrieval signal." If this basolateral retrieval signal were permanently active, pIgR might continuously recycle to the basolateral surface and never be transcytosed to the apical surface. However, we have found multiple mechanisms that promote transcytosis. First, Ser664, which is located in the 17-residue basolateral sorting signal, is phosphorylated (Casanova *et al.*, 1990). Mutation of Ser664 to a nonphosphorylatable alanine decreases transcytosis and increases recycling. Mutation to an aspartic acid, whose negative charge may mimic a phosphate, increases transcytosis and also increases TGN-to-apical sorting. The effect of this aspartic acid mutation is very similar to the alanine scanning mutations described above that weaken the basolateral targeting signal. We suggest that the nonphosphorylated pIgR is initially targeted to the basolateral surface. Once reaching that surface (or perhaps after endocytosis), pIgR is phosphorylated on Ser664, thereby weakening the basolateral sorting signal and allowing pIgR to be transcytosed.

A second major control mechanism for transcytosis is binding of the ligand, pIgA (Song *et al.*, 1994) (reviewed in Mostov *et al.*, 2003). Although a significant rate of transcytosis occurs when pIgR is not bound to its ligand, binding of pIgA augments this rate of transcytosis. This stimulation does not depend on phosphorylation of Ser664. The finding that pIgA binding to pIgR stimulates transcytosis suggests that pIgR is capable of transducing a signal across the plasma membrane to the cytoplasmic sorting machinery **(Fig. 12.6)**. A broad outline of this signal transduction pathway is beginning to emerge, although much remains to be learned.

Binding of pIgA to pIgR apparently causes dimerization of the pIgR, although the evidence on this point is somewhat indirect (Singer and Mostov, 1998). Within 10 seconds of pIgA binding, several proteins become tyrosine-phosphorylated (Luton *et al.*, 1998). The pIgR is not itself a tyrosine kinase and is not phosphorylated on tyrosine. Rather, the pIgR somehow recruits p62yes, a nonreceptor tyrosine kinase of the Src family, although p62yes apparently does not bind directly to pIgR (Luton *et al.*, 1999). Mice with deletions in both alleles for p62yes have a small deficiency in basal transport of pIgA from blood to bile and a much greater (40-fold) deficiency in hepatic transport of pIgA when challenged with a large bolus of intravenous pIgA (Luton *et al.*, 1999). The direct downstream substrates of p62yes are not known. However, one of the proteins that becomes phosphorylated is a phosphatidylinositol-specific phospholipase Cγ1 (PLCγ1). This enzyme causes hydrolysis of phosphatidylinositol-4,5-bisphosphate (PIP2) to diacylglyceride and inositol 1,4,5-trisphosphate (IP3). The diacylglyceride in turn leads to activation of protein kinase C (PKC). Activation of PKC by phorbol esters stimulates transcytosis, so it is likely that activation of PKC by pIgA binding to pIgR also stimulates transcytosis (Cardone *et al.*, 1994, 1996). The production of IP3 probably causes the release of Ca^{2+} from intracellular stores and an increase in intracellular free Ca^{2+} ($[Ca^{++}]i$). Artificially increasing $[Ca^{++}]i$ rapidly stimulates transcytosis, so it is likely that the increase in $[Ca^{++}]i$ caused by pIgA binding to pIgR also stimulates transcytosis (Cardone *et al.*, 1996; Luton and Mostov, 1999).

The stimulation of transcytosis by pIgA binding to pIgR has been observed for rabbit pIgR cDNA exogenously expressed in MDCK cells and in rat liver *in vivo* (Giffroy *et al.*, 1998). It is interesting that ligand-mediated stimulation of pIgR transcytosis was not observed in MDCK cells express-

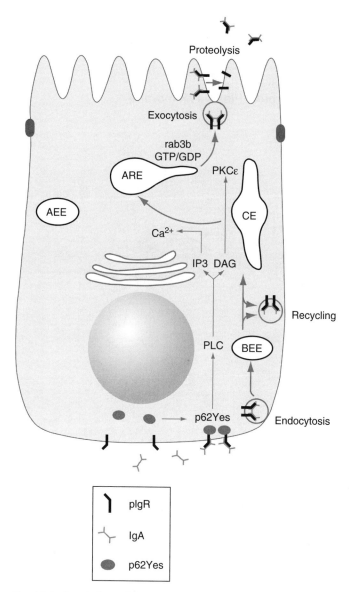

Fig. 12.6. Regulation of transcytosis of pIgR by binding of dIgA. When dIgA binds to the pIgR, the pIgR apparently dimerizes and recruits the nonreceptor tyrosine kinase p62Yes. The p62yes activates a phospholipase C-g1 (PLC). The PLC hydrolyzes phosphatidylinositol 4,5-bisphosphate, which leads to the production of inositol 1,4,5 trisphosphate (IP3) and diacylglyceride (DAG). The IP3 leads to an increase of intracellular free calcium, which promotes transcytosis. The DAG activates protein kinase Ce, which also promotes transcytosis. The pIgR also associates with the small GTPase rab3b in the ARE. Binding of dIgA to the pIgR promotes transcytosis of the pIgR.

ing human pIgR (Natvig *et al.*, 1997; Giffroy *et al.*, 2001) (reviewed in Brandtzaeg and Johansen, 2001). Binding of pIgA to the exogenously expressed human pIgR was found to cause production of the IP3 signal; however, human pIgR appeared to be unable to respond to this signal (Giffroy *et al.*, 2001). One possible explanation for this species difference in ligand-stimulated transcytosis is that rodent and rabbit pIgR, but not human pIgR, is expressed at high levels in hepatocytes (see subsequent section, Species Differences in

Hepatobiliary Transport of IgA). We can speculate that blood to bile transport of pIgA in rodents and rabbits may require the ability to cope with large changes in the amount of pIgA presented to the basolateral surface of the hepatocyte, which is mediated by the ability of pIgR transcytosis to be regulated by pIgA binding. This may play a poorly understood role in immune protection in rodents. In contrast, transport of pIgA by nonhepatic tissues in humans may not require this type of regulation, perhaps because the level of pIgA presented to the basolateral surface may not vary as rapidly or dramatically. In any case, the regulation of pIgR traffic by pIgA binding has proven to be an excellent model system for regulation of membrane traffic in polarized epithelial cells and how signaling information can move across such cells.

Transcytosis of pIgR and pIgA is also regulated by small GTPases of the rab family. Rab proteins regulate every step of membrane traffic and appear to act in a number of ways (reviewed in Pfeffer, 2001). A surprising finding is that the pIgR interacts directly with rab3b, illustrating a novel way in which rab proteins can regulate traffic (Van Ijzendoorn et al., 2002). Rab3b apparently interacts with pIgR when the rab3b is in the GTP-bound form. In this situation, the rab3b prevents the transcytosis of pIgR and instead directs the pIgR to recycle. When pIgA binds to the pIgR, the rab3b hydrolyzes its GTP and dissociates from the pIgR, and the complex of pIgR and pIgA is transcytosed to the apical surface. We had previously found that stimulation of transcytosis by pIgA binding required that the pIgR be sensitized by binding of pIgA at the basolateral surface (Luton and Mostov, 1999). It now appears that this sensitization corresponds to the binding of rab3b to the pIgR (Van Ijzendoorn et al., 2002).

Finally, pIgR transcytosis has been shown to be regulated by extracellular signals other than pIgA. For example, binding of bradykinin or cholinergic drugs to their receptors stimulates transcytosis, possibly by activation of PKC and increasing $[Ca^{++}]I$ (Kelleher et al., 1991). Activation of the heterotrimeric Gs protein also stimulates transcytosis, as well as delivery from the TGN to the apical surface (Bomsel and Mostov, 1993). Part of this stimulation is apparently due to activation of adenylate cyclase by Gs.

HEPATOBILIARY TRANSPORT OF IgA

Species differences in hepatobiliary transport of IgA

In humans, pIgR does not appear to be expressed at significant levels on hepatocytes, and S-IgA in hepatic bile is a relatively minor constituent of the total IgA output in intestinal secretions (see previous section, Tissue-Specific Expression of pIgR). It has been estimated that 50% of the pIgA in human bile is serum derived, whereas the remaining 50% is derived from transport of locally synthesized pIgA across bile duct and gall bladder epithelium (Nagura et al., 1981; Delacroix et al., 1982b; Dooley et al., 1982; Nagura et al., 1983; Brandtzaeg, 1985). Although pIgR-mediated hepatobiliary transport of pIgA is a minor pathway in humans, other pathways appear to exist for hepatic clearance of IgA

and IgA-containing immune complexes (see subsequent section, Hepatic Uptake and Clearance of IgA and IgA Immune Complexes).

By contrast, S-IgA and free SC were found to be two of the three most abundant proteins of rat bile, exceeded only by albumin (Lemaitre-Coelho et al., 1977; Mullock et al., 1978; Acosta-Altamirano et al., 1980). Studies of the clearance of intravenously administered IgA in rats demonstrated rapid transport of pIgA from blood to bile (Jackson et al., 1978; Mullock et al., 1978; Orlans et al., 1978, 1979; Fisher et al., 1979; Lemaitre-Coelho et al., 1981). A similar pathway was observed during perfusion of normal rat liver, where pIgA was transported into bile across a strong concentration gradient (Jackson et al., 1978; Chintalacharuvu et al., 1994). Evidence of the role of pIgR in hepatobiliary transport of pIgA in rats came from the observation that purified rabbit IgG anti-rat SC was efficiently transported into bile and that this transport could be completed with excess free SC or pIgA (Lemaitre-Coelho et al., 1981; Limet et al., 1983). It was subsequently demonstrated that circulating pIgA stimulates pIgR transcytosis in rat liver in vivo (Giffroy et al., 1998). Although most of the pIgA transported into rat bile appears to be derived from serum, secretion of antigen-specific S-IgA in bile during perfusion of livers from immunized animals demonstrated that migratory antibody-forming cells within the liver can also contribute to biliary S-IgA (Jackson et al., 1992).

In the studies of rat liver described above, hepatobiliary transport of IgA was selective for pIgA, which was transported into bile much more rapidly and efficiently than monomeric IgA, S-IgA, IgG, IgE, or even IgM. The lack of transport of IgM was later explained by the demonstration that rat but not human pIgR binds poorly to rodent IgM (Underdown et al., 1992) (see previous section, Binding of pIg to pIgR). The investigators suggested that the apparent discrepancy between the IgM binding capacity of human vs. rat pIgR could be explained on an evolutionary basis by the fact that rats but not humans express pIgR on hepatocytes. In rats, binding of IgM to pIgR on hepatic parenchymal cells could compromise the immune function of IgM by removing it from the systemic circulation, whereas hepatic clearance of IgM would not be an issue for humans and other species that do not express pIgR on hepatocytes.

A similar although less efficient pIgR-mediated pathway for selective hepatobiliary transport of pIgA has been demonstrated in mice, rabbits, chickens, and hamsters (Jackson et al., 1977; Delacroix et al., 1982a; Orlans et al., 1983; Phillips et al., 1984; Delacroix et al., 1984; Peppard et al., 1986; Vaerman and Langendries, 1997) but not in guinea pigs, sheep, dogs, or nonhuman primates (Orlans et al., 1983; Delacroix et al., 1984; Moldoveanu et al., 1990). Evidence that pIgR is the rate-limiting factor in pIgA transport came from cross-species comparisons, where hepatobiliary transport of pIgA correlated with the level of expression of pIgR by hepatocytes (Delacroix et al., 1984). The phenotype of mice with disruptions in genes for either pIgR or J chain (elevated serum IgA and markedly reduced IgA in bile) demonstrated that pIgR-mediated transcytosis is the only significant pathway for hepatobiliary transport of IgA in mice (Johansen *et al.*, 1999; Shimada *et al.*, 1999; Hendrickson *et al.*, 1995, 1996; Lycke *et al.*, 1999).

The pathway of transcytosis of pIgR in rat hepatocytes

Immunohistochemical and ultrastructural studies of rat liver demonstrated that pIgR is expressed abundantly on the sinusoidal surface of hepatocytes, where it would have access to circulating pIgA (Mullock *et al.*, 1979; Renston *et al.*, 1980; Wilson *et al.*, 1980; Takahashi *et al.*, 1982; Hoppe *et al.*, 1985; Limet *et al.*, 1985). Transport of pIgR or pIgR-pIgA complexes was shown to involve a vesicular pathway to the canalicular face (Mullock *et al.*, 1980; Renston *et al.*, 1980; Takahashi *et al.*, 1982; Courtoy *et al.*, 1983; Geuze *et al.*, 1984; Hoppe *et al.*, 1985; Pol *et al.*, 1997), where release into bile is effected by proteolytic cleavage of pIgR (Kloppel and Brown, 1984; Solari *et al.*, 1986). Cleavage of pIgR to SC has been shown to be mediated by a leupeptin-sensitive protease localized to the bile canalicular membrane (Musil and Baenziger, 1987a, 1988; Solari *et al.*, 1989). Following cleavage, the membrane-anchoring domain and cytoplasmic tail of pIgR appear to be partially degraded and ultimately released into bile (Solari *et al.*, 1989).

The pathway of pIgR transcytosis has been been studied on a molecular level both *in vivo* and in cultured rat hepatocytes (Sztul *et al.*, 1983, 1985a,b; Hoppe *et al.*, 1985; Larkin *et al.*, 1986; Solari *et al.*, 1986; Musil and Baenziger, 1987b; Buts *et al.*, 1992). Pulse labeling of rat liver with [^{35}S]-cysteine followed by immunoprecipitation with antibodies to pIgR revealed that newly translated and core glycosylated SC in the endoplasmic reticulum had an M_r of about 105 kDa. Following 15 to 30 minutes of chase with unlabeled cysteine, the 105-kDa form was converted successively to two molecular species of about 115 kDa and 120 kDa, the former representing terminal glycosylation of pIgR in the Golgi complex and the latter representing phosphorylated mature pIgR. It has been reported that endosomal fractions from rat liver are enriched in the phosphorylated form of pIgR, suggesting that phosphorylation may occur after endocytosis of pIgR from the sinusoidal membrane (Enrich *et al.*, 1995). This scenario is consistent with the regulation of pIgR transcytosis in MDCK cells, where phosphorylation of Ser664 on the cytoplasmic tail of pIgR may signal entry into the transcytotic pathway (see previous section, Pathway of pIgR Transcytosis).

The use of rat liver as a model for studying the regulation of pIgR transcytosis provides a complementary approach to studies of MDCK cells (see previous section, IgR Trafficking and Signals), since hepatocytes appear to utilize a unique sorting pathway and may differ in the composition and function of endosomal compartments (van Ijzendoorn and Hoekstra, 1999; Van Ijzendoorn *et al.*, 2000; Tuma *et al.*, 2001, 2002). In hepatocytes, all newly synthesized plasma membrane proteins (including pIgR) are initially targeted to the sinusoidal surface, equivalent to the basolateral surface of columnar epithelial cells (Hubbard *et al.*, 1989). Proteins destined for the bile canalicular membrane (equivalent to the

apical surface of columnar epithelial cells) are internalized from the sinusoidal surface and re-sorted to their final destination. A tubular endosomal compartment, found to be highly enriched in recycling receptors as well as pIgR, appears to be a common destination before segregation of enodocytosed proteins into distinct recycling and transcytotic pathways (Verges *et al.*, 1999). Because the sorting pathway for most apically targeted proteins involves a "detour" to the basolateral surface of hepatocytes, it is not clear whether the basolateral targeting signal of pIgR is utilized in the same way as in MDCK cells (see previous section, Basolateral Sorting Signal of pIgR). Although rat liver does not lend itself as well as MDCK cells to a mutational approach for studying pIgR targeting, the availability of large amounts of tissue has facilitated the isolation of intracellular vesicular carriers involved in targeting and transcytosis of pIgR. Sztul *et al.* (1991) first described the isolation of "transcytotic vesicles" by a combination of sucrose density gradient centrifugation and immunoisolation with antibodies to the cytoplasmic domain of pIgR. These vesicles were enriched in the mature 120-kDa form of pIgR as well as pIgA and were depleted in elements of the secretory pathway, Golgi, sinusoidal plasma membrane, and early endosomal components; thus they appeared to represent a unique compartment specialized for transcytosis to the bile canaliculus. This conclusion was supported by the observation that transcytotic vesicles containing mature, phosphorylated SC and pIgA accumulated in the pericanalicular cytoplasm of rat hepatocytes following bile duct ligation (Larkin and Palade, 1991; Barr and Hubbard, 1993). A similar immunoisolation approach has subsequently been used to identify at least three classes of carrier vesicles involved in various stages of pIgR targeting and transcytosis in rat hepatocytes (Saucan and Palade, 1994; Barr *et al.*, 1995).

Two classes of proteins have been shown to participate in vesicular transport of pIgR in rat liver: p22, a novel Ca2^{++}-binding protein (Barroso *et al.*, 1996); and several members of the Rab family of small GTP-binding proteins (Jin *et al.*, 1996). It is important to note that these cytosolic proteins participate in multiple vesicular fusion events and do not appear to interact directly with the cytoplasmic domain of pIgR. By contrast, the Rab3D isoform has recently been shown to colocalize with the transcytosed form of pIgR but not the precursor form associated with the secretory pathway and other Golgi markers (Larkin *et al.*, 2000). Bile duct ligation caused rab3D to accumulate in the pericanalicular cytoplasm of hepatocytes, suggesting that it may play a role in the regulation of apically directed transcytosis. Other studies have implicated the cytoplasmic protein cellubrevin in regulating the apical transcytosis pathway in rat liver (Calvo *et al.*, 2000). The investigators reported that pIgR coimmunoprecipitated with cellubrevin and that pIgA loading caused cellubrevin to redistribute into endosomal fractions enriched in transcytotic structures. Finally, it has been demonstrated that pIgR is a major calmodulin-binding protein in rat liver endosomes (Chapin *et al.*, 1996; Enrich *et al.*, 1996). Because calmodulin has been shown to bind to the cytoplasmic domain of pIgR and to regulate its transcytosis in MDCK cells (see previous section, Regulation of pIgR Traffic), it is likely to carry out a similar function in rat hepatocytes.

Hepatic uptake and clearance of IgA and IgA immune complexes

Although hepatobiliary transport of pIgA appears to correlate best with pIgR expression on hepatocytes, other cell surface receptors may also participate in the uptake of IgA by the liver parenchyma. For example, purified asialoglycoprotein receptor (ASGP-R) from rat liver was shown to bind IgA (predominantly monomeric) from normal human serum (Stockert et al., 1982). In mice, uptake of mIgA by hepatic ASGP-R was shown to account for more catabolism of mIgA than all other tissues combined (Mestecky et al., 1989). Several lines of evidence suggest that the ASGP-R recognition sites on IgA are the O-linked oligosaccharides in the hinge region of the IgA1 subclass. Human monomeric IgA1 and S-IgA (which cannot bind pIgR) were as effective as pIgA in binding to ASGP-R (Tomana et al., 1985). Furthermore, binding of asialoorosomucoid by rat or mouse liver in vivo (Schiff et al., 1984) or by plasma membrane-enriched fractions from rat, monkey, and human liver (Daniels et al., 1989) was inhibited by human IgA1 but not by rat IgA, which lacks O-linked oligosaccharides. Hepatic uptake by the ASGP-R generally results in delivery of the ligand to lysosomes for degradation. However, Schiff et al. (1986) demonstrated in rat liver that human IgA endocytosed via ASGP-R could dissociate within endosomes and become associated with pIgR and thus be targeted to the transcytotic pathway for secretion into bile as S-IgA. Because expression of pIgR by human hepatocytes is insignificant, endocytosis of IgA1 by the ASGP-R may represent an important pathway for hepatic clearance of this major IgA subclass in human blood. Although the bulk of endocytosed IgA would presumably be catabolized in lysosomes, some of the pIgA could possibly end up as biliary S-IgA. Experiments involving nonhuman primates did not reveal any difference in hepatic clearance of intravenously injected human IgA1 versus IgA2, although pIgA of both classes was cleared more efficiently than monomeric IgA (Moldoveanu et al., 1990). There is thus probably an as-yet-undefined binding site for IgA on hepatocytes distinct from the ASGP-R and with preferential affinity for pIgA regardless of subclass; this has been suggested previously on the basis of in vitro experiments with rat as well as human hepatocytes (Tolleshaug et al., 1981; Brandtzaeg, 1985; Tomana et al., 1988).

Kupffer cells in human liver have been shown to express FcαRI, which binds both monomeric and polymeric IgA (reviewed in Monteiro and van De Winkel, 2003). Although mice do not appear to expresses a homolog for FcαRI, mice transgenic for human FcαRI have been used to study the function of this receptor in vivo (van Egmond et al., 2000). Treatment of these mice with granulocyte colony stimulating factor induced expression of FcαRI in Kupffer cells, which mediated phagocytosis of bacteria coated with serum IgA but not S-IgA. The investigators later reported that serum but not S-IgA could induce phagocytosis in human neutrophils, suggesting that bound SC may inhibit proinflammatory actions of pIgA (Vidarsson et al., 2001) (see previous section, Unique Functions of pIg and pIgR in Mucosal Epithelia). In nonhuman primates, Kupffer cells have been shown to contribute to uptake and catabolism of circulating IgA (Moldoveanu et al., 1990), suggesting that this mechanism may be operative in humans as well.

Hepatic clearance of IgA-containing immune complexes (IC) has been studied mainly with regard to systemic mechanisms for removal of circulating IC of all classes. In humans (Rifai et al., 1989) and rodents (Socken et al., 1981; Russell et al., 1981; Brown et al., 1982; Harmatz et al., 1982; Brown et al., 1983; Phillips et al., 1988), intravenously administered IgA IC or heat-aggregated IgA are cleared primarily by the liver, presumably via the same receptors that mediate uptake of IgA. In mice, pIgR-mediated hepatobiliary clearance of circulating IgA IC has been shown to be involved in clearance of intestinally absorbed and bacterial antigens (Russell et al., 1983; Brown et al., 1984). However, this pathway is probably of little or no significance in humans. Kupffer cells contribute to the clearance of IgA IC by phagocytosis (Rifai and Mannik, 1984) and, for IC containing IgG as well as IgA, by Fcγ and complement receptors (Roccatello et al., 1992). Because the systemic mechanisms for clearance of IgA IC are saturable (Russell et al., 1981; Rifai and Mannik, 1984), high concentrations of IgA IC in the circulation may lead to their deposition in extrahepatic tissues, as has been implicated in the pathogenesis of IgA nephropathy (Emancipator and Lamm, 1989).

CONCLUSIONS

The polymeric immunoglobulin receptor plays a unique role in the mucosal immune system, acting both as an epithelial transporter and as an integral component of secretory immunoglobulins. Major advances in the past 40 years with use of the approaches of immunology, protein chemistry, cell biology, and molecular biology have increased our understanding of the structure, function, and regulation of pIgR. Production of mice genetically deficient in pIgR expression has allowed a more defined characterization of its biological functions. Molecular characterization of the gene encoding pIgR in humans and several animal species has provided important insights into the mechanisms by which its transcription is regulated by the immune and endocrine systems. Further characterization of molecular mechanisms of pIgR regulation, at the level of both synthesis and transcytosis, will increase our understanding of the integration of this important molecule with other effectors of the mucosal immune system.

REFERENCES

Abdou, N. I., Schumacher, H. R., Colman, R. W., Sagawa, A., Herbert, J., Pascual, E., Carrol, E. T., Miller, M., South, M. A., and Abdou, N. L. (1978). Behçet's disease: possible role of secretory component deficiency, synovial inclusions, and fibrinolytic abnormality in the various manifestations of the disease. *J. Lab. Clin. Med.* 91, 409–422.

Abreu, M. T., Thomas, L. S., Tesfay, S. Y., Lukasek, K., Michelsen, K. S., Zhou, Y., Hu, B., Wada, A., Hirayama, T., and Arditi, M. (2003). Regulation of TLR4 and MD-2 in the intestinal epithelium: evidence for dysregulated LPS signaling in human inflammatory bowel disease. *American Association of Immunologists 90th Annual Meeting, Denver, CO.* Abstract 36.34.

Ackermann, L. W., Wollenweber, L. A., and Denning, G. M. (1999). IL-4 and IFN-γ increase steady state levels of polymeric Ig receptor mRNA in human airway and intestinal epithelial cells. *J. Immunol.* 162, 5112–5118.

Acosta-Altamirano, G., Barranco-Acosta, C., Van Roost, E., and Vaerman, J.-P. (1980). Isolation and characterization of secretory IgA (sIgA) and free secretory component (FSC) from rat bile. *Mol. Immunol.* 17, 1525–1537.

Adamski, F. M., and Demmer, J. (1999). Two stages of increased IgA transfer during lactation in the marsupial, *Trichosurus vulpecula* (brushtail possum). *J. Immunol.* 162, 6009–6015.

Adamski, F. M., and Demmer, J. (2000). Immunological protection of the vulnerable marsupial pouch young: two periods of immune transfer during lactation in *Trichosurus vulpecula* (brushtail possum). *Dev. Comp Immunol.* 24, 491–502.

Ahlstedt, I., Lindholm, C., Lonroth, H., Hamlet, A., Svennerholm, A. M., and Quiding-Jarbrink, M. (1999). Role of local cytokines in increased gastric expression of the secretory component in *Helicobacter pylori* infection. *Infect. Immun.* 67, 4921–4925.

Allansmith, M. R., and Gillette, T. E. (1980). Secretory component in human ocular tissues. *Am. J. Ophthal.* 89, 353–361.

Allansmith, M. R., Kajiyama, G., Abelson, M. B., and Simon, M. A. (1976). Plasma cell content of main and accessory lacrimal glands and conjunctiva. *Am. J. Ophthal.* 82, 819–826.

Alonso de Velasco, E., Verheul, A. F., Verhoef, J., and Snippe, H. (1995). *Streptococcus pneumoniae*: virulence factors, pathogenesis, and vaccines. *Microbiol. Rev.* 59, 591–603.

Anderson, M. S., Venanzi, E. S., Klein, L., Chen, Z., Berzins, S. P., Turley, S. J., von Boehmer, H., Bronson, R., Dierich, A., Benoist, C., and Mathis, D. (2002). Projection of an immunological self shadow within the thymus by the aire protein. *Science* 298, 1395–1401.

Aoki, T., Koch, K. S., and Leffert, H. L. (1997). Attenuation of gene expression by a trinucleotide repeat-rich tract from the terminal exon of the rat hepatic polymeric immunoglobulin receptor gene. *J. Mol. Biol.* 267, 229–236.

Apodaca, G. (2001). Endocytic traffic in polarized epithelial cells: role of the actin and microtubule cytoskeleton. *Traffic* 2, 149–159.

Apodaca, G., Cardone, M. H., Whiteheart, S. W., DasGupta, B. R., and Mostov, K. E. (1996). Reconstitution of transcytosis in SLO-permeabilized MDCK cells: Existence of an NSF-dependent fusion mechanism with the apical surface of MDCK cells. *EMBO J.* 15, 1471–1481.

Apodaca, G., Katz, L. A., and Mostov, K. E. (1994). Receptor-mediated transcytosis of IgA in MDCK cells is via apical recycling endosomes. *J. Cell Biol.* 125, 67–86.

Arends, J. W., Wiggers, T., Thijs, C. T., Verstijnen, C., Swaen, G. J. V., and Bosman, F. T. (1984). The value of secretory component (SC) immunoreactivity in diagnosis and prognosis of colorectal carcinomas. *Am. J. Clin. Pathol.* 82, 267–274.

Aroeti, B., Kosen, P. A., Kuntz, I. D., Cohen, F. E., and Mostov, K. E. (1993). Mutational and secondary structural analysis of the basolateral sorting signal of the polymeric immunoglobulin receptor. *J. Cell Biol.* 123, 1149–1160.

Aroeti, B., and Mostov, K. E. (1994). Polarized sorting of the polymeric immunoglobulin receptor in the exocytotic and endocytotic pathways is controlled by the same amino acids. *EMBO J.* 13, 2297–2304.

Asahi, Y., Yoshikawa, T., Watanabe, I., Iwasaki, T., Hasegawa, H., Sato, Y., Shimada, S., Nanno, M., Matsuoka, Y., Ohwaki, M., Iwakura, Y., Suzuki, Y., Aizawa, C., Sata, T., Kurata, T., and Tamura, S. (2002). Protection against influenza virus infection in polymeric Ig receptor knockout mice immunized intranasally with adjuvant-combined vaccines. *J. Immunol.* 168, 2930–2938.

Baklien, K., Brandtzaeg, P., and Fausa, O. (1977). Immunoglobulins in jejunal mucosa and serum from patients with adult coeliac disease. *Scand. J. Gastroenterol.* 12, 149–159.

Bakos, M. -A., Kurosky, A., and Goldblum, R. M. (1991a). Characterization of a critical binding site for human polymeric Ig on secretory component. *J. Immunol.* 147, 3419–3426.

Bakos, M. -A., Kurosky, A., Woodard, C. S., Denney, R. M., and Goldblum, R. M. (1991b). Probing the topography of free and polymeric Ig-bound human secretory component with monoclonal antibodies. *J. Immunol.* 146, 162–168.

Bakos, M. -A., Widen, S. G., and Goldblum, R. M. (1994). Expression and purification of biologically active domain I of the human polymeric immunoglobulin receptor. *Mol. Immunol.* 31, 165–168.

Ball, J. M., Moldoveanu, Z., Melsen, L. R., Kozlowski, P. A., Jackson, S., Mulligan, M. J., Mestecky, J., and Compans, R. W. (1995). A polarized human endometrial cell line that binds and transports polymeric IgA. *In Vitro Cell. Dev. Biol. Anim.* 31, 196–206.

Banting, G., Brake, B., Braghetta, P., Luzio, J. P., and Stanley, K. K. (1989). Intracellular targetting signals of polymeric immunoglobulin receptors are highly conserved between species. *FEBS Lett.* 254, 177–183.

Barr, V. A., and Hubbard, A. L. (1993). Newly synthesized hepatocyte plasma membrane proteins are transported in transcytotic vesicles in the bile duct–ligated rat. *Gastroenterol.* 105, 554–571.

Barr, V. A., Scott, L. J., and Hubbard, A. L. (1995). Immunoadsorption of hepatic vesicles carrying newly synthesized dipeptidyl peptidase IV and polymeric IgA receptor. *J. Biol. Chem.* 270, 27834–27844.

Barroso, M., Bernd, K. K., DeWitt, N. D., Chang, A., Mills, K., and Sztul, E. S. (1996). A novel Ca^{2+}-binding protein, p22, is required for constitutive membrane traffic. *J. Biol. Chem.* 271, 10183–10187.

Barton, G. M., and Medzhitov, R. (2003). Toll-like receptor signaling pathways. *Science* 300, 1524–1525.

Beale, D. (1988). Cyanogen bromide cleavage of bovine secretory component and its tryptic fragments. *Int. J. Biochem.* 20, 873–879.

Beckmann, H., Su, L.-K., and Kadesch, T. (1990). TFE3: A helix-loop-helix protein that activates transcription through the immunoglobulin enhancer muE3 motif. *Genes Dev.* 4, 167–179.

Berget, S. M. (1995). Exon recognition in vertebrate splicing. *J. Biol. Chem.* 270, 2411–2414.

Bienenstock, J., and Strauss, H. (1970). Evidence for synthesis of human colostral γA as 11S dimer. *J. Immunol.* 105, 274–277.

Bienenstock, J., and Tomasi, T. B. (1968). Secretory γA in normal urine. *J. Clin. Invest.* 47, 1162–1171.

Bjercke, S., and Brandtzaeg, P. (1993). Glandular distribution of immunoglobulins, J chain, secretory component, and HLA-DR in the human endometrium throughout the menstrual cycle. *Hum. Reprod.* 8, 1420–1425.

Bjerke, K., and Brandtzaeg, P. (1988). Lack of relation between expression of HLA-DR and secretory component (SC) in follicle-associated epithelium of human Peyer's patches. *Clin. Exp. Immunol.* 71, 502–507.

Blanch, V. J., Piskurich, J. F., and Kaetzel, C. S. (1999). Cutting edge: coordinate regulation of IFN regulatory factor–1 and the polymeric Ig receptor by proinflammatory cytokines. *J. Immunol.* 162, 1232–1235.

Bomsel, M., Heyman, M., Hocini, H., Lagaye, S., Belec, L., Dupont, C., and Desgranges, C. (1998). Intracellular neutralization of HIV transcytosis across tight epithelial barriers by anti-HIV envelope protein dIgA or IgM. *Immunity.* 9, 277–287.

Bomsel, M., and Mostov, K. (1992). Role of heterotrimeric G proteins in membrane traffic. *Mol. Biol. Cell* 3, 1317–1328.

Bomsel, M., and Mostov, K. E. (1993). Possible role of both the α and βγ subunits of the heterotrimeric G protein, G_s, in transcytosis of the polymeric immunoglobulin receptor. *J. Biol. Chem.* 268, 25824–25835.

Braathen, R., Sorensen, V., Brandtzaeg, P., Sandlie, I., and Johansen, F. E. (2002). The carboxy-terminal domains of IgA and IgM direct isotype-specific polymerization and interaction with the polymeric immunoglobulin receptor. *J. Biol. Chem.* 277, 42755–42762.

Brandtzaeg, P. (1973). Structure, synthesis and external transfer of mucosal immunoglobulins. *Ann. Immunol. (Paris)* 124, 417–438.

Brandtzaeg, P. (1974a). Mucosal and glandular distribution of immunoglobulin components: differential localization of free and bound SC in secretory epithelial cells. *J. Immunol.* 112, 1553–1559.

Brandtzaeg, P. (1974b). Mucosal and glandular distribution of immunoglobulin components: Immunohistochemistry with a cold ethanol-fixation technique. *Immunol.* 26, 1101–1114.

Brandtzaeg, P. (1974c). Presence of J chain in human immunocytes containing various immunoglobulin classes. *Nature* 252, 418–420.

Brandtzaeg, P. (1975a). Blocking effect of J chain and J-chain antibody on the binding of secretory component to human IgA and IgM. *Scand. J. Immunol.* 4, 837–842.

Brandtzaeg, P. (1975b). Human secretory immunoglobulin M. An immunochemical and immunohistochemical study. *Immunol.* 29, 559–570.

Brandtzaeg, P. (1977). Human secretory component. VI. Immunoglobulin-binding properties. *Immunochemistry.* 14, 179–188.

Brandtzaeg, P. (1978). Polymeric IgA is complexed with secretory component (SC) on the surface of human intestinal epithelial cells. *Scand. J. Immunol.* 8, 39–52.

Brandtzaeg, P. (1983a). Immunohistochemical characterization of intracellular J-chain and binding site for secretory component (SC) in human immunoglobulin (Ig)–producing cells. *Mol. Immunol.* 20, 941–966.

Brandtzaeg, P. (1983b). The secretory immune system of lactating human mammary glands compared with other exocrine organs. *Ann. N.Y. Acad. Sci.* 409, 353–382.

Brandtzaeg, P. (1984). Immune functions of human nasal mucosa and tonsils in health and disease. In *Immunology of the Lung and Upper Respiratory Tract* (ed. J. Bienenstock), 28–95. New York: McGraw-Hill Book Co.

Brandtzaeg, P. (1985). Role of J chain and secretory component in receptor-mediated glandular and hepatic transport of immunoglobulins in man. *Scand. J. Immunol.* 22, 111–146.

Brandtzaeg, P. (1988). Immunopathological alterations in tonsillar disease. *Acta Otolaryngol (Stockh)* Suppl. 454, 64–69.

Brandtzaeg, P. (1991). Immunologic basis for celiac disease, inflammatory bowel disease, and type B chronic gastritis. *Curr. Opin. Gastroenterol.* 7, 450–462.

Brandtzaeg, P., and Baklien, K. (1976). Immunohistochemical studies of the formation and epithelial transport of immunoglobulins in normal and diseased human intestinal mucosa. *Scand. J. Gastroenterol.* 11, Suppl. 36, 1–45.

Brandtzaeg, P., Halstensen, T. S., Huitfeldt, H. S., Krajci, P., Kvale, D., Scott, H., and Thrane, P. S. (1992). Epithelial expression of HLA, secretory component (poly-Ig receptor), and adhesion molecules in the human alimentary tract. *Ann. N. Y. Acad. Sci.* 664, 157–179.

Brandtzaeg, P., Jahnsen, F. L., and Farstad, I. N. (1996). Immune functions and immunopathology of the mucosa of the upper respiratory pathways. *Acta Otolaryngol (Stockholm)* 116, 149–159.

Brandtzaeg, P., and Johansen, F. E. (2001). Confusion about the polymeric Ig receptor. *Trends Immunol.* 22, 545–546.

Brandtzaeg, P., and Korsrud, F. R. (1984). Significance of different J chain profiles in human tissues: generation of IgA and IgM with binding site for secretory component is related to the J chain expressing capacity of the total local immunocyte population, including IgG and IgD producing cells, and depends on the clinical state of the tissue. *Clin. Exp. Immunol.* 58, 709–718.

Brandtzaeg, P., Nilssen, D. E., Rognum, T. O., and Thrane, P. S. (1991). Ontogeny of the mucosal immune system and IgA deficiency. *Gastroenterol. Clin. North Am.* 20, 397–439.

Brandtzaeg, P., and Prydz, H. (1984). Direct evidence for an integrated function of J chain and secretory component in epithelial transport of immunoglobulins. *Nature* 311, 71–73.

Breitfeld, P. P., Harris, J. M., and Mostov, K. E. (1989). Postendocytotic sorting of the ligand for the polymeric immunoglobulin receptor in Madin-Darby canine kidney cells. *J. Cell Biol.* 109, 475–486.

Brock, S. C., McGraw, P. A., Wright, P. F., and Crowe, J. E. (2002). The human polymeric immunoglobulin receptor facilitates invasion of epithelial cells by *Streptococcus pneumoniae* in a strain-specific and cell type–specific manner. *Infect. Immun.* 70, 5091–5095.

Brooks, J. J., and Ernst, C. S. (1984). Immunoreactive secretory component of IgA in human tissues and tumors. *Am. J. Clin. Pathol.* 82, 660–665.

Brown, P. S., Wang, E., Aroeti, B., Chapin, S. J., Mostov, K. E., and Dunn, K. W. (2000). Definition of distinct compartments in polarized Madin-Darby canine kidney (MDCK) cells for membrane-volume sorting, polarized sorting and apical recycling. *Traffic* 1, 124–140.

Brown, R. W., Clark, G. M., Tandon, A. K., and Allred, D. C. (1993). Multiple-marker immunohistochemical phenotypes distinguishing malignant pleural mesothelioma from pulmonary adenocarcinoma. *Hum. Pathol.* 24, 347–354.

Brown, T. A., Russell, M. W., Kulhavy, R., and Mestecky, J. (1983). IgA-mediated elimination of antigens by the hepatobiliary route. *Fed. Proc.* 42, 3218–3221.

Brown, T. A., Russell, M. W., and Mestecky, J. (1982). Hepatobiliary transport of IgA immune complexes: molecular and cellular aspects. *J. Immunol.* 128, 2183–2186.

Brown, T. A., Russell, M. W., and Mestecky, J. (1984). Elimination of intestinally absorbed antigen into the bile by IgA. *J. Immunol.* 132, 780–782.

Brown, W. R., Isobe, K., Nakane, P. K., and Pacini, B. (1977). Studies on translocation of immunoglobulins across intestinal epithelium IV. Evidence for binding of IgA and IgM to secretory component in intestinal epithelium. *Gastroenterol.* 73, 1333–1339.

Brown, W. R., Isobe, Y., and Nakane, P. K. (1976). Studies on translocation of immunoglobulins across intestinal epithelium. II. Immunoelectron-microscopic localization of immunoglobulins and secretory component in human intestinal mucosa. *Gastroenterol.* 71, 985–995.

Brown, W. R., and Kloppel, T. M. (1989). The liver and IgA: immunological, cell biological and clinical implications. *Hepatology* 9, 763–784.

Bruce, S. R., Kaetzel, C. S., and Peterson, M. L. (1999). Cryptic intron activation within the large exon of the mouse polymeric immunoglobulin receptor gene: cryptic splice sites correspond to protein domain boundaries. *Nucleic Acids Res.* 27, 3446–3454.

Bruce, S. R., and Peterson, M. L. (2001). Multiple features contribute to efficient constitutive splicing of an unusually large exon. *Nucleic Acids Res.* 29, 2292–2302.

Bruno, M. E. C., and Kaetzel, C. S. (2003). Regulation of the polymeric Ig receptor in HT29 cells by prolonged exposure to TNF. *American Association of Immunologists 90th Anniversary Annual Meeting.* Abstract 118.14.

Bruno, M. E. C., West, R. B., Schneeman, T. A., Bresnick, E. H., and Kaetzel, C. S. (2004). Upstream stimulatory factor but not c-Myc enhances transcription of the human polymeric immunoglobulin receptor gene. *Mol. Immunol.*, 40, 695–708.

Bucher, P. (1990). Weight matrix descriptions of four eukaryotic RNA polymerase II promoter elements derived from 502 unrelated promoter sequences. *J. Mol. Biol.* 212, 563–578.

Burgio, G. R., Lanzavecchia, A., Plebani, A., Jayakar, S., and Ugazio, A. G. (1980). Ontogeny of secretory immunity: levels of secretory IgA and natural antibodies in saliva. *Pediatr. Res.* 14, 1111–1114.

Burns, J. W., Siadat-Pajouh, M., Krishnaney, A. A., and Greenberg, H. B. (1996). Protective effect of rotavirus VP6-specific IgA monoclonal antibodies that lack neutralizing activity. *Science* 272, 104–107.

Buts, J.-P., Bernasconi, P., Vaerman, J.-P., and Dive, C. (1990). Stimulation of secretory IgA and secretory component of immunoglobulins in small intestine of rats treated with *Saccharomyces boulardii*. *Dig. Dis. Sci.* 35, 251–256.

Buts, J.-P., De Keyser, N., Kolanowski, J., Sokal, E., and Van Hoof, F. (1993). Maturation of villus and crypt cell functions in rat small intestine: Role of dietary polyamines. *Dig. Dis. Sci.* 38, 1091–1098.

Buts, J.-P., Vaerman, J.-P., and Lescoat, G. (1992). Ontogeny of the receptor for polymeric immunoglobulins in rat hepatocytes. *Gastroenterol.* 102, 949–955.

Calvo, M., Pol, A., Lu, A., Ortega, D., Pons, M., Blasi, J., and Enrich, C. (2000). Cellubrevin is present in the basolateral endocytic compartment of hepatocytes and follows the transcytotic pathway after IgA internalization. *J. Biol. Chem.* 275, 7910–7917.

Cardone, M. H., Smith, B. L., Mennitt, P. A., Mochly-Rosen, D., Silver, R. B., and Mostov, K. E. (1996). Signal transduction by the polymeric immunoglobulin receptor suggests a role in regulation of receptor transcytosis. *J. Cell Biol.* 133, 997–1005.

Cardone, M. H., Smith, B. L., Song, W., Mochly-Rosen, D., and Mostov, K. E. (1994). Phorbol myristate acetate–mediated stimulation of transcytosis and apical recycling in MDCK cells. *J. Cell Biol.* 124, 717–727.

Cario, E., and Podolsky, D. K. (2000). Differential alteration in intestinal epithelial cell expression of toll-like receptor 3 (TLR3) and TLR4 in inflammatory bowel disease. *Infect. Immun.* 68, 7010–7017.

Carpenter, G. H., Garrett, J. R., Hartley, R. H., and Proctor, G. B. (1998). The influence of nerves on the secretion of immunoglobulin A into submandibular saliva in rats. *J. Physiol* 512, 567–573.

Casanova, J. E., Apodaca, G., and Mostov, K. E. (1991). An autonomous signal for basolateral sorting in the cytoplasmic domain of the polymeric immunoglobulin receptor. *Cell* 66, 65–75.

Casanova, J. E., Breitfeld, P. P., Ross, S. A., and Mostov, K. E. (1990). Phosphorylation of the polymeric immunoglobulin receptor required for its efficient transcytosis. *Science* 248, 742–745.

Casanova, J. E., Wang, X., Kumar, R., Bhartur, S. G., Navarre, J., W., Woodrum, J. E., Altschuler, Y., Ray, G. S., and Goldenring, J. R. (1999). Association of Rab25 and Rab11a with the apical recycling system of polarized Madin-Darby canine kidney cells. *Mol. Biol. Cell* 10, 47–61.

Chapin, S. J., Enrich, C., Aroeti, B., Havel, R. J., and Mostov, K. E. (1996). Calmodulin binds to the basolateral targeting signal of the polymeric immunoglobulin receptor. *J. Biol. Chem.* 271, 1336–1342.

Chen, S. -T., and Tobe, T. (1974). Cellular sites of immunoglobulins. IV. Studies of antral mucosa of human stomachs. *Digestion* 10, 177–183.

Chen, S. C., Fynan, E. F., Robinson, H. L., Lu, S., Greenberg, H. B., Santoro, J. C., and Herrmann, J. E. (1997). Protective immunity induced by rotavirus DNA vaccines. *Vaccine* 15, 899–902.

Chintalacharuvu, K. R., and Morrison, S. L. (1997). Production of secretory immunoglobulin A by a single mammalian cell. *Proc. Natl. Acad. Sci. USA* 94, 6364–6368.

Chintalacharuvu, K. R., Tavill, A. S., Louis, L. N., Vaerman, J.-P., Lamm, M. E., and Kaetzel, C. S. (1994). Disulfide bond formation between dimeric immunoglobulin A and the polymeric immunoglobulin receptor during hepatic transcytosis. *Hepatology* 19, 162–173.

Chintalacharuvu, K. R., Vuong, L. U., Loi, L. A., Larrick, J. W., and Morrison, S. L. (2001). Hybrid IgA2/IgG1 antibodies with tailor-made effector functions. *Clin. Immunol.* 101, 21–31.

Cleveland, M. G., Bakos, M.-A., Pyron, D. L., Rajaraman, S., and Goldblum, R. M. (1991). Characterization of secretory component in amniotic fluid: Identification of new forms of secretory IgA. *J. Immunol.* 147, 181–188.

Colombel, J. F., Rambaud, J. C., Vaerman, J. P., Galian, A., Delacroix, D. L., Nemeth, J., Duprey, F., Halphen, M., Godeau, P., and Dive, C. (1988). Massive plasma cell infiltration of the digestive tract. Secretory component as the rate-limiting factor of immunoglobulin secretion in external fluids. *Gastroenterol.* 95, 1106–1113.

Conley, M. E., and Delacroix, D. L. (1987). Intravascular and mucosal immunoglobulin A: two separate but related systems of immune defense? *Ann. Intern. Med.* 106, 892–899.

Courtoy, P. J., Limet, J. N., Quintart, J., Schneider, Y. J., Vaerman, J. P., and Baudhuin, P. (1983). Transfer of IgA into rat bile: ultrastructural demonstration. *Ann. N.Y. Acad. Sci.* 409, 799–802.

Coutinho, H.B., Robalinho, T. I., Coutinho, V. B., Almeida, J. R., Filho, J. T. O., King, G., Jenkins, D., Mahida, Y., Sewell, H. F., and Wakelin, D. (1996a). Immunocytochemistry of mucosal changes in patients infected with the intestinal nematode *Strongyloides stercoralis*. *J. Clin. Pathol.* 49, 717–720.

Coutinho, H. B., Robalinho, T. I., Coutinho, V. B., Amorin, A. M. S., Almeida, J. R., Filho, J. T. O., Walker, E., King, G., Sewell, H. F., and Wakelin, D. (1996b). Immunocytochemical demonstration that human duodenal Brunner's glands may participate in intestinal defence. *J. Anat.* 189, 193–197.

Coyne, R. S., Siebrecht, M., Peitsch, M. C., and Casanova, J. E. (1994). Mutational analysis of polymeric immunoglobulin receptor/ligand interactions. Evidence for the involvement of multiple complementarity determining region (CDR)-like loops in receptor domain I. *J. Biol. Chem.* 269, 31620–31625.

Crago, S. S., Kulhavy, R., Prince, S. J., and Mestecky, J. (1978). Secretory component on epithelial cells is a surface receptor for polymeric immunoglobulins. *J. Exp. Med.* 147, 1832–1837.

Crago, S. S., Kutteh, W. H., Moro, I., Allansmith, M. R., Radl, J., Haaijman, J. J., and Mestecky, J. (1984). Distribution of IgA1-, IgA2-, and J chain-containing cells in human tissues. *J. Immunol.* 132, 16–18.

Crottet, P., and Corthesy, B. (1998). Secretory component delays the conversion of secretory IgA into antigen-binding competent F(ab')2: a possible implication for mucosal defense. *J. Immunol.* 161, 5445–5453.

Crottet, P., and Corthesy, B. (1999). Mapping the interaction between murine IgA and murine secretory component carrying epitope substitutions reveals a role of domains II and III in covalent binding to IgA. *J. Biol. Chem.* 274, 31456–31462.

Crottet, P., Peitsch, M. C., Servis, C., and Corthesy, B. (1999). Covalent homodimers of murine secretory component induced by epitope substitution unravel the capacity of the polymeric Ig receptor to dimerize noncovalently in the absence of IgA ligand. *J. Biol. Chem.* 274, 31445–31455.

Cruz, J. R., Cano, F., and Cáceres, P. (1991). Association of human milk SIgA antibodies with maternal intestinal exposure to microbial antigens. *Adv. Exp. Med. Biol.* 310, 193–199.

Dallas, S. D., and Rolfe, R. D. (1998). Binding of *Clostridium difficile* toxin A to human milk secretory component. *J Med. Microbiol.* 47, 879–888.

Daniele, R. P. (1990). Immunoglobulin secretion in the airways. *Annu. Rev. Physiol.* 52, 177–195.

Daniels, C. K., Schmucker, D. L., and Jones, A. L. (1989). Hepatic asialoglycoprotein receptor–mediated binding of human polymeric immunoglobulin A. *Hepatology* 9, 229–234.

Davidson, M. K., Le Beau, M. M., Eddy, R. L., Shows, T. B., DiPietro, L. A., Kingzette, M., and Hanly, W. C. (1988). Genetic mapping of the human polymeric immunoglobulin receptor gene to chromosome region 1q31–q41. *Cytogenet. Cell Genet.* 48, 107–111.

de Oliveira, I. R., de Araujo, A. N., Bao, S. N., and Giugliano, L. G. (2001). Binding of lactoferrin and free secretory component to enterotoxigenic *Escherichia coli*. *FEMS Microbiol. Lett.* 203, 29–33.

Deitcher, D. L., and Mostov, K. E. (1986). Alternate splicing of rabbit polymeric immunoglobulin receptor. *Mol. Cell. Biol.* 6, 2712–2715.

Delacroix, D. L., Denef, A. M., Acosta, G. A., Montgomery, P. C., and Vaerman, J.-P. (1982a). Immunoglobulins in rabbit hepatic bile: Selective secretion of IgA and IgM and active plasma-to-bile transfer of polymeric IgA. *Scand. J. Immunol.* 16, 343–350.

Delacroix, D. L., Furtado-Barreira, G., Rahier, J., Dive, C., and Vaerman, J.-P. (1984). Immunohistochemical localization of secretory component in the liver of guinea pigs and dogs versus rats, rabbits, and mice. *Scand. J. Immunol.* 19, 425–434.

Delacroix, D. L., Hodgson, H. J. F., McPherson, A., Dive, C., and Vaerman, J. P. (1982b). Selective transport of polymeric immunoglobulin A in bile. Quantitative relationships of monomeric and polymeric immunoglobulin A, immunoglobulin M, and other proteins in serum, bile, and saliva. *J. Clin. Invest.* 70, 230–241.

Denning, G. M. (1996). IL-4 and IFN-γ synergistically increase total polymeric IgA receptor levels in human intestinal epithelial cells. Role of protein tyrosine kinases. *J. Immunol.* 156, 4807–4814.

Dobrin, R. S., Knudson, F. E., and Michael, A. F. (1975). The secretory immune system and renal disease. *Clin. Exp. Immunol.* 21, 318–328.

Dooley, J. S., Potter, B. J., Thomas, H. C., and Sherlock, S. (1982). A comparative study of the biliary secretion of human dimeric and monomeric IgA in the rat and in man. *Hepatology* 2, 323–327.

Dunne, A., and O'Neill, L. A. (2003). The interleukin-1 receptor/Toll-like receptor superfamily: signal transduction during inflammation and host defense. *Sci. STKE.* 2003, re3.

Eckman, E. A., Mallender, W. D., Szegletes, T., Silski, C. L., Schreiber, J. R., Davis, P. B., and Ferkol, T. W. (1999). In vitro transport of active α(1)-antitrypsin to the apical surface of epithelia by targeting the polymeric immunoglobulin receptor. *Am J Respir. Cell Mol. Biol.* 21, 246–252.

Eiffert, H., Quentin, E., Decker, J., Hillemeir, S., Hufschmidt, M., Klingmuller, D., Weber, M. H., and Hilschmann, N. (1984). The primary structure of the human free secretory component and the arrangement of the disulfide bonds. *Hoppe-Seyler's Z. Physiol. Chem.* 365, 1489–1495.

El Kaissouni, J., Bene, M. C., and Faure, G. C. (1996). Investigation of activation markers demonstrates significant overexpression of the secretory component on salivary glands epithelial cells in Sjögren's syndrome. *Clin. Immunol. Immunopath.* 79, 236–243.

Elm, C., Ranveig, B., Bergmann, S., Frank, R., Vaerman, J.-P., Kaetzel, C. S., Chhatwal, G. S., Johansen, F.-E. and Hammerschmidt, S. (2004). Ectodomains 3 and 4 of human polymeric immunoglobulin receptor (hpIgR) mediate invasion of *Streptococcus pneumoniae* into the epithelium. *J. Biol. Chem.* 279, 6296–6304.

Emancipator, S. N., and Lamm, M. E. (1989). IgA nephropathy: Overproduction or decreased clearance of immune complexes? *Lab. Invest.* 61, 365–367.

Enrich, C., Jäckle, S., and Havel, R. J. (1996). The polymeric immunoglobulin receptor is the major calmodulin-binding protein in an endosome fraction from rat liver enriched in recycling receptors. *Hepatology* 24, 226–232.

Enrich, C., Vergés, M., and Evans, W. H. (1995). Functional identification of three major phosphoproteins in endocytic fractions from rat liver. A comparative *in vivo* and *in vitro* study. *Eur. J. Biochem.* 231, 802–808.

Espinoza, C. G., Balis, J. U., Saba, S. R., Paciga, J. E., and Shelley, S. A. (1984). Ultrastructural and immunohistochemical studies of bronchiolo-alveolar carcinoma. *Cancer* 54, 2182–2189.

Fahey, J. V., Humphrey, S. L., Stern, J. E., and Wira, C. R. (1998). Secretory component production by polarized epithelial cells from the human female reproductive tract. *Immunol. Invest* 27, 167–180.

Fallgreen-Gebauer, E., Gebauer, W., Bastian, A., Kratzin, H. D., Eiffert, H., Zimmermann, B., Karas, M., and Hilschmann, N. (1993). The covalent linkage of secretory component to IgA. Structure of sIgA. *Biol. Chem. Hoppe-Seyler* 374, 1023–1028.

Feltelius, N., Hvatum, M., Brandtzaeg, P., Knutson, L., and Hällgren, R. (1994). Increased jejunal secretory IgA and IgM in ankylosing spondylitis: normalization after treatment with sulfasalazine. *J. Rheumatol.* 21, 2076–2081.

Feng, N., Lawton, J. A., Gilbert, J., Kuklin, N., Vo, P., Prasad, B. V., and Greenberg, H. B. (2002). Inhibition of rotavirus replication by a non-neutralizing, rotavirus VP6-specific IgA mAb. *J. Clin. Invest* 109, 1203–1213.

Ferkol, T., Cohn, L. A., Phillips, T. E., Smith, A., and Davis, P. B. (2003). Targeted delivery of antiprotease to the epithelial surface of human tracheal xenografts. *Am. J. Respir. Crit Care Med* 167, 1374–1379.

Ferkol, T., Eckman, E., Swaidani, S., Silski, C., and Davis, P. (2000). Transport of bifunctional proteins across respiratory epithelial cells via the polymeric immunoglobulin receptor. *Am. J. Respir. Crit. Care Med.* 161, 944–951.

Ferkol, T., Kaetzel, C. S., and Davis, P. B. (1993). Gene transfer into respiratory epithelial cells by targeting the polymeric immunoglobulin receptor. *J. Clin. Invest.* 92, 2394–2400.

Ferkol, T., Pellicena-Palle, A., Eckman, E., Perales, J. C., Trzaska, T., Tosi, M., Redline, R., and Davis, P. B. (1996). Immunologic responses to gene transfer into mice via the polymeric immunoglobulin receptor. *Gene Ther.* 3, 669–678.

Ferkol, T., Perales, J. C., Eckman, E., Kaetzel, C. S., Hanson, R. W., and Davis, P. B. (1995). Gene transfer into the airway epithelium of animals by targeting the polymeric immunoglobulin receptor. *J. Clin. Invest.* 95, 493–502.

Fernandez, M. I., Pedron, T., Tournebize, R., Olivo-Marin, J. C., Sansonetti, P. J., and Phalipon, A. (2003). Anti-inflammatory role for intracellular dimeric immunoglobulin A by neutralization of lipopolysaccharide in epithelial cells. *Immunity* 18, 739–749.

Fichorova, R. N., and Anderson, D. J. (1999). Differential expression of immunobiological mediators by immortalized human cervical and vaginal epithelial cells. *Biol. Reprod.* 60, 508–514.

Fichorova, R. N., Rheinwald, J. G., and Anderson, D. J. (1997). Generation of papillomavirus-immortalized cell lines from normal human ectocervical, endocervical, and vaginal epithelium that maintain expression of tissue-specific differentiation proteins. *Biol. Reprod.* 57, 847–855.

Fiedler, M. A., Kaetzel, C. S., and Davis, P. B. (1991). Sustained production of secretory component by human tracheal epithelial cells in primary culture. *Am. J. Physiol. (Lung Cell Mol. Physiol.)* 261, L255–L261.

Finkbeiner, W. E., Carrier, S. D., and Teresi, C. E. (1993). Reverse transcription–polymerase chain reaction (RT-PCR) phenotypic analysis of cell cultures of human tracheal epithelium, tracheobronchial glands, and lung carcinomas. *Am. J. Respir. Cell Mol. Biol.* 9, 547–556.

Fisher, D. E., Carr, C. S., Parent, L. A., and Sharp, P. A. (1991). TFEB has DNA-binding and oligomerization properties of a unique helix-loop-helix/leucine-zipper family. *Genes Dev.* 5, 2342–2352.

Fisher, M. M., Nagy, B., Bazin, H., and Underdown, B. J. (1979). Biliary transport of IgA: Role of secretory component. *Proc. Natl. Acad. Sci. USA* 76, 2008–2012.

Fodor, E., Feren, A., and Jones, A. (1997). Isolation and genomic analysis of the rat polymeric immunoglobulin receptor gene terminal domain and transcriptional control region. *DNA Cell Biol.* 16, 215–225.

Folsch, H., Ohno, H., Bonifacino, J. S., and Mellman, I. (1999). A novel clathrin adaptor complex mediates basolateral targeting in polarized epithelial cells. *Cell* 99, 189–198.

Foss-Bowman, C., Jones, A. L., Dejbakhsh, S., and Goldman, I. S. (1983). Immunofluorescent and immunocytochemical localization of secretory component and immunoglobulins in human liver. *Ann. N.Y. Acad. Sci.* 409, 822–823.

Franklin, R. M., Kenyon, K. R., and Tomasi, T. B. (1973). Immunohistologic studies of human lacrimal gland: Localization of immunoglobulins, secretory component and lactoferrin. *J. Immunol.* 110, 984–992.

Frutiger, S., Hughes, G. J., Hanly, W. C., Kingzette, M., and Jaton, J. C. (1986). The amino-terminal domain of rabbit secretory component is responsible for noncovalent binding to immunoglobulin A dimers. *J. Biol. Chem.* 261, 16673–16681.

Futter, C. E., Gibson, A., Allchin, E. H., Maxwell, S., Ruddock, L. J., Odorizzi, G., Domingo, D., Trowbridge, I. S., and Hopkins, C. R. (1998). In polarized MDCK cells basolateral vesicles arise from clathrin-γ-adaptin-coated domains on endosomal tubules. *J. Cell Biol.* 141, 611–623.

Gan, Y. -J., Chodosh, J., Morgan, A., and Sixbey, J. W. (1997). Epithelial cell polarization is a determinant in the infectious outcome of immunoglobulin A–mediated entry by Epstein-Barr virus. *J. Virol.* 71, 519–526.

Gan, Y., McGraw, T. E., and Rodriguez-Boulan, E. (2002). The epithelial-specific adaptor AP1B mediates post-endocytic recycling to the basolateral membrane. *Nat. Cell Biol.* 4, 605–609.

Gangopadhyay, N. N., Moldoveanu, Z., and Stephensen, C. B. (1996). Vitamin A deficiency has different effects on immunoglobulin A production and transport during influenza A infection in BALB/c mice. *J. Nutr.* 126, 2960–2967.

Gao, J., Lambert, R. W., Wickham, L. A., Banting, G., and Sullivan, D. A. (1995). Androgen control of secretory component mRNA levels in the rat lacrimal gland. *J. Steroid Biochem.* 52, 239–249.

Gehrke, I., and Pabst, R. (1990). The epithelium overlying rabbit bronchus-associated lymphoid tissue does not express the secretory component of immunoglobulin A. *Cell and Tissue Res.* 259, 397–399.

Geuze, H. J., Slot, J. W., Strous, G. J. A. M., Peppard, J., von Figura, K., Hasilik, A., and Schwartz, A. L. (1984). Intracellular receptor sorting during endocytosis: Comparative immunoelectron microscopy of multiple receptors in rat liver. *Cell* 37, 195–204.

Gibson, A., Futter, C. E., Maxwell, S., Allchin, E. H., Shipman, M., Kraehenbuhl, J. P., Domingo, D., Odorizzi, G., Trowbridge, I. S., and Hopkins, C. R. (1998). Sorting mechanisms regulating membrane protein traffic in the apical transcytotic pathway of polarized MDCK cells. *J. Cell Biol.* 143, 81–94.

Giffroy, D., Courtoy, P. J., and Vaerman, J. P. (2001). Polymeric IgA binding to the human pIgR elicits intracellular signalling, but fails to stimulate pIgR-transcytosis. *Scand. J. Immunol.* 53, 56–64.

Giffroy, D., Langendries, A., Maurice, M., Daniel, F., Lardeux, B., Courtoy, P. J., and Vaerman, J. P. (1998). *In vivo* stimulation of polymeric Ig receptor transcytosis by circulating polymeric IgA in rat liver. *Int. Immunol.* 10, 347–354.

Giugliano, L. G., Ribeiro, S. T. G., Vainstein, M. H., and Ulhoa, C. J. (1995). Free secretory component and lactoferrin of human milk inhibit the adhesion of enterotoxigenic *Escherichia coli. J. Med. Microbiol.* 42, 3–9.

Goldblum, R. M., and Goldman, A. S. (1994). Immunological components of milk: formation and function. In *Handbook of Mucosal Immunology* (eds. P. L. Ogra, J. Mestecky, M. E. Lamm, W. Strober, J. R. McGhee, and J. Bienenstock), 643–652. San Diego, CA: Academic Press.

Greenwell, D., Petersen, J., Kulvicki, A., Harder, J., Goldblum, R., and Neal, D. E. (1995). Urinary secretory immunoglobulin A and free secretory component in pyelonephritis. *Am. J. Kid. Dis.* 26, 590–594.

Gupta, S., Eastman, J., Silski, C., Ferkol, T., and Davis, P. B. (2001). Single chain Fv: a ligand in receptor-mediated gene delivery. *Gene Ther.* 8, 586–592.

Gurevich, P., Zusman, I., Moldavsky, M., Szvalb, S., Elhayany, A., Halperin, R., Gurevich, E., and Ben Hur, H. (2003). Secretory immune system in human intrauterine development: immunopathomorphological analysis of the role of secretory component (pIgR/SC) in immunoglobulin transport (review). *Int. J. Mol. Med.* 12, 289–297.

Ha, C. L., and Woodward, B. (1997). Reduction in the quantity of the polymeric immunoglobulin receptor rs sufficient to account for the low concentration of intestinal secretory immunoglobulin a in a weanling mouse model of wasting protein-energy malnutrition. *J. Nutr.* 127, 427–435.

Ha, C. L., and Woodward, B. (1998). Depression in the quantity of intestinal secretory IgA and in the expression of the polymeric immunoglobulin receptor in caloric deficiency of the weanling mouse. *Lab Invest* 78, 1255–1266.

Haelens, A., Verrijdt, G., Callewaert, L., Peeters, B., Rombauts, W., and Claessens, F. (2001). Androgen-receptor-specific DNA binding to an element in the first exon of the human secretory component gene. *Biochem. J.* 353, 611–620.

Haelens, A., Verrijdt, G., Schoenmakers, E., Alen, P., Peeters, B., Rombauts, W., and Claessens, F. (1999). The first exon of the human sc gene contains an androgen responsive unit and an interferon regulatory factor element. *Mol. Cell Endocrinol.* 153, 91–102.

Hahn-Zoric, M., Carlsson, B., Jalil, F., Mellander, L., Germanier, R., and Hanson, L. A. (1989). The influence on the secretory IgA antibody levels in lactating women of oral typhoid and parenteral cholera vaccines given alone or in combination. *Scand. J. Infect. Dis.* 21, 421–426.

Halpern, M. S., and Koshland, M. E. (1970). Novel subunit in secretory IgA. *Nature* 228, 1276–1278.

Hammerschmidt, S., Talay, S. R., Brandtzaeg, P., and Chhatwal, G. S. (1997). SpsA, a novel pneumococcal surface protein with specific binding to secretory immunoglobulin A and secretory component. *Mol. Microbiol.* 25, 1113–1124.

Hammerschmidt, S., Tillig, M. P., Wolff, S., Vaerman, J. P., and Chhatwal, G. S. (2000). Species-specific binding of human secretory component to SpsA protein of *Streptococcus pneumoniae* via a hexapeptide motif. *Mol. Microbiol.* 36, 726–736.

Hamza, M., Ayed, K., and Makni, S. (1991). Acquired and transitory IgA deficiency in Behçet's disease. *Clin. Exp. Rheumatol.* 9, 208–209.

Hamza, M., and Makni, S. (1995). Secretory component deficiency in Behçet's disease. *Clin. Rheumatol.* 14, 227–228.

Hansen, G. H., Niels-Christiansen, L. L., Immerdal, L., Hunziker, W., Kenny, A. J., and Michael, Danielsen E. (1999). Transcytosis of Immunoglobulin A in the mouse enterocyte occurs through glycolipid Raft- and Rab17-containing compartments. *Gastroenterology* 116, 610–622.

Hanson, L. A. (1982). The mammary gland as an immunological organ. *Immunol. Today* 3, 168–173.

Harmatz, P. R., Kleinman, R. E., Bunnell, B. W., Bloch, K. J., and Walker, W. A. (1982). Hepatobiliary clearance of IgA immune complexes formed in the circulation. *Hepatology* 2, 328–333.

Harris, J. P., Caleb, M. H., and South, M. A. (1975). Secretory component in human mammary carcinoma. *Cancer Res.* 35, 1861–1864.

Harris, J. P., and South, M. A. (1981). Secretory component: a glandular epithelial cell marker. *Am. J. Pathol.* 105, 47–53.

Hausmann, M., Kiessling, S., Mestermann, S., Webb, G., Spottl, T., Andus, T., Scholmerich, J., Herfarth, H., Ray, K., Falk, W., and Rogler, G. (2002). Toll-like receptors 2 and 4 are up-regulated during intestinal inflammation. *Gastroenterology* 122, 1987–2000.

Hayakawa, T., Kondo, T., Shibata, T., Murase, T., Harada, H., Ochi, K., and Tanaka, J. (1993). Secretory component and lactoferrin in pure pancreatic juice in chronic pancreatitis. *Dig. Dis. Sci.* 38, 7–11.

Hayani, K. C., Guerrero, M. L., Ruiz-Palacios, G. M., Gomez, H. F., and Cleary, T. G. (1991). Evidence for long-term memory of the mucosal immune system: Milk secretory immunoglobulin A against *Shigella* lipopolysaccharides. *J. Clin. Microbiol.* 29, 2599–2603.

Hayashi, Y., Kurashima, C., Takemura, T., and Hirokawa, K. (1989). Ontogenic development of the secretory immune system in human fetal salivary glands. *Pathol. Immunopathol. Res.* 8, 314–320.

Hehlgans, T., and Mannel, D. N. (2002). The TNF-TNF receptor system. *Biol. Chem.* 383, 1581–1585.

Hempen, P. M., Phillips, K. M., Conway, P. S., Sandoval, K. H., Schneeman, T. A., Wu, H. J., and Kaetzel, C. S. (2002). Transcriptional regulation of the human polymeric Ig receptor gene: Analysis of basal promoter elements. *J. Immunol.* 169, 1912–1921.

Hendrickson, B. A., Conner, D. A., Ladd, D. J., Kendall, D., Casanova, J. E., Corthesy, B., Max, E. E., Neutra, M. R., Seidman, C. E., and Seidman, J. G. (1995). Altered hepatic transport of immunoglobulin A in mice lacking the J chain. *J. Exp. Med.* 182, 1905–1911.

Hendrickson, B. A., Rindisbacher, L., Corthesy, B., Kendall, D., Waltz, D. A., Neutra, M. R., and Seidman, J. G. (1996). Lack of association of secretory component with IgA in J chain-deficient mice. *J. Immunol.* 157, 750–754.

Hexham, J. M., White, K. D., Carayannopoulos, L. N., Mandecki, W., Brisette, R., Yang, Y. S., and Capra, J. D. (1999). A human immunoglobulin (Ig)A Cα3 domain motif directs polymeric Ig receptor–mediated secretion. *J. Exp. Med.* 189, 747–752.

Hirata, H., Noguchi, M., Shimosato, Y., Uei, Y., and Goya, T. (1990). Clinicopathologic and immunohistochemical characteristics of bronchial gland cell type adenocarcinoma of the lung. *Am. J. Clin. Pathol.* 93, 20–25.

Hirunsatit, R., Kongruttanachok, N., Shotelersuk, K., Supiyaphun, P., Voravud, N., Sakuntabhai, A., and Mutirangura, A. (2003). Polymeric immunoglobulin receptor polymorphisms and risk of nasopharyngeal cancer. *BMC Genet.* 4, 3.

Hooper, L. V., Wong, M. H., Thelin, A., Hansson, L., Falk, P. G., and Gordon, J. I. (2001). Molecular analysis of commensal host–microbial relationships in the intestine. *Science* 291, 881–884.

Hopf, U., Brandtzaeg, P., Hutteroth, T. H., and Meyer zum Buschenfelde, K. H. (1978). In vivo and in vitro binding of IgA to the plasma membrane of hepatocytes. *Scand. J. Immunol.* 8, 543–549.

Hoppe, C. A., Connolly, T. P., and Hubbard, A. L. (1985). Transcellular transport of polymeric IgA in the rat hepatocyte: Biochemical and morphological characterization of the transport pathway. *J. Cell Biol.* 101, 2113–2123.

Hsu, S. M., and Hsu, P. L. (1980). Demonstration of IgA and secretory component in human hepatocytes. *Gut* 21, 985–989.

Huang, Z., Lambert, R. W., Wickham, A., and Sullivan, D. A. (1996). Analysis of cytomegalovirus infection and replication in acinar epithelial cells of the rat lacrimal gland. *Invest. Ophthalmol. Vis. Sci.* 37, 1174–1186.

Hubbard, A. L., Stieger, B., and Bartles, J. R. (1989). Biogenesis of endogenous plasma membrane proteins in epithelial cells. *Annu. Rev. Physiol.* 51, 755–770.

Hughes, G. ., Frutiger, S., Savoy, L. A., Reason, A. J., Morris, H. R., and Jaton, J. C. (1997). Human free secretory component is composed of the first 585 amino acid residues of the polymeric immunoglobulin receptor. *FEBS Letters* 410, 443–446.

Huling, S., Fournier, G. R., Feren, A., Chuntharapai, A., and Jones, A. L. (1992). Ontogeny of the secretory immune system: Maturation of a functional polymeric immunoglobulin receptor regulated by gene expression. *Proc. Natl. Acad. Sci. USA* 89, 4260–4264.

Hunt, S., Spitznas, M., Seifert, P., and Rauwolf, M. (1996). Organ culture of human main and accessory lacrimal glands and their secretory behaviour. *Exp. Eye Res.* 62, 541–554.

Imayama, S., Shimozono, Y., Hoashi, M., Yasumoto, S., Ohta, S., Yoneyama, K., and Hori, Y. (1994). Reduced secretion of IgA to skin surface of patients with atopic dermatitis. *J. Allergy Clin. Immunol.* 94, 195–200.

Imayama, S., Shimozono, Y., Urabe, A., and Hori, Y. (1995). A simple method for measuring the amount of immunoglobulin A secreted onto the skin surface. *Acta Derm. Venereol.* 75, 212–217.

Isaacson, P. (1982a). Immunoperoxidase study of the secretory immunoglobulin system and lysozyme in normal and diseased gastric mucosa. *Gut* 23, 578–588.

Isaacson, P. (1982b). Immunoperoxidase study of the secretory immunoglobulin system in colonic neoplasia. *J. Clin. Pathol.* 35, 14–25.

Ishida, T., Kaneko, S., Tateishi, M., Oka, T., Mitsudomi, T., Sugimachi, K., Hara, N., and Ohta, M. (1990a). Large cell carcinoma of the lung. Prognostic implications of histopathologic and immunohistochemical subtyping. *Am. J. Clin. Pathol.* 93, 176–182.

Ishida, T., Tateishi, M., Kaneko, S., Yano, T., Mitsudomi, T., Sugimachi, K., Hara, N., and Ohta, M. (1990b). Carcinosarcoma and spindle cell carcinoma of the lung. Clinicopathologic and immuno-histochemical studies. *J. Thorac. Cardiovasc. Surg.* 100, 844–852.

Jackson, G. D. F., Hanson, P. G. C., and Underdown, B. J. (1992). Further evidence that hepatic sources confer biliary antibody in the rat. *Immunol.* 76, 397–401.

Jackson, G. D. F., Lemaitre-Coelho, I., and Vaerman, J.-P. (1977). Transfer of MOPC-315 IgA to secretions in MOPC-315 tumour-bearing and normal BALB/c mice. *Protides Biol. Fluids* 25, 919–922.

Jackson, G. D. F., Lemaitre-Coelho, I., Vaerman, J. P., Bazin, H., and Beckers, A. (1978). Rapid disappearance from serum of intravenously injected rat myeloma IgA and its secretion into bile. *Eur. J. Immunol.* 8, 123–126.

Jenkins, S. L., Wang, J., Vazir, M., Vela, J., Sahagun, O., Gabbay, P., Hoang, L., Diaz, R. L., Aranda, R., and Martin, M. G. (2003). Role of passive and adaptive immunity in influencing enterocyte-specific gene expression. *Am. J. Physiol. Gastrointest. Liver Physiol.* 285, G714–G725.

Jin, M., Saucan, L., Farquhar, M. G., and Palade, G. E. (1996). Rab1a and multiple other Rab proteins are associated with the transcytotic pathway in rat liver. *J. Biol. Chem.* 271, 30105–30113.

Johansen, F. E., Bosloven, B. A., Krajci, P., and Brandtzaeg, P. (1998). A composite DNA element in the promoter of the polymeric immunoglobulin receptor regulates its constitutive expression. *Eur. J. Immunol.* 28, 1161–1171.

Johansen, F. E., Braathen, R., and Brandtzaeg, P. (2000). Role of J chain in secretory immunoglobulin formation. *Scand. J. Immunol.* 52, 240–248.

Johansen, F. E., Braathen, R., and Brandtzaeg, P. (2001). The J chain is essential for polymeric Ig receptor–mediated epithelial transport of IgA. *J. Immunol.* 167, 5185–5192.

Johansen, F. E., Pekna, M., Norderhaug, I. N., Haneberg, B., Hietala, M. A., Krajci, P., Betsholtz, C., and Brandtzaeg, P. (1999). Absence of epithelial immunoglobulin A transport, with increased mucosal leakiness, in polymeric immunoglobulin receptor/secretory component–deficient mice. *J. Exp. Med.* 190, 915–922.

Johansson, M., and Lycke, N. Y. (2003). Immunology of the human genital tract. *Curr. Opin. Infect. Dis.* 16, 43–49.

Jonard, P. P., Rambaud, J. C., Vaerman, J. P., Galian, A., and Delacroix, D. L. (1984). Secretion of immunoglobulins and plasma proteins from the jejunal mucosa. Transport rate and origin of polymeric immunoglobulin A. *J. Clin. Invest.* 74, 525–535.

Kaetzel, C. S. (2001). Polymeric Ig receptor: defender of the fort or Trojan horse? *Curr. Biol.* 11, R35–R38.

Kaetzel, C. S., Blanch, V. B., Hempen, P. M., Phillips, K. M., Piskurich, J. F., and Youngman, K. R. (1997a). The polymeric Ig receptor: structure and synthesis. *Biochem. Soc. Trans.* 25, 475–480.

Kaetzel, C. S., Robinson, J. K., Chintalacharuvu, K. R., Vaerman, J.-P., and Lamm, M. E. (1991). The polymeric immunoglobulin receptor (secretory component) mediates transport of immune complexes across epithelial cells: A local defense function for IgA. *Proc. Natl. Acad. Sci. USA* 88, 8796–8800.

Kaetzel, C. S., Robinson, J. K., and Lamm, M. E. (1994). Epithelial transcytosis of monomeric IgA and IgG cross-linked through antigen to polymeric IgA: A role for monomeric antibodies in the mucosal immune system. *J. Immunol.* 152, 72–76.

Kaushic, C., Richardson, J. M., and Wira, C. R. (1995). Regulation of polymeric immunoglobulin A receptor messenger ribonucleic acid expression in rodent uteri: effect of sex hormones. *Endocrinol.* 136, 2836–2844.

Kawai, T., Torikata, C., and Suzuki, M. (1988). Immunohistochemical study of pulmonary adenocarcinoma. *Am. J. Clin. Pathol.* 89, 455–462.

Kelleher, R. S., Hann, L. E., Edwards, J. A., and Sullivan, D. A. (1991). Endocrine, neural, and immune control of secretory component output by lacrimal gland acinar cells. *J. Immunol.* 146, 3405–3412.

Khattar, N. H., Osterhage, J., and Kaetzel, C. S. (2003). Regulation of the polymeric Ig receptor by pro-inflammatory cytokines in mucosal epithelial cell lines. *American Association of Immunologists 90th Anniversary Annual Meeting,* Abstract 118.15.

Kiermaier, A., Gawn, J. M., Desbarats, L., Saffrich, R., Ansorge, W., Farrell, P. J., Eilers, M., and Packham, G. (1999). DNA binding of USF is required for specific E-box dependent gene activation in vivo. *Oncogene* 18, 7200–7211.

Kim, K. J., and Malik, A. B. (2003). Protein transport across the lung epithelial barrier. *Am. J. Physiol. Lung Cell Mol. Physiol.* 284, L247–L259.

Kloppel, T. M., and Brown, W. R. (1984). Rat liver membrane secretory component is larger than free secretory component in bile: Evidence for proteolytic conversion of membrane form to free form. *J. Cell. Biochem.* 24, 307–317.

Koch, K. S., Gleiberman, A. S., Aoki, T., Leffert, H. L., Feren, A., Jones, A. L., and Fodor, E. J. (1995). Discordant expression and variable numbers of neighboring GGA- and GAA-rich triplet repeats in the 3′ untranslated regions of two groups of messenger RNAs encoded by the rat polymeric immunoglobulin receptor gene. *Nucl. Acids Res.* 23, 1098–1112.

Kodama, T., Shimosato, Y., Koide, T., Watanabe, S., and Teshima, S. (1985). Large cell carcinoma of the lung: ultrastructural and immunohistochemical studies. *Jpn. J. Clin. Oncol.* 15, 431–441.

Kondi-Paphitis, A., and Addis, B. J. (1986). Secretory component in pulmonary adenocarcinoma and mesothelioma. *Histopathology* 10, 1279–1287.

Koretz, K., Schlag, P., Quentmeier, A., and Moller, P. (1994). Evaluation of the secretory component as a prognostic variable in colorectal carcinoma. *Int. J. Cancer* 57, 365–370.

Korsrud, F. R., and Brandtzaeg, P. (1980). Quantitative immunohistochemistry of immunoglobulin- and J-chain-producing cells in human parotid and submandibular salivary glands. *Immunol.* 39, 129–140.

Korsrud, F. R., and Brandtzaeg, P. (1982). Characterization of epithelial elements in human major salivary glands by functional markers: Localization of amylase, lactoferrin, lysozyme, secretory component, and secretory immunoglobulins by paired immunofluorescence staining. *J. Histochem. Cytochem.* 30, 657–666.

Kozak, M. (1987). An analysis of 5′-noncoding sequences from 699 vertebrate messenger RNAs. *Nucl. Acids Res.* 15, 8125–8148.

Kraehenbuhl, J. P., Racine, L., and Galardy, R. E. (1975). Localization of secretory IgA, secretory component, and alpha chain in the mammary gland of lactating rabbits by immunoelectron microscopy. *Ann. N.Y. Acad. Sci.* 254, 190–202.

Krajci, P., Gedde-Dahl, T., Hoyheim, B., Rogde, S., Olaisen, B., and Brandtzaeg, P. (1992a). The gene encoding human transmembrane secretory component (locus PIGR) is linked to D1S58 on chromosome 1. *Hum. Genet.* 90, 215–219.

Krajci, P., Grzeschik, K. H., Geurts van Kessel, A. H. M., Olaisen, B., and Brandtzaeg, P. (1991). The human transmembrane secretory component (poly-Ig receptor): molecular cloning, restriction fragment length polymorphism and chromosomal sublocalization. *Hum. Genet.* 87, 642–648.

Krajci, P., Kvale, D., Tasken, K., and Brandtzaeg, P. (1992b). Molecular cloning and exon-intron mapping of the gene encoding human transmembrane secretory component (the poly-Ig receptor). *Eur. J. Immunol.* 22, 2309–2315.

Krajci, P., Meling, G. I., Andersen, S. N., Hofstad, B., Vatn, M. H., Rognum, T. O., and Brandtzaeg, P. (1996). Secretory component mRNA and protein expression in colorectal adenomas and carcinomas. *Br. J. Cancer* 73, 1503–1510.

Krajci, P., Solberg, R., Sandberg, M., Oyen, O., Jahnsen, T., and Brandtzaeg, P. (1989). Molecular cloning of the human transmembrane secretory component (poly-Ig receptor) and its mRNA expression in human tissues. *Biochem. Biophys. Res. Comm.* 158, 783–789.

Krajci, P., Tasken, K., Kvale, D., and Brandtzaeg, P. (1993). Interferon-γ stimulation of messenger RNA for human secretory component (poly-Ig receptor) depends on continuous intermediate protein synthesis. *Scand. J. Immunol.* 37, 251–256.

Kubagawa, H., Bertoli, L. F., Barton, J. C., Koopman, W. J., Mestecky, J., and Cooper, M. D. (1987). Analysis of paraprotein transport into the saliva by using anti-idiotype antibodies. *J. Immunol.* 138, 435–439.

Kuhn, L. C., Kocher, H. P., Hanly, W. C., Cook, L., Jaton, J. C., and Kraehenbuhl, J. P. (1983). Structural and genetic heterogeneity of the receptor mediating translocation of immunoglobulin A dimer antibodies across epithelia in the rabbit. *J. Biol. Chem.* 258, 6653–6659.

Kuhn, L. C., and Kraehenbuhl, J. P. (1979a). Interaction of rabbit secretory component with rabbit IgA dimer. *J. Biol. Chem.* 254, 11066–11071.

Kuhn, L. C., and Kraehenbuhl, J. P. (1979b). Role of secretory component, a secreted glycoprotein, in the specific uptake of IgA dimer by epithelial cells. *J. Biol. Chem.* 254, 11072–11081.

Kulseth, M. A., Krajci, P., Myklebost, O., and Rogne, S. (1995). Cloning and characterization of two forms of bovine polymeric immunoglobulin receptor. *DNA Cell Biol.* 14, 251–256.

Kulseth, M. A., Toldo, S. S., Fries, R., Womack, J., Lien, S., and Rogne, S. (1994). Chromosomal localization and detection of DNA polymorphisms in the bovine polymeric immunoglobulin receptor gene. *Anim. Genet.* 25, 113–117.

Kumura, B. H., Sone, T., Shimazaki, K., and Kobayashi, E. (2000). Sequence analysis of porcine polymeric immunoglobulin receptor from mammary epithelial cells present in colostrum. *J. Dairy Res.* 67, 631–636.

Kushiro, A., and Sato, T. (1997). Polymeric immunoglobulin receptor gene of mouse: sequence, structure and chromosomal location. *Gene* 204, 277–282.

Kutteh, W. H., Blackwell, R. E., Gore, H., Kutteh, C. C., Carr, B. R., and Mestecky, J. (1990). Secretory immune system of the female reproductive tract. II. Local immune system in normal and infected fallopian tube. *Fertil. Steril.* 54, 51–55.

Kutteh, W. H., Hatch, K. D., Blackwell, R. E., and Mestecky, J. (1988). Secretory immune system of the female reproductive tract: I. Immunoglobulin and secretory component–containing cells. *Obstet. Gynecol.* 71, 56–60.

Kutteh, W. H., and Mestecky, J. (1994). Secretory immunity in the female reproductive tract. *Am. J. Reprod. Immunol.* 31, 40–46.

Kutteh, W. H., Prince, S. J., Hammond, K. R., Kutteh, C. C., and Mestecky, J. (1996). Variations in immunoglobulins and IgA subclasses of human uterine cervical secretions around the time of ovulation. *Clin. Exp. Immunol.* 104, 538–542.

Kutteh, W. H., Prince, S. J., and Mestecky, J. (1982). Tissue origins of human polymeric and monomeric IgA. *J. Immunol.* 128, 990–995.

Kvale, D., and Brandtzaeg, P. (1995). Constitutive and cytokine induced expression of HLA molecules, secretory component, and intercellular adhesion molecule-1 is modulated by butyrate in the colonic epithelial cell line HT-29. *Gut* 36, 737–742.

Kvale, D., Brandtzaeg, P., and Lovhaug, D. (1988). Up-regulation of the expression of secretory component and HLA molecules in a human colonic cell line by tumour necrosis factor-α and γ interferon. *Scand. J. Immunol.* 28, 351–357.

Laird, A. R., Gentsch, J. R., Nakagomi, T., Nakagomi, O., and Glass, R. I. (2003). Characterization of serotype G9 rotavirus strains isolated in the United States and India from 1993 to 2001. *J. Clin. Microbiol.* 41, 3100–3111.

Lambert, R. W., Kelleher, R. S., Wickham, L. A., Vaerman, J.-P., and Sullivan, D. A. (1994). Neuroendocrinimmune modulation of secretory component production by rat lacrimal, salivary, and intestinal epithelial cells. *Invest. Ophthalmol. Vis. Sci.* 35, 1192–1201.

Lamm, M. E., and Greenberg, J. (1972). Human secretory component. Comparison of the form occurring in exocrine immunoglobulin A to the free form. *Biochem.* 11, 2744–2750.

Larkin, J. M., and Palade, G. E. (1991). Transcytotic vesicular carriers for polymeric IgA receptors accumulate in rat hepatocytes after bile duct ligation. *J. Cell Sci.* 98, 205–216.

Larkin, J. M., Sztul, E. S., and Palade, G. E. (1986). Phosphorylation of the rat hepatic polymeric IgA receptor. *Proc. Natl. Acad. Sci. USA* 83, 4759–4763.

Larkin, J. M., Woo, B., Balan, V., Marks, D. L., Oswald, B. J., LaRusso, N. F., and McNiven, M. A. (2000). Rab3D, a small GTP-binding protein implicated in regulated secretion, is associated with the transcytotic pathway in rat hepatocytes. *Hepatology* 32, 348–356.

Lawton, A. R., and Mage, R. G. (1969). The synthesis of secretory IgA in the rabbit. I. Evidence for synthesis as an 11S dimer. *J. Immunol.* 102, 693–697.

Lemaitre-Coelho, I., Altamirano, G. A., Barranco-Acosta, C., Meykens, R., and Vaerman, J.-P. (1981). In vivo experiments involving secretory component in the rat: hepatic transfer of polymeric IgA from blood into bile. *Immunol.* 43, 261–270.

Lemaitre-Coelho, I., Jackson, G. D. F., and Vaerman, J. P. (1977). Rat bile as a convenient source of secretory IgA and free secretory component. *Eur. J. Immunol.* 7, 588–590.

Leung, S. M., Ruiz, Wily, G., and Apodaca, G. (2000). Sorting of membrane and fluid at the apical pole of polarized Madin-Darby canine kidney cells. *Mol. Biol. Cell* 11, 2131–2150.

Li, T. W., Wang, J., Lam, J. T., Gutierrez, E. M., Solorzano-Vargus, R. S., Tsai, H. V., and Martín, M. G. (1999). Transcriptional control of the murine polymeric IgA receptor promoter by glucocorticoids. *Am. J. Physiol.* 276, G1425–G1434.

Limet, J. N., Quintart, J., Courtroy, P. J., Vaerman, J. P., and Schneider, Y. J. (1983). Hepatic uptake and transfer into bile of polymeric IgA, anti-secretory component IgG, haptoglobin-hemoglobin complex, galactosylated serum albumin, and horseradish peroxidase: A comparative biochemical study in the rat. *Ann. N.Y. Acad. Sci.* 409, 838–840.

Limet, J. N., Quintart, J., Schneider, Y., and Courtoy, P. J. (1985). Receptor-mediated endocytosis of polymeric IgA and galactosylated serum albumin in rat liver: Evidence for intracellular ligand sorting and identification of distinct endosomal compartments. *Eur. J. Biochem.* 146, 539–548.

Lin, C. -T., Lin, C.-R., Tan, G.-K., Chen, W., Dee, A. N., and Chan, W.-Y. (1997). The mechanism of Epstein-Barr virus infection in nasopharyngeal carcinoma cells. *Am. J. Pathol.* 150, 1745–1756.

Lin, C. T., Kao, H. J., Lin, J. L., Chan, W. Y., Wu, H. C., and Liang, S. T. (2000). Response of nasopharyngeal carcinoma cells to Epstein-Barr virus infection in vitro. *Lab Invest* 80, 1149–1160.

Lindh, E. (1975). Increased resistance of immunoglobulin A dimers to proteolytic degradation after binding of secretory component. *J. Immunol.* 1975, 284–286.

Loman, S., Jansen, H. M., Out, T. A., and Lutter, R. (1999). Interleukin-4 and interferon-γ synergistically increase secretory component gene expression, but are additive in stimulating secretory immunoglobulin A release by Calu-3 airway epithelial cells. *Immunol.* 96, 537–543.

Loman, S., Radl, J., Jansen, H. M., Out, T. A., and Lutter, R. (1997). Vectorial transcytosis of dimeric IgA by the Calu-3 human lung epithelial cell line: Upregulation by IFN-γ. *Am. J. Physiol. Lung Cell. Mol. Physiol.* 272, L951–L958.

Loosli, H., and Hurlimann, J. (1984). Immunohistological study of malignant diffuse mesotheliomas of the pleura. *Histopathology* 8, 793–803.

Lu, L., Lamm, M. E., Li, H., Corthesy, B., and Zhang, J. R. (2003). The human polymeric immunoglobulin receptor binds to *Streptococcus pneumoniae* via domains 3 and 4. *J. Biol. Chem.* 278, 48178–48187.

Lullau, E., Heyse, S., Vogel, H., Marison, I., von Stockar, U., Kraehenbuhl, J. P. and Corthesy, B. (1996). Antigen binding properties of purified immunoglobulin A and reconstituted secretory immunoglobulin A antibodies. *J. Biol. Chem.* 271, 16300–16309.

Luton, F., Verges, M., Vaerman, J. P., Sudol, M., and Mostov, K. E. (1999). The SRC family protein tyrosine kinase p62*yes* controls polymeric IgA transcytosis in vivo. *Mol. Cell* 4, 627–632.

Luton, F., Cardone, M. H., Zhang, M., and Mostov, K. E. (1998). Role of tyrosine phosphorylation in ligand-induced regulation of transcytosis of the polymeric Ig receptor. *Mol. Biol. Cell* 9, 1787–1802.

Luton, F., and Mostov, K. E. (1999). Transduction of basolateral-to-apical signals across epithelial cells: ligand-stimulated transcytosis of the polymeric immunoglobulin receptor requires two signals. *Mol. Biol. Cell* 10, 1409–1427.

Lüscher, B., and Larsson, L. G. (1999). The basic region/helix-loop-helix/leucine zipper domain of Myc proto-oncoproteins: function and regulation. *Oncogene* 18, 2955–2966.

Lycke, N., Erlandsson, L., Ekman, L., Schon, K., and Leanderson, T. (1999). Lack of J chain inhibits the transport of gut IgA and abrogates the development of intestinal antitoxic protection. *J. Immunol.* 163, 913–919.

Ma, J. K. C., Hikmat, B. Y., Wycoff, K., Vine, N. D., Chargelegue, D., Yu, L., Hein, M. B., and Lehner, T. (1998). Characterization of a recombinant plant monoclonal secretory antibody and preventive immunotherapy in humans. *Nature Med.* 4, 601–606.

Marshall, L. J., Perks, B., Ferkol, T., and Shute, J. K. (2001). IL-8 released constitutively by primary bronchial epithelial cells in culture forms an inactive complex with secretory component. *J. Immunol.* 167, 2816–2823.

Martín, M. G., Gutierrez, E. M., Lam, J. T., Li, T. W., and Wang, J. (1997). Genomic cloning and structural analysis of the murine polymeric IgA receptor (pIgR) gene and promoter region. *Gene* 201, 189–197.

Martín, M. G., Wang, J., Li, T. W., Lam, J. T., Gutierrez, E. M., Solorzano-Vargas, R. S., and Tsai, A. H. (1998a). Characterization of the 5′-flanking region of the murine polymeric IgA receptor gene. *Am. J. Physiol.* 275, G778–G788.

Martín, M. G., Wang, J., Li, T. W., Lam, J. T., Gutierrez, E. M., Solorzano-Vargas, R. S., and Tsai, A. H. (1998b). Characterization of the 5′-flanking region of the murine polymeric IgA receptor gene. *Am. J. Physiol.* 275, G778–G788.

Mazanec, M. B., Coudret, C. L., and Fletcher, D. R. (1995). Intracellular neutralization of influenza virus by immunoglobulin A anti-hemagglutinin monoclonal antibodies. *J. Virol.* 69, 1339–1343.

Mazanec, M. B., Kaetzel, C. S., Lamm, M. E., Fletcher, D., and Nedrud, J. G. (1992). Intracellular neutralization of virus by immunoglobulin A antibodies. *Proc. Natl. Acad. Sci. USA* 89, 6901–6905.

Meier, J. L., Luo, X., Sawadogo, M., and Straus, S. E. (1994). The cellular transcription factor USF cooperates with varicella-zoster virus immediate-early protein 62 to symmetrically activate a bidirectional viral promoter. *Mol. Cell Biol.* 14, 6896–6906.

Menge, A. C., and Mestecky, J. (1993). Surface expression of secretory component and HLA class II DR antigen on glandular epithelial cells from human endometrium and two endometrial adenocarcinoma cell lines. *J. Clin. Immunol.* 13, 259–264.

Mestecky, J., Lue, C., and Russell, M. W. (1991). Selective transport of IgA. Cellular and molecular aspects. *Gastroenterol. Clin. North Am.* 20, 441–471.

Mestecky, J., Moldoveanu, Z., Tomana, M., Epps, J. M., Thorpe, S. R., Phillips, J. O., and Kulhavy, R. (1989). The role of the liver in catabolism of mouse and human IgA. *Immunol. Invest.* 18, 313–324.

Mestecky, J., Russell, M. W., Jackson, S., and Brown, T. A. (1986). The human IgA system: A reassessment. *Clin. Immunol. Immunopath.* 40, 105–114.

Mestecky, J., Zikan, J., and Butler, W. T. (1971). Immunoglobulin M and secretory immunoglobulin A: Presence of a common polypeptide chain different from light chains. *Science* 171, 1163–1165.

Miller, M. A., and McCann, L. (2000). Policy analysis of the use of hepatitis B, *Haemophilus influenzae* type b–, *Streptococcus pneumoniae*-conjugate and rotavirus vaccines in national immunization schedules. *Health Econ.* 9, 19–35.

Moldoveanu, Z., Moro, I., Radl, J., Thorpe, S. R., Komiyama, K., and Mestecky, J. (1990). Site of catabolism of autologous and heterologous IgA in non-human primates. *Scand. J. Immunol.* 32, 577–583.

Momotani, E., Ishikawa, Y., and Yoshino, T. (1986). Immunohistochemical distribution of immunoglobulin and secretory component in the ileum of normal and paratuberculosis-infected cattle. *J. Comp. Path.* 96, 659–669.

Monteiro, R. C., and van De Winkel, J. G. (2003). IgA Fc receptors. *Annu. Rev. Immunol.* 21, 177–204.

Moro, I., Saito, I., Asano, M., Takahashi, T., and Iwase, T. (1991). Ontogeny of the secretory IgA system in humans. In: *Immunology of Milk and the Neonate* (eds. J. Mestecky, C. Blair, and P. L. Ogra), 51–57. New York: Plenum Press.

Mostov, K., Su, T., and ter Beest, M. (2003). Polarized epithelial membrane traffic: conservation and plasticity. *Nat. Cell Biol.* 5, 287–293.

Mostov, K. E., and Deitcher, D. L. (1986). Polymeric immunoglobulin receptor expressed in MDCK cells transcytoses IgA. *Cell* 46, 613–621.

Mostov, K. E., Friedlander, M., and Blobel, G. (1984). The receptor for transepithelial transport of IgA and IgM contains multiple immunoglobulin-like domains. *Nature* 308, 37–43.

Mostov, K. E., Kraehenbuhl, J.-P., and Blobel, G. (1980). Receptor-mediated transcellular transport of immunoglobulin: synthesis of secretory component as multiple and larger transmembrane forms. *Proc. Natl. Acad. Sci. USA* 77, 7257–7261.

Mostov, K. E., Verges, M., and Altschuler, Y. (2000). Membrane traffic in polarized epithelial cells. *Curr. Opin. Cell Biol.* 12, 483–490.

Motegi, Y., and Kita, H. (1998). Interaction with secretory component stimulates effector functions of human eosinophils but not of neutrophils. *J. Immunol.* 161, 4340–4346.

Motegi, Y., Kita, H., Kato, M., and Morikawa, A. (2000). Role of secretory IgA, secretory component, and eosinophils in mucosal inflammation. *Int. Arch. Allergy Immunol.* 122 Suppl 1, 25–27.

Mullock, B. M., Dobrota, M., and Hinton, R. H. (1978). Sources of the proteins of rat bile. *Biochim. Biophys. Acta* 543, 497–507.

Mullock, B. M., Hinton, R. H., Dobrota, M., Peppard, J., and Orlans, E. (1979). Endocytic vesicles in liver carry polymeric IgA from serum to bile. *Biochim. Biophys. Acta* 587, 381–391.

Mullock, B. M., Jones, R. S., and Hinton, R. H. (1980). Movement of endocytic shuttle vesicles from the sinusoidal to the bile canalicular face of hepatocytes does not depend on occupation of receptor sites. *FEBS Letters* 113, 201–205.

Musil, L. S., and Baenziger, J. U. (1987a). Cleavage of membrane secretory component to soluble secretory component occurs on the cell surface of rat hepatocyte monolayers. *J. Cell Biol.* 104, 1725–1733.

Musil, L. S., and Baenziger, J. U. (1987b). Intracellular transport and processing of secretory component in cultured rat hepatocytes. *Gastroenterol.* 93, 1194–1204.

Musil, L. S., and Baenziger, J. U. (1988). Proteolytic processing of rat liver membrane secretory component. Cleavage activity is localized to bile canalicular membranes. *J. Biol. Chem.* 263, 15799–15808.

Muthukumar, A. R., Jolly, C. A., Zaman, K., and Fernandes, G. (2000). Calorie restriction decreases proinflammatory cytokines and polymeric Ig receptor expression in the submandibular glands of autoimmune prone (NZB x NZW)F1 mice. *J. Clin. Immunol.* 20, 354–361.

Nagura, H., Brandtzaeg, P., Nakane, P. K., and Brown, W. R. (1979a). Ultrastructural localization of J chain in human intestinal mucosa. *J. Immunol.* 123, 1044–1050.

Nagura, H., Nakane, P. K., and Brown, W. R. (1978). Breast milk IgA binds to jejunal epithelium in suckling rats. *J. Immunol.* 120, 1333–1339.

Nagura, H., Nakane, P. K., and Brown, W. R. (1979b). Translocation of dimeric IgA through neoplastic colon cells in vitro. *J. Immunol.* 123, 2359–2368.

Nagura, H., Smith, P. D., Nakane, P. K., and Brown, W. R. (1981). IgA in human bile and liver. *J. Immunol.* 126, 587–595.

Nagura, H., Tsutsumi, Y., Hasegawa, H., Watanabe, K., and Nakane, P. K. (1983). IgA plasma cells in biliary mucosa: a likely source of locally synthesized IgA in human hepatic bile. *Clin. Exp. Immunol.* 54, 671–680.

Natvig, I. B., Johansen, F. E., Nordeng, T. W., Haraldsen, G., and Brandtzaeg, P. (1997). Mechanism for enhanced external transfer of dimeric IgA over pentameric IgM. Studies of diffusion, binding to the human polymeric Ig receptor, and epithelial transcytosis. *J. Immunol.* 159, 4330–4340.

Nelson, W. J., and Yeaman, Charles (2001). Protein trafficking in the exocytic pathway of polarized epithelial cells. *Trends Cell Biol.* 11, 483–486.

Nihei, Y., Maruyama, K., Endo, Y., Sato, T., Kobayashi, K., and Kaneko, F. (1996). Secretory component (polymeric immunoglobulin receptor) expression on human keratinocytes by stimulation with interferon-γ and differences in response. *J. Dermatol. Sci.* 11, 214–222.

Nilsen, E. M., Johansen, F. E., Kvale, D., Krajci, P., and Brandtzaeg, P. (1999). Different regulatory pathways employed in cytokine-enhanced expression of secretory component and epithelial HLA class I genes. *Eur. J. Immunol.* 29, 168–179.

Norderhaug, I. N., Johansen, F. E., Krajci, P., and Brandtzaeg, P. (1999a). Domain deletions in the human polymeric Ig receptor disclose differences between its dimeric IgA and pentameric IgM interaction. *Eur. J. Immunol.* 29, 3401–3409.

Norderhaug, I. N., Johansen, F. E., Schjerven, H., and Brandtzaeg, P. (1999b). Regulation of the formation and external transport of secretory immunoglobulins. *Crit. Rev. Immunol.* 19, 481–508.

O'Daly, J. ., Craig, S. W., and Cebra, J. J. (1971). Localization of b markers, alpha-chain and SC of SIgA in epithelial cells lining Lieberkuhn crypts. *J. Immunol.* 106, 286–288.

Obara, W., Iida, A., Suzuki, Y., Tanaka, T., Akiyama, F., Maeda, S., Ohnishi, Y., Yamada, R., Tsunoda, T., Takei, T., Ito, K., Honda, K., Uchida, K., Tsuchiya, K., Yumura, W., Ujiie, T., Nagane, Y., Nitta, K., Miyano, S., Narita, I., Gejyo, F., Nihei, H., Fujioka, T., and Nakamura, Y. (2003). Association of single-nucleotide polymorphisms in the polymeric immunoglobulin receptor gene with immunoglobulin A nephropathy (IgAN) in Japanese patients. *J. Hum. Genet.* 48, 293–299.

Ogra, S. S., Ogra, P. L., Lippes, J., and Tomasi, T. B. (1972). Immunohistologic localization of immunoglobulins, secretory component, and lactoferrin in the developing human fetus. *Proc. Soc. Exp. Biol. Med.* 139, 570–574.

Okada, T., Konishi, H., Ito, M., Nagura, H., and Asai, J. (1988). Identification of secretory immunoglobulin A in human sweat and sweat glands. *J. Invest. Dermatol.* 90, 648–651.

Okamoto, C. T., Shia, S.-P., Bird, C., Mostov, K. E., and Roth, M. G. (1992). The cytoplasmic domain of the polymeric immunoglobulin receptor contains two internalization signals that are distinct from its basolateral sorting signal. *J. Biol. Chem.* 267, 9925–9932.

Ordonez, N. G. (1989). The immunohistochemical diagnosis of mesothelioma. Differentiation of mesothelioma and lung adenocarcinoma. *Am. J. Surg. Pathol.* 13, 276–291.

Orlans, E., Peppard, J., Fry, J. F., Hinton, R. H., and Mullock, B. M. (1979). Secretory component as the receptor for polymeric IgA on rat hepatocytes. *J. Exp. Med.* 150, 1577–1581.

Orlans, E., Peppard, J., Reynolds, J., and Hall, J. (1978). Rapid active transport of immunoglobulin A from blood to bile. *J. Exp. Med.* 147, 588–592.

Orlans, E., Peppard, J. V., Payne, A. W. R., Fitzharris, B. M., Mullock, B. M., Hinton, R. H., and Hall, J. G. (1983). Comparative aspects of the hepatobiliary transport of IgA. *Ann. N. Y. Acad. Sci.* 409, 411–427.

Orzech, E., Cohen, S., Weiss, A., and Aroeti, B. (2000). Interactions between the exocytic and endocytic pathways in polarized Madin-Darby canine kidney cells. *J. Biol. Chem.* 275, 15207–15219.

Pahud, J. -J., and Mach, J.-P. (1972). Equine secretory IgA and secretory component. *Int. Arch. Allergy* 42, 175–186.

Pal, K., Kaetzel, C. S., and Cuff, C. F. (2003). Regulation of polyimmunoglobulin receptor expression following reovirus infection. *American Association of Immunologists 90th Annual Meeting, Denver, CO.* Abstract 42.10.

Pappo, J., and Owen, R. L. (1988). Absence of secretory component expression by epithelial cells overlying rabbit gut–associated lymphoid tissue. *Gastroenterol.* 95, 1173–1177.

Parr, M. B., and Parr, E. L. (1989a). Immunohistochemical investigation of secretory component and immunoglobulin A in the genital tract of the female rat. *J. Reprod. Fert.* 85, 105–113.

Parr, M. B., and Parr, E. L. (1989b). Immunohistochemical localization of secretory component and immunoglobulin A in the urogenital tract of the male rodent. *J. Reprod. Fert.* 85, 115–124.

Peppard, J. V., Hobbs, S. M., Jackson, L. E., Rose, M. E., and Mockett, A. P. A. (1986). Biochemical characterization of chicken secretory component. *Eur. J. Immunol.* 16, 225–229.

Perez, J. H., Wight, D. G. D., Wyatt, J. I., Van Schaik, M., Mullock, B. M., and Luzio, J. P. (1989). The polymeric immunoglobulin A receptor is present on hepatocytes in human liver. *Immunol.* 68, 474–478.

Perry, M. E. (1994). The specialised structure of crypt epithelium in the human palatine tonsil and its functional significance. *J. Anat.* 185, 111–127.

Peters, I. R., Helps, C. R., Batt, R. M., Day, M. J., and Hall, E. J. (2003). Quantitative real-time RT-PCR measurement of mRNA encoding alpha-chain, pIgR and J-chain from canine duodenal mucosa. *J. Immunol. Methods* 275, 213–222.

Pfeffer, S. R. (2001). Rab GTPases: specifying and deciphering organelle identity and function. *Trends Cell Biol.* 11, 487–491.

Phalipon, A., Cardona, A., Kraehenbuhl, J. P., Edelman, L., Sansonetti, P. J., and Corthesy, B. (2002). Secretory component: a new role in secretory IgA-mediated immune exclusion in vivo. *Immunity* 17, 107–115.

Phalipon, A., and Corthesy, B. (2003). Novel functions of the polymeric Ig receptor: well beyond transport of immunoglobulins. *Trends Immunol.* 24, 55–58.

Phalipon, A., and Sansonetti, P. J. (1999). Microbial-host interactions at mucosal sites. Host response to pathogenic bacteria at mucosal sites. *Curr. Top. Microbiol. Immunol* 236, 163–189.

Phillips-Quagliata, J.M., Patel, S., Han, J. K., Arakelov, S., Rao, T. D., Shulman, M. J., Fazel, S., Corley, R. B., Everett, M., Klein, M. H., Underdown, B. J., and Corthesy, B. (2000). The IgA/IgM receptor expressed on a murine B cell lymphoma is poly-Ig receptor. *J. Immunol.* 165, 2544–2555.

Phillips, J. O., Everson, M. P., Moldoveanu, Z., Lue, C., and Mestecky, J. (1990). Synergistic effect of IL-4 and IFN-γ on the expression of polymeric Ig receptor (secretory component) and IgA binding by human epithelial cells. *J. Immunol.* 145, 1740–1744.

Phillips, J. O., Komiyama, K., Epps, J. M., Russell, M. W., and Mestecky, J. (1988). Role of hepatocytes in the uptake of IgA and IgA-containing immune complexes in mice. *Mol. Immunol.* 25, 873–879.

Phillips, J. O., Russell, M. W., Brown, T. A., and Mestecky, J. (1984). Selective hepatobiliary transport of human polymeric IgA in mice. *Mol. Immunol.* 21, 907–914.

Pilette, C., Godding, V., Kiss, R., Delos, M., Verbeken, E., Decaestecker, C., De Paepe, K., Vaerman, J. P., Decramer, M., and Sibille, Y. (2001). Reduced epithelial expression of secretory component in small airways correlates with airflow obstruction in chronic obstructive pulmonary disease. *Am. J. Respir. Crit Care Med.* 163, 185–194.

Pilette, C., Ouadrhiri, Y., Dimanche, F., Vaerman, J. P., and Sibille, Y. (2003). Secretory component is cleaved by neutrophil serine proteinases but its epithelial production is increased by neutrophils through NF-kappa B- and p38 mitogen-activated protein kinase-dependent mechanisms. *Am. J. Respir. Cell Mol. Biol.* 28, 485–498.

Piskurich, J. F., Blanchard, M. H., Youngman, K. R., France, J. A., and Kaetzel, C. S. (1995). Molecular cloning of the mouse polymeric Ig receptor. Functional regions of the molecule are conserved among five mammalian species. *J. Immunol.* 154, 1735–1747.

Piskurich, J. F., France, J. A., Tamer, C. M., Willmer, C. A., Kaetzel, C. S., and Kaetzel, D. M. (1993). Interferon-γ induces polymeric immunoglobulin receptor mRNA in human intestinal epithelial cells by a protein synthesis dependent mechanism. *Mol. Immunol.* 30, 413–421.

Piskurich, J. F., Youngman, K. R., Phillips, K. M., Hempen, P. M., Blanchard, M. H., France, J. A., and Kaetzel, C. S. (1997). Transcriptional regulation of the human polymeric immunoglobulin receptor gene by interferon-γ. *Mol. Immunol.* 34, 75–91.

Poger, M. E., Hirsch, B. R., and Lamm, M. E. (1976). Synthesis of secretory component by colonic neoplasms. *Am. J. Pathol.* 82, 327–338.

Poger, M. E., and Lamm, M. E. (1974). Localization of free and bound secretory component in human intestinal epithelial cells. A model for the assembly of secretory IgA. *J. Exp. Med.* 139, 629–642.

Pol, A., Ortega, D., and Enrich, C. (1997). Identification and distribution of proteins in isolated endosomal fractions of rat liver: Involvement in endocytosis, recycling and transcytosis. *Biochem. J.* 323, 435–443.

Popper, H., Wirnsberger, G., Hoefler, H., and Denk, H. (1987). Immunohistochemical and histochemical markers of primary lung cancer, lung metastases, and pleural mesotheliomas. *Cancer Detect. Prev.* 10, 167–174.

Prabhala, R. H., and Wira, C. R. (1991). Cytokine regulation of the mucosal immune system: *In vivo* stimulation by interferon-γ of secretory component and immunoglobulin A in uterine secretions and proliferation of lymphocytes from spleen. *Endocrinology* 129, 2915–2923.

Prigent-Delecourt, L., Coffin, B., Colombel, J. F., Dehennin, J. P., Vaerman, J.-P., and Rambaud, J. C. (1995). Secretion of immunoglobulins and plasma proteins from the colonic mucosa: an *in vivo* study in man. *Clin. Exp. Immunol.* 99, 221–225.

Proctor, G. B., and Carpenter, G. H. (2001). Chewing stimulates secretion of human salivary secretory immunoglobulin A. *J. Dent. Res.* 80, 909–913.

Proctor, G. B., Carpenter, G. H., and Garrett, J. R. (2000). Sympathetic decentralization abolishes increased secretion of immunoglobulin A evoked by parasympathetic stimulation of rat submandibular glands. *J. Neuroimmunol.* 109, 147–154.

Pudney, J., and Anderson, D. J. (1995). Immunobiology of the human penile urethra. *Am. J. Pathol.* 147, 155–165.

Quesnel, A., Cu-Uvin, S., Murphy, D., Ashley, R. L., Flanigan, T., and Neutra, M. R. (1997). Comparative analysis of methods for collection and measurement of immunoglobulins in cervical and vaginal secretions of women. *J. Immunol. Methods* 202, 153–161.

Reich, V., Mostov, K., and Aroeti, B. (1996). The basolateral sorting signal of the polymeric immunoglobulin receptor contains two functional domains. *J. Cell Sci.* 109, 2133–2139.

Remington, J. S., and Schafer, I. A. (1968). Transport piece in the urines of premature infants. *Nature* 217, 364–365.

Renegar, K. B., Jackson, G. D., and Mestecky, J. (1998). In vitro comparison of the biologic activities of monoclonal monomeric IgA, polymeric IgA, and secretory IgA. *J. Immunol.* 160, 1219–1223.

Renston, R. H., Jones, A. L., Christiansen, W. D., Hradek, G. T., and Underdown, B. J. (1980). Evidence for a vesicular transport mechanism in hepatocytes for biliary secretion of immunoglobulin A. *Science* 208, 1276–1278.

Rice, J. C., Spence, J. S., Megyesi, J., Goldblum, R. M., and Safirstein, R. L. (1999). Expression of the polymeric immunoglobulin receptor and excretion of secretory IgA in the postischemic kidney. *Am. J. Physiol* 276, F666–F673.

Rice, J. C., Spence, J. S., Megyesi, J., Safirstein, R. L., and Goldblum, R. M. (1998). Regulation of the polymeric immunoglobulin receptor

by water intake and vasopressin in the rat kidney. *Am. J. Physiol.* 274, F966–F977.

Richardson, J., Kaushic, C., and Wira, C. R. (1993). Estradiol regulation of secretory component: Expression by rat uterine epithelial cells. *J. Steroid Biochem. Mol. Biol.* 47, 143–149.

Richardson, J. M., Kaushic, C., and Wira, C. R. (1995). Polymeric immunoglobulin (Ig) receptor production and IgA transcytosis in polarized primary cultures of mature rat uterine epithelial cells. *Biol. Reprod.* 53, 488–498.

Rifai, A., and Mannik, M. (1984). Clearance of circulating IgA immune complexes is mediated by a specific receptor on Kupffer cells in mice. *J. Exp. Med.* 160, 125–137.

Rifai, A., Schena, F. P., Montinaro, V., Mele, M., D'Addabbo, A., Nitti, L., and Pezzullo, J. C. (1989). Clearance kinetics and fate of macromolecular IgA in patients with IgA nephropathy. *Lab. Invest.* 61, 381–388.

Rincheval-Arnold, A., Belair, L., Cencic, A., and Djiane, J. (2002a). Upregulation of polymeric immunoglobulin receptor mRNA in mammary epithelial cells by IFN-γ. *Mol. Cell Endocrinol.* 194, 95–105.

Rincheval-Arnold, A., Belair, L., and Djiane, J. (2002b). Developmental expression of pIgR gene in sheep mammary gland and hormonal regulation. *J. Dairy Res.* 69, 13–26.

Robinson, J. K., Blanchard, T. G., Levine, A. D., Emancipator, S. N., and Lamm, M. E. (2001). A mucosal IgA-mediated excretory immune system in vivo. *J. Immunol.* 166, 3688–3692.

Roccatello, D., Picciotto, G., Ropolo, R., Coppo, R., Quattrocchio, G., Cacace, G., Molino, A., Amoroso, A., Baccega, M., Isidoro, C., Cardosi, R., Sena, L. M., and Piccoli, G. (1992). Kinetics and fate of IgA-IgG aggregates as a model of naturally occurring immune complexes in IgA nephropathy. *Lab. Invest.* 66, 86–95.

Roe, M., Norderhaug, I. N., Brandtzaeg, P., and Johansen, F. E. (1999). Fine specificity of ligand-binding domain 1 in the polymeric Ig receptor: importance of the CDR2-containing region for IgM interaction. *J. Immunol.* 162, 6046–6052.

Rognum, T., Elgjo, K., Brandtzaeg, P., Orjasaeter, H., and Bergan, A. (1982). Plasma carcinoembryonic antigen concentrations and immunohistochemical patterns of epithelial marker antigens in patients with large bowel carcinoma. *J. Clin. Pathol.* 35, 922–933.

Rognum, T. O., Brandtzaeg, P., Elgjo, K., and Fausa, O. (1987). Heterogeneous epithelial expression of class II (HLA-DR) determinants and secretory component related to dysplasia in ulcerative colitis. *Br. J. Cancer* 56, 419–424.

Rognum, T. O., Brandtzaeg, P., Orjasaeter, H., Elgjo, K., and Hognestad, J. (1980). Immunohistochemical study of secretory component, secretory IgA and carcinoembryonic antigen in large bowel carcinomas. *Path. Res. Pract.* 170, 126–145.

Rojas, R., and Apodaca, G. (2002). Immunoglobulin transport across polarized epithelial cells. *Nat. Rev. Mol. Cell. Biol.* 3, 944–955.

Rosato, R., Jammes, H., Belair, L., Puissant, C., Kraehenbuhl, J.-P., and Djiane, J. (1995). Polymeric-Ig receptor gene expression in rabbit mammary gland during pregnancy and lactation: evolution and hormonal regulation. *Mol. Cell. Endocrinol.* 110, 81–87.

Rossel, M., Brambilla, E., Billaud, M., Vuitton, D. A., Blanc-Jouvan, F., Biichle, S., and Revillard, J. P. (1993). Nonspecific increased serum levels of secretory component in lung tumors: Relationship to the gene expression of the transmembrane receptor form. *Am. J. Respir. Cell Mol. Biol.* 9, 341–346.

Rossen, R. D., Morgan, M., Hsu, K. C., Butler, W. T., and Rose, H. M. (1968). Localization of 11 S external secretory IgA by immunofluorescence in tissues lining the oral and respiratory passages in man. *J. Immunol.* 100, 706–717.

Ruggeri, F. M., Johansen, K., Basile, G., Kraehenbuhl, J. P., and Svensson, L. (1998). Antirotavirus immunoglobulin A neutralizes virus in vitro after transcytosis through epithelial cells and protects infant mice from diarrhea. *J. Virol.* 72, 2708–2714.

Russell, M. W., Brown, T. A., Claflin, J. L., Schroer, K., and Mestecky, J. (1983). Immunoglobulin A–mediated hepatobiliary transport constitutes a natural pathway for disposing of bacterial antigens. *Infect. Immun.* 42, 1041–1048.

Russell, M. W., Brown, T. A., and Mestecky, J. (1981). Role of serum IgA. Hepatobiliary transport of circulating antigen. *J. Exp. Med.* 153, 968–976.

Rümke, P. (1974). The origin of immunoglobulins in semen. *Clin. Exp. Immunol.* 17, 287–297.

Saito, H., Kasajima, T., and Nagura, H. (1985). An immunocytochemical study on secretory mechanism of IgA in human pancreas. *Acta Pathol. Jpn.* 35, 87–101.

Sarkar, J., Gangopadhyay, N. N., Moldoveanu, Z., Mestecky, J., and Stephensen, C. B. (1998). Vitamin A is required for regulation of polymeric immunoglobulin receptor (pIgR) expression by interleukin-4 and interferon-γ in a human intestinal epithelial cell line. *J. Nutr.* 128, 1063–1069.

Sato, T. (1998). Mapping of mouse polymeric immunoglobulin receptor (PIgR) gene using simple sequence length polymorphism markers. *Genes Genet. Syst.* 73, 271–273.

Saucan, L., and Palade, G. E. (1994). Membrane and secretory proteins are transported from the Golgi complex to the sinusoidal plasmalemma of hepatocytes by distinct vesicular carriers. *J. Cell Biol.* 125, 733–741.

Schiff, J. M., Fisher, M. M., Jones, A. L., and Underdown, B. J. (1986). Human IgA as a heterovalent ligand: Switching from the asialoglycoprotein receptor to secretory component during transport across the rat hepatocyte. *J. Cell Biol.* 102, 920–931.

Schiff, J. M., Fisher, M. M., and Underdown, B. J. (1984). Receptor-mediated biliary transport of immunoglobulin A and asialoglycoprotein: sorting and missorting of ligands revealed by two radiolabeling methods. *J. Cell Biol.* 98, 79–89.

Schjerven, H., Brandtzaeg, P., and Johansen, F. E. (2000). Mechanism of IL-4-mediated up-regulation of the polymeric Ig receptor: role of STAT6 in cell type–specific delayed transcriptional response. *J. Immunol.* 165, 3898–3906.

Schjerven, H., Brandtzaeg, P., and Johansen, F. E. (2001). A novel NF-kappa B/Rel site in intron 1 cooperates with proximal promoter elements to mediate TNF-α-induced transcription of the human polymeric Ig receptor. *J. Immunol.* 167, 6412–6420.

Schjerven, H., Brandtzaeg, P., and Johansen, F. E. (2003). Hepatocyte NF-1 and STAT6 cooperate with additional DNA-binding factors to activate transcription of the human polymeric Ig receptor gene in response to IL-4. *J. Immunol.* 170, 6048–6056.

Schneeman, T. A., and Kaetzel, C. S. (2003). Regulation of the polymeric Ig receptor by Toll-like receptors. American Association of Immunologists 90th Anniversary Annual Meeting, Abstract 118.16.

Schwartz-Cornil, I., Benureau, Y., Greenberg, H., Hendrickson, B. A., and Cohen, J. (2002). Heterologous protection induced by the inner capsid proteins of rotavirus requires transcytosis of mucosal immunoglobulins. *J. Virol.* 76, 8110–8117.

Scott, H., Brandtzaeg, P., Solheim, B. G., and Thorsby, E. (1981). Relation between HLA-DR-like antigens and secretory component (SC) in jejunal epithelium of patients with coeliac disease or dermatitis herpetiformis. *Clin. Exp. Immunol.* 44, 233–238.

Sharp, P. A. (1992). TATA-binding protein is a classless factor. *Cell* 68, 819–821.

Sheff, D. R., Kroschewski, Ruth and Mellman, Ira (2002). Actin Dependence of polarized receptor recycling in Madin-Darby canine kidney cell endosomes. *Mol. Biol. Cell* 13, 262–275.

Sheldrake, R. F., Husband, A. J., Watson, D. L., and Cripps, A. W. (1984). Selective transport of serum-derived IgA into mucosal secretions. *J. Immunol.* 132, 363–368.

Shimada, S., Kawaguchi-Miyashita, M., Kushiro, A., Sato, T., Nanno, M., Sako, T., Matsuoka, Y., Sudo, K., Tagawa, Y., Iwakura, Y., and Ohwaki, M. (1999). Generation of polymeric immunoglobulin receptor-deficient mouse with marked reduction of secretory IgA. *J. Immunol.* 163, 5367–5373.

Simmen, T., Honing, S., Icking, A., Tikkanen, R., and Hunziker, W. (2002). AP-4 binds basolateral signals and participates in basolateral sorting in epithelial MDCK cells. *Nat. Cell Biol.* 4, 154–159.

Singer, K. L., and Mostov, Keith E. (1998). Dimerization of the polymeric immunoglobulin receptor controls Its transcytotic trafficking. *Mol. Biol. Cell* 9, 901–915.

Sirito, M., Lin, Q., Deng, J. M., Behringer, R. R., and Sawadogo, M. (1998). Overlapping roles and asymmetrical cross-regulation of the USF proteins in mice. *Proc. Natl. Acad. Sci. USA* 95, 3758–3763.

Sixbey, J. W., and Yao, Q. Y. (1992). Immunoglobulin A–induced shift of Epstein-Barr virus tissue tropism. *Science* 255, 1578–1580.

Socken, D. J., Simms, E. S., Nagy, B. R., Fisher, M. M., and Underdown, B. J. (1981). Secretory component–dependent hepatic transport of IgA antibody-antigen complexes. *J. Immunol.* 127, 316–319.

Socken, D. J., and Underdown, B. J. (1978). Comparison of human, bovine and rabbit secretory component–immunoglobulin interactions. *Immunochem.* 15, 499–506.

Solari, R., Racine, L., Tallichet, C., and Kraehenbuhl, J.-P. (1986). Distribution and processing of the polymeric immunoglobulin receptor in the rat hepatocyte: Morphological and biochemical characterization of subcellular fractions. *J. Histochem.* Cytochem. 34, 17–23.

Solari, R., Schaerer, E., Tallichet, C., Braiterman, L. T., Hubbard, A. L., and Kraehenbuhl, J.-P. (1989). Cellular location of the cleavage event of the polymeric immunoglobulin receptor and fate of its anchoring domain in the rat hepatocyte. *Biochem. J.* 257, 759–768.

Sollid, L. M., Kvale, D., Brandtzaeg, P., Markussen, G., and Thorsby, E. (1987). Interferon-γ enhances expression of secretory component, the epithelial receptor for polymeric immunoglobulins. *J. Immunol.* 138, 4303–4306.

Solorzano-Vargas, R. S., Wang, J., Jiang, L., Tsai, H. V., Ontiveros, L. O., Vazir, M. A., Aguilera, R. J., and Martín, M. G. (2002). Multiple transcription factors in 5′-flanking region of human polymeric Ig receptor control its basal expression. *Am. J. Physiol Gastrointest. Liver Physiol.* 283, G415–G425.

Song, W., Bomsel, M., Casanova, J., Vaerman, J.-P., and Mostov, K. (1994). Stimulation of transcytosis of the polymeric immunoglobulin receptor by dimeric IgA. *Proc. Natl. Acad. Sci. USA* 91, 163–166.

Spohn, M., and McColl, I. (1979a). Studies on human gastric mucosal immunoglobulin A. *Biochim. Biophys. Acta* 576, 1–8.

Spohn, M., and McColl, I. (1979b). Studies on human gastric mucosal immunoglobulin A II. Further evidence for the absence of the secretory component from the predominant immunoglobulin A of human gastric mucus. *Biochim. Biophys. Acta* 576, 9–16.

Stern, J. E., Gardner, S., Quirk, D., and Wira, C. R. (1992). Secretory immune system of the male reproductive tract: effects of dihydrotestosterone and estradiol on IgA and secretory component levels. *J. Reprod. Immunol.* 22, 73–85.

Stern, J. E., and Wira, C. R. (1986). Immunoglobulin and secretory component regulation in the rat uterus at the time of decidualization. *Endocrinol.* 119, 2427–2432.

Stern, J. E., and Wira, C. R. (1988). Progesterone regulation of secretory component (SC): uterine SC response in organ culture following in vivo hormone treatment. *J. Steroid Biochem.* 30, 233–237.

Stockert, R. J., Kressner, M. S., Collins, J. C., Sternlieb, I., and Morell, A. G. (1982). IgA interaction with the asialoglycoprotein receptor. *Proc. Natl. Acad. Sci. USA* 79, 6229–6231.

Sullivan, D. A., Bloch, K. J., and Allansmith, M. R. (1984a). Hormonal influence on the secretory immune system of the eye: Androgen regulation of secretory component levels in rat tears. *J. Immunol.* 132, 1130–1135.

Sullivan, D. A., Richardson, G. S., MacLaughlin, D. T., and Wira, C. R. (1984b). Variations in the levels of secretory component in human uterine fluid during the menstrual cycle. *J. Steroid Biochem.* 20, 509–513.

Sullivan, D. A., Underdown, B. J., and Wira, C. R. (1983). Steroid hormone regulation of free secretory component in the rat uterus. *Immunol.* 49, 379–386.

Sullivan, D. A., Vaerman, J.-P., and Soo, C. (1993). Influence of severe protein malnutrition on rat lacrimal, salivary and gastrointestinal immune expression during development, adulthood and ageing. *Immunol.* 78, 308–317.

Sullivan, D. A., and Wira, C. R. (1983). Variations in free secretory component levels in mucosal secretions of the rat. *J. Immunol.* 130, 1330–1335.

Sun, F. J., Kaur, S., Ziemer, D., Banerjee, S., Samuelson, L. C., and De Lisle, R. C. (2003). Decreased gastric bacterial killing and up-regulation of protective genes in small intestine in gastrin-deficient mouse. *Dig. Dis. Sci.* 48, 976–985.

Svanborg Edén, C., Kulhavy, R., Prince, S. J., and Mestecky, J. (1985). Urinary immunoglobulins in healthy individuals and children with acute pyelonephritis. *Scand. J. Immunol.* 21, 305–313.

Sztul, E. S., Howell, K. E., and Palade, G. E. (1983). Intracellular and transcellular transport of secretory component and albumin in rat hepatocytes. *J. Cell Biol.* 97, 1582–1591.

Sztul, E. S., Howell, K. E., and Palade, G. E. (1985a). Biogenesis of the polymeric IgA receptor in rat hepatocytes. II. Localization of its intracellular forms by cell fractionation studies. *J. Cell Biol.* 100, 1255–1261.

Sztul, E. S., Howell, K. E., and Palade, G. E. (1985b). Biogenesis of the polymeric IgA receptor in rat hepatocytes. I. Kinetic studies of its intracellular forms. *J. Cell Biol.* 100, 1248–1254.

Takahashi, I., Nakane, P. K., and Brown, W. R. (1982). Ultrastructural events in the translocation of polymeric IgA by rat hepatocytes. *J. Immunol.* 128, 1181–1187.

Takeda, K., and Akira, S. (2003). Toll receptors and pathogen resistance. *Cell Microbiol.* 5, 143–153.

Takemura, T., and Eishi, Y. (1985). Distribution of secretory component and immunoglobulins in the developing lung. *Am. Rev. Respir. Dis.* 131, 125–130.

Takenouchi-Ohkubo, N., Takahashi, T., Tsuchiya, M., Mestecky, J., Moldoveanu, Z., and Moro, I. (2000). Role of nuclear factor-kappaB in the expression by tumor necrosis factor-α of the human polymeric immunoglobulin receptor (pIgR) gene. *Immunogenetics* 51, 289–295.

Tamer, C. M., Lamm, M. E., Robinson, J. K., Piskurich, J. F., and Kaetzel, C. S. (1995). Comparative studies of transcytosis and assembly of secretory IgA in Madin-Darby canine kidney cells expressing human polymeric Ig receptor. *J. Immunol.* 155, 707–714.

Taylor, C. L., Harrison, G. A., Watson, C. M., and Deane, E. M. (2002). cDNA cloning of the polymeric immunoglobulin receptor of the marsupial *Macropus eugenii* (tammar wallaby). *Eur. J. Immunogenet.* 29, 87–93.

Thrane, P. S., Rognum, T. O., and Brandtzaeg, P. (1991). Ontogenesis of the secretory immune system and innate defence factors in human parotid glands. *Clin. Exp. Immunol.* 86, 342–348.

Thrane, P. S., Rognum, T. O., and Brandtzaeg, P. (1994). Up-regulated epithelial expression of HLA-DR and secretory component in salivary glands: reflection of mucosal immunostimulation in sudden infant death syndrome. *Ped. Res.* 35, 625–628.

Thrane, P. S., Sollid, L. M., Haanes, H. R., and Brandtzaeg, P. (1992). Clustering of IgA-producing immunocytes related to HLA-DR-positive ducts in normal and inflamed salivary glands. *Scand. J. Immunol.* 35, 43–51.

Tolleshaug, H., Brandtzaeg, P., and Holte, K. (1981). Quantitative study of the uptake of IgA by isolated rat hepatocytes. *Scand. J. Immunol.* 13, 47–56.

Tomana, M., Kulhavy, R., and Mestecky, J. (1988). Receptor-mediated binding and uptake of immunoglobulin A by human liver. *Gastroenterol.* 94, 762–770.

Tomana, M., Phillips, J. O., Kulhavy, R., and Mestecky, J. (1985). Carbohydrate-mediated clearance of secretory IgA from the circulation. *Mol. Immunol.* 22, 887–892.

Tomasi, T. B., Tan, E. M., Solomon, A., and Prendergast, R. A. (1965). Characteristics of an immune system common to certain external secretions. *J. Exp. Med.* 121, 101–124.

Tomasi, T. B., and Yurchak, A. M. (1972). The synthesis of secretory component by the human thymus. *J. Immunol.* 108, 1132–1135.

Tourville, D. R., Adler, R. H., Bienenstock, J., and Tomasi, T. B. (1969). The human secretory immunoglobulin system: immunohistological localization of γA, secretory piece and lactoferrin in normal human tissues. *J. Exp. Med.* 129, 411–429.

Tourville, D. R., Ogra, S. S., Lippes, J., and Tomasi, T. B. (1970). The human female reproductive tract: Immunohistological localization of gA, gG, gM, secretory "piece," and lactoferrin. *Amer. J. Obstet. Gynecol.* 108, 1102–1108.

Traicoff, J. L., De Marchis, L., Ginsburg, B. L., Zamora, R. E., Khattar, N. H., Blanch, V. J., Plummer, S., Bargo, S. A., Templeton, D. J., Casey, G., and Kaetzel, C. S. (2003). Characterization of the human polymeric immunoglobulin receptor (*PIGR*) 3'UTR and differential expression of *PIGR* mRNA during colon tumorigenesis. *J. Biomed. Sci.*, 10, 792–804.

Tuma, P. L., Nyasae, Lydia K., Backer, Jonathan M., and Hubbard, Ann L. (2001). Vps34p differentially regulates endocytosis from the apical and basolateral domains in polarized hepatic cells. *J. Cell Biol.* 154, 1197–1208.

Tuma, P. L., Nyasae, Lydia K., and Hubbard, Ann L. (2002). Nonpolarized cells selectively sort apical proteins from cell surface to a novel compartment, but lack apical retention mechanisms. *Mol. Biol. Cell* 13, 3400–3415.

Uehling, D. T. (1971). Secretory IgA in seminal fluid. *Fertil. Steril.* 22, 769–773.

Uehling, D. T., and Steihm, E. R. (1971). Elevated urinary secretory IgA in children with urinary tract infection. *Pediatrics* 47, 40–46.

Underdown, B. J., Switzer, I., and Jackson, G. D. F. (1992). Rat secretory component binds poorly to rodent IgM. *J. Immunol.* 149, 487–491.

Uren, T. K., Johansen, F. E., Wijburg, O. L., Koentgen, F., Brandtzaeg, P., and Strugnell, R. A. (2003). Role of the polymeric Ig receptor in mucosal B cell homeostasis. *J. Immunol.* 170, 2531–2539.

Vaerman, J. P., and Langendries, A. (1997). Hepatobiliary transport of IgA in the golden Syrian hamster (*Mesocricetus auratus*). *Immunol. Lett.* 55, 19–26.

Vaerman, J. P., Langendries, A., Giffroy, D., Brandtzaeg, P., and Kobayashi, K. (1998a). Lack of SC/pIgR-mediated epithelial transport of a human polymeric IgA devoid of J chain: in vitro and in vivo studies. *Immunol.* 95, 90–96.

Vaerman, J. P., Langendries, A. E., Giffroy, D. A., Kaetzel, C. S., Fiani, C. M., Moro, I., Brandtzaeg, P., and Kobayashi, K. (1998b). Antibody against the human J chain inhibits polymeric Ig receptor–mediated biliary and epithelial transport of human polymeric IgA. *Eur. J. Immunol.* 28, 171–182.

Valnes, K., Brandtzaeg, P., Elgjo, K., and Stave, R. (1984). Specific and nonspecific humoral defense factors in the epithelium of normal and inflamed gastric mucosa. Immunohistochemical localization of immunoglobulins, secretory component, lysozyme, and lactoferrin. *Gastroenterology* 86, 402–412.

van der Feltz, M. J., de Groot, N., Bayley, J. P., Lee, S. H., Verbeet, M. P., and De Boer, H. A. (2001). Lymphocyte homing and Ig secretion in the murine mammary gland. *Scand. J. Immunol.* 54, 292–300.

van Egmond, M., van Garderen, E., van Spriel, A. B., Damen, C. A., van Amersfoort, E. S., van Zandbergen, G., van Hattum, J., Kuiper, J., and van De Winkel, J. G. (2000). FcαRI-positive liver Kupffer cells: reappraisal of the function of immunoglobulin A in immunity. *Nat. Med.* 6, 680–685.

van Ijzendoorn, S. C., Maier, O., Van Der Wouden, J. M., and Hoekstra, D. (2000). The subapical compartment and its role in intracellular trafficking and cell polarity. *J Cell Physiol* 184, 151–160.

van Ijzendoorn, S. C., Tuvim, M. J., Weimbs, T., Dickey, B. F., and Mostov, K. E. (2002). Direct interaction between Rab3b and the polymeric immunoglobulin receptor controls ligand-stimulated transcytosis in epithelial cells. *Dev. Cell* 2, 219–228.

van Ijzendoorn, S. C. D., and Hoekstra, Dick (1999). The subapical compartment: a novel sorting centre? *Trends Cell Biol.* 9, 144–149.

Vanaken, H., Vercaeren, I., Claessens, F., De, Vos R., Dewolf-Peeters, C., Vaerman, J. P., Heyns, W., Rombauts, W., and Peeters, B. (1998). Primary rat lacrimal cells undergo acinar-like morphogenesis on reconstituted basement membrane and express secretory component under androgen stimulation. *Exp. Cell Res.* 238, 377–388.

Verbeet, M. P., Vermeer, H., Warmerdam, G. C. M., De Boer, H. A., and Lee, S. H. (1995a). Cloning and characterization of the bovine polymeric immunoglobulin receptor–encoding cDNA. *Gene* 164, 329–333.

Verbeet, M. P., Vollebregt, E., van Amersfoorth, S., Kaetzel, C., He Lee, S., and De Boer, H. A. (1995b). Cloning and genome structure of the murine polymeric immunoglobulin receptor gene. *J. Cell. Biochem.* Suppl.19A, 252.

Vergés, M., Havel, R. J., and Mostov, K. E. (1999). A tubular endosomal fraction from rat liver: biochemical evidence of receptor sorting by default. *Proc. Natl. Acad. Sci. USA* 96, 10146–10151.

Vergés, M., Havel, R. J., and Mostov, K. E. (1999). A tubular endosomal fraction from rat liver: Biochemical evidence of receptor sorting by default. *Proc. Natl. Acad. Sci. USA* 96, 10146–10151.

Verrijdt, G., Schoenmakers, E., Alen, P., Haelens, A., Peeters, B., Rombauts, W., and Claessens, F. (1999). Androgen specificity of a response unit upstream of the human secretory component gene is mediated by differential receptor binding to an essential androgen response element. *Mol. Endocrinol.* 13, 1558–1570.

Verrijdt, G., Schoenmakers, E., Haelens, A., Peeters, B., Verhoeven, G., Rombauts, W., and Claessens, F. (2000). Change of specificity mutations in androgen-selective enhancers. Evidence for a role of differential DNA binding by the androgen receptor. *J. Biol. Chem.* 275, 12298–12305.

Verrijdt, G., Swinnen, J., Peeters, B., Verhoeven, G., Rombauts, W., and Claessens, F. (1997). Characterization of the human secretory component gene promoter. *Biochim. Biophys. Acta* 1350, 147–154.

Vidarsson, G., Der Pol, W. L., van Den Elsen, J. M., Vile, H., Jansen, M., Duijs, J., Morton, H. C., Boel, E., Daha, M. R., Corthesy, B., and van De Winkel, J. G. (2001). Activity of human IgG and IgA subclasses in immune defense against *Neisseria meningitidis* serogroup B. *J. Immunol.* 166, 6250–6256.

Wang, E., Brown, P. S., Aroeti, B., Chapin, S. J., Mostov, K. E., and Dunn, K. W. (2000). Apical and basolateral endocytic pathways of MDCK cells meet in acidic common endosomes distinct from a nearly-neutral apical recycling endosome. *Traffic* 1, 480–493.

Watts, C. L., and Bruce, M. C. (1995). Comparison of secretory component for immunoglobulin A with albumin as reference proteins in tracheal aspirate from preterm infants. *J. Pediatr.* 127, 113–122.

White, K. D., and Capra, J. D. (2002). Targeting mucosal sites by polymeric immunoglobulin receptor–directed peptides. *J. Exp. Med.* 196, 551–555.

Wickham, L. A., Huang, Z., Lambert, R. W., and Sullivan, D. A. (1997). Effect of sialodacryoadenitis virus exposure on acinar epithelial cells from the rat lacrimal gland. *Ocul. Immunol. Inflamm.* 5, 181–195.

Wiggers, T., Arends, J. W., Schutte, B., Volovics, L., and Bosman, F. T. (1988). A multivariate analysis of pathologic prognostic indicators in large bowel cancer. *Cancer* 61, 386–395.

Williams, A. F., and Barclay, A. N. (1988). The immunoglobulin superfamily: domains for cell surface recognition. *Annu. Rev. Immunol.* 6, 381–405.

Wilson, I. D., Wong, M., and Erlandsen, S. L. (1980). Immunohistochemical localization of IgA and secretory component in rat liver. *Gastroenterol.* 79, 924–930.

Wira, C. R., Bodwell, J. E., and Prabhala, R. H. (1991). In vivo response of secretory component in the rat uterus to antigen, IFN-γ, and estradiol. *J. Immunol.* 146, 1893–1899.

Wira, C. R., and Colby, E. M. (1985). Regulation of secretory component by glucocorticoids in primary cultures of rat hepatocytes. *J. Immunol.* 134, 1744–1748.

Wira, C. R., and Rossoll, R. M. (1991). Glucocorticoid regulation of the humoral immune system. Dexamethasone stimulation of secretory component in serum, saliva and bile. *Endocrinology* 128, 835–842.

Wira, C. R., Stern, J. E., and Colby, E. (1984). Estradiol regulation of secretory component in the uterus of the rat: evidence for involvement of RNA synthesis. *J. Immunol.* 133, 2624–2628.

Wira, C. R., and Sullivan, D. A. (1985). Estradiol and progesterone regulation of immunoglobulin A and G and secretory component in cervicovaginal secretions of the rat. *Biol. Reproduct.* 32, 90–95.

Witkin, S. S., Zelikovsky, G., Good, R. A., and Day, N. K. (1981). Demonstration of 11S IgA antibody to spermatozoa in human seminal fluid. *Clin. Exp. Immunol.* 44, 368–374.

Yan, H., Lamm, M. E., Bjorling, E., and Huang, Y. T. (2002). Multiple functions of immunoglobulin A in mucosal defense against viruses: an in vitro measles virus model. *J. Virol.* 76, 10972–10979.

Youngman, K. R., Fiocchi, C., and Kaetzel, C. S. (1994). Inhibition of IFN-γ activity in supernatants from stimulated human intestinal mononuclear cells prevents up-regulation of the polymeric Ig receptor in an intestinal epithelial cell-line. *J. Immunol.* 153, 675–681.

Zhang, J. R., Mostov, K. E., Lamm, M. E., Nanno, M., Shimida, S., Ohwaki, M., and Tuomanen, E. (2000). The polymeric immunoglobulin receptor translocates pneumococci across human nasopharyngeal epithelial cells. *Cell* 102, 827–837.

Fc Receptors

Chapter 13

Jenny M. Woof

Division of Pathology and Neuroscience, University of Dundee Medical School, Dundee, United Kingdom

Marjolein van Egmond

Departments of Molecular Cell Biology and Surgical Oncology, VU University Medical Center, Amsterdam, The Netherlands

Michael A. Kerr

Department of Clinical Biochemistry and Immunology, General Infirmary at Leeds, Leeds, United Kingdom

The different classes of human immunoglobulins (Ig), once they have recognized a pathogen via specific antigen-binding sites in their Fab regions, elicit potent elimination mechanisms mediated through their Fc regions. Triggering of these effector functions usually involves one of three main possibilities, depending on antibody isotype: recognition by C1q, the initial component of the classic pathway of complement; interaction with mannose binding lectin, which activates complement via the lectin pathway; or binding to specific receptors (Fc receptors) on the surface of leukocytes and other cell types. Leukocyte receptors for IgG and IgE have been studied extensively for many years, whereas IgA receptors have emerged as a focus of attention more recently. The majority of Fc receptors have evolved as structurally related members of the Ig gene superfamily with either two or three extracellular Ig-like domains in their unique ligand binding chains (α chains), the transmembrane region of which is often complexed with more promiscuous γ signaling chains.

Three different classes of human leukocyte receptors for IgG have been characterized, each with multiple variant forms. FcγRI (CD64) is a high-affinity ($K_a \sim 5 \times 10^8$ M^{-1}) receptor present on monocytes and macrophages and inducible on neutrophils following treatment with interferon-γ (IFNγ). FcγRII (CD32) is a medium-affinity ($K_a \sim 10^6$ M^{-1}) receptor binding predominantly to aggregated IgG and is found chiefly on neutrophils, macrophages, B cells, and eosinophils. FcγRIII (CD16) is a low- to medium-affinity receptor that binds poorly to monomer IgG but binds avidly to aggregated IgG. It is present on neutrophils, macrophages, and natural killer (NK) cells. The structure,

function, and expression of these receptors have been reviewed elsewhere (Hulett and Hogarth, 1994; Ravetch, 1997).

The high-affinity receptor for IgE (FcεRI) is found on mast cells and basophils. This complex molecule contains the α-chain which is structurally related to FcγR ligand-binding chains, the β chain and a γ-chain dimer. An unrelated, low affinity IgE receptor (FcεRII, CD23) is found on B cells, activated macrophages, and eosinophils. This receptor is a member of the C-type lectin superfamily. Both classes of IgE receptors have also been studied extensively (Gould et al., 2003).

Fc receptors for IgA have been recognized functionally for many years (Spiegelberg et al., 1974; Lawrence et al., 1975; Fanger et al., 1980). The myeloid receptor, FcαRI (CD89), is the most thoroughly characterized (reviewed in van Egmond et al., 2001a; Monteiro and van de Winkel, 2003). It is structurally related to the FcγRs and FcεRI and also associates with the FcR γ chain dimer. The general properties and cellular distribution of FcαRI, along with those of the FcγRs and FcεRs, are presented in **Table 13.1**.

In recent years it has become increasingly apparent that another class of Fc receptor, FcRn, plays important roles in the transport of IgG across the epithelial layer at mucosal surfaces (Spiekermann et al., 2002; Roopenian et al., 2003). FcRn shares only limited homology with other FcR and is distantly related to the MHC class I family, dimerizing with β$_2$-microglobulin (β$_2$m), the obligate subunit of all class I molecules. Its role in IgG homeostasis and transport has been recently reviewed (Ghetie and Ward, 2002).

Table 13.1. Molecular Properties and Cellular Distribution of Important Human Leukocyte Fc Receptors

Property	FcαRI	FcγRI	FcγRII	FcγRII	FcγRII	FcγRIII	FcγRIII	FcεRI	FcεRII	FcεRII
CD number	CD89	CD64	CD32			CD16			CD23	
Molecular weight (kDa)	50–70	50–70	40			50–80		45–65	45–50	
Chief isoforms expressed	FcαRIA	FcγRIA	FcγRIIA	FcγRIIB	FcγRIIC	FcγRIIIA	FcγRIIIB	FcεRI	FcεRIIα	FcεRIIβ
Allotypes			LR	HR			NA1 and NA2			
Binding affinity for monomer Ig (M^{-1})	Medium (10^7)	High (10^8–10^9)	Low ($<10^7$)	Low ($<10^7$)	Low ($<10^7$)	Low ($<10^7$)	Medium (10^7)	Very high (10^{10})	Low (10^7)	Low
Specificity for human Ig	Serum IgA1=2, S-IgA1=S-IgA2	IgG1=3>4 IgG2 doesn't bind	IgG3≥1 =2 IgG4 doesn't bind	IgG3 ≥1>>>2 IgG4 doesn't bind	IgG3≥1 >>2>4	ND	IgG1=3 >>>2=4	IgE	IgE	IgE
Specificity for mouse Ig	Mouse IgA doesn't bind	IgG2a=3 >>>1=2b	IgG2a =2b >>1	IgG2a =2b =1	IgG2a=2b≥1	ND	IgG3>2a>2b >>1	IgE	IgE	IgE
Signalling motif	γ chain ITAM	γ chain ITAM	α chain ITAM	α chain ITIM	α chain ITAM	γ chain ITAM	GPI-linked	γ chain ITAM	C-type lectin	C-type lectin
Cellular distribution	Neutrophils monocytes, some MØ, eosinophils, Kupffer cells, some DC	Monocytes, MØ, neutrophils (IFNγ stim), eosinophils (IFNγ stim)	Monocytes, MØ, neutrophils, platelets, Langerhans cells	Monocytes, MØ, B cells	Monocytes, MØ, neutrophils, B cells	MØ, NK cells, γδ T cells, some monocytes	Neutrophils, eosinophils (IFNγ stim)	Mast cells, basophils, Langerhans cells, activated monocytes	B cells	B cells, T cells, monocytes, eosinophils, MØ

Some receptors signal directly through activatory or inhibitory motifs in their ligand binding (α) chain, while others rely on membrane association with the γ chain to allow signaling via the γ chain ITAM signalling motif. Abbreviations: ND, not determined; GPI, glycerophosphoinositol; ITAM, immunoreceptor tyrosine-based activation motif; ITIM, immunoreceptor tyrosine-inhibition motif; MØ, macrophages; IFNγ stim, after IFNγ stimulation.

CD89

It is established that FcαRI is constitutively expressed on neutrophils, monocytes, some macrophages (tonsillar, splenic, and alveolar), eosinophils, and also a number of related cell lines (Table 13.1). It has also been shown that the receptor is present on interstitial dendritic cells (Geissemann et al., 2001; Heystek et al., 2002) and Kupffer cells (van Egmond et al., 2000). A recent study of *in vivo* expression concluded that most CD89-positive cells identified in both blood and tissue were neutrophils displaying high levels of CD89, while recently emigrated monocytes/macrophages in the tissues tended to have lower levels of CD89 than those in blood (Hamre et al., 2003).

The expression levels of FcαRI on a number of cell types can be upregulated or downregulated by certain cytokines or other stimuli (reviewed in Monteiro and van de Winkel, 2003). Increased expression is seen on monocytes and macrophages on treatment with calcitriol, phorbol myristate acetate (PMA), tumor necrosis factor-α (TNF-α), interleukin 1-β (IL-1β), granulocyte-macrophage colony stimulating factor (GM-CSF), and lipopolysaccharide (LPS), whereas decreased expression is reportedly driven by transforming growth factor-β (TGF-β), IFNγ, suramin, and polymeric IgA (pIgA). Both eosinophils and neutrophils show increased expression with ionomycin treatment. Neutrophil expression can also be enhanced by factors such as IL-8, TNF-α, GM-CSF, formyl-methionyl-leucyl-phenylalanine (FMLP), and zymosan-activated serum.

Molecular characterization

Genetics

The cDNA for FcαRI, originally isolated by expression cloning with use of the anti-FcαRI mAb My43, codes for a protein of 287 amino acids, including a leader sequence of 21 amino acids cleaved during membrane insertion. The remaining 266 amino acids comprise two Ig-like domains, a transmembrane region, and a short cytoplasmic tail. The two Ig-like domains show sequence homology (~20%) with those of the three classes of FcγR and FcεRI α-chain, although at a lower level than that shared by these other FcR classes (Maliszewski et al., 1990). The cytoplasmic tail contains no recognized signalling motifs.

The gene for FcαRI has five exons: the first (S1) contains the 5′ untranslated region, initiation codon, and most of the signal peptide; the second mini-exon (S2) encodes the remainder of the signal peptide; the third and fourth (EC1 and EC2) encode the two Ig-like domains (D1 and D2; 206 amino acids in total); and the final exon (TM/C) encodes the transmembrane region (19 amino acids) and the cytoplasmic tail (41 amino acids). The overall structure of the gene is similar to that of other Fc receptors, but it is only distantly related (de Wit et al., 1995). Whereas the α chains of the three classes of FcγR and FcεRI map to chromosome 1q32.3, that of FcαRI lies on chromosome 19q13.4, alongside members of a family including natural killer cell inhibitory receptors (KIRs), LAIR-1 and -2, leukocyte Ig-

like receptors (LILR), and the platelet-specific collagen receptor (GPVI), with which it shares greater homology (~35%) (Kremer et al., 1992; Jandrot-Perrus et al., 2000). The various receptors in this so-called leukocyte receptor cluster (LRC) differ markedly with regard to function and expression, presumably because of functional differentiation after duplication of a common ancestral gene.

Despite rigorous efforts, no murine equivalent of FcαRI has been found, but human FcαRI shares considerable homology with a bovine IgG receptor, Fcγ2R (Zhang et al., 1995). Recently, the first true orthologue of human FcαRI has been cloned from cattle (Morton et al., 2003). Bovine FcαRI shares a very high degree of homology with the human receptor and binds both human and bovine IgA. Reminiscent of its human equivalent, bovine FcαRI maps close to the bovine KIR genes on chromosome 18. Phylogenetic analysis shows that the human and bovine FcαRI and bovine Fcγ2R, along with other members of the LRC, form a cluster distinct from other FcR (Morton et al., 2003).

It is known that the human FcαRI promoter region, lying between 59 and 197 bp downstream of the major transcription start site, possesses a number of consensus-binding sites for transcription factors implicated in myeloid-specific gene expression (Shimokawa et al., 2000; Shimokawa and Ra, 2003). Two C-T transition polymorphisms (lying at 114 bp upstream and 56 bp downstream of the transcription start site) that result in differential promoter activity have been identified. The -114CC genotype appears to be associated with an increased disposition to IgA nephropathy (IgAN) (Tsuge et al., 2001).

cDNAs for numerous alternatively spliced variants of FcαRI have been characterized in a number of laboratories (Patry et al., 1996; Pleass et al., 1996; Morton et al., 1996a; Reterink et al., 1996; Toyabe et al., 1997; Togo et al., 2003). Translation products of the full-length transcript, termed FcαRI a.1, and a shorter version (a.2 lacking 66 bp from EC2) have been demonstrated *in vivo*. The a.1 protein expression profile is given in Table 13.1. The a.2 protein appears to be exclusively expressed on alveolar macrophages (Patry et al., 1996). A novel variant of CD89 in eosinophils and neutrophils, termed FcαRb, in which the transmembrane/cytoplasmic region is replaced by 23 new amino acids, has also been reported (van Dijk et al., 1996). Protein products corresponding to the other splice variants have not been readily identified.

Structure

The FcαRI α chain protein core of around 30 kDa carries five potential *N*-linked sugars and a number of possible *O*-glycosylation sites. The mature cell surface receptor has a final mass ranging from 50 to 100 kDa, depending on cell type, with variable glycosylation accounting for the heterogeneity (Monteiro et al., 1992). The extracellular region of the α chain is arranged into two Ig-like domains, for which crystal structures have recently been resolved (Herr et al., 2003a; Ding et al., 2003). The domains are orientated at roughly 90° to each other and display a similar overall topology and domain orientation to the domains of the leukocyte

Ig-like receptor LIR-1 and KIR receptors. While the FcγRII, FcγRIII, and FcεRI receptors also have bent structures, their relative D1–D2 orientations are inverted. N-linked glycans are visible in the FcαRI crystal structures at four potential sites (Asn44, Asn58, Asn120, and Asn156). A degree of moderate flexibility appears to exist between the domains with the interdomain angle varying between 97° and 88° in the three different crystal structures obtained.

The short cytoplasmic tail of FcαRI does not bear any known signaling motifs, and signaling via FcαR is dependent on association with the FcR γ chain subunit, forming the FcαRI/γγ complex (Pfefferkorn and Yeaman, 1994). FcR γ chain has also been shown to constitute a component of IgG and IgE Fc receptors (Ravetch, 1997). However, the interaction of FcαRI and FcR γ chain is particularly strong because of an electrostatic interaction due to the presence of a positively charged arginine residue (Arg209) in the transmembrane region of FcαRI, which was shown to be essential for association with the FcR γ chain (Morton et al., 1995). It has previously been reported that FcαRI and FcRγIIIa can compete for FcR γ chain in mast cells (Dombrowicz et al., 1997). No evidence was found, however, that FcαRI and FcγRI cross-compete for FcR γ chain in neutrophils, either in vitro or in vivo (van Egmond et al., 2001b).

Recently it was reported that FcαRI can be expressed without FcR γ chain—the so-called γ-less receptor—on monocytes and neutrophils, despite the presence of abundant amounts of intracellular FcR γ chain (Launay et al., 1999; Honorio-Franca et al., 2001). In contrast, FcαRI expression in human FcαRI transgenic (Tg) mice required the presence of FcR γ chain, and neutrophils and monocytes/macrophages of these animals no longer expressed FcαRI when crossed with FcR γ chain–deficient mice (van Egmond et al., 1999). Taken together, these data suggest that in humans FcαRI might associate with other—as yet undefined—molecules that are absent in mice.

Soluble forms of FcαRI may be generated by proteolysis or shedding from the cell surface. FcR γ chain–dependent proteolysis has been described as one means to produce a 30-kDa soluble product, which is found covalently associated with pIgA in normal serum (van Zandbergen et al., 1999; van der Boog et al., 2002). In serum from IgAN patients, an alternative 50–70-kDa soluble form has been identified (Launay et al., 2000).

Ligand binding

Earlier Scatchard analysis of the binding of IgA to neutrophil cell-surface FcαRI estimated the K_D of the interaction to be around 21 nm (Weisbart et al., 1988). Recent biosensor experiments using a soluble ectodomain of FcαRI and a recombinant Fc of IgA1 indicate that the binding data are most consistent with a bivalent mechanism where two FcαRI molecules bind one IgA Fc molecule sequentially, with respective equilibrium dissociation constants of 180 nm and 431 nM for the two events (Herr et al., 2003b). The affinity of one binding site appears to be little influenced by binding to the other. A decrease in binding affinity at low pH was noted, consistent with the involvement of a histidine residue in the binding site.

Equilibrium gel-filtration and analytical ultracentrifugation data were also consistent with a 2:1 stoichiometry.

On the basis of mutagenesis studies, the interaction site on IgA was postulated to occupy a site lying at the interface of the Cα2 and Cα3 domains, with critical contributions from one loop in the Cα2 domain (Leu257, Leu258) and another in the Cα3 domain (Pro440-Phe443) (Carayannopoulos et al., 1996; Pleass et al., 1999). The interaction site on FcαRI was also localized, through a series of mutagenesis studies, to a number of close-lying residues forming a surface on the membrane distal D1 domain (Wines et al., 1999; Wines et al., 2001). Residues Tyr35, Tyr81, and Arg82 were particularly implicated, with some contributions also from Arg52 and Gly84, His85, and Tyr86. Both these site localizations have very recently been confirmed through resolution of the crystal structure of the tailpieceless Fc of IgA1 (residues Cys242–Lys454) complexed with the extracellular domains of FcαRI (residues Gln1–Thr195) (Herr et al., 2003a). The structure of the complex, solved at 3.1Å resolution, shows that the interface between receptor and Fc comprises a central hydrophobic core involving residues Leu257, Leu258, Met433, Leu441, Ala442, and Phe443 and the aliphatic portion of Arg382 of IgA and Tyr35, Leu54, Phe56, Gly84, and His85 and the aliphatic portion of Lys55 of FcαRI, with contributions from a number of surrounding charged residues (Arg382, Glu389, and Glu437 in IgA and Arg52, Arg53, Lys55, and Arg82 in FcαRI) **(Fig. 13.1)**. These peripheral interactions may include hydrogen bond interactions, but no salt bridges are observed, in keeping with the predicted minor contribution of electrostatic interactions to the free energy of binding (Herr et al., 2003b; Pleass et al., 2003). Whereas an N-linked sugar attached to Asn58 of FcαRI forms potential hydrogen bonds and a van der Waals contact with IgA Fc, the N-linked sugar attached to Asn263 of the Cα2 domain of IgA is not involved in the interaction, con-

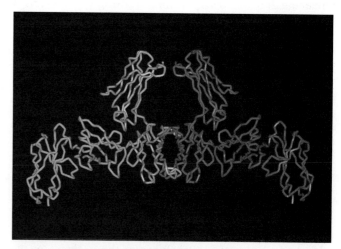

Fig. 13.1. X-ray crystal structure of the complex of human IgA1 Fc with the extracellular domains of human FcαRI (coordinates from Herr et al., 2003a; PDB code 1OW0). **(See page 7 of the color plates.)** One IgA Fc heavy chain is shown in red, the other in orange. The FcαRI molecules are shown in blue and green-blue.

sistent with the findings of earlier functional studies (Mattu et al., 1998).

Despite structural similarities between both receptors and their ligands, the mode of interaction between IgA and FcαRI differs markedly from those of IgG with FcγR and IgE with FcεRI. The FcγR receptors (FcγRI, FcγRII, and FcγRIII) all interact with a hinge-proximal site at the top of the Cγ2 domains (Burton and Woof, 1992; Sondermann et al., 2000) while FcεRI binds to an equivalent position at the top of the Cε3 domains in IgE (Garman et al., 2000). In addition, although the interaction site on FcαRI occupies a very similar position to the ligand-binding site on the structurally related inhibitory receptor LIR-1 (Chapman et al., 2000), it is very different from those on the FcγR and FcεRI for their Ig ligands. On FcαRI, the site lies on the membrane distal domain, whereas the FcγR and FcεRI ligand sites are in their membrane proximal D2 domains (Sondermann et al., 2000; Garman et al., 2000).

Moreover, there are important differences in stoichiometry. X-ray crystallographic studies (Herr et al., 2003a) confirmed the FcαRI:IgA 2:1 stoichiometry revealed by analytical ultracentrifugation and equilibrium gel-filtration experiments (Herr et al., 2003b). In contrast, X-ray crystal structures reveal one molecule of IgG Fc binds only one FcγRIII, and similarly one molecule of IgE binds only one FcεRI receptor (Sondermann et al., 2000; Garman et al., 2000). One can speculate that this "alternative" Fc receptor binding site in the interdomain region of IgA may have been favored during evolution because of steric restrictions imposed by the more rigid conformation most likely adopted by the IgA1 hinge region. In comparison, the hinge of IgG is very flexible and the IgE Fc accommodates a considerable degree of bending on receptor engagement (Wan et al., 2002), thereby circumventing any potential steric hindrance by the Fab arms.

Although the IgA Fc can bind two FcαRI molecules simultaneously in solution, presumably under normal physiologic conditions binding of one IgA molecule to two cell-membrane receptors does not occur or is not sufficient to trigger a signaling cascade. A number of possible explanations have been offered (Herr et al., 2003). First, the distance between the receptors (predicted to be ~124 Å at the cell surface) may be too great to initiate subsequent signaling steps. Close clustering of numerous receptors by IgA immune complexes may be necessary to elicit such downstream events. Second, the receptors may be tethered to elements of the cytoskeleton, which may not be triggered to undergo necessary rearrangements compatible with receptor clustering below a certain level of receptor engagement or prior to cell priming by other factors such as cytokines. Third, the concentration of circulating IgA is sufficiently high to drive the equilibrium toward 1:1 complexes, which would presumably be displaced by incoming IgA immune complexes. Multivalent interactions with the latter would result in slow off-rates and subsequent triggering events.

The 2:1 stoichiometry may also offer explanations for two intriguing facets of IgA-mediated immune responses, namely, the ability of cytokine stimulation to enhance the affinity of the FcαRI-IgA interaction without increasing receptor expression (see signalling section) and the inability of S-IgA to trigger phagocytosis (van Egmond et al., 2000). It is suggested that the binding of SC to the IgA Fc region in S-IgA may occlude the FcαRI site, resulting in an inability to activate the cell via FcαRI (Herr et al., 2003a). A requirement for the integrin coreceptor Mac-1 (CR3; CD11b/CD18) in binding of S-IgA to FcαRI has been demonstrated (van Spriel et al., 2001), and possibly this coreceptor may help overcome the decreased binding capacity for FcαRI, offering an explanation for the ability of S-IgA to elicit neutrophil respiratory bursts via FcαRI (Stewart and Kerr, 1990).

Signalling

FcR γ chains bear an immunoreceptor tyrosine (Tyr)–based activation motif (ITAM) in their cytoplasmic regions, consisting of two Tyr-containing "YxxL" boxes interspaced by seven amino acids, which is essential for initiation of activatory signals (Reth, 1989). Mutation of either of the tyrosines diminishes or abrogates signaling. FcαRI cross-linking triggers phosphorylation of ITAMs by the Src protein Tyr kinase (PTK) p56[lyn] (Gulle et al., 1998). The subsequent steps involve association of p72[Syk] with phosphorylated ITAM and modulation of a multimolecular adaptor complex—containing Cbl, Shc, SHIP, Grb2, Sos, SLP-76, and CrkL—that might regulate signaling (Launay et al., 1998; Park et al., 1999) (Fig. 13.2). FcαRI triggering was shown to activate the NADPH oxidase complex, which is dependent on the release of calcium from intracellular stores in human neutrophils. Furthermore, NADPH oxidase activation can be blocked by addition of phosphoinositide 3-kinase inhibitors (Lang and Kerr, 1997; Lang and Kerr, 2000).

Following cross-linking, FcαRI was shown to relocate to specialized sphingolipid-cholesterol-rich microdomains in the plasma membrane, which are rich in signaling molecules (including p56[lyn]) and are hypothesized to serve as platforms for the initiation of signal transduction (Lang et al., 1999). Redistribution of FcαRI was associated with phosphorylation of FcR γ chain, p56[lyn], and Btk and recruitment of Blk and Syk. Additionally, both phosphoinositide kinases, such as 3-phosphoinositide 3-kinase and phospholipase Cγ2, and serine/threonine kinases like protein kinase C (PKC) α, PKCε, and PKBα were recruited to rafts, suggesting that lipid rafts function as platforms for recruitment of multiple classes of signaling molecules initiated by FcαRI cross-linking (Lang et al., 2002).

It has long been established that GM-CSF can rapidly increase the affinity of IgA binding to neutrophils without increasing surface expression of FcαRI (Weisbart et al., 1988). In a similar way, in human eosinophils Th2-derived cytokines interleukin (IL)-4 and IL-5 were demonstrated to regulate FcαRI activation, leading to increased ligand binding without affecting levels of FcαR expression (Bracke et al., 1997). These findings suggest that cytokine stimulation results in alteration of either receptor affinity or avidity. Substitution of a single C-terminal residue (Ser263) in the

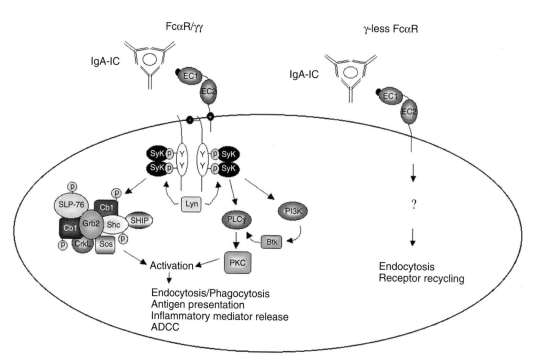

Fig. 13.2. Signaling pathways triggered by FcαRI. IgA-mediated cellular activation is shown in a schematic model that depends on clustering of FcαRI-γγ complexes (IC, immune complexes).

FcαRI α-chain resulted in constitutive IgA binding, indicating that Ser263 is responsible for receptor modulation upon cytokine stimulation (Bracke *et al.*, 2001). Thus the ligand-binding subunit of the FcαRI/γγ complex does not simply play a passive role in IgA binding, but inside-out signaling of FcαRI requires the intracellular domain of the α-chain to modulate interactions between FcαRI and the cytoskeleton. A possible mechanism for the cytokine-induced affinity switch has been suggested on the basis of regulation of the stoichiometry of the FcαRI-IgA interaction by cytoskeletal interactions (Herr *et al.*, 2003b). In an unstimulated state, the spatial movements of many FcαRI may be restricted by cytoskeletal interactions, thereby preventing two receptors from simultaneously binding to a single IgA molecule. After cytokine stimulation, dephosphorylation of Ser263 disrupts the interaction with the cytoskeleton such that two receptors become sufficiently mobile or optimally orientated to enable them to bind to the same IgA molecule, generating a higher avidity interaction.

Additionally, a role for the β_2 integrin Mac-1 (CR3; CD11b/CD18) in FcαRI function has been implicated. FcαRI efficiently induces antibody-mediated cellular cytotoxicity (ADCC), but the capacity to lyse tumor cells was abolished in neutrophils of FcαRI Tg mice that were deficient in Mac-1, indicating that Mac-1 is essential for FcαRI-mediated tumor cell killing (van Egmond *et al.*, 1999). Recent studies demonstrated that Mac-1$^{-/-}$ neutrophils were unable to spread on antibody-coated tumor targets, leading to impaired immunological synapse formation between FcαRI/Mac-1$^{-/-}$ neutrophils and tumor cells. Extracellular

lysis therefore may be absent because of abnormal interactions between Mac-1$^{-/-}$ effector cells and target cells (van Spriel *et al.*, 2001). Furthermore, Mac-1 was required for binding of S-IgA to neutrophil FcαRI and as such functions as a novel accessory protein, possibly by binding to the secretory component (SC) of S-IgA (van Spriel *et al.*, 2002).

Biological effects

Several conflicting reports addressing the putative function of IgA receptors have been described. Early data demonstrated suppression of neutrophil chemotaxis by human myeloma IgA proteins and failure of IgA to induce phagocytosis by human neutrophils (van Epps and Williams, 1976). These studies, accentuated by the poor ability of IgA in activating complement, led to the view of IgA receptors as anti-inflammatory molecules. However, the tide began to turn when it was shown that serum IgA antiyeast antibodies were more efficient than IgG antibodies at triggering phagocytosis by unstimulated neutrophils in the absence of complement (Yeaman and Kerr, 1987). Others confirmed IgA-mediated phagocytosis by neutrophils (Weisbart *et al.*, 1988), and recently data supporting the capacity of IgA to trigger a plethora of inflammatory functions by interacting with FcαRI have been accumulating (for review, see Morton *et al.*, 1996b; Monteiro and van de Winkel, 2003).

Most cellular functions triggered via FcαRI—such as calcium mobilization, cytokine release, phagocytosis, and antigen presentation—depend on tyrosine kinase activity of FcR γ chain, which was shown with the use of transfectants expressing either FcαRI or FcαRI/γγ (Morton *et al.*, 1995;

van Egmond *et al.*, 1999; and own unpublished data). However, no difference in endocytosis rate between FcαRI/γγ complexes or γ-less FcαRI was observed, indicating that endocytosis of IgA complexes occurs regardless of FcR γ chain presence (Launay *et al.*, 1999). IgA complexes internalized via γ-less FcαRI are recycled and thereby protected from degradation, which might lead to serum homeostasis (Launay *et al.*, 1999).

A recent study, in which the antigen-presenting capacity of transfectants expressing FcαRI/γγ was compared with that of cells expressing FcαRI and FcR γ chains in which the ITAM motifs were altered, confirmed that signaling-competent FcR γ chain was not required for endocytosis of IgA-ovalbumin complexes (Shen *et al.*, 2001). However, transport of ligated FcαRI to lamp-1⁺ late endocytic compartments, remodeling and activation of these compartments, degradation of IgA complexes, and efficient antigen presentation were dependent on FcR γ chain (Shen *et al.*, 2001).

FcαRI has been shown to mediate phagocytosis of beads, bacteria, and yeast particles. Whereas unstimulated neutrophils clearly mediate FcαRI-directed phagocytosis (Yeaman and Kerr, 1987), the phagocytic capacity of neutrophils and monocytes may be enhanced by priming with cytokines such as GM-CSF and IL-8 or with IL-1, TNF-α, and GM-CSF, respectively (Morton *et al.*, 1996; Weisbart *et al.*, 1988; Shen *et al.*, 1994). Priming with GM-CSF, IL-4, or IL-5 appears essential for eosinophil-mediated phagocytosis of IgA-coated beads (Bracke *et al.*, 1997). In contrast to human serum IgA, some reports have found human S-IgA to be incapable of triggering phagocytosis by either neutrophils *in vitro* or Kupffer cells *in vivo* (van Egmond *et al.*, 2000). However, others have found S-IgA able to compete with serum IgA for binding to preparations of purified FcαRI (Mazengera and Kerr, 1990). The obtained K_i value of 500 nM lies close to the recent equilibrium dissociation constant values reported for the IgA-FcαRI interaction (Herr *et al.*, 2003a). Therefore, the suggested blockade of the FcαRI-binding site on IgA by SC may not account for all observations, and we must await a more detailed structural understanding of the IgA-SC interaction in order to clarify the situation.

There is, however, a consensus that S-IgA is capable of initiating respiratory burst activity by neutrophils (Stewart and Kerr, 1990; Stewart *et al.*, 1994). This activity has been shown to be dependent on Mac-1 (van Egmond *et al.*, 2000; van Spriel *et al.*, 2002). Furthermore, S-IgA provides the most potent stimulus for degranulation of eosinophils, which might also be linked to expression of a unique receptor for "SC" on eosinophils (Abu-Ghazaleh *et al.*, 1989; Lamkhioued *et al.*, 1995) (see below). Cross-linking of FcαRI on monocytes, either by IgA immune complexes or anti-FcαRI monoclonal antibodies, induces release of superoxide production as well (Shen and Collins, 1989; Shen *et al.*, 1989). Furthermore, release of prostaglandins, leukotrienes, and the cytokines IL-6 and TNF-α upon FcαRI cross-linking has been documented (Ferreri *et al.*, 1986; Deviere *et al.*, 1991; Patry *et al.*, 1995).

FcαRI was additionally shown to efficiently induce ADCC by neutrophils and macrophages (Valerius *et al.*, 1997; Keler *et al.*, 2000; van Egmond *et al.*, 1999b). On neutrophils, FcαRI proved to represent the most effective Fc receptor for the induction of tumor cell lysis (Stockmeyer *et al.*, 2000; van Egmond *et al.*, 2001b; Huls *et al.*, 1999).

OTHER LEUKOCYTE IgA RECEPTORS

Fcα/μR

A receptor termed Fcα/μR, which binds IgA and IgM with intermediate to high affinity, has been noted in both mice and humans. In mice, it is expressed constitutively on the majority of B lymphocytes and macrophages (Shibuya *et al.*, 2000) and is abundant in lymph nodes, appendix, kidney, and intestine (Sakamoto *et al.*, 2001). Recently it has also been demonstrated on oligodendrocytes (Nakahara *et al.*, 2003). In humans, expression of receptor protein has been less well studied, but Fcα/μR transcripts have been found in mesangial cells, suggesting a possible role in IgAN (McDonald *et al.*, 2002). The gene for the human receptor lies on chromosome 1 near genes for the polymeric immunoglobulin receptor (pIgR), FcεRI, and FcγR (Shimizu *et al.*, 2001).

Murine Fcα/μR is a type I transmembrane protein with an extracellular portion of 432 amino acids, a 20–amino acid transmembrane region, and a cytoplasmic tail of 60 amino acids. Human Fcα/μR shares around 49% identity with the murine receptor. In both cases, the membrane distal part of the EC region is thought to fold up into an Ig-like domain that contains a conserved motif, also present in the first EC domains of human, bovine, and murine pIgR, that has been implicated in binding to IgA and IgM (Shibuya *et al.*, 2000). The receptor is expressed on mature B cells and appears to acquire the ability to bind IgA and IgM after B cell stimulation (Sakamoto *et al.*, 2001). Not only has cross-linking of mouse Fcα/μR by IgM-coated microparticles been shown to result in internalization of the receptor, but also Fcα/μR has been shown to mediate B cell endocytosis of IgM-coated *Staphylococcus aureus* targets (Shibuya *et al.*, 2000), suggesting the receptor may play an important role in the primary response to various microbes.

SC receptor on eosinophils

Eosinophils in mucosal tissues play a key role in the defense against parasite infection and in the pathophysiology of allergic inflammation. The role of Igs in the stimulation of these mucosal cells remains unclear. The paucity of FcγR and continuing controversy about the function of FcεR on human eosinophils (Kita *et al.*,1999) contrast with the details that have emerged concerning the function of FcαRI on these cells (Abu-Ghazaleh *et al.*, 1989; Dunne *et al.*, 1993; Monteiro *et al.*, 1993). Although aggregated serum IgA is a potent stimulator of eosinophils, S-IgA is even more potent. This is because eosinophils but not neutrophils appear to express a receptor for SC (Lamkhioued *et al.*, 1995). CD89 is expressed in both cell types. Flow cytometric analysis revealed that purified human SC could bind to a subpopulation (4%–59%) of blood eosinophils from patients with eosinophilia (Lamkhioued et al., 1995). The binding of radiolabeled human SC could be competitively inhibited with unlabeled SC or S-IgA but not with serum IgA or IgG. Immunoprecipitation and immunosorbent chromatography with use of human SC revealed the presence of a major SC-binding component at 15 kDa in eosinophil extracts, but this molecule has not been characterized further. The same study went on to show that the binding of cross-linked human SC or S-IgA caused the release of granule proteins and generated a respiratory burst. When eosinophils were stimulated with immobilized S-IgA, degranulation and superoxide production were greater than when stimulated with serum IgA. In contrast, neutrophils responded similarly to S-IgA and serum IgA. S-IgA-mediated superoxide production by eosinophils was enhanced by some cytokines but was abolished by anti-CD18 monoclonal antibody (mAb), suggesting that β2 integrins might be crucial for this reaction (Motegi and Kita, 1998).

Other IgA receptors

M-cell receptor

Specialized epithelial cells, termed M cells, located within the follicle-associated epithelium that overlies organized mucosa-associated lymphoid tissues, mediate selective transport of antigens across the epithelial barrier. Such antigen sampling is essential to ensure an appropriate S-IgA response at mucosal surfaces. A receptor for Igs on the surface of M cells was first suggested by the selective accumulation of milk-derived IgA on the apical surfaces of Peyer's patch M cells in rabbit neonates (Roy and Varvayanis, 1987) and the association of S-IgA with M cells in adult rabbits (Kato, 1990; Lelouard et al., 1999). Moreover, IgA-coated particles were observed not only to bind mouse Peyer's patch M cells but also to be taken up into cytoplasmic vesicles and to cross the cell into the underlying space (Weltzin et al., 1989), suggesting that the receptor may be involved in transepithelial transport of IgA and IgA-antigen complexes. Recently, the mouse M-cell receptor has been further characterized (Mantis et al., 2002). It is specific for IgA, recognizing both mouse and human IgA2 with or without SC but showing no binding to mouse serum IgG, mouse monoclonal IgM, or human IgA1. The difference in specificity for human IgA1 and IgA2 appears to result from the extended hinge of IgA1 rendering critical sites in the Cα1 and Cα2 domains too far apart for optimal receptor engagement. The same study (Mantis et al., 2002) showed that the M-cell receptor is distinct from other receptors present on intestinal epithelial cells or cell lines, including the pIgR, the asialoglycoprotein receptor (ASGP-R), β-1,4-galactosyl transferase (Tomana et al., 1993), and other lectin-like receptors, and its specificity profile indicates that it is neither FcαRI nor a novel IgA receptor on the HT-29 human colonic carcinoma cell line (Kitamura et al., 2000). However, at this stage the possibility that the receptor is a form of Fcα/μR cannot be

ruled out formally. Endogenous S-IgA has also been shown on the surfaces of pediatric human M cells in the lamina propria and lymphoid follicles of normal terminal ileum, indicating that an M-cell receptor is also present in humans (Mantis et al., 2002).

Transferrin receptor (CD71)

The transferrin receptor (TfR or CD71) was identified as an IgA binding molecule when the antigen recognized by mAb A24, an antibody capable of blocking IgA1 binding to epithelial and B cell lines, was found to be CD71 (Moura et al., 2001). This receptor is a disulphide-linked homodimer of total molecular mass 180 kDa that also binds transferrin and the hemochromatosis protein. The binding of IgA1 is inhibitable by transferrin. CD71 binds human IgA1 but not IgA2 and shows a preference for pIgA1 over the monomeric form (Monteiro et al., 2002). The selectivity for IgA1 suggests that binding is most likely influenced by the extended hinge region carrying O-linked glycan moieties that are present in IgA1 but lacking in IgA2. This binding profile is reminiscent of that described earlier for T cells (Rudd et al., 1994), raising the possibility that IgA1 binding to T cells might be accounted for by CD71 (Monteiro and van de Winkel, 2003).

CD71 expression has been demonstrated on some lymphocytic cell lines such as Daudi cells (B cell line) and Jurkat cells (T cell line), on the myeloid cell line U937 (unstimulated), and on the HT-29 epithelial cell line. In vivo, it has been found on mononuclear hematopoietic cells in fetal liver and bone marrow, but it is not readily seen on adult blood mononuclear and polymorphonuclear cells (Moura et al., 2001). Perhaps most important, it has been demonstrated on cultured human mesangial cells and in mesangial areas of renal biopsy specimens from patients with IgAN. Indeed, the expression is enhanced in patients with IgAN (Berger's disease and Henoch-Schönlein nephritis) (Haddad et al., 2003), and it has been postulated that the receptor plays a role in the pathogenesis of IgAN (see below).

Asialoglycoprotein receptor (ASGP-R)

Another receptor with ability to bind IgA is the ASGP-R. On hepatocytes, ASGP-R binds, in the presence of calcium, the terminal Gal or GalNac residues of desialylated glycoproteins and triggers their subsequent internalization and degradation (Stockert, 1995). Earlier studies using myeloma IgA proteins implicated both pIgR and ASGP-R on liver cells in the regulation of serum IgA levels. However, a limited number of human studies have shown that liver pIgR does not play an important role in regulating serum IgA levels in humans, in contrast to the situation in some rodents (see Chapters 11 and 12). Recently, investigators have looked at clearance of intravenously administered human IgA (produced in mouse Sp2/0 cells) in a mouse model (Rifai et al., 2000). Liver ASGP-R was shown to rapidly clear the IgA2 subclasses and to mediate some clearance of IgA1. In this system, it appeared that the O-linked sugars in the IgA1 hinge were not critical for the interaction but that the N-linked glycan moieties engaged ASGP-R. However, care should be taken in interpretation of work with heterologous ligands and receptors, particularly since other studies using the human hepatoma cell line HepG2 showed that ASGP-R bound human IgA1 better than IgA2 (Tomana *et al.*, 1988). A description of the role of ASGP-R in catabolism of IgA is provided in Chapter 9.

IgA RECEPTORS IN DISEASE

IgAN is the commonest form of glomerulonephritis, characterized by the deposition of complexed IgA1 in the mesangium, mesangial cell proliferation, and increased synthesis of extracellular matrix (Chapter 92). IgA1 deposition in the mesangium is also a secondary phenomenon associated with a range of diseases in which IgA metabolism is abnormal (e.g., alcoholic liver disease). The granular IgA1 deposits are readily detected by immunohistochemistry or by electron microscopy. They are characteristically pIgA1 derived from serum IgA1, but the reason for their deposition remains unknown. The appearance of deposits in normal kidneys after transplantation into patients with previous IgAN suggests that the abnormalities are in the IgA itself or in receptors found on other tissues involved in removal of IgA from the circulation, rather than in the kidney (Berger *et al.*, 1975). Nevertheless, mesangial cells have been shown to express a number of types of IgA receptor that might play a role in the subsequent pathology of the disease (Monteiro *et al.*, 2002).

An extensive literature has detailed many observations of abnormalities in the serum IgA1 of patients with IgAN. Most recently this has centered on the abnormal glycosylation of IgA1 in the disease. *In vitro* aggregation of IgA1 deficient in galactose at high temperatures has been described. If glycosylation abnormalities cause similar aggregation *in vivo*, this could lead to circulating IgA immune complexes and subsequent deposition in the kidneys (Chapter 92). Such aggregation of the IgA will clearly have a marked effect on the interaction of the IgA with its receptors.

IgA from patients with IgAN appears to bind better to FcαRI than normal IgA. Leukocyte FcαRI expression is altered in patients with IgAN, although the quantitation of receptor is complicated by the fact that the receptors can be lost from the surface of leukocytes by internalization and/or shedding (Grosstete *et al.*, 1998). Several studies have shown that FcαRI shed from the surface of leukocytes can bind to IgA in serum, leading to its aggregation (Launay *et al.*, 2000; van der Boog *et al.*, 2002). Although these complexes were first detected in IgAN, a recent report suggests that they are not specific to IgAN (van der Boog *et al.*, 2003).

Reports that CD89 is expressed on mesangial cells have now been largely discounted (Novak *et al.*, 2001). A human FcαRI Tg mouse has been shown to develop IgAN-like disease associated with deposition of mouse pIgA. The significance is unclear because the binding of mouse pIgA to human FcαRI appears weak at best (Launay *et al.*, 2000).

This reported binding of mouse IgA to FcαRI is difficult to reconcile with the fact that the amino acid sequence of human and mouse IgA differ markedly around the FcαRI-binding site. Indeed, when the human sequence is mutated to resemble that of the mouse, the resultant antibody no longer binds human FcαRI (Pleass *et al.*, 1999).

Recently, the transferrin receptor (CD71) has been shown to act as an IgA receptor. This receptor is a marker of cell proliferation, for example, being expressed on proliferating leukocytes but not on circulating cells. It is also expressed on cultured mesangial cells, although not in normal glomeruli. Glomerular expression appears to be increased in patients with IgAN, allowing detection by immunohistochemistry. This overexpression of CD71 has been suggested to play a role in the progression of IgAN (reviewed by Monteiro *et al.*, 2002). Other IgA receptors have been postulated to play a role in the disease. These include the Fcα/μR, which shows increased mRNA expression in human mesangial cells on IL-1 stimulation (McDonald *et al.*, 2003) and an as-yet-uncharacterized IgA receptor demonstrated on mesangial cells that binds pIgA better than monomeric forms (Barratt *et al.*, 2000).

IgA RECEPTORS IN INFECTIOUS DISEASE

FcαRI and mucosal defense

At mucosal sites, S-IgA is abundantly present. Because it is important to balance responses against foreign pathogens and indigenous microflora and dietary antigens, in the past it was believed that S-IgA functioned as a noninflammatory antibody by blocking the entry of microorganisms. The role of FcαRI in mucosal defense is therefore not fully understood. Isolated intestinal lamina propria macrophages were shown to lack FcαRI expression, which is suggestive of an anti-inflammatory role protecting mucosal wall integrity (Smith *et al.*, 2001; Hamre *et al.*, 2003). However, a detailed survey of various tissues revealed some level of FcαRI expression (albeit often low) in all tissues examined (tonsils, appendix, kidney, intestinal mucosa, lymph nodes, and liver) (Hamre *et al.*, 2003). It is interesting that the only distinct FcαRI+ cells observed in the tissue sections were either neutrophils with high FcαRI expression or newly emigrated monocytes/macrophages with much lower expression levels. Peritoneal fluid and bronchoalveolar lavage fluid also contained these weakly positive newly emigrated macrophages. Inflamed intestinal and recently transplanted liver showed large influxes of FcαRI+ cells, which were chiefly neutrophils (Hamre *et al.*, 2003).

Although no FcαRI expression was observed on epidermal CD1a+ dendritic cells (DC) in skin sections (Hamre *et al.*, 2003), others have found low levels of FcαRI expression on monocyte-derived interstitial-type DC that are located *in vivo* beneath the epithelium. The function of FcαRI on DC remains controversial (Geissmann *et al.*, 2001; Heystek *et al.*, 2002). One study reported active FcαRI-mediated uptake of IgA immune complexes leading to upregulation of MHC class II molecules and costimulatory molecule CD86, suggesting that FcαR+ DC play a role in mounting immune responses against mucosal antigens (Geissmann et al., 2001). Another report, however, showed endocytosis of S-IgA immune complexes without induction of DC maturation, which was hypothesized to represent a mechanism for maintaining peripheral self-tolerance (Heystek et al., 2002). Uptake of immune complexes was attributed to binding to carbohydrate-recognizing receptors rather than to FcαRI.

To further investigate the *in vivo* role of FcαRI, Tg mouse models were generated in which cells of the myeloid lineage express FcαRI (van Egmond et al., 1999a, 1999b; Launay et al., 2000). Treatment with anti-*Streptococcus pneumoniae* IgA antibodies was shown to protect FcαRI Tg mice against the development of pneumonia and sepsis after infection with *S. pneumoniae* (G. Vidarsson and E. Saeland, unpublished). Similarly, targeting to FcαRI decreased bacterial colonization of *Bordetella pertussis* in the lungs of FcαRI Tg mice (Hellwig et al., 2001). Although the precise protective mechanisms in these models still have to be established, involvement of FcαRI in IgA-mediated immunity is implicated.

One observation made in FcαRI Tg mice directly linked FcαRI to mucosal immunity. Kupffer cells, which are essential for elimination of invasive bacteria that have entered via the gut, were shown to express FcαRI (van Egmond et al., 2000). Furthermore, FcαRI+ Kupffer cells vigorously ingested human serum IgA–opsonized *Escherichia coli* bacteria *in vivo*. In contrast, human S-IgA was unable to initiate phagocytosis. Although it is yet unknown if this mechanism plays a role for other pathogens, *in vitro* experiments showed phagocytosis of human serum IgA- but not S-IgA-coated *S. aureus*, *Candida albicans*, *Bordetella pertussis*, and *S. pneumoniae* by human neutrophils or neutrophils from human FcαRI Tg mice (van Spriel et al., 1999; van der Pol et al., 2000; Hellwig et al., 2001). On the basis of these results, a hypothesis was formulated that proposes a noninflammatory role for S-IgA as "antiseptic coating" of the mucosa by preventing adherence and invasion of microorganisms in the absence of inflammatory processes (van Egmond et al., 2000). However, in case mucosal integrity is breached, resulting in invasion of microorganisms into the circulation (which are then exposed to serum IgA), FcαRI+ Kupffer cells can prevent septicemia and disease by phagocytosing serum IgA-coated microorganisms. Interactions between FcαRI and serum IgA may therefore provide a "second line of defense," designating serum IgA an inflammatory antibody.

Cleavage of IgA

The importance of IgA in the defense against infection is underlined by the finding that numerous important pathogens have developed ways of specifically avoiding the effects of this Ig by producing IgA-cleaving proteases or IgA-binding proteins. The secretion of highly specific IgA1-cleaving proteases by important bacterial pathogens that invade mucosal surfaces, particularly species of *Streptococcus*, *Haemophilus*, and *Neisseria*, has been recognized for many years (Kilian et al., 1996). These enzymes are well characterized (Chapter 15). Other pathogens, including certain *Pseudomonas*, *Serratia*, and *Proteus* species and some parasites, secrete less-specific proteases that cleave IgA1, IgA2, and IgG. In both cases, active enzyme and characteristic fragments of IgA have been detected in body fluids of patients infected with these pathogens.

Although the biological significance of the cleavage of IgA by these enzymes is not fully understood, the effects of cleavage of serum and S-IgA by proteinases from *Proteus mirabilis* and *Neisseria meningitidis* on the ability to bind to FcαRI have recently been investigated (Almogren et al., 2003). The cleavage of S-IgA1 by the *N. meningitidis* proteinase was found to be as rapid as that of serum IgA1, occurring only in the hinge region and resulting in the separation of Fab and Fc fragments. The Fab fragments retain the ability to bind to antigens but cannot trigger effector functions. Indeed, a bacterium coated with Fab fragments of IgA may be protected from other antibody- or complement-mediated events (Kilian et al., 1996). Although it is unlikely to be of significance *in vivo*, the purified Fc fragment from serum IgA1, when aggregated artificially by binding to a microtiter well, stimulated a respiratory burst in neutrophils through binding to FcαRI. In contrast, the (Fcα)$_2$-SC fragment from digested S-IgA1 did not (Almogren et al., 2003).

The same study showed that cleavage of serum IgA1 by the *P. mirabilis* proteinase occurred at several sites, starting with the removal of the tailpiece and followed by the removal of the CH3 domain and then the CH2 domain. The loss of the tailpiece had little effect on the ability of the cleaved serum IgA to bind to FcαRI, consistent with the findings of an earlier mutagenesis study (Pleass et al., 1999), but the loss of the CH3 domain removed all activity. The α1 chain in S-IgA1 was much more resistant to cleavage by the *P. mirabilis* proteinase than serum IgA1, although the enzyme did cleave SC of S-IgA1. Whether cleaved or not, SC appeared to protect the *Proteus* proteinase cleavage sites in the S-IgA1 heavy chain. S-IgA1, treated with *P. mirabilis* proteinase under conditions that would result in degradation of serum IgA1, retained the ability to bind to FcαRI. These results are consistent with the localization of the FcαRI binding site to the CH2-CH3 interface of IgA. These data shed further light on the structure of S-IgA1 and suggest that the binding site for FcαRI in S-IgA is protected by SC, thus prolonging its potential to activate phagocytic cells at the mucosal surface.

Streptococcal IgA-binding proteins

Bacterial IgA binding proteins (IgA-BP) have been described, particularly in many strains of the important human pathogens group A streptococcus (*Streptococcus pyogenes*) and group B streptococcus and, to a limited extent, in a few other species (Hammerschmidt et al., 1997; Sandt and Hill, 2001). IgA-binding proteins expressed by group A streptococcus include proteins Arp4 and Sir22, members of the M protein family, a group of coiled-coil proteins implicated in virulence (Frithz et al., 1989; Stenberg et al., 1994). Certain group B streptococcal strains express an IgA-binding protein, unrelated to those of *S. pyogenes*, termed β protein (Hédén *et al.* 1991; Jerlström *et al.*, 1991). All these streptococcal IgA-BP appear to share the same interaction site on IgA (Pleass *et al.*, 2001). It is remarkable that the IgA residues involved are largely the same as those bound by human FcαRI. In fact, the streptococcal proteins have been shown to be capable of inhibiting the binding of IgA to human FcαRI, and the Arp4 protein inhibited the ability of IgA to trigger a respiratory burst via FcαRI (Pleass *et al.*, 2001). Thus, the streptococcal IgA-BP may be capable of perturbing IgA function during a bacterial infection. The outcome may be that the bacterium evades the elimination processes that would normally be triggered via FcαRI ligation.

FcRn-MEDIATED IgG TRANSEPITHELIAL TRANSPORT

Some human secretions contain IgG as well as IgA (see Chapter 9). The mechanism by which IgG crosses the epithelia to reach the secretions has not been fully elucidated, but increasing evidence suggests that the so-called neonatal Fc receptor (FcRn) plays an important role. FcRn, which was originally characterized as the receptor responsible for the transport of milk-derived IgG across the intestinal epithelium in neonatal rodents, has evolved as a distantly related member of the MHC class I protein family. It binds IgG in the interdomain region of the Fc, interacting with loops on both Cγ2 and Cγ3 (Burmeister *et al.*, 1994). The interaction is pH-dependent, with low pH favoring association and neutral pH favoring dissociation. This pH dependency facilitates binding of IgG in the intestinal lumen and subsequent release in the tissues and plasma after transport across the epithelial barrier. It has also been established that FcRn regulates the persistence of IgG in the circulation, ensuring that specific IgG remains available for long-term protection (Ghetie and Ward, 2002). This homeostatic mechanism provides half-lives of greater than 20 days for most human IgGs. Experiments with FcRn-deficient mice have recently confirmed the dual role of FcRn in perinatal IgG transport and IgG homeostasis (Roopenian *et al.*, 2003). In humans, FcRn is found in the placental syncytiotrophoblast, where it plays a role in mediating transfer of maternal IgG to the fetus, possibly via IgG transfer from a novel FcγR of 55 kDa (Gafencu *et al.*, 2003). It is also found in human fetal intestine, suggesting that it may play an additional role in fetal uptake of IgG present in ingested amniotic fluid (Shah *et al.*, 2003).

It is now apparent that FcRn is expressed on adult epithelial tissue in both rodents and humans as well as in neonates. Thus, in human adults it has been demonstrated on intestinal epithelium (Israel *et al.*, 1997), bronchial epithelium (Spiekermann *et al.*, 2002), and renal proximal tubular epithelium (Kobayashi *et al.*, 2002), as well as on monocytes, macrophages, and DC (Zhu *et al.*, 2001). In rodents, the receptor has also been shown to be expressed at the blood-brain barrier (Schlachetzki *et al.*, 2002).

A number of recent studies indicate that human and rodent FcRn can transport IgG across epithelial cells bidirectionally, i.e., from basolateral surface to apical surface (mucosal lumen) and in the opposite direction, from lumen to basolateral surface (Dickinson *et al.*, 1999; Praetor *et al.*, 1999; McCarthy *et al.*, 2002; Spiekermann *et al.*, 2002; Kobayashi *et al.*, 2002). Thus the possibility exists that FcRn undergoes multiple rounds of transcytosis, transporting IgG in both lumenal and ablumenal directions (Dickinson *et al.*, 1999). Hence FcRn may have multiple transport roles: to transport ingested IgG from the lumen, to transport maternal IgG to fetus, to transfer IgG out into the secretions, and to carry IgG complexed with lumenal antigens back across the epithelium. This latter function represents a novel means of immunosurveillance whereby ingested or inhaled antigens can be retrieved and delivered to immunocompetent cells underlying the epithelium for initiation of an appropriate specific immune response, whether active immunity or tolerance (Blumberg *et al.*, 2001; Spiekermann *et al.*, 2002).

Acknowledgments
The authors acknowledge support from the Leukaemia Research Fund, MRC, and the Wellcome Trust.

REFERENCES

Abu-Ghazaleh, R.I., Fujisawa, T., Mestecky, J., Kyle, R.A., and Gleich, G.J. (1989). IgA-induced eosinophil degranulation. *J. Immunol.* 142, 2393–2400.

Almogren, A., Senior, B.W., Loomes, L.M., and Kerr, M.A. (2003). Structural and functional consequences of cleavage of human secretory and serum immunoglobulin A1 by proteinases from *Proteus mirabilis* and *Neisseria meningitidis*. *Infect. Immun.* 71, 3349–3356.

Barratt, J., Greer, M.R., Pawluczyk, I.Z., Allen, A.C., Bailey, E.M., Buck, K.S., and Feehally, J. (2000). Identification of a novel Fcα receptor expressed by human mesangial cells. *Kidney Int.* 57, 1936–1948.

Berger, J., Yaneva, H., Nabarra, B., and Barbanel, C. (1975). Recurrence of mesangial deposition of IgA after renal transplantation. *Kidney Int.* 7, 232–241.

Blumberg, R.S., van de Wal, Y., Claypool, S., Corazza, N., Dickinson, B., Nieuwenhuis, E., Pitman, R., Spiekermann, G., Zhu, X., Colgan, S., and Lencer, W.I. (2001). The multiple roles of major histocompatibility complex class-I-like molecules in mucosal immune function. *Acta Odontol. Scand.* 59, 139–144.

Bracke, M., Dubois, G.R., Bolt, K., Bruijnzeel, P.L., Vaerman, J.P., Lammers, J.W., and Koenderman, L. (1997). Differential effects of the T helper cell type 2-derived cytokines IL-4 and IL-5 on ligand binding to IgG and IgA receptors expressed by human eosinophils. *J. Immunol.* 159, 1459–1465.

Bracke, M., Lammers, J.W., Coffer, P.J., and Koenderman, L. (2001). Cytokine-induced inside-out activation of FcαR (CD89) is mediated by a single serine residue (S263) in the intracellular domain of the receptor. *Blood* 97, 3478–3483.

Burmeister, W.P., Huber, A.H., and Bjorkman, P.J. (1994). Crystal structure of the complex of rat neonatal Fc receptor with Fc. *Nature* 372, 379–383.

Burton, D.R., and Woof, J.M. (1992). Human antibody effector function. *Adv. Immunol.* 51, 1–84.

Carayannopoulos, L., Hexham, J.M., and Capra, J.D. (1996). Localization of the binding site for the monocyte immunoglobulin (Ig) A-Fc receptor (CD89) to the domain boundary between Cα2 and Cα3 in human IgA1. *J. Exp. Med.* 183, 1579–1586.

Chapman, T.L., Heikema, A.P., West, A.P., and Bjorkman, P.J. (2000). Crystal structure and ligand binding properties of the D1D2 region of the inhibitory receptor LIR-1 (ILT2). *Immunity* 13, 727–736.

Deviere, J., Vaerman, J.P., Content, J., Denys, C., Schandene, L., Vandenbussche, P., Sibille, Y., and Dupont, E. (1991). IgA triggers tumor necrosis factor α secretion by monocytes: a study in normal subjects and patients with alcoholic cirrhosis. *Hepatology* 13, 670–675.

de Wit, T.P., Morton, H.C., Capel, P.J., and van de Winkel, J.G. (1995). Structure of the gene for the human myeloid IgA Fc receptor (CD89). *J. Immunol.* 155, 1203–1209.

Dickinson, B.L., Badizadegan, K., Wu, Z., Ahouse, J.C., Zhu, X., Simister, N.E., Blumberg, R.S., and Lencer, W.I. (1999). Bidirectional FcRn-dependent IgG transport in a polarized human intestinal epithelial cell line. *J. Clin. Invest.* 104, 903–911.

Ding, Y., Xu, G., Yang, M., Yao, M., Gao, G.F., Zhang, W., and Rao, Z. (2003). Crystal structure of the ectodomain of human FcαRI. *J. Biol. Chem.* 278, 27966–27970.

Dombrowicz, D., Flamand, V., Miyajima, I., Ravetch, J.V., Galli, S.J., and Kinet, J.P. (1997). Absence of FcεRI α chain results in upregulation of FcγRIII-dependent mast cell degranulation and anaphylaxis. Evidence of competition between FcεRI and FcγRIII for limiting amounts of FcR β and γ chains. *J. Clin. Invest.* 99, 915–925.

Dunne, D.W., Richardson, B.A., Jones, F.M., Clark, M., Thorne, K.J., and Butterworth, A.E. (1993). The use of mouse/human chimaeric antibodies to investigate the roles of different antibody isotypes, including IgA2, in the killing of *Schistosoma mansoni* schistosomula by eosinophils. *Parasite Immunol.* 15, 181–185.

Fanger, M.W., Shen, L., Pugh, J., and Bernier, G.M. (1980). Subpopulations of human peripheral granulocytes and monocytes express receptors for IgA. *Proc. Natl. Acad. Sci. USA* 77, 3640–3644.

Ferreri, N.R., Howland, W.C., and Spiegelberg, H.L. (1986). Release of leukotrienes C4 and B4 and prostaglandin E2 from human monocytes stimulated with aggregated IgG, IgA, and IgE. *J. Immunol.* 136, 4188–4193.

Frithz, E., Hedén, L.-O., and Lindahl, G. (1989). Extensive sequence homology between IgA receptor and M proteins in *Streptococcus pyogenes*. *Mol. Microbiol.* 3, 1111–1119.

Gafencu, A., Heltianu, C., Burlacu, A., Hunziker, W., and Simionescu, M. (2003). Investigation of IgG receptors expressed on the surface of human placental endothelial cells. *Placenta* 24, 664–676.

Garman, S.C., Wurzburg, B.A., Tarchevskaya, S.S., Kinet, J.P., and Jardetzky, T.S. (2000). Structure of the Fc fragment of human IgE bound to its high-affinity receptor FcεRIa. *Nature* 406, 259–266.

Geissmann, F., Launay, P., Pasquier, B., Lepelletier, Y., Leborgne, M., Lehuen, A., Brousse, N., and Monteiro, R.C. (2001). A subset of human dendritic cells expresses IgA Fc receptor (CD89), which mediates internalization and activation upon cross-linking by IgA complexes. *J. Immunol.* 166, 346–352.

Ghetie, V., and Ward, E.S. (2002). Transcytosis and catabolism of antibody. *Immunol. Res.* 25, 97–113.

Gould H.J., Sutton B.J., Beavil A.J., Beavil R.L., McCloskey N., Coker H.A., Fear D., and Smurthwaite L. (2003). The biology of IgE and the basis of allergic disease. *Annu. Rev. Immunol.* 21, 579–628.

Grossetete, B., Launay, P., Lehuen, A., Jungers, P., Bach, J.F., and Monteiro, R.C. (1998). Down-regulation of Fcα receptors on blood cells of IgA nephropathy patients: evidence for a negative regulatory role of serum IgA. *Kidney Int.* 53, 1321–1335.

Gulle, H., Samstag, A., Eibl, M.M., and Wolf, H.M. (1998). Physical and functional association of FcαR with protein tyrosine kinase Lyn. *Blood* 91, 383–391.

Haddad, E., Moura, I.C., Arcos-Fajardo, M., Macher, M.A., Baudouin, V., Alberti, C., Loirat, C., Monteiro, R.C., and Peuchmaur, M. (2003). Enhanced expression of the CD71 mesangial IgA1 receptor in Berger disease and Henoch-Schönlein nephritis: association between CD71 expression and IgA deposits. *J. Am. Soc. Nephrol.* 14, 327–337.

Hammerschmidt, S., Talay, S.R., Brandtzaeg, P., and Chhatwal, G.S.(1997). SpsA, a novel pneumococcal surface protein with specific binding to secretory immunoglobulin A and secretory component. *Mol. Microbiol.* 25, 1113–1124.

Hamre, R., Farstad, I.N., Brandtzaeg, P., and Morton, H.C. (2003). Expression and modulation of the human immunoglobulin A Fc receptor (CD89) and the FcR γ chain on myeloid cells in blood and tissue. *Scand. J. Immunol.* 57, 506–516.

Hedén, L.-O., Frithz, E., and Lindahl, G.(1991). Molecular characterization of an IgA receptor from group B streptococci: sequence of the gene, identification of a proline-rich region with unique structure and isolation of N-terminal fragments with IgA-binding capacity. *Eur. J. Immunol.* 21, 1481–1490.

Hellwig, S.M., van Spriel, A.B., Schellekens, J.F., Mooi, F.R., and van de Winkel, J.G.J. (2001). Immunoglobulin A-mediated protection against *Bordetella pertussis* infection. *Infect. Immun.* 69, 4846–4850.

Herr, A.B., Ballister, E.R., and Bjorkman, P.J. (2003a). Insights into IgA-mediated immune responses from the crystal structures of human FcαRI and its complex with IgA1-Fc. *Nature* 423, 614–620.

Herr, A.B., White, C.L., Milburn, C., Wu, C., and Bjorkman, P.J. (2003b). Bivalent binding of IgA1 to FcαRI suggests a mechanism for cytokine activation of IgA phagocytosis. *J. Mol. Biol.* 327, 645–657.

Heystek, H.C., Moulon, C., Woltman, A.M., Garonne, P., and van Kooten, C. (2002). Human immature dendritic cells efficiently bind and take up secretory IgA without the induction of maturation. *J. Immunol.* 168, 102–107.

Honorio-Franca, A.C., Launay, P., Carneiro-Sampaio, M.M., and Monteiro, R.C. (2001). Colostral neutrophils express Fcα receptors (CD89) lacking γ chain association and mediate noninflammatory properties of secretory IgA. *J. Leukoc. Biol.* 69, 289–296.

Huls, G., Heijnen, I.A., Cuomo, E., van der Linden, J., Boel, E., van de Winkel, J.G.J., and Logtenberg, T. (1999). Antitumor immune effector mechanisms recruited by phage display-derived fully human IgG1 and IgA1 monoclonal antibodies. *Cancer Res.* 59, 5778–5784.

Hulett, M.D., and Hogarth, P.M. (1994). Molecular basis of Fc receptor function. *Adv. Immunol.* 57, 1–127.

Israel, E.J., Taylor, S., Wu, Z., Mizoguchi, E., Blumberg, R.S., Bhan, A., and Simister, N.E. (1997). Expression of the neonatal Fc receptor, FcRn, on human intestinal epithelial cells. *Immunology* 92, 69–74.

Jandrot-Perrus, M., Busfield, S., Lagrue, A.H., Xiong, X., Debili, N., Chickering, T., Le Couedic, J.P., Goodearl, A., Dussault, B., Fraser, C., Vainchenker, W., and Villeval, J.L. (2000). Cloning, characterization, and functional studies of human and mouse glycoprotein VI: a platelet-specific collagen receptor from the immunoglobulin superfamily. *Blood* 96, 1798–1807.

Jerlström, P.G., Chhatwal, G.S., and Timmis, K.N.(1991). The IgA-binding beta antigen of the c protein complex of Group B streptococci: sequence determination of its gene and detection of two binding regions. *Mol. Microbiol.* 5, 843–849.

Kato, T. (1990). A study of secretory immunoglobulin A on membranous epithelial cells (M cells) and adjacent absorptive cells of rabbit Peyer's patches. *Gastroenterol. Jpn.* 25, 15–23.

Keler, T., Wallace, P.K., Vitale, L.A., Russoniello, C., Sundarapandiyan, K., Graziano, R.F., and Deo, Y.M. (2000). Differential effect of cytokine treatment on Fcα receptor I- and Fcγ receptor I-mediated tumor cytotoxicity by monocyte-derived macrophages. *J. Immunol.* 164, 5746–5752.

Kilian, M., Reinholdt, J., Lomholt, H., Poulsen, K., and Frandsen, E.V.G. (1996). Biological significance of IgA1 proteases in bacterial colonization and pathogenesis: critical evaluation of experimental evidence. *APMIS* 104, 321–338.

Kita, H., Kaneko, M., Bartemes, K.R., Weiler, D.A., Schimming, A.W., Reed, C.E., and Gleich, G.J. (1999). Does IgE bind to and activate eosinophils from patients with allergy? *J. Immunol.* 162, 6901–6911.

Kitamura, T., Garofalo, R.P., Kamijo, A., Hammond, D.K., Oka, J.A., Caflisch, C.R., Shenoy, M., Casola, A., Weigel, P.H., and Goldblum, R.M. (2000). Human intestinal epithelial cells express a novel receptor for IgA. *J. Immunol.* 164, 5029–5034.

Kobayashi, N., Suzuki, Y., Tsuge, T., Okumura, K., Ra, C., and Tomino, Y. (2002). FcRn-mediated transcytosis of immunoglobulin G in human renal proximal tubular epithelial cells. *Am. J. Physiol. Renal Physiol.* 282, F358–365.

Kremer, E.J., Kalatzis, V., Baker, E., Callen, D.F., Sutherland, G.R., and Maliszewski, C.R. (1992). The gene for the human IgA Fc receptor maps to 19q13.4. *Hum. Genet.* 89,107–108.

Lang, M.L., and Kerr, M.A. (1997). Neutrophil Fc receptors signal through PI 3-kinase to trigger a respiratory burst. *Biochem. Soc. Trans.* 25, S603.

Lang, M.L., and Kerr, M.A. (2000). Characterization of FcαR-triggered Ca(2+) signals: role in neutrophil NADPH oxidase activation. *Biochem. Biophys. Res. Commun.* 276, 749–755.

Lang, M.L., Shen, L., and Wade, W.F. (1999). γ-chain dependent recruitment of tyrosine kinases to membrane rafts by the human IgA receptor FcαR. *J. Immunol.* 163, 5391–5398.

Lang, M.L., Chen, Y.W., Shen, L., Gao, H., Lang, G.A., Wade, T.K., and Wade, W.F. (2002). IgA Fc receptor (FcαR) cross-linking recruits tyrosine kinases, phosphoinositide kinases and serine/threonine kinases to glycolipid rafts. *Biochem. J.* 364, 517–525.

Lamkhioued, B., Gounni, A.S., Gruart, V., Pierce, A., Capron, A., and Capron, M. (1995). Human eosinophils express a receptor for secretory component. Role in secretory IgA-dependent activation. *Eur. J. Immunol.* 25, 117–125.

Launay, P., Lehuen, A., Kawakami, T., Blank, U., and Monteiro, R.C. (1998). IgA Fc receptor (CD89) activation enables coupling to syk and Btk tyrosine kinase pathways: differential signalling after IFN-γ or phorbol ester stimulation. *J. Leukoc. Biol.* 63, 636–642.

Launay, P., Patry, C., Lehuen, A., Pasquier, B., Blank, U., and Monteiro, R.C. (1999). Alternative endocytic pathway for immunoglobulin A Fc receptors (CD89) depends on the lack of FcRα association and protects against degradation of bound ligand. *J. Biol. Chem.* 274, 7216–7225.

Launay, P., Grossetete, B., Arcos-Fajardo, M., Gaudin, E., Torres, S.P., Beaudoin, L., Patey-Mariaud de Serre, N., Lehuen, A., and Monteiro, R.C. (2000). Fcα receptor (CD89) mediates the development of immunoglobulin A (IgA) nephropathy (Berger's disease). Evidence for pathogenic soluble receptor-IgA complexes in patients and CD89 transgenic mice. *J. Exp. Med.* 191, 1999–2009.

Lawrence, D.A., Weigle, W.O., and Spiegelberg, H.L. (1975). Immunoglobulins cytophilic for human lymphocytes, monocytes, and neutrophils. *J. Clin. Invest.* 55, 368–387.

Lelouard, H., Reggio, H., Mangeat, P., Neutra, M., and Montcourrier, P. (1999). Mucin-related epitopes distinguish M cells and enterocytes in rabbit appendix and Peyer's patches. *Infect. Immun.* 67, 357–367.

Maliszewski, C.R., March, C.J., Schoenborn, M.A., Gimpel, S., and Shen, L. (1990). Expression cloning of a human Fc receptor for IgA. *J. Exp. Med.* 172, 1665–1672.

Mantis, N.J., Cheung, M.C., Chintalacharuvu, K.R., Rey, J., Corthesy, B., and Neutra, M.R. (2002). Selective adherence of IgA to murine Peyer's patch M cells: evidence for a novel IgA receptor. *J. Immunol.* 169,1844–1851.

Mattu, T.S., Pleass, R.J., Willis, A.C., Kilian, M., Wormald, M.R., Lellouch, A.C., Rudd, P.M., Woof, J.M., and Dwek, R.A. (1998). The glycosylation and structure of human serum IgA1, Fab and Fc regions and the role of N-glycosylation on FcαR interactions. *J. Biol. Chem.* 273, 2260–2272.

Mazengera, R.L., and Kerr, M.A. (1990). The specificity of the IgA receptor purified from human neutrophils. *Biochem. J.* 272, 159–165.

McCarthy, K.M., Yoong, Y., and Simister, N.E. (2000). Bidirectional transcytosis of IgG by the rat neonatal Fc receptor expressed in a rat kidney cell line: a system to study protein transport across epithelia. *J. Cell Sci.* 113, 1277–1285.

McDonald, K.J., Cameron, A.J., Allen, J.M., and Jardine, A.G. (2002). Expression of Fcα/μ receptor by human mesangial cells: a candidate receptor for immune complex deposition in IgA nephropathy. *Biochem. Biophys. Res. Commun.* 290, 438–442.

Monteiro, R.C., Cooper, M.D., and Kubagawa, H. (1992). Molecular heterogeneity of Fcα receptors detected by receptor-specific monoclonal antibodies. *J. Immunol.* 148, 1764–1770.

Monteiro, R.C., Hostoffer, R.W., Cooper M.D., Bonner, J.R., Gartland, G.L., and Kubagawa, H. (1993). Definition of immunoglobulin A receptors on eosinophils and their enhanced expression in allergic individuals. *J. Clin. Invest.* 92, 1681–1685.

Monteiro, R.C., Moura, I.C., Launay, P., Tsuge, T., Haddad, E., Benhamou, M., Cooper, M.D., and Arcos-Fajardo, M. (2002). Pathogenic significance of IgA receptor interactions in IgA nephropathy. *Trends Mol. Med.* 8, 464–468.

Monteiro, R.C., and van de Winkel, J.G.J. (2003). IgA Fc Receptors. *Annu. Rev. Immunol.* 21,177–204.

Morton, H.C., van den Herik-Oudijk, I.E., Vossebeld, P., Snijders, A., Verhoeven, A.J., Capel, P.J.A., and van de Winkel, J.G.J. (1995). Functional association between the human myeloid immunoglobulin A Fc receptor (CD89) and FcR γ chain. Molecular basis for CD89/FcR γ chain association. *J. Biol. Chem.* 270, 29781–29789.

Morton, H.C., Schiel, A.E., Janssen, S.W., and van de Winkel, J.G.J. (1996a). Alternatively spliced forms of the human myeloid Fcα receptor (CD89) in neutrophils. *Immunogenetics* 43, 246–247.

Morton, H.C., van Egmond, M., and van de Winkel, J.G.J. (1996b). Structure and function of human IgA Fc receptors (FcαR). *Crit. Rev. Immunol.* 16, 423–440.

Morton, H.C., Pleass, R.J., Storset, A.K., Dissen, E., Williams, J.L., Brandtzaeg, P., and Woof, J.M. (2003). Cloning and characterization of an IgA Fc receptor from cattle (bFcαR). *Immunology* 111, 204–211.

Motegi, Y., and Kita, H. (1998). Interaction with secretory component stimulates effector functions of human eosinophils but not of neutrophils. *J. Immunol.* 161, 4340–4346.

Moura, I.C., Centelles, M.N., Arcos-Fajardo, M., Malheiros, D.M., Collawn, J.F., Cooper, M.D., and Monteiro, R.C. (2001). Identification of the transferrin receptor as a novel immunoglobulin (Ig)A1 receptor and its enhanced expression on mesangial cells in IgA nephropathy. *J. Exp. Med.* 194, 417–425.

Nakahara, J., Seiwa, C., Shibuya, A., Aiso, S., and Asou, H. (2003). Expression of Fc receptor for immunoglobulin M in oligodendrocytes and myelin of mouse central nervous system. *Neurosci. Lett.* 337, 73–76.

Novak, J., Julian, B.A., Tomana, M., and Mestecky, J. (2001). Progress in molecular and genetic studies of IgA nephropathy. *J. Clin. Immunol.* 21, 310–327.

Park, R.K., Izadi, K.D., Deo, Y.M., and Durden, D.L. (1999). Role of Src in the modulation of multiple adaptor proteins in FcαRI oxidant signalling. *Blood* 94, 2112–2120.

Patry, C., Herbelin, A., Lehuen, A., Bach, J.F., and Monteiro, R.C. (1995). Fcα receptors mediate release of tumour necrosis factor-α and interleukin-6 by human monocytes following receptor aggregation. *Immunology* 86, 1–5.

Patry, C., Sibille, Y., Lehuen, A., and Monteiro, R.C. (1996). Identification of Fcα receptor (CD89) isoforms generated by alternative splicing that are differentially expressed between blood monocytes and alveolar macrophages. *J. Immunol.* 156, 4442–4448.

Pfefferkorn, L.C., and Yeaman, G.R. (1994). Association of IgA-Fc receptors (FcαR) with FcεRI γ2 subunits in U937 cells: Aggregation induces the tyrosine phosphorylation of γ2. *J. Immunol.* 153, 3228–3236.

Pleass, R.J., Andrews, P.D., Kerr, M.A., and Woof, J.M. (1996). Alternative splicing of the human IgA Fc receptor CD89 in neutrophils and eosinophils. *Biochem. J.* 318, 771–777.

Pleass, R.J., Dunlop, J.I., Anderson, C.M., and Woof, J.M. (1999). Identification of residues in the CH2/CH3 domain interface of IgA essential for interaction with the human Fcα receptor (FcαR) CD89. *J. Biol. Chem.* 274, 23508–23514.

Pleass, R.J., Areschoug, T., Lindahl, G., and Woof, J.M. (2001). Streptococcal IgA-binding proteins bind in the Cα2-Cα3 interdomain region and inhibit binding of IgA to human CD89. *J. Biol. Chem.* 276, 8197–8204.

Pleass, R.J., Dehal, P.K., Lewis, M.J., and Woof, J.M. (2003). Limited role of charge matching in the interaction of human immunoglobulin A (IgA) with the IgA Fc receptor (FcαRI) CD89. *Immunology* 109, 331–335.

Praetor, A., Ellinger, I., and Hunziker, W. (1999). Intracellular traffic of the MHC class I-like IgG Fc receptor, FcRn, expressed in epithelial MDCK cells. *J. Cell Sci.* 112, 2291–2299.

Ravetch, J.V. (1997). Fc receptors. *Curr. Opin. Immunol.* 9, 121–125.

Reterink, T.J., Verweij, C.L., van Es, L.A., and Daha, M.R. (1996). Alternative splicing of IgA Fc receptor (CD89) transcripts. *Gene* 175, 279–280.

Reth, M. (1989). Antigen receptor tail clue. *Nature* 338, 383–384.

Rifai, A., Fadden, K., Morrison, S.L., and Chintalacharuvu, K.R. (2000). The *N*-glycans determine the differential blood clearance and hepatic uptake of human immunoglobulin (Ig)A1 and IgA2 isotypes. *J. Exp. Med.* 191, 2171–2182.

Roopenian, D.C., Christianson, G.J., Sproule, T.J., Brown, A.C., Akilesh, S., Jung, N., Petkova, S., Avanessian, L., Choi, E.Y., Shaffer, D.J., Eden, P.A., and Anderson, C.L. (2003). The MHC Class I-like IgG receptor controls perinatal IgG transport, IgG homeostasis, and fate of IgG-Fc-coupled drugs. *J. Immunol.* 170, 3528–3533.

Roy, M.J., and Varvayanis, M. (1987). Development of dome epithelium in gut associated lymphoid tissues: association of IgA with M cells. *Cell Tissue Res.* 248, 645–651.

Rudd, P.M., Fortune, F., Patel, T., Parekh, R.B., Dwek, R.A., and Lehner, T. (1994). A human T-cell receptor recognizes 'O'-linked sugars from the hinge region of human IgA1 and IgD. *Immunology* 83, 99–106.

Sakamoto, N., Shibuya, K., Shimizu, Y., Yotsumoto, K., Miyabayashi, T., Sakano, S., Tsuji, T., Nakayama, E., Nakauchi, H., and Shibuya, A. (2001). A novel Fc receptor for IgA and IgM is expressed on both hematopoietic and non-hematopoietic tissues. *Eur. J. Immunol.* 31, 1310–1316.

Sandt, C.H., and Hill, C.W. (2001). Nonimmune binding of human immunoglobulin A (IgA) and IgG Fc by distinct sequence segments of the EibF cell surface protein of *Escherichia coli. Infect. Immun.* 69, 7293–7303.

Schlachetzki, F., Zhu, C., and Pardridge, W.M. (2002). Expression of the neonatal Fc receptor (FcRn) at the blood-brain barrier. *J. Neurochem.* 81, 203–206.

Shah, U., Dickinson, B.L., Blumberg, R.S., Simister, N.E., Lencer, W.I., and Walker, W.A. (2003). Distribution of the IgG Fc receptor, FcRn, in the human fetal intestine. *Pediatr. Res.* 53, 295–301.

Shen, L., and Collins, J. (1989). Monocyte superoxide secretion triggered by human IgA. *Immunology*, 68, 491–496.

Shen, L., Lasser, R., and Fanger, M.W. (1989). My 43, a monoclonal antibody that reacts with human myeloid cells inhibits monocyte IgA binding and triggers function. *J. Immunol.* 143, 4117–4122.

Shen, L., Collins, J.E., Schoenborn, M.A., and Maliszewski, C.R. (1994). Lipopolysaccharide and cytokine augmentation of human monocyte IgA receptor expression and function. *J. Immunol.* 152, 4080–4086.

Shen, L., van Egmond, M., Siemasko, K., Gao, H., Wade, T., Lang, M.L., Clark, M., van de Winkel, J.G.J., and Wade, W.F. (2001). Presentation of ovalbumin internalized via the immunoglobulin-A Fc receptor is enhanced through Fc receptor γ-chain signaling. *Blood* 97, 205–213.

Shibuya, A., Sakamoto, N., Shimizu, Y., Shibuya, K., Osawa, M., Hiroyama, T., Eyre, H.J., Sutherland, G.R., Endo, Y., Fujita, T., Miyabayashi, T., Sakano, S., Tsuji, T., Nakayama, E., Phillips, J.H., Lanier, L.L., and Nakauchi, H. (2000). Fcα/μ receptor mediates endocytosis of IgM-coated microbes. *Nat. Immunol.* 1, 441–446.

Shimokawa, T., Tsuge, T., Okumura, K., and Ra, C. (2000). Identification and characterization of the promoter for the gene encoding the human myeloid IgA Fc receptor (FcαR, CD89). *Immunogenetics* 51, 945–954.

Shimokawa, T., and Ra, C. (2003). C/EBPα and Ets protein family members regulate the human myeloid JgA Fc receptor (FcαR, CD89) promoter. *J. Immunol.* 170, 2564–2572.

Shimizu, Y., Honda, S., Yotsumoto, K., Tahara-Hanaoka, S., Eyre, H.J., Sutherland, G.R., Endo, Y., Shibuya, K., Koyama, A., Nakauchi, H., and Shibuya A. (2001). Fcα/μ receptor is a single gene-family member closely related to polymeric immunoglobulin receptor encoded on Chromosome 1. *Immunogenetics* 53, 709–711.

Smith, P.D., Smythies, L.E., Mosteller-Barnum, M., Sibley, D.A., Russell, M.W., Merger, M., Sellers, M.T., Orenstein, J.M., Shimada, T., Graham, M.F., and Kubagawa, H. (2001). Intestinal macrophages lack CD14 and CD89 and consequently are down-regulated for LPS- and IgA-mediated activities. *J. Immunol.* 167, 2651–2656.

Sondermann, P., Huber, R., Oosthuizen, V., and Jacob, U. (2000). The 3.2-Å crystal structure of the human IgG1 Fc fragment-FcγRIII complex. *Nature* 406, 267–273.

Spiekermann, G.M., Finn, P.W., Ward, E.S., Dumont, J., Dickinson, B.L., Blumberg, R.S., and Lencer, W.I. (2002). Receptor-mediated immunoglobulin G transport across mucosal barriers in adult life: functional expression of FcRn in the mammalian lung. *J. Exp. Med.* 196, 303–310.

Spiegelberg, H.L., Lawrence, D.A., and Henson, P. (1974). Cytophilic properties of IgA to human neutrophils. *Adv. Exp. Med. Biol.* 44, 67–74.

Stenberg, L., O'Toole, P.W., Mestecky, J., and Lindahl, G. (1994). Molecular characterization of protein Sir, a streptococcal cell surface protein that binds both immunoglobulin A and immunoglobulin G. *J. Biol. Chem.* 269, 13458–13464.

Stewart, W.W., and Kerr, M.A. (1990). The specificity of the human neutrophil IgA receptor (FcαR) determined by measurement of chemiluminescence induced by serum or secretory IgA1 or IgA2. *Immunology* 71, 328–334.

Stewart, W.W., Mazengera, R.L., Shen, L., and Kerr, M.A. (1994). Unaggregated serum IgA binds to neutrophil FcαR at physiological concentrations and is endocytosed but cross-linking is necessary to elicit a respiratory burst. *J. Leukoc. Biol.* 56, 481–487.

Stockert, R.J. (1995). The asialoglycoprotein receptor: relationships between structure, function and expression. *Physiol. Rev.* 75, 591–609.

Stockmeyer, B., Dechant, M., van Egmond, M., Tutt, A.L., Sundarapandiyan, K., Graziano, R.F., Repp, R., Kalden, J.R., Gramatzki, M., Glennie, M.J., van de Winkel, J.G.J., and Valerius, T. (2000). Triggering Fcα-receptor I (CD89) recruits neutrophils as effector cells for CD20-directed antibody therapy. *J. Immunol.* 165, 5954–5961.

Togo, S., Shimokawa, T., Fukuchi, Y., and Ra, C. (2003). Alternative splicing of myeloid IgA Fc receptor (FcαR, CD89) transcripts in inflammatory responses. *FEBS Lett.* 535, 205–209.

Tomana, M., Kulhavy, R., and Mestecky, J. (1988). Receptor-mediated binding and uptake of immunoglobulin A by human liver. *Gastroenterology* 94, 762–770.

Tomana, M., Zikan, J., Kulhavy, R., Bennett, J.C., and Mestecky, J. (1993). Interactions of galactosyltransferase with serum and secretory immunoglobulins and their component chains. *Mol. Immunol.* 30, 277–286.

Toyabe, S., Kuwano, Y., Takeda, K., Uchiyama, M., and Abo, T. (1997). IgA nephropathy-specific expression of the IgA Fc receptors (CD89) on blood phagocytic cells. *Clin. Exp. Immunol.* 110, 226–232.

Tsuge, T., Shimokawa, T., Horikoshi, S., Tomino, Y., and Ra, C. (2001). Polymorphism in promoter region of Fcα receptor gene in patients with IgA nephropathy. *Hum. Genet.* 108, 128–133.

Valerius, T., Stockmeyer, B., van Spriel, A.B., Graziano, R.F., van den Herik-Oudijk, I.E., Repp, R., Deo, Y.M., Lund, J., Kalden, J.R., Gramatzki, M., and van de Winkel, J.G.J. (1997). FcαRI (CD89) as a novel trigger molecule for bispecific antibody therapy. *Blood* 90, 4485–4492.

van der Boog, P.J., van Zandbergen, G., de Fijter, J.W., Klar-Mohamad, N., van Seggelen, A., Brandtzaeg, P., Daha, M.R., and van Kooten, C. (2002) FcαRI/CD89 circulates in human serum covalently linked to IgA in a polymeric state. *J. Immunol.* 168, 1252–1258.

van der Boog, P.J., de Fijter, J.W., van Kooten, C., van der Holst, R., van Seggelen, A., van Es, L.A., and Daha, M.R. (2003). Complexes of IgA with FcαRI/CD89 are not specific for primary IgA nephropathy. *Kidney Int.* 63, 514–521.

van der Pol, W., Vidarsson, G., Vile, H.A., van de Winkel, J.G.J., and Rodriguez, M.E. (2000). Pneumococcal capsular polysaccharide-specific IgA triggers efficient neutrophil effector functions via FcαRI (CD89). *J. Infect. Dis.* 182, 1139–1145.

van Dijk, T.B., Bracke, M., Caldenhoven, E., Raaijmakers, J.A., Lammers, J.W., Koenderman, L., and de Groot, R.P. (1996). Cloning and characterization of FcαRb, a novel Fcα receptor (CD89) isoform expressed in eosinophils and neutrophils. *Blood* 88, 4229–4238.

van Egmond, M., van Vuuren, A.J., Morton, H.C., van Spriel, A.B., Shen, L., Hofhuis, F.M., Saito, T., Mayadas, T.N., Verbeek, J.S., and van de Winkel, J.G.J. (1999a). Human immunoglobulin A receptor (FcαRI, CD89) function in transgenic mice requires both FcR γ chain and CR3 (CD11b/CD18). *Blood* 93, 4387–4394.

van Egmond, M., van Vuuren, A.J., and van de Winkel, J.G.J. (1999b). The human Fc receptor for IgA (FcαRI, CD89) on transgenic peritoneal macrophages triggers phagocytosis and tumor cell lysis. *Immunol. Lett.* 68, 83–87.

van Egmond, M., van Garderen, E., van Spriel, A.B., Damen, C.A., van Amersfoort, E.S., van Zandbergen, G., van Hattum, J., Kuiper, J., and van de Winkel, J.G.J. (2000). FcαRI-positive liver Kupffer cells: reappraisal of the function of immunoglobulin A in immunity. *Nat. Med.* 6, 680–685.

van Egmond, M., Damen, C.A., van Spriel, A.B., Vidarsson, G., van Garderen, E., and van de Winkel, J.G.J. (2001a). IgA and the IgA Fc receptor. *Trends Immunol.* 22, 205–211.

van Egmond, M., van Spriel, A.B., Vermeulen, H., Huls, G., van Garderen, E., and van de Winkel, J.G.J. (2001b). Enhancement of polymorphonuclear cell-mediated tumour cell killing on simultaneous engagement of FcγRI (CD64) and FcαRI (CD89). *Cancer Res.* 61, 4055–4060.

van Epps, D.E., and Williams, R.C. Jr. (1976). Suppression of leukocyte chemotaxis by human IgA myeloma components. *J. Exp. Med.* 144, 1227–1242.

van Spriel, A.B., van den Herik-Oudijk, I.E., van Sorge, N.M., Vile, H.A., van Strijp, J.A., and van de Winkel, J.G.J. (1999). Effective phagocytosis and killing of *Candida albicans* via targeting FcγRI (CD64) or FcαRI (CD89) on neutrophils. *J. Infect. Dis.* 179, 661–669.

van Spriel, A.B., Leusen, J.H., van Egmond, M., Dijkman, H.B., Assmann, K.J., Mayadas, T.N., and van de Winkel, J.G.J. (2001). Mac-1 (CD11b/CD18) is essential for Fc receptor-mediated neutrophil cytotoxicity and immunologic synapse formation. *Blood* 97, 2478–2486.

van Spriel, A.B., Leusen, J.H., Vile, H., and van de Winkel, J.G.J. (2002). Mac-1 (CD11b/CD18) as accessory molecule for FcαR (CD89) binding of IgA. *J. Immunol.*, 169, 3831–3836.

van Zandbergen, G., Westerhuis, R., Mohamad, N.K., van de Winkel, J.G., Daha, M.R., and van Kooten, C. (1999). Crosslinking of the human Fc receptor for IgA (FcαRI/CD89) triggers FcR gamma-chain-dependent shedding of soluble CD89. *J. Immunol.* 163, 5806–5812.

Wan, T., Beavil, R.L., Fabiane, S.M., Beavil, A.J., Sohi, M.K., Keown, M., Young, R.J., Owens, R.J., Gould, H.J., and Sutton, B.J. (2002). The crystal structure of IgE reveals an asymmetrically bent conformation. *Nat. Immunol.* 3, 681–686.

Weisbart, R.H., Kacena, A., Schuh, A., and Golde, D.W. (1988). GM-CSF induces human neutrophil IgA-mediated phagocytosis by an IgA Fc receptor activation mechanism. *Nature* 332, 647–648.

Weltzin, R., Lucia-Jandris, P., Michetti, P., Fields, B.N., Kraehenbuhl, J.P., and Neutra, M.R.(1989). Binding and transepithelial transport of immunoglobulins by intestinal M cells: demonstration using monoclonal IgA antibodies against enteric viral proteins. *J. Cell. Biol.* 108, 1673–1685.

Wines, B.D., Hulett, M.D., Jamieson, G.P., Trist, H.M., Spratt, J.M., and Hogarth, P.M. (1999). Identification of residues in the first domain of human Fcα receptor essential for interaction with IgA. *J. Immunol.* 1622, 2146–2153.

Wines, B.D., Sardjono, C.T., Trist, H.M., Lay, C.-S., and Hogarth, P.M. (2001). The interaction of FcαRI with IgA and its implications for ligand binding by immunoreceptors of the leukocyte receptor cluster. *J. Immunol.* 166, 1781–1789.

Yeaman, G.R., and Kerr, M.A. (1987). Opsonization of yeast by human serum IgA anti-mannan antibodies and phagocytosis by human polymorphonuclear leucocytes. *Clin. Exp. Immunol.* 68, 200–208.

Zhang, G., Young, J.R., Tregaskes, C.A., Sopp, P., and Howard, C.J. (1995). Identification of a novel class of mammalian Fcγ receptor. *J. Immunol.* 155, 1534–1541.

Zhu, X., Meng, G., Dickinson, B.L., Li, X., Mizoguchi, E., Miao, L., Wang, Y., Robert, C., Wu, B., Smith, P.D., Lencer, W.I., and Blumberg, R.S. (2001). MHC class I-related neonatal Fc receptor for IgG is functionally expressed in monocytes, intestinal macrophages, and dendritic cells. *J. Immunol.* 166, 3266–3276.

Biological Activities of IgA

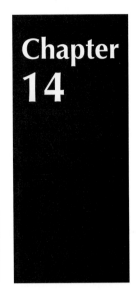

Chapter 14

Michael W. Russell

Department of Microbiology and Immunology, and of Oral Biology, University at Buffalo, Buffalo, New York

Mogens Kilian

Department of Medical Microbiology and Immunology, University of Aarhus, Aarhus, Denmark

INTRODUCTION

Two different environments

Secretory IgA (S-IgA) is the principal immunoglobulin on mucosal surfaces of humans and most other mammals. In addition, IgA is the second most abundant immunoglobulin class in the human circulation. To understand the biological significance of these forms of IgA, it is important to recognize that S-IgA operates in an environment that is very different from the circulation and tissues in which other immunoglobulin isotypes operate, including its plasma counterpart, sometimes referred to as serum IgA. The mucosal surfaces of the body provide an extensive interface that physically separates the interior of the body and the outside world. The host defense problems in the two environments are completely different: the interior of this interface is normally sterile, and the presence of a microorganism indicates a potentially life-threatening invasion. In contrast, the mucosal surfaces are colonized by a commensal microbiota having many beneficial properties and are constantly exposed to environmental antigens such as the daily food intake and other macromolecules, including potential allergens. Superimposed on this normal activity are periodic encounters with potentially pathogenic microorganisms and viruses. Thus, while the systemic immune system must react forcefully to any invasion, S-IgA and the mucosal immune system in general must keep a balance with the normal microbiota while maintaining the ability to respond vigorously to potential pathogens (Shroff *et al.*, 1995). An important aspect of the balancing act with the normal microbiota may be the role played by maternal milk S-IgA antibodies in promoting the establishment of an appropriate intestinal microbiota in neonates (see Chapter 104). This process may be of paramount importance not only for the local microenvironment but also for priming the immune system in general with regard to the future pattern of immune reactivity (Kalliomaki *et al.*, 2003; Sudo *et al.*, 1997).

Other immunoglobulins are found in mucosal secretions to varying extents **(Table 14.1)**. However, apart from IgM, which can also be transported through epithelia by pIgR to form secretory (S-) IgM (Brandtzaeg *et al.*, 1986a; Thompson, 1970), it is generally assumed that these reach the secretions by paracellular transudation, as no specific transport mechanisms are known. A notable exception to this is the transport of IgG1 from the circulation into milk in ruminants, possibly by means of the Brambell Fc receptor (Junghans, 1997). In these animals, which do not transport IgG through the placenta, the colostrum contains large quantities of IgG, which is absorbed through the intestine into the circulation of the newborn to provide initial passive immunity. Human genital tract secretions contain typically more IgG than IgA (see Chapter 99), but the mechanisms by which it is secreted—if other than by passive transudation—are not known. IgG also transudes from the plasma into the lung alveolar fluid; thus the terminal airways are protected more by systemic than by mucosal immune defense mechanisms.

The functions of other immunoglobulin isotypes in mucosal protection are assumed to be reflections of their respective systemic defense activities (Table 14.1). Only S-IgM, by virtue of its bound secretory component (SC), displays structural differences from its circulating counterpart, but whether this confers any distinctive properties has not been explored. Presumably SC helps to protect S-IgM from proteolytic degradation, as it does in S-IgA, although this has not actually been demonstrated. Other isotypes, compared with S-IgA, may not survive intact for long in the enzymatically hostile environment represented especially by the gastrointestinal tract.

It has become clear that the microorganisms present at mucosal surfaces form complex multispecies communities known as biofilms, which possess characteristics, including resistance to host defense systems (or exogenous therapeutic agents), that are very different from those of planktonic organisms. Thus comprehension of mucosal defense will require investigation of the interaction of factors such as

Table 14.1. Isotypes and Functions of Mucosal Immunoglobulins

Isotype	Occurrence	Functions
S-IgA	Major form of Ig in most secretions of humans and many other mammals	Noninflammatory mucosal protection[a]
(S-)IgM	Second most abundant Ig in most secretions; S-IgM compensates for lack of S-IgA in IgA deficiency	Probably similar to plasma IgM or S-IgA; activates complement
IgG	Normally minor component; relatively abundant in nasal, respiratory, and genital tract secretions; probably transudes from plasma; increased in inflammatory conditions	Neutralization; potentially inflammatory; activates complement and phagocytes
IgA (plasma-type)	Found in human bile and other secretions; transudes from plasma or transported by alternative mechanisms	Possibly similar to S-IgA; poor complement activation, or inhibitory[a]
IgD	Significant minor component of nasal secretions and milk	Unknown
IgE	Normally insignificant; elevated in atopic allergies and helminth infections	Adverse hypersensitivity states (atopy); parasite expulsion

[a]See text for additional discussion.

S-IgA with biofilms, an area that is likely to assume great importance in the future. A recent publication has suggested that S-IgA may facilitate biofilm development, at least as demonstrated by the ability of *Escherichia coli* to grow on fixed epithelial cell monolayers (Bollinger *et al.*, 2003).

The two very different situations in which IgA antibodies operate are also reflected in the presence or absence of ancillary factors (notably the complement system, phagocytic or other cells, and innate defense factors) and of other macromolecules. In the mucosal secretions there is no compelling evidence for the presence of a biologically active complement system; nor are significant numbers of live phagocytes normally present. Although in the presence of mucosal inflammation with its attendant increase in permeability and chemotactic factors, both complement components and leukocytes can be found in mucosal fluids, the functional significance of this is still not clear.

Protective potential of IgA antibodies

Numerous studies in animal models and in humans have provided convincing evidence that protection against a variety of bacterial, parasitic, and viral mucosal pathogens can be achieved by oral or intranasal immunization. Although antibody responses to infection and deliberate immunization are diverse, never being restricted to the IgA class, many studies have demonstrated strong correlations between titers of specific S-IgA antibodies in secretions and resistance to infection (e.g., Clements *et al.*, 1986; Coulson *et al.*, 1992; Haque *et al.*, 2001; Jertborn *et al.*, 1986; Johnson *et al.*, 1986; Keren *et al.*, 1988; Ogra *et al.*, 1968; Onorato *et al.*, 1991; Reuman *et al.*, 1990; Watt *et al.*, 1990). Several groups have taken advantage of monoclonal antibody technology to study

the protective effects of IgA antibodies against both viral and bacterial pathogens. In addition to providing insight into the protective potential of isolated IgA antibodies, several of these studies have compared the protective effects of IgA antibodies directed against different epitopes on the infecting agents. **Table 14.2** provides an overview of studies in which IgA antibodies were delivered in two ways: by direct application onto a mucosal surface, e.g., by instilling into the respiratory or gastrointestinal tracts, often together with the infectious inoculum; or indirectly (e.g., by systemic injection or by means of "backpack" tumors). In this elegant model, hybridoma cells producing the relevant monoclonal IgA antibody in polymeric form are injected subcutaneously into the back of a mouse; as the tumor enlarges, the IgA antibody appears in both plasma and gut mucosal secretions as a result of the efficient transport of polymeric (p) IgA from the circulation into the bile through the liver in this species. Table 2 also includes reference to two studies in which IgA monoclonal antibodies against capsular polysaccharides of *Streptococcus pneumoniae* and *Streptococcus agalactiae* were shown to have protective abilities comparable to those of IgG and IgM when applied systemically to mice together with the respective bacterial pathogens. Most studies that have compared the mucosal protective ability of IgA and IgG antibodies against the same antigenic determinant on a mucosal pathogen have demonstrated the superiority of IgA antibodies, provided they are in polymeric form (Table 14.2).

It is important to note that the effect of passive immunization against mucosal infections *in vivo* does not always correlate with the *in vitro* neutralizing effects of the antibodies employed. This can be explained by the fact that viral and bacterial surface epitopes are often altered *in vivo* by prote-

Table 14.2 Passive Protection of Animals against Microbial Pathogens by Monoclonal IgA Antibodies

Pathogen	Site	Model	Result	Reference
Viruses				
Sendai	Respiratory	Mouse	pIgA = IgG protects	Mazanec et al., 1987, 1992
Influenza	Respiratory	Mouse	IgA > IgG protects	Renegar and Small, 1991
	Respiratory	Mouse IgA-ko	pIgA = IgM = IgG protects	Mbawuike et al., 1999
Respiratory syncytial	Respiratory	Mouse, rhesus monkey	Intranasal IgA mAb protects	Weltzin et al., 1994, 1996
		Mouse	IgA = IgG protects	Fisher et al., 1999
Rotavirus	Gastrointestinal	Mouse "backpack" tumor	"Nonneutralizing" IgA mAb protects across epithelium	Burns et al., 1996
			IgA mAb protects	Ruggeri et al., 1998
Rotavirus	Gastrointestinal	Mouse	S-IgA > IgG protects orally	Offit and Clark, 1985
			IgA protects	Feng et al., 2002
Reovirus	Gastrointestinal	Mouse "backpack" tumor	Only IgA mAb protects against peroral infection	Kraehenbuhl and Neutra, 1992
Bacteria				
Streptococcus pyogenes	Respiratory	Mouse	Topical S-IgA > IgG protects	Bessen and Fischetti, 1988
Streptococcus agalactiae	Systemic	Mouse	IgA mAb protects against i.p. infection	Egan et al., 1983
Streptococcus pneumoniae	Systemic	Mouse	Human IgA Ab protects mice against lethal infection	Steinitz et al., 1986
Streptococcus pneumoniae	Respiratory	Mouse	Human IgA2 > IgA1 protects against lethal infection	Janoff et al., 2002
Vibrio cholerae	Gastrointestinal	Mouse "backpack" tumor	pIgA protects against oral challenge	Winner et al., 1991
Salmonella typhimurium	Gastrointestinal	Mouse "backpack" tumor	pIgA protects against oral challenge	Michetti et al., 1992
Helicobacter felis	Gastrointestinal	Mouse	IgA mAb protects against gastric infection	Czinn et al., 1993
Shigella flexneri	Pulmonary	Mouse	S-IgA > IgA protects	Blanchard et al., 1995
		Mouse "backpack" tumor		Phalipon et al., 1995, 2002
Chlamydia trachomatis	Vaginal	Mouse	IgA and IgG mAbs prevent colonization	Cotter et al., 1995
			IgA mAb protects	Pal et al., 1997
Protozoa				
Cryptosporidium parvum	Gastrointestinal	Neonatal mouse	pIgA protects	Enriquez and Riggs, 1998
Acanthamoeba castellanii	Ocular	Hamster	pIgA protects	Leher et al., 1999

i.p., intraperitoneal; ko, knockout; mAb, monoclonal antibody.

olysis. For example, the VP3 protein of poliovirus is altered by proteases as the virus passes through the intestine. The neoepitopes exposed as a result of this change induce IgA antibodies that have no counterparts in the IgG response to injected virus (Zhaori *et al.*, 1989). Another example is one of the major outer capsid proteins of reovirus. In contrast to the μ1c protein, which remains intact, the σ3 protein is cleaved during intestinal passage by luminal proteases (Sharpe and Fields, 1985). Accordingly, only monoclonal IgA antibodies against the μ1c protein protect mice against an oral dose of reovirus, although antibodies against both proteins neutralize the virus *in vitro* (Kraehenbuhl and Neutra, 1992). Thus, to provide protection, S-IgA antibodies must recognize the surface of the pathogen even after it has been altered by luminal enzymes.

The studies summarized above clearly illustrate the protective potential of an IgA response even to a single epitope on the infectious agent, provided that the epitope is exposed *in vivo*. Under natural conditions a mucosal immune response would be polyclonal, with antibodies directed to multiple epitopes rather than the single determinant recognized by a monoclonal antibody and consequently should be even more protective. In most of the quoted studies, protection is undoubtedly mediated by S-IgA either on the mucosal surface or within epithelial cells, but some studies demonstrate protection against systemic challenge with capsule-forming bacterial pathogens. Although circulating IgA must be responsible for this protection in the mouse model, it is important to stress that there is no consensus on this (Schreiber *et al.*, 1986), and there is as yet no evidence for plasma IgA-mediated protection against microbial pathogens in humans. In this context it must be noted that there are significant differences in the physiology of IgA between mice and humans, as revealed for example by the apparent absence of FcαRI (CD89) in mice. The significance of this factor is revealed by the recent demonstration that intraperitoneal administration of human anticapsular IgA1 antibodies protects mice from lethal intranasal challenge provided that the mice are transgenic for human FcαR (van der Pol *et al.*, 2000). Furthermore, humans and anthropoid apes have evolved a novel subclass of IgA, IgA1, which circulates at relatively high concentrations predominantly in monomeric form, whereas in mice and other mammals, the major form of systemic IgA more closely resembles human IgA2 and circulates at lower concentrations in polymeric form. In addition, mice and other rodents have an active pIgR-dependent hepatobiliary transport of pIgA from the plasma into bile, which does not occur in humans (see Chapter 11).

Table 14.3 summarizes protective functions of IgA as revealed by studies of mice in which IgA, J chain, or pIgR has been genetically deleted or by studies of IgA-deficient humans. IgA deficiency is relatively common in humans (see Chapter 63) and is associated with increased frequency of upper respiratory and gastrointestinal tract infections, although individuals with this condition are not necessarily severely compromised. Reasons ascribed for this include compensation by other adaptive or innate mechanisms of immunity, especially

the substitution of S-IgM for S-IgA in secretions (Brandtzaeg *et al.*, 1986a; Thompson, 1970). The defect underlying IgA deficiency remains unclear, but it is plainly regulatory in nature, and moreover, the lack of IgA, although profound, is not always absolute and it may be accompanied by deficiencies in other isotypes that confound interpretation of the consequences. However, those who do not compensate for a total absence of IgA tend to be most seriously affected. Mice in which the Cα chain is genetically inactivated and are therefore unable to produce IgA (IgA-knockout mice) (Harriman *et al.*, 1999) have yielded conflicting results with regard to their susceptibility to various infections or even to the same infection in different studies (Table 14.3). Remarkably, IgA-knockout mice also display alterations in the expression of other isotypes as well as immune response defects (Harriman *et al.*, 1999; Arulanandam *et al.*, 2001), which complicate the conclusions drawn. Perhaps more informative, therefore, is the J chain deletion that abrogates the assembly of polymeric Igs and thereby prevents the transport and formation of S-IgA. Such animals display defective mucosal immunity (Lycke *et al.*, 1999; Schwartz-Cornil *et al.*, 2002). Mice with a deletion in the pIgR gene also lack S-IgA (and S-IgM) and have impaired epithelial barrier functions (Johansen *et al.*, 1999), but otherwise these animals have not been examined for defects in immune defense. Deficiency of SC in humans has been reported (Strober *et al.*, 1976), but this has been subsequently questioned, and the extreme rarity of the condition perhaps implies that it may be lethal.

The mechanisms by which IgA antibodies interfere with various infectious processes have been demonstrated in numerous *in vitro* experimental models (**Table 14.4**). In many of these it has been found that pIgA is superior to mIgA, according to its ability to interact with pIgR and possibly because of greater capacity to cross-link and thereby activate receptors such as FcαRI. These aspects of IgA function are discussed more fully in the section on Biological Activity of IgA in Tissues.

BIOLOGICAL PROPERTIES OF IgA

Relationship of IgA structure to function

IgA is the most heterogeneous of immunoglobulin isotypes, as it occurs in a variety of molecular forms as well as subclasses and allotypes. However, the patterns of heterogeneity vary significantly between different species of mammals and birds (see Chapter 11). In humans, chimpanzees, gorillas, and gibbons, there are two unique subclasses (IgA1 and IgA2), whereas most other animals that have been investigated have only one, with the remarkable exception of the lagomorphs (rabbits and their allies), which have 13 IgA subclasses. Two, possibly more, allotypes of human IgA2 have been described, and they appear to represent different combinations of constant-region domains of the α-heavy chains (see Chapter 9). In humans and other primates, the predominant molecular form of circulating (serum) IgA is monomeric, in contrast to the pIgA that is produced in

Table 14.3. Active Protection against Microbial Pathogens by S-IgA Antibodies in Animals and Humans: Examples from Immunodeficiency States

Pathogen	Site	Model	Result	Reference
Viruses				
Influenza	Respiratory	Mouse IgA-ko	Increased susceptibility in immunized IgA-ko mice	Arulanandam et al., 2001
			Conflicting results	Benton et al., 2001
				Mbawuike et al., 1999
Influenza	Respiratory	Mouse, total parenteral nutrition	Diminished S-IgA responses, diminished immunity	Renegar et al., 2001
Rotavirus	Gastrointestinal	Mouse IgA-ko	IgA not required for protection	O'Neal et al., 2000
Herpes simplex 2	Genital	Mouse IgA-ko	IgA not required for protection	Parr et al., 1998
Reovirus	Gastrointestinal	Mouse IgA-ko	IgA-ko mice cleared primary but not secondary infection	Silvey et al., 2001
Rotavirus	Gastrointestinal	Mouse J chain-ko	Mucosally immunized ko mice show impaired immunity	Schwartz-Cornil et al., 2002
Bacteria				
Escherichia coli	Gastrointestinal	Human IgA deficiency	Increased frequency of E. coli strains in IgA-deficient humans	Friman et al., 2002
Cholera toxin	Gastrointestinal	Mouse J chain ko	Diminished protection against toxin in immunized ko mice	Lycke et al., 1999
Protozoan				
Giardia	Gastrointestinal	Mouse IgA-ko, IgM-ko, B cell-deficient	IgA important for protection	Langford et al., 2002
Other				
(n/a)	Gastrointestinal	Mouse pIgR-ko	Increased mucosal leakiness	Johansen et al., 1999

mucosal tissues and transported into the secretions as S-IgA. Further levels of heterogeneity arise from the variable number and composition of the oligosaccharide side-chains present on α-heavy chains (see Chapter 9).

How all of this structural heterogeneity is reflected in the functional properties of IgA antibodies is not fully understood. The two subclasses show differences in their ability to interact with certain receptors and bacterial proteins, in some cases as a result of differences in glycosylation. However, human IgA1 and IgA2 and the allotypes of IgA2 have few distinct biological properties; a notable exception is the different susceptibility of IgA subclasses to bacterial IgA1 proteases (see Chapter 15). A different distribution of antibody specificities between IgA1 and IgA2 has often been described, but this is not absolute and the regulatory mechanisms responsible are not known. For example, parenteral immunization with protein antigens tends to elicit serum IgA1, whereas polysaccharides tend to induce IgA2 antibodies (Brown and Mestecky, 1985; Heilman et al., 1988; Lue et al., 1988; reviewed in Russell et al., 1992). However, naturally occurring serum IgA antibodies to bacterial capsular polysaccharides are mainly IgA1 (Engström et al., 1990), and protein-conjugated capsular polysaccharides induce IgA1 (and IgG1)

responses (Barington et al., 1994; Kauppi-Korkeila et al., 1998). These disparities suggest that different IgA subclass responses may depend on various factors, including the type of antigen and its molecular context, site of induction (parenteral or mucosal), age of the subject, and whether they result from primary or secondary antigen exposure. It is not currently known if these differences are reflected in the functional activities of the resulting IgA antibodies. The different molecular forms of IgA, however, are known to have functional significance, particularly with regard to their ability to interact with receptors for IgA. In this context, it should be noted that serum IgA antibody responses usually commence with pIgA and progress subsequently to the monomeric form (reviewed in Russell et al., 1992), but the biological significance of this is not well understood. Indeed, whereas the functions of S-IgA in protecting mucosal surfaces are quite well known, those of serum IgA remain poorly understood, and it is possible that the heterogeneity of serum IgA not only has functional significance but also may account for some of the controversies that have arisen.

As is true for other antibody isotypes, whereas some effects of IgA antibodies result directly from their binding to antigen, most biological functions depend on the Fc domains

Table 14.4. Protective Functions of IgA Antibodies Demonstrated *in vitro*

Pathogen	System	Result	Reference
Toxin Neutralization			
Clostridium difficile toxin	T84 colon carcinoma EC	pIgA > mIgA = IgG neutralizes	Stubbe *et al.*, 2000
Streptococcal superantigen	Human PBMC	IgA inhibits mitogenicity	Norrby-Teglund et al., 2000
Shigella flexneri LPS	Polarized mouse intestinal EC	pIgA mAb inhibits NF-κB activation	Fernandez *et al.*, 2003
Virus Neutralization or Inhibition			
Influenza	Hemagglutination inhibition	pIgA/S-IgA > mIgA inhibit	Renegar *et al.*, 1998
Rotavirus	Polarized pIgR-expressing MDCK cells	pIgA mAbs inhibit infection	Ruggeri *et al.*, 1998
Sendai	Polarized pIgR-expressing MDCK cells	pIgA mAbs inhibit infection	Mazanec *et al.*, 1992
Measles	Polarized pIgR-expressing EC	pIgA mAbs inhibit replication	Yan *et al.*, 2002
Rotavirus	Lipofected EC	IgA mAb inhibits replication	Feng *et al.*, 2002
Antibacterial, Complement/Phagocyte-Dependent			
Streptococcus pneumoniae	HL-60 cells, human PMN	IgA ± C opsonizes, CD89-dependent	Janoff *et al.*, 1999 van der Pol *et al.*, 2000
Streptococcus pneumoniae	Human PMN	S-IgA + C opsonizes	Finn *et al.*, 2000
Neisseria meningitidis	Human PMN	p/mIgA mAbs opsonize	Vidarsson *et al.*, 2001
Bordetella pertussis	Human PMN, CD89-transfected mouse PMN	IgA opsonizes, CD89-dependent	Hellwig *et al.*, 2001
Inhibition of Adherence/Invasion			
Streptococcus mutans	Adherence to saliva-coated hydroxyapatite	S-IgA > mIgA = IgG inhibits adherence	Hajishengallis et al., 1992
Salmonella enterica	Polarized Hep-2 cells	IgA mAbs inhibit adhesion/invasion	Iankov *et al.*, 2002
Naegleria fowleri	Adherence to collagen	Human S-IgA Abs inhibit adherence	Shibayama *et al.*, 2003

EC, epithelial cells; mAb, monoclonal antibody; PBMC, peripheral blood mononuclear cells; PMN, polymorphonuclear neutrophils.

and, in the case of S-IgA, the attached secretory component (SC), as well as the interactions of these with other molecules (Kilian *et al.*, 1988). The Fc.SC region of S-IgA is hydrophilic and negatively charged as compared with the Fc of IgG, due to the abundance and exposure of N-linked oligosaccharides with terminal sialic acid residues in both Fcα and SC, in contrast to the smaller number, size, and hidden location of glycans in IgG-Fc (Mattu *et al.*, 1997; Royle *et al.*, 2003), and the predominance of hydrophilic amino acids in the Fc of IgA. It has been suggested that the disposition of glycan chains in S-IgA, which contains approximately 20% carbohydrate, contributes to innate defense by interaction with bacterial lectin-like adhesins (Royle *et al.*, 2003), although the availability of the necessary determinants may depend upon enzymic activity (such as sialidase) or denaturing conditions to expose otherwise hidden sugar residues.

The hinge region that links Fab to Fc in human IgA1 possesses some unusual structural features that are reminiscent of mucin, including the presence of O-linked oligosaccharides (see Chapter 9). While the biological significance of these is not fully understood, they have been implicated in carbohydrate-dependent interactions of IgA1 with cellular receptors (Tomana *et al.*, 1988) and may impart resistance to many proteolytic enzymes. The elongated hinge region of IgA1 confers greater flexibility on its Fab arms relative to those of both IgA2 and IgG (Boehm *et al.*, 1999; Mattu *et al.*, 1997), although it has been suggested that this may be somewhat reduced by the O-linked oligosaccharides (Jentoft, 1990). Whether an extended hinge region facilitates divalent binding to adjacent epitopes, e.g., in polysaccharide antigens, which typically have repeating epitopes, is not known. In contrast, the hinge region of human IgA2 is short, consisting of eight residues, including five prolines, and more similar in length to the hinge in IgA of most other animals. Recent studies indicate that as a result, IgA2 is more compact and has substantially less segmental flexibility than IgA1 (Whitty *et al.*, 2002), but the biological implications of this are at present unclear. The situation in lagomorphs, which have genes for 13 IgA subclasses with hinge regions ranging from 6 to 21 amino acid residues in length, remains enigmatic. However, not all of these are normally expressed; their relative abundance and expression vary, for example, in different segments of the gut and during ontogeny (see Chapter 11), and their differential functional properties, if any, are not understood.

Among the immunoglobulins that reach mucosal surfaces whether through active transport or passive transudation, S-IgA is particularly stable. While other isotypes are rapidly degraded, intact S-IgA molecules can be regularly demonstrated in samples from mucosal surfaces, even in the presence of large numbers of microorganisms. This stability of S-IgA depends largely on SC, which is covalently bonded to Fcα and masks potential proteolytic cleavage sites in that region (Lindh, 1975; Crottet and Corthésy, 1998). These properties make S-IgA particularly well suited to function in the enzymatically hostile environment that prevails on mucosal surfaces.

It has been proposed that S-IgA originates from two distinct cellular sources: the B-1 cells that constitute a self-renewing population and are responsible for the production of "natural" antibodies to common microbial determinants, and conventional B-2 cells that produce most antibodies as a result of antigenic stimulation and T cell help (Lamm and Phillips-Quagliata, 2002). Whether IgA antibodies from these different sources have structural differences (for example, in glycosylation) that might confer functional differences is not known, but it is likely that they display different spectra of antibody specificities.

Mechanisms of protection by S-IgA at mucosal surfaces

Inhibition of adherence

Concomitant with the recognition that adherence of a microorganism to a mucosal surface is a critical first step in colonization (see Chapter 3) has been the concept that inhibition of adherence by antibodies is a major protective function of mucosal immunity (Williams and Gibbons, 1972; Abraham and Beachey, 1985). Even before the molecular nature of many bacterial adhesin-receptor interactions was known, S-IgA antibodies to microbial surfaces had been demonstrated to inhibit adherence to pharyngeal, intestinal, and genitourinary tract epithelia and to tooth surfaces (Carbonare *et al.*, 1995; Cravioto *et al.*, 1991; Fubara and Freter, 1973; Hajishengallis *et al.*, 1992; Kilian *et al.*, 1981; Svanborg-Eden and Svennerholm, 1978; Tramont, 1977; Williams and Gibbons, 1972). The important contribution of SC in the defense functions of S-IgA has been revealed in a comparative study of protection against shigella infection of the respiratory tract in mice by monoclonal pIgA antibody

to *Shigella* lipopolysaccharide (LPS) and the same antibody coupled to recombinant SC (Phalipon *et al.*, 2002).

While any isotype of a relevant antibody may be capable of interfering with the interaction between a microbial adhesin and its host receptor, S-IgA antibodies have advantageous properties that are not shared by other isotypes, due to the hydrophilic and negatively charged Fc.SC part of the molecule (see above). Thus S-IgA appears to surround a microbe and other particulate antigens with a hydrophilic shell that repels attachment to a mucosal surface. It is possible that S-IgM, which compensates for S-IgA in many IgA-deficient subjects, can exert a similar effect, but specific evidence of this is not available. In contrast, IgG, which has considerably fewer carbohydrate residues that are not exposed, is more hydrophobic and less charged in the Fc region and may substitute the specific adhesin-receptor binding with other (less specific) hydrophobic interactions.

Another important mechanism of antibody-mediated inhibition of microbial colonization is agglutination. This is undoubtedly the mechanism behind the colonization-inhibiting activity of S-IgA antibodies to the capsular polysaccharide of *Haemophilus influenzae* serotype b observed in a rat model (Kauppi-Korkeila *et al.*, 1996). Both *in vitro* and *in vivo* studies have demonstrated that dimeric F(ab')2 fragments of effective antibodies can inhibit attachment of bacteria to the gut mucosa or tooth surfaces, whereas monomeric Fab fragments lack this ability (Cisar *et al.*, 1991; Kauppi-Korkeila *et al.*, 1996; Ma *et al.*, 1990; Steele *et al.*, 1975). Although pIgA and S-IgA antibodies are particularly adept at agglutinating microorganisms, monomeric (m) IgA antibodies agglutinate (and precipitate) poorly (Heremans, 1974), possibly because their hydrophilic Fcα regions are less able to participate in Fc-Fc interactions. Analysis of antigen-antibody complexes by two-phase liquid partition chromatography has shown that IgA1 and IgA2 complexes display different surface properties than those made from IgG or IgM (Wingren and Hansson, 1997). It would be of interest to determine if these properties relate to their respective abilities to form immune precipitates and aggregates.

In addition to specific antibody-mediated inhibition of adherence, human IgA and in particular S-IgA bind to many bacterial species and antigens through their carbohydrate chains (see section on Biological Activity of IgA in Tissues and Chapter 15). It has been suggested that S-IgA in secretions, including human milk, may thus be able to interfere with the adherence and penetration of bacteria and potential allergens (Davin *et al.*, 1991; Royle *et al.*, 2003; Schroten *et al.*, 1998; Wold *et al.*, 1990, 1994). As an example, IgA2, which can agglutinate *E. coli* through its type 1 (mannose-dependent) pili by means of mannose-rich glycan chains, may inhibit type 1 pilus-dependent adherence of *E. coli* to epithelial cells (Wold *et al.*, 1990, 1994). The *in vivo* significance of this is supported by the observation that IgA-deficient individuals show lower frequencies of *E. coli*–carrying genes for type 1 fimbriae in their gut microflora (68% versus 90%) (Friman *et al.*, 2002). It has also been shown that adhesion of S-fimbriated *E. coli* to human epithelial cells is inhibited by interactions with sialyl-oligosaccharides on S-IgA (Schroten et al, 1998). Likewise, several bacterial species, including *Helicobacter pylori* and *S. pneumoniae*, have surface-exposed proteins that recognize carbohydrates of S-IgA, an interaction that is suggested to inhibit their attachment to epithelial cells (Borén *et al.*, 1993; Royle *et al.*, 2003; Falk *et al.*, 1993; Hammerschmidt *et al.*, 1997). However, other observations have led to the alternative interpretation that bacteria may exploit such carbohydrate-dependent interactions with S-IgA to enhance their ability to colonize mucosal surfaces (Friman *et al.*, 1996). It is conceivable that the size of agglutinates determines whether such interactions tend to promote or prevent microbial colonization (Liljemark *et al.*, 1979).

Conversely, it has been suggested that *S. pneumoniae* can exploit binding to SC to enhance its own invasion of epithelial cells, by a mechanism that involves retrograde reuptake of SC (Zhang *et al.*, 2000). Another study of the phenomenon, however, indicates that it is dependent upon both the strain of pneumococcus and the particular epithelial cell line (Brock *et al.*, 2002).

Mucus trapping

It has been speculated that S-IgA may be able to associate specifically with mucins, possibly through interactions between mucin and the mucin-like hinge region of IgA1, or even by forming disulphide bonds (Clamp, 1977). However, more recent studies have demonstrated that S-IgA diffuses freely through mucus (Saltzman *et al.*, 1994), which contradicts the old concept that S-IgA antibody molecules are lined up at the surface of mucus layers on mucosal membranes and act as an immunological "fly-paper." Nevertheless, several observations indicate that microorganisms or other particulate antigens coated with S-IgA antibodies are entrapped in mucus. If the binding of S-IgA to bacteria renders them more "mucophilic" (Magnusson and Stjernström, 1982) or reduces their hydrophobicity (Edebo *et al.*, 1985), this would help to entrap the microbes within the mucus layer. The finding that high-molecular-weight fractions of saliva contain both mucins and small amounts of S-IgA suggests an interaction between them, and the binding of S-IgA to salivary mucin MG2 has been described (Biesbrock *et al.*, 1991). An interaction between the Fc.SC region of antigen-complexed S-IgA and mucus is also implied by the finding that spermatozoa coated with S-IgA show impaired penetration of cervical mucus and that selective removal of the Fc.SC regions by IgA1 protease treatment restores this ability (Bronson *et al.*, 1987). However, this effect is not confined to IgA antibodies, although the polymeric configuration may be important, and it depends upon the presence of the Fc region, as well as complex formation.

Virus neutralization

A considerable body of evidence shows that S-IgA antibodies to various viruses can effectively neutralize them (Table 14.4). While inhibition of viral binding to cellular receptors is a plausible mechanism in many cases, inhibition of viral replication may occur by other means, depending upon the epitope specificity, isotype, and concentration of antibody as well as the virus and cells involved. High concentrations of S-IgA or IgM antibodies to influenza virus hemagglutinin inhibit cellular attachment, whereas IgG or lower concentrations of pIgA antibodies that permit attachment may inhibit internalization or intracellular replication (Armstrong and Dimmock, 1992). The isotype and molecular form of antiviral antibody may be especially important in view of evidence that S-IgA antibodies are more effective than IgG in mediating cross-protective immunity against different antigenic variants of influenza virus (Liew *et al.*, 1984), and a recombinant dimeric IgA antibody against transmissible gastroenteritis virus was found to neutralize the virus 50-fold more effectively than a recombinant monomeric IgG having the same antigen-binding site (Castilla *et al.*, 1997). Likewise, monoclonal pIgA and S-IgA antibodies to influenza virus are more effective than mIgA in hemagglutination inhibition (Renegar *et al.*, 1998). However, one mechanism of viral uptake can be replaced by another: human antibodies of any isotype against the surface gp340 of Epstein-Barr virus (EBV) neutralize its infectivity for B cells (via complement receptor CR2), but pIgA antibodies promote infection of pIgR-expressing colonic carcinoma cells, thereby changing its tissue tropism (Sixbey and Yao, 1992). The outcome depends also upon the state of the epithelial cells, as polarized epithelial cells in culture transport pIgA-complexed EBV from the basal to the apical surface without becoming infected by the virus, in apparently the same fashion as mouse hepatocytes transport pIgA-complexed EBV *in vivo*, whereas unpolarized pIgR-expressing cells become infected by pIgA-complexed EBV (Gan *et al.*, 1997). A similar phenomenon is potentially important in connection with HIV infection: IgA antibodies to gp120 may neutralize HIV infection of T cells (Burnett *et al.*, 1994), whereas IgA antibodies enhance HIV infection of FcαR-expressing monocytes (Janoff *et al.*, 1995; Kozlowski *et al.*, 1995). S-IgA or plasma IgA from HIV-1-exposed but -uninfected individuals is especially effective in inhibiting the uptake and transcytosis of HIV-1 in epithelial cells (Devito *et al.*, 2000). S-IgA antibodies to gp41, in particular the ELDKWA epitope, have been shown to prevent epithelial cell uptake of HIV-1 by inhibiting binding to galactosyl ceramide receptors (Alfsen *et al.*, 2001). pIgA (and IgM) antibodies to these determinants were earlier found to re-export viral particles to the apical surface of pIgR-expressing epithelial cells through apical recycling endosomes (Bomsel *et al.*, 1998), in a process resembling those described in the next paragraph for the intracellular neutralization of viruses and the removal of absorbed antigens.

An additional mechanism of viral neutralization may be mediated by pIgA antibodies within epithelial cells during their pIgR-mediated transepithelial transport. If the same epithelial cells are infected with a virus, it may be possible for transcytosing antivirus IgA antibodies to inhibit intracellular viral replication. The effectiveness of such neutralizing interactions probably depends on the replication mechanisms of particular viruses and the reactivity of IgA antibodies for different viral components (Mazanec *et al.*, 1996). For example, during vesicular transport across epithelial cells, IgA antibodies are more likely to encounter viral envelope glycoproteins that follow the vesicular exocytic pathway after synthesis in the rough endoplasmic reticulum than to encounter internal viral components that are synthesized on cytoplasmic ribosomes. Evidence of intraepithelial cell neutralization of viruses by IgA antibodies has been obtained both *in vitro* and *in vivo*. IgA antibodies to viral proteins can inhibit the replication of Sendai, influenza, and measles viruses as well as the transport of HIV-1 *in vitro* in polarized epithelial monolayers that express pIgR (Mazanec *et al.*, 1992, 1995; Wolbank *et al.*, 2003; Yan *et al.*, 2002). Studies of epithelial cells lipofected with nonneutralizing IgA antibodies against VP6 capsid protein suggest that such antibodies can inhibit viral RNA transcription (Feng *et al.*, 2002). Conversely, another study indicated that only pIgA antibody to VP8 could protect infant mice from rotaviral diarrhea and neutralize rotavirus infection of pIgR-transfected epithelial cells (Ruggeri *et al.*, 1998). Evidence obtained with antibodies to murine rotavirus and murine hepatitis virus applied by different routes to infected mice supports the concept that IgA antibodies can neutralize viruses *in vivo* inside intestinal epithelial cells and hepatocytes, respectively (Burns *et al.*, 1996; Huang *et al.*, 1997). The extent to which this mechanism operates under natural conditions will depend upon the availability of IgA antibody–secreting cells of appropriate specificity in the vicinity of the viral invasion. Furthermore, viruses that invade through M cells or even the villi may not encounter pIgA, which is transported largely through intestinal crypt cells.

Neutralization of enzymes and toxins

Specific examples of S-IgA antibodies that inhibit enzymes or toxins include intestinal antibodies to cholera and related heat-labile enterotoxins (Lycke *et al.*, 1987; Majumdar and Ghose, 1981); salivary antibodies to neuraminidases, hyaluronidase, and chondroitin sulfatase from oral bacteria (Fukui *et al.*, 1973); salivary antibodies to the glycosyltransferases of *Streptococcus mutans* and *Streptococcus sobrinus*, which synthesize adherent glucans from sucrose and enable these cariogenic bacteria to adhere to tooth surfaces (Smith *et al.*, 1985); and antibodies against IgA proteases (see Chapter 15). pIgA antibodies against *Clostridium difficile* enterotoxin A neutralize this toxin more effectively than equivalent mIgA or IgG antibodies (Johnson *et al.*, 1995; Stubbe *et al.*, 2000). Since the latter report was based on experiments using genetically engineered antibodies having the same antigen-binding variable domains, such neutralization is unlikely to be due simply to steric blocking of binding to the substrate or to a conformational change that affects toxicity, because this would be expected to be independent of the antibody isotype, the presence of the Fc region, or molecular conformation. However, as divalent F(ab')$_2$ fragments of IgA antibody retain neutralizing activity, it appears that multivalent binding to the toxin is important for neutralization, even if the Fc region is not required (Johnson *et*

al., 1995). Polymeric forms of antibody, either pIgA or IgM, have also been found effective in neutralizing group A streptococcal superantigens (Norrby-Teglund *et al.*, 2000). Conversely, the univalent Fab fragments of IgA1 antibodies against bacterial IgA1 proteases retain inhibitory activity, implying that in this instance inhibition is independent of Fc-associated properties (Gilbert *et al.*, 1983).

A novel finding akin to the intraepithelial inhibition of viral replication described above is that pIgA antibody to *Shigella* LPS can inhibit the induction of inflammatory responses of epithelial cells by LPS (Fernandez *et al.*, 2003). The IgA was shown to colocalize with LPS in apical recycling endosomes and to inhibit the nuclear translocation of NF-κB.

Inhibition of antigen penetration

The intestinal uptake of antigenically intact food substances is diminished by S-IgA antibodies arising from prior enteric exposure to them (Walker *et al.*, 1972), and it has been shown that such intestinal immunity can inhibit the absorption of environmental carcinogens (Silbart and Keren, 1989). Likewise, absorption of antigen instilled into the airway is inhibited by the simultaneous administration of IgA antibody (Stokes *et al.*, 1975). The importance of S-IgA-mediated immune exclusion for the protection of the host against excessive antigenic challenge from environmental macromolecules is suggested by the findings that IgA-deficient subjects show increased absorption of food antigens and formation of circulating immune complexes (Cunningham-Rundles *et al.*, 1978), as well as statistically increased susceptibility to atopic allergies or autoimmune disease. An early report of a deficiency of allergen-specific IgA antibodies in patients with IgE-mediated atopic disease is frequently cited as evidence of the significance of S-IgA antibodies for the prevention of allergen penetration through mucosal membranes (Stokes *et al.*, 1974). However, more recent studies show that allergic patients are characterized by having high levels of not only allergen-specific IgE antibodies but also IgA, including S-IgA, and IgG antibodies, in contrast to healthy individuals, in whom such antibodies are barely detectable (Benson *et al.*, 2003; Peebles *et al.*, 2001; Platts-Mills *et al.*, 1976; Reed *et al.*, 1991). The reason for this apparent functional insufficiency of IgA antibodies in sensitized patients is unclear but may be the receptor-mediated uptake of allergens (Campbell *et al.*, 1998; Yang *et al.*, 1999) and the enhanced local release of bacterial IgA1 proteases in these patients (Kilian *et al.*, 1995).

The mechanisms underlying the immune exclusion activity of S-IgA conceivably are a combination of the properties described above, including hydrophilicity, agglutination, and mucus entrapment. In addition, it has been suggested that the pIgR-mediated transport of pIgA by enterocytes may also serve to re-export absorbed antigens if they become complexed with pIgA antibody in the lamina propria (see the section on Interaction with Epithelial Cells) in a process analogous to the previously described hepatobiliary transport of pIgA-complexed antigens (Brown *et al.*, 1984; Peppard *et al.*, 1981; Russell *et al.*, 1981, 1983; Socken *et al.*, 1981).

It is intriguing that, conversely, enteric S-IgA antibodies may be able to promote uptake of antigen through the M cells of Peyer's patches and consequently enhance the mucosal immune response to that antigen (Weltzin *et al.*, 1989), although another report from the same laboratory describes inhibition of reovirus infection of M cells by S-IgA antibodies (Silvey *et al.*, 2001). S-IgA-mediated uptake of antigen into Peyer's patches has been proposed as a strategy of mucosal immunization by the incorporation of epitopes into recombinant IgA molecules (Corthésy *et al.*, 1996). IgA receptors distinct from pIgR or the asialoglycoprotein receptor but possibly lectinlike have been noted on murine M cells (Mantis *et al.*, 2002), and human IgA2, not IgA1, appeared to bind selectively. Another receptor for IgA has been noted on HT-29 intestinal epithelial cells (Kitamura *et al.*, 2000), but its nature and physiological function are unknown.

Interaction with innate antimicrobial factors

The secretions of most mucosal surfaces contain an array of innate defense factors that are highly effective in killing or inhibiting a broad range of microorganisms (see Chapter 5). Because S-IgA is able to interact with some of the protein components of these systems, there is ample opportunity for synergism in which S-IgA antibodies might introduce an element of specificity. However, few such interactions have been described in molecular detail. The bacteriostatic synergy of lactoferrin and S-IgA antibodies (Funakoshi *et al.*, 1982; Stephens *et al.*, 1980) may be due to antibody-mediated interference with alternative channels of iron uptake that many mucosal organisms possess. Lactoferrin can form covalent complexes with S-IgA (Watanabe *et al.*, 1984), but the physiological significance of this is not known. An enhancement of the inhibitory effect of lactoperoxidase-H_2O_2-SCN^- on *S. mutans* metabolism by myeloma IgA1 and IgA2 proteins and by S-IgA but not by IgG or IgM has been attributed to the binding of lactoperoxidase to IgA, presumably by the Fc region, and a stabilizing effect on the enzyme activity (Tenovuo *et al.*, 1982). Recent studies show that S-IgA interacts with human secretory leukocyte protease inhibitor, which is present in mucosal secretions, and that this may play a protective role (Hirano *et al.*, 1999). The ability of human colostral S-IgA antibody, in concert with complement and lysozyme, to lyse *E. coli* (Adinolfi *et al.*, 1966), a once-seminal finding, is now thought to be due to the presence of undetected components.

Biological activity of IgA in tissues

Interaction with complement

The question of whether and how IgA activates complement has been a controversial issue that has still not been completely resolved. Early findings that IgA is incapable of binding C1q and activating the classical complement pathway (CCP) have been generally accepted; IgA molecules do not have the C1q-binding motif that is present in IgG. Reports that some Fcα fragments of myeloma IgA, but not the intact IgA molecules can deplete the early components of the CCP (Burritt *et al.*, 1977), or that rat pIgA can bind C1q without activating it (Hiemstra *et al.*, 1990), remain unexplained. In contrast, numerous texts state that IgA activates the alternative complement pathway (ACP), but this view is not justified by primary research reports and the conditions under which most experiments were performed.

Thus, several reports show that artificially aggregated, chemically cross-linked, or denatured human serum polyclonal or monoclonal (myeloma) IgA or colostral S-IgA can activate the ACP (Boackle *et al.*, 1974; Götze and Müller-Eberhard, 1971; Hiemstra *et al.*, 1987, 1988), although others were not able to demonstrate this (Vaerman and Heremans, 1968, and see references therein). A chimeric human IgA2/rat antibody produced in a mouse transfectoma cell line activated the ACP when complexed with a haptenated protein antigen (Valim and Lachmann, 1991). In contrast, human monoclonal and polyclonal IgA antibodies physiologically complexed with antigen failed to activate the ACP (Colten and Bienenstock, 1974; Imai *et al.*, 1988; Romer *et al.*, 1980; Russell and Mansa, 1989). Furthermore, IgA antibodies that did not activate the ACP when bound to antigen instead activated the ACP when interfacially aggregated on a plastic surface or when complexed with antigen after chemical cross-linking or deglycosylation (Nikolova *et al.*, 1994b; Russell and Mansa, 1989; Zhang and Lachmann, 1994). An interesting finding is that ACP activation by interfacially aggregated IgA seems to be associated with the Fc (or Fc.SC) region rather than Fab, which is involved in ACP activation by IgG (Nikolova *et al.*, 1994b). Heat-aggregated mixtures of human IgG and IgA activate the ACP in proportion to the content of IgG, and analysis of the C3b-containing complexes showed that C3b became covalently coupled to the IgG and not to the IgA component (Waldo and Cochran, 1989). A potent regulatory activity of IgA against complement (C4) deposition has been suggested to be advantageous in intravenous administration of IgA-enriched preparations of immunoglobulin for certain conditions, including graft-versus-host disease and endotoxemia (Miletic *et al.*, 1996). The lower ability of IgA immune complexes, compared with IgG complexes, to bind to primate erythrocytes *in vivo* may also be a reflection of their inability to fix complement and hence to bind to complement receptors (mainly CR1) on erythrocytes (Waxman *et al.*, 1986). Several studies of animal (mouse, rat, rabbit) IgA antihapten antibodies have shown that when complexed with a haptenated protein antigen, IgA antibodies activate the ACP (Pfaffenbach *et al.*, 1982; Rits *et al.*, 1988; Schneiderman *et al.*, 1990). A series of studies of mouse monoclonal antibodies of different isotypes showed that the precipitability of immune complexes in the presence of fresh human serum, or the resolubilization of precipitated immune complexes, is related to their ability to fix complement, and whereas IgM and IgG complexes fix C4 and C3 and are solubilized, IgA complexes are not (Stewart *et al.*, 1990).

All these conflicting results may be due to a number of factors, including the conformational integrity of IgA after exposure to denaturing conditions during purification, abnormal glycosylation of proteins produced in hybridoma or transfectoma cells, and direct activation of the ACP by heavily haptenated proteins, all of which could materially affect the experimental findings. Nevertheless, it remains possible that human and animal IgA, which are structurally different in amino acid sequence, especially in the hinge region as well as in glycosylation and display important physiological differences *in vivo*, differ also in ACP-activating properties.

In contrast, IgA antibody to the capsular polysaccharide inhibits IgG or IgM antibody–dependent complement-mediated lysis of *Neisseria meningitidis*, thereby theoretically accounting for the exacerbation of meningococcal infection in certain patients (Griffiss *et al.*, 1975). A similar observation was made earlier on the lysis of *Brucella abortus* by rabbit antisera (Hall *et al.*, 1971). Likewise, murine IgA antibodies inhibit IgG antibody–dependent complement-mediated hemolysis *in vitro* and the Arthus reaction *in vivo* (Russell-Jones *et al.*, 1980, 1981). Human monoclonal and polyclonal IgA1 antibodies inhibit IgG antibody–dependent CCP activation *in vitro*, and furthermore, Fab fragments of IgA1 antibodies have the same inhibitory activity as intact IgA antibodies (Nikolova *et al.*, 1994a; Russell *et al.*, 1989). Fab fragments of IgA antibodies to meningococci, which produce IgA1 protease, also inhibit IgG- and complement-mediated cytolysis of these bacteria (Jarvis and Griffiss, 1991). The precise specificity of the antibodies may be a factor, as IgA antibody to meningococcal capsular polysaccharide inhibits IgG- and complement-mediated lysis, whereas IgA antibody to outer-membrane proteins induces lysis of meningococci by an unexplained mechanism requiring C1q (Jarvis and Griffiss, 1989; Jarvis and Li, 1997). Recombinant human IgA monoclonal antibodies against meningococcal porin, however, failed to mediate complement-dependent lysis, although IgG antibodies with identical antigen-binding domains could readily do so, and IgA antibodies blocked lysis induced by IgG (Vidarsson *et al.*, 2001).

It has become evident in recent years that a third major pathway of complement activation involves lectins such as the mannose-binding lectin (MBL), a member of the collectin family that resembles C1q in molecular structure. MBL binds to terminal mannose, fucose, or *N*-acetylglucosamine residues in a calcium-dependent manner and then recruits serine proteases homologous to C1r/s, which lead into the remainder of the classical pathway from C4 onward (Møller-Kristensen *et al.*, 2003). Solid-phase-deposited pIgA (but not mIgA) can initiate this pathway (Roos *et al.*, 2001), and it is noteworthy that MBL and other collectins may be found in some secretions (see Chapter 5). It is possible that some of the controversy surrounding complement activation by IgA results from this activity, which has only recently become elucidated. However, the conditions necessary for its activation *in vivo* and the relative importance of its contribution to IgA-mediated protection against infections remain to be clarified.

Despite some unexplained exceptions, it generally appears that human IgA antibodies have poor to no complement-activating ability by the CCP or ACP when bound physiologically to antigen. However, the ACP-activating properties of IgA depend on some degree of denaturation or conformational change that does not ensue directly from binding to antigen or possibly on abnormal structure, including that of the oligosaccharide side chains. Such changes may occur under physiological or pathological circumstances *in vivo*, as a result of either aberrant synthesis or microbial degradation, and thereby contribute to inflammatory conditions in which IgA is implicated. In IgA nephropathy, for example, defective glycosylation of IgA1 may be a factor allowing it to deposit in the glomerular mesangium and activate the ACP (see Chapter 92). Cleavage of carbohydrate residues by bacterial glycosidases diminishes the ability of IgA antibodies to interfere with complement activation (Nikolova *et al.*, 1994a). The anti-inflammatory property of IgA antibodies with respect to complement activation may be of physiological significance in controlling inflammation at or beneath mucosal surfaces where IgA is abundant and where maintenance of the mucosal barrier is important.

Interaction with leukocytes

Several early studies indicated that IgA had a negative or inhibitory effect on phagocytosis, bactericidal activity, or chemotaxis by neutrophils, monocytes, and macrophages (reviewed in Kilian *et al.*, 1988). In some cases, results obtained with specific IgA antibody suggested that it competes with IgG antibody for binding to the target antigen, but in most experiments myeloma IgA proteins or colostral S-IgA, regardless of antibody activity, were used. A recent study indicates that solid-phase IgA (or S-IgA) can induce apoptosis in neutrophils, dependent also on Mac-1 (Schettini *et al.*, 2002). Other studies, particularly using neutrophils, monocytes, or macrophages derived from a mucosal environment (the gingival crevice or colostrum) or cultured *in vitro* with purified myeloma IgA or colostral S-IgA, reveal an opsonizing effect of IgA antibodies, sometimes in synergy with IgG antibodies (Fanger *et al.*, 1983; Gorter *et al.*, 1987; Honorio-França *et al.*, 1997; Lowell *et al.*, 1980). Several instances of heat-stable (i.e., complement-independent) opsonization or antibody-dependent cell-mediated cytotoxicity by IgA antibodies (reviewed in Kerr, 1990) have now been reported, including the postphagocytic respiratory burst and intracellular killing.

FcαRI (CD89) has been demonstrated on human neutrophils, monocytes/macrophages, and eosinophils (reviewed in Monteiro and van de Winkel, 2003; see also Chapter 13). It binds both subclasses of serum IgA equally and with moderate affinity at the junction of the Cα2 and Cα3 domains but not, it now appears, S-IgA. Unusually among Fc receptors, the IgA-binding site on FcαRI has been located on the membrane-distal domain 1, and recent studies show that a single Fcα region can bind two receptors cooperatively but in a pH-dependent manner (Herr *et al.*, 2003a,b). Although constitutively expressed on neutrophils and monocytes, FcαRI is upregulated on exudative neutrophils (e.g., from the gingival crevice) or by exposure of cells to activating agents such as phorbol esters, cytokines, bacterial LPS, chemotactic factors, and even IgA itself (Fanger *et al.*, 1983;

Hostoffer *et al.*, 1994; Maliszewski *et al.*, 1985). Among cytokines, TNF-α, IL-8, and GM-CSF have been found to enhance the surface expression of FcαRI on neutrophils, whereas IFN-γ and TGF-β downregulate it (Gessl *et al.*, 1994; Nikolova and Russell, 1995; Reterink *et al.*, 1996; Shen *et al.*, 1994; Weisbart *et al.*, 1988). Because FcαRI itself has no cytoplasmic signaling domain, association with the signal-transducing FcR-γ chain is important for its function (Morton *et al.*, 1995), but this appears to be highly variable in different cell types, their precise location, and state of activation or differentiation (Hamre *et al.*, 2003). Remarkably, mice appear to lack FcαRI, again pointing to important differences in the physiological functions of IgA in mice and humans. Although experiments performed on transgenic mice that express human FcαRI have yielded interesting insights into the function of the receptor (van der Pol *et al.*, 2000; van Egmond *et al.*, 2000), it must be remembered that this is an artificial situation.

The presence of IgA receptors on lymphocytes has been somewhat controversial, although several reports describe IgA (Fc) binding by T cells (Lum *et al.*, 1979a; Millet *et al.*, 1988; Sandor *et al.*, 1992) and by B cells (Bonner and Kerr, 1997; Lum *et al.*, 1979b; Millet *et al.*, 1989; Rao *et al.*, 1992). Although these putative receptors were never defined in molecular terms, recently a receptor for IgA and IgM (Fcα/μR) that appears to be related to pIgR has been identified on human and murine lymphocytes and may possibly account for some of the earlier observations (Phillips-Quagliata *et al.*, 2000; Sakamoto *et al.*, 2001; Shimizu *et al.*, 2001). The transferrin receptor (CD71) has also been implicated as a receptor for IgA1 on B cells as well as on epithelial cells (Moura *et al.*, 2001). IgA-mediated killing of bacteria by intestinal T cells has been described (Tagliabue *et al.*, 1986). IgA, especially IgA2, interacts with NK cells in a manner that suggests binding to carbohydrate-specific receptors that are distinct from either FcαRI or the mannose receptor (Komiyama *et al.*, 1986; Mota *et al.*, 2003). It has been proposed that a minor subset of NK cells expressing receptors for IgA that are upregulated by exposure to IgA complexed with IgG antibody regulates isotype-specific immunoglobulin secretion by B cells (Kimata, 1988).

It is now clear that human IgA can mediate phagocytosis and related processes by neutrophils, monocytes, or macrophages **(Fig. 14.1)** and induce postphagocytic intracellular events, at least *in vitro*. Although plasma IgA concentrations are sufficient to saturate FcαRI, the cells are not triggered unless the receptors are cross-linked, and pIgA is more effective in this than mIgA (Stewart *et al.*, 1994). Moreover, association of FcαRI with signaling γ chain is necessary for phagocytosis and cell activation (Honorio-França *et al.*, 2001; van Egmond *et al.*, 1999), and in its absence IgA may be taken up and recycled without inducing inflammatory responses (Launay *et al.*, 1999). It is interesting that Mac-1 (CD11b/CD18) has been identified as an accessory molecule involved in the binding of S-IgA (but not serum IgA) in murine neutrophils transgenically expressing human FcαRI (van Spriel *et al.*, 2002).

Several studies have shown that human serum (polyclonal) or monoclonal IgA antibodies can promote phagocytic uptake and killing of bacteria such as *S. pneumoniae* or *N. meningitidis* by human neutrophils *in vitro*. In some cases dependence on complement was shown (Janoff *et al.*, 1999), but not in others (van der Pol *et al.*, 2000; Vidarsson *et al.*, 2001). However, the precise role of complement in these experiments is unclear, although nonclassical pathway and complement receptors CR1 or CR3 were implicated, and the requirement for complement was diminished when neutrophils were preactivated with C5a or TNF-α (Janoff *et al.*, 1999). IgA-mediated protection against infection has been shown *in vivo* in mice that transgenically express human FcαRI, presumably involving opsonophagocytic mechanisms (Hellwig *et al.*, 2001; van der Pol *et al.*, 2000; van Egmond *et al.*, 2000).

It is evident that numerous factors influence the ability of IgA antibodies to mediate opsonophagocytic defense *in vivo*. Critical among these are whether relevant phagocytes express FcαRI and whether the receptor is associated with signaling γ chain. It is clear that these are highly variable even within the same type of cell at different locations and under different states of activation or differentiation. Thus, although neutrophils express high levels of FcαRI, they express relatively low levels of γ chain (Hamre *et al.*, 2003). Furthermore, monocytes and macrophages downregulate FcαRI expression as they mature, and both intestinal lamina propria and gingival macrophages appear to lack FcαRI altogether (Hamre *et al.*, 2003; Smith *et al.*, 2001; Yuan *et al.*, 2000). If IgA antibodies lack the ability to fix complement as discussed previously, the contribution of complement to opsonophagocytic defense mediated by IgA is difficult to comprehend. Possibly, enhanced fluid-phase turnover of the ACP could yield cleavage products such as C3a and C5a that might activate phagocytes by upregulating FcαRI or its association with γ chain. It may be postulated that expression of FcαRI by mucosal neutrophils, but not macrophages, would allow the former to dispose of invading, IgA-opsonized pathogens without major induction of inflammatory responses.

Reports that IgA could downregulate the release of inflammatory cytokines and induce the production of IL-1 receptor antagonist in human monocytes stimulated with bacterial LPS (Wolf *et al.*, 1994, 1996) were consistent with the concept of IgA as an anti-inflammatory isotype and with the oral administration of an IgA-enriched immunoglobulin preparation for therapy (albeit controversial) against necrotizing enterocolitis (Eibl *et al.*, 1988). Although this effect was dependent on FcαRI, subsequent studies revealed that the intracellular signaling mechanisms induced by IgA involved Src-family kinases, similar to those induced through other γ-chain-dependent Fc receptors (Gulle *et al.*, 1998). A more complex situation, however, is revealed by studies of human alveolar macrophages: whereas pIgA or S-IgA downregulated the respiratory burst induced by LPS through inhibition of the ERK1/2 pathway, they enhanced the response to phorbol ester in association with ERK1/2 phosphorylation and enhanced TNF-α release by an ERK1/2-independent

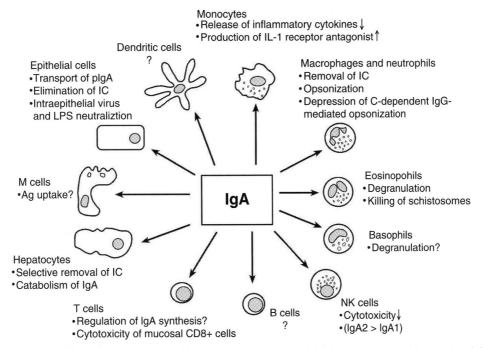

Fig. 14.1. Interactions of IgA with various cell types. Human cells of the myeloid lineage (neutrophils, eosinophils, monocytes, and macrophages) express FcαRI (CD89), through which they can be activated by serum IgA, especially in polymeric form or when aggregated or complexed with antigen. Binding of S-IgA (at least by neutrophils) requires Mac-1 as a co-receptor. Expression of FcαRI varies according to the cell type, its state of differentiation or activation, and location. Signal transduction and hence cellular responses depend on association of FcαRI with FcR γ chain. Eosinophils bind and respond especially well to S-IgA (or SC), but the nature of the receptor is not clear. Basophils are also reported to degranulate in response to S-IgA. Fcα/μR occurs on T and B lymphocytes, but its physiological function remains uncertain. The interaction of IgA with NK cells may be mediated by lectin-like receptors for carbohydrate determinants. Dendritic cells variably express FcαRI or another receptor for IgA, but their response to IgA is controversial. Epithelial cells, including hepatocytes of certain nonprimate animal species, express pIgR, which binds pIgA and thereby transports it to the apical surface, where it is released as S-IgA. Antigens complexed to pIgA antibodies can be similarly transported by hepatocytes into bile or by intestinal epithelial cells into the gut lumen. pIgA antibodies may also be able to interfere with intracellular viral replication or inhibit responses to LPS within epithelial cells. Enterocytes and M cells are also reported to bind IgA by other, possibly lectinlike, receptors. Serum IgA is catabolized by hepatocytes, probably after uptake mediated by the asialoglycoprotein receptor. For further details, see text.

mechanism (Ouadrhiri *et al.*, 2002). Studies on the partitioning of ligand-bound FcαRI into membrane lipid rafts with recruitment of tyrosine kinases have suggested that there are temporally regulated signaling events associated with IgA binding (Lang *et al.*, 2002).

IgA is particularly effective in stimulating the degranulation of eosinophils (Abu-Ghazaleh *et al.*, 1989) and in mediating the killing of schistosomes by eosinophils (Dunne *et al.*, 1993; Grezel *et al.*, 1993). Human eosinophils are also reported to bind S-IgA and SC by a 15-kDa receptor that is distinct from FcαRI and that mediates degranulation (Lamkhioued *et al.*, 1995). Stimulation of eosinophils by S-IgA or SC also involves β2 integrins, since it is inhibited by anti-CD18 antibody (Motegi and Kita, 1998). Complexes of S-IgA can induce IL-10 secretion and inhibit IL-2 and IFN-γ release from eosinophils (Woerly *et al.*, 1999), suggesting an immunoregulatory role. Immobilized S-IgA, but not mIgA, has been reported to induce degranulation of basophils (Iikura *et al.* 1998), possibly suggesting a role in allergic reactions. In contrast, IgA antibodies were long ago

shown to inhibit IgE-mediated hypersensitivity (Ishizaka *et al.*, 1963; Russell-Jones *et al.*, 1981). The interaction of IgA with these systems and its role both in defense against parasites and in allergic responses deserve more attention.

FcαRI has recently been identified on human interstitial dermal and gingival dendritic cells (DC), but not on Langerhans cells (Geissman *et al.*, 2001), as well as on DC derived from monocytes *in vitro* by culture with GM-CSF and IL-4. Triggering with pIgA complexes induced endocytosis and the production of IL-10 as well as functional activation of monocyte-derived DC, suggesting that interstitial DC may be able to take up and process IgA-opsonized antigens. Conversely, Heystek *et al.* (2002) found that CD89 expression was greatly diminished upon differentiation of monocytes into DC, whereas monocyte-derived DC bound S-IgA independently of FcαRI, possibly through carbohydrate recognition, but were not thereby activated. These authors suggested that immature DC may serve to modulate immune responses to S-IgA-complexed antigens at mucosal surfaces.

On most mucosal surfaces where S-IgA is the predominant immunoglobulin, functionally active leukocytes and complement are not normally present, so that S-IgA will have little opportunity to activate either system. Where the mucosal barrier is breached or inflammation occurs, both mucosal S-IgA and submucosal pIgA secreted by resident plasma cells could have an important role in a complex interplay of immunological effectors that may provide not only immune defense but also damage-limiting capability through the regulation of immune and inflammatory responses.

Other examples of IgA functioning as a regulatory isotype include the observations that IgA antibodies to HLA class I determinants enhance the survival of kidney allografts (Koka et al., 1993) and that IgA antibodies block cytotoxicity against melanoma cells or antibody-dependent cellular cytotoxicity against EBV-related nasopharyngeal carcinoma (Mathew et al., 1981; O'Niell and Romsdahl, 1974). Further investigation of these intriguing findings seems warranted.

Interaction with epithelial cells

pIgA-mediated elimination of antigen from the circulation by hepatobiliary transport (Peppard et al., 1981; Russell et al., 1981, 1983; Socken et al., 1981) has been demonstrated to occur, notably in certain rodents and rabbits in which there is rapid active transport of pIgA from the circulation to the bile by means of pIgR expressed on the sinusoidal surface of hepatocytes (see Chapter 11). However, despite a few reports to the contrary, it is now accepted that human hepatocytes do not express pIgR or transport pIgA and pIgA immune complexes in this manner. Nevertheless, other receptors such as the asialoglycoprotein receptor (or possibly membrane galactosyltransferase), which normally mediates the vesicular uptake of IgA and other desialylated glycoproteins for catabolism by hepatocytes (Mestecky et al., 1991), may allow a proportion of the IgA that is taken up, together with any complexed antigen, to be diverted into the biliary secretory pathway instead of the lysosomal degradative pathway (Schiff et al., 1986). The ability of serum IgA to interact with such alternative receptors, however, is greatly dependent upon the exposure of appropriate sugar residues on the molecular surface (Basset et al., 1999), and this is subject not only to posttranslational modification during synthesis but also to deglycosylation by microbial or other enzymes.

IgA antibodies can also bind antigens within the mucosal lamina propria, as even under normal conditions, small quantities of antigens from the lumen can penetrate the epithelium by transcytosis or diffusion, and during an infection microbial pathogens or their antigens may be present. Immune complexes formed in the lamina propria could then be taken up locally by phagocytic cells or might enter the blood or lymph, but another possible mechanism for disposing of them is local excretion through the epithelial cells by the same pIgR-mediated transcytosis that transports pIgA to the apical surface. Because IgA interacts with pIgR through its Fc region, transport can occur whether or not the antigen-binding sites in the Fab arms are occupied. Evidence

supporting this idea is the demonstration in vitro that immune complexes containing pIgA antibody can be transported intact across polarized epithelial cell monolayers that express pIgR (Gan et al., 1997; Kaetzel et al., 1991). Because pIgA is the dominant mucosal immunoglobulin and because IgA immune complexes that also contain other isotypes of antibody can be transported across epithelial cells (Kaetzel et al., 1994), local excretion through the epithelium offers a simple and direct means of ridding the mucosa of potentially noxious immune complexes, while helping to protect the circulation from an overload of them. Moreover, since cytokines produced during mucosal inflammation can upregulate the synthesis and expression of epithelial pIgR (Phillips et al., 1990; Sollid et al., 1987), the capacity of the epithelium to transport both free IgA and IgA immune complexes during times of stress can be increased. Although most intestinal antigen uptake probably occurs through the villi and S-IgA transport largely occurs in the crypts, evidence supporting the possibility that pIgA-mediated excretion of antigen can take place in vivo has been provided by experiments performed on transgenic mice expressing T cell receptors that recognize a peptide derived from ovalbumin (Robinson et al., 2001). In mice that had been mucosally immunized with ovalbumin to generate a vigorous S-IgA response and then challenged intravenously with the antigen, ovalbumin was detected in intestinal epithelial cells, in accordance with the distribution of pIgA transport. Hepatobiliary excretion of intestinally absorbed antigen was previously demonstrated in mice injected with pIgA antibody (Brown et al., 1984).

Because of their relatively nonphlogistic nature, IgA antibodies, in comparison with other isotypes, can form immune complexes and participate in host defense functions without inciting inflammatory reactions that might cause bystander damage to normal tissues (Brandtzaeg and Tolo, 1977; Brown et al., 1982). This property of IgA is especially valuable in mucous membranes, where the immune system continuously interacts with foreign substances. The ability of pIgA antibody to inhibit viral replication or LPS-induced inflammatory responses in epithelial cells during its pIgR-mediated transcytosis has already been discussed previously in this section.

IgA AND HOMEOSTASIS

Despite the considerable advances that have been made in unraveling the complexities of the immune system, it is remarkable that the biological activities and physiological functions of IgA are still so poorly comprehended, especially with respect to the circulating plasma form of IgA. It has been suggested that the role of plasma IgA is that of the "discreet housekeeper," implying a background regulatory activity for which there is evidence in terms of its interference with complement activation and modulation of phagocytic activity, as well as allergic reactions. S-IgA can be viewed in a similar way, except that perhaps it is the "discreet gatekeeper" whose job is to keep undesirables out. The abundance of IgA beneath as well as on mucosal surfaces may be of critical importance for maintaining the integrity of the mucosae by limiting the collateral damage inflicted by other immune defense mechanisms. In addition, S-IgA antibody may regulate the initiation of the immune response, as suggested by observations that preexisting mucosal antibody responses can interfere with the use of live bacterial or viral vectors for the delivery of mucosal vaccines and the demonstration that antibody responses in neonatal mice to reovirus are suppressed by suckling on immune foster mothers (Kramer and Cebra, 1995). New developments in this area comprise the interaction of S-IgA with epithelial cells, M cells, or DC, as discussed previously in this chapter. Likewise, the low level of mucosal antibodies elicited by commensal bacteria may serve to prevent overstimulation of the immune system by essentially harmless organisms, while permitting continuation of the relationship between commensal and host (Shroff et al., 1995).

Nevertheless, there may be situations in which IgA becomes inflammatory, as it can be involved in pathological conditions such as IgA nephropathy (see Chapter 92) or IgA immune complex–induced lung injury in rats (Mulligan et al., 1992). The question that must be asked, however, is whether these are the pathological manifestations of derangements in normal IgA structure and function or a consequence, albeit exaggerated, of normal physiological IgA activity. Conversely, other mucosal diseases may be associated with an apparent failure of IgA to maintain adequate anti-inflammatory control, for example, in periodontal disease in which infection-driven chronic inflammation results in destruction of the structures supporting the teeth. The balance between IgA and IgG antibodies may be the important factor (Brandtzaeg et al., 1977; Lim and Rowley, 1982). This raises the question of whether the anti-inflammatory effects of IgA can be exploited to ameliorate these conditions (Russell et al., 1997).

It might be expected that deficiency of IgA would manifest itself in profound disturbances, but this is generally not the case. Selective IgA deficiency occurs in Western populations with a frequency as high as 1 in 400 individuals (but it is 40-fold rarer in Japan), and yet the subjects do not inevitably suffer serious consequences, although as a group they have increased susceptibility to upper respiratory tract and oral infections, atopy, and other conditions (see also Chapter 63). It has been suggested that IgA deficiency would have more serious consequences in populations lacking modern hygienic facilities, where the antigenic and infectious challenge to mucosal surfaces is much greater. However, data supporting this hypothesis are lacking; the prevalence of IgA deficiency among blood donors in Sao Paulo (Brazil) or in KwaZulu-Natal (South Africa) is comparable with that in Western populations (Carneiro-Sampaio et al., 1989; Hattingh et al., 1996), but arguably these are self-selected healthy individuals, and it remains unknown what the frequency of IgA deficiency may be in undeveloped rural areas.

Curiously, significant numbers of IgD-secreting plasma cells also occur in certain submucosae, such as the nasal pas-

sages (Brandtzaeg et al., 1991), but there is no known mechanism for the secretion of this poorly understood isotype. Furthermore, IgD is highly susceptible to proteolysis, thus placing it at a disadvantage in secretions where proteases occur, and it appears that IgD cannot compensate for lack of IgA in IgA deficiency (Brandtzaeg et al., 1986a). IgG-secreting cells are also numerically increased in the mucosae of IgA-deficient subjects, and higher concentrations of IgG may be found in their secretions (Brandtzaeg et al., 1986b). However, there is no known transport mechanism for secretion of IgG through mucosal epithelia, and it probably reaches the surface by paracellular diffusion. Nasal secretions, as well as the genital tract, normally contain relatively more IgG than most other secretions, and there is some local production of IgG in the genital tract (see Chapter 99). The mechanisms by which these responses are generated and their significance for protection of the genital tract mucosae remain to be established.

In many respects, although it is the most abundant isotype of immunoglobulin in humans, IgA remains an enigma. Despite its abundance and the physiological energy expended in its production, IgA may seem to be dispensable, as IgA deficiency is relatively common and subjects are not always seriously immunocompromised. That view, however, is inconsistent with the notion that IgA has persisted through at least 250 million years of evolution, as it is found in both birds and mammals (see Chapter 11). As reviewed in this chapter, IgA straddles the interior and mucosal environments and can exert mucosal and systemic protection, and even if it may not always be essential in this role, especially against viruses, a great deal of evidence demonstrates its importance in mucosal defense. Conventional wisdom has ascribed a non-inflammatory and perhaps anti-inflammatory role for IgA, and much evidence supports this concept. However, in other contexts it can be inflammatory, although whether this is a physiological or pathological effect is debatable. In the gut and elsewhere, IgA can inhibit antigen uptake, but some reports suggest it may enhance the uptake of antigens for the promotion of immune responses in the inductive sites. Some of these paradoxes may be resolved by recognizing that IgA is highly variable in its structure: thus IgA subclass, molecular form, glycosylation, and structural integrity all impinge on its biological functions. Moreover, the receptors by which IgA interacts with a large variety of cell types are also multiple and variable, particularly in the case of FcαRI. Finally, there are subtle but significant differences in IgA and its receptors between humans and other mammals, notably mice, that confound the extrapolation of findings from one species to another. Defining the functions of IgA therefore requires defining the context of the question.

REFERENCES

Abraham, S.N., and Beachey, E.H. (1985). Host defenses against adhesion of bacteria to mucosal surfaces. In *Advances in Host Defense Mechanisms* (eds. J. F. Gallin and A. S. Fauci), Vol. 4, 63–88. New York: Raven Press.

Abu-Ghazaleh, R.I., Fujisawa, T., Mestecky, J., Kyle, R.A., and Gleich, G.J. (1989). IgA-induced eosinophil degranulation. *J. Immunol.* 142, 2393–2400.

Adinolfi, M., Glynn, A.A., Lindsay, M., and Milne, C.M. (1966). Serological properties of IgA antibodies to *Escherichia coli* present in human colostrum. *Immunology* 10, 517–526.

Alfsen, A., Iniguez, P., Bouguyon, E., and Bomsel, M. (2001). Secretory IgA specific for a conserved epitope on gp41 envelope glycoprotein inhibits epithelial transcytosis of HIV-1. *J. Immunol.* 166, 6257–6265.

Armstrong, S.J., and Dimmock, N.J. (1992). Neutralization of influenza virus by low concentrations of hemagglutinin-specific polymeric immunoglobulin A inhibits viral fusion activity, but activation of the ribonucleoprotein is also inhibited. *J. Virol.* 66, 3823–3832.

Arulanandam, B.P., Raeder, R.H., Nedrud, J.G., Bucher, D.J., Le, J.H., and Metzger, D.W. (2001). IgA immunodeficiency leads to inadequate Th cell priming and increased susceptibility to influenza virus infection. *J. Immunol.* 166, 226–231.

Barington, T., Juul, L., Gyhrs, A. and Heilman, C. (1994). Heavy-chain isotype patterns of human antibody-secreting cells induced by *Haemophilus influenzae* type b conjugate vaccines in relation to age and preimmunity. *Infect. Immun.* 62, 3066–3074.

Basset, C., Devauchelle, V., Durand, V., Jamin, C., Pennec, Y.L., Youinou, P., and Dueymes, M. (1999). Glycosylation of immunoglobulin A influences its receptor binding. *Scand. J. Immunol.* 50, 572–579.

Benson, M., Reinholdt, J., and Cardell, L.O. (2003). Allergen-reactive antibodies are found in nasal fluids from patients with birch pollen-induced intermittent allergic rhinitis, but not in healthy controls. *Allergy* 58, 386–392.

Benton, K.A., Misplon, J.A., Lo, C.Y., Brutkiewicz, R.R., Prasad, S.A., and Epstein, S.L. (2001). Heterosubtypic immunity to influenza A virus in mice lacking IgA, all Ig, NKT cells, or γδ T cells. *J. Immunol.* 166, 7437–7445.

Bessen, D., and Fischetti, V.A. (1988). Passive acquired mucosal immunity to group A streptococci by secretory immunoglobulin A. *J. Exp. Med.* 167, 1945–1950.

Biesbrock, A.R., Reddy, M.S., and Levine, M.J. (1991). Interaction of a salivary mucin-secretory immunoglobulin A complex with mucosal pathogens. *Infect. Immun.* 59, 3492–3497.

Blanchard, T.G., Czinn, S.J., Maurer, R., Thomas, W.D., Soman, G., and Nedrud, J.G. (1995). Urease-specific monoclonal antibodies prevent *Helicobacter felis* infection in mice. *Infect. Immun.* 63, 1394–1399.

Boackle, R.J., Pruitt, K.M., and Mestecky, J. (1974). The interactions of human complement with interfacially aggregated preparations of human secretory IgA. *Immunochemistry* 11, 543–548.

Boehm, M.K., Woof, J.M., Kerr, M.A., and Perkins, S.J. (1999). The Fab and Fc fragments of IgA1 exhibit a different arrangement from that in IgG: A study by X-ray and neutron solution scattering and homology modelling. *J. Mol. Biol.* 286, 1421–1447.

Bollinger, R.R., Everett, M.L., Palestrant, D., Love, S.D., Lin, S.S., and Parker, W. (2003). Human secretory immunoglobulin A may contribute to biofilm formation in the gut. *Immunology* 109, 580–587.

Bomsel, M., Heyman, M., Hocini, H., Lagaye, S., Belec, L., Dupont, C., and Desgranges, C. (1998). Intracellular neutralization of HIV transcytosis across tight epithelial barriers by anti-HIV envelope protein dIgA or IgM. *Immunity* 9, 277–287.

Bonner, B.C., and Kerr, M.A. (1997). Purification of high *Mr* forms of IgA1 from human serum: demonstration of binding to human B-lymphocytes. *Biochem. Soc. Trans.* 25, 331S.

Borén, T., Falk, P., Roth, K.A., Larson, G., and Normark, S. (1993). Attachment of *Helicobacter pylori* to human gastric epithelium mediated by blood group antigens. *Science* 262, 1892–1895.

Brandtzaeg, P., Karlsson, G., Hansson, G., Petruson, B., Bjorkander, J., and Hanson, L. A. (1986a). The clinical condition of IgA-deficient patients is related to the proportion of IgD- and IgM-producing cells in their nasal mucosa. *Clin. Exp. Immunol.* 67, 626–636.

Brandtzaeg, P., Kett, K., and Rognum, T.O. (1986b). Distribution of mucosal IgA and IgG subclass-producing immunocytes and alterations in various disorders. *Monogr. Allergy* 20, 179–194.

Brandtzaeg, P., Nilssen, D.E., Rognum, T.O., and Thrane, P.S. (1991). Ontogeny of the mucosal immune system and IgA deficiency. *Gastroenterol. Clin. N. Amer.* 20, 397–439.

Brandtzaeg, P., and Tolo, K. (1977). Mucosal penetrability enhanced by serum-derived antibodies. *Nature* 266, 262–263.

Brock, S.C., McGraw, P.A., Wright, P.F., and Crowe, J.E. (2002). The human polymeric immunoglobulin receptor facilitates invasion of epithelial cells by *Streptococcus pneumoniae* in a strain-specific and cell type–specific manner. *Infect. Immun.* 70, 5091–5095.

Bronson, R.A., Cooper, G.W., Rosenfeld, D.L., Gilbert, J.V. and Plaut, A.G. (1987). The effect of an IgA1 protease on immunoglobulins bound to the sperm surface and sperm cervical mucus penetrating ability. *Fertil. Steril.* 47, 985–991.

Brown, T.A., and Mestecky, J. (1985). Immunoglobulin A subclass distribution of naturally occurring salivary antibodies to microbial antigens. *Infect. Immun.* 49, 459–462.

Brown, T.A., Russell, M.W., and Mestecky, J. (1982). Hepatobiliary transport of IgA immune complexes: molecular and cellular aspects. *J. Immunol.* 128, 2183–2186.

Brown, T.A., Russell, M.W., and Mestecky, J. (1984). Elimination of intestinally absorbed antigen into the bile by IgA. *J. Immunol.* 132, 780–782.

Burnett, P.R., VanCott, T.C., Polonis, V R., Redfield, R.R., and Birx, D.L. (1994). Serum IgA-mediated neutralization of HIV type 1. *J. Immunol.* 152, 4642–4648.

Burns, J.W., Siadat-Pajouh, M., Krishnaney, A.A., and Greenberg, H.B. (1996). Protective effect of rotavirus VP6-specific IgA monoclonal antibodies that lack neutralizing activity. *Science* 272, 104–107.

Burritt, M.F., Calvanico, N.J., Mehta, S., and Tomasi, T.B. (1977). Activation of the classical complement pathway by Fc fragment of human IgA. *J. Immunol.* 118, 723–725.

Campbell, A.M., Vachier, I., Chanez, P., Vignola, A.M., Lebel, B., Kochan, J., Godard, P., and Bousquet, J. (1998). Expression of the high-affinity receptor for IgE on bronchial epithelial cells of asthmatics. *Am. J. Respir. Cell Mol. Biol.* 19, 92–97.

Carbonare, S.B., Silva, M.L. M., Trabulsi, L.R., and Carneiro-Sampaio, M.M.S. (1995). Inhibition of HEp-2 cell invasion by enteroinvasive *Escherichia coli* by human colostrum IgA. *Int. Arch. Allergy Immunol.* 108, 113–118.

Carneiro-Sampaio, M., Carbonare, S., Rozentraub, R.B., Mamede, M.N., Ribeiro, M.A., and Porto, M.H. (1989). Frequency of selective IgA deficiency among Brazilian blood donors and healthy pregnant women. *Allergol. Immunopathol.* 17, 213–216.

Castilla, J., Sola, I., and Enjuanes, L. (1997). Interference of coronavirus infection by expression of immunoglobulin G (IgG) or IgA virus-neutralizing antibodies. *J. Virol.* 71, 5251–5258.

Cisar, J.O., Barsumian, E.L., Siraganian, R.P., Clark, W.B., Yeung, M.K., Hsu, S.D., Curl, S.H., Vatter, A.E., and Sandberg, A.L. (1991). Immunochemical and functional studies of *Actinomyces viscosus* T14V type 1 fimbriae with monoclonal and polyclonal antibodies directed against the fimbrial subunit. *J. Gen. Microbiol.* 137, 1971–1979.

Clamp, J.R. (1977). The relationship between secretory immunoglobulin A and mucus. *Biochem. Soc. Trans.* 5, 1579–1581.

Clements, M.L., Betts, R.F., Tierney, E.L., and Murphy, B.R. 1986. Serum and nasal wash antibodies associated with resistance to experimental challenge with influenza A wild-type virus. *J. Clin. Microbiol.* 24, 157–160.

Colten, H.R., and Bienenstock, J. (1974). Lack of C3 activation through classical or alternate pathways by human secretory IgA antiblood group A antibody. *Adv. Exp. Med. Biol.* 45, 305–308.

Corthésy, B., Kaufmann, M., Phalipon, A., Peitsch, M., Neutra, M.R., and Kraehenbuhl, J.P. (1996). A pathogen-specific epitope inserted into recombinant secretory immunoglobulin A is immunogenic by the oral route. *J. Biol. Chem.* 271, 33670–33677.

Cotter, T.W., Meng, Q., Shen, Z.-L., Zhang, Y.-X., Su, H., and Caldwell, H.D. (1995). Protective efficacy of major outer membrane protein–specific immunoglobulin A (IgA) and IgG monoclonal antibodies in a murine model of *Chlamydia trachomatis* genital tract infection. *Infect. Immun.* 63, 4704–4714.

Coulson, B.S., Grimwood, K., Hudson, I.L., Barnes, G.L., and Bishop, R.F. (1992). Role of coproantibody in clinical protection of children during reinfection with rotavirus. *J. Clin. Microbiol.* 30, 1678–1684.

Cravioto, A., Tello, A., Villafan, H., Ruiz, J., del Vedovo, S., and Neeser, J.-R. (1991). Inhibition of localized adhesion of enteropathogenic *Escherichia coli* to HEp-2 cells by immunoglobulin and oligosaccharide fractions of human colostrum and breast milk. *J. Infect. Dis.* 163, 1247–1255.

Crottet, P., and Corthésy, B. (1998). Secretory component delays the conversion of secretory IgA into antigen-binding competent F(ab')₂: A possible implication for mucosal defense. *J. Immunol.* 161, 5445–5453.

Cunningham-Rundles, C., Brandeis, W.E., Good, R.A., and Day, N.K. (1978). Milk precipitins, circulating immune complexes, and IgA deficiency. *Proc. Natl. Acad. Sci. U.S.A.* 75, 3387–3389.

Czinn, S.J., Cai, A., and Nedrud, J.G. (1993). Protection of germ-free mice from infection by *Helicobacter felis* after active oral or passive IgA immunization. *Vaccine* 11, 637–642.

Davin, J.C., Senterre, J., and Mahieu, P.R. (1991). The high lectin-binding capacity of human secretory IgA protects nonspecifically mucosae against environmental antigens. *Biol Neonate* 59, 121–125.

Devito, C., Broliden, K., Kaul, R., Svensson, L., Johansen, K., Kiama, P., Kimani, J., Lopalco, L., Piconi, S., Bwayo, J.J., Plummer, F., Clerici, M., and Hinkula, J. (2000). Mucosal and plasma IgA from HIV-1-exposed uninfected individuals inhibit HIV-1 transcytosis across human epithelial cells. *J. Immunol.* 165, 5170–5176.

Dunne, D.W., Richardson, B.A., Jones, F. M., Clark, M., Thorne, K.J.I., and Butterworth, A.E. (1993). The use of mouse/human chimaeric antibodies to investigate the roles of different antibody isotypes, including IgA2, in the killing of *Schistosoma mansoni* schistosomula by eosinophils. *Parasite Immunol.* 15, 181–185.

Edebo, L., Richardson, N., and Feinstein, A. (1985). The effects of binding mouse IgA to dinitrophenylated *Salmonella typhimurium* on physicochemical properties and interaction with phagocytic cells. *Int. Arch. Allergy Appl. Immunol.* 78, 353–357.

Egan, M.L., Pritchard, D.G., Dillon, H.G., and Gray, B.M. (1983). Protection of mice from experimental infection with type III group B *Streptococcus* using monoclonal antibodies. *J. Exp. Med.* 158, 1006–1011.

Eibl, M., Wolf, H.M., Furnkranz, H., and Rosenkranz, A. (1988). Prevention of necrotizing enterocolitis in low-birth-weight infants by IgA-IgG feeding. *N. Engl. J. Med* 319, 1–7.

Engström, P.-E., Norhagen, G.E., Bottaro, A., Carbonara, A.O., Lefranc, G., Steinitz, M., Söder, P.Ö., Smith, C.I.E. and Hammerström, L. (1990). Subclass distribution of antigen-specific IgA antibodies in normal donors and individuals with homozygous Cα1 or Cα2 gene deletions. *J. Immunol.* 145, 109–116.

Enriquez, F.J., and Riggs, M.W. (1998). Role of immunoglobulin A monoclonal antibodies against P23 in controlling murine *Cryptosporidium parvum* infection. *Infect. Immun.* 66, 4469–4473.

Falk, P, Roth, K.A., Borén, T., Westblom, T.U., Gordon, J.I., and Normark, S. (1993). An *in vitro* adherence assay reveals that *Helicobacter pylori* exhibits cell lineage–specific tropism in the human gastric epithelium. *Proc. Natl. Acad. Sci. USA* 90, 2035–2039.

Fanger, M.W., Goldstine, S.N., and Shen, L. (1983). Cytofluorographic analysis of receptors for IgA on human polymorphonuclear cells and monocytes and the correlation of receptor expression with phagocytosis. *Molec. Immunol.* 20, 1019–1027.

Feng, N.G., Lawton, J.A., Gilbert, J., Kuklin, N., Vo, P., Prasad, B.V.V., and Greenberg, H.B. (2002). Inhibition of rotavirus replication by a non-neutralizing rotavirus VP6-specific IgA mAb. *J. Clin. Invest.* 109, 1203–1213.

Fernandez, M.I., Pedron, T., Tournebize, R., Olivo-Marin, J.C., Sansonetti, P.J., and Phalipon, A. (2003). Anti-inflammatory role for intracellular dimeric immunoglobulin A by neutralization of lipopolysaccharide in epithelial cells. *Immunity* 18, 739–749.

Finn, A., Zhang, Q.B., Seymour, L., Fasching, C., Pettitt, E., and Janoff, E.N. (2002). Induction of functional secretory IgA responses in breast milk, by pneumococcal capsular polysaccharides. *J. Infect. Dis.* 186, 1422–1429.

Fisher, R.G., Crowe, J.E., Jr., Johnson, T.R., Tang, Y.W., and Graham, B.S. (1999). Passive IgA monoclonal antibody is no more effective than IgG at protecting mice from mucosal challenge with respiratory syncytial virus. *J. Infect. Dis.* 180, 1324–1327.

Friman, V., Adlerberth, I., Connell, H., Svanborg, C., Hanson, L.-Å., and Wold, A.E. (1996). Decreased expression of mannose-specific adhesins by *Escherichia coli* in the colonic microflora of immunoglobulin A–deficient individuals. *Infect. Immun.* 64, 2794–2798.

Friman, V., Nowrouzian, F., Adlerberth, I., and Wold, A.E. (2002). Increased frequency of intestinal *Escherichia coli* carrying genes for S fimbriae and haemolysin in IgA-deficient individuals. *Microb. Pathog.* 32, 35–42.

Fubara, E.S., and Freter, R. (1973). Protection against enteric bacterial infection by secretory IgA antibodies. *J. Immunol.* 111, 395–403.

Fukui, Y., Fukui, K., and Moriyama, T. (1973). Inhibition of enzymes by human salivary immunoglobulin A. *Infect. Immun.* 8, 335–340.

Funakoshi, S., Dot, T., Nakajima, T., Suyama, T., and Tokuda, M. (1982). Antimicrobial effect of human serum IgA. *Microbiol. Immunol.* 26, 227–239.

Gan, Y.J., Chodosh, J., Morgan, A., and Sixbey, J.W. (1997). Epithelial cell polarization is a determinant in the infectious outcome of immunoglobulin A–mediated entry by Epstein-Barr virus. *J. Virol.* 71, 519–526.

Geissmann, F., Launay, P., Pasquier, B., Lepelletier, Y., Leborgne, M., Lehuen, A., Brousse, N., and Monteiro, R.C. (2001). A subset of human dendritic cells expresses IgA Fc receptor (CD89), which mediates internalization and activation upon cross-linking by IgA complexes. *J. Immunol.* 166, 346–352.

Gessl, A., Willheim, M., Spittler, A., Agis, H., Krugluger, W., and Boltz-Nitulescu, G. (1994). Influence of tumor-necrosis factor-α on the expression of Fc IgG and IgA receptors, and other markers by cultured human blood monocytes and U937 cells. *Scand. J. Immunol.* 39, 151–156.

Gorter, A., Hiemstra, P.S., Leijh, P.C.J., van der Sluys, M.E., van den Barselaar, M.T., van Es, L.A., and Daha, M.R. (1987). IgA- and secretory IgA–opsonized *S. aureus* induce a respiratory burst and phagocytosis by polymorphonuclear leucocytes. *Immunology* 61, 303–309.

Götze, O., and Müller-Eberhard, H.J. (1971). The C3-activator system: an alternative pathway of complement activation. *J. Exp. Med.* 134, 90s–108s.

Grezel, D., Capron, M., Grzych, J.-M., Fontaine, J., Lecocq, J.-P., and Capron, A. (1993). Protective immunity induced in rat schistosomiasis by a single dose of the Sm28GST recombinant antigen: effector mechanisms involving IgE and IgA antibodies. *Eur. J. Immunol.* 23, 454–460.

Griffiss, J.M., Broud, D., and Bertram, M.A. (1975). Bactericidal activity of meningococcal antisera. Blocking by IgA of lytic antibody in human convalescent sera. *J. Immunol.* 114, 1779–1784.

Gulle, H., Samstag, A., Eibl, M.M., and Wolf, H.M. (1998). Physical and functional association of FcαR with protein tyrosine kinase Lyn. *Blood* 91, 383–391.

Hajishengallis, G., Nikolova, E., and Russell, M.W. (1992). Inhibition of *Streptococcus mutans* adherence to saliva-coated hydroxyapatite by human secretory immunoglobulin A (S-IgA) antibodies to cell surface protein antigen I/II: reversal by IgA1 protease cleavage. *Infect. Immun.* 60: 5057–5064.

Hall, W.M., Manion, R.E., and Zinneman, H.H. (1971). Blocking serum lysis of *Brucella abortus* by hyperimmune rabbit immunoglobulin A. *J. Immunol.* 107, 41–46.

Hammerschmidt, S., Talay, S.R., Brandtzaeg, P., and Chhatwal, G.S. (1997). SpsA, a novel pneumococcal surface protein with specific binding to secretory immunoglobulin A and secretory component. *Mol. Microbiol.* 25, 1113–1124.

Hamre, R., Farstad, I.N., Brandtzaeg, P., and Morton, H.C. (2003). Expression and modulation of the human immunoglobulin A Fc receptor (CD89) and the FcR γ chain on myeloid cells in blood and tissue. *Scand. J. Immunol.* 57, 506–516.

Haque, R., Ali, I.M., Sack, R.B., Farr, B.M., Ramakrishnan, G., and Petri, W.A. (2001). Amebiasis and mucosal IgA antibody against the *Entamoeba histolytica* adherence lectin in Bangladeshi children. *J. Infect. Dis.* 183, 1787–1793.

Harriman, G.R., Bogue, M., Rogers, P., Finegold, M., Pacheco, S., Bradley, A., Zhang, Y.X., and Mbawuike, I.N. (1999). Targeted deletion of the IgA constant region in mice leads to IgA deficiency with alterations in expression of other Ig isotypes. *J. Immunol.* 162, 2521–2529.

Hattingh, C., Green, F., Bubb, M.O., and Conradie, J.D. (1996). The incidence of IgA deficiency amongst blood donors in KwaZulu-Natal. *S. Afr. J. Sci.* 92, 206–209.

Heilman, C., Barington, T. and Sigsgaard, T. (1988). Subclass of individual IgA-secreting human lymphocytes. Investigation of *in vivo* pneumococcal polysaccharide-induced and *in vitro* mitogen-induced blood B cells by monolayer plaque-forming cell assays. *J. Immunol.* 140, 1496–1499.

Hellwig, S.M.M., Van Spriel, A.B., Schellekens, J.F.P., Mooi, F.R., and Van de Winkel, J.G.J. (2001). Immunoglobulin A–mediated protection against *Bordetella pertussis* infection. *Infect. Immun.* 69, 4846–4850.

Heremans, J.F. (1974). Immunoglobulin A. In *The Antigens* (ed. M. Sela), Vol. 2, pp. 365–522. New York: Academic Press Inc.

Herr, A.B., Ballister, E.R., and Bjorkman, P.J. (2003a). Insights into IgA-mediated immune responses from the crystal structures of human FcαRI and its complex with IgA1-Fc. *Nature* 423, 614–620.

Herr, A.B., White, C.L., Milburn, C., Wu, C., and Bjorkman, P.J. (2003b). Bivalent binding of IgA1 to FcαRI suggests a mechanism for cytokine activation of IgA phagocytosis. *J. Mol. Biol.* 327, 645–657.

Heystek, H.C., Moulon, C., Woltman, A.M., Garonne, P., and van Kooten, C. (2002). Human immature dendritic cells efficiently bind and take up secretory IgA without induction of maturation. *J. Immunol.* 168, 102–107.

Hiemstra, P.S., Gorter, A., Stuurman, M.E., van Es, L.A., and Daha, M.R. (1987). Activation of the alternative pathway of complement by human serum IgA. *Eur. J. Immunol.* 17, 321–326.

Hiemstra, P.S., Biewenga, J., Gorter, A., Stuurman, M.E., Faber, A., Van Es, L.A., and Daha, M.R. (1988). Activation of complement by human serum IgA, secretory IgA and IgA1 fragments. *Molec. Immunol.* 25, 527–533.

Hiemstra, P.S., Rits, M., Gorter, A., Stuurman, M.E., Hoekzema, R., Bazin, H., Vaerman, J.-P., Van Es, L.A., and Daha, M.R. (1990). Rat polymeric IgA binds C1q, but does not activate C1. *Molec. Immunol.* 27, 867–874.

Hirano, M., Kamada, M., Maegawa, M., Gima, H., and Aono, T. (1999). Binding of human secretory protease inhibitor in uterine cervical mucus to immunoglobulins: pathophysiology in immunologic infertility and local immune defense. *Fertil. Steril.* 71, 1108–1114.

Honorio-França, A.C., Carvalho, M.P.S.M., Isaac, L., Trabulsi, L.R., and Carneiro-Sampaio, M.M.S. (1997). Colostral mononuclear phagocytes are able to kill enteropathogenic *Escherichia coli* opsonized with colostral IgA. *Scand. J. Immunol.* 46, 59–66.

Honorio-França, A.C., Launay, P., Carneiro-Sampaio, M.M.S., and Monteiro, R.C. (2001). Colostral neutrophils express Fcα receptors (CD89) lacking γ chain association and mediate noninflammatory properties of secretory IgA. *J. Leukocyte Biol.* 69, 289–296.

Hostoffer, R.W., Krukovets, I., and Berger, M. (1994). Enhancement by tumor necrosis factor-α of Fcα receptor expression and IgA-mediated superoxide generation and killing of *Pseudomonas aeruginosa* by polymorphonuclear leukocytes. *J. Infect. Dis.* 170, 82–87.

Huang, D.S., Emancipator, S.N., Lamm, M.E., Karban, T.L., Blatnik, F.H., Tsao, H.M., and Mazanec, M.B. (1997). Virus-specific IgA reduces hepatic viral titers *in vivo* on mouse hepatitis virus (MHV) infection. *Immunol. Cell Biol.* 75 (Suppl. 1), A12.

Iankov, I.D., Petrov, D.P., Mladenov, I.V., Haralambieva, I.H., and Mitov, I.G. (2002). Lipopolysaccharide-specific but not anti-flagellar immunoglobulin A monoclonal antibodies prevent *Salmonella enterica* serotype enteritidis invasion and replication within HEp-2 cell monolayers. *Infect. Immun.* 70, 1615–1618.

Iikura, M., Yamaguchi, M., Fujisawa, T., Miyamasu, M., Takaishi, T., Morita, Y., Iwase, T., Moro, I., Yamamoto, K., and Hirai, K. (1998). Secretory IgA induces degranulation of IL-3-primed basophils. *J. Immunol.* 161, 1510–1515.

Imai, H., Chen, A., Wyatt, R.J., and Rifai, A. (1988). Lack of complement activation by human IgA immune complexes. *Clin. Exp. Immunol.* 73, 479–483.

Ishizaka, K., Ishizaka, T., and Hornbrook, M.M. (1963). Blocking of Prausnitz-Kustner sensitization with reagin by normal human β2A globulin. *J. Allergy* 34, 395–403.

Janoff, E.N., Wahl, S.M., Thomas, K., and Smith, P.D. (1995). Modulation of human immunodeficiency virus type 1 infection of human monocytes by IgA. *J. Infect. Dis.* 172, 855–858.

Janoff, E.N., Fasching, C., Orenstein, J.M., Rubins, J.B., Opstad, N.L., and Dalmasso, A.P. (1999). Killing of *Streptococcus pneumoniae* by capsular polysaccharide–specific polymeric IgA, complement, and phagocytes. *J. Clin. Invest.* 104, 1139–1147.

Janoff, E.N., Rubins, J.B., Fasching, C., Plaut, A., and Weiser, J.N. (2002). Inhibition of IgA-mediated killing of *S. pneumoniae* (Spn) by IgA1 protease (IgA1P). 11th International Congress of Mucosal Immunology, *Mucosal Immunology Update*, vol. 10, Abst. 2839.

Jarvis, G.A., and Griffiss, J.M. (1989). Human IgA1 initiates complement-mediated killing of *Neisseria meningitidis*. *J. Immunol.* 143, 1703–1709.

Jarvis, G.A., and Griffiss, J.M. (1991). Human IgA1 blockade of IgG-initiated lysis of *Neisseria meningitidis* is a function of antigen-binding fragment binding to the polysaccharide capsule. *J. Immunol.* 147, 1962–1967.

Jarvis, G.A., and Li, J. (1997). IgA1-initiated killing of *Neisseria meningitidis*: requirement for C1q and resistance to IgA1 protease. *Immunol. Cell Biol.* 75 (Suppl. 1), A12.

Jentoft, N. (1990). Why are proteins O-glycosylated? *Trends Biochem. Sci.* 15, 291–294.

Jertborn, M., Svennerholm, A.M., and Holmgren, J. (1986). Saliva, breast milk, and serum antibody responses as indirect measures of intestinal immunity after oral cholera vaccination or natural disease *J. Clin. Microbiol.* 24, 203–209.

Johansen, F.E., Pekna, M., Norderhaug, I.N., Haneberg, B., Hietala, M.A., Krajci, P., Betsholtz, C., and Brandtzaeg, P. (1999). Absence of epithelial immunoglobulin A transport, with increased mucosal leakiness, in polymeric immunoglobulin receptor/secretory component-deficient mice. *J. Exp. Med.* 190, 915–921.

Johnson, P.R., Feldman, S., Thompson, J.M., Mahoney, J.D., and Wright, P. (1986). Immunity to influenza A virus infection in young children: a comparison of natural infection, live cold-adapted vaccine, and inactivated vaccine. *J. Infect. Dis.* 154, 121–127.

Johnson, S., Sypura, W.D., Gerding, D.N., Ewing, S.L., and Janoff, E.N. (1995). Selective neutralization of a bacterial enterotoxin by serum immunoglobulin A in response to mucosal disease. *Infect. Immun.* 63, 3166–3173.

Junghans, R.P. (1997). Finally! The Brambell receptor (FcRB) — Mediator of transmission of immunity and protection from catabolism for IgG. *Immunol. Res.* 16, 29–57.

Kaetzel, C.S., Robinson, J.K., Chintalacharuvu, K.R., Vaerman, J.-P., and Lamm, M.E. (1991). The polymeric immunoglobulin receptor (secretory component) mediates transport of immune complexes across epithelial cells: A local defense function for IgA. *Proc. Natl. Acad. Sci. USA* 88, 8796–8800.

Kaetzel, C.S., Robinson, J.K., and Lamm, M.E. (1994). Epithelial transcytosis of monomeric IgA and IgG cross-linked through antigen to polymeric IgA. A role for monomeric antibodies in the mucosal immune system. *J. Immunol.* 152, 72–76.

Kalliomaki, M., Salminen, S., Poussa, T., Arvilommi, H., and Isolauri, E. (2003). Probiotics and prevention of atopic disease: 4-year follow-up of a randomised placebo-controlled trial. *Lancet* 361, 1869–1871.

Kauppi-Korkeila, M., van Alphen, L., Madore, D., Saarinen, L., and Käyhty, H. (1996). Mechanism of antibody-mediated reduction of nasopharyngeal colonization by *Haemophilus influenzae* type b studied in an infant rat model. *J. Infect. Dis.* 174, 1337–1340.

Kauppi-Korkeila, M., Saarinen, L., Eskola, J., and Käyhty, H. (1998). Subclass distribution of IgA antibodies in saliva and serum after immunization with *Haemophilus influenzae* type b conjugate vaccines. *Clin. Exp. Immunol.* 111, 237–242.

Keren, D.F., McDonald, R.A., Carey, J.L. (1988). Combined parenteral and oral immunization results in an enhanced mucosal immunoglobulin A response to *Shigella flexneri*. *Infect. Immun.* 56, 910–915.

Kerr, M.A. (1990). The structure and function of human IgA. *Biochem. J.* 271, 285–296.

Kilian, M., Roland, K., and Mestecky, J. (1981). Interference of secretory immunoglobulin A with sorption of oral bacteria to hydroxyapatite. *Infect. Immun.* 31, 942–951.

Kilian, M., Mestecky, J., and Russell, M.W. (1988). Defense mechanisms involving Fc-dependent functions of immunoglobulin A and their subversion by bacterial immunoglobulin A proteases. *Microbiol. Rev.* 52, 296–303.

Kilian, M., Husby, S., Høst, A., and Halken, S. (1995). Increased proportions of bacteria capable of cleaving IgA1 in the pharynx of infants with atopic disease. *Pediatr. Res.* 38, 182–186.

Kimata, H., and Saxon, A. (1988). Subset of natural killer cells is induced by immune complexes to display Fc receptors for IgE and IgA and demonstrates isotype regulatory function. *J. Clin. Invest.* 82, 160–167.

Kitamura, T., Garofalo, R.P., Kamijo, A., Hammond, D.K., Oka, J.A., Caflisch, C.R., Shenoy, M., Casola, A., Weigel, P.H., and Goldblum, R.M. (2000). Human intestinal epithelial cells express a novel receptor for IgA. *J. Immunol.* 164, 5029–5034.

Koka, P., Chia, D., Terasaki, P.I., Chan, H., Chia, J., Ozawa, M., and Lim, E. (1993). The role of IgA anti-HLA class I antibodies in kidney transplant survival. *Transplantation* 56, 207–211.

Komiyama, K., Crago, S. S., Itoh, K., Moro, I., and Mestecky, J. (1986). Inhibition of natural killer cell activity by IgA. *Cell. Immunol.* 101, 143–155.

Kozlowski, P.A., Black, K.P., Shen, L., and Jackson, S. (1995). High prevalence of serum IgA HIV-1 infection-enhancing antibodies in HIV-infected persons: masking by IgG. *J. Immunol.* 154, 6163–6173.

Kraehenbuhl, J.-P., and Neutra M.R. (1992). Molecular and cellular basis of immune protection of mucosal surfaces. *Physiol. Rev.* 72, 853–879.

Kramer, D.R., and Cebra, J.J. (1995). Role of maternal antibody in the induction of virus specific and bystander IgA responses in Peyer's patches of suckling mice. *Internat. Immunol.* 7, 911–918.

Lamkhioued, B., Gounni, A.S., Gruart, V., Pierce, A., Capron, A., and Capron, M. (1995). Human eosinophils express a receptor for secretory component. Role in secretory IgA-dependent activation. *Eur. J. Immunol.* 25, 117–125.

Lamm, M.E., and Phillips-Quagliata, J.M. (2002). Origin and homing of intestinal IgA antibody–secreting cells. *J. Exp. Med.* 195, F5–F8.

Lang, M.L., Chen, Y.W., Shen, L., Gao, H., Lang, G.A., Wade, T.K., and Wade, W.F. (2002). IgA Fc receptor (FcαR) cross-linking recruits tyrosine kinases, phosphoinositide kinases and serine/threonine kinases to glycolipid rafts. *Biochem. J.* 364, 517–525.

Langford, T.D., Housley, M.P., Boes, M., Chen, J.Z., Kagnoff, M.F., Gillin, F.D., and Eckmann, L. (2002). Central importance of immunoglobulin A in host defense against *Giardia* spp. *Infect. Immun.* 70, 11–18.

Launay, P., Patry, C., Lehuen, A., Pasquier, B., Blank, U., and Monteiro, R.C. (1999). Alternative endocytic pathway for immunoglobulin A Fc receptors (CD89) depends on the lack of FcRγ association and protects against degradation of bound ligand. *J. Biol. Chem.* 274, 7216–7225.

Leher, H., Zaragoza, F., Taherzadeh, S., Alizadeh, H., and Niederkorn, J.Y. (1999). Monoclonal IgA antibodies protect against *Acanthamoeba* keratitis. *Exp. Eye Res.* 69, 75–84.

Liew, F.Y., Russell, S.M., Appleyard, G., Brand, C.M., and Beale, J. (1984). Cross protection in mice infected with influenza A virus by the respiratory route is correlated with local IgA antibody rather than serum antibody or cytotoxic T cell reactivity. *Eur. J. Immunol.* 14, 350–356.

Liljemark, W.F., Bloomquist, C.G., and Ofstehage, J.C. (1979). Aggregation and adherence of *Streptococcus sanguis*: role of human salivary immunoglobulin A. *Infect. Immun.* 26, 1104–1110.

Lim, P.L., and Rowley, D. (1982). The effect of antibody on the intestinal absorption of macromolecules and on intestinal permeability in adult mice. *Int. Arch. Allergy Appl. Immunol.* 68, 41–46.

Lindh, E. (1975). Increased resistance of immunoglobulin A dimers to proteolytic degradation after binding secretory component. *J. Immunol.* 14, 284–286.

Lowell, G.H., Smith, L.F., Griffiss, J.M., and Brandt, B.L. (1980). IgA-dependent, monocyte-mediated, antibacterial activity. *J. Exp. Med.* 152, 452–457.

Lue, C., Tarkowski, A., and Mestecky, J. (1988). Systemic immunization with pneumococcal polysaccharide vaccine induces a predominant IgA2 response of peripheral blood lymphocytes and increases of both serum and secretory antipneumococcal antibodies. *J. Immunol.* 140, 3793–3800.

Lum, L.G., Muchmore, A.V., Keren, D., Decker, J., Koski, I., Strober, W., and Blaese, R.M. (1979a). A receptor for IgA on human T lymphocytes. *J. Immunol.* 122, 65–69.

Lum, L.G., Muchmore, A.V., O'Connor, N., Strober, W., and Blaese, R.M. (1979b). Fc receptors for IgA on human B, and human non-B, non-T lymphocytes. *J. Immunol.* 123, 714–719.

Lycke, N., Eriksen, L., and Holmgren, J. (1987). Protection against cholera toxin after oral immunization is thymus-dependent and associated with intestinal production of neutralizing IgA antitoxin. *Scand. J. Immunol.* 25, 413–419.

Lycke, N., Erlandsson, L., Ekman, L., Schön, K., and Leanderson, T. (1999). Lack of J chain inhibits the transport of gut IgA and abrogates the development of intestinal antitoxic protection. *J. Immunol.* 163, 913–919.

Ma, J.K.-C., Hunjan, M., Smith, R., Kelly, C. and Lehner, T. (1990). An investigation into the mechanism of protection by local passive immunization with monoclonal antibodies against *Streptococcus mutans*. *Infect. Immun.* 58, 3407–3414.

Magnusson, K.-E., and Stjernstrom, I. (1982). Mucosal barrier mechanisms. Interplay between secretory IgA (SIgA), IgG and mucins on the surface properties and association of salmonellae with intestine and granulocytes. *Immunology* 45, 239–248.

Majumdar, A.S., and Ghose, A.C. (1981). Evaluation of the biological properties of different classes of human antibodies in relation to cholera. *Infect. Immun.* 32, 9–14.

Maliszewski, C.R., Shen, L., and Fanger, M.W. (1985). The expression of receptors for IgA on human monocytes and calcitriol-treated HL-60 cells. *J. Immunol.* 135, 3878–3881.

Mantis, N.J., Cheung, M.C., Chintalacharuvu, K.R., Rey, J., Corthésy, B., and Neutra, M.R. (2002). Selective adherence of IgA to murine Peyer's patch M cells: evidence for a novel IgA receptor. *J. Immunol.* 169, 1844–1851.

Mathew, G.D., Qualtiere, L.F., Neel, H.B., and Pearson, G.R. (1981). IgA antibody, antibody-dependent cellular cytotoxicity and prognosis in patients with nasopharyngeal carcinoma. *Int. J. Cancer* 27, 175–180.

Mattu, T.S., Pleass, R.J., Willis, A.C., Kilian, M., Wormald, M.R., Lellouch, A.C., Rudd, P.M., Woof, J.M., and Dwek, R.A. (1998). The glycosylation and structure of human serum IgA1, Fab, and Fc regions and the role of N-glycosylation on Fcα receptor interactions. *J. Biol. Chem.* 273, 2260–2272.

Mazanec, M.B., Nedrud, J.G., and Lamm, M.E. (1987). Immunoglobulin A monoclonal antibodies protect against Sendai virus. *J. Virol.* 61, 2624–2626.

Mazanec, M.B., Kaetzel, C.S., Lamm, M.E., Fletcher, D., and Nedrud, J.G. (1992). Intracellular neutralization of virus by immunoglobulin A antibodies. *Proc. Natl. Acad. Sci. USA.* 89, 6901–6905.

Mazanec, M.B., Coudret, C.L., and Fletcher, D.R. (1995). Intracellular neutralization of influenza virus by immunoglobulin A anti-hemagglutinin monoclonal antibodies. *J. Virol.* 69, 1339–1343.

Mazanec, M.B., Huang, Y.T., Pimplikar, S.W., and Lamm, M.E. (1996). Mechanisms of inactivation of respiratory viruses by IgA, including intraepithelial neutralization. *Semin. Virol.* 7, 285–292.

Mbawuike, I.N., Pacheco, S., Acuna, C.L., Switzer, K.C., Zhang, Y.X., and Harriman, G.R. (1999). Mucosal immunity to influenza without IgA: An IgA knockout mouse model. *J. Immunol.* 162, 2530–2537.

Mestecky, J., Lue, C., and Russell, M.W. (1991). Selective transport of IgA: cellular and molecular aspects. *Gastroenterol. Clin. N. Am.* 20, 441–471.

Michetti, P., Mahan, M.J., Slauch, J.M., Mekalanos, J.J., and Neutra, M.R. (1992). Monoclonal secretory immunoglobulin A protects mice against oral challenge with the invasive pathogen *Salmonella typhimurium*. *Infect. Immun.* 60, 1786–1792.

Miletic, V.D., Hester, C.G., and Frank, M.M. (1996). Regulation of complement activity by immunoglobulin I. Effect of immunoglobulin isotype on C4 uptake on antibody-sensitized sheep erythrocytes and solid-phase immune complexes. *J. Immunol.* 156, 749–757.

Millet, I., Panaye, G., and Revillard, J.P. (1988). Expression of receptors for IgA on mitogen-stimulated human T lymphocytes. *Eur. J. Immunol.* 18, 621–626.

Millet, I., Brière, F., Vincent, C., Pousset, F., Andreoni, C., de Vries, J.E., and Revillard, J.P. (1989). Spontaneous expression of a low affinity Fc receptor for IgA (FcαR) on human B cell lines. *Clin. Exp. Immunol.* 76, 268–273.

Møller-Kristensen, M., Thiel, S., Hansen, A.G., and Jensenius, J.C. (2003). On the site of C4 deposition upon complement activation via the mannan-binding lectin pathway or the classical pathway. *Scand. J. Immunol.* 57, 556–561.

Monteiro, R.C., and van de Winkel, J.G.J. (2003). IgA Fc receptors. *Annu. Rev. Immunol.* 21, 177–204.

Morton, H.C., van den Herik-Oudijk, I.E., Vossebeld, P., Snijders, A., Verhoeven, A.J., Capel, P.J.A., and van de Winkel, J.G.J. (1995). Functional association between the human myeloid immunoglobulin A Fc receptor (CD89) and FcR γ chain—Molecular basis for CD89/FcR γ chain association. *J. Biol. Chem.* 270, 29781–29787.

Mota, G., Manciulea, M., Cosma, E., Popescu, I., Hirt, M., Jensen-Jarolim, E., Calugaru, A., Galatiuc, C., Regalia, T., Tamandl, D., Spittler, A., and Boltz-Nitulescu, G. (2003). Human NK cells express Fc receptors for IgA which mediate signal transduction and target cell killing. *Eur. J. Immunol.* 33, 2197–2205.

Motegi, Y., and Kita, H. (1998). Interaction with secretory component stimulates effector functions of human eosinophils but not of neutrophils. *J. Immunol.* 161, 4340–4346.

Moura, I.C., Centelles, M.N., Arcos-Fajardo, M., Malheiros, D.M., Collawn, J.F., Cooper, M.D., and Monteiro, R.C. (2001). Identification of the transferrin receptor as a novel immunoglobulin (Ig)A1 receptor and its enhanced expression on mesangial cells in IgA nephropathy. *J. Exp. Med.* 194, 417–425.

Mulligan, M.S., Warren, J.S., Smith, C.W., Anderson, D.C., Yeh, C.G., Rudolph, A.R., and Ward, P.A. (1992). Lung injury after deposition of IgA immune complexes. Requirements for CD18 and L-arginine. *J. Immunol.* 148, 3086–3092.

Nikolova, E.B., and Russell, M.W. (1995). Dual function of human IgA antibodies: inhibition of phagocytosis in circulating neutrophils and enhancement of responses in IL-8-stimulated cells. *J. Leukocyte Biol.* 57, 875–882.

Nikolova, E.B., Tomana, M., and Russell, M.W. (1994a). All forms of human IgA antibodies bound to antigen interfere with complement (C3) fixation induced by IgG or by antigen alone. *Scand. J. Immunol.* 39, 275–280.

Nikolova, E.B., Tomana, M., and Russell, M.W. (1994b). The role of the carbohydrate chains in complement (C3) fixation by solid-phase-bound human IgA. *Immunology* 82, 321–327.

Norrby-Teglund, A., Ihendyane, N., Kansal, R., Basma, H., Kotb, M., Andersson, J., and Hammarström, L. (2000). Relative neutralizing activity in polyspecific IgM, IgA, and IgG preparations against group A streptococcal superantigens. *Clin. Infect. Dis.* 31, 1175–1182.

O'Neal, C.M., Harriman, G.R., and Conner, M.E. (2000). Protection of the villus epithelial cells of the small intestine from rotavirus infection does not require immunoglobulin A. *J. Virol.* 74, 4102–4109.

O'Niell, P.A., and Romsdahl, M.M. (1974). IgA as a blocking factor in human malignant melanoma. *Immunol. Commun.* 3, 427–438.

Offit, P.A., and Clark, H.F. (1985). Protection against rotavirus-induced gastroenteritis in a murine model by passively acquired gastrointestinal but not circulating antibodies. *J. Virol.* 54, 58–64.

Ogra, P.L., Karzon, D.T., Righthand, F., and McGillivray, M. (1968). Immunoglobulin response in serum and secretions after immunization with live and inactivated polio vaccine and natural infection. *N. Engl. J. Med.* 279, 893–900.

Onorato, I.M., Modlin, J.F., McBean, A.M., Thomas, M.L., Losonsky, G.A., and Bernier R.H., (1991). Mucosal immunity induced by enhanced-potency inactivated and oral polio vaccines. *J. Infect. Dis.* 163, 1–6.

Ouadrhiri, Y., Pilette, C., Monteiro, R.C., Vaerman, J.P., and Sibille, Y. (2002). Effect of IgA on respiratory burst and cytokine release by human alveolar macrophages: Role of ERK1/2 mitogen-activated protein kinases and NF-κB. *Am. J. Respir. Cell. Mol. Biol.* 26, 315–332.

Pal, S., Theodor, I., Peterson, E. M., and De la Maza, L. M. (1997). Monoclonal immunoglobulin A antibody to the major outer membrane protein of the *Chlamydia trachomatis* mouse pneumonitis biovar protects mice against a chlamydial genital challenge. *Vaccine* 15, 575–582.

Parr, M.B., Harriman, G.R., and Parr, E.L. (1998). Immunity to vaginal HSV-2 infection in immunoglobulin A knockout mice. *Immunology* 95, 208–213.

Peebles, R.S., Hamilton, R.G., Lichtenstein, L.M., Schlosberg, M, Liu, MC, Proud, D., and Togias, A. (2001). Antigen-specific IgE and IgA antibodies in bronchoalveolar lavage fluid are associated with stronger antigen-induced late phase reactions. *Clin. Exp. Allergy* 31, 239–248.

Peppard, J., Orlans, E., Payne, A.W., and Andrew, E. (1981). The elimination of circulating complexes containing polymeric IgA by excretion in the bile. *Immunology* 42, 83–89.

Pfaffenbach, G., Lamm, M.E., and Gigli, I. (1982). Activation of the guinea pig alternative complement pathway by mouse IgA immune complexes. *J. Exp. Med.* 155, 231–247.

Phalipon, A., Kaufmann, M., Michetti, P., Cavaillon, J.M., Huerre, M., Sansonetti, P., and Kraehenbuhl, J.P. (1995). Monoclonal immunoglobulin A antibody directed against serotype-specific epitope of *Shigella flexneri* lipopolysaccharide protects against murine experimental shigellosis. *J. Exp. Med.* 182, 769–778.

Phalipon, A., Cardona, A., Kraehenbuhl, J.P., Edelman, L., Sansonetti, P.J., and Corthésy, B. (2002). Secretory component: A new role in secretory IgA-mediated immune exclusion *in vivo*. *Immunity* 17, 107–115.

Phillips, J.O., Everson, M.P., Moldoveanu, Z., Lue, C., and Mestecky, J. (1990). Synergistic effect of IL-4 and IFN-γ on the expression of polymeric Ig receptor (secretory component) and IgA binding by human epithelial cells. *J. Immunol.* 145, 1740–1744.

Phillips-Quagliata, J.M., Patel, S., Han, J.K., Arakelov, S., Rao, T.D., Shulman, M.J., Fatal, S., Corley, R.B., Everett, M., Klein, M.H., Underdown, B.J., and Corthésy, B. (2000). The IgA/IgM receptor expressed on a murine B cell lymphoma is poly-Ig receptor. *J. Immunol.* 165, 2544–2555.

Platts-Mills, T.A., von Maur, R.K., Ishizaka, K., Norman, P.S., and Lichtenstein, L.M. (1976). IgA and IgG anti-ragweed antibodies in nasal secretions. Quantitative measurements of antibodies and correlation with inhibition of histamine release. *J. Clin. Invest.* 57, 1041–1050.

Rao, T.D., Maghazachi, A.A., González, A.V., and Phillips-Quagliata, J.M. (1992). A novel IgA receptor expressed on a murine B cell lymphoma. *J. Immunol.* 149, 143–153.

Reed, C.E., Bubak, M., Dunnette, S., Blomgren, J., Pfenning, M., Wentz-Murtha, P., Wallen N, Keating M, and Gleich GJ. (1991). Ragweed-specific IgA in nasal lavage fluid of ragweed-sensitive allergic rhinitis patients: increase during the pollen season. *Int. Arch. Allergy Appl. Immunol.* 94, 275–277.

Renegar, K.B., and Small, P. (1991). Passive transfer of local immunity to influenza virus infection by IgA antibody. *J. Immunol.* 146, 1972–1978.

Renegar, K.B., Jackson, G.D.F., and Mestecky, J. (1998). *In vitro* comparison of the biologic activities of monoclonal monomeric IgA, polymeric IgA, and secretory IgA. *J. Immunol.* 160, 1219–1223.

Renegar, K.B., Johnson, C.D., Dewitt, R.C., King, B.K., Li, J., Fukatsu, K., and Kudsk, K.A. (2001). Impairment of mucosal immunity by total parenteral nutrition: Requirement for IgA in murine nasotracheal anti-influenza immunity. *J. Immunol.* 166, 819–825.

Reterink, T.J.F., Levarht, E.W.N., Klar-Mohamad, N., Van Es, L.A., and Daha, M.R. (1996). Transforming growth factor-beta 1 (TGF-β1) down-regulates IgA Fc-receptor (CD89) expression on human monocytes. *Clin. Exp. Immunol.* 103, 161–166.

Reuman, P.D., Bernstein, D.I., Keely, S.P., Sherwood, J.R., Young, E.C., and Schiff, G.M. (1990). Influenza-specific ELISA IgA and IgG predict severity of influenza disease in subjects pre-screened with hemagglutination inhibition. *Antiviral Res.* 13, 103–110.

Rits, M., Hiemstra, P.S., Bazin, H., Van Es, L.A., Vaerman, J.-P., and Daha, M.R. (1988). Activation of rat complement by soluble and insoluble rat IgA immune complexes. *Eur. J. Immunol.* 18, 1873–1880.

Robinson, J.K., Blanchard, T.G., Levine, A.D., Emancipator, S.N., and Lamm, M.E. (2001). A mucosal IgA-mediated excretory immune system *in vivo*. *J. Immunol.* 166, 3688–3692.

Romer, W., Rothke, U., and Roelcke, D. (1980). Failure of IgA cold agglutinin to activate C. *Immunobiology* 157, 41–46.

Roos, A., Bouwman, L.H., van Gijlswijk-Janssen, D.J., Faber-Krol, M.C., Stahl, G.L., and Daha, M.R. (2001). Human IgA activates the complement system via the mannan-binding lectin pathway. *J. Immunol.* 167, 2861–2868.

Royle, L., Roos, A., Harvey, D.J., Wormald, M.R., van Gijlswijk-Janssen, D., Redwan, E.-R.M., Wilson, I.A., Daha, M.R., Dwek, R.A., and Rudd, P.M. (2003). Secretory IgA N- and O-glycans provide a link between the innate and adaptive immune systems. *J. Biol. Chem.* 278, 20140–20153.

Ruggeri, F.M., Johansen, K., Basile, G., Kraehenbuhl, J.-P., and Svensson, L. (1998). Antirotavirus immunoglobulin A neutralizes virus *in vitro* after transcytosis through epithelial cells and protects infant mice from diarrhea. *J. Virol.* 72, 2708–2714.

Russell, M.W., and Mansa, B. (1989). Complement-fixing properties of human IgA antibodies: alternative pathway complement activation by plastic-bound, but not by specific antigen-bound IgA. *Scand. J. Immunol.* 30, 175–183.

Russell, M.W., and Sibley, D.A. (1999). IgA as an anti-inflammatory regulator of immunity. *Oral Dis.* 5, 55–56.

Russell, M.W., Brown, T.A., and Mestecky, J. (1981). Role of serum IgA: Hepatobiliary transport of circulating antigen. *J. Exp. Med.* 153, 968–976.

Russell, M.W., Brown, T.A., Claflin, J.L., Schroer, K., and Mestecky, J. (1983). Immunoglobulin A-mediated hepatobiliary transport constitutes a natural pathway for disposing of bacterial antigens. *Infect. Immun.* 42, 1041–1048.

Russell, M.W., Reinholdt, J., and Kilian, M. (1989). Anti-inflammatory activity of human IgA antibodies and their Fabα fragments: inhibition of IgG-mediated complement activation. *Eur. J. Immunol.* 19, 2243–2249.

Russell, M.W., Lue, C., van den Wall Bake, A.W.L., Moldoveanu, Z., and Mestecky, J. (1992). Molecular heterogeneity of human IgA antibodies during an immune response. *Clin. Exp. Immunol.* 87, 1–6.

Russell-Jones, G.J., Ey, P.L., and Reynolds, B.L. (1980). The ability of IgA to inhibit the complement-mediated lysis of target red blood cells sensitized with IgG antibody. *Molec. Immunol.* 17, 1173–1180.

Russell-Jones, G.J., Ey, P.L., and Reynolds, B.L. (1981). Inhibition of cutaneous anaphylaxis and Arthus reactions in the mouse by antigen-specific IgA. *Int. Arch. Allergy Appl. Immunol.* 316–325.

Sakamoto, N., Shibuya, K., Shimizu, Y., Yotsumoto, K., Miyabayashi, T., Sakano, S., Tsuji, T., Nakayama, E., Nakauchi, H., and Shibuya, A. (2001). A novel Fc receptor for IgA and IgM is expressed on both hematopoietic and non-hematopoietic tissues. *Eur. J. Immunol.* 31, 1310–1316.

Saltzman, W.M., Radomsky, M.L., Whaley, K.J., and Cone, R.A. (1994). Antibody diffusion in human cervical mucus. *Biophys. J.* 66, 508–515.

Sandor, M., Houlden, B., Bluestone, J., Hedrick, S.M., Weinstock, J., and Lynch, R.G. (1992). *In vitro* and *in vivo* activation of murine γ/δ T cells induces the expression of IgA, IgM, and IgG Fc receptors. *J. Immunol.* 148, 2363–2369.

Schettini, J., Salamone, G., Trevani, A., Raiden, S., Gamberale, R., Vermeulen, M., Giordano, M., and Geffner, J.R. (2002). Stimulation of neutrophil apoptosis by immobilized IgA. *J. Leukocyte Biol.* 72, 685–691.

Schiff, J.M., Huling, S.L., and Jones, A.L. (1986). Receptor-mediated uptake of asialoglycoprotein by the primate liver initiates both lysosomal and transcellular pathways. *Hepatology* 6, 837–847.

Schneiderman, R.D., Lint, T.F., and Knight, K.L. (1990). Activation of the alternative pathway of complement by twelve different rabbit-mouse chimeric transfectoma IgA isotypes. *J. Immunol.* 145, 233–237.

Schreiber, J.R., Barrus, V., Cates, K.L., and Siber, G.R. (1986). Functional characterization of human IgG, IgM, and IgA antibody directed to the capsule of *Haemophilus influenzae* type b. *J. Infect. Dis.* 153, 8–16.

Schroten, H., Stapper, C., Plogmann, R., Köhler, H., Hacker, J., and Hanisch, F.-G. (1998). Fab-independent antiadhesion effects of secretory immunoglobulin A on S-fimbriated *Escherichia coli* are mediated by sialyloligosaccharides. *Infect. Immun.* 66, 3971–3973.

Schwartz-Cornil, I., Benureau, Y., Greenberg, H., Hendrickson, B.A., and Cohen, J. (2002). Heterologous protection induced by the inner capsid proteins of rotavirus requires transcytosis of mucosal immunoglobulins. *J. Virol.* 76, 8110–8117.

Sharpe, A.H., and Fields, B.N. (1985). Pathogenesis of viral infections. Basic concepts derived from the reovirus model. *N. Engl. J. Med.* 312, 486–497.

Shen, L., Collins, J.E., Schoenborn, M.A., and Maliszewski, C.R. (1994). Lipopolysaccharide and cytokine augmentation of human monocyte IgA receptor expression and function. *J. Immunol.* 152, 4080–4086.

Shibayama, M., Serrano-Luna, J.D.J., Rojas-Hernández, S., Campos-Rodríguez, R., and Tsutsumi, V. (2003). Interaction of secretory immunoglobulin A antibodies with *Naegleria fowleri* trophozoites and collagen type I. *Can. J. Microbiol.* 49, 164–170.

Shimizu, Y., Honda, S., Yotsumoto, K., Tahara-Hanaoka, S., Eyre, H.J., Sutherland, G.R., Endo, Y., Shibuya, K., Koyama, A., Nakauchi, H., and Shibuya, A. (2001). Fcα/μ receptor is a single gene-family member closely related to polymeric immunoglobulin receptor encoded on Chromosome 1. *Immunogenetics* 53, 709–711.

Shroff, K.E., Meslin, K., and Cebra, J.J. (1995). Commensal enteric bacteria engender a self-limiting humoral mucosal immune response while permanently colonizing the gut. *Infect. Immun.* 63, 3904–3913.

Silbart, L.K., and Keren, D.F. (1989). Reduction of intestinal carcinogen absorption by carcinogen-specific secretory immunity. *Science* 243, 1462–1464.

Silvey, K.J., Hutchings, A.B., Vajdy, M., Petzke, M.M., and Neutra, M.R. (2001). Role of immunoglobulin A in protection against reovirus entry into murine Peyer's patches. *J. Virol.* 75, 10870–10879.

Sixbey, J.W., and Yao, Q. (1992). Immunoglobulin A–induced shift of Epstein-Barr virus tissue tropism. *Science* 255, 1578–1580.

Smith, D.J., Taubman, M.A., and Ebersole, J.L. (1985). Salivary IgA antibody to glucosyltransferase in man. *Clin. Exp. Immunol.* 61, 416–424.

Smith, P.D., Smythies, L.E., Mosteller-Barnum, M., Sibley, D.A., Russell, M.W., Merger, M., Sellers, M.T., Orenstein, J.M., Shimada, T., Graham, M.F., and Kubagawa, H. (2001). Intestinal macrophages lack CD14 and CD89 and consequently are down-regulated for LPS- and IgA-mediated activities. *J. Immunol.* 167, 2651–2656.

Socken, D.J., Simms, E.S., Nagy, B.R., Fisher, M.M., and Underdown, B.J. (1981). Secretory component-dependent hepatic transport of IgA antibody-antigen complexes. *J. Immunol.* 127, 316–319.

Sollid, L.M., Kvale, D., Brandtzaeg, P., Markussen, G., and Thorsby, E. (1987). Interferon-γ enhances expression of secretory component, the epithelial receptor for polymeric immunoglobulins. *J. Immunol.* 138, 4303–4306.

Steele, E.J., Chaicumpa, W., and Rowley, D. (1975). Further evidence for cross-linking as a protective factor in experimental cholera: Properties of antibody fragments. *J. Infect. Dis.* 132, 175–180.

Steinitz, M., Tamir, S., Ferne, M., and Goldfarb, A. (1986). A protective human monoclonal IgA antibody produced *in vitro*: anti-pneumococcal antibody engendered by Epstein-Barr virus-immortalized cell line. *Eur. J. Immunol.* 16, 187–193.

Stephens, S., Dolby, J.M., Montreuil, J., and Spik, G. (1980). Differences in inhibition of the growth of commensal and enteropathogenic strains of *Escherichia coli* by lactotransferrin and secretory immunoglobulin A isolated from human milk. *Immunology* 41, 597–603.

Stewart, W.W., Johnson, A., Steward, M.W., Whaley, K., and Kerr, M.A. (1990). The effect of antibody isotype on the activation of C3 and C4 by immune complexes formed in the presence of serum: correlation with the prevention of immune precipitation. *Molec. Immunol.* 27, 423–428.

Stewart, W.W., Mazengera, R.L., Shen, L., and Kerr, M.A. (1994). Unaggregated serum IgA binds to neutrophil FcαR at physiological concentrations and is endocytosed but cross-linking is necessary to elicit a respiratory burst. *J. Leukocyte Biol.* 56, 481–487.

Stokes, C.R., Taylor, B., and Turner, M.W. (1974). Association of house-dust and grass-pollen allergies with specific IgA antibody deficiency. *Lancet* ii, 485–488.

Stokes, C.R., Soothill, J.F., and Turner, M.W. (1975). Immune exclusion is a function of IgA. *Nature.* 255, 745–746.

Strober, W., Krakauer, R., Klaeveman, H.L., Reynolds, H.Y., and Nelson, D.L. (1976). Secretory component deficiency. A disorder of the IgA immune system. *N. Engl. J. Med.* 294, 351–356.

Stubbe, H., Berdoz, J., Kraehenbuhl, J.P., and Corthésy, B. (2000). Polymeric IgA is superior to monomeric IgA and IgG carrying the same variable domain in preventing *Clostridium difficile* toxin A damaging of T84 monolayers. *J. Immunol.* 164, 1952–1960.

Sudo, N., Sawamura, S.-A., Tanaka, K, Aiba, Y., Kubo, C., and Koga, Y. (1997). The requirement of intestinal bacterial flora for the development of an IgE production system fully susceptible to oral tolerance induction. *J. Immunol.* 159, 1739–1745.

Svanborg-Eden, C., and Svennerholm, A.-M. (1978). Secretory immunoglobulin A and G antibodies prevent adhesion of *Escherichia coli* to human urinary tract epithelial cells. *Infect. Immun.* 22, 790–797.

Tagliabue, A., Villa, L., De Magistris, M. T., Romano, M., Silvestri, S., Boraschi, D., and Nencioni, L. (1986). IgA-driven T cell–mediated anti-bacterial immunity in man after live oral Ty21a vaccine. *J. Immunol.* 137, 1504–1510.

Tenovuo, J., Moldoveanu, Z., Mestecky, J., Pruitt, K.M., and Mansson-Rahemtulla, B. (1982). Interaction of specific and innate factors of immunity: IgA enhances the antimicrobial effect of the lactoperoxidase system against *Streptococcus mutans*. *J. Immunol.* 128, 726–731.

Thompson, R.A. (1970). Secretory piece linked to IgM in individuals deficient in IgA. *Nature* 226, 946–948.

Tomana, M., Kulhavy, R., and Mestecky, J. (1988). Receptor-mediated binding and uptake of immunoglobulin A by human liver. *Gastroenterology* 94, 762–770.

Tramont, E.C. (1977). Inhibition of adherence of *Neisseria gonorrhoeae* by human genital secretions. *J. Clin. Invest.* 59, 117–124.

Vaerman, J.-P., and Heremans, J.F. (1968). Effect of neuraminidase and acidification on complement-fixing properties of human IgA and IgG. *Int. Arch. Allergy Appl. Immunol.* 34, 49–52.

Valim, Y.M.L., and Lachmann, P.J. (1991). The effect of antibody isotype and antigenic epitope density on the complement-fixing activity of immune complexes: a systematic study using chimaeric anti-NIP antibodies with human Fc regions. *Clin. Exp. Immunol.* 84, 1–8.

Van der Pol, W.L., Vidarsson, G., Vilé, H.A., Van de Winkel, J.G.J., and Rodriguez, M.E. (2000). Pneumococcal capsular polysaccharide-specific IgA triggers efficient neutrophil effector functions via FcαRI (CD89). *J. Infect. Dis.* 182, 1139–1145.

Van Egmond, M., Van Vuuren, A.J.H., Morton, H.C., Van Spriel, A.B., Shen, L., Hofhuis, F.M.A., Saito, T., Mayadas, T.N., Verbeek, J.S., and Van de Winkel, J.G.J. (1999). Human immunoglobulin A receptor (FcαRI, CD89) function in transgenic mice requires both FcR γ chain and CR3 (CD11b/CD18). *Blood* 93, 4387–4394.

Van Egmond, M., Van Garderen, E., Van Spriel, A.B., Damen, C.A., Van Amersfoort, E.S., Van Zandbergen, G., Van Hattum, J., Kuiper, J., and Van de Winkel, J.G.J. (2000). FcαRI-positive liver Kupffer cells: Reappraisal of the function of immunoglobulin A in immunity. *Nature Med.* 6, 680–685.

Van Spriel, A.B., Leusen, J.H.W., Vilé, H., and Van de Winkel, J.G.J. (2002). Mac-1 (CD11b/CD18) as accessory molecule for FcαR (CD89) binding of IgA. *J. Immunol.* 169, 3831–3836.

Vidarsson, G., van der Pol, W.-L., van den Elsen, J.M.H., Vilé, H., Jansen, M., Duijs, J., Morton, H.C., Boel, E., Daha, M.R., Corthésy, B., and Van de Winkel, J.G.J. (2001). Activity of human IgG and IgA subclasses in immune defense against *Neisseria meningitidis* serogroup B. *J. Immunol.* 166, 6250–6256.

Waldo, F.B., and Cochran, A.M. (1989). Mixed IgA-IgG aggregates as a model of immune complexes in IgA nephropathy. *J. Immunol.* 142, 3841–3846.

Walker, W.A., Isselbacher, K.J., and Bloch, K.J. (1972). Intestinal uptake of macromolecules: effect of oral immunization. *Science* 177, 608–610.

Watanabe, T., Nagura, H., Watanabe, K., and Brown, W.R. (1984). The binding of human milk lactoferrin to immunoglobulin A. *FEBS Lett.* 168, 203–207.

Watt, P.J., Robinson, B.S., Pringle, C.R., and Tyrrell, D.A.J. (1990). Determinants of susceptibility to challenge and the antibody response of adult volunteers given experimental respiratory syncytial virus vaccines. *Vaccine* 8, 231–236.

Waxman, F.J., Hebert, L.A., Cosio, F.G., Smead, W.L., Van Aman, M.E., Taguiam, J.M., and Birmingham, D. J. (1986). Differential binding of immunoglobulin A and immunoglobulin G1 immune complexes to primate erythrocytes *in vivo*. *J. Clin. Invest.* 77, 82–89.

Weisbart, R.H., Kacena, A., Schuh, A., and Golde, D.W. (1988). GM-CSF induces human neutrophil IgA-mediated phagocytosis by an IgA Fc receptor activation mechanism. *Nature* 332, 647–648.

Weltzin, R., Hsu, S.A., Mittler, E.S., Georgakopoulos, K., and Monath, T.P. (1994). Intranasal monoclonal immunoglobulin A against respiratory syncytial virus protects against upper and lower respiratory tract infections in mice. *Antimicrob. Agents Chemother.* 38, 2785–2791.

Weltzin, R., Lecia-Jandris, P., Michetti, P., Fields, B.N., Kraehenbuhl, J.P., and Neutra, M.R. (1989). Binding and transepithelial transport of immunoglobulins by intestinal M cells: demonstration using monoclonal IgA antibodies against enteric viral proteins. *J. Cell Biol.* 108, 1673–1685.

Weltzin, R., Traina-Dorge, V., Soike, K., Zhang, J.-Y., Mack, P., Soman, G., Drabik, G., and Monath, T.P. (1996). Intranasal monoclonal IgA antibody to respiratory syncytial virus protects rhesus monkeys against upper and lower respiratory tract infection. *J. Infect. Dis.* 174, 256–261.

Whitty, P.W., Robertson, A., Kerr, M.A., Woof, J.M., and Perkins, S.J. (2002). Human IgA2 displays a more compact structural configuration than human IgA1. 11th International Congress of Mucosal Immunology, *Mucosal Immunology Update*, vol. 10, abst. 2626.

Williams, R.C., and Gibbons, R.J. (1972). Inhibition of bacterial adherence by secretory immunoglobulin A: a mechanism of antigen disposal. *Science* 177, 697–699.

Wingren, C., and Hansson, U.-B. (1997). Surface of properties of antigen-antibody complexes. *Scand. J. Immunol.* 46, 159–167.

Winner, L., Mack, J., Weltzin, R., Mekalanos, J.J., Kraehenbuhl, J.-P., and Neutra, M.R. (1991). New model for analysis of mucosal immunity: intestinal secretion of specific monoclonal immunoglobulin A from hybridoma tumors protects against *Vibrio cholerae* infection. *Infect. Immun.* 59, 977–982.

Woerly, G., Roger, N., Loiseau, S., Dombrowicz, D., Capron, A., and Capron, M. (1999). Expression of CD28 and CD86 by human eosinophils and role in the secretion of type 1 cytokines (interleukin 2 and interferon γ): Inhibition by immunoglobulin A complexes. *J. Exp. Med.* 190, 487–495.

Wolbank, S., Kunert, R., Stiegler, G., and Katinger, H. (2003). Characterization of human class–switched polymeric (immunoglobulin M [IgM] and IgA) anti-human immunodeficiency virus type 1 antibodies 2F5 and 2G12. *J. Virol.* 77, 4095–4103.

Wold, A., Mestecky, J., Tomana, M., Kobata, A., Ohbayashi, H., Endo, T., and Svanborg Eden, C. (1990). Secretory immunoglobulin A carries oligosaccharide receptors for *Escherichia coli* type 1 fimbrial lectin. *Infect. Immun.* 58, 3073–3077.

Wold, A.E., Motas, C., Svanborg, C., and Mestecky, J. (1994). Lectin receptors on IgA isotypes. *Scand. J. Immunol.* 39, 195–201.

Wolf, H.M., Fischer, M.B., Puhringer, H., Samstag, A., Vogel, E., and Eibl, M.M. (1994). Human serum IgA downregulates the release of inflammatory cytokines (tumor necrosis factor-α, interleukin-6) in human monocytes. *Blood* 83, 1278–1288.

Wolf, H.M., Hauber, I., Gulle, H., Samstag, A., Fischer, M.B., Ahmad, R.U., and Eibl, M.M. (1996). Anti-inflammatory properties of human serum IgA: induction of IL-1 receptor antagonist and FcαR (CD89)-mediated down regulation of tumor necrosis factor-alpha (TNF-α) and IL-6 in human monocytes. *Clin. Exp. Immunol.* 105, 537–543.

Yan, H.M., Lamm, M.E., Björling, E., and Huang, Y.T. (2002). Multiple functions of immunoglobulin A in mucosal defense against viruses: an *in vitro* measles virus model. *J. Virol.* 76, 10972–10979.

Yang, P.C., Berin, M.C., and Perdue, M.H. (1999). Enhanced antigen transport across rat tracheal epithelium induced by sensitization and mast cell activation. *J. Immunol.* 163, 2769–2776.

Yuan, Z.N., Gjermo, P., Helgeland, K., and Schenk, K. (2000). Fcα receptor I (CD89) on neutrophils in periodontal lesions. *J. Clin. Periodontol.* 27, 489–493.

Zhang, W., and Lachmann, P. J. (1994). Glycosylation of IgA is required for optimal activation of the alternative complement pathway by immune complexes. *Immunology* 81, 137–141.

Zhaori, G., Sun, M., Faden, H.S., and Ogra, P.L. (1989). Nasopharyngeal secretory antibody response to poliovirus type 3 virion proteins exhibit different specificities after immunization with live or inactivated poliovirus vaccines. *J. Infect. Dis.* 159, 1018–1024.

Microbial Evasion of IgA Functions

Chapter
15

Mogens Kilian

Department of Medical Microbiology and Immunology, University of Aarhus, Aarhus, Denmark

Michael W. Russell

Department of Microbiology and Immunology, and of Oral Biology, University at Buffalo, Buffalo, New york

One of the common themes of host–parasite relationships is that microorganisms that are successfully associated with their respective host, either as pathogens or as commensals, possess properties that allow them to evade host immune factors. At mucosal surfaces evasion of both innate and adaptive immune factors is necessary for successful colonization. This chapter focuses on microbial strategies specifically related to evasion of IgA functions, in particular in humans. The most convincing evidence in this context relates to bacterial IgA1 proteases, which have evolved independently in several mucosal pathogens and members of the commensal microbiota of the human respiratory tract, presumably with the primary purpose of evading functions of human IgA1. Other strategies employed to evade adaptive immunity in general may also apply to IgA antibodies in secretions and in the circulation. These more general evasion mechanisms include variation and diversity of surface antigens, as well as masking of critical surface epitopes by chemical or structural modification, molecular mimicry, or absorption of host components. Several reviews have covered this subject in detail (Marrack and Kappler, 1994; Finlay and Falkow, 1997).

SPECIFIC IgA PROTEASES

The elongated hinge region in IgAl of humans, chimpanzees, gorillas, and orangutans (see Chapter 9) allows the Fab regions of this subclass greater conformational freedom relative to corresponding domains of other immunoglobulin isotypes. The ensuing theoretical ability of IgA1 antibodies to interact with a larger range of spatially diverse epitopes has been achieved at the expense of introducing an open stretch, which, like other interdomain areas of immunoglobulin molecules, is potentially more susceptible to proteolytic attack.

In the IgA1 hinge region this problem is counteracted by the unusual amino acid sequence combined with O-glycosylation of several serine and threonine residues (Mattu *et al.*, 1998) **(Fig. 15.1)**. As a result, the extended IgA1 hinge is not susceptible to cleavage by traditional proteolytic enzymes of host or microbial origin at physiological conditions. However, a number of important mucosal pathogens and selected members of the commensal microbiota of the human upper respiratory tract have developed unique proteases that allow them to cleave the IgA1 hinge region. In this way, the bacteria not only circumvent all the Fc-mediated functions of IgA1 antibodies described in Chapter 14 but, in addition, take advantage of the released Fab fragments. Besides their function in host–parasite relationships, the IgA1 proteases constitute important tools for generating defined fragments of IgA1, including its hinge region.

Comprehensive screenings of bacteria, fungi, parasites, and viruses have revealed that IgA1 proteases are produced by a limited number of bacterial species that successfully colonize or infect mucosal membranes of humans. It is particularly striking that IgA1 protease production is a characteristic of all three principal causes of bacterial meningitis, *Neisseria meningitidis*, *Haemophilus influenzae*, and *Streptococcus pneumoniae* (Plaut *et al.*, 1975; Kilian *et al.*, 1979; Male, 1979). Virtually all members of these three species produce IgA1 protease, including isolates from patients with respiratory tract and middle ear infections and healthy carriers. Other IgA1 protease–producing members of the genus *Haemophilus* are the eye-pathogenic *H. aegyptius* and *H. influenzae* biogroup aegyptius, both of which are closely related but not identical to *H. influenzae* (Kilian *et al.*, 2002), and *H. parahaemolyticus*, a species of undefined pathogenic potential (Male, 1979). *H. influenzae* biogroup aegyptius is the cause of a fulminant septicemic disease in children called Brazilian

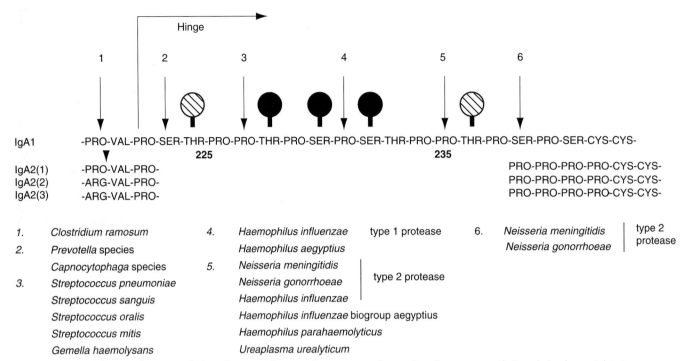

Fig. 15.1. Hinge region of IgA1 and the allotypes of IgA2. The arrows refer to the cleavage specificity of the bacterial IgA proteases. The *O*-glycosidically linked carbohydrate side chains in the IgA1 hinge region are according to results published for serum IgA1 by Mattu *et al.* (1998). The hatched circles denote side chains that are variably present.

purpuric fever (Brenner *et al.*, 1988). Two important uro-genital pathogens, *Neisseria gonorrhoeae* and *Ureaplasma urealyticum,* also produce IgA1 protease (Plaut *et al.*, 1975; Kilian *et al.*, 1984; Robertson *et al.*, 1984). However, IgA1 protease activity is not restricted to pathogenic bacteria but is present in several dominant members of the commensal microbiota of the oral cavity and pharynx, i.e., *Streptococcus sanguis, Streptococcus mitis, Streptococcus oralis,* and *Gemella haemolysans* (Plaut *et al.*, 1974a; Kilian and Holmgren, 1981; Lomholt and Kilian, 2001). Likewise, all species of *Capnocytophaga* and *Prevotella* associated with humans have IgA1 protease activity (Kilian, 1981; Frandsen *et al.*, 1986). These bacteria have their primary habitat in the human oral cavity, primarily in dental plaques, and it has been suggested that some of the *Prevotella* species potentially are implicated in the pathogenesis of periodontal diseases.

Among the highly specific bacterial proteases that cleave human IgA, an enzyme produced by *Clostridium ramosum* is unique in being able to cleave both IgA1 and the A2m(1) allotype of IgA2 (Fujiyama *et al.*, 1985; Senda *et al.*, 1985). *C. ramosum* is a regular inhabitant of the human gut.

IgA protease activity is a stable characteristic of all members of the mentioned species. The only exceptions are *S. mitis,* in which IgA1 protease activity and the corresponding gene may or may not be present (Reinholdt *et al.*, 1990; Poulsen *et al.*, 1998), and *C. ramosum,* of which only <3% of examined isolates from human feces produce the protease; in contrast to original expectations, no association with inflammatory bowel disease has been observed (Senda *et al.*, 1985).

Enzymatic properties of IgA proteases

The IgA1 proteases constitute an enzymatically diverse but functionally identical group of proteolytic enzymes that are unique in several respects. They belong to the very rare examples of postproline endopeptidases and, in most cases, attack a peptide bond immediately adjacent to a carbohydrate side chain. Each IgA1 protease cleaves one of several prolyl–seryl or prolyl–threonyl peptide bonds present within the hinge region of human IgA1 but lacking in human IgA2 (Fig. 15.1) (Plaut *et al.*, 1974b, 1975; Kilian *et al.*, 1980, 1983a; Mulks *et al.*, 1980a, 1982; Mortensen and Kilian, 1984; Spooner *et al.*, 1992). Recent studies using recombinant IgA1 molecules with various mutations in the hinge revealed remarkable differences in the amino acid sequence requirements of streptococcal IgA1 proteases. Particularly, the *S. pneumoniae* IgA1 protease seems to lack an absolute requirement for either proline or threonine at residues 227 and 228 (Batten *et al.*, 2003).

Attempts to sequentially cleave the IgA1 hinge with enzymes attacking different sites (Fig. 15.1) show that efficient cleavage occurs only when the target sequence is associated with the Fc part of the heavy chain (Lomholt et al, 1995), suggesting that structural properties, including glycosylation of the substrate (Reinholdt *et al.*, 1990), are important. However, decapeptides identical to the relevant hinge sequence may be cleaved by serine-type IgA1 protease at a significantly lower catalytic efficiency (10%) (Wood and Burton, 1991). Studies using various hybrids of IgA as substrate show that most but not all IgA1 proteases will cleave a postproline peptide bond in one-half of the IgA1 hinge, even when seen in the context of the IgA2 Fc (Senior *et al.*, 2000).

The IgA protease of *C. ramosum* cleaves the prolyl–valyl bond just before the hinge within a sequence shared by IgA1 and the A2m(1) allotype (Fig. 15.1) (Fujiyama *et al.*, 1985, 1986). This peptide bond is lacking in the A2m(2) allotype and in an additional variant of IgA2 that may constitute a third allotype (Chintalacharuvu *et al.*, 1994). The protease also cleaves the identically located Arg-Val bond in gorilla IgA1, showing that proline is not a strict substrate requirement of this protease (Qui *et al.*, 1996).

Cleavage of IgA by IgA1 proteases or by the IgA protease of *C. ramosum* results in the release of intact monomeric Fab fragments that retain antigen-binding activity (Mallett *et al.*, 1984; Mansa and Kilian, 1986; Tyler and Cole, 1998) and Fc fragments, or Fc$_2$-secretory component (SC) fragments when S-IgA is cleaved. SC of S-IgA1 molecules confers no resistance to cleavage by IgA1 protease (Kilian *et al.*, 1980), but purified S-IgA is often relatively resistant because of the presence of neutralizing antibodies against IgA proteases (see later in this chapter).

All IgA1 proteases examined in detail are constitutively expressed. The serine-type IgA1 proteases of *N. gonorrhoeae*, *N. meningitidis*, and *H. influenzae* are synthesized as an ~170-kDa precursor, which includes a pore-forming autosecretion system, and eventually undergoes autoproteolysis at three sites (Pohlner *et al.*, 1987; Poulsen *et al.*, 1989; Lomholt *et al.*, 1995; Veiga *et al.*, 2002). The secreted, mature IgA1 protease of these bacteria has a size of 100 kDa. The IgA1 protease of the *Streptococcus* species is close to 200 kDa. These are unusually large sizes for proteases.

Phylogeny of IgA1 proteases

Although the IgA1 proteases display virtually identical enzymatic activity, they do so by at least three different catalytic mechanisms. Some of the IgA1 proteases are serine-type proteases, others are metalloproteinases, and yet others are

thiol (cysteine) proteinases **(Fig. 15.2)**. As a result of detailed characterization of most of the IgA1 proteases shown in Figure 15.1, at gene or enzyme levels, one may conclude that IgA1 protease activity is a consequence of at least five independent lines of evolutionary events (Fig. 15.2) (Koomey *et al.*, 1982; Bricker *et al.*, 1983; Koomey and Falkow, 1984; Mortensen and Kilian, 1984; Frandsen *et al.*, 1987; Gilbert *et al.*, 1988, 1991; Poulsen *et al.*, 1988, 1996; Bachovchin *et al.*, 1990; Spooner *et al.*, 1992; Lomholt *et al.*, 1995; Wani *et al.*, 1996; Kosowska *et al.*, 2002). Thus, the IgA proteases are a striking example of convergent evolution of a highly specialized enzymatic activity, which by itself provides strong evidence of their biological significance. The relationships illustrated in Figure 15.2 reflect gene homologies (for reviews, see Lomholt, 1996, and Poulsen *et al.*, 1998).

The serine type IgA1 proteases are the prototypes (Pohlner *et al.*, 1987) of a growing family of IgA1 protease–like, autotransporter proteins in gram-negative bacteria. Other members of this family include the Hap protein in *H. influenzae* and proteins in a variety of gram-negative bacteria. Among these proteins the IgA1 protease (Poulsen *et al.*, 1989; Bachovchin *et al.*, 1990), the Hap surface protein of *H. influenzae* (St. Geme *et al.*, 1994) and the corresponding protein of *N. meningitidis* (van Ulsen *et al.*, 2001), the Sep A protein of *Shigella flexneri* (Benjjelloun-Touimi *et al.*, 1995), the Ssp protein of *Serratia marcescens* (Yanagida *et al.*, 1986), the Tsh protein of avian-pathogenic *Escherichia coli* (Provence and Curtiss, 1994), and the EspC and EspP proteins of enteropathogenic and enterohemorrhagic *E. coli* (Stein *et al.*, 1996; Brunder *et al.*, 1997) have putative serine protease motifs, which in some of the proteins is crucial for autoproteolytic cleavage (Pohlner *et al.*, 1987; Hendrixon *et al.*, 1997; Yanagida *et al.*, 1986). However, only the IgA1 proteases are capable of cleaving human IgA1.

Also, the IgA1 protease of *S. pneumoniae* is one of several proteins encoded by genes that have arisen by gene duplication. Thus, screening of the available genome sequences of

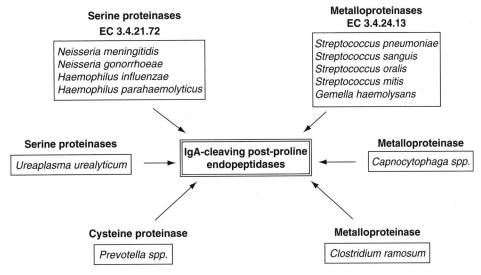

Fig. 15.2. Evolutionary relationships of bacterial IgA1 proteases.

several strains of *S. pneumoniae* reveals up to three genes with a high degree of homology to the IgA1 protease (*iga*) gene. In some databases and publications, these genes have been termed *iga* 1, 2, 3, but there is no indication that the additional genes encode proteases with IgA1-cleaving activity. Thus, inactivation of the *iga* gene that was identified by cloning in *E. coli* results in loss of IgA1 protease activity (Poulsen, K., unpublished observations).

in vivo activity

The substrate specificity of IgA1 proteases is in complete agreement with the predominance of that subclass in the normal habitat of IgA1 protease–producing bacteria and with regard to subclass distribution of specific antibodies against relevant surface antigens such as bacterial polysaccharide capsules (Barington *et al.*, 1994; Delacroix *et al.*, 1982; Crago *et al.*, 1984; Brown and Mestecky, 1985; Kett *et al.*, 1986; Mestecky and Russell, 1986). The same applies to the IgA protease of *C. ramosum*, which, in its normal habitat (the human gut), is exposed to an even distribution of the two subclasses. One exception is *N. gonorrhoeae*, which in its primary habitat encounters IgA1 and IgA2 in approximately equal proportions. A likely explanation to this seeming lack of optimal adaptation is that the common ancestor of meningococci and gonococci belonged in the upper respiratory tract and that the selection pressure on gonococci for further adaptation has been limited because of an abundance of other immune escape mechanisms employed by this species (Meyer, 1990).

Physiological protease inhibitors such as α2-macroglobulin and α1-protease inhibitor do not affect IgA1 proteases. Resistance to β_2-macroglobulin can be explained by the exquisite substrate specificity of IgA1 proteases, which precludes activation by cleavage of the bait region of the inhibitor. Accordingly, there is evidence that IgA1 proteases are active *in vivo*. Thus, characteristic intact cleavage fragments of S-IgA1 can be detected in nasopharyngeal, oral, and intestinal secretions of subjects colonized or infected with IgA1 protease–producing bacteria at the respective sites of the body (Mehta *et al.*, 1973; Kilian, 1981; Sørensen and Kilian, 1984; Ahl and Reinholdt, 1991). Extensive cleavage of S-IgA1 was demonstrated in a study of secretions collecting in the nasal cavity of children (<5 years of age) during surgical anesthesia. Characteristic Fab and Fc_2-SC fragments were detected in 18 of 97 children (18.6%), with a significantly increased prevalence in children with a history of atopic diseases (61.5% versus 11.9%; $P < 0.001$) (Sørensen and Kilian, 1984). A longitudinal follow-up study of the nasopharyngeal microbiota in infants developing atopic diseases compared with that in healthy infants revealed that the former were indeed colonized with higher proportions of IgA1 protease–producing bacteria, the most significant of which, surprisingly, was *S. mitis* 1 (Kilian *et al.*, 1995).

In vivo release of IgA1 protease is also evident from the enzyme activity that may be detected in the cerebrospinal fluid of patients with bacterial meningitis caused by *H.*

influenzae type b (Insel *et al.*, 1982) and in vaginal secretions of women with gonococcal infection (Blake *et al.*, 1979). Indirect evidence of *in vivo* cleavage of IgA1 induced by the oral *Prevotella* and *Capnocytophaga* species has been obtained by detection of serum antibodies to a neoepitope exposed on Fabα fragments released from IgA1 upon cleavage with these proteases (Frandsen *et al.*, 1995).

More recent studies of vaginal secretions of women with gonococcal infection failed to demonstrate IgA1 cleavage fragments, although addition of IgA1 protease did result in cleavage *in vitro* (Hedges *et al.*, 1998). Likewise, no detectable cleavage of IgA1 was evident in nasal washes of two adults who carried IgA1 protease–producing *S. mitis* in the absence of detectable inhibitory antibodies (Kirkeby *et al.*, 2000). Thus, it is possible that the extensive cleavage of IgA1 detected in nasopharyngeal secretions from anesthetized children (Sørensen and Kilian, 1984) was a result of prolonged exposure of the secreted IgA to IgA1 proteases due to the anesthesia and that cleavage of S-IgA1 under normal conditions is restricted to the microenvironment of the actual IgA1 protease–producing bacteria.

The extent of IgA1 cleavage conceivably depends on several factors associated with the bacteria as well as the host. When carried by healthy individuals, potential pathogens such as *H. influenzae*, *N. meningitidis*, and *S. pneumoniae* constitute a minor part of the microbiota in the respiratory tract, and the resulting release of IgA1 protease is consequently limited. However, in subjects who develop local or invasive infection, these bacteria become predominant and may release substantial amounts of IgA1 protease. In this context, it is important also that there are significant interspecies and intraspecies differences in the amount of IgA1 protease released by bacteria (Simpson *et al.*, 1988; Reinholdt and Kilian, 1997). Although there is no overall relationship between invasive potential at the species level and the amount of protease released, meningococci generally show levels of activity that may be several hundred times higher than that of some of the oral streptococci. However, significant variations may also be seen among strains of *S. mitis*, and some strains show activity comparable to that of strains of *S. pneumoniae* (Reinholdt and Kilian, 1997). An interesting finding in recent examinations of comprehensive collections of *N. meningitidis* and *H. influenzae* is that disease-associated strains tend to produce more IgA1 protease than isolates from healthy individuals (Vitovski *et al.*, 1999, 2002). Also relevant to the extent of IgA1 cleavage detectable in the secretion is that the majority of IgA1 protease produced by streptococci remains associated with the cell wall (Poulsen *et al.*, 1996; Wani *et al.*, 1996; Reinholdt and Kilian, 1997) and therefore is less likely to affect the integrity of IgA1 remote from the bacteria. Finally, as discussed subsequently, the possible presence of enzyme-neutralizing antibodies is an important factor.

Biological consequences of IgA1 protease activity

By cleaving a peptide bond in the IgA hinge region, IgA proteases separate the Fc part from monomeric antigen-binding fragments. Consequently, the proteases are capable of interfering with the cross-linking activity as well as all Fc-mediated secondary effector functions of IgA antibodies (see Chapter 14). Several *in vitro* studies have supported this conclusion and have elucidated the various mechanisms by which protease-producing bacteria may benefit from this activity *in vivo*.

Loss of antibody-mediated agglutination is undoubtedly a functionally significant consequence of IgA protease activity, as several *in vivo* studies have demonstrated that cross-linking is important for the antibody-mediated prevention of bacterial colonization of mucosal membranes and tooth surfaces (Steele *et al.*, 1975; Ma *et al.*, 1990). *In vitro* studies involving gonococci and oral streptococci revealed that IgA1 protease activity is able to reverse the inhibitory effect of S-IgA on adherence of these bacteria, or purified bacterial adhesins, to epithelial cells and saliva-coated hydroxyapatite, respectively (Mulks *et al.*, 1980b; Reinholdt and Kilian, 1987; Hajishengallis *et al.*, 1992; Tyler and Cole, 1998). Although the bacteria become coated with Fabα fragments as a result of IgA1 protease activity, this does not interfere with their ability to adhere to the target surface. Further studies are required to explain this phenomenon. It is possible that the hydrophobic nature of Fabα fragments *per se* facilitates association with the respective surface. This hypothesis is supported by the recent interesting demonstration that encapsulated *S. pneumoniae*, which normally does not adhere to epithelial cells because of the hydrophilic surface, adheres well in the presence of capsule-specific IgA1 antibodies and that this enhancement is dependent on IgA1 protease activity (Weiser *et al.*, 2003).

Longitudinal studies of noncapsulate *H. influenzae* in the pharynxes of healthy children have provided further support for the hypothesis that an active IgA1 protease is important for the successful colonization of these bacteria. Thus, successive clones of *H. influenzae* colonizing an individual produce antigenically different IgA1 proteases that are not inhibited by antibodies induced by previously colonizing clones (Lomholt *et al.*, 1993). Likewise, the fact that 80% to 90% of the streptococci that initiate the colonization of tooth enamel after cleaning produce IgA1 protease (Nyvad and Kilian, 1990) indirectly suggests that this property is important for their ability to colonize in the presence of specific IgA antibodies in saliva. This property may be particularly important early in life, when the oral microbiota becomes established under the influence of S-IgA antibodies in mother's milk (Cole *et al.*, 1994). Studies involving selectively IgA-deficient adults have suggested that IgA1 proteases of oral streptococci have limited significance later in life. The colonization pattern of tooth surfaces in adults shows no difference between normal and selectively IgA-deficient adults who compensate with S-IgM in saliva, despite the possibility that IgA1 protease–producing streptococci may have lost their selective advantage in the latter group (Reinholdt *et al.*, 1993). Further studies are required to understand fully the relationship between members of the resident microbiota and mucosal S-IgA antibodies and the significance of IgA1 proteases in this balance.

As discussed in Chapter 14, interactions between mucus and immune complexes containing S-IgA conceivably contribute to the barrier function of mucous membranes. Although S-IgA diffuses freely through mucus, multiple S-IgA antibodies bound on the surface of microorganisms may mediate trapping and ensuing prevention of penetration of the surface (Biesbrock *et al.*, 1991; Saltzman *et al.*, 1994). Studies of this phenomenon performed with human sperm suggest that IgA1 proteases can interfere with this protective mechanism. Sperm coated with S-IgA antibodies are unable to penetrate a layer of cervical mucus, but the ability may be restored by selective removal of the Fcα_2-SC moieties by IgA1 protease treatment (Bronson *et al.*, 1987; Kutteh *et al.*, 1994). If these results can be extrapolated to the relationship between IgA1 protease–producing bacteria and mucus, it may explain, in part, the ability of some of these bacteria to penetrate the superficial parts of the mucosal barrier.

In the event of successful penetration, loss of the Fcα portion of IgA1 antibodies bound to the surface of the pathogen will preclude all antigen-elimination mechanisms associated with this immunoglobulin isotype (see Chapter 14). At the same time, Fabα fragments coating the bacterial surface will conceivably block access of intact antibodies of other isotypes and may mask relevant epitopes for the immune system. *In vitro* studies indicate that surface-bound Fabα fragments can interfere with complement activation and complement-mediated lysis in the presence of IgM and IgG antibodies (Russell *et al.*, 1989; Jarvis and Griffiss, 1991).

Two studies have attempted to elucidate the biological significance of IgA1 proteases in human organ culture models. Isogenic strains of *N. gonorrhoeae* and *H. influenzae* with or without IgA1 protease activity (as a result of gene deletion) were used to infect human fallopian tube and nasopharyngeal organ cultures. No differences in the ability to attach to or penetrate the mucosal tissues were observed (Cooper *et al.*, 1984; Farley *et al.*, 1986). Although these studies indicate that cleavage of other potential substrates of IgA1 proteases may not be important for infection, they do not elucidate any effect related to IgA, as the models lacked specific IgA1 antibodies. The same reservation applies to the observation that an *N. gonorrhoeae* IgA1 protease mutant has unaltered infectious potential in the human challenge model of urethral infection (Johannsen *et al.*, 1999). Furthermore, as discussed previously in this section, it is possible that the IgA1-cleaving activity has become obsolete in the gonococcus.

Neutralizing antibodies against IgA1 proteases

Like other bacterial virulence factors, IgA1 proteases induce antibodies, some of which have enzyme-neutralizing activity. Such antibodies can be experimentally induced in rabbits or other animals injected with protease preparations and may be detected in sera and secretions of humans colonized or infected by IgA1 protease–producing bacteria (Gilbert *et al.*, 1983; Kilian *et al.*, 1983b; Brooks *et al.*, 1992; Devenyi *et al.*, 1993; Reinholdt and Kilian, 1995). In general, human milk contains neutralizing antibodies to bacterial IgA1 proteases, with the consequence that S-IgA1 purified from human colostrum is resistant to most IgA1 proteases unless they are added in excessive amounts (Kobayashi *et al.*, 1987).

Studies of the antibody response to the IgA1 protease of *N. meningitidis* group A have shown that IgA1 proteases are strongly immunogenic and that serum antibodies to the protease are more long-lasting than antibodies to the capsular polysaccharide. Furthermore, the same level of serum antibodies develops in healthy carriers and infected subjects (Brooks *et al.*, 1992; Thiesen *et al.*, 1997). Besides inhibiting IgA1 protease activity, neutralizing antibodies block the release of the enzyme from *H. influenzae*, meningococci, and gonococci, by inhibition of the autocatalytic cleavage responsible for this process (Pohlner *et al.*, 1987). As a result, antibodies against IgA1 proteases may agglutinate the bacteria through interaction with the surface-bound protease, which constitutes a novel surface antigen (Plaut *et al.*, 1992).

Specific T-cell responses in humans to *Neisseria* IgA1 proteases have also been detected (Tsirpouchtsidis *et al.*, 2002).

Antigenic diversity of IgA1 proteases

Comprehensive serological examinations of IgA1 proteases produced by members of species listed in Figure 15.1 have disclosed a remarkable antigenic diversity, most notably among *H. influenzae* and *S. pneumoniae* IgA1 proteases (Kilian *et al.*, 1983a; Lomholt *et al.*, 1992; Lomholt and Kilian, 1994; Lomholt, 1995). Thus, more than 30 antigenic variants ("inhibition types") of *H. influenzae* IgA1 proteases have been found (Kilian *et al.*, 1983a; Lomholt *et al.*, 1993). IgA1 proteases of the two pathogenic *Neisseria* species show less diversity detectable with neutralizing antisera and share the same protease "inhibition types" in agreement with their close genetic relationship (Lomholt *et al.*, 1992; Lomholt and Kilian, 1995). Sequence analyses of the IgA1 protease genes (*iga*) in *H. influenzae* and the two pathogenic *Neisseria* species reveal that the antigenic diversity is generated by recombination between and within these species and affecting particular regions of the gene (Halter *et al.*, 1989; Poulsen *et al.*, 1992; Morelli *et al.*, 1994; Lomholt *et al.*, 1995). It is conceivable that this antigenic diversity increases the immune escape potential of IgA1 proteases.

IgA1 proteases of most of the commensal oral bacteria (i.e., *S. sanguis*, *S. oralis*, *Prevotella*, and *Capnocytophaga* species), in comparison, show a remarkable lack of antigenic diversity (Frandsen *et al.*, 1987; Reinholdt *et al.*, 1987), paralleled by a general paucity of neutralizing antibody activity in secretions and sera against IgA1 proteases of these bacteria (Gilbert *et al.*, 1983; Reinholdt and Kilian, 1995; Frandsen *et al.*, 1997). The apparent lack of antibody response to the IgA protease of *C. ramosum* (Kobayashi *et al.*, 1987) may be another example of a more subtle relationship between commensal bacteria and their host. High titers of neutralizing salivary antibodies against IgA1 proteases of viridans streptococci observed in occasional subjects (Reinholdt and Kilian, 1995) may have been induced by pneumococci with antigenically related IgA1 proteases (Lomholt and Kilian, 1994). Likewise, once viridans streptococci penetrate beyond the mucosal barrier and cause systemic infection, as in subacute bacterial endocarditis, high serum titers of neutralizing antibodies against the IgA1 protease of the bacteria develop (Reinholdt and Kilian, 1995).

IgA protease–producing bacteria take advantage of IgA antibodies

One enigma related to an understanding of the biological significance of IgA1 proteases concerns the relationship between cleavage-relevant IgA1 antibodies and IgA1 protease–neutralizing antibodies. Although there are no studies comparing the kinetics of antibody responses to surface epitopes of potential pathogens and to their IgA1 proteases, it is conceivable that they develop concurrently. Thus, once a human host has responded to an acquired IgA1 protease–producing bacterium with IgA1 antibodies, the cleavage of which would be beneficial to the bacterium, neutralizing antibodies against its IgA1 protease are likely to be present too. However, in this balance, the total amount of secreted IgA1 protease, as discussed above, is conceivably of paramount significance. The demonstrated coating of protease-producing bacteria with Fabα fragments is clear evidence that the balance between the different specificities of antibodies sometimes does allow relevant IgA1 antibodies to be cleaved *in vivo*.

IgA1 protease activity may have particular consequences if a potential pathogen colonizes a human host who already has IgA1 antibodies to surface epitopes of the bacteria but no antibodies to its IgA1 protease. This scenario constitutes the basis of a hypothetical model for invasive infections with IgA1 protease–producing bacteria (Kilian and Reinholdt, 1987).

The fact that the three principal causes of bacterial meningitis all produce an IgA1 protease is hardly a coincidence and suggests that the IgA1 protease is a virulence factor that plays a role in the pathogenesis of this particular invasive disease. According to the hypothesis, acquisition of *H. influenzae* serotype b, *N. meningitidis*, or *S. pneumoniae* and the subsequent temporary nasopharyngeal colonization, as it occurs in the majority of infants and children, results in the concurrent induction of S-IgA antibodies to surface antigens and the IgA1 protease of the bacteria. The protease-neutralizing antibodies prevent cleavage of IgA1 antibodies and, hence, coating of the pathogen with Fabα fragments. The concurrent induction of these antibodies results in immunity to invasive infection and subsequent attacks by bacteria expressing the same combination of capsular surface epitopes and IgA1 protease "inhibition type." By contrast, invasive infection in occasional individuals is a result of nonsynchronized induction of the two types of antibodies caused by successive encounters with two different microorganisms: first is colonization in the gut or upper respiratory tract with bacteria expressing surface epitopes similar or identical to those of the respective pathogen (e.g., *E. coli* K100 in the case of *H. influenzae* type b, and *E. coli* K1 or *Moraxella nonliquefaciens* in the case of *N. meningitidis* group B), and second is subsequent colonization with the actual pathogen. As a result of the prior colonization with a cross-reactive microorganism, the pathogen encounters preexisting IgA1 antibodies to its surface epitopes but no antibodies that will neutralize its IgA1 protease. This situation enables the pathogen to become coated with Fabα fragments, allowing adherence in spite of the hydrophilic capsule, masking of the surface for other components of the immune system, and prevention of complement activation and phagocytosis. As discussed elsewhere, this hypothetical model is in agreement with several hitherto-unexplained observations in both humans and animal models (Kilian and Reinholdt, 1987).

Host specificity of IgA protease–producing bacteria

Infections caused by *H. influenzae*, meningococci, and gonococci occur naturally only in humans but have been occasionally observed or experimentally induced in chimpanzees and gorillas (McClure, 1980). The exclusive susceptibility of IgA1 of these host species to the IgA1 proteases (Plaut *et al.*, 1974b; Plaut, 1978; Cole and Hale, 1991; Qui *et al.*, 1996) is conceivably part of the explanation of this clinical fact. As a consequence, this substrate specificity precludes studies of the biological significance of IgA1 proteases in traditional experimental animal models.

In attempts to identify potential animal models, numerous animal-specific pathogens have been examined for their ability to cleave IgA of their respective hosts. Early studies revealed that *Actinobacillus* (formerly *Haemophilus*) *pleuropneumoniae*, which causes fatal lower respiratory tract infections in pigs, induces extensive degradation of porcine IgA (Kilian *et al.*, 1979). This finding has been confirmed (Negrete-Abascal *et al.*, 1994), but the patterns of cleavage and hence the potential consequences are not similar to those observed with specific IgA1 proteases. By contrast, screening of a large number of animal pathogenic *Mycoplasma* and *Ureaplasma* species have identified a protease capable of inducing specific cleavage in the hinge region of canine IgA in *Ureaplasma* strains associated with infections in dogs (Kapatais-Zoumbos *et al.*, 1985). So far, this potential model has not been employed in studies of the biological significance of IgA proteases.

Alternative functions of IgA1 proteases

Search for protein sequences with similarity to the susceptible hinge region of IgA1 resulted in the demonstration of a number of potential alternative substrates of IgA1 proteases (Hauck and Meyer, 1997; Lin *et al.*, 1997; Senior *et al.*, 2001). Of particular interest is the finding that the lysosomal/phagosomal membrane protein Lamp1 is cleaved by the type 2 gonococcal IgA1 protease, thereby promoting intracellular survival of the bacteria (Hauck and Meyer, 1997; Lin *et al.*, 1997). The significance of this activity is further supported by the demonstration that *iga* mutants have a statistically significant and reproducible defect in their ability to traverse monolayers of polarized epithelial cells *in vitro* (Hopper *et al.*, 2000).

The unusual molecular size of the IgA1 proteases raises the question of whether the proteins have additional functions unrelated to the proteolytic activity. Indeed, recent studies demonstrated significant immunomodulatory properties of IgA1 protease, some of which are unrelated to the protease activity. Thus, native gonococcal type 2 IgA1 protease, but not denatured protein, induces release of proin-flammatory cytokines such as TNF-α, IL-1β, IL-6, and IL-8 from peripheral blood mononuclear cells (Lorenzen *et al.*, 1999). Furthermore, the same protease is capable of inhibiting TNF-α-mediated apoptosis of the human myelomonocytic cell line, an effect conceivably related to the concurrent cleavage by the protease of TNF-α receptor II (Beck and Meyer, 2000).

The concept that IgA1 proteases play a role in infections, in addition to cleaving IgA1, is suggested by the finding that inactivation of one *iga* gene in *S. pneumoniae* leads to significantly reduced virulence in a mouse infection model, despite the fact that the protease does not cleave murine IgA (Polissi *et al.*, 1998). However, it cannot be excluded that the mutations examined affected a paralogous "*iga*" gene and not the gene encoding the IgA1 protease (see discussion above).

Further studies are needed to fully elucidate the spectrum of potential substrates and other properties of IgA proteases. So far experiments have been performed exclusively with gonococcal type 2 IgA1 protease, and it is not clear if these findings apply to all IgA1 proteases.

OTHER MICROBIAL PROTEASES WITH IgA-CLEAVING ACTIVITY

Several microorganisms produce broad-spectrum proteases that can degrade immunoglobulins, complement factors, and many other proteins involved in the protection of the human body. Broad-spectrum proteases capable of cleaving immunoglobulins, including IgA, have been demonstrated in *Porphyromonas gingivalis*, *Pseudomonas aeruginosa*, *Proteus mirabilis*, *Pasteurella multocida*, *Serratia marcescens*, *Staphylococcus aureus*, *Streptococcus pyogenes*, *Candida albicans*, and the parasites *Entamoeba histolytica*, *Trichomonas vaginalis*, and *Paragonimus westermani*, among many others (Kilian *et al.*, 1983b; Rüchel, 1986; Quezada-Cavillo and Lopez-Revillo, 1987; Reinholdt *et al.*, 1987; Molla *et al.*, 1988; Pouedras *et al.*, 1992; Prokesová *et al.*, 1992; Kelsall and Ravdin, 1993; Provenzano and Alderete, 1995; Shin *et al.*, 2001; Collin and Olsen, 2001). However, to what extent these proteases are able to function in the presence of physiological protease inhibitors is not clear, although some are capable of degrading protease inhibitors too. The potential sites of cleavage in IgA have not always been determined but appear to lie outside the hinge region of IgA. Few such enzymes have been characterized, and in some cases their wide activity spectrum may be due to several enzymes working in concert. This is probably the case with the putative periodontal pathogen *Porphyromonas gingivalis* (*Bacteroides asaccharolyticus*), which degrades IgA1 and IgA2 as well as other immunoglobulin isotypes and many other host proteins into small fragments (Kilian, 1981). *Pseudomonas aeruginosa*, a notable opportunistic pathogen that has significant hydrolytic activity, cleaves IgA, S-IgA, SC, and IgG. Among several proteases secreted by this bacterium, the elastase completely degrades the Fab fragment of IgA (Döring *et al.*, 1981; Heck *et al.*, 1990). Although such broad-spectrum activity may play a significant role in infectious diseases, the biological consequences of IgA cleavage are entirely different from those discussed previously in this section for IgA1 proteases.

Of potential importance is the finding that some members of the family *Enterobacteriaceae* are capable of cleaving human IgA (Metha *et al.*, 1973; Milazzo and Delisle, 1984). This activity has been detected only in fresh isolates from human feces or from patients with urinary tract infections and is lost on subcultivation of the bacteria. Similar strains from culture collections have not disclosed IgA-cleaving activity, nor has it been possible to restore lost activity; hence, nothing is known about the specificity of the enzyme(s) involved. An exception is an IgA-cleaving protease from *Proteus mirabilis*, which is stable, has a pepsin-like activity on IgA, and cleaves initially between the CH2 and CH3 domains, whereas it cleaves IgG initially at either side of the hinge region (Loomes *et al.*, 1990; Senior *et al.*, 1991). Such proteases may be responsible for the fragmentation of IgA that can be demonstrated in extracts of human stools (Mehta *et al.*, 1973; Bouvet *et al.*, 1993). The cross-linking activity of fragments that include Fab may be retained or even enhanced by interaction with protein Fv secreted from the liver to the gut (Bouvet *et al.*, 1990, 1993).

GLYCOSIDASES

IgA and, in particular, S-IgA are heavily glycosylated with both N-linked and O-linked glycan chains (see Chapter 9), which may be attacked by bacterial glycosidases. As an example, *S. pneumoniae* and the oral streptococcal species *S. oralis* and *S. mitis* are capable of stripping IgA1 molecules of all their carbohydrate side chains (Kilian *et al.*, 1980; Reinholdt *et al.*, 1990). Other microorganisms selectively remove part of the oligosaccharide chains such as the terminal sialic acid residues (Reinholdt *et al.*, 1990; Frandsen, 1994).

The carbohydrates of IgA molecules are important for their conformation, net charge, and hydrophilicity and for their resistance to proteolytic enzymes (Tao and Morrison, 1989; Reinholdt *et al.*, 1990; Jefferis, 1993). Studies involving IgA as well as IgG have furthermore disclosed significant effects of carbohydrate depletion on antibody functions (Nose and Wigzell, 1983; Tao and Morrison, 1989; Jefferis, 1993; Nikolova *et al.*, 1994a; Chuang and Morrison 1997; Rifai *et al.*, 2000; Rudd *et al.*, 2001). Some of the carbohydrate-dependent functions of IgA molecules are discussed in Chapter 14. Thus, it is conceivable that bacteria-induced alterations of the glycosylation of IgA molecules can interfere with their antibody function. However, the *in vivo* significance of this hypothesis has not been examined.

IgA-BINDING PROTEINS

Several species of bacteria express proteins on their surface that bind to IgA molecules in an antibody-independent manner. The most extensively studied are those expressed by some pathogenic streptococci. Proteins Arp and Sir are members of the heterogeneous M-protein family of surface proteins of *Streptococcus pyogenes*, and β-protein (Bac) is an unrelated conserved protein expressed by strains of *Streptococcus agalactiae* (group B streptococci). These proteins bind to Fcα of both subclasses of IgA, including both serum IgA and S-IgA, and recognize sequences in the Cα2–Cα3 interdomain region (Pleass *et al.*, 2001). Although they share binding specificity, they are structurally and immunologically unrelated (Lindahl and Åkerström, 1989; Lindahl *et al.*, 1990; Hedén *et al.*, 1991; Jerlström *et al.*, 1991; Stenberg *et al.*, 1994). The IgA-binding domain of M proteins, present in approximately 50% of all *S. pyogenes* strains (Lindahl et al., 1990), has been identified as 29 amino acid residues. Lindahl and his group have demonstrated that a 50-residue synthetic peptide (Sap) that includes this sequence of 29 amino acids is an efficient tool for affinity purification of IgA and for specific detection of IgA bound in immune complexes (Sandin *et al.*, 2002).

By analogy with the IgG-binding protein A on *Staphylococcus aureus*, it is believed that the streptococcal IgA receptors serve an immune escape function at mucosal surfaces, but the precise mechanism of action is not yet known. The complexity of this biological phenomenon is emphasized by the fact that both proteins Arp and Sir, in addition, bind to the C4b-binding protein (C4BP), which is an inhibitor of the classical pathway C3 convertase C4bC2a (Thern *et al.*, 1995). The function of IgA-binding in this context, if any, is unknown. However, recent studies demonstrate that interaction of streptococcal proteins with IgA interferes with binding of the antibody with the Fcα receptor on phagocytic cells (CD89) (Pleass *et al.*, 2001).

Several species of *Enterobacteriaceae*, including *E. coli*, express type 1 fimbriae, which enable them to bind to mannose-containing carbohydrate structures on host cells. Type 1 fimbriae also bind to exposed mannose residues on incomplete N-linked carbohydrate side chains of IgA and especially of the IgA2 subclass (Wold *et al.*, 1990, 1994). Strains of the oral bacteria *Streptococcus gordonii* and *Actinomyces naeslundii* express a lectin that recognizes the O-linked carbohydrate side chains in the hinge region of IgA1 (Ruhl *et al.*, 1996). Both *Helicobacter pylori* and *S. pneumoniae* express surface proteins that bind S-IgA through the secretory component (Borén *et al.*, 1993; Hammerschmidt *et al.*, 1997). Studies of the binding specificities of *H. pylori* revealed that this gastric pathogen can interact with fucose residues on S-IgA molecules but not with serum IgA (Borén *et al.*, 1993). The surface proteins (SpsA and CbpA) of *S. pneumoniae* that interact with SC belong to the group of choline-binding proteins and are expressed by most strains (Hammerschmidt *et al.*, 1997; Zhang et al., 2000). This interaction may promote pneumococcal cell invasion *in vitro* (Zhang *et al.*, 2000), but as it depends upon a postulated retrograde p-IgR-mediated uptake from the luminal side as well as upon both the strain of *S. pneumoniae* and certain pIgR-expressing epithelial cell lines, its biological significance is questionable (Brock *et al.*, 2002).

It has been suggested that such lectin-mediated interactions with microorganisms represent antibody-independent (innate) protective abilities of IgA (Royle *et al.*, 2003). Thus, the interaction between type 1 fimbriae on *E. coli* and IgA results in agglutination of the bacteria and in inhibition of their attachment to colonic epithelial cells *in vitro* (Wold *et al.*, 1990). Likewise, the attachment of *H. pylori* to gastric surface mucus cells *in vitro* is inhibited by human colostral S-IgA. The inhibition is reduced when S-IgA is treated with α-L-fucosidase (Falk *et al.*, 1993). However, it is still an open question whether the interactions are beneficial to the host or to the bacteria. In support of the latter view is the observation that selectively IgA-deficient individuals show reduced carriage in the gut of *E. coli* that express type 1 fimbriae (Friman *et al.*, 1996) and that S-IgA in the acquired pellicle forming on tooth surfaces promotes attachment of some oral streptococci (Liljemark *et al.*, 1979; Kilian *et al.*, 1981).

CONCLUSIONS

Like most other immune factors, IgA is the target of several microbial evasion strategies. Among these, IgA1 proteases are unique in their specific ability to cleave human IgA1. By attacking a single peptide bond in the IgA1 hinge region, IgA1 proteases eliminate all secondary effector functions of IgA1 antibodies while enabling the bacteria to take advantage of the released monomeric antigen-binding fragments for colonization and evasion of other parts of the immune system. Several lines of direct and indirect evidence indicate that the activity of IgA1 proteases secreted by bacteria colonizing the upper respiratory tract may result in a local functional IgA1 deficiency that facilitates penetration or alternative processing of potential allergens. However, because of the lack of a satisfactory animal model, full appreciation of the biological significance of IgA1 proteases must await successful strategies to prevent their activity, for example, by active or passive immunization. Likewise, further studies are necessary to understand how bacterial IgA binding proteins and glycosidases that attack the carbohydrate moiety of IgA may interfere with its protective functions.

REFERENCES

Ahl, T., and Reinholdt, J. (1991). Detection of immunoglobulin A1 protease–induced Fab alpha fragments on dental plaque bacteria. *Infect. Immun.* 59, 563–569.

Bachovchin, W.W., Plaut, A.G., Flentke, G.R., Lynch, M., and Kettner, C.A. (1990). Inhibition of IgA1 proteinases from *Neisseria gonorrhoeae* and *Haemophilus influenzae* by peptide prolyl boronic acids. *J. Biol. Chem.* 265, 3738–3743.

Barington, T., Juul, L., Gyhrs, A., and Heilman, C. (1994). Heavy-chain isotype patterns of human antibody-secreting cells induced by *Haemophilus influenzae* type b conjugate vaccines in relation to age and preimmunity. *Infect. Immun.* 62, 3066–3074.

Batten, M.R., Senior, B.W., Kilian, M., and Woof, J.M. (2003). Amino acid sequence requirements in the hinge of human immunoglobulin A1 (IgA1) for cleavage by streptococcal IgA1 proteases. *Infect. Immun.* 71, 1462–1469.

Beck, S.C., and Meyer, T.F. (2000). IgA1 protease from *Neisseria gonorrhoeae* inhibits TNF alpha-mediated apoptosis of human monocytic cells. *FEBS Lett.* 472, 287–292.

Benjelloun-Touimi, Z., Sansonetti, P.J., and Parsot, C. (1995). SepA, the major extracellular protein of *Shigella flexneri*: autonomous secretion and involvement in tissue invasion. *Mol. Microbiol.* 62, 123–135.

Biesbrock, A.R., Reddy, M.S., and Levine, M.J. (1991). Interaction of a salivary mucin-secretory immunoglobulin A complex with mucosal pathogens. *Infect. Immun.* 59, 3492–3497.

Blake, M., Holmes, K.K., and Swanson, J. (1979). Studies on gonococcus infection. XVII. IgA1-cleaving protease in vaginal washings from women with gonorrhoea. *J. Infect. Dis.* 139, 89–92.

Borén, T., Falk, P., Roth, K.A., Larson, G., and Normark, S. (1993). Attachment of *Helicobacter pylori* to human gastric epithelium mediated by blood group antigens. *Science* 262, 1892–1895.

Bouvet, J.-P., Pirés, R., Iscaki, S., and Pillot, J. (1993). Nonimmune macromolecular complexes of Ig in human gut lumen. *J. Immunol.* 151, 2562–2571.

Bouvet, J.-P., Pires, R., Lunel-Fabiani, F., Crescenzo-Chaigne, B., Maillard, P., Valla, D., Opolon, P., and Pillot, J. (1990). Protein F: a novel F(ab)-binding factor, present in normal liver, and largely released in the digestive tract during hepatitis. *J. Immunol.* 145, 1176–1180.

Brenner, D.J., Mayer, L.W., Carlone, G.M., Harrison, L.H., Bibb, W.F., Brandileone, M.C., Sottnek, F.O., Irino, K., Reeves, M.W., Swenson, J.M., Birkness, K.A., Weyant, R.S., Berkley, S.F., Woods, T.C., Steigerwalt, A.G., Grimont, P.A.D., McKinney, R.M., Fleming, D.W., Gheesling, L.L., Cooksey, R.C., Arko, R.J., Broome, C.V., and the Brazilian Purpuric Fever Study Group. (1988). Biochemical, genetic, and epidemiologic characterization of *Haemophilus influenzae* biogroup aegyptius (*Haemophilus aegyptius*) strains associated with Brazilian purpuric fever. *J. Clin. Microbiol.* 1988, 26, 1524–1534.

Bricker, J., Mulks, M.H., Plaut, A.G., Moxon, E.R., and Wright, A. (1983). IgA1 proteases of *Haemophilus influenzae*: cloning and characterization in *Escherichia coli* K-12. *Proc. Natl. Acad. Sci. USA* 80, 2681–2685.

Brock, S.C., McGraw, P.A., Wright, P.F., and Crowe Jr., J.E. (2002). The human polymeric immunoglobulin receptor facilitates invasion of epithelial cells by Streptococcus pneumoniae in a strain-specific and cell type-specific manner. *Infect. Immun.* 70, 5091–5095.

Bronson, R.A., Cooper, G.W., Rosenfeld, D.L., Gilbert, J.V., and Plaut, A.G. (1987). The effect of an IgA1 protease on immunoglobulins bound to the sperm surface and sperm cervical mucus penetrating ability. *Fertil. Steril.* 47, 985–991.

Brooks, G.F. Lammel, C.J., Blake, M.S., Kusecek, B., and Achtman, M. (1992). Antibodies against IgA1 protease are stimulated both by clinical disease and asymptomatic carriage of serogroup A *Neisseria meningitidis*. *J. Infect. Dis.* 166, 1316–1321.

Brown, T.A., and Mestecky, J. (1985). Immunoglobulin A subclass distribution of naturally occurring salivary antibodies to microbial antigens. *Infect. Immun.* 49, 459–462.

Brunder, W., Schmidt, H., and Karch, H. (1997). EspP, a novel extracellular serine protease of enterohaemorrhagic *Escherichia coli* O157:H7 cleaves human coagulation factor V. *Mol. Microbiol.* 24, 767–778.

Chintalacharuvu, K.R., Raines, M., and Morrison, S.L. (1994). Divergence of human α-chain constant region gene sequences: a novel recombinant α2 gene. *J. Immunol.* 152, 5299–5304.

Chuang, P.D., and Morrison, S.L. (1997). Elimination of N-linked glycosylation sites from the human IgA1 constant region. *J. Immunol.* 158, 724–732.

Cole, M.F., Evans, M., Fitzsimmons, S., Johnson, J., Pearce, C., Sheridan, M.J., Wientzen, R., and Bowden, G. (1994). Pioneer oral streptococci produce immunoglobulin A1 protease. *Infect. Immun.* 62, 2165–2168.

Cole, M.F., and Hale, C.A. (1991). Cleavage of chimpanzee, secretory immunoglobulin A by *Haemophilus influenzae* IgA1 protease. *Microb. Pathog.* 11, 39–46.

Collin, M., and Olsen, A. (2001). Effect of SpeB and EndoS from *Streptococcus pyogenes* on human immunoglobulins. *Infect. Immun.* 69, 7187–7189.

Cooper, M.D., McGee, Z.A., Mulks, M.H., Koomey, J.M., and Hindman, T.L. (1984). Attachment to and invasion of human fallopian tube mucosa by an IgA1 protease–deficient mutant of *Neisseria gonorrhoeae* and its wild-type parent. *J. Infect. Dis.* 150, 737–744.

Crago, S.S., Kutteh, W.H., Moro, I., Allansmith, M.R., Radl, J., Haaijman, J.J., and Mestecky, J. (1984). Distribution of IgA1-, IgA2- and J chain-containing cells in human tissues. *J. Immunol.* 132, 16–18.

Delacroix, D.L., Dive, C., Rambaud, J.C., and Vaerman, J.P. (1982). IgA subclasses in various secretions and in serum. *Immunology* 47, 383–385.

Devenyi, A.G., Plaut, A.G., Grundy, F.J., and Wright, A. (1993). Postinfectious human serum antibodies inhibit IgA1 proteinases by interaction with the cleavage site specificity determinant. *Mol. Immunol.* 30, 1243–1248.

Döring, G., Obernesser, H.J., and Botzenhart, K. (1981). Extracellular toxins of *Pseudomonas aeruginosa* II. Effect of two proteases on human immunoglobulin IgG, IgA and secretory IgA. *Zentralbl. Bakteriol.* 249, 89–98.

Falk, P, Roth, K.A., Borén, T., Westblom, T.U., Gordon, J.I., and Normark, S. (1993). An *in vitro* adherence assay reveals that *Helicobacter pylori* exhibits cell lineage-specific tropism in the human gastric epithelium. *Proc. Natl. Acad. Sci. USA* 90, 2035–2039.

Farley, M.M., Stephens, D.S., Mulks, M.H., Cooper, M.D., Bricker, J.V., Mirra, S.S., and Wright, A. (1986). Pathogenesis of IgA1 protease–producing and nonproducing *Haemophilus influenzae* in human naso-pharyngeal organ cultures. *J. Infect. Dis.* 154, 752–759.

Finlay, B.B., and Falkow, S. (1997). Common themes in microbial pathogenicity revisited. *Microbiol. Mol. Biol. Rev.* 61, 136–169.

Frandsen, E.V.G. (1994). Carbohydrate depletion of immunoglobulin A1 by oral species of gram-positive rods. *Oral Microbiol. Immunol.* 9, 352–358.

Frandsen, E.V.G., Kjeldsen, M., and Kilian, M. (1997). Inhibition of *Prevotella* and *Capnocytophaga* immunoglobulin A1 protease by human serum. *Clin. Diagn. Lab. Immunol.* 4, 458–464.

Frandsen, E.V.G., Reinholdt, J., and Kilian, M. (1987). Enzymatic and antigenic characterization of immunoglobulin A1 proteases from *Bacteroides* and *Capnocytophaga* spp. *Infect. Immun.* 55, 631–638.

Frandsen, E.V.G., Reinholdt, J., and Kilian, M. (1995). In vivo cleavage of immunoglobulin A1 by immunoglobulin A1 proteases from *Prevotella* and *Capnocytophaga* species. *Oral Microbiol. Immunol.* 10, 291–296.

Frandsen, E.V.G., Theilade, E., Ellegaard, B., and Kilian, M. (1986). Proportions and identity of IgA1-degrading bacteria in periodontal pockets from patients with juvenile and rapidly progressive periodontitis. *J. Periodont. Res.* 21, 613–623.

Friman, V., Adlerberth, I., Connell, H., Svanborg, C., Hanson, L.-A., and Wold, A.E. (1996). Decreased expression of mannose-specific adhesins by *Escherichia coli* in the colonic microflora of immunoglobulin A-deficient individuals. *Infect. Immun.* 64, 2794–2798.

Fujiyama, Y., Iwaki, M., Hodohara, K., Hosoda, S., and Kobayashi, K. (1986). The site of cleavage in human alpha chains of IgA1 and IgA2: A2m(1) allotype paraproteins by the clostridial IgA protease. *Mol. Immunol.* 23, 147–150.

Fujiyama, Y., Kobayashi, K., Senda, S., Benno, Y., Bamba, T., and Hosoda, S. (1985). A novel IgA protease from *Clostridium* sp. capable of cleaving IgA1 and IgA2 A2m(1) but not IgA2 A2m(2) allotype paraproteins. *J. Immunol.* 134, 573–576.

Gilbert, J.V., Plaut, A.G., Fishman, Y., and Wright, A. (1988). Cloning of the gene encoding streptococcal immunoglobulin A protease and its expression in *Escherichia coli*. *Infect. Immun.* 56, 1961–1966.

Gilbert, J.V., Plaut, A.G., and Wright, A. (1991). Analysis of the immunoglobulin A protease gene of *Streptococcus sanguis*. *Infect. Immun.* 59, 7–17.

Gilbert, J.V., Plaut, A.G., Longmaid, B., and Lamm, M.E. (1983). Inhibition of microbial IgA proteases by human secretory IgA and serum. *Mol. Immunol.* 20, 1039–1049.

Hajishengallis, G., Nikolova, E., and Russell, M.W. (1992). Inhibition of *Streptococcus mutans* adherence to saliva-coated hydroxyapatite by human secretory immunoglobulin A (S-IgA) antibodies to cell surface protein antigen I/II: reversal by IgA1 protease cleavage. *Infect. Immun.* 60, 5057–5064.

Halter, R., Pohlner, J., and Meyer, T.F. (1989). Mosaic-like organization of IgA protease genes in *Neisseria gonorrhoeae* generated by horizontal genetic exchange in vivo. *EMBO J.* 8, 2737–2744.

Hammerschmidt, S., Talay, S.R., Brandtzaeg, P., and Chhatwal, G.S. (1997). SpsA, a novel pneumococcal surface protein with specific binding to secretory immunoglobulin A and secretory component. *Mol. Microbiol.* 25, 1113–1124.

Hauck, C.R., and Meyer, T.F. (1997). The lysosomal/phagosomal membrane protein h-lamp-1 is a target of the IgA1 protease of *Neisseria gonorrhoeae*. *FEBS Lett.* 405, 86–90.

Heck, L.W., Alarcon, P.O., Kulhavy, R.M., Morihara, K., Russell, M.W., and Mestecky, J.F. (1990). Degradation of IgA proteins by *Pseudomonas aeruginosa* elastase. *J. Immunol.* 144, 2253–2257.

Hedén, L.O. Frithz, E., and Lindahl, G. (1991). Molecular characterization of an IgA receptor from group B streptococci: sequence of the gene, identification of a proline-rich region with unique structure and isolation of N-terminal fragments with IgA-binding capacity. *Eur. J. Immunol.* 21, 1481–1490.

Hedges, S.R., Mayo, M.S., Kallman, L., Mestecky, J., Hook, E.W. 3rd, and Russell, M.W. (1998). Evaluation of immunoglobulin A1 (IgA1) protease and IgA1 protease–inhibitory activity in human female genital infection with *Neisseria gonorrhoeae*. *Infect. Immun.* 66, 5826–5832.

Hendrixson, D.R., de la Morena, M.L., Stathopoulos, C., and St. Geme, III, J.W. (1997) Structural determinants of processing and secretion of *Haemophilus influenzae* Hap protein. *Mol. Microbiol.* 26, 505–518.

Hopper, S., Vasquez, B., Merz, A., Clary, S., Wilbur, J.S., and So, M. (2000). Effects of the immunoglobulin A1 protease on *Neisseria gonorrhoeae* trafficking across polarized T84 epithelial monolayers. *Infect. Immun.* 68, 906–911.

Insel, R.A., Alien, P.Z., and Berkoitz, I.D. (1982). Types and frequency of *Haemophilus influenzae* IgA1 proteases. In *Seminars in Infectious Disease. Vol. IV: Bacterial Vaccines* (eds. J. B. Robbins, J. C. Hill, and J. C. Sadoff), 225–231. New York: Thieme-Stratton.

Jarvis, G.A., and Griffiss, J.M. (1991). Human IgA1 blockade of IgG-initiated lysis of *Neisseria meningitidis* is a function of antigen-binding fragment binding to the polysaccharide capsule. *J. Immunol.* 147, 1962–1967.

Jefferis, R. (1993). The glycosylation of antibody molecules: functional significance. *Glycoconj. J.* 10, 358–361.

Jerlström, P.G., Chhatwal, G.S., and Timmis, K.N. (1991). The IgA-binding beta-antigen of the c protein complex of group B streptococci: sequence determination of its gene and detection of two binding regions. *Mol. Microbiol.* 5, 843–849.

Johannsen, D.B., Johnston, D.M/, Koymen, H.O., Cohen, M.S., and Cannon, J.G. (1999). A *Neisseria gonorrhoeae* immunoglobulin A1 protease mutant is infectious in the human challenge model of urethral infection. *Infect. Immun.* 67, 3009–3013.

Jose, J., Wolk, U., Lorenzen, D., Wenschuh, H., and Meyer, T.F. (2000). Human T-cell response to meningococcal immunoglobulin A1 protease associated alpha-proteins. *Scand. J. Immunol.* 51, 176–185.

Kapatais-Zoumbos, K., Chandler, D.K., and Barile, M.F. (1985). Survey of immunoglobulin A protease activity among selected species of *Ureaplasma* and *Mycoplasma* specificity for host immunoglobulin A. *Infect. Immun.* 47, 704–709.

Kelsall, N.L., and Ravdin, J.I. (1993). Degradation of human IgA by *Entamoeba histolytica*. *J. Infect. Dis.* 168, 1319–1322.

Kett, K., Brandtzaeg, P., Radl, J., and Haaijman, J.T. (1986). Different subclass distribution of IgA-producing cells in human lymphoid organs and various secretory tissues. *J. Immunol.* 136, 3631–3635.

Kilian, M. (1981). Degradation of immunoglobulins A1, A2, and G by suspected principal periodontal pathogens. *Infect. Immun.* 34, 757–765.

Kilian, M., Brown, M.B., Brown, T.A., Freundt, E.A., and Cassell, G.H. (1984). Immunoglobulin A1 protease activity in strains of *Ureaplasma urealyticum*. *Acta. Pathol. Microbiol. Immunol. Scand. B* 92, 61–64.

Kilian, M., and Holmgren, K. (1981). Ecology and nature of immunoglobulin A1 protease–producing streptococci in the human oral cavity and pharynx. *Infect. Immun.* 31, 868–873.

Kilian, M., Husby, S., Høst, A., and Halken, S. (1995). Increased proportions of bacteria capable of cleaving IgA1 in the pharynx of infants with atopic disease. *Pediatr. Res.* 38, 182–186.

Kilian, M., Mestecky, J., and Schrohenloher, R.E. (1979). Pathogenic species of *Haemophilus* and *Streptococcus pneumoniae* produce immunoglobulin A1 protease. *Infect. Immun.* 26, 143–149.

Kilian, M., Mestecky, J., Kulhavy, R., Tomana, M., and Butler, W.T. (1980). IgA1 proteases from *Haemophilus influenzae, Streptococcus pneumoniae, Neisseria meningitidis,* and *Streptococcus sanguis:* comparative immunochemical studies. *J. Immunol.* 124, 2596–2600.

Kilian, M., Mikkelsen, L., and Henrichsen, J. (1989). Taxonomic study of viridans streptococci: Description of *Streptococcus gordonii* sp. nov. and emended descriptions of *Streptococcus sanguis* (White and Niven 1946), *Streptococcus oralis* (Bridge and Sneath 1982), and *Streptococcus mitis* (Andrewes and Horder 1906). *Int. J. Syst. Bacteriol.* 39, 471–484.

Kilian, M., Poulsen, K., and Lomholt, H. (2002). Evolution of the paralogous *hap* and *iga* genes in *Haemophilus influenzae*: evidence for a conserved hap pseudogene associated with microcolony formation in the recently diverged *Haemophilus aegyptius* and *H. influenzae* biogroup aegyptius. *Mol. Microbiol.* 46, 1367–1380.

Kilian, M., and Reinholdt, J. (1987). A hypothetical model for the development of invasive infection due to IgA1 protease–producing bacteria. *Adv. Exp. Med. Biol.* 216B, 1261–1269.

Kilian, M., Roland, K., and Mestecky, J. (1981). Interference of secretory immunoglobulin A with sorption of oral bacteria to hydroxyapatite. *Infect. Immun.* 31, 942–951.

Kilian, M., Thomsen, B., Petersen, T.E., and Bleeg, H. (1983a). Molecular biology of *Haemophilus influenzae* IgA1 proteases. *Mol. Immunol.* 20, 1051–1058.

Kilian, M., Thomsen, B., Petersen, T.E., and Bleeg, H.S. (1983b). Occurrence and nature of bacterial IgA proteases. *Ann. N. Y. Acad. Sci.* 409, 612–624.

Kirkeby, L., Rasmussen, T.T., Reinholdt, J., and Kilian, M. (2000). Immunoglobulins in nasal secretions of healthy humans: structural integrity of secretory immunoglobulin A1 (IgA1) and occurrence of neutralizing antibodies to IgA1 proteases of nasal bacteria. *Clin. Diagn. Lab. Immunol.* 7, 31–39.

Kobayashi, K., Fujiyama, Y., Hagiwara, K., and Kondoh, H. (1987). Resistance of normal serum IgA and secretory IgA to bacterial IgA proteases: evidence for the presence of enzyme-neutralizing antibodies in both serum and secretory IgA, and also in serum IgG. *Microbiol. Immunol.* 31, 1097–1106.

Koomey, J.M., and Falkow, S. (1984). Nucleotide sequence homology between the immunoglobulin A1 protease genes of *Neisseria gonorrhoeae, Neisseria meningitidis,* and *Haemophilus influenzae. Infect. Immun.* 43, 101–107.

Koomey, J.M., Gill, R.E., and Falkow, S. (1982). Genetic and biochemical analysis of gonococcal IgA1 protease: cloning in *Escherichia coli* and construction of mutants of gonococci that fail to produce the activity. *Proc. Natl. Acad. Sci. USA* 79, 7881–7885.

Kosowska, K., Reinholdt, J., Rasmussen, L.K., Sabat, A., Potempa, J., Kilian, M., and Poulsen, K. (2002). The *Clostridium ramosum* IgA proteinase represents a novel type of metalloendopeptidase. *J. Biol. Chem.* 277, 11987–11994.

Kutteh, W.H., Kilian, M., Ermel L.D., Byrd, E.W., Mestecky, J. (1994). Antisperm antibodies (ASAs) in infertile males: Subclass distribution of IgA antibodies and the effect of an IgA1 protease on sperm-bound antibodies. *Am. J. Reprod. Immunol.* 31, 77–83.

Liljemark, W.F., Bloomquist, C.G., and Ofstehage, J.C. (1979). Aggregation and adherence of *Streptococcus sanguis*: role of human salivary immunoglobulin A. *Infect. Immun.* 26, 1104–1110.

Lin, L., Ayala, P., Larson, J., Mulks, M., Fukuda, M., Carlsson, S.R., Enns, C., and So, M. (1997). The *Neisseria* type 2 IgA1 protease cleaves LAMP1 and promotes survival of bacteria within epithelial cells. *Mol. Microbiol.* 24, 1083–1094.

Lindahl, G., and Åkerström, B. (1989). Receptor for IgA in group A streptococci: cloning of the gene and characterization of the protein expressed in *Escherichia coli. Mol. Microbiol.* 3, 239–247.

Lindahl, G., Åkerström, B., Vaerman, J.P., and Stenberg, L. (1990). Characterization of an IgA receptor from group B streptococci: specificity for serum IgA. *Eur. J. Immunol.* 20, 2241–2247.

Lomholt, H. (1995). Evidence of recombination and an antigenically diverse immunoglobulin A1 protease among strains of *Streptococcus pneumoniae. Infect. Immun.* 63, 4238–4243.

Lomholt, H. (1996). Molecular biology and vaccine aspects of bacterial immunoglobulin A1 proteases. *Acta Pathol. Microbiol. Immunol. Scand.* 104, S1–S28.

Lomholt, H., and Kilian, M. (1994). Antigenic relationships among immunoglobulin A1 proteases from *Haemophilus, Neisseria,* and *Streptococcus* species. *Infect. Immun.* 62, 3178–3183.

Lomholt, H., and Kilian, M. (1995). *Neisseria gonorrhoeae* IgA1 proteases share epitopes recognized by neutralizing antibodies. *Vaccine* 13, 1213–1220.

Lomholt, H., Poulsen, K., and Kilian, M. (1995). Comparative characterization of the *iga* gene encoding IgA1 protease in *Neisseria meningitidis, Neisseria gonorrhoeae* and *Haemophilus influenzae. Mol. Microbiol.* 15, 495–506.

Lomholt, H., Poulsen, K., Caugant, D.A., and Kilian, M. (1992). Molecular polymorphism and epidemiology of *Neisseria meningitidis* immunoglobulin A1 proteases. *Proc. Natl. Acad. Sci. USA* 89, 2120–2124.

Lomholt, H., van Alphen, L., and Kilian, M. (1993). Antigenic variation of immunoglobulin A1 proteases among sequential isolates of *Haemophilus influenzae* from healthy children and patients with chronic obstructive pulmonary disease. *Infect. Immun.* 61, 4575–4581.

Lomholt, J.A., and Kilian, M. (2000). Immunoglobulin A1 protease activity in *Gemella haemolysans. J. Clin. Microbiol.* 38, 2760–2762.

Loomes, L.M., Senior, B.W., and Kerr, M.A. (1990). A proteolytic enzyme secreted by *Proteus mirabilis* degrades immunoglobulins of the immunoglobulin A1 (IgA1), IgA2, and IgG isotypes. *Infect. Immun.* 58, 1979–1985.

Lorenzen, D.R., Dux, F., Wolk, U., Tsirpouchtsidis, A., Haas, G., and Meyer, T.F. (1999). Immunoglobulin A1 protease, an exoenzyme of pathogenic *Neisseriae,* is a potent inducer of proinflammatory cytokines. *J. Exp. Med.* 190, 1049–1058.

Ma, J.K.-C., Hunjan, M., Smith, R., Kelly, C., and Lehner, T. (1990). An investigation into the mechanism of protection by local passive immunization with monoclonal antibodies against *Streptococcus mutans. Infect. Immun.* 58, 3407–3414.

Male, C.J. (1979). Immunoglobulin A1 protease production by *Haemophilus influenzae* and *Streptococcus pneumoniae. Infect. Immun.* 26, 254–261.

Mallett, C.P., Boylan, R.J., and Everhart, D.L. (1984). Competent antigen-binding fragments (Fab) from secretory immunoglobulin A using *Streptococcus sanguis* immunoglobulin A protease. *Caries Res.* 18, 201–208.

Mansa, B., and Kilian, M. (1986). Retained antigen-binding activity of Fab alpha fragments of human monoclonal immunoglobulin A1 (IgA1) cleaved by IgA1 protease. *Infect. Immun.* 52, 171–174.

Marrack, P., and Kappler, J. (1994). Subversion of the immune system by pathogens. *Cell* 76, 323–332.

Mattu, T.S., Pleass, R.J., Willis, A.C., Kilian, M., Wormald, M.R., Lellouch, A.C., Rudd, P.M., Woof, J.M., and Dwek, R.A. (1998). The glycosylation and structure of human serum IgA1, Fab and Fc regions and the role of N-glycosylation on Fcα receptor interactions. *J. Biol. Chem.* 273, 2260–2272.

McClure, H. (1980). Bacterial diseases of nonhuman primates. In *The Comparative Pathology of Zoo Animals* (eds. R. J. Montali and G. Migaki), 197–218. Washington, DC: Smithsonian Institution Press.

Mestecky, J., and Russell, M.W. (1986). IgA subclasses. *Monogr. Allergy* 19, 277–301.

Mehta, S., Plaut, A.G., Calvanico, N.J., and Tomasi, T.B. (1973). Human immunoglobulin A: production of an Fc fragment by an enteric microbial proteolytic enzyme. *J. Immunol.* 111, 1274–1276.

Meyer, T.F. (1990). Pathogenic neisseriae—a model of bacterial virulence and genetic flexibility. *Int. J. Med. Microbiol.* 274, 135–154.

Milazzo, F.H., and Delisle, G.J. (1984). Immunoglobulin A proteases in gram-negative bacteria isolated from human urinary tract infections. *Infect. Immun.* 43, 11–13.

Molla, A., Kagimoto, T., and Maeda, H. (1988). Cleavage of immunoglobulin G (IgG) and IgA around the hinge region by proteases from *Serratia marcescens*. *Infect. Immun.* 56, 916–920.

Morelli, G., del Valle, J., Lammel, C.J., Pohlner, J., Müller, K., Blake, M., Brooks, G.F., Meyer, T.F., Koumare, B., Brieske, N., and Achtman, M. (1994). Immunogenicity and evolutionary variability of epitopes within IgA1 protease from serogroup A *Neisseria meningitidis*. *Mol. Microbiol.* 11, 175–187.

Mortensen, S.B., and Kilian, M. (1984). Purification and characterization of an immunoglobulin A1 protease from *Bacteroides melaninogenicus*. *Infect. Immun.* 45, 550–557.

Mulks, M.H., and Kornfeld, S.J., Frangione, B., and Plaut, A.G. (1982). Relationship between the specificity of IgA proteases and serotypes in *Haemophilus influenzae*. *J. Infect. Dis.* 146, 266–274.

Mulks, M.H., Plaut, A.G., Feldman, H.A., and Frangione, B. (1980a). IgA proteases of two distinct specificities are released by *Neisseria meningitidis*. *J. Exp. Med.* 152, 1442–1447.

Mulks, M.H., Plaut, A.G., and Lamm, M. (1980b). Gonococcal IgA protease reduces inhibition of bacterial adherence by human secretory IgA. In *Genetics and Immunobiology of Pathogenic Neisseria* (eds. S. Normark and D. Danielsson), 217–220. Umea, Sweden: University of Umea.

Negrete-Abascal, E., Tenorio, V.R., Serrano, J.J., Garcia, C.C., and de la Garza, M. (1994). Secreted proteases from *Actinobacillus pleuropneumoniae* serotype 1 degrade porcine gelatin hemoglobin and immunoglobulin A. *Can. J. Vet. Res.* 58, 83–86.

Nikolova, E.B., Tomana, M. and Russell, M.W. (1994). All forms of human IgA antibodies bound to antigen interfere with complement (C3) fixation induced by IgG or by antigen alone. *Scand. J. Immunol.* 39, 275–280.

Nose, M., and Wigzell H. (1983). Biological significance of carbohydrate chains on monoclonal antibodies. *Proc. Natl. Acad. Sci. USA* 80, 6632–6636.

Nyvad, B., and Kilian, M. (1990). Comparison of the initial streptococcal microflora on dental enamel in caries-active and in caries-inactive individuals. *Caries Res.* 24, 267–272.

Plaut, A.G. (1978). Microbial IgA proteases. *N. Engl. J. Med.* 298, 1459–1463.

Plaut, A.G., Genco, R.J., and Tomasi, T.B. Jr. (1974a). Isolation of an enzyme from *Streptococcus sanguis* which specifically cleaves IgA. *J. Immunol.* 113, 289–291.

Plaut, A.G., Wistar, R. Jr., and Capra, J.D. (1974b). Differential susceptibility of human IgA immunoglobulins to streptococcal IgA protease. *J. Clin. Invest.* 54, 1295–1300.

Plaut, A.G., Gilbert, J.V., Artenstein, M.S., and Capra, J.D. (1975). *Neisseria gonorrhoeae* and *Neisseria meningitidis*: extracellular enzyme cleaves human immunoglobulin A. *Science* 193, 1103–1105.

Plaut, A.G., Qiu, J., Grundy, F., and Wright, A. (1992). Growth of *Haemophilus influenzae* in human milk: synthesis, distribution and activity of IgA protease as determined by study of iga+ and mutant iga− cells. *J. Infect. Dis.* 166, 43–52.

Pleass, R.J., Areschough, T., Lindahl, G., and Woof, J.M. (2001). Streptococcal IgA-binding proteins bind in the Cα2-Cα3 interdomain region and inhibit binding of IgA to human CD89. *J. Biol. Chem.* 276, 8197–8204.

Pohlner, J., Halter, R., Bayreuther, K., and Meyer, T.F. (1987). Gene structure and extracellular secretion of *Neisseria gonorrhoeae* IgA protease. *Nature* 325, 452–462.

Polissi, A., Pontiggia, A., Feger, G., Altieri, M., Mottl, H., Ferrari, L. and Simon, D. (1998). Large-scale identification of virulence genes from *Streptococcus pneumoniae*. *Infect. Immun.* 66, 5620–5629.

Pouedras, P., Andre, P.M., Donnio, P.Y., and Avril, J.L. (1992). Cleavage of immunoglobulin A1, A2 and G by proteases from clinical isolates of *Pasteurella multocida*. *J. Med. Microbiol.* 37, 128–132.

Poulsen, K., Brandt, J., Hjorth, J.P., Thogersen, H.C., and Kilian, M. (1989). Cloning and sequencing of the immunoglobulin A1 protease gene (iga) of *Haemophilus influenzae* serotype b. *Infect Immun.* 57, 3097–3105.

Poulsen, K., Hjorth, J.P., and Kilian, M. (1988). Limited diversity of the immunoglobulin A1 protease gene (iga) among *Haemophilus influenzae* serotype b strains. *Infect. Immun.* 56, 987–992.

Poulsen, K., Reinholdt, J., Jespersgaard, C., Boye, K., Brown, T.A., Hauge, M., and Kilian, M. (1998). A comprehensive genetic study of streptococcal IgA1 protease: evidence for recombination within and between species. *Infect. Immun.* 66, 181–190.

Poulsen, K., Reinholdt, J., and Kilian, M. (1992). A comparative genetic study of serologically distinct *Haemophilus influenzae* type 1 immunoglobulin A1 proteases. *J. Bacteriol.* 174, 2913–2921.

Poulsen, K., Reinholdt, J., and Kilian, M. (1996). Characterization of the *Streptococcus pneumoniae* immunoglobulin A1 protease gene (iga) and its translation product. *Infect. Immun.* 64, 3957–3966.

Provence, D.L., and Curtiss, R. III. (1994). Isolation and characterization of a gene involved in hentagglutination by an avian pathogenic *Escherichia coli* strain. *Infect. Immun.* 62, 1369–1380.

Provenzano, D., and Alderete, J.F. (1995). Analysis of human immunoglobulin-degrading cysteine proteinases of *Trichomonas vaginalis*. 63, 3388–3395.

Qiu, J., Brackee, G.P., and Plaut, A.G. (1996). Analysis of the specificity of bacterial immunoglobulin A (IgA) protease by a comparative study of ape serum IgAs as substrates. *Infect. Immun.* 64, 933–937.

Quezada-Calvillo, R., and Lopez-Revilla, R. (1987). IgA protease in *Entamoeba histolytica* trophozoites. *Adv. Exp. Med. Biol.* 216B, 1283–1288.

Reinholdt, J., Friman, V., and Kilian, M. (1993). Similar proportions of immunoglobulin A1 (IgA1) protease–producing streptococci in initial dental plaque of selectively IgA-deficient and normal individuals. *Infect. Immun.* 61, 3998–4000.

Reinholdt, J., and Kilian, M. (1987). Interference of IgA protease with the effect of secretory IgA on adherence of oral streptococci to saliva-coated hydroxyapatite. *J. Dent. Res.* 66, 492–497.

Reinholdt, J., and Kilian, M. (1997). Comparative analysis of immunoglobulin A1 protease activity among bacteria representing different genera, species, and strains. *Infect. Immun.* 65, 4452–4459.

Reinholdt, J., and Kilian, M. (1995). Titration of inhibiting antibodies to bacterial IgA1 proteases in human sera and secretions. *Adv. Exp. Med. Biol.* 371A, 605–608.

Reinholdt, J., Krogh, P., and Holmstrup, P. (1987). Degradation of IgA1, IgA2, and S-IgA by *Candida* and *Torulopsis* species. *Acta Pathol. Microbiol. Immunol. Scand. C.* 95, 265–274.

Reinholdt, J., Tomana, M., Mortensen, S.B., and Kilian, M. (1990). Molecular aspects of immunoglobulin A1 degradation by oral streptococci. *Infect. Immun.* 58, 1186–1194.

Rifai A, Fadden K, Morrison SL, Chintalacharuvu KR. (2000). The N-glycans determine the differential blood clearance and hepatic uptake of human immunoglobulin (Ig)A1 and IgA2 isotypes. *J. Exp. Med.* 191, 2171–2182.

Robertson, J.A., Stemler, M.E., and Stemke, G.W. (1984). Immunoglobulin A protease activity of *Ureaplasma urealyticum*. *J. Clin. Microbiol.* 19, 255–258.

Royle, L., Roos, A., Harvey, D.J., Wormald, M.R., Van Gijlswijk-Janssen, D.J., Redwan, E.R., Wilson, I.A., Daha, M.R., Dwek, R.A., and Rudd, P.M.. (2003). Secretory IgA N- and O-glycans provide a link between the innate and adaptive immune systems. *J. Biol. Chem.* 278, 20140–20153.

Rüchel, R. (1986). Cleavage of immunoglobulins by pathogenic yeasts of the genus *Candida*. *Microbiol. Sci.* 3, 316–319.

Rudd, P.M., Elliott, T., Cresswell, P., Wilson, I.A., and Dweck, R.A. (2001). Glycosylation and the immune system. *Science* 291, 2368–2376.

Ruhl, S., Sandberg, A.L., Cole, M.F., and Cisar, J.O. (1996). Recognition of immunoglobulin A1 by oral actinomyces and streptococcal lectins. *Infect. Immun.* 64, 5421–5424.

Russell, M.W., Reinholdt, J., and Kilian, M. (1989). Anti-inflammatory activity of human IgA antibodies and their Fabα fragments: inhibition of IgG-mediated complement activation. *Eur. J. Immunol.* 19, 2243–2249.

Sandin, C., Linse, S., Areschoug, T., Woof, J.M., Reinholdt, J., and Lindahl, G. (2002). Isolation and detection of human IgA using a streptococcal IgA-binding peptide. *J. Immunol.* 169, 1357–1364.

Saltzman, W.M., Radomsky, M.L., Whaley, K.J., and Cone, R.A. (1994). Antibody diffusion in human cervical mucus. *Biophys. J.* 66, 508–515.

Senda, S., Fujiyama, Y., Ushijima, T., Hodohara, K., Bamba, T., Hosoda, S., and Kobayashi, K. (1985). *Clostridium ramosum,* and IgA protease–producing species and its ecology in the human intestinal tract. *Microbiol. Immunol.* 29, 203–207.

Senior, B.W., Dunlop, J.I., Batten, M.R., Kilian, M., and Woof, J.M. (2000). Cleavage of a recombinant human immunoglobulin A2 (IgA2)-IgA1 hybrid antibody by certain bacterial IgA1 proteases. *Infect. Immun.* 68, 463–469.

Senior, B.W., Loomes, L.M., and Kerr, M.A. (1991). The production and activity in vivo of *Proteus mirabilis* IgA protease in infections of the urinary tract. *J. Med. Microbiol.* 35, 203–207.

Senior, B.W., Stewart, W.W., Galloway, C., and Kerr, M.A. (2001). Cleavage of the hormone human chorionic gonadotropin, by the Type 1 IgA1 protease of *Neisseria gonorrhoeae,* and its implications. *J. Infect. Dis.* 184, 922–925.

Simpson, D.A., Hausinger, R.P., and Mulks, M.H. (1988). Purification, characterization, and comparison of the immunoglobulin A1 proteases of *Neisseria gonorrhoea. J. Bacteriol.* 170, 1866–1873.

Sørensen, C.H., and Kilian, M. (1984). Bacterium-induced cleavage of IgA in nasopharyngeal secretions from atopic children. *Acta Pathol. Microbiol. Immunol. Scand. C* 92, 85–87.

Spooner, R.K., Russell, W.C., and Thirkell, D. (1992). Characterization of the immunoglobulin A protease of *Ureaplasma urealyticum. Infect. Immun.* 60, 2544–2546.

Steele, E.J., Chaicumpa, W., and Rowley, D. (1975). Further evidence for cross-linking as a protective factor in experimental cholera: properties of antibody fragments. *J. Infect. Dis.* 132, 175–180.

Stein, M., Kenny, B., Stein, M.A., and Finlay, B.B. (1996). Characterization of EspC, a 110-kilo dalton protein secreted by enteropathogenic *Escherichia coli* which is homologous to members of the immunoglobulin A protease–like family of secreted proteins. *J. Bacteriol.* 178, 6546–6554.

Stenberg, L., O'Toole, P.W., Mestecky, J., and Lindahl, G. (1994). Molecular characterization of protein Sir, a streptococcal cell surface protein that binds both IgA and IgG. *J. Biol. Chem.* 269, 13458–13464.

St. Geme, J.W., 3rd, de la Morena, M.L., and Falkow, S. (1994). A *Haemophilus influenzae* IgA protease–like protein promotes intimate interaction with human epithelial cells. *Mol. Microbiol.* 14, 217–233.

Tao, M.-H., and Morrison, S.L. (1989). Studies of a glycosylated chimeric mouse-human IgG. Role of carbohydrate in the structure and effector functions mediated by the human IgG constant region. *J. Immunol.* 143, 2595–2601.

Thern, A., Stenberg, L., Dahlback, B., and Lindahl, G. (1995). Ig-binding surface proteins of *Streptococcus pyogenes* also bind human C4b-binding protein (C4BP), a regulatory component of the complement system. *J. Immunol.* 154, 375–386.

Thiesen, B., Greenwood, B., Brieske, N., and Achtman, M. (1997). Persistence of antibodies to meningococcal IgA1 protease versus decay of antibodies to group A polysaccharide and Opc protein. *Vaccine* 15, 209–219.

Tsirpouchtsidis, A., Hurwitz, R., Brinkmann, V., Meyer, T.F., and Haas, G. (2002). Neisserial immunoglobulin A1 protease induces specific T-cell responses in humans. *Infect. Immun.* 70, 335–344.

Tyler, B.M., and Cole, M.F. (1998). Effect of IgA1 protease on the ability of secretory IgA1 antibodies to inhibit the adherence of *Streptococcus mutans. Microbiol. Immunol.* 42, 503–508.

Yanagida, N., Uozumi, T., and Beppu, T. (1986). Specific excretion of *Serratia marcescens* protease through the outer membrane of *Escherichia coli. J. Bacteriol.* 166, 937–944.

van Ulsen, P., van Alphen, L., Hopman, C.T., van der Ende, A., and Tommassen, J. (2001). In vivo expression of *Neisseria meningitidis* proteins homologous to the *Haemophilus influenzae* Hap and Hia autotransporters. *FEMS Immunol. Med. Microbiol.* 32, 53–64.

Veiga, E., Sugawara, E., Nikaido, H., de Lorenzo, V., and Fernandez, L.A. (2002). Export of autotransported proteins proceeds through an oligomeric ring shaped by C-terminal domains. *EMBO J.* 21, 2122–2131.

Vitovski, S., Dunkin, K.T., Howard, A.J., and Sayers, J.R. (2002). Nontypeable *Haemophilus influenzae* in carriage and disease: a difference in IgA1 protease activity levels. *J. Am. Med. Assoc.* 287, 1699–1705.

Vitovski, S., Read, R.C., and Sayers, J.R. (1999). Invasive isolates of *Neisseria meningitidis* possess enhanced immunoglobulin A1 protease activity compared to colonizing strains. *FASEB J.* 13, 331–337.

Wani, J.H., Gilbert, J.V., Plaut, A.G., and Weiser, J.N. (1996). Identification, cloning, and sequencing of the immunoglobulin A1 protease gene of *Streptococcus pneumoniae. Infect. Immun.* 64, 3967–3974.

Weiser, J.N., Bae, D., Fasching, C., Scamurra, R.W., Ratner, A.J., Janoff, E.N. (2003). Antibody-enhanced pneumococcal adherence requires IgA1 protease. *Proc. Natl. Acad. Sci. USA* 100: 4215–4220.

Wold, A., Mestecky, J., Tomana, M., Kobata, A., Ohbayashi, H., Endo, T., and Svanborg-Edén, C. (1990). Secretory immunoglobulin A carries oligosaccharide receptors for *Escherichia coli* type 1 fimbrial lectin. *Infect. Immun.* 58, 3073–3077.

Wold, A.E., Motas, C., Svanborg, C., and Mestecky, J. (1994). Lectin receptors in IgA isotypes. *Scand. J. Immunol.* 39, 195–201.

Wood, S.G., and Burton, J. (1991). Synthetic peptide substrates for the immunoglobulin A1 protease from *Neisseria gonorrhoeae* (type 2). *Infect. Immun.* 59, 1818–1822.

Zhang, J.R., Mostov, K.E., Lamm, M.E., Nanno, M., Shimida, S., Ohwaki, M., and Tuomanen, E. (2000). The polymeric immunoglobulin receptor translocates pneumococci across human nasopharyngeal epithelial cells. *Cell* 102, 827–837.

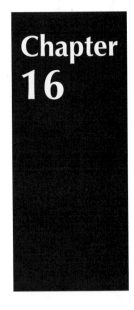

Ontogeny of Mucosal Immunity and Aging

Allan W. Cripps
School of Medicine, Griffith University, Queensland, Australia

Maree Gleeson
Hunter Area Pathology Services, Newcastle, New South Wales, Australia

Chapter 16

This chapter provides an overview of the ontogeny and aging of the human mucosal immune system. In some instances, reference is made to studies involving animals to support preliminary findings that have been observed in the human. Studies of ontogeny and aging of mucosal immunity in humans have always been complicated by experimental design difficulties, ethical considerations, and the sensitivities of the various technologies used. In the prenatal period, this is further complicated by the small number of normal fetuses available for study and the difficulty of determining the precise gestational age. In the postnatal period and in the elderly, many researchers have focused on the measurement of salivary parameters to provide an insight into the ontogeny of the mucosal immune network. This approach has two major advantages. First, it provides a simple noninvasive sample collection procedure, and second, saliva is a suitable secretion that can be relatively easily analyzed by routine laboratory procedures in large numbers (Gleeson *et al.*, 1995). The salivary glands have long been recognized as part of the common mucosal immune system (Bienenstock and Befus, 1980); as such, salivary secretions are probably indicative of the mucosal immune system. A criticism of the use of saliva to draw conclusions about the mucosal immune network has been that the antibodies in saliva most likely reflect the end result of the mucosal immune response following migration of plasma cells from mucosal germinal centers to the salivary glands rather than the induction phase of the mucosal immune response (Gleeson *et al.*, 1995). Another consideration when using saliva is the influence of physiological variations such as flow rate on the concentrations of the parameters being measured. This factor also applies to any other mucosal secretion and, in particular, tears. A number of approaches have been used to overcome physiological factors. These include measuring the levels of osmolality (Blannin *et al*, 1998), albumin, or total protein and applying a correction factor; determining actual flow rates; and collecting samples at a defined time each day. Despite these limitations, analysis of salivary parameters has provided considerable useful information on the ontogeny, aging, and competence of the mucosal immune system in humans.

This chapter focuses only on human research, and the reader is directed to a number of excellent review articles for further reading. [For ontogeny, see Hanson *et al.* (1986), Brandtzaeg *et al.* (1991), MacDonald (1994, 1996), Goldblum *et al.* (1996), Husband and Gleeson (1996), and Spencer *et al.* (1997), and for aging, see Gardner (1980), Effros and Walford (1987), and Wade and Szewczuk (1987).] An understanding of ontogeny, or normality, provides the foundation for investigations of disease states or factors that modify the human mucosal immune system. This chapter focuses on some of the factors that influence the maturation of mucosal immunocompetence or modify the mucosal immune response. This knowledge has been essential to the development of intervention strategies, such as oral vaccines, for the prevention of diseases resulting in high mortality and morbidity.

Studies of ontogeny have also shown that in humans the mucosal and systemic components of the immune system, while interrelated, develop and age independently and at different rates.

ONTOGENY OF MUCOSAL IMMUNOLOGY

Prenatal development of mucosal immunity

Lymphoid structures

The communicating network of lymphatic vessels essential to achieve dissemination of lymphomyeloid cells develops in the early stage of fetal growth. Lymphatic vessels in humans begin to differentiate at 35 to 42 days of gestation (Yoffey and Courtice, 1970). In the human fetal intestine, clusters of lymphocytes that may represent early Peyer's patches can be microscopically detected between 100 and 110 days of gestation (Spencer *et al.*, 1986, 1987), and Peyer's patches can be macroscopically seen at 200 days of gestation (Cornes, 1965). Discrete primary B-cell follicles, T-cell zones with high endothelial venules, a dome region, and a follicle-associated epithelium are observed in the human fetal intestine around 130 to 140 days of gestation (Spencer *et al.*, 1997).

MHC class I antigens (HLA-A-B) are expressed on human intestinal epithelial cells from 120 to 140 days of gestation (the earliest time studied) (Russell *et al.*, 1990a; Rognum *et al.*, 1992). The high endothelial venules express intercellular adhesion molecules and vascular cell adhesion molecules (Dohan *et al.*, 1993), and Peyer's patch lymphocytes have been reported to express HLA-DR (MacDonald *et al.*, 1988). Although it is likely that small amounts of HLA-DR are expressed by human fetal gastrointestinal tissue (Oliver *et al.*, 1988; MacDonald *et al.*, 1988), significant HLA-DR expression occurs only after birth in normal neonates (Russell *et al.*, 1990a; Rognum *et al.*, 1992).

In the human fetal lung, organized lymphoid aggregates called bronchus-associated lymphoid tissue (BALT) are present only occasionally prior to birth in the absence of any identifiable underlying infection. In normal fetuses, ill-defined lymphoid aggregates are seen at 110 days of gestation with well-defined aggregates at 140 days of gestation (Gould and Isaacson, 1993). However, in contrast to the intestine, the development of BALT is largely dependent on infection or antigenic stimulus and is not naturally present in fetal life.

B lymphocytes and the IgA secretory mechanism

The ontogeny of the mucosal B-cell and secretory S-IgA apparatus is somewhat confused because of differences in methods and mucosal sites examined as well as inherent difficulties in determining the precise age of the fetus. In the fetal human intestine, B cells located in lymphoid aggregates are sIgM+, sIgD+, and CD5+ (Spencer *et al.*, 1986, 1987). Occasionally IgA+ and IgG+ cells are present. However, in the lamina propria, no IgA+ or IgG+ cells are present at birth (Spencer *et al.*, 1986; Russell *et al.*, 1990a; Rognum *et al.*, 1992). The omentum appears to be an important source of CD5+ B cells in the developing fetus (Solvason and Kearney, 1992). In mice, the B-1 cells play an important role in the production of IgA plasma cells in the intestinal mucosa (Kroese *et al.*, 1996). and the close proximity of the omentum to the developing gut may be an important factor in the ontogeny of the mucosal defense system. The B-cell maturation process commences at about 100 days of gestation with the appearance of sIgM+, sIgD+, and CD5+ cells (Spencer *et al.*, 1986, 1997), whereas sIgA expression occurs from about 120 days of gestation (Russell *et al.*, 1990a). In the bronchi and major salivary glands, IgM+ cells have been reported from 140 days of gestation, and in the minor salivary glands and bronchioles, a few IgM+ cells have been observed from 175 days of gestation. IgA+ cells have also been reported in association with the bronchi and salivary glands at 180 days of gestation (Iwase *et al.*, 1987). However, sensitive polymerase chain reaction (PCR) methods have shown that IgA and IgM synthesis may occur in the lung and intestine as early as 110 days of gestation (Moro *et al.*, 1991).

Ig-containing lymphocytes do not occur in the lung prior to birth in normal circumstances (Takemura and Eishi, 1985). The numbers and distribution of IgM+ or IgA+ cells observed at the various fetal mucosal sites examined do not alter after 200 days of gestation (Iwase *et al.*, 1987).

In the human fetal parotid salivary gland, occasional IgM- and IgA-producing cells occur from 170 days of gestation (Iwase *et al.*, 1987). IgA-producing cells are predominantly of the IgA1 subclass and are also joining (J) chain–positive (Thrane *et al.*, 1991). Crypts develop in the neonatal palatine tonsils at about 120 days of gestation, and the crypt epithelium is rapidly populated by dendritic cells and lymphocytes (van Gaudecker and Müller-Hemelink, 1982).

The ontogeny of the expression of polymeric Ig receptor (pIgR) has been restricted by the availability of postmortem fetal tissue, and comparisons between studies have not been able to provide precise data for the earliest detection of pIgR in mucosal epithelium. The consensus of the studies suggests that pIgR expression appears in the respiratory tract earlier than in the intestinal epithelium, but by 200 days of gestation, expression rapidly increases at both sites. In the lung, pIgR has been reported in the bronchial surface epithelium and between the epithelial cells as early as 56 days of gestation (Ogra *et al.*, 1972), although more recent studies suggest that pIgR expression in the lung may occur later than this, between 90 and 100 days of gestation (Takemura and Eishi, 1985; Moro *et al.*, 1991). A marked increase in pIgR expression occurs in the columnar epithelium of the large bronchi at 140 days of gestation (Iwase *et al.*, 1987, Moro *et al.*, 1991). pIgR can be detected in the apical cytoplasm of a few epithelial cells of duct-like structures in salivary glands by 143 days of gestation (Iwase *et al.*, 1987). Two investigations showed that pIgR expression in salivary gland ducts increased from 175 days of gestation to approximately 200 days of gestation, after which no further changes were seen in either the intensity or the distribution of expression (Iwase *et al.*, 1987; Thrane *et al.*, 1991). pIgR synthesis in the intestine may occur as early as 40 days of gestation (Moro *et al.*, 1991). However, pIgR expression in the small intestine is usually present by about 90 to 120 days of gestation (Ogra *et al.*, 1972; Crago *et al.*, 1978; Moro *et al.*, 1991). Immunofluorescence studies show that pIgR expression by intestinal epithelial cells occurs in relatively small amounts by 200 days of gestation and thereafter increases rapidly to show an adult distribution pattern by 1 week post partum (Rognum *et al.*, 1992). The early studies by Crago *et al.* (1978) indicate that the appearance of pIgR in the developing fetal intestine coincides with the potential of the epithelium to bind polymeric Ig.

The third of the component proteins of secretory immunoglobulins is the J chain, which may participate in the intracellular polymerization of IgA and IgM. J-chain expression in the human fetus is an early event in B-cell ontogeny and precedes the expression of μ-chain (Moro *et al.*, 1991). J chain is expressed in the fetal liver at 40 days of gestation but is not detected in spleen, thymus, lung, and small intestine until 110 days of gestation (Moro *et al.*, 1991). A study by Isawe *et al.* (1987), in which the youngest fetal age was 110 days of gestation, also noted J-chain-positive cells in the liver, spleen, and bone marrow at this time.

T lymphocytes

T cells are observed in the human terminal ilium as early as 100 days of gestation. By 140 days, these cells are organized around distinct B-cell follicular areas (Spencer *et al.*, 1986). There is some confusion concerning the exact phenotype of the developing T-cell repertoire. However, in the lamina propria it appears that both the helper/inducer (CD3+/CD4+) and suppressor/cytotoxic (CD3+/CD8+) phenotypes are present at 140 days of gestation (Spencer *et al.*, 1986; Russell *et al.*, 1990a), but the helper/inducer phenotype predominates. Intraepithelial lymphocytes (IEL) are observed in the fetal intestine from around 100 days of gestation. In contrast to T cells in the lamina propria, a high proportion of fetal IEL are CD3+ or CD4–/CD8– and, in contrast to the postnatal intestine, T-cell receptor (TCR)γδ (Spencer *et al.*, 1989). The significance of these differences is unknown (Spencer *et al.*, 1997). As the immune system is established in the first trimester of pregnancy, there is the possibility of abnormalities developing *in utero* if the pregnancy is exposed to adverse conditions, such as infection or chemical toxicity, during this critical phase. The prenatal development of mucosal lymphoid structures and cell populations is shown in **Table 16.1**.

Prenatal immunocompetence

Innate defenses

Innate defense factors afford nonspecific protection in fetal life and at the time of birth in the absence of adaptive specific immunity. Amylase, lysozyme, and lactoferrin are all present in the human salivary gland by 200 days of gestation at levels similar to those observed in the postnatal period (Ogra *et al.*, 1972; Thrane *et al.*, 1991; Brandtzaeg *et al.*, 1991). All three proteins show a dramatic decrease at birth (Thrane *et al.*, 1991). The cause of this depletion is unknown. However, it has been suggested that cellular stores of these proteins are depleted as a result of suckling (Thrane *et al.*, 1991).

Specific immunity

The mucosal immune apparatus is anatomically in place prior to birth, with all components identified by 200 days of gestation. Although the mucosal immune system is not usually activated by antigen challenge until birth, there is good evidence that the fetal mucosal immune system is capable of mounting a response that, in some circumstances, may be protective in postnatal life. Immune stimulation in these cases arises from intrauterine infection and possibly as an anti-idiotypic response to maternal antibody. However, antigen-independent B-cell differentiation is an additional possibility (Table 16.1).

In the human fetal lung, the development of BALT *in vitro* is seen following infection. In addition, in premature infants who develop pulmonary infection, IgA- or IgM-containing plasma cells appear in association with the bronchial glands

Table 16.1. Prenatal Development (in days of gestation) of Mucosal Lymphoid Structures and Cell Population (Consensus of Studies on Human Fetuses)

Development	Earliest Detection
Lymphoid structures	
Lymphatic vessels	35–42
Diffuse lymphoid cluster	100–110
Defined lymphoid aggregates	130–140
Organized lymphoid aggregates	
Peyer's patches	200
BALT	Post partum
Lymphoid cells	
Mucosal B cells	
sIgM+ , IgD, CD5+ in	
intestinal aggregates	~100
IgA+ in intestinal aggregates	~120
IgM+ in lung	~140
IgA+ in lung and salivary glands	~175
Mucosal epithelium: pIgR expression	
Lung	90–110
Small intestine	40
Salivary glands	175–200
J-chain expression	
Small intestine	~110
Lung	~110
Mucosal T cells	
Terminal ilium	~100
Intestinal IEL	~100
Tonsils	~120

at the equivalent of the 39th gestational week. IgG-containing cells appear 1 to 2 weeks later in association with the submucosal layer of the bronchi (Takemura and Eishi, 1985). Mellander *et al.* (1984) reported salivary IgA and IgM antibodies to *Escherichia coli* and poliovirus antigens in saliva and most meconium samples taken during the first day of life from Swedish infants. It is quite probable that these secretory antibodies are of fetal origin, as fetal exposure to poliovirus in Sweden is highly unlikely (Mellander *et al.*, 1984). In one case, antibodies were detected in the infant of a hypogammaglobulinemic mother who was being administered intravenous immunoglobulin that contained only IgG antibodies against *E. coli* and poliovirus, thus excluding the possibility that the antibodies were of maternal origin.

Postnatal development of mucosal immunity: anatomical factors

In the normal full-term infant, in the absence of any intrauterine infection, the essential components of the mucosal immune system are present and have the potential to respond to antigenic stimulation. The mucosal system is essentially devoid of IgA-containing lymphocytes, and there are no reactive B cells in the intestinal lymphoid follicles. Germinal centers appear in the intestinal mucosa after birth (Bridges *et al.*, 1959; Gebbers and Laissue, 1990), and pIgR expression in the epithelium increases rapidly to about 8 weeks of age, when an adult distribution pattern is observed (Thrane *et al.*, 1991; Rognum *et al.*, 1992). Prenatally, most of the germinal center cells stain immunohistochemically for cytoplasmic IgM or IgG, not IgA (Bjerke and Brandtzaeg, 1986). This is rapidly reversed after birth in response to antigenic challenge (Brandtzaeg *et al.*, 1991). Ig-containing cells are not present in normal bronchial walls at birth (Takemura and Eishi, 1985). IgA-containing cells appear around the bronchial glands at 10 days after birth and IgM-containing cells in lesser numbers about 1 month of age; IgG-containing cells are rare under normal conditions (Takemura and Eishi, 1985).

In the parotid salivary gland, IgA- and IgD-producing immunocytes increase in number from about 4 weeks of age; IgG-producing cells initially increase, reaching a peak at about 12 weeks of age and then plateau at lower numbers after 24 weeks of age (Thrane *et al.*, 1991). The numbers of IgA immunocytes approach the lower normal adult range at about 15 months, and only small increases occur throughout early childhood (Korsrud and Brandtzaeg, 1980). IgA1-positive cells predominate in the salivary gland at birth, although the proportion of IgA2-positive cells increases in the first 3 months of age to near-adult levels (Thrane *et al.*, 1991). In the intestine, IgM-containing cells predominate up to 1 month of age (Perkkio and Savilahti, 1980; Knox, 1986). Thereafter, IgA-containing cells predominate, and although the numbers remain low, they continue to increase up to 2 years of age (Perkkio and Savilahti, 1980). Plasma cells are present in tonsillar tissue by 8 weeks of age (Davis, 1912). There is a rise in both IgA- and IgM-producing cells in the appendix between 2 and 4 weeks of age, but after a few months, the IgG-producing cells expand in the appendix

lamina propria to represent 50% of the immunocytes (Gebbers and Laissue, 1990).

Few studies have examined the postnatal development of T cells at mucosal sites in the human. The number of IEL expands after birth, reaching adult levels at 2 years of age. This expansion primarily relates to TCRαβ-positive cells, which undergo a 10-fold expansion. However, TCRγδ-positive cells expand by twofold to threefold. It is thought that the expansion of TCRαβ-positive cells is more dependent on antigenic stimuli than that of TCRγδ-positive cells (Cerf-Bensussan and Guy-Grand, 1991). Phenotypically, the IEL remain predominantly CD3+/CD8+ from birth to adulthood (Russell *et al.*, 1990a; Cerf-Bensussan and Guy-Grand, 1991). It has been suggested that the predominance of the TCRαβ+/CD8+ subset and the location of the IEL support the concept that these T cells are involved in oral tolerance to dietary antigens (Brandtzaeg *et al.*, 1991). MHC class II antigen expression (HLA-DR) appears to occur primarily postnatally (Russell *et al.*, 1990a; Rognum *et al.*, 1992), between birth and 2 weeks of age, when HLA-DR expression is well established (Rognum *et al.*, 1992). However, it is likely that small amounts are expressed by human fetal tissue (MacDonald *et al.*, 1988; Oliver *et al.*, 1988). Dendritic cells are also reported to appear postnatally (MacDonald, 1996). The perinatal development of human mucosal lymphoid structures in summarized in **Table 16.2**.

Postnatal development of mucosal immunity: immunocompetence at birth

Innate defenses

At birth, the concentrations of saliva, lysozyme, and lactoferrin decrease temporarily, probably because of depletion of cellular stores as a result of suckling (Thrane *et al.*, 1991). The importance of this observation in relation to defense mechanisms in the immediate postpartum period is unclear, and further studies are required. However, these proteins increase again after delivery, reaching a peak between 6 and

Table 16.2. Perinatal Development of Human Mucosal Lymphoid Structures

Lymphoid Structure	Earliest Detection	Perinatal Changes
Intestinal lymphoid follicles	~10 days	Germinal centers appear pIgR expression increases IgA- and IgM-containing cells appear IEL T-cell numbers increase (predominantly CD3+/CD8+/TCRαβ+ population) Dendritic cells appear
Lung	~2 weeks	Organized lymphoid aggregates (BALT) appear in association with submucosal layer of the bronchi
Appendix	~3 weeks	IgA- and IgM-producing cells appear IgG-producing cells predominate by 3 months
Salivary glands	~4 weeks	IgA- and IgD-producing immunocytes appear IgM immunocytes decrease after first month
Tonsillar tissue	~8 weeks	Plasma cells are present

20 weeks of age. Stable levels are observed after 28 weeks of age (Thrane *et al.*, 1991). The "window" of depletion of these antimicrobial factors immediately after birth may be significant if the infant is exposed to pathogens during this period, when the specific immune system is also incapable of responding with immediate effective defense mechanisms.

Specific immunity

The normal full-term infant is born virtually IgA-deficient. It takes several weeks before GALT responds effectively to antigenic challenge; during this period, the neonate is susceptible to infections. The unresponsiveness of the mucosal immune system is due to the combined effects of hormonal influences during the birthing process, the immaturity of the antigen-presenting cells, and the immunosuppressive effects of maternally derived serum IgG antibodies and colostral S-IgA antibodies (Husband and Gleeson, 1996). A rapid upregulation of HLA-DR expression after birth is consistent with the concept that postnatal exposure to antigen is important in determining the repertoire of immunologically determined epitopes. This upregulation of HLA-DR expression is almost certainly cytokine-driven, suggesting that mucosal T cells and macrophages are competent in achieving this maturation process. Tumor necrosis factor-α and interferon-γ (INF-γ) are known to upregulate HLA molecule expression. Postnatal human mucosal T cells have not been studied in this context, although fetal lamina propria T cells have been reported to secrete interleukin-2 (IL-2) and INF-γ when stimulated with bacterial superantigens (Lionetti *et al.*, 1993). Other studies on fetal intestinal explants (Dohan *et al.*, 1993) have shown that the adhesion molecules ICAM-1, VCAM-1, and E-selection can also be induced by activated T cells in the lamina propria endothelium. Hence, at birth, it is likely that the appropriate endothelial adhesion molecules required to direct phagocyte cells to the intestine are present.

Development of mucosal immunity

Ontogeny

The mucosal immune system is rapidly stimulated at birth by bacterial colonization of the mucosal and external surfaces. The development of effective mucosal immunity is essential for protection against infection and allergen exposure in the postnatal period. This period is characterized by two important components of the neonate's immune development: the closure of mucosal epithelial membranes and the appearance of secretory antibodies.

The immediate postnatal period is characterized by increased intestinal permeability to intact macromolecules (Roberton *et al.*, 1982). Ingestion of colostrum promotes membrane maturation in the gastrointestinal tract, leading to closure within 48 hours of birth (Bines and Walker, 1991). A similar pattern of membrane closure is also observed at other mucosal sites, and the maturation process can be monitored by the disappearance of IgG from saliva (Gleeson *et al.*, 1986, 1995). Rapid closure of membranes is an important process in limiting systemic exposure to antigens, which,

if handled inappropriately, could lead to overwhelming infection, atopy, or subsequent tolerance.

Consistent with stimulation of the mucosal immune system, pIgR expression in the salivary gland and intestinal epithelium increases between 1 to 2 weeks after birth (Hayashi *et al.*, 1989; Thrane *et al.*, 1991). Levels equivalent to those in adults continue to be expressed in the intestinal crypts (Brandzaeg *et al.*, 1991), but the expression of pIgR declines in the salivary glands, to the perinatal level, around 6 months (Hayashi *et al.*, 1989; Thrane *et al.*, 1991). The free extracellular portion of pIgR, secretory component, can be detected in the saliva of newborn infants (Seidel *et al.*, 2001). The availability of pIgR is essential for the transport of S-IgA and S-IgM across the epithelium to external secretions and hence is one of the prerequisites for the development of mucosal defense (mechanism reviewed in Goldblum *et al.*, 1996).

In a healthy neonate the pattern of appearance of antibodies in mucosal secretions is consistent with the rapid population of the neonatal intestine with initially IgM- and then IgA-containing plasma cells (Perkkio and Savilahti, 1980). Although S-IgA has been reported to be present at birth in saliva (Gross and Buckley, 1980; Seidel *et al.*, 2001) and nasal secretions (Roberts and Freed, 1977), most investigators report the first detection of S-IgA in mucosal secretions between 1 week and 2 months of age (Haworth and Dilling, 1966; South *et al.*, 1967; Sellner *et al.*, 1968; Ostergaard and Blom, 1997; Burgio *et al.*, 1980; Hanson *et al.*, 1980; Gleeson *et al.*, 1982; 1986; Mellander *et al.*, 1984).

IgA antibodies secreted at extraintestinal mucosal sites begin to increase during the first few weeks of life (Hanson *et al.*, 1980; Gleeson *et al.*, 1982; 1986; Taylor and Toms, 1984; Cripps *et al.*, 1987; Sennhauser *et al.*, 1990; Smith and Taubman, 1992; Fitzsimmons *et al.*, 1994). Salivary IgA levels increase rapidly in the neonatal period to peak levels between 4 and 6 weeks of age (Gleeson *et al.*, 1986). The initial peak in S-IgA in saliva has been reported to decline to lower levels between 3 and 6 months of age (Burgio *et al.*, 1980; Gahnberg *et al.*, 1985; Gleeson *et al.*, 1986). However, this has not been observed in other studies of ontogeny in the neonate (Mellander *et al.*, 1984; Fitzsimmon *et al.*, 1994). Studies of preterm infants are inconsistent but do demonstrate the readiness of the mucosal immune system by 210 days of gestation. Both Seidel *et al.* (2000) and Kuitunen and Savilahti (1995) report the presence of IgA in saliva early in the neonatal period. Whilst Seidel *et al.* (2000) demonstrated no significant differences in salivary IgA levels between term and preterm infants in the first 9 months of life, Kuitunen and Savilahti (1995) reported significantly lower levels of IgA and cow's milk antibodies in the saliva of preterm infants than in that of full-term infants. Salivary IgA levels remain relatively consistent until exposure to increased antigenic loads, such as when children are hospitalized (Mellander *et al.*, 1984) or when they begin school at 4 to 5 years of age (Gleeson *et al.*, 1987a). Adult levels of S-IgA in saliva are reached around 7 years of age (Burgio *et al.*, 1980; Gleeson *et al.*, 1987a). The inconsistencies reported for the ontogeny patterns of total S-IgA in saliva reflect differences in study populations, frequency of testing, and collection protocols, including the source of saliva. The best indicators of ontogeny of S-IgA come from the longitudinal as opposed to cross-sectional studies, and it must be acknowledged that these are difficult to undertake in human infants.

Ontogeny studies of the IgA subclasses in mucosal secretions are limited, but both IgA subclasses are present in saliva, and the proportions are characteristic of adult saliva by 6 months of age (Smith and Taubman, 1992; Fitzsimmons et al., 1994). The study by Fitzsimmon et al. (1994) indicated that S-IgA1 was the dominant subclass in saliva at birth, that the proportion of S-IgA2 increased linearly to 6 months of age, and that the rate of increase of both total S-IgA concentrations and S-IgA1 and S-IgA2 concentrations was greater in breastfed than formula-fed infants. The high proportion of S-IgA1 in saliva may not necessarily reflect the situation in other mucosal secretions, as the distribution of subclasses in the IgA plasma cells at mucosal sites varies (Brandtzaeg et al., 1986). The ontogeny of plasma cells of IgA subclasses has not been established postnatally in human mucosal tissues, and at present it can only be speculated that the proportions in mucosal secretions are reflecting the plasma cell distributions in these tissues.

The appearance of specific S-IgA antibodies in infants is dependent on the degree of vaccination or natural exposure to antigen. Antibodies to pathogenic organisms such as poliovirus in nonendemic countries will appear only after first vaccination (Smith et al., 1986), and conversely, in endemic countries, the ontogeny patterns indicate the early appearance of mucosal antibodies (Hanson et al., 1987). Another example of these differences is the early appearance of antibodies to Haemophilus influenzae in infants in endemic areas of Papua New Guinea (Clancy et al., 1987).

Recent studies of mucosal responses to Streptococcus pneumoniae in children aged 2 to 24 months have provided some interesting findings on the possible relationships between vaccination, carriage, and specific salivary IgA responses. Two studies have now shown that type-specific salivary IgA antibodies are boosted following secondary systemic immunization with conjugate pneumococcal polysaccharide conjugate vaccines (Nurkka et al., 2001; Choo et al., 2000). These and other studies have led to the suggestion that some antigens may induce mucosal IgA memory when administered systemically. This would certainly appear to be the case for pneumococcus. In unvaccinated children, higher pneumococcal polysaccharide–type antibodies have been found in the saliva of children who carried these types in the nasopharynx or middle ear, prior to sampling, than in the saliva of children who did not (Simell et al., 2002). Further studies are urgently required to determine if these early mucosal responses to natural colonization have any bearing on the poor efficacy of systemic immunization against pneumococcal otitis media.

Antigenic exposure is also important in the ontogeny of S-IgA responses to common enteric organisms. E. coli–specific S-IgA antibodies to E. coli somatic antigens appear in the intestine during the first weeks of life (Lodinova et al., 1973), but in this period very low levels of S-IgA antibodies against

E. coli adhesions are detected (Hanson et al., 1983). Artificial colonization of the intestine of newborns with nonpathogenic E. coli strains stimulated the production of both IgA and IgM antibodies in stool and saliva (Lodinová-Zádníková et al., 1989) and reduced the number of infections and mortality among high-risk infants. In a cohort of normal Australian children, S-IgA antibodies to E. coli O antigen were not detected in saliva until 1 to 2 months of age and gradually increased with age (Gleeson et al., 1987a). Bronchial aspirates from premature neonates showed a similar pattern of appearance of S-IgA anti-E. coli antibodies (Sennhauser et al., 1990). These studies indicate a tightly controlled mucosal immune response to a major colonizing antigen. The studies by Mellander et al. (1984) in a Swedish community revealed higher levels of E. coli antibodies in the saliva of children attending day-care centers or exposed to hospitalization than in children under total home care, suggesting a greater antigenic load or attenuating factors in these environments.

Salivary antibodies to organisms that colonize the oral cavity are also detected by 1 to 2 months of age and increase during the first few years of life (Smith and Taubman, 1992). Salivary IgA antibodies to streptococci, such as Streptococcus sanguis and Streptococcus mutans, generally appear after tooth eruption and the loss of maternally derived antibody to these microbiota (Gahnberg et al., 1985; Alaluusua, 1983).

S-IgM, the other major class of secretory antibodies, is often forgotten (Gleeson et al., 1997) and is not well studied, as S-IgM is not routinely detected in mucosal secretions (Gleeson et al., 1986). S-IgM is absent from saliva at birth in healthy full-term neonates but appears transiently between 1 and 6 months of age (Gleeson et al., 1986; Smith et al., 1989). IgM is occasionally detected in nasopharyngeal secretions in the first week of life but is routinely present at weeks of age (Taylor and Toms, 1984). The concentration of IgM in bronchial washings also increases during the first week of life (Sennhauser et al., 1990). Total salivary IgM (Gleeson et al., 1990) and specific IgM antibodies (Mellander et al., 1984; Smith and Taubman, 1992) are occasionally observed in infants and adults in a pattern consistent with the concept that IgM antibodies in mucosal secretions reflect immune responses to novel antigens presented at mucosal sites, particularly the gastrointestinal tract. S-IgM is usually present in high concentrations in mucosal secretions of IgA-deficient subjects, in whom S-IgM and IgG appear to play a compensatory role (Gleeson et al., 1993; Norhagen et al., 1989; Brandtzaeg et al., 1987; Nilssen et al., 1992).

Markers of immunocompetence

The first 12 months of life appear to be critical for the maturation of the mucosal immune system, and several markers in saliva have been identified to determine mucosal immunocompetence. There is increasing evidence to suggest that the integrity of the mucosal epithelium is an important factor in mucosal immunity. The loss of IgG from mucosal secretions (Gleeson et al., 1986; Taylor and Toms, 1984; Sennhauser et al., 1990) in the immediate postnatal period is indicative of membrane closure. Subsequent detection of IgG in saliva, with the exception of IgA-deficiency states, provides a marker for disrupted epithelial integrity (Gleeson et al., 1995).

The most important attribute for assessing immunocompetence is the ability to produce secretory antibodies. Longitudinal studies in children indicate that, in saliva, the switch from producing monomeric IgA to S-IgA occurs at varying times during the first year of life (Cripps et al., 1989), although a cross-sectional study failed to confirm these findings (Smith et al., 1989). Comparison of the distribution of polymeric IgA and IgA subclasses in serum of infants and adults supports the concept of a maturation process occurring during the first year of life (Conley et al., 1983; Delacroix et al., 1983). The immaturity of the mucosal apparatus is also reflected by the presence of IgD in saliva in a significant proportion of the infant population during the first year of life (Gleeson et al., 1987b; Seidel et al., 2001). For the first 6 months after birth, there is a significant proportion of IgD-producing cells in the salivary glands, at the same time as the rapid increase in IgA immunocytes (Thrane et al., 1991). The loss of IgD and the appearance of S-IgA in saliva, concomitant with the changes in plasma cell populations in the salivary glands over the first year of life, provide two markers of mucosal immunocompetence. The inverse relationship between IgA and IgD in infancy (Gleeson et al., 1987b) and in IgA-deficient subjects (Nilssen et al., 1992) probably reflects the role of IgD in isotype switching and the preferential clonal differentiation to IgA-producing cells at mucosal sites.

In a longitudinal study, with frequent sampling of saliva in the first year of life, transient absences of salivary IgA were observed, and in a follow-up study the absences have been shown to be associated with an increased susceptibility to bronchial hyperactivity, but not asthma, later in life (Gleeson et al., 1996). The transient absences have been shown to have a negative association with atopy, suggesting a hypoimmune mucosal immune response during the maturation period. This hyporesponsiveness in the respiratory tract appears to be associated with defective antigen processing by the local dendritic cells (Nelson and Holt, 1995) and is another indicator that the mucosal immune system undergoes a maturation process in the first year of life. Factors that influence the development of mucosal immunity are discussed in the next sections.

Although it has not been demonstrated in humans, it is also likely that the passive acquisition of maternal antibodies in colostrum has the same suppressive effect on the development of specific immune responses in the neonate as that observed in animals (Kramer and Cebra, 1995). The delay in appearance of IgA in the saliva of breastfed infants, observed by Gleeson et al. (1986), is consistent with this concept. However, a study by Fitzsimmon et al. (1994) indicated a greater rate of increase of S-IgA in saliva of breastfed infants.

Factors that affect mucosal immune development
Feeding practices early in life
The role of infant feeding practices in the development of mucosal immunity cannot be underestimated. Human colostrum not only provides the newborn infant with optimal nutrition but also confers passive protection and maturational factors. There are significant associations between neonatal feeding patterns and mucosal immunological maturation and long-term health outcomes.

Infant feeding regimens are an important determinant of the maturation of the mucosal immune system. Oral feeding per se provides a stimulus for mucosal immune development. Intravenously fed full-term infants are devoid of IgA- and IgM-containing plasma cells in the gut lamina propria at an age when infants receiving oral feeds have normal numbers of immunocytes (Knox, 1986). This delayed immune development in intravenously fed infants reflects the lack of immune stimulation by food or bacterial antigens. The initial bacterial colonization patterns in the gastrointestinal tract differ between breast- and formula-fed infants (Bullen and Tearle, 1976); hence, so do the degree and nature of antigenic stimulation of the mucosal immune system.

Colostrum deprivation has been shown to delay closure of mucosal membranes (Bines and Walker, 1991; Gleeson et al., 1986). This protracted period of increased membrane permeability may contribute to the higher incidence of infections (Fergusson et al., 1981; Myers et al., 1984; Forman et al., 1984; Goldblum et al., 1996) and atopic disease (Fallstrom et al., 1984) observed in non-breastfed infants. A factor in colostrum that suppresses IgE synthesis may also contribute to the lower risk of atopy in breastfed neonates (Sarfati et al., 1986).

Maternally acquired immunity is essential for survival in the neonatal period until endogenous immunity develops. However, the presence of exogenous antibodies acquired prenatally by transplacental transfer or postnatally via colostrum has a suppressive effect on the development of mucosal immune responses. In animal models the presence of maternal IgA in milk delays the onset of maturation of the mucosal immune system (Beh et al., 1974; Kramer and Cebra, 1995). In human studies, the data on the potential immunosuppressive effect of colostral IgA are conflicting. In humans, ingestion of colostrum has been reported to delay the appearance of IgA and IgM in saliva of totally breastfed infants in the first 3 months of life (Gleeson et al., 1986). These observations were later confirmed by Avanzini et al. (1992), who reported significantly lower levels of salivary IgA in breastfed children in the first months of life. However, Fitzsimmons et al. (1994) reported a more rapid increase in salivary IgA over the first 6 months in breastfed infants than in formula-fed infants. With the current interest in oral tolerance, it is important to clarify whether breast-feeding delays activation of the mucosal immune system in the perinatal period during membrane maturation and affords protection from systemic tolerance.

Breast-feeding
Whether or not colostrum has an immunosuppressive effect in the perinatal period on the initial appearance of S-IgA and S-IgM, breast-feeding has been shown to enhance vaccine responses. Breast-feeding enhances the secretory antibody

responses to parental and oral vaccines (Hahn-Zoric et al., 1990), with infants showing significantly higher salivary S-IgA and stool IgA1 responses to tetanus toxoid and poliovirus. The long-term influence of breast-feeding on immune development and health outcomes is now becoming evident. The enhanced immune response to vaccines is also observed in older children (Hahn-Zoric et al., 1990; Pabst et al., 1989; Pabst and Spady, 1990), and breastfed infants have long-term protection against H. influenzae infection (reviewed by Hanson et al., 1997). Breastfed infants also produce higher levels of total S-IgA in urine than do formula-fed infants (Goldblum et al., 1989).

The induction of immunological tolerance, by the transfer of immunocytes in breast milk, may also explain the protective long-term effect of breast-feeding on the decreased risk of developing autoimmune type 1 diabetes (Dosch et al., 1993), atopic dermatitis (Sigurs et al., 1992), lymphomas (Davis et al., 1988), and Crohn's disease (Koletzko et al., 1989), as well as the improved survival of maternal renal transplants (Campbell et al., 1984). This evidence suggests that the initial handling of antigens by the mucosal immune system in the gut is critical in the development of effective immunity and subsequent immune responses. The modifying effect of breast milk is important not only in determining protective immunity but also in reducing adverse immune responses, resulting in atopy and autoimmune and lymphoproliferative disorders.

Nutrition and diet

Impairment of systemic immune responses in children small for gestational age has been well described (Chandra, 1992), but studies of the effect on mucosal immunity are lacking. However, because children born below 80% weight for age who have increased infections also have fewer Ig-producing cells and lower amounts of Ig secreted (Chandra, 1992), it could be assumed that the ontogeny of mucosal immunity will also be compromised. The effect of nutritional status on the ontogeny of mucosal IgA responses has been examined in a cross-sectional study of Papua New Guinea children (Clancy et al., 1987; Cripps et al., 1991). The total level of salivary IgA and the specific IgA responses to E. coli and H. influenzae were lower in children below 80% weight for age. The immunological abnormalities resulting from intrauterine malnutrition persist for several months after birth (Puri and Chandra, 1985), at a time when the mucosal immune system is maximally challenged and maturing.

The risk of undernourishment is heightened in children who are not totally breastfed. As well as providing less than optimum nutrition, non-breastfed infants have increased risks of infection, particularly diarrhea, adding to the complication of undernutrition. One of the consequences of the poor nutrition associated with frequent diarrhea is vitamin A deficiency (Hanson et al., 1997). In rats, vitamin A deficiency results in a 90% reduction in intestinal S-IgA responses to oral cholera vaccine (Wiederman et al., 1993).

The outcome of pilot studies of vitamin A supplementation via breast milk will be of interest (Hanson et al., 1997). In a comparison of British and West African children (the latter having considerably lower nutritional and hygiene status), there was no significant difference in the IgA output in intestinal secretions of well children (Croft et al., 1997). However, during infections, the secretion rates of intestinal IgA and IgM were increased in the West African children with acute watery diarrhea.

Malnutrition during the immediate postnatal period may impair an already immature immune system and further compromise host resistance to infection by reducing the availability of essential vitamins and trace minerals (Schlesinger and Uauy, 1991). Protein malnutrition is associated with decreased IgA responses to oral antigens (McGee and McMurray, 1988) and an increase in eye infections associated with decreased ocular IgA responses (Sullivan et al., 1993). Mild malnutrition reduces the IgA response to dietary antigens but has little effect on the response to common enteric pathogens (Nagao et al., 1995). Even temporary dietary inadequacies, such as fasting for several days, can have subtle effects on mucosal function and potentially mucosal immunity (Ottaway and Husband, 1994).

A study of caloric supplementation of undernourished Guatemalan mothers concluded that moderate undernutrition did not impair the levels of S-IgA in milk (Herias et al., 1993). However, the S-IgA levels and daily output were decreased in low-caloric compared with high-caloric supplementation and prevented the deterioration of milk S-IgA output. These findings emphasize the importance of breast-feeding, even by undernourished mothers, as a source of passive mucosal protection for the neonate and the prevention of infections in infancy.

Maternal factors

In addition to the role of maternal antibodies in the maturation of mucosal immunity in the offspring, there is some evidence to suggest that maternal emotional stress may reduce immune defenses in the neonate (Groer et al., 1994) through the transfer of maternal corticosteroids via breast milk. However, the data from this study, showing an inverse correlation between cortisol levels in maternal milk and S-IgA levels in term infants, were not conclusive, as preterm mothers had positive correlations of anger and vigor with S-IgA levels in milk. The endogenous production of stress hormones around the time of birth may also result in immunosuppression. There are few reports on the effects of maternal stress or toxins on the development of mucosal immunity in humans. Many of the conclusions must be inferred from animal models and known effects on systemic immunity.

Exposure during pregnancy to toxic chemicals that cross the placenta can result in developmental disorders, causing immune suppression (Halliday et al., 1994). Maternal ethanol consumption impairs in utero development of immunity and postnatally modulates proliferation responses (Taylor et al., 1993) and cytokine production by rat milk cells (Na and Seelig, 1994). Maternal smoking is also associated with impaired gastrointestinal function (Cryer et al., 1992) and lower salivary IgA levels (Barton et al., 1990). The lower levels of S-IgA in mothers who smoke and are breast-feeding will lead to reduced passive protection in the neonate; this may account, in part, for the increased respiratory morbidity and atopy in exposed children (Di Benedetto, 1995; Bakoula et al., 1995). Each of these toxins will impact on the development of effective mucosal immunity in children and may determine many of the clinical outcomes in later life.

Infection

The development of mucosal immunity is profoundly effected by exposure to infections. The degree of antigenic exposure determines the ontogeny patterns for mucosal antibodies. As expected, in countries with lower standards of hygiene and health, mucosal antibodies appear in children earlier and at higher levels than in developed countries (Hanson et al., 1986; Cripps et al., 1991). Even in developed countries, increased antigenic exposure of infants through hospitalization or daycare attendance results in high levels of antibodies in saliva (Mellander et al., 1984). The same development pattern was also observed in older children following first attendance at school (Gleeson et al., 1987a), which again is a period of high exposure to novel antigens and greater antigenic burden. In a longitudinal study of children aged 3.5 to 5 years attending preschool, high levels of salivary IgA were correlated with the incidence of upper respiratory tract infection systems and low ambient air temperatures (Cripps et al., unpublished observations). Children with cystic fibrosis, who have significantly higher rates of mucosal infection, have higher intestinal output of S-IgA than do well children (Croft et al., 1997).

Respiratory infections in early life can also cause immune dysregulation and have been associated with sudden infant death syndrome (Thrane et al., 1990; Stoltenberg et al., 1992; Gleeson et al., 1993) and the induction of IgA deficiency (Gleeson et al., 1994). Respiratory infections during the periods of transient IgA deficiency in the first year of life may also be a cause of the subsequent increased bronchial hyperreactivity observed in these children (Gleeson et al., 1996).

Factors that influence mucosal immunocompetence at birth and markers of mucosal immunocompetence in the neonate are presented in **Tables 16.3** and **16.4**.

AGING

Aged individuals are more susceptible to infections at mucosal sites such as the respiratory tract (Dhar et al., 1976; Verghese and Berk, 1983; Ershler et al., 1984; Smith, 1985), the gastrointestinal tract (Schmucker and Daniels, 1986), and the urinary tract (Yoshikawa, 1983). In the eye, bacterial colonization increases with age in the conjunctival sac (McClellan et al., 1997). Increased disease susceptibility is most likely to be multifactorial and to include factors such as nutritional deficiencies, poor hygiene, stress, greater exposure to pathogens in hospitals and care facilities for the aged, and generally poorer living conditions, as well as a decline in mucosal immunocompetence. However, at this stage, few studies have been conducted that assess mucosal immunocompetence with age in humans. Hence, a causal

Table 16.3. Factors Influencing Immunocompetence in the Human Neonate at the Time of Birth

Factor	Effects
Interuterine toxicity	Toxic chemicals, including smoking and ethanol consumption, cause immune suppression in the neonate
Interuterine infection and immunization	Activates mucosal immune mechanisms in utero and can have adverse (infection) or beneficial (preimmunization) effects in the neonate
Gestation	Maternally acquired passive immunity is reduced in preterm infants
Endogenous hormones	Corticosteroids released at the time of birth and in colostrum may be immunosuppressive in the neonate
Nutritional status	Malnutrition during pregnancy impairs immune responses in the neonate
	Protein malnutrition and vitamin A deficiency are both associated with reduced SIgA responses in the neonate
Feeding practices	Colostrum deprivation will delay maturation of mucosal membranes and increase the risk of infection and atopy
	Colostrum may delay maturation of specific mucosal antibody responses in the neonate
Innate defenses	Antimicrobial actions are compromised by a temporary fall in salivary amylase, lysozyme, and lactoferrin in the neonate during the birthing process
Postnatal infection	Mucosal antibodies appear earlier in neonates exposed to high antigenic loads
	Early infections are a cause of increased mortality and may be a cause of immune dysregulation in the neonate
Mucosal immune system	The mucosal immune apparatus is in place prior to birth but not activated until postnatal antigenic stimulation occurs
	The immaturity results in a "window" of impaired effective immune defense

Table 16.4. Markers of Mucosal Immunocompetence in the Human Neonate

Mucosal Immunocompetence	Maturation Markers
Mucosal membrane maturation	The loss of IgG from mucosal secretions is indicative of mucosal membrane closure after birth
	Permeability studies can confirm epithelial integrity
Production of secretory antibodies	The appearance of S-IgA in mucosal secretions is indicative of maturation of mucosal immunity
	The loss of IgD from secretions and IgD-positive immunocytes at mucosal sites is indicative of the referential switch to IgA-producing B cells at mucosal sites
Specific immune response	The appearance of specific S-IgA or S-IgM antibodies in response to infection or vaccination indicates effective mucosal immunity
Innate defense	Adequate levels of antimicrobial agents in mucosal secretions (e.g., lactoferrin, lysozyme) ensure appropriate defense mechanisms at mucosal surfaces

relationship between decline in mucosal immune function and infection has not been established.

Nutritional inadequacy in aged persons is widespread, and a causal relationship between infection and malnutrition is now well recognized. Nutritional deficiencies have also been associated with less-than-optimal mucosal immune function. Hence, in the elderly, environmental factors may be the major contributing factors leading to increased susceptibility to infection. Further studies are required to examine the importance of age-related mucosal immune dysfunction, given that the human ileal Peyer's patches regress with age (Cornes, 1965). However, in animal studies, despite some age-related changes in T-cell phenotypes, in contrast to systemic immunity, current evidence indicates that there is little impairment of mucosal immune function, with the stem cell, B-cell, and T-cell compartments retaining their ability to function normally in the aged animal (Wade and Szewczuk, 1984, 1987). For example, in mice, mesenteric lymph node responses to antigens such as tri-nitro-phenol (TNP)–bacillus Calmette-Guerin (Szewczuk *et al.*, 1981), the α(1–3) glucan determinant on dextran B1355 (Rivier *et al.*, 1983), and TNP-keyhole limpet hemocyanin (KLH) (Wade and Szewczuk, 1984) are unaffected by age.

The most significant observation in aged animals is that antigen-specific B cell responses to cholera toxin at mucosal effector sites are lower than in healthy adults (Fujihashi *et al.*, 2000). This could be as a result of altered T cell regulatory mechanisms as well as homing deficiencies of IgA+ immunoblasts from mucosal induction sites (Schmucker, 2002). Whilst there is some suggestion that CD4+ T helper cell function declines earlier in the mucosal immune system of mice than does the systemic compartment (Koga *et al.*, 2000), further studies are necessary to confirm these observations and to determine the extent of the age-related deficiency with respect to antigens other than cholera toxin.

Studies in humans suggest that there is no impairment of antibody-mediated immunity in adulthood (Smith *et al.*, 1992; Ganguly, 1987; Gleeson *et al.*, 1990; Russell *et al.*, 1990b; Doshi and Barton, 1997; McClellan *et al.*, 1997).

Studies of human saliva have not detected major differences in total Ig levels between elderly subjects and younger adults (Ganguly, 1987; Russell *et al.*, 1990b), although this may be gland-determined, and the overall levels of immunoglobulin in saliva are determined by the relative flow rates. For example, Smith *et al.* (1992) showed a significant age-related decline in the output of IgA from the lower labial glands but not the parotid glands. Total salivary IgA1 and IgA2 levels have been reported to be higher in elderly subjects than in younger adults, and this was reflected in higher specific-antibody levels against some antigens, particularly *Streptococcus mutans* surface protein antigen and pneumococcal polysaccharide type 23 (Russell *et al.*, 1990b). In the eye, the levels of total IgA and IgA *H. influenzae*–specific antibodies in tears increase with age (McClellan *et al.*, 1997). The level of IgA in gastric juice does not change with age, whereas the level of urinary IgA has been reported to decrease with age (Doshi and Barton 1997). At this stage, a causal link between lower levels of IgA in the urinary tract and increased urinary tract infections in the elderly has not been established.

Studies on innate immune mechanisms in the elderly have been limited to lysozyme. In healthy elderly subjects, the level of salivary lysozyme is reduced (Ganguly, 1987). In elderly patients with chronic bronchitis, an association has been drawn between infection and the level of salivary lysozyme (Taylor *et al.*, 1992). Patients who were prone to acute respiratory infections had significantly lower levels of salivary lysozyme than did patients who were not prone to infection. The level of lysozyme in tears has also been reported to fall with increasing age (Pietsch and Pearlman, 1973; McGill *et al.*, 1984; McClellan *et al.*, 1997). Bacterial colonization of the conjunctival sac increases with age, and it has been hypothesized that this is a result of reduced innate defenses in the eye (McClellan *et al.*, 1997). However, the increase in specific IgA antibodies observed in tears with age may protect the eye against infection despite impaired innate mechanisms. Studies of lysozyme levels in mucosal secretions suggest that innate mucosal immune defenses may decline with age. Certainly, lower lysozyme levels in mucosal secretions would reduce both the opsonic and bactericidal capacity of these secretions. The effect of aging on other innate immune mechanisms at the mucosal level requires examination.

The data currently available suggest that in the healthy human, acquired mucosal immune function is maintained with age, although there may be some loss of innate defense mechanisms such as lysozyme or secondary to anatomical and physiological changes. This is in contrast to the systemic immune mechanisms and raises the possibility of utilizing mucosal immunization for vaccination of elderly populations to provide immune protection at the mucosal level or to boost systemic immunity against infections such as influenza, bacterial pneumonia, *Helicobacter pylori*, or malignant disease, which are significant causes of morbidity and mortality in the elderly. In this context, the coadministration of a live attenuated influenza A virus vaccine intranasally with an inactivated vaccine intramuscularly significantly enhanced IgA antibody responses in nasal washings of elderly subjects (Gorse *et al.*, 1996). However, if a choice has to be made, intranasal administration induces better mucosal IgA antibody responses (Muszkat *et al.*, 2000).

The increased incidence of infection observed in elderly persons is most likely to be associated with the "aged environment" and its interaction with immune mechanisms as well as increased exposure to potential pathogens. It is well established that many environmental factors can alter mucosal immunocompetence throughout life (Gleeson *et al.*, 1995; Cripps *et al.*, 1997). **Table 16.5** summarizes the effect of aging on mucosal immune parameters.

ASSOCIATION OF ONTOGENY PROFILES WITH DISEASE

Recent studies have focused on whether or not the profiles of mucosal immune parameters can be used to predict disease outcomes or to identify subjects who are at risk of infection or disease.

The salivary IgA levels in infants born to atopic parents have been studied (Van Asperen *et al.*, 1985). There was a significantly higher prevalence of transitory salivary IgA deficiency in infants aged 4 to 20 months born to atopic parents, and total salivary IgA levels were significantly lower at 8 and 12 months of age than in infants of nonatopic parents. However, in those infants born to atopic parents who developed atopic disease, there was no greater prevalence of IgA deficiency than in infants born to nonatopic parents, even though total salivary IgA levels were significantly lower at 4 months of age. These observations suggest that mucosal IgA deficiency early in life could lead to the development of atopic disease (Van Asperen *et al.*, 1985), possibly by failure of antigen exclusion (Taylor *et al.*, 1973). However, the failure to correlate transient salivary IgA deficiency with the development of atopy in infancy and the fact that not all IgA-deficient adults (reportedly 5% to 58%) develop atopy strongly argue against a causal association (Van Asperen *et al.*, 1985). Consistent with these findings, the incidence of transient salivary IgA deficiency in the first year of life was found to be associated with bronchial hyperreactivity but not atopy (Gleeson *et al.*, 1996), although there is no apparent association between salivary IgA levels and wheezing (Hoelzer *et al.*, 2002).

IgA deficiency is the most common variant of immunodeficiency, with an incidence of approximately 1 per 700 in the population (Hanson *et al.*, 1983). In a prospective study of the ontogeny of the mucosal immune system in which salivary Ig levels were monitored (Gleeson *et al.*, 1994), one child with a family history of organ-specific autoimmune disease developed IgA deficiency at 3.5 years of age. The acquired IgA deficiency was associated with two recent episodes of acute respiratory infections and significantly elevated salivary IgM levels. In the same prospective study, an infant died of sudden infant death syndrome (SIDS) at 10 weeks of age, following a mild upper respiratory tract infection at 3.5 weeks (Gleeson *et al.*, 1993). The levels of salivary IgA and IgM continued to increase following the infection episode; the level of salivary IgM was 10 times the age-related median

Table 16.5. Effect of Aging on Mucosal Immune Parameters in Humans

Mucosal Secretion	Parameter	Outcome
Saliva	Total IgA, IgA1, IgA2	Increased (may be gland-dependent)
	Other immunoglobulin isotopes	No change
	IgA-specific antibody	No change or increased; antigen-dependent
	Lysozyme	Decreased, associated with proneness to respiratory infections in subjects with chronic bronchitis
Tears	Total IgA	Increased
	IgA-specific antibody	No change or increased; antigen-dependent
	Lysozyme	Decreased; may be related to increased bacterial colonization of the conjunctival sac
Gastric juice	Total IgA	No change
Urine	Total IgA	Decreased

level just prior to death. More recently, elevated salivary IgA and IgM levels have also been observed in infants admitted to the hospital because of acute life-threatening events suspected of being "near-miss SIDS" (Gleeson *et al.*, unpublished observations). These studies suggest an association between upper respiratory infections and the induction of immune disorders at mucosal surfaces and the potential diagnostic role for measurement of salivary immunoglobulins for predicting mucosal immune dysfunction.

In this context, salivary IgA has been shown to be a useful diagnostic marker for monitoring exercise-induced mucosal immunosuppression in high-performance athletes (Gleeson and Pyne, 2000). Low levels of salivary IgA are associated with an increased risk of upper respiratory illness (Gleeson *et al.*, 1999) and have also been used as an indication for overtraining (Mackinnon and Hooper, 1994). The mucosal response to exercise has demonstrated a consistent pattern across age groups, from young children (Dorrington and Gleeson, unpublished observations) to the elderly (Akimoto *et al.*, 2003), showing increases in salivary IgA with moderate exercise and significant decreases after maximal exercise training (Williams *et al.*, 2001).

S-IgA has also been used to monitor responses to psychological stressors, which results in enhanced IgA levels (Hucklebridge *et al.*, 2000; Reid *et al.*, 2001), while chronic stressors induce suppression of salivary IgA (McClelland, 1989). The lower levels of salivary IgA following chronic stress have also been associated with an increased incidence of upper respiratory illness (Jemmott and McClelland, 1989).

There is now good evidence that S-IgA has a protective role against the development of allergy. Böttcher and colleagues (Böttcher *et al.*, 2002) recently reported that children who were skin prick test–positive to either cat allergen

(Fel d 1) or β-lactoglobulin and developed allergic symptoms had lower levels of S-IgA in their saliva than children who did not develop allergy.

Interactions occur between the mucosal immune system and a range of other factors in addition to those already discussed in this chapter; these include climate, pollution, sleep deprivation, obesity, and immunological stress associated with antigen load (Gleeson *et al.*, 1995; Cripps *et al.*, 1997, Pallaro *et al.*, 2002). How these factors interact with the mucosal immune compartment is complex. Little is known about how they might modify immune profiles of ontogeny and aging or disease susceptibility. However, it has been reported that an infective insult can result in impaired immunoglobulin gene regulation, rendering a child IgA-deficient in the early states of ontogeny (Gleeson *et al.*, 1994). Systematic studies are required to enhance our understanding of these associations and their impact on the efficacy of vaccines or other therapeutic interventions. Factors that have the potential to modify immune profiles of ontogeny and aging are presented in **Table 16.6**.

CONCLUSIONS

Anatomically, the human mucosal immune system begins to develop early in gestation. Components of the system can be histologically recognized as early as 40 days of gestation. The system continues to develop throughout fetal life and into early childhood. At birth all the essential components of the mucosal immune system are present and have the potential to respond to antigenic stimulation. The development of effective mucosal immunity essentially occurs in the postnatal period. After birth the ontogeny of mucosal immunity is

Table 16.6. Factors that Modify Mucosal Immune Parameters and Have the Potential to Alter Ontogeny and Aging Immune Profiles (Age Groups of Reported Research Indicated)

Factor	Modification
Protein-caloric malnutrition	Reduced levels of S-IgA in nasal washings: children
Obesity	Suppressed salivary IgA levels in children 6–13 years old
Infections	Downregulation of IgA responses by some infections. Potential induction of IgA deficiencies: children
Moderate exercise	Enhanced mucosal immunity: all ages
High-intensity exercise	Suppressed salivary IgA responses: all ages and particularly smaller, prepubertal children
Acute psychological stress	Increased salivary IgA responses: adolescents, adults, and elderly
Chronic psychological stress	Suppressed salivary IgA responses: adolescents, adults, and elderly
Sleep deprivation	Impaired salivary IgA and IgM responses to oral vaccination: adults
Climate	Suppressed salivary IgA and enhanced salivary IgM responses associated with reduced daylight hours: adults
Cigarette smoking	Reduced levels of S-IgA in bronchoalveolar lavage fluids. Decreased levels of salivary IgA levels: adult smokers
Passive cigarette exposure	Enhanced levels of salivary IgA: children from birth to age 1 year

influenced by a number of factors, including neonatal feeding practices, nutrition and diet, vaccination, and exposure to infection, as well as maternal factors that occurred *in utero* and postnatally. Events during the first year of life determine the development of mucosal immunity, and links between ontogeny profiles and clinical disease are emerging. Salivary IgA and IgM levels and the incidence of transient salivary IgA deficiency in ontogeny have potential diagnostic value in predicting disease outcomes. In the elderly the acquired mucosal immune system remains competent; however, some loss of innate defenses occurs, such as decreased lysozyme levels in secretions and diminished function secondary to the physiological changes of aging. It appears that increased susceptibility to infection in the aged is primarily a consequence of environmental factors and declining systemic immunity.

ACKNOWLEDGMENT

The authors gratefully acknowledge the secretarial assistance of Diane Williamson.

REFERENCES

Akimoto, T., Kumai, Y., Akama, T., Hayashi, E., Murakami, H., Soma, R., Kuno, S., and Kono I. (2003). Effects of 12 months of exercise training on salivary secretory IgA levels in elderly subjects. *Br. J. Sports Med.* 37, 76–79.

Alaluusua, S. (1983). Longitudinal study of salivary IgA in children from 1 to 4 years old with reference to dental caries. *Scand. J. Dent. Res.* 91, 163–168.

Avanzini, M.A., Plebani, A., Monafo, V., Pasinetti, G., Teani, M., Colombo, A., Mellander, L., Carlsson, B., Hanson L.Å., Ugazio, A.G., and Burgio, G R. (1992). A comparison of secretory antibodies in breast-fed and formula-fed infants over the first six months of life. *Acta Paediatr.* 81, 296–301.

Bakoula, C.G., Kafritsa, Y.J., Kavadias, G.D., Lazopoulou, D.D., Theodoridou, M.C., Marvalius, K.P., and Matsaniotis, N.S. (1995). Objective passive smoking indicators and respiratory morbidity in young children. *Lancet* 346, 280–281.

Barton, J.R., Riad, M.A., Gaze, M.N., Maran, A.G., and Ferguson, A. (1990). Mucosal immunodeficiency in smokers, and in patients with epithelial head and neck tumours. *Gut* 31, 378–382.

Beh, K.J., Watson, D.L., and Lascelles, A.K. (1974). Concentrations of immunoglobulins and albumin in lymph collected from various regions of the body of sheep. *Aust. J. Exp. Biol. Med. Sci.* 52, 81–86.

Bienenstock, J., and Befus, A.D. (1980). Mucosal immunology. *Immunology* 41, 249–270.

Bines, J.E., and Walker, W.A. (1991). Growth factors and the development of neonatal host defence. *Adv. Exp. Med. Biol.* 310, 31–39.

Bjerke, K., and Brandtzaeg, P. (1986). Immunoglobulin- and J chain-producing cells associated with lymphoid follicles in the human appendix, colon and ileum. including Peyer's patches. *Clin. Exp. Immunol.* 64, 432–441.

Blannin, A.K., Robson, P.J., Walsh, N.P., Clark, A.M., Glennon, L, and Gleeson, M (1998). The effect of exercising to exhaustion at different intensities on saliva immunoglobulin A, protein and electrolyte secretion. *Int. J. Sports Med.* 19, 547–552.

Böttcher, M.F., Häggström, P., Björkstén, B., and Jenmalm, M.C. (2002). Total and allergen-specific immunoglobulin A levels in saliva in relation to the development of allergy in infants up to 2 years of age. *Clin. Exp. Allergy* 32, 1293–1298.

Brandtzaeg, P., Karlsson, C., Hansson, G., Petruson, B., Björkander, J., and Hanson, L.Å. (1987). The clinical condition of IgA-deficient patients is related to the proportion of IgD- and IgM-producing cells in the nasal mucosa. *Clin. Exp. Immunol.* 67, 626–636.

Brandtzaeg, P., Kelt, K., Rognum, T. O., Söderstrom, R., Björkander, J., Söderstrom, T., Petruson, B., and Hanson, L.Å. (1986). Distribution of mucosal IgA and IgG subclass-producing immunocytes and alterations in various disorders. *Monogr. Allergy* 20, 179–194.

Brandtzaeg, P., Nilssen, D.E., Rognum, T.O., and Thrane, P.S. (1991). Ontogeny of the mucosal immune system and IgA deficiency. *Gastroenterol. Clin. North. Am.* 20, 397–439.

Bridges, R.A., Condie, R.M., Zak, S.J., and Good, R.A. (1959). The morphologic basis of antibody formation development during the neonatal period. *J. Lab. Clin. Med.* 53, 331–357.

Bullen, C.L., and Tearle, P.V. (1976). Bifidobacteria in the intestinal tract of infants: an *in vitro* study. *J. Med. Microbiol.* 9, 335–344.

Burgio, G.R., Lanzavecchia, A., Plebani, A., Jayakar, S., and Ugazio, A.G. (1980). Ontogeny of secretory immunity: levels of secretory IgA and natural antibodies in saliva. *Pediatr. Res.* 14, 1111–1114.

Campbell, D.A., Lorber, M.I., Sweeten, J.C., Turcoite, J.C., Niederhuber, J., and Beer, A.E. (1984). Breast-feeding and maternal-donor renal allografts. *Transplantation* 37, 340–344.

Cerf-Bensussan. N., and Guy-Grand, N. (1991). Intestinal intraepithelial lymphocytes. *Gastroenterol. Clin. North. Am.* 20, 549–576.

Chandra, R. (1992). Nutritional immunology comes of age. In *Nutrition and Immunology*, 3–4. ARTS Biomedical, St. Johns, Newfoundland, Canada.

Choo, S., Zhang, Q., Seymour, L., Akhtar, S., and Finn, A. (2000). Primary and booster salivary antibody responses to a 7-valent pneumococcal conjugate vaccine in infants. *J. Infect. Dis.* 182, 1260–1263.

Clancy, R.L., Cripps, A.W., Yeung, S., Standish-White, S., Pang, G., Gratten, H.. Koki, G., Smith D., and Alpers, M. (1987). Salivary and serum antibody responses to *Haemophilus influenzae* infection in Papua New Guinea. *Papua New Guinea Med. J.* 30, 271–274.

Conley, M.E., Arbeter, A., and Douglas, S.D. (1983). Serum levels of IgA1 and IgA2 in children and in patients with IgA deficiency. *Mol. Immunol.* 20, 977–981.

Cornes, J.S. (1965). Number, size and distribution of Peyer's patches in the human small intestine. *Gut* 6, 225.

Crago, S.S., Kulhavy, R., Prince, S.J., and Mestecky, J. (1978). Secretory component on epithelial cells is a surface receptor for polymeric immunoglobulins. *J. Exp. Med.* 147, 1832–1837.

Cripps, A.W., Clancy, R.L., Gleeson, M., Hensley, M.J., Dobson, A.J., Firman, D.W., Wlodarcyk, J., and Pang, G.T. (1987). Mucosal immunocompetence in man—the first five years. *Adv. Exp. Med. Biol.* 216B, 1369–1396.

Cripps, A.W., Gleeson, M., and Clancy, R.L. (1989). Molecular characteristics of IgA in infant saliva. *Scand. J. Immunol.* 29, 317–324.

Cripps, A.W., Gleeson, M., and Clancy, R.L. (1991). Ontogeny of the mucosal immune response in children. *Adv. Exp. Med. Biol.* 310, 87–91.

Cripps, A.W., Gleeson, M., Ewing, T., and Horn, P. (1997). Environmental influences on the mucosal immune system. In *Mucosal Solutions: Advances in Mucosal Immunology* (eds. A. J. Husband, K. W. Beagley, R. L. Clancy, A. M. Collins, A. W. Cripps, and D. L. Emery), vol. 2, 3–16. Sydney, Australia: University of Sydney Press.

Croft, N.M., Marshall, T.G., Hodges, M., Ferguson A., and Kabba, L.H. (1997). Intestinal secretion rates of immunoglobulins A and M in British and African children. *Immunol. Cell Biol.* 75 (Suppl. 1), A61.

Cryer, B., Lee, E., and Feldman, M. (1992). Factors influencing gastroduodenal mucosal prostaglandin concentrations: roles of smoking and aging. *Ann. Intern. Med.* 116, 636–640.

Davis, D.J. (1912). On plasma cells in the tonsils. *J. Infect. Dis.* 10, 142–161.

Davis, M.K., Savitz, D.A., and Graurford B. (1988). Infant feeding in childhood. *Lancet* ii, 365–368.

Delacroix, D.L., Liroux, E., and Vaerman, J.-P. (1983). High proportion of polymeric IgA in young infants' sera and independence between IgA-size and IgA-subclass distributions. *J. Clin. Immunol.* 3, 51–56.

Dhar, S., Shastri, S.R., and Lenora, R.A.K. (1976). Aging and the respiratory system. *Med. Clin. North Am.* 60, 1121–1139.

Di Benedetto, G. (1995). Passive smoking in childhood. *J. Royal Soc. Health* 115, 13–16.

Dohan, A., MacDonald, T.T., and Spencer, J. (1993). The ontogeny of adhesion molecule expression in the human intestine. *Clin. Exp. Immunol.* 91, 532–537.

Dosch, H.M., Martin, J.M., Bobinson, B.H., Akerblom, H.K., and Karjalainen, J. (1993). An immune basis for disproportionate diabetes risks in children with a type I diabetic mother or father. *Diabetes Care* 16, 949–951.

Doshi, M.K., and Barton, J.R. (1997). Effect of aging on human secretory immunity. *Immunol. Cell Biol.* 75 (Suppl. 1), A54.

Effros, R.B., and Walford, R.L. (1987). Infection and immunity in relating to aging. In *Aging and the Immune Response. Cellular and Humoral Aspect*, 45–65. New York: Marcel Dekker.

Ershler, W.V., Moore, A.L., and Socinski, M.A. (1984). Influenza and aging: age related changes and the effects of thymosin on the antibody response to influenza vaccine. *J. Clin. Immunol.* 4, 445.

Fallstrom, S.P., Ahlstedt, S., Carlsson, B., Wettergren, B., and Hanson, L.Å. (1984). Influence of breast feeding on the development of cow's milk protein antibodies and the IgE level. *Int. Arch. Allergy. Appl. Immunol.* 75, 87–91.

Fergusson, D.M., Horwood, L.J., Shannon, F.T., and Taylor, B. (1981). Breast-feeding, gastrointestinal and lower respiratory illness in the first two years. *Aust. Paediatr. J.* 17, 191–195.

Fitzsimmons, S.P., Evans, M.K., Pearce, C.L., Sheridan, M.J., Wientzen, R., and Cole, M.F. (1994). Immunoglobulin A subclasses in infants' saliva and in saliva and milk from their mothers. *J. Pediatr.* 124, 566–573.

Forman, M.R., Graubard, B.I., Hoffman, H.J., Beren, R., Harley, E.E., and Bennett, P. (1984). The Pima infant feeding study: breast-feeding and respiratory infections during the first year of life. *Int. J. Epidemiol.* 13, 447–453.

Fujihashi, K., Koga, T., and McGhee J.R. (2000). Mucosal vaccination and immune responses in the elderly. *Vaccine* 18, 1675–1680.

Gahnberg, L., Smith. D.J., Taubman, M.A., and Ebersole, J.L. (1985). Salivary IgA antibody to glucosyltransferase of oral microbial origin in children. *Arch. Oral Biol.* 30, 551–556.

Ganguly, R (1987). Oropharyngeal tract host defences in aging. *Adv. Exp. Med. Biol.* 216B, 1409–1416.

Gardner, I.D. (1980). The effect of aging on susceptibility to infection. *Rev. Infect. Dis.* 2, 801–810.

Gebbers, J-O., and Laissue, J.A. (1990). Postnatal immunomorphology of the gut. In *Inflammatory Bowel Disease and Coeliac Disease in Children* (eds. F. Hadziselimovic, B. Herzog, A. Burgin-Wolff), 3–44. Dordrecht: Kluwer Academic Publishers.

Gleeson. M., Clancy R.L., and Cripps, A.W. (1993). Mucosal immune response in a case of sudden infant death syndrome. *Pediatr. Res.* 33, 554–556.

Gleeson, M., Clancy, R.L., Cripps, A.W., Henry, R.L., Hensley, M.J., and Wlodarczyk, J.H. (1994). Acquired IgA deficiency. *Pediatr. Allergy Immunol.* 5, 157–161.

Gleeson, M., Clancy, R.L., Hensley, M.J., Cripps, A.W., Henry, R.L., Wlodarczyk, J.I., and Gibson, P.G. (1996). Development of bronchial hyperreactivity following transient absence of salivary IgA. *Am. J. Respir. Crit. Care Med.* 153, 1785–1789.

Gleeson, M., Cripps, A.W., and Clancy, R.L. (1995). Modifiers of the human mucosal immune system. *Immunol. Cell Biol.* 73, 397–404.

Gleeson, M., Cripps, A.W., Clancy, R.L., and Geraghty, S.B. (1990). The variability of immunoglobulins and albumin in saliva of normal and IgA deficient adults. In *Advances in Mucosal Immunology* (eds. T. T. MacDonald, S. J. Challacombe, P. W. Bland, C. R. Stokes, R. V. Heatley, A. McL. Mowat), 500–501. Lancaster: Kluwer Academic Publishers.

Gleeson, M., Cripps, A.W., Clancy, R.L. Hensley, M.J., Dobson., A.J., and Firman, D.W. (1986). Breast feeding conditions a differen-

tial pattern of mucosal immunity. *Clin. Exp. Immunol.* 66, 216–222.

Gleeson, M., Cripps, A.W., Clancy, R.L., Husband, A.J., Hensley, M.J., and Leeder, S.R. (1982). Ontogeny of the secretory immune system in man. *Aust. N. Z. J. Med.* 12, 255–258.

Gleeson, M., Cripps, A.W., Clancy, R.L., Wlodarczyk, J.H., Dobson, A.J., and Hensley, M.J. (1987a). The development of IgA specific antibodies to *Escherichia coli* O antigen in children. *Scand. J. Immunol.* 26, 639–643.

Gleeson, M., Cripps, A.W., Clancy, R.L., Wlodarczyk, J., and Hensley, M.J. (1987b). IgD in infant saliva. *Scand. J. Immunol.* 26, 55–57.

Gleeson, M., Hall, S., Cripps, A.W., and Clancy, R.L. (1997). Secretory IgM—the forgotten mucosal immunoglobulin. In *Mucosal Solutions: Advances in Mucosal Immunology* (eds. A. J. Husband, K. W. Beagley, R. L. Clancy, A. M. Collins, A. W. Cripps, and D. L. Emery), vol. 2, 197–205. Sydney, Australia: University of Sydney Press.

Gleeson, M., McDonald, W., Pyne, D., Cripps, A.W., Francis, J.L., Fricker, P.A., and Clancy, R.L. (1999). Salivary IgA levels and infection risk in elite swimmers. *Med. Sci. Sports Exercise* 31, 67–73.

Gleeson, M., and Pyne, D.B. (2000). Exercise effects on mucosal immunity. *Immun. Cell Biol.* 78, 536–544.

Goldblum, R.M., Hanson, L.Å., and Brandtzaeg, P. (1996). The mucosal defence system. In *Immunologic Disorders in Infants and Children*, 4th ed. (ed. R. T. Stiehm), 159–199. Philadelphia: WB Saunders.

Goldblum, R.M., Schandler, R.J., Garza, C., and Goldman, A.S. (1989). Human milk feeding enhances the urinary excretion of immunologic factors in low birth weight infants. *Pediatr. Res.* 25, 184–188.

Gorse, G.J., Otto, E.E., Powers, D.C., Chambers, G.W., Eickhoff, C.S. and Newman, F.K. (1996). Induction of mucosal antibodies by live attenuated and inactivated influenza virus vaccines in the chronically ill elderly. *J. Infect. Dis.* 173, 285–290.

Gould, S.J., and Isaacson, P.G. (1993). Bronchus associated lymphoid tissue (BALT) in human fetal and infant lung. *J. Pathol.* 169, 229–234.

Groer, M.W., Humenick, S., and Hill, P.D. (1994). Characterizations and psychoneuroimmunologic implications of secretory immunoglobulin A and cortisol in pre-term and term breast milk. *J. Perinatol. Neonat. Nurs.* 7, 42–51.

Gross, S.J., and Buckley, R.H. (1980). IgA in saliva of breast fed and bottle fed infants. *Lancet* ii, 543.

Hahn-Zoric, M., Fulconis, F., Minoli, I., Moro, C., Carlsson, B., Bötiger, M., Räïhä, N., and Hanson, L.Å. (1990). Antibody responses to parenteral and oral vaccines are impaired by conventional and low protein formulas as compared to breastfeeding. *Acta Paediatr. Scand.* B79, 1137–1142.

Halliday, S.D., Comment, C.E., Kwon, J., and Luster, M.I. (1994). Fetal hematopoietic alterations after maternal exposure to ethylene glycol monomethyl ether; prelymphoid cell targeting. *Toxicol. Appl. Pharmacol.* 129, 53–60.

Hanson, L.Å., Bjorkander, J., and Oxelius, U.A. (1983). Selective IgA deficiency. In *Primary and Secondary Immunodeficiency Disorders* (ed. R. K. Chandra), 62–84. Edinburgh: Churchill Livingstone.

Hanson, L.Å., Carlsson, B., Dahlgren, U., Jalil, F., Mellander, L., Wold, A., and Zaman, S. (1987). Vaccination and the ontogeny of the secretory IgA response. *Adv. Exp. Med. Biol.* 216B, 1353–1358.

Hanson, L.Å., Carlsson, B., Dahlgren, U., Mellander, L., and Svanborg-Eden, C. (1980). The secretory IgA in the neonatal period. *Ciba Found. Symp.* 77, 187–204.

Hanson, L.Å., Carlsson, B., Jalil, F., Mellander, L., Söderström, T., and Zaman, S. (1986). Ontogeny of mucosal immunity. In *Frontiers of Gastrointestinal Research. 13. Pediatric Gastroenterology: Aspects of Immunology and Infections* (eds. D. Branski, G. Dinari, P. Rozen, and J. A. Walker-Smith), 1–9. Basel: Karger.

Hanson, L.Å., Soderstrom, T., Brinton, C., Carlsson, B., Larsson, P., Mellander, L., and Svanborg-Eden, C. (1983). Neonatal colonisation with *Escherichia coli* and the ontogeny of the antibody response. *Prog. Allergy* 33, 40–52.

Hanson, L.Å., Wiedermann, U., Ashraf, R., Zaman, S., Alderberth, I., Dahlgren, D., Wold, A., and Jalil, F. (1997). *The Effect of*

Breastfeeding on the Baby and Its Immune System. The Vatican: Pontifical Academy of Science.

Haworth, J.C., and Dilling, L. (1966). Concentration of γA-globulin in serum, saliva and nasopharyngeal secretions of infants and children. *J. Lab. Clin. Med.* 67, 922–933.

Hayashi, Y., Kuirashima, C., Takemura, T., and Hirokawa, K. (1989). Ontogenic development of the secretory immune system in human fetal salivary glands. *Pathol. Immunopathol. Res.* 8, 314–320.

Herias, M.V., Cruz, J.R., Gonzalez-Cossio, T., Nave, F., Carlsson, B., and Hanson, L.Å. (1993). The effect of caloric supplementation on selected milk protective factors in undernourished Guatamalan mothers. *Pediatr. Res.* 34, 217–221.

Hoelzer, J., Stiller-Winkler, R., Lemm, F., Ewers, U., Idel, H., and Wilhelm, M. (2002). Prevalence of respiratory symptoms in school children and salivary IgA: An epidemiological study in a rural area of Northrhine-Westphalia, Germany. *Int. J. Hyg. Env. Health* 205, 309–319.

Hucklebridge, F., Lambert, S., Clow, A., Warburton, D.W., Evans, P.D., and Sherwood, N. (2000). Modulation of secretory immunoglobulin A in saliva; response to manipulation of mood. *Biol.Psych.* 53, 25–35.

Husband, A.J., and Gleeson, M. (1996). Ontogeny of mucosal immunity—environmental and behavioral influences. *Brain Behav. Immun.* 10, 188–204.

Iwase, T., Moro, I., and Mestecky, J. (1987). Immunohistochemical study of the ontogeny of the secretory immune system. *Adv. Exp. Med. Biol.* 216B, 1359–1368.

Jemmott, J.B., and McClelland, D.C. (1989). Secretory IgA as a measure of resistance to infectious disease: Comments on Stone, Cox, Valdimarsdottir, and Neale. *Behavioral Med.* 15, 63–70.

Knox, W.F. (1986). Restricted feeding and human intestinal plasma cell development. *Arch. Dis. Child.* 61, 744–749.

Koga, T., McGhee, J.R., Kato, H., Kato, R., Kiyono, H., and Fuihashi, K. (2000). Evidence for early aging in the mucosal immune system. *J. Immunol.* 165, 5352–5359.

Koletzko, S., Sherman, P., Corem, M., Griffiths, A., and Smith C. (1989). Role of infant feeding practices in Crohn's disease in childhood. *Br. Med. J.* 298, 1617–1618.

Korsrud, F.R., and Brandtzaeg, P. (1980). Quantitative immunohistochemistry of immunoglobulin- and J-chain-producing cells in human parotid and submandibular glands. *Immunology* 39, 129–140.

Kramer, D.R., and Cebra, J.J. (1995). Role of maternal antibody in the induction of virus specific and bystander IgA responses in Peyer's patches of suckling mice. *Int. Immunol.* 7, 911–918.

Kroese, F.G.M., de Waard, R., Bos, N.A. (1996). B-1 cells and their reactivity with the murine intestinal microflora. *Seminars in Immunology* 8, 11–18

Kuitunem, M., and Savilahti, E (1995). Mucosal IgA, mucosal cows milk antibodies, scrum cow's milk antibodies and gastrointestinal permeability in infants. *Pediatr. Allergy Immunol.* 6, 30–35.

Lionetti, P., Breese, E., Spencer, J., March, S.H., Taylor, J., and MacDonald, T.T. (1993). Activation of Vbeta3 + T cells and tissue damage in human small intestine induced by the bacterial superantigen, *Staphylococcus aureus* enterotoxin B. *Eur. J. Immunol.* 23, 664–668.

Lodinová, R., Jouja, V., and Wagner, V. (1973). Serum immunoglobulins and coproantibody formation in infants after artificial intestinal colonisation with *Escherichia coli* 083 and oral lysozyme administration. *Pediatr. Res.* 7, 659–669.

Lodinová-Zádniková, R., Tlaskalová, H., and Bartáková, Z. (1989). The antibody response in infants after colonization of the intestine with *E. coli* 083. Artificial colonization used as a prevention against nosocomial infections. *Adv. Exp. Med. Biol.* 310, 329–335.

MacDonald, T.T. (1994). Development of mucosal immune function in man: potential for GI disease states. *Acta Paediatr. Jpn.* 36, 532–536.

MacDonald, T.T. (1996). Accessory cells in the human gastrointestinal tract. *Histopathology* 29, 89–92.

MacDonald, T.T., Weinel, A., and Spencer, J. (1988). HLA-DR expression in human fetal intestinal epithelium. *Gut* 29, 1342–1348.

McClellan, K.A., Cripps, A.W., Clancy, R.L., and Bilson, F.A. (1997). A study in normal subjects of the effect of age on the defences of the outer eye, with reference to the common mucosal immune system, by assay of IgA isotype specific antibody in tears, saliva and serum and lysozyme in tears. In *Mucosal Solutions: Advances in Mucosal Immunology* (eds. A. J. Husband, K. W. Beagley, R. L. Clancy, A. M. Collins, A. W. Cripps, and D. L. Emery), vol. 1, 355–367. Sydney, Australia: University of Sydney Press.

McClelland, D.C. (1989). Motivational factors in health and disease. *Am. Psychol.* 22, 132–137.

McGee, D.W., and McMurray, D.N. (1988). Protein malnutrition reduces the IgA immune response to oral antigen by altering B-cell and suppressor T-cell functions. *Immunology* 64, 697–702.

McGill, J.I., Liakos, G.M., Goulding, N., and Seal, D.V. (1984). Normal tear protein profiles and age-related changes. *Br. J. Ophthalmol.* 68, 316–320.

Mackinnon, L.T., and Hooper, S. (1994). Mucosal (secretory) immune system responses to exercise of varying intensity and during overtraining. *Int. J. Sports Med.* 15B, S179–S183.

Mellander, L., Carlsson, B., and Hanson, L.Å (1984). Appearance of secretory IgM and IgA antibodies to *Escherichia coli* in saliva during early infancy and childhood. *J. Pediatr.* 104, 564–568.

Moro, I., Saito, I., Asano, M., Takahashi, T., and Iwase, T. (1991). Ontogeny of the secretory IgA system in humans. *Adv. Exp. Med. Biol.* 310, 51–57.

Muszkat, A., Yehuda, B., Schein, M.H., Friedlander, Y., Naveh, P., Greenbaum, E., Schlesinger, M., Levy, R., Zakay-Rones, Z., and Friedman, G. (2000). Local and systemic immune response in community-dwelling elderly after intranasal or intramuscular immunization with inactivated influenza. *J Med. Virol.* 6, 100–106.

Myers, M.G., Fomon, S.H., Koontz, P.P., McGuinness, G.A., Lachenbruch, P.A., and Hollingshead, R. (1984). Respiratory and gastrointestinal illness in breast and formula-fed infants. *Am. J. Dis. Child.* 138, 629–632.

Na, H.R., and Seelig, L.L. (1994). Effect of maternal ethanol consumption on *in vitro* tumor necrosis factor, interleukin-6 and interleukin-2 production by rat milk and blood leukocytes. *Alcohol Clin. Exp. Res.* 18, 398–402.

Nagao, A.T., Carneiro-Sampaio, M.D., Carlson, B., and Hanson, L.Å. (1995). Antibody titre and avidity in saliva and serum are not impaired in mildly to moderately undernourished children. *J. Trop. Pediatr.* 41, 153–157.

Nelson, D.J., and Holt, P.G. (1995) Defective regional immunity in the respiratory tract of neonates is attributable to hyporesponsiveness of local dendritic cell to activation signals. *J. Immunol.* 155, 3517–3524.

Nilssen, D.E., Brandtzaeg, P., Froland, S.S., and Fausa, O. (1992). Subclass composition and J-chain expression of the 'compensatory' gastrointestinal IgG cell population in selective IgA deficiency. *Clin. Exp. Immunol.* 87, 237–245.

Norhagen, G., Engström, P.E., Hammerström, L., Soder, P.O., and Smith, C.J. (1989). Immunoglobulin levels in saliva in individuals with selective IgA deficiency: compensatory IgM secretion and its correlation with HLA and susceptibility to infections. *J. Clin. Immunol.* 9, 279–286.

Nurkka, A., Ahman, H., Yaich, M., Eskola, J., and Kayhty, H. (2001). Serum and salivary anti-capsular antibodies in infants and children vaccinated with octavalent pneumococcal conjugate vaccines, PncD and PncT. *Vaccine* 20, 194–201.

Ogra, S.S., Ogra, P.L., Lippes, J., and Tomasi, T.B. (1972). Immunohistologic localisation of immunoglobulins, secretory component and lactoferrin in the developing human fetus. *Proc. Soc. Exp. Biol. Med.* 139, 570–574.

Oliver, A.M., Thomson, A.W., Sewell, H.F., and Abramovich, D.R. (1988). Major histocompatibility complex (MHC) class II antigen (HLA-DR, DR and DP) expression in human fetal endocrine organs and gut. *Scand. J. Immunol.* 27, 731–737.

Ostergard, P.A., and Blom, M. (1977). Whole salivary immunoglobulin levels in 60 healthy children: determined by a sensitive electroimmuno technique after prior carbamylation. *J. Clin. Chem. Clin. Biochem.* 15, 393–396.

Ottaway, C.A., and Husband, A.J. (1994). The influence of neuro-endocrine pathways on lymphocyte migration. *Immunol. Today* 15, 511–517.

Pabst, H., Grace, M., Godel, J., Cho, H., and Spady, D. (1989). Effect of breastfeeding on immune response to BCG vaccination. *Lancet* i, 295–297.

Pabst, H.F., and Spady, D.W. (1990). Effect of breastfeeding on antibody response to conjugate vaccine. *Lancet* 336, 269–270.

Pallaro, A., Barbeito, S., Taberner, P., Marino, P., Franchello, A., Strasnoy, I., Ramos, O., and Slobodianik, N. (2002) Total salivary IgA, serum C3c and IgA in obese school children. *J. Nutr. Biochem.* 13, 539–542.

Perkkio, M., and Savilahti, E. (1980). Time of appearance of immunoglobulin-containing cells in the mucosa of the neonatal intestine. *Pediatr. Res.* 14, 953–955.

Pietsch, R.L., and Pearlman, M.E. (1973). Human tear lysozyme variables. *Arch. Ophthalmol.* 90, 94–96.

Puri, S., and Chandra, R.K. (1985). Nutritional regulation of host resistance and predictive value of immunologic test in assessment of outcome. *Pediatr. Clin. North Am.* 32, 499–516.

Reid, M.R., Drummond, P.D., and Mackinnon, L.T (2001). The effect of moderate exercise and relation to secretory immunoglobulin A. *Int. J. Sports Med.*, 22, 132–137.

Rivier, D.A., Trefts, P.E., and Kagnoff, M.F. (1983). Age-dependence of the IgA anti-α (1→3) dextran B1355 response in vitro. *Scand. J. Immunol.* 17, 115–121.

Roberton, D.M., Paganelli, R., Dinwiddie, R., and Levinsky, R.J. (1982). Milk antigen absorption in the preterm and term neonate. *Arch. Dis. Child.* 57, 369.

Roberts, S.A., and Freed, D.L.J. (1977). Neonatal IgA secretion enhanced by breast feeding. *Lancet* ii, 1131.

Rognum, T.O., Thrane, P.S., Stoltenberg, L., Vege, A., and Brandtzaeg, P. (1992). Development of intestinal mucosal immunity in fetal life and in the first postnatal months. *Pediatr. Res.* 32, 145–149.

Russell, G.J., Bhan, A.K., and Winter, H.S. (1990a). The distribution of T and B lymphocyte populations and MHC class II expression in human fetal and post-natal intestine. *Pediatr. Res.* 27, 239–244.

Russell, M.W., Prince, S.J., Ligthart, G.J., Mestecky, J., and Radl, J. (1990b). Comparison of salivary and serum antibodies to common environmental antigens in elderly, edentulous, and normal adult subjects. *Aging: Immunol. Infect. Dis.* 2, 275–286.

Sarfati, M., Vanderbeeken, Y., Rubio-Trujillo, M., Duncan, D., and Delespesse, G. (1986). Presence of IgE suppressor factors in human colostrum. *Eur. J. Immunol.* 16, 1005–1008.

Schlesinger, L., and Uauy, R. (1991). Nutrition and neonatal immune function. *Semin. Perinatol.* 15, 469–477.

Schmucker, D.L. (2002). Intestinal mucosal immunosenescence in rats. *Exp. Gerontol.* 37 197–203.

Schmucker, D., and Daniels, C. (1986). Aging, gastrointestinal infections and mucosal immunity. *J. Am. Geriatr. Soc.* 34, 377–384.

Seidel, B.M., Schulze, B., Schubert, S., and Borte, M. (2000). Oral mucosal immunocompetence in preterm infants in the first 9 months of life. *Eur. J. Pediatr.* 159, 789.

Seidel, B.M., Schubert, S., Schulze, B., and Borte, M. (2001). Secretory IgA, free secretory component and IgD in saliva of newborn infants. *Early Hum. Dev.* 62, 159–164.

Sellner, J.C., Merrill, D.A., and Claman, H.N. (1968). Salivary immunoglobulin and albumin: development during the newborn period. *J. Pediatr.* 72, 685–689.

Sennhauser, F., Balloch, A., Shelton, M.J., Doyle, L.W., Yu, V.Y., and Roberton, D.M. (1990). Immunoglobulin and anti *Escherichia coli* antibody in lower respiratory tract secretions from infants weighing less than 1500g at birth. *Arch. Dis. Child.* 65, 48–53.

Sigurs, N., Hattevig, G., and Kjellman, B. (1992). Maternal avoidance of eggs, cow's milk and fish during lactation: effect on allergic manifestations, skin-prick tests and specific IgE antibodies in children at age 4 hours. *Paediatrics* 89, 735–739.

Simell, B., Kilpi, T.M, and Kayhty, H. (2002). Pneumococcal carriage and otitis media induce salivary antibodies and pneumococcal capsular polysaccharides in children. *J. Infect. Dis.* 186(8), 1106–1114.

Smith, D.J., Gahnberg, L., Taubman, M.A., and Ebersole, J.L. (1986). Salivary antibody responses to oral and parenteral vaccines in children. *J. Clin. Immunol.* 6, 43–49.

Smith, D.J., Joshipura, K., Kent, R., and Taubman, M.A. (1992). Effect of age on immunoglobulin content and volume of human labial gland saliva. *J. Dent. Res.* 71, 1891–1894.

Smith, D.J., King, W.F., and Taubman, M.A. (1989). Isotype, subclass and molecular size of immunoglobulins in saliva from young infants. *Clin. Exp. Immunol.* 76, 97–102.

Smith, D.J., and Taubman, M.A. (1992). Ontogeny of immunity to oral microbiota in human. *Crit. Rev. Oral Biol. Med.* 3, 109–133.

Smith, I.M. (1985). Pneumonia and the aging lung. In *Relations Between Normal Aging and Disease* (ed. H. A. Johnson), 101–115. Philadelphia: Lippincott-Raven.

Solvason, N., and Kearney, J.F. (1992). The human fetal omentum: a site of B cell generation. *J. Exp. Med.* 175, 397–404.

South, M.A., Wardck, W.J., Wollheim, F.A., and Good, R.A. (1967). The IgA system. III IgA levels in the serum and saliva of paediatric patients—evidence for a local immunological system. *J. Pediatr.* 71, 645–653.

Spencer, J., Dunn-Walters, D.J., Dogan, A., and MacDonald, T.T. (1997). Ontogeny of human mucosal immunity and the original of mucosal effector cells. In *Mucosal Solutions: Advances in Mucosal Immunology*, vol. 1 (eds. A. J. Husband, R. L. Clancy, A. M. Collins, A. W. Cripps, and D. L. Emery), 229–241, Sydney, Australia: University of Sydney Press.

Spencer, J., Isaacson, P.G., Diss, T.C., and MacDonald, T.T. (1989). Expression of disulfide-linked and non-disulfide-linked forms of T cell receptor gamma/delta heterodimer in human intestinal intraepithelial lymphocytes. *Eur. J. Immunol.* 19, 1335–1338.

Spencer, J., MacDonald, T.T., Finn, T., and Isaacson, P.G. (1986). The development of gut associated lymphoid tissue in the terminal ileum of fetal human intestine. *Clin. Exp. Immunol.* 64, 536–543.

Spencer, J., MacDonald, T.T., and Isaacson, P.G. (1987). Development of human gut-associated lymphoid tissue. *Adv. Exp. Med. Biol.* 216B, 1421–1430.

Stoltenberg, L., Saugstad, O.D., and Rognum, T.O. (1992). Sudden infant death syndrome victims show local immunoglobulin M response in tracheal wall and immunoglobulin A response in duodenal mucosa. *Pediatr. Res.* 31, 372–375.

Sullivan, D.A., Vaeman, J.P., and Soo, C. (1993). Influences of severe protein malnutrition on rat lacrimal, salivary and gastrointestinal immune expression during development, adulthood and aging. *Immunology* 78, 308–311.

Szewczuk, M.R., Campbell, R.J., and Jung, L.K. (1981). Lack of age-associated immune dysfunction in mucosal associated lymph nodes. *J. Immunol.* 126, 2200–2204.

Takemura, T., and Eishi, Y. (1985). Distribution of secretory component and immunoglobulins in the developing lung. *Am. Rev. Respir. Dis.* 131, 125–130.

Taylor, A.N., Ben-Eliyahn, S., Yirmiya, R., Chang, M.P., Norman, D.C., and Chiappelli, F. (1993). Actions of alcohol on immunity and neoplasia in fetal alcohol exposed and adult rats. *Alcohol 2* (Suppl. 1), 69–74.

Taylor, B., Norman, A.P., Orgel, H.A., Stokes, C.R., Turner, M.W., and Soothill, J.F. (1973). Transient IgA deficiency and pathogenesis of infantile atopy. *Lancet* ii, 111–120.

Taylor, C.E., and Toms, G.L. (1984). Immunoglobulin concentrations in nasopharyngeal secretions. *Arch. Dis. Child.* 59, 48–53.

Taylor, D.C., Cripps, A.W., and Clancy, R.L. (1992). Measurement of lysozyme by an enzyme-linked immunosorbent assay. *J. Immunol. Methods* 146, 55–61.

Thrane, P.S., Rognum, T.O., and Brandtzaeg, P. (1990). Increased immune response in upper respiratory and digestive tract in SIDS. *Lancet* i, 229–230.

Thrane, P.S., Rognum, T.O., and Brandtzaeg, P. (1991). Ontogenesis of the secretory immune system and innate defence factors in human parotid glands. *Clin. Exp. Immunol.* 86, 342–348.

Van Asperen, P.P., Gleeson, M., Kemp, A.S., Cripps, A.W., Geraghty, S.B., Mellis, C.M., and Clancy, R.L. (1985). The relationship between atopy and salivary IgA deficiency in infancy. *Clin. Exp. Immunol.* 62, 753–757.

van Gaudecker, B., and Müller-Hermelink, H.K. (1982). The development of the human tonsilla palatina. *Cell Tissue Res.* 224, 579–600.

Verghese, A., and Berk, S.L. (1983). Bacterial pneumonia in the elderly. *Medicine* 62, 271–285.

Wade, A.W., and Szewcsuk, M.R. (1984). Aging, idiotype repertoire shifts and compartmentalization of the mucosal-associated lymphoid system. *Adv. Immunol.* 36, 143–188.

Wade, A.W., and Szewcsuk, M.R. (1987) Changes in the mucosal-associated B-cell response with age. In *Aging and the Immune Response. Cellular and Humoral Aspects* (ed. E. A Goide), 95–122. New York: Marcel Dekker.

Wiederman, U., Dahlgren, U., Holmgren, J., and Hanson, L.Å. (1993). Impaired mucosal antibody response to cholera toxin in vitamin A-deficient rats immunised with oral cholera vaccine. *Infect. Immun.* 61, 3952–3957.

Williams, N., Gleeson, M., Callister, R., Fitzgerald, P.E, Reid, V.L., and Clancy, R.L. (2001). Effect of exercise intensity on mucosal immunity in competitive athletes suffering fatigue and recurrent infections. *Med. Sci. Sports Exercise* 33(5) Suppl, ISEI Addendum, Abstract 39.

Yoffey, J.M., and Courtice, F.C. (1970). *Lymphatics, Lymph and Lymphomyeloid Complex*. London: Academic Press.

Yoshkikawa, T.T. (1983). Geriatric infectious diseases: an emerging problem. *J. Am. Geriatr. Soc.* 31, 34–39.

Phylogeny of the Gut-Associated Lymphoid Tissue (GALT)

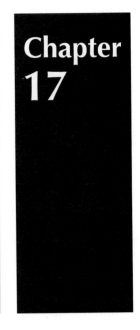

Thomas T. MacDonald

Division of Infection, Inflammation, and Repair, University of Southampton School of Medicine, Southampton, United Kingdom

Robert D. Miller

Department of Biology, University of New Mexico, Albuquerque, New Mexico

Even primitive vertebrates have to eat, and the necessity of a thin epithelium to facilitate nutrient absorption has meant that the gut has always been a weak point in host defenses. As vertebrates took on more complex forms, specialization of both the gut and the immune system occurred. The gut immune system, at the forefront of interaction with endogenous microbes, pathogens, and food antigens, has therefore played a crucial role in vertebrate evolution.

In this review we have decided to include a brief primer on the phylogeny of the immune system itself, since this is clearly crucial for our understanding of the inductive and effector mechanisms that operate at mucosal surfaces in more primitive animals. We will then move up the evolutionary tree. However, it must be emphasized that the literature is rather sparse, and knowledge of GALT in lower vertebrates is fragmentary.

THE PHYLOGENY OF ADAPTIVE IMMUNITY

Phylogenetic considerations

Jawed vertebrates do not comprise an entire phylum alone but are a subset of just one of the 20-plus phyla of animals on the planet. The jawed vertebrates can be divided into two basic groups: the Chondrichthyans (cartilaginous fish such as ratfishes, sharks, and rays) and the Euteleostomi (bony vertebrates, including bony fish and tetrapods; **Fig. 17.1**). Within the Euteleostomi there are two major lineages: the Actinopterygii (ray-finned fishes) and Sarcopterygii (lobe-finned fishes). Tetrapods, the land-dwelling animals (amphibians, reptiles, birds, and mammals), are derived from within the Sarcopterygii. Since mammals are among the best studied of the vertebrates, particular attention will be given here to the major mammalian lineages.

The common ancestors of all modern mammals gave rise to three lineages or subclasses of mammals between 120 and 170 million years ago (MYA) (Retief *et al.*, 1993; Belov *et al.*, 2002). These three lineages are the prototherians, the metatherians, and the eutherians. Prototherians, also commonly called the monotremes, are the egg-laying mammals. Although they reproduce by egg-laying, they are true mammals, have fur, and feed their young milk. Once more widespread (Pascual *et al.*, 1992), the monotremes are now restricted to three species in Australasia: the duckbill platypus (*Ornithorhyncus anatinus*), the short-beaked echidna (*Tachyglossus aculeatus*), and the long-nosed echidna (*Zaglossus bruijni*). The metatherians, commonly called the marsupials, were also once more widespread but are now restricted to two regions, Australasia and South America. The North American or Virginia opossum is a relatively new immigrant into North America, having migrated from South America around 3 MYA. The third mammalian lineage is the eutherians, which are the placental mammals, distinguished by longer gestation times resulting in the birth of more highly developed young.

The overall relationship between the monotremes, marsupials, and placentals is, surprisingly, still a matter of debate. The classic view maintains that the two viviparous lineages, marsupials and placentals, are sister taxa and that the monotremes are an ancient divergence (Huxley 1880). This view is supported by most molecular phylogenetic analyses using nuclear gene data (Killian *et al.*, 2001; Miska *et al.*, 2003). The alternative hypothesis, called the Marsupionta hypothesis, proposes that the monotremes and marsupials are sister groups, with the eutherians diverging separately first. The Marsupionta hypothesis has been supported by molecular analyses using mitochondrial DNA sequence (Janke *et al.*, 1996). The resolution of this debate has significance for mucosal immunology, particularly with regard to maternal immune protection of offspring.

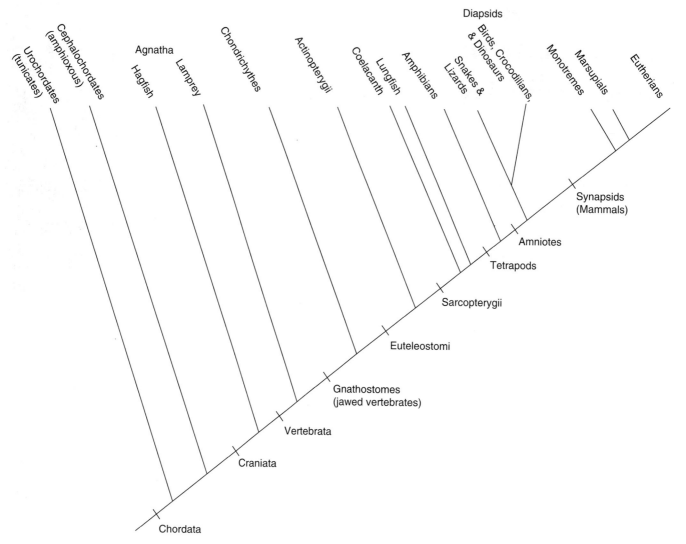

Fig. 17.1. The phylogenetic tree of vertebrates.

Evolutionary origins of the adaptive immune response

The characteristic that distinguishes the vertebrate immune system from that of all other animals is the presence of antigen receptors encoded by genes assembled somatically by DNA recombination and expressed on the surface of specialized cells called lymphocytes. This recombination, the so-called V(D)J recombination, assembles the immunoglobulin (Ig) and T cell receptors (TCR) encoding loci in developing lymphocytes. Ig and TCR, along with the third class of antigen receptors, the molecules of the major histocompatibility complex (MHC), compose the adaptive immune system. The term adaptive immunity is used to distinguish the antigen-specific components of an immune response that leads to memory (immunity) from the more ancient, innate immune mechanisms that vertebrates share with invertebrates.

The challenge to those who wish to investigate the origins of the adaptive immune system is to piece together the evolutionary events that resulted in this complex and integrated system. Although much remains to be determined, one thing is clear: the genes of the adaptive immune system (Ig, TCR, and MHC) are present in their entirety in the extant, jawed vertebrates and entirely absent in the agnatha (jawless fish, *e.g.*, hagfish and lampreys) and the invertebrates **(Table 17.1)**. The timing of the appearance of the adaptive immune system, therefore, clearly coincides with other important changes during vertebrate evolution, namely, the appearance of a lower jaw.

Jawed vertebrates are members of the phylum *Chordata*, which also includes some invertebrates, namely, the Urochordates (the tunicates, *e.g.*, *Botryllus schlosseri*) and Cephalochordates (lancelets, *e.g.*, amphioxus), and jawless vertebrates (Fig. 17.1). Within chordate evolution, approximately 550 MYA, appeared the Craniata, animals that

Table 17.1. Summary of Immunoglobulin Classes, T-Cell Receptor, and MHC Molecules in Different Orders of Vertebrates

Major Lineage	MYA[a]	Igh	Igl[c]	TCR	MHC	Rag1/Rag2
Agnatha (hagfish)	550	—	—	—	—	—
Agnatha (lamprey)	530	—	—	—	—	—
Chondrichthyes (sharks, rays, skates)	500	IgM, IgW[b]	3 classes	αβ, γδ	Class I, Class II	+
Actinopterygii (bony, ray-finned fish)	450	IgM, IgD	Igσ?, 2 classes	αβ, γδ	Class I, Class II	+
Amphibians (frogs, toads, salamanders)	360	IgM, IgY, IgX	Igλ, Igκ, Igσ	αβ, γδ	Class I, Class II	+
Lepidosaurians (snakes, lizards)	300	IgM, IgY, ?	n.d.	n.d.	Class I, Class II	+
Archosaurians (birds, crocodiles, alligators)	300	IgM, IgA, IgY	Igλ	αβ, γδ	Class I, Class II	+
Monotremes	170	IgM, IgG, IgE, IgA	Igλ, Igκ	αβ, γδ	Class I, Class II	+
Marsupials	120	IgM, IgG, IgE, IgA	Igλ, Igκ	αβ, γδ	Class I, Class II	+
Eutherians	0	IgM, IgD, IgG, IgE, IgA	Igλ, Igκ	αβ, γδ	Class I, Class II	+

The presence of a particular gene class is noted when it has been reported from at least one representative in the group.
[a]Approximate time in millions of years since last common ancestor with the eutherians. Dates adapted from a variety of sources (Carrol, 1988; Kumar and Hedges, 1998; Belov et al., 2002).
[b]IgW is used to indicate the class of Ig found in Chondrichythes that includes IgNARC, IgX, and IgW.
[c]From the amphibians on, there are clear Igλ and Igκ homologues and a third class called Igσ. In the fishes, the relationship to Igλ and Igκ is much less clear (for recent review on this, see Pilstrom, 2002).
n.d., no data.

encase nervous tissue within a cranium. The only surviving Craniata that are not vertebrates are the eel-like hagfish, of which there are roughly 40 living species. Hagfish are agnatha that lack a vertebral column and hence are not true vertebrates. The most ancient, true vertebrates are the lampreys, which also are eel-like fish that lack a lower jaw. There are approximately 40 extant species of lampreys. Around 500 MYA, the vertebrates gained multiple important innovations, including a lower jaw and an adaptive immune system.

What changes occurred within the vertebrates that allowed for such innovations? Current theory ties these changes, in part, to genome duplication. Genome duplications create the genetic fodder that allows for the divergence of genes and the concomitant invention of new functions. The evidence of a genome duplication that separates the lampreys and more ancient chordates from the jawed vertebrates comes from many analyses, including the multiple HOX developmental gene clusters and, intriguingly, four apparently paralogous genomic regions, one of which includes the MHC region itself (discussed later in this chapter).

The origins of the V(D)J recombination system

Genomic duplications alone, however, cannot explain all the innovations associated with the adaptive immune system. We will therefore consider some of the genes and gene systems that are necessary for adaptive immunity and the current theory on their origins. The somatic assembly of mature immunoglobulin (Ig) and T cell receptor (TCR) genes in B and T cells, respectively, can be divided into two processes. The first is a site-specific, endonuclease activity associated with the recombination activating genes, Rag-1 and Rag-2. The second are DNA repair systems that resolve the DNA breaks created by Rag-1 and Rag-2.

Genes encoding Rag-1 and Rag-2 have been described from all major lineages of jawed vertebrates, from sharks to mammals. They are highly conserved, and isolating Rag-1 and Rag-2 from novel vertebrate species is not difficult. In fact, their conservation and slow evolution have made them informative for vertebrate molecular phylogenetic studies (Groth and Barrowclough, 1999). All reported attempts to isolate Rag-1 and Rag-2 homologues from agnathans have been negative. Current theory on the origin of Rag-1 and Rag-2 holds they are genes that invaded the vertebrate genome via transposition, coincident with the appearance of the lower jaw. This theory is supported by evidence that Rag-1 and Rag-2 can catalyze DNA similarly to transposases, including the formation of DNA hairpins as a mechanism of DNA cleavage (Agrawal *et al.*, 1998; Hiom *et al.*, 1998). Furthermore, Rag-1 and Rag-2 appear to have greatest similarity to prokaryotic transposases rather than any other genes known from eukaryotic genomes (Bernstein *et al.*, 1996). The enzymes that are involved in the movement of transposons are encoded on the transposable element itself and, in all species so far examined, Rag-1 and Rag-2 are in linked pairs, suggesting that they moved into the genome as a unit. In conclusion, Rag-1 and Rag-2 are part of the V(D)J recombination machinery that appear to have "jumped" *de*

novo into the genome of an ancestor common to all living jawed vertebrates (for a more detailed review, see Hansen and McBlane, 2000).

The resolution of the DNA break created by Rag-1 and Rag-2 involves many different proteins, including the DNA-dependent protein kinase (DNA-PK). DNA-PK is activated by double-strand DNA breaks and activates other DNA repair components and arrests cell cycle by phosphorylating various regulatory factors such as p53. DNA-PK is composed of three protein subunits: Ku70, Ku80, and the DNA-PK catalytic subunit (DNA-Pkcs). The connection between DNA-PK and V(D)J recombination was confirmed when the gene encoding DNA-Pkcs was linked to the *scid* mutation in mice (Miller *et al.*, 1995). The Ku proteins, which directly bind the ends of double-strand breaks, are ancient, and their appearance in yeast as well as higher eukaryotes has been described (Tuteja and Tuteja, 2000). Clear homologues of DNA-Pkcs outside of vertebrates have not been described; however, it is a member of an ancient family of kinases that includes the ATM (ataxia telangiectasia mutated) gene in mammals and the Tel-1 and Mec-1 genes in fungi (Rouse and Jackson, 2002). Although this review is not comprehensive, it demonstrates that some enzymatic components used in the V(D)J recombination system were already present in the ancestors of vertebrates, whereas others were novel introductions into the vertebrate genome.

The origins of the antigen receptor genes

Important questions remain unresolved, such as what are the substrates of V(D)J recombination, what are the evolutionary origins of the Ig and TCR genes, and where did the MHC come from? There are no clear answers to these questions, but there are many intriguing observations. Ig, TCR, and MHC all contain Ig protein domains. Ig domains in vertebrate antigen receptors are characterized as V-type or C-type, corresponding to the variable and constant region domains of Ig and TCR, respectively, or as intermediate type. The intermediate type Ig domain is ancient in evolution and predates the existence of vertebrates. V-types are thought to be unique to Ig and TCR genes, but the description of V-like Ig domains in snails (Adema *et al.*, 1997), Cephalochordates (Cannon *et al.*, 2002), and other invertebrates (Du Pasquier 2000) suggests that these domain types were present prior to the appearance of jawed vertebrates and the adaptive immune response. To create the substrate for the V(D)J recombination system, the exons encoding Ig domains were fragmented to create the variable (V), diversity (D), and joining (J) segments, flanked by the recombination signal sequences (RSS). The explanation for the fragmentation and insertion of the RSS appears to fall on the transposon model again. RSS resemble the site-specific sequences flanking some transposable elements (Agrawal *et al.*, 1998). The insertion of a transposable element containing RSS along with the genes encoding the transposases (Rag-1 and Rag-2) directly into the genome of the ancestor of jawed vertebrates would have simultaneously introduced both elements. This insertion could have been directly into an exon encoding an

Ig domain or later as a secondary transposition event. Ultimately the Rag-1 and Rag-2 genes would have had to be relocated elsewhere in the genome to prevent them from being deleted whenever V(D)J recombination was initiated (Hanson and McBlane, 2000).

MHC and antigen processing

The origins of the MHC are speculative at best, and true homologues of the MHC appear to be altogether absent in jawless fish and invertebrates. Much investigation of the origins of the vertebrate MHC has focused on the paralogous regions of vertebrate genomes that include the MHC. Characterization of duplicated genes or regions (paralogues) can help to reconstruct the evolutionary history of genes. These paralogous regions reflect either entire or partial genome duplications in common ancestors, the most famous of which are the duplications of the HOX developmental genes (Ruddle *et al.*, 1994). Four clusters of HOX genes on human chromosomes 2, 7, 12, and 17 suggest that two rounds of genome duplication occurred during the transition from protochordates to vertebrates, resulting in the current vertebrate genome content. The human MHC on chromosome 6 contains genes duplicated on chromosomes 1, 9, and 19, suggesting that this region is also the product of two rounds of duplication in the ancestors of modern vertebrates (Kasahara, 2000). Other components of the antigen-presenting system, the proteasomes, are part of the normal housekeeping machinery that would have already been in place when vertebrates appeared. Two of the MHC-linked peptide processing elements, the LMP and TAP genes, also have ancestral relationships to proteins that predate the appearance of jawed vertebrates. The LMP proteins are a class of proteasome β-subunits, and the TAP proteins are related to ABC peptide transporters. Genes related to the TAP genes found in vertebrate MHC have been recently uncovered in lampreys (Uinuk-ool *et al.*, 2003).

Adaptation within the jawed vertebrates

All the major genetic components of the adaptive immune system can be found in both Chondrichthyans and Euteleostomi. Of the most ancient living jawed vertebrates, the elasmobranches (sharks and rays) are the best studied. They have been found to contain all the basic antigen receptor types described in mice and humans. Elasmobranchs have genes encoding TCR α and β chains and TCR γ and δ chains, Ig heavy and light chains, and MHC class I and class II molecules (Rast *et al.*, 1997; Flajnik and Rumfelt 2000). Although there are certainly major evolutionary lineages for which there are few data, it is expected that all of these classes of antigen receptor genes will be found in all jawed vertebrates. What did occur within the jawed vertebrates were continued gene duplication and divergence and the evolution of new functions in some of the antigen receptor genes.

Ig heavy chains

Ig heavy chain (Igh) evolution is apparent with the appearance of new isotypes with novel functions in different vertebrate groups. IgM is the most ancient of the Igh and has been described from all the jawed vertebrate lineages, Chondrichthyans and Euteleostomi. A second Igh, called IgW, has been described in Chondrichthyans (Flajnik and Rumfelt 2000). The nomenclature for IgW is confusing, and this isotype is also known as IgX, IgR, IgNAR, and IgNARC, depending upon the species studied (Bengten *et al.*, 2000). This isotype was thought to be restricted to the Chondrichthyans until recent reports of an IgW-like heavy chain from the African lungfish (Ota *et al.*, 2003). This result is significant, given that lungfish (the Dipnoi) are thought to be the Sarcopterygii most closely related to the ancestor of the tetrapods, and suggests that this isotype might have been more widespread in vertebrate evolution.

Unique Igh isotypes evolved in tetrapods: IgY, IgG and IgE. IgY is found in amphibians, reptiles, and birds and is most abundant during secondary antibody responses. IgG and IgE are exclusively found in mammals and are present in all three mammalian subclasses: monotremes, marsupials, and eutherians (Miller and Belov 2000, Vernersson *et al.*, 2002). IgG and IgE appear to be derived from a duplication of the IgY constant region found in the nonmammalian tetrapods.

Also restricted to the tetrapods is IgA, the most significant isotype to mammalian mucosal immunology. IgA has been unequivocally found only in mammals and birds so far and appears to have evolved from a duplication of the IgM constant region. The presence of IgA in both the synapsids (mammals) and diapsids (birds) suggests that it was present in the last common ancestor of these lineages and should be expected to be found in at least some if not all of the reptilian and crocodilian lineages. Reptiles, however, are among the least-studied vertebrate groups with regard to their immune system.

Ig light chains

The Ig light chains (Igl) are classified with respect to mammalian Igκ and Igλ. There are three general classes of Igl among the vertebrates: those that are Igκ-like, those that are Igλ-like, and those that are neither and are called Igσ by some investigators (Pilstrom 2002). Igσ is a catch-all for light chains that are clearly neither Igκ-like nor Igλ-like and is probably not a single evolutionary lineage. All three mammalian subclasses have both Igκ and Igλ (Miller *et al.*, 1999, Lucero *et al.*, 1998, and unpublished data). Birds have only Igλ. Amphibians have all three types, Igσ, Igκ, and Igλ. Fish also have multiple Igl classes; however, their relationship to the mammalian Igκ and Igλ is still a matter of some debate (Pilstrom 2002).

Evolutionary origins of lymphoid tissues

It is generally accepted that jawless fish lack Ig, TCR, and MHC genes and the Rag genes in their genome. The jawless fish also lack true lymphoid organs. True lymphoid organs, including the thymus and spleen, appear in the jawed vertebrates. The most ancient of the jawed vertebrates, the Chondrichthyans, have a thymus and spleen that are histologically similar to the mammalian equivalents.

The thymus and spleen

The thymus and spleen occur in all jawed vertebrates, appearing to have the same function in T cell development as in mice and humans. The thymus, therefore, likely gives rise to both αβ and γδ T cells in all jawed vertebrates. There are minor anatomical differences in thymus structure among different lineages. In most fish the two lobes of the thymus are separated on either side of the body cavity. In some marsupials—koalas for example—there is both a thoracic thymus and a cervical thymus, the latter being a second set of thymic lobes above the thoracic cavity. What function this second thymus serves remains unknown.

It has also been suggested that the thymus evolved from specialized GALT (Matsunaga and Rahman, 2001). The mammalian thymus is derived from the third pharyngeal pouch. The second pharyngeal pouch becomes GALT in the form of the palatine tonsil. The second pharyngeal pouch develops into thymus in some fish, whereas other species have six pharyngeal pouches, all of which develop into a thymus. The fish thymus is therefore in contact with the external environment and is anatomically linked to the gills. These data suggest that GALT developed first and that it was only subsequently that higher animals subordinated its activity from GALT into a primary lymphoid organ.

THE PHYLOGENY OF GALT

GALT in fish (including lampreys and hagfish)

Fish differ from all other vertebrates in that they do not have lungs. Instead, they obtain oxygen directly through their skin and principally via the gills. Water constantly passes over the gill surfaces, which are also exposed to the external environment, so like the gut, the gills are a site where there is only a thin barrier between the internal and external milieu.

The jawless fishes do not have an adaptive immune system and lack T and B cell antigen receptors and cell-surface major histocompatibility molecules. However, their gut does contain cells with lymphocyte-like morphology (Mayer et al., 2002). Analysis of cDNA from these cells reveals the presence of transcripts associated with lymphocyte function, such as CD45 and CD81 (Uinuk-ool et al., 2002). The absence of these genes from other tissues in the lamprey suggests strongly that the adaptive immune system began to evolve in the gut but that jawless vertebrates still lack the machinery to generate diverse antigen receptors.

The cartilaginous fishes (sharks, rays, and skates) have an adaptive immune system and a spleen but no true lymph nodes. However there is only limited information on their GALT. Dogfish have lymphocytes and macrophages in their gut at hatching, and their number increases with age. Plasma cells appear in their gut at 6 months of age (Hart et al., 1986). Cells in the intestine secreting Ig have been noted in sharks, along with "lymphocyte-like" cells in the gut lining (Tomonaga et al., 1986) .

There is more information on the gut immune system of bony fishes, and some reagents are available for more detailed immunohistochemical studies (**Fig. 17.2**). Fish do not have Peyer's patches. A monoclonal antibody to sea bass thymocytes showed positive immunoreactivity in the gut (Romano et al., 1997). More detailed analysis showed that starting at 6 weeks post-hatching, positively staining cells were present in the gut epithelium and thymus but in no other tissue (Picchietti et al., 1997). Positive selection of cells recognized by this antibody showed that they contained transcripts with some homology to trout T cell receptor β chain, so it is probable that the antibody recognizes T cells (Scapigliati et al., 2000). Very few immunoglobulin-positive cells were seen in sea bass by 11 weeks post-hatching (Picchietti et al., 1997). Functional studies of mucosal immunity in sea bass have also been carried out. Intraperitoneal immunization with DNP-KLH or two bacteria (*Vibrio anguillarum* and *Photobacterium damselae* spp. *piscida*) revealed an increase in antibody-secreting cells in the gut (dos Santos et al., 2001a). More relevant studies examined the antibody response following immersion of the fish in *Photobacterium damselae* spp. *piscida* bacterin. By far the largest antibody response was in the gills (dos Santos et al., 2001b).

Carp intestine contains many immunoglobulin-positive leukocytes, some with plasma-cell-like morphology (Rombout et al., 1993), as does the gut of the turbot (Fournier-Betz et al., 2000). However, there may be species differences because few B cells are present in the gut of the channel catfish; the main immune cells isolated are neutrophils (Hebert et al., 2002). A monoclonal antibody to carp intestinal T cells labeled 50% to 70% of the lymphoid cells from gut, gills, or skin, and some of the cells were large granular leukocytes (Rombout et al., 1998). The antibody labeled few peripheral T cells. The antigen recognized appeared to be a 76-kd protein made up of two 38-kd homodimers, but its identity is unknown. Nonetheless, this result suggests that like mammals, fish might have a unique population of T cells in the gut.

Amphibians and reptiles

There is virtually no information on GALT in these classes of vertebrates. B cells have been identified in the gut of Xenopus (Du Pasquier and Flajnik, 1990). Reptiles have intraepithelial lymphocytes in their gut and accumulations of lymphocytes, which may be primitive Peyer's patches (Zapata and Solas, 1979; Solas and Zapata, 1980).

Birds

Chickens were of importance in highlighting the major role of primary lymphoid organs for immune competence following the discovery that removal of the bursa of Fabricius (a blind sac of lymphoid tissue invaginating from the cloaca near the anus, named after Hieronymus Fabricius, who described it in the 16th century in young chickens) led to antibody deficiency. No such equivalent organ exists in humans (although the appendix and ileal Peyer's patches are primary lymphoid organs in rabbits and sheep, respectively), but the discovery of the immunological role of the bursa was at the forefront in the development of immunology as a

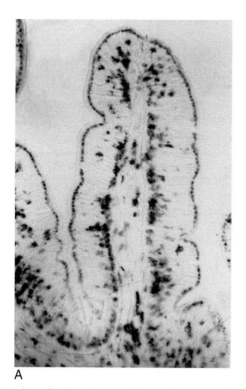 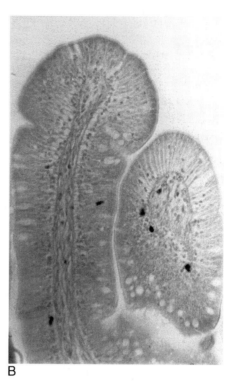

A   B

Fig. 17.2. T cells (**A**) and B cells (**B**) in the gut of the sea bass. Note that T cells are abundant in the lamina propria and especially in the epithelium and far outnumber B cells. Immunoperoxidase immunohistochemistry; original magnification, x100. Image courtesy of Dr. Guiseppe Scapigliati, University della Tuscia, Italy.

discipline in the 1950s. Chickens are also a major commercial source of protein of economic importance. In crowded conditions, as occur at megafarms, outbreaks of infection caused by the intestinal coccidians of the *Eimeria* species can devastate flocks. Accordingly, there has been a considerable amount of investigation of chicken GALT, because the ideal vaccine against coccidia would be one that elicits mucosal immunity (Yun *et al.*, 2000).

Chickens have Peyer's patches, although fewer than rodents or humans. Young chickens have about five Peyer's patches scattered along the bowel, but by 1 year of age, only a single patch is visible near the ileocecal valve (Befus *et al.*, 1980). Above the follicle there is a specialized epithelium that contains M cells and that can take up particles from the gut lumen (Jeurissen *et al.*, 1999). However, the epithelial cells in the FAE also take up luminal particles in chickens (Jeurissen *et al.*, 1999). Uptake of particles from the lumen is not associated with just Peyer's patches. Particles are also taken up by the bursa of Fabricius (Bockman and Stevens, 1977), although it is not clear if the bursal epithelium contains M cells. In addition, although the bursa is clearly a primary lymphoid organ and is the same size in germ-free and conventional chickens (Honjo *et al.*, 1993), ligation of the bursa at day 18 *in ovo* to prevent gut contents from entering the bursal lumen after birth has been reported to reduce bursal development and prevent the appearance of germinal centers in the spleen (Ekino *et al.*, 1985, 1995). Chickens

also have GALT not present in mammals, such as the cecal tonsils (aggregates of lymphoid tissue at the distal end of each of the two cecal tonsils) and Meckels diverticulum (a derivative of the yolk sac). These are secondary lymphoid tissues and have an FAE that contains M cells (Jeurissen *et al.*, 1999). Consistent with this, the lymphoid follicles in the cecal tonsils of germ-free chickens are smaller than the follicles in conventional chickens (Honjo *et al.*, 1993).

There have also been descriptive studies of the cell types in chicken GALT. The FAE of cecal tonsils contains large numbers of CD8 T cells (Jeurissen *et al.*, 1999). CD4 T cells are present in cecal tonsils, primarily between the follicles, and their numbers rapidly increase after hatching. By 6 weeks of age, however, CD8 cells exceed CD4 cells. The majority of the T cells express the αβ T cell receptor. Cecal tonsil follicles contain germinal centers and IgA-positive cells (Gomez del Moral *et al.*, 1998, Bar-Shira *et al.*, 2003). The lamina propria of the small intestine of chickens contains large numbers of antibody-secreting cells, presumably IgA plasma cells (Arnaud-Battandier *et al.*, 1980). The majority of T cells express CD4 (Rothwell *et al.*, 1995). Similar to all mammalian species so far examined, CD8 T cells exceed CD4 T cells in the gut epithelium of the chicken (Lillehoj and Chung 1992). A large number of αβ and γδ T cells in chicken gut epithelium express the CD8αα homodimer; however, both T cell types are thymus-derived (Imhof *et al.*, 2000). IEL are present, and although there are few at hatching, their numbers increase rapidly in young chickens (Lillehoj and Chung, 1992). There are at least as many γδ IEL as αβ IEL, but the ratio varies between chicken strains and with age (Lillehoj and Chung, 1992; Lillehoj, 1993). Approximately 30% of chicken IEL express CD8 but lack T and B cell markers and have natural-killer-cell activity (Gobel *et al.*, 2001).

There has been interest in following the changes in IEL that occur after infection with *Eimeria* species, because these parasites are obligate intracellular pathogens of gut epithelial cells. They also infect CD8 T cells. *Eimeria acervulina* infects the duodenum, and infection elicits a rather modest increase in CD4, CD8, and γδ T cells in the epithelium (Bessay *et al.*, 1996). *Eimeria tenella* infects the cecum and also elicits a modest increase in CD4 and CD8 cells, but there is no increase in γδ IEL at this site (Bessay *et al.*, 1996). Following infection with *E. tenella* there is an increase in interferon-γ transcripts in the small bowel IEL (Yun *et al.*, 2000), which is puzzling since the parasite infects the cecum. Cecal tonsil lymphocytes also express more interferon-γ transcripts, and there appears to be preferential expression in CD4 cells (Yun *et al.*, 2000). Interferon-γ may be involved in protective immunity to coccidia (Yun *et al.*, 2000).

GALT in metatherian and prototherian mammals

Information on the immune system of prototheria or monotremes (platypus and echidnas) is very sparse. Monotremes have IgA, and there are at least two IgA subclasses in the platypus (Belov *et al.*, 2002a). Although they have no obvious macroscopic GALT, histology reveals that they have Peyer's patches and cecal lymphoid follicles (Connolly *et al.*, 1999). This organization is consistent with the rest of the monotreme lymphoid tissues where lymph nodules are present, containing only a single follicle (Connolly *et al.*, 1999).

More investigations have been done on metatherian mammals or marsupials. However, it must be emphasized that there is considerable variation between marsupial species, as would be expected from a class that ranges from large animals like the red kangaroo to small marsupial mice. Indeed, this is very much like the case in eutherian mammals, where there is a huge range of different GALT with different functions in mice, humans, and sheep. Marsupials are as old an evolutionary lineage as the eutherians.

The first publication on gut lymphoid tissue in marsupials appeared in 1975 and noted that Peyer's patches were not identifiable histologically until 6 months of age in the quokka, a small wallabylike animal (Ashman and Papadimitriou, 1975). In 1984 Peyer's patches were examined in two species of marsupial mice (*Antechinus swainsonii* and *A. stuartii*). Both species lack a cecum and appendix (Poskitt *et al.*, 1984). In comparison with eutherian mice, marsupial mice have fewer Peyer's patches, with more numerous follicles. The South American white-bellied opossum (*Didelphis albiventris*) also has Peyer's patches, but they are unusual in that they do not have a conspicuous dome and the M cells are at the bases of the villi around the follicles (Coutinho *et al.*, 1990). Subsequent immunohistology in the same species showed that there were T cells in the epithelium

and in the Peyer's patches and that the patches were well formed while the newborn opossums were still in the pouch (Coutinho *et al.*, 1994). In a detailed study of GALT in koalas, brushtail possums, and common ringtailed possums, Peyer's patches were identified in all three species, as well as a large amount of lymphoid tissue in the cecum (Hemsley *et al.*, 1996a). Single follicles and aggregates of follicles were also seen in the colon. Immunohistology revealed that T and B cells had largely the same distribution in the Peyer's patches of these marsupials as in eutherian mammals (**Fig. 17.3**), with T cells between the lymphoid follicles (Hemsley *et al.*, 1996b), although there appear to be more B cells in the dome regions of the Peyer's patches than in mammals (Fig. 17.3). It is not clear why a previous publication found a paucity of lymphoid tissue in the gut of the koala (Hanger and Heath, 1994).

In an extensive analysis of the development of lymphoid tissue in the brushtail possum, CD3+ cells were detectable in the small intestine only, beginning at day 2 postpartum. By day 28, CD3+ cells were detectable in both the large and small intestine, but few Ig+ cells were present at this time. By day 73, there were extensive Ig+ and CD3+ cells throughout the intestine (**Fig. 17.4**), however, clear Peyer's patches were not visible until after day 73 (Baker *et al.*, 1999).

The adult Tammar wallaby (*Macropus eugenii*) GALT has also been investigated, and T cells were identified in the mucosal lamina propria and epithelium (Basden *et al.*, 1997). The Peyer's patches of Tammar wallabies contain T and B cells with the same distribution as eutherian mammals, namely, a large follicle center with T cells in the interfollicular zones (Old and Deane, 2002a). In juvenile eastern grey kangaroos, the distribution of T and B cells was also essentially similar to that in eutherian mammals (Old and Deane, 2001). In the northern brown bandicoot, two types of lymphoid follicles in the gut were described: those that had a linear appearance in histological sections and those that were aggregates of follicles (Old and Deane, 2002b). T cells were abundant between the follicles, and there were large follicle centers. Many of the Peyer's patches had clearly defined domes. T cells were again abundant in the mucosa.

Very little molecular analysis of mucosal immunity in marsupials has been done. The polymeric immunoglobulin receptor of the brushtail possum has been cloned, and it is expressed in the mammary gland along with IgA transcripts (Adamski and Demmer, 1999). This makes it highly likely that the poly-Ig receptor is expressed in the gut and transports IgA into the lumen later in life. This speculation would be consistent with the evidence of transfer of Ig into circulation of suckling opossums from immune mothers (Samples *et al.*, 1986).

PHYLOGENY OF MATERNAL TRANSPORT OF IMMUNOGLOBULINS

The hallmark of marsupial reproduction is the birth of relatively immature young that complete embryonic development

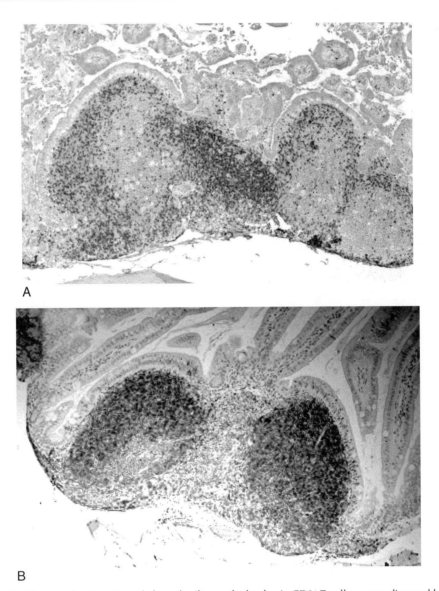

Fig. 17.3. Immunohistological image of a Peyer's patch from the ileum of a koala. **A,** CD3⁺ T cells surrounding and between the follicles and penetrating into the dome region; **B,** B cells, identifiable by expression of CD79. They predominate at the tops of the follicles and are also abundant in the FAE. Images courtesy of Dr. Paul Canfield and Dr. Susan Hemsley, Faculty of Veterinary Science, University of Sydney.

while attached to the teat within a pouch or marsupium. Similar to the variation in the transfer of maternal Ig in eutherian mammals, there are also differences in the transfer of maternal Ig in marsupials. In the grey short-tailed opossum (*Monodelphis domestica*), the quokka (*Setonix brachyurus*), and the brushtail possum (*T. vulpecula*), there is no apparent transfer of maternal Ig *in utero* (Adamski and Demmer, 2000; Samples *et al.*, 1986; Yadav and Eadie, 1973). In the tammar wallaby, maternal Ig is detectable in the yolk sac, fetal serum, and newborn serum (Deane *et al.*, 1990). These differences do not follow phylogenetic patterns since both the wallaby and the quokka are macropods (kangaroo family).

Marsupials have a more complex lactation than eutherian mammals. Following a colostrum phase, there is an early milk phase corresponding to the time when the pouch young are always attached to the teats, followed by a switch phase in which the milk protein composition changes to create a late-phase milk that resembles eutherian milk. Immediately following birth of the brushtail possum, there is a high level of secretory IgA in the colostrum and milk and concomitant expression of the polymeric Ig receptor (pIgR) in the possum mammary gland. The levels of IgA steadily decline throughout the remainder of lactation; however, there is a large increase in IgG in the late milk phase (Adamski and Demmer, 2000). The presence of both IgG and IgA in this marsupial is similar to eutherian ungulates that also lack prenatal transfer of maternal Ig. The pIgR has been cloned from both the brushtail possum and the tammar wallaby, providing the opportunity to study transfer of Ig at mucosal sites (Adamski and Demmer, 2000; Taylor *et al.*, 2002).

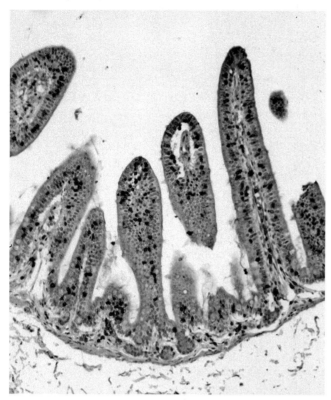

Fig. 17.4. Immunohistological demonstration of CD3[+] T cells in the mucosa of the brush-tailed possum. Positive cells are present in the epithelium and lamina propria. Image courtesy of Dr. Paul Canfield and Dr. Susan Hemsley, Faculty of Veterinary Science, University of Sydney.

CONCLUSIONS

The immune systems of animals other than mice and humans remain underinvestigated, and thus it is not particularly surprising that information on GALT in species other than mice and humans is even less investigated. Nonetheless, piecing together the fragmentary data, it is possible to come to some conclusions. Fish do not have Peyer's patches; they have T and B cells scattered along their guts. There are no solid data on reptiles and amphibians. The warm-blooded vertebrates clearly have a well-evolved mucosal immune system. Birds and marsupials have Peyer's patches that appear to differ very little from those of eutherian mammals in that they have follicle-associated epithelium with M cells, large germinal centers, and T cells and plasma cells secreting IgA in the mucosa between the organized GALT.

REFERENCES

Adamski, F.M., Demmer, J. (1999) Two stages of increased IgA transfer during lactation in the marsupial, trichosurus vulpecula (Brushtail possum). *J. Immunol.* 162, 6009–6015.

Adamski, F.M., Demmer, J. (2000) Immunological protection of the vulnerable marsupial pouch young: two periods of immune transfer during lactation in Trichosurus vulpecula (brushtail possum). *Dev. Comp. Immunol.* 24, 491–502.

Adema, C.M., Hertel, L.A., Miller, R.D., and Loker, E.S. (1997) A family of fibrinogen-related proteins that precipitates parasite-derived molecules is produced by an invertebrate after infection. *Proc. Natl. Acad. Sci. USA*, 94, 8691–8696.

Agrawal, A., Eastman, Q.M., and Schatz, D.G. (1998) Transposition mediated by RAG1 and RAG2 and its implications for the evolution of the immune system. *Nature* 394, 744–751.

Arnaud-Battandier, F., Lawrence, E.C., and Blaese, R.M. (1980) Lymphoid populations of gut mucosa in chickens. *Dig. Dis. Sci.* 25, 252–259.

Ashman, R.B., Papadimitriou, J.M. (1975) Development of lymphoid tissue in a marsupial, Setonix brachyurus (quokka). *Acta Anat. (Basel)* 91, 594–611.

Baker, M.L., Gemmell, E., and Gemmell, R.T. (1999) Ontogeny of the immune system of the brushtail possum, Trichosurus vulpecula. *Anat. Rec.* 256, 354–365.

Bar-Shira, E., Sklan, D., and Friedman, A. (2003) Establishment of immune competence in the avian GALT during the immediate post-hatch period. *Dev. Comp. Immunol.* 27, 147–157.

Basden, K., Cooper, D.W., and Deane, E.M. (1997) Development of the lymphoid tissues of the tammar wallaby Macropus eugenii. *Reprod. Fertil. Dev.* 9, 243–254.

Befus, A.D., Johnston, N., Leslie, G.A., and Bienenstock, J. (1980) Gut-associated lymphoid tissue in the chicken. I. Morphology, ontogeny, and some functional characteristics of Peyer's patches. *J. Immunol.* 125, 2626–2632.

Belov, K., Zenger, K.R., Hellman, L., and Cooper, D.W. (2002a) Echidna IgA supports mammalian unity and traditional Therian relationship. *Mamm. Genome* 13, 656–663.

Belov, K., Hellman, L., and Cooper, D.W. (2002b) Characterisation of echidna IgM provides insights into the time of divergence of extant mammals. *Dev. Comp. Immunol.* 26, 831–839.

Bengten, E., Wilson, M., Miller, N., Clem, L.W., Pilstrom, L., and Warr, G.W. (2000) Immunoglobulin isotypes: structure, function, and genetics. *Curr. Top. Microbiol. Immunol.* 248, 189–219.

Bernstein, R.M., Schluter, S.F., Bernstein, H., and Marchalonis, J.J. (1996) Primordial emergence of the recombination activating gene 1 (RAG1): sequence of the complete shark gene indicates homology to microbial integrates. *Proc. Natl. Acad. Sci. USA* 93, 9454–9459.

Bessay, M., Le Vern, Y., Kerboeuf, D., Yvore, P., and Quere, P. (1996) Changes in intestinal intra-epithelial and systemic T-cell subpopulations after an Eimeria infection in chickens: comparative study between E acervulina and E tenella. *Vet. Res.* 27, 503–514.

Bockman, D.E., Stevens, W. (1977) Gut-associated lymphoepithelial tissue: bidirectional transport of tracer by specialized epithelial cells associated with lymphoid follicles. *J. Reticuloendothel. Soc.* 21, 245–254.

Cannon, J.P., Haire, R.N., and Litman, G.W. (2002) Identification of diversified genes that contain immunoglobulin-like variable regions in a protochordate. *Nat. Immunol.* 3, 1200–1207.

Carrol, R. L. (1998) Vertebrate paleontology and evolution. New York: WH Freeman and Co.

Connolly, J.H., Canfield, P.J., McClure, S.J., and Whittington, R.J. (1999) Histological and immunohistological investigation of lymphoid tissue in the platypus (Ornithorhynchus anatinus). *J. Anat.* 195 (Pt 2), 161–171.

Coutinho, H.B., Nogueira, J.C., King, G., Coutinho, V.B., Robalinho, T.I., Amorim, A.M., Cavalcanti, V.M., Robins, R.A., and Sewell, H.F. (1994) Immunocytochemical study of the ontogeny of Peyer's patches in the Brazilian marsupial Didelphis albiventris. *J. Anat.* 185 (Pt 2), 347–354.

Coutinho, V.B., Coutinho, H.B., Robalinho, T.I., Silva, E.S., Sewell, H.F., and McKinnon, A.D. (1990) Histological and ultrastructural studies of the marsupial Didelphis albiventris Peyer's patches. *Mem. Inst. Oswaldo Cruz* 85, 435–443.

Deane, E.M., Cooper, D.W., and Renfree, M.B. (1990) Immunoglobulin G levels in fetal and newborn tammar wallabies (Macropus eugenii). *Reprod. Fertil. Dev.* 2, 369–375.

dos Santos, N.M., Taverne-Thiele, J.J., Barnes, A.C., van Muiswinkel, W.B., Ellis, A.E., and Rombout, J.H. (2001) The gill is a major organ for antibody secreting cell production following direct immersion of sea bass (Dicentrarchus labrax, L.) in a

Photobacterium damselae ssp. piscicida bacterin: an ontogenetic study. *Fish Shellfish Immunol.* 11, 65–74.

dos Santos, N.M., Taverne-Thiele, J.J., Barnes, A.C., Ellis, A.E., and Rombout, J.H. (2001) Kinetics of juvenile sea bass (Dicentrarchus labrax, L.) systemic and mucosal antibody secreting cell response to different antigens (Photobacterium damselae spp. piscicida, Vibrio anguillarum and DNP). *Fish. Shellfish Immunol.* 11, 317–331.

Du, P.L., Flajnik, M.F. (1990) Expression of MHC class II antigens during Xenopus development. *Dev. Immunol.* 1, 85–95.

Du, P.L. (2000) The phylogenetic origin of antigen-specific receptors. *Curr. Top. Microbiol. Immunol.* 248, 160–185.

Ekino, S., Urano, T., Fujii, H., and Kotani, M. (1985) The bursa of Fabricius as a trapping mechanism for environmental antigens. *Adv. Exp. Med. Biol.* 186, 487–493.

Ekino, S., Riwar, B., Kroese, F.G., Schwander, E.H., Koch, G., and Nieuwenhuis, P. (1995) Role of environmental antigen in the development of IgG+ cells in the bursa of Fabricius. *J. Immunol.* 155, 4551–4558.

Flajnik, M.F., Rumfelt, L.L. (2000) The immune system of cartilaginous fish. *Curr. Top. Microbiol. Immunol.* 248, 249–270.

Fournier-Betz, V., Quentel, C., Lamour, F., and LeVen, A. (2000) Immunocytochemical detection of Ig-positive cells in blood, lymphoid organs and the gut associated lymphoid tissue of the turbot (Scophthalmus maximus). *Fish. Shellfish Immunol.* 10, 187–202.

Gobel, T.W., Kaspers, B., and Stangassinger, M. (2001) NK and T cells constitute two major, functionally distinct intestinal epithelial lymphocyte subsets in the chicken. *Int. Immunol.* 13, 757–762.

Gomez, D.M., Fonfria, J., Varas, A., Jimenez, E., Moreno, J., and Zapata, A.G. (1998) Appearance and development of lymphoid cells in the chicken (Gallus gallus) caecal tonsil. *Anat. Rec.* 250, 182–189.

Groth, J.G., Barrowclough, G.F. (1999) Basal divergences in birds and the phylogenetic utility of the nuclear RAG-1 gene. *Mol. Phylogenet. Evol.* 12, 115–123.

Hanger, J.J., Heath, T.J. (1994) The arrangement of gut-associated lymphoid tissues and lymph pathways in the koala (Phascolarctos cinereus). *J. Anat.* 185 (Pt 1), 129–134.

Hansen, J.D., McBlane, J.F. (2000) Recombination-activating genes, transposition, and the lymphoid-specific combinatorial immune system: a common evolutionary connection. *Curr. Top. Microbiol. Immunol.* 248, 111–135.

Hart, S., Wrathmell, A.B., and Harris, J.E. (1986) Ontogeny of gut-associated lymphoid tissue (GALT) in the dogfish Scyliorhinus canicula L. *Vet. Immunol. Immunopathol.* 12, 107–116.

Hebert, P., Ainsworth, A.J., and Boyd, B. (2002) Histological enzyme and flow cytometric analysis of channel catfish intestinal tract immune cells. *Dev. Comp Immunol.* 26, 53–62.

Hemsley, S.W., Canfield, P.J., and Husband, A.J. (1996) The distribution of organised lymphoid tissue in the alimentary tracts of koalas (Phascolarctos cinereus) and possums (Trichosurus vulpecula and Pseudocheirus peregrinus). *J. Anat.* 188 (Pt 2), 269–278.

Hemsley, S.W., Canfield, P.J., and Husband, A.J. (1996) Histological and immunohistological investigation of alimentary tract lymphoid tissue in the koala (Phascolarctos cinereus), brushtail possum (Trichosurus vulpecula) and ringtail possum (Pseudocheirus peregrinus). *J. Anat.* 188 (Pt 2), 279–288.

Hiom, K., Melek, M., and Gellert, M. (1998) DNA transposition by the RAG1 and RAG2 proteins: a possible source of oncogenic translocations. *Cell* 94, 463–470.

Honjo, K., Hagiwara, T., Itoh, K., Takahashi, E., and Hirota, Y. (1993) Immunohistochemical analysis of tissue distribution of B and T cells in germfree and conventional chickens. *J. Vet. Med. Sci.* 55, 1031–1034.

Huxley, TH. On the application of laws of evolution to the arrangement of the Vertebrata, and more particularly of the Mammalia. *Proc. Zoo. Soc. Lond.* 1880;43:649–662.

Imhof, B.A., Dunon, D, Courtois, D., Luhtala, M., and Vainio, O. (2000) Intestinal CD8 alpha alpha and CD8 alpha beta intraepithelial lymphocytes are thymus derived and exhibit subtle differences in TCR beta repertoires. *J. Immunol.* 165:6716–6722.

Iwata, A., Iwase, T., Ogura, Y., Takahashi, T., Matsumoto, N., Yoshida, T., Kamei, N., Kobayashi, K., Mestecky, J., and Moro, I. (2002) Cloning and expression of the turtle (Trachemys scripta) immunoglobulin joining (J)-chain cDNA. *Immunogenetics* 54, 513–519.

Janke, A., Gemmell, N.J., Feldmaier-Fuchs, G., von Haeseler, A., and Paabo, S. (1996) The mitochondrial genome of a monotreme: the platypus (Ornithorhynchus anatinus). *J. Mol. Evol.* 42, 153–159.

Jeurissen, S.H., Wagenaar, F., and Janse, E.M. (1999) Further characterization of M cells in gut-associated lymphoid tissues of the chicken. *Poult. Sci.* 78, 965–972.

Kasahara, M. (2000) Genome paralogy: a new perspective on the organization and origin of the major histocompatibility complex. *Curr. Top. Microbiol. Immunol.* 248, 53–66.

Killian, J.K., Buckley, T.R., Stewart, N., Munday, B.L., and Jirtle, R.L. (2001) Marsupials and Eutherians reunited: genetic evidence for the Theria hypothesis of mammalian evolution. *Mamm. Genome* 12, 513–517.

Kumar, S. and Hedges, S.B. (1998) A molecular timescale for vertebrate evolution. *Nature* 392, 917–919.

Lillehoj, H.S., Chung, K.S. (1992) Postnatal development of T-lymphocyte subpopulations in the intestinal intraepithelium and lamina propria in chickens. *Vet. Immunol. Immunopathol.* 31, 347–360.

Lillehoj, H.S. (1993) Avian gut-associated immune system: implication in coccidial vaccine development. *Poult. Sci.* 72, 1306–1311.

Lucero, J.E., Rosenberg, G.H., and Miller, R.D. (1998) Marsupial light chains: complexity and conservation of lambda in the opossum Monodelphis domestica. *J. Immunol.* 161, 6724–6732.

Matsunaga, T., Rahman, A. (2001) In search of the origin of the thymus: the thymus and GALT may be evolutionarily related. *Scand. J. Immunol.* 53, 1–6.

Mayer, W.E., Uinuk-Ool, T., Tichy, H., Gartland, L.A., Klein, J., and Cooper, M.D. (2002) Isolation and characterization of lymphocyte-like cells from a lamprey. *Proc. Natl. Acad. Sci. USA* 99, 14350–14355.

Miller, R.D., Hogg, J., Ozaki, J.H., Gell, D., Jackson, S.P., and Riblet, R. (1995) Gene for the catalytic subunit of mouse DNA-dependent protein kinase maps to the scid locus. *Proc. Natl. Acad. Sci. USA* 92, 10792–10795.

Miller, R.D., Bergermann, E.R., and Rosenberg, G.H. (1999). Marsupial light chains: Igκ with four V families in the opossum *Monodelphis domestics. Immunogenetics* 50:329–335.

Miller, R.D., Belov, K. (2000) Immunoglobulin genetics of marsupials. *Dev. Comp. Immunol.* 24, 485–490.

Miska, K.B., Hellman, L., and Miller, R.D. (2003) Characterization of beta(2)-microglobulin coding sequence from three non-placental mammals: the duckbill platypus, the short-beaked echidna, and the grey short-tailed opossum. *Dev. Comp. Immunol.* 27, 247–256.

Old, J.M., Deane, E.M. (2001) Histology and immunohistochemistry of the gut-associated lymphoid tissue of the eastern grey kangaroo, Macropus giganteus. *J. Anat.* 199, 657–662.

Old, J.M., Deane, E.M. (2002) Immunohistochemistry of the lymphoid tissues of the tammar wallaby, Macropus eugenii. *J. Anat.* 201, 257–266.

Old, J.M., Deane, E.M. (2002) The gut-associated lymphoid tissues of the northern brown bandicoot (Isoodon macrourus). *Dev. Comp. Immunol.* 26, 841–848.

Ota, T., Rast, J.P., Litman, G.W., and Amemiya, C.T. (2003) Lineage-restricted retention of a primitive immunoglobulin heavy chain isotype within the Dipnoi reveals an evolutionary paradox. *Proc. Natl. Acad. Sci. USA* 100, 2501–2506.

Pascual, R., Archer, M., Jaureguizar, E.O., Prado, J.L., Godthelp, H., and Hand, S.J. (1992) First discovery of monotremes in South America. *Nature* 356, 704–706.

Picchietti, S., Terribili, F.R., Mastrolia, L., Scapigliati, G., and Abelli, L. (1997) Expression of lymphocyte antigenic determinants in developing gut-associated lymphoid tissue of the sea bass Dicentrarchus labrax (L.). *Anat. Embryol. (Berl.)* 196, 457–463.

Pilstrom, L. (2002) The mysterious immunoglobulin light chain. *Dev. Comp. Immunol.* 26, 207–215.

Poskitt, D.C., Duffey, K., Barnett, J., Kimpton, W.G., and Muller, H.K. (1984) The gut-associated lymphoid system of two species of Australian marsupial mice, Antechinus swainsonii and Antechinus stuartii. Distribution, frequency and structure of Peyer's patches and lymphoid follicles in the small and large intestine. *Aust. J. Exp. Biol. Med. Sci.* 62 (Pt 1), 81–88.

Rast, J.P., Anderson, M.K., Strong, S.J., Luer, C., Litman, R.T., and Litman, G.W. (1997) alpha, beta, gamma, and delta T cell antigen receptor genes arose early in vertebrate phylogeny. *Immunity* 6, 1–11.

Retief, J.D., Winkfein, R.J., and Dixon, G.H. (1993) Evolution of the monotremes. The sequences of the protamine P1 genes of platypus and echidna. *Eur. J. Biochem.* 218, 457–461.

Romano, N., Abelli, L., Mastrolia, L., and Scapigliati, G. (1997) Immunocytochemical detection and cytomorphology of lymphocyte subpopulations in a teleost fish Dicentrarchus labrax. *Cell Tissue Res.* 289, 163–171.

Rombout, J.H., Taverne-Thiele, A.J., and Villena, M.I. (1993) The gut-associated lymphoid tissue (GALT) of carp (Cyprinus carpio L.): an immunocytochemical analysis. *Dev. Comp. Immunol.* 17, 55–66.

Rombout, J.H., Joosten, P.H., Engelsma, M.Y., Vos, A.P., Taverne, N., and Taverne-Thiele, J.J. (1998) Indications for a distinct putative T cell population in mucosal tissue of carp (Cyprinus carpio L.). *Dev. Comp. Immunol.* 22, 63–77.

Rothwell, L., Gramzinski, R.A., Rose, M.E., and Kaiser, P. (1995) Avian coccidiosis: changes in intestinal lymphocyte populations associated with the development of immunity to Eimeria maxima. *Parasite Immunol.* 17, 525–533.

Rouse, J., Jackson, S.P. (2002) Interfaces between the detection, signaling, and repair of DNA damage. *Science* 297, 547–551.

Ruddle, F.H., Bentley, K.L., Murtha, M.T., and Risch, N. (1994) Gene loss and gain in the evolution of the vertebrates. *Dev. Suppl.* 155–161.

Samples, N.K., Vandeberg, J.L., and Stone, W.H. (1986) Passively acquired immunity in the newborn of a marsupial (Monodelphis domestica). *Am. J. Reprod. Immunol. Microbiol.* 11, 94–97.

Scapigliati, G., Romano, N., Abelli, L., Meloni, S., Ficca, A.G., Buonocore, F., Bird, S., and Secombes, C.J. (2000) Immunopurification of T-cells from sea bass Dicentrarchus labrax (L.). *Fish Shellfish Immunol.* 10, 329–341.

Solas, M.T., Zapata, A. (1980) Gut-associated lymphoid tissue (GALT) in reptiles: intraepithelial cells. *Dev. Comp. Immunol.* 4, 87–97.

Taylor, C.L., Harrison, G.A., Watson, C.M., and Deane, E.M. (2002) cDNA cloning of the polymeric immunoglobulin receptor of the marsupial Macropus eugenii (tammar wallaby). *Eur. J. Immunogenet*, 29, 87–93.

Tomonaga, S., Kobayashi, K, Hagiwara, K, Yamaguchi, K, and Awaya, K. (1986) Gut associated lymphoid tissue in elasmobranches. *Zool. Sci.* 3, 453–458.

Tuteja, R., Tuteja, N. (2000) Ku autoantigen: a multifunctional DNA-binding protein. *Crit. Rev. Biochem. Mol. Biol.* 35, 1–33.

Uinuk-Ool, T., Mayer, W.E., Sato, A., Dongak, R., Cooper, M.D., and Klein, J. (2002) Lamprey lymphocyte-like cells express homologs of genes involved in immunologically relevant activities of mammalian lymphocytes. *Proc. Natl. Acad. Sci. USA* 99, 14356–14361.

Uinuk-Ool, T.S., Mayer, W.E., Sato, A., Takezaki, N., Benyon, L., Cooper, M.D., and Klein, J. (2003) Identification and characterization of a TAP-family gene in the lamprey. *Immunogenetics* 55, 38–48.

Vernersson, M., Aveskogh, M., Munday, B., and Hellman, L. (2002) Evidence for an early appearance of modern post-switch immunoglobulin isotypes in mammalian evolution (II); cloning of IgE, IgG1 and IgG2 from a monotreme, the duck-billed platypus, Ornithorhynchus anatinus. *Eur. J. Immunol.* 32, 2145–2155.

Willett, C.E., Cortes, A., Zuasti, A., and Zapata, A.G. (1999) Early hematopoiesis and developing lymphoid organs in the zebrafish. *Dev. Dyn.* 214, 323–336.

Yadav, M and Eadie, M. (1973) Passage of maternal immunoglobulin to the pouch young of a marsupial, Setonix brachyurus. *Aust. J. Zool.* 21, 171–181.

Yun, C.H., Lillehoj, H.S., and Choi, K.D. (2000) Eimeria tenella infection induces local gamma interferon production and intestinal lymphocyte subpopulation changes. *Infect. Immun.* 68, 1282–1288.

Yun, C.H., Lillehoj, H.S., and Lillehoj, E.P. (2000) Intestinal immune responses to coccidiosis. *Dev. Comp. Immunol.* 24, 303–324.

Zapata, A., Solas, M.T. (1979) Gut-associated lymphoid tissue (GALT) in reptilia: structure of mucosal accumulations. *Dev. Comp. Immunol.* 3, 477–487.

The Role of Mucosal Microbiota in the Development, Maintenance, and Pathologies of the Mucosal Immune System

John J. Cebra, Han-Qing Jiang

Department of Biology, University of Pennsylvania, Philadelphia, Pennsylvania

Nadiya Boiko

Department of Biology, University of Pennsylvania, Philadelphia, Pennsylvania, and Department of Genetics and Plant Physiology, Uzhhorod National University, Uzhhorod, Ukraine

Helena Tlaskalova-Hogenova

Department of Gnotobiology and Immunology, Institute of Microbiology, Czech Academy of Sciences, Prague, Czech Republic

DEVELOPMENT OF THE SYSTEMIC IMMUNE SYSTEM: ROLE OF ENVIRONMENTAL ANTIGENS

A comprehensive review of the history and role of intestinal microflora is given in the version of this chapter presented in the previous edition of this volume (Cebra et al., 1999). The pioneering studies concerned whether the presence of bacteria in the intestine was essential for the life of the host (see Leidy, 1849). The general approaches involved either deriving mammals with a sterile intestinal tract (axenic or "germ-free" [GF]), which could then be deliberately colonized with known members of the intestinal microbiota (gnotobiotic mammals), or analyzing newborns, born essentially GF, as they developed and naturally acquired a "normal" microbiota. Early on, changes in the systemic immune system were monitored, since the somewhat separate mucosal immune system had not yet been properly

defined and appreciated. The early pioneers in GF/gnotobiotic studies of mammals included Glimstedt (1932) and Gustafsson (1948) in Sweden, Reyniers (1932), Pleasants, Wostmann, and Pollard at the Lobund Institute, in the United States (see Carter and Pollard, 1971); Miyakawa *et al.* (1958) in Japan; and Sterzl, Mandel *et al.* (1960) in Czechoslovakia. Pleasants, Wostmann, and their coworkers further minimized microbial and food antigen stimulation of mice by developing "antigen-free" (AF) mice fed a chemically defined (CD) diet of water-soluble, low-molecular-weight nutrients plus soy oil containing vitamins (Pleasants *et al.*, 1986). From earlier times (van der Waaij, 1969) up to the present (Fagarasan *et al.*, 2002), investigators have sought to simplify the elimination of gut microbes and circumvent the intricate, complex, and expensive procedures used to derive and maintain GF or AF rodents by decontaminating them with "cocktails" of orally administered antibiotics. Usually, the "physiologically normal" state of hypertrophy and inflammation of the lymphoid system is somewhat reversed but there is little information of the effects on the developmental status and functional activity of particular elements of the immune system. However, the many analyses of the effects of intestinal colonization with microbes of GF or AF mice and of natural colonization of neonates on the systemic immune system can be generalized as follows (see Cebra *et al.*, 1999, for a more detailed account).

Conventionally reared (CNV) neonates develop "natural" plaque-forming cells (PFC) or antibody-secreting cells (ASC) in spleen and peripheral lymph nodes (PLN) against autoantigens, bacterial antigens (Ags) (especially lipopolysaccharide [LPS]), and sheep red blood cells (SRBC), whereas GF neonates are greatly retarded in this development (Tlaskalova *et al.*, 1970, 1983; Tlaskalova and Stepankova, 1980).

GF and AF adults can and do respond to active parenteral immunization with SRBC, protein Ags, and hapten-protein conjugates and to colonization by gut bacteria with splenic PFC or ASC, often at higher frequencies or titers than their CNV counterparts (Berg and Savage, 1975; Kim, 1979; Bos and Ploplis, 1994).

GF neonates, especially colostrum-deprived piglets, show a profound hypotrophy of PLN and spleen and a marked diminution of peripheral lymphoid cells reactive versus mitogens or polyclonal stimuli (Tlaskalova *et al.*, 1970; Tlaskalova and Stepankova, 1980; Kim, 1979). The hypotrophy persists into adulthood for both GF and especially AF mice, although the latter do show nearly normal numbers of splenic marginal zone and peritoneal cavity (PeC) B cells relative to their CNV counterparts (Bos *et al.*, 2003). The GF neonates also respond poorly to deliberate Ag stimulation (Tlaskalova and Stepankova, 1980; Kim, 1979; Tlaskalova *et al.*, 1994). The neonatal hyporesponsiveness of GF and even CNV mammals, especially versus microbial polysaccharide Ags, has often been attributed to immaturity of B cells and the time lag in transition of recently arrived B cells in the periphery ("virgin B cells") to B cells positively responsive to cross-linking of BCRs (primary B cells). It has long been proposed that gut microbial stimulation, especially via LPS, can drive this process. Recently, Monroe and his students have shown a delay in the development of competence of neonatal B cells (until 18–23 days of life), to respond to *in vitro* cross-linking of their BCRs with $F(ab')_2$ anti-mouse IgM (Monroe *et al.*, 1993; Yellin-Shaw and Monroe, 1992). Neonatal and adult peripheral B cells are about equally responsive to mitogenic stimulation with LPS. Finally, this group further found that addition of LPS to cultures of neonatal B cells unresponsive to the presence of $F(ab')_2$ anti-IgM markedly enhanced their reactivity (Wechsler-Reya and Monroe, 1996). Thus, microbial products such as LPS may naturally enhance specific B cell responsiveness to cross-linking of their BCRs *in vivo* during neonatal development via microbial colonization of the gut.

DEVELOPMENT OF THE MUCOSAL IMMUNE SYSTEM: ROLE OF MICROFLORA

Most mucosal sites of lymphoid tissue—respiratory tract, adenoids, salivary glands, urogenital tract—in healthy mammals are in a quiescent state and generally resemble the status of lymphoid areas in spleen and most PLN. The intestinal tract, palatine tonsils, and occasionally the nasal-associated lymphoid tissue (NALT) are the exceptions. These mucosal lymphoid tissues are in a "physiologically normal state of inflammation" (Weinstein *et al.*, 1991; Liu *et al.*, 1991). Indeed, Prof. Hall (1984) has pointed out that were the respiratory tract–associated lymphoid tissues (RALT) in the same state as the gut-associated lymphoid tissue (GALT), we would all suffer from chronic pneumonia and bronchitis. It is the thesis of this chapter that intestinal microbes drive the development of GALT during neonatal life and act to maintain its physiologically normal steady state of inflammation. Specific and adaptive, "natural" and semispecific, and aspecific elements of the mucosal immune systems may benefit and be activated by host interactions with environmental Ags. To provide the experimental rationale for implicating intestinal or oral/nasal microflora in the development of GALT, palatine tonsil, and sometimes NALT and their steady state of inflammation, we must briefly contrast the status of systemic lymphoid tissue in healthy mammals—spleen, PLN—with GALT, palatine tonsils, and NALT.

GALT compartments

Early on, the term *GALT* was meant to include only the "inductive" sites in gut-associated lymphoid tissues, for lymphoid cell activation and proliferation (Brandtzaeg and Farstad, 1999), following the earlier usage of BALT (bronchus-associated lymphoid tissues). Recently, the inclusion of appreciable numbers of lymphoid cells from solitary follicles in typically isolated single-cell suspensions from gut lamina propria (LP) has been appreciated, blurring the distinctions between "inductive" and "effector" sites (see Hiroi *et al.*, 2000). Perhaps, future directed immunohistochemical analyses, microdissection (see Hamada *et al.*, 2002), and analyses using gene arrays on microchips after laser capture of cells will permit clear distinctions between cells in solitary follicles and those in the loose connective tissue of the gut LP itself. Thus, we feel that the inclusion of gut LP as one of the divisions of GALT is presently appropriate. The recognition of "atypical" subsets of T cells, natural killer (NK) cells, and NK-like cells in the intraepithelial spaces and the rather broad or "aspecific" reactivity of some of them with microbial products make their local activation likely and their inclusion as a compartment of GALT likewise appropriate.

Peyer's patches (PP) and solitary follicles (SF)

Peyer's patches (about 8–10) and SF are found in the walls of the small intestine or both small and large intestine, respectively. About 30,000 SF occur in the human intestine, and about 10–20 SF occur in the murine small intestine, as just recently described (Brandtzaeg and Farstad, 1999; Hamada *et al.*, 2002). These organized lymphoid structures are composed conspicuously or mainly of spherical B lymphoid follicles, including chronically present B lymphoblasts embedded in a meshwork of follicular dendritic cells (DC). Both GALT and palatine tonsillar B cell follicles are secondary and display chronic germinal center reactions (GCR) (Weinstein *et al.*, 1991; Liu *et al.*, 1991). The predominant non-IgM isotype expressed on GC B blasts in the PP and SF of most mammalian species is IgA; B blasts in human tonsillar GC mainly express IgG isotypes (Lebman *et al.*, 1987; Pascuel *et al.*, 1994). Both these tissues normally contain relatively large numbers of IgA (Peyer's patches) or IgG (tonsils) "memory" B cells. Thus, the B cell follicles of these mucosal tissues differ from those of spleen and lymph node, which are ordinarily quiescent and "primary," displaying no GCR with dividing B blasts and being composed of IgM/IgD-positive primary B cells. The B cell follicles of PP, SF, and also murine NALT contain microfold (M) cells, scattered through their follicle-associated epithelium (FAE). These M cells act as "efferent lymphatics," transporting samples of foreign antigen from the gut lumen or airways into the organized lymphoid tissue (Weltzin *et al.*, 1989; Hamada *et al.*, 2002; Zuercher and Cebra, 2002; Zuercher *et al.*, 2002). Although the SF of mice share many characteristics of PP and differ from "cryptopatches" (see Kanamori *et al.*, 1996), they appear to also contain some of the cells characteristic of cryptopatches, especially the c-kit[+], IL-7R[+], Thy1[+] cells involved in lymphopoiesis of some gut T cells (Hamada *et al.*, 2002).

Most of the T lymphocytes in PP reside in the wedge-shaped, interfollicular regions and include both CD4[+] and CD8[+] T cells (London *et al.*, 1990). Both of these subsets generally include a higher proportion of cells displaying activated phenotypes, such as CD45RB[low], CD69[+], and CD62L[low] (Talham *et al.*, 1999; Jump and Levine, 2002), than corresponding subsets from quiescent spleen or lymph nodes. Recently, *in vitro* culture of PP T cells in anti-CD3-coated plates has shown that a "naturally activated" population of CD45RB[low], CD4[+] T cells can be stimulated via TCR to produce much greater amounts of IL-10, but not IFNγ, IL-4, or IL-12, in comparison with MLN and PLN (Jump and Levine, 2002). Thus, the PP seems to contain a set of T cells that express similar properties to those that may mediate oral tolerance or downregulation of peripheral T cells.

Interdigitating DC from PP of CNV mice (CD11c[+] DC) have been shown to selectively induce production of IL-4 and IL-10 by naïve CD4[+] T cells from TCR-transgenic mice (Iwasaki and Kelsall, 1999). Such DC are likely also found in gut LP and MLN (see the section on Gut Lamina Propria). Recently, Iwasaki and Kelsall (2001) have distinguished three subsets of DCs in PPs. The CD11b[+]/CD8α[–] (myeloid) DCs, localized to the subepithelial dome, appear

to be the subset that produces IL-10 upon stimulation with CD40-ligand trimer and that can present Ag-peptide to stimulate CD4[+] T cells to produce IL-4 and IL-10.

Gut lamina propria

The gut LP is a meshwork of connective tissue underlying the gut epithelium and containing a broad spectrum of myeloid, lymphoid, and mesenchymal cells. With respect to B cell status, this gut compartment is roughly equivalent to medullary cords of lymph nodes. However, the B blasts and plasma cells in the LP of GALT in most mammalian species mostly secrete IgA antibodies (Crabbe *et al.*, 1965; Crandall *et al.*, 1967), whereas the splenic and lymph node plasmablasts largely express other immunoglobulin isotypes. Because of the recent recognition of SFs in the mouse small intestine and the usual manner of preparing dispersed cell suspensions with collagenase, dispase, and other enzymes, which includes the contents of the SFs in "LP preparations," the whereabouts and preferential localization of B220[+], IgM[+] B cells within this compartment is presently unclear. Certainly SF are rich in such cells (Hamada *et al.*, 2002).

The turnover or half-life of IgA plasmablasts in the gut LP was determined in neonatal mice (days 15 to 35 after birth) by chronic injection of ^{3}H-thymidine at a time when this compartment was filling with these cells (Mattioli and Tomasi, 1973). A half-life of 4.7 days, under normal conditions of gut colonization of neonates with microbes, was found. However, given the influence of suckled maternal antibodies on forestalling gut colonization with some bacteria and the consequent delay in expressing the normal steady-state of IgA production in the gut until after weaning (days 22–24) (Jiang *et al.*, 2001), these periweaning estimations should be revisited in adult mice. We believe this reanalysis is especially important in view of the identification of long-lived plasma cells, functional in systemic antibody production (Slifka *et al.*, 1998; O'Connor *et al.*, 2002), and the long-term persistence of LP IgA-forming cells after the disappearance of PP GCR provoked by gut colonization with microbes (Shroff *et al.*, 1995) or the elimination of a gut-colonizing microbe by a shift from conventional to chemically defined diet (see below).

The CD4[+] T cells of gut LP are generally more activated than splenic or lymph node counterparts, and they tend to express locally lymphokines associated with the Th2 subset of CD4[+] T cells (Taguchi *et al.*, 1990). Recently, the construction of TCR transgenic mice expressing a receptor for ovalbumin peptide, responsive to class II molecule presentation, has provided a convincing example of the activation stimuli that are effective in the gut and are likely microbial products: the transgenic mice contain large numbers of dividing, activated CD4[+] T cells in their gut LP that are expressing endogenous TCRs, i.e., their own TCRs, not the transgenic TCR (Saparov *et al.*, 1999). If these transgenic mice are crossed onto a RAG-2 (–/–) background, such activated gut CD4[+] T cells are not present.

Both T and B cells that express their effector function (memory T cells, IgA-committed B blasts, etc.) in the gut LP "home" to this tissue via HEV-like blood vessels (Jeurisseen *et al.*, 1987). This "homing" is initially accidental via the recirculation in blood but leads to selective lodging in mucosal tissue based mainly on lymphocyte expression of α4β7 integrin (the so-called homing receptor) and its ligand on vessel endothelial cells in mucosal tissue, mucosal vascular addressin (MAdCAM-1) (Nakache *et al.*, 1989; Williams and Butcher, 1997; Butcher *et al.*, 1999). At least IgA blasts then respond to the chemokine TECK (thymus-expressing chemokine), or CCL25 as it is presently named, a chemotactic factor made by gut epithelial cells. Thus, after "docking" via an α4/β7-MadCAM-dependent process, the IgA blasts are motivated directionally by a CCL25 gradient (Bowman *et al.*, 2002). A further factor in selective lodging of these cells in gut LP, leading to eventual local IgA production by IgM⁻, IgA⁺ or IgM⁺, IgA⁻ (already expressing I-Cα transcripts) B cells, is their responsiveness to IL-15 to promote IgA expression (Hiroi *et al.*, 2000). This particular responsiveness, which involves upregulation of IL-15R expression, is especially attributed to B-1 cells. The distinction between B-1 and B-2 cells in the gut LP is based on level of B220 (CD45R) expression. However, in the gut B220 expression may be more of a developmental marker rather than a B-subset marker. This matter may be resolved by distinguishing SF cells from bona fide LP cells. At any rate, IL-15 is also a product of gut epithelial cells (Reinecker *et al.*, 1996), like CCL25, and it remains to be determined whether gut microbial colonization induces the expression of either of these factors, since AF mice show negligible numbers of either B-1- or B-2-derived IgA plasmablasts in their gut LP (Bos *et al.*, 2003). A final likely candidate for facilitating the accumulation of IgA blasts in gut LP, pIgR, seems not to fulfill this function, as shown in pIgR (–/–) mice (Uren *et al.*, 2003).

Finally, the gut LP appears to contain DC that can be exposed to gut luminal Ags and act as antigen-presenting cells (APC) locally or emigrate to draining MLN, where they may prime T cells against gut-derived Ags (Liu and MacPherson, 1993). Such DC, recovered from CNV mouse MLN, can selectively stimulate naïve CD4⁺ T cells from TCR-transgenic mice to produce IL-4, IL-10, and TGFβ (Alpan *et al.*, 2001; Akbari *et al.*, 2001).

Intraepithelial leukocyte (IEL) spaces

The intraepithelial leukocyte (IEL) spaces, found between absorptive epithelial cells and above basement membrane, are populated by a variety of small round cells, especially NK cells, NK-like T (NK-T) cells, and many CD8⁺ T cell subsets (Guy-Grand *et al.*, 1991; Goodman and Lefrancois, 1989; Bannai *et al.*, 2001). IELs are supposed to lodge between epithelial cells (EC) via their surface αᴱβ⁷ integrin, reactive with the E-cadherin on the EC (Cepek *et al.*, 1994). Of particular interest as mediators of innate immunity are NK and NK-T cells. The former NK cells from IEL spaces are in a more activated state (based on killer-target ratios to achieve a given level of cytotoxicity) and target cell range than are NK cells from spleen or lymph nodes. It is interesting that the NK cells of the IEL spaces of CNV severe combined immunodeficient (*scid*) mice are more numerous and in a higher state of activation than those corresponding cells from CNV immunocompetent (*imcomp*) mice (these observations are shown in **Figs. 18.1** and **18.2**). The CD8⁺ T cells of the IEL spaces, unlike those from spleen and lymph nodes, display a much higher level of "constitutive" cytotoxicity without deliberate *in vitro* or *in vivo* activation (Lefrancois and Goodman, 1989). These findings are based on an assay, redirected cytotoxicity, which depends on coupling of putative cytotoxic T cells with target cells via antibody versus T-cell receptor (TCR) that also reacts with Fcγ receptors on target cells (Leo *et al.*, 1986). The abundance of "activated" NK

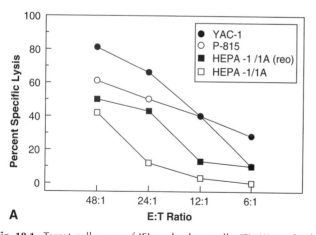

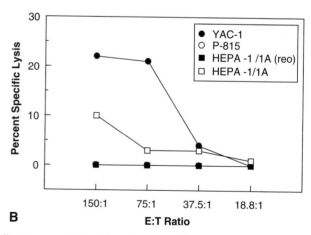

Fig. 18.1. Target cell range of IEL and spleen cells. IEL **(A)**, and spleen cells **(B)**, were isolated from C.B17 *scid* and assayed against YAC-1 (closed circles), P-815 (open circles), reovirus-infected HEPA-1/1A (closed squares), and noninfected HEPA-1/1A (open squares) in 6-hour ⁵¹Cr release assay at various E:T ratios. Spleen cells did not kill either virus-infected HEPA-1/1A or P-815 cells. Results shown are representative of five separate similar experiments (Cuff, C., and Cebra, J., unpublished data).

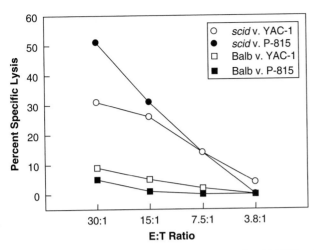

Fig. 18.2. Cytotoxic activity of IEL from CB.17 *scid* and BALB/c mice. IEL were isolated from groups of uninfected C.B17 *scid* (circles) and BALB/c mice (squares) and assayed against YAC-1 cells (open symbols) or P-815 cells (closed symbols) in 6-hour ^{51}Cr release assay at various E:T ratios. Typical results from one of four separate experiments are shown (Cuff, C., and Cebra, J., unpublished data).

and CD8$^+$ T cells in the gut relative to those in spleen or lymph nodes suggests a chronic stimulation, likely by food and microbial Ags, and this matter will be considered below.

There is also an abundance of both conventional and unconventional NK-T cells in the IEL spaces of the large intestine (Bannai *et al.*, 2001; Heller *et al.*, 2002). These NK-T cells are either CD4$^+$/CD8$^-$ or CD4$^-$/CD8$^-$/α/β TCR$^+$ and express NK1.1. Some of these express the invariant chain Vα 14, Jα 281, are restricted by the CD1 element (Bleicher *et al.*, 1990), and are responsive to α-galactosyl ceramide-type ligands (conventional) (see Heller *et al.*, 2002). Others of this NK-T subset are neither restricted by CD1 nor classical MHC class I Ags and are much more diverse in expression of TCRs (Bannai *et al.*, 2001).

Finally, ever since it was shown that DCs can extend processes from the LP, through the basement membrane, into the IEL spaces (Maric *et al.*, 1996), their role in facilitating microbial translocation and as APCs to directly activate B cells (Wykes *et al.*, 1998) and influence mucosal T cell differentiation (Alpan *et al.*, 2001; Akbari *et al.*, 2001) has been the focus of intense analyses (see next section).

INTERACTIONS OF THE INTESTINAL MICROFLORA WITH THE HOST: MAMMALIAN MODELS

Joseph Leidy (1849) wrote that "from the opinion so frequently expressed that contagious diseases and some others might have their origin and reproductive character through the agency of cryptogamic spores . . . I was led to reflect upon the possibility of plants of this description existing in healthy animals, as a natural condition; or at least apparently so, as in

the case of *Entozoa*." Leidy reasoned that the wet epithelial surfaces of the body could provide a rich culture medium for commensal microbes. Perhaps the first systematic analyses of these commensal microbes was provided by Schaedler, Dubos, and their coworkers (Schaedler *et al.*, 1965a, 1965b; Dubos *et al.*, 1965). They stated that "mice and other mammals normally harbor an extensive bacterial flora, not only in the large intestine, but also in the stomach and small intestine. Although this flora plays an essential role in the development and well-being of its host, its exact composition is not known" (Schaedler *et al*, 1965a). Unfortunately, their final lament is still true, although there have been significant advances in classifying and quantitating gut bacteria without *in vitro* cultivation. The most widely used methods for such classification rely on 16S rRNA sequence analysis via cDNA (see Amann *et al.*, 1995), and the use of distinctive oligonucleotides based on these sequences, either labeled for detection or used in microarray methodology, have allowed quantitation of particular fecal bacteria (see Amann *et al.*, 1995; Harmsen *et al.*, 1999; Rigottier-Gois *et al.*, 2003; Wang *et al.*, 2002). Promising novel approaches for "cultivating the uncultured" bacteria are also being developed (Zengler *et al.*, 2002).

The three seminal papers of Schaedler, Dubos, and coworkers offered the first comprehensive characterization of a portion of the gut microflora (using both aerobic and anaerobic *in vitro* culture) and employing the very models we still depend on today to assess the interactions of gut microbes with the GALT—the natural colonization of neonates and the deliberate colonization of axenic (GF) mice with particular gut commensal bacteria. The pioneering studies identified or established that the gut microflora included facultative anaerobes and obligate anaerobes such as lactobacilli, enterococci, and enterobacilli (including lactose-slow-fermenting *Escherichia coli*) in the former group and *Bacteroides* species and *Clostridium* species in the latter; that colonies of mice differed in the composition of those bacteria that could be cultured *in vitro*; and that there was a normal succession of colonization of the small and large gut with first lactobacilli, then enterococci, and then bacteroides in the large gut. Gram-negative enterobacilli were usually a minor component in the presence of the "complete" gut flora. These investigators also noted that certain populations of enterobacilli and enterococci decreased precipitously after having reached a maximum level. They found similarities between naturally colonized neonates and deliberately colonized GF mice with respect to succession of colonization and eventual localization in the gastrointestinal tract of particular microbial forms. Although no systemic or mucosal host immune responses were studied, these investigators speculated that the eventual outcomes of colonization with particular members of the indigenous microbiota might also allow a division between *normal microbiota* and *autochthonous microbiota*. The latter were supposed to have coevolved in a way that precluded a host response against self. Presently, immunological evidence that substantiates the concept of autochthonous microbiota remains inconclusive; rather, it would appear that the gut mucosal response to some luminal microbes does not particularly compromise their continued, successful colonization (van der Waaij et al., 1994; Friman et al., 1996). For instance, a high proportion of the normal bacterial commensals of the human gut are found to be coated with "natural" IgA secreted into the gut lumen.

These early studies have led to the development of mice with a defined intestinal flora—"altered Schaedler's flora"— and these represent oligo-associated, gnotobiotic mice carrying eight benign commensal enteric bacteria (Dewhirst et al., 1999). Further definition of the normal intestinal microbiota of mice has led to discovery of a major colonizer, segmented filamentous bacteria (SFB) (Davis and Savage, 1974). These SFB have been shown to be related to clostridia (Snel et al., 1995), and variants have been found in rats, pigs, chickens, and trout (Snel et al., 1995; Meyerholz et al., 2002; Yamauchi and Snel, 2000; Urdaci et al., 2001). So far, these obligate anaerobic SFB remain uncultivatable. Another notable normal commensal, Helicobacter muridarum, has been described by Phillips and Lee (1983) as a major colonizer of the murine colonic crypts. Finally, analysis of 16S rRNA libraries of mouse intestinal microbiota has revealed a large new group of intestinal bacteria (Salzman et al., 2002). Further treatment of the microbiota of mice (Schaedler and Orcutt, 1983) and of humans (Mackie et al., 1999; Savage, 1999) is available in excellent reviews.

Most of our present understanding of the role of gut microbes in stimulating the development of the host's gut mucosal immune system and maintaining its "normally inflamed" steady state has come from combining elements of the original studies by Schaedler, Dubos, and coworkers but adding to these approaches contemporary in vivo and in vitro assays for the status of all the elements of both the mucosal immune system and the systemic immune system. Thus we divide this section into consideration of each element of the innate and adaptive mucosal immune system as it is perturbed in neonates by natural or deliberate microbial colonization, or in GF mice, deliberately colonized with known members of the gut flora, to yield "gnotobiotic" hosts.

Humoral mucosal immune system (adaptive and "natural")

Shortly after the gut LP of several mammalian species (humans, rabbits, rats, and mice) was found to contain an abundance of secretory plasma cells (Crabbe et al., 1965; Crandall et al., 1967; Pierce and Gowans, 1975; Cebra et al., 1977), most of which made IgA, it was noted that both GF adult mice (Crabbe et al., 1970) and neonatal mice (Parrott and MacDonald, 1990) have a paucity of such cells. More recently, antigen-minimized mice (referred to as antigen-free [AF]) fed a liquid diet of hydrolyzed nutrients were found to have even fewer IgA blasts in their gut LP (Bos et al., 2003). Thus, the absence of gut microbes seemed to forestall the natural development of the abundant population of IgA plasma cells normally present in gut LP. In the case of mice, the stimulatory effects of gut microbial products appears to apply to both B-2- and B-1-cell-derived IgA plasmablasts that accumulate in mouse gut LP (Bos et al., 2003).

As early as 1968, Crabbe et al. (1968) were able to show that colonization of formerly GF mice with normal intestinal flora could stimulate the development of IgA plasma cells to normal levels within 4 weeks; in 1970, they showed that oral administration of the protein antigen ferritin to GF mice led to the appearance of antigen-specific IgA plasma cells in gut LP (Crabbe et al., 1969). Pollard and his coworkers, in 1970 to 1971, made the significant observations that Peyer's patches of GF mice contained mainly "primary" (quiescent) B-lymphoid follicles but that some enteric bacteria could activate GC reactions, while others were less effective (Pollard and Sharon, 1970; Carter and Pollard, 1971). Pollard and coworkers, Foo and Lee (1972), and Berg and Savage (1975) all agreed that some enteric bacteria were more effective than others in stimulating the development of specific circulating antibodies. Thus, they tended to support the notion of autochthonous versus normal gut microbiota. Of relevance is the somewhat more recent finding that the specificities of IgA antibodies in human milk seem to reflect the gut microbes that were present in a mother's gut during the third trimester (Carlsson and Hanson, 1994). Many of the mammary IgA plasma cells seem to have been initially primed in GALT.

Coincident with these observations, in 1971 PPs were found to be sites for the preferred generation and accumulation of precursors for IgA plasma cells (Craig and Cebra, 1971), which could emigrate to and selectively populate all mucosal tissues (Cebra et al., 1977). We now recognize that SF in both the small and large intestine may play a role similar to that of PPs (Brandtzaeg and Farstad, 1999; Hamada et al., 2002). Thus, it became relevant to link the development of specific, IgA-committed B cells in PP and SF to the appearance and accumulation of specific IgA plasmablasts in the gut LP or elsewhere in mucosal tissues and to try to implicate particular gut microbes as effective stimuli of these perturbations.

Thus far we have established a set of general principles concerning gut microbial stimulation of the humoral mucosal immune system, while leaving some unresolved issues, as outlined in the next section.

IgA plasma cells and effective stimulators among the gut microbiota

Some commensal gut bacteria of the mouse stimulate the appearance of IgA plasma cells in gut LP of formerly GF mice better than others, and certain mixtures lead to gnotobiotic mice with almost two-thirds of the IgA plasmablasts that are found in CNV mice. Although no specific IgA responses in the gut or IgA plasmablasts in gut LP were addressed, Bacteroides and Escherichia species were found to be more effective than a variety of other microbes, including lactobacilli, enterococci, clostridia, corynebacteria, and actinobacilli. A mixture of four different gut microbes, used to colonize GF mice, came closest to simulating the development of a steady state of IgA plasma cells, comparable to that in the LP of CNV mice over a 4-week period (Moreau et al., 1978).

These observations raise the following two questions. Are particular members of the normal gut microflora especially effective at driving the development and maintaining the steady state of the humoral mucosal immune system in the gut? Do particular members of the normal gut microflora differ in stimulating specific versus polyclonal (aspecific) IgA production?

Although mixtures of gut microbial species, each successfully cultivated *in vitro*, have been shown to stimulate the development of IgA plasma cells in gut LP of formerly GF mice to roughly one-half to two-thirds of the levels from that in conventionally reared mice (Moreau *et al.*, 1978), most associations with single gut commensals are far less effective, quantitatively and temporally (Carter and Pollard, 1971; Foo and Lee, 1972; Berg and Savage, 1975; Moreau *et al.*, 1978; **Table 18.1**). In the last decade, we have appreciated that major elements of the gut flora of mice and of many other animals were obligate anaerobes that have not yet been cultured *in vitro* (Tannock *et al.*, 1987). Indeed, Joseph Leidy (1849) described a dominant gut morphotype, segmented filamentous bacteria (SFB), which he found in the midgut of termites. This SFB was tentatively named *Arthromitis* (jointed thread), and similar morphotypes have been found in the chicken, rat, mouse, pig, and trout (Snel *et al*, 1995; Meyerholz *et al.*, 2003; Yamauchi and Snel, 2000; Urdaci *et al.*, 2001). The vertebrate

versions of this morphotype are gram-positive, segmented, obligate anaerobes that are spore formers (Davis and Savage, 1974). Savage and coworkers recognized SFB as a major component of the gut microbiota of mice and were able to enrich for these noncultivatable bacteria by isolating intestinal epithelial cells, to which the 5- to 20-μm SFB attached firmly via a holdfast segment that interdigitated with but did not penetrate the brush border (Davis and Savage, 1974; Tannock *et al.*, 1987). The SFB of mice has recently been isolated by the Nijmegen group, using treatment of fecal material with organic solvents to kill vegetative organisms, followed by limiting dilution to colonize formerly GF mice (Klaasen *et al.*, 1991). The latter limiting dilution was made possible by the finding that the vast majority of spore-forming, obligate anaerobes in postweanling to young adult mice were SFB. Snel *et al.* (1995) have used sequencing of 16S RNA to position the SFB of mice, rat, and chicken as a closely related group *within* the larger cluster of *Clostridium* species. Their relationship with Leidy's *Arthromitis* is still not clear.

Perhaps of greater relevance, the Nijmegen group has found that monoassociation of formerly GF mice with spores of this single gut commensal, SFB, provides a profound stimulus for the development of IgA ASC in the gut LP (Klaasen

Table 18.1. Natural IgA And Specific IgA Production in Germ-Free Mice Monoassociated with Individual Bacteria

Bacterium	Mouse Strain	Days after Colonization[a]	Total IgA (ng/ml)[b]	Specific IgA (ng/ml)[c]	% Specific IgA
Listeria monocytogenes actA(−) [d]	GF C3H	21	2200	322	14.6
Morganella morganii	GF C3H	28	924	44	4.8
Segmented filamentous	GF C3H	14	2460	33	1.3
Ochrobactrum anthropi	GF BALB/c	54	560	0	0
Helicobacter muridarum	GF BALB/c	14	491	4	0.8
Escherichia coli, Schaedler	GF BALB/c	30	462 (SI) 648 (PP)	118 (SI) 80 (J) 67 (I)	25.5 (D) 17.3 (J) 14.5 (I)
ASF	GF BALB/c	70	2250 (SI) 2150 (PP)	na	—

[a]Time of maximal specific antibody output after colonization.
[b]IgA production was determined in Peyer's patches (PP) and small intestinal (SI) fragment cultures by radioimmunoassay. Typical values for output of total IgA from PP and SI fragments cultures are: 3000–4000 ng/ml for CNV mice and 100–200 ng/ml for GF mice.
[c]Specific IgA production was determined by radioimmunoassay on plates that were coated with lysates derived from the involved bacteria.
[d]*L. monocytogenes* act A(−) is a mutant strain of *Listeria* in which the actA gene is inactive. The actA gene is important in translocation of *Listeria* across epithelial cells. *M. morganii* is a gram-negative commensal bacterium that can translocate into the host but has not been shown to be pathogenic. Segmented filamentous bacterium is a strictly anaerobic commensal bacterium that cannot be grown outside of the host. *O. anthropi* is an aerobic gram-negative bacterial strain that grows poorly in the intestinal tract and almost does not translocate into the host. *H. muridarum* is a commensal bacterium that has been described as living in the crypts of the large intestine and has no history of pathogenic properties. *E. coli* Schaedler is gram-negative representative of commensal mouse flora with slow fermentative activities. ASF (altered Schaedler flora): eight microorganisms including *Lactobacillus acidophilus* (ASF 360), *Lactobacillus salivarius* (ASF 361), *Bacteroides distasonis* (ASF 519), *Flexistipes phylum* (spiral-shaped ASF 457), *Clostridium* cluster strains, and extremely oxygen-sensitive fusiform bacteria (ASF 356, ASF 492, ASF 502, and ASF 500). Abbreviations: na = not applicable; D = duodenum; J = jejunum; I = ileum (from Bos *et al.*, 2001; Boiko, N., and Cebra, J., unpublished).

et al., 1993). The magnitude of the response suggests that it is polyclonal, composed of much "natural" IgA; however, the rapid but delayed rise to preeminence of SFB attached to epithelial cells of the small intestine between 4 and 12 weeks of age, followed by exclusion of SFB to the cecum and large bowel (mostly unattached), suggests a specific component of the host's response (Snel et al., 1998). Indeed, we find that formerly GF scid mice, monoassociated with SFB, do not clear SFB from their small intestine for up to 1 year. We have collaborated with the Nijmegen group to evaluate SFB-specific versus polyclonal ("natural") IgA plasmablast development driven by gut association of formerly GF mice with SFB and to quantitate how effective this stimulus was compared with "normal" expression of IgA by CNV mice with a "complete" microbiota (Snel et al., 1998; Talham et al., 1999). Our findings were that GC reactions occurred in Peyer's patches by 14 to 21 days postinfection, and these gradually waned over about 100 days of colonization; "natural" IgA production by GALT fragment culture followed GC reactions in PP and reached levels of 70% of that found from GALT of CNV mice; and specific anti-SFB IgA antibodies did develop over 7 to 12 weeks, but these never exceeded 0.5% to 1.0% of the total "natural" IgA output. Thus, it appears that SFB may be a major stimulus for the development of the "natural" IgA system. We do not yet know how the host's specific immune response to SFB effects its disappearance from the small gut; the bacteria do take on a coat of endogenous IgA (see following section). However, the level of "natural" IgA remains rather constant for up to 100 days of colonization as GC reactions subside. Thus, mechanisms for maintenance of IgA plasmablasts in gut LP should be investigated. One mechanism that may account for the maintenance of IgA plasmablasts for over 100 days is bacterial DNA–mediated survival. Unmethylated CpG dinucleotide motifs in bacterial DNA seem to rescue splenic B cells from apoptosis (Yi et al., 1998; Yi et al., 1999).

We have sought to extend the analyses by Moreau et al. (1978) to include seven innocuous enteric organisms as monoassociates of formerly GF mice as well as the eight commensal microbes in the altered Schaedler's flora (ASF) (Dewhirst et al., 1999). We compared their ability to stimulate the expression of "natural" IgA in the gut as well as specific antibodies reactive with sonicates of the organisms. Although there may be only a "thin line" between gut commensal and pathogen (Gilmore and Ferretti, 2003), we defined an enteric species as innocuous if it caused no detectable pathogenesis after monoassociating formerly GF scid mice and did not interfere with normal breeding. We used organ fragment cultures of various sections of gut and of PP to evaluate total and specific IgA production (Logan et al., 1991; Weinstein and Cebra, 1991). Table 18.1 shows that each particular enteric microbe induced a particular level and ratio of "natural" and specific IgA production in the gut. Some organisms (Morganella morganii, Listeria monocytogenes mutant) resulted in a relatively high proportion of specific antibody while others did not (H. muridarum, SFB). In agreement with Moreau et al. (1978), a cocktail of gut commensals (the eight members of ASF) stimulated nearly normal levels of total IgA production, as did the single microbial colonizer, SFB.

Germinal center reactions (GCR) in PP

B lymphoid follicles in PLN and spleen of healthy animals are normally in a "quiescent" state, being composed of mainly primary, sIgM[+], nondividing B cells. So too are the B cell follicles of PPs in GF or AF mice (Weinstein and Cebra, 1991; Bos et al., 2003). Gut colonization of GF or AF mice leads to the development of chronic GCR in the core of B cell follicles of PP, composed of rapidly dividing B cell blasts enmeshed in a three-dimensional web of follicular dendritic cells. GC of peripheral lymphoid organs are sites of isotype-switching and of the accumulation of point mutations in the V(D)J region of productive genes encoding Igs, leading to "affinity maturation" of the antibodies expressed by the B blasts (see Liu et al., 1992). These GCR have been generally supposed to be dependent on CD4[+] T cells (see Kelly et al. 1995), cognate T/B interactions, and cells of the B2 lineage in mice (Linton et al. 1992). Similar processes have been supposed to occur in the chronic GCR of PP, but there are few data concerning this matter. Milstein's group has used transgenic mice expressing a transgene for a kappa chain that participates in binding 2-phenyl oxazolone (Gonzalez-Fernandez and Milstein, 1993; Gonzalez-Fernandez et al., 1994). They find extensive point mutations in the Vκ/Jκ of this transgene of clonotypically related GC B cells from PP of unimmunized donors. However, these do not show the type of selection processes associated with affinity maturation among transgenes of peripheral B cells in secondarily immunized mice. They suppose the transgene in PP B cells acts as a "passenger" gene, accompanying B cells expressing endogenous Vκ/Jκ genes of antibody reactive with environmental Ag in the gut. Certainly, deliberate oral immunization with effective TD Ag, such as cholera toxin (Fuhrman and Cebra, 1981) and reovirus type 1 (Weinstein and Cebra, 1991), results in accumulation of IgA-committed, memory B cells and in GCR in PP, but the specific GC B blasts have not been examined for pattern of point mutations in V-genes that could result in affinity maturation.

Recently, we have examined unselected B cells from PP and gut LP differing or not in their expected membership in the B2 or B1 cell lineages taken from a variety of CNV mice (Stoel et al., in press). Our findings were similar in all cases: the CDR3 spectrotypes of Vα-genes showed pauciclonality; the individual Vα/D$_H$/J$_H$ genes expressed gave sequences with few point mutations and short N-additions with respect to documented GL genes; and a surprisingly high incidence of clonotypically related sequences was noted in some samples, which exhibited few but unrelated point mutations. These observations are different from those with use of unselected or specific B cells from spleen (Berek et al., 1991; Stoel et al., in press) and suggest that many PP and gut LP B cells derive from a process different from clonal selection, expansion, and secondary Ag selection in GCR.

Both B2 and B1 cells likely contribute to the process generating gut IgA blasts expressing near GL genes (Stoel *et al.*, in press). Recently, TI-2 type Ags such as $\alpha(1 \rightarrow 6)$ dextran and (4-hydroxy-3-nitrophenyl) acetyl-Ficoll have been found to stimulate GCR in spleen, albeit rather vestigial, and the specific B cells showed few point mutations and no evidence of their clustering in CDR (Wang *et al.*, 1994; Lentz and Manser, 2001; Toellner *et al.*, 2002). Presumably these small GCR were initiated by cells of the B2 lineage in the absence of cognate T-cell interaction. These observations of splenic GCR raise the possibility that the sequences of expressed V-genes in IgA blasts from the gut that we have found may be due to B2 cell–initiated, vestigial GCR in PP, occurring in the absence of cognate T/B interactions. Indeed, with use of influenza virus challenge of the respiratory tract in chimeric mice carrying B cells lacking class II molecule expression (Sangster *et al.*, in press) or of reovirus challenge of the gut of TCR (−/−) mice (Zuercher and Cebra, unpublished), specific antibody was produced of non-IgM isotypes by mucosal-associated lymphoid tissue in the absence of appreciable increase in "natural" Ig. In the case of the reovirus challenge of TCR (−/−) mice, vestigial GCR were observed in PP. A possible mechanism for such apparently T-independent responses is the "presentation" of multivalent Ags by interdigitating and/or follicular DC to B cells in conjunction with their secretion of B lymphocyte stimulator protein (BLyS) or "a proliferation inducing ligand" (APRIL) to stimulate modest expansion and isotype-switching (MacLennon and Vinuesa, 2002; Litinskiy *et al.*, 2002). Microbial polysaccharide Ag or "rafts" of Ag determinants on the surface of microbes might be especially functional stimulants of gut lymphoid tissues, especially since the ability of interdigitating DC extending through IEL spaces to transport bacteria from the gut lumen has been recognized (Rescigno *et al.*, 2001).

We also do not know whether continued presence of specific IgA plasmablasts in gut LP depends upon continued colonization by the particular microbe. We have found that the waxing and waning of GCR in PP is commonly observed upon monoassociation of formerly GF mice with many different commensal enteric microbes such as SFB (Talham *et al.*, 1999). To support the need for continuous restimulation of PP with novel microbial Ag in order to maintain the chronic GCR, we find that supercolonization of SFB monoassociated mice with *M. morganii* after their GCR have waned results in a new cycle of GCR (Talham *et al.*, 1999).

Contribution of cells of the B2 versus B1 lineage to IgA production in the gut LP

This subject has been comprehensively reviewed in this volume (Chapter 33), but here we emphasize a few points relevant to gut microbial/B cell interactions and comment on the specificities of these interactions.

The contributions of B1 versus B2 cells to the composition of gut IgA plasmablasts and to IgA secreted into the gut lumen have been estimated at greater than 50% (Kroese *et al.*, 1989) to less than 5% (Thurnheer *et al.*, 2003). Both

studies used transfer of congenic, Ig-allotype distinct B1 cells from adult PeC into recipients that were CNV adults and immunocompromised (Kroese *et al.*, 1989; Bos *et al.*, 2000)—*scid*, X-irradiated—or were GF neonates, treated with anti-host IgM allotype to delay B cell development (Thurnheer *et al.*, 2003). The latter pups, upon maturation, were monoassociated with one of three common gut commensal microbes. We believe that the latter mouse model is likely closer to the normal physiologic state of CNV neonates when the balance of their IgA plasmablasts is established in the gut. However, the contributions of B2 versus B1 cells to IgA plasmablasts can clearly be compensatory, if one or the other B cell lineage is impaired (Snider *et al.*, 1999).

Although we believe that B1 cells can populate the gut with IgA plasmablasts and some of these make IgA that reacts with a particular pattern of microbial Ags (Bos *et al.*, 1996), we have so far found little substantial evidence that indicates that these cells arise by specific Ag selection and stimulation to divide and/or differentiate into secretory plasma cells. Recently, Macpherson *et al.* (2000) have shown that TCR (−/−) mice can exhibit an antimicrobial IgA response in the gut and that a complex radiation chimera seems to express a predominance of IgA plasmablasts with the allotype of the transferred, semipurified PeC B1 cells; no specific responses were measured in the latter case. Unfortunately, TI responses are not acceptable criteria for B1-derived, gut IgA responses, and the radiation chimera—comparing transferred PeC versus BM B cells—suffers from the same criticisms as the original model (Kroese *et al.* 1989. see Thurnheer *et al.*, 2003). Furthermore, the latter chimeric model (Macpherson *et al.*, 2000) does not address specific Ag stimulation of B1 cells.

Recently, we have found that upon transfer of extensively purified, CD4+ T cell–free B1 cells into CNV *scid* recipients, no IgA plasmablasts develop in gut LP over 8–10 weeks unless CD4+ T cells are cotransferred (Jiang *et al.*, 2004). This synergy requires colonization of the host with enteric microbes, and apparently both B1 and CD4+ T cells benefit from the colonization. Apparently the T cell effect is of the "bystander" type since monoclonal DO11.10 (ovalbumin-peptide specific) TCR transgenic, RAG-2 (−/−) T cells are effective at facilitating B1-mediated IgA production in the gut. This effect occurs only if the transgenic cells are activated in the donor or, by ovalbumin feeding, in the recipient, and is not successful in GF recipients. Although the latter observation suggests T cell activation via TCR, either by ovalbumin or microbial Ags, it does not indicate whether the requirement of B1 cells for microbial colonization is specific or not.

It has previously been shown that LPS, given orally or intraduodenally, can activate peripheral B1 cells to secrete antibody (Murakami *et al.*, 1994). This is presumably a polyclonal activation that could be acting via the B1 cell LPS-R (TLR-4/CD14) or indirectly via activation of gut Tr1-type, CD4+ T cells through their TLR-4 to produce IL-10, a B1 cell growth and differentiation factor (O'Garra *et al.*, 1992; Caramalho *et al.*, 2003). Finally, IL-15 seems to be involved in accumulation of B1 lineage-derived IgA plasmablasts in the gut LP (Hiroi *et al.*, 2000). Since gut epithelial cells (EC) can make IL-15 (Fehninger and Caligiuri, 2001), it is possible that enteric gut commensals can upregulate this synthesis. At any rate, the specific Ag selection and stimulation of B1 cells remain problematic.

Suckled maternal antibodies

Suckled maternal antibodies can forestall the natural development of active mucosal immune responses in neonates against gut microbes. It has been known for some time that the gut LP of newborns shows a paucity of IgA plasmablasts (Parrott and MacDonald, 1990) and that specific antigen-reactive B cells in PP committed to IgA (IgA memory cells) against the microbial determinants phosphocholine, β2→1 fructosyl (inulin [In]), and β-galactosyl take weeks after birth to rise to adult frequencies (Cebra, 1999). We speculated that "it seems plausible that changes in gut flora accompanying weaning or a decline in passively acquired maternal antibodies to In or both could result in increased natural stimulation of In-reactive cells at 3 to 5 weeks" (Shahin and Cebra, 1981).

To address whether neonatal mice had an underdeveloped or competent humoral mucosal immune system, we infected 10-day-old pups with reovirus 1 by the oral/intragastric route (Kramer and Cebra, 1995a). Reovirus 1 is a potent stimulator of both cellular and humoral mucosal immune responses in adult mice and is normally absent from our specific-pathogen-free (SPF) mouse colonies (London *et al.*, 1987). Thus, dams in our colonies have no circulating or mucosal antibodies against reovirus. Given orally to either 10-day-old pups or adults, reovirus 1 causes a transient intestinal infection without clinical symptoms. We found that pups expressed prompt, specific IgA antibody responses in 3 to 5 days, using the method of PP and small intestine organ fragment culturing. These responses were accompanied by distinct GC reactions in PP, with many IgA blasts, at a time, 14 to 17 days after birth, when nonimmunized pups still had quiescent B-cell follicles in PP. We also found that immunized pups expressed about 20 times more "natural" IgA than virus-specific IgA, whereas noninfected control pups made neither specific nor "natural" IgA. Apparently, 14- to 17-day-old pups are able to develop "natural" IgA responses but ordinarily do not do so until 22 to 25 days of age, unless challenged with an infectious enteric virus not commonly associated with the mouse colonies (Kramer and Cebra, 1995a).

We sought to evaluate possible effects of the immune system of both birth and nurse mothers on development of the neonatal mucosal immune system, especially on the expression of "natural" IgA (Kramer and Cebra, 1995b). We reciprocally crossed *imcomp* mice with coisogeneic *scid* mice. The homozygous *scid/scid* mouse cannot express any form of specific, adaptive immunity, whereas the heterozygous F$_1$ mice (*scid/+*) are fully competent. Thus, the only difference between the two groups of F$_1$ mice, born to parents exposed to the same SPF flora, is whether they were born of *scid* or

imcomp mothers. F$_1$ mice could also be swapped at birth, so that pups born of *scid* mothers could be nursed on *imcomp* dams and vice versa. Without using any *deliberate* gut mucosal stimulus, we made a number of principal findings:

- F$_1$ pups born to and nursed on *scid* dams show a precocious rise in "natural" IgA production in PP and small intestine on days 15 to 16 after birth, with concomitant GCR in PP, whereas such expression of IgA is delayed at least until days 22 to 25 in pups born to *imcomp* mothers;
- This difference between the two groups of F$_1$ pups is reflected by IgA-secreting cells from PP, MLN, and gut LP; for instance, pups born of *scid* mothers have about 200 IgA ASC/10^6 in PP and 2000 IgA ASC/10^6 in the LP, whereas at day 16, pups born of *imcomp* dams have negligible ASC;
- The F$_1$ pups born of *imcomp* mothers have high levels of suckled, maternal IgA in their stomach contents, whereas it is absent from pups born of *scid* mothers; and
- The bacteria isolated from the intestine of pups born and nursed on *imcomp* dams are "coated" with IgA at an early age, whereas bacteria from pups of *scid* dams are initially "uncoated" but gradually, beginning on day 16 after birth, acquire an IgA coating via active production of IgA (Kramer and Cebra, 1995b).

The implication of these findings is that suckled, maternal IgA antibodies coat gut commensal bacteria in the neonatal intestines, blocking active mucosal immunization against members of the normal gut flora until weaning. In the absence of the shielding effects of passively acquired, maternal antibodies, neonates born of *scid* mothers are fully capable of developing gut IgA responses, PP GCRs, and gut LP IgA ASC against environmental antigens.

To directly implicate passively acquired, suckled maternal immune elements in forestalling the development of active, humoral mucosal immunity in the neonatal gut, we deliberately immunized some of the *imcomp* dams orally with reovirus (Kramer and Cebra, 1995a; Periwal *et al.*, 1997). Offspring of immune, nonimmune but *imcomp*, and *scid* mothers were also swapped for nursing. We took advantage of the stimulatory effect of enteric reovirus not only for virus-specific IgA antibodies but also for the development of "natural" IgA. The findings were rather consistent: oral vaccination of *imcomp* nurse dams had the greatest effect in preventing or retarding both virus-specific and "natural" IgA responses by the nursing pups; oral immunization of birth mothers had only subtle suppressive effects if the pups were then suckled on *scid* or nonimmune *imcomp* dams. We have sought to immunize neonates born of mucosally immune mothers actively by the oral route (Periwal *et al.* 1997). The aim was to allow the pups to benefit from the potentially protective effects of passively acquired maternal antibodies while still being actively immunized via the mucosal route. We have found that "live" reovirus 1, a protective vaccine against oral challenge with reovirus type 3 (Cuff *et al.*, 1990), can be encapsulated with spermine/alginate compounds. The small (about 5 µm) capsules can be given orally to avoid neutralization by coincidently suckled maternal antibodies, and these stimulate both active systemic and mucosal immune responses in the pups (Periwal *et al.*, 1997). It has been known for some time that lactating human mothers contain antibodies in their milk reactive with their own gut microbes, especially those present during the outset of the last trimester of pregnancy, and these could protect their nursing neonates against potential enteric pathogens (Carlsson and Hanson, 1987). Using a mouse model involving *imcomp* or *scid* dams, we have found that their immunologic competence is a factor in forestalling the development of the neonatal mucosal immune system of their nursing pups and that it is also associated with a delay in colonization by certain gut commensals, such as SFB (Jiang *et al.*, 2001).

Cellular mucosal immune system (innate and adaptive)

The most conspicuous compartments of the cellular mucosal immune system of the gut include the IEL spaces, the PP, and the gut LP. There is considerably less information concerning the role of gut microflora in the development and activation of the elements of the cellular versus humoral immune system. Generally, the approaches have used comparisons between neonates and adults and of GF or AF adults, before and after deliberate colonization with commensal microbes.

IEL compartment cells

The cells in the IEL compartment change in number and proportions of phenotypically/functionally distinct subsets during normal development and after colonization of formerly GF adult mice with gut microbes.

NK cells in the IEL spaces

NK cells (large granular lymphocytes) comprise a significant proportion of IELs in CNV rodents (Tagliabue *et al.*, 1982). Generally, their target cell range and potency (E:T ratio) is greater than that of NK cells in spleen or peripheral lymph nodes (see Fig. 18.1 for CNV *scid* mice). Gut infection of *imcomp* mice with coronavirus (Carmen *et al.*, 1996) and of *scid* mice with reovirus **(Table 18.2)** results in activation of gut NK cells in the IEL spaces. The CNV *scid* mice actually have IEL NK cells that display an activation state much greater than that of CNV *imcomp* mice before deliberate infection, that is, show greater potency in cytotoxic assays using YAC-1 targets or P815 (Fig. 18.2). Unlike CNV *scid* mice, the cytotoxic potency of NK cells in the IEL compartment of CNV *imcomp* mice is low and similar to that in their GF counterparts **(Fig. 18.3)**. Colonization of the GF *imcomp* mice (C3H/HeJ) with SFB results in a marked increase in NK potency over a 14- to 23-day period postinfection, as measured with YAC-1, P815, and P388 target cells (Lee, 1995; Fig. 18.3 and **Fig. 18.4**). The mouse *E. coli* (Schaedler's), when used to monoassociate GF *scid* mice, also is associated with a rise in pan-NK-positive cells in IEL spaces, compared with the cohort in AF *imcomp* mice, but they do not reach the level of those in CNV *scid* mice **(Fig. 18.5)**. The functional poten-

Table 18.2. Effects of Reovirus Infection on the Cytotoxic Activity of IEL from *scid* Mice

Group[a]	Weeks Postinfection			
	1	2	3	4
Noninfected	13.3[b]	17.2	10.5	20.0
Infected	5.5	16.6	66.6	<5.0[c]

[a]Groups of 4–6 *scid* mice received 10^7 plaque forming units of reovirus serotype 1/L by the oral route. One to 4 weeks after infection, groups of infected and noninfected mice were killed, and isolated IEL were assayed for cytotoxic activity against ^{51}Cr-labeled YAC-1 targets in a 6-hour assay.
[b]Results are expressed as LU/10^6 cells to achieve 30% specific lysis.
[c]Significant morbidity and mortality are observed at 4 weeks postinfection.

tial and number of NK cells in the IEL compartment of GF *scid* mice have not yet been reliably determined. Thus, it seems likely that normal gut microbes can be partly responsible for the activated state of NK cells in the IEL compartment, relative to those in spleen and peripheral lymph nodes.

Mechanisms for the interaction of microbial products with NK cells in the IEL spaces have not been well studied. However, some possibly relevant observations have been made with use of splenic NK cells assessed *in vitro* or *in vivo*. Wherry *et al.* (1991) found that a heat-killed *L. monocytogenes* vaccine, along with macrophage-produced TNFα and another unknown factor, could stimulate splenic NK cells *in vitro* to produce IFNγ. Likely, the "unknown factor" was IL-12 (Hunter, 1996; Chace *et al.*, 1997). Further, differentiation of bone marrow precursors of NK cells requires IL-15, but so does the survival and maintenance of transferred, mature splenic NK cells as detected later in spleen, blood, and liver (Cooper *et al.*, 2002). Perhaps, NK cells in IEL spaces likewise require IL-15, made by gut EC (Fehninger and Caligiuri, 2001) and possibly induced by microbial products, for their maintenance. Also, microbial products originating in the gut possibly can activate NK cells and their expression of IFNγ. Finally, it is not clear why *imcomp* mice have less NK potency contributed by IEL cells than *scid* mice. Possibly, *imcomp* mice have secretory antibodies that can more effectively exclude gut microbial products from the various sites of the gut where NK cells are found.

T cells in the IEL compartment

The major set of T cells in the IEL spaces is CD8⁺, although many subsets of these are often present (Goodman and Lefrancois, 1989; Guy-Grand *et al.*, 1991). The CD8⁺ T cells in neonatal mice and in GF and AF mice include a much higher proportion of cells expressing γ/δ TCR than is commonly found in IELs from CNV adult mice (Lefrancois and Goodman, 1989; Guy-Grand *et al.*, 1991; Hooper *et al.*,

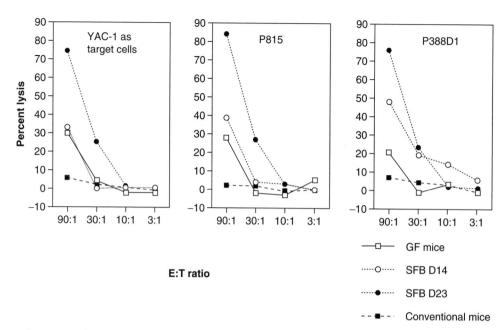

Fig. 18.3. Upon gut colonization of GF BALB/c mice with segmented filamentous bacteria, the cells of the IEL compartment show an increase in cytotoxicity versus NK- and NC-cell targets (YAC-1, P-815, and P-388 D1 cells) (Lee, F., and Cebra, J., unpublished data).

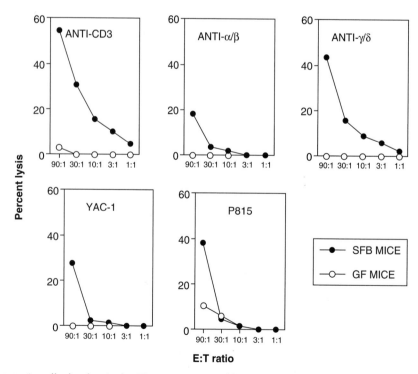

Fig. 18.4. Constitutively cytotoxic cells develop in the IEL compartment of formerly GF C3H/HeN mice following oral/gut colonization with SFB. IELs from GF mice were compared with those from formerly GF mice colonized for 60 days with SFB. Target cells were hybridoma lines making anti-CD3, anti-α/β TCR, or anti-γ/δ TCR (to detect various subsets of constitutively cytotoxic T-cells) and YAC-1 and P-815 (to detect NK and NC cells, respectively) (Lee, F., and Cebra, J., unpublished data).

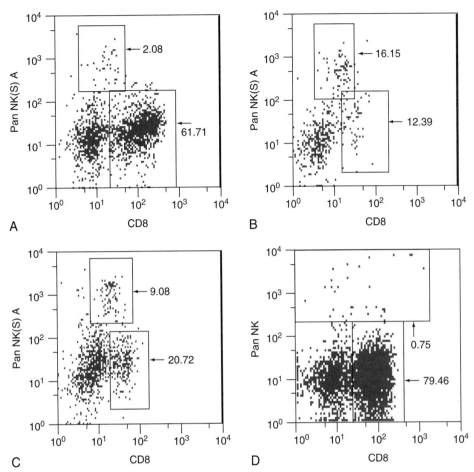

Fig. 18.5. FACS analyses of cells from IEL compartment of **(A)**, AF *imcomp* BALB/c mice; **(B)**, CNV *scid* mice; **(C)**, GF *scid* mice after 24 days of monoassociation with Schaedler's *E. coli* (mouse commensal coliform bacterium); and **(D)**, CNV *imcomp* BALB/c. (Boiko, N., and Cebra, J., unpublished data).

1995). Most of the CD8[+] T cells in these latter rodents are Thy-1 negative and express the α/α rather than the α/β form of the CD8 molecule. The constitutive (redirected) cytotoxicity of these T cells is generally low (Lefrancois and Goodman, 1989). With maturation of mice, and especially after deliberate oral infection of adult GF mice with reovirus or gut commensal bacteria, the proportion of α/β TCR[+], Thy-1[+], and α/β CD8[+] T cells increases (Cuff *et al.*, 1992, 1993; Umesaki *et al.*, 1993; Kawaguchi *et al.*, 1993). This increasing subset, which accounts for a twofold to fivefold increase in cellularity in the IEL compartment, includes both antigen-specific and constitutive cytotoxic and precytotoxic T cells. GF mice have very low levels of CD8[+] T cell–mediated constitutive cytotoxicity (Lefrancois and Goodman, 1989). However, colonization of either formerly GF BALB/c mice (Umesaki *et al.*, 1995) or C3H (Lee, 1995) mice with SFB results in the progressive increase of Thy-1[+], α/β TCR[+], CD8[+] T cells in the IEL spaces, which express the α/β CD8 heterodimer. These newly arising T cells appear to contain the constitutive cytotoxicity that increases among the IELs (Fig. 18.4). It is not clear what specificities are expressed by these T cells, apparently stimulated by SFB colonization.

Although reovirus-specific, CD8[+] cytotoxic T cells seem to be generated in PP following viral entry via M cells and these then appear to migrate to IEL spaces (Cuff *et al.*, 1993), it is not clear how gut commensal bacterial colonizers mediate the accumulation of constitutively cytotoxic, α/β TCR[+], α/β CD8[+] T cells in IEL spaces. Perhaps gut interdigitating DC that extend their processes through IEL spaces to penetrate the gut EC monolayer can "sample" gut bacterial colonizers and their microbial products (Rescigno *et al.*, 2001). At any rate, following gut colonization of GF mice with members of their normal microbiota, continuous BrdU-labeling shows a preferential increase and labeling of these cells or their immediate precursors (Imaoka *et al.*, 1996). It is still not clear whether these CD8[+] T cells in the IEL compartment respond specifically or polyclonally to microbial Ags and/or products such as TLR ligands.

Although the deliberate colonization of GF mice with commensal gut bacteria or infection with reovirus increases the α/β CD8[+], α/β TCR[+] IEL cells twofold to fivefold, molecular analyses of the Vβ genes expressed by this subset of IEL cells reveals that the population is oligoclonal but idiosyncratic for any given mouse (Regnault *et al.*, 1994). A comparison of this subset of IEL T cells from CNV versus GF mice reveals the same degree of oligoclonality in each group, although the GF mice had 10-fold fewer of such cells (Regnault *et al.*, 1996). The generalization from this and other findings is that intestinal, microbial Ags are not a main selective stimulus for the development of this oligoclonality, and particular gut colonizers (SFB) may increase the number of these α/β TCR⁺, CD8⁺ T cells in the IEL spaces, but they do not appreciably alter the pattern of Vβ-gene expression when used to colonize formerly GF mice (Bousso *et al.*, 1999; Umesaki *et al.*, 1999).

Both the α/β and α/α CD8⁺, α/β TCR⁺ T cells in IEL spaces seem to require both IL-2 and IL-15 for their expansion and survival (Gelfanov *et al.*, 1995; Lodoice *et al.*, 1998; Lai *et al.*, 1999). The α/β CD8⁺, α/β TCR⁺ T cells seem to be a source for the local IL-2, while gut EC likely provide the IL-15 (Reinecker *et al.*, 1996). Only the α/β CD8⁺, α/β TCR⁺ T cells can mediate perforin-based cytotoxicity, while both they and α/α CD8⁺, α/β TCR⁺ T cells can kill via a Fas/FasL-based mechanism (Gelfanov *et al.*, 1996). However, we still do not know how benign bacterial colonizers stimulate the accumulation, survival, and activation of these T cells in the IEL spaces. Perhaps part of this process involves the upregulation of IL-15 production by gut EC.

The γ/δ TCR⁺ T cells appear to develop and then accumulate in the IEL spaces independent of gut microbial colonization (Bandeira *et al.*, 1990). Thus, this subset could be considered the T-cell counterpart of B1 cells, which develop and accumulate in the peritoneal and pleural cavities, although not in the gut LP (Bos *et al.*, 2003), independently of exogenous environmental antigens (Guy-Grand *et al.*, 1991; Hardy and Hayakawa, 1992). Although the γ/δ TCR⁺ T cells in the IEL spaces are prone to activation-induced death upon stimulation via their TCR, these cells also show enhanced survival promoted by exogenous IL-15 (Chu *et al.*, 1999). Perhaps microbial products can contribute to their activation, if not accumulation in IEL spaces, and also to their continued survival via EC-produced IL-15.

Responsiveness of CD4⁺ T cells in PP and gut LP

Gut microbial antigens may stimulate and activate CD4⁺ T cells in the PP and the gut LP. This topic is particularly relevant to the next section of this chapter, chronic noninfectious diseases, and will be addressed further there. Not many convincing studies have been published concerning the development of *specific* responsiveness of GALT CD4⁺ T cells to commensal microbial antigens. The difficulties include the polyclonal and/or mitogenic stimulants that accompany bacterial extracts and sonicates (MacDonald, 1995). However, the few studies in GF or AF rodents and their colonized gnotobiotic counterparts indicate the following. First, AF mice, deprived of exogenous stimulation, develop a normal repertoire of functional T cells (Vos *et al.*, 1992). Second, CD4⁺ T cells from PP of CNV *imcomp* mice exhibit "spontaneous" proliferation (autologous mixed lymphocyte reactions, or AMLR) to endogenous or exogenous APC; either GF or AF CD4⁺ T cells or APCs in cocultures

with their APC or CD4⁺ T cell counterparts from CNV mice respectively show diminished AMLR. These observations suggest that the GALT ordinarily contains both APCs charged with microbial antigenic determinants and reactive CD4⁺ T cells (Hooper *et al.*, 1994, 1995). Third, generally, the *in vitro* CD4⁺ T cell reactivity to microbial antigens is not manifest *in vivo*, although in patients with inflammatory bowel disease (IBD) or in animal models exhibiting IBD lesions, there is evidence that GALT CD4⁺ T cells do react with antigens of the endogenous microbial flora (Duchmann *et al.*, 1999). Fourth, we have found that CD4⁺ T cells in PP of CNV mice have a majority of CD45RB^low cells, indicative of prior exposure to antigens (Talham *et al.*, 1999). Spleen and PLN of such mice have CD4⁺ T cells that are mostly CD45RB^high, indicative of naive or unprimed T cells. In GF mice, the majority of PP CD4⁺ T cells are CD45RB^high. However, colonization of these mice with SFB activates their PP CD4⁺ T cells and shifts this population in 4 to 8 weeks to a CD45RB^low majority (Talham *et al.*, 1999). This observation suggests a nonspecific role for commensal gut organisms in activating GALT CD4⁺ T cells.

The specificities expressed by gut CD4⁺ T cells, via their TCR, for gut commensal bacteria have long been enigmatic. Attempts to implicate gut commensal bacteria as provocateurs of inflammatory bowel disease (IBD) in various mouse models have involved comparisons among fecal/bacterial extracts, medium alone, or extracts of food pellets and PMA/ionomycin to try to demonstrate bacterial product–driven proliferation or lymphokine production (usually IFN-γ or IL-2) by gut LP CD4⁺ T cells recovered from mice developing IBD (Brimnes *et al.*, 2001; Cong *et al.*, 1998). Generally, these T cell responses seemed to be dependent on MHC class II molecule expression and could be inhibited *in vitro* with specific anti–class II antibody. Also, the IBD development failed to occur in otherwise susceptible class II gene "knockout" mice (Matsuda *et al.*, 2000). In further support of specific stimulation by the gut microbial Ag was the finding of oligoclonality, albeit single-mouse unique, among TCR expressed by CD4⁺ T cells from mice with IBD, in CDR3-β spectrotype analysis (Matsuda *et al.*, 2000). Other observations that indirectly support TCR/bacterial Ag interaction in the activation of gut CD4⁺ T cells come from analyses of the DO11.10 transgenic mouse. This mouse is transgenic for TCR reactive with an ovalbumin peptide in the context of I-A^d. While DO11.10 transgenic mice with a RAG-2 (−/−) background had few and quiescent (naïve phenotype) gut CD4⁺ T cells, the transgenic mice lacking knockout of the RAG-2 gene had plentiful, activated T cells in their gut LP, expressing many nonclonatypic, endogenous TCR (Saparov *et al.*, 1999).

Another example of the interaction of gut microbial products with T cells, either directly or indirectly, is seen in the phenomenon of "homeostatic proliferation" in irradiated *imcomp* mice, CNV *scid* mice, or GF *scid* mice. **Fig. 18.6** shows that splenic fluorescent dye (CFSE)–labeled CD4⁺, CD8⁺, or C4 transgenic CD8⁺ T cells, transferred separately to the CNV recipients, exhibit rapid homeostatic proliferation

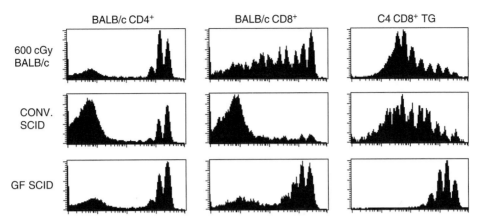

Fig. 18.6. An inoculum of 1×10^6 purified CD4+, CD8+, or C4 (monoclonal TCR) CD8+ T cells, fluorochrome-labeled with CFSE, was injected intravenously into irradiated *imcomp* BALB/c, CNV *scid* or GF *scid* mice. Four days later, splenocytes were analyzed by FACS for green fluorescence of the infected T cells. The abcissae show increasing intensity of fluorescence, from left to right (Suhr, C., Shen, H., Troy, A., Jiang, H.-Q., and Cebra, J., unpublished data).

over 4 days, while proliferation is minimal in GF *scid* recipients (Suhr, Shen, and Cebra, unpublished). Again, the specificities of TLR or TCR expressed by the responding T cells are unknown.

It has been difficult to demonstrate TCR-based specificity for a particular gut bacterium, even in monoassociated mice with IBD (Jiang, H.-Q., and Cebra, J. J., unpublished). Perhaps the findings of Caramalho *et al.* (2003) that CD4+ T cells may be activated by microbial products such as LPS, CpG, PG, and flagella via their TLR and that this stimulus can act synergistically with engagement of the TCR could support a rather broad specificity for T cells reactive with some microbial Ag. Examples of possibly broadly cross-reactive Ag expressed by bacteria include flagella, the N-formyl-methionyl peptides (Kerksiek *et al.*, 2001), and the S-polypeptides (Sleytr and Beveridge, 1999). It seems that a systematic comparison of individual gut microbial species bearing a variety of TLR ligands for reactivity with gut CD4+ T cells from monoassociated mice is in order.

Role of gut microbes in regulating oral tolerance
Although the systemic and mucosal immune systems are somewhat discrete, it seems that Ag in the gut lumen can affect elements of both systems. A profound effect of gut Ag is to induce "oral tolerance." Oral tolerance is a phenomenon that has most convincingly been defined by the oral ingestion/administration of protein ("dietary") Ag, resulting in a decreased systemic response to local "priming" with the Ag, as reflected in diminished *in vivo* or *in vitro* response to specific Ag challenge. Usually, the diminished response assessed is of Th1 cells or of T-dependent systemic antibody responses (Dahlman-Hoglund *et al.*, 1995; Lundin *et al.*, 1996; Alpan *et al.*, 2001). Presently, oral tolerance itself is considered by most as a positive, specific immune response that has downregulatory consequences for these previously mentioned aspects of the multifaceted immune response. One opera-

tionally defined lymphoid mediator of this downregulatory effect has been termed Tr1 (or Treg) cells, which can be described as follows: CD4+ T cells that are CD25+, produce IL-10 and/or TGF-β, disseminate from the gut mucosa, proliferate only minimally or not at all *in vitro* to Ag/APC, and are capable of downregulating responses *in vivo* to Ag corresponding to their own specificity as well as to irrelevant Ag that are stimulating other specific T cells in their presence (bystander effect) (Dahlman-Hoglund *et al.*, 1995; Thorstenson and Khoruts, 2001; Lundin *et al.*, 1999; Shevach, 2001; Chen *et al*, 1998).

One of the first examples of the effects of the gut microflora on the development of oral tolerance was given by Wannemuehler *et al.* (1982), who used feeding of sheep erythrocytes, a classical oral toleragen (Mattingly and Waksman, 1978), to show that convincing oral tolerance developed in CNV but not GF mice. More recently, this finding has been extended to use of ovalbumin as an oral toleragen by Moreau *et al.* (1999), and this group also showed that formerly GF mice monoassociated with *E. coli* did develop oral tolerance to ovalbumin while similar mice monoassociated with bifidobacteria did not. This latter report highlighted the problems of achieving effective systemic priming in Trexler-type isolators; this step almost precludes the use of parenterally administered Ag in CFA. We have overcome this problem by using maleylated (MA) Ag (Singh *et al.*, 1998), which can be filter-sterilized and easily introduced in glass ampules into the isolator. **Figure 18.7** shows the use of MA-Ag to compare the development of oral tolerance in GF versus CNV mice fed dietary Ag and the facilitation of oral tolerance upon monoassociating formerly GF mice with Schaedler's *E. coli*.

Presently, a principal question is how gut microbes affect the development of oral tolerance to dietary proteins. Kiyono *et al.* (1982) gave suggestive evidence of the role of a microbial product, LPS, in the induction of oral tolerance by showing that LPS-responder mice, such as C3H/HeN-strain

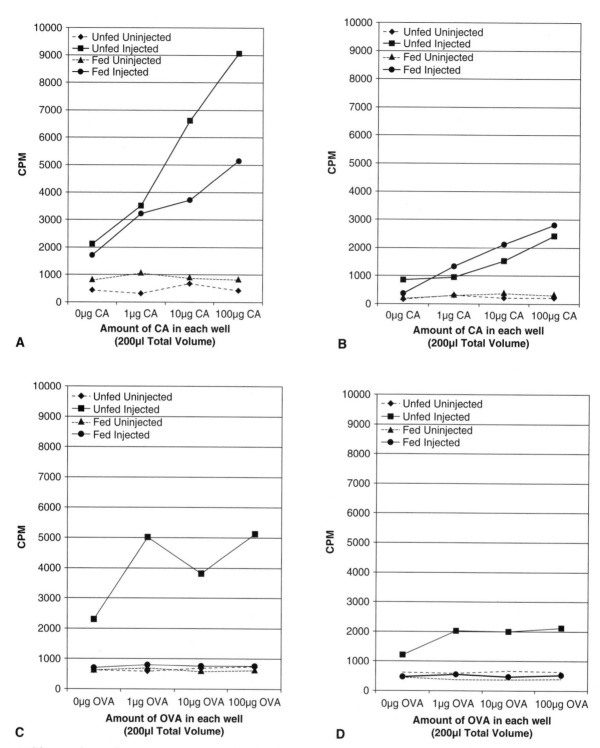

Fig. 18.7. Proliferation data with use of β-emission from 3H-thymidine incorporated into mouse spleen cells cultured for 4 days with varying concentrations of proteins. **A,** CNV mice fed, injected, and cultured with conalbumin (CA); **B,** GF mice fed, injected, and cultured with CA; **C,** CNV mice fed, injected, and cultured with OVA; **D,** *E. coli*–monoassociated mice fed, injected, and cultured with OVA (George, A., Boiko, N., and Cebra, J., unpublished data).

mice, developed prolonged and profound oral tolerance to sheep erythrocytes, while LPS-nonresponder mice (C3H/HeJ) did not. However, Moreau and Corthier (1988) found that GF C3H/HeJ mice did develop convincing oral tolerance after feeding with ovalbumin, but it was maintained for a shorter period than in CNV C3H/HeJ mice. Perhaps microbial products other than LPS, found in mice with a complete microflora, can facilitate oral tolerance. Why

GF C3H/HeJ mice do exhibit oral tolerance, albeit for a shorter duration than their CNV counterparts (Moreau and Corthier, 1988), while LPS-responder GF mice do not (Moreau *et al.*, 1999; Fig. 18.6) is unclear.

The development of "suppressor T cells," now called *downregulatory* or *Tr1* cells, that disseminate systemically and mediate oral tolerance has been recognized for many years (Mattingly and Waksman, 1978). It seems likely that these Tr1 cells depend upon Ag presented by interdigitating DC for their selective development, possibly including those that extend through the IEL spaces and interface with the gut lumen (Viney *et al.*, 1998; Akbari *et al.*, 2001; Alpan *et al.*, 2001; Maric *et al.*, 1996; Rescigno *et al.*, 2001). Since Caramalho *et al.* (2003) have recently shown that LPS can selectively activate Tr1 cells via their TLR and that this activation is synergistic with activation via TCR, it remains to be shown whether particular protein Ag from enteric bacteria can possibly activate Tr1 cells via their TCR and whether various microbial products, such as LPS, can synergize this activation via TLR. To involve such a mechanism to explain the effects of gut bacteria on the development of oral tolerance would require that Tr1 cells act in a bystander fashion in the periphery, but this has already been demonstrated (Dahlman-Hoglund *et al.*, 1995; Lundin *et al.*, 1996).

Finally, here we address whether mice and rats become orally tolerant, via the gut mucosal, to members of their normal gut microbiota and, if so, when they develop this oral tolerance. Perhaps the most informative experiments performed thus far involve the comparison of rats colonized at birth or at 6 weeks of age with an *E. coli* expressing plasmid-encoded ovalbumin. Streptomycin/ampicillin was given prior to oral colonization of young rats and near-term pregnant dams, and administration of ampicillin was continued via the drinking water of both young rats and naturally colonized neonates. The latter showed oral tolerance to both ovalbumin and pillus Ag when challenged 6 weeks after colonization, while the adults exhibited an exaggerated systemic response, indicative of oral priming (Karlsson *et al.*, 1999). In a mouse model, adults displayed oral tolerance after oral administration of sonicates of *Leishmania major* and *Staphylococcus aureus*; however, similar treatment with sonicates of *E. coli* and *Salmonella typhimurium* indicated no development of oral tolerance but development of priming for an exaggerated response to challenge (Garg *et al.*, 1999). More work needs to be done to assess whether commensal microbes induce specific, Tr1-mediated oral tolerance and why the time window seems to be restricted to the postnatal period. It is also not clear whether GF young adults may or may not be orally tolerized versus members of the normal microbiota upon monoassociation or oligoassociation.

Mechanisms for the interactions of commensal bacteria with intestinal epithelial cells and dendritic cells and consequent effects on lymphoid elements

The complex microbiota in mammals is sequentially developed after birth and dynamically maintained throughout life (Savage, 1999). Evolutionarily, commensal relationships are established through host-microbial interactions. At the front line of the interactions are the mucosal surfaces, which are in direct contact with varieties of members of microbiota. In the gastrointestinal tract, the cross-talk between mucosal microbiota and intestinal epithelial cells is physiologically significant in maintaining the homeostasis of the micro-ecosystem. Yet little is known about the interplay and how it influences the physiology of the gastrointestinal tract.

Because of the complexity of the microbiota (about 400 bacterial species, the majority of which are obligate anaerobes) and the difficulty in maintaining live primary gut ECs *ex vivo*, most of our limited understanding of microbial-EC interactions is entirely based on the information obtained from *in vitro* culture of cell lines with pathogenic bacteria (Elewaut *et al.*, 1999; Eckmann *et al.*, 2000). Gnotobiotic animals provide a unique model for investigating host-microbial interactions *in vivo* (Gordon and Pesti, 1971). This valuable approach generally starts with a comparative study of conventionally reared and GF animals. To further pinpoint the member(s) of microbiota that may be responsible for certain effects on the host cells, the dissected member(s) of microbiota are further examined by analyzing formerly GF animals associated with a single bacterium or a defined group of bacteria and comparing these with GF and CNV reared animals. There are two general approaches to profiling gene expression upon host-microbial interactions (Kagnoff and Eckmann, 2001). One approach is to identify differentially expressed mRNAs and then further define the identity of the respective genes and their function. The other approach is to analyze global gene expression by assessing changes in large numbers of defined genes with DNA microarray technology. The latter is a powerful tool for discovery-oriented studies of host-microbial interactions, as a broad range of host cell activities are monitored. New discoveries through such analyses may serve as guidance for further elucidating the function and significance of the differentially expressed genes. Combined with the technology of laser-capture microdissection, which can isolate a single cell type from a complex tissue sample, it becomes possible to characterize the effects of members of microbiota on a particular host cell population (Stappenbeck *et al.*, 2002a).

Role of intestinal microbiota in the development and physiology of the intestine

The pioneering work on this subject had showed the importance of intestinal microbiota in the development of normal morphology and function of the gastrointestinal tract (Gustafsson *et al.*, 1982). Compared to conventionally reared counterparts, GF rodents showed a greatly enlarged cecum, thinner intestinal wall, reduced overall cell mass, and less IgA plasma cells in the gut (Gordon and Pesti, 1971; Thompson and Trexler, 1971; Crabbe *et al.*, 1968). Without microbiota, the EC cycle is significantly changed, being characterized by slower epithelial renewal, lower mitotic index of crypt ECs, and prolonged transit process of EC differentiation (Abrams *et al.*, 1963; Lesher *et al.*, 1964; Cook and Bird, 1973). The impact of intestinal microflora on other aspects of intestinal function has also been observed. GF rodents showed reduced intestinal motility (Abrams and Bishop, 1967) and distinct patterns of enzyme production by ECs, different from those of CNV mice (DeBoth and Plaisier, 1974).

In recent years, advances of modern technology have led to a fine example of intestinal EC-commensal bacterial interactions (Bry et al., 1996). As a sensitive marker of gut epithelial differentiation, fucosylated glycoconjugate expression on ECs has been monitored and compared in GF versus CNV reared neonatal mice. Intestinal microbiota are required for the production of fucosylated glycoconjugate on intestinal ECs, as it was not expressed in GF mice. However, the expression could be initiated in formerly GF young adult mice upon monoassociation with *Bacteroides thetaiotaomicron*, a member of the microbiota in the ileum of humans and rodents. The production of fucosylated glycoconjugates was associated with accumulation of $\alpha1$, 2-fucosyl-transferase gene transcripts in ECs. An interesting finding is that the production of fucosylated glycoconjugates depended on the density of the bacterial population and the ability of the colonizer to use fucose as a carbon source, as isogenic strains of *B. thetaiotaomicron* that had disrupted fucose utilization regulon were not able to induce ECs to produce fucosylated glycoconjugates. Umesaki et al. (1995) have previously shown that another single indigenous intestinal bacterium, SFB, could induce production of fucosyl asialo GM1 glycolipids on small intestinal ECs in monoassociated formerly GF mice, similar to that observed in conventionalized mice. With use of DNA microarray, analysis of *B. thetaiotaomicron*-monoassociated mice revealed effects of this single member of the microbiota in modulating gene expression involved in multiple intestinal functions, including nutrient absorption, mucosal barrier fortification, xenobiotic metabolism, angiogenesis, and postnatal intestinal maturation (Hooper et al., 2001). For instance, it was further demonstrated that *B. thetaiotaomicron*, like intestinal microbiota in CNV reared mice, could initiate the development of intestinal angiogenesis through interaction with Paneth cells in the intestinal epithelium and induce the development of normal intestinal vasculature in formerly GF mice (Stappenbeck et al., 2002b). Moreover, a family member of mouse angiogenins, angiogenin 4, which is a member of the RNase superfamily like other angiogenins, was found to have microbicidal activity and be specifically produced and secreted into the gut lumen by Paneth cells in the crypt of the small intestine (Hooper et al., 2003). The expression and secretion of angiogenin 4 were induced and regulated by commensal bacteria and bacterial products, such as *B. thetaiotaomicron* and LPS in the intestine, representing one of the mechanisms by which the balance or homeostasis of the microecosystem is maintained through the delicate host–microbial interactions. Most recently, another study showed that a colon-specific gene expression that encoded for the production of a secreted protein called RELMβ was regulated by microbial colonization in the gut, as conventionalized formerly GF mice had dramatically enhanced expression and secretion of RELMβ into the stool in comparison with the very low level

prior to the introduction of the normal microbiota (He et al., 2003). In mice, RELMβ was produced specifically by goblet cells throughout the large intestine, with the highest level in the cecum and the distal half of the colon. The mRNA for RELMβ was solely expressed in the crypt epithelium, suggesting the activation of the RELMβ gene occurs in the crypt. It is not known yet which specific member(s) of the microbiota or their products induce RELMβ expression and what the significance is of the RELMβ production in the large intestine.

The profiles of the host gene-expression changes modulated by various indigenous members of microbiota were somewhat different. It is likely that the outcome of the host-microbial interactions under conventional conditions results from the collective effects of the members of microbiota, of which the composition is continuously varying.

Impact of the interactions between intestinal microbiota and ECs on innate and adaptive immunity

It becomes apparent that the dialogue between intestinal microbiota and ECs has great impact on innate and adaptive immunity. Intestinal ECs are more actively participating in regulating immune responses beyond just being a passive barrier at the interface between external and internal environment (Kato and Owen, 1999). It has been demonstrated that intestinal ECs constitutively express several members of transmembrane receptors called toll-like receptors (TLRs) (Cario et al., 2002). TLR family members recognize and respond to different microbial-associated molecular patterns (Barton and Medzhitov, 2002). Recognition by TLRs initiates a signaling pathway that leads to activation of NF-κB transcription factors and members of the MAP kinase family, thereby initiating the innate immune response (Medzhitov, 2001). The transcription factor NF-κB is a major player in the inflammatory immune response of the gut (Tak and Firestein, 2001). Activation of NF-κB in intestinal ECs by proinflammatory stimuli or pathogenic bacteria results in expression of various genes encoding inflammatory cytokines and chemokines (Elewaut et al., 1999; Gewritz et al., 2000). A recent study showed that a nonpathogenic strain of *Salmonella* was able to interfere with the NF-κB activation pathway elicited by diverse proinflammatory stimuli. Through direct interaction with model human epithelia, the nonpathogenic bacteria could block IκB degradation, an inhibitor of NF-κB, thereby abrogating synthesis of inflammatory mediators (Neish et al., 2000). It is reasonable to speculate that this may also be the mechanism for the homeostatic state maintained at the intestinal mucosal surface under normal conditions (Xavier and Podolsky, 2000).

TLRs were also expressed on macrophages and DCs (Janeway and Medzhitov, 2002; Akira et al., 2001), in which the impact of TLR signaling on homeostasis of the microecosystem may also be critical through innate immune responses and hence indirectly through adaptive immune responses. Moreover, recent studies showed that TLR signaling can serve as a direct link between the innate and adaptive immune system through TLRs expressed on B and T lymphocytes (Barton and Medzhitov, 2002; Matsuguchi *et al.*, 2000; Mokuno *et al.*, 2000). Furthermore, it was demonstrated that regulatory T cells (Tr1, CD4$^+$CD25$^+$) selectively expressed TLRs and could respond directly to proinflammatory bacterial products such as LPS, resulting in the increase of Tr1 survival/proliferation and the enhancement of their *in vitro* suppressive function (Caramalho *et al.*, 2003), which suggests that microbial products can directly modulate an adaptive immune response. Therefore, TLR signaling may represent another mechanism whereby the homeostasis of the microecosystem is maintained through host-microbial interactions.

Intestinal ECs can function as APCs and regulate T cell responses and other immune cells in the intestinal mucosa, thereby participating in adaptive immune responses (Kato and Owen, 1999). Besides the highly specialized M cells that overlie PP and can internalize and transport luminal Ags to the underlying lymphoid tissue, villous ECs are capable of uptaking and presenting antigen to T cells. Differing substantially from professional APCs, intestinal ECs can present unique and classical antigen-presenting molecules (classical and nonclassical MHC), costimulatory molecules (CD58, CD86), and some molecules that may facilitate antigen uptake (FcRγ, Ganglioside M1). In addition, most of these molecules are expressed in a polarized fashion, more on the basolateral or apical surface of the intestinal ECs, suggesting the complexity of ECs as APCs (Blumberg *et al.*, 1999; Hershberg and Mayer, 2000). These features enable ECs to interact with T cells in the mucosa. Overcoming the technical difficulties in isolating and maintaining primary intestinal ECs *ex vivo* for a relatively long period of time (14 days), Telega *et al.* (2000) showed that small intestinal and colonic ECs are both able to uptake protein Ag in a dose-dependent fashion, with a higher capacity shown by the latter. In comparison with wild-type mice, Ag uptake by colonic ECs from IL-2$^{-/-}$ mice was increased, in parallel with higher expression of MHC class II molecules. Consistent with the increased levels of Ag uptake, Ag-pulsed colonic ECs from IL2$^{-/-}$ mice were able to induce the highest levels of specific T cell activation in an MHC class II restricted way. Very little is known about how intestinal ECs, as APCs, deal with the tremendous amounts of Ags from intestinal microbiota and modulate immune response at mucosal sites. Indigenous bacteria, such as SFB, can induce expression of MHC class II molecules on small intestinal ECs and strongly stimulate the mucosal immune system (Umesaki *et al.*, 1995; Klaasen *et al.*, 1993; Talham *et al.*, 1999). SFB are in intimate contact with intestinal ECs, and the attachment induces apparent morphological changes at the apical surface of ECs, including indented, thickened, and more electron-dense membrane and accumulation of actin filaments (Davis and Savage, 1974; Jepson *et al.*, 1993). Recently, Yamauchi and Snel (2000) have presented evidence strongly suggesting that SFB are phagocytosed and intracellularly processed in intestinal ECs of chicken ileum. Alternatively, according to the findings of Rescigno *et al.* (2001), SFB may also be sampled into the LP from the surface of the epithelium by the protruding dendrites of the DCs from the LP, which can open the tight junction between the ECs and meanwhile are able to express tight-junction proteins to preserve the integrity of the epithelial barrier. In addition, it was recently observed that porcine SFB could pass by M cells to the subepithelial region, which overlies PP (Meyerholz *et al.*, 2002). These findings may show part of the mechanisms by which SFB act as a potent stimulus of the mucosal immune system. Through interactions with normal microbiota at the front line, ECs may be an important modulator for maintaining homeostasis and for preventing a pathological inflammation.

Probiotics

Confronted by increasing amounts of antibiotics over the past 60 years, bacteria have responded with the propagation of progeny no longer susceptible to them. We currently face multiresistant infectious disease organisms that are difficult and sometimes impossible to treat against successfully. Today we can list a number of organisms in both hospitals and the community that thwart treatment because they are resistant to not one but many different antibiotics. The term "multidrug resistance," which initially described resistant mammalian tumor cells and later strains of *Mycobacterium tuberculosis*, now can describe *any* multiresistant microorganism—bacterium, fungus, or parasite (van der Waaij and Nord, 2000). Among these opportunistic pathogens are the enterococci, the coagulase-negative staphylococci, *Pseudomonas aeruginosa*, *Klebsiella pneumoniae*, *Proteus vulgaris*, *Clostridium perfringens*, and *Acinetobacter baumanii*. Those physicians attending medical school 20–30 years ago probably did not even discuss these organisms as important pathogens, although today they cause prominent, even potentially lethal problems in hospitals worldwide.

The majority of research to date has focused on the mechanisms by which pathogenic bacteria achieve their detrimental effects. It was even possible to develop a new infectious model by using a hypertoxigenic enterohemorrhagic *E. coli* strain in GF mice (Taguchi *et al.*, 2002). However, more recently, attention has turned to the indigenous nonpathogenic microorganisms and the ways in which they benefit the host (Hart *et al.*, 2002). The mammalian intestinal tract contains a complex, dynamic, diverse society of nonpathologic bacteria. Indeed, the number of bacteria that colonize the human body is so large that researchers have estimated that the human body contains 10^{14} cells, only 10% of which are not bacteria and belong to the human body proper (Teitelbaum and Walker, 2002). Further understanding of the beneficial effects of developing a normal bacterial flora is achieved by the analysis of GF animal models.

Documentation of the health benefits of bacteria in food dates back to as early as the Persian version of the Old Testament (Genesis 18:8), which states "Abraham owed his longevity to the consumption of sour milk." Plinius, a Roman historian in 76 B.C., recommended the use of fermented milk products for the treatment of gastroenteritis (Schrezenenmeir and deVrese, 2001). In 1908 Nobel Prize–winning Russian scientist Elie Metchnikoff suggested that the ingestion of lactobacillus-containing yogurt decreases the number of toxin-producing bacteria in the intestine and thus contributes to the longevity of Bulgarian peasants (Metchnikoff, 1907; Sanders, 2000). He proposed that the ingestion of saccharolytic organisms in the form of fermented milk was reversing the effect of the proteolytic organisms, which caused autointoxication of the host. He isolated microorganisms from fermented milk. One strain he called the Bulgarian bacillus (this was *Lactobacillus bulgaricus*, which is now called *L. delbrueckii* subsp. *bulgaricus* and with *Streptococcus salivarius* subsp. *thermophilus* is used to ferment milk to yogurt).

It was these observations that led to the concept of a "probiotic," derived from the Greek, meaning "for life." The term was first used (Lilley and Stillwell, 1965) in contrast to the word antibiotic and defined as "a substance secreted by one microorganism, which stimulates the growth of another." Later (Sperti, 1971) this word was used to describe tissue extracts that stimulate bacterial growth. The origin of the term (as microbial feed/food supplement) is attributed to Alan Parker (Parker, 1974), who defined probiotics as "organisms and substances which contribute to intestinal microbial balance." Roy Fuller (1989) modified this term as a "live microbial feed supplement which beneficially affects the host animal or human by improving its intestinal microbial balance."

A probiotic should

- be of animal host origin (the attachment to ECs is very host-specific, which means in practical terms that a strain that is suitable for development in one animal may not be active in another);
- be nonpathogenic in nature;
- be resistant to destruction by technical processing;
- be resistant to destruction by gastric acid and bile;
- adhere to intestinal epithelial tissue;
- colonize the gastrointestinal tract, if even for a short time;
- produce antimicrobial substances;
- modulate immune responses; and
- influence gut metabolic activities (e.g., cholesterol assimilation, vitamin production) (Gibson and Fuller, 2000).

According to Roy Fuller (1989), the species currently being used as probiotics include the following: *L. bulgaricus, L. acidophilus, L. plantarum, L. casei, L. helveticus, L. lactis, L. salivarius, S. thermophilus, Enterococcus faecium, E. faecalis, Bifidobacterium* species, *and E. coli*.

Some commercial probiotic preparations contain a *Bacillus subtilis* strain or *B. cereus* as one of their components (Kirchgessner *et al.*, 1993; Hoa *et al.*, 2000). Therefore, *B. subtilis* and *B. cereus* are two *Bacillus* species that may have potential value as probiotics (Maruta *et al.*, 1996). Other microorganisms also can be used or considered for use as probiotics in humans or animals, including various *Bacteroides* species, *Propionibacterium* species (Zarate *et al.*, 2002), and fungi. For example, *Saccharomyces boulardii* is a patented yeast preparation that has been shown to inhibit the growth of pathogenic bacteria both *in vivo* and *in vitro*. It can prevent antibiotic-associated diarrhea, live at an optimum temperature of 37°C, be resistant to digestion, and thus reach the colon in a viable state. However, once therapy is completed, the yeast is rapidly eliminated (Surawics *et al.*, 1989).

Probiotics in veterinary practice

We shall consider only certain of the most promising microorganisms as efficacious probiotics. Oral dosage of poultry with native gut microorganisms to prevent infection with *Salmonella* was first examined by Nurmi and Rantala (1973). Prophylactic inoculation of GF chicks with *L. acidophilus* was shown to reduce shedding of pathogenic *E. coli* from 100% to 47% (Watkins *et al.*, 1982). For instance, the use of an avian-specific probiotic containing *L. acidophilus* and *S. faecium* for reducing the shedding and colonization of *Clostridium jejuni* in the chicken intestinal tract has been evaluated (Morishita *et al.*, 1997). Reducing (to 27%) the *C. jejuni* colonization level in chickens can potentially decrease the incidence of *C. jejuni* infections in humans. Nowadays, more attention is being paid to selection of promising probiotic strains according to the criteria mentioned previously. From a total of 112 strains of lactic acid bacteria of duck origin, only two—*L. animalis* and *L. salivarius*, on the basis of tests for aggregation, coaggregation, tolerance to acidic pH, detection of inhibitory activity, characterization of adhesion, and *in vivo* persistence—were proposed for use in poultry (Ehrmann *et al.*, 2002). It is interesting that 18 of 1200 bacterial isolates from cattle feces and intestinal tissue samples, which were screened and determined to inhibit the growth *E. coli* O157:H7 *in vitro*, were identified as other strains of *E. coli*, and one other strain was *Proteus mirabilis*. All 19 of these strains are nonproducers of Shiga toxin. Those selected probiotic bacteria, orally administered to cattle prior to exposure to *E. coli* O157:H7, can reduce the level of carriage of *E. coli* O157:H7 in most animals (Zhao *et al.*, 1998). Another set of data suggests that *L. salivarius* 51R, which was isolated from chicken caeca and administered orally to newly hatched broiler chickens, can significantly lower counts of enterococci and coliforms in the crop during the whole experimental period (Rada and Rychly, 1995). Recently presented results (La Ragione *et al.*, 2001) confirm that a single oral inoculum of 2.5×10^8 *B. subtilis* spores sufficiently suppressed all aspects of infection with *E. coli* O78:K80 (a known virulent strain associated with an avian colibacillosis).

Gnotobiotic and GF studies: models and approaches

In CNV animals, a study of the specific role of microorganisms as well as their interactions is difficult to achieve, given the complexity of the microbial ecosystem of the gastrointestinal tract. Although numerous data have been published on the dynamics of different representative constituents in CNV young, still little is known concerning gnotobiotic animals with a limited and defined microflora of the digestive tract. However, it has long been appreciated that the levels of several biochemical indices in the blood as well as immune responses of CNV versus gnotobiotic animals differed substantially. Only four various species of bacteria (but five strains) isolated from rumen of adult sheep—*S. bovis* C277, *Prevotella ruminicola* B14, *Butyrivibrio fibrisolvens* SH1, *B. fibrisolvens* JW2, and *Selenomonas ruminantium* Z108, which each were used in quantities of 1×10^6 microbial cells for inoculation of GF lambs—can significantly influence the level of the digestive processes as well as intensiveness of nutrient metabolism (Bomba *et al.*, 1995). In general, these results enable us to state that differences in the ecosystem of the digestive tract influenced both nitrogen and energy metabolism in CNV and gnotobiotic lambs. Rumen contents of gnotobiotic lambs showed significantly higher α-amylase and cellulase activities than in CNV lambs. This finding could be due to the composition of the inoculum, which presented a uniform population of amylolytic and cellulotic bacterial strains. Since the ecosystem of the CNV animals contained a whole range of metabolic groups of microorganisms, the proportions of amylytic and cellolytic bacteria are decreased through competition. Total serum protein levels and urea levels in CNV animals were also increased. Glucose levels did not differ significantly between groups. Total lipids in gnotobiotic lambs were substantially elevated. These differences between the groups persisted until the end of the investigation, although daily weight gains were similar. Another set of experimental data suggests that inoculation only by a single bacterium (*L. casei*) in gnotobiotic lambs (Bomba *et al.*, 1997), as in gnotobiotic chicks (*L. acidophilus*) (Watkins *et al.*, 1982), can protect against enterotoxigenic *E. coli* infection. Three other species (*L. acidophilus*, *Saccharomyces boulardii*, and *E. coli*) each are individually used (Figueiredo *et al.*, 1996) also as probiotic strains to protect against enteropathogenic agents. In order to determine if there was a synergistic effect of individual microbes, organisms were orally administered to GF mice (*L. acidophilus* and *E. coli* intragastrically in a single dose of 10^8 viable cells; *S. boulardii* orally, every 2 days throughout experiment, 10^9 viable cells at each administration). Ten days after colonization of the digestive tract, groups of animals associated with these microorganisms or not (control) were challenged orally with streptomycin-resistant or -susceptible strains of *Shigella flexneri* or *S. enteritidis* subsp. *typhimurium*. All possible dissociations and monoassociations of the three probiotics with gnotobiotic mice were also performed, and these experiments led to the conclusion that only in mice in which *E. coli* was present could antagonism be obtained (Figlo-Lima, 2000).

Probiotics in medicine

The presence of the indigenous flora is crucial not only for maturation of the immune system but also for the development of normal intestinal morphology and maintenance of a chronic and immunologically balanced intestinal inflammatory response—so-called physiological inflammation. Probiotics appear to be useful in the prevention or treatment of several gastrointestinal disorders of humans, including infectious diarrhea, antibiotic diarrhea, and traveler's diarrhea

(Salminen *et al.*, 1996; Gionchetti *et al.*, 2000). Results of preliminary human studies suggest that patients with IBD and even irritable bowel syndrome may benefit from probiotic therapy (Vanderhoof and Young, 1998). Most important is that each proposed probiotic must be studied individually and extensively to determine its efficacy and safety in each disorder for which its use may be considered. A double-blind, placebo-controlled study has shown that treatment with *Lactobacillus GG*, administered orally, was able to significantly reduce the incidence and duration of rotavirus diarrhea in comparison with a placebo (Isolauri *et al.*, 1991). Saavedra *et al.* (1994) have shown that supplementing an infant formula with *Bifidobacterium bifidum* and *S. thermophilus* can reduce the incidence of acute diarrhea and rotavirus shedding in infants admitted to the hospital. Only two other examples are known of probiont bacteria—*Lactobacillus GG* (Biller *et al.*, 1995) and *S. boulardii* (McFarland *et al.*, 1994)—successful in the treatment of diarrhea in relapsing colitis due to *Clostridium difficile*. Oral bacteriotherapy with *Lactobacillus GG* in Crohn's disease indicates that such probiotic bacteria may have the potential to increase gut IgA and thereby promote the gut immunological barrier, irrespective of the course of the main disease (Malin *et al.*, 1996). Probiotics have been examined and therefore reviewed (Rolfe, 2000) for their effectiveness in the prevention and treatment of other gastrointestinal disorders such as antibiotic-associated and infectious diarrhea (including those caused by *Shigella*, *Salmonella*, enterotoxigenic *E. coli*, and *Klebsiella*) and *H. pylori* gastroenteritis. It is interesting that *Lactobacillus* has been shown to be antagonistic to *H. pylori* both *in vitro* and in a gnotobiotic murine model (Kabir *et al.*, 1997; Aiba *et al.*, 1998). Unfortunately, the results of a few studies involving *Lactobacillus* and humans are conflicting.

Two really promising practical applications of *E. coli* nonpathogenic strain O83:K24:H31 (Lodinova-Zadnikova *et al.*, 1991, 2000, 2003) or O6:K5:H1 (Kruiz *et al.*, 1997) have been recently reported. *E. coli* serotype O6:K5:H1 was examined for its ability to prevent relapses of ulcerative colitis. Preliminary data look promising and suggest that this may be another option in maintenance therapy for such diseases. The other *E. coli* strain was used in order to determine whether the common mucosal immune system was triggered (on tested inoculated healthy full-term infants) and to investigate effectiveness of artificial colonization of the intestine on the occurrence of nosocomial infections, presence of bacterial pathogens, and infant mortality (among high-risk infants in an intensive care unit). The most important advantage of this long-term presence of probiont bacteria in the intestine is probably stable protection of formula-fed infants from nosocomial infectious agents by an early induction of IgA antibodies that appeared in stool and saliva (partially compensating for their lack in maternal milk). In high-risk premature infants, preventive colonization was even more significant and resulted in a decrease in the number of infections, infant mortality, presence of pathogens in the intestine and other body locations, and need for antibiotics.

Clinicians should pay special attention to investigations of probiotic efficacy in the prevention of colon cancer. Studies that have explored the cause–effect relationship directly have used animal models. The general conclusion of these studies is that probiotics have an inhibitory effect on the development of aberrant crypts and tumors (Brady et al., 2000).

Two final examples of successful use of probiotics are the treatment of food-allergy diseases (Paganelli et al., 2002) and the prevention of atopic diseases such as eczema, allergic rhinitis, and asthma (Kalliomaki et al., 2001).

Postulated mechanisms of probiotic activity

Possible mechanisms of probiotic activity are still mostly enigmatic. However, nowadays a largely accepted hypothesis is that effective probiotics initiate a complex, multifaceted process. For example, proven phenomena of so-called colonization resistance (the sum of all processes by which benign bacteria can inhibit the colonization by other mainly pathogenic strains) could not explain the mechanisms of action of particular probiotics against particular pathogens. Sometimes the same probiotic may inhibit different pathogens by different mechanisms. Here are brief descriptions of some nonspecific and specific mechanisms by which probiotics can protect the host against various diseases.

One mechanism involves the production of inhibitory substances against both gram-positive and gram-negative microorganisms (organic acids, especially produced by Lactobacillus species as metabolic substances; hydrogen peroxide and bacteriocins). Antibiotics, as substantially important products of probiotic-based bacteria, can also be responsible for their antibacterial properties (Pinchuk et al., 2001). B. subtilis strain 3 is known to have antagonistic properties against some species of the family Enterobacteriaceae, but it has been shown to also inhibit H. pylori in vitro. One of the compounds of cell-free supernatant from B. subtilis to which H. pylori cultures were susceptible was identified as amicoumacin A, an antibiotic with anti-inflammatory properties.

A second mechanism involves the blocking of adhesion sites. Competition for bacterial adhesion sites on intestinal epithelial surfaces is a proven mechanism of action for probiotics, which is why it is so important to select potentially effective strains according to their ability to adhere to host epithelial cells.

Competition for nutrients has also been proposed as a mechanism of probiotic action, but in vivo evidence of this is lacking (Rolfe, 2000).

A fourth mechanism is degradation of toxin receptor. The best example of this is S. boulardii, which can protect animals against C. difficile intestinal diseases through degradation of the toxin receptor on the intestinal mucosa (Castagliuolo et al., 1996, 1999). Properties of some probiont bacteria to neutralize the effect of enterotoxins were also mentioned as possible mechanisms of their activity (Sissons, 1989; Boiko, 2000).

Fifth is stimulation of immunity. Recent evidence suggests that stimulation of specific as well as nonspecific systemic and secretory immunity may be a basic mechanism by which probiotics can protect the host, especially against enteropathogens (Perdigon et al., 1995; Cukrowska et al., 2002). The underlying mechanisms of immune stimulation are not well understood yet, but specific cell wall components or even cell layers may act as adjuvants and significantly increase humoral immune responses. An interesting observation was that L. casei induced translocation of the normal flora to the liver in malnourished mice. Usually treatment with Lactobacillus or Bifidobacterium (Yasui et al., 1992) was associated with an enhancement of specific antibody–secreting cells to pathogens. Therefore, it was suggested that certain strains of lactic acid bacteria, particularly Lactobacillus GG, promote both systemic and local immune responses. It is interesting that comparison of the immunological effects of viable and heat-inactivated lactic acid bacteria (Majamaa et al., 1995) shows that Lactobacillus GG, administered as a viable preparation during acute rotavirus gastroenteritis, resulted in a significantly increased rotavirus specific IgA response at convalescence; the heat-inactivated form was clinically as efficient, but the increased IgA response was not detected. Probiotic modulation of humoral, cellular, and nonspecific immunity has been generally reviewed (Erickson and Hubbard, 2000). In addition, recently it was shown that B. bifidum but not C. perfringens can significantly induce total IgA and IgM synthesis by both MLN and PP mucosal B cells. Mucosal antibody production following oral administration of B. bifidum to mice caused increased numbers of IgG, IgM, and IgA in the culture of splenic cells, but such bacteria did not induce their own specific antibody response.

Recently it has been shown that a human intestinal microflora strain, Lactobacillus GG (ATCC 53103), promotes local antigen-specific immune responses (particularly of the IgA class), prevents permeability defects, and confers controlled antigen absorption. In that study the concentration of fecal α1-antitrypsin, tumor necrosis factor α, and eosinophil cationic protein were determined as markers of intestinal inflammation before and after probiotic intervention. The clinical score of atopic dermatitis improved significantly in infants treated with Lactobacillus GG. The concentration of α1-antitrypsin decreased in this group, but not in the group without treatment. In parallel, the median (lower-quartile to upper-quartile) concentration of fecal TNF-α decreased significantly in this group in comparison with those receiving the extensively hydrolyzed whey formula only. The concentration of fecal eosinophil cationic protein remained unaltered during therapy. These results suggest that probiotic bacteria may promote endogenous barrier mechanisms in patients with atopic dermatitis and food allergy, and by alleviating intestinal inflammation, they may be a useful tool in the treatment of food allergy (Majamaa and Isolauri, 1997).

Finally, some protective mechanisms of probiotics in the development of colon tumors have been postulated: prevention of mutations and antigenotoxic activity (decreased DNA damage in colon cells); decreased procarcinogenic enzyme activity; binding of mutagens and/or a decrease in their excretion; and decrease in the proliferation of transformed cells and their apoptosis (Wollowski et al., 2001).

Involvement of infectious components present on mucosal surfaces in etiology and pathogenic mechanisms of idiopathic, inflammatory, and autoimmune diseases

While the major cause of death in the less-developed world remains infectious diseases, the major killers in the developed world are cardiovascular disease and cancer. High morbidity is caused by chronic disorders such as allergy, arthritic diseases, and other inflammatory and autoimmune diseases.

The main characteristics of inflammatory and autoimmune diseases are tissue destruction and functional impairment as a consequence of immunologically mediated mechanisms that are principally the same as those functioning against dangerous (pathogenic) infections. In the case of autoimmune diseases, a major effort has been made to understand the pathogenic mechanisms leading to the loss of tolerance to self-components (autoantigens) (Bach, 2002; Shoenfeld et al., 2002).

Despite the fact that target antigens and the genetic bases of several autoimmune diseases are now better understood, the initial events leading to a loss of tolerance toward self-components remain unknown. One of the most popular explanations for autoimmune phenomena has always centered on various infections as possible natural events capable of initiating the process in genetically predisposed individuals (Tlaskalova-Hogenova et al., 1998; Rose and Mackay, 2000; Shoenfeld et al., 2002). Increased interest in infectious agents as causes of chronic diseases was awakened by the discovery of H. pylori as a causative agent of stomach ulcers, chronic gastritis, and probably gastric cancer.

A number of defined microorganisms have been shown to evoke autoimmunity. Infection with intestinal microbial pathogens such as Salmonella, Shigella, and Yersinia can trigger autoimmune reactions in joints and other organs (Toivanen and Toivanen, 2000). Diseases with autoimmune features such as rheumatic fever and acute glomerulonephritis may develop after a streptococcal infection. Also, viral infections can bring about autoimmune reactions; for instance, infection with coxsackievirus is accompanied by severe autoimmune myocarditis. Although there are several autoimmune disease models with well-defined initiating infections, for most autoimmune diseases the pathogenic role of plausible environmental agents is still being investigated.

The most accepted hypothesis about how infectious components cause autoimmunity is based on the concept of cross-reactive "molecular mimicry." This hypothesis assumes a similarity between the epitopes of an autoantigen present in the afflicted organism and the epitopes in the environmental antigen. The latter may consist of a microorganism or another external antigen that causes the autoimmune response (Oldstone, 1987). Moreover, in identical twins, autoimmune disease does not necessarily develop in both individuals. This may be explained by a genetically based susceptibility to disease development and by changes in the immune regulatory mechanisms ("dysregulation") as a consequence of environmental stimuli. With use of specific T-cell clones and a broad spectrum of peptides derived from basic myelin protein, it was demonstrated that the activation of autoaggressive cells can be the consequence of a binding of structurally related but not necessarily identical peptides (Wucherpfennig, 2002). From this finding one can conclude that the stimulation of specific autoreactive cells can take place following a binding of structurally similar peptides originating from different environmental sources, i.e., viral, bacterial, and/or food. Sequentially appearing responses to autoantigen epitopes or to autoantigenic molecules (epitope spreading) is a characteristic feature of developing autoimmune diseases. "Bystander" activation of immune cells was recently shown to be another mechanism by which autoimmune reactivity can spread.

Infectious stimuli may participate in the development of autoimmune conditions by inadequate activation of components of the innate immune system. Antigen-presenting cells, mainly DCs, could be activated (leading to maturation) by microbial components through TLRs to mediate the interaction of innate and adaptive immune systems. Adjuvant activity of microbial components or their synthetic substitutes has been found to correspond to the degree of activation of DCs. During activation of DCs, expression of costimulatory molecules increases, which can lead to changes in the presentation of self-antigens.

Increased synthesis and expression of heat stress proteins (hsp), chaperones, and transplantation antigens (molecules which could become target structures for autoimmune response) lead to abnormal processing and presentation of self-antigens by changing the transport and processing of intracellular peptides. Abnormal presentation of antigens can then evoke a response to cryptic self-epitopes, equal to the response to a dominant autoantigen. Superantigens are considered to be one of the most effective bacterial components to induce inflammatory reactions; they are believed to take part in the induction and course of autoimmune mechanisms (Oldstone, 1987; vanEden, 1991; Kotzin et al., 1993; Tlaskalova-Hogenova et al., 1998; Wucherpfennig, 2002).

The main contemporary approaches used to support the idea of the participation of microorganisms in the etiology of idiopathic, chronic, complex (polygenic) diseases are the following:

- Determination of prevalence of the disease in correlation with the occurrence of infection (epidemiology),
- Determination of antibodies directed to a certain (suspicious) infectious agent in sera of patients (serology), and
- Detection of an infectious agent in blood or biopsy samples of the affected tissues by PCR or another sensitive method.

Unfortunately, the tests for identification of the infectious component are usually applied after diagnosis has been determined, that is, after a delay. This fact represents the main difficulty in characterizing the environmental triggering agent, because a long time has elapsed from the triggering event to the clinical onset of these idiopathic, chronic diseases. Patients usually come to the clinic after their disease has become symptomatic and advanced, and this has made understanding of the early events leading to the disease very difficult. This is why experimental animal models of human diseases are used to elucidate the etiological and pathogenic aspects of these polygenic diseases.

In this connection it is interesting to note that experimental models of autoimmune disease induced by immunization with autoantigens practically all use complete Freund adjuvant containing mycobacteria (with strong immunostimulating activity) for immunization; moreover, some of them also use suspensions of killed bacteria, *e.g.*, *Bordetella pertussis*. Thus, for induction of autoimmune reactions in animals, it is necessary to activate DCs with microbial components to achieve activation of autoaggressive cells.

Genetically based or environmentally induced changes in mechanisms regulating mucosal immunity and tolerance can lead to impaired mucosal barrier function, increased penetration of microbial components into the circulation, and consequently, exaggeration of aberrant immune responses and inflammation. In fact, increased permeability of the gut mucosa was demonstrated in patients or their relatives with some autoimmune diseases (Yacyshyn *et al.*, 1996).

Some examples of chronic inflammatory and autoimmune diseases and the possible participation of infectious agents, including components from the normal microflora, in their etiology are presented next.

Inflammatory bowel diseases: IBD

Inflammatory bowel diseases (IBD) (*e.g.*, Crohn's disease and ulcerative colitis) are severe chronic disorders that affect approximately 0.2% of the human population. Despite the long-lasting interest of investigators, their etiology and pathogenesis remain unclear. IBD seem to involve interactions among immune, environmental, and genetic factors; the combination of these factors results in induction of inflammation, subsequent mucosal lesions, and then repair. Various specific microorganisms have been implicated in the etiology of these diseases.

Recently, experimental animal models of intestinal inflammation induced chemically or developing spontaneously have been described that make it possible to examine the early events (during induction) of the disease, to control all steps in disease progression, and to develop new preventive and therapeutic strategies. Several murine and rat models of spontaneously developing colitis suggest that disruption of T-lymphocyte regulatory functions or mucosal barrier defects could lead to chronic intestinal inflammation. Mice with a null mutation in the IL-2, IL-10, transforming growth factor β1 (TGF-β1), MHC class II, T-cell-receptor (TCR) α chain, and TCR-β chain and mice lacking signaling G protein subunit α-2 chain were shown to develop spontaneous chronic intestinal inflammation. When these mouse models of human disease were reared in GF conditions, the disease did not appear (Sadlack *et al.*, 1993; Hudcovic *et al.*, 2001; Kuhn *et al.*, 1993; Elson and Cong, 2002; Jiang *et al.*, 2002; Strober *et al.*, 2002). Therefore, it was suggested that dysreg-

ulation of the intestinal immune response to normal bacterial flora plays a crucial role. A loss of physiologically normal regulatory mechanisms of the local immune system, perhaps a breakdown of oral tolerance to environmental antigens (commensal gut bacteria), is probably involved in the pathogenic mechanism. Findings from experimental models of IBD indicate that T cells are responsible for the regulation of the intestinal immunological response to luminal antigens. Direct evidence of the participation of a subpopulation of CD4+ T cells in gut immunoregulation came from the finding that colitis in *scid* mice, developing after the transfer of a "pathogenic" CD45RB^{high} CD4+ T-cell subpopulation isolated from spleen of conventional BALB/c mice, could be prevented by simultaneous transfer of a "regulatory" CD45RB^{low} CD4+ T-cell population; these T cells express CD25 marker (Powrie, 1995). Surprisingly, the regulatory T-cell population isolated from GF mice was also able to suppress the inflammatory reaction when transferred together with pathogenic T cells (Singh *et al.*, 2001). In this model as well as in others, the important role of normal flora in disease development was confirmed, and the potential members of microflora responsible for intestinal inflammation were analyzed.

The finding that there is an abnormal T-cell responsiveness against indigenous microflora in human inflammatory bowel disease and its experimental models awakened interest in the possibility that commensal bacteria may initiate and/or maintain IBD lesions (Duchman *et al.*, 1995). Under conditions of an immunoregulatory disorder, the common intestinal flora is obviously capable of evoking stimulation leading to a chronic intestinal or systemic inflammation. A loss of physiological regulatory mechanisms of the local immune system or a lack of induction or breakdown of oral tolerance to commensal gut bacteria could be involved. The answer to the questions of which and how gut bacteria and which cells are involved in induction and maintenance of chronic intestinal inflammation is of great importance because it could bring about a new approach to therapy for and/or prevention of this severe disease (Xavier and Podolsky, 2000).

At present only three commensal enteric microbes have been shown to contribute to the initiation of IBD in each of three different animal models: *Bacteroides vulgatus* in HLA-B27 transgenic rats (Rath *et al.*, 1999); *H. muridarum* upon monoassociation of formerly GF *scid* mice then given CD45RB^{high}, CD4+ T cells (Jiang *et al.*, 2002); and *E. faecalis* in IL-10 (−/−) mice (Balish and Warner, 2002). Unfortunately, none of the effective strains of these bacteria has been used reciprocally to attempt to initiate IBD in the opposite animal model. The specificity or lack of specificity of any of these effective bacteria has not been defined; nor have the mechanisms for initiating CD4+ T cell–dependent IBD been clarified in any of these cases. Finally, there is some controversy as to whether *H. hepaticus* induces or potentiates colitis in IL-10 (−/−) mice (Dieleman *et al.*, 2000; Kuhlberg *et al.*, 1998). At any rate, *H. hepaticus* must be considered a frank pathogen, since it appears to initiate enterocolitis upon colonization of GF, *imcomp* mice (Fox *et al.*, 1996).

Periodontal disease

Periodontitis is a chronic inflammatory disease affecting the connective tissues and bone housing the teeth. The prevalence of the disease is high; a moderate form of this disease affects about 50% of adults, while the progressive, destructive form of periodontal disease occurs in a smaller proportion of the population (5%–15%). Periodontitis is a multifactorial disease in which immunological mechanisms, poorly understood genetic factors, and microbial etiology play a major role. The presence of subgingival flora is essential but not sufficient for the disease to occur. Periodontopathic bacteria that have been implicated in the etiology of the disease are *Porphyromonas gingivalis*, *Bacterioides forsythus*, *Actinobacillus actinomycetem comitans*, *Fusobacterium nucleatum*, and others (Seymour *et al.*, 1993; Henderson *et al.*, 1999; Wilson *et al.*, 2002). The possible involvement of these bacteria in periodontitis corresponds to the findings of increased levels of antibodies to these microbes in the patients and the pathological effects of these bacteria in animal models of this disease. Experimental models of the disease include GF rats monoassociated with *P. gingivalis*, mice infected with *P. gingivalis*, and ligated rat or hamster teeth. Most of these microorganisms are gram-negative bacteria, thus containing LPS that could induce polyclonal B cell activation. The essential role of bacterial involvement was demonstrated by the finding that induction of the disease by ligating the teeth was possible only in animals with an oral microflora. Periodontitis with bone loss did not occur in animals reared in GF conditions (Seymour *et al.*, 1993; Henderson *et al.*, 1999; Wilson *et al.*, 2002).

Rheumatic diseases

In recent years the relationship between the rheumatic diseases and the potential infectious components and elements of both innate and adaptive immune systems has been elucidated at the molecular level. Most forms of human diseases affecting connective tissues of the joints as well as experimental animal models of these diseases involve participation of microbial components. It is not only in reactive arthritis that intestinal bacteria were found to play the triggering role in disease development. The presence of microbial degradation products in the joint tissue was demonstrated in patients with rheumatoid arthritis, and the normal intestinal flora of these patients differs in composition from that of control healthy people (van Eden, 1991; de Keyser *et al.*, 1998; Rose and Mackay, 2000; Toivanen and Toivanen, 2000). In an animal model of human spondyloarthropathy, *i.e.*, in HLA-B27 transgenic rats or in BR10 mice, it was demonstrated that disease develops only in the presence of normal microflora; when these animals were kept in GF conditions, the disease did not develop (Rehakova *et al.*, 2000).

Type I diabetes, insulin-dependent diabetes mellitus (IDDM)

Insulin-dependent diabetes mellitus (IDDM) is one of the most studied organ-specific autoimmune diseases. It develops as a consequence of the selective destruction of β cells, the pancreatic insulin-producing cells in the islets of Langerhans. It is generally accepted that autoimmunity against β cells may arise from activation of the immune system in genetically predisposed individuals by environmental factors bearing epitopes similar to those in the β cell. Candidate environmental antigens in IDDM include various microbial and food components. In particular, the most diabetogenic factors seem to be dietary proteins—in particular, cow's milk proteins. All these antigens are usually introduced to the body via mucosal surfaces. An increased risk for the development of IDDM has been associated with triggering of the immune system by enterovirus infection and cow's milk proteins. Moreover, enhanced immune responsiveness to dietary proteins has been noted in patients with newly diagnosed IDDM (Karjaleinen et al. 1992). Animal models that are being used to help elucidate the pathogenesis of this disease are BB rats and NOD mice spontaneously developing diabetes (Rose and Mackay, 2000; Bach, 2002; Shoenfeld *et al.*, 2002).

It was shown that in these animal models, autoimmune diabetes could be inhibited by dietary manipulations and induction of oral tolerance by feeding autoantigens. Our findings demonstrating that a gluten-free diet in NOD mice prevents onset of diabetes suggest the role of the gut in induction of diabetes (Funda *et al.*, 1999). NOD mice were derived in our laboratory into a GF condition, and the effect of microflora components is being assessed. It is interesting that in our preliminary experiments, it seems that autoimmune diabetes is developing also in GF NOD mice.

Atherosclerosis

Recently, atherosclerosis was shown to begin as an inflammatory disease affecting endothelial cells and other compartments of arterial wall. This inflammatory reaction, characterized by accumulation of macrophages and T and B lymphocytes, is accompanied by fatty depositions on the walls of the blood vessels, leading to their occlusion. During the past several years, various bacteria have been implicated in the etiology of this disease (Bachmaier *et al.*, 2000; Kiechl *et al.*, 2001): the intracellular bacterium *Chlamydia pneumoniae*, *H. pylori*, and various oral bacteria, suggested also as causative agents of periodontitis (*P. gingivalis*, *Prevotella intermedia*, *Actinobacillus actinomycetemcomitans*).

Increased levels of antibodies to Hsp 60 in the population of the people exhibiting atherosclerotic changes in their vessels and experiments on animal models indicate that infection leading to increased production of Hsp 60 antibodies could, by similarity with human Hsp 60 expressed under stress in bifurcation of the vessels, trigger the inflammatory disease (Bachmaier *et al.*, 2000; Kiechl *et al.*, 2001; Wilson *et al.*, 2002). Thus far, one mouse model prone to developing atherosclerosis, the apolipoprotein (apo) E –/– mouse, has been derived and maintained in GF conditions (Wright *et al.*, 2000). These GF mice show no detectable differences from their CNV-reared conterparts in the time course of development or severity of the atherosclerotic symptoms.

Allergy

A sudden increase in allergies occurring in recent years and a continuation of this trend in economically developed countries have triggered interest in factors in the external environment. The results of recent epidemiological studies showed that their incidence today is almost three times higher than it was in 1970. This increase, which concerns mainly economically well-developed countries, was not found in the former socialist countries (Russia, Romania, Bulgaria). A search for an explanation for this trend resulted in a hypothetical statement that exaggerated hygienic conditions in developed countries decreased the quantity of natural infectious stimuli from the external environment, disturbing well-balanced development of subpopulations of T cells (the so-called hygienic hypothesis about the increase in allergies).

In early infancy the immune system and functions are not yet fully developed. At birth, Th2 cells are predominantly active, but this changes in favor of Th1 cells, providing a normal course of early postnatal development. Because the microorganisms colonizing the intestinal tract of newborn infants are the first microbial stimuli to which they are exposed soon after birth, it stands to reason that intestinal flora may be one of the principal candidates for providing an explanation for this phenomenon. Recent microbiological analyses pointed out differences in the composition of intestinal microflora between children from highly developed and underdeveloped countries. The former are born under controlled conditions in nursing homes under maximal care and observance of all hygienic measures. Consequently, the spectrum of microbes of their intestinal tract is much more limited than that of children in less-developed countries (Bjorksten *et al.*, 2001; Tlaskalova-Hogenova *et al.*, 2002; Kaliomaki and Isolauri, 2003). Unfortunately, there is still little understanding of the role played by intestinal lymphatic tissue and mucosal immunity in these processes, and there is a paucity of animal models for food allergies that could be manipulated to assess the effects of the "normal" intestinal microbiota.

ACKNOWLEDGMENTS

The authors' work on and in the field of this treatise was supported by grants (to JJC) from the United States National Institute of Health (AI-37108) and the Crohn's and Colitis Foundation and grants (to HT-H) from the Grant Agency of the Czech Republic (320/01/0933), the Czech Academy of Sciences (A 5020205, S 5020203), and the Ministry of Health of the Czech Republic (NK6742-3) The authors thank Mrs. Ethel Cebra for preparing the manuscript, editing it, and providing extensive help in referencing it.

REFERENCES

Abrams, G. D., Bauer, H., and Sprinz. H. (1963). Influence of the normal flora on mucosal morphology and cellular renewal in ileum. A comparison of germfree and conventional mice. *Lab. Invest.* 12, 335–364.

Akbari, O., DeKruyff, R. H., and Umetsu, D. T. (2001). Pulmonary dendritic cells producing IL-10 mediate tolerance induced by respiratory exposure to antigen. *Nature Immunol.* 2, 725–731.

Akira, S., Takeda, K., and Kaisho, K. (2001). Toll-like receptors: critical proteins linking innate and acquired immunity. *Nature Immunol.* 2:675–680.

Aiba, Y., Suzuki, N., Kabir, A. M., Talkagi, A., and Koga, Y. (1998). Lactic acid mediated suppression of *Helicobacter pylori* by the oral administration of *Lactobacillus salivarius* as a probiotic in a gnotobiotic murine model. *Am. J. Gastroenterol.* 93, 2097–2101.

Alpan, O., Rudomen, G., and Matzinger, P. (2001). The role of dendritic cells, B cells, and M cells in gut-oriented immune responses. *J. Immunol.* 166, 4843–4852.

Amann, R. I., Ludwig, W., and Schleifer, K.-H. (1995). Phylogenetic identification and in situ detection of individual microbial cells without cultivation. *Microbiol. Rev.* 59, 143–169.

Bach, J. F. (2002). Current concepts of autoimmunity. *Rev. Neurol.* (Paris) 158, 881–886.

Bachmaier, K., Le, J., and Penninger, J. M. (2000). "Catching heart disease": antigenic mimicry and bacterial infections. *Nature Med.* 6, 841–842.

Balish, E., and Warner, T. (2002). *Enterococcus faecalis* induces inflammatory bowel disease to interleukin-10 knockout mice. *Am. J. Pathol.* 160, 2253–2257.

Bandeira, A., Mota-Santos, T., Itohara, S., Degermann, S., Heusser, C., Tonegawa, S., and Coutinho, A. (1990). Localization of γ/δ T cells to the intestinal epithelium is independent of normal bacterial colonization. *J. Exp. Med.* 172, 239–244.

Bannai, M., Kawamura, T., Naito, T., Kameyama, H., Abe, T., Kaawamura, H., Tsukada, C., Watanabe, H., Hatakeyama, K., Hamada, H., Nishiyama, Y., Ishikawa, H., Takeda, K., Okumura, K., Taniguchi, M., and Abo, T. (2001). Abundance of unconventional CD8+ natural killer T cells in the large intestine. *Eur. J. Immunol.* 31, 3361–3369.

Barton. G. M., and Medzhitov. R. (2002). Toll-like receptors and their ligands. *Curr. Topics Microbiol. Immunol.* 270, 81–92.

Berek, C., Berger, A., and Apel, A. (1991). Maturation of the immune response in germinal centers. *Cell* 67, 1121–1129.

Berg, R. D., and Savage, D. C. (1975). Immune responses of specific pathogen-free and gnotobiotic mice to antigens of indigenous and nonindigenous microorganisms. *Infect. Immun.* 11, 1010–1020.

Biller, J. A., Katz, A. J., Flores, A. F., Buie, T. M., and Gorbach, S. L. (1995). Treatment of recurrent *Clostridium difficile* colitis with Lactobacillus GG. *J. Pediatr. Gastroenterol. Nutr.* 21, 224–226.

Bjorksten, B., Sepp, E., Julge, K., Voor, T., and Mikelsaar, M. (2001). Allergy development and the intestinal microflora during the first year of life. *J. Allergy Clin. Immunol.* 108, 516–520.

Bleicher, P. A., Balk, S. P., Hagen, S. J., Blumberg, R. S., Flotte, T. J., and Terhorst, C. (1990). Expression of murine CD1 on gastrointestinal epithelium. *Science* 250, 679–682.

Blumberg, R. S., Lencer, W. I., Zhu, X., Kim, H-S., Claypool, S., Balk, S. P., Saubermann, L. J., and Colgan, S. P. (1999). Antigen presentation by intestinal epithelial cells. *Immunol. Letters* 69, 7–11.

Boiko, N. V. (2000). Anti-toxic effectiveness of the *Bacillus subtilis* strain 090 as a basis of a new probiotic "Monosporine-PK" *Sci. Bull. UzNU, Ser. Biol.* 8, 18–22.

Bomba, A., Zitnan, R., Koniarova, I., Laukova, A., Sommer, A., Posivak, J., Bucko, V., and Pataky, J. (1995). Rumen fermentation and metabolic profile in conventional and gnotobiotic lambs. *Arch. Anim. Nutr.* 48, 231–243.

Bomba, A., Kravjanskc, I., Kastel, R., Herich, R., Juna-Sova, Z., Cizek, M., and Kapitancik, B. (1997). Inhibitory effect of *Lactobacillus casei* upon the adhesion of enterotoxigenic *Escherichia coli* K 99 to the intestinal mucosa in gnotobiotic lambs. *Small Ruminant Res.* 23, 199–206.

Bos, N. A., and Ploplis, V. A. (1994). Humoral immune response to DNP-KLH in antigen-free, germfree and conventional BALB/c mice. *Eur. J. Immunol.* 24, 59–65.

Bos, N. A., Bun, J. C., Popma, S. H., Cebra, E. R., Deenen, G. J., van der Cammen, M. J. F., Kroese, F. G. M., and Cebra, J. J. (1996). Monoclonal immunoglobulin A derived from peritoneal B cells is encoded by both germ line and somatically mutated V_H genes and is reactive with commensal bacteria. *Infect. Immun.* 64, 616–523.

Bos, N. A., Jiang, H.-Q., and Cebra, J. J. (2001). T cell control of the gut IgA response against commensal bacteria. *Gut* 48, 762–764.

Bos, N. A., Cebra, J. J., and Kroese, F. G. M. (2000). B-1 cells and the intestinal microflora. *Curr. Topics Microbiol. Immunol.* 252, 211–220.

Bos, N. A., Bun, J. C., Meedendorp, B., Wubbena, A. S., Kroese, F. G. M., Ploplis, V. A., and Cebra, J. J. (2003). B cell populations in antigen-free mice. In *Old Herborn University Symposium Monograph 6: The Ontogeny of the Immune System.* 7–19.

Bousso, P., Lemaitre, F., Laouini, D., Kanellopoulos, J., and Kourilsky, P. (2000). The peripheral CD8 T cell repertoire is largely independent of the presence of intestinal flora. *Int. Immunol.* 12, 425–430.

Bowman, E. P., Kuklin, N. A., Youngman, K. R., Lazarus, N. H., Kunkel, E. J., Pan, J., Greenberg, H. B., and Butcher, E. C. (2002). The intestinal chemokine thymus-expressed chemokine (CCL25) attracts IgA antibody–secreting cells. *J. Exp. Med.* 195, 269–275.

Brady, L. J., Gallaher, D. D., and Busta, F. F. (2000). The role of probiotic cultures in the prevention on colon cancer. Symposium. Probiotic bacteria: implication for human health. *J. Nutr.* 130, 410–414.

Brandtzaeg, P., and Farstad, I. N. (1999). The human mucosal B-cell system. In *Mucosal Immunology*, 2nd ed. (eds. P. L. Ogra, J. Mestecky, M. E. Lamm, W. Strober, J. Bienenstock, and J. R. McGhee). 439–468. San Diego: Academic Press.

Brimnes, J., Reimann, J., Nissen, M. H., and Claesson, M. H. (2001). Enteric bacterial antigens activate CD4+ T cells from *scid* mice with inflammatory bowel disease. *Eur. J. Immunol.* 31, 23–31.

Bry, L., Falk, P. G., Midtvedt, T., and Gordon, J. I. (1996). A model of host-microbial interactions in an open mammalian ecosystem. *Science* 273, 1380–1383.

Butcher, E. C., Williams, M., Youngman, K., Rott, L., and Briskin, M. (1999). Lymphocyte trafficking and regional immunity. *Adv. Immunol.* 72, 209–253.

Caramalho, I., Lopes-Carvalho, T., Ostler, D., Zelenay, S., Haury, M., and Demengeot, J. (2003). Regulatory T cells selectively express toll-like receptors and are activated by lipopolysaccharide. *J. Exp. Med.* 197, 403–411.

Cario, E., Brown, D., McKee, M., Lynch-Devaney, K., Gerken, G., and Podolsky, D. (2002). Commensal-associated molecular patterns induce selective toll-like receptor-trafficking from apical membrane to cytoplasmic compartments in polarized intestinal epithelium. *Am. J. Pathol.* 160, 165–173.

Carlsson, B., and Hanson, L. A. (1994). Immunologic effects of breast-feeding on the infant. In *Handbook of Mucosal Immunology* (eds. P. L. Ogra, M. E. Lamm, J. R. McGhee, W. Strober, and J. Bienenstock), 653–660, San Diego, Academic Press.

Carmen, P. S., Ernst, P. B., Rosenthal, K. L., Clark, D. A., Befus, A. D., and Bienenstock, J. (1996). Intraepithelial leukocytes contain a unique subpopulation of NK-like cytotoxic cells active in the defense of gut epithelium to enteric murine coronavirus. *J. Immunol.* 136, 1548–1553.

Carter, P. B., and Pollard, M. (1971). Host responses to "normal" microbial flora in germ-free mice. *J. Reticuloendothel. Soc.* 9, 580–587.

Castagliuolo, I., LaMont, J. T., Nikulasson, S. T., and Pothoulakis, C. (1996). *Saccharomyces boulardii* protease inhibits *Clostridium difficile* toxins A effects in the rat ileum. *Infect. Immun.* 64, 5225–5232.

Castagliuolo, I., Riegler, M. F., Valenick, L., LaMont, J. T., and Pothoulakis, C. (1999). *Saccharomyces boulardii* protease inhibits the effect of *Clostridium difficile* toxins A and B in human colonic mucosa. *Infect. Immun.* 67, 302–307.

Cebra, J. J., Gearhart, P. J., Kamat, R., Robertson, S. M., and Tseng, J. (1977). Origins and differentiation of lymphocytes involved in the secretory IgA response. In *Origins of Lymphocyte Diversity* XLI, 201–215. Cold Spring Harbor, NY: Cold Spring Harbor Laboratory.

Cebra, J. J. (1999). Influences of microbiota on intestinal immune system development. *Am. J. Clin. Nutr.* 69, 1046s–1051s.

Cebra, J. J., Jiang, H.-Q., Sterzl, J., and Tlaskalova-Hogenova, H. (1999). The role of mucosal microbiota in the development and maintenance of the mucosal immune system. In *Mucosal Immunology*, 2nd ed. (eds. P. L. Ogra, M. E. Lamm, J. Bienenstock, J. Mestecky, W. Strober, and J. R. McGhee), 267–280. San Diego, Academic Press.

Cepek, K. L., Shaw, S. K., Parker, C. M., Russell, G. J., Morrow, J. S., Rimm, D. L., and Brenner, M. B. (1994). Adhesion between epithelial cells and T lymphocytes mediated by E-cadherin and the alpha E beta 7 integrin. *Nature* 372, 190–193.

Chace, J. H., Hooker, N. A., Mildenstein, K. L., Krieg, A. M., and Cowdery, J. S. (1997). Bacterial DNA-induced NK cell IFN-production is dependent on macrophage secretion of IL-12. *Clin. Immunol. Immunopathol.* 84, 185–193.

Chen, W., Jin, W., and Wahl, S. M. (1998). Engagement of cytotoxic T lymphocyte–associated antigen 4 (CTLA-4) induces transforming growth factor β (TGF-β) production by murine CD4+ T cells. *J. Exp. Med.* 188, 1849–1857.

Chu, C.-L., Chen, S.-S., Wu, T.-S., Kuo, S.-C., and Liao, N.-S. (1999). Differential effects of IL-2 and IL-15 on the death and survival of activated TCRγδ+ intestinal intraepithelial lymphocytes. *J. Immunol.* 162, 1896–1903.

Cong, Y., Brandwein, S. L., McCabe, R. P., Lazenby, A., Birkenmeier, E. H., Sundberg, J. P., and Elson, C. O. (1998). CD4+ T cells reactive to enteric bacterial antigens in spontaneously colitic C3H/HeKBir mice: Increased T helper cell type 1 response and ability to transfer disease. *J. Exp. Med.* 187, 855–864.

Cook, R. H., and Bird, F. H. (1973). Duodenal villus area and epithelial migration in conventional and germfree chicks. *Poultry Sci.* 52, 2776–2780.

Cooper, M. A., Bush, J. E., Fehniger, T. A., VanDeusen, J. B., Waite, R. E., Liu, Y., Aguila, H. L., and Caligiuri, M. A. (2002). In vivo evidence for a dependence on interleukin 15 for survival of natural killer cells. *Blood* 100, 3633–3638.

Crabbe, P. A., Carbonara, A. O., and Heremans, J. E. (1965). The normal human intestinal mucosa as a major source of plasma cells containing γA-immunoglobulin. *Lab. Invest.* 14, 235–248.

Crabbe, P. A., Bazin, H., Eyssen, H., and Heremans, J. F. (1968). The normal microbial flora as a major stimulus for proliferation of plasma cells synthesizing IgA in the gut. *Int. Arch. Allergy Appl. Immunol.* 34, 362–375.

Crabbe, P. A., Nash, D. R., Bazin, H., Eyssen, H., and Heremans, J. E. (1969). Antibodies of the IgA type in intestinal plasma cells of germfree mice after oral or parenteral immunization with ferritin. *J. Exp. Med.* 130, 723–744.

Crabbe, P. A., Nash, D. R., Bazin, H., Eyssen, H., and Heremans, J. E. (1970). Immunohistochemical observations on lymphoid tissues from conventional and germ-free mice. *Lab. Invest.* 22, 448–457.

Craig, S. W., and Cebra, J. J. (1971). Peyer's patches: An enriched source of precursors for IgA-producing immunocytes in the rabbit. *J. Exp. Med.* 134, 188–200.

Crandall, R. B., Cebra, J. J., and Crandall, C. A. (1967). The relative proportions of IgG-, IgA-, and IgM-containing cells in rabbit tissues during experimental trichinosis. *Immunology* 12, 147–158.

Cuff, C. F., Lavi, E., Cebra, C. K., Cebra, J. J., and Rubin, D. H. (1990). Passive immunity to fatal reovirus serotype 3–induced meningoencephalitis in neonatal mice is mediated by both secretory and transplacental factors. *J. Virol.* 64, 1256–1263.

Cuff, C. F., Hooper, D. C., Kramer, D., Rubin, D. H., and Cebra, J. J. (1992). Functional and phenotypic analyses of the mucosal immune response in mice: Approaches to studying the immunogenicity of antigens applied by the enteric route. *Vaccine Res.* 1, 175–182.

Cuff, C. F., Cebra, C. K., Rubin, D. H., and Cebra, J. J. (1993). Developmental relationship between cytotoxic α/β T cell receptor–positive intraepithelial lymphocytes and Peyer's patch lymphocytes. *Eur. J. Immunol.* 23, 1333–1339.

Cukrowska, B., Lodinova-Zadnikova, R., Enders, C., Sonnenborn, U., Schulze, J., and Tlaskalova-Hogenova, H. (2002). Specific proliferative and antibody responses of premature infants to intestinal colonization with nonpathogenic probiotic *E. coli* strain Nissle 1917. *Scand. J. Immunol.* 55, 204–209.

Dahlman-Hoglund, A., Dahlgren, U., Ahlstedt, S., Hanson, L. A., and Telemo, E. (1995). Bystander suppression of the immune response to human serum albumin in rats fed ovalbumin. *Immunology* 86, 128–133.

Davis C. P., and Savage, D. C. (1974). Habitat, succession, attachment, and morphology of segmented, filamentous microbes indigenous to the murine gastrointestinal tract. *Infect. Immun.* 10, 948–956.

DeBoth, N. J., and Plaisier, H. (1974). The influence of changing cell kinetics on functional differentiation in small intestine of the rat. A study of enzymes involved in carbohydrate metabolism. *J. Histochem. Cytochem.* 22, 352–360.

De Keyser, F., Elewaut, D., De Vos, M., De Vlam, K., Cuvelier, C., Mielants, H., and Veys, E. M. (1998). Bowel inflammation and the spondyloarthropathies. *Rheum. Dis. Clin. N. Amer.* 24, 785–813.

Dewhirst, F. E., Chien, C.-C., Paster, B. J., Ericson, R. L., Orcutt, R. P., Schauer, D. B., and Fox, J. G. (1999). Phylogeny of the defined murine microbiota: Altered Schaedler flora. *Appl. Environ. Microbiol.* 65, 3287–3292.

Dieleman, L. A., Arends, A., Tonkonogy, S. L., Goerres, M. S., Craft, D. W., Grenther, W., Sellon, R. K., Balish, E., and Sartor, R. B. (2000). *Helicobacter hepaticus* does not induce or potentiate colitis in interleukin-10-deficient mice. *Infect. Immun.* 68, 5107–5113.

Dubos, R., Schaedler, R. W., Costello, R., and Hoet, P. (1965). Indigenous, normal, and autochthonous flora of the gastrointestinal tract. *J. Exp. Med.* 122, 67–75.

Duchmann, R., Kaiser, I., Hermann, E., Mayet, W., Ewe, K., and Meyer zum Buschenfelde, K.-H. (1995). Tolerance exists towards resident intestinal flora but is broken in active inflammatory bowel disease (IBD). *Clin. Exp. Immunol.* 102, 448–455.

Duchmann, R., May, E., Heike, M., Knolle, P., Neurath, M., and Meyer zum Buschenfelde, K-H. (1999). T cell specificity and cross reactivity towards enterobacteria, *Bacteroides*, *Bifidobacterium*, and antigen from resident intestinal flora in humans. *Gut* 44, 812–818.

Eckmann, L., Smith, J. R., Housley, M. P., Dwinell, M. B., and Kagnoff, M. F. (2000). Analysis by high density cDNA arrays of altered gene expression in human intestinal epithelial cells in response to infection with the invasive enteric bacteria *Salmonella. J. Biol. Chem.* 275, 14084–14094.

Ehrmann, M.A., Kurzak, P., Bauer, J., and Vogel, R.F. (2002). Characterization of lactobacilli towards their use as probiotics adjuncts in poultry. *J. Appl. Microbiol.* 92, 966–975.

Elewaut, D., DiDonato, J. A., Kim, J. M., Truong, F., Eckmann, L., and Kagnoff, M. F. (1999). NF-κB is a central regulator of the intestinal epithelial cell innate immune response induced by infection with enteroinvasive bacteria. *J. Immunol.* 163, 1457–1466.

Elson, C. O., and Cong, Y. (2002). Understanding immune-microbial homeostasis in intestine. *Immunol. Res.* 26, 87–94.

Erickson, K. L., and Hubbard, N. E. (2000). Probiotic immunomodulation in health and disease. *Symposium:* Probiotic bacteria: implication for human health. *J. Nutr.* 130, 403–409.

Fagarasan, S., and Honjo, T. (2002). Intestinal IgA synthesis regulation of front-line body defences. *Nature Rev. Immunol.* 3, 63–72.

Fagarasan, S., Muramatsu, M., Suzuki, K., Nagaoka, H., Hiai, H., and Honjo, T. (2002). Critical roles of activation-induced cytidine deaminase in the homeostasis of gut flora. *Science* 298, 1424–1427.

Fehninger, T. A., and Caligiuri, M. A. (2001). Interleukin 15: biology and relevance to human disease. *Blood* 97, 14–32.

Figlo-Lima, J. V. M., Vieira, E. C., and Nicoli, J. R. (2000). Antagonistic effect of *Lactobacillus acidophilus, Saccharomyces boulardii* and *Escherichia coli* combination against experimental infection with *Shigella flexneri* and *Salmonella enteritidis* subsp. *typhimurium* in gnotobiotic mice. *J. Appl. Microbiol.* 88, 365–370.

Figueiredo, P. P., Lobo, B. M., and Nicoli, J. R. (1996). Oral inoculation of *Escherichia coli* EMO in human new-borns as probiotic against diarrhoea during the first year of life. *Microecology Therapy* 24, 301–305.

Foo, M. C., and Lee, A. (1972). Immunological response of mice to members of the autochthonous intestinal microflora. *Infect. Immun.* 6, 525 –532.

Fox, J. G., Yan, L., Shames, B., Campbell, J., Murphy, J. C., and Li, X. (1996). Persistent hepatitis and enterocolitis in germfree mice infected with *Helicobacter hepaticus. Infect. Immun.* 64, 3673–3681.

Friman, V., Adlerberth, L., Connell, H., Svanborg, C., Hanson, L. A., and Wold, A. E. (1996). Decreased expression of mannose-specific adhesions by *Escherichia coli* in the colonic microflora of immunoglobulin A-deficient individuals. *Infect. Immun.* 64, 2794–2798.

Fuhrman, J. A., and Cebra, J. J. (1981). Special features of the priming process for a secretory IgA response. B cell priming with cholera toxin. *J. Exp. Med.* 153, 534–544.

Fuller, R. (1989). Probiotics in man and animals. A review. *J. Appl. Bacteriol.* 66, 365–378.

Funda, D. P., Kaas, A., Bock, T., Tlaskalova-Hogenova, H., and Buschard, K. (1999). Gluten-free diet prevents diabetes in NOD mice. *Diabetes Metab. Res. Rev.* 15, 323–327.

Garg, S., Bal, V., Rath, S., and George, A. (1999). Effect of multiple antigenic exposures in the gut on oral tolerance and induction of antibacterial systemic immunity. *Infect. Immun.* 67, 5917–5924.

Gelfanov, V., Lai, Y.-G., Gelfanova, V., Dong, J.-Y., Su, J.-P., and Liao, N.-S. (1995). Differential requirement of CD28 costimulation for activation of murine CD8⁺ intestinal intraepithelial lymphocyte subsets and lymph node cells. *J. Immunol.* 155, 76–82.

Gelfanov, V., Gelfanova, V., Lai, Y.-G., and Liao, N.-S. (1996). Activated αβ-CD8⁺, but not αα-CD8⁺, TCR-αβ⁺ murine intestinal intraepithelial lymphocytes can mediate perforin-based cytotoxicity, whereas both subsets are active in Fas-based cytotoxicity. *J. Immunol.* 156, 35–41.

Gewritz, A., Rao, A., Simon, P., Merlin, D., Carnes, D., Madara, J. L., and Neish, A. S. (2000). *Salmonella typhimurium* induces epithelial IL-8 expression via Ca⁺²-mediated activation of the NF-κB pathway. *J. Clin. Invest.* 105, 79–92.

Gibson, G. R., and Fuller, R. (2000). Aspects of *in vitro* and *in vivo* research approaches directed toward identifying probiotics and prebiotics for human use. *Symposium:* Probiotic bacteria: implication for human health. *J. Nutr.* 130, 391–395.

Gilmore, M. S., and Ferretti, J. J. (2003). The thin line between gut commensal and pathogen. *Science* 299, 1999–2002.

Gionchetti, P., Rizzello, F., Venturi, A., and Campieri, M. (2000). Probiotic in infective diarrhoea and inflammatory bowel diseases. *J. Gastr. Hepat.* 15, 489–493.

Glimstedt, G. (1932). Das Leben ohne Bakterien. Steile Aufziehung von Meerschweinchen. *Verhandl. Anat. Ges. Anat. Anz.* 75, 78–89.

Gonzalez-Fernandez, A., and Milstein, C. (1993). Analysis of somatic hypermutation in mouse Peyer's patches using immunoglobulin κ light-chain transgenes. *Proc. Natl. Acad. Sci. USA* 90, 9862–9866.

Gonzalez-Fernandez, A., Gilmore, D., and Milstein, C. (1994). Age-related decrease in the proportion of germinal center B cells from mouse Peyer's patches is accompanied by an accumulation of somatic mutations in their immunoglobulin genes. *Eur. J. Immunol.* 24, 2918–2921.

Goodman, T., and Lefrancois, L. (1989). Intraepithelial lymphocytes. Anatomical site, not T cell receptor form, dictates phenotype and function. *J. Exp. Med.* 170, 1569–1581.

Gordon, H. A., and Pesti, L. (1971). The gnotobiotic animal as a tool in the study of host microbial relationships. *Bacteriol. Rev.* 35, 390–429.

Gustafsson, B. (1948). Germfree rearing of rats. *Acta Pathol. Microbiol. Scand.* 22 (Suppl. 1), 1–132.

Gustafsson, B. E. (1982). The physiological importance of the colonic microflora. *Scand. J. Gastroenterol.* 17 (Suppl. 77), 117–131.

Guy-Grand, D., Cerf-Bensussan, N., Malessen, B., Malassis-Seris, M., Briottet, C., and Vassalli, P. (1991). Two gut intraepithelial CD8⁺ lymphocyte populations with different T cell receptors: a role for the gut epithelium in T cell differentiation. *J. Exp. Med.* 173, 471–481.

Hall, J. (1984). Review: immunology of the lung and upper respiratory tract. *Immunol. Today* 5, 305.

Hamada, H., Hiroi, T., Nishiyama, Y., Takahashi, H., Masunaga, Y., Hachimura, S., Kaminogawa, S., Takahashi-Iwanaga, H.,

Iwanaga, T., Kiyono, H., Yamamoto, H., and Ishikawa, H. (2002). Identification of multiple isolated lymphoid follicles on the antimesenteric wall of the mouse small intestine. *J. Immunol* 168, 57–64.

Hardy, R. R., and Hayakawa, K. (1992). Developmental origins, specificities and immunoglobulin gene biases of murine Ly-1 B cells. *Int. Rev. Immunol.* 8, 189–207.

Harmsen, H. J. M., Elfferich, P., Schut, F., and Welling, G. W. (1999). A 16S rRNA-targeted probe for detection of Lactobacilli and Enterococci in faecal samples by fluorescent *in situ* hybridization. *Microb. Ecol. Health Dis.* 11, 3–12.

Hart, A.L., Stagg, A.J., Frame, M., Graffner, H., Glise, H., Falk, P., and Kamm, M.A. (2002). Review article: the role of the gut flora in health and disease, and its modification as therapy. *Aliment. Pharmacol. Ther.* 16, 1383–1393.

He, W., Wang, M.-L., Jiang, H.-Q., Steppan, C. M., Thurnheer, M. C., Cebra, J. J., Lazar, M. A., and Wu, G. D. (2003). Bacterial colonization leads to the colonic secretion of RELMβ/FIZZ2, a novel goblet cell-specific protein. *Gastroenterology* 125, 1388–1397.

Heller, F., Fuss, I. J., Nieuwenhuis, E. E., Blumberg, R. S., and Strober, W. (2002). Oxazolone colitis, a Th2 colitis model resembling ulcerative colitis, is mediated by IL-13-producing NK-T cells. *Immunity* 17, 629–638.

Henderson, B., Wilson, M., McNab, R., and Lax, A. J. (1999). *Cellular Microbiology.* Chichester: John Wiley & Sons.

Hershberg, R. M., and Mayer, L. (2000). Antigen processing and presentation by intestinal epithelial cells-polarity and complexity. *Immunol. Today* 21, 123–128.

Hiroi, T., Yanagita, M., Ohta, N., Sakaue, G., and Kiyono, H. (2000). IL-15 and IL-15 receptor selectively regulate differentiation of common mucosal immune system-independent B-1 cells for IgA responses. *J. Immunol.* 165, 4329–4337.

Hoa, N. T., Baccigalupi, L., Huxham, A., Smertenko, A., Van, P. H., Ammendola, S., Ricca, E., and Cutting, S. M. (2000). Characterization of *Bacillus* species used for oral bacteriotherapy and bacterioprophylaxis of gastrointestinal disorders. *Appl. Environ. Microbiol.* 66, 5241–5247.

Hooper, D. C., Rubin, D. H., and Cebra, J. J. (1994). Spontaneous proliferation of Peyer's patch cells *in vitro. Int. Immunol.* 6, 873–880.

Hooper, D. C., Molowitz, E. H., Bos, N. A., Ploplis, V. A., and Cebra, J. J. (1995). Spleen cells from antigen-minimized mice are superior to spleen cells from germ-free and conventional mice in the stimulation of primary *in vitro* proliferative responses to nominal antigens. *Eur. J. Immunol.* 25, 212–217.

Hooper, L. V., Wong, M. H., Thelin, A., Hansson, L., Falk, P. G., and Gordon, J. I. (2001). Molecular analysis of commensal host-microbial relationships in the intestine. *Science* 291, 881–884.

Hooper, L. V., Stappenbeck, T. S., Hong, C. V., and Gordon, J. I. (2003). Angiogenins: a new class of microbicidal proteins involved in innate immunity. *Nature Immunol.* 4, 269–273.

Hudcovic, T., Stepankova, R., Cebra, J., and Tlaskalova-Hogenova, H. (2001). The role of microflora in the development of intestinal inflammation: acute and chronic colitis induced by dextran sulfate in germ-free and conventionally reared immunocompetent and immunodeficient mice. *Folia Microbiol.* 46, 565–572.

Hunter, C. A. (1996). How are NK cell responses regulated during infection? *Ex. Parasitol.* 84, 444–448.

Imaoka, A., Matsumoto, S., Setoyama, H., Okada, Y., and Umesaki, Y. (1996). Proliferative recruitment of intestinal intraepithelial lymphocytes after microbial colonization of germ-free mice. *Eur. J. Immunol.* 26, 945–948.

Isolauri, E., Juntunen, M., Rautanen, T, Sillanaukee, P., and Koivula, T. (1991). A human *Lactobacillus* strain (*Lactobacillus casi sp GG*) promotes recovery from acute diarrhea in children. *Pediatrics* 88, 90–97.

Iwasaki, A., and Kelsall, B. L (1999). Freshly isolated Peyer's patch, but not spleen, dendritic cells produce interleukin 10 and induce the differentiation of T helper type 2 cells. *J. Exp. Med.* 190, 229–239.

Iwasaki, A., and Kelsall, B. L. (2001). Unique functions of CD11b⁺, CD8α⁺, and double-negative Peyer's patch dendritic cells. *J. Immunol.* 166, 4884–4890.

Janeway, C. A., Jr., and Medzhitov, R. (2002). Innate immune recognition. *Annu. Rev. Immunol.* 20, 197–216.

Jepson, M. A., Clark, A. C., Simmons, N. L., and Hirst, B. H. (1993). Actin accumulation at sites of attachment of indigenous apathogenic segmented filamentous bacteria to mouse ileal epithelial cells. *Infect. Immun.* 61, 4001–4004.

Jeurissen, S. H. M., Duijvestijn, A. M., Sontag, Y., and Kraal, G. (1987). Lymphocyte migration into the lamina propria of the gut is mediated by specialized HEV-like blood vessels. *Immunology* 62, 273–277.

Jiang, H.-Q., Bos, N. A., and Cebra, J. J. (2001). Timing, localization, and persistence of colonization by segmented filamentous bacteria in the neonatal mouse gut depend on immune status of mothers and pups. *Infect. Immun.* 69, 3611–3617.

Jiang, H-Q., Kushnir, N., Thurnheer, M. C. Bos, N. A., and Cebra, J. J. (2002). Monoassociation of SCID mice with Helicobacter muridarum, but not four other enterics, provokes IBD upon receipt of T cells. *Gastroenterol.* 122, 1346–1354.

Jiang, H-Q., Thurnheer, M. C., Zuercher, A. W., Boiko, N. V., Bos, N. A., Cebra, J. J. (2004). Interactions of commensal gut microbes with subsets of B- and T-cells in the murine host. *Vaccine* 22, 805–811.

Jump, R. L., and Levine, A. D. (2002) Murine Peyer's patches favor development of an IL-10-secreting, regulatory T cell population. *J. Immunol.* 168, 6113–6119.

Kabir, A. M., Aiba, Y., Takagi, A., Kamiya, S., Miwa, T., and Koga, Y. (1997). Prevention of *Helicobacter pylori* infection by *Lactobacilli* in a gnotobiotic murine model. *Gut* 41, 49–55.

Kagnoff, M. F., and Eckmann, L. (2001). Analysis of host responses to microbial infection using gene expression profiling. *Curr. Opin. Microbiol.* 4, 246–250.

Kalliomaki, M., Salminen, S., Arvilommi, H., Kero, P., Koskinen, P., and Isolauri, E. (2001). Probiotic in primary prevention of atopic diseases; a randomized placebo-controlled trial. *Lancet* 357, 1076–1079.

Kalliomaki, M., and Isolauri, E. (2003). Role of intestinal flora in the development of allergy. *Curr. Opin. Allergy Clin. Immunol.* 3, 15–20.

Kanamori, Y., Ishimaru, K., Nanno, M., Maki, K., Ikuta, K., Nariuchi, H., and Ishikawa, H. (1996). Identification of novel lymphoid tissues in murine intestinal mucosa where clusters of c-kit⁺ IL-7R⁺ Thy1⁺ lympho-hemopoietic progenitors develop. *J. Exp. Med.* 184, 1449–1459.

Karjalainen, J., Saukkonen, T., Savilahti, E., and Dosch, H. M. (1992). Disease-associated anti-bovine serum albumin antibodies in type 1 (insulin-dependent) diabetes mellitus are detected by particle concentration fluoroimmunoassay, and not by enzyme linked immunoassay. *Diabetologia* 35, 985–990.

Karlsson, M. R., Kahu, H., Hanson, L. A., Telemo, E., and Dahlgren, U. I. H. (1999). Neonatal colonization of rats induces immunological tolerance to bacterial antigens. *Eur. J. Immunol.* 29, 109–118.

Kato, Y., and Owen, R. L. (1999). Structure and function of intestinal mucosal epithelium. *Mucosal Immunology* (eds. P. L. Ogra, M. E. Lamm, J. Bienenstock, J. Mestecky, W. Strober, and J. R. McGhee). 115–132. San Diego, Academic Press.

Kawaguchi, M., Nanno, M., Umesaki, Y., Matsumoto, S., Okada, Y., Cai, Z., Shimamura, T., Matsuoka, Y., Ohwaki, M., and Ishikawa, H. (1993). Cytolytic activity of intestinal intraepithelial lymphocytes in germ-free mice is strain dependent and determined by T cells expressing γδ T-cell antigen receptors. *Proc. Natl. Acad. Sci. USA* 90, 8591–8594.

Kelly, K. A., Bucy, R. P., and Nahm, M. H. (1995). Germinal center T cells exhibit properties of memory helper T cells. *Cell. Immunol.* 163, 206–214.

Kerksiek, K. M., Busch, D. H., and Pamer, E. G. (2001). Variable immunodominance hierarchies for H2-M3-restricted N-formyl peptides following bacterial infection. *J. Immunol.* 166, 1132–1140.

Kim, Y. B. (1979). Role of antigen in ontogeny of the immune response. In *Microbiology—1979.* Schlessinger, D. (ed.), American Society for Microbiology, 343–348.

Kiechl, S., Egger, G., Mayr, M., Wiedermann, C. J., Bonora, E., Oberhollenzer, F., Muggeo, M., Xu, Q., Wick, G., Poewe, W., and Willeit, J. (2001). Chronic infections and the risk of carotid atherosclerosis: prospective results from a large population study. *Circulation* 103, 1064–1070.

Kirchgessner, M., Roth, F. X., Eidelsburger, U., and Gedek, B. (1993). The nutritive efficiency of *Bacillus cereus* as a probiotic in the raising of piglets. 1. Effect on the grows parameters and gastrointestinal environment. *Arch. Anim. Nutr.* 44, 111–121.

Kiyono, H., McGhee, J. R., Wannemuehler, J., and Michalek, S. M. (1982). Lack of oral tolerance in C3H/HeJ mice. *J. Exp. Med.* 155, 605–610.

Klaasen, H. L. M. B., Koopman, J. P., Van den Brink, M. E., Van Wezel, H. P. N., and Beynen, A. C. (1991). Mono-association of mice with non-cultivable, intestinal, segmented, filamentous bacteria. *Arch. Microbiol.* 156, 148–151.

Klaasen, H. L. B. M., Van der Heijden, P. J., Stok, W., Poelma, F. J. G., Koopman, J. P., Van der Brink, M. E., Bakker, M. H., Eling, W. M. C., and Beynen, A. C. (1993). Apathogenic, intestinal, segmented, filamentous bacteria stimulate the mucosal immune system of mice. *Infect. Immun.* 61, 303–306.

Kotzin, B. L., Leung, D. Y, Kappler, J., and Marrack, P. (1993). Superantigens and their potential role in human disease. *Adv. Immunol.* 54, 99–166.

Kramer, D. R., and Cebra, J. J. (1995a). Role of maternal antibody in the induction of virus specific and bystander IgA responses in Peyer's patches of suckling mice. *Int. Immunol.* 7, 911–918.

Kramer, D. R., and Cebra, J. J. (1995b). Early appearance of "natural" mucosal IgA responses and germinal centers in suckling mice developing in the absence of maternal antibodies. *J. Immunol.* 154, 2051–2062.

Kroese, F. G. M., Butcher, E. C., Stall, A. M., Adams, S., and Herzenberg, L. A. (1989). Many of the IgA producing plasma cells in murine gut are derived from self-replenishing precursors in the peritoneal cavity. *Int. Immunol.* 1, 75–84.

Kruiz, W., Schutz, E., Fric, P., Fixa, B., Judmaier, G., and Stolte, M. (1997). Double-blind comparison of an oral *Escherichia coli* preparation and mesalazine in maintaining remission of ulcerative colitis. *Aliment. Pharmacol. Ther.* 11, 853–858.

Kuhn, R., Lohler. J., Rennick, D., Rajewsky. K., and Muller, W. (1993). Interleukin 10–deficient mice develop chronic enterocolitis. *Cell* 75, 263–274.

Kullberg, M. C., Ward, J. M., Gorelick, P. L., Caspar, P., Hieny, S., Cheever, A. W., Jankovic, D., and Sher, A. (1998). *Helicobacter hepaticus* triggers colitis in specific-pathogen-free interleukin-10 (IL-10)-deficient mice through an IL-12 and gamma interferon-dependent mechanism. *Infect. Immun.* 66, 5157–5166.

La Ragione, R. M., Casula, G., Cutting, S. M., and Woodward, M. J. (2001). *Bacillus subtilis* spores competitively exclude *Escherichia coli* O78:K80 in poultry. *Vet. Microbiol.* 79, 133–142.

Lai, Y.-G., Gelfanov, V., Gelfanova, V., Kulik, L., Chu, C.-L., Jeng, S.-W., and Liao, N.-S. (1999). IL-15 promotes survival but not effector function differentiation of CD8+ TCR αβ+ intestinal intraepithelial lymphocytes. *J. Immunol.* 163, 5843–5850.

Lebman, D. A., Griffin, P. M., and Cebra, J. J. (1987). Relationship between expression of IgA by Peyer's patch cells and functional IgA memory cells. *J. Exp. Med.* 166, 1405–1418.

Lee, F. (1995). Oral listeriosis: murine models for the study of pathogenesis—including central nervous system disease—and for the development of oral vaccines. Thesis. Philadelphia: University of Pennsylvania.

Lefrancois, L., and Goodman, T. (1989). In vivo modulation of cytolytic activity and Thy-1 expression in TCR-γδ+ intraepithelial lymphocytes. *Science* 243, 1716–1718.

Leidy, J. (1849). On the existence of entophyta in healthy animals in a natural condition. *Proc. Acad. Natl. Sci. Phila.* 4, 225–233.

Lentz, V. M., and Manser, T. (2001). Cutting edge: Germinal centers can be induced in the absence of T cells. *J. Immunol.* 167, 15–20.

Leo, O., Sachs, D. H., Samelson, L. E., Foo, M., Quinones, R., Gress, R., and Blusestone, J. A. (1986). Identification of monoclonal antibodies specific for the T cell receptor complex by Fc receptor-mediated CTL lysis. *J. Immunol.* 137, 3874–3880.

Lesher. S., Walburg, H. E., and Sacher, G. A. (1964). Generation cycle in the duodenal crypt cells of germfree and conventional mice. *Nature* 202, 884–886.

Lilley, D.M., and Stillwell, R.H. (1965). Probiotics: growth-promoting factors produced by microorganisms. *Science* 147, 747–748.

Litinskiy, M. B., Nardelli, B., Hilbert, D. M., He, B., Schaffer, A., Casali, P., and Cerutti. A. (2002). DCs induce CD40-independent immunoglobulin class switching through BLyS and APRIL. *Nature Immunol.* 3, 822–829.

Linton, P.-J., Lo, D., Lai, J., Thorbecke, G. J., and Klinman, N. R. (1992). Among naïve precursor cell subpopulations only progenitors of memory B cells originate germinal centers. *Eur. J. Immunol.* 22, 1293–1297.

Liu, Y.-J., Cairns, J. A., Holder, M. J., Abbot, S. D., Jansen, K. U., Bonnefoy, J.-Y., Gordon, J., and MacLennan, I. C. M. (1991). Recombinant 25-kDa CD23 and interleukin 1α promote the survival of germinal center B cells: evidence for bifurcation in the development of centrocytes rescued from apoptosis. *Eur. J. Immunol.* 21, 1107–1114.

Liu, Y.-J., Johnson, G. D., Gordon, J., and MacLennan, I. C. M. (1992). Germinal centres in T-cell-dependent antibody responses. *Immunol. Today* 13, 17–21.

Liu, L. M., and MacPherson, G. G. (1993). Antigen acquisition by dendritic cells: intestinal dendritic cells acquire antigen administered orally and can prime naïve T cells *in vivo. J. Exp. Med.* 177, 1299–1307.

Lodoice, J. P., Boone, D. L., Chai, S., Swain, R. E., Dassopoulos, T., Trettin, S., and Ma, A. (1998). IL-15 receptor maintains lymphoid homeostasis by supporting lymphocyte homing and proliferation. *Immunity* 9, 669–676.

Lodinova-Zadnikova, R., Tlaskalova, H., and Bartakova, Z. (1991). The antibody response in infants after colonization of the intestine with *E. coli* O83. Artificial colonization used as prevention against nosocomial infection. *Adv. Exp. Med. Biol.* 310, 329–335..

Lodinova-Zadnikova, R., Cukrowska, B., and Tlaskalova, H. (2000). Reducing risk of nosocomial infection by oral colonization of infants after birth with a probiotic *E. coli* strain and its influence on the frequency of infections and allergies: 10 and 20 years after. In *International Probiotic Conference: The Prospects of Probiotics Prevention and Therapy of Diseases of Young. Conference Proceedings*, 24. Slovak Republic: High Tetras.

Lodinova-Zadnikova, R., Cukrowska, B., and Tlaskalova-Hogenova, H. (2003). Oral administration of probiotic *Escherichia coli* after birth reduces frequency of allergies and repeated infections later in life (after 10 and 20 years). *Int. Arch. Allergy Appl. Immunol.* 131, 209–211.

Logan, A. C., Chow, K.-P. N., George, A., Weinstein, P. D., and Cebra, J. J. (1991). Use of Peyer's patch and lymph node fragments cultures to compare local immune responses to *Morganella morganii. Infect. Immun.* 59, 1024–1031.

London, S. D., Rubin, D. H., and Cebra, J. J. (1987). Gut mucosal immunization with Reovirus serotype 1/L stimulates viral specific cytotoxic T cell precursors as well as IgA memory cells in Peyer's patches. *J. Exp. Med.* 165, 830–847.

London, S. D., Cebra-Thomas, J. A., Rubin, D. H., and Cebra, J. J. (1990). CD8 lymphocyte subpopulations in Peyer's patches induced by reovirus serotype 1 infection. *J. Immunol.* 144, 3187–3194.

Lundin, B. S., Dahlgren, U. I. H., Hanson, L. A., and Telemo, E. (1996). Oral tolerization leads to active suppression and bystander tolerance in adult rats while anergy dominates in young rats. *Scand. J. Immunol.* 43, 56–63.

Lundin, B. S., Karlsson, M. R., Svensson, L. A., Hanson, L. A., Dahlgren, U. I. H., and Telemo, E. (1999). Active suppression in orally tolerized rats coincides with *in situ* transforming growth factor-beta (TGF-β) expression in the draining lymph nodes. *Clin. Exp. Immunol.* 116, 181–187.

MacDonald, T.T. (1995). Breakdown of tolerance to the intestinal bacterial flora in inflammatory bowel disease (IBD). *Clin. Exp. Immunol.* 102, 445–447.

Mackie, R. I., Sghir, A., and Gaskins, H. R. (1999). Developmental microbial ecology of the neonatal gastrointestinal tract. *Am. J. Clin. Nutr.* 69, 1035S–1045S.

MacLennan, I. C. M., and Vinuesa, C. G. (2002). Dendritic cells, BAFF, and APRIL: Innate players in adaptive antibody responses. *Immunity* 17, 235–238.

Macpherson, A. J., Gatto, D., Sainsbury, E., Harriman, G. R., Hengartner, H., and Zinkernagel, R. M. (2000). A primitive T cell–independent mechanism of intestinal mucosal IgA responses to commensal bacteria. *Science* 288, 2222–2226.

Majamaa, H., and Isolauri, E. (1997). Probiotics: a novel approach in the management of food allergy. *J. Allergy Clin. Immunol.* 99, 179–185.

Majamaa, H., Isolauri, E., Saxelin, M., and Vesikari, T. (1995). Lactic acid bacteria in the treatment of acute rotavirus gastroenteritis. *J. Ped. Gastroenter. Nutr.* 20, 333–338.

Malin, M., Suomaqlainen, H., Saxelin, M., and Isolauri, E. (1996). Promotion of IgA immune response in patients with Crohn's disease by oral bacteriotherapy with *Lactobacillus GG. Ann. Nutr. Metab.* 40, 137–145.

Maric, I., Holt, P. G., Perdue, M. H., and Bienenstock, J. (1996). Class II MHC antigen (Ia)-bearing dendritic cells in the epithelium of the rat intestine. *J. Immunol.* 156, 1408–1414.

Maruta, K., Miyazaki, H., Masuda, S., Takahasahi, M., Marubashi, T., Tadano, Y., and Takahashi, H. (1996). Exclusion of intestinal pathogens by continuous feeding with *Bacillus subtilis* C-3102 and its influence on the intestinal microflora in broilers. *Anim. Sci. Technol.* 67, 273–280.

Matsuda, J. L., Gapin, L., Sydora, B. C., Byrne, F., Binder, S., Kronenberg, M., and Aranda, R. (2000). Systemic activation and antigen-driven oligoclonal expansion of T cells in a mouse model of colitis. *J. Immunol.* 164, 2797–2806.

Matsuguchi, T., Takagi, K., Musikacharoen, T., and Yoshikai, Y. (2000). Gene expressions of lipopolysaccharide receptors, toll-like receptors 2 and 4, are differently regulated in mouse T lymphocytes. *Blood* 95:1378–1385.

Mattingly, J. A., and Waksman, B. (1978). Immunologic suppression after oral administration of antigen. I. Specific suppressor cells formed in rat Peyer's patches after oral administration of sheep erythrocytes and their systemic migration. *J. Immunol.* 121, 1878–1883.

Mattioli, C. A., and Tomasi, T. B. (1973). The life span of IgA plasma cells from the mouse intestine. *J. Exp. Med.* 138, 452–460.

McFarland, L.V., Surawicz, C.M., Greenberg, R.N., Fekety, R., Elmer, G.W., Moyer, K.A., Melcher, S.A., Bowen, K.E., Cox, J.L., and Noorani, Z. (1994). A randomized placebo controlled trial of *Saccharomyces boulardii* in combination with standard antibiotics for *Clostridium difficile* diseases. *J. Am. Med. Assoc.* 271, 224–226.

Medzhitov, R. (2001). Toll-like receptors and innate immunity. *Nature Rev. Immunol.* 1, 135–145.

Mechnikoff, E. (1907). In: *The Prolongation of Life: Optimistic Studies* (ed. Mitchell, C.), 161–183. London: William Heinemann.

Meyerholz, D. K., Stabel, T. J., and Cheville, N. F. (2002). Segmented filamentous bacteria interact with intraepithelial mononuclear cells. *Infect. Immun.* 70, 3277–3280.

Miyakawa, M., Iijima, S., Kishimoto, H., Kobayashi, R., Tajima, M., Isomura, N., Asano, M., and Hong, C. (1958). Rearing germfree guinea pigs. *Acta Pathol. Jpn.* 8, 55.

Mokuno, Y., Matsuguchi, T., Takano, M., Nishimura, H., Washizu, J., Ogawa, T., Takeuchi, O., Akira, S., Nimura, Y., and Yoshikai, Y. (2000). Expression of toll-like receptor 2 on gamma delta T cells bearing invariant V gamma 6/V delta 1 induced by *Escherichia coli* infection in mice. *J. Immunol.* 165:931–940.

Monroe, J. G., Yellen-Shaw, A. J., and Seyfert, V. L. (1993). Molecular basis for unresponsiveness and tolerance induction in immature stage B lymphocytes. *Adv. Mol. Cell. Immunol.* 18, 1–32.

Moreau, M. C., and Corthier, G. (1988). Effect of the gastrointestinal microflora on induction and maintenance of oral tolerance to ovalbumin in C3H/HeJ mice. *Infect. Immun.* 56, 2766–2768.

Moreau, M. C., Ducluzeau, R., Guy-Grand, D., and Muller, M. C. (1978). Increase in the population of duodenal immunoglobulin A plasmacytes in axenic mice associated with different living or dead bacterial strains of intestinal origin. *Infect. Immun.* 21, 532–539.

Moreau, M. C., Gaboriau-Routhiau, V., Dubuquoy, C., Bisteei, N., and Bouley, C. (1999). Modulating properties of two bacterial strains present in the gut of babies, *Escherichia coli* and *Bifidobacterium* on oral tolerance to ovalbumin and intestinal IgA anti-rotavirus response, in gnotobiotic mice. *10th Int. Congress Mucosal Immunol.*, Abs. 40.5.

Morishita, T. Y., Aye, P. P., Harr, B. S., Cobb, C. W., and Clifford, J. R. (1997). Evaluation of an avian specific probiotic to reduce the colonization and shedding of *Campylobacter jejuni* in broilers. *Avian Dis.* 41(4), 850–855.

Murakami, M., Tsubata, T., Shinkura, R., Nisitani, S., Okamoto, M., Yoshioka, H., Usui, T., Miyawaki, S., and Honjo, T. (1994). Oral administration of lipopolysaccharides activates B-1 cells in the peritoneal cavity and lamina propria of the gut and induces autoimmune symptoms in an autoantibody transgenic mouse. *J. Exp. Med.* 180, 111–121.

Nakache, M., Berg, E. L., Streeter, P. R., and Butcher, E. C. (1989). The mucosal vascular addressin is a tissue-specific endothelial cell adhesion molecule for circulating lymphocytes. *Nature* 337, 179–181.

Neish, A. S., Gewirtz, A. T., Zeng, H., Young, A. N., Hobert, M. E., Karmali, V., Rao, A. S., and Madara, J. L. (2000). Prokaryotic regulation of epithelial responses by inhibition of IκB-α ubiquitination. *Science* 289, 1560–1563.

Nurmi, E., and Rantata, M. (1973). New aspects of *Salmonella* infection in broiler production. *Nature* 241, 210–211.

O'Garra, A., Chang, R., Go, N., Hastings, R., Haughton, G., and Howard, M. (1992). Ly-1 B (B-1) cells are the main source of B cell–derived interleukin 10. *Eur. J. Immunol.* 22, 711–717.

O'Connor, B. P., Cascalho, M., and Noelle, R. J. (2002). Short-lived and long-lived bone marrow plasma cells are derived from a novel precursor population. *J. Exp. Med.* 195, 737–745.

Oldstone, M. B. (1987). Molecular mimicry and autoimmune disease. *Cell* 50, 819–820.

Paganelli, R., Ciuffreda, S., Verna, N., Cavallucci, E., Paolini, F., Ramondo, S., and Gioacchino, M.Di. (2002). Probiotic and food allergic diseases. *Allergy* 57(Suppl. 72), 97–99.

Parker R.B. (1974). Probiotics: the other half of the antibiotics story. *Anim. Nutr. Health.* 29, 4–8.

Parrott, D., and MacDonald, T. T. (1990). The ontogeny of the mucosal immune system in rodents. In *Ontogeny of the Immune System of the Gut.* (ed. T. T. MacDonald), 51–67, Boca Raton, FL: CRC Press.

Pascuel, V., Liu, Y.-J., Magalski, A., de Bouteiller, O., Bancherau, J., and Capra, J. D. (1994). Analysis of somatic mutation in five B cell subsets of human tonsil. *J. Exp. Med.* 180, 329–339.

Perdigon, G., Alvarez, S., Rachid, M., Aguero, G., and Gobbato, N. (1995). Immune system stimulation by probiotics. Symposium. Probiotic bacteria for humans: clinical systems for evaluation of effectiveness. *J. Dairy. Sci.* 78, 1597–1606.

Periwal, S. B., Speaker, T. J., and Cebra, J. J. (1997). Orally administered microencapsulated reovirus can bypass suckled, neutralizing maternal antibody that inhibits active immunization of neonates. *J. Virol.* 71, 2844–2850.

Phillips, M. W., and Lee, A. (1983). Isolation and characterization of a spiral bacterium from the crypts of rodent gastrointestinal tracts. *Appl. Environ. Microbiol.* 45, 675–683.

Pierce, N. F., and Gowans, J. L. (1975). Cellular kinetics of the intestinal immune response to cholera toxoid in rats. *J. Exp. Med.* 142, 1550–1563.

Pinchuk, I. V., Bressollier, P., Verneuil, B., Fenet, B., Sorokulova, I. B., Megraud, F., and Urdaci M. C. (2001). *In vitro* anti-*Helicobacter pylori* activity of the probiotic strain *Bacillus subtilis* 3 is due to secretion of antibiotics. *Antimicrob. Agents Chemother.* 45, 3156–3161.

Pleasants, J. R., Johnson, M. H., and Wostmann, B. S. (1986). Adequacy of chemically defined, water-soluble diet for germfree BALB/c mice through successive generations and litters. *J. Nutr.* 116, 1949–1964.

Pollard, M., and Sharon, S. (1970). Responses of the Peyer's patches in germ-free mice to antigenic stimulation. *Infect. Immun.* 2, 96–100.

Powrie, F. (1995). T cells in inflammatory bowel disease: protective and pathogenic roles. *Immunity* 3, 171–174.

Rada, V., and Rychly, I. (1995). The effect of *Lactobacillus salivarius* administration on coliform bacteria and enterococci in the crop and cecum of broiler chickens. *Vet. Med.* 40, 311–315.

Rath, H. C., Schultz, M., Freitag, R., Dieleman, L. A., Li, F., Linde, H., Scholmerich, J., and Sartor, R. B. (1999). Different subsets of enteric bacteria induce and perpetuate experimental colitis in rats and mice. *Infect. Immun.* 69, 2277–2285.

Regnault, A., Cumano, A., Vassalli, P., Guy-Grand, D., and Kourilsky, P. (1994). Oligoclonal repertoire of the CD8αα and the CD8αβ TCR-α/β murine intestinal intraepithelial T lymphocytes: Evidence for the random emergence of T cells. *J. Exp. Med.* 180, 1345–1358.

Regnault, A., Levraud, J. P., Lim, A., Six, A., Moreau, C., Cumano, A., and Kourilsky, P. (1996). The expansion and selection of T cell receptor alpha beta intestinal intraepithelial T cell clones. *Eur. J. Immunol.* 26, 914–921.

Rehakova, Z., Capkova, J., Stepankova, R., Sinkora, J., Louzecka, A., Ivanyi, P., and Weinreich, S. (2000). Germ-free mice do not develop ankylosing enthesopathy, a spontaneous joint disease. *Hum. Immunol.* 61, 555–558.

Reinecker, H. C., MacDermott, R. P., Mirau, S., Dignass, A., and Podolsky, D. K. (1996). Intestinal epithelial cells both express and respond to interleukin 15. *Gastroenterology* 111, 1706–1713.

Rescigno, M., Urbano, M., Valzasina, B., Francolini, M., Rotta, G., Bonasio, R., Granucci, F., Kraehenbuhl, J.-P., and Ricciardi-Castagnoli, P. (2001). Dendritic cells express tight junction proteins and penetrate gut epithelial monolayers to sample bacteria. *Nature Immunol.* 2, 361–367.

Reyniers, J. A. (1932). The use of germfree guinea pigs in bacteriology. *Proc. Indiana Acad. Sci.* 42, 35–37.

Rigottier-Gois, L., Le Bourhis, A.-G., Gramet, G., Rochet, V., and Dore, J. (2003). Fluorescent hybridization combined with flow cytometry and hybridization of total RNA to analyze the composition of microbial communities in human faeces using 16S rRNA probes. *FEMS Microbiol Ecol.* 43, 237–245.

Rolfe, D.R. (2000). The role of probiotic cultures in the control of gastrointestinal health. *Symposium:* Probiotic bacteria: implication for human health. *J. Nutr.* 130, 396–402.

Rose, N. R., and Mackay, I. R. (2000). Molecular mimicry: a critical look at exemplary instances in human diseases. *Cell. Mol. Life Sci.* 57, 542–551.

Saavedra, J.M., Bauman, N.A., Oung, I., Perman J.A., and Yolken, R.H. (1994). Feeding of *Bifidobacterium bifidum* and *Streptococcus thermophilus* to infants in hospital for prevention of diarrhoea and shedding rotavirus. *Lancet.* 344, 1046–1049.

Sadlack, B., Merz. H., Schorle H., Schimpl. A., Feller, A. C., and Horak, I. (1993). Ulcerative colitis-like disease in mice with a disrupted interleukin-2 gene. *Cell* 75, 253–261.

Salminen, S., Isolauri, E., and Salminen, E. (1996). Clinical uses of probiotics for stabilizing the gut mucosal barrier: successful strains and future challenges. *Antonie van Leeuwenhoek J. Microbiol.* 70, 347–358.

Salzman, N. H., de Jong, H., Paterson, Y., Harmsen, H. J. M., Welling, G. W., and Bos, N. A. (2002). Analysis of 16S libraries of mouse gastrointestinal microflora reveals a large new group of mouse intestinal bacteria. *Microbiology* 148, 3651–3660.

Sanders, M.E. (2000). Consideration for use of probiotic bacteria to modulate human health. *J. Nutr.* 130, 384–390.

Sangster, M. Y., Riberdy, J. M., Gonzalez, M., Topham, D. J., Baumgarth, N., and Doherty, P. C. (2003). An early CD4+ T cell–dependent IgA response to influenza infection in the absence of key cognate T-B interactions. *J. Exp. Med.* 198, 1011–1021.

Saparov, A., Kraus, L. A., Cong, Y., Marwill, J., Xu, X.-Y., Elson, C. O., and Weaver, C. T. (1999). Memory/effector T cells in TCR transgenic mice develop via recognition of enteric antigens by a second, endogenous TCR. *Int. Immunol.* 11, 1253–1263.

Savage, D. (1999). Mucosal microbiota. In *Mucosal Immunology* (eds. P. L. Ogra, J. Mestecky, W. Strober, J. Bienenstock and J. R. McGhee) 19–30. San Diego: Academic Press.

Schaedler, R.W., and Orcutt, R. P. (1983). Gastrointestinal microflora. In *The Mouse in Biomedical Research*, vol. III. (eds. H. L. Foster, J. D. Small, and J. G. Fox), 327–345. New York: Academic Press.

Schaedler, R. W., Dubos, R., and Costello, R. (1965a). The development of the bacterial flora in the gastrointestinal tract of mice. *J. Exp. Med.* 122, 59–66.

Schaedler, R. W., Dubos, R., and Costello, R. (1965b). Association of germ-free mice with bacteria isolated from normal mice. *J. Exp. Med.* 122, 77–83.

Schrezenenmeir, J., and deVrese, M. (2001). Probiotics, prebiotics, and synbiotics—approaching a definition. *Am. J. Clin. Nutr.* 73, 361–364.

Seymour, G. J., Gemmell, E., Reinhardt, R. A, Eastcott, J., and Taubman, M. A. (1993). Immunopathogenesis of chronic inflammatory periodontal disease: cellular and molecular mechanisms. *J. Periodontal Res.* 28, 478–486.

Shahin, R. D., and Cebra, J. J. (1981). The rise in inulin-sensitive B cells during ontogeny can be prematurely stimulated by thymus-dependent and thymus-independent antigens. *Infect. Immun.* 32, 211–215.

Shevach, E. M. (2001). Certified professionals: CD4+ CD25+ suppressor T cells. *J. Exp. Med.* 193, F41–F45.

Shoenfeld, Y., Sherer, Y., and Kalden, J. R. (2002). The expanding world of autoimmunity. *Trends Immunol.* 23, 278–279.

Shroff, K. E., Meslin, K., and Cebra, J. J. (1995). Commensal enteric bacteria engender a self-limiting humoral mucosal immune response while permanently colonizing the gut. *Infect. Immun.* 63, 3904–3913.

Singh, B., Read, S., Asseman, C., Malmstrom, V., Mottet, C., Stephens, L. A,, Stepankova, R., Tlaskalova, H., and Powrie, F. (2001). Control of intestinal inflammation by regulatory T cells. *Immunol. Rev.* 182, 190–200.

Singh, N., Bhatia, S., Abraham, R., Basu, S. K., George, A., Bal, V., and Rath, S. (1998). Modulation of T cell cytokine profiles and peptide-MHC complex availability in vivo by delivery to scavenger receptors via antigen maleylation. *J. Immunol.* 160, 4860–4880.

Sissons, J.W. (1989). Potential of probiotic organisms to prevent diarrhoea and promote digestion in farm animals: a review. *J. Sci. Food Agric.* 49, 1–13.

Sleytr, U. B., and Beveridge, T. J. (1999). Bacterial S-layers. *Trends Microbiol.* 7, 253–260.

Slifka, M. K., Antia, R., Whitmire, J. K., and Ahmed, R. (1998). Humoral immunity due to long-lived plasma cells. *Immunity* 8, 363–372.

Snel, J., Heinen, P. P., Blok, H. J., Carmen, R. J., Duncan, A. J., Allen, P. C., and Collins, M. D. (1995). Comparison of 16S rRNA sequences of segmented filamentous bacteria isolated from mice, rats, and chickens and proposal of "*Candidatus arthromitus.*" *Int. J. Syst. Bacteriol.* 45, 780–782.

Snel, J., Hermsen, C. C., Smits, H. J., Bos, N. A., Eling, W. M. C., Cebra, J. J., and Heidt, P. J. (1998). Interactions between gut-associated lymphoid tissue and colonization levels of indigenous, segmented, filamentous bacteria in the small intestine of mice. *Can. J. Microbiol.* 44, 1177–1182.

Snider, D. P., Liang, H., Switzer, I., and Underdown, B. J. (1999). IgA production in MHC class II-deficient mice is primarily a function of B-1a cells. *Int. Immunol.* 11, 191–198.

Sperti, G.S. (1971). *Probiotics.* West Point, Connecticut: A VI Publishing Co.

Stappenbeck, T. S., Hooper, L. V., Manchester, J. K., Wong, M. H., and Gordon, J. I. (2002a). Laser capture microdissection of mouse intestine: characterizing mRNA and protein expression, and profiling intermediary metabolism in specified cell populations. *Methods Enzymol.* 356, 167–196.

Stappenbeck, T. S., Hooper, L. V., and Gordon, J. I. (2002b). Developmental regulation of intestinal angiogenesis by indigenous microbes via Paneth cells. *Proc. Natl. Acad. Sci. USA* 99, 15454–15455.

Sterzl, J., Kostka, J., and Mandel, L. (1960). Attempts to determine the formation and character of gamma globulin and of natural and immune antibodies in young piglets reared without colostrum. *Folia Microbiol.* 5, 29–45.

Stoel, M., Jiang, H.-Q., van Diemen, C. C., Bun, J. C. A. M., Dammers, P. M., Thurnheer, M. C., Kroese, F. G. M., Cebra, J. J., and Bos,

N. A. (2004). Restricted IgA repertoire in both B-1 and B-2 cell derived gut plasmablasts. *J. Immunol.* (in press)

Strober, W., Fuss, I. J., and Blumberg, R. S. (2002). The immunology of mucosal models of inflammation. *Annu. Rev. Immunol.* 20, 495–549.

Surawics, C.M., Elmer, G.W., Speelman, P., McFarland, L.V., Chinn J., and van Belle G. (1989). Prevention of antibiotic-associated diarrhea by *Saccharomyces boulardii*: a prospective study. *Gastroenterology* 96, 981–988.

Tagliabue, A., Befus, A. D., Clark, D. A., and Bienenstock, J. (1982). Characteristics of natural killer cells in the murine intestinal epithelium and lamina propria. *J. Exp. Med.* 155, 1785–1796.

Taguchi, T., McGhee, J. R., Coffman, R. L., Beagley, K. W., Eldridge, J. H., Takatsu, K., and Kiyono, H. (1990). Analysis of Th1 and Th2 cells in murine gut-associated tissues. Frequencies of CD4+ and CD8+ T cells that secrete IFN-γ and IL-5. *J. Immunol.* 145, 68–77.

Taguchi, H., Takahashi, M., Yamaguchi, H., Osaki, T., Komatsu, A., Fujioka, Y., and Kamiya, S. (2002). Experimental infection of germ free mice with hyper-toxigenic enterohaemorrhagic *Escherichia coli* O157:H7, strain 6. *J. Med. Microbiol.* 51, 336–343.

Tak, P. P., and Firestein, G. S. (2001). NF-κB: a key role in inflammatory diseases. *J. Clin. Invest.* 107, 7–11.

Talham, G. L., Jiang, H-Q., Bos, N. A., and Cebra, J. J. (1999). Segmented filamentous bacteria are potent stimuli of a physiologically normal state of the murine gut mucosal immune system. *Infect. Immun.* 67, 1992–2000.

Tannock, G. W., Crichton, C. M., and Savage, D. C. (1987). A method for harvesting non-cultivable filamentous segmented microbes inhabiting the ileum of mice. *FEMS Microbiol. Ecol.* 45, 329–332.

Teitelbaum, J.E., and Walker, W.A. (2002). Nutritional impact of pre- and probiotics as protective gastrointestinal organisms. *Annu. Rev. Nutr.* 22, 107–138.

Telega, G. W., Baumgart, D. C., and Carding, S. R. (2000). Uptake and presentation of antigen to T cells by primary colonic epithelial cells in normal and diseased states. *Gastroenterology* 119, 1548–1559.

Thompson, G. R., and Trexler, P. C. (1971). Gastrointestinal structure and function in germ free or gnotobiotic animals. *Gut* 12, 230–235.

Thorstenson, K. M., and Khoruts, A. (2001). Generation of anergic and potentially immunoregulatory CD25+ CD4 T cells in vivo after induction of peripheral tolerance with intravenous or oral antigen. *J. Immunol.* 167, 188–195.

Thurnheer, M. C., Zuercher, A. W., Cebra, J. J., and Bos, N. A. (2003). B1 cells contribute to serum IgM, but not to intestinal IgA, production in gnotobiotic Ig allotype chimeric mice. *J. Immunol.* 170, 4564–4571.

Tlaskalova, H., Sterzl, J., Hajek, P., Pospisil, M., Riha, I., Marvanova, H., Kamarytova, V., Mandel, L., Kruml, J., and Kovaru, F. (1970). The development of antibody formation during embryonal and postnatal periods. In *Developmental Aspects of Antibody Formation and Structure* (eds. J. Sterzl and I. Riha), 767–790. Prague: Academic Publishing House.

Tlaskalova-Hogenova, H., and Stepankova, R. (1980). Development of antibody formation in germ-free and conventionally reared rabbits: the role of intestinal lymphoid tissue in antibody formation to *E. coli. Folia Biol.* 26, 81–93.

Tlaskalova-Hogenova, H., Sterzl, J., Stepankova, R., Vetvicka, V., Rossmann, P., Mandel, L., and Rejnek, J. (1983). Development of immunological capacity under germfree and conventional conditions. *Ann. N.Y. Acad. Sci.* 409, 96–113.

Tlaskalova-Hogenova, H., Mandel, L., Trebichavsky, I., Kovaru, F., Barot, R., and Sterzl, J. (1994). Development of immune responses in early pig ontogeny. *Vet. Immunol. Immunopathol.* 43, 135–142.

Tlaskalova-Hogenova, H., Stepankova, R., Tuckova, L., Farre, M. A., Funda, D. P., Verdu, E. F., Sinkora, J., Hudcovic, T., Rehakova, Z., Cukrowska, B., Kozakova, H., and Prokesova, L. (1998). Autoimmunity, immunodeficiency and mucosal infections: chronic intestinal inflammation as a sensitive indicator of immunoregulatory defects in response to normal luminal microflora. *Folia Microbiol.* 43, 545–550.

Tlaskalova-Hogenova, H., Tuckova, L., Lodinova-Zadnikova, R., Stepankova, R., Cukrowska, B., Funda, D. P., Striz, I., Kozakova, H., Trebichavsky, I., Sokol, D., Rehakova, Z., Sinkora, J., Fundova, P., Horakova, D., Jelinkova, L., and Sanchez, D. (2002). Mucosal immunity: its role in defense and allergy. *Int. Arch. Allergy Immunol.* 128, 77–89.

Toellner, K. M., Jenkinson, W. E., Taylor, D. R., Khan, M., Sze, D. M., Sansom, D. M., Vinuesa, C. G., and MacLennan, I. C. (2002). Low-level hypermutation in T cell–independent germinal centers compared with high mutation rates associated with T cell-dependent germinal centers. *J. Exp. Med.* 195, 383–389.

Toivanen, A., and Toivanen, P. (2000). Reactive arthritis. *Curr. Opin. Rheumatol.* 12, 300–305.

Umesaki, Y., Setoyama, H., Matsumoto, S., and Okada, Y. (1993). Expansion of αβ T-cell receptor-bearing intestinal intraepithelial lymphocytes after microbial colonization in germ-free mice and its independence from thymus. *Immunology* 79, 32–37.

Umesaki, Y., Okada, Y., Matsumoto, S., Imaoka, A., Setoyama, H. (1995). Segmented filamentous bacteria are indigenous intestinal bacteria that activate intraepithelial lymphocytes and induce MHC class II molecules and fucosyl asialo GM1 glycolipids on the small intestinal epithelial cells in the ex-germ-free mouse. *Microbiol. Immunol.* 39, 555–562.

Umesaki, Y., Setoyama, H. Matsumoto, S., Imaoka, A., and Itoh, K. (1999). Differential roles of segmented filamentous bacteria and *Clostridia* in development of the intestinal immune system. *Infect. Immun.* 67, 3504–3511.

Urdaci, M. C., Regnault, B., and Grimont, P. A. D. (2001). Identification by in situ hybridization of segmented filamentous bacteria in the intestine of diarrheic rainbow trout (*Oncorhynchus mykiss*). *Res. Microbiol.* 152, 67–73.

Uren, T. K., Johansen, F.-J., Wijburg, O. L. C., Koentgen, F., Brandtzaeg, P., and Strugnell, R. A. (2003). Role of the polymeric Ig receptor in mucosal B cell homeostasis. *J. Immunol.* 170, 2531–2539.

Vanderhoof, J.A., and Young, R.J. (1998). Use of probiotics in childhood gastrointestinal disorders. *J. Pediatr. Gastroenterol. Nutr.* 27, 323–332.

van der Waaij, D. (1969). Similarities between germfree mice and mice with an antibiotic decontaminated digestive tract. In *Germ-free Biology*, 181–189. New York: Plenum Press.

van der Waaij, L. A., Mesander, G., Limberg, P. C., and van der Waaij, D. (1994). Direct flow cytometry of anaerobic bacteria in human feces. *Cytometry* 16, 270–279.

van der Waaij, D., and Nord, C.E. (2000). *Int. J. Antimicrob. Agents* 16, 191–197.

van Eden, W. (1991). Heat-shock proteins as immunogenic bacterial antigens with the potential to induce and to regulate autoimmune arthritis. *Immunol. Rev.* 121, 5–28.

Viney, J. L., Mowat, A. M., O'Malley, J. M., Williamson, E., and Fanger, N. A. (1998). Expanding dendritic cells in vivo enhances the induction of oral tolerance. *J. Immunol.* 160, 5815–5825.

Vos, Q., Jones, L. A., and Kruisbeek, A. M. (1992). Mice deprived of exogenous antigenic stimulation develop a normal repertoire of functional T cells. *J. Immunol.* 149, 1204–1210.

Wang, D., Wells, S. M., Stall, A. M., and Kabat, E. A. (1994). Reaction of germinal centers in the T-cell-independent response to the bacterial polysaccharide α(1→6)dextran. *Proc. Natl. Acad. Sci. USA* 91, 2502–2506.

Wang, R.-F., Beggs, M. L., Robertson, L. H., and Cerniglia, C. E. (2002). Design and evaluation of oligonucleotide-microarray method for the detection of human intestinal bacteria in fecal samples. *FEMS Microbiol. Lett.* 213, 175–182.

Wannemuehler, M. J., Kiyono, H., Babb, J. L., Michalek, S. M., and McGhee, J. R. (1982). Lipopolysaccharide (LPS) regulation of the immune response: LPS converts germfree mice to sensitivity to oral tolerance induction. *J. Immunol.* 129, 959–965.

Watkins, B.A., Miller, B.F., and Neil, D.H. (1982). In vivo inhibitory effect of *Lactobacillus acidophilus* against pathogenic *Escherichia coli* in gnotobiotic chicks. *Poultry Sci.* 61, 1298–1308.

Wechsler-Reya, R. J., and Monroe, J. G. (1996). Lipopolysaccharide prevents apoptosis and induces responsiveness to antigen receptor cross-linking in immature B cells. *Immunology* 89, 356–362.

Weinstein, P. D, and Cebra, J. J. (1991). The preference for switching to IgA expression by Peyer's patch germinal center B cells is likely due to the intrinsic influence of their microenvironment. *J. Immunol.* 147, 4126–4135.

Weinstein, P. D., Schweitzer, P. A., Cebra-Thomas, J. A., and Cebra, J. J. (1991). Molecular genetic features reflecting the preference for isotype switching to IgA expression by Peyer's patch germinal center B cells. *Int. Immunol.* 3, 1253–1263.

Weltzin, R., Lucia-Jandris, P., Michetti, P., Fields, B. N., Kraehenbuhl, J. P., and Neutra, M. R. (1989). Binding and transepithelial transport of immunoglobulins by intestinal M cells: Demonstration using monoclonal IgA antibodies against enteric viral proteins. *J. Cell Biol.* 108, 1673–1685.

Wherry, J. C., Schreiber, R. D., and Unanue, E. R. (1991). Regulation of gamma interferon production by natural killer cells in *scid* mice: Roles of tumor necrosis factor and bacterial stimuli. *Infect. Immun.* 59, 1709–1715.

Williams, M. B., and Butcher, E. C. (1997). Homing of naïve and memory T lymphocyte subsets to Peyer's patches, lymph nodes, and spleen. *J. Immunol.* 159, 1746–1752.

Wilson, M., McNab, R., and Henderson, B. (2002). *Bacterial Disease Mechanisms.* Cambridge: Cambridge University Press.

Wollowski, I., Rechkemmer, G., and Pool-Zobel, B.L. (2001). Protective role of probiotics and prebiotics in colon cancer. *Am. J. Clin. Nutr.* 73 (Suppl), 451–455.

Wright, S. D., Burton, C. Hernandez, M., Hassing, H., Montenegro, J., Mundt, S., Patel, S., Card, D. J., Hermanowski-Vosatka, A., Bergstorm, J. D., Sparrow, C. P., Detmers, P. A., and Chao, Y-S. (2000). Infectious agents are not necessary for murine atherosclerosis. *J. Exp. Med.* 191, 1437–1441.

Wucherpfennig, K. W. (2002). Infectious triggers for inflammatory neurological diseases. *Nature Med.* 8, 455–457.

Wykes, M., Pombo, A., Jenkins, C., and MacPherson, G. G. (1998). Dendritic cells interact directly with naïve B lymphocytes to transfer antigen and initiate class switching in a primary T-dependent response. *J. Immunol.* 161, 1313–1319.

Xavier, R. J., and Podolsky, D. K. (2000). How to get along: Friendly microbes in a hostile world. *Science* 289, 1483–1484.

Yacyshyn, B., Meddings, J., Sadowski, D., and Bowen-Yacyshyn, M. B. (1996). Multiple sclerosis patients have peripheral blood CD45RO⁺ B cells and increased intestinal permeability. *Dig. Dis. Sci.* 41, 2493–2498.

Yamauchi, K.-E., and Snel, J. (2000). Transmission electron microscopic demonstration of phagocytosis and intracellular processing of segmented filamentous bacteria by intestinal epithelial cells of the chick ileum. *Infect. Immun.* 68, 6496–6504.

Yasui, H., Nagaoka, N., Mike, A., Hayakawa, K., and Ohwaki, M. (1992). Detection of Bifidobacterium strains that induce large quantities of IgA. *Microbial. Ecol. Health Dis.* 5, 155–162.

Yellin-Shaw, A., and Monroe, J. G. (1992). Differential responsiveness of immature- and mature-stage B cells to anti-IgM reflects both FcR-dependent and -independent mechanisms. *Cell. Immunol.* 145, 339–350.

Yi, A. K., Peckham, D. W., Ashman, R. F., and Krieg, A. M. (1999). CpG DNA rescues B cells from apoptosis by activating NFkappaB and preventing mitochondrial membrane potential disruption via a chloroquine-sensitive pathway. *Int. Immunol.* 11, 2015–2024.

Yi, A. K., Chang, M., Peckham, D. W., Krieg, A. M., and Ashman, R. F. (1998). CpG oligodeoxyribonucleotides rescue mature spleen B cells from spontaneous apoptosis and promote cell cycle entry. *J. Immunol.* 160, 5898–5906.

Zarate, G., Morata De Ambrosini V., Perez Chaia A., and Gonzalez, S. (2002). Some factors affecting the adhere of probiotic *Propionibacterium acidopropionici* CRL 1198 to intestinal epithelial cells. *Can. J. Microbiol.* 48, 449–457.

Zengler, K., Toledo, G., Rappe, M., Elkins, J., Mathur, E. J., Short, J. M., and Keller, M. (2002). Cultivating the uncultured. *Proc. Natl. Acad. Sci. USA* 99, 15681–15686.

Zhao, T., Doyle, M. P., Harmon, B. G., Brown, C. A., Mueller, P. O., and Parks, A. H. (1998). Reduction of carriage of enterohemorrhagic *Escherichia coli* O157:H7 in cattle by inoculation with probiotic bacteria. *J. Clin. Microbiol.* 36,3. 641–647.

Zuercher, A. W., and Cebra, J. J. (2002). Structural and functional differences between putative mucosal inductive sites of the rat. *Eur. J. Immunol.* 32, 3191–3196.

Zuercher, A. W., Jiang, H.-Q., Thurnheer, M. C., Cuff, C. F., and Cebra, J. J. (2002). Distinct mechanisms for cross-protection of the upper versus lower respiratory tract through intestinal priming. *J. Immunol.* 169, 3920–3925.

SECTION B

Inductive and Effector Tissues and Cells of the Mucosal Immune System

Inductive and Effector Tissues and Cells of the Mucosal Immune System: An Overview

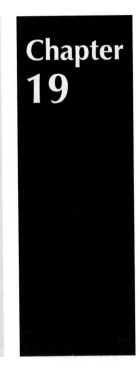

Chapter 19

Warren Strober

Mucosal Immunology Section, Laboratory of Host Defense, National Institute of Allergy and Infectious Disease, National Institutes of Health, Bethesda, Maryland

Jerry R. McGhee

Department of Microbiology, University of Alabama at Birmingham, Birmingham, Alabama

As the reader will quickly appreciate, Section B chapters deal with many of the fundamental aspects of mucosal immunology. First, it includes chapters that address the organization and function of the major parts of the mucosal system as a whole, such as the bronchus-associated lymphoid tissue, the gut-associated lymphoid tissue, and the nasopharyngeal-associated lymphoid tissue (BALT, GALT, and NALT). Second, it contains chapters that focus on individual cell systems such as mucosal dendritic cells, T cells, B cells, mast cells, and eosinophils. Third, it contains chapters dealing with major processes of the mucosal immune system, namely, the process of oral tolerance and the process of mucosal cellular traffic. These chapters provide in-depth reviews of their respective areas of concentration and thus when read *in toto* provide an excellent starting point for potential students of various areas of mucosal immunology. In addition, they can be read in part to obtain up-to-date background information for those whose major interests lie outside the areas of concentration. Finally, they form an essential background for the more "applied" areas of mucosal immunology dealt with later on in the book, such as mucosally related diseases.

The reader will also find that a number of important questions in the study of mucosal immunity are addressed several times by these chapters. At first this may appear to be unnecessary redundancy. Closer inspection, however, will indicate that these topics are approached from different directions in the various chapters and thus provide the serious reader with different perspectives on the same issues. This is as it should be in the discussion of as complex a topic as mucosal immunology.

If one would compare the chapters written here with similar chapters written in the second edition of *Mucosal Immunology* one would find that the last several years has seen enormous growth in our knowledge of mucosal immune processes in virtually every area of mucosal immunity. This development has rendered the comparable chapters in the second edition more or less obsolete and has necessitated the almost total revamping of the chapters in this section. In the following overview we will touch on these new developments as we briefly introduce the chapters in Section B.

The section opens with a series of chapters addressing the major components of the mucosal immune system, namely, BALT, GALT, and NALT. These components are discussed as integrated systems of cells by Bienenstock and Clancy (BALT); by Ishisaka, Kiyono, Fujihashi, and Nishikawa (GALT); by MacDonald and Monteleone (Human GALT); and by Kraal (NALT). The reader will note that each system manifests a commonality with other major mucosal immune components as well as unique features found only in that component.

One of the major new developments in the understanding of these systems is the elucidation of the molecular events governing the organogenesis of mucosal lymphoid follicles. Thus, as lucidly discussed by Ishikawa and his colleagues, we learn of the symphonic interplay of lymphotoxins and tumor necrosis factor in this process and, in turn, how these factors interact with the expression of chemokines and adhesion molecules, leading to the assembly of Peyer's patches as mature mucosal effector sites. In this context, we learn of the factors affecting the development of totally unappreciated mucosal effector sites, the isolated lymphoid nodules; these are mini-follicles of microscopic size that develop after birth of the animal as a result of antigen exposure. Finally, we learn of the cryptopatches, tiny progenitor sites that may be the origin of mucosal cells that populate the intraepithelial compartment. The recognition of these new types of "organized" mucosal tissues has greatly expanded our concepts of how mucosal inductive sites interact with mucosal effector sites.

In the interrelated chapters, Mayer and Blumberg (Epithelial Cell in Antigen Presentation) and Vijaykumar and Gewirtz (Epithelial Cells and the Generation of Mucosal Cytokines) explore the expanding universe of epithelial cell function in the mucosal immune system. In these chapters, the authors lay out a new story of how epithelial cells function as antigen-presenting cells, as protein transporters, as cytokine and chemokine factories, as producers of antimicrobial substances, and as a firewall against the entry of undesirable bacteria into the underlying lamina propria. As a result of this new work, epithelial cells are now considered an integral part of the mucosal immune system and one that not only plays a key role in mucosal host defense but also participates in the development of mucosal inflammation.

It is fair to say that until the last several years, knowledge of mucosal dendritic cells (DCs) and macrophages (MØ) (mucosal antigen-presenting cells) was embryonic. On the contrary, this area is now one that attracts intense interest, as we have come to better appreciate that these cells take part in the uptake of mucosal antigens and in the regulation of the immune response to these antigens. As thoroughly discussed by Kelsall and Smith in Chapter 26, we now appreciate that a wide array of DCs are present in mucosal tissues and that these cells in some instances differ from their counterparts in systemic lymphoid tissues. A newly emerging concept is that certain DCs lead to the development of mucosal regulatory cells and therefore underlie the development of mucosal tolerance. Another new and potentially important development is the discovery that DCs extend out processes between epithelial cells to sample antigens in the mucosal lumen. This opens up a totally new concept as to how antigens gain entrance to the mucosal immune system.

The nerve centers of the mucosal immune system are the mucosal T cells, and for this reason the function of these cells is considered in no less than three chapters in this section. Fujihashi and McGhee lead off in a chapter in which they clearly delineate the various classes of CD4+ T cells that participate in mucosal responses. As much as now possible, these authors define the mucosal T cells that are dedicated to switch differentiation, to terminal differentiation, and to regulatory function. In doing so they define the cytokine environment that controls the development of mucosal B cell function and thus the conditions necessary for optimal mucosal vaccination. In addition, they provide the foundation for the understanding of negative or tolerogenic responses in the mucosal immune system. Chapters on mucosal CD8+ cytotoxic cells by LeFrancois and on intraepithelial cells by Kronenberg and Cheroute round out the picture. LeFrancois lays out a new synthesis of how CD8+ cytotoxic cells function in relation to epithelial cells infected with virus and thus how these function as key host defense elements. On the other hand, Kronenberg and Cheroute focus on the hitherto mysterious intraepithelial cells, T cells

that are truly in the front line of the mucosal immune system. It is now clear that intraepithelial cells are a somewhat diverse population of T cells with a variety of key duties in the mucosal system. In particular, they discuss the fact that these cells are long-lived memory cells that exhibit effector functions in relation to antigens presented by epithelial cells and, as such, mediate host-defense functions or functions related to maintenance of epithelial cells.

B cells of the mucosal immune system are also considered in this section in great detail. In a comprehensive chapter on the development of IgA B cells in the mucosal immune system, Strober, Fagarasan, and Lycke discuss the development of IgA B cells in the mucosal immune system. This topic, of course, touches on one of the historically important concerns of mucosal immunologists, and, indeed, one of the major advances in the understanding of mucosal immunity is the body of work that has established that Peyer's patches are beehives of IgA B cell development in which IgA B cells arising from T cell–dependent adaptive immune responses are the norm. As fully discussed in this chapter, however, in more recent work it has been shown that IgA B cells can develop in a T cell–independent manner as part of an innate immune response. While the quantitative importance of this innate response is still controversial, these new data add another dimension to the IgA story and its role in mucosal immunity.

To add depth to this key issue, Cebra, Bos, and Kroese discuss B cell development in the mucosal immune system with a special emphasis on the innate IgA response. In this chapter, a full examination of the role of this response in relation to commensal flora of the gastrointestinal tract is presented and the quantitative importance of this innate IgA response to the overall IgA response is addressed. Finally, Brandtzaeg, Carlsen, and Farstad concentrate on B cell development in the mucosal immune system from the point of view of the human system. This allows them to discuss human diseases involving abnormalities of IgA B cell development.

This section of the book also contains several outstanding chapters that address key processes or functions of the mucosal immune system rather than specific cells or cell systems. In an encyclopedic chapter, Mowat, Faria, and Weiner take on the topic of oral tolerance. Here they draw on their vast experience in this area to address the general question of why the mucosal immune system has a finely tuned mechanism of turning off responses, not only in the mucosal immune system but in the systemic immune system as well. In this chapter, the authors build on the extensive data showing that oral tolerance has two components: a passive component involving induction of clonal anergy or deletion and an active component involving induction of suppressor T cells. New concepts as to why these components are so prominent in mucosal immune responses and the related question as to why suppressor T cells are evoked by oral antigens are discussed in great detail. This discussion allows them to address the question of oral tolerance in disease, from the point of view of both pathogenesis and treatment.

A second chapter focusing on mucosal immune function is that of Butcher, Youngman, and Lazarus on lymphocyte trafficking in the mucosal immune system. The contents of this chapter bear on a major feature of the mucosal immune system, namely, the fact that cells in the system are linked to mucosal tissues by cell surface mucosa–specific homing molecules. It has been known for some time that these surface molecules are composed of integrins that interact with mucosa-specific "addressins." In the last several years, however, it has become clear that these integrins are aided and abetted by chemokine receptors that respond to mucosal specific ligands (chemokines). Thus the picture that emerges is that mucosal trafficking is a complex process involving many combinations of molecules on the cell surface interacting with an equally large group of molecules on endothelial cells in the mucosal tissues. The chapter encompasses this complexity.

Yet another process-oriented chapter is contributed by Sartor and Hoentjen, who provide an excellent discussion of the inflammatory cytokines secreted by mucosal cells in the gastrointestinal tract, the mechanisms that are involved in induction of these cytokines, and the mechanisms that lead to the inhibition of such induction. These authors give us valuable insight into the intracellular biochemical pathways involved in the induction of cytokine production and thus add an important molecular dimension to mucosal immune function.

The section concludes with two excellent chapters addressing nonlymphoid cells of the mucosal immune system, mast cells and eosinophils, that play important roles in normal mucosal homeostasis and in the mechanism of inflammatory mucosal diseases. These chapters provide a nice prospective on the lymphocyte-centered or epithelial cell–centered focus of preceding chapters and thus remind the student of mucosal immunology that mucosal immune responses are indeed a microcosm of immunity in general.

Bronchus-Associated Lymphoid Tissues

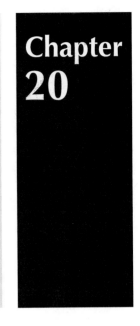

Chapter
20

John Bienenstock

Departments of Medicine & Pathology and Molecular Medicine, McMaster University, Hamilton, Ontario, Canada

Robert L. Clancy

Department of Pathology, University of Newcastle, Newcastle, New South Wales, Australia

The immune system in mucosal tissues is found in the form of organized lymphoid tissue or a diffuse collection of cellular elements either in the epithelium above the basement membrane or in the lamina propria or interstitium. Where the lymphoid tissue is organized, it occurs as isolated lymphoid follicles or follicles that are aggregated together to form larger units. Ham (1969) described the presence of subepithelial lymphoid follicles as a characteristic of epithelial surfaces bathed by glandular mucosal secretions. The term "mucosa-associated lymphoid tissue" (MALT) was first coined to emphasize the concept that mucosal lymphoid follicles and aggregates have some common features (Bienenstock *et al.*, 1979) and may be linked in what has been termed a common mucosal immune system (McDermott and Bienenstock, 1979).

Intraepithelial T lymphocytes (IEL) can be found in all epithelia of the body. Particular characteristics of intestinal IEL have been described that render them different in ontogeny, phenotype, and function from other T-cell subsets (Sim, 1995). There are also considerable species differences in terms of phenotype; for example, in the rodent, the intestinal IEL mostly express γδ T-cell receptors, whereas the human counterparts mostly express αβ T-cell receptors. The IEL in bronchial epithelium of normal, healthy nonsmoking subjects have been described (Fournier *et al.*, 1989). They were increased in number in smokers and predominantly expressed CD8. Subsequent characterization of human bronchial xenografts in SCID mice showed that bronchial IEL survived much longer (different half-life) than T cells in the lamina propria (Goto *et al.*, 2000). Almost all bronchial IEL (99.5%) expressed the αβ T-cell receptor, and 35.8% expressed the αεβ7 integrin, generally considered a marker of IEL since more than 95% of human intestinal IEL express this integrin (Cerf-Bensussan *et al.*, 1987). Others have suggested that human bronchial IEL may have a continuing sustaining relationship in terms of growth factors such as IL-7 and stem cell factor made by bronchial epithelium and molecules expressed by epithelial cells, such as ICAM-1 and HLA-DR (Goto *et al.*,

2000). Despite the predominance of the αβ phenotype in IEL, γδ cells have been found in human bronchoalveolar lavage fluid in a variety of diseases (see Wisnewski *et al.*, 2001), and these expressed, as expected, a limited immunological repertoire. In addition, γδ T cell lines have been derived from human airway biopsy specimens from both normal and atopic individuals (Wisnewski *et al.*, 2001), but whether these cells originate from the epithelium or lamina propria is not clear. What was clear from this study was that airways provided an enriched source of γδ T cells in comparison with peripheral blood from the same individuals. It is likely that bronchial IEL are similar to intestinal IEL and that their lineage and development may be different from the majority of T cells found elsewhere in the body. In this sense, it is important to emphasize that they would bear little relationship to T cells found in the organized lymphoid tissue of the lung.

Mucosal lymphoid follicles have several characteristics in common wherever they occur, including an overlying specialized epithelium originally termed follicle-associated epithelium by Bockman and Cooper (1973) and subsequently M (microfold) cells by Owen (1977). This epithelium differs from nearby mucosal epithelium because it is attenuated and often infiltrated by lymphocytes from the underlying follicles (Kraehenbuhl and Neutra, 1992). This epithelium does not contain goblet or other specialized cells found commonly in epithelium; it often has lymphocytes enfolded by the M cells to form nests or clusters of lymphocytes (Owen and Bhalla, 1983; Racz *et al.*, 1977), and it occasionally contains "nurse cells" (Nieuwenhuis, 1971; Wekerle *et al.*, 1980) in which T lymphocytes appear to be within the cytoplasm of macrophage-like cells. Nurse cells have also been noted at the periphery of rat bronchus-associated lymphoid tissue (BALT) (Otsuki *et al.*, 1989). The epithelium does not express secretory component or the polymeric immunoglobulin receptor. It is derived from renewable stem cells, which are found in the crypts in the intestine, and from glandular epithelium or basal epithelial cells in the respiratory tract. These stem cells appear to be directly transformed by interactions with the underlying lymphoid tissue. The actual number of transformed epithelial cells that overlie the lymphoid follicles may be small since it is only where the lymphoid tissue itself is apposed directly to the epithelium that the lymphoepithelium is found. In the murine intestine, glycosylated structures on the M-cell surface appear to bind preferentially to ulex lectin (Clark *et al.*, 1995), thus suggesting special surface modification during differentiation. Similar observations have been made in the mouse that BALT and gut-associated lymphoid tissue (GALT) share ulex-reactive M cells and that these cells appear in development before lymphoid accumulation (Tango *et al.*, 2000). The epithelium has the selective capacity to take up molecules including proteins from the luminal environment. This activity is not limited to molecules but includes viruses such as the reovirus and extends to particulate structures, including mycoplasma and bacteria, such as the tubercle bacillus and *Vibrio cholerae*. Molecules or particulates that include carbon particles are transported and exocytosed by these cells onto their basal aspects. Lymphocytes and macrophages that are thought to have come from the underlying follicles can sometimes be seen overlying M cells and particulate matter, and even cells that are found on the luminal surface have been described as penetrating these lymphoid follicles from the luminal aspects (Pabst and Binns, 1995).

Although the follicles and aggregates lack afferent lymphatics, they all possess efferent lymphatics draining to the regional lymph node and thus differ considerably from other nonmucosal lymphoid tissues. Mucosal and nonmucosal postcapillary high endothelial venules (HEV) differ in that they facilitate predominantly surface IgM-positive and IgA-positive B cells to localize or accumulate mucosally. These HEV are always found in or adjacent to the follicles, and the organization of the follicles and especially the aggregates is such that predominantly T- or B-cell areas can often be identified in relatively distinct anatomic positions. These are not necessarily constant in relation to the lumen. When the populations of B lymphocytes within the follicles are further characterized, there is predominant surface expression of IgA and IgM. Plasma cells are not found within the follicles or lymphoid aggregates. Nerve fibers that most frequently contain neuropeptides characteristic of cholinergic or adrenergic nerves are invariably found within or adjacent to these lymphoid structures, and the follicles or germinal centers do not regularly contain nerve fibers (Nohr and Weihe, 1991).

Lymphoid follicles can be found before birth in most mucosal tissues, but these are usually primitive and expand and mature upon exposure to antigen or microbial colonization. In the germ-free state, lymphoid follicles are rare but are present in the intestine and can be identified occasionally in the respiratory tract.

Initially, MALT was described on the basis of repopulation experiments with B lymphocytes obtained from BALT and GALT as well as the lamina propria in surrounding tissues (Rudzik *et al.*, 1975a). Subsequently, the concept was extended to include mucosal T lymphocytes and described a propensity of these cells to selectively localize in other mucosal tissues. The concept still provides a useful structural conceptual framework that is constantly being improved as more information on the determinants of localization becomes clearer (Butcher and Picker, 1996). It is important to emphasize that these lymphoid collections undergo considerable maturation when subjected to the consequences of mild to moderate inflammation, as may be induced, for example, by cigarette smoke in the human lung (Richmond *et al.*, 1993). Germinal center formation, significant expansion of the lymphoid tissue and dendritic cell components, upregulation, and change in expression of endothelial ligands such as MAdCAM-1, ICAM-1, and integrins responsible for binding to these mucosal addressins occur rapidly upon significant acute and chronic stimulation. Expression of NK-1 receptors specific for substance P is found in this tissue only in chronic inflammatory states (Mantyh *et al.*, 1988). Thus, a great deal of care must be taken in assessing the functional activity of this type of lymphoid tissue at any given point in time, and one must take into account the state of normal activation consequent to exposure to irritants, antigens, and microbial products (Butcher and Picker, 1996).

One of the proofs that the concept of MALT is operational comes from a study of mucosa-associated lymphomas that form a distinct subgroup of non-Hodgkin's lymphoma (Thieblemont *et al.*, 1995). While this condition most commonly arises in lymphoid tissue in the gastrointestinal tract, it also can extend or arise from and be found in the lung, breast, conjunctiva, salivary glands, respiratory tract, and gallbladder. The lymphoma arises from the lymphoid tissue and secondarily invades the epithelial tissue to form characteristic lymphoepithelial lesions. When this involves the lung, multifocal or diffuse lymphoid hyperplasia of BALT is seen and termed "lymphoid interstitial pneumonitis" (Koss, 1995).

BRONCHIAL LYMPHOID TISSUE

Bronchial lymphoid tissue is linked primarily to mucosal defense against inhaled microbes and therefore is one of many integrated lymphoid mechanisms that help to ensure the sterility of the gas exchange apparatus while avoiding sensitization to inhaled antigens. The cooperative activity of these different mechanisms and their ability to downregulate inflammatory responses within the bronchopulmonary system underscore the value of studying the bronchial mucosal lymphoid tissue in relation to these additional lymphoid mechanisms. Furthermore, the relationship between the bronchial lymphoid aggregates originally termed the BALT (Bienenstock, 1984) and the less-organized lymphoid tissue that predominates in humans and others (Emery and Dinsdale, 1973; 1974; Kyriazis and Esterly, 1970) deserves consideration.

T- and B-cell effector mechanisms are generated from bronchial lymphoid tissue and delivered into the bronchial lumen. For example, secretory-IgA (S-IgA) was one of the first well-studied mucosal defense mechanisms. Luminal antigen-specific S-IgA plays a key role in local control of microbial colonization (Waldman and Henney, 1971). The susceptibility of S-IgA responses to high zone tolerance induction (Clancy *et al.*, 1987), the rather poor immunological memory associated with this isotype (Clancy and Bienenstock, 1974), and the good health of most IgA-deficient individuals suggest that other mechanisms are crucial to pulmonary mucosal defense. The carpet of mucus contains mostly bronchoalveolar cells, of which 90% are bone-marrow-derived macrophages and the rest are lymphocytes (Young and Reynolds, 1984). This indicates strong luminal representation of effector cells. The exact relationships between the bronchoalveolar lymphocytes and macrophages, the large pools of lymphocytes within the lung interstitium, and those in the pulmonary circulation are not known (Pabst and Tschernig, 1995), but these latter sources certainly play a role in determining the activities of the bronchoalveolar cell population. The vascular and interstitial cells represent selective contributions from the systemic pool, whereas half of the resident macrophage population is derived from local cell proliferation (Mezzetti *et al.*, 1991). About 10% to 20% of the interstitial lymphocyte pool is composed of T cells, and the nonrandom expansion of T cells bearing v-chain determinants is consistent with further restrictive elements operating in the lung interstitium (Augustin *et al.*, 1989).

Communication between the bronchial lymphoid tissue and distant mucosae via intermucosal cell traffic, termed the common mucosal immune system (McDermott and Bienenstock, 1979), involves predominantly a "gut to bronchus" flow of cells from Peyer's patches (Scicchitano *et al.*, 1984). Depending on antigen dose and previous immunological experience, antigen-reactive T cells (Husband *et al.*, 1984) and B cells (Rudzik *et al.*, 1975a; Scicchitano *et al.*, 1984) from Peyer's patches can populate the bronchial mucosa to modulate immunity, a principle used successfully to develop an oral vaccine against acute bronchitis (Clancy *et al.*, 1985; Lehmann *et al.*, 1991). The vigorous T-cell response to inhaled antigen (Clancy and Bienenstock, 1974) and the capacity of CD4$^+$ T cells to transfer immunity between animals (Wallace *et al.*, 1991) support T-cell control of persistent infection or in circumstances where the inhaled antigen dose is large. Studies of animal models in which activated T cells contribute to mucosal defense indicate that T-cell-dependent neutrophil recruitment is important (Wallace *et al.*, 1991), although additional mechanisms—for example, lysozyme secretion from T-cell-activated macrophages (Taylor *et al.*, 1990)—have also been implicated.

The normal operation of these effector mechanisms, with minimal inflammation within the bronchial lumen or mucosa, depends on two factors. First, downregulating mechanisms restrict cell division and recruitment of nonspecific inflammatory cells (Sedgwick and Holt, 1985). Second, regional lymph nodes rather than the mucosa are primary sites for antigen handling (Yoshizawa *et al.*, 1989) and induction of responses (van der Brugge-Gamelkoorn *et al.*, 1986). The downregulating mechanisms are linked to antigen dep-

osition sites. Thus, allergens in the nasopharynx initiate suppressor cell responses within regional lymph nodes that control immediate and delayed hypersensitivity reactions (Sedgwick and Holt, 1985), whereas colonization of the bronchial mucosa is associated with an expansion of T cells, which can inhibit antigen-induced T-cell proliferation (Puci *et al.*, 1982). Whether T suppressor cells such as Tr1 are found within the bronchus and are activated by the presentation of antigen on MHC class II–bearing epithelial cells, as has been suggested for the gut (Pang *et al.*, 1990), or through the BALT is not clear. It has now been shown that under certain circumstances, inhaled antigen can promote tolerance through γδ-expressing T cells (Holt *et al.*, 1990). This has been called into question more recently (Lahn *et al.*, 1999). However, it is likely that "respiratory tolerance" exists. Whether it represents a mechanism similar to that proposed for oral tolerance, through TGF-β and IL-10, cannot be concluded at present (Strobel and Mowat, 1998; Weiner, 1997). The lumen is protected from inflammation by the antiproliferative effect of T-cell-activated alveolar macrophages, which export antigen either away from the mucosa to regional lymph nodes (Warner *et al.*, 1981) or over the epiglottis into the gut, where aspirated antigen may interact with Peyer's patches.

The bronchial lymphocyte compartment therefore has a complex relationship with various lymphocytes that are important in the activation and regulation of bronchial immunity, including antigen-reactive, effector, and regulatory lymphocytes, as well as ancillary cells derived from mucosal and systemic sources. Early studies on bronchial lymphoid tissue used animal species with organized BALT and facilitated an understanding of function, in part, by analogy with Peyer's patches (Bienenstock *et al.*, 1973a, b). Interspecies differences in the degree of organization of bronchial lymphoid tissue led to the idea that early studies on nonhuman aggregated lymphoid tissue may not be relevant to bronchial immune function, at least in humans, where major BALT development is relatively poorly represented in health (Pabst and Gehrke, 1990). However, failure to detect BALT in some studies (Pabst, 1992; Sminia *et al.*, 1989) may reflect sampling error, since BALT in normal human bronchus has been well described (Richmond *et al.*, 1993). Indeed, the presence of BALT or the isolated follicles termed bronchus-associated lymphoid units (BALU) by Sminia and van der Brugge-Gamelkoorn (1989) may to a large extent depend on how clean the inspired air is and how effectively the upper airways perform (Holt, 1993). Since a network of MHC II$^+$ dendritic cells are present in the epithelium and immediately below it (Holt *et al.*, 1990, 1993, 1994), a classic lymphoepithelium with M cells may not be essential for antigen processing.

CLASSIC BRONCHUS-ASSOCIATED LYMPHOID TISSUE

The existence of lymphoid aggregates in the bronchial wall was noted as early as 1870 by Burdon-Sanderson (1870), and these were described to be analogous to the lymphoid

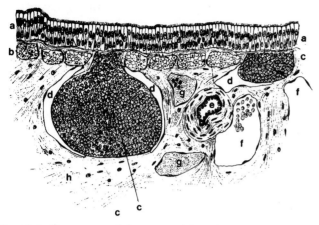

Fig. 20.1. The nature of the mucosal lymphoid follicle and the epithelial relationship are seen clearly. Reprinted from Klein (1875).

follicles found in other mucosal sites such as the tonsil and intestine (Klein, 1875) (**Fig. 20.1** and Bienenstock *et al.*, 1982; Bienenstock, 1984). Interest in the lymphoid tissue of the bronchial mucosa reawakened in 1973 with a systematic study of lymphoid aggregates in animals (Bienenstock *et al.*, 1973a, b), when the similarity to Peyer's patches was noted. Subsequently, descriptions were published of classic BALT in several species, including rats (Bienenstock *et al.*, 1973a), rabbits (Bienenstock *et al.*, 1973a, b; Bienenstock and Johnston, 1976; Tenner-Racz *et al.*, 1979), mice (Milne *et al.*, 1975), sheep, chickens (Bienenstock *et al.*, 1982), and guinea pigs; best characterized was BALT in rats and rabbits. Other species, such as healthy pigs, cats, and humans, have few classic BALT aggregates (Daniele, 1988; Jeffery and Corrin, 1984), although in pigs, mycoplasma infection was linked to regular BALT development (Chu *et al.*, 1989). These and other studies (Weisz-Carrington *et al.*, 1987) emphasize the importance of antigenic stimulation in the full expression of organized BALT, although there is considerable species variation. Since much of the current understanding of bronchial lymphoid tissue comes from either direct study of BALT aggregates or indirect study by isolation of lymphocytes from bronchial tissues containing BALT aggregates, review of this work on structure and function provides an excellent approach to understanding bronchial lymphoid tissue.

BALT develops in early postnatal life in most species (Bienenstock *et al.*, 1973a; Milne *et al.*, 1975). Antigen is not necessary for this development since BALT is present in germ-free rats (Bienenstock *et al.*, 1973a) and mice. In a study of the development of BALT in rats, it was concluded that BALT contained all necessary T-cell phenotypes already at day 4 after birth (Marquez *et al.*, 2000). It is also seen in fetal lungs transplanted into syngeneic adults (Bienenstock *et al.*, 1982; Milne *et al.*, 1975). BALT development under these circumstances is primitive when compared with that in conventionally raised animals (Bienenstock *et al.*, 1973a), and antigenic exposure (Rudzik *et al.*, 1975a) induces early, hyperplastic BALT. Lymphoreticular aggregates appear at one week of age in humans (Weisz-Carrington *et al.*, 1987),

although larger, more confluent aggregates are described with a lymphoepithelium in sudden infant death syndrome (Emery and Dinsdale, 1974), in which intercurrent infection is common. Lymphoepithelium in the lung has been noted as early as 20 weeks of gestation (Gould and Isaacson, 1993). BALT was identified in an autopsy study in 77% of infant lungs examined, with and without infection, and was present in 10% (5) of 51 fetuses without infection. BALT can be macroscopically identified in rabbits, rats, guinea pigs, and chickens (Bienenstock *et al.*, 1973a, 1982). Thirty of 50 BALT aggregates concentrated around bifurcations in the major bronchus divisions were seen in adult rats (Plesch, 1982) at sites of inhaled particle impaction.

Others have studied the development of BALT by implanting human fetal bronchial tissue into SCID mice with or without various other tissues, including bone marrow, thymus, peripheral lymph nodes, and liver (Tirouvanziam *et al.*, 2002). Only the cotransplantation of peripheral lymph nodes resulted in this model in the appearance of BALT. Bronchus-PLN implants could mount a vigorous αβ and γδ T-cell-mediated immune response to pseudomonas and chemical challenge. These authors suggest that PLN are responsible for the lymphocyte population of BALT follicles.

Although classical BALT is structurally similar to Peyer's patches, division into distinct structural and functional areas is less apparent. The epithelium overlying BALT aggregates is often less specialized and is heavily infiltrated with lymphocytes but contains M cells similar to those noted in the Peyer's patches and the bursa of Fabricius (**Fig. 20.2**) (Bienenstock *et al.*, 1973a, b; Bockman and Cooper, 1973). BALT cells cluster within a reticulin framework as a "dome" beneath the epithelium and a follicle that is usually single

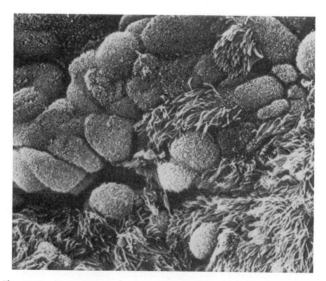

Fig. 20.2. A scanning electron micrograph showing the junction between the ciliated and nonciliated lymphoepithelium overlying the BALT follicle immediately below. Note the microprojections on the M cells and the crevices between cells (× 378). Reprinted with permission from Bienenstock and Johnston (1976).

(Bienenstock *et al.*, 1973a; Bienenstock and Johnston, 1976; Sminia *et al.*, 1989). In mammals, BALT germinal centers are usually found only after antigenic stimulation (Bienenstock *et al.*, 1973a). Tenner-Racz *et al.* (1979) described a perifollicular T-cell area after immunization.

Extensive collections of BALT are present in chickens, a species that has no lymph nodes. Neither bursectomy nor thymectomy alone at hatching caused noticeable effects in BALT. However, combined bursectomy and thymectomy, which led to deficient serum and S-IgA, normal IgM, and decreased IgG (Perey and Bienenstock, 1973), caused complete disruption of the BALT architecture and loss of germinal centers (Bienenstock *et al.*, 1982). This procedure did not result in changes in germinal centers found in cecal tonsils. This indicates the involvement of BALT in the IgA system and its incorporation into the MALT concept.

Plasma cells are found only around the BALT periphery (Bienenstock *et al.*, 1973a; Milne *et al.*, 1975), whereas cells capable of presenting antigen, including macrophages (Owen, 1977) and dendritic cells (Holt *et al.*, 1993; 1994; Milne *et al.*, 1975), reside within BALT. Only efferent lymphatic vessels are described (van der Brugge-Gamelkoorn and Kraal, 1985). In rabbit BALT, ~ 20% of lymphocytes have the T-cell marker rabbit thymic lymphocyte antigen (RTLA), a percentage similar to that in the Peyer's patches, but location in a distinct perifollicular area can be recognized only after antigenic stimulation (Bienenstock *et al.*, 1973b). The presence of HEV and interdigitating dendritic cells is characteristic of T-dependent areas in other lymphoid structures. Quantitation of cells within rat BALT HEV showed a distribution typical of MALT: T, 54.7%; S-IgG, 2.4%; S-IgM, 28.4%; and S-IgA, 27.3% (Otsuki *et al.*, 1989). These results are similar to those described for rabbit BALT (Rudzik *et al.*, 1975b).

Study of the function of BALT has focused on the analogy with Peyer's patches: induction of a mucosal immune response and use of the common mucosal immune system to deliver this response. Horseradish peroxidase is taken up preferentially by BALT epithelium, a process that is enhanced after stimulation with bacillus Calmette-Guerin (BCG) and causes hypertrophy of the specialized epithelium (Tenner-Racz *et al.*, 1979). In the Tenner-Racz *et al.* (1979) study, bacteria occurred within BALT macrophages, supporting the findings of Bienenstock *et al.* (1982), who identified BALT as an early site for the uptake of particulate material. BALT can be stimulated to proliferate also by chemical irritants since inhalation of ozone promoted increased thymidine uptake within BALT follicles and vacuolization of the lymphoepithelium (Dziedzic *et al.*, 1990). Other studies have shown that epithelial cells can present soluble antigen (Pang *et al.*, 1990) and that a layer of major histocompatibility complex (MHC) II–bearing dendritic cells lies within and beneath the respiratory epithelium (Holt *et al.*, 1993, 1994). This raises important questions about the qualitative and quantitative contributions of BALT to the development of local immunity. The clear link between the amount of BALT and antigenic stimulus (Delventhal *et al.*, 1992a; Meuwissen and

Hussain, 1982; Pabst, 1992; Pabst and Gehrke, 1990) supports the view that classic BALT is, in part, an adaptation to antigen load, with variable amounts of lymphoid aggregates expressed constitutively. The transformation of young, mature epithelial cells into M cells induced by lymphocyte-epithelial contact (Craig and Cebra, 1971) supports this view. Of particular interest with respect to human BALT was a study on chronically inflamed human lungs, in which classical BALT was noted in 8% of 100 patients; in those with an occlusive tumor, BALT was confined to the poststenotic segments (Delventhal *et al.*, 1992b). However, BALT is also present in healthy young adult elite skiers (64%) (Sue-Chu *et al.*, 1998). Although the skiers had a prevalence of asthma-like symptoms (exercise-induced asthma), the presence of lymphoid aggregates was not associated with this or with respiratory allergy.

In a classic study, Craig and Cebra (1971) first indicated the major role mucosal lymphoid aggregates play in generating mucosal immunity. Allotypic markers and adoptive transfer of Peyer's patch cells in rabbits were used to demonstrate that this tissue was an enriched source of IgA plasma cell precursors. Environmental factors, including antigen and bacterial lipopolysaccharide (LPS), were suggested to drive B-cell differentiation during antigen-stimulated clonal expansion, a concept consistent with oral immunization, inducing increased numbers of B cells expressing surface IgA in the Peyer's patches (Fuhrman and Cebra, 1981). Subsequently, Elson *et al.* (1979) demonstrated that IgA "switch" T-helper cells within Peyer's patches directed clonal expansion of IgA plasma cell precursors. T-cell clones from the Peyer's patches (Kawanishi *et al.*, 1983; Kiyono *et al.*, 1982) bearing IgA receptors suggest that T-lymphocyte populations may be involved in mucosal immunoregulation, possibly by secreting isotype-specific immunoglobulin-binding factors (Kiyono *et al.*, 1985). There is evidence that dendritic cells from different lymphoid tissues have different and selective functions in terms of promotion of IgA synthesis. The Peyer's patch dendritic cells primarily promote Th2-type responses, whereas those from the spleen promote primarily Th1 type (Everson *et al.*, 1996). Whether the same preferential capacity to switch the T-cell class response exists in dendritic cells from other than intestinal mucosal tissue is not known.

The repopulation studies of Rudzik *et al.* (1975a, c), in which bronchial lamina propria cells were transferred to lethally irradiated rabbits, demonstrated IgA-containing plasma cells repopulating the gut and bronchial mucosa. These studies identified the BALT as analogous to the Peyer's patch and provided the information on which the concept of a common mucosal immune system was developed (McDermott and Bienenstock, 1979). Inhaled-antigen-stimulated T-cell proliferation within the bronchial lymphocyte population correlated with the appearance of proliferating T cells in the bronchial lumen (Clancy and Bienenstock, 1974; Waldman and Henney, 1971), as well as T cells secreting cytokines (Clancy *et al.*, 1977) and cytotoxic T cells (Clancy *et al.*, 1983). The contribution of specific T lymphocytes to the common mucosal immune system (Clancy et al., 1977), as well as the specific relocation of influenza-specific T-cell clones to the lung (Bienenstock et al., 1983), is consistent with the observed circulation pathway of T lymphoblasts from mediastinal lymph nodes via the thoracic duct to mucosal surfaces (Guy-Grand et al., 1974; Sprent, 1976) and their origin, in part, from Peyer's patches. The role of BALT in the localization of T cells and B cells in bronchial mucosa is uncertain. The functions localized to aggregated lymphoid tissue in the bronchus may be restricted to the generation and distribution of specific T- and B-cell responses to inhaled antigen. The potential for aggregated lymphoid structures to generate suppression within mucosal (Puci et al., 1982) or systemic tissues (Ngan and Kind, 1978; Richman et al., 1981) is raised by the appearance of antigen-specific suppressor T cells within Peyer's patches. Downregulation within bronchopulmonary tissues suggests that a similar function exists in BALT, typified by nonresponsiveness in mucosal T-cell populations after antigen inhalation (Clancy and Bienenstock, 1974).

BRONCHUS-ASSOCIATED LYMPHOID TISSUE REVISITED

BALT is classically defined as an aggregated lymphoid structure separated from the bronchial lumen by a specialized lymphoepithelium. The availability of this relatively organized structure has allowed structural and functional analysis, focusing in particular on its role in the development of a local immune response to inhaled antigen (Rudzik et al., 1975a). The similarity in structural relationships between BALT and Peyer's patches has allowed a better understanding of respiratory tract immunity. Certain differences observed between the gut and lung mucosal lymphoid structures, often quantitative in nature, can be explained in terms of environmental stimuli associated with gut content (dietary and microbial stimulation). The similarity of structure, however, led to the concept of a common mucosal immune system when the morphological similarities between Peyer's patches and BALT were extended to include enriched IgA plasma cell precursor populations (Rudzik et al., 1975a). Subsequent studies in sheep (Scicchitano et al., 1984) and rats (van der Brugge-Gamelkoorn et al., 1986) modified our general concept to emphasize a "gut to bronchus" directional flow of activated lymphocytes. On the basis of these observations, an orally administered, killed, nontypeable *Haemophilus influenzae* vaccine was shown to be protective against recurrent episodes of acute bronchitis in carriers of this bacteria by reducing bronchial colonization (Clancy et al., 1985, 1989; Lehmann et al., 1991). This protection was transferred with primed thoracic duct T cells (Lehmann et al., 1991; Wallace et al., 1989). Recent work by Sato et al. (2000) has emphasized the gut-to-bronchus pathway. These investigators examined the effect of intratracheal immunization on GALT in thoracic duct lymphocyte traffic from both intestinally immunized and unimmunized donors. Clear

conclusions could be drawn. Prior intratracheal immunization increased traffic into BALT. This was most pronounced when the donor cells came from orally immunized animals. It is reasonable to conclude that intratracheal immunization promoted HEV binding in BALT of both nonantigen as well as antigen-specific activated GALT and TDL. BALT has expanded after direct immunization. These observations raise the question of the role played by BALT in localizing gut-derived T and B lymphocytes. Since there are no afferent lymphatics in BALT, most lymphocytes are likely to reach the bronchial mucosa via binding of specific integrins to addressins on post-capillary venular endothelium (Sminia et al., 1989), which is a mechanism used by lymphocytes for entry into other lymphoid organs. Adherence *in vitro* by lymphocytes to the HEV in BALT differs from that in the Peyer's patches, where the majority of adhering cells are B cells (Kieran et al., 1989). The BALT HEV functions more like that in mesenteric lymph nodes (van der Brugge-Gamelkoorn and Kraal, 1985), with equal numbers of T and B lymphocytes adhering.

BALT is likely involved in the localization of both T and B lymphocytes within the moderately inflamed bronchial mucosa, where additional regulatory T cells (Iwata and Sato, 1991) and a transport epithelium, allowing migration into the bronchial lumen (Bienenstock et al., 1973a, b), are sited conveniently. A regulatory role for BALT (Clancy and Bienenstock, 1974) has been extended by infection and immunization models, confirming the narrow antigen dose and temporal range that stimulate a local antibody response and T-cell help followed by immune suppression (Iwata and Sato, 1991). Thus, in rats, pulmonary infection with *Pseudomonas aeruginosa* elicits an early dominance of sIgA$^+$ cells correlated with a predominance of W3/25$^-$ T cells, giving way to a dominance of OX8$^+$ suppressor T cells after 2 weeks and correlating with a decrease in both sIgA$^+$ cells and inflammatory changes in the lung (Iwata and Sato, 1991). Proinflammatory cytokines detected by messenger ribonucleic acid (mRNA) expression and cytokine secretion by T cells cloned from sputum in subjects with chronic bronchial inflammation (G. Pang and R. Clancy, unpublished observations) indicates that T cells derived from bronchial mucosa migrating into the bronchial lumen may play a more prominent role in mucosal defense under circumstances of high dose and/or chronic antigenic stimulation.

That BALT is actively involved in T-cell-mediated responses is further evidenced by the fact that it appears to be the primary site of acute rejection of lung allografts (Prop et al., 1985). Subsequent studies showed that the BALT became smaller and defective in mounting a local immune response to viruses and uptake of inhaled carbon particles (Winter et al., 1995), presumably as a result of local graft-versus-host immune processes.

There is a regional distribution of peptidergic nerve fibers within classic BALT. Localization of immunoreactive neuropeptides (substance P, VIP, CGRP) known to influence lymphocyte physiology are found in different zones of the

BALT (Nohr and Weihe, 1991; Pascual *et al.*, 1999). This suggests the existence of important neuroimmunological control mechanisms in the bronchial mucosa. The close connection between BALT and regional lymph nodes, involving efferent lymphatics (van der Brugge-Gamelkoorn *et al.*, 1986), is reflected in the compartmentalized response to bronchial infection that includes both lymphoid structures (Weisz-Carrington *et al.*, 1987). The regional lymph nodes relating to BALT appear to have several important roles. The migratory patterns of lymphocytes in efferent lymphatics are more eclectic than those from mesenteric nodes (Joel and Chanana, 1987; Rudzik *et al.*, 1975a; Scicchitano *et al.*, 1988). Clearly, despite the potential of BALT B cells to populate intestinal mucosa (Scicchitano *et al.*, 1988), respiratory tract immunization has little influence on the intestinal immune response (Bice and Shopp, 1988; Scicchitano *et al.*, 1984). The regional node, however, has an important role establishing a generalized immune response within the lung (Scicchitano *et al.*, 1984) as well as providing systemic sensitization (Butler *et al.*, 1982; Kaltreider *et al.*, 1987). A second role relates to the generation of an immune response to inhaled antigen. Macrophage-associated antigen transported from the lumen requires local cytokine activation of dendritic cells before emigration occurs to the regional nodes. Downregulation of IgE- and T-cell-dependent hyposensitization by allergen inhalation involves the generation of a suppressor T-cell population in regional nodes of the upper respiratory tract (Holt *et al.*, 1981).

The detection of T-cell populations in Peyer's patches capable of downregulation (Clancy and Pucci, 1978; Kiyono *et al.*, 1980) and the switch toward a T-suppressor phenotype (Iwata and Sato, 1991) in chronic lung infection indicate a regulatory role for BALT, but the relative contribution compared with that of the regional lymph node is not clear.

Much of the discussion heretofore is based on studies involving a variety of species, including humans, that vary considerably in their expression of organized BALT. Several general observations can be made. First, regardless of the relative presence or absence in health of organized BALT, major interspecies differences are not found in the mucosal handling of antigen, in the development of local immune responses and the participation in a gut-driven, common mucosal immune system. Second, most if not all species (including humans) can develop classic BALT structures, including a lymphoepithelium under conditions of increased antigen load. In species with little BALT, under normal conditions, an adaptive immune function would focus the elements of an immune response into an efficient mechanism for the induction, capture, and delivery of a local mucosal immune response, as well as its control and integration within a broader defense network of lymphoid structures. Third, study of aggregated BALT and cells obtained essentially from these aggregates has given much insight into mechanisms of mucosal defense, both within the bronchopulmonary system and within mucosal tissues in general.

The presence of additional antigen-handling mechanisms within the bronchial mucosa that involve DC and epithelial cells and the presence of T- and B-cell effector and regulatory lymphocytes, however, require a dissection of the various components of mucosal immunity to determine the degree to which BALT in its classic form encompasses all these functions in one efficient unit. Further, the interdependence of various "pools" of lymphocytes within the lungs **(Fig. 20.3)** and their functional interaction in health and disease must be studied carefully. Perhaps particular insight into these interactions could come from careful analysis of cell traffic through the often forgotten regional lymph node, which not only represents a crossroad for lymphocyte traffic but appears to be central to the generation of mucosa-related

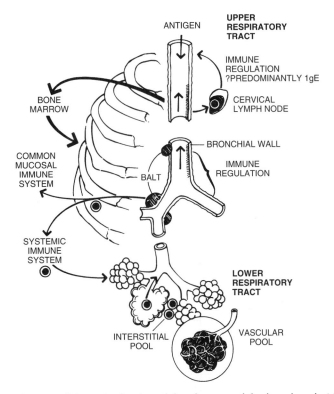

Fig. 20.3. Schematic drawing of the elements of the lung lymphoid tissue. An immune regulation loop involves cervical lymph nodes, particularly relevant to the downregulation of IgE (Holt *et al.*, 1981). The immune regulation loop involving mucosal T lymphocytes is particularly relevant to the inhibition of T-cell proliferation (Pucci *et al.*, 1982). The bronchus-associated lymphoid tissue (BALT) is a mechanism for effectively generating both T- and B-lymphocyte immunity in response to luminal antigen, both locally and at distinct mucosal sites. The role of the mesenteric regional lymph node appears crucial to the expansion of mucosal-associated immunity. The exact role of the bronchial and mediastinal nodes is less clear. The interstitial lymphocyte pool is modified in function from that of the circulating blood pool and is at least as large as the latter. Its role within the lung and its relationship to other "pulmonary lymphocyte" pools are undefined (Pabst, 1990). The vascular lymphocyte pool has been identified on the basis of cell sequestration studies. Whether this pool represents more than differential cell sequestration or has an important modulatory effect on cell traffic within other lymphocyte pools is not known (Pabst and Tschernig, 1995). The bronchoalveolar cell pool contains 5% to 10% lymphocytes, whose functions probably involve immunoregulating activities that range from afferent to efferent limbs of the inflammatory response.

immune responses, the upregulation and downregulation of immune pathways, and the expansion of lung-specific immunity.

REFERENCES

Augustin, A., Kubo, R. T., and Sim, G. K. (1989). Resident pulmonary lymphocytes expressing the gamma/delta T-cell receptor. *Nature* 340, 239-241.

Bice, D. E. and Shopp, G. M. (1988). Antibody responses after lung immunization. *Exp. Lung. Res.* 14, 133-155.

Bienenstock, J. (1984). Bronchus-associated lymphoid tissue. In *Immunology of the Lung and Upper Respiratory Tract* (ed. Bienenstock, J.), 96-118. New York: McGraw-Hill.

Bienenstock, J., Befus, A. D., McDermott, M., Mirski, S., Rosenthal, K., and Tagliabue, A. (1983). The mucosal immunological network: compartmentalization of lymphocytes, natural killer cells, and mast cells. *Ann. N.Y. Acad. Sci.* 409, 164-170.

Bienenstock, J. and Johnston, N. (1976). A morphologic study of rabbit bronchial lymphoid aggregates and lymphoepithelium. *Lab. Invest.* 35, 343-348.

Bienenstock, J., Johnston, N., and Perey, D. Y. (1973). Bronchial lymphoid tissue. I. Morphologic characteristics. *Lab. Invest.* 28, 686-692.

Bienenstock, J., Johnston, N., and Perey, D. Y. (1973). Bronchial lymphoid tissue. II. Functional characteristics. *Lab. Invest.* 28, 693-698.

Bienenstock, J., McDermott, M., and Befus, D. (1979). A common mucosal immune system. In *Immunology of Breast Milk* (eds. Ogra, P. L., and Dayton, D.), 91-104. New York: Raven Press.

Bienenstock, J., McDermott, M. R., and Befus, A. D. (1982). The significance of bronchus-associated lymphoid tissue. *Bull. Eur. Physiopathol. Respir.* 18, 153-177.

Bockman, D. E. and Cooper, M. D. (1973). Pinocytosis by epithelium associated with lymphoid follicles in the bursa of Fabricius, appendix, and Peyer's patches. An electron microscopic study. *Am. J. Anat.* 136, 455-477.

van der Brugge-Gamelkoorn, G. J., Claassen, E., and Sminia, T. (1986). Anti-TNP-forming cells in bronchus-associated lymphoid tissue (BALT) and paratracheal lymph node (PTLN) of the rat after intratracheal priming and boosting with TNP-KLH. *Immunology* 57, 405-409.

van der Brugge-Gamelkoorn, G. J. and Kraal, G. (1985). The specificity of the high endothelial venule in bronchus-associated lymphoid tissue (BALT). *J. Immunol.* 134, 3746-3750.

Burdon-Sanderson, J. (1870). Recent researches on tuberculosis. *Edinburgh Med. J.* 15, 385.

Butcher, E. C. and Picker, L. J. (1996). Lymphocyte homing and homeostasis. *Science* 272, 60-66.

Butler, J. E., Swanson, P. A., Richerson, H. B., Ratajczak, H. V., Richards, D. W., and Suelzer, M. T. (1982). The local and systemic IgA and IgG antibody responses of rabbits to a soluble inhaled antigen: measurement of responses in a model of acute hypersensitivity pneumonitis. *Am. Rev. Respir. Dis.* 126, 80-85.

Cerf-Bensussan, N., Jarry, A., Brousse, N., Lisowska-Grospierre, B., Guy-Grand, D., and Griscelli, C. (1987). A monoclonal antibody (HML-1) defining a novel membrane molecule present on human intestinal lymphocytes. *Eur. J. Immunol.* 17, 1279-1285.

Chu, R. M., Huange, Y. T., and Wang, C. N. (1989). Changes in epithelial cells covering the intrapulmonary airway-associated lymphoid tissues after *Mycoplasma hypopneumoniae* inoculation. *Immunobiology* 4, 75.

Clancy, R. and Bienenstock, J. (1974). The proliferative response of bronchus-associated lymphoid tissue after local and systemic immunization. *J. Immunol.* 112, 1997-2001.

Clancy, R., Cripps, A., Murree-Allen, K., Yeung, S., and Engel, M. (1985). Oral immunisation with killed *Haemophilus influenzae* for protection against acute bronchitis in chronic obstructive lung disease. *Lancet* 2, 1395-1397.

Clancy, R. L., Cripps, A. W., and Gebski, V. (1990). Protection against recurrent acute bronchitis after oral immunization with killed *Haemophilus influenzae*. *Med. J. Aust.* 152, 413-416.

Clancy, R., Cripps, A. W., Husband, A. J., and Gleeson, M. (1983). Restrictions on mucosal B-lymphocyte function in man. *Ann. N.Y. Acad. Sci.* 409, 745-750.

Clancy, R. and Pucci, A. (1978). Human mucosal lymphocytes — memory for "recall" antigens and non-specific suppression by T-lymphocytes. *Adv. Exp. Med. Biol.* 107, 575-582.

Clancy, R., Rawls, W. E., and Jagannath, S. (1977). Appearance of cytotoxic cells within the bronchus after local infection with herpes simplex virus. *J. Immunol.* 119, 1102-1105.

Clancy, R. L., Cripps, A. W., Yeung, S., Standish-White, S., Pang, G., Gratten, H., Koki, G., Smith, D., and Alpers, M. P. (1987). Salivary and serum antibody responses to *Haemophilus influenzae* infection in Papua New Guinea. *P. N. G. Med. J.* 30, 271-276.

Clark, M. A., Jepson, M. A., Simmons, N. L., and Hirst, B. H. (1995). Selective binding and transcytosis of *Ulex europaeus* 1 lectin by mouse Peyer's patch M-cells in vivo. *Cell Tissue Res*, 282, 455-461.

Craig, S. W. and Cebra, J. J. (1971). Peyer's patches: an enriched source of precursors for IgA-producing immunocytes in the rabbit. *J. Exp. Med.* 134, 188-200.

Daniele, R. P. (1988). The secretory immune system of the lung. In *Immunology and Immunologic Diseases of the Lung.* 115-126. New York: McGraw-Hill.

Delventhal, S., Brandis, A., Ostertag, H., and Pabst, R. (1992). Low incidence of bronchus-associated lymphoid tissue (BALT) in chronically inflamed human lungs. *Virchows Arch. B Cell Pathol. Incl. Mol. Pathol.* 62, 271-274.

Delventhal, S., Hensel, A., Petzoldt, K., and Pabst, R. (1992). Effects of microbial stimulation on the number, size and activity of bronchus-associated lymphoid tissue (BALT) structures in the pig. *Int. J. Exp. Pathol.* 73, 351-357.

Dziedzic, D., Wright, E. S., and Sargent, N. E. (1990). Pulmonary response to ozone: reaction of bronchus-associated lymphoid tissue and lymph node lymphocytes in the rat. *Environ. Res.* 51, 194-208.

Elson, C. O., Heck, J. A., and Strober, W. (1979). T-cell regulation of murine IgA synthesis. *J. Exp. Med.* 149, 632-643.

Emery, J. L. and Dinsdale, F. (1973). The postnatal development of lymphoreticular aggregates and lymph nodes in infants' lungs. *J. Clin. Pathol.* 26, 539-545.

Emery, J. L. and Dinsdale, F. (1974). Increased incidence of lymphoreticular aggregates in lungs of children found unexpectedly dead. *Arch. Dis. Child.* 49, 107-111.

Everson, M. P., McDuffie, D. S., Lemak, D. G., Koopman, W. J., McGhee, J. R., and Beagley, K. W. (1996). Dendritic cells from different tissues induce production of different T cell cytokine profiles. *J. Leukoc. Biol.* 59, 494-498.

Fournier, M., Lebargy, F., Le Roy Ladurie, F., Lenormand, E., and Pariente, R. (1989). Intraepithelial T-lymphocyte subsets in the airways of normal subjects and of patients with chronic bronchitis. *Am. Rev. Respir. Dis.* 140, 737-742.

Fuhrman, J. A. and Cebra, J. J. (1981). Special features of the priming process for a secretory IgA response. B cell priming with cholera toxin. *J. Exp. Med.* 153, 534-544.

Goto, E., Kohrogi, H., Hirata, N., Tsumori, K., Hirosako, S., Hamamoto, J., Fujii, K., Kawano, O., and Ando, M. (2000). Human bronchial intraepithelial T lymphocytes as a distinct T-cell subset: their long-term survival in SCID-Hu chimeras. *Am. J. Respir. Cell Mol. Biol.* 22, 405-411.

Gould, S. J. and Isaacson, P. G. (1993). Bronchus-associated lymphoid tissue (BALT) in human fetal and infant lung. *J. Pathol.* 169, 229-234.

Guy-Grand, D., Griscelli, C., and Vassalli, P. (1974). The gut-associated lymphoid system: nature and properties of the large dividing cells. *Eur. J. Immunol.* 4, 435-443.

Ham, A. W. (1969). *Histology.* Philadelphia: Lippincott.

Holt, P. G. (1993). Development of bronchus associated lymphoid tissue (BALT) in human lung disease: a normal host defence mechanism awaiting therapeutic exploitation? *Thorax* 48, 1097-1098.

Holt, P. G., Batty, J. E., and Turner, K. J. (1981). Inhibition of specific IgE responses in mice by pre-exposure to inhaled antigen. *Immunology* 42, 409-417.

Holt, P. G., Haining, S., Nelson, D. J., and Sedgwick, J. D. (1994). Origin and steady-state turnover of class II MHC-bearing dendritic cells in the epithelium of the conducting airways. *J. Immunol.* 153, 256-261.

Holt, P. G., Oliver, J., Bilyk, N., McMenamin, C., McMenamin, P. G., Kraal, G., and Thepen, T. (1993). Downregulation of the antigen presenting cell function(s) of pulmonary dendritic cells in vivo by resident alveolar macrophages. *J. Exp. Med.* 177, 397-407.

Holt, P. G., Schon-Hegrad, M. A., and McMenamin, P. G. (1990). Dendritic cells in the respiratory tract. *Int. Rev. Immunol.* 6, 139-149.

Husband, A. J., Dunkley, M. L., Cripps, A. W., and Clancy, R. L. (1984). Antigen-specific response among T lymphocytes following intestinal administration of alloantigens. *Aust. J. Exp. Biol. Med. Sci.* 62 (Pt 6), 687-699.

Iwata, M. and Sato, A. (1991). Morphological and immunohistochemical studies of the lungs and bronchus-associated lymphoid tissue in a rat model of chronic pulmonary infection with *Pseudomonas aeruginosa*. *Infect. Immun.* 59, 1514-1520.

Jeffery, P. K. and Corrin, B. (1984). Structural analysis of the respiratory tract. In *Immunology of the Lung and Upper Respiratory Tract* (ed. Bienenstock, J.), 1-27. New York: McGraw-Hill.

Joel, D. D., and Chanana, A. D. (1987). Distribution of lung-associated lymphocytes from the caudal mediastinal lymph node: effect of antigen. *Immunology* 62, 641-646.

Kaltreider, H. B., Curtis, J. L., and Arraj, S. M. (1987). The mechanism of appearance of specific antibody-forming cells in lungs of inbred mice after immunization with sheep erythrocytes intratracheally. II. Dose-dependence and kinetics of appearance of antibody-forming cells in hilar lymph nodes and lungs of unprimed and primed mice. *Am. Rev. Respir. Dis.* 135, 87-92.

Kawanishi, H., Saltzman, L. E., and Strober, W. (1983). Mechanisms regulating IgA class-specific immunoglobulin production in murine gut-associated lymphoid tissues. I. T cells derived from Peyer's patches that switch sIgM B cells to sIgA B cells in vitro. *J. Exp. Med.* 157, 433-450.

Kieran, M. W., Blank, V., le Bail, O., and Israel, A. (1989). Lymphocyte homing. *Res. Immunol.* 140, 399-450.

Kiyono, H., Babb, J. L., Michalek, S. M., and McGhee, J. R. (1980). Cellular basis for elevated IgA responses in C3H/HeJ mice. *J. Immunol.* 125, 732-737.

Kiyono, H., McGhee, J. R., Mosteller, L. M., Eldridge, J. H., Koopman, W. J., Kearney, J. F., and Michalek, S. M. (1982). Murine Peyer's patch T cell clones. Characterization of antigen-specific helper T cells for immunoglobulin A responses. *J. Exp. Med.* 156, 1115-1130.

Kiyono, H., Mosteller-Barnum, L. M., Pitts, A. M., Williamson, S. I., Michalek, S. M., and McGhee, J. R. (1985). Isotype-specific immunoregulation. IgA-binding factors produced by Fc alpha receptor-positive T cell hybridomas regulate IgA responses. *J. Exp. Med.* 161, 731-747.

Klein, E. (1875). The anatomy of the lymphatic system. In *The Lung*. London: Smith Elder and Co.

Koss, M. N. (1995). Pulmonary lymphoid disorders. *Semin. Diagn. Pathol.* 12, 158-171.

Kraehenbuhl, J. P. and Neutra, M. R. (1992). Molecular and cellular basis of immune protection of mucosal surfaces. *Physiol. Rev.* 72, 853-879.

Kyriazis, A. A. and Esterly, J. R. (1970). Development of lymphoid tissues in the human embryo and early fetus. *Arch. Pathol.* 90, 348-353.

Lahn, M., Kanehiro, A., Takeda, K., Joetham, A., Schwarze, J., Kohler, G., O'Brien, R., Gelfand, E. W., Born, W., and Kanehio, A. (1999). Negative regulation of airway responsiveness that is dependent on gammadelta T cells and independent of alphabeta T cells. *Nat. Med.* 5, 1150-1156.

Lehmann, D., Coakley, K. J., Coakley, C. A., Spooner, V., Montgomery, J. M., Michael, A., Riley, I. D., Smith, T., Clancy, R. L., and Cripps, A. W. (1991). Reduction in the incidence of acute bronchitis by an oral Haemophilus influenzae vaccine in patients with chronic bronchitis in the highlands of Papua New Guinea. *Am. Rev. Respir. Dis.* 144, 324-330.

Mantyh, C. R., Gates, T. S., Zimmerman, R. P., Welton, M. L., Passaro, E. P., Jr., Vigna, S. R., Maggio, J. E., Kruger, L., and Mantyh, P. W. (1988). Receptor binding sites for substance P, but not substance K or neuromedin K, are expressed in high concentrations by arterioles, venules, and lymph nodules in surgical specimens obtained from patients with ulcerative colitis and Crohn's disease. *Proc. Natl. Acad. Sci. USA* 85, 3235-3239.

Marquez, M. G., Sosa, G. A., and Roux, M. E. (2000). Developmental study of immunocompetent cells in the bronchus-associated lymphoid tissue (BALT) from Wistar rats. *Dev. Comp. Immunol.* 24, 683-689.

McDermott, M. R. and Bienenstock, J. (1979). Evidence for a common mucosal immunologic system. I. Migration of B immunoblasts into intestinal, respiratory, and genital tissues. *J. Immunol.* 122, 1892-1898.

Meuwissen, H. J. and Hussain, M. (1982). Bronchus-associated lymphoid tissue in human lung: correlation of hyperplasia with chronic pulmonary disease. *Clin. Immunol. Immunopathol.* 23, 548-561.

Mezzetti, M., Soloperto, M., Fasoli, A., and Mattoli, S. (1991). Human bronchial epithelial cells modulate CD3 and mitogen-induced DNA synthesis in T cells but function poorly as antigen-presenting cells compared to pulmonary macrophages. *J. Allergy Clin. Immunol.* 87, 930-938.

Milne, R. W., Bienenstock, J., and Perey, D. Y. (1975). The influence of antigenic stimulation on the ontogeny of lymphoid aggregates and immunoglobulin-containing cells in mouse bronchial and intestinal mucosa. *J. Reticuloendothel. Soc.* 17, 361-369.

Ngan, J. and Kind, L. S. (1978). Suppressor T cells for IgE and IgG in Peyer's patches of mice made tolerant by the oral administration of ovalbumin. *J. Immunol.* 120, 861-865.

Nieuwenhuis, P. *On the Origin And Fate of Immunologically Competent Cells.* Thesis/dissertation. (1971) Groningen, The Netherlands: University Groningen.

Nohr, D. and Weihe, E. (1991). The neuroimmune link in the bronchus-associated lymphoid tissue (BALT) of cat and rat: peptides and neural markers. *Brain Behav. Immun.* 5, 84-101.

Otsuki, Y., Ito, Y., and Magari, S. (1989). Lymphocyte subpopulations in high endothelial venules and lymphatic capillaries of bronchus-associated lymphoid tissue (BALT) in the rat. *Am. J. Anat.* 184, 139-146.

Owen, R. C. and Bhalla, D. H. (1983). Lympho-epithelial organs and lymph nodes. *Blamed Res. Appl. Sem.* 3, 79-169.

Owen, R. L. (1977). Sequential uptake of horseradish peroxidase by lymphoid follicle epithelium of Peyer's patches in the normal unobstructed mouse intestine: an ultrastructural study. *Gastroenterology* 72, 440-451.

Pabst, R. (1990). Compartmentalization and kinetics of lymphoid cells in the lung. *Reg. Immunol.* 3, 62-71.

Pabst, R. (1992). Is BALT a major component of the human lung immune system? *Immunol. Today* 13, 119-122.

Pabst, R. and Binns, R. M. (1995). Lymphocytes migrate from the bronchoalveolar space to regional bronchial lymph nodes. *Am. J. Respir. Crit. Care Med.* 151, 495-499.

Pabst, R. and Gehrke, I. (1990). Is the bronchus-associated lymphoid tissue (BALT) an integral structure of the lung in normal mammals, including humans? *Am. J. Respir. Cell Mol. Biol.* 3, 131-135.

Pabst, R. and Tschernig, T. (1995). Lymphocytes in the lung: an often neglected cell. Numbers, characterization and compartmentalization. *Anat. Embryol. (Berl.)* 192, 293-299.

Pang, G., Clancy, R., and Saunders, H. (1990). Dual mechanisms of inhibition of the immune response by enterocytes isolated from the rat small intestine. *Immunol. Cell Biol.* 68 (Pt 6), 387-396.

Pascual, D. W., Stanisz, A. M., Bienenstock, J., and Bost, K. L. (1999). Neural Intervention in Mucosal Immunity. In *Mucosal Immunology* (eds. Ogra, P., Mestecky, J., Lamm, M., Strober, W., Bienenstock, J., and McGhee, J.), 631-642. San Diego, Academic Press.

Perey, D. Y., and Bienenstock, J. (1973). Effects of bursectomy and thymectomy on ontogeny of fowl IgA, IgG, and IgM. *J. Immunol.* 111, 633-637.

Plesch, B. E. (1982). Histology and immunohistochemistry of bronchus associated lymphoid tissue (BALT) in the rat. *Adv. Exp. Med. Biol.* 149, 491-497.

Prop, J., Wildevuur, C. R., and Nieuwenhuis, P. (1985). Lung allograft rejection in the rat. III. Corresponding morphological rejection phases in various rat strain combinations. *Transplantation* 40, 132-136.

Pucci, A., Clancy, R., and Jackson, G. (1982). Quantitation of T-lymphocyte subsets in human bronchus mucosa. *Am. Rev. Respir. Dis.* 126, 364-366.

Racz, P., Tenner-Racz, K., Myrvik, Q. N., and Fainter, L. K. (1977). Functional architecture of bronchial associated lymphoid tissue and lymphoepithelium in pulmonary cell-mediated reactions in the rabbit. *J. Reticuloendothel. Soc.* 22, 59-83.

Richman, L. K., Graeff, A. S., Yarchoan, R., and Strober, W. (1981). Simultaneous induction of antigen-specific IgA helper T cells and IgG suppressor T cells in the murine Peyer's patch after protein feeding. *J. Immunol.* 126, 2079-2083.

Richmond, I., Pritchard, G. E., Ashcroft, T., Avery, A., Corris, P. A., and Walters, E. H. (1993). Bronchus associated lymphoid tissue (BALT) in human lung: its distribution in smokers and non-smokers. *Thorax* 48, 1130-1134.

Rudzik, R., Clancy, R. L., Perey, D. Y., Day, R. P., and Bienenstock, J. (1975). Repopulation with IgA-containing cells of bronchial and intestinal lamina propria after transfer of homologous Peyer's patch and bronchial lymphocytes. *J. Immunol.* 114, 1599-1604.

Rudzik, O., Clancy, R. L., Perey, D. Y., Bienenstock, J., and Singal, D. P. (1975). The distribution of a rabbit thymic antigen and membrane immunoglobulins in lymphoid tissue, with special reference to mucosal lymphocytes. *J. Immunol.* 114, 1-4.

Rudzik, O., Perey, D. Y., and Bienenstock, J. (1975). Differential IgA repopulation after transfer of autologous and allogeneic rabbit Peyer's patch cells. *J. Immunol.* 114, 40-44.

Sato, J., Chida, K., Suda, T., Sato, A., and Nakamura, H. (2000). Migratory patterns of thoracic duct lymphocytes into bronchus-associated lymphoid tissue of immunized rats. *Lung* 178, 295-308.

Scicchitano, R., Husband, A. J., and Clancy, R. L. (1984). Contribution of intraperitoneal immunization to the local immune response in the respiratory tract of sheep. *Immunology* 53, 375-384.

Scicchitano, R., Stanisz, A., Ernst, P., and Bienenstock, J. (1988). A common mucosal immune system revisited. In *Migration and Homing of Lymphoid Cells* (ed. Husband, A. J.), 1-34. Boca Raton, Florida: CRC Press.

Sedgwick, J. D. and Holt, P. G. (1985). Down-regulation of immune responses to inhaled antigen: studies on the mechanism of induced suppression. *Immunology* 56, 635-642.

Sim, G. K. (1995). Intraepithelial lymphocytes and the immune system. *Adv. Immunol.* 58, 297-343.

Sminia, T., van der Brugge-Gamelkoorn, G. J., and Jeurissen, S. H. (1989). Structure and function of bronchus-associated lymphoid tissue (BALT). *Crit. Rev. Immunol.* 9, 119-150.

Sprent, J. (1976). Fate of H2-activated T lymphocytes in syngeneic hosts. I. Fate in lymphoid tissues and intestines traced with ^{3}H-thymidine, ^{125}I-deoxyuridine and ^{51}chromium. *Cell. Immunol.* 21, 278-302.

Strobel, S. and Mowat, A. M. (1998). Immune responses to dietary antigens: oral tolerance. *Immunol. Today* 19, 173-181.

Sue-Chu, M., Karjalainen, E. M., Altraja, A., Laitinen, A., Laitinen, L. A., Naess, A. B., Larsson, L., and Bjermer, L. (1998). Lymphoid aggregates in endobronchial biopsies from young elite cross-country skiers. *Am. J. Respir. Crit. Care Med.* 158, 597-601.

Tango, M., Suzuki, E., Gejyo, F., and Ushiki, T. (2000). The presence of specialized epithelial cells on the bronchus-associated lymphoid tissue (BALT) in the mouse. *Arch. Histol. Cytol.* 63, 81-89.

Taylor, D. C., Cripps, A. W., and Clancy, R. (1990). Interaction of bacteria and the epithelial surface in chronic bronchitis. In *Advances in Mucosal Immunology* (eds. MacDonald, T. T., and Challacombe, S. J.), 806-807. London: Kluwer Academic Publishers.

Tenner-Racz, K., Racz, P., Myrvik, Q. N., Ockers, J. R., and Geister, R. (1979). Uptake and transport of horseradish peroxidase by lymphoepithelium of the bronchus-associated lymphoid tissue in normal and bacillus Calmette-Guerin-immunized and challenged rabbits. *Lab. Invest.* 41, 106-115.

Thieblemont, C., Berger, F., and Coiffier, B. (1995). Mucosa-associated lymphoid tissue lymphomas. *Curr. Opin. Oncol.* 7, 415-420.

Tirouvanziam, R., Khazaal, I., N'Sonde, V., Peyrat, M. A., Lim, A., de Bentzmann, S., Fournie, J. J., Bonneville, M., and Peault, B. (2002). *Ex vivo* development of functional human lymph node and bronchus-associated lymphoid tissue. *Blood* 99, 2483-2489.

Waldman, R. H. and Henney, C. S. (1971). Cell-mediated immunity and antibody responses in the respiratory tract after local and systemic immunization. *J. Exp. Med.* 134, 482-494.

Wallace, F. J., Clancy, R. L., and Cripps, A. W. (1989). An animal model demonstration of enhanced clearance of nontypable *Haemophilus influenzae* from the respiratory tract after antigen stimulation of gut-associated lymphoid tissue. *Am. Rev. Respir. Dis.* 140, 311-316.

Wallace, F. J., Cripps, A. W., Clancy, R. L., Husband, A. J., and Witt, C. S. (1991). A role for intestinal T lymphocytes in bronchus mucosal immunity. *Immunology* 74, 68-73.

Warner, L. A., Holt, P. G., and Mayrhofer, G. (1981). Alveolar macrophages. VI. Regulation of alveolar macrophage-mediated suppression of lymphocyte proliferation by a putative T cell. *Immunology* 42, 137-147.

Weiner, H. L. (1997). Oral tolerance: immune mechanisms and treatment of autoimmune diseases. *Immunol Today* 18, 335-343.

Weisz-Carrington, P., Grimes, S. R., Jr., and Lamm, M. E. (1987). Gut-associated lymphoid tissue as source of an IgA immune response in respiratory tissues after oral immunization and intrabronchial challenge. *Cell. Immunol.* 106, 132-138.

Wekerle, H., Ketelsen, U. P., and Ernst, M. (1980). Thymic nurse cells. Lymphoepithelial cell complexes in murine thymuses: morphological and serological characterization. *J. Exp. Med.* 151, 925-944.

Winter, J. B., Prop, J., Groen, M., Petersen, A. H., Uyama, T., Meedendorp, B., and Wildevuur, C. R. (1995). Defective bronchus-associated lymphoid tissue in long-term surviving rat lung allografts. *Am. J. Respir. Crit. Care Med.* 152, 1367-1373.

Wisnewski, A. V., Cain, H., Magoski, N., Wang, H., Holm, C. T., and Redlich, C. A. (2001). Human gamma/delta T-cell lines derived from airway biopsies. *Am. J. Respir. Cell Mol. Biol.* 24, 332-338.

Yoshizawa, I., Noma, T., Kawano, Y., and Yata, J. (1989). Allergen-specific induction of interleukin-2 (IL-2) responsiveness in lymphocytes from children with asthma. I. Antigen specificity and initial events of the induction. *J. Allergy Clin. Immunol.* 84, 246-255.

Young, K. R. and Reynolds, H. Y. (1984). Bronchoalveolar washings: proteins and cells from normal lungs. In *Immunology of the Lung and Upper Respiratory Tract* (ed. Bienenstock, J.), 157-173. New York: McGraw-Hill.

Development and Function of Organized Gut-Associated Lymphoid Tissues

Chapter 21

Hiromichi Ishikawa

Department of Microbiology and Immunology, Keio University School of Medicine, Tokyo, Japan

Yutaka Kanamori

Department of Microbiology and Immunology, Keio University School of Medicine, and Department of Pediatric Surgery, Graduate School of Medicine, The University of Tokyo, Tokyo, Japan

Hiromasa Hamada

Department of Microbiology and Immunology, Keio University School of Medicine, Tokyo, Japan

Hiroshi Kiyono

Division of Mucosal Immunology, Department of Microbiology and Immunology, Institute of Medical Science, The University of Tokyo, Tokyo, Japan; Departments of Microbiology and Oral Biology, The Immunobiology Vaccine Center, University of Alabama at Birmingham, Birmingham, Alabama

INTRODUCTION

The mucosal immune system provides a first line of defense against invading pathogens and creates an appropriate cohabitant situation between the host and outside environments. To understand how it induces and regulates antigen-specific immune responses at the surface barrier, its anatomic and functional uniqueness must be appreciated. Because foreign antigens and pathogens are generally encountered through normal physiologic functions such as ingestion and inhalation, the host has evolved a cluster of uniquely organized lymphoid tissues known as mucosa-associated lymphoid tissues (MALT) in those regions to facilitate the initiation of antigen-specific immune responses. Of MALT, two of the most important are the gut-associated lymphoid tissues (GALT) of the gastrointestinal (GI) tract and the nasopharyngeal-associated lymphoid tissues (NALT) of the respiratory tract (see Chapters 17, 20, 21, and 23). MALT, including GALT and NALT, are known to

be IgA-inductive sites and contain all of the immunocompetent cells, including antigen-presenting cells (APCs), B cells, Th cells, and cytotoxic T lymphocytes (CTLs), necessary for the development of effector and memory B and T cells upon antigen presentation by APCs including dendritic cells (DCs) and macrophages. Once developed, these antigen-specific B-cell and T-cell populations emigrate from the inductive site via lymphatic drainage, circulate through the bloodstream, and home to distant mucosal effector sites, including the lamina propria (LP) regions of the intestinal, respiratory, and reproductive tracts. In these more diffuse LP regions, as at other mucosal effector sites, antigen-specific IgA-committed B, Th1, and Th2 cells communicate with one another through an array of regulatory cytokines to generate secretory IgA (S-IgA) antibody responses, which in turn provide a first line of protection at mucosal surfaces (McGhee *et al.* 1989; Mestecky *et al.* 2003). For example, oral immunization of protein antigen together with cholera toxin as mucosal adjuvant induces antigen-specific Th2 cell–mediated

IgA B-cell responses (Xu-Amano *et al.* 1993). Oral immunization has also been shown to enhance antigen-specific CTL responses (London *et al.* 1987). The common mucosal immune system (CMIS), as the IgA inductive (e.g., organized MALT, including GALT and NALT) and effector (e.g., diffuse LP region) sites together are known to be integral in the induction and regulation of antigen-specific immune responses.

UNIQUE CHARACTERISTICS OF GALT

Peyer's patches (PP), the appendix, and solitary lymphoid nodules, major components of GALT, serve as the mucosal inductive sites for the GI tract, and the tonsils and adenoids, collectively identified as NALT, do the same for the upper respiratory tract and the nasal/oral cavity (Iijima *et al.* 2001). In addition, a recent study has provided direct evidence that isolated lymphoid follicles (ILF) are equipped with immunologic characteristics that are in some respects similar to those of PP (Hamada *et al.* 2002) and thus should be considered as a part of GALT (see the following text).

Of all the GALT, murine PP has been the most extensively characterized as a mucosal inductive tissue (Iijima *et al.* 2001; Mowat 2003). The surface of PP is covered by a unique epithelial layer known as the follicle-associated epithelium (FAE). The FAE is enriched with specialized antigen-sampling cells known as microfold (M) cells, so named because of the irregular and shortened microvilli that uniquely characterize them (Owen and Jones 1974). At the basal membrane site, M cells form an apparent pocket, which contains T cells, B cells, macrophages, and DCs. The M cells, characterized by small cytoplasmic vesicles and few lysosomes, are adept at the uptake and transport of luminal antigens (Owen *et al.* 1988). It is believed that antigen uptake by M cells does not result in the degradation of the antigen, but rather in the delivery of the intact antigen to the underlying APC (Owen and Bhalla 1983). In addition to the transport of luminal antigens, M cells serve as a port of entry for pathogens. For example, invasive strains of *Salmonella* and reovirus initiate infection by invading the M cells of PP (Wolf *et al.* 1981; Weinstein *et al.* 1998). Therefore, M cells can be considered as a gateway to the mucosal immune system (Neutra *et al.* 1996a).

Anatomically, PP are characterized by a dome configuration, with the area just below the FAE known to be enriched with IgA-committed B cells, Th1 and Th2 lymphocytes, macrophages, and DCs, all necessary for the induction of antigen-specific immune responses. After uptake and delivery by M cells, antigens are immediately processed and presented by DCs as APCs (Kelsall and Stober 1996). At least three DC subpopulations have been described in PP: myeloid (CD11b[+]), lymphoid (CD8α[+]), and double negative (Iwasaki and Kelsall 2000, 2001) (see Chapter 26). Myeloid DCs in the subepithelial dome (SED) lack maturation markers such as DEC-205 and so appear to be immature. Lymphoid and double-negative DCs induce the Th1 differentiation necessary for the subsequent development of cell-mediated immunity (CMI), and myeloid DCs induce the Th2 cells required for the generation of IgA immune responses at mucosal effector sites. Lymphoid and double-negative DCs are classified as belonging to the DC1 subtype, and myeloid DCs belong to the DC2 subtype (Banchereau *et al.* 2000). Following exposure to innocuous food antigens, the myeloid DCs produce IL-10 and TGF-β and may contribute for the induction of systemic unresponsiveness to orally administered antigen known as oral tolerance or mucosal tolerance by mediating the T-cell differentiation of Th3 or T regulatory (Tr) cells (Iwasaki and Kelsall 1999, 2000). Myeloid DCs in the SED region express the chemokine receptor CCR6, whose ligand, CCL20, is expressed by the FAE. Mature myeloid DCs express enhanced levels of the chemokine receptor CCR7, which migrates from the SED to the interfollicular region (IFR), where it interacts with T cells (see Chapters 26 and 34).

Distinct follicles (B-cell zones), which contain germinal centers for B-cell division are located directly below the FAE region. Because these PP germinal centers are considered to be the site of affinity maturation and of frequent B-cell isotype switches from IgM to IgA (Sonoda *et al.* 1989), they are thought to contain the majority of surface IgA positive (sIgA[+]) B cells. Adjacent to the B-cell zones are found T cell–dependent zones, constituted of mature T cells expressing all major T-cell subsets but almost wholly belonging to TCR[+] αβ T cells (αβ T cells). Approximately 65% of the αβ T cells are CD4[+] CD8[−] and exhibit properties of Th cells. After antigen presentation by the relevant DCs described in the preceding text, these Th cells differentiate into the Th1 and Th2 type cells required for the induction and regulation of antigen-specific CMI and IgA responses, respectively. Approximately 30% of αβ T cells are CD4[−] CD8[+] and contain precursors of CTL (London *et al.* 1987). Thus the organized inductive tissues (e.g., PP) are equipped with all of the immunocompetent cells necessary for the initiation of antigen-specific mucosal immune responses.

ORGANOGENESIS OF PEYER'S PATCHES (PP)

Initial studies of the role of molecular events in the organogenesis of PP

The first step toward understanding the molecular events driving the organogenesis of PP was taken with the characterization of a unique mouse mutation of alymphoplasia (*aly*) (Miyawaki *et al.* 1994). *aly/aly* mice, which possess two copies of the *aly* mutation, were found to exhibit no sign of PP development in the intestinal wall, to have grossly disorganized splenic T-cell and B-cell zones, and to lack all peripheral lymph nodes (LN). Soon after *aly/aly* mice were discovered to be deficient in PP and LN, it was found that a similar PP and LN deficiency and a parallel disorganization of the splenic architecture could be caused by an LT-α gene deletion (De Togni *et al.* 1994). The *aly* allele encoded a single mutation in the C-terminal interaction domain of

NF-κB–inducing kinase (NIK) (Matsumoto *et al.* 1999; Shinkura *et al.* 1999). Thus the deletion of the NIK gene resulted in a deficiency in PP similar to that seen in *aly/aly* mice (Yin *et al.* 2001). Since NIK was shown to be a downstream-signaling molecule for inflammatory cytokine receptors such as LTβR (Stancovski and Baltimore 1997; Yin *et al.* 2001), an obvious expectation was that the deficiency of the LTβR gene would lead to the lack of PP formation. When LTβR⁻/⁻ mice were examined, PP were indeed found to be absent (Futterer *et al.* 1998; Rennert *et al.* 1996). Taken together, these findings suggest the important role played by the inflammatory cytokine-signaling cascade between LTβR and downstream NIK in the formation of PP.

Initiation of PP genesis at the embryonic stage

As early as embryonic day 15 (E15)–15.5 (Adachi *et al.* 1997), when the transition from endoderm to epithelium had already begun and the simultaneous appearance of lymphatic vessels and mesenchymal cells had already occurred (Wells and Melton 1999), the first PP anlagen were recognized (Adachi *et al.,* 1997) **(Fig. 21.1)**. First identified as vascular cell adhesion molecule 1 (VCAM-1), positive spots at the proximal end of small intestine with the colocalization of intercellular adhesion molecule 1 (ICAM-1) expression, the PP anlagen sequentially developed toward the distal end (Adachi *et al.* 1997). The development of these early VCAM-1⁺ spots/clusters of stromal cells are presumed to be regulated by the IL-7R-signaling and LTβR-signaling pathways, because the blockade of such signaling during embryogenesis is known to lead to PP deficiency in mice (Rennert *et al.* 1996; Yoshida *et al.* 1999). In fact, the formation of these stromal cell spots can be suppressed by a single administration of anti-IL-7R mAb at E15. Within one and one-half days (E16.5–17.0) after the formation of the spots, the clusters of VCAM-1/ICAM-1 anlagen are colonized by CD3⁻ CD4⁺ CD45⁺ IL-7R⁺ cells, known as inducer cells (Adachi *et al.* 1997, 1998; Yoshida *et al.* 1999) **(Fig. 21.2)**. Those inducer cells must express IL-7R if PP are to be formed, as evidenced by experiments showing that no PP genesis was seen in gene-

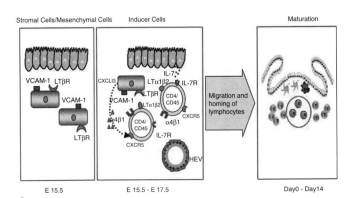

Fig. 21.2. Cytokine regulation of organogenesis program for PP. **(See page 7 of the color plates.)** Signal exchanges between inducer cells (CD3⁻CD4⁺CD45⁺) and stromal/mesenchymal cells are operated by an array of cytokine/ cytokine receptor, chemokine/chemokine receptor, and adhesion molecules/homing receptor interactions. Among these, IL-7/IL-7R and LTα1β2/LTβR interactions are essential for the initiation of PP organogenesis during the time window between embryonic 15.5 and 17.5 days.

manipulated mice lacking the receptor or its downstream JAK-3 (DiSanto *et al.* 1995; Cao *et al.* 1995). Further, successive administration of anti-IL-7R mAb during the period of E15–17.5 affected the numbers of PP as well as their sequential development from the proximal to the distal parts of the small intestine (Yoshida *et al.* 1999). Interestingly, the injection of anti-IL-7R mAb on E18.5 failed to block the formation of PP.

These findings demonstrate that the embryonic days between E15 and E17.5 are the key window for the initiation of PP organogenesis (Figs. 21.1 and 21.2). At E16.5, the expression of MAdCAM-1 is first recognized in the PP as they develop anlagen for the recruitment of immunocompetent cells (Hashi *et al.* 2001). Prior to the wave of lymphocyte migration occurring after birth, the first of those immunocompetent cells to arrive at the developing PP are the CD11c⁺ DC (Honda *et al.* 2001; Hashi *et al.* 2001). Thus a triangular interaction among VCAM-1⁺/ICAM-1⁺ organizer cells, CD3⁻CD4⁺ CD45⁺ inducer cells, and DC seems to initiate PP tissue genesis. Mature lymphocytes begin to migrate into PP within two days after birth, and within four days a fully matured architecture of PP with a follicular DC (FDC) network, a B-cell follicle region, and a T cell–dependent area is evident (see Chapter 34).

Inflammatory cytokine regulation of the tissue genesis program for PP

As discussed in the preceding text, the cytokine-signaling cascade mediated via IL-7R is critical for the initiation of tissue genesis during the targeted gestational period. In addition, inflammatory cytokine family members are also key players in the development of PP. LT has been demonstrated to be a critical signaling molecule for the secondary lymphoid genesis including PP and LN since experiments showing that the deletion of a specific gene for LTα resulted in the lack of organized lymphoid tissues (De Togni *et al.* 1994).

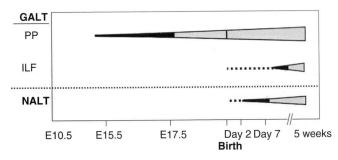

Fig. 21.1. Chronology of the tissue genesis for mucosa-associated lymphoid tissues. Among gut-associated lymphoid tissues (GALT), the organogenesis of Peyer's patches (PP) is initiated during the gestational period, and the tissue genesis of isolated lymphoid follicles (ILF) is begun after the birth. For the development of nasopharyngeal associated lymphoid tissues (NALT), the organogenesis program is also initiated during the early postnatal period.

LTα forms membrane-bound LTα1β2 heterotrimers that can transduce an activation signal through LTβR for the organization of PP and LN (Crowe *et al.* 1994; Rennert *et al.* 1996, 1998). Not surprisingly, then, the gene-manipulated, LT receptor–deficient mice developed no PP (Futterer *et al.* 1998). When mice were treated with a fusion protein of LTβR-Ig, an antagonist of the receptor *in utero*, they likewise showed no signs of PP genesis (Rennert *et al.* 1997; Yamamoto *et al.* 2000) **(Fig. 21.3)**. Like LTα-deficient mice, LTβ−/− mice showed no PP development (Koni *et al.* 1997). LIGHT (or herpes virus entry mediator ligand), a member of the TNF family, has been shown to bind to LTβR (Mauri *et al.* 1998), but in its absence PP develop just as do any other LN (Scheu *et al.* 2002). These findings convincingly demonstrate that an inflammatory cytokine interaction between LTα1β2 and LTβR is another essential programming element in the genesis of PP.

In contrast, the role played in PP development by another known inflammatory cytokine, TNF, remains a subject of controversy. One study recorded an absence of PP in TNFR-I (or TNFRp55) knock-out mice (Neumann *et al.* 1996), but others have shown that TNF-deficient mice and TNFR-I knock-out mice did not demonstrate the loss of PP organogenesis (Koni and Flavell 1998; Pasparakis *et al.* 1997). Further, *in utero* administration of TNFR-I-Ig fusion protein had no impact on PP development (Rennert *et al.* 1996). The mouse strain difference was suggested for the explanation of opposite findings. These findings suggest that TNFR-I plays some role in PP formation, but it is a secondary one to that played by LTβR. Furthermore, both LTβR-signaling blockade models of the specific gene deletion and *in utero* LTβR-Ig treatment resulted in PP deficiency, and these effects were clearly strain independent. TRANCE (TNF-related activation induced cytokine) and RANK (receptor

activator of NF-κB), another group of ligands and receptors belonging to the TNF family, did not influence PP genesis, but their removal resulted in deficient LN formation (Kong *et al.* 1999; Dougall *et al.* 1999). Among the member of the TNF family, PP genesis is totally dependent on the signal provided via LTβR.

In summary, then, two cytokine-mediated pathways, namely IL-7R and LTβR, are essential for the tissue genesis of PP, a major compartment of GALT. However, recent studies have shown that these pathways are not involved in the organogenesis of NALT in the respiratory immune compartment (see Chapters 20 and 23). NALT is known to develop even under PP-deficient conditions (Fukuyama *et al.* 2002; Harmsen *et al.* 2002). For example, NALT formation was initiated in PP-deficient IL-7R−/− and LTα−/− mice (Fukuyama *et al.* 2002). *In utero* treatment with LTβR-Ig suppressed PP formation but did not adversely affect NALT initiation. Taken together, these findings show that NALT tissue genesis is independent of IL-7R and LTβR-mediated lymphoid tissue development. The distinctions between NALT and PP genesis may also be seen in the chronology of development, with PP genesis beginning as early as embryonic day 15, although NALT genesis is not observed until after birth (Fukuyama *et al.* 2002). However, Id-2 deficiency resulted in the lack of CD3− CD4+ CD45+ inducer cells and thereby in the lack of both NALT and PP development (Fukuyama *et al.* 2002). These findings suggest that PP and NALT share a common set of the inducer cell population, but require distinct cytokine cascades for tissue genesis.

Critical role of the LTβR-mediated signaling cascade in PP formation

Following specific ligand binding, LTβR is believed to specifically activate NF-κB via NIK (Matushima *et al.* 2001). NIK then activates I-κB kinase, such as IKKα and IKKβ, which involves the degradation of I-κB and thereby transforms inactive NF-κB into an active form of NF-κB (Dejardin *et al.* 2002; Yilmaz *et al.* 2003). The active form of NF-κB, the heterodimers of p52 and RelB, then moves to nucleus and stimulates the production of the lymphoid chemokines necessary for the recruitment of lymphocytes to the site for lymphoid tissue development (Dejardin *et al.* 2002; Weih *et al.* 2001) (see the following text). The absence of these heterodimers disrupts PP genesis, as evidenced by studies using IKKα−/−, p52−/−, and RelB−/− mice (Weih *et al.* 1995; Matsushima *et al.* 2001; Paxian *et al.* 2002; Yilmaz *et al.* 2003). The characterization of *aly/aly* mice that harbor a natural point mutation in the specific gene encoded for NIK (Miyawaki *et al.* 1994; Shinkura *et al.* 1999; Yin *et al.* 2001), discussed in the preceding text, also provides further support for the importance of this signaling pathway in PP genesis. Like the NIK-dependent pathway, the LTβR-signaling cascade also leads to the formation of p50-RelA heterodimers (Dejardin *et al.* 2002), which are important signaling molecules for the induction of vascular cell adhesion molecules (VCAM-1) (Weih *et al.* 2001; Dejardin *et al.* 2002).

In Utero Blockade of LTβR Signaling Pathway
Results in the Lack of Peyer's Patches

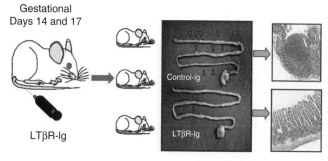

Fig. 21.3. Treatment of pregnant mice with the chimeric fusion protein of LTβR-Ig results in the delivery of PP-deficient mice. **(See page 7 of the color plates.)** Pregnant mice are injected with 200 μg LTβR-Ig at gestational days 14 and 17. Newborn mice delivered from the fusion protein–treated mothers are not able to develop PP. On the other hand, newborn mice delivered from the control Ig fusion protein–treated mothers develop PP.

Roles for chemokines and adhesion molecules in PP development

During PP organogenesis, the early expression of adhesion molecules is thought to be required to attract and retain migrating cells for the formation of clusters of cells so essential to tissue genesis. The cluster creates a conducive atmosphere for the paracrine triggering of receptors and thus for the sequential cell-to-cell interactions needed for tissue development. For example, LTβR$^+$ mesenchymal cells express VCAM-1 following ligation with the heterotrimeric form of LTα1β2 at E15.5 (Honda et al. 2001). Because their specific messages were detected by RT-PCR analysis, lymphoid chemokines such as CXCL13 and CCL19 are thought to be produced by these VCAM-1$^+$ and LTβR$^+$ mesenchymal cells. VCAM-1 expression is also to be expected on LTβR$^+$ stromal cells and endothelial cells. Thus the expression of VCAM-1 in early PP anlagen could play a key role in retaining the incoming inducer cells of CD3$^-$ CD4$^+$ CD45$^+$, so that they will be in place to interact with stromal and hematopoietic cells and thereby to initiate the necessary cellular communications for PP formation. This CD3$^-$ CD4$^+$ CD45$^+$ inducer population is known to express CXCR5 (Mebius et al. 1997) and the active form of α4β1, a specific ligand of VCAM-1 resulting from the activation of β1 integrin via CXCL13 and CXCR5 interaction (Finke et al. 2002). Thus the removal of the CXCR5-specific gene or the blockade of the β1 integrin results in the reduction of VCAM-1 spots on the embryonic intestine and thereby to reduced numbers of PP in young adult mice (Ansel et al. 2000; Finke et al. 2002). A similar change in PP development was also seen in CXCL13 knock-out mice (Ansel et al. 2000). The inducer cells in embryonic PP also express CCR7 (Hashi et al. 2001) and thus are qualified to respond to the CCL19 and CCL21 produced by VCAM-1$^+$ cells. However, PP developed normally in mice from which CCR7 had been genetically deleted and in those exhibiting a *ptl* mutation causing CCL19 and CCL21 deficiency (Forster et al. 1996). This finding could be explained by the transient expression of CCR7 on the CD3$^-$ CD4$^+$ CD45$^+$ subset. Thus the responsiveness of the elected group of chemokines and adhesion molecules is the key mechanism that drives PP genesis. Inducer cells express CCR5 and α4β1, and the VCAM-1$^+$ organizer cells are capable of producing CXCL13 in an LTα1β2/LTβR-dependent manner (Honda et al. 2001). This mutually beneficial positive feedback loop mediated by chemokines and adhesion molecules drives PP genesis forward.

Role played by the intestinal microbial flora in PP maturation

The indigenous intestinal microflora provide the most potent environmental stimulation for the postnatal phase of intestinal development. These indigenous antigens exert a significant biologic influence on the anatomic, functional, and immunologic development of the mucosal immune system. For example, it has been shown that environmental antigens and stimuli can influence the development of PP (Neutra *et al.* 1996b). Under germfree conditions, fully developed PP still exhibit immature histologic/anatomic characteristics. The well-developed dome-shaped architecture characterizing PP in conventional mice is flattened in germfree mice, where the PP is embedded in the intestinal wall. After the introduction of germfree mice to conventional or specific pathogen-free conditions, PP development returned to normal (Smith *et al.* 1987). Oral exposure of germfree mice to a single pathogenic or nonpathogenic microorganism resulted in the maturation of PP and an increase in their numbers (Savidge *et al.* 1991). In addition, oral administration of germfree mice with lipopolysaccharide (LPS) or a monoinfection of *Escherichia coli* resulted in the acceleration of the immunologic and functional development of PP (Kiyono *et al.* 1980).

This evidence suggests that intestinal microbial stimulation may lead to the generation of an optimal inflammatory signaling environment for the maturation and maintenance of GALT. Indeed, inflammatory cytokine signals submitted via LTβR have been shown to be important in the maintenance of secondary lymphoid tissue in adult mice (Mackay and Browning 1998; Fu and Chaplin 1999). When this LTβR-signaling cascade was blocked in young adult mice via weekly treatment with a soluble form of the receptor, macroscopic analysis revealed a flattened appearance in PP (Dohi *et al.* 2001). Macroscopically visible PP were only half as frequent in treated as in untreated mice. Following the discontinuation of the receptor blockade treatment, PP recovered both their cellularity and size. The indigenous intestinal microflora provide the optimal activation for the induction of physiologically relevant inflammatory cytokine signaling for the maturation and maintenance of PP. This evidence further emphasizes the importance of inflammatory cytokine-signaling cascades (e.g., LTα1β2/LTαR) in at least two distinct stages of PP development, that is, the gestational and postnatal periods. Thus LTβR signaling is essential both for the initiation of PP genesis in the specific gestational phase and for the maintenance of the fully developed tissue after birth.

ISOLATED LYMPHOID FOLLICLES (ILF)

As stated in the preceding text, PP are congregations of lymphocytes in the intestine that are visible without magnification and contain many follicles packed with proliferating B cells. It is also evident that PP are the major sites of luminal antigen and microorganism sampling, which leads to continuous immune responses (Kelsall and Strober 1996; Gebert et al. 1996; Banchereau and Steinman 1998; Iwasaki and Kelsall 1999; Neutra et al. 2001). Other forms of lymphoid follicles, termed "isolated lymphoid follicles (ILF)" or "solitary lymphoid follicles," have been identified in the intestinal wall of human (Shorter and Tomasi 1982; Price 1985; Moghaddami et al. 1998), rabbit (Keren et al. 1978), and guinea pig (Rosner and Keren 1984). These ILF are macroscopically invisible from the serosal or mucosal surface of the small intestine. In humans, ILF are distributed throughout the intestine and increase in frequency in the distal ileum and colon, especially in the rectum and in dead-ended extensions of the intestinal lumen, such as the cecum and appendix, where the microflora are particularly abundant (O'Leary and Sweeney 1986; Neutra *et al.* 2001).

Like PP, ILF also contain spherical B-cell clusters, including B-cell blasts embedded in a meshwork of follicular DCs. B-cell clusters in PP and ILF are usually secondary, rather than primary, follicles displaying germinal center (GC) reactions (Weinstein *et al.* 1991; Liu *et al.* 1991), and epithelia overlying the follicles contain M cells (Rosner and Keren 1984; Gebert *et al.* 1996; Neutra *et al.* 2001). Although most of the T cells in PP reside in the wedge-shaped interfollicular regions (Kelsall and Strober 1996) and include both CD4+ and CD8+ T cells (London *et al.* 1990), ILF lack such T cell–enriched compartments. Overall, ILF are structurally similar to the B cell–enriched follicular units that compose PP.

Histologic and immunologic comparison of ILF and PP

Although readily seen upon histologic examination of the rabbit and human intestines, ILF have been virtually ignored in immunologic literature. One impediment to our understanding has been the lack of cellular-level knowledge about lymphocytes residing in ILF, perhaps because the extremely small size of the ILF makes it difficult to isolate them for analysis. As described in the preceding text, however, immunohistochemical and electron microscopic analyses show ILF to be composed of a large B-cell area including a germinal center and the epithelia overlying them to contain M cells. These findings indicate that ILF are an equivalent or complementary system to PP for the induction of the intestinal IgA Ab responses that are important for the first line of defense against the dangerous gut environment (reviewed by Fagarasan and Honjo 2003). A number of experimental observations lend support to this notion. First, in a chronically isolated ileal loop model, a vigorous IgA Ab response can be elicited to an invasive microorganism in segments of rabbit intestine lacking grossly identifiable PP (Keren *et al.* 1978). Second, even when PP are surgically removed from the intestine of rats, no change in the number of IgA-containing cells in the LP of the small intestine is observed, and subsequent intestinal immunization of PP-deficient rats with a lipid-conjugated solution of human serum albumin elicits a comparatively normal secondary Ab response to this antigen (Heatley *et al.* 1981). These findings strongly indicate but do not prove that ILF represent an organized GALT that contains precursors of IgA-producing cells and are therefore functionally similar to the follicular units of PP where humoral immune responses to luminal antigens are continuously taking place. However, since ILF are devoid of the interfollicular T-cell congregations present in PP, it remains to be determined whether these two types of GALT participate in exactly the same intestinal immune responses.

Identification of ILF in the mouse small intestine

Although ILF have been widely acknowledged as a type of GALT found in the intestines of humans, rabbits, and guinea pigs, their existence in mice, the most important laboratory

animals, has not been described in the immunologic literature to date. In fact, very recent histochemical studies describing multiple tiny clusters filled with closely packed B220+ B cells in the small intestinal LP of BALB/c **(Figs. 21.4A, B,** and **C),** C57BL/6, DBA/2, and C3H mice mark the first time that ILF have been identified in the mouse small intestine (Hamada *et al.* 2002). Although absolute numbers of these B-cell clusters vary among adult animals of different mouse strains, in BALB/c mouse, they are more abundant in the small intestine (150–200 per small intestine) than in the large intestine (~50 per large intestine). Remarkably, in the small intestine of BALB/c mice (Hamada *et al.* 2002), most of these B-cell clusters are aligned at roughly regular intervals along the antimesenteric wall of the gut mucosa (Fig. 21.4A), whereas those of the large intestine are situated at random around the circumference of the gut wall. In C57BL/6 mice, ILF can be found throughout the small intestinal mucosa, but those localized at the antimesenteric wall are bigger than those interspersed elsewhere. Detailed immunohistochemical and electron microscopic analyses have revealed that the B-cell clusters include a GC (Fig. 21.4D) and that epithelia overlying them contain M cells **(Fig. 21.5).** These findings provide direct evidence that the novel B-cell clusters identified in the mouse small intestine fulfill the criteria of the

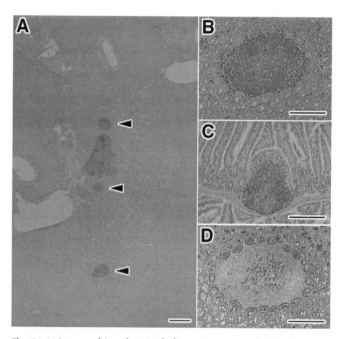

Fig. 21.4. Immunohistochemical characterization of ILF in the small intestine of BALB/c mice. **A,** A horizontal section was stained with anti-B220 mAb. Three ILF are aligned along the antimesenteric wall of the mucosa (arrowheads). Bar, 500 μm. **B,** A magnified horizontal view of the ILF colonized with the B220+ cells. Bar, 100 μm. **C,** A representative longitudinal view of the ILF colonized with the B220+ cells. Note that the villus that contains ILF is thicker and shorter than the surrounding classical villi. Bar, 100 μm. **D,** A cluster of peanut agglutinin–binding (PNA-binding) cells is compartmentalized in the center of B220+ cell aggregation, indicating the germinal center formation in ILF. Bar, 100 μm.

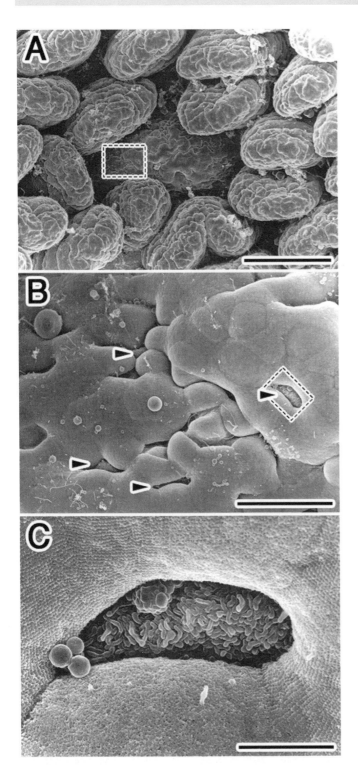

Fig. 21.5. Scanning electron microscopic analysis of the epithelium adjacent to an ILF. **A,** Among the classical villi, a thick and shorter villus containing ILF is seen. Bar, 150 μm. **B,** Magnified view of the *inset* in Figure 21.5A shows the presence of four M cells (arrowheads). Bar, 20 μm. **C,** Magnified view of the *inset* in Figure 21.5B. The M cell in the center is surrounded by absorptive enterocytes that possess numerous closely packed regular and tall microvilli on their apices. Note the short, wide, and irregular microvilli of the M cell. Bar, 3 μm.

aforementioned human, rabbit, and guinea pig ILF. On the whole, identification of mouse ILF offers a great advantage in dissecting the developing B cells that reside in ILF because a murine model makes available a set of monoclonal antibodies (mAbs) to various cell surface molecules on lymphoid cells and makes possible cellular study at the genetic level.

ILF are B cell–enriched organized lymphoid tissues

In order to study the B cells concentrated in mouse ILF in depth, a sufficiently pure population of ILF lymphocytes must be isolated. To do this, ILF in sections (~10 mm in length) of longitudinally opened small intestine were located by a transillumination stereomicroscope, and subsequently, a tiny fragment of the small intestine containing one ILF was extracted with the aid of an amputated and tapered 18-gauge or 21-gauge needle (Hamada *et al.* 2002). The results of this study show that both ILF and PP harbor a large population of $B220^+CD19^+IgM^+$ B cells along with a significant population of IgA^+ B cells, and mesenteric lymph nodes (MLN) contain few IgA^+ B cells.

IgA is a predominant Ig, which is secreted mainly across mucosal membranes. Most IgA-producing plasma cells are found in the LP of intestines (McIntyre and Strober 1999) and have been shown to derive either from conventional Ag-specific IgA-committed B-2 B cells originated from PP (Craig and Cebra 1971; Husband and Gowans 1978; Hiroi *et al.* 1999, 2000) or from, most likely, B-1 B cells (Hayakawa *et al.* 1983; Macpherson *et al.* 2000; Fagarasan and Honjo 2000; Hiroi *et al.* 1999, 2000) that are enriched among B cells compartmentalized in the peritoneal cavity (PEC) (Kroese, *et al.* 1989). Given the potential importance of B-1 B cells in the development of IgA-producing plasma cells, it is of considerable interest to determine whether B-1 B cells or B-2 B cells are differentiating in these mouse ILF. B cells isolated from ILF, PP, and MLN display the $IgM^{low}IgD^{high}$ phenotype, and the majority of those recovered from PEC display the $IgM^{high}IgD^{low}$ phenotype. Two-thirds of $B220^+$ cells from PEC express CD5 and Mac-1 molecules, but such $B220^+CD5^+$ cells and $B220^+Mac-1^+$ cells are minimal in ILF, PP, and MLN compartments. Moreover, most $B220^+$ cells from ILF and PP are $CD23^+$, whereas those from PEC remain $CD23^-$ (Hamada *et al.* 2002). Since mucosal B cells have been classified into B-1 and B-2 categories based on the differential expression of B220, IgM, IgD, CD5, Mac-1, and CD23 molecules (Hardy and Hayakawa 1994; Hiroi *et al.* 1999, 2000), these results indicate that mouse ILF are inductive sites for the initiation of IgA-committed B-2 B cell responses in the GI tract. In any event, the missing link between B-1 B cells in PEC and such B-1 B cell–derived IgA-producing plasma cells in the LP of mouse intestine, that is, how these B cells are activated, migrate, and differentiate into IgA-producing plasma cells, still remains to be explored. However, this scenario has recently been challenged by showing that intestinal IgA production induced by commensal bacteria is mainly performed by B-2, not B-1, B cells (Thurnheer *et al.* 2003).

Biologic role of ILF in the mucosal immune system

Mouse ILF structurally resemble the follicular units that comprise PP both in that they contain a GC, IgM-positive and IgA-positive B cells, and M cells in the overlying epithelium. Mouse ILF and PP also exhibit some functional similarities, in that both are anatomic sites where the development of Ag-specific IgA-committed B-2 B cells appears to take place. Although a B-cell follicle of ILF is smaller than that of PP (Hamada et al. 2002), ILF of BALB/c mice outnumber (150–200 per small intestine) PP (6–12 per small intestine) 10 to 1 (Hamada et al. 2002). Thus, from a functional point of view, ILFs appear to be just as or even potentially much more efficient than PP in inducing humoral immune responses to luminal antigens. Recently, however, it has been reported that a conspicuous ILF hyperplasia associated with a 100-fold expansion of anaerobic flora is induced (Fagarasan et al. 2002) in the small intestine of activation-induced cytidine deaminase-deficient (AID$^{-/-}$) young adult mice (Muramatsu et al. 2000), indicating that normal B cells in ILF play a major and probably a distinctive role in maintaining gut homeostasis. The same studies (Fagarasan et al. 2002; Fagarasan and Honjo 2003) also demonstrated that a critical event causing anaerobe expansion and the resultant development of hyperplasia of ILF was the blockade on somatic hypermutation of IgM Abs in AID$^{-/-}$ mice that inhibits the diversification of local B cells. Offering further support for this finding, a recent study showed that mature ILF formation in the small intestine of normal C57BL/6 mice is triggered by luminal stimuli, including normal bacterial flora (Lorenz et al. 2003). Thus somatic hypermutation of ILF B cells appears to play a critical role in regulating commensal microbes in the mouse small intestine.

As far as organogenesis is concerned, ILF are not detectable until day 7 of postnatal life in BALB/c mouse and until day 25 of postnatal life in C57BL/6 mice and thereafter increase gradually in numbers and average size (Hamada et al. 2002; Lorenz et al. 2003). As mentioned in the preceding text, the organogenesis of PP involves at least three distinct steps in the late embryonic stage (Yoshida et al. 1999). Notably, organogenesis commences on gestational day 14.5 to 15.5 fetuses and is completed just before birth on gestational day 20 to 21, offering only a short but critical time window for PP formation. It is also noteworthy that in utero treatment with anti-IL-7R mAb (Yoshida et al. 1999) or LTβR-Ig chimeric protein (Rennert et al. 1997; Yamamoto et al. 2000) abrogates the formation of PP but has no effect on that of ILF (Hamada et al. 2002). However, when the progeny of anti-IL-7R mAb-treated (unpublished observation) or LTβR-Ig-treated (Yamamoto et al. 2000) mice lacking PP but retaining ILF are orally immunized with ovalbumin (OVA) plus cholera toxin as mucosal adjuvant, OVA-specific intestinal IgA Ab responses were induced. In the context of these findings and given that PP evolved earlier than ILF, it is conceivable that the development of ILF in the mouse small intestine is a fail-safe system. Conversely, if ILF evolved earlier than PP, the development of PP could

be regarded as a complementary system to the lack of ILFs during the early postnatal life. In conclusion, in terms of their structural, cellular, and functional properties, mouse ILF bear all the hallmarks of inductive sites for intestinal B-cell responses. It is therefore of considerable importance to continuously elucidate their precise role in gut immunity.

CRYPTOPATCHES (CP)

Since the middle of the 19th century, it has been known that intestinal intraepithelial lymphocytes (IEL) are interspersed among the intestinal epithelial cells (IEC) that form a layer on the basement membrane of the intestinal mucosa (Weber 1847). Genes and molecular structures of the TCR were already evident in the 1980s. Thereafter, studies using mAb to TCR revealed the surprising fact that almost all mouse IEL are T cells (Klein 1998; Lefrancois and Puddington 1999; Aranda et al. 1999). The interior of the basement membrane consists of LP that contains IgA-producing B cells, various T cells, and many lympho-myeloid cells. The marked differences between the inside and outside of the basement membrane are very important in connection with clarification of the in vivo physiologic functions and the development of IEL on the frontline of intestinal mucosa. In research over the past 25 years, IEL in mice and humans, especially IEL distributed in the small intestine, have been found to be remarkably different from the main players in cellular immunity, the T cells of good pedigree, which are distributed in the peripheral lymphoid tissues such as the spleen and LN after development in the thymus (for review, see Hayday et al. 2001) (see Chapter 30). The vast majority of T cells distributed in the peripheral lymphoid tissues of mice and humans are αβ T cells, with a few γδ T cells seen. In contrast, IEL in mice and humans include large numbers of both αβ-IEL and γδ-IEL and are appreciated to be highly atypical T-cell clusters **(Table 21.1)**.

As shown in Table 21.1 (line 7), CD8αα$^+$ T cells, a major T-cell subset in mouse IEL, are present in sufficient numbers in congenitally athymic nu/nu mice and thymectomized, lethally irradiated, bone marrow-reconstituted (BM-reconstituted) mice, suggesting that substantial numbers of IEL develop without passing through the thymus and are therefore thymus-independent T cells (TI IEL) (Klein 1996). A number of explanations have been offered for such thymus independence. For instance, the IEL may develop elsewhere, possibly within the liver (Sato et al. 1995) and then home to the intestine. However, as early as 1967, the intestinal IEC layer was proposed as a lymphocyte-producing organ (Fichtelius 1968). GALT, which contain ~60% of all peripheral lymphocytes, monitor and defend the intestinal mucosa in most vertebrates. T cells and antibodies, the key players in adaptive immunity, have not been found in Agnatha or Cyclostom, the oldest phylogenic vertebrates lacking thymus, spleen, and LN (Du Pasguier 1993; Matsunaga 1998; Du Pasguier and Flajnik 1999). Importantly, however, GALT characterized by many lymphoid cells is found in

Table 21.1. Distinctive T-cell Features of Mouse and Human IELs

IELs contain many γδ T cells with γδ-TCR (γδ-IEL) in addition to αβ-IEL.	Goodman and Lefrancois 1988; Bonneville *et al.* 1988; Deusch *et al.* 1991; Lundqvist *et al.* 1995
A large fraction of γδ-IELs and many αβ-IELs express CD8α homodimer and use, as part of CD3 complex, Fc receptor γ-chain in place of the ζ-chain.	Lefrancois 1991a; Guy-Grand *et al.* 1991a; Jarry *et al.* 1990; Deusch *et al.* 1991; Kawaguchi *et al.* 1993; Ohno *et al.* 1993 ; Liu *et al.* 1993; Malissen *et al.* 1993; Lundqvist *et al.* 1995
IELs are exceptional among peripheral T cells in that they consist of more than 14 discriminable subpopulations when sorted on the basis of expression of TCR (αβ vs. γδ), Thy-1, CD4, CD5, CD8αα, and/or CD8αβ molecules.	Goodman and Lefrancois 1989; Mosley *et al.* 1990a, b; Lefrancois 1991b; Guy-Grand *et al.* 1991a; Camerini *et al.* 1993; Kawaguchi *et al.* 1993; Ibraghimov and Lynch 1994; Nanno *et al.* 1994
The majority of IELs are terminally differentiated and activated T cells, which possess a granular cytoplasmic structure and are capable of killing Fc receptor–bearing target cells after bridging them with anti-CD3 or anti-TCR antibody.	Davies and Parrott 1980; Klein and Kagnoff 1984; Ernst *et al.* 1986; Lefrancois and Goodman 1989; Viney *et al.* 1990; Guy-Grand *et al.* 1991b; Sydora *et al.* 1993; Kawaguchi *et al.* 1993; Ishikawa *et al.* 1993
IEL express constitutively $\alpha_E\beta_7$ integrin and its ligand is E-cadherin expressed by IECs (intestinal epithelial cells).	Cepek *et al.* 1994; Karecla *et al.* 1995; Austrup *et al.* 1995
IELs use a limited number of junctional sequences in TCR genes (oligoclonality) as compared with the diverse usage of junctional sequences by the other peripheral T cells.	Balk *et al.* 1991; Van Kerckhove *et al.* 1992; Blumberg *et al.* 1993; Chowers *et al.* 1994; Regnault *et al.* 1994; Gross *et al.* 1994
Most γδ-IELs and many αβ-IELs develop most likely in the intestinal mucosa without passing through the thymus.	Mosley *et al.* 1990b; Lefrancois *et al.* 1990; Guy-Grand *et al.* 1991a; Lefrancois 1991b; Rocha *et al.* 1991; Bandeira *et al.* 1991; Poussier *et al.* 1992, 1993

Agnatha such as lampreys and hagfish, and the intestinal mucosa appear to serve as the lymphocyte production plant in such animals (Du Pasguier 1993; Du Pasguier and Flajnik 1999). Furthermore, bursa of Fabricus, a GALT of birds, and PP of sheep are also well known to be the primary lymphoid tissues responsible for the development of B cells (Greibel and Hein 1996).

The question of where mouse and human IEL develop in the intestinal mucosa has received considerable research attention. Screening of surface antigens has revealed small numbers of progenitor T cells in IEL (Guy-Grand *et al.* 1992; Lin *et al.* 1994; Mowat and Viney 1997; Hamad *et al.* 1997; Page *et al.* 1998; Lefrancois and Puddington 1999), and transcripts of the RAG-1 (Guy-Grand *et al.* 1992; Lin *et al.* 1994) and RAG-2 (Boll *et al.* 1995; Lefrancois and Puddington 1999) genes have been detected in IEL. Therefore, it is possible that development of IEL is localized in the IEC layer. In consideration of the fact that GALT is present in Agnatha, the most ancient of vertebrates, and that the intestinal mucosa is the most high-risk location in the host, it follows that TI IEL, T cells that develop in the intestines, serve as vigilantes to protect the intestinal mucosa.

However, the question of whether or not these TI IEL actually develop in the IEC layer *in situ* has remained an open one.

Discovery of cryptopatches (CP) in the mouse intestine

Screening of cryosections of the mouse alimentary canal using hematoxylin-eosin staining has shown that many small groups of lymphocytes in the shape of minute rugby balls **(Fig. 21.6A)** are scattered throughout the small intestinal LP in crypts (called cryptopatches [CP]) from the base of the villi (Figs. 21.6A, B, and C) (Kanamori *et al.* 1996). CP are not present in the gastric mucosa but are found throughout the small (~1500) and large (~150) intestinal mucosa, with the total number estimated at 1500 to 1700. One CP contains about 1000 lymphoid cells, and the diameter of most CP is about 100–150 μm. Unlike PP and ILF, which are characterized by well-developed GC (Weinstein *et al.* 1991; Liu *et al.* 1991; McIntyre and Strober 1999; Hamada *et al.* 2002) and are covered by distinct M-cell containing FAE, CP do not display either GC or FAE formation (Hamada *et al.* 2002).

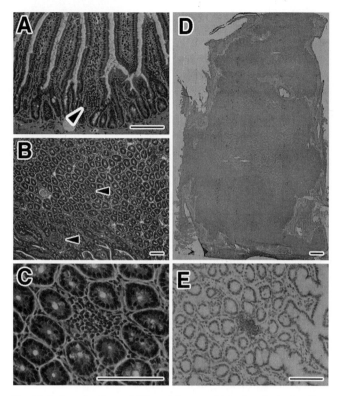

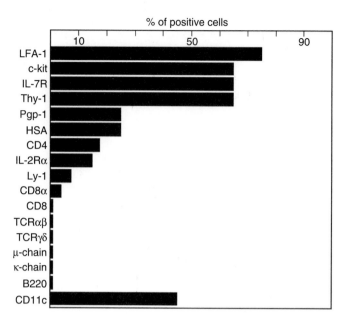

Fig. 21.7. Expression of lymphocyte cell surface molecules by resident cells in the small intestinal CP of C57BL/6 mice. Geometric average of positive cell fractions obtained by more than five independent immunohistochemical studies on the small intestinal CP from 8–20-week-old mice.

Fig. 21.6. Localization of CP and immunohistochemical visualization of CP filled with c-kit[+] cells in the small intestine of C57BL/6 mouse. **A,** Hematoxylin/eosin-stained longitudinal tissue section of the small intestine shows a small cluster of lymphocytes in the shape of minute rugby balls in crypt lamina propria from the base of villus (CP, arrowhead). Bar, 100 μm. **B,** Two CP are seen in a hematoxylin/eosin-stained horizontal tissue section of the crypt lamina propria (arrowheads). Bar, 100 μm. **C,** Magnified view of one CP shown in Fig. 21.6B. Bar, 100 μm. **D,** Horizontally sectioned jejunal tissue was stained immunohistochemically by using anti-c-kit mAb. Note that numerous tiny CP are interspersed throughout the mucosa. Bar, 500 μm. **E,** Magnified view of one CP shown in **D.** Bar, 100 μm.

Immunohistochemical analysis of cells sojourning in CP

To investigate the properties of lymphocytes congregating at CP, immunohistochemical (Kanamori *et al.* 1996; Oida *et al.* 2000; Laky *et al.* 2000; Suzuki *et al.* 2000; Onai *et al.* 2002) analysis using mAbs for various lymphocyte surface antigens has been conducted. A large number of CP cells express receptor-type tyrosine kinase (c-kit; ligand is stem cell factor [SCF]) (Figs. 21.6D and E) and IL-7R, as well as Thy-1, which is mainly expressed by mouse T cells and the lymphocyte function–associated antigen-1 (LFA-1), a lymphocyte marker. Most of them, however, do not express CD3, TCR-αβ, TCR-γδ, sIgM, and B220 molecules, which are expressed by mature T and B cells **(Fig. 21.7).** Because many Thy-1-positive B220-negative cells are present among CP cells, it is conceivable that CP cells are T cell–type rather than B cell–type undifferentiated lymphocytes. In this context, the c-kit[+]IL-7R[+]Thy1[+] phenotype of CP lymphocytes is reminiscent of the c-kit[low]IL-7R[+]Thy1[+] phenotype deter-

mined for the mouse fetal blood prothymocyte population, which is T lineage–committed prior to thymus colonization (Rodewald *et al.* 1994). In addition, various populations of lymphocyte in CP express CD44 (Pgp-1), CD25 (IL-2Rα), and CD24 (heat-stable antigen, HSA) molecules (20% to 50%), and the composition of CD8[+], Ly-1[+], and CD4[+] subsets is smaller but also variable (3% to 20%) (Fig. 21.7). When the expression of these cell surface antigens by CP are compared with that of earlier and/or the earliest T-cell precursors in the thymus (Wu *et al.* 1991a, b; Godfrey *et al.* 1993, 1994), it becomes clear that T lineage–committed precursors consisting of cells at various maturational stages are present among CP lymphocytes. Although CP cells consist of several percent CD8[+] cells, CD4[+] cells account for 15% to 20% of all cells (Fig. 21.7). Therefore, CD3[−]CD4[+]CD8[−] cells are also present. If these lymphocytes are equivalent to CD3[−] CD4[low]CD8[−] T cells, the earliest precursor cells in the thymus (Wu *et al.* 1991a, b), they can be considered to be the most undifferentiated cells in the gut CP.

Many CD11c/CD18 integrin-positive DCs (Kanamori *et al.* 1996) are also found in CP (Fig. 21.7). Double immunofluorescence visualization of CP has revealed that c-kit[+] CP cells, most of which simultaneously express IL-7R and Thy-1 molecules (Kanamori *et al.* 1996; Suzuki *et al.* 2000), and CD11c/CD18[+] DCs constitute two discrete nonoverlapping populations (Kanamori *et al.* 1996). Importantly, the CD11c/CD18[+] DCs settle mainly at the margins of CP, and it is in a mesh structure of these DCs that the c-kit[+] CP cells are found clustered (Kanamori *et al.* 1996; Nanno *et al.* 1998).

Electron microscopic examination of CP

CP can be visualized from the serosa in the longitudinally opened small intestinal tissue using transillumination stereomicroscopy. Tissue containing one CP was excised under stereomicroscopy using a polished 21-gauge syringe (inner diameter: 570 μm) (Saito et al. 1998; Hamada et al. 2002). Electron microscopic examination of the intestinal tissue containing CP showed many small lymphocytes in the center of a CP surrounded by macrophage-like cells (Ishikawa et al. 1999). It also showed blood vessels along with reticulocytes with dendritic processes acting as support tissue in CP (Ishikawa et al. 1999). These findings indicate that CP are not simply accumulations of lymphocytes but have structural and histologic features characteristic of small lymphoid tissues (Saito et al. 1998; Ishikawa et al. 1999). Using scanning electron microscopy, transit images of lymphocytes with basement membrane in contact with the CP was observed **(Fig. 21.8)**, but not with basement membrane in other sites (Saito et al. 1998). These findings suggest that the basement membrane adjacent to the CP is a busy portal line of the mouse small intestine where migration of lymphocytes into the epithelium takes place.

c-kit^{high} CP cells as precursors of IEL

CP lymphocytes were carefully isolated from excised intestinal tissue containing one CP **(Fig. 21.9A)** using forceps for microsurgery in 100% fetal calf serum (FCS) at 4° C via stereomicroscopy (Fig. 21.9A). This procedure allowed 600 to 2000 lymphocytes to be obtained from each CP$^+$ tissue. Among lymphocytes isolated from both CP-containing (CP$^+$) and CP-deficient (CP$^-$) small intestinal tissues as well as from epithelial layers (IEL), PP, and MLN, only those from CP$^+$ tissue possessed a large population (~30%) of c-kit^{high}α$_E$β$_7$$^-Lin^-$ cells (Lin; lineage markers) (CD3, B220, Mac-1, Gr-1 and TER119) (c-kit^{high}) (Fig. 21.9B). These c-kit^{high} CP cells also express IL-7R and CD44 and contain Thy-1$^{+/-}$, CD4$^{+/-}$, and/or CD25$^{low/-}$ cells (Suzuki et al. 2000). Thus, a substantial number of c-kit^{high}IL-7R$^+$CD44$^+$Thy-1$^{+/-}$CD4$^{+/-}$CD25$^{low/-}$α$_E$β$_7$$^-Lin^-$ lymphocytes appear to settle exclusively in CP, not in other GALT. As mentioned earlier, the characteristics of c-kit^{high} CP cells are almost identical to those of immature thymocytes (Wu et al. 1991a, b; Godfrey et al. 1993; Godfrey and Zlotnik 1993; Godfrey et al. 1994; Zuniga-Pflucker and Lenardo 1996; Shortman et al. 1998).

To examine whether c-kit^{high} CP cells express CD3ε and pre-Tα specific mRNA like immature thymocytes, c-kit^{high} CP cells and c-kit$^{low/-}$ and α$_E$β$_7$$^+$, and/or Lin$^+$ (c-kit$^{low/-}$), were purified by flow cytometry (Fig. 21.9C). CD3ε transcripts were found in c-kit^{high} CP cells, although at levels five-fold below those found in c-kit$^{low/-}$ CP cells, IEL, MLN cells, and thymocytes (Fig. 21.9D). In contrast to IEL and c-kit$^{low/-}$ CP cells, c-kit^{high} CP cells were found to have no or a drastically reduced number of pre-Tα transcripts (Fig. 21.9D). These findings appear to support the notion that progenitor T cells, which match the developmental stage of c-kit$^+$CD44$^+$CD25$^{low/-}$ thymocytes before pre-Tα gene transcription (Saint-Ruf et al. 1994; Wilson and MacDonald 1995; Koyasu et al. 1997) but after expression of CD3ε specific mRNA (Wilson and MacDonald 1995; Wang et al. 1999), are present in the gut CP. Further, the fact that germline TCR-γ and TCR-β but not rearranged TCR-γ and TCR-β gene-specific mRNA are detected in c-kit^{high} CP cells (Fig. 21.9D) is also consistent with the compartmentalization of T lineage–committed precursors in the gut CP, because TCR genes retain their germline configuration in c-kit$^+$CD44$^+$CD25$^-$ and c-kit$^+$CD44$^+$CD25$^+$ thymocytes (Godfrey and Zlotnik 1993; Godfrey et al. 1994; Zuniga-Pflucker and Lenardo 1996; Hozumi et al. 1996; Shortman et al. 1998).

Cytokine regulation of CP and IEL development

The IL-7/IL-7R–mediated signaling pathway is indispensable for the development of PP (Adachi et al. 1998) as well as for the V-J rearrangement of the TCR-γ gene (Maki et al. 1996). Thus neither IL-7R$^{-/-}$ mice (Maki et al. 1996) nor IL-7$^{-/-}$ mice (Moore et al. 1996) possess PP and γδ T cells. In the small intestine of IL-7R$^{-/-}$ mice, CP are reduced drastically in numbers and average size (Oida et al. 2000), and γδ-IEL are absent from the epithelial compartment (Maki et al. 1996; Oida et al. 2000). In contrast, αβ-IEL number only two-fold less in IL-7R$^{-/-}$ than in wild type (WT) B6 mice and contain all five discriminable (Kawaguchi et al. 1993) thymus-dependent (TD) and TI IEL subsets (Oida et al. 2000). These findings demonstrate that the small CP present in IL-7R$^{-/-}$ mice are functionally normal and suggest that TI αβ-IEL develop by passing through these CP. Mouse IEC are known to produce IL-7 and SCF (Fujihashi et al. 1996; Puddington et al. 1994; Laky et al. 1997) and human IEC to produce IL-7 (Watanabe et al. 1995). IL-7 produced by IEC has also been shown to play an important role in the development of TI αβ-IELs (Laky et al. 1998). Based on these findings,

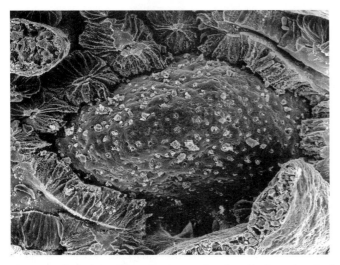

Fig. 21.8. Scanning electron micrograph of epithelium-detached basement membrane extending over a CP. The detachment of epithelium reveals the highly perforated basement membrane, and these holes most likely facilitate the migration of CP lymphocytes into the epithelial compartment.

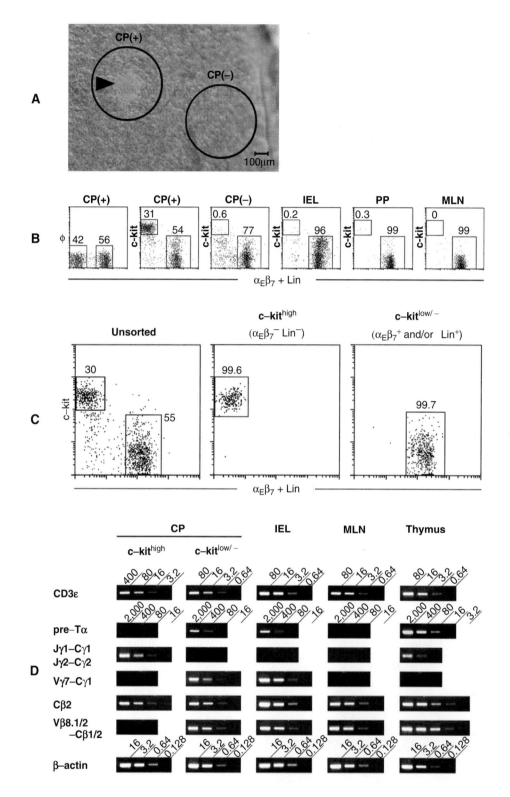

Fig. 21.9. Flow cytometric and semiquantitative RT-PCR analyses of lymphocytes that settle in CP. (Reprinted from an article [Suzuki *et al.* 2000] with permission from Elsevier.) **A,** Stereomicroscopic view of the small intestinal mucosa. Circles indicate the CP⁺ and CP⁻ fragments to be extracted with the aid of an amputated and tapered 21-gauge needle (inner diameter, 570 μm). **B,** Flow cytometric profiles of CP⁺ cells (735 ± 175 per fragment), CP⁻ cells (80.1 ± 29.5 per fragment), IEL, PP cells, and MLN cells. Lin (lineage markers; CD3, B220, Mac-1, Gr-1, and TER119). Note that only CP⁺ cells contain a large population of c-kit^{high}α_Eβ_7⁻Lin⁻ (c-kit^{high}) lymphocytes. **C,** Flow cytometric profiles of CP⁺ cells before and after purification by FACS Vantage. **D,** Serial five-fold dilutions of RNAs equivalent to RNAs extracted from the indicated numbers of cells were reverse transcribed, and the cDNA products were PCR amplified. Although the signal is five-fold reduced in c-kit^{high} CP cells, all cells express substantial levels of CD3ε gene. In contrast, although the signal for pre-Tα is detected in c-kit$^{low/-}$ CP cells, IEL, and thymus cells, the same signal is almost undetectable in c-kit^{high} CP and MLN cells. Germline Jγ1-Cγ1–specific and Jγ2-Cγ2–specific mRNA are detectable only in c-kit^{high} CP and thymus cells, whereas rearranged Vγ7-Cγ1–specific mRNA are detectable only in c-kit$^{low/-}$ CP cells and IEL. All cells express comparable levels of Cβ gene, but in contrast to the other cells, c-kit^{high} CP fail to express any detectable Vβ8.1/2-Cβ1/2–specific signal, indicating that the Cβ signal in c-kit^{high} CP cells is most likely from germline transcripts of TCR-β gene.

transgenic (Tg) mice producing IL-7 only by IEC were created from IL-7$^{-/-}$ mice by inserting IL-7 cDNA in the promoter of IEC-specific fatty acid–binding protein (IL-7 Tg mice) (Laky *et al.* 2000). In contrast to IL-7$^{-/-}$ mice, which were observed to express less than 30 small CP in the small intestine, IL-7 Tg mice expressed about ~750 ordinary CP as well as γδ-IEL development (Laky *et al.* 2000). These findings support the fact that the IL-7 produced by IEC is essential in the normal development of CP and localized IEL in the intestine.

By contrast, IL-2Rβ$^{-/-}$ mice in which signal transmission from IL-2/IL-2R and IL-15/IL-15R has been compromised (Giri *et al.* 1994; Suzuki *et al.* 1995, 1997) express clusters of c-kit$^+$ cells, that is, CP in the intestinal mucosa that are only slightly less numerous than those in WT mice (Oida *et al.* 2000). Strikingly, however, the population size of the major TI CD8αα$^+$ IEL subset is drastically reduced in the IL-2Rβ$^{-/-}$ condition (Oida *et al.* 2000). An analysis of lymphocytes in IL-2Rβ$^{-/-}$ mice (Suzuki *et al.* 1997; Ohteki *et al.* 1997) and in IL-15Rα$^{-/-}$ mice (Lodolce *et al.* 1998) have shown that signal transmission from IL-15/IL-15R is important for the development of NK cells, NKT cells, and CD8αα$^+$ IEL. Therefore, although the CP of IL-2Rβ$^{-/-}$ mice appear to be normal immunohistochemically, they are either functionally crippled or, because of the absence of IL-15/IL-15R–mediated signaling, lead to an impaired final step of TI-IEL development in the intestinal epithelium.

The cytokine receptor γ-chain is a signal transmission molecule common to IL-2R, IL-4R, IL-7R, IL-9R, and IL-15R. The γ-chain mutant male (IL-2Rγ$^{-/Y}$) mice are PP deficient and suffer from developmental disorders in various lymphoid tissues as well as from immunologic abnormalities (Cao *et al.* 1995; DiSanto *et al.* 1995). A detailed examination of the small intestinal mucosa of mice bearing a mutation of the membrane-penetrating exon of the γ-chain gene (IL-2Rγ$^{-/Y}$ mice) (Ohbo *et al.* 1996) has shown that CP levels are below the detection limit and no CD8αα$^+$ IEL are present (Oida *et al.* 2000) **(Fig. 21.10)**. Very few thymus-dependent (TD) Thy-1$^+$CD4$^+$ αβ-IEL and TD Thy-1$^+$CD8αβ$^+$αβ-IEL but no γδ-IEL were detected because the mice are IL-7/IL-7R– signal transmission deficient (Maki *et al.* 1996; Oida *et al.* 2000). When IEL were examined in athymic nu/nu IL-2Rγ$^{-/Y}$ mice deficient in PP and CP, the TD αβ-IEL observed in the euthymic IL-2Rγ$^{-/Y}$ mice had completely disappeared (Fig. 21.10), and IEL expressing c-kit, Thy-1, CD4, or CD8αβ molecules were present only in small numbers in the CD3$^-$ (TCR$^-$) population. Notably, however, the CD3$^-$CD8αα$^+$ subset levels were below the detection limit (Fig. 21.10). Next, in a comparative study of TCR$^-$ IELs in nu/nu IL-2Rγ$^{-/Y}$ mice and those in nu/nu SCID mice that are both TCR$^+$ IEL-deficient and athymic in the same way as nu/nu IL-2Rγ$^{-/Y}$ mice but have normal CP c-kit$^+$Lin$^-$ cells (Fig. 21.10), the following findings concerning the physiologic functions of CP were obtained: development of CD8αα$^+$ TI IEL, expression of IEL-inherent αEβ7 integrin (Cepek *et al.* 1994; Karecla *et al.* 1995; Austrup *et al.* 1995), recombination of TCR gene V(D)J and transcription of the

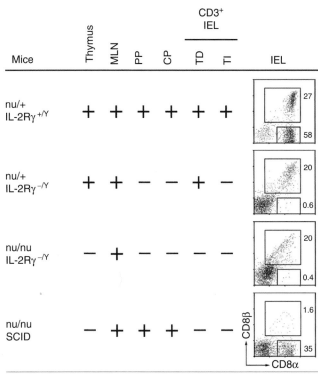

Fig. 21.10. Presence and absence of thymus, MLN, PP, CP, CD3$^+$ TD IEL, and/or CD3$^+$ TI IEL in wild-type, nu/+ interleukin 2 receptor γ-chain–deficient (IL-2Rγ$^{-/Y}$), nu/nu IL-2Rγ$^{-/Y}$ and nu/nu SCID mice, and two-color (CD8α vs. CD8β) flow cytometric profiles of IEL from these four different mice. It was reported that PP and ILF were absent from the small intestine of *aly/aly* mutant mice (Nanno *et al.* 1994; Hamada *et al.* 2002) and that histogenesis of CP and intestinal development of IEL that had derived from c-kit$^+$ CP cells were maintained in *aly/aly* mutant mice (Nanno *et al.* 1994; Kanamori *et al.* 1996), so PP are not an absolute requirement for the development of extrathymic IEL expressing CD8αα homodimers. Thus the findings depicted in this figure strongly indicate that CP are indispensable anatomic sites for the generation of such CD8αα$^+$ IEL.

CD3ε gene (Oida *et al.* 2000). However, since the appropriateness of these findings is based on the premise that there is no impairment of the physiologic function in the IEC layer, further exploration is necessary before any final conclusion can be reached.

Control of CP and IEL development by a CC chemokine

Through the rapid progress that has been made in recent years in research on chemokine/chemokine receptors, it is now evident that interactions among chemokine/chemokine receptors are very important in such processes as development, motility, localization, and the functional expression of various lymphocytes (Yoshie *et al.* 2001). The CC chemokine CCL25 (TECK) has been shown to be expressed in stromal cells in the thymus and crypt epithelium in the small intestine (Kunkel *et al.* 2000; Wurbel *et al.* 2000), and α4β7 integrin-positive intestinal homing T and B cells have been shown to express CCR9, a ligand of CCL25 (Zabel *et al.*

1999). It has recently been shown that CCL25 is a potent and selective chemoattractant for IgA Ab–producing cells, efficiently recruiting IgA-producing but not IgG-producing and IgM-producing cells to LP from spleen, PP, and MLN (Bowman *et al.*, 2002). These findings suggest that interaction of CCL25 and CCR9 might be important for the specialized localization of T and B cells engaged in the gut-oriented immune response. Accordingly, the CCL25 gene has been introduced into c-kit+ BM cells *in vitro* (intrakine, IK) using retrovirus-expressing vector containing an internal ribosomal entry site (IRES) (Onai *et al.* 2000). These c-kit+ BM cells were transplanted into mice given a lethal dose of irradiation. In lymphoid and myeloid cells developed from IK-introduced stem cells, CCR9 was trapped by the IRES-IK (CCL25), and transfer of CCR9 to the cell surface was inhibited. The results of a detailed investigation of intestines reconstituted with IK cells showed that CP were markedly reduced, that the remaining CP are small in size, and that the population size of CD8αα+ TI IEL was sharply attenuated (Onai *et al.*, 2002). In contrast, the IK cell–derived CD8αβ+ T cells distributed in the thymus and spleen were found to maintain levels comparable to those of the controls (Onai *et al.* 2002). Furthermore, an analysis of normal CP by a laser scanning microscope revealed that c-kit+ cells express CCR9 and CD11c+ DC express CCL25 (Onai *et al.* 2002). These findings support the importance in the normal development of CP of the interaction between CCR9 on the c-kit+ cells and CCL25 produced by the CD11c+ DC distributed

in the intestinal mucosa. Consistent with this notion, it has been reported that the total count of IEL is reduced by half because of the marked decrease in γδ-IEL in the small intestine of CCR9−/− mice (Wurbel *et al.* 2001).

The sequential cellular events in the development of TI IEL in the gut mucosa

To more thoroughly understand the development of CP and TI IEL in the gut mucosa, 6 Gy-irradiated athymic IL-2Rγ−/Y mutant mice (Ly5.2+) that lack thymus, PP, CP, and TCR+ IEL (Oida *et al.* 2000) were reconstituted with T cell–depleted wild-type Ly5.1+ BM cells (Suzuki *et al.* 2000). The results show that the cluster of BM-derived CD11c+ DC, namely CP anlage, is first detected in the crypt region of 6 Gy-irradiated athymic IL-2Rγ−/Y hosts, but at this stage, very few c-kit+ cells are present in these DC aggregates. Thereafter, a rapid and marked increase of these clusters both in number and size is observed (Suzuki *et al.* 2000), and with this increase, BM-derived c-kit+ cells start to accumulate in these CP anlagen. Simultaneously, at this posttransplantation period, BM-derived TCR− IEL are first detected in the epithelial cell layers of villi around the regenerated CP. Soon thereafter, these TCR− IEL repopulate all of the epithelial cell layers, and with the rapid increase in this population, the generation of BM-derived αβ-IEL and γδ-IEL starts to take place sluggishly (Suzuki *et al.* 2000). These distinctive cellular events in the reconstitution of TI IEL in BM chimeric mice are depicted in **Figure 21.11**.

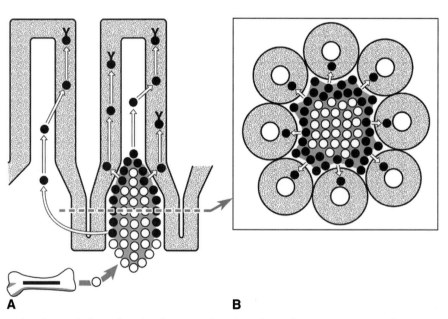

A **B**

Fig. 21.11. Cartoons show that thymus-independent development of IEL in radiation bone-marrow (BM) chimeric mice proceeds through at least four successive steps. Lethally irradiated interleukin 2 receptor γ-chain–deficient Ly5.2+ mice that lack the thymus, PP, CP, and TCR+ IEL were reconstituted with wild-type Ly5.1+ BM cells. **A,** First, BM-derived c-kit+ cells (open circle) accumulate in the regenerating CP anlagen. Second, c-kit−TCR− IEL precursors (closed circle) differentiated from BM-derived c-kit+ cells in the regenerated CP appear within villous epithelia of small intestine overlying the regenerated CP. Third, these TCR− IEL subsequently emerge throughout the epithelia. Fourth, TCR+ IEL (closed circle with V [TCR]) increase slowly to a comparable number to that in athymic mice and consist of both TCR-γδ and TCR-αβ IEL. **B,** Horizontal view of the CP shown in Figure 21.11A. Note that one CP is capable of providing eight adjacent villi with c-kit−TCR− IEL precursors (closed circle).

As described in the preceding text, CP have been identified in the crypt region of the mouse intestinal LP. It has also become possible to analyze CP in the context of the anatomic site where c-kit$^+$ IEL progenitors develop. However, important goals of future research must be the dissection at the subcellular level of CP histogenesis and TI IEL development and differentiation from c-kit$^+$ CP cells as well as exploration of hematopoietic progenitors for lympho-myeloid descendants other than TI IEL that might reside in gut CP (Lambolez et al. 2002).

In any event, a coherent picture of IEL immunobiology is gradually emerging, but much more remains to be explored. For instance, very important and related points meriting consideration in the context of TI IEL development are as follows. A recent study has shown that extrathymic T-cell lymphopoiesis such as development of TI IEL is a minor pathway of T-cell differentiation, taking place mostly in the MLN but not in the CP and operating only when thymopoiesis is defective (Guy-Grand et al. 2003). Also eagerly awaited are detailed studies of CP or CP-like lymphoid structures in human and rat intestines because the growing evidence indicates the development of T cells, mainly IEL, in the intestinal mucosa of humans (Deusch et al. 1991; Lundqvist et al. 1995; Jarry et al. 1990; Latthe et al. 1994; Lynch et al. 1995; Koningsberger et al. 1997; Howie et al. 1998) and rats (Ramanathan et al. 2002).

SUMMARY

The gut is an essential organ for the intake of nutrients, and even primitive animals with primitive brains and nervous systems have a well-developed intestine. Intestinal mucosa, which is continuously invaded by many food-derived extrinsic antigens and allergens as well as by toxins and pathogenic organisms, is the highest risk site in the body. Therefore, it is defended by intestinal immune tissue composed of large numbers of immunocompetent cells that represent 60% of the entire peripheral lymphocyte population. It is also evident that immune control of the intestinal mucosa is subject to specific conditions not seen in other parts of the body, because various dangerous substances, whose excretion should be triggered by immune defenses, are present together with foreign substances that should be physiologically and nutritionally taken into the body without invoking immune response in the intestine. Thus the gut is not only a digestive and absorptive organ but also the most advanced immune organ in the body. To this end, the gut mucosal immune system has developed uniquely organized lymphoid tissue such as PP, ILF, and CP to deliver both innate and acquired immunity.

Among the numerous luminal antigens, commensal microbes constitute the largest antigenic load in the gut lumen (Neutra et al. 2001; Elson et al. 2001). In fact, about one trillion microbes inhabit our intestines and show specific and nonspecific control of intestinal physiologic and immunologic functions (Abrams et al. 1963; Elson et al. 2001; Simmons et al. 2001; Hooper and Gordon 2001). Even in mice reared under specific pathogen-free conditions, large numbers of T and B cells in the intestinal mucosa remain constantly activated, and GC formation occurs constantly in PP and ILF. In spite of the presence of this volcanic immune reaction, the intestinal mucosa is considered as "disease free" or "activated yet resting" (Elson et al. 2001). Since no pathophysiology or lesions are observed, this condition is called "physiologic inflammation" (Abrams et al. 1963; Elson et al. 2001). However, this "physiologic inflammation" maintained by a complex, delicate balance is actually a glass house that can easily be shattered as is evident from the high incidence of inflammatory bowel disease observed in mice with mutations caused by genes involved in immune function (Strober and Ehrhard 1993; MacDonald 1994; Powrie 1995). Obviously, the distinctive features of the immune surveillance of the GI tract are becoming clear, but there are still many riddles concerning the labyrinthine intestinal immune system that will require our unstinted efforts to solve.

ACKNOWLEDGMENTS

We would like to thank the many members of our laboratories, and Drs. T. Iwanaga and H. Takahasi-Iwanaga for their excellent electron microscope analysis, all of whom have contributed to portions of our work embodied in this chapter. The data provided in the preparation of this chapter were supported in part by Grant-in-Aid for Creative Scientific Research, the Japan Society for the Promotion of Science (13GS0015), by Special Coordination Fund for Promoting Science and Technology from the Ministry of Education, Culture, Sports, Science and Technology, and by a Health Sciences Research Grant, Ministry of Health Labour and Welfare (H. I.) and by grants from the Ministry of Education, Science, Sports and Culture, Ministry of Health Labour and Welfare and Core Research of Evolutionary Science and Technology of Japan Science and Technology Agency, Japan (H. K.).

REFERENCES

Abrams, G. D., Bauer, H., and Sprinz, H. (1963). Influence of the normal flora on mucosal morphology and cellular renewal in the ileum. A comparison of germ-free and conventional mice. *Lab. Invest.* 12, 355–364.

Adachi, S., Yoshida, H., Kataoka, H., and Nishikawa, S. (1997). Three distinctive steps in Peyer's patch formation of murine embryo. *Int. Immunol.* 9, 507–514.

Adachi, S., Yoshida, H., Honda, K., Maki, K., Saijo, K., Ikuta, K., Saito, T., and Nishikawa, S.-I. (1998). Essential role of IL-7 receptor α in the formation of Peyer's patch anlage. *Int. Immunol.* 10, 1–6.

Ansel, K. M., Ngo, V. N., Hyman, P. L., Luther, S. A., Forster, R., Sedgwick, J. D., Browning, J. L., Lipp, M., and Cyster, J. G. (2000). A chemokine-driven positive feedback loop organizes lymphoid follicles. *Nature* 406, 309–314.

Aranda, R., Sydora, B. C. and Kronenberg, M. (1999). Intraepithelial lymphocytes: Function. In *Mucosal Immunology*, ed 2. (eds. P. L. Ogra, J. Mestecky, M. E. Lamm, W. Strober, J. Bienenstock, and J. R. McGhee), 429–437. San Diego: Academic Press.

Austrup, F., Rebstock, S., Kilshaw, P. J., and Hamann, A. (1995). Transforming growth factor-β 1-induced expression of the mucosa-related integrin αE on lymphocytes is not associated with mucosa-specific homing. *Eur. J. Immunol.* 25, 1487–1491.

Balk, S. P., Ebert, E. C., Blumenthal, R. L., McDermott, F. V., Wucherpfennig, K. W., Landau, S. B., and Blumberg, R. S. (1991). Oligoclonal expansion and CD1 recognition by human intestinal intraepithelial lymphocytes. *Science* 253, 1411–1415.

Bancherau, J., and Steinman, R. M. (1998). Dendritic cells and the control of immunity. *Nature* 392, 245–252.

Bancherau, J., Briere, F., Caux, C., Davoust, J., Lebecque, S., Liu, Y. J., Pulendran, B., and Palucka, K. (2000). Immunobiology of dendritic cells. *Annu. Rev. Immunol.* 18, 767–811.

Bandeira, A., Itohara, S., Bonneville, M., Burlen-Defranoux, O., Mota-Santos, T., Coutinho, A., and Tonegawa, S. (1991). Extrathymic origin of intestinal intraepithelial lymphocytes bearing T-cell antigen receptor γδ. *Proc. Natl. Acad. Sci. USA* 88, 43–47.

Blumberg, R. S., Yockey, C. E., Gross, G. G., Ebert, E. C. and Balk, S. P. (1993). Human intestinal intraepithelial lymphocytes are derived from a limited number of T cell clones that utilize multiple Vβ T cell receptor genes. *J. Immunol.* 150, 5144–5153.

Boll, G., Rudolphi, A., Spiess, S., and Reimann, J. (1995). Regional specialization of intraepithelial T cells in the murine small and large intestine. *Scand. J. Immunol.* 41, 103–113.

Bonneville, M., Janeway, C. A. Jr., Ito, K., Haser, W., Ishida, I., Nakanishi, N., and Tonegawa, S. (1988). Intestinal intraepithelial lymphocytes are a distinct set of γδ T cells. *Nature* 336, 479–481.

Bowman, E. P., Kuklin, N. A., Youngman, K. R., Lazarus, N. H., Kunkel, E. J., Pan, J., Greenberg, H. B., and Butcher, E. C. (2002). The intestinal chemokine thymus-expressed chemokine (CCL25) attracts IgA antibody-secreting cells. *J. Exp. Med.* 195, 269–275.

Camerini, V., Panwala, C., and Kronenberg, M. (1993). Regional specialization of the mucosal immune system: Intraepithelial lymphocytes of the large intestine have a different phenotype and function than those of the small intestine. *J. Immunol.* 151, 1765–1776.

Cao, X., Shores, E. W., Hu-Li, J., Anver, M. R., Kelsall, B. L., Russell, S. M., Drago, J., Noguchi, M., Grinberg, A., and Bloom, E. T. (1995). Defective lymphoid development in mice lacking expression of the common cytokine receptor γ chain. *Immunity* 2, 223–238.

Cepek, K. L., Shaw, S. K., Parker, C. M., Russell, G. J., Morrow, J. S., Rimm, D. L., and Brenner, M. B. (1994). Adhesion between epithelial cells and T lymphocytes mediated by E-cadherin and the αEβ7 integrin. *Nature* 372, 190–193.

Chowers, Y., Holtmeier, W., Harwood, J., Morzycka-Wroblewska, E., and Kagnoff, M. F., (1994). The Vδ 1 T cell receptor repertoire in human small intestine and colon. *J. Exp. Med.* 180, 183–190.

Craig, S. W., and Cebra, J. J. (1971). Peyer's patches: An enriched source of precursors for IgA-producing immunocytes in the rabbit. *J. Exp. Med.* 134, 188–200.

Crowe, P. D., VanArsdale, T. L., Walter, B. N., Ware, C. F., Hession, C., Ehrenfels, B., Browning, J. L., Din, W. S., Goodwin, R. G., and Smith, C.A. (1994). A lymphotoxin-β-specific receptor. *Science*, 264, 707–710.

Davies, M. D., and Parrott, D. M. (1980). The early appearance of specific cytotoxic T cells in murine gut mucosa. *Clin. Exp. Immunol.* 42, 273–279.

Dejardin E., Droin, N. M., Delhase, M., Haas, E., Cao, Y., Makris, C., Li, Z. W., Karin, M., Ware, C. F., and Green, D. R. (2002). The lymphotoxin-beta receptor induces different patterns of gene expression via two NF-kappaB pathways. *Immunity* 17, 525–535.

De Togni, P., Goellner, J., Ruddle, N. H., Streeter, P. R., Fick, A., Mariathasan, S., Smith, S. C., Carlson, R., Shornick, L. P., Strauss-Schoenberger, J., Russell, J. H., Karr, R., and Chaplin, D. D. (1994). Abnormal development of peripheral lymphoid organs in mice deficient in lymphotoxin. *Science* 264, 703–707.

Deusch, K., Luling, F., Reich, K., Classen, M., Wagner, H., and Pfeffer, K. (1991). A major fraction of human intraepithelial lymphocytes simultaneously expresses the γ/δ T cell receptor, the CD8 accessory molecule and preferentially uses the Vdelta1 gene segment. *Eur. J. Immunol.* 21, 1053–1059.

DiSanto, J. P., Muller, W., Guy-Grand, D., Fischer, A., and Rajewsky, K. (1995). Lymphoid development in mice with a targeted deletion of the interleukin 2 receptor γ chain. *Proc. Natl. Acad. Sci. USA* 92, 377–381.

Dohi, T., Rennert, P. D., Fujihashi, K., Kiyono, H., Shirai, Y., Kawamura., Y. I., Browning, J. L., and McGhee, J. R. (2001). Elimination of colonic patches with lymphotoxin β-receptor-Ig prevents Th2 cell-type colitis. *J. Immunol.* 167, 2781–2790.

Dougall, W. C., Glaccum, M., Charrier, K., Rohrbach, K., Brasel, K., De Smedt, T., Daro, E., Smith, J., Tometsko, M. E., Maliszewski, C. R., Armstrong, A., Shen, V., Bain, S., Cosman, D., Anderson, D., Morrissey, P. J., Peschon, J. J., and Schuh, J. (1999). RANK is essential for osteoclast and lymph node development. *Genes Dev.* 13, 2412–2424.

Du Pasguier, L. (1993). Evolution of the immune system. In *Fundamental Immunology* (ed. W. Paul), 199–234. New York: Raven Press.

Du Pasguier, L., and Flajnik, M. (1999). Origin and evolution of the vertebrate immune system. In *Fundamental Immunology* (ed. W. Paul), 605–650. Philadelphia, New York: Lippincott-Raven Publishers.

Elson, C. O., Cong, Y., Iqbal, N., and Weaver, C. T. (2001). Immuno-bacterial homeostasis in the gut: New insights into an old enigma. *Semin. Immunol.* 13, 187–194.

Ernst, P. B., Clark, D. A., Rosenthal, K. L., Befus, A. D., and Bienenstock, J. (1986). Detection and characterization of cytotoxic T lymphocyte precursors in the murine intestinal intraepithelial leukocyte population. *J. Immunol.* 136, 2121–2126.

Fagarasan, S., and Honjo, T. (2000). T-Independent immune response: New aspects of B cell biology. *Science* 290, 89–92.

Fagarasan, S., and Honjo, T. (2003). Intestinal IgA synthesis: Regulation of front-line body defences. *Nat. Rev. Immunol.* 3, 63–72.

Fagarasan, S., Muramatsu, M., Suzuki, K., Nagaoka, H., Hiai, H., and Honjo, T. (2002). Critical roles of activation-induced cytidine deaminase in the homeostasis of gut flora. *Science* 298, 1424–1427.

Fichtelius, K. E. (1968). The gut epithelium—A first level lymphoid organ? *Exp. Cell. Res.* 49, 87–104.

Finke, D., Acha-Orbea, H., Mattis, A., Lipp, M., and Kraehenbuhl, J. (2002). CD4+ CD3− cells induce Peyer's patch development: Role of alpha4beta1 integrin activation by CXCR5. *Immunity* 17, 363–373.

Forster, R., Mattis, A. E., Kremmer, E., Wolf, E., Brem, G., and Lipp, M. (1996). A putative chemokine receptor, BLR1, directs B cell migration to defined lymphoid organs and specific anatomic compartments of the spleen. *Cell* 87, 1037–1047.

Fu, Y. X., and Chaplin, D. D. (1999). Development and maturation of secondary lymphoid tissues. *Annu Rev Immunol.* 17, 399–433.

Fujihashi, K., Kawabata, S., Hiroi, T., Yamamoto, M., McGhee, J. R., Nishikawa, S., and Kiyono, H. (1996). IL-2 and IL-7 reciprocally induce IL-7 and IL-2 receptors on γδ TCR+ intraepithelial lymphocytes. *Proc. Natl. Acad. Sci. USA* 93, 3613–3618.

Fukuyama, S., Hiroi, T., Yokota, Y., Rennert, P. D., Yanagita, M, Kinoshita, N., Terawaki, S., Shikina, T., Yamamoto, M., Kurono, Y., and Kiyono, H. (2002). Initiation of NALT organogenesis is independent of the IL-7R, LTβR, and NIK signaling pathways but requires the Id2 gene and CD3− CD4+ CD45+ cells. *Immunity* 17, 31–40.

Futterer, A., Mink, K., Luz, A., Kosco-Vilbois, M. H., and Pfeffer, K. (1998). The lymphotoxin beta receptor controls organogenesis and affinity maturation in peripheral lymphoid tissues. *Immunity* 9, 59–70.

Gebert, A., Rothkotter, H. J., and Pabst, R.(1996). M cells in Peyer's patches of the intestine. *Int. Rev. Cytol.* 167, 91–159.

Giri, J. G., Ahdieh, M., Eisenman, J., Shanebeck, K., Grabstein, K., Kumaki, S., Namen, A., Park, L. S., Cosman, D., and Anderson, D. (1994). Utilization of the β and γ chains of the IL-2 receptor by the novel cytokine IL-15. *EMBO J.* 13, 2822–2830.

Godfrey, D. I., and Zlotnik, A. (1993). Control points in early T-cell development. *Immunol. Today* 14, 547–553.

Godfrey, D. I., Kennedy, J., Suda, T., and Zlotnik, A. (1993). A developmental pathway involving four phenotypically and functionally distinct subsets of CD3−CD4−CD8− triple-negative adult mouse thymocytes defined by CD44 and CD25 expression. *J. Immunol.* 150, 4244–4252.

Godfrey, D. I., Kennedy, J., Mombaerts, P., Tonegawa, S., and Zlotnik, A. (1994). Onset of TCR-β gene rearrangement and role of TCR-β expression during CD3⁻ CD4⁻ CD8⁻ thymocyte differentiation. *J. Immunol.* 152, 4783–4792.

Goodman, T., and Lefrancois, L. (1988). Expression of the γδ TCR on intestinal CD8⁺ intraepithelial lymphocytes. *Nature* 333, 855–858.

Goodman, T., and Lefrancois, L. (1989). Intraepithelial lymphocytes: Anatomical site, not T cell receptor form, dictates phenotype and function. *J. Exp. Med.* 170, 1569–1581.

Griebel, P. J., and Hein, W. R. (1996). Expanding the role of Peyer's patches in B-cell ontogeny. *Immunol. Today* 17, 30–39.

Gross, G. G., Schwartz, V. L., Stevens, C., Ebert, E. C., Blumberg, R. S., and Balk, S. P. (1994). Distribution of dominant T cell receptor β chains in human intestinal mucosa. *J. Exp. Med.* 180, 1337–1344.

Guy-Grand, D., Cerf-Bensussan, N., Malissen, B., Malassis-Seris, M., Briottet, C., and Vassalli, P. (1991a). Two gut intraepithelial CD8⁺ lymphocyte populations with different T cell receptors: A role for the gut epithelium in T cell differentiation. *J. Exp. Med.* 173, 471–481.

Guy-Grand, D., Malassis-Seris, M., Briottet, C., and Vassalli, P. (1991b). Cytotoxic differentiation of mouse gut thymodependent and independent intraepithelial T lymphocytes is induced locally. Correlation between functional assays, presence of perforin and granzyme transcripts, and cytoplasmic granules. *J. Exp. Med.* 173, 1549–1552.

Guy-Grand, D., Vanden Broecke, C., Briottet, C., Malassis-Seris, M., Selz, F., and Vassalli, P. (1992). Different expression of the recombination activity gene RAG-1 in various populations of thymocytes, peripheral T cells and gut thymus-independent intraepithelial lymphocytes suggests two pathways of T cell receptor rearrangement. *Eur. J. Immunol.* 22, 505–510.

Guy-Grand, D., Azogui, O., Celli, S., Darche, S., Nussenzweig, M. C., Kourilsky, P. and Vassalli, P. (2003). Extrathymic T cell lymphopoiesis: Ontogeny and contribution to gut intraepithelial lymphocytes in athymic and euthymic mice. *J. Exp. Med.* 197, 333–341.

Hamad, M., Whetsell, M., Wang, J., and Klein, J. R. (1997). T cell progenitors in the murine small intestine. *Dev. Comp. Immunol.* 21, 435–442.

Hamada, H., Hiroi, T., Nishiyama, Y., Takahashi, H., Masunaga, Y., Hachimura, S., Kaminogawa, S., Takahashi-Iwanaga, H., Iwanaga, T., Kiyono, H., Yamamoto, H., and Ishikawa, H. (2002). Identification of multiple isolated lymphoid follicles on the antimesenteric wall of the mouse small intestine. *J. Immunol.* 168, 57–64.

Hardy, R. R., and Hayakawa, K. (1994). CD5 B cells, a fetal B cell lineage. *Adv. Immunol.* 55, 297–339.

Harmsen, A., Kusser, K., Hartson, L., Tighe, M., Sunshine, M. J., Sedgwick, J. D., Choi, Y., Littman, D. R., and Randall, T. D. (2002) Cutting edge: Organogenesis of nasal-associated lymphoid tissue (NALT) occurs independently of lymphotoxin-α (LT α) and retinoic acid receptor-related orphan receptor-γ, but the organization of NALT is LT α dependent. *J. Immunol.* 168, 986–990.

Hashi, H., Yoshida, H., Honda, K., Fraser, S., Kubo, H., Awane, M., Takabayashi, A., Nakano, H., Yamaoka, Y., and Nishikawa, S. (2001). Compartmentalization of Peyer's patch anlagen before lymphocyte entry. *J. Immunol.* 166, 3702–3709.

Hayakawa, K., Hardy, R. R., Parks, D. R., and Herzenberg, L. A. (1983). The "Ly-1 B" cell subpopulation in normal immunodefective, and autoimmune mice. *J. Exp. Med.* 157, 202–218.

Hayday, A., Theodoridis, E., Ramsburg, E., and Shires, J. (2001), Intraepithelial lymphocytes: Exploring the Third Way in immunology. *Nat. Immunol.* 2, 997–1003.

Heatley, E. V., Stark, J. M., Horsewood, P., Bandouvas, E., Cole, F., and Bienenstock, J. (1981). The effects of surgical removal of Peyer's patches in rat on systemic antibody responses to intestinal antigen. *Immunology* 44, 543–548.

Hiroi, T., Yanagita, M., Iijima, H., Iwatani, K., Yoshida, T., Takatsu, K., and Kiyono, H. (1999). Deficiency of IL-5 receptor alpha-chain

selectively influences the development of the common mucosal immune system independent IgA-producing B-1 cell in mucosa-associated tissues. *J. Immunol.* 162, 821–828.

Hiroi, T., Yanagita, M., Ohta, N., Sakaue, G., and Kiyono, H. (2000). IL-15 and IL-15 receptor selectively regulate differentiation of common mucosal immune system-independent B-1 cells for IgA responses. *J. Immunol.* 165, 4329–4337.

Honda, K., Nakano, H., Yoshida, H., Nishikawa, S., Rennert, P., Ikuta, K., Tamechika, M., Yamaguchi, K., Fukumoto, T., Chiba, T., and Nishikawa, S. I. (2001). Molecular basis for hematopoietic/mesenchymal interaction during initiation of Peyer's patch organogenesis. *J. Exp. Med.* 193, 621–630.

Hooper, L. V., and Gordon, J. I. (2001). Commensal host-bacterial relationships in the gut. *Science* 292, 1115–1118.

Howie, D., Spencer, J., DeLord, D., Pitzalis, C., Wathen, N. C., Dogan, A., Akbar, A. and MacDonald, T. T. (1998). Extrathymic T cell differentiation in the human intestine early in life. *J. Immunol.* 161, 5862–5872.

Hozumi, K., Kobori, A., Sato, T., Nishimura, T., and Habu, S. (1996). Transcription and demethylation of TCR β gene initiate prior to the gene rearrangement in c-kit⁺ thymocytes with CD3 expression: Evidence of T cell commitment in the thymus. *Int. Immunol.* 8, 1473–1481.

Husband, A. J., and Gowans, J. L. (1978). The origin and antigen-dependent distribution of IgA-containing cells in the intestine. *J. Exp. Med.* 148, 1146–1160.

Ibraghimov, A. R., and Lynch, R. G. (1994). Heterogeneity and biased T cell receptor αβ repertoire of mucosal CD8⁺ cells from murine large intestine: implications for functional state. *J. Exp. Med.* 180, 433–444.

Iijima, H., Takahashi, I., and Kiyono, H. (2001). Mucosal immune network in the gut for the control of infectious diseases. *Rev. Med. Virol.* 11, 117–133.

Ishikawa, H., Li, Y., Abeliovich, A., Yamamoto, S., Kaufmann, S. H., and Tonegawa, S. (1993). Cytotoxic and interferon γ-producing activities of γδ T cells in the mouse intestinal epithelium are strain dependent. *Proc. Natl. Acad. Sci. USA* 90, 8204–8208.

Ishikawa, H., Saito, H., Suzuki, K., Oida, T., and Kanamori, Y. (1999). New gut associated lymphoid tissue "cryptopatches" breed murine intestinal intraepithelial T cell precursors. *Immunol. Res.* 20, 243–250.

Iwasaki, A., and Kelsall, B. L. (1999). Freshly isolated Peyer's patch, but not spleen, dendritic cells produce interleukin 10 and induce the differentiation of T helper type 2 cells. *J. Exp. Med.* 190, 229–240.

Iwasaki, A., and Kelsall, B. L. (2000). Localization of distinct Peyer's patch dendritic cell subsets and their recruitment by chemokines macrophage inflammatory protein (MIP)-3alpha, MIP-3beta, and secondary lymphoid organ chemokine. *J. Exp. Med.* 191, 1381–1394.

Iwasaki, A., and Kelsall, B. L. (2001). Unique functions of CD11b⁺, CD8α⁺, and double-negative Peyer's patch dendritic cells. *J. Immunol.* 166, 4884–4890.

Jarry, A., Cerf-Bensussan, N., Brousse, N., Selz, F., and Guy-Grand, D. (1990). Subsets of CD3⁺ (T cell receptor α/β or γ/δ) and CD3⁻ lymphocytes isolated from normal human gut epithelium display phenotypical features different from their counterparts in peripheral blood. *Eur. J. Immunol.* 20, 1097–1103.

Kanamori, Y., Ishimaru, K., Nanno, M., Maki, K., Ikuta, K., Nariuchi, H., and Ishikawa, H. (1996). Identification of novel lymphoid tissues in murine intestinal mucosa where clusters of c-kit⁺ IL-7R⁺ Thy1⁺ lympho-hemopoietic progenitors develop. *J. Exp. Med.* 184, 1449–1459.

Karecla, P. I., Bowden, S. J., Green, S. J., and Kilshaw, P. J. (1995). Recognition of E-cadherin on epithelial cells by the mucosal T cell integrin α M290 β7 (αEβ7). *Eur. J. Immunol.* 25, 852–856.

Kawaguchi, M., Nanno, M., Umesaki, Y., Matsumoto, S., Okada, Y., Cai, Z., Shimamura, T., Matsuoka, Y., Ohwaki, M., and Ishikawa, H. (1993). Cytolytic activity of intestinal intraepithelial lymphocytes in germ-free mice is strain dependent and determined by T cells expressing γδ T-cell antigen receptors. *Proc. Natl. Acad. Sci. USA* 90, 8591–8594.

Kelsall, B. L., and Strober, W. (1996). Distinct populations of dendritic cells are present in the subepithelial dome and T cell regions of the murine Peyer's patch. *J. Exp. Med.* 183, 237–247.

Keren, D. F., Holt, P. S., Collins, H. H., Gemski, P., and Formal, S. B. (1978). The role of Peyer's patches in the local immune response of rabbit ileum to live bacteria. *J. Immunol.* 120, 1892–1896.

Kiyono, H., McGhee, Jerry R., and Michalek, S. M. (1980). Lipopolysaccharide regulation of the immune response: Comparison of responses to LPS in germfree, *Escherichia coli*-monoassociated and conventional mice. *J. Immunol.* 124, 36–41.

Klein, J. R. (1996). Whence the intestinal intraepithelial lymphocyte? *J. Exp. Med.* 184, 1203–1206.

Klein, J. R. (1998). Thymus-independent development of gut T cells. *Chem. Immunol.* 71, 88–102.

Klein, J. R., and Kagnoff, M. F. (1984). Nonspecific recruitment of cytotoxic effector cells in the intestinal mucosa of antigen-primed mice. *J. Exp. Med.* 160, 1931–1936.

Kong, Y. Y., Yoshida, H., Sarosi, I., Tan, H. L., Timms, E., Capparelli, C., Morony, S., Oliveira-dos-Santos, A. J., Van, G., Itie, A., Khoo, W., Wakeham, A., Dunstan, C. R., Lacey, D. L., Mak, T. W., Boyle, W. J., and Penninger, J. M. (1999). OPGL is a key regulator of osteoclastogenesis, lymphocyte development and lymph-node organogenesis. *Nature* 397, 315–323.

Koni, P. A., and Flavell, R. A. (1998). A role for tumor necrosis factor receptor type 1 in gut-associated lymphoid tissue development: Genetic evidence of synergism with lymphotoxin beta. *J. Exp. Med.* 187, 1977–1983.

Koni, P. A., Sacca, R., Lawton, P., Browning, J. L., Ruddle, N. H., and Flavell, R. A. (1997). Distinct roles in lymphoid organogenesis for lymphotoxins alpha and beta revealed in lymphotoxin beta-deficient mice. *Immunity* 6, 491–500.

Koningsberger, J. C., Chott, A., Logtenberg, T., Wiegman, L. J., Blumberg, R. S., van Berge Henegouwen, G. P., and Balk, S. P. (1997). TCR expression in human fetal intestine and identification of an early T cell receptor β-chain transcript. *J. Immunol.* 159, 1775–1782.

Koyasu, S., Clayton, L. K., Lerner, A., Heiken, H., Parkes, A., and Reinherz, E. L. (1997). Pre-TCR signaling components trigger transcriptional activation of a rearranged TCR α gene locus and silencing of the pre-TCR α locus: Implications for intrathymic differentiation. *Int. Immunol.* 9, 1475–1480.

Kroese, F. G., Butcher, E. C., Stall, A. M., Lalor, P. A., Adams, S., and Herzenberg, L. A. (1989). Many of the IgA producing plasma cells in murine gut are derived from self-replenishing precursors in the peritoneal cavity. *Int. Immunol.* 1, 75–84.

Kunkel, E. J., Campbell, J. J., Haraldsen, G., Pan, J., Boisvert, J., Roberts, A. I., Ebert, E. C., Vierra, M. A., Goodman, S. B., Genovese, M. C., Wardlaw, A. J., Greenberg, H. B., Parker, C. M., Butcher, E. C., Andrew, D. P., and Agace, W. W. (2000). Lymphocyte CC chemokine receptor 9 and epithelial thymus-expressed chemokine (TECK) expression distinguish the small intestinal immune compartment: Epithelial expression of tissue-specific chemokines as an organizing principle in regional immunity. *J. Exp. Med.* 192, 761–768.

Laky, K., Lefrancois, L., and Puddington, L. (1997). Age-dependent intestinal lymphoproliferative disorder due to stem cell factor receptor deficiency: Parameters in small and large intestine. *J. Immunol.* 158, 1417–1427.

Laky, K., Lefrancois, L., von Freeden-Jeffry, U., Murray, R., and Puddington, L. (1998). The role of IL-7 in thymic and extrathymic development of TCR γδ cells. *J. Immunol.* 161, 707–713.

Laky, K., Lefrancois, L., Lingenheld, E. G., Ishikawa, H., Lewis, J. M., Olson, S., Suzuki, K., Tigelaar, R. E., and Puddington, L. (2000). Enterocyte expression of interleukin 7 induces development of γδ T cells and Peyer's patches. *J. Exp. Med.* 191, 1569–1580.

Lambolez, F., Azogui, O., Joret, A-M., Garcia, C., von Boehmer, H., Di Santo, J., Ezine, S., and Rocha, B. (2002). Characterization of T cell differentiation in the murine gut. *J. Exp. Med.* 195, 437–449.

Latthe, M., Terry, L., and MacDonald, T. T. (1994). High frequency of CD8αα homodimer-bearing T cells in human fetal intestine. *Eur. J. Immunol.* 24, 1703–1705.

Lefrancois, L. (1991a). Extrathymic differentiation of intraepithelial lymphocytes: Generation of a separate and unequal T-cell repertoire? *Immunol. Today* 12, 436–438.

Lefrancois, L. (1991b). Phenotypic complexity of intraepithelial lymphocytes of the small intestine. *J. Immunol.* 147, 1746–1751.

Lefrancois, L., and Goodman, T. (1989). *In vivo* modulation of cytolytic activity and Thy-1 expression in TCR-γδ+ intraepithelial lymphocytes. *Science* 243, 1716–1718.

Lefrancois, L., and Puddington, L. (1999). Basic aspects of intraepithelial lymphocyte immunobiology. In *Mucosal Immunology*, ed. 2. (eds. P. L. Ogra, J. Mestecky, M. E. Lamm, W. Strober, J. Bienenstock, and J. R. McGhee), 413–428. San Diego: Academic Press.

Lefrancois, L., LeCorre, R., Mayo, J., Bluestone, J. A., and Goodman, T. (1990). Extrathymic selection of TCR γ/δ+ T cells by class II major histocompatibility complex molecules. *Cell* 63, 333–340.

Lin, T., Matsuzaki, G., Yoshida, H., Kobayashi, N., Kenai, H., Omoto, K., and Nomoto, K. (1994). CD3−CD8+ intestinal intraepithelial lymphocytes (IEL) and the extrathymic development of IEL. *Eur. J. Immunol.* 24, 1080–1087.

Liu, Y-J., Cairns, J. A., Holder, M. J., Abbot, S. D., Jansen, K. U., Bonnefoy, J-Y., Gordon, J. and MacLennan, I. C. (1991). Recombinant 25-kDa CD23 and interleukin 1 α promote the survival of germinal center B cells: Evidence for bifurcation in the development of centrocytes rescued from apoptosis. *Eur. J. Immunol.* 21, 1107–1114.

Liu, C. P., Ueda, R., She, J., Sancho, J., Wang, B., Weddell, G., Loring, J., Kurahara, C., Dudley, E. C., Hayday, A., Terhorst, C., and Huang, M. (1993). Abnormal T cell development in CD3ζ−/− mutant mice and identification of a novel T cell population in the intestine. *EMBO J.* 12, 4863–4875.

Lodolce, J. P., Boone, D. L., Chai, S., Swain, R. E., Dassopoulos, T., Trettin, S., and Ma, A. (1998). IL-15 receptor maintains lymphoid homeostasis by supporting lymphocyte homing and proliferation. *Immunity* 9, 669–676.

London, S. D., Rubin, D. H., and Cebra, J. J. (1987). Gut mucosal immunization with reovirus serotype 1/L stimulates virus-specific cytotoxic T cell precursors as well as IgA memory cells in Peyer's patches. *J. Exp. Med.* 165, 830–847.

London, S. D., Cebra-Thomas, J. A., Rubin, D. H., and Cebra, J. J. (1990). CD8 lymphocyte subpopulations in Peyer's patches induced by reovirus serotype 1 infection. *J. Immunol.* 144, 3187–3194.

Lorenz, R. G., Chaplin, D. D., McDonald, K. G., McDonough, J. S., and Newberry, R. D. (2003). Isolated lymphoid follicle formation is inducible and dependent upon lymphotoxin-sufficient B lymphocytes, lymphotoxin β receptor, and TNF receptor I function. *J. Immunol.* 170, 5475–5482.

Lundqvist, C., Baranov, V., Hammarstrom, S., Athlin, L., and Hammarstrom, M. L. (1995). Intra-epithelial lymphocytes. Evidence for regional specialization and extrathymic T cell maturation in the human gut epithelium. *Int. Immunol.* 7, 1473–1487.

Lynch, S., Kelleher, D., McManus, R., and O'Farrelly, C. (1995). RAG1 and RAG2 expression in human intestinal epithelium: Evidence of extrathymic T cell differentiation. *Eur. J. Immunol.* 25, 1143–1147.

MacDonald, T. T. (1994). Gastrointestinal inflammation: Inflammatory bowel disease in knockout mice. *Curr. Biol.* 4, 261–263.

Mackay, F., and Browning, J. L. (1998). Turning off follicular dendritic cells. *Nature* 395, 26–27

Macpherson, A. J., Gatto, D., Sainsbury, E., Harriman, G. R., Hengartner, H. Zinkernagel, R. M. (2000). A primitive T cell-independent mechanism of intestinal mucosal IgA responses to commensal bacteria. *Science* 288, 2222–2226.

Maki, K., Sunaga, S., and Ikuta, K. (1996). The V-J recombination of T cell receptor-γ genes is blocked in interleukin-7 receptor-deficient mice. *J. Exp. Med.* 184, 2423–2427.

Malissen, M., Gillet, A., Rocha, B., Trucy, J., Vivier, E., Boyer, C., Kontogen, F., Brun, N., Mazza, G., Spanopoulou, E., Guy-Grand, D., and Malissen, B. (1993). T cell development in mice lacking the CD3-ζ/μ gene. *EMBO J.* 12, 4347–4355.

Matsumoto, M., Iwamasa, K., Rennert, P. D., Yamada, T., Suzuki, R., Matsushima, A., Okabe, M., Fujita, S., and Yokoyama, M. (1999). Involvement of distinct cellular compartments in the abnormal lymphoid organogenesis in lymphotoxin-α-deficient mice and alymphoplasia (aly) mice defined by the chimeric immune analysis. *J. Immunol.* 163, 1584–1591.

Matsunaga, T. (1998). Did the first adaptive immunity evolve in the gut of ancient jawed fish? *Cytogenet. Cell. Genet.* 80, 138–141.

Matsushima, A., Kaisho, T., Rennert, P. D., Nakano, H., Kurosawa, K., Uchida, D., Takeda, K., Akira, S., and Matsumoto, M. (2001). Essential role of nuclear factor (NF)-κB-inducing kinase and inhibitor of κB (IκB) kinase α in NF-κB activation through lymphotoxin β-receptor, but not through tumor necrosis factor receptor I. *J. Exp. Med.* 193, 631–636.

Mauri, D. N., Ebner, R., Montgomery, R. I., Kochel, K. D., Cheung, T. C., Yu, G. L., Ruben, S., Murphy, M., Eisenberg, R. J., Cohen, G. H., Spear, P. G., and Ware, C. F. (1998). LIGHT, a new member of the TNF superfamily, and lymphotoxin alpha are ligands for herpesvirus entry mediator. *Immunity* 8, 21–30.

McGhee, J. R., Mestecky, J., Elson, C. O., and Kiyono, H. (1989). Regulation of IgA synthesis and immune response by T cells and interleukins. *J. Clin. Immunol.* 9, 175–199.

McIntyre, T. M., and Strober, S. (1999). Gut-associated lymphoid tissue: Regulation of IgA B-cell development. In *Mucosal Immunology*, ed. 2. (eds. R. L. Ogra, J. Mestecky, M. E. Lamm, W. Strober, J. Bienenstock, and J. R. McGhee), 319–356. San Diego: Academic Press.

Mebius, R. E., Rennert, P., and Weissman, I. L. (1997). Developing lymph nodes collect CD4⁺CD3⁻ LT-β⁺ cells that can differentiate to APC, NK cells, and follicular cells but not T or B cells. *Immunity* 7, 493–504.

Mestecky, J., Blumberg, R., Kiyono, H., and McGhee, J. R. (2003). The mucosal immune system. In *Fundamental Immunology*, ed. 5. (ed. W. E. Paul), pp. 965–1020. New York: LWW.

Miyawaki, S., Nakamura, Y., Suzuka, H., Koba, M., Yasumizu, R., Ikehara, S., and Shibata, Y. (1994). A new mutation, aly, that induces a generalized lack of lymph nodes accompanied by immunodeficiency in mice. *Eur. J. Immunol.* 24, 429–434.

Moghaddami, M., Cummins, A., and Mayrhofer, G. (1998). Lymphocyte-filled villi: Comparison with other lymphoid aggregations in the mucosa of the human small intestine. *Gastroenterology* 115, 1414–1425.

Moore, T. A., von Freeden-Jeffry, U., Murray, R., and Zlotnik, A. (1996). Inhibition of γδ T cell development and early thymocyte maturation in IL-7⁻/⁻ mice. *J. Immunol.* 157, 2366–2373.

Mosley, R. L., Styre, D., and Klein, J. R. (1990a). CD4⁺CD8⁺ murine intestinal intraepithelial lymphocytes. *Int. Immunol.* 2, 361–365.

Mosley, R. L., Styre, D., and Klein, J. R. (1990b). Differentiation and functional maturation of bone marrow-derived intestinal epithelial T cells expressing membrane T cell receptor in athymic radiation chimeras. *J. Immunol.* 145, 1369–1375.

Mowat, A. M. (2003). Anatomical basis of tolerance and immunity to intestinal antigens. *Nat. Rev. Immunol.* 3, 331–341.

Mowat, A. M., and Viney, J. L. (1997). The anatomical basis of intestinal immunity. *Immunol. Rev.* 156, 145–166.

Muramatsu, M., Kinoshita, K., Fagarasan, S., Yamada, S., Shinkai, Y., and Honjo, T. (2000). Class switch recombination and hypermutation require activation-induced cytidine deaminase (AID), a potential RNA editing enzyme. *Cell* 102, 553–563.

Nanno, M., Matsumoto, S., Koike, R., Miyasaka, M., Kawaguchi, M., Masuda, T., Miyawaki, S., Cai, Z., Shimamura, T., Fujiura, Y., and Ishikawa, H. (1994). Development of intestinal intraepithelial T lymphocytes is independent of Peyer's patches and lymph nodes in aly mutant mice. *J. Immunol.* 153, 2014–2020.

Nanno, M., Kanamori, Y., Saito, H., Kawaguchi-Miyashita, M., Shimada, S., and Ishikawa, H. (1998). Intestinal intraepithelial T lymphocytes: Our T cell horizons are expanding. *Immunol. Res.* 18, 41–53.

Neumann, B., Luz A., Pfeffer K., and Holzmann B. (1996). Defective Peyer's patch organogenesis in mice lacking the 55-kD receptor for tumor necrosis factor. *J. Exp. Med.* 184, 259–264.

Neutra, M. R., Frey, A. and Kraehenbuhl, J. P. (1996a). Epithelial M Cells: Gateways for mucosal infection and immunization. *Cell* 86, 345–348.

Neutra, M. R., Pringault, E., and Kraehenbuhl, J. P. (1996b). Antigen sampling across epithelial barriers and induction of mucosal immune responses. *Annu. Rev. Immunol.* 14, 275–300.

Neutra, M. R., Mantis, N. J., and Kraehenbuhl, J-P. (2001). Collaboration of epithelial cells with organized mucosal lymphoid tissues. *Nat. Immunol.* 2, 1004–1009.

Ohbo, K., Suda, T., Hashiyama, M., Mantani, A., Ikebe, M., Miyakawa, K., Moriyama, M., Nakamura, M., Katsuki, M., Takahashi, K., Yamamura, K., and Sugamura, K. (1996). Modulation of hematopoiesis in mice with a truncated mutant of the interleukin-2 receptor γ chain. *Blood* 87, 956–967.

Ohno, H., Aoe, T., Taki, S., Kitamura, D., Ishida, Y., Rajewsky, K., and Saito, T. (1993). Developmental and functional impairment of T cells in mice lacking CD3ζ chains. *EMBO J.* 12, 4357–4366.

Ohteki, T., Ho, S., Suzuki, H., Mak, T. W., and Ohashi, P. S. (1997). Role for IL-15/IL-15 receptor β-chain in natural killer 1.1⁺ T cell receptor-αβ⁺ cell development. *J. Immunol.* 159, 5931–5935.

Oida, T., Suzuki, K., Nanno, M., Kanamori, Y., Saito, H., Kubota, E., Kato, S., Itoh, M., Kaminogawa, S., and Ishikawa, H. (2000). Role of gut cryptopatches in early extrathymic maturation of intestinal intraepithelial T cells. *J. Immunol.* 164, 3616–3626.

O'Leary, A. D., and Sweeney, E. C. (1986). Lymphoglandular complexes of the colon: Structure and distribution. *Histopathology* 10, 267–283.

Onai, N., Zhang, Y., Yoneyama, H., Kitamura, T., Ishikawa, S., and Matsushima, K. (2000). Impairment of lymphopoiesis and myelopoiesis in mice reconstituted with bone marrow-hematopoietic progenitor cells expressing SDF-1-intrakine. *Blood* 96, 2074–2080.

Onai, N., Kitabatake, M., Zhang, Y. Y., Ishikawa, H., Ishikawa, S., and Matsushima, K. (2002). Pivotal role of CCL25 (TECK)–CCR9 in the formation of gut cryptopatches and consequent appearance of intestinal intraepithelial T lymphocytes. *Int. Immunol.* 14, 687–694.

Owen, R. L., and Bhalla, D. K. (1983). Cytochemical analysis of alkaline phosphatase and esterase activities and of lectin-binding and anionic sites in rat and mouse Peyer's patch M cells. *Am. J. Anat.* 168, 199–212.

Owen, R. L., and Jones, A. L. (1974). Epithelial cell specialization within human Peyer's patches: An ultrastructural study of intestinal lymphoid follicles. *Gastroenterology* 66, 189–203.

Owen, R. L., Cray, W. C. Jr., Ermak, T. H., and Pierce, N. F. (1988). Bacterial characteristics and follicle surface structure: Their roles in Peyer's patch uptake and transport of *Vibrio cholerae*. *Adv. Exp. Med. Biol.* 237, 705–715.

Page, S. T., Bogatzki, L. Y., Hamerman, J. A., Sweenie, C. H., Hogarth, P. J., Malissen, M., Perlmutter, R. M., and Pullen, A. M. (1998). Intestinal intraepithelial lymphocytes include precursors committed to the T cell receptor αβ lineage. *Proc. Natl. Acad. Sci. USA* 95, 9459–9464.

Pasparakis, M., Alexopoulou, L., Grell, M., Pfizenmaier, K., Bluethmann, H., and Kollias, G. (1997). Peyer's patch organogenesis is intact yet formation of B lymphocyte follicles is defective in peripheral lymphoid organs of mice deficient for tumor necrosis factor and its 55-kDa receptor. *Proc. Natl. Acad. Sci. USA* 94, 6319–6323.

Paxian, S., Merkle, H., Riemann, M., Wilda, M., Adler, G., Hameister, H., Liptay, S., Pfeffer, K., and Schmid, R. M. (2002). Abnormal organogenesis of Peyer's patches in mice deficient for NF-kappaB1, NF-kappaB2, and Bcl-3. *Gastroenterology* 122, 1853–1868.

Poussier, P., Edouard, P., Lee, C., Binnie, M., and Julius, M. (1992). Thymus-independent development and negative selection of T cells expressing T cell receptor α/β in the intestinal epithelium: Evidence for distinct circulation patterns of gut- and thymus-derived T lymphocytes. *J. Exp. Med.* 176, 187–199.

Poussier, P., Teh, H. S., and Julius, M. (1993). Thymus-independent positive and negative selection of T cells expressing a major histocompatibility complex class I restricted transgenic T cell receptor α/β in the intestinal epithelium. *J. Exp. Med.* 178, 1947–1957.

Powrie, F. (1995). T cells in inflammatory bowel disease: protective and pathogenic roles. *Immunity* 3, 171–174.

Price, A. B. (1985). Small intestinal biopsy. In *Disorders of the Small Intestine* (eds. C. C. Booth and G. Neale), 12–21. Oxford, England: Blackwell Scientific.

Puddington, L., Olson, S., and Lefrancois, L. (1994). Interactions between stem cell factor and c-kit are required for intestinal immune system homeostasis. *Immunity* 1, 733–739.

Ramanathan, S., Marandi, L., and Poussier, P. (2002). Evidence for the extrathymic origin of intestinal TCRγδ+ T cells in normal rats and for an impairment of this differentiation pathway in BB rats. *J. Immunol.* 168, 2182–2187.

Regnault, A., Cumano, A., Vassalli, P., Guy-Grand, D., and Kourilsky, P. (1994). Oligoclonal repertoire of the CD8αα and the CD8αβ TCR-α/β murine intestinal intraepithelial T lymphocytes: evidence for the random emergence of T cells. *J. Exp. Med.* 180, 1345–1358.

Rennert, P. D., Browning, J. L., Mebius, R., Mackay, F., and Hochman, P. S. (1996). Surface lymphotoxin alpha/beta complex is required for the development of peripheral lymphoid organs. *J. Exp. Med.* 184, 1999–2006.

Rennert, P. D., Browning, J. L., and Hochman, P. S. (1997). Selective disruption of lymphotoxin ligands reveals a novel set of mucosal lymph nodes and unique effects on lymph node cellular organization. *Int. Immunol.* 9, 1627–1639.

Rennert, P. D., James, D., Mackay, F., Browning, J. L., and Hochman, P. S. (1998). Lymph node genesis is induced by signaling through the lymphotoxin β receptor. *Immunity* 9, 71–79.

Rocha, B., Vassalli, P., and Guy-Grand, D. (1991). The Vβ repertoire of mouse gut homodimeric α CD8+ intraepithelial T cell receptor α/β+ lymphocytes reveals a major extrathymic pathway of T cell differentiation. *J. Exp. Med.* 173, 483–486.

Rodewald, H.-R., Kretzschmar, K., Takeda, S., Hohl, C., and Dessing, M. (1994). Identification of pro-thymocytes in murine fetal blood: T lineage commitment can precede thymus colonization. *EMBO J.* 13, 4229–4240.

Rosner, A. J., and Keren, D. F. (1984). Demonstration of M cells in the specialized follicle-associated epithelium overlying isolated lymphoid follicles in the gut. *J. Leukoc. Biol.* 35, 397–404.

Saint-Ruf, C., Ungewiss, K., Groettrup, M., Bruno, L., Fehling, H. J., and von Boehmer, H. (1994). Analysis and expression of a cloned pre-T cell receptor gene. *Science* 266, 1208–1212.

Saito, H., Kanamori, Y., Takemori, T., Nariuchi, H., Kubota, E., Takahashi-Iwanaga, H., Iwanaga, T., and Ishikawa, H. (1998). Generation of intestinal T cells from progenitors residing in gut cryptopatches. *Science* 280, 275–278.

Sato, K., Ohtsuka, K., Hasegawa, K., Yamagiwa, S., Watanabe, H., Asakura, H., and Abo, T. (1995). Evidence for extrathymic generation of intermediate T cell receptor cells in the liver revealed in thymectomized, irradiated mice subjected to bone marrow transplantation. *J. Exp. Med.* 182, 759–767.

Savidge, T. C., Smith, M. W., James, P. S., and Aldred, P. (1991). *Salmonella*-induced M-cell formation in germ-free mouse Peyer's patch tissues. *Am. J. Pathol.* 139, 177–184.

Scheu, S., Alferink, J., Potzel, T., Barchet, W., Kalinke, U., and Pfeffer, K. (2002). Targeted disruption of LIGHT causes defects in co-stimulatory T cell activation and reveals cooperation with lymphotoxin beta in mesenteric lymph node genesis. *J. Exp. Med.* 195, 1613–1624.

Shinkura, R., Kitada, K., Matsuda, F., Tashiro, K., Ikuta, K., Suzuki, M., Kogishi, K., Serikawa, T., and Honjo, T. (1999). Alymphoplasia is caused by a point mutation in the mouse gene encoding NF-kappa β-inducing kinase. *Nat. Genet.* 22, 74–77.

Shorter, R. G., and Tomasi, T. B. (1982). Immune mechanisms in the small intestine: Part 1. In *Gastroenterology 2* (eds. V. S. Chadwick and S. F. Phillips), 73–79. London: Butterworth Scientific.

Shortman, K., Vremec, D., Corcoran, L. M., Georgopoulos, K., Lucas, K., and Wu, L. (1998). The linkage between T-cell and dendritic cell development in the mouse thymus. *Immunol. Rev.* 165, 39–46.

Simmons, C. P., Clare, S., and Dougan, G. (2001). Understanding mucosal responsiveness: Lessons from enteric bacterial pathogens. *Semin. Immunol.* 13, 201–209.

Smith, M. W., James, P. S., and Tivey, D. R. (1987). M cell numbers increase after transfer of SPF mice to a normal animal house environment. *Am. J. Pathol.* 128, 385–389.

Sonoda, E., Matsumoto, R., Hitoshi, Y., Ishii, T., Sugimoto, M., Araki, S., Tominaga, A., Yamaguchi, N., and Takatsu, K. (1989). Transforming growth factor beta induces IgA production and acts additively with interleukin 5 for IgA production. *J. Exp. Med.* 170, 1415–1420.

Stancovski, I., and Baltimore, D. (1997). NF-κB activation: The I κB kinase revealed? *Cell* 91, 299–302.

Strober, W., and Ehrhardt, R. O. (1993). Chronic intestinal inflammation: An unexpected outcome in cytokine or T cell receptor mutant mice. *Cell* 75, 203–205.

Suzuki, H., Kundig, T. M., Furlonger, C., Wakeham, A., Timms, E., Matsuyama, T., Schmits, R., Simard, J. J., Ohashi, P. S., Griesser, T., Taniguchi, T., Paige, C. J., and Mak, T. W. (1995). Deregulated T cell activation and autoimmunity in mice lacking interleukin-2 receptor β. *Science* 268, 1472–1476.

Suzuki, H., Duncan, G. S., Takimoto, H., and Mak, T. W. (1997). Abnormal development of intestinal intraepithelial lymphocytes and peripheral natural killer cells in mice lacking the IL-2 receptor β chain. *J. Exp. Med.* 185, 499–505.

Suzuki, K., Oida, T., Hamada, H., Hitotsumatsu, O., Watanabe, M., Hibi, T., Yamamoto, H., Kubota, E., Kaminogawa, S., and Ishikawa, H. (2000). Gut cryptopatches: direct evidence of extrathymic anatomical sites for intestinal T lymphopoiesis. *Immunity* 13, 691–702.

Sydora, B. C., Mixter, P. F., Holcombe, H. R., Eghtesady, P., Williams, K., Amaral, M. C., Nel, A., and Kronenberg, M. (1993). Intestinal intraepithelial lymphocytes are activated and cytolytic but do not proliferate as well as other T cells in response to mitogenic signals. *J. Immunol.* 150, 2179–2191.

Thurnheer, M. C., Zuercher, A. W., Cebra, J. J., and Bos, N. A. (2003). B1 cells contribute to serum IgM, but not to intestinal IgA, production in gnotobiotic Ig allotype chimeric mice. *J. Immunol.* 170, 4564–4571.

Van Kerckhove, C., Russell, G. J., Deusch, K., Reich, K., Bhan, A. K., DerSimonian, H. and Brenner, M. B. (1992). Oligoclonality of human intestinal intraepithelial T cells. *J. Exp. Med.* 175, 57–63.

Viney, J. L., Kilshaw, P. J., and MacDonald, T. T. (1990). Cytotoxic α/β+ and γ/δ+ T cells in murine intestinal epithelium. *Eur. J. Immunol.* 20, 1623–1626.

Wang, B., Wang, N., Whitehurst, C. E., She, J., Chen, J., and Terhorst, C. (1999). T lymphocyte development in the absence of CD3ε or CD3γδεζ. *J. Immunol.* 162, 88–94.

Watanabe, M., Ueno, Y., Yajima, T., Iwao, Y., Tsuchiya, M., Ishikawa, H., Aiso, S., Hibi, T., and Ishii, H. (1995). Interleukin 7 is produced by human intestinal epithelial cells and regulates the proliferation of intestinal mucosal lymphocytes. *J. Clin. Invest.* 95, 2945–2953.

Weber, E. (1847). Uber den Mechanismus der Einsaugung des Speisesaftes beim Menschen und bei einigen tieren. *Physiol. Wissenschaftliche Med. Archiv Anat.* 400–402.

Weih, F., Carrasco, D., Durham, S. K., Barton, D. S., Rizzo, C. A., Ryseck, R. P., Lira, S. A., and Bravo, R. (1995). Multiorgan inflammation and hematopoietic abnormalities in mice with a targeted disruption of RelB, a member of the NF-kappa B/Rel family. *Cell* 80, 331–340.

Weih, D. S., Yilmaz, Z. B., and Weih, F. (2001). Essential role of RelB in germinal center and marginal zone formation and proper expression of homing chemokines. *J. Immunol.* 167, 1909–1919.

Weinstein, D. L., O'Neill, B. L., Hone, D. M., and Metcalf, E. S. (1998). Differential early interactions between *Salmonella enterica* serovar Typhi and two other pathogenic *Salmonella* serovars with intestinal epithelial cells. *Infect. Immun.* 66, 2310–2318.

Weinstein, P. D., Schweitzer, P. A., Cebra-Thomas, J. A., and Cebra, J. J. (1991). Molecular genetic features reflecting the preference for isotype switching to IgA expression by Peyer's patch germinal center B cells. *Int. Immunol.* 3, 1253–1263.

Wells, J. M., and Melton, D. A. (1999). Vertebrate endoderm development. *Annu. Rev. Cell. Dev. Biol.* 15, 393–410.

Wilson, A., and MacDonald, H. R. (1995). Expression of genes encoding the pre-TCR and CD3 complex during thymus development. *Int. Immunol.* 7, 1659–1664.

Wolf, J. L., Rubin, D. H., Finberg, R., Kauffman, R. S., Sharpe, A. H., Trier, J. S., and Fields, B. N. (1981). Intestinal M cells: A pathway for entry of reovirus into the host. *Science* 212, 471–472.

Wu, L., Antica, M., Johnson, G. R., Scollay, R., and Shortman, K. (1991a). Developmental potential of the earliest precursor cells from the adult mouse thymus. *J. Exp. Med.* 174, 1617–1627.

Wu, L., Scollay, R., Egerton, M., Pearse, M., Spangrude, G. J., and Shortman, K. (1991b). CD4 expressed on earliest T-lineage precursor cells in the adult murine thymus. *Nature* 349, 71–74.

Wurbel, M. A., Philippe, J. M., Nguyen, C., Victorero, G., Freeman, T., Wooding, P., Miazek, A., Mattei, M. G., Malissen, M., Jordan, B. R., Malissen, B., Carrier, A., and Naquet, P. (2000). The chemokine TECK is expressed by thymic and intestinal epithelial cells and attracts double- and single-positive thymocytes expressing the TECK receptor CCR9. *Eur. J. Immunol.* 30, 262–271.

Wurbel, M. A., Malissen, M., Guy-Grand, D., Meffre, E., Nussenzweig, M. C., Richelme, M., Carrier, A., and Malissen, B. (2001). Mice lacking the CCR9 CC-chemokine receptor show a mild impairment of early T- and B-cell development and a reduction in T-cell receptor γδ⁺ gut intraepithelial lymphocytes. *Blood* 98, 2626–2632.

Xu-Amano, J., Kiyono, H., Jackson, R. J., Staats, H. F., Fujihashi, K., Burrows, P. D., Elson, C. O., Pillai, S., and McGhee, J. R. (1993). Helper T cell subsets for immunoglobulin A responses: Oral immunization with tetanus toxoid and cholera toxin as adjuvant selectively induces Th2 cells in mucosa associated tissues. *J. Exp. Med.* 178, 1309–1320.

Yamamoto, M., Rennert, P., McGhee, J. R., Kweon, M.-N., Yamamoto, S., Dohi, T., Otake, S., Bluethmann, H., Fujihashi, K., and Kiyono, H. (2000). Alternate mucosal immune system: Organized Peyer's patches are not required for IgA responses in the gastrointestinal tract. *J. Immunol.* 164, 5184–5191.

Yilmaz, Z. B., Weih, D. S., Sivakumar, V., and Weih, F. (2003). RelB is required for Peyer's patch development: Differential regulation of p52-RelB by lymphotoxin and TNF. *EMBO J.* 22, 121–130.

Yin, L., Wu, L., Wesche, H., Arthur, C. D., White, J. M., Goeddel, D. V., and Schreiber, R. D. (2001). Defective lymphotoxin-beta receptor-induced NF-kappaB transcriptional activity in NIK-deficient mice. *Science* 291, 2162–2165.

Yoshida, H., Honda, K., Shinkura, R., Adachi, S., Nishikawa, S., Maki, K., Ikuta, K., and Nishikawa, S.-I. (1999). IL-7 receptor α⁺ CD3⁻ cells in the embryonic intestine induces the organizing center of Peyer's patches. *Int. Immunol.* 11, 643–655.

Yoshie, O., Imai, T., and Nomiyama, H. (2001). Chemokines in immunity. *Adv. Immunol.* 78, 57–110.

Zabel, B. A., Agace, W. W., Campbell, J. J., Heath, H. M., Parent, D., Roberts, A. I., Ebert, E. C., Kassam, N., Qin, S., Zovko, M., LaRosa, G. J., Yang, L. L., Soler, D., Butcher, E. C., Ponath, P. D., Parker, C. M., and Andrew, D. P. (1999). Human G protein-coupled receptor GPR-9-6/CC chemokine receptor 9 is selectively expressed on intestinal homing T lymphocytes, mucosal lymphocytes, and thymocytes and is required for thymus-expressed chemokine-mediated chemotaxis. *J. Exp. Med.* 190, 1241–1256.

Zuniga-Pflucker, J. C., and Lenardo, M. J. (1996). Regulation of thymocyte development from immature progenitors. *Curr. Opin. Immunol.* 8, 215–224.

Human Gut-Associated Lymphoid Tissues

Chapter 22

Thomas T. MacDonald

Division of Infection, Inflammation, and Repair, University of Southampton School of Medicine, Southampton, United Kingdom

Giovanni Monteleone

Cattedra di Gastroenterologia, Department Medicina Interna, Università Tor Vergata, Rome, Italy

INTRODUCTION

The true gut-associated lymphoid tissues (GALT) in humans are the Peyer's patches (PP), small intestinal isolated lymphoid follicles, the appendix, and colonic lymphoid follicles. GALT also appears in the stomach as a consequence of *Helicobacter pylori* infection. The oropharyngeal lymphoid tissues and the mesenteric lymph nodes show features of both systemic and mucosal lymphoid tissues. It needs to be emphasized that many of the paradigms of mucosal immunology are derived from rodents, yet huge differences exist between the mucosal immune sytem of rodents, humans, and other species such as sheep. Examples include the fact that mice have 8–10 PP, whereas humans have hundreds; mice have thousands of small aggregates of lymphoid cells, cryptopatches, which function as primary lymphoid tissues, whereas humans have none; at birth the mucosal immune system of a mouse is virtually nonexistent, whereas humans have a well-developed gut immune system from 19 weeks' gestation; and finally, γδ cells are abundant in the gut epithelium of mice, but make up only a small percentage of normal human intraepithelial lymphocytes (IEL). These phenotypic and structural differences are worthy of mention, but more important are the functional differences, which are becoming increasingly apparent.

There is only a limited literature on human GALT, and much of it is descriptive. The reason for this is that, although the literature contains illustrations of the gross morphology of human PP as seen from the lumen, if one examines a specimen of small intestine taken from a patient, PP are not visible. The most common surgical specimens available for functional studies are colons resected for carcinoma. Colonic follicles are also not visible because the follicle is submucosal and the dome region is small. Because the human gut wall is thick, the white areas of lymphoid tissue do not stand out as they do in mice. Interestingly, there may be 5–10 follicles per

square centimeter of colonic mucosa (Dukes and Bussey 1926; Langman and Rowland 1986), so when a cell suspension is made of colonic mucosa, it is a mixture of lymphocytes from the follicles and cells from the lamina propria. Right hemicolectomies from patients with carcinoma are also a source of normal ileum, but if one examines this tissue, even with a dissecting microscope, the PP cannot be seen. If the tissue is fixed in acetic acid, the follicle become very obvious as white areas on a translucent background, but this precludes functional studies.

One way to sample human PP is to biopsy them during ileoscopy (MacDonald *et al.* 1987). However this requires skilled endoscopists, and it biases the samples obtained toward children and adolescents, because like all lymphoid tissue, GALT is larger in children than it is in adults (Cornes 1965). **Figure 22.1** illustrates the endoscopic appearance of PP as seen through the endoscope in a normal child and in a child with ileal lymphoid hyperplasia.

Strictly speaking, the lamina propria and gut epithelium are not "lymphoid tissues"; their function is primarily nutrient absorption, but because the gut is constantly exposed to antigens, and because mucosal immune responses must be expressed along the length of the bowel and not just in organized GALT, in healthy people the lamina propria and epithelium are filled with T cells, plasma cells, mast cells, macrophages (MØ), and dendritic cells (DCs). This has been termed "physiologic inflammation," but it is really a diffuse, largely mononuclear, infiltrate.

DISTRIBUTION AND STRUCTURE OF ORGANIZED GALT IN HUMANS

The organized lymphoid structures of the gastrointestinal (GI) tract have anatomic features in common that distinguish

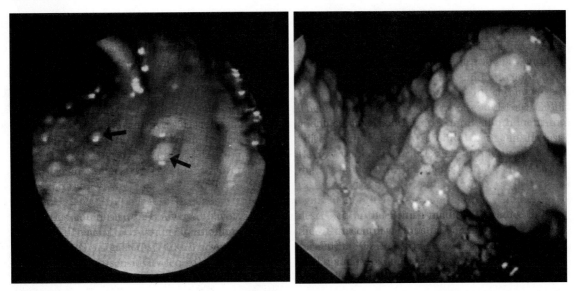

Fig. 22.1. Endoscopic images of Peyer's patches in the terminal ileum. The image on the left shows Peyer's patches as small white protuberances. The image on the right is a healthy child who has ileal lymphoid hyperplasia, a condition of unknown origin in immunologically normal children.

them from other secondary lymphoid tissues such as the lymph nodes in the groin and neck. The most obvious of these common features is the lack of a defined fibrous tissue capsule around the lymphoid tissue or afferent lymphatics. Thus, whereas in lymph nodes the demarcation between lymphocytes and surrounding tissues is easily visible because of the barrier of the capsule, in the gut lymphoid tissue the lateral aspects of the follicles diffuse into the surrounding lamina propria, and what might appear to be an accumulation of lymphocytes in the lamina propria (i.e., inflammation) in fact may be the edge of a follicle.

Structurally PP are organized areas of lymphoid tissue in the mucosa of the small bowel. They are overlain by a specialized lymphoepithelium (the follicle-associated epithelium, FAE) without crypts or villi. There are about 100–300 PP in the whole small intestine by late adolescence, and this decreases with increasing age (Cornes 1965). However, Cornes only counted PP with more than five follicles and there are many hundreds, probably tens of thousands more that have only one to four follicles. More recently, PP have been counted in the last 2 m of the human small bowel (Van Kruiningen et al. 2002). In this study a PP was defined as having at least three follicles, and only around 30 were identified, which is considerably less than Cornes demonstrated. It is unlikely that these differences are attributable to the difference in the size of specimen examined. The colon also contains many thousands of isolated lymphoid follicles (Dukes and Bussey 1926; Langman and Rowland 1986) with the highest density in the rectum. The normal human jejunum also contains structures that have been termed "lymphocyte-filled villi" (Moghaddami et al. 1998). On histologic sections they appear as short squat villi filled with T cells and a variable number of B cells. They have an FAE, which is infiltrated with CD4-positive (CD4+) T cells.

A spectacular exuberance of human GALT is seen in a condition termed "ileal lymphoid hyperplasia" (ILH, Fig. 22.1). ILH is not a pathologic, inflammatory condition, and it should not be confused with ileitis, which is inflammation of the ileal mucosa, as in Crohn's disease. The histologic appearance of the enlarged follicles in ILH is identical to that seen in the follicles of patients without gut disease, and both show extensive immune reactivity (such as large germinal centers containing tingible body MØ) (Webster et al. 1977). The classical association of ILH in the gut is with antibody deficiency states (Heremans et al. 1966; Adjukiewicz et al. 1972). These patients display nodular lymphoid hyperplasia of the upper and lower small bowel and colon, and often are infected with the parasite *Giardia lamblia* (Eidelman 1976). It is not known why patients with antibody deficiencies show ILH, although the infection with *G. lamblia* is probably because these patients do not secrete IgM or IgA, which is needed to prevent this microbe from binding to the surface of gut epithelial cells. Very recently mice have been made who are only able to make IgM antibody responses and cannot make IgG or IgA responses (Fagarasan et al. 2002). A striking feature of these animals is that they also develop hyperplastic lymphoid follicles with large germinal centers, and this is associated with a massive increase in the numbers of bacteria in their small intestines. If the bacteria are cleared with antibiotics, the hyperplasia subsides. The genetic defect in these mice produces very much the same immunologic effects as are seen in patients with common variable immunodeficiency. Taken together, the mouse data give an indication that ILH seen in patients may be driven by colonization of the small intestine with large numbers of bacteria. Consistent with this, there is evidence that patients with antibody deficiencies also show increased colonization of the small bowel with bacteria

(Brown *et al.* 1972). Very recently, Kokkonen and Kartunnen (2002) reported that 85% of children who had no evidence of colonic inflammation had ILH, and this was weakly associated with food allergy.

There is very little difference between mice and humans in the histology of PP or colonic follicles **(Fig. 22.2)**. Each is overlain by a dome epithelium with M cells. Below the epithelium, there is the dome region, which contains DCs, T cells, B cells, and MØ. Dendritic cells in the dome are CD11c$^+$ and so probably correspond to myeloid DCs, whereas plasmacytoid DCs, identified by expression of CD123, are not found in the dome, but are common in the T-cell zones between the follicles (Jameson *et al.* 2002). The B cells become more dense in the mantle zone, and there is almost invariably a large germinal center in a PP (Spencer *et al.* 1986). This is different from the colonic follicles, only a minority of which have germinal centers (O'Leary and Sweeney 1986). The T cells (mostly CD4$^+$ T cells) lie between the follicles surrounding the high endothelial venules, which express MAdCAM-1 **(Fig. 22.3)**. In a very detailed study, Farstad and colleagues (1997) identified activated T cells near the microlymphatics draining the PP, which may represent T cells responding to luminal antigens leaving the PP and trafficking to the mucosa.

IMMUNE FUNCTION IN HUMAN GALT

The PP are clearly the site for induction of the secretory-IgA (S-IgA) response (Chapter 21). However, there has been very little functional work on T cells in human GALT. Several years ago, we observed that it was possible to visualize PP in the ileums of children undergoing colonoscopy for suspected inflammatory bowel disease (MacDonald *et al.* 1987). The PP could be selectively biopsied and compared with biopsies

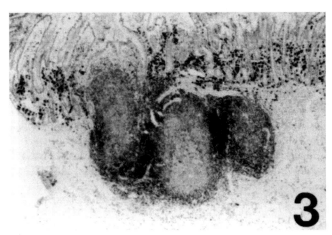

Fig. 22.3. T cells in a normal human Peyer's patch. Note that they predominate between the follicles. Immunoperoxidase with anti-CD3 antibody, original magnification ×10.

taken of adjacent mucosa. Thus it was possible to sample both the inductive and effector phases of the human mucosal immune response.

If a comparison is made of the spontaneous cytokine production by enzyme-linked immunospot (ELISPOT) of peripheral blood T cells, the PP T cells, and mucosal lamina propria T cells from normal children, several striking features emerge (Hauer *et al.* 1998). As expected, blood cells show virtually no cytokine-secreting cells. The PP, however, show a very high percentage of cells that continue to secrete cytokines when taken from the patient and cultured overnight. The response is dominated by interferon-γ–secreting cells, with few interleukin-4–secreting (IL-4–secreting), IL-5–secreting, or IL-10–secreting cells **(Fig. 22.4)**. The same pattern is seen with lamina propria T cells, and if anything, the interferon-γ response is greater. When PP cells are placed in culture, they spontaneously release large amounts of interferon-γ (IFN-γ) into the culture supernatant and only trace amounts of IL-2, IL-4, IL-5, or IL-10 (Monteleone *et al.* 2003).

In an effort to determine if antigen-specific Th1-type responses also occurred, PP cells were stimulated with cow's milk protein antigens *in vitro*, in an effort to generate a recall response (Nagata *et al.* 2000). Surprisingly, PP T cells gave strong antigen-specific response to β-lactoglobulin (β-lg), whereas peripheral blood T cells gave weak responses. Responsiveness was verified by the observation that β-lg induced a large increase in the number of CD4$^+$, CD25$^+$ in cultures of PP, but not in peripheral blood. These results were also verified by polymerase chain reaction (PCR). In seeking an explanation for this response, it was observed that PP contained abundant transcripts for IL-12 p40, that PP cells secreted IL-12 p70 into culture supernatants, and that IL-12 p70 could be visualized in cells below the dome epithelium.

The abundance of IL-12 in the PP therefore means that when a T cell responds to a nominal peptide antigen, it does so in an environment biased toward Th1 cells, which explains

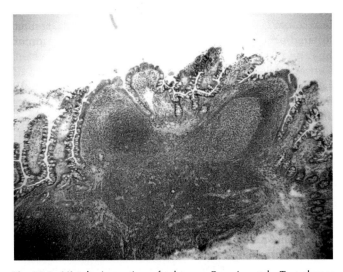

Fig. 22.2. Histologic section of a human Peyer's patch. Two domes are clearly visible, and there is a large germinal center in the follicle on the right. H&E, original magnification ×10.

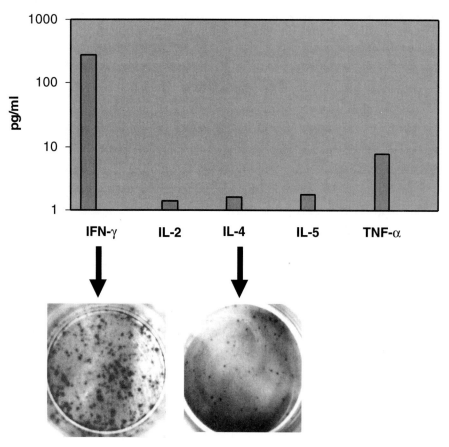

Fig. 22.4. When normal human Peyer's patch cells are placed in culture overnight, there is spontaneous production of IFN-γ and negligible production of IL-2, IL-4, IL-5, or TNF-α. To emphasize this, ELISPOT data on normal human Peyer's patch cells are also shown. The IFN-γ ELISPOT well contained 5000 cells, whereas the IL-4 well contained 40,000 cells, and yet it is clear that the response is dominated by IFN-γ. (Data adapted from Hauer *et al.* 1998 and Monteleone *et al.* 2003.)

the high level of spontaneous interferon-γ–secreting cells and the interferon-γ dominated response to β-lg.

By Western blotting, IL-12 p70 was easily demonstrable in protein extracts of human PP. The T-cell response to IL-12 is dependent on the expression of high-affinity IL-12 receptor (IL-12R) composed by two subunits, IL-12Rβ1 and IL-12Rβ2, with the IL-12Rβ2 chain being the critical signaling component. IL-12Rβ2 RNA was consistently detected in CD4+ and CD8+ PP and lamina propria lymphocytes (LPL) but not peripheral blood leukocytes (PBL) (Monteleone *et al.*, 2003). The effect of IL-12 on Th1 cell differentiation depends specifically on rapid phosphorylation and activation of signal transducer and activator of transcription 4 (STAT4). Activated STAT4 was seen in all PP and mucosal biopsies analyzed, but not in freshly isolated human PBL. In contrast, active STAT6, a transcription factor induced by IL-4 and associated with the development of Th2 cells, was weakly expressed in PP and ileal mucosal biopsies. STAT4 was detectable in nuclear extracts of PP T cells and EMSA analysis demonstrated

specific STAT4 binding to target DNA. The new transcription factor, T-bet, is sufficient in initiating Th1 differentiation and repressing Th2 cell responses. Nuclear proteins extracted from PPL all show immunoreactivity with anti-T-bet (Monteleone *et al.*, 2003).

Anti-IL-12 antibody almost completely inhibited the increase in interferon-γ production induced by superantigen activated PP T cells. Overall, therefore, the evidence is quite overwhelming that the default T-cell response in the PP of the human terminal ileum is along the Th1 pathway.

FACTORS THAT MAY INDUCE IL-12 IN HUMAN PP

The key issue therefore is the identification of the factors that induce the high expression of IL-12 in human PP, probably in subepithelial DCs and MØ. IL-12 is produced by monocytes and DCs in response to bacteria or bacterial products (Trinchieri and Scott 1999), and the M cells in the

FAE are almost certainly constantly transporting bacterial products and other luminal bioactive molecules, such as bacterial DNA containing CpG motifs, into the dome region of the PP. The human ileum has an abundant and diverse indigenous microflora (Peach *et al.* 1978; Keighley *et al.* 1978), and even in the upper bowel, where there are fewer PP, *H. pylori* in the stomach of many individuals, oral microbes, and microbes in foods must also be transported in the jejunal follicles.

Subepithelial DCs will almost certainly express toll-like receptors (TLRs), although this has not yet been studied in human or in experimental animals. Peptidoglycans and lipoproteins from gram-positive bacteria can activate DCs through TLR2. Lipopolysaccharide from gram-negative bacteria can activate through TLR4 and CpG DNA through TLR9 (Kaisho and Akira 2001). Although the interest in TLRs has arisen through their roles as pathogen recognition molecules, in the gut with an abundant indigenous microbial flora, there is no *a priori* reason why peptidoglycans, lipopolysaccharide, and lipoteichoic acids from this source should not also be capable of acting as ligands for TLRs. Engagement of TLRs by products of the normal flora would then activate nuclear factor (NF)-κB and the p38 mitogen-activated protein kinase via the adapter protein MyD88 and increase IL-12 production (O'Neil and Dinarello 2000; Thomas-Uszynski *et al.* 2000). IL-12 would then drive any T cell responding to antigen in the PP along a Th1 pathway **(Fig. 22.5)**.

ARE PP INVOLVED IN INFLAMMATORY BOWEL DISEASE?

The classical early sign of Crohn's disease is the punched out aphthoid ulcer in an otherwise endoscopically normal mucosa (Rickert and Carter 1980). Histology of these ulcers shows disintegration of the FAE and ulceration of the dome region overlying a colonic or ileal lymphoid follicle (Fujimura *et al.* 1992). There is no satisfactory observation for this finding, although it is universally observed. However, there are two possible ways in which it could tie in with the immunology of Crohn's disease as we now know it (a strongly polarized Th1 response with abundant mucosal IL-12 (MacDonald and Monteleone 2003). First, the patchy lesions may have their origins in the follicles, and as it becomes more severe, the follicle is obliterated. Since the normal ileal PP is a strong Th1 environment anyway, with abundant IL-12, perhaps merely a quantitative increase in the PP Th1 response, to a member of the flora that has entered the dome region and persisted, may be sufficient to induce enough local TNF-α and IFN-γ production to increase adhesion molecule expression and allow the emigration of blood-borne cells into the PP. TNF-α could also activate PP myofibroblasts to secrete matrix metalloproteinases, which could digest the basement membrane, and the epithelium would fall off (MacDonald and Pender 2003). There is some evidence that the *NOD2* mutation makes epithelial cells at least less able to kill bacteria

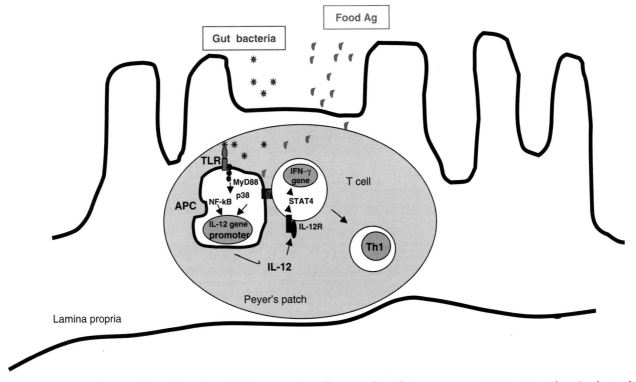

Fig. 22.5. Illustration of the possible pathway by which the normal gut flora can drive Th1-type responses in Peyer's patches. Products of the normal flora signal to Peyer's patch DCs through TLRs and induce IL-12 production. IL-12 then activates STAT4 in virgin T cells responding to luminal antigens. Importantly, once the T cells make IFN-γ in the Peyer's patches, this also maintains the Th1-type environment because IFN-γ induces T-bet in T cells, the major transcription factor involved in Th1 differentiation.

(Hisamatsu *et al.* 2003), and it may also be the case that it renders PP MØ less capable of killing bacteria. Bacteria may therefore persist and engender a large Th1-cell response. This is not likely to be the whole story because aphthous ulcers occur in Crohn's patients at a much higher frequency than those with the *NOD2* mutation.

The second notion is that the ulcer reflects enhanced immune activity to luminal antigens, and activation of CD4[+] T cells. These T cells would then migrate to the lamina propria in quantitatively higher numbers, increasing the chance that they may reencounter the same antigen in the lamina propria, secrete proinflammatory cytokines, and begin a local response.

THE APPENDIX

Although the appendix (like the tonsil) is readily available, there are no recent published reports on the function of appendix lymphocytes. However, for many years it has been observed that, in patients with distal colitis, there was often reddening at the mouth of the appendix (Yang *et al.* 1999). There has now been a number of studies that show clearly that appendectomy protects against the development of ulcerative colitis. Moreover, patients who were appendectomized but did develop ulcerative colitis (UC) have less severe disease (Radford-Smith *et al.* 2002; Cosnes *et al.* 2002). The protective effect may also occur in Crohn's disease (Radford-Smith *et al.* 2002). These results are fascinating, given the role that the appendix plays in generating B-cell diversity in other species such as the rabbit (Mage *et al.* 1998), taken together with the fact that the most prominent immunologic feature of UC is a massive IgG plasma cell infiltrate and local complement activation (Kett *et al.* 1987; Halstensen *et al.* 1992). Whether UC is an autoimmune disease or an antibody-mediated hypersensitivity response to the flora, these data strongly suggest the involvement of the appendix in sensitization, and this area deserves more research.

CONCLUSIONS

Despite the importance of the organized lymphoid tissue of the gut wall in the genesis of mucosal immune responses, our understanding of the biology of these tissues in humans is still rudimentary. However, there is absolutely no doubt that as far as T cells are concerned, the default pathway of lamina propria T cells in normal individuals is along the Th1 pathway (Fuss *et al.* 1996; Hauer *et al.* 1997, 1998; Carol *et al.* 1998). The reason for this polarization almost certainly lies in the fact that human PP contain IL-12 and interferon-γ, which induces T-bet and STAT4 activation in virgin T cells when they encounter immunogenic peptides in the PP microenvironment. Once activated in PP, these cells then migrate to the lamina propria. At this site in healthy individuals, there is an absence of IL-12, IL-18, and IFN-α, which

promote Th1-cell survival and a relative abundance of TGF-β1, IL-10, and prostaglandin E2 (PGE2). In the generally immunosuppressive environment of the normal lamina propria, it appears that most T cells then die by apoptosis (Bu *et al.* 2001).

ACKNOWLEDGMENTS

The authors wish to thank the Biotechnology and Biological Sciences Research Council for their continuing support of this work and Kirsteen Coombs for assistance in preparing the manuscript. We also wish to thank all our valued colleagues who have supplied biopsies of PP and who participated in this work, notably Christopher Williams, Jo Spencer, Simon Murch, Rob Heuschkel, Mark Beattie, Mike Thompson, Nick Croft, Peter Fairclough, Catriona McKenzie, and Satoru Nagata.

REFERENCES

Ajdukiewicz, A. B., Youngs, G. R., and Bouchier, I. A. (1972). Nodular lymphoid hyperplasia with hypogammaglobulinaemia. *Gut* 13, 589–595.

Brown, W. R., Savage, D. C., Dubois, R. S., Alp, M. H., Mallory, A., and Kern, F., Jr. (1972). Intestinal microflora of immunoglobulin-deficient and normal human subjects. *Gastroenterology* 62, 1143–1152.

Bu, P., Keshavarzian, A., Stone, D. D., Liu, J., Le, P. T., Fisher, S., and Qiao, L. (2001). Apoptosis: One of the mechanisms that maintains unresponsiveness of the intestinal mucosal immune system. *J. Immunol.* 166, 6399–6403.

Carol, M., Lambrechts, A., Van Gossum, A., Libin, M., Goldman, M., and Mascart-Lemone, F. (1998). Spontaneous secretion of interferon gamma and interleukin 4 by human intraepithelial and lamina propria gut lymphocytes. *Gut* 42, 643–649.

Cornes, J. S. (1965). Number, size, and distribution of Peyer's patches in the human small intestine. l. Part I. (1965). *Gut* 6, 225–233.

Cosnes, J., Carbonnel, F., Beaugerie, L., Blain, A., Reijasse, D., and Gendre, J. P. (2002). Effects of appendicectomy on the course of ulcerative colitis. *Gut* 51, 803–807.

Dukes, C. and Bussey, H. J. R. (1926). The number of lymphoid follicles of the human large intestine. *J. Pathol. Bact.* 111–116.

Eidelman, S. (1976). Intestinal lesions in immune deficiency. *Hum. Pathol.* 7, 427–434.

Fagarasan, S., Muramatsu, M., Suzuki, K., Nagaoka, H., Hiai, H., and Honjo, T. (2002). Critical roles of activation-induced cytidine deaminase in the homeostasis of gut flora. *Science* 298, 1424–1427.

Farstad, I. N., Norstein, J., and Brandtzaeg, P. (1997). Phenotypes of B and T cells in human intestinal and mesenteric lymph. *Gastroenterology* 112, 163–173.

Fujimura, Y., Hosobe, M., and Kihara, T. (1992). Ultrastructural study of M cells from colonic lymphoid nodules obtained by colonoscopic biopsy. *Dig. Dis. Sci.* 37, 1089–1098.

Fuss, I. J., Neurath, M., Boirivant, M., Klein, J. S., de la Motte C., Strong, S. A., Fiocchi, C., and Strober, W. (1996). Disparate CD4+ lamina propria (LP) lymphokine secretion profiles in inflammatory bowel disease: Crohn's disease LP cells manifest increased secretion of IFN-gamma, whereas ulcerative colitis LP cells manifest increased secretion of IL-5. *J. Immunol.* 157, 1261–1270.

Halstensen, T. S., Mollnes, T. E., Garred, P., Fausa, O., and Brandtzaeg, P. (1992). Surface epithelium related activation of complement differs in Crohn's disease and ulcerative colitis. *Gut* 33, 902–908.

Hauer, A. C., Breese, E. J., Walker-Smith, J. A., and MacDonald, T. T. (1997). The frequency of cells secreting interferon-gamma and interleukin-4, -5, and -10 in the blood and duodenal mucosa of children with cow's milk hypersensitivity. *Pediatr. Res.* 42, 629–638.

Hauer, A. C., Bajaj-Elliott, M., Williams, C. B., Walker-Smith, J. A., and MacDonald, T. T. (1998). An analysis of interferon gamma, IL-4, IL-5 and IL-10 production by ELISPOT and quantitative reverse transcriptase-PCR in human Peyer's patches. *Cytokine* 10, 627–634.

Hermans, P. E., Huizenga, K. A., Hoffman, H. N., Brown, A. L., Jr., and Markowitz, H (1966). Dysgammaglobulinemia associated with nodular lymphoid hyperplasia of the small intestine. *Am. J. Med.* 40, 78–89.

Hisamatsu, T., Suzuki, M., Reinecker, H. C., Nadeau, W. J., McCormick, B. A., and Podolsky, D. K. (2003). CARD15/NOD2 functions as an antibacterial factor in human intestinal epithelial cells. *Gastroenterology* 124, 993–1000.

Jameson, B., Baribaud, F., Pohlmann, S., Ghavimi, D., Mortari, F., Doms, R. W., and Iwasaki, A. (2002). Expression of DC-SIGN by dendritic cells of intestinal and genital mucosae in humans and rhesus macaques. *J. Virol.* 76, 1866–1875.

Kaisho, T., and Akira, S. (2001). Dendritic-cell function in Toll-like receptor- and MyD88-knockout mice. *Trends Immunol.* 22, 78–83.

Keighley, M. R., Arabi, Y., Dimock, F., Burdon, D. W., Allan, R. N., and Alexander-Williams, J. (1978). Influence of inflammatory bowel disease on intestinal microflora. *Gut* 19, 1099–1104.

Kett, K., Rognum, T. O., and Brandtzaeg, P. (1987). Mucosal subclass distribution of immunoglobulin G-producing cells is different in ulcerative colitis and Crohn's disease of the colon. *Gastroenterology* 93, 919–924.

Kokkonen, J., and Karttunen, T. J. (2002). Lymphonodular hyperplasia on the mucosa of the lower gastrointestinal tract in children: An indication of enhanced immune response? *J. Pediatr. Gastroenterol. Nutr.* 34, 42–46.

Langman, J. M., and Rowland, R. (1986). The number and distribution of lymphoid follicles in the human large intestine. *J. Anat.* 149, 189–194.

MacDonald, T. T., and Monteleone, G. (2004). Role of the immune system in the pathogenesis of IBD. In *Immune Mechanisms in IBD* (eds. M. Neurath and R. Blumberg). New York, Landes, in press.

MacDonald, T. T., and Pender, S. L. (2004). Mechanisms of tissue injury. In *Kirsner's Inflammatory Bowel Disease* (eds. R B. Sartor and W. Sandborn), St. Louis, Elsevier, pp.163–178.

MacDonald, T. T., Spencer, J., Viney, J. L., Williams, C. B., and Walker-Smith, J. A. (1987). Selective biopsy of human Peyer's patches during ileal endoscopy. *Gastroenterology* 93, 1356–1362.

Mage, R. G. (1998). Diversification of rabbit VH genes by gene-conversion-like and hypermutation mechanisms. *Immunol. Rev.* 162, 49–54.

Moghaddami, M., Cummins, A., and Mayrhofer, G. (1998). Lymphocyte-filled villi: Comparison with other lymphoid aggregations in the mucosa of the human small intestine. *Gastroenterology* 115, 1414–1425.

Monteleone, G., Holloway, J., Salvati, V. M., Pender, S. L., Fairclough, P. D., Croft, N., and MacDonald, T. T. (2003). Activated STAT4 and a functional role for IL-12 in human Peyer's patches. *J. Immunol.* 170, 300–307.

Nagata, S., McKenzie, C., Pender, S. L., Bajaj-Elliott, M., Fairclough, P. D., Walker-Smith, J. A., Monteleone, G., and MacDonald, T. T. (2000). Human Peyer's patch T cells are sensitized to dietary antigen and display a Th cell type 1 cytokine profile. *J. Immunol.* 165, 5315–5321.

O'Leary, A. D., and Sweeney, E. C. (1986). Lymphoglandular complexes of the colon: Structure and distribution. *Histopathology* 10, 267–283.

O'Neill, L. A., and Dinarello, C. A. (2000). The IL-1 receptor/toll-like receptor superfamily: Crucial receptors for inflammation and host defense. *Immunol. Today* 21, 206–209.

Peach, S., Lock, M. R., Katz, D., Todd, I. P., and Tabaqchali, S. (1978). Mucosal-associated bacterial flora of the intestine in patients with Crohn's disease and in a control group. *Gut* 19, 1034–1042.

Radford-Smith, G. L., Edwards, J. E., Purdie, D. M., Pandeya, N., Watson, M., Martin, N. G., Green, A., Newman, B., and Florin, T. H. (2002). Protective role of appendicectomy on onset and severity of ulcerative colitis and Crohn's disease. *Gut* 51, 808–813.

Rickert, R. R., and Carter, H. W. (1980). The "early" ulcerative lesion of Crohn's disease: Correlative light- and scanning electron-microscopic studies. *J. Clin. Gastroenterol.* 2, 11–19.

Spencer, J., Finn, T., and Isaacson, P. G. (1986). Human Peyer's patches: An immunohistochemical study. *Gut* 27, 405–410.

Thoma-Uszynski, S., Kiertscher, S. M., Ochoa, M. T., Bouis, D. A., Norgard, M. V., Miyake, K., Godowski, P. J., Roth, M. D., and Modlin, R. L. (2000). Activation of toll-like receptor 2 on human dendritic cells triggers induction of IL-12, but not IL-10. *J. Immunol.* 165, 3804–3810.

Trinchieri, G., and Scott, P. (1999). Interleukin-12: basic principles and clinical applications. *Curr. Top. Microbiol. Immunol.* 238, 57–78.

Van Kruiningen, H. J., West, A. B., Freda, B. J., and Holmes, K. A. (2002). Distribution of Peyer's patches in the distal ileum. *Inflamm. Bowel. Dis.* 8, 180–185.

Webster, A. D., Kenwright, S., Ballard, J., Shiner, M., Slavin, G., Levi, A. J., Loewi, G., and Asherson, G. L. (1977). Nodular lymphoid hyperplasia of the bowel in primary hypogammaglobulinaemia: Study of *in vivo* and *in vitro* lymphocyte function. *Gut* 18, 364–372.

Yang, S. K., Jung, H. Y., Kang, G. H., Kim, Y. M., Myung, S. J., Shim, K. N., Hong, W. S., and Min, Y. I. (1999). Appendiceal orifice inflammation as a skip lesion in ulcerative colitis: An analysis in relation to medical therapy and disease extent. *Gastrointest. Endosc.* 49, 743–747.

Nasal-Associated Lymphoid Tissue

Georg Kraal

Department of Molecular Cell Biology, VU University Medical Center, Amsterdam, The Netherlands

LYMPHOID ORGANS OF THE RESPIRATORY TRACT

The upper and lower respiratory airways are continuously exposed to antigenic challenges. This is reflected in the presence of specialized cells and lymphoid organs in the nasal and buccal mucosae and in the lungs. However, the organization of these structures may differ in different species.

In the human pharynx, a set of lymphoid tissues surrounds the nasal and oral passages into the pharynx. They are collectively called Waldeyer's ring and include the adenoids and other tonsils (Perry and Whyte 1998).

In contrast to this highly organized and strategically positioned oronasal complex of lymphoid tissue, in lungs of humans only poorly developed lymphoid tissue can be found. Such lymphoid aggregates in the bronchial wall, with high similarity to the Peyer's patches in the small intestines, have been described in several other animal species, such as mice, rats, guinea pigs, and rabbits and are referred to as bronchus-associated lymphoid tissue (BALT) (Sminia *et al.* 1989). They are concentrated at the bifurcations of the larger bronchi, correlating with areas of high antigen impact. It remains to be seen whether in species with small and seemingly underdeveloped BALT the structure is part of the ontogenetic development or reflects a tertiary lymphoid structure resulting from local chronic inflammation (Tschernig and Pabst 2000). Species that do show well-developed BALT usually do not have a complex ring of Waldeyer, but will show lymphoid aggregates in the nasal cavity at the entrance to the pharyngeal duct. Such aggregates are referred to as nasal-associated lymphoid tissue (NALT) (Kuper *et al.* 1992). It may well be that these anatomic differences reflect differences in breathing patterns. Animals with predominant or exclusive nose breathing, such as rodents, have well-developed NALT and BALT, whereas in species with mixed breathing through nose and mouth, tonsillar structures in the pharynx can be seen, associated with absence or minimal development of BALT.

STRUCTURE OF THE NALT

The organization and structure of the NALT have been studied most extensively in small rodents such as rats and mice (Koornstra *et al.* 1993; Kuper *et al.* 1992; Spit *et al.* 1989). It is situated in the floor of the nasal cavity as a paired organ, slightly bulging out into the nasal cavity, right at the entrance of the pharyngeal duct **(Figures 23.1 and 23.2)**. In addition to these well-organized lymphoid structures, many lymphocytes can be found in and underneath the epithelium lining the nasal passages into the pharynx. They probably represent a population of effector cells at the site where antigenic deposition is high, and although it is not lymphoid tissue *in sensu stricto*, it is sometimes referred to as diffuse NALT (Kuper *et al.* 1992; Liang *et al.* 2001).

The most proximal regions of the nasal cavity of the rodent are lined with stratified squamous epithelium. Further into the cavities, pseudostratified epithelium is found on the ventral surfaces that line the entrance to and the length of the nasopharyngeal duct. In addition to ciliated columnar cells, this respiratory epithelium also contains numerous goblet cells, which are involved in the production of the protective glycocalyx. At those places where the respiratory epithelium covers the NALT, it is characterized by the presence of specialized microfold (M) cells (Karchev and Kabakchiev 1984). These M cells are found in all mucosal epithelia covering lymphoid aggregates, such as tonsils, Peyer's patches, and BALT **(Figure 23.3)**. These epithelia are therefore often referred to as follicle-associated epithelium (FAE) (Spit *et al.* 1989). In addition to M cells, which can be found in small clusters or alone, the epithelium covering the NALT also contains a few mucous goblet cells.

Whereas most of the epithelial cells lining the nasal cavity are determined to keep antigens and microorganisms out, being protected by a mucus layer and constant activity of their microvilli, the M cells have evolved special mechanisms to transport macromolecules and particles across the epithelium. The basolateral surface of M cells is deeply invaginated

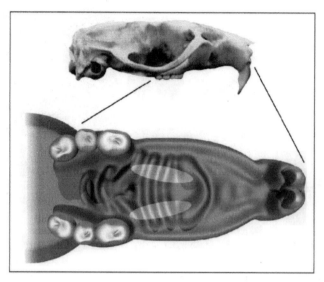

Fig. 23.1. Anatomic position of nasal-associated lymphoid tissue (NALT) in the mouse. The ventral view of the palate is shown with its relative position to the skull. The ellipsoid areas represent the position of the NALT in the nasal cavities. Adapted from Heritage *et al.* 1997.

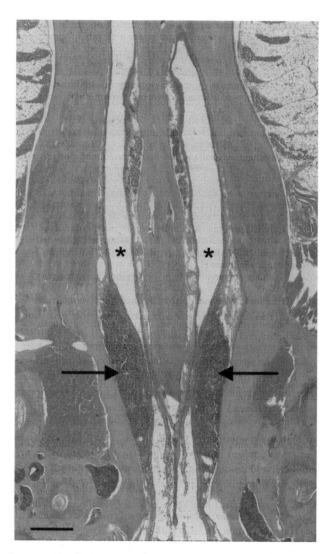

Fig. 23.2. Histologic position location of the paired conglomerates of nasal-associated lymphoid tissue (NALT) (arrow) in the nasal cavity (asterisk) of a BALB/c mouse. **(See page 7 of the color plates.)** Hematoxylin-eosin staining. Scale bar: 500 µm. Courtesy of Dr. Pascale Gueirard (Pasteur Institute, Paris).

whereby large intraepithelial pockets are formed, which serve as an initial collection site for transcytosed material. Together with extensive arrays of intermediate filaments, this pocket forms the cardinal characteristic of the M cell. Inside the pocket, lymphocytes as well as macrophages can be found, in close association with the M-cell membrane, suggestive for some sort of interaction. Furthermore, M cells form long basal processes that are found to extend deeper into the lymphoid tissue underneath the epithelium, where they can associate with other cells such as antigen-presenting cells. Most of the knowledge we have on M cells is based on observations made in the lymphoepithelium overlying the domes of Peyer's patches. However, based on the overall similarities in structure and occurrence, it is likely that most characteristics found for Peyer's patch M cells are attributable to those in NALT (Fujimura 2000), with perhaps slight regional differences, such as binding patterns of lectins. Both rat and hamster M cells in the NALT stain rather specifically with GSI-B4, a lectin from *Griffonia simplicifolia*, directed against α-linked galactoses (Giannasca *et al.* 1997; Takata *et al.* 2000). The importance of these findings may lie in the application of such lectins in targeting drugs or vaccines to the NALT.

M cells seem to be specialized in transcytosis (Kraehenbuhl and Neutra 2000; Neutra *et al.* 2001). Bound particles such as bacteria and viruses induce changes in the apical membrane and cytoskeleton, after which phagocytosis takes place. Reorganization of the cell membrane and extension of cellular processes around the particles have been described, and the particles are transported through the cell in a phagocytic vesicle (Owen 1999). Smaller particles and macromolecules are taken up through clathrin-coated pits or by receptor-mediated phagocytosis. All material that has been

taken up is released again in the basolateral pocket, but it is unclear whether any degradation of the transported material or particles has taken place during the transit and whether the cells play an active role in antigen presentation. Nevertheless there seems to be an active interaction between the M cells and underlying lymphocytes because after depletion of lymphocytes by irradiation the intraepithelial pocket of the M cells in Peyer's patches is lost (Ermak *et al.* 1989). That the activity of M cells in the NALT is influenced by antigenic stimuli was found in a comparison of NALT epithelium from normally reared and specific pathogen-free (SPF) rats (Jeong *et al.* 2000). First, the number of M cells was lower and remained lower in SPF rats, but the cells also showed a more uniform morphology. In conventionally reared animals, the number of M cells increased with age, and their morphology altered, leading to extensive cytoplas-

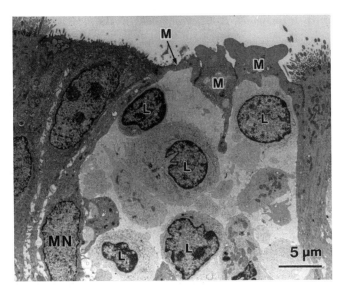

Fig. 23.3. A transmission electron micrograph showing M cells (M) that have enfolded many lymphoid cells (L) in the covering epithelium of adenoid tissue. MN, nucleus of M cell. Reprinted from Fujimura 2000, with permission of Springer-Verlag, Germany.

mic interfoliation and wide intercellular spaces filled with amorphous material.

Data on the phenotype of the lymphocytes that reside in the pockets of the M cells in NALT are limited (Hameleers *et al.* 1989), but in Peyer's patches the majority of cells that are localized in the M-cell pockets are $CD4^+$ T cells. They can have characteristics of naive T cells, but also are found to show activation markers such as CD69 and CD45RO. B cells are also found in the pockets, and both naive B cells, based on CD45RA expression, as well as more activated cells have been described (Farstad *et al.* 1994). The presence of B cells has led to the speculation that these cells are involved in the actual antigen presentation to T cells in these special epithelial niches.

The overall composition of NALT tissue in mice with respect to lymphocyte distribution has been studied in more detail by several groups (Asanuma *et al.* 1997; Heritage *et al.* 1997). The number of B lymphocytes in the NALT roughly equaled the number of T cells or was found to be about twice as much, probably related to the housing conditions of the animals **(Table 23.1)**. When $CD4^+$ and $CD8^+$ T cells were compared, a preponderance of $CD4^+$ cells was found, reflecting the normal distribution of these cell types in lymphoid tissue of the mouse (Kraal *et al.* 1983).

Less than two decades ago, NALT was described for the first time, and the apparent resemblance in structure with Peyer's patches of the small intestines has been emphasized by many investigators (Kuper *et al.* 1992; Spit *et al.* 1989). Both organs are situated directly underneath an epithelial layer and characterized by the absence of afferent lymphatic vessels. Both are composed of B-cell follicles with alternating

Table 23.1   Comparison of Features of NALT, Peyer's Patches (PP), and BALT

	NALT	PP	BALT
Ontogeny			
Presence of tissue	At birth	Before birth	At day 4 after birth
First lymphocytes to appear	T cells	T cells	B cells
Involvement of lymphotoxin	Not for anlage	Essential	?
Role for $CD4^+$, $CD3^-$ cells	No	Yes	?
Formation of T-cell and B-cell compartments	At day 10 after birth	At day 10 after birth	After 3 weeks following birth
Structure			
Follicle-associated epithelium	+	+	+
M cells	+	+	+
Intraepithelial lymphocytes	+	+	+
Germinal centers	±	++	±
Follicular dendritic cells	+	+	+
Tingible body macrophages	±	+	±
High endothelial venules			
—expressing mucosal vascular addressin (MAdCAM-1)	+	+	?
—expressing peripheral vascular addressin (PNAd)	+	−	?
T-cell and B-cell areas	T = B	T < B	T = B
T : B cell ratio	0.9	0.2	0.7
CD4 : CD8 ratio	2.4	5.0	2.6

T-lymphocyte compartments. In the T-cell areas, discrete high endothelial venules can be seen through which lymphocyte immigration takes place. In the case of the NALT, efferent lymphatics drain into the cervical lymph nodes of the upper thorax region, whereas the Peyer's patches drain into the mesenteric lymph nodes. Studies on lymphocyte trafficking revealed interesting differences between NALT and Peyer's patches (Csencsits *et al.* 1999). When the expression of vascular addressins was studied on high endothelial venules (HEV) in NALT of mice, a unique expression profile was found with a predominant expression of the peripheral node addressin (PNAd) and fewer HEV expressing the mucosal addressin MAdCAM-1. In Peyer's patches, all HEV express both addressins. This was reflected in the binding capacity of lymphocytes on NALT tissue that was primarily mediated by PNAd–L selectin interaction (Csencsits *et al.* 1999). In addition, it was found that in NALT HEV could also be found in the B-cell areas, in contrast to Peyer's patches where HEV are more restricted to the interfollicular T-cell compartments. These findings point to clear differences in organization between NALT and Peyer's patches. Interestingly, this is also reflected in the ontogenetic development of the two organs (see the following text).

DEVELOPMENT OF THE NALT

At birth, the NALT of rodents is composed of only small aggregates of predominantly T cells and nonlymphoid cells (Hameleers *et al.* 1989; van der Ven and Sminia 1993; van Poppel *et al.* 1993). During the first days after birth, the number of lymphocytes increases, and after 7 days, the first signs of compartmentalization in discrete B-cell follicles and T-cell areas are seen. In the T-cell areas, distinct HEV develop and over time a steady increase of dendritic major histocompatibility complex (MHC) class II–positive cells as well as macrophages can be found. During aging, the structure of the NALT remains the same, but the overall size of the organ diminishes (Koornstra *et al.* 1993). This also correlates with the situation in humans, where the tonsils are most active in childhood, but start to involute after puberty (Brandtzaeg 1988). Recently, the molecular pathways that are involved in the organogenesis of lymphoid tissues have been elucidated in great detail (Banks *et al.* 1995; De Togni *et al.* 1994; Rennert *et al.* 1996). A large set of obligatory genes are needed that are expressed in well-regulated, sequential steps on multiple cell types. For lymph nodes and Peyer's patch development, many of these steps have been worked out, but for the development of the NALT, only limited, yet exciting information has emerged (Harmsen *et al.* 2002). For the proper development of lymph nodes and Peyer's patches members of the tumor necrosis factor (TNF) family, Lymphotoxin α (LTα), LTβ, and the receptor for LTβ are obligatory (Banks *et al.* 1995; De Togni *et al.* 1994; Rennert *et al.* 1996). LT is likely to be important for the induction of adhesion molecules and chemokines on stromal cells expressing LTβR in the anlage of the organs. The first cells

of hematopoietic origin to localize at the site of a developing organ are cells that express CD4$^+$, but lack CD3, and express receptors for IL-7 (Mebius *et al.* 1997). It is proposed that for Peyer's patch formation IL-7R ligands induce the expression of LT on these CD4$^+$CD3$^-$ inducer cells, which will then lead to an organizing center by induction of adhesion molecules and chemokines on LTβR expressing stromal elements such as endothelial cells and reticular fibroblasts (Honda *et al.* 2001). This leads to the formation of reticular networks, after which the recruitment of lymhocytes can take place. The importance of the CD4$^+$CD3$^-$ cells can be inferred from the total absence of lymph node and Peyer's patches in mice that are mutated in the retinoic acid receptor–related orphan receptor-γ (RORγ) or the transcription factor Id2 and are unable to generate these cells (Sun *et al.* 2000).

Interestingly, when in light of the many data on the development of the Peyer's patch the early development of the murine NALT was studied, a different picture emerged (Harmsen *et al.* 2002). Mice mutated in RORγ and thus not having CD4$^+$CD3$^-$ cells developed a normal NALT structure. This suggested that these cells that seem so crucial for the formation of lymph nodes and Peyer's patches are not necessary for the formation of NALT and also that the role of LT is questionable.

However, when NALT formation was studied in LTα$^{-/-}$ mice, a disorganized and lymphopenic structure was found, clearly suggesting that LT signaling does play a role in the NALT development. This was confirmed in experiments in which bone marrow cells from wild-type animals were transferred into LTα$^{-/-}$ mice, and a normal structure and function of NALT were restored. Such restoration by bone marrow cells does not occur for Peyer's patches and lymph nodes (Rennert *et al.* 1996). Together this demonstrates that in spite of the overall similarities in structure and function, the initial anlage of the NALT is quite different from that of Peyer's patches, which may have implications for the function of NALT.

FUNCTION OF THE NALT

Although comparisons of NALT with tonsillar structures in humans can only be made with great care, it is interesting to see that many aspects of the actual functioning of these organs are still unclear. Descriptions of tonsillectomy have already been given by the ancient Greeks, and many accurate and clear descriptions have been made since on the structure of tonsils, the cell types present, and the deposition of IgA (Perry and Whyte 1998). However, how the organs are to be positioned in the overall assembly of lymphoid organs that make up the immune system and whether they function as inductive or effector sites, or both, is still rather elusive. Nevertheless, in the past years, evidence has been accumulating that NALT is an important inducive site of immune responses after nasal immunization. In fact, immunization via the nose is an effective way to induce mucosal immune responses at remote effector sites, and a role for the NALT in the induction of these responses has been recognized. Tracking of antigens such as microspheres and viruses made it clear that these antigens are rapidly deposited in NALT after nasal administration and that cellular activation can take place (Carr *et al.* 1996; Eyles *et al.* 2001; Kuper *et al.* 1992; Velin *et al.* 1997).

A scheme with the function and position of the NALT in its relationship with nose-draining lymph nodes and the nasal epithelium is shown in **Figure 23.4** and is based on the work of Kuper *et al.* (1992). An important feature is that a distinction is made between the uptake of soluble antigens and particulate antigens, such that the latter are predominantly taken up by the M cells in the FAE of the NALT, whereas soluble antigens can also pass directly through the nasal epithelium not associated with NALT. Soluble antigens then gain access to nose-draining lymph node such as the superficial cervical lymph node (SCLN), either freely

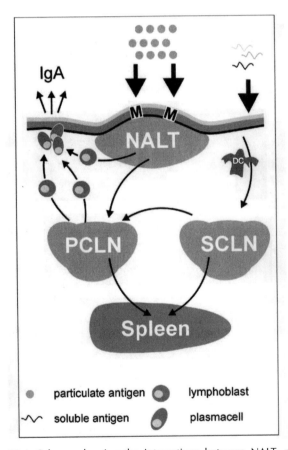

Fig. 23.4. Scheme showing the interactions between NALT, nose-draining lymph nodes, and the spleen. Particulate antigen is predominantly taken up by the M cells of the follicle-associated epithelium of the NALT, whereas soluble, smaller antigens are taken up by the nasal epithelium and drain into lymph nodes, either directly, or associated with dendritic cells (DC). In the lymphoid organs, B cells will preferentially switch to IgA plasmablasts, after which they leave the lymphoid tissue to localize as effector plasma cells in and underneath the epithelium of the nasal passages. SCLN, superficial cervical lymph node; PCLN, posterior cervical lymph node. Adapted from Kuper *et al.* 1992.

through the lymphatics or taken up and transported by antigen-presenting dendritic cells. Soluble antigens can also enter the NALT via the lymphoepithelium or indirectly via submucosal passage.

In a detailed analysis of the responses after nasal immunization with influenza virus, antigen-specific IgA-forming cells in the NALT could be detected early after immunization, with similar or even slightly earlier kinetics and higher cell numbers than in cervical lymph nodes (Liang *et al.* 2001). Interestingly, predominantly IgA antibody– forming cells were found in NALT, whereas other isotypes could readily be detected in the lymph nodes. In the same article, a long-term analysis was performed that showed that the presence of antibody-forming cells waned over time in both NALT and cervical lymph nodes, but remained detectable for as long as 18 months in the diffuse NALT, the area lining the nasal passages (Liang *et al.* 2001). These data clearly suggest that NALT is an inductive site for IgA switching and that IgA blasts will migrate from NALT into effector sites such as the nasal passages. In addition, they may be able to migrate to other effector sites in the oropharyngeal and respiratory tract based on the presence of IgA antibodies in nasal washes (Heritage *et al.* 1997), in lung lavage (Hou *et al.* 2002), in serum, and also in saliva and tears (Carr *et al.* 1996; Hou *et al.* 2002; Liang *et al.* 2001). That NALT is very well capable of inducing immune responses may also be deduced from the interesting observations made by Hou and coworkers, who were able to inject bacterial antigens directly into the mouse NALT, leading to a rapid and protective response (Hou *et al.* 2002).

The preferential switching to IgA is an apparent characteristic of humoral immune responses elicited through the nose and is reflected by the presence of IL-6–producing T cells in the NALT after immunization (Hiroi *et al.* 1998; Matsuo *et al.* 2000). In addition, it is suggested that the NALT is equipped with a unique machinery to enrich for high-affinity IgA cells in the memory compartment. This is based on studies in which somatic mutations in germinal centers of NALT were compared for the IgG and IgA isotypes using antihapten responses. Cells from NALT were sorted for germinal center (CD38[dull]) and memory (CD38[+]) phenotype and analyzed for isotype and accumulation of somatic mutations. Interestingly, germinal center B cells showed mutations in both IgG and IgA cells, whereas memory cells predominantly showed mutations and therefore affinity maturation in IgA cells (Shimoda *et al.* 2001). The precise mechanism behind this phenomenon is unclear; neither is it known whether similar preferential switching and affinity maturation takes place at other mucosal sites. The advantage is, of course, obvious, providing mucosal sites with highly affine, noninflammatory antibodies that have the unique capacity to be secreted over the mucosal epithelia to exert their protective function.

Evidence that the NALT is not only an important site for IgA induction, but is also capable of generating cytotoxic activity has lately accumulated (Porgador *et al.* 1998; Wiley *et al.* 2001; Zuercher *et al.* 2002). Using a peptide that is an epitope for cytotoxic T cells, Porgador and coworkers (1998) have studied the activity of dendritic cells removed from either NALT or cervical lymph nodes after immunization with this peptide. Both sources of dendritic cells could stimulate a peptide-specific hybridoma *in vitro*, indicating that nasal immunization with the peptide led to uptake and presentation of the particular epitope by antigen-presenting cells in both organs (Porgador *et al.* 1998). However, this was only seen when the peptide was administered together with cholera toxin as adjuvant. Without the adjuvants, only cervical lymph node dendritic cells displayed activity, indicating that the peptide had not reached the NALT. In **Figure 23.5**, a nice example of the presence and expansion of dendritic cells in the NALT is shown after nasal immunization with *Bordetella bronchiseptica*.

These data touch upon the important issue of the differential uptake of antigen as shown in Figure 23.4 where soluble antigens in the nasal cavity are primarily taken up through the epithelium that is not covering the NALT. In fact, in all the literature on nasal immunizations and NALT activation cited in the preceding text, the antigen is either a particle such as a virus or bacterium or administered in combination with cholera toxin to enhance epithelium passage. This may explain the conflicting data on nasal immunization and nasal tolerance induction. Through the induction of

mucosal tolerance, the body is prevented from harmful inflammatory reactions against nondangerous proteins such as food components. This naturally occuring immunologic phenomenon has been described for the mucosae of the upper and lower airways and the gastrointestinal tract (Faria and Weiner 1999; Hoyne *et al.* 1993) and involves clonal deletion and anergy of T cells, but also active T cell–mediated suppression (Harrison *et al.* 1996; Tsitoura *et al.* 1999; van Halteren *et al.* 1997). The latter is especially found when tolerance is induced via the nasal mucosa. This site may therefore be favorable when therapeutic applications of mucosal tolerance are considered to prevent allergies and autoimmune disorders, since both IgE production and delayed type hypersensivity (DTH) can be efficiently downregulated by nasal tolerance (van Halteren *et al.* 1997; Wolvers *et al.* 1997, 1999).

The initial steps leading to the induction of tolerance after antigen is deposited on the mucosal surfaces are still largely unknown. In case of nasal tolerance, we demonstrated in mice the absolute requirement for the organized lymphoid tissue of the nose-draining lymph nodes (Wolvers *et al.* 1999). In a series of experiments in which the nose-draining cervical lymph nodes were either removed or replaced by other lymph nodes through transplantation, we could not only demonstrate that the presence of cervical lymph nodes

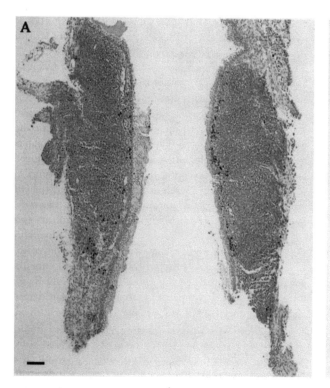 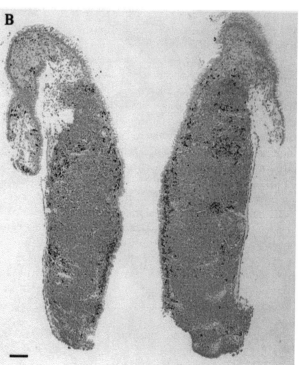

Fig. 23.5. Histologic examination of NALT tissues after intranasal instillation of *Bordetella bronchiseptica* into BALB/c mice. **(See page 8 of the color plates.)** The NALT sections were stained with CD11c to reveal the position and numbers of dendritic cells as antigen-presenting cells. **A,** NALT tissue of naïve BALB/c mice. **B,** NALT tissue of mice 48 hours after nasal instillation with 5.5×10^5 CFU of 9.73H[+] *B. bronchiseptica* parental strain. The increase in number of CD11c dendritic cells in the NALT is impressive, and their position in the T-cell area could reflect their involvement in immunologic reactions taking place in the organ. Scale bar: 100 μm. Courtesy of Dr. Pascale Gueirard (Pasteur Institute, Paris) who would like to acknowledge the fruitful collaboration with Drs. P. Ave, S. Thiberge, and N. Guiso.

was necessary for tolerance induction, but that this function could not be taken over by peripheral lymph nodes when transplanted to this site (Wolvers *et al.* 1999).

Consequently, neither the uptake of antigen through the mucosal surface nor the uptake and transport of antigen by the antigen-presenting cells from the mucosal surface to the draining cervical lymph nodes is sufficient to determine whether tolerance is induced or not. Rather, intrinsic capacities of cervical lymph nodes, the superficial cervical and internal jugular in particular, are instrumental for the mode of antigen presentation by specialized antigen-presenting cells to T cells, eventually leading to active immunologic tolerance. Together, these data make it unlikely that NALT is involved in the induction of tolerance to soluble antigens, but is specialized through its anatomic features to react to particulate and therefore more often pathogenic antigens. Such differentiation of functions between lymphoid structures in the oropharynx emphasizes the fascinating complexity of the immune system.

ACKNOWLEDGMENTS

I am greatly indebted to Dr. Pascale Gueirard (Pasteur Institute, Paris) for the use of the microphotographs in Figures 23.2 and 23.5, and to Dr. Yoshinori Fujimura (Kawasaki Medical School, Kurashiki, Japan) for permission to use Figure 23.3.

REFERENCES

Asanuma, H., Thompson, A. H., Iwasaki, T., Sato, Y., Inaba, Y., Aizawa, C., Kurata, T., and Tamura, S. (1997). Isolation and characterization of mouse nasal-associated lymphoid tissue, *J. Immunol. Methods* 202, 123–131.

Banks, T. A., Rouse, B. T., Kerley, M. K., Blair, P. J., Godfrey, V. L., Kuklin, N. A., Bouley, D. M., Thomas, J., Kanangat, S., and Mucenski, M. L. (1995). Lymphotoxin-alpha-deficient mice: Effects on secondary lymphoid organ development and humoral immune responsiveness. *J. Immunol.* 155, 1685–1693.

Brandtzaeg, P. (1988). Immunobarriers of the mucosa of the upper respiratory and digestive pathways. *Acta Otolaryngol.* 105, 172–180.

Carr, R. M., Lolachi, C. M., Albaran, R. G., Ridley, D. M., Montgomery, P. C., and O'Sullivan, N. L. (1996). Nasal-associated lymphoid tissue is an inductive site for rat tear IgA antibody responses. *Immunol. Invest.* 25, 387–396.

Csencsits, K. L., Jutila, M. A., and Pascual, D. W. (1999). Nasal-associated lymphoid tissue: Phenotypic and functional evidence for the primary role of peripheral node addressin in naive lymphocyte adhesion to high endothelial venules in a mucosal site. *J. Immunol.* 163, 1382–1389.

De Togni, P., Goellner, J., Ruddle, N. H., Streeter, P. R., Fick, A., Mariathasan, S., Smith, S. C., Carlson, R., Shornick, L. P., Strauss-Schoenberger, J., Russell, J. H., Karr, R., and Chaplin, D. (1994). Abnormal development of peripheral lymphoid organs in mice deficient in lymphotoxin. *Science* 264, 703–707.

Ermak, T. H., Steger, H. J., Strober, S., and Owen, R. L. (1989). M cells and granular mononuclear cells in Peyer's patch domes of mice depleted of their lymphocytes by total lymphoid irradiation. *Am. J. Pathol.* 134, 529–537.

Eyles, J. E., Bramwell, V. W., Williamson, E. D., and Alpar, H. O. (2001). Microsphere translocation and immunopotentiation in systemic tissues following intranasal administration. *Vaccine* 19, 4732–4742.

Faria, A. M., and Weiner, H. L. (1999). Oral tolerance: Mechanisms and therapeutic applications. *Adv. Immunol.* 73, 153–264.

Farstad, I. N., Halstensen, T. S., Fausa, O., and Brandtzaeg, P. (1994). Heterogeneity of M-cell-associated B and T cells in human Peyer's patches. *Immunology* 83, 457–464.

Fujimura, Y. (2000). Evidence of M cells as portals of entry for antigens in the nasopharyngeal lymphoid tissue of humans. *Virchows Arch.* 436, 560–566.

Giannasca, P. J., Boden, J. A., and Monath, T. P. (1997). Targeted delivery of antigen to hamster nasal lymphoid tissue with M-cell-directed lectins. *Infect. Immun.* 65, 4288–4298.

Hameleers, D. M., van der Ende, M., Biewenga, J., and Sminia, T. (1989). An immunohistochemical study on the postnatal development of rat nasal-associated lymphoid tissue (NALT). *Cell Tissue Res.* 256, 431–438.

Harmsen, A., Kusser, K., Hartson, L., Tighe, M., Sunshine, M. J., Sedgwick, J. D., Choi, Y., Littman, D. R., and Randall, T. D. (2002). Cutting edge: Organogenesis of nasal-associated lymphoid tissue (NALT) occurs independently of lymphotoxinalpha (LT alpha) and retinoic acid receptor-related orphan receptor-gamma, but the organization of NALT is LT alpha dependent. *J. Immunol.* 168, 986–990.

Harrison, L. C., Dempsey-Collier, M., Kramer, D. R., and Takahashi, K. (1996). Aerosol insulin induces regulatory CD8 gamma delta T cells that prevent murine insulin-dependent diabetes. *J. Exp. Med.* 184, 2167–2174.

Heritage, P. L., Underdown, B. J., Arsenault, A. L., Snider, D. P., and McDermott, M. R. (1997). Comparison of murine nasal-associated lymphoid tissue and Peyer's patches. *Am. J. Respir. Crit. Care Med.* 156, 1256–1262.

Hiroi, T., Iwatani, K., Iijima, H., Kodama, S., Yanagita, M., and Kiyono, H. (1998). Nasal immune system: Distinctive Th0 and Th1/Th2 type environments in murine nasal-associated lymphoid tissues and nasal passage, respectively. *Eur. J. Immunol.* 28, 3346–3353.

Honda, K., Nakano, H., Yoshida, H., Nishikawa, S., Rennert, P., Ikuta, K., Tamechika, M., Yamaguchi, K., Fukumoto, T., Chiba, T., and Nishikawa, S. I. (2001). Molecular basis for hematopoietic/mesenchymal interaction during initiation of Peyer's patch organogenesis. *J. Exp. Med.* 193, 621–630.

Hou, Y., Hu, W. G., Hirano, T., and Gu, X. X. (2002). A new intra-NALT route elicits mucosal and systemic immunity against *Moraxella catarrhalis* in a mouse challenge model. *Vaccine* 20, 2375–2381.

Hoyne, G. F., O'Hehir, R. E., Wraith, D. C., Thomas, W. R., and Lamb, J. R. (1993). Inhibition of T cell and antibody responses to house dust mite allergen by inhalation of the dominant T cell epitope in naive and sensitized mice. *J. Exp. Med.* 178, 1783–1788.

Jeong, K. I., Suzuki, H., Nakayama, H., and Doi, K. (2000). Ultrastructural study on the follicle-associated epithelium of nasal-associated lymphoid tissue in specific pathogen-free (SPF) and conventional environment-adapted (SPF-CV) rats. *J. Anat.* 196, 443–451.

Karchev, T., and Kabakchiev, P. (1984). M-cells in the epithelium of the nasopharyngeal tonsil. *Rhinology* 22, 201–210.

Koornstra, P. J., Duijvestijn, A. M., Vlek, L. F., Marres, E. H., and van Breda Vriesman, P. J. (1993). Immunohistochemistry of nasopharyngeal (Waldeyer's ring equivalent) lymphoid tissue in the rat. *Acta Otolaryngol.* 113, 660–667.

Kraal, G., Weissman, I. L., and Butcher, E. C. (1983). Genetic control of T-cell subset representation in inbred mice. *Immunogenetics* 18, 585–592.

Kraehenbuhl, J. P., and Neutra, M. R. (2000). Epithelial M cells: Differentiation and function. *Annu. Rev. Cell Dev. Biol.* 16, 301–332.

Kuper, C. F., Koornstra, P. J., Hameleers, D. M., Biewenga, J., Spit, B. J., Duijvestijn, A. M., van Breda Vriesman, P. J., and Sminia, T. (1992). The role of nasopharyngeal lymphoid tissue. *Immunol. Today* 13, 219–224.

Liang, B., Hyland, L., and Hou, S. (2001). Nasal-associated lymphoid tissue is a site of long-term virus-specific antibody production following respiratory virus infection of mice. *J. Virol.* 75, 5416–5420.

Matsuo, K., Iwasaki, T., Asanuma, H., Yoshikawa, T., Chen, Z., Tsujimoto, H., Kurata, T., and Tamura, S. S. (2000). Cytokine mRNAs in the nasal-associated lymphoid tissue during influenza virus infection and nasal vaccination. *Vaccine* 18, 1344–1350.

Mebius, R. E., Rennert, P., and Weissman, I. L. (1997). Developing lymph nodes collect CD4+CD3−LTbeta+ cells that can differentiate to APC, NK cells, and follicular cells but not T or B cells. *Immunity* 7, 493–504.

Neutra, M. R., Mantis, N. J., and Kraehenbuhl, J. P. (2001). Collaboration of epithelial cells with organized mucosal lymphoid tissues. *Nat. Immunol.* 2, 1004–1009.

Owen, R. L. (1999). Uptake and transport of intestinal macromolecules and microorganisms by M cells in Peyer's patches: A personal and historical perspective. *Semin. Immunol.* 11, 157–163.

Perry, M., and Whyte, A. (1998). Immunology of the tonsils. *Immunol. Today* 19, 414–421.

Porgador, A., Staats, H. F., Itoh, Y., and Kelsall, B. L. (1998). Intranasal immunization with cytotoxic T-lymphocyte epitope peptide and mucosal adjuvant cholera toxin: Selective augmentation of peptide-presenting dendritic cells in nasal mucosa-associated lymphoid tissue. *Infect. Immun.* 66, 5876–5881.

Rennert, P. D., Browning, J. L., Mebius, R., Mackay, F., and Hochman, P. S. (1996). Surface lymphotoxin alpha/beta complex is required for the development of peripheral lymphoid organs. *J. Exp. Med.* 184, 1999–2006.

Shimoda, M., Nakamura, T., Takahashi, Y., Asanuma, H., Tamura, S., Kurata, T., Mizuochi, T., Azuma, N., Kanno, C., and Takemori, T. (2001). Isotype-specific selection of high affinity memory B cells in nasal-associated lymphoid tissue. *J. Exp. Med.* 194, 1597–1607.

Sminia, T., van der Brugge-Gamelkoorn, G. J., and Jeurissen, S. H. (1989). Structure and function of bronchus-associated lymphoid tissue (BALT). *Crit. Rev. Immunol.* 9, 119–150.

Spit, B. J., Hendriksen, E. G., Bruijntjes, J. P., and Kuper, C. F. (1989). Nasal lymphoid tissue in the rat. *Cell Tissue Res.* 255, 193–198.

Sun, Z., Unutmaz, D., Zou, Y. R., Sunshine, M. J., Pierani, A., Brenner-Morton, S., Mebius, R. E., and Littman, D. R. (2000). Requirement for RORgamma in thymocyte survival and lymphoid organ development. *Science* 288, 2369–2373.

Takata, S., Ohtani, O., and Watanabe, Y. (2000). Lectin binding patterns in rat nasal-associated lymphoid tissue (NALT) and the influence of various types of lectin on particle uptake in NALT. *Arch. Histol. Cytol.* 63, 305–312.

Tschernig, T., and Pabst, R. (2000). Bronchus-associated lymphoid tissue (BALT) is not present in the normal adult lung but in different diseases. *Pathobiology* 68, 1–8.

Tsitoura, D. C., DeKruyff, R. H., Lamb, J. R., and Umetsu, D. T. (1999). Intranasal exposure to protein antigen induces immunological tolerance mediated by functionally disabled CD4+ T cells. *J. Immunol.* 163, 2592–2600.

van der Ven, I., and Sminia, T. (1993). The development and structure of mouse nasal-associated lymphoid tissue: An immuno- and enzyme-histochemical study. *Reg. Immunol.* 5, 69–75.

van Halteren, A. G., van der Cammen, M. J., Cooper, D., Savelkoul, H. F., Kraal, G., and Holt, P. G. (1997). Regulation of antigen-specific IgE, IgG1, and mast cell responses to ingested allergen by mucosal tolerance induction. *J. Immunol.* 159, 3009–3015.

van Poppel, M. N., van den Berg, T. K., van Rees, E. P., Sminia, T., and Biewenga, J. (1993). Reticulum cells in the ontogeny of nasal-associated lymphoid tissue (NALT) in the rat. *Cell Tissue Res.* 273, 577–581.

Velin, D., Fotopoulos, G., Luthi, F., and Kraehenbuhl, J. P. (1997). The nasal-associated lymphoid tissue of adult mice acts as an entry site for the mouse mammary tumor retrovirus. *J. Exp. Med.* 185, 1871–1876.

Wiley, J. A., Hogan, R. J., Woodland, D. L., and Harmsen, A. G. (2001). Antigen-specific CD8(+) T cells persist in the upper respiratory tract following influenza virus infection. *J. Immunol.* 167, 3293–3299.

Wolvers, D. A., van der Cammen, M. J., and Kraal, G. (1997). Mucosal tolerance is associated with, but independent of, up-regulation Th2 responses. *Immunology* 92, 328–333.

Wolvers, D. A., Coenen-de Roo, C. J., Mebius, R. E., van der Cammen, M. J., Tirion, F., Miltenburg, A. M., and Kraal, G. (1999). Intranasally induced immunological tolerance is determined by characteristics of the draining lymph nodes: studies with OVA and human cartilage gp-39. *J. Immunol.* 162, 1994–1998.

Zuercher, A. W., Coffin, S. E., Thurnheer, M. C., Fundova, P., and Cebra, J. J. (2002). Nasal-associated lymphoid tissue is a mucosal inductive site for virus-specific humoral and cellular immune responses. *J. Immunol.* 168, 1796–1803.

Role of Epithelium in Mucosal Immunity

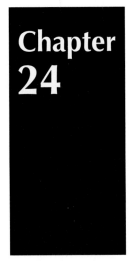

Chapter 24

Matam Vijay-Kumar and Andrew T. Gewirtz

Epithelial Pathobiology Division, Department of Pathology and Laboratory Medicine, Emory University, Atlanta, Georgia

INTRODUCTION

Microbes seeking to colonize mammalian hosts will initially encounter the host at mucosal epithelial surfaces. Thus, it is not surprising that mucosal immunity begins in the epithelium and that the epithelial cell itself takes center stage in that it uses substantial and complex mechanisms to protect the host from these potential microbial onslaughts. Such mechanisms include formation of a difficult to penetrate physical barrier, direct antibacterial activity, and coordination of both innate and adaptive immune responses. Current understanding of these various mechanisms is summarized in this chapter.

EPITHELIAL BARRIER FUNCTION

Mucosal surfaces, especially those that serve as absorptive surfaces such as the intestinal epithelium can be quite vast (intestinal epithelium has a surface area of 200 m² [Ogra et al. 1999], the approximate size of a tennis court) and are in contact with vast quantities of a diverse population of microbes and their metabolites, which include immunostimulatory/proinflammatory products such as lipopolysaccharide (LPS) and flagellin. The vast majority of these microbes and their metabolites are excluded from internal access to the host by the physical barrier formed by the single layer of epithelial cells that line mucosal surfaces. This barrier includes the epithelial cells themselves, their intercellular tight junctions, and the mucus that covers the epithelial surface. Further, this barrier is bathed in a milieu of antibacterial proteins to keep the microbial population in check.

Epithelial cells

The cellular portion of the epithelium consists of a single layer of tightly packed, interconnected, highly polarized epithelial cells, which are separated from the connective and supportive tissue surrounding various types of cells in the lamina propria (Madara 1990). The vast majority of these epithelial cells are absorptive cells referred to as *enterocytes*. While the tight packing of these cells is important in allowing for efficient cellular absorption of nutrients, it also permits a high degree of barrier function from the bacteria and their metabolites in the intestinal lumen (**Fig. 24.1**). Enterocytes originate from stem cells in epithelial crypts and migrate up the villus until they are shed, which on average occurs 18 hours later, making it one of the most rapidly regenerating cell systems in the body (Gordon et al. 1992). Such continual supply of new cells is important for maintenance of the epithelial barrier. This rapid turnover is achieved by a high rate of proliferation, which is matched by a high rate of apoptosis allowing for maintenance of epithelial cell homeostasis (Varedi et al. 1999) and permits the epithelium to heal rapidly following injury. Furthermore, observations that apoptosis of epithelial cells is accelerated in response to infection suggest that such apoptosis may be a mechanism of host clearance of pathogens (Kim et al. 1998).

In addition to enterocytes, the intestinal epithelium has other specialized cell types that make crucial contributions to mucosal immunity. Goblet cells, the next most numerous intestinal epithelial cell type, are interspersed throughout the gut epithelium and are characterized by their brandy goblet shape and pale-stained mucin-filled granules (Antonioli et al. 1992). These cells produce the mucus layer that coats the gastrointestinal (GI) tract (discussed in the following text). Paneth cells are specialized epithelial cells located only at the base of the crypts in the small intestine (Malinin 1975). This location positions them adjacent to the intestinal stem cells that are thought to protect via their secretions of antibacterial peptides (discussed in the following text). Morphologically, these cells are characterized by the unusually large apical defensin-rich secretory granules. These granules are released into narrow epithelial crypts and are thought to maintain a near-sterile window around stem cells. Paneth cells live much longer than enterocytes, having an average lifespan of 20 days (Gordon et al. 1992). M cells are another structurally distinct epithelial cell type, characterized by

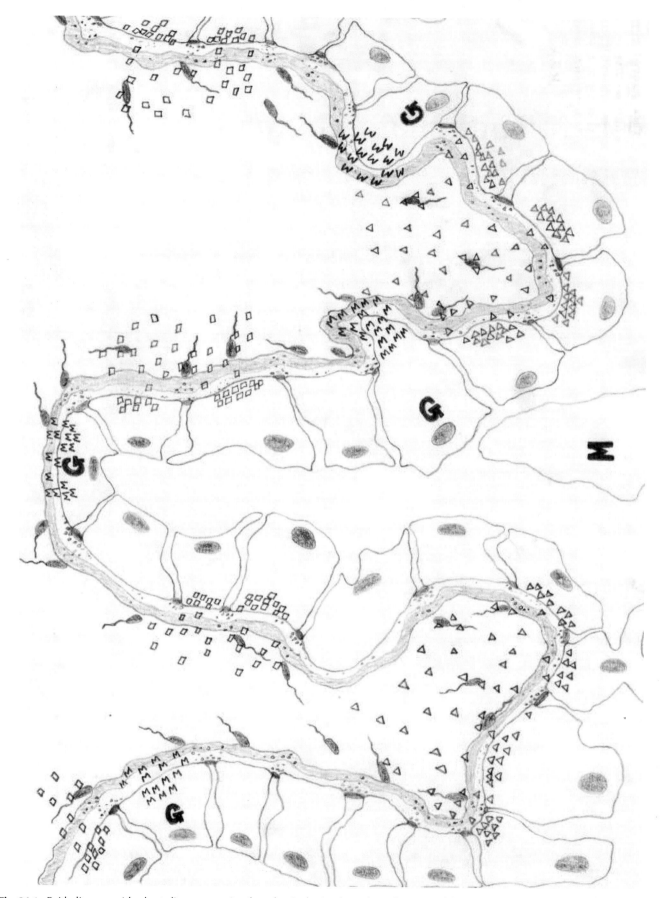

Fig. 24.1. Epithelium provides host direct protection from luminal microbes. This schematic of the intestinal surface shows the mucus layer, produced by mucin-secreting (m) goblet (G) cells minimizes bacterial–epithelial cell contact while epithelial tight junctions restrict soluble bacterial products from internal access to the host including lamina propria macrophages (M). Paneth cells (in crypt bases) secrete α-defensins (triangles), while enterocytes secrete β-defensins (squares) to limit bacterial growth.

microfolding plasma membrane. As discussed extensively elsewhere in this volume, they play an important role in adaptive mucosal immunity, especially in immunosurveillance. Finally, beyond host epithelial cells, the other cellular constituents of the GI epithelium are the approximately 10^{14} commensal bacteria, composed of over 500 different species (Hooper et al. 1998). Although the major portion of this microbiota is not thought to be in direct physical contact with epithelial cells, these bacteria nonetheless appear to play a substantial role in host defense by preventing pathogen colonization by competing for attachment sites and nutrients as well as by secreting toxins against pathogens collectively referred to as competitive exclusion (Fig. 24.1) (Ogra et al. 1999). Furthermore, they likely have a variety of additional roles in a variety of metabolic and immunologic processes that have only begun to be appreciated.

Mucus layer

Most microbes in the intestinal lumen do not have direct access to epithelial cells, but rather, the epithelial surface is covered with a slippery, viscoelastic gel that lubricates the intestinal tract. This mucus layer has long been regarded as the first line of intestinal defense against microbial pathogens (Fig. 24.1). The ability of the mucus layer to protect underlying epithelial cells relies on its gel-forming properties of its highly complex glycoproteins, ranging from 200–2000 kDa. Further, a structurally distinct glycolipid layer, the glycocalyx, underlies the mucus layer and is in direct contact with epithelial cells. The major components of the mucus layer are mucins, secreted by goblet cells that are interspersed among enterocytes throughout the epithelium. Mucins are composed of a peptide backbone to which sugar moieties are attached to serine or threonine residues by *O*-glycosidic bonds. Consistent with its role in protecting epithelial cells from luminal microbes, it has been suggested that changes in mucin composition might underlie the etiology of some diseases such as ulcerative colitis and *Helicobacter pylori* gastritis (Jass and Walsh 2001). The carbohydrates found on mucin are extraordinarily diverse and provide potential binding sites for the commensals and invaded pathogens. Therefore the intestinal mucus layer serves as a niche for microbial colonization. Although, as discussed in the preceding text, such colonization by commensal microbes is generally beneficial, the mucus layer nonetheless protects the epithelium from these microbes by minimizing direct bacterial–epithelial contact and colonization. The mucus greatly reduces epithelial access to pathogens and thus provides protection against invasion by pathogens; however, it also provides a transient foothold for pathogens that allows them to subsequently adhere or invade epithelial cells and thus exert deleterious effects. Nonetheless, restriction of pathogens to the mucus layer may enhance their removal by intestinal characteristic peristaltic flow. Thus the outcome of pathogen–mucus interaction likely depends on the specific type and quantity of mucins, intestinal motility, other secretions, and the rate of intestinal fluid flow. If the rate of pathogen proliferation exceeds that of removal, infection is likely to occur.

Several specific mucin domains that interact with bacterial components have been identified. For example, Gal-GalNAc serves as receptors for *Entamoeba histolytica* trophozoites (Chadee et al. 1987), oligomannosides of mucin N-glycans bind type I pili of certain *Escherichia coli* (Sajjan and Forstner 1990), fucose-containing receptors provide recognition sites for *Salmonella typhimurium* (Ensgraber et al. 1992) and *Campylobacter jejuni* (McSweegan and Walker 1986), and saccharides are recognized by several pili on enterotoxigenic *E. coli* (Mouricout and Julien 1987). Determining roles of localized variation in mucins in infectious events *in vivo* remains an important research challenge in this area.

Intercellular junctions

Although the mucus layer is important for preventing access to relatively large objects such as bacteria, the epithelial cells themselves (i.e., the transcellular pathway) are relatively impervious to most nonlipophilic molecules. The rate-limiting barrier to most molecules of 200–200,000 daltons is the paracellular pathway, whose permeability is specifically thought to be limited by the intercellular junctions between epithelial cells (Anderson 2001). Thus such junctions prevent subepithelial cells from contacting microbial products that are abundant in the intestinal lumen (Fig. 24.1). As such products include toxins and immunostimulatory compounds, these junctions protect the host from bacterial toxins and from excessive immune responses. Consistent with this role, disruption of intracellular junctions drastically alters paracellular permeability and is a hallmark of inflammation. The effectiveness and stability of this epithelial barrier depend on a complex of proteins composing different intercellular junctions, which include tight junctions, adherens junctions, and desmosomes (Mitic and Anderson 1998). These junctions completely surround the subapical region of epithelial cells and maintain the structural integrity and physiologic function of the epithelium. Whereas tight junctions are limiting to permeability, the other junction types are likely important for barrier integrity/stability. Tight junctions and adherens junctions have a common structural organization, and their junctional complexes consists of both transmembrane components with adhesive function and cytosolic adaptor proteins that provide a direct or indirect link to the cytoskeleton. Tight junctions are the most apical cell–cell junctions and seal epithelial cells together in a way that prevents leaking of even small molecules between cells. Tight junctions are composed of zona occludens (ZO-1), ZO-2, and claudins. Of these molecules, claudins are exclusively responsible for the formation of tight-junction strands and are connected with the actin cytoskeleton mediated by ZO-1 (Schneeberger and Lynch 1992). Transepithelial resistance (TER), although specifically a measure of impermeability to charged particles, functions as a commonly used indicator of tight junction integrity in general (Madara et al. 1992).

Adherens junctions are positioned immediately below the tight junctions, and their formation is prerequisite for the formation of tight junctions between epithelial cells; thus alteration of these junctions modulates tight junction formation and subsequently epithelial paracellular barrier function (Troxell *et al.* 2000). E-cadherin is an important component of adherens junctions and is the major cadherin expressed in epithelial cells. E-cadherin is a transmembrane protein containing an extracellular domain with Ca^{2+}-binding sequence repeat and a conserved C-terminal cytoplasmic domain (Takeichi 1990). The other proteins of the adherens junction are intracellular α-catenins and β-catenins. β-catenin directly associates with E-cadherin and mediates cell–cell contacts (Gumbiner 1996). The cadherin and catenin complex is linked through α-catenin either directly or indirectly to the actin cytoskeleton through the actin-binding protein α-catenin or vinculin (Rimm *et al.* 1995). The expression of adheren junction proteins E-cadherin and α-catenin in some types of chronic inflammation such as inflammatory bowel disease (IBD) is reduced in epithelial cells (Dogan *et al.* 1995), whereas tight and desmosomal junctions are expressed at normal levels, suggesting an important role for this junctional molecule in regulating mucosal immunity.

Epithelial intercellular junctions also play a role in regulating leukocyte migration (diapedesis) across the intestinal epithelium. Leukocyte transepithelial migration is triggered by pathogenic microbes and is the defining hallmark of active mucosal inflammation. It is initiated after the cells adhere to basolateral surface of the epithelium in response to chemokines, which in turn signals the opening of the tight junctions (Parkos *et al.* 1991). This process seems to occur without global localization changes to tight junction structural elements. However, a significant increase in tyrosine phophorylation occurs at the area of tight junctions, suggesting an active cross-talk between leukocytes and epithelial cells (Parkos *et al.* 1991). As discussed in the following text, such neutrophil migration is important in pathogen clearance but can also lead to epithelial injury.

DIRECT INNATE IMMUNE ACTIVITY OF THE EPITHELIUM

Beyond serving as a physical barrier to microbes, the epithelium produces, both constitutively and inducibly, a variety of antimicrobial molecules designed to protect the host from the microbial biomass that resides in the mucosal lumen (Ganz 2003). Although some of these molecules are secreted by enterocytes themselves, the expression of others is exclusive to, or highly enriched in, Paneth cells residing in intestinal crypts. Epithelial antimicrobial secretions include antimicrobial lytic enzymes such as lysozyme, nutrient-binding proteins such as lactoferrin, or proteins such as lactoperoxidase that kill microbes via oxidative mechanisms. More recently, it has been recognized that the epithelium also secretes a panel of smaller antimicrobial peptides with less than 100 amino acids. In general, these peptides interact with anionic part of the microbial membrane because of their cationic charge. This leads to their insertion into the microbial membranes and the creation of pores resulting in cell lysis (Grandjean *et al.* 1987). The major class of such antimicro-

bial peptides is the defensins, although the roles of more recently recognized classes are beginning to emerge.

Defensins

Defensins are a family of evolutionarily related arginine rich, small cationic peptides of 3.5–4.5 kDa molecular mass with 29–35 amino acid residues. They have a typical triple-stranded β-sheet containing six disulfide-linked cysteines. They are abundant in cells of both hematopoietic and somatic origin that are involved in host defense against microbial infections (Fig. 24.1). Data from experimental animals indicate that defensins make up around 15% of the total antimicrobial activity of the gut in both gnotobiotic and conventional mice. This suggests that the expression of defensin is not highly dependent upon gut microflora (Putsep *et al.* 2000). Concentration of defensins in intestinal crypts can be quite high, reaching >10 mg ml^{-1} (Ayabe *et al.* 2000). Defensins are subclassified into two subfamilies, the α-defensins and β-defensins, based on their specific placement of the disulfide bonds (Ganz 2003). To date, six α-defensins have been identified in humans. Four of these, designated as human neutrophil peptides (HNP) 1, 2, 3, and 4, form part of the armory of neutrophils' oxygen-independent killing of phagocytosed microbes and participate in systemic innate immunity. The other two α-defensins, human defensins 5 and 6 (HD-5 and HD-6), are expressed in intestinal Paneth cells of the small intestine at the crypt bases and contribute to innate defense of the GI mucosal surface.

α-defensins are synthesized as tripartite prepropeptide sequences, in which a 90–100 amino acid precursor contains ~19 amino acid N-terminal signal sequence, an anionic propiece of ~45 amino acid, and a ~30 amino acid C-terminal mature cationic defensin (Valore and Ganz 1992). The anionic charge of many α-defensins precursor prosegment has been suggested to neutralize the basic charge of the functional peptide (Michaelson *et al.* 1992), which is essential for the proper folding and/or preventing of intracellular interactions with the membrane (Valore *et al.* 1996). The key enzymes essential for the processing of intestinal prodefensin HD-5 are the three forms of trypsin that are expressed by the same Paneth cells that synthesize, store, and secrete HD-5. In the case of mouse Paneth cell defensins, which are called cryptidins, the metalloproteinase matrilysin (MMP7) is required for the processing. In humans, Paneth cell defensins are stored as proforms that undergo processing during or after release from Paneth cells, regulated by α1-antitrypsin (Ghosh *et al.* 2002).

The expression pattern of α-defensins in the small intestine, where bacterial populations are maintained at much lower levels than in the colon, suggests a significant role of these peptides in local host defense. HD-5 has antimicrobial activity against *Listeria monocytogenes*, *E. coli*, and *Candida albicans* over a wide range of salt concentration and pH values (Porter *et al.* 1997). Interestingly, it has been shown that *S. typhimurium* inhibits α-defensin expression, possibly as a pathogenic mechanism. Consistent with the notions that defensins might be a substantial hindrance to *Salmonella* species, HD-5 transgenic mice were markedly resistant to oral challenge with virulent *S. typhimurium* (Saltzman *et al.* 2001). These findings provide further support for a critical *in vivo* role of epithelial-derived defensins in mammalian host defense.

Human β-defensins, in contrast to α-defensins, are not restricted to Paneth cells but rather are expressed more widely within the GI tract. The structure of β-defensin precursor is simpler than α-defensin. It consists of a signal sequence, a short or absent anionic propiece, and a mature defensin at the C-terminus. In humans, three β-defensins have been identified: hBD-1, hBD-2 and hBD-3. hBD-1 was originally isolated from hemodialysate (Bensch *et al.* 1995) and is constitutively expressed by enterocytes. It appears not to be upregulated by proinflammatory cytokines (O'Neil *et al.* 1999). In contrast, hBD-2 is expressed by enterocytes, but only in response to proinflammatory cytokines or infection with enteric pathogens such as *S. typhimurium*.

Interestingly, the antimicrobial peptide activity of defensins is not confined to the killing of microorganisms (Yang *et al.* 2002). By using chemokine receptors on dendritic cells and T cells, defensins also regulate host adaptive immunity against microbial invasion. Defensins have significant immunologic adjuvant activity. Although defensins show similarity in tertiary structure and activity with chemokines, the evolutionary relationship between them remains to be elucidated (Yang *et al.* 2002). hBD-2 has been reported to serve as a ligand for TLR4 (Biragyn *et al.* 2002), and thus this receptor–ligand interaction may underlie some of these other bioactivities.

Cathelecidins, histones, and angiogenins

The last several years have seen a substantial number of new discoveries relating to some previously unappreciated classes of antibacterial peptides. Cathelecidins are linear, α-helical peptides without cysteine residues. In humans, at least one cathelecidin, LL-37/human cationic antimicrobial peptide 18 (hCAP-18), is expressed by enterocytes on the surface and upper crypts of normal human colon (Hase *et al.* 2002). It has bactericidal activity against gram-positive and gram-negative bacteria, consistent with the observation that its expression is upregulated by infection with *Salmonella enteriditis* or enteroinvasive *E. coli*. Interestingly, some enteric pathogens such as *Shigella* species downregulate LL-37/hCAP-18 and hBD-2, possibly as a mechanism of bacterial virulence.

Histones are highly conserved basic (H1, H2A, H2B, H3, and H4) proteins. In addition to their major role in organizing the structure of DNA, histones have long been known to have antibacterial activity (Miller *et al.* 1942). Suggesting such a role in the intestinal epithelium, H1 has been shown to be present not only within the nuclei but also in the cytoplasm of villus epithelial cells (Rose *et al.* 1998). The cytoplasmic histone H1 may help protect against invading pathogens, whereas the histone H1 released from exfoliated apoptotic villus cells may provide broader protection against luminal microorganisms. Recently, angiogenin (Ang4), another member of the family of endogenous antimicrobial proteins, has been discovered in mouse Paneth cells (Hooper

et al. 2003). Ang4 belongs to RNase superfamily and is composed of 144 amino acids. Unlike defensins, Ang4 expression depends on the commensal microflora with *Bacteroides thetaiotaomicron* being one specific member of the gut flora that can induce Ang4 expression. Thus defining the direct antimicrobial activities of enterocytes and specialized epithelial cells remains an active area of investigation.

COORDINATION OF MUCOSAL IMMUNE RESPONSE

Although the previously described mechanisms play an important role in preventing bacterial overgrowth at mucosal surfaces and in protecting against large numbers of bacteria in general, they are insufficient to defend against a number of bacteria, especially pathogens. Thus the epithelium has evolved the ability to coordinate immune responses by regulating the "professional" immune cells of both the innate and adaptive immune systems. Specifically, via both secretion of soluble molecules and expression of surface molecules, the epithelium can direct movement and functional responsiveness of immune cells **(Fig. 24.2)**.

Chemokines and adhesion molecules

Epithelial cells secrete an extensive panel of cytokines that regulate immune cells (Fig. 24.2). The specific list has grown recently, primarily because of development of large-scale analytical techniques such as cDNA microarray analysis and thus outpaced knowledge regarding functional significance. Nonetheless the list includes cytokines that are known to direct movement and regulate function of innate and adaptive immune cells. Cytokine secretion by epithelial cells has been observed in a large number of epithelial cell lines, primary cells, and *in vivo* by intracellular cytokine staining and *in situ* hybridization (Jung *et al.* 1995; Cromwell *et al.* 1992; Mazzucchelli *et al.* 1994). However, as most of these cytokines are also secreted by immune cells, the relative importance of epithelial cytokines has not been clearly discerned, although the fact that epithelial cells are by far the most numerous cells at mucosal surfaces suggests that, even though their cytokine output on a per cell basis tends to be somewhat less than immune cells (e.g., macrophages), their level of expression of these cytokines will have a dominant effect on the local cytokine concentrations. Use of chimeric mice in which either the somatic cells, including the epithelium, or the hematopoietic cells, including immune cells, are lacking specific genes will likely make the relative role of these cell types in setting local and systemic concentrations of these cytokines much more clear in coming years.

Such caveats notwithstanding, epithelial cells secrete a number of chemotactic cytokines (i.e., chemokines) that direct the movement and thus control mucosal populations of both innate and adaptive immune cells. Epithelial-secreted chemokines demonstrated to regulate neutrophil movement include interleukin-8 (IL-8) (McCormick *et al.*

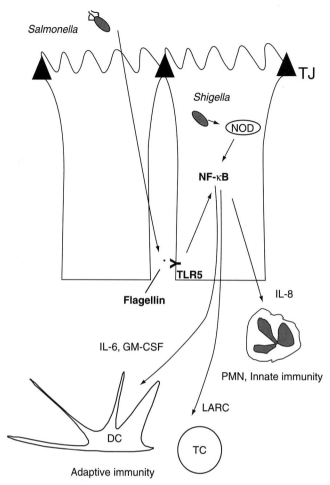

Fig. 24.2. Pathogen-induced epithelial cytokine secretion regulates innate and adaptive immune cells. TLR5 detects basolateral flagellin while NODs detect intracellular bacterial muramyl-dipeptides, both resulting in NF-κB–mediated gene expression. Such genes include chemokines (e.g., IL-8 and LARC) that recruit innate and adaptive immune cells and cytokines that regulate these cells responses.

1993), epithelial neutrophil attractant-78 (ENA-78) (Keates *et al.* 1997), Groα, and Groβ (CXCL8, CXCL5, CXCL1, and CXCL2 respectively) (Dwinell *et al.* 2003). Interestingly, although these chemokines might seem to perform similarly in recruiting neutrophils, their expression patterns can differ, for example, expression of ENA-78 is considerably delayed and longer lasting than that of IL-8, suggesting different specific roles for these chemokines in responding to infections or other stimuli. Epithelial recruitment of monocytes appears to be driven primarily by monocyte chemotactic protein 1 (MCP-1), macrophage inflammatory protein 1α (MIP1α), and regulated upon activation, normal T cell expressed, and presumably secreted (RANTES) (CCL2, CCL3, and CCL5 respectively) (Lin *et al.* 1998). MIP-1α also appears to play a particularly important role in recruitment of mucosal dendritic cells (Sierro *et al.* 2001). Finally, although less well studied *in vitro* or *in vivo*, epithelial cells also secrete a variety of chemokines that direct the movement of macrophages, mast cells, basophils, and eosinophils (Dwinell *et al.* 2003).

The epithelium also secretes chemokines that direct movement of various populations of T cells in the mucosa. Chemokines thought to be important for directing the movement of intraepithelial lymphocytes (IEL) include interferon-inducible protein 10 (IP-10) and the monokine induced by interferon-γ (MIG) (Shibahara *et al.* 2001). Consistent with the fact that IEL, unlike neutrophils, are normally present in the mucosa, these chemokines are constitutively expressed by epithelial cells, although their expression can nonetheless be significantly upregulated by cytokines or other proinflammatory stimuli (Shibahara *et al.* 2001; Shaw *et al.* 1998). These same chemokines also regulate movement of CD4+ T cells, although the fact that increased numbers of these cells are associated with inflammation and that other T-cell chemoattractants such as MIP1α and liver and activation-regulated chemokine (LARC) are among the epithelial genes most upregulated by proinflammatory stimuli suggest a more prominent role for these latter chemokines in being more dynamic regulators of T-cell movement (Gewirtz *et al.* 2002; Zeng *et al.* 2003).

Beyond orchestrating the movement of immune cells, the epithelium also secretes a number of proinflammatory cytokines, TNFα and IL-6 being the best examples (Cromwell et al. 1992; Sitaraman et al. 2001). While epithelial secretion of these cytokines would seem certainly to affect the local milieu, they may also exhibit a substantial effect over overall levels of serum cytokines. These cytokines can have profound effects on both epithelial cells and immune cells. TNFα strongly promotes expression of other proinflammatory cytokines and chemokines, thus tending to amplify these responses. Further, TNFα will prime effector functions of innate immune cells, for example, causing neutrophils to make more superoxide and release more granule content when encountering bacterial stimuli. As these innate immune effector mechanisms can have potent effects on both microbes and host cells, the levels of these immunomodulating cytokines would seem to have a profound effect upon the outcome of host–microbial interactions that occur routinely in mucosal surfaces.

In addition to soluble factors, the epithelium also regulates a number of adhesion molecules that will affect the interaction of the epithelium with immune cells. Epithelial cells express basal levels of several ligands for IEL, of which αεβ7 integrin plays a particularly prominent role (Shaw et al. 1994), as well as upregulate several other T-cell ligands (e.g., ICAM-1, CD54, LFA-3, and CD58) (Cruickshank et al. 1998). Moreover, epithelial expression of neutrophil ligands is thought to play a major role in regulating both the adherence and transepithelial migration of neutrophils. Particularly important roles of epithelial CD47 and signal regulatory protein (SIRP) 1a in regulating the transmigration process have been reported (Liu et al. 2002; Parkos et al. 1996). Intercellular adhesion molecule 1 (ICAM-1) is markedly upregulated in inflammatory conditions and likely plays a role in the increased neutrophil–epithelial adherence associated with IBD (Colgan et al. 1993). Overall, regulation of epithelial expression of immune cell ligands and chemokines likely work in concert in coordinating immune responses, consistent with observations that many genes appear to be co-regulated in these cells in inflammatory clusters (Zeng et al. 2003).

Regulation of innate immune activation

A key aspect of the epithelium's role in mucosal immunity is its ability to appropriately regulate immune cell function. In considering the importance of such regulation, it is instructive to first consider the potential consequences if some of these functions were inappropriately regulated. Insufficient expression of basal mediators of epithelial immunity such as hBD-1 would seem to render the mucosa susceptible to bacterial overgrowth while overexpression might be metabolically wasteful or might have a detrimental effect on the normal mucosal microflora, which may, in itself, lead to metabolic problems or may render the host more susceptible to attack by pathogens. The consequences of improper regulation of inducible epithelial genes that regulate immune function seem more acute. For example, the inability to

recruit immune cells rapidly in response to pathogens would make the host more susceptible to systemic infection. Conversely, recruitment of immune cells, especially neutrophils, in the absence of a perturbing pathogen is likely detrimental because it can lead to substantial damage of host tissue (discussed in the following text), as is thought to occur in chronic inflammatory diseases. Thus, the epithelium exerts tight control over its immunomodulating genes, especially those associated with acute inflammation such as the neutrophil chemoattractant IL-8.

A number of the epithelial genes that regulate immune cells can be classified as proinflammatory genes in that their bioaction promote inflammation and their expression levels are changed dramatically with proinflammatory stimuli. Like proinflammatory genes in other cell systems, their expression is largely regulated by three major signal transduction pathways, namely the NF-κB, mitogen-activated kinase (MAPK), and signal transducer and activator of transcription (STAT) pathway. While the NF-κB and STAT pathways effect gene expression primarily by acting as transcription factors, MAPK members, particularly p38, also effect translation and/or message stability (Kontoyiannis et al. 1999). In general, these transcription factors seem to function in epithelial cells in a manner similar to that described in other cell types, and thus we need not digress into details of their function. Although these pathways are all clearly important in regulating epithelial proinflammatory gene expression, NF-κB-regulated genes appear to be the most upregulated in response to proinflammatory stimuli and thus studying the on/off switches for NF-κB activation seems the clearest way of understanding of how epithelial immunomodulatory genes are regulated (Gewirtz et al. 2002; Zeng et al. 2003).

The primary activation of NF-κB in the course of a mucosal infection is via the direct interaction of a microbe or microbial component with epithelial cells, the first cells encountered by most pathogens. Such activation of NF-κB can result from microbial products ligating pattern recognition receptors on the epithelial surface or in response to intracellular detection of bacteria. A key component of such pattern recognition receptors are the "toll-like receptors" (TLRs) 1–10, which recognize a panel of microbial molecules. Known TLR ligands (and their receptors in parentheses) include LPS (TLR4), lipopeptide (TLR2), flagellin (TLR5), bacterial DNA (i.e., DNA with unmethylated CpG motifs) (TLR9), and viral RNA (i.e., double stranded) (TLR3) (Akira et al. 2003). A common feature of these molecules in different bacteria is that they tend to be somewhat invariant, at least in select regions, thus permitting a relatively small number of TLRs to recognize a large number of different microbes. While such broad recognition is an important aspect of innate immunity, it also precludes these receptors from being able to distinguish between commensal and pathogenic microbes because they are structurally very similar to each other. Thus, although the bacterial features recognized by the innate immune system are collectively referred to as pathogen-associated molecular patterns (PAMPs), this term is somewhat confusing in that these molecular patterns are also found in commensal bacteria. Although phagocytes might reasonably consider any microbes they encounter to be potentially pathogenic, intestinal epithelial cells that perpetually live in close proximity to large numbers of commensal bacteria exhibit considerably more restraint. Nonetheless, epithelia appear to utilize these TLRs to detect microbes.

Epithelial cells without a large bacterial load, such as airway epithelial cells, have been reported to exhibit a TLR4-mediated response to LPS (Wang et al. 2002; Schwartz 2001). In contrast, under normal (i.e., noninflamed) conditions, human intestinal epithelial cells appear to express little TLR4 (Naik et al. 2001), and most intestinal epithelial cell lines do not exhibit significant responses to LPS (Gewirtz et al. 2001b; Eckmann et al. 1993; Savkovic et al. 1997; Eaves-Pyles et al. 1999). However, epithelial TLR4 appears to be upregulated in inflamed mucosa, consistent with observations that TLR4 and its associated signaling apparatus are upregulated by interferon-γ in cell culture (Abreu et al. 2001, 2002). Thus expressing TLR4 only under "high alert" status may be one way of guarding against inappropriate epithelial expression of immunoactivating molecules.

Another means by which epithelia appear to use restraint in using pattern recognition receptors to activate proinflammatory gene expression is via the selective positioning of these receptors. The most dramatic example of this strategy is the case of TLR5, the receptor for flagellin, which is the molecular subunit of flagella (Fig. 24.2). Epithelial cell expression of TLR5 is highly polarized to the basolateral surface so that these cells exhibit a more than 1000-fold greater response to flagellin added basolaterally than to an equal amount added apically (Gewirtz et al. 2001a). Thus, on intestinal epithelial cells, TLR5 will only become activated when the epithelium has been breeched either by a flagellated microbe or its soluble flagellar component (i.e., flagellin). Basolaterally polarized expression of TLRs may be a general paradigm in epithelial-mediated innate immunity because responses to LPS have also been shown to be highly preferentially polarized to the basolateral surface (Abreu et al. 2003). Epithelial cells also respond, at least in cell culture, to TLR9 ligands. However, this receptor is not on the cell surface but intracellular (endosomal or cell organelle) and thus would seem to be less available to soluble bacterial products (Takeshita et al. 2001). Although not yet reported, one would imagine that these TLRs might be more likely to be activated in response to a microbe that has invaded the cells.

A recently appreciated related class of pattern recognition receptors, currently referred to as nucleotide-binding site and leucine-rich repeat (NBS-LRR), appears to function as intracellular detectors (Chamaillard et al. 2003). Specifically, nucleotide-binding oligomerization domains (NOD) 1 and 2 respond to specific glycopeptide components of gram-negative bacteria that attain intracellular access to epithelia by invading these cells (Fig. 24.2). Although these pattern recognition receptors do not signal as robustly as TLRs, they may be essential in activating epithelial orchestration of immune cells in response to pathogens that do not activate

other TLRs. For example, Shigella flexneri is a flagellate and does not activate TLR5, but rather activates NF-κB following invasion (Girardin et al. 2003). The potential importance of these intracellular pattern recognition receptors can be seen for NOD2, in which individuals homozygous for two nonfunctional NOD2 alleles exhibit increased susceptibility to Crohn's disease (Ogura et al. 2001). Although the reason NOD2 deficiency leads to Crohn's is unknown, it highlights the importance of pattern recognition receptors in mucosal immunity.

Another means by which epithelia activate proinflammatory gene expression in response to bacterial colonization results from specialized bacterial secretion systems. Specifically, bacterial species such as Salmonella, Yersinia, Pseudomonas, and enteropathogenic E. coli (EPEC) are able to translocate (i.e., inject) proteins into epithelia that directly activate host-signaling pathways. For example, Salmonella inserts SopB protein into epithelial cells that activate small guanosine triphosphate–binding (GTP-binding) proteins (Zhou, 2001), perhaps eventuating in activation of the MAPK cascade (Hobbie, 1997). Although a direct signaling link between these prokaryotic proteins and the NF-κB pathway has not been demonstrated under physiologic conditions, it is likely that mechanisms of activating host signals exist and play a role in activation of this proinflammatory transcription factor. The translocation of gram-negative effector proteins is accomplished by a type III secretion apparatus (Galan, 1998). EPEC uses a very similar apparatus to activate tyrosine kinase pathways, necessary for the pedestal-like interaction this bacteria generates with its host and may also play a role in the subsequent NF-κB activation (Kenny, 1997). Although it is not clear whether type III secretion–mediated activation of proinflammatory gene expression represents a host response to these injected proteins or a deliberate attempt by bacteria to activate these pathways, they may nonetheless appear to play a role in activating epithelial immune responses. Further, bacterial secretion systems probably underlie bacterial ability to breech epithelia and thus may underlie responses by basolateral TLR5 and intracellular pattern recognition receptors.

CONSEQUENCES OF EPITHELIAL PROINFLAMMATORY SIGNALING

Two facts—(1) that so many in vitro studies demonstrate pronounced upregulation of proinflammatory gene expression in response to mucosal pathogens; and (2) that a subset of these extend the upregulated gene expression to showing functional effects on human immune cells added ex vivo—strongly suggest that epithelium is playing a prominent role in coordinating mucosal immune responses in vivo. However, because of the caveats described in the preceding text, discerning the relative role of the epithelium in coordinating these responses has been difficult, but studies strongly suggest an important role. For example, Karin and colleagues showed that, although mice lacking ability to upregulate NF-κB (because of knockout of a critical kinase in the NF-κB cascade) in their hematopoietic cells have a substantial immune deficiency, mice lacking NF-κB in their somatic cells exhibit massive infections and die within days of birth as a result (Egan *et al.* 2002). Speaking more to the role of epithelial NF-κB in particular, these investigators further showed that mice lacking ability to activate NF-κB only in the intestinal epithelial cells exhibit less inflammation in an ischemia-reperfusion injury model consistent with an important role for the epithelium in coordinating an immune response *in vivo*.

The primary initial consequence of epithelial proinflammatory gene expression will be increased recruitment of immune cells. In acute response to infection, this will most predominantly consist of neutrophils to be followed by a prolonged increase in mucosal T cells. It has been shown in animal models of infection that neutralization of chemokines reduces the neutrophil influx and leads to increased bacterial dissemination to peripheral tissues (Sansonetti *et al.* 1999). The influx of neutrophils will directly clear and kill invading pathogens. Furthermore, this influx of neutrophils will induce epithelial ion transport, resulting in the movement of isotonic fluid into the intestinal lumen. Specifically, neutrophils will secrete the nucleoside 5′ adenosine monophosphate (AMP) (Madara *et al.* 1993) that is converted to adenosine by epithelial 5′ ectonucleotidase CD73, a glycosylphosphotidylinositol (GPI) anchored protein (Strohmeier *et al.* 1997). Such adenosine will potently induce epithelial chloride secretion that will serve as the driving force for the secretory diarrhea associated with this state. This epithelial-driven secretion of fluid is thought to serve as a nonspecific method of clearing both pathogenic bacteria and their toxins from the intestinal mucosa. Because of the importance of this flushing of the intestine in response to pathogens, antidiarrhea drugs are generally avoided in these infectious states.

Aside from being unpleasant to the host, activation of epithelial proinflammatory gene expression can have negative consequences. Neutrophil transepithelial migration also results in a reduction of epithelial barrier function (Nash *et al.* 1987), which can lead to opportunistic infections of microorganisms that would not normally be able to breach the epithelial barrier. For example, neutrophil-mediated disruption of epithelial barrier function has been specifically demonstrated to allow *Shigella* (Sansonetti 2001) and *Yersinia* (McCormick *et al.* 1997) to breach mucosal defenses. Furthermore, such epithelial disruption will allow the noxious (PAMP-laden) contents of the intestinal lumen to reach the basolateral epithelial surface, leading to further NF-κB activation/inflammation. In addition to the risk of opportunistic infection and dehydration, the oxidants and proteases released by neutrophils can cause lasting tissue damage and likely play a role in the early development of neoplasia. Therefore it is extremely important for the host to activate the inflammatory process sparingly. Interestingly though, some degree of low level "surveillance" NF-κB activation may be physiologic. The one IBD susceptibility gene (*NOD2*) cloned to date is a null version of an NBS-LRR (discussed in the preceding text). Thus it is possible that

the failure to activate low levels of NF-κB in response to normally harmless intracellular pathogens leads to chronic infection with subsequent severe and global proinflammatory activation.

Role of epithelium in adaptive immunity

In addition to its previously described role in regulating innate immunity, the epithelium also likely regulates mucosal adaptive immune responses. One way by which this occurs is simply that, via its barrier function, the epithelium regulates what luminal antigens are seen by lamina propria antigen-presenting cells and thus subsequently mucosal T cells. The fact that there is increased epithelial permeability in IBD (Hollander 1999), a disease characterized by chronically increased numbers of mucosal T cells, suggests a role for epithelial permeability as a physiologic regulator of mucosal T cells. In addition to simply regulating what antigens are seen, it is also quite likely that the epithelium plays a role in determining whether the response to antigens will be immunity or tolerance. Specifically, considering that the epithelium secretes cytokines such as IL-6 and granulocyte-macrophage colony-stimulating factor (GM-CSF) with potential to activate dendritic cell maturation (Zou and Tam 2002), and more generally, in light of its potentially dominant role in setting the cytokine environment in the lamina propria based on whether it has activated an innate immune response to a milieu of antigens, the epithelial cells likely play a major role in dictating whether an adaptive immune response will be mounted to given antigens (i.e., antigens that contain bacteria or bacterial products that are able to activate epithelial cell proinflammatory gene expression will likely produce far more robust adaptive immune responses). Although such responses are appropriate to pathogenic bacteria, in the case of a dysfunctional epithelia, they may occur in response to normally harmless bacteria, or their products such as may occur in IBD. In addition to these potential mechanisms, as reviewed elsewhere in this volume, epithelial cells may also be important mucosal antigen-presenting cells.

CONCLUSIONS

The intestinal epithelium is a remarkable and complex structural barrier that permits absorption of life-sustaining nutrients but yet protects its host from microbial onslaught. The epithelium is not a passive barrier but rather a very active interface between bacteria, antigens, epithelial cells, and immune cells. Via its regulation of mucosal permeability, secretion of innate immune effectors, and coordination of immune cells, the epithelial cells generally maintain this interface in a functional state, and in addition, possess mechanisms to clear perturbing microbes and restore the functional state. Further study should allow understanding of how this is achieved and how it might go awry in disease states characterized by seemingly inappropriate mucosal immune responses such as IBD.

REFERENCES

Abreu, M. T., Vora, P., Faure, E., Thomas, L. S., Arnold, E. T., and Arditi, M. (2001). Decreased expression of Toll-like receptor-4 and MD-2 correlates with intestinal epithelial cell protection against dysregulated proinflammatory gene expression in response to bacterial lipopolysaccharide. *J. Immunol.* 167, 1609–1616.

Abreu, M. T., Arnold, E. T., Thomas, L. S., Gonsky, R., Zhou, Y., Hu, B., and Arditi, M. (2002). TLR4 and MD-2 expression is regulated by immune-mediated signals in human intestinal epithelial cells. *J. Biol. Chem.* 277, 20431–20437.

Abreu, M. T., Thomas, L. S., Arnold, E. T., Lukasek, K., Michelsen, K. S., and Arditi, M. (2003). TLR signaling at the intestinal epithelial interface. *J. Endotoxin Res.* 9, 322–330.

Akira, S., and Hemmi, H. (2003). Recognition of pathogen-associated molecular patterns by TLR family. *Immunol. Lett.* 85, 85–95.

Anderson, J. M. (2001). Molecular structure of tight junctions and their role in epithelial transport. *News Physiol. Sci.* 16, 126–130.

Antonioli, D. A., and Madara, J. L. (1992). Functional anatomy of the gastrointestinal tract. In *Pathology of the Gastrointestinal Tract* (eds. S. Ming and H. Goldman), 14. Philadelphia: Saunders.

Ayabe, T., Satchell, D. P., Wilson, C. L., Parks, W. C., Selsted, M. E., and Ouellette, A. J. (2000). Secretion of microbicidal alpha-defensins by intestinal Paneth cells in response to bacteria. *Nat. Immunol.* 1, 113–118.

Bensch, K. W., Raida, M., Magert, H. J., Schulz-Knappe, P., and Forssmann, W. G. (1995). hBD-1: A novel beta-defensin from human plasma. *FEBS Lett.* 368, 331–335.

Biragyn, A., Ruffini, P. A., Leifer, C. A., Klyushnenkova, E., Shakhov, A., Chertov, O., Shirakawa, A. K., Farber, J. M., Segal, D. M., Oppenheim, J. J., and Kwak, L. W. (2002). Toll-like receptor 4-dependent activation of dendritic cells by beta-defensin 2. *Science* 298, 1025–1029.

Chadee, K., Petri, W. A., Jr., Innes, D. J., and Ravdin, J. I. (1987). Rat and human colonic mucins bind to and inhibit adherence lectin of *Entamoeba histolytica*. *J. Clin. Invest.* 80, 1245–1254.

Chamaillard, M., Girardin, S. E., Viala, J., and Philpott, D. J. (2003). Nods, Nalps and Naip: Intracellular regulators of bacterial-induced inflammation. *Cell Microbiol.* 5, 581–592.

Colgan, S. P., Parkos, C. A., Delp, C., Arnaout, M. A., and Madara, J. L. (1993). Neutrophil migration across cultured intestinal epithelial monolayers is modulated by epithelial exposure to IFN-gamma in a highly polarized fashion. *J. Cell Biol.* 120, 785–798.

Cromwell, O., Hamid, Q., Corrigan, C. J., Barkans, J., Meng, Q., Collins, P. D., and Kay, A. B. (1992). Expression and generation of interleukin-8, IL-6 and granulocyte-macrophage colony-stimulating factor by bronchial epithelial cells and enhancement by IL-1 beta and tumour necrosis factor-alpha. *Immunology* 77, 330–337.

Cruickshank, S. M., Southgate, J., Selby, P. J., and Trejdosiewicz, L. K. (1998). Expression and cytokine regulation of immune recognition elements by normal human biliary epithelial and established liver cell lines *in vitro*. *J. Hepatol.* 29, 550–558.

Dogan, A., Wang, Z. D., and Spencer, J. (1995). E-cadherin expression in intestinal epithelium. *J. Clin. Pathol.* 48, 143–146.

Dwinell, M. B., Johanesen, P. A., and Smith, J. M. (2003). Immunobiology of epithelial chemokines in the intestinal mucosa. *Surgery* 133, 601–607.

Eaves-Pyles, T., Szabo, C., and Salzman, A. L. (1999). Bacterial invasion is not required for activation of NF-κB in enterocytes. *Infect. Immun.* 67, 800–804.

Eckmann, L., Kagnoff, M., and Fierer, J. (1993). Epithelial cells secrete the chemokine interleukin-8 in response to bacterial entry. *Infect. Immun.* 61, 4569–4574.

Ensgraber, M., Genitsariotis, R., Storkel, S., and Loos, M. (1992). Purification and characterization of a *Salmonella typhimurium* agglutinin from gut mucus secretions. *Microb. Pathog.* 12, 255–266.

Galan, J. E. (1998). Interactions of Salmonella with host cells: encounters of the closest kind. *Proc. Natl. Acad. Sci. USA.* 95, 14006–14008.

Ganz, T. (2003). Defensins: Antimicrobial peptides of innate immunity. *Nat. Rev. Immunol.* 3, 710–720.

Gewirtz, A. T., Navas, T. A., Lyons, S., Godowski, P. J., and Madara, J. L. (2001a). Cutting edge: bacterial flagellin activates basolaterally expressed TLR5 to induce epithelial proinflammatory gene expression. *J. Immunol.* 167, 1882–1885.

Gewirtz, A. T., Simon, P. O., Jr., Schmitt, C. K., Taylor, L. J., Hagedorn, C. H., O'Brien, A. D., Neish, A. S., and Madara, J. L. (2001b). *Salmonella typhimurium* translocates flagellin across intestinal epithelia, inducing a proinflammatory response. *J. Clin. Invest.* 107, 99–109.

Gewirtz, A. T., Collier-Hyams, L. S., Young, A. N., Kucharzik, T., Guilford, W. J., Parkinson, J. F., Williams, I. R., Neish, A. S., and Madara, J. L. (2002). Lipoxin a(4) analogs attenuate induction of intestinal epithelial proinflammatory gene expression and reduce the severity of dextran sodium sulfate-induced colitis. *J. Immunol.* 168, 5260–5267.

Ghosh, D., Porter, E., Shen, B., Lee, S. K., Wilk, D., Drazba, J., Yadav, S. P., Crabb, J. W., Ganz, T., and Bevins, C. L. (2002). Paneth cell trypsin is the processing enzyme for human defensin-5. *Nat. Immunol.* 3, 583–590.

Girardin, S. E., Boneca, I. G., Carneiro, L. A., Antignac, A., Jehanno, M., Viala, J., Tedin, K., Taha, M. K., Labigne, A., Zahringer, U., Coyle, A. J., DiStefano, P. S., Bertin, J., Sansonetti, P. J., and Philpott, D. J. (2003). Nod1 detects a unique muropeptide from gram-negative bacterial peptidoglycan. *Science* 300, 1584–1587.

Gordon, J. I., Schmidt, G. H., and Roth, K. A. (1992). Studies of intestinal stem cells using normal, chimeric, and transgenic mice. *FASEB J.* 6, 3039–3050.

Grandjean, V., Vincent, S., Martin, L., Rassoulzadegan, M., and Cuzin, F. (1997). Antimicrobial protection of the mouse testis: Synthesis of defensins of the cryptdin family. *Biol. Reprod.* 57, 1115–1122.

Gumbiner, B. M. (1996). Cell adhesion: The molecular basis of tissue architecture and morphogenesis. *Cell* 84, 345–357.

Hase, K., Eckmann, L., Leopard, J. D., Varki, N., and Kagnoff, M. F. (2002). Cell differentiation is a key determinant of cathelicidin LL-37/human cationic antimicrobial protein 18 expression by human colon epithelium. *Infect. Immun.* 70, 953–963.

Hobbie, S., Chen, L. M., Davis, R. J., and Galan, J. E. (1997). Involvement of mitogen-activated protein kinase pathways in the nuclear responses and cytokine production induced by Salmonella typhimurium in cultured intestinal epithelial cells. *J. Immunol.* 159, 5550–5559.

Hollander, D. (1999). Intestinal permeability, leaky gut, and intestinal disorders. *Curr. Gastroenterol. Rep.* 1, 410–416.

Hooper, L. V., Bry, L., Falk, P. G., and Gordon, J. I. (1998). Host-microbial symbiosis in the mammalian intestine: Exploring an internal ecosystem. *Bioessays* 20, 336–343.

Hooper, L. V., Stappenbeck, T. S., Hong, C. V., and Gordon, J. I. (2003). Angiogenins: A new class of microbicidal proteins involved in innate immunity. *Nat. Immunol.* 4, 269–273.

Jass, J. R., and Walsh, M. D. (2001). Altered mucin expression in the gastrointestinal tract: A review. *J. Cell Mol. Med.* 5, 327–351.

Jung, H. C., Eckmann, L., Yang, S.-K., Panja, A., Fierer, J., Morzycka-Wroblewska, E., and Kagnoff, M. F. (1995). A distinct array of proinflammatory cytokines is expressed in human colon epithelial cells in response to bacterial invasion. *J. Clin. Invest.* 95, 55–65.

Keates, S., Keates, A. C., Mizoguchi, E., Bhan, A., and Kelly, C. P. (1997). Enterocytes are the primary source of the chemokine ENA-78 in normal colon and ulcerative colitis. *Am. J. Physiol.* 273, G75–G82.

Kenny, B., De Vinney, R., Stein, M., Reinscheid, D. J., Frey, E. A., Finlay, B. B. (1997). Enteropathogenic *E. coli* (EPEC) transfers its receptor for intimate adherence into mammalian cells. *Cell* 91, 511–520.

Kim, J. M., Eckmann, L., Savidge, T. C., Lowe, D. C., Witthoft, T., and Kagnoff, M. F. (1998). Apoptosis of human intestinal epithelial cells after bacterial invasion. *J. Clin. Invest.* 102, 1815–1823.

Kontoyiannis, D., Pasparakis, M., Pizarro, T. T., Cominelli, F., and Kollias, G. (1999). Impaired on/off regulation of TNF biosynthesis in mice lacking TNF AU-rich elements: Implications for joint and gut-associated immunopathologies. *Immunity* 10, 387–398.

Lin, Y., Zhang, M., and Barnes, P. F. (1998). Chemokine production by a human alveolar epithelial cell line in response to *Mycobacterium tuberculosis*. *Infect. Immun.* 66, 1121–1126.

Liu, Y., Buhring, H. J., Zen, K., Burst, S. L., Schnell, F. J., Williams, I. R., and Parkos, C. A. (2002). Signal regulatory protein (SIRPalpha), a cellular ligand for CD47, regulates neutrophil transmigration. *J. Biol. Chem.* 277, 10028–10036.

Madara, J. L. (1990). Warner-Lambert/Parke-Davis Award Lecture: Pathobiology of the intestinal epithelial barrier. *Am. J. Pathology* 137, 1273–1281.

Madara, J. L., Colgan, S. P., Nusrat, A., Delp, C., and Parkos, C. A. (1992). A simple approach to measurement of electrical parameters of cultured epithelial monolayers: Use in assessing neutrophil epithelial interactions. *J. Tissue Culture Meth.* 15, 209.

Madara, J. L., Patapoff, T. W., Gillece-Castro, B., Colgan, S. P., Parkos, C. A., Delp, C., and Mrsny, R. J. (1993). 5′-Adenosine monophosphate is the neutrophil-derived paracrine factor that elicits chloride secretion from T84 intestinal epithelial cells. *J. Clin. Invest.* 91, 2320–2325.

Malinin, G. I. 1975. Direct quantitative estimation of Paneth and total cell populations in the jejunal glands of Lieberkuhn. *Am. J. Anat.* 142, 201–204.

Mazzucchelli, L., Hauser, C., Zgraggen, K., Wagner, H., Hess, M., Laissue, J. A., and Mueller, C. 1994. Expression of interleukin-8 gene in inflammatory bowel disease is related to the histological grade of active inflammation. *Am. J. Pathol.* 144, 997–1007.

McCormick, B. A., Colgan, S. P., Delp-Archer, C. D., Miller, S. I., Madara, J. L. (1993). *Salmonella typhimurium* attachment to human intestinal epithelial monolayers: transcellular signalling to subepithelial neutrophils. *J. Cell Biol.* 123, 895–907.

McCormick, B. A., Nusrat, A., Parkos, C. A., D'Andrea, L., Hofman, P. M., Carnes, D., Liang, T. W., and Madara, J. L. (1997). Unmasking of intestinal epithelial lateral membrane beta1 integrin consequent to transepithelial neutrophil migration *in vitro* facilitates inv-mediated invasion by *Yersinia pseudotuberculosis*. *Infect. Immun.* 65, 1414–1421.

McSweegan, E., and Walker, R. I. (1986). Identification and characterization of two *Campylobacter jejuni* adhesins for cellular and mucous substrates. *Infect. Immun.* 53, 141–148.

Michaelson, D., Rayner, J., Couto, M., and Ganz, T. (1992). Cationic defensins arise from charge-neutralized propeptides: A mechanism for avoiding leukocyte autocytotoxicity? *J. Leukoc. Biol.* 51, 634–639.

Miller, B. F., Abrams, R., Dorfman, A., and Klein, M. (1942). Antibacterial properties of protamines and histone. *Science* 96, 428–430.

Mitic, L. L., and Anderson, J. M. (1998). Molecular architecture of tight junctions. *Annu. Rev. Physiol.* 60, 121–142.

Mouricout, M. A., and Julien, R. A. (1987). Pilus-mediated binding of bovine enterotoxigenic *Escherichia coli* to calf small intestinal mucins. *Infect. Immun.* 55, 1216–1223.

Naik, S., Kelly, E. J., Meijer, L., Pettersson, S., and Sanderson, I. R. (2001). Absence of Toll-like receptor 4 explains endotoxin hyporesponsiveness in human intestinal epithelium. *J. Pediatr. Gastroenterol. Nutr.* 32, 449–453.

Nash, S., Stafford, J., and Madara, J. L. (1987). Effects of polymorphonuclear leukocyte transmigration on barrier function of cultured intestinal epithelial monolayers. *J. Clin. Invest.* 80, 1104–1113.

Nusrat, A., Parkos, C. A., Liang, T. W., Carnes, D. K., and Madara, J. L. (1997). Neutrophil migration across model intestinal epithelia: Monolayer disruption and subsequent events in epithelial repair. *Gastroenterology* 113, 1489–1500.

Ogra, P. L., Mestecky, J., Lamm, M. E., Strober, W., BienStock, J., and McGhee, J. (1999). *Mucosal Immunology.* New York: Academic Press.

Ogura, Y., Bonen, D. K., Inohara, N., Nicolae, D. L., Chen, F. F., Ramos, R., Britton, H., Moran, T., Karaliuskas, R., Duerr, R. H., Achkar, J. P., Brant, S. R., Bayless, T. M., Kirschner, B. S., Hanauer, S. B., Nunez, G., and Cho, J. H. (2001). A frameshift mutation in NOD2 associated with susceptibility to Crohn's disease. *Nature* 411, 603–606.

O'Neil, D. A., Porter, E. M., Elewaut, D., Anderson, G. M., Eckmann, L., Ganz, T., and Kagnoff, M. F. (1999). Expression and regulation of the human beta-defensins hBD-1 and hBD-2 in intestinal epithelium. *J. Immunol.* 163, 6718–6724.

Parkos, C. A., Delp, C., Arnaout, M. A., and Madara, J. L. (1991). Neutrophil migration across a cultured intestinal epithelium: Dependence on a CD1lb/CD18-mediated event and enhanced efficiency in physiologic direction. *J. Clin. Invest.* 88, 1605–1612.

Parkos, C. A., Colgan, S. P., Liang, T. W., Nusrat, A., Bacarra, A. E., Carnes, D. K., and Madara, J. L. (1996). CD47 mediates postadhesive events required for neutrophil migration across polarized intestinal epithelia. *J. Cell Biol.* 132, 437–450.

Porter, E. M., van Dam, E., Valore, E. V., and Ganz, T. (1997). Broadspectrum antimicrobial activity of human intestinal defensin 5. *Infect. Immun.* 65, 2396–2401.

Putsep, K., Axelsson, L. G., Boman, A., Midtvedt, T., Normark, S., Boman, H. G., and Andersson, M. (2000). Germ-free and colonized mice generate the same products from enteric prodefensins. *J. Biol. Chem.* 275, 40478–40482.

Rimm, D. L., Koslov, E. R., Kebriaei, P., Cianci, C. D., and Morrow, J. S. (1995). Alpha 1(E)-catenin is an actin-binding and -bundling protein mediating the attachment of F-actin to the membrane adhesion complex. *Proc. Natl. Acad. Sci. USA* 92, 8813–8817.

Rose, F. R., Bailey, K., Keyte, J. W., Chan, W. C., Greenwood, D., and Mahida, Y. R. (1998). Potential role of epithelial cell-derived histone H1 proteins in innate antimicrobial defense in the human gastrointestinal tract. *Infect. Immun.* 66, 3255–3263.

Sajjan, S. U., and Forstner, J. F. (1990). Role of the putative "link" glycopeptide of intestinal mucin in binding of piliated *Escherichia coli* serotype O157:H7 strain CL-49. *Infect. Immun.* 58, 868–873.

Salzman, N. H., Ghosh, D., Huttner, K. M., Paterson, Y., and Bevins, C. L. (2003). Protection against enteric salmonellosis in transgenic mice expressing a human intestinal defensin. *Nature* 422, 522–526.

Sansonetti, P. J. (2001). Rupture, invasion and inflammatory destruction of the intestinal barrier by *Shigella*, making sense of prokaryote-eukaryote cross-talks. *FEMS Microbiol.* Rev. 25, 3–14.

Savkovic, S. D., Koutsouris, A., and Hecht, G.. (1997). Activation of NF-κB in intestinal epithelial cells by enteropathogenic *Escherichia coli. Am. J. Physiol.* 273, C1160–C1167.

Schneeberger, E. E., and Lynch, R. D. (1992). Structure, function, and regulation of cellular tight junctions. *Am. J. Physiol.* 262, L647–661.

Schwartz, D. A. (2001). The role of TLR4 in endotoxin responsiveness in humans. *J. Endotoxin Res.* 7, 389–393.

Shaw, S. K., Cepek, K. L., Murphy, E. A., Russell, G. J., Brenner, M. B., and Parker, C. M. (1994). Molecular cloning of the human mucosal lymphocyte integrin alpha E subunit: Unusual structure and restricted RNA distribution. *J. Biol. Chem.* 269, 6016–6025.

Shaw, S. K., Hermanowski-Vosatka, A., Shibahara, T., McCormick, B. A., Parkos, C. A., Carlson, S. L., Ebert, E. C., Brenner, M. B., and Madara, J. L. (1998). Migration of intestinal intraepithelial lymphocytes into a polarized epithelial monolayer. *Am. J. Physiol.* 275, G584–G591.

Shibahara, T., Wilcox, J. N., Couse, T., and Madara, J. L. (2001). Characterization of epithelial chemoattractants for human intestinal intraepithelial lymphocytes. *Gastroenterology* 120, 60–70.

Sierro, F., Dubois, B., Coste, A., Kaiserlian, D., Kraehenbuhl, J. P., and Sirard, J. C. (2001). Flagellin stimulation of intestinal epithelial cells triggers CCL20-mediated migration of dendritic cells. *Proc. Natl. Acad. Sci. USA* 98, 13722–13727.

Sitaraman, S. V., Merlin, D., Wang, L., Wong, M., Gewirtz, A. T., Si-Tahar, M., and Madara, J. L. (2001). Neutrophil-epithelial crosstalk at the intestinal lumenal surface mediated by reciprocal secretion of adenosine and IL-6. *J. Clin. Invest.* 107, 861–869.

Strohmeier, G. R., Lencer, W. I., Patapoff, T. W., Thompson, L. F., Carlson, S. L., Moe, S. J., Carnes, D. K., Mrsny, R. J., and Madara, J. L. (1997). Surface expression, polarization, and functional significance of CD73 in human intestinal epithelia. *J. Clin. Invest.* 99, 2588–2601.

Takeichi, M. (1990). Cadherins: A molecular family important in selective cell-cell adhesion. *Annu. Rev. Biochem.* 59, 237–252.

Takeshita, F., Leifer, C. A., Gursel, I., Ishii, K. J., Takeshita, S., Gursel, M., and Klinman, D. M. (2001). Cutting edge: Role of Toll-like receptor 9 in CpG DNA-induced activation of human cells. *J. Immunol.* 167, 3555–3558.

Troxell, M. L., Gopalakrishnan, S., McCormack, J., Poteat, B. A., Pennington, J., Garringer, S. M., Schneeberger, E. E., Nelson, W. J., and Marrs, J. A. (2000). Inhibiting cadherin function by dominant mutant E-cadherin expression increases the extent of tight junction assembly. *J. Cell Sci.* 113 (Pt 6), 985–996.

Valore, E. V., and Ganz, T. (1992). Posttranslational processing of defensins in immature human myeloid cells. *Blood* 79, 1538–1544.

Valore, E. V., Martin, E., Harwig, S. S., and Ganz, T.. (1996). Intramolecular inhibition of human defensin HNP-1 by its propiece. *J. Clin. Invest.* 97, 1624–1629.

Varedi, M., Greeley, G. H., Jr., Herndon, D. N., and Englander, E. W. (1999). A thermal injury-induced circulating factor(s) compromises intestinal cell morphology, proliferation, and migration. *Am. J. Physiol.* 277, G175–G182.

Wang, X., Moser, C., Louboutin, J. P., Lysenko, E. S., Weiner, D. J., Weiser, J. N., and Wilson, J. M. (2002). Toll-like receptor 4 mediates innate immune responses to *Haemophilus influenzae* infection in mouse lung. *J. Immunol.* 168, 810–815.

Yang, D., Biragyn, A., Kwak, L. W., and Oppenheim, J. J. (2002). Mammalian defensins in immunity: More than just microbicidal. *Trends Immunol.* 23, 291–296.

Zeng, H., Carlson, A. Q., Guo, Y., Yu, Y., Collier-Hyams, L. S., Madara, J. L., Gewirtz, A. T., and Neish, A. S. (2003). Flagellin is the major proinflammatory determinant of enteropathogenic *Salmonella. J. Immunol.* 171, 3668–3674.

Zhou, D., Chen, L. M., Hernandez, L., Shears, S. B., and Galan, J. E. (2001). A Salmonella inositol polyphosphatase acts in conjunction with other bacterial effectors to promote host cell actin cytoskeleton rearrangements and bacterial internalization. *Mol. Microbiol.* 39, 248–259.

Zou, G. M., and Tam, Y. K. (2002). Cytokines in the generation and maturation of dendritic cells: recent advances. *Eur. Cytokine Netw.* 13, 186–199.

Role of Epithelial Cells in Mucosal Antigen Presentation

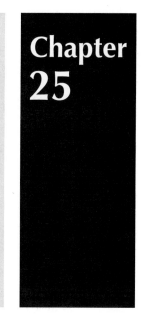

Chapter 25

Lloyd Mayer

Immunology Center, Mount Sinai Medical Center, New York, New York

Richard S. Blumberg

Division of Gastroenterology, Harvard Medical School, Brigham and Women's Hospital, Boston, Massachusetts

INTRODUCTION

In addition to its role in barrier function, which may, in turn, be tightly regulated by mucosal lymphocytes through the production of cytokines such as interleukin-4 (IL-4), interferon-γ (IFN-γ) and keratinocyte growth factor (Kaoutzani *et al.* 1994; Colgan *et al.* 1994), the intestinal epithelial cell (IEC) plays a broad role in regional immunologic function. It is convenient to broadly define immunologic functions in terms of innate and acquired immune responses to capture the immediacy of the response in the former and the adaptive nature of the latter. Although somewhat arbitrary in its application, if considered in this manner, it is clear that the epithelium participates in both types of immunologic responses that are often applied to the classical immune system **(Table 25.1)**. IECs function as direct participants in innate immunity through the secretion of a variety of factors that contribute to functional barrier formation. In contrast, IECs participate in acquired immune responses through local immunoregulation of acquired immune functions of subjacent lymphoid tissue. They play a sentinel role in immune surveillance as the first potential antigen-presenting (Ag-presenting) cell type to come in contact with luminal Ag. This chapter will begin with a discussion on the innate effector functions of IECs and immunoregulatory functions and conclude with an extensive discussion on the potential Ag presentation functions of IECs.

EFFECTOR FUNCTIONS OF IECs IN INNATE IMMUNITY

In addition to the barrier function contributed by the tight junctions and the associated structures of the epithelial cells, which, as noted, may be modulated by cytokines from regional lymphocytes [such as the closely adherent intestinal intraepithelial lymphocyte (IEL)], the IEC contributes significantly to barrier function. This is accomplished by the IEC contributing directly to the formation of the closely adherent glycocalyx and associated proteins such as secreted intestinal trefoil (ITF) factor (Kindon *et al.* 1995). The ITFs are small, compact proteins that are secreted by goblet cells, which establish a close biophysical interaction with the mucin glycoproteins of the glycocalyx. Mammalian ITFs form protease-resistant dimers that, as defined by x-ray crystallography, form a potential binding pocket that theoretically interacts with structures on the mucin glycoprotein. Work performed in *in vivo* and *in vitro* model systems clearly show the important role of these molecules in both epithelial repair and in providing natural resistance to mucosal injury (Mashimo *et al.* 1996).

The epithelial layer lies between luminal bacteria and the mucosal immune system. The IEC's ability to sense luminal flora has always been questioned. In fact, most studies have shown that IECs are resistant to lipopolysaccharide (LPS), thought to be caused by the absence of CD14, a critical component of the LPS receptor, and MD2, a surface molecule associated with Toll-like receptor (TLR) 4 signal transduction. However, more recently, several groups have described the presence of pattern recognition receptors on or inside IECs. Cario *et al.* (2000) demonstrated that both IEC lines as well as IECs *in vivo* expressed TLR2, TLR3, and TLR4 by mRNA but less apparent by protein. TLR3 and TLR4 were upregulated in inflammatory bowel disease (IBD) (Cario and Podolsky 2000). The functional consequence of such expression is less clear since IECs still fail to activate nuclear factor-κB (NF-κB) in response to LPS (downstream of TLR-signaling pathway) (Cario *et al.* 2002). Other TLRs recognize peptidoglycans (TLR2), lipoteichoic acids (TLR2), flagellin from *Salmonella* TLR5), bacterial DNA (TLR9), and so forth. However, the response of normal IECs to these bacterial products is also less clear-cut. IECs have the

Table 25.1. Comparison of Human MHC Class I, MHC Class II, and CD1

	MHC Class I	MHC Class II	CD1
Structure			
Gene locus	Chromosome 6	Chromosome 6	Chromosome 1
N-glycosylation	Yes	Yes	Yes/No (CD1d)
Cytoplasmic tail	Long-3 exons	Variable lengths—one	Short-two exons with motif for endosomal targeting in CD1b, c, and d (YXXZ)[a]
Genomic structure	Exons 2–4 encode the domains	Exons 2–3 encode the (β1, β2) domains	Exons 2–4 encode the α1, α2, α3 domains
Homology in α1, α2, α3 domains	—	—	15% with α1, 25% with α2; 28% with α3 domain of MHC Class I; 30–35% with β2 domain of MHC class II
Allelic polymorphism in α1–α2 domains	Polymorphic	Polymorphic	Nonpolymorphic
Crystal structure, Antigen	Closed end groove; Ag always present	Open ended groove; Ag always present	Narrow, deep hydrophobic groove
Biosynthesis/Assembly			
β_2-microglobulin dependence	Yes	No	Exists with and without (CD1d); weak (CD1a,b)
TAP dependence	Yes	No	No
Associated chaperones	Calnexin	Invariant chain	Calnexin (CD1b)
Function			
Cellular expression	Ubiquitous	B-cells, dendritic cells, Langerhans cells, Intestinal epithelial cells, macrophages	CD1a–c: thymocytes, B-cells, Langerhans cells, monocytes, intestinal IELs CD1d: intestinal epithelial cells, dendritic cells, hepatocytes, B-cells
Peptide presentation	9 amino acids	14–22 amino acids	22 amino acids (murine CD1d)?
Lipoglycan presentation	No	No	Yes (CD1b, c, d)
T-cell recognition	CD8+, TCR $\alpha\beta^+$	CD4+, TCR $\alpha\beta^+$	CD8-CD4-, TCR $\alpha\beta^+$ (CD1a, b, c, d) CD8-CD4-, TCR $\gamma\delta$+ (CD1c) CD8+, TCR $\alpha\beta$+ iIELs (CD1a, c, d)

[a] YXXZ, Tyrosine–amino acid–amino acid–hydrophobic amino acid.

signaling machinery to respond to TLR ligation because transfection of TLRs into IEC lines can restore responses (e.g., IL-8 secretion) to these ligands (Bocker *et al.* 2003; Abreu *et al.* 2003; Naik *et al.* 2001; Bogunovic *et al.* 2003). Two studies have suggested that TLR-4 is expressed in a limited fashion by the IECs *in vivo*. Enteroendocrine cells produce somatostatin in response to peptidoglycan (TLR1/2) (Bogunovic *et al.* 2003). These latter findings make sense in terms of the control of innate responses to luminal bacteria. Both of these cell types contribute to normal homeostasis in the gut.

The nucleotide-binding oligomerization domain (NOD) family of proteins are intracellular pattern recognition recep-

tors. NOD1 and NOD2 belong to the caspase-recruitment domain (CARD) family bearing a leucine-rich repeat (LRR) involved in binding muramyl dipeptide (MDP), a nuclear-binding domain, and two CARD domains that in other family members are involved in control of apoptotic pathways. It is thought that NODs play a role in the control of intracellular infections. Initially, NODs were thought to be present only in cells of the monocyte/macrophage lineage. Mutations in NOD2 (in the LRR region) have been associated with Crohn's disease (CD). Three common mutations have been reported in the LRR domain, each associated with a loss of function and binding to MDP (decreased NF-κB activation).

Homozygous and compound heterozygous mutations occur in roughly a quarter of Crohn's patients (Ogura *et al.* 2001; Hugot *et al.* 2001). However, having the mutation alone is not sufficient to induce disease. The initial conundrum related to the fact that CD is a disease characterized by increased NF-κB expression. If the NOD2 mutations described result in decreased activation of NF-κB, the correlation was not obvious. Hisamatsu *et al.* (2003) were the first to detect NOD2 in IECs (isolated cells and lines). This raised the question as to whether their function was different in IECs from their function in monocytes. Bonen *et al.* (2003) transfected mutant *NOD2* genes into monocyte lines and measured NF-κB activation and bacterial persistence intracellularly. Bacteria persisted abnormally within these mutant cells. This correlates well with reports that epithelial cells from Crohn's patients display intracellular bacteria with greater frequency than normal control IECs (Glasser *et al.* 2001). Thus one component of CD may be a defect in innate immunity at the level of the epithelium (Berrebi *et al.* 2003; Rosenstiel *et al.* 2003; Gutierrez *et al.* 2002). There is increasing experimental evidence to support such a concept. For example, Paneth cells express NOD and secrete cryptins in response to TLR-mediated signaling (Lala *et al.* 2003).

IECs also secrete soluble molecules that are often considered to be part of the innate immune response, which may theoretically play a role in the neutralization and/or inactivation of microorganisms and their toxins. Most notably, these secreted molecules include complement components and cryptins. Model epithelial cell lines have been shown to secrete C3, C4, and factor B which can, in turn, be upregulated by cytokines such as IL-1β, IL-6, tumor necrosis factor-α (TNF-α) and IFN-γ (Andoh *et al.* 1993). Deposition of these complement components can occur under pathologic circumstances on the apical cell surface of the epithelial cell (Halstensen *et al.* 1990). Cryptins, which are approximately 35 amino acid antimicrobial peptides homologous to the defensins of neutrophils, are secreted by Paneth cells, a subtype of IEC, in the small intestine (Ouellette *et al.* 1989; Eisenhauer *et al.* 1992). These antimicrobial peptides not only have broad pathogen specificity, but they may also directly regulate epithelial cell function in an autocrine manner (Lencer *et al.* 1997). Finally, although classically a part of the adaptive immune response, it is convenient to consider secretory immunoglobulin A (S-IgA) in the context of this discussion on the innate immune functions of IECs. Although they do not play a primary role in immunoglobulin synthesis, IECs play a crucial role in the uptake and transport of secretory IgA into the lumen (Mestecky *et al.* 1991).

IMMUNOREGULATORY FUNCTIONS OF INTESTINAL EPITHELIAL CELLS

It is also increasingly evident that IECs participate, both directly and indirectly, in regulating local immunologic functions of IELs and the subjacent lymphocytes and mononuclear cells contained within the lamina propria. This cross-talk that exists is accomplished through both direct mechanisms, involving cell surface molecules that are displayed on the epithelial cells, as well as soluble molecules secreted by the epithelial cell that may influence the epithelial cell itself, in an autocrine manner. These factors also are capable of influencing leukocytes and other parenchymal cells in a paracrine manner. As such, the epithelial cell may participate directly in regulating its own integrity and barrier function, cell growth and renewal, and the immune response of subjacent leukocytes and lymphoid elements. Moreover, these cell surface and secreted molecules are likely to be directly regulated by luminal bacterial Ags, as well as other inflammatory events that might occur during the pathogenesis of a clinically relevant disorder. It might also be argued that because of lymphocyte and dendritic cell trafficking, these events, which are regulated by epithelial cells, may have a consequence not only for the immediate epithelial and subepithelial surface, but also for the peripheral compartments. Thus, as a member of the immunologic community, the epithelial cell may influence important phenomena such as oral tolerance.

As noted, IECs express a number of molecules that are either constitutively expressed by the epithelial cell or induced on the cell surface of the epithelial cell and which may directly influence the function of adjacent leukocytes, lymphocytes, and macrophages. IECs express E-cadherin, which is an important ligand for the mucosal integrin, αEβ7 (Cepek *et al.* 1993, 1994; Roberts *et al.* 1993; Sarnacki *et al.* 1992). E-cadherin, a major ligand for αEβ7, plays a direct role in the localization of IEL to the basolateral surface of the epithelial cell. These interactions between E-cadherin and αEβ7 are not only important in adhesion between the IEC and local T cells, but also likely provide important regulatory intracellular signals both to the T cell and presumably to the IEC. For example, anti-CD3–mediated signals are modulated by ligation of αEβ7 on IELs (Sarnacki *et al.* 1992), suggesting an important potential costimulatory function for IELs, which are largely CD28 negative. On the other hand, it is equally likely that αEβ7 ligation of E-cadherin on the IEC may modulate important epithelial functions in view of the known interaction of E-cadherin and intracellular catenins, which bind the gene product of the *APC* gene (Dogan *et al.* 1995; Peifer 1993; Rubinfield *et al.* 1993). IECs also constitutively express members of the CD66 serologic cluster such as a novel carcinoembryonic Ag–related (CD66e-related) molecule called gp180 (Yio and Mayer 1997). Interestingly, gp180 expression on normal IECs likely plays a role in activating CD8[+] T cells through direct binding and activation of the CD8-associated tyrosine kinase, p56lck (Li *et al.* 1995). As discussed further in the following text, gp180 may be another novel, costimulatory molecule for the largely CD28[−] T cells that populate this compartment and which may be functionally linked to generation of local suppression of immune responses at the epithelial interface. It is also of interest that the cognate restriction element for gp180-induced activation is neither a classical major histocompatibility complex (MHC) class I nor MHC class II molecule and may be a nonclassical MHC class I molecule with which gp180 may coassociate (Panja *et al.* 1995).

IECs are also induced to express a variety of molecules that play an important role in leukocyte and lymphocyte adhesion and regulation of function. IECs, *in vitro* and *in vivo*, can be induced to express intracellular adhesion molecule 1 (ICAM-1) or CD54, lymphocyte-associated antigen-3 (LFA-3), and B7-2 (CD86). ICAM-1 is an important ligand for the β2 integrin, αLβ2 (LFA-1). Interestingly, when expressed, ICAM-1 is localized apically, suggesting that IECs may actively segregate particular immunoregulatory molecules to specific subcellular compartments (Parkos *et al.* 1996). Such immunorestriction of immunoregulatory molecule function may have an important role in regulating and/or limiting particular leukocyte–epithelial cell interactions. LFA-3, a ligand for CD2 on T cells, is potentially very important because of the known importance of CD2 in comparison with CD3 pathways in regulating T-cell function in the epithelial compartment (Kvale *et al.* 1992). IELs exhibit a decreased response to anti-CD3 signals in comparison with anti-CD2 signals, which are preserved (Ebert 1989; Liang *et al.* 1991; Pirzer *et al.* 1990). CD86 is not expressed on normal epithelial cells but can be expressed in certain inflammatory conditions of the intestine, suggesting that, under appropriate circumstances (Nakazawa *et al.* 1999), IEC can provide signals requisite for full T-cell activation (Ye *et al.* 1997). Although the vast majority of IELs are CD28⁻, lymphocytes within the lamina propria as well as CD4-bearing lymphocytes within the epithelium of the colon do express CD28, making this an important potential pathway for regulating T-cell activation (Lundqvist *et al.* 1995). IECs subjected to stress express the MHC class I–related molecules A and B (MICA and MICB), which bind to and activate the cytolytic function of Vδ1-bearing γ/δ T cells (Groh *et al.* 1998).

IECs also secrete a large variety of soluble factors and cytokines that regulate local immune functions. Some of these soluble factors remain to be identified and include, importantly, soluble mediators that downregulate the function of T cells. It is well known from a variety of studies that epithelial cells secrete factors that inhibit CD3-mediated proliferation of T lymphocytes *in vitro* (Qiao *et al.* 1993; Ebert *et al.* 1990; Christ *et al.* 1996). These factors have been identified from a variety of IEC lines, such as HT29, T84, and CaCo₂ as well as primary epithelial tumor cell lines. Importantly, these secreted factors inhibit anti-CD3–mediated signals of not only mucosal T cells but also T cells from peripheral blood. Taken together with the tendency of IECs to stimulate CD8⁺ T cells, the secretion of such factors may play an important role in minimizing the response of T lymphocytes to Ag-mediated activation, thus limiting the promiscuous response of mucosal T cells to Ag-mediated activation along the mucosal surfaces.

IECs have also recently been shown to produce a wide variety of cytokines. The cytokines that IECs secrete can be categorized as three varieties: (1) those that are involved in regulating lymphocyte development and propagation, (2) those that are involved in regulation of local inflammatory responses, and (3) those that are involved in causing the attraction of cells into the epithelium in response to luminal

pathogens. The group of cytokines that are involved in regulating lymphocyte development and growth include TGF-β (Ciacci *et al.* 1993b), stem cell factor (Laky *et al.* 1997), thyroid-stimulating hormone (TSH) (Wang and Klein 1994), IL-6 (Eckmann *et al.* 1993a), IL-7 (Watanabe *et al.* 1995), and IL-15 (Reinecker *et al.* 1996). Transforming growth factor-β (TGF-β) may be involved in many aspects of IEC function and may play an important downregulatory role in lymphocyte responses as well as regulate the expression of molecules that are involved in IEC–lymphocyte interactions such as αEβ7 (Cepek *et al.* 1994). IECs express stem cell factor, which upon binding its ligand on T cells, c-kit, regulates the growth and differentiation of mucosal T-cell subsets such as γδ T cells (Laky *et al.* 1997). IECs secrete TSH, which may be under the influence of thyroid-releasing hormone (Wang and Klein 1994). TSH released from IECs likely binds and regulates the growth and/or differentiation of local IELs, which express TSH receptors. These observations provide a novel rationale for the manner in which extrathymic sites, such as the intestine, may influence T-cell development. IL-6, IL-7, and IL-15 are likely constitutively made by IECs and, in the case of IL-6, regulated by IL-1β in humans (Panja *et al.* 1995) and TGF-β, prostaglandin E2 (PGE₂), LPS, cholera toxin, IL-1β and TNF-α in rat (McGee *et al.* 1992; Meyer *et al.* 1994; McGee *et al.* 1993). These cytokines may be important growth factors for IELs. Moreover, production of IL-6 and TGF-β may be important regulators of regional B-cell responses, especially in the differentiation of lamina propria B cells into plasma cells.

IECs express a variety of inflammatory mediators that are synthesized downstream of a variety of other cell surface events and that may further modulate local immune interactions. Rabbit, rodent, and human IECs constitutively express, or are induced to express, a wide variety of prostanoids including PGE₂ and 6-ketoprostaglandin F1α (Hata *et al.* 1993). Prostanoid synthesis is upregulated by bradykinin (Le Duc *et al.* 1994) and downregulated by indomethacin and 5-aminosalicylic acid (Hata *et al.* 1993). Prostanoids, especially PGE2, have important effects on epithelial cell growth and differentiation and, as such, function in an autocrine manner, as well as having an inhibitory effect on local T cells. IECs can also be induced to express the inducible form of nitric oxide synthetase and, consequently, NO production (Dignass *et al.* 1995), although the data supporting this finding are controversial. Metabolic products from this pathway can be readily identified in the lumen in a variety of inflammatory conditions, which presumably represent, in part, secretion of NO from epithelial cells. The function of NO produced by epithelial cells is unknown but presumably has a wide variety of effects on local inflammatory cells and vascular structures, including the possibility that it influences leukocyte and lymphocyte trafficking into the lamina propria.

Finally, IECs produce a wide range of chemotactic proteins in response to a variety of viral, bacterial, and protozoan infections. As such, it has rapidly become clear that IECs function as a sentinel cell of the innate immune system.

Although early studies suggested that this production of chemokines by IECs may, in fact, require invasion of the epithelial cell by bacterial pathogens (Eckmann *et al.* 1993b), it has become clear through studies with organisms, such as noninvasive enteropathogenic *Eshcerichia coli* and *Helicobacter pylori*, that this, in fact, is not necessarily the case (Crabtree *et al.* 1995). Both C-C chemokines [monocyte chemoattractant protein (MCP) and regulated on activation normal T cell expressed and secreted (RANTES)] and C-X-C chemokines [IL-8, gro-α, gro-β, and epithelial-neutrophil–activating peptide–78 (ENA-78)] are all secreted by epithelial cells as a consequence of pathogen interactions with the epithelial cell (Jung *et al.* 1995). In addition to these chemoattractants, the IEC, in response to pathogen invasion, also secretes a number of proinflammatory cytokines, including IL-6, TNF-α, and granulocyte-macrophage colony–stimulating factor (GMCSF), which, together with the chemokines, regulate the influx of inflammatory cells and the activity of these inflammatory cells as a consequence of pathogen invasion (Jung, *et al.* 1995; Fierer *et al.* 1993). Importantly, the release of these soluble factors is coordinated, which presumably ensures regulated entry and activation of cellular elements. For example, MCP, IL-8, gro-α, and gro-β are secreted at early time points, whereas RANTES and ENA-78 are secreted later during pathogenic bacterial infection (Yang *et al.* 1997). These factors also arm submucosal effector cells and feedback and regulate themselves, such as the ability of IL-1β and TNF-α production to regulate IL-8 secretion (Eckmann *et al.* 1995). Finally, this pathogen-induced regulation of secretion also involves the secretion of prostaglandins and leukotrienes, which are also important to the function of this response to pathogens.

As a corollary of this ability to secrete a variety of cytokines, IECs also express a variety of cytokine receptors, which can be influenced by IEC-secreted cytokines in an autocrine fashion as well as by cytokines secreted by local leukocytes and lymphocytes. IEC cell lines and freshly isolated IECs express mRNA for the common γ-chain of the IL-2 receptor as well as the specific α-chains of the IL-2 receptor, IL-4 receptor, IL-7 receptor, IL-9 receptor, and the IL-15 receptor as defined by polymerase chain reaction amplification and/or binding studies (Reinecker and Podolsky 1995; Reinecker *et al.* 1996; Stevens *et al.* 1997; Ciacci *et al.* 1993a). In the case of the IL-2 and IL-15 receptors, these cytokine receptors are likely functional. The functional consequences of these for epithelial cell growth and development as well as barrier function are unknown at this time. Functional IL-1 receptors are also expressed by IECs (Sutherland *et al.* 1994; McGee *et al.* 1996).

INTRODUCTION TO ANTIGEN PRESENTATION AND FUNCTION IN ADAPTIVE IMMUNITY

The vast surface area of the bowel covered by a single layer of epithelium has access to a wide variety of Ags; dietary pro-

teins, carbohydrates, and lipids as well as luminal bacteria and viruses. A number of chemical and physical barriers both alter these Ags prior to their interaction with the epithelium or actively prevent their access. Still it has been documented that up to 2% of dietary proteins can be found intact in the portal venous system after a meal, suggesting that transepithelial trafficking does occur. This may be aided by what has been termed "luminal preprocessing," reflecting the effect of gastric acid, gastric enzymes (e.g., pepsin), and pancreatic proteases. In the normal digestive process, these result in the breakdown of complex proteins into small dipeptides and tripeptides capable of being rapidly absorbed from the lumen, yet too small to evoke an immune response. Thus a large percentage of the potential Ag pool is rendered nonimmunogenic. The physical barriers cannot be ignored either. The glycocalyx, alluded to earlier, produced by the epithelium, may serve as a physical rather than as a chemical barrier. Interestingly, the glycocalyx overlying the absorptive epithelium differs from that seen overlying M cells. Clearly the types of Ags sampled by these two cell types are different, soluble proteins by the former and large particulate Ags by the latter. Although these differences may reflect other properties of these cell types, the role of the surface glycocalyx cannot be ignored. The efficiency of soluble protein uptake by M cells has not been directly measured, but it is less efficient than that reported for particulate Ags. The opposite appears to be the case for the epithelium. In a study by So *et al.* (2000), insoluble proteins were excluded from uptake by a variety of epithelial cell lines while their soluble counterparts were taken up in a slow but consistent manner. What the effects of luminal processing are on the nature of the Ag has not been quantified. It can be assumed that some of the more hostile conditions within the lumen might favor aggregation and insolubility. Such a mechanism may be an extremely effective way of reducing the antigenic load in the gut. However, there has to be a balance between physical exclusion of Ags and the need to absorb nutrients that could be antigenic. If the gut were to exclude all Ags, the host would slowly starve. Thus there is a requirement for potential Ags to be taken up from the lumen. Other factors would then be in play to control the subsequent immune response.

Overview of antigen presentation

The most important feature of the immune system is its ability to distinguish between self and nonself. The network of defense against nonself is maintained by an intricate communication system between specialized cells that are stationed throughout the body. These cells, T and B lymphocytes, interact to fend off foreign pathogens that gain access to the host. T and B cells possess specialized receptor molecules on their surfaces that are capable of recognizing and responding to foreign Ags, B cells by their surface immunoglobulin and T cells by their Ag receptor. Surface immunoglobulin (sIg) is capable of binding to Ag in solution. However, unlike B cells, T cells can interact only with Ag that is cell bound and presented in association with products of the MHC on an antigen-presenting cell (APC) (Ziegler and Unanue 1981). One group of

MHC glycoproteins, known as class I molecules, arms the immune system to help eradicate cells that have been altered secondary to infection or malignant degeneration. These molecules are expressed on virtually all nucleated cells in the body. The other group of MHC glycoproteins, known as class II molecules, binds processed peptides that had been taken up exogenously by APCs and presents them to helper T cells. In peripheral blood, lymph nodes, and spleen, helper T cells (CD4$^+$) recognize Ag bound to MHC class II molecules on dendritic cells, macrophages and B cells. Cytotoxic T cells (CD8$^+$), on the other hand, are restricted to recognizing Ag bound to MHC class I molecules. Given the general characteristics of this system, we must realize that regulation of immune responses depends on the nature of Ag handling by the APCs through appropriate cellular and molecular mechanisms.

Types of antigen-presenting cells

Several distinct cell types have been documented to function as APCs for T-cell activation (Rosenthal and Shevach 1973; Nussenzweig and Steinman 1980; Ziegler and Unanue 1981; Pober *et al.* 1983; Geppert and Lipsky 1985). Although most of our knowledge is limited to *in vitro* systems, clear differences exist among various APCs relating to their mechanism(s) of Ag presentation as well as to other accessory functions. Monocytes and macrophages are APCs located in blood, lymph nodes, spleen, and interstitium. These cells are large, with active lysosomes, endosomes, and hydrolytic enzymes. These phagocytes are not only vital for the initiation of immune responses, but also play a crucial role in T-cell activation through their ability to produce potent accessory cytokines. B cells, apart from their major function as antibody-producing cells, also possess phagocytic capacity, most effectively via interaction of specific Ag with sIg receptors. When Ag is encountered by sIg on the B cell, the Ag is internalized in an endocytic vacuole and subsequently processed and presented, complexed to MHC class II determinants, to the helper T cell. This activated T cell in turn secretes the necessary cytokines required for B cells to become antibody-producing plasma cells. Steinman and Cohn (1973) described a novel cell isolated from the mouse spleen that appears to be one of the most potent APCs, the dendritic cell (DC). Distinct from the macrophages and B cells, DCs are irregularly shaped cells with abundant class II Ags but no Fc receptors (FcR) (Steinman and Nussenzweig 1980). These cells are potent stimulators in a mixed lymphocyte reaction and, on a cell per cell basis, are probably the most effective APCs described to date. Terminally differentiated DCs are no longer phagocytic and therefore require earlier, more immature forms to process proteins into peptides that can complex with MHC molecules. However, less differentiated DCs have phagocytic potential and have been reported to carry processed peptides for prolonged periods of time. These cells are ubiquitous and are found within lymph nodes, spleen, thymus, and the gastrointestinal (GI) tract. Depending on location, DCs are part of a family of APCs that promote local immune responses. In the skin, these are the classical Langerhans cells; in the gut, they are represented by the "veiled cells" in the Peyer's patch (PP) (see subsequent discussion).

These three cell types (B cells, monocytes, DCs) constitute the group termed the "professional APCs," because they express class II molecules, typically process and present Ag to T cells, and as will be described, provide the conventional accessory signals required for T-cell activation. However, several investigators have described other cells capable of expressing class II molecules (when activated) and presenting peptides to T cells. However, the results of T-cell interactions with these "nonprofessional APCs" are quite distinct from the interactions described previously. Activated human T cells are such a cell type that can express class II molecules (Lanzavecchia *et al.* 1988; Siliciano *et al.* 1988). These cells are capable of taking up, processing, and presenting human immunodeficiency virus (HIV) gp120 protein to other T cells, for example. However, in contrast to professional APCs, activated T cells are unable to present soluble Ag (e.g., tetanus toxoid) (Lanzavecchia *et al.* 1988) and generally result in the induction of anergy (La Salle *et al.* 1992). Class II Ag expression has been induced on fibroblasts, endothelial cells, and a variety of epithelial cells, and although the class II molecules can be recognized by the T-cell receptors, these cells are either poorly stimulatory or evoke a unique type of immune response. The neoexpression of class II molecules on epithelial cells in the thyroid or the pancreatic islets has been invoked to explain the induction of autoimmunity (Botazzo *et al.* 1983; Piccinini *et al.* 1987), with the presentation of self-peptides to previously tolerized self-reactive T cells. Clearly this area of research is growing rapidly, and our knowledge base relating to the regulation of immune responses using such cells is expanding. One such cell, the IEC, is described in greater detail in a subsequent section.

Mechanisms of antigen uptake

For foreign Ag to be placed into a form that can be recognized by the T-cell Ag receptor, it must be taken up and processed within intracytoplasmic organelles. Mechanisms of Ag uptake include those that are nonspecific, random, and therefore less efficient and those mediated by receptor interactions, which have higher efficiency. First, we discuss receptor-mediated uptake, which is different for various APCs.

sIg-mediated uptake of antigen

Ag uptake by B cells was reported first by Chesnut and Grey (1981). In this study, these investigators demonstrated the capacity of rabbit IgG-specific B cells to present processed rabbit IgG to T cells. Clearly this way of generating a specific immune response is extremely effective. If Ag-specific B cells are presenting to Ag-specific T cells, help for clonal growth or differentiation (specific or nonspecific) can be focused on these activated B cells. In such an Ag-driven system, the requirement for the high concentrations of Ags needed to activate T cells would be less. Studies by Rock and colleagues (1984) have demonstrated that hapten-specific B lymphocytes are extremely efficient at presenting processed carrier to T cells via hapten binding to surface Ig molecules. In contrast to the nonspecific Ag uptake by B cells, maximal stimulation of responding T lymphocytes can be achieved with a minimum of Ag (Chesnut *et al.* 1982). Thus, within a lymph node, Ag carried to the primary follicles may interact with sIg on B cells and be presented as peptides to parafollicular T cells.

Fc receptor–mediated antigen uptake

All professional APCs (including less mature dendritic cells) express FcR. These receptors are specific for distinct Ig isotypes and vary in their ability to bind immune complexes. FcR appears to play a major role in the immune response by facilitating Ag uptake after binding to an immune complex. In this respect, initial evidence was provided by Cohen and coworkers (1973), who showed that cytophilic antibodies in the serum of immune animals could enhance the Ag-presenting capacity of naive macrophages. Further, a similar phenomenon was demonstrated by Celis and Chang (1984), documenting that the presence of FcR+ APCs could reduce 10-fold to 100-fold the concentration requirement of hepatitis B virus surface antigen (HBsAg) to trigger an HBsAg-specific T-cell clone. This phenomenon was supported further by studies by Kehry and Yamashita (1990), in which they described that presentation of trinitrophenol (TNP) carrier conjugates by mouse B cells could be enhanced 100-fold to 1000 fold if TNP-specific IgE is bound to FcR on mouse B cells.

Uptake by complement components

Complement (C) is the clearest example of the incorporation of the innate (nonspecific) immune system with adaptive (specific) immunity. Bacterial products can trigger the alternative pathway of complement activation, resulting in the generation of C3b fragments. C3b fragments coat bacteria, rendering them accessible to complement receptors on B cells and monocytes. Thus, in the absence of an adaptive immune response (i.e., antibody), bacteria can be opsonized by macrophages, processed, and presented to T cells, initiating a specific immune response.

Immune complexes also can bind C (IgG and IgM), and therefore be susceptible to uptake through C3b receptors. Studies by Daha and van Es (1984) demonstrated, in a guinea pig model, that receptors for C3b are present on red blood cells, which seem to bind C-coated immune complexes and deliver them to the Kupffer cells in the liver. Arvieux and colleagues (1988) showed that triggering of tetanus toxoid Ag-specific T cells by Epstein-Barr virus–transformed (EBV-transformed) B cells can be enhanced by binding C3b or C4b components to the Ag. Thus, through a number of interactions, complement can play an important role in Ag uptake.

Antigen uptake by phagocytosis

To this point, we have discussed specific mechanisms for Ag uptake, yet a very important mechanism is the one that occurs before any immune response has been generated, non-specific phagocytosis. As the term suggests, B cells, immature DCs, and monocytes can sample their environment by engulfing macromolecules through pinocytosis or by uptake of molecules in clathrin-coated pits. By either mechanism, the process is relatively inefficient; only a small fraction of the Ag is taken up. However, by any of these processes, Ag is incorporated into the endosomal compartment, where processing begins in an effort to generate a specific response.

Antigen uptake by intestinal epithelial cells

The first step in the process of Ag presentation is the uptake of Ag from outside the cell. As described in the preceding text, in a professional APC, Ag is taken up by one of the several mechanisms. In the case of IECs, the mechanisms are more limited. Several groups have documented that Ag can be taken up by IEC by fluid phase pinocytosis. Gonnella and Neutra (1984) documented this phenomenon *in vivo* in an isolated rat intestinal loop model. Ovalbumin was injected into the lumen and uptake and trafficking were monitored by electron microscopy. Ag appeared to be taken up apically into endosomal vesicles and finally colocalized within class II–bearing compartments. This process was rather slow, and no attempt to define processing of the protein was made. Brandeis *et al.* (1994) fed rats Class II peptides in an effort to promote oral tolerance to alloantigen. This group was able to document the presence of these fed peptides in small bowel epithelium 6 hours after ingestion. These studies were followed by a number of *in vitro* studies using a variety of malignant epithelial cell lines. The results varied depending upon the cell line used. Ag pulsed HT29 cells, analyzed by confocal microscopy, localized Ag in endosomal compartments with eventual trafficking through major histocompatibility class II–positive compartments compartments (MHC) and finally into lysosomes (So *et al.* 2000a, b). The path of the Ag appeared to be from the apex to the basal surface, although these cells were not truly polarized. In polarized CaCo$_2$ cells, the Ag appeared to hang up in the supranuclear region and eventually diffused laterally to the intercellular space. No transcytosis was noted. Thus *in vitro* studies relating to Ag trafficking within epithelium are highly dependent upon the cell line used. Although *in vitro*, epithelial cell lines are able to take up Ag. Studies in T-cell deficient mice suggest that such processes are highly dependent upon T cells, and in their absence, Ag uptake is diminished (Telega *et al.* 2000). *In vivo* experiments support transcellular transport of soluble protein Ags, although the kinetics of this passage vary. Berin *et al.* (1997) suggested a mechanism for this variable transport. In mice immunized systemically with the fed Ag, transepithelial transport was markedly enhanced. Thus some Ag-specific facilitated entry and trafficking must occur.

The nature of the Ag also plays a role in whether it is taken up or excluded. As alluded to earlier, insoluble protein Ags are excluded by absorptive epithelial cell lines. Particulate Ags as well as specific bacteria and viruses may be selectively sampled via the M cell (see the following text). Entry of Ag via the M cells has been well characterized. Bacteria, viruses, and protozoa can pass through the M cell intact into the subepithelial pocket where macrophages and CD4[+] T cells reside. The M cell has either no or limited numbers of lysosomal compartments, making intracellular processing unlikely. However, the requirement for processing may be negated by the focusing of Ag into the underlying PP. This inductive site of mucosal immunity possesses all of the requisite cellular components to appropriately process and present Ag to T cells (DCs, macrophages, and B cells). In fact, this is the site of IgA induction, a process clearly regulated by PP T cells.

The proximity of the M cell to the PP is no accident. Some very elegant recent studies have demonstrated that this is an active process. Through a series of cognate and possibly noncognate interactions with the overlying epithelium, PP lymphocytes induce the differentiation of the overlying epithelium into M cells. This process would essentially guarantee that sites of active immunity within the mucosa would have selective access to the Ag pool in the lumen. Such a finding is consistent with the observation that the distribution of M cells in the gut is limited, found mainly in the distal small bowel and rectum. This may reflect differences in the antigenic load in the different sites along the GI tract and potentially distinct requirements for immune responses. These issues remain to be resolved.

Returning to the fate of soluble proteins, we need to redirect our attention back to the epithelial cell. Both *in vitro* and *in vivo* studies have documented apical uptake of soluble proteins. The kinetics of uptake has been variable but slow in most studies utilizing cell lines. However, one older and one more recent study have suggested that, depending upon the immune status of the host, kinetics of uptake can be altered (Berin *et al.* 1997). These two *in vivo* studies used soluble proteins (OVA and HRP) to which the animal had been previously immunized systemically. Compared with uptake and transcytosis in the unimmunized animals, uptake and transcytosis of the specific Ag were very rapid, completing the process in two minutes (the unimmunized controls had Ag in the apical portion of the cell only). Thus there must be some Ag-specific factors facilitating uptake and transcytosis. Interestingly, even if the animal had been immunized with an irrelevant Ag, uptake was still more rapid, suggesting an Ag-nonspecific facilitator (cytokine?) as well.

Two other pathways of Ag uptake have been described for IEC. Early studies had supported the existence of an FcR for IgG on neonatal rat IECs. More recently, this neonatal FcR (FcRn) has been shown to share homology with a series of nonclassical Class I molecules and is reportedly expressed on adult human IEC. The FcRn is also functional in that it is capable of binding IgG albeit at low pH (~5.5–6). Rodent and human FcRn exhibit bidirectionality in their transport of IgG (Dickinson *et al.* 1999) in contrast to pIgR, which only works in a unidirectional manner. The ability of FcRn to transport IgG bidirectionally may allow for its ability to facilitate Ag transport from the lumen into the subjacent lamina propria (Claypool *et al.* 2002). It is intriguing to note that there is increasing evidence for the presence of IgG in the gut lumen, especially in disease states. This IgG may form complexes with luminal Ags and promote facilitated transport of Ags into the IEC. The second pathway involves another Ig receptor, that being the polymeric Ig receptor (pIgR) or secretory component (SC). The pIgR is expressed only on the basolateral surface of the polarized epithelial cell and has long been known to serve as the major transport pathway for secretory IgA (S-IgA). However, recent studies by Mazanec *et al.* have demonstrated that the pIgR can bind sIgA/Ag (virus in these studies) complexes and facilitate their transport from the basolateral surface to the apex. In this setting, virus that enters the cell from the lamina propria would be effectively removed into the lumen. Alternatively, virus that enters the cell apically can meet with vacuolar compartments containing sIgA and viral neutralization can occur within the cell. The pIgR may also be capable of transport from a luminal to abluminal direction across the IEC.

Finally, bacteria and viruses can enter the IEC, but their intracellular pathway may be quite distinct from that of soluble proteins. Invasive pathogenic microorganisms may bypass the class I–containing or class II–containing vesicular compartments and enter the lamina propria unchanged. In the lamina propria, these pathogens can encounter professional APCs and inflammatory cells.

Antigen uptake by dendritic cells

DCs are the most potent APCs described. Distinct immune responses occur depending upon whether the DC presenting the Ag is mature or immature. Rescigno *et al.* (2001) recently described a novel property of DCs. They are able to express tight junction proteins (e.g., ZO1) and intercalate their dendrites between the epithelium and into the lumen, potentially sampling Ag directly from the lumen and presenting these to cells in the lamina propria. Although this has not been shown to be functionally relevant, it is of interest that measures used to increase DCs in the gut are associated with an increase in oral tolerance induction (Viney *et al.* 1998).

Mechanisms of antigen processing

As mentioned in the introduction, Ags must be processed before they are presented to and recognized by T cells. Conventionally, APCs (monocytes, B cells) internalize exogenous Ags through phagocytosis (a phenomenon first described by Metchnikoff in 1884) as described earlier. Within the endosome, limited proteolysis results in the generation of fragments that subsequently are expressed on the cell surface in combination with MHC class II molecules (Germain 1986). Endogenous Ags (viral proteins) utilize a distinct pathway described subsequently and typically associate with MHC class I molecules. Endogenous Ags can also enter MHC class I molecules via a pathway that has been coined "cross-priming."

The numerous steps and mechanisms of these cytosolic phenomena (processing) are not completely understood. The endosomal compartment develops an acidic pH that facilitates proteolytic enzyme activity that digests pinocytosed material (Braciale *et al.* 1987). After digestion in the endosome, the Ag fragments have one of two fates: they can bind to class II molecules in multivesicular bodies and be recycled back to the membrane as a complex or the endosome can fuse with a lysosome, resulting in further proteolysis and loss of immunogenicity or potential recycling to the surface. The signals that direct the choice of one pathway or the other are unknown. However, class II molecules produced in the Golgi are associated with a third chain, the invariant chain (Cresswell 1992). This chain stabilizes the class II molecule so it can exit the Golgi, but will be processed by proteases (cathepsin S) in an acidic compartment allowing peptide to bind to the MHC molecule. Once bound to peptide, which is facilitated by HLA-DM and inhibited by HLA-DO, the class II molecule is targeted to the surface. Fusion of multiple endosomes or Golgi vesicles with endosomes forms multi-vesicular bodies that may be important in signaling recycling.

Peptides generated by processing associate with the Ag-binding groove in the MHC. Typically, for macrophage-, DC-, and B-cell–derived peptides, these peptides are between 8 and 14 amino acids in length (Sette and Grey 1992). Thus potential differences in processing machinery may alter the types of immune response generated. Association of peptides with MHC class I molecules is different from association with class II. Class I molecules formed in the endoplasmic reticulum (ER) associate with cytoplasmic peptides that are carried to the ER by transporters associated with Ag presentation (TAP) (Monaco 1992). Peptides of shorter length (compared with class II MHC) are generally the rule (8–10 mers) (Braciale 1992). Class I–peptide complexes traffic to the membrane, where they can be recognized by T-cell receptors on CD8[+] T cells. One additional intracytoplasmic transporter has been identified that may be relevant in the GI tract. The family of heat-shock proteins bind peptides and can transfer these peptides to class I (and maybe class II) molecules within the cell (Vanbuskirk et al. 1989).

It has recently become clear that a third pathway of Ag presentation exists for presentation of lipid and glycolipid Ags of mycobacteria and mammalian cells (Beckman 1994; Sieling 1995, 1997a, b; Joyce et al. 1998) (Table 1). This pathway is associated with the CD1 family of proteins (Caide 1995a, b). Although the proteins are MHC class I–like in structure, and associate with β2 microglobulin, their pathway of biosynthesis is TAP independent and involves an endocytic cycle through the MIIC compartment by virtue of a YXXZ (tyrosine–amino acid–amino acid–hydrophobic amino acid) motif in the cytoplasmic tail of CD1b, c, and d (Blumberg 1996). This pathway is therefore inhibitable by chloroquine and concanamycin A. The CD1 family of proteins fall into two groups: CD1a–c, which are expressed predominantly by professional APCs such as dendritic cells, monocytes activated by GM-CSF and IL-4 and B cells, and CD1d, which is expressed primarily by B cells, hepatocytes, and epithelial cells including IECs, making these cell types important potential APCs for CD1 molecules.

Antigen processing by IECs

Although it is well documented that Ags are taken up apically by IEC traffic in Class II–containing compartments,

surprisingly little is known about the fate of these Ags within these compartments. That appropriate processing occurs can be inferred from the early studies documenting that IEC could process and present proteins to either CD4[+] T-cell hybridomas or alloreactive T cells (Kaiserlian et al. 1993; Mayer et al. 1990). That processing was not optimal can be inferred from the studies documenting that the level of T-cell activation was lower when compared with that of professional APCs. Bland and co-workers (1987) directly demonstrated that OVA processed by IEC failed to evoke a T-cell response when that Ag mixture was used to pulse fixed macrophages. This suggested that the action of processing of Ag was distinct in the different APCs. This concept was strengthened by the finding that leupeptin, a conventional endosomal protease inhibitor, failed to block processing and presentation of OVA by rat IECs to primed T cells. Several groups focused on the expression of endosomal proteases in IEC. Many of the cathepsins were shown to be present, including cathepsin B, D, H, and L; however, in many studies the levels of these critical enzymes were lower than those reported for professional APCs. Clearly more critical analyses of not only the existence but also the function of these proteases are required to definitively establish the degree of processing capability of the normal IEC.

Antigen presentation in the mucosal tissues

Because of differences in the antigenic microenvironment of the different organs, the responsibilities of the local immune systems must also be different. To coordinate these diverse responsibilities, the mechanisms of Ag handling must also be diverse. Among the mucosal tissues, the intestinal mucosa is the largest and is exposed continuously to food Ags, viruses, bacteria, parasites, or the by-products of these organisms. For this reason, it is appropriate that Ag presentation, interactions between immunocompetent T cells and APCs, and other immunologic phenomena are also very specialized.

Although other mucosal sites (lung, bladder) are also exposed chronically to Ag, the magnitude of exposure is much less. Therefore, let us first discuss mechanisms of Ag entry into the GI mucosa. Early reports suggested that specialized epithelial cells, M cells, were responsible for Ag handling in the gut. M cells are believed to derive from epithelial cells and reside over PP (Shimizu and Andrew 1967; Wolf and Bye 1984). Some variability has been seen in the reports that these cells express class II molecules on their surface (Bjerke and Brandtzaeg 1988; Bland and Kambarage 1991). Large particulate Ags seem particularly well suited for uptake by M cells (Owen 1977), and some viruses bind to M cells via a specific receptor (e.g., poliovirus, reovirus III) (Wolf et al. 1981; Sicinski et al. 1990). However, the number of M cells in the intestine is limited when compared with the vast array of immunogenic substances encountered in the lumen. M cells appear to transport Ag by transcytosis without any processing of the Ag (Owen et al. 1986), so the immune response relies on macrophages lying below the M cells. Major evidence for this concept has been provided by the studies of Owen and Jones (1974) documenting that these cells lack lysosomes, an important source of proteolytic enzymes in their cytoplasm.

The transport of large macromolecules has been demonstrated clearly by many researchers. Although controversy exists over whether M cells express class II molecules (Hirata et al. 1986; Bjerke and Brandtzaeg 1990), the general feeling is that these cells do not interact with T cells in the lamina propria. Instead, Ags pass through in pinocytotic vesicles untouched or unprocessed. One group of investigators has documented the presence of acidic vesicles (lysosomes possibly) in these cells, but formal proof is still required (Allen et al. 1992). M cells predominate in the small bowel where Ag entry is greatest, but also exist in the colon and rectum. In fact, some investigators have suggested that these cells may be the site of entry for HIV (Lehner et al. 1991).

The next obvious question is what happens to Ag after passage through the M cell. This question raises the issue of the role of macrophages in the GI tract. Macrophages are quite heterogeneous, and subpopulations localize to distinct areas in the GI tract, where they express different functional properties. Much of the information regarding intestinal macrophages comes from immunohistochemical studies, unfortunately with some degree of disparity. However, the disparate findings can be explained. Most studies come to a general consensus on location and functional properties. Researchers generally agree on the location of intestinal macrophages: the villus core of the small bowel, the subepithelial space in the crypt, under the dome (M cell) epithelium overlying PP, and in the patch itself (Golder and Doe 1983; Selby et al. 1983; Winter et al. 1983; Beeken et al. 1987; Harvey and Jones 1991). Most groups report that macrophages are greater in number in the small bowel, underscoring a role in Ag sampling, detoxification via release of chemical mediators (superoxides, etc.), and scavenging of potentially harmful substances (with possible release into the lumen). This latter point has been suggested by the finding of large amounts of carbon particles in carbon-fed mice within subepithelial macrophages and little free carbon elsewhere (including the patch) (Joel et al. 1978). Several types of material have been found within macrophages, including DNA from damaged cells (Sawicki et al. 1977). Colonic macrophages may be increased because of the numbers of enteric Ags that pass through or between the epithelium.

With respect to M-cell transport of Ag, subepithelial macrophages take up the transported Ag and presumably "carry" it to the PP. The actual transfer of Ag has not been elucidated, especially since the number of macrophages within the patch is limited and Ag transfer has never been visualized. Within the villous core, the observations have been more clear. Macrophages reside near plasma cells in the subepithelial layer. Non-M-cell–transported Ag may be processed and presented by the macrophage, although formal proof of this behavior is required. Macrophages in the small and large bowel have been reported to be suppressive, secreting PGE2, and inhibiting immune responses (Pavli et al. 1990) in a manner similar to alveolar macrophages (in a mixed lymphocyte reaction). These cells do express nonspe-

cific esterase and acid phosphatase, consistent with conventional APCs, but the level of expression is lower than that of peripheral monocytes in some studies (Mahida et al. 1989). These enzymes, however, render the cells functional as APCs.

Functionally, gut macrophages are also quite heterogeneous. Generally, they are poorly adherent to plastic, although this characteristic may relate to isolation by Ficoll-Hypaque (Verspaget and Beeken 1985). These cells do adhere to fibronectin-coated plates, however, and can be enriched by this method. Gut macrophages express FcR and take up immune complexes (coated red blood cells, toxin–antitoxin complexes). Phagocytosis can stimulate the respiratory burst, which is less active than that of peripheral monocytes but present nonetheless. Gut macrophages also express MHC class II and CD1 Ags. Finally, these cells produce complement components C3 and C4 and express complement receptors. However, as stated earlier, they may be suppressive in mixed lymphocyte reactions; macrophages within the patch are poorly stimulatory (Le Fevre et al. 1979). This latter point is important because, with the potential for a large Ag load in the patch, priming but not active immune response is consistent with the histology of the patch, which differs from a reactive lymph node. Thus, in summary, much is still unknown about intestinal macrophages.

Antigen presentation by intestinal epithelial cells

We are, therefore, left with one cell (B cells have not been studied carefully for their APC function in the gut) that has been proposed as a major player in Ag presentation in the gut, the IEC. Several groups studying different model systems have documented that intestinal epithelium, especially in the small bowel, constitutively expresses class II molecules (Wiman et al. 1978; Mason et al. 1981; Selby et al. 1981; Kaiserlian et al. 1990; Mayer et al. 1990). Further, as alluded to earlier, subsequent studies revealed that these cells could function as APCs, processing and presenting Ag to primed T cells (Bland and Warren 1986a, b; Mayer and Shlien 1987; Kaiserlian et al. 1989). However, the unique feature is that these cells appear to activate CD8+ suppressor T cells selectively by direct activation (Bland and Warren 1986a, b; Mayer and Shlien 1987) or by suppression by soluble factors (PGE2) (Santos et al. 1990; Christ et al. 1997). Such findings concur with the phenomenon of oral tolerance, in which the mechanisms of suppressor cell activation were previously unclear. However, epithelial cells are capable of stimulating CD4− T cells as well (Kaiserlian et al. 1989; Mayer and Eisenhardt 1990) via classical class II–mediated pathways. Under most circumstances, suppression would predominate, whereas in other situations (e.g., inflammatory states), helper T-cell activation could occur.

The expression of class II molecules by IECs had been somewhat controversial. With the use of more sensitive techniques, this controversy has ended with strong evidence that IECs do express MHC class II molecules. Although researchers generally agree that small bowel IECs constitutively express class II molecules, identification of these molecules on colonocytes has been more variable. With sensitive techniques, class II molecules can be detected with expression that may be patchy. Expression appears to relate to the presence of intraepithelial lymphocytes (IELs) (Cerf-Bensussan *et al.* 1984) and is enhanced in states in which IFN-γ is produced or passively administered (Ouyang *et al.* 1988; Steiniger *et al.* 1989; Masson and Perdue 1990; Zhang and Michael 1990). The distribution of class II molecules on the IECs is also of interest. Presumably because of the overlapping membranes on the microvillus border, class II molecules are highly expressed on the luminal side. Intuitively, this situation makes little sense since cell interactions (i.e., T cell–IEC) do not occur in the lumen. However, Bland (1990) has suggested that the class II molecules may serve as "peptide receptors" for predigested (or preprocessed) peptides that result from proteolysis within the stomach and upper small bowel. Peptides bound to class II molecules then would be internalized and presented to lamina propria T cells (via fenestrations in the basement membrane) or even potentially to IELs.

IEC also express classical class I molecules, although the functional integrity of this set of restriction elements has not really been explored. There is little evidence for widespread cytotoxic T lymphocyte (CTL) activity against virally infected IECs and no data to support that there is leakage of Ag from the classical class II pathway into the class I pathway (cross-priming). This has been described in a limited fashion in professional APCs where pulsing with bacterial Ags exogenously can result in the generation of antibacterial CTL. Using a transgenic model system where OVA peptide is expressed by small intestinal IECs (driven by the intestinal fatty acid binding promoter), it is clear that MHC class I–restricted Ag presentation can occur. However, it is of interest that in the absence of a viral infection, no destruction of IECs is seen despite the presence of anti-OVA CTLs. These findings suggest that class I–restricted immune responses related to the IEC are tightly regulated, perhaps as a defense mechanism against producing large holes in the epithelial barrier. Other model systems confirm the ability of IECs to process and present Ag in an MHC class II–restricted fashion (Hershberg *et al.* 1997) and possibly *in vivo* (Vezys *et al.* 2001). Moreover, in intestinal inflammation, IEC uptake and presentation by this pathway may be increased (Telega *et al.* 2000) The functional relevance of these pathways remains to be established. However, it is of interest that IECs are apparently capable of cross-priming MHC class II pathways by the ability to form exosomes (van Niel *et al.* 2001). Exosomes are class II/peptide-bearing vacuoles that are secreted by B cells and IECs. These can be picked up by classical APCs, processed, and presented to local or distant T-cell populations.

Human IECs also express several nonclassical class I molecules, such as the FcRn, MICA, and HLA-E. However, the most abundantly expressed class Ib molecule, which is relevant to Ag presentation, is CD1d. This nonpolymorphic molecule may exist in several forms on the IEC including a β2 microglobulin associated (48 kDa), which is fully glycosylated as well as an unassociated form (37 kDa), which is nonglycosylated. Initial studies suggested that IELs might recognize

Ags presented by CD1d, especially cytolytic IELs. The nature of the Ag presented to these cytolytic IEL by CD1d is unknown. As mentioned earlier, members of the CD1 family have been shown to bind glycolipid Ags consistent with the crystal structure of CD1d. One study by Castano *et al.*, however, did document that CD1 could bind hydrophobic protein Ags, although the size of the peptide tended to be larger than those capable of binding to classical class I or class II molecules. Moreover, Panja *et al.* (1993) demonstrated that antibodies to CD1d inhibited the proliferation of CD1d-reactive T cells in peripheral T cell–IEC cocultures. Thus nonclassical presentation may be a dominant form of Ag presentation in the gut. Campbell *et al.* (1999) further demonstrated that gp180 and CD1d form a complex on the IEC surface and that a subpopulation of CD8+CD28− IEC–activated cells are CD1d restricted (Allez *et al.* 2002). *In vivo* studies are really required to define the pathway utilized most efficiently. However, it is now clear that immune cells, both human and mouse, exhibit CD1d-restricted glycolipid Ag presentation (van de Wal *et al.* 2003) that is similar in nature to class II pathways (Hershberg *et al.* 1998).

An issue related to this unique form of presentation is the fact that the IEC, which is a class II MHC–bearing cell, stimulates CD8+ T cells. The majority of IELs are typically CD8+. The data on this topic are only now becoming available; some suggest a non-class II–CD8 interaction between IECs and T cells (Mayer *et al.* 1990), and potentially a nonclassical class I molecule such as either CDld, demonstrated to be present on human and murine IECs (Bleicher *et al.* 1990; Blumberg *et al.* 1991, Balk *et al.* 1994), or TL in the mouse (Hershberg *et al.* 1990). The interaction of a class I–like molecule with CD8+ T cells may overshadow the "typical" interaction of class II with CD4. These speculations are just that, and although IECs are tempting cells to evoke in normal Ag presentation in the gut, no consistent *in vivo* model has been generated, and no clear evidence exists that these cells clearly function as APCs in a physiologic system.

SUMMARY

Given the nature of the GI tract and its continuous Ag exposure, obviously unique systems of Ag handling must be developed. Clearly typical APCs do not function typically in the GI tract and atypical (nonprofessional) APCs may play a more dominant role. However, a clear understanding of this entire process awaits the development of physiologic model systems in which these hypotheses can be tested.

REFERENCES

Abreu, M. T., Vora, P., Faure, E., Thomas, L. S., Arnold, E. T., and Arditi, M. (2001). Decreased expression of Toll-like receptor-4 and MD-2 correlates with intestinal epithelial cell protection against dysregulated proinflammatory gene expression in response to bacterial lipopolysaccharide. *J. Immunol.* 167(3), 1609–1616.

Allen, C. H., Mendrick, D. L., and Trier, J. S. (1992). M cells contain acidic compartments and express class II MHC determinants. *Gastroenterology* 102, A589.

Allez, M., Brimnes, J., Dotan, I., and Mayer, L. (2002). Expansion of CD8[+] T cells with regulatory function after interaction with intestinal epithelial cells. *Gastroenterology* 123(5), 1516–1526.

Andoh, A., Fujiyama, Y., Bamba, T., and Hosoda, S. (1993). Differential cytokine regulation of complement C3, C4 and factor B synthesis in human intestinal epithelial cell line, Caco-2. *J. Immunol.* 151, 4239–4247.

Arvieux, J., Yssel, H., and Colomb, M. G. (1988). Antigen bound C3b and C4b enhance antigen-presenting cell function in activation of human T-cell clones. *Immunology* 65, 229–235.

Beeken, W., Northwood, I., Beliveau, C., and Gump, D. (1987). Phagocytes in cell suspensions of human colon mucosa. *Gut* 28, 976–980.

Berin, M. C., Kiliaan, A. J., Yang, P. C., Groot, J. A., Taminiau, J. A., and Perdue, M. H. (1997). Rapid transepithelial antigen transport in rat jejunum: Impact of sensitization and the hypersensitivity reaction. *Gastroenterology* 113(3), 856–864.

Berrebi, D., Maudinas, R., Hugot, J. P., Chamaillard, M., Chareyre, F., De Lagausie, P., Yang, C., Desreumaux, P., Giovannini, M., Cezard, J. P., Zouali, H., Emilie, D., and Peuchmaur, M. (2003). Card15 gene overexpression in mononuclear and epithelial cells of the inflamed Crohn's disease colon. *Gut* 52(6), 840–846.

Bjerke, K., and Brandtzaeg, P. (1988). Lack of relation between expression of HLA-DR and secretory component (SC) in follicle associated epithelium of human Peyer's patches. *Clin. Exp. Immunol.* 71, 502–507.

Bland, P. W., and Kambarage, D. M. (1991). Antigen handling by the epithelium and lamina propria macrophages. *Gastroenterol. Clin. North Am.* 20, 577–596.

Bland, P. W., and Warren, L. G. (1986a). Antigen presentation by epithelial cells of the rat small intestine. I. Kinetics, antigen specificity and blocking by anti-Ia antisera. *Immunology* 58, 1–7.

Bland, P. W., and Warren, L. G. (1986b). Antigen presentation by epithelial cells of the rat small intestine. II. Selective induction of suppressor T cells. *Immunology* 58, 9–14.

Bland, P. W., and Whiting, C. V. (1989). Antigen processing by isolated rat intestinal villus enterocytes. *Immunology* 68(4), 497–502.

Bleicher, P. A., Balk, S. P., Hagen, S. J., Blumberg, R. S., Flotte, T. J., and Terhorst, C. (1990). Expression of murine CD1 on gastrointestinal epithelium. *Science* 250, 679–682.

Blumberg, R. S., Terhorst, C., Bleicher, P., McDermott, F. V., Allan, C. H., Landau, S. B., Trier, J. S., and Balk, S. P. (1991). Expression of a nonpolymorphic MHC class I-like molecule, CDlD, by human intestinal epithelial cells. *J. Immunol.* 147, 2518–2524.

Bocker, U., Yezerskyy, O., Feick, P., Manigold, T., Panja, A., Kalina, U., Herweck, F., Rossol, S., and Singer, M. V. (2003). Responsiveness of intestinal epithelial cell lines to lipopolysaccharide is correlated with Toll-like receptor 4 but not Toll-like receptor 2 or CD14 expression. *Int. J. Colorectal Dis.* 18(1), 25–32.

Bonen, D. K., Ogura, Y., Nicolae, D. L., Inohara, N., Saab, L., Tanabe, T., Chen, F. F., Foster, S. J., Duerr, R. H., Brant, S. R., Cho, J. H., and Nunez, G. (2003). Crohn's disease-associated NOD2 variants share a signaling defect in response to lipopolysaccharide and peptidoglycan. *Gastroenterology* 124(1),140–146.

Botazzo, G. F., Pujol-Borrell, R., Hanafusa, T., and Feldmann, M. (1983). Role of aberrant HLA-DR expression and antigen presentation in induction of endocrine autoimmunity. *Lancet* 2, 1115–1119.

Braciale, T. J. (1992). Antigen processing for presentation by MHC class I molecules. *Curr. Opin. Immunol.* 4, 59–62.

Braciale, T. J., Morrison, L. A., Sweetser, M. T., Sambrook, J., Gething, M. J., and Braciale, V. L. (1987). Antigen presentation pathways to class I and class 11 MHC-restricted T lymphocytes. *Immunol. Rev.* 98, 95–114.

Brandeis, J. M., Sayegh, M. H., Gallon, L., Blumberg, R. S., and Carpenter, C. B. (1994). Rat intestinal epithelial cells present major histocompatibility complex allopeptides to primed T cells. *Gastroenterology* 107(5), 1537–1542.

Brandtzaeg, P., and Bjerke, K. (1990). Immunomorphological characteristics of human Peyer's patches. *Digestion* 46(Suppl. 2), 262–273.

Campbell, N. A., Kim, H. S., Blumberg, R. S., and Mayer, L. (1999). The nonclassical class I molecule CD1d associates with the novel CD8 ligand gp180 on intestinal epithelial cells. *J. Biol. Chem.* 274(37), 26259–26265.

Campbell, N. A., Park, M. S., Toy, L. S., Yio, X. Y., Devine, L., Kavathas, P., and Mayer, L. (2002). A non-class I MHC intestinal epithelial surface glycoprotein, gp180, binds to CD8. *Clin. Immunol.* 102(3), 267–274.

Cario, E., and Podolsky, D. K. (2000). Differential alteration in intestinal epithelial cell expression of toll-like receptor 3 (TLR3) and TLR4 in inflammatory bowel disease. *Infect. Immun.*, 68(12), 7010–7017.

Cario, E., Rosenberg, I. M., Brandwein, S. L., Beck, P. L., Reinecker, H. C., and Podolsky, D. K. (2000). Lipopolysaccharide activates distinct signaling pathways in intestinal epithelial cell lines expressing Toll-like receptors. *J. Immunol.* 164(2), 966–972.

Cario, E., Gerken, G., and Podolsky, D. K. (2002). "For whom the bell tolls!"—Innate defense mechanisms and survival strategies of the intestinal epithelium against lumenal pathogens. *Z. Gastroenterol.* 40(12), 983–990.

Celis, E., and Chang, T. W. (1984). Antibodies to hepatitis B surface antigen potentiate the response of human T lymphocyte clones to the same antigen. *Science* 224, 297–299.

Cepek, K. L., Parker, C. M., Madara, J. L., and Brenner, M. B. (1993). Integrin αEβ7 mediates adhesion of T lymphocytes to epithelial cells. *J. Immunol.* 150, 3459–3470.

Cepek, K. L., Shaw, S. K., Parker, C. M., Russell, G. J., Morrow, J. S., Rimm, D. L., and Brenner, M. B. (1994). Adhesion between epithelial cells and T lymphocytes mediated by E-cadherin and the αEβ7 integrin. *Nature* 372, 190–193.

Cerf-Bensussan, N., Quaroni, A., Kurnick, J. T., and Bhan, A. K. (1984). Intraepithelial lymphocytes modulate Ia expression by intestinal epithelial cells. *J. Immunol.* 132, 2244–2251.

Chesnut, R. W., and Grey, H. M. (1981). Studies on the capacity of B cells to serve as antigen presenting cells. *J. Immunol.* 126, 1075–1079.

Chesnut, R. W., Colon, S. M., and Grey, H. M. (1982). Antigen presentation by normal B cells, B cell tumors, and macrophages: Functional and biochemical comparison. *J. Immunol.* 128, 1764–1768.

Christ, A. D., Colgan, S. P., Probert, C. S. J., Balk, S. P., and Blumberg, R. S. (1996). CD3-mediated proliferation of human lymphocytes is modulated by soluble factor(s) from a human intestinal epithelial cell (IEC) line. *Gastroenterology* 110, A883.

Ciacci, C., Mahida, Y. R., Dignass, A., Koizumi, M., and Podolsky, D. C. (1993a). Functional interleukin-2 receptors on intestinal epithelial cells. *J. Clin. Invest.* 92, 527–532.

Ciacci, C., Lind, S. E., and Podolsky, D. K. (1993b). Transforming growth factor b regulation of migration in wounded rat intestinal epithelial monolayers. *Gastroenterology* 105, 93–101.

Claypool, S. M., Dickinson, B. L., Yoshida, M., Lencer, W. I., and Blumberg, R. S. (2002). Functional reconstitution of human FcRn in Madin-Darby canine kidney cells requires co-expressed human beta 2-microglobulin. *J. Biol. Chem.* 277(31), 28038–28050.

Cohen, B. E., Rosenthal, A. S., and Paul, W. E. (1973). Antigen macrophage interaction. II. Relative roles of cytophilic antibody and other membrane sites. *J. Immunol.* 111, 820–828.

Colgan, S. P., Resnick, M. B., Parkos, C. A., Delp-Archer, C., McGuirk, D., Bacarra, A. E., Weller, P. F., and Madara, J. L. (1994). IL-4 directly modulates function of a model human intestinal epithelium. *J. Immunol.* 153, 2122–2129.

Crabtree, J. E., Xiang, Z., Lindley, I. J., Tompkins, D. S., Rappuoli, R., and Covacci, A. (1995). Induction of interleukin-8 secretion from gastric epithelial cells by a cagA negative isogenic mutant of *Helicobacter pylori. J. Clin. Pathol.* 48, 967–969.

Cresswell, P. (1992). Chemistry and functional role of the invariant chain. *Curr. Opin. Immunol.* 4, 87–92.

Daha, M. R., and van Es, L. A. (1984). Fc- and complement receptor dependent degradation of soluble immune complexes and stable immunoglobulin aggregates by guinea pig monocytes, peritoneal macrophages, and Kupffer cells. *J. Leukoc. Biol.* 36, 569–579.

Darfeuille-Michaud, A. (2002). Adherent-invasive *Escherichia coli*: A putative new *E. coli* pathotype associated with Crohn's disease. *Int. J. Med. Microbiol.* 292(3–4), 185–93.

Dickinson, B. L., Badizadegan, K., Wu, Z., Ahouse, J. C., Zhu, X., Simister, N. E., Blumberg, R. S., and Lencer, W. I. (1999). Bidirectional FcRn-dependent IgG transport in a polarized human intestinal epithelial cell line. *J. Clin. Invest.* 104(7), 903–911.

Dignass, A. U., Podolsky, D. K., and Rachmilewitz, D. (1995). NO chi generation by cultured small intestinal epithelial cells. *Dig. Dis. Sci.* 40, 1859–1865.

Dogan, A., Wang, Z. D., and Spencer, J. (1995). E-cadherin expression in intestinal epithelium. *J. Clin. Pathol.* 48, 143–146.

Ebert, E. C. (1989). Proliferative responses of human intraepithelial lymphocytes to various T-cell stimuli. *Gastroenterology* 97, 1372–1381.

Ebert, E. C., Roberts, A. I., Devereux, D., and Nagase, H. (1990). Selective immunosuppressive action of a factor produced by colon cancer cells. *Cancer Res.* 50, 6158–6161.

Eckmann, L., Jung, H. C., Schurer-Maly, C., Panja, A., Morzycka-Wroblewska, E., and Kagnoff, M. F. (1993a). Differential cytokine expression by human intestinal epithelial cell lines: Regulated expression of interleukin 8. *Gastroenterology* 105, 1689–1697.

Eckmann, L., Kagnoff, M. F., and Fierer, J. (1993b). Epithelial cells secrete the chemokine interleukin-8 in response to bacterial entry. *Infect. Immun.* 61, 4569–4574.

Eckmann, L., Reed, S. L., Smith, J. R., and Kagnoff, M. F. (1995). *Entamoeba histolytica* trophozoites induce an inflammatory cytokine response by cultured human cells through the paracrine action of cytolytically released interleukin-1 alpha. *J. Clin. Invest.* 96, 1269–1279.

Eckmann, L., Stenson, W. F., Savidge, T. C., Lowe, D. C., Barrett, K. E., Fierer, J., Smith, J. R., and Kagnoff, M. F. (1997). Role of intestinal epithelial cells in the host secretory response to infection by invasive bacteria: Bacterial entry induces epithelial prostaglandin h synthase-2 expression and prostaglandin E2 and F2 alpha production. *J. Clin. Invest.* 100, 296–309.

Eisenhauer, P. B., Harwig, S. S., and Lehrer, R. I. (1992). Cryptdins: Antimicrobial defensins of the murine small intestine. *Infect. Immun.* 60, 3556–3565.

Fierer, J., Eckmann, L., and Kagnoff, M. (1993). IL-8 secreted by epithelial cells invaded by bacteria. *Infect. Agents Dis.* 2, 255–258.

Geppert, T. D., and Lipsky, P. E. (1985). Antigen presentation by interferon γ-treated endothelial cells and fibroblasts: Differential ability to function as antigen presenting cells despite comparable Ia expression. *J. Immunol.* 135, 3750–3762.

Germain, R. N. (1986). Immunology. The ins and outs of antigen processing and presentation. *Nature* 322, 687–689.

Glasser, A. L., Boudeau, J., Barnich, N., Perruchot, M. H., Colombel, J. F., and Darfeuille-Michaud, A. (2001). Adherent invasive *Escherichia coli* strains from patients with Crohn's disease survive and replicate within macrophages without inducing host cell death. *Infect. Immun.* 69(9), 5529–5537.

Golder, J. P., and Doe, W. F. (1983). Isolation and preliminary characterization of human intestinal macrophages. *Gastroenterology* 84, 795–802.

Gonnella, P. A., and Neutra, M. R. (1984). Membrane-bound and fluid-phase macromolecules enter separate prelysosomal compartments in absorptive cells of suckling rat ileum. *J. Cell Biol.* 99(3), 909–917.

Gonnella, P. A., and Wilmore, D. W. (1993). Co-localization of class II antigen and exogenous antigen in the rat enterocyte. *J. Cell Sci.* 106(Pt. 3), 937–940.

Groh, V., Steinle, A., Bauer, S., and Spies, T. (1998). Recognition of stress-induced MHC molecules by intestinal epithelial gamma delta T cells. *Science* 279, 1737–1740.

Gutierrez, O., Pipaon, C., Inohara, N., Fontalba, A., Ogura, Y., Prosper, F., Nunez, G., and Fernandez-Luna, J. L. (2002). Induction of Nod2 in myelomonocytic and intestinal epithelial cells via

nuclear factor-kappa B activation. *J. Biol. Chem.* 277(44), 41701–41705.

Halstensen, T. S., Mollnes, T. E., Garred, P., Fausa, O., and Brandtzaeg, P. (1990). Epithelial deposition of immunoglobulin G1 and activated complement (C3b and terminal complement complex) in ulcerative colitis. *Gastroenterology* 98, 1264–1271.

Harvey, J., and Jones, D. B. (1991). Human mucosal T-lymphocyte and macrophage subpopulations in normal and inflamed intestine. *Clin. Exp. Allergy* 21, 549–560.

Hata, Y., Ota, S., Nagata, T., Uehara, Y., Terano, A., and Sugimoto, T. (1993). Primary colonic epithelial cell culture of the rabbit producing prostaglandins. *Prostaglandins* 45, 129–141.

Hershberg, R., Eghtesady, P., Sydora, B., Brorson, K., Cheroutre, H., Modlin, R., and Kronenberg, M. (1990). Expression of the thymus leukemia antigen in mouse intestinal epithelium. *Proc. Natl. Acad. Sci. USA* 87, 9727–9731.

Hershberg, R. M., Framson, P. E., Cho, D. H., Lee, L. Y., Kovats, S., Beitz, J., Blum, J. S., and Nepom, G. T. (1997). Intestinal epithelial cells use two distinct pathways for HLA class II antigen processing. *J. Clin. Invest.* 100(1), 204–215.

Hershberg, R. M., Cho, D. H., Youakim, A., Bradley, M. B., Lee, J. S., Framson, P. E., and Nepom, G. T. (1998). Highly polarized HLA class II antigen processing and presentation by human intestinal epithelial cells. *J. Clin. Invest.* 102(4), 792–803.

Hirata, I., Austin, L. L., Blackwell, W. H., Weber, J. R., and Dobbins, W. O. 3rd (1986). Immunoelectron microscopic localization of HLA-DR antigen in control small intestine and colon and in inflammatory bowel disease. *Dig. Dis. Sci.* 31, 1317–1330.

Hisamatsu, T., Suzuki, M., Reinecker, H. C., Nadeau, W. J., McCormick, B. A., and Podolsky, D. K. (2003). CARD15/NOD2 functions as an antibacterial factor in human intestinal epithelial cells. *Gastroenterology* 124(4), 993–1000.

Hugot, J. P., Chamaillard, M., Zouali, H., Lesage, S., Cezard, J. P., Belaiche, J., Almer, S., Tysk, C., O'Morain, C. A., Gassull, M., Binder, V., Finkel, Y., Cortot, A., Modigliani, R., Laurent-Puig, P., Gower-Rousseau, C., Macry, J., Colombel, J. F., Sahbatou, M., and Thomas, G. (2001). Association of NOD2 leucine-rich repeat variants with susceptibility to Crohn's disease. *Nature* 411(6837), 599–603.

Joel, D. D., Laissue, J. A., and LeFevre, M. E. (1978). Distribution and fate of ingested carbon particles in mice. *J. Reticuloendothel. Soc.* 24(5), 477–487.

Joyce, S., Woods, A. S. Yewdell, J. W., Bennink, J. R., DeSilva, A. D., Boesteanu, A., Balk, S. P., Cotter, R. J., Brutkiewicz, R. R. (1998). Natural ligand of mouse CD1d1: Cellular glycosylphosphatidylinositol. *Science* 279, 1541–1544.

Jung, H. C., Eckmann, L., Yang, S. K., Panja, A., Fierer, J., Morzycka-Wroblewska, E., and Kagnoff, M. F. (1995). A distinct array of proinflammatory cytokines is expressed in human colon epithelial cells in response to bacterial invasion. *J. Clin. Invest.* 95, 55–65.

Kaiserlian, D., Vidal, K., and Reveillard, J. P. (1989). Murine enterocytes can present soluble antigen to specific class II-restricted CD4⁺ T cells. *Eur. J. Immunol.* 19(8), 1513–1516.

Kaiserlian, D., Nicolas, J. F., and Revillard, J. P. (1990). Constitutive expression of Ia molecules by murine epithelial cells: A comparison between keratinocytes and enterocytes. *J. Invest. Dermatol.* 94(3), 385–386.

Kaoutzani, P., Colgan, S. P., Cepek, K. L., Burkhard, P. G., Carlson, S., Delp-Archer, C., Brenner, M. B., and Madara, J. L. (1994). Reconstitution of cultured intestinal epithelial monolayers with a mucosal-derived T lymphocyte cell line. Modulation of epithelial phenotype dependent on lymphocyte–basolateral membrane apposition. *J. Clin. Invest.* 94, 788–796.

Kehry, M. R., and Yamashita, L. C. (1990). Role of the low affinity Fc epsilon receptor in B lymphocyte antigen presentation. *Immunology* 141, 77–81.

Kindon, H., Pothoulakis, C., Thim, L., Lynch-Devaney, K., and Podolsky, D. K. (1995). Trefoil peptide protection of intestinal epithelial barrier function: Cooperative interaction with mucin glycoprotein. *Gastroenterology* 109, 516–523.

Kvale, D., Krajci, P., and Brandtzaeg, P. (1992). Expression and regulation of adhesion molecules ICAM-1 (CD54) and LFA-3

(CD58) in human intestinal epithelial cell lines. *Scand. J. Immunol.* 35, 669–676.

Laky, K., Lefrancois, L., and Puddington, L. (1997). Age-dependent intestinal lymphoproliferative disorder due to stem cell factor receptor deficiency: Parameters in small and large intestine. *J. Immunol.* 158, 1417–1427.

Lala, S., Ogura, Y., Osborne, C., Hor, S. Y., Bromfield, A., Davies, S., Ogunbiyi, O., Nunez, G., and Keshav, S. (2003). Crohn's disease and the NOD2 gene: A role for Paneth cells. *Gastroenterology* 125(1), 47–57.

Lanzavecchia, A., Roosnek, E., Gregory, T., Berman, P., and Abrignani, S. (1988). T cells can present antigens such as HIV gp120 targeted to their own surface molecules. *Nature* 334, 530–532.

LaSalle, J. M., Tolentino, P. J., Freeman, G. J., Nadler, L. M., and Hafler, D. A. (1992). Early signaling defects in human T cells anergized by T cell presentation of autoantigen. *J. Exp. Med.* 176, 177–186.

Le Duc, L. E., Brown, L., and Vidrich, A. (1994). Bradykinin and FMLP stimulate prostanoid production by adult rabbit colonocytes in culture. *Am. J. Physiol.* 267, G778–G785.

LeFevre, M. E., Hammer, R., and Joel, D. D. (1979). Macrophages of the mammalian small intestine: A review. *J. Reticuloendothel. Soc.* 26, 553–573.

Lehner, T., Hussain, L., Wilson, J., and Chapman, M. (1991). Mucosal transmission of HIV. *Nature* 353, 709.

Lencer, W. I., Cheung, G., Strohmeier, G. R., Currie, M. G., Ouellette, A. J., Selsted, M. E., and Madara, J. L. (1997). Induction of epithelial chloride secretion by channel-forming cryptdins 2 and 3. *Proc. Natl. Acad. Sci. USA* 94, 8585–8589.

Li, Y., Yio, X. Y., and Mayer, L. (1995). Human intestinal epithelial cell-induced CD8+ T cell activation is mediated through CD8 and the activation of CD8-associated p56lck. *J. Exp. Med.* 182, 1079–1088.

Lundqvist, C., Baranov, V., Hammarstrom, S., Athlin, L., and Hammarstrom, M. L. (1995). Intraepithelial lymphocytes. Evidence for regional specialization and extrathymic T-cell maturation in the human gut epithelium. *Int. Immunol.* 7, 1473–1487.

Mahida, Y. R., Wu, K. C., and Jewell, D. P. (1988). Characterization of antigen-presenting activity of intestinal mononuclear cells isolated from normal and inflammatory bowel disease colon and ileum. *Immunology* 65, 543–549.

Mahida, Y. R., Patel, S., Gionchetti, P., Vaux, D., and Jewell, D. P. (1989). Macrophage subpopulations in lamina propria of normal and inflamed colon and terminal ileum. *Gut* 30, 826–834.

Mashimo, H., Wu, D. C., Podolsky, D. K., and Fishman, M. C. (1996). Impaired defense of intestinal mucosa in mice lacking intestinal trefoil factor. *Science* 274, 262–265.

Mason, D. W., Dallman, M., and Barclay, A. N. (1981). Graft-versus-host disease induces expression of Ia antigen in rat epidermal cells and gut epithelium. *Nature* 293, 150–151.

Masson, S. D., and Perdue, M. H. (1990). Changes in distribution of Ia antigen on epithelium of the jejunum and ileum in rats infected with *Nippostrongylus brasiliensis*. *Clin. Immunol. Immunopathol.* 57(1), 83–95.

Mayer, L., and Eisenhardt, D. (1990). Lack of induction of suppressor T cells by intestinal epithelial cells from patients with inflammatory bowel disease. *J. Clin. Invest.* 86, 1255–1260.

Mayer, L., and Shlien, R. (1987). Evidence for function of Ia molecules on gut epithelial cells in man. *J. Exp. Med.* 166, 1471–1483.

Mayer, L., Eisenhardt, D., Salomon, P., Bauer, W., Plous, R., and Piccinini, L. (1991). Expression of class 11 molecules on intestinal epithelial cells in humans: Differences between normal and inflammatory bowel disease. *Gastroenterology* 100, 3–12.

Mayer, L., Siden, E. Becker, S., and Eisenhardt, D. (1990). Antigen handling in the intestine mediated by normal enterocytes. *Adv. Mucosal Immunol.* 23–28.

McGee, D. W., Beagley, K. W., Aicher, W. K., and McGhee, J. R. (1992). Transforming growth factor-beta enhances interleukin-6 secretion by intestinal epithelial cells. *Immunology* 77, 7–12.

McGee, D. W., Elson, C. O., and McGhee, J. R. (1993). Enhancing effect of cholera toxin on interleukin-6 secretion by IEC-6 intestinal epithelial cells: Mode of action and augmenting effect of inflammatory cytokines. *Infect. Immun.* 61, 4637–4644.

McGee, D. W., Vitkus, S. J., and Lee, P. (1996). The effect of cytokine stimulation on IL-1 receptor mRNA expression by intestinal epithelial cells. *Cell Immunol.* 168, 276–280.

Melmed, G., Thomas, L. S., Lee, N., Tesfay, S. Y., Lukasek, K., Michelsen, K. S., Zhou, Y., Hu, B., Arditi, M., and Abreu, M. T. (2003). Human intestinal epithelial cells are broadly unresponsive to Toll-like receptor 2-dependent bacterial ligands: implications for host-microbial interactions in the gut. *J. Immunol.* 170(3), 1406–1415.

Mestecky, J., Lue, C., and Russell, M. W. (1991). Selective transport of IgA: Cellular and molecular aspects. *Gastroenterol. Clin. North Am.* 20, 441–471.

Meyer, T. A., Noguchi, Y., Ogle, C. K., Tiao, G., Wang, J. J., Fischer, J. E., and Hasselgreen, P. O. (1994). Endotoxin stimulates interleukin-6 production in intestinal epithelial cells: A synergistic effect with prostaglandin E2. *Arch. Surg.* 129, 1290–1294.

Monaco, J. J. (1992). Genes in the MHC that may affect antigen processing. *Curr. Opin. Immunol.* 4, 70–73.

Naik, S., Kelly, E. J., Meijer, L., Pettersson, S., and Sanderson, I. R. (2001). Absence of Toll-like receptor 4 explains endotoxin hyporesponsiveness in human intestinal epithelium. *J. Pediatr. Gastroenterol. Nutr.* 32(4), 449–453.

Nakazawa, A., Watanabe, M., Kanai, T., Yajima, T., Yamazaki, M., Ogata, H., Ishii, H., Azuma, M., and Hibi, T. (1999). Functional expression of costimulatory molecule CD86 on epithelial cells in the inflamed colonic mucosa. *Gastroenterology* 117(3), 536–545.

Nussenzweig, M. C., and Steinman, R. M. (1980). Contribution of dendritic cells to stimulation of the murine syngeneic mixed leukocyte reaction. *J. Exp. Med.* 151, 1196–1212.

Ogura, Y., Bonen, D. K., Inohara, N., Nicolae, D. L., Chen, F. F., Ramos, R., Britton, H., Moran, T., Karaliuskas, R., Duerr, R. H., Achkar, J. P., Brant, S. R., Bayless, T. M., Kirschner, B. S., Hanauer, S. B., Nunez, G., and Cho, J. H. (2001). A frameshift mutation in NOD2 associated with susceptibility to Crohn's disease. *Nature* 411(6837), 603–606.

Ouellette, A. J., Greco, R. M., James, M., Frederick, D., Naftilan, J., and Fallon, J. T. (1989). Developmental regulation of cryptdin, a corticostatin/defensin precursor mRNA in mouse small intestinal crypt epithelium. *J. Cell Biol.* 108, 1687–1695.

Owen, R. L. (1977). Sequential uptake of horseradish peroxidase by lymphoid follicle epithelium of Peyer's patches in the normal unobstructed mouse intestine: An ultrastructural study. *Gastroenterology* 72, 440–451.

Owen, R. L., and Jones, A. L. (1974). Epithelial cell specialization within human Peyer's patches: An ultrastructural study of intestinal lymphoid follicles. *Gastroenterology* 66, 189–203.

Owen, R. L., Pierce, N. F., Apple, R. T., and Cray, W. C., Jr. (1986). M cell transport of *Vibrio cholerae* from the intestinal lumen into Peyer's patches: A mechanism for antigen sampling and for microbial transepithelial migration. *J. Infect. Dis.* 153, 1108–1118.

Panja, A., Siden, E., and Mayer, L. (1995). Synthesis and regulation of accessory/proinflammatory cytokines by intestinal epithelial cells. *Clin. Exp. Immunol.* 100, 298–305.

Parkos, C. A., Colgan, S. P., Diamond, M. S., Nusrat, A., Liang, T. W., Springer, T. A., and Madara, J. L. (1996). Expression and polarization of intracellular adhesion molecule-I on human intestinal epithelia: consequences for CD11b/CD18-mediated interactions with neutrophils. *Mol. Med.* 2, 489–505.

Pavli, P., Woodhams, C. E., Doe, W. F., and Hume, D. A. (1990). Isolation and characterization of antigen-presenting dendritic cells from the mouse intestinal lamina propria. *Immunology* 70, 40–47.

Peifer, M. (1993). Cancer, catenins, and cuticle pattern: A complex connection. *Science* 262, 1667–1668.

Piccinini, L. A., Goldsmith, N. K., Roman, S. H., and Davies, T. F. (1987). HLA-DP, DQ and DR gene expression in Graves disease and normal thyroid epithelium. *Tissue Antigens* 30, 145–154.

Pirzer, U. C., Schurmann, G., Post, S., Betzler, M., and Meuer, S. C. (1990). Differential responsiveness to CD3-Ti vs. CD2-dependent activation of human intestinal T lymphocytes. *Eur. J. Immunol.* 20, 2339–2342.

Pober, J. S., Collins, T., Gimbrone, M. A., Jr., Cotran, R. S., Gitlin, J. D., Fiers, W., Clayberger, C., Krensky, A. M., Burakoff, S. J., and

Reiss, C. S. (1983). Lymphocytes recognize human vascular endothelial and dermal fibroblast Ia antigens induced by recombinant immune interferon. *Nature* 305, 726–729.

Qiao, L., Schurmann, G., Autschbach, F., Wallich, R., Meuer, S. C. (1993). Human intestinal mucosa alters T-cell reactivities. *Gastroenterology* 105, 814–819.

Qiao, L., Schurmann, G., Betzler, M., and Meuer, S. C. (1991). Activation and signaling status of human lamina propria T lymphocytes. *Gastroenterology* 101, 1529–1536.

Qin, O.Y., el Youssef, M., Yen-Lieberman, B., Sapatnekar, W., Youngman, K. R., Kusugami, K., and Fiocchi, C. (1988). Expression of HLA-DR antigens in inflammatory bowel disease mucosa: Role of intestinal lamina propria mononuclear cell derived interferon gamma. *Dig. Dis. Sci.* 33, 1528–1536.

Reinecker, H. C., and Podolsky, D. K. (1995). Human intestinal epithelial cells express functional cytokine receptors sharing the common gamma c chain of the interleukin 2 receptor. *Proc. Natl. Acad. Sci. USA* 92, 8353–8357.

Reinecker, H. C., MacDermott, R. P., Mirau, S., Dignass, A., and Podolsky, D. K. (1996). Intestinal epithelial cells both express and respond to interleukin 15. *Gastroenterology* 111, 1706–1713.

Rescigno, M., Urbano, M., Valzasina, B., Francolini, M., Rotta, G., Bonasio, R., Granucci, F., Kraehenbuhl, J. P., and Ricciardi-Castagnoli, P. (2001). Dendritic cells express tight junction proteins and penetrate gut epithelial monolayers to sample bacteria. *Nat. Immunol.* 2(4), 361–367.

Roberts A. I., O'Connell, S. M., and Ebert, E. C. (1993). Intestinal intraepithelial lymphocytes bind to colon cancer cells by HML-1 and CD11a. *Cancer Res.* 53, 1608–1611.

Rock, K. L., Benacerraf, B., and Abbas, A. K. (1984). Antigen presentation by hapten-specific B lymphocytes. 1. Role of surface immunoglobulin receptors. *J. Exp. Med.* 160, 1102–1113.

Rosenstiel, P., Fantini, M., Brautigam, K., Kuhbacher, T., Waetzig, G. H., Seegert, D., and Schreiber S. (2003). TNF-alpha and IFN-gamma regulate the expression of the NOD2 (CARD15) gene in human intestinal epithelial cells. *Gastroenterology* 124(4), 1001–1009.

Rosenthal, A. S., and Shevach, E. M. (1973). Function of macrophages in antigen recognition by guinea pig T lymphocytes. I. Requirement for histocompatible macrophages and lymphocytes. *J. Exp. Med.* 138, 1194–1212.

Rubinfeld, B., Souza, B., Albert, I., Muller, O., Chamberlain, S. H., Masiarz, F. R., Munemitsu, S., and Polakis, P. (1993). Association of the APC gene product with beta-catenin. *Science* 262, 1731–1734.

Santos, L. M., Lider, O., Audette, J., Khoury, S. J., and Weiner, H. L. (1990). Characterization of immunomodulatory properties and accessory cell function of small intestinal epithelial cells. *Cell. Immunol.* 127, 26–34.

Sarnacki, S., Begue, B., Buc, H., Le Deist, F., and Cerf-Bensussan, N. (1992). Enhancement of CD3-induced activation of human intestinal intraepithelial lymphocytes by stimulation of the β7-containing integrin defined by HML-1 monoclonal antibody. *Eur. J. Immunol.* 22, 2887–2892.

Sawicki, W., Kucharczyk, K., Szymanska, K., and Kujawa, M. (1977). Lamina propria macrophages of intestine of the guinea pig. Possible role in phagocytosis of migrating cells. *Gastroenterology* 73, 1340–1344.

Selby, W. S., Janossy, G., Goldstein, G. and Jewell, D. P. (1981). T lymphocyte subsets in human intestinal mucosa: the distribution and relationship to MHC-derived antigens. *Clin. Exp. Immunol.* 44, 453–458.

Selby, W. S., Poulter, L. W., Hobbs, S., Jewell, D. P., and Janossy, G. (1983). Heterogeneity of HLA-DR-positive histiocytes in human intestinal lamina propria: A combined histochemical and immunohistological analysis. *J. Clin. Pathol.* 36, 379–384.

Sette, A., and Grey, H. (1992). Chemistry of peptide interactions with MHC proteins. *Curr. Opin. Immunol.* 4, 79–86.

Shimizu, Y., and Andrew, W. (1967). Studies on the rabbit appendix. I. Lymphocyte-epithelial relations and the transport of bacteria from lumen to lymphoid nodule. *J. Morphol.* 123, 231–249.

Sicinski, P., Rowinski, J., Warchol, J. B., Jarzabek, Z., Gut, W., Szcygiel, B., Bielecki, K., and Koch, G. (1990). Poliovirus type 1 enters the human host through intestinal M cells. *Gastroenterology* 98, 56–58.

Siliciano, R. F., Lawton, T., Knall, C., Karr, R. W., Berman, P., Gregory, T., and Reinherz, E. L. (1988). Analysis of host-virus interactions in AIDS with anti-gp12O T cell clones: Effect of HIV sequence variation and a mechanism for CD4+ cell depletion. *Cell* 54, 561–575.

Sminia, T., and Jeurissen, S. (1986). The macrophage population of the gastrointestinal tract of the rat. *Immunobiology* 172, 72–80.

So, L. P., Pelton-Henrion, K., Small, G., Becker, K., Dei, E., Tyorkin, M., Sperber, K., Mayer, L. (2000a). Antigen uptake and trafficking in human intestinal epithelial cells. *Dig. Dis. Sci.* 45, 1451–1461.

So, L. P., Small, G., Sperber, K., Becker, K., Dei, E., Tyorkin, M., Mayer, L. (2000b). Factors affecting antigen uptake by human intestinal epithelial cell lines. *Dig. Dis. Sci.* 45, 1130–1137.

Soesatyo, M., Biewenga, J., Kraal, G., and Sminia, T. (1990). The localization of macrophage subsets and dendritic cells in the gastrointestinal tract of the mouse with special reference to the presence of high endothelial venules. An immuno- and enzyme-histochemical study. *Cell Tissue Res.* 259, 587–593.

Spalding, D. M., and Griffin, J. A. (1986). Different pathways of differentiation of pre-B cell lines are induced by dendritic cells and T cells from different lymphoid tissues. *Cell* 44, 507–515.

Spalding, D. M., Williamson, S. I., Koopman, W. J., and McGhee, J. R. (1984). Preferential induction of polyclonal IgA secretion by murine Peyer's patch dendritic cell-T cell mixtures. *J. Exp. Med.* 160, 941–946.

Steiniger, B., Falk, P., Lohmuller, M., and van der Meide, P. H (1989). Class II MHC antigens in the rat digestive system: Normal distribution and induced expression after interferon-gamma treatment *in vivo. Immunology* 68(4), 507–513.

Steinman, R. M., and Cohn, Z. A. (1973). Identification of a novel cell type in peripheral lymphoid organs of mice. I. Morphology, quantitation, tissue distribution. *J. Exp. Med.* 137, 1142–1162.

Steinman, R. M., and Nussenzweig, M. C. (1980). Dendritic cells: Features and functions. *Immunol. Rev.* 53, 127–147.

Stevens, A. C., Matthews, J., Andres, P., Baffis, V., Zheng, X. X., Chae, D-W., Smith, J., Strom, T. B., Maslinski, W. (1997). Interleukin 15 signals T84 colonic epithelial cells in the absence of the interleukin 2 receptor β chain. *Am. J. Physiol.* 272(5, Pt. 1), G1201-1208.

Sutherland, D. B., Varilek, G. W., and Neil, G. A. (1994). Identification and characterization of the rat intestinal epithelial cell (IEC-18) interleukin-1 receptor. *Am. J. Physiol.* 266, C1198–C1203.

Telega, G. W., Baumgart, D. C., and Carding, S. R. (2000). Uptake and presentation of antigen to T cells by primary colonic epithelial cells in normal and diseased states. *Gastroenterology* 119(6), 1548–1559.

Vanbuskirk, A., Crump, B. L., Margoliash, E., and Pierce, S. K. (1989). A peptide binding protein having a role in antigen presentation is a member of the HSP70 heat shock family. *J. Exp. Med.* 170, 1799–1809.

van de Wal, Y., Corazza, N., Allez, M., Mayer, L. F., Iijima, H., Ryan, M., Cornwall, S., Kaiserlian, D., Hershberg, R., Koezuka, Y., Colgan, S. P., and Blumberg, R. S. (2003). Delineation of a CD1d-restricted antigen presentation pathway associated with human and mouse intestinal epithelial cells. *Gastroenterology* 124(5), 1420–1431.

van Niel, G., Raposo, G., Candalh, C., Boussac, M., Hershberg, R., Cerf-Bensussan, N., and Heyman, M. (2001). Intestinal epithelial cells secrete exosome-like vesicles. *Gastroenterology* 121(2), 337–349.

Verspaget, H., and Beeken, W. (1985). Mononuclear phagocytes in the gastrointestinal tract. *Acta Chir. Scand. (Suppl.)* 525, 113–126.

Vezys, V, Olson, S., and Lefrancois, L. (2000). Expression of intestine-specific antigen reveals novel pathways of CD8 T cell tolerance induction. *Immunity* 12(5), 505–514.

Viney, J. L., Mowat, A. M., O'Malley, J. M., Williamson, E., and Fanger, N. A. (1998). Expanding dendritic cells *in vivo* enhances the induction of oral tolerance. *J. Immunol.* 160(12), 5815–5825.

Wang, J., and Klein, J. R. (1994). Thymus-neuroendocrine interactions in extrathymic T cell development. *Science* 265, 1860–1862.

Watanabe, M., Ueno, Y., Yajima, T., Iwao, Y., Tsuchiya, M., Ishikawa, H., Aiso, S., Hibi, T., and Ishii, H. (1995). Interleukin 7 is produced by human intestinal epithelial cells and regulates the proliferation of intestinal mucosal lymphocytes. *J. Clin. Invest.* 95, 2945–2953.

Wiman, K., Curman, B., Forsum, U., Klareskog, L., Malmas Tjernlund, U., Rask, L., Tragardh, L., and Peterson, P. A. (1978). Occurrence of Ia antigens on tissues of non-lymphoid origin. *Nature* 276, 711–713.

Winter, H. S., Cole, F. S., Huffer, L. M., Davison, C. B., Katz, A. J., and Edelson, P. J. (1983). Isolation and characterization of resident macrophages from guinea pig and human intestine. *Gastroenterology* 85, 358–363.

Wolf, J. L., and Bye, W. A. (1984). The membranous epithelial (M) cell and the mucosal immune system. *Ann. Rev. Med.* 35, 95–112.

Wolf, J. L., Rubin, D. H., Finberg, R., Kauffman, R. S., Sharpe, A. H., Trier, J., and Fields, B. N. (1981). Intestinal M cells: A pathway for entry of reovirus into the host. *Science* 212, 471–472.

Yang, S. K., Eckmann, L., Panja, A., and Kagnoff, M. F. (1997). Differential and regulated expression of c-x-c, c-c, and c- chemokines by human colon epithelial cells. *Gastroenterology* 113, 1214–1223.

Ye, G., Barrera, C., Fan, X., Gourley, W. K., Crowe, S. E., Ernst, P. B., and Reyes, V. E. (1997). Expression of B7-1 and B7-2 costimulatory molecules by human gastric epithelial cells: Potential role in CD4+ T cell activation during *Helicobacter pylori* infection. *J. Clin. Invest.* 99(7), 1628–1636.

Yio, X. Y., and Mayer, L. (1997) Characterization of a 180-kDa intestinal epithelial cell membrane glycoprotein, gp180. A candidate molecule mediating T cell-epithelial cell interactions. *J. Biol. Chem.* 272, 12786–12792.

Zhang, Z. Y., and Michael, J. G. (1990). Orally inducible immune unresponsiveness is abrogated by IFN-gamma treatment *J. Immunol.* 144(11), 4163–4165.

Ziegler, K., and Unanue, E. R. (1981). Identification of a macrophage antigen-processing event required for I-region-restricted antigen presentation to T lymphocytes, *J. Immunol.* 127, 1869–1875.

Antigen Handling and Presentation by Mucosal Dendritic Cells and Macrophages

Brian L. Kelsall and Francisco Leon

Laboratory of Clinical Investigation, National Institute of Allergy and Infectious Disease, National Institutes of Health, Bethesda, Maryland

Lesley E. Smythies

Division of Gastroenterology and Hepatology, Department of Medicine, University of Alabama at Birmingham, Birmingham, Alabama

Phillip D. Smith

Division of Gastroenterology and Hepatology, Department of Medicine, University of Alabama at Birmingham, and The Research Service, Veterans Administration Medical Center, Birmingham, Alabama

INTRODUCTION

The purpose of this chapter is to review the currently available data regarding the role of dendritic cells (DCs) and macrophages in the induction and regulation of immune responses at mucosal surfaces, in particular how each cell type plays a role in the maintenance of the balance between tolerance and immunity. The initial section will focus on DCs, which have unique properties that allow them to process antigens efficiently and bind and activate naive T cells. Mucosal DCs have a particular capacity to induce regulatory T-cell differentiation in the steady (noninfected, nonimmunized) state, but allow for the induction of effector T-cell responses, depending on both the particular subpopulation involved and the surface receptors engaged during DC activation and T-cell priming. In addition, mucosal DCs may contribute to innate defense by the production of cytokines, such as type 1 interferons (type 1 IFNs) and interleukin-12 (IL-12), following direct exposure to pathogens, as well as contribute to the maintenance of secondary T-cell responses within inflamed mucosa. The second section will address mucosal macrophages, in particular those in the intestine. Resident intestinal macrophages have unique functions in that they do not appear to act as antigen-presenting cells

(APCs) or produce inflammatory cytokines, but avidly scavenge, phagocytose, and kill pathogens and macromolecules. Thus they are noninflammatory specialized cells for mucosal defense against pathogens. In contrast, during active mucosal inflammation, as occurs in inflammatory bowel disease (IBD), fully inflammatory monocytes are recruited from the blood, which can contribute to tissue injury and damage.

Our discussion emphasizes DCs and macrophages in the intestine and respiratory tracts, because these organs constitute the major mucosal surfaces of the body. However, recent progress has been made with regards to the understanding of DC function within the genitourinary tract, in particular with regard to their roles in the pathogenesis and immunity to viral pathogens, such as herpes simplex virus (HSV), type 2, and human immunodeficiency virus (HIV) (for reviews, see Iwasaki 2003; Steinman *et al.* 2003a).

MUCOSAL DENDRITIC CELLS

DCs can be divided into follicular and nonfollicular DCs. Follicular DCs develop from a non–bone marrow–derived precursor and express high levels of receptors for immunoglobulin and complement. Antigen expressed on follicular DCs may be important for the germinal center reaction and for the maintenance of B-cell memory (see Kosco-Vilbois 2003). In contrast, non-follicular DCs comprise a family of cells that develop from bone marrow–derived stem cells under the influence of flt-3 ligand, granulocyte-macrophage colony-stimulating factor (GM-CSF) and other cytokines. These cells are present in three immunologic compartments: (1) in lymph where they have extensive processes (veiled cells); (2) in non-lymphoid tissues, such as the interstitium of internal organs (tissue, or nonlymphoid DCs), or the epidermis (Langerhans cells) and dermis of the skin (dermal DCs); and (3) in lymphoid tissues, such as the T-cell regions of draining lymph nodes (LNs), where they have been referred to as interdigitating dendritic cells. This chapter will only discuss nonfollicular DCs, simply referred to as DCs.

DCs are APCs that are uniquely capable of efficiently stimulating the differentiation of naive T cells. DCs are present in a less than fully mature (or activated) form within all vascularized tissues and at distant or peripheral sites, such as the skin and mucosal surfaces. There, they efficiently capture or sample foreign as well as self-antigens. Upon direct exposure to microbial products or inflammatory signals, DCs mature and migrate to T-cell areas of organized lymphoid tissues, where they interact with and activate migrating naive T cells. During migration and maturation (or activation), DCs undergo significant changes in morphology, decrease their ability to process new antigens, and enhance their ability to present antigenic peptides to CD4 and CD8[+] T cells. The increased ability to present antigens is the consequence of the upregulated surface expression of major histocompatibility complex (MHC)/antigen complexes, costimulatory and adhesion molecules, and enhanced production of cytokines. This allows for efficient binding and priming of naive T cells with antigens selectively acquired at distant sites. Because of their unique localization and biology, a primary function of DCs is to detect and induce immune responses to invading pathogens encountered at skin and mucosal surfaces.

What has become clear in the past 5–10 years, however, is that the DC system is much more complex than what is described by this well-established paradigm of DC function (see Banchereau et al. 2000; Kapsenberg 2003; Moser 2003; Shortman and Liu 2002; Steinman et al. 2003b). For example, multiple DC subpopulations have now been identified in mice and humans. These subpopulations have several maturational stages, are present at unique anatomic sites, and have discrete phenotypic and functional characteristics (see Ardavin 2003; Shortman and Liu 2002). In addition, not all antigens are processed at "distant" sites by DCs that then migrate to lymphoid tissues to induce immunity. DC populations reside within discrete regions of organized lymphoid tissues in immature form and process and present systemically administered or blood-borne antigens (Wilson et al. 2003). Such resident DCs may be important for inducing T-cell tolerance to innocuous antigens and in processing cell-associated foreign or self-antigens for presentation to T cells, by a process termed "cross-presentation" (Belz et al. 2002b; Larsson et al. 2003). Furthermore, it is now recognized that DC apoptosis acts to

limit "normal" immune responses functionally (Semnani et al. 2003) and is regulated by discrete signaling pathways.

Despite this increasingly recognized complexity of DC biology, recent studies have continued to shed light on the role of DCs in the induction and regulation of mucosal immune responses. Following in this section is a brief discussion of factors known to affect DC function, including the current definition of DC subpopulations in mouse and man, which will be followed by more specific information regarding mucosal DCs. The latter will include information on mucosal DC subsets, antigen uptake by mucosal DCs, DC trafficking, and the role of DC populations in immunity to pathogens, oral tolerance, and the induction and maintenance of abnormal mucosal inflammation, as occurs in allergy and IBDs.

Factors affecting dendritic cell function

The factors affecting the ability of dendritic cells to induce T-cell responses are schematically depicted in **Figure 26.1**. These include the state of DC maturation, the existence of subpopulations of DCs, and the particular signals or stimuli to which DCs are exposed during maturation and T-cell priming.

Dendritic cell maturation

Because the half-life of most DC populations in both lymphoid and nonlymphoid tissues under steady-state conditions is quite short (on the order of days) (Kamath et al. 2002; Pugh et al. 1983), DCs are postulated to migrate continuously from nonlymphoid and peripheral sites, such as the gut, to organized lymphoid tissues where they present self-antigens, for the induction and maintenance of self-tolerance (see Steinman et al. 2003b). The precise nature of constitutively migrating DCs is not yet clear. One hypothesis is that DC precursors continuously enter tissues, where they differentiate into immature DC populations and process self-antigens in the absence of activating signals. These immature DCs become tolerogenic DCs by default (lack of activation) following migration to LNs. A second hypothesis is that immature tissue DCs process self-antigen in the form of apoptotic cells or bodies (see Larsson et al. 2003; Savill et al. 2002). The latter are processed via DC receptors, such as CD36 (Albert et al. 1998), CD47 (Tada et al. 2003), and CR3 (Verbovetski et al. 2002) that do not activate and, indeed, can inhibit DC maturation in terms of MHC antigen upregulation and production of cytokines, such as IL-12i (Demeure et al., 2000; Latour et al. 2001; Urban et al. 2001). However, at the same time, apoptotic cells can induce the expression of CCR7 (Hirao et al. 2000; Verbovetski et al. 2002), which responds to CCL21 expressed in T-cell zones of LNs. The end result would be a "quiescent" DC that migrates toward interfollicular T-cell zones in the absence of classical maturation. Finally, antigen presentation by immature or "quiescent" DCs may be facilitated by the presence of local tissue factors that prevent active DC maturation, such as IL-10, TGF-β, or thrombospondin (Buelens et al. 1995; Demeure et al. 2000; Doyen et al. 2003; Sato et al.

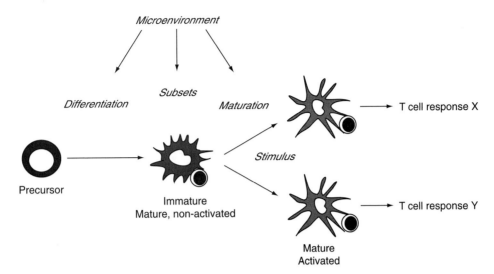

Fig. 26.1. Factors affecting dendritic cell function.

2003b; Steinbrink *et al.* 1997). These inhibitory factors may be present at particularly high levels in certain tissue microenvironments, such as the gut, and are produced by dying apoptotic cells (W. Chen *et al.* 2001), or released by macrophages after surface receptor ligation by apoptotic cells (Savill *et al.* 2002; Voll *et al.* 1997).

In contrast to immature or "quiescent" DCs that migrate in the steady state, resident or newly recruited immature DCs may be induced to migrate to draining LNs after activation and maturation into fully immunostimulatory DCs. This can occur in response to pathogens via interactions of pattern recognition receptors (PRR), such as Toll-like receptors (TLRs) with "pathogen-associated molecular patterns" (PAMPs) expressed by organisms (Kaisho and Akira 2003), or from indirect sensing of infection or inflammation, via recognition of inflammatory cytokines (e.g., TNF-α), IL-1, or type I IFNs (Honda *et al.* 2003), intracellular compounds (e.g., uric acid) (Shi *et al.* 2003), and ongoing specific immune responses (e.g., via CD40–CD40L interactions) (see Bancherau *et al.* 2000; Kapsenberg 2003; Reis e Sousa *et al.* 2003; Rescigno 2002). The maturation process is associated with the loss of endocytic and phagocytic receptors, the upregulation of costimulatory molecules, and the extension of dendrites that increase the surface area available for interaction with T cells (see Banchereau *et al.* 2000). Maturation also results in a shift in lysosomal compartments with downregulation of CD68 and upregulation of DC-lysosome–associated membrane protein (DC-LAMP), increased expression of MHC/antigen complexes, and a shift in chemokine receptor expression (e.g., from CCR6 to CCR7) that allows for DC migration to lymphoid tissues. These mature or activated cells are well suited to binding and activating naive T cells.

Dendritic cell subpopulations

To date, eight subsets of DCs and DC precursors have been defined in the mouse **(Fig. 26.2)** (Iwasaki and Kelsall 2001;

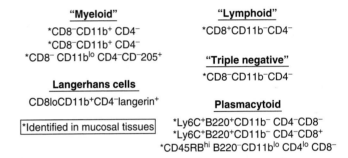

"Myeloid"
*$CD8^-CD11b^+$ $CD4^-$
*$CD8^-CD11b^+$ $CD4^-$
*$CD8^-$ $CD11b^{lo}$ $CD4^-CD^-205^+$

Langerhans cells
$CD8loCD11b^+CD4^-$langerin$^+$

*Identified in mucosal tissues

"Lymphoid"
*$CD8^+CD11b^-CD4^-$

"Triple negative"
*$CD8^-CD11b^-CD4^-$

Plasmacytoid
*$Ly6C^+B220^+CD11b^-$ $CD4^-CD8^-$
*$Ly6C^+B220^+CD11b^-$ $CD4^-CD8^+$
*$CD45RB^{hi}$ $B220^-CD11b^{lo}$ $CD4^{lo}$ $CD8^-$

Fig. 26.2. Intestinal dendritic cell subpopulations currently defined in the mouse. Populations that have been identified in mucosal tissues are identified with an asterisk.

Shortman and Liu 2002; Wakkach *et al.* 2003). Three main DC subsets exist in the spleen ($CD11c^+/CD11b^+/CD4^+/CD8^-$; $CD11c^+/CD11b^+/CD4^-/CD8^-$ ("double negative"); and $CD11c^+/CD11b^-/CD4^-/CD8\alpha^+$), while skin-draining LNs contain two additional populations ($CD11c^+/CD11b^+CD4^-/CD8^-/CD205^+$, and $CD11c^+/CD11b^+/CD8\alpha^{lo}/CD4^-/langerin^+$). The relationship of these subsets in the spleen and LNs was addressed using continuous BrdU labeling of DC precursors, *in vivo*, which demonstrated that all five DC subsets arise from independent precursors, at least as far back as the dividing cell (i.e., that one subset does not appear to mature into another under steady-state conditions) (Kamath *et al.* 2002). These populations are short lived (on the order of 3–5 days) in lymphoid tissues (Kamath *et al.* 2002); the three common DC subpopulations arising from blood precursors, whereas the additional lymph node populations are thought to represent migrating dermal DC and Langerhans cells (LC). Mesenteric lymph nodes (MLNs) and Peyer's patches (PP) contain three predominant populations: $CD11c^+/CD11b^+/CD4^-/CD8^-$ ("double negative"), $CD11c^+/CD11b^-/CD4^-/CD8\alpha^+$, and $CD11c^+/CD11b^-/CD4^-/CD8\alpha^-$ ("triple negative") cells (Iwasaki and Kelsall 2000, 2001).

Three populations of plasmacytoid DC precursors (pDCs) have also been described in lymphoid tissues and blood (Asselin-Paturel et al. 2001, 2003; Bilsborough et al. 2003; P. Martin et al. 2002; Nakano et al. 2001; O'Keeffe et al. 2002; Wakkach et al. 2003). pDCs morphologically resemble plasma cells, but lack most B-cell markers and do not produce immunoglobulins. They express intermediate levels of CD11c and Ly6C. Two populations additionally express B220, with one expressing CD8 (CD11c^{int}/B220$^+$/CD8$^-$, CD11c^{int}/B220$^+$/CD8$^+$), the latter of which may represent a more mature form of the former (Asselin-Paturel et al. 2001; Bilsborough et al. 2003; P. Martin et al. 2002; Nakano et al. 2001; O'Keeffe et al. 2002). Finally, a pDC-like subset expressing intermediate levels of CD11c and Ly6C, but lacking B220 has recently been described (Wakkach et al. 2003). This population additionally expresses CD45RB (CD11c^{int}/CD45RB^{hi}). Upon activation in vitro, pDCs become fully immunostimulatory DCs. Thus, pDCs may have unique roles as precursors in innate immune responses (e.g., by the production of type 1 IFN) and as mature immunostimulatory DCs in the induction of acquired immunity. In addition, B220$^+$/CD8$^+$ and CD11c^{int}/CD45RB^{hi} pDCs may have unique capacities to induce IL-10-producing T cells (Bilsborough et al. 2003; P. Martin et al. 2002; Wakkach et al. 2003) (see the following text). Ontologic relationships between DCs present in mucosal tissues and the three types of pDCs are not well understood.

It had been proposed that different DC subsets were related to "lymphoid" or "myeloid" cell lineages based primarily on cell surface marker expression (e.g., CD8 or CD11b, respectively) and the common development of CD8$^+$ DCs and lymphocytes from CD4^{low} early thymic precursors. Further studies have supported or refuted this concept (see Shortman and Liu 2002 and Ardavin 2003); however, it is now clear that the major classes of splenic murine DCs [CD8$^+$ DCs, CD8$^-$ DCs (which includes CD11b$^+$ CD4$^+$ and CD11b$^+$ CD4$^-$ DCs) and B220$^+$ plasmacytoid pre-DCs] can be derived from either common lymphoid or common myeloid bone marrow precursors, as well as from a novel specific DC precursor from the peripheral blood (del Hoyo et al. 2002). In addition, it has recently been suggested that CD8$^-$ and CD8$^+$ murine DCs may arise from blood monocytes upon extravasation into tissues (Leon et al. 2003), similar to what has been proposed for DC differentiation from monocytes upon migration into the lymph in humans (Randolph et al. 1998, 1999, 2002). Therefore at present there is little support for the designations of DC subpopulations as "lymphoid" or "myeloid."

Whether all murine DC subpopulations have phenotypic and functional equivalents in humans is also not yet clear (Shortman and Liu 2002). This is because most studies of human DCs, out of experimental necessity, have been carried out not with cells freshly isolated from tissues but with DCs generated in vitro from blood monocytes or CD34$^+$ precursors from either cord blood or bone marrow treated with cytokines. In addition, surface markers of human cell subsets

are not analogous to those of the mouse. In particular, CD11c, which is a key marker to identify DCs in the mouse is broadly expressed by many human hematopoietic cells, and is present only on certain subpopulations of human DCs.

Despite these limitations, however, studies of human and mouse DCs generated in vitro and the few studies of DCs in situ, or directly isolated from human tissue, suggest that functional equivalents will be identified (O'Keeffe et al. 2003). Human DCs generated from CD34$^+$/CLA$^+$ precursors in the presence of TGF-β resemble LC (equivalent to LC in mouse), those derived from CD34$^+$/CLA-precursors and human monocytes may be most akin to interstitial DCs (equivalent to CD11b$^+$ DCs in the mouse), and those derived from pDC may be equivalent to CD123$^+$ DCs found in tissues (equivalent to murine pDCs). As yet, no clear equivalent of the CD8$^+$ murine DC subset has been identified, although DCs are localized to T-cell zones in human lymphoid tissues. An indication that more DC subtypes will be identified in human tissue is the recent findings of multiple putative DC precursor populations in human peripheral blood. These findings have relied on studies of HLA-DR^{hi} peripheral blood mononuclear cells that do not express typical markers of T cells, B cells, monocytes, and natural killer (NK) cells ["lineage negative" (lin$^-$)]. HLA-DR^{hi}/lin$^-$ cells include three nonoverlapping subsets of classical CD11c^{hi} precursor DCs (expressing CD1b/CD1c, CD16, or BDCA3) and CD11c^{lo} precursor plasmacytoid DCs that express CD123, BDCA2, and BDCA4. These cells also differ in their expression of immunoglobulin-like transcript (ILT) (CD85) family members, costimulatory and adhesion molecules, and C-type lectins (see Banchereau et al. 2000; Shortman and Liu 2002).

The question of whether the functional diversity of DCs as a whole results from functionally independent DC subpopulations (as defined by surface marker expression) has been the focus of significant effort over the past several years (Ardavin 2003). The collective data support the conclusion that there is considerable functional specialization of murine DC subpopulations, although, as mentioned in the following text, this is not absolute. First, different DC subsets localize to specific sites, suggesting that they interact with external antigens or with T and B cells to differing degrees. In this regard, CD8$^-$ DCs (which may include CD11b$^+$/CD8$^-$/CD4$^+$, CD11b$^+$/CD8$^-$/CD4$^-$, or CD11b$^-$/CD8$^-$/CD4$^-$ DCs) are present at sites of antigen exposure in the spleen and PP, in B-cell follicles in the PP, and at T–B junctions in PPs, LNs, and the spleen, while CD8$^+$ DCs are restricted to T-cell zones. Consistent with this localization, CD8$^-$, not CD8$^+$, DCs have the ability to directly induce B-cell activation and plasmablast differentiation (Balazs et al. 2002).

Second, although CD8$^-$ DCs have a higher phagocytic capacity (Kamath et al. 2002; Leenen et al. 1998), recent evidence suggests that CD8$^+$, but not CD8$^-$, DCs can internalize apoptotic cells (Iyoda et al. 2002) and are the major cells responsible for T-cell tolerance following intravenous injection of antigen-loaded apoptotic cells (Iyoda et al. 2002; Liu et al. 2002) and for the cross-presentation of self-antigens to CD8$^+$

T cells *in vivo* (Belz *et al.* 2002a, b; den Haan *et al.* 2000). In addition, CD8$^+$ DCs in T-cell zones are extremely effective at inducing T-cell tolerance following the targeting of soluble antigens to the C-type lectin antigen processing receptor DEC-205, which is expressed constitutively by CD8$^+$ and not CD8$^-$ DCs (Bonifaz *et al.* 2002; Hawiger *et al.* 2001).

Third, in addition to substantial evidence demonstrating a role for CD8$^+$ DCs in tolerance induction, early studies demonstrated that the adoptive transfer of antigen-pulsed CD8$^+$ DCs to naive recipient mice preferentially induced Th1 responses, while CD8$^-$ DCs induce Th2 responses (Maldonado-Lopez *et al.* 1999; Pulendran *et al.* 1999). Consistent with this role in Th-cell induction, CD8$^+$ produce much higher amounts of IL-12p70 than CD8$^-$ DCs upon stimulation *in vivo* and *in vitro* with microbial products (Maldonado-Lopez *et al.* 1999; Pulendran *et al.* 1999; Iwasaki and Kelsall 2001). These findings resulted in the original designation of CD8$^+$ DCs at "DC1" cells and CD8$^-$ (or CD11b$^+$) DCs as "DC2." Furthermore, the ability of CD8$^+$ DCs to induce Th1 responses following adoptive transfer is dependent on their production of IL-12p40 (thus either IL-12-p70 or IL-23), as well as IFN-γ, while CD8$^-$ DC induction of Th2 responses was dependent to some degree on autocrine production of IL-10 (Maldonado-Lopez *et al.* 2001).

Similarly, studies of human DCs provide some support for functional specialization and separate "DC1" and "DC2" lineages. CD154-activated mature DCs derived from monocytes in culture with GM-CSF and IL-4 were initially found to preferentially induce Th1 responses *in vitro*, while mature plasmacytoid DCs derived upon culture of CD123$^+$ blood precursors with IL-3 and CD154-activated preferentially induced Th2 responses (Shortman and Liu 2002). Functional specialization is also suggested by the expression of different TLR receptors on different subpopulations of DC (Boonstra *et al.* 2003; Kaisho and Akira 2003).

Plasticity of dendritic cell function

Despite evidence for DCs specialization in the ability to induce T-cell responses, recent studies indicate significant "plasticity" in the function of DC subsets (reviewed in Kapsenberg 2003; Mazzoni and Segal 2004; Reis e Sousa *et al.* 2003; Shortman and Liu 2002). These studies argue that the induction of T-cell differentiation by DCs is directly influenced by the signals DCs receive during antigen uptake, activation, and T-cell priming. First, in contrast to the studies mentioned in the preceding text, murine CD8$^+$ DCs can produce IL-10 and little IL-12 *in vitro* under certain conditions, such as following stimulation with the yeast *Schizosaccharomyces pombe* or zymosan and CD40L, whereas CD8$^-$ DCs can produce substantial amounts of IL-12 p70, such as after TLR combined with CD40L signaling, or in the absence of endogenous DC IL-10 production (Schultz *et al.* 2000; Edwards *et al.* 2002; Manickasingham *et al.* 2003). In addition, murine CD11b$^+$ DCs have recently been shown to initiate Th1 responses following vaginal infection with HSV 2 (Iwasaki 2003), and

skin infection with *Leishmania major* (Von Stebut *et al.* 2003), possibly because of CD11b$^+$ DC activation by local IL-1 (Von Stebut *et al.* 2003). Furthermore, certain microbial products, including cholera toxin (Braun *et al.* 1999; Gagliardi *et al.* 2000), *Porphyromonas gingivalis* lipopolysaccharide (LPS) (M. Martin *et al.* 2003; Pulendran *et al.* 2001), *Schistosoma mansoni* egg antigens (Pearce *et al.* 1991), or *Candida albicans* hyphae (Romani *et al.* 2004) and inflammatory mediators, such as histamine (Caron *et al.* 2001; Mazzoni *et al.* 2001), prostaglandin E-2 (PGE-2) (Kalinski *et al.* 1997), or thymic stromal lymphopoietin (TSLP) (IL-50) (Soumelis *et al.* 2002) can promote a Th2 phenotype, at least partially via direct effects on DCs (for example, by suppression of IL-12 production). Alternatively, many TLR ligands can induce IL-12 production by the same DC populations *in vitro* and drive Th1 responses *in vivo*.

Second, the T-cell phenotype appears to vary depending on the antigen dose and the ratio of DCs and T cells put in the original culture (Boonstra *et al.* 2003; Manickasingham *et al.* 2003). Studies suggest that high antigen doses or DC/T-cell ratios favor Th1 responses, while low antigen doses and ratios favor Th2 responses.

Third, the ability of DCs to mediate either tolerance or immunization depends on their state of activation, which in turn, depends on the form of antigen (e.g., soluble, apoptotic body–associated, or CD205-directed vs. pathogen-associated) and the presence or absence of activating tissue factors, such as inflammatory cytokines, or products of damaged cells, or ongoing acquired immune responses. Furthermore, exposure of DCs to certain cytokines or growth factors (such as IL-10 or TGF-β) or to certain pathogens or their products such as *Plasmodium falciparum* (Urban *et al.* 1999, 2001), the *Bordetella pertussis* fimbrial hemagglutinin (FHA) (McGuirk *et al.* 2002), or the lysophosphatidylserine from *S. mansoni* (van der Kleij *et al.* 2002) can promote tolerogenic responses via active engagement of regulatory receptors expressed by DCs. Tolerance in these cases may result from active inhibition of DC maturation (e.g., *P. falciparum* binding to CD36 and CD51) or direct activation of DCs to produce IL-10 while suppressing IL-12, resulting in the induction of IL-10-producing regulatory T cells (IL-10-producing Treg) (e.g., *B. pertussis* FHA or *C. albicans* hyphae binding to CD11b). Therefore, in addition to directing different Th-cell responses, DCs are also flexible in their ability to induce tolerance or immunity.

What has emerged from these data is the fact that the immunoregulatory role of DCs is complex, and to date, only partially understood. Although there is a predisposition of certain DC lineages for certain types of immune responses (e.g., CD8$^+$ for the induction of Th1 responses), the ligation of specific receptors that initiate and modulate DC maturation and cytokine production can result in the development of functionally different effector DCs populations that selectively promote Th1, Th2, or T-cell tolerance via the induction of anergy, deletion or regulatory T-cell differentiation.

Intestinal dendritic cells

The importance of DCs in the induction of mucosal immune responses was initially suggested by studies performed prior to the availability of specific reagents to identify DCs. These studies focused on MHC class II–positive cells with the morphology of DCs in PPs (Bjerke *et al.* 1993; Bland and Whiting 1993; Brandtzaeg and Bjerke 1990; Mahida *et al.* 1989b; Mayrhofer *et al.* 1983; Nagura *et al.* 1991; Pavli *et al.* 1990; Sminia *et al.* 1982; Sminia and van der Ende 1991; Soesatyo *et al.* 1990, 1992; Wilders *et al.* 1985, 1983), the lamina propria (LP) of the intestine (Bland and Whiting 1993; Liu and MacPherson 1995; Maric *et al.* 1996; Mayrhofer *et al.* 1983; Pavli *et al.* 1990, 1993), and in the lymph draining the intestine (Liu and MacPherson 1991, 1993, 1995; MacPherson 1989; MacPherson *et al.* 1995; Pugh *et al.* 1983). These studies indicated the presence and location of DCs in intestinal tissues, as well as their ability to act as APCs, primarily via their ability to stimulate a mixed lymphocyte reaction (MLR). Since these early studies, significant progress has been made in understanding the role for DCs in the induction and regulation of mucosal immune responses. The following discussion will be focused primarily on studies done in the mouse and rat, because very few studies have addressed the role of human DCs in the mucosal immune system.

Subpopulations of intestinal dendritic cells

Peyer's patch. The PP, the primary site for antigen processing in the intestine, is divided into regions according to histology and cell types **(Fig. 26.3)**. Luminal antigens gain access to the PP via transfer across specialized epithelial cells, known as M (microfold) cells, which are scattered among the columnar epithelial cells in the follicle-associated epithelium (FAE) above the PP (Owen 1977). M cells express MHC II antigens (Allan *et al.* 1993; Nagura *et al.* 1991) and are capable of producing IL-1 (Pappo and Mahlman 1993), and it has been suggested that these cells may present antigens directly to underlying PP T cells. However, because M cells are physically limited from the bulk of the PP T-cell population, the antigen-presenting function of these cells is probably limited. After transport into the PP, DCs likely play a key role in antigen processing. MHC class II^{hi} putative DCs were identified in PPs in mice, rats, pigs, and humans. Early studies in the mouse also demonstrated that PP accessory function, as measured by the proliferation of periodate-treated T cells, was present in a non-B–cell, non-T–cell, Fc receptor$^-$, Ia$^+$ PP, 33D1$^+$ population with low buoyant density and dendritic morphology (Spalding *et al.* 1983). Other early studies supported the ability of PP DCs to act as APCs for T-cell responses. DCs purified from the murine PP by adherence to irradiated, periodate-treated T cells, when cultured with nonirradiated periodate-treated T cells, were capable of supporting polyclonal IgA production by B cells (Spalding *et al.* 1984), and when added with antigen-specific Th2 clones and antigen to clonal microcultures, were essential for the induction of large numbers of IgA-producing B-cell clones (George and Cebra 1991). In addition, early studies of human PPs identified

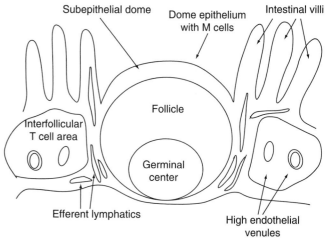

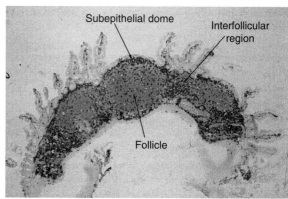

Fig. 26.3. Intestinal CD11c$^+$ dendritic cells in the murine Peyer's patch. Above is a schematic diagram of a Peyer's patch for orientation purposes, and shown below is a immunohistologic section of a murine Peyer's patch stained with anti-CD11c antibodies (Kelsall and Strober 1996).

MHC class II$^+$, S-100 protein$^+$ cells in the PP interfollicular regions (IFR) and subepithelial dome (SED) with cytoplasmic processes that extended into the dome epithelium that are most likely DCs (Bjerke *et al.* 1993; Nagura *et al.* 1991; Spencer *et al.* 1986). These reports suggested that PP DCs were important APCs for T-cell proliferation and T-cell help for B-cell responses in the PP.

In more recent studies, DCs have been identified with dendritic cell–reactive monoclonal antibodies. DCs were initially directly identified in PPs of normal (Witmer and Steinman 1984) and osteopetrotic (op/op) mice (Witmer-Pack *et al.* 1993). In initial studies from our laboratory, staining of frozen sections of murine PPs revealed a striking concentration of CD11c$^+$ DCs in the SED and IFR that coexpressed an intracellular antigen of murine DCs and B cells and MHC class II (Kelsall and Strober 1996) (Fig. 26.3). A subpopulation in the SED expressed low levels of CD11b, while those in the IFR expressed CD205 (DEC-205). Furthermore, total PP DC populations isolated from mice fed ovalbumin (OVA) stimulated OVA-specific T-cell receptor transgenic (TCR-transgenic) T cells (Kelsall and Strober 1996). Similar findings were reported by Ruedl and colleagues (Ruedl *et al.*

1996). PP DCs are primarily immature in phenotype and mature to fully immunostimulatory cells upon activation *in vitro* (Ruedl and Hubele 1997). These studies established DCs as major APCs in the PP and indicated their capacity to process oral antigen *in vivo*.

Subsequent studies addressed whether PP DCs are unique in their capacity to induce T cells that mediate IgA B-cell switching or oral tolerance. Highly purified PP DCs induced the differentiation of T cells, that upon *in vitro* restimulation produced high levels of IL-4 and IL-10 and lower levels of IFN-γ compared with T cells primed with spleen DCs, which produced predominantly IFN-γ (Iwasaki and Kelsall 1999). In addition, IFN-γ production by T cells primed with PP, but not splenic, DCs was enhanced by the addition of neutralizing antibody to either TGF-β or IL-10 to the priming cultures (Iwasaki and Kelsall 1999). Furthermore, PP, but not splenic, DCs secreted IL-10 after overnight stimulation *in vitro* (Iwasaki and Kelsall 1999). Similarly, preferential induction of T cells producing IL-4 and IL-6 by PP DCs was reported by Everson and colleagues (Everson *et al.* 1996, 1998). Finally, PP DCs produce IL-10 in response to activation via the costimulatory molecule RANK (receptor activator of NF-κB), whereas similarly stimulated spleen DCs produce IL-12 (Williamson *et al.* 2002). Taken together, these studies support the hypothesis that IL-10 and possibly TGF-β are produced by PP DCs upon interaction with naive T cells and that these cytokines either directly or indirectly drive T cells to differentiate into T cells producing IL-4, IL-10, and TGF-β. As discussed in the following text, similar findings have been reported for lung DCs (Akbari *et al.* 2001, 2002; Stumbles *et al.* 1998), suggesting that the production of IL-10, and the induction of IL-10-producing T cells appears to be a fundamental characteristic of DCs at mucosal sites under steady-state conditions.

Five of the eight murine DC populations listed in Figure 26.2 are present in the PP. Three express high levels of CD11c and can be defined by their coexpression of CD8α and CD11b (Iwasaki and Kelsall 2001). CD11c^hi PP DCs were found to be either CD8α⁺CD4⁻CD11b⁻, CD8α⁻ CD4⁻CD11b⁺, or CD8α⁻,CD4⁻,CD11b⁻. The latter population, while present in the spleen and peripheral LNs, was highly overrepresented in both the PP and MLN. Following isolation, these three DC subsets expressed similar low levels of MHC II and costimulatory markers, with enhanced expression upon activation. In addition, all maintained their CD8α and CD11b expression on activation, suggesting one population is not simply a more differentiated or activated form of another population.

In functional assays, PP CD11b⁺ DCs produced low levels of bioactive IL-12p70, similarly to the spleen CD11b⁺ DC upon stimulation with CD40-ligand alone, or with SAC and IFN-γ. However, when compared with either the CD8α⁺ or CD8α⁻CD4⁻CD11b⁻ PP DCs, or with CD11b⁺ DCs from the spleen or peripheral LNs, PP CD11b⁺ DCs produced high levels of IL-10 (Iwasaki and Kelsall 2001). In addition, CD11b⁺ PP DCs induced naive T cells to differentiate into cells that produced much higher levels of IL-10 than T cells

primed with any other DC subset. In contrast, both CD8α⁺ and CD8α⁻CD4⁻CD11b⁻ PP DCs produced IL-12 and little to no IL-10 and induced the differentiation of T cells producing only IFN-γ, similarly to the CD8α⁺ spleen DCs. These studies identified CD8α⁻CD4⁻CD11b⁻ DCs at mucosal sites of antigen exposure and showed they were particularly capable of inducing Th1 responses. The studies also showed that the CD11b⁺ DCs from the PP are unique in their ability to induce IL-10 producing T cells and thus may have a role in the induction of Treg or the induction of IgA B-cell responses. The latter was recently supported by studies demonstrating that when compared with SP DCs, freshly isolated PP CD11b⁺ DCs induced higher levels of IgA secretion from naive B cells in a DC–T cell–B cell coculture system. (Sato *et al.* 2003a).

CD11c^hi,CD11b⁺ DCs, such as skin LC, DCs resident in nonlymphoid tissues, and DCs present in the marginal zones of the spleen and LNs were found to be localized to the SED, whereas CD8α⁺ DCs were localized exclusively in the T-cell zone IFRs (Iwasaki and Kelsall 2000). CD11b⁻CD8α⁻CD4⁻ were present in both SED and IFR and scattered throughout the B-cell follicle, except the germinal centers. Furthermore, a population of CD8α⁻CD4⁻CD11b⁻ DCs present within the epithelial layer of the FAE expressed high levels of intracellular (rather than surface) MHC class II antigens, indicating an immature phenotype (Iwasaki and Kelsall 2001). Some of these cells coassociated with UEA⁺ M cells, suggesting at least some reside in M-cell pockets. Similarly, MHC class II⁺ cells were also identified within the FAE in the rat (Maric *et al.* 1996) and human (Nagura *et al.* 1991). Finally, PP DCs have been shown to express the integrin-ligand mucosal addressin-cell adhesion molecule-1 (MAdCAM-1), which preferentially binds the integrin molecule most associated with mucosal homing, α4β7 (Szabo *et al.* 1997), suggesting that SED DCs express surface molecules that facilitate interactions with mucosal T and B cells.

Recently, CD11c^int B220⁺ plasmacytoid pre-DCs also were identified in the murine PP (Asselin-Paturel *et al.* 2003; Bilsborough *et al.* 2003). Using an antibody (120G8), which is reactive with pDCs, and when administered *in vivo* depletes IFN-α-producing pDCs, Asselin-Paturel and colleagues have identified pDCs in the IFR of PPs (Asselin-Paturel *et al.* 2003). In addition, pDCs were isolated from PPs of mice treated with flt-3-ligand, which dramatically and preferentially increases the numbers of DCs, including pDCs (Bilsborough *et al.* 2003). These cells expressed the typical markers of pDCs, including B220 and ly6C, but also expressed CD8, a marker typically associated with mature plasmacytoid DCs (Bilsborough *et al.* 2003). Functional studies showed the cells produce IFN-α, similarly to pDCs from the blood and other tissues. However, these cells were particularly capable of inducing IL-10-producing T cells (Bilsborough *et al.* 2003), similarly to a CD8⁺ pDC subset described from the spleen (P. Martin *et al.* 2002). In unpublished data from our laboratory, we have identified both CD8a⁺ and CD8a⁻ CD11c^int B220⁺, Ly6C⁺ pDCs in the PP and have confirmed the localization of 120G8+ cells in the IFR and SED (Kelsall, unpublished observation).

Similar to those in studies of mice, PP DCs in the human and rhesus macaque have been demonstrated in the IFR, SED, and follicle SED (Jameson *et al.* 2002). DCs in the IFR and some in the SED expressed DC-SIGN (Jameson *et al.* 2002), suggesting that these cells may be targets of HIV and other mucosal pathogens that attach to this lectin receptor (van Kooyk and Geijtenbeek 2003). In addition, M-DC8+ cells that most likely represent DCs were also found in the SED region of tonsils and PPs from inflamed tissues (de Baey *et al.* 2003). The latter produced high levels of TNF-α and may have a role in driving T-cell responses during inflammation.

Chemokines and chemokine receptors that govern the localization and migration of DC populations in the intestine are just beginning to be unraveled. In murine PP in the steady state, CD11b+ DCs appear to be recruited to SED by a number of chemokines expressed constitutively by epithelial cells in the FAE, including CCL9 (Zhao *et al.* 2003) and possibly CCL20 (Iwasaki and Kelsall 2000); the chemokines that attract CD8α⁻CD4⁻CD11b-DCs to this site have not been identified. Upon activation *in vivo* with a soluble tachyzoite antigen preparation from *Toxoplasma gondii* trophozoites (STAg), the SED CD11b+, and possibly some CD8α⁻,CD4⁻,CD11b⁻, DCs migrated to the PP IFR (Iwasaki and Kelsall 2000). This correlated with an upregulation upon overnight culture of CCR7, the receptor for CCL7 and CCL8, which are constitutively expressed in the IFR. These studies support the hypothesis that activation of DCs in the SED, as would occur following exposure to organisms entering via M cells, results in their migration to the IFR where T-cell priming could occur. In contrast, CD8α+ DCs constitutively expressed CCR7 and not CCR6 and migrated toward CCL7, but not CCL20, *in vitro*, suggesting that CD8α+ DCs are resident in the IFR throughout much of their life cycle.

Finally, one additional unique feature of PP DCs has recently been identified. PP and MLN but not spleen or LN DCs can induce the mucosal homing receptor α4β7 as well as the chemokine receptor CCR9 on T cells *in vitro* (Mora *et al.* 2003). Upon adoptive transfer to naive mice, PP-primed CD8+ T cells preferentially migrate to mucosal lymphoid tissues. These studies demonstrated that DCs from different tissues have the capacity to imprint T cells with tissue-specific homing receptors.

Mesenteric lymph node. In classic studies, "veiled cells" were described in the thoracic duct lymph from mesenteric lymph-adenectomized rats (Liu and MacPherson 1991, 1993, 1995; MacPherson 1989; MacPherson *et al.* 1995; Pugh *et al.* 1983). Veiled cells are a heterogeneous population of cells that migrate from all regions of the intestinal tract to draining MLNs, where they are normally trapped (MacPherson 1989; Pugh *et al.* 1983). These veiled cells process fed antigen (Liu and MacPherson 1993) or antigen delivered by direct intestinal injection (Liu and MacPherson 1991, 1993), are capable of stimulating primed T cells

in vitro, and when transferred to the footpad of an unprimed mouse, prime naive T cells *in vivo* (Liu and MacPherson 1993). Although the site of antigen acquisition cannot be precisely determined from these studies, the antigen-loaded DCs likely came from the intestinal tract, because thoracic duct cells from nonlymphadenectomized rats contain very few DCs (<0.2%), when compared with lymphadenectomized rats (8% to 10%) (MacPherson *et al.* 1995). These migrating DCs have a short half-life in tissues (on the order 2–3 days) similarly to most other DC populations, which is significantly shortened following the induction of TNF-α production by systemically administered LPS (MacPherson *et al.* 1995).

In further studies of their ability to stimulate an MLR (Liu and MacPherson, 1995), LP and PP DCs stimulated only a modest MLR, compared with MLN and thoracic duct lymph DCs, which induced a potent MLR. In addition, following overnight culture with GM-CSF, PP and LP DCs had significantly increased potency in the MLR, equivalent to that of lymph or MLN DCs, which did not have enhanced accessory cell activity following culture. These studies thus suggest that PP and LP DCs are less activated than DCs that have migrated to the MLN and support the general concept that DCs become more capable of inducing T-cell differentiation after migration from sites of antigen acquisition. Furthermore, the studies provide evidence that under steady-state conditions DCs constitutively migrate from the intestine to the MLNs, and pathogen products enhance this migration.

Rat intestinal lymph contains at least two DC populations that have typical DC morphology, are major histocompatibility complex class II^hi, and express OX62, CD11c, and CD80. One population, CD4+/OX41 (SIRPα)+ DCs, are strong APCs in MLRs, whereas the other population, CD4⁻/OX41⁻ DCs are weak APCs (see Yrlid and MacPherson 2003). Both DC populations are also present in rat MLNs, where CD4⁻ DCs are localized to T-cell zones and CD4+ DCs are found outside the T-cell zone in the parafollicular regions. Many MLN CD4⁻ DCs contain cytoplasmic apoptotic DNA, epithelial cell–restricted cytokeratins, and nonspecific esterase-positive inclusions, suggesting the cells carry material from apoptotic enterocytes to T-cell zones of the MLN (Huang *et al.* 2000). In addition, CD4⁻ DCs from the rat spleen produce IL-12 after stimulation *in vitro*, while the CD4+ DCs do not. These studies suggest that rat CD4⁻ DCs are similar to mouse CD8+ DCs, whereas rat CD4+ DCs resemble mouse CD11b+CD4+ DCs.

Many of the features of MLN DCs are similar to those of the PP DCs. In the mouse, the MLN contains the same five populations of DCs present in the PP, with an increased proportion of C11b⁻CD8⁻CD4⁻ DCs (Iwasaki and Kelsall, 2001). CD8a+, CD11b⁻CD8⁻CD4⁻ and pDCs have been localized to the T-cell zones (Asselin-Paturel *et al.* 2003; Iwasaki and Kelsall 2000), whereas CD11b+ DCs are located primarily outside the T-cell zones. Whether the population we describe as CD11b⁻CD8⁻CD4⁻ corresponds to a CD8⁻CD11b^lo CD205^int DC population described in the MLN by others (see Shortman and Liu 2002) has not yet been resolved. Interestingly, the CD11b⁻CD8⁻CD4⁻ DCs that we described in the PP do not express CD205 or higher levels of MHC class II molecules than the other subsets following isolation, although both surface antigens could be upregulated after overnight incubation with CD40L-trimer. Thus the CD8$^-$CD11b^{lo}CD205^{int} DCs in the MLNs may represent more "mature" (at least with regards to MHC class II expression) CD11b$^-$CD8$^-$CD4$^-$ DCs that have migrated from the PP or possibly the intestinal LP under steady-state conditions.

Functional studies have also demonstrated similarities between murine MLN and PP DCs. Similarly to PP DCs, MLN DCs from antigen-fed mice produce IL-10, and possibly TGF-β and preferentially stimulate antigen-specific CD4$^+$ T cells to produce IL-4, IL-10, and TGF-β (Akbari et al. 2001; Alpan et al. 2001). Similar results were obtained with both wild-type and uMT mice, which lack B cells and well-developed PPs, allowing the argument that soluble antigen-loaded MLN DCs do not necessarily originate in the PP (Alpan et al. 2001). An additional feature shared by MLN and PP DCs, as mentioned in the preceding text, is the capacity to induce the α4β7 integrin on T cells (Johansson-Lindbom et al. 2003; Stagg et al. 2002).

Finally, in humans, DCs in the MLN are HLA-DR^{hi}, large dendriform cells in the T-cell areas that coexpress CD40, CD54, CD80, CD83, CD86, and the S-100 protein, but lack CD1a. These DCs are attached to numerous CD4$^+$ T cells and IgD$^+$ naive B cells *in vivo* and preferentially formed clusters with IgD$^+$ and IgM$^+$, but not IgA$^+$ or IgG$^+$ B cells *in vitro*. These findings suggest that human MLN DCs may induce T-cell help for primary B-cell responses.

Intestinal lamina propria (LP). DCs are a major antigen-presenting cell population in the intestinal LP of the mouse (Pavli et al. 1990), rat (Maric et al. 1996; Mayrhofer et al. 1983; Liu and MacPherson 1995), and human (Pavli et al. 1993). Irregularly shaped, strongly MHC class II–positive LP DCs cells have been described primarily in the LP just below the basement membrane. In the rat, DCs have also been described within the epithelium of the intestine (Maric et al. 1996). There they formed an organized network that extended dendrites between epithelial cells. Although similar intraepithelial DCs have not yet been described in the LP–associated epithelium in other species in the steady state, murine small bowel DCs may be induced to migrate into the epithelium and extend their processes into the intestinal lumen to sample bacteria by a well-orchestrated process (Rescigno et al. 2001b) (see discussion in the following text). Recently, DCs were found to be a dominant cell in the LP of the small bowel in mice but rare in the colon, except in isolated lymphoid follicles (Becker et al. 2003).

The phenotype of LP DCs is not as well defined as that of PP DCs. Mowat and colleagues recently detected the same three 3 CD11c^{hi} DC subsets in the LP that had been defined in the PP, as well as pDCs (Mowat 2003). Others found a predominance of CD11b$^-$ CD8$^-$ DCs, especially in the terminal ileum (Becker et al. 2003). In contrast, studies by our laboratory show a predominance of CD11b$^+$ and fewer CD11b$^-$CD8$^-$CD4$^-$ and no CD8$^+$ DCs in the small

bowel and colonic LP of mice (Kelsall, unpublished observations). In addition, we have confirmed the concentration of colonic DCs within organized follicles. In humans, one study suggests that DCs are present in the LP and in poorly defined lymphoid aggregates in the small bowel, which do not have the structure of PPs (Moghaddami et al. 1998). CD11c$^+$HLA-DR$^+$lin$^-$ (CD3$^-$CD14$^-$CD16$^-$CD19$^-$CD34$^-$) DCs in colonic and rectal biopsies have been reported to be of an immature phenotype, but to mature into fully immunostimulatory DCs upon migration out of tissues following overnight culture (Bell et al. 2001). Similarly, CD83$^+$ and DC-SIGN$^+$ cells have been identified in the LP and may produce IL-12 and IL-18 during intestinal inflammation from Crohn's disease (CD) (te Velde et al. 2003). Finally, DC-SIGN-expressing cells are found diffusely throughout the human and rhesus macaque rectal LP, and some of these cells coexpress CCR5 andCD4, suggesting they could be targets of HIV infection (Jameson et al. 2002).

Studies of chemokines responsible for the migration of DCs to the LP in the steady state are lacking, although epithelial cell–expressed CCL25, the ligand for CCR9 or CCR10, is a possible candidate chemokine in the small bowel, and CCL28, the ligand for CCR3 or CCR10, may be important in the colon (see Ajuebor and Swain 2002; Caux et al. 2002; Kunkel et al. 2003; Papadakis 2004; Zhao et al. 2003). During inflammation, however, a large number of inflammatory chemokines are produced by epithelial cells that could attract DCs, including CCL20/CCR6, CCL2/CCR2, CCL5/CCR5 or CCR1, and CXCL-12/CXCR4 (see Caux et al. 2002). The most studied of these is CCL20 (Dieu et al. 1998; Greaves et al. 1997; Homey et al. 2000; Izadpanah et al. 2001; Kwon et al. 2002, 2003; Scheerens et al. 2001; Tanaka et al. 1999; Vanbervliet et al. 2002), which, as mentioned in the preceding text, is constitutively expressed only by the FAE. However, CCL20 mRNA expression and protein production were upregulated in intestinal epithelial cells *in vitro* by stimulation with LPS, TNF-α, or IL-1α or infection with the enteric bacterial pathogens *Salmonella* or enteroinvasive *Escherichia coli* (Tanaka et al. 1999; Izadpanah et al. 2001). In addition, MIP-3α was shown to function as an NFκB target gene (Izadpanah et al. 2001). *In vitro* findings were paralleled *in vivo* by increased expression of CCL20 in the epithelium of cytokine-stimulated or bacteria-infected human intestinal xenografts and in the epithelium of inflamed human colon (Izadpanah et al. 2001). Therefore CCL20 could act to attract CCR6-expressing immature DCs to lymphoid follicle in the steady state and more broadly to inflamed tissues. Because CCR6 is expressed by more immature DCs and is downregulated following activation, coincident with an upregulation of CCR7 (Dieu et al. 1998; see Caux et al. 2002), immature DCs may be attracted to epithelial tissues as immature cells and upon activation by local signals, which are increased with inflammation, migrate to the PP IFRs or to MLNs for priming of naive, or activation of central memory T cells. However, given the redundancy of the chemokine system, and the likely need for signals for both cell extravasation and localization within tissues, multiple chemokines/receptors will certainly be involved in DC migration in inflamed and noninflamed mucosae. For example, data were recently provided to support a sequential role for CCR2 and CCR6 in immature DC migration into epithelial tissues (Vanbervliet *et al.* 2002).

Functional studies of LP DCs from all species have confirmed that these cells are potent inducers of the MLR (Liu and MacPherson 1995; Mayrhofer *et al.* 1983; Pavli *et al.* 1990, 1993). The aforementioned DCs in the terminal ileum of mice (but not of the more proximal small intestine) were shown to express IL-12p40 in the steady state, as well as mRNA for p19 (much greater than IL-12p35), suggesting that they constitutively express IL-23 (Becker *et al.* 2003). In addition, these cells were associated with bacteria *in vivo* suggesting that DCs in the terminal ileum may normally process endogenous bacterial microflora. Finally, it has been suggested that DCs from the LP may be particularly capable of inducing oral tolerance (Mowat 2003). However, there are no published studies to date of antigen-induced (vs. MLR-induced) T-cell responses specifically using well-defined LP DCs as APCs available to address this possibility.

Antigen handling by intestinal dendritic cells

Fundamental to understanding how mucosal immune responses are induced and regulated is where different types of antigens are processed and presented by DCs to T and B cells. As mentioned in the preceding text, intestinal DCs are present in several regions where antigens may be processed. From these sites, DCs constitutively traffic to draining LNs in the steady state and are induced to migrate at higher rates following exposure to microorganisms or proinflammatory cytokines. Less clear are the mechanisms for the uptake and processing of particular antigens and pathogens by intestinal DCs.

Luminal antigens are transported into the PP via specialized epithelial cells known as "M cells" or microfold cells, which are scattered among conventional epithelial cells overlying the dome of the PP follicle (reviewed in Kraehenbuhl and Neutra 2000). Compared with absorptive epithelial cells, with whom they share a common progenitor cell, M cells have poorly developed brush borders, reduced enzymatic activity, and a thin overlying glycocalyx. These features, possibly combined with a unique cytoskeleton and a pronounced capacity to form endocytic vesicles, facilitate the ability of M cells to transport microorganisms and macromolecules from the mucosal lumen to the SED of the PP. M cells likely do not have APC function because of their limited numbers and limited contact with T cells in the PP. Rather, DCs in the PP, and in particular, the SED, are likely to be important for the induction of immune responses to a large number of invading pathogens that gain entry via M-cell uptake. In this regard, it has been shown, for instance, that DCs in the SED phagocytose orally administered *Salmonella typhimurium* (Daniels *et al.* 1996; Hopkins and Kraehenbuhl

1997; Hopkins *et al.* 2000) and are the first targets of *Listeria monocytogenes* infection in rats (Pron *et al.* 2001). In addition, a population of CD11c$^+$ CD8$^-$ CD11b$^-$ cells in the SED was shown to take up 0.2 μm fluorescent latex beads given orally (Shreedhar *et al.* 2003). These cells remained in the SED for up to 14 days and rapidly migrated to the IFR following the administration of cholera toxin, suggesting that they may represent a resident population of long-lived cells particularly capable of processing particulate antigens.

Recent studies from our laboratory demonstrate that CD11c$^+$CD8$^-$CD4$^-$CD11b$^-$ DCs process antigens from type 1 *Reovirus,* at least some of which is in the form of apoptotic bodies from infected epithelial cells from the FAE (Fleeton *et al.* 2004). Whether this "cross-presentation" pathway applies to other organisms shown to induce apoptosis of enterocytes, such as *Salmonella* (Kim *et al.* 1998), is not clear. Direct sampling of antigens or organisms by the aforementioned immature intraepithelial DCs in the FAE has not yet been demonstrated. However, such sampling is supported by studies demonstrating the uptake of antigens by MHC Class II^{high}, non-B, non-T-cell pocket lymphocytes in the rabbit (Ermak *et al.* 1994). Finally, antigen uptake by M cells can be enhanced by the presence of specific IgA (Neutra and Kraehenbuhl 1993; Weltzin *et al.* 1989), suggesting that local immunoglobulin will direct antigens to PPs. Since DCs have been shown to express IgA receptors, which increase their uptake of antigens (Geissmann *et al.* 2001; Heystek *et al.* 2002), local antigen-specific IgA may enhance uptake of luminal antigens by PP (or LP) DC. Taken together, these findings suggest that DCs in the SED and FAE directly sample antigens and microorganisms transported into the PP by overlying M cells and from apoptotic epithelial cells of the FAE.

Microorganisms may also gain access to DCs in the LP directly across the normally exclusive intestinal epithelium following epithelial barrier disruption by infection and/or inflammation, as occurs in IBD. The DCs identified within the LP epithelium (Maric *et al.* 1996) suggest that a population of DCs may be the first APCs to come into contact with luminal antigens that cross the glycocalyx/mucous coat overlying epithelial cells of the LP. These DCs may compete with epithelial cells in the processing and presentation of luminal or self-antigens to αβ, or γδ-TCR IEL populations.

In addition, DCs may sample luminal contents by a unique mechanism described by Rescigno and colleagues (Rescigno *et al.* 2001a, b). DCs are capable of opening tight junctions between enterocytes and sending dendrites into the intestinal lumen to directly sample bacteria. This sampling process appears to require signals from luminal bacteria, which result not only in DC migration but also in the coordinated expression of tight junction proteins by DCs. The latter allows DCs to form adhesive interactions with enterocytes resulting in the maintenance of the epithelial barrier. This mechanism was also suggested in studies of bacterial uptake *in vivo* using *S. typhimurium,* as well as nonpathogenic *E. coli* (Rescigno *et al.* 2001b) Whether this is a generalized mechanism by which mucosal pathogens or normal flora gain access to the mucosal immune system is not yet clear. However, as mentioned in the preceding text, bacteria have been associated with DCs in the terminal ileum of normal mice *in vivo*, suggesting that this may be a location where direct DC sampling of normal intestinal flora bacteria may occur.

In contrast to these studies demonstrating uptake of microbial organisms by DCs in the PP and LP, there are few studies demonstrating the direct uptake of soluble antigens by mucosal DCs. Soluble antigens can be transported by a receptor-mediated mechanism from the lumen to the LP by conventional absorptive epithelial cells. Although this transport may result in the degradation of proteins into fragments that are nonimmunogenic, there may be particular receptors that translocate more intact antigenic fragments. One such receptor is the "neonatal" Fc-receptor for IgG that is present on epithelial cells on both the apical and basolateral membranes not only during the neonatal period, where it plays a vital role in the absorption of maternal IgG following the ingestion of breast milk, but also during adulthood (Israel *et al.* 1997). Antigens transported by this mechanism may be taken up by DCs, because DCs as well as LP macrophages express this receptor (Zhu *et al.* 2001).

In addition, it is clear that following high doses of oral antigen, protein can be found in the peripheral blood, possibly in an "altered" form that may be particularly tolerogenic (Bruce and Ferguson 1986; Furrie *et al.* 1995). Consistent with these studies, very high doses (100–250 mg) of oral antigen result in simultaneous activation of antigen-specific T cells in multiple sites, including the LP, PPs, and MLNs. In addition, such doses result in peripheral T-cell activation and anergy induction similar to what has been shown with intravenous antigen administration (Blanas *et al.* 2000; Gutgemann *et al.* 1998; Kobets *et al.* 2003; K. M. Smith *et al.* 2002; Sun *et al.* 1999; Van Houten and Blake 1996; Williamson *et al.* 1999). Studies of lower doses of oral antigen (1–60 mg), demonstrated that transferred T cells are activated preferentially in MLN and PP (rather than systemic lymphoid tissue), but that such activation occurs with virtually identical kinetics, even at the 1-mg dose (Blanas *et al.* 2000), suggesting that antigens are simultaneously processed in the PP and LP, with migration of the LP DCs to the MLNs. Although none of these studies formally addresses the initial site of antigen uptake (FAE vs. absorptive enterocyte), they suggest that at both high and low doses antigen is processed by DCs at both sites and that only with very high doses does antigen get distributed via the bloodstream for presentation by DCs at systemic sites. Whether specific subsets of DCs preferentially process soluble mucosal antigens is not clear. Although following very high oral antigen doses, CD8$^-$ DCs in MLNs and PLNs were found to preferentially present antigen/MHC complexes (Kobets *et al.* 2003), targeting of specific antigen to CD8$^+$/CD205$^+$ DCs is particularly effective in inducing systemic tolerance (Bonifaz *et al.* 2002; Hawiger *et al.* 2001).

Intestinal dendritic cells in the induction and regulation of immune responses

Based on the information presented in the preceding text, it is possible to present models of how DCs play a role in the induction of oral tolerance and immunity to mucosal pathogens. Under steady-state conditions, precursor DCs continuously enter the mucosal LP and PP, develop into immature DCs, and become localized to different regions by the local constitutive expression of specific chemokines, such as CCL9, and CCL19, CCL20, and CCL21 in the murine PP. After transport of antigens across M cells, or epithelial cells, or possibly via uptake of antigen associated with apoptotic bodies from epithelial cells, DCs migrate from the LP to the MLN or from the PP SED to the PP IFR in the steady state **(Fig. 26.4)**. This is accompanied by an upregulation of chemokine receptors for T-cell zone chemokines, such as CCR7, but low levels of costimulatory molecules and cytokines. Migration from the PP to the MLN is less likely since the PP contains T-cell zone chemokines, such as CCL19 and CCL21, which will attract activated or possibly "quiescent" DCs.

Following migration of antigen-loaded, "quiescent" DCs to T-cell zones in the PP or MLN, such DCs stimulate T cells to differentiate into Treg that can mediate bystander tolerance following subsequent antigen encounter. Although the precise nature of these regulatory cells in relation to the CD25$^+$ Treg originally described by Sakaguchi and colleagues (Sakaguchi *et al.* 1985) is not clear, they seem to suppress primarily via a cytokine-dependent mechanism *in vitro* and *in vivo*, involving TGF-β, IL-10, and possibly IL-4 (Th2/Th3/TR1) (see Weiner 2001; Wu and Weiner 2003). This is in contrast to Treg generated in the lung following inhalation of innocuous antigens that do not appear to produce TGF-β (Akbari *et al.* 2001).

The induction of regulatory cells most likely involves one of three DC populations. CD11b$^+$ DCs are ideally located for antigen capture in the PP SED and LP, produce IL-10, and induce IL-4, IL-10, and likely TGF-β-producing cells *in vitro*. PP DCs could either induce CD4$^+$ T cells to differentiate in the SED or migrate to the IFR to induce CD4 or CD8 responses, while LP DCs could drive memory responses in the LP or migrate to the MLN to prime or tolerize CD4$^+$ or CD8$^+$ T cells **(Fig. 26.5A)**. In the PP or LP, it is possible that innocuous antigens are also processed by the CD8$^-$CD11b$^-$CD4$^-$ DCs, but that in the absence of a strong activating signal, such as an adjuvant, these cells produce little IL-12, and induce T-cell deletion (similar to high-dose antigen feeding as discussed in the following text) or contribute to regulatory T-cell differentiation under the influence of bystander IL-10 or TGF-β. In addition to CD11b$^+$ DCs, another candidate for Treg induction is the pDC, which as mentioned in the preceding text, is also located within the PP SED and IFR and LP. In particular, CD8α^+ B220$^+$ pDCs from the PP were shown to induce IL-10-producing Treg cells *in vitro*, which could mediate suppression. Finally, the population of murine

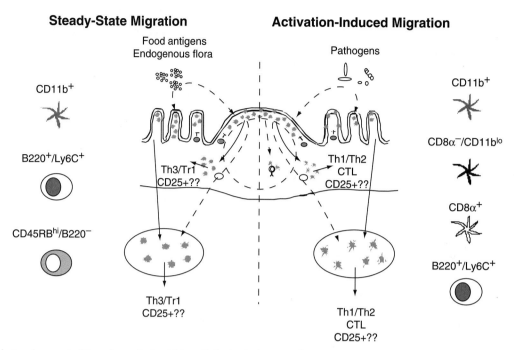

Fig. 26.4. Possible involvement of Peyer's patch dendritic cells in the induction of immune responses. This schematic presents a working model for how dendritic cells may be involved in the induction of tolerance and immunity. In steady-state conditions, innocuous antigens are taken up by dendritic cells (DCs) in either the Peyer's patch or lamina propria by one of several possible mechanisms. DCs constitutively migrate to the Peyer's patch interfollicular region (IFR) or to the mesenteric lymph node (MLN), where they induce the differentiation or expansion of regulatory T cells, which produce interleukin-10 and possibly transforming growth factor-β. Based primarily on *in vitro* studies, the DC subsets most likely involved in this process are indicated on the left. Not depicted here is the possibility that DCs (likely CD8α+) in either the Peyer's patch or MLN may simultaneously be involved in the induction of T-cell anergy or deletion, as depicted in Fig. 26.5B (see text for further discussion). In contrast, following activation by pathogens or by inflammatory signals, DCs are activated into fully immunostimulatory cells that will migrate at an increased rate to either the IFR or MLN for the induction of effector T-cell responses. The phenotype of the effector response will depend on the DC population and the pathogen involved and the microenvironment in which DC activation and T-cell priming occur. All DC populations can be activated to mature into immunostimulatory DCs, shown on the right.

pDC that is CD11c^int but B220− and CD45RB^hi and induces IL-10-producing T cells may contribute to the induction of Treg. These pDCs are present in the PP and peripheral lymphoid organs. The phenotype of the PP and MLN DCs that induce Treg may be influenced by local stromal factors, such as TGF-β and prostaglandin E 2 (PGE2) (Barnard *et al.* 1993; Newberry *et al.* 1999, 2001). Thus, intestinal stromal cells stromal cells may promote a suppressive environment that conditions DCs to induce Treg cells.

After oral administration of high doses of antigens, LP and PP DCs take up antigens, and a certain portion of antigen will gain access to the bloodstream for systemic dissemination (Figure 26.5B). The consequence of systemic dissemination is the induction of T-cell anergy or deletion, similar to that which follows the intravenous injection of antigen. In the mouse, the DCs most likely involved in this process are CD8+ DCs in the T-cell zones of the spleen and LN, although the spleen may be the most important site. The implication that CD8+ DCs are involved in this induction is made based on the finding that CD8+ DCs are in continuous contact with the majority of T cells and may process antigens for presentation in the absence of activation or migration, and thus in

the absence of high levels of costimulatory molecules and cytokines. In the event of low levels of costimulation that may preferentially engage inhibitory coreceptors (see Sharpe and Freeman 2002) and the absence of IL-12 (Marth *et al.* 1996, 1999; Zhang *et al.* 2002) and possibly IL-18 (Eaton *et al.* 2003), T cells that may initially produce IFN-γ upon activation are deleted or induced into an anergic state. The most likely fate of anergic T cells is dissemination to peripheral tissues and death (Reinhardt *et al.* 2001), although it is possible that some may become Treg cells, which are poorly proliferative. In support of this possibility, high antigen doses, which when administered once will result in T-cell anergy/deletion, when given repeatedly can also result in the generation of regulatory cells (albeit likely less efficiently than repeated low doses) that can mediate bystander tolerance (Y. Chen *et al.* 1995; DePaolo *et al.* 2003). The induction of Treg cells may be more limited following systemic antigen administration, because this may restrict the precursors available for the generation of Treg cells at mucosal sites.

In contrast to tolerogenic responses to innocuous antigens, mucosal pathogens induce active local and systemic immunity. Initial encounter of pathogens with the cellular components of the innate mucosal barrier, epithelial cells and underlying DCs and macrophages, involves the recognition of microbial PAMPs by pattern recognition receptors (PRRs), such as TLR receptors (Barton and Medzhitov 2002; Didierlaurent *et al.* 2002; Gewirtz 2003; Kaisho and Akira 2003). TLR signaling of epithelial cells results in the production of proinflammatory cytokines and chemokines, such as IL-1, IL-8, IL-6, TNF-α, IFN-α, CCL5, and CCL20, which can recruit and activate neutrophils, macrophages, and DCs (Kagnoff and Eckmann 1997). In addition to this indirect mechanism of DC activation by

epithelial cell–derived cytokines, DCs may be directly activated by invading pathogens via TLRs and other surface receptors. In the mouse, CD11b⁺, or CD8⁻CD11b⁻ CD4⁻ DCs in the SED or LP are most likely involved in the initial interaction and uptake of invading pathogens, whereas CD8⁺ DCs may be involved in the direct presentation of pathogens that are disseminated or through cross-presenting antigens carried to the IFRs by DCs or macrophages or exosomes from epithelial cells. Direct activation of pDCs in the PP or LP by viruses will result in type 1 IFN production, which can activate innate defense mechanisms, as well as contribute to

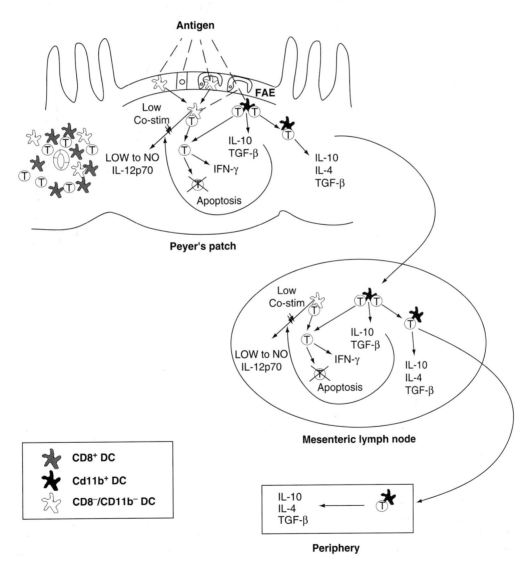

Fig. 26.5. Theoretical model for the role of DC subpopulations in the induction of oral tolerance. **A,** Repeated low doses of oral antigen. CD11b⁺ and CD8⁻CD11b⁻ DCs in the Peyer's patch or intestinal lamina propria take up antigen. Under nonadjuvanted/noninfectious conditions, CD8⁻CD11b⁻ DCs will present antigen to T cells in the absence of high levels of IL-12 or costimulation. CD40 ligation by responding T-cell expressed CD40L is inadequate to induce cytokine production alone. In addition, IL-12 production and DC maturation may be inhibited by bystander IL-10 or possibly TGF-β produced by neighboring CD11b⁺ DCs, which make IL-10 in response to CD40 ligation alone (Iwasaki and Kelsall 2001). The end result will be the induction of regulatory T cells and possibly the deletion of some cells stimulated by CD8⁻, CD11b⁻ DCs in the absence of IL-12 and high levels of costimulation.

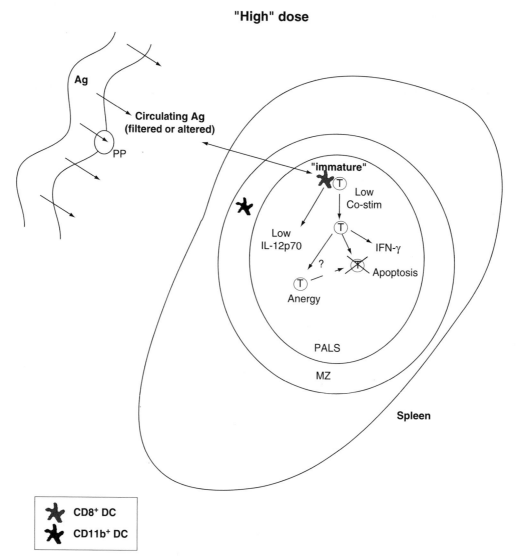

Fig. 26.5. (cont'd.) **B,** High antigen doses. Following high antigen doses, one mechanism of T-cell tolerance is the induction of T-cell anergy and deletion. A likely mechanism involved, at least for "very high" dose oral antigens (see text) is the distribution of soluble filtered or possibly "altered" antigen to systemic sites via the bloodstream. Such antigen is likely processed by CD8α⁺ DCs within the T-cell zones of lymphoid organs. Here the spleen is depicted because splenectomy may prevent the induction of high-dose oral tolerance. However, a similar mechanism is likely involved in other lymphoid tissues, including the Peyer's patch and MLN. Following antigen distribution, DCs process antigens for the induction of activation, and T cells are induced to proliferate initially and produce low levels of IFN-γ. In the absence of IL-12 and high levels of costimulation, such activation is followed by anergy, migration, and eventual deletion. It must be stressed that these are very hypothetical models. In addition, it is likely that some degree of both anergy/deletion and regulatory T-cell generation is occurring at all antigen doses, but the particular sites where this occurs as well as the degree of one response over another will depend on antigen dose and the repetitive nature of antigen exposure (see text for discussion).

the activation of non-plasmacytoid DCs. pDCs may also be driven to mature into immunostimulatory DCs by viral pathogens, such as influenza and HSV. As discussed in the preceding text, the induction or expansion of specific T-cell responses by mucosal DCs following infection will depend on the subset of DCs involved, the particular compilation of surface receptors engaged by the pathogen, microenvironmental factors such as cytokines, chemokines, prostaglandins, complement, heat shock proteins, uric acid, for example, and the combined effects of antigen dose and dura-

tion and/or frequency of T cell–DC contacts. Finally, DCs may be directly involved in the induction of IgA responses to pathogens or following immunization with mucosal adjuvants such as cholera toxin **(Fig. 26.6)**.

Intestinal dendritic cells and disease: A focus on inflammatory bowel disease
Intestinal DCs sample enteric antigens and present them to the immune system, shaping the host response toward tolerance versus immunity (see Stagg *et al.* 2003). The involvement

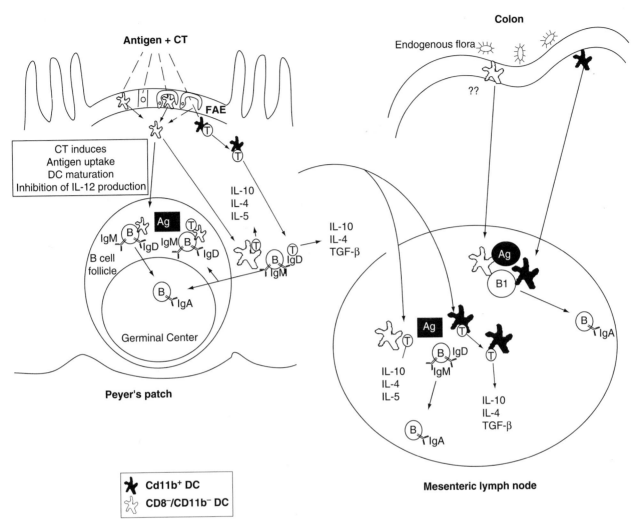

Fig. 26.6. Intestinal Theoretical model for the role of DC subpopulations in the induction of IgA responses in the intestine. Foreign antigens and vaccines need to be delivered to mucosal surfaces with an adjuvant for effective induction of IgA responses. This schematic depicts a possible direct role for DCs in this regard. Either CD11b⁺ or CD8⁻CD11b⁻ DCs that process antigens in the Peyer's patches (PP) or lamina propria will be induced to migrate to T-cell zones and T–B cell zones of the PP or MLN. In addition, CD8⁻CD11b⁻ DCs may migrate into the B-cell follicle, where they can directly interact with B cells or with B cells and T cells. Cholera toxin (CT) may act directly on DCs to induce maturation and to suppress the production of IL-12. Under these conditions, T cells producing TGF-β, IL-4, and IL-10 will predominate and help B-cell switching to IgA. In addition, DC production of IL-6 may be important for the differentiation of IgA B cells (Sato *et al.* 2003a). In contrast, in the absence of adjuvant, either CD11b⁺ or CD8⁻CD11b⁻ DCs from the colon or terminal ileum may be involved in the uptake of endogenous flora for the induction of IgA production from B1 or B2 B cells in the MLN or perhaps locally in the lamina propria (see discussion elsewhere in this volume).

of DCs in IBD may be two-fold. First, DCs are likely involved in the priming of the initial T-cell immune response in organized lymphoid tissue (PP, colonic follicles, or MLN) after antigen uptake, activation, and migration to sites rich in T cells. In addition, activated DCs may help maintain T-cell reactivity by restimulation of central memory T cells within organized lymphoid tissues. Second, DC may promote the persistence of the inflammatory T-cell responses by direct interactions with LP T cells *in situ*. This interaction would likely involve DCs that are induced to mature within the tissues, but that do not migrate following activation. Local activated DCs could enhance ongoing T-cell responses by direct cognate interaction and by the production of cytokines such

as IL-12 or IL-23 that could expand effector T-cell populations and/or prolong their survival. This latter possibility is supported by recent research in allergic respiratory disease and other chronic inflammatory diseases, such as in chronic periodontitis (Jotwani *et al.* 2001; Cirrincione *et al.* 2002), gastritis (Ninomiya *et al.* 2000), transplant-rejection nephritis (Sonderbye *et al.* 1998), and affected glands in Sjogren's syndrome (Ozaki *et al.* 2001), in which mature DCs (fascin⁺ or CD86⁺) have been found in inflamed T cell–rich tissues.

DCs in animal models and humans with IBD. Rodent models of colitis have provided strong evidence that the interaction between commensal bacteria flora and the mucosal immune system plays an essential role in pathogenesis of experimental IBD (reviewed in Strober *et al.* 2002; Uhlig and Powrie 2003). Consistent with the potential role of DCs both in abnormal mucosal immune responses in these models, DC activation has been demonstrated in both the organized lymphoid structures (MLN and colonic follicles) and in the nonorganized LP. In the "SCID/transfer" model of colitis (Powrie *et al.* 1994), the number of DCs in the MLN was increased and activated and likely induced the onset of colitis through interaction between DC-expressed CD134L with CD134 on T cells (Malmstrom *et al.* 2001). In addition, in the "RAG-KO/transfer" model of colitis, non-reconstituted RAG1-deficient mice have clusters of subepithelial CD11c+ DC in the colon. Upon reconstitution, naive CD4+ T cells appear in these clusters, where they may expand prior to the onset of colitis (Leithauser *et al.* 2001). The degree of expansion within the clusters was proportional to the severity of the resultant intestinal inflammation, suggesting a role for DCs in the pathogenesis of inflammation in this model (Leithauser *et al.* 2001). In addition, coincident with disease development in this model, LP DCs increase in number, are of a mature/activated phenotype, and likely produce IL-23 (Krajina *et al.* 2003). These data are consistent with the findings mentioned in the preceding text that CD11c+ CD8α- CD11b- DCs in the terminal ileum produced IL-23 in response to the bacterial flora (Becker *et al.* 2003).

Finally, our laboratory has investigated the localization and phenotype of DC subsets in intestinal inflammation in the Giα2−/− model of colitis and has a major increase in activated CD11b+ DCs within inflamed tissue (Kelsall, unpublished observations). Taken together, these studies in mice argue for an important role for DCs in intestinal inflammation, both in the induction and expansion of T cells within organized lymphoid tissues and in the maintenance of T-cell responses at the site of disease.

Human studies of IBD have also documented increased numbers and activation of mucosal DCs in IBD. Because of the difficulty in obtaining secondary lymphoid tissue from human gut, most human studies have focused on the LP, where DCs may be present (Pavli *et al.* 1993). The early literature described an increase in the number and/or maturation of LP DCs in IBD (Selby *et al.* 1983; Wilders *et al.* 1984; Oshitani *et al.* 1997, 1998; Seldenrijk *et al.* 1989; Waraich *et al.* 1997). The interpretation of these studies is complicated by the fact that most markers used in the studies (CD68, S-100, HLA class II, CD83, CD11c, CD86, CD-14-negativity) were not DC-specific (reviewed in MacDonald 2003 and Stagg *et al.* 2003). In particular, CD83 and CD11c can be found on activated T cells, CD86 can be found on plasma cells, and human intestinal macrophages are CD14- (Rogler *et al.* 1998; P. D. Smith *et al.* 2001b). More recently, immature CD11c+ ("myeloid") DCs have been clearly identified in the human colon by flow cytometry after collagenase digestion of biopsies (Bell *et al.* 2001). This lineage-negative HLA-DR+ CD11c+ CD83lo CD80- DC subset constitutes about 0.6% of mononuclear cells in the uninflamed LP and a slightly increased percentage in tissues from patients with CD. Whereas DCs from diseased tissues expressed elevated levels of CD40, which is reduced after treatment with anti-TNF-α (Stagg *et al.* 2003) and consistent with elevated levels of CD40-L on LP T cells in CD (Liu *et al.* 1999), the DCs did not display a phenotype typical of mature DCs with high levels of HLA-DR or CD86 (Bell *et al.* 2001).

In contrast, several groups have shown an increase in the number of LP DCs expressing high levels of costimulatory markers in IBD tissues. One group described an increase in the number of CD83+ CD80- cells in cell aggregates in the LP of CD tissues, as well as an increase in IL-12-producing and IL-18-producing CD83- CD80+ DC-SIGN+ cells, which may be DC or macrophages (te Velde *et al.* 2003). The number of lineage-negative CD86+ and CD40+ LP DCs was also elevated in CD (Vuckovic *et al.* 2001). In ulcerative colitis (UC), there is also an increase in the number of CD83+ and CD86+ LP cells. These cells produced macrophage inhibitory factor (MIF), and MIF induced significant levels of IL-1 and IL-8 in monocytes and DC from UC and CD patients (Murakami *et al.* 2002). In addition, DC generated *in vitro* from peripheral monocytes from UC patients showed an increased immunostimulatory capacity (Ikeda *et al.* 2001). Our own unpublished studies demonstrate a relative increase in the number of CD86+ CD11c+ in peripheral blood and of fascinhi DC in the colonic LP in CD (Leon *et al.*, manuscript in preparation). Finally, M-DC8+ monocytes, which may be precursors of DC (de Baey *et al.* 2001) with a high potential to secrete TNF-α, are also elevated in the colonic LP of CD (de Baey *et al.* 2003), suggesting an additional pathogenic mechanism in IBD.

Finally, although the exact mechanisms by which oral tolerance fails in food allergy remain to be defined (reviewed in Brandtzaeg 2002), the critical role of DC in allergic airway disease (see the following text) predicts an important involvement of DCs in this process. A particular type of hypersensitivity, celiac disease (CeD) or gluten-sensitive enteropathy, is one of the commonest gastrointestinal and genetic disorders, with a prevalence of 1% in the Western world (Schuppan and Hahn 2002). CeD is an immune-mediated intolerance to gluten, a cereal protein, and DC may potentially be involved in both the induction and the effector phases of its pathogenesis. On the one hand, CeD is likely initiated by an abnormal presentation of gluten peptides by HLA-DQ2/DQ8 on APCs, possibly DCs, to CD4+ LP T cells. On the other hand, CeD is characterized by an increase in IL-15 that induces the expansion and survival of intraepithelial lymphocytes with a capacity to lyse epithelial cells and induce enteropathy. In addition to epithelial-bound IL-15, cells with monocytic and dendritic morphology express high levels of IL-15 in the LP in CeD (Maiuri *et al.* 2000; Mention *et al.* 2003), suggesting that DC may contribute to the effector mechanisms of intestinal epithelial atrophy (Ruckert *et al.* 2003).

Dendritic cells as therapeutic targets in IBD. In addition to experimental therapies that target DC and APC function, such as anti-IL12 or anti-CR3 antibodies that reduce IL-12 and are therapeutic in murine experimental colitis (Leon *et al.*, unpublished observations) or aim to increase "regulatory" DCs (such as granulocyte colony-stimulating factor [G-CSF], which increases pDC [Leon *et al.*, manuscript in preparation]), the therapeutic use of probiotic agents in IBD may also affect DCs. Because microbial products play a critical role in modulating gut DC function, the demonstrated effect of probiotic bacteria in IBD (Mimura *et al.* 2004) may function, at least in part, by modulating the function of DC.

Dendritic cells of the respiratory system

The epithelium of the lung and airways is exposed to a myriad of environmental antigens. Much as in the gut, most are innocuous plant-derived or animal-derived antigens such as pollens, but the respiratory system is also a prime source of contact with potentially pathogenic microorganisms. As a result, the respiratory immune system faces the task of adequately responding to harmful pathogens while controlling the intensity of the reactions to prevent damage to the fragile epithelial surfaces where essential gas exchange takes place.

Subpopulations of respiratory tract dendritic cells

DC are distributed throughout the respiratory system, from the nasal mucosa to the pleura in all species studied (reviewed in Stumbles *et al.* 2003; Novak *et al.* 2004). DC appear first in the nasal mucosa at birth and then, after antigen encounter, they populate the rest of the airways (Nelson *et al.* 1994). Langerhans cells (LC) and "myeloid" DC (CD11c$^+$), as well as plasmacytoid DC [CD123 (IL-3R)$^+$], have been found in human nasal mucosa (Godthelp *et al.* 1996; Novak *et al.* 2004). In the oral mucosa, langerin$^+$ LC express unusually high levels of FcεR (Novak *et al.* 2004). In the lower respiratory tract, DC are very prominent in the conducting airways (500–1000/mm^2 in the rat), where they form a dense mesh of MHC-class II$^+$ cells, as illustrated in rodents by the tangential section immunohistochemistry method developed by Holt (Holt *et al.* 1989; Schon-Hegrad *et al.* 1991; see Stumbles *et al.* 2003). This network is similar to the one formed by LC in the epidermis. In the lung parenchyma, interstitial DC are located in the alveolar wall, mainly at the interseptal junctions between alveoli (Holt *et al.* 1988, 1993). The DC of the lower respiratory tract have been reported as immature CD1a$^+$ "myeloid" DC both in the human (CD11c$^+$) (Jahnsen *et al.* 2000) and in the mouse (CD11b$^+$) (Wang *et al.* 2000), with a notable absence of murine lymphoid CD8α^+ DC (Dodge *et al.* 2003) and human plasmacytoid DC (Jahnsen *et al.* 2001).

DC reach the lung from peripheral blood, where they are present as bone marrow–derived DC precursors. The interaction between CCR6 in immature DC and CCL20/MIP-3α produced by pneumocytes is important in DC homing to the lung (Power *et al.* 1997; Reibman *et al.* 2003). It has been proposed that airway DC can additionally develop from alveolar DC, which have the potential of entering the mucosa (Havenith *et al.* 1993).

Antigen handling by respiratory dendritic cells

Respiratory DCs are found in a resting or steady state until they face antigenic contact. As with those in other organs, immature respiratory DCs are characterized by lower levels of MHC and costimulatory molecules and a high capacity to uptake inhaled antigen. This is achieved by several mechanisms (see Lambrecht 2001), including macropinocytosis (Noirey *et al.* 2000), receptor-mediated endocytosis, phagocytosis (including the uptake of apoptotic cells that allows for cross-priming), and likely, passive transfer from resident macrophages (Gong *et al.* 1994). An additional mechanism that may play a role in atopic or allergic diseases is the "focusing" of antigen by IgE that subsequently binds to the high-affinity IgE receptors present in respiratory DCs (Foster *et al.* 2003; Maurer *et al.* 1998).

The more efficient and more relevant antigen uptake mechanism in the lung is receptor-mediated endocytosis involving clathrin-coated pits, and immature respiratory DCs express many specialized receptors such as C-type lectin carbohydrate receptors (langerin as in LC, DC-SIGN, dectin, mannose receptor, and CD205; see Lambrecht 2001). The main receptor seems to be the mannose receptor (Cochand *et al.* 1999). DC-SIGN has gained recent attention because it acts as the entry receptor for *Mycobacterium tuberculosis* (Tailleux *et al.* 2003), as well as other microorganisms, into DCs, which may result in immune suppression by the induction of IL-10 production by DCs (see van Kooyk and Geijtenbeek, 2003). Interestingly, similar to what has been postulated for the intestine (Maric *et al.* 1996; Rescigno *et al.* 2001a, b), airway DCs have been found to extend dendrites into the lumen, which may constitute a means of antigenic sampling (Sertl *et al.* 1986; Holt *et al.* 1992).

Isolated murine respiratory DCs have been shown to present antigen *in vitro* to primed T cells after exposure *in vivo* to aerosol or intratracheal administered particulate matter, viruses, bacteria, and fungi (reviewed in Stumbles *et al.* 2003). Furthermore, respiratory DCs have been shown to retain antigen for prolonged periods of time in two rodent models of respiratory antigenic exposure to *Leishmania* (Julia *et al.* 2002) and *Listeria* (Vu *et al.* 2002). This raises the interesting possibility that respiratory DCs may maintain a pool of chronically activated T cells within the airways.

Respiratory dendritic cells in the induction and regulation of immune responses

In the steady state, respiratory DCs circulate to regional LN where their initial low capacity to present antigens (Holt *et al.* 1988) increases significantly (Xia *et al.* 1995), a phenomenon dependent on maturation signals such as the one provided by GM-CSF produced by airway epithelial cells (Christensen *et al.* 1995; Holt *et al.* 1988; Tazi *et al.* 1993).

The turnover of resting respiratory DCs is very high, comparable to gut DCs: 2 days in the epithelium of the airways, 7–10 days in the lung wall (Holt *et al.* 1994). Under these steady-state conditions, DC promote either tolerance or Th2 responses to aeroantigens and self-antigens.

One possible mechanism that can explain the steady-state tolerizing capacity of airway-derived DC is that upon exposure to respiratory antigen, murine pulmonary CD86$^+$ DC transiently express IL-10 (Stumbles *et al.* 1998), which drives the generation of IL-10-producing Treg (Tr1) in the draining LN (Akbari *et al.* 2001). The induction of Tr1 cells is dependent on the engagement of inducible costimulator (ICOS) on T cells by ICOS-ligand on DC (Akbari *et al.* 2002), though ICOS is also essential for the development of dysregulated Th2 allergic responses (Gonzalo *et al.* 2001).

In other models, Th2 priming rather than tolerance occurs following inhalation and airway rechallenge (Herrick *et al.* 2000). Freshly isolated antigen-pulsed unmanipulated rat lung DC prime Th2 responses (Stumbles *et al.* 1998), and this mirrors the "Th2 default," which is observed in initial responses to inhaled antigen *in vivo* (McMenamin and Holt 1993). The murine lung lacks both CD8α$^+$ and CD11B/ CD4$^+$ DC and, consistently, lacks DC-derived IL-12 production that, in addition to the effect of DC-derived IL-6, results in Th2 skewing (Dodge *et al.* 2003). Interestingly, in LTα knockout mice, which lack normal LN, respiratory DC are capable of Th2 priming and activation *in situ* (Constant *et al.* 2002; Julia *et al.* 2002), which may play a role in responses to chronic antigen exposure and recall responses.

The precise rules establishing whether regulatory or Th2 responses will be mounted are not yet fully elucidated, though some insight has been recently gained. Lung DC-produced IL-10 is necessary for the development of the Tr1-cell response (Akbari *et al.* 2001), lung DC-produced IL-6 may contribute to the Th2 skewing in the respiratory system (Dodge *et al.* 2003), and the activation of peroxisome proliferator-activated receptors (PPAR) in lung DC prevents the induction of Th2-dependent eosinophilic airway inflammation in a murine model of asthma, suggesting that PPAR contributes to immune homeostasis in the lung (Hammad *et al.* 2004). It remains to be seen to what extent these mechanisms play a role in the human lung. In addition, further research is needed to determine whether human respiratory "myeloid" DC are able to promote Tr/Th2 responses, the logical inference from rodent models.

A different scenario ensues in the context of inflammation. Blood DCs are recruited to the airways by means of chemokine gradients. Bronchial epithelium and alveolar macrophages express IL-8 and human type II pneumocytes express ENA-78. Both factors are CXC chemokines that may recruit CXCR2$^+$ DCs into the respiratory system. In response to allergic challenge, myeloid blood DCs are recruited by the release of chemotactic factors such as CCL20, CCL17, CCL22, and CCL5 (Novak *et al.* 2004), as will be addressed in the following text. Similar to what likely occurs in the intestine, upon exposure to activating signals (e.g., microbial pathogens, inflammatory cytokines, products of stressed or dying cells), resident and recruited DC increase their expression of MHC and costimulatory molecules, as well as change their pattern of expression of chemokine receptors. CCR6 expression is shut down, and expression of CCR7 and CXCR4 is increased, resulting in migration to afferent lymphatics and T-cell areas of regional LN, where CCL21 is expressed (Gunn *et al.* 1999; Hammad *et al.* 2002 and where DCs fully mature and stimulate the differentiation of naive T cells.

The already rapid steady-state turnover of respiratory DC is greatly accelerated in inflammation. In response to inhaled bacterial antigens or viral infection, DCs are recruited within 1 hour, sample local antigen, and migrate to draining LNs (McWilliam *et al.* 1994, 1997). The presentation of inhaled protein to primed T cells by DCs isolated from airway draining LN occurs within 2–24 hours after antigen exposure (Huh *et al.* 2003). It has been proposed that after priming T cells in the LN some DCs recirculate to the lung, although it is difficult to conceive of a mechanism for this recirculation. Suffice it to say that the accumulation of mature DCs following secondary antigen challenge is regulated by chemokines, cytokines [IL-2 has a direct chemotactic activity on rat lung DCs *in vitro* and *in vivo* (Kradin *et al.* 1996)], and neuropeptides (such as substance P). Depletion of tachykinins abrogates the secondary antigen challenge-induced accumulation of DCs around lung venules (Kradin *et al.* 1997). These mature DCs may now induce the chronicity of the response by local stimulation of T cells, similarly to what was proposed in the preceding text for IBD.

The lung is protected from the entry of pathogens by non-specific mechanisms, such as antibacterial peptides (defensins). If the initial barrier is breached, the innate immune system is the next line of defense, but its responses are tightly controlled to avoid excessive damage to the gas-exchange system. Accordingly, alveolar macrophages are weak APC that suppress T-cells and DC function by means of NO production (Bilyk and Holt 1995; Holt *et al.* 1993). DCs are particularly relevant APC for respiratory infections *in vivo* (reviewed in Lambrecht *et al.* 2001). Their position at the interface between the innate and the adaptive immune system is clearly illustrated by the fact that human β-defensin-2 has a strong chemotactic activity for immature DC (Yang *et al.* 1999). Exposure of rodents to inhaled bacteria, fungi, and viruses induces marked increases in the numbers and activation status of airways DCs (Lambrecht *et al.* 2001).

DCs sample antigen in the airway and migrate to LN to prime T cells. An accelerated migration of murine respiratory DCs to the peribronchial LN takes place during the first 24 hours after pulmonary influenza virus infection (Legge and Braciale 2003). Interestingly, following the initial emigration of DCs to draining LN in this model, resident DCs are refractory to further migration despite ongoing viral replication and pulmonary inflammation and become refractory to a secondary inflammatory stimulus. This paralysis of DC migration results in depressed immune responses to new antigenic/viral challenge and may help explain the increased susceptibility to secondary bacterial infections seen following clinical influenza infection. Despite the mentioned default Th2/Tr1-cell response promoted by lung DCs, the response can be modulated and adapted to host defense. The change in the response is driven by the characteristics of the pathogen (Kalinski *et al.* 1999), as is beautifully illustrated by the functional plasticity of murine airway DCs in response to different forms of *Aspergillus fumigatus*: DCs produce IL-12 if stimulated with conidia and IL-4/IL-10 if challenged with hyphae *in vivo* (Bozza *et al.* 2002).

In addition to the capacity of activated pulmonary DCs to promote Th1 responses, DCs can directly activate the cytotoxic activity of NK cells (reviewed in Lambrecht *et al.* 2001), and their interaction with B cells and IL-5-producing epithelial cells leads to extralymphoid production of secretory IgA (Fayette *et al.* 1997). Immunity to mycobacteria is mediated via macrophages, TcR-γδ+ Tc and also DCs, which are able to induce a protective Th1 immunity against *M. tuberculosis* challenge *in vivo* (Demangel *et al.* 1999; Lagranderie *et al.* 2003).

Current active areas of research include the potential role of type I IFN–producing pDC in immunity to respiratory viruses and the potential use of DCs as cellular vaccines for infectious diseases (Lambrecht *et al.* 2001).

Pulmonary dendritic cells and disease: A focus on asthma

Respiratory DCs are increased in smokers, in idiopathic interstitial fibrosis, and in the obliterative bronchiolitis seen in chronic lung graft rejection (reviewed in Holt 2000). Lung DC have also an important role in tumor surveillance (Furukawa *et al.* 1985), and there are lung DC tumors (histiocytosis X or LC histiocytosis) (Tazi *et al.* 1993). However, the main role of respiratory DCs in human pathology concerns allergic disease, particularly asthma, and that has led to an intense research effort in the recent years.

Respiratory tract DC and allergic airway disease. As discussed before, the pulmonary immune response is biased not to react overtly with inhaled soluble antigen, which will be either ignored after nonspecific clearance mechanisms or will elicit tolerance. However, these mechanisms occasionally fail, and at the core of allergic diseases such as atopic dermatitis, rhinitis, and asthma, a dysregulated Th2-driven eosinophil-rich inflammation is found. Sensitization to allergens takes place early in life (even transplacentally), and the predominant response in newborns is Th2. Nonatopic individuals experience a protective shift toward a Th1 response to allergens later in life, but this seems to fail in atopic individuals (Holt *et al.* 1999). Indeed, a polymorphism in the IL-12 promoter that results in a decreased production of this key Th1 cytokine is associated with the severity of childhood asthma (Morahan *et al.* 2002). A decreased skewing to Th1-mediated inflammation following a lower frequency of infectious diseases has been suggested to account for the increased incidence of allergic diseases in the developed

world (the so-called "hygiene hypothesis") (Yazdanbakhsh *et al.* 2002). However, there is also an increase in Th1-mediated autoimmunity in developed countries. Therefore a more plausible explanation is that populations in developed countries have a reduced induction of regulatory T-cell responses to self-antigens and ubiquitous antigens that are required to control inflammation during responses to infectious agents and which can limit both Th1-mediated and Th2-mediated immune responses.

DCs in animal models and humans with asthma. The critical initial stages in the allergic immune response are defined at the APC level, and respiratory DCs play a fundamental role. In rodent models of asthma (e.g., OVA-induced eosinophilic airway inflammation), CCR5+ CCR6+ CD11b+ DCs from peripheral blood are recruited to the lung within hours in response to an allergic challenge (Novak *et al.* 2004), a phenomenon dependent on matrix metalloproteinase-9 (Vermaelen *et al.* 2003). This is accompanied by the release of chemokines that may attract DCs as well as other immune cells. For example, the major house dust mite allergen, Der-p1, has been shown to induce release of IL-8 and CCL5. In addition, mast cells release a number of chemokines after IgE cross-linking (reviewed in Lambrecht and Hammad 2003a). CD11b+ DCs then capture the inhaled antigen and present it to T cells in mediastinal LN, where Th2 sensitization takes place (Lambrecht *et al.* 2000b). The presence of OX40L on APC in the lung is necessary for the development of allergic inflammation (Jember *et al.* 2001). The role of DCs in the sensitization phase of asthma is further supported by the fact that eosinophilic airway inflammation can be adoptively transferred by OVA-pulsed DCs instilled intratracheally (Lambrecht *et al.* 2000a).

It has been proposed that a limited IL-10 (and thus reduced Tr1 generation) and enhanced IL-4 and IL-13 production may result in the Th2-driven deviated response seen in allergic asthma (Akbari *et al.* 2003). Indeed, allergen-induced production of IL-13 by human monocyte–derived DCs activates signal transducer and activator of transcription 6 (STAT-6) in T cells *in vitro* and may contribute to the generation of Th2 cells (Bellinghausen *et al.* 2003). IL-13 also has a direct effect on epithelial cells and induces airway hyperreactivity (Kuperman *et al.* 2002). The reported production of IL-6 by lung DCs may have a double effect in this regard, on one hand by contributing to the Th2 response as mentioned (Dodge *et al.* 2003; Rincon *et al.* 1997), on the other by abrogating the regulatory function of CD4+ CD25+ Treg (Pasare and Medzhitov 2003). The expression of proallergic cytokine IL-50/TSLP (thymic stromal lymphopoietin) (Gilliet *et al.* 2003) in asthma has not been reported, but its strong expression in lesional skin of atopic dermatitis patients (Soumelis *et al.* 2002) supports a potential involvement in allergic airway disease. Finally, the administration of IL-25 to mice has been described to induce all features of asthma (Fort *et al.* 2001; Hurst *et al.* 2002), and its potential implication in allergic sensitization remains to be elucidated.

In addition to the sensitization phase, T-cell activation during the late-phase allergic airway response is associated with upregulation of CD86 on DCs and their migration to regional LN after allergen exposure (Huh *et al.* 2003). It has been proposed that airway DCs may not only be crucial for sensitization to inhaled allergens and for stimulation of recirculating central memory T cells within draining LNs, but also may have a role in established inflammation by directly interacting with and restimulating T cells locally within the airways (Huh *et al.* 2003; Lambrecht and Hammad 2003b; Reinhardt *et al.* 2003).

Human studies are still in the descriptive phase and have shown that DCs are increased in number in the nasal mucosa of rhinitic patients after allergenic exposure (Fokkens *et al.* 1989; Godthelp *et al.* 1996). In addition, in the bronchial mucosa of atopic asthmatics, recruited DCs also have an activated phenotype (Jahnsen *et al.* 2001; Moller *et al.* 1996), with an enhanced expression of FcεR (Tunon-De-Lara *et al.* 1996). Consistent with a possible involvement of plamacytoid DCs in type 2 responses (human "DC2," see preceding discussion), pDCs that are present at low levels in the nasal mucosa of atopic individuals increase considerably after allergen exposure (Jahnsen *et al.* 2000). However, this does not occur in the bronchial mucosa following short-term allergen challenge (Jahnsen *et al.* 2001). pDCs are also relatively increased in peripheral blood of asthmatics (Matsuda *et al.* 2002; Reider *et al.* 2002). A novel experimental approach for the study of allergic inflammation is the reconstitution of SCID mice with peripheral blood cells from asthmatic humans. In these chimeric animals, adoptive transfer of allergen-pulsed monocyte-derived DCs induces allergen-specific IgE and airway infiltration by allergen-specific T cells (Hammad *et al.* 2000). Taken together, these findings suggest a pivotal role of DCs in allergen-induced immune responses.

In addition to a genetic bias toward a Th2 response, some relevant allergens can directly modify the function of human DCs. Der-p1 induces monocyte-derived DC from sensitized individuals to produce IL-10, TNF-α, IL-1β, and IL-6, while it induces IL-12 production from DCs from nonsensitized subjects (Hammad *et al.* 2001). Most aeroallergens are proteases capable of cleaving the proteinase-activated receptor-2 (PAR-2) from the surface of respiratory epithelial cells. This increases the production of eotaxin and GM-CSF, which induce eosinophil migration and DC maturation, respectively (Fields *et al.* 2003; Vliagoftis *et al.* 2001).

Dendritic cells as therapeutic targets in allergic disease. Together, all of these studies suggest that DC may constitute a therapeutic target in allergic disease. Indeed, systemic depletion of CD11b+ DCs (Lambrecht *et al.* 1998) and airway-selective depletion of DCs (Lambrecht and Hammad 2003b) during allergen challenge of sensitized mice abrogated the symptoms and reduced the Th2 response. Along these lines, CpG oligonucleotides that act via TLR-9 on APCs have been successfully used to inhibit allergic inflammation by means of promoting a Th1 response (Kline *et al.* 1998).

INTESTINAL MACROPHAGES

The gastrointestinal (GI) tract mucosa is the largest body surface to interface with the external environment (Brandtzaeg 1989). Unique for its close proximity to huge numbers of luminal bacteria and antigenic stimuli, this important interface tissue and immunologic organ contains the largest reservoir of macrophages in the body (Lee *et al.* 1985). Gastrointestinal macrophages are present exclusively in the subepithelial LP of the small intestine and colon (Hume *et al.* 1984) and are referred to here as intestinal macrophages. The major functions of intestinal macrophages are to: (a) regulate inflammatory responses to stimulatory bacteria and antigens that have breached the epithelium, (b) protect the mucosa against harmful pathogens, and (c) scavenge dead cells and noxious macromolecules. These goals are achieved through a series of cellular events in which monocytes are recruited to the mucosa and then undergo downregulation of their innate receptors, proinflammatory activities, and antigen presentation capabilities but retain avid host defense and scavenger functions through strong phagocytic and cytotoxic activities (P. D. Smith *et al.* 1997, 2001a; Smythies *et al.* 2003). Thus intestinal macrophages are phenotypically and functionally distinct from blood monocytes.

Origin of intestinal macrophages

Intestinal macrophages are derived from bone marrow stem cells through a highly regulated cascade of differentiation events (Gordon *et al.* 1995; Valledor *et al.* 1998). In the bone marrow, IL-1, IL-3, and IL-6 induce heteromitosis of stem cells into a pluripotent granulocyte-erythrocyte-megakaryocyte-macrophage colony–forming unit. In the continued presence of IL-1 and IL-3, this precursor becomes a progenitor of both granulocytes and macrophages, referred to as a granulocyte–macrophage colony–forming unit. IL-3 and GM-CSF induce proliferation of both of these myeloid precursors, whereas IL-1, IL-3, and macrophage colony–stimulating factor (M-CSF) induce the proliferation and differentiation of monocyte precursors. The continued presence of M-CSF, GM-CSF, and IL-3 induces further differentiation of the monocyte precursor into a monoblast, then promonocyte, and finally a monocyte. In addition to cytokine growth factors, transcription factors are involved in macrophage differentiation (McKercher *et al.* 1996). These factors include PU.1 and AML1, which control myeloid cell development. PU.1 is particularly important, because it regulates the expression of the receptor for M-CSF, which is critical for M-CSF-dependent differentiation (Voso *et al.* 1994). The transcription factors GATA-2, SCL, and c-Myb regulate myeloid cell survival. Additional transcription factors, including NF-M/C/EBPα, HOXB7, and c-Myc regulate the intermediate stages of myeloid differentiation, and C/EBPβ EBR-1, IRF-1, NF-Y, and some Jun/Fos and Stat proteins regulate monocyte maturation. Monocytes leave the bone marrow and enter the blood compartment, where they circulate for approximately 72 hours before entering the tissue. In the tissue, monocytes mature into macrophages, and they grow in size and increase their lysosomal content, amount of hydrolytic enzymes, number and size of mitochondria, and energy requirements. After a period of weeks to possibly several months, tissue macrophages undergo programmed cell death and are replaced by newly recruited blood monocytes.

Recruitment of blood monocytes to the intestinal mucosa

Unlike lymphocytes, blood monocytes and macrophages do not proliferate. Increasing evidence indicates that intestinal macrophages are derived from blood monocytes. Initial studies showed that the phenotype of intestinal macrophages in normal mucosa differs from that of blood monocytes, but during active IBD, the intestinal macrophage phenotype more closely resembles that of blood monocytes (Allison and Poulter 1991; Burgio et al. 1995; Mahida et al. 1989a; Rogler et al. 1998; Rugtveit et al. 1994). Together, these studies suggest that the majority of mononuclear phagocytes present in inflamed (IBD) mucosa are newly recruited blood monocytes. The higher percentage of CD14+ mononuclear phagocytes in the lesions than in normal, uninflamed intestinal tissue (Grimm et al. 1995a) and the preferential localization of experimentally inoculated, radiolabeled CD14+ monocytes to regions of intestinal inflammation (Grimm et al. 1995b) further support the concept that blood monocytes populate the intestinal mucosa, particularly inflammatory lesions. Detailed immunohistochemical analysis of CD lesions showed that the endothelial cells lining small blood vessels in the mucosa display high levels of CD34, which promotes the rolling of L-selectin+ monocytes in high endothelial venules, and increased levels of intercellular adhesion molecule 1 (ICAM-1) and CD31, which facilitate transendothelial migration of circulating monocytes (Burgio et al. 1995). These findings suggest that the endothelial cells in mucosal vessels in CD tissue express molecules that promote the rolling and subsequent transendothelial migration of circulating L-selectin+ monocytes into the LP. The factor(s) that initiate monocyte recruitment to inflamed mucosa likely include inflammatory CC chemokines (MIP-1α,β, RANTES, MCP-1,2,3,4,5 and TGF-β), noncysteine-containing chemotactic ligands (C5a, C3a, and TGF-β), and pathogen-derived peptides (Helicobacter pylori urease and f-met-leu-phe). The factors that induce recruitment of monocytes to normal tissue have not yet been identified.

Role of intestinal macrophages in mucosal inflammation

Macrophages, along with neutrophils, are the prototypic effector cells of the innate immune system, the evolutionarily primitive system of initial defense mechanisms through which the host rapidly responds to microorganisms and their products (P. D. Smith et al. 2001c). The first step in this response, the recognition of microorganisms and their products, is achieved through monocyte expression of highly

conserved molecules, termed pathogen recognition receptors, which recognize carbohydrate and lipid structures on microorganisms or their products. Key pathogen recognition receptors include CD14, the high affinity receptor for complexes of bacterial LPS and LPS-binding protein; Toll-like receptors 2 and 4 (TLR 2 and TLR 4), which participate in the recognition of peptidoglycan in gram-positive bacteria and LPS in gram-negative bacteria, respectively; and Fc Ig receptors, which link adaptive (antibody-specific) responses to innate monocyte effector activities. In contrast to blood monocytes, which express an extensive array of innate receptors as well as integrins, intestinal macrophages lack or are markedly downregulated for most innate response receptors, notably CD14, Fcγ and Fcα **(Table 26.1)** (P. D. Smith et al. 2001a; Smythies et al. 2003), and TLR 2 and TLR 4 (Hausmann et al. 2002). However, a subset express surface neonatal Fc receptor (FcRn) (Zhu et al. 2001), suggesting the presence of novel IgG binding functions on some intestinal macrophages. The downregulation of CD14 (and likely other innate response receptors) extends to colonic macrophages as well (Grimm et al. 1995a; Rogler et al. 1998). Because the innate response receptors are germ-line encoded, their absence on lamina propria macrophages is likely the consequence of local factors produced by LP mast and mesenchymal cells, which downregulate the receptors on newly recruited blood monocytes (Martinez-Pomares et al. 1996; Smythies et al. 2003).

After recognition of a microorganism or foreign molecule, tissue macrophages orchestrate an inflammatory response

Table 26.1. Expression of Surface Antigens and Receptors on Purified Matched Intestinal Macrophages and Blood Monocytes[a]

	Intestinal Macrophages	Blood Monocytes
HLA-DR	85.1	87.9
CD13 (aminopeptidase N)	90.8	94.7
CD83 (dendritic cells)	0.1	0.0
CD14 (LPS-R)	0.2	93.6
CD89 (FcαR)	0.5	91.4
CD16 (FcγRIII)	1.4	19.8
CD32 (FcγRII)	0.1	78.6
CD64 (FcγRI)	0.7	49.1
CD11a (integrin α, LFA-1)	0.2	95.0
CD11b (integrin α, MAC-1)	0.6	75.2
CD11c (integrin α)	0.2	86.6
CD18 (integrin β2)	0.2	93.6
CD25 (IL-2R)	0.3	3.7
CD25+ LPS[b]	0.2	24.7
CD123 (IL-3Rα)	0.1	19.2
CD36 (scavenger R B)	9.9	73.8

[a] Percent of cells positive.
[b] Cells incubated with LPS (1 μg/ml) for 24 hours.

through the production and release of cytokines such as IL-1, IL-6, IL-8, and TNF-α. Based on studies of tissue macrophages and monocyte-derived macrophages, LP macrophages are presumed to direct intestinal inflammatory responses through the elaboration of cytokines (Sartor 1994). However, study of isolated macrophages from normal human intestine indicates that resident intestinal macrophages do not produce, or are markedly downregulated for the production of, IL-1, IL-6, IL-8, and TNF-α in response to LPS **(Fig. 26.7)**. Although the absence of CD14, the LPS receptor, on intestinal macrophages offers an explanation for this profound downregulation, the inability of intestinal macrophages to produce cytokines in response to multiple stimuli of bacterial and non-bacterial origin **(Fig. 26.8)** indicates a global, stimulus-independent downregulation of normal intestinal macrophages to produce proinflammatory and immunoregulatory cytokines. The inability of resident intestinal macrophages to produce these cytokines, as well as IL-10, IL-12, RANTES, and TGF-β, indicates that intestinal macrophages are functionally, as well as phenotypically, distinct from blood monocytes.

Intestinal macrophages exhibit strong phagocytic and cytotoxic activities

Early studies of isolated but nonpurified mononuclear phagocytes from the human intestine and colon suggested that mucosal macrophages were capable of phagocytosing red blood cells (Golder and Doe 1983; Winter *et al.* 1983) and bacteria (Beeken *et al.* 1987). The phagocytic activity of intestinal macrophages has been confirmed using purified human jejunal macrophages, which avidly phagocytose FITC-labeled microspheres **(Fig. 26.9)**, *Candida albicans* (P. D. Smith *et al.* 1997), and both *S. typhimurium* and *E. coli*, achieving >99% killing within 30 to 60 minutes. (Fig. 26.9C, D). Intestinal macrophages appear to be more bacteriocidal for *Salmonella* and *E. coli* than for monocytes (Fig. 26.9C, D). The mechanism of this bacteriocidal activity may not involve reactive oxygen intermediates, because CD14⁻ intestinal macrophages appear incapable of respiratory burst activity (Rugtveit *et al.* 1995). Importantly, phagocytosis itself induces blood monocytes, but not intestinal macrophages, to release abundant levels of cytokines (Fig. 26.9). Thus resident macrophages in normal intestine are downregulated for the expression of proinflammatory receptors and the production of cytokines but express normal (or increased) phagocytic and bacteriocidal activity, ideal for downmodulating mucosal inflammation while protecting the mucosa against invading microorganisms. In contrast to macrophages from uninflamed intestine, macrophages from infected or inflamed tissue are often CD14⁺, likely representing newly recruited monocytes that respond to local stimulatory signals by producing cytokines that promote tissue inflammation (Rugtveit *et al.* 1997b).

Intestinal macrophage accessory cell function

Intestinal macrophages are constantly exposed to a rich array of antigenic stimuli. In view of their strategic location and

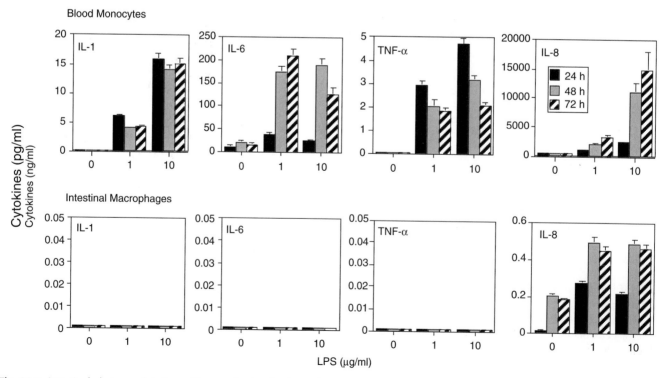

Fig. 26.7. Intestinal downregulated cytokine production by lipopolysaccharide-stimulated (LPS-stimulated) intestinal macrophages. Blood monocytes and intestinal macrophages (2×10⁶/ml) were incubated with or without LPS for 24, 48, and 72 hours, and supernatants were assayed for IL-1, IL-6, TNF-α, and IL-8. Mean + SD (N = 3). (From Smythies *et al.* 2003.)

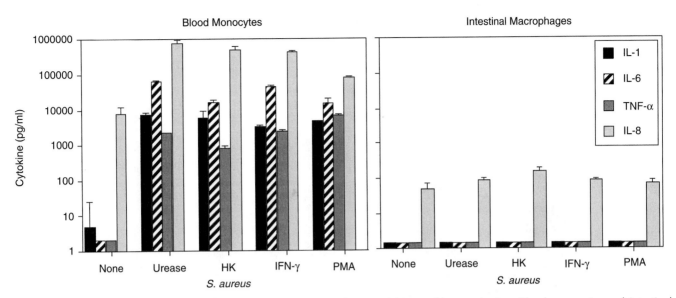

Fig. 26.8. Intestinal stimulus-independent downregulation of intestinal macrophage cytokine production. Blood monocytes and intestinal macrophages (2×10^6 per ml) were incubated with and without *Helicobacter pylori* urease (10 µg/ml), Hong Kong *Staphylococcus aureus* (10^7 cfu/ml), interferon-γ (IFN-γ) (100 U/ml), and phorbol myristate acetate (PMA) (40 ng/ml) for 24 hours, and supernatants were assayed for IL-1, IL-6, TNF-α, and IL-8. Mean + SD (N = 3). (From Smythies *et al.* 2003.)

phagocytic activity, intestinal macrophages are presumed to participate in accessory cell function. Analysis of accessory cell function by human intestinal macrophages is now possible because of the development of techniques for the isolation and purification of LP macrophages (P. D. Smith *et al.* 1997). In contrast to blood monocytes, intestinal macrophages lack constitutive and inducible expression of CD80 (B7.1), CD86 (B7.2), and CD40, costimulatory molecules that play a key role in accessory cell costimulation. As summarized in **Table 26.2**, isolated intestinal macrophages do not constitutively express CD80, CD86, or CD40, and the expression of these costimulatory molecules could not be induced by exposure to GM-CSF or cholera toxin. Immunohistochemical analysis of intestinal and colonic tissue for costimulatory molecules support the low level of expression of CD80 and CD86 on LP macrophages from uninflamed mucosa (Rugtveit *et al.* 1997a). Intestinal macrophages also lack the ability to produce costimulatory cytokines, including IL-1, IL-10, and IL-12, which participate in the priming and expansion of both antigen-specific and helper T cells.

Consistent with the absence of costimulatory molecule expression and costimulatory cytokine production, intestinal macrophages pulsed with mitogen (PHA) or antigens (tetanus toxoid and cecal bacterial antigen) and then cultured with intestinal T cells resulted in markedly reduced T-cell cytokine responses compared with similarly pulsed blood monocytes cultured with blood T cells **(Fig. 26.10)**. Thus intestinal macrophages do not function as antigen-presenting cells, at least *in vitro* for intestinal T cells. Moreover, preliminary studies suggest that factors within the LP stroma downregulate the antigen-presenting capability of blood

monocytes. These findings suggest that *in vivo* monocytes recruited to the LP stroma encounter factors that downregulate the antigen handling, as well as proinflammatory, function of blood monocytes as they differentiate into intestinal macrophages. Thus, in normal mucosa, resident macrophages display strong phagocytic and microbicidal activity but lack, or are strongly downregulated for, responses to immunostimulatory microorganisms and antigens. These features serve the host well, downmodulating mucosal inflammation while protecting the mucosa from commensal bacteria and foreign pathogens.

CONCLUDING COMMENTS

In conclusion, the past 5–10 years have witnessed remarkable progress in our understanding of the roles of DCs and macrophages in the induction, regulation, and maintenance of mucosal immune responses. We now have a better understanding of the basic biology of these cells and have begun to appreciate their function in host defense and inflammation, both in animal models and human disease. The preceding discussion highlights significant parallels between the immunology of the intestinal and pulmonary tracts, which together strengthen our understanding of how a host can be immunologically tolerant to the myriad of harmless environmental antigens and flora, yet remain capable of mounting effective defense against invading pathogens. First, one of the most apparent similarities between respiratory and intestinal DCs is that in the absence of inflammation they are constitutive migratory cells that produce IL-10 upon stimulation and have a propensity to induce the differentiation of regula-

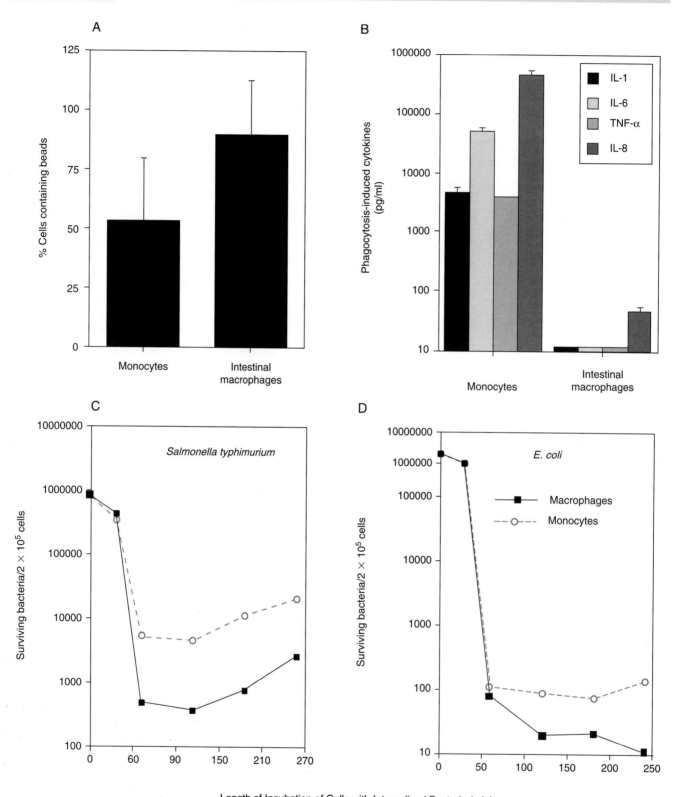

Fig. 26.9. Intestinal phagocytic and bacteriocidal activity of blood monocytes and intestinal macrophages. **A,** Blood monocyte and intestinal macrophage phagocytosis. Phagocytosis was measured as the percent of cells that contained fluorescein isothiocyanate–labeled (FITC-labeled) beads after 1-hour incubation. Mean + SD (N = 3). **B,** Phagocytosis-induced cytokine production by blood monocytes and intestinal macrophages. Blood monocytes and intestinal macrophages were incubated with latex beads for 2 hours, washed, cultured for 24 hours, and the supernatants assayed for IL-1, IL-6, TNF-α, and IL-8. Mean + SD (N = 4). **C,D,** Killing of gram-negative bacteria by blood monocytes and intestinal macrophages. Intestinal macrophages and blood monocytes (2×10^5 cells/250 μl) were incubated with **(C)** *Salmonella typhimurium* (8×10^6 CFU/ml) or **(D)** *E. coli* (4×10^6 CFU/ml), and intracellular killing was determined by enumerating the number of live bacteria in lysed cells. (Adapted from Smythies *et al.* 2003.)

tory T cells, thereby allowing for induction of regulatory cells against external antigens. Although it is likely that similar microenvironments exist in the intestine and lung that condition common DC precursors to differentiate into "regulatory" DCs, the precise nature of this environment, the

mucosal DCs involved, and the Treg induced by mucosal DCs need further elucidation.

Second, during inflammation, DCs can be activated and induced to migrate more rapidly in response to inflammatory signals and to induce positive immune responses. The nature of

Table 26.2. Expression of Macrophage-Specific and Costimulatory Molecules on Matched Intestinal Macrophages and Blood Monocyte

	Medium	GM-CSF[a]	CT[b]	CT-B[c]
Intestinal macrophages				
HLA-DR	85.1[d]	87.9	86.4	85.2
CD14	0.2	0.2	0.3	0.6
CD80	0.6	0.2	0.3	0.7
CD86	6.8	4.5	3.2	4.6
CD40	2.0	0.9	1.3	2.7
Blood monocytes				
HLA-DR	91.2	98.0	63.9	97.6
CD14	87.4	94.1	96.2	94.7
CD80	8.9	16.2	2.4	8.2
CD86	49.3	70.3	55.7	58.1
CD40	38.0	57.9	3.3	55.7

[a] GM-CSF, granulocyte-macrophage colony-stimulating factor, 500 U/ml for 48 hours.
[b] CT, cholera toxin, 100 ng/ml for 48 hours.
[c] CT-B, cholera toxin B subunit, 100 ng/ml for 48 hours.
[d] Percent of cells positive.

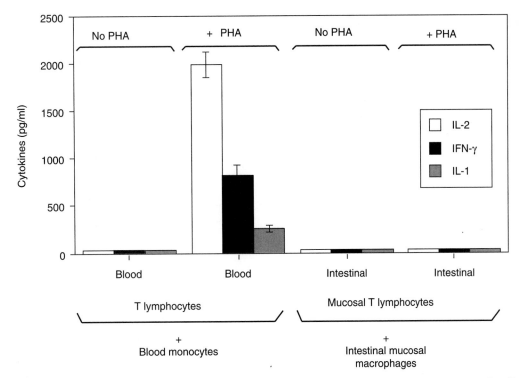

Fig. 26.10. Intestinal macrophage accessory cell function. Intestinal macrophages or homologous monocytes (2×10^5/well) were incubated with intestinal lymphocytes or blood lymphocytes (5×10^4/well), respectively, which had been preincubated for 48 hours with GM-CSF (500 U/ml) and 3 hours with PHA (5 μg/ml). IL-2 and IL-1 were measured in culture supernatant on day 2, IFN-γ was measured on day 3.

these ensuing immune responses depends on the signals to which DCs are exposed during their activation and interaction with T cells. Such signals include cytokines, chemokines, prostaglandins, PAMPs, costimulatory molecules, such as CD40L, complement fragments, immunoglobulins, and products from damaged cells, such as uric acid. Understanding how these signals influence DC function during infection or immunologic insult is a demanding challenge for the future studies that will require the use of well-defined animal models.

Third, it is now clear that in addition to their well-established role in T-cell priming and tolerance induction within organized lymphoid tissues, both in the lung and likely the gut, DCs may act to enhance (or possibly suppress) T-cell responses at sites of inflammation. In the past, this function was ascribed solely to macrophages. Determining the importance of DCs in this regard, as well as establishing a potential role for DCs in continuous activation of naive or central memory cells in LNs draining inflammatory sites may focus attention on the DC as a potential therapeutic target for chronic inflammatory diseases, such as IBD.

Fourth, it is now quite clear that macrophages play an important role in host defense in both the intestine and lung by acting as effector cells that efficiently clear invading pathogens. Remarkably, as mucosal macrophages perform this task, they are not activated to produce proinflammatory cytokines and, in fact, in the lung may be antiinflammatory via their production of nitric oxide. In addition, they do not present antigen. This common feature of mucosal macrophages also suggests common developmental environments in the lung and gut. Finally, a change in the tissue microenvironment during active inflammation appears to promote the recruitment of monocytes and their development into inflammatory macrophages.

Thus, both mucosal DCs and macrophages during steady-state conditions function to prevent untoward immune responses, DCs by inducing regulatory cells and macrophages by acting in silent fashion to clear harmless self-antigens and environmental antigens. However, in responding to infection, DCs can become activated and induce both innate and adaptive responses, while newly recruited monocytes can contribute to the production proinflammatory cytokines that are important for pathogen clearance. In this sense, mucosal DCs and macrophages have evolved functional niches that fully complement one another.

ACKNOWLEDGMENTS

L.E.S. and P.D.S. were supported by NIH grants DK-47322, DK-54495, HD-41361, DK-64400, and the Research Service of the Veterans Affairs.

REFERENCES

Ajuebor, M. N., and Swain, M. G. (2002). Role of chemokines and chemokine receptors in the gastrointestinal tract. *Immunology* 105, 137–143.

Akbari, O., DeKruyff, R. H., and Umetsu, D. T. (2001). Pulmonary DCs producing IL-10 mediate tolerance induced by respiratory exposure to antigen. *Nat. Immunol.* 2, 725–731.

Akbari, O., Freeman, G. J., Meyer, E. H., Greenfield, E. A., Chang, T. T., Sharpe, A. H., Berry, G., DeKruyff, R. H., and Umetsu, D. T. (2002). Antigen-specific regulatory T cells develop via the ICOS-ICOS-ligand pathway and inhibit allergen-induced airway hyper-reactivity. *Nat. Med.* 8, 1024–1032.

Akbari, O., Stock, P., DeKruyff, R. H., and Umetsu, D. T. (2003). Role of regulatory T cells in allergy and asthma. *Curr. Opin. Immunol.* 15, 627–633.

Albert, M. L., Pearce, S. F., Francisco, L. M., Sauter, B., Roy, P., Silverstein, R. L., and Bhardwaj, N. (1998). Immature dendritic cells phagocytose apoptotic cells via alphavbeta5 and CD36, and cross-present antigens to cytotoxic T lymphocytes. *J. Exp. Med.* 188, 1359–1368.

Allan, C. H., Mendrick, D. L., and Trier, J. S. (1993). Rat intestinal M cells contain acidic endosomal-lysosomal compartments and express class II major histocompatibility complex determinants. *Gastroenterology* 104, 698–708.

Allison, M. C., and Poulter, L. W. (1991). Changes in phenotypically distinct mucosal macrophage populations may be a prerequisite for the development of inflammatory bowel disease. *Clin. Exp. Immunol.* 85, 504–509.

Alpan, O., Rudomen, G., and Matzinger, P. (2001). The role of dendritic cells, B cells, and M cells in gut-oriented immune responses. *J. Immunol.* 166, 4843–4852.

Ardavin, C. (2003). Origin, precursors and differentiation of mouse dendritic cells. *Nat. Rev. Immunol.* 3, 582–590.

Asselin-Paturel, C., Boonstra, A., Dalod, M., Durand, I., Yessaad, N., Dezutter-Dambuyant, C., Vicari, A., O'Garra, A., Biron, C., Briere, F., and Trinchieri, G. (2001). Mouse type I IFN-producing cells are immature APCs with plasmacytoid morphology. *Nat. Immunol.* 2, 1144–1150.

Asselin-Paturel, C., Brizard, G., Pin, J. J., Briere, F., and Trinchieri, G. (2003). Mouse strain differences in plasmacytoid dendritic cell frequency and function revealed by a novel monoclonal antibody. *J. Immunol.* 171, 6466–6477.

Balazs, M., Martin, F., Zhou, T., and Kearney, J. (2002). Blood dendritic cells interact with splenic marginal zone B cells to initiate T-independent immune responses. *Immunity* 17, 341–352.

Banchereau, J., Briere, F., Caux, C., Davoust, J., Lebecque, S., Liu, Y. J., Pulendran, B., and Palucka, K. (2000). Immunobiology of dendritic cells. *Annu. Rev. Immunol.* 18, 767–811.

Barnard, J. A., Warwick, G. J., and Gold, L. I. (1993). Localization of transforming growth factor beta isoforms in the normal murine small intestine and colon. *Gastroenterology* 105, 67–73.

Barton, G. M., and Medzhitov, R. (2002). Toll-like receptors and their ligands. *Curr. Top. Microbiol. Immunol.* 270, 81–92.

Becker, C., Wirtz, S., Blessing, M., Pirhonen, J., Strand, D., Bechthold, O., Frick, J., Galle, P. R., Autenrieth, I., and Neurath, M. F. (2003). Constitutive p40 promoter activation and IL-23 production in the terminal ileum mediated by dendritic cells. *J. Clin. Invest.* 112, 693–706.

Beeken, W., Northwood, I., Beliveau, C., and Gump, D. (1987). Phagocytes in cell suspensions of human colon mucosa. *Gut* 28, 976–980.

Bell, S. J., Rigby, R., English, N., Mann, S. D., Knight, S. C., Kamm, M. A., and Stagg, A. J. (2001). Migration and maturation of human colonic dendritic cells. *J. Immunol.* 166, 4958–4967.

Bellinghausen, I., Brand, P., Bottcher, I., Klostermann, B., Knop, J., and Saloga, J. (2003). Production of interleukin-13 by human dendritic cells after stimulation with protein allergens is a key factor for induction of T helper 2 cytokines and is associated with activation of signal transducer and activator of transcription-6. *Immunology* 108, 167–176.

Belz, G. T., Behrens, G. M., Smith, C. M., Miller, J. F., Jones, C., Lejon, K., Fathman, C. G., Mueller, S. N., Shortman, K., Carbone, F. R., and Heath, W. R. (2002a). The CD8alpha(+) dendritic cell is responsible for inducing peripheral self-tolerance to tissue-associated antigens. *J. Exp. Med.* 196, 1099–1104.

Belz, G. T., Carbone, F. R., and Heath, W. R. (2002b). Cross-presentation of antigens by dendritic cells. *Crit. Rev. Immunol.* 22, 439–448.

Bilsborough, J., George, T. C., Norment, A., and Viney, J. L. (2003). Mucosal CD8alpha+ DC, with a plasmacytoid phenotype, induce differentiation and support function of T cells with regulatory properties. *Immunology* 108, 481–492.

Bilyk, N., and Holt, P. G. (1995). Cytokine modulation of the immunosuppressive phenotype of pulmonary alveolar macrophage populations. *Immunology* 86, 231–237.

Bjerke, K., Halstensen, T. S., Jahnsen, F., Pulford, K., and Brandtzaeg, P. (1993). Distribution of macrophages and granulocytes expressing L1 protein (calprotectin) in human Peyer's patches compared with normal ileal lamina propria and mesenteric lymph nodes. *Gut* 34, 1357–1363.

Blanas, E., Davey, G. M., Carbone, F. R., and Heath, W. R. (2000). A bone marrow-derived APC in the gut-associated lymphoid tissue captures oral antigens and presents them to both CD4+ and CD8+ T cells. *J. Immunol.* 164, 2890–2896.

Bland, P. W., and Whiting, C. V. (1993). Differential control of major histocompatibility complex class II I-Ek alpha protein expression in the epithelium and in subsets of lamina propria antigen-presenting cells of the gut. *Immunology* 79, 107–111.

Bonifaz, L., Bonnyay, D., Mahnke, K., Rivera, M., Nussenzweig, M. C., and Steinman, R. M. (2002). Efficient targeting of protein antigen to the dendritic cell receptor DEC-205 in the steady state leads to antigen presentation on major histocompatibility complex class I products and peripheral CD8+ T cell tolerance. *J. Exp. Med.* 196, 1627–1638.

Boonstra, A., Asselin-Paturel, C., Gilliet, M., Crain, C., Trinchieri, G., Liu, Y. J., and O'Garra, A. (2003). Flexibility of mouse classical and plasmacytoid-derived dendritic cells in directing T helper type 1 and 2 cell development: Dependency on antigen dose and differential toll-like receptor ligation. *J. Exp. Med.* 197, 101–109.

Bozza, S., Gaziano, R., Spreca, A., Bacci, A., Montagnoli, C., di Francesco, P., and Romani, L. (2002). Dendritic cells transport conidia and hyphae of *Aspergillus fumigatus* from the airways to the draining lymph nodes and initiate disparate Th responses to the fungus. *J. Immunol.* 168, 1362–1371.

Brandtzaeg, P. (1989). Overview of the mucosal immune system. *Curr. Top. Microbiol. Immunol.* 146, 13–25.

Brandtzaeg, P., and Bjerke, K. (1990). Immunomorphological characteristics of human Peyer's patches. *Digestion* 46(Suppl. 2), 262–273.

Brandtzaeg, P. E. (2002). Current understanding of gastrointestinal immunoregulation and its relation to food allergy. *Ann. N. Y. Acad. Sci.* 964, 13–45.

Braun, M. C., He, J., Wu, C. Y., and Kelsall, B. L. (1999). Cholera toxin suppresses interleukin (IL)-12 production and IL-12 receptor beta1 and beta2 chain expression. *J. Exp. Med.* 189, 541–552.

Bruce, M. G., and Ferguson, A. (1986). Oral tolerance to ovalbumin in mice: Studies of chemically modified and 'biologically filtered' antigen. *Immunology* 57, 627–630.

Buelens, C., Willems, F., Delvaux, A., Pierard, G., Delville, J. P., Velu, T., and Goldman, M. (1995). Interleukin-10 differentially regulates B7-1 (CD80) and B7-2 (CD86) expression on human peripheral blood dendritic cells. *Eur. J. Immunol.* 25, 2668–2672.

Burgio, V. T., Fais, S., Boirivant, M., Perrone, A., and Pallone, F. (1995). Peripheral monocyte and naive T-cell recruitment and activation in Crohn's disease. *Gastroenterology* 109, 1029–1038.

Caron, G., Delneste, Y., Roelandts, E., Duez, C., Bonnefoy, J. Y., Pestel, J., and Jeannin, P. (2001). Histamine polarizes human dendritic cells into Th2 cell-promoting effector dendritic cells. *J. Immunol.* 167, 3682–3686.

Caux, C., Vanbervliet, B., Massacrier, C., Ait-Yahia, S., Vaure, C., Chemin, K., Dieu, N., Mc, and Vicari, A. (2002). Regulation of dendritic cell recruitment by chemokines. *Transplantation* 73, S7–S11.

Chen, W., Frank, M. E., Jin, W., and Wahl, S. M. (2001). TGF-beta released by apoptotic T cells contributes to an immunosuppressive milieu. *Immunity* 14, 715–725.

Chen, Y., Inobe, J., Marks, R., Gonnella, P., Kuchroo, V. K., and Weiner, H. L. (1995). Peripheral deletion of antigen-reactive T cells in oral tolerance. *Nature* 376, 177–180.

Christensen, P. J., Armstrong, L. R., Fak, J. J., Chen, G. H., McDonald, R. A., Toews, G. B., and Paine, R., 3rd (1995). Regulation of rat pulmonary dendritic cell immunostimulatory activity by alveolar epithelial cell-derived granulocyte macrophage colony-stimulating factor. *Am. J. Respir. Cell Mol. Biol.* 13, 426–433.

Cirrincione, C., Pimpinelli, N., Orlando, L., and Romagnoli, P. (2002). Lamina propria dendritic cells express activation markers and contact lymphocytes in chronic periodontitis. *J. Periodontol.* 73, 45–52.

Cochand, L., Isler, P., Songeon, F., and Nicod, L. P. (1999). Human lung dendritic cells have an immature phenotype with efficient mannose receptors. *Am. J. Respir. Cell Mol. Biol.* 21, 547–554.

Constant, S. L., Brogdon, J. L., Piggott, D. A., Herrick, C. A., Visintin, I., Ruddle, N. H., and Bottomly, K. (2002). Resident lung antigen-presenting cells have the capacity to promote Th2 T cell differentiation in situ. *J. Clin. Invest.* 110, 1441–1448.

Daniels, J. J., Autenrieth, I. B., Ludwig, A., and Goebel, W. (1996). The gene slyA of *Salmonella typhimurium* is required for destruction of M cells and intracellular survival but not for invasion or colonization of the murine small intestine. *Infect. Immun.* 64, 5075–5084.

de Baey, A., Mende, I., Riethmueller, G., and Baeuerle, P. A. (2001). Phenotype and function of human dendritic cells derived from M-DC8(+) monocytes. *Eur. J. Immunol.* 31, 1646–1655.

de Baey, A., Mende, I., Baretton, G., Greiner, A., Hartl, W. H., Baeuerle, P. A., and Diepolder, H. M. (2003). A subset of human dendritic cells in the T cell area of mucosa-associated lymphoid tissue with a high potential to produce TNF-alpha. *J. Immunol.* 170, 5089–5094.

del Hoyo, G. M., Martin, P., Vargas, H. H., Ruiz, S., Arias, C. F., and Ardavin, C. (2002). Characterization of a common precursor population for dendritic cells. *Nature* 415, 1043–1047.

Demangel, C., Bean, A. G., Martin, E., Feng, C. G., Kamath, A. T., and Britton, W. J. (1999). Protection against aerosol *Mycobacterium tuberculosis* infection using *Mycobacterium bovis* Bacillus Calmette Guerin-infected dendritic cells. *Eur. J. Immunol.* 29, 1972–1979.

Demeure, C. E., Tanaka, H., Mateo, V., Rubio, M., Delespesse, G., and Sarfati, M. (2000). CD47 engagement inhibits cytokine production and maturation of human dendritic cells. *J. Immunol.* 164, 2193–2199.

den Haan, J. M., Lehar, S. M., and Bevan, M. J. (2000). CD8(+) but not CD8(–) dendritic cells cross-prime cytotoxic T cells *in vivo*. *J. Exp. Med.* 192, 1685–1696.

DePaolo, R. W., Rollins, B. J., Kuziel, W., and Karpus, W. J. (2003). CC chemokine ligand 2 and its receptor regulate mucosal production of IL-12 and TGF-beta in high dose oral tolerance. *J. Immunol.* 171, 3560–3567.

Didierlaurent, A., Sirard, J. C., Kraehenbuhl, J. P., and Neutra, M. R. (2002). How the gut senses its content. *Cell Microbiol.* 4, 61–72.

Dieu, M. C., Vanbervliet, B., Vicari, A., Bridon, J. M., Oldham, E., Ait-Yahia, S., Briere, F., Zlotnik, A., Lebecque, S., and Caux, C. (1998). Selective recruitment of immature and mature dendritic cells by distinct chemokines expressed in different anatomic sites. *J. Exp. Med.* 188, 373–386.

Dodge, I. L., Carr, M. W., Cernadas, M., and Brenner, M. B. (2003). IL-6 production by pulmonary dendritic cells impedes Th1 immune responses. *J. Immunol.* 170, 4457–4464.

Doyen, V., Rubio, M., Braun, D., Nakajima, T., Abe, J., Saito, H., Delespesse, G., and Sarfati, M. (2003). Thrombospondin 1 is an autocrine negative regulator of human dendritic cell activation. *J. Exp. Med.* 198, 1277–1283.

Eaton, A. D., Xu, D., and Garside, P. (2003). Administration of exogenous interleukin-18 and interleukin-12 prevents the induction of oral tolerance. *Immunology* 108, 196–203.

Edwards, A. D., Manickasingham, S. P., Sporri, R., Diebold, S. S., Schulz, O., Sher, A., Kaisho, T., Akira, S., and Reis e Sousa, C. (2002). Microbial recognition via Toll-like receptor-dependent and -independent pathways determines the cytokine response of murine dendritic cell subsets to CD40 triggering. *J. Immunol.* 169, 3652–3660.

Ermak, T. H., Bhagat, H. R., and Pappo, J. (1994). Lymphocyte compartments in antigen-sampling regions of rabbit mucosal lymphoid organs. *Am. J. Trop. Med. Hyg.* 50, 14–28.

Everson, M. P., McDuffie, D. S., Lemak, D. G., Koopman, W. J., McGhee, J. R., and Beagley, K. W. (1996). Dendritic cells from different tissues induce production of different T cell cytokine profiles. *J. Leukoc. Biol.* 59, 494–498.

Everson, M. P., Lemak, D. G., McDuffie, D. S., Koopman, W. J., McGhee, J. R., and Beagley, K. W. (1998). Dendritic cells from Peyer's patch and spleen induce different T helper cell responses. *J. Interferon Cytokine Res.* 18, 103–115.

Fayette, J., Dubois, B., Vandenabeele, S., Bridon, J. M., Vanbervliet, B., Durand, I., Bancherau, J., Caux, C., and Briere, F. (1997). Human dendritic cells skew isotype switching of CD40-activated naive B cells towards IgA1 and IgA2. *J. Exp. Med.* 185, 1909–1918.

Fields, R. C., Schoenecker, J. G., Hart, J. P., Hoffman, M. R., Pizzo, S. V., and Lawson, J. H. (2003). Protease-activated receptor-2 signaling triggers dendritic cell development. *Am. J. Pathol.* 162, 1817–1822.

Fleeton, M. N., Contractor, N., Leon, F., Wetzel, J. D., Dermody, T. S., Kelsall, B. L. (2004). Peyer's patch dendritic cells process viral antigen from apoptotic epithelial cells in the intestine of reovirus-infected mice. *J. Exp. Med.* 200, 235–245.

Fokkens, W. J., Vroom, T. M., Rijntjes, E., and Mulder, P. G. (1989). Fluctuation of the number of CD-1(T6)-positive dendritic cells, presumably Langerhans cells, in the nasal mucosa of patients with an isolated grass-pollen allergy before, during, and after the grass-pollen season. *J. Allergy Clin. Immunol.* 84, 39–43.

Fort, M. M., Cheung, J., Yen, D., Li, J., Zurawski, S. M., Lo, S., Menon, S., Clifford, T., Hunte, B., Lesley, R., Muchamuel, T., Hurst, S. D., Zurawski, G., Leach, M. W., Gorman, D. M., and Rennick, D. M. (2001). IL-25 induces IL-4, IL-5, and IL-13 and Th2-associated pathologies *in vivo. Immunity* 15, 985–995.

Foster, B., Metcalfe, D. D., and Prussin, C. (2003). Human dendritic cell 1 and dendritic cell 2 subsets express FcepsilonRI: Correlation with serum IgE and allergic asthma. *J. Allergy Clin. Immunol.* 112, 1132–1138.

Furrie, E., Turner, M. W., and Strobel, S. (1995). Partial characterization of a circulating tolerogenic moiety which, after a feed of ovalbumin, suppresses delayed-type hypersensitivity in recipient mice. *Immunology* 86, 480–486.

Furukawa, T., Watanabe, S., Kodama, T., Sato, Y., Shimosato, Y., and Suemasu, K. (1985). T-zone histiocytes in adenocarcinoma of the lung in relation to postoperative prognosis. *Cancer* 56, 2651–2656.

Gagliardi, M. C., Sallusto, F., Marinaro, M., Langenkamp, A., Lanzavecchia, A., and De Magistris, M. T. (2000). Cholera toxin induces maturation of human dendritic cells and licenses them for Th2 priming. *Eur. J. Immunol.* 30, 2394–2403.

Geissmann, F., Launay, P., Pasquier, B., Lepelletier, Y., Leborgne, M., Lehuen, A., Brousse, N., and Monteiro, R. C. (2001). A subset of human dendritic cells expresses IgA Fc receptor (CD89), which mediates internalization and activation upon cross-linking by IgA complexes. *J. Immunol.* 166, 346–352.

George, A., and Cebra, J. J. (1991). Responses of single germinal-center B cells in T-cell-dependent microculture. *Proc. Natl. Acad. Sci. USA* 88, 11–15.

Gewirtz, A. T. (2003). Intestinal epithelial toll-like receptors: To protect. And serve? *Curr. Pharm. Des.* 9, 1–5.

Gilliet, M., Soumelis, V., Watanabe, N., Hanabuchi, S., Antonenko, S., de Waal-Malefyt, R., and Liu, Y. J. (2003). Human dendritic cells activated by TSLP and CD40L induce proallergic cytotoxic T cells. *J. Exp. Med.* 197, 1059–1063.

Godthelp, T., Fokkens, W. J., Kleinjan, A., Holm, A. F., Mulder, P. G., Prens, E. P., and Rijntes, E. (1996). Antigen presenting cells in the nasal mucosa of patients with allergic rhinitis during allergen provocation. *Clin. Exp. Allergy* 26, 677–688.

Golder, J. P., and Doe, W. F. (1983). Isolation and preliminary characterization of human intestinal macrophages. *Gastroenterology* 84, 795–802.

Gong, J. L., McCarthy, K. M., Rogers, R. A., and Schneeberger, E. E. (1994). Interstitial lung macrophages interact with dendritic cells to present antigenic peptides derived from particulate antigens to T cells. *Immunology* 81, 343–351.

Gonzalo, J. A., Tian, J., Delaney, T., Corcoran, J., Rottman, J. B., Lora, J., Al-garawi, A., Kroczek, R., Gutierrez-Ramos, J. C., and Coyle, A. J. (2001). ICOS is critical for T helper cell-mediated lung mucosal inflammatory responses. *Nat. Immunol.* 2, 597–604.

Gordon, S., Clarke, S., Greaves, D., and Doyle, A. (1995). Molecular immunobiology of macrophages: recent progress. *Curr. Opin. Immunol.* 7, 24–33.

Greaves, D. R., Wang, W., Dairaghi, D. J., Dieu, M. C., Saint-Vis, B., Franz-Bacon, K., Rossi, D., Caux, C., McClanahan, T., Gordon, S., Zlotnik, A. and Schall T. J. (1997). CCR6, a CC chemokine receptor that interacts with macrophage inflammatory protein 3alpha and is highly expressed in human dendritic cells. *J. Exp. Med.* 186, 837–844.

Grimm, M. C., Pavli, P., and Doe, W. F. (1995a). Evidence for a CD14+ population of monocytes in inflammatory bowel disease mucosa: Implications for pathogenesis. *Clin. Exp. Immunol.* 100, 291–297.

Grimm, M. C., Pullman, W. E., Benner, G. M., Sullivan, P. J., Pavli, P., and Doe, W. F. (1995b). Direct evidence of monocyte recruitment to inflammatory bowel disease mucosa. *J. Gastroenterol. Hepatol.* 10, 387–395.

Gunn, M. D., Kyuwa, S., Tam, C., Kakiuchi, T., Matsuzawa, A., Williams, L. T., and Nakano, H. (1999). Mice lacking expression of secondary lymphoid organ chemokine have defects in lymphocyte homing and dendritic cell localization. *J. Exp. Med.* 189, 451–460.

Gutgemann, I., Fahrer, A. M., Altman, J. D., Davis, M. M., and Chien, Y. H. (1998). Induction of rapid T cell activation and tolerance by systemic presentation of an orally administered antigen. *Immunity* 8, 667–673.

Hammad, H., Duez, C., Fahy, O., Tsicopoulos, A., Andre, C., Wallaert, B., Lebecque, S., Tonnel, A. B., and Pestel, J. (2000). Human dendritic cells in the severe combined immunodeficiency mouse model: Their potentiating role in the allergic reaction. *Lab. Invest.* 80, 605–614.

Hammad, H., Charbonnier, A. S., Duez, C., Jacquet, A., Stewart, G. A., Tonnel, A. B., and Pestel, J. (2001). Th2 polarization by Der p 1-pulsed monocyte-derived dendritic cells is due to the allergic status of the donors. *Blood* 98, 1135–1141.

Hammad, H., Lambrecht, B. N., Pochard, P., Gosset, P., Marquillies, P., Tonnel, A. B., and Pestel, J. (2002). Monocyte-derived dendritic cells induce a house dust mite-specific Th2 allergic inflammation in the lung of humanized SCID mice: Involvement of CCR7. *J. Immunol.* 169, 1524–1534.

Hammad, H., De Heer, H. J., Soullie, T., Angeli, V., Trottein, F., Hoogsteden, H. C., and Lambrecht, B. N. (2004). Activation of peroxisome proliferator-activated receptor-gamma in dendritic cells inhibits the development of eosinophilic airway inflammation in a mouse model of asthma. *Am. J. Pathol.* 164, 263–271.

Hausmann, M., Kiessling, S., Mestermann, S., Webb, G., Spöttl, T., Andus, T., Schölmerich, J., Herfarth, H., Ray, K., Falk, W., and Rogler, G. (2002). Toll-like receptors 2 and 4 are up-regulated during intestinal inflammation. *Gastroenterology* 122, 1987–2000.

Havenith, C. E., van Miert, P. P., Breedijk, A. J., Beelen, R. H., and Hoefsmit, E. C. (1993). Migration of dendritic cells into the draining lymph nodes of the lung after intratracheal instillation. *Am. J. Respir. Cell Mol. Biol.* 9, 484–488.

Hawiger, D., Inaba, K., Dorsett, Y., Guo, M., Mahnke, K., Rivera, M., Ravetch, J. V., Steinman, R. M., and Nussenzweig, M. C. (2001). Dendritic cells induce peripheral T cell unresponsiveness under steady state conditions in vivo. *J. Exp. Med.* 194, 769–779.

Herrick, C. A., MacLeod, H., Glusac, E., Tigelaar, R. E., and Bottomly, K. (2000). Th2 responses induced by epicutaneous or inhalational protein exposure are differentially dependent on IL-4. *J. Clin. Invest.* 105, 765–775.

Heystek, H. C., Moulon, C., Woltman, A. M., Garonne, P., and van Kooten, C. (2002). Human immature dendritic cells efficiently bind and take up secretory IgA without the induction of maturation. *J. Immunol.* 168, 102–107.

Hirao, M., Onai, N., Hiroishi, K., Watkins, S. C., Matsushima, K., Robbins, P. D., Lotze, M. T., and Tahara, H. (2000). CC chemokine receptor-7 on dendritic cells is induced after interaction with apoptotic tumor cells: Critical role in migration from the tumor site to draining lymph nodes. *Cancer Res.* 60, 2209–2217.

Holt, P. G. (2000). Antigen presentation in the lung. *Am. J. Respir. Crit. Care Med.* 162, S151–S156.

Holt, P. G., Schon-Hegrad, M. A., and Oliver, J. (1988). MHC class II antigen-bearing dendritic cells in pulmonary tissues of the rat: Regulation of antigen presentation activity by endogenous macrophage populations. *J. Exp. Med.* 167, 262–274.

Holt, P. G., Schon-Hegrad, M. A., Phillips, M. J., and McMenamin, P. G. (1989). Ia-positive dendritic cells form a tightly meshed network within the human airway epithelium. *Clin. Exp. Allergy* 19, 597–601.

Holt, P. G., Oliver, J., McMenamin, C., and Schon-Hegrad, M. A. (1992). Studies on the surface phenotype and functions of dendritic cells in parenchymal lung tissue of the rat. *Immunology* 75, 582–587.

Holt, P. G., Oliver, J., Bilyk, N., McMenamin, C., McMenamin, P. G., Kraal, G., and Thepen, T. (1993). Downregulation of the antigen presenting cell function(s) of pulmonary dendritic cells in vivo by resident alveolar macrophages. *J. Exp. Med.* 177, 397–407.

Holt, P. G., Haining, S., Nelson, D. J., and Sedgwick, J. D. (1994). Origin and steady-state turnover of class II MHC-bearing dendritic cells in the epithelium of the conducting airways. *J. Immunol.* 153, 256–261.

Holt, P. G., Macaubas, C., Stumbles, P. A., and Sly, P. D. (1999). The role of allergy in the development of asthma. *Nature* 402, B12–17.

Homey, B., Dieu-Nosjean, M. C., Wiesenborn, A., Massacrier, C., Pin, J. J., Oldham, E., Catron, D., Buchanan, M. E., Muller, A., deWaal Malefyt, R., Deng, G., Orozco, R., Ruzicka, T., Lehmann, P., Lebecque, S., Caux, C., and Zlotnik, A. (2000). Up-regulation of macrophage inflammatory protein-3 alpha/CCL20 and CC chemokine receptor 6 in psoriasis. *J. Immunol.* 164, 6621–6632.

Honda, K., Sakaguchi, S., Nakajima, C., Watanabe, A., Yanai, H., Matsumoto, M., Ohteki, T., Kaisho, T., Takaoka, A., Akira, S., Seya, T., and Taniguchi, T. (2003). Selective contribution of IFN-alpha/beta signaling to the maturation of dendritic cells induced by double-stranded RNA or viral infection. *Proc. Natl. Acad. Sci. USA* 100, 10872–10877.

Hopkins, S. A., and Kraehenbuhl, J. P. (1997). Dendritic cells of the murine Peyer's patches colocalize with *Salmonella typhimurium* avirulent mutants in the subepithelial dome. *Adv. Exp. Med. Biol.* 417, 105–109.

Hopkins, S. A., Niedergang, F., Corthesy-Theulaz, I. E., and Kraehenbuhl, J. P. (2000). A recombinant *Salmonella typhimurium* vaccine strain is taken up and survives within murine Peyer's patch dendritic cells. *Cell Microbiol.* 2, 59–68.

Huang, F. P., Platt, N., Wykes, M., Major, J. R., Powell, T. J., Jenkins, C. D., and MacPherson, G. G. (2000). A discrete subpopulation of dendritic cells transports apoptotic intestinal epithelial cells to T cell areas of mesenteric lymph nodes. *J. Exp. Med.* 191, 435–444.

Huh, J. C., Strickland, D. H., Jahnsen, F. L., Turner, D. J., Thomas, J. A., Napoli, S., Tobagus, I., Stumbles, P. A., Sly, P. D., and Holt, P. G. (2003). Bidirectional interactions between antigen-bearing respiratory tract dendritic cells (DCs) and T cells precede the late phase reaction in experimental asthma: DC activation occurs in the airway mucosa but not in the lung parenchyma. *J. Exp. Med.* 198, 19–30.

Hume, D. A., Perry, V. H., and Gordon, S. (1984). The mononuclear phagocyte system of the mouse defined by immunohistochemical localisation of antigen F4/80: Macrophages associated with epithelia. *Anat. Rec.* 210, 503–512.

Hurst, S. D., Muchamuel, T., Gorman, D. M., Gilbert, J. M., Clifford, T., Kwan, S., Menon, S., Seymour, B., Jackson, C., Kung, T. T., Brieland, J. K., Zurawski, S. M., Chapman, R. W., Zurawski, G., and Coffman, R. L. (2002). New IL-17 family members promote Th1 or Th2 responses in the lung: *In vivo* function of the novel cytokine IL-25. *J. Immunol.* 169, 443–453.

Ikeda, Y., Akbar, F., Matsui, H., and Onji, M. (2001). Characterization of antigen-presenting dendritic cells in the peripheral blood and colonic mucosa of patients with ulcerative colitis. *Eur. J. Gastroenterol. Hepatol.* 13, 841–850.

Israel, E. J., Taylor, S., Wu, Z., Mizoguchi, E., Blumberg, R. S., Bhan, A., and Simister, N. E. (1997). Expression of the neonatal Fc receptor, FcRn, on human intestinal epithelial cells. *Immunology* 92, 69–74.

Iwasaki, A. (2003). The role of dendritic cells in immune responses against vaginal infection by herpes simplex virus type 2. *Microbes Infect.* 5, 1221–1230.

Iwasaki, A., and Kelsall, B. L. (1999). Freshly isolated Peyer's patch, but not spleen, dendritic cells produce interleukin 10 and induce the differentiation of T helper type 2 cells. *J. Exp. Med.* 190, 229–239.

Iwasaki, A., and Kelsall, B. L. (2000). Localization of distinct Peyer's patch dendritic cell subsets and their recruitment by chemokines macrophage inflammatory protein (MIP)-3alpha, MIP-3beta, and secondary lymphoid organ chemokine. *J. Exp. Med.* 191, 1381–1394.

Iwasaki, A., and Kelsall, B. L. (2001). Unique functions of CD11b+, CD8 alpha+, and double-negative Peyer's patch dendritic cells. *J. Immunol.* 166, 4884–4890.

Iyoda, T., Shimoyama, S., Liu, K., Omatsu, Y., Akiyama, Y., Maeda, Y., Takahara, K., Steinman, R. M., and Inaba, K. (2002). The CD8+ dendritic cell subset selectively endocytoses dying cells in culture and *in vivo*. *J. Exp. Med.* 195, 1289–1302.

Izadpanah, A., Dwinell, M. B., Eckmann, L., Varki, N. M., and Kagnoff, M. F. (2001). Regulated MIP-3alpha/CCL20 production by human intestinal epithelium: Mechanism for modulating mucosal immunity. *Am. J. Physiol. Gastrointest. Liver Physiol.* 280, G710–719.

Jahnsen, F. L., Lund-Johansen, F., Dunne, J. F., Farkas, L., Haye, R., and Brandtzaeg, P. (2000). Experimentally induced recruitment of plasmacytoid (CD123high) dendritic cells in human nasal allergy. *J. Immunol.* 165, 4062–4068.

Jahnsen, F. L., Moloney, E. D., Hogan, T., Upham, J. W., Burke, C. M., and Holt, P. G. (2001). Rapid dendritic cell recruitment to the bronchial mucosa of patients with atopic asthma in response to local allergen challenge. *Thorax* 56, 823–826.

Jameson, B., Baribaud, F., Pohlmann, S., Ghavimi, D., Mortari, F., Doms, R. W., and Iwasaki, A. (2002). Expression of DC-SIGN by dendritic cells of intestinal and genital mucosae in humans and rhesus macaques. *J. Virol.* 76, 1866–1875.

Jember, A. G., Zuberi, R., Liu, F. T., and Croft, M. (2001). Development of allergic inflammation in a murine model of asthma is dependent on the costimulatory receptor OX40. *J. Exp. Med.* 193, 387–392.

Jensen, V. B., Harty, J. T., and Jones, B. D. (1998). Interactions of the invasive pathogens *Salmonella typhimurium*, *Listeria monocytogenes*, and *Shigella flexneri* with M cells and murine Peyer's patches. *Infect. Immun.* 66, 3758–3766.

Johansson-Lindbom, B., Svensson, M., Wurbel, M. A., Malissen, B., Marquez, G., and Agace, W. (2003). Selective generation of gut tropic T cells in gut-associated lymphoid tissue (GALT): requirement for GALT dendritic cells and adjuvant. *J. Exp. Med.* 198, 963–969.

Jotwani, R., Palucka, A. K., Al-Quotub, M., Nouri-Shirazi, M., Kim, J., Bell, D., Banchereau, J., and Cutler, C. W. (2001). Mature dendritic cells infiltrate the T cell-rich region of oral mucosa in chronic periodontitis: *In situ, in vivo*, and *in vitro* studies. *J. Immunol.* 167, 4693–4700.

Julia, V., Hessel, E. M., Malherbe, L., Glaichenhaus, N., O'Garra, A., and Coffman, R. L. (2002). A restricted subset of dendritic cells captures airborne antigens and remains able to activate specific T cells long after antigen exposure. *Immunity* 16, 271–283.

Kagnoff, M. F., and Eckmann, L. (1997). Epithelial cells as sensors for microbial infection. *J. Clin. Invest.* 100, 6–10.

Kaisho, T., and Akira, S. (2003). Regulation of dendritic cell function through toll-like receptors. *Curr. Mol. Med.* 3, 759–771.

Kalinski, P., Hilkens, C. M., Snijders, A., Snijdewint, F. G., and Kapsenberg, M. L. (1997). IL-12-deficient dendritic cells, generated in the presence of prostaglandin E2, promote type 2 cytokine production in maturing human naive T helper cells. *J. Immunol.* 159, 28–35.

Kalinski, P., Hilkens, C. M., Wierenga, E. A., and Kapsenberg, M. L. (1999). T-cell priming by type-1 and type-2 polarized dendritic cells: The concept of a third signal. *Immunol. Today* 20, 561–567.

Kamath, A. T., Henri, S., Battye, F., Tough, D. F., and Shortman, K. (2002). Developmental kinetics and lifespan of dendritic cells in mouse lymphoid organs. *Blood* 100, 1734–1741.

Kapsenberg, M. L. (2003). Dendritic-cell control of pathogen-driven T-cell polarization. *Nat. Rev. Immunol.* 3, 984–993.

Kelsall, B. L., and Strober, W. (1996). Distinct populations of dendritic cells are present in the subepithelial dome and T cell regions of the murine Peyer's patch. *J. Exp. Med.* 183, 237–247.

Kim, J. M., Eckmann, L., Savidge, T. C., Lowe, D. C., Witthoft, T., and Kagnoff, M. F. (1998). Apoptosis of human intestinal epithelial cells after bacterial invasion. *J. Clin. Invest.* 102, 1815–1823.

Kline, J. N., Waldschmidt, T. J., Businga, T. R., Lemish, J. E., Weinstock, J. V., Thorne, P. S., and Krieg, A. M. (1998). Modulation of airway inflammation by CpG oligodeoxynucleotides in a murine model of asthma. *J. Immunol.* 160, 2555–2559.

Kobets, N., Kennedy, K., and Garside, P. (2003). An investigation of the distribution of antigen fed in tolerogenic or immunogenic forms. *Immunol. Lett.* 88, 147–155.

Kosco-Vilbois, M. H. (2003). Are follicular dendritic cells really good for nothing? *Nat. Rev. Immunol.* 3, 764–769.

Kradin, R. L., Xia, W., Pike, M., Byers, H. R., and Pinto, C. (1996). Interleukin-2 promotes the motility of dendritic cells and their accumulation in lung and skin. *Pathobiology* 64, 180–186.

Kradin, R., MacLean, J., Duckett, S., Schneeberger, E. E., Waeber, C., and Pinto, C. (1997). Pulmonary response to inhaled antigen: neuroimmune interactions promote the recruitment of dendritic cells to the lung and the cellular immune response to inhaled antigen. *Am. J. Pathol.* 150, 1735–1743.

Kraehenbuhl, J. P., and Neutra, M. R. (2000). Epithelial M cells: differentiation and function. *Annu. Rev. Cell Dev. Biol.* 16, 301–332.

Krajina, T., Leithauser, F., Moller, P., Trobonjaca, Z., and Reimann, J. (2003). Colonic lamina propria dendritic cells in mice with CD4+ T cell-induced colitis. *Eur. J. Immunol.* 33, 1073–1083.

Kunkel, E. J., Campbell, D. J., and Butcher, E. C. (2003). Chemokines in lymphocyte trafficking and intestinal immunity. *Microcirculation* 10, 313–323.

Kuperman, D. A., Huang, X., Koth, L. L., Chang, G. H., Dolganov, G. M., Zhu, Z., Elias, J. A., Sheppard, D., and Erle, D. J. (2002). Direct effects of interleukin-13 on epithelial cells cause airway hyperreactivity and mucus overproduction in asthma. *Nat. Med.* 8, 885–889.

Kweon, M. N., Fujihashi, K., Wakatsuki, Y., Koga, T., Yamamoto, M., McGhee, J. R., and Kiyono, H. (1999). Mucosally induced systemic T cell unresponsiveness to ovalbumin requires CD40 ligand-CD40 interactions. *J. Immunol.* 162, 1904–1909.

Kwon, J. H., Keates, S., Bassani, L., Mayer, L. F., and Keates, A. C. (2002). Colonic epithelial cells are a major site of macrophage inflammatory protein 3alpha (MIP-3alpha) production in normal colon and inflammatory bowel disease. *Gut* 51, 818–826.

Kwon, J. H., Keates, S., Simeonidis, S., Grall, F., Libermann, T. A., and Keates, A. C. (2003). ESE-1, an enterocyte-specific Ets transcription factor, regulates MIP-3alpha gene expression in Caco-2 human colonic epithelial cells. *J. Biol. Chem.* 278, 875–884.

Lagranderie, M., Nahori, M. A., Balazuc, A. M., Kiefer-Biasizzo, H., Lapa e Silva, J. R., Milon, G., Marchal, G., and Vargaftig, B. B. (2003). Dendritic cells recruited to the lung shortly after intranasal delivery of *Mycobacterium bovis* BCG drive the primary immune response towards a type 1 cytokine production. *Immunology* 108, 352–364.

Lambrecht, B. N. (2001). Allergen uptake and presentation by dendritic cells. *Curr. Opin. Allergy Clin. Immunol.* 1, 51–59.

Lambrecht, B. N., and Hammad, H. (2003a). The other cells in asthma: dendritic cell and epithelial cell crosstalk. *Curr. Opin. Pulm. Med.* 9, 34–41.

Lambrecht, B. N., and Hammad, H. (2003b). Taking our breath away: Dendritic cells in the pathogenesis of asthma. *Nat. Rev. Immunol.* 3, 994–1003.

Lambrecht, B. N., Salomon, B., Klatzmann, D., and Pauwels, R. A. (1998). Dendritic cells are required for the development of chronic eosinophilic airway inflammation in response to inhaled antigen in sensitized mice. *J. Immunol.* 160, 4090–4097.

Lambrecht, B. N., De Veerman, M., Coyle, A. J., Gutierrez-Ramos, J. C., Thielemans, K., and Pauwels, R. A. (2000a). Myeloid dendritic cells induce Th2 responses to inhaled antigen, leading to eosinophilic airway inflammation. *J. Clin. Invest.* 106, 551–559.

Lambrecht, B. N., Pauwels, R. A., and Fazekas De St Groth, B. (2000b). Induction of rapid T cell activation, division, and recirculation by intratracheal injection of dendritic cells in a TCR transgenic model. *J. Immunol.* 164, 2937–2946.

Lambrecht, B. N., Prins, J. B., and Hoogsteden, H. C. (2001). Lung dendritic cells and host immunity to infection. *Eur. Respir. J.* 18, 692–704.

Larsson, M., Fonteneau, J. F., and Bhardwaj, N. (2003). Cross-presentation of cell-associated antigens by dendritic cells. *Curr. Top. Microbiol. Immunol.* 276, 261–275.

Latour, S., Tanaka, H., Demeure, C., Mateo, V., Rubio, M., Brown, E. J., Maliszewski, C., Lindberg, F. P., Oldenborg, A., Ullrich, A., Delespesse G, and Sarfati M. (2001). Bidirectional negative regulation of human T and dendritic cells by CD47 and its cognate receptor signal-regulator protein-alpha: down-regulation of IL-12 responsiveness and inhibition of dendritic cell activation. *J. Immunol.* 167, 2547–2554.

Lee, S. H., Starkey, P. M., and Gordon, S. (1985). Quantitative analysis of total macrophage content in adult mouse tissues: Immunochemical studies with monoclonal antibody F4/80. *J. Exp. Med.* 161, 475–489.

Leenen, P. J., Radosevic, K., Voerman, J. S., Salomon, B., van Rooijen, N., Klatzmann, D., and van Ewijk, W. (1998). Heterogeneity of mouse spleen dendritic cells: *In vivo* phagocytic activity, expression of macrophage markers, and subpopulation turnover. *J. Immunol.* 160, 2166–2173.

Legge, K. L., and Braciale, T. J. (2003). Accelerated migration of respiratory dendritic cells to the regional lymph nodes is limited to the early phase of pulmonary infection. *Immunity* 18, 265–277.

Leithauser, F., Trobonjaca, Z., Moller, P., and Reimann, J. (2001). Clustering of colonic lamina propria CD4(+) T cells to subepithelial dendritic cell aggregates precedes the development of colitis in a murine adoptive transfer model. *Lab. Invest.* 81, 1339–1349.

Leon, B., Martinez Del Hoyo, G., Parrillas, V., Hernandez Vargas, H., Sanchez-Mateos, P., Longo, N., Lopez-Bravo, M., and Ardavin, C. (2003). Dendritic cell differentiation potential of mouse monocytes: Monocytes represent immediate precursors of CD8− and CD8+ splenic dendritic cells. *Blood* 100, 383–390.

Liu, L. M., and MacPherson, G. G. (1991). Lymph-borne (veiled) dendritic cells can acquire and present intestinally administered antigens. *Immunology* 73, 281–286.

Liu, L. M., and MacPherson, G. G. (1993). Antigen acquisition by dendritic cells: intestinal dendritic cells acquire antigen administered orally and can prime naive T cells *in vivo*. *J. Exp. Med.* 177, 1299–1307.

Liu, L. M., and MacPherson, G. G. (1995). Rat intestinal dendritic cells: immunostimulatory potency and phenotypic characterization. *Immunology* 85, 88–93.

Liu, Z., Colpaert, S., D'Haens, G. R., Kasran, A., de Boer, M., Rutgeerts, P., Geboes, K., and Ceuppens, J. L. (1999). Hyperexpression of CD40 ligand (CD154) in inflammatory bowel disease and its contribution to pathogenic cytokine production. *J. Immunol.* 163, 4049–4057.

Liu, K., Iyoda, T., Saternus, M., Kimura, Y., Inaba, K., and Steinman, R. M. (2002). Immune tolerance after delivery of dying cells to dendritic cells *in situ*. *J. Exp. Med.* 196, 1091–1097.

MacDonald, T. T. (2003). The mucosal immune system. *Parasite Immunol.* 25, 235–246.

MacPherson, G. G. (1989). Properties of lymph-borne (veiled) dendritic cells in culture. I. Modulation of phenotype, survival and function: partial dependence on GM-CSF. *Immunology* 68, 102–107.

MacPherson, G. G., Jenkins, C. D., Stein, M. J., and Edwards, C. (1995). Endotoxin-mediated dendritic cell release from the intestine: Characterization of released dendritic cells and TNF dependence. *J. Immunol.* 154, 1317–1322.

Mahida, Y. R., Patel, S., Gionchetti, P., Vaux, D., and Jewell, D. P. (1989a). Macrophage subpopulations in lamina propria of normal and inflamed colon and terminal ileum. *Gut* 30, 826–834.

Mahida, Y. R., Patel, S., and Jewell, D. P. (1989b). Mononuclear phagocyte system of human Peyer's patches: An immunohistochemical study using monoclonal antibodies. *Clin. Exp. Immunol.* 75, 82–86.

Maiuri, L., Ciacci, C., Auricchio, S., Brown, V., Quaratino, S., and Londei, M. (2000). Interleukin 15 mediates epithelial changes in celiac disease. *Gastroenterology* 119, 996–1006.

Maldonado-Lopez, R., De Smedt, T., Michel, P., Godfroid, J., Pajak, B., Heirman, C., Thielemans, K., Leo, O., Urbain, J., and Moser, M. (1999). CD8alpha+ and CD8alpha− subclasses of dendritic cells direct the development of distinct T helper cells *in vivo*. *J. Exp. Med.* 189, 587–592.

Maldonado-Lopez, R., Maliszewski, C., Urbain, J., and Moser, M. (2001). Cytokines regulate the capacity of CD8alpha(+) and

CD8alpha(−) dendritic cells to prime Th1/Th2 cells *in vivo*. *J. Immunol.* 167, 4345–4350.

Malmstrom, V., Shipton, D., Singh, B., Al-Shamkhani, A., Puklavec, M. J., Barclay, A. N., and Powrie, F. (2001). CD134L expression on dendritic cells in the mesenteric lymph nodes drives colitis in T cell-restored SCID mice. *J. Immunol.* 166, 6972–6981.

Manickasingham, S. P., Edwards, A. D., Schulz, O., and Reis e Sousa, C. (2003). The ability of murine dendritic cell subsets to direct T helper cell differentiation is dependent on microbial signals. *Eur. J. Immunol.* 33, 101–107.

Maric, I., Holt, P. G., Perdue, M. H., and Bienenstock, J. (1996). Class II MHC antigen (Ia)-bearing dendritic cells in the epithelium of the rat intestine. *J. Immunol.* 156, 1408–1414.

Marth, T., Strober, W., and Kelsall, B. L. (1996). High dose oral tolerance in ovalbumin TCR-transgenic mice: Systemic neutralization of IL-12 augments TGF-beta secretion and T cell apoptosis. *J. Immunol.* 157, 2348–2357.

Marth, T., Zeitz, M., Ludviksson, B. R., Strober, W., and Kelsall, B. L. (1999). Extinction of IL-12 signaling promotes Fas-mediated apoptosis of antigen-specific T cells. *J. Immunol.* 162, 7233–7240.

Martin, M., Schifferle, R. E., Cuesta, N., Vogel, S. N., Katz, J., and Michalek, S. M. (2003). Role of the phosphatidylinositol 3 kinase-Akt pathway in the regulation of IL-10 and IL-12 by *Porphyromonas gingivalis* lipopolysaccharide. *J. Immunol.* 171, 717–725.

Martin, P., Del Hoyo, G. M., Anjuere, F., Arias, C. F., Vargas, H. H., Fernandez, L. A., Parrillas, V., and Ardavin, C. (2002). Characterization of a new subpopulation of mouse CD8alpha⁺ B220⁺ dendritic cells endowed with type 1 interferon production capacity and tolerogenic potential. *Blood* 100, 383–390.

Martinez-Pomares, L., Platt, N., McKnight, A. J., da Silva, R. P., and Gordon, S. (1996). Macrophage membrane molecules: Markers of tissue differentiation and heterogeneity. *Immunobiology* 195, 407–416.

Matsuda, H., Suda, T., Hashizume, H., Yokomura, K., Asada, K., Suzuki, K., Chida, K., and Nakamura, H. (2002). Alteration of balance between myeloid dendritic cells and plasmacytoid dendritic cells in peripheral blood of patients with asthma. *Am. J. Respir. Crit. Care Med.* 166, 1050–1054.

Maurer, D., Fiebiger, E., Reininger, B., Ebner, C., Petzelbauer, P., Shi, G. P., Chapman, H. A., and Stingl, G. (1998). Fc epsilon receptor I on dendritic cells delivers IgE-bound multivalent antigens into a cathepsin S-dependent pathway of MHC class II presentation. *J. Immunol.* 161, 2731–2739.

Mayrhofer, G., Pugh, C. W., and Barclay, A. N. (1983). The distribution, ontogeny and origin in the rat of Ia-positive cells with dendritic morphology and of Ia antigen in epithelia, with special reference to the intestine. *Eur. J. Immunol.* 13, 112–122.

Mazzoni, A., and Segal, D. M. (2004). Controlling the Toll road to dendritic cell polarization. *J. Leukoc. Biol.* 75, 721–730.

Mazzoni, A., Young, H. A., Spitzer, J. H., Visintin, A., and Segal, D. M. (2001). Histamine regulates cytokine production in maturing dendritic cells, resulting in altered T cell polarization. *J. Clin. Invest.* 108, 1865–1873.

McGuirk, P., McCann, C., and Mills, K. H. (2002). Pathogen-specific T regulatory 1 cells induced in the respiratory tract by a bacterial molecule that stimulates interleukin 10 production by dendritic cells: A novel strategy for evasion of protective T helper type 1 responses by *Bordetella pertussis*. *J. Exp. Med.* 195, 221–231.

McKercher, S. R., Torbett, B. E., Anderson, K. L., Henkel, G. W., Vestal, D., Baribault, H., Klemsz, M., Feeney, A. J., Wu, G. E., Paige, C. J., and Maki, R. A. (1996). Targeted disruption of the PU.1 gene results in multiple hematopoietic abnormalities. *EMBO J.* 15, 5647–5658.

McMenamin, C., and Holt, P. G. (1993). The natural immune response to inhaled soluble protein antigens involves major histocompatibility complex (MHC) class I-restricted CD8⁺ T cell-mediated but MHC class II-restricted CD4⁺ T cell-dependent immune deviation resulting in selective suppression of immunoglobulin E production. *J. Exp. Med.* 178, 889–899.

McWilliam, A. S., Nelson, D., Thomas, J. A., and Holt, P. G. (1994). Rapid dendritic cell recruitment is a hallmark of the acute inflammatory response at mucosal surfaces. *J. Exp. Med.* 179, 1331–1336.

McWilliam, A. S., Marsh, A. M., and Holt, P. G. (1997). Inflammatory infiltration of the upper airway epithelium during Sendai virus infection: Involvement of epithelial dendritic cells. *J. Virol.* 71, 226–236.

Mention, J. J., Ben Ahmed, M., Begue, B., Barbe, U., Verkarre, V., Asnafi, V., Colombel, J. F., Cugnenc, P. H., Ruemmele, F. M., McIntyre, E., Brousse, N., Cellier, C., Cerf-Bensussan, N. (2003). Interleukin 15: A key to disrupted intraepithelial lymphocyte homeostasis and lymphomagenesis in celiac disease. *Gastroenterology* 125, 730–745.

Mimura, T., Rizzello, F., Helwig, U., Poggioli, G., Schreiber, S., Talbot, I. C., Nicholls, R. J., Gionchetti, P., Campieri, M., and Kamm, M. A. (2004). Once daily high dose probiotic therapy (VSL#3) for maintaining remission in recurrent or refractory pouchitis. *Gut* 53, 108–114.

Moghaddami, M., Cummins, A., and Mayrhofer, G. (1998). Lymphocyte-filled villi: comparison with other lymphoid aggregations in the mucosa of the human small intestine. *Gastroenterology* 115, 1414–1425.

Moller, G. M., Overbeek, S. E., Van Helden-Meeuwsen, C. G., Van Haarst, J. M., Prens, E. P., Mulder, P. G., Postma, D. S., and Hoogsteden, H. C. (1996). Increased numbers of dendritic cells in the bronchial mucosa of atopic asthmatic patients: Downregulation by inhaled corticosteroids. *Clin. Exp. Allergy* 26, 517–524.

Mora, J. R., Bono, M. R., Manjunath, N., Weninger, W., Cavanagh, L. L., Rosemblatt, M., and Von Andrian, U. H. (2003). Selective imprinting of gut-homing T cells by Peyer's patch dendritic cells. *Nature* 424, 88–93.

Morahan, G., Huang, D., Wu, M., Holt, B. J., White, G. P., Kendall, G. E., Sly, P. D., and Holt, P. G. (2002). Association of IL12B promoter polymorphism with severity of atopic and non-atopic asthma in children. *Lancet* 360, 455–459.

Moser, M. (2003). Dendritic cells in immunity and tolerance: Do they display opposite functions? *Immunity* 19, 5–8.

Mowat, A. M. (2003). Anatomical basis of tolerance and immunity to intestinal antigens. *Nat. Rev. Immunol.* 3, 331–341.

Murakami, H., Akbar, S. M., Matsui, H., Horiike, N., and Onji, M. (2002). Macrophage migration inhibitory factor activates antigen-presenting dendritic cells and induces inflammatory cytokines in ulcerative colitis. *Clin. Exp. Immunol.* 128, 504–510.

Nagura, H., Ohtani, H., Masuda, T., Kimura, M., and Nakamura, S. (1991). HLA-DR expression on M cells overlying Peyer's patches is a common feature of human small intestine. *Acta Pathol. Jpn.* 41, 818–823.

Nakano, H., Yanagita, M., and Gunn, M. D. (2001). CD11c(+)B220(+)Gr-1(+) cells in mouse lymph nodes and spleen display characteristics of plasmacytoid dendritic cells. *J. Exp. Med.* 194, 1171–1178.

Nelson, D. J., McMenamin, C., McWilliam, A. S., Brenan, M., and Holt, P. G. (1994). Development of the airway intraepithelial dendritic cell network in the rat from class II major histocompatibility (Ia)-negative precursors: differential regulation of Ia expression at different levels of the respiratory tract. *J. Exp. Med.* 179, 203–212.

Neutra, M. R., and Kraehenbuhl, J. P. (1993). The role of transepithelial transport by M cells in microbial invasion and host defense. *J. Cell Sci. (Suppl.)* 17, 209–215.

Newberry, R. D., Stenson, W. F., and Lorenz, R. G. (1999). Cyclooxygenase-2-dependent arachidonic acid metabolites are essential modulators of the intestinal immune response to dietary antigen. *Nat. Med.* 5, 900–906.

Newberry, R. D., McDonough, J. S., Stenson, W. F., and Lorenz, R. G. (2001). Spontaneous and continuous cyclooxygenase-2-dependent prostaglandin E2 production by stromal cells in the murine small intestine lamina propria: Directing the tone of the intestinal immune response. *J. Immunol.* 166, 4465–4472.

Ninomiya, T., Matsui, H., Akbar, S. M., Murakami, H., and Onji, M. (2000). Localization and characterization of antigen-presenting dendritic cells in the gastric mucosa of murine and human autoimmune gastritis. *Eur. J. Clin. Invest.* 30, 350–358.

Noirey, N., Rougier, N., Andre, C., Schmitt, D., and Vincent, C. (2000). Langerhans-like dendritic cells generated from cord blood progenitors internalize pollen allergens by macropinocytosis, and part of the molecules are processed and can activate autologous naive T lymphocytes. *J. Allergy Clin. Immunol.* 105, 1194–1201.

Novak, N., Allam, J. P., Betten, H., Haberstok, J., and Bieber, T. (2004). The role of antigen presenting cells at distinct anatomic sites: They accelerate and they slow down allergies. *Allergy* 59, 5–14.

O'Keeffe, M., Hochrein, H., Vremec, D., Caminschi, I., Miller, J. L., Anders, E. M., Wu, L., Lahoud, M. H., Henri, S., Scott, B., Hertzog, P., Tatarczuch, L., and Shortman, K. (2002). Mouse plasmacytoid cells: Long-lived cells, heterogeneous in surface phenotype and function, that differentiate into CD8(+) dendritic cells only after microbial stimulus. *J. Exp. Med.* 196, 1307–1319.

O'Keeffe, M., Hochrein, H., Vremec, D., Scott, B., Hertzog, P., Tatarczuch, L., and Shortman, K. (2003). Dendritic cell precursor populations of mouse blood: identification of the murine homologues of human blood plasmacytoid pre-DC2 and CD11c⁺ DC1 precursors. *Blood* 101, 1453–1459.

Oshitani, N., Sawa, Y., Hara, J., Adachi, K., Nakamura, S., Matsumoto, T., Arakawa, T., and Kuroki, T. (1997). Functional and phenotypical activation of leucocytes in inflamed human colonic mucosa. *J. Gastroenterol. Hepatol.* 12, 809–814.

Oshitani, N., Kitano, A., Kakazu, Y., Hara, J., Adachi, K., Nakamura, S., Matsumoto, T., and Kobayashi, K. (1998). Functional diversity of infiltrating macrophages in inflamed human colonic mucosa ulcerative colitis. *Clin. Exp. Pharmacol. Physiol.* 25, 50–53.

Owen, R. L. (1977). Sequential uptake of horseradish peroxidase by lymphoid follicle epithelium of Peyer's patches in the normal unobstructed mouse intestine: An ultrastructural study. *Gastroenterology* 72, 440–451.

Ozaki, Y., Amakawa, R., Ito, T., Iwai, H., Tajima, K., Uehira, K., Kagawa, H., Uemura, Y., Yamashita, T., and Fukuhara, S. (2001). Alteration of peripheral blood dendritic cells in patients with primary Sjogren's syndrome. *Arthritis Rheum.* 44, 419–431.

Papadakis, K. A. (2004). Chemokines in inflammatory bowel disease. *Curr. Allergy Asthma Rep.* 4, 83–89.

Pappo, J., and Mahlman, R. T. (1993). Follicle epithelial M cells are a source of interleukin-1 in Peyer's patches. *Immunology* 78, 505–507.

Parronchi, P., Romagnani, P., Annunziato, F., Sampognaro, S., Becchio, A., Giannarini, L., Maggi, E., Pupilli, C., Tonelli, F., and Romagnani, S. (1997). Type 1 T-helper cell predominance and interleukin-12 expression in the gut of patients with Crohn's disease. *Am. J. Pathol.* 150, 823–832.

Pasare, C., and Medzhitov, R. (2003). Toll-like receptors: Balancing host resistance with immune tolerance. *Curr. Opin. Immunol.* 15, 677–682.

Pavli, P., Woodhams, C. E., Doe, W. F., and Hume, D. A. (1990). Isolation and characterization of antigen-presenting dendritic cells from the mouse intestinal lamina propria. *Immunology* 70, 40–47.

Pavli, P., Hume, D. A., Van De Pol, E., and Doe, W. F. (1993). Dendritic cells, the major antigen-presenting cells of the human colonic lamina propria. *Immunology* 78, 132–141.

Pearce, E. J., Caspar, P., Grzych, J. M., Lewis, F. A., and Sher, A. (1991). Downregulation of Th1 cytokine production accompanies induction of Th2 responses by a parasitic helminth, *Schistosoma mansoni. J. Exp. Med.* 173, 159–166.

Podolsky, D. K. (2002). Inflammatory bowel disease. *N. Engl. J. Med.* 347, 417–429.

Power, C. A., Church, D. J., Meyer, A., Alouani, S., Proudfoot, A. E., Clark-Lewis, I., Sozzani, S., Mantovani, A., and Wells, T. N. (1997). Cloning and characterization of a specific receptor for the novel CC chemokine MIP-3alpha from lung dendritic cells. *J. Exp. Med.* 186, 825–835.

Powrie, F., Correa-Oliveira, R., Mauze, S., and Coffman, R. L. (1994). Regulatory interactions between CD45RBhigh and CD45RBlow CD4⁺ T cells are important for the balance between protective and pathogenic cell-mediated immunity. *J. Exp. Med.* 179, 589–600.

Pron, B., Boumaila, C., Jaubert, F., Berche, P., Milon, G., Geissmann, F., and Gaillard, J. L. (2001). Dendritic cells are early cellular targets of *Listeria monocytogenes* after intestinal delivery and are involved in bacterial spread in the host. *Cell Microbiol.* 3, 331–340.

Pugh, C. W., MacPherson, G. G., and Steer, H. W. (1983). Characterization of nonlymphoid cells derived from rat peripheral lymph. *J. Exp. Med.* 157, 1758–1779.

Pulendran, B., Smith, J. L., Caspary, G., Brasel, K., Pettit, D., Maraskovsky, E., and Maliszewski, C. R. (1999). Distinct dendritic cell subsets differentially regulate the class of immune response *in vivo. Proc. Natl. Acad. Sci. USA* 96, 1036–1041.

Pulendran, B., Kumar, P., Cutler, C. W., Mohamadzadeh, M., Van Dyke, T., and Banchereau, J. (2001). Lipopolysaccharides from distinct pathogens induce different classes of immune responses *in vivo. J. Immunol.* 167, 5067–5076.

Randolph, G. J., Beaulieu, S., Lebecque, S., Steinman, R. M., and Muller, W. A. (1998). Differentiation of monocytes into dendritic cells in a model of transendothelial trafficking. *Science* 282, 480–483.

Randolph, G. J., Inaba, K., Robbiani, D. F., Steinman, R. M., and Muller, W. A. (1999). Differentiation of phagocytic monocytes into lymph node dendritic cells *in vivo. Immunity* 11, 753–761.

Randolph, G. J., Sanchez-Schmitz, G., Liebman, R. M., and Schakel, K. (2002). The CD16(+) (FcgammaRIII(+)) subset of human monocytes preferentially becomes migratory dendritic cells in a model tissue setting. *J. Exp. Med.* 196, 517–527.

Reibman, J., Hsu, Y., Chen, L. C., Bleck, B., and Gordon, T. (2003). Airway epithelial cells release MIP-3alpha/CCL20 in response to cytokines and ambient particulate matter. *Am. J. Respir. Cell Mol. Biol.* 28, 648–654.

Reider, N., Reider, D., Ebner, S., Holzmann, S., Herold, M., Fritsch, P., and Romani, N. (2002). Dendritic cells contribute to the development of atopy by an insufficiency in IL-12 production. *J. Allergy Clin. Immunol.* 109, 89–95.

Reinhardt, R. L., Khoruts, A., Merica, R., Zell, T., and Jenkins, M. K. (2001). Visualizing the generation of memory CD4 T cells in the whole body. *Nature* 410, 1–105.

Reinhardt, R. L., Bullard, D. C., Weaver, C. T., and Jenkins, M. K. (2003). Preferential accumulation of antigen-specific effector CD4 T cells at an antigen injection site involves CD62E-dependent migration but not local proliferation. *J. Exp. Med.* 197, 751–762.

Reis e Sousa, C., Diebold, S. D., Edwards, A. D., Rogers, N., Schulz, O., and Sporri, R. (2003). Regulation of dendritic cell function by microbial stimuli. *Pathol. Biol. (Paris)* 51, 67–68.

Rescigno, M. (2002). Dendritic cells and the complexity of microbial infection. *Trends Microbiol.* 10, 425–461.

Rescigno, M., Rotta, G., Valzasina, B., and Ricciardi-Castagnoli, P. (2001a). Dendritic cells shuttle microbes across gut epithelial monolayers. *Immunobiology* 204, 572–581.

Rescigno, M., Urbano, M., Valzasina, B., Francolini, M., Rotta, G., Bonasio, R., Granucci, F., Kraehenbuhl, J. P., and Ricciardi-Castagnoli, P. (2001b). Dendritic cells express tight junction proteins and penetrate gut epithelial monolayers to sample bacteria. *Nat. Immunol.* 2, 361–367.

Rincon, M., Anguita, J., Nakamura, T., Fikrig, E., and Flavell, R. A. (1997). Interleukin (IL)-6 directs the differentiation of IL-4-producing CD4⁺ T cells. *J. Exp. Med.* 185, 461–469.

Rogler, G., Hausmann, M., Vogl, D., Aschenbrenner, E., Andus, T., Falk, W., Andreesen, R., Scholmerich, J., and Gross, V. (1998). Isolation and phenotypic characterization of colonic macrophages. *Clin. Exp. Immunol.* 112, 205–215.

Romani, L., Montagnoli, C., Bozza, S., Perruccio, K., Spreca, A., Allavena, P., Verbeek, S., Calderone, R. A., Bistoni, F., and Puccetti, P. (2004). The exploitation of distinct recognition receptors in dendritic cells determines the full range of host immune relationships with *Candida albicans. Int. Immunol.* 16, 149–161.

Ruckert, R., Brandt, K., Bulanova, E., Mirghomizadeh, F., Paus, R., and Bulfone-Paus, S. (2003). Dendritic cell-derived IL-15 controls the induction of CD8 T cell immune responses. *Eur. J. Immunol.* 33, 3493–3503.

Ruedl, C., and Hubele, S. (1997). Maturation of Peyer's patch dendritic cells *in vitro* upon stimulation via cytokines or CD40 triggering. *Eur. J. Immunol.* 27, 1325–1330.

Ruedl, C., Rieser, C., Bock, G., Wick, G., and Wolf, H. (1996). Phenotypic and functional characterization of CD11c⁺ dendritic cell population in mouse Peyer's patches. *Eur. J. Immunol.* 26, 1801–1806.

Rugtveit, J., Brandtzaeg, P., Halstensen, T. S., Fausa, O., and Scott, H. (1994). Increased macrophage subset in inflammatory bowel disease: Apparent recruitment from peripheral blood monocytes. *Gut* 35, 669–674.

Rugtveit, J., Haraldsen, G., Hogasen, A. K., Bakka, A., Brandtzaeg, P., and Scott, H. (1995). Respiratory burst of intestinal macrophages in inflammatory bowel disease is mainly caused by CD14+L1+ monocyte derived cells. *Gut* 37, 367–373.

Rugtveit, J., Bakka, A., and Brandtzaeg, P. (1997a). Differential distribution of B7.1 (CD80) and B7.2 (CD86) costimulatory molecules on mucosal macrophage subsets in human inflammatory bowel disease (IBD). *Clin. Exp. Immunol.* 110, 104–113.

Rugtveit, J., Nilsen, E. M., Bakka, A., Carlsen, H., Brandtzaeg, P., and Scott, H. (1997b). Cytokine profiles differ in newly recruited and resident subsets of mucosal macrophages from inflammatory bowel disease. *Gastroenterology* 112, 1493–1505.

Sakaguchi, S., Fukuma, K., Kuribayashi, K., and Masuda, T. (1985). Organ-specific autoimmune diseases induced in mice by elimination of T cell subset. I. Evidence for the active participation of T cells in natural self-tolerance; deficit of a T cell subset as a possible cause of autoimmune disease. *J. Exp. Med.* 161, 72–87.

Sartor, R. B. (1994). Cytokines in intestinal inflammation: pathophysiological and clinical considerations. *Gastroenterology* 106, 533–539.

Sato, A., Hashiguchi, M., Toda, E., Iwasaki, A., Hachimura, S., and Kaminogawa, S. (2003a). CD11b+ Peyer's patch dendritic cells secrete IL-6 and induce IgA secretion from naive B cells. *J. Immunol.* 171, 3684–3690.

Sato, K., Yamashita, N., Baba, M., and Matsuyama, T. (2003b). Regulatory dendritic cells protect mice from murine acute graft-versus-host disease and leukemia relapse. *Immunity* 18, 367–379.

Savill, J., Dransfield, I., Gregory, C., and Haslett, C. (2002). A blast from the past: Clearance of apoptotic cells regulates immune responses. *Nat. Rev. Immunol.* 2, 965–975.

Scheerens, H., Hessel, E., de Waal-Malefyt, R., Leach, M. W., and Rennick, D. (2001). Characterization of chemokines and chemokine receptors in two murine models of inflammatory bowel disease: IL-10–/– mice and Rag-2–/– mice reconstituted with CD4+CD45RBhigh T cells. *Eur. J. Immunol.* 31, 1465–1474.

Schon-Hegrad, M. A., Oliver, J., McMenamin, P. G., and Holt, P. G. (1991). Studies on the density, distribution, and surface phenotype of intraepithelial class II major histocompatibility complex antigen (Ia)-bearing dendritic cells (DC) in the conducting airways. *J. Exp. Med.* 173, 1345–1356.

Schulz, O., Edwards, A. D., Schito, M., Aliberti, J., Manickasingham, S., Sher, A., and Reis e Sousa, C. (2000). CD40 triggering of heterodimeric IL-12 p70 production by dendritic cells in vivo requires a microbial priming signal. *Immunity* 13, 453–462.

Schuppan, D., and Hahn, E. G. (2002). Biomedicine: Gluten and the gut-lessons for immune regulation. *Science* 297, 2218–2220.

Selby, W. S., Poulter, L. W., Hobbs, S., Jewell, D. P., and Janossy, G. (1983). Heterogeneity of HLA-DR-positive histiocytes in human intestinal lamina propria: A combined histochemical and immunohistological analysis. *J. Clin. Pathol.* 36, 379–384.

Seldenrijk, C. A., Drexhage, H. A., Meuwissen, S. G., Pals, S. T., and Meijer, C. J. (1989). Dendritic cells and scavenger macrophages in chronic inflammatory bowel disease. *Gut* 30, 486–491.

Semnani, R. T., Liu, A. Y., Sabzevari, H., Kubofcik, J., Zhou, J., Gilden, J. K., and Nutman, T. B. (2003). *Brugia malayi* microfilariae induce cell death in human dendritic cells, inhibit their ability to make IL-12 and IL-10, and reduce their capacity to activate CD4+ T cells. *J. Immunol.* 171, 1950–1960.

Sertl, K., Takemura, T., Tschachler, E., Ferrans, V. J., Kaliner, M. A., and Shevach, E. M. (1986). Dendritic cells with antigen-presenting capability reside in airway epithelium, lung parenchyma, and visceral pleura. *J. Exp. Med.* 163, 436–451.

Sharpe, A. H., and Freeman, G. J. (2002). The B7-CD28 superfamily. *Nat. Rev. Immunol.* 2, 116–126.

Shi, Y., Evans, J. E., and Rock, K. L. (2003). Molecular identification of a danger signal that alerts the immune system to dying cells. *Nature* 425, 516–521.

Shortman, K., and Liu, Y. J. (2002). Mouse and human dendritic cell subtypes. *Nat. Rev. Immunol.* 2, 151–161.

Shreedhar, V. K., Kelsall, B. L., and Neutra, M. R. (2003). Cholera toxin induces migration of dendritic cells from the subepithelial dome region to T- and B-cell areas of Peyer's patches. *Infect. Immun.* 71, 504–509.

Sminia, T., and van der Ende, M. B. (1991). Macrophage subsets in the rat gut: An immunohistochemical and enzyme-histochemical study. *Acta Histochem.* 90, 43–50.

Sminia, T., Janse, E. M., and Wilders, M. M. (1982). Antigen-trapping cells in Peyer's patches of the rat. *Scand. J. Immunol.* 16, 481–485.

Smith, K. M., Davidson, J. M., and Garside, P. (2002). T-cell activation occurs simultaneously in local and peripheral lymphoid tissue following oral administration of a range of doses of immunogenic or tolerogenic antigen although tolerized T cells display a defect in cell division. *Immunology* 106, 144–158.

Smith, P. D., Janoff, E. N., Mosteller-Barnum, M., Merger, M., Orenstein, J. M., Kearney, J. F., and Graham, M. F. (1997). Isolation and purification of CD14-negative mucosal macrophages from normal human small intestine. *J. Immunol. Meth.* 202, 1–11.

Smith, P. D., Smythies, L. E., Mosteller-Barnum, M., Sibley, D. A., Russell, M. W., Merger, M., Graham, M. F., Shimada, T., and Kubagawa, H. (2001a). Intestinal macrophages lack CD14 and CD89 and consequently are down-regulated for LPS- and IgA-mediated activities. *J. Immunol.* 167, 2651–2656.

Smith, P. D., Smythies, L. E., Mosteller-Barnum, M., Sibley, D. A., Russell, M. W., Merger, M., Sellers, M. T., Orenstein, J. M., Shimada, T., Graham, M. F., and Kubagawa, H. (2001b). Intestinal macrophages lack CD14 and CD89 and consequently are down-regulated for LPS- and IgA-mediated activities. *J. Immunol.* 167, 2651–2656.

Smith, P. D., Smythies, L. E., and Wahl, S. M. (2001c). Macrophage effector function. In Clinical Immunology (ed. H. W. J. Schroeder), 19.11–19.19. London: Harcourt Health Sciences.

Smythies, L. E., Sellers, M., Mosteller-Barnum, M., Meng, G., and Smith, P. D. (2003). Matrix and mesenchymal cells from the intestinal lamina propria release TGF-β which is chemotactic for blood monocytes: mechanism for monocyte recruitment to the mucosa, manuscript submitted.

Soesatyo, M., Biewenga, J., Kraal, G., and Sminia, T. (1990). The localization of macrophage subsets and dendritic cells in the gastrointestinal tract of the mouse with special reference to the presence of high endothelial venules. An immuno- and enzyme-histochemical study. *Cell Tissue Res.* 259, 587–593.

Soesatyo, M., van den Berg, T. K., van Rees, E. P., Biewenga, J., and Sminia, T. (1992). Ontogeny of reticulum cells in the rat intestine and their possible role in the development of the lymphoid microenvironment. *Reg. Immunol.* 4, 46–52.

Sonderbye, L., Meehan, S., Palsson, R., Ahsan, N., Ladefoged, J., and Langhoff, E. (1998). Immunohistochemical study of actin binding protein (p55) in the human kidney. *Transplantation* 65, 1004–1008.

Soumelis, V., Reche, P. A., Kanzler, H., Yuan, W., Edward, G., Homey, B., Gilliet, M., Ho, S., Antonenko, S., Lauerma, A., Smith, K., Gorman, D., Zurawski, S., Abrams, J., Menon, S., McClanahan, T., de Waal-Malefyt, Rd. R., Bazan, F., Kastelein, R. H., and Liu, Y. J. (2002). Human epithelial cells trigger dendritic cell mediated allergic inflammation by producing TSLP. *Nat. Immunol.* 3, 673–680.

Spalding, D. M., Koopman, W. J., Eldridge, J. H., McGhee, J. R., and Steinman, R. M. (1983). Accessory cells in murine Peyer's patch. I. Identification and enrichment of a functional dendritic cell. *J. Exp. Med.* 157, 1646–1659.

Spalding, D. M., Williamson, S. I., Koopman, W. J., and McGhee, J. R. (1984). Preferential induction of polyclonal IgA secretion by murine Peyer's patch dendritic cell-T cell mixtures. *J. Exp. Med.* 160, 941–946.

Spencer, J., Finn, T., and Isaacson, P. G. (1986). Human Peyer's patches: An immunohistochemical study. *Gut* 27, 405–410.

Stagg, A. J., Kamm, M. A., and Knight, S. C. (2002). Intestinal dendritic cells increase T cell expression of alpha4beta7 integrin. *Eur. J. Immunol.* 32, 1445–1454.

Stagg, A. J., Hart, A. L., Knight, S. C., and Kamm, M. A. (2003). The dendritic cell: Its role in intestinal inflammation and relationship with gut bacteria. *Gut* 52, 1522–1529.

Steinbrink, K., Wolfl, M., Jonuleit, H., Knop, J., and Enk, A. H. (1997). Induction of tolerance by IL-10-treated dendritic cells. *J. Immunol.* 159, 4772–4780.

Steinman, R. M., Granelli-Piperno, A., Pope, M., Trumpfheller, C., Ignatius, R., Arrode, G., Racz, P., and Tenner-Racz, K. (2003a). The interaction of immunodeficiency viruses with dendritic cells. *Curr. Top. Microbiol. Immunol.* 276, 1–30.

Steinman, R. M., Hawiger, D., and Nussenzweig, M. C. (2003b). Tolerogenic dendritic cells. *Annu. Rev. Immunol.* 21, 685–711.

Strober, W., Fuss, I. J., and Blumberg, R. S. (2002). The immunology of mucosal models of inflammation. *Annu. Rev. Immunol.* 20, 495–549.

Stumbles, P. A., Thomas, J. A., Pimm, C. L., Lee, P. T., Venaille, T. J., Proksch, S., and Holt, P. G. (1998). Resting respiratory tract dendritic cells preferentially stimulate T helper cell type 2 (Th2) responses and require obligatory cytokine signals for induction of Th1 immunity. *J. Exp. Med.* 188, 2019–2031.

Stumbles, P. A., Upham, J. W., and Holt, P. G. (2003). Airway dendritic cells: co-ordinators of immunological homeostasis and immunity in the respiratory tract. *APMIS* 111, 741–755.

Sun, J., Dirden-Kramer, B., Ito, K., Ernst, P. B., and Van Houten, N. (1999). Antigen-specific T cell activation and proliferation during oral tolerance induction. *J. Immunol.* 162, 5868–5875.

Szabo, M. C., Butcher, E. C., and McEvoy, L. M. (1997). Specialization of mucosal follicular dendritic cells revealed by mucosal addressin-cell adhesion molecule-1 display. *J. Immunol.* 158, 5584–5588.

Tada, K., Tanaka, M., Hanayama, R., Miwa, K., Shinohara, A., Iwamatsu, A., and Nagata, S. (2003). Tethering of apoptotic cells to phagocytes through binding of CD47 to Src homology 2 domain-bearing protein tyrosine phosphatase substrate-1. *J. Immunol.* 171, 5718–5726.

Tailleux, L., Schwartz, O., Herrmann, J. L., Pivert, E., Jackson, M., Amara, A., Legres, L., Dreher, D., Nicod, L. P., Gluckman, J. C., Lagrange, P. H., Gicquel, B., and Neyrolles, O. (2003). DC-SIGN is the major *Mycobacterium tuberculosis* receptor on human dendritic cells. *J. Exp. Med.* 197, 121–127.

Tanaka, Y., Imai, T., Baba, M., Ishikawa, I., Uehira, M., Nomiyama, H., and Yoshie, O. (1999). Selective expression of liver and activation-regulated chemokine (LARC) in intestinal epithelium in mice and humans. *Eur. J. Immunol.* 29, 633–642.

Tazi, A., Bouchonnet, F., Grandsaigne, M., Boumsell, L., Hance, A. J., and Soler, P. (1993). Evidence that granulocyte macrophage-colony-stimulating factor regulates the distribution and differentiated state of dendritic cells/Langerhans cells in human lung and lung cancers. *J. Clin. Invest.* 91, 566–576.

te Velde, A. A., van Kooyk, Y., Braat, H., Hommes, D. W., Dellemijn, T. A., Slors, J. F., van Deventer, S. J., and Vyth-Dreese, F. A. (2003). Increased expression of DC-SIGN+IL-12+IL-18+ and CD83+IL-12-IL-18-dendritic cell populations in the colonic mucosa of patients with Crohn's disease. *Eur. J. Immunol.* 33, 143–151.

Tunon-De-Lara, J. M., Redington, A. E., Bradding, P., Church, M. K., Hartley, J. A., Semper, A. E., and Holgate, S. T. (1996). Dendritic cells in normal and asthmatic airways: expression of the alpha subunit of the high affinity immunoglobulin E receptor (Fc epsilon RI -alpha). *Clin. Exp. Allergy* 26, 648–655.

Uhlig, H. H., and Powrie, F. (2003). Dendritic cells and the intestinal bacterial flora: A role for localized mucosal immune responses. *J. Clin. Invest.* 112, 648–651.

Urban, B. C., Ferguson, D. J., Pain, A., Willcox, N., Plebanski, M., Austyn, J. M., and Roberts, D. J. (1999). *Plasmodium falciparum*-infected erythrocytes modulate the maturation of dendritic cells. *Nature* 400, 73–77.

Urban, B. C., Willcox, N., and Roberts, D. J. (2001). A role for CD36 in the regulation of dendritic cell function. *Proc. Natl. Acad. Sci. USA* 98, 8750–8755.

Valledor, A. F., Borras, F. E., Cullell-Young, M., and Celada, A. (1998). Transcription factors that regulate monocyte/macrophage differentiation. *J. Leukoc. Biol.* 63, 405–417.

van der Kleij, D., Latz, E., Brouwers, J. F., Kruize, Y. C., Schmitz, M., Kurt-Jones, E. A., Espevik, T., de Jong, E. C., Kapsenberg, M. L., Golenbock, D. T., and Tielens AG, Yazdanbakhsh M. (2002). A novel host-parasite lipid cross-talk: Schistosomal lyso-phosphatidylserine activates toll-like receptor 2 and affects immune polarization. *J. Biol. Chem.* 277, 48122–48129.

Van Houten, N., and Blake, S. F. (1996). Direct measurement of anergy of antigen-specific T cells following oral tolerance induction. *J. Immunol.* 157, 1337–1341.

van Kooyk, Y., and Geijtenbeek, T. B. (2003). DC-SIGN: Escape mechanism for pathogens. *Nat. Rev. Immunol.* 3, 697–709.

Vanbervliet, B., Homey, B., Durand, I., Massacrier, C., Ait-Yahia, S., de Bouteiller, O., Vicari, A., and Caux, C. (2002). Sequential involvement of CCR2 and CCR6 ligands for immature dendritic cell recruitment: possible role at inflamed epithelial surfaces. *Eur. J. Immunol.* 32, 231–242.

Verbovetski, I., Bychkov, H., Trahtemberg, U., Shapira, I., Hareuveni, M., Ben-Tal, O., Kutikov, I., Gill, O., and Mevorach, D. (2002). Opsonization of apoptotic cells by autologous iC3b facilitates clearance by immature dendritic cells, down-regulates DR and CD86, and up-regulates CC chemokine receptor 7. *J. Exp. Med.* 196, 1553–1561.

Vermaelen, K. Y., Cataldo, D., Tournoy, K., Maes, T., Dhulst, A., Louis, R., Foidart, J. M., Noel, A., and Pauwels, R. (2003). Matrix metalloproteinase-9-mediated dendritic cell recruitment into the airways is a critical step in a mouse model of asthma. *J. Immunol.* 171, 1016–1022.

Vliagoftis, H., Befus, A. D., Hollenberg, M. D., and Moqbel, R. (2001). Airway epithelial cells release eosinophil survival-promoting factors (GM-CSF) after stimulation of proteinase-activated receptor 2. *J. Allergy Clin. Immunol.* 107, 679–685.

Voll, R. E., Herrmann, M., Roth, E. A., Stach, C., Kalden, J. R., and Girkontaite, I. (1997). Immunosuppressive effects of apoptotic cells. *Nature* 390, 350–351.

Von Stebut, E., Ehrchen, J. M., Belkaid, Y., Kostka, S. L., Molle, K., Knop, J., Sunderkotter, C., and Udey, M. C. (2003). Interleukin 1alpha promotes Th1 differentiation and inhibits disease progression in *Leishmania major*-susceptible BALB/c mice. *J. Exp. Med.* 198, 191–199.

Voso, M. T., Burn, T. C., Wulf, G., Lim, B., Leone, G., and Tenen, D. G. (1994). Inhibition of hematopoiesis by competitive binding of transcription factor PU.1. *Proc. Natl. Acad. Sci. USA* 91, 7932–7936.

Vu, Q., McCarthy, K. M., McCormack, J. M., and Schneeberger, E. E. (2002). Lung dendritic cells are primed by inhaled particulate antigens, and retain MHC class II/antigenic peptide complexes in hilar lymph nodes for a prolonged period of time. *Immunology* 105, 488–498.

Vuckovic, S., Florin, T. H., Khalil, D., Zhang, M. F., Patel, K., Hamilton, I., and Hart, D. N. (2001). CD40 and CD86 upregulation with divergent CMRF44 expression on blood dendritic cells in inflammatory bowel diseases. *Am. J. Gastroenterol.* 96, 2946–2956.

Wakkach, A., Fournier, N., Brun, V., Breittmayer, J. P., Cottrez, F., and Groux, H. (2003). Characterization of dendritic cells that induce tolerance and T regulatory 1 cell differentiation in vivo. *Immunity* 18, 605–617.

Wang, J., Snider, D. P., Hewlett, B. R., Lukacs, N. W., Gauldie, J., Liang, H., and Xing, Z. (2000). Transgenic expression of granulocyte-macrophage colony-stimulating factor induces the differentiation and activation of a novel dendritic cell population in the lung. *Blood* 95, 2337–2345.

Waraich, T., Sarsfield, P., and Wright, D. H. (1997). The accessory cell populations in ulcerative colitis: a comparison between the colon and appendix in colitis and acute appendicitis. *Hum. Pathol.* 28, 297–303.

Weiner, H. L. (2001). Oral tolerance: Immune mechanisms and the generation of Th3-type TGF-beta-secreting regulatory cells. *Microbes Infect.* 3, 947–954.

Weltzin, R., Lucia-Jandris, P., Michetti, P., Fields, B. N., Kraehenbuhl, J. P., and Neutra, M. R. (1989). Binding and transepithelial transport of immunoglobulins by intestinal M cells:

Demonstration using monoclonal IgA antibodies against enteric viral proteins. *J. Cell Biol.* 108, 1673–1685.

Wilders, M. M., Sminia, T., Plesch, B. E., Drexhage, H. A., Weltevreden, E. F., and Meuwissen, S. G. (1983). Large mononuclear Ia-positive veiled cells in Peyer's patches. II. Localization in rat Peyer's patches. *Immunology* 48, 461–467.

Wilders, M. M., Drexhage, H. A., Kokje, M., Verspaget, H. W., and Meuwissen, S. G. (1984). Veiled cells in chronic idiopathic inflammatory bowel disease. *Clin. Exp. Immunol.* 55, 377–387.

Wilders, M. M., Drexhage, H. A., Sminia, T., Mullink, H., Weltevreden, E. F., Plesh, B. E., and Meuwissen, S. G. (1985). Veiled cells in the gastrointestinal tract. *Acta Chir. Scand. Suppl.* 525, 93–111.

Williamson, E., O'Malley, J. M., and Viney, J. L. (1999). Visualizing the T-cell response elicited by oral administration of soluble protein antigen. *Immunology* 97, 565–572.

Williamson, E., Bilsborough, J. M., and Viney, J. L. (2002). Regulation of mucosal dendritic cell function by receptor activator of NF-kappa B (RANK)/RANK ligand interactions: impact on tolerance induction. *J. Immunol.* 169, 3606–3612.

Wilson, N. S., El-Sukkari, D., and Villadangos, J. A. (2003). Dendritic cells constitutively present self antigens in their immature state *in vivo*, and regulate antigen presentation by controlling the rates of MHC class II synthesis and endocytosis. *Blood* 102, 2187–2194.

Winter, H. S., Cole, F. S., Huffer, L. M., Davidson, C. B., Katz, A. J., and Edelson, P. J. (1983). Isolation and characterization of resident macrophages from guinea pig and human intestine. *Gastroenterology* 85, 358–363.

Witmer, M. D., and Steinman, R. M. (1984). The anatomy of peripheral lymphoid organs with emphasis on accessory cells: Light-microscopic immunocytochemical studies of mouse spleen, lymph node, and Peyer's patch. *Am. J. Anat.* 170, 465–481.

Witmer-Pack, M. D., Hughes, D. A., Schuler, G., Lawson, L., McWilliam, A., Inaba, K., Steinman, R. M., and Gordon, S.

(1993). Identification of macrophages and dendritic cells in the osteopetrotic (op/op) mouse. *J. Cell Sci.* 104 (Pt. 4), 1021–1029.

Wu, H. Y., and Weiner, H. L. (2003). Oral tolerance. *Immunol. Res.* 28, 265–284.

Xia, W., Pinto, C. E., and Kradin, R. L. (1995). The antigen-presenting activities of Ia+ dendritic cells shift dynamically from lung to lymph node after an airway challenge with soluble antigen. *J. Exp. Med.* 181, 1275–1283.

Yang, D., Chertov, O., Bykovskaia, S. N., Chen, Q., Buffo, M. J., Shogan, J., Anderson, M., Schroder, J. M., Wang, J. M., Howard, O. M., and Oppenheim, J. J. (1999). Beta-defensins: Linking innate and adaptive immunity through dendritic and T cell CCR6. *Science* 286, 525–528.

Yazdanbakhsh, M., Kremsner, P. G., and van Ree, R. (2002). Allergy, parasites, and the hygiene hypothesis. *Science* 296, 490–494.

Yrlid, U., and Macpherson, G. (2003). Phenotype and function of rat dendritic cell subsets. *APMIS* 111, 756–765.

Zhang, G. X., Xu, H., Kishi, M., Calida, D., and Rostami, A. (2002). The role of IL-12 in the induction of intravenous tolerance in experimental autoimmune encephalomyelitis. *J. Immunol.* 168, 2501–2507.

Zhao, X., Sato, A., Dela Cruz, C. S., Linehan, M., Luegering, A., Kucharzik, T., Shirakawa, A. K., Marquez, G., Farber, J. M., Williams, I., and Iwasaki, A. (2003). CCL9 is secreted by the follicle-associated epithelium and recruits dome region Peyer's patch CD11b+ dendritic cells. *J. Immunol.* 171, 2797–2803.

Zhu, X., Meng, G., Dickinson, B. L., Li, X., Mizoguchi, E., Miao, L., Wang, Y., Robert, C., Wu, B., Smith, P. D., Lencer, W. I., and Blumberg, R. S. (2001). MHC class I-related neonatal Fc receptor for IgG is functionally expressed in monocytes, intestinal macrophages, and dendritic cells. *J. Immunol.* 166, 3266–3276.

Oral Tolerance: Physiologic Basis and Clinical Applications

Chapter 27

Allan McI. Mowat

Department of Immunology and Bacteriology, Division of Immunology, Infection, and Inflammation, University of Glasgow, and Western Infirmary, Glasgow, Scotland, United Kingdom

Ana M. C. Faria

Departamento de Bioquímica e Imunologia, Instituto de Ciências Biológicas, Universidade Federal de Minas Gerais, Belo Horizonte, Brazil

Howard L. Weiner

Center for Neurologic Diseases, Brigham and Women's Hospital, Harvard Medical School, Boston, Massachusetts

INTRODUCTION

The diet of all animals consists of a complex mixture of animal and vegetable products, most of which are nonself in immunologic terms and, hence, are potentially antigenic. As other chapters in this volume describe, the gut-associated lymphoid tissue (GALT) is the largest immune tissue mass in the body and contains a wide array of different effector mechanisms to counter continual bombardment by potential pathogens. Mobilization of this powerful battery of responses against food antigens would be undesirable, partly because it would limit their uptake and metabolic usefulness but more importantly because hypersensitivity to foods can produce intestinal pathology, as typified by celiac disease and other food-sensitive enteropathies (FSE).

These conditions are rare, not because intestinal digestion destroys all immunologically relevant food antigens, but because the intestinal immune system can discriminate between food antigens and those of pathogenic importance. Contrary to the widespread belief among immunologists, a substantial proportion of ingested protein reaches the GALT and systemic immune tissues in an immunologically relevant form. Thus each meal results in the absorption of significant amounts of intact protein and/or protein fragments that are capable of stimulating immune responses if administered by other routes (Swarbrick *et al.*, 1979; Kilshaw and Cant, 1984; Husby *et al.*, 1986, 1987; Harmatz *et al.*, 1989). Interestingly, there is a two-way dialogue between food antigens and the immune system, because the continuous and physiologic stimulation provided by food antigens plays an important role in the full maturation of the immune system. As a result, animals weaned on to a protein-free, amino acid–based diet are normal by nutritional standards but have low levels of IgG and IgA antibodies and poor Th1 type immune responses as adults (Menezes *et al.*, 2003). Additional large sources of antigens in the normal intestine are the bacterial flora. Once again, these organisms are essential for normal life, yet they constitute a potential challenge to the integrity of the individual. Commensal bacteria may provoke similar homeostatic mechanisms, and a breakdown in this physiologic state may underlie inflammatory bowel diseases (IBD) such as Crohn's disease and ulcerative colitis (Strober *et al.*, 2002; Elson *et al.*, 2001).

In this chapter, we review the immunoregulatory mechanisms that normally prevent the induction of hypersensitivity by this formidable antigenic challenge and discuss the exploitation of oral tolerance to proteins as a means of delivering therapy against inflammatory and autoimmune conditions.

IMMUNE RESPONSES TO INTESTINALLY DERIVED ANTIGENS

The intestinal immune system can react in three principal ways to a novel antigen (**Fig. 27.1**). First, a local secretory IgA (S-IgA) antibody response may occur in the mucosa; second, the systemic immune system may be primed, with the generation of serum antibodies and cell-mediated immunity (CMI); and finally, a state of systemic and/or local

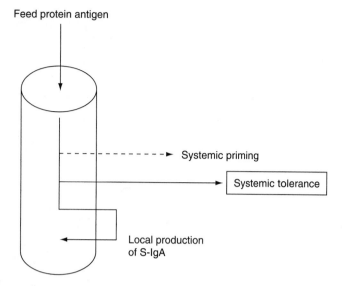

Feed protein antigen

Systemic priming

Systemic tolerance

Local production of S-IgA

Fig. 27.1. The immunologic responses to intestinal antigen. Depending on the antigen, the animal model, and the circumstances involved, oral administration of antigen may stimulate production of S-IgA antibodies in the intestine, may induce a primary systemic immune response, or may result in systemic unresponsiveness to subsequent challenge with the antigen. In practice, this systemic tolerance is the default response to dietary proteins and commensal bacteria.

immunologic tolerance may develop, preventing the induction of potentially damaging active immunity when the offending antigen is encountered on subsequent occasions. The first two of these comprise the protective immune response to invasive pathogens, whereas dietary proteins and commensal bacteria predominantly induce tolerance and do not provoke injurious local or systemic immune responses.

As we shall discuss, the position with local IgA production to these antigens is less clear. Experimental evidence suggests that the production of local IgA antibodies to food antigens may mediate a specific immune exclusion mechanism that, thereafter, prevents the uptake of the appropriate antigen (Swarbrick et al., 1979; Challacombe and Thomasi, 1980). That this mechanism is one means of preventing clinical food hypersensitivity is consistent with the higher frequency of serum antibodies and hypersensitivity to food proteins that occur in individuals with selective IgA deficiency (Crabbe and Heremans, 1967; Walker, 1987). Nevertheless, most patients with this common form of immune deficiency are entirely normal and have no evidence of food sensitivity. The relative importance of intestinal IgA in the prevention of food sensitivity is challenged further by the fact that inducing IgA antibodies by immunizing normal animals orally with conventional protein antigens is difficult (Elson and Ealding, 1984; Lycke and Holmgren, 1986; Wilson et al., 1989; Van der Heijden et al., 1991; McGhee et al., 1992; Mowat et al., 1993). Further, normal humans have little or no intestinal IgA antibody against food antigens (O'Mahony et al., 1991). Thus production of S-IgA antibodies alone is unlikely to account for the absence of hypersensitivity

reactions to food antigens, although this mechanism seems likely to provide a useful backup to other, more potent, immunoregulatory mechanisms.

ORAL TOLERANCE

Tolerance is a state of specific immunologic unresponsiveness to antigens that, under other circumstances, are capable of inducing a protective or injurious immune response. One of the most reliable means of inducing immunologic tolerance in experimental animals is to present noninvasive antigen by the oral route. The resulting phenomenon of oral tolerance has been studied predominantly in laboratory rodents, but it has also been described in several other animal species including pigs (Miller et al., 1984; Stokes et al., 1987), dogs (Deplazes et al., 1995; Zemann et al., 2003), guinea pigs (Heppell and Kilshaw, 1982), and rabbits (Bhogal et al., 1986). Importantly, longstanding circumstantial evidence for its existence in humans (Korenblatt et al., 1968; Lowney, 1968; Walker, 1987) has been confirmed by studies in which volunteers have been tolerized by oral administration of keyhole limpet hemocyanin (KLH) (Husby et al., 1994; Matsui et al., 1996; Kraus et al., 2004). Treatment of atopic humans by induction of oral tolerance to Dermatophagoides extract has also been reported (Suko et al., 1995), as has oral desensitization to nickel (Bagot et al., 1995) and decreased T-cell responses in thyroiditis patients fed porcine thyroid extracts (S. Lee et al., 1998). Normal humans also do not have significant antibody or T-cell proliferative responses against food proteins, despite evidence of recognition of these antigens by T cells (Zivny et al., 2001). Species differences do occur, however. Inducing oral tolerance in rabbits or guinea pigs (Peri and Rothberg, 1981; Silverman et al., 1982; Heppell and Kilshaw, 1982) is relatively difficult, whereas ruminants (Stokes, 1984) and chickens (C. C. Miller and Cook, 1994) may not develop significant tolerance to dietary constituents at all.

The phenomenon is illustrated readily by feeding mice a protein such as ovalbumin (OVA) some time before immunizing the animals with the antigen in adjuvant via an immunogenic route. In most experiments of this type, antigen-fed animals have almost complete suppression of their immune response to the challenge immunizations **(Fig. 27.2)**. An equivalent phenomenon can also be induced by intranasal or aerosol exposure of animals to soluble antigen (see the following text) and also by injection of antigen into the anterior chamber of the eye (Streilein, 1999), suggesting that the mucosal surfaces share common immunoregulatory mechanisms that ensure that tolerance is the default response to harmless antigens at these sites.

Historical perspectives

The possibility that ingestion of antigen might have immunologic consequences different from those associated with systemic immunization was alluded to by Besredka in 1909 (Besredka, 1909) and detailed first by Wells and

A

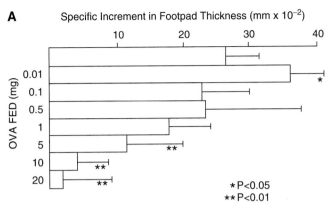

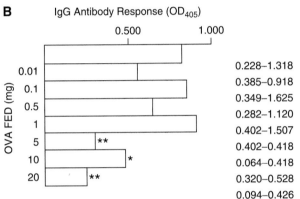

Fig. 27.2. Induction of oral tolerance by feeding the protein antigen ovalbumin (OVA) to normal adult mice. Dose-dependent suppression of systemic delayed type hypersensitivity (DTH) **(A)** and IgG antibody **(B)** responses to subcutaneous challenge with OVA in adjuvant in mice fed OVA. Systemic T-cell responses (DTH) are more sensitive to the effects of antigen feeding, but also show evidence of priming when the lowest doses of OVA are used.

Osborne in 1911. Their experiments showed that anaphylactic reactions to OVA and other proteins in guinea pigs could be inhibited by prior feeding of the appropriate material (Wells and Osborne, 1911). The immunologic nature of the phenomenon first was established by the much later experiments of Chase (1946), using contact sensitizing agents. Exploiting the knowledge that was emerging at that time on cellular immunity and on the induction of tolerance in other systems, Chase's work demonstrated the antigen specificity of oral tolerance and recognized how readily the immune system could be downregulated by what came to be known as the Sulzberger-Chase phenomenon. Since then, protocols for inducing oral tolerance and the mechanisms involved have attracted considerable attention, not only from mucosal immunologists, but also from others interested in using the phenomenon as a model of immunoregulation or as a means of inhibiting immune responses to antigens of immunopathologic importance.

Scope

The induction of systemic tolerance by feeding antigen has been demonstrated with a wide range of nonreplicating anti-

gens. In addition to the many proteins that have been studied, these antigens include heavy metals (Waldo *et al.*, 1994; Van Hoogstraten *et al.*, 1993; Artik *et al.*, 2001), contact sensitizing agents (Glaister, 1973; Asherson *et al.*, 1977, 1979; Newby *et al.*, 1980; Elson *et al.*, 1996), normal or haptenized self proteins (Neurath *et al.*, 1996; Dasgupta *et al.*, 2001), superantigens (Migita and Ochi, 1994; Migita *et al.*, 1995; Nishimura *et al.*,. 2002; heterologous red blood cells (Kagnoff, 1978a, 1978b, 1980; Mattingly and Waksman, 1978, 1980; Kiyono *et al.*, 1982; MacDonald, 1983), allogeneic leukocytes (Sayegh *et al.*, 1992a; Ilan *et al.*, 2000), extracts of pollen (Aramaki *et al.*, 1994) or *Dermatophagoides* and *Blomia* mites (Suko *et al.*, 1995; M. N. Sato *et al.*, 2002), and inactivated viruses or bacteria (Stokes *et al.*, 1979; Challacombe and Tomasi, 1980; Rubin *et al.*, 1981; Chen *et al.*, 1998a). Interestingly, from the practical point of view, protein antigens expressed in plants are also tolerogenic when eaten (Ma *et al.*, 1997; Arakawa *et al.*, 1998).

In addition to traditional model antigens such as sheep red blood cells (SRBC) and proteins such as OVA, many of the advances made in the field during the past decade have come from the use of proteins of immunopathologic importance, including several autoantigens and foreign proteins. These are discussed in detail in the following text. It is also possible to induce oral tolerance to peptides containing defined T-cell epitopes, thus allowing more detailed analysis of the immunologic basis of the phenomenon (A. Miller *et al.*, 1993; Gregerson *et al.*, 1993; Al-Sabbagh *et al.*, 1994; Khare *et al.*, 1995; Javed *et al.*, 1995; Wildner *et al.*, 1996; Hoyne *et al.*, 1994). However, variable results have been reported using different peptides. Although this could reflect true differences in the ability of individual epitopes to induce oral tolerance, it seems more likely that the lack of knowledge on the physiologic factors regulating the intestinal uptake and handling of short peptides has limited development of optimal dosage regimes. A similar caveat may apply to apparent immunologic differences obtained using different intact proteins, where size-related or charge-related differences in uptake by the intestine as well as inherent differences in immunogenicity will influence the outcome of feeding.

Virtually all proteins examined have been found to induce oral tolerance. Exceptions to this are cholera toxin (CT) and the related heat-stable enterotoxin from *Escherichia coli* (LT) (Elson and Ealding, 1984; Lycke and Holmgren, 1986; Wilson *et al.*, 1989; Van der Heijden *et al.*, 1991; McGhee *et al.*, 1992; Gaboriau-Routhiau and Moreau, 1996) (reviewed in Eriksson and Holmgren, 2002). As detailed elsewhere in this volume, CT and LT have the unusual abilities to stimulate primary local humoral and cell-mediated immune responses, as well as to act as adjuvants by preventing the induction of oral tolerance to other coadministered proteins. As the enzymatically inactive cholera toxin B (CT-B) fragment greatly enhances oral tolerance (Sun *et al.*, 1994; and see the following text), these effects of CT and LT appear to reflect their pharmacologic ability to activate G proteins and other intracellular signaling pathways. Certain plant lectins such as mistletoe lectin also stimulate active immunity via the intestine and act as local adjuvants for other proteins (Lavelle *et al.*, 2000, 2001). The reasons for these effects are unknown, but may be caused by pharmacologic activation of antigen-presenting cells (APC), or because the lectins target M cells in Peyer's patches (PP).

Immunologic consequences of oral tolerance

Feeding protein antigen can tolerize all aspects of the subsequent systemic immune response, including IgM, IgG, and IgE antibodies (Hanson *et al.*, 1977; Vaz *et al.*, 1977; Ngan and Kind, 1978; Richman *et al.*, 1978; Swarbrick *et al.*, 1979; Challacombe and Tomasi, 1980; Titus and Chiller, 1981; Mowat *et al.*, 1982; Thompson and Staines, 1990), as well as CMI responses measured by lymphocyte proliferation (Challacombe and Tomasi, 1980; Titus and Chiller, 1981; Higgins and Weiner, 1988; Lider *et al.*, 1989) and delayed-type hypersensitivity (DTH) or contact sensitivity *in vivo* (Asherson *et al.*, 1977, 1979; S. D. Miller and Hanson, 1979; Newby *et al.*, 1980; Titus and Chiller, 1981; Mowat *et al.*, 1982; Gautam and Battisto, 1985; Kay and Ferguson, 1989a, b). In addition, the clonal expansion and migration of antigen-specific CD4$^+$ T cells are reduced on challenge (Williamson *et al.*, 1999a; Viney *et al.*, 1998; Shi *et al.*, 2000; Smith *et al.*, 2002b). Oral tolerance to proteins exhibits classical carrier specificity (Hanson *et al.*, 1977; Richman *et al.*, 1978; Titus and Chiller, 1981; Cowdrey and Johlin, 1984), and recent elegant studies using the cotransfer of T-cell receptor (TcR) and B-cell receptor (BcR) transgenic T and B cells have proven directly that helper T-cell function is inhibited in orally tolerized animals (Smith *et al.*, 2002b). B cells may be primed by feeding even high doses of antigen (Franco *et al.*, 1998), and tolerance of antibody production *in vivo* can be broken if the defective helper T cells are bypassed using an unrelated carrier or are stimulated with lipopolysaccharide (LPS) (Titus and Chiller, 1981; Mowat *et al.*, 1986). When B cells are tolerized by feeding antigen, they recover much more quickly than T cells (Vives *et al.*, 1980).

One consequence of this is that *in vivo* CMI responses are generally easier to tolerize than are humoral immune responses, requiring less antigen, and the tolerance persists much longer (Fig. 27.2) (Heppell and Kilshaw, 1982; Mowat *et al.*, 1982, 1986; Strobel and Ferguson, 1987; Kay and Ferguson, 1989a, b; Ke and Kapp, 1996; Christensen *et al.*, 2003). Indeed, small primary serum antibody responses have been reported after feeding tolerogenic doses of proteins (Franco *et al.*, 1998). DTH and T-cell proliferative responses are also more susceptible to oral tolerance in man (Husby *et al.*, 1994; Kraus *et al.*, 2004; S. Lee *et al.*, 1998). These *in vivo* differences have often been considered to reflect a dichotomy in the susceptibility of individual subsets of CD4$^+$ T cell to oral tolerance and indeed Th1-dependent cytokines such as interleukin-2 (IL-2) and interferon-γ (IFN-γ) are frequently easier to inhibit by feeding antigen than Th2-dependent cytokines such as IL-4, IL-5 and IL-10 (Weiner *et al.*, 1994; Gregerson *et al.*, 1993; Melamed and Friedman, 1994; Fishman-Lobell *et al.*, 1994; Melamed *et al.*, 1996; von

Herrath *et al.*, 1996; Franco *et al.*, 1998). In parallel, IL-4-dependent IgG1 antibody responses may be more resistant to tolerance than IFN-γ-dependent IgG2a responses (Melamed and Friedman, 1994; Claessen *et al.*, 1996). These effects on individual Th responses may be dose dependent, with high doses of antigen suppressing the production of all Th1- and Th2-dependent cytokines (Friedman and Weiner, 1994; Garside *et al.*, 1995b; Y. Chen *et al.*, 1995a; Melamed *et al.*, 1996; Franco *et al.*, 1998), whereas multiple, low doses of antigen may preferentially upregulate production of IL-4 and IL-10, with concomitant inhibition of IL-2 and IFN-γ (Y. Chen *et al.*, 1997; Friedman and Weiner, 1994; Melamed *et al.*, 1996).

Whether this apparent distinction between classical Th1 dependence and Th2 dependence is a hard-wired property of oral tolerance seems unlikely, because recent findings show that the susceptibility of the different Th subsets may reflect the nature of the adjuvant used to challenge fed animals. Thus Th2 responses are much more readily tolerized when mice are immunized using the Th2-polarizing adjuvants alum (Tobagus *et al.*, 2004) or CT (Kato *et al.*, 2001), whereas parenteral challenge with complete Freund's adjuvant (CFA) reveals better tolerance of Th1-dependent responses. In addition, it has long been known that systemic IgE antibody responses are remarkably sensitive to inhibition by feeding antigen before or after parenteral immunization (Vaz *et al.*, 1977; Ngan and Kind, 1978; Jarrett and Hall, 1984; Saklayen *et al.*, 1984; Pecquet *et al.*, 1999; M. N. Sato *et al.*, 2002; Christensen *et al.*, 2003). Similar findings have been made in human infants, in whom Th2-mediated IL-4 and IL-13 responses appear to be preferentially suppressed in children who acquire oral tolerance to peanut allergen (Turcanu *et al.*, 2003). Furthermore, antigen feeding can inhibit Th2-mediated models of asthma and eosinophil recruitment in the lung of mice (Nakao *et al.*, 1998; Haneda *et al.*, 1997) and dogs (Zemann *et al.*, 2003), as well as allergic conjunctivitis in dogs (Zemann *et al.*, 2003). Together, these results support the idea that the suppressive mechanisms induced by oral tolerance can be tailored to the type of systemic immune response that has been induced. It is interesting to note that the effector functions that are most susceptible to oral tolerance *in vivo* (IgE and DTH), are also the mechanisms most frequently associated with pathologic food hypersensitivity. These ideas are also consistent with recent findings on regulatory CD4$^+$ T cells in other systems, which are able to suppress most forms of immune response *in vivo*, responding to the nature of the inflammation and perhaps to signals from the innate immune system, rather than inhibiting distinct subsets of T cell (Maloy *et al.*, 2003; Higgins *et al.*, 2003; Sakaguchi, 2003).

CD8$^+$ T-cell dependent responses can also be tolerized by feeding soluble antigens, but this is a somewhat controversial area, with different groups reporting tolerance, priming, or no effect on systemic T-cell responses after feeding antigen to either normal mice, or mice transferred with antigen-specific TcR transgenic CD8$^+$ T cells (Garside *et al.*, 1995a; Ke and Kapp, 1996; Blanas *et al.*, 1996, 2000; Kim *et al.*, 1998;

Lefrançois *et al.*, 1999; Vezys *et al.*, 2000; Desvignes *et al.*, 1996, 2000; von Herrath *et al.*, 1996; Hänninen *et al.*, 2001) (reviewed in Garside and Mowat, 2001). These discrepancies may reflect whether CD4+ T cells are required for the CD8+ CTL responses under study, because we found that only CD4-dependent CTL responses could be tolerized by oral administration of antigen (Garside *et al.*, 1995a; P. Garside, M. Steel, and A. McI Mowat, unpublished observations). However, others have reported that both CD4-dependent and CD4-independent CTL can be tolerized completely by feeding OVA (Ke and Kapp, 1996), although there are several reports that OVA-specific CD8+ CTL can be primed directly by feeding tolerogenic doses of antigen (Blanas *et al.*, 1996; Hänninen *et al.*, 2000, 2001). The reasons for these discrepant results are unclear, but given the evidence that feeding antigen may induce a population of CD8+ regulatory T cells (Treg) (see the following text), it may be that some regimens of antigen feeding may induce a state of "split tolerance" in CD8+ T cells, with CTL being tolerized or unaffected in the face of priming of IL-4/IL-10-producing Treg (Ke and Kapp, 1996; von Herrath *et al.*, 1996; Zhou *et al.*, 2000). Split tolerance of mucosal CD8+ T-cell responses has been described in other models of peripheral tolerance (Tanchot *et al.*, 1998), as well as in animals expressing OVA only on intestinal epithelial cells and transferred with OVA-specific TcR transgenic T cells (Vezys *et al.*, 2000). In this model, CTL activity was preserved, but other functions such as clonal expansion and the production of IFN-γ and tumor necrosis factor-α (TNF-α) were tolerant. Thus CD8+ T cells of different functions may be differentially susceptible to oral tolerance.

The status of mucosal immune responses in orally tolerized animals remains controversial, despite the fact that prevention of local hypersensitivity would seem to be the most likely physiologic role of the phenomenon. Early reports suggested that the degree of tolerance of systemic immunity induced by feeding antigen correlated directly with the concomitant development of S-IgA antibody responses and IgA-mediated immune exclusion (Swarbrick *et al.*, 1979; Challacombe and Tomasi, 1980). However, strain differences in immune exclusion among protein-fed mice do not correlate with their susceptibility to oral tolerance (Stokes *et al.*, 1983b), while IgA antibodies against food antigens are absent in normal individuals. In addition, examination of mice with knockouts of different immunoregulatory molecules including the IFN-γ receptor has shown that local IgA production and oral tolerance appear to be regulated independently (Kjerrulf *et al.*, 1997).

Conflicting findings have been reported on the effects of feeding antigen on local IgA production and most workers have examined only the levels of primary IgA antibodies during the induction phase, rather than after subsequent mucosal challenge. As we have noted, some studies have shown the production of specific S-IgA antibodies in the gut after feeding tolerogenic doses of protein (Challacombe and Tomasi, 1980; Husby *et al.*, 1994; Franco *et al.*, 1998; Y. Chen *et al.*, 2002), but this is not a universal finding. It may be related to the dose of antigen fed, with low doses generating Treg (see the following text) and priming IgA production, perhaps via the induction of transforming growth factor-β (TGF-β), whereas higher doses of antigen may inhibit all responses, including mucosal IgA (Franco *et al.*, 1998; Strober *et al.*, 1997; Faria and Weiner, 1999). Secondary IgA antibody responses have also been reported to be both normal (Kelly and Whitacre, 1996; Elson *et al.*, 1996; Pecquet *et al.*, 1999) or suppressed in tolerized mice (Elson *et al.*, 1996; Kiyono *et al.*, 1982; MacDonald, 1983; Lycke *et al.*, 1995; Kato *et al.*, 2001; Christensen *et al.*, 2003). These discrepancies are difficult to resolve at present, and there is a need for detailed studies of the effects of different feeding regimens on mucosal IgA responses to challenge under defined conditions.

Even less is known of mucosal T-cell responsiveness to local challenge in orally tolerant animals. It is now clear that some degree of T-cell priming occurs in PP and other GALT soon after the induction of tolerance (see the following text). This was first suggested by early studies that reported the concomitant induction of PP T cells that suppressed IgG production but helped the synthesis of IgA antibodies after feeding soluble antigen (Richman *et al.*, 1981a). More surprisingly, priming of IFN-γ-producing T cells also occurs in PP very soon after feeding tolerogenic doses of antigen to mice (Marth *et al.*, 1996; Y. Chen *et al.*, 1997), and studies in humans suggest that the normal PP contains relatively high numbers of food antigen–specific T cells capable of producing IFN-γ (Nagata *et al.*, 2000). It has also been reported that expansion of antigen-specific CD4+ T cells occurs in lamina propria (LP) after induction of tolerance in TcR transgenic mice (Whitacre *et al.*, 1996; Smith *et al.*, 2002a), although food antigen–specific effector T cells cannot be cloned from normal human mucosa (Beyer *et al.*, 2002). Thus there is clear evidence that antigen-specific T cells recognize orally administered tolerogen, responding by cell division, functional differentiation, and migration to the LP. However, the absence of productive immunity or immunopathology under these conditions indicates that this T-cell response is limited in scope, and it would be important to define the functional capacities of the differentiated T cells found in GALT or LP under these circumstances. It might be predicted that some of these T cells are either IgA-specific helper T cells or are Treg whose function is to maintain mucosal homeostasis. That tolerance of local T cells can be induced under appropriate circumstances is suggested by the fact that feeding tolerizing dose of OVA greatly inhibits subsequent proliferative and cytokine responses by PP CD4+ T cells in response to oral challenge with antigen plus CT (Kato *et al.*, 2001). In addition, the experimental colitis caused by activation of mucosal IFN-γ-producing lymphocytes by rectal administration of haptens can be suppressed by feeding haptenated colonic proteins. This is accompanied by reduced local production of IFN-γ and increased levels of TGF-β (Neurath *et al.*, 1996). Local immune responses to adenovirus can also be suppressed by feeding viral antigens (Ilan *et al.*, 1997, 1998).

Locomotor activity is a further aspect of lymphocyte function that can be inhibited by the effects of oral tolerance. This can be demonstrated after systemic challenge by defective migration of peripheral lymph node antigen-specific CD4+ T lymphocytes in response to chemokinetic stimuli *in vitro* (**Fig. 27.3**). *In vivo*, orally tolerized antigen-specific CD4+ T lymphocytes fail to migrate into the B-cell follicles of draining lymphoid organs after clonal expansion in the T-cell area (Smith *et al.*, 2002b). This contrasts to what is found when T cells are primed by feeding or systemic immunization with antigen plus adjuvant and is consistent with the behavior of T cells that have been tolerized by other routes (Kearney *et al.*, 1994; Smith *et al.*, 2002b). It will be interesting to determine whether this related to the recent findings that T lymphocytes that have been anergized *in vitro* fail to show chemokine-driven migration across endothelial monolayers, because of expression of the extracellular dipeptidyl-peptidase CD26 (James *et al.*, 2003). Not all locomotory functions are inhibited in tolerant lymphocytes, as antigen-specific CD4+ T cells in the mesenteric lymph nodes (MLN) of orally tolerized mice acquire responsiveness to the CCR9 ligand thymus-expressed chemokine (TECK), consistent with the ability of these cells to accumulate subsequently in the LP (Fig. 27.3). In addition, orally tolerized

antigen-specific CD4+ T cells can migrate from TDA into B-cell follicles in response to parenteral challenge with antigen in adjuvant, despite their failure to exhibit subsequent helper T-cell activity (see the preceding text) (Smith *et al.*, 2002b). Defective patterns of migration *in vivo* may contribute to the poor effector functions seen in tolerant animals.

Time course and duration of oral tolerance

Systemic tolerance can be demonstrated very soon after a feed of protein. Significantly suppressed responses to systemic challenge with OVA are observed within 1–2 days of feeding the antigen (Challacombe and Tomasi, 1980; M. Steel, P. Garside, and A. McI Mowat, unpublished observations). The maximum degree of unresponsiveness then occurs during the first weeks after feeding, although in most experimental protocols, a 1–2 week gap between feeding and challenge has been found to be the most appropriate. At least some aspects of the resulting tolerance are then remarkably persistent, although different components of the systemic immune response behave differently with time. Work with OVA has shown that tolerance of DTH responses remains essentially intact up to at least 18 months after a single feed of high-dose OVA (Strobel and Ferguson, 1987; M. Steel, P. Garside, and A. McI Mowat, unpublished observations).

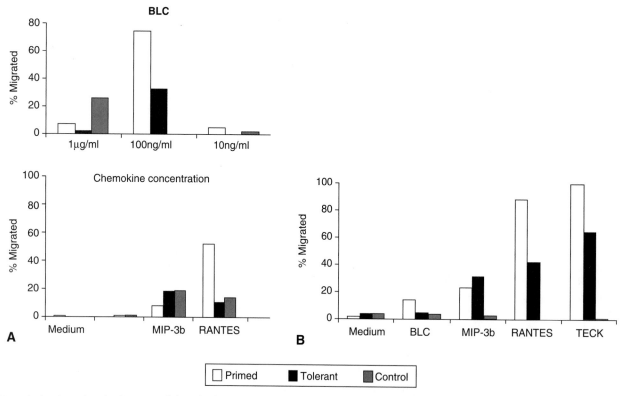

Fig. 27.3. Induction of oral tolerance inhibits the locomotor activity of lymphocytes. **A,** Adoptively transferred, OVA-specific TcR transgenic CD4+ T cells were obtained from the peripheral lymph node of mice fed OVA and challenged subcutaneously with OVA in CFA and allowed to migrate in chemotaxis chambers *in vitro*. T cells from mice fed soluble OVA to induce tolerance do not migrate in response to RANTES or B-lymphocyte chemoattractant (BLC), unlike cells from mice primed with the same dose of OVA fed with CT as a mucosal adjuvant. **B,** Both tolerant and primed CD4+ T cells acquire responsiveness to the small intestine–specific chemokine thymus-expressed chemokine (TECK) when taken from the MLN 7 days after feeding.

This is remarkable given that the average life span of a laboratory mouse is little more than 2 years. However, other immune functions return more quickly in the tolerant animal, and in the experimental autoimmune encephalitis (EAE) model, myelin basic protein–fed (MBP-fed) animals are protected for only 1–2 months after multiple low-dose feeding (Higgins and Weiner, 1988). Using OVA, tolerance of serum IgG antibody responses persists for only 3–6 months after a single feed of OVA (Strobel and Ferguson, 1987; Moreau and Gaboriau-Routhiau, 1996), as do the suppressed IL-3, IL-5, and IL-10 responses in vitro (M. Steel et al., unpublished observations). Proliferative responses begin to return to normal after 3–6 weeks, but may remain significantly inhibited for up to 6–9 months (M. Steel et al., unpublished observations; Melamed and Friedman, 1993). A requirement for antigen to persist for tolerance to be maintained has been implied by studies that show that much more profound tolerance is retained for longer if mice are challenged with antigen in the depot adjuvant CFA, rather than rested for long periods after the feeding of soluble antigen (Melamed and Friedman, 1993).

Tolerance induced by feeding other antigens such as heterologous red cells may not develop so rapidly, since multiple feeds of SRBC over a period of >2 weeks often are required for unresponsiveness to be demonstrable. This result may reflect the fact that SRBC may induce a sustained primary immune response when given orally and that this priming first must be overcome before tolerance ensues (Kagnoff, 1978a, b; David, 1979; Mattingly and Waksman, 1980).

FACTORS THAT INFLUENCE THE INDUCTION AND MAINTENANCE OF ORAL TOLERANCE

Nature of antigen

As we have discussed, a wide range of antigens is capable of inducing oral tolerance. Proteins are particularly easy to induce tolerance to, probably reflecting the physiologic purpose of the phenomenon. However, heat or chemically denatured proteins do not induce oral tolerance, possibly because they are destroyed rapidly in the gut and are not absorbed efficiently (Mowat, 1985; Peng et al., 1995).

Certain types of antigens are more likely to provoke active immunity rather than tolerance by the oral route, particularly viable organisms such as viruses and bacteria (Stokes et al., 1979; Rubin et al., 1981; Pope et al., 2001). This difference in response is not dependent on the structure of the antigens involved, because the same organisms will induce oral tolerance if killed or inactivated (Rubin et al., 1981). It is probable that the critical factor is not the viability of the antigenic vector, but its ability to persist in local tissues and perhaps invade more widely. Thus normally tolerogenic soluble proteins induce active immunity by the oral route when expressed as gene products in invasive (Dahlgren et al., 1991), but not noninvasive (Singh

et al., 1996) E. coli. This phenomenon may explain why commensal bacteria (Duchmann et al., 1995, 1996) and certain strains of probiotic organisms (Karlsson et al., 1999) also appear to induce specific tolerance.

Inducing tolerance by feeding thymus-independent antigens also is generally impossible (Stokes et al., 1979; Titus and Chiller, 1981), even if these are administered in association with a thymus-dependent antigen. Thus, mice fed killed E. coli develop tolerance to the thymus-dependent K antigen but acquire local and systemic immunity to the thymus-independent 0 antigen on the same organism (Stokes et al., 1979). Particulate antigens are also generally less able than soluble antigens to induce oral tolerance, because OVA coated on to polyglycoside microspheres or incorporated into particulate immunostimulating complexes (ISCOMs) stimulates active immunity by the oral route (McGhee et al., 1992; Maloy et al., 1994). Particulate antigens may be immunogenic because they may be taken up and processed more efficiently by targeting M cells in PP, as has been shown directly for several live organisms, as well as microparticles, ISCOMs, and lectins (Owen, 1994; Ermak et al., 1995; Jones, 1995; Lavelle et al., 2000, 2001; Kim et al., 2002). Interestingly, extremely low doses of antigen in the form of polylactide-coglycolide microparticles may induce tolerance, rather than priming by the oral route (Pecquet et al., 2000; Kim et al., 2002). Therefore such agents may act by increasing the delivery of fed antigens to the immune system and the induction of tolerance may have an upper dose threshold which has not been achieved using the proteins themselves (see the following text).

Together, these findings may help explain the ability of the intestinal immune system to discriminate between harmless and pathogenic antigens, as most harmful organisms will be invasive, particulate, and rich in thymus-independent antigens such as LPS.

Dose and frequency of antigen feeding

A wide range of antigen doses will induce significant oral tolerance; a single feed of a few milligrams of protein is sufficient in mice [Fig. 27.2; (Hanson et al., 1977; Mowat et al., 1986]. The exact dose required for the optimal effect depends on the protein under study, and the different limbs of the systemic immune response are differentially susceptible. Maximal immune suppression after feeding OVA occurs with doses ranging from 1–20 mg of protein, but DTH responses can be tolerized reproducibly by doses of as little as 100 µg OVA, whereas at least 5–10 mg are necessary to inhibit humoral immunity (Fig. 27.2). In most studies, tolerance cannot be overcome by feeding larger doses of native proteins, but as we have noted in the preceding text, incorporation of antigen into more efficient delivery vehicles may reveal loss of tolerance at supramaximal doses (Pecquet et al., 2000). This may not be of physiologic importance in the context of food protein consumption, but does raise important issues for vaccine development and also for the understanding the potential effects of increased intestinal permeability on oral tolerance.

At doses immediately below those that induce tolerance, feeding antigen has no effect on systemic immunity, whereas even lower amounts actually may prime the immune response [Fig. 27.2 (Lamont *et al.*, 1989; Meyer *et al.*, 1996; Viney *et al.*, 1998)]. In mice, systemic priming occurs after feeding single doses of 1–50 μg protein and, *in vivo*, affects CMI effector responses more than humoral immunity. A similar phenomenon has been noted in piglets in which large amounts of weaning diet produce tolerance and low amounts prime the animals to develop food sensitivity (B. G. Miller *et al.*, 1984). Interestingly, initial exposure to low amounts of food antigens has also been suggested to predispose to eczema in children (Jarrett, 1984).

Much interest has focused on the possibility that the exact immunologic consequences of oral tolerance may be determined by the nature of the feeding regimen **(Fig. 27.4)**. Compared with single feeds of antigen, continuous administration of antigen in drinking water or in the diet produces more profound tolerance. This also now affects more aspects of the systemic immune response, including those such as IL-4 and IgG1 production that are normally difficult to tolerize (Hirahara *et al.*, 1995; Melamed *et al.*, 1996; Lundin *et al.*, 1996). Similar findings have been made in previously primed animals (Peng *et al.*, 1989a; Meyer *et al.*, 1996) and in ageing mice that are normally refractory to tolerance (Faria *et al.*, 1998, 2003). These effects of continuous feeding appear to reflect the continuous exposure to antigen, rather than the total dose administered. The regulatory mechanisms induced by induction of oral tolerance may also depend on the feeding regime. Thus, several workers have shown that repeated administration of relatively low doses of protein (<5 mg in normal mice) appears to induce active Treg cells that demonstrate "bystander suppressor" functions via production of cytokines such as IL-4, IL-10, and TGF-β. Continuous feed-

ing is also associated with upregulation of regulatory cytokines such as IL-10 and TGF-β (Lundin *et al.*, 1996, 1999; Faria *et al.*, 2003; Marth *et al.*, 2000). In contrast, single high doses of protein may induce clonal anergy or deletion of T cells, without involvement of regulatory cells. A further difference between such feeding regimens appears to be the involvement of the chemokine macrophage chemotactic protein 1 (MCP-1; CCL2) and its receptor CCR2. Mice depleted of MCP-1, and CCR6 knockout (KO) or CCL2 KO mice have defective tolerance to single high doses of protein, but not to low doses (Gonnella *et al.*, 2003; DePaolo *et al.*, 2003). These regimens are often referred to as "low-dose" and "high-dose" tolerance, but in practice, few studies have compared regimens that use the same antigen given in different doses at different frequencies. Thus it remains unclear exactly how antigen dose or timing of administration influences the immunologic consequences of tolerance. This is an important issue to be clarified if oral tolerance is to be successful in clinical practice.

Genetic background of the host

Since the commonest form of clinical food hypersensitivity, celiac disease, is linked closely to the *HLA-DQ2* locus of the human major histocompatibility complex (MHC) (Sollid, 2002), it seems reasonable to predict that genetic factors will influence experimental oral tolerance. Strain differences in the susceptibility of mouse strains to the induction of oral tolerance by feeding OVA have been noted by several workers, although most of these differences have not been investigated systematically (Lafont *et al.*, 1982; Stokes *et al.*, 1983b; Tomasi *et al.*, 1983; Faria *et al.*, 1993). In more detailed analyses, we and others have found that most mouse strains are tolerized readily by feeding OVA, with no consistent effects of genes such as those encoding the idiotypic regions of immunoglobulins (Lamont *et al.*, 1988b; Ishii *et al.*, 1993).

Nevertheless, one aspect to emerge from this work was that mice carrying the H-2^d MHC haplotype were particularly susceptible to the induction of tolerance, whereas the H-2^b haplotype frequently was associated with less profound tolerance. This was illustrated very clearly by the fact that BALB/b (H-2^b) mice were much more difficult to tolerize than the congenic BALB/c (H-2^d) strain (Mowat *et al.*, 1987; Lamont *et al.*, 1988b), supporting a possible role for MHC genes in regulating oral tolerance to protein antigens. These strain differences did not reflect differences in the processing of protein in the intestine, but were the result of the inability of the BALB/B immune system to be regulated by tolerogenic protein coming from the intestine (Mowat *et al.*, 1987). H-2^b mice on the C57 background may share this relative resistance to oral tolerance (Lamont *et al.*, 1988b; A. Lamont and A. Mowat, unpublished observations), a finding that has implications for studies in transgenic and KO mice, many of which are on an H-2^b background. The immunologic basis of this MHC-linked effect remains to be established, and other, non-MHC-linked genes have also been implicated in oral tolerance (Tomasi *et al.*, 1983). In another study, these did

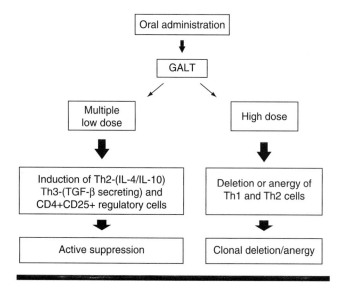

Oral Tolerance

Fig. 27.4. Proposed dose-dependent mechanisms of oral tolerance.

not appear to operate via the immune exclusion function of S-IgA antibody, but resistance to tolerance induction correlated with unusually rapid clearance of absorbed antigen from the circulation (Stokes *et al.*, 1983b). In our own work, susceptibility to induction of oral tolerance did not correlate with differences in tolerance induced by the intravenous route, but more recent findings suggest that these two phenomena may be under common genetic control (Kamphorst *et al.*, 2004a,b). Thus tolerance to fed antigens may involve a variety of genetic mechanisms, some of which are distinct from those that control immunity to parenterally administered antigen and others that are the same. One could imagine that these include genes that may influence general immune responsiveness, as well as factors more selective to the intestine, such as intestinal absorption, protein clearance, and catabolism. The recent description of tolerance susceptible (TS) and resistant (TR) mice derived by equilibrated intercrossing of eight separate mouse strains and which show opposite phenotypes for oral tolerance induction for several antigens may offer important insights into the polygenic control of the phenomenon (A. C. da Silva *et al.*, 1998; M. F. da Silva *et al.*, 2001).

One additional level of genetic control that has been noted is that strains of mice with genetically determined systemic lupus erythematosus (SLE)–like autoimmune disease are unusually resistant to the induction of tolerance by feeding some, but not all, protein antigens (Cowdrey *et al.*, 1982; M. L. Miller *et al.*, 1983; Carr *et al.*, 1985; and see the following text). Thus different mechanisms may be involved in oral tolerance to different antigens.

Influence of host age on susceptibility to oral tolerance

Food hypersensitivities are most common in infants, particularly at or near the time of weaning. It is interesting to note, therefore, that early studies indicated that neonatal and weaning rodents exhibited defects in the induction of tolerance by feeding protein antigens (Hanson, 1981; Strobel and Ferguson, 1984; Peng *et al.*, 1989b; B. G. Miller *et al.*, 1994; Pecquet *et al.*, 1999). In these reports, animals fed antigen on the first day or two of life did not develop the tolerance of systemic immunity found in adults fed the same weight-related dose and showed evidence of systemic priming when challenged parenterally as adults. This particularly affected T cell–dependent responses such as DTH or EAE (Hanson, 1981; Strobel and Ferguson, 1984; Peng *et al.*, 1989b; B. G. Miller *et al.*, 1994), but defective tolerance of IgE responses has also been noted (Pecquet *et al.*, 1999). Similar findings have been reported in neonatal mice exposed early in lactation to gluten present in the milk of mothers fed a gluten-containing diet (Troncone and Ferguson, 1988). In addition, the ability to sensitize calves or piglets by feeding antigen during the preweaning period further supports an age-related defect in oral tolerance at this time (Stokes *et al.*, 1987; Stokes, 1984; B. G. Miller *et al.*, 1984; Barratt *et al.*, 1987). In mice, the adult pattern of susceptibility to tolerance developed after 4 days of age

and was established fully around 7 days. However, even then, the neonatal and adult immune systems may respond differently to fed antigen. Thus equivalent feeding regimens induce mainly clonal anergy in late neonatal rats, but active regulation in adults (Lundin *et al.*, 1996). One explanation for these differences between animals of different ages could be that differences in antigen uptake by the neonatal intestine lead to different amounts of antigen entering the immune system. However, the defective tolerance in the newborn mouse does not correlate directly with differences in the amount of protein absorbed by the neonatal intestine and can be corrected by transfer of mature lymphocytes (Hanson, 1981; Peng *et al.*, 1989b). Thus the infant immune system may respond by inducing distinctive regulatory mechanisms to intestinally derived tolerogen. Very recent studies have contested the idea that there may be a defect in oral tolerance in newborn mice and suggested that neonatal and adult animals are equally sensitive to weight-related doses of fed antigen (Tobagus *et al.*, 2004). Interestingly, these latter studies used a feeding regimen in which antigen was given into the oral cavity, rather than by the intragastric route that was used in earlier work, and it is possible that the different mechanisms of antigen uptake that operate in these sites may have influenced the immunologic outcome of feeding. Given the fact that the oral route is the more physiologic route by which the neonate will usually first encounter food antigens, these issues warrant further investigation.

An additional transient defect in tolerance induction occurs in the days around weaning (Hanson, 1981; Strobel and Ferguson, 1984, A. Miller *et al.*, 1994). This is not related to the age of the animal, but is influenced by the process of weaning itself and is likely to be determined by the alterations in intestinal microenvironment or in systemic hormone levels associated with weaning.

At the other end of the age spectrum, ageing mice have been reported to become increasingly resistant to the induction of oral tolerance by feeding OVA (Faria *et al.*, 1993, 1998, 2003; Moreau and Gaboriau-Routhiau, 1996; Kato *et al.*, 2003). This phenomenon correlates with a reduced ability to prime mice by oral immunization with CT as an adjuvant and with deficiencies in the numbers of T cells and dendritic cells (DC) in PP, suggesting it is part of a more generalized impairment of mucosal immunity in senescence (Koga *et al.*, 2000; Kato *et al.*, 2003).

Influence of intestinal flora

Evidence from both human and veterinary work suggests that clinical FSE may develop subsequent to intestinal infection. As we have noted, the changes in gut flora at the time of weaning may be associated with a period of defective oral tolerance. One of several possible explanations for these findings is that bacterial products may influence the regulation of immune responses to dietary antigens.

The immunomodulatory effects of LPS and other bacterial products are well known. Germfree mice have defective systemic and intestinal immune competence (Moreau and

Corthier, 1988; MacDonald and Carter, 1979; Collins and Campbell, 1980) and cannot be tolerized by feeding SRBC (Wannemuehler et al., 1982). In addition, it is impossible to induce tolerance by feeding SRBC to C3H/HeJ mice that have a mutation in TLR 4 and so cannot respond to LPS (Kiyono et al., 1982; Michalek et al., 1982; Mowat et al., 1986; Kitamura et al., 1987). Unlike normal congenic C3H mice, LPS-unresponsive animals are primed by feeding SRBC and develop systemic antibody and DTH responses as well as local IgA antibodies. These effects were originally associated with a defect in the induction of Treg cells and a parallel appearance of T cells that assisted IgA production and that appeared to localize preferentially among $\alpha\beta$ TcR$^+$ intraepithelial lymphocytes (IEL) (Suzuki et al., 1986a, b; Kitamura et al., 1987; Fujihashi et al., 1989).

This influence of LPS on tolerance to SRBC may reflect the strong thymus-independent component of this antigen, and the effects of bacterial LPS on the induction of oral tolerance to protein antigens are less clear. This develops entirely normally in LPS-unresponsive C3H/HeJ mice (Saklayen et al., 1983; Mowat et al., 1986) and tolerance to haptens and autochthonous gut flora is also normal in these animals (Duchmann et al., 1996; Elson et al., 1996). Exogenous LPS cannot break established T-cell tolerance as it can B-cell tolerance in OVA-fed mice (Mowat et al., 1986). However, if given at the time of feeding, LPS may enhance the induction of T-cell tolerance in normal mice fed OVA (Kim and Ohsawa, 1995; Mowat et al., 1986; Khoury et al., 1990; Khoury et al., 1992), and although significant oral tolerance to proteins can be achieved in germfree mice, certain aspects of the phenomenon are reduced in comparison with conventional animals. Thus tolerance to OVA may be relatively weak or short-lived (Moreau and Corthier, 1988; Moreau and Gaboriau-Routhiau, 1996; Maeda et al., 2001) and may be relatively easy to abrogate with the E. coli LT adjuvant (Matysiak-Budnik et al., 2003b); systemic Th2-mediated IgE responses may also be unusually difficult to tolerize under germfree conditions (Sudo et al., 1997). In addition, there is considerable anecdotal evidence that it has become more difficult to induce oral tolerance in laboratory rodents because the microbiologic status of animal-handling facilities has improved throughout the world. How the germfree state may influence oral tolerance has not been determined, but in the case of systemic Th2 responses, it has been suggested that the immune system in germfree animals has not matured sufficiently to be able to generate the normal balance between Th1 and Th2 functions that allows tolerance to be induced by feeding antigen (Sudo et al., 1997). In addition, the lack of mature T cells in the PP of germfree mice appears to correlate with the failure to induce oral tolerance in these animals (Maeda et al., 2001). A defect in general lymphocyte development or immune responsiveness of this kind is supported by the fact that the uptake of tolerogenic antigen into serum is normal in germfree mice (Furrie et al., 1994). The exact nature of the component of the microflora responsible for allowing full development of oral tolerance is unknown, and it is controversial whether the physiologic state can be restored with single bacterial species such

as Bifidobacterium (Sudo et al., 1997) or whether a more complex flora is required (Matysiak-Budnik et al., 2003b). However, colonization must begin during the neonatal period, emphasizing the close relationship between the intestinal flora and the maturation and maintenance of normal immune homeostasis in the gut. One attractive hypothesis is that LPS or other microbial products present in the microenvironment of the intestine and GALT stimulate the production of immunomodulatory mediators that are required for the generation of tolerogenic mechanisms. In support of this idea, recent studies suggest that exposure to physiologic amounts of LPS may induce intestinal stromal cells to produce immunoregulatory amounts of prostaglandin E_2 (PGE$_2$) (Newberry et al., 1999, 2001) (see the following text).

Role of intestinal absorption and antigen uptake

As we shall discuss, oral tolerance to protein antigens reflects the manner in which the protein is processed in the intestine (see subsequent text). Thus one might predict that any factor that alters either the amount or the chemical nature of the antigen absorbed from the intestine also will influence the immunologic consequences of this material. This idea is supported by the high levels of food-specific antibodies that occur in individuals with disorders that cause increased intestinal permeability to macromolecules, for example, Crohn's disease and celiac disease (Cunningham-Rundles, 1987; Walker, 1987). Experimental factors that increase the amount of protein entering the circulation frequently are associated with prevention of tolerance induction (Louis et al., 1996; Hanson et al., 1993; Furrie et al., 2002). In addition, experimental infection with Helicobacter felis in mice prevents the induction of oral tolerance to OVA in association with increased gastric permeability, and both effects are reversed by rebamipide, a mucosal stabilizing agent (Matysiak-Budnik et al., 1998, 2003b). Nevertheless, no direct correlation between intestinal uptake of antigen and the degree of tolerance and/or active immunity has been established.

The role of proteolytic processing in the intestine is also ill defined, although many workers routinely coadminister agents that inhibit the activity of stomach acid and intestinal proteases. In addition, inhibition of gastric acid production enhances the immunogenicity of proteins in mouse models of IgE-mediated food allergy (Untersmayr et al., 2003). However, partially hydrolyzed fragments comprising as few as 20 amino acids of milk proteins are fully capable of inducing oral tolerance (Pecquet et al., 2000). In addition, it has been reported that administration of the protease inhibitors aprotinin or soya trypsin inhibitor prevents the induction of tolerance by feeding single doses of either MBP or OVA to mice (Hanson et al., 1993; Meyer et al., 1996). Further conflicting evidence comes from reports that trypsin inhibitors may have no effect (Saklayen et al., 1984) or even enhance tolerance associated with both anergy (Migita and Ochi, 1994) and bystander suppression (A. Miller et al., 1993). These discrepancies may partly reflect a species difference between rats and mice, as it is suggested that the absence of a gallbladder in rats inhibits effective absorption of proteins, necessitating the use of protease inhibitors to ensure survival of sufficient protein in the lumen (Meyer *et al.*, 1996). Additionally, individual T-cell epitopes that may be required for inducing different mechanisms of tolerance may also vary in their sensitivity to proteolysis.

Nutritional influences on oral tolerance

The function of the immune system is highly dependent on the nutritional status of the host and there are several reports that protein-calorie malnutrition compromises the ability of animals to make mucosal immune responses (Chandra *et al.*, 1987). Nutritional deficiencies are most likely to occur in the early neonatal period, when the risk of disordered regulation of immunity to fed antigens is also at its highest. It is often difficult to distinguish between the effects of malnutrition itself and those that are the result of secondary complications, such as intestinal abnormalities or infection. One carefully controlled study has shown that mice on an isocaloric low-protein diet have defective induction of tolerance after feeding of OVA and that this defect is related to a primary effect of malnutrition on the immune system (Lamont *et al.*, 1987). If this finding extends to other forms of malnutrition, particularly in developing animals, poor nutritional status could predispose to food hypersensitivity in infancy.

Immunologic status of the host

The ability to suppress established disease will be essential if oral tolerance is to be exploited for treatment of autoimmune disease. Although initial work suggested that a similar effect of priming extended to oral tolerance (Hanson *et al.*, 1979b), several investigators have shown since that oral tolerance can be induced in parenterally primed mice (Lafont *et al.*, 1982; Higgins and Weiner, 1988; Lider *et al.*, 1989; Lamont *et al.*, 1988a; Peng *et al.*, 1989a; Thompson and Staines, 1990; Melamed and Friedman, 1993; Meyer *et al.*, 1996; Leishman *et al.*, 1998, 2000). In addition, as we discuss in the following text, it is also possible to suppress ongoing disease in several experimental models. However, larger doses of fed antigen or more frequent feeds are often required to induce tolerance equivalent to that found in naive animals. In addition, there is only a short time window after systemic priming during which oral tolerance is inducible by a single feed of antigen. This period is generally less than 7 days (Peng *et al.*, 1989a; Melamed and Friedman, 1993; Leishman *et al.*, 1998), although some workers found that this can be extended using repeated feeds of antigen (Peng *et al.*, 1989a; Meyer *et al.*, 1996; Melamed and Friedman, 1993; Y. Chung *et al.*, 1999). However, our own experience was that repeated feeds of even large doses of antigen did not substantially alter the scope or timing of tolerance in primed mice (Leishman *et al.*, 1998, 2000). Tolerance to protein antigens in primed animals can affect all aspects of T-cell mediated immune responses, including DTH, proliferation and the production of both Th1 and Th2 cytokines including IFN-γ production. However, serum antibody responses are unaffected or enhanced, even using doses of antigen equivalent to or greater than those that tolerize these responses in naive animals (Lamont *et al.*, 1988a; Peng *et al.*, 1989a; Leishman *et al.*, 1998, 2000; Y. Chung *et al.*, 1999), with prolonged and continuous feeding of high doses of antigen soon after primary immunization being the only regimen reported to suppress antibody production (Conde *et al.*, 1998). Thus the immune system may only be susceptible to intestinally derived tolerogenic signals during the early expansion and effector stages, but not once stable priming has been achieved. The mechanisms regulating tolerance in primed animals may be distinct from those induced by the same regimens in naive animals, although in both cases, tolerance is intact in IL-4 KO mice (Leishman *et al.*, 1998). The reasons for the resistance of primed mice to the induction of may include the appearance of primary serum antibodies (Leishman *et al.*, 1998), which are known to interfere with the induction of oral tolerance (Hanson *et al.*, 1979b; Melamed and Friedman, 1993), as well as inherent resistance of primed antigen-specific T cells to tolerance induction (Leishman *et al.*, 2000; Y. Chung *et al.*, 1999). These factors, together with the selectivity of the tolerance induced in primed animals, will be important considerations in designing clinically useful therapeutic regimens. Recent studies showing that coupling a number of antigens to CT-B enhances the induction of oral tolerance in primed animals offer one possible approach to this problem (J. B. Sun *et al.*, 1996; Rask *et al.*, 2000). The β2 adrenergic agonist salbutamol has also been shown to increase the tolerogenic potential of feeding proteins to primed mice (Cobelens *et al.*, 2002b), and these strategies are discussed in more detail in the following text.

MECHANISMS OF ORAL TOLERANCE

Introduction

Oral tolerance is one of a number of forms of peripheral tolerance in which administration of nominal antigen to mature animals induces immunologic unresponsiveness, presumably without gaining access to central lymphoid organs such as the thymus. The understanding of peripheral tolerance has been revolutionized in recent years by the application of new techniques in molecular and cellular immunology, and these approaches have enabled considerable advances to be made in the field of oral tolerance.

Immunoregulation and peripheral tolerance

The mechanisms that have been derived as a result can be classified broadly as those involving direct inactivation of antigen-specific lymphocytes via clonal deletion or anergy or those requiring interactions between regulatory and effector T cells, principally of the CD4$^+$ subset **(Table 27.1)**. Although once these were considered to be entirely distinct mechanisms, there is now substantial evidence that clonal anergy and active regulation may be related properties of the same cell, and many older studies of these topics need to be reconsidered carefully in this light. In addition, it is likely

Table 27.1. Potential Mechanisms of Tolerance (see text for details)

Clonal deletion	Self antigens in thymus
	Very high doses peripheral antigens?
	Apoptosis after ligation of TcR
Clonal anergy	? self antigens in thymus
	Self-antigens in periphery
	Harmless foreign antigens in periphery (foods, commensals, etc.)
	TcR ligation in absence of costimulation (or with dominant negative costimulation by, for example, CTLA-4, PD-1) → partial activation, failure to transcribe IL-2 gene, defective clonal expansion, and no proliferation/IL-2 production on challenge
Regulatory T cells	T cells actively inhibit priming/functions of other, naive T cells
	Self-antigens in thymus—CD4$^+$CD25$^+$ T cells
	Self or foreign antigens in periphery
	CD4$^+$CD25$^+$ T cells generated by aberrant selection in thymus
	Regulatory T cells induced in periphery by resting APC or APC conditioned by, for example, IL-10
	CD4$^+$CD25$^+$ T cells act by cytokines, cell–cell contact
	Peripheral Treg cells act by producing IL10/TGF-β (T_R1, T_H3)

that more than one mechanism may be operating at any one time under different conditions.

Clonal deletion is the principal mechanism involved in the elimination of self-reactive T cells in the thymus and has also been observed after peripheral exposure to tolerogenic antigen. It involves the permanent removal of antigen-specific T cells via an apoptotic pathway and generally requires high-affinity T-cell recognition. Clonal anergy was first described *in vitro* and is the consequence of inappropriate presentation of antigen, either because of a lack of any costimulatory molecules on the APC or because of the selective involvement of inhibitory costimulatory molecules such as cytotoxic T-lymphocyte-associated protein 4 (CTLA-4) (Schwartz, 2003). It has also been reported in a number of models of peripheral tolerance *in vivo*, and its critical feature is that antigen-specific T cells survive the encounter with tolerogen, but are subsequently unable to proliferate or produce IL-2 in response to immunogenic stimuli. Until recently, it was believed that anergic T cells were bereft of all functions, but it is now clear that they may retain a number of activities, including the production of cytokines such as IL-4 and IL-10 (Buer *et al.*, 1998; Lanoue *et al.*, 1997; Ryan and Evavold, 1998). Furthermore, there are a number of instances in which anergic CD4$^+$ T cells appear to act as suppressor cells *in vivo* and *in vitro* (Lombardi *et al.*, 1994; Hirahara *et al.*, 1995; Lombardi *et al.*, 1997; Cauley *et al.*, 1997; Thornton and Shevach, 1998; Takahashi *et al.*, 1998; Taams *et al.*, 1998). This has led to a blurring between the distinction between "anergic" T cells and Treg cells, with many of the latter being similarly unable to proliferate or produce IL-2 when stimulated via their TcR.

Treg cells were first described in the 1970s, when they were considered to be mainly CD8$^+$ and were referred to as "suppressor" T cells. After falling into disrepute during the 1980s and 1990s, the idea that certain T cells could have the specific

function of preventing or modulating immune responses has been resurrected in recent years and indeed the study of such Treg cells is currently one of the most rapidly moving topics in immunology. The majority of the newer generation of Treg cells are CD4$^+$ T cells, but a large number of different subsets have been described under different conditions. The relationships between them are not always clear. The current view is that there may be two major groups, "innate" and "adaptive," the former arising principally in the thymus as a result of T-cell selection by self-antigens and the latter differentiating from naive CD4$^+$ T cells in response to external antigen (Bluestone and Abbas, 2003; Bach and Bach, 2003). The best understood of the innate Treg cells are those characterized by expression of the IL-2 receptor α chain (CD25), which first came to light during studies of the autoimmune disorder that occurs after neonatal thymectomy of rodents (Hori *et al.*, 2003b; Bach and Bach, 2003). This disease can be prevented by the transfer of CD4$^+$CD25$^+$ T cells, and many subsequent studies have shown that this subset of T cell has potent immunosuppressive properties *in vitro* and *in vivo*. CD4$^+$CD25$^+$ Treg cells are anergic to TcR stimulation *in vitro*, but can proliferate efficiently *in vivo*, and their suppressive activities are completely dependent on triggering via the TcR. The mechanisms involved in their suppressive activities are controversial and may require cell–cell contact *in vitro*, but the production of cytokines such as IL-10 and TGF-β *in vivo* (Hori *et al.*, 2003b; Bach and Bach, 2003). One unifying suggestion is that this apparent discrepancy reflects the expression of membrane-bound TGF-β (Nakamura *et al.*, 2001, 2004). CD4$^+$CD25$^+$ Treg cells express self-reactive TcR of very high affinity and appear to be the product of aberrant selection in the thymus under the control of a unique transcription factor, Foxp-3 (Jordan *et al.*, 2001; Hori *et al.*, 2003a, b). It has proved difficult to identify other specific markers of CD4$^+$CD25$^+$ Treg cells, although they express glucocorticoid inducible TNF-related receptor (GITR), a member of the TNF receptor family (Hori *et al.*, 2003b). Although the subset is believed to be important in regulating autoimmune diseases, it is controversial whether this subset can recognize foreign antigens and be involved in models of tolerance such as oral tolerance. However, there are accumulating reports that CD4+CD25+ Treg cells may regulate immune responses to exogenous antigen in, for example, infectious disease, chronic inflammation, and allergy in animal models and humans, including IBD (Takahashi *et al.*, 1998; McHugh and Shevach, 2002; Maloy *et al.*, 2003; Xu *et al.*, 2003). As we shall discuss, it has also been suggested that CD4+CD5+ Treg cells be induced during oral tolerance. Recent work suggests that CD4+CD25+ Treg cells may not only produce TGF-β themselves, but that this cytokine can induce FOXP3-mediated differentiation of naive CD4+ T cells into CD4+CD25+ Treg cells (W. Chen *et al.*, 2003), supporting other suggestions that this subset may develop in the periphery in response to antigen (Thorstenson and Khoruts, 2001).

Another population of "innate" Treg cells is characterized by the expression of the natural killer (NK) cell marker, NK1.1. These are also the products of thymic selection by self-antigens, but many of the Treg cells express oligoclonal TcR, and they are restricted mainly by the nonclassical MHC molecule CD1; as a result, the nature of the antigens they recognize is unclear. NK T cells of this kind have been shown to be important in regulating several models of autoimmune disease including type 1 diabetes, often via the production of the cytokines IL-4 and IL-10 (Bach and Francois Bach, 2003; Bluestone and Abbas, 2003). They have also been implicated in oral tolerance.

The group of "adaptive" Treg cells contains a variety of subsets, all of which seem to be the result of exposure to exogenous antigens in the peripheral immune system and which are distinguished by the profile of cytokines they produce. In this way, they are analogous to the well-known Th1 and Th2 subsets of CD4+ helper cells, with their differentiation from naive T cells being determined by the local immunomodulatory microenvironments or the nature of the APC. Like CD4+CD25+ Treg cells adaptive Treg cells are mostly anergic *in vitro*, but have potent immunosuppressive functions *in vivo* and *in vitro*. Of these, the most well described are the Th3 and Tr1 cells. As we shall see, Th3 cells were first described in oral tolerance and are characterized by the production of TGF-β and to a lesser extent, IL-10 (Y. Chen *et al.*, 1994; Faria and Weiner, 1999). Although similar cells have been noted in other systems, the factors regulating their differentiation are generally unclear. Tr1 cells, on the other hand, have been studied mainly *in vitro*, where they differentiate under the specific influence of the cytokines IL-10, type 1 IFN, and IL-15 and are characterized by the production of IL-10, together with smaller amounts of IFN-γ (Roncarolo *et al.*, 2001; Groux, 2003). Tr1 have also been implicated in the regulation of allograft responses *in vivo* (Hara *et al.*, 2001), and *in vitro*–generated Tr1 cells have been shown to inhibit experimental colitis in mice (Groux *et al.*, 1997; and see the following text). A further population of CD4+ Treg cells is the CD45RB^lo subset identified by its

ability to modulate rodent models of IBD via the production of IL-10 and/or TGF-β (Powrie *et al.*, 1996; Maloy and Powrie, 2001). Although a substantial proportion of the regulatory activity of these cells is associated with the CD25+ subset (Mottet *et al.*, 2003), it appears that they may be more similar to the adaptive group of Treg cells, as they seem to recognize gut bacteria, rather than self-antigens.

Thus a number of different CD4+ Treg cells have been described, with a variety of different properties and mechanisms for suppressing immune responses. As many of them have been identified under different experimental conditions, it has been difficult to determine if each subset truly represents an independent population of T cell, or if their functional differences simply reflect the study of cells at distinct stages of differentiation.

Bystander suppression

One of the most important properties of all the Treg cells that have been described is their ability to mediate bystander suppression, in which T cells specific for one antigen can suppress the function of T cells of other specificities, providing both antigens are present together. The phenomenon was first described when it was shown that cells from animals fed low doses of MBP could suppress the proliferation of an OVA-specific T-cell line providing both antigens were present in the restimulation culture (A. Miller *et al.*, 1991). The suppression was active across a Transwell membrane and was at least partly dependent on TGF-β. Since then, the phenomenon has been studied in a number of situations during oral tolerance *in vivo*, and the practical implications of the phenomenon are discussed in detail in the following text. However, an appreciation of the fundamental principles involved is also important for a fuller understanding of how mucosal immune responses are regulated.

Work on individual populations of Treg cells has attempted to determine the mechanisms responsible for bystander suppression, but no consensus has emerged. With a few exceptions (Carvalho *et al.*, 1994, 1997), the phenomenon *in vivo* requires the two antigens to be present in the same anatomic site, and in all cases, the Treg cells have to be triggered via its TcR. One obvious way to explain these findings is that the Treg cells and the target T cell interact indirectly via an APC that is presenting both antigens simultaneously. This idea is supported by several reports that APC are necessary for bystander suppression to be effective *in vitro* (Taams *et al.*, 1998; Cobbold *et al.*, 2003) and that Treg cells can inhibit the APC function of DC (Cederbom *et al.*, 2000; Vendetti *et al.*, 2000; Min *et al.*, 2003). In addition, recent studies have shown that Treg cells induced by feeding nickel salts can induce APC to become tolerogenic *in vivo* (Roelofs-Haarhuis *et al.*, 2003). These effects would be analogous to the way in which CD4+ helper T cells can assist the activation of CD8+ T cells by "licensing" DC to express appropriate costimulatory molecules (Lanzavecchia, 1998; Schoenberger *et al.*, 1998). However, others have contested the need for APC in the delivery of bystander suppression, and the molecular basis is unknown, with controversy over whether it requires cell–cell contact or the production of cytokines such as IL-10 and TGF-β (Bach and Bach, 2003; Thornton and Shevach, 2000; Hori *et al.*, 2003b). Irrespective of the precise mechanisms involved, bystander suppression is potentially central to the use of oral tolerance in most disease-related models of autoimmune disease, where the antigen initiating disease is usually not the one used to induce tolerance and may in fact not be known at all. However, the ability to induce bystander effects may allow functional tolerance against tissue antigens to be induced by feeding an unrelated, but defined antigen.

Clonal anergy and deletion of T cells in oral tolerance

Several early studies reported that T-cell tolerance in antigen-fed mice did not necessarily correlate with the presence of Treg cells (Titus and Chiller, 1981; Hanson and Miller, 1982; Tomasi *et al.*, 1983), and tolerance of humoral immunity was frequently not transferable by Treg cells (Mowat, 1987). More detailed experiments using limiting dilution analysis then showed that mice fed MBP had reduced frequencies of antigen-specific IL-2 and IFN-γ-producing T cells in the absence of transferable Ts (Whitacre *et al.*, 1991). These results indicated that antigen-specific T cells could be inactivated directly by fed antigen, which could reflect deletion or functional anergy of individual T cells.

Clonal deletion

Clonal deletion is the principal mechanism responsible for tolerance of self-reactive T cells in the thymus, but is rarely seen after induction of peripheral tolerance using nominal antigen in mature animals. Experiments in fully TcR transgenic mice have suggested that feeding high doses of OVA can induce clonal deletion of antigen-specific CD4+ T cells in the PP (Y. Chen *et al.*, 1995a; Marth *et al.*, 1996, 1999; Meyer *et al.*, 2001) and other tissues including the spleen, thymus, and peripheral lymph nodes (LN) (Y. Chen *et al.*, 1995a; Meyer *et al.*, 2001; Marth *et al.*, 1999). In addition, a very recent study observed increased caspase activity and decreased levels of caspase-sensitive proteins in antigen-specific CD4+ T cells after long-term feeding of OVA to TcR transgenic mice, findings consistent with apoptosis of the T cells (Kaji *et al.*, 2003). Nevertheless, very high amounts of high antigen (up to 500 mg daily) or additional neutralization of anti-IL-12 (Marth *et al.*, 1999) were required to induce T-cell deletion in some of these studies, and clonal deletion was not observed in one further study of this kind (Y. Chen *et al.*, 1996). In addition, it is now appreciated that fully TcR transgenic mice are not appropriate models to study immunoregulation *in vivo*, because of the very high proportion of identical, high-affinity specific T cells present. Similar reservations apply to experiments in which clonal deletion was detected in wild-type mice fed the superantigen staphylococcal enterotoxin B (SEB) (Migita and Ochi, 1994; Migita *et al.*, 1995; Nishimura *et al.*, 2002). One further proviso is that several of the studies that concluded that deletion of TcR transgenic T cells was occurring were based on the disappearance of TcR-expressing lymphocytes. This could reflect downregulation of the TcR consequent on cellular activation rather than true disappearance of the cells.

Clonal deletion has not been demonstrated directly in normal animals after feeding antigen or in models using the adoptive transfer of limited numbers of identifiable TcR transgenic T cells into wild-type mice (Van Houten and Blake, 1996). One study using this latter approach found that the number of transgenic cells in peripheral tissues decreased below that of unfed controls 20 days after feeding high doses of OVA peptide, as did experiments in which animals transgenic only for the TcRβ gene were fed high doses of cytochrome c (Gütgemann *et al.*, 1998). Nevertheless, neither of these studies examined for apoptotic cells, and the possibility that the apparent disappearance of cells simply reflected anatomic redistribution of antigen-specific cells was not excluded (Y. Chen *et al.*, 1997). Nevertheless, it should be noted that feeding antigen to normal animals does increase the susceptibility of their lymphocytes to die by apoptosis after systemic challenge with antigen in adjuvant (Garside *et al.*, 1996). In these experiments, lymphocytes from mice fed single, high doses of OVA died rapidly when cultured *in vitro* in the absence of antigen, showing morphologic and cytologic evidence of apoptosis. However, this phenomenon affected both CD4+ and CD8+ T cells and frequently resulted in the loss of up to 90% of the starting population, a proportion too high to be accounted for by the numbers of antigen-specific T cells. Together with the fact that oral tolerance is normal in fas-deficient lpr mice **(Fig. 27.5)**, these findings argue against the involvement of conventional fas-mediated clonal deletion of T cells in oral tolerance under normal conditions. Although it has been reported that oral tolerance may be defective in mice lacking the p55 type 1 TNF receptor (Gardine *et al.*, 2001), this is more likely to reflect the abnormalities in lymphoid anatomy in these mice, and the role of other mechanisms of apoptosis in oral tolerance has not been studied in detail.

Clonal anergy

The possibility that clonal anergy occurs in oral tolerance was first suggested by low-dose antigen studies and by experiments in which T-cell tolerance could be reversed *in vitro* by exogenous IL-2 (Whitacre *et al.*, 1991). Responsiveness to IL-2 and the absence of transferable suppression were then used as the criteria for defining clonal anergy as the principal mechanism underlying oral tolerance to high doses of fed antigen (reviewed in Weiner *et al.*, 1994). This conclusion has been confirmed more directly in work using adoptively transferred TcR transgenic T cells (Williamson *et al.*, 1999a; Van Houten and Blake, 1996; J. Sun *et al.*, 1999; Shi *et al.*, 2000). In these experiments, antigen-specific CD4+ T cells undergo transient activation and clonal expansion *in vivo* after feeding tolerogenic doses of antigen. These responses are initially similar to those found after priming with antigen in adjuvant, but are more limited and transient. After feeding, the antigen-specific T cells go through fewer cell divisions and then become unre-

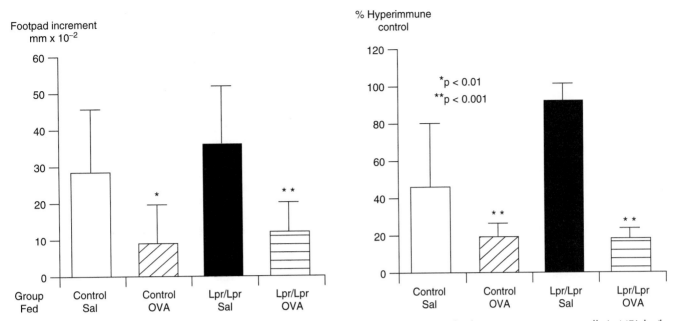

Fig. 27.5. Oral tolerance does not require fas. Suppression of systemic DTH and serum IgG antibody responses occurs normally in MRL lpr/lpr mice fed 25 mg OVA before immunization.

sponsive to subsequent restimulation with antigen (J. Sun *et al.*, 2003). Similar abortive priming of T cells occurs in normal animals fed proteins (Gautam *et al.*, 1990; Hoyne and Thomas, 1995; Hoyne *et al.*, 1993a; Y. Chen *et al.*, 1997; Mowat *et al.*, 1999), and together, these features are similar to those reported in other models of tolerance in which T-cell anergy predominates (Pape *et al.*, 1997; Mueller and Jenkins, 1995; Sloan-Lancaster and Allen, 1996). In addition, antigen-specific T cells in fully TcR transgenic mice fed continuous high doses of antigen show intracellular signaling abnormalities similar to those seen in models of T-cell anergy *in vitro*, including failure of nuclear factor of activated T cells (NF-AT) nuclear localization and accumulation of the cell cycle inhibitor p27^{kip} (Asai *et al.*, 2002). Similar findings have been made in mice fed SEB, where antigen-specific T cells show an identical defect in signaling to that found after induction of clonal anergy by intravenous injection of antigen (Migita and Ochi, 1994; Migita *et al.*, 1995; Nishimura *et al.*, 2002). Finally, there is evidence for clonal anergy of food antigen-specific T cells in humans, as restimulation of peripheral blood lymphocytes induces upregulation of the IL-2 receptor α chain (CD25) in the absence of proliferation (Zivny *et al.*, 2001).

Initial studies led to the idea that clonal anergy was the tolerogenic mechanism induced preferentially by feeding high doses of antigen, but as we have noted, all these findings now need to be interpreted in the light of the evidence that anergic cells may function as active Treg cells. Indeed, it has been shown that T cells "anergized" by feeding antigen can survive for long periods in secondary recipients (Hirahara *et al.*, 1995) and act as regulatory cells under such circumstances (Artik *et al.*, 2001; Hirahara *et al.*, 1995). *In vitro*

cultures of food antigen–specific human anergic lymphocytes also show some evidence of bystander suppression of responses to unrelated antigens (Zivny *et al.*, 2001). In view of the fact that it is now clear that there is significant repopulation of the immune system by naive cells emigrating from the thymus, even in adults, survival of anergic cells with regulatory function would be a much more useful means of maintaining tolerance. It will be important to reexamine the relationship between anergic and Treg cells in tolerized animals.

Regulatory T cells and bystander suppression

The earliest mechanistic studies viewed oral tolerance as an example of a "suppressor" cell–mediated phenomenon, which could be transferred by CD8$^+$ T cells and prevented by agents that were believed to deplete these cells, such as cyclophosphamide (reviewed in Mowat, 1987). Although much of this work was never substantiated at the molecular level and the CD8$^+$ Treg cells were not well characterized, the field has recently returned to the idea that Treg cells are the principal mechanisms involved. Initially associated primarily with tolerance induced by multiple low doses of antigen (Weiner *et al.*, 1994; Franco *et al.*, 1998), Treg cells may play an even wider role in oral tolerance, and a number of such cells have been proposed.

CD4$^+$ T cells

In common with many other systems, current work has emphasized the possibility that CD4$^+$ T cells are the principal Treg cells involved in oral tolerance. Depletion of CD8$^+$ T cells using genetically engineered CD8 or β2m KO mice (Lycke *et al.*, 1995; Vistica *et al.*, 1996; Gardine *et al.*, 2001) or treatment of mice with anti-CD8 antibodies (Garside *et al.*,

1995a; Y. Chen *et al.*, 1995b; Barone *et al.*, 1995; Vistica *et al.*, 1996) has no effect on the induction of systemic tolerance by feeding antigen. Conversely, depletion of CD4+ T cells at the time of feeding antigen prevents the induction of tolerance to OVA (Garside *et al.*, 1995a; Barone *et al.*, 1995), and CD4 KO mice do not become tolerant to contact sensitizing agents, even when the effector response is mediated by CD8+ T cells (Desvignes *et al.*, 1996; Dubois *et al.*, 2003). Oral tolerance can also be transferred by CD4+ T cells (Hirahara *et al.*, 1995; Y. Chen *et al.*, 1995b, 1996; Artik *et al.*, 2001). The exact nature of the regulatory CD4+ T cells remains unclear. They were originally thought to be classical Th2 cells that could suppress Th1-dependent immune responses via the production of IL-4 and IL-10 (Khoury *et al.*, 1992; Weiner *et al.*, 1994; Fishman-Lobell *et al.*, 1994; Y. Chen *et al.*, 1994, 1996; Melamed and Friedman, 1994; Melamed *et al.*, 1996; Neurath *et al.*, 1996), but most workers find that oral tolerance can be induced normally in IL-4 or stat 6 KO mice that lack Th2 cells (Garside *et al.*, 1995b; Wolvers *et al.*, 1997; Mowat, 1999b; Shi *et al.*, 1999b; Rizzo *et al.*, 1999) and also in mice treated with anti-IL-4 antibodies (Wolvers *et al.*, 1997). The exceptions to these findings appear to be restricted to models of disease that are particularly susceptible to modulation by IL-4, such as experimental arthritis (Yoshino, 1998; Yoshino and Yoshino, 1998) and type 1 diabetes (Homann *et al.*, 1999). In addition, the possibility that IL-4 acts as specific growth and differentiation factor for TGF-β-producing T cells complicates interpretation of such work (Inobe *et al.*, 1998). For these reasons, more recent ideas have centered on the possible involvement of one or other of the subsets of CD4+ Treg cells alluded to in the preceding text.

CD4+CD25+ Treg cells. This is currently the most highly studied cell in T-cell immunology and is believed to play a central role in many forms of immune regulation. It is therefore not surprising that several workers have attempted to define a role for CD4+CD25+ Treg cells in oral tolerance. The first evidence that this might be the case came from studies in which OVA-specific TcR transgenic CD4+ T cells were adoptively transferred into normal recipients that were fed tolerogenic doses of OVA (Thorstenson and Khoruts, 2001). Under these conditions, the transgenic T cells expanded clonally in the MLN and peripheral tissues, but a few days after clonal expansion had terminated, a small population of antigen-specific CD4+CD25+ T cells remained present. These did not produce IL-2 when restimulated *in vitro*, and there was no selective production of any cytokines. Similar cells were generated after intravenous induction of tolerance using low doses of peptide, and in this case, these were shown directly to have Treg cell activity, suggesting that their induction was a specific consequence of tolerance induction. Interestingly, the CD4+CD25+ T cells did not undergo full clonal expansion during the initial response to fed antigen, and it was suggested that their generation requires failure to undergo an adequate number of cell divisions after primary contact with antigen. A more recent study using the same adoptive transfer model has also provided evidence that a population of CD4+CD25+ Treg cells arises in the GALT after feeding a high dose of tolero-

genic antigen (Hauet-Broere *et al.*, 2003). However, in this case, the regulatory activity was not restricted to the CD4+CD25+ population, but was a function of all antigen-specific T cells that had divided in response to antigen, irrespective of whether they were CD25+ or CD25−. In addition, these Treg cells arose within 2–3 days of feeding antigen, rather than after the primary response had waned. As in the initial work, the Treg cells did not produce cytokines such as IL-10, but expressed CTLA-4, a costimulatory molecule that has been associated with the function of anergic Treg cells in other systems (Bluestone and Abbas, 2003). These are clearly antigen-induced T cells, but whether their properties genuinely reflect a distinct subset of regulatory T cell rather than unusual functions of a recently divided cell remains to be ascertained. In studies using fully TcR transgenic DO11.10 mice, it has also been found that oral administration of high doses of OVA resulted in a relative increase of CD4+CD25+ Treg cells in the PP (X. Zhang *et al.*, 2001; Nagatani *et al.*, 2004). These express CTLA-4 (X. Zhang *et al.*, 2001) and also FOXP-3, the transcription factor associated with the development of CD4+CD25+ Treg cells (Nagatani *et al.*, 2004). The CD4+CD25+ Treg cells, persisted for up to 4 weeks after feeding, were anergic *in vitro*, and secreted high levels of IL-10 and TGF-β. In addition, they were capable of suppressing DTH responses in naive recipients (X. Zhang *et al.*, 2001; Nagatani *et al.*, 2004). They also acted as Treg cells *in vitro*, an activity that was partly inhibited by blocking IL-10, TGF-β, or CTLA-4 (X. Zhang *et al.*, 2001). As yet, there is only one study of CD4+CD25+ Treg cell activity during oral tolerance in unmanipulated mice. In this work, depletion of CD4+CD25+ T cells from normal mice prevented the tolerance of CD8+ T cell–mediated contact sensitivity induced by feeding hapten (Dubois *et al.*, 2003). Furthermore, the defect in this tolerance that occurs in invariant chain KO mice because of a lack of CD4+ T cells can be restored by transfer of CD4+CD25+ T cells from normal mice (Dubois *et al.*, 2003). Although it is not clear what antigen is recognized by the CD4+CD25+ Treg cells in these experiments, they appear to act by directly inhibiting the clonal expansion and differentiation of hapten-specific CD8+ T cells. The question of antigen specificity of CD4+CD25+ Treg cells in oral tolerance has been partly addressed by another recent report in which antigen-specific Treg cells were cloned from the PP of mice fed multiple low doses of β lactoglobulin; the cloned Treg cells were CD4+CD25+, produced TGF-β, and were anergic (Tsuji *et al.*, 2003; Tsuji and Nowak, 2004). Preliminary work suggests that an unusual feature of these cells was that they were IL-18 responsive and this model of oral tolerance was defective in IL-18 KO mice (Tsuji and Nowak, 2004). The significance of these findings is unclear, and as with the study by Hauet-Broere *et al.*, (Hauet-Broere *et al.*, 2003), it is important to emphasize that all activated CD4+ T cells express CD25, as expression of this molecule by recently activated or cloned T cells cannot be taken as a stable phenotypic marker of Treg cell function. It is also controversial whether CD4+CD25+ Treg cells can be generated *de novo* after exposure to exogenous antigen and several workers believe that they are entirely self-reactive T cells that develop in the thymus (Bluestone and Abbas, 2003; Hori *et al.*, 2003b). Thus experiments ascribing a role for CD4+CD25+ Treg cells in antigen-specific oral tolerance need to be interpreted with great caution.

Th3 and TGF-β. As we have noted, Th3 cells were first isolated and cloned from the lymphoid tissues of mice tolerized by feeding low doses of antigen (Khoury *et al.*, 1992; Weiner *et al.*, 1994; Y. Chen *et al.*, 1994, 1997; Fukaura *et al.*, 1996). Although they have some similarities to Th2 cells, producing variable amounts of characteristic Th2 products such as IL-4 and IL-10, they have a unique ability to produce TGF-β, a cytokine that has been widely implicated in oral tolerance and other forms of immunoregulation.

There is considerable evidence that TGF-β is involved in the regulation of intestinal immune responses, although the cell involved has not been identified with certainty. Initial studies indicated that the ability of tolerized CD8+ T cells to mediate bystander suppression after feeding MBP is dependent on production of TGF-β (A. Miller *et al.*, 1992). Subsequently it was demonstrated that natural recovery from EAE and its prevention by feeding MBP were accompanied by upregulated TGF-β production *in vivo* (Khoury *et al.*, 1992). As we have noted earlier, increased production of TGF-β has been identified directly in the PP, LP, and draining lymphoid tissues after induction of oral tolerance and also in lymphoid tissues that have been restimulated after induction of tolerance (Y. Chen *et al.*, 1995a; Gonnella *et al.*, 1998, 2001; Weiner, 1997; Pecquet *et al.*, 1999; Lundin *et al.*, 1999; DePaolo *et al.*, 2003). This appears to be associated mainly with CD4+ T cells, but TGF-β-secreting CD4+ and CD8+ T cells can be isolated and cloned from the PP and MLN of orally tolerized mice (Y. Chen *et al.*, 1994, 1996; Santos *et al.*, 1994; Wang *et al.*, 1994; Alpan *et al.*, 2001), as well as from the peripheral blood of humans fed MBP (Fukaura *et al.*, 1996) and mice fed streptococcal cell wall antigens (W. Chen *et al.*, 1998a). Further circumstantial evidence that local production of TGF-β is important in regulating immune responses to food proteins comes from a recent work that food allergic children have decreased numbers of TGF-β-secreting cells in the duodenal mucosa compared with normal controls (Perez-Machado *et al.*, 2003). TGF-β production is also preserved preferentially in transgenic mice with T-cell deletion or anergy induced by feeding high doses of OVA or OVA peptide (Y. Chen *et al.*, 1995a, 1997; Marth, 1996; Marth *et al.*, 2000), a phenomenon markedly enhanced by depletion of IL-12 *in vivo* (Marth *et al.*, 1996). Finally, the absence of high dose oral tolerance in MCP-1 (CCL2) or CCR2 KO mice is associated with failure to upregulate TGF-β production in the PP, as is seen in normal animals (DePaolo *et al.*, 2003). The source of TGF-β under these conditions is uncertain, given that the majority of antigen-specific T cells are deleted in antigen-fed transgenic mice, but again was believed to be CD4+ T cells. However, it should be noted that many other cell types found in the mucosa produce TGF-β, including macrophages and enterocytes (Barnard *et al.*, 1993). How these cells could contribute to antigen-specific tolerance is unclear, although one study has suggested that antigen-pulsed epithelial cells

may inhibit T-cell activation via production of TGF-β (Galliaerde *et al.*, 1995). A recent study of oral tolerance of IgE-mediated immunopathology in dogs has provided evidence for an additional potential source of TGF-β after the induction of oral tolerance, as it demonstrated preferential upregulation of its mRNA in CD14+ monocyte/macrophages in bronchoalveolar lavage fluid (Zemann *et al.*, 2003). Nevertheless, a specific failure of T cells to respond to TGF-β is associated with similar immune dysfunction to that seen in the complete absence of the cytokine (Gorelik and Flavell, 2000; Lucas *et al.*, 2000).

Several aspects of oral tolerance can be inhibited by anti-TGF-β antibody *in vitro* or *in vivo* (Neurath *et al.*, 1996; Weiner, 1997; Haneda *et al.*, 1997). The general importance of TGF-β in immune regulation is supported by the fact that TGF-β KO mice die soon after birth because of widespread inflammatory disease. One group attempted to overcome this problem by treating TGF-β KO mice from birth with anti-LFA-1 antibody to prevent inflammation and showed that these animals can be tolerized by feeding high (10–20 mg) or low (1 mg) doses of OVA (Barone *et al.*, 1998). However, certain aspects of systemic tolerance were less pronounced in the TGF-β KO mice, and some KO mice fed lower doses of OVA exhibited no tolerance or even priming of systemic proliferative responses. These experiments suggest that TGF-β may play an important role in oral tolerance, but the complicating effects of anti-LFA-1 treatment make this study difficult to interpret definitively.

The evidence that TGF-β may play a critical role in oral tolerance is consistent with findings from other models of tolerance and Treg cell activity. In particular, the ability of CD4+CD45RB^lo T cells to prevent colitis in scid mice given CD4+CD45RB^hi T cells is dependent on the production of TGF-β by CD4+CD25+ Treg cells (Maloy *et al.*, 2003; Xu *et al.*, 2003; Nakamura *et al.*, 2004; Powrie *et al.*, 1996; Groux and Powrie, 1999; Oida *et al.*, 2003), as is the protective effect of feeding antigen on the colitis induced by local administration of contact sensitizing agents to normal animals (Neurath *et al.*, 1996). The regulation of type 1 insulin-dependent diabetes mellitus (IDDM) by CD4+CD25+ Treg cells (Green *et al.*, 2003) and the induction of tolerance via the anterior chamber of the eye (Streilein, 1999; Takeuchi *et al.*, 1998; D'Orazio and Niederkorn, 1998a) are also dependent on TGF-β. Nevertheless, the exact role of TGF-β in immunoregulation remains controversial, and the cellular basis of its induction and actions is unclear. There is some evidence that TGF-β secretion by CD4+ T cells may be controlled by distinctive processes or is a feature shown by T cells at a unique stage of differentiation. The Th3 cells cloned from tolerized mice appear to be dependent on IL-4, rather than IL2, for their growth, and some Th3 clones produce IL-4 and/or IL-10 together with TGF-β (Inobe *et al.*, 1998). TGF-β itself can also enhance the differentiation of Th3 cells, a process that can be enhanced by IL-10 or anti-IL-12 (Paul and Seder, 1994; Weiner, 1997). Local production of TGF-β is also absent in B-cell KO mice (Gonnella *et al.*, 2001), although how B cells control T-cell differentiation to a TGF-β-producing phenotype is unclear. As discussed in the following text, there is evidence that DC in PP may selectively enhance TGF-β production in a manner dependent on MCP-1/CCR2 (DePaolo *et al.*, 2003).

Recent studies have highlighted the idea that TGF-β production is a feature of anergic Treg cells (Groux, 2003; Bach and Bach, 2003), and recent work has suggested that murine CD4⁺CD25⁺ Treg cells express TGF-β and its latency-associated peptide (LAP) on the surface after activation. The regulatory function of these cells *in vitro* is reported to be dependent on TGF-β (Nakamura *et al.*, 2001, 2004). If confirmed, this finding might help explain the apparent controversy between whether Treg cells act via cell–cell contact or by production of cytokines. We have also found that latency-associated peptide-expressing (LAP-expressing) T cells are a critical component of the population of CD45RB^lo cells that regulate CD4⁺CD45RB^hi-induced colitis (Oida *et al.*, 2003). In this system, LAP was expressed on both CD4⁺CD25⁺ and CD4⁺CD25⁻ cells, and the LAP⁺ cells were also positive for thrombospondin, a natural converter of latent TGF-β to its active form. Their regulatory function *in vivo* was abrogated by treatment with anti-TGF-β monoclonal antibodies (Oida *et al.*, 2003). It would be important to investigate the role of TGF-β/LAP⁺ T cells in oral tolerance.

A further link between active regulation via TGF-β and mechanisms more traditionally associated with clonal anergy is suggested by the report that cross-linking CTLA-4 on T cells may induce the production of TGF-β (W. Chen *et al.*, 1998b). CTLA-4 is thought to be one of the main costimulatory molecules involved in the induction of T-cell anergy and tolerance (Greenwald *et al.*, 2002; Sharpe and Freeman, 2002), is expressed by many subsets of Treg cells (see the preceding text), and has been implicated in the regulation of both inflammation and tolerance in the intestine (Read *et al.*, 2000; X. Zhang *et al.*, 2001; Barone *et al.*, 2002; Y. Chen *et al.*, 2002; Fowler and Powrie, 2002). Again these findings suggest that active regulation and anergy may be overlapping mechanisms in oral tolerance. TGF-β could also be involved in regimens that appear to induce clonal deletion in oral tolerance. In addition to the fact that uptake of apoptotic cells by phagocytic cells stimulates the production of TGF-β (Fadok *et al.*, 1998), apoptotic T cells themselves release TGF-β because of redistribution of existing cytokine into the cytosol following loss of mitochondrial membrane potential (W. Chen *et al.*, 2001). Thus clonal deletion of T cells may foster active mechanisms of suppression.

A particularly attractive feature of TGF-β as a central mediator of immunoregulation in the gut is that its class switching properties could explain the findings that oral tolerance may be accompanied by upregulation of IgA synthesis. In this way, the TGF-β-rich microenvironment of the gut can be seen as an appropriate means of maintaining noninflammatory responses to harmless antigens in the diet or flora. Nevertheless, it must be acknowledged that enhanced TGF-β production is by no means a universal finding in all models of mucosal tolerance, including that found in humans (Husby *et al.*, 1994). In addition, a study on a mouse model of experimental acute uveitis (EAU) showed that anti-TGF-β antibody had no effect on oral tolerance where IL-4 and IL-10 were upregulated (Rizzo *et al.*, 1999). Therefore other mechanisms may also play a role.

Tr1 cells and IL-10. Tr1 cells, characterized by selective production of IL-10, have not been identified formally in oral tolerance, but administration of IL-10 can restore tolerance to indigenous flora in mice with IBD (Marth *et al.*, 1996). Furthermore, IL-10 KO mice develop spontaneous IBD in association with abnormal T-cell activation (Kuhn *et al.*, 1993), while *in vitro*–generated Tr1 cells can prevent CD4⁺CD45RB^hi T cell–mediated colitis in scid mice in a bystander manner, providing the cognate antigen for the Tr1 cells is fed to mice (Groux *et al.*, 1997; Groux and Powrie, 1999; Foussat *et al.*, 2003). Enhanced IL-10 production has also been reported in mice tolerized by feeding low doses of protein or peptide (Y. Chen *et al.*, 1994, 1995b, 1996, 1997; Neurath *et al.*, 1996; Marth *et al.*, 1996), while IL-10-producing cells with regulatory activity can be isolated from the PP of mice fed low doses of β-lactoglobulin (Tsuji *et al.*, 2001). However, tolerance of IL-10 responses has also been demonstrated in mice fed antigen, even when low doses are used (Garg *et al.*, 1999), while oral tolerance to single feeds of antigen can be induced normally in mice depleted with anti-IL-10 antibodies and anti-IL-10 cannot abrogate established tolerance *in vivo* (Aroeira *et al.*, 1995). In one report, tolerance after multiple feeding of antigen was defective in IL-10-deficient mice, but only if the animals had also been treated with recombinant IL-2. Without this additional treatment, oral tolerance developed normally (Rizzo *et al.*, 1999), and there have been no subsequent studies in which IL-10 has been neutralized in models of feeding multiple low doses of antigen. As with TGF-β, the use of IL-10 KO mice in studies of oral tolerance is limited by their spontaneous development of colitis, but by crossing IL-10 KO mice on to the DO11.10 OVA-specific TcR transgenic strain, one group has shown that IL-10 KO CD4⁺ T cells are inherently susceptible to the induction of tolerance by feeding OVA (Fowler and Powrie, 2002). Thus the role of IL-10 in oral tolerance remains to be confirmed, and it is unclear whether T cells themselves need to be the source of this regulatory cytokine. One recent article has suggested that TGF-β may induce the differentiation of IL-10 producing Treg cells, indicating there may be cross-talk between these different populations of Treg cells (Kitani *et al.*, 2003). Nevertheless, several other cell types can produce IL-10 such as DC (see the following text), and the upregulation of IL-10 found in the lung of dogs fed antigen is associated mainly with CD14⁺ non-T cells (Zemann *et al.*, 2003).

NK1.1⁺ T cells. As we have noted, the idea that NK T cells can play an important role in immunoregulation has received considerable attention recently, including in models that are apparently analogous to oral tolerance, such as that induced via the anterior chamber of the eye (Sonoda *et al.*, 1999; Bach and Chatenoud, 2001; Bach and Francois Bach, 2003). Two reports have suggested that oral tolerance induced by feeding haptenized colonic proteins or alloantigens can be transferred by NK T cells from the liver (Trop *et al.*, 1999; Margenthaler *et al.*, 2002), but other workers have shown normal oral tolerance in mice lacking NK T cells because of a KO of the Jα 281 component of the invariant TcR found on most of these cells (Ishimitsu *et al.*, 2003).

CD8+ T cells

The proposed CD8+ suppressor T cells that were implicated many years ago were not characterized adequately, and it became difficult to understand how such cells could recognize exogenous protein antigens derived from the gut. However, it is now clear that orally administered protein antigens can be processed and presented to CD8+ T cells, both for the induction of tolerance and priming (see the preceding text). There are reports that a population of CD8+ Treg cells that may produce IL-4 or IL-10 may be primed by feeding antigen (Ke and Kapp, 1996; von Herrath *et al.*, 1996; Gardine *et al.*, 2001; Zhou *et al.*, 2001), and one study has reported that low-dose oral tolerance to thyroglobulin may require CD8+ T cells (Gardine *et al.*, 2001). However, most workers have found that systemic tolerance can be induced and maintained normally in CD8 KO or β2m KO mice (Grdic *et al.*, 1998) and in mice treated with anti-CD8 antibodies (Garside *et al.*, 1995a; W. Chen *et al.*, 1995b; Barone *et al.*, 1995; Vistica *et al.*, 1996). Interestingly, however, orally induced tolerance of *mucosal* immune responses may be defective in CD8 KO mice (Grdic *et al.*, 1998), indicating that, although there may be no absolute requirement for CD8+ T cells in the systemic consequences of oral tolerance, these cells may play a role in certain sites such as the mucosa itself.

γδ T cells

One possible explanation for the possible role of regulatory CD8+ T cells is that they may be γδ T cells. This was first suggested by work showing that aerosol induced tolerance of serum IgE responses in rats could be transferred with very small numbers of splenic CD8α+ γδ T cells that produced IFN-γ (McMenamin *et al.*, 1991, 1994, 1995). Diabetes in nonobese diabetic (NOD) mice can also be prevented by CD8+ γδ T cells induced by aerosol administration of insulin (Harrison *et al.*, 1996; Hanninen and Harrison, 2000), and subsequent studies have shown that γδ T cells can transfer orally induced tolerance (Wildner *et al.*, 1996; Hanninen and Harrison, 2000). Oral tolerance to proteins can be prevented or even abrogated by depleting γδ T cells with antibody *in vivo* (Mengel *et al.*, 1995; Ke *et al.*, 1997) and cannot be induced in δ TcR KO mice that lack γδ T cells (Ke *et al.*, 1997). This defect seems to apply particularly to low-dose tolerance (Spahn *et al.*, 1999; Gardine *et al.*, 2001). The effects of γδ T cells in oral tolerance have been shown to be antigen specific, but little is known of the molecular basis of how these cells can recognize conventional antigens or of the restriction specificities involved. As discussed elsewhere in this volume, work in other models has suggested that γδ. T cells may play a regulatory role in mucosal immunity, being able to inhibit inflammation in spontaneous and infectious models of colitis in mice (Roberts, 1996; Bhan *et al.*,

1999). However, in these cases, the γδ T cells appear to act by sustaining mucosal repair, rather than by inhibiting specific immune responses. One study suggested that the γδ Treg cells induced by feeding antigen may recognize antigenic peptide when presented by an αβ T cell bearing the appropriate TcR (Wildner *et al.*, 1996), but this has not been confirmed. The antigen recognition properties of γδ T cells is not well understood in general.

Although it is tempting to speculate that they are derived from the intraepithelial compartment, where CD8+ γδ T cells are relatively enriched, the transferable γδ T cells that have been described have been obtained from organized systemic lymphoid tissues. Although CD8αα+ IEL have been shown to act as Treg cells in experimental IBD, this has been associated with the αβ T-cell subset of IEL (Poussier *et al.*, 2002; Das *et al.*, 2003), and the role of γδ IEL in intestinal homeostasis remains an important area for future study.

Bystander suppression in oral tolerance

Bystander suppression solves a major conceptual problem in the design of antigen-specific or T cell–specific therapy for inflammatory autoimmune diseases such as multiple sclerosis (MS), type 1 diabetes, and rheumatoid arthritis in which the autoantigen is unknown or where there are reactivities to multiple autoantigens in the target tissue. During the course of chronic inflammatory autoimmune processes in animals, there is intraantigenic and interantigenic spread of autoreactivity at the target organ (Cross *et al.*, 1993; Kaufman *et al.*, 1993, Lehmann *et al.*, 1992; McCarron *et al.*, 1990; Tisch *et al.*, 1993). Similarly, in human autoimmune diseases, there are reactivities to multiple autoantigens in the target tissue. For example, in MS, there is immune reactivity to at least three myelin antigens: MBP, proteolipid protein (PLP) and myelin oligodendrocyte glycoprotein (MOG) (Kerlero de Rosbo *et al.*, 1993; J. Zhang *et al.*, 1993). In type 1 diabetes, there are multiple islet-cell antigens that could be the target of autoreactivity including glutamic acid decarboxylase (GAD), insulin, and heat shock proteins (Harrison, 1992). Because regulatory cells induced by oral antigen secrete antigen-nonspecific cytokines after being triggered by the fed antigen, they suppress inflammation in the microenvironment where the fed antigen is localized. Thus for a human organ–specific inflammatory disease, it is not necessary to know the specific antigen that is the target of an autoimmune response, but only to feed an antigen capable of inducing regulatory cells, which then migrate to the target tissue and suppress inflammation.

Bystander suppression has been demonstrated in a number of autoimmune disease models in which oral tolerance has been induced. For instance, PLP-induced EAE can be suppressed by feeding MBP (Al-Sabbagh *et al.*, 1994; Y. Chen *et al.*, 1994) or by administering TGF-β-secreting MBP-specific T-cell clones from orally tolerized animals (Y. Chen *et al.*, 1994). In the Lewis rat model of EAE, disease induced by MBP peptide 71-90 can be suppressed by feeding peptide 21-40 (A. Miller *et al.*, 1993). In arthritis models, adjuvant- and antigen-induced disease can be suppressed by feeding collagen (Yoshino *et al.*, 1995; J. Zhang *et al.*, 1990). In a virus-induced model of diabetes, whereby a lymphocytic choriomeningitis virus (LCMV) protein is expressed on the insulin promoter and the animal is then infected with the LCMV, diabetes can be suppressed by feeding insulin (von Herrath *et al.*, 1996). Moreover, adjuvants for oral tolerance, such as CT-B, also enhance bystander suppression when administered with insulin in this virus-induced model of diabetes (Bregenholt *et al.*, 2003). Allogeneic responses, including graft rejection and allospecific DTH and cytokine production can also be suppressed by feeding either OVA before challenging animals with both OVA and the allospe-

cific stimulus **(Fig. 27.6)**. This raises the possibility that readily available nominal antigens could be used to induce bystander tolerance to complex antigens such as allografts.

Induction of tolerance toward antigens that drive susceptibility or pathology may be considered a new mode of treatment for the inflammatory injury associated with several infections. Hepatitis B virus, for example, is a noncytopathic virus. Bystander suppression induced by oral administration of hepatitis B virus–envelope (HBV-envelope) proteins was shown to be effective in decreasing antibody responses to other virus antigens, in alleviating the immune-mediated liver damage while enhancing Th1-mediated antiviral immunity in

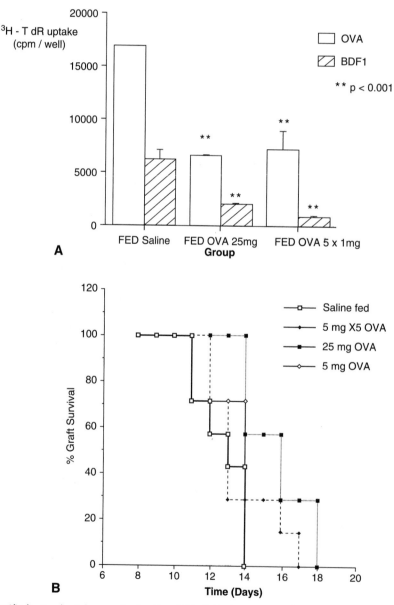

Fig. 27.6. Induction of allospecific bystander tolerance by feeding OVA. BALB/c mice (H-2d) fed differing amounts of OVA on one occasion or daily for 5 days have suppressed proliferative responses both to OVA and fully allogeneic BDF1 (H-2^b × H-2^d)F$_1$ cells when challenged systemically with both OVA/CFA and BDF1 cells **(A)**. Rejection of BDF$_1$ skin grafts is also delayed in OVA-fed mice challenged with OVA/CFA at the time of grafting **(B)**.

chronically infected patients (Ilan, 2002). In a mouse model of *Schistosoma* infection, oral administration of OVA also showed bystander modulation of lung granulomas after coinjection of *S. mansoni* eggs and OVA. Granuloma modulation is an important phenomenon *in vivo* that correlates with decrease in tissue damage and in disease severity (Carvalho *et al.*, 2002). One question that remains in the attempts to induce tolerance to infectious agents is whether protective immune responses will be affected by the same bystander effect. In hepatitis B infection, this is not the case, and suppression of a set of T cells seems to boost the activity of others that provide protective immunity (Ilan, 2002). In other infections, such as human filariasis, tolerance induction by exposure during early life protects from pathology upon reexposure to the parasite; yet tolerized patients possess a larger reservoir of the parasite.

Bystander suppression *in vitro* has recently been shown in humans by using common dietary proteins (OVA, bovine γ globulin) to stimulate cells *in vitro* and then using these cells to suppress *in vitro* tetanus toxoid responses (Zivny *et al.*, 2001). However, bystander suppression may be more difficult to induce in uveitis models (Wildner and Thurau, 1995), and feeding OVA has been reported to induce bystander suppression in adults animals but anergy in young animals (Lundin *et al.*, 1996).

In theory, bystander suppression could be applied in the treatment of organ-specific inflammatory conditions that are not classic autoimmune diseases, such as psoriasis, or could be used to target anti-inflammatory cytokines to an organ in which inflammation may play a role in disease pathogenesis even if the disease is not primarily inflammatory in nature. For example, oral MBP decreased stroke size in a rat stroke model, presumably by decreasing inflammation associated with ischemic injury (Becker *et al.*, 1997). Induction of nasal tolerance in mice to a peptide of the myelin antigen MOG also reduces ischemic injury following stroke. Regulatory cells are generated in tolerant wild-type but not in IL-10-deficient mice. These cells can transfer tolerance to naive recipients (Frenkel *et al.*, 2003). Bystander suppression achieved by oral antigen in nonimmune pathologic conditions may mimic a physiologic protective reaction to self-antigens in response to inflammatory insult as observed in the experimental model of central nervous system (CNS) axonal injury in EAE-susceptible and resistant rat strains. Oral treatment with low-dose MBP is beneficial for posttraumatic survival of retinal ganglion cells in Lewis rats following optic nerve injury (Monsonego *et al.*, 2003). Heat-shock proteins, known to be upregulated in inflammatory situations, are also a suitable target for bystander suppression strategies. Oral as well as nasal administration of hsp65 in LDL-R-deficient mice fed a high-cholesterol diet inhibits IL-2 and IFN-γ production and aortic plaque development. Production of IL-10 but not TGF-β is upregulated in hsp-tolerized mice (Maron *et al.*, 2002b; Harats *et al.*, 2002).

Other mechanisms of tolerance

IFN-γ. Suppression of IFN-γ production in response to systemic challenge is an almost universal finding in orally induced tolerance. However, the development of tolerance is frequently preceded by priming of antigen-specific IFN-γ production (Hoyne *et al.*, 1993a; Hoyne and Thomas, 1995; Marth *et al.*, 1996; Y. Chen *et al.*, 1997; Mowat *et al.*, 1999; Hauet-Broere *et al.*, 2003), while IFN-γ producing, food antigen–specific T cells are present in normal human blood and PP (Nagata *et al.*, 2000; Schmidt *et al.*, 2001). Indeed, studies on peanut allergic children have suggested that their skewing towards a Th2-mediated immune response is associated with an absence of the IFN-γ and TNF-α–producing T cells that dominate the response to peanut in normal, orally tolerized children (Turcanu *et al.*, 2003).

Similar enhancement or preservation of IFN-γ production has long been known to occur in other models of T-cell anergy *in vivo* and *in vitro* (Mueller *et al.*, 1989), and reversal of tolerance by depleting IFN-γ has also been reported in such circumstances (Y. Liu and Janeway, 1990). The γδ T cell–dependent tolerance of IgE antibody production that is induced by aerosol administration of proteins appears to be mediated by IFN-γ (McMenamin *et al.*, 1995), and IFN-γ is produced transiently by antigen-specific CD4+ T cells that can subsequently transfer tolerance to orally administered OVA (Hauet-Broere *et al.*, 2003). Although we and others found that depletion of IFN-γ *in vivo* did not influence the induction of oral tolerance (Mowat *et al.*, 1999) and that oral tolerance could be induced normally in IFN-γ receptor KO or IL-12 KO mice (Mowat *et al.*, 1999; Kjerrulf *et al.*, 1997), others have reported that oral tolerance cannot be induced in IFN-γ-deficient mice (Kweon *et al.*, 1998; H. O. Lee *et al.*, 2000; Niederkorn, 2002). The latter of these studies also showed that oral tolerance could not be induced in adoptively transferred TcR transgenic T cells on a IFN-γ KO background, and it was suggested that IFN-γ was necessary for the expression of adhesion molecules and chemokines involved in recruiting Treg cells into the immune system or other tissues (H. O. Lee *et al.*, 2000). The reasons for these discrepancies are unknown, especially as similar experimental models were used in many cases and the role of IFN-γ in oral tolerance clearly warrants further investigation.

Non-T cell–dependent mechanisms. Although active mechanisms of oral tolerance are mainly T cell–mediated, other regulatory mechanisms have been reported. Isolated reports suggest that tolerance to SRBC and certain contact sensitizing agents can be transferred using serum from antigen-fed mice (Kagnoff, 1978b; Andre *et al.*, 1975; Chalon *et al.*, 1979; Bhogal *et al.*, 1986). Regulation of immunity by antiidiotypic antibody also has been described in mice tolerized by portal vein inoculation of allogeneic lymphocytes (S. Sato *et al.*, 1988). Although it is generally not possible to transfer tolerance to proteins using immunoglobulin (Hanson *et al.*, 1979a), milk from mice tolerized orally or parenterally during pregnancy can induce tolerance in the neonate by transfer of antiidiotypic antibody (Wannemuehler *et al.*, 1982; Jarrett and Hall, 1984). Blocking and cross-reactive antibodies have also been demonstrated as a suppressive mechanism in a recent report on oral tolerance to grass pollen (de Weerd *et al.*, 2003). Thus the possibility remains that this mechanism provides an additional means of conferring tolerance on the neonate at a time when susceptibility to food sensitivity is high.

PRESENTATION AND PROCESSING OF INTESTINALLY DERIVED ANTIGEN

It is now generally accepted that the way in which it is presented to T lymphocytes determines whether administration of antigen induces active immunity or tolerance. This may reflect the involvement of specific antigen-presenting cells and their cell surface molecules or mediators, or it may be a function of the anatomic site in which these processes occur. As we have discussed, oral tolerance appears to involve anergy or functional deviation of CD4$^+$ T cells, and this is preceded by partial activation of these T cells, followed by abortive clonal expansion (J. Sun et al., 1999, 2003; Thorstenson and Khoruts, 2001; Smith et al., 2002a). These features are consistent with the possibility that the initial event in the process is presentation of fed antigen by APC that lack costimulatory molecules or which possess unusual costimulatory properties (Mowat, 1999b). This idea is consistent with older evidence that feeding one antigen to naive mice causes transient activation of the reticuloendothelial system (RES) and interferes with the induction of tolerance by feeding a second antigen (Stokes et al., 1983a). Oral tolerance in mice fed OVA also can be prevented by in vivo administration of agents that activate APC functions of the RES, including estrogen, muramyl dipeptide (MDP), IFN-γ, and a graft-versus-host reaction (Mowat and Parrott, 1983; Strobel et al., 1985; Strobel and Ferguson, 1986; Z. Zhang and Michael, 1990).

In turn, these events reflect where fed antigen interacts with APCs and T cells, as well as the nature of the cellular processes involved.

Routes of antigen uptake from the intestine
Peyer's patches and the induction of oral tolerance
A number of sites for the uptake and presentation of orally administered antigen have been suggested, including local tissues such as the intestinal epithelium, the LP, the PP, or MLN, and more distal tissues including the spleen, liver, and peripheral lymph nodes. As discussed elsewhere in this volume, it is generally considered that living and particulate antigens are taken up preferentially by M cells in the follicle-associated epithelium (FAE) of PP, before being passed on to professional APC and thence to T cells in the underlying lymphoid tissues. There is less direct evidence for the uptake of soluble antigens by this route, and recent morphologic studies have shown that orally administered OVA enters endosomal vesicles in villus enterocytes, suggesting that a substantial proportion of protein antigen enters via the conventional villus epithelium (Zimmer et al., 2000). Indeed, it has been proposed that this dichotomy in antigen uptake by M cells and villus enterocytes may be the principal factor in determining whether immunity or tolerance occurs after oral administration of antigen, based on the possibility that class

II MHC expressing, costimulatory molecule–negative enterocytes might be expected to present antigen to CD4$^+$ T cells in a tolerogenic manner (Schwartz, 2003).

Experiments designed to examine directly the role of M cells and PP in oral tolerance have provided conflicting results. The conventional idea that PP are the first place where T cells recognize fed antigen was derived partly from older studies that showed that Treg cells could be identified in the PP before appearing in peripheral tissues such as the spleen (Mattingly and Waksman, 1978). Antigen-loaded APC can be isolated from the PP soon after feeding either intact protein or peptide (Richman et al., 1981b; Galliaerde et al., 1995; Kunkel et al., 2003; DePaolo et al., 2003), and experiments in which tolerogenic doses of protein antigen have been fed to mice containing TcR transgenic T cells have shown rapid activation and/or clonal deletion of antigen-specific CD4$^+$ (Chen et al., 1995a, 1997; Marth et al., 1996, 2000; H. O. Lee et al., 2000; Meyer et al., 2001; Smith et al., 2002a; Gonnella et al., 1998; Hauet-Broere et al., 2003) and CD8$^+$ T cells in the PP (Blanas et al., 2000). Human PP also contain T cells that are responsive to dietary antigens in vitro (Nagata et al., 2000). There is also production of regulatory cytokines (Gonnella et al., 1998; Marth et al., 2000; Hauet-Broere et al., 2003; DePaolo et al., 2003) and generation of antigen-specific Treg cells in the PP of fed mice (Tsuji et al., 2003). Together with evidence that the normal PP has been reported to have a cytokine profile dominated by IL-4, IL-10, and TGF-β, as well as possessing a generally immunosuppressive environment that can affect newly arrived lymphocytes (Daynes et al., 1990; Premier and Meeusen, 1998; Kellermann and McEvoy, 2001; Jump and Levine, 2002; DePaolo et al., 2003), these findings would be entirely consistent with a role for PP in determining the induction of Treg cells and tolerance after feeding antigen.

Despite this, it has been difficult to define whether M cells and PP are essential for oral tolerance. It has been reported that oral tolerance to proteins may be defective in mice with no PP because of genetic KO of the type 1 TNF receptor (Gardine et al., 2001) or after prenatal neutralization of lymphotoxin β receptor (LTβR) by intrauterine administration of soluble LTβR-Fc fusion protein (Fujihashi et al., 2001). Interestingly, however, the latter workers reported normal oral tolerance induction when the hapten trinitrobenzene sulfonate (TNBS) was used as the antigen, and others have reported entirely normal oral tolerance to either low-dose or high-dose OVA in LTβR-Fc fusion protein–treated mice (Spahn et al., 2001, 2002), as well as in other mouse models with relatively selective defects in PP development, including TNF-α KO, LTβ KO, and (LTα$^{+/-}$ LTβ$^{+/-}$) mice, or mice depleted of TNF-α and LTα by neutralizing antibodies in vivo. Oral tolerance to protein antigens also appears to be normal in B-cell KO mice that have only rudimentary PP and lack virtually all M cells (Golovkina et al., 1999; Peng et al., 2000; Hashimoto et al., 2001; Alpan et al., 2001; Gonnella et al., 2001). Although these experiments can be criticized on the basis that the KO strategies used can alter other components of the immune system, including lymph node development, germinal center formation, and splenic architecture, an older study also reported that surgical removal of PP from rats had no effect on oral tolerance (Enders *et al.*, 1986). Taken together, the balance of evidence therefore suggests that M cells and PP may not be necessary for the uptake and processing of antigens for the induction of oral tolerance.

A critical role for the mesenteric lymph node

In contrast to the rather contradictory evidence on PP, the MLN clearly play a critical role in the induction of mucosal immune responses. Antigen-loaded APC can be isolated readily from the MLN of antigen-fed animals (Blanas *et al.*, 2000; Alpan *et al.*, 2001; Akbari *et al.*, 2001; Kunkel *et al.*, 2003), and indeed, low doses of peptide appear to localize preferentially in MLN, rather than PP (Kunkel *et al.*, 2003). All studies using adoptively transferred transgenic T cells agree that antigen recognition occurs in MLN within a few hours of feeding protein antigen (Y. Chen *et al.*, 1997; Williamson *et al.*, 1999a; Van Houten and Blake, 1996; J. Sun *et al.*, 1999; Gütgemann *et al.*, 1998; Meyer *et al.*, 2001; Shi *et al.*, 2000; Blanas *et al.*, 2000; H.O. Lee *et al.*, 2000; Lefrancois *et al.*, 2000; Smith *et al.*, 2002a). It is also impossible to induce oral tolerance in LTα KO or (LTα × TNFα) KO mice that lack MLN, whereas MLN are present in all the models of PP-null mice in which tolerance is usually maintained (Spahn *et al.*, 2001, 2002).

This critical role for MLN in determining the fate of food antigen–specific T cells is not surprising, given the known importance of draining lymph nodes in initiating responses to most antigens that emanate from tissues. In addition, it is now clear that there is regional specialization of secondary lymphoid organs in different anatomic sites, and that this may program the nature of local immune responses. Work on the respiratory tract indicates that the lymph nodes draining the mucosal tissues may differ from lymph nodes in other anatomic sites and may provide specialized microenvironments for the induction of tolerance. Thus, the draining cervical lymph node is necessary for the tolerant state induced by nasal administration of antigen, and the absence of tolerance that occurs when this node is removed can be restored by transplantation of the appropriate lymph node but not by other, peripheral lymph nodes (Wolvers *et al.*, 1999). The basis of this effect is unknown and whether a similar phenomenon occurs in the MLN has never been studied. Nevertheless, the MLN shares many of the unusual immunomodulatory properties of PP, favoring the generation of Th2 or T_{reg} (Daynes *et al.*, 1990; Premier and Meeusen, 1998), features that may relate to local differences in responsiveness to steroid hormones (Daynes *et al.*, 1990).

The question arises of whether naive T cells first encounter antigen in the MLN itself and where the antigen gains access to the APC involved. Early studies of suppressor T cells induced by feeding antigen indicated that these may migrate from PP to MLN (Mattingly and Waksman, 1978), and more recent work using adoptively transferred TcR transgenic CD4+ T cells has also suggested Treg cells may appear in PP before MLN (Hauet-Broere *et al.*, 2003). Nevertheless, as we have discussed, PP may not be essential for oral tolerance,

and it has been shown that even low doses of orally administered peptide gain access to APC in the MLN entirely normally in the absence of PP (Kunkel *et al.*, 2003). In addition, presentation of antigen to T cells in the PP should only generate lymphocyte populations that recirculate preferentially to mucosal sites, meaning that systemic unresponsiveness would be difficult to attain. As the MLN is believed to be a crossover point between the mucosal and systemic immune systems, presentation to T cells in the MLN could account for the combined local and systemic consequences of oral tolerance.

The APC involved in T-cell presentation in the MLN may acquire antigen that traffics there from the intestine directly in the bloodstream or draining lymph. Alternatively, as discussed elsewhere in this volume, antigen taken up by APC in the gut wall can be carried to the MLN in lymph-borne APC (L. Liu and MacPherson, 1991, 1993, 1995; MacPherson and Liu, 1999). Under normal circumstances, at least a proportion of these APC may be derived from the PP, but it is known that lymph-borne DC in intestinal lymph also emanate from the villus mucosa (L. Liu and MacPherson, 1991, 1993, 1995; MacPherson and Liu, 1999). The conventional epithelium covering the villi represents a much larger surface area than that of the PP, and as we have noted, this epithelium is capable of transporting immunologically relevant antigen (Galliaerde *et al.*, 1995; Zimmer *et al.*, 2000). In addition, it has been shown that APC in villus LP are loaded by fed antigen (Zimmer *et al.*, 2000), and our own recent work suggests that this accounts for the majority of uptake of fed protein antigens (Chirdo, F. G., Millington, O. P., Beacock-Sharp, H., Parker, L. A., and Mowat, A., submitted for publication). Therefore both PP and LP may be sources of both antigen and APC for the induction of oral tolerance in the MLN.

Systemic dissemination of orally administered antigen

One mechanism that could explain the systemic effects of intestinal antigen is that immunologically relevant amounts of fed antigen can be disseminated throughout the mucosal and peripheral immune systems. After the feeding of proteins to humans or animals, immunologically intact antigen can be detected rapidly in the bloodstream (Strobel *et al.*, 1983; Peng *et al.*, 1990; Furrie *et al.*, 1995; Strobel and Mowat, 1998; Husby *et al.*, 1987), and antigen-loaded APC are found in the spleen of mice fed protein (Gütgemann *et al.*, 1998, 2002). In rodents, the material found in the serum of protein-fed animals can induce tolerance when transferred to naive recipients (Strobel *et al.*, 1983; Peng *et al.*, 1990; Furrie *et al.*, 1995; Strobel and Mowat, 1998). In addition, antigen-specific T-cell activation can be seen simultaneously in the GALT and peripheral lymphoid tissues of mice fed large doses of antigen, although this is less extensive than in the MLN (Gütgemann *et al.*, 1998, 2002; Williamson *et al.*, 1999a; Van Houten and Blake, 1996; J. Sun *et al.*, 1999; Smith *et al.*, 2002a). Unlike other models of tolerance (D'Orazio and Niederkorn, 1998b), the induction of oral tolerance does not require the spleen **(Fig. 27.7)**. The effects of fed antigen on systemic T cells could reflect an effect of circulating antigen or the redistribution of antigen-loaded APC from the intes-

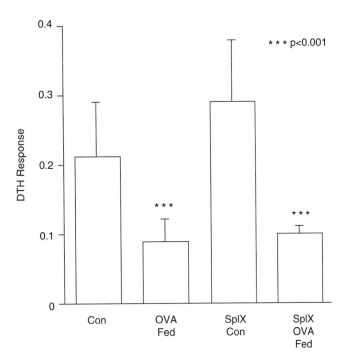

Fig. 27.7. Splenectomy does not affect the induction of tolerance by feeding protein antigen. Mice fed OVA have suppressed systemic DTH responses on challenge with OVA in CFA, irrespective of the presence of a spleen.

tine to other lymphoid organs. Thus it seems possible that both local and systemic effects may contribute to the functional tolerance found after feeding antigen, with presentation of antigen to T cells occurring in the LP, PP, MLN, and periphery. Such widely distributed events may be necessary to provide overlapping layers of immunoregulation that can ensure complete integrity of this physiologically critical phenomenon. The extent to which each layer is involved may depend on the dose of antigen used. Low doses of antigen may penetrate no further than the mucosa, PP, and perhaps the MLN, where the local microenvironment and specialized APC determine that activation of Treg cells is the result. In contrast, higher doses of antigen may gain direct access to the more conventional APC and T cells in peripheral lymphoid organs, ensuring that generalized T-cell anergy predominates over any local regulatory T-cell activity that is induced. That distinct regulatory mechanisms could operate in different sites is suggested by the fact that although feeding antigen can tolerize both systemic and mucosal immune responses, systemic tolerance is intact in the absence of $CD8^+$ T cells, whereas the local tolerance is not (Grdic et al., 1998).

Intestinal processing of antigen generates tolerogenic moieties

As we have noted, small amounts of immunologically intact protein are absorbed from the intestine, and there is substantial evidence that this circulating material is critically important in tolerance. Passive administration of antibody blocks the induction of tolerance (Hanson et al., 1979b; Melamed

and Friedman, 1994), and serum removed from mice fed OVA 1 hour beforehand induces systemic tolerance when transferred intraperitoneally to naive syngeneic recipients. This intestinally processed material inhibits systemic DTH responses selectively in recipient mice (Strobel et al., 1983; Bruce and Ferguson, 1986a, b), and similar findings have been made with other protein antigens (Kay and Ferguson, 1989a; S. Strobel, unpublished observations), as well as in primed recipients (Karlsson et al., 2000). The tolerance induced by serum from fed mice requires a cyclophosphamide-sensitive regulatory cell (Strobel et al., 1983), and one recent study in rats suggests that the suppression may be mediated by $CD4^+CD25^+ T_{reg}$ (Karlsson et al., 2000).

The events involved in the generation of this material are unclear, and its exact nature is controversial. As serum taken from mice given equivalent doses of protein by other parenteral routes does not reproduce the phenomenon (Bruce and Ferguson, 1986b), it seems that the tolerogen must be generated in the intestine. This is a rapid process, as tolerogenic material appears in serum within 20–30 minutes of feeding and therefore is unlikely to involve any immunologically active molecule (Peng et al., 1990). However, it is not generated in immunodeficient scid or irradiated mice, a defect that can be restored by transferring normal lymphoid cells (Bruce and Ferguson, 1986a; Furrie et al., 1994). These results suggest a role for hemopoietic cells in processing gut-derived antigen, and until recently, the consensus was that the tolerogen consisted of the protein itself. Initial work showed that it reacted with antibodies directed at native OVA (Bruce and Ferguson, 1986a) and eluted on gel filtration columns or high performance liquid chromatography (HPLC) with the native molecule (Bruce and Ferguson, 1986a; Peng et al., 1990; Furrie et al., 1995). These findings suggest that a simple filtration mechanism in the intestine may produce deaggregated monomers of protein that are known to be tolerogenic in other systems. However, the ability of serum to transfer tolerance does not correlate directly with the absolute amount of intact protein present (Peng et al., 1990; Furrie et al., 1995), supporting the view that intestinal processing could involve alterations in antigenic structure. Other work suggested that the presence or absence of tolerogenic OVA in serum of normal or scid mice correlates with the appearance of immunogenic moieties with a molecular weight approximately half that of intact OVA (Furrie et al., 1995). It is also feasible that small peptides that cannot be detected by antibody could contribute.

A further intriguing possible explanation for the presence of tolerogenic material in the serum of fed animals is that it may be in the form of lipid vesicles ("tolerosomes") that contain antigen bound to class II MHC molecules and which are derived from enterocytes (Karlsson et al., 2001). Class II MHC–positive vesicles of this kind can be identified inside enterocytes and lying free in the LP of normal animals. In addition, vesicles of the appropriate density that induce tolerance in T cells appear in the supernatants of class II MHC–expressing epithelial cells cultured with OVA (Karlsson et al., 2001). Analogous class II MHC–expressing vesicles (exosomes) that can be recognized directly by T cells have been found to be released by other APC such as DC and B cells (Thery *et al.*, 2002). Further, it has been suggested that fed antigen complexes with class II MHC in enterocytes, with membrane fragments then being released as tolerosomes into the circulation. The nature of these novel tolerosomes must be considered in the light of the fact that antigenic material bound to class II MHC in this way should be in the form of peptide, while the original descriptions of the serum tolerogen showed that it was reactive with antibodies against native molecule. In addition, recent work that has confirmed the ability of enterocytes to produce class II MHC–expressing, antigen-loaded exosomes *in vitro* showed that they were not tolerogenic *in vivo*, but primed systemic antibody responses in naive recipients (van Niel *et al.*, 2001, 2003). Thus the nature and role of tolerosomes needs further characterization.

That proteolytic digestion may be involved in oral tolerance is suggested by reports that inhibiting pancreatic enzyme activity prevents the induction of tolerance (Hanson *et al.*, 1993; Meyer *et al.*, 1996). However, opposing results have been reported (Saklayen *et al.*, 1984), and increasing the susceptibility of OVA to digestion by carboxymethylation completely prevents the induction of tolerance (Peng *et al.*, 1995). As tolerance can be induced using peptides, it seems that limited proteolysis in the intestine may be essential for tolerance to be induced by intact proteins. This may reflect enhanced availability of antigen to APC or differences in the absolute amounts of antigen in serum.

APC–T cell interactions in oral tolerance
Nature of APC involved in oral tolerance

The APC populations that have been implicated in oral tolerance are class II MHC–expressing enterocytes, B lymphocytes, and DCs. Although the villus epithelium has always been considered an impermeable barrier to macromolecules, recent work shows that proteins such as OVA can be taken up and processed by enterocytes *in situ* (Zimmer *et al.*, 2000). Intestinal epithelial cell lines can also process apically absorbed antigen and present it from the basal surface to CD4[+] T cells *in vitro* (Hershberg and Mayer, 2000; Hershberg *et al.*, 1998). This presentation could occur in the form of direct recognition of class II MHC–peptide complexes on the epithelial membrane or after release of the tolerosomes discussed in the preceding text. Because enterocytes are class II MHC–positive in most species, but normally do not express the costimulatory molecules required for full T-cell activation (Sanderson *et al.*, 1993; Bloom *et al.*, 1995; Dippold *et al.*, 1993), presentation of antigen by epithelial cells might be expected to result in anergy of CD4[+] T cells, a phenomenon that has been reported using hapten-pulsed enterocytes in mice (Galliaerde *et al.*, 1995). In addition, there is evidence that enterocytes may present antigen selectively to CD8[+] T cells with regulatory activity (Bland and Warren, 1986; Mayer and Schlien, 1987; Li *et al.*, 1995; Hershberg and Mayer, 2000). However, these pathways have never been examined *in vivo*, and because naive T cells are

rare in the LP and LP T cells do not migrate out of the gut (MacDonald and Pender, 1998), it seems unlikely that direct presentation of antigen by enterocytes to local T cells could contribute to the induction of systemic tolerance. Furthermore, it has been shown that bone marrow–derived APC are alone necessary for presentation of orally administered antigens to CD4[+] T cells (Blanas *et al.*, 2000). Despite these reservations, it is possible that presentation of antigen to CD4[+] T cells by class II MHC–expressing enterocytes could be involved in maintaining the survival and activity of already primed Treg cells in the mucosa.

Resting B cells are capable of inducing tolerance in T cells *in vivo* and *in vitro* (Eynon and Parker, 1992; Fuchs and Matzinger, 1992; Buhlmann *et al.*, 1995), and B lymphocytes are required for the induction of T-cell tolerance that occurs after administration of soluble antigen into the anterior chamber of the eye (D'Orazio and Niederkorn, 1998b). In addition, B cells are among the principal APC loaded by tolerogenic antigen in the spleen of fed mice, where they are found close to naive T cells (Gütgemann *et al.*, 2002). Antigen-presenting B cells from mice fed nickel salts have also been found to be capable of inducing infectious tolerance by activation of Treg cells (Roelofs-Haarhuis *et al.*, 2003). However, a number of studies show that oral tolerance is essentially normal in B-cell deficient mice (Peng *et al.*, 2000; Alpan *et al.*, 2001; Hashimoto *et al.*, 2001; Yoshida *et al.*, 1998, 2001; Gonnella, 2001), and it appears that B cells do not play an essential role in the phenomenon. However, one recent report has suggested that the mechanisms of tolerance may be different in B-cell KO mice (Gonnella *et al.*, 2001). In particular, these animals may have a defect in the local production of the cytokines required for the generation of active Treg cells after feeding of multiple low doses of antigen. This is associated with the uptake of more antigen from the intestine and the development of a more anergic pattern of T-cell dysfunction. However, it is important to note that it is not known how B cells could account for these differences, and other work has found that B-cell KO mice can generate Treg cells normally after feeding low doses of antigen (Alpan *et al.*, 2001).

The current consensus is that DCs are the principal population of APC that controls whether orally administered antigen induces tolerance or active immunity. DC in PP and MLN account for the largest proportion of uptake of orally administered peptide (Kunkel *et al.*, 2003), and expansion of DC numbers *in vivo* using the cytokine flt3 ligand (flt3L) enhances the susceptibility of mice to the induction of oral tolerance by feeding OVA (Viney *et al.*, 1998; Williamson *et al.*, 1999a), as well as increasing the abortive activation of CD4[+] T cells that occurs in mucosal and peripheral lymphoid tissues after feeding antigen (Williamson *et al.*, 1999a). More recently, the enhancing effects of flt3L on oral tolerance have been extended to a model of experimental autoimmune encephalomyelitis in mice (Whitacre *et al.*, 2004). The nature and location of the DC involved remain to be ascertained. As discussed elsewhere in this volume, several subsets of DC are present in all the tissues that have been implicated in the induction phase of oral tolerance, including the PP, MLN, and peripheral lymphoid organs, as well as the intestinal mucosa itself. Of particular note, the PP contains DC that produce IL-10 and TGF-β (Iwasaki and Kelsall, 1999, 2001; Akbari *et al.*, 2001), and the dominant CD11b⁺CD8α subset preferentially stimulates naive T cells to secrete IL-10 and IL-4 when compared with DC from nonmucosal sites (Iwasaki and Kelsall, 2001). Recent studies suggest that feeding high doses of protein antigen induces the expression of MCP-1 (CCL2) in PP and that this chemokine costimulates the ability of local antigen-loaded DC to stimulate the differentiation of TGF-β- producing T cells (DePaolo *et al.*, 2003).

Immunoregulatory DC of this kind are not unique to the PP, as it has been shown that MLN DC may present fed proteins to T cells in a way that favors the production of IL-4, IL-10, and TGF-β (Alpan *et al.*, 2001; Akbari *et al.*, 2001). Like the PP, MLN also contains a population of CD8α⁺ "plasmacytoid" DC that can induce the generation of Treg cells (Bilsborough *et al.*, 2003). DC are also present in the LP of the villus mucosa (Mayrhofer, 1983; Viney *et al.*, 1998), and we have found that LP DC avidly take up proteins from the intestine in mice (F. Chirdo *et al.*, submitted for publication). These DC can present orally administered antigens to CD4⁺ T cells *in vivo* and *in vitro*, but interestingly, this appears to induce tolerance in naive recipients. Other *in vivo* loaded DC do not possess this ability, and together, these results suggest that LP DC may play a central role in the induction of oral tolerance, probably after migration to meet naive CD4⁺T cells in the MLN. These findings are consistent with older work that showed the presence of a tolerogenic, but unidentified APC in the LP of protein-fed mice (Harper *et al.*, 1996). The nature of the DC involved in this process has not been determined, but we found a number of subsets in LP, including the CD11b⁺CD8α, CD11b⁻CD8α,⁻ and CD11b⁻CD8α⁺ cells found in PP and MLN. In addition, there is a small subset of CD11c^lo class II MHC^lo B220⁺ DC, analogous to the recently described subset of "plasmacytoid" DC in mice, which stimulates Treg cell differentiation in other tissues (P. Martin *et al.*, 2002; Wakkach *et al.*, 2003). Interestingly, LP DC constitutively express mRNA for IL-10 and type 1 IFN and do not produce substantial amounts of proinflammatory cytokines such as IL-12 p70 or TNF-α, again supporting the view that their physiologic function may be to present antigen to Tr1 or other Treg cells (F. Chirdo *et al.*, submitted for publication).

One further way in which mucosal DC could contribute to tolerance is suggested by the recent discovery of a subpopulation of DC in the intestinal lymph that contains fragments of apoptotic enterocytes and that these DC have relatively low stimulatory activity for T cells (Huang *et al.*, 2000). It is suggested that intestinal DC may be able to induce tolerance to self-antigens, or to luminal antigens that have been taken up by the enterocytes before dying. In support of this mechanism, findings indicate that mice expressing OVA only in enterocytes are tolerant to the antigen, even when the OVA construct used cannot be secreted and so can only be presented to T cells by an indirect route (Vezys *et al.*, 2000). It

is possible that food proteins taken up by effete enterocytes in this way could be presented by local DC for the induction of tolerance.

Costimulatory events in oral tolerance

The molecular basis of how antigen-loaded DC may trigger tolerance to antigens such as food proteins is contentious, but may include the presence of independent subsets with distinctive roles in tolerance or immunity, the maturation status of the DC, and the expression of distinctive costimulatory molecules (Steinman *et al.*, 2003; Guermonprez *et al.*, 2002). As we have noted, there is evidence for unusual subsets of DC in the mucosa and GALT that may stimulate Treg cells. In addition, it has been proposed that immature or resting DC may present antigen in a tolerogenic fashion because of the lack of costimulatory molecules such as CD80, CD86, and CD40, whereas mature (activated) DC drive T-cell immunity. Consistent with this idea, freshly isolated DC from the GALT may show relatively low expression of costimulatory molecules (F. Chirdo *et al.*, submitted for publication; Viney *et al.*, 1998; Williamson *et al.*, 1999b; Iwasaki and Kelsall, 1999) and overexpression of CD80 in PP partially abrogates the induction of oral tolerance (Y. Chen *et al.*, 2000). However, more recent work indicates that the induction of tolerance requires some degree of DC maturation, with a role for both conventional costimulatory molecules and for others that are preferentially associated with inhibitory functions, including CTLA-4 and PD-1 (Sharpe and Freeman, 2002; Greenwald *et al.*, 2002). The idea that oral tolerance may require expression of these molecules on APC is supported by the fact that the enhanced tolerance found in mice infected with *Heligmosomoides polygyrus* is associated with increased expression of CD86 and to a lesser extent CD80 in MLN and PP (Shi *et al.*, 2000). Under physiologic conditions, "quiescent" DCs may be the result of alternative forms of activation, perhaps because the presence of factors such as IL-10, TGF-β, or PGE₂ (Steinman *et al.*, 2003; Guermonprez *et al.*, 2002). As noted in the preceding text, MCP-1 may be one further factor involved in modulating the function of GALT DC in oral tolerance (DePaolo *et al.*, 2003).

The relative importance of these factors in oral tolerance remains to be established, and the role of individual costimulatory molecules is still uncertain. A number of studies indicate that recognition of CD80/CD86 on APC by CTLA-4 on T cells is important for the induction of anergy and tolerance (Perez *et al.*, 1997; Sharpe and Freeman, 2002; Greenwald *et al.*, 2002). As with oral tolerance, these models involve transient activation of T cells before tolerance ensues and is believed to reflect the fact that CTLA-4 has a higher affinity than activating molecule CD28 for low levels of CD80/CD86 on "quiescent" or immature APC. Interestingly, most populations of anergic Treg cells described in other systems have been shown to express high levels of CTLA-4 (Maloy and Powrie, 2001; Bach and Francois Bach, 2003; Bluestone and Abbas, 2003), and cross-linking CTLA-4 may induce the production of TGF-β by T cells (W. Chen *et al.*, 1998b). Consistent with these ideas, continuous feeding of OVA to intact DO11.10 TcR transgenic mice leads to reduced expression of CD80/CD86 on APC, perhaps because of negative feedback mechanisms induced by tolerized T cells (X.-M. Wu *et al.*, 1998), and blocking CTLA-4 function *in vivo* inhibits the induction of oral tolerance after feeding high doses of antigen (Samoilova *et al.*, 1998). CTLA-4 has also been implicated in the tolerance of antigen-specific CD4[+] T cells induced by feeding antigen (Fowler and Powrie, 2002), and blocking CTLA-4 is associated with a loss of the unblocked clonal expansion normally found under these conditions, as well as the appearance of primary serum and intestinal IgA responses to the fed antigen (Y. Chen *et al.*, 2002). Blocking CTLA-4 has little or no effect on low-dose oral tolerance (Barone *et al.*, 2002), and together, these findings support the idea that CTLA-4 plays an important role in oral tolerance that is mediated by anergy of CD4[+] T cells.

Initial studies on the role of CD80 and CD86 in immune responses suggested that the induction of systemic Th2-dependent CD4[+] T-cell responses required ligation of CD86, while Th1 responses were dependent on costimulation via CD80 (Kuchroo *et al.*, 1995). Thus it seemed unsurprising that blocking CD86 *in vivo* was reported to inhibit the induction of low-dose tolerance that might require IL-4-dependent Th3 cells (L. Liu *et al.*, 1999), whereas inhibiting CD80 only prevented high-dose tolerance that seems to involve anergy of Th1 cells (Samoilova *et al.*, 1998). However, studies of CD80/CD86 KO mice do not support a clear association between these molecules and specific CD4[+] T-cell subsets, and it seems more likely that CD86 is critically important for the priming of all CD4[+] T-cell functions, while CD80 plays a relatively minor role (McAdam *et al.*, 1998; Sharpe and Freeman, 2002). The role of CD80 and CD86 in oral tolerance needs to be reevaluated with these findings in mind.

One of the most critical accessory events in the activation and expression of CD4[+] T-cell function is the ligation of CD40L on T cells by CD40 on APC. In DC, this induces expression of costimulatory molecules, as well as the production of IL-12 and other mediators (Banchereau and Steinman, 1998; Guermonprez *et al.*, 2002), and DC lacking CD40 have been shown to be tolerogenic (E. Martin *et al.*, 2003). Although it has been reported that it is impossible to induce high-dose oral tolerance in CD40L-deficient mice (Kweon *et al.*, 1999), these animals have severe immune abnormalities and more recent results have shown that inhibiting the CD40–CD40L interaction *in vivo* does not interfere with oral tolerance induction, despite its ability to prevent the concomitant priming of CD8[+] T cells (Hanninen *et al.*, 2001). Furthermore, two recent reports show that activating DC by cross-linking CD40 does not prevent the induction of oral tolerance to either low or high doses of antigen (J. Sun and Van Houten, 2002; Y. Chung *et al.*, 2004). Overall, it appears that a lack of CD40–CD40L–mediated costimulation is not a critical event in the induction of oral tolerance.

An additional costimulatory interaction that has been implicated in oral tolerance is that involving RANK-RANK ligand (TNF-related activation-induced cytokine [TRANCE]) (Williamson *et al.*, 2002). Receptor activator of NF-κB (RANK) is expressed by DC in most tissues, including PP and MLN, and its ligation by TRANCE on T cells is thought to be an important survival signal for antigen-presenting in lymphoid tissues *in vivo* (Wong *et al.*, 1997). Cross-linking RANK on most populations of DC enhances the production of IL-12, but selectively stimulates IL-10 production by DC from PP. In parallel, *in vivo* administration of TRANCE as an agonist enhances the induction of oral tolerance (Williamson *et al.*, 2002). These intriguing results suggest that this unique, inhibitory costimulatory event may be central to the interaction between regulatory DC and T cells in the GALT that underlie oral tolerance.

Role of the liver in oral tolerance

The majority of blood draining from the intestine goes to the liver via the portal venous system, and large amounts of antigen are likely to enter the liver rapidly after oral administration. The liver is the largest tissue of the RES, raising the possibility that this organ may be a major site of the antigen-processing events that determine the immunologic consequences of antigen feeding. It has been known for many years that direct administration of antigen into the portal vein induces a state of systemic unresponsiveness that has many similarities to oral tolerance (Qian *et al.*, 1985; Fujiwara *et al.*, 1986; S. Sato *et al.*, 1988; Mowat, 1999a). These include the deletion and anergy of antigen-specific T cells (Wrenshall *et al.*, 2001), preferential suppression of DTH and IFN-γ responses, with concomitant upregulation of IL4, IL-10, and TGF-β production (Gorczynski *et al.*, 1994, 1995, 1996a, b, c; S. W. Chung *et al.*, 1995). In combination with anti-IL-10, anti-TGF-β antibody prevents the induction of portal vein tolerance (Gorczynski *et al.*, 1997). Furthermore, portal vein tolerance can be transferred by T cells expressing the γδTcR (Gorczynski, 1994, 1996a, c) and appears to involve distinct mechanisms from those involved in tolerance induced by injection of antigen into other veins (S. W. Chung *et al.*, 1995; Gorczynski *et al.*, 1996a). Like the intestine, the liver contains large numbers of natural Treg cells, such as γδ T cells and NK1.1[+] CD4[+] T cells (Crispe and Mehal, 1996). Together with its size and anatomic position, these features mean it is difficult to exclude a role for the liver in tolerance to antigens emanating from the intestine.

Despite these parallels, it is still unclear how much the liver contributes to the phenomenon of oral tolerance (Mowat, 1999a). Conflicting results have been reported from studies of oral tolerance in which the liver was bypassed by a porto-caval shunt (Thomas *et al.*, 1976; Yang *et al.*, 1994), and the many side effects of this surgical maneuver make interpretation of the results difficult. Recent studies have shown that feeding high doses of antigen to intact TcR transgenic mice induces the generation of a Th2/Th3-like population of Treg cells in the liver that produce IL-4, IL-10, and TGF-β and which cause deletion of antigen-specific Th1 cells via a fas-fasL mediated mechanism (Watanabe *et al.*, 2002, 2003). It is unknown why antigen delivered via the portal tracts induces tolerance so effectively, although it is assumed that this reflects association with a tolerogenic population of

APC (Mowat, 1999a). Allografts of liver are rejected only slowly, and it is has been suggested that this is because of the presence of regulatory DC that can tolerize invading T cells (Steptoe and Thomson, 1996; Thomson *et al.*, 2002). Again, this process is analogous to that we have suggested may occur in the intestine, and these DC may be an additional APC population that takes up orally administered soluble antigen for the induction of tolerance. Indeed, the induction of fasL⁺ Treg cells in the liver of TcR transgenic mice fed antigen is dependent on antigen loaded, IL-18 producing DC that polarize T-cell differentiation *in vivo* and *in vitro* (Watanabe *et al.*, 2003). Whether these processes in the liver play an essential role in oral tolerance under normal conditions remains to be determined. That Kupffer cells are not involved is suggested by the fact that, although orally administered haptenized protein can be found on Kupffer cells in the liver, Kupffer cell depletion did not affect oral tolerance induction (Ju and Pohl, 2001).

Modulation of oral tolerance

The initiation of clinical trials has raised interest in finding agents that can enhance the induction of oral tolerance. As oral tolerance mainly affects Th1 responses in the periphery, anything that favors Th1 versus Th2 or Th3 responses might be expected to abrogate oral tolerance and the converse **(Table 27.2)**. This is consistent with the ability of exogenous IFN-γ, IL-18 or IL-12 to abrogate oral tolerance (Z. Zhang and Michael, 1990; Marinaro *et al.*, 1997; Eaton *et al.*, 2003) and with the enhanced tolerance found after administration of anti-IL-12 to OVA TCR transgenic mice. This last effect is associated both with increased TGF-β secretion and T-cell apoptosis (Marth *et al.*, 1996). Transgenic overexpression of IL-12 in the PP also partially prevents oral tolerance induction, especially for Th1 cell

tolerance (Y. Chen *et al.*, 2000). The ability of exogenous IL-12 and IL-18 to prevent oral tolerance is accompanied by enhanced CD80 expression on DC (Eaton *et al.*, 2003). In uveitis, IL-2 potentiates oral tolerance in association with increased production of TGF-β, IL-4, and IL-10 in PP (Rizzo *et al.*, 1994). Furthermore, the ability of LPS to enhance oral tolerance to MBP is associated with increased expression of IL-4 in the brain (Khoury *et al.*, 1990, 1992), and oral administration of IL-4 itself (Inobe *et al.*, 1998) or of IL-10 (Slavin *et al.*, 2001) can enhance oral tolerance in EAE. The β and τ forms of type 1 IFN have similar effects in MBP-fed mice in association with upregulated production of IL-10 and TGF-β (Nelson *et al.*, 1996; Soos *et al.*, 2002). Certain commonly used drugs for autoimmune diseases such as methotrexate may also enhance oral tolerance (Al-Sabbagh *et al.*, 1997), while nondepleting anti-CD4 monoclonal antibodies and oral alloantigens have synergistic effects in inducing tolerance of cardiac allografts (Niimi *et al.*, 2000). Other exogenous agents that have been reported to enhance oral tolerance when given orally include infection with the helminth *H. polygyrus* (Shi *et al.*, 2000), soluble egg antigens (SEA) from *Schistosoma mansoni* (Maron *et al.*, 1998), the β2-adrenergic agonist salbutamol (Cobelens *et al.*, 2002b), dietary polyunsaturated fatty acids (Harbige and Fisher, 2001), and polysaccharide AZ9 from *Klebsiella oxytoca* (Sugihara *et al.*, 2002). The basis of these effects is unknown, although SEA induces the differentiation of DC that polarize T cells to a Th2/Th3 phenotype (Sher *et al.*, 2003).

One of the most potent means of enhancing oral tolerance is to couple antigen to the B subunit of CT-B, contrasting with the mucosal adjuvant properties of the intact CT holotoxin (Holmgren *et al.*, 2003). This has been achieved using a number of different antigens, including SRBC, but has been studied particularly with proteins and peptides of pathologic importance, such as insulin and heat shock protein (J. B. Sun *et al.*, 1994, 1996; Arakawa *et al.*, 1998; Bergerot *et al.*, 1997; Ploix *et al.*, 1999; Phipps *et al.*, 2003; Sadeghi *et al.*, 2002, Bregenholt *et al.*, 2003; Petersen *et al.*, 2003). This approach requires extremely low doses of antigen and can increase the tolerogenic potential of fed antigens by many fold, as well as allow suppression of ongoing immune responses in primed animals (Rask *et al.*, 2000). Induction of oral tolerance with CT-B is associated with the generation of bystander suppression and may be mediated by IL-10, IL-4, or TGF-β producing Treg cells (J.B. Sun *et al.*, 2000; Phipps *et al.*, 2003). Although it is not known how CT-B enhances oral tolerance, it is known to increase the uptake of antigen by APC via its ability to bind to GM1 ganglioside (Eriksson *et al.*, 2003). Because of its lack of enzymatic activity, CT-B may therefore enhance presentation in the absence of inflammation with resulting induction of anergy or Treg cells. This is consistent with the evidence discussed in the preceding text that oral antigen delivery using noninflammatory, biodegradable microparticles such as a multiple emulsion system (Pecquet *et al.*, 2000; Kim *et al.*, 2002), liposomes (Masuda *et al.*, 2002), entrapping polymers such as

Table 27.2. Modulation of Oral Tolerance[a]

Augments	Prevents
IL-2	IFN-γ
IL-4/IL-10	IL-12, IL-18
Helminth infection	CD80 overexpression
Anti-CD4	
Anti-IL-12	CT
CT-B	Anti-MCP-1 (CCL2)
LPS	Anti γδ-Ab
Type 1 IFNs	GVHR
Multiple emulsions	CY, 2'-dGuo
Liposomes	Estradiol
PLGA	

[a] Abbreviations: CT-B, cholera toxin B subunit; IFN, interferon; IL, interleukin; LPS, lipopolysaccharide; MCP, monocyte chemotactic protein 1; CY, cyclophosphamide; 2'-dGuo, 2'-deoxyguanosine.

polylactic-coglycolic acid (PLGA) (Kim *et al.*, 2002), or dietary polyunsaturated fatty acids (Harbige and Fisher, 2001) also enhances oral tolerance. On the other hand, coupling of OVA to other slow delivery systems such as cyclodextrins has no effect on oral tolerance induction (Kamphorst *et al.*, 2004b). Possibly these systems that improve tolerance induction enhance tolerogenic antigen presentation.

A number of agents can interfere with the induction of oral tolerance, including drugs that deplete regulatory cells, such as cyclophosphamide and 2′-deoxyguanosine (Mowat *et al.*, 1982; Mowat, 1986), as well as the factors that enhance generalized APC functions (see the preceding text). The abrogation of oral tolerance by CT may reflect selective pharmacologic effects on Treg cells. Alternatively, the strong mucosal Th1 responses induced by orally administered CT (Wilson *et al.*, 1991; Hörnquist and Lycke, 1993) may make it impossible to suppress subsequent systemic Th1 responses after peripheral challenge. It has also been reported that antibodies to the chemokine MCP-1 abrogate oral tolerance, perhaps by interfering with the development or chemotaxis of the Th2-type or Th3-type regulatory cells generated in the gut (Karpus and Lukacs, 1996). Oral tolerance is completely blocked when residues of palmitate are covalently bound to the fed antigen. Moreover, oral administration of OVA-palmitate can boost and/or prime mice for both cellular and antibody responses (Oliveira *et al.*, 2002). Infectious agents may also break oral tolerance by cross-presentation of tolerated antigens in an inflammatory context by APCs. Links between the development of autoimmunity and infection have been frequently observed. In a recent report on a model system in which transgenic OVA is expressed by enterocytes, oral tolerance was readily abrogated by either concomitant infection with vesicular stomatitis virus encoding OVA, oral CT administration, or CD40 triggering (Vezys and Lefrancois, 2002).

INDUCTION OF TOLERANCE BY THE NASAL ROUTE

Other forms of mucosal tolerance have recently been investigated, specifically the administration of antigen via the nasal or aerosol route. These routes appear equally efficient and in some instances may be more effective in suppressing autoimmune diseases in animal models (Al-Sabbagh *et al.*, 1996a; Daniel and Wegmann, 1996; Harrison *et al.*, 1996; Dick *et al.*, 1993, 1994, 2001; Hoyne *et al.*, 1993b; Ma *et al.*, 1995; Metzler and Wraith, 1993; Staines *et al.*, 1996; Tian *et al.*, 1996; Zou *et al.*, 1999; Barchan *et al.*, 1999; Garcia *et al.*, 1999; Laliotou and Dick, 1999; Derry *et al.*, 2001; Kaya *et al.*, 2002; Monfardini *et al.*, 2002; Prakken *et al.*, 2002; Bardos *et al.*, 2002; H. Y. Wu *et al.*, 2002). Nasal administration of major allergens such as *Dermatophagoides* proteins (Derp1) or microencapsulated immunodominant peptides of Derp1 is effective in inhibiting specific IgE production and airway inflammation (Hall *et al.*, 2003). Nasal tolerance in these models is linked to the production of IL-10 by antigen-specific

CD4[+] T cells, although clonal deletion has been suggested to be the mechanism of the tolerance induced by intranasal administration of peptides from phospholipase A2, a major bee venom allergen (Astori *et al.*, 2000). Although most immune responses seem to be sensitive to nasal tolerance, including Th1-mediated and Th2-mediated inflammatory conditions, as well as IFN-γ, IL-4, and IL-13 production and specific IgE antibodies, IgG1 antibody production appears to be resistant (Akbari *et al.*, 2001; Maron *et al.*, 2002b).

As with oral tolerance, the induction of nasal tolerance is influenced by the dose and frequency of antigen administration (Jiang *et al.*, 2001), as well as by the genetic background (Quinn *et al.*, 2001) and age of the animal (Mucida *et al.*, 2004). T cells from NOD mice appear to be resistant to tolerization by this route, a property linked to the expression of the I-A^{g7} class II MHC molecule on APC (Quinn *et al.*, 2001). Nasal tolerance also depends on the full development of the immune system, and neonatal animals are less susceptible to nasally induced tolerance (Menezes *et al.*, 2003; Mucida *et al.*, 2004). Intranasal tolerance has been demonstrated to have beneficial effects in humans with allergic rhinitis (van Hage-Hamsten *et al.*, 2002; Bellussi *et al.*, 2002; Bertoni *et al.*, 1999).

There are obvious advantages of using the nasal route for tolerance induction, especially the fact that smaller doses of antigen can be used, perhaps because there is less degradation of proteins in the respiratory tract. Similarities and differences can be observed in the mechanisms involved in the two forms of tolerance. Although IL-10 is usually reported to be the key regulatory mediator, increased TGF-β production has also been detected in some systems (Takeda *et al.*, 2002; Im *et al.*, 2000a; Shi *et al.*, 1999a; Xiao *et al.*, 1998). Moreover, CD4[+] T cells engineered to produce either IL-10 (Oh *et al.*, 2002) or TGF-β1 (Hansen *et al.*, 2000) can reverse allergen-induced airway hyperreactivity and inflammation induced by OVA-specific Th2 effector cells *in vivo*. A role for antigen-specific CD4[+]CD25[+] Treg cells (Unger *et al.*, 2003) and IFN-γ-producing γδ CD8α[+] T cells (McMenamin *et al.*, 1991, 1994, 1995; Hanninen and Harrison, 2000) has also been defined. Bystander suppression can also be achieved by nasal administration of antigens, and this has been exploited therapeutically in experimental models of atherosclerosis (Maron *et al.*, 2002b), Alzheimer's disease (Weiner *et al.*, 2000), and stroke (Takeda *et al.*, 2002; Frenkel *et al.*, 2004). IL-10 and TGF-β have been the regulatory mechanisms implicated in these models.

Recent studies comparing nasal and oral administration of antigen have suggested that the nature of the local DC populations determines a bias toward IL-10-dependent mechanisms in nasal tolerance, compared with mixed, or TGF-β-dependent regulation in the intestine (Akbari *et al.*, 2001). This reflects the polarizing effects of DC isolated from the draining lymphoid organs of each tissue, leading to the induction of Treg cells with different cytokine patterns. In the case of nasal tolerance, mucosal DC produce mainly IL-10 (Stumbles *et al.*, 1998; Akbari *et al.*, 2001) and express the inducible costimulatory molecule (ICOS), leading to a population of IL-10-producing T_{reg} (Akbari *et al.*, 2002).

CLINICAL APPLICATIONS OF ORAL TOLERANCE

Treatment of animal models of autoimmune disease by induction of oral tolerance

Many studies have demonstrated the effectiveness of orally administered myelin antigens in rat and mouse models of autoimmune disease (Table 27.3).

Experimental autoimmune encephalomyelitis

Acute EAE in rats and mice can be suppressed by feeding MBP, with high doses of MBP resulting in clonal anergy in the Lewis rat (Bitar and Whitacre, 1988; Whitacre *et al.*, 1991; Javed *et al.*, 1995), whereas lower doses induce transferable cellular suppression (Higgins and Weiner, 1988; A. Miller *et al.*, 1993; J. E. A. P. Miller and Heath, 1993). In the nervous system of low-dose-fed animals, inflammatory cytokines such as TNF and IFN-γ are downregulated, and TGF-β is upregulated (Khoury *et al.*, 1992). Oral MBP

can also partially suppress serum antibody responses, especially at higher doses (Higgins and Weiner, 1988; Kelly and Whitacre, 1996). Administration of myelin to sensitized animals in the chronic guinea pig model, or of larger doses of MBP in the murine EAE model is protective and does not exacerbate disease (Brod *et al.*, 1991; Meyer *et al.*, 1996), and long-term administration over a 6-month period of myelin in mice with chronic was beneficial (Al-Sabbagh *et al.*, 1996b). EAE can also be suppressed in animals transgenic for an MBP-specific TCR following feeding with MBP (Y. Chen *et al.*, 1996). A variety of MBP or PLP peptides can also suppress EAE (A. Miller *et al.*, 1993; Al-Sabbagh *et al.*, 1994; Karpus and Luckacs, 1996), as can nasally administered MBP (Al-Sabbagh *et al.*, 1996a) and MBP peptides (Metzler and Wraith, 1993). Oral administration of glatiramer acetate (Cop1, Copaxone), a copolymer that appears to act as an altered peptide ligand for MBP, induces tolerance to EAE in both the mouse and the rat models (Teitelbaum *et al.*, 1999; Maron *et al.*, 2002a). It also suppresses EAE and induces the upregulation of TGF-β in MBP TcR transgenic mice (Maron *et al.*, 2002a) and is currently being used parenterally to treat multiple sclerosis.

Table 27.3. Suppression of Autoimmunity by Oral Tolerance[a]

| (a) Animal Models | |
Model	Protein Fed
EAE	MBP, PLP, Copaxone
Arthritis (CII, AA)	CII
Uveitis	S-Ag, IRBP
Neuritis	PNS-myelin
Experimental	Myelin, P2 peptide
Autoimmune neuritis	
Myasthenia gravis	AChR
Diabetes (NOD mouse)	Insulin, GAD
Transplantation	Alloantigen, MRC peptide, type V collagen
Thyroiditis	Thyroglobulin
Colitis	Haptenized or normal cononic proteins
Atopic disease	Derp1, cedar pollen
Antiphospholipid syndrome	Immunoglobulins
(b) Human Disease Trials	
Disease Trial	Protein Fed
Multiple sclerosis	Bovine myelin
Rheumatoid arthritis	Chicken, bovine type II collagen
Uveitis	Bovine S-Ag
Type 1 diabetes	Human insulin, GAD65
Contact allergy	Nickel salts
Systemic sclerosis	Bovine type I collagen

[a] Abbreviations: AChR, acetylcholine receptor; CII, type II collagen; EAE, experimental allergic encephalomyelitis; IRBP, interphotoreceptor binding protein; MBP, myelin basic protein; MHC, major histocompatibility complex; NOD, nonobese diabetic; PLP, proteolipid protein.

Arthritis

Oral administration of type II collagen suppresses several models of arthritis including collagen-induced arthritis (CIA) (Nagler-Anderson *et al.*, 1986; Thompson and Staines, 1986; Thompson *et al.*, 1993b), adjuvant arthritis (J. Zhang *et al.*, 1990), pristane arthritis (Thompson *et al.*, 1993a), and antigen-induced arthritis (Yoshino *et al.*, 1995; Inada *et al.*, 1996). Interestingly, it was reported that systemic anti-IL-4 treatment during oral administration of collagen II blocked the suppression of CIA by oral tolerance (Yoshino and Yoshino, 1998). Aerosol administration of type II collagen suppressed CIA in rats to a degree similar to that seen with oral administration (Al-Sabbagh *et al.*, 1996). Oral administration of an immunodominant human collagen peptide modulates CIA in mice (Khare *et al.*, 1995), and type II collagen peptides given nasally also suppresses CIA in mice (Staines *et al.*, 1996). Oral administration of collagen II is effective for tolerization in adjuvant-induced arthritis (AA) in rats (J. Zhang *et al.*, 1990) and in pristane-induced arthritis (Thompson *et al.*, 1993). Other animal models of arthritis that have been successfully treated by mucosal tolerance include streptococcal cell wall arthritis (W. Chen *et al.*, 1998a), silicone-induced arthritis (Yoshino *et al.*, 1995), and avridine-induced arthritis (Prakken *et al.* 1997). A synergistic suppressive effect in the AA model was observed using methotrexate (a widely used drug in rheumatoid arthritis) and oral administration of collagen II (Weiner and Komagata, 1998). Oral mycobacterial 65-kD heat shock protein also suppresses AA (Haque *et al.*, 1996), an effect that is associated with expansion of CD4+CD25+ T_{reg} in the spleen (Cobelens *et al.*, 2002a).

Experimental autoimmune uveitis

Oral administration of S antigen (S-Ag), a retinal autoantigen that induces EAU or S-Ag peptides prevents or markedly diminishes the clinical appearance of S-Ag-induced disease as measured by ocular inflammation (Nussenblatt *et al.*, 1990; Singh *et al.*, 1992; Thurau *et al.*, 1996; Vrabec *et al.*, 1992). Feeding interphotoreceptor binding protein (IRBP) suppresses IRBP-induced disease, and this is potentiated by IL-2 (Rizzo *et al.*, 1994; Wildner and Thurau, 1995). As we have noted earlier, this IL-2-induced tolerance is dependent on IL-4 and IL-10 (Rizzo *et al.*, 1999). Recent studies show that feeding a peptide derived from HSP60 linked to CT-B can suppress EAU in rats, suggesting a novel approach to treating this condition using defined stress proteins (Phipps *et al.*, 2003).

Experimental autoimmune myasthenia gravis

Although myasthenia gravis is an antibody-mediated disease, oral (Okumura *et al.*, 1994; Wang *et al.*, 1993a, b, 1995) and nasal (Ma *et al.*, 1995) administration of the Torpedo acetylcholine receptor (AChR) to Lewis rats prevents or delays the onset of experimental autoimmune myasthenia gravis (EAMG). Although large doses of antigen were required to achieve these effects, oral administration by oral route of a nonmyasthenogenic recombinant fragment of the AchR α-subunit inhibits ongoing acute and chronic experimental

myasthenia gravis in rats by an active suppressive mechanism (Im *et al.*, 1999, 2000b). Experimental autoimmune myasthenia gravis can also be suppressed by nasally administered AchR (Ma *et al.*, 1995) and AchR peptides (Karachunski *et al.*, 1997).

Insulin-dependent diabetes mellitus

Oral insulin has been shown to delay and, in some instances, prevent diabetes in the NOD mouse model. Such suppression is transferable, primarily by CD4+ cells (J. Zhang *et al.*, 1991; Bergerot *et al.*, 1994). Immunohistochemistry of pancreatic islets of Langerhans isolated from insulin-fed animals demonstrates decreased insulitis associated with decreased IFN-γ, as well as increased expression of TNF, IL-4, IL-10, TGF-β, and PGE$_2$ (Hancock *et al.*, 1995). Interestingly, oral tolerance is a more effective therapy for IDDM in neonates compared with adult NOD mice, suggesting that the ideal period for a prophylactic use of oral tolerance in high-risk human populations may be very early in life (Maron *et al.*, 2001). Some reports on oral tolerance support a beneficial role for Th2 cytokines in the suppression of diabetes. Oral dosing with bacterial stimulants such as LPS and *E. coli* extract OM-89 in NOD mice induces a Th2 shift in the gut cytokine gene expression, and concomitantly, improves diabetes prevention by oral insulin administration (Hartmann *et al.*, 1997). Regulatory Th2-type T-cell lines against insulin and glutamic acid decarboxylase (GAD) peptides derived from orally and nasally treated NOD mice suppress diabetes (Maron *et al.* 1999). Conjugation of insulin to CT-B produces extremely potent oral tolerance of experimental IDDM, and this is associated with upregulation of IL-4 and TGF-β (Ploix *et al.*, 1999; Bregenholt *et al.*, 2003; Petersen *et al.*, 2003; Sadeghi *et al.*, 2002). Nasal administration of the insulin B chain or GAD and aerosol insulin suppresses diabetes in the NOD mouse (Daniel and Wegmann, 1996; Harrison *et al.*, 1996; Tian *et al.*, 1996; Maron *et al.*, 1999; Hanninen and Harrison, 2000).

A note of caution must be added to these findings, which is that it is possible to prime CD8+ T cell–dependent IDDM by feeding antigen to mice expressing OVA on pancreatic islets (Blanas *et al.*, 1996; Hänninen *et al.*, 2001). These findings indicate that care may need to be taken in designing therapeutic regimes of oral tolerance in IDDM. This priming effect has not been noted with insulin, and indeed, it has been shown that feeding insulin suppresses diabetes in a virally induced, CD8+ T cell–dependent model of diabetes in which LCMV was expressed under the insulin promoter and animals infected with LCMV to induce diabetes (von Herrath *et al.*, 1996). Under these conditions, protection was associated with a shift toward production of IL-4, IL-10 and TGF-β in the islets.

Transplantation and other models of immunopathology

Oral administration of allogeneic cells to mice sensitized by skin grafts modulates accelerated rejection of vascularized cardiac allografts such that they are now rejected in a manner more similar to the acute response seen in unsensitized recipients (Sayegh *et al.*, 1992b). Orally administered allopeptides in the Lewis rat reduces DTH responses to the peptide (Sayegh et al., 1992a). Oral, but not intravenous, alloantigen was accompanied by elevation of intragraft levels of IL-4 (Sayegh et al., 1992b). Oral alloantigen has also been shown to enhance corneal allograft survival even in preimmune hosts (He et al., 1996). This tolerance is absent in IL-4 KO and IFN-γ KO mice (Niederkorn and Mayhew, 2002). Lung allograft rejection can be prevented by oral treatment with an autoantigen, type V collagen, and this bystander suppressor effect is dependent on TGF-β (Haque et al., 2002; Yasufuku et al., 2001).

Allergy and other models of immunopathology

Suppression of Th2-mediated experimental asthma can also be achieved by oral tolerance (Russo et al., 1998; Nakao et al., 1998; Y. Chung et al., 2002), and optimal oral regimens such as continuous feeding reduce specific IgE/IgG1 responses and airway eosinophilic inflammation even in IL-5 transgenic mice (Russo et al., 2001). TGF-β appears to be the critical regulatory factor involved (Haneda et al., 1997). As we have noted earlier, the beneficial effects of oral tolerance in IgE-mediated atopy extend to major allergens such as Derp1 (M. N. Sato et al., 2002) and its peptides (Hoyne et al., 1994) as well as to cedar pollen antigens in rhinitis (Yoshitomi et al., 2002) and milk allergens in atopic conjunctivitis in dogs (Zemann et al., 2003).

Other organ-specific autoimmune or inflammatory conditions that are susceptible to oral tolerance include autoimmune thyroiditis, which can be suppressed by feeding thyroglobulin (Guimaraes et al., 1995a, b; Peterson and Braley-Mullen, 1995). Experimental autoimmune neuritis (EAN), a model of human inflammatory demyelinating neuropathies, which is induced by immunization with bovine peripheral nervous system (PNS)-myelin or a neuritogenic P2 peptide, can be inhibited by feeding either of these antigens (Jung et al., 2001). Feeding of glomerular basement membrane prevents the development of experimental autoimmune glomerulonephritis in WKY rats (Reynolds and Pusey, 2001). Experimental granulomatous colitis in mice can be prevented by feeding normal colonic proteins (Dasgupta et al., 2001), or in the case of hapten-induced colitis, by feeding the hapten itself (Elson et al., 1996) or haptenized colonic proteins (Neurath et al., 1996). In the latter case, the tolerance is dependent on TGF-β. In addition to these organ-specific conditions, more generalized autoimmune disease has also been prevented by oral tolerance, with the anti-phospholipid syndrome being suppressed by induction of CD8+ T cells producing IL-10 and TGF-β by oral administration of polyclonal immunoglobulins ((Krause et al., 2002). Oral tolerization to adenoviral antigens permitted long-term gene expression using recombinant adenoviral vectors (Ilan et al., 1997).

Human disease

The initial indication that oral tolerance could occur in humans came from studies showing that exposure to a contact-sensitizing agent via the mucosa prior to subsequent skin challenge led to unresponsiveness in a portion of patients studied (Lowney, 1968). Subsequently it was reported that KLH administered orally to human subjects decreased subsequent cell-mediated immune responses, although antibody responses were not affected (Husby et al., 1994). Nasal KLH has also been reported to induce tolerance in humans (Waldo et al., 1994). On the basis of the long history of oral tolerance and the safety of the approach, human trials were initiated in MS, retinal angiopathy (RA), uveitis, and diabetes (see Table 27.3). These initial trials suggested that there was no systemic toxicity or exacerbation of disease. Although positive effects were observed, consistent clinical efficacy has yet to be demonstrated. Results in humans, however, have paralleled several aspects of what has been observed in animals.

In MS patients, MBP-specific and PLP-specific TGF-β-secreting Th3-type cells have been observed in the peripheral blood of patients treated with an oral bovine myelin preparation and not in patients who were untreated (Fukaura et al., 1996). There was no increase in MBP-specific or PLP-specific IFN-γ-secreting cells in treated patients. These results demonstrate that it is possible to induce autoantigen-specific TGF-β-secreting cells in a human autoimmune disease by oral administration of the autoantigen. A pilot study of oral myelin in MS suggested positive effects related to DR type or sex (Weiner et al., 1993). However, a subsequent 515-patient, placebo-controlled, double-blind Phase III trial of single-dose bovine myelin in relapsing-remitting MS randomized for DR type and sex did not show differences between placebo and treated groups in the number relapses, a large placebo effect being observed (AutoImmune, Inc., Lexington, MA, USA). Preliminary analysis of magnetic resonance imaging data from this trial, however, showed significant changes favoring oral myelin in certain of the prospectively defined and randomized patient subgroups. Based on the results of oral tolerance in uveitis in humans (Nussenblatt et al., 1997) and in animal models (Benson et al., 1999), it appears that protein mixtures, such as the ones used in MS trials, may not be as effective oral tolerogens as purified proteins.

In rheumatoid arthritis, a single center double-blind study of oral collagen showed statistically significant effects of feeding collagen (Trentham et al., 1993). A 274-patient double-blind phase II dosing trial of chicken type II collagen in doses ranging from 20 μg–2500 μg demonstrated statistically significant positive effects in the group treated with the lowest dose (Barnett et al., 1998). Oral administration of larger doses of bovine type II collagen (1–10 mg) did not show a significant difference between tested and placebo groups, although a higher prevalence of responders was reported for the groups treated with type II collagen (Sieper et al., 1996). These results are consistent with animal studies of orally administered type II collagen in which protection against adjuvant-induced and antigen-induced arthritis and bystander suppression was observed only at the lower doses

(Yoshino *et al.*, 1995; Z. Zhang and Michael, 1990). An open-label pilot study of oral collagen in juvenile RA gave positive results with no toxicity (Barnett *et al.*, 1996). This lack of systemic toxicity is an important feature for the clinical use of oral tolerance, especially in children for whom the long-term effects of immunosuppressive drugs is unknown. Results from a further phase II dosing trial of oral collagen in 360 patients showed substantial differences from baseline in patients receiving 60 μg but no statistically significant differences between treated and placebo groups (again, a large placebo effect was observed). However, additional recently completed phase II trials have shown that a significant number of patients receiving 20 μg oral collagen do better than when treated previously with methotrexate (AutoImmune, Inc.). Recent studies with small numbers of patients with rheumatoid arthritis have shown clinical improvement of disease and downmodulation of proinflammatory cytokines after oral treatment with low doses of bovine collagen type II for 3 months. Increase in TGF-β production was also observed in orally treated patients (Myers *et al.*, 2001).

Induction of immune tolerance to human type I collagen (CI) in patients with systemic sclerosis was reported by oral administration of bovine type I collagen. The oral treatment with 0.1 mg of solubilized native bovine CI daily for one month was followed by 0.5 mg daily for 11 months. Improvement in skin thickness scores and lung carbon monoxide diffusing capacity was observed in treated patients (McKown *et al.*, 1999).

Trials have also been initiated in new-onset diabetes in which recombinant human insulin and GAD65 were administered orally, and a recent trial was conducted in 372 subjects at risk for diabetes as part of the diabetes prevention trial (DPT-1). Preliminary data from the DPT-1 Oral Insulin Trial, presented in oral form, showed that oral insulin did not delay or prevent type 1 diabetes in relatives of patients with type 1 diabetes selected by the presence of CIA and insulin autoantibodies (Skyler, 2004). A two-dose oral insulin tolerance trial was also performed recently in diagnosed diabetic patients with positive CIA. Preliminary results from this study indicated that oral insulin resulted in improved endogenous insulin secretion in patients diagnosed over age 20 years. In patients diagnosed under age 20, feeding doses of 1 mg did not alter insulin secretion, and the 10-mg dose worsened the outcome (MacLaren *et al.*, 2004). If confirmed, these findings suggests that dose and age of diagnosis are important parameters for the design of future trials on diabetes.

In uveitis, a pilot trial of S-Ag and an S-Ag mixture performed at the National Eye Institute (Bethesda, MD, USA) showed positive trends with oral bovine S-Ag, but not with a mixture of retinal antigens (Nussenblatt *et al.*, 1997). Feeding a peptide derived from a patient's own HLA antigen appeared to have an effect on uveitis, in that patients could discontinue their steroids because of reduced intraocular inflammation mediated by oral tolerance (Thurau *et al.*, 1999). Oral desensitization to nickel allergy in humans induces a decrease in nickel-specific T cells and affects cutaneous eczema (Bagot *et al.*, 1995).

It is clear from the trials that have already been conducted in humans that there are important parameters to be considered for mucosal tolerance to be effective in human diseases. These include the dose and degree of purity of the antigen, and in some cases, nasal treatment may be more suitable. Mucosal adjuvants with properties to deviate immune responses toward Th2/Th3 type and the use of a combined therapy with conventional immunosuppressive drugs may also help to increase efficiency.

Although it is clear that oral antigen can suppress autoimmunity in animals, much remains to be learned. Under certain experimental conditions, worsening of autoimmune diseases in animals by oral antigen has been reported (Blanas *et al.* 1996; Meyer *et al.* 1996; C. C. Miller *et al.* 1994; Terato *et al.* 1996), emphasizing the need to understand the molecular events underlying the induction of tolerance and immunity via the gut. As these become understood better, the ability to apply mucosal tolerance successfully for the treatment of human autoimmune and other diseases will be further enhanced.

Consequences of breakdown in oral tolerance
The strength and persistence of oral tolerance indicate its potential physiologic importance in preventing hypersensitivity to food proteins and commensal bacteria. This hypothesis is supported by the relative infrequency of naturally occurring immunologic responsiveness to dietary antigens and IBD, as well as by evidence from experimental studies.

In experimental situations when oral tolerance has been prevented, subsequent oral challenge of the mice with antigen results in the development of mucosal pathology in the jejunum, which consists of crypt hyperplasia, crypt hypertrophy, and increased infiltration of the epithelium by lymphocytes (Mowat and Ferguson, 1981; Mowat and Parrott, 1983; Mowat, 1986; Lamont *et al.*, 1989; Strobel and Ferguson, 1986; Stokes *et al.*, 1987). These features are accompanied by a local cell-mediated immune response in the draining mesenteric lymph nodes (Mowat and Ferguson, 1982; Mowat and Parrott, 1983) and are consistent with the presence of Th1-mediated intestinal immunopathology (Mowat, 1997). The features of the mucosal pathology induced in the absence of oral tolerance are also qualitatively similar to those found in naturally occurring FSE and in the early lesions of IBD such as Crohn's disease (Mowat, 1984; Ferguson, 1987). That a defect in oral tolerance may account for the development of food-sensitive enteropathy (FSE) under natural conditions is suggested by studies in weaning piglets that have shown that the development of postweaning diarrhea is influenced by the age of introduction of novel antigens and can be prevented by artificially inducing oral tolerance to the antigens to be fed at weaning (B. G. Miller *et al.*, 1984; Stokes *et al.*, 1987). Neonatal calves exhibit a similar susceptibility to developing systemic hypersensitivity and enteropathy in response to dietary proteins such as soy protein (Barratt *et al.*,

1987). These findings are consistent with the evidence that there are decreased numbers of TGF-β–secreting cells in the mucosa of food allergic children (Perez-Machado et al., 2003) and that celiac disease is associated with increased levels of IFN-γ production (Nilsen et al., 1998; Monteleone et al., 2001b), supporting the view that a loss of normal regulatory responses to food proteins predisposes to inflammatory immunopathology.

We have discussed the evidence that this homeostasis is mediated by the fact that intestinal DCs are normally in a "quiescent" state and propose that this is maintained by the presence of the high levels of modulatory cytokines such as TGF-β and IL-10. In addition, recent studies have suggested that intestinal macrophages and stromal cells produce cyclo-oxygenase 2 (COX-2) dependent PGE_2 constitutively under the influence of the physiologic levels of LPS absorbed from intestinal flora (Newberry et al., 1999, 2001). DC themselves may also express COX-2 and produce PGE_2 in response to LPS (Harizi et al., 2002). As PGE_2 is known to polarize DC differentiation toward an IL-10-producing, inhibitory phenotype (Kalinski et al., 1998, 1999; Harizi et al., 2002), this could also help explain the prevalence of such DC in the normal gut. The result of these interactions between intestinal contents, unique anatomic features, immune and non-immune cells is an environment that favors the induction of IgA antibodies and regulatory T cell–dependent tolerance. This ensures that a homeostatic balance is maintained between the intestinal immune system and its antigen load, retaining the ability to recognize both dangerous and harmless antigens as foreign, while preventing hypersensitivity reactions. Clearly, pathogen-derived danger signals and other inflammatory stimuli can override the normally inhibitory phenotype of mucosal DC (Williamson et al., 1999b), allowing protective immunity to develop when necessary, and one might predict that similar innate immune stimuli may predispose to the development of celiac disease and other food hypersensitivities. Interference with the PGE_2-mediated regulatory activity in the intestine produces a celiac-like condition in TcR transgenic mice fed specific antigen (Newberry et al., 1999). Sensitizing agents such as trinitrobenzene sulfonate (TNBS) (Elson et al., 1996) and alcohol (Andrade et al., 2003) as well as ablation of regulatory T-cell subsets (Morrisey et al., 1993; Kuhn et al., 1993; Powrie, 1995) also result in oral tolerance breakdown and colitis. It has been shown that rodents and humans are normally tolerant to their own microbiota, and a breakdown in this state is accompanied by the development of IL-12/IFN-γ-dependent IBD (Duchmann et al., 1995, 1996). In addition, there has long been circumstantial evidence that intestinal infection precedes the onset of celiac disease and recent findings have implicated type 1 IFN in initiating the Th1-mediated pathogenesis of celiac disease (Monteleone et al., 2001a, b). Furthermore, certain fragments of gliadin, the causal antigen in celiac disease can activate several aspects of innate immunity in the mucosa, including local DCs (Maiuri et al., 2003), and the celiac epithelium shows increased permeability to such material (Matysiak-Budnik

et al., 2003a). Together with the association between polymorphisms in the CTLA-4 gene and celiac disease (Popat et al., 2002), these results support the experimental data we have discussed on how oral tolerance to dietary antigens reflects a complex interplay between intestinal absorption, regulation of specific immune responses, and innate immunity. Dissecting how these pathways are maintained and can be disturbed will provide new insight into the pathogenesis of disease and perhaps the more efficient use of oral tolerance as a therapeutic tool.

REFERENCES

Akbari, O., DeKruyff, R. H., and Umetsu, D.T. (2001). Pulmonary dendritic cells producing IL-10 mediate tolerance induced by respiratory exposure to antigen. *Nat. Immunol.* 2, 725–731.

Akbari, O., Freeman, G. J., Meyer, E. H., Greenfield, E. A., Chang, T. T., Sharpe, A. H., Berry, G., DeKruyff, R. H., and Umetsu, D.T. (2002). Antigen-specific regulatory T cells develop via the ICOS-ICOS-ligand pathway and inhibit allergen-induced airway hyperreactivity. *Nat. Med.* 8, 1024–1032.

Alpan, O., Rudomen, G., and Matzinger, P. (2001). The role of dendritic cells, B cells and M cells in gut-oriented immune responses *J. Immunol.* 166, 4843–4852.

Al-Sabbagh, A., Miller, A., Santos, L. M. B., and Weiner, H. L. (1994). Antigen-driven tissue-specific suppression following oral tolerance: Orally administered myelin basic protein suppresses proteolipid induced experimental autoimmune encephalomyelitis in the SJL mouse. *Eur. J. Immunol.* 24, 2104–2109.

Al-Sabbagh, A., Nelson, P., Sobel, R. A., and Weiner, H. L. (1996a). Antigen-driven peripheral immune tolerance: Suppression of experimental autoimmune encephalomyelitis and collagen induced arthritis by aerosol administration of myelin basic protein or type II collagen. *Cell. Immunol.* 171, 111–119.

Al-Sabbagh, A. M., Goad, M. E. P., Weiner, H. L., and Nelson, P. A. (1996b). Decreased CNS inflammation and absence of clinical exacerbation of disease after six months oral administration of bovine myelin in diseased SJL/J mice with chronic relapsing experimental autoimmune encephalomyelitis. *J. Neurol. Res.* 45, 424–429.

Al-Sabbagh, A., Garcia, G., Slavin, A., Weiner, H. L., and Nelson, P. (1997). *Neurology* 48, A421.

Andrade M.C., Vaz, N.M., and Faria, A.M.C. (2003). Ethanol-induced colitis prevents oral tolerance induction in mice. *Braz. J. Med. Biol. Res.* 36: 1227–1232.

Andre, C., Heremans, J. F., Vaerman, J., and Cambiasco, C. L. (1975). A mechanism for the induction of immunological tolerance by antigen feeding: Antigen-antibody complexes. *J. Exp. Med.* 142, 1509–1519.

Arakawa, T., Yu, J., Chong, D. K., Hough, J., Engen, P. C., and Langridge, W. H. (1998). A plant-based cholera toxin B subunit-insulin fusion protein protects against the development of autoimmune diabetes. *Nat. Biotechnol.* 16, 934–938.

Aramaki, Y., Fujii, Y., Suda, H., Suzuki, I., Yadomae, T., and Tsuchiya., S. (1994). Induction of oral tolerance after feeding of ragweed pollen extract in mice. *Immunol. Lett.* 40, 21–25.

Aroeira, L. S., Cardillo, F., De-Albuquerque, D., Vaz, N. M., and Mengel, J. (1995). Anti-IL-10 treatment does not block either the induction or the maintenance of orally induced tolerance to OVA. *Scand. J. Immunol.* 44, 319–323.

Artik, S., Haarhuis, K., Wu, X., Begerow, J., Gleichmann, E. (2001). Tolerance to nickel: oral nickel administration induces a high frequency of anergic T cells with persistent suppressor activity. *J. Immunol.* 15, 167, 6794–803.

Asai, K., Hachimura, S., Kimura, M., Toraya, T., Yamashita, M., Nakayama, T., and Kaminogawa, S. (2002). T cell hyporesponsiveness induced by oral administration of ovalbumin is associated with impaired NFAT nuclear translocation and p27^{kip1} degradation. *J. Immunol.* 169, 4723–4731.

Asherson, G. L., Zembala, M., Perera, M. A. C. C., Mayhew, B., and Thomas, W. R. (1977). Production of immunity and unresponsiveness in the mouse by feeding contact sensitizing agents and the role of suppressor cells in the Peyer's Patches, mesenteric lymph nodes and other lymphoid tissues. *Cell. Immunol.* 33, 145–155.

Asherson, G. L., Perera, M. A. C. C., and Thomas, W. R. (1979). Contact sensitivity and the DNA response in mice to high and low doses of oxazolone: Low dose unresponsiveness following painting and feeding and its prevention by pretreatment with cyclophosphamide. *Immunology* 36, 449–459.

Astori, M., von Garnier, C., Kettner, A., Dufour, N., Corradin, G., and Spertini, F. (2000). Inducing tolerance by intranasal administration of long peptides in naive and primed CBA/J mice. *J. Immunol.* 165, 3497–3505.

Bach, J. F., and Chatenoud, L. (2001). Tolerance to islet autoantigens in type 1 diabetes. *Annu. Rev. Immunol.* 19, 131–161.

Bach, J. F., and Francois Bach, J. (2003). Regulatory T cells under scrutiny. *Nat. Rev. Immunol.* 3, 189–198.

Bagot, M., Charue, D., Flechet, M. L., Terki, N., Toma, A., and Revuz, J. (1995). Oral desensitization in nickel allergy induces a decrease in nickel-specific T-cells. *Eur. J. Dermatol.* 5, 614–617.

Banchereau, J., and Steinman, R. L. (1998). Dendritic cells and the control of immunity. *Nature* 392, 245–252.

Barchan, D., Souroujon, M. C., Im, S. H., Antozzi, C., and Fuchs, S. (1999). Antigen-specific modulation of experimental myasthenia gravis: Nasal tolerization with recombinant fragments of the human acetylcholine receptor α-subunit. *Proc. Natl. Acad. Sci. USA* 96, 8086–8091.

Bardos, T., Czipri, M., Vermes, C., Zhang, J., Mikecz, K., and Glant, T. T. (2002). Continuous nasal administration of antigen is critical to maintain tolerance in adoptively transferred autoimmune arthritis in SCID mice. *Clin. Exp. Immunol.* 129, 224–231.

Barnard, J. A., Warwick, G. J., and Gold, L. .I. (1993). Localization of transforming growth factor β isoforms in the normal murine small intestine and colon. *Gastroenterology* 105, 67–73.

Barnett, M. L., Combitchi, D., and Trentham, D. E. (1996). A pilot trial of oral type II collagen in the treatment of juvenile rheumatoid arthritis. *Arth. Rheumat.* 39, 623–628.

Barnett, M. L., Kremer, J. M., St Clair, E. W., Clegg, D. O., Furst, D., Weisman, M., Fletcher, M. J., Chasan-Taber, S., Finger, E., Morales, A., Le, C. H., and Trentham, D. E. (1998). Treatment of rheumatoid arthritis with oral type II collagen: Results of a multicenter, double-blind, placebo-controlled trial. *Arth. Rheumat.* 41, 290–297.

Barone, K. S., Jain, S. L., and Michael, J. G. (1995). Effect of *in vivo* depletion of CD4+ and CD8+ cells on the induction and maintenance of oral tolerance. *Cell. Immunol.* 163, 19–29.

Barone, K. S., Tolarova, D. D., Ormsby, I., Doetschman, T., and Michael, J. G. (1998). Induction of oral tolerance in TGF-β1 null mice. *J. Immunol.* 161, 154–160.

Barone, K. S., Herms, B., Karlosky, L., Murray, S., and Qualls, J. (2002). Effect of *in vivo* administration of anti-CTLA-4 mAb and IL-12 on the induction of low dose oral tolerance. *Clin. Exp. Immunol.* 130, 196–203.

Barratt, M. E. J., Powell, J. R., Allen, W. D., and Porter, P. (1987). Immunopathology of intestinal disorders in farm animals. In *Immunopathology of the Small Intestine* (ed. M. N. Marsh), 253–258. Chichester, UK: John Wiley and Sons..

Becker, K. J., McCarron, R. M., and Hallenbeck, J. M. (1997). Oral tolerance to myelin basic protein decreases stroke size. *Stroke* 28, 246.

Bellussi L., Bologna, M., Di Stanislao, C., Lauriello, M., Mezzedimi C., Muzi, P., Passali, G. C., and Passali, D. (2002). Simplified local nasal immunotherapy in mite dust allergic rhinitis. *J. Investig. Allergol. Clin. Immunol.* 12, 42–47.

Benson, J. M., Stuckman, S. S., Cox, K. L., Wardrop, R. M., Gienapp, I. E., Cross, A. H., Trotter, J. L., and Whitacre, C. C. (1999). Oral administration of myelin basic protein is superior to myelin in suppressing established relapsing experimental autoimmune encephalomyelitis. *J. Immunol.* 162, 6247–6254.

Bergerot, J., Fabien, N., Maguer, V., and Thivolet, C. (1994). Oral administration of human insulin to NOD mice generates CD4+ T cells that suppress adoptive transfer of diabetes. *J. Autoimmun.* 7, 655–663.

Bergerot, I., Fioix, C., Peterson, J., Moulin, V., Rask, C., Fabien, N., Lindblad, M., Mayer, A., Czerkinsky, C., Holmgren, J., and Thivolet, C. (1997). A cholera toxoid-insulin conjugate as an oral vaccine against spontaneous autoimmune diabetes. *Proc. Natl. Acad. Sci. USA* 94, 4610–4614.

Bertoni, M., Cosmi, F., Bianchi, I., and Di Bernardino, L. (1999). Clinical efficacy and tolerability of a steady dosage schedule of local nasal immunotherapy: Results of preseasonal treatment in grass pollen rhinitis. *Ann. Allergy Asthma Immunol.* 82, 47–51.

Besredka, A. (1909). De L'Anaphylaxie: Sixieme memoire de l'anaphylaxie lactique. *Ann. Instit. Pasteur* 23, 166–176.

Beyer, K., Castro, R., Birnbaum, A., Benkov, K., Pittman, N., and Sampson, H. A. (2002). Human milk-specific mucosal lymphocytes of the gastrointestinal tract display a TH2 cytokine profile. *J Allergy Clin. Immunol.* 109, 707–713.

Bhan, A. K., Mizoguchi, E., Smith, R. N., and Mizoguchi, A. (1999). Colitis in transgenic and knockout animals as models of human inflammatory bowel disease. *Immunol. Rev.* 169, 195–207.

Bhogal, B. S., Karkhanis, Y. D., Bell, M. K., Sanchez, P., Zemcik, B., Siskind, G. W., and Thorbecke, G. J. (1986). Production of auto-anti-idiotypic antibody during the normal immune response. XII. Enhanced auto-anti-idiotypic antibody production as a mechanism for apparent B cell tolerance in rabbits after feeding antigens. *Cell Immunol.* 101, 93–104.

Bilsborough, J., George, T. C., Norment, A., and Viney, J. L. (2003). Mucosal CD8α+ DC, with a plasmacytoid phenotype, induce differentiation and support function of T cells with regulatory properties. *Immunology* 108, 481–492.

Bitar, D., and Whitacre, C. C. (1988). Suppression of experimental autoimmune encephalomyelitis by the oral administration of myelin basic protein. *Cell Immunol.* 112, 364–370.

Blanas, E., Carbone, F. R., Allison, J., Miller, J. F. A. P., and Heath, W. R. (1996). Induction of autoimmune diabetes by oral administration of autoantigen. *Science* 274, 1707–1709.

Blanas, E., Carbone, F. R., and Heath, W. R. (2000). A bone marrow-derived APC in the gut-associated lymphoid tissue captures oral antigens and presents them to both CD4+ and CD8+ T cells. *J. Immunol.* 164, 2890–2896.

Bland, P. W., and Warren, L. G. (1986). Antigen presentation by epithelial cells of rat small intestine. II. Selective induction of suppressor T cells. *Immunology* 58, 9–14.

Bloom, S., Simmons, D., and Jewell, D. P. (1995). Adhesion molecules intercellular adhesion molecule-1 (ICAM-1), ICAM-3 and B7 are not expressed by epithelium in normal or inflamed colon. *Clin. Exp. Immunol.* 101, 157–163.

Bluestone, J. A., and Abbas, A. K. (2003). Natural versus adaptive regulatory T cells. *Nat. Rev. Immunol.* 3, 253–257.

Bregenholt, S., Wang, M., Wolfe, T., Hughes, A., Baerentzen, L., Dyrberg, T., von Herrath, M. G., and Petersen, J. S. (2003). The cholera toxin B subunit is a mucosal adjuvant for oral tolerance induction in type 1 diabetes. *Scand. J. Immunol.* 57, 432–438.

Brod, S. A., Al-Sabbagh, A., Sobel, R. A., Hafler, D. A., and Weiner, H. L. (1991). Suppression of experimental autoimmune encephalomyelitis by oral administration of myelin antigens. IV. Suppression of chronic relapsing disease in the Lewis rat and strain 13 guinea pig. *Ann. Neurol.* 29, 615–622.

Bruce, M. G., and Ferguson, A. (1986a). The influence of intestinal processing on the immunogenicity and molecular size of absorbed, circulating ovalbumin in mice. *Immunology* 59, 295–300.

Bruce, M. G., and Ferguson, A. (1986b). Oral tolerance to ovalbumin in mice: Studies of chemically modified and of "biologically filtered" antigen. *Immunology* 57, 627–630.

Buer, J., Lanoue, A., Franzke, A., Garcia, C., von Boehmer, H., and Sarukhan, H. (1998). Interleukin 10 secretion and impaired effector function of major histocompatibility complex class II-restricted T cells anergized *in vivo*. *J. Exp. Med.* 187, 177–183.

Buhlmann, J. E., Foy, T. M., Aruffo, A., Crassi, K. M., Ledbetter, J. A., Green, W. R., Xu, J. C., Schultz, L. D., Roopesian, D., Flavell,

R. A., Fast, L., Noelle, R. J., and Durie, F. H. (1995). In the absence of a CD40 signal, B cells are tolerogenic. *Immunity* 2, 645–653.

Carr, R. I., Etherbridge, P. D., and Tilley, D. (1985). Failure of oral tolerance in NZB/W mice is antigen dependent and parallels antibody patterns in human systemic lupus erythematosus (SLE). *Fed. Proc.* 44, 1542.

Carvalho, C. R., Verdolin, B. A., de Souza, A. V., and Vaz, N. M. (1994). Indirect effects of oral tolerance in mice. *Scand. J. Immunol.* 39, 533–538.

Carvalho, C. R., Verdolin, B. A., and Vaz, N. M. (1997). Indirect effects of oral tolerance cannot be ascribed to bystander suppression. *Scand. J. Immunol.* 45, 276–281.

Carvalho, C. R., Lenzi, H. L., Correa-Oliveira, R., and Vaz, N. M. (2002). Indirect effects of oral tolerance to ovalbumin interfere with the immune responses triggered by *Schistosoma mansoni* eggs. *Braz. J. Med. Biol. Res.* 35, 1195–1199.

Cauley, L. S., Cauley, K. A., Shub, F., Huston, G., and Swain, S. L. (1997). Transferable anergy: superantigen treatment induces CD4+ T cell tolerance that is reversible and requires CD4-CD8- cells and interferon γ. *J. Exp. Med.* 186, 71–81.

Cederbom, L., Hall, H., and Ivars, F. (2000). CD4+CD25+ regulatory T cells down-regulate co-stimulatory molecules on antigen-presenting cells. *Eur. J. Immunol.* 30, 1538–1543.

Challacombe, S. J., and Thomasi, T. B. (1980). Systemic tolerance and secretory immunity after oral immunisation. *J. Exp. Med.* 152, 1459–1472.

Chalon, M.-P., Milne, R. W., and Vaerman, J.-P. (1979). *In vitro* immunosuppressive effect of serum from orally immunised mice. *Eur. J. Immunol.* 9, 747–750.

Chandra, R. K., Puri, S., and Vyas, D. (1987) Malnutrition and intestinal immunity. In *Immunopathology of the Small Intestine* (ed. M. N. Marsh), 105–119. Chichester, UK: John Wiley and Sons.

Chase, M. W. (1946). Inhibition of experimental drug allergy by prior feeding of the sensitivity agent. *Proc. Soc. Exp. Biol. Med.* 61, 257–259.

Chen, W., Jin, W., Cook, M., Weiner, H. L., and Wahl, S. M. (1998a). Oral delivery of group A streptococcal cell walls augments circulating TGF-β and suppresses streptococcal cell wall arthritis. *J. Immunol.* 161, 6297–6304.

Chen, W., Jin, W., and Wahl, S. M. (1998b). Engagement of cytotoxic T lymphocyte-associated antigen 4 (CTLA-4) induces transforming growth factor β (TGF-β) production by murine CD4+ T cells. *J. Exp. Med.* 188, 1849–1857.

Chen, W., Jin, W., Tian, H., Sicurello, P., Frank, M., Orenstein, J. M., and Wahl, S. M. (2001). Requirement for transforming growth factor β1 in controlling T cell apoptosis. *J. Exp. Med.* 194, 439–453.

Chen, W., Jin, W., Hardegen, N., Lei, K. J., Li, L., Marinos, N., McGrady, G., and Wahl, S. M. (2003). Conversion of peripheral CD4+CD25- naive T cells to CD4+CD25+ regulatory T cells by TGF-β induction of transcription factor Foxp3. *J. Exp. Med.* 198, 1875–1886.

Chen, Y., Kuchroo, V. K., Inobe, J.-I., Hafler, D. A., and Weiner, H. L. (1994). Regulatory T cell clones induced by oral tolerance: suppression of autoimmune encephalomyelitis. *Science* 265, 1237–1240.

Chen, Y., Inobe, J.-I., Marks, R., Gonnella, P., Kuchroo, V. K., and Weiner, H. L. (1995a). Peripheral deletion of antigen-reactive T cells in oral tolerance. *Nature* 376, 177–180.

Chen, Y., Inobe, J.-I., and Weiner, H. L. (1995b). Induction of oral tolerance to myelin basic protein in CD8- depleted mice: Both CD4+ and CD8+ cells mediate active suppression. *J. Immunol.* 155, 910–916.

Chen, Y., Inobe, J.-I., Kuchroo, V. K., Baron, J. L., Janeway, C. A., and Weiner, H. L. (1996). Oral tolerance in myelin basic protein T-cell receptor transgenic mice: Suppression of autoimmune encephalomyelitis and dose-dependent induction of regulatory cells. *Proc. Natl. Acad. Sci. USA* 93, 388–391.

Chen, Y., Inobe, J.-I., and Weiner, H. L. (1997). Inductive events in oral tolerance in the TcR transgenic adoptive transfer model. *Cell. Immunol.* 178, 62–68.

Chen, Y., Song, K., and Eck, S. L. (2000). An intra-Peyer's patch gene transfer model for studying mucosal tolerance: distinct roles of B7 and IL-12 in mucosal T cell tolerance. *J. Immunol.* 165, 3145–3153.

Chen, Y., Ma, Y., and Chen, Y. (2002). Roles of CTLA-4 in the inductive phase of oral tolerance *Immunology* 105, 171–180.

Christensen, H. R., Kjaer, T. M., and Frokiaer, H. (2003). Low-dose oral tolerance due to antigen in the diet suppresses differentially the cholera toxin-adjuvantized IgE, IgA, and IgG response. *Int. Arch. Allergy Immunol.* 132, 248–257.

Chung, S. W., Gorczynski, R. M., Dziadkowiec, I., and Levy, G. A. (1995). Induction of T-cell hyporesponsiveness by intrahepatic modulation of donor antigen-presenting cells. *Immunology* 85, 582–590.

Chung, Y., Chang, S.-Y., and Kang, C.-Y. (1999). Kinetic analysis of oral tolerance: memory lymphocytes are refractory to oral tolerance. *J. Immunol.* 163, 3692–3698.

Chung, Y., Choi, J., Chang, Y.-S., Cho, S.-H., and Kang, C.-Y. (2002). Preventive and therapeutic effects of oral tolerance in a murine model of asthma. *Immunobiology* 206, 408–423.

Chung, Y., Kim, D.-H., Lee, S.-H., and Kang, C.-Y. (2004). Activation of APCs by CD40 ligation does not abrogate the induction of oral tolerance. *Immunology* 111, 19–26.

Claessen, A. M. E., Von Blomberg, B. M. E., De Groot, J., Wolvers, D. A. E., Kraal, G., and Scheper, R. J. (1996). Reversal of mucosal tolerance by subcutaneous administration of interleukin-12 at the site of attempted sensitization. *Immunology* 88, 363–367.

Cobbold, S. P., Nolan, K. F., Graca, L., Castejon, R., Le Moine, A., Frewin, M., Humm, S., Adams, E., Thompson, S., Zelenika, D., Paterson, A., Yates, S., Fairchild, P. J., and Waldmann, H. (2003). Regulatory T cells and dendritic cells in transplantation tolerance: Molecular markers and mechanisms. *Immunol. Rev.* 196, 109–124.

Cobelens, P. M., Kavelaars, A., van der Zee, R., van Eden, W., and Heijnen, C. J. (2002a). Dynamics of mycobacterial HSP65-induced T-cell cytokine expression during oral tolerance induction in adjuvant arthritis. *Rheumatology (Oxford)* 41, 775–779.

Cobelens, P. M., Kavelaars, A., Vronn, A., Ringeling, M., van der Zee, R., van Eden, W., and Heijnen, C. J. (2002b). The β2-adrenergic agonist salbutamol potentiates oral induction of tolerance suppressing adjuvant arthritis and antigen-specific immunity. *J. Immunol.* 169, 5028–5035.

Collins, S. R., and Campbell, J. B. (1980). Development of delayed hypersensitivity in gnotobiotic mice. *Int. Arch. Allergy Appl. Immunol.* 61, 165–170.

Conde, A. A., Stransky, B., Faria, A. M. C., and Vaz, N. M. (1998). Interruption of recently induced immune responses by oral administration of antigen. *Braz. J. Med. Biol. Res.* 31, 377–380.

Cowdrey, J. S., and Johlin, B. J. (1984). Regulation of the primary *in vitro* response to TNP-polymerised ovalbumin by T suppressor cells induced by ovalbumin feeding. *J. Immunol.* 132, 2783–2789.

Cowdrey, J. S., Curtin, M. F., and Steinberg, A. D. (1982). Effect of prior intragastric antigen administration on primary and secondary anti-ovalbumin responses of C57Bl/6 and NZB mice. *J. Exp. Med.* 156, 1256–1261.

Crabbe, P. A., and Heremans, J. F. (1967). Selective IgA deficiency with steatorrhoea: A new syndrome. *Am. J. Med.* 42, 319.

Crispe, I. N., and Mehal, W. Z. (1996). Strange brew: T cells in the liver. *Immunol. Today* 17, 522–525.

Cross, A. H., Tuohy, V. K., and Raine, C. S. (1993). Development of reactivity to new myelin antigens during chronic relapsing autoimmune demyelination. *Cell Immunol.* 146, 261–270.

Cunningham-Rundles, C. (1987) Failure of antigen exclusion. In *Food Allergy and Intolerance* (eds. J. Brostoff and S. J. Challacombe), 223–226. Eastbourne, UK: W. B. Saunders.

da Silva, A. C., de Souza, K. W., Machado, R. C., da Silva, M. F., and Sant'Anna, O. A. (1998). Genetics of immunological tolerance: I. Bidirectional selective breeding of mice for oral tolerance. *Res. Immunol.* 149, 151–161.

da Silva, M. F., da Costa, S. C., Ribeiro, R. C., Sant'Anna, O. A., and da Silva, A. C. (2001). Independent genetic control of B- and T-cell tolerance in strains of mouse selected for extreme phenotypes of oral tolerance. *Scand. J. Immunol.* 53, 148–154.

Dahlgren, U. I. H., Wold, A. E., Hanson, L. A., and Midtvedt, T. (1991). Expression of dietary protein in *E. coli* renders it strongly antigenic to gut lymphoid tissue. *Immunology* 73, 394–397.

Daniel, D., and Wegmann, D. R. (1996). Protection of nonobese diabetic mice from diabetics by intranasal or subcutaneous administration of insulin peptide B-(9-23) *Proc. Natl. Acad. Sci. USA* 93, 956–960.

Das, G., Augustine, M. M., Das, J., Bottomly, K., Ray, P., and Ray, A. (2003). An important regulatory role for CD4⁺CD8αα T cells in the intestinal epithelial layer in the prevention of inflammatory bowel disease. *Proc. Natl. Acad. Sci. USA* 100, 5324–5329.

Dasgupta, A., Kesari, K. V., Ramaswamy, K. K., Amenta, P. S., and Das, K. M. (2001). Oral administration of unmodified colonic but not small intestinal antigens protects rats from hapten-induced colitis. *Clin. Exp. Immunol.* 125, 41–47.

David, M. F. (1979). Induction of hyporesponsiveness to particulate antigen by feeding: The sequence of immunologic response to fed antigen. *J. Allergy Clin. Immunol.* 64, 164–170.

Daynes, R. A., Araneo, B. A., Dowell, T. A., Huang, K., and Dudley, D. (1990). Regulation of murine lymphokine production in vivo. III. The lymphoid tissue microenvironment exerts regulatory influences over T helper cell function. *J. Exp. Med.* 171, 979–996.

DePaolo, R. W., Rollins, B. J., Kuziel, W., and Karpus, W. J. (2003). CC chemokine ligand 2 and its receptor regulate mucosal production of IL-12 and TGF-β in high dose oral tolerance. *J. Immunol.* 171, 3560–3567.

Deplazes, P., Penhale, W. J., Greene, W. K., and Thompson, R. C. (1995). Effect on humoral tolerance (IgG and IgE) in dogs by the oral administration of ovalbumin and Der pI. *Vet. Immunol. Immunopathol.* 45, 361–367.

Derry, C. J., Harper, N., Davies, D. H., Murphy, J. J., and Staines, N. A. (2001). Importance of dose of type II collagen in suppression of collagen-induced arthritis by nasal tolerance. *Arth. Rheumat.* 44, 1917–1927.

Desvignes, C., Bour, H., Nicholas, J. F., and Kaiserlian, D. (1996). Lack of oral tolerance but oral priming for contact sensitivity to dinitrofluorobenzene in major histocompatibility antigen deficient mice and in CD4⁺ T cell-depleted mice. *Eur. J. Immunol.* 26, 1756–1761.

Desvignes, C., Etchart, N., Kehren, J., Akiba, I., Nicolas, J. F., and Kaiserlian, D. (2000). Oral administration of hapten inhibits in vivo induction of specific cytotoxic CD8⁺ T cells mediating tissue inflammation: A role for regulatory CD4⁺ T cells. *J. Immunol.* 164, 2515–2522.

de Weerd, N., Bhalla, P. L., and Singh, M. B. (2003). Oral immunization with a recombinant major grass pollen allergen induces blocking antibodies in mice. *Int. Arch. Allergy Immunol.* 130, 119–124.

Dick, A. D., Cheng, Y. F., McKinnon, A., Liversidge, J., and Forrester, J. V. (1993). Nasal administration of retinal antigens suppresses the inflammatory response in experimental allergic uveoretinitis: A preliminary report of intranasal induction of tolerance with retinal antigens. *Br. J. Ophthalmol.* 77, 171–175.

Dick, A. D., Cheng, Y. F., Liversidge, J., and Forrester, J. V. (1994). Intranasal administration of retinal antigens suppresses retinal antigen-induced experimental autoimmune uveoretinitis. *Immunology* 82, 625–631.

Dick, A. D., Sharma, V., and Liversidge, J. (2001). Single dose intranasal administration of retinal autoantigen generates a rapid accumulation and cell activation in draining lymph node and spleen: Implications for tolerance therapy. *Br. J. Ophthalmol.* 85, 1001–6100.

Dippold, W., Wittig, B., Schwaeble, W., Mayet, W., and Meyer zum Buschenfelde, K. H. (1993). Expression of intercellular adhesion molecule 1 (ICAM-1, CD54) in colonic epithelial cells. *Gut* 34, 1593–1597.

D'Orazio, T. J., and Niederkorn, J. Y. (1998a). A novel role for TGF-β and IL-10 in the induction of immune privilege. *J. Immunol.* 160, 2089–2098.

D'Orazio, T. J., and Niederkorn, J. Y. (1998b). Splenic B cells are required for tolerogenic antigen presentation in the induction of anterior chamber-associated immune deviation (ACAID). *Immunology* 95, 47–55.

Dubois, B., Chapat, L., Goubier, A., Papiernik, M., Nicolas, J. F., and Kaiserlian, D. (2003). Innate CD4⁺CD25⁺ regulatory T cells are required for oral tolerance and control CD8⁺ T cells mediating skin inflammation. *Blood* 102, 3295–3301.

Duchmann, R., Kaiser, I., Hermann, E., Mayet, W., Ewe, K., and Meyer zum Büschenfelde, K. H. (1995). Tolerance exists towards resident intestinal flora but is broken in active inflammatory bowel disease (IBD). *Clin. Exp. Immunol.* 102, 448–455.

Duchmann, R., Schmitt, E., Knolle, P., Meyer zum Büschenfelde, K. H., and Neurath, M. (1996). Tolerance towards resident intestinal flora in mice is abrogated in experimental colitis and restored by treatment with interleukin-10 or antibodies to interleukin-12. *Eur. J. Immunol.* 26, 934–938.

Eaton, A. D., Xu, D., and Garside, P. (2003). Administration of exogenous interleukin-18 and interleukin-12 prevents the induction of oral tolerance. *Immunology* 108, 196–203.

Elson, C. O., and Ealding, W. (1984). Generalised systemic and mucosal immunity in mice after mucosal stimulation with cholera toxin. *J. Immunol.* 132, 2736–2741.

Elson, C., Beagley, K., Sharmanov, A., Fujihashi, K., Kiyono, H., Tennyson, G., Cong, Y., Black, C., Ridwan, B., and McGhee, J. (1996). Hapten-induced model of murine inflammatory bowel disease: Mucosa immune responses and protection by tolerance. *J. Immunol.* 157, 2174–2185.

Elson, C., Cong, Y., Iqbal, N., and Weaver, C. T. (2001). Immuno-bacterial homeostasis in the gut: New insights into an old enigma. *Semin. Immunol.* 13, 187–194.

Enders, G., Gottwald, T., and Brendel, W. (1986). Induction of oral tolerance in rats without Peyer's patches. *Immunology* 58, 311–314.

Eriksson, K., and Holmgren, J. (2002). Recent advances in mucosal vaccines and adjuvants. *Curr. Opin. Immunol.* 14, 666–672.

Eriksson, K., Fredriksson, M., Nordstrom, I., and Holmgren, J. (2003). Cholera toxin and its B subunit promote dendritic cell vaccination with different influences on Th1 and Th2 development. *Infect. Immun.* 71, 1740–1747.

Ermak, T., Dougherty, E. P., Bhagat, H. R., Kabok, Z., Pappo, J. (1995). Uptake and transport of copolymer biodegradable microspheres by rabbit Peyer's patch M cells. *Cell Tissue Res.* 279, 433–436.

Eynon, E. E., and Parker, D. C. (1992). Small B cells as antigen-presenting cells in the induction of tolerance to soluble protein antigens. *J. Exp. Med.* 175, 131.

Fadok, V. A., Bratton, D. L., Konowal, A., Freed, P. W., Westcott, J. Y., and Henson, P. M. (1998). Macrophages that have ingested apoptotic cells in vitro inhibit proinflammatory cytokine production through autocrine/paracrine mechanisms involving TGF-β, PGE2, and PAF. *J. Clin. Invest.* 101, 890–898.

Faria, A. M. C., and Weiner, H. L. (1999). Oral tolerance: Mechanisms and therapeutic applications. *Adv. Immunol.* 73, 153–264.

Faria, A. M. C., Garcia, G., Rios, M. J., Michalaros, C. L., and Vaz, N. M. (1993). Decrease in susceptibility to oral tolerance induction and occurrence of oral immunization to ovalbumin in 20–38-week-old mice: The effect of interval between oral exposures and rate of antigen intake in the oral immunization. *Immunology* 78, 147–151.

Faria A. M. C., Ficker, S. M., Speziali E., Menezes, J. S., Stransky, B., Rodrigues, V. S., and Vaz, N. M. (1998). Aging affects oral tolerance induction but not its maintenance in mice. *Mech. Ageing Dev.* 102, 67–80.

Faria, A. M., Maron, R., Ficker, S. M., Slavin, A. J., Spahn, T., and Weiner, H. L. (2003). Oral tolerance induced by continuous feeding: Enhanced up-regulation of transforming growth factor-β/interleukin-10 and suppression of experimental autoimmune encephalomyelitis. *J. Autoimmun.* 20, 135–145.

Ferguson, A. (1987). Models of immunologically-driven small intestinal damage. In *Immunopathology of the Small Intestine* (ed. M. N. Marsh), 225–252. Chichester, UK: John Wiley and Sons.

Fishman-Lobell, J., Friedman, A., and Weiner, H. L. (1994). Different kinetic patterns of cytokine gene expression in vivo in orally tolerant mice. *Eur. J. Immunol.* 24, 2720–2724.

Foussat, A., Cottrez, F., Brun, V., Fournier, N., Breittmayer, J. P., and Groux, H. (2003). A comparative study between T regulatory Type 1 and CD4⁺CD25⁺ T cells in the control of inflammation. *J. Immunol.* 171, 5018–5026.

Fowler, S., and Powrie, F. (2002). CTLA-4 expression on antigen-specific cells but not IL-10 secretion is required for oral tolerance. *Eur. J. Immunol.* 32, 2997–3006.

Franco, L., Benedetti, R., Ferek, G. A., Massouh, E., and Flo, J. (1998). Priming or tolerization of the B and Th2 dependent immune response by the oral administration of OVA-DNP is determined by the antigen dosage. *Cell Immunol.* 190, 1–11.

Frenkel, D., Huang, Z., Maron, R., Koldzic, D. N., Hancock, W. W., Moskowitz, M. A., and Weiner, H. L. (2003). Nasal vaccination with myelin oligodendrocyte glycoprotein reduces stroke size by inducing Il-10 producing CD4+ T cells. *J. Immunol.* 171, 6549-6555.

Friedman, A., and Weiner, H. L. (1994). Induction of anergy or active suppression following oral tolerance is determined by antigen dosage. *Proc. Natl. Acad. Sci. USA* 91, 6688–6692.

Fuchs, E. J., and Matzinger, P. (1992). B cells turn off virgin but not memory T cells. *Science*, 258, 1156.

Fujihashi, K., Kiyono, H., Aicher, W. K., Green, D. R., Singh, B., Eldrige, J. G., and McGhee, J. R. (1989). Immunoregulatory function of CD3+, CD4− and CD8− T cells: γδ T cell receptor-positive T cells from nude mice abrogate oral tolerance. *J. Immunol.* 143, 3415–3422.

Fujihashi, K., Dohi, T., Rennert, P. D., Yamamoto, M., Koga Y., Kiyono, H., and McGhee, J. R. (2001). Peyer's patches are required for oral tolerance to proteins *Proc. Natl. Acad. Sci. USA* 98, 3310–3315.

Fujiwara, H., Qian, J.-H., Satoh, S., Kokudo, S., Ikegama, R., and Hamacka, T. (1986). Studies on the induction of tolerance to alloantigens. II. The generation of serum factor(s) able to transfer alloantigen-specific tolerance for delayed-type hypersensitivity by postal venous inoculation with allogeneic cells. *J. Immunol.* 136, 2763–2768.

Fukaura, H., Kent, S. C., Pietrusewicz, M. L., Khoury, S. J., Weiner, H. L., and Hafler, D. A. (1996). Induction of circulating myelin basic protein and proteolipid protein-specific transforming growth factor-β1-secreting Th3 cells by oral administration of myelin in multiple sclerosis. *J. Clin. Invest.* 98, 70–77.

Furrie, E., Turner, M. W., and Strobel, S. (1994). Failure of scid mice to generate an oral tolerogen after a feed of ovalbumin: A role for a functioning gut-associated lymphoid system. *Immunology* 83, 562–567.

Furrie, E., Turner, M. W., and Strobel, S. (1995). Partial characterization of a circulating tolerogenic moiety which, after a feed of ovalbumin, suppresses delayed-type hypersensitivity in recipient mice. *Immunology* 86, 480–486.

Furrie, E., Smith, R. E., Turner, M. W., Strobel, S., and Mowat, A. McI. (2002). Induction of local innate immune responses and modulation of antigen uptake as mechanisms underlying the mucosal adjuvant properties of Immune Stimulating Complexes (ISCOMS). *Vaccine* 20, 2254–2262.

Gaboriau-Routhiau, V., and Moreau, M. C. (1996). Gut flora allows recovery of oral tolerance to ovalbumin in mice after transient breakdown mediated by cholera toxin or *Escherichia coli* heat-labile enterotoxin. *Pediatr. Res.* 39, 625–629.

Galliaerde, V., Desvignes, C., Peyron, E., and Kaiserlian, D. (1995). Oral tolerance to haptens: intestinal epithelial cells from 2,4-dinitrochlorobenzene-fed mice inhibit hapten-specific T cell activation *in vitro*. *Eur. J. Immunol.* 25, 1385–1390.

Garcia, G., Komagata, Y., Slavin, A. J., Maron, R., and Weiner, H. L. (1999). Suppression of collagen-induced arthritis by oral or nasal administration of type II collagen. *J. Autoimmun.* 13, 315–324.

Gardine, C. A., Kouki, T., and DeGroot, L. (2001). Characterization of the T lymphocyte subsets and lymphoid populations involved in the induction of low dose tolerance to human thyroglobulin. *Cell. Immunol.* 212, 1–15.

Garg, S., Bal, V., Rath, S., and George, A. (1999). Effect of multiple antigenic exposures in the gut on oral tolerance and induction of antibacterial systemic immunity. *Infect. Immun.* 67, 5917–5924.

Garside, P., and Mowat, A. McI. (2001). Oral tolerance. *Semin. Immunol.* 13, 177–185.

Garside, P., Steel, M., Liew, F. Y., and Mowat, A. McI. (1995a). CD4+ but not CD8+ T cells are required for the induction of oral tolerance. *Int. Immunol.* 7, 501–504.

Garside, P., Steel, M., Worthey, E. A., Satoskar, A., Alexander, J., Bluethmann, H., Liew, F. Y., and Mowat, A. McI. (1995b). Th2 cells are subject to high dose oral tolerance and are not essential for its induction *J. Immunol.* 154, 5649–5655.

Garside, P., Steel, M., Worthey, E. A., Kewin, P. J., Howie, S. E. M., Harrison, D. J., Bishop, D., and Mowat, A. McI. (1996). Oral tolerance in mice is associated with increased susceptibility of challenged lymphocytes to undergo apoptosis *in vivo*. *Am. J. Pathol.* 149, 1971–1980.

Gautam, S. C., and Battisto, J. R. (1985). Orally induced tolerance generates an efferently acting suppressor T cell and an acceptor T cell that together down-regulate contact sensitivity. *J. Immunol.* 135, 2975–2983.

Gautam, S. C., Chikkala, N. F., and Battisto, J. R. (1990). Oral administration of the contact sensitizer trinitrochlorobenzene: Initial sensitization and subsequent appearance of a suppressor population. *Cell Immunol.* 125, 437–448.

Glaister, J. R. (1973). Some effects of oral administration of oxazolone to mice. *Int. Arch. Allergy Appl. Immunol.* 45, 828–843.

Golovkina, T. V., Shlomchik, M., Hannum, L., and Chervonsky, A. (1999). Organogenic role of B lymphocytes in mucosal immunity. *Science* 286, 1965–1968.

Gonnella, P. A., Chen, Y., Inobe, J.-I., Komagata, Y., Quartulli, M., and Weiner, H. L. (1998). *In situ* immune response in gut-associated lymphoid tissue (GALT) following oral antigen in TCR-transgenic mice. *J. Immunol.* 160, 4708–4718.

Gonnella, P. A., Waldner, H. P., and Weiner, H. L. (2001). B cell deficient (μMT) mice have alterations in the cytokine microenvironment of the gut associated lymphoid tissue (GALT) and a defect in the low dose mechanism of oral tolerance. *J. Immunol.* 166, 4456–4464.

Gorczynski, R. M. (1994). Adoptive transfer of unresponsiveness to allogeneic skin grafts with hepatic γδ+ T cells. *Immunology* 81, 27–35.

Gonnella, P. A., Kodali, D., and Weiner, H. L. (2003). Induction of low dose oral tolerance in monocyte chemotactic protein-1- and CCR2-deficient mice. *J. Immunol.* 170, 2316–2322.

Gorczynski, R. M., Hozumi, N., Wolf, S., and Chen, Z. (1995). Interleukin 12 in combination with anti-interleukin 10 reverses graft prolongation after portal venous immunization. *Transplantation* 60, 1337–1341.

Gorczynski, R. M., Chen, Z., Hoang, Y., and Rossi-Bergman, B. (1996a). A subset of γδ T-cell receptor positive cells produce T-helper type 2 cytokines and regulate mouse skin graft rejection following portal venous pretransplant preimmunization. *Immunology* 87, 381–389.

Gorczynski, R. M., Cohen, Z., Leung, Y., and Chen, Z. (1996b). γδ TcR+ hybridomas derived from mice preimmunized via the portal vein adoptively transfer increased skin allograft survival *in vivo*. *J. Immunol.* 157, 574–581.

Gorczynski, R. M., Cohen, Z., Levy, G., and Fu, X. M. (1996c). A role for γ(δ)TCR+ cells in regulation of rejection of small intestinal allografts in rats. *Transplantation* 62, 844–851.

Gorczynski, R. M., Chen, Z., Zeng, H., and Fu, X. M. (1997). Specificity for *in vivo* graft prolongation in γδ T cell receptor+ hybridomas derived from mice given portal vein donor-specific preimmunization and skin allografts. *J. Immunol.* 159, 3698–3706.

Gorelik, L., and Flavell, R. A. (2000). Abrogation of TGF β signalling in T cells leads to spontaneous T cell differentiation and autoimmune disease. *Immunity* 12, 171–181.

Grdic, D., Hornquist, E., Kjerrulf, M., and Lycke, N. (1998). Lack of local suppression in orally tolerant CD8-deficient mice reveals a critical regulatory role of CD8+ T cells in the normal gut mucosa. *J. Immunol.* 160, 754–762.

Green, E. A., Gorelik, L., McGregor, C. M., Tran, E. H., and Flavell, R. A. (2003). CD4+CD25+ T regulatory cells control anti-islet CD8+ T cells through TGF-β–TGF-β receptor interactions in type 1 diabetes. *Proc. Natl. Acad. Sci. USA* 100, 10878–10883.

Greenwald, R. J., Latchman, Y. E., and Sharpe, A. H. (2002). Negative co-receptors on lymphocytes. *Curr. Opin. Immunol.* 14, 391–396.

Gregerson, D. S., Obritsch, W. F., and Donoso, L. A. (1993). Oral tolerance in experimental autoimmune uveoretinitis: Distinct mechanisms of resistance are induced by low versus high dose feeding protocols. *J. Immunol.* 151, 5751–5761.

Groux, H., and Powrie, F. (1999). Regulatory T cells in inflammatory bowel disease. *Immunol. Today* 20, 442–446.

Groux, H., O'Garra, A., Bigler, M., Rouleau, M., Antonenko, S., de Vries, J. E., and Roncarlo, M. G. (1997). A CD4+ T-cell subset inhibits antigen-specific T-cell responses and prevents colitis. *Nature* 389, 737–742.

Groux, H. (2003). Type 1 T-regulatory cells: their role in the control of immune responses *Transplantation* 75, 8S–12S.

Guermonprez, P., Valladeau, J., Zitvogel, L., Thery, C., and Amigorena, S. (2002). Antigen presentation and T cell stimulation by dendritic cells. *Annu. Rev. Immunol.* 20, 621–667.

Guimaraes, V. C., Quintans, J., Fisfalen, M. E., Straus, F. H., Fields, P. E., Neto, G. M., and DeGroot, L. J. (1995a). Immunosuppression of thyroiditis. *Endocrinology* 137, 2199–2207.

Guimaraes, V. C., Quintans, J., Fisfalen, M. E., Straus, F. H., Wilhelm, K., Medeiros-Neto, G. A., and DeGroot, L. J. (1995b). Suppression of experimental autoimmune thyroiditis by oral administration of thyroglobulin. *Endocrinology* 136, 3353–3359.

Gütgemann, I., Fahrer, A. M., Davis, M. M., and Chien, Y.-H. (1998). Induction of rapid T cell activation and tolerance by systemic presentation of an orally administered antigen. *Immunity* 8, 667–673.

Gütgemann, I., Darling, J. M., Greenberg, H. B., Davis, M. M., and Chien, Y. H. (2002). A blood-borne antigen induces rapid T-B cell contact: A potential mechanism for tolerance induction. *Immunology* 107, 420–425.

Hall, G., Houghton, C. G., Rahbek. J. U., Lamb, J. R., and Jarman, E. R. (2003). Suppression of allergen reactive Th2 mediated responses and pulmonary eosinophilia by intranasal administration of an immunodominant peptide is linked to IL-10 production. *Vaccine* 21, 549–561.

Hancock, W. W., Polanski, M., Zhang, J., Blogg, N., and Weiner, H. L. (1995). Suppression of insulitis in non-obese diabetic (NOD) mice by oral insulin is associated with selective expression of interleukin-4 and -10, transforming growth factor-β, and prostaglandin-E. *Am. J. Pathol.* 147, 1193–1199.

Haneda, K., Sano, K., Tamura, G., Sato, T., Habu, S., and Shirato, K. (1997). TGF-β induced by oral tolerance ameliorates experimental tracheal eosinophilia. *J. Immunol.* 159, 4484–4490.

Hanninen, A., and Harrison, L. C. (2000). γδ T cells as mediators of mucosal tolerance: The autoimmune diabetes model. *Immunol. Rev.* 173, 109–119.

Hanninen, A., Braakhuis, A., Heath, W. R., and Harrison, L. C. (2001). Mucosal antigen primes diabetogenic cytotoxic T-lymphocytes regardless of dose or delivery route. *Diabetes* 50, 771–775.

Hansen, G., McIntire, J. J., Yeung, V. P., Berry, G., Thorbecke, G. J., Chen, L., DeKruyff, R. H., and Umetsu, D. T. (2000). CD4(+) T helper cells engineered to produce latent TGF-β1 reverse allergen-induced airway hyperreactivity and inflammation. *J. Clin. Invest.* 105, 61–70.

Hanson, D. G. (1981). Ontogeny of orally induced tolerance in newborns. *J. Immunol.* 127, 1518–1522.

Hanson, D. G., and Miller, S. D. (1982). Inhibition of specific immune responses by feeding protein antigens. V. Induction of the tolerant state in the absence of specific suppressor T cells. *J. Immunol.* 128, 2378–2381.

Hanson, D. G., Vaz, N. M., and Maia, L. C. S. (1977). Inhibition of specific immune responses by feeding protein Ag's. *Int. Arch. Allergy Appl. Immunol.* 55, 526–532.

Hanson, D. G., Vaz, N. M., Maia, L. C. S., and Lynch, J. M. (1979a). Inhibition of specific immune responses by feeding protein antigens. III. Evidence against maintenance of tolerance to ovalbumin by orally induced antibodies. *J. Immunol.* 123, 2337–2343.

Hanson, D. G., Vaz, N. M., Rawlings, L. A., and Lynch, J. M. (1979b). Inhibition of specific immune responses by feeding protein Ag's II. Effects of prior passive and active immunisation. *J. Immunol.* 122, 2261–2266.

Hanson, D. G., Roy, M. J., Green, G. M., and Miller, S. D. (1993). Inhibition of orally-induced immune tolerance in mice by prefeeding an endopeptidase inhibitor. *Reg. Immunol.* 5, 76–84.

Haque, M. A., Mizobuchi, T., Yasufuku, K., Fujisawa, T., Brutkiewicz, R. R., Zheng, Y., Woods, K., Smith, G. N., Cummings, O. W., Heidler, K. M., Blum, J. S., and Wilkes, D. S. (2002). Evidence for immune responses to a self-antigen in lung transplantation: Role of type V collagen-specific T cells in the pathogenesis of lung allograft rejection. *J. Immunol.* 169, 1542–1549.

Haque, M. A., Yoshino, S., Inada, S., Nomaguchi, H., Tokunaga, O., and Kohashi, O. (1996). Suppression of adjuvant arthritis in rats by induction of oral tolerance to mycobacterial 65-kDa heat shock protein. *Eur. J. Immunol.* 26, 2650–2656.

Hara, M., Kingsley, C. L., Niimi, M., Read, S., Turvey, S. E., Bushell, A. R., Morris, P. J., Powrie, F., and Wood, K. J. (2001). IL-10 is required for regulatory T cells to mediate tolerance to alloantigens *in vivo*. *J. Immunol.* 166, 3789–3796.

Harats, D., Yacov, N., Gilburd, B., Shoenfeld, Y., and George, J. (2002). Oral tolerance with heat shock protein 65 attenuates *Mycobacterium tuberculosis*-induced and high-fat-diet-driven atherosclerotic lesions. *J. Am. Coll Cardiol.* 40, 1333–1338.

Harbige, L. S., and Fisher, B. A. (2001). Dietary fatty acid modulation of mucosally-induced tolerogenic immune responses. *Proc. Nutr. Soc.* 60, 449–456.

Harizi, H., Juzan, M., Pitard, V., Moreau, J. F., and Gualde, N. (2002). Cyclooxygenase-2-issued prostaglandin e(2) enhances the production of endogenous IL-10, which down-regulates dendritic cell functions. *J. Immunol.* 168, 2255–2263.

Harmatz, P. R., Bloch, K. J., Brown, M., Walker, W. A., and Kleinman, R. E. (1989). Intestinal adaptation during lactation in the mouse. I. Enhanced intestinal uptake of dietary protein antigen. *Immunology* 67, 92–95.

Harper, H., Cochrane, L, and Williams, NA (1996). The role of small intestinal antigen-presenting cells in the induction of T-cell reactivity to soluble protein antigens: Association between aberrant presentation in the lamina propria and oral tolerance. *Immunology* 89, 449–456.

Harrison, L. C. (1992). Islet cell antigens in insulin-dependent diabetes: Pandora's box revisited *Immunol. Today* 13, 348–352.

Harrison, L. C., Dempsey-Collier, M., Kramer, D. R., and Takahashi, K. (1996). Aerosol insulin induces regulatory CD8 γδ T cells that prevent murine insulin-dependent diabetes. *J. Exp. Med.* 184, 2167–2174.

Hartmann, B., Bellmann, K., Ghiea, I., Kleemann, R., and Kolb, H. (1997). Oral insulin for diabetes prevention in NOD mice: Potentiation by enhancing Th2 cytokine expression in the gut through bacterial adjuvant. *Diabetologia*, 40, 902–909.

Hashimoto, A., Yamada, H., Matsuzaki, G., and Nomoto, K. (2001). Successful priming and tolerization of T cells to orally administered antigens in B cell deficient mice. *Cell. Immunol.* 207, 36–40.

Hauet-Broere, F., Unger, W. W. J., Garssen, J., Hoijer, M. A., Kraal, G., and Samsom, J. N. (2003). Functional CD25⁻ and CD25⁺ mucosal regulatory T cells are induced in gut draining lymphoid tissue within 48 hours after oral antigen application. *Eur. J. Immunol.* 33, 2801–2810.

He, Y. G., Mellon, J., and Niederkorn, J. Y. (1996). The effect of oral immunization on corneal allograft survival. *Transplantation* 61, 920–926.

Heppell, L. M., and Kilshaw, P. J. (1982). Immune responses in guinea pigs to dietary protein. I. Induction of tolerance by feeding ovalbumin. *Int. Archs. Allergy Appl. Immunol.* 68, 54–61.

Hershberg, R. M., and Mayer, L. M. (2000). Antigen processing and presentation by intestinal epithelial cells—polarity and complexity. *Immunol. Today* 21, 123–128.

Hershberg, R. M., Cho, D. H., Youakim, A., Bradley, M. B., Lee, J. S., Framson, P. E., and Nepom, G. T. (1998). Highly polarized HLA class II antigen processing and presentation by human intestinal epithelial cells. *J. Clin. Invest.* 102, 792–803.

Higgins, P. J., and Weiner, H. (1988). Suppression of experimental autoimmune encephalomyelitis by oral administration of myelin basic protein and its fragments. *J. Immunol.* 140, 440–445.

Higgins, S. C., Lavelle, E. C., McCann, C., Keogh, B., McNeela, E., Byrne, P., O'Gorman, B., Jarnicki, A., McGuirk, P., and Mills, K. H. (2003). Toll-like receptor 4-mediated innate IL-10 activates antigen-specific regulatory T cells and confers resistance to *Bordetella pertussis* by inhibiting inflammatory pathology. *J. Immunol.* 171, 3119–3127.

Hirahara, K., Hisatune, T., Nishijima, K.-I., Kato, H., Shiho, O., and Kaminogowa, S. (1995). CD4+ T cells anergized by high dose feeding establish oral tolerance to antibody responses when transferred in SCID and nude mice. *J. Immunol.* 154, 6238–6245.

Holmgren, J., Czerkinsky, C., Eriksson, K., and Mharandi, A. (2003). Mucosal immunisation and adjuvants: A brief overview of recent advances and challenges. *Vaccine*, 21(Suppl. 2), S89–S95.

Homann, D., Holz, A., Bot, A., Coon, B., Wolfe, T., Petersen, J., Drybrg, T. P., Grusby, M. J., and von Herrath, M. G. (1999). Autoreactive CD4+ T cells protect from autoimmune diabetes via bystander suppression using the IL-4/Stat 6 pathway. *Immunity* 11, 463–472.

Hori, S., Nomura, T., and Sakaguchi, S. (2003a). Control of regulatory T cell development by the transcription factor Foxp3. *Science* 299, 1057–1061.

Hori, S., Takahashi, T., and Sakaguchi, S. (2003b). Control of autoimmunity by naturally arising regulatory CD4+ T cells. *Adv. Immunol.* 81, 331–371.

Hörnquist, E., and Lycke, N. (1993). Cholera toxin adjuvant greatly promotes antigen priming of T cells. *Eur. J. Immunol.* 23, 2136–2143.

Hoyne, G. F., Callow, M. G., Kuhlman, J., and Thomas, W. R. (1993a). T-cell lymphokine response to orally administered proteins during priming and unresponsiveness. *Immunology* 78, 534–540.

Hoyne, G. F., O'Hehir, R. E., Wraith, D. C., Thomas, W. R., and Lamb, J. R. (1993b). Inhibition of T cell and antibody responses to house dust mite allergen by inhalation of the dominant T cell epitope in naive and sensitized mice. *J. Exp. Med.* 178, 1783–1788.

Hoyne, G. F., and Thomas, W. R. (1995). T-cell responses to orally administered antigens: Study of the kinetics of lymphokine production after single and multiple feeding. *Immunology* 84, 304–309.

Hoyne, G. F., Callow, M. G., Kuo, M. C., and Thomas, W. R. (1994). Inhibition of T-cell responses by feeding peptides containing major and cryptic epitopes: studies with the Der p I allergen. *Immunology* 83, 190–195.

Huang, F. P., Platt, N., Wykes, M., Major, J. R., Powell, T. J., Jenkins, C. D., and MacPherson, G. G. (2000). A discrete subpopulation of dendritic cells transports apoptotic intestinal epithelial cells to T cell areas of mesenteric lymph nodes. *J. Exp. Med.* 191, 435–444.

Husby, S., Jensenius, J. C., and Svehag, S.-E. (1986). Passage of undergraded dietary antigen into the blood of healthy adults: Further characterization of the kinetics of uptake and the size distribution of the antigen. *Scand. J. Immunol.* 24, 447–452.

Husby, S., Foged, N., Host, A., and Svehag, S.-E. (1987). Passage of dietary antigens into the blood of children with coeliac disease: Quantification and size distribution of absorbed antigens. *Gut* 28, 1062–1072.

Husby, S., Mestecky, J., Moldoveanu, Z., Holland, S., and Elson, C. O. (1994). Oral tolerance in humans: T cell but not B cell tolerance after antigen feeding. *J. Immunol.* 152, 4663–4670.

Ilan, Y. (2002). Immune downregulation leads to upregulation of an antiviral response: A lesson from the hepatitis B virus. *Microbes Infect.* 4, 1317–1326.

Ilan, Y., Prakash, R., Davidson, A., Jona, V., Droguett, G., Horwitz, M., Chowdhury, N. R., and Chowdhury, J. R. (1997). Oral tolerization to adenoviral antigens permits long-term gene expression using recombinant adenoviral vectors. *J. Clin. Invest.* 99, 1098–1106.

Ilan, Y., Sauter, B., Chowdhury, N. R., Reddy, B. V., Thumalla, N. R., Droguett, G., Davidson, A., Ott, M., Horwitz, M. S., and Chowdhury, J. R. (1998). Oral tolerization to adenoviral proteins permits repeated adenovirus-mediated gene therapy in rats with pre-existing immunity to adenoviruses *Hepatology* 27, 1368–1376.

Ilan, Y., Gotsman, I., Pines, M., Beinart, R., Zeira, M., Ohana, M., Rabbani, E., Engelhardt, D., and Nagler, A. (2000). Induction of oral tolerance in splenocyte recipients towards pretransplant antigens ameliorates chronic graft versus host disease in a murine model. *Blood* 95, 3613–3619.

Im, S. H., Barchan, D., Fuchs, S., and Souroujon, M. C. (1999). Suppression of ongoing experimental myasthenia by oral treatment with an acetylcholine receptor recombinant fragment. *J. Clin. Invest.* 104, 1723–1730.

Im, S. H., Barchan, D., Fuchs, S., and Souroujon, M. C. (2000a). Mechanism of nasal tolerance induced by a recombinant fragment of acetylcholine receptor for treatment of experimental myasthenia gravis. *J. Neuroimmunol.* 111, 161–168.

Im, S. H., Barchan, D., Souroujon, M. C., and Fuchs, S. (2000b). Role of tolerogen conformation in induction of oral tolerance in experimental autoimmune myasthenia gravis. *J. Immunol.* 165, 3599–3605.

Inada, S., Yoshino, S., Haque, M. A., Ogata, Y., and Kohashi, O. (1996). Clonal anergy is a potent mechanism of oral tolerance in the suppression of acute antigen-induced arthritis in rats by oral administration of the inducing antigen. *Cell. Immunol.* 175, 67–75.

Inobe, J.-I., Slavin, A. J., Komagata, Y., Chen, Y., Liu, L., and Weiner, H. L. (1998). IL-4 is a differentiation factor for transforming growth factor-β secreting Th3 cells and oral administration of IL-4 enhances oral tolerance in experimental allergic encephalomyelitis. *Eur. J. Immunol.* 28, 2780–2790.

Ishii, N., Moriguchi, N., Sugita, Y., Nakajima, H., Tanaka, S., and Aoki, I. (1993). Analysis of responsive cells in tolerance by the oral administration of ovalbumin. *Immunol. Invest.* 22, 451–462.

Ishimitsu, R., Yajima, T., Nishimura, H., Kawauchi, H., and Yoshikai, Y. (2003). NKT cells are dispensable in the induction of oral tolerance but are indispensable in the abrogation of oral tolerance by prostaglandin E. *Eur. J. Immunol.* 33, 183–193.

Iwasaki, A., and Kelsall, B. L. (1999). Freshly isolated Peyer's patch, but not spleen, dendritic cells produce interleukin 10 and induce the differentiation of T helper type 2 cells. *J. Exp. Med.* 190, 229–239.

Iwasaki, A., and Kelsall, B. L. (2001). Unique functions of CD11b+, CD8α+ and double negative Peyer's patch dendritic cells. *J. Immunol.* 166, 4884–4890.

James, M. J., Belaramani, L., Prodromidou, K., Datta, A., Nourshargh, S., Lombardi, G., Dyson, J., Scott, D., Simpson, E., Cardozo, L., Warrens, A., Szydlo, R. M., Lechler, R. I., and Marelli-Berg, F. M. (2003). Anergic T cells exert antigen-independent inhibition of cell:cell interactions via chemokine metabolism. *Blood* 102: 2173-2179.

Jarrett, E. E. (1984). Perinatal influences on IgE responses. *Lancet* 2, 797–799.

Jarrett, E. E., and Hall, E. (1984). The development of IgE-suppressive immunocompetence in young animals: Influence of exposure to antigen in the presence or absence of maternal immunity. *Immunology* 53, 365–373.

Javed, N. H., Gienapp, I. E., Cox, K. L., and Whitacre, C. C. (1995). Exquisite peptide specificity of oral tolerance in experimental autoimmune encephalomyelitis. *J. Immunol.* 155, 1599–1605.

Jiang, H. R., Taylor, N., Duncan, L., Dick, A. D., and Forrester, J. V. (2001). Total dose and frequency of administration critically affect success of nasal mucosal tolerance induction. *Br. J. Ophthalmol.* 85, 739–744.

Jones, B., Pascopella, L, and Falkow, S. (1995). Entry of microbes into the host: using M cells to break the mucosal barrier. *Curr. Opin. Immunol.* 7, 474–478.

Jordan, M. S., Boesteanu, A., Reed, A. J., Petrone, A. L., Holenbeck, A. E., Lerman, M. A., Naji, A., and Caton, A. J. (2001). Thymic selection of CD4+CD25+ regulatory T cells induced by an agonist self-peptide. *Nat. Immunol.* 2, 301–306.

Ju, C., and Pohl, L. R. (2001). Immunohistochemical detection of protein adducts of 2,4-dinitrochlorobenzene in antigen presenting cells and lymphocytes after oral administration to mice: Lack of a role of Kupffer cells in oral tolerance. *Chem. Res. Toxicol.* 14, 1209–1217.

Jump, R. L., and Levine, A. D. (2002). Murine Peyer's patches favor development of an IL-10-secreting, regulatory T cell population. *J. Immunol.* 168, 6113–6119.

Jung, S., Gaupp, S., Hartung, H. P., and Toyka, K. V. (2001). Oral tolerance in experimental autoimmune neuritis (EAN) of the Lewis rat. II. Adjuvant effects and bystander suppression in P2 peptide-induced EAN. *J. Neuroimmunol.* 116, 21–28.

Kagnoff, M. F. (1978a). Effects of antigen-feeding on intestinal and systemic immune responses. II. Suppression of delayed type hypersensitivity reactions. *J. Immunol.* 120, 1509–1513.

Kagnoff, M. F. (1978b). Effects of antigen-feeding on intestinal and systemic immune responses. III. Antigen-specific serum-mediated suppression of humoral antibody responses after antigen-feeding. *Cell. Immunol.* 40, 186–203.

Kagnoff, M. F. (1980). Effects of antigen-feeding on intestinal and systemic immune responses. IV. Similarity between the suppressor factor in mice after erythrocyte-lysate injection and erythrocyte feeding. *Gastroenterology* 79, 54–61.

Kaji, T., Hachimura, S., Ise, W., and Kaminogawa, S. (2003). Proteome analysis reveals caspase activation in hyporesponsive CD4 T lymphocytes induced *in vivo* by the oral administration of antigen *J. Biol. Chem.* 278, 27836–27843.

Kalinski, P., Schuitemaker, J. H., Hilkens, C. M., and Kapsenberg, M. L. (1998). Prostaglandin E2 induces the final maturation of IL-12-deficient CD1a⁺CD83⁺ dendritic cells: the levels of IL-12 are determined during the final dendritic cell maturation and are resistant to further modulation. *J. Immunol.* 161, 2804–2809.

Kalinski, P., Hilkens, C. M. U., Wierenga, E. A., and Kapsenberg, M. L. (1999). T-cell priming by type-1 and type-2 polarized dendritic cells: the concept of a third signal. *Immunol. Today* 20, 561–567.

Kamphorst, A. O., da Silva, M. F. S., da Silva, A. C., Carvalho, C. R., and Faria, A. M. C. (2004a). Selection for resistance or susceptibility to oral tolerance using OVA affects general mechanisms of tolerance induction. *Ann. N. Y. Acad. Sci.*, 1, 38.

Kamphorst, A. O., Mendes, I., Faria, A. M. C., and Sinisterra, R. (2004b). Association complexes between ovalbumin and cyclodextrins have no effect on the immunological properties of ovalbumin. *Eur. J. Pharmac. Biopharmac.* 57, 199–205.

Karachunski, P. I., Ostlie, N. S., Okita, D. K., and Conti-Fine, B. M. (1997). Prevention of experimental myasthenia gravis by nasal administration of synthetic acetylcholine receptor T epitope sequences. *J. Clin. Invest.* 100, 3027–3035.

Karlsson, M. R., Kahu, H., Hanson, L. A., Telemo, E., and Dahlgren, U. I. (1999). Neonatal colonization of rats induces immunological tolerance to bacterial antigens. *Eur. J. Immunol.* 29, 109–218.

Karlsson, M. R., Kahu, H., Hanson, L. A., Telemo, E., and Dahlgren, U. I. (2000). Tolerance and bystander suppression, with involvement of CD25-positive cells, is induced in rats receiving serum from ovalbumin-fed donors. *Immunology* 100, 326–333.

Karlsson, M., Lundin, S., Dahlgren, U., Kahu, H., Pettersson, I., and Telemo, E. (2001). "Tolerosomes" are produced by intestinal epithelial cells. *Eur. J. Immunol.* 31, 2892–2900.

Karpus, W. J., and Lukacs, N. W. (1996). The role of chemokines in oral tolerance: Abrogation of nonresponsiveness by treatment with antimonocyte chemotactic protein-1. *Ann. N. Y. Acad. Sci.* 778, 133–144.

Kato, H., Fujihashi, K., Kato, R., Yuki, Y., and McGhee, J. R. (2001). Oral tolerance revisited: Prior oral tolerization abrogates cholera toxin-induced mucosal IgA responses. *J. Immunol.* 166, 3114–3121.

Kato, H., Fujihashi, K., Kato, R., and McGhee, J. R. (2003). Lack of oral tolerance in aging is due to sequential loss of T cell responses in Peyer's patches. *Int. Immunol.* 15, 145–158.

Kaufman, D. I., Clare-Salzler, M., Tian, J., Forsthuber, T., Ting, G. S. P., Robinson, P., Atkinson, M. A., Sercaz, E. E., Tobin, A. J., and Lehmann, P. V. (1993). Spontaneous loss of T-cell tolerance to glutamic acid decarboxylase in murine insulin-dependent diabetes. *Nature* 366, 69–72.

Kay, R., and Ferguson, A. (1989a). The immunological consequences of feeding cholera toxin. II. Mechanisms responsible for the induction of oral tolerance for DTH. *Immunology* 66, 416–421.

Kay, R., and Ferguson, A. (1989b). The immunological consequences of feeding cholera toxin. I. Feeding cholera toxin suppresses the induction of systemic delayed-type hypersensitivity but not humoral immunity. *Immunology* 66, 410–415.

Kaya, Z., Dohmen, K. M., Wang, Y., Schlichting, J., Afanasyeva, M., Leuschner, F., and Rose, N. R. (2002). Cutting edge: A critical role for IL-10 in induction of nasal tolerance in experimental autoimmune myocarditis. *J. Immunol.* 168, 1552–1556.

Ke, Y., and Kapp, J. A. (1996). Oral antigen inhibits priming of CD8⁺ CTL, CD4⁺ T cells and antibody responses while activating CD8⁺ suppressor T cells. *J. Immunol.* 156, 916–921.

Ke, Y., Pearce, K., Lake, J. P., Ziegler, H. K., and Kapp, J. A. (1997). γδ T lymphocytes regulate the induction of oral tolerance. *J. Immunol.* 158, 3610–3618.

Kearney, E. R., Pape, K. A., Loh, D. Y., and Jenkins, M. K. (1994). Visualization of peptide-specific T cell immunity and peripheral tolerance induction *in vivo*. *Immunity* 1, 327–339.

Kellermann, S. A., and McEvoy, L. M. (2001). The Peyer's patch microenvironment suppresses T cell responses to chemokines and other stimuli. *J. Immunol.* 167, 682–690.

Kelly, K. A., and Whitacre, C. C. (1996). Oral tolerance in EAE: reversal of tolerance by T helper cell cytokines. *J. Neuroimmunol.* 66, 77–84.

Kerlero de Rosbo, N., Milo, R., Lees, M. B., Burger, D., Bernard, C. C. A., and Ben-Nun, A. (1993). Reactivity to myelin antigens in multiple sclerosis: Peripheral blood lymphocytes respond predominantly to myelin oligodendrocyte glycoprotein. *J. Clin. Invest.* 92, 2602–2608.

Khare, S. D., Krco, C. J., Griffiths, M. M., Luthra, H. S., and David, C. S. (1995). Oral administration of an immunodominant human collagen peptide modulates collagen-induced arthritis. *J. Immunol.* 155, 3653–3659.

Khoury, S. J., Lider, O., Al-Sabbagh, A., and Weiner, H. L. (1990). Suppression of experimental autoimmune encephalomyelitis by oral administration of myelin basic protein. III. Synergistic effect of lipopolysaccharide. *Cell Immunol.* 131, 302–310.

Khoury, S. J., Hancock, W. W., and Weiner, H. L. (1992). Oral tolerance to myelin basic protein and natural recovery from experimental autoimmune encephalomyelitis are associated with downregulation of inflammatory cytokines and differential upregulation of transforming growth factor β, interleukin 4, and prostaglandin E expression in the brain. *J. Exp. Med.* 176, 1355–1364.

Kilshaw, P. J., and Cant, A. J. (1984). The passage of maternal dietary proteins into human breast milk. *Int. Arch. Allergy Appl. Immunol.* 75, 8–15.

Kim, J. H., and Ohsawa, M. (1995). Oral tolerance to ovalbumin in mice as a model for detecting modulators of the immunologic tolerance to a specific antigen. *Biol. Pharm. Bull.* 18, 854–858.

Kim, S.-K., Reed, D. S., Olson, S., Schnell, M. J., Rose, J. K., Morton, P. A., and Lefrançois, L. (1998). Generation of mucosal cytotoxic T cells against soluble protein by tissue-specific environmental and costimulatory signals. *Proc. Natl. Acad. Sci. USA* 95, 10814–10819.

Kim, W. U., Lee, W. K., Ryoo, J. W., Kim, S. H., Kim, J., Youn, J., Min, S. Y., Bae, E. Y., Hwang, S. Y., Park, S. H., Cho, C. S., Park, J. S., and Kim, H. Y. (2002). Suppression of collagen-induced arthritis by single administration of poly(lactic-co-glycolic acid) nanoparticles entrapping type II collagen: A novel treatment strategy for induction of oral tolerance. *Arth. Rheumat.* 46, 1109–1120.

Kitamura, K., Kiyono, H., Fujihashi, K., Eldbridge, J. H., Green, D. R., and McGhee, J. R. (1987). Contrasuppressor cells that break oral tolerance are antigen-specific T cells distinct from T helper (L3T4⁺), T suppressor (Lyt2⁺) and B cells. *J. Immunol.* 139, 3251–3259.

Kitani, A., Fuss, I., Nakamura, K., Kumaki, F., Usui, T., and Strober, W. (2003). Transforming growth factor (TGF)-β1-producing regulatory T cells induce Smad-mediated interleukin 10 secretion that facilitates coordinated immunoregulatory activity and amelioration of TGF-β1-mediated fibrosis. *J. Exp. Med.* 198, 1179–1188.

Kiyono, H., McGhee, J. R., Wannemuehler, M. J., and Michalek, S. M. (1982). Lack of oral tolerance in C3H/HeJ mice. *J. Exp. Med.* 155, 605–610.

Kjerrulf, M., Grdic, D., Ekman, L., Schon, K., Vajdy, M., and Lycke, N. Y. (1997). Interferon-γ receptor-deficient mice exhibit impaired gut mucosal immune responses but intact oral tolerance. *Immunology* 92, 60–68.

Koga, T., McGhee, J. R., Kato, H., Kato, R., Kiyono, H., and Fujihashi, K. (2000). Evidence for early aging in the mucosal immune system. *J. Immunol.* 165, 5352–5359.

Korenblatt, P. E., Rothberg, R. M., Minden, P., and Farr, R. S. (1968). Immune responses of adult humans after oral and parenteral exposure to bovine serum albumin. *J. Allergy* 41, 226–235.

Kraus, T., Toy, L., Chan, L., Childs, J., and Mayer, L. (2004). Failure to induce oral tolerance to a soluble protein in patients with inflammatory bowel disease. *Gastroenterology* 126, 1771–1778.

Krause, I., Blank, M., Sherer, Y., Gilburd, B., Kvapil, F., and Shoenfeld, Y. (2002). Induction of oral tolerance in experimental antiphospholipid syndrome by feeding with polyclonal immunoglobulins *Eur. J. Immunol.* 32, 3414–3424.

Kuchroo, V. K., Das, J. A., Brown, A. M., Zamvil, S. S., Sobel, R. A., Weiner, H. L., Nabavi, N., and Glimcher, L. H. (1995). B7-1 and

B7-2 costimulatory molecules activate differentially the Th1/Th2 developmental pathways: application to autoimmune disease therapy. *Cell* 80, 707–718.

Kuhn, R., Lohler, J., Rennick, D., Rajewsky, K., and Muller, W. (1993).Interleukin-10-deficient mice develop chronic enterocolitis. *Cell* 75, 263–279.

Kunkel, D., Kirchhoff, D., Nishikawa, S., Radbruch, A., and Scheffold, A. (2003). Visualization of peptide presentation following oral application of antigen in normal and Peyer's patches-deficient mice. *Eur. J. Immunol.* 33, 1292–1301.

Kweon, M.-N., Fujihashi, K., VanCott, J. L., Higuchi, K., Yamamoto, M., McGhee, J. R., and Kiyono, H. (1998). Lack of orally induced systemic unresponsiveness in IFN-γ knockout mice. *J. Immunol.* 160, 1687–1693.

Kweon, M.-N., Fujihashi, K., Wakatsuki, Y., Yamamoto, M., McGhee, J. R., and Kiyono, H. R. (1999). Mucosally induced systemic T cell unresponsiveness to ovalbumin requires CD40 ligand–CD40 interactions. *J. Immunol.* 162, 1904–1909.

Lafont, S., Andre, C., Andre, F., Gillon, J., and Fargier, M. C. (1982). Abrogation by subsequent feeding of antibody response, including IgE in parenterally immunised mice. *J. Exp. Med.* 155, 1573–1578.

Laliotou, B., and Dick, A. D. (1999). Modulating phenotype and cytokine production of leucocytic retinal infiltrate in experimental autoimmune uveoretinitis following intranasal tolerance induction with retinal antigens. *Br. J. Ophthalmol.* 83, 478–485.

Lamont, A. G., Gordon, M., and Ferguson, A. (1987). Oral tolerance in protein-deprived mice. I. Profound antibody tolerance but impaired DTH tolerance after antigen feeding. *Immunology* 61, 333–337.

Lamont, A. G., Bruce, M. G., Watret, K. C., and Ferguson, A. (1988a). Suppression of an established DTH response to ovalbumin in mice by feeding antigen after immunization. *Immunology* 64, 135–140.

Lamont, A. G., Mowat, A., McI., Browning, M. J., and Parrott, D. M. V. (1988b). Genetic control of oral tolerance to ovalbumin in mice. *Immunology* 63, 737–739.

Lamont, A. G., Mowat, A. McI., and Parrott, D. M. V. (1989). Priming of systemic and local delayed-type hypersensitivity responses by feeding low doses of ovalbumin to mice. *Immunology* 66, 595–599.

Lanoue, A., Bona, C., von Boehmer, H., and Sarukhan, A. (1997). Conditions that induce tolerance in mature CD4+ T cells. *J. Exp. Med.* 185, 405–414.

Lanzavecchia, A. (1998). Licence to kill. *Nature* 393, 413–414.

Lavelle, E. C., Grant, G., Pusztai, A., Pfüller, U., and O'Hagan, D. T. (2000). Mucosal immunogenicity of plant lectins in mice. *Immunology* 99, 30–37.

Lavelle, E. C., Grant, G., Pusztai, A., Pfuller, U., and O'Hagan, D. T. (2001). The identification of plant lectins with mucosal adjuvant activity. *Immunology* 102, 77–86.

Lee, H. O., Miller, S. D., Hurst, S. D., Tan, L. J., Cooper, C. J., and Barrett, T. A. (2000). Interferon γ induction during oral tolerance reduces T-cell migration to sites of inflammation. *Gastroenterology* 119, 129–138.

Lee, S., Scherberg, N., and DeGroot, L. J. (1998). Induction of oral tolerance in human autoimmune thyroid disease. *Thyroid* 8, 229–234.

Lefrancois, L., Altman, J. D., Williams, K., and Olson, S. (2000). Soluble antigen and CD40 triggering are sufficient to induce primary and memory cytotoxic T cells. *J. Immunol.* 164, 725–732.

Lefrançois, L., Olson, S., and Masopust, D. (1999). A critical role for CD40–CD40 ligand interactions in amplification of the mucosal CD8 T cell response *J. Exp. Med.* 190, 1275–1283.

Lehmann, P., Forsthuber, T., Miller, A., and Sercarz, E. (1992). Spreading of T-cell autoimmunity to cryptic determinants of an autoantigen. *Nature* 358, 155–157.

Leishman, A. J., Garside, P., and Mowat, A. McI. (1998). Intervention in established immune responses by induction of oral tolerance. *Cell Immunol.* 183, 137–148.

Leishman, A. J., Garside, P., and Mowat, A. McI. (2000). Induction of oral tolerance in the primed immune system: Influence of antigen persistence and adjuvant form. *Cell Immunol.* 202, 71–78.

Li, Y., Yio, X. Y., and Mayer, L. (1995). Human intestinal epithelial cell-induced CD8+ T cell activation is mediated through CD8 and the activation of CD8- associated p56lck. *J. Exp. Med.* 182, 1079–1088.

Lider, O., Santos, L. M. B., Lee, C. S. Y., Higgins, P. J., and Weiner, H. L. (1989). Suppression of experimental autoimmune encephalomyelitis by oral administration of myelin basic protein. II. Suppression of disease and *in vitro* immune responses is mediated by antigen-specific CD8+ T lymphocytes. *J. Immunol.* 142, 748–752.

Liu, L. M., and MacPherson, G. G. (1991). Lymph-borne (veiled) dendritic cells can acquire and present intestinally administered antigens. *Immunology* 73, 281.

Liu, L., and MacPherson, G. (1993). Antigen acquisition by dendritic cells: Intestinal dendritic cells acquire antigen administered orally and can prime naive T cells *in vivo. J. Exp. Med.* 177, 1299–1307.

Liu, L., and MacPherson, G. G. (1995). Rat intestinal dendritic cells: immunostimulatory potency and phenotypic characterisation. *Immunology* 85, 88–93.

Liu, L., Kuchroo, V. K., and Weiner, H. L. (1999). B7.2 (CD86) but not B7.1 (CD80) costimulation is required for the induction of low dose oral tolerance. *J. Immunol.* 163, 2284–2290.

Liu, Y., and Janeway, C. A. (1990). Interferon γ plays a critical role in induced cell death of effector T cells: A possible third mechanism of self-tolerance. *J. Exp. Med.* 172, 1735–1739.

Lombardi, G., Sidhu, S., Batchelor, R., and Lechler, R. (1994). Anergic T cells as suppressor cells *in vitro. Science* 264, 1587–1589.

Lombardi, G., Arnold, K., Uren, J., Marelli-Berg, F., Hargreaves, R., Imami, N., Weetman, A., and Lechler, R. (1997). Antigen presentation by interferon-γ-treated thyroid follicular cells inhibits interleukin-2˙ (IL-2) and supports IL-4 production by B7-dependent human T cells. *Eur. J. Immunol.* 27, 62–71.

Louis, E., Franchimont, D., Deprez, M., Lamproye, A., Schaaf, N., Mahieu, P., and Belaiche, J. (1996). Decrease in systemic tolerance to fed ovalbumin in indomethacin-treated mice. *Int. Arch. Allergy. Appl. Immunol.* 109, 21–26.

Lowney, E. D. (1968). Immunologic unresponsiveness to a contact sensitizer in man. *J. Invest. Dermatol.* 51, 411–417.

Lucas, P. J., Kim, S.-J., Melby, S. J., and Gress, R. E. (2000). Disruption of T cell homeostasis in mice expressing a T cell-specific dominant negative transforming growth factor β II receptor. *J. Exp. Med.* 191, 1187–1196.

Lundin, B. S., Dahlgren, U. I., Hanson, L. A., and Telemo, E. (1996). Oral tolerization leads to active suppression and bystander tolerance in adult rats, while anergy dominates in young rats. *Scand. J. Immunol.* 43, 56–63.

Lundin, B. S., Karlsson, M. R., Svensson, L. A., Hanson, L. A., Dahlgren, U. I., and Telemo, E. (1999). Active suppression in orally tolerized rats coincides with *in situ* transforming growth factor-β (TGF-β) expression in the draining lymph nodes. *Clin. Exp. Immunol.* 116, 181–187.

Lycke, N., and Holmgren, J. (1986). Strong adjuvant properties of cholera toxin on gut mucosal immune responses to orally presented antigens. *Immunology* 59, 301–308.

Lycke, N., Bromander, A., Ekman, L., Grdic, D., Hörnquist, E., Kjerrulf, M., Kopf, M., Kosco-Vilbois, M., Schon, K., and Vajdy, M. (1995). The use of knock-out mice in studies of induction and regulation of gut mucosal immunity. *Mucosal Immunol. Update* 3, 1–8.

Ma, C.-G., Zhang, G.-X., Xiao, B.-G., Link, J., Olsson, T., and Link, H. (1995). Suppression of experimental autoimmune myasthenia gravis by nasal administration of acetylcholine receptor. *J. Neuroimmunol.* 58, 51–60.

Ma, S.-W., Zhao, D.-L., Mukherjee, R., Singh, H. B., Qin, H.-Y., Stiller, C. R., and Jevnikar, A. M. (1997). Transgenic plants expressing autoantigens fed to mice to induce oral tolerance. *Nat. Med.* 3, 793–796.

MacDonald, T. T. (1983). Immunosuppression caused by antigen feeding. II. Suppressor T cells mask Peyer's patch B cell priming to orally administered antigen. *Eur. J. Immunol.* 13, 138–142.

MacDonald, T. T., and Carter, P. B. (1979). Requirement for a bacterial flora before mice generate cells capable of mediating the DTH reaction to sheep red blood cells. *J. Immunol.* 122, 2624–2629.

MacDonald, T. T., and Pender, S. L. F. (1998). Lamina propria T cells. *Chem. Immunol.* 71, 103–117.

MacLaren, N. K., Krischer, J., Crockett, S., Deeb, L., and Marks, J. (2004). Age and dose affects oral insulin tolerance therapy on endogenous insulin retention in new-onset immune-mediated (Type-1) diabetes: oral insulin therapy in Type-1 diabetes. *Ann. N. Y. Acad. Sci.*, in press.

MacPherson, G. G., and Liu, L. M. (1999). Dendritic cells and Langerhans cells in the uptake of mucosal antigens. *Curr. Top. Microbiol. Immunol,* 236, 33–53.

Maeda, Y., Noda, S., Tanaka, K., Sawamura, S., Aiba, Y., Ishikawa, H., Hasegawa, H., Kawabe, N., Miyasaka, M., and Koga, Y. (2001). The failure of oral tolerance induction is functionally coupled to the absence of T cells in Peyer's patches under germfree conditions. *Immunobiology* 204, 442–457.

Maiuri, L., Ciacci, C., Ricciardelli, I., Vacca, L., Raia, V., Auricchio, S., Picard, J., Osman, M., Quaratino, S., and Londei, M. (2003). Association between innate response to gliadin and activation of pathogenic T cells in coeliac disease. *Lancet* 362, 30–37.

Maloy, K. J., and Powrie, F. (2001). Regulatory T cells in the control of immune pathology. *Nat. Immunol.* 2, 816–822.

Maloy, K. J., Donachie, A. M., Ohagan, D. T., and Mowat, A. McI. (1994). Induction of mucosal and systemic immune-responses by immunization with ovalbumin entrapped in poly(lactide-co-glycolide) microparticles. *Immunology* 81, 661–667.

Maloy, K. J., Salaun, L., Cahill, R., Dougan, G., Saunders, N. J., and Powrie, F. (2003). CD4+CD25+ T(R) cells suppress innate immune pathology through cytokine-dependent mechanisms. *J. Exp. Med.* 197, 111–119.

Margenthaler, J. A., Landeros, K., Kataoka, M., and Flye, M. W. (2002). CD1-dependent natural killer (NK1.1(+)) T cells are required for oral and portal venous tolerance induction. *J. Surg. Res.* 104, 29–35.

Marinaro, M., Boyaka, P. N., Finkelman, F. D., Kiyono, H., Jackson, R. J., Jirillo, E., and McGhee, J. R. (1997). Oral but not parental interleukin (IL)-12 redirects T helper 2 (Th2)-type responses to an oral vaccine without altering mucosal IgA responses. *J. Exp. Med.* 185, 415–427.

Maron, R., Palanivel, V., Weiner, H. L., and Harn, D. A. (1998). Oral administration of schistosome egg antigens and insulin B-chain generates and enhances Th2-type responses in NOD mice. *Clin. Immunol. Immunopathol.* 87, 85–92.

Maron, R., Melican, N. S., and Weiner, H. L. (1999). Regulatory Th2-type T cell lines against insulin and GAD peptides derived from orally- and nasally-treated NOD mice suppress diabetes. *J. Autoimmun.* 12, 251–258.

Maron, R., Guerau-de-Arellano, M., Zhang, X., and Weiner, H. L. (2001). Oral administration of insulin to neonates suppresses spontaneous and cyclophosphamide induced diabetes in the NOD mouse *J. Autoimmun.* 16, 21–28.

Maron, R., Slavin, A. J., Hoffmann, E., Komagata, Y., and Weiner, H. L. (2002a). Oral tolerance to copolymer 1 in myelin basic protein (MBP) TCR transgenic mice: Cross-reactivity with MBP-specific TCR and differential induction of anti-inflammatory cytokines. *Int. Immunol.* 14, 131–138.

Maron, R., Sukhova, G., Faria, A. M., Hoffmann, E., Mach, F., Libby, P., and Weiner, H. L. (2002b). Mucosal administration of heat shock protein-65 decreases atherosclerosis and inflammation in aortic arch of low-density lipoprotein receptor-deficient mice. *Circulation* 106, 1708–1715.

Marth, T., Strober, W., and Kelsall, B. L. (1996). High dose oral tolerance in ovalbumin TcR-transgenic mice: systemic neutralisation of interleukin 12 augments TGFβ secretion and T cell apoptosis. *J. Immunol.* 157, 2348–2357.

Marth, T., Zeitz, M., Ludviksson, B. R., Strober, W., and Kelsall, B. L. (1999). Extinction of IL-12 signaling promotes Fas-mediated apoptosis of antigen-specific T cells. *J. Immunol.* 162, 7233–7240.

Marth, T., Ring, S., Schulte, D., Klensch, N., Strober, W., Kelsall, B. L., Stallmach, A., and Zeitz, M. (2000). Antigen-induced mucosal T cell activation is followed by Th1 T cell suppression in continuously fed ovalbumin TCR-transgenic mice. *Eur. J. Immunol.* 30, 3478–3486.

Martin, E., O'Sullivan, B., Low, P., and Thomas, R. (2003). Antigen-specific suppression of a primed immune response by dendritic cells mediated by regulatory T cells secreting interleukin-10. *Immunity* 18, 155–167.

Martin, P., Del Hoyo, G. M., Anjuere, F., Arias, C. F., Vargas, H. H., Fernandez, L. A., Parrillas, V., and Ardavin, C. (2002). Characterization of a new subpopulation of mouse CD8α+ B220+ dendritic cells endowed with type 1 interferon production capacity and tolerogenic potential. *Blood* 100, 383–390.

Masuda, K., Horie, K., Suzuki, R., Yoshikawa, T., and Hirano, K. (2002). Oral delivery of antigens in liposomes with some lipid compositions modulates oral tolerance to the antigens. *Microbiol. Immunol.* 46, 55–58.

Matsui, M., Hafler, D. A., and Weiner, H. L. (1996). Pilot study of oral tolerance to keyhole limpet hemocyanin in humans: Down regulation of KLH-reactive precursor-cell frequency. *Ann. N. Y. Acad. Sci.* 778, 398–404.

Mattingly, J. A., and Waksman, B. H. (1978). Immunologic suppression after oral administration of antigen. I. Specific suppressor cells formed in rat Peyer's patches after oral administration of sheep erythrocytes and their systemic migration. *J. Immunol.* 121, 1878–1883.

Mattingly, J. A., and Waksman, B. H. (1980). Immunologic suppression after oral administration of antigen. II. Antigen specific helper and suppressor factors produced by spleen cells of rats fed sheep erythrocytes. *J. Immunol.* 125, 1044–1047.

Matysiak-Budnik, T., Terpend, K., Alain, S., Sanson le Pors, M. J., Desjeux, J. F., Megraud, F., and Heyman, M. (1998). *Helicobacter pylori* alters exogenous antigen absorption and processing in a digestive tract epithelial cell line model. *Infect Immun.* 66, 5785–5791.

Matysiak-Budnik, T., Candalh, C., Dugave, C., Namane, A., Cellier, C., Cerf-Bensussan, N., and Heyman, M. (2003a). Alterations of the intestinal transport and processing of gliadin peptides in celiac disease. *Gastroenterology* 125, 696–707.

Matysiak-Budnik, T., van Niel, G., Megraud, F., Mayo, K., Bevilacqua, C., Gaboriau-Routhiau, V., Moreau, M. C., and Heyman, M. (2003b). Gastric *Helicobacter* infection inhibits development of oral tolerance to food antigens in mice. *Infect Immun.* 71, 5219–5324.

Mayer, L., and Shlien, R. (1987). Evidence for function of Ia molecules on gut epithelial cells in man *J. Exp. Med.* 166, 1471–1483.

Mayrhofer, G., Pugh, C. W., Barclay, A. N. (1983). The distribution, ontogeny and origin in the rat of Ia-positive cells with dendritic morphology and of Ia antigen in epithelia, with special reference to the intestine. *Eur. J. Immunol.* 13, 112–122.

McAdam, A. J., Schweitzer, A. N., and Sharpe, A. H. (1998). The role of B7 co-stimulation in activation and differentiation of CD4+ and CD8+ T cells. *Immunol. Rev.* 165, 231–247.

McCarron, R., Fallis, R., and McFarlin, D. (1990). Alterations in T cell antigen specificity and class II restriction during the course of chronic relapsing experimental allergic encephalomyelitis. *J. Neuroimmunol.* 29, 73–79.

McGhee, J. R., Mestecky, J., Dertzbaugh, M. T., Eldridge, J. H., Hirasawa, M., and Kiyono, H. (1992). The mucosal immune system: From fundamental concepts to vaccine development. *Vaccine* 10, 75–88.

McHugh, R. S., and Shevach, E. M. (2002). The role of suppressor T cells in regulation of immune responses. *J Allergy Clin. Immunol.* 110, 693–702.

McKown, K. M., Carbone, L. D., Kaplan, S. B., Aelion, J. A., Lohr, K. M., Cremer, M. A., Bustillo, J., Gonzalez, M., Kaeley, G., Steere, E. L., Somes, G. W., Myers, L. K., Seyer, J. M., Kang, A. H., and Postlethwaite, A. E. (1999). Lack of efficacy of oral bovine type II collagen added to existing therapy in rheumatoid arthritis. *Arth. Rheumat.* 42, 1204–1208.

McMenamin, C., Oliver, J., Girn, B. J., Kees, U. R., Thomas, W. R., and Holt, P. G. (1991). Regulation of T-cell sensitization at epithelial surfaces in the respiratory tract: Suppression of IgE responses to inhaled antigens by CD3+TcRα/β lymphocytes (putative γ/T cells). *Immunology* 74, 234–239.

McMenamin, C., Pimm, C., McKersey, M., and Holt, P. G. (1994). Regulation of IgE responses to inhaled antigen in mice by antigen-specific γ/δ T cells. *Science,* 265, 1869–1871.

McMenamin, C., McKersey, M., Kuhnlein, P., Hunig, T., and Holt, P. G. (1995). γ δ T cells down-regulate primary IgE responses in rats to inhaled soluble protein antigens. *J. Immunol.* 154, 4390–4394.

Melamed, D., and Friedman, A. (1993). Modification of the immune response by oral tolerance: Antigen requirements and interaction with immunogenic stimuli. *Cell Immunol.* 146, 412–420.

Melamed, D., and Friedman, A. (1994). *In vivo* tolerization of Th1 lymphocytes following a single feed with ovalbumin: Anergy in the absence of suppression. *Eur. J. Immunol.* 24, 1974–1981.

Melamed, D., Fischmann-Lobell, J., Uni, Z., Weiner, H. L., and Friedman, A. (1996). Peripheral tolerance of Th2 lymphocytes induced by continuous feeding of ovalbumin. *Int. Immunol.* 8, 717–724.

Menezes, J. da S., Mucida, D. de S., Cara, D. C., Alvarez-Leite, J. I., Russo, M., Vaz, N. M., and Faria, A. M. (2003). Stimulation by food proteins plays a critical role in the maturation of the immune system *Int. Immunol.* 15, 447–455.

Mengel, J., Cardillo, F., Aroeira, L. S., Williams, O., Russo, M., and Vaz, N. M. (1995). Anti-γδ T cell antibody blocks the induction and maintenance of oral tolerance to ovalbumin in mice. *Immunol. Lett.* 48, 97–102.

Metzler, B., and Wraith, D. C. (1993). Inhibition of experimental autoimmune encephalomyelitis by inhalation but not oral administration of the encephalitogenic peptide: Influence of MHC binding affinity. *Int. Immunol.* 5, 1159–1165.

Meyer, A. L., Benson, J. M., Gienapp, I. E., Cox, K. L., and Whitacre, C. C. (1996). Suppression of murine chronic relapsing autoimmune encephalomyelitis by the oral administration of myelin basic protein. *J. Immunol.* 157, 4230–4238.

Meyer, A. L., Benson, J., Song, F., Javed, N., Gienapp, I. E., Goverman, J., Brabb, T. A., Hood, L., Whitacre, C. C., and Iglewski, B. H. (2001). Rapid depletion of peripheral antigen-specific T cells in TcR-transgenic mice after oral administration of myelin basic protein. *J. Immunol.* 166, 5773–5782.

Michalek, S. M., Kiyono, H., Wannemuehler, M. J., Mosteller, L. M., and McGhee, J. R. (1982). Lipopolysaccharide (LPS) regulation of the immune response: LPS influence on oral tolerance induction. *J. Immunol.* 128, 1992–1998.

Migita, K., and Ochi, A. (1994). Induction of clonal anergy by oral administration of staphylococcal enterotoxin B. *Eur. J. Immunol.* 24, 2081–2086.

Migita, K., Eguchi, K., Kawabe, Y., Tsukada, T., Ichinose, Y., and Nagataki, S. (1995). Defective TCR-mediated signaling in anergic T cells. *J. Immunol.* 155, 5083–5087.

Miller, A., Lider, O., and Weiner, H. L. (1991). Antigen-driven bystander suppression following oral administration of antigens. *J. Exp. Med.* 174, 791–798.

Miller, A., Lider, O., Roberts, A. B., Sporn, M. B., and Weiner, H. L. (1992). Suppressor T cells generated by oral tolerization to myelin basic protein suppress both *in vitro* and *in vivo* immune responses by the release of transforming growth factor β after antigen-specific triggering. *Proc. Natl. Acad. Sci. USA* 89, 421–425.

Miller, A., Al-Sabbagh, A., Santos, L. M. B., Das, M. P., and Weiner, H. L. (1993). Epitopes of myelin basic protein that trigger TGF-β release after oral tolerization are distinct from encephalitogenic epitopes and mediate epitope-driven bystander suppression. *J. Immunol.* 151, 7307–7315.

Miller, A., Lider, O., Abramsky, O., and Weiner, H. L. (1994). Orally administered myelin basic protein in neonates primes for immune responses and enhances experimental autoimmune encephalomyelitis in adult animals. *Eur. J. Immunol.* 24, 1026–1032.

Miller, B. G., Newby, T. J., Stokes, C. R., and Bourne, F. J. (1984). Influence of diet on postweaning malabsorption and diarrhoea in the pig. *Res. Vet. Sci.*, 36, 187–193.

Miller, B. G., Whittemore, C. T., Stokes, C. R., and Telemo, E. (1994). The effects of delayed weaning on the development of oral tolerance to soya-bean protein in pigs. *Br. J. Nutr.* 71, 615–625.

Miller, C. C., and Cook, M. E. (1994). Evidence against the induction of immunological tolerance by feeding antigens to chickens. *Poultry Sci.* 73, 106–112.

Miller, J. E. A. P., and Heath, W. R. (1993). Self-ignorance in the peripheral T-cell pool. *Immunol. Rev.* 133, 131–150.

Miller, M. L., Cowdrey, J. S., and Curtin, M. F. (1983). Gastrointestinal tolerance in autoimmune mice. *Fed. Proc.* 42, 942.

Miller, S. D., and Hanson, D. G. (1979). Inhibition of specific immune responses by feeding protein antigens. IV. Evidence for tolerance and specific active suppression of cell-mediated immune responses to ovalbumin. *J. Immunol.* 123, 2344–2350.

Min, W. P., Zhou, D., Ichim, T. E., Strejan, G. H., Xia, X., Yang, J., Huang, X., Garcia, B., White, D., Dutartre, P., Jevnikar, A. M., and Zhong, R. (2003). Inhibitory feedback loop between tolerogenic dendritic cells and regulatory T cells in transplant tolerance. *J. Immunol.* 170, 1304–1312.

Monfardini, C., Milani, M., Ostlie, N., Wang, W., Karachunski, P. I., Okita, D. K., Lindstrom, J., and Conti-Fine, B. M. (2002). Adoptive protection from experimental myasthenia gravis with T cells from mice treated nasally with acetylcholine receptor epitopes. *J. Neuroimmunol.* 123, 123–134.

Monsonego, A., Beserman, Z. P., Kipnis, J., Yoles, E., Weiner, H. L., and Schwartz, M. (2003). Beneficial effect of orally administered myelin basic protein in EAE-susceptible Lewis rats in a model of acute CNS degeneration. *J. Autoimmun.* 21, 131–138.

Monteleone, G., Pender, S. L., Wathen N.C., and MacDonald, T. T. (2001a). Interferon-α drives T cell-mediated immunopathology in the intestine. *Eur. J. Immunol.* 31, 2247–2255.

Monteleone, G., Pender, S. L. F., Alstead, E., Hauer, A. C., Lionetti, P., and MacDonald, T. T. (2001b). Role of interferon α in promoting T helper cell type 1 responses in the small intestine in coeliac disease. *Gut* 48, 425–429.

Moreau, M. C., and Corthier, G. (1988). Effect of the gastrointestinal microflora on induction and maintenance of oral tolerance to ovalbumin in C3H/HeJ mice. *Infect. Immunol.* 56, 2766–2768.

Moreau, M., and Gaboriau-Routhiau, V. (1996). The absence of gut flora, the doses of antigen ingested and ageing affect the long-term peripheral tolerance induced by ovalbumin feeding in mice. *Res. Immunol.* 147, 49–59.

Morrissey, P., Charrier, K., Braddy, S., Liggitt, D., and Watson, J. (1993). CD4+ T cells that express high levels of CD45RB induce wasting disease when transferred into congenic severe combined immunodeficient mice: Disease development is prevented by cotransfer of purified CD4+ T cells. *J. Exp. Med.* 178, 237–244.

Mottet, C., Uhlig, H. H., and Powrie, F. (2003). Cutting edge: cure of colitis by CD4+CD25+ regulatory T cells. *J. Immunol.* 170, 3939–3943.

Mowat, A. McI. (1984). The immunopathogenesis of food sensitive enteropathies. In *Local Immune Responses of the Gut* (eds. T. J. Newby and C. R. Stokes), 199–225. Boca Raton, FL: CRC Press.

Mowat, A. McI. (1985). The role of antigen recognition and suppressor cells in mice with oral tolerance to ovalbumin. *Immunology* 56, 253–260.

Mowat, A. McI. (1986). Depletion of suppressor T cells by 2'-deoxyguanosine abrogates tolerance in mice fed ovalbumin and permits the induction of intestinal delayed-type-hypersensitivity. *Immunology* 58, 179–184.

Mowat, A. McI. (1987). The regulation of immune responses to dietary protein antigens. *Immunol. Today* 8, 93–95.

Mowat, A. McI. (1997). Intestinal graft-versus-host disease. In *Graft Versus Host Disease* (eds. J. M. Ferrara, J. H. Deeg., and S. J. Burakoff), 337–384. New York: Marcel Dekker.

Mowat, A. McI. (1999a). Induction of peripheral tolerance by portal vein administration of antigen. In *The Immunology of the Liver* (ed. I. N. Crispe), 101–115. New York: John Wiley & Sons.

Mowat, A. McI. (1999b). Oral tolerance; physiology, and clinical implications. *Curr. Opin. Gastroenterol.* 15, 546–556.

Mowat, A. McI., and Ferguson, A. (1981). Hypersensitivity in the small intestinal mucosa. V. Induction of cell mediated immunity to a dietary antigen. *Clin. Exp. Immunol.* 43, 574–582.

Mowat, A. McI., and Ferguson, A. (1982). Migration inhibition of lymph node lymphocytes as an assay for regional cell-mediated immunity in the intestinal lymphoid tissues of mice immunised orally with ovalbumin. *Immunology* 47, 365–370.

Mowat, A. McI. I., and Parrott, D. M. V. (1983). Immunological responses to fed protein antigens in mice. IV. Effects of stimulating the reticuloendothelial system on oral tolerance and intestinal immunity to ovalbumin. *Immunology* 50, 547–554.

Mowat, A. McI., Strobel, S., Drummond, H. E., and Ferguson, A. (1982). Immunological responses to fed protein antigens in mice. I. Reversal of oral tolerance to ovalbumin by cyclophosphamide. *Immunology* 45, 104–113.

Mowat, A. McI., Thomas, M. J., Mackenzie, S., and Parrott, D. M. V. (1986). Divergent effects of bacterial lipopolysaccharide on immunity to orally administered protein and particulate antigens in mice. *Immunology* 58, 677–684.

Mowat, A. McI., Lamont, A. G., and Bruce, M. G. (1987). A genetically determined lack of oral tolerance to ovalbumin is due to failure of the immune system to respond to intestinally derived tolerogen. *Eur. J. Immunol.* 17, 1673–1676.

Mowat, A. McI., Maloy, K. J., and Donachie, A. M. (1993). Immune stimulating complexes as adjuvants for inducing local and systemic immunity after oral immunization with protein antigens *Immunology* 80, 527–534.

Mowat, A. McI., Steel, M., Leishman, A. J., and Garside, P. (1999). Normal induction of oral tolerance in the absence of a functional IL12 dependent γ interferon signalling pathway. *J. Immunol.* 163, 4728–4736.

Mucida, D. S., Rodrigues, D., Keller, A. C., Gomes, E., Faria, A. M. C., and Russo, M. (2004). Decreased nasal tolerance to allergic asthma in mice fed an amino acid-based protein-free diet. *Ann. N. Y. Acad. Sci.*, in press.

Mueller, D. L., and Jenkins, M.K. (1995). Molecular mechanisms underlying functional T-cell unresponsiveness. *Curr. Opin. Immunol*, 7, 375–381.

Mueller, D. L., Jenkins, M. K., and Schwartz, R. H. (1989). Clonal expansion versus functional clonal inactivation: A costimulatory signalling pathway determines the outcome of T cell antigen receptor occupancy. *Ann. Rev. Immunol.* 7, 445–480.

Myers, L. K., Higgins, G. C., Finkel, T. H., Reed, A. M., Thompson, J. W., Walton, R. C., Hendrickson, J., Kerr, N. C., Pandya-Lipman, R. K., Shlopov, B. V., Stastny, P., Postlethwaite, A. E., and Kang, A. H. (2001). Juvenile arthritis and autoimmunity to type II collagen. *Arth. Rheumat.* 44, 1775–1781.

Nagata, S., McKenzie, C., Pender, S. L. F., Bajaj-Elliott, M., Fairclough, P. D., Walker-Smith, J., Monteleone, G., and MacDonald, T. T. (2000). Human Peyer's patch T cells are sensitised to dietary antigens and display a T helper cell type 1 cytokine profile. *J. Immunol.* 165, 5315–5321.

Nagatani, K., Komagata, Y., and Yamamoto, K. (2004). Peyer's patch dendritic cells capturing oral antigen interact with antigen specific T cells and induce gut-homing CD4+ CD25+ regulatory T cells in Peyer's patch. *Ann. N. Y. Acad. Sci. USA* in press.

Nagler-Anderson, C., Bober, L. A., Robinson, M. E., Siskind, G. W. A., and Thorbecke, G. J. (1986). Suppression of type II collagen-induced arthritis by intragastric administration of soluble type II antigen. *Proc. Natl. Acad. Sci. USA* 83, 7443–7446.

Nakamura, K., Kitani, A., and Strober, W. (2001). Cell contact-dependent immunosuppression by CD4(+)CD25(+) regulatory T cells is mediated by cell surface-bound transforming growth factor β. *J. Exp. Med.* 194, 629–644.

Nakamura, K., Kitani, A., Fuss, I., Pedersen, A., Harada, N., Nawata, H., and Strober, W. (2004). TGF-β1 plays an important role in the mechanism of CD4+CD25+ regulatory T cell activity in both humans and mice. *J. Immunol.* 172, 834–842.

Nakao, A., Kasai, M., Kumano, K., Nakajima, H., Kurasawa, K., and Iwamoto, I. (1998). High-dose oral tolerance prevents antigen-induced eosinophil recruitment into the mouse airways. *Int. Immunol.* 104, 387–394.

Nelson, P. A., Akselband, Y., Dearborn, S., Al-Sabbagh, A., Tian, Z. J., Gonnella, P., Zamvil, S., Chen, Y., and Weiner, H. L. (1996). Effect of oral β interferon on subsequent immune responsiveness. *Ann. N. Y. Acad. Sci.* 778, 145–155.

Neurath, M. F., Fuss, I., Kelsall, B. L., Presky, D. H., Waegell, W., and Strober, W. (1996). Experimental granulomatous colitis in mice is abrogated by induction of TGF-β-mediated oral tolerance. *J. Exp. Med.* 183, 2605–2616.

Newberry, R. D., Stenson, W. P., and Lorenz, R. G. (1999). Cyclooxygenase-2-dependent arachidonic acid metabolites are

essential modulators of the intestinal immune response to dietary antigen. *Nat. Med.* 5, 900–906.

Newberry, R. D., McDonough, J. S., Stenson, W. F., and Lorenz, R. G. (2001). Spontaneous and continuous cyclooxygenase-2-dependent prostaglandin E2 production by stromal cells in the murine small intestinal lamina propria: Directing the tone of the intestinal immune response. *J. Immunol.* 166, 4465–4472.

Newby, T. J., Stokes, C. R., and Bourne, F. J. (1980). Effects of feeding bacterial lipopolysaccharide and dextran sulphate on the development of oral tolerance to contact sensitizing agents. *Immunology* 41, 617–621.

Ngan, J., and Kind, L. S. (1978). Suppressor T cells for IgE and IgG in Peyer's patches of mice made tolerant by the oral administration of ovalbumin. *J. Immunol.* 120, 861–865.

Niederkorn, J. Y. (2002). Immunology and immunomodulation of corneal transplantation. *Int. Rev. Immunol.* 21, 173–196.

Niederkorn, J. Y., and Mayhew, E. (2002). Phenotypic analysis of oral tolerance to alloantigens: evidence that the indirect pathway of antigen presentation is involved. *Transplantation* 73, 1493–1500.

Niimi, M., Takashina, M., Ikeda, Y., Shirasugi, N., Shatari, T., Takami, H., Kodaira, S., Kameyama, K., Matsumoto, K., Hamano, K., and Esato, K. (2000). Mice treated with anti-CD4 monoclonal antibody accept fully allogeneic thyroid grafts but reject second-donor-type thyroid grafts in maintenance phase. *Transplant. Proc.* 32, 2086.

Nilsen, E. M., Jahnsen, F. L., Lundin, K. E., Johansen, F. E., Fausa, O., Sollid, L. M., Jahnsen, J., Scott, H., and Brandtzaeg, P. (1998). Gluten induces an intestinal cytokine response strongly dominated by interferon γ in patients with celiac disease. *Gastroenterology* 115, 551–563.

Nishimura, M., Fujiyama, Y., Niwakawa, M., Sasaki, T., and Bamba, T. (2002). *In vivo* cytokine responses in gut-associated lymphoid tissue (GALT) and spleen following oral administration of staphylococcal enterotoxin B. *Immunol. Lett.* 81, 77–85.

Nussenblatt, R. B., Caspi, R. R., Mahdi, R., Chan, C.-C., Roberge, F., Lider, O., and Weiner, H. L. (1990). Inhibition of S-antigen induced experimental autoimmune uveoretinitis by oral induction of tolerance with S-antigen. *J. Immunol.* 144, 1689–1696.

Nussenblatt, R. B., Gery, I., Weiner, H. L., Ferris, F., Shiloach, J., Ramaley, N., Perry, C., Caspi, R., Hafler, D. A., Foster, S., and Whitcup, S. M. (1997). Treatment of uveitis by oral administration of retinal antigens: Results of a phase I/II randomized masked trial. *Am. J. Ophthal.* 123, 583–592.

Oh, J. W., Seroogy, C. M., Meyer, E. H., Akbari, O., Berry, G., Fathman, C. G., Dekruyff, R. H., and Umetsu, D. T. (2002). CD4 T-helper cells engineered to produce IL-10 prevent allergen-induced airway hyperreactivity and inflammation. *J. Allergy Clin. Immunol.* 110, 460–468.

Oida, T., Zhang, X., Goto, M., Hachimura, S., Totsuka, M., Kaminogawa, S., and Weiner, H. L. (2003). CD4+CD25− T cells that express latency-associated peptide on the surface suppress CD4+CD45RBhigh-induced colitis by a TGF-β-dependent mechanism. *J. Immunol.* 170, 2516–2522.

Okumura, S., McIntosh, K., and Drachman, D. B. (1994). Oral administration of acetylcholine receptor: Effects on experimental myasthenia gravis. *Ann. Neurol.* 36, 704–713.

Oliveira, F.M., Santos, E.M., Mota-Santos, T.A., Ruiz-De- Souza, V., and Gontijo, C.M. (2002). Covalent coupling of palmitate to ovalbumin inhibits and blocks the induction of oral tolerance. *Scand. J. Immunol.* 55, 570–576.

O'Mahony, S., Arranz, E., Barton, J. R., and Ferguson, A. (1991). Dissociation between systemic and mucosal humoral immune responses in coeliac disease. *Gut* 32, 29–35.

Owen, R. L. (1994). M cells: entryways of opportunity for enteropathogens. *J. Exp. Med.* 180, 7–9.

Pape, K. A., Kearney, E. R., Khoruts, A., Mondino, A., Merica, R., Chen, Z.-M., Ingulli, E., White, J., Johnson, J. G., and Jenkins, M. K. (1997). Use of adoptive transfer of T-cell-antigen-receptor-transgenic T cells for the study of T-cell activation *in vivo*. *Immunol. Rev.* 156, 67–78.

Paul, W. E., and Seder, R. A. (1994). Lymphocyte responses and cytokines. *Cell*, 76, 241–251.

Pecquet, S., Pfeifer, A., Gauldie, S., and Fritsché, R. (1999). Immunoglobulin E suppression and cytokine modulation in mice orally tolerized to β-lactoglobulin. *Immunology* 96, 278–285.

Pecquet, S., Leo, E., Fritsche, R., Pfeifer, A., Couvreur, P., and Fattal, E. (2000). Oral tolerance elicited in mice by β-lactoglobulin entrapped in biodegradable microspheres. *Vaccine* 18, 1196–1202.

Peng, H.-J., Turner, M. W., and Strobel, S. (1989a). The kinetics of oral hyposensitisation to a protein antigen are determined by immune status and the timing, dose, and frequency of antigen administration. *Immunology* 67, 425–430.

Peng, H.-J., Turner, M. W., and Strobel, S. (1989b). Failure to induce oral tolerance to protein antigens in neonatal mice can be corrected by transfer of adult spleen cells. *Pediatr. Res.* 26, 486–490.

Peng, H.-J., Turner, M. W., and Strobel, S. (1990). The generation of a "tolerogen" after the ingestion of ovalbumin is time-dependent and unrelated to serum levels of immunoreactive antigen. *Clin. Exp. Immunol.* 81, 510–515.

Peng, H.-J., Chang, Z.-N., Han, S.-H., Won, M.-H., and Huang, B.-T. (1995). Chemical denaturation of ovalbumin abrogates the induction of oral tolerance of specific IgG antibody and DTH responses in mice. *Scand. J. Immunol.* 42, 297–304.

Peng, H.-J., Chang, Z.-N., Lee, C.-C., and Kuo, S.-W. (2000). B-cell depletion fails to abrogate the induction of oral tolerance of specific Th1 immune responses in mice. *Scand. J. Immunol.* 51, 454–460.

Perez, V. L., Parijs, L. V., Biuckians, A., Zheng, X. X., Strom, T. B., and Abbas, A. K. (1997). Induction of peripheral T cell tolerance *in vivo* requires CTLA-4 engagement. *Immunity* 6, 411–417.

Perez-Machado, M. A., Ashwood, P., Thomson, M. A., Latcham, F., Sim, R., Walker-Smith, J. A., and Murch, S. H. (2003). Reduced transforming growth factor-β1-producing T cells in the duodenal mucosa of children with food allergy. *Eur. J. Immunol.* 33, 2307–2315.

Peri, B. A., and Rothberg, R. M. (1981). Circulating antitoxin in rabbits after ingestion of diphtheria toxin. *Infect. Immunity* 32, 1148–1154.

Petersen, J. S., Bregenholt, S., Apostolopolous, V., Homann, D., Wolfe, T., Hughes, A., De Jongh, K., Wang, M., Dyrberg, T., and Von Herrath, M. G. (2003). Coupling of oral human or porcine insulin to the B subunit of cholera toxin (CTB) overcomes critical antigenic differences for prevention of type I diabetes. *Clin. Exp. Immunol.* 134, 38–45.

Peterson, K. E., and Braley-Mullen, H. (1995). Suppression of murine experimental autoimmune thyroiditis by oral administration of porcine thyroglobulin. *Cell Immunol.* 166, 123–130.

Phipps, P. A., Stanford, M. R., Sun, J. B., Xiao, B. G., Holmgren, J., Shinnick, T., Hasan, A., Mizushima, Y., and Lehner, T. (2003). Prevention of mucosally induced uveitis with a HSP60-derived peptide linked to cholera toxin B subunit. *Eur. J. Immunol.* 33, 224–232.

Ploix, C., Bergerot, I., Durand, A., Czerkinsky, C., Holmgren, J., and Thivolet, C. (1999). Oral administration of cholera toxin B-insulin conjugates protects NOD mice from autoimmune diabetes by inducing CD4+ regulatory T-cells. *Diabetes* 48, 2150–2156.

Popat, S., Hearle, N., Hogberg, L., Braegger, C. P., O'Donoghue, D., Falth-Magnusson, K., Holmes, G. K., Howdle, P. D., Jenkins, H., Johnston, S., Kennedy, N. P., Kumar, P. J., Logan, R. F., Marsh, M. N., Mulder, C. J., Torinsson Naluai, A., Sjoberg, K., Stenhammar, L., Walters, J. R., Jewell, D. P., and Houlston, R. S. (2002). Variation in the CTLA4/CD28 gene region confers an increased risk of coeliac disease. *Ann. Hum. Genet.* 66, 125–137.

Pope, C., Kim, S. K., Marzo, A., Masopust, D., Williams, K., Jiang, J., Shen, H., and Lefrancois, L. (2001). Organ-specific regulation of the CD8 T cell response to *Listeria monocytogenes* infection. *J. Immunol.* 166, 3402–3409.

Poussier, P., Ning, T., Banerjee, D., and Julius, M. (2002). A unique subset of self-specific intraintestinal T cells maintains gut integrity. *J. Exp. Med.* 195, 1491–1497.

Powrie, F. (1995). T cells in inflammatory bowel disease: protective and pathogenic roles. *Immunity* 3, 171–174.

Powrie, F., Carlino, J., Leach, M. W., Mauze, S., and Coffman, R. L. (1996). A critical role for transforming growth factor-β but not

interleukin 4 in the suppression of T helper type 1-mediated colitis by CD45RBlow CD4+ T cells. *J. Exp. Med.* 183, 2669–2674.

Prakken B.J., van der Zee, R., Anderton, S.M., van Kooten, P.J., Kuis, W., and van Eden, W. (1997). Peptide-induced nasal tolerance for a mycobacterial heat shock protein 60 T cell epitope in rats suppresses both adjuvant arthritis and nonmicrobially induced experimental arthritis. *Proc. Natl. Acad. Sci. USA* 94, 3284–3289.

Prakken, B. J., Roord, S., van Kooten, P. J., Wagenaar, J. P., van Eden, W., Albani, S., and Wauben, M. H. (2002). Inhibition of adjuvant-induced arthritis by interleukin-10-driven regulatory cells induced via nasal administration of a peptide analog of an arthritis-related heat-shock protein 60 T cell epitope *Arth. Rheumat.* 46, 1937–1946.

Premier, R. R., and Meeusen, E. N. T. (1998). Lymphocyte surface marker and cytokine expression in peripheral and mucosal lymph nodes. *Immunology* 94, 363–367.

Qian, J.-H., Hashimoto, T., Fujiwara, H., and Hamaoka, T. (1985). Studies on the induction of tolerance to alloantigens. 1. The abrogation of potentials for delayed-type hypersensitivity responses to alloantigens by portal venous inoculation with allogeneic cells. *J. Immunol.* 134, 3656–3661.

Quinn, A., Melo, M., Ethell, D., and Sercarz, E. E. (2001). Relative resistance to nasally induced tolerance in non-obese diabetic mice but not other I-A(g7)-expressing mouse strains. *Int. Immunol.* 13, 1321–1333.

Rask, C., Holmgren, J., Fredriksson, M., Lindblad, M., Nordström, I., Sun, J.-B., and Czerkinsky, C. (2000). Prolonged oral treatment with low doses of allergen conjugated to cholera toxin B subunit suppresses immunoglobulin E antibody responses in sensitized mice. *Clin Exp Allergy*, 30, 1024–1032.

Read, S., Malmstrom, V., and Powrie, F. (2000). Cytotoxic T lymphocyte-associated antigen 4 plays an essential role in the function of CD25(+)CD4(+) regulatory cells that control intestinal inflammation. *J. Exp. Med.* 192, 295–302.

Reynolds, J., and Pusey, C. D. (2001). Oral administration of glomerular basement membrane prevents the development of experimental autoimmune glomerulonephritis in the WKY rat. *J. Am. Soc. Nephrol.* 12, 61–70.

Richman, L. K., Chiller, J. M., Brown, W. R., Hanson, D. G., and Vaz, N. M. (1978). Enterically induced immunologic tolerance. I. Induction of suppressor T lymphocytes by intragastric administration of soluble proteins. *J. Immunol.* 121, 2429–2434.

Richman, L. K., Graeff, A. S., Yarchoan, R., and Strober, W. (1981a). Simultaneous induction of antigen-specific IgA helper T cells and IgA suppressor T cells in the murine Peyer's patch after protein feeding. *J. Immunol.* 126, 2079–2083.

Richman, L. K., Graeff, A. S, Strober, W (1981b). Antigen presentation by macrophage-enriched cells from the mouse Peyer's patch. *Cell Immunol.* 62, 110–118.

Rizzo, L. V., Miller-Rivero, N. E., Chan, C.-C., Wiggert, B., Nussenblatt, R. B., and Caspi, R. R. (1994). Interleukin-2 treatment potentiates induction of oral tolerance in a murine model of autoimmunity. *J. Clin. Invest.* 94, 1668–1672.

Rizzo, L. V., Morawetz, R. A., Miller-Rivero, N. E., Choi, R., Wiggert, B., Chan, C.-C., Morse, H. C., Nusenblatt, R. B., and Caspi, R. R. (1999). IL-4 and IL-10 are both required for the induction of oral tolerance. *J. Immunol.* 162, 2613–2622.

Roberts, S. J., Smith, A. L., West, A. B., Wen, L., Findly, R. C., Owen, M. J., Hayday, A. C. (1996). T-cell α β+ and γ δ+ deficient mice display abnormal but distinct phenotypes toward a natural, widespread infection of the intestinal epithelium. *Proc. Natl. Acad. Sci. USA* 93, 11774–11779.

Roelofs-Haarhuis, K., Wu, X., Nowak, M., Fang, M., Artik, S., and Gleichmann, E. (2003). Infectious nickel tolerance: A reciprocal interplay of tolerogenic APCs and T suppressor cells that is driven by immunization. *J. Immunol.* 171, 2863–2872.

Roncarolo, M. G., Bacchetta, R., Bordignon, C., Narula, S., and Levings, M. K. (2001). Type 1 T regulatory cells. *Immunol. Rev.* 182, 68–79.

Rubin, D., Weiner, H. L., Fields, B. N., and Greene, M. I. (1981). Immunologic tolerance after oral administration of reovirus: Requirement for two viral gene products for tolerance induction. *J. Immunol.* 127, 1697–1701.

Russo, M., Jancar, S., Pereira de Siqueira, A. L., Mengel, J., Gomes, E., Ficker, S. M., and Caetano de Faria, A. M. (1998). Prevention of lung eosinophilic inflammation by oral tolerance. *Immunol. Lett.* 61, 15–23.

Russo, M., Nahori, M. A., Lefort, J., Gomes, E., de Castro Keller, A., Rodriguez, D., Ribeiro, O. G., Adriouch, S., Gallois, V., de Faria, A. M., and Vargaftig, B. B. (2001). Suppression of asthma-like responses in different mouse strains by oral tolerance. *Am. J. Respir. Cell Mol. Biol.* 24, 518–526.

Ryan, K. R., and Evavold, B. D. (1998). Persistence of peptide-induced CD4+ T cell anergy *in vitro. J. Exp. Med.* 187, 89–96.

Sadeghi, H., Bregenholt, S., Wegmann, D., Petersen, J. S., Holmgren, J., and Lebens, M. (2002). Genetic fusion of human insulin B-chain to the B-subunit of cholera toxin enhances in vitro antigen presentation and induction of bystander suppression *in vivo. Immunology* 106, 237–45.

Sakaguchi, S. (2003). Control of immune responses by naturally arising CD4+ regulatory T cells that express toll-like receptors. *J. Exp. Med.* 197, 397–401.

Saklayen, M. G., Pesce, A. J., Pollak, V. E., and Michael, J. G. (1983). Induction of oral tolerance in mice unresponsive to bacterial lipopolysaccharide. *Infect. Immun.* 41, 1383–1385.

Saklayen, M. G., Pesce, A. J., Pollak, V. E., and Michael, J. G. (1984). Kinetics of oral tolerance: Study of variables affecting tolerance induced by oral administration of antigen. *Int. Arch. Allergy Appl. Immunol.* 73, 75–79.

Samoilova, E. B., Horton, J. L., Zhang, H., Khoury, S. J., Weiner, H. L., and Chen, Y. (1998). CTLA-4 is required for the induction of high dose oral tolerance. *Int. Immunol.* 10, 491–498.

Sanderson, I., Ouellette, AJ, Carter, EA, Walker, WA, and Harmatz, PR (1993). Differential regulation of B7 mRNA in enterocytes and lymphoid cells. *Immunology* 79, 434–438.

Santos, L. M. B., Al-Sabbagh, A., Londono, A. A., and Weiner, H. L. (1994). Oral tolerance to myelin basic protein induces regulatory TGR-β secreting cells in Peyer's patches of SJL mice. *Cell Immunol*, 157, 439–447.

Sato, M. N., Oliveira, C. R., Futata, E. A., Victor, J. R., Maciel, M., Fusaro, A. E., Carvalho, A. F., and Duarte, A. J. (2002). Oral tolerance induction to *Dermatophagoides pteronyssinus* and *Blomia tropicalis* in sensitized mice: occurrence of natural autoantibodies to immunoglobulin E. *Clin. Exp. Allergy* 32, 1667–1674.

Sato, S., Qian, J.-H., Kokudo, S., Ikegami, R., Suda, T., Hamaoka, T., and Fujiwara, H. (1988). Studies on the induction of tolerance to alloantigens. III. Induction of antibodies directed against alloantigen-specific delayed-type hypersensitivity T cells by a single injection of allogeneic lymphocytes via portal venous route. *J. Immunol*, 140, 717–722.

Sayegh, M. H., Khoury, S. J., Hancock, W. H., Weiner, H. L., and Carpenter, C. B. (1992a). Induction of immunity and oral tolerance with polymorphic class II major histocompatibility complex allopeptides in the rat. *Proc. Natl. Acad. Sci. USA* 89, 7762–7766.

Sayegh, M. H., Zhang, Z. J., Hancock, W. W., Kwok, C. A., Carpenter, C. B., and Weiner, H. L. (1992b). Down-regulation of the immune response to histocompatibility antigen and prevention of sensitization by skin allografts by orally administered alloantigen. *Transplantation* 53, 163–166.

Schoenberger, S. P., Toes, R. E. M., van der Voort, E. I. H., Offringa, R., and Melief, C. J. M. (1998). T-cell help for cytotoxic T lymphocytes is mediated by CD40-CD40L interactions. *Nature* 393, 480–483.

Schwartz, R. H. (2003). T cell anergy. *Annu. Rev. Immunol.* 21, 305–334.

Sharpe, A. H., and Freeman, G. J. (2002). The B7-CD28 superfamily. *Nat. Rev. Immunol.* 2, 116–226.

Sher, A., Pearce, E., and Kaye, P. (2003). Shaping the immune response to parasites: Role of dendritic cells. *Curr. Opin. Immunol.* 15, 421–429.

Shi, F. D., Li, H., Wang, H., Bai, X., van der Meide, P. H., Link, H., and Ljunggren, H. G. (1999a). Mechanisms of nasal tolerance induction in experimental autoimmune myasthenia gravis: Identification of regulatory cells. *J. Immunol.* 162, 5757–5763.

Shi, H. N., Grusby, M. J., and Nagler-Anderson, C. (1999b). Orally induced peripheral nonresponsiveness is maintained in the absence of functional Th1 or Th2 cells. *J. Immunol.* 162, 5143–5148.

Shi, H. N., Liu, H. Y., and Nagler-Anderson, C. (2000). Enteric infection as an adjuvant for the response to a model food antigen. *J. Immunol.* 165, 6174–6182.

Sieper, J., Kary, S., Sörensen, H., Alten, R., Eggens, U., Hüge, W., Hiepe, F., Kühne, A., Listing, J., Ulbrich, N., Braun, J., Zink, A., and Mitchison, N. A. (1996). Oral type II collagen treatment in early rheumatoid arthritis: A double blind, placebo-controlled, randomized trial. *Arth. Rheumat.* 39, 41–51.

Silverman, G. A., Peri, B. A., and Rothberg, R. M. (1982). Systemic antibody responses of different species following ingestion of soluble protein antigens. *Dev. Comp. Immunol.* 6, 737–746.

Singh, V. K., Kalra, H. K., Yamaki, K., and Shinohara, T. (1992). Suppression of experimental autoimmune uveitis in rats by the oral administration of the uveitopathogenic S-antigen fragment or a cross-reactive homologous peptide. *Cell Immunol.* 139, 81–90.

Singh, V. K., Anand, R., Sharma, K., and Agarwal, S. (1996). Suppression of experimental autoimmune uveitis in Lewis rats by oral administration of recombinant *Escherichia coli* expressing retinal S-antigen. *Cell. Immunol.* 172, 158–162.

Skyler, J. S. (2004). The effects of oral insulin in relatives of patients with type 1 diabetes. *Ann. N.Y. Acad. Sci.*, in press.

Slavin, A. J., Maron, R., and Weiner, H. L. (2001). Mucosal administration of IL-10 enhances oral tolerance in autoimmune encephalomyelitis and diabetes. *Int. Immunol.* 13, 825–833.

Sloan-Lancaster, J., and Allen, P. M. (1996). Altered peptide ligand-induced partial T cell activation: molecular mechanisms and role in T cell biology. *Ann. Rev. Immunol.* 14, 1–27.

Smith, K. M., Davidson, J. M., and Garside, P. (2002a). T-cell activation occurs simultaneously in local and peripheral lymphoid tissue following oral administration of a range of doses of immunogenic or tolerogenic antigen although tolerized T cells display a defect in cell division. *Immunology* 106, 144–158.

Smith, K. M., McAskill, F., and Garside, P. (2002b). Orally tolerized T cells are only able to enter B cell follicles following challenge with antigen in adjuvant, but they remain unable to provide B cell help. *J. Immunol.* 168, 4318–4325.

Sollid, L. M. (2002). Coeliac disease: Dissecting a complex inflammatory disorder. *Nat. Rev. Immunol.* 2, 647–655.

Sonoda, K. H., Exley, M., Snapper, S., Balk, S. P., and Stein-Streilein, J. (1999). CD1-reactive natural killer T cells are required for development of systemic tolerance through an immune privileged site. *J. Exp. Med.* 190, 1215–1226.

Soos, J. M., Stuve, O., Youssef, S., Bravo, M., Johnson, H. M., Weiner, H. L., and Zamvil, S. S. (2002). Cutting edge: oral type I IFN-tau promotes a Th2 bias and enhances suppression of autoimmune encephalomyelitis by oral glatiramer acetate. *J. Immunol.* 169, 2231–2235.

Spahn, T. W., Issazadah, S., Salvin, A. J., and Weiner, H. L. (1999). Decreased severity of myelin oligodendrocyte glycoprotein peptide 33-35-induced experimental autoimmune encephalomyelitis in mice with a disrupted TCR δ chain gene. *Eur. J. Immunol.* 29, 4060–4071.

Spahn, T. W., Fontana, A., Faria, A. M., Slavin, A. J., Eugster, H. P., Zhang, X., Koni, P. A., Ruddle, N. H., Flavell, R. A., Rennert, P. D., and Weiner, H. L. (2001). Induction of oral tolerance to cellular immune responses in the absence of Peyer's patches. *Eur. J. Immunol.* 31, 1278–1287.

Spahn, T. W., Weiner, H. L., Rennert, P. D., Lugering, N., Fontana, A., Domschke, W., and Kucharzik, T. (2002). Mesenteric lymph nodes are critical for the induction of high-dose oral tolerance in the absence of Peyer's patches. *Eur. J. Immunol.* 32, 1109–1113.

Staines, N. A., Harper, N., Ward, F. J., Malmström, V., Holmdahl, R., and Bansal, S. (1996). Mucosal tolerance and suppression of collagen-induced arthritis (CIA) induced by nasal inhalation of synthetic peptide 184-198 of bovine type II collagen (CII) expressing a dominant T cell epitope. *Clin. Exp. Immunol.* 103, 368–375.

Steinman, R. M., Hawiger, D., and Nussenzweig, M. C. (2003). Tolerogenic dendritic cells. *Annu. Rev. Immunol.* 21, 685–711.

Steptoe, R. J., and Thomson, A. W. (1996). Dendritic cells and tolerance induction. *Clin. Exp. Immunol.* 105, 397–402.

Stokes, C. R. (1984) Induction and control of intestinal immune responses. In *Local Immune Responses of the Gut* (eds. C. R. Stokes and T. J. Newby), 97–141. Boca Raton, FL: CRC Press.

Stokes, C. R., Newby, T. J., Huntley, J. H., Patel, D., and Bourne, F. J. (1979). The immune response of mice to bacterial antigens given by mouth. *Immunology* 38, 497–502.

Stokes, C. R., Newby, T. J., and Bourne, F. J. (1983a). The influence of oral immunization on local and systemic immune responses to heterologous antigens. *Clin. Exp. Immunol.* 52, 399–406.

Stokes, C. R., Swarbrick, E. T., and Soothill, J. F. (1983b). Genetic differences in immune exclusion and partial tolerance to ingested antigens. *Clin. Exp. Immunol.* 52, 678–684.

Stokes, C. R., Miller, B. G., and Bourne, F. J. (1987) Animal models of food sensitivity. In *Food Allergy and Intolerance* (eds. J. Brostoff and S. J. Challacombe), 286–300. Eastbourne, UK: W. B. Saunders.

Streilein, J. W. (1999). Immunologic privilege of the eye. *Springer Semin. Immunopathol.* 21, 95–111.

Strobel, S., and Ferguson, A. (1986). Modulation of intestinal and systemic immune responses to a fed protein. *Gut* 27, 829–837.

Strobel, S., and Ferguson, A. (1987). Persistence of oral tolerance in mice fed ovalbumin is different for humoral and cell mediated immune responses. *Immunology* 60, 317–318.

Strobel, S., and Mowat, A. McI. (1998). Immune responses to dietary antigens: Oral tolerance. *Immunol. Today* 19, 173–181.

Strobel, S., Mowat, A. McI., Drummond, H. E., Pickering, M. G., and Ferguson, A. (1983). Immunological responses to fed protein antigens in mice. 2. Oral tolerance for CMI is due to activation of cyclophosphamide sensitive cells by gut processed antigen. *Immunology* 49, 451–456.

Strobel, S., and Ferguson, A. (1984). Immune responses to fed protein antigens in mice. III. Systemic tolerance or priming is related to age at which antigen is first encountered. *Pediatr. Res.* 18, 588–594.

Strobel, C., Mowat, A. McI., and Ferguson, A. (1985). Prevention of oral tolerance induction to ovalbumin and enhanced antigen presentation during a graft-versus-host reaction in mice. *Immunology* 56, 57–64.

Strober, W., Fuss, I. J., and Blumberg, R. S. (2002). The immunology of mucosal models of inflammation. *Annu. Rev. Immunol.* 20, 495–549.

Strober, W., Kelsall, B., Fuss, I., Marth, T., Ludviksson, B., Ehrhardt, R., and Neurath, M. (1997). Reciprocal IFN-γ and TGF-β responses regulate the occurrence of mucosal inflammation. *Immunol. Today* 18, 61–64.

Stumbles, P. A., Thomas, J. A., Pimm, C. L., Lee, P. T., Venaille, T. J., Proksch, S., and Holt, P. G. (1998). Resting respiratory tract dendritic cells preferentially stimulate helper cell type 2 (Th2) responses and require obligatory cytokine signals for induction of Th1 immunity. *J. Exp. Med.* 188, 2019–2031.

Sudo, N., Sawamura, S., Tanaka, K., Aiba, Y., Kubo, C., and Koga, Y. (1997). The requirement of intestinal bacterial flora for the development of an IgE production system fully susceptible to oral tolerance induction. *J. Immunol.* 159, 1739–1745.

Sugihara, R., Matsumoto, Y., and Ohmori, H. (2002). Suppression of IgE antibody response in mice by a polysaccharide, AZ9, produced by *Klebsiella oxytoca* strain TNM3. *Immunopharmacol. Immunotoxicol.* 24, 245–254.

Suko, M., Mori, A., Ito, K., and Okudaira, H. (1995). Oral immunotherapy may induce T cell anergy. *Int. Arch. Allergy Immunol.* 107, 278–281.

Sun, J., and Van Houten, N. (2002). CD40 stimulation *in vivo* does not inhibit CD4+ T cell tolerance to soluble antigens. *Immunol. Lett.* 84, 125–132.

Sun, J., Dirden-Kramer, B., Ito, K., Ernst, P. B., and Van Houten, N. (1999). Antigen-specific T cell activation and proliferation during oral tolerance induction. *J. Immunol.* 162, 5865–5875.

Sun, J., Stalls, M. A., Thompson, K. L., and Fisher Van Houten, N. (2003). Cell cycle block in anergic T cells during tolerance induction. *Cell Immunol.* 225, 33–41.

Sun, J.-B., Holmgren, J., and Czerkinsky, C. (1994). Cholera toxin B subunit: An efficient transmucosal carrier-delivery system for induction of peripheral immunological tolerance. *Proc. Natl. Acad. Sci. USA* 91, 10795–10799.

Sun, J.-B., Rask, C., Olsson, T., Holmgren, J., and Czerkinsky, C. (1996). Treatment of experimental autoimmune encephalomyelitis by feeding myelin basic protein conjugated to cholera toxin B subunit. *Proc. Natl. Acad. Sci. USA* 93, 7196–7201.

Sun, J.-B., Xiao, B.-G., Lindblad, M., Li, H., Link, H., Czerkinsky, C., and Holmgren, J. (2000). Oral administration of cholera toxin B subunit conjugated to myelin basic protein protects against acute and chronic experimental autoimmune encephalomyelitis by inducing TGF-β secreting cells and suppressing chemokine expression. *Int. Immunol.*, in press.

Suzuki, I., Kitamura, K., Kiyono, H., Kurita, T., Green, D. R., and McGhee, J. R. (1986a). Isotype-specific immunoregulation: Evidence for a distinct subset of T contrasuppressor T cells for IgA responses in murine Peyer's patches. *J. Exp. Med.* 164, 501–516.

Suzuki, I., Kiyono, H., Kitamura, K., Green, D. R., and McGhee, J. R. (1986b). Abrogation of oral tolerance by contrasuppressor T cells suggests the presence of regulatory networks in the mucosal immune system. *Nature* 320, 451–454.

Swarbrick, E. T., Stokes, C. R., and Soothill, J. F. (1979). Absorption of antigens after oral immunization and the simultaneous induction of specific systemic tolerance. *Gut* 20, 121–125.

Taams, L. S., van Rensen, A. J. M. L., Poelen, M. C. M., van Els, C. A. C. M., Besseling, A. C., Wagenaar, J. P. A., van Eden, W., and Wauben, M. H. M. (1998). Anergic T cells actively suppress T cell responses via the antigen-presenting cell. *Eur. J. Immunol.* 28, 2902–2912.

Takahashi, T., Kuniyasu, Y., Toda, M., Sakaguchi, N., Itoh, M., Iwata, M., Shimizu, J., and Sakaguchi, S. (1998). Immunologic self-tolerance maintained by CD25+CD4+ naturally anergic and suppressive T cells: Induction of autoimmune disease by breaking their anergic/suppressive state. *Int. Immunol.* 10, 1969–1980.

Takeda, H., Spatz, M., Ruetzler, C., McCarron, R., Becker, K., and Hallenbeck, J. (2002). Induction of mucosal tolerance to E-selectin prevents ischemic and hemorrhagic stroke in spontaneously hypertensive genetically stroke-prone rats. *Stroke* 33, 2156–2163.

Takeuchi, M., Alard, P., and Streilein, J. W. (1998). TGF-β promotes immune deviation by altering accessory signals of antigen-presenting cells. *J. Immunol.* 160, 1589–1597.

Tanchot, C., Guillaume, S., Delon, J., Bourgeois, C., Franzke, A., Sarukhan, A., Trautmann, A., and Rocha, B. (1998). Modifications of CD8+ T cell function during *in vivo* memory or tolerance induction. *Immunity* 8, 581–590.

Teitelbaum, D., Arnon, R., and Sela, M. (1999). Immunomodulation of experimental autoimmune encephalomyelitis by oral administration of copolymer 1. *Proc. Natl. Acad. Sci. USA* 96, 3842–3847.

Terato, K., Xiu, J. Y., Miyahara, H., Cremer, M. A., and Griffiths, M. M. (1996). Induction of chronic autoimmune arthritis in DBA/1 mice by oral administration of type II collagen and *Escherichia coli* lipopolysaccharide. *Br. J. Rheumatol.* 35, 1–11.

Thery, C., Duban, L., Segura, E., Veron, P., Lantz, O., and Amigorena, S. (2002). Indirect activation of naive CD4+ T cells by dendritic cell-derived exosomes. *Nat. Immunol.* 3, 1156–1162.

Thomas, H. C., Ryan, C. J., Benjamin, I. S., Blumgart, L. H., and MacSween, R. N. M. (1976). The immune system response in cirrhotic rats: The induction of tolerance to orally administered protein antigens. *Gastroenterology* 71, 114–117.

Thompson, H. S., and Staines, N. A. (1990). Could specific oral tolerance be a therapy for autoimmune disease? *Immunol. Today* 11, 396–399.

Thompson, H. S. G., and Staines, N. A. (1986). Gastric administration of type II collagen delays the onset and severity of collagen-induced arthritis in rats. *Clin. Exp. Immunol.* 64, 581–586.

Thompson, H. S. G., Harper, N., Bevan, D. J., and Staines, N. A. (1993a). Suppression of collagen induced arthritis by oral administration of type II collagen: Changes in immune and arthritic responses mediated by active peripheral suppression. *Autoimmunity* 16, 189–199.

Thompson, S. J., Thompson, H. S. G., Harper, N., Day, M. J., Coad, A. J., Elson, C. J., and Staines, N. A. (1993b). Prevention of pristane-induced arthritis by the oral administration of type II collagen. *Immunology* 79, 152–157.

Thomson, A. W., O'Connell, P. J., Steptoe, R. J., and Lu, L. (2002). Immunobiology of liver dendritic cells. *Immunol. Cell Biol.* 80, 65–73.

Thornton, A. M., and Shevach, E. M. (1998). CD4+CD25+ immunoregulatory T cells suppress polyclonal T cell activation *in vitro* by inhibiting interleukin 2 production. *J. Exp. Med.* 188, 287–296.

Thornton, A. M., and Shevach, E. M. (2000). Suppressor effector function of CD4+CD25+ immunoregulatory T cells is antigen nonspecific. *J. Immunol.* 164, 183–190.

Thorstenson, K. M., and Khoruts, A. (2001). Generation of anergic and potentially immunoregulatory CD25+CD4+ T cells *in vivo* after induction of peripheral tolerance with intravenous or oral antigen. *J. Immunol.* 167, 188–195.

Thurau, S. R., Chan, C.-C., Nusenblatt, R. B., and Caspi, R. R. (1996). Oral tolerance in a murine model of relapsing experimental autoimmune uveoretinitis (EAU): Induction of protective tolerance in primed animals. *Clin. Exp. Immunol.* 109, 370–376.

Thurau, S. R., Diedrichs-Mohring, M., Fricke, H., Burchardi, C., and Wildner, G. (1999). Oral tolerance with an HLA-peptide mimicking retinal autoantigen as a treatment of autoimmune uveitis. *Immunol. Lett.* 68, 205–212.

Tian, J., Atkinson, M. A., Clare-Salzler, M., Herschenfeld, A., Forsthuber, T., Lehmann, P. V., and Kaufman, D. L. (1996). Nasal administration of glutamate decarboxylase (GAD65) peptides induces Th2 responses and prevents murine insulin-dependent diabetes. *J. Exp. Med.* 183, 1561–1567.

Tisch, R., Yang, X.-D., Singer, S. M., Liblau, R. S., Fugger, L., and McDevitt, H. O. (1993). Immune response to glutamic acid decarboxylase correlates with insulitis in non-obese diabetic mice. *Nature* 366, 72–75.

Titus, R. G., and Chiller, J. M. (1981). Orally-induced tolerance: Definition at the cellular level. *Int. Arch. Allergy Appl. Immunol.* 65, 323–338.

Tobagus, I. T., Thomas, W. R., and Holt, P. G. (2004). Adjuvant costimulation during secondary antigen challenge directs qualitative aspects of oral tolerance induction, particularly during the neonatal period. *J. Immunol.* 172, 2274–2285.

Tomasi, T. B., Barr, W. G., Challacombe, S. J., and Curran, G. (1983). Oral tolerance and accessory cell function of Peyer's patches. *Ann. N.Y. Acad. Sci.* 409, 145–163.

Trentham, D. E., Dynesius-Trentham, R. A., Orav, E. J., Combitchi, D., Lorenzo, C., Sewell, K. L., Hafler, D. A., and Weiner, H. L. (1993). Effects of oral administration of collagen on rheumatoid arthritis. *Science,* 261, 1727–1730.

Troncone, R., and Ferguson, A. (1988). In mice, gluten in maternal diet primes systemic immune responses to gliadin in offspring. *Immunology* 64, 533–537.

Trop, S., Samsonov, D., Gotsman, I., Alper, R., Diment, J., and Ilan, Y. (1999). Liver-associated lymphocytes expressing NK1.1 are essential for oral immune tolerance induction in a murine model. *Hepatology* 29, 746–755.

Tsuji, N. M., Mizumachi, K., and Kurisaki, J. (2001). Interleukin-10-secreting Peyer's patch cells are responsible for active suppression in low-dose oral tolerance. *Immunology* 103, 458–464.

Tsuji, N. M., Mizumachi, K., and Kurisaki, J., (2003). Antigen-specific, CD4(+)CD25(+) regulatory T cell clones induced in Peyer's patches. *Int. Immunol.* 15, 525–534.

Tsuji, N. M., and Nowak, B. (2004). IL-18 and antigen-specific CD4+ regulatory T cells in Peyer's patches. *Ann. N.Y. Acad. Sci.,* in press.

Turcanu, V., Maleki, S. J., and Lack, G. (2003). Characterization of lymphocyte responses to peanuts in normal children, peanut-allergic children, and allergic children who acquired tolerance to peanuts. *J. Clin. Invest.* 111, 1065–1072.

Unger, W. W. J., Hauet-Broere, F., Jansen, W., van Berkel, L. A., Kraal, G., and Samsom, J. N. (2003). Early events in peripheral regulatory T cell induction via the nasal mucosa. *J. Immunol.* 171, 4592–4603.

Untersmayr, E., Scholl, I., Swoboda, I., Beil, W. J., Forster-Waldl, E., Walter, F., Riemer, A., Kraml, G., Kinaciyan, T., Spitzauer, S., Boltz-Nitulescu, G., Scheiner, O., and Jensen-Jarolim, E. (2003). Antacid medication inhibits digestion of dietary proteins and causes food allergy: A fish allergy model in BALB/c mice. *J. Allergy Clin. Immunol.* 112, 616–623.

Van der Heijden, P. J., Bianchi, A. T. J., Dol, M., Pals, J. W., Stok, W., and Bokhout, B. A. (1991). Manipulation of intestinal immune responses against ovalbumin by cholera toxin and its B subunit in mice. *Immunology* 72, 89–93.

van Hage-Hamsten, M., Johansson, E., Roquet, A., Peterson, C., Andersson, M., Greiff, L., Vrtala, S., Valenta, R., and Gronneberg, R. (2002). Nasal challenges with recombinant derivatives of the major birch pollen allergen Bet v 1 induce fewer symptoms and lower mediator release than rBet v 1 wild-type in patients with allergic rhinitis. *Clin. Exp. Allergy* 32, 1448–1453.

Van Hoogstraten, I. M., Boos, C., Boden, D., Von Blumberg, M. E., Scheper, R. J., and Kraal, G. (1993). Oral induction of tolerance to nickel sensitization in mice. *J. Invest. Dermatol.* 101, 26–31.

Van Houten, N., and Blake, S. F. (1996). Direct measurement of anergy of antigen-specific T cells following oral tolerance induction. *J. Immunol.* 157, 1337–1341.

van Niel, G., Raposo, G., Candalh, C., Boussac, M., Hershberg, R., Cerf-Bensussan, N., and Heyman, M. (2001). Intestinal epithelial cells secrete exosome-like vesicles. *Gastroenterology* 121, 337–349.

Van Niel, G., Mallego, l. J., Bevilacqua, C., Candalh, C., Brugiere, S., Tomaskovic-Crook, E., Heath, J. K., Cerf-Bensussan, N., and Heyman, M. (2003). Intestinal epithelial exosomes carry MHC class II/peptides able to inform the immune system in mice. *Gut* 52, 1690–1697.

Vaz, N. M., Maia, L. C. S., Hanson, D. G., and Lynch, J. M. (1977). Inhibition of homocytotropic antibody responses in adult inbred mice by previous feeding of the specific antigen. *J. Allergy Clin. Immunol.* 60, 110–115.

Vendetti, S., Chai, J. G., Dyson, J., Simpson, E., Lombardi, G., and Lechler, R. (2000). Anergic T cells inhibit the antigen-presenting function of dendritic cells. *J. Immunol.* 165, 1175–1178.

Vezys, V., and Lefrancois, L. (2002). Cutting edge: inflammatory signals drive organ-specific autoimmunity to normally cross-tolerizing endogenous antigen. *J. Immunol.* 169, 6677–6680.

Vezys, V., Olson, S., and Lefrancois, L. (2000). Expression of intestine-specific antigen reveals novel pathways of CD8 T cell tolerance induction. *Immunity* 12, 505–514.

Viney, J. L., Mowat, A. McI., O'Malley, J. M., Williamson, E., and Fanger, N. (1998). Expanding dendritic cells *in vivo* enhances the induction of oral tolerance. *J. Immunol.* 160, 5815–5825.

Vistica, B. P., Chanaud, N. P., Felix, N., Caspi, R. R., Rizzo, I. V., Nussenblatt, R. B., and Gery, I. (1996). CD8 T-cells are not essential for the induction of "low dose" oral tolerance. *Clin. Immunol. Immunopathol.* 78, 196–202.

Vives, J., Parks, D. E., and Weigle, W. O. (1980). Immunologic unresponsiveness after gastric administration of human γ-globulin: antigen requirements and cellular parameters. *J. Immunol.* 125, 1811.

von Herrath, M. G., Dyrberg, T., and Oldstone, M. B. A. (1996). Oral insulin treatment suppresses virus-induced antigen-specific destruction of β cells and prevents autoimmune diabetes in transgenic mice. *J. Clin. Invest.* 98, 1324–1331.

Vrabec, T. R., Gregerson, D. S., Dua, H. S., and Donoso, L. A. (1992). Inhibition of experimental autoimmune uveoretinitis by oral administration of s-antigen and synthetic peptides. *Autoimmunity* 12, 175–184.

Wakkach, A., Fournier, N., Brun, V., Breittmayer, J. P., Cottrez, F., and Groux, H. (2003). Characterization of dendritic cells that induce tolerance and T regulatory 1 cell differentiation *in vivo*. *Immunity* 18, 605–617.

Waldo, F. B., Van Den Wall Bake, A. W. L., Mestecky, J., and Husby, S. (1994). Suppression of the immune response by nasal immunization. *Clin. Immunol. Immunopathol.* 72, 30–34.

Walker, W. A. (1987). Role of the mucosal barrier in antigen handling by the gut. In *Food Allergy and Intolerance* (eds. J. Brostoff and S. J. Challacombe), 209–222. Eastbourne, UK: W. B. Saunders.

Wang, Z. Y., Qiao, J., and Link, H. (1993a). Suppression of experimental autoimmune myasthenia gravis by oral administration of acetylcholine receptor. *J. Neuroimmunol.* 44, 209–214.

Wang, Z. Y., Qiao, J., Melms, A., and Link, H. (1993b). T cell reactivity to acetylcholine receptor in rats orally tolerized against experimental autoimmune myasthenia gravis. *Cell Immunol.* 152, 394–404.

Wang, Z. Y., Link, H., Ljungdahl, A., Hojeberg, B., Link, J., He, B., Qiao, J., Melms, A., and Olsson, T. (1994). Induction of interferon-γ, interleukin-4, and transforming growth factor-β in rats orally tolerized against autoimmune myaesthenia gravis. *Cell Immunol.* 157, 353–368.

Wang, Z. Y., He, B., Qiao, J., and Link, H. (1995). Suppression of experimental autoimmune myasthenia gravis and experimental allergic encephalomyelitis by oral administration of acetylcholine receptor and myelin basic protein: Double tolerance. *J. Neuroimmunol.* 63, 79–86.

Wannemuehler, M. J., Kiyono, H., Babb, J. L., Michalek, S. M., and McGhee, J. R. (1982). Lipopolysaccharide (LPS) regulation of the immune response: LPS converts germfree mice to sensitivity to oral tolerance induction. *J. Immunol.* 129, 959–965.

Watanabe, T., Yoshida, M., Shirai, Y., Yamori, M., Yagita, H., Itoh, T., Chiba, T., Kita, T., and Wakatsuki, Y. (2002). Administration of an antigen at a high dose generates regulatory CD4⁺ T cells expressing CD95 ligand and secreting IL-4 in the liver. *J. Immunol.* 168, 2188–2199.

Watanabe, T., Katsukura, H., Shirai, Y., Yamori, M., Nishi, T., Chiba, T., Kita, T., and Wakatsuki, Y. (2003). A liver tolerates a portal antigen by generating CD11c⁺ cells, which select Fas ligand+ Th2 cells via apoptosis. *Hepatology* 38, 403–412.

Weiner, H. L. (1997). Oral tolerance: immune mechanisms and treatment of autoimmune diseases. *Immunol. Today* 18, 335–343.

Weiner, H. L., and Komagata, Y. (1998). Oral tolerance and the treatment of rheumatoid arthritis. *Springer Semin. Immunopathol.* 20, 289–308.

Weiner, H. L., Mackin, G. A., Matsui, M., Orav, E. J., Khoury, S. J., Dawson, D. M., and Hafler, D. A. (1993). Double-blind pilot trial of tolerization with myelin antigens in multiple sclerosis. *Science,* 259, 1321–1324.

Weiner, H. L., Friedman, A., Miller, A., Khoury, S. J., Al-Sabbagh, A., Santos, L., Sayegh, M., Nussenblatt, R. B., Trentham, D. E., and Hafler, D. A. (1994). Oral tolerance: immunologic mechanisms and treatment of animal and human organ-specific autoimmune diseases by oral administration of autoantigens. *Ann. Rev. Immunol.* 12, 809–838.

Weiner, H. L., Lemere, C. A., Maron, R., Spooner, E. T., Grenfell, T. J., Mori, C., Issazadeh, S., Hancock, W. W., and Selkoe, D. J. (2000). Nasal administration of amyloid-β peptide decreases cerebral amyloid burden in a mouse model of Alzheimer's disease. *Ann. Neurol.* 48, 567–579.

Wells, H. G., and Osborne, T. B. (1911). The biological reactions of the vegetable proteins. I. Anaphylaxis. *J. Infect. Dis.* 8, 66–124.

Whitacre, C. C., Gienapp, I. E., Orosz, C. G., and Bitar, D. M. (1991). Oral tolerance in experimental autoimmune encephalitis. III. Evidence for clonal anergy. *J. Immunol.* 147, 2155–2163.

Whitacre, C. C., Gienapp, I. E., Meyer, A., Cox, K. L., and Javed, N. (1996). Oral tolerance in experimental autoimmune encephalomyelitis. *Ann. N. Y. Acad. Sci.* 778, 217–227.

Whitacre, C. C., Song, F., Wardrop, R., Campbell, K., McLain, M., Benson, J., and Gienapp, I. E. (2004). Regulation of autoreactive T cell function by oral tolerance to self antigens. *Ann. N. Y. Acad. Sci.,* in press.

Wildner, G., and Thurau, S. R. (1995). Orally induced bystander suppression in experimental autoimmune uveoretinitis occurs only in the periphery and not in the eye. *Eur. J. Immunol.* 25, 1292–1297.

Wildner, G., Hünig, T., and Thurau, S. R. (1996). Orally induced, peptide-specific γδ TcR+ cells suppress experimental autoimmune uveitis. *Eur. J. Immunol.* 26, 2140–2148.

Williamson, E., O'Malley, J. M., and Viney, J. L. (1999a). Defining the role of dendritic cells in oral tolerance induction by visualizing the T cell response elicited by oral administration of soluble protein antigen. *Immunology* 97, 565–572.

Williamson, E., Westrich, G. M., and Viney, J. L. (1999b). Modulating dendritic cells to optimize mucosal immunization protocols. *J. Immunol.* 163, 3668–3675.

Williamson, E., Bilsborough, J. M., and Viney, J. L. (2002). Regulation of mucosal dendritic cell function by receptor activator of NF-κ B (RANK)/RANK ligand interactions: Impact on tolerance induction. *J. Immunol.* 169, 3606–3612.

Wilson, A. D., Stokes, C. R., and Bourne, F. J. (1989). Adjuvant effect of cholera toxin on the mucosal immune response to soluble proteins: Differences between mouse strains and protein antigens. *Scand. J. Immunol.* 29, 739–745.

Wilson, A. D., Bailey, M., Williams, N. A., and Stokes, C. R. (1991). The *in vitro* production of cytokines by mucosal lymphocytes immunized by oral administration of keyhole limpet hemocyanin using cholera toxin as an adjuvant. *Eur. J. Immunol.* 21, 2333–2339.

Wolvers, D. A. W., van der Cammen, M. J. F., and Kraal, G. (1997). Mucosal tolerance is associated with, but independent of, upregulation of Th2 responses. *Immunology* 92, 328–333.

Wolvers, D. A. W., Coenen-De Roo, C. J. J., Mebius, R. E., Van Der Cammen, M. J. F., Tirion, F., Miltenburg, A. M. M., and Kraal, G. (1999). Intranasally induced immunological tolerance is determined by characteristics of the draining lymph nodes: Studies with OVA and human cartilage gp39. *J. Immunol.* 162, 1994–1998.

Wong, B. R., Josien, R., Lee, S. Y., Sauter, B., Li, H. L., Steinman, R. M., and Choi, Y. (1997). TRANCE (tumor necrosis factor [TNF]-related activation-induced cytokine), a new TNF family member predominantly expressed in T cells, is a dendritic cell-specific survival factor. *J. Exp. Med.* 186, 2075–2080.

Wrenshall, L. E., Ansite, J. D., Eckman, P. M., Heilman, M. J., Stevens, R. B., and Sutherland, D. E. (2001). Modulation of immune responses after portal venous injection of antigen. *Transplantation* 71, 841–850.

Wu, H. Y., Ward, F. J., and Staines, N. A. (2002). Histone peptide-induced nasal tolerance: Suppression of murine lupus. *J. Immunol.* 169, 1126–1134.

Wu, X.-M., Nakashima, M., and Watanabe, T. (1998). Selective suppression of antigen-specific Th2 cells by continuous micro-dose oral tolerance. *Eur. J. Immunol.* 28, 134–142.

Xiao, B. G., Zhang, G. X., Shi, F. D., Ma, C. G., and Link, H. (1998). Decrease of LFA-1 is associated with upregulation of TGF-β in CD4(+) T cell clones derived from rats nasally tolerized against experimental autoimmune myasthenia gravis. *Clin. Immunol. Immunopathol.* 89, 196–204.

Xu, D., Liu, H., Komai-Koma, M., Campbell, C., McSharry, C., Alexander, J., and Liew, F. Y. (2003). CD4⁺CD25⁺ regulatory T cells suppress differentiation and functions of Th1 and Th2 cells, *Leishmania major* infection, and colitis in mice. *J. Immunol.* 170, 394–399.

Yang, R., Liu, Q., Grosfeld, J. L., and Pescovitz, M. D. (1994). Intestinal drainage through liver is a pre-requisite for oral tolerance induction. *J. Paediatr. Surg,* 29, 1145–1148.

Yasufuku, K., Heidler, K. M., O'Donnell, P. W., Smith, G. N., Jr., Cummings, O. W., Foresman, B. H., Fujisawa, T., and Wilkes, D. S. (2001). Oral tolerance induction by type V collagen downregulates lung allograft rejection. *Am. J. Respir. Cell Mol. Biol.* 25, 26–34.

Yoshida, H., Hachimura, S., Hirahara, K., Hisatsune, T., Shiraishi, A., and Kaminogawa, S. (1998). Induction of oral tolerance in splenocyte-reconstituted SCID mice. *Clin. Immunol. Immunopathol,* 87, 282–291.

Yoshino, S. (1998). Treatment with anti-IL4 monoclonal antibody blocks suppression of collagen-induced arthritis in mice by oral administration of type II collagen. *J. Immunol.* 160, 3067–3071.

Yoshino, S., and Yoshino, J. (1998). Effect of a monoclonal antibody against interleukin-4 on suppression of antigen-induced arthritis in mice by oral administration of the inducing antigen. *Cell Immunol.* 187, 139–144.

Yoshino, S., Quattrocchi, E., and Weiner, H. L. (1995). Oral administration of type II collagen suppresses antigen-induced arthritis in Lewis rats. *Arth. Rheumat.* 38, 1092–1096.

Yoshitomi, T., Hirahara, K., Kawaguchi, J., Serizawa, N., Taniguchi, Y., Saito, S., Sakaguchi, M., Inouye, S., and Shiraishi, A. (2002). Three T-cell determinants of Cry j 1 and Cry j 2, the major

Japanese cedar pollen antigens, retain their immunogenicity and tolerogenicity in a linked peptide. *Immunology* 107, 517–522.

Zemann, B., Schwaerzler, C., Griot-Wenk, M., Nefzger, M., Mayer, P., Schneider, H., de Weck, A., Carballido, J. M., and Liehl, E. (2003). Oral administration of specific antigens to allergy-prone infant dogs induces IL-10 and TGF-β expression and prevents allergy in adult life.. *J Allergy Clin. Immunol.* 111, 1069–1075.

Zhang, J., Lee, C. S.Y., Lider, O., and Weiner, H. L. (1990). Suppression of adjuvant arthritis in Lewis rats by oral administration of type II collagen. *J. Immunol.* 145, 2489–2493.

Zhang, J., Davidson, L., Eisenbarth, G., and Weiner, H. L. (1991). Suppression of diabetes in NOD mice by oral administration of porcine insulin. *Proc. Natl. Acad. Sci. USA* 88, 10252–10256.

Zhang, J., Markovic, S., Raus, J., Lacet, B., Weiner, H. L., and Hafler, D. A. (1993). Increased frequency of IL-2 responsive T cells specific for myelin basic protein and proteolipid protein in peripheral blood and cerebrospinal fluid of patients with multiple sclerosis. *J. Exp. Med.* 179, 973–984.

Zhang, X., Izikson, L., Liu, L., and Weiner, H. L. (2001). Activation of CD25⁺CD4⁺ regulatory T cells by oral antigen administration. *J. Immunol.* 167, 4245–4253.

Zhang, Z., and Michael, J. G. (1990). Orally inducible immune unresponsiveness is abrogated by IFNγ treatment. *J. Immunol.* 144, 4163–4165.

Zhou, J., Carr, R. I., Liwski, R. S., Stadnyk, A. W., and Lee, T. D. G. (2001). Oral exposure to alloantigen generates intragraft CD8⁺ regulatory cells. *J. Immunol.* 167, 107–113.

Zimmer, K. P., Buning, J., Weber, P., Kaiserlian, D., and Strobel, S. (2000). Modulation of antigen trafficking to MHC class II-positive late endosomes of enterocytes. *Gastroenterology* 118, 128–137.

Zivny, J. H., Moldoveanu, Z., Vu, H. L., Russell, M.W., Mestecky, J., and Elson, C. O. (2001). Mechanisms of immune tolerance to food antigens in humans. *Clin. Immunol.*, 101, 158–168.

Zou, L. P., Ma, D. H., Levi, M., Wahren, B., Wei, L., Mix, E., van der Meide, P. H., Link, H., and Zhu, J. (1999). Antigen-specific immunosuppression: Nasal tolerance to P0 protein peptides for the prevention and treatment of experimental autoimmune neuritis in Lewis rats. *J. Neuroimmunol.* 94, 109–121.

Th1/Th2/Th3 Cells for Regulation of Mucosal Immunity, Tolerance, and Inflammation

Kohtaro Fujihashi

Departments of Oral Biology and Microbiology, and The Immunobiology Vaccine Center, University of Alabama at Birmingham, Birmingham, Alabama

Jerry R. McGhee

Department of Microbiology, University of Alabama at Birmingham, Birmingham, Alabama

The development of mucosal immunity, inflammation, or tolerance to protein-based vaccines, viral and bacterial pathogens, allergens, and autoantigens requires T cells, including CD4-positive (CD4+) T helper (Th) cells, including Th1-/Th2-cell subsets, CD8+ cytotoxic T lymphocytes (CTLs), and other T-cell subpopulations. In addition, these three types of mucosal immune responses are also regulated by other cell subsets, termed T regulatory (Treg) cells. Of course, B-cell commitment (μ → α switching) and B cell–CD4+ Th cell interactions that result in the induction of plasma cells producing polymeric IgA (pIgA) are of central importance in mucosal immunity. Cytokines produced by CD4+ and CD8+ T-cell subsets and by classical antigen (Ag)-presenting cells (APCs) (*e.g.*, dendritic cells, MØ, and B cells), as well as by nonclassical APCs (*e.g.*, epithelial cells) contribute to all aspects of normal mucosal immunity, tolerance, and inflammation in the immune response. In this chapter, we will focus only on CD4+ Th1/Th2/Th3 and Treg cells in mucosal immunoregulation. The roles of mucosal CD8+ CTLs are covered elsewhere in this book.

Regulatory T cells, which normally exhibit a CD4+ phenotype, can be classified as: (1) naive, or those that have not yet encountered antigen; (2) activated (effector); and (3) memory, in which both effector and memory T cells have engaged in the immune response. The mucosal migration patterns of these three subsets, along with the homing of B lymphocytes, form the cellular basis of the common mucosal immune system (CMIS). Naive CD4+ precursors of Th cells (pTh) normally recognize foreign peptide in association with MHC class II on APCs and express an αβ TCR+, CD3+, CD4+, CD8− phenotype. Thus, mucosal encounters with foreign Ag (peptides) will result in development of effector CD4+ T cells, which are either Th1 cells for cell-mediated immunity (CMI) or CD4+ Th2 cells for mucosal and peripheral antibody (Ab) responses. Thus, the mucosal inductive sites (*i.e.*, the mucosa-associated lymphoreticular tissues [or MALT]) should be considered as significant reservoirs of pTh cells such that encounter with bacterial or viral pathogens will result in the induction of effector CD4+ Th-cell subset responses.

MUCOSAL CD4+ T HELPER CELL SUBSETS

CD4+ Th1 and Th2 cells

The seminal observation in 1986 that CD4+ Th-cell clones could be divided into two distinct groups or subsets based upon the cytokines produced (Mosmann *et al.*, 1986) has led to an incredible interest in defining immune responses, tolerance, and inflammation based upon the presence of two major cell subsets, Th1 and Th2 (Mosmann *et al.*, 1986; Mosmann and Coffman, 1989). As CD4+ Th cells mature in response to foreign antigens, they assume unique characteristics such as production of distinct cytokine arrays. The pTh cells first produce IL-2 in response to stimuli and develop into T cells producing multiple cytokines (including both IFN-γ and IL-4), a stage first termed Th0 (Paliard *et al.*,

1988; Frestein *et al.*, 1989; Andersson *et al.*, 1990). The environment and cytokine milieu greatly influence the further differentiation of these Th0 cells **(Fig. 28.1)**. For example, stimulation by certain pathogens such as intracellular bacteria leads to the differentiation of CD4$^+$ Th1 cells producing IFN-γ, IL-2, and tumor necrosis factors (TNFs). These cells often develop following production of IL-12 by DCs or MØ (Hsieh *et al.*, 1993; Trinchieri, 1995) activated through the ingestion of intracellular pathogens (Fig. 28.1). There is compelling evidence that secreted IL-12 induces NK and other cells to produce IFN-γ (Kobayashi *et al.*, 1989; Chan *et al.*, 1991), which, together with IL-12, upregulates IL-12 receptor β (IL-12Rβ) expression on differentiating Th1-type cells (Fig. 28.1). Further, murine CD4$^+$ Th1-type responses are associated with development of CMI as manifested by delayed type hypersensitivity (DTH) as well as by B-cell Ab responses with characteristic IgG subclass patterns. For example, Th1 cell–derived IFN-γ induces $\mu \rightarrow 2\alpha$ switches (Snapper and Paul, 1987) and production of complement-fixing IgG2a Abs in mice.

On the other hand, exogenous Ag in mucosal environments can trigger CD4$^+$, NK1.1$^+$ T cells (Yoshimoto and Paul, 1994; Yoshimoto *et al.*, 1995; Arase *et al.*, 1993) as well

as other precursor cells that produce IL-4 for initiation of Th2-type responses (presumably from Th0 cells). CD4$^+$ Th2-type cells also produce IL-4 for expansion of this subset as well as IL-5, IL-6, IL-9, IL-10, and IL-13 (Seder, 1994; Mosmann and Coffman, 1989; Coffman *et al.*, 1991) (Fig. 28.1). This Th2-cell array may include production of IL-4 with other Th2-type cytokines; however, individual cytokines are regulated through different signal transduction pathways so that all Th1- or Th2-type cells do not produce the entire array of cytokines. The production of IL-4 by Th2 cells is supportive of B-cell switches from surface IgM (sIgM) expression to sIgG1 and to sIgE (Coffman *et al.*, 1988; Esser and Radbruch, 1990; Finkelman *et al.*, 1990). Further, the Th2-cell subset is considered the major helper phenotype for supporting the mucosal IgA Ab isotype in addition to plasma IgG1, IgG2b, and IgE Ab responses in the mouse system (McGhee and Kiyono, 1999).

Our focus here is on CD4+ Th- and Treg-cell subsets; however, it is clear that dendritic cell precursors and derived subsets clearly influence Th1- or Th2-cell development. These DC subsets influence Th-cell subsets in different ways. For example, DCs in Peyer's patches, an IgA inductive site, produce IL-10 and little IL-12, which allows predominant

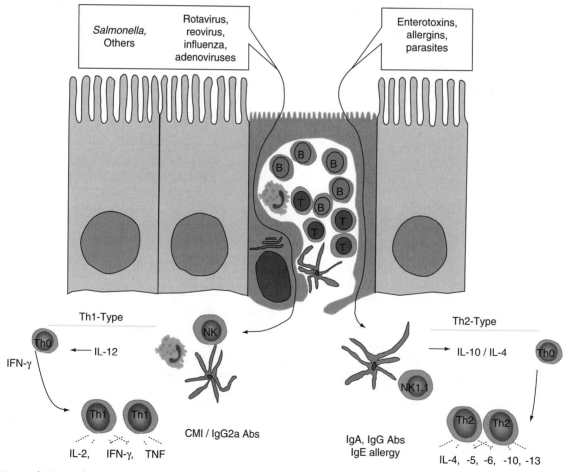

Fig. 28.1. Mucosal CD4$^+$ T helper cell subsets. The environmental and cytokine milieu greatly influences the differentiation of Th1 and Th2 cells. Interleukin-12 and IL-4 production is of central importance in the induction of mucosal CD4$^+$ Th1 and Th2 cells.

CD4+ Th2-type development (Iwasaki and Kelsall, 1999). Only myeloid DCs from GALT produced IL-10, whereas lymphoid DCs, such as DCs from spleen, produced IL-12 (Iwasaki and Kelsall, 2001) **(Fig. 28.2)**. In peripheral lymphoid sites, pDCs produce IL-1, which of course favors CD4+ Th1-type development (Iwasaki and Kelsall, 2001). In addition, human monocyte–derived DCs favor Th1s and are thus named DC1s, whereas plasmacytoid DCs favor Th2s and are often termed DC2 (Rissoan *et al.*, 1999). The DC1 versus DC2 influence was independent of either IL-4 or IL-12 (Rissoan *et al.*, 1999).

Before focusing on Th1 and Th2 subsets in the mucosal immune system, several other concepts should also be mentioned. Initially, it was speculated that humans may differ from mice in the absence of Th1- or Th2-type cells; however, it is now quite clear that humans indeed bear regulatory T-cell subsets (Romagnani, 1991). This became evident from studies of predominant Th1 or Th2 responses in human inflammatory and allergic diseases (Romagnani, 1991). Another misconception is that the presence of a predominant Th1- or Th2-cell response would influence other immune responses, especially in situations of inflammation. However, studies have now shown that Th1 responses to an Ag and Th2 responses to a second Ag may occur simultaneously (Ismali and Bretscher, 1999). This clearly emphasizes

the importance of the mucosal microenvironment of T-B cell interactions for clonal CD4+ Th1/Th2 B-cell responses.

Early evidence that two T-cell subsets regulate IgA

Clones of Ag-specific, Peyer's patch CD4+ Th cells were shown to support proliferation and differentiation of sIgA+ B cells into IgA-producing plasma cells (Kiyono *et al.*, 1982, 1984). These Th-cell clones were derived from Peyer's patches of mice fed sheep erythrocytes (SRBC), and SRBC-specific Th-cell clones were categorized based upon the Ab response induced. The first category supported IgM, IgG1, and high IgA anti-SRBC Ab responses, and although these studies preceded discovery of Th1 and Th2 subsets, in retrospect these clones would have properties of Th2-type cells. A second group of clones that supported only IgA anti-SRBC Ab responses (Xu *et al.*, 1993) may be considered as level 2 Th2-type cells producing IL-6 and IL-10 (Bottaro *et al.*, 1994). For example, CD4+ Th cells preferentially producing IgA-enhancing cytokines (*e.g.*, IL-6 and IL-10) were induced in a Th1-type environment following oral immunization with recombinant *S. typhimurium* (Bottaro *et al.*, 1994). Further, several studies have shown that both GALT and effector site CD4+ T cells produce IL-5, IL-6, and IFN-γ (Harriman *et al.*, 1996; Coffman *et al.*, 1989), and this cytokine array may also support induction of sIgA+ B cells to

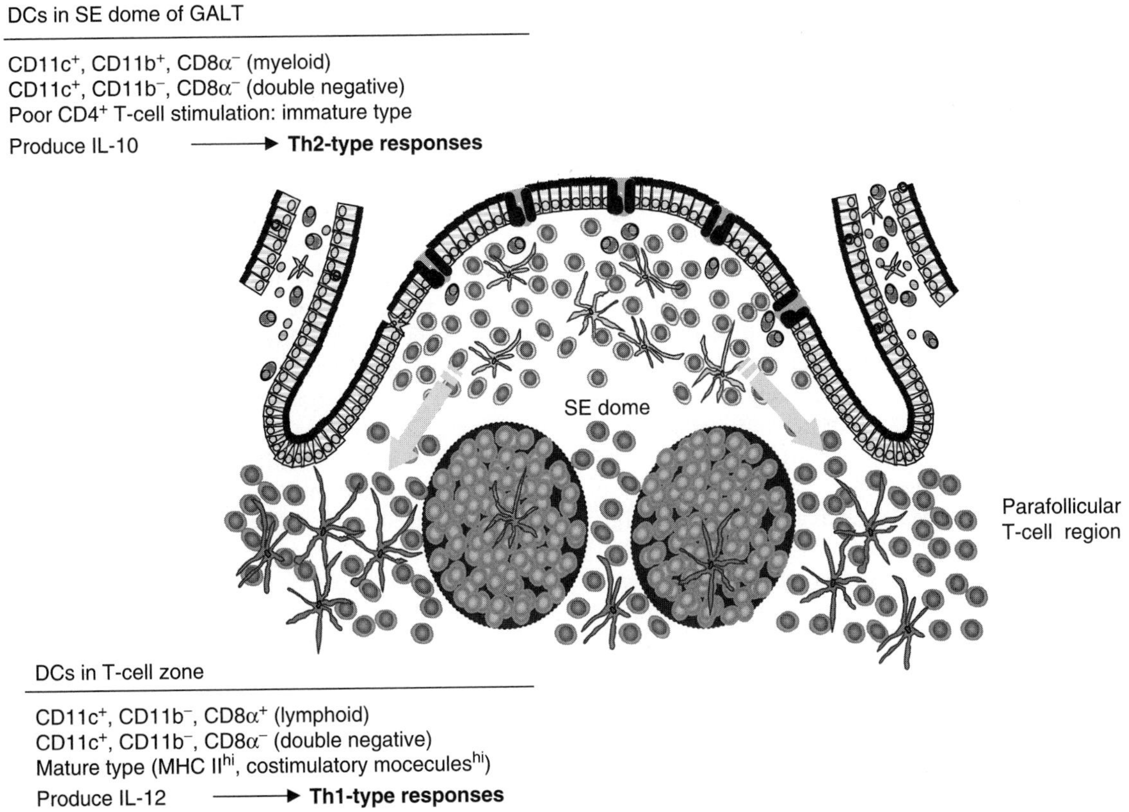

DCs in SE dome of GALT

CD11c+, CD11b+, CD8α− (myeloid)
CD11c+, CD11b−, CD8α− (double negative)
Poor CD4+ T-cell stimulation: immature type

Produce IL-10 ⟶ **Th2-type responses**

SE dome

Parafollicular T-cell region

DCs in T-cell zone

CD11c+, CD11b−, CD8α+ (lymphoid)
CD11c+, CD11b−, CD8α− (double negative)
Mature type (MHC II^hi, costimulatory mocecules^hi)

Produce IL-12 ⟶ **Th1-type responses**

Fig. 28.2. Mucosal Dendritic Cells (DCs) for Th1 and Th2 cell induction. **(See page 8 of the color plates.)** The subepithelial dome area of Peyer's patches contains myeloid type DCs, which favor induction of Th2 cells. On the other hand, parafollicular T-cell regions are enriched in lymphoid type DCs, which preferentially promote Th1-cell induction.

differentiate into IgA-secreting plasma cells. More recent studies have formally shown that most GALT CD4$^+$ Th clones induced in mice by oral immunization with SRBC indeed exhibit a Th2 phenotype (Lebman et al., 1990a).

Regulation of mucosal IgA by Th1- versus Th2-cell subsets

It is now established that CD4$^+$ Th cells are required for mucosal IgA responses to protein-based antigens (McGhee et al., 1989; Mega et al., 1991; Hörnqvist et al., 1991). Further, as discussed subsequently, both CD4$^+$ Th1 and Th2 cells can support mucosal IgA Ab responses; however, most agree that Th2-type cells are more efficient because they are for other Ig isotypes. As already discussed, Th1 and Th2 cells are sensitive to cross-regulation in which IFN-γ produced by Th1 cells inhibit proliferation of Th2 cells. This cytokine facilitates the isotype switch from IgM to IgG2a (Snapper and Paul, 1987; Revy et al., 2000) and inhibits isotype switching induced by IL-4 (Gajewski and Fitch, 1988). As indicated, Th2 cells regulate the effects of Th1 cells by secreting IL-4, which inhibits cytokine secretion by Th1 cells (Seder, 1994; Mosmann and Coffman, 1989; Coffman et al., 1991; Murphy et al., 2000) (e.g., IFN-γ production), in turn decreasing IFN-γ-mediated inhibition of Th2 cells. Despite this polarization, IL-4 can enhance ongoing Th1 responses, whereas IL-12 also acts as adjuvant for ongoing Th2-type responses (Oriss et al., 1999; Germann et al., 1995; Marinaro et al., 1999). Therefore, it is important to determine the Ag-specific cytokine secretion profile as well as the outcome of antigen-specific responses. This may include analysis of IgG subclasses, IgE, and IgA Ab responses to fully characterize immune responses induced by mucosal antigen delivery.

Cholera toxin as mucosal adjuvant normally induces Th2-type immunity

Earlier studies had shown that oral immunization with a combined vaccine containing protein Ags (e.g., tetanus toxoid, ovalbumin, or lysozyme) together with the mucosal adjuvant cholera toxin resulted in protein-specific CD4$^+$ T cells in GALT and spleen that preferentially produce IL-4 and IL-5, but not IFN-γ or IL-2 (Xu-Amano et al., 1993). This immunization protocol also induced serum IgG responses characterized by high IgG1 Ab titers with low or undetectable IgG2a Abs, as well as increased Ag-specific IgE Ab responses (Marinaro et al., 1995). Thus, oral immunization with soluble proteins and cholera toxin as adjuvant resulted in the induction of CD4$^+$ Th2-type responses. Others have also found that oral immunization of other mouse strains with two doses of lysozyme and cholera toxin separated by 3 weeks induces Ag-specific IgG (predominantly IgG1), IgA, and IgE Ab responses (Snider et al., 1994). Additionally, systemic challenge of orally immunized mice with lysozyme led to a fatal anaphylactic reaction because of the high levels of Ag-specific IgE (Snider et al., 1994). Oral immunization of C57BL/6 mice with keyhole limpet hemocyanin and cholera toxin and its B subunit (CT-B)

on three occasions at 10-day intervals resulted in both Peyer's patch and lamina propria T-lymphocyte populations that produced low levels of IL-2, IFN-γ, and higher levels of IL-4 and IL-5 (Wilson et al., 1991). These early results support the notion that oral immunization with a soluble protein antigen and cholera toxin as an adjuvant induces Th2-type immune responses. As discussed in a subsequent section, nasal immunization for NALT-based mucosal immunity has become the most common current mode of mucosal vaccination. Numerous studies with various protein vaccine Ags and cholera toxin as nasal adjuvant have also revealed that CD4$^+$ Th2-type responses are normally seen (Fig. 28.3).

The precise mechanism for mucosal adjuvanticity by cholera toxin is not known; however, this adjuvant clearly acts on APCs, including DCs. Cholera toxin was shown to inhibit IL-12 production by myeloid DCs as well as suppress IL-12 receptor β1 and β2 chain expression by T cells (Braun et al., 1999). In contrast, the labile toxin of E. coli as adjuvant upregulates IL-12R β1 and β2 expression on CD4$^+$ T cells and results in Th1-cell production of IFN-γ (Boyaka et al., 2003). It is also known that cholera toxin increases T-cell responses to unrelated Ags presumably through enhanced permeability of the mucosal epithelium (Hornquist and Lycke, 1995).

As indicated, the heat labile toxin of enterotoxigenic E. coli is also an effective immunogen and adjuvant for the induction and regulation of Ag-specific IgA responses (Walker and Clements, 1993; Takahashi et al., 1996). Oral immunization with labile toxin resulted in the induction of Ag-specific serum IgG as well as mucosal IgA Ab responses (Takahashi et al., 1996), and assessment of labile toxin B subunit (LT-B)-specific IgG subclass responses revealed high IgG2a with IgG1 and IgG2b anti-LT-B Abs, which contrasted with IgG subclass responses induced by cholera toxin (e.g., dominant IgG1 without IgG2a anti-CT-B Abs). Further, much lower IgE responses were seen following oral immunization with labile than with cholera toxin (Takahashi et al., 1996). With regard to the profile of isotype and subclass of Ag-specific responses induced by these two orally administered enterotoxins, both supported mucosal IgA responses, although labile and cholera toxin behaved differently for the induction of serum IgG subclass and IgE Ab responses. Large amounts of IFN-γ and IL-5 but little IL-4 were detected in LT-B-specific CD4$^+$ T cells from Peyer's patches and spleen of mucosally immunized mice. In marked contrast to cholera toxin, the labile toxin induced both Th1- and Th2-type responses. The production of IFN-γ by mucosally induced LT- specific Th1-type cells may lead to the induction of level 2 Th2-type cells where the IgA enhancing cytokine, IL-5, is produced without IL-4. In this regard, the labile toxin could be used as a mucosal adjuvant for induction of both Th1- and Th2-type responses following mucosal immunization, whereas cholera toxin could be considered as a selective Th2 inducer in the murine system. These findings suggest that one can manipulate the outcome of Th1- and/or Th2-type responses following mucosal immunization using cholera and labile enterotoxins.

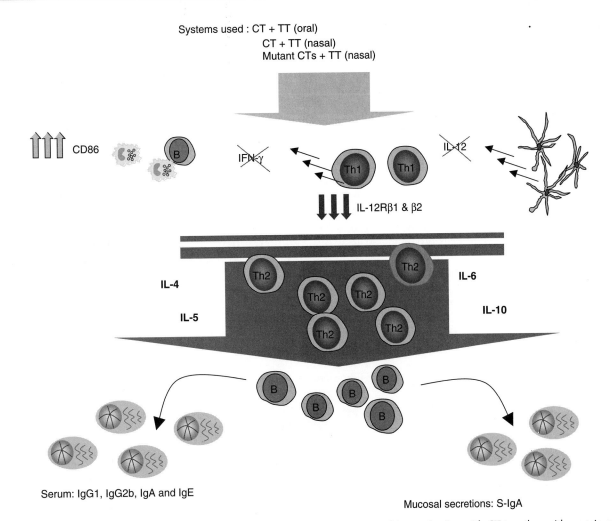

Fig. 28.3. Cholera toxin (CT) as mucosal adjuvant induces Th2-type immunity. Mucosal immunization with CT together with protein antigens such as tetanus toxoid or ovalbumin induces Th2 cell–mediated, Ag-specific Ab responses in both systemic and mucosal sites. IgM, IgG, IgA, and IgE isotype and IgG1 an d IgG2b subclass responses were induced in plasma. Secretory IgA Ab responses were high in mucosal secretions. Th2 cells preferentially produce IL-4, IL-5, IL-6, IL-10, and IL-13 for the induction Ag-specific immunity.

Attenuated bacteria/viruses usually induce a Th1 type of mucosal immunity

Attenuated avirulent *Salmonella* strains have received considerable attention as mucosal vaccine delivery vectors for recombinant proteins associated with virulence (Curtiss *et al.*, 1993; Roberts *et al.*, 1994; Chatfield *et al.*, 1993; Doggett and Brown, 1996). Following oral administration, *Salmonella* replicate directly in the mucosa-associated tissues (*e.g.*, the Peyer's patches) and thereafter disseminate *via* the GALT to systemic sites (*e.g.*, spleen). This characteristic dissemination pattern of growth in both mucosal and systemic sites allows *Salmonella* to induce broad-based immune responses, including CD4+ Th1 CMI as well as serum IgG2a and mucosal S-IgA Ab responses. Although a large number of genes from bacteria, viruses, parasites, and mammalian species have been expressed in attenuated *Salmonella* (Curtiss *et al.*, 1993; Roberts *et al.*, 1994), few studies have fully characterized both T- and B-cell responses to the expressed protein Ag. In particular, the balance between Ag-

specific CD4+ Th1 and Th2 cells and their subsequent influence on subclass-specific IgG and mucosal S-IgA responses has received less attention in these systems. Such clarity is paramount to the development of delivery protocols that will provide the appropriate immune response to a given pathogen.

A pioneering study in this area showed that mice given an oral attenuated *S. typhimurium* (expressing *Leishmania* surface protein gp63) elicited CD4+ T cells that produced IFN-γ and IL-2, but not IL-4 (Yang *et al.*, 1990). The results at first might appear puzzling. Because it had appeared that mucosal S-IgA Ab responses were completely dependent upon Th2 cells and cytokines such as IL-5, IL-6, and IL-10, by what mechanisms do these attenuated r*Salmonella* expressing foreign protein antigen induce S-IgA responses? Recent studies have addressed this issue by use of r*Salmonella* expressing the Tox C gene of tetanus toxin. Oral administration of r*Salmonella* Tox C resulted in predominant plasma IgG2a and IgG2b as well as mucosal S-IgA anti-tetanus toxoid (TT) Ab responses (VanCott et al., 1996) **(Fig. 28.4)**. Additionally, splenic and Peyer's patch CD4+ T cells selectively produced IFN-γ and IL-2 as well as the Th2-cytokine IL-10 (VanCott et al., 1996). Further, MØ from these mice produced heightened levels of IL-6 (VanCott et al., 1996) (Fig. 28.4). Clear verification that IL-4 was not involved was shown by oral immunization of IL-4 knockout (IL-4⁻/⁻) mice with rSalmonella Tox C, which produced serum IgG2a and mucosal S-IgA Abs. Interestingly, CD4+ T cells in these mice exhibited two cytokine patterns, a Th1 phenotype as well as T cells that produced IL-6 and IL-10, but not IL-5 (Okahashi et al., 1996) (Fig. 28.4). The latter subset of Th2 cells, which produce only IgA-enhancing cytokines, have been termed level 2 Th2-type cells in contrast to so-called level 1 Th2-type cells producing an array of IL-4, IL-5, IL-6, and IL-10.

A number of studies have shown that nasal delivery of attenuated bacterial or viral vectors also induces predominant mucosal CD4+ Th1-type responses. For example, a recent study showed that nasal delivery of rSalmonella expressing urease elicited Th1-type responses with IgG2a antiurease Abs (Londoño-Arcila et al., 2002). Interestingly, parenteral boosting with urease in alum adjuvant induced a balanced Th1/Th2 response profile, suggesting the potential to alter the type of mucosal immune response desired. Nasal administration of Shigella mutants to mice has been a useful model for study of pathogenesis (Mallett et al., 1993; VandeVerg et al., 1995). This has naturally led to development of attenuated Shigella expressing vaccine components (Mallett et al., 1993; Noriega et al., 1996), a response pattern also associated with Th1-type responses (Mallett et al., 1993; Noriega et al., 1996). In addition, a highly attenuated Shigella vector expressing measles virus DNA also elicited CD4+ Th1-type and CD8+ CTL responses (Sizemore et al., 1995; Fennelly et al., 1999).

Interestingly, infections in 2-month-old infants by *Bordetella pertussis*, the etiologic agent of whooping cough, also resulted in CD4+ Th1-type responses even though neonates are more prone toward Th2-type responses (Mascart et al., 2003). Nasal administration of inactivated respiratory syncytial virus (RSV) with cholera toxin resulted in nasal IgA and serum IgG anti-RSV Ab responses (Reuan

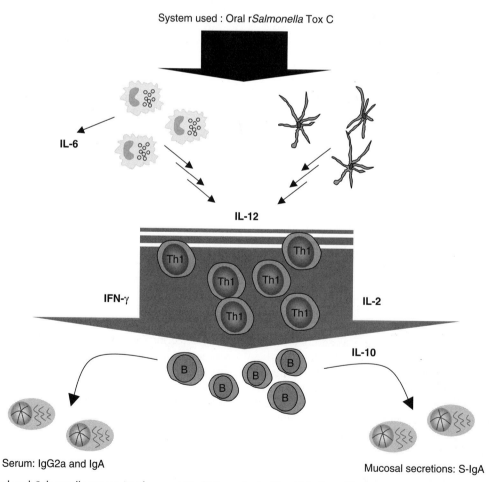

Fig. 28.4. Attenuated oral *Salmonella* expressing fragment C of tetanus toxin (Tox C) induces Th1-type mucosal immunity. Oral immunization of rSalmonella-Tox C induces Th1 cell–mediated Ag-specific immune responses in both mucosal and systemic lymphoid tissues. Marked increases of IFN-γ production by CD4+ Th1 cells is noted. Antigen-specific IgG2a and IgA Abs in plasma and S-IgA Abs in mucosal secretions were seen.

et al., 1991). Analysis of IgG subclasses suggested that both IgG1 and IgG2a were induced (Reuan *et al.*, 1991). Interestingly, infection with RSV and subsequent Th1-type responses are characterized by a favorable outcome, whereas Th2-type responses are associated with significant pathology (Graham *et al.*, 1991a, 1991b).

It has been proposed that adenovirus (Ad) vectors may be used for gene therapy with the development of replication-deficient mutants (Rosenfeld *et al.*, 1992; Zabner *et al.*, 1993; Jaffe *et al.*, 1992; Kay *et al.*, 1995). However, despite the obvious importance of the potential use of Ad vectors for gene therapy, for example, in cystic fibrosis, the nature of immune responses in the lungs and associated respiratory lymphoid tissues has not been studied in detail. CTL responses, which are largely induced to viral early proteins associated with replication (E1) and to DNA-binding protein E2a, thus play a role in developing immunity to Ad (Ada and Blanden, 1994; Riddell and Greenberg, 1995; Rawle *et al.*, 1991; Mullbacher *et al.*, 1989). In addition, the Ad vectors induced $CD4^+$ T-cell responses. Thus, studies have shown that Ad vector delivery to the respiratory tract induces $CD4^+$ T cells and neutralizing anti-Ad Abs (Kolls *et al.*, 1996; Yang *et al.*, 1995; van Ginkel *et al.*, 1995). The use of Ad vectors for development of mucosal vaccines has also received considerable attention. It has now been established that oral immunization with Ad4 and Ad7 limits respiratory diseases in military personnel (Takafuji *et al.*, 1979; Imler, 1995; Gaydos and Gaydos, 199). However, the nature of the responsive $CD4^+$ T cells, especially pulmonary-associated $CD4^+$ T cells, was not established. It has been shown that both $CD4^+$ and $CD8^+$ T cells migrate into the lung following sequential intratracheal Ad5 transgene instillations. In this regard, the IL-4-producing T cells were largely $CD4^+$, whereas IFN-γ expression was associated with both $CD4^+$ and $CD8^+$ T cells (van Ginkel *et al.*, 1997). Thus, Ad5-specific $CD4^+$ T cells produced both Th1 (IFN-γ and IL-2)- and Th2 (IL-4, IL-5 and IL-6)-type cytokines, whereas β gal-specific $CD4^+$ T cells secreted IFN-γ and IL-6 (van Ginkel *et al.*, 1997). This study provides direct evidence for the concomitant induction of Th2- with Th1-type responses in both the pulmonary systemic and mucosal immune compartments to the Ad5 vector as well as a Th1-dominant response to the transgene.

CpG DNA induces mucosal $CD4^+$ Th1-type responses

Another well-established mucosal adjuvant that clearly programs host $CD4^+$ Th1-type responses is CpG DNA. The finding that these immunostimulatory DNA sequences promote Th1-cell responses (Roman *et al.*, 1997) has led to its worldwide use as a mucosal adjuvant (Moldoveanu *et al.*, 1998; McCluskie and Davis, 1999, 1998; Horner *et al.*, 1998; McCluskie *et al.*, 2000). Thus, CpG ODN administered by the nasal route induces mucosal and peripheral immunity to influenza virus (Moldoveanu *et al.*, 1998), hepatitis B Ag (McCluskie and Davis, 1999, 1998), and the model Ag β-galactosidase (Horner *et al.*, 1998). It is also an effective mucosal adjuvant for both hepatitis B Ag and TT

given orally (McCluskie *et al.*, 2000). This CpG DNA adjuvant is so potent that it may even change a predominant Th2- into a Th1-type response (Weeratna *et al.*, 2001). The precise mechanisms for CpG DNA adjuvanticity are not yet known; however, CpG DNA upregulates MAP kinases associated with IL-12 production by APCs (Yi *et al.*, 2002). What is emerging from numerous studies is that mucosal inductive sites are especially enriched in naive, precursor Th cells with a potential to differentiate into either Th1- or Th2-type pathways. Unfortunately, only one study has addressed this at the single T-cell level and concluded that NALT (an inductive site) is enriched for Th0 (Thp) cells, whereas nasal passages (an effector site) are enriched in more differentiated Th1- or Th2-type cells (Hiroi *et al.*, 1998).

Despite the fact that bacterial and viral vectors and adjuvants like labile toxin and CpG DNA induce potent mucosal $CD4^+$ Th1-type responses, the mucosal inductive sites themselves are generally more prone to $CD4^+$ Th2-type responses. A full explanation for this is not yet complete; however, it appears that mucosal DCs provide clues to this paradox. In the rat model, it has been shown that respiratory tract DCs exhibit an immature phenotype and produce IL-10 (Stumbles *et al.*, 1998). When pulsed with Ag and adoptively transferred, these DCs supported strong Th2-type responses (Stumbles *et al.*, 1998). Similar findings have been put forth for mouse GALT. Thus, murine DCs from Peyer's patches but not spleen produce IL-10 and support $CD4^+$ Th2 responses, whereas splenic DCs produce IL-12 for $CD4^+$ Th1 responses (Iwasaki and Kelsall, 1999). Additional studies have now defined at least three subpopulations of DCs in murine Peyer's patches (Iwasaki and Kelsall, 2001; Iwasaki and Kelsall, 2000). Further, it now appears that myeloid DCs produce IL-10 and support Th2-type responses, whereas lymphoid DCs produce IL-12 for Th1-type responses (Iwasaki and Kelsall, 2001).

MUCOSAL Th3 CELLS AND OTHER REGULATORY T CELLS

Mucosal lymphoid tissues are enriched in $CD4^+$ Treg cells, which downregulate $CD4^+$ Th1- or Th2-type responses. As will be emphasized, they have been characterized by expression of surface molecules (*i.e.*, $CD25^+$), CTLA-4 binding, and by production of regulatory cytokines, especially IL-10 and TGF-β1. All of these T-cell subsets later described remain incompletely characterized in terms of Ag specificity, their pathway of development in the thymus, and their mode of regulation *in vivo*. The Treg cells appear to control mucosal immunity, tolerance, and inflammation to a much higher degree than comparable Treg cell types in peripheral lymphoid tissues. The areas where their existence and function are best described are in oral tolerance induction and in normal control of intestinal homeostasis and prevention of IBD development. One subset, Th3, which responds to and produces TGF-β1, may be the putative switch T cell for $\mu \rightarrow \alpha$ switching. Unfortunately, the T cells that may mediate these functions have somewhat different regulatory characteristics and have been given separate designations (Th3 cells, Tr1 cells, and Treg cells).

Th3 cells may be the T switch cell for IgA

The presence of CD3+, CD4+ T cells producing TGF-β1 were actually first described in studies of oral tolerance. For example, CD4+ T-cell clones were generated after the induction of oral tolerance to myelin basic protein (MBP) and led to the characterization of a new phenotype of Treg cell. Clones of CD4+ T cells were MBP specific, and of 48 clones assessed, 42 produced the active form of TGF-β1 (Chen et al., 1994). Six clones produced high levels of TGF-β1 with essentially no IL-4 or IL-10 (Takafuji et al., 1979). On the other hand, five clones produced high IL-4 and IL-10; that is, of course, typical of Th2-type cells. The authors suggested the existence of a TGF-β1-producing, regulatory T cell involved in control of mucosal immune responses and named it Th3 (Chen et al., 1994). There is only circumstantial evidence that Th3 cells are indeed involved in regulation of the mucosal IgA response. Unfortunately, it has become dogma that Th3 cells producing TGF-β1 actually direct μ → α switches in the germinal centers of mucosal inductive sites. There is no direct evidence for this and thus this area represents an important frontier for research. What is known regarding T-cell and cytokine regulation of IgA class switching is presented in the following section.

T cells for μ → α switching

Clear evidence was presented that clones of T cells from murine GALT, when mixed with noncommitted sIgM+ B cells, induced isotype switching to B cells expressing membrane or surface IgA (sIgA) (Kawanishi et al., 1983a, b). The initial studies with murine T switch (Tsw) cells used T-cell clones derived by mitogen stimulation and IL-2-supported outgrowth, and when Tsw cells were added to sIgM+, sIgA− B cell cultures resulted in marked increases in sIgA+ cells (Kawanishi et al., 1983a). GALT Tsw cells did not induce IgA synthesis, even when incubated with sIgA+ B cell–enriched cultures; however, addition of B-cell growth and differentiation factors readily induced IgA secretion (Kawanishi et al., 1983b). Additional experiments showed that Tsw cells were autoreactive and suggested that continued uptake of gut lumenal antigens in GALT resulted in a unique microenvironment for T–B cell interactions and subsequent IgA responses (Kawanishi et al., 1985). This result suggests that cognate interactions between Tsw and B cells were required for induction of the IgA class switch. It remains to be formally proven that Tsw cells respond to and produce TGF-β1 and thus are indeed Th3 cells.

Other studies have revealed that T–B cell interactions support B-cell switches and have postulated a major role for the CD40 receptor on germinal center B cells with CD40L on activated T cells (Fuleihan et al., 1993; Banchereau et al., 1994; MacLennan, 1994). In the presence of antigen, the B cells may alter the affinity and functions of the antibody receptor through somatic mutation of variable region genes,

with cytokines such as IL-4 (for IgG1 and IgE) and TGF-β1 (for IgA) directing heavy chain (isotype) switching. Further, the environment of the B cell may play a role in switching (Weinstein and Cebra, 1991). Germane to this discussion are studies with an effective APC, the DC, which resides in the dome region as well as T-cell zones of the Peyer's patches, and influences switching to IgA. For example, coculture of activated T cells and DC from GALT with purified sIgM+, sIgA− B cells resulted in the synthesis of large amounts of IgA, whereas DC-T cells isolated from spleen were less effective (Spalding and Griffin, 1986). Additional studies showed that a DC–T cell mixture from GALT also induced isotype switching to IgA in a pre-B cell line, whereas DC–T cell mixtures from spleen were without effect. Although these studies purported to show that the DC was the major cell type promoting B-cell switches to IgA, it remains possible that the GALT DC–T cell mixtures harbored contaminating B cells producing IgA, and thus more definitive proof that the DC is directly involved in B-cell switches to IgA is required. This is another fertile area for investigation.

Evidence for Tsw cells in human IgA responses has stemmed from an earlier study with malignant T cells from a patient RAC (T_{RAC} cells) who suffered from a mycosis fungoides/Sézary-like syndrome. The T_{RAC} cells induced tonsillar sIgM+ B cells to switch and secrete IgG and IgA (Mayer et al., 1986). Furthermore, T_{RAC} cells, when added to B-cell cultures obtained from patients with hyper-IgM immunodeficiency, induced eight of nine cultures to secrete IgG and three of nine to produce IgA (Benson and Strober, 1988). T-cell clones have also been obtained from human appendix, and these clones and their derived culture supernatants exhibited preferential help for IgA synthesis (Benson and Strober, 1988). Direct evidence was also provided that CD3+, CD4+, CD8- T-cell clones induced μ → α B-cell switches as well as terminal differentiation of sIgA+ B cells into IgA-producing plasma cells (Benson and Strober, 1988).

TGF-β1 is the major IgA switch cytokine

Definitive studies now suggest that TGF-β1 is the major cytokine for B-cell switching to IgA (Coffman et al., 1989; Lebman et al., 1990a, 1990b; Islam et al., 1991; Nilsson et al., 1991; Stavnezer, 1995; Sonoda et al., 1989). The first studies showed that addition of TGF-β1 to LPS-triggered mouse splenic B-cell cultures resulted in switching to IgA, and IgA synthesis was markedly enhanced by IL-2 (Coffman et al., 1991) or IL-5 (Sonoda et al., 1989). The effect of TGF-β1 was on sIgM+, sIgA− B cells and was not due to selective induction of terminal B-cell differentiation. It was shown that TGF-β1 induced sterile Cα germline transcripts (Coffman et al., 1989; Lebman et al., 1990b), an event that clearly precedes actual switching to IgA. Interestingly, deficient Iα mice apparently lose their requirement for TGF-β1-induced switching, presumably because the Cα locus is constitutively activated and LPS alone is sufficient for induction of μ → α B-cell switches (Harriman et al., 1996). Later work showed that TGF-β1 also induced human B cells to switch to either IgA1 or IgA2, an event preceded by formation of Cα1 and Cα2 germline transcripts (Islam *et al.*, 1991; Nilsson *et al.*, 1991). It can be presumed that TGF-β1 induces μ → α switches in normal physiologic circumstances, because sIgM⁺, sIgD⁺ B cells triggered through CD40 were induced to switch to IgA by TGF-β and to secrete IgA in the presence of IL-10 (DeFrance *et al.*, 1992; Rousset *et al.*, 1991).

It should be emphasized that almost all studies to date with TGF-β1-induced switches have been done in B-cell cultures stimulated with mitogens or *via* coreceptor signaling (Coffman *et al.*, 1989; Lebman *et al.*, 1990a, 1990b; Islam *et al.*, 1991; Nilsson *et al.*, 1991; Stavnezer, 1995). These studies reveal that only 2% to 5% of B cells actually switch to IgA, making it difficult to explain the high rate of switching that normally occurs in GALT germinal centers (>60%). This point was specifically addressed in a system in which B cells were triggered with anti-CD40 and antidextran Abs, both of which mimic T-dependent and T-independent stimuli, respectively. It was shown that TGF-β1 together with IL-4 and IL-5 induced sIgA⁺ B-cell populations of up to 15% to 20% (McIntyre *et al.*, 1995). Although one would predict that deletion of the TGF-β1 gene would lead to a negative influence on the IgA immune system, the TGF-β1 gene knockout mice unfortunately die from a generalized lymphoproliferative disease 3 to 5 weeks after birth, making it difficult to use this model to investigate the role of TGF-β1 in IgA regulation *in vivo*. Nevertheless, TGF-β1⁻/⁻ mice exhibit low levels of IgA plasma cells in effector sites and of S-IgA in external secretions (van Ginkel *et al.*, 1999), providing evidence that TGF-β1 is also important for μ → α switching *in vivo*. In a recent study, conditional mutagenesis (Cre/LoxP) was used to knock out the TGF-β receptor in B cells (Cazac and Roes, 2000). These mice exhibited expanded peritoneal B-1 cells and B-cell hyperplasia in Peyer's patches and a complete absence of serum IgA (Cazac and Roes, 2000).

Th1/Th2/Th3 CELLS REGULATE MUCOSAL TOLERANCE

Oral administration of a single high dose or repeated oral delivery of low doses of proteins has been shown to induce systemic unresponsiveness, presumably in the presence of mucosal IgA Ab responses (Weiner *et al.*, 1994; Czerkinsky *et al.*, 1999; Mayer, 2000; Fujihashi *et al.*, 2001). These immunologically distinct responses in mucosa-associated versus systemic-associated lymphoid tissues were originally termed oral tolerance (Tomasi, 1980). More recent studies have shown that the nasal administration of proteins also induces systemic unresponsiveness (McMenamin and Holt, 1993; Hoyne *et al.*, 1993; Tian *et al.*, 1996; Higuchi *et al.*, 2000) and has led to the more general term mucosal tolerance to include nasal or oral Ag induction of unresponsiveness (Fig. 28.4) (see Chapter 27). The development of mucosal tolerance is an important natural physiologic mechanism whereby the host presumably avoids hypersensitivity

reactions to many ingested food proteins and other antigens (Garside *et al.*, 1999). Thus, mucosal tolerance (or mucosal/systemic unresponsiveness) represents the most common response of the host to our environment. The continuous ingestion of several thousand different food proteins is but one important example, whereas tolerance to our indigenous microflora, which colonizes the large intestine, represents another major example. It is also useful to consider that induction of mucosal and systemic immunity by oral immunization is rather difficult and requires use of potent mucosal adjuvants, vectors, or other special delivery systems (see previous discussion) **(Fig. 28.5)**. Further, the development of mucosal tolerance against pollen and dust antigens could also be essential for the inhibition of allergic reactions, including IgE-mediated hypersensitivity.

Most now agree that mucosal tolerance is mediated by T cells, which are involved in the generation of active suppression or clonal anergy and/or deletion (Friedman and Weiner, 1994). For example, high doses of antigen given by the oral route induced clonal deletion or anergy (Whitacre *et al.*, 1991; Chen *et al.*, 1995a, 1995b; Melamed and Friedman, 1993; Chen *et al.*, 1995b) characterized by the absence of T-cell proliferation and diminished IL-2 production as well as IL-2R expression. Frequent low oral Ag doses result in CD4⁺ T cells that respond to and secrete TGF-β1 that appear to downregulate host responses (Kawanishi *et al.*, 1983). Although not yet clear just how this occurs, these Th3 cells regulate both TGF-β1-induced unresponsiveness (Kawanishi *et al.*,1983) as well as potentially supporting μ → α B-cell switches for mucosal immunity. It is also known that cholera toxin and perhaps other adjuvants can prevent induction of mucosal tolerance, which normally occurs when the protein Ag is given alone. Further, one cannot normally overcome an existing Th1 or Th2 immune response by mucosal tolerance, even by oral delivery of enormous amounts of antigen (Leishman *et al.*, 2000). An interesting corollary to this was the finding that a Th2-biased environment in the gastrointestinal (GI) tract to a parasite resulted in failure to induce a Th2-type of oral tolerance to OVA (Leishman *et al.*, 2000). However, unresponsiveness at the level of OVA-specific, Th1 responses was fully intact (Shi *et al.*, 1998).

T-cell anergy

Anergy is defined as a state of T-cell unresponsiveness characterized by the lack of proliferation and of IL-2 synthesis, with diminished IL-2R expression (Schwartz, 1990), a condition reversed by preculturing T cells with IL-2 (DeSilva *et al.*, 1991). Oral tolerance to a large dose of OVA Ag induced anergy in OVA-specific T cells (Weiner *et al.*, 1994) **(Fig. 28.6)**. Further, oral myelin basic protein (MBP) diminished IL-2 and IFN-γ synthesis (Whitacre *et al.*, 1991). These findings suggest that Th1-type T cells may be susceptible to the induction of anergy after oral feeding. To support this, it has been shown that Th1-type cells appear to be more sensitive to the induction of tolerance *in vitro* than Th2-type cells (Williams *et al.*, 1990). *In vivo* evidence has demonstrated

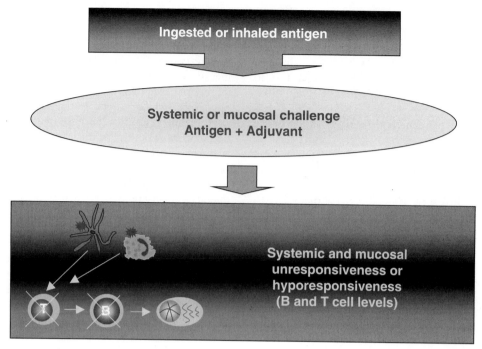

Fig. 28.5. The concept of mucosal tolerance. Prolonged mucosally administered antigens induce both systemic and mucosal unresponsiveness to the same Ag when challenged in the presence of adjuvant.

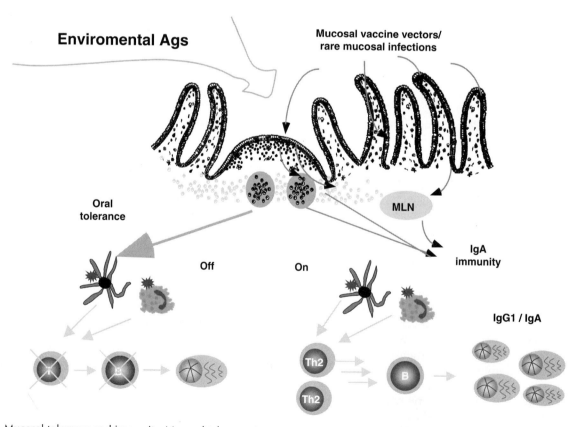

Fig. 28.6. Mucosal tolerance and immunity. Mucosal tolerance is a common immune response required to maintain homeostasis in the host. On the other hand, induction of Ag-specific mucosal immunity is a special case because this type of response is rarely seen, and mucosal adjuvants and special delivery systems are required for its induction.

that Th1 cells are likely to be anergized in oral tolerance (Burstein and Abbas, 1993). This may be an oversimplification because it has been shown that oral tolerance can be induced in mice defective in Th1 (STAT4$^{-/-}$) or Th2 (STAT6$^{-/-}$) cells (Shi et al., 1999). Further, to identify which lymphocyte compartment (e.g., CD4$^+$ versus CD8$^+$ T cells) preferentially mediates the induction of oral tolerance, cell transfer experiments were also performed using SCID and nu/nu mice (Hirahara et al., 1995). Adoptive transfer of splenic lymphocytes from mice orally tolerized with bovine α-casein resulted in the induction of tolerance in these immunocompromised mice. It was shown that oral tolerance was induced by anergized CD4$^+$ but not CD8$^+$ T cells.

An imbalanced Th1/Th2 cytokine network

The induction of oral tolerance can also be explained by dysregulation of homeostasis between Th1- and Th2-type cells. For example, preferential activation of Th2 cells may lead to downregulation of Th1–CMI responses by Th2 cytokines such as IL-4 and IL-10 (Burstein and Abbas, 1993). In addition, Th1-type cells appear to be more sensitive to anergy induction following oral administration of protein antigens. For example, conjugation of a *Leishmania* antigen LACK with CT-B was quite efficient at inducing nasal tolerance in mice (McSorley et al., 1998). Further, this resulted in diminished CD4$^+$ Th1 cells and IFN-γ, whereas Th2 cytokines were normal (McSorley et al., 1998). These findings suggest that oral tolerance is associated with selective downregulation of Th1 cells by Th2 cells *via* their respective cytokines in the systemic immune compartment. This possibility is consistent with the fact that oral tolerance has more profound effects on Th1-regulated CMI responses than on Th2-mediated Ab responses. However, studies have shown that feeding a single high dose of OVA inhibited production of both Th1 (IL-2 and IFN-γ) and Th2 (IL-4, IL-5, and IL-10-type) cytokines and resulted in the reduction of IFN-? γ- and IL-4-dependent antigen-specific IgG2a and IgG1 antibody responses, respectively (Garside et al., 1995). These findings indicate that both subsets of Th cells can be downregulated by oral OVA. In a separate study, oral OVA induced brisk IFN-γ production with inhibition of the IgG-enhancing cytokine IL-4 by Th2 cells, leading to reduced B-cell responses, whereas no oral tolerance was seen in IFN-γ knockout mice (Kweon et al., 1998). These two studies are not conflicting, because it appears that initial production of IFN-γ, perhaps by Th1 cells, precedes oral tolerance development and, in the absence of IFN-γ, this does not occur. Further, repeated oral administration of high doses of OVA to OVA-specific TCR Tg mice resulted in IFN-γ-dominated Th1-type responses in the Peyer's patches (Marth et al., 1996). Taken together, the immunologic consequences of systemic B-cell tolerance induced by a high dose of oral Ag may be due to IFN-γ-mediated immune regulation, with significant suppression of Th2-type cells. The CD4$^+$ CD25$^+$ Treg-cell subset can inhibit the development of EAE in MBP-Tg mice (Olivares-Villagomez et al., 1998) in a manner analogous to prevention of EAE by oral tolerance to MBP, and it is likely that Treg cells mediate some forms of oral tolerance. Thus, one possibility is that Th1 cell–derived IFN-γ downregulates Th2 responses and the Th1 cells may then become anergic. Other possibilities are that both Th1 and Th2 cells become anergic and subsets may switch to Treg cells producing IL-10 and/or TGF-β1.

The regulation by Th1, Th2, and other cells may differ depending upon whether mucosal tolerance is induced by either oral or nasal routes. For example, oral OVA induced tolerance as manifested by lower IgG1 and IgE anti-OVA Abs, whereas nasal OVA only inhibited IgE anti-OVA Abs (van Halteren et al., 1997). Both oral and nasal tolerance blocked mast cell function and anti-IFN-γ mAb treatment blocked tolerance suggesting that Th1-derived IFN-γ blocks Th2 responses differentially for IgE when compared with IgG1 Ab responses (van Halteren et al., 1997).

Treg cells in mucosal tolerance

Several groups have recently focused on naturally occurring "T suppressor" cells using various models of organ-specific autoimmune or infectious diseases. In general, the suppressive activity is found in a rather large subset of CD3, αβTCR$^+$ CD4$^+$, CD25$^+$ T cells (Roncarolo and Levings, 2000). It is quite likely that Treg cells control mucosal immunity, tolerance, and inflammation to a higher degree than comparable Treg cells in peripheral lymphoid tissues. Generally speaking, Treg cells do not proliferate well *in vitro*, a characteristic reminiscent of anergic T cells. In fact, cloned anergic T cells can suppress the immune response *in vivo* and this appears to be in part due to effects on APCs (Chai et al., 1999; Taams et al., 1998; Vendetti et al., 2000). Thus, anergic T cells downregulate DC expression of CD80 and CD86 in a contact-specific fashion (Vendetti et al., 2000). Further, anergic T cells have been shown to produce IL-10, which is a major characteristic of some CD4$^+$ CD25$^+$ Treg cells (Sundstedt et al., 1997; Buer et al., 1998; Shevach, 2000; Sakaguchi, 2000) **(Fig. 28.7)**. Thus, it appears that anergic T cells, through production of IL-10 (and perhaps through other mechanisms), develop into Treg cells that suppress immune responses to other antigens (Buer et al., 1998), a process sometimes termed "infectious tolerance" or "bystander suppression." This may not be a universal pathway, however, because it was recently shown in an adoptive transfer model that CTLA-4 but not IL-10 expression was necessary for CD4$^+$ T-cell tolerance (Fowler and Powrie, 2002) (Fig. 28.7). Despite their poor proliferative responses to Ag, it has been possible to induce populations of T-cell clones after incubation with IL-10 and alloantigen in humans (Groux et al., 1996) or to OVA peptide in DO11.10 mice (Groux et al., 1997). The T-cell clones obtained had similar properties, including secretion of high levels of IL-10, some production TGF-β1, with no IL-4 synthesis and poor proliferative responses (Maloy and Powrie, 2001) (Fig. 28.7). The precise locale for induction of anergic T cells is not known; however, the liver itself may contribute to this. For example, protein Ags given orally in high doses perfuse the liver. Further, oral delivery of a large OVA dose to OVA-Tg mice resulted in high numbers of apoptotic, OVA-specific

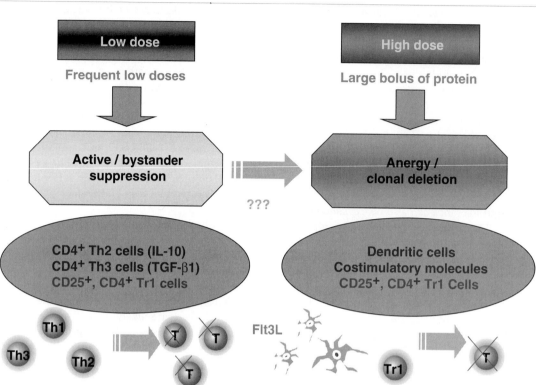

Fig. 28.7. Current proposed mechanisms of mucosal tolerance induction. For low dose tolerance induction, regulatory types of CD4⁺ T cells including TGF-β1 producing Th3 and CD25 positive Tr1 cells play central roles for active/bystander suppression. Meanwhile, anergy/clonal deletion of Ag-specific CD4⁺ T cells were induced by dendritic cell–mediated responses. CD4⁺, CD25⁺ Treg cells were also involved in these immune responses.

CD4⁺ T cells in the liver (Watanabe *et al.*, 2002). This led to the presence of CD4⁺ T cells secreting TGF-β1, IL-4, and IL-10, which could suppress T-cell proliferative responses (Watanabe *et al.*, 2003). Cells with these characteristics are now termed Tr1 cells. The CD4⁺ CD25⁺ Treg-cell subset can inhibit the development of EAE in MBP-Tg mice (Olivares-Villagomez *et al.*, 1998) in a manner analogous to prevention of EAE by oral tolerance to MBP, and it is likely that Treg cells mediate some forms of oral tolerance. Thus far, Tr1 and Th3 cells have in common the production of TGF-β1 (Th3) or TGF-β1 plus IL-10 (Tr1) with suppressive-type properties.

Th1/Th2 AND Treg CELLS IN MUCOSAL INFLAMMATION

Th1 and/or Th2 cell–mediated colitis

Human inflammatory bowel diseases (IBDs) are characterized by episodes of abdominal pain, diarrhea, bloody stools, weight loss, and intestinal inflammation. It is generally agreed that human IBDs are multifactorial with immunologic, environmental, and genetic contributions making systematic studies difficult. The IBDs represent chronic,

relapsing, and tissue-destructive diseases. Although the etiologies of these IBDs remain unknown, there is supportive evidence to link them to the mucosal immune system's failure to attenuate immunity to luminal antigens (Braegger and MacDonald, 1994; Brandtzaeg *et al.*, 1997). A recent study has shown a primary role for T cells in IBD by demonstrating that anti-CD4 mAbs were effective in treating the disease (Emmrich *et al.*, 1991). Chronic enteric inflammation is experimentally induced in mice by manipulating T cells and/or cytokines by gene targeting. Various experimental murine models of IBD also support a central role for T cells in chronic intestinal inflammation (Morrissey *et al.*, 1993; Mizoguchi *et al.*, 1996a, 1996b; Mombaerts *et al.*, 1993; Takahashi *et al.*, 1997). These models are generally characterized by an imbalance in regulatory cytokines, most notably by excessive production of IFN-γ. Chronic intestinal inflammation has been shown to develop in IL-2 knockout mice that exhibited abnormal B-cell responses, including colon autoAbs (Sadlack *et al.*, 1993). IL-10 knockout mice develop severe focal inflammation in both the small and large intestine, and these mice exhibit an elevated production of the Th1 cytokine IFN-γ (Kuhn *et al.*, 1993). Another well-characterized model involves adoptive transfer of CD45RB^Hi (naive) T cells into SCID mouse recipients, which subsequently develop a colitis characterized by expansion of CD4⁺ T cells producing IFN-γ (Powrie *et al.*, 1994). It is interesting that TGF- β1 is corrective in the CD45RB^Hi transfer system as well as in the TNBS (2, 4, 6-trinitrobenzene sulfonic acid) colitis model (Powrie *et al.*, 1996; Neurath *et al.*, 1996), suggesting that TGF-β1 downregulates mucosal inflammation, perhaps through the induction of tolerance. Yet another model involves the adoptive transfer of T cell–depleted bone marrow in normal mice into TCR-defective CD3ε transgenic mice (Höllander *et al.*, 1995). Additional studies have now shown that both CD4⁺ αβ⁺ and γδ⁺ T cells producing IFN-γ and TNF-α characterize the colonic lesion of CD3ε transgenic mice (Simpson *et al.*, 1997). Thus, compelling evidence is at hand to suggest that dysregulated T-cell responses are associated with murine IBD, and that exaggerated Th1-type cells producing IFN-γ are the major effector population that has been incriminated thus far. These effector T cells respond to autoantigens and intestinal flora, to which they are normally tolerant (Duchmann *et al.*, 1996). In this regard, abrogation of tolerance may be an important aspect in Th1-type dysregulation in the various IBD models **(Fig. 28.8)**.

Mice have been treated with chemical haptens or modified immunologically to induce colonic inflammation. In these models, some mouse strains exhibit greater susceptibility, suggesting significant genetic control in the development of IBD. One of these models is based on local exposure of colonic mucosa to the contact-sensitizing agent 2, 4, 6-trinitrobenzene sulfonic acid (TNBS), first established in rats (Morris *et al.*, 1989) and more recently in mice (Neurath *et al.*, 1995; Elson *et al.*, 1996). The colonic administration of a single dose of TNBS in 50% ethanol induces chronic distal colitis in rats that could persist for 2 months or more (Morris *et al.*, 1989), and a similar, single dose also induces colitis in mice (Neurath *et al.*, 1995; Elson *et al.*, 1996). Contact-sensitizing agents such as TNBS are covalently reactive compounds that attach to autologous proteins and stimulate a DTH response to hapten (TNP)-modified self-Ags, a reaction that is regulated by complex interactions among various functional subsets of CD4⁺ T cells (Miller and Butler, 1983; Greene *et al.*, 1982). This model was used to contrast the potential roles for Th1-inducing cytokines in stimulating development of IBD or in ameliorating the disease. It was first shown that T cells from mice with TNBS-induced colitis produced both IL-2 and IFN-γ (Th1 type), and *in situ* analysis of IBD lesions revealed

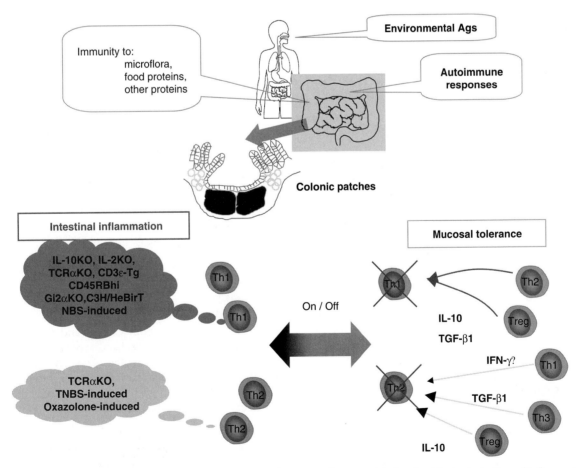

Fig. 28.8. Both Th1 and Th2 cells mediate intestinal inflammation. Th1-type cells are mainly involved in the induction of inflammatory bowel diseases (IBDs). In some cases, Th2 cells are also responsible for the induction of colitis. The regulatory T (Treg) cells, which produce IL-10 and/or TGF-β1, control the induction of these IBDs.

increased IFN-γ production (Neurath et al., 1995). Treatment of mice with anti-IL-12 mAb markedly decreased the severity of TNBS-induced colitis (Neurath et al., 1995).

Thus, most mouse IBD models are associated with activated T cells producing cytokines characteristic of a Th1 phenotype, a finding in agreement with the clinical observations in Crohn's disease (Niessner et al., 1995; Breese et al., 1993; Autschbach et al., 1995). However, because the production of Th1-type cytokines is not as pronounced in ulcerative colitis as it is in Crohn's disease (Fuss et al., 1996; Monteleone et al., 1997), it is still possible that a Th2-type response is also operative in the ulcerative colitis-type of chronic intestinal inflammation. In support of this, recent studies have suggested that exaggerated Th2-type responses also result in murine IBD. For example, studies in other models such as T-cell receptor (TCR) α gene knockout mice suggested a significant role for IL-4 in the spontaneous development of intestinal inflammation (Mizoguchi et al., 1996b; Mombaerts et al., 1993; Takahashi et al., 1997). These TCRα-chain knockout mice develop a chronic colitis accompanied by enhanced production of IFN-γ and IL-4 by gut-associated T cells (Mizoguchi et al., 1996b; Mombaerts et al., 1993). Further, it has been shown that the development of IL-4 producing α⁻ β⁺ T cells is associated with formation of chronic colitis in TCRα knockout mice (Takahashi et al., 1997). Hapten-induced colitis with colonic administration of oxazolone was also induced by an IL-4-mediated pathway (Boirivant et al., 1998). Thus, chronic intestinal inflammation may occur in immunologically altered conditions in which either Th1- or Th2-type responses are dominant. Moreover, it was demonstrated that hapten-induced, typical Th1-type colitis model with TNBS was characterized as both Th1- and Th2-type cytokine-mediated colitis (Dohi et al., 1999, 2000) (Fig. 28.8).

In comparison to various specific gene-deleted murine IBD models, one advantage of the TNBS-induced system is the use of normal mice with an intact immune system whereby one can investigate the exact role of individual immune competent cells for the development of mucosal inflammation. Further, it should be emphasized that immunologic and immunopathologic investigations can be performed in a TNBS-specific manner. In this regard, the development of TNBS-induced inflammation in cytokine-deficient mice was examined to determine the possible development of Th2-type, cytokine-associated colitis. These studies clearly showed that TNBS colitis could be induced in the absence of IFN-γ in BALB/c mice (Dohi et al., 1999). This result allows determination of pathophysiologic differences between Th1 and Th2 cell–mediated colonic inflammation.

To further define the role of Th2-type cells and derived cytokines, TNBS colitis in IL-12 gene-disrupted (IL-12⁻/⁻) mice were examined to eliminate the possibility of a Th1-driven immune response, and this was directly compared with IL-4-deficient (IL-4⁻/⁻) mice in which Th2-type responses are absent. Because BALB/c mice are known to favor Th2-type immune responses, the C57BL/6 mouse strain was chosen for this study to ensure that Th2-type

responses associated with IBD were not inherent to the mouse strain itself. These studies demonstrated that both IL-12⁻/⁻ and IFN-γ⁻/⁻ C57BL/6 mice develop significant TNBS colitis, whereas IL-4⁻/⁻ mice of the same C57BL/6 background showed a different pattern of disease (Dohi et al., 2000). The comparative study of normal, IL-12⁻/⁻, IFN-γ⁻/⁻, and IL-4⁻/⁻ mice is the first to illustrate the differential roles for Th1-type and Th2-type cytokines in the pathogenesis of intestinal inflammation. These results clearly showed that Th2-type cytokine responses were also involved in Ag-specific colitis. The most recent study also showed that OVA-specific colitis models are clearly associated with either Th1 or Th2 pathway (Iqbal et al., 2002) (Fig. 28.8).

Treg (CD4⁺, CD25⁺) cells in mucosal inflammation

It has been shown that adoptive transfer of CD4⁺ CD45RB^Hi T cells into SCID mice resulted in wasting disease and colitis (Morrissey et al., 1993; Powrie et al., 1994). On the other hand, CD4⁺, CD45RB^Low T-cell transfer not only failed to induce colitis but also prevented development of wasting disease when cotransferred (Morrissey et al., 1993; Powrie et al., 1993). This evidence indicates that Treg cells control inflammatory responses in the large intestine (Fig. 28.8). CD4⁺, CD25⁺ Treg cells were initially identified as a CD4⁺ T-cell subset that prevented the development of organ-specific autoimmune disease (Asano et al., 1996; Sakaguchi et al., 1995). In this regard, follow-up studies showed that CD4⁺, CD45RB^Low CD25⁺ T cells were mainly responsible for prevention CD4⁺, CD45RB^Hi T cell–induced colitis; however, a subset CD25⁻ population also possessed Treg-cell function (Read et al., 2000; Annacker et al., 2001). Several studies have now shown that IL-10 and TGF-β1 produced by Treg cells are both involved in the prevention of colitis development (Groux et al., 1997; Kuhn et al., 1993; Powrie et al., 1996; Hagenbaugh et al., 1997; Asseman et al., 1999). Further, it was recently shown that the small intestine–specific IL-10 transgenic mice resulted in increased levels of IL-10 and TGF-β1 production as well as elevated numbers of CD4⁺, CD25⁺ Treg cells in the small intestine (De Winter et al., 2002). Thus, these mice were resistant to induction of dextran sodium sulfate (DSS)–induced colitis (De Winter et al., 2002). In addition, prevention of TNBS-induced colitis by oral tolerance development was totally abolished by either anti-IL-10, or anti-TGF-β1, Ab treatment (Fuss et al., 2002). On the other hand, it was reported that IL-10, but not TGF-β1, produced by both CD25⁺ and CD25⁻ subsets in CD4⁺, CD45RB^Low Treg cells downregulated Helicobacter hepaticus–induced colitis (Kullbert et al., 2002). These results indicate that the regulatory mechanisms provided by Treg cells for the prevention of colitis induction may differ in each of the experimental colitis models.

SUMMARY AND FUTURE NEEDS

Studies over the last 2 decades have clearly shown that CD4⁺ T cells and their derived cytokines play essential roles in the maintenance of mucosal immune responses. In this regard, Th1- and Th2-type cytokine-producing CD4$^+$ T helper cells are involved in the induction of both CMI and Ab immune responses. Futher, bacterial and viral infections have been controlled by Th1-type cytokines such as IFN-γ producing mucosal CD4$^+$ T cells in addition to CD8$^+$ CTLs. On the other hand, IL-4, IL-5, IL-6, IL-10, and IL-13 played a central role in the induction of Ag-specific mucosal IgA Ab responses. Despite the induction of mucosal immunity, it is essential to have mechanisms that control and subsequently terminate these responses to avoid hyperimmune responses or inflammation. Mucosal tolerance is one of the major immune regulatory mechanisms for the maintenance host homeostasis. Thus, both Th1- and Th2-type CD4$^+$ T cells are involved in the induction and regulation of oral tolerance. In addition, IL-10 and/or TGF-β1 from Th3 or Treg CD4$^+$ T cells are essential cytokines to induce oral tolerance. Along this same line, it was recently shown that Th3 and Treg CD4$^+$ T cells downregulated mucosal inflammation, autoimmune, and hyperimmune responses for the maintenance of homeostasis. It is thus logical to have both up (Th1 and Th2) and down (Th3 and Treg) CD4$^+$ T cells for the induction and regulation of effective immune responses. To further explore the precise roles of these up- and downregulatory CD4$^+$ T cells, one should directly investigate Ag-specific CD4$^+$ T-cell responses by using state-of-the-art approaches. In this regard, postgenome projects including proteomics research may be key in clarifying existing and unsolved problems. Indeed, most recent reports showed that Foxp3 gene is of central importance in the development of CD4$^+$, CD25$^+$ Treg cells (O'Garra and Vieira, 2003; Fontenot *et al.*, 2003; Khattri *et al.*, 2003).

REFERENCES

Ada, G. L. and Blanden, R. V. (1994). CTL immunity and cytokine regulation in viral infection. *Res. Immunol.* 145, 625–628.

Andersson, U., Anderson, J., Lindfors, A., Wagner, K., Moller, G., and Heusser, C. H. (1990). Simultaneous production of interleukin 2, interleukin 4, and inferferon-γ by activated human blood lymphocytes. *Eur. J. Immunol.* 20, 591–596.

Annacker, O, Pimenta-Araujo, R., Burlen-Defranoux, O., Barbosa, T. C., Cumano, A., and Bandeira, A. (2001). CD25 CD4 T cells regulate the expansion of peripheral CD4 T cells through the production of IL-10. *J. Immunol.* 166, 3008–3018.

Arase, H., Arase, N., Nakagawa, K., Good, R. A., and Onoe, K. (1993). NK1.1$^+$ CD4$^+$ CD8- thymocytes with specific lymphokine secretion. *Eur. J. Immunol.* 23, 307–310.

Asano, M., Toda, M., Sakaguchi, N., and Sakaguchi, S. (1996). Autoimmune disease as consequence of developmental abnormality of a T cell subpopulation. *J. Exp. Med.* 184, 387–396.

Asseman, C., Mauze, S., Leach, M. W., Coffman, R. L., and Powrie, F. (1999). An essential role for interleukin 10 in the function of regulatory T cells that inhibit intestinal inflammation. *J. Exp. Med.* 190, 995–1004.

Autschbach, F., Schurmann, G., Qiao, L., Merz, H., Wallich, R., and Meuer, S. C. (1995). Cytokine messenger RNA expression and proliferation status of intestinal mononuclear cells in noninflamed gut and Crohn's disease. *Virchows Arch.* 426, 51–60.

Bancereau, J., Bazan, F., Blanchard, D., Biere, F., Galizzi, J. P., van Kooten, C., Liu, Y. J., Rousset, F., and Saeland, S. (1994). The CD40 antigen and its ligand. *Annu. Rev. Immunol.* 12, 881–922.

Benson, E. B. and Strober, W. (1988). Regulation of IgA secretion by T cell clones derived from the human gastrointestinal tract. *J. Immunol.* 140, 1874–1882.

Boirivant, M., Fuss, I. J., Chu, A., and Strober, W. (1998). Oxazolone colitis: A murine model of T helper cell type 2 colitis treatable with antibodies to interleukin 4. *J. Exp. Med.* 188, 1929–1939.

Bottaro, A., Lansford, R., Xu, L., Zhang, J., Rothman, P., and Alt, F. W. (1994). S region transcription per se promotes basal IgE class switch recombination but additional factors regulate the efficiency of the process. *EMBO J.* 13, 665–674.

Boyaka, P. N., Ohmura, M., Fujihashi, K., Koga, T., Yamamoto, M., Kweon, M.-N., Takeda, Y., Jackson, R. J., Kiyono, H., Yuki, Y., and McGhee, J. R. (2003). Chimeras of labile toxin one and cholera toxin retain mucosal adjuvanticity and direct Th cell subsets via their B subunit. *J. Immunol.* 170, 454–462.

Braegger, C. P. and MacDonald, T. T. (1994). Immune mechanisms in chronic inflammatory bowel disease. *Ann. Allergy* 72, 135–141.

Brandtzaeg, P., Haraldsen, G., and Rugtveit, J. (1997). Immunopathology of human inflammatory bowel disease. *Springer Semin. Immunopathol.* 18, 555–589.

Braun, M. C., He, J., Wu, C.-Y., and Kelsall, B. L. (1999). Cholera toxin suppresses interleukin (IL)-12 production and IL-12 receptor β1 and β2 chain expression. *J. Exp. Med.* 189, 541–552.

Breese, E., Braegger, C. P., Corrigan, C. J., Walker-Smith, J. A., and MacDonald, T. T. (1993). Interleukin-2 and interferon-γ-secreting T cells in normal and diseased human intestinal mucosa. *Immunology* 78, 127–131.

Buer, J., Lanoue, A., Franzke, A., Garcia, C., von Boehmer, H., and Sarukhan, A. (1998). Interleukin 10 secretion and impaired effector function of major histocompatibility complex class II-restricted T cells anergized *in vivo*. *J. Exp. Med.* 187, 177–183.

Burstein, H. J. and Abbas, A. K. (1993). *In vivo* role of interleukin 4 in T cell tolerance induced by aqueous protein antigen. *J. Exp. Med.* 177, 457–463.

Cazac, B. B. and Roes, J. (2000). TGF-β receptor controls B cell responsiveness and induction of IgA *in vivo*. *Immunity* 13, 443–451.

Chai, J. G., Bartok, I., Chandler, P., Vendetti, S., Antoniou, A., Dyson, J., and Lechler, R. (1999). Anergic T cells act as suppressor cells *in vitro* and *in vivo*. *Eur. J. Immunol.* 29, 686–692.

Chan, S. H., Perussia, B., Gupta. J. W., Kobayashi, M., Pospisil, M., Young, H. A., Wolf, S. F., Young, D., Clark, S. C., and Trinchieri, G. (1991). Induction of interferon gamma production by natural killer cell stimulatory factor: Characterization of the responder cells and synergy with other inducers. *J. Exp. Med.* 173, 869–879.

Chatfield, S., Roberts, M., Londono, P., Cropley, I., Douce, G., and Dougan, G. (1993). The development of oral vaccines based on live attenuated *Salmonella* strains. *FEMS Immunol. Med. Microbiol.* 7, 1–7.

Chen, Y., Inobe, J., Marks, R., Gonnella, P., Kuchroo, V. K., and Weiner, H. L. (1995a). Peripheral deletion of antigen- reactive T cells in oral tolerance. *Nature* 376, 177–180.

Chen, Y., Inobe, J., and Weiner, H. L. (1995b). Induction of oral tolerance to myelin basic protein in CD8-depleted mice: Both CD4$^+$ and CD8$^+$ cells mediate active suppression. *J. Immunol.* 155, 910–916.

Chen, Y., Kuchroo, V. K., Inobe, J., Hafler, D. A., and Weiner, H. L. (1994). Regulatory T cell clones induced by oral tolerance: Suppression of autoimmune encephalomyelitis. *Science* 265, 1237–1240.

Coffman, R. L., Lebman, D. A., and Schrader, B. (1989). Transforming growth factor β specifically enhances IgA production by lipopolysaccharide-stimulated murine B lymphocytes. *J. Exp. Med.* 170, 1039–1044.

Coffman, R. L., Seymour, B. W., Lebman, D. A., Hiraki, D. D., Christiansen, J. A., Shrader, B., Cherwinksi, H. M., Savelkoul, H. F., Finkelman, F. D., and Bond, M. W. (1988). The role of helper T cell products in mouse B cell differentiation and isotype regulation. *Immunol. Rev.* 102, 5–28.

Coffman, R. L., Varkila, K., Scott, P., and Chatelain, R. (1991). Role of cytokines in the differentiation of CD4$^+$ T-cell subsets *in vivo*. *Immunol. Rev.* 123, 189–207.

Curtiss, R. III, Kelley, S. M., and Hassan, J. O. (1993). Live oral avirulent *Salmonella* vaccines. *Vet. Microbiol.* 37, 397–405.

Czerkinsky, C., Anjuere, F., McGhee, J. R., George-Chandy, A., Holmgren, J., Kieny, M.-P., Fujihashi, K., Mestecky, J. F., Pierrefite-Carle, V., Rak, C., and Sun, J.-B. (1999). Mucosal immunity and tolerance: relevance to vaccine development. *Immunol. Rev.* 170, 197–222.

DeFrance, T., Vanbervliet, B., Briere, F., Durand, I., Rousset, F., and Banchereau, J. (1992). Interleukin 10 and transforming growth factor beta cooperate to induce anti-CD40-activated naive human B cells to secrete immunoglobulin A. *J. Exp. Med.* 175, 671–682.

DeSilva, D. R., Urdahl, K. B., and Jenkins, M. K. (1991). Clonal anergy is induced *in vitro* by T cell receptor occupancy in the absence of proliferation. *J. Immunol.* 147, 3261–3267.

De Winter, H., Elewaut, D., Turovskaya, O., Huflejt, M., Shimeld, C., Hagenbaugh, A., Binder, S., Takahashi, I., Kronenberg, M., and Cheroutre, H. (2002). Regulation of mucosal immune responses by recombinant interleukin 10 produced by intestinal epithelial cells in mice. *Gastroenterology* 122, 1829–1841.

Doggett, T. A. and Brown, P. K. (1996). Attenuated *Salmonella* as vectors for oral immunization. In *Mucosal Vaccines* (ed. H. Kiyono), 105–108. San Diego, CA: Academic Press.

Dohi, T., Fujihashi, K., Kiyono, H., Elson, C. O., and McGhee, J. R. (2000). Mice deficient in Th1- and Th2-type cytokines develop distinct forms of hapten-induced colitis. *Gastroenterology* 119, 724–733.

Dohi, T., Fujihashi, K., Rennert, P. D., Iwatani, K., Kiyono, H., and McGhee, J. R. (1999). Hapten-induced colitis is associated with colonic patch hypertrophy and T helper cell 2-type responses. *J. Exp. Med.* 189, 1169–1180.

Duchmann, R., Schmitt, E., Knolle, P., Meyer zum Büschenfelde, K. H., and Neurath, M. (1996). Tolerance towards resident intestinal flora in mice is abrogated in experimental colitis and restored by treatment with interleukin-10 or antibodies in interleukin-12. *Eur. J. Immunol.* 26, 934–938.

Elson, C. O., Beagley, K. W., Sharmanov, A. T., Fujihashi, K., Kiyono, H,. Tennyson, G. S., Cong, Y., Black, C. A., Ridwan, B. W., and McGhee, J. R. (1996). Hapten-induced model of murine inflammatory bowel disease: Mucosa immune responses and protection by tolerance. *J. Immunol.* 157, 2174–2185.

Emmrich, J., Seyfarth, M., Fleig, W. E., and Emmrich, F. (1991). Treatment of inflammatory bowel disease with anti-CD4 monoclonal antibody. *Lancet* 338, 570–571.

Esser, C. and Radbruch, A. (1990). Immunoglobulin class switching: Molecular and cellular analysis. *Annu. Rev. Immunol.* 8, 717–735.

Fennelly, G. J., Khan, S. A., Abadi, M. A., Wild, T. F., and Bloom, B. R. (1999). Mucosal DNA vaccine immunization against measles with a highly attenuated *Shigella flexeri* vector. *J. Immunol.* 162, 1603–1610.

Finkelman, F. D., Holmes, J., Katona, I. M., Urban, J. F., Jr., Beckmann, M. P., Park, L. S., Schooley, K. A., Coffman, R. L., Mosmann, T. R., and Paul, W. E. (1990). Lymphokine control of *in vivo* immunoglobulin isotype selection. *Annu. Rev. Immunol.* 8, 303–333.

Firestein, G. S., Roeder, W. D., Laxer, J. A., Townsend, K. S., Weaver, C. T., Hom, J. T., Linton, J., Torbett, B. E., and Glasebrook, A. L. (1989). A new murine CD4+ T cell subset with an unrestricted cytokine profile. *J. Immunol.* 143, 518–525.

Fontenot, J. D., Gavin, M. A., and Rudensky, A. Y. (2003). Foxp3 programs the development and function of CD4+ CD25+ T regulatory cells. *Nat. Immunol.* 4, 330–336.

Fowler, S. and Powrie, F. (2002). CTLA-4 expression on antigen-specific cells but not IL-10 secretion is required for oral tolerance. *Eur. J. Immunol.* 32, 2997–3006.

Friedman, A. and Weiner, H. L. (1994). Induction of anergy or active suppression following oral tolerance is determined by antigen dosage. *Proc. Natl. Acad. Sci. U.S.A.* 91, 6688–6692.

Fujihashi, K., Kato, H., and McGhee, J. R. (2001). A revisit of current dogma for the cellular and molecular basis of oral tolerance. In *The Intestinal Mucosa and Dietary Antigens. Oral Tolerance* (ed. O. Morteau) Chapter 3, 1–13. Austin, TX: Landes Biosciences.

Fuleihan, R., Ramesh, N., and Geha, R. S. (1993). Role of CD40-CD40-ligand interaction in Ig-isotype switching. *Curr. Opin. Immunol.* 5, 963–967.

Fuss, I. J., Neurath, M., Boirivant, M., Klein, J. S., de la Motte, C., Strong, S. A., Fiocchi, C., and Strober, W. (1996). Disparate CD4+ lamina propria (LP) lymphokine secretion profiles in inflammatory bowel disease. *J. Immunol.* 157, 1261–1270.

Fuss, I. J., Boirivant, M., Lacy, B., and Strober, W. (2002). The interrelated roles of TGF-β and IL-10 in the regulation of experimental colitis. *J. Immunol.* 168, 900–908.

Gajewski, T. F. and Fitch, F. W. (1988). Anti-proliferative effect of IFN-γ in immune regulation. I. IFN-γ inhibits the proliferation of Th2 but not Th1 murine helper T lymphocyte clones. *J. Immunol.* 40, 4245–4252.

Garside, P., Mowat, A. M., and Khoruts, A. (1999). Oral tolerance in disease. *Gut* 44, 137–142.

Garside, P., Steel, M., Worthey, E. A., Satoskar, A., Alexander, J., Bluethmann, H., Liew, F. Y., and Mowat, A. M. (1995). T helper 2 cells are subject to high dose oral tolerance and are not essential for its induction. *J. Immunol.* 154, 5649–5655.

Gaydos, C. A. and Gaydos, J. C. (1995). Adenovirus vaccines in the U.S. military. *Mil. Med.* 160, 300–304.

Germann, T., Guckes, S., Bongartz, M., Dlugonska, H., Schmitt, E., Kolbe, L., Kolsch, E., Podlaski, F. J., Gately, M. K., and Rude, E. (1995). Administration of IL-12 during ongoing immune responses fails to permanently suppress and can even enhance the synthesis of antigen-specific IgE. *Int. Immunol.* 7, 1649–1657.

Graham, B. S., Bunton, L. A., Rowland, J., Wright, P. F., and Karzon, D. T. (1991b). Respiratory syncytial virus infection in anti-μ treated mice. *J. Virol.* 65, 4936–4942.

Graham, B. S., Bunton, L. A., Wright, P. F., and Karzon, D. T. (1991a). Role of T lymphocyte subsets in the pathogenesis of primary infection and rechallenge with respiratory syncytial virus in mice. *J. Clin. Invest.* 88, 1026–1033.

Greene, M. I., Ginsburg, C. H., and Benacerraf, B. (1982). The regulation of hapten-specific granuloma formation. *Clin. Immunol. Immunopathol.* 23, 275–285.

Groux, H., Bigler, M., de Vries, J. E., and Roncarolo, M. G. (1996). Interleukin-10 induces a long-term antigen-specific anergic state in human CD4+ T cells. *J. Exp. Med.* 184, 19–29.

Groux, H., O'Garra, A., Bigler, M., Rouleau, M., Antonenko, S., de Vries, J. E., and Roncarolo, M. G. (1997). A CD4+ T-cell subset inhibits antigen-specific T-cell responses and prevents colitis. *Nature* 389, 737–742.

Hagenbaugh, A., Sharma, S., Dubinett, S. M., Wei, S. H., Aranda, R., Cheroutre, H., Fowell, D J., Binder, S., Tsao, B., Locksley, R. M., Moore, K. W., and Kronenberg, M. (1997). Altered immune responses in interleukin 10 transgenic mice. *J. Exp. Med.* 185, 2101–2110.

Harriman, G. R., Bradley, A., Das, S., Rogers-Fani, P., and Davis, A. C. (1996). IgA class switch in Iα exon-deficient mice. Role of germline transcription in class switch recombination. *J. Clin. Invest.* 97, 477–485.

Higuchi, K., Kweon, M. N., Fujihashi, K., McGhee, J. R., and Kiyono, H. (2000). Comparison of nasal and oral tolerance for the prevention of collagen induced murine arthritis. *J. Rheumatol.* 27, 1038–1044.

Hirahara, K., Hisatsune, T., Nishijima, K., Kato, H., Shiho, O., and Kaminogawa, S. (1995). CD4+ T cells anergized by high dose feeding establish oral tolerance to antibody responses when transferred in SCID and nude mice. *J. Immunol.* 154, 6238–6245.

Hiroi, T., Iwatani, K., Iijima, H., Kodama, S., Yanagita, M., and Kiyono, H. (1998). Nasal immunize system: Distinctive Th0 and Th1/Th2 type environments in murine nasal-associated lymphoid tissues and nasal passage, respectively. *Eur. J. Immunol.* 28, 3346–3353.

Höllander, G. A., Simpson, S. J., Mizoguchi, E., Nichogiannopoulou, A., She, J., Gutierrez-Ramos, J.-C., Bhan, A. K., Burakoff, S. J., Wang, B., and Terhorst, C. (1995). Severe colitis in mice with aberrant thymic selection. *Immunity* 3, 27–38.

Horner, A. A., Ronaghy, A., Cheng, P.-M., Nguyen, M.-D., Cho, H. J., Broide, D., and Raz, E. (1998). Immunostimulatory DNA is a potent mucosal adjuvant. *Cell. Immunol.* 190, 77–82.

Hörnqvist, E., Goldschmidt, T. J., Holmdahl, R., and Lycke, N. (1991). Host defense against cholera toxin is strongly CD4+ T cell dependent. *Infect. Immun.* 59, 3630–3638.

Hornquist, E. and Lycke, N. (1995). Cholera toxin increases T lympho-cyte responses to unrelated antigens. In *Advances in Mucosal Immunology* (eds. J. Mestecky *et al.*), 1507–1512. New York: Plenum Press.

Hoyne, G. F., O'Hehir, R. E., Wraith, D. C., Thomas, W. R., and Lamb, J. R. (1993). Inhibition of T cell and antibody responses to house dust mite allergen by inhalation of the dominant T cell epitope in naive and sensitized mice. *J. Exp. Med.* 178, 1783–1788.

Hsieh, C. S., Macatonia, S. E., Tripp, C. S., Wolf, S. F., O'Garra, A., and Murphy, K. M. (1993). Development of Th1 CD4⁺ T cells through IL-12 produced by *Listeria*-induced macrophages. *Science* 260, 547–549.

Imler, J. L. (1995). Adenovirus vectors as recombinant viral vaccines. *Vaccines* 13, 1143-1151.

Iqbal, N., Oliver, J. R., Wagner, F. H., Lazenby, A. S., Elson, C. O., and Weaver, C. T. (2002). T helper 1 and T helper 2 cells are patho-genic in an antigen-specific model of colitis. *J. Exp. Med.* 195, 71–84.

Islam, K. B., Nilsson, L., Sideras, P., Hammarstrom, L., and Smith, C. I. (1991). TGF-β1 induces germ-line transcripts of both IgA subclasses in human B lymphocytes. *Int. Immunol.* 3, 1099–1106.

Ismail, N. and Bretscher, P. A. (1999). The Th1/Th2 nature of concur-rent immune responses to unrelated antigens can be indepen-dent. *J. Immunol.* 163, 4842–4850.

Iwasaki, A. and Kelsall, B. L. (1999). Freshly isolated Peyer's patch, but not spleen, dendritic cells produce interleukin 10 and induce the differentiation of T helper type 2 cells. *J. Exp. Med.* 190, 229–239.

Iwasaki, A. and Kelsall, B. L. (2000). Localization of distinct Peyer's patch dendritic cell subsets and their recruitment by chemokines macrophage inflammatory protein (MIP)-3α, MIP-3β, and sec-ondary lymphoid organ chemokine. *J. Exp. Med.* 191, 1381–1393.

Iwasaki, A. and Kelsall, B. L. (2001). Unique functions of CD11b⁺, CD8alpha⁺ and double-negative Peyer's patch dendritic cells. *J. Immunol.* 166, 4884–4890.

Jaffe, H.-A., Danel, C., Longenecker, G., Metzger, M., Setoguchi, Y., Rosenfeld, M. A., Gant, T. W., Thorgeirsson, S. S., Stratford-Perricaudet, L. D., and Perricaudet,, M. (1992). Adenovirus-mediated *in vitro* gene transfer and expression in normal rat liver. *Nat. Genet.* 1, 372–378.

Kawanishi, H., Ozato, K., and Strober, W. (1985). The profilerative response of cloned Peyer's patch T cells to syngeneic and allogeneic stimuli. *J. Immunol.* 134, 3586–3591.

Kawanishi, H., Saltzman, L. E., and Strober, W. (1983a). Mechanisms regulating IgA class-specific immunoglobulin production in murine gut-associated lymphoid tissues. I. T cells derived from Peyer's patches that switch sIgM B cells to sIgA B cells *in vitro*. *J. Exp. Med.* 157, 433–450.

Kawanishi, H., Saltzman, L., and Strober, W. (1983b). Mechanisms reg-ulating IgA class-specific immunoglobulin production in murine gut-associated lymphoid tissues. II. Terminal differentiation of postswitch sIgA-bearing Peyer's patch B cells. *J. Exp. Med.* 158, 649–669.

Kay. M. A., Graham, F., Leland, F., and Woo, S. L. (1995). Therapeutic serum concentrations of human alpha-I-antitrypsin after adeno-viral-mediated gene transfer into mouse hepatocytes. *Hepatology* 21, 815–819.

Khattri, R., Cox, T., Yasayko, S.-A., and Ramsdell, F. (2003). An essen-tial role for scurfin in CD4⁺ CD25⁺ T regulatory cells. *Nat. Immunol.* 4, 337–342.

Kiyono, H., McGhee, J. R., Mosteller, L. M., Eldridge, J. H., Koopman, W. J., Kearney, F. J., and Michalek, S. M. (1982). Murine Peyer's patch T cell clones. Characterization of antigen-specific helper T cells for immunoglobulin A responses. *J. Exp. Med.* 156, 1115–1130.

Kiyono, H., Cooper, M. D., Kearney, J. F., Mosteller, L. M., Michalek, S. M., Koopman, W. J., and McGhee, J. R. (1984). Isotype-speci-ficity of helper T cell clones. Peyer's patch Th cells preferentially collaborate with mature IgA B cells for IgA responses. *J. Exp. Med.* 159, 798–811.

Kobayashi, M., Fitz, L., Ryan, M., Hewick, R.M., Clark, S.C., Chan, S., Loudon, R., Sherman, F., Perussia, B., and Trinchieri, G. (1989). Identification and purification of natural killer cell stimulatory

factor (NKSF), a cytokine with multiple biologic effects on human lymphocytes. *J. Exp. Med.* 170, 827–845.

Kolls, J. K., Lei, D., Odom, G., Nelson, S., Summer, W. R., Gerber, M. A., and Shellito, J. E. (1996). Use of transient CD4 lymphocyte depletion to prolong transgene expression of E1-deleted adeno-viral vectors. *Hum. Gene Ther.* 7, 489–197.

Kuhn, R., Lohler, J., Rennick, D., Rajewsky, K., and Muller, W. (1993). Interleukin-10-deficient mice develop chronic enterocolitis. *Cell* 75, 263–274.

Kullberg, M. C., Jankovic, D., Gorelick, P. L., Caspar, P., Letterio, J. J., Cheever, A. W., and Sher, A. (2002). Bacteria-triggered CD4⁺ T regulatory cells suppress *Helicobacter hepaticus*-induced colitis. *J. Exp. Med.* 196, 505–515.

Kweon, M. N., Fujihashi, K., VanCott, J. L., Higuchi, K., Yamamoto, M., McGhee, J. R., and Kiyono, H. (1998). Lack of orally induced systemic unresponsiveness in IFN-γ knockout mice. *J. Immunol.* 160, 1687–1693.

Lebman, D. A., Nomura, D. Y., Coffman, R. L., and Lee, F. D. (1990a). Molecular characterization of germ-line immunoglobulin A tran-scripts produced during transforming growth factor type β-induced isotype switching. *Proc. Natl. Acad. Sci. USA* 87, 3962–3966.

Lebman, D. A., Lee, F. D., and Coffman, R. L. (1990b). Mechanism for transforming growth factor β and IL-2 enhancement of IgA expression in lipopolysaccharide-stimulated B cell cultures. *J. Immunol.* 144, 952–959.

Leishman, A. J., Garside, P., and Mowat, A. M. (2000). Induction of oral tolerance in the primed immune system: Influence of antigen persistence and adjuvant form. *Cell. Immunol.* 202, 71–78.

Londoño-Arcila, P., Freeman, D., Kleanthous, H., O'Dowd, A. M., Lewis, S., Turner, A. K., Rees, E. L., Tibbitts, T. J., Greenwood, J., Monath, T. P., and Darsley, M. J. (2002). Attenuated *Salmonella enterica* serovar typhi expressing urease effectively immunizes mice against *Helicobacter pylori* challenge as part of heterologous mucosal priming-parenteral boosting vaccination regimen. *Infect. Immun.* 70, 5096–5106.

MacLennan, I. C. (1994). Germinal centers. *Annu. Rev. Immunol.* 12, 117–139.

Mallett, C. P., VanDeVerg, L., Collins, H. H., and Hale, T. L. (1993). Evaluation of *Shigella* vaccine safety and efficacy in an intranasally challenged mouse model. *Vaccine* 11, 190–196.

Maloy, K. J. and Powrie, F. (2001). Regulatory T cells in the control of immune pathology. *Nat. Immunol.* 2, 816–822.

Marinaro, M., Boyaka, P. N., Jackson, R. J., Finkelman, F. D., Kiyono, H., Jirillo, E., and McGhee, J. R. (1999). Use of intranasal IL-12 to target predominantly Th1 responses to nasal and Th2 responses to oral vaccines given with cholera toxin. *J. Immunol.* 162, 114–121.

Marinaro, M., Staats, H. F., Hiroi, T., Jackson, R. J., Coste, M., Boyaka, P. N., Okahashi, N., Yamamoto, M., Kiyono, H., Bluethmann, H., Fujihashi, K., and McGhee, J. R. (1995). Mucosal adjuvant effect of cholera toxin in mice results from induction of T helper 2 (Th2) cells and IL-4. *J. Immunol.* 155, 4621–4629.

Marth, T., Strober, W., and Kelsall, B. L. (1996). High dose oral toler-ance in ovalbumin TCR-transgenic mice: Systemic neutralization of IL-12 augments TGF-β secretion and T cell apoptosis. *J. Immunol.* 157, 2348–2357.

Mascart, F., Verscheure, V., Malfroot, A., Hainaut, M., Pierard, D., Temerman, S., Peltier, A., Debrie, A.-S., Levy, J., Del Giudice, G., and Locht, C. (2003). *Bordetella pertussis* infection in 2-month old infants promotes type 1 T cell responses. *J. Immunol.* 170, 1504–1509.

Mayer, L., Kwan, S. P., Thompson, C., Ko, H. S., Chiorazzi, N., Waldmann, T., and Rosen, F. (1986). Evidence for a defect in "switch" T cells in patients with immunodeficiency and hyper-immunoglobulinemia M. *N. Engl. J. Med.* 314, 409–413.

Mayer, L. (2000). Oral tolerance: new approaches, new problems. *Clin. Immunol.* 94, 1–8.

McCluskie, M. J., Weeratna, R. D., Krieg, A. M., and Davis, H. L. (2000). CpG DNA is an effective oral adjuvant to protein anti-gens in mice. *Vaccine* 19, 950–957.

McCluskie, M. J. and Davis, H. L. (1999). CgG DNA as mucosal adju-vant. *Vaccine* 18, 231–237.

McCluskie, M. J. and Davis, H. L. (1998). Cutting edge. CpG DNA is a potent enhancer of systemic and mucosal immune responses against hepatitis B surface antigen with intranasal administration to mice. *J. Immunol.* 161, 4463–4466.

McGhee, J. R. and Kiyono, H. (1999). The mucosal immune system. In *Fundamental Immunology* 4th ed. (ed. W. E. Paul), 909–945. Philadelphia/New York: Lippincott-Raven Publishers.

McGhee, J. R., Mestecky, J., Elson, C. O., and Kiyono, H. (1989). Regulation of IgA synthesis and immune response by T cells and interleukins. *J. Clin. Immunol.* 9, 175–199.

McIntyre, T. M., Kehry, M. R., and Snapper, C. M. (1995). Novel *in vitro* model for high-rate IgA class switching. *J. Immunol.* 154, 3156–3161.

McMenamin, C. and Holt, P. G. (1993). The natural immune response to inhaled soluble protein antigens involves major histocompatibility complex (MHC) class I-restricted CD8+ T cell-mediated but MHC class II-restricted CD4+ T cell-dependent immune deviation resulting in selective suppression of immunoglobulin E production. *J. Exp. Med.* 178, 889–899.

McSorley, S. J., Rask, C., Pichot, R., Julia, V., Czerkinsky, C., and Glaichenhaus, N. (1998). Selective tolerization of Th1-like cells after nasal administration of a cholera toxoid-LACK conjugate. *Eur. J. Immunol.* 28, 424–432.

Mega, J., Bruce, M. G., Beagley, K. W., McGhee, J. R., Taguchi, T., Pitts, A. M., McGhee, M. L., Bucy, R. P., Eldridge, J. H., and Mestecky, J. (1991). Regulation of mucosal responses by CD4+ T lymphocytes: Effects of anti-L3T4 treatment on the gastrointestinal immune system. *Int. Immunol.* 3, 793–805.

Melamed, D. and Friedman, A. (1993). Direct evidence for anergy in T lymphocytes tolerized by oral administration of ovalbumin. *Eur. J. Immunol.* 23, 935–942.

Miller, S. D. and Butler, L. D. (1983). T cell responses induced by the parenteral injection of antigen-modified syngeneic cells. I. Induction, characterization, and regulation of antigen-specific T helper cells involved in delayed-type hypersensitivity responses. *J. Immunol.* 131, 77–85.

Mizoguchi, A., Mizoguchi, E., Chiba, C., Spiekermann, G. M., Tonegawa, S., Nagler-Anderson, C., and Bhan, A. K. (1996a). Cytokine imbalance and autoantibody production in T cell receptor-α mutant mice with inflammatory bowel disease. *J. Exp. Med.* 183, 847–856.

Mizoguchi, A., Mizoguchi, E., Tonegawa, S., and Bhan, A. K. (1996b). Alteration of a polyoclonal to an oligoclonal immune response to cecal aerobic bacterial antigens in TCRα mutant mice with inflammatory bowel disease. *Int. Immunol.* 8, 1387–1394.

Moldoveanu, Z., Love-Homan, L., Huang, W. Q., and Krieg, A. M. (1998). CpG DNA, a novel immune enhancer for systemic and mucosal immunization with influenza virus. *Vaccine* 16, 1216–1224.

Mombaerts, P., Mizoguchi, E., Grusby, M. J., Glimcher, L. H., Bhan, A. K., and Tonegawa, S. (1993). Spontaneous development of inflammatory bowel disease in T cell receptor mutant mice. *Cell* 75, 274–282.

Monteleone, G., Biancone, L., Marasco, R., Morrone, G., Marasco, O., Luzza, F., and Pallone, F. (1997). Interleukin 12 is expressed and actively released by Crohn's disease intestinal lamina propria mononuclear cells. *Gastroenterology* 112, 1169–1178.

Morris, G. P., Beck, P. L., Herridge, M. S., Depew, W. T., Szewczuk, M. R., and Wallace, J. L. (1989). Hapten-induced model of chronic inflammation and ulceration in the rat colon. *Gastroenterology* 96, 795–803.

Morrissey, P. J., Charrier, K., Braddy, S., Liggitt, D., and Watson, J. D. (1993). CD4+ T cells that express high levels of CD45RB induce wasting disease when transferred into congenic severe combined immunodeficient mice. Disease development is prevented by cotransfer of purified CD4+ T cells. *J. Exp. Med.* 178, 237–244.

Mosmann, T. R., Cherwinski, H., Bond, M. W., Giedlin, M. A., and Coffman, R. L. (1986). Two types of murine helper T cell clone. I. Definition according to profiles of lymphokine activities and secreted proteins. *J. Immunol.* 136, 348–357.

Mosmann, T. R. and Coffman, R. L. (1989). Th1 and Th2 cells: Different patterns of lymphokine secretion lead to different functional properties. *Annu. Rev. Immunol.* 7, 145–173.

Mosmann, T. R. and Coffman, R. L. (1989). Th1 and Th2 cells: Different patterns of lymphokine secretion lead to different functional properties. *Annu. Rev. Immunol.* 7, 145–173.

Mullbacher, A., Bellett, A. J., and Hla, R. T. (1989). The murine cellular immune response to adenovirus type 5. *Immunol. Cell Biol.* 67, 31–39.

Murphy, K. M., Ouyang, W., Farrar, J. D., Yang, J., Ranganath, S., Asnagli, H., Afkarian, M., and Murphy, T. L. (2000). Signaling and transcription in T helper development. *Annu. Rev. Immunol.* 18, 451–494.

Neurath, M. F., Fuss, I., Kelsall, B. L., Presky, D. H., Waegell, W., and Strober, W. (1996). Experimental granulomatous colitis in mice is abrogated by induction of TGF-β-mediated oral tolerance. *J. Exp. Med.* 183, 2605–2616.

Neurath, M. F., Fuss, I., Kelsall, B. L., Stuber, E., and Strober, W. (1995). Antibodies to interleukin 12 abrogate established experimental colitis in mice. *J. Exp. Med.* 182, 1281–1290.

Niessner, M. and Vold, B. A. (1995). Altered Th1/Th2 cytokine profiles in the intestinal mucosa of patients with inflammatory bowel disease as assessed by quantitative reversed transcribed polymerase chain reaction (RT-PCR). *Clin. Exp. Immunol.* 101, 428–435.

Nilsson, L., Islam, K. B., Olafsson, O., Zalcberg, I., Samakovlis, C., Hammarstrom, L., Smith, C. I., and Sideras, P. (1991). Structure of TGF-β1-induced human immunoglobulin Cαα1 and Cα2 germ-line transcripts. *Int. Immunol.* 3, 1107–1115.

Noriega, F. R., Losonsky, G., Wang, J. Y., Formal, S. B., and Levine, M. M. (1996). Further characterization of ΔaroA ΔvirG *Shigella flexeri* 2a strain CVD 1203 as a mucosal *Shigella* vaccine and as a live-vector vaccine for delivering antigens of enterotoxigenic *Escherichia coli*. *Infect. Immun.* 64, 23–27.

O'Garra, A. and Vieira, P. (2003). Twenty-first century Foxp3. *Nat. Immunol.* 4, 304–306.

Okahashi, N., Yamamoto, M., VanCott, J. L., Chatfield, S. N., Roberts, M., Bluethmann, H., Hiroi, T., Kiyono, H., and McGhee, J. R. (1996). Oral immunization of interleukin-4 (IL-4) knockout mice with a recombinant *Salmonella* strain or cholera toxin reveals that CD4+ Th2 cells producing IL-6 and IL-10 are associated with mucosal immunoglobulin A responses. *Infect. Immun.* 64, 1516–1525.

Olivares-Villagomez, D., Wang, Y., and Lafaille, J. J. (1998). Regulatory CD4+ T cells expressing endogenous T cell receptor chains protect myelin basic protein-specific transgenic mice from spontaneous autoimmune encephalomyelitis. *J. Exp. Med.* 188, 1883–1894.

Oriss, T. B., McCarthy, S. A., Campana, M. A., and Morel, P. A. (1999). Evidence of positive cross-regulation on Th1 by Th2 and antigen-presenting cells: Effects on Th1 induced by IL-4 and IL-12. *J. Immunol.* 162, 1999–2007.

Paliard, X., de Waal Malefijt, R., Yssel, H., Blanchard, D., Chretien, I., Abrams, J., de Vries, J., and Spits, H. (1988). Simultaneous production of IL-2, IL-4, and IFN-γ by activated human CD4+ and CD8+ T cell clones. *J. Immunol.* 141, 849–855.

Powrie, F., Carlino, J., Leach, M. W., Mauze, S., and Coffman, R. L. (1996). A critical role for transforming growth factor-β but not interleukin 4 in the suppression of T helper type 1-mediated colitis by CD45RBlow CD4+ T cells. *J. Exp. Med.* 183, 2669–2674.

Powrie, F., Leach, M. W., Mauze, S., Caddle, L. B., and Coffman, R. L. (1993). Phenotypically distinct subsets of CD4+ T cells induce or protect from chronic intestinal inflammation in C.B-17 SCID mice. *Intern. Immunol.* 5, 1461–1471.

Powrie, F., Leach, M. W., Mauze, S., Menon, S., Caddle, L. B., and Coffman, R. L. (1994). Inhibition of Th1 responses prevents inflammatory bowel disease in SCID mice reconstituted with CD45RBhi CD4+ T cells. *Immunity* 1, 553–562.

Rawle, F. C., Knowles, B. B., Ricciardi, R. P., Brahmacheri, V., Duerken-Hughes, P., Wold, W. S., and Gooding, L. R. (1991). Specificity of the mouse cytotoxic T lymphocyte response to adenovirus 5.E1A is immunodominant in H-2b, but not in H-2d or H2k mice. *J. Immunol.* 146, 3977–3984.

Read, S., Malmsrom, V., and Powrie, F. (2000). Cytotoxic T lymphocyte-associated antigen 4 plays an essential role in the function of CD25+ CD4+ regulatory cells that control intestinal inflammation. *J. Exp. Med.* 192, 295–302.

Reuman, P. D., Keely, S. P., and Schiff, G. M. (1991). Similar subclass antibody responses after intranasal immunization with UV-inactivated RSV mixed with cholera toxin or live RSV. *J. Med. Virol.* 35,192–197.

Revy, P., Muto, T., Levy, Y., Geissman, F., Plebani, A., Sanal, O., Catalan, N., Forveille, M., Dufourcq-Labelouse, R., Gennery, A., Tezcan, I., Ersoy, F., Kayserili, H., Ugazio, A. G., Brousse, N., Muramatsu, M., Notarangelo, L. D., Kinoshita, K., Honjo, T., Fischer, A., and Durnady, A. (2000). Activation-induced cytidine deaminase (AID) deficiency causes the autosomal recessive form of the Hyper-IgM syndrome (HIGM2). *Cell* 102, 565–575.

Riddell. S. R. and Greenberg, P. D. (1995). Principles of adoptive T cell therapy of human viral diseases. *Annu. Rev. Immunol.* 13, 545–586.

Rissoan, M.-C., Soumelis, V., Kadowaki, N., Grouard, G., Briere, F., de Waal Malefyt, R., and Liu, Y.-J. (1999). Reciprocal control of T helper cell and dendritic cell differentiation. *Science* 283, 1183–1186.

Roberts, M., Chatfield, S. N., and Dougan, G. (1994). *Salmonella* as carriers of heterologous antigens. In *Novel Delivery Systems for Oral Vaccines* (ed. D. T. O'Hagan), 27–35. Boca Raton, FL: CRC Press.

Romagnani, S. (1991). Human Th1 and Th2 subsets: Doubt no more. *Immunol. Today* 12, 256–257.

Roman, M. E., Martin-Orozco, E., Goodman, J. S., Nguyen, M. D., Sato, Y., Ronaghy, A., Kornbluth, R. S., Richman, D. D., Carson, D. A., and Raz, E. (1997). Immunostimulatory DNA sequences function as T helper 1-promoting adjuvants. *Nat. Med.* 3, 849–854.

Roncarolo, M. G. and Levings, M. K. (2000). The role of different subsets of T regulatory cells in controlling autoimmunity. *Curr. Opin. Immunol.* 12, 676–683.

Rosenfeld, M. A., Yoshimura, K., Trapnell, B. C., Yoneyama. K., Rosenthal, E. R., Dalemans, W., Fukayama, M., Bargon, J., Stier, L. E., and Stratford-Perricaudet, L. (1992). *In vivo* transfer of the human cystic fibrosis transmembrane conductance regulator gene to the airway epithelium. *Cell* 68, 143–155.

Rousset, F., Garcia, E., and Banchereau, J. (1991). Cytokine-induced proliferation and immunoglobulin production of human B lymphocytes triggered through their CD40 antigen. *J. Exp. Med.* 173, 705–710.

Sadlack, B., Merz, H., Schorle, A., Schimpl, A., Feller, A. C., and Horak, I. (1993). Ulcerative colitis-like disease in mice with a disrupted interleukin-2 gene. *Cell* 75, 253–261.

Sakaguchi, S., Sakaguchi, N., Asano, M., Ito, M., and Toda, M. (1995). Immunologic self-tolerance maintained by activated T cells expressing IL-2 receptora-chain (CD25). Breakdown of a single mechanism of self-tolerance causes various autoimmune diseases. *J. Immunol.* 155, 1151–1164.

Sakaguchi, S. (2000). Animal models of autoimmunity and their relevance to human diseases. *Curr. Opin. Immunol.* 12, 684–690.

Schwartz, R. H. (1990). A cell culture model for T lymphocyte clonal anergy. *Science* 248, 1349–1356.

Seder, R. A. (1994). Acquisition of lymphokine-producing phenotype by CD4+ T cells. *J. Allergy Clin. Immunol.* 94, 1195–1202.

Shevach, E. M. (2000). Regulatory T cells in autoimmunity. *Annu. Rev. Immunol.* 18, 423–449.

Shi, H. N., Ingui, C. J., Dodge, I., and Nagler-Anderson, C. (1998). A helminth-induced mucosal Th2 response alters nonresponsiveness to oral administration of a soluble antigen. *J. Immunol.* 160, 2449–2455.

Shi, H. N., Grusby, M. J., and Nagler-Anderson, C. (1999). Orally induced peripheral nonresponsiveness is maintained in the absence of functional Th1 or Th2 cells. *J. Immunol.* 162, 5143–5148.

Simpson, S. J., Hollander, G. A., Mizoguchi, E., Allen, D., Bhan, A. K., Wang, B., and Terhorst, C. (1997). Expression of pro-inflammatory cytokines by TCR αβ+ and TCR γδ+ T cells in an experimental model of colitis. *Eur. J. Immunol.* 27, 17–25.

Sizemore, D. R., Branstromm, A. A., and Sadoff, J. C. (1995). Attenuated *Shigella* as a DNA delivery vehicle for DNA-mediated immunization. *Science* 270, 299–302.

Snapper, C. M. and Paul, W. E. (1987). Interferon-gamma and B cell stimulatory factor-1 reciprocally regulate Ig isotype production. *Science* 236, 944–947.

Snider, D. P., Marshall, J. S., Perdue, M. H., and Liang, H. (1994). Production of IgE antibody and allergic sensitization of intestinal and peripheral tissues after oral immunization with protein Ag and cholera toxin. *J. Immunol.* 153, 647–657.

Sonoda, E., Matsumoto, R., Hitoshi, Y., Ishii, T., Sugimoto, M., Araki, S., Tominaga, A., Yamaguchi, N., and Takatasu, K. (1989). Transforming growth factor β induces IgA production and acts additively with interleukin 5 for IgA production. *J. Exp. Med.* 170, 1415–1420.

Spalding, D. M. and Griffin, J. A. (1986). Different pathways of differentiation of pre-B cell lines are induced by dendritic cells and T cells from different lymphoid tissues. *Cell* 44, 507–515.

Stavnezer, J. (1995). Regulation of antibody production and class switching by TGF-β. *J. Immunol.* 155, 1647–1651.

Stumbles, P. A., Thomas, J. A., Pimm, C. L., Lee, P. T., Venaille, T. J., Proksch, S., and Holt, P. G. (1998). Resting respiratory tract dendritic cells preferentially stimulate T helper cell type 2 (Th2) responses and require obligatory cytokine signals for induction of Th1 immunity. *J. Ex. Med.* 188, 2019–2031.

Sundstedt, A., Höidén, I., Rosendahl, A., Kalland, T., van Rooijen, N., and Dohlsten, M. (1997). Immunoregulatory role of IL-10 during superantigen-induced hyporesponsiveness *in vivo. J. Immunol.* 158, 180–186.

Taams, L. S., van Rensen, A. J., Poelen, M. C., van Els, C. A., Besseling, A. C., Wagenaar, J. P., van Eden, W., and Wauben, M. H. (1998). Anergic T cells actively suppress T cell responses via the antigen-presenting cell. *Eur. J. Immunol.* 28, 2902–2912.

Takafuji. E. T., Gaydos, J. C., Allen, R. G., and Top, F. H., Jr. (1979). Simultaneous administration of live, enteric-coated adenovirus types 4, 7 and 21 vaccines: safety and immunogenicty. *J. Infect. Dis.* 140, 48–53.

Takahashi, I., Kiyono, H., and Hamada, S. (1997). CD4+ T-cell population mediates development of inflammatory bowel disease in T-cell receptor α chain-deficient mice. *Gastroenterology* 112, 1876–1886.

Takahashi, I., Marinaro, M., Kiyono, H., Jackson, R. J., Nakagawa, I., Fujihashi, K., Hamada, S., Clements, J. D., Bost, K. L., and McGhee, J. R. (1996). Mechanisms for mucosal immunogenicity and adjuvancy of *Escherichia coli* labile enterotoxin. *J. Infect. Dis.* 173, 627–635.

Tian, J., Atkinson, M. A., Clare-Salzler, M., Herschenfeld, A., Forsthuber, T., Lehmann, P. V., and Kaufman, D. L. (1996). Nasal administration of glutamate decarboxylase (GAD65) peptides induces Th2 responses and prevents murine insulin-dependent diabetes. *J. Exp. Med.* 183, 1561–1567.

Tomasi, T. B. Jr. (1980). Oral tolerance. *Transplantation* 29, 353–356.

Trinchieri G. (1995). Interleukin-12: A proinflammatory cytokine with immunoregulatory functions that bridge innate resistance and antigen-specific adaptive immunity. *Annu. Rev. Immunol.* 13, 251–276.

VanCott, J. L., Staats, H. F., Pascual, D. W., Roberts, M., Chatfield, S. N., Yamamoto, M., Coste, M., Carter, P. B., Kiyono, H., and McGhee, J. R. (1996). Regulation of mucosal and systemic antibody responses by T helper cell subsets, macrophages and derived cytokines following oral immunization with live recombinant *Salmonella. J. Immunol.* 156, 1504–1514.

van Ginkel. F. W., Liu, C., Simecka, J. W., Dong, J.-Y., Greenway, T., Frizzell, R. A., Kiyono, H., McGhee, J. R., and Pascual, D. W. (1995). Intratracheal gene delivery with adenoviral vector induces elevated systemic IgG and mucosal IgA antibodies to adenovirus and β-galactosidase. *Hum. Gene Ther.* 6, 895–903.

van Ginkel, F. W., McGhee, J. R., Liu, C., Simecka, J. W., Yamamoto, M., Frizzell, R. A., Scorscher, E. J., Kiyono, H., and Pascual, D. W. (1997). Adenovirus gene delivery elicits distinct pulmonary-associated T helper cell responses to the vector and its transgene. *J. Immunol.* 159, 685–693.

van Ginkel, F. W., Wahl, S. M., Kearney, J. F., Kweon, M. N., Fujihashi, K., Burrows, P. D., Kiyono, H., and McGhee, J. R. (1999). Partial IgA-deficiency with increased Th2-type cytokines in TGF-β1 knockout mice. *J. Immunol.* 163, 1951–1957.

van Halteren, A. G., vander Cammen, M. J., Cooper, D., Savelkoul, H. F., Kraal, G., and Holt, P. B. (1997). Regulation of antigen-specific IgE, IgG1 and mast cell responses to ingested allergen by mucosal tolerance induction. *J. Immunol.* 159, 3009–3015.

VandeVerg, L. L., Mallett, C. P., Collins, H. H., Larsen, T., Hammack, C., and Hale, T. L. (1995). Antibody and cytokine responses in a mouse pulmonary model of *Shiella flexneri* serotype 2a infection. *Infect. Immun.* 63, 1947–1954.

Vendetti, S, Chai, J.-G., Dyson. J., Simpson, E., Lombardi, G., and Lechler, R. (2000). Anergic T cells inhibit the antigen-presenting function of dendritic cells. *J. Immunol.* 165, 1175–1181.

Walker, R. I. and Clements, J.D. (1993). Use of heat-labile toxin of enterotoxigenic *Escherichia coli* to facilitate mucosal immunization. *Vaccine Research* 2, 1.

Watanabe, T., Yoshida, M., Shirai, Y., Yamori, M., Yagita, H., Itoh, T., Chiba, T., Kita, T., and Wakatsuki, Y. (2002). Administration of an antigen at a high dose generates regulatory CD4+ T cells expressing CD95 ligand and secreting IL-4 in the liver. *J. Immunol.* 168, 2188–2199.

Weeratna, R. D., Brazolot-Millan, C. L., McCluskie, M. J., and Davis, H. L. (2001). CpG ODN can re-direct the Th bias of established Th2 immune responses in adult and young mice. *FEMS Immunol. Med. Microbiol.* 32, 65–71.

Weiner, H. L., Friedman, A., Miller, A., Khoury, S. J., al-Sabbagh, A., Santos, L., Sayegh, M., Nussenblatt, R. B., Trentham, D. E., and Hafler, D. A. (1994). Oral tolerance: Immunologic mechanisms and treatment of animal and human organ- specific autoimmune diseases by oral administration of autoantigens. *Annu. Rev. Immunol.* 12, 809–837.

Weinstein, P. D. and Cebra, J. J. (1991). The preference for switching to IgA expression by Peyer's patch germinal center B cells is likely due to the intrinsic influence of their microenvironment. *J. Immunol.* 147, 4126–4135.

Whitacre, C. C., Gienapp, I. E., Orosz, C. G., and Bitar, D. M. (1991). Oral tolerance in experimental autoimmune encephalomyelitis III. Evidence for clonal anergy. *J. Immunol.* 147, 2155–2163.

Williams, M. E., Lichtman, A. H., and Abbas, A. K. (1990). Anti-CD3 antibody induces unresponsiveness to IL-2 in Th1 clones but not in Th2 clones. *J. Immunol.* 144, 1208–1214.

Wilson, A. D., Bailey, M., Williams, N. A., and Stokes, C. R. (1991). The *in vitro* production of cytokines by mucosal lymphocytes immunized by oral administration of keyhole limpet hemocyanin using cholera toxin as an adjuvant. *Eur. J. Immunol.* 21, 2333–2339.

Xu, L., Groham, B., Li, S. C., Bottaro, A., Alt, F. W., and Rothman, P. (1993). Replacement of germ-line epsilon promoter by gene targeting alters control of immunoglobulin heavy chain class switching. *Proc. Natl. Acad. Sci. USA* 90, 3705–3709.

Xu-Amano, J., Kiyono, H., Jackson, R. J., Staats, H. F., Fujihashi, K., Burrows, P. D., Elson, C. O., Pillai, S., and McGhee, J. R. (1993). Helper T cell subsets for immunoglobulin A responses: Oral immunization with tetanus toxoid and cholera toxin as adjuvant selectively induces Th2 cells in mucosa associated tissues. *J. Exp. Med.* 178, 1309–1320.

Yang, D. M., Fairweather, N., Button, L. L., McMaster, W. R., Kahl, L. P., and Liew, F. Y. (1990). Oral *Salmonella typhimurium* (AroA-) vaccine expressing a major *Leishmanial* surface protein (gp63) preferentially induces T helper 1 cells and protective immunity against Leishmaniasis. *J. Immunol.* 145, 2281–2285.

Yang, Y., Trinchieri, G., and Wilson, J. M. (1995). Recombinant IL-12 prevents formation of blocking IgA antibodies to recombinant adenovirus and allows repeated gene therapy to mouse lung. *Nat. Med.* 1, 890–893.

Yi, A.-K., Yoon, J.-G., Yeo, S.-J., Hong, S.-C., English, B. K., and Krieg, A. M. (2002). Role of mitogen-activated protein kinases in CpG DNA-mediated IL-10 and IL-12 production: Central role of extra cellular signal-regulated kinase in negative feedback loop of the CpG DNA-mediated Th1 response. *J. Immunol.* 168, 4711–4720.

Yoshimoto, T., Bendelac, A., Watson, C., Hu-Li, J., and Paul, W. E. (1995). Role of NK1.1+ T cells in a Th2 response and in immunoglobulin E production. *Science* 270, 1845–1847.

Yoshimoto, T. and Paul, W. E. (1994). CD4POS NK1.1POS T cells promptly produce interleukin 4 in response to *in vivo* challenge with anti-CD3. *J. Exp. Med.* 179, 1285–1295.

Zabner, J., Couture, L. A., Gregory, R. J., Graham, S. M., Smith, A. E., and Welsh, M. J. (1993). Adenovirus-mediated gene transfer transiently corrects the chloride transport defect in nasal epithelia of patients with cystic fibrosis. *Cell* 75, 207–216.

Cytotoxic T Cells of the Mucosal Immune System

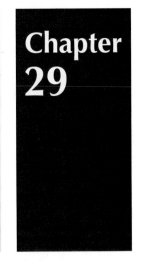

Chapter 29

Leo Lefrançois

Division of Immunology, Department of Internal Medicine, University of Connecticut Health Center, Farmington, Connecticut

The effector sites of the intestinal mucosa are composed of loosely organized lymphoid tissue. There are two main anatomical compartments containing primarily intestinal mucosal effector lymphocytes: the lamina propria (LP), and the epithelium, containing intraepithelial lymphocytes (IEL) (Mowat and Viney, 1997). The LP contains CD4 and CD8 T cells as well as memory B cells and plasma cells mainly producing IgA. There are major phenotypic and functional distinctions between T cells residing in the LP or IEL compartments. Whereas the LP is home to T cells resembling subsets found outside of the intestine, IEL consist of tissue-specific subsets. The latter include CD4⁻CD8αα TCRγδ and TCRαβ T cells and CD4⁺ CD8αα⁺ TCRαβ⁺ T cells (Goodman and Lefrançois, 1989; Lefrançois, 1991). Resident in the epithelium as well as in the LP is a substantial population of "conventional" CD8αβ⁺ TCRαβ⁺ T cells. This chapter will focus chiefly on the origin and function of this population of T cells.

HISTORICAL BACKGROUND

That IEL and LP T cells possess phenotypic characteristics of activated or memory cells has been known for many years (Parrott *et al.*, 1983; Mowat *et al.*, 1986). The origin and specificity of these cells also have been debated for some time (Fichtelius, 1968; Guy-Grand *et al.*, 1978; Lefrançois and Puddington, 1995). Early hypotheses suggested that activated IEL originated in Peyer's patch (PP) (Guy-Grand *et al.*, 1978), likely in response to bacterial antigens derived from the gut lumen. This possibility was supported by the finding that gnotobiotic mice lacking bacterial flora have a poorly developed intestinal mucosal immune system and low numbers of IEL (Imaoka *et al.*, 1996). Direct *ex vivo* cytotoxic activity by mucosal CD8 T cells was initially demonstrated using an antigen nonspecific redirected lysis assay in which anti-TCR mAb are used to trigger lytic activity directed at Fc-receptor-bearing target cells (Lefrançois and Goodman, 1989). More recent data suggest that, although

cytolytic, IEL exhibit characteristics of partially activated T cells (Wang *et al.*, 2002). This is reminiscent of memory cells, although the phenotype of IEL does not always correlate precisely with the classical memory phenotype (Wang *et al.*, 2002). Both TCRγδ and TCRαβ mouse IEL exhibit constitutive lytic activity, and this activity is dependent on the presence of bacterial flora (Lefrançois and Goodman, 1989). Indeed, sole colonization of the mouse gut by an apparently ubiquitous strain of bacteria, termed "segmented filamentous bacteria," results in an increase in TCRαβ IEL and in induction of lytic activity (Okada *et al.*, 1994; Umesaki *et al.*, 1995). Whether this response is antigen specific and whether other bacterial species possess this activity are unclear. In the case of TCRγδ IEL, it appears that microbial flora are not required to induce lytic activity, but that food antigens may be important in the process (Kawaguchi-Miyashita *et al.*, 1996). Furthermore, in the mouse, TCRγδ lytic activity and interferon-gamma (IFN-γ) production are strain dependent (Kawaguchi *et al.*, 1993). Thus, TCRγδ IEL from C57BL/6 mice exhibit lytic activity and produce IFN-γ whereas TCRγδ IEL from most other strains do not, and these findings are not different using IEL from germfree C57BL/6 mice (Kawaguchi *et al.*, 1993; Ishikawa *et al.*, 1993). The antigen specificity of TCRγδ IEL remains obscure, although it is generally assumed that bacterial products or cellular ligands induced by them are being recognized. Human IEL and LP lymphocytes (LPL) also mediate redirected lysis, which is attributable to a small population of CD8 TCRαβ T cells (Lundqvist *et al.*, 1996; Melgar *et al.*, 2002). In the case of CD8αβ TCRαβ LP and IEL, recent evidence has shed light on their origin and specificity.

Tracking antigen-specific CD8 T cells in the intestinal mucosa

Early work showed that TCRαβ IEL can be primed against alloantigen, and against viral, bacterial, and parasite antigens (London *et al.*, 1989; Offit and Dudzik, 1989; Yamamoto *et al.*, 1993; Cuff *et al.*, 1993b; Chardes *et al.*, 1994; Emoto *et al.*, 1996). *In vivo* priming experiments demonstrate that intestinal primary and memory CD8[+] T cells can be induced by virus infection. Antigen-specific cytotoxic T lymphocytes (CTL) are detected within the LP and IEL compartments, as well as in secondary lymphoid tissue of mice following oral rotavirus infection (Offit *et al.*, 1991). However, CTL are present in the LP but not in the IEL following footpad immunization, indicating discordance of the response even within mucosal effector sites. Additionally, memory cytotoxic T lymphocyte precursors (CTLp), as determined by limiting dilution analysis (LDA), are detected in the LP up to 21 days after oral infection but could not be detected in the IEL at any time. The latter result points out the inherent problems with *in vitro* culture of mucosal T cells because IEL lytic activity is present at a time point at which CTLp are not found. Oral reovirus infection results in the generation of MHC-restricted virus-specific cytolytic Thy1[+] TCRαβ IEL (London *et al.*, 1989; Cuff *et al.*, 1993; Chardes *et al.*, 1994). Belyakov *et al.* (1998) analyzed CTL induction in response to an HIV combinatorial peptide and showed that intrarectal immunization leads to primary and memory CTL within the LP, IEL, and spleen. In contrast, and unlike the results with subcutaneous rotavirus infection (Offit *et al.*, 1991), subcutaneous immunization with the peptide leads to CTL activity in spleen but not mucosa (Belyakov *et al.*, 1998). Overall, these studies imply that induction of mucosal primary and memory CTL can depend on the route of infection as well as the form of the immunogen.

In those studies and others, it was not possible to directly visualize and quantify antigen-specific CD8 T cells in the intestinal mucosal compartments or in other sites. Such studies are also complicated by the relative inability of mucosal T cells to be activated to proliferate *in vitro* (Mosley *et al.*, 1991; Gramzinski *et al.*, 1993; Sydora *et al.*, 1993). However, technologic advances now allow the identification of antigen-specific T cells directly *ex vivo* by flow cytometry and even *in vivo* using histologic and imaging methodology. In particular, the transfer of small numbers of identifiable antigen-specific TCR transgenic T cells to normal hosts followed by immunization (Kearney *et al.*, 1994) has provided a detailed description of the pathway that activated, effector CD8[+] T cells follow to the LP and epithelium (Kim *et al.*, 1997, 1998, 1999; Lefrançois *et al.*, 1999b; Svensson *et al.*, 2002). In these studies, trackable OT-I CD8 T cells specific for ovalbumin in the context of H-2K[b] are transferred to normal mice. One of the strengths of the adoptive transfer system for this type of analysis is the ability to determine the location of naive T cells before immunization. It should also be noted that TCR transgenic T cells deficient in the ability to rearrange endogenous TCRs (*i.e.*, RAG[−/−]) should be employed because ligation of endogenous TCRs can result in activation and subsequent generation of activated/memory T cells in the transgenic donor before transfer. Using this system, the results show that few naive CD8 T cells are present in the intestinal mucosa before immunization, whereas small populations are detected in the spleen, lymph nodes (LN), and PP. In addition, nearly all IEL and LP CD8 T cells express molecules associated with activated or memory phenotypes. Thus, it is unlikely that the LP or epithelium is a site for primary activation of naive T cells.

Activation of transferred OT-I cells by feeding soluble ovalbumin does not induce lytic activity in nonintestinal OT-I cells, but upon migration into the intestinal mucosa, OT-I cells become highly lytic (Kim *et al.*, 1998). Similar results are obtained when OT-I cells are transferred to transgenic mice expressing ovalbumin only in the intestinal epithelium. Moreover, optimal activation of mucosal T cells requires the costimulator B7-1, although this molecule plays a minimal role in lymphoid T-cell activation (Kim *et al.*, 1998). In addition, CD40L expressed by CD8 T cells is important for optimal expansion of CD8 T cells in the LP in response to virus infection (Lefrançois *et al.*, 1999a). These results illustrate that: (1) CD8 T-cell activation results in migration to the intestinal LP and epithelium; (2) secondary activation in the mucosa occurs perhaps upon secondary encounter with antigen; (3) environmental cues in the mucosa, possibly antigen nonspecific, drive T-cell activation even in response to tolerogenic forms of antigen; and (4) costimulatory elements may specifically regulate intestinal T-cell responses. This example of secondary control of mucosal responses holds important implications for generation of effective mucosal vaccines and for induction and control of autoimmune diseases affecting the gastrointestinal system.

Mucosal CD8 responses to infection have also been studied using the adoptive transfer system. Systemic infection of OT-I-transferred mice with a recombinant vesicular stomatitis virus encoding ovalbumin (ova) (VSV-ova) results in rapid and robust expansion of the ova-specific CD8 T cells, with the peak of the expansion phase in the lymphoid tissues ~4 days after infection. However, activated OT-I cells are detectable in the LP and IEL compartments starting at ~day 3 post infection, indicating an ~48–72-hour lag between initial activation of naive T cells and entry of effector cells into the intestinal mucosa. Furthermore, in contrast to the results using soluble antigen, VSV infection results in induction of CTL in secondary lymphoid tissues as well as in the intestinal mucosa, demonstrating that inflammatory signals generated by infection promote effector CD8[+] T-cell induction. By analogy, the induction of CTL in the intestinal mucosa in response to soluble protein could be driven by inflammatory mediators constitutively present in the gut, which may serve to activate mucosal dendritic cells or perhaps activate T cells *via* soluble mediators.

Endogenous CD8 T-cell responses to infection

The advent of MHC tetramers or multimers coupled with the ability to detect cytokine production *ex vivo* provided tools for visualization of antigen-specific CD4 and CD8 T cells throughout an immune response. Because of the generally much greater magnitude of CD8 versus CD4 T-cell responses, and because of the relative ease of production of MHC class I tetramers (Altman *et al.*, 1996), a large literature has developed around the analysis of CD8 T-cell responses to infection. This includes analysis of mucosal immune responses to HIV/SIV, which are covered in detail in another chapter (and for a review, see Douek *et al.*, 2003). In mouse experimental systems, the intestinal mucosal CD8 T-cell response has been characterized to varying degrees following systemic VSV and *Listeria monocytogenes* (LM) infections (Masopust *et al.*, 2001a, b), and oral LM (Pope *et al.*, 2001; Huleatt *et al.*, 2001) and rotavirus infections (Rose *et al.*, 1998; Kuklin *et al.*, 2000). VSV infection results in CD8 T-cell activation followed by migration of effector cells to all non-lymphoid tissues (including lung, liver, kidney, intestinal mucosa, etc.) (Masopust *et al.*, 2001a,b). The magnitude of the response in the LP and IEL compartments is substantially larger than that observed in the spleen, with ~30% of the intestinal CD8 T cells specific for the major immunodominant VSV peptide derived from the nucleoprotein. The peak of the response is also sustained as compared with that detected in the spleen, with the former remaining at apogee for 2 to 3 days versus 1 day in the spleen.

The contraction phase of the response occurs in all tissues but again with distinct kinetics when lymphoid versus non-lymphoid tissues are compared (Masopust *et al.*, 2001a,b). Interestingly, the CD8 T-cell response in the lamina propria and epithelium undergoes a protracted decline, with stable memory populations established only after ~1 month. In parallel with the prolonged contraction phase of the CD8 T-cell response, a sustained effector phase was also evident. Even 20 days after infection with VSV, high levels of antigen-specific lytic activity are detected in the LP (Masopust *et al.*, 2001b). Indeed, even at much later times when memory cell levels are stable, lytic activity remains detectable (see the following section).

The CD8 T-cell response to enteric infection with *Listeria monocytogenes* (LM) largely parallels that observed after systemic infection with some notable differences (Pope *et al.*, 2001; Huleatt *et al.*, 2001). With oral LM infection, bacteria can be detected in the spleen, liver, mesenteric LN (MLN), and intestinal tissue. In contrast, intravenous infection results in infection in the same tissues with the exception of the intestine (Huleatt *et al.*, 2001). Nevertheless, either route of infection generates antigen-specific CD8 and CD4 T cells, which appear in the LP and IEL compartments. Enteric infection appears to induce larger numbers of LM-reactive T cells in the mucosa than does intravenous infection. Moreover, the TCR Vβ repertoire of splenic versus intestinal LM-specific CD8 T cells is distinct (Huleatt *et al.*, 2001), indicating either differential migration or expansion of CD8 T-cell subpopulations. Secondary oral infection with LM also induces a robust CD8 and CD4 T-cell recall response resulting in generation of a greatly increased population of long-term memory cells. The costimulatory requirements for induction of LM-specific CD8 T cells in the LP are distinct from those of splenic CD8 T cells. Thus, CD40 is required to mount an optimal anti-LM LP CD8 T-cell response, whereas absence of CD40 had little effect on the induction of the splenic CD8 T-cell response (Pope *et al.*, 2001). Once again, these data suggest a second level of regulation of primary response induction in which intestinal mucosa-specific regulatory factors come into play. Whether the effects are mediated at the level of migration, APC function or cytokine production remains to be seen. With regard to the latter, it is interesting to note that autocrine IL-2 preferentially regulates the nonlymphoid (including LP) CD8 T-cell response by limiting the magnitude of the expansion phase (D'Souza *et al.*, 2002).

CD8 T-CELL MEMORY IN THE INTESTINAL MUCOSA

The response to a variety of pathogens administered either systemically or enterically results in the generation of antigen-specific memory cells in many tissues, including the intestinal LP (Masopust *et al.*, 2001b; Lefrançois and Masopust, 2002). Enteric rotavirus infection appears to induce memory cells (detected in the spleen), which preferentially express the α4β7 integrin (Rose *et al.*, 1998; Kuklin *et al.*, 2000). By analogy with primary activated CD8 T cells (Lefrançois *et al.*, 1999b), the assumption is that memory cells migrating to the LP utilize the α4β7 integrin to traverse mucosal endothelium, but this remains to be proven. In fact, α4β7 expression by rotavirus memory cells is not required for protection against mucosal infection (Kuklin *et al.*, 2000) although it should be noted that the requirement for α4β7 integrin for migration of primary effectors to the mucosa is not absolute (Lefrançois *et al.*, 1999b; Masopust *et al.*, 2001a). The magnitude of the primary response to oral rotavirus infection is small in comparison with the responses to infection with several other viruses and bacteria, perhaps because of the limited nature of the infection. This has hampered direct identification of rotavirus-specific memory cells in the mucosa. In the case of VSV or LM infection, memory cells are readily detectable in the LP throughout the life of the animal. Interestingly, the presence of CD8 memory cells in the LP is not always an indication that memory cells are present in the epithelium. Thus, in some animals a substantial LP memory cell population in the absence of a memory IEL population has been observed (Masopust *et al.*, 2001a). In addition, LP and IEL memory cells are phenotypically distinct from each other as well as from memory cells in other organs. These results again point up the distinct nature of the LP and IEL compartments with respect to migration and function.

Recent results suggest that two populations of memory CD4 and CD8 T cells exist: central memory cells residing in secondary lymphoid tissue and requiring reactivation, and effector memory cells residing in nonlymphoid tissues with immediate effector function (Sallusto *et al.*, 1999; Reinhardt *et al.*, 2001; Masopust *et al.*, 2001b). This distinction extends to memory cells in the intestinal LP (Masopust *et al.*, 2001b). VSV- or LM-specific LP memory cells are constitutively lytic as are their counterparts in the liver and lung, whereas splenic memory cells are weakly lytic. Although the original distinction in human central and effector memory cells also extended to cytokine production, in the mouse most CD8 memory cells regardless of location produce IFN-γ upon stimulation *in vitro* (Masopust *et al.*,

2001b). Locating effector memory cells in mucosal tissues makes teleologic sense if a rapid, cell-autonomous response is important for an immediate attack against a secondary assault by a pathogen. Whether LP or epithelial memory cells are directly involved in this type of protection remains to be proven.

PATHOGENIC RESPONSES BY MUCOSAL CYTOLYTIC T CELLS

In general, inflammatory bowel diseases are thought to be mediated by dysregulation of CD4 T-cell responses (Strober et al., 2002). However, it remains possible that CD8 T cells are involved at some level and their involvement in other autoimmune diseases is now becoming well established (Liblau et al., 2002). CD8 T cells could be pathogenic themselves via cell-damaging mechanisms including lysis or inflammatory cytokine production, and this likely occurs in the intestinal mucosa during graft-versus-host disease (GVHD). Lytic pathways may include perforin or FAS/FAS-L-mediated destruction of IEC or other cell types. It should also be noted that CD4 T cells can display cytotoxic activity (Williams and Engelhard, 1996), which is in fact regulated by CD8 T cells (Williams and Engelhard, 1997). In at least one model of colitis, CD4 T cells may display lytic activity (Simpson et al., 1998, 2000). Nonetheless, there is reasonable evidence that CD8 T cells may play a role in ulcerative colitis (UC) or Crohn's disease (CD). For example, CTL clones with apparent specificity for colonic epithelial cells can be isolated from UC patients (Yonamine et al., 1999; Sunagawa et al., 2001).

Mouse-based experimental systems have also been employed, and the results further support the possibility that CD8 T cells could play a pathogenic role in inflammatory bowel disease (IBD). Intestinal inflammation is induced when hsp60-specific CD8 T cells are transferred to TCRβ$^{-/-}$ mice, and the inflammation is largely dependent on TNFα receptor expression but, unlike in other IBD models, is not dependent on the presence of bacterial flora (Steinhoff et al., 1999). Interestingly, additional studies suggest that there may be preferential presentation of hsp60-derived peptides (and by analogy other proteins as well) because of tissue-specific antigen processing by 20S proteasomes (Kuckelkorn et al., 2002). If this is the case, then one can envision the production, and perhaps the pathogenic recognition under appropriate circumstances, of organ-specific epitopes by CD8 as well as CD4 T cells.

In another interesting system, CD8 T-cell reactivity with a neoself antigen expressed in enteric glial cells results in their destruction (Cornet et al., 2001). As a result, severe intestinal inflammation characterized by infiltration of CD8 T cells occurs. Importantly, the loss of the enteric glial cell network in this model parallels that observed in intestinal tissue of CD, but not of UC, patients. It is proposed that the loss of glial cells leads to disruption of the epithelial barrier because of alterations in blood vessel permeability (Cornet et al.,

2001). These results provide an excellent example of how indirect effects on intestinal integrity may lead to IBD.

In a model in which a neoself antigen is expressed primarily in intestinal epithelial cells, adoptively transferred antigen-specific CD8 T cells (OT-I) can also mediate small intestinal disease via IEC damage (Vezys et al., 2000). However, triggering disease requires inflammatory signals, which can be provided by nonspecific agents including virus infection or cholera toxin (Vezys and Lefrançois, 2002). In this system, primary T-cell activation occurs in MLN and PP, demonstrating that IEC-derived antigen can gain access to secondary lymphoid tissues perhaps via acquisition of effete IEC by DC and their migration to MLN (Huang et al., 2000). Subsequent to activation, CD8 T-cell migration to the intestinal mucosa occurs followed by apparent in situ expansion. Interestingly, in the absence of inflammation, the OT-I cells isolated from the IEL compartment exhibit potent perforin-dependent lytic activity in vitro but do not cause epithelial injury. However, these cells are poor producers of cytokines unless additional inflammatory signals are provided (Vezys and Lefrançois, 2002). This result suggests that IEC damage in this scenario is mediated through cytokines. Indeed, preliminary results indicate that lymphotoxin and FAS are the important mediators of IEC insult in this model. Although models such as this do not directly demonstrate a role for CD8 T cells in IBD or IBD-like diseases, the findings demonstrate that: (1) presentation of antigen derived from IEC is normally a cross-tolerizing event; (2) products of infection or perhaps of normal bacterial flora can provide secondary signals which under certain circumstances may induce cross-reactive or self-reactive T cells to become pathogenic; and (3) factors either present or lacking in the intestinal epithelium allow "resistance" of IEC to perforin-mediated lysis even in the face of IEC-presented antigen.

SUMMARY AND CONCLUSIONS

The data available at this writing provide ample evidence that intestinal effector CD8 T cells play an important role in protection against mucosal viral and bacterial infections. It is also apparent that tissue-specific regulation of intestinal T-cell responses is mediated at the level of cytokines and costimulation. Questions remain regarding important details of the system, including whether antigen-specific intestinal memory T cells are responsible for rapid protection against secondary infection, and whether these cells constitute a fixed population of memory cells resident in the intestine, distinct from the recirculating pool. With regard to intestinal autoimmune mechanisms, CD8 T cells are likely to play integral roles, largely unappreciated as yet, in pathogenesis as well as perhaps in regulation of intestinal diseases. These areas will provide fertile ground for continued research that will promote the production of more effective vaccines against mucosal pathogens and therapies for amelioration of intestinal disease.

ACKNOWLEDGMENTS

I would like to thank the many members of my laboratory who have contributed to our work described in this chapter. Our studies were supported by grants from NIDDK and NIAID.

REFERENCES

Altman, J. D., Moss, P. A., Goulder, P. J., Barouch, D. H., McHeyzer-Williams, M. G., Bell, J. I., McMichael, A. J., and Davis, M. M. (1996). Phenotypic analysis of antigen-specific T lymphocytes. *Science* 274, 94–96.

Belyakov, I. M., Derby, M. A., Ahlers, J. D., Kelsall, B. L., Earl, P., Moss, B., Strober, W., and Berzofsky, J. A. (1998). Mucosal immunization with HIV-1 peptide vaccine induces mucosal and systemic cytotoxic T lymphocytes and protective immunity in mice against intrarectal recombinant HIV-vaccinia challenge. *Proc. Natl. Acad. Sci. USA* 95, 1709–1714.

Chardes, T., Buzoni-Gatel, D., Lepage, A., Bernard, F., and Bout, D. (1994). *Toxoplasma gondii* oral infection induces specific cytotoxic CD8 α/β(+) Thy-1(+) gut intraepithelial lymphocytes, lytic for parasite-infected enterocytes. *J. Immunol.* 153, 4596–4603.

Cornet, A., Savidge, T. C., Cabarrocas, J., Deng, W. L., Colombel, J. F., Lassmann, H., Desreumaux, P., and Liblau, R. S. (2001). Enterocolitis induced by autoimmune targeting of enteric glial cells: A possible mechanism in Crohn's disease? *Proc. Natl. Acad. Sci. USA* 98, 13306–13311.

Cuff, C. F., Cebra, C. K., Rubin, D. H., and Cebra, J. J. (1993). Developmental relationship between cytotoxic α/β T cell receptor-positive intraepithelial lymphocytes and Peyer's patch lymphocytes. *Eur. J. Immunol.* 23, 1333–1339.

Douek, D. C., Picker, L. J., and Koup, R. A. (2003). T cell dynamics in HIV-1 infection. *Annu. Rev. Immunol.* 21, 265–304.

D'Souza, W. N., Schluns, K. S., Masopust, D., and Lefrançois, L. (2002). Essential role for IL-2 in the regulation of antiviral extralymphoid CD8 T cell responses. *J. Immunol.* 168, 5566–5572.

Emoto, M., Neuhaus, O., Emoto, Y., and Kaufmann, S. H. (1996). Influence of β2-microglobulin expression on γ interferon secretion and target cell lysis by intraepithelial lymphocytes during intestinal *Listeria monocytogenes* infection. *Infect. Immun.* 64, 569–575.

Fichtelius, K. E. (1968). The gut epithelium—a first level lymphoid organ? *Exp. Cell. Res.* 49, 87–104.

Goodman, T. and Lefrançois, L. (1989). Intraepithelial lymphocytes. Anatomical site, not T cell receptor form, dictates phenotype and function. *J. Exp. Med.* 170, 1569–1581.

Gramzinski, R. A., Adams, E., Gross, J. A., Goodman, T. G., Allison, J. P., and Lefrançois, L. (1993). T cell receptor-triggered activation of intraepithelial lymphocytes *in vitro*. *Int. Immunol.* 5, 145–153.

Guy-Grand, D., Griscelli, C., and Vassalli, P. (1978). The mouse gut T lymphocyte, a novel type of T cell. Nature, origin, and traffic in mice in normal and graft-versus-host conditions. *J. Exp. Med.* 148, 1661–1677.

Huang, F-P., Platt, N., Wykes, M., Major, J. R., Powell, T. J., Jenkins, C. D., and MacPherson, G. G. (2000). A discrete subpopulation of dendritic cells transports apoptotic intestinal epithelial cells to T cell areas of mesenteric lymph nodes. *J. Exp. Med.* 191, 435–444.

Huleatt, J. W., Pilip, I., Kerksiek, K., and Pamer, E. G. (2001). Intestinal and splenic T cell responses to enteric *Listeria monocytogenes* infection: Distinct repertoires of responding CD8 T lymphocytes. *J. Immunol.* 166, 4065–4073.

Imaoka, A., Matsumoto, S., Setoyama, H., Okada, Y., and Umesaki, Y. (1996). Proliferative recruitment of intestinal intraepithelial lymphocytes after microbial colonization of germ-free mice. *Eur. J. Immunol.* 26, 945–948.

Ishikawa, H., Li, V., Abeliovich, A., Yamamoto, S., Kaufmann, S. H., and Tonegawa, S. (1993). Cytotoxic and interferon γ-producing activ-ities of γδ T cells in the mouse intestinal epithelium are strain dependent. *Proc. Natl. Acad. Sci. USA* 90, 8204–8208.

Kawaguchi, M., Nanno, M., Umesaki, Y., Matsumoto, S., Okada, Y., Cai, Z., Shimamura, T., Matsuoka, Y., Ohwaki, M., and Ishikawa, H. (1993). Cytolytic activity of intestinal intraepithelial lymphocytes in germ-free mice is strain dependent and determined by T cells expressing γδ-T-cell antigen receptors. *Proc. Natl. Acad. Sci. USA* 90, 8591–8594.

Kawaguchi-Miyashita, M., Shimizu, K., Nanno, M., Shimada, S., Watanabe, T., Koga, Y., Matsuoka, Y., Ishikawa, H., Hashimoto, K., and Ohwaki, M. (1996). Development and cytolytic function of intestinal intraepithelial T lymphocytes in antigen-minimized mice. *Immunology* 89, 268–273.

Kearney, E. R., Pape, K. A., Loh, D. Y., and Jenkins, M. K. (1994). Visualization of peptide-specific T cell immunity and peripheral tolerance induction *in vivo*. *Immunity* 1, 327–339.

Kim, S. K., Reed, D. S., Heath, W. R., Carbone, F., and Lefrançois, L. (1997). Activation and migration of CD8 T cells in the intestinal mucosa. *J. Immunol.* 159, 4295–4306.

Kim, S. K., Reed, D. S., Olson, S., Schnell, M. J., Rose, J. K., Morton, P. A., and Lefrançois, L. (1998). Generation of mucosal cytotoxic T cells against soluble protein by tissue-specific environmental and costimulatory signals. *Proc. Natl. Acad. Sci. USA* 95, 10814–10819.

Kim, S. K., Schluns, K. S., and Lefrançois, L. (1999). Induction and visualization of mucosal memory CD8 T cells following systemic virus infection. *J. Immunol.* 163, 4125–4132.

Kuckelkorn, U., Ruppert, T., Strehl, B., Jungblut, P. R., Zimny-Arndt, U., Lamer, S., Prinz, I., Drung, I., Kloetzel, P. M., Kaufmann, S. H., and Steinhoff, U. (2002). Link between organ-specific antigen processing by 20S proteasomes and CD8(+) T cell-mediated autoimmunity. *J. Exp. Med.* 195, 983–990.

Kuklin, N. A., Rott, L., Darling, J., Campbell, J. J., Franco, M., Feng, N., Muller, W., Wagner, N., Altman, J., Butcher, E. C., and Greenberg, H. B. (2000). α(4)β(7) independent pathway for CD8(+) T cell-mediated intestinal immunity to rotavirus. *J. Clin. Invest.* 106, 1541–1552.

Lefrançois, L. (1991). Phenotypic complexity of intraepithelial lymphocytes of the small intestine. *J. Immunol.* 147, 1746–1751.

Lefrançois, L. and Goodman, T. (1989). *In vivo* modulation of cytolytic activity and Thy-1 expression in TCR-γδ+ intraepithelial lymphocytes. *Science* 243, 1716–1718.

Lefrançois, L. and Masopust, D. (2002). T cell immunity in lymphoid and non-lymphoid tissues. *Curr. Opin. Immunol.* 14, 503–508.

Lefrançois, L., Olson, S., and Masopust, D. (1999a). A critical role for CD40-CD40 ligand interactions in amplification of the mucosal CD8 T cell response. *J. Exp. Med.* 190, 1275–1284.

Lefrançois, L., Parker, C. M., Olson, S., Muller, W., Wagner, N., Schon, M.P., and Puddington, L. (1999b). The role of β7 integrins in CD8 T cell trafficking during an antiviral immune response. *J. Exp. Med.* 189, 1631–1638.

Lefrançois, L. and Puddington, L. (1995). Extrathymic intestinal T-cell development: Virtual reality? *Immunol. Today* 16, 16–21.

Liblau, R. S., Wong, F. S., Mars, L. T., and Santamaria, P. (2002). Autoreactive CD8 T cells in organ-specific autoimmunity: Emerging targets for therapeutic intervention. *Immunity* 17, 1–6.

London, S. D., Cebra, J. J., and Rubin, D. H. (1989). Intraepithelial lymphocytes contain virus-specific, MHC-restricted cytotoxic cell precursors after gut mucosal immunization with reovirus serotype 1/Lang. *Reg. Immunol.* 2, 98–102.

Lundqvist, C., Melgar, S., Yeung, M. M., Hammarstrom, S., and Hammarstrom, M. L. (1996). Intraepithelial lymphocytes in human gut have lytic potential and a cytokine profile that suggest T helper 1 and cytotoxic functions. *J. Immunol.* 157, 1926–1934.

Masopust, D., Jiang, J., Shen, H., and Lefrançois, L. (2001a). Direct analysis of the dynamics of the intestinal mucosa CD8 T cell response to systemic virus infection. *J. Immunol.* 166, 2348–2356.

Masopust, D., Vezys, V., Marzo, A. L., and Lefrançois, L. (2001b). Preferential localization of effector memory cells in nonlymphoid tissue. *Science* 291, 2413–2417.

Melgar, S., Bas, A., Hammarstrom, S., and Hammarstrom, M. L. (2002). Human small intestinal mucosa harbours a small population of cytolytically active CD8$^+$ αβ T lymphocytes. *Immunology* 106, 476–485.

Mosley, R. L., Whetsell, M., and Klein, J. R. (1991). Proliferative properties of murine intestinal intraepithelial lymphocytes (IEL): IEL expressing TCRαβ or TCR γδ are largely unresponsive to proliferative signals mediated via conventional stimulation of the CD3-TCR complex. *Int. Immunol.* 3, 563–569.

Mowat, A. M., MacKenzie, S., Baca, M. E., Felstein, M. V., and Parrott, D. M. (1986). Functional characteristics of intraepithelial lymphocytes from mouse small intestine. II. *In vivo* and *in vitro* responses of intraepithelial lymphocytes to mitogenic and allogeneic stimuli. *Immunology* 58, 627–634.

Mowat, A. M. and Viney, J. L. (1997). The anatomical basis of intestinal immunity. *Immunol. Rev.* 156, 145–166.

Offit, P. A., Cunningham, S. L., and Dudzik, K. I. (1991). Memory and distribution of virus-specific cytotoxic T lymphocytes (CTLs) and CTL precursors after rotavirus infection. *J. Virol.* 65, 1318–1324.

Offit, P. A. and Dudzik, K. I. (1989). Rotavirus-specific cytotoxic T lymphocytes appear at the intestinal mucosal surface after rotavirus infection. *J. Virol.* 63, 3507–3512.

Okada, Y., Setoyama, H., Matsumoto, S., Imaoka, A., Nanno, M., Kawaguchi, M., and Umesaki, Y. (1994). Effects of fecal microorganisms and their chloroform-resistant variants derived from mice, rats, and humans on immunological and physiological characteristics of the intestines of ex-germfree mice. *Infect. Immun.* 62, 5442–5446.

Parrott, D. M., Tait, C., MacKenzie, S., Mowat, A. M., Davies, M. D., and Micklem, H. S. (1983). Analysis of the effector functions of different populations of mucosal lymphocytes. *Ann. N. Y. Acad. Sci.* 409, 307–320.

Pope, C., Kim, S.-K., Marzo, A., Masopust, D., Williams, K., Jiang, J., Shen, H., and Lefrançois, L. (2001). Organ-specific regulation of the CD8 T cell response to *Listeria monocytogenes* infection. *J. Immunol.* 166, 3402–3409.

Reinhardt, R. L., Khoruts, A., Merica, R., Zell, T., and Jenkins, M. K. (2001). Visualizing the generation of memory CD4 T cells in the whole body. *Nature* 410, 101–105.

Rose, J. R., Williams, M. B., Rott, L. S., Butcher, E. C., and Greenberg, H. B. (1998). Expression of the mucosal homing receptor α4β7 correlates with the ability of CD8$^+$ memory T cells to clear rotavirus infection. *J. Virol.* 72, 726–730.

Sallusto, F., Lenig, D., Forster, R., Lipp, M., and Lanzavecchia, A. (1999). Two subsets of memory T lymphocytes with distinct homing potentials and effector functions. *Nature* 401, 708–712.

Simpson, S. J., de Jong, Y. P., Comiskey, M., and Terhorst, C. (2000). Pathways of T cell pathology in models of chronic intestinal inflammation. *Int. Rev. Immunol.* 19, 1–37.

Simpson, S. J., de Jong, Y. P., Shah, S. A., Comiskey, M., Wang, B., Spielman, J. A., Podack, E. R., Mizoguchi, E., Bhan, A. K., and Terhorst, C. (1998). Consequences of Fas-ligand and perforin

expression by colon T cells in a mouse model of inflammatory bowel disease. *Gastroenterology* 115, 849–855.

Steinhoff, U., Brinkmann, V., Klemm, U., Aichele, P., Seiler, P., Brandt, U., Bland, P. W., Prinz, I., Zugel, U., and Kaufmann, S. H. (1999). Autoimmune intestinal pathology induced by hsp60-specific CD8 T cells. *Immunity* 11, 349–358.

Strober, W., Fuss, I. J., and Blumberg, R. S. (2002). The immunology of mucosal models of inflammation. *Annu. Rev. Immunol.* 20, 495–549.

Sunagawa, T., Yonamine, Y., Kinjo, F., Watanabe, M., Hibi, T., and Saito, A. (2001). HLA class-I-restricted and colon-specific cytotoxic T cells from lamina propria lymphocytes of patients with ulcerative colitis. *J. Clin. Immunol.* 21, 381–389.

Svensson, M., Marsal, J., Ericsson, A., Carramolino, L., Broden, T., Marquez, G., and Agace, W. W. (2002). CCL25 mediates the localization of recently activated CD8αβ(+) lymphocytes to the small-intestinal mucosa. *J. Clin. Invest.* 110, 1113–1121.

Sydora, B. C., Mixter, P. F., Holcombe, H. R., Eghtesady, P., Williams, K., Amaral, M. C., Nel, A., and Kronenberg, M. (1993). Intestinal intraepithelial lymphocytes are activated and cytolytic but do not proliferate as well as other T cells in response to mitogenic signals. *J. Immunol.* 150, 2179–2191.

Umesaki, Y., Okada, Y., Matsumoto, S., Imaoka, A., and Setoyama, H. (1995). Segmented filamentous bacteria are indigenous intestinal bacteria that activate intraepithelial lymphocytes and induce MHC class II molecules and fucosyl asialo GM1 glycolipids on the small intestinal epithelial cells in the ex-germ-free mouse. *Microbiol. Immunol.* 39, 555–562.

Vezys, V. and Lefrançois, L. (2002). Cutting edge: Inflammatory signals drive organ-specific autoimmunity to normally cross-tolerizing endogenous antigen. *J. Immunol.* 169, 6677–6680.

Vezys, V., Olson, S., and Lefrançois, L. (2000). Expression of intestine-specific antigen reveals novel pathways of CD8 T cell tolerance induction. *Immunity* 12, 505–514.

Wang, H. C., Zhou, Q., Dragoo, J., and Klein, J. R. (2002). Most murine CD8$^+$ intestinal intraepithelial lymphocytes are partially but not fully activated T cells. *J. Immunol.* 169, 4717–4722.

Williams, N. S. and Engelhard, V. H. (1996). Identification of a population of CD4$^+$ CTL that utilizes a perforin-rather than a Fas ligand-dependent cytotoxic mechanism. *J. Immunol.* 156, 153–159.

Williams, N. S. and Engelhard, V. H. (1997). Perforin-dependent cytotoxic activity and lymphokine secretion by CD4$^+$ T cells are regulated by CD8$^+$ T cells. *J. Immunol.* 159, 2091–2099.

Yamamoto, S., Russ, F., Teixeira, H. C., Conradt, P., and Kaufmann, S. H. (1993). *Listeria monocytogenes*-induced γ interferon secretion by intestinal intraepithelial γ/δ T lymphocytes. *Infect. Immun.* 61, 2154–2161.

Yonamine, Y., Watanabe, M., Kinjo, F., and Hibi, T. (1999). Generation of MHC class I-restricted cytotoxic T cell lines and clones against colonic epithelial cells from ulcerative colitis. *J. Clin. Immunol.* 19, 77–85.

Development, Function, and Specificity of Intestinal Intraepithelial Lymphocytes

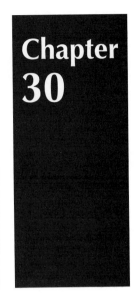

Chapter
30

Mitchell Kronenberg and Hilde Cheroutre

La Jolla Institute for Allergy & Immunology, San Diego, California

Intestinal intraepithelial lymphocytes (IEL) are a distinctive population of predominantly T lymphocytes dispersed as single cells among the luminal epithelial cells. Although they are located at the basolateral side of the epithelium, they are likely to be exposed to a diverse range of food-derived and bacterial antigens. IEL therefore are located at the front lines between the interior of the body and the antigen-rich external world. Regardless of the species analyzed, or the section of the intestine they were obtained from, IEL exhibit several distinguishing characteristics, including the expression of activation markers, an oligoclonal repertoire of T-cell antigen receptors (TCRs), and particularly in the small intestine, a predominance of CD8 T cells. Despite this, IEL are heterogeneous with regard to phenotype, and they contain subpopulations with diverse functions. Immune memory provides a unifying hypothesis for understanding all subpopulations of IEL, although their memory phenotype and behavior may be acquired centrally in the thymus, as well as by more conventional means in the periphery. Here we summarize the properties and functions of IEL and highlight the ways in which they resemble and differ from memory and other T cells of the systemic immune system.

SUBSETS OF IEL IDENTIFIED BY PHENOTYPE

Intraepithelial lymphocytes (IELs) are found along the length of the digestive tract (Wang *et al.*, 1994) and in other epithelia (Boyaka *et al.*, 2000; Gould *et al.*, 2001). IEL are most numerous in the intestine, however, and in this chapter we focus our discussion on intestinal IEL. The presence of lymphocytes in the intestine epithelium has been recognized for decades (Fichtelius, 1968; Fichtelius *et al.*, 1968), but their contemporary study began in the 1980s with the availability of monoclonal antibodies that could identify T-cell subpopulations (Cerf-Bensussan *et al.*, 1985; Dillon and MacDonald,

1986; Goodman and Lefrancois, 1988; Klein *et al.*, 1985). By immunohistology there is at least one IEL for every 10 epithelial cells (Ferguson, 1977; Mysorekar *et al.*, 2002), making IEL among the most numerous T cells. Despite this, less than 5×10^6 IEL can be obtained in suspension from the intestine epithelium of mice (Camerini *et al.*, 1993), substantially less than the number of T cells that can be obtained from a spleen.

IEL of the mouse small intestine have been the most thoroughly studied population (reviewed in Beagley and Husband, 1998; Cheroutre, 2004; Guy-Grand and Vassalli, 1993; Hayday *et al.*, 2001; Lefrancois *et al.*, 1997). The majority express CD8, and most of them appear to be activated, as evidenced by expression of CD69, cytolytic activity (Cerf-Bensussan *et al.*, 1985; Goodman and Lefrancois, 1989) and the presence of activated MAP kinases (Sydora *et al.*, 1993). IEL are not predominantly CD25 (IL-2 receptor α chain) positive (Wang *et al.*, 2002), although they express CD122, the IL-2Rβ chain. The expression of other activation markers is not consistently observed (Wang *et al.*, 2002).

IEL of the mouse small intestine can be divided into four categories based upon TCR and coreceptor expression (**Table 30.1**). Category I are IEL that express CD8$\alpha\beta$ heterodimers, which are characteristic of cells that react to peptides presented by MHC class I molecules. Less numerous are the category II cells, which are $\alpha\beta$ TCR$^+$ IEL that express CD4, typical of MHC class II reactive lymphocytes. Additionally, there are substantial numbers of $\alpha\beta$ TCR$^+$ IEL that do not express either typical coreceptor (category III), and a very substantial representation of $\gamma\delta$ TCR$^+$ lymphocytes (category IV).

A common feature of all mouse small intestine IEL subsets is their expression of CD8$\alpha\alpha$ homodimers. Most of the category III and IV IEL, including the great majority of the $\gamma\delta$ TCR$^+$ lymphocytes and a major subset of $\alpha\beta$ TCR$^+$ IEL, express CD$\alpha\alpha$ exclusively (Guy-Grand *et al.*, 1994). CD8$\alpha\alpha$ homodimers are also expressed, however, by some CD4$^+$

Table 30.1. Populations of Mouse Intestinal IEL

Category	Phenotype	TCR Repertoire	Specificity	Function
I	αβ TCR⁺ CD8αβ (CD8αα)	Oligoclonal	Peptides presented by MHC class I	Effector/memory Host protection
II	αβ TCR⁺ CD4 (CD8αα)	Oligoclonal (?)	Peptides presented by MHC class II	Effector/memory Host protection
III	αβTCR⁺ DN (CD8αα)	Oligoclonal	?? (self–reactive)	Natural memory: regulation of inflammation in the intestine (?)
IV	γδ TCR⁺ DN (CD8αα)	Restricted V regions, diverse CDR3	MICA (human) ?? (mouse)	Natural memory: Epithelial maintenance (?)

DN, CD4 and CD8αβ double negative. (CD8αα), variable percentages, usually the majority, of each population shown express CD8αα homodimers.

IEL (Mosley *et al.*, 1990), and they are coexpressed by the majority of the CD8αβ⁺ IEL (Leishman *et al.*, 2001).

In a recent review, IEL were divided into two subsets (Hayday *et al.*, 2001). The type a IEL correspond to categories I and II here as they express one of the typical coreceptors. The type b IEL include the more unconventional αβ TCR⁺ or γδ TCR⁺ lymphocytes of categories III and IV. This is a very reasonable distinction, because both αβ TCR⁺ CD8αα and γδ TCR⁺ IEL have a greatly reduced expression of a number of surface proteins characteristic of conventional T cells, including Thy-1 (Klein, 1986), CD28 (Ohteki and MacDonald, 1993), and CD2 (Van Houten *et al.*, 1993). Furthermore, the analysis of the gene expression profiles of αβ TCR⁺ CD8αα IEL and γδ TCR⁺ CD8αα IEL demonstrated a high degree of similarity (Pennington *et al.*, 2003). There are, however, some important differences that have been reported to distinguish these two CD8αα expressing cell populations (Hayday *et al.*, 2001). These include the secretion of keratinocyte growth factor (KGF) by γδ TCR⁺ IEL (Boismenu and Havran, 1994), the dependence of the αβTCR⁺ CD8αα subset on β2m expression (Correa *et al.*, 1992), and their ability to prevent colitis (Poussier *et al.*, 2002).

IEL in the mouse may not closely resemble those in humans. As for peripheral T cells, the ratio of γδ to αβ TCRs in IEL also varies among species. In humans, TCRγδ⁺ IEL are a relatively small (~10%) percentage (Faure *et al.*, 1988), although their numbers increase significantly during celic disease (Spencer *et al.*, 1991). Similarly, αβ TCR⁺ CD8αα⁺ IEL are infrequent in humans, although they are more prevalent during the fetal period. Humans may be exceptional, because αβ TCR⁺ CD8αα⁺ IEL are abundant in most other species (Sonea *et al.*, 2000; Torres-Nagel *et al.*, 1992; Tregaskes *et al.*, 1995; Tschetter *et al.*, 1998). The mouse–human interspecies comparison is complicated by several factors, including the source of the IEL. Most analyses of human IEL used material derived from the colon,

whereas studies in mice focused on the small intestine. However, we (Camerini *et al.*, 1993) and subsequently several other groups (Beagley *et al.*, 1995; Boll *et al.*, 1995; Ibraghimov and Lynch, 1994) showed that mouse IEL from the large intestine also have a decreased representation of the category III and IV subsets. There is even evidence for regional variation in the mouse small intestine, with the ileum having a reduced representation of αβ TCR⁺ CD8αα IEL (Suzuki *et al.*, 2000a; Suzuki *et al.*, 2000b). Therefore, some of the differences between species may depend on the different locations from which the IEL were collected, as well as the age of the subjects, diet, and exposure to microbes.

DEVELOPMENTAL ORIGIN OF IEL

Lymphocyte precursors in the intestine

Many studies of IEL have been driven by the underlying hypothesis that IEL are entirely different from mainstream T lymphocytes. This hypothesis is highlighted by the widely held belief that IEL subpopulations differentiate by an extra thymic pathway in the intestine (Poussier *et al.*, 1992; Rocha *et al.*, 1992a). There is evidence for lymphopoiesis of B cells in mucosal-associated lymphoid tissues of the sheep (Miyasaka *et al.*, 1984) and chicken (Glick and Whatley, 1967), but the idea that the single layer of epithelium in the intestine can direct mucosal T-cell development is striking. It has been known for years, however, that activated T-cell blasts from the systemic immune system can home to the intestine (Guy-Grand *et al.*, 1978; Sprent and Miller, 1972), providing a connection between systemic immunity and IEL, and that the conventional T cells that take residence there exhibit many of the specialized properties of IEL such as the expression of CD8αα (Morrissey *et al.*, 1995), activation antigens, and the exhibition of cytolytic activity (Camerini *et al.*, 1998).

Interestingly, there is evidence for lymphocyte precursor activity in the intestine. In an immunohistochemical search for anatomical sites of lymphopoiesis within the gut, small clusters of lymphoid precursors called cryptopatches (CP) were discovered within the lamina propria adjacent to the epithelial crypts in the mouse small intestine (Saito et al., 1998). Similar structures in other species, however, have not been described (Lefrancois and Puddington, 1998). In congenitally athymic (nu/nu) nude mice, which have a mutation in the winged-helix transcription factor Whn required for differentiation of thymic epithelial cells (Nehls et al., 1994), none of these CP clusters contains CD3+ TCR+ cells (Saito et al., 1998), there is relatively little cell turnover in CP, and very few CP cells express RAG mRNA (Lambolez et al., 2002). These data do not fit the properties that might be expected of a major site of extrathymic T-cell differentiation, but they do not rule it out. CP lin− cells express GATA-2, a transcription factor found in pluripotent hematopoietic progenitor cells (Tsai et al., 1994), and it is also possible that CP cells are predominantly precursors of other hematopoietic cells.

In addition to CP cells, precursor activity also may be found in IEL, which in mice express mRNA for pre-Tα (Bruno et al., 1995), although it is present in very few cells (Lambolez et al., 2002). mRNA for RAG-1 and -2 could be isolated from human IEL (Lynch et al., 1995) although terminal deoxynucleotidyl transferase was undetectable (Taplin et al., 1996). Human fetal intestine contains T cells in the LP and epithelium beginning from 12 to 14 weeks gestation (Spencer et al., 1986), but the fetal thymus is already exporting T cells at this stage. This stands in contrast to mouse IEL, which develop in the postnatal period, with the biggest population increases around the time of weaning (Kuo et al., 2001; Manzano et al., 2002). The majority of fetal human IEL express an activated phenotype, and unlike adult IEL, they are actively proliferating (Howie et al., 1998). It is highly unlikely that IEL in the fetal intestine have migrated there as effectors in response to non-self antigens. Interestingly, diverse TCR β gene transcripts have been found in fetal IEL, but few α gene transcripts (Koningsberger et al., 1997), suggesting that fetal human IEL are differentiating T lymphocytes that have rearranged TCRβ but not TCRα genes. Precursor activity in IEL also could be demonstrated functionally in mice. Coculture of CD3− CD8− Ig− CD45+ IEL in reaggregate cultures with newborn thymic stromal cells, which had been depleted of CD45+ thymocytes, led to the generation of αβ TCR+ double positive (DP) cells and single positive (SP) CD4+ cells and CD8αβ+ cells (Woodward and Jenkinson, 2001).

All IEL subsets can be obtained from the thymus

A controversial issue is the extent to which the lymphocyte precursors in the intestine can make a significant, extrathymic contribution to the mature IEL population in normal mice. The results from several experiments provide a strong challenge to the extrathymic pathway. First, neonatal thymectomy of mice causes a drastic decrease in all IEL subpopulations (Lin et al., 1995). Second, nude mice have a greatly reduced αβ TCR+ IEL population, although there is a residual γδ TCR+ IEL population (Yoshikai et al., 1986). Nude rats have greatly reduced IEL numbers (Helgeland et al., 1997) and chicken IEL are thymus derived (Dunon et al., 1993a,b; Imhof et al., 2000). Additionally, early thymectomy results in decreased IEL in Xenopus (Horton et al., 1998). Therefore, the extra thymic pathway is not phylogenetically conserved. Third, the putative extrathymic category III and IV CD8αα+ mouse IEL can originate from thymic transplants (Leishman et al., 2002; Lin et al., 1996), and the evidence indicates that the αβ TCR+ CD8αα cells require positive selection in the thymus (see the section, Positive Selection of TCRαβ+ CD8αα IEL Based Upon Self-Reactivity) (Leishman et al., 2002).

By contrast with these results, transfer of precursors obtained from either CP (Saito et al., 1998; Suzuki et al., 2000c), bone marrow, or fetal liver (Poussier et al., 1992; Rocha et al., 1992b) to athymic mice could give rise to several IEL subpopulations, and not necessarily just the CD8αα cells. In nearly all of these experiments, however, the recipients were irradiated. When precursors were transferred into thymectomized c-kit mutant mice, which because of reduced hematopoiesis did not require irradiation for engraftment of the donor cells, most of the IEL that were generated were γδ TCR+ cells (Lefrancois and Olson, 1997), similar to the observations made with nude mice.

A unifying hypothesis for thymic and extrathymic IEL generation

The results from most experiments support the hypothesis that the positive selection of αβ TCR+ IEL is thymus dependent in normal mice. The requirement of γδ TCR+ IEL for a functional thymus is much less clearly established, and in fact, the requirement for the positive selection of γδ TCR+ T cells is controversial (Guehler et al., 1999; Schweighoffer and Fowlkes, 1996). The data support the hypothesis that the intestine epithelium and/or CP have lymphocyte precursor activity, and in the absence of a thymus and under lymphopenic conditions, they can support the differentiation of some lymphocytes. This activity may not be so different, however, from the reported activity of bone marrow precursors (Dejbakhsh-Jones et al., 1995) and liver mononuclear cells (Shimizu et al., 1999) to give rise to extrathymic T cells. In each of these organs, however, it remains to be proven that the extrathymic TCR+ lymphocytes are functional, and that they have been subjected to positive selection based upon the specificity of their αβ TCRs, a process that probably only occurs efficiently in the thymus.

The results from the recent analysis of transgenic mice, which carry a green fluorescent protein reporter gene driven by the RAG-2 promoter, are consistent with the views outlined above (Guy-Grand et al., 2003). Cells expressing high levels of GFP in these mice indicate recent transcription of RAG-2, reflecting recent TCR or Ig gene rearrangements in developing cells (Yu *et al.*, 1999). Using this reporter system, it was demonstrated that athymic mice had recent antigen receptor gene rearrangements predominantly in the mesenteric lymph nodes and Peyer's patches, but not in CP (Guy-Grand *et al.*, 2003). Interestingly, this pathway was totally suppressed in euthymic mice, except under conditions of severe lymphopenia. Nevertheless, in euthymic TCRβ$^{-/-}$ mice, which have only mature γδ T cells, GFP$^+$ cells were still present (Guy-Grand *et al.*, 2003). This indicated that the lack of extrathymic T-cell development in euthymic mice is not due merely to the presence of a thymus, but rather that the presence of the thymus-derived TCRαβ T cells themselves actively downmodulated T lymphopoiesis in the intestine, as it may do in other sites as well.

POSITIVE SELECTION OF TCRαβ$^+$ CD8αα IEL BASED UPON SELF-REACTIVITY

The naive repertoire of αβ TCRs expressed in the periphery is imprinted by the interactions of TCRs with complexes of self-peptide plus MHC during positive selection in the thymus (Savage and Davis, 2001). The affinity/avidity-based model for selection proposes that TCR signal strength is central to the outcome of thymic selection, with a relatively weak TCR signal resulting in positive selection, and strong TCR-mediated signals leading to deletion or negative selection. Although similar rules may hold true for the αβ TCR CD8αα IEL subset, they are governed by a different avidity cutoff than the conventional T cells. In mice bearing an endogenous retroviral superantigen encoded by the Mtv-7 provirus, T cells expressing Mtv7 reactive TCR β chains (Vβ6, Vβ8.1, or Vβ11) are deleted from the conventional repertoire. These TCRs are present, however, in αβ TCR$^+$ CD8αα IEL (Rocha *et al.*, 1991). Similar results were obtained in several other studies (Croitoru *et al.*, 1994; Murosaki *et al.*, 1991; Poussier *et al.*, 1992) **(Table 30.2)**.

Potentially self-reactive T cells were also found in multiple experimental systems in which TCR transgenic mice also express the cognate antigen recognized by that TCR transgene (Cruz *et al.*, 1998; Guehler *et al.*, 1996; Leishman *et al.*, 2002; Levelt *et al.*, 1999; Podd *et al.*, 2001; Poussier *et al.*, 1992; Rocha *et al.*, 1992b) (see Table 30.2). The generation of αβ TCR$^+$ CD8αα IEL, when conventional αβ TCR$^+$ T cells could not develop and were mostly deleted, clearly demonstrated the distinct selection requirements for the category III IEL. The ratio of category III αβ TCR$^+$ CD8αα IEL to CD8β$^+$ or category I IEL expressing the same TCR transgene depended upon the affinity or avidity for the peptide/MHC complex (Table 30.2). For example, H-Y TCR transgenic male mice had a higher percentage of category III IEL when they were homozygous for the D^b molecule that presents the H-Y self-peptide than when the mice were heterozygous for D^b (Podd *et al.*, 2001). Similarly, the percentage of category III IEL was increased in the flu-specific F5 TCR transgenic system when the mice also expressed a transgene encoding a high-affinity agonist as opposed to an antagonist peptide (Levelt *et al.*, 1999).

Thymus transplants demonstrated that the αβ TCR CD8αα IEL originated most from a thymus in which the self-agonist peptide also is expressed (Leishman *et al.*, 2002). For example, transplants of the thymus tissue from male antigen-specific H-Y TCR transgenic mice generated αβ TCR CD8αα IEL more effectively when the donor tissue was male (antigen expressing) than when it was female (Leishman *et al.*, 2002). Analysis of male H-Y TCR transgenic mice crossed to the nude mutation likewise indicated that the potentially self-reactive H-Y TCR$^+$ CD8αα IEL required a thymus (Guy-Grand *et al.*, 2001). The transplant data indicated that not only can αβ TCR$^+$ CD8αα IEL derive from thymus tissue, but that they require recognition of a self-agonist peptide in the thymus. Consistent with this, αβ TCR CD8αα thymocytes could be generated by fetal thymic organ culture dosed with agonist peptides (Barnden *et al.*, 1997; Chidgey and Boyd, 1998). Cells with this phenotype are rare in the intact thymus, however, and it remains uncertain if CD8αα expression normally is induced after emigration from the thymus, or if thymocytes with this phenotype never reach substantial numbers because they are exported from the thymus rapidly *in vivo*. Positive selection of CD4$^+$ CD25$^+$ regulatory T cells (Jordan *et al.*, 2001) and NKT cells (Bendelac, 1995; Capone *et al.*, 2001; Legendre *et al.*, 1999) also may depend upon the relatively high affinity recognition of self-agonists. This type of selection might enable the immune system to make use of T cells that recognize self-antigens, for specialized functions.

MIGRATION OF LYMPHOCYTES TO THE INTESTINE

Conditioning by dendritic cells

The T cells in the intestine epithelium have some characteristics of antigen-experienced lymphocytes, a property they share with T lymphocytes in other nonlymphoid tissues such as the liver and lung. This antigen-experienced phenotype might be acquired by peripheral exposure to antigens, but in other cases it might be acquired during development in the thymus (αβ TCR$^+$ CD8αα T cells) or even by development in extrathymic sites (possibly γδ TCR$^+$ IEL). Recently, it has been shown that culture with dendritic cells (DCs) from mucosal sites conditions CD8 T cells for migration to the intestine using short-term homing assays, compared to culture with DCs from other sites. CD8 T cells cultured with Peyer's patch or mesenteric lymph node DC were shown to express higher levels of gut-homing integrins and chemokine receptors (Johansson-Lindbom *et al.*, 2003; Mora *et al.*, 2003; Stagg *et al.*, 2002), and those cultured with Peyer's patch DC migrated more efficiently in response to CCL25, a chemokine that promotes homing to the small intestine. Antigenic stimulation in the presence of Peyer's patch DC led to preferential homing to the small but not the large intestine (Mora *et al.*, 2003). The molecular basis for this DC conditioning is not known, but it has been shown previously that myeloid DC from Peyer's patches have distinct properties such as the ability to produce IL-10 following stimulation as well as

Table 30.2. Self–Reactive T Cells That Give Rise to αβ TCR⁺ CD8αα IEL

TCR Specificity	Self–Antigen	Peripheral Cells	IEL Phenotype	Comments	References
Vβ3, Vβ6, Vβ8.1, Vβ11	Mtv (endogenous retroviruses)	Majority deleted	CD8αα		Rocha et al., 1991; Murosaki et al., 1991; Poussier et al., 1992; Croitoru et al., 1994
Transgene H–Y/D^b	Male D^b mice	Aberrant CD8^{low} T cells present	CD8αα	Female mice have few IEL	Poussier et al., 1992; Rocha et al., 1992; Cruz et al., 1998; Leishmann et al., 2002
Transgene H–Y/D^b	Male D^b/D^d heterozygotes	CD8⁺ cells present	CD8αβ and CD8αα		Podd et al., 2001
Transgene 2C (L^d alloreactive)	L^d expressing mice	Deleted	CD8αα some DN	Th2 cytokine deviation	Guehler et al., 1996
F5 (flu peptide + D^b)	NP68 flu antigen transgene	Deleted	CD8αα some DN	Antigen is a strong agonist	Levelt et al., 1999
F5 (flu peptide + D^b)	NP34 antigen transgene	Failure of positive selection	CD8αβ and CD8αα	Antigen is an antagonist	Levelt et al., 1999
Transgene OT–I (OVA peptide/K^b)	RIP–mOVA transgenic mice	Deleted	CD8αα, fewer CD8αβ	RIP–mOVA expression in the thymus is required for CD8 αα	Leishman et al., 2002
Transgene 3BMM74 (A^{bm12} alloreactive)	A^{bm12} expressing mice	Deleted	CD8αα	Requires ERK interacting part of TCR α	Leishman et al., 2002
Transgene AND (cytochrome c + E^k)	E^k expressing mice	Thymus small, CD4⁺ peripheral cells present	CD8	Not present in mice that express A^b, which also positively selects this TCR	Leishman et al., 2002

CD8αβ IEL includes cells that coexpress CD8αα.

the ability to induce T-cell production of IL-4 and IL-10 (Iwasaki and Kelsall, 2001). By contrast with these short-term assays, in the steady state mice with a mutation in the NF-κB inducing kinase (NIK), which disrupts Peyer's patch and lymph node differentiation, nearly normal numbers of all subpopulations of IEL are present (Nanno et al., 1994), demonstrating that organized lymphoid structures are not an absolute requirement for IEL generation.

Integrins

Not surprisingly, the interactions of integrins with mucosal addressins play a role in the localization of lymphocytes to the intestinal epithelium. Studies on mice deficient for the genes encoding integrin subunits indicate that LFA-1 (Huleatt and Lefrancois, 1996), which interacts with ICAM molecules, and VLA-1, which binds to collagen (Meharra et al., 2000),

are important for the generation of normal IEL numbers. The β$_7$ integrins also have attracted interest because they are highly expressed by mucosal lymphocytes. β$_7$ can pair with two α subunits. The α$_4$β$_7$ heterodimer binds to an Ig-like domain in the MAdCAM-1 addressin expressed by endothelium in Peyer's patches, intestinal lamina propria, and elsewhere (Berlin et al., 1993; Briskin et al., 1993). It is expressed by LP lymphocytes, but not by most IEL. The α$_E$β$_7$ heterodimer, by contrast, is expressed by most IEL, and it binds to E-cadherin expressed by intestinal epithelial cells and other cell types (Cepek et al., 1994). Mice deficient for β$_7$ integrins have a greatly reduced number of IEL (Wagner et al., 1996). Mice defective for the α$_E$ subunit also have decreased IEL (Schon et al., 1999), although the decrease is less dramatic. This highlights the importance of the α$_4$β$_7$ integrin, which may be involved in allowing IEL precursors to enter the intestinal tissue, although continued expression of this integrin by IEL is not required. SMAD7 transgenic mice deficient for TGFβ signaling in mature T cells also have reduced IEL, suggesting a connection between TGFβ cytokine and $β_7$ integrin expression (Suzuki *et al.*, 2002).

One attractive model is that $α_4β_7$ is required for extravasation and localization, whereas $α_Eβ_7$ is most important for tethering IEL to the epithelial cells. Consistent with the importance of $α_4β_7$ for migration, the ability of transferred IEL to adhere to villus microvessels was inhibited by antibodies to $β_7$ integrin or MAdCAM-1, but not by anti-$α_E$ antibody (Koseki *et al.*, 2001). The function of the $α_Eβ_7$ integrin, however, remains to be determined. In a model system in which the response to vesicular stomatitis virus (VSV) carrying an OVA epitope was followed, the $α_E^{-/-}$ OVA reactive T cells were maintained as effectively in the epithelial compartment as $α_E$ wild type T cells (Lefrancois *et al.*, 1999). It is possible that this integrin has some other function in IEL, such as acting as a costimulatory molecule.

Chemokines and their receptors

The chemokine CCL25 (TECK) is produced in the thymus and by epithelial cells in the small intestine, but not by those in the large intestine (Campbell and Butcher, 2002; Kunkel *et al.*, 2003; Wurbel *et al.*, 2000), and its receptor CCR9 likewise is found on small intestine IEL and LPL (Papadakis *et al.*, 2000) and thymocytes. Recent data suggest that this chemokine may be involved in the selective homing of conventional T cells to the small intestine (Hosoe *et al.*, 2003; Papadakis *et al.*, 2003; Svensson *et al.*, 2002), although the analysis of CCR9$^{-/-}$ mice (Uehara *et al.*, 2002; Wurbel *et al.*, 2001) indicated only modest decreases in IEL, with the knockout having the strongest effect on γδ TCR$^+$ IEL. Treatment with CCR9 blocking antibodies likewise only partially decreased IEL numbers, particularly the category III and IV IEL (Svensson *et al.*, 2002). It is therefore likely that there is redundancy in this chemokine/chemokine-receptor system, especially when intact, gene-deficient mice are analyzed that could build up their IEL populations using a relatively minor pathway. Consistent with redundancy, it has been reported that TECK also can bind to CCR11 (Gosling *et al.*, 2000; Schweickart *et al.*, 2000, 2001). Furthermore, additional chemokines are likely to be important. There is evidence for a role for CCR6 in the balance between different IEL subpopulations (Lugering *et al.*, 2003), and for CCR5 in CD8 IEL migration to the intestine of mice in the context of *Toxoplasma* infection (Luangsay *et al.*, 2003), as well as *in vitro* evidence suggesting CXCR3 expression by human IEL could be important for chemotaxis mediated by IP-10 (CXCL10) and Mig (CXCL9) (Shibahara *et al.*, 2001).

Are IEL stationary?

Parabiotic mice have been used by several groups to study the recirculation of IEL. When the parabionts are congenic for the CD45 locus, cells from each partner can be distinguished with monoclonal antibodies. Because of extensive recirculation, lymphocytes in the spleen and lymph nodes equilibrate quickly, so that in the CD45.2 parabiont 50% of the cells are from the CD45.1 parabiont in a matter of days. By contrast, IEL from the small intestine retain the genotype of the original parabiont for weeks, indicating that IEL are mostly not recirculating, and not dependent on frequent output from the thymus (Poussier *et al.*, 1992; Suzuki *et al.*, 1998).

Survival and homeostasis of IEL

Although they have a surface phenotype similar to activated effector cells, most IEL are in the G0/G1 phase of the cell cycle. They are resistant to cell death induced by corticosteroids and irradiation and have high levels of expression of survival-promoting factors such as Bcl-2 (Van Houten *et al.*, 1997). This may permit them to survive under conditions of chronic activation *in vivo*. The results from BrdU labeling experiments indicate that mouse IEL have a relatively long half-life, approximately 3 weeks (Penney *et al.*, 1995). There are data emerging indicating that the CD8αα molecule expressed by IEL may promote survival under conditions of activation. CD8αα interacts preferentially with the thymus leukemia (TL) antigen (Leishman *et al.*, 2001; Liu *et al.*, 2003), a nonclassical class I molecule expressed constitutively by small intestine epithelial cells of the mouse. When the TCR is signaled, the simultaneous interaction of CD8αα with TL modulates the TCR signal to decrease proliferation while increasing cytokine production and survival (Leishman *et al.*, 2001).

Intestinal epithelial cells originate from dividing precursors in the crypts and migrate up the villus to the tip where they are exfoliated (reviewed in Brittan and Wright, 2002; Stappenbeck *et al.*, 1998). This process takes approximately 3 days, and therefore the half-life of IEL is substantially longer. IEL are solitary cells located at the basolateral aspect of the epithelial layer. The difference in half-life leads to the notion that the epithelial cells migrate over the longer-lived IEL, which might maintain attachments to the basement membrane or to dendritic cells (DCs) located just beneath the epithelial layer (Rescigno *et al.*, 2001). This arrangement might permit individual IEL to survey a significant number of epithelial cells.

IEL are likely to be dependent upon cytokines as well as cell–cell interactions for their survival. Memory CD8$^+$ T cells are dependent upon IL-15 and IL-7 for their maintenance (Schluns and Lefrancois, 2003). Both cytokines also are important for IEL, IL-7 deficiency has a greater effect on γδ TCR$^+$ IEL than on αβ TCR$^+$ IEL (Fujihashi *et al.*, 1997; Porter and Malek, 1999), whereas IL-15 deficiency has a greater effect on categories III and IV IEL (Lodolce *et al.*, 1998). Data indicate that IL-15 is important for cell survival as opposed to IEL development (Lai *et al.*, 1999).

SPECIFICITY OF IEL

Oligoclonality

A striking feature of the αβ TCR repertoires expressed by mouse, rat, and human IEL, as revealed by CDR3 length analysis, is their oligoclonality (Blumberg *et al.*, 1993;

Helgeland *et al.*, 1999; Regnault *et al.*, 1994). Interestingly, the repertoires of the CD8αβ and CD8αα αβ TCR$^+$ IEL are different (Regnault *et al.*, 1994). The TCRs expressed by αβ TCR$^+$ CD8αβ$^+$ IEL also can be detected in lamina propria T cells and in the blasts circulating in the thoracic duct lymph of the same mouse, whereas the clones expressed by CD8αα$^+$ IEL cannot (Arstila *et al.*, 2000). This indicates that the αβ TCR$^+$ CD8αβ$^+$ are likely to be derived from conventional T cells activated in the periphery. Consistent with this, following systemic infection with lymphocytic choriomeningitis virus (LCMV), virus-specific cytotoxic T cells (CTL) could be detected, predominantly in the CD8αβ$^+$ IEL (Muller *et al.*, 2000). The predominant clones in IEL are different even when genetically identical mice housed in the same cage were compared (Regnault *et al.*, 1994). This indicates that the oligoclonal IEL are not responding to a monomorphic determinant, but more likely to recent antigenic stimuli, with the different repertoires resulting from subtle differences in antigenic stimulation or somatic rearrangement of antigen receptor genes. Furthermore, oligoclonality is not the result of microbial colonization, because it is also observed in germfree mice (Regnault *et al.*, 1996).

Response to pathogens

IEL can respond following infection with viruses such as LCMV (Muller *et al.*, 2000; Sydora *et al.*, 1996b), reovirus (London *et al.*, 1989), rotavirus (Offit and Dudzik, 1989), vesicular stomatitis virus (VSV) (Masopust *et al.*, 2001a), and vaccinia virus (Masopust *et al.*, 2001a), and protozoa such as *Toxoplasma gondii* (Chardes *et al.*, 1994), *Eimeria vermformis* (Findly *et al.*, 1993), *Cryptosproidum sporis* (McDonald *et al.*, 1996), and *Giardia* (Ebert, 1998; Kanwar *et al.*, 1986). The antigen-specific IEL response to the bacteria *Listeria monocytogenes* could be followed using bacteria expressing the model antigen OVA (Masopust *et al.*, 2001a). In the case of the viruses and *Toxoplasma*, antigen-specific CD8 T-cell responses are in the CD8αβ subset, although for *Cryptosporidium* the response involved predominantly CD4$^+$ IEL (McDonald *et al.*, 1996).

Specificity of αβ TCR$^+$ CD8αα IEL

The specificity of category III αβ TCR$^+$ IEL CD8αα IEL is not known. The number of αβ TCR$^+$ CD8αα IEL is drastically reduced in β2-microglobulin (β2m)-deficient mice (Correa *et al.*, 1992; Fujiura *et al.*, 1996; Neuhaus *et al.*, 1995; Sydora *et al.*, 1996a), but they are present in mice deficient for either the transporter associated with antigen processing (TAP) gene (Sydora *et al.*, 1996a) or in animals deficient for the genes encoding the classical class I molecules (K$^{b-/-}$D$^{b-/-}$) (Das and Janeway, 1999; Gapin *et al.*, 1999; Park *et al.*, 1999). This suggests that category III IEL require a TAP-independent nonclassical or class Ib molecule.

It has been reported that mice deficient in the nonclassical MHC class I molecule, Qa-2, which is for the most part TAP dependent (Tabaczewski and Stroynowski, 1994), had fewer CD8αα IEL, suggesting Qa-2 reactivity for some αβ TCR$^+$ CD8αα IEL (Das *et al.*, 2000). By comparing BALB/c mice with the Qa-2^{null} Bailey substrain (BALB/cByJ), we were unable to confirm these findings (L. Gapin, M. K., and H.C., unpublished data). Two other nonclassical class I molecules, the TL antigen (Hershberg *et al.*, 1990; Wu *et al.*, 1991) and CD1d (Bleicher *et al.*, 1990), have been reported to be expressed by mouse intestinal epithelial cells, although this is controversial in the case of mouse CD1d (Brossay *et al.*, 1997). Both TL and CD1d are TAP independent, but they require β2m expression (Brutkiewicz *et al.*, 1995; Holcombe *et al.*, 1995; Teitell *et al.*, 1997), similar to the αβ TCR$^+$ CD8αα IEL. There is no evidence, however, indicating that either class Ib molecule is recognized by the TCRs of this IEL subset in mice. Recent structural data indicate that the TL antigen has a very narrow and closed groove that is not likely to be capable of interacting with αβ TCRs (Liu *et al.*, 2003).

Surprisingly, using several MHC class II restricted TCR transgenic systems (Guy-Grand *et al.*, 2001; Leishman *et al.*, 2002) it could be shown that CD8αα expressing IEL were generated when agonist self-peptides were present, as in the MHC class I restricted systems. Despite this, the systemic T cells in these same MHC class II restricted TCR transgenic mice were CD4$^+$. These observations indicate that CD8αα does not function as a TCR coreceptor, and therefore expression of CD8αα by αβ TCR$^+$ IEL does not necessarily imply MHC class I reactivity. Based on these results, we propose that αβ TCR$^+$ CD8αα IEL are self-reactive but not selected for self-reactivity to a single self-antigen, and that they may include cells reactive to classical class I molecules, nonclassical class I molecules, and MHC class II molecules. Mouse-to-mouse variation, and compensatory increases in IEL with different specificities when one antigen-presenting molecule is removed (Fujiura *et al.*, 1996), make it difficult to estimate the fraction of cells reactive to different types of antigen-presenting molecules. The reduction in αβ TCR$^+$ CD8αα IEL in β$_2$m$^{-/-}$ mice therefore may only in part reflect the absence of MHC class I molecules responsible for the positive selection of some of these cells, but it also may reflect the absence of the TL molecule, which by interacting with CD8αα might allow for the maintenance of category III IEL with different specificities.

Specificity of γδ TCR$^+$ IEL

The specificity of γδ TCR$^+$ IEL in mice also is not known. These IEL have a predominant use of the Vγ5 (also known as Vγ7) gene segment together with several Vδ genes (Allison and Havran, 1991). Their CDR3 regions are relatively diverse compared with the invariant γδ TCRs expressed in the skin and reproductive tracts (Asarnow *et al.*, 1989). Although the great majority of these cells express CD8αα, their numbers are not reduced in β$_2$m$^{-/-}$ mice (Fujiura *et al.*, 1996; Neuhaus *et al.*, 1995). In humans, the γδ TCRs expressed by IEL predominantly use Vδ1 (Halstensen *et al.*, 1989), and they have oligoclonal CDR3 repertoire that can be sustained over a period of many months (Chowers *et al.*, 1994). These TCRs recognize MIC molecules, MICA and MICB, class I-like molecules that are induced by heat shock or stress on epithelial cells (Groh *et al.*, 1998; Steinle *et al.*, 1998; Wu *et al.*, 2002). MIC molecules, similar to the TL antigen in mice, are not capable of presenting peptides or other ligands (Li *et al.*, 1999). Interestingly, MIC molecules also are recognized by NKG2D, a C type lectin NK receptor that is expressed by IEL, as well as natural killer (NK) cells and systemic T cells (Bauer *et al.*, 1999). Mice do not have a functional MIC gene ortholog, but they do have NKG2D receptors that recognize class I-like molecules such as H-60 and the members of the RAE class I-like family (Cerwenka *et al.*, 2000; Diefenbach *et al.*, 2000). There are so far no reports, however, indicating that significant populations of γδ TCR⁺ IEL or other mouse γδ TCR⁺ cells recognize these class I-like molecules.

ARE IEL GOVERNED BY UNIQUE MOLECULAR INTERACTIONS?

A number of molecular interactions have been characterized that appear to set IEL subpopulations apart from other T lymphocytes, including those involving antigen receptors, chemokines, integrins, and molecules involved in immune regulation. Most of these involve the interaction of an IEL surface molecule with a molecule on epithelial cells. Several examples have been discussed in the preceding sections, and these along with additional ones are listed in **Table 30.3**. For example, in humans, CD1d together with gp180, which is so far defined only at the serologic level, interact with CD8 molecules to promote the induction of suppressive T cells (Campbell *et al.*, 1999). Interestingly, several of the molecular interactions reported to be characteristic for IEL are also typical of memory cells. For example, CD8αα⁺ IEL require IL-15 mediated signals, as do peripheral CD8 memory cells. The interaction of the thymus leukemia (TL) antigen with CD8αα provides a second example, as recent evidence indicates that the CD8αα-TL interaction is important for CD8⁺ memory cells as well as IEL (Madakamutil *et al.*, 2004). IEL (Fahrer *et al.*, 2001; Shires *et al.*, 2001) and CD8⁺ memory cells (Swanson *et al.*, 2002) both have high levels of transcripts of the RANTES chemokine when analyzed *ex vivo* without TCR activation, and they both express high levels of survival-promoting Bcl-2 family molecules.

The epithelium has very little expression of B7 costimulatory molecules in the absence of inflammation, and some IEL

Table 30.3. Molecular Interactions Typical of IEL

Receptor (IEL)	Function	Ligand	Ligand Type
Antigen receptors			
Vδ1 (human)	Response to antigens	MICA (epithelium)	Class I–like, stress induced
Vγ5 (mice)	Response to antigens	??	
Homing			
α_Eβ_7 integrin	Adhesion to epithelium	E cadherin (epithelium)	Adhesion molecule
CCR9 chemokine receptor	Migration to the small intestine	TECK (CCL25)	Chemokine made by thymus and small intestine
Regulation			
CD8αα (mouse)	Modulation of IEL function when activated	TL (epithelium)	Mouse class I molecule—does not present antigens
CD8 (human)	Generation of suppressor T cells	gp180 + CD1d (epithelium)	CD1d presents lipids gp180(?)
OX40 (mouse) TNF receptor superfamily	Costimulation	OX40L (IEL)	TNF superfamily ligand
CD43 (mouse) Sialoglycoprotein	Costimulation	Siglec–1 (?) (macrophages)	Sialic acid–binding immunoglobulin–like lectin (Siglec)
NKG2D (human) C–type lectin activating NK receptor	Costimulation	MICA (epithelium)	Class I–like, stress induced
CD160 (human) Ig family inhibitory NK receptor	Inhibition	MHC class I (epithelium and elsewhere)	Antigen presenting molecules
CD66a (human) carcino–embryonic antigen family	Inhibition	Homotypic interaction with CD66a (epithelium, lymphocytes)	Carcinoembryonic antigen family

do not express CD28. Based upon *in vitro* studies, alternative costimulatory pathways for IEL have been proposed. Using mouse cells, it has been reported that the coengagement of CD43 with the TCR costimulates mouse IEL (Bagriacik *et al.*, 2001). Like many other T cells, mouse IEL have been reported to express the TNF family cytokine OX40 after activation, but surprisingly, they also express OX40L, providing another potential costimulatory pathway (Wang and Klein, 2001). 4-1BB, a member of the TNF superfamily, also has been reported to be induced by activated IEL and to costimulate their activity (Zhou *et al.*, 1994). It is consistent with the partially activated nature of IEL, however, that late-acting members of the array of defined T-cell costimulatory molecules (Croft, 2003), such as OX40 and 4-1BB, are expressed by IEL, whereas the earlier-acting CD28 costimulatory molecule is expressed to a lesser extent.

In human IEL, an important costimulatory role has been reported for BY55 (CD160) (Nikolova *et al.*, 2002). CD160 is an Ig family member with broad specificity for class I molecules (Anumanthan *et al.*, 1998; Le Bouteiller *et al.*, 2002). It is expressed by all human IEL, and a subset of NK cells and CD8 T cells (Anumanthan *et al.*, 1998). A costimulatory role for NKG2D interacting with MICA and MICB proteins has been reported for human IEL (Roberts *et al.*, 2001); a similar role for NKG2D also has been found for CD8 memory cells (Groh *et al.*, 2001).

IEL FUNCTION

Cytokines and effector functions

IEL can produce a variety of cytokines immediately after TCR activation. IFN γ has been reported in a number of studies, but Th2 cytokines also have been detected in some cases (Barrett *et al.*, 1992; Fujihashi *et al.*, 1993). Microarray analyses of gene expression of IEL analyzed *ex vivo* indicated these cells are producing abundant mRNA for granzymes, the chemokine RANTES, and lymphotoxin β (Fahrer *et al.*, 2001; Shires *et al.*, 2001), which is important for the homeostasis of lamina propria B cells (Newberry *et al.*, 2002). Further activation is required to induce IEL to produce interferon γ and other cytokines (Hayday *et al.*, 2001). Mouse IEL exhibit cytotoxic activity *ex vivo* (Cerf-Bensussan *et al.*, 1985; Goodman and Lefrancois, 1989), whereas conventional CD8 T cells require activation before they will kill targets. Both Fas ligand-mediated and perforin-mediated cytotoxicity can be detected in mouse IEL subpopulations (Corazza *et al.*, 2000; Gelfanov *et al.*, 1996). Human IEL contain a cytotoxic subset, but unlike the mouse, the cytotoxic cells are a reduced percentage of the total population (Melgar *et al.*, 2002).

In addition to antigen-specific cytotoxicity, IEL preparations include natural killer (NK) cytotoxic activity (Guy-Grand *et al.*, 1996; Leon *et al.*, 2003). Diverse NK receptors are expressed by human IEL including killer inhibitory receptors (KIRs), NKR-P1A, CD94 (Jabri *et al.*, 2000), and NKG2D (Roberts *et al.*, 2001). IEL also express carcinoem-

bryonic antigen cell adhesion molecule 1 (CEACAM1), also known as biliary glycoprotein (CD66a) (Morales *et al.*, 1999). CD66a contains an immune receptor tyrosine-based inhibitory motif. Antibodies to CD66a inhibited the cytolytic activity of IEL derived from the human small intestine (Morales *et al.*, 1999). This receptor is also expressed by some NK cells and activated T cells outside the intestine. Interestingly, unlike other NK-type inhibitory receptors, CD66a does not recognize class I molecules, but it engages in homotypic interactions (Markel *et al.*, 2002). Mouse IEL also express NK receptors and exhibit NK killing activity. The expression of several NK receptors is enriched in the αβ TCR$^+$ CD8αα population or this population together with the γδ TCR$^+$ IEL (Guy-Grand *et al.*, 1996), and functional NK activity is detected primarily in the αβ TCR$^+$ CD8αα population.

Overview of biologic functions of IEL

Several biologic functions have been proposed for IEL including: (1) surveillance of the epithelial layer for detection of invasive pathogens; (2) elimination of damaged, stressed, or transformed epithelial cells; (3) maintenance of epithelial integrity *via* secretion factors that promote epithelial growth; and (4) regulation of local or systemic immune responses (reviewed in Aranda *et al.*, 1999).

Microbial surveillance by memory cells

A microbial surveillance function for IEL is well established. The specificity of IEL for a number of microbial antigens was summarized in the section, Specificity of IEL. Moreover, transfer of IEL from infected mice to recipients can be protective in the context of infections *via* the oral route, including the responses to parasites such as *Toxoplasma gondii* (Buzoni-Gatel *et al.*, 1997) and *Cryptosporidium muris* (McDonald *et al.*, 1996) and viruses such as rotavirus (Dharakul *et al.*, 1990) and reovirus (Cebra *et al.*, 1991). The protective cells were αβ TCR$^+$ in every case, and CD8$^+$ except in the case of *Cryptosporidium*, which required CD4$^+$ IEL. The CD8β$^+$ cells were most likely to be the important effectors following *Toxoplasma* infection (Buzoni-Gatel *et al.*, 1997; Lepage *et al.*, 1998) and as noted in the section, Specificity of IEL, LCMV-specific CTL also were CD8β$^+$ cells (Corazza *et al.*, 2000). It is therefore reasonable to conclude that TCR αβ$^+$ IEL that are either CD4$^+$ or CD8αβ$^+$ are memory cells derived from conventional T cells primed in the periphery but adapted to the intestine environment. These cells constitute an effector/memory population. This is consistent with the early studies showing that in the context of a response to MHC-encoded alloantigens, blast cells collected from the thoracic duct lymph home to the intestine upon transfer to secondary recipients (Sprent and Miller, 1972). Given that the antigen-specific cells persist for weeks (Lepage *et al.*, 1998; Kim *et al.*, 1999), memory would be an accurate characterization for many of these cells.

Are intestinal memory cells exceptional?

Experimental data indicate that the gut-seeking, antigen-experienced T cells have some differences from those residing in the spleen, including an initial dependence upon CD40–CD40L interactions (Masopust *et al.*, 2001a), effector function that can readily be measured *in vitro* (Kim *et al.*, 1999), and longer survival than the memory cells in the spleen (Kim *et al.*, 1999). It has recently become apparent, however, that antigen-experienced T cells migrate to a variety of tertiary sites, including the lung and liver, as well as the intestine (Masopust *et al.*, 2001b; Reinhardt *et al.*, 2001). This has led to the concept that there are two types of memory T cells that can be distinguished by expression of CCR7 and other molecules (Sallusto *et al.*, 1999). Central memory cells are localized to lymphoid organs, whereas effector memory cells are found in different tissues. There are differences, however, between the intestine and other tissue sites with regard to requirements for class II positive cells and CD40 expression, and taking these data into consideration, it would be unwise to consider all tissue localized effector/memory cells as equivalent.

Natural memory T cells

We put forward the hypothesis here that all IEL subpopulations are in a distinct state, which, considering their cell surface phenotype, is related to memory or effector cells of the systemic immune system. From a functional point of view, however, IEL are most similar to memory cells, including their slow turnover, expression of survival-promoting proteins of the Bcl-2 family, and rapid cytokine secretion. For CD4+ and CD8β+ lymphocytes exposed to antigen in peripheral lymphoid organs, this resemblance is expected. We speculate that the γδ TCR+ IEL are essentially self-reactive T cells, whereas the data indicate that this is true for the αβ TCR+ CD8αα subset. The encounter of these cells with self-antigen during development in central lymphoid organs, such as the thymus for αβ TCR+ CD8αα IEL, dictates their activated phenotype. Self-reactivity is controlled in part by the expression of inhibitory NK receptors and by the interaction of CD8αα with the TL antigen. The expression of the FcεR γ chain as part of the TCR signaling module of these IEL subpopulations might also be related to the control of their responses. The resemblance of category III IEL to CD1d-dependent or Vα14 invariant NKT cells is noteworthy. These NKT cells have self-reactivity to CD1d expressing antigen-presenting cells (Ikarashi *et al.*, 2001), they express inhibitory NK receptors (Bendelac *et al.*, 1997), and they rapidly exhibit effector functions when activated (Matsuda *et al.*, 2000). Recent data indicate that Vα14 invariant NKT cells are poised to produce both IL-4 and IFN-γ (Matsuda *et al.*, 2003; Stetson *et al.*, 2003), and this is initiated relatively early in their thymus differentiation, when first the IL-4 and then the IFN-γ locus transition to the open state (Stetson *et al.*, 2003).

γδ TCR+ IEL and epithelial maintenance

The synthesis of KGF by γδ TCR+ IEL has led to the hypothesis that these cells are important for the integrity and healing of the epithelium. Consistent with this, the epithelium of

the intestine in TCR δ−/− mice had reduced numbers of crypts, and a reduced turnover and migration of enterocytes (Komano *et al.*, 1995). By contrast, the epithelium had a higher mitotic index in the presence of a γδ TCR transgene (Matsumoto *et al.*, 1999). Additionally, TCR δ−/− mice have increased susceptibility to epithelial damage induced by dextran sodium sulfate and slower tissue repair (Chen *et al.*, 2002). They also have increased epithelial damage following infection with *Eimeria vermiformis* (Roberts *et al.*, 1996). It remains to be determined if the effect of γδ TCR+ IEL on epithelial cells is mediated solely by KGF, or if other factors are involved. γδ TCR+ IEL synthesize mRNA for TGF-β1 (Shires *et al.*, 2001) and TGF-β3 (Fahrer *et al.*, 2001), and TGF-β has been reported to aid in the healing of epithelial damage (Beck *et al.*, 2003). γδ TCR+ IEL also were found to have abundant levels of mRNA encoding prothymosin β4 (Shires *et al.*, 2001), a multifunctional molecular that has been reported to aid in epithelial wound healing (Malinda *et al.*, 1999).

Are αβ TCR+ CD8αα IEL regulatory T cells?

In several experimental models, the development of inflammation in the intestine of mice is associated with a decrease in γδ TCR+ IEL and αβ TCR+ CD8αα+ IEL and the loss of cryptopatches, and an increase in CD4+ and CD8αβ+ cells (Eisenbraun *et al.*, 2000; Kronenberg and Cheroutre, 2000; Panwala *et al.*, 1998; Poussier *et al.*, 2000). It remained to be determined, however, if this was merely correlative, resulting from the increased infiltration of activated peripheral T cells during inflammation, or if the category III or IV IEL have an active regulatory function. In a subsequent study, it was shown that pretransfer of αβ TCR+ CD8αα+ IEL to immune-deficient mice could prevent the colitis that is induced by the transfer of CD4+ CD45RB^Hi T cells to immune-deficient recipients (Poussier *et al.*, 2002). Transfer of either γδ TCR+ IEL or αβ TCR+ CD8αβ+ IEL did not prevent disease. It is surprising that the αβ TCR+ CD8αα+ IEL could prevent inflammation in the colon, although this population is most prevalent in the small intestine, and the small intestine was the source of the transferred cells (Poussier *et al.*, 2002). Interestingly, all subpopulations of small intestine–derived IEL were able to populate the colon in the immune-deficient recipients, but the αβ TCR+ CD8αα+ IEL were uniquely able to prevent the full expansion of the pathogenic CD4+ donor T cells there (Poussier *et al.*, 2002). It has also been reported that the αβ TCR+ CD4+ CD8αα+ IEL have a regulatory function (Das *et al.*, 2003), and in rats these cells are capable of producing TGF-β. (Yamada *et al.*, 1999).

Prevention of colitis by the αβ TCR+ CD8αα+ IEL required activation in the recipients, and when the cells were obtained from IL-10−/− mice, they were ineffective (Poussier *et al.*, 2002). Despite this, *in vitro* TCR stimulation of αβ TCR+ CD8αα+ IEL did not lead to detectable IL-10 protein synthesis. Although it is possible that the proper conditions were not used to activate these cells *in vitro*, there remains little information as to how these IEL might prevent inflammation and regulate mucosal immune responses.

Interestingly, CD4+CD25+ regulatory T cells (Jordan *et al.*, 2001) and Vα14 invariant NKT cells (Bendelac *et al.*, 1997) are selected by self-agonists in the thymus, like αβ TCR+ CD8αα+ IEL, and it has been proposed that all three populations have a regulatory role, albeit in different contexts. We speculate that thymocytes expressing antigen receptors with a higher than normal degree of self-reactivity are preserved during selection, and that these cells subsequently differentiate into various types of specialized regulatory populations.

SUMMARY

IEL have long been considered enigmatic lymphocytes, but they have begun to yield their secrets as a result of the development of genetic technologies and *in vivo* models. The lymphocyte populations in the epithelium are dominated by long-lived, antigen-experienced CD8+ cells that share some features with CD8+ memory T cells. They have an oligoclonal TCR repertoire, and they exhibit rapid effector functions, consistent with the hypothesis that they survey epithelial cells migrating from the crypts. It is now certain that conventional T cells activated in the periphery can migrate to the intestine and give rise to IEL that can protect the host from oral or systemic microbial infections. Although there are similarities between IEL and memory T cells of the systemic immune system, unique adaptations to the intestinal environment take place. IEL also may contain lymphocyte populations that are to some extent self-reactive and that function to regulate epithelial cell homeostasis or local immune responses. The memory-like phenotype and behavior of some of these cells may be acquired centrally during development. Furthermore, the molecular interactions that govern the behavior of these cells are distinct, although to some extent they are found in other cell types including activated/effector CD8 T cells, NKT cells, or NK cells.

REFERENCES

Allison, J. P., and Havran, W. L. (1991). The immunobiology of T cells with invariant γ δ antigen receptors. *Annu. Rev. Immunol.* 9, 679–705.

Anumanthan, A., Bensussan, A., Boumsell, L., Christ, A. D., Blumberg, R. S., Voss, S. D., Patel, A. T., Robertson, M. J., Nadler, L. M., and Freeman, G. J. (1998). Cloning of BY55, a novel Ig superfamily member expressed on NK cells, CTL, and intestinal intraepithelial lymphocytes. *J. Immunol.* 161, 2780–2790.

Aranda, R., Sydora, B. C., and Kronenberg, M. (1999). Intraepithelial lymphocytes: Function. In *Mucosal Immunology* (eds. P. L. Ogra, J. Mestecky, M. E. Lamm, W. Strober, J. Bienenstock, and J. R. McGhee), 429–437. San Diego, CA: Academic Press.

Arstila, T., Arstila, T. P., Calbo, S., Selz, F., Malassis-Seris, M., Vassalli, P., Kourilsky, P., and Guy-Grand, D. (2000). Identical T cell clones are located within the mouse gut epithelium and lamina propia and circulate in the thoracic duct lymph. *J. Exp. Med.* 191, 823–834.

Asarnow, D. M., Goodman, T., LeFrancois, L., and Allison, J. P. (1989). Distinct antigen receptor repertoires of two classes of murine epithelium-associated T cells. *Nature* 341, 60–62.

Bagriacik, E. U., Tang, M., Wang, H. C., and Klein, J. R. (2001). CD43 potentiates CD3-induced proliferation of murine intestinal intraepithelial lymphocytes. *Immunol. Cell. Biol.* 79, 303–307.

Barnden, M. J., Heath, W. R., and Carbone, F. R. (1997). Down-modulation of CD8 β-chain in response to an altered peptide ligand enables developing thymocytes to escape negative selection. *Cell. Immunol.* 175, 111–119.

Barrett, T. A., Gajewski, T. F., Danielpour, D., Chang, E. B., Beagley, K. W., and Bluestone, J. A. (1992). Differential function of intestinal intraepithelial lymphocyte subsets. *J. Immunol.* 149, 1124–1130.

Bauer, S., Groh, V., Wu, J., Steinle, A., Phillips, J. H., Lanier, L. L., and Spies, T. (1999). Activation of NK cells and T cells by NKG2D, a receptor for stress-inducible MICA. *Science* 285, 727–729.

Beagley, K. W., Fujihashi, K., Lagoo, A. S., Lagoo-Deenadaylan, S., Black, C. A., Murray, A. M., Sharmanov, A. T., Yamamoto, M., McGhee, J. R., Elson, C. O., *et al.* (1995). Differences in intraepithelial lymphocyte T cell subsets isolated from murine small versus large intestine. *J. Immunol.* 154, 5611–5619.

Beagley, K. W. and Husband, A. J. (1998). Intraepithelial lymphocytes: origins, distribution, and function. *Crit. Rev. Immunol.* 18, 237–254.

Beck, P. L., Rosenberg, I. M., Xavier, R. J., Koh, T., Wong, J. F., and Podolsky, D. K. (2003). Transforming growth factor-β mediates intestinal healing and susceptibility to injury in vitro and in vivo through epithelial cells. *Am. J. Pathol.* 162, 597–608.

Bendelac, A. (1995). Positive selection of mouse NK1+ T cells by CD1-expressing cortical thymocytes. *J. Exp. Med.* 182, 2091–2096.

Bendelac, A., Rivera, M. N., Park, S. H., and Roark, J. H. (1997). Mouse CD1-specific NK1 T cells: development, specificity, and function. *Annu. Rev. Immunol.* 15, 535–562.

Berlin, C., Berg, E. L., Briskin, M. J., Andrew, D. P., Kilshaw, P. J., Holzmann, B., Weissman, I. L., Hamann, A., and Butcher, E. C. (1993). α4 β7 integrin mediates lymphocyte binding to the mucosal vascular addressin MAdCAM-1. *Cell* 74, 185–185.

Bleicher, P. A., Balk, S. P., Hagen, S. J., Blumberg, R. S., Flotte, T. J., and Terhorst, C. (1990). Expression of murine CD1 on gastrointestinal epithelium. *Science* 250, 679–682.

Blumberg, R. S., Yockey, C. E., Gross, G. G., Ebert, E. C., and Balk, S. P. (1993). Human intestinal intraepithelial lymphocytes are derived from a limited number of T cell clones that utilize multiple Vβ T cell receptor genes. *J. Immunol.* 150, 5144–5153.

Boismenu, R., and Havran, W. L. (1994). Modulation of epithelial cell growth by intraepithelial γ δ T cells. *Science* 266, 1253–1255.

Boll, G., Rudolphi, A., Spiess, S., and Reimann, J. (1995). Regional specialization of intraepithelial T cells in the murine small and large intestine. *Scand. J. Immunol.* 41, 103–113.

Boyaka, P. N., Wright, P. F., Marinaro, M., Kiyono, H., Johnson, J. E., Gonzales, R. A., Ikizler, M. R., Werkhaven, J. A., Jackson, R. J., Fujihashi, K., *et al.* (2000). Human nasopharyngeal-associated lymphoreticular tissues. Functional analysis of subepithelial and intraepithelial B and T cells from adenoids and tonsils. *Am. J. Pathol.* 157, 2023–2035.

Briskin, M. J., McEvoy, L. M., and Butcher, E. C. (1993). MAdCAM-1 has homology to immunoglobulin and mucin-like adhesion receptors and to IgA1. *Nature* 363, 461–464.

Brittan, M. and Wright, N. A. (2002). Gastrointestinal stem cells. *J. Pathol.* 197, 492–509.

Brossay, L., Jullien, D., Cardell, S., Sydora, B. C., Burdin, N., Modlin, R. L., and Kronenberg, M. (1997). Mouse CD1 is mainly expressed on hemopoietic-derived cells. *J. Immunol.* 159, 1216–1224.

Bruno, L., Rocha, B., Rolink, A., von Boehmer, H., and Rodewald, H. R. (1995). Intra- and extra-thymic expression of the pre-T cell receptor α gene. *Eur. J. Immunol.* 25, 1877–1882.

Brutkiewicz, R. R., Bennink, J. R., Yewdell, J. W., and Bendelac, A. (1995). TAP-independent, β 2-microglobulin- dependent surface expression of functional mouse CD1.1. *J. Exp. Med.* 182, 1913–1919.

Buzoni-Gatel, D., Lepage, A. C., Dimier-Poisson, I. H., Bout, D. T., and Kasper, L. H. (1997). Adoptive transfer of gut intraepithelial lymphocytes protects against murine infection with *Toxoplasma gondii*. *J. Immunol.* 158, 5883–5889.

Camerini, V., Panwala, C., and Kronenberg, M. (1993). Regional specialization of the mucosal immune system. Intraepithelial lymphocytes of the large intestine have a different phenotype and function than those of the small intestine. *J. Immunol.* 151, 1765–1776.

Camerini, V., Sydora, B. C., Aranda, R., Nguyen, C., MacLean, C., McBride, W. H., and Kronenberg, M. (1998). Generation of intestinal mucosal lymphocytes in SCID mice reconstituted with mature, thymus-derived T cells. *J. Immunol.* 160, 2608–2618.

Campbell, D. J. and Butcher, E. C. (2002). Intestinal attraction: CCL25 functions in effector lymphocyte recruitment to the small intestine. *J. Clin. Invest.* 110, 1079–1081.

Campbell, N. A., Kim, H. S., Blumberg, R. S., and Mayer, L. (1999). The nonclassical class I molecule CD1d associates with the novel CD8 ligand gp180 on intestinal epithelial cells. *J. Biol. Chem.* 274, 26259–26265.

Capone, M., Troesch, M., Eberl, G., Hausmann, B., Palmer, E., and MacDonald, H. R. (2001). A critical role for the T cell receptor α-chain connecting peptide domain in positive selection of CD1-independent NKT cells. *Eur. J. Immunol.* 31, 1867–1875.

Cebra, J. J., Cuff, C. F., and Rubin, D. H. (1991). Relationship between α/β T cell receptor/CD8+ precursors for cytotoxic T lymphocytes in the murine Peyer's patches and the intraepithelial compartment probed by oral infection with reovirus. *Immunol. Res.* 10, 321–323.

Cepek, K. L., Shaw, S. K., Parker, C. M., Russell, G. J., Morrow, J. S., Rimm, D. L., and Brenner, M. B. (1994). Adhesion between epithelial cells and T lymphocytes mediated by E-cadherin and the αeβ7 integrin. *Nature* 372, 190–193.

Cerf-Bensussan, N., Guy-Grand, D., and Griscelli, C. (1985). Intraepithelial lymphocytes of human gut: Isolation, characterisation and study of natural killer activity. *Gut* 26, 81–88.

Cerwenka, A., Bakker, A. B., McClanahan, T., Wagner, J., Wu, J., Phillips, J. H., and Lanier, L. L. (2000). Retinoic acid early inducible genes define a ligand family for the activating NKG2D receptor in mice. *Immunity* 12, 721–727.

Chardes, T., Buzoni-Gatel, D., Lepage, A., Bernard, F., and Bout, D. (1994). *Toxoplasma gondii* oral infection induces specific cytotoxic CD8 α/β+ Thy-1+ gut intraepithelial lymphocytes, lytic for parasite-infected enterocytes. *J. Immunol.* 153, 4596–4603.

Chen, Y., Chou, K., Fuchs, E., Havran, W. L., and Boismenu, R. (2002). Protection of the intestinal mucosa by intraepithelial γδ T cells. *Proc. Natl. Acad. Sci. USA* 99, 14338–14343.

Cheroutre, H. (2004). Starting at the beginning: new perspectives on the biology of mucosal T cells. *Ann. Rev. Immunol.* 22, 217–246.

Chidgey, A. P. and Boyd, R. L. (1998). Positive selection of low responsive, potentially autoreactive T cells induced by high avidity, non-deleting interactions. *Int. Immunol.* 10, 999–1008.

Chowers, Y., Holtmeier, W., Harwood, J., Morzycka-Wroblewska, E., and Kagnoff, M. F. (1994). The V δ 1 T cell receptor repertoire in human small intestine and colon. *J. Exp. Med.* 180, 183–190.

Corazza, N., Muller, S., Brunner, T., Kagi, D., and Mueller, C. (2000). Differential contribution of Fas- and perforin-mediated mechanisms to the cell-mediated cytotoxic activity of naive and in vivo-primed intestinal intraepithelial lymphocytes. *J. Immunol.* 164, 398–403.

Correa, I., Bix, M., Liao, N. S., Zijlstra, M., Jaenisch, R., and Raulet, D. (1992). Most γδ T cells develop normally in β 2-microglobulin-deficient mice. *Proc. Natl. Acad. Sci. USA* 89, 653–657.

Croft, M. (2003). Co-stimulatory members of the TNFR family: Keys to effective T-cell immunity. *Nat. Rev. Immunol.* 3, 609–620.

Croitoru, K., Bienenstock, J., and Ernst, P. B. (1994). Phenotypic and functional assessment of intraepithelial lymphocytes bearing a 'forbidden' αβ TCR. *Int. Immunol.* 6, 1467–1473.

Cruz, D., Sydora, B. C., Hetzel, K., Yakoub, G., Kronenberg, M., and Cheroutre, H. (1998). An opposite pattern of selection of a single T cell antigen receptor in the thymus and among intraepithelial lymphocytes. *J. Exp. Med.* 188, 255–265.

Das, G., Augustine, M. M., Das, J., Bottomly, K., Ray, P., and Ray, A. (2003). An important regulatory role for CD4+CD8αα T cells in the intestinal epithelial layer in the prevention of inflammatory bowel disease. *Proc. Natl. Acad. Sci. USA* 100, 5324–5329.

Das, G., Gould, D. S., Augustine, M. M., Fragoso, G., Sciutto, E., Stroynowski, I., Van Kaer, L., Schust, D. J., Ploegh, H., Janeway, C. A., Jr., and Scitto, E. (2000). Qa-2- dependent selection of CD8α/α T cell receptor α/β(+) cells in murine intestinal intraepithelial lymphocytes. *J. Exp. Med.* 192, 1521–1528.

Das, G. and Janeway, C. A., Jr. (1999). Development of CD8α/α and CD8α/β T cells in major histocompatibility complex class I-deficient mice. *J. Exp. Med.* 190, 881–884.

Dejbakhsh-Jones, S., Jerabek, L., Weissman, I. L., and Strober, S. (1995). Extrathymic maturation of αβ T cells from hemopoietic stem cells. *J. Immunol.* 155, 3338–3344.

Dharakul, T., Rott, L., and Greenberg, H. B. (1990). Recovery from chronic rotavirus infection in mice with severe combined immunodeficiency: virus clearance mediated by adoptive transfer of immune CD8+ T lymphocytes. *J. Virol.* 64, 4375–4382.

Diefenbach, A., Jamieson, A. M., Liu, S. D., Shastri, N., and Raulet, D. H. (2000). Ligands for the murine NKG2D receptor: expression by tumor cells and activation of NK cells and macrophages. *Nat. Immunol.* 1, 119–126.

Dillon, S. B. and MacDonald, T. T. (1986). Functional characterization of Con A-responsive Lyt2-positive mouse small intestinal intraepithelial lymphocytes. *Immunology* 59, 389–396.

Dunon, D., Cooper, M. D., and Imhof, B. A. (1993a). Migration patterns of thymus-derived γδ T cells during chicken development. *Eur. J. Immunol.* 23, 2545–2550.

Dunon, D., Cooper, M. D., and Imhof, B. A. (1993b). Thymic origin of embryonic intestinal γδ T cells. *J. Exp. Med.* 177, 257–263.

Ebert, E. C. (1998). Tumour necrosis factor-α enhances intraepithelial lymphocyte proliferation and migration. *Gut* 42, 650–655.

Eisenbraun, M. D., Mosley, R. L., Teitelbaum, D. H., and Miller, R. A. (2000). Altered development of intestinal intraepithelial lymphocytes in P-glycoprotein-deficient mice. *Dev. Comp. Immunol.* 24, 783–795.

Fahrer, A. M., Konigshofer, Y., Kerr, E. M., Ghandour, G., Mack, D. H., Davis, M. M., and Chien, Y. H. (2001). Attributes of γδ intraepithelial lymphocytes as suggested by their transcriptional profile. *Proc. Natl. Acad. Sci. USA* 98, 10261–10266.

Faure, F., Jitsukawa, S., Triebel, F., and Hercend, T. (1988). Characterization of human peripheral lymphocytes expressing the CD3-γδ complex with anti-receptor monoclonal antibodies. *J. Immunol.* 141, 3357–3360.

Ferguson, A. (1977). Intraepithelial lymphocytes of the small intestine. *Gut* 18, 921–937.

Fichtelius, K. E. (1968). The gut epithelium—a first level lymphoid organ? *Exp. Cell. Res.* 49, 87–104.

Fichtelius, K. E., Yunis, E. J., and Good, R. A. (1968). Occurrence of lymphocytes within the gut epithelium of normal and neonatally thymectomized mice. *Proc. Soc. Exp. Biol. Med.* 128, 185–188.

Findly, R. C., Roberts, S. J., and Hayday, A. C. (1993). Dynamic response of murine gut intraepithelial T cells after infection by the coccidian parasite Eimeria. *Eur. J. Immunol.* 23, 2557–2564.

Fujihashi, K., McGhee, J. R., Yamamoto, M., Peschon, J. J., and Kiyono, H. (1997). An interleukin-7 internet for intestinal intraepithelial T cell development: knockout of ligand or receptor reveal differences in the immunodeficient state. *Eur. J. Immunol.* 27, 2133–2138.

Fujihashi, K., Yamamoto, M., McGhee, J. R., and Kiyono, H. (1993). αβ T cell receptor-positive intraepithelial lymphocytes with CD4+, CD8– and CD4+, CD8+ phenotypes from orally immunized mice provide Th2-like function for B cell responses. *J. Immunol.* 151, 6681–6691.

Fujiura, Y., Kawaguchi, M., Kondo, Y., Obana, S., Yamamoto, H., Nanno, M., and Ishikawa, H. (1996). Development of CD8αα+ intestinal intraepithelial T cells in β2-microglobulin- and/or TAP1-deficient mice. *J. Immunol.* 156, 2710–2715.

Gapin, L., Cheroutre, H., and Kronenberg, M. (1999). Cutting edge: TCR αβ+ CD8αα+ T cells are found in intestinal intraepithelial lymphocytes of mice that lack classical MHC class I molecules. *J. Immunol.* 163, 4100–4104.

Gelfanov, V., Gelfanova, V., Lai, Y. G., and Liao, N. S. (1996). Activated αβ-CD8+, but not αα-CD8+, TCR-αβ+ murine intestinal intraepithelial lymphocytes can mediate perforin-based cytotoxicity, whereas both subsets are active in Fas-based cytotoxicity. *J. Immunol.* 156, 35–41.

Glick, B. and Whatley, S. (1967). The presence of immunoglobulin in the bursa of Fabricius. *Poult. Sci.* 46, 1587–1589.

Goodman, T. and Lefrancois, L. (1988). Expression of the γ-δ T-cell receptor on intestinal CD8+ intraepithelial lymphocytes. *Nature* 333, 855–858.

Goodman, T. and Lefrancois, L. (1989). Intraepithelial lymphocytes. Anatomical site, not T cell receptor form, dictates phenotype and function. *J. Exp. Med.* 170, 1569–1581.

Gosling, J., Dairaghi, D. J., Wang, Y., Hanley, M., Talbot, D., Miao, Z., and Schall, T. J. (2000). Cutting edge: Identification of a novel chemokine receptor that binds dendritic cell- and T cell-active chemokines including ELC, SLC, and TECK. *J. Immunol.* 164, 2851–2856.

Gould, D. S., Ploegh, H. L., and Schust, D. J. (2001). Murine female reproductive tract intraepithelial lymphocytes display selection characteristics distinct from both peripheral and other mucosal T cells. *J. Reprod. Immunol.* 52, 85–99.

Groh, V., Rhinehart, R., Randolph-Habecker, J., Topp, M. S., Riddell, S. R., and Spies, T. (2001). Costimulation of CD8αβ T cells by NKG2D via engagement by MIC induced on virus-infected cells. *Nat. Immunol.* 2, 255–260.

Groh, V., Steinle, A., Bauer, S., and Spies, T. (1998). Recognition of stress-induced MHC molecules by intestinal epithelial γδ T cells. *Science* 279, 1737–1740.

Guehler, S. R., Bluestone, J. A., and Barrett, T. A. (1996). Immune deviation of 2C transgenic intraepithelial lymphocytes in antigen-bearing hosts. *J. Exp. Med.* 184, 493–503.

Guehler, S. R., Bluestone, J. A., and Barrett, T. A. (1999). Activation and peripheral expansion of murine T-cell receptor γδ intraepithelial lymphocytes. *Gastroenterology* 116, 327–334.

Guy-Grand, D., Azogui, O., Celli, S., Darche, S., Nussenzweig, M. C., Kourilsky, P., and Vassalli, P. (2003). Extrathymic T cell lymphopoiesis: Ontogeny and contribution to gut intraepithelial lymphocytes in athymic and euthymic mice. *J. Exp. Med.* 197, 333–341.

Guy-Grand, D., Cuenod-Jabri, B., Malassis-Seris, M., Selz, F., and Vassalli, P. (1996). Complexity of the mouse gut T cell immune system: Identification of two distinct natural killer T cell intraepithelial lineages. *Eur. J. Immunol.* 26, 2248–2256.

Guy-Grand, D., Griscelli, C., and Vassalli, P. (1978). The mouse gut T lymphocyte, a novel type of T cell. Nature, origin, and traffic in mice in normal and graft-versus-host conditions. *J. Exp. Med.* 148, 1661–1677.

Guy-Grand, D., Pardigon, N., Darche, S., Lantz, O., Kourilsky, P., and Vassalli, P. (2001). Contribution of double-negative thymic precursors to CD8αα (+) intraepithelial lymphocytes of the gut in mice bearing TCR transgenes. *Eur. J. Immunol.* 31, 2593–2602.

Guy-Grand, D., Rocha, B., Mintz, P., Malassis-Seris, M., Selz, F., Malissen, B., and Vassalli, P. (1994). Different use of T cell receptor transducing modules in two populations of gut intraepithelial lymphocytes are related to distinct pathways of T cell differentiation. *J. Exp. Med.* 180, 673–679.

Guy-Grand, D. and Vassalli, P. (1993). Gut intraepithelial T lymphocytes. *Curr. Opin. Immunol.* 5, 247–252.

Halstensen, T. S., Scott, H., and Brandtzaeg, P. (1989). Intraepithelial T cells of the TcR γ/δ+ CD8– and Vδ1/Jδ1+ phenotypes are increased in coeliac disease. *Scand. J. Immunol.* 30, 665–672.

Hayday, A., Theodoridis, E., Ramsburg, E., and Shires, J. (2001). Intraepithelial lymphocytes: exploring the Third Way in immunology. *Nat. Immunol.* 2, 997–1003.

Helgeland, L., Brandtzaeg, P., Rolstad, B., and Vaage, J. T. (1997). Sequential development of intraepithelial γδ and αβ T lymphocytes expressing CD8αβ in neonatal rat intestine: requirement for the thymus. *Immunology* 92, 447–456.

Helgeland, L., Johansen, F. E., Utgaard, J. O., Vaage, J. T., and Brandtzaeg, P. (1999). Oligoclonality of rat intestinal intraepithelial T lymphocytes: overlapping TCR β-chain repertoires in the CD4 single-positive and CD4/CD8 double-positive subsets. *J. Immunol.* 162, 2683–2692.

Hershberg, R., Eghtesady, P., Sydora, B., Brorson, K., Cheroutre, H., Modlin, R., and Kronenberg, M. (1990). Expression of the thymus leukemia antigen in mouse intestinal epithelium. *Proc. Natl. Acad. Sci. USA* 87, 9727–9731.

Holcombe, H. R., Castaño, A. R., Cheroutre, H., Teitell, M., Maher, J. K., Peterson, P. A., and Kronenberg, M. (1995). Nonclassical behavior of the thymus leukemia antigen: Peptide transporter-independent expression of a nonclassical class I molecule. *J. Exp. Med.* 181, 1433–1443.

Horton, J. D., Horton, T. L., Dzialo, R., Gravenor, I., Minter, R., Ritchie, P., Gartland, L., Watson, M. D., and Cooper, M. D. (1998). T-cell and natural killer cell development in thymectomized *Xenopus*. *Immunol. Rev.* 166, 245–258.

Hosoe, N., Miura, S., Watanabe, C., Tsuzuki, Y., Hokari, R., Oyama, T., Fujiyama, Y., Nagata, H., and Ishii, H. (2003). Demonstration of functional role of TECK/CCL25 in T lymphocyte-endothelium interaction in inflamed and uninflamed intestinal mucosa. *Am. J. Physiol. Gastrointest. Liver Physiol.* 286, 6458–6466.

Howie, D., Spencer, J., DeLord, D., Pitzalis, C., Wathen, N. C., Dogan, A., Akbar, A., and MacDonald, T. T. (1998). Extrathymic T cell differentiation in the human intestine early in life. *J. Immunol.* 161, 5862–5872.

Huleatt, J. W. and Lefrancois, L. (1996). β2 integrins and ICAM-1 are involved in establishment of the intestinal mucosal T cell compartment. *Immunity* 5, 263–273.

Ibraghimov, A. R., and Lynch, R. G. (1994). Heterogeneity and biased T cell receptor α/β repertoire of mucosal CD8+ cells from murine large intestine: implications for functional state. *J. Exp. Med.* 180, 433–444.

Ikarashi, Y., Mikami, R., Bendelac, A., Terme, M., Chaput, N., Terada, M., Tursz, T., Angevin, E., Lemonnier, F. A., Wakasugi, H., and Zitvogel, L. (2001). Dendritic cell maturation overrules H-2D-mediated natural killer T (NKT) cell inhibition: critical role for B7 in CD1d-dependent NKT cell interferon γ production. *J. Exp. Med.* 194, 1179–1186.

Imhof, B. A., Dunon, D., Courtois, D., Luhtala, M., and Vainio, O. (2000). Intestinal CD8αα and CD8αβ intraepithelial lymphocytes are thymus derived and exhibit subtle differences in TCR β repertoires. *J. Immunol.* 165, 6716–6722.

Iwasaki, A. and Kelsall, B. L. (2001). Unique functions of CD11b+, CD8α+, and double-negative Peyer's patch dendritic cells. *J. Immunol.* 166, 4884–4890.

Jabri, B., de Serre, N. P., Cellier, C., Evans, K., Gache, C., Carvalho, C., Mougenot, J. F., Allez, M., Jian, R., Desreumaux, P., *et al.* (2000). Selective expansion of intraepithelial lymphocytes expressing the HLA-E-specific natural killer receptor CD94 in celiac disease. *Gastroenterology* 118, 867–879.

Johansson-Lindbom, B., Svensson, M., Wurbel, M. A., Malissen, B., Marquez, G., and Agace, W. (2003). Selective generation of gut tropic T cells in gut-associated lymphoid tissue (GALT): requirement for GALT dendritic cells and adjuvant. *J. Exp. Med.* 198, 963–969.

Jordan, M. S., Boesteanu, A., Reed, A. J., Petrone, A. L., Holenbeck, A. E., Lerman, M. A., Naji, A., and Caton, A. J. (2001). Thymic selection of CD4+CD25+ regulatory T cells induced by an agonist self-peptide. *Nat. Immunol.* 2, 301–306.

Kanwar, S. S., Ganguly, N. K., Walia, B. N., and Mahajan, R. C. (1986). Direct and antibody dependent cell mediated cytotoxicity against *Giardia lamblia* by splenic and intestinal lymphoid cells in mice. *Gut* 27, 73–77.

Kim, S. K., Schluns, K. S., and Lefrancois, L. (1999). Induction and visualization of mucosal memory CD8 T cells following systemic virus infection. *J. Immunol.* 163, 4125–4132.

Klein, J. R. (1986). Ontogeny of the Thy-1–, Lyt-2+ murine intestinal intraepithelial lymphocyte. Characterization of a unique population of thymus-independent cytotoxic effector cells in the intestinal mucosa. *J. Exp. Med.* 164, 309–314.

Klein, J. R., Lefrancois, L., and Kagnoff, M. F. (1985). A murine cytotoxic T lymphocyte clone from the intestinal mucosa that is antigen specific for proliferation and displays broadly reactive inducible cytotoxic activity. *J. Immunol.* 135, 3697–3703.

Komano, H., Fujiura, Y., Kawaguchi, M., Matsumoto, S., Hashimoto, Y., Obana, S., Mombaerts, P., Tonegawa, S., Yamamoto, H., Itohara, S., *et al.* (1995). Homeostatic regulation of intestinal epithelia by intraepithelial γδ T cells. *Proc. Natl. Acad. Sci. USA* 92, 6147–6151.

Koningsberger, J. C., Chott, A., Logtenberg, T., Wiegman, L. J., Blumberg, R. S., van Berge Henegouwen, G. P., and Balk, S. P. (1997). TCR expression in human fetal intestine and identification of an early T cell receptor β-chain transcript. *J. Immunol.* 159, 1775–1782.

Koseki, S., Miura, S., Fujimori, H., Hokari, R., Komoto, S., Hara, Y., Ogino, T., Nagata, H., Goto, M., Hachimura, S., et al. (2001). In situ demonstration of intraepithelial lymphocyte adhesion to villus microvessels of the small intestine. *Int. Immunol.* 13, 1165–1174.

Kronenberg, M. and Cheroutre, H. (2000). Do mucosal T cells prevent intestinal inflammation? *Gastroenterology* 118, 974–977.

Kunkel, E. J., Campbell, D. J., and Butcher, E. C. (2003). Chemokines in lymphocyte trafficking and intestinal immunity. *Microcirculation* 10, 313–323.

Kuo, S., El Guindy, A., Panwala, C. M., Hagan, P. M., and Camerini, V. (2001). Differential appearance of T cell subsets in the large and small intestine of neonatal mice. *Pediatr. Res.* 49, 543–551.

Lai, Y. G., Gelfanov, V., Gelfanova, V., Kulik, L., Chu, C. L., Jeng, S. W., and Liao, N. S. (1999). IL-15 promotes survival but not effector function differentiation of CD8+ TCRαβ+ intestinal intraepithelial lymphocytes. *J. Immunol.* 163, 5843–5850.

Lambolez, F., Azogui, O., Joret, A. M., Garcia, C., von Boehmer, H., Di Santo, J., Ezine, S., and Rocha, B. (2002). Characterization of T cell differentiation in the murine gut. *J. Exp. Med.* 195, 437–449.

Le Bouteiller, P., Barakonyi, A., Giustiniani, J., Lenfant, F., Marie-Cardine, A., Aguerre-Girr, M., Rabot, M., Hilgert, I., Mami-Chouaib, F., Tabiasco, J., et al. (2002). Engagement of CD160 receptor by HLA-C is a triggering mechanism used by circulating natural killer (NK) cells to mediate cytotoxicity. *Proc. Natl. Acad. Sci. USA* 99, 16963–16968.

Lefrancois, L., Fuller, B., Huleatt, J. W., Olson, S., and Puddington, L. (1997). On the front lines: intraepithelial lymphocytes as primary effectors of intestinal immunity. *Springer Semin. Immunopathol.* 18, 463–475.

Lefrancois, L., Parker, C. M., Olson, S., Muller, W., Wagner, N., Schon, M. P., and Puddington, L. (1999). The role of β7 integrins in CD8 T cell trafficking during an antiviral immune response. *J. Exp. Med.* 189, 1631–1638.

Lefrancois, L. and Olson, S. (1997). Reconstitution of the extrathymic intestinal T cell compartment in the absence of irradiation. *J. Immunol.* 159, 538–541.

Lefrancois, L. and Puddington, L. (1998). Anatomy of T-cell development in the intestine. *Gastroenterology* 115, 1588–1591.

Legendre, V., Boyer, C., Guerder, S., Arnold, B., Hammerling, G., and Schmitt-Verhulst, A. M. (1999). Selection of phenotypically distinct NK1.1+ T cells upon antigen expression in the thymus or in the liver. *Eur. J. Immunol.* 29, 2330–2343.

Leishman, A. J., Gapin, L., Capone, M., Palmer, E., MacDonald, H. R., Kronenberg, M., and Cheroutre, H. (2002). Precursors of functional MHC class I- or class II-restricted CD8αα(+) T cells are positively selected in the thymus by agonist self-peptides. *Immunity* 16, 355–364.

Leishman, A. J., Naidenko, O. V., Attinger, A., Koning, F., Lena, C. J., Xiong, Y., Chang, H. C., Reinherz, E., Kronenberg, M., and Cheroutre, H. (2001). T cell responses modulated through interaction between CD8αα+ and the nonclassical MHC class I molecule, TL. *Science* 294, 1936–1939.

Leon, F., Roldan, E., Sanchez, L., Camarero, C., Bootello, A., and Roy, G. (2003). Human small-intestinal epithelium contains functional natural killer lymphocytes. *Gastroenterology* 125, 345–356.

Lepage, A. C., Buzoni-Gatel, D., Bout, D. T., and Kasper, L. H. (1998). Gut-derived intraepithelial lymphocytes induce long term immunity against *Toxoplasma gondii*. *J. Immunol.* 161, 4902–4908.

Levelt, C. N., de Jong, Y. P., Mizoguchi, E., O'Farrelly, C., Bhan, A. K., Tonegawa, S., Terhorst, C., and Simpson, S. J. (1999). High- and low-affinity single-peptide/MHC ligands have distinct effects on the development of mucosal CD8αα and CD8αβ T lymphocytes. *Proc. Natl. Acad. Sci. USA* 96, 5628–5633.

Li, P., Willie, S. T., Bauer, S., Morris, D. L., Spies, T., and Strong, R. K. (1999). Crystal structure of the MHC class I homolog MIC-A, a γδ T cell ligand. *Immunity* 10, 577–584.

Lin, T., Matsuzaki, G., Yoshida, H., Kenai, H., Omoto, K., Umesue, M., Singaram, C., and Nomoto, K. (1996). Thymus ontogeny and the development of TCR αβ intestinal intraepithelial lymphocytes. *Cell. Immunol.* 171, 132–139.

Lin, T., Takimoto, H., Matsuzaki, G., and Nomoto, K. (1995). Effect of neonatal thymectomy on murine small intestinal intraepithelial

lymphocytes expressing T cell receptor αβ and "clonally forbidden Vβ s." *Adv. Exp. Med. Biol.* 371A, 129–131.

Liu, Y., Xiong, Y., Naidenko, O. V., Liu, J. H., Zhang, R., Joachimiak, A., Kronenberg, M., Cheroutre, H., Reinherz, E. L., and Wang, J. H. (2003). The crystal structure of a TL/CD8αα complex at 2.1 A° resolution: Implications for modulation of T cell activation and memory. *Immunity* 18, 205–215.

Lodolce, J. P., Boone, D. L., Chai, S., Swain, R. E., Dassopoulos, T., Trettin, S., and Ma, A. (1998). IL-15 receptor maintains lymphoid homeostasis by supporting lymphocyte homing and proliferation. *Immunity* 9, 669–676.

London, S. D., Cebra, J. J., and Rubin, D. H. (1989). Intraepithelial lymphocytes contain virus-specific, MHC-restricted cytotoxic cell precursors after gut mucosal immunization with reovirus serotype 1/Lang. *Reg. Immunol.* 2, 98–102.

Luangsay, S., Kasper, L. H., Rachinel, N., Minns, L. A., Mennechet, F. J., Vandewalle, A., and Buzoni-Gatel, D. (2003). CCR5 mediates specific migration of *Toxoplasma gondii*-primed CD8 lymphocytes to inflammatory intestinal epithelial cells. *Gastroenterology* 125, 491–500.

Lugering, A., Kucharzik, T., Soler, D., Picarella, D., Hudson, J. T., 3rd, and Williams, I. R. (2003). Lymphoid precursors in intestinal cryptopatches express CCR6 and undergo dysregulated development in the absence of CCR6. *J. Immunol.* 171, 2208–2215.

Lynch, S., Kelleher, D., McManus, R., and O'Farrelly, C. (1995). RAG1 and RAG2 expression in human intestinal epithelium: Evidence of extrathymic T cell differentiation. *Eur. J. Immunol.* 25, 1143–1147.

Madakamutil, L. T., Christen, U., Wang-Zhu, Y., Attinger, A., Sundarrajan, M., Ellmeier, W., von Herrath, M. G., Jensen, P., Littman, D. R., and Cheroutre, H. (2004). CD8αα-mediated survival and differentiation of CD8 memory T cell precursors. *Science* 304, 590–593.

Malinda, K. M., Sidhu, G. S., Mani, H., Banaudha, K., Maheshwari, R. K., Goldstein, A. L., and Kleinman, H. K. (1999). Thymosin β4 accelerates wound healing. *J. Invest. Dermatol.* 113, 364–368.

Manzano, M., Abadia-Molina, A. C., Garcia-Olivares, E., Gil, A., and Rueda, R. (2002). Absolute counts and distribution of lymphocyte subsets in small intestine of BALB/c mice change during weaning. *J. Nutr.* 132, 2757–2762.

Markel, G., Lieberman, N., Katz, G., Arnon, T. I., Lotem, M., Drize, O., Blumberg, R. S., Bar-Haim, E., Mader, R., Eisenbach, L., and Mandelboim, O. (2002). CD66a interactions between human melanoma and NK cells: A novel class I MHC-independent inhibitory mechanism of cytotoxicity. *J. Immunol.* 168, 2803–2810.

Masopust, D., Jiang, J., Shen, H., and Lefrancois, L. (2001a). Direct analysis of the dynamics of the intestinal mucosa CD8 T cell response to systemic virus infection. *J. Immunol.* 166, 2348–2356.

Masopust, D., Vezys, V., Marzo, A. L., and Lefrancois, L. (2001b). Preferential localization of effector memory cells in nonlymphoid tissue. *Science* 291, 2413–2417.

Matsuda, J. L., Gapin, L., Baron, J. L., Sidobre, S., Stetson, D. B., Mohrs, M., Locksley, R. M., and Kronenberg, M. (2003). Mouse Vα14i natural killer T cells are resistant to cytokine polarization in vivo. *Proc. Natl. Acad. Sci. USA* 100, 8395–8400.

Matsuda, J. L., Naidenko, O. V., Gapin, L., Nakayama, T., Taniguchi, M., Wang, C. R., Koezuka, Y., and Kronenberg, M. (2000). Tracking the response of natural killer T cells to a glycolipid antigen using CD1d tetramers. *J. Exp. Med.* 192, 741–754.

Matsumoto, S., Nanno, M., Watanabe, N., Miyashita, M., Amasaki, H., Suzuki, K., and Umesaki, Y. (1999). Physiological roles of γδ T-cell receptor intraepithelial lymphocytes in cytoproliferation and differentiation of mouse intestinal epithelial cells. *Immunology* 97, 18–25.

McDonald, V., Robinson, H. A., Kelly, J. P., and Bancroft, G. J. (1996). Immunity to *Cryptosporidium muris* infection in mice is expressed through gut CD4+ intraepithelial lymphocytes. *Infect. Immun.* 64, 2556–2562.

Meharra, E. J., Schon, M., Hassett, D., Parker, C., Havran, W., and Gardner, H. (2000). Reduced gut intraepithelial lymphocytes in VLA1 null mice. *Cell. Immunol.* 201, 1–5.

Melgar, S., Bas, A., Hammarstrom, S., and Hammarstrom, M. L. (2002). Human small intestinal mucosa harbours a small population of cytolytically active CD8+ αβ T lymphocytes. *Immunology* 106, 476–485.

Miyasaka, M., Dudler, L., Bordmann, G., Leiserson, W. M., Gerber, H. A., Reynolds, J., and Trnka, Z. (1984). Differentiation of B lymphocytes in sheep. I. Phenotypic analysis of ileal Peyer's patch cells and the demonstration of a precursor population for sIg+ cells in the ileal Peyer's patches. *Immunology* 53, 515–523.

Mora, J. R., Bono, M. R., Manjunath, N., Weninger, W., Cavanagh, L. L., Rosemblatt, M., and Von Andrian, U. H. (2003). Selective imprinting of gut-homing T cells by Peyer's patch dendritic cells. *Nature* 424, 88–93.

Morales, V. M., Christ, A., Watt, S. M., Kim, H. S., Johnson, K. W., Utku, N., Texieira, A. M., Mizoguchi, A., Mizoguchi, E., Russell, G. J., et al. (1999). Regulation of human intestinal intraepithelial lymphocyte cytolytic function by biliary glycoprotein (CD66a). *J. Immunol.* 163, 1363–1370.

Morrissey, P. J., Charrier, K., Horovitz, D. A., Fletcher, F. A., and Watson, J. D. (1995). Analysis of the intra-epithelial lymphocyte compartment in SCID mice that received co-isogenic CD4+ T cells. Evidence that mature post-thymic CD4+ T cells can be induced to express CD8 α in vivo. *J. Immunol.* 154, 2678–2686.

Mosley, R. L., Styre, D., and Klein, J. R. (1990). CD4+CD8+ murine intestinal intraepithelial lymphocytes. *Int. Immunol.* 2, 361–365.

Muller, S., Buhler-Jungo, M., and Mueller, C. (2000). Intestinal intraepithelial lymphocytes exert potent protective cytotoxic activity during an acute virus infection. *J. Immunol.* 164, 1986–1994.

Murosaki, S., Yoshikai, Y., Ishida, A., Nakamura, T., Matsuzaki, G., Takimoto, H., Yuuki, H., and Nomoto, K. (1991). Failure of T cell receptor Vβ negative selection in murine intestinal intraepithelial lymphocytes. *Int. Immunol.* 3, 1005–1013.

Mysorekar, I. U., Lorenz, R. G., and Gordon, J. I. (2002). A gnotobiotic transgenic mouse model for studying interactions between small intestinal enterocytes and intraepithelial lymphocytes. *J. Biol. Chem.* 277, 37811–37819.

Nanno, M., Matsumoto, S., Koike, R., Miyasaka, M., Kawaguchi, M., Masuda, T., Miyawaki, S., Cai, Z., Shimamura, T., Fujiura, Y., et al. (1994). Development of intestinal intraepithelial T lymphocytes is independent of Peyer's patches and lymph nodes in aly mutant mice. *J. Immunol.* 153, 2014–2020.

Nehls, M., Pfeifer, D., Schorpp, M., Hedrich, H., and Boehm, T. (1994). New member of the winged-helix protein family disrupted in mouse and rat nude mutations. *Nature* 372, 103–107.

Neuhaus, O., Emoto, M., Blum, C., Yamamoto, S., and Kaufmann, S. H. (1995). Control of thymus-independent intestinal intraepithelial lymphocytes by β2-microglobulin. *Eur. J. Immunol.* 25, 2332–2339.

Newberry, R. D., McDonough, J. S., McDonald, K. G., and Lorenz, R. G. (2002). Postgestational lymphotoxin/lymphotoxin β receptor interactions are essential for the presence of intestinal B lymphocytes. *J. Immunol.* 168, 4988–4997.

Nikolova, M., Marie-Cardine, A., Boumsell, L., and Bensussan, A. (2002). BY55/CD160 acts as a co-receptor in TCR signal transduction of a human circulating cytotoxic effector T lymphocyte subset lacking CD28 expression. *Int. Immunol.* 14, 445–451.

Offit, P. A. and Dudzik, K. I. (1989). Rotavirus-specific cytotoxic T lymphocytes appear at the intestinal mucosal surface after rotavirus infection. *J. Virol.* 63, 3507–3512.

Ohteki, T. and MacDonald, H. R. (1993). Expression of the CD28 costimulatory molecule on subsets of murine intestinal intraepithelial lymphocytes correlates with lineage and responsiveness. *Eur. J. Immunol.* 23, 1251–1255.

Panwala, C. M., Jones, J. C., and Viney, J. L. (1998). A novel model of inflammatory bowel disease: mice deficient for the multiple drug resistance gene, mdr1a, spontaneously develop colitis. *J. Immunol.* 161, 5733–5744.

Papadakis, K. A., Landers, C., Prehn, J., Kouroumalis, E. A., Moreno, S. T., Gutierrez-Ramos, J. C., Hodge, M. R., and Targan, S. R. (2003). CC chemokine receptor 9 expression defines a subset of peripheral blood lymphocytes with mucosal T cell phenotype and Th1 or T-regulatory 1 cytokine profile. *J. Immunol.* 171, 159–165.

Papadakis, K. A., Prehn, J., Nelson, V., Cheng, L., Binder, S. W., Ponath, P. D., Andrew, D. P., and Targan, S. R. (2000). The role of thymus-expressed chemokine and its receptor CCR9 on lymphocytes in the regional specialization of the mucosal immune system. *J. Immunol.* 165, 5069–5076.

Park, S. H., Guy-Grand, D., Lemonnier, F. A., Wang, C. R., Bendelac, A., and Jabri, B. (1999). Selection and expansion of CD8α/α TCRα/β+ intestinal intraepithelial lymphocytes in the absence of both classical major histocompatibility complex class I and nonclassical CD1 molecules. *J. Exp. Med.* 190, 885–890.

Penney, L., Kilshaw, P. J., and MacDonald, T. T. (1995). Regional variation in the proliferative rate and lifespan of αβ TCR+ and γδ TCR+ intraepithelial lymphocytes in the murine small intestine. *Immunology* 86, 212–218.

Pennington, D. J., Silva-Santos, B., Shires, J., Theodoridis, E., Pollitt, C., Wise, E. L., Tigelaar, R. E., Owen, M. J., and Hayday, A. C. (2003). The inter-relatedness and interdependence of mouse T cell receptor γδ+ and αβ+ cells. *Nat. Immunol.* 4, 991–998.

Podd, B. S., Aberg, C., Kudla, K. L., Keene, L., Tobias, E., and Camerini, V. (2001). MHC class I allele dosage alters CD8 expression by intestinal intraepithelial lymphocytes. *J. Immunol.* 167, 2561–2568.

Porter, B. O. and Malek, T. R. (1999). IL-2Rβ/IL-7Rα doubly deficient mice recapitulate the thymic and intraepithelial lymphocyte (IEL) developmental defects of γc-/- mice: roles for both IL-2 and IL-15 in CD8αα IEL development. *J. Immunol.* 163, 5906–5912.

Poussier, P., Edouard, P., Lee, C., Binnie, M., and Julius, M. (1992). Thymus-independent development and negative selection of T cells expressing T cell receptor α/β in the intestinal epithelium: evidence for distinct circulation patterns of gut- and thymus-derived T lymphocytes. *J. Exp. Med.* 176, 187–199.

Poussier, P., Ning, T., Banerjee, D., and Julius, M. (2002). A unique subset of self-specific intraintestinal T cells maintains gut integrity. *J. Exp. Med.* 195, 1491–1497.

Poussier, P., Ning, T., Chen, J., Banerjee, D., and Julius, M. (2000). Intestinal inflammation observed in IL-2R/IL-2 mutant mice is associated with impaired intestinal T lymphopoiesis. *Gastroenterology* 118, 880–891.

Regnault, A., Cumano, A., Vassalli, P., Guy-Grand, D., and Kourilsky, P. (1994). Oligoclonal repertoire of the CD8 αα and the CD8 αβ TCR-α/β murine intestinal intraepithelial T lymphocytes: evidence for the random emergence of T cells. *J. Exp. Med.* 180, 1345–1358.

Regnault, A., Levraud, J. P., Lim, A., Six, A., Moreau, C., Cumano, A., and Kourilsky, P. (1996). The expansion and selection of T cell receptor αβ intestinal intraepithelial T cell clones. *Eur. J. Immunol.* 26, 914–921.

Reinhardt, R. L., Khoruts, A., Merica, R., Zell, T., and Jenkins, M. K. (2001). Visualizing the generation of memory CD4 T cells in the whole body. *Nature* 410, 101–105.

Rescigno, M., Urbano, M., Valzasina, B., Francolini, M., Rotta, G., Bonasio, R., Granucci, F., Kraehenbuhl, J. P., and Ricciardi-Castagnoli, P. (2001). Dendritic cells express tight junction proteins and penetrate gut epithelial monolayers to sample bacteria. *Nat. Immunol.* 2, 361–367.

Roberts, A. I., Lee, L., Schwarz, E., Groh, V., Spies, T., Ebert, E. C., and Jabri, B. (2001). NKG2D receptors induced by IL-15 costimulate CD28-negative effector CTL in the tissue microenvironment. *J. Immunol.* 167, 5527–5530.

Roberts, S. J., Smith, A. L., West, A. B., Wen, L., Findly, R. C., Owen, M. J., and Hayday, A. C. (1996). T-cell αβ+ and γδ+ deficient mice display abnormal but distinct phenotypes toward a natural, widespread infection of the intestinal epithelium. *Proc. Natl. Acad. Sci. USA* 93, 11774–11779.

Rocha, B., Vassalli, P., and Guy-Grand, D. (1991). The V β repertoire of mouse gut homodimeric α CD8+ intraepithelial T cell receptor α/β + lymphocytes reveals a major extrathymic pathway of T cell differentiation. *J. Exp. Med.* 173, 483–486.

Rocha, B., Vassalli, P., and Guy-Grand, D. (1992a). The extrathymic T-cell development pathway. *Immunol. Today* 13, 449–454.

Rocha, B., von Boehmer, H., and Guy-Grand, D. (1992b). Selection of intraepithelial lymphocytes with CD8 α/α co-receptors by self–antigen in the murine gut. *Proc. Natl. Acad. Sci. USA* 89, 5336–5340.

Saito, H., Kanamori, Y., Takemori, T., Nariuchi, H., Kubota, E., Takahashi–Iwanaga, H., Iwanaga, T., and Ishikawa, H. (1998). Generation of intestinal T cells from progenitors residing in gut cryptopatches. *Science* 280, 275–278.

Sallusto, F., Lenig, D., Forster, R., Lipp, M., and Lanzavecchia, A. (1999). Two subsets of memory T lymphocytes with distinct homing potentials and effector functions. *Nature* 401, 708–712.

Savage, P. A. and Davis, M. M. (2001). A kinetic window constricts the T cell receptor repertoire in the thymus. *Immunity* 14, 243–252.

Schluns, K. S. and Lefrancois, L. (2003). Cytokine control of memory T–cell development and survival. *Nat. Rev. Immunol.* 3, 269–279.

Schon, M. P., Arya, A., Murphy, E. A., Adams, C. M., Strauch, U. G., Agace, W. W., Marsal, J., Donohue, J. P., Her, H., Beier, D. R., *et al.* (1999). Mucosal T lymphocyte numbers are selectively reduced in integrin α E (CD103)–deficient mice. *J. Immunol.* 162, 6641–6649.

Schweickart, V. L., Epp, A., Raport, C. J., and Gray, P. W. (2000). CCR11 is a functional receptor for the monocyte chemoattractant protein family of chemokines. *J. Biol. Chem.* 275, 9550–9556.

Schweickart, V. L., Epp, A., Raport, C. J., and Gray, P. W. (2001). CCR11 is a functional receptor for the monocyte chemoattractant protein family of chemokines. *J. Biol. Chem.* 276, 856.

Schweighoffer, E. and Fowlkes, B. J. (1996). Positive selection is not required for thymic maturation of transgenic γ δ T cells. *J. Exp. Med.* 183, 2033–2041.

Shibahara, T., Wilcox, J. N., Couse, T., and Madara, J. L. (2001). Characterization of epithelial chemoattractants for human intestinal intraepithelial lymphocytes. *Gastroenterology* 120, 60–70.

Shimizu, T., Sugahara, S., Oya, H., Maruyama, S., Minagawa, M., Bannai, M., Hatakeyama, K., and Abo, T. (1999). The majority of lymphocytes in the bone marrow, thymus and extrathymic T cells in the liver are generated in situ from their own preexisting precursors. *Microbiol. Immunol.* 43, 595–608.

Shires, J., Theodoridis, E., and Hayday, A. C. (2001). Biological insights into TCRγδ+ and TCRαβ+ intraepithelial lymphocytes provided by serial analysis of gene expression (SAGE). *Immunity* 15, 419–434.

Sonea, I. M., Jergens, A. E., Sacco, R. E., Niyo, Y., Merten, E., Kauffman, L. K., and Moore, P. F. (2000). Flow cytometric analysis of colonic and small intestinal mucosal lymphocytes obtained by endoscopic biopsy in the healthy dog. *Vet. Immunol. Immunopathol.* 77, 103–119.

Spencer, J., Isaacson, P. G., MacDonald, T. T., Thomas, A. J., and Walker–Smith, J. A. (1991). Γ/δ T cells and the diagnosis of coeliac disease. *Clin. Exp. Immunol.* 85, 109–113.

Spencer, J., MacDonald, T. T., Finn, T., and Isaacson, P. G. (1986). The development of gut associated lymphoid tissue in the terminal ileum of fetal human intestine. *Clin. Exp. Immunol.* 64, 536–543.

Sprent, J. and Miller, J. F. (1972). Interaction of thymus lymphocytes with histoincompatible cells. II. Recirculating lymphocytes derived from antigen–activated thymus cells. *Cell. Immunol.* 3, 385–404.

Stagg, A. J., Kamm, M. A., and Knight, S. C. (2002). Intestinal dendritic cells increase T cell expression of α4β7 integrin. *Eur. J. Immunol.* 32, 1445–1454.

Stappenbeck, T. S., Wong, M. H., Saam, J. R., Mysorekar, I. U., and Gordon, J. I. (1998). Notes from some crypt watchers: regulation of renewal in the mouse intestinal epithelium. *Curr. Opin. Cell Biol.* 10, 702–709.

Steinle, A., Groh, V., and Spies, T. (1998). Diversification, expression, and γ δ T cell recognition of evolutionarily distant members of the MIC family of major histocompatibility complex class I–related molecules. *Proc. Natl. Acad. Sci. USA* 95, 12510–12515.

Stetson, D. B., Mohrs, M., Reinhardt, R. L., Baron, J. L., Wang, Z. E., Gapin, L., Kronenberg, M., and Locksley, R. M. (2003). Constitutive cytokine mRNAs mark natural killer (NK) and NK T cells poised for rapid effector function. *J. Exp. Med.* 198, 1069–1076.

Suzuki, H., Jeong, K. I., Okutani, T., and Doi, K. (2000a). Regional variations in the distribution of small intestinal intraepithelial lymphocytes in three inbred strains of mice. *J. Vet. Med. Sci.* 62, 881–887.

Suzuki, H., Jeong, K. I., Okutani, T., and Doi, K. (2000b). Regional variations in the number and subsets of intraepithelial lymphocytes in the mouse small intestine. *Comp. Med.* 50, 39–42.

Suzuki, K., Oida, T., Hamada, H., Hitotsumatsu, O., Watanabe, M., Hibi, T., Yamamoto, H., Kubota, E., Kaminogawa, S., and Ishikawa, H. (2000c). Gut cryptopatches: Direct evidence of extrathymic anatomical sites for intestinal T lymphopoiesis. *Immunity* 13, 691–702.

Suzuki, R., Nakao, A., Kanamaru, Y., Okumura, K., Ogawa, H., and Ra, C. (2002). Localization of intestinal intraepithelial T lymphocytes involves regulation of αEβ7 expression by transforming growth factor–β. *Int. Immunol.* 14, 339–345.

Suzuki, S., Sugahara, S., Shimizu, T., Tada, T., Minagawa, M., Maruyama, S., Watanabe, H., Saito, H., Ishikawa, H., Hatakeyama, K., and Abo, T. (1998). Low level of mixing of partner cells seen in extrathymic T cells in the liver and intestine of parabiotic mice: Its biological implication. *Eur. J. Immunol.* 28, 3719–3729.

Svensson, M., Marsal, J., Ericsson, A., Carramolino, L., Broden, T., Marquez, G., and Agace, W. W. (2002). CCL25 mediates the localization of recently activated CD8αβ(+) lymphocytes to the small– intestinal mucosa. *J. Clin. Invest.* 110, 1113–1121.

Swanson, B. J., Murakami, M., Mitchell, T. C., Kappler, J., and Marrack, P. (2002). RANTES production by memory phenotype T cells is controlled by a posttranscriptional, TCR–dependent process. *Immunity* 17, 605–615.

Sydora, B. C., Brossay, L., Hagenbaugh, A., Kronenberg, M., and Cheroutre, H. (1996a). TAP–independent selection of CD8+ intestinal intraepithelial lymphocytes. *J. Immunol.* 156, 4209–4216.

Sydora, B. C., Jamieson, B. D., Ahmed, R., and Kronenberg, M. (1996b). Intestinal intraepithelial lymphocytes respond to systemic lymphocytic choriomeningitis virus infection. *Cell. Immunol.* 167, 161–169.

Sydora, B. C., Mixter, P. F., Holcombe, H. R., Eghtesady, P., Williams, K., Amaral, M. C., Nel, A., and Kronenberg, M. (1993). Intestinal intraepithelial lymphocytes are activated and cytolytic but do not proliferate as well as other T cells in response to mitogenic signals. *J. Immunol.* 150, 2179–2191.

Tabaczewski, P. and Stroynowski, I. (1994). Expression of secreted and glycosylphosphatidylinositol–bound Qa–2 molecules is dependent on functional TAP–2 peptide transporter. *J. Immunol.* 152, 5268–5274.

Taplin, M. E., Frantz, M. E., Canning, C., Ritz, J., Blumberg, R. S., and Balk, S. P. (1996). Evidence against T–cell development in the adult human intestinal mucosa based upon lack of terminal deoxynucleotidyltransferase expression. *Immunology* 87, 402–407.

Teitell, M., Holcombe, H. R., Brossay, L., Hagenbaugh, A., Jackson, M. J., Pond, L., Balk, S. P., Terhorst, C., Peterson, P. A., and Kronenberg, M. (1997). Nonclassical behavior of the mouse CD1 class I–like molecule. *J. Immunol.* 158, 2143–2149.

Torres–Nagel, N., Kraus, E., Brown, M. H., Tiefenthaler, G., Mitnacht, R., Williams, A. F., and Hunig, T. (1992). Differential thymus dependence of rat CD8 isoform expression. *Eur. J. Immunol.* 22, 2841–2848.

Tregaskes, C. A., Kong, F. K., Paramithiotis, E., Chen, C. L., Ratcliffe, M. J., Davison, T. F., and Young, J. R. (1995). Identification and analysis of the expression of CD8αβ and CD8αα isoforms in chickens reveals a major TCR–γδ CD8 αβ subset of intestinal intraepithelial lymphocytes. *J. Immunol.* 154, 4485–4494.

Tsai, F. Y., Keller, G., Kuo, F. C., Weiss, M., Chen, J., Rosenblatt, M., Alt, F. W., and Orkin, S. H. (1994). An early haematopoietic defect in mice lacking the transcription factor GATA–2. *Nature* 371, 221–226.

Tschetter, J. R., Davis, W. C., Perryman, L. E., and McGuire, T. C. (1998). CD8 dimer usage on α β and gama δ T lymphocytes from equine lymphoid tissues. *Immunobiology* 198, 424–438.

Uehara, S., Grinberg, A., Farber, J. M., and Love, P. E. (2002). A role for CCR9 in T lymphocyte development and migration. *J. Immunol.* 168, 2811–2819.

Van Houten, N., Blake, S. F., Li, E. J., Hallam, T. A., Chilton, D. G., Gourley, W. K., Boise, L. H., Thompson, C. B., and Thompson, E. B. (1997). Elevated expression of Bcl–2 and Bcl–x by intestinal intraepithelial lymphocytes: Resistance to apoptosis by glucocorticoids and irradiation. *Int. Immunol.* 9, 945–953.

Van Houten, N., Mixter, P. F., Wolfe, J., and Budd, R. C. (1993). CD2 expression on murine intestinal intraepithelial lymphocytes is bimodal and defines proliferative capacity. *Int. Immunol.* 5, 665–672.

Wagner, N., Lohler, J., Kunkel, E. J., Ley, K., Leung, E., Krissansen, G., Rajewsky, K., and Muller, W. (1996). Critical role for β7 integrins in formation of the gut–associated lymphoid tissue. *Nature* 382, 366–370.

Wang, H. C. and Klein, J. R. (2001). Multiple levels of activation of murine CD8(+) intraepithelial lymphocytes defined by OX40 (CD134) expression: Effects on cell–mediated cytotoxicity, IFN–γ, and IL–10 regulation. *J. Immunol.* 167, 6717–6723.

Wang, H. C., Zhou, Q., Dragoo, J., and Klein, J. R. (2002). Most murine CD8+ intestinal intraepithelial lymphocytes are partially but not fully activated T cells. *J. Immunol.* 169, 4717–4722.

Wang, H. H., Mangano, M. M., and Antonioli, D. A. (1994). Evaluation of T–lymphocytes in esophageal mucosal biopsies. *Mod. Pathol.* 7, 55–58.

Woodward, J. and Jenkinson, E. (2001). Identification and characterization of lymphoid precursors in the murine intestinal epithelium. *Eur. J. Immunol.* 31, 3329–3338.

Wu, J., Groh, V., and Spies, T. (2002). T cell antigen receptor engagement and specificity in the recognition of stress–inducible MHC class I–related chains by human epithelial γ δ T cells. *J. Immunol.* 169, 1236–1240.

Wu, M., van Kaer, L., Itohara, S., and Tonegawa, S. (1991). Highly restricted expression of the thymus leukemia antigens on intestinal epithelial cells. *J. Exp. Med.* 174, 213–218.

Wurbel, M. A., Malissen, M., Guy–Grand, D., Meffre, E., Nussenzweig, M. C., Richelme, M., Carrier, A., and Malissen, B. (2001). Mice lacking the CCR9 CC–chemokine receptor show a mild impairment of early T– and B–cell development and a reduction in T–cell receptor γδ(+) gut intraepithelial lymphocytes. *Blood* 98, 2626–2632.

Wurbel, M. A., Philippe, J. M., Nguyen, C., Victorero, G., Freeman, T., Wooding, P., Miazek, A., Mattei, M. G., Malissen, M., Jordan, B. R., et al. (2000). The chemokine TECK is expressed by thymic and intestinal epithelial cells and attracts double– and single–positive thymocytes expressing the TECK receptor CCR9. *Eur. J. Immunol.* 30, 262–271.

Yamada, K., Kimura, Y., Nishimura, H., Namii, Y., Murase, M., and Yoshikai, Y. (1999). Characterization of CD4+ CD8αα+ and CD4– CD8αα+ intestinal intraepithelial lymphocytes in rats. *Int. Immunol.* 11, 21–28.

Yoshikai, Y., Reis, M. D., and Mak, T. W. (1986). Athymic mice express a high level of functional γ–chain but greatly reduced levels of α– and β–chain T–cell receptor messages. *Nature* 324, 482–485.

Yu, W., Nagaoka, H., Jankovic, M., Misulovin, Z., Suh, H., Rolink, A., Melchers, F., Meffre, E., and Nussenzweig, M. C. (1999). Continued RAG expression in late stages of B cell development and no apparent re–induction after immunization. *Nature* 400, 682–687.

Zhou, Z., Pollok, K. E., Kim, K. K., Kim, Y. J., and Kwon, B. S. (1994). Functional analysis of T–cell antigen 4–1BB in activated intestinal intra–epithelial T lymphocytes. *Immunol. Lett.* 41, 177–184.

IgA B Cell Development

Chapter 31

Warren Strober

Mucosal Immunity Section, Laboratory of Host Defense, National Institute of Allergy and Infectious Disease, National Institutes of Health, Bethesda, Maryland

Sidonia Fagarasan

Laboratory of Mucosal Immunology, RIKEN Research Center for Allergy and Immunology, Yokohama City, Japan

Nils Lycke

Department of Medical Microbiology and Immunology, Göteborg University, Göteborg, Sweden

One of the key effector functions of the gut-associated lymphoid tissue (GALT) is the elaboration of B cells with the capacity to synthesize IgA, the major mucosal immunoglobulin (Ig). In this chapter, we concern ourselves with the cellular and molecular events that take place in the GALT that lead to such B cells. To this end, we address the organogenesis and structure of the anatomic sites at which B cells become committed to the expression of IgA, as well as the microenvironmental conditions within these sites that facilitate this process. In addition, we consider the contribution of the various adhesion molecules and chemokines to the homing of B cells to mucosal tissues and thus to the topography of the mucosal immune system. Finally and most fundamentally, we provide an in-depth discussion of the intercellular interactions and intracellular biochemical events that govern B cell differentiation in general, as well as IgA B cell differentiation in particular, with the view of providing insight into the regulation of IgA B cell development during both adaptive and innate mucosal immune responses.

B CELL DEVELOPMENT AND IMMUNOGLOBULIN CLASS SWITCHING

Early B cell maturation

The bone marrow, in both the adult mouse and the human being, is the primary site of early B cell maturation (Kincade and Gimble, 1993). At this location, B cells pass through a series of antigen-independent maturational stages defined by the presence or absence of certain surface and cytoplasmic markers and by specific stages of Ig variable region heavy and light chain gene rearrangement and expression (Hardy *et al.*, 1991; Li *et al.*, 1993; Ehlich *et al.*, 1993; Loffert *et al.*,

1994). In each B cell, the selection and assembly of the genes encoding the variable region of the Ig molecule occur as a result of a random recombination process in which selected variable (V), diversity (D), and joining (J) gene segments come together to form a single variable region gene complex. The heavy chain V region gene is formed by two rearrangements. First is the joining of D and J genes, followed by the joining of a V gene to the fused DJ sequence, whereas the light chain variable region gene is formed by a single rearrangement joining V and J genes (Brack *et al.*, 1978). These variable region recombinations ultimately result in the production of specific heavy and light chain proteins that can then be assembled to produce the unique Ig molecules that characterize each B cell and its progeny. V(D)J recombination is tightly controlled by transcriptional regulation of the recombinase genes that encode the RAG-1 and RAG-2 proteins (Schatz *et al.*, 1989; Oettinger *et al.*, 1990; Mombaerts *et al.*, 1992; Shinkai *et al.*, 1992).

The most immature B cells contain unrearranged heavy and light chain variable region genes (*i.e.*, genes in germline configuration). Upon recombination of the heavy chain variable region genes, μ heavy chains encoded by the rearranged variable genes linked to the downstream Cμ gene are present in the cytoplasm and on the cell surface in combination with "surrogate" light chains. Then, following completion of the light chain gene rearrangement, both heavy and light chains are produced, and a complete IgM or IgD molecule can be assembled from the organized variable region genes linked to Cμ or Cδ. heavy chain genes, respectively. The immature IgM⁺ B cell can then be formed that coexpresses high levels of surface IgM and low levels of surface IgD. These immature B cells leave the bone marrow and pass via the circulation to various peripheral lymphoid tissues, including the spleen, Peyer's patches (PPs) of the intestine, and lymph nodes. Further maturation to a mature, naïve, immunocompetent surface IgM^{lo}/IgD^{hi} B cell is thought to occur in the periphery. Once B cells reach the destination of their secondary lymphoid organ, the most mature, resting, conventional B cells are found either in primary follicles or in the mantle zone of secondary follicles. In the spleen, however, resting B cells are also found in the marginal zone.

Upon specific immune challenge, a humoral immune response can be induced that is characterized by the formation of activated B cells. Thus, once antigen combines with the specific antigen receptor on the B cell surface, B cell clones committed to producing antigen-specific Ig are selectively expanded. In the spleen, loci of activated B cells are found in the outer region of the periarteriolar lymphoid sheath (PALS). After these loci are formed, activated B cells seed germinal centers in nearby follicles. At this point, surface IgM$^+$ (sIgM$^+$) B cells may undergo either terminal differentiation to IgM-secreting plasma cells or class-switch recombination (CSR) into B cells producing another Ig isotype. Somatic hypermutation (SHM) may also take place at this stage of B cell development, resulting in intraclonal diversity and enhanced antibody affinity and/or specificity. Finally, the initial encounter of a host with a particular antigenic array serves to enhance the host's state of readiness for its immune response to successive encounters with the same antigenic stimuli. This is accomplished by providing a memory B cell response characterized by B cells that possess antigen receptors with enhanced affinity for antigen and that produce classes of Ig with more specialized effector functions through a mechanism termed Ig class or isotype switching.

Immunoglobulin class switching: molecular events

During the early stages of both B and T cell differentiation, V(D)J recombination allows the assembly of variable (V), diversity (D), and joining (J) segments of the V exon of the immunoglobulin and T cell receptor genes, giving rise to diverse repertoires of B and T cells, each expressing receptors for specific antigens.

Mature B cells that have completed functional V(D)J recombination of both heavy (H) and light (L) chain genes and expressing IgM on the surface migrate to the secondary lymphoid organs, where they encounter antigens. Appropriately activated B cells proliferate and differentiate into plasma cells or memory B cells. It is during this process of peripheral differentiation that B cells undergo a second wave of remodeling the immunoglobulin loci, namely, the aforementioned CSR and SHM, which are responsible for isotype switching and affinity maturation, respectively. As is discussed more completely below, these two different recombination events have recently been found to be regulated by a single molecule, activation-induced cytidine deaminase (AID) (Muramatsu et al., 2000).

Outline of molecular mechanisms for CSR

The immunoglobulin C$_H$ locus consists of an ordered array of C$_H$ genes, which, except for Cδ, are flanked at their 5′ region

by unique repetitive sequences called S regions (Honjo and Kataoka, 1978; Kataoka et al., 1980; Davis et al., 1980; Rabbitts et al., 1980; Cory et al., 1980; Shimizu et al., 1982) **(Fig. 31.1)**. The presence of S regions is absolutely required for CSR, as shown by the fact that artificial switch substrates lacking S sequences are completely unable to undergo class switch recombination (Leung and Maizels, 1992; Lepse et al., 1994; Daniels and Lieber, 1995; Kinoshita et al., 1998; Stavnezer et al., 1999; Petry et al., 1999). CSR takes place between two S regions (region specific S-S recombination). It requires double strand breakages, one in Sμ and the other in one of the downstream S regions, and it results in a looped-out deletion of the intervening DNA segments (Iwasato et al., 1990; Matsuoka et al., 1990; von Schwedler et al., 1990). It is followed by repair and ligation of the broken DNA ends and by activation of the ubiquitously expressed nonhomologous end-joining (NHEJ) repair system (Rolink et al., 1996; Casellas et al., 1998; Manis et al., 1998). The looped-out circular DNA contains an I promoter that is still responsive to cytokines and directs production of I-Cμ transcripts called circle transcripts (CTs). These CTs serve as a hallmark for active CSR in vitro and in vivo (Kinoshita et al., 2001; Fagarasan et al., 2001) (Fig. 31.1).

The Cμ gene is located at the V$_H$ proximal end of the C$_H$ gene cluster, so that CSR between Sμ and another S region located 5′ to a C$_H$ gene brings that particular C$_H$ gene adjacent to the V$_H$ exon. The result is a "switch" of the immunoglobulin isotype from IgM/IgD to IgG, IgA, or IgE having the same antigenic specificity but with different biological properties.

The molecular processes that underlie switch differentiation are not random events but are induced by external environmental factors (McIntyre and Strober, 1999). Initiation of CSR requires B cell activation by antigens and cytokines secreted by a variety of cells, such as activated T cells, dendritic cells, or macrophages. Generally, switching to a particular Ig isotype can be said to depend on the type of the activation signal delivered to the B cells and the cytokine milieu to which the B cells are exposed (Lycke, 1998; McIntyre and Strober, 1999). Some antigens and some anatomic locations promote isotype-restricted responses, as shown by the preference for IgA development in GALT (Cebra et al., 1998).

Signal transduction through surface IgM, Toll-like receptors, CD40, other TNF family member receptors (BCMA, TACI, BAFF-R), and cytokine receptors on B cells induces two essential events that are required for CSR: selection of a target S region and induction of AID (Zelazowski et al., 1995; Nakamura et al., 1996; Muramatsu et al., 1999; Litinskiy et al., 2002).

Factors necessary for germline transcription

CSR is preceded by the expression of RNA species encoded by different C$_H$ genes in the germline (Stavnezer-Nordgren and Sirlin, 1986; Yancopoulos et al., 1986). The "germline" transcription initiates upstream of the S region within a promoter located 5′ to the I exon, proceeds through the S

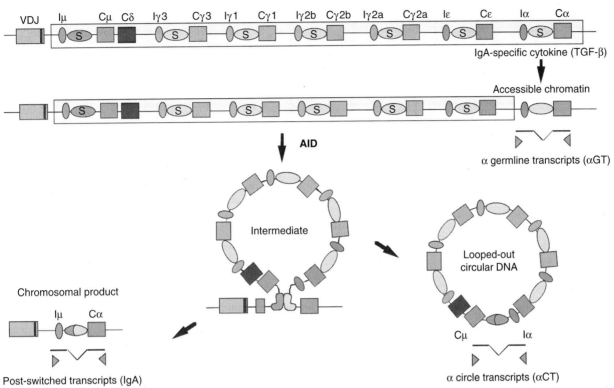

Fig 31.1. Events and markers in IgA switch recombination. **(See page 9 of the color plates.)** The organization of the mouse immunoglobulin heavy-chain locus after completion of V(D)J recombination is shown. Class switch recombination to IgA takes place between the Sμ and downstream Sα regions, and it results in a looped-out deletion of the intervening DNA segments. It requires expression of germline α transcripts, which are initiated from the Iα intronic promoter located upstream of the Sα region upon cytokine stimulation, such as TGF-β. Germline transcription opens the chromatin structure of the Sα region and renders it accessible to the putative switch recombinase. Activation-induced cytidine deaminase (AID), which is induced after B cell stimulation, appears to be the only B-cell-specific marker absolutely required for class-switch recombination and is probably involved in recognition and cleavage of the target DNA. Class-switch recombination to IgA is accompanied by looping-out deletion of the DNA fragment containing Cμ and CH genes located upstream of Cα from the chromosome, and it is followed by repair and ligation of the broken ends by the nonhomologous end-joining repair system (NHEJ). The Iα promoter located on the circular DNA is still active and responsive to cytokines and directs the production of Iα-Cμ transcripts called α circle transcripts. These α circle transcripts are detected after induction of AID, simultaneously with expression of IgA on the surface of B cells, and they disappear more quickly than α germline transcripts, AID, or circular DNAs after removal of switch stimulation. Thus, α circle transcripts are the best available molecule markers for active IgA switch recombination.

region, and terminates at the 3′ end of the C_H gene. Splicing out of the S region creates the final germline C_H RNA (Lutzker and Alt, 1988; Gaff and Gerondakis, 1990; Gerondakis, 1990; Lebman *et al.*, 1990; Radcliffe *et al.*, 1990; Rothman *et al.*, 1990). In mature B cells, the Sμ region is constitutively transcribed, whereas transcription of downstream S regions is induced only after cytokine stimulation.

The close association between isotype specificity of germline transcription and the recombination targeting of S regions by stimulation with a certain cytokine has led some investigators to propose an "accessibility model" of isotype recombination. In this model, transcribed germline genes become "accessible" to the recombination machinery and thus are preferentially rearranged and expressed when cells are exposed to certain cytokines or other influences (Stavnezer-Nordgren and Sirlin, 1986; Yancopoulos *et al.*, 1986). For example, TGF-β induces increased accessibility to DNA encoding the germline α gene and this, in turn, leads to an increase in steady-state levels of germline α (Lebman *et al.*, 1990; Lebman *et al.*, 1990) and γ2b (McIntyre *et al.*,

1993) RNA in activated mouse B cells. Similarly, the combination of IL-4 and TGF-β induces increased access to DNA encoding for the germline α gene (Islam *et al.*, 1991; Nilsson *et al.*, 1991) and the germline ε gene (Gascan *et al.*, 1991; Shapira *et al.*, 1992; Jabara *et al.*, 1993) in human B cells.

The selectivity of the germline transcription process lies in the presence of unique sequences located 5′ to each I exon, capable for binding of a series of regulatory proteins, whose expression may be influenced by the activation conditions. Gene-targeting studies have demonstrated that transcription from I promoters is a necessary prerequisite to CSR (Jung *et al.*, 1993; Zhang *et al.*, 1993; Bottaro *et al.*, 1994; Lorenz *et al.*, 1995). Furthermore, the appearance and quantity of germline transcripts correlate with the efficiency of CSR (Lee *et al.*, 2001; Lundgren *et al.*, 1995; Qiu and Stavnezer, 1998). Although the transcripts are present in the cytoplasm and some have open reading frames (Radcliffe *et al.*, 1990; Bachl *et al.*, 1996), there is no evidence of their translation *in vivo*. Experiments using mice with targeted deletions or mutations in the I exons or their promoters (Bottaro *et al.*, 1994; Seidl *et al.*, 1998; Harriman *et al.*, 1996; Qiu *et al.*, 1999; Xu *et al.*, 1993) and also artificial switch constructs (Kinoshita *et al.*, 1998; Petry *et al.*, 1999; Li *et al.*, 1997; Ballantyne *et al.*, 1998; Okazaki *et al.*, 2002) have shown that the I promoter is dispensable and replaceable by any of a number of promoters. On the other hand, the splice donor site of the I exon has been shown to be critical to its function, as replacement or deletion of the I exon splice site upstream of Sγ region severely inhibited CSR (Lorenz and Radbruch, 1996; Hein *et al.*, 1998). The requirement for the splice donor suggests that splicing machinery might be required for the recombination itself, and/or splicing releases the intron sequences that hybridize with the S region DNA sequences and form an R-loop structure. On the basis of *in vitro* experiments which have shown that S region RNA can form R-loop with S region DNA, it was proposed that the RNA-DNA heteroduplex may be a recognition target for switch recombination (Reaban and Griffin, 1990; Daniels and Lieber, 1995; Tian and Alt, 2000). However, the existence of such structures *in vivo* remains to be demonstrated. Finally, it is important to note that regulatory regions of many I promoters have been extensively studied and shown to contain binding motifs of transcription factors that are regulated by specific cytokines (Iciek *et al.*, 1997; Jumper *et al.*, 1996; Lin and Stavnezer, 1996; Messner *et al.*, 1997; Pan *et al.*, 2000; Pardali *et al.*, 2000; Warren *et al.*, 1999; Xie *et al.*, 1999).

IgA B cell development is particularly associated with TGF-β. TGF-β is a pleiotropic cytokine, having both inhibitory and stimulatory effects on the differentiation of many cell types and suppressive effects on growth (Massague, 1990). We shall discuss the influence of this cytokine on IgA B cell development in great detail. Here we confine ourselves to the effects of TGF-β on the recombination machinery.

TGF-β-induced IgA B cell switching is explained as alluded to previously, by the ability of this cytokine to induce transcription from germline Cα genes. The ligand TGF-β assembles a receptor complex that activates Smads, and the Smads form multisubunit complexes that regulate transcription. Genomic segments encompassing about 130 base pairs upstream of the human and mouse Iα transcription initiation sites appear to be sufficient for expression and TGF-β responsiveness of a reporter gene in B cell lines (Nilsson *et al.*, 1991; Lin and Stavnezer, 1992). The region within these segments (TβRE) that could transfer TGF-β responsiveness to an unrelated promoter contains binding sites for Smad and transcription factors of the acute myeloid leukemia (AML/CBFα/Runx). AML proteins cooperate with transcription factors of the Ets family or directly interact with Smads to activate the Iα promoter (Pardali *et al.*, 2000; Xie *et al.*, 1999). Other transcription factors that bind to the Iα promoter either activate (AYF/CREB) or inhibit (BSAP) α germline transcription (Shi *et al.*, 2001).

It is well known that LPS induces germline transcripts and CSR of both Cγ3 and Cγ2b by mouse B cells. Production of IgG3 after LPS stimulation may be due to the presence

within the Iγ3 promoter of a binding site for NF-κB together with a PU-box (Gerondakis *et al.*, 1991). Various motifs are found within the Iγ2b promoter sequence, including ETS-1, C/EBP, and AP-1 sites (Laurencikiene *et al.*, 2001).

Addition of IL-4 during B cell stimulation by LPS suppresses the Cγ3/Cγ2b transcription and instead promotes switching to IgG1 and IgE. The mouse Iγ1 promoter includes binding sites for signal transducers and activators of transcription 6 (STAT6), C/EBP, PU-1, an AP-3 site, and a TGF-β inhibitory element (TIE) (Xu and Stavnezer, 1992). Although STAT6 binds to both Iγ1 and Iε promoters, the affinity binding to Iγ1 promoter is much lower as compared with that for Iε promoter, which would imply that Iγ1 is less inducible and less dependent on IL-4 stimulation than Iε (Mao and Stavnezer, 2001). Somewhat paradoxically, IL-4 has a greater stimulatory effect on switching to IgG1 than to IgE. This apparent paradox was recently explained by the demonstration that Id2, a negative regulator of basic helix-loop-helix (bHLH) transcription factors, such as E2A proteins, has an inhibitory effect on transcription from the Iε promoter, which appears to be stronger than the effect on Iγ1 promoter (Sugai *et al.*, 2003). The promoter region for Sε germline transcription contains sites for E2A, C/EBP, STAT6, NF-κB, and Pax-5 (BSAP). Id2, which is induced in the presence of TGF-β, acts as a negative regulator of Sε transcription, by sequestering E2A and thus preventing its interaction with E-box motifs of the Iε promoter (Sugai *et al.*, 2003).

Some I promoters are regulated by interferons (IFNs). For example, IFNγ induces specifically the Iε2 promoter while inhibiting the Iε promoter (Xu and Rothman, 1994; Ezernieks *et al.*, 1996). IFNγ induction of germline transcripts involves JAK1 and STAT-1 and a transcription factor specific for Th1 commitment, T-bet (Szabo *et al.*, 2000), which is active in inducing IgG2α switching in B cells (Peng *et al.*, 2002).

Role of AID in class switch recombination

As discussed previously, the selection of a target S region is mediated by transcription from the particular I promoter of that S region, and this event is an absolute requirement for CSR. However, artificial constructs containing constitutive promoters for Sμ and Sα regions introduced into CH12F3-2 B cell lymphoma line (which undergo IgA switching almost exclusively after stimulation with CD40L, IL-4, and TGF-β) (Nakamura *et al.*, 1996) were unable to switch unless cytokine stimulation was given (Kinoshita *et al.*, 1998). Furthermore, cycloheximide, a protein synthesis inhibitor, blocked cytokine-induced CSR, implying that *de novo* protein synthesis is also required for CSR (Muramatsu *et al.*, 1999). Therefore, cytokine stimulation induces not only germline transcription associated with chromatin opening but also activation of new genes involved in CSR, such as AID (Kinoshita *et al.*, 1998; Muramatsu *et al.*, 1999).

AID was identified by cDNA subtractive hybridization between cDNA libraries of stimulated and nonstimulated CH12F3-2, and AID transcripts were observed only in activated B cells that undergo CSR upon *in vitro* stimulation (Muramatsu *et al.*, 1999). When AID is overexpressed in

CH12F3-2 cells, which constitutively synthesize α germline transcripts, these cells undergo IgA switching without any additional stimulation (Muramatsu *et al.*, 2000). Furthermore, when ectopically expressed in fibroblasts, AID was found to induce CSR in artificial switch constructs (Okazaki *et al.*, 2002). This would imply that AID is the only B cell-specific factor required for CSR and that all other trans-acting factors are probably ubiquitously expressed. Although the molecular mechanism for AID function is still uncertain, it is probably involved in the cleavage step during CSR (Kinoshita and Honjo, 2001; Honjo *et al.*, 2002).

In vivo, AID is strongly expressed in B cells located in the germinal center, the anatomic site where CSR and SHM take place with high efficiency (Muramatsu *et al.*, 1999; MacLennan, 1994). The essential role of AID on CSR was revealed by loss-of-function studies in both mice and humans (Muramatsu *et al.*, 2000; Revy *et al.*, 2000). Mice deficient in AID cannot produce any Ig isotype other than IgM, which is abundantly secreted under both immunized and nonimmunized conditions. CSR is not detected in AID-deficient B cells even after *in vitro* stimulation, although these B cells proliferate normally and express normal germline transcripts of all downstream S regions in response to cytokine stimulation.

One of the surprising characteristics of AID deficiency is the almost complete lack of SHM. Sequence analysis of the $V_H186.2$ gene in *aid*$^{-/-}$ mice after immunization with 4-hydroxy-3-nitrophenylacetyl (NP) conjugated with chicken γ-globulin (CGG) revealed that the mutation frequency was no more than the error rate of the *Taq* polymerase used for the experiment. Human AID deficiency, called hyper-IgM syndrome type II, shows an identical phenotype to AID deficiency in mouse, clearly indicating that AID is absolutely required for both CSR and SHM (Durandy and Honjo, 2001). As discussed next, AID deficiency in mice leads to drastic changes in the ability of the animals to control the growth of the mucosal microflora.

Immunoglobulin class switching: role of cytokines
Considerable data have accumulated indicating that the molecular processes underlying switch differentiation are not stochastic events but rather processes induced by influences acting from outside the cell. This external control first became apparent when research performed independently by the laboratories of Severinson and Vitetta uncovered the ability of T cell supernatants, when added to LPS-stimulated B cells *in vitro*, to enhance IgG1 production selectively while inhibiting the synthesis of IgG3 and IgG2 (Isakson *et al.*, 1982; Vitetta *et al.*, 1985; Sideras *et al.*, 1985; Bergstedt-Lindqvist *et al.*, 1984). The activity in these supernatants was termed B cell differentiation factor for IgG (BCDF-γ) and was later found to be identical to B cell growth factor-I (BCGF-I), a factor shown to enhance proliferation of anti-Ig-activated B cells. After cloning of these factors, they were later renamed interleukin-4 (IL-4) (Noma *et al.*, 1986; Lee *et al.*, 1986).

Further studies have shown that LPS-stimulated murine B cells cultured in the absence of IL-4 produce mainly IgG3 and IgG2b, whereas these same cells, cultured in the presence of IL-4, produce large amounts of IgG1 and decreased amounts of IgG3 and IgG2b (Bergstedt-Lindqvist *et al.*, 1984; Snapper and Paul, 1987b; Coffman and Carty, 1986; Layton *et al.*, 1984; Isakson *et al.*, 1982). In addition, IL-4 was shown to induce purified sIgM$^+$ B cells to produce IgG1; increase the precursor frequency of IgG1-secreting B cells in limiting dilution studies; and induce molecular events involving the Cγ1 gene segment that precede the onset of B cell proliferation. These studies ruled out the possibility that IL-4 merely promotes the selective proliferation of B cells that already had switched to IgG1 expression, and they focused attention on the ability of this lymphokine to induce IgG1 switch differentiation (Coffman and Carty, 1986; Snapper *et al.*, 1988a; Coffman *et al.*, 1986). Finally, it was shown that at high concentrations IL-4 also induces IgE switch differentiation. Although this effect was quantitatively small in comparison with the IgG1 effect, it was critical to IgE production since mice treated with anti-IL-4 had greatly reduced or even absent IgE responses when challenged with an IgE antibody–inducing stimulus (Lebman and Coffman, 1988). Recently it has been shown that not only primary IgE responses but also secondary IgE responses are at least partially dependent on IL-4. In this case, the IgE cells arise from sIgG1$^+$ B cells (rather than sIgM$^+$ B cells) that are induced to undergo sequential switching under the influence of CD40L and IL-4 signaling (Sudowe *et al.*, 2000).

Additional support for the concept that Ig class switching is a process directed by cytokines comes from studies of the effects of IFN-γ, IL-5, and TGF-β on class switching. Thus, it has been shown that IFN-γ induces anti-IgD-dextran-activated (Snapper *et al.*, 1992) and T-cell-activated (Croft and Swain, 1991) B cells to switch to IgG3 and induces LPS-, anti-IgD-dextran-(Snapper *et al.*, 1992), T-cell-(Stevens *et al.*, 1988), and CD40L-activated (Snapper, 1996) B cells to switch to IgG2α. It has also been shown that IFN-γ and IL-4 have a somewhat reciprocal relationship with regard to class-switch differentiation (Snapper and Paul, 1987). Thus, IFN-γ is inhibitory for many IL-4-induced activities such as IgG1 and IgE class switching, whereas IL-4 inhibits IFN-γ-induced activities such as switching to IgG2α. Along similar lines, IL-5, although better known as a terminal differentiation factor, can also serve as a switch factor under appropriate circumstances. In particular, if sIgM$^+$ B cells are stimulated with CD38 ligation in the presence of IL-5, they undergo switching to sIgG1$^+$ B cells. Finally, as discussed in much greater detail below, TGF-β has been shown to regulate the switch to LPS-activated B cells to IgA (Coffman *et al.*, 1989; Lebman *et al.*, 1990a,b) and IgG2b (McIntyre *et al.*, 1993). Suffice it to say here that TGF-β is the only cytokine that has clearly been established as an isotype switch factor for both mouse and human IgA B cells. Thus, while other cytokines such as IL-4 and IL-10 have been proposed as IgA switch factors and can clearly magnify *in vitro* IgA responses, they cannot cause purified sIgM$^+$ B cells or B cell lines to become sIgA$^+$ B cells in culture systems in which TGF-β is not present (Cerutti *et al.*, 1998). In addition, neither of these cytokines is essential for *in vivo* IgA responses. Thus, while IL-4-deficient mice mount poor IgA responses following stimulation with soluble proteins, they mount normal IgA responses when stimulated by cholera toxin or *Salmonella* organisms (Vajdy *et al.*, 1995; Okahashi *et al.*, 1996). Similarly, IL-10-deficient mice manifest normal or even increased IgA responses (Justice *et al.*, 2001). The true role of IL-4 in IgA B cell differentiation may thus lie in the fact that this cytokine is necessary for Th2 T cell differentiation and that Th2 T cells favor IgA B cell differentiation at the post-switch level via production of cytokines that are known to be important terminal B-cell differentiation factors, such as IL-6 (Okahashi, *et al.*, 1996). Likewise, IL-10 itself is a potent terminal differentiation factor for IgA (Zan *et al.*, 1998).

The cytokine effects on class switching discussed previously may underlie the capacity of different murine strains to express various Ig classes during an antibody response. This follows from the fact that, as discussed below, mouse strains differ in their ability to produce IL-4 via a Th2 response and IFN-γ via a Th1 response. Thus, given the opposing effects of these cytokines on various types of switch differentiation, these mouse strains differ in their capacities to produce IgG1 (IL-4 dependent) and IgG2a (IFN-γ dependent). There is also some evidence that mouse strains differ with respect to endogenous TGF-β production. This is suggested by studies showing that *in vitro* LPS stimulation of B cells from one mouse strain (BALB/c) leads to IgG2b production in the absence of exogenous TGF-β, whereas B cells from another mouse strain (DBA/2) require exogenous TGF-β (McIntyre *et al.*, 1993).

Finally, the above studies of the effects of cytokines on class-switch differentiation of murine B cells are complemented by studies of human B cells. In one notable set of studies conducted with a monoclonal sIgM+/sIgD+ B cell line (CL-01) that is capable of undergoing isotype switching *in vitro*, it has been shown that switching to all downstream isotypes (verified by various molecular markers) is readily obtained with CD40L signaling in the presence of IL-4 (Cerruti *et al.*, 1998). In this system, TGF-β, but not IL-10, produced by the B cells is necessary for switching to IgA. The lack of effect of IL-10 runs counter to a previous report that IL-10 is an IgA switch factor in humans (Malison *et al.*, 1996). This apparent discrepancy is probably resolved by the fact that IL-10 is a potent terminal differentiation factor and thus can expand small numbers of cells already switched to IgA that are not apparent initially.

Innate and adaptive IgA B cell differentiation

In recent years our concept of IgA B cell differentiation has undergone a paradigm shift in that we can no longer consider the IgA response as related exclusively to adaptive immunity, in which the IgA B cell is strictly dependent on a T cell both for its differentiation into an IgA B cell (class-switch differentiation) and for its differentiation into an antibody-producing plasma cell (terminal differentiation). Instead, we recognize that IgA B cells develop under a dual regime, one encompassing the adaptive immune response occurring in the organized mucosal follicles and another comprising the

innate immune response and occurring in the nonorganized lymphoid tissues of the lamina propria. The first or adaptive response is in fact a highly T-cell–dependent response and in murine systems is said to involve B-2 B cells, whereas the second or innate response occurs in the absence of T cells and is driven by factors derived from either antigen-presenting cells or stromal cells; in murine systems this latter response is said to involve B-1 B cells. In the discussion to follow we initially consider the factors regulating the adaptive IgA system in the PPs and other organized lymphoid follicles. We then turn our attention to the innate system and the development of IgA B cells in the lamina propria in the absence of T cells.

Organization of mucosal inductive sites

The structure and cellular organization of mucosal inductive sites have been extensively discussed in a preceding chapter (Chapter 21). Here we concern ourselves mainly with those aspects that relate to B cell development.

The organized lymphoid tissues of the mucosal immune system, *i.e.*, the inductive sites, consist of large nodules visible to the naked eye, such as the PPs, and the recently described microscopic nodules, the isolated lymphoid follicles (ILF) (see further discussion in the next section). Both are found along the antimesenteric side of the intestinal wall, either in the terminal ileum and/or in other areas of the intestine associated with high concentrations of bacteria. In addition, they are found in other mucosal tissues such as the bronchus-associated and nasal-associated mucosal lymphoid tissues. These lymphoid structures are unique in that antigen enters via specialized epithelial cells, termed M cells, which are adapted for antigen uptake and transport across the epithelium. Such antigen transport is followed by uptake by interdigitating dendritic cells forming a dense cellular net just beneath the epithelial cell layer (Kelsall and Strober, 1996). Some DCs then migrate to interfollicular areas, where they present antigen to CD8+ T cells and induce the latter to become CD8+ T cell effector cells, such as CTLs. Others migrate to adjacent subepithelial dome (SED) areas or to deeper, follicular zones, where they interact with CD4+ T cells that secrete cytokines and act as helper cells for B cells via CD40L signaling. In the last several years it has been shown that PP dendritic cells consist of several different subsets defined by their cell surface markers. These subsets can have functions that are unique to the mucosal immune system (Iwasaki and Kelsall, 1999). Finally, it is now known that dendritic cells can insert cellular arms in between epithelial cells and thus directly sample antigen in the intestinal lumen (Rescigno *et al.*, 2001). This mode of antigen acquisition is not limited to the PPs and, at least theoretically, could occur anywhere in the lamina propria.

B cells that ultimately form germinal centers are activated in T-cell-rich regions containing the aforementioned interdigitating DCs and CD4+ T cells. These B cells first undergo massive clonal expansion to form the outer "dark zone" of a nascent germinal center; they then migrate into an inner "light zone," where they assume the form of centroblasts, *i.e.*, large B cells, that are not in cell cycle. Within germinal centers of the PP, as in germinal centers of other lymphoid tissues, B cells undergo somatic mutation, positive and negative selection, and isotype switch differentiation and develop into memory B cells. However, B cell differentiation in the germinal centers of the PPs differ from that in peripheral lymphoid follicles in two critical ways. First, isotype switch differentiation in these lymphoid structures is heavily skewed toward IgA switching so that, as shown by Butcher *et al.*, >70% of all B cells in PP germinal centers develop into IgA B cells; by contrast, very few, if any, B cells differentiate into IgA B cells in peripheral follicles (Butcher *et al.*, 1982). Second, mature B cells in PP germinal centers do not undergo terminal differentiation into plasma cells and move into medullary cords as in peripheral lymph nodes (PLNs). Instead, mature (memory) B cells are either retained in the PP (in the SED region) or migrate to draining lymph nodes or to distant mucosal effector sites before they begin terminal differentiation (Tseng *et al.*, 1988). In the latter regard, mature B cells in the PPs retain the ability to express L-selectin, the surface antigen that allows migration through high endothelial venules (HEVs) of PLNs and other lymphoid tissues (Moller *et al.*, 1991).

Recently it has been reported that B cells bearing memory cell markers and spatially related to underlying germinal centers may also occur near M cell "pockets," usually adjacent to memory T cells (Yamanaka *et al*, 2001). From their location and phenotype it is reasonable to suppose that such cells have emerged from germinal centers and act as rapid response elements to newly arriving antigens.

The germinal center also contains follicular dendritic cells (FDCs)—dendritic cells that are quite separate in origin from interdigitating dendritic cells and have very different functions. In contrast to the latter cells, these dendritic cells are localized to germinal centers and interact with B cells rather than T cells. In this regard, it has been shown that PP FDCs, but not peripheral node FDCs, display MAdCAM-1 on their surface, an integrin that facilitates binding of mucosal B cells (Szabo *et al*, 1997). The main function of FDCs appears to be the display of antigen and the continued stimulation of B cells in the germinal centers. Recent work has disclosed that direct cell-to-cell interactions between FDCs or between FDCs and B cells within germinal centers occur at connexin 43 gap junctions that arise in FDCs in response to antigen stimulation (Krenacs *et al.*, 1997). Most of these gap junctions are localized to the light zone of germinal centers, where FDCs interact with maturing B cells and CD4$^+$/CD57$^+$ T cells that are thought to regulate B cell differentiation. Thus, it is possible that germinal center B cells are stimulated by both T cells and FDCs, an idea that we return to later. Finally, a small number of CD4$^+$/CD11c$^+$/CD3$^-$ dendritic cells are present in germinal centers that are similar, if not identical, to interdigitating DCs found in other locations (Grouard *et al.*, 1996). The function of these cells in the germinal center is unclear, although it is possible that they maintain germinal center T cells in an activated state necessary to affect B cell isotype switching.

T cells in germinal centers produce a variety of cytokines detectable at the mRNA or protein level with *in situ* detection techniques; whereas T cells containing IL-4 mRNA have been consistently observed (Butcher *et al.*, 1993; Krenacs *et al.*, 1997), those containing IL-2, IL-10, IFN-γ, and TNF-α mRNA have also been occasionally seen. This would be consistent with the necessary role of Th2 cytokines in the support of B cell differentiation. On the other hand, IL-7 mRNA and protein are produced by human tonsillar FDCs (Kröncke *et al.*, 1996), and both IL-5 and TGF-β protein have been found in germinal centers without precise cellular location (Imal and Yamakawa, 1996; Krenacs *et al.*, 1997). As we shall see, these cytokines may play critical roles in IgA B-cell switch differentiation.

The organogenesis of lymphoid structures supporting adaptive IgA responses

IgA B cells develop within a complex cellular milieu such as the PPs, the isolated lymphoid follicles, or the lamina propria. On this basis the organogenesis of the follicular tissue is a major requirement for IgA production (as it is for the production of other immunoglobulins as well). Recent studies have shown that PP development is dependent on the combined effects of cytokines, integrins, and chemokines (and their respective receptors) acting on progenitor cells and, later, on B cells and T cells in the primitive gut. Initially, a CD3$^-$CD4$^+$ progenitor cell makes its appearance in the developing intestinal wall and is stimulated by IL-7α to express surface LT α1β2, which acts on stromal cells via LTβR to synthesize CXCL13 (Honda *et al.*, 2001). This produces conditions leading to a possible feedback loop for CD3$^-$CD4$^+$ cell accumulation in which the stromal cell–derived CXCL13 attracts additional CD3$^-$CD4$^+$ cells via its CXCR5 receptor and the latter cells induce additional stromal CXCL13 (Müller and Lipp, 2003). Activation of α4β1 on the surface of CD3$^-$CD4$^+$ cells by chemokine signaling (CXCR5 signaling) leads to activation of α4β1 and subsequent interactions between α4β1 on CD3$^-$CD4$^+$ cells and VCAM-1 on stromal cells, which also facilitate this proposed loop by promoting the expression of LTα1β2 on the cell surface (Finke *et al.*, 2002). Finally, the secretion of CXCL13 attracts mature B cells into the developing PP while other stromal cell–derived chemokines, CCL19 and CCL21, attract T cells (acting via CCR7 [Muller and Lipp, 2003]).

A key feature of this organogenesis is the signaling of stromal cells by LTα1β2. Such signaling has recently been shown to be mediated by various components of the NF-κB pathway (Yilmaz *et al.*, 2003). Thus, signaling via LTβR leads to NF-κB-inducing cytokine (NIK) activation, IKKα activation, and p100/RelB activation that, in turn, lead to production of CXCL13, CCL19, and CCL21; this explains the fact that NIK mutations characteristic of aly/aly mice are associated with defective PP development (Miyanoki *et al.*, 1994). Alternatively, LTβR signaling proceeds through IKKγ (NEMO) and p50 or REL A complexes and, in turn, leads to production of CCLR and VCAM-1.

The CD3⁻CD4⁺ progenitor cell is present in RAG-2-deficient mice and thus has not undergone TCR rearrangement. This accords with the fact that these cells can develop into NK cells or CD11c⁺ APCs but not into T cells or B cells (Mebius et al., 1997). The stimulus acting on CD3⁻CD4⁺ cells to initiate PP organogenesis is unknown, but, as mentioned, a factor acting via the IL-7Rα is undoubtedly involved. Since the common γ chain is also necessary for PP development (DiSanto et al., 1995) and this chain combines with IL-7Rα to form the IL-7 receptor, it is likely that IL-7 itself or another factor acting via the IL-7 receptor such as thymic stromal lymphopoietin is involved (Müller and Lipp, 2003).

The above discussion bears on recent insights into the role of lymphotoxin-α (LTα) and TNF in mucosal follicular development derived from mice deficient in these cytokines or their receptors or mice in which such signaling is blocked. LTα forms secreted homotrimers (LTα3) that react with TNFR I and II or membrane-bound heterotrimers containing LTβ (LTα$_1$β$_2$) that react with LTβ-R (Chaplin and Fu, 1998). Targeted deletion of LTα leads to mice lacking lymph nodes and PPs and disrupted splenic white pulp architecture characterized by poorly delineated T and B cell areas and lack of marginal zones (De Togni et al., 1994). On the other hand, targeted disruption of TNF or TNF-RI (p55TNF-R) leads to mice that can develop at least rudimentary PPs and PLN containing segregated T cells, B cells, and dendritic cells to which B cells can home; however, these lymphoid structures are defective in that they lack B cell follicles, follicular dendritic cell networks, and germinal centers (Neuman et al., 1996; Pasparakis et al., 1997). This indicates that LT αβ signaling via LTβR and LTα signaling via TNF-RI is not sufficient for normal organogenesis and that the latter requires TNF-α signaling via TNF-RI as well.

PPs and recently described "isolated lymphoid follicles" (ILFs) differ somewhat with relation to LTα/LTβR signaling (Hamada et al., 2002; Lorenz et al., 2003). Thus, development of PPs requires LTα/LTβR signaling during fetal life, and mice deficient in such signaling because of treatment in utero with LTβR-Fc (an agent that blocks LT α/LTβR signaling) and thus lacking PPs cannot develop patches if such signaling is restored after birth by cessation of LT-βR-Fc treatment. In contrast, while ILFs also require LT α/LTβR signaling for their development, this requirement is manifest postnatally and ILFs can develop in mice treated in utero with LT βR-Fc. Such postnatal ILF development is in keeping with the fact that ILFs do not occur under germ-free conditions and thus require factors in the normal mucosal microflora. Finally, it should be noted that ILFs are similar to PPs in that immature or rudimentary ILFs occur in the absence of TNF-RI signaling, but mature ILFs require such signaling.

LT and LTβR are expressed by different types of cells: LT is produced by B cells, T cells, and NK cells, and LTβR by non-bone-marrow-derived cells, such as stromal cells and a subset of monocytes. With respect to ILF formation, various bone marrow repletion studies using cells from LTα-deficient mice and LT βR-deficient recipients disclosed that ILF formation requires B cells expressing LTα and stromal cells expressing LTβR for formation of immature ILFs and TNF-RI signaling for formation of mature ILFs. Assuming the same requirements exist for PPs, one can say that organized mucosal lymphoid tissues are dependent on B cell–stromal cell interactions.

Since development of organized lymphoid tissues is sequential, it is possible to obtain mice lacking PPs but having intact mesenteric lymph nodes (as well as other lymph nodes) by treating them with LTβR-Fc in utero at a late gestational age. It is interesting that such mice have virtually normal numbers of IgA plasma cells in their lamina propria and respond to orally administered antigen (plus adjuvant) with a virtually normal IgA antibody response (Yamamoto et al., 2002). In contrast, mice deficient in both TNF and LTα and thus lacking both PPs and mesenteric nodes display poor IgA responses to the same type of antigenic challenge. These results suggest that mesenteric lymph nodes can sustain IgA responses even in the absence of PPs (Yamamoto et al., 2002). However, this conclusion is subject to the caveat that LTβR-Fc treatment in utero does not impair the development of ILFs, and therefore ILFs, rather than mesenteric nodes, are the source of the IgA response. Complete ablation of lymphoid development in mice deficient in TNF and LTα also prevents ILF development, so that mice lacking all organized lymphoid tissue cannot mount normal IgA responses, at least responses to specific antigens (Lorenz et al., 2003).

With regard to IgA production by nonfollicular tissue in the lamina propria, it has been shown that mice deficient in LTα or LTβ (the latter lacking membrane LTβ) and thus lacking both PPs and mesenteric lymph nodes have greatly reduced levels of IgA in serum and intestinal washes (Kang et al., 2002). However, while this deficiency was not found in LTα-deficient mice reconstituted with normal bone marrow, it was found in LTβR-deficient mice reconstituted with normal bone marrow, suggesting that interactions between normal B cells expressing LTα and stromal cells in the lamina propria expressing LTβR were sufficient for nonfollicular IgA production (Kang et al., 2002). This conclusion was confirmed by the fact that transplantation of a segment of intestine from RAG-2-deficient mice into LT α-deficient mice led to normal IgA production. On the basis of these results it is apparent that not only IgA responses in organized (follicular) tissues of the mucosal immune system (involving B-2 B cells) but also IgA responses in diffuse (nonfollicular) tissues (involving B-1 B cells) require LTα/LTβR interactions. It should be noted, however, that this requirement relates to the development of the milieu where IgA cells can develop, not to the process of B cell switching to IgA. This is clearly shown by the fact that normal mice treated with LTβR-Ig or TNFRI-Ig in the postnatal period, i.e., mice treated after formation of mucosal follicles, have completely normal IgA responses following oral antigen challenge (Yamamoto et al., 2000).

Site of commitment of B cells to IgA B cell differentiation

The preponderance of data relating to T-cell-dependent IgA B cell development supports the concept that all the essential events relating to such development occur in PPs and other inductive mucosal sites and have, as their substrate, uncommitted (naïve) sIgM$^+$ B cells (see discussion below). However, the possibility must also be considered that IgA B cells develop in PPs primarily because this type of lymphoid site selectively accumulates B cell precursors already precommitted to IgA development at the time of their entry into the patches. Such precommitment occurs in primary lymphoid organs (*i.e.*, the bone marrow) and results in sIgM$^+$ B cells that are phenotypically indistinguishable from other, uncommitted sIgM$^+$ B cells, at least in relation to their surface markers. This notion finds support from the existence of two lymphoma B cell lines, CH12.LX and I.29, which spontaneously switch to IgA and therefore may be examples of precommitted B cells ready for further development in PPs. However, the biological relevance of these cells must be viewed in relation to the fact that CH12.LX B cells were obtained in mice subjected to repeated systemic immunization, and thus these B cells probably did not arise in primary lymphoid tissues but rather in secondary nodal tissues. Further support for precommitment of B cells to IgA expression at a primary lymphoid site comes from the demonstration, in humans, that a significant number of IgA-producing B cells are found in the bone marrow (Alley, 1987). Thus, although such bone marrow IgA B cells may have originated in PPs and may be undergoing terminal differentiation at this site, the reverse can also be envisaged; *i.e.*, bone marrow IgA B cell development may be completed in the PP. If this latter theory were true, however, one would expect to find evidence that a certain fraction of bone marrow cells manifest a "marker" of cells precommitted to IgA differentiation—for example, a tendency to produce Cα germline transcripts—but no such tendency has been reported.

Also relating to the possibility that B cells can be precommitted to IgA expression prior to their entry into a mucosal site is the fact that, at least in mice, the B cell pool has been shown to consist of B-2 B cells and B-1 B cells that have different requirements for differentiation and activation, particularly with respect to their dependence on T cell signaling. We will return to a comprehensive discussion of these cells below. Suffice it to say here that in contrast to the B-2 B cell population, the B-1 B cell population may not develop in PP and other inductive mucosal sites, and thus the possibility arises that these B cells are precommitted to IgA differentiation before they enter mucosal sites. Arguing against this interpretation, however, is the fact that B-1 B cells are exclusively sIgM$^+$ B cells in their premucosal sites and thus, like B-2 B cells, do not seem precommitted to IgA B cell development. Rather, these cells appear to develop into IgA B cells when present in the mucosa and under the influence of mucosal-tissue-specific stimulation.

Homing of B lymphocytes to PPs

The question of whether PPs contain B cells precommitted to IgA-specific differentiation also relates to the question of lymphocyte homing, since one can hardly entertain the notion of precommitment in the absence of a PP-specific homing mechanism. Lymphocyte homing involves a cascade of interactions between specific homing receptors on migrating lymphocytes and counter-receptors (addressins) on vascular endothelium (high endothelial venules [HEVs]) (Holzmann *et al.*, 1989; Bargatze *et al.*, 1995; De Keyser *et al.*, 1996; Pabst and Rothkotter, 1997). In addition, it involves interactions between chemokines expressed on lymphocytes and their respective receptors on endothelial cells, which occur subsequent to adhesin–addressin interactions and which lead to changes in integrin configuration and chemotaxis that allow movement of cells across the endothelium and into the tissue proper.

In mice, the integrin molecule known as lymphocyte PP HEV adhesion molecule (LPAM-1)—identical to the α4β7 integrin in humans (Kilshaw and Murant, 1991)—has been shown to be a PP-specific homing receptor (Holzmann *et al.*, 1989; Hu *et al.*, 1992). Thus, homing of lymphocytes to PPs, but not to PLNs, is inhibited by various antibodies to α4β7 (Hamann *et al.*, 1991, 1994), and β7-chain gene-deficient mice do not form the various tissue components of GALT (Wagner *et al.*, 1996). The counter-receptor for LPAM-1 (α4β7) is a molecule expressed on mucosal HEVs called mucosal addressin cell adhesion molecule-1 (MAdCAM-1), and studies with transfectants of a B cell lymphoma cell line that express the β-chain of α4β7 have established that LPAM-1-MAdCAM-1 interactions are the functionally dominant adhesion pathway for lymphocyte homing to mucosal sites (Berlin *et al.*, 1993; Strauch *et al.*, 1994). Murine and human MAdCAM-1 are structurally and functionally similar in their integrin binding domain but diverge in other domains (Shyjan *et al.*, 1996).

T cells also express α4β7 and use this integrin for entry into mucosal tissues (Kilshaw and Murant, 1991). Thus, whereas α4β7 expression on T cells is not as high on B cells, α4β7^{hi} CD4$^+$ T cells are enriched in PPs (Andrew *et al.*, 1996). In addition, CD44^{hi}/α4β7^{hi} naïve T cells home to PPs as efficiently as CD44^{lo} naïve T cells, whereas α4β7–memory T cells tend to home to PLNs (Williams and Butcher, 1997).

Although α4β7 is the main receptor used by lymphocytes for mucosa-specific homing to PPs, L-selectin (MEL-14) may also contribute to this process. This view is supported by studies showing that administration of anti-L-selectin antibody inhibits the homing of purified naïve CD4$^+$ cells to PPs (as well as to PLNs) (Bradley *et al.*, 1997). In addition, studies of lymphocyte subsets in human PPs show that naïve cells (CD45RA$^+$ T cells and sIgD$^+$ B cells) in follicular mantle zones often express abundant L-selectin but only intermediate levels of α4β7. By contrast, more mature T cells and B cells (CD45RO$^+$ T cells and sIgD-B cells) express L-selectin, and most such cells also express α4β7 (Farstad *et al.*, 1997). It should be noted, however, that PPs contain a normal complement of naïve cells even when L-selectin is blocked, indicating that naïve cells may gain entry to PP even in the absence of L-selectin. In contrast, blockade of both L-selectin and α4β7 results in profound depletion of naïve cells in the PP (Bradley *et al.*, 1998).

In recent years it has become increasingly apparent that entry of cells into PPs (and other lymphoid tissues) is specified by chemokines as well as integrins. B cell entry into PPs involves cell adhesion to PP HEVs via CXCR5, CCR7, and CXCR4 since adhesion is substantially reduced when all of these receptors are blocked (Okada *et al.*, 2002). In addition, CCR6, the receptor for MIP-3α/CCL20, may also be involved in localization of dendritic cells to PPs (Kunkel *et al.*, 2003). Whereas CXCL12 is expressed by HEVs in multiple tissues, CXCL13, the ligand for CXCR5, is selectively expressed in the PP HEVs. A somewhat different picture obtains for T cells, since in this case CCR7, the receptor for secondary lymphoid tissue chemokine (SLC) as well as MIP-3β/CCL19, appears to play a major role (Warnock *et al.*, 2000). The described differences in the chemokine mechanisms used by B and T cells for PP entry are underscored by the fact that the receptors associated with these cells are segregated in the PPs (Warnock *et al.*, 2000). Thus, while B cells can arrest in areas of high SLC expression (interfollicular areas), they tend to arrest in areas of low SLC expression that are in or adjacent to follicular sites. Conversely, T cells arrest only in areas of high SLC expression.

Chemokines and their receptors also play an important role in the trafficking of lymphocytes that develop in mucosal follicle tissues (mucosal inductive sites) to lamina propria areas (mucosal effector sites). Thus, it has been shown that activation of both CD4+ T cells and B cells in mesenteric lymph nodes undergo selective upregulation of CCR9, the latter endowing the cells with responsiveness to TECK/CCL25 (Campbell *et al.*, 2002), and sIgA B cells manifest increased expression of CCR10, thus increasing their responsiveness to MEC/CCL28 (Kunkel *et al.*, 2000). Congruent with such upregulation, CCR9 is preferentially expressed in small intestinal T cells, and synthesis of its ligand, TECK/CCL25, is restricted to small intestinal epithelial cells (Kunkel *et al.*, 2000; Papadakis *et al.*, 2000). It should be noted, however, that CCR9-deficient mice exhibit surprisingly little defect in the migration of T cells to the small intestine. This is probably due to compensatory expression of other chemokine receptors such as CCR6 (Agace *et al.*, 2000). At least a proportion of migrating B cells also use the CCR9 system for migration back to the small intestinal lamina propria (Bowman *et al.*, 2002). However, in mucosal areas where TECK/CCL25 is not expressed (such as the large intestine), B cell localization may occur via CCR10, the other receptor upregulated in mesenteric nodes (Kunkel *et al.*, 2003).

Homing receptors such as α4β7 (LPAM-1) and L-selectin may be differentially expressed on cells, depending on the state of activation of local cytokine environments (Huang *et al.*, 1990; Postigo *et al.*, 1993). In this context, it has been shown that TNF-α, IFN-γ, granulocyte-macrophage colony-stimulating factor (GM-CSF), TGF-β, and IL-4 have varying and complex effects on lymphocyte adhesion to HEVs *in vitro* (Chin *et al.*, 1990; 1992). Of particular interest with regard to IgA B cells is the finding that TGF-β, a cytokine essential to IgA B cell switch differentiation (see subsequent discussion), influences adhesion of lymphocytes to HEVs in multiple ways, perhaps the most important being its ability to upregulate the expression of α4β7 (Chin *et al.*, 1990, 1992, 1996).

Having discussed the factors relating to the recruitment of cells to mucosal inductive sites, we can now return to the question posed initially concerning whether or not localization of B cells to such sites reflects the fact that certain naïve B cell subpopulations are precommitted to IgA B cell differentiation. The only evidence relevant to this question available so far is that, as discussed earlier, CXCR5 (and its ligand, BLC/CXCL13) appears to be specific for B cell recruitment to PPs. Thus, it is possible that indeed a B cell differentiation event occurs prior to mucosal recruitment that results in both B cell localization in the mucosal inductive sites and a predisposition to undergo IgA-specific differentiation. This specificity of localization involving CXCR5 does not unequivocally imply precommitment to IgA-specific differentiation, however, since the specificity of B cell localization may in reality be due to local factors that cause rapid upregulation of CXCR5 rather than premucosal differentiation events.

PPs and other organized mucosal lymphoid tissues serve as unique inductive sites for the generation of IgA responses

Our present knowledge of IgA B cell development in PPs and other mucosal follicular tissues can be said to have begun with the studies of Craig and her colleagues, who established that PPs were the major inductive sites for mucosal IgA B cell responses. Using adoptive transfer techniques, these investigators showed that transfer of donor cells obtained from PPs or appendix into irradiated recipients were a major source of precursors of IgA B cells, whereas cells obtained from other tissues were a poor source of such precursors (Craig and Cebra, 1981). Initially, these data were obtained in studies utilizing rabbits in which cells were transferred to allogeneic recipients, but later similar results were obtained in studies of mice in which cells were transferred to syngeneic recipients (Tseng, 1981). Thus, these data strongly suggested that PPs were important sites for the development of IgA B cells and, in addition, were the source of IgA B cells found at other sites, namely, the nonfollicular areas of the mucosal immune system, *i.e.*, the lamina propria.

Subsequent to this ground-breaking work, attention shifted to the nature of germinal centers in PP follicular tissue. In this context it was recognized that these T-cell-dependent structures showed a preferential commitment to IgA B cell development, which was manifest not only in the fraction of cells developing into IgA B cells versus cells of other isotypes and in comparison with germinal centers in peripheral lymphoid tissues but also in the prompt appearance of IgA B cells after a new antigenic challenge; here again, the response differed from that in peripheral tissue in that the first response in the latter was an IgG response (Butcher *et al.*, 1982; Weinstein and Cebra, 1991). That this preferential appearance of IgA cells in mucosal follicular tissue was in fact the major source of cells in nonfollicular mucosal tissues was later convincingly shown by the fact that the clonality of the IgA B cell population in the PP germinal centers is mirrored in the clonality of the cells in the lamina propria (Dunn-Walters *et al.*, 1997). In other words, the cells in the lamina propria bear the molecular markers of the cells in the Peyer's patches and are thus derived from cells in the former tissue.

In the next several subsections we explore the features of mucosal germinal centers in greater detail in order to better explain the process of IgA B cell differentiation in these structures. Our first concern is the role of T cells in PPs in the development of IgA B cells; specifically, we explore the data establishing their role as IgA-specific switch T cells. In this context we focus on the costimulatory role of T cells in IgA B cell development as well as on the role of T cells as a source of TGF-β and other cytokines necessary for such development. We then turn our attention to PP dendritic cells and the role they play in the IgA B cell development. An important aspect of the discussion here is whether dendritic cells can function independently of T cells and whether they can function in nonfollicular as well as follicular sites to influence IgA B cell development. Additionally, since PPs are in close juxtaposition to epithelial cells that are themselves capable of producing cytokines (such as IL-10 and TGF-β), we discuss how these cells can influence dendritic cell differentiation in relation to IgA B cells. Finally, we draw upon this discussion, as well as other relevant findings, to construct a model of IgA B cell development occurring in mucosal follicles.

T cell dependence of IgA B cell differentiation in PPs and other organized mucosal lymphoid tissues

Early concepts of IgA B cell differentiation in PPs centered on whether the development of IgA B cells from IgM B cells occurred simply because the B cells in mucosal tissues were exposed to massive and unrelenting antigen stimulation or whether such differentiation was critically dependent on T cells. In the former view, class switching to IgA occurred in the PPs because the superabundant B cell stimulation characteristic of this site inevitably drove the B cells to express their most 3' C_H gene, the Cα gene in mouse, and the most 3' C_H gene of each Ig gene cassette in humans. However, this theory was at odds with the fact that the cells in PPs do not overexpress relatively downstream Cγ genes and, in fact, IgA B cells make an early appearance in the PPs of germ-free mice monoinfected with a reovirus that were not exposed to massive antigenic stimulation (Weinstein and Cebra, 1991). On the other hand, the view that T cells were essential components of IgA B cell differentiation associated with IgA responses in the organized mucosal tissues obtained support from a variety of studies. In initial studies of this possibility

it was shown that both mice and rabbits lacking thymic function manifested decreased IgA levels or IgA antibody responses (Clough *et al.*, 1971; Pritchard *et al.*, 1973). Later, it was shown that such deficiency could be related to PP T cell activity. Thus, Elson *et al.* observed that whereas mitogen-activated T cells derived from PPs enhance LPS-driven IgA production, they suppress LPS-driven IgM and IgG production; in contrast, splenic T cells activated in the same way suppress LPS-driven Ig responses of any isotype (Elson *et al.*, 1979). This characteristic of IgA responses was later corroborated in studies by Mongini *et al.*, utilizing a "splenic focus technique" to evaluate class switching in clonal B cells that were repopulating the spleen of irradiated mice transferred with various cell populations (Mongini *et al.*, 1983). Here it was shown that the addition of T cells to the transferred cells enhanced the frequency of IgA-expressing clones and that such clones did not usually coexpress any of the various IgG subclasses. Taken together, these studies established that IgA B cell differentiation is regulated by T cells and that such regulation is at least in part separate from that governing IgG B cell differentiation.

In further studies by Kawanishi *et al.*, the question of whether the T cell regulation of IgA B cell development was manifest at the level of switch differentiation or terminal differentiation was explored (Kawanishi *et al.*, 1983). These authors prepared mitogen-activated T cell clones from either the PPs or the spleen and then cocultured the clones with LPS-stimulated sIgM$^+$ B cells. They found that such B cells cocultured with T cell clones derived from the PPs frequently differentiated into sIgA$^+$ B cells, whereas the same B cells cocultured with T cell clones derived from the spleen frequently differentiated into sIgG$^+$ B cells. Additional findings to emerge from this study included the fact that the clones did not induce increased B cell proliferation or Ig-secreting plasma cells, suggesting that switch differentiation and terminal differentiation were separate processes. However, switched sIgA$^+$ B cells occurring in cultures containing clonal T cells from PPs could be induced to differentiate into IgA-secreting plasma cells by coculture with helper T cells producing cytokines. Finally, studies by Benson *et al.* showed that similar findings could be obtained with human T cells (Benson and Strober, 1988). These investigators showed that mitogen-activated T cell clones derived from human appendix had a greater capacity to enhance IgA production than similar T cell clones derived from human peripheral blood. In addition, several of these lines had a greater capacity to enhance IgA production of sIgM$^+$/sIgA$^-$ B cells than in sIgM$^-$/sIgA$^+$ B cells, suggesting that some of these lines were indeed inducing switch differentiation. Collectively, these data provided strong evidence that IgA B cell differentiation is a T-cell-directed process and that, indeed, one could point to a population of T cells in these tissues that could be called IgA-specific switch T cells.

Support for the general concept that T cells are intimately involved in B cell isotype differentiation subsequently came from Mayer *et al.*, who showed that T cells from a patient with Sezary syndrome (a type of lymphoma) were capable of inducing IgG and IgA secretion in cultures of normal tonsillar sIgM[+] B cells or sIgM[+] B cells from patients with hyper-IgM syndrome, who normally cannot produce IgG and IgA (Mayer *et al.*, 1985; Mayer *et al.*, 1986). Several years later it was shown that most patients with hyper-IgM syndrome have a genetic defect that renders them deficient in CD40L, a key costimulatory molecule on activated T cells (Aruffo *et al.*, 1993). Thus, it became evident that the lack of B cell switch differentiation in hyper-IgM patients was due to a lack of B cell stimulation via CD40L and that this molecule is one component by which T cells bring about B cell switching. However, since the switch activity of T cells discovered by Mayer *et al.* brought about both IgG and IgA production, it was evident that CD40L could be not the only factor involved in IgA B cell switching.

Subsequent studies in which IgA B cell–specific switch T cells have been sought have yielded equivocal results. Thus, a notable series of studies along these lines by Philips-Quagliata and her colleagues showed that antigen-specific T cell clones from a variety of tissues, not just PPs, could support IgA responses (Al Maghazachi and Phillips-Quagliata, 1988; Arny *et al.*, 1984). However, these studies did not distinguish between effects of T cells on switch differentiation and terminal differentiation, since the starting B cell population under study were not naïve B cells and could potentially have been cells already committed to a particular pathway of isotype development. Nevertheless, the questions raised by these studies are real, and it is clear that many aspects of the phenotype and function of putative IgA-specific switch T cells remain to be defined.

In other studies addressing the role of T cells in IgA B cell differentiation, Kiyono *et al.* reported the identification of T cells that express Fc receptors for IgA and that preferentially induce the proliferation and differentiation of sIgA[+] (post-switch) B cells (Kiyono *et al.*, 1982; Kiyono *et al.*, 1984). Later studies by these and other investigators provided data suggesting that these T cells produced soluble Fc factors that specifically bind IgA and induce IgA B cell differentiation. However, in the light of our present knowledge that various Th2 T-cell-derived cytokines fulfill this function (particularly IL-5 and IL-6), it now seems likely that the role of these Fc factors in terminal IgA B cell differentiation is marginal at best.

The role of CD40L and costimulatory molecules in IgA B cell differentiation

It is now well-established that germinal centers are T-cell-dependent structures in which T cells exert their influence on B cells via costimulatory molecules involving interactions between CD80/86 and CD28/CTLA-4, OX40L and OX40, B7RP and ICOS, and CD40 and CD40L on B cells and T cells, respectively (Kawabe *et al.*, 1994; Fay *et al.*, 1994; Walker *et al.*, 1997; Dong *et al.*, 2001; Tafuri *et al.*, 2001). Indeed, mice that are deficient in any of these components manifest impaired or even totally absent GC development in either the spleen or PLNs following immunization with a

T-cell-dependent (TD) antigen (Kawabe *et al.*, 1994; Fay *et al.*, 1994; Ferguson *et al.*, 1996; Han *et al.*, 1995). The role of CD40/CD40L may be particularly important in this regard since it has been shown that mice lacking either of these molecules are unable to develop germinal centers or to exhibit isotype-switched (IgG) antibody responses following immunization or infection (Kawabe *et al.*, 1994; Fay *et al.*, 1994).

The importance of CD40L in IgA B cell differentiation first became evident in *in vitro* studies in which it was shown that CD40L-expressing T cells and certain cytokines were shown to promote strong IgA B cell differentiation (Reusset *et al.*, 1991; Dubois *et al.*, 1997). However, other B cell mitogens also had this effect, and it was not until CD40-deficient mice became available that the role of the CD40–CD40L interaction in IgA B cell differentiation could be assessed under *in vivo* conditions. Studies of these mice showed that in the absence of CD40L stimulation of B cells, T-cell-dependent IgM responses assessed in both serum and gut lavage fluids were substantially higher than in wild-type mice, while IgG1 and IgG2 responses were virtually absent (Gardby, E., and Lycke, N., unpublished information; Garbdy, E., Thesis, ISBN 91-628-4288-9). However, this picture suggesting that CD40L deficiency is associated with a complete absence of class-switch differentiation was belied by the fact that while mucosal IgA responses were severely impaired, they were still present (roughly 20% of normal) (Chirmule *et al.*, 2000; Gardby, R., Ph.D. Thesis; ISBN 91-628-4288-9). Further studies revealed that CD40L-deficient mice had no detectable germinal centers in their PPs (or in other lymphoid tissues), and the PP contained IgM but not IgA B cells (Gardby, R., Ph.D. Thesis; ISBN 91-628-4288-9). Thus, the residual IgA response did not originate from cells undergoing differentiation in the PP. As alluded to previously and discussed more fully below, the response may have originated from B cells undergoing class switching in the absence of direct activation by T cells.

In discussing the role of CD40L in the development of IgA B cells, it is also important to mention that CD40L-signaling in B cells leads to expression of costimulatory molecules, notably CD80 and CD86, which then "back-stimulate" T cells via CD28 and CTLA-4 (Chirmule *et al.*, 2000). The importance of such "back stimulation" of T cell function by CD40 is evident from the fact that without it, T cell cytokine production is severely curtailed and there is no germinal center formation and B cell differentiation. Thus, CD40L-deficient mice with poor IgA responses exhibit restored IgA responses following administration of an agonistic anti-CD28 antibody (Chirmule *et al.*, 2000).

The role of costimulation in IgA B cell development has also been extensively studied with the use of mice bearing a transgene expressing CTLA-4Hγ1 and therefore secreting a protein that blocks CD28/CTLA-4 interactions with CD80 and CD86 (Gardby *et al.*, 1998). It was found that such mice exhibited germinal center formation in the PPs but not in the spleen or PLNs and that total IgA production as measured by IgA levels in gut lavage fluids and in the serum were normal, whereas total IgG levels in the serum were depressed. This seemingly unaffected IgA production, however, was belied by the fact that oral immunization of the transgenic mice (with antigen plus cholera toxin adjuvant) led to a greatly impaired response compared to that of wild-type mice; thus, induction of conventional IgA responses requires CD80 and CD86 costimulation, as does induction of systemic IgG responses. Why, then, do transgenic mice bearing a CTLA-4Hγ1 transgene manifest normal total amounts of IgA? One possibility is that such IgA arises from cell–cell interactions in PPs that are dependent on unique costimulatory molecules that are not blocked by CTLA-4Hγ1. In this context, it is worth mentioning that costimulation via ICOS (which signals the B cell via B7RP1) may play an enhanced role in IgA responses under some conditions. Evidence in support of this possibility comes from several studies showing this form of costimulation is particularly important in CD40-mediated isotype switching and Th2 responses, as well as a recent finding that ICOS signaling was necessary for IgE production at mucosal sites (McAdam et al., 2001; Gonzalo et al., 2001).

Additional insight into the role of costimulation in the generation of IgA responses came from subsequent study of CD28-deficient mice (Gardby et al., 2003). In this case, PPs were devoid of GC, as were other lymphoid organs, and while serum IgA levels were reduced, gut lavage IgA levels were still normal and the lamina propria contained normal numbers of IgA plasma cells. Moreover, IgA in lavage fluid from these mice was modified by somatic mutation, albeit at a lower rate than IgA in wild-type mice. Finally, CD28-deficient mice, in contrast to CTLA-4Hγ1 transgenic mice, exhibited normal oral antigen responses (again administered with the adjuvant, cholera toxin). Since the only difference between the CD28-deficient mice and the CTLA-4Hγ1 transgenic mice, as far as T cell signaling is concerned, is that signaling via CTLA-4 (or some as-yet-unidentified costimulatory molecule) is intact in the former but not in the latter, these studies imply that co-stimulation via CTLA-4 is all that is required for mucosal IgA responses. At first sight, this possibility seems unlikely, given previous studies in which it has been shown that costimulation via this molecule provides a negative rather than a positive signal to the T cell and, in fact, CTLA-4-deficient mice exhibit excessive immune responses (Chambers et al., 1997). It should be noted, however, that CTLA-4 signaling leads to enhanced TGF-β secretion, which, as discussed below, is a key IgA-switching cytokine (Chen et al., 1998). Thus, the possibility that comes into view is that IgA responses are to some extent unique in their costimulatory requirements because of the need for TGF-β signaling.

Another unanswered question arising from studies with CD28-deficient mice relates to the observation that T-cell-dependent IgA responses can occur in the absence of germinal centers in the PP. The possibility that in this situation IgA switching occurs in the mesenteric lymph node is unlikely because nodal germinal centers are also absent in CD28-deficient mice. However, if we assume that IgA-specific switch T cells actually arise in the thymus, then the possibility emerges that IgA switching can occur in non-

organized mucosal tissues. A final point concerning CD28 costimulation is that serum IgA responses are greatly reduced in CD28-deficient mice (Gardby et al., 2003). This argues that serum IgA has its origin in systemic tissues rather than in the mucosa and that serum IgA is more dependent on CD28 costimulation than mucosal IgA.

It should also be noted that CD40L stimulation may act through dendritic cells to induce "B lymphocyte stimulator" protein (BLyS) and "a proliferation-inducing ligand" (APRIL) that act in concert with TGF-β and possibly IL-10 to induce/support IgA class-switch recombination (Litinskiy et al., 2002). Such secretion would not only affect T-cell-dependent IgA B cell differentiation but also T-cell-independent responses in the same cellular microenvironment. This is shown by the fact that in BLyS-deficient mice both T-cell-dependent and T-cell-independent IgA responses are impaired.

TGF-β: a key cytokine in the induction of IgA-specific B cell switch differentiation

Historically, the notion that IgA B cell switching requires a cytokine signal (later identified as a TGF-β signal) had its origin in the recognition that B cell switch differentiation to various IgG isotypes or IgE requires the presence of Ig class–specific factors or cytokines such as IL-4 in the case of IgG1 and IgE. However, early studies of switch T cells or dendritic cells involved in IgA switching failed to reveal the presence of a secreted factor, and the idea that a switch factor existed therefore lay dormant until solid evidence emerged from two groups that showed that TGF-β could induce LPS-activated mouse splenocytes to switch from IgM to IgA production. In particular, these groups showed that TGF-β augmented LPS-induced IgA production 10-fold or more, especially in cultures also containing terminal differentiation factors such as IL-5 and IL-2 (Coffman et al., 1989; Sonoda et al., 1989). Thus, whereas IgA constitutes only 0.1% of the total Ig produced by LPS-stimulated B cell cultures in the absence of TGF-β, the percentage increases to 15% to 25% in LPS-stimulated cultures containing TGF-β plus IL-2. This striking finding in murine B cell systems was confirmed by others and, in addition, was extended to human B cell systems (Islam et al., 1991; Nilsson et al., 1991; Defrance et al., 1992; van Vlasselaer et al., 1992), in which B cells were stimulated with pokeweed mitogen in the presence of CD4+ T cells.

The final proof that TGF-β was necessary for IgA switch differentiation came from in vivo studies of IgA levels and/or IgA antibody responses in TGF-β1−/− mice and TGF-βRII−/− mice, i.e., mice that do not produce TGF-β1 or do not respond to TGF-β. Studies of TGF-β1−/− mice indicated that both serum and secretory IgA levels (as well as cells secreting IgA) are greatly reduced (but not absent) in the deficient mice, whereas IgG and IgE levels (particularly the latter) were greatly increased. Similarly, in mice lacking the TGF-βRII receptor, IgA levels were decreased about 10-fold in young mice and were virtually absent in older (8-month-old) mice, whereas IgG levels and antibody responses were increased. In addition, IgA plasma cells were rare in all lymphoid tissues, including the PPs, and IgA antibody responses were undetectable. The fact that very low but still detectable levels of IgA were present in both types of mice can be attributed either to the effects of TGF-β2 or TGF-β3 on B cell differentiation in the TGF-β1$^{-/-}$ mice or to leakiness of the knockout in the TGF-βRII$^{-/-}$ mice that is manifest early but not late in life because of selective survival of mutant B cells.

From the outset, strong evidence was presented that the TGF-β effect on B cells manifests itself at the level of switch differentiation rather than terminal differentiation. First were the findings that TGF-β acts on sIgM$^+$/sIgA$^-$ B cells rather than on sIgA$^+$ B cells and that TGF-β increases the frequency of B cell clones secreting IgA rather than increasing the number of IgA B cells per clone (Kim and Kagnoff, 1990). Second was the observation that TGF-β has no selective effect on B cell viability and produces its maximal effect on IgA production if it is added early in the culture period and then removed (Kim and Kagnoff, 1990). Third was the demonstration that TGF-β actually inhibits IgA production by already switched sIgA$^+$ B cells (Ehrhardt et al., 1996a, b). Fourth and most important was the evidence that in both murine and human B cells, TGF-β induces the production of Cα germline transcripts, an early and essential molecular step in the IgA switch process, as mentioned previously (Lebman et al., 1990a, b; Kitani et al., 1994). Collectively, these data establish beyond question that, under in vitro conditions, TGF-β does act as an IgA switch factor.

With respect to the molecular mechanisms involved in TGF-β-regulated switch activity, it is now clear that in the mouse TGF-β induces transcription factors that interact with TGF-β-responsive elements in the promoter region upstream of the Cα germline transcription initiation site (Shi and Stavnezer, 1998). These factors include at least one member of the acute myeloid leukemia transcription factor family (AML-2), Smad3/4, and a cAMP-response element-binding protein (CREB), which bind to the promoter at separate sites and collaborate to provide maximal promoter activation (Shi and Stavnezer, 1998; Zhang and Derynck, 2000; Park et al., 2001). In addtion, Ets proteins NF-κB also take part in this process (Shi et al., 2001). It should be noted, however, that the regulation of Cα transcription is complex, since it may also involve TGF-β regulation of negative response elements (Edmiston and Lebman, 1997) and, in humans, 3′ enhancer elements that are not under the control of TGF-β (Hu et al., 2000). In addition, TGF-β-responsive elements are found in the regulatory regions of several C$_H$ germline genes, not only those governing IgA, and these regions can also be active in certain settings (Lin and Stavnezer, 1992).

TGF-β may also lead to IgA switching and Cα transcription by regulating a process even more proximal than germline transcription, namely, the accessibility of the region 5′ to C$_H$ genes to transcription factors. The need for such accessibility in the context of IgA switch differentiation comes from the observation that TGF-β does not induce Cα germline transcription in CH1 B cells, a murine lymphoma sIgM$^+$ B cell line with a methylated and therefore inaccessi-

ble Cα locus (Whitmore et al., 1990). However, the existing data on whether TGF-β regulates Cα accessibility is somewhat equivocal since studies of this question are usually conducted in the presence of a B-cell stimulant such as LPS or CD40L (Lebman et al., 1990a, b; Islam et al., 1991; Nilsson et al., 1991; Lin and Stavnezer, 1992), which can itself induce accessibility, albeit in an Ig class–nonspecific fashion. In addition, studies of murine B cell lines that may be relevant to this question do not provide clear answers, since it is possible that such cells have achieved a level of Cα accessibility prior to their immortalization; thus, the effects of TGF-β on their capacity to undergo IgA switching may be a reflection of its ability to induce germline transcription, not accessibility. In the light of these considerations, it becomes clear that conclusions as to whether TGF-β affects accessibility await new studies in which the effects of TGF-β on biochemical concomitants of accessibility such as histone acetylation and DNAase hypersensitivity are assessed.

A final set of data relating to effects of TGF-β on Cα accessibility come from studies of human IgA switch differentiation. In two such studies in which the effects of TGF-β on Cα germline transcription were evaluated in sIgA$^-$ B cells by measuring the production of Cα germline transcripts with use of a sensitive reverse transcriptase–polymerase chain reaction assay, it was found that Cα1 germline transcription can probably be induced and Cα2 germline transcription can definitely be induced by TGF-β alone in the absence of a B cell stimulant (Islam et al., 1991). These studies establish the capacity of TGF-β to induce Cα accessibility, but as alluded to previously, the magnitude of this effect may be insignificant in the absence of concomitant B cell stimulation.

Another consideration relevant to the role of TGF-β in isotype switching, one that complements the discussion on the locus of the TGF-β effect, relates to the magnitude of this effect. In the earliest studies by Lebman and colleagues (1990a) relating to the ability of TGF-β to affect IgA switching, TGF-β was shown to induce only a small fraction of LPS-stimulated sIgM$^+$ B cells to switch to sIgA$^+$ B cells (3.2%). From these data one might conclude that, although TGF-β does indeed induce IgA switching, it does so only at a minor nonphysiologic rate that is in no way comparable to the rate observed at in vivo IgA induction sites, at which the frequency of Ig switching is at the 70% to 85% level (Butcher et al., 1982). However, LPS is not a physiological B cell stimulant, so one can argue that when B cells are stimulated in other ways, a more significant TGF-β-mediated IgA induction can be seen. To examine this question, Ehrhardt et al. (1992) stimulated highly purified sIgM$^+$/sIgD$^+$ B cells (containing <0.2% sIgA$^+$ B cells) with T cells in a cognate interaction (using a T-cell clone that recognized rabbit Ig determinants and B cells treated with IgG rabbit anti-IgM) or in a noncognate interaction (using irradiated anti-CD3-activated T-cell clones in the absence of additional mitogens or antigens), all in the presence or absence of TGF-β. They found that even though the B cells were being stimulated in a highly physiological fashion, TGF-β still induced only a small fraction of the B cells (1% to 3%) to undergo IgA switch differentiation. Furthermore, they showed that the amount of IgA secreted from such switched (sIgA⁺) cells was quite low in comparison with the amount secreted by the number of sIgM⁺ cells equal to the number of B cells in the culture if such sIgA⁺ cells were stimulated under optimal conditions, indicating that indeed only a small fraction of the B cells in the culture ultimately became IgA-secreting cells.

These results demonstrating the relative ineffectiveness of TGF-β-induced IgA switching were in sharp contrast to subsequent findings of McIntyre *et al.* (1995), who showed that TGF-β could induce much more efficient IgA switching under certain circumstances. In these studies, highly enriched populations of high-density (naïve) splenic B cells were stimulated not with a single stimulus, as in the Ehrhardt *et al.* (1992) studies, but with a dual stimulus, either LPS plus anti-IgD linked to dextran (anti-IgD-dextran) or soluble CD40L (trimer) plus anti-IgD-dextran in the presence or absence of TGF-β (and with the B cell helper factors IL-4 and IL-5). In this case, it was found that up to nearly 25% of B cells in culture switched to IgA, a level of switching eight times higher than that observed previously and much more comparable to that observed within the PPs *in vivo*. Similarly, far higher levels of IgA secretion were observed in such cultures. Two potential explanations of this result can be put forward. The first is that by providing the B cell with a second activation signal via the Ig receptor, one renders the cell more receptive to the TGF-β switch signal. Moreover, since B cells in PP germinal centers are in fact subject to stimulation via the Ig receptor by antigens arrayed on the filamentous arms of FDCs, one can say this dual *in vitro* stimulation is quite physiological, and thus *in vivo*, TGF-β is a highly efficient switch factor. The second explanation relies on the additional fact that in the studies of McIntyre *et al.* (1995) the concentration of TGF-β necessary to induce the high-level switching was far greater than that used in previous studies (10 ng/ml versus 0.5 to 2 ng/ml). Thus, the effect of the stimulation via the Ig receptor was not necessary for switching *per se* but rather for maintaining survival of the cell in the face of the high TGF-β concentration. This explanation finds resonance in the fact that, in studies by Banchereau and colleagues, it was shown that IL-10, a factor now known to enhance B cell survival via induction of the anti-apoptotic factor Bcl-2, also enhanced IgA secretion by human B cells stimulated by anti-CD40 in the presence of TGF-β (Defrance *et al.*, 1992).

Two additional considerations relating to the role of TGF-β in IgA switch differentiation concern the sites of TGF-β secretion relative to IgA–B cell differentiation and the general inhibitory effect of TGF-β on lymphoid cells. With regard to the first issue, it is known that TGF secretion is widespread in lymphoid tissues and that many lymphoid and nonlymphoid cells produce this cytokine. This presents a problem, since such widespread production would lead to the prediction that IgA switch differentiation should occur everywhere, when in fact it occurs only within PPs. The resolution to this problem may lie in the level of ubiquitous TGF-β secretion relative to the level of secretion necessary for induction of switch differentiation. Thus, it is possible that whereas TGF-β secretion occurs in many lymphoid tissues, such secretion is below the

level necessary for IgA switch differentiation, particularly in view of the fact mentioned above that such differentiation occurs *in vitro* only at levels comparable to that occurring in PPs when TGF-β concentrations are quite high. Another factor to consider in this context is that it is possible that for TGF-β to be effective in IgA switch differentiation, it must be secreted at or on the B cell surface, very close to cell surface TGF-β receptors, and that any other, more distant TGF-β secretion is irrelevant to switching. Two possible sources of such proximal TGF-β are T cells interacting with B cells as "switch T cells" or the B cell itself.

With regard to the second issue—that TGF-β is a potent inhibitory factor—one must mention that even before the effect of TGF-β on IgA switch differentiation was recognized, TGF-β was shown to have profound negative effects on both B- and T-cell proliferation (Kehrl *et al.*, 1986, 1987, 1991; Wahl *et al.*, 1988; Moses *et al.*, 1990). While this suppressive effect was most evident in relation to IgM and IgG secretion, it was also seen in relation to IgA secretion (Kehrl *et al.*, 1991). In addition, although TGF-β is necessary for IgA switch differentiation, it inhibits B cells after the switching event occurs. Thus, higher IgA secretion is routinely obtained in B cell cultures if anti-TGF-β is added 1 to 2 days after initiation of the culture. In addition, post-switch sIgA⁺ B cells, optimally activated by T cells to produce IgA, produce less IgA in the presence of TGF-β than in its absence (Ehrhardt *et al.*, 1996a, b). Finally, B cells in cultures containing low concentrations of TGF-β (0.1 ng/ml) secrete 15 times less IgA than do B cells in cultures containing higher concentrations of TGF-β (1.0 ng/ml, unless additional cofactors are added), even though the higher TGF-β concentration induces a higher number of sIgA⁺ B cells. These data, taken together, indicate that the presence of TGF-β in a lymphoid milieu is a double-edged sword and can clearly inhibit IgA B cell development as well as enhance it. This too represents a problem but one that may be resolved by the fact, as mentioned previously, that certain forms of cell stimulation may protect the cell from death (apoptosis) and thus may allow the cell to withstand the negative effects of TGF-β on cell proliferation while allowing the positive effects of TGF-β on switch differentiation.

The role of dendritic cells in IgA B cell differentiation
While the role of T cells in adaptive IgA responses were first being explored, studies on the role of dendritic cells in this process also appeared. Thus, in studies by Spalding *et al.* (1984), it was shown that mixtures of periodate-activated T cells and dendritic cells (T cell–DC clusters) derived from the PPs had a far greater propensity to induce IgA secretion in B cells derived from PPs or spleen than clusters derived from the spleen. That this phenomenon represented switch differentiation rather than terminal differentiation was subsequently shown by the fact that the clusters derived from PP cells, not those derived from the spleen, preferentially induced IgA production in a pre–B cell line (Spalding and Griffin, 1986). Finally, in these studies the source of the dendritic cell was more important than the source of the

T cell, since clusters composed of DC from the PPs could induce IgA secretion when they were admixed with either T cells from PPs or the spleen, and conversely, clusters composed of DC from the spleen could not induce IgA secretion when they were admixed with T cells from either the PPs or the spleen.

Cebra and his colleagues subsequently conducted additional studies of the role of dendritic cells in IgA B cell differentiation (George and Cebra, 1991). These authors cultured antigen-specific B cells at limiting dilution with a Th2 T cell line in the presence and absence of purified splenic dendritic cells. They found that B cells cultured with T cells alone produced only IgM antibody, whereas those cultured with dendritic cells produced IgG and IgA antibody as well, including cells that produced only IgG or IgA. Similar results were obtained with sIgD$^+$ cells, i.e., naïve B cells that had not yet switched. These studies thus appeared to contradict those of Spalding et al. (1984) showing that dendritic cells do not have to come from PPs to induce IgA B cells. It should be noted, however, that these studies cannot be compared with those of Spalding, since it was not clear if the magnitude of the responses in the Cebra studies correspond to those obtained by Spalding or, indeed, those seen in vivo.

Yet another series of studies on the role of dendritic cells in IgA B cell differentiation has been conducted by Fayette and his colleagues (Fayette et al., 1997). In an initial series of studies, these investigators found that the human dendritic cells generated from CD34$^+$ cells by culture of the latter in the presence of GM-CSF and TNF-α induced about 10% of sIgD$^+$ B cells (naïve B cells) to switch to sIgA$^+$ cells in the absence of additional stimuli and induced 40% to 50% of these B cells to switch to sIgA$^+$ cells (consisting of both sIgA1 and sIgA2 cells) in the presence of IL-10 and TGF-β. In addition, while dendritic cells alone did not induce IgA secretion, dendritic cells plus IL-10 did induce secretion, confirming once again the ability of IL-10 to act as a terminal differentiation factor. While these data suggested that some IgA class switching could occur in the absence of TGF-β, it was still possible that the latter cytokine could arise from the B cells themselves. In a follow-up study by these investigators, it was shown that CD40-signaled naïve B cells cultured in the presence of DCs produce low levels of Ig in an initial culture, even in the presence of IL-2/IL-10; these cells went on to produce high levels of Ig in a second culture in which the CD40 signaling was removed and IL-2 or IL-2/IL-10 was present (Fayette et al., 1998). These studies were noteworthy in that they showed that the effect of the DCs on B cell differentiation were related to class switching rather than terminal differentiation, and, perhaps more important, affected class switching to all isotypes, not just IgA, as implied in the previous study.

Recently, a possible molecular basis of this DC effect on class switching has come into view with the discovery that DCs may induce such differentiation via the secretion of two B cell stimulatory factors, BLyS and APRIL. BLyS (a TNF family member also known as BAFF and TALL-1) and APRIL (a proliferation-inducing ligand) bind to B cells via several receptors, including B cell maturation antigen (BCMA) (Rolink and Melchers, 2002). BlyS induces B Ig production to both TI and TD antigens, whereas APRIL induces Ig production to TI antigens but not TD antigens. However, neither effect is isotype-specific. Both BlyS and APRIL are produced by dendritic cells (as well as by monocytes and macrophages) following stimulation with LPS, IFN-α, IFN-γ, or CD40L; thus, they can be induced via induction of innate or adaptive immune responses (Litinskiy et al., 2002). Finally, the ability of dendritic cells to influence B cell differentiation, as discussed previously, is mediated by BLyS and APRIL since culture of DCs with B cells in the presence of antibodies to BlyS or BCMA blocks the effects of DCs on B cell differentiation.

Further studies of the effects of BlyS and APRIL on B cell differentiation show that these factors affect B cells in the absence of CD40 signaling and are synergistic (Litinskiy et al., 2002). In addition, molecular analysis reveals that these factors induce class-switch differentiation but that such differentiation requires the concomitant effect of other cytokines. Thus, IgA switching requires the presence of TGF-β or IL-10 and raises the question of whether BlyS and APRIL act, at least in part, through the induction of these cytokines. Finally, BlyS and APRIL promote the binding of NF-κB-Rel to the CD40-responsive element of the Cγ3 germline promoter, an effect which is enhanced by BCR engagement. Thus, these factors also have direct molecular effects on class-switch differentiation.

The role of the intestinal epithelium, intra-epithelial lymphocytes and IL-7 in the development of IgA B cell responses

The role of the intestinal epithelium in promoting the development of T cells producing TGF-β requires further comment with respect to γδ-TCR intraepithelial lymphocytes and IL-7, given the considerable body of work showing that these factors also impact on IgA B cell differentiation (Fujihashi et al, 1992; Yamamoto and Kiyono, 1999). With regard to the role of IELs, it has been shown that TCR δ-chain knock-out mice exhibit substantially reduced numbers of both IgA-secreting cells in PPs and lamina propria (Itohara et al, 1993). The mechanism of these effects is not yet clear. The possibility that the γδ T cells directly interact with naïve B cells to induce IgA-specific switching seems remote, given the physical separation of the two types of cells in mucosal tissues. Another and perhaps more likely possibility is that γδ T cells produce cytokines that promote development of IgA B cells that diffuse into the PPs. In this regard, γδ T cells have been shown to produce Th1 and Th2 cytokines as well as TGF-β, which could favor the development of more proximal IgA-specific regulatory cells (Takaguchi et al., 1991). Along these lines, it has recently been reported that γδ T cells are increased in the peripheral blood of patients with IgA nephropathy, and this correlates with the proportion of sIgA$^+$ cells present (Toyale et al., 2001). In addition, purified γδ T cells from patients (but not normal individuals) produce considerably increased amounts of TGF-β and induce naïve IgD⁺ B cells to undergo IgA-specific switching. Finally, there is some evidence that γδ T cells enhance IgA responses by blocking suppressor cell responses normally elicited by oral antigen administration (Fujihashi, *et al.*, 1992). However, this evidence is from cell transfer studies that may not reflect physiologic conditions.

The effect of γδ T cells on IgA responses brings up the question of the role of IL-7 in IgA B cell development, since in addition to its growth-enhancing effect on precursor B cells, IL-7 has several effects on T cells, particularly γδ T cells. Thus, this cytokine promotes the expansion of mature γδ T cells and inhibits the expansion of mature αβ T cells in fetal thymus cultures; in addition, along with IL-2, IL-7 is necessary for the proliferation of γδ^dim T cells in the IEL compartment and thus is necessary for the development of γδ T cells as a whole (Fujihashi *et al.*, 1996). The latter fact accounts for the observation that IL-7R-deficient mice are specifically lacking in γδ T cells. One further point that deserves mention with regard to IL-7 is that the latter cytokine and another factor affecting intraepithelial cell growth, stem cell factor, have been shown to arise from epithelial cells and, in turn, intraepithelial cells

produce factors that sustain epithelial cell growth (Yamamoto *et al.*, 1999). By the same token, such reciprocal interaction could impact on terminal IgA B cell differentiation by leading to the production of various factors that support such differentiation.

A working hypothesis of IgA B cell differentiation in the PPs and other organized mucosal lymphoid tissues

The time has come in our discussion of IgA B cell differentiation in the organized mucosal lymphoid tissues to draw together the various strands of relevant data concerning APCs, T cells, and B cells in these tissues in order to construct a working hypothesis of how and why such differentiation comes about. In doing so, we will create a picture of the factors controlling the adaptive IgA response to mucosal antigens **(Fig. 31.2)**.

IgA B cell differentiation can be said to begin when inductive T cells (*i.e.*, the IgA-specific switch T cells presaged by the early studies of Elson *et al.*, and Kawanishi *et al.*) interact with sIgM⁺ (naïve) B cells localized in the follicular corona to

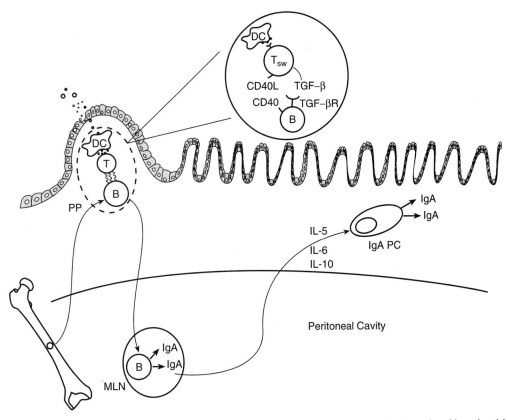

Fig 31.2. In the adaptive IgA B cell response, B-2 B cells arising in the bone marrow migrate to the PPs (or isolated lymphoid follicles) and enter the latter via integrin and chemokine receptor/ligand interactions. In PPs, the B cells, initially in a naïve state, are stimulated by T cells via antigen/TCR and various costimulatory interactions, especially involving CD40L/CD40. A critical step in IgA B cell differentiation occurring at this point is stimulation of B cells with TGF-β, a cytokine unique in its ability to initiate IgA-specific switch differentiation. TGF-β is provided in the form of either a cell-membrane or secreted molecule. Following initial differentiation, the nascent IgA B cell migrates out of the PP and mesenteric lymph node and then back to the unorganized mucosal immune system in the lamina propria areas. Such trafficking back to the mucosal areas is also under integrin/chemokine control. Terminal differentiation of IgA B cells into plasma cells requires additional cytokines, including IL-5, IL-6, and IL-10. In addition, newly described factors produced by APCs, such as BlyS, may also play a role at this stage.

initiate the molecular events that lead to IgA class-switch differentiation (Elson et al., 1979; Kawanishi et al., 1983). The first requirement of such T cells is the expression of CD40L and the ability of the T cells to interact with B cells via a CD40L–CD40 interaction. This is shown by the fact that mice lacking CD40L have a greatly reduced capacity to mount IgA responses to T-cell-dependent antigens (Gardby, R., Ph.D. Thesis; ISBN 91-628-4288-9)). In addition, purified human sIgD+ cells stimulated with a B cell mitogen alone (such as anti-IgM or SAC) in the presence of TGF-β produce little IgA, whereas the same cells stimulated by one of these mitogens in the presence of TGF-β and a CD40L signal produce large amounts of IgA (De France et al., 1992). Similar results are obtained in murine B cell stimulation systems in that purified B cells stimulated by anti-IgD-dextran plus a CD40L signal in the presence of TGF-β produce large amounts of IgA (McIntyre et al., 1995), whereas the same stimulus lacking CD40L produces small amounts of IgA. Recent studies of CD40L signaling provide some insight into the molecular mechanisms that account for the importance of such signaling in class switching (A. Jain, 2004, personal communication). These studies strongly suggest that CD40L signaling is necessary for activation of Iκκγ (NF-κB essential modulator or NEMO), which, in turn, is essential to the activation of c-Rel and thus the induction of c-Rel-dependent transcription factors that are essential for switch differentiation.

If indeed T cells in the mucosal follicles are the proximal inducers of IgA-specific switch differentiation, what are the characteristics of such cells that distinguish them from non-mucosal T cells that induce IgG-specific switch differentiation and therefore account for the fact that adaptive IgA responses occur largely in mucosal follicles and not in other lymphoid tissues? Given the key role of TGF-β in the initiation of IgA switch differentiation, one possible answer to this question is that IgA switching depends on PP T cells that are uniquely capable of providing a TGF-β signal to B cells during the initial stages of B cell activation. Evidence in support of this possibility consists first of the well-established fact that regulatory cells producing TGF-β are induced in PPs by oral antigen administration and that such cells are indeed T cells since they do not occur in mice lacking CD4+ T cells, either because of gene deletion or because of administration of anti-CD4 antibodies (Desvignes et al., 1996; Strober et al., 1998). These T cells are in fact the so-called Th3 T cells that are thought to mediate oral tolerance (Weiner, 2001).

Further support for the concept that PPs containing T cells producing TGF-β are responsible for IgA B cell switching relates to recent studies suggesting that, at least in part, regulatory T cells induced in PPs comprise CD4+CD25+ T cells that exercise regulatory function in the periphery via expression of TGF-β (Zhang et al., 2001; Nakamura et al., 2001). Since it is now known that such CD25+ T cells initially develop in the thymus as a result of high-affinity interactions with self-antigens (Jordan et al., 2001), one might postulate that Th3 T cells begin life as a subset of intrathymic CD25+ T (precursor) cells as a result of stimulation by mucosal antigens that have gained access to the internal

milieu and that are treated as self-antigens in the thymus. Following such intrathymic development, the nascent Th3 (CD25+) T cells return to the mucosa, where they are expanded by restimulation with mucosal antigens. The Th3 (CD25+) T cells thus formed then mediate oral tolerance and/or act as regulatory cells that prevent mucosal inflammation upon exposure to mucosa microflora (Motet et al., 2003). That these regulatory T cells also act as IgA-specific switch T cells is favored by recent findings that these cells not only secrete TGF-β but, in addition, express cell-membrane TGF-β. Thus, these cells can directly target naïve sIgM+ B cells for IgA-specific switch differentiation (Nakamura et al., 2001). In retrospect, this idea is consonant with the fact that the switch T cells described previously were in fact autoreactive T cells that could respond to self-antigens and had a tendency to suppress Ig synthesis of IgG B cells even as they supported Ig syntheses by IgA B cells (Elson et al., 1979; Kawanishi et al., 1985).

Additional support for the idea that a T cell is the source of the TGF-β necessary for IgA-specific switch differentiation is the lack of evidence that such TGF-β arises from either a mucosal APC or B cell themselves. Thus, in extensive studies of the conditions under which T cells develop into TGF-β-producing cells, it was shown that APCs (even those derived from the PPs) were not a source of measurable amounts of TGF-β (Marth et al., 1997); it was also shown that cytokines inhibiting the differentiation of T cells producing TGF-β (IFN-γ) are stimulants of cytokine production by APCs, whereas those favoring such T cell differentiation (IL-4, IL-10) are inhibitors of cytokine production by APCs (Corinti et al., 2001). Finally, in direct studies of PP dendritic cells, it has been shown that while addition of anti-TGF-β to cultures of PP DCs (but not spleen DCs) and T cells led to enhanced T-cell-cytokine production, the DCs could not be shown to secrete TGF-β (although they expressed increased amounts of TGF-β mRNA in comparison with spleen DCs) (Iwasaki et al., 1999). These findings suggest that PP DCs do not secrete TGF-β, but they may have special effects on regulatory T cells that enable the latter to express TGF-β. As for whether B cells themselves are the source of the TGF-β, again, there is considerable evidence that whereas this cell type may produce small amounts of this cytokine, it is unlikely to produce enough to support the level of IgA-specific switch differentiation found in PPs. This is validated by the fact that T cell/B cell cultures do not result in significant IgA B cell development in the absence of exogenous TGF-β.

Expanding on the latter point relating to the concentration of TGF-β necessary for IgA-specific switch differentiation, we should note that concentrations of TGF-β optimal for cell survival induce only a small fraction of sIgM+ B cells to become sIgA+ B cells. One possible explanation of this difficulty is that additional factors are necessary that act in concert with TGF-β to promote high levels of IgA differentiation. A second possible explanation, however, is suggested by the findings of McIntyre et al., who showed that concentrations of TGF-β sufficient to induce substantial levels of IgA differentiation could be introduced into B cell cultures, provided the B cells were stimulated with LPS or CD40L (or a combination of these stimulators) and costimulated with anti-IgD (in the form of anti-IgD-dextran) (McIntyre et al., 1995). Their studies raised the question of whether certain forms of B cell stimulation (in this case involving signaling via the B cell Ig receptor) lead to increased survival of B cells in the face of high TGF-β levels. Indeed, this seems to be the case, as in other studies in which McIntyre and Strober showed that after such stimulation, B cells exhibited decreased rather than increased apoptosis following exposure to TGF-β (McIntyre and Strober, unpublished observations).

A final set of observations supporting the role of TGF-β-producing T cells in the development of IgA B cells in PP concern the fact that the PP microenvironment is conducive to the expansion of such cells. Thus, it has been shown that the development of TGF-β-producing T cells in vitro is inhibited in the presence of concomitantly induced Th1 responses and, conversely, are enhanced in the presence of concomitant, induced Th2 responses, including IL-10 responses (Seder et al., 1998). These findings fit with the fact that OVA-TCR transgenic mice fed OVA initially develop a Th1 response in their PPs, not accompanied by cells producing TGF-β; however, if the mice are treated with anti-IL-12 at the time of feeding, cells producing TGF-β and cells producing IL-10 are observed (Marth et al., 1997). In addition, they are consonant with the findings that DCs in PPs have been shown to be different from spleen DCs in their greatly increased tendency to produce IL-10 and thus their potential to support TGF-β-producing cells by downregulating Th1 responses (Iwasaki et al., 1999). Along these lines, it has been shown that the mucosal epithelium produces IL-10 that may also contribute to the expansion of TGF-β-producing T cells either directly, by suppressing Th1 responses, or indirectly, by inducing DCs that produce copious amounts of IL-10. In this regard, we have already mentioned the fact that the mice bearing a transgene encoding IL-10 in the epithelium exhibit greatly increased mucosal TGF-β production (De Winter, 2002).

Taken together, these observations paint a picture of a PP microenvironment that is favorable to the development of TGF-β-producing T cells by virtue of the cytokines produced at this site, particularly IL-10. It finds further validation in the recent observation that in studies of TGF-β-producing regulatory T cells developing in relation to experimentally induced colitis, IL-10 was essential for such development either because it could downregulate opposing (Th1) cytokines or because it has direct growth-inducing effects on the regulatory T cells (Fuss et al., 2002). Finally, the concept that IL-10 plays a role in TGF-β-producing T cells that support IgA B cell differentiation fits neatly with the fact that in many systems, IL-10 and TGF-β seem to play a role in such differentiation (Malison et al., 1996).

The aforementioned accounting of IgA B cell differentiation during the adaptive IgA response in mucosal follicles and involving B-2 B cells in murine systems is obviously

focused on a specialized T cell that delivers a "generic" switching signal to B cells via CD40L as well as an IgA-specific signal in the form of TGF-β. The origin of this view is the repeated observation that it is possible to generate IgA responses from naïve B cells in in vitro culture systems in which the only B cell signal is a T-cell-derived signal (McIntyre et al., 1995). Given what we now know concerning the innate IgA response occurring in the lamina propria (see subsequent discussion), however, we must consider an alternative hypothesis for the adaptive IgA response. In this alternative hypothesis, the T cell still remains to deliver the generic switching signal, but the TGF-β signal arises from other cells, notably, stromal cells in the mucosal environment (there is little evidence that it arises from dendritic cells, as discussed previously) (Fagarasan et al., 2003). Furthermore, this TGF-β is induced by factors such as the previously discussed BLyS and APRIL that are in fact synthesized by non-T cells such as dendritic cells or macrophages (Litinskiy et al., 2002). Thus, in this alternative view, the unique capacity of the mucosal tissues to manifest adaptive IgA responses is shifted from a T cell to other cells, namely, dendritic cells and stromal cells. Further work will be necessary to decide between this alternative hypothesis and the older, T-cell-centered view. A clear goal for such research is the better identification of T cells performing the function of IgA-specific switch cells, as defined previously, or the identification of non-T cells that are unique to mucosal tissues and that produce TGF-β under conditions of T cell stimulation.

IgA B cell differentiation in the innate IgA B cell response

Overview

In the late 1980s studies by Kroese et al. showed that IgA B cells in the lamina propria could arise from B cell populations present in the peritoneal cavity that are distinct from those in the PPs both in origin and in phenotype (Kroese et al., 1989). These IgA cells were shown to be part of a class of B cells, termed B-1 B cells, that were later shown to recognize self- and commensal antigens and to undergo isotype switching in the absence of T cells; as such, B-1 B cells were said to be the origin of "natural" IgA antibodies that provide an early and "innate" immune response against bacterial and viral invaders (Macpherson et al. 2000). B-1 B cells were thus distinct from the B-2 B cells that populate most follicular lymphoid tissues, including the PPs, since the latter B cells participate in T-cell-dependent events and are part of the adaptive immune response (vide infra).

The nature of B-1 B cells

B-1 B cells initially arise in the bone marrow from newly formed B cells that ultimately differentiate into marginal zone B cells, follicular B cells (B-2 B cells), or peritoneal/pleural cavity B cells (B-1 B cells) (Martin and Kearney, 2001). In contrast to B-2 B cells that recognize exogenous, non-self-antigens with high affinity and exquisite specificity, B-1 B cells recognize endogenous self-antigens with relatively low specificity (Lalor and Morahan, 1990). Convincing evidence in support of this distinction is that mice expressing a V_H transgene specific for a self-antigen develop both B-1 and B-2 B cells expressing the transgene, but only the B-1 B cells produce antibody against the self-antigen, and these B cells are enriched in the peritoneal cavity (Hayakawa et al., 1999). In addition, in mice expressing a V_H transgene that do not express the self-antigen, B-1 B cells producing anti-self antibody are not found, although B-2 B cells with the transgene (associated with a diverse set of light chains) persist. Perhaps because antigens in the mucosal microflora are functional self-antigens, B-1 B cells also react with these antigens and thus are a major source of IgM antibodies that form part of the innate immune response against commensal organisms.

In one hypothesis concerning the origin of B-1 B cells, these cells constitute a separate cell lineage exhibiting a unique antibody repertoire and a unique set of surface markers (IgM^{hi}, IgD^{lo}, CD23$^-$, CD43$^+$, IL-5R, and either CD5$^+$ [B-la] or CD5$^-$ [B-lb] cells) (Su and Tarakhovsky, 2000; Martin and Kearney, 2001). Other evidence of their separate lineage is that they occupy a particular anatomic niche, the peritoneal and pleural cavities, possibly because they express unique chemokine receptors that mediate traffic to this site (Ansel et al., 2002). In addition, they appear to be a self-renewing population that is relatively independent of replenishment by bone marrow precursors. In another hypothesis, B-1 B cells are not a separate lineage and instead diverge from B-2 B cells only because of their specificity for self-antigens and the phenotypic changes imposed on them by interaction with such antigens. In this view, the observation that B-1 B cells are found in the peritoneal and pleural cavities is explained by the fact that while B-1 B cells are resistant to antigen-induced deletion (see subsequent discussion), they are nevertheless more subject to such deletion than B cells that recognize non-self-antigens if only because self-antigens are more or less ubiquitous; in the peritoneal and pleural cavities, however, they avoid contact with self-antigens and thus preferentially accumulate at this site. In addition, their apparent self-renewing properties are due not to their independence from bone marrow precursors but rather to their relative resistance to Fas-mediated apoptosis following CD40 signaling (probably due to decreased CD40L-induced Fas expression) and thus their survival following certain forms of stimulation and proliferation.

As implied previously, the question of whether B-1 B cells have a separate cell lineage comes down to the matter of whether the phenotype of B-1 B cells is antigen-induced. Recent evidence suggests that this is in fact the case, in that mice bearing a transgenic V_H chain associated with B-1 B cells do not express CD5 early in life but do express CD5 later on, presumably after interaction with self-antigen (Cong et al., 1991). Thus, the expression of the most specific marker of B-1 B cells, CD5, is dependent on antigen stimulation. In addition, cells bearing two V_H transgenes, one associated with B-1 B cells and one associated with B-2 B cells,

have the phenotype of B-2 B cells, presumably because in the presence of a B-2-associated V_H chain the B-1-associated V_H chain is not expressed at a high enough density to signal the cell and induce B-1-type differentiation (Lam and Majewsky, 1999). Thus, in this case, the type of B cell that develops is dependent on the type of BCR (and type of antigen) that is recognized by the cell. Finally, B-1 B cells have a higher threshold for BCR activation than do B-2 B cells and, in addition, exhibit no proliferation in response to anti-IgM signaling (i.e., proliferation induced by antigen alone) (Martin and Kearney, 2001). This distinctive property of B-1 B cells also appears to be antigen-driven in that antigen-induced expression of CD5 leads to inhibition of BCR signaling via SHP-1 phosphatases associated with its cytoplasmic tail (Sen et al., 1999). Taken together, these data suggest that B-1 B cells develop their distinctive features not because of an intrinsic developmental program but rather because of their encounter with certain antigens that then determine a particular cellular phenotype.

Recent studies by Hayakawa et al. (2003) support and extend these conclusions. These authors found that in mice with B cells bearing μ and κ transgenes that allow reactivity to a given self-antigen, the B cells undergo negative selection in the bone marrow, and those B cells that do emerge from the bone marrow and go to the spleen do not progress beyond an immature B cell stage, although they do express CD5. Nevertheless, these mice did exhibit high levels of autoantibody specific for the recognized antigen, indicating that positive selection of autoreactive cells was occurring somewhere within the lymphoid system. Indeed, large numbers of plasma cells were found in the mucosal lamina propria, and the authors suggested on the basis of in vitro studies that exposure of the B cells first to antigen and then to LPS (the latter in the intestine) allows the cells to escape deletion. Although these authors did not suggest it, these studies indicate that the lamina propria is a primary site of B-1 B cell development (see subsequent discussion).

T-cell–independent IgA B-1 B cells

That IgA B cells can develop independently of T cells was indicated initially by the finding that mice that lack T cells or that lack costimulatory molecules necessary for T cell–B cell interactions can nevertheless produce IgA (Mombaerts et al., 1994; Gardby et al., 1998). This idea was later crystallized in a study by Macpherson et al. (2000), in which it was shown that:

- monoinfection of germ-free mice led to prompt IgA antibody responses that then prevented the penetration of the bacteria into the circulation and the induction of an IgG response;
- such IgA was induced by the introduction of an SPF flora into gnotobiotic mice that were T-cell-deficient by a number of mechanisms, indicating that the B cells were T-cell-independent (the level of IgA induced under these circumstances was about one-half that in normal mice but could be augmented by repeated antigen stimulation);

- such IgA was induced in mice lacking well-developed PPs because of TNF-receptor-1 deficiency, indicating that PPs were not the source of the B cells; however, mice totally lacking lymphoid structures, *i.e.*, lymphotoxin-A-deficient mice, manifested greatly reduced IgA responses (<1/100 of controls);
- the IgA responses observed were specific for bacterial antigens as well as new antigens contained in engineered intestinal organisms, indicating that responses are not simply against a stereotypic group of bacterial antigens; and
- the cells producing the IgA were in fact B-1 B cells, since reconstitution of irradiated T-cell-deficient mice with peritoneal B cells and bone marrow cells from T-cell-deficient mice led to repopulation with cells from mice bearing the allotype of the peritoneal B cell donor.

These data thus corroborate an earlier finding by Kroese *et al.* (1993), showing that B cells of mice carrying μ and κ transgenes that concomitantly express endogenous IgM genes are B-1 cells by phenotypic criteria, and location in the peritoneal cavity give rise to IgA cells in the lamina propria. Taken together, these findings offer powerful evidence that B cells producing IgA in the lamina propria can arise from a B-1 B cell population and in a T-cell-independent fashion that does not require the presence of PPs, follicular dendritic cells, and germinal centers. Thus, Macpherson *et al.* (2001) concluded that IgA responses formed part of a "primitive" immune response system that others would classify as an innate immune response. In later studies, the authors showed that mice lacking μ or δ chains because of a pro-B-cell developmental block, μMT mice, can produce small amounts of IgA but not other immunoglobulins independently of T cells. Although such production could not be tied to B-1 B cells or indeed to mucosal responses in particular, these data were taken as additional evidence that IgA responses are primitive responses.

Sites of activation and differentiation of B1-B cells in mucosal tissues

If indeed B-1 B cells develop into IgA B cells that constitute a substantial fraction of all of the IgA cells in the lamina propria and virtually all of the IgA cells that mediate innate IgA responses, as suggested previously, one must be able to visualize when and where a peritoneal B cell population interacts with antigen and how these cells migrate into mucosal tissues. The answers to these questions are not known, although it is perhaps generally thought that B-1 B cells initially develop into self-antigen-reactive sIgM+ cells in the bone marrow rather than in the peritoneal cavity, given the fact that the latter site is not amenable to efficient cell–cell interactions. Depending on which theory of B-1 B cell development one ascribes to, either they migrate specifically to the peritoneal cavity as a result of lineage-specific chemokine expression or they disseminate widely and then accumulate in the peritoneal cavity as a refuge from self-antigen-induced deletion. In the former case, they may specifically respond to

CXCL13, a chemokine produced by peritoneal macrophages and cells in the omentum (Ansel *et al.*, 2002).

In the peritoneal cavity, B-1 B cells are sIgM+ and must migrate to mucosal tissues to undergo differentiation into plasma cells. This is shown in studies of aly/aly mice that have defective NF-κB activation due to a mutation of NIK (NF-κB-inducing kinase), a mediator of NF-κB activation regulated by the TNF receptor family (Shinkura *et al.*, 1999; Faragasan *et al.*, 2000). As a result, these mice lack PPs and lymph nodes and, in addition, exhibit poor chemotactic responses due to defective activation of NF-κB by chemokines. While aly/aly mice have B-1 B cells in the peritoneal cavity, they do not have Ig-producing plasma cells in mucosal tissues; similarly, RAG-2-deficient mice with B-1 cells transferred from aly/aly mice do not develop plasma cells in mucosal tissues. One explanation of these findings, put forward by Faragasan *et al.* (1999 and 2000), is that in the absence of an intact chemotactic response, B-1 B cells cannot migrate out of the peritoneal cavity and cannot differentiate into plasma cells. As shown by Watanabe *et al.* (2000), one stimulus for such migration can arise from noncognate interactions with T cells. Thus, in mice bearing a BCR specific for a self-antigen (RBCs), the only B cells that are not deleted are B-1 B cells in the peritoneal cavity; nevertheless, these mice do not develop anti-RBC autoantibodies, presumably because, as noted previously, these cells must migrate out of the peritoneal cavity to differentiate and this requires some form of stimulation. If, however, the mice are crossed with mice expressing a γδ TCR specific for the MHC-related thymus leukemia (TL) antigen, B-1 B cells are found in the mesenteric nodes that differentiate into cells that produce anti-RBC antibodies. Presumably, the γδ TCR-bearing T cells facilitate such migration by secretion of B-1 B cell–attracting chemokines or, alternatively, by the stimulation of macrophages to secrete such chemokines. Thus, in this view, B-1 B cells migrate out of the peritoneal cavity in response to chemotactic factors secreted by cells in the mucosal tissues proper.

While this explanation is not unreasonable, it falls short because it postulates an as-yet-unproven mechanism of cellular migration that relies on T cells that can interact with B cells, albeit in a noncognate fashion. The latter is inconsistent with the presumed activity of B-1 B cells in the absence of T cells. An alternative hypothesis is one based on the idea, already alluded to above, that B-1 B cells are activated in mucosal tissues and either migrate to or accumulate in the peritoneal cavity because they are shielded from the deleting effects of self-antigens in this space. In this hypothesis, B-1 B cells needn't migrate from the peritoneal cavity to mucosal tissues under the influence of chemokines because they are already present in these tissues and merely await appropriate activation. The failure of B-1 B cells to differentiate into plasma cells in aly/aly mice in this view is due to a general inability of mice with an NF-kB to support B cell terminal differentiation, consistent with the lack of general lymphoid development in these mice. Similarly, the ability of γδ T cells to support B-1 B cell differentiation into plasma cells can be attributed not to the elaboration of chemokines but rather to the stimulation of B-1 B cells already present in the mucosal tissues and thus the induction of B cell changes that render the cell more resistant to apoptosis by self-antigens. This could take the form of changes in the affinity of the differentiating B-1 B cell for its cognate antigen or changes in the way such B cells respond to various apoptosis-inducing factors. In the latter regard, it has already been reported that B-1 B cells may be more resistant to Fas-mediated apoptosis by its ability to downregulate Fas ligand (Goodnow, 1996).

Quite aside from the question of whether B-1 B cells migrate into mucosal tissues or are present in such tissues to begin with is the question of the mechanism by which these cells differentiate outside of PPs and in the absence of T cells into Ig-secreting B cells, some of which are IgA-secreting cells that reflect IgA-specific class switch recombination. It has been conclusively shown that sIgA$^+$ B cells extracted from the lamina propria manifest various molecular concomitants of switching, namely, Ca germline transcripts, AID activation, and switch circles containing germline Ca (Faragasan, et al., 2001). It should be noted, however, that this does not necessarily imply switching in the lamina propria, since this molecular evidence of switch differentiation could arise from partially switched B cells that could have recently emigrated to the lamina propria from the PPs. In addition, the switching could involve B cells that developed in isolated lymphoid follicles under the influence of T cells, since cells from such nodules are difficult or impossible to separate from lamina propria. These possibilities are in fact favored by the observation that lamina propria sIgM$^+$ B cells differentiate into sIgA$^+$ cells more readily than sIgM$^+$ B cells in PPs, presumably because they are new arrivals from the PPs that have in fact already undergone initial switch differentiation steps at the latter inductive sites (Faragasan et al., 2001).

If indeed T-cell-independent IgA-class-specific switching does occur in the lamina propria, the question arises as to the stimuli that induce and support such switching. In discussing how this may come about, one must first be aware that entry of antigens and other possible stimulants into the mucosal milieu is not restricted to the PPs and its overlying M cells, as formerly thought. On the contrary, it is now clear that dendritic cells can sample antigens all along the mucosal epithelium by processes that reach into the lumen of the mucosal structures between epithelial cells (Rescigno et al., 2001). This opens up the potential of dendritic cell presentation of antigen directly to B cells in the absence of a T cell intermediate. Taking these observations as a starting point, Fagarasan et al. (2001) first showed that sIgM$^+$ B cells from lamina propria undergo switching to sIgA$^+$ B cells in vitro when cultured with LPS, TGF-β, and IL-5, whereas PP sIgM$^+$ B cells did not undergo such switching and instead required the presence of T cells. Fagarasan et al. then showed that in fact sIgM$^+$ B cells (from a variety of organs) that overexpress retroviral AID can undergo switching to sIgA$^+$ B cells in vitro (in the absence of CD40L stimulation) when cultured with LPS, IL-5, and, perhaps most important, lamina propria stromal cells but not bone marrow stromal cells. The key role of lamina propria stromal cells relates to the fact that these cells serve

as an all-important source of TGF-β, as shown by the fact that they can be replaced in the culture by supernatants derived from cultured stromal cells and the activity of these supernatants is abolished by the addition of anti-TGF-β. In addition, they secrete other, as-yet-unidentified terminal differentiation factors (other than IL-10 or IL-6). One caveat to these striking findings, however, is that the studies were performed with sIgM$^+$ B cells expressing retroviral AID, which had been shown previously to have a heightened tendency to undergo switching to sIgA$^+$ B cells. Finally, in studies that corroborated the aforementioned finding in an in vivo system, these authors showed that repletion of RAG-2-deficient mice (which lack T cells) with lamina propria sIgM$^+$ B cells results in repopulation of mesenteric lymph nodes and lamina propria with sIgA$^+$ B cells, and this source of B cells led to more sIgA$^+$ B cells than repletion with cells from the PPs or mesenteric lymph nodes. On this basis the authors concluded that the lamina propria contains all of the cellular and molecular elements necessary for the differentiation of sIgM$^+$ B cells into sIgA$^+$ B cells and that this process may be critically dependent on the lamina propria stromal cells.

The quantitative importance of the innate (B-1 B cell) response in normal mice

The above studies, particularly those of Macpherson et al., and Faragasan et al., provide strong support for the existence of an alternative (innate) IgA B cell differentiation program based on B-1 B cells and occurring in the lamina propria, i.e., an IgA B cell system that is quite independent of the previously described system in PPs and other organized (germinal center–containing) tissues (Macpherson et al., 2001; Faragasan and Honjo, 2003) **(Fig. 31.3)**. In addition, in the previous discussion we mentioned a number of situations involving mice with impaired T cells—such as mice with CD40L deficiency or with defective costimulatory function—that nevertheless manifest the ability to produce substantial amounts of IgA. Thus, it now seems incontrovertible that T-cell-independent IgA switching can occur in the lamina propria and that this switching for the most part involves B-1 B cells. This conclusion, however, does not speak to the question of whether this sort of switching does occur with substantial frequency under certain physiologic conditions (particularly in humans).

Several observations need to be considered in this context. First, the vast majority of the data supporting the extrafollicular (T-cell-independent) development of IgA B cells from B-1 B cells comes mainly from studies of lethally irradiated or otherwise impaired mice that are then repleted with B-1 B cells. Thus, the development of the latter in mucosal tissues takes place in a highly unphysiologic environment that may not reflect normal IgA B cell development. Evidence that cell expansion in normal tissue under competition from preexisting cells differs from that in abnormal tissue lacking other cells comes from recent studies, in which cells bearing a RAG-green fluorescence protein transgene to mark sites of Ig or TCR rearrangement, showing extrathymic T cell development, do not occur in the mucosal tissues in a euthymic

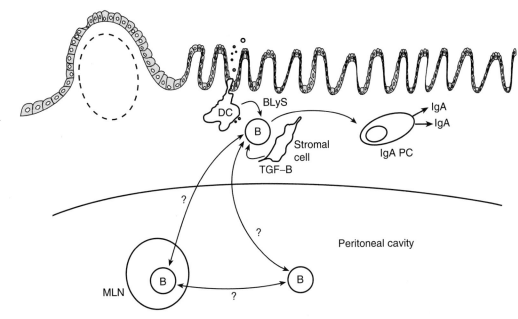

Fig 31.3. In the innate IgA B cell response, B-1 B cells initially arising in the bone marrow migrate to the unorganized mucosal areas in the form of sIgM⁺ B cells with specificity for self-antigens and antigens in the mucosal microflora. These cells may then migrate to the peritoneal cavity, where they form a pool of cells that may migrate back to the mesenteric nodes or lamina propria. In any case, these cells are subject to IgA-specific differentiation via interaction with dendritic cells and/or stromal cells. The former are a source of stimulatory antigen and co-stimulatory factors such as BlyS. The latter are a source of TGF-β, as are the B cells themselves. Terminal differentiation of these cells may involve particular cytokines such as IL-5 and IL-15.

host but do occur in a host lacking a thymus (D. Guy-Grand, personal communication). Second, studies in which the magnitude of the B-1 B cell contribution to IgA B cell development utilizing data do not rely on studies involving reconstitution of a T-cell-depleted host are either equivocal or negative. In the former category are the studies of Kiyono and his colleagues showing that B-1 B cell differentiation is more dependent on IL-5 and IL-15 than B-2 B cell differentiation and that depletion of these cytokines by administration of anti-IL-5 or anti-IL-15 results in a 30% to 50% diminution is mucosal IgA production (and little or no effect on systemic IgA levels). In addition, a comparable number of B-1 B cells could be identified in lamina propria B cell populations by marker studies (Hiroi et al., 1999; Hiroi et al., 2000) On the face of it, these data would imply a large contribution of B-1 B cells to the normal IgA B cell population; however, problems arise because of uncertainties of distinguishing B-1 and B-2 B cells with use of existing markers and thus of overestimating B-1 B cell numbers and of attributing anti-IL-5 and anti-IL-15 effects only to blockade of B-1 B cell function, when the same treatment could be affecting the B-2 B cell population as well. In the latter category, i.e., the category of studies clearly against identifying a large B-1 B cell–derived IgA B cell population in the normal lamina propria, are recent studies by Thurnheer et al. in which the level of IgA responses to commensal bacterial were measured in germ-free mice that were stable chimeras containing B-1 and B-2 B cells marked by different immunoglobulin allotypes. These authors found that the vast

majority of the response was in fact attributable to B-2 B cells and that the B-1 B cells contributed a very insignificant part of the response. This fits with an older study showing that clearance of rotavirus infection depended on B-2 B cells (along with CD4⁺ T cells), not B-1 B cells (Kushnir et al., 2001). Finally, the concept of a substantial B-1 B cell component in the IgA response runs into particular difficulties in human models. In this species there is scant evidence that B-1 B cells even exist, since CD5⁺, the most characteristic marker of B-1 B cells, cannot be found on B cells in the human lamina propria (Farstad et al., 2000); in addition, Brandtzaeg et al. (2001) have indicated that very few B cells are found in the human lamina propria, outside of organized (inductive) structures. On the other hand, evidence in humans that IgA B cells do in fact originate in germinal centers of inductive tissues is inherent in the finding that both human IgM and human IgA plasma cells manifest a V gene profile that reflects a high degree of somatic mutation and, in addition, B cells from human PPs display a clonal pattern that is mirrored in lamina propria lymphocytes (Dunn-Walters et al., 1997). Thus, the cellular and molecular basis of an alternative system has not been identified in humans, at least as yet.

From these various studies, we would have to conclude that while a T-cell-independent, B-1 B cell–mediated pathway leading to IgA production certainly exists, at least in the mouse, much more remains to be done to prove its quantitative importance and/or its indispensability in dealing with pathogens or commensal organisms.

Terminal differentiation of IgA B cells

As we have seen, IgA switch differentiation is the B cell differentiation process that is responsible for the unique association of IgA B cells with mucosal tissues. Nevertheless, it is only the first stage of IgA B cell development, and further stages—such as clonal IgA B cell expansion, IgA memory cell formation, and terminal differentiation of IgA B cells into plasma cells—must be considered as well. In general, these processes are more generic in the sense that similar processes also apply to the differentiation of other B cell isotypes; as will become apparent, however, aspects of this process do, in fact, distinguish IgA B cell differentiation from that of other Ig isotypes.

The sIgA⁺ B cells emerging from the isotype switch process are available for further stimulation and expansion in the light zone of the germinal centers. It is interesting that these cells respond poorly, if at all, to stimulation by LPS or antibodies that cross-link the antigen (IgA) receptor (Ehrhardt et al., 1996b); furthermore, such unresponsiveness extends to both proliferation and differentiation into IgA-producing plasma cells, although some proliferation is seen if the antigen receptor is cross-linked in the presence of cytokines. This pattern of unresponsiveness is in sharp contrast to the responsiveness of sIgM⁺ B cells to the same stimuli and is akin to the partial responsiveness of other (postswitch) sIgG⁺ B cells. A very different picture is obtained with respect to stimulation via CD40 (by T cells or T-cell membranes expressing CD40L). With this stimulus, sIgA⁺ B cells exhibit excellent proliferative and differentiative responses, whereas sIgM⁺ cells are only modestly responsive. A further point, and one that may explain the lack of differentiation of sIgA⁺ B cells into plasma cells in PPs, is that sIgA⁺ B cells are not only unresponsive to antigen receptor cross-linking but also are actually rendered unresponsive to other stimuli by this form of stimulation. Thus, sIgA⁺ B cells stimulated initially by anti-IgA-dextran are then unresponsive to stimulation via CD40, unless the latter is quite persistent.

The aforementioned facts concerning the responsiveness of postswitch sIgA⁺ B cells allow us to draw a picture concerning the course of events in IgA B cell development in PPs. Initially, naïve sIgM⁺/sIgD⁺ B cells are induced to undergo IgA isotype switch differentiation by IgA-specific switch T cells, as defined by the conditions described in detail previously. This occurs *pari passu* with initial rounds of cell proliferation and somatic mutation and leads to the formation of a nascent germinal center. It should be noted again that this stage of IgA B cell development is facilitated by, if not dependent on, the presence of antigen arrayed on FDCs, which provide the switching B cells with a second signal necessary for survival. The end result of the isotype switch process is the generation of a large number of postswitch sIgA⁺ B cells that accumulate in the germinal center light zones. As mentioned previously, these cells not only are unresponsive to stimulation via the antigen receptor but also are actually turned off by such stimulation. This, along with the fact that the light zones lack interdigitating dendritic cells and thus lack activated T cells expressing high

levels of CD40L, can explain the observation that sIgA⁺ B cells do not differentiate into IgA plasma cells at this site. For the latter to occur, they require restimulation by activated T cells expressing CD40L, presumably at other mucosal sites.

The scenario cited above endows the IgA B cell response with certain features that allow it to function more effectively at the mucosal surface. First, it ensures that LPS and other T-cell-independent B cell mitogens that are present in high concentrations in the mucosal environment and that might therefore diffuse into the mucosal tissues and cause inappropriate IgA B cell stimulation are unable to do so because, as mentioned, sIgA⁺ B cells are unresponsive to this kind of stimulus. Second, because it places the locus of control of B cell stimulation on the mucosal T cell, it ensures that only appropriately stimulated T cells that have escaped tolerance induction are actually capable of initiating adaptive IgA responses. Third, since the unresponsiveness of the sIgA⁺ B cells is broken only by persistent CD40L expression on highly activated T cells, sIgA⁺ B cells are not inadvertently stimulated by T cells in a noncognate interaction, because such interactions are not likely to provide the intense CD40L stimulation needed to overcome the anti-antigen-receptor-induced unresponsiveness.

Finally, it is important to discuss the various cytokine and/or cell–cell interactions that induce terminal differentiation of sIgA⁺ B cells into plasma cells. As mentioned, earlier work had postulated the existence of IgA-Fc-receptor-bearing T cells that regulated terminal differentiation either by cell–cell interactions (via IgA-Fc on the T cells and sIgA on the B cells) or by secretion of soluble IgA-binding factors (Kiyono et al., 1990). However, it now seems doubtful that T cells with high-affinity IgA–Fc receptors exist in sufficient numbers under physiologic conditions and thus that such cells play a meaningful role in normal terminal IgA B cell differentiation. On the other hand, it has recently been shown that terminal B cell differentiation, not just of IgA B cells but also of other postswitch B cells, is probably dependent on interactions between OX40 on T cells and OX40L on B cells (Stüber et al., 1995; Stüber and Strober, 1996). In the relevant studies, it has been shown that both *in vitro* and *in vivo*, terminal differentiation of B cells, particularly of postswitch IgG and IgA B cells, is greatly inhibited if antibodies block the OX40–OX40L interaction. In addition, it was shown at the molecular level that this interaction is responsible for the abrogation of the negative regulation of BSAP sites with the 3′αE. Finally, in the *in vivo* studies referred to above, it appears that the signal to the B cell via OX40L may render the differentiation signals delivered by cytokines (discussed later) virtually superfluous; cytokines, however, may be necessary for terminal B cell differentiation in areas of the lamina propria where T-cell signaling may be less sustainable or less acceptable.

As for the effects of various cytokines on terminal IgA B cell differentiation, the best studies are those that focus on terminal differentiation of B cells cultured with cytokines in the absence of exogenous stimuli such as LPS, which would itself induce cytokine production and thus obscure the effects of exogenous cytokines. In one such study, it was shown with PP B cells that IL-5 and IL-6 are the most effective cytokines for the support of IgA B cell terminal differentiation, and these cytokines exert their largest effects in concert with one another; thus IgA B cells differ from IgM B cells or even IgG B cells in that the latter respond better to IL-6 alone or to a combination of IL-1 and IL-6 (Kunimoto et al., 1989). In another study of this kind, of a number of different cytokines (including IL-2, IL-4, and IL-7) tested, only IL-5 and IL-6 were found to be potent differentiation factors, with IL-6 having a greater effect than IL-5 (Beagley et al., 1989). Along these lines, there is one report that IL-6 knockout mice mount particularly poor IgA antibody responses (as well as poor IgG antibody responses) (Ramsay et al., 1994). The significance of this finding, however, is mitigated by the fact that it was not reproducible in studies of IL-6 knock-out mice using other types of antigenic stimuli (Bromander et al., 1996). Finally, while we often assume that cytokines involved in B cell differentiation such as IL-6 arise from APCs, it is important to note that in the mucosa they can also be produced by epithelial cells. This is supported by data showing that epithelial cell–derived IL-6 and TGF-β enhance IgA production and suppress IgM production induced by LPS (Goodrich and McGee, 1999).

Other cytokines potentially involved in postswitch IgA differentiation in murine systems are IL-10 and IL-15. Evidence of IL-10 involvement in this process comes from a study of mice with intestinal epithelial cells that overexpress IL-10 due to the presence of a transgene that expresses IL-10 under an epithelial cell–specific (fatty acid binding protein) promoter (De Winter et al., 2002). Such mice, it was shown, contain mucosal lymphocytes that manifest considerably increased TGF-β production following anti-CD3 stimulation as well as modestly increased numbers of IgA-producing B cells but not increased numbers of IgG-producing B cells (as detected by ELISPOT assay). It should be noted, however, that it was not clear that the increase in IgA was a secondary effect of the increased TGF-β production (rather than the IL-10 overexpression).

Whereas IL-5 and IL-6 appear to be the major cytokines involved in the terminal differentiation of murine IgA B cells, it appears that IL-10 is perhaps the most important in the terminal differentiation of human IgA B cells. Thus, in studies of human B cells stimulated with both CD40L and the B cell mitogen *Staphylococcus aureus* Cowan 1 (SAC), it was shown that IL-4 and IL-10, but especially the latter, produced the highest amount of IgA secretion (Briere et al., 1994; Defrance et al., 1992). Moreover, peripheral cells from patients with isolated IgA deficiency could be induced to produce IgA by SAC and/or CD40 stimulation if IL-10 was added to the cultures (Briere et al., 1994). These studies clearly implicated IL-10 in human IgA B cell differentiation but did not distinguish an effect of IL-10 on switch differentiation from an effect on terminal differentiation. Moreover, these studies did not rule out a concomitant effect of IL-6 on IgA B cell terminal differentiation, even though this cytokine

was not added to the culture system, since B cells themselves produce IL-6.

In other and perhaps more definitive studies of terminal IgA B cell differentiation in humans, it has been shown that stimulation of naïve sIgM⁺ B cells by SAC plus IL-10 (the latter produced by the B cell itself) induces the production of mature Cα1 transcripts (a marker of such differentiation) and that the induction of mature Cα2 transcripts requires a T cell stimulus (CD40L) and IL-10. Furthermore, the addition of exogenous IL-10 enhanced mature transcript generation, whereas the addition of anti-IL-10 abrogated such generation (Kitani and Strober, 1994). In yet other studies, in this case utilizing a unique sIgM⁺/sIgD⁺ B cell lymphoma line derived from a human Burkett lymphoma (CL0-1 cells) that is capable of undergoing both class-switch and terminal differentiation *in vivo*, it was shown that CD40L stimulation induces the B cell line to undergo class-switch differentiation, indicated by the generation of "switch circles" (DNA excision products resulting from class switch recombination) and the generation of mature Cα1 and Cα2 transcripts (Zan et al., 1998). Moreover, such stimulation was accompanied by the production of TGF-β and IL-10 and class-switch differentiation was inhibited by the addition of anti-TGF-β but not by the addition of anti-IL-10. Taken together, these studies provide excellent proof that while IL-10 is an important IgA differentiation factor for human B cells, it is a factor that does not in itself bring about class-switch differentiation; more likely, it acts either as a facilitator of TGF-β-mediated class-switch differentiation or, more likely, as a postswitch terminal differentiation factor.

So far in our discussion of factors influencing IgA B cell terminal differentiation, we have focused on differentiation of B cells derived from PPs that are T-cell-dependent B-2 B cells. A different set of rules regarding terminal differentiation may apply to T-cell-independent B-1 B cells. Thus, IL-5, a cytokine that, as indicated previously, plays a role along with IL-6 in terminal differentiation of IgA B-2 B cells, appears to be an obligate cytokine for IgA B-1 B cells, since IL-5 deficient mice exhibit selective depletion of B cells bearing B-1 lineage markers and a defect in the capacity to mount responses to a T-cell-independent antigen (phosphoryl choline). In contrast, such mice have only a modest reduction in overall IgA levels and respond normally to a T-cell-dependent antigen (OVA) (Bao et al., 1998; Hiroi et al., 1999). Another cytokine that appears to be important for the terminal differentiation of B-1 IgA B cells is IL-15. In the relevant studies it was shown that B-1 B cells contained much higher levels of IL-15R mRNA than did B-2 B cells, and indeed IL-15 induced greater proliferation and IgA production in B-1 cells than in B-2 cells (Hiroi et al., 2000). Of interest, IL-15 acts on sIgM⁺/sIgA⁻ B cells to induce IgA production but nevertheless cannot be considered an IgA switch factor, since this cell population can be shown to contain Cα germline transcripts. Nevertheless, the authors suggested that IL-15 acted on B-1 B cells at an earlier stage than IL-5, another cytokine that induces differentiation of B-1 B cells, as mentioned above.

Another type of differentiation factor involved in terminal B cell differentiation in general and that therefore impacts on terminal IgA B cell differentiation are the factors mentioned previously in relation to dendritic cell effects, namely, BlyS and APRIL. These factors are induced via both T-cell-dependent interactions involving CD40L and T-cell-independent interactions involving type I interferons (Litinskiy *et al.*, 2002). Thus, they may affect differentiation of both B-1 and B-2 B cells. However, mice with TACI deficiency, *i.e.*, deficiency of one of the receptors for BlyS, manifest impaired IgG and IgA responses to T-cell-independent antigens but not T-cell-dependent antigens. Thus, it is likely that BlyS has a greater impact on B-1 B cells than B-2 B cells. In any case, the effects of BlyS and APRIL are dependent on stimulation of B cells via the BCR and on the presence of conventional cytokines such as IL-15. Thus, they affect B cell differentiation at another level.

Finally, it should not go unnoticed in this discussion of cytokines supporting the terminal differentiation of IgA B cells that the cytokines active in this context are in fact now known as Th2 cytokines. This brings us inevitably to the question of the role of IL-4 in IgA B cell terminal differentiation. The data relating to this question derive mainly from the study of IL-4-deficient mice and provide a fairly clear answer: while responses to protein antigens are clearly decreased in IL-4-deficient mice, the latter do produce IgA antibodies in response to strong antigens such as cholera toxin and *Salmonella* organisms and maintain normal IgA levels in both serum and secretions. Moreover, while cholera toxin acting as an adjuvant induces robust IL-4 secretion in its support of IgA responses, another adjuvant, heat-labile *Escherichia coli* toxin, induces a mixed Th1 and Th2 response that also gives rise to IgA responses. The latter ability of IgA responses to occur in a Th1 environment is underscored by the observation that antigen plus adjuvant results in a strong IgA response, even if exogenous IL-12 is administered and a Th1 response is induced (Marinelli *et al.* 1997). Thus, IL-4 is permissive of IgA responses probably because of its ability to induce "secondary" Th2 cytokines (such as IL-10 and IL-6) that actually can be produced in the absence of IL-4; thus, IgA responses can be mounted in its absence.

The significance of IgA B cell development to mucosal homeostasis: mucosal phenotype of AID-deficient mice

Throughout this discussion we have not concerned ourselves with the consequences of defective IgA B cell differentiation. In humans, the not-infrequent syndrome of selective IgA deficiency and the rarer condition known as common variable immunodeficiency (CVI) could conceivably provide insight into this question, but in such patients either the deficiency is relative rather than absolute or certain compensatory mechanisms supervene that mitigate the full effects of IgA immunodeficiency. Perhaps a better test of IgA immunodeficiency involves mice lacking AID and thus having B cells that are unable to undergo either class-switch recombination or somatic hypermutation; thus, their IgA deficiency cannot

be compensated by other immunoglobulins. Before we discuss these mice further, it is important to point out that AID deficiency would impair IgA B cell development involving both the B-2 B cell or adaptive IgA response and the B-1 B cell or innate IgA response. Thus, the phenotype of these mice does not reflect the importance of one or the other of these IgA components.

Recent studies of *aid*[-/-] mice by Fagarasan *et al.* (2001) showed that the complete absence of CSR and SHM due to AID deficiency leads to an enormous enlargement of germinal centers in all lymphoid tissues and accumulation of activated B cells and IgM plasma cells, especially in the gut lamina propria (Muramatsu *et al.*, 2000; Fagarasan *et al.*, 2001). The presence of IgM plasma cells in the intestine of these mice is explained by the finding that in the absence of AID, class-switch differentiation is not possible, and thus B cell development culminates in IgM B cell and plasma cell development. Within a few weeks of life, accumulation of such IgM B cells leads to hypertrophy of isolated lymphoid follicles, which become macroscopically visible all along the small intestine (Fagarasan *et al.*, 2002) **(Fig. 31.4)**. The follicular hyperplasia in *aid*[-/-] mice appears to be induced by a sustained activation in the gut, caused by a profound disregulation of the gut microflora, with a significant expansion of anaerobic bacteria in the absence of normal intestinal IgA. The anaerobes detected in all segments of *aid*[-/-] small intestine are nonpathogenic, commensal strains that usually are found in flora of the large intestine. An antibiotic treatment inhibiting anaerobes abolishes both gut hyperplasia and induction of GC formation in peripheral lymphoid tissue. Thus, it appears that continuous antigenic stimulation by an excessive population of intestinal anaerobic bacteria is responsible for both local and systemic B cell activation. The theory that antigenic pressure leads to the massive expansion of B cells and induction of hypertrophic organized structures in lamina propria of *aid*[-/-] mice is supported by repertoire studies of the B cells isolated from mucosal and peripheral tissues. The repertoire of B cells isolated from gut follicles and spleen of *aid*[-/-] mice is diverse, with many V genes and VDJ combinatorial diversity. Furthermore, individual gut isolated follicles contain different predominant V genes, which may suggest that selection and expansion of B cells took place *in situ*, possibly depending on the prevailing antigenic diversity of local bacteria (Fagarasan *et al.*, 2002). Thus, it seems that the IgA that is normally secreted into the gut lumen functions not only to protect against bacterial or viral antigens (Russell *et al.*, 1999) but also in the homeostasis of the gut flora, which is essential to prevent overstimulation of the nonmucosal immune system (Fagarasan *et al.*, 2002).

It is of interest that the mucosal phenotype in *aid*[-/-] mice resembles the nodular lymphoid hyperplasia seen in humans with common variable immunodeficiency syndrome (CVID) (Bastlein *et al.*, 1988; Levy *et al.*, 1998; Burt and Jacoby, 1999). These patients also have low levels of IgA and IgG as well as a marked reduction in SHM (Levy *et al.*, 1998) and suffer from frequent gastrointestinal infections and malab-

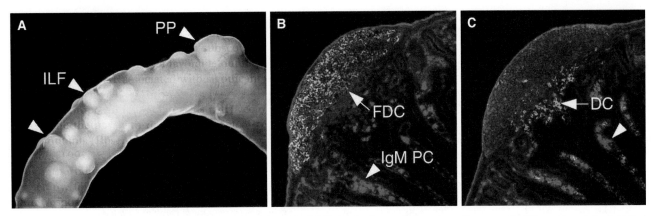

Fig 31.4. AID deficiency leads to hyperplasia of isolated lymphoid follicles in the small intestine. **(See page 9 of the color plates.) A,** A duodenal segment of the small intestine of *aid⁻/⁻* mouse showing many protruding follicles (ILF) and an enlarged Peyer's patch (PP). **B, C,** Adjacent sections of an isolated lymphoid follicle, consisting of many B cells on a follicular dendritic cell (FDC) network (*arrow*, **B**). Dendritic cells (DC) are located in a region equivalent to the subepithelial dome of the Peyer's patches (*arrow*, **C**). Lamina propria contains many IgM plasma cells (IgM PC) (*arrowheads*, **B** and **C**).

sorption. The mechanisms for the development of follicular hyperplasia in humans remain unknown, although it is likely to occur as a result of exacerbated local immune responses to gut antigens (Burt and Jacoby, 1999), possibly derived from anaerobic bacteria (Fagarasan *et al.*, 2002; Fagarasan and Honjo, 2003).

CONCLUDING REMARKS

The IgA humoral immune response characteristic of GALT was, from the first, recognized as the most unique feature of the mucosal immune system. It was in fact the discovery that IgA B cells were concentrated in mucosal tissues and that IgA antibodies predominated in mucosal fluids that led immunologists to define mucosal immunity as a separate field of immunologic study. Thus, it is both satisfying and useful that some of the main features of IgA B cell development have now been defined and can be recounted here with some degree of understanding. Nevertheless, this advance in knowledge has led to a new appreciation of the complexity of the IgA system, and we recognize that several key questions concerning the development of IgA B cells still await definitive answers. We therefore look forward to further research into this still-unfolding area of immunobiology.

REFERENCES

Ahsel, K., Harris, R., and Cyster, J. (2002). CXCL13 is required for B1-cell homing, natural antibody production and body-cavity immunity. *Immunity* 16, 67–76.

Agace, W., Roberts, A., Wu, L., Greineder, C., Ebert, E., and Parker, C. (2000). Human intestinal lamina propria and intraepithelial lymphocytes express receptors specific for chemokines induced by inflammation. *Eur. J. Immunol.* 30, 819–826.

Alley, C. (1987). Human bone marrow–derived IgA is produced by IgA-committed B cells in vitro. *J. Clin. Immunol.* 7, 151–158.

Al Maghazachi, A., and Phillips-Quagliata, J. (1988). Con A–propogated, auto-reactive T cell clones that secrete factors promoting high IgA responses. *Int. Arch. Allergy Appl. Immunol.* 86, 147–156.

Al Maghazachi, A., and Phillips-Quagliata, J. (1988). Keyhole limpet hemocyanin-propagated Peyer's patch T cell clones that help IgA responses. *J. Immunol.* 140, 3380–3388.

Arny, M., Kelly-Hatfield, P., Lamm, M., and Phillips-Quagliata, J. (1984). T-cell help for the IgA response: the function of T cells from different lymphoid organs in regulating the proportions of plasma cells expressing various isotypes. *Cell. Immunol.* 89, 95–112.

Aruffo, A., Farrington, M., Hollenbaugh, D., Li, X., Milatovich, A., Nonoyama, S., Ledbetter, J., Francke, U., and Ochs, H. (1993). The CD40 ligand, gp39, is defective in activated T cells from patients with X-linked hyper-IgM syndrome. *Cell.* 72, 291–300.

Bachl, J., Turck, C., and Wahl, M. (1996). Translatable germ-line transcript. *Eur. J. Immunol.* 26, 870–874.

Ballantyne, J., Henry, D., Muller, J., Briere, F., Snapper, C., Kehry, M., and Marcu, K. (1998). Efficient recombination of a switch substrate retrovector in CD40-activated B lymphocytes: implications for the control of CH gene switch recombination. *J. Immunol.* 161, 1336–1347.

Bao, S., Beagley, K., Murray, A., Cariso, V., Matthaei, K., Young, I., and Husband, A. (1998). Intestinal IgA plasma cells of the B1 lineage are IL-5 dependent. *Immunology* 94, 181–188.

Bastlein, C., Burlefinger, R., Holzberg, E., Voeth, C., Garbrecht, M., and Ottenjann, R. (1988). Common variable immunodeficiency syndrome and nodular lymphoid hyperplasia in the small intestine. *Endoscopy* 20, 272–275.

Beagley, K., Eldridge, J., Lee, F., Kiyono, H., Everson, M., Koopman, W., Hirano, T., Kishimoto, T., and McGhee, J. (1989). Interleukin and IgA synthesis. Human and murine interleukin 6 induce high rate IgA secretion in IgA-committed B cells. *J. Exp. Med.* 169, 2133–2148.

Benson, E., and Strober, W. (1988). Regulation of IgA secretion by T cell clones derived from the human gastrointestinal tract. *J. Immunol.* 140, 1874–1882.

Bottaro, A., Lansford, R., Xu, L., Zhang, J., Rothman, P., and Alt, F. (1994). I region transcription (*per se*) promotes basal IgE class switch recombination but additional factors regulate the efficiency of the process. *EMBO J.* 13, 665–674.

Bowman, E., Kuklin, N., Youngman, K., Lazarus, N., Kunkel, E., Pan, J., Greenberg, H., and Butcher, E. (2002). The intestinal chemokine thymus-expressing chemokine (CCL 25) attracts IgA antibody-secreting cells. *J. Exp. Med.* 195, 269–275.

Bradley, L., Malo, M., Fong, S., Tonkonogy, S., and Watson, S. (1998). Blockade of both L-selectin and alpha4 integrins abrogates naïve CD4 cell trafficking and responses in gut-associated lymphoid organs. *Int. Immunol.* 10, 961–968.

Bradley, L., Malo, M., Tonkonogy, S., and Watson, S. (1997). L-selectin is not essential for naïve CD4 cell trafficking or development of primary responses in Peyer's patches. *Eur. J. Immunol.* 27, 1140–1146.

Brandtzaeg, P., Baekkevold, E., and Morton, C. (2001). From B to A the mucosal way. *Nat. Immunology.* 2, 1093–1094.

Briere, F., Bridon, J., Chevet, D., Souillet, G., Bienvenu, F., Guret, C., Martinez-Valdez, H., and Bancherau, J. (1994). Interleukin 10 induces B lymphocytes from IgA-deficient patients to secrete IgA. *J. Clin. Invest.* 94, 97–104.

Burrows, P., Stephan, R., Wang, Y., Lassoued, K., Zhang, Z., and Cooper, M.D. (2002). The transient expression of pre–B cell receptors governs B cell development. *Semin. Immunol.* 14, 343–349.

Burt, R., and Jacoby, R. (1999). Polyposis Syndromes. In *Textbook of Gastroenterology* (eds. T. Yamada, D. Alpers, L. Laine, C. Owyang, and D. Powell), Vol. II, 1995–2022. Philadelphia: Lippincott Williams & Wilkins.

Butcher, E., Rouse, R., Coffman, R., Nottenburg, C., Hardy, R., and Weissman, I. (1982). Surface phenotype of Peyer's patch germinal center cells: implications for the role of germinal centers in B cell differentiation. *J. Immunol.* 129, 2698–2707.

Campbell, D., and Butcher, E. (2002). Rapid acquisition of tissue-specific homing phenotypes by CD4$^+$ T cells activated in cutaneous or mucosal lymphoid tissues. *J. Exp. Med.* 195, 135–141.

Cassellas, R., Nussenzweig, A., Wuerffel, R., Pelanda, R., Reichlin, A., Suh, H., Qin, X., Besmer, E., Kenter, A., Rajewsky, K., and Nussenzweig, M. (1998). Ku80 is required for immunoglobulin isotype switching. *EMBO J.* 17, 2404–2411.

Cazac, B., and Roes, J. (2000). TGF-β receptor controls B cell responsiveness and induction of IgA *in vivo*. *Immunity* 13, 443–451.

Cebra, J., Periwal, S., Lee, G., Lee, F., and Shroff, K. (1998). Development and maintenance of the gut-associated lymphoid tissue (GALT): the roles of enteric bacteria and viruses. *Dev. Immunol.* 6, 13–18.

Cerutti, A., Zan, H., Schaffer, A., Bergsagel, L., Hardindranath, N., Max, E., and Casali, P. (1998). CD40 ligand and appropriate cytokines induce switching to IgG, IgA, and IgE and coordinated germinal center and plasmacytoid phenotypic differentiation in a human monoclonal IgM$^+$IgD$^+$ B cell line. *J. Immunol.* 160, 2145–2157.

Chambers, C., Sullivan, T., and Allison, J. (1997). Lymphoproliferation in CTLA-4-deficient mice is mediated by costimulation-dependent activation of CD4$^+$ T cells. *Immunity* 7, 885–895.

Chaplin, D., and Fu, Y. (1998). Cytokine regulation of secondary lymphoid organ development. *Curr. Opin. Immunol.* 10, 289.

Chen, W., Jin, W., and Wahl, S. (1998). Engagement of cytotoxic T lymphocyte–associated antigen 4 (CTLA-4) induces transforming growth factor beta (TGF-beta) production by murine CD4$^+$ T cells. *J. Exp. Med.* 188, 1849–1857.

Chirmule, N., Tazelaar, J., and Wilson, J. (2000). Th2-dependent B cell responses in the absence of CD40–CD40 ligand interactions. *J. Immunol.* 164, 248–255.

Chung, J., Silverman, M., and Monroe, J. (2003). Transitional B cells: step by step towards immune competence. *Trends Immunol.* 24, 343–349.

Clough, J., Mims, L., and Strober, W. (1971). Deficient IgA antibody response to arsonilic acid bovine serum albumin (BSA) in neonatally thymectomized rabbits. *J. Immunol.* 106, 1624–1629.

Coffman, R., Lebman, D., and Shrader, B. (1989). Transforming growth factor beta specifically enhances IgA production by lipopolysaccharide-stimulated murine B lymphocytes. *J. Exp. Med.* 170, 1039–1044.

Cong, Y., Rabin, E., and Wortis, H. (1991). Treatment of murine CD5$^-$ B cells with anti-Ig, but not LPS, induces surface CD5: two B-cell activation pathways. *Int. Immunol.* 3, 467–476.

Cory, S., Jackson, J., and Adams, J. (1980). Deletions in the constant region locus can account for switches in immunoglobulin heavy chain expression. *Nature* 285, 450–456.

Craig, S., and Cebra, J. (1981). Peyer's patches: an enriched source of precursors for IgA-producing immunocytes in the rabbit. *J. Exp. Med.* 134, 188–200.

Daniels, G., and Lieber, M. (1995). RNA:DNA complex formation upon transcription of immunoglobulin switch regions: implications for the mechanism and regulation of class switch recombination. *Nucleic Acids Res.* 23, 5006–5011.

Daniels, G., and Lieber, M. (1995). Strand specificity in the transcriptional targeting of recombination at immunoglobulin switch sequences. *Proc. Natl. Acad. Sci. USA* 92, 5625–5629.

Davis, I., Knight, K., and Rouse, B. (1998). The spleen and organized lymph nodes are not essential for the development of gut-induced mucosal immune responses in lymphotoxin-α deficient mice. *Clin. Immunol., and Immunopathology* 89, 150–159.

Davis, M., Kim, S., and Hood, L. (1980). DNA sequences mediating class switching in α-immunoglobulins. *Science.* 209, 1360–1365.

Defrance, T., Vanbervliet, B., Briere, F., Durand, I., Rousett, F., and Bancherau, J. (1992). Interleukin-10 and transforming growth factor β cooperate to induce anti-CD40-activated naïve human B cells to secrete immunoglobulin A. *J. Exp. Med.* 175, 671–682.

Desvignes, C., Bour, H., Nicolas, J., and Kaiserlian, D. (1996). Lack of oral tolerance but oral priming for contact sensitivity to dinitrofluorobenzene in major histocompatibility complex class II–deficient mice and in CD4$^+$ T cell–depleted mice. *Eur. J. Immunol.* 26, 1756–1761.

De Togni, P., Goellner, T., Ruddle, N., Streeter, P., Fick, A., Mariathasan, S., Smith, S., Carlson, R., Shornick, L., Strauss-Schoenberger, J., Russell, J., Karr, R., and Chaplin, D. (1994). Abnormal development of peripheral lymphoid organs in mice deficient in lymphotoxin. *Science* 264, 703–707.

De Winter, H., Elewaut, D., Turovskaya, O., Huflejit, M., Shimeld, C., Hagenbaugh, A., Binder, S., Takashi, I., Kronenberg, M., and Cheroute, H. (2002). Regulation of mucosal immune responses by recombinant interleukin 10 produced by intestinal epithelial cells in mice. *Gastroenterology* 122, 1829–1841.

DiSanto, J., Muller, W., Guy-Grand, D., Fischer, A., and Rajewsky, K. (1995). Lymphoid development in mice with a targeted deletion of the interleukin 2 receptor gamma chain. *Proc. Nat. Acad. Sci. USA* 92, 377–381.

Dong, C., Temann, U., and Flavell, R. (2001). Cutting edge: critical role of inducible costimulator in germinal center reactions. *J. Immunol.* 166, 3659–3662.

Dubois, B., Vanbervliet, B., Fayette, J., Massacrier, C., Van Kooten, C., Briere, F., Bancherau, J., and Caux, C. (1997). Dendritic cells enhance growth and differentiation of CD40-activated B lymphocytes. *J. Exp. Med.* 185, 941–951.

Dunn-Walters, D., Isaacson, P., and Spencer, J. (1997). Sequence analysis of human IgVH genes indicates that ileal lamina propria plasma cells are derived from Peyer's patches. *Eur. J. Immunol.* 27, 463–467.

Durandy, A., and Honjo, T. (2001). Human genetic defects in class-switch recombination (hyper-IgM syndromes). *Curr. Opin. Immunol.* 13, 543–548.

Edmiston, J., and Lebman, D. (1997). A transforming growth factor–beta regulatable RNA-binding protein interacts specifically with germline Ig alpha transcripts. *Int. Immunol.* 9, 427–433.

Ehrhardt, R., Strober, W., and Harriman, G. (1992). Effect of transforming growth factor (TGF)–beta 1 on IgA isotype expression. TGF–beta 1 induces a small increase in sIgA$^+$ B cells regardless of the method of B cell activation. *J. Immunol.* 148, 3830–3836.

Elson, C., Heck, J., and Strober, W. (1979). T cell regulation of murine IgA synthesis. *J. Exp. Med.* 149, 632–643.

Estes, D., Tuo, W., Brown, W., and Goin, J. (1998). Effects of type I/type II interferons and transforming growth factor–beta on B-cell differentiation and proliferation. Definition of costimulation and cytokine requirements for immunoglobulin synthesis and expression. *Immunology* 95, 604–611.

Ezernieks, J., Schnarr, B., Metz, K., and Duschl, A. (1996). The human IgE germline promoter is regulated by interleukin-4, interleukin-13, interferon-alpha and interferon-gamma via an interferon-gamma-activated site and its flanking regions. *Eur. J. Biochem.* 240, 667–673.

Fagarasan, S., Shinkura, R., Kamata, T., Nogaki, F., Ikuta, K., Tashiro, K., and Honjo, T. (2000). Alymphoplasia (aly)–type nuclear factor kappaB–inducing kinase (NIK) causes defects in secondary lymphoid tissue chemokine receptor signaling and homing of peritoneal cells to the gut-associated lymphatic tissue system. *J. Exp. Med.* 191, 1477–1486.

Fagarasan, S., Kinoshita, K., Muramatsu, M., Ikuta, K., and Honjo, T. (2001). *In situ* class switching and differentiation to IgA-producing cells in the gut lamina propria. *Nature* 413, 639–643.

Fagarasan, S., Muramatsu, M., Suzuki, K., Nagaoka, H., Hiai, H., and Honjo, T. (2002). Critical roles of activation-induced cytidine deaminase (AID) in the homeostasis of gut flora. *Science* 298, 1424–1427.

Fagarasan, S., and Honjo, T. (2003). Intestinal IgA synthesis: regulation of front-line body defenses. *Nat. Rev. Immunology* 3, 63–72.

Fagarasan, S., and Honjo, T. (2000). T-independent immune response: new aspects of B cell biology. *Science* 290, 89–92.

Fayette, J., Durand, I., Bridon, J., Arpin, C., Dubois, B., Cauz, C., Liu, J., Banchereau, J., and Briere, F. (1998). Dendritic cells enhance the differentiation of naïve B cells into plasma cells *in vitro*. *Scand. J. Immunol.* 48, 563–570.

Fayette, J., Dubois, B., Vandenabeele, S., Bridon, J., Vanbervliet, B., Durand, I., Banchereau, J., Caux, C., and Brière, F. (1997). Human dendritic cells skew isotype switching of CD40-activated naïve B cells towards IgA₁ and IgA₂. *J. Exp. Med.* 185, 1909–1918.

Ferguson, S., Han, S., Kelsoe, G., and Thompson, C. (1996). CD28 is required for germinal center formation. *J. Immunol.* 156, 457–481.

Finke, D., Acha-Orbea, H., Mattis, A., Lipp, M., and Kraehlenbuhl, J. (2002). CD4⁺CD3⁻ cells induce Peyer's patch development: role of α4β1 integrin activation by CXCR5. *Immunity* 17, 363–373.

Foy, T., Laman, J., Ledbetter, J., Aruffo, A., Claassen, E., and Noelle, R. (1994). Gp39–CD40 interactions are essential for germinal center formation and the development of B cell memory. *J. Exp. Med.* 180, 157–163.

Fujihashi, K., Taguchi, T., Aicher, W., McGhee, J., Bluestone, J., Eldridge, J., and Kiyono, H. (1992). Immunoregulatory functions for murine intraepithelial lymphocytes: γ/δ T cell receptor–positive (TCR⁺) T cells abrogate oral tolerance while α/β TCR⁺ T cells provide B cell help. *J. Exp. Med.* 175, 695–707.

Fuss, I., Boirivant, M., Lacy, B., and Strober, W. (2002). The interrelated roles of TGF-beta and IL-10 in the regulation of experimental colitis. *J. Immunol.* 168, 900–908.

Gaff, C., and Gerondakis, S. (1990). RNA splicing generates alternate forms of germline immunoglobulin alpha heavy chain transcripts. *Int. Immunol.* 2, 1143–1148.

Gardby, E., Lane, P., and Lycke, N. (1998). Requirements for B7–CD28 costimulation in mucosal IgA responses: paradoxes observed in CTLA4-H gamma 1 transgenic mice. *J. Immunol.* 161, 45–59.

Gardby, E., Wrammert, J., Schön, K., Ekman, L., Leanderson, T., and Lycke, N. (2003). Strong differential regulation of serum and mucosal IgA responses as revealed in CD28-deficient mice using cholera toxin adjuvant. *J. Immunol.* 170, 55–63.

Gascan, H., Gauchat, J., Aversa, G., Van Vlasselaer, P., and de Vries, J. (1991). Anti-CD40 monoclonal antibodies or CD4⁺ T cell clones and IL-4 induce IgG4 and IgE switching in purified human B cells via different signaling pathways. *J. Immunol.* 147, 8–13.

George, A., and Cebra, J. (1991). Response of single germinal-center B cells in T-cell-dependent microculture. *Proc. Natl. Acad. Sci. USA* 88, 11–15.

Gerondakis, S. (1990). Structure and expression of murine germ-line immunoglobulin epsilon heavy chain transcripts induced by interleukin 4. *Proc. Natl. Acad. Sci. USA* 87, 1581–1585.

Gerondakis, S., Gaff, C., Goodman, D., and Grumont, R. (1991). Structure and expression of mouse germline immunoglobulin gamma 3 heavy chain transcripts induced by the mitogen lipopolysaccharide. *Immunogenetics* 34, 392–400.

Gonzalo, J., Tian, J., Delaney, T., Corcoran, J., Rottman, J., Lora, J., Algarawi, A., Kroczek, R., Gutierrez-Ramos, J., and Coyle, A. (2001). ICOS is critical for T helper cell–mediated lung mucosal inflammatory responses. *Nat. Immunol.* 2, 597–604.

Goodrich, M., and McGhee, D. (1999). Effect of intestinal epithelial cell cytokines on mucosal B-cell IgA secretion: enhancing effect of epithelial-derived IL-6 but not TGF-beta on IgA⁺ B cells. *Immunol. Lett.* 67, 11–14.

Goodrich, M., and McGhee, D. (1999). Preferential enhancement of B cell IgA secretion by intestinal epithelial cell–derived cytokines and interleukin-2. *Immunol. Invest.* 28, 67–75.

Goodrich, M., and McGhee, D. (1998). Regulation of mucosal B cell immunoglobulin secretion by intestinal epithelial cell–derived cytokines. *Cytokine* 10, 948–955.

Hamada, H., Hiroi, T., Nishiyama, Y., Takahashi, H., Masunaga, Y., Hachimura, S., Kaminogawa, S., Takahashi-Iwanaga, H., Iwanaga, T., Kiyono, H., Yamamoto, H., and Isikawa, H. (2002). Identification of multiple isolated lymphoid follicles on the antimesenteric wall of the mouse small intestine. *J. Immunol.* 168, 57–64.

Han, S., Hathcock, K., Zheng, B., Kepler, T., Hodes, R., and Kelsoe, G. (1995). Cellular interaction in germinal centers. Roles of CD40 ligand and B7-2 in established germinal centers. *J. Immunol.* 155, 556–567.

Harriman, G., Bradley, A., Das, S., Rogers-Fani, P., and Davis, A. (1996). IgA class switch in Iα exon deficient mice. Role of germline transcription in class switch recombination. *J. Clin. Invest.* 97, 477–485.

Hayakawa, K., Asano, M., Shinton, S., Gui, M., Wen, L., Dashoff, J., and Hardy, R. (2003). Positive selection of anti-Thy-1 autoreactive B-1 cells and natural serum autoantibody production independent from bone marrow B cell development. *J. Exp. Med.* 197, 87–99.

Hein, K., Lorenz, M., Siebenkotten, G., Petry, K., Christine, R., and Radbruch, A. (1998). Processing of switch transcripts is required for targeting of antibody class switch recombination. *J. Exp. Med.* 188, 2369–2374.

Hiroi, T., Yanagita, M., Iijima, H., Iwatani, K., Yoshida, T., Takatsu, K., and Kiyono, H. (1999). Deficiency of IL-5 receptor α-chain selectively influences the development of the common mucosal immune system independent IgA-producing B-1 cell in mucosa associated tissues. *J. Immunol.* 162, 821–828.

Hiroi, T., Yanagita, M., Ohta, N., Sakaue, G., and Kiyono, H. (2000). IL-15 and IL-15 receptor selectively regulate differentiation of common mucosal immune system–independent B-1 cells for IgA responses. *J. Immunol.* 165, 4329–4337.

Honda, K., Nakano, H., Yoshida, H., Nishikawa, S., Rennert, P., Ikuta, K., Tamechika, M., Yamaguchi, K., Fukumoto, T., Chiba, T., and Nishikawa, S. (2001). Molecular basis for hematopoietic/mesenchymal interaction during initiation of Peyer's patch organogenesis. *J. Exp. Med.* 193, 621–630.

Honjo, T., and Kataokoa, T. (1978). Organization of immunoglobulin heavy chain genes and allelic deletion model. *Proc. Natl. Acad. Sci. USA* 75, 2140–2144.

Honjo, T., Kinoshita, K., and Muramatsu, M. (2002). Molecular mechanisms of class switch recombination: linkage with somatic hypermutation. *Annu. Rev. Immunol.* 20, 165–196.

Horikawa, K., Kaku, H., Nakajima, H., Davey, H., Hennighausen, L., Iwamoto, I., Yasue, T., Kariyone, A., and Takatsu, K. (2001). Essential role of STAT5 for IL-5 dependent IgH switch recombination in mouse B cells. *J. Immunol.* 167, 5018–5026.

Hu, Y., Pan, Q., Pardalli, E., Mills, F., Bernstein, R., Max, E., Sideras, P., and Hammarstrom, L. (2000). Regulation of germline promotors by the two human Ig heavy chain 3' alpha enhancers. *J. Immunol.* 164, 6380–6386.

Iciek, L., Delphin, S., and Stavnezer, J. (1997). CD40 cross-linking induces Ig epsilon germline transcripts in B cells via activation of NF-kappaB: synergy with IL-4 induction. *J. Immunol.* 158, 4769–4779.

Islam, K., Nilsson, L., Sideras, P., Hammarstrom, L., and Smith, C. (1991). TGF-beta 1 induces germ-line transcripts of both IgA subclasses in human B lymphocytes. *Int. Immunol.* 3, 1099–1106.

Iwasaki, A., and Kelsall, B. (1999). Freshly isolated Peyer's patch, but not spleen, dendritic cells produce interleukin 10 and induce the differentiation of T helper type 2 cells. *J. Exp. Med.* 190, 229–239.

Iwasata, T., Shimizu, A., Honjo, T., and Yamagishi, H. (1990). Circular DNA is excised by immunoglobulin class switch recombination. *Cell* 62, 143–149.

Jabara, H., Loh, R., Ramesh, N., Vercelli, D., and Geha, R. (1993). Sequential switching from mu to epsilon via gamma 4 in human

B cells stimulated with IL-4 and hydrocortisone. *J. Immunol.* 151, 4528–4533.

Jordan, M., Boesteanu, A., Reed, A., Petrone, A., Holenbeck, A., Lerman, M., Naji, A., and Caton, A. (2001). Thymic selection of CD4+CD25+ regulatory T cells induced by an agonist self-peptide. *Nat. Immunol.* 2, 301–306.

Jumper, M., Fujita, K., Lipsky, P., and Meek, K. (1996). A CD30 responsive element in the germline epsilon promoter that is distinct from and inhibitory to the CD40 response element. *Mol. Immunol.* 33, 965–972.

Jung, S., Rajewsky, K., and Radbruch, A. (1993). Shutdown of class switch recombination by deletion of a switch region control element. *Science* 259, 984–987.

Justice, J., Shibata, Y., Sur, S., Mustafa, J., Fan, M., and Van Scott, M. (2001). IL-10 gene knockout attenuates allergen-induced airway hyperresponsiveness in C57BL/6 mice. *Am. J. Physiol. Lung Cell Mol. Physiol.* 280, L363–L368.

Kang, H., Chin, R., Wang, Y., Yu, P., Wang, J., Newell, K., and Fu, Y. (2002). Signaling via LTβR on the lamina propria stromal cells of the gut is required for IgA production. *Nat. Immunol.* 3, 576–582.

Kataoka, T., Kawakami, T., Takahashi, N., and Honjo, T. (1980). Rearrangement of immunoglobulin γ1-chain gene and mechanism for heavy-chain class switch. *Proc. Natl. Acad. Sci. USA* 77, 919–923.

Kawabe, T., Naka, T., Yoshida, K., Tanaka, T., Fujiwara, H., Suematsu, S., Yoshida, N., Kishimoto, T., and Kikutani, H. (1994). The immune responses in CD40-deficient mice: impaired immunoglobulin class switching and germinal center formation. *Immunity* 1, 167–178.

Kawanishi, H., Saltzman, L., and Strober, W. (1983). Mechanisms regulating IgA class–specific immunoglobulin production in murine gut-associated lymphoid tissues. I. T cells derived from Peyer's patches that switch sIgM B cells to sIga B cells *in vitro. J. Exp. Med.* 157, 433–450.

Kawanishi, H., Saltzman, L., and Strober, W. (1983). Mechanisms regulating IgA class–specific immunoglobulin production in murine gut-associated lymphoid tissues. II. Terminal differentiation of postswitch sIgA-bearing Peyer's patch B cells. *J. Exp. Med.* 158, 649–669.

Kawanishi, H., Saltzman, L, and Strober, W. (1983). Characteristics and regular function of murine con A–induced, cloned T cells obtained from Peyer's patches and spleen. Mechanisms regulating isotype-specific immunoglobulin production by Peyer's patch B cells. *J. Immunol.* 129, 475–483.

Kawanishi, H., Ozato, K., and Strober, W. (1985). The proliferative response of cloned Peyer's patch switch T cells to syngeneic and allogeneic stimuli. *J. Immunol.* 134, 3586–3591.

Kelsoe, G., and Zheng, B. (1993). Sites of B-cell activation *in vivo. Curr. Opin. Immunol.* 5, 418–422.

Kihira, T., and Kawanishi, H. (1995). Induction of IgA B cell differentiation of bone marrow–derived B cells by Peyer's patch autoreactive helper T cells. *Immunol. Invest.* 24, 701–711.

Kim, P., and Kagnoff, M. (1990). Transforming growth factor beta 1 increases IgA isotype switching at the clonal level. *J. Immunol.* 145, 3773–3778.

Kim, P., Eckmann, L., Lee, W., Han, W., and Kagnoff, M. (1998). Cholera toxin and cholera toxin B subunit induce IgA switching through the action of TGF-beta 1. *J. Immunol.* 160, 1198–1203.

Kinoshita, K., Tashiro, J., Tomita, S., Lee, C., and Honjo, T. (1998). Target specificity of immunoglobulin class switch recombination is not determined by nucleotide sequences of S regions. *Immunity* 9, 849–858.

Kinoshita, K., Harigai, M., Fagarasan, S., Muramatsu, M., and Honjo, T. (2001). A hallmark of active class switch recombination: transcripts directed by I promoters on looped-out circular DNAs. *Proc. Natl. Acad. Sci. USA* 98, 12620–12623.

Kinoshita, K., and Honjo, T. (2001). Linking class-switch recombination with somatic hypermutation. *Nat. Rev. Mol. Cell. Biol.* 2, 493–503.

Kitani, A., and Strober, W. (1994). Differential regulation of C alpha 1 and C alpha 2 germ-line and mature mRNA transcripts in human peripheral blood B cells. *J. Immunol.* 153, 1466–1477.

Kroese, F., Ammerlaan, W., Kantor, A. (1993). Evidence that intestinal IgA plasma cells in mu, kappa transgenic mice are derived from B-1 (Ly-1 B) cells. *Int. Immunol.* 5, 1317–1327.

Kunkel, E., Campbell, D., and Butcher, E. (2003). Chemokines in lymphocyte trafficking and intestinal immunity. *Microcirculation* 10, 313–323.

Kunkel, E., Campbell, J., Haraldsen, G., Pan, J., Boisvert, J., Roberts, A., Ebert, E., Vierra, M., Goodman, S., Genovese, M., Wardlaw, A., Greenberg, H., Parker, C., Butcher, E., Andrew, D., and Agace, W. (2000). Lymphocyte CC chemokine receptor 9 and epithelial thymus-expressed chemokine (TECK) expression distinguish the small intestinal immune compartment: epithelial expression of tissue-specific chemokines as an organizing principle in regional immunity. *J. Exp. Med.* 192, 761–768.

Kunkel, E., Kim, C., Lazarus, N., Vierra, M., Soler, Bowman, E., and Butcher, E. (2003). CCR10 expression is a common feature of circulating and mucosal epithelial tissue IgA Ab–secreting cells. *J. Clin. Invest.* 111, 1001–1010.

Kunimoto, D., Nordan, R., and Strober, W. (1989). IL-6 is a potent cofactor of IL-1 in IgM synthesis and IL-5 in IgA synthesis. *J. Immunol.* 143, 2230–2235.

Kushnir, N., Bos, N., Zuercher, A., Coffin, S., Moser, C., Offitt, P., and Cebra, J. (2001). B2 but not B1 cells can contribute to CD4+ T-cell-mediated clearance of rotavirus in SCID mice. *J. Virol.* 75, 5482–5490.

Lalor, P.A., and Morahan, G. (1990). The peritoneal Ly-1 (CD5) B cell repertoire is unique among murine B cell repertoires. *Eur. J. Immunol.* 20, 485–492.

Lam, K.P., and Rajewsky, K. (1999). B cell antigen receptor specificity and surface density together determine B-1 versus B-2 cell development. *J. Exp. Med.* 190, 471–477.

Laurencikiene, J., Deveikaite, V., and Severinson, E. (2001). HS1,2 enhancer regulation of germline epsilon and gamma2b promoters in murine B lymphocytes: evidence for specific promoter–enhancer interactions. *J. Immunol.* 167, 3257–3265.

Lebman, D., Lee, F., and Coffman, R. (1990). Mechanism for transforming growth factor beta and IL-2 enhancement of IgA expression in lipopolysaccharide-stimulated B cell cultures. *J. Immunol.* 144, 952–959.

Lebman, D., Nomura, D., Coffman, R., and Lee, F. (1990). Molecular characterization of germ-line immunoglobulin A transcripts produced during transforming growth factor type beta–induced isotype switching. *Proc. Nat. Acad. Sci. USA* 87, 3962–3966.

Lebman, D., and Edmiston, J. (1999). The role of TGF-β in growth, differentiation, and maturation of B lymphocytes. *Microbes Infection* 1, 1297–1304.

Lee, C., Kinoshita, K., Arudchandran, A., Cerritelli, S., Crouch, R., and Honjo, T. (2001). Quantitative regulation of class switch recombination by switch region transcription. *J. Exp. Med.* 194, 365–374.

Lepse, C., Kumar, R., and Ganea, D. (1994). Extrachromosomal eukaryotic DNA substrates for switch recombination: analysis of isotype and cell specificity. *DNA Cell Biol.* 13, 1151–1161.

Leung, H., and Maizels, N. (1992). Transcriptional regulatory elements stimulate recombination in extrachromosomal substrates carrying immunoglobulin switch-region sequences. *Proc. Natl. Acad. Sci. USA* 89, 4154–4158.

Levy, Y., Gupta, N., Le Deist, F., Garcia, C., Fischer, A., Weill, J., and Reynaud, C. (1998). Defect in IgV gene somatic hypermutation in common variable immuno-deficiency syndrome. *Proc. Natl. Acad. Sci. USA* 95, 13135–13140.

Li, M., Chung, W., and Maizels, N. (1997). Developmental specificity of immunoglobulin heavy chain switch region recombination activities. *Mol. Immunol.* 34, 201–208.

Lin, S., and Stavnezer, J. (1996). Activation of NF-kappaB/Rel by CD40 engagement induces the mouse germ line immunoglobulin Cgamma1 promoter. *Mol. Cell. Biol.* 16, 4591–4603.

Lin, Y., and Stavnezer, J. (1992). Regulation of transcription of the germ-line Ig alpha constant region gene by an ATF element and by novel transforming growth factor–beta 1-responsive elements. *J. Immunol.* 149, 2914–2925.

Litinskiy, M., Nardelli, B., Hilbert, D., He, B., Schaffer, A., Casali, P., and Cerutti, A. (2002). DCs induce CD40-independent immunoglobulin class switching through BlyS and APRIL. *Nat. Immunology* 3, 822–829.

Lorenz, M., Jung, S., and Radbruch, A. (1995). Switch transcripts in immunoglobulin class switching. *Science* 267, 1825–1828.

Lorenz, M., and Radbruch, A. (1996). Developmental and molecular regulation of immunoglobulin class switch recombination. *Curr. Top. Microbiol. Immunol.* 217, 151–169.

Lorenz, R., Chaplin, D., McDonald, K., McDonough, J., and Newberry, R. (2003). Isolated lymphoid follicle formation is inducible and dependent upon lymphotoxin-sufficient B lymphocytes, lymphotoxin β receptor, and TNF receptor 1 function. *J. Immunol.* 170, 5475–5482.

Lundgren, M., Strom, L., Bergqvist, L., Skog, S., Heiden, T., Stavnezer, J., and Severinson, E. (1995). Cell cycle regulation of germline immunoglobulin transcription: potential role of Ets family members. *Eur. J. Immunol.* 25, 2042–2051.

Lutzker, S., and Alt, F. (1988). Structure and expression of germ line immunoglobulin gamma 2b transcripts. *Mol. Cell. Biol.* 8, 1849–1852.

Lycke, N. (1998). T cell and cytokine regulation of the IgA response. In *Mucosal T Cells* (ed. T. MacDonald), 209–234. Basel: Karger.

MacLennan, I. (1994). Germinal centers. *Annu. Rev. Immunol.* 12, 117–139.

Macpherson, A., Gatto, D., Sainsbury, E., Harriman, G., Hengartner, H., and Zinkernagel, R. (2000). A primitive T cell–independent mechanism of intestinal mucosal IgA responses to commensal bacteria. *Science* 288, 2222–2226.

Macpherson, A., Hunziker, L., McCoy, K., and Lamarre, A. (2001). IgA responses in the intestinal mucosa against pathogenic and non-pathogenic microorganisms. *Microbes Infection* 3, 1021–1035.

Macpherson, A., Lamarre, A., McCoy, K., Harriman, G., Odermatt, B., Dougan, G., Hengartner, H., and Zinkernagel, R. (2001). IgA production without μ or δ chain expression in developing B cells. *Nat. Immunology* 2, 625–631.

Malisan, F., Briere, F., Bridon, J., Harindranath, N., Mills, F., Max, E., and Banchereau, J., Martinez-Valdez, H. (1996). Interleukin-10 induces immunoglobulin G isotype switch recombination in human CD40–activated naïve B lymphocytes. *J. Exp. Med.* 183, 937–947.

Manis, J., Gu, Y., Lansford, R., Sonoda, E., Ferrini, R., Davidson, L., Rajewsky, K., and Alt, F. (1998). Ku70 is required for late B cell development and immunoglobulin heavy chain switching. *J. Exp. Med.* 187, 2081–2089.

Mao, C., and Stavnezer, J. (2001). Differential regulation of mouse germline Ig gamma 1 and epsilon promoters by IL-4 and CD40. *J. Immunol.* 167, 1522–1534.

Marth, T., Strober, W., Seder, R., and Kelsall, B. (1997). Regulation of transforming growth factor–beta production by interleukin-12. *Eur. J. Immunol.* 27, 1213–1220.

Martin, F., and Kearney, J. (2001). B1 cells: similarities and differences with other B cell subsets. *Curr. Opin. Immunol.* 13, 195–201.

Martin, F., and Kearney, J. (2002). Marginal-zone B cells. *Nat. Rev. Immunol.* 2, 323–335.

Massague, J. (1990). Transforming growth factor–alpha. A model for membrane-anchored growth factors. *J. Biol. Chem.* 265, 21393–21396.

Matsuoda, M., Yoshida, K., Maeda, T., Usuda, S., and Sakano, H. (1990). Switch circular DNA formed in cytokine-treated mouse splenocytes: evidence for intramolecular DNA deletion in immunoglobulin class switching. *Cell* 62, 135–142.

Mayer, L., Posnett, D., and Kunkel, H. (1985). Human malignant T cells capable of inducing an immunoglobulin class switch. *J. Exp. Med.* 161, 134–144.

Mayrhofer, G. (1997). Peyer's patch organogenesis: cytokines rule, OK? *Gut* 41, 707–709.

McAdam, A., Greenwald, R., Levin, M., Chernova, T., Malenkovich, N., Ling, V., Freeman, G., and Sharpe, A. (2001). ICOS is critical for CD40-mediated antibody class switching. *Nature* 409, 102–105.

McIntyre, T., Klinman, D., Rothman, P., Lugo, M., Dasch, J., Mond, J., and Snapper, C. (1993). Transforming growth factor beta 1 selectivity stimulates immunoglobulin G2b secretion by lipopolysaccharide-activated murine B cells. *J. Exp. Med.* 177, 1031–1037.

McIntyre, T., Kehry, M., and Snapper, C. (1995). Novel *in vitro* model for high-rate IgA class switching. *J. Immunol.* 154, 3156–3161.

McIntyre, T., and Strober, W. (1999). Gut-associated lymphoid tissue: regulation of IgA B-cell development. In *Mucosal Immunology* (eds. P. Ogra, J. Mestecky, M. Lamm, W. Strober, J. Bienenstock, and J. McGhee), 319–356. San Diego: Academic Press.

Mebius, R., Rennert, P., and Weissman, I. (1997). Developing lymph nodes collect CD4+CD3−LTβ+ cells that can differentiate to APC, NK cells, and follicular cells but not T or B cells. *Immunity* 7, 493–504.

Mega, J., Bruce, M., Beagley, K., McGhee, J., Taguchi, T., Pitts, A., McGhee, M., Bucy, R., Eldridge, J., Mestecky, J., and Kiyono, H. (1991). Regulation of mucosal responses by CD4+ T lymphocytes: effects of anti-L3T4 treatment on the gastrointestinal immune system. *Int. Immunol.* 3, 793–805.

Messner, B., Stutz, A., Albrecht, B., Peiritsch, S., and Woisetschlager, M. (1997). Cooperation of binding sites for STAT6 and NF kappa B/rel in the IL-4-induced up-regulation of the human IgE germline promoter. *J. Immunol.* 159, 3330–3337.

Moller, P., Eichelmann, A., Mechtersheimer, G., and Koretz, K. (1991). Expression of beta 1-integrins, H-CAM (CD44) and LECAM-1 in primary gastro-intestinal B-cell lymphomas as compared to the adhesion receptor profile of the gut-associated lymphoid system, tonsil and peripheral lymph node. *Int. J. Cancer* 49, 846–855.

Mombaerts, P., Iacomini, J., Johnson, R., Herrup, K., Tonegawa, S., and Papaioannou, V. (1992). RAG-1-deficient mice have no mature B and T lymphocytes. *Cell* 68, 869–877.

Mombaerts, P., Mizoguchi, E., Ljunggren, H., Iacomini, J., Ishikawa, H., Wang, L., Grusby, M.J., Glimcher, L., Winn, H., Bhan, A.K., et al. (1994). Peripheral lymphoid development and function in TCR mutant mice. *Int. Immunol.* 6, 1061–1070.

Mongini, P., Paul, W., and Metcalf, E. (1983). IgG subclass IgE, and IgA anti-trinitrophenol antibody production within trinitrophenol-Ficoll-responsive B cell clones. Evidence in support of three distinct switching pathways. *J. Exp. Med.* 157, 69–85.

Mottet, C., Uhlig, H., and Powrie, F. (2003). Cutting edge: cure of colitis by CD4+CD25+ regulatory T cells. *J. Immunol.* 170, 3939–3943.

Müller, G., and Lipp, M. (2003). Concerted action of the chemokine and lymphotoxin system in secondary lymphoid-organ development. *Curr. Opin. Immunol.* 15, 217–224.

Muramatsu, M., Sankaranand, V., Anant, S., Sugai, M., Kinoshita, K., Davidson, N., and Honjo, T. (1999). Specific expression of activation-induced cytidine deaminase (AID), a novel member of the RNA-editing deaminase family in germinal center B cells. *J. Biol. Chem.* 274, 18470–18476.

Muramatsu, M., Kinoshita, K., Fagarasan, S., Yamada, S., Shinkai, Y., and Honjo, T. (2000). Class switch recombination and hypermutation require activation-induced cytidine deaminase (AID), a potential RNA editing enzyme. *Cell* 102, 553–563.

Nakagawa, I., Takahashi, I., Kiyono, H., McGhee, J.R., and Hamada, S. (1996). Oral immunization with the B subunit of the heat-labile enterotoxin of Escherichia coli induces early Th1 and late Th2 cytokine expression in Peyer's patches. *J. Infect. Dis.* 173, 1428–1436.

Nakamura, K., Kitani, A., and Strober, W. (2001). Cell contact–dependent immunosuppression by CD4+CD25+ regulatory T cells is mediated by cell surface–bound transforming growth factor beta. *J. Exp. Med.* 194, 629–644.

Nakamura, M., Kondo, S., Sugai, M., Nazarea, M., Imamura, S., and Honjo, T. (1996). High frequency class switching of an IgM+ B lymphoma clone CH12F3 to IgA+ cells. *Int. Immunol.* 8, 193–201.

Neumann, B., Luz, A., Pfeffer, K., and Holzmann, B. (1996). Defective Peyer's patch organogenesis in mice lacking the 55-kD receptor for tumor necrosis factor. *J. Exp. Med.* 184, 259–264.

Nilsson, L., Islam, K., Olafsson, O., Zalcberg, I., Samakovlis, C., Hammarstrom, L., Smith, C., and Sideras, P. (1991). Structure of TGF-beta 1–induced human immunoglobulin C alpha 1 and C alpha 2 germ-line transcripts. *Int. Immunol.* 3, 1107–1115.

Oettinger, M., Schatz, D., Gorka, C., and Baltimore, D. (1990). RAG-1 and RAG-2, adjacent genes that synergistically activate V(D)J recombination. *Science* 248, 1517–1523.

Okahashi, N., Yamamoto, M., Vancott, J., Chatfield, S., Roberts, M., Bluethmann, H., Hiroi, T., Kiyono, H., and McGhee, J. (1996). Oral immunization of interleukin-4 (IL-4) knockout mice with a recombinant Salmonella strain or cholera toxin reveals that CD4+ Th2 cells producing IL-6 and IL-10 are associated with mucosal immunoglobulin A responses. *Infect. Immun.* 64, 1516–1525.

Okada, T., Ngo, V., Ekland, E., Forster, R., Lipp, M., Littman, D., and Cyster, J. (2002). Chemokine requirements for B cell entry to lymph nodes and Peyer's patches. *J. Exp. Med.* 196, 67–75.

Ozaki, I., Kinoshita, K., Muramatsu, M., Yoshikawa, K., and Honjo, T. (2002). The AID enzyme induces class switch recombination in fibroblasts. *Nature* 416, 340–345.

Pan, Q., Petit-Frere, C., Stavnezer, J., and Hammarstrom, L. (2000). Regulation of the promoter for human immunoglobulin gamma3 germ-line transcription and its interactions with the 3' alpha enhancer. *Eur. J. Immunol.* 30, 1019–1029.

Papadakis, K., Prehn, J., Nelson, V., Cheng, L., Binder, S., Ponath, P., Andrew, D., and Targan, S. (2000). The role of thymus-expressed cytokines and its receptor CCR9 on lymphocytes in the regional specialization of the mucosal immune system. *J. Immunol.* 165, 5069–5076.

Pardali, E., Xie, X., Tsapogas, P., Itoh, S., Arvanitidis, K., Heldin, C., ten Dijke, P., Grundstrom, T., and Sideras, P. (2000). Smad and AML proteins synergistically confer transforming growth factor beta1 responsiveness to human germ-line IgA genes. *J. Biol. Chem.* 275, 3552–3560.

Park, S., Lee, J., and Kim, P. (2001). Smad3 and Smad4 mediate transforming growth factor-beta1-induced IgA expression in murine B lymphocytes. *Eur. J. Immunol.* 31, 1706–1715.

Pasparakis, M., Alexopoulou, L., Grell, M., Pfizenmaier, K., Bluethmann, H., and Kollias, G. (1997). Peyer's patch organogenesis is intact yet formation of B lymphocyte follicles is defective in peripheral lymphoid organs of mice deficient for tumor necrosis factor and its 55-kDa receptor. *Proc. Natl. Acad. Sci. USA* 94, 9510.

Peng, S., Szabo, S., and Glimcher, L. (2002). T-beta regulates IgG class switching and pathogenic autoantibody production. *Proc. Natl. Acad. Sci. USA* 99, 5545–5550.

Petry, K., Siebenkotten, G., Christine, R., Hein, K., and Radbruch, A. (1999). An extrachromosomal switch recombination substrate reveals kinetics and substrate requirements of switch recombination in primary murine B cells. *Int. Immunol.* 11, 753–763.

Pritchard, H., Riddaway, J., and Micklem, H. (1973). Immune responses in congenitally thymusless mice. II. Quantitative studies of serum immunoglobulin, the antibody response to sheep erythrocytes, and the effect of thymus allografting. *Clin. Exp. Immunol.* 13, 125–138.

Qui, G., and Stavnezer, J. (1998). Over-expression of BSAP/Pax-5 inhibits switching to IgA and enhances switching to IgE in the 1.29μ B cell line. *J. Immunol.* 161, 2906–2918.

Qiu, G., Harriman, G., and Stavnezer, J. (1999). Iα exon-replacement mice synthesize a spliced HPRT-Cα transcript which may explain their ability to switch to IgA: inhibition of switching to IgG in these mice. *Int. Immunol.* 11, 37–46.

Rabbits, T., Forster, A., Dunnick, W., and Bentley, D. (1980). The role of gene deletion in the immunoglobulin heavy chain switch. *Nature* 283, 351–356.

Radcliffe, G., Lin, Y., Julius, M., Marcu, K., and Stavnezer, J. (1990). Structure of germ line immunoglobulin alpha heavy-chain RNA and its location on polysomes. *Mol. Cell. Biol.* 10, 382–386.

Reaban, M., and Griffin, J. (1990). Induction of RNA-stabilized DNA conformers by transcription of an immunoglobulin switch region. *Nature* 348, 342–344.

Renshaw, B., Fanslow, W., Armitage, R., Campbell, K., Ligitt, D., Wright, B., Davison, B., and Maliszewski, C. (1994). Humoral immune responses in CD40 ligand-deficient mice. *J. Exp. Med.* 180, 1889–1900.

Rescigno, M., Rotta, G., Valzasina, B., and Ricciardi-Castagnoli, P. (2001). Dendritic cells shuttle microbes across gut epithelial monolayers. *Immunobiology* 204, 572–581.

Revy, P., Muto, T., Levy, Y., Geissmann, F., Plebani, A., Sanal, O., Catalan, N., Forveille, M., Dufourcq-Labelouse, R., Gennery,

A., Tezcan, I., Ersoy, F., Kayserili, H., Ugazio, A., Brousse, N., Muramatsu, M., Notarangelo, L., Kinoshita, K., Honjo, T., Fischer, A., and Durandy, A. (2000). Activation-induced cytidine deaminase (AID) deficiency causes the autosomal recessive form of the hyper-IgM syndrome (HIGM2). *Cell.* 102, 565–575.

Rolink, A., Melchers, F., and Andersson, J. (1996). The SCID but not the RAG-2 gene product is required for S mu-S epsilon heavy chain class switching. *Immunity* 5, 319–330.

Rolink, A., Haasner, D., Melchers, F., and Andersson, J. (1996). The surrogate light chain in mouse B-cell development. *Int. Rev. Immunol.* 13, 341–356.

Rolink, A., and Melchers, F. (2002). BAFFled B cells survive and thrive: roles of BAFF in B-cell development. *Curr. Opin. Immunol.* 14, 266–275.

Rothman, P., Chen, Y., Lutzker, S., Li, S., Stewart, V., Coffman, R., and Alt, F. (1990). Structure and expression of germ line immunoglobulin heavy-chain epsilon transcripts: interleukin-4 plus lipopolysaccharide-directed switching to C epsilon. *Mol. Cell. Biol.* 10, 1672–1679.

Rousset, F., Garcia, E., and Banchereau, J. (1991). Cytokine-induced proliferation and immunoglobulin production of human B lymphocytes triggered through their CD40 antigen. *J. Exp. Med.* 173, 705–710.

Russell, M., Kilian, M., and Lamm, M. (1999). Biological activities of IgA. In *Mucosal Immunology* (eds. P. Ogra, J. Mestecky, M. Lamm, W. Strober, J. Bienenstock, and J. McGhee), 225–240. San Diego: Academic Press.

Sato, A., Hashiguchi, M., Toda, E., Iwasaki, A., Hachimura, S., and Kaminogawa, S. (2003). CD11b+ Peyer's patch dendritic cells secrete IL-6 and induce IgA secretion from naïve B cells. *J. Immunol.* 171, 3684–3690.

Schaffer, A., Cerutti, A., Shah, S., Zan, H., and Casali, P. (1999). The evolutionarily conserved sequence upstream of the human Ig heavy chain S gamma 3 region is an inducible promoter: synergistic activation by CD40 ligand and IL-4 via cooperative NK-κB and STAT-6 binding sites. *J. Immunol.* 162, 5327–5336.

Schatz, D., Oettinger, M., and Baltimore, D. (1989). The V(D)J recombination activating gene, RAG-1. *Cell* 59, 1035–1048.

Schneider, P., Takatsuka, H., Wilson, A., Mackay, F., Tardivel, A., Lens, S., Cachero, T., Finke, D., Beermann, F., and Tschopp, J. (2001). Maturation of marginal zone and follicular B cells requires B cells activating factor of the tumor necrosis factor family and is independent of B cell maturation antigen. *J. Exp. Med.* 194, 1691–1697.

Seder, R., Marth, T., Sieve, M., Strober, W., Letterio, J., Roberts, A., and Kelsall, B. (1998). Factors involved in the differentiation of TGF-β-producing cells from naïve CD4+ T cells: IL-4 and IFN-gamma have opposing effects while TGF-beta positively regulates its own production. *J. Immunol.* 160, 5719–5728.

Seidl, K., Bottaro, A., Vo., A., Zhang, J., Davidson, L., and Alt, F. (1998). An expressed neo(r) cassette provides required functions of the I gamma2b exon for class switching. *Int. Immunol.* 10, 1683–1692.

Sen, G., Bikah, G., Venkataraman, C., and Bondada, S. (1999). Negative regulation of antigen receptor–mediated signaling by constitutive association of CD5 with the SHP-1 protein tyrosine phosphatase in B-1 B cells. *Eur. J. Immunol.* 29, 3319–3328.

Shapira, S., Vercelli, D., Japara, H., Fu, S., and Geha, R. (1992). Molecular analysis of the induction of immunoglobulin E synthesis in human B cells by interleukin 4 and engagement of CD40 antigen. *J. Exp. Med.* 175, 289–292.

Shi, M., Stavenezer, J. (1998). CBF alpha3 (AML2) is induced by TGF-beta1 to bind and activate the mouse germline Ig alpha promotor. *J. Immunol.* 161, 6751–6760.

Shi, M., Park, S., Kim, P., and Stavnezer, J. (2001). Roles of Ets proteins, NF-kappa B and nocodazole in regulating induction of transcription of mouse germline Ig alpha RNA by transforming growth factor-beta 1. *Int. Immunol.* 13, 733–746.

Shimizu, A., Takahashi, N., Yaoita, Y., and Honjo, T. (1982). Organization of the constant-region gene family of the mouse immunoglobulin heavy chain. *Cell* 28, 499–506.

Shinkai, Y., Rathbun, G., Lam, K., Oltz, E., Stewart, V., Mendelsohn, M., Charron, J., Datta, M., Young, F., Stall, A., et al. (1992). RAG-2-deficient mice lack mature lymphocytes owing to inability to initiate V(D)J rearrangement. *Cell* 68, 855–867.

Shinkura, R., Kitada, K., Matsuda, F., Tashiro, K., Ikuta, K., Suzuki, M., Kogishi, K., Serikawa, T., and Honjo, T. (1999). Alymphoplasia is caused by a point mutation in the mouse gene encoding NF-kappa b–inducing kinase. *Nat. Genet.* 22, 74–77.

Sonoda, E., Matsumoto, R., Hitoshi, Y., Ishii, T., Sugimoto, M., Araki, S., Tominaga, A., Yamaguchi, N., and Takatsu, K. (1989). Transforming growth factor beta induces IgA production and acts additively with interleukin 5 for IgA production. *J. Exp. Med.* 170, 1415–1420.

Spalding, D., and Griffin, J. (1986). Different pathways of differentiation of pre–B cell lines are induced by dendritic cells and T cells from different lymphoid tissues. *Cell* 44, 507–515.

Spalding, D., Williamson, S., Koopman, W., and McGhee, J. (1984). Preferential induction of polyclonal IgA secretion by murine Peyer's patch dendritic cell–T cell mixtures. *J. Exp. Med.* 160, 941–946.

Stavnezer-Nordgren, J., and Sirlin, S. (1986). Specificity of immunoglobulin heavy chain switch correlates with activity of germline heavy chain genes prior to switching. *EMBO J.* 5, 95–102.

Stavnezer, J., Bradley, S., Rousseau, N., Pearson, T., Shanmugam, A., Waite, D., Rogers, P., and Kenter, A. (1999). Switch recombination in a transfected plasmid occurs preferentially in a B cell line that undergoes switch recombination of its chromosomal Ig heavy chain genes. *J. Immunol.* 163, 2028–2040.

Strober, W., Kelsall, B., and Marth, T. (1998). Oral tolerance. *J. Clin. Immunol.* 18, 1–30.

Su, I., and Tarakhovsky, A. (2000). B-1 cells: orthodox or conformist? *Curr. Opin. Immunol.* 12, 191–194.

Sudowe, S., Arps, V., Vogel, T., and Kolsch, E. (2000). The role of interleukin-4 in the regulation of sequential isotype switch from immunoglobulin G1 to immunoglobulin E antibody production. *Scand. J. Immunol.* 51, 461–471.

Sugai, M., Gonda, H., Kusunoki, T., Katakai, T., Yokota, Y., and Shimizu, A. (2003). Essential role of Id2 in negative regulation of IgE class switching. *Nat. Immunol.* 4, 25–30.

Szabo, M., Butcher, E., and McEvoy, L. (1997). Specialization of mucosal follicular dendritic cells revealed by mucosal addressin-cell adhesion molecule-1 display. *J. Immunol.* 158, 5584–5588.

Szabo, S., Kim, S., Costa, G., Zhang, X., Fathaman, C., and Glimcher, L. (2000). A novel transcription factor, T-bet, directs Th1 lineage commitment. *Cell* 100, 655–669.

Tafuri, A., Shahinian, A., Bladt, F., Yoshinaga, S., Jordana, M., Wakeham, A., Boucher, L., Bouchard, D., Chan, V., Duncan, G., Odermatt, B., Ho, A., Itie, A., Horan, T., Whoriskey, J., Pawson, T., Penninger, J., Ohashi, P., and Mak, T. (2001). ICOS is essential for effective T-helper-cell responses. *Nature* 409, 105–109.

Takachika, H., Yanagita, M., Ohta, N., Sakaue, G., and Kiyono, H. (2000). IL-15 and IL-15 receptor selectively regulate differentiation of common mucosal immune system–independent B-1 cells for IgA responses. *J. Immunol.* 165, 4329–4337.

Takaguchi, T., Aicher, W., Fujihashi, K., Yamamoto, M., McGhee, J., Bluestone, J., and Kiyono, H. (1991). Novel function for intestinal intraepithelial lymphocytes: murine CD3+ γ/δ TCR+ T cells produce IFN-γ and IL-5. *J. Immunol.* 147, 3736–3744.

Thurnheer, M., Zuercher, Z., Cebra, J., and Bos, N.A. (2003). B1 cells contribute to serum IgM, but not to intestinal IgA, production in gnotobiotic Ig allotype chimeric mice. *J. Immunol.* 170, 4564–4571.

Tian, M., and Alt, F. (2000). Transcription-induced cleavage of immunoglobulin switch regions by nucleotide excision repair nucleases in vitro. *J. Biol. Chem.* 275, 24163–24172.

Toyabe, S., Harada, W., and Uchiyama, M. (2001). Oligoclonally expanding γ δ T lymphocytes induce IgA switching in IgA nephropathy. *Clin. Exp. Immunol.* 124, 110–117.

Tseng, J. (1981). Transfer of lymphocytes of Peyer's patches between immunoglobulin allotype congenic mice: repopulation of the IgA plasma cells in the gut lamina propria. *J. Immunol.* 127, 2039–2043.

Vajdy, M., Kosco-Vilbois, M., Kopf, M., Kohler, G., and Lycke, N. (1995). Impaired mucosal immune responses in interleukin 4–targeted mice. *J. Exp. Med.* 181, 41–53.

van Essen, D., Kikutani, H., and Gray, D. (1995). CD40 ligand–transduced co-stimulation of T cells in the development of helper function. *Nature* 378, 620–623.

van Ginkel, F., Wahl, S., Kearney, J., Kweon, M., Fujihashi, K., Burrow, P., Kiyono, H., and McGhee, J. (1999). Partial IgA-deficiency with increased Th2-type cytokines in TGF-β1 knockout mice. *J. Immunol.* 163, 1951–1957.

von Schwedler, U., Jack, H., and Wabl, M. (1990). Circular DNA is a product of the immunoglobulin class switch rearrangement. *Nature* 345, 452–456

Walker, L., Gulbranson-Judge, A., Flynn, S., Brocker, T., Raykundalia, C., Goodall, M., Forster, R., Lipp, M., and Lane, P. (1999). Compromised OX40 function in CD28-deficient mice is linked with failure to develop CXC chemokine receptor 5–positive CD4 cells and germinal centers. *J. Exp. Med.* 190, 1115–1122.

Watanabe, N., Ikuta, K., and Fagarasan, S. (2000). Migration and differentiation of autoreactive B-1 cells induced by activated γ/δ T cells in antierythrocyte immunoglobulin transgenic mice. *J. Exp. Med.* 192, 1577–1586.

Warnock, R., Campbell, J., Dorf, M., Matsuzawa, A., McEvoy, L., and Butcher, E. (2000). The role of chemokines in the microenvironmental control of T versus B cell arrest in Peyer's patch high endothelial venules. *J. Exp. Med.* 191, 77–88.

Warren, W., Roberts, K., Linehan, L., and Berton, M. (1999). Regulation of the germline immunoglobulin Cγ1 promoter by CD40 ligand and IL-4: dual role for tandem NF-κB binding sites. *Mol. Immunol.* 36, 31–44.

Weiner, H. (2001). Induction and mechanism of action of transforming growth factor-beta–secreting Th3 regulatory cells. *Immunol. Rev.* 182, 207–214.

Weinstein, P., and Cebra, J. (1991). The preference for switching to IgA expression by Peyer's patch germinal center B cells is likely due to the intrinsic influence of their microenvironment. *J. Immunol.* 147, 4126–4135.

Xie, X., Pardali, E., Holm, M., Sideras, P., and Grundstrom, T. (1999). AML and Ets proteins regulate the I alpha1 germ-line promoter. *Eur. J. Immunol.* 29, 488–498.

Yamamoto, M., Rennert, P., McGhee, J., Kweon, M., Yamamoto, S., Dohi, T., Otake, S., Bluethmann, H., Fujihashi, K., and Kiyono, H. (2000). Alternate mucosal immune system: organized Peyer's patches are not required for IgA responses in the gastrointestinal tract. *J. Immunol.* 164, 5184–5191.

Yamamoto, M., and Kiyono, H. (1999). Immunoregulatory functions of mucosal γδ T cells. *Microbes and Infection* 1, 241–246.

Yamanaka, T., Straumfors, A., Morton, H., Fausa, O., Brandtzaeg, P., and Farstad, I. (2001). M cell pockets of human Peyer's patches are specialized extensions of germinal centers. *Eur. J. Immunol.* 31, 107–117.

Yancopoulos, G., DePinho, R., Zimmerman, K., Lutzker, S., Rosenberg, N., and Alt, F. (1986). Secondary genomic rearrangement events in pre-B cells: VHDJH replacement by a LINE-1 sequence and directed class switching. *EMBO J.* 5, 3259–3266.

Yasue, T., Baba, M., Mori, S., Mizoguchi, C., Uehara, S., and Takatsu, K. (1999). IgG1 production by sIgD+ splenic B cells and peritoneal B-1 cells in response to IL-5 and CD38 ligation. *Int. Immunol.* 11, 915–923.

Yilmaz, Z., Weib, D., Sivakumar, V., and Weih, F. (2003). RelB is required for Peyer's patch development: differential regulation of p52–RelB by lymphotoxin and TNF. *EMBO J.* 22, 121–130.

Yoshida, H., Naito, A., Inoue, J., Satoh, M., Santee-Cooper, S., Ware, C., Togawa, A., Nishikawa, S., and Nishikawa, S. (2002). Different cytokines induce surface lymphotoxin-alphabeta on IL-7 receptor-alpha cells that differentially engender lymph nodes and Peyer's patches. *Immunity* 17, 823–833.

Xu, M., and Stavnezer, J. (1992). Regulation of transcription of immunoglobulin germ-line gamma 1 RNA: analysis of the promoter/enhancer. *EMBO J.* 11, 145–155.

Xu, L., Gorham, B., Li, S., Bottaro, A., Alt, F., and Rothman, P. (1993). Replacement of germ-line epsilon promoter by gene targeting alters control of immunoglobulin heavy chain class switching. *Proc. Natl. Acad. Sci. USA* 90, 3705–3709.

Xu, L., and Rothman, P. (1994). IFN-gamma represses epsilon germline transcription and subsequently down-regulates switch recombination to epsilon. *Int. Immunol.* 6, 515–521.

Xu, J., Foy, T., Laman, J., Elliott, E., Dunn, J., Waldschmidt, T., Elsemore, J., Noelle, R., and Flavell, R. (1994). Mice deficient for the CD40 ligand. *Immunity.* 1, 423–431.

Zan, H., Cerutti, A., Dramitinos, P., Schaffer, A., and Casali, P. (1998). CD40 engagement triggers switching to IgA1 and IgA2 in human B cells through induction of endogenous TGF-beta: evidence for TGF-beta but not IL-10-dependent direct Sμ → Sα and sequential Sμ → Sγ, Sγ → Sα DNA recombination. *J. Immunol.* 161, 5217–5225.

Zelazowski, P., Collins, J., Dunnick, W., and Snapper, C. (1995). Antigen receptor cross-linking differentially regulates germ-line CH ribonucleic acid expression in murine B cells. *J. Immunol.* 154, 1223–1231.

Zhang, J., Bottaro, A., Li, S., Stewart, V., and Alt, F. (1993). A selective defect in IgG2b switching as a result of targeted mutation of the Iγ2b promoter and exon. *EMBO J.* 12, 3529–3537.

Zhang, Y., and Derynck, R. (2000). Transcriptional regulation of the transforming growth factor-beta-inducible mouse germ line Ig alpha constant region gene by functional cooperation of Smad, CREB, and AML family members. *J. Biol. Chem.* 275, 16979–16985.

Zhang, Y., Izikson, L., Liu, L., and Weiner, H. (2001). Activation of CD25$^+$CD4$^+$ regulatory T cells by oral antigen administration. *J. Immunol.* 167, 4245–4253.

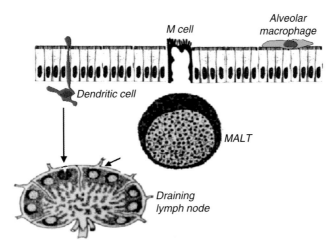

Fig. 7.1. Antigen sampling across simple epithelia. Dendritic cells (DCs) migrate into stratified epithelia in the skin and the vagina (Langerhans cells) or into simple epithelia in the airways and intestine. Some DCs *(shown at left)* may open tight junctions, sample antigens and microorganisms, and then migrate to local organized lymphoid tissues or draining lymph nodes. In the epithelium associated with mucosal lymphoid follicles, specialized M cells *(center)* take up and transport antigens to intraepithelial and subepithelial lymphocytes and DCs. In the lung, macrophages located on the surface of the alveolar epithelium *(right)* can phagocytose antigens, particles, and microorganisms.

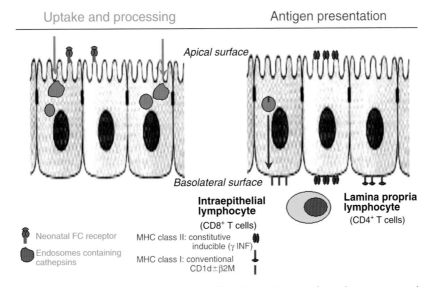

Fig. 7.2. Antigen uptake, processing, and presentation by intestinal epithelial cells. Antigen uptake and processing: In the small intestine, villus enterocytes can endocytose antigens from the lumen and direct them into endosomes where they may be processed and loaded onto presentation molecules. Membrane components such as neonatal Fc receptors may enhance internalization of antigens (Spiekerman *et al.* 2002). Antigens are transported from early apical endosomes to a late endosomal compartment common to incoming apical and basolateral endocytic pathways. The late endosomes contain proteolytic enzymes, for example, cathepsins, that process antigens. Antigen presentation: Intestinal enterocytes express both class I and class II MHC molecules. These include conventional MHC 1 and CD1d, a nonclassical member of the MHC gene family, which may or may not be associated with $\beta2$ microglobulin ($\beta2M$). Conventional MHC II is synthesized with invariant chain in response to inflammatory signals such as γ-interferon (γ-IFN). Unconventional MHC II not associated with invariant chain is constitutively expressed on enterocytes.

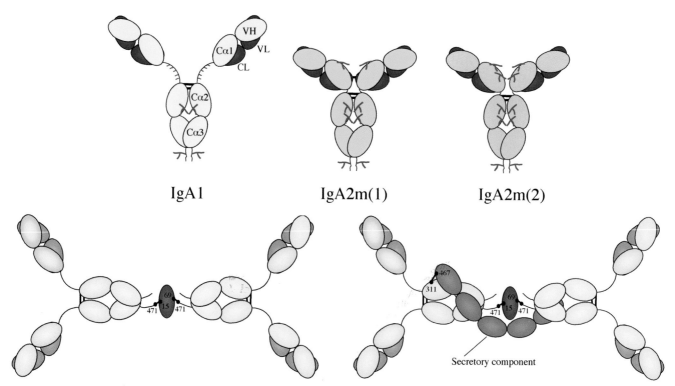

IgA1   IgA2m(1)   IgA2m(2)

Secretory component

Fig. 9.1. **(A–C)** A schematic representation of the human IgA of various molecular forms. Light chains are shown in dark orange, with the different heavy chains in shades of yellow/gold. Carbohydrates are shown in blue; *N*-linked glycans are branched, and *O*-glycans on the IgA1 hinge are shorter unbranched structures. In IgA2m(1) the usual heavy–light chain disulfide bonds are missing, and instead a disulfide bridge forms between the two light chains. **(A)** mIgA. **(B)** A schematic representation of human dIgA (J chain in red). For clarity, the distance separating the IgA monomers and J chain has been purposefully increased. Disulfide bridges between α-chain tailpieces and J chain are highlighted with the position of the cysteine residues involved labeled. Cys 471 in the tailpiece of one IgA monomer binds Cys 15 of J chain, while Cys 471 in the tailpiece of the other monomer binds Cys 69 of J chain. The Cys 471 residues of the remaining tailpieces, shown unbound, may interact with other free Cys residues such as Cys 311 (Prahl *et al.*, 1971). **(C)** Schematic representation of human S-IgA (SC in blue). J chain–IgA disulfide bridges are highlighted as in **(B)**. In addition, the disulfide bridge between Cys 311 of a heavy chain of one IgA monomer and Cys 467 in domain V of SC is indicated.

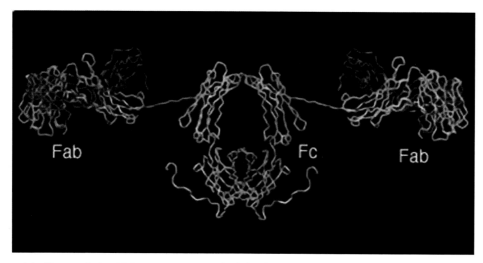

Fig. 9.2. Molecular model of human IgA1 (PDB accession 1iga). The light chains are shown in red, one heavy chain in blue and the other in orange.

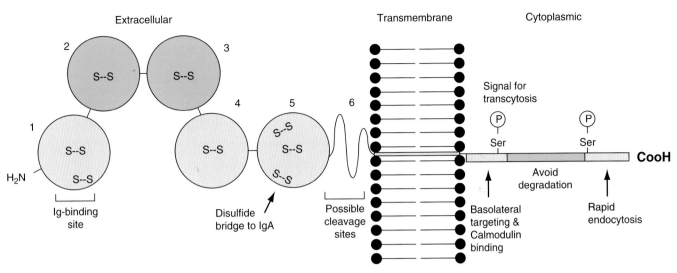

Fig. 12.2. Model of pIgR structure. The extracellular region of pIgR (which is cleaved at the apical surface to form SC) comprises five immunoglobulinlike domains and a sixth domain of unrelated structure. Domains 1, 4, and 5 (yellow) are encoded by single exons that are always included in pIgR mRNA. Domains 2 and 3 (blue) are encoded by a single exon that is sometimes deleted by alternative splicing of rabbit pIgR mRNA. Intradomain disulfide bonds that are conserved in all known pIgR sequences are noted. Multiple sites of SC cleavage in domain 6 have been proposed. The cytoplasmic domain of pIgR contains highly conserved signals for intracellular sorting, endocytosis, and transcytosis.

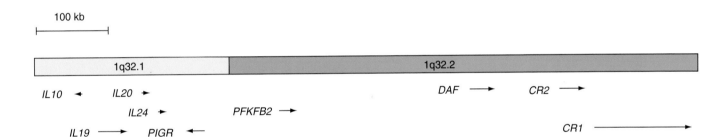

Fig. 12.4. Chromosomal localization of the human *PIGR* gene and binding sites for transcription factors. **A,** Localization of the *PIGR* gene in band q32.1 of chromosome 1, in a cluster of immunologically relevant genes (National Center for Biotechnology Information, USA). Other genes in this region include interleukin (*IL*) 10, 19, 20, and 24; regulator of Fas-induced apoptosis (*TOSO*); Fcαμ receptor (*FcαμR*); 6-phosphofructo-2-kinase/fructose-2,6-bisphosphatase 2 (*PFKFB2*); complement component 4 binding proteins (*C4BP*) A and B; decay-accelerating factor (*DAF*), and complement receptors (*CR*) 1 and 2. Arrows indicate relative size and direction of transcription of individual genes. **B,** Binding sites for regulatory transcription factors in the 5'-flanking, promoter, exon 1, and intron 1 regions of the human *PIGR* gene. Abbreviations: AR, androgen receptor; NF-κB, nuclear factor κB; USF, upstream stimulatory factor; AP, activator protein; IRF, interferon regulatory factor; HNF, hepatocyte nuclear factor; STAT, signal transducer and activator of transcription.

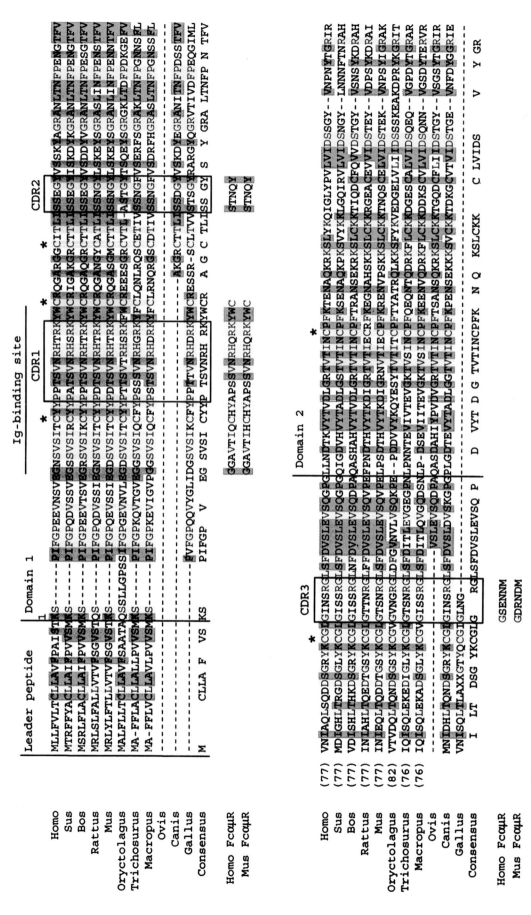

Fig. 12.3. Interspecies alignment of pIgR protein sequences. Full-length sequences were aligned for *Homo sapiens* (X73079), *Sus scrofa* (AB032195), *Bos taurus* (X81371), *Rattus norvegicus* (X15741), *Mus musculus* (U06431), *Oryctolagus cuniculus* (X00412), *Trichosurus vulpecula* (AF091137), and *Macropus eugenii* (AF317205). Partial sequences were aligned for *Ovis aries* (AJ313189), *Canis familiaris* (AY081057), and *Gallus gallus* (BM426916 and BG712734). Numbering of amino acids begins with the first residue of the mature protein (domain 1). Yellow shading indicates sequence identity among all species (excluding those species with no overlapping sequence at that position). Blue shading indicates sequence identity among six or more species. Sequences of the three complementarity-determining regions (CDRs) in domain 1 are boxed. Also shown are homologous sequences within the Ig-binding site and CDRs for the Fcαμ receptor (FcαμR) from *Homo sapiens* (AY063125) and *Mus musculus* (AB048834). Asterisks denote conserved cysteine residues involved in intrachain and interchain disulfide bonding. The arrows in domain 6 indicate potential sites of SC cleavage. Plus signs denote conserved residues in the cytoplasmic domain that have been shown to be required for basolateral targeting and rapid endocytosis. Conserved serine residues known to be phosphorylated are denoted "P." See text for explanation of domain structure and conserved motifs.

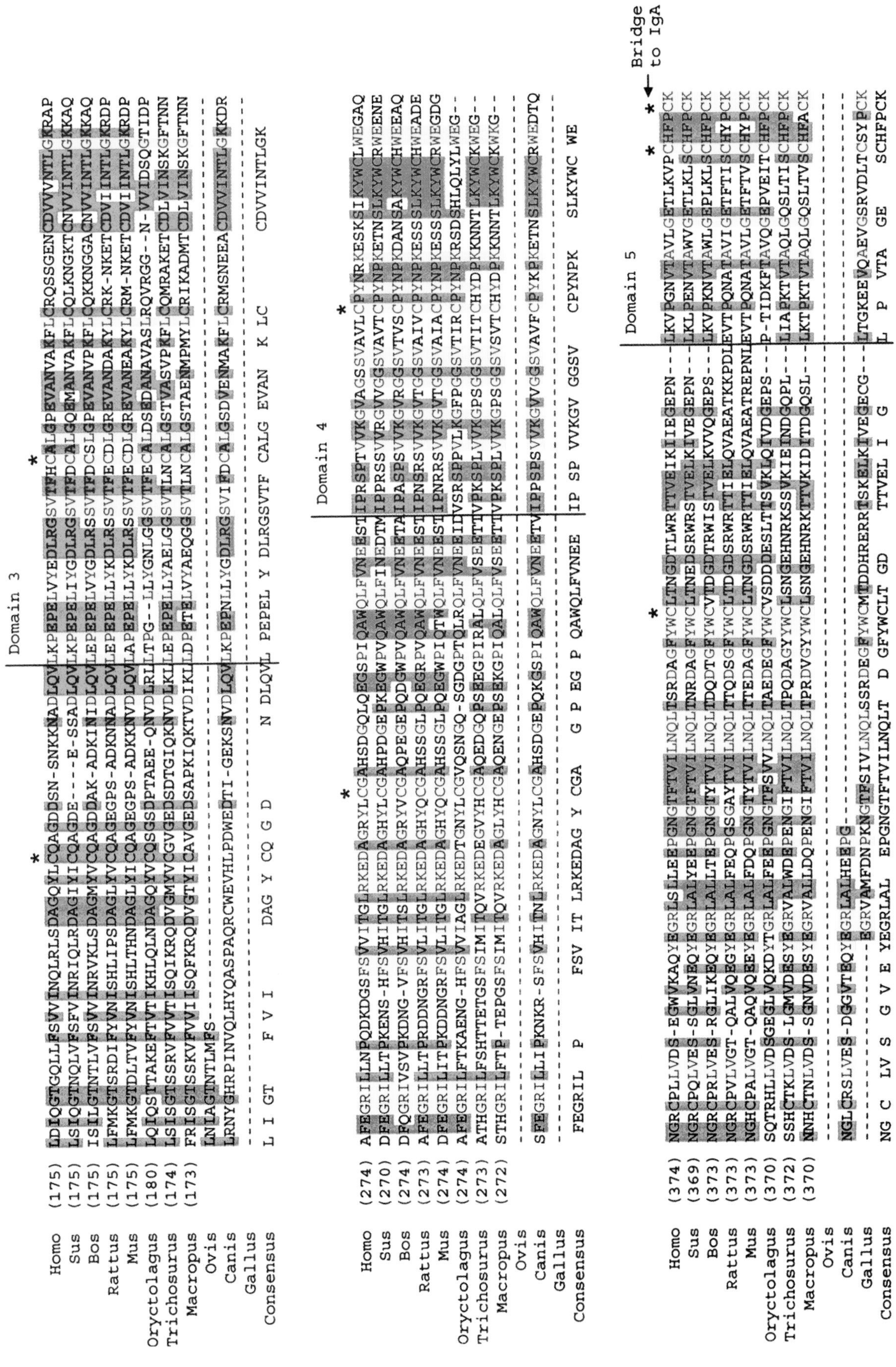

Bridge
to IgA

Domain 3

Domain 4

Domain 5

Continued

Homo
Sus
Bos
Rattus
Mus
Oryctolagus
Trichosurus
Macropus
Ovis
Canis
Gallus
Consensus

Fig. 12.3. *Cont'd*

Domain 6

```
Homo         (470) FSSYEKYWCKWNNTGCQALPSQDEGPSKAFVNCDENSRLVSLTLNLVTRADEGWYWCGVKQGHFYGETAAVVAVERKAAGSRD-
Sus          (465) FYSYQKYWCKWSNTGCRALPSQDEGQSQAFVNCDKKSQIISINLNPVRKEDEGWYWCGVKDGLHYGETGAVYVAV-EQKAKGSGD-
Bos          (469) FYSFEKYWCKWSNRGCSALPTQNDGPSQAFVSCDQNSQVVSLNLDTVTKEDEGWYWCGVKEGPRYGETAAVYVAV-ESRVKGS--
Rattus       (472) FYSQEKYWCKWSNDGCHILPSHDEGARQSSVSCDQSSQISMTLNPVKKEDEGWYWCGVKEGQVYGETTAIYIAVEERTRGSPHINPT-
Mus          (472) FYSQEKYWCKWSNKGCHILPSHDEGARQSSVSCDQSSQISMTLNPVSKEDEGWYWCGVKQGQTYGETTAIYIAVEERTRGSSHVNPT-
Oryctolagus  (466) YFSSYEKYWCKWNDHGCEDLPTKLS-SSGDLVKCN-NNLVLTLTLDSVSEDDEGWYWCGAKDGHEFEVAAVRVELTEPAKVVEPAKVPVDPAKAAPAPA
Trichosurus  (468) FYSYEKYWCKWSNQGCETLPTQEEGSQAFVDCNQNSRNVSLTLNSVTRDHEGWYWCGVNGQNYGETIAVSVSVEE---EVSG-
Macropus     (466) LYSYEKYWCKWSNQGCENLPTQEEGSQAFVDCNQDSRIVSLTLNPVTRAHEGWYWCGAKKGQNYGQTTAVFVSVEE---KVSR-
Ovis
Canis              ---
Gallus             YISYEKYWCKWSRDGCTPLTSSDQSHPGLDVSCDTANKTLILSLDPVTVEDQGWYWCGVK KHNGHYGETMAVSLQVDGGKAANISPELLD
Consensus          FYS EKYWCKWSN GC LP EG SQ V CD S VSLTLN V DEGWYWCGVK G YGET AV V E
```

A/V   Transmembrane Domain

```
Homo         (555) -VSLAKADAAPDFKVLDSGFREIENKAIQDPRLFAEEKAVADTRDQADGSRASVDGSSEEQG--GSSRALVSTLVPLGLVLAVGAVAVGVA
Sus          (549) -ARLANAPAPAEDAIEPRARETENEVLLDPSLIAEDRAVKDGEGPASGSGVPAPASSVGQG--GGSKAVVSTLVPLALVMLVGAVTIGVL
Bos          (551) -QGAKQVKAPAGAAIQSRAGEIQNKALLDPSFFAKESVKDAAGGPG---APADPGRPTGYS--GSKAIVSTLVPLALVLTVAGVVAIGVV
Rattus       (560) -DANARAKDAPEEEAMESSVREDENKANLDPRLFADEREIQNAGDQAQENRASGNAGSAGQS--GSSKVLFSTLVPLGLVLAVGLVAVWVA
Mus          (560) -DANARAKVALEEEVVDSSISEKENKAIPNPGPFANEREIQNVRDQAQENRASGDAGSADGQSRSSSSKVLFSTLVPLGLVLAVGAIAVWVA
Oryctolagus  (564) EEKAKAAVPSAQEKAVVPIVKEANKVVQKPRLLAEEVAVQSAEDPASGSRASVDASSASGQS--GSAKVLISTLVPLGLVLAAGAMAVAIA
Trichosurus  (554) -NAIQPTNAVLNEDAVEPKVRGKEIEVV---PTDL-----------------------------GSTEEHS--GGSSVIVSTLVPLALVLTVGAVALGII
Macropus     (552) -KDVKPANSVLNEDSVEPKVRAKEPEVV--PTDL------------------------------VSKEEQG--GGSLLVSTVVPVALVLTVGAVALGVI
Ovis
Canis
Gallus             -LEASNAAAAPDEAVPQ-------------------------------
Consensus          A A E        E EN    P   A          D GS      Q    G S   L STLVPL LVL VGAVA  V
```

Cytoplasmic Domain

BL Targeting/Calmodulin Binding   Avoid Degradation   Rapid Endocytosis

```
Homo         (644) RARHRKNVDRVSIRSYRTDISMSDFE-NSREFGANDNMGASSITQETSLGKEEFVATTESTTETKEPKKAKRSSKEEAEMAYKDFLLQSSTVAAE-AQDGPQEA
Sus          (638) RARHRKNVDRISIRSYRTDISMSDFE-SSRDFGAHDNAGATLDTQETSLGKDRFTTTTENIMEDKEPKRAKRSSKEEADKAFTTFLLQANSIIAA-TQNGPREA
Bos          (636) RARHRKNVDRISIRSYRTDISMSDFE-NSRDFEGRDNMGASPEAQETSLGKDEFATTTEDTVESKEPKKAKRSSKEEADEAFTTFLLQAKNLASAATQNGPTEA
Rattus       (649) RVRHRKNVDRMSISSYRTDISMGDFR-NSRDLGGNDNMGATPDTQETVLEGKDEIETTTECTTEPEESKKAKRSSKEEADMAYSAFLWQSSTIAAQ-VHDGPQEA
Mus          (651) RVRHRKNVDRMSISSYRTDISMADFK-NSRDLGGNDNMGASPDTQQTVIEGKDEIVTTTECTAEPEESKKAKRSSKEEADMAYSAFLLQSSTIAAQ-VHDGPQEA
Oryctolagus  (654) RARHRRNVDRVSIGSYRTDISMSDLE-NSREFGAIDNPSACPDARETALGGKDELATATESTVEIEEPKKAKRSSKEEADLAYSAFLLQSNTIAAE-HQDGPKEA
Trichosurus  (613) KARRWRFSDRVSVGSYRTDLSMSELENNPRQFGANENMDAS--VQETTLGGEDEIIIQTENPEEIQQPKQVKRSSKEEADMAYTAFLLQSNNMANEIPLDDPSNA
Macropus     (611) KARRGRFSDRVSIGSYRTDISMSELERNPRQFGANDNMGSS--IQESTLEGEIEFIIQTENPEEIQEPKQVKRSSKEEADMAYTAFLLQANNMASEIPLDGHSDA
Ovis
Canis
Gallus
Consensus          RARHR NVDR SI SYRTDISMSD E NSR FG DNMGA        QET L GKDE T TE T E EPK AKRSSKEEAD AY  FLLQ A    DGP EA
```

Fig. 12.3. *Contd*

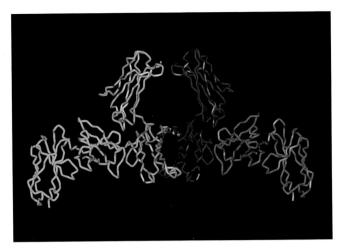

Fig. 13.1. X-ray crystal structure of the complex of human IgA1 Fc with the extracellular domains of human FcαRI (coordinates from Herr *et al.*, 2003a; PDB code 1OW0). One IgA Fc heavy chain is shown in red, the other in orange. The FcαRI molecules are shown in blue and green-blue.

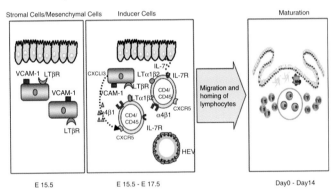

Fig. 21.2. Cytokine regulation of organogenesis program for PP. Signal exchanges between inducer cells (CD3⁻CD4⁺CD45⁺) and stromal/mesenchymal cells are operated by an array of cytokine/ cytokine receptor, chemokine/chemokine receptor, and adhesion molecules/homing receptor interactions. Among these, IL-7/IL-7R and LTα1β2/LTβR interactions are essential for the initiation of PP organogenesis during the time window between embryonic 15.5 and 17.5 days.

In Utero Blockade of LTbr Signaling Pathway
Results in the Lack of Peyer's Patches

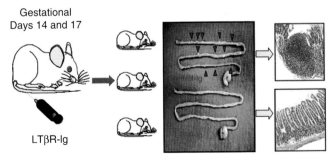

Fig. 21.3. Treatment of pregnant mice with the chimeric fusion protein of LTβR-Ig results in the delivery of PP-deficient mice. Pregnant mice are injected with 200 μg LTβR-Ig at gestational days 14 and 17. Newborn mice delivered from the fusion protein–treated mothers are not able to develop PP. On the other hand, newborn mice delivered from the control Ig fusion protein–treated mothers develop PP.

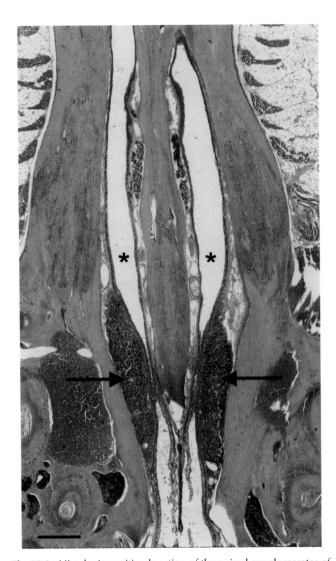

Fig. 23.2. Histologic position location of the paired conglomerates of nasal-associated lymphoid tissue (NALT) (arrow) in the nasal cavity (asterisk) of a BALB/c mouse. Hematoxylin-eosin staining. Scale bar: 500 μm. Courtesy of Dr. Pascale Gueirard (Pasteur Institute, Paris).

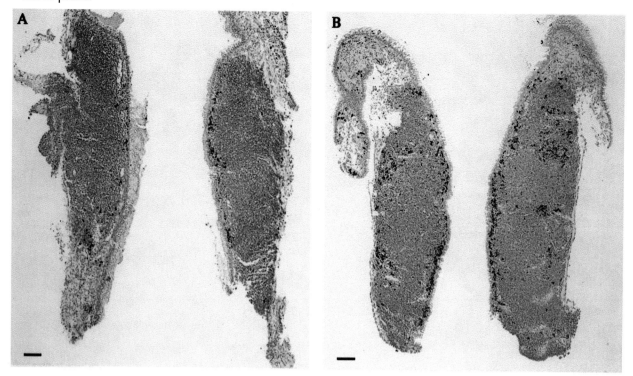

Fig. 23.5. Histologic examination of NALT tissues after nasal instillation of *Bordetella bronchiseptica* into BALB/c mice. The NALT sections were stained with CD11c to reveal the position and numbers of dendritic antigen-presenting cells. **A,** NALT tissue of naïve BALB/c mice. **B,** NALT tissue of mice 48 hours after nasal instillation with 5.5×10^5 CFU of $9.73H^+$ *B. bronchiseptica* parental strain. The increase in number of CD11c dendritic cells in the NALT is impressive, and their position in the T-cell area could reflect their involvement in immunologic reactions taking place in the organ. Scale bar: 100 μm. Courtesy of Dr. Pascale Gueirard (Pasteur Institute, Paris) who would like to acknowledge the fruitful collaboration with Drs. P. Ave, S. Thiberge, and N. Guiso.

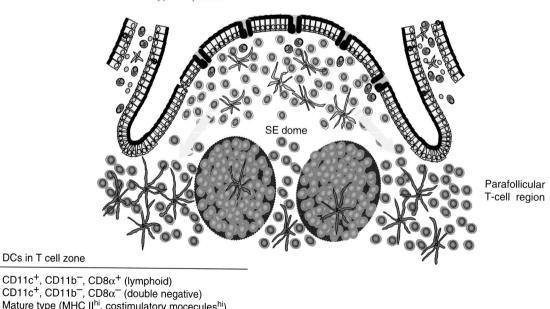

DCs in SE dome of GALT

CD11c⁺, CD11b⁺, CD8α⁻ (myeloid)
CD11c⁺, CD11b⁻, CD8α⁻ (double negative)
Poor CD4⁺ T cell Stimulation: immature type

Produce IL-10   ▶ Th2-type responses

SE dome

Parafollicular
T-cell region

DCs in T cell zone

CD11c⁺, CD11b⁻, CD8α⁺ (lymphoid)
CD11c⁺, CD11b⁻, CD8α⁻ (double negative)
Mature type (MHC II^hi, costimulatory mocecules^hi)

Produce IL-12   Th1-type responses

Fig. 28.2. Mucosal Dendritic Cells (DCs) for Th1 and Th2 cell induction. The subepithelial dome area of Peyer's patches contains myeloid type DCs, which favor induction of Th2 cells. On the other hand, parafollicular T-cell regions are enriched in lymphoid type DCs, which preferentially promote Th1-cell induction.

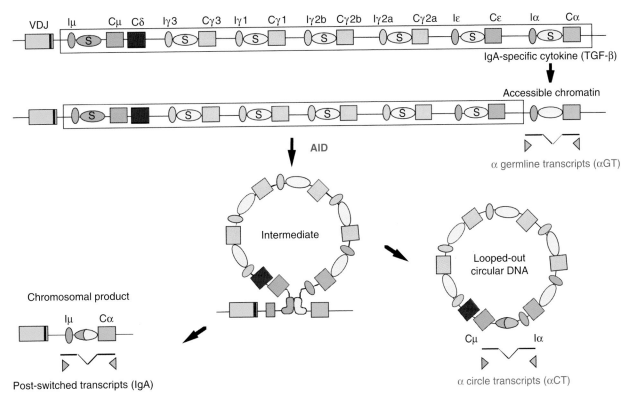

Fig. 31.1. Events and markers in IgA switch recombination. The organization of the mouse immunoglobulin heavy-chain locus after completion of V(D)J recombination is shown. Class switch recombination to IgA takes place between the Sμ and downstream Sα regions, and it results in a looped-out deletion of the intervening DNA segments. It requires expression of germline α transcripts, which are initiated from the Iα intronic promoter located upstream of the Sα region upon cytokine stimulation, such as TGF-β. Germline transcription opens the chromatin structure of the Sα region and renders it accessible to the putative switch recombinase. Activation-induced cytidine deaminase (AID), which is induced after B cell stimulation, appears to be the only B-cell-specific marker absolutely required for class-switch recombination and is probably involved in recognition and cleavage of the target DNA. Class-switch recombination to IgA is accompanied by looping-out deletion of the DNA fragment containing Cμ and CH genes located upstream of Cα from the chromosome, and it is followed by repair and ligation of the broken ends by the nonhomologous end-joining repair system (NHEJ). The Iα promoter located on the circular DNA is still active and responsive to cytokines and directs the production of Iα-Cμ transcripts called α circle transcripts. These α circle transcripts are detected after induction of AID, simultaneously with expression of IgA on the surface of B cells, and they disappear more quickly than α germline transcripts, AID, or circular DNAs after removal of switch stimulation. Thus, α circle transcripts are the best available molecule markers for active IgA switch recombination.

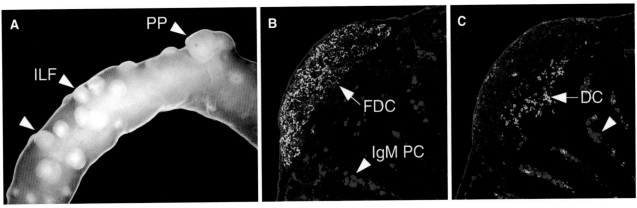

Fig. 31.4. AID deficiency leads to hyperplasia of isolated lymphoid follicles in the small intestine. (A) A duodenal segment of the small intestine of *aid⁻/⁻* mouse showing many protruding follicles (ILF) and an enlarged Peyer's patch (PP). (B, C) Adjacent sections of an isolated lymphoid follicle, consisting of many B cells on a follicular dendritic cell (FDC) network (*arrow*, B). Dendritic cells (DC) are located in a region equivalent to the subepithelial dome of the Peyer's patches (*arrow*, C). Lamina propria contains many IgM plasma cells (IgM PC) (*arrowheads*, B and C).

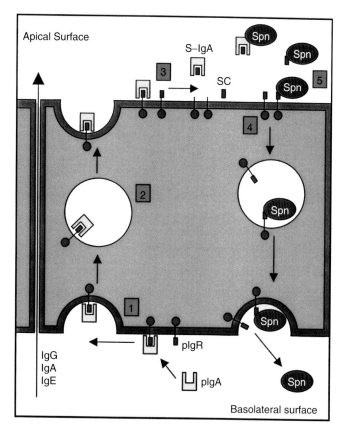

Fig. 40.1. Pneumococcal transcytosis. (1) The polymeric immuno-globulin receptor (pIgR) on the basolateral surface of epithelial cells binds to polymeric IgA (pIgA) or IgM and is endocytosed. (2) During transcytosis pIgR, pIgR-pIgA is sorted into vesicles for transport to the apical surface. (3) On the apical surface a protease cleaves pIgR, releasing S-IgA or free secretory component (SC). (4) Uncleaved pIgR can be internalized and subsequently recycled to the apical surface or transcytosed to the basolateral side. (5) *Streptococcus pneumoniae* that binds to uncleaved pIgR can take advantage of the recycling of pIgR and along with pIgR transcytose across the epithelial cell to the basolateral surface.

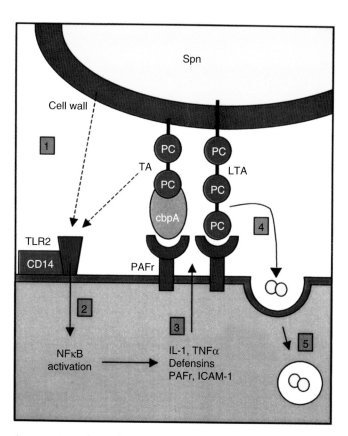

Fig. 40.3. PAFr-dependent adhesion and invasion. (1) Gram-positive cell wall components such as peptidoglycan and teichoic acid bind their cognate pattern recognition protein (CD14/TLR2). (2) The CD14:cell wall complex binds to TLR2, initiating intracellular signaling that ultimately results in NF-κB activation. (3) NF-κB activation results in transcription and *de novo* production of inflammatory cytokines such as IL-1, TNFα, defensins, and surface receptors such as PAFr. (4) Enhanced expression of PAFr allows bacteria with phosphorylcholine to bind the PAFr. (5) In some bacteria such as the pneumococcus, binding of PAFr potentiates cell invasion in a cbpA-dependent manner.

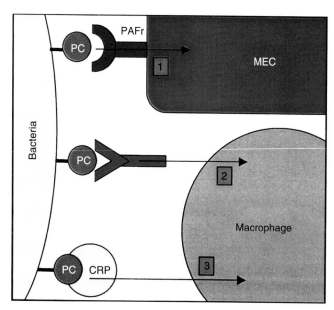

Fig. 40.2. Binding events mediated by phosphorylcholine. Phosphorylcholine (PC) residues on bacteria allow the bacteria to (1) adhere to and invade mucosal epithelial cells expressing PAFr. Expression of PC on the bacterial surface allows opsonization of the bacteria either by (2) antibodies to PC or (3) CRP. Both activate complement deposition and subsequently further opsonize the bacteria for phagocytosis.

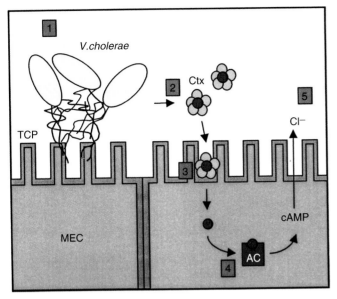

Fig. 40.4. Cholera toxin. (1) *Vibrio cholerae* initially forms micro-colonies and associates with the apical surface of the mucosal epithelial cell (MEC) through a type IV pilus called the toxin coregulated pilus (TCP). (2) Cholera toxin (Ctx), which is composed of one enzymatic A subunit (*red circles*) and five B subunits (*orange circles*), is coordinately expressed with TCP and secreted. (3) After the B subunits bind to the GM1 gangliosides on the MEC surface, the A subunit is translocated inside the cell. (4) Through the ADP-ribosylation activity, the A subunit constitutively activates adenylate cyclase (AC). (5) The resulting increase in intracellular cAMP causes efflux of chloride ions and secretory diarrhea.

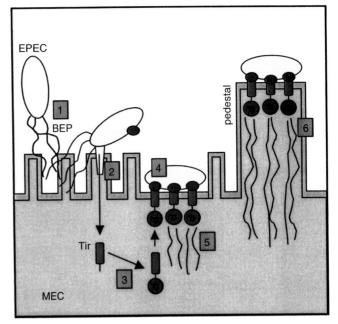

Fig. 40.5. EPEC formation of pedestals. (1) Enteropathogenic *Escherichia coli* (EPEC) associates with the apical surface of MEC using a pilus called the bundle-forming pilus (BFP). (2) Using a type III secretion system (TTSS), the EPEC-derived protein Tir is injected into the MEC cytosol. Tir is a receptor for the EPEC outer-membrane protein intimin (*blue circles*). (3) Once inside the cytosol, Tir is phosphorylated by MEC kinases and inserted into the apical membrane. (4) Intimin on the bacteria binds tightly with Tir on the MEC to form "intimate attachment." (5) The cytosolic domains of Tir interact with host actin nucleation complexes after binding to intimin. The resulting actin polymerization causes the formation of protruding structures called pedestals and the subsequent effacement of the surrounding membrane surface.

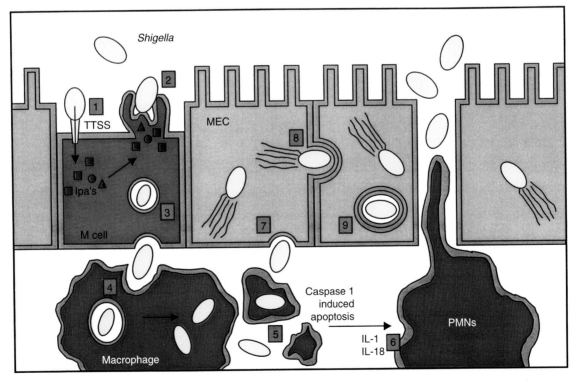

Fig. 40.6. *Shigella* invasion. (1) *Shigella* interacts with M cells and injects the Ipa effector proteins into the cytosol through a TTSS. (2) The Ipa effectors stimulate membrane ruffling at the apical surface, and the bacterium is engulfed. (3) Once inside, the M cell translocates the membrane-bound bacteria to the lamina propria. (4) Resident macrophages engulf the *Shigella* and (5) are induced to undergo apoptosis through activation of caspase 1. (6) This also causes the release of inflammatory cytokines that recruit polymorphonuclear cells (PMNs) into the area. This inflammation creates a breach in the MEC barrier that allows more bacteria to infiltrate. (7) Shigella can efficiently infect the MEC from their basolateral surfaces. (8) Intracellular bacteria exit their vacuoles and propel themselves around the cytosol, using an actin-based motility. (9) Some bacteria are capable of moving into adjacent cells and are enclosed in a double membrane that is quickly destroyed by the bacterium.

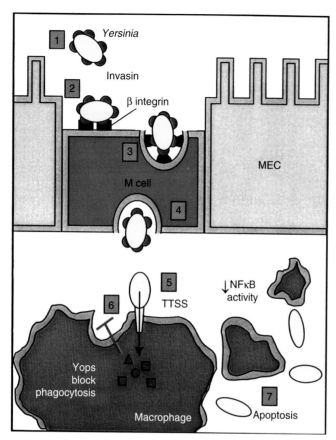

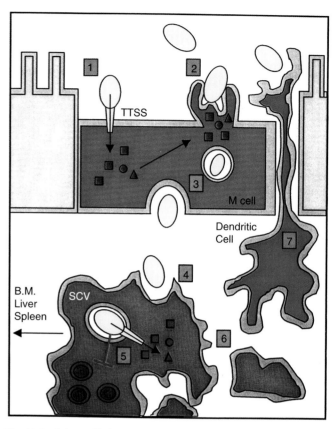

Fig. 40.7. *Yersinia* invasion. (1) *Yersinia* has an outer-membrane protein called invasin. (2) Invasin can bind to β1-integrins on the surface of M cells. (3) Through a zippering mechanism, the bacteria are engulfed by the M cell. (4) The bacteria are translocated across the M cell and delivered to the lamina propria. (5) Plasmid-encoded effector proteins called *Yops* are transferred to the resident macrophage via a TTSS. (6) Through interference with host cell signaling cascades and interactions with the cytoskeleton, the Yops block phagocytosis. (7) In addition, another Yop inhibits NF-κB activity, which leads to apoptosis and allows the bacteria to remain extracellular and spread to the regional lymph nodes.

Fig. 40.8. *Salmonella* invasion. (1) *Salmonella* interacts with the apical membrane of M cells and injects bacterial effector proteins into the M cells via the Inv-Spa TTSS. (2) These effectors induce membrane ruffling, and the bacterium is engulfed. (3) The M cell translocates the bacterium to the lamina propria. (4) Resident macrophages phagocytose the bacteria, where they are retained in a special compartment called the *Salmonella* containing vacuole (SCV). (5) From inside the SCV, *Salmonella* secretes another set of effector proteins into the macrophage cytosol, via the SPI-2 TTSS, that modulates expression of a large set of virulence genes controlled by the PhoP/PhoQ regulon and blocks the trafficking of the SCV to the endosome and lysosome. Retained bacteria replicate within the macrophage and are transported to the organs of the reticuloendothelial cell system. (6) Another fate of the resident macrophages is death shortly after infection, mediated by a caspase 1 pathway, or late-onset death after migration to distant sites through genes encoded by the SPI-2. (7) Uptake may also be mediated via dendritic cells, which sample luminal contents by sending dendrites between epithelial cells.

The Human Mucosal B-Cell System

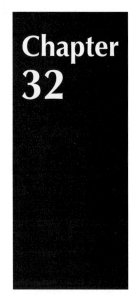

Chapter 32

Per Brandtzaeg, Hege S. Carlsen, Inger Nina Farstad

Laboratory for Immunohistochemistry and Immunopathology (LIIPAT), Institute of Pathology, University of Oslo, The National Hospital, Rikshospitalet, Oslo, Norway

Secretory immunity is the best defined effector mechanism of the mucosal immune system. This first line of adaptive humoral defense depends on a fascinating cooperation between B cells and secretory epithelia (Brandtzaeg *et al.*, 1999a). Effector cells of the mucosal immune system occur mainly as terminally differentiated immunocytes (plasmablasts and plasma cells) in exocrine tissues, where they preferentially produce dimers and larger polymers of IgA (collectively called pIgA). Because pIgA contains a 15-kD polypeptide termed the "joining" or J chain (Mestecky and McGhee, 1987), it can bind avidly to a 100-kD-transmembrane glycoprotein called secretory component (SC) that is expressed as a basolateral receptor on secretory epithelial cells (Brandtzaeg 1974a, 1985). Membrane SC is generally referred to as the polymeric Ig receptor (pIgR) because it can export to the lumen both pIgA and pentameric IgM with incorporated J chain (Brandtzaeg and Prydz, 1984). The J chain and the pIgR are hence to be considered as two key proteins in secretory immunity.

This chapter deals with activation of mucosal B cells and their unique immunoregulation that results in high levels of J-chain expression, regardless of concurrent Ig isotype production (Brandtzaeg, 1974b, 1985; Brandtzaeg and Korsrud, 1984). The obvious functional goal of this regulatory mechanism is abundant generation of Ig polymers at mucosal effector sites, where these molecules can readily be subjected to external transport and become operative as secretory antibodies (S-IgA and S-IgM). Homing mechanisms involved in the preferential migration of B cells with J-chain expression from their inductive sites to secretory effector sites also is discussed in this chapter.

Early experiments in rats showed that the large lymphocytes (or blasts) that normally enter the bloodstream from the thoracic duct migrate extensively into the intestinal lamina propria, where they terminate as plasma cells (Gowans and Knight, 1964; Hall and Smith, 1970). Many of these thoracic duct cells were reported to express surface (s)IgA, and those homing massively to the gut also contained cytoplasmic IgA (Williams and Gowans, 1975). Such plasmablasts were thought to be derived mainly from Peyer's patches, because transfer studies demonstrated that these structures, as well as the mesenteric lymph nodes, were enriched precursor sources for IgA-producing immunocytes in comparison with peripheral lymph nodes and the spleen (Craig and Cebra, 1971; McWilliams et al., 1977; McDermott and Bienenstock, 1979). These findings gave rise to the term *IgA cell cycle* (Lamm, 1976), but later studies showed that also B cells of other Ig isotypes and T cells induced in Peyer's patches exhibit gut-seeking properties.

Because experiments generally cannot be performed in humans, most mechanistic information with regard to cellular regulation and homing within the mucosal immune system is necessarily derived from animal studies (Brandtzaeg *et al.*, 1987a; Fagarasan and Honjo, 2003). Nevertheless, the clinical significance of both the unique inductive and preferential migratory properties of mucosal B cells is emphasized by the fact that more than 80% of all human immunocytes are located in secretory tissues and 80% to 90% of them produce pIgA (Brandtzaeg *et al.*, 1989). The mucosae and related exocrine glands thus harbor by far the quantitatively most important activated B-cell system of the human body.

STIMULATION OF MUCOSAL B CELLS

Inductive lymphoepithelial tissue

Lymphoid cells are located in three histologically distinct tissue compartments at mucosal surfaces: immune-inductive organized mucosa-associated lymphoid tissue (MALT), the lamina propria or glandular stroma, and the surface epithelia.

Peyer's patches in the distal small intestine **(Fig. 32.1 A)** are typical MALT structures believed to be a main source of conventional (B2) sIgA-expressing primed mucosal B cells. The lamina propria is principally an effector site but is also important in terms of expansion and terminal differentiation of B cells. In fact, differentiation of sIgA+ B cells takes place when they migrate from Peyer's patches to distant effector sites (Guy-Grand et al., 1974; Roux et al., 1981); the fraction with cytoplasmic IgA increases from 2% initially to 50% in mesenteric lymph nodes, 75% in thoracic duct lymph, and finally 90% in the intestinal lamina propria (Parrott, 1976).

MALT structures resemble lymph nodes with B-cell follicles (Fig. 32.1 B,C), intervening T-cell areas, and a variety of antigen-presenting cells (APCs), but they lack afferent lymphatics (Brandtzaeg et al., 1999a). All such structures therefore sample exogenous antigens directly from the mucosal surface through a characteristic follicle-associated epithelium (FAE), which contains "membrane" (M) cells **(Fig. 32.2)**. These thin epithelial cells have been shown to be effective in the uptake of live and dead (especially particulate) antigens from the gut lumen, and many enteropathogenic bacterial (e.g., *Salmonella* species, *Vibrio cholerae*) and viral (e.g., poliovirus, HIV-1, reovirus) infectious agents use the M cells as portals of entry (Neutra et al., 2001).

Gut-associated lymphoid tissue

Gut-associated lymphoid tissue (GALT) includes Peyer's patches, the appendix, and scattered solitary or isolated lymphoid follicles (ILFs). Peyer's patches occur mainly in the ileum (less frequently in the jejunum) and consist of at least five aggregated lymphoid follicles (Fig. 32.1 A,B) but can contain up to 200 such structures (Cornes, 1965). Human Peyer's patch *anlagen*, composed of CD4+ dendritic cells (DCs), can be seen at 11 weeks of gestation, and discrete T- and B-cell areas occur at 19 weeks; however, no germinal centers appear until shortly after birth, reflecting dependency on antigenic stimulation, which also induces some follicular hyperplasia (Spencer and MacDonald, 1990). The number of macroscopically visible human Peyer's patches increases from some 50 at the beginning of the last trimester to 100 at birth and 250 in the midteens and then diminishes to become approximately 100 between 70 and 95 years of age (Cornes, 1965).

Human intestinal mucosa harbors at least 30,000 ILFs (Fig. 32.2), increasing in density distally (Trepel, 1974). Thus, the normal small intestine contains only one follicle per 269 villi in the jejunum but one per 28 villi in the ileum (Moghaddami et al., 1998). In the normal large bowel, the density of ILFs is likewise relatively small; their numbers in

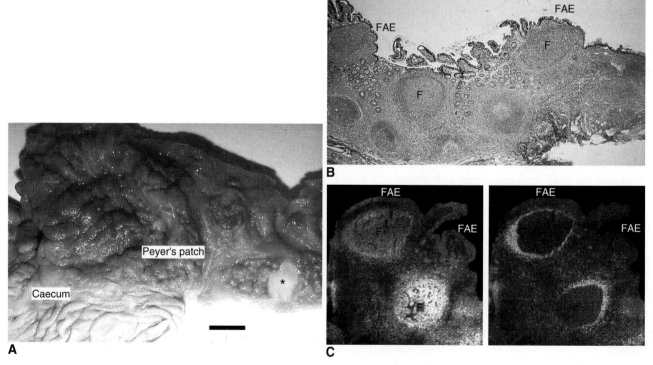

Fig. 32.1. A, Peyer's patches in the terminal ileum of a 10-year-old girl. A specimen has been excised from one of the patches (*). Bar represents 1 cm. **B,** Histology of excised specimen from normal human Peyer's patch (hematoxylin–eosin staining) containing several activated lymphoid follicles (F) with germinal centers beneath specialized dome epithelium that lacks villi (× 25; FAE = follicle-associated epithelium). **C,** Two-color immunofluorescence staining (same field) for B cells (CD20, *left*) and IgD (*right*) in a section from human Peyer's patch. Note that IgD (marker of naïve B cells) is mainly expressed on B cells in the mantle zones of the lymphoid follicles (F) and to some extent on B cells scattered in the extrafollicular areas, whereas CD20 also decorates the germinal centers (×25; FAE = follicle-associated epithelium).

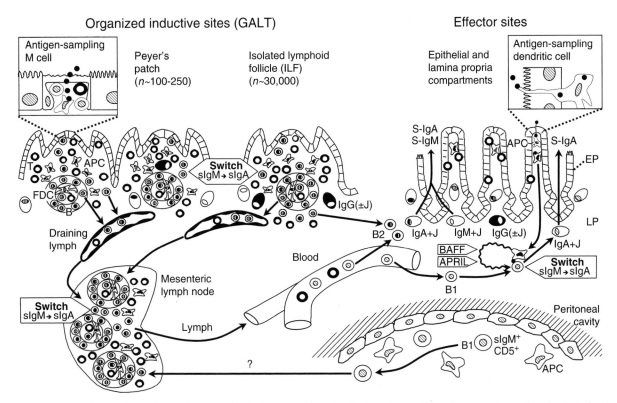

Fig. 32.2. Antigen-sampling and B-cell-switching sites for induction of intestinal IgA responses. Dots denote antigen. The classic inductive sites are constituted by gut-associated lymphoid tissue (GALT), which is equipped with antigen-sampling M cells, T-cell areas (T), B-cell follicles (B), and antigen-presenting cells (APC). Switch of conventional B-2 cells from surface (s)IgM to sIgA occurs in GALT and mesenteric lymph nodes; from here primed B and T cells home to the lamina propria (LP) via lymph and blood. T cells end up mainly in the epithelium (EP), whereas sIgA⁺ B cells differentiate to LP plasma cells producing dimeric IgA with J chain (IgA⁺J), which then is exported as secretory IgA (S-IgA). Primed B cells may also migrate from Peyer's patches and isolated lymphoid follicles directly into the LP as indicated, whereas those differentiating to plasma cells just outside of a follicle often show reduced J-chain expression and a propensity for IgG production (IgG ± J). B-2 cells also give rise to plasma cells producing pentameric IgM (IgM+J), which becomes secretory IgM (SIgM). B1 cells (CD5⁺) from the peritoneal cavity reach the LP by an unknown route (?), perhaps via mesenteric lymph nodes. These sIgM⁺ cells are particularly abundant in mice and may switch to sIgA within the LP under the influence of APCs that have sampled microbial antigens as dendritic cells within the epithelium and become activated to secrete stimulatory factors (*waved arrow*), such as BAFF and APRIL. The sIgA⁺ B-1 cells differentiate to plasma cells that provide SIgA directed mainly against the commensal gut flora.

tissue sections increase from 0.02 per millimeter of muscularis mucosae in the ascending colon to 0.06 per millimeter in the rectosigmoid (O'Leary and Sweeney, 1986). ILFs have recently been characterized immunologically in mice, showing features compatible with induction of B cells for intestinal IgA responses (Hamada *et al.*, 2002). An interesting finding was that the organogenesis of murine ILFs commences after birth, in contrast to Peyer's patches.

Nasopharynx-associated lymphoid tissue

Although GALT is the largest and best defined part of MALT, other potentially inductive sites for mucosal B-cell responses are bronchus-associated lymphoid tissue (BALT) and nasopharynx-associated lymphoid tissue (NALT)—in humans, particularly the unpaired nasopharyngeal tonsil (often called adenoids) and the paired palatine tonsils (Brandtzaeg, 1987; Brandtzaeg and Halstensen, 1992; Perry and Whyte, 1998). These organs make up most of Waldeyer's pharyngeal lymphoid ring and may play a major role for

mucosal immunity in human airways, because BALT structures are not present in normal lungs of adults and in only 40% of healthy adolescents and children (Tschering and Pabst, 2000).

Rodents lack tonsils, whereas two paired NALT structures occur laterally to the nasopharyngeal duct dorsal to the cartilaginous soft palate (Kuper *et al.*, 1992). A regionalized protective IgA response has been shown to be induced by nasal vaccine application in mice (Yanagita *et al.*, 1999). Indeed, murine NALT can drive an IgA-specific enrichment of high-affinity memory B cells but in addition gives rise to a major germinal center population of IgG-producing cells (Shimoda *et al.*, 2001)—quite similar to the situation in human tonsils (Brandtzaeg, 1987; Brandtzaeg *et al.*, 1999b). In contrast to tonsils, however, the *anlagen* of which appears at the same fetal age as that of Peyer's patches (von Gaudecker and Müller-Hermelink, 1982), the organogenesis of murine NALT begins after birth, like murine ILFs (Fukuyama *et al.*, 2002; Hamada *et al.*, 2002; Mebius, 2003).

Other sources of mucosal B cells

In mice, proliferating T cells rapidly obtain gut-homing properties during antigen priming in mesenteric lymph nodes (Campbell and Butcher, 2002). Most likely, therefore, regional lymph nodes generally share immune-inductive properties with related MALT structures from which they receive antigens via afferent lymph and antigen-transporting DCs. Numerous DCs are found at epithelial surfaces, where they can pick up luminal antigens by penetrating tight junctions with their processes (Rescigno et al., 2001). The human nasal mucosa is extremely rich in various DC types, both within and beneath the epithelium (Jahnsen et al., 2004), and a subepithelial band of putative APCs is seen below the surface epithelium as well as the FAE in the human gut (Rugtveit et al., 1997; Yamanaka et al., 2001).

The peritoneal cavity is recognized as yet another source of mucosal B cells in mice, actually providing 40% to 50% of the intestinal IgA immunocytes (Kroese et al., 1989). The precursors are self-renewing sIgM$^+$ B1 (CD5$^+$) cells, which give rise to polyreactive ("natural") SIgA antibodies (Fig. 32.2), particularly directed against commensal bacteria as a result of T cell–independent responses (Macpherson et al., 2000). How and where this subset differentiates to the IgA phenotype remains uncertain, but it has recently been suggested that the lamina propria is an important class switch site (Fagarasan et al., 2001; Fagarasan and Honjo, 2003). Notably, though, no evidence exists to suggest that B1 cells are significantly involved in intestinal IgA production in humans (Brandtzaeg et al., 2001; Boursier et al., 2002), despite considerable levels of polyreactive S-IgA antibodies recognizing both self- and microbial antigens in human secretions (Bouvet and Fischetti, 1999).

B-cell activation in MALT structures

Antigen encounter via follicle-associated epithelium

The bell-shaped M cells characteristic of FAE can sample luminal antigens unspecifically or by receptor-mediated uptake (Neutra et al., 2001); their pockets represent an intimate interface between the external environment and the mucosal immune system (Fig. 32.2). However, there is no convincing evidence that this specialized epithelial cell type has an antigen-presenting function. Although M cells show lysosomal enzyme activity by which they to some extent may degrade or process antigens (Savidge, 1996), their expression of MHC class II (HLA-DR) in humans is normally faint, at most (Bjerke and Brandtzaeg, 1988).

Various MHC class II–expressing putative APCs are present immediately underneath the FAE (Bjerke and Brandtzaeg, 1988; Bjerke et al., 1993), but the M-cell pockets are dominated by memory T and B lymphocytes **(Fig. 32.3 A)** in approximately equal distribution (Farstad et al., 1994; Yamanaka et al., 2001). Some interesting experimental results suggest that lymphoid interaction, particularly involving activated B cells, can induce the epithelial M-cell phenotype (Kernéis et al., 1997). Studies in germ-free and conventionalized rats have furthermore demonstrated that bacterial colonization drives the accumulation and dif-

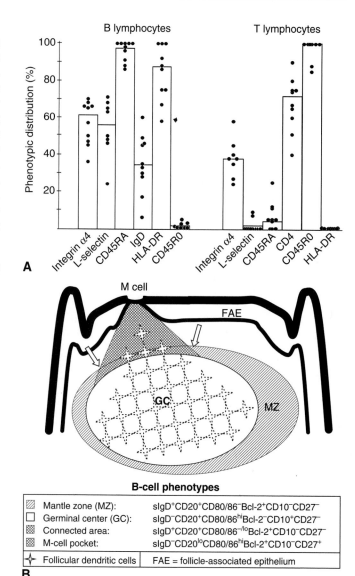

B-cell phenotypes

▨	Mantle zone (MZ):	sIgD$^+$CD20$^+$CD80/86$^-$Bcl-2$^+$CD10$^-$CD27$^-$
☐	Germinal center (GC):	sIgD$^-$CD20$^+$CD80/86^{hi}Bcl-2$^-$CD10$^+$CD27$^-$
▨	Connected area:	sIgD$^+$CD20$^+$CD80/86$^{-/lo}$Bcl-2$^+$CD10$^-$CD27$^-$
▨	M-cell pocket:	sIgD$^-$CD20^{lo}CD80/86^{hi}Bcl-2$^+$CD10$^-$CD27$^+$
✧	Follicular dendritic cells	FAE = follicle-associated epithelium

B

Fig. 32.3. A, Phenotypic distribution of B and T lymphocytes within M-cell pockets of human Peyer's patches. Columns indicate median percentages. Adapted from Farstad et al. (1994). **B,** Schematic depiction of relationship between elements of secondary (activated) B-cell follicle and M-cell pocket in human Peyer's patch. The germinal center (GC) is mostly surrounded by the mantle zone (MZ) and filled with sIgD$^-$CD20$^+$CD80/86^{hi}Bcl-2$^-$CD10$^+$ CD27$^-$ B cells. The MZ consists of naïve sIgD$^+$CD20$^+$ CD80/86$^-$Bcl-2$^+$ CD10$^-$CD27$^-$ B cells but is broken (*open arrows*) beneath the M-cell pocket. This connected area is seen only in a restricted part of the follicle, as defined by reduced immunostaining for sIgD toward the M-cell pocket. A follicular-dendritic cell network defined as CD21$^+$CD20$^-$ phenotype shows a topographically similar extension but does not reach inside the pocket. The M-cell pocket contains both naïve sIgD$^+$CD20$^+$ CD80/86$^{-/lo}$Bcl-2$^+$CD10$^-$CD27$^-$ and memory (or recently stimulated) sIgD$^-$CD20^{lo}CD80/86^{hi}Bcl-2$^+$CD10$^-$CD27$^+$ B-cell phenotypes, the latter being predominant. Adapted from Yamanaka et al. (2001).

ferentiation of T and B cells in the M-cell pockets, apparently with an initial involvement of antigen-transporting DCs, followed by germinal center formation (Yamanaka et al., 2003).

Specialization of M-cell pockets

The M-cell pockets may in fact represent specialized germinal-center extensions designed for rapid recall responses (Fig. 32.3B). The most likely cell type to mediate MHC class II interaction with cognate T cells in these microcompartments is the long-lived sIgD⁻IgM⁺Bcl-2⁺CD27⁺ memory B cells that express costimulatory molecules (Yamanaka *et al.*, 2001). In human tonsils, memory B cells have been shown to colonize the antigen-transporting reticular crypt epithelium; by rapid upregulation of costimulatory B7 molecules, they acquire potent antigen-presenting properties (Liu *et al.*, 1995). Likewise, we have found that memory B cells present in the M-cell areas of human Peyer's patches relatively often express B7.2 (CD86) and sometimes B7.1 (CD80), which would be a prerequisite for stimulation of productive immunity (Figs. 32.3 and **32.4**).

It is known that B cells can internalize cognate antigen by their sIg, a mechanism that is some 10,000-fold more efficient than the nonspecific uptake by conventional APCs; it has been postulated that this is useful for diversification of immune responses (Mamula and Janeway, 1993). Therefore,

the antigen-transporting (and processing?) M cells may provide an efficient opportunity for juxtaposed sIgD⁻ IgM⁺/IgA⁺HLA-DR⁺ memory B cells to present luminal antigens to adjacent cognate CD28-expressing memory as well as naïve T cells; this interaction likely leads to interleukin (IL)-2 secretion, promotion of T-cell survival (Boise *et al.*, 1995), and enhanced diversification of mucosal immune responses (Fig. 32.4). Evidence does exist that SIgA antibodies show a broader specificity than comparable serum antibodies (Waldman *et al.*, 1970; Shvartsman *et al.*, 1977), which would be important to cope with the antigenic drift of the microbial flora of the various mucosae.

It is more difficult to visualize what might happen if naïve B cells without the necessary costimulatory molecules capture antigens in competition with a smaller number of conventional APCs in the M-cell areas (Fig. 32.4). One possibility is induction of T-cell anergy and hence tolerance. However, the outcome would probably depend on the differentiation of the interacting T cells as well as on the amount of available antigens (Zhong *et al.*, 1997). The alternative high-affinity CD28-homologue B7 receptor, cytotoxic T-lymphocyte antigen-4

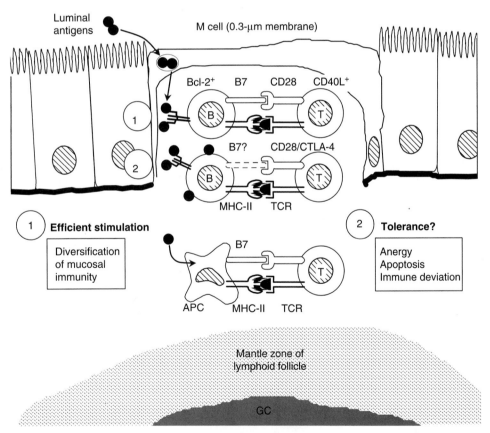

Fig. 32.4. Hypothetical scheme for positive and negative immune regulation taking place in M-cell area of gut-associated lymphoid tissue. Long-lived memory B cell (Bcl-2⁺) internalizes specific antigen efficiently and provides efficient cognate stimulation of adjacent CD4⁺ CD40L⁺ T cell by antigen presentation and B7-CD28 ligation; this interaction likely leads to a diversified T-cell response that can further diversify the B-cell response (1). In competition with ordinary antigen-presenting cell (APC), naïve B cell with low or absent level of costimulatory molecules (B7?) internalizes antigen either specifically or nonspecifically (depending on the dose?) and presents it to T cell that might become tolerized. Interaction of B (naïve or memory) and T cell via B7-CTLA-4 might also result in tolerance (2). B, B cell; T, T cell; GC, germinal center; MHC-II, major histocompatibility complex class II molecule; TCR, T-cell receptor.

(CTLA-4), can be expressed transiently by activated T cells, and its engagement may provide negative signals that lead to apoptosis (Boise *et al.*, 1995; Chambers and Allison, 1997). Murine experiments with feeding of large amounts of soluble antigens have suggested that one mechanism for induction of oral tolerance is clonal deletion by apoptosis after T-cell activation in Peyer's patches (Chen *et al.*, 1995).

Germinal center B-cell response
Role of lymphotoxins and molecular interactions in germinal center formation
Primary lymphoid follicles contain recirculating naïve B lymphocytes (sIgD⁺IgM⁺), which pass into the network formed by antigen-capturing follicular dendritic cells (FDCs). The origin of FDCs remains obscure (Kapasi *et al.*, 1998), but both their development and the clustering that allows follicle formation depend on lymphotoxin (LT) signaling (Gommerman *et al.*, 2002). Experimental evidence suggests that B cells are one important LT source (Fu *et al.*, 1998; Tumanov *et al.*, 2002). Among the known actions of the soluble homotrimer LTα, previously termed tumor necrosis factor (TNF)-β, is augmentation of B-cell proliferation and adhesion molecule expression. Knockout mice deficient in LTα virtually lack lymph nodes and have no detectable Peyer's patches. Moreover, a membrane-associated form of LT exists as a heterotrimeric complex containing LTα, together with a transmembrane protein designated LTβ (α1 β2). Knockout mice deficient in LTβ

have no detectable FDCs, and they lack Peyer's patches, peripheral lymph nodes and organized splenic germinal centers (Chaplin and Fu, 1998).

Primary follicles are turned into secondary follicles by the germinal center reaction. In humans, this process has been extensively studied in tonsils (MacLennan, 1994; Liu and Arpin, 1997), but much relevant mechanistic information relies on observations of lymph nodes and spleen from immunized animals (MacLennan *et al.*, 1997). Germinal centers are of vital importance for T cell–dependent generation of conventional (B2) memory B cells, affinity maturation of the B-cell receptor (BCR), and Ig class switching. It has been shown that naïve B cells are first stimulated at the edge of the primary follicle by cognate interaction with activated CD4⁺ T cells, which have previously been presented with processed antigen by MHC class II–expressing interdigitating DCs (Garside *et al.*, 1998). The B cells then re-enter the follicle to become proliferating sIgD⁺IgM⁺CD38 germinal center "founder cells" (**Fig. 32.5**), as noted in human tonsils (Liu and Arpin, 1997; Lebecque *et al.*, 1997). Such initially stimulated B cells produce unmutated IgM (and some IgG) antibody of low affinity that can bind circulating antigen; the resulting soluble immune complexes subsequently become deposited on the FDCs, where antigen is retained for prolonged periods to maintain B-cell memory (Ahmed and Gray, 1996; Lindhout *et al.*, 1997; MacLennan *et al.*, 1997). Such a role for IgM in the induction of

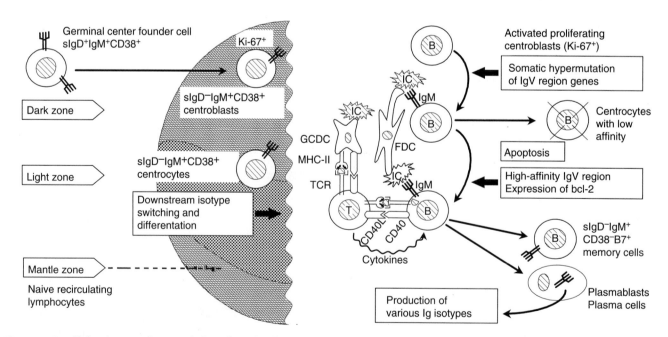

Fig. 32.5. B-cell developmental events believed to take place in the dark and light zones of germinal centers, leading to the generation of extrafollicular or distant plasma cells of various isotypes. The germinal center founder cell is activated in the extrafollicular compartment (see Fig. 32.6) and then migrates to the dark zone, where it proliferates and differentiates (see Fig. 32.8). The molecular cell-cell interactions and immune events taking place in the germinal center reaction are schematically depicted on the right. Further details are discussed in the text. B, B cell; T, T cell; GCDC, germinal center dendritic cell; IC, immune complex; Ki-67, proliferation marker; MHC-II, major histocompatibility complex class II molecule; TCR, T-cell receptor.

secondary immune responses with antibody affinity maturation has been strongly supported by observations in knock-out mice lacking natural ("nonspecific") background IgM antibodies (Ehrenstein et al., 1998).

The complement receptors CR1/CR2 (CD35/CD21) are considered among the cell-surface molecules that play a crucial role in the germinal center reaction. CD21 is expressed abundantly on both FDCs and B cells and may function by localizing antigen to the FDC network and/or by lowering the threshold of B-cell activation via recruitment of CD19 into the BCR (Tarlinton, 1998). Activation of complement on FDCs is controlled by regulatory factors when these cells retain immune complexes, but some release of inflammatory mediators may cause edema that facilitates dispersion of FDC-derived "immune complex–coated bodies," or iccosomes, thereby enhancing the BCR-mediated uptake of their contained antigens by B cells (Brandtzaeg and Halstensen, 1992).

Role of chemokines and their receptors

Several homeostatic chemokines have been identified as major cues for lymphocyte trafficking and positioning in organized lymphoid tissue (Cyster, 1999; Moser and Loetscher, 2001). The CXC chemokine BCA-1 (B cell–attracting chemokine-1)/CXCL13 (CXC chemokine ligand 13) is an attractant for naïve human B cells in vitro and has been shown to be produced in follicles of human lymph nodes (Legler et al., 1998). This chemokine was concurrently described in mice and called BLC (B-lymphocyte chemoattractant) (Gunn et al., 1998a). Several lines of evidence suggest that CXCL13 and its receptor CCR5 are directly involved in the formation of organized lymphoid tissue of mice (Förster et al., 1996; Luther et al., 2000). It is interesting that CXCL13 upregulates LT $\alpha 1\beta 2$ on B cells, and a positive feedback loop may thereby be established (Ansel et al., 2000). The follicular expression of murine CXCL13 is reportedly more consistent in Peyer's patches than peripheral lymph nodes (Gunn et al., 1998a). Alternative B cell–attracting chemokines may also operate in human lymphoid tissue. Indeed, stromal cell–derived factor 1 (SDF-1)/CXCL12, which appears to be produced by cells lining tonsillar germinal centers, has been shown by an in vitro assay to attract naïve and memory B cells expressing CXCR4 (Bleul et al., 1998).

CXCL13 (BCA-1) and CXCR5 were found to be expressed in normal human GALT structures, in the ileum (Peyer's patches) and colon (ILFs) as well as in irregular lymphoid aggregates of inflammatory bowel disease (IBD) lesions (Carlsen et al., 2002). The general expression of CXCR5 seen in follicular mantle zones **(Fig. 32.6)** agreed with the notion that CXCL13 is a selective chemoattractant for naïve B cells from human blood in vitro, although with moderate effect (Legler et al., 1998), paralleling the relatively low receptor level observed in the mantle zones.

Scattered T cells with strong CXCR5 expression are seen within GALT follicles (Carlsen et al., 2002), and the CXCR5+CD4+ phenotype has been functionally described as "follicular B-helper T cells," or T_{FH} cells (Fig. 32.6), because it shows all the characteristics required for efficient B-cell help within tonsillar follicles (Schaerli et al., 2000; Breitfeld et al., 2000; Moser et al., 2002). Nevertheless, flow-cytometric analysis of lymphoid cells from murine Peyer's patches and human tonsils has revealed a much higher proportion of CXCR5+ T cells, implying the presence of this phenotype also in the extrafollicular areas (Schaerli et al., 2000; Breitfeld et al., 2000). However, a small T_{FH}-cell subset, identified as CXCR5+CD57+ and termed germinal center T-helper (GC-Th) cells, appears to be essential for B-cell differentiation and antibody production (Kim et al., 2001); its exclusive germinal-center localization agrees with our immunohistochemical observations in tonsils, normal GALT, and IBD-associated lymphoid aggregates (Carlsen et al., 2002).

The partial overlap produced by immunostaining for CXCL13 and several traditional FDC markers in human tissues suggested that this chemokine is deposited on peripheral extensions of FDCs (Fig. 32.6) after secretion by another cell type (Carlsen et al., 2002). Indeed, the main source of CXCL13 appeared to be the previously identified germinal center dendritic cell (GCDC) reported to stimulate T cells in this compartment (Grouard et al., 1996). It is interesting that both GCDCs and large CXCL13-producing cells in IBD-associated B-cell aggregates were found to exhibit a phenotype compatible with macrophage derivation, sometimes expressing CD14 as evidence of recent extravasation (Carlsen et al., 2004). Our observations implied that monocyte-derived cells may play an early and important role in lymphoid neogenesis. CXCL13 produced by such activated innate cells and LT expressed by B cells and/or other cell types (Gonzales et al., 1998; Endres et al., 1999; Tumanov et al., 2002) could together provide the microenvironment required for formation of organized follicles with FDCs **(Fig. 32.7)**.

Differentiation and dispersion of germinal-center B cells

Positive selection and plasma-cell induction

Germinal centers can be divided into different compartments in which antigen-dependent selection of B cells takes place (Fig. 32.5). Stimulation in the dark zone produces exponential growth of B-cell blasts positive for the Ki-67 nuclear proliferation marker (Brandtzaeg and Halstensen, 1992). The resulting centroblasts somatically hypermutate their Ig-variable (V) region genes and give rise to sIgD⁻IgM+CD38+ centrocytes. This process changes the affinity as well as specificity of the BCR and will likely induce some self-reactivity. However, mechanisms exist to eliminate autoreactive B-cell clones (Liu and Arpin, 1997; Lindhout et al., 1997; Pulendran et al., 1997). Also, centrocytes with specificity for exogenous antigens undergo apoptosis unless selected by high-affinity binding to FDCs via their sIgM/BCR (Fig. 32.5). The centrocytes may actually pick up antigen from iccosomes (Brandtzaeg and Halstensen, 1992), process it, and present foreign peptide to cognate CD4+ T_{FH} cells (Fig. 32.5).

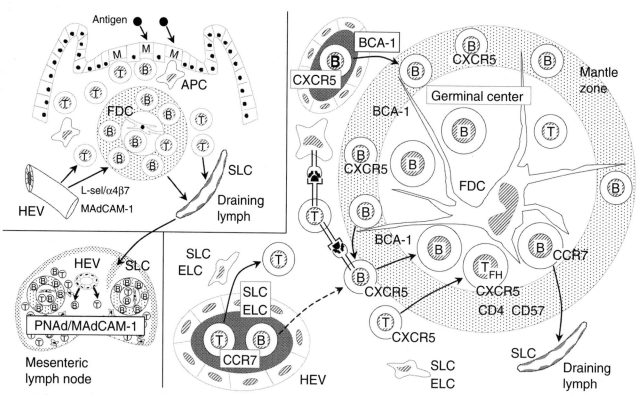

Fig. 32.6. Schematic depiction of adhesion molecule– and chemokine-regulated steps of T- and B-cell migration to, and positioning within, organized gut-associated lymphoid tissue (GALT) compartments. Antigens (*dots*) are sampled from the gut lumen by M cells (M) in GALT, whereas mesenteric lymph nodes receive antigens via draining lymph (either in soluble form or carried by dendritic cells; not shown). Naïve T and B cells enter both GALT and mesenteric lymph nodes (*left*) via high endothelial venules (HEV), by interactions principally between L-selectin (L-sel) and endothelial MAdCAM-1 or PNAd distributed as indicated. Primed (memory/effector) T and B cells may to some extent re-enter these sites by leukointegrin α4β7-MAdCAM-1 interactions. The chemokines involved (*right*) at the level of HEVs are SLC (CCL21) and ELC (CCL19), provided by stromal cells and redistributed to the HEV endothelium as indicated to attract preferentially CCR7+ naïve T cells and less actively B cells (*broken arrow*); SLC may also be involved in the exit of lymphoid cells from GALT via draining lymphatics. Naïve B cells are CXCR5+ and extravasate mainly via modified HEVs presenting CXCL13 (called BCA-1 in humans) juxtaposed to, or inside of, the lymphoid follicles; they are next attracted to the mantle zone, where BCA-1 is deposited on dendritic elements such as the follicular dendritic cell (FDC) tips. Also, follicular B-helper T (T_{FH}) cells (CXCR5+CD4+CD57+) are attracted to the follicle by similar interactions. B cells are primed just outside of the lymphoid follicle by interaction with cognate T cells and antigen-presenting cells (APC); they then re-enter the follicle and end up as CCR7+ germinal center cells after interactions with FDCs and T_{FH} cells. The B cells may thereafter leave the follicle as memory or effector cells.

The importance of cognate interaction between B and T cells is documented by the fact that no germinal centers are formed when CD40–CD40L (CD154) ligation is experimentally blocked (Lindhout *et al.*, 1997). Moreover, this ligation promotes switching of the Ig heavy-chain constant-region (C_H) genes from Cμ to downstream isotypes, while apparently representing a negative signal for terminal B-cell differentiation within the follicles (MacLennan *et al.*, 1997; Randall *et al.*, 1998). The mechanisms contributing to the continuation of primed B cells down the memory pathway rather than leaving it and differentiating along the effector pathway remain elusive (Ahmed and Gray, 1996; Arpin *et al.*, 1997). However, interaction between CD27 on CD38+ germinal center B cells and CD27L (CD70) on T cells may be a determining event (Agematsu *et al.*, 2000; Jung *et al.*, 2000).

Exit of B cells from germinal centers

Emigration of activated B cells from germinal centers is most likely directed by chemokines, and the actual cues may be extrafollicular ligands for CCR7 (Fig. 32.6). Thus, activated germinal center B cells downregulate CXCR5 and upregulate CCR7, which in animal experiments have profound consequences for their positioning (Reif *et al.*, 2002). In fact, most MALT-induced sIgD−IgM+CD38− putative memory B cells migrate continuously out of the germinal centers to sites such as the tonsillar crypt epithelium (Liu *et al.*, 1995) or Peyer's patch M-cell pockets (Yamanaka *et al.*, 2001), where they presumably present recall antigens to cognate memory T cells (Fig. 32.4). Likewise, most plasma cell precursors (CD20−CD38hi) become rapidly dispersed in juxtaposed extrafollicular compartments or migrate via lymph and blood to distant effector sites, where

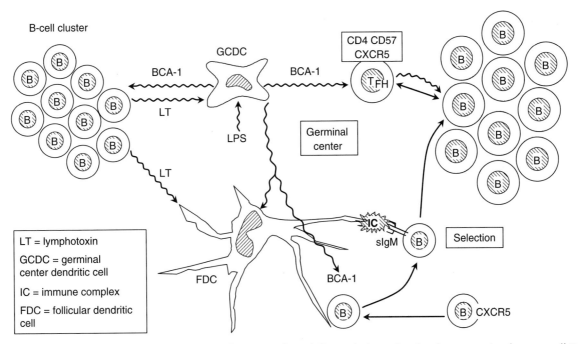

Fig. 32.7. Simplified model of lymphoid neogenesis in inflammatory bowel disease lesions, showing the progression from a small B-cell cluster to an organized follicle containing FDCs. As discussed in the text, the major source of CXCL13 (BCA-1) appears to be GCDCs, which most likely represent activated macrophages. B cells (B), and probably T cells (T) and other cell types, produce LT, which may exert a reciprocal effect on germinal center and FDC formation. Both follicular B-helper T (T$_{FH}$) cells and B cells with a high level of CXCR5 expression are attracted to the follicle by BCA-1, but germinal center B cells downregulate CXCR5 after proliferation and selection for high antigen affinity on IC-bearing FDCs via their surface receptor (sIgM). Such affinity maturation is followed by Ig-class switch (see Fig. 32.8).

they undergo terminal differentiation **(Fig. 32.8)**, as discussed below.

REGULATION OF B-CELL ISOTYPE SWITCHING AND J-CHAIN EXPRESSION

The switching process

Following activation, naïve B cells usually first change their BCR composition from sIgD$^+$IgM$^+$ to become sIgD$^-$ IgM$^+$ memory cells and may then switch to another class such as IgG or IgA **(Fig. 32.9)**. During plasma-cell differentiation, the BCR is gradually lost, together with several other B-cell markers, particularly CD20 and then CD19 (in mice, also B220). Activation-induced cytidine deaminase (AID) plays an essential role in this process (Kinoshita and Honjo, 2001). This enzyme is present during class-switch recombination (CSR) and may link CSR to somatic hypermutation of IgV-gene segments, which takes place during the germinal center reaction. Fagarasan *et al.* (2001) used AID-knockout mice with defective CSR to study the accumulated switching potential of intestinal B cells harvested outside of Peyer's patches. Like IgA-deficient humans (see subsequent discussion), AID-deficient mice had numerous lamina propria IgM–producing immunocytes (B220$^-$), which gave rise to abundant sIgM. When sIgM$^+$B220$^+$ intestinal B cells from these mice were transformed with retrovirus to overexpress

AID, they displayed a strong IgA-switch propensity after *in vitro* stimulation with lipopolysaccharide (LPS), transforming growth factor (TGF)-β and IL-5. The same tendency was observed for similarly harvested sIgM$^+$B220$^+$ B cells from normal mice in conjunction with AID upregulation, whereas cells of the same phenotype obtained from Peyer's patches showed a lower IgA-switch efficiency under identical conditions.

During CSR, the DNA between the switch sites is looped out and excised, thereby deleting Cμ (Fig. 32.9), which is followed either sequentially or directly by loss of other C$_H$ genes (Kinoshita and Honjo, 2001). After direct switch to IgA expression, the Iα-Cμ circular transcripts (αCTs), derived from the excised recombinant DNA, are gradually lost through dilution from progeny cells during proliferation (Fagarasan and Honjo, 2003). Therefore, readily detectable αCTs are considered a marker of recent CSR. It is interesting that αCTs are detectable in murine intestinal sIgA$^+$B220$^+$ B cells located outside of Peyer's patches, which might suggest that lamina propria IgA immunocytes are derived directly from sIgM$^+$B220$^+$ B cells *in situ* (Fagarasan *et al.*, 2001). This CSR is not believed to require CD40–CD40L interaction, therefore most likely involving T cell–independent B1 cells in a process engaging the BlyS/BAFF (B cell–activating factor of the TNF family) receptor (Litinskiy *et al.*, 2002; Fagarasan and Honjo, 2003). BAFF or other proliferation-inducing ligands such as APRIL

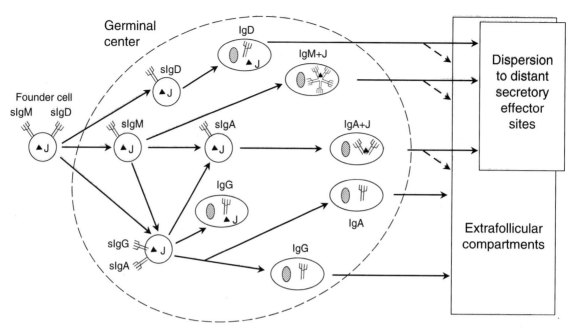

Fig. 32.8. Schematic representation of putative B-cell developmental stages in germinal center of MALT follicle. The pathways to terminal plasma-cell differentiation may include coexpression of cytoplasmic J chain and any of the four Ig classes depicted, but the J chain can combine only with cytoplasmic IgA and IgM to form polymers (IgA+J, dimeric IgA; IgM+ J, pentameric IgM). The B cells will to a variable extent terminate their differentiation topically in extrafollicular compartments (*broken arrows*), but those with a mucosal phenotype (J chain–expressing) preferentially migrate to distant secretory effector sites. Further details are discussed in the text.

(Mackay and Browning, 2002) are secreted by activated DCs (*e.g.*, after LPS exposure in the gut) and may thus operate in the intestinal lamina propria (Fig. 32.2).

It is of note, however, that AID-deficient mice show a dramatic hyperplasia of ILFs in response to intestinal overgrowth of the indigenous microbiota (Fagarasan *et al.*, 2002). This could reflect an inadequate compensatory antibody repertoire in the gut due to lack of somatic hypermutation in the S-IgM that replaces the missing S-IgA in these mice. It cannot be excluded, therefore, that Fagarasan *et al.* (2001) actually observed a difference in IgA-switching capacity between Peyer's patches and hyperplastic ILFs rather than CSR outside of such GALT structures (Brandtzaeg *et al.*, 2001).

Differences among immune-inductive sites
Isotype switching and J-chain expression
B-cell differentiation involves downstream (5′→3′) switching of C_H genes on chromosome 14 (Fig. 32.9), from IgM (Cμ) to other isotypes (Flanagan and Rabbits, 1982). The tonsillar germinal center reaction involves extensive switching and also some terminal differentiation of effector B cells (Dahlenborg *et al.*, 1997). Thus, immunohistochemical studies have revealed a substantial although variable number of intrafollicular Ig-producing plasmablasts, predominantly with cytoplasmic IgG (55% to 72%) or IgA (13% to 18%), the latter isotype being more frequent in children than in adults (Brandtzaeg, 1987). Both these germinal center immunocyte classes, and also those producing IgM and IgD,

are often associated with detectable cytoplasmic J-chain expression (IgG, 36%; IgA, 29%; IgM, 55%; and IgD, 82%) in normal palatine tonsils as well as adenoids from children (Korsrud and Brandtzaeg, 1981a). In children, moreover, tonsillar CSR gives rise to an even higher percentage of extrafollicular IgA immunocytes with J-chain expression (51%), whereas only a small proportion (~2%) of the dominating extrafollicular IgG subset is J chain–positive (**Figs. 32.10 and 32.11**).

The germinal center reaction of human Peyer's patches and the appendix generates relatively more intrafollicular IgA immunocytes with J-chain expression than seen in tonsillar germinal centers; and in the juxtaposed lamina propria and dome zones, immunocytes that produce IgA are numerically equal to, or dominate over, those producing IgG (Bjerke and Brandtzaeg, 1986, 1990a). Like in the tonsils, the IgG isotype is associated with much less J-chain expression than is IgA, which contrasts with the striking overall IgA immunocyte dominance (see subsequent discussion) and high level of J-chain expression associated with both isotypes in normal secretory effector tissues, such as the intestinal lamina propria (Figs. 32.10 and 32.11).

Different J-chain expression in putative early and mature effector clones
To support secretory immunity, B-cell regulation in MALT must give rise to dispersion of primed cells with prominent J-chain expression (Fig. 32.8), thereby providing pIgA and pentameric IgM for export by pIgR at distant effector sites,

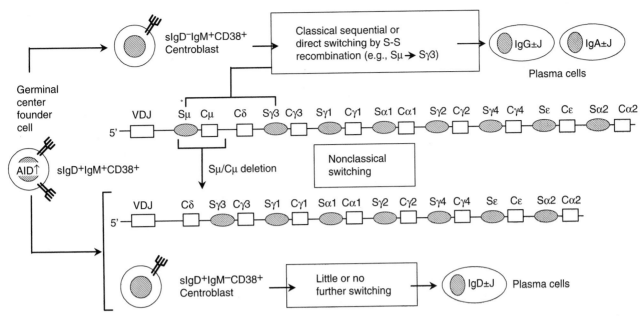

Fig. 32.9. Predicted events in class-switch recombination leading to differentiation of B cells in mucosa-associated lymphoid tissue. This complex process takes place after activation of germinal center founder cells, resulting in elevated levels of activation-induced cytidine deaminase (AID), as indicated. In the classic pathway, the centroblast progeny changes its Ig heavy-chain constant-region (C_H) gene expression from $C\mu$ to one of the downstream C_H genes, either sequentially or directly by recombination between switch (S) regions (comprising repetitive sequences of palindrome-rich motifs), followed by looping-out of the intervening DNA fragment containing $C\mu$ and other C_H genes from the chromosome. This pathway gives rise to plasma cells of various IgG and IgA subclasses (and IgE, not shown), with or without concurrent J-chain expression (±J). A minor fraction of tonsillar centroblasts undergo nonclassical switching by deleting a variable part of $S\mu$ and the complete $C\mu$ region. This pathway selectively gives rise to IgD-producing plasma cells.

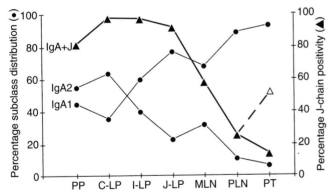

Fig. 32.10. Subclass distribution and J-chain expression of IgA-producing cells in various normal extrafollicular tissue compartments from adults. PP, Peyer's patch; C-LP, I-LP, and J-LP, distant colonic, ileal, and jejunal lamina propria, respectively; MLN, mesenteric lymph nodes; PLN, peripheral lymph nodes; and PT, palatine tonsils. For the latter organ, J-chain data from healthy children are also indicated (*open triangles connected by broken line*). Based on published data from the authors' laboratory, as referred to in the text.

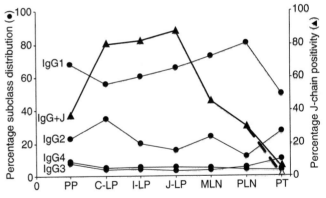

Fig. 32.11. Subclass distribution and J-chain expression of IgG-producing cells in various normal extrafollicular tissue compartments, as defined in the legend to Fig. 32.10. Based on published data from the authors' laboratory, as referred to in the text.

as discussed in the next section. Remarkably, B cells that undergo terminal differentiation juxtaposed to MALT follicles show prominent IgG production and downregulated J-chain expression **(Fig. 32.12)**; this could reflect that they have been through several rounds of stimulation in germinal

centers, thus belonging to relatively exhausted effector clones compared with those rapidly migrating to distant secretory sites (Fig. 32.8). Local retention of "mature" clones would fit with the "decreasing potential hypothesis," implying reduced potential for generation of new memory cells and enhanced potential for terminal differentiation and apoptosis (Ahmed and Gray, 1996). Our immunohistochemical studies indicate increased extrafollicular accumulation of

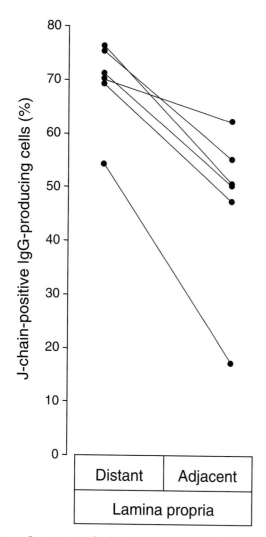

Fig. 32.12. Comparison of J-chain expression shown by IgG-producing immunocytes in lamina propria of normal appendix mucosa distant from and adjacent to lymphoid follicles, as indicated. Adapted from Bjerke and Brandtzaeg (1986).

nal center cells (see previous discussion), as well as circulating IgG-, IgD-, and IgA-producing plasmablasts (Brandtzaeg, 1976), show prominent J-chain expression supports the notion that this is a feature of relatively early effector clones. Moreover, the reduced J-chain expression seen in extrafollicular IgA immunocytes of normal palatine tonsils from adults, compared with counterparts from children (Fig. 32.10), and the strikingly reduced J-chain expression of tonsillar IgA cells in children with recurrent tonsillitis (Korsrud and Brandtzaeg, 1981b) do support the idea that downregulation of the J-chain gene is part of the decreased potential of mature effector clones.

Regulation of J-chain expression

Little is known about factors causing the high level of J-chain expression in putative early effector B cells that home from MALT to secretory tissue sites (Fig. 32.8). Transcriptional regulation of the J-chain gene involving cytokines such as IL-2, IL-4, IL-5, and IL-6 has been described in mice, and both positive and negative regulatory elements appear to be present in the promoter region (Tigges et al., 1989; Takayasu and Brooks, 1991; Randall et al., 1992; Shin and Koshland, 1993; Turner et al., 1994; Kang et al., 1998; Rao et al., 1998). Contrary to the situation in mice, transcription of the human J-chain gene is apparently initiated during early stages of B-lineage differentiation, even before Ig production takes place (McCune et al., 1981; Hajdu et al., 1983; Max and Korsmeyer, 1985; Kubagawa et al., 1988). Altogether, therefore, how the human J-chain is induced and regulated to provide a mucosal B-cell phenotype remains an enigma.

Regional isotype-switch mechanisms differ

The cytokine profiles and other microenvironmental factors that determine isotype differentiation of B cells are likewise obscure. The fact that the IgA1 subclass dominates IgA responses both in tonsils and in the regionally related exocrine tissues supports the notion that mucosal B-cell differentiation in this body region mainly takes place from sIgD⁻IgM⁺CD38⁺ centrocytes by sequential downstream C_H gene switching (Brandtzaeg, 1987; Brandtzaeg et al., 1999b). Conversely, the relatively enhanced IgA2 expression in Peyer's patches and the distal gut altogether (Fig. 32.10), including the mesenteric lymph nodes (Kett et al., 1986; Bjerke and Brandtzaeg, 1990a,b), could reflect direct switching from Cμ to Cα2 with excision of intervening C_H gene segments (Fig. 32.9). B cells from murine Peyer's patches are able to switch directly from Cμ to Cα, and in human B cells this pathway may preferentially lead to IgA2 production (Conley and Bartelt, 1984). Molecular evidence of autocrine TGF-β-mediated switch region (S) recombination, either direct (Sμ→ Sα) or sequential (Sμ→ Sγ, Sγ→ Sα), has been obtained in naïve human B cells after engagement of CD40 (Zan et al., 1998). However, although it is known that IgA expression induced by TGF-β involves mobilization of the transcription factor (TF) core-binding factor (CBF)α3 (AML2), the critical role of this pleiotropic cytokine in IgA regulation remains elusive (Cazac and Roes, 2000).

putative mature B-cell clones with downregulated J-chain expression in the order of GALT, mesenteric lymph nodes, peripheral lymph nodes, and palatine tonsils from adults (Figs. 32.10 and 32.11). These differences might to some extent depend on the magnitude of persistent immune stimulation (topical antigenic load), which is probably much higher in palatine tonsils (with deep antigen-retaining crypts) than in GALT.

According to our idea, the functional role of J chain in secretory immunity is sufficient biological justification for its expression also by MALT-derived B cells terminating with IgG or IgD production; these immunocytes may be considered "spin-offs" from recently generated effector clones that through downstream C_H switching are on their way to pIgA production (Brandtzaeg and Korsrud, 1984; Brandtzaeg et al., 1999b). The fact that IgG- and IgD-producing germi-

As mentioned previously, the germinal center reaction generates relatively more intrafollicular J chain–positive IgA cells in human Peyer's patches and the appendix than in tonsils (Brandtzaeg *et al.*, 1999b). Also, in juxtaposed extrafollicular GALT compartments, IgA immunocytes are equal to or exceed in numbers their IgG counterparts (Bjerke and Brandtzaeg, 1986; Bjerke *et al.*, 1986), whereas in tonsils there is a more than twofold dominance of IgG immunocytes outside of the follicles (Brandtzaeg, 1987). Therefore, the drive for switching to IgA and expression of J chain is much more pronounced in GALT than in tonsils. Perhaps GALT is distinct from other MALT structures because of special accessory cells or a particular cytokine profile (see subsequent discussion). Alternatively, the continuous superimposition of new exogenous stimuli in the gut may enhance the development of early effector B-cell clones with an increased potential for IgA and J-chain expression (Brandtzaeg *et al.*, 1999b).

A regionalized microbial impact on mucosal B-cell differentiation may be exemplified by the unique sIgD⁺IgM⁻CD38⁺ subset identified in the dark zone of palatine tonsillar germinal centers (Liu and Arpin, 1997). These centroblasts show deletion of the Cμ and Sμ gene segments (Fig. 32.9), therefore giving rise selectively to IgD immunocytes by nonclassical switching (Arpin *et al.*, 1998). We have obtained molecular evidence of preferential occurrence of B cells with Cμ deletion also in normal adenoids and secretory effector tissues of the upper aerodigestive tract but virtually never in small intestinal mucosa (Brandtzaeg *et al.*, 2002). Such compartmentalized B-cell dispersion explains the relatively high frequency of IgD immunocytes normally occurring in this region, particularly the large IgD-positive replacement subset that often is seen at regional secretory sites in IgA deficiency (see next section). Most strains of *Haemophilus influenzae* and *Moraxella catarrhalis*, which are frequent colonizers of the nasopharynx, produce an IgD-binding factor (protein D) that can crosslink sIgD/BCR (Ruan *et al.*, 1990; Janson *et al.*, 1991). In this manner it is possible that sIgD⁺ tonsillar centrocytes are stimulated to proliferate and differentiate polyclonally, thereby driving IgVᵥ gene hypermutation and Cμ deletion (Liu *et al.*, 1996; Arpin *et al.*, 1998).

Such regional microbial influence on B-cell differentiation is supported by our observation that Cμ deletion is more frequently detected in diseased than in clinically normal tonsils and adenoids (Brandtzaeg *et al.*, 2002), and there is an increased number of extrafollicular IgD immunocytes in recurrent tonsillitis and adenoid hyperplasia (Brandtzaeg, 1987). Molecular evidence strongly suggests that these extrafollicular plasma cells are indeed derived from the sIgD⁺IgM⁻ centroblast subset (Arpin et al., 1998). IgD-deficient mice are sensitive to tolerance induction because sIgD protects B cells against deletion (Carsetti *et al.*, 1993), whereas sIgM is associated with prohibitin and a prohibitin-related protein that transduce negative signals (Terashima *et al.*, 1994). Therefore, sIgD⁺IgM⁻ cells could in addition have a particular proliferative advantage when stimulated

through their BCR. Conversely, LPS that is abundantly present in the distal gut may inhibit selective expression of IgD (Parkhouse and Cooper, 1977).

Identified IgA-promoting stimuli

Schrader *et al.* (1990) first reported that DCs from murine Peyer's patches and spleen enhanced preferentially IgA production in a microculture system based on cognate interactions between B and T cells. A similar role for DCs was later observed in a human *in vitro* system not including T cells but employing CD40-activated naïve B cells (Fayette *et al.*, 1997). As mentioned earlier, TGF-β appears to be a crucial IgA switch factor for activated (AID⁺) B cells, whereas IL-2, IL-5, and IL-10 may be important for their expansion and terminal differentiation, perhaps with support from IL-6 and interferon-γ **(Fig. 32.13)**. All these cytokines are known to be produced by antigen-activated CD4⁺ T cells from human intestinal mucosa (Nilsen *et al.*, 1995) and are also expressed in human Peyer's patches (Hauer *et al.*, 1998; MacDonald and Monteleone, 2001). IL-6 has furthermore been reported to enhance preferentially IgA production (IgA2 > IgA1) by human appendix B cells (Fujihashi *et al.*, 1991), and a central role for IL-10 is supported by the fact that this cytokine can release the differentiation block of IgA-committed B cells from IgA-deficient patients (Brière *et al.*, 1994). Human naïve B cells activated through CD40 can be pushed toward IgA production by TGF-β and IL-10 in combination (Defrance *et al.*, 1992). It is interesting that DCs enhance synergistically the effect of both TGF-β and IL-10 on IgA expression and, via unknown signals, may be essential for the IgA2 phenotype (Fayette *et al.*, 1997).

Neuroendocrine peptides may furthermore be involved in mucosal B-cell differentiation. Thus, human fetal B cells activated *in vitro* through CD40 were shown to be selectively induced by vasoactive intestinal polypeptide (VIP) to produce both IgA1 and IgA2 (Kimata et al., 1995). Similarly treated sIgM⁻CD19⁺ pre-B cells from human fetal bone marrow were likewise induced to produce the two IgA subclasses in addition to IgM. These results suggested that VIP can act as a true switch factor (Fig. 32.13), which is interesting in view of its relatively high concentration in the gut. In cultures of intestinal mononuclear cells, VIP was also reported to enhance the number of IgA precursors, increase the synthesis of IgA, and decrease IgG production (Boirivant *et al.*, 1994). Finally, substance P has been shown to promote both IgA and IgM production by murine B-cell lines, the latter isotype particularly in the presence of LPS (Pascual *et al.*, 1991).

Switch to IgA outside of germinal centers

Natural antibodies secreted by B-1 cells are generally encoded in germline (unmutated IgV) genes, but when produced in response to commensal gut bacteria, such murine IgA often shows somatic mutation, which suggests a germinal center event (Bos *et al.*, 1996). Nevertheless, although microbial colonization is a prerequisite to induce S-IgA antibodies in mice, implying an antigen-induced process, no

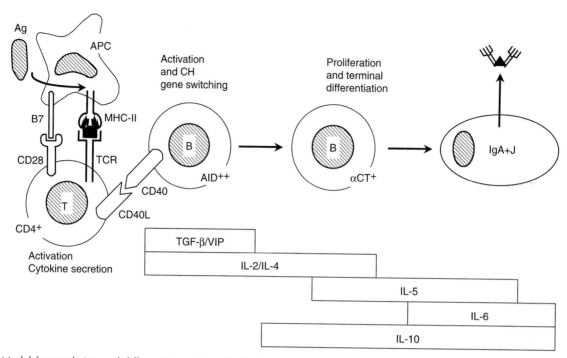

Fig. 32.13. Model for regulation and differentiation of B cells (B) in inductive mucosa-associated lymphoid tissue (*left*) leading to generation of plasma cells that mainly produce dimeric IgA with J chain (IgA+J) at secretory effector site (*right*). Antigen (Ag) is processed by antigen-presenting cells (APC) at inductive site and presented to naïve CD4$^+$ T cells (T) in the context of MHC class II molecules (MHC-II); this step is highly dependent on the costimulatory molecules B7 (CD80/86) and CD28. Activated T lymphocytes and other cells in the microenvironment secrete immunoregulatory factors such as cytokines and vasoactive intestinal polypeptide (VIP), which are important for various steps in mucosal B-cell differentiation, as indicated (*boxes at the bottom*). The costimulatory molecules CD40 and CD40L are crucial for the initiation of the switching process of Ig–heavy chain constant region (C_H)-genes in sIgM$^+$ cells to become IgA-expressing by looping-out of Iα -Cμ circular transcripts (αCT), which thereafter are gradually lost. The class switch is facilitated by activation-induced cytidine deaminase (AID), which is highly upregulated in activated B cells, as indicated (AID^{++}). Information obtained in experimental animals suggests that productive transcription of the J-chain gene depends on IL-2, IL-5, and IL-6, whereas IL-4 may have an opposing effect.

clear dependency on germinal centers or T cells has been revealed (Fagarasan and Honjo, 2000; Macpherson *et al.*, 2000). Under certain conditions, IgA differentiation driven by gut bacteria may even bypass the usual sIgM (or sIgD) BCR requirement (Macpherson *et al.*, 2001); and the intestinal lamina propria is suggested, but not directly proven (see prior discussion), to be a potent site for switch to IgA (Fagarasan *et al.* 2001). The possibility remains that this could be true for B1 cells derived from the murine peritoneal cavity (Fig. 32.2), but it appears to be of little or no relevance to the human gut, where both IgA and IgM immunocytes have highly mutated IgV genes, which is consistent with precursor selection in germinal centers (Dunn-Walters *et al.*, 1997a; Fischer *et al.*, 1998). Sequences of heavy-chain V$^-$ gene segments from human Peyer's patch B cells are in fact clonally related to ileal lamina propria immunocytes (Dunn-Walters *et al.*, 1997b), in accordance with a predominant derivation from GALT (Fig. 32.2). Conversely, in the human peritoneal cavity, IgM genes are mostly unmutated, and the mutated ones exhibit fewer mutations than corresponding genes from intestinal B cells (Boursier *et al.*, 2002). Likewise, the IgV$_H$4-34 genes used by IgG and IgA in human peritoneal B cells show significantly fewer mutations than their mucosal counterparts.

Altogether, there is no reason to believe that switching to IgA takes place to any significant degree in the human lamina propria and recent evidence suggests that the same is true for the murine lamina propria (Shikima *et al.*, 2004). Even for murine B-1 cells, the possibility remains that their precommitment to IgA is induced in the peritoneal cavity, because freshly isolated sIgM$^+$IgA$^-$ cells from this site are reportedly class-switched at the DNA level (Hiroi *et al.*, 2000). Notably, although some studies have suggested that murine B1 cells may depend on the microenvironment of mesenteric lymph nodes for plasma cell differentiation, the actual route and speed of migration of such cells to the intestinal lamina propria remain elusive (Fagarasan and Honjo, 2000).

RECRUITMENT OF B CELLS TO MUCOSAL INDUCTIVE SITES AND EFFECTOR SITES

Adhesion molecules and chemokines operating in GALT

Certain adhesion molecules guiding immune-cell extravasation are more strongly expressed on naïve than on primed (memory/effector) subsets, and *vice versa*, and some are relatively tissue-specific in their function. Counter-receptors expressed by endothelial cells may likewise show tissue specificity (Butcher and Picker, 1996). Thus, in human GALT and mesenteric lymph nodes, but not in peripheral lymph nodes, mucosal addressin cell adhesion molecule (MAdCAM)-1 is abundantly expressed by high endothelial venules (HEVs) (Brandtzaeg *et al.*, 1999a). However, the microenvironmental factors that explain such preferential expression in the gut remain elusive (Denis *et al.*, 1996; Brandtzaeg *et al.*, 1999c). It is well documented in mice that this complex multidomain adhesion molecule plays a major role in intestinal extravasation of immune cells (Streeter *et al.*, 1988). Human MAdCAM-1 has also been cloned and characterized (Shyjan *et al.*, 1996).

When MAdCAM-1 is expressed by HEVs in murine GALT, the glycosylation of its mucin-like domain promotes binding of L-selectin (CD62L) that is present at a high level on naïve lymphocytes (Berg *et al.*, 1993). This initial endothelial adherence (tethering), together with binding of leukointegrin α4β7 to the two N-terminal Ig-like domains

of MAdCAM-1, is crucial for the preferential emigration of naïve lymphocytes into GALT structures such as Peyer's patches, whereas mesenteric lymph nodes in addition employ mucinlike domains on peripheral lymph node addressin, or PNad (Figs. 32.6 and **32.14**). The less prominent GALT endowment with primed immune cells (α4β7[hi]L-selectin[lo]) may be mediated selectively by MAdCAM-1, because its interaction with α4β7 also supports tethering (Berlin *et al.*, 1995). It is interesting that under flow conditions, the secondary lymphoid tissue chemokine (SLC/CCL21) stimulates α4β7-mediated human lymphocyte adhesion to MAdCAM-1, in contrast to other CC chemokines tested (Pachynski *et al.*, 1998). Regardless of tissue site, an additional contribution to the emigration of both naïve and memory cells is provided by other more generalized adhesion molecules such as leukocyte function–associated molecule (LFA)-1 (αLβ2 or CD11a/CD18) that binds to intercellular adhesion molecule (ICAM)-1 (CD54) and ICAM-2 (CD120) on the endothelium (Butcher and Picker, 1996).

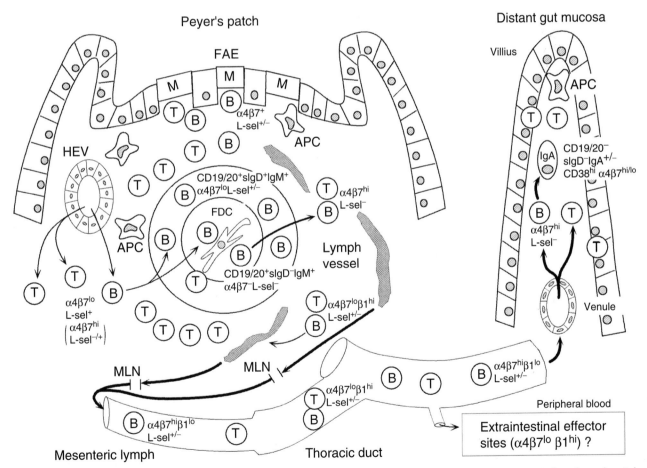

Fig. 32.14. Distribution of leukocyte adhesion molecules in various human intestinal tissue compartments, mesenteric lymph, and peripheral blood. The predominant expression pattern is indicated (positive, +; high intensity, hi; low intensity, lo; or negative, –) with regard to α4β7, α4β1, and L-selectin (L-sel) expressed by B cells (B) and T cells (T). Phenotype given in parentheses indicates low priority. MLN marks location of mesenteric lymph nodes, FDC represents follicular dendritic cells in germinal center of secondary lymphoid follicle, HEV depicts high endothelial venule located in T-cell zone of Peyer's patch, ATC represents putative antigen-presenting cells, and the parafollicular microlymphatics are shaded. The migration routes of the lymphoid cells are indicated by arrows, the heavy ones marking the GALT–lamina propria axis preferentially followed by primed (memory and effector) α4β7[hi]L-sel[–] subsets, mostly B cells that become IgA-producing mucosal plasma cells. Further details are discussed in the text.

The phenotype-related distribution of adhesion molecules has been analyzed in human Peyer's patches and appendix both by flow cytometry and by immunohistochemistry (**Table 32.1**). The naïve B cells constituting follicular mantle zones generally express abundantly L-selectin but variably α4β7 and usually no β1 (CD29). Also, lymphocytes positive for L-selectin found around or within the parafollicular HEVs are generally weakly positive or negative for α4β7. Notably, they are mostly naïve T cells (CD3⁺CD45RA⁺); only some are B cells, again usually of the naïve (sIgD⁺) phenotype (Farstad et al., 1995, 1996, 1997a). Therefore, these vessels do not appear to be a major entrance site for B cells, as discussed in the next section (Fig. 32.6).

The initial tethering of leukocytes to the endothelium is relatively loose until they are stopped by chemokine signaling through G protein–coupled seven-transmembrane receptors (Baggiolini, 1998; Kunkel and Butcher, 2002). SLC/CCL21 and Epstein-Barr virus–induced molecule 1 ligand chemokine (ELC)/CCL19 are produced by stromal cells in secondary lymphoid tissue and become transcytosed by HEV cells to be presented at the vascular surface

(Fig. 32.6). Both chemokines attract preferentially CCR7-expressing T cells, which are retained in the parafollicular areas (Gunn et al., 1998b; Campbell et al., 1998; Willimann et al., 1998; Baekkevold et al., 2001).

The chemokines responsible for B-cell recruitment via HEVs are more unclear. A recent mouse study indicated that although CCR7 ligands operating together with the CXCR4 ligand SDF-1/CXCL12 are crucial for endothelial B-cell adhesion in lymph nodes, B-cell entry in Peyer's patches depends in addition significantly on CXCR5 (Okada et al., 2002). CXCR5–CXCL13 interaction appeared to mediate extravasation of B cells directly into the follicles via HEV-like vessels and not into the parafollicular zone via ordinary HEVs. The importance of this alternative extravasation pathway was supported by intravital microscopy demonstrating T- and B-cell positioning at various vascular levels in murine Peyer's patches (Fig. 32.6), with B cells mainly adhering to SLC-negative vessels near or within the follicles (Warnock et al., 2000). CXCL13-positive vessels are also present in human tonsils and GALT structures (Schaerli et al., 2000; Carlsen et al., 2002).

Table 32.1. Flow-Cytometric Analysis of the Phenotypic Distribution of B and T Cells in Two Human Gut Compartments[a]

	Coexpression Pattern[b]	
Phenotype Proportion[c]	**Small Cells[b]**	**Large Cells[b]**
Organized GALT		
B cells		
50% CD19⁺CD38⁻α4β7^int	25% L-selectin⁺	
	50% sIgD⁺ (40% L-selectin⁺)	
	30% sIgA⁺ (15% L-selectin⁺)	
	14% sIgG⁺ (25% L-selectin⁺)	
<5% CD19^{+/−} CD38^hi α4β7^{int/hi}		L-selectin⁻
T cells		
45% CD3⁺α4β7^{int/hi}	40% L-selectin⁺	Only few cells
	70% CD4⁺αEβ7⁻	
	20% CD8⁺αEβ7^{−/+}	
Mucosal Lamina Propria		
B cells		
10% CD19⁺CD38⁻α4β7^{int/hi}	L-selectin⁻	L-selectin⁻
25% CD19^{+/−}CD38^hi α4β7^hi	>80% sIgA⁺	>90% s/cIgA^{+d}
T cells		
60% CD3⁺α4β7^int	L-selectin⁻	
	65% CD4⁺αEβ7^{−/+}	
	30% CD8⁺αEβ7⁺	
4% CD3⁺α4β7^hi		L-selectin⁻αEβ7⁻
		90% CD4⁺ <5% CD8⁺

[a]Adapted from Farstad et al. (1995, 1996, 1997a) and unpublished data from the authors' laboratory.
[b]Calculated from all B or T cells.
[c]Dispersed mononuclear cells gated according to size and analyzed for surfaces markers and fluorescence intensity (positive, +; negative, −; low, lo; intermediate, int; high, hi).
[d]Cytoplasmic IgA (cIgA) determined by immunohistochemistry.

Traffic of naïve and primed B cells from GALT

Immune cells exit from GALT through draining microlymphatics (Figs. 32.6 and 32.14). In human Peyer's patches and the appendix, these vessels are seen as thin-walled spaces lacking endothelial expression of von Willebrand factor (Farstad *et al.*, 1997a,b). Similar lymph vessels have been noted in human tonsils (Fujisaka *et al.*, 1996). Draining microlymphatics are believed to start blindly with a fenestrated endothelium, and the lymphoid cells probably enter them by selective mechanisms. Thus, lymph endothelium shares with HEVs expression of both SLC and certain adhesion molecules (Gunn *et al.*, 1998b; Irjala *et al.*, 2003).

In human GALT, memory B (sIgD⁻) and T (CD45R0⁺) cells with strong expression of α4β7 are often located near and also within the draining microlymphatics (Fig. 32.14), together with some CD19⁺CD38^hi α4β7^hi blasts (Farstad *et al.*, 1997a,b). However, the lymph vessels contain mainly naïve lymphocytes with low levels of α4β7. Cytochemical and flow-cytometric analyses of human mesenteric lymph have provided similar marker profiles; notably, the small fraction of identified B-cell blasts (2%–6%) contained cytoplasmic IgA, IgM, and IgG in the proportions 5:1:<0.5 (Farstad *et al.*, 1997b). Altogether, the α4β7^hi subsets identified at exit through lymphatics in human GALT may be taken to signify the first homing step to populate particularly the intestinal lamina propria with primed lymphoid cells (Fig. 32.14). Relatively few memory cells concurrently expressed high levels of L-selectin in intestinal and mesenteric lymph (Farstad *et al.*, 1997b); those that did, might likely either re-enter GALT or extravasate in mesenteric lymph nodes, peripheral lymphoid organs, or Waldeyer's ring, together with naïve cells, by binding to PNAd expressed by HEVs (Bradley *et al.*, 1996). A flow-cytometric study of circulating human lymphocytes supported such a fundamental subdivision according to vascular adhesion properties (Rott *et al.*, 1996).

Adhesion molecules and chemokines operating in gut lamina propria

There is a general consensus that homing of primed lymphoid cells to the intestinal lamina propria depends on their high level of α4β7 in the absence of L-selectin (Fig. 32.14), which allows binding to unmodified MAdCAM-1 on the lamina propria microvasculature (Butcher and Picker, 1996; Brandtzaeg *et al.*, 1999a,c). This phenotype is predominantly expressed by antigen-specific B cells appearing in human peripheral blood after enteric stimulation, whereas such cells elicited by systemic immunization show preferentially L-selectin but relatively little α4β7 expression (Quiding-Järbrink *et al.*, 1995a; 1997; Kantele *et al.*, 1996; 1997). Although interaction of MAdCAM-1 with L-selectin has apparently been explored only in mice, the virtual absence in human intestinal lamina propria of lymphoid cells bearing L-selectin (Table 32.1) strongly suggests that it does not bind to MAdCAM-1 outside of GALT (Brandtzaeg *et al.*, 1999a,c). It is interesting that many large B cells retain high levels of α4β7 after migration into the human intestinal lamina propria, despite abundant coexpression of CD38 and cytoplasmic IgA (Table 32.1). Therefore, it is possible that α4β7,

in addition to mediating extravasation, together with CD44 contributes to local retention of effector cells (see below).

The thymus-expressed chemokine (TECK/CCL25) appears to have a decisive role in migration of both T and B cells into (and/or retention within) the small intestinal lamina propria **(Fig. 32.15)**. Notably, this chemokine that interacts with CCR9 is selectively produced by the crypt epithelium in this part of the gut (Kunkel *et al.*, 2000; Papadakis *et al.*, 2000; Bowman *et al.*, 2002, Kunkel and Butcher, 2002). In the large intestine, the mucosae-associated chemokine (MEC/CCL28) has recently been identified as a decisive cue for attracting IgA plasmablasts, which express high levels of the corresponding receptor, CCR10 (Kunkel *et al.*, 2003). It is surprising that T cells are not directed by this chemokine. Because the epithelial expression of MEC is much higher in the colon than in the appendix and small intestine (Pan *et al.*, 2002; Wang *et al.*, 2000), this chemokine probably plays a compartmentalized role in intestinal B-cell homing.

The cues that determine extravasation of GALT-derived circulating B cells in gut mucosa may also be involved in migration of primed cells from GALT structures directly into the lamina propria. There are direct although limited vascular connections from Peyer's patches to the villi immediately surrounding them, and these channels can be used for trafficking of B cells (Parrott, 1976). Such a mechanism could explain that when germ-free mice are transferred to conventional conditions, the first IgA immunocytes occur around Peyer's patches (Crabbe *et al.*, 1970). It seems likely that there are similar direct pathways from ILFs to the surrounding lamina propria (Fig. 32.2). This notion is strongly supported by the report that the intestinal immunocyte population was remarkably well retained in rats when the B-cell traffic through the thoracic duct was diverted by lymph cannulation (Mayrhofer and Fisher, 1979). However, as discussed earlier, many of those B cells that normally settle immediately adjacent to GALT follicles apparently belong to "exhausted clones" (Ahmed and Grey, 1996) with decreased J-chain–expressing potential and disproportionately increased class switch to IgG (Figs. 32.2 and 32.12).

Mucosal homing molecules operating beyond the gut

While GALT-derived dissemination of secretory immunity to extraintestinal effector sites is well documented, migration to the gut of B cells induced in NALT or BALT appears to be quite limited, as revealed by immunization or infection experiments in rodents and pigs (McDermott and Bienenstock, 1979; Sminia *et al.*, 1989; Van Cott *et al.*, 1994). On the other hand, considerable indirect evidence summarized elsewhere suggests that dispersion of primed pIgA precursor cells takes place from Waldeyer's ring (human NALT) to regional secretory effector sites (Brandtzaeg, 1999). Even more convincing results have been obtained by immunization of murine NALT (Yanagita *et al.*, 1999) and rabbit palatine tonsils (Inoue *et al.*, 1999). Such putative B-cell homing dichotomy between the upper and lower body regions is

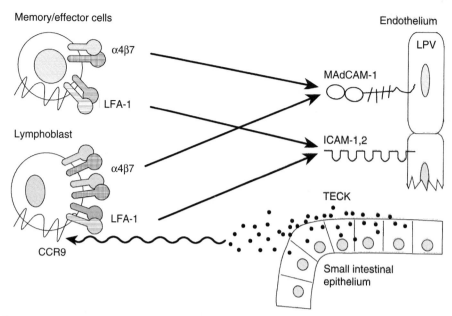

Fig. 32.15. Schematic depiction of putative homing mechanisms that attract preferentially gut-associated lymphoid tissue (GALT)–derived T and B memory/effector cells to human small intestinal lamina propria. Interaction between unmodified (containing no L-selectin-binding O-linked carbohydrates) MAdCAM-1 expressed on ordinary flat lamina propria venules (LPV) is important for the targeting of primed α4β7-bearing cells to all segments of the gut. The level of this activated integrin is particularly high on lymphoblasts. Adherence to the endothelium is strengthened by interactions between generalized adhesion molecules such as LFA-1 and ICAM-1/ICAM-2, as indicated. Selectively produced by the epithelium of the small intestine, the chemokine TECK (CCL25) attracts GALT-derived lymphoid cells that express CCR9 only to this segment of the gut.

supported by the disparate dispersion of human tonsillar sIgD⁺IgM⁻CD38⁺ centroblasts, identified by tracking of their Cμ-gene deletion (Fig. 32.9). We believe that their distribution reflects the homing properties of all B cells with a mucosal phenotype (J chain–expressing) primed in Waldeyer's ring (Brandtzaeg et al., 2002). In keeping with this notion, activated human tonsillar B cells transferred intraperitoneally to mice with severe combined immunodeficiency migrated to the lung but not to gut mucosa (Nadal et al., 1991).

Several studies have suggested that α4β7 is not an important homing receptor for lymphoid cells in the airways of humans (Picker et al., 1994), mice (Wagner et al., 1996), or sheep (Abitorabi et al., 1996). Intranasal immunization in humans induced an insufficient level of α4β7 on specific B cells to make them gut-seeking, whereas antibody production was evoked in both adenoids and nasal mucosa (Quiding-Järbrink et al., 1995b). Notably, the circulating specific B cells showed substantial coexpression of L-selectin and α4β7, in contrast to the high level of α4β7 induced on antibody-producing cells by enteric immunization (Quiding-Järbrink et al., 1997).

A nonintestinal homing receptor profile might also explain B-cell migration from NALT to the urogenital tract. This putative link is reflected by particularly high levels of specific IgA and IgG antibodies in cervicovaginal secretions of mice and monkeys after intranasal immunization with a variety of antigens (Brandtzaeg, 1997; Johansson et al., 2001). A relatively consistent level of L-selectin on NALT-derived B cells, allowing them to bind to PNAd on lymph node HEVs, could

furthermore explain substantial integration between mucosal immunity in the upper aerodigestive tract and the systemic immune system (Rudin et al., 1998; Johansson et al., 2001). B-cell migration to secretory tissues beyond the gut might also involve α4β1 (CD49d/CD29) interactions (Fig. 32.14). The chief counter-receptor for this integrin is vascular-cell adhesion molecule (VCAM)-1, which is expressed on microvascular endothelium in human bronchial and nasal mucosa (Bentley et al., 1993; Jahnsen et al., 1995). However, no evidence exists to suggest that high expression of β1 integrin consistently directs primed B cells to the upper aerodigestive tract, lungs, or urogenital tract.

A unifying chemokine receptor for primed mucosal B cells (but not T cells) affording homing to intestinal as well as extraintestinal secretory effector sites appears to be CCR10. This receptor has recently been shown to be expressed by human IgA plasmablasts (and less so by plasma cells) at every studied mucosal effector site (Kunkel et al., 2003). The corresponding ligand MEC is produced by secretory epithelia all over the body and at relatively high levels in the upper aerodigestive tract (Pan et al., 2000; Wang et al., 2000). It is interesting that MEC (but not TECK) was shown to attract tonsillar IgA plasmablasts in an in vitro assay (Kunkel et al., 2003). Therefore, graded tissue–dependent CCR10-MEC interactions, together with insufficient levels of classical gut-homing molecules, most likely explain the observed dispersion dichotomy for effector B cells derived from Waldeyer's ring **(Fig. 32.16)**.

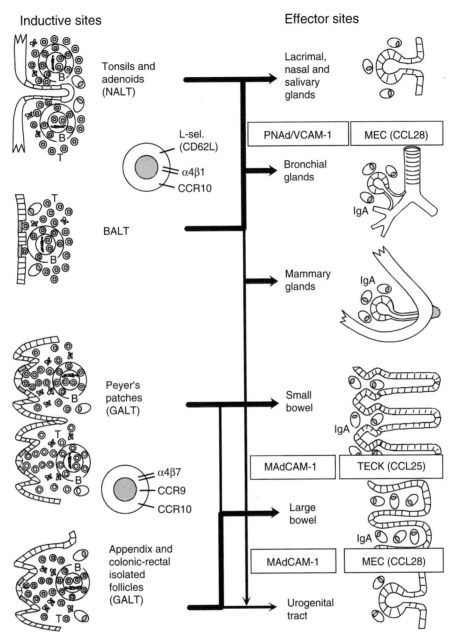

Fig. 32.16. Proposed model for homing of primed B cells from mucosal inductive sites with activated lymphoid follicles to secretory effector sites in the integrated human mucosal immune system. The specialized follicle–associated epithelium contains M cells with antigen-transporting properties (see Fig. 32.2). Putative compartmentalization in the trafficking from inductive to effector sites is indicated, the heavier arrows representing preferential B-cell migration pathways. Homing from GALT is believed to be determined mainly by integrin $\alpha 4\beta 7$ on primed cells, interacting with MAdCAM-1 expressed on the microvascular endothelium in the intestinal lamina propria. In the small intestinal lamina propria, attraction and/or retention of CCR9-expressing cells is mediated by the chemokine TECK (see Fig. 32.15), while CCR10-MEC interactions appear to be important in the large bowel. Other adhesion molecules such as L-selectin (L-sel) and $\alpha 4\beta 1$ that bind to endothelial PNAd and VCAM-1, respectively, may be employed mainly by B cells primed in bronchus-associated (BALT) and nasopharynx-associated (NALT) lymphoid tissue. Human NALT comprises the various lymphoepithelial structures of Waldeyer's ring, including the palatine tonsils and the nasopharyngeal tonsil (adenoids). In this region, abundantly produced epithelial MEC attracts primed B cells via CCR10. The urogenital tract may employ molecular homing mechanisms similar to those of the upper aerodigestive tract and the large bowel, therefore probably receiving primed cells from inductive sites in both these regions. Also, lactating mammary glands appear to receive primed cells from NALT as well as GALT, and much more efficiently so than the urogenital tract.

Signals for B-cell retention, proliferation, and terminal differentiation

Experiments in gene-manipulated mice have indicated that signaling through LTβR on lamina propria stromal cells is necessary for the presence of B cells and IgA immunocytes in gut mucosa (Kang *et al.*, 2002; Newberry *et al.*, 2002), and adhesion molecules as well as chemokines/chemokine receptors may also be involved in cellular retention. One interesting but unproven candidate in this respect is the extracellular matrix receptor CD44, which is expressed at high levels on post–germinal center B cells (Kremmidiotis and Zola, 1995). Likewise, there is little decisive knowledge about factors triggering terminal B-cell differentiation at secretory effector sites, although it has been suggested that IL-5, IL-6, and IL-10 are particularly important (Fig. 32.6). Notably, topical exposure to antigen appears to have a marked impact on site-specific accumulation of IgA-producing cells (see later in the chapter), thereby influencing the observed homing pattern but without imposing any selectivity on the extravasation step. Thus, GALT-derived blasts home to presumably antigen-free neonatal intestinal mucosa (Halstead and Hall, 1972) and to fetal gut grafted under the adult kidney capsule of experimental animals (Guy-Grand *et al.*, 1974; Parrott and Ferguson, 1974).

The impact of exogenous antigens on the conventional B2 cell–dependent effector arm of the SIgA system is most likely mediated largely via "second signals" from activated cognate T cells. However, several other factors may contribute to site-specific survival and restimulation of memory T cells (Bode *et al.*, 1997). Compartmentalized variables could be a high density of MHC class II molecules (Matis *et al.*, 1983), allowing only trace amounts of foreign antigens or anti-idiotypic antibodies to elicit sufficient second signals for B cells. It is interesting that in human salivary and lactating mammary glands, IgA immunocytes accumulate preferentially adjacent to HLA-DR-expressing epithelial ducts (Newman *et al.*, 1980; Brandtzaeg, 1983a; Thrane *et al.*, 1992).

Site-specific survival differences of IgA immunocytes might directly or indirectly (via activated T cells) be influenced by similar variables, including rescue from apoptosis by contact with stromal cells (Merville *et al.*, 1996). It has been suggested that the half-life of plasma cells varies from a few days to several months, and those ending up in the gut may be particularly short-lived (Ahmed and Grey, 1996; Slifka and Ahmed, 1998).

Role of topical antigen exposure

Substantial antigen-driven proliferation of IgA cells has been observed in intestinal lamina propria of experimental animals (Pierce and Gowans, 1975; Lange *et al.*, 1980), especially in the crypt regions (Husband, 1982). This is the level where most IgA immunocytes occur also in the human gut (Brandtzaeg and Baklien, 1976), and scattered sIgA⁺ memory cells with a proliferative potential are present in human intestinal lamina propria (Farstad *et al.*, 2002).

Although a stimulatory effect of topical antigen outside of Peyer's patches has been demonstrated in terms of localiza-

tion, magnitude, and persistence of human SIgA antibody responses (Ogra and Karzon, 1970), the role of ILFs is difficult to evaluate in such experiments. Thus, rectal immunization elicits particularly high levels of IgA antibodies in colorectal secretions and feces, in both experimental animals (Hopkins *et al.*, 1995) and humans (Kantele *et al.*, 1998), apparently reflecting enhanced stimulation by combined exposure of ILFs and the lamina propria to the same antigen. Repeated vaginal or rectal immunization in monkeys has likewise demonstrated local accumulation of effector B cells at the respective sites (Eriksson *et al.*, 1998). Altogether, it appears that primed immune cells tend to accumulate preferentially at effector sites that correspond to the inductive site where they were initially stimulated.

Rapid and widespread dissemination of fed antigen (perhaps partially carried by DCs), followed by extravasation and activation of specific T cells at sites of cognate antigen presentation, has been observed in T-cell-receptor transgenic mice (Gütgemann *et al.*, 1998). This observation, together with previous results of adoptive B-cell transfer in syngeneic rats (Dunkley and Husband, 1990), supports the notion that local antigen-driven T-cell activation provides important second signals for retention, proliferation, and terminal differentiation of Ig-producing immunocytes at secretory effector sites, even at a long distance from mucosal surfaces. Nevertheless, the density of immunocytes at a particular effector site (see later in the chapter) generally reflects the level of topical antigen exposure, being seven times higher in human colonic mucosa (which has an enormous microbial load) than in parotid and lactating mammary glands (Brandtzaeg, 1983a). It is not likely that live or dead exogenous material normally gains direct access to the latter sites, whereas the lacrimal gland, which is connected by many short ducts to the excessively aeroantigen-exposed conjunctiva, shows an IgA immunocyte density approaching that of the colon (Brandtzaeg, 1983a).

DISTRIBUTION OF Ig-PRODUCING IMMUNOCYTES IN HUMAN EXOCRINE TISSUES

Methodology for quantification of immunocytes at mucosal effector sites

Studies of the B-cell system in the intestinal lamina propria based on flow cytometry are hampered by two important pitfalls. First, it is impossible to ensure that ILFs are not included in the dispersed cell populations. On average, we found only about 10% of small CD19⁺CD20⁺CD38⁻ B cells in this mucosal compartment (Table 32.1), but the wide range suggested that contamination from ILFs sometimes occurred **(Fig. 32.17)**. Second, a selective loss of large, activated B cells has to be considered when cell suspensions are prepared (Fossum *et al.*, 1979). In our opinion, therefore, flow-cytometric investigation of the mucosal B-cell system should be supported by phenotypic *in situ* "maps" obtained by immunohistochemistry (Brandtzaeg, 1998).

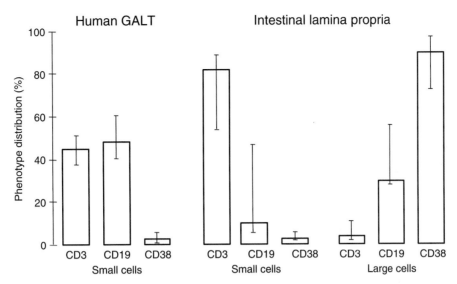

Fig. 32.17. Phenotypic proportions (%) of T lymphocytes (CD3), B lymphocytes (CD19), and B-cell blasts and plasma cells (CD38) obtained by flow cytometry with small mononuclear cells obtained from human gut–associated lymphoid tissue (GALT) represented by Peyer's patches and the appendix, or with normal human intestinal lamina propria small and large mononuclear cells, as indicated. Medians (*columns*) and observed ranges (*vertical lines*) are depicted. Adapted from Farstad *et al.* (1995) and including unpublished data representative of 10 additional samples.

Tissue specimens can principally be prepared for immunohistochemistry in three different ways: fresh-frozen for cryosections; subjection to a precipitating or coagulative fixative (*e.g.*, ethanol), followed by paraffin wax embedding; or subjection to a cross-linking fixative (*e.g.*, formaldehyde), followed by embedding (Brandtzaeg, 1982). Cryosections are usually best suited for membrane-anchored glycoproteins, whereas formaldehyde-fixed tissue is preferred for easily diffusible components of low molecular weight. However, masking of antigenic determinants is a problem in studies of glycoproteins that have been subjected to cross-linking fixatives, although various unmasking procedures are now available (Brandtzaeg *et al.*, 1997a).

For reliable demonstration of interstitial and epithelial Ig distribution, ethanol fixation is undoubtedly the method of choice (Brandtzaeg, 1982). Modification of this approach by including a prefixation tissue-washing period is often necessary for visualization of Ig-producing and particularly Ig-bearing cells against a fairly unstained background (Brandtzaeg, 1974c). The antigenic determinants of certain molecules, such as IgA-associated cytoplasmic J chain, are masked even in ethanol-fixed tissue; denaturation of tissue sections in acid urea is therefore necessary for its reliable detection (Brandtzaeg, 1983b).

In addition to these important precautions, quantification of Ig-producing cells must be based on appropriate morphometric methods to provide meaningful data that can be compared among various laboratories. Immunocyte densities should preferably be reported as the number of counted cells per square millimeter section area or in a defined tissue compartment. However, most exocrine tissues beyond the gut show a strikingly heterogeneous immunocyte density, so evaluated fields must be selected in a well-defined manner

(Korsrud and Brandtzaeg, 1980). Paired staining of two or three Ig isotypes in the same tissue section is always preferable to obtain reliable phenotype ratios (Brandtzaeg 1974c, 1982; Brandtzaeg *et al.*, 1997a). In the intestinal lamina propria, counts of immunocytes per length unit of the gut, including the full height of the mucosa **(Fig. 32.18)**, provide the best measure of local B-cell effector activity (Brandtzaeg and Baklien, 1976). Quantitation of IgA subclass ratios in normal parotid secretions (Müller *et al.*, 1991) fits remarkably well with the immunohistochemical IgA1 and IgA2 cell counts obtained in normal parotid glands, both being on average close to 64:36 (see next section). Moreover, as reviewed elsewhere (Brandtzaeg *et al.*, 1992), our immunohistochemical enumeration of IgG-producing cells in normal colonic mucosa displays a subclass distribution well in agreement with the ratios obtained between spontaneous secretion of IgG1, IgG2, IgG3, and IgG4 by isolated lamina propria mononuclear cells *in vitro* (Scott *et al.*, 1986).

Immunocytes in exocrine tissues of normal adults
IgA-producing immunocytes are remarkably abundant
All secretory effector sites in normal human adults contain a striking preponderance (70%–90%) of IgA-producing immunocytes **(Figs. 32.19 and 32.20)**. Accordingly, most large lymphoid cells dispersed from the lamina propria belong to the terminally differentiated phenotype (CD38+CD27+CD19+/−CD20−) with IgA on the surface and/or in the cytoplasm, whereas most small lymphoid cells are T lymphocytes (Table 32.1). This is in contrast to the flow-cytometric data obtained from GALT compartments such as Peyer's patches and the appendix, where small B lymphocytes (CD19+) and T lymphocytes (CD3+) dominate (Fig. 32.17). These results accord with parallel immunohistochemical

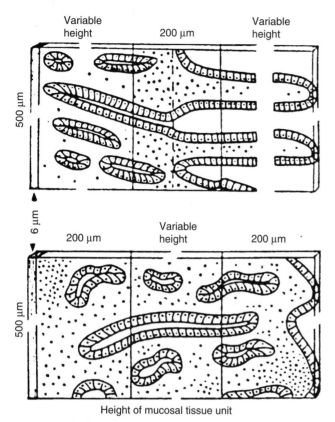

Fig. 32.18. Schematic representation of normal (*top*) and diseased (*bottom*) "tissue unit" defined in a 6-μm-thick section (small intestine illustrated) prepared for immunohistochemical analysis. The lamina propria area included varies among different specimens, depending on the height of the tissue unit; the total number of Ig-producing immunocytes per unit is determined by this variable as well as by the actual cell density. The distribution of dots indicates heterogeneity in cell density. The highest immunocyte density is normally found around the base of the villi in the normal small intestine or close to the lumen in "flat" lesions or normal colonic mucosa. The definition of the corresponding 200-μm zones, which may be used for quantitative comparisons within or between units, is shown by vertical lines. Adapted from Brandtzaeg and Baklien, 1976.

observations, which show that small naïve B lymphocytes (sIgD⁺IgM⁺CD19⁺CD20⁺) in the human gut are almost exclusively present in follicular mantle zones of GALT (Farstad *et al.*, 2000). The proportion of small B lymphocytes in dispersed lamina propria samples varies from 4% to 42%, and 5% to 50% of these cells show a naïve phenotype (sIgD⁺), reflecting a highly variable contamination from GALT structures such as ILFs.

The human lamina propria contains only few and scattered sIgA⁺CD27⁺ memory cells with low levels of CD40. Following CD40 ligation, these cells proliferate *in vitro* and constitutively secrete IgA, thus signifying a capacity for local recall responses (Farstad *et al.*, 2000). Notably, lamina propria CD19⁺ cells are negative for CD5, which supports the notion that B1 cells do not contribute significantly to the human IgA immunocyte population (Boursier *et al.*, 2000).

By immunohistochemistry we have estimated that almost 10^{10} IgA-producing immunocytes occur per meter of adult bowel (Brandtzaeg and Baklien, 1976), with a predominance proximally and distally **(Fig. 32.21)**. Absolute figures are difficult to obtain for other exocrine tissues in which the immunocytes are more heterogeneously distributed throughout the stroma. Nevertheless, on the basis of our quantitative data **(Fig. 32.22)**, it appears clear that the gut is the most active exocrine B cell organ (Brandtzaeg, 1983a). Moreover, the magnitude of its immunocyte population is impressive in view of the comparable figure (2.5×10^{10}) estimated collectively for bone marrow, spleen, and lymph nodes (Turesson, 1976). Indeed, at least 80% of all human Ig-producing immunocytes are located in the gut (Brandtzaeg *et al.*, 1989), and a similar estimate has been reported for mice (van der Heijden *et al.*, 1987). Aging does not appear to reduce the remarkable IgA-producing capacity of the intestinal mucosa (Penn *et al.*, 1991), although specific mucosal immunity may be compromised in the geriatric population (Schmucker *et al.*, 1996).

MALT-derived B cells also enter lactating mammary glands (Fig. 32.16), and human colostrum contains some 300 times more SIgA than stimulated parotid saliva. Nevertheless, the tissue density of IgA immunocytes is similar in human salivary and lactating mammary glands and actually six to seven times less than in lacrimal glands and colonic mucosa (Fig. 32.22). Therefore, the large organ size, combined with capacity for storage of locally produced pIgA in the epithelium and duct system of mammary glands, explains the striking output of SIgA during breast-feeding (Brandtzaeg, 1983a).

Disparate IgA subclass distribution

The remarkably heterogeneous distribution of locally produced IgA subclasses supports the existence of regional immunoregulatory differences in the human mucosal immune system **(Fig. 32.23)**. IgA immunocytes show a relatively large IgA2 proportion (29% to 64%) in gut mucosa in comparison with peripheral lymphoid tissue and upper airways (7% to 25%), but IgA2 dominates (64%) only in the large bowel (Crago *et al.*, 1984; Jonard *et al.*, 1984; Kett *et al.*, 1986; Burnett *et al.*, 1987). A skewing toward S-IgA2 may be important for the stability of secretory antibodies, because this isotype is resistant to several IgA1-specific bacterial proteases (Kilian *et al.*, 1996). The concentration ratio of the two S-IgA subclasses in various secretions (Jonard *et al.*, 1984; Müller *et al.*, 1991; Feltelius *et al.*, 1994) corresponds to the immunocyte proportions at the related secretory tissues, supporting the notion that both isotypes of pIgA are equally well exported by the pIgR (Brandtzaeg, 1977).

The molecular events underlying preferential IgA1 or IgA2 responses remain unclear. Secretory antibodies to LPS are generally of the S-IgA2 subclass, whereas protein antigens stimulate predominantly S-IgA1 (Mestecky and Russell, 1986; Tarkowski *et al.*, 1990). The fact that jejunal IgA immunocytes are mainly of the IgA1 subclass (~77%), in contrast to the IgA2 dominance (~64%) in the colon (Kett

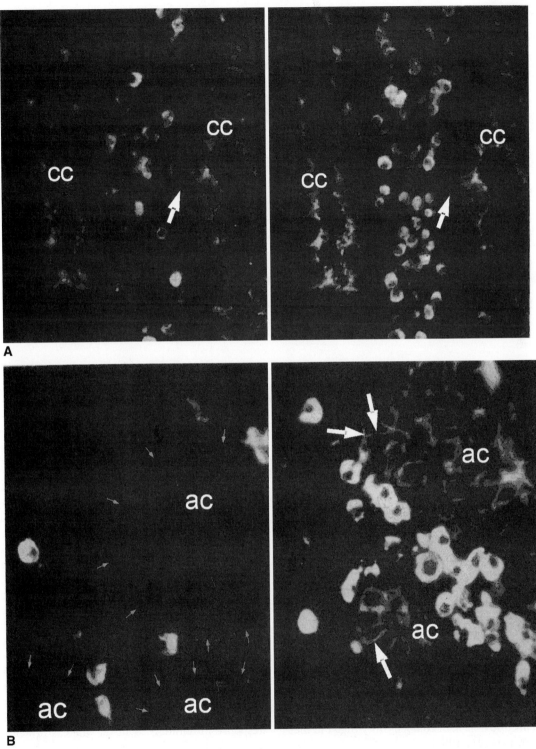

Fig. 32.19. Immunofluorescence localization of **(A)** IgM (*left*) and IgA (*right*) in human intestinal mucosa (paired staining), and **(B)** IgG (*left*) and IgA (*right*) in nasal mucosa (comparable fields). Diffusible extracellular Ig components have been removed from the interstitium and basement membrane zones by extraction of the tissue samples before fixation. Note general dominance of IgA-producing immunocytes. IgA and IgM are present along the basolateral peripheries (*arrows*) and in the cytoplasm of crypt cells (cc) and acinar cells (ac) as a sign of pIgR-mediated export. No such transcytosis takes place for IgG, despite considerable local production of this isotype in nasal mucosa. Original magnification: × 300.

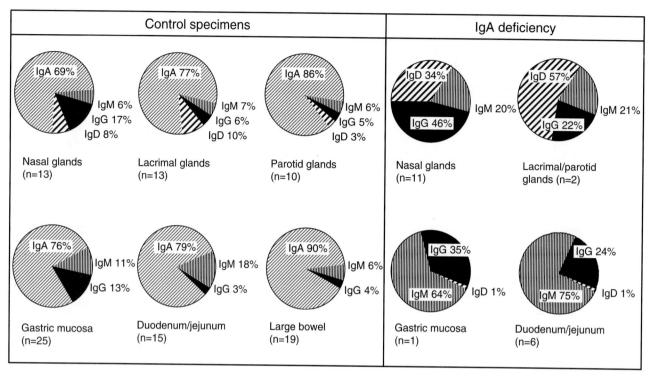

Fig. 32.20. Average percentage distribution of immunocytes producing different Ig classes in various secretory tissues from controls and subjects with IgA deficiency. Based on immunohistochemical data from the authors' laboratory, as referred to in the text.

et al., 1986), may hence reflect the disparate luminal distribution of food antigens *versus* gram-negative bacteria. Bacterial overgrowth in bypassed jejunal segments alters the immunocyte composition with an increase of IgA2 and a decrease of IgM production (Kett *et al.*, 1995), suggesting LPS-induced direct isotype switching from Cμ to Cα2 or progressive sequential downstream switching of the C_H genes (Fig. 32.9).

Disparate isotype distribution of other immunocytes
IgM-producing cells constitute a substantial but variable immunocyte fraction in the adult human gut (Figs. 32.20 and 32.21). The relatively high proportion of this isotype (~18%) in the proximal small intestine may be related to the low levels of LPS (see above) and is in striking contrast to a much lower frequency in the upper aerodigestive tract (Brandtzaeg *et al.*, 1979). This disparity is remarkably accentuated in IgA-deficient patients (Fig. 32.20), who may have clinical problems due to lack of compensatory SIgM in their airways (Brandtzaeg *et al.*, 1987b).

IgG-producing cells normally constitute only 3% to 4% of human intestinal immunocytes, but there is a considerably larger proportion in gastric and nasal mucosae (Fig. 32.20), which often show some low-grade inflammation (Valnes *et al.*, 1986). In IBD, the IgG fraction is dramatically increased (Brandtzaeg *et al.*, 1989; 1992; 1997b). Moreover, although IgA immunocytes remain dominating in both ulcerative colitis and Crohn's disease, the cells are aberrant

by showing an increased IgA1 subclass proportion (Kett and Brandtzaeg, 1987) and decreased J-chain expression (Brandtzaeg and Korsrud, 1984; Kett *et al.*, 1988).

Immunohistochemical studies of human upper airways (Brandtzaeg *et al.*, 1987b) as well as normal jejunal (Nilssen *et al.*, 1991), ileal (Bjerke and Brandtzaeg, 1990b), and colonic (Helgeland *et al.*, 1992) mucosae have demonstrated that IgG1 is the predominating locally produced IgG subclass (56% to 69%), similar to its dominance in serum. However, IgG2 immunocytes are generally more frequent (20% to 35%) than IgG3 cells (4% to 6%) in the distal gut (Fig. 32.11), whereas the reverse is often true in airway mucosae (Brandtzaeg *et al.*, 1987b). Such IgG-subclass disparity supports the idea that isotype-switching pathways may differ in various body regions (Fig. 32.9). It is interesting that the Cγ2 and Cα2 genes are located on the same DNA segment (Flanagan and Rabbits, 1982), and many carbohydrate and bacterial antigens preferentially induce an IgG2 response in addition to IgA2, whereas proteins (which are clearly T cell–dependent antigens) primarily generate IgG1 responses together with IgA1 (Papadea and Check, 1989). Such response differences might be reflected in the variable subclass patterns of intestinal IgA and IgG immunocytes (Figs. 32.10 and 32.11).

IgD-producing cells are only occasionally encountered in the human gut, while they normally constitute a significant fraction (3% to 10%) at secretory sites in the upper aerodigestive tract (Brandtzaeg *et al.*, 1979; 1987b; Korsrud and

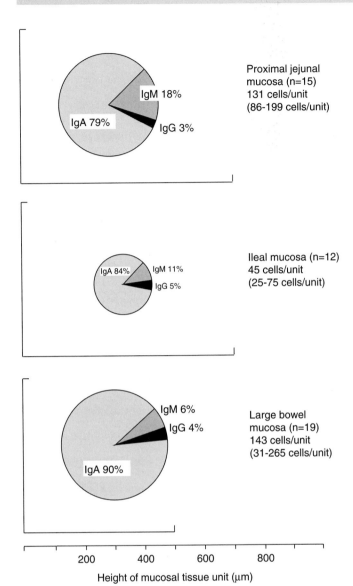

Proximal jejunal
mucosa (n=15)
131 cells/unit
(86-199 cells/unit)

Ileal mucosa (n=12)
45 cells/unit
(25-75 cells/unit)

Large bowel
mucosa (n=19)
143 cells/unit
(31-265 cells/unit)

Height of mucosal tissue unit (μm)

Fig. 32.21. Pie charts depicting average percentage and numerical distribution of immunocytes producing different Ig classes in the normal proximal jejunum, ileum, and large bowel. Median numbers (and observed ranges) of immunocytes (IC) per mucosal tissue unit (see Fig. 32.18) are given on the right. All units are 500-μm wide (*vertical axis*), and the median height (*horizontal axis*) for each specimen category is indicated (n = number of subjects). Based on immunohistochemical data from the authors' laboratory, as referred to in the text.

Brandtzaeg, 1980). In IgA deficiency, this disparity is even more striking for IgD than that noted for IgM immunocytes (Fig. 32.20), which may reflect compartmentalized differences in immune regulation and homing mechanisms (see earlier discussion).

IgE-producing cells are virtually absent from human mucosae, with rare exceptions only in allergic patients, whereas IgE-bearing mast cells are commonly found (Rognum and Brandtzaeg et al., 1989).

J-Chain expression is a characteristic of mucosal immunocytes

To support secretory immunity, MALT must favor the development and dispersion of B cells with prominent expression of J chain, which is a prerequisite for production of pIgA and pentameric IgM that can be exported by the pIgR (Fig. 32.2). Although this peptide is not absolutely required for IgA and IgM polymerization, the cellular expression level of J chain determines the production of dimers *versus* monomers of IgA and of pentamers *versus* J chain-deficient hexamers of IgM (Brandtzaeg, 1985; Brewer *et al.*, 1994; Wiersma *et al.*, 1998; Sørensen *et al.*, 1999; Johansen *et al.*, 2000; Braathen *et al.*, 2002). Notably, only J chain–containing polymers show spontaneous noncovalent interaction with pIgR or its cleaved extracellular portion, the so-called free SC (Brandtzaeg, 1973; 1974b; 1985; Eskeland and Brandtzaeg, 1974; Brandtzaeg and Prydz, 1984; Johansen *et al.*, 2001).

Most IgA1 (~90%) and virtually all IgA2 immunocytes in normal gut mucosa express substantial levels of cytoplasmic J chain (Crago *et al.*, 1984; Kett *et al.*, 1988), and the same is true for IgA immunocytes in other secretory tissues (Brandtzaeg and Korsrud, 1984; Bjerke and Brandtzaeg, 1990a). Most mucosal IgM immunocytes likewise produce J chain (Brandtzaeg, 1983b; 1985). By contrast, IgA immunocytes present in mesenteric and particularly in typical systemic-type lymphoid tissue such as peripheral lymph nodes show a much lower expression level of J chain (Fig. 32.10).

Direct evidence that J chain–positive IgA immunocytes do in fact produce pIgA was first obtained by a binding test on human tissue sections performed with free SC (Brandtzaeg, 1973; 1974b; 1985). Subsequent immunoelectron-microscopical localization of J chain in intestinal IgA immunocytes suggested that the IgA dimerization process begins in the rough endoplasmic reticulum (Nagura *et al.*, 1979), a notion that was supported by similar studies of transformed normal lymphoid cells (Moro *et al.*, 1990).

As discussed earlier (Fig. 32.11), 80% to 90% of the IgG immunocytes in normal intestinal mucosa produce J chain (Brandtzaeg and Korsrud, 1984; Bjerke and Brandtzaeg, 1990a; Nilssen *et al.*, 1992), although it is not secreted from these cells but degraded intracellularly (Mosmann *et al.*, 1978). The same is probably true for J chain produced by mucosal IgD immunocytes, which are almost 100% positive for this polypeptide (Brandtzaeg *et al.*, 1979; Korsrud and Brandtzaeg, 1980; Brandtzaeg, 1983b). We have proposed that J chain–expressing mucosal IgG and IgD immunocytes represent "spin-offs" from MALT-derived early effector B-cell clones during their class switch and differentiation to pIgA production (Brandtzaeg *et al.*, 1999a,b). This notion is strongly supported by the observation (Fig. 32.20) that J chain–positive IgM, IgG, and IgD immunocytes numerically replace the normal immunocyte population in secretory tissues of IgA-deficient subjects (Brandtzaeg *et al.*, 1979; Brandtzaeg and Korsrud, 1984). Thus, differentiation and homing properties reflecting

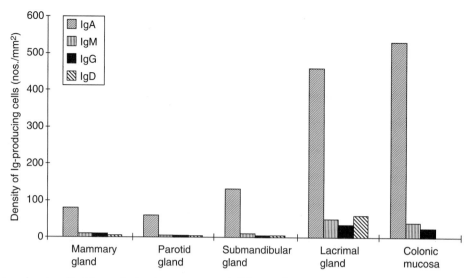

Fig. 32.22. Densities (numbers/mm²) of Ig-producing immunocytes of different classes in tissue sections of various normal human exocrine glands and colonic mucosa, as indicated. Based on immunohistochemical data from the authors' laboratory, as referred to in the text.

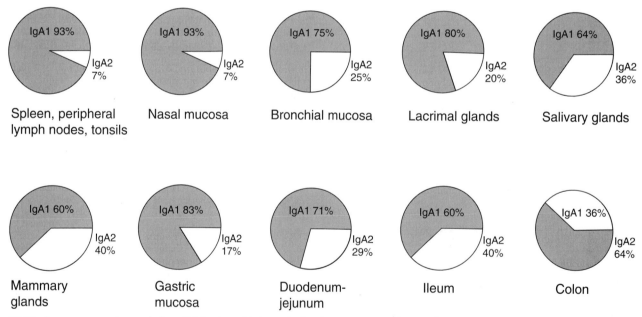

Fig. 32.23. Average percentage subclass distribution of IgA-producing immunocytes in human lymphoid and normal secretory tissues. Based on immunohistochemical data from the authors' laboratory, as referred to in the text, and from Burnett *et al.* (1987) for bronchial mucosa.

a mucosal B-cell phenotype are more closely related to J-chain than to IgA expression *per se*. This is further in keeping with the fact that J-chain expression is dramatically decreased in nonsecretory tissues (Figs. 32.10 and 32.11), the only exception being the mesenteric lymph nodes and germinal centers of MALT structures (see earlier discussion).

ONTOGENY OF MUCOSAL IMMUNOCYTES

Perinatal development

Scattered B and T lymphocytes are seen in the human fetal gut lamina propria from 14 weeks of gestation (Spencer *et al.*, 1986). A few IgM- and IgG-producing cells have been reported to appear somewhat later and remain in small numbers until birth, whereas IgA immunocytes are either absent or extremely rare (Brandtzaeg et al., 1991). By contrast, human fetal salivary glands may contain a few scattered IgA-producing cells, especially after 30 weeks of gestation (Hayashi et al., 1989); approximately 90% of these immunocytes are of the IgA1 subclass, and virtually all express J chain (Thrane et al., 1991). This apparent difference in immunological activation between salivary glands and gut mucosa is intriguing (Brandtzaeg et al., 1991).

GALT is certainly immunocompetent at least during the final trimester, because numerous plasma cells can appear in the intestinal mucosa in response to intrauterine infection (Silverstein and Lukes, 1962). However, very few B-cell blasts with IgA-producing capacity normally circulate in peripheral blood of newborns (<8 per million mononuclear cells), although this number is remarkably increased already after 1 month (~600 per million mononuclear cells), reflecting progressive stimulation of GALT with homing of primed immune cells to mucosal effector sites (Nahmias et al. 1991). Accordingly, a couple of weeks after birth, the numbers of IgA- and IgM-producing cells increase rapidly in the gut (including the appendix) and salivary glands; the IgA class becomes predominant at 1–2 months **(Fig. 32.24)**. For the first 6 months there is often a striking admixture of IgD-producing cells in parotid glands (Thrane et al., 1991), and many infants (about 50%) have detectable IgD in their saliva during the same period (Gleeson et al., 1987). This IgD reaches the secretion by passive diffusion because of increased epithelial permeability in the postnatal period.

During the first 3 months after birth, the IgA1:IgA2 immunocyte ratio in salivary glands approaches the normal adult value of approximately 64:36 (Kett et al., 1986). This change might reflect increased postnatal influx of IgA precursor cells from GALT in the distal gut, where the IgA2 isotype normally predominates (Figs. 32.10 and 32.23). At the same time the high J-chain-expression level (94% to 97%) is maintained for both subclasses of the developing IgA immunocytes (Thrane et al., 1991).

Childhood development

The normal state

At an average age of 15 months (Fig. 32.24), the density of IgA immunocytes in salivary glands has approached the lower normal adult range (Korsrud and Brandtzaeg, 1980), and throughout early childhood, it appears to increase very little (Hayashi et al., 1989). Also the number of intestinal IgA-producing cells has been reported to become fairly stable after 1 year, while IgM-producing cells may decrease (Blanco et al., 1976). However, others have reported a continuing increase of intestinal IgA immunocytes, even after 2 years (Savilahti, 1972; Maffei et al., 1979), although the number is apparently stabilized in the appendix after 5 months (Gebbers and Laissue, 1990). As discussed elsewhere (Brandtzaeg et al., 1991), a faster maturation of the intestinal immune system is usually seen in developing countries with extensive microbial exposure.

Notably, the number of IgG-producing cells becomes quite sizable in the appendix after a few months (Gebbers and Laissue, 1990), reflecting that this subset constitutes almost

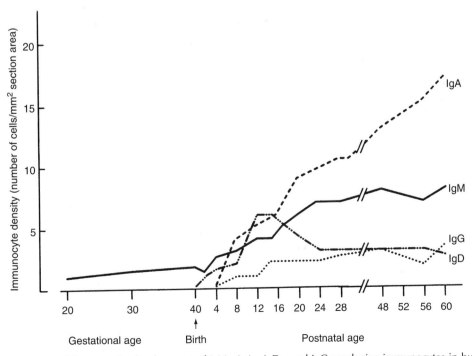

Fig. 32.24. Schematic depiction of the numeric development of IgM-, IgA-, IgD-, and IgG-producing immunocytes in human parotid glands, according to age in weeks. Based on immunohistochemical data from Thrane et al. (1991).

50% of the lamina propria immunocytes adjacent to the numerous lymphoid follicles (Bjerke et al., 1986). As discussed earlier, the markedly downregulated J-chain expression in such GALT-associated lamina propria IgG immunocytes (Fig. 32.12) probably indicates that they belong to exhausted effector clones with decreased potential for migration to distant sites (Fig. 32.8). The potency of a MALT structure to function as a precursor source for the secretory immune system may hence be inversely related to its extrafollicular IgG-cell density, in harmony with the major role suggested for Peyer's patches in mucosal immunity. Clinical data suggest that early appendectomy may protect against subsequent development of ulcerative colitis; perhaps some regional dispersion of IgG precursor cells with specificity for indigenous bacteria may precipitate proinflammatory immune reactions in the large bowel mucosa (Brandtzaeg et al., 1997b). This idea is supported by the observation that appendectomy protects against spontaneous IBD in TCR-α mutant mice (Mizoguchi et al., 1996).

Effect of antigenic exposure

The mucosal antigen load appears to be decisive for the postnatal development of local immunity. The indigenous microbial flora is probably of utmost importance, as suggested by the fact that the intestinal IgA system of germ-free or specific pathogen–free mice is normalized after about 4 weeks of conventionalization (Crabbé et al., 1970; Horsfall et al., 1978). Bacteroides species and Escherichia coli are considered particularly stimulative for the development of intestinal IgA immunocytes (Moreau et al., 1978). Also, antigenic constituents of food probably exert a stimulatory effect (Sagie et al., 1974). It follows that geographic variations have a striking impact on the mucosal immune system. In contrast to the situation in Sweden, infants in a developing country exposed to poliovirus often show substantial salivary levels of SIgA antibodies to this virus as early as 1 month after birth, and these generally approach adult levels by the age of 6 months (Carlsson et al., 1985). In infants heavily exposed to E. coli from birth on, salivary SIgA antibody increases significantly by 2 to 3 weeks of age and rapidly reaches adult levels (Mellander et al., 1985).

Alterations associated with SIDS

The incidence of sudden infant death syndrome (SIDS) is significantly correlated with respiratory viral isolation in the general pediatric population, and it appears to be especially high in cold weather (Milner and Ruggins, 1989). Furthermore, there is evidence of an intensified immune response in the upper aerodigestive tract. Thus, elevated concentrations of IgM and IgA have been found in bronchial lavage fluid from SIDS victims, together with an increased number of the three major immunocyte classes in their interstitial lung tissue (Forsyth et al., 1989). Also, they show overstimulated tonsillar germinal centers, with numerous IgG and IgA immunocytes (Stoltenberg et al., 1995), and activated B cells are apparently distributed to regional effector sites; increased numbers of all the three major immunocyte

classes occur in their parotid glands, on an absolute basis in the order IgA>IgM>IgG (Thrane et al., 1990). The idea of intensified local immunostimulation is supported by the fact that the parotid glands from the same SIDS victims showed enhanced epithelial HLA class II and SC expression (Thrane et al., 1994).

IMPACT OF IMMUNODEFICIENCY ON THE MUCOSAL B-CELL SYSTEM

Selective IgA deficiency and related clinical problems

The activity of the secretory immune system in IgA-deficient subjects is fairly unpredictable on the basis of individual serum IgA levels (Brandtzaeg et al., 1991; Brandtzaeg and Nilssen, 1995). A decreased intestinal IgA:IgM immunocyte ratio reflects immaturity of the secretory immune system and also appears to be a good indicator of a significant IgA deficiency after infancy. Thus, the intestinal IgA immunocyte population is commonly intact when serum IgA concentrations are above 18% of the normal average, while between 5% and 18%, the number of jejunal IgA-producing cells is usually decreased, whereas the IgM subset is increased (Savilahti, 1974). A dichotomy between the immunocyte patterns in jejunal and rectal mucosa is seen in some subjects (Savilahti and Pelkonen, 1979; Brandtzaeg et al., 1981).

Enhanced intestinal production and export of IgM in selective IgA deficiency may partly explain the fact that most subjects with this disorder have no or few gastrointestinal symptoms (Brandtzaeg and Nilssen, 1995); rather, their problems are related to the upper respiratory tract (Brandtzaeg et al., 1987b). In a group of 14 IgA-deficient patients (serum IgA levels <0.1 g/l) who underwent immunohistochemical studies of the jejunal mucosa in this laboratory, celiac disease was diagnosed in two children and four adults (Nilssen et al., 1992); a good response on gluten-free diet was noted in four of them. A few patients suffered from other types of food intolerance, irritable colon, gastric ulcer, atopic eczema, asthmatic bronchitis, or periodic depression. Autoimmune disease was observed in one patient with systemic lupus erythematosus and in another with Reynaud's disease. Malignancies such as gastrointestinal non-Hodgkin's lymphoma occurred later on in one patient. Only few of them suffered from chronic lung disease, except bronchitis, which was quite common; 12 of the patients suffered from recurrent infections, mostly of the upper respiratory tract.

It is interesting that the total number of jejunal IgM- and IgG-producing cells per defined mucosal tissue unit (Fig. 32.18) in subjects who completely lack IgA cells was found to be distributed within a range (40–227 cells/unit) that overlapped with values for the total local immunocyte population in normal controls (86–199 cells/unit) and adults with treated celiac disease (144–335 cells/unit) examined in this laboratory (Brandtzaeg et al., 1979; Nilssen et al., 1992). Also, the IgD, IgG, and IgM immunocyte density in normal parotid tissue from an IgA-deficient subject was within the normal range (29 versus 26–98 cells/mm²), and the same was true in the normal lacrimal gland of another IgA-deficient patient (432 versus 307–789 cells/mm²). Thus, mucosal B cells without IgA-secreting capacity are able to migrate efficiently from MALT to secretory effector sites and undergo local terminal differentiation, apparently because of their CCR10 expression (our unpublished observations). However, the regional isotype difference in the immunocyte replacement, with numerous IgD-producing cells (25%–80%) often occurring in the upper aeroalimentary tract (Fig. 32.20), appears to be of clinical significance. Thus, patients with an abundancy of IgD but relatively few IgM immunocytes in their nasal mucosa were clinically similar to those with no replacement of their lacking IgA immunocytes; they were prone to have upper respiratory tract infections, recurrent tonsillitis, and even pneumonia (Brandtzaeg et al., 1987b).

Immune exclusion is clearly suboptimal also in the intestine of IgA-deficient subjects, because more than half of them have raised levels of IgG antibodies to bovine milk proteins and circulating immune complexes containing such antigens (Cunningham-Rundles et al., 1979; Cunningham-Rundles, 1981). These findings signify increased gastrointestinal permeability, which may explain the relatively high incidence of autoimmunity in IgA deficiency (Cunningham-Rundles et al., 1981). Moreover, the incidence of this deficiency is considerably higher among patients with celiac disease than in the general population (Brandtzaeg and Nilssen, 1995), and food allergy may be associated with a defect of the mucosal IgA system in infancy (Brandtzaeg, 2002).

It is intriguing that up to 40% of the jejunal immunocytes in IgA deficiency may produce IgG without causing overt clinical signs of disturbed mucosal homeostasis (Nilssen et al., 1992). Indeed, the jejunal IgG cells expand more than the IgM cells in response to oral cholera vaccination in IgA-deficient subjects (Nilssen et al., 1993; Friman et al., 1994). Therefore, intestinal SIgM together with IgG antibodies usually afford satisfactory mucosal protection of the gut with preserved local homeostasis in IgA-deficient subjects as long as the innate defense mechanisms and cell-mediated immunity are functioning adequately (McLoughlin et al., 1978). Nevertheless, the proinflammatory properties of IgG antibodies render them potentially deleterious for the epithelial barrier function (Brandtzaeg and Tolo, 1977).

Effect of generalized B Cell deficiency
It is still more intriguing that gastrointestinal disorders are quite rare in patients with infantile X-linked (Bruton-type) B-cell deficiency leading to agammaglobulinemia (Eidelman, 1976; Ochs and Ament, 1976; Brandtzaeg and Nilssen, 1995). Conversely, 20%–50% of the patients with common variable immunodeficiency (hypogammaglobulinemia) develop diarrhea and malabsorption. The intestinal lesions vary over a wide range, from showing more or less villous atrophy to mimicking Crohn's disease. Most likely, the common intestinal-disease diagnoses should generally not be applied in these cases because immunodeficiency apparently by "imitation" may result in a variety of mucosal lesions.

The intestinal mucosa of patients with generalized B-cell deficiency contains no or very little interstitial IgG unless substitution therapy has been given (Brandtzaeg, 1974c; Brandtzaeg and Baklien, 1976). However, some mucosal plasma cells (mainly of the IgM class) are often seen in hypogammaglobulinemia (Brandtzaeg, 1974c; Broom et al., 1975), particularly associated with solitary lymphoid follicles (see next paragraph). The expression of pIgR/SC shows a normal epithelial distribution (Brandtzaeg and Baklien, 1976), so the small amounts of locally produced IgM may contribute to immune exclusion. It appears paradoxical, therefore, that hypogammaglobulinemic patients often have strikingly raised levels of bovine milk proteins in their blood, whereas the agammaglobulinemic ones reportedly do not have higher than normal levels (Cunningham-Rundles et al., 1984).

Some patients with hypogammaglobulinemia who present with diarrhea have a markedly increased number of ILFs in their gastrointestinal mucosa, mainly in the small intestine (Eidelman, 1976). These follicles contain a distinct mantle zone of sIgD⁺IgM⁺ naïve B lymphocytes. The B-cell maturation defect is to some extent overcome under the influence of antigens from the lumen, as signified by the development of a few IgM-producing immunocytes between the follicles and the surface epithelium. It is possible that such nodular lymphoid hyperplasia reflects immune stimulation due to an excessive influx of antigens from the lumen (Cunningham-Rundles et al., 1984), but there is no apparent relationship between this mode of reaction and the development of intestinal B-cell (MALT) lymphoma.

CONCLUSIONS

The mucosal immune system is quantitatively the most important activated B-cell system of the body. Indeed, secretory tissues contain more than 80% of all Ig-producing cells, and the major product of these immunocytes is normally pIgA with associated J chain. It is well established that the human mucosal B-cell system responds to an infection with local IgA and IgM production (Söltoft and Söberg, 1972). The level of this response appears to determine whether clinical symptoms will occur or not (Agus et al., 1974; Brandtzaeg and Johansen, 2003). However, there are many open questions regarding the nature and regulation of this large antibody system (Johansen and Brandtzaeg, 2004). Mechanistic information about mucosal B cells is to a great extent based on animal experiments, with the inherent problem of species differences. The following facts and puzzles related to the human secretory antibody system can be listed.

- Secretory immunity depends on an intimate cooperation between mucosal B cells and exocrine epithelia. The biological significance of the striking J-chain expression shown by MALT-derived immunocytes dispersed to secretory effector sites is thus that pIgA and pentameric IgM with high affinity for pIgR are produced locally and become readily available for export to the mucosal surface. This important functional goal in terms of clonal differentiation appears to explain why J chain is also expressed by mucosal B cells terminating their differentiation with IgG or IgD production; such immunocytes may be considered "spin-offs" from early effector clones that, through class switch, are on their way to pIgA production.

- There is considerable evidence to support the notion that intestinal immunocytes are largely derived from B cells initially induced in GALT. However, there is insufficient knowledge concerning the relative importance of M cells, MHC class II–expressing epithelial cells, B cells, and other professional APCs in the transport, processing, and presentation of luminal antigens that take place in GALT to accomplish the extensive and continuous priming and expansion of mucosal B cells. Also, it is not clear how the germinal-center reaction in GALT so strikingly promotes class switch to IgA and expression of J chain.

- Although the B-cell migration to the intestinal lamina propria is guided by rather well-defined adhesion molecules and chemokines/chemokine receptors, better definition of chemotactic stimuli determining homing mechanisms in different segments of the gut is required. This is even more true for homing of mucosal B cells to secretory effector sites beyond the gut, and in this respect the role of Waldeyer's ring as a regional inductive tissue needs further characterization.

- In addition to homing molecules, retention and accumulation of B cells extravasated at secretory effector sites are influenced by antigen-driven local proliferation and differentiation. However, the role of cognate T cells, MHC class II–expressing APCs, and epithelial cells in providing the necessary stimulatory signals remains poorly defined.

- Compartmentalization of the mucosal immune system must be taken into account in the development of effective local vaccines to protect the airways, the eyes, the oral cavity, and the urogenital tract. Even without employing the classic gut-homing receptors, selective migration of putative early effector B-cell clones with preferential expression of J chain and pIgA is just as remarkable to secretory tissues in the upper aerodigestive tract as to the intestinal lamina propria. It is hoped that future studies will help to elucidate the complexity of molecular mechanisms underlying this basic principle of secretory immunity.

- It is also important to point out that clinical observations in immunodeficient patients have shown that S-IgA, S-IgM, and IgG antibodies are not the only important components of the mucosal immune system. Evidence is accumulating that innate defense mechanisms are much more crucial and complex than previously believed. The cooperation between innate and adaptive immunity needs to be further explored to enable better understanding of how the homeostasis of mucous membranes is normally maintained.

ACKNOWLEDGMENTS

Studies in the authors' laboratory are supported by the University of Oslo, Norwegian Cancer Society, Research Council of Norway, Anders Jahres Fund, and Otto Kr. Bruun's Legacy. Ms. Hege Eliassen and Mr. Erik Kulø Hagen are gratefully acknowledged for excellent assistance with the manuscript.

REFERENCES

Abitorabi, M.A., Mackay, C.R., Jerome, E.H., Osorio, O., Butcher, E.C., and Erle, D.J. (1996). Differential expression of homing molecules on recirculating lymphocytes from sheep gut, peripheral, and lung lymph. *J. Immunol.* 156, 3111–3117.

Agematsu, K., Hokibara, S., Nagumo, H., and Komiyama, A. (2000). CD27: a memory B-cell marker. *Immunol. Today* 21, 204–206.

Agus, S.G., Falchuk, Z.M., Sessoms, C.S., Wyatt, R.G., and Dolin, R. (1974). Increased jejunal IgA synthesis in vitro during acute infectious non-bacterial gastroenteritis. *Am. J. Dig. Dis.* 19, 127–131.

Ahmed, R., and Gray, D. (1996). Immunological memory and protective immunity: understanding their relation. *Science* 272, 54–60.

Ansel, K.M., Ngo, V.N., Hyman, P.L., Luther, S.A., Forster, R., Sedgwick, J.D., Browning, J.L., Lipp, M., and Cyster, J.G. (2000). A chemokine-driven positive feedback loop organizes lymphoid follicles. *Nature* 406, 309–314.

Arpin, C., Banchereau, J., and Liu, Y.J. (1997). Memory B cells are biased towards terminal differentiation: a strategy that may prevent repertoire freezing. *J. Exp. Med.* 186, 931–940.

Arpin, C., de Bouteiller, O., Razanajaona, D., Fugier-Vivier, I., Briere, F., Banchereau, J., Lebecque, S., and Liu, Y.J. (1998). The normal counterpart of IgD myeloma cells in germinal center displays extensively mutated IgVH gene, Cμ-Cδ switch, and λ light chain expression. *J. Exp. Med.* 187, 1169–1178.

Baggiolini, M. (1998). Chemokines and leukocyte traffic. *Nature* 392, 565–568.

Baekkevold, E.S., Yamanaka, T., Palframan, R.T., Carlsen, H.S., Reinholt, F.P., von Andrian, U.H., Brandtzaeg, P., and Haraldsen, G. (2001). The CCR7 ligand ELC (CCL19) is transcytosed in high endothelial venules and mediates T cell recruitment. *J. Exp. Med.* 193, 1105–1111.

Bentley, A.M., Durham, S.R., Robinson, D.S., Menz, G., Storz, C., Cromwell, O., Kay, A.B., and Wardlaw, A.J. (1993). Expression of endothelial and leukocyte adhesion molecules, intercellular adhesion molecule-1, E-selectin, and vascular cell adhesion molecule-1 in the bronchial mucosa in steady-state and allergen-induced asthma. *J. Allergy Clin. Immunol.* 92, 857–868.

Berg, E.L., McEvoy, L.M., Berlin, C., Bargatze, R.F., and Butcher, E.C. (1993). L-selectin-mediated lymphocyte rolling on MAdCAM-1. *Nature* 366, 695–698.

Berlin, C., Bargatze, R.F., Campbell, J.J., von Andrian, U.H., Szabo, M.C., Hasslen, S.R., Nelson, R.D., Berg, E.L., Erlandsen, S.L., and Butcher, E.C. (1995). α4 integrins mediate lymphocyte attachment and rolling under physiologic flow. *Cell* 80, 413–422.

Bjerke, K., and Brandtzaeg, P. (1986). Immunoglobulin- and J-chain-producing cells associated with the lymphoid follicles of human appendix, colon and ileum, including the Peyer's patches. *Clin. Exp. Immunol.* 64, 432–441.

Bjerke, K., and Brandtzaeg, P. (1988). Lack of relation between expression of HLA-DR and secretory component (SC) in follicle-associated epithelium of human Peyer's patches. *Clin. Exp. Immunol.* 71, 502–507.

Bjerke, K., and Brandtzaeg, P. (1990a). Terminally differentiated human intestinal B cells. J chain expression of IgA and IgG subclass-producing immunocytes in the distal ileum compared with mesenteric and peripheral lymph nodes. *Clin. Exp. Immunol.* 82, 411–415.

Bjerke, K., and Brandtzaeg, P. (1990b). Terminally differentiated human intestinal B cells. IgA and IgG subclass-producing immunocytes in the distal ileum, including Peyer's patches, compared with lymph nodes and palatine tonsils. *Scand. J. Immunol.* 32, 61–67.

Bjerke, K., Brandtzaeg, P., and Rognum, T.O. (1986). Distribution of immunoglobulin producing cells is different in normal human appendix and colon mucosa. *Gut* 27, 667–674.

Bjerke, K., Halstensen, T.S., Jahnsen, F., Pulford, K., and Brandtzaeg, P. (1993). Distribution of macrophages and granulocytes expressing L1 protein (calprotectin) in human Peyer's patches compared with normal ileal lamina propria and mesenteric lymph nodes. *Gut* 34, 1357–1363.

Blanco, A., Linares, P., Andion, R., Alonso, M., and Villares, E.S. (1976). Development of humoral immunity system of the small bowel. *Allergol. Immunopathol.* 4, 235–240.

Bleul, C.C., Schultze, J.L., and Springer, T.A. (1998). B lymphocyte chemotaxis regulated in association with microanatomic localization, differentiation state, and B cell receptor engagement. *J. Exp. Med.* 187, 753–762.

Bode, U., Wonigeit, K., Pabst, R., and Westermann, J. (1997). The fate of activated T cells migrating through the body: rescue from apoptosis in the tissue of origin. *Eur. J. Immunol.* 27, 2087–2093.

Boirivant, M., Fais, S., Annibale, B., Agostini, D., Delle Fave G., and Pallone F. (1994). Vasoactive intestinal polypeptide modulates the in vitro immunoglobulin A production by intestinal lamina propria lymphocytes. *Gastroenterology* 106, 576–582.

Bos, N.A., Bun, J.C., Popma, S.H., Cebra, E.R., Deenen, G.J., van der Cammen, M.J., Kroese, F.G., and Cebra, J.J. (1996). Monoclonal immunoglobulin A derived from peritoneal B cells is encoded by both germ line and somatically mutated VH genes and is reactive with commensal bacteria. *Infect. Immun.* 64, 616–623.

Boursier, L., Farstad, I.N., Mellembakken, J.R., Brandtzaeg, P., and Spencer, J. (2002). IgVH gene analysis suggests that peritoneal B cells do not contribute to the gut immune system in man. *Eur. J. Immunol.* 32, 2427–2436.

Bouvet, J.P., and Fischetti, V.A. (1999). Diversity of antibody-mediated immunity at the mucosal barrier. *Infect. Immun.* 67, 2687–2691.

Bowman, E.P., Kuklin, N.A., Youngman, K.R., Lazarus, N.H., Kunkel, E.J., Pan, J., Greenberg, H.B., and Butcher, E.C. (2002). The intestinal chemokine thymus-expressed chemokine (CCL25) attracts IgA antibody-secreting cells. *J. Exp. Med.* 195, 269–275.

Braathen, R., Sørensen, V., Brandtzaeg, P., Sandlie, I., and Johansen, F.-E. (2002). The carboxyl-terminal domains of IgA and IgM direct isotype-specific polymerization and interaction with the polymeric immunoglobulin receptor. *J. Biol. Chem.* 277, 42755–42762.

Bradley, L.M., and Watson, S.R. (1996). Lymphocyte migration into tissue: the paradigm derived from CD4 subsets. *Curr. Opin. Immunol.* 8, 312–320.

Brandtzaeg, P. (1973). Two types of IgA immunocytes in man. *Nature New Biol.* 243, 142–143.

Brandtzaeg, P. (1974a). Mucosal and glandular distribution of immunoglobulin components. Differential localization of free and bound SC in secretory epithelial cells. *J. Immunol.* 112, 1553–1559.

Brandtzaeg, P. (1974b). Presence of J chain in human immunocytes containing various immunoglobulin classes. *Nature* 252, 418–420.

Brandtzaeg, P. (1974c). Mucosal and glandular distribution of immunoglobulin components. Immunohistochemistry with a cold ethanol-fixation technique. *Immunology* 26, 1101–1114.

Brandtzaeg, P. (1976). Studies on J chain and binding site for secretory component in circulating human B cells. II. The cytoplasm. *Clin. Exp. Immunol.* 25, 59–66.

Brandtzaeg, P. (1977). Human secretory component. VI. Immunoglobulin-binding properties. *Immunochemistry* 14, 179–188.

Brandtzaeg, P. (1982). Tissue preparation methods for immunohistochemistry. In *Techniques in Immunocytochemistry* (eds. G.R. Bullock and P. Petrusz), Vol. 1, 1-75. London: Academic Press.

Brandtzaeg, P. (1983a). The secretory immune system of lactating human mammary glands compared with other exocrine organs. *Ann. N.Y. Acad. Sci.* 409, 353–381.

Brandtzaeg, P. (1983b). Immunohistochemical characterization of intracellular J-chain and binding site for secretory component (SC) in human immunoglobulin (Ig)-producing cells. *Mol. Immunol.* 20, 941–966.

Brandtzaeg, P. (1985). Role of J chain and secretory component in receptor-mediated glandular and hepatic transport of immunoglobulins in man. *Scand. J. Immunol.* 22, 111–146.

Brandtzaeg, P. (1987). Immune functions and immunopathology of palatine and nasopharyngeal tonsils. In *Immunology of the Ear* (eds. J.M. Bernstein and P.L. Ogra), 63-106. New York: Raven Press.

Brandtzaeg, P. (1997). Mucosal immunity in the female genital tract. *J. Reprod. Immunol.* 36, 23–50.

Brandtzaeg, P. (1998). The increasing power of immunohistochemistry and immunocytochemistry. *J. Immunol. Meth.* 216, 49–67.

Brandtzaeg, P. (1999). Regionalized immune function of tonsils and adenoids. *Immunol. Today* 20, 383–384.

Brandtzaeg, P. (2002). Current understanding of gastrointestinal immunoregulation and its relation to food allergy. *Ann. N.Y. Acad. Sci.* 964, 13–45.

Brandtzaeg, P., and Baklien, K. (1976). Immunohistochemical studies of the formation and epithelial transport of immunoglobulins in normal and diseased human intestinal mucosa. *Scand. J. Gastroenterol.* 11 (Suppl. 36), 1–45.

Brandtzaeg, P., and Halstensen, T.S. (1992). Immunology and immunopathology of tonsils. *Adv. Otorhinolaryngol.* 47, 64–75.

Brandtzaeg, P., and Johansen, F.-E. (2003). Immunology of the gut. In *Perspectives in Medical Virology* (eds. A.J. Zuckerman and L.K. Mushahwar). *Viral Gastroenteritis* (eds. U. Desselberger and J. Gray), 69–91. Amsterdam: Elsevier.

Brandtzaeg, P., and Korsrud, F.R. (1984). Significance of different J chain profiles in human tissues: generation of IgA and IgM with binding site for secretory component is related to the J chain expressing capacity of the total local immunocyte population, including IgG and IgD producing cells, and depends on the clinical state of the tissue. *Clin. Exp. Immunol.* 58, 709–718.

Brandtzaeg, P., and Nilssen, D.E. (1995). Mucosal aspects of primary B-cell deficiency and gastrointestinal infections. *Curr. Opin. Gastroenterol.* 11, 532–540.

Brandtzaeg, P., and Prydz, H. (1984). Direct evidence for an integrated function of J chain and secretory component in epithelial transport of immunoglobulins. *Nature* 311, 71–73.

Brandtzaeg, P., and Tolo, K. (1977). Mucosal penetrability enhanced by serum-derived antibodies. *Nature* 266, 262–263.

Brandtzaeg, P., Gjeruldsen, S.T., Korsrud, F., Baklien, K., Berdal, P., and Ek, J. (1979). The human secretory immune system shows striking heterogeneity with regard to involvement of J chain positive IgD immunocytes. *J. Immunol.* 122, 503–510.

Brandtzaeg, P., Guy-Grand, D., and Griscelli, C. (1981). Intestinal, salivary, and tonsillar IgA and J-chain production in a patient with severe deficiency of serum IgA. *Scand. J. Immunol.* 13, 313–325.

Brandtzaeg, P., Baklien, K., Bjerke, K., Rognum, T.O., Scott, H., and Valnes, K. (1987a). Nature and properties of the human gastrointestinal immune system. In *Immunology of the Gastrointestinal Tract*, Vol. I (eds. K. Miller and S. Nicklin), 1-86. Boca Raton, Florida: CRC Press.

Brandtzaeg, P., Karlsson, G., Hansson, G., Petruson, B., Björkander, J., and Hanson, L.Å. (1987b). The clinical condition of IgA-deficient patients is related to the proportion of IgD- and IgM-producing cells in their nasal mucosa. *Clin. Exp. Immunol.* 67, 626–636.

Brandtzaeg, P., Halstensen, T. S., Kett, K., Krajci, P., Kvale, D., Rognum, T. O., Scott, H., and Sollid, L. M. (1989). Immunobiology and immunopathology of human gut mucosa: humoral immunity and intraepithelial lymphocytes. *Gastroenterology* 97, 1562–1584.

Brandtzaeg, P., Nilssen, D.E., Rognum, T.O., and Thrane, P.S. (1991). Ontogeny of the mucosal immune system and IgA deficiency. *Gastroenterol. Clin. North Am.* 20, 397–439.

Brandtzaeg, P., Halstensen, T.S., Helgeland, L., and Kett, K. (1992). The mucosal immune system in inflammatory bowel disease. In *Immunology of Gastrointestinal Disease* (ed. T.T. MacDonald), 19-39. London: Kluwer Academic Publishers.

Brandtzaeg, P., Halstensen, T.S., Huitfeldt, H., and Valnes, K. (1997a). Immunofluorescence and immunoenzyme histochemistry. In *Immunochemistry 2: A Practical Approach* (eds. A.P. Johnstone and M.W. Turner), 71-130. Oxford: Oxford University Press.

Brandtzaeg, P., Haraldsen, G., and Rugtveit, J. (1997b). Immunopathology of human inflammatory bowel disease. *Springer Semin. Immunopathol.* 18, 555–589.

Brandtzaeg, P., Farstad, I.N., Johansen, F.-E., Morton, H.C., Norderhaug, I.N., and Yamanaka, T. (1999a). The B-cell system of human mucosae and exocrine glands. *Immunol. Rev.* 171, 45–87.

Brandtzaeg, P., Baekkevold, E.S., Farstad, I.N., Jahnsen, F.L., Johansen, F.-E., Nilsen, E.M., and Yamanaka, T. (1999b). Regional specialization in the mucosal immune system: what happens in the microcompartments? *Immunol. Today* 20, 141–151.

Brandtzaeg, P., Farstad, I.N., and Haraldsen, G. (1999c). Regional specialization in the mucosal immune system: primed cells do not always home along the same track. *Immunol. Today* 20, 267–277.

Brandtzaeg, P., Baekkevold, E.S., and Morton, H.C. (2001). From B to A the mucosal way. *Nat. Immunol.* 2, 1093–1094.

Brandtzaeg, P., Johansen, F.-E., Baekkevold, E.S., and Farstad, I.N. (2002). Direct tracking of mucosal B-cell migration in humans reveals distinct effector-site differences. 11th International Congress of Mucosal Immunology (ICMI), Orlando, Florida. *Mucosal Immunology Update 10*, abstract 2476.

Breitfeld, D., Ohl, L., Kremmer, E., Ellwart, J., Sallusto, F., Lipp, M., and Forster, R. (2000). Follicular B helper T cells express CXC chemokine receptor 5, localize to B cell follicles, and support immunoglobulin production. *J. Exp. Med.* 192, 1545–1552.

Brewer, J.W., Randall, T.D., Parkhouse, R.M., and Corley, R.B. (1994). IgM hexamers? *Immunol. Today* 15, 165–168.

Briére, F., Bridon, J.M., Chevet, D., Souillet, G., Bienvenu, F., Guret, C., Martinez-Valdez, H., and Bancheereau, J. (1994). Interleukin 10 induces B lymphocytes from IgA-deficient patients to secrete IgA. *J. Clin. Invest.* 94, 97–104.

Broom, B.C., de la Concha, E.G., Webster, A.D., Loewi, G., and Asherson, G.L. (1975). Dichotomy between immunoglobulin synthesis by cells in gut and blood of patients with hypogamma-globulinaemia. *Lancet* 2, 253–256.

Burnett, D., Crocker, J., and Stockley, R.A. (1987). Cells containing IgA subclasses in bronchi of subjects with and without chronic obstructive lung disease. *Clin. Pathol.* 40, 1217–1220.

Butcher, E.C., and Picker, L.J. (1996). Lymphocyte homing and homeostasis. *Science* 272, 60–66.

Campbell, D.J., and Butcher, E.C. (2002). Rapid acquisition of tissue-specific homing phenotypes by CD4⁺ T cells activated in cutaneous or mucosal lymphoid tissues. *J. Exp. Med.* 195, 135–141.

Campbell, J.J., Bowman, E.P., Murphy, K., Youngman, K.R., Siani, M.A., Thompson, D.A., Wu, L., Zlotnik, A., and Butcher, E.C. (1998). 6-C-kine (SLC), a lymphocyte adhesion-triggering chemokine expressed by high endothelium, is an agonist for the MIP-3beta receptor CCR7. *J. Cell. Biol.* 141, 1053–1059.

Carlsen, H.S., Baekkevold, E.S., Johansen, F.-E., Haraldsen, G., and Brandtzaeg, P. (2002). B cell attracting chemokine 1 (CXCL13) and its receptor CXCR5 are expressed in normal and aberrant gut associated lymphoid tissue. *Gut* 51, 364–371.

Carlsen, H.S., Baekkevold, E.S., Morton, H.C., Haraldsen, G., and Brandtzaeg, P. (2004). Monocyte-like and mature macrophages produce CXCL13 (B-cell-attracting chemokine 1) in inflammatory lesions with lymphoid neogenesis. *Blood* (prepublished online July 29, 2004; DOI 10.1182/blood-2004-02-0701).

Carlsson, B., Zaman, S., Mellander, L., Jalil, F., and Hanson, L.A. (1985). Secretory and serum immunoglobulin class-specific antibodies to poliovirus after vaccination. *J. Infect. Dis.* 152, 1238–1244.

Carsetti, R., Kohler, G., and Lamers, M.C. (1993). A role for immunoglobulin D: interference with tolerance induction. *Eur. J. Immunol.* 23, 168–178.

Cazac, B.B., and Roes, J. (2000). TGF-β receptor controls B cell responsiveness and induction of IgA in vivo. *Immunity* 13, 443–451.

Chambers, C.A., and Allison, J.P. (1997). Co-stimulation in T cell responses. *Curr. Opin. Immunol.* 9, 396–404.

Chaplin, D.D., and Fu, Y. (1998). Cytokine regulation of secondary lymphoid organ development. *Curr. Opin. Immunol.* 10, 289–297.

Chen, Y., Inobe, J., Marks, R., Gonnella, P., Kuchroo, V.K., and Weiner, H.L. (1995). Peripheral deletion of antigen-reactive T cells in oral tolerance. *Nature* 376, 177–180.

Conley, M.E., and Bartelt, M.S. (1984). In vitro regulation of IgA subclass synthesis. II. The source of IgA2 plasma cells. *J. Immunol.* 133, 2312–2316.

Cornes, J.S. (1965). Number, size and distribution of Peyer's patches in the human small intestine. *Gut* 6, 225–233.

Crabbé, P.A., Nash, D.R., Bazin, H., Eyssen, H., and Heremans JF. (1970). Immunohistochemical observations on lymphoid tissues from conventional and germ-free mice. *Lab. Invest.* 22, 448–457.

Crago, S.S., Kutteh, W.H., Moro, I., Allansmith, M.R., Radl, J., Haaijman, J.J., and Mestecky, J. (1984). Distribution of IgA1-, IgA2-, and J chain-containing cells in human tissues. *J. Immunol.* 132, 16–18.

Craig, S.W., and Cebra, J.J. (1971). Peyer's patches: an enriched source of precursors for IgA-producing immunocytes in the rabbit. *J. Exp. Med.* 134, 188–200.

Cunningham-Rundles, C. (1981). The identification of specific antigens in circulating immune complexes by an enzyme-linked immunosorbent assay: detection of bovine κ-casein IgG complexes in human sera. *Eur. J. Immunol.* 11, 504–509.

Cunningham-Rundles, C., Brandeis, W.E., Good, R.A., and Day, N.K. (1979). Bovine antigens and the formation of circulating immune complexes in selective immunoglobulin A deficiency. *J. Clin. Invest.* 64, 272–279.

Cunningham-Rundles, C., Carr, R.I., and Good, R.A. (1984). Dietary protein antigenemia in humoral immunodeficiency. Correlation with splenomegaly. *Am. J. Med.* 76, 181–185

Cyster, J.G. (1999). Chemokines and cell migration in secondary lymphoid organs. *Science* 286, 2098–2102.

Dahlenborg, K., Pound, J.D., Gordon, J., Borrebaeck, C.A., and Carlsson, R. (1997). Terminal differentiation of human germinal center B cells in vitro. *Cell Immunol.* 175, 141–149.

Defrance, T., Vanbervliet, B., Briere, F., Durand, I., Rousset, F., and Bancheereau, J. (1992). Interleukin 10 and transforming growth factor beta cooperate to induce anti-CD40-activated naive human B cells to secrete immunoglobulin A. *J. Exp. Med.* 175, 671–682.

Denis, V., Dupuis, P., Bizouarne, N., de O Sampaio, S., Hong, L., Lebret, M., Monsigny, M., Nakache, M., and Kieda, C. (1996). Selective induction of peripheral and mucosal endothelial cell addressins with peripheral lymph nodes and Peyer's patch cell-conditioned media. *J. Leukoc. Biol.* 60, 744–752.

Dunkley, M.L., and Husband, A.J. (1990-91). The role of non-B cells in localizing an IgA plasma cell response in the intestine. *Reg. Immunol.* 3, 336–340.

Dunn-Walters, D.K., Boursier, L., and Spencer, J. (1997a). Hypermutation, diversity and dissemination of human intestinal lamina propria plasma cells. *Eur. J. Immunol.* 27, 2959–2964.

Dunn-Walters, D.K., Isaacson, P.G., and Spencer, J. (1997b). Sequence analysis of human IgVH genes indicates that ileal lamina propria plasma cells are derived from Peyer's patches. *Eur. J. Immunol.* 27, 463–467.

Ehrenstein, M.R., O'Keefe, T.L., Davies, S.L., and Neuberger, M.S. (1998). Targeted gene disruption reveals a role for natural secretory IgM in the maturation of the primary immune response. *Proc. Natl. Acad. Sci. USA* 95, 10089–10093.

Eidelman, S. (1976). Intestinal lesions in immune deficiency. *Hum. Pathol.* 7, 427–434.

Endres, R., Alimzhanov, M.B., Plitz, T., Futterer, A., Kosco-Vilbois, M.H., Nedospasov, S.A., Rajewsky, K., and Pfeffer, K. (1999). Mature follicular dendritic cell networks depend on expression of lymphotoxin β receptor by radioresistant stromal cells and of lymphotoxin β and tumor necrosis factor by B cells. *J. Exp. Med.* 189, 159–168.

Eriksson, K., Quiding-Järbrink, M., Osek, J., Moller, A., Björk, S., Holmgren, J., and Czerkinsky, C. (1998). Specific-antibody-secreting cells in the rectums and genital tracts of nonhuman primates following vaccination. *Infect. Immun.* 66, 5889–5896.

Eskeland, T., and Brandtzaeg, P. (1974). Does J chain mediate the combination of 19S IgM and dimeric IgA with the secretory component rather than being necessary for their polymerization? *Immunochemistry* 11, 161–163.

Fagarasan, S., and Honjo, T. (2000). T-Independent immune response: new aspects of B cell biology. *Science* 290, 89–92.

Fagarasan, S., and Honjo, T. (2003). Intestinal IgA synthesis: regulation of front-line body defences. *Nat. Rev. Immunol.* 3, 63–72.

Fagarasan, S., Kinoshita, K., Muramatsu, M., Ikuta, K., and Honjo, T. (2001). In situ class switching and differentiation to IgA-producing cells in the gut lamina propria. *Nature* 413, 639–643.

Fagarasan, S., Muramatsu, M., Suzuki, K., Nagaoka, H., Hiai, H., and Honjo, T. (2002). Critical roles of activation-induced cytidine deaminase in the homeostasis of gut flora. *Science.* 298: 1424–1427.

Farstad, I.N., Halstensen, T.S., Fausa, O., and Brandtzaeg, P. (1994). Heterogeneity of M-cell-associated B and T cells in human Peyer's patches. *Immunology* 83, 457–464.

Farstad, I.N., Halstensen, T.S., Lazarovits, A.I., Norstein, J., Fausa, O., and Brandtzaeg, P. (1995). Human intestinal B-cell blasts and plasma cells express the mucosal homing receptor integrin α4β7. *Scand. J. Immunol.* 42, 662–672.

Farstad, I.N., Halstensen, T.S., Lien, B., Kilshaw, P.J., Lazarovits, A.I., and Brandtzaeg, P. (1996). Distribution of β7 integrins in human intestinal mucosa and organized gut-associated lymphoid tissue. *Immunology* 89, 227–237.

Farstad, I.N., Halstensen, T.S., Kvale, D., Fausa, O., and Brandtzaeg, P. (1997a). Topographic distribution of homing receptors on B and T cells in human gut-associated lymphoid tissue. Relation of L-selectin and integrin α 4β7 to naive and memory phenotypes. *Am. J. Pathol.* 150, 187–199.

Farstad, I.N., Norstein, J., and Brandtzaeg, P. (1997b). Phenotypes of B and T cells in human intestinal and mesenteric lymph. *Gastroenterology* 112, 163–173.

Farstad, I.N., Carlsen, H., Morton, H.C., and Brandtzaeg, P. (2000). Immunoglobulin A cell distribution in the human small intestine: phenotypic and functional characteristics. *Immunology* 101, 354–363.

Fayette, J., Dubois, B., Vandenabeele, S., Bridon, J.M., Vanbervliet, B., Durand, I., Bancherau, J., Caux, C., and Briere, F. (1997). Human dendritic cells skew isotype switching of CD40-activated naive B cells towards IgA1 and IgA2. *J. Exp. Med.* 185, 1909–1918.

Feltelius, N., Hvatum, M., Brandtzaeg, P., Knutson, L., and Hällgren, R. (1994). Increased jejunal secretory IgA and IgM in ankylosing spondylitis: normalization after treatment with sulfasalazine. *J. Rheumatol.* 21, 2076–2081.

Fischer, M., and Kuppers, R. (1998). Human IgA- and IgM-secreting intestinal plasma cells carry heavily mutated V$_H$ region genes. *Eur. J. Immunol.* 28, 2971–2977.

Flanagan, J.G., and Rabbitts, T.H. (1982). Arrangement of human immunoglobulin heavy chain constant region genes implies evolutionary duplication of a segment containing γ, ε and α genes. *Nature* 300, 709–713.

Förster, R., Mattis, A.E., Kremmer, E., Wolf, E., Brem, G., and Lipp, M. (1996). A putative chemokine receptor, BLR1, directs B cell migration to defined lymphoid organs and specific anatomic compartments of the spleen. *Cell* 87, 1037–1047.

Forsyth, K.D., Weeks S.C., Koh, L., Skinner, J., and Bradley, J. (1989). Lung immunoglobulins in the sudden infant death syndrome. *Br. Med. J.* 298, 23–26.

Fossum, S., Rolstad, B., and Tjernshaugen, H. (1979). Selective loss of S-phase cells when making cell suspensions from lymphoid tissue. *Cell. Immunol.* 48, 149–154.

Friman, V., Quiding, M., Czerkinsky, C., Nordström, I., Larsson, L., Ericson, D., Björkander, J., Theman, K., Kilander, A., Holmgren, J., *et al.* (1994). Intestinal and circulating antibody-forming cells in IgA-deficient individuals after oral cholera vaccination. *Clin. Exp. Immunol.* 95, 222–226.

Fu, Y.X., Huang, G., Wang, Y., and Chaplin, D.D. (1998). B lymphocytes induce the formation of follicular dendritic cell clusters in a lymphotoxin α-dependent fashion. *J. Exp. Med.* 187, 1009–1018.

Fujihashi, K., McGhee, J.R., Lue, C., Beagley, K.W., Taga, T., Hirano, T., Kishimoto, T., Mestecky, J., and Kiyono, H. (1991). Human appendix B cells naturally express receptors for and respond to

interleukin 6 with selective IgA1 and IgA2 synthesis. *J. Clin. Invest.* 88, 248–252.

Fujisaka, M., Ohtani, O., and Watanabe, Y. (1996). Distribution of lymphatics in human palatine tonsils: a study by enzyme-histochemistry and scanning electron microscopy of lymphatic corrosion casts. *Arch. Histol. Cytol.* 59, 273–280.

Fukuyama, S., Hiroi, T., Yokota, Y., Rennert, P.D., Yanagita, M., Kinoshita, N., Terawaki, S., Shikina, T., Yamamoto, M., Kurono, Y., and Kiyono, H. (2002). Initiation of NALT organogenesis is independent of the IL-7R, LTβR, and NIK signaling pathways but requires the Id2 gene and CD3⁻CD4⁺CD45⁺ cells. *Immunity* 17, 31–40.

Garside, P., Ingulli, E., Merica, R.R., Johnson, J.G., Noelle, R.J., and Jenkins, M.K. (1998). Visualization of specific B and T lymphocyte interactions in the lymph node. *Science* 281, 96–99.

Gebbers, J.-O., and Laissue, J.A. (1990). Postnatal immunomorphology of the gut. In *Inflammatory Bowel Disease and Coeliac Disease in Children* (eds. F. Hadziselimovic, B. Herzog, and A. Bürgin-Wolff), 3–44. Dordrecht: Kluwer Academic Publishers.

Gleeson, M., Cripps, A.W., Clancy, R.L., Wlodarczyk, J.D., and Hensley, M.J. (1987). IgD in infant saliva. *Scand. J. Immunol.* 26, 55–57.

Gommerman, J.L., Mackay, F., Donskoy, E., Meier, W., Martin, P., and Browning, J.L. (2002). Manipulation of lymphoid microenvironments in nonhuman primates by an inhibitor of the lymphotoxin pathway. *J. Clin. Invest.* 110, 1359–1369.

Gonzalez, M., Mackay, F., Kosco-Vilbois, M.H., and Noelle. R.J. (1998). The sequential role of lymphotoxin and B cells in the development of splenic follicles. *J. Exp. Med.* 187, 997–1007.

Gowans, J.L., and Knight, E.J. (1964). The route of re-circulation of lymphocytes in the rat. *Proc. R. Soc. London, Ser. B* 159, 257–282.

Grouard, G., Durand, I., Filgueira, L., Banchereau, J., Liu, Y.-J. (1996). Dendritic cells capable of stimulating T cells in germinal centres. *Nature* 384, 364–367.

Gunn, M.D., Ngo, V.N., Ansel, K.M., Ekland, E.H., Cyster, J.G., and Williams, L.T. (1998a). A B-cell-homing chemokine made in lymphoid follicles activates Burkitt's lymphoma receptor-1. *Nature* 391, 799–803.

Gunn, M.D., Tangemann, K., Tam, C., Cyster, J.G., Rosen, S.D., and Williams, L.T. (1998b). A chemokine expressed in lymphoid high endothelial venules promotes the adhesion and chemotaxis of naive T lymphocytes. *Proc. Natl. Acad. Sci. USA* 95, 258–263.

Gütgemann, I., Fahrer, A.M., Altman, J.D., Davis, M.M., and Chien, Y.H. (1998). Induction of rapid T cell activation and tolerance by systemic presentation of an orally administered antigen. *Immunity* 8, 667–673.

Guy-Grand, D., Griscelli, C., and Vassalli, P. (1974). The gut-associated lymphoid system: nature and properties of the large dividing cells. *Eur. J. Immunol.* 4, 435–443.

Hajdu, I., Moldoveanu, Z., Cooper, M.D., Mestecky, J. (1983). Ultrastructural studies of human lymphoid cells: μ and J chain expression as a function of B cell differentiation. *J. Exp. Med.* 158, 1993–2006.

Hall, J.G., and Smith, M.E. (1970). Homing of lymph-borne immunoblasts to the gut. *Nature* 226, 262–263.

Halstead, T.E., and Hall, J.G. (1972). The homing of lymph-borne immunoblasts to the small gut of neonatal rats. *Transplantation* 14, 339–346.

Hamada, H., Hiroi, T., Nishiyama, Y., Takahashi, H., Masunaga, Y., Hachimura, S., Kaminogawa, S., Takahashi-Iwanaga, H., Iwanaga, T., Kiyono, H., Yamamoto, H., and Ishikawa, H. (2002). Identification of multiple isolated lymphoid follicles on the antimesenteric wall of the mouse small intestine. *J. Immunol.* 168, 57–64.

Hauer, A.C., Bajaj-Elliott, M., Williams, C.B., Walker-Smith, J.A., and MacDonald, T.T. (1998). An analysis of interferon γ, IL-4, IL-5 and IL-10 production by ELISPOT and quantitative reverse transcriptase-PCR in human Peyer's patches. *Cytokine* 10, 627–634.

Hayashi, Y., Kurashima, C., Takemura, T., and Hirokawa, K. (1989). Ontogenic development of the secretory immune system in human fetal salivary glands. *Pathol. Immunopathol. Res.* 8, 314–320.

Helgeland, L., Tysk, C., Järnerot, G., Kett, K., Lindberg, E., Danielsson, D., Andersen, S.N., and Brandtzaeg, P. (1992). The IgG subclass distribution in serum and rectal mucosa of monozygotic twins with or without inflammatory bowel disease. *Gut* 33, 1358–1364.

Hiroi, T., Yanagita, M., Ohta, N., Sakaue, G., and Kiyono, H. (2000). IL-15 and IL-15 receptor selectively regulate differentiation of common mucosal immune system-independent B-1 cells for IgA responses. *J. Immunol.* 165, 4329–4337.

Hopkins, S., Kraehenbuhl, J.P., Schodel, F., Potts, A., Peterson, D., de Grandi, P., and Nardelli-Haefliger, D. (1995). A recombinant *Salmonella typhimurium* vaccine induces local immunity by four different routes of immunization. *Infect. Immun.* 63, 3279–3286.

Horsfall, D.J., Cooper, J.M., and Rowley, D. (1978). Changes in the immunoglobulin levels of the mouse gut and serum during conventionalisation and following administration of Salmonella typhimurium. *Aust. J. Exp. Biol. Med. Sci.* 56, 727–735.

Husband, A.J. (1982). Kinetics of extravasation and redistribution of IgA-specific antibody-containing cells in the intestine. *J. Immunol.* 128, 1355–1359.

Inoue, H., Fukuizumi, T., Tsujisawa, T., and Uchiyama, C. (1999). Simultaneous induction of specific immunoglobulin A-producing cells in major and minor salivary glands after tonsillar application of antigen in rabbits. *Oral Microbiol. Immunol.* 14, 21–26.

Irjala, H., Elima, K., Johansson, E.L., Merinen, M., Kontula, K., Alanen, K., Grenman, R., Salmi, M., and Jalkanen, S. (2003). The same endothelial receptor controls lymphocyte traffic both in vascular and lymphatic vessels. *Eur. J. Immunol.* 33, 815–824.

Jahnsen, F.L., Haraldsen, G., Aanesen, J.P., Haye, R., and Brandtzaeg, P. (1995). Eosinophil infiltration is related to increased expression of vascular cell adhesion molecule-1 in nasal polyps. *Am. J. Respir. Cell Molec. Biol.* 12, 624–632.

Jahnsen, F.L., Gran, E., Haye, R., and Brandtzaeg, P. (2004). Human nasal mucosa contains antigen-presenting cells of strikingly different functional phenotypes. *Am. J. Respir. Cell Mol.* 30, 31–37.

Janson, H., Hedén, L.-O., Grubb, A., Ruan, M., and Forsgren, A. (1991). Protein D, an immunoglobulin D-binding protein of *Haemophilus influenzae*: cloning, nucleotide sequence, and expression in *Escherichia coli*. *Infect. Immun.* 59, 119–125.

Johansen, F.-E., Braathen, R., and Brandtzaeg, P. (2000). Role of J chain in secretory immunoglobulin formation. *Scand. J. Immunol.* 52, 240–248.

Johansen, F.-E. and Brandtzaeg, P. (2004). Transcriptional regulation of the mucosal IgA system. *Trends Immunol.* 25, 150–157.

Johansen, F.-E., Braathen, R., and Brandtzaeg, P. (2001). The J chain is essential for polymeric Ig receptor-mediated epithelial transport of IgA. *J. Immunol.* 167, 5185–5192.

Johansson, E.L., Wassén, L., Holmgren, J., Jertborn, M., and Rudin, A. (2001). Nasal and vaginal vaccinations have differential effects on antibody responses in vaginal and cervical secretions in humans. *Infect. Immun.* 69, 7481–7486.

Jonard, P.P., Rambaud, J.C., Dive, C., Vaerman, J.P., Galian, A., and Delacroix, D.L. (1984). Secretion of immunoglobulins and plasma proteins from the jejunal mucosa. Transport rate and origin of polymeric immunoglobulin A. *J. Clin. Invest.* 74, 525–535.

Jung, J., Choe, J., Li, L., and Choi, Y.S. (2000). Regulation of CD27 expression in the course of germinal center B cell differentiation: the pivotal role of IL-10. *Eur. J. Immunol.* 30, 2437–2443.

Kang, C.J., Sheridan, C., and Koshland, M.E. (1998). A stage-specific enhancer of immunoglobulin J chain gene is induced by interleukin-2 in a presecretor B cell stage. *Immunity* 8, 285–295.

Kang, H.S., Chin, R.K., Wang, Y., Yu, P., Wang, J., Newell, K.A., and Fu, Y.X. (2002). Signaling via LTβR on the lamina propria stromal cells of the gut is required for IgA production. *Nat. Immunol.* 3, 576–582.

Kantele, J.M., Arvilommi, H., Kontiainen, S., Salmi, M., Jalkanen, S., Savilahti, E., Westerholm, M., and Kantele, A. (1996). Mucosally activated circulating human B cells in diarrhea express homing receptors directing them back to the gut. *Gastroenterology* 110, 1061–1067.

Kantele, A., Kantele, J.M., Savilahti, E., Westerholm, M., Arvilommi, H., Lazarovits, A., Butcher, E.C., and Makela, P.H. (1997). Homing potentials of circulating lymphocytes in humans depend on the site of activation: oral, but not parenteral, typhoid vaccination induces circulating antibody-secreting cells that all bear homing receptors directing them to the gut. *J. Immunol.* 158, 574–579.

Kantele, A., Hakkinen, M., Moldoveanu, Z., Lu, A., Savilahti, E., Alvarez, R.D., Michalek, S., and Mestecky, J. (1998). Differences in immune responses induced by oral and rectal immunizations with *Salmonella typhi* Ty21a: evidence for compartmentalization within the common mucosal immune system in humans. *Infect. Immun.* 66, 5630–5635.

Kapasi, Z.F., Qin, D., Kerr, W.G., Kosco-Vilbois, M.H., Shultz, L.D., Tew, J.G., and Szakal, A.K. (1998). Follicular dendritic cell (FDC) precursors in primary lymphoid tissues. *J. Immunol.* 160, 1078–1084.

Kernéis, S., Bogdanova, A., Kraehenbuhl, J.-P., and Pringault, E. (1997). Conversion by Peyer's patch lymphocytes of human enterocytes into M cells that transport bacteria. *Science* 277, 949–952.

Kett, K., and Brandtzaeg, P. (1987). Local IgA subclass alterations in ulcerative colitis and Crohn's disease of the colon. *Gut* 28, 1013–1021.

Kett, K., Brandtzaeg, P., Radl, J., and Haaijman, J.J. (1986). Different subclass distribution of IgA-producing cells in human lymphoid organs and various secretory tissues. *J. Immunol.* 136, 3631–3635.

Kett, K., Brandtzaeg, P., and Fausa, O. (1988). J-chain expression is more prominent in immunoglobulin A2 than in immunoglobulin A1 colonic immunocytes and is decreased in both subclasses associated with inflammatory bowel disease. *Gastroenterology* 94, 1419–1425.

Kett, K., Baklien, K., Bakken, A., Kral, J.G., Fausa, O., and Brandtzaeg, P. (1995). Intestinal B-cell isotype response in relation to local bacterial load: evidence for immunoglobulin A subclass adaptation. *Gastroenterology* 109, 819–825.

Kilian, M., Reinholdt, J., Lomholt, H., Poulsen, K., and Frandsen, E.V. (1996). Biological significance of IgA1 proteases in bacterial colonization and pathogenesis: critical evaluation of experimental evidence. *APMIS* 104, 321–338.

Kim, C.H., Rott, L.S., Clark-Lewis, I., Campbell, D.J., Wu, L., and Butcher, E.C. (2001). Subspecialization of CXCR5+ T cells: B helper activity is focused in a germinal center-localized subset of CXCR5+ T cells. *J. Exp. Med.* 193, 1373–1381.

Kimata, H., and Fujimoto, M. (1995). Induction of IgA1 and IgA2 production in immature human fetal B cells and pre-B cells by vasoactive intestinal peptide. *Blood* 85, 2098–2104.

Kinoshita, K., and Honjo, T. (2001). Linking class-switch recombination with somatic hypermutation. *Nat. Rev. Mol. Cell. Biol.* 2, 493–503.

Korsrud, F.R., and Brandtzaeg, P. (1980). Quantitative immunohistochemistry of immunoglobulin- and J-chain-producing cells in human parotid and submandibular glands. *Immunology* 39, 129–140.

Korsrud, F.R., and Brandtzaeg, P. (1981a). Immunohistochemical evaluation of J-chain expression by intra- and extra-follicular immunoglobulin-producing human tonsillar cells. *Scand. J. Immunol.* 13, 271–280.

Korsrud, F.R., and Brandtzaeg, P. (1981b). Influence of tonsillar disease on the expression of J-chain by immunoglobulin-producing cells in human palatine and nasopharyngeal tonsils. *Scand. J. Immunol.* 13, 281–287.

Kremmidiotis, G., and Zola, H. (1995). Changes in CD44 expression during B cell differentiation in the human tonsil. *Cell. Immunol.* 161, 147–157.

Kroese, F.G., Butcher, E.C., Stall, A.M., Lalor, P.A., Adams, S., and Herzenberg, L.A. (1989). Many of the IgA producing plasma cells in murine gut are derived from self-replenishing precursors in the peritoneal cavity. *Int. Immunol.* 1, 75–84.

Kubagawa, H., Burrows, P. D., Grossi, C. E., Mestecky, J., and Cooper, M. D. (1988). Precursor B cells transformed by Epstein-Barr virus undergo sterile plasma-cell differentiation: J-chain expression without immunoglobulin. *Proc. Natl. Acad. Sci. USA* 85, 875–879.

Kunkel, E.J., and Butcher, E.C. (2002). Chemokines and the tissue-specific migration of lymphocytes. *Immunity* 16, 1–4.

Kunkel, E.J., Campbell, J.J., Haraldsen, G., Pan, J., Boisvert, J., Roberts, A.I., Ebert, E.C., Vierra, M.A., Goodman, S.B., Genovese, M.C., Wardlaw, A.J., Greenberg, H.B., Parker, C.M., Butcher, E.C., Andrew, D.P., and Agace, W.W. (2000). Lymphocyte CC chemokine receptor 9 and epithelial thymus-expressed chemokine (TECK) expression distinguish the small intestinal immune compartment: Epithelial expression of tissue-specific chemokines as an organizing principle in regional immunity. *J. Exp. Med.* 192, 761–768.

Kunkel, E.J., Kim, C.H., Lazarus, N.H., Vierra, M.A., Soler, D., Bowman, E.P., and Butcher, E.C. (2003). CCR10 expression is a common feature of circulating and mucosal epithelial tissue IgA Ab-secreting cells. *J. Clin. Invest.* 111, 1001–1010.

Kuper, C.F., Koornstra, P.J., Hameleers, D.M.H., Biewenga, J., Spit, B.J., Duijvestijn, A.M., van Breda Vriesman, P.J., and Sminia, T. (1992). The role of nasopharyngeal lymphoid tissue. *Immunol. Today* 13, 219–224.

Lamm, M.E. (1976). Cellular aspects of immunoglobulin A. *Adv. Immunol.* 22, 223–290.

Lange S, Nygren H, Svennerholm A-M, Holmgren J. Antitoxic cholera immunity in mice: influence of antigen deposition on antitoxin-containing cells and protective immunity in different parts of the intestine. *Infect. Immun.* 1980; 28: 17–23.

Lebecque, S., de Bouteiller, O., Arpin, C., Banchereau, J., and Liu, Y.-J. (1997). Germinal center founder cells display propensity for apoptosis before onset of somatic mutation. *J. Exp. Med.* 185, 563–571.

Legler DF, Loetscher M, Roos RS, Clark-Lewis I, Baggiolini M, Moser B. (1998) B cell-attracting chemokine 1, a human CXC chemokine expressed in lymphoid tissues, selectively attracts B lymphocytes via BLR1/CXCR5. *J. Exp. Med.* 187: 655–660.

Lindhout E, Koopman G, Pals ST, de Groot C. (1997) Triple check for antigen specificity of B cells during germinal centre reactions. *Immunol. Today* 18: 573–577.

Litinskiy, M.B., Nardelli, B., Hilbert, D.M., He, B., Schaffer, A., Casali, P., and Cerutti, A. (2002). DCs induce CD40-independent immunoglobulin class switching through BLyS and APRIL. *Nat. Immunol.* 3, 822–829.

Liu, Y.-J., and Arpin, C. (1997). Germinal center development. *Immunol. Rev.* 156, 111–126.

Liu Y.-J., Barthélémy C., de Bouteiller O., Arpin C., Durand I., and Banchereau J. (1995). Memory B cells from human tonsils colonize mucosal epithelium and directly present antigen to T cells by rapid up-regulation of B7-1 and B7-2. *Immunity* 2, 239–248.

Liu, Y.-J., Arpin, C., de Bouteiller, O., Guret, C., Banchereau, J., Martinez-Valdez, H., and Lebecque, S. (1996). Sequential triggering of apoptosis, somatic mutation and isotype switch during germinal center development. *Sem. Immunol.* 8, 169–177.

Luther, S.A., Lopez, T., Bai, W., Hanahan, D., and Cyster, J.G. (2000). BLC expression in pancreatic islets causes B cell recruitment and lymphotoxin-dependent lymphoid neogenesis. *Immunity* 12, 471–481.

MacDonald, T.T., and Monteleone, G. (2001). IL-12 and Th1 immune responses in human Peyer's patches. *Trends Immunol.* 22, 244–247.

Mackay, F., and Browning, J.L. (2002). BAFF: a fundamental survival factor for B cells. *Nature Rev. Immunol.* 2, 465–475.

MacLennan, I.C.M. (1994). Germinal centers. *Annu. Rev. Immunol.* 12, 117–139.

MacLennan, I.C.M., Gulbranson-Judge, A., Toellner, K.M., Casamayor-Palleja, M., Chan, E., Sze, D.M., Luther, S.A., and Orbea, H.A. (1997). The changing preference of T and B cells for partners as T-dependent antibody responses develop. *Immunol. Rev.* 156, 53–66.

Macpherson, A.J., Gatto, D., Sainsbury, E., Harriman, G.R., Hengartner, H., and Zinkernagel, R.M. (2000). A primitive T cell-independent mechanism of intestinal mucosal IgA responses to commensal bacteria. *Science* 288, 2222–2226.

Macpherson, A.J., Lamarre, A., McCoy, K., Harriman, G.R., Odermatt, B., Dougan, G., Hengartner, H., and Zinkernagel, R.M. (2001). IgA production without mu or delta chain expression in developing B cells. *Nat. Immunol.* 2, 625–631.

Maffei, H.V.L., Kingston, D., Hill, I.D., and Shiner, M. (1979). Histopathologic changes and the immune response within the jejunal mucosa in infants and children. *Pediatr. Res.* 13, 733–736.

Mamula, M.J., and Janeway, C.A. (1993). Do B cells drive the diversification of immune responses? *Immunol. Today* 14, 151–152.

Matis, L.A., Glimcher, L.H., Paul, W.E., and Schwartz, R.H. (1983). Magnitude of response of histocompatibility-restricted T-cell clones is a function of the product of the concentrations of antigen and Ia molecules. *Proc. Natl. Acad. Sci. USA* 80, 6019–6023.

Max, E.E., and Korsmeyer, S.J. (1985). Human J chain gene. Structure and expression in B lymphoid cells. *J. Exp. Med.* 161, 832–849.

Mayrhofer, G., and Fisher, R. (1979). IgA-containing plasma cells in the lamina propria of the gut: failure of a thoracic duct fistula to deplete the numbers in rat small intestine. *Eur. J. Immunol.* 9, 85–91.

McCune, J.M., Fu, S.M., and Kunkel, H.G. (1981). J chain biosynthesis in pre-B cells and other possible precursor B cells. *J. Exp. Med.* 154, 138–145.

McDermott, M.R., and Bienenstock, J. (1979). Evidence for a common mucosal immunologic system. I. Migration of B immunoblasts into intestinal, respiratory, and genital tissues. *J. Immunol.* 122, 1892–1898.

McLoughlin, G.A., Hede, J.E., Temple, J.G., Bradley, J., Chapman, D.M., and McFarland, J. (1978). The role of IgA in the prevention of bacterial colonization of the jejunum in the vagotomized subject. *Br. J. Surg.* 65, 435–437.

McWilliams, M., Phillips-Quagliata, J.M., and Lamm, M.E. (1977). Mesenteric lymph node B lymphoblasts which home to the small intestine are precommitted to IgA synthesis. *J. Exp. Med.* 145, 866–875.

Mellander, L., Carlsson, B., Jalil, F., Soderstrom, T., and Hanson, L.A. (1985). Secretory IgA antibody response against Escherichia coli antigens in infants in relation to exposure. *J. Pediatr.* 107, 430–433.

Merville, P., Dechanet, J., Desmouliere, A., Durand, I., de Bouteiller, O., Garrone, P., Banchereau, J., and Liu, Y.J. (1996). Bcl-2+ tonsillar plasma cells are rescued from apoptosis by bone marrow fibroblasts. *J. Exp. Med.* 183, 227–236.

Mestecky, J., and Russell, M.W. (1986). IgA subclasses. *Monogr. Allergy* 19, 277–301.

Mestecky, J., and McGhee, J.R. (1987). Immunoglobulin A (IgA): Molecular and cellular interactions involved in IgA biosynthesis and immune response. *Adv. Immunol.* 40, 153–245.

Milner, A.D., and Ruggins, M. (1989). Sudden infant death syndrome. Recent focus on the respiratory system. *Br. Med. J.* 298, 689–690.

Mizoguchi, A., Mizoguchi, E., Chiba, C., and Bhan, A.K. (1996). Role of appendix in the development of inflammatory bowel disease in TCR-alpha mutant mice. *J. Exp. Med.* 184, 707–715.

Moghaddami, M., Cummins, A., and Mayrhofer, G. (1998). Lymphocyte-filled villi: comparison with other lymphoid aggregations in the mucosa of the human small intestine. *Gastroenterology* 115, 1414–1425.

Moreau, M.C., Ducluzeau, R., Guy-Grand, D., and Muller, M.C. (1978). Increase in the population of duodenal immunoglobulin A plasmocytes in axenic mice associated with different living or dead bacterial strains of intestinal origin. *Infect. Immun.* 121, 532–539.

Moro, I., Iwase, T., Komiyama, K., Moldoveanu, Z., and Mestecky, J. (1990). Immunoglobulin A (IgA) polymerization sites in human immunocytes: immunoelectron microscopic study. *Cell Struct. Funct.* 15, 85–91.

Moser, B., and Loetscher, P. (2001). Lymphocyte traffic control by chemokines. *Nat. Immunol.* 2, 123–128.

Moser, B., Schaerli, P., and Loetscher, P. (2002). CXCR5+ T cells: follicular homing takes center stage in T-helper-cell responses. *Trends Immunol.* 23, 250–254.

Mosmann, T.R., Gravel, Y., Williamson, A. R., and Baumal, R. (1978). Modification and fate of J chain in myeloma cells in the presence and absence of polymeric immunoglobulin secretion. *Eur. J. Immunol.* 8, 94–101.

Müller, F., Frøland, S. S., Hvatum, M., Radl, J., and Brandtzaeg, P. (1991). Both IgA subclasses are reduced in parotid saliva from patients with AIDS. *Clin. Exp. Immunol.* 83, 203–209.

Nadal, D., Albini, B., Chen, C.Y., Schläpfer, E., Bernstein, J.M., and Ogra, P.L. (1991). Distribution and engraftment patterns of human tonsillar mononuclear cells and immunoglobulin-secreting cells in mice with severe combined immunodeficiency: role of the Epstein-Barr virus. *Int. Arch. Allergy Appl. Immunol.* 95, 341–351.

Nagura, H., Brandtzaeg, P., Nakane, P. K., and Brown, W. R. (1979). Ultrastructural localization of J chain in human intestinal mucosa. *J. Immunol.* 23, 1044–1050.

Nahmias, A., Stoll, B., Hale, E., Ibegbu, C., Keyserling, H., Innis-Whitehouse, W., Holmes, R., Spira, T., Czerkinsky, C., and Lee, F. (1991). IgA-secreting cells in the blood of premature and term infants: normal development and effect of intrauterine infections. *Adv. Exp. Med. Biol.* 310, 59–69.

Neutra, M.R., Mantis, N.J., and Kraehenbuhl, J.P. (2001). Collaboration of epithelial cells with organized mucosal lymphoid tissues. *Nat. Immunol.* 2, 1004–1009.

Newberry, R.D., McDonough, J.S., McDonald, K.G., and Lorenz, R.G. (2002). Postgestational lymphotoxin/lymphotoxin beta receptor interactions are essential for the presence of intestinal B lymphocytes. *J. Immunol.* 168, 4988–4997.

Newman, R.A., Ormerod, M.G., and Greaves, M.F. (1980). The presence of HLA-DR antigens on lactating human breast epithelium and milk fat globule membranes. *Clin. Exp. Immunol.* 41, 478–486.

Nilsen, E.M., Lundin, K.E.A., Krajci, P., Scott, H., Sollid, L.M., and Brandtzaeg, P. (1995). Gluten-specific, HLA-DQ restricted T cells from coeliac mucosa produce cytokines with Th1 or Th0 profile dominated by interferon γ. *Gut* 37, 766–776.

Nilssen, D. E., Söderström, R., Brandtzaeg, P., Kett, K., Helgeland, L., Karlsson, G., Söderström, T., and Hanson, L. Å. (1991). Isotype distribution of mucosal IgG-producing cells in patients with various IgG-subclass deficiencies. *Clin. Exp. Immunol.* 83, 17–24.

Nilssen, D. E., Brandtzaeg, P., Frøland, S. S., and Fausa, O. (1992). Subclass composition and J-chain expression of the "compensatory" IgG-cell population in selective IgA deficiency. *Clin. Exp. Immunol.* 87, 237–245.

Nilssen, D.E., Friman, V., Theman, K., Björkander, J., Kilander, A., Holmgren, J., Hanson, L.Å., and Brandtzaeg, P. (1993). B-cell activation in duodenal mucosa after oral cholera vaccination in IgA deficient subjects with or without IgG subclass deficiency. *Scand. J. Immunol.* 38, 201–208.

Ochs, H.D., and Ament, M.E. (1976). Gastrointestinal tract and immunodeficiency. In *Immunological Aspects of the Liver and Gastrointestinal Tract* (eds. A. Ferguson and R.N.M. MacSween), 82–120. Lancaster: MTP Press.

Ogra, P.L., and Karzon, D.T. (1970). The role of immunoglobulins in the mechanism of mucosal immunity to virus infection. *Pediatr. Clin. North Am.* 17, 385–400.

Okada, T., Ngo, V.N., Ekland, E.H., Forster, R., Lipp, M., Littman, D.R., and Cyster, J.G. (2002). Chemokine requirements for B cell entry to lymph nodes and Peyer's patches. *J. Exp. Med.* 196, 65–75.

O'Leary, A.D., and Sweeney, E.C. (1986). Lymphoglandular complexes of the colon: structure and distribution. *Histopathology* 10, 267–283.

Pachynski, R.K., Wu, S.W., Gunn, M.D., and Erle, D.J. (1998). Secondary lymphoid-tissue chemokine (SLC) stimulates integrin α4β7-mediated adhesion of lymphocytes to mucosal addressin cell adhesion molecule-1 (MAdCAM-1) under flow. *J. Immunol.* 161, 952–956.

Pan, J., Kunkel, E.J., Gosslar, U., Lazarus, N., Langdon, P., Broadwell, K., Vierra, M.A., Genovese, M.C., Butcher, E.C., Soler, D. (2000). A novel chemokine ligand for CCR10 and CCR3 expressed by epithelial cells in mucosal tissues. *J. Immunol.* 165, 2943–2949.

Papadakis, K.A., Prehn, J., Nelson, V., Cheng, L., Binder, S.W., Ponath, P.D., Andrew, D.P., and Targan, S.R. (2000). The role of thymus-expressed chemokine and its receptor CCR9 on lymphocytes in the regional specialization of the mucosal immune system. *J. Immunol.* 165, 5069–5076.

Papadea, C., and Check, I.J. (1989). Human immunoglobulin G and immunoglobulin G subclasses: biochemical, genetic, and clinical aspects. *Crit. Rev. Clin. Lab. Sci.* 27, 27–58.

Parkhouse, R.M.E., and Cooper, M.D. (1977). A model for the differentiation of B lymphocytes with implications for the biological role of IgD. *Immunol. Rev.* 37, 105–126.

Parrott, D.M. (1976). The gut as a lymphoid organ. *Clin. Gastroenterol.* 5, 211–228.

Parrott, D.M., and Ferguson, A. (1974). Selective migration of lymphocytes within the mouse small intestine. *Immunology* 26, 571–588.

Pascual, D.W., Xu-Amano, J.C., Kiyono, H., McGhee, J.R., and Bost, K.L. (1991). Substance P acts directly upon cloned B lymphoma cells to enhance IgA and IgM production. *J. Immunol.* 146, 2130–2136.

Penn, N. D., Purkins, L, Kelleher, J., Heatley, R. V., and Mascie-Taylor, B. H. (1991). Ageing and duodenal mucosal immunity. *Age Ageing* 20, 33–36.

Perry, M., and Whyte, A. (1998). Immunology of the tonsils. *Immunol. Today* 19, 414–421.

Persson, C.G., Erjefält, J.S., Greiff, L., Erjefält, I., Korsgren, M., Linden, M., Sundler, F., Andersson, M., and Svensson, C. (1998). Contribution of plasma-derived molecules to mucosal immune defence, disease and repair in the airways. *Scand. J. Immunol.* 47, 302–313.

Picker, L.J., Martin, R.J., Trumble, A., Newman, L.S., Collins, P.A., Bergstresser, P.R., and Leung, D.Y.M. (1994). Differential expression of lymphocyte homing receptors by human memory/effector T cells in pulmonary versus cutaneous immune effector sites. *Eur. J. Immunol.* 24, 1269–1277.

Pierce, N.F., and Gowans, J.L. (1975). Cellular kinetics of the intestinal immune response to cholera toxoid in rats. *J. Exp. Med.* 142, 1550–1563.

Pulendran, B., van Driel, R., and Nossal, G.J.V. (1997). Immunological tolerance in germinal centres. *Immunol. Today* 18, 27–32.

Quiding-Järbrink, M., Lakew, M., Nordström, I., Banchereau, J., Butcher, E., Holmgren, J., and Czerkinsky, C. (1995a). Human circulating specific antibody-forming cells after systemic and mucosal immunizations: differential homing commitments and cell surface differentiation markers. *Eur. J. Immunol.* 25, 322–327.

Quiding-Järbrink, M., Granström, G., Nordström, I., Holmgren, J., and Czerkinsky, C. (1995b). Induction of compartmentalized B-cell responses in human tonsils. *Infect. Immun.* 63, 853–857.

Quiding-Järbrink, M., Nordström, I., Granström, G., Kilander, A., Jertborn, M., Butcher, E.C., Lazarovits, A.I., Holmgren, J., and Czerkinsky, C. (1997). Differential expression of tissue-specific adhesion molecules on human circulating antibody-forming cells after systemic, enteric, and nasal immunizations. A molecular basis for the compartmentalization of effector B cell responses. *J. Clin. Invest.* 99, 1281–1286.

Randall, T.D., Parkhouse, R.M.E., and Corley, R.B. (1992). J chain synthesis and secretion of hexameric IgM is differentially regulated by lipolysaccharide and interleukin 5. *Proc. Natl. Acad. Sci. USA* 89, 962–966.

Randall, T.D., Heath, A.W., Santos-Argumedo, L., Howard, M.C., Weissman, I.L., and Lund, F.E. (1998). Arrest of B lymphocyte terminal differentiation by CD40 signaling: mechanism for lack of antibody-secreting cells in germinal centers. *Immunity* 8, 733–742.

Rao, S., Karray, S., Gackstetter, E.R., and Koshland, M.E. (1998). Myocyte enhancer factor-related B-MEF2 is developmentally expressed in B cells and regulates the immunoglobulin J chain promoter. *J. Biol. Chem.* 273, 26123–26129.

Reif, K., Ekland, E.H., Ohl, L., Nakano, H., Lipp, M., Forster, R., and Cyster, J.G. (2002). Balanced responsiveness to chemoattractants from adjacent zones determines B-cell position. *Nature* 416, 94–99.

Rescigno, M., Urbano, M., Valzasina, B., Francolini, M., Rotta, G., Bonasio, R., Granucci, F., Kraehenbuhl, J.P., and Ricciardi-Castagnoli, P. (2001). Dendritic cells express tight junction proteins and penetrate gut epithelial monolayers to sample bacteria. *Nat. Immunol.* 2, 361–367.

Rognum, T.O., and Brandtzaeg, P. (1989). IgE-positive cells in human intestinal mucosa are mainly mast cells. *Int. Arch. Allergy Appl. Immunol.* 89, 256–260.

Rott, L.S., Briskin, M.J., Andrew, D.P., Berg, E.L., and Butcher, E.C. (1996). A fundamental subdivision of circulating lymphocytes defined by adhesion to mucosal addressin cell adhesion molecule-1. Comparison with vascular cell adhesion molecule-1 and correlation with β7 integrins and memory differentiation. *J. Immunol.* 156, 3727–3736.

Roux, M.E., McWilliams, M., Phillips-Quagliata, J.M., Weisz-Carrington, P., and Lamm, M.E. (1977). Origin of IgA-secreting plasma cells in the mammary gland. *J. Exp. Med.* 146, 1311–1322.

Roux, M.E., McWilliams, M., Phillips-Quagliata, J.M., and Lamm, M.E. (1981). Differentiation pathway of Peyer's patch precursors of IgA plasma cells in the secretory immune system. *Cell. Immunol.* 61, 141–153.

Ruan, M., Akkoyunlu, M., Grubb, A., and Forsgren, A. (1990). Protein D of Haemophilus influenzae. A novel bacterial surface protein with affinity for human IgD. *J. Immunol.* 145, 3379–3384.

Rudin, A., Johansson, E.L., Bergquist, C., and Holmgren, J. (1998). Differential kinetics and distribution of antibodies in serum and nasal and vaginal secretions after nasal and oral vaccination of humans. *Infect. Immun.* 66, 3390–3396.

Rugtveit, J., Bakka, A., and Brandtzaeg, P. (1997). Differential distribution of B7.1 (CD80) and B7.2 (CD86) co-stimulatory molecules on mucosal macrophage subsets in human inflammatory bowel disease (IBD). *Clin. Exp. Immunol.* 110, 104–113.

Sagie, E., Tarabulus, J., Maeir, D. M., and Freier, S. (1974). Diet and development of intestinal IgA in the mouse. *Isr. J. Med.* Sci. 10, 532–534.

Savidge, T.C. (1996). The life and times of an intestinal M cell. *Trends Microbiol.* 4, 301–306.

Savilahti, E. (1972). Immunoglobulin-containing cells in the intestinal mucosa and immunoglobulins in the intestinal juice in children. *Clin. Exp. Immunol.* 11, 415–425.

Savilahti, E. (1974). Workshop on secretory immunoglobulins. In *Progress in Immunology* (eds. L. Brent and J. Holborow), 238–243. Amsterdam: North/Holland Publishing Co.

Savilahti, E., and Pelkonen, P. (1979). Clinical findings and intestinal immunoglobulins in children with partial IgA deficiency. *Acta Paediatr. Scand.* 68, 513–519.

Schaerli, P., Willimann, K., Lang, A.B., Lipp, M., Loetscher, P., and Moser, B. (2000). CXC chemokine receptor 5 expression defines follicular homing T cells with B cell helper function. *J. Exp. Med.* 192, 1553–1562.

Schmucker, D.L., Heyworth, M.F., Owen, R.L., and Daniels, C.K. (1996). Impact of aging on gastrointestinal mucosal immunity. *Dig. Dis. Sci.* 41, 1183–1193.

Schrader, C.E., George, A., Kerlin, R.L., and Cebra, J.J. (1990). Dendritic cells support production of IgA and other non-IgM isotypes in clonal microculture. *Int. Immunol.* 2, 563–570.

Scott, M. G., Nahm, M. H., Macke, K., Nash, G. S., Bertovich, M. J., and MacDermott, R. P. (1986). Spontaneous secretion of IgG subclasses by intestinal mononuclear cells: differences between ulcerative colitis, Crohn's disease, and controls. *Clin. Exp. Immunol.* 66, 209–215.

Shikina, T., Hiroi, T., Iwatani, K., Jang, M.H., Fukuyama, S., Tamura, M., Kubo, T., Ishikawa, H., Kiyono, H. (2004). IgA class switch occurs in the organized nasopharynx- and gut-associated lymphoid tissue, but not in the diffuse lamina propria of airways and gut. *J. Immunol.* 172, 6259–6294.

Shimoda, M., Nakamura, T., Takahashi, Y., Asanuma, H., Tamura, S., Kurata, T., Mizuochi, T., Azuma, N., Kanno, C., and Takemori, T. (2001). Isotype-specific selection of high affinity memory B cells in nasal-associated lymphoid tissue. *J. Exp. Med.* 194, 1597–1607.

Shin, M.K., and Koshland, M.E. (1993). Ets-related protein PU.1 regulates expression of the immunoglobulin J-chain gene through a novel Ets-binding element. *Genes Dev.* 7, 2006–2015.

Shvartsman, Y.S., Agranovskaya, E.N., and Zykov, M.P. (1977). Formation of secretory and circulating antibodies after immunization with live and inactivated influenza virus vaccines. *J. Infect. Dis.* 135, 697–705.

Shyjan, A.M., Bertagnolli, M., Kenney, C.J., and Briskin, M.J. (1996). Human mucosal addressin cell adhesion molecule-1 (MAdCAM-1) demonstrates structural and functional similarities to the α4β7-integrin binding domains of murine MAdCAM-

1, but extreme divergence of mucin-like sequences. *J. Immunol.* 156, 2851–2857.

Silverstein, A.M., and Lukes, R.J. (1962). Fetal response to antigenic stimulus. I. Plasmacellular and lymphoid reactions in the human fetus to intrauterine infection. *Lab. Invest.* 11, 918–932.

Slifka, M.K., and Ahmed, R. (1998). Long-lived plasma cells: a mechanism for maintaining persistent antibody production. *Curr. Opin. Immunol.* 10, 252–258.

Sminia, T., van der Brugge-Gamelkoorn, G.J., and Jeurissen, S.H. (1989). Structure and function of bronchus-associated lymphoid tissue (BALT). *Crit. Rev. Immunol.* 9, 119–150.

Söltoft, J., and Söeberg, B. (1972). Immunoglobulin-containing cells in the small intestine during acute enteritis. *Gut* 13, 535–538.

Spencer, J., Dillon, S.B., Isaacson, P.G., and MacDonald, T.T. (1986). T cell subclasses in fetal human ileum. *Clin. Exp. Immunol.* 65, 553–558.

Sørensen, V., Sundvold, V., Michaelsen, T.E., and Sandlie, I. (1999). Polymerization of IgA and IgM: roles of Cys^{309}/Cys^{414} and the secretory tailpiece. *J. Immunol.* 162, 3448–3455.

Spencer, J., and MacDonald, T.T. (1990). Ontogeny of human mucosal immunity. In *Ontogeny of the Immune System of the Gut* (ed. T.T. MacDonald), 23–50. Boca Raton, Florida: CRC Press.

Stoltenberg, L., Vege, A., Saugstad, O.D., and Rognum, T.O. (1995). Changes in the concentration and distribution of immunoglobulin-producing cells in SIDS palatine tonsils. Pediatr. *Allergy Immunol.* 6, 48–55.

Streeter, P.R., Berg, E.L., Rouse, B.T., Bargatze, R.F., and Butcher, E.C. (1988). A tissue-specific endothelial cell molecule involved in lymphocyte homing. *Nature* 331, 41–46.

Takayasu, H., and Brooks, K. H. (1991). IL-2 and IL-5 both induce μ_s and J chain mRNA in a clonal B cell line, but differ in their cell-cycle dependency for optimal signaling. *Cell. Immunol.* 136, 472–485.

Tarkowski, A., Lue, C., Moldoveanu, Z., Kiyono, H., McGhee, J.R., and Mestecky, J. (1990). Immunization of humans with polysaccharide vaccines induces systemic, predominantly polymeric IgA2-subclass antibody responses. *J. Immunol.* 144, 3770–3778.

Tarlinton, D. (1998). Germinal centers: form and function. *Curr. Opin. Immunol.* 10, 245–251.

Terashima, M., Kim, K.M., Adachi, T., Nielsen, P.J., Reth, M., Kohler, G., and Lamers, M.C. (1994). The IgM antigen receptor of B lymphocytes is associated with prohibitin and a prohibitin-related protein. *EMBO J.* 13, 3782–3792.

Thrane, P. S., Rognum, T. O., and Brandtzaeg, P. (1990). Increased immune response in upper respiratory and digestive tracts in SIDS. *Lancet* 335, 229–230.

Thrane, P. S., Rognum, T. O., and Brandtzaeg, P. (1991): Ontogenesis of the secretory immune system and innate defence factors in human parotid glands. *Clin. Exp. Immunol.* 86, 342–348.

Thrane, P.S., Sollid, L.M., Haanes, H.R., and Brandtzaeg, P. (1992). Clustering of IgA-producing immunocytes related to HLA-DR-positive ducts in normal and inflamed salivary glands. *Scand. J. Immunol.* 35, 43–51.

Thrane, P. S., Rognum, T. O., and Brandtzaeg, P. (1994). Up-regulated epithelial expression of HLA-DR and secretory component in salivary glands: reflection of mucosal immunostimulation in sudden infant death syndrome. *Pediatr. Res.* 35, 625–628.

Tigges, M.A., Casey, L.S., and Koshland, M.E. (1989). Mechanism of interleukin-2 signaling: mediation of different outcomes by a single receptor and transduction pathway. *Science* 243, 781–786.

Trepel, F. (1974). Number and distribution of lymphocytes in man. A critical analysis. *Klin Wochenschr.* 52, 511–515.

Tschernig, T., and Pabst, R. (2000). Bronchus-associated lymphoid tissue (BALT) is not present in the normal adult lung but in different diseases. *Pathobiology* 68, 1–8.

Tumanov, A., Kuprash, D., Lagarkova, M., Grivennikov, S., Abe, K., Shakhov, A., Drutskaya, L., Stewart, C., Chervonsky, A., and Nedospasov, S. (2002). Distinct role of surface lymphotoxin expressed by B cells in the organization of secondary lymphoid tissues. *Immunity* 17, 239–250.

Turesson, I. (1976). Distribution of immunoglobulin-containing cells in human bone marrow and lymphoid tissues. *Acta Med. Scand.* 199, 293–304.

Turner, C.A., Mack, D.H., and Davis, M.M. (1994). Blimp-1, a novel zinc finger-containing protein that can drive the maturation of B lymphocytes into immunoglobulin-secreting cells. *Cell* 77, 297–306.

Valnes, K., Brandtzaeg, P., Elgjo, K., and Stave, R. (1986). Quantitative distribution of immunoglobulin-producing cells in gastric mucosa: relation to chronic gastritis and glandular atrophy. *Gut* 27, 505–514.

Van Cott, J.L., Brim, T.A., Lunney, J.K., and Saif, L.J. (1994). Contribution of antibody-secreting cells induced in mucosal lymphoid tissues of pigs inoculated with respiratory or enteric strains of coronavirus to immunity against enteric coronavirus challenge. *J. Immunol.* 152, 3980–3990.

van der Heijden, P. J., Stok, W., and Bianchi, T. J. (1987). Contribution of immunoglobulin-secreting cells in the murine small intestine to the "background" immunoglobulin production. *Immunology* 62, 551–555.

von Gaudecker, B., and Muller-Hermelink, H.K. (1982). The development of the human tonsilla palatina. *Cell. Tissue Res.* 224, 579–600.

Wagner, N., Löhler, J., Kunkel, E.J., Ley, K., Leung, E., Krissansen, G., Rajewsky, K., and Müller, W. (1996). Critical role for β7 integrins in formation of the gut-associated lymphoid tissue. *Nature* 382, 366–370.

Waldman, R.H., Wigley, F.M., and Small, P.A. (1970). Specificity of respiratory secretion antibody against influenza virus. *J. Immunol.* 105, 1477–1483.

Wang, W., Soto, H., Oldham, E.R., Buchanan, M.E., Homey, B., Catron, D., Jenkins, N., Copeland, N.G., Gilbert, D.J., Nguyen, N., Abrams, J., Kershenovich, D., Smith, K., McClanahan, T., Vicari, A.P., and Zlotnik, A. (2000). Identification of a novel chemokine (CCL28), which binds CCR10 (GPR2). *J. Biol. Chem.* 275, 22313–22323.

Warnock, R.A., Campbell, J.J., Dorf, M.E., Matsuzawa, A., McEvoy, L.M., and Butcher, E.C. (2000). The role of chemokines in the microenvironmental control of T versus B cell arrest in Peyer's patch high endothelial venules. *J. Exp. Med.* 191, 77–88.

Wiersma, E.J., Collins, C., Fazel, S., and Shulman, M.J. (1998). Structural and functional analysis of J chain-deficient IgM. *J. Immunol.* 160, 5979–5989.

Williams, A.F., and Gowans, J.L. (1975). The presence of IgA on the surface of rat thoracic duct lymphocytes which contain internal IgA. *J. Exp. Med.* 141, 335–345.

Willimann, K., Legler, D.F., Loetscher, M., Roos, R.S., Delgado, M.B., Clark-Lewis, I., Baggiolini, M., and Moser, B. (1998). The chemokine SLC is expressed in T cell areas of lymph nodes and mucosal lymphoid tissues and attracts activated T cells via CCR7. *Eur. J. Immunol.* 28, 2025–2034.

Yamanaka, T., Straumfors, A., Morton, H.C., Fausa, O., Brandtzaeg, P., and Farstad, I.N. (2001). M cell pockets of human Peyer's patches are specialized extensions of germinal centers. *Eur. J. Immunol.* 31, 107–117.

Yamanaka, T., Helgeland, L., Farstad, I.N., Midtvedt, T., Fukushima, H., and Brandtzaeg, P. (2003). Microbial colonization drives lymphocyte accumulation and differentiation in the follicle-associated epithelium of Peyer's patches. *J. Immunol.* 170, 816–822.

Yanagita, M., Hiroi, T., Kitagaki, N., Hamada, S., Ito, H.O., Shimauchi, H., Murakami, S., Okada, H., and Kiyono, H. (1999). Nasopharyngeal-associated lymphoreticular tissue (NALT) immunity: fimbriae-specific Th1 and Th2 cell-regulated IgA responses for the inhibition of bacterial attachment to epithelial cells and subsequent inflammatory cytokine production. *J. Immunol.* 162, 3559–3565.

Zan, H., Cerutti, A., Dramitinos, P., Schaffer, A., and Casali, P. (1998). CD40 engagement triggers switching to IgA1 and IgA2 in human B cells through induction of endogenous TGF-β: evidence for TGF-β but not IL-10-dependent direct Sμ→ Sα and sequential Sμ →Sγ, Sγ →Sα DNA recombination. *J. Immunol.* 161, 5217–5225.

Zhong, G., Reis e Sousa, C., and Germain, R.N. (1997). Antigen-unspecific B cells and lymphoid dendritic cells both show extensive surface expression of processed antigen-major histocompatibility complex class II complexes after soluble protein exposure in vivo or in vitro. *J. Exp. Med.* 186, 673–682.

B-1 Cells and the Mucosal Immune System

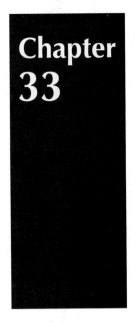

Nicolaas A. Bos and Frans G. M. Kroese

Department of Cell Biology, Immunology Section, University of Groningen, Groningen, The Netherlands

John J. Cebra

Department of Biology, University of Pennsylvania, Philadelphia, Pennsylvania

INTRODUCTION

B-1 cells are a small but unique subpopulation of B cells, with features that differ from the majority B cell population of mature, recirculating follicular B cells (conventional B cells, or B-2 cells; for reviews see, *e.g.*, (Berland and Wortis, 2002; Hardy and Hayakawa, 2001; Hayakawa and Hardy, 2000; Herzenberg, 2000; Wortis and Berland, 2001). B-1 cells have a distinct phenotype and are IgM^{hi}, IgD^{lo}, CD23$^-$, CD43$^+$, CD45/B220^{lo} cells. B-1 cells can further be subdivided into B-1a cells, which express CD5 (B-1a cells), and cells that lack this marker (B-1b cells). B-1 cells are the most abundant B cell population in the peritoneal and pleural cavities, represent only a small fraction of the B cells in spleen, and are virtually absent from lymph nodes and Peyer's patches. The antibodies produced by B-1 cells are frequently reactive with autoantigens and polysaccharide (TI-2) antigens of microorganisms and are generally encoded by relatively unmutated Ig V-genes. Despite the fact that B-1 cells constitute only a minor fraction of all B cells in the mouse, they appear to produce much of the IgM and probably a significant proportion of the natural antibodies in serum and at mucosal sites. Natural antibodies can be defined as those antibodies that are present naturally before any deliberate immunization. B-1 cells arise early during ontogeny; in the adult mouse these cells appear to be a self-replenishing population of cells that maintain themselves in the absence of replenishment by bone marrow precursor cells. There are many excellent recent review articles available on B-1 cells (*e.g.*, Berland and Wortis, 2002; Hardy and Hayakawa, 2001; Hayakawa and Hardy, 2000; Herzenberg, 2000; Wortis and Berland, 2001). For this reason we do not attempt here to review extensively the B-1 cell literature but summarize those issues that are necessary to understand the role of these cells in the mucosal immune system.

ORIGIN OF B-1 CELLS

IgA-producing cells usually arise from IgM precursors, except for the development of IgA plasma cells in mice without IgM expression (μMT mice) that still show some development of IgA plasma cells (Macpherson *et al.*, 2001). Whether the repertoire of IgA plasma cells in μMT mice has similarities with the IgM repertoire is unclear. Selective forces that drive these cells directly toward differentiation into IgA plasma cells could be different than the selective forces during primary B cell development or activation and isotype switching of IgM precursors.

The differences between B-1 cells and B-2 cells in early development and selection as IgM precursors can have consequences on the repertoire of IgA-producing cells arising from these precursors. The origin of B-1 cells has been an area of much controversy (for extensive discussions see, *e.g.*, Berland and Wortis, 2002; Hardy and Hayakawa, 2001; Hayakawa and Hardy, 2000; Herzenberg, 2000; Wortis and Berland, 2001). Originally, Herzenberg and colleagues proposed that B-1 cells belong to a separate B cell lineage, with their own committed fetal/neonatal progenitor cells (as reviewed in Hardy and Hayakawa, 2001; Herzenberg, 2000). According to this lineage hypothesis, the unique characteristics of the B-1 cells are developmentally predetermined before the pre–B cell stage. The lineage model is largely based on cell transfer experiments and B cell chimeras. In essence, adoptive transfer of adult bone marrow into irradiated recipient animals does not lead to generation of appreciable numbers of B-1 cells but results in full reconstitution of B-2 cells; B-1 cell repopulation in these animals requires the cotransfer of sIgM$^+$ B-1 cells. Precursor cells for B-1 cells are predominantly of fetal origin. Fetal omentum and embryonic paraaortic splanchnopleura contain progenitor cells that give rise to exclusively B-1 cells upon transfer into SCID recipients (Solvason *et al.*, 1991). Fetal liver cells appear to reconstitute both B-1 cells and B-2 cells (Hayakawa *et al.*, 1999). Once B-1 cells are produced in the neonate, they maintain themselves by their self-renewing capacity, as was originally shown in a variety of transfer experiments. In mice where the recombination activation gene (RAG)-2 could be inducibly deleted, the RAG-2 gene was deleted in adult animals (Hao and Rajewsky, 2001). In these mice the follicular type B-2 cells were gradually lost over time, whereas levels of peritoneal B-1 cells were not affected. These findings also support the concept that, in the adult mouse, B-1 cells are a self-replenishing population of cells that do not require RAG-2 gene expression for their maintenance. In addition to lack of B-1 cell progenitors in the adult animal, *de novo* development from progenitor cells is also prevented by the existence of feedback inhibition by mature B-1 cells. There are some indications that the precursor cells for B-1 cells and B-2 cells may differ phenotypically from each other (Lu *et al.*, 2002) and may exhibit differences in pre–B-cell receptor (BCR) signaling (Hardy and Hayakawa, 2001). In summary, there is considerable evidence that progenitor cells for B-1 and B-2 cells are present in distinct cell sources and that B-1 cells and B-2 cells belong to separate developmental B cell lineages.

In contrast, work initiated by Wortis and colleagues suggested that there is only one B cell lineage and that, in principle, any B cell can become a B-1 cell (for reviews see Berland and Wortis, 2002; Wortis and Berland, 2001). According to this induced differentiation hypothesis, B-1 cells arise from B (B-2) cells in response to surface IgM ligation by (self-) antigen in the absence of T cell help. Several lines of evidence are given that would favor such a model of B-1 cell genesis.

First, *in vitro* stimulation of splenic B (B-2) cells with anti-IgM antibodies results in the generation of B cells with a (partial) B-1a phenotype and a responsiveness to PMA, similar to B-1 cells. Second, studies with gene-disrupted mice and transgenic animals further show that BCR signaling is critical for B-1 cell development. Disruption of genes that positively regulate BCR signaling (*e.g.*, Btk [Khan *et al.*, 1995], CD19 [Inaoki *et al.*, 1997], CD21 [Ahearn *et al.*, 1996], Oct-2 [Humbert and Corcoran, 1997], vav-1 [Tarakhovsky *et al.*, 1995; Zhang *et al.*, 1995]) lead to weakening of the BCR signal. These mice generally have reduced numbers of B-1a cells. Transgenic expression of CD19 (Sato *et al.*, 1996) and some mutations of negative regulators of BCR signaling (*e.g.*, SHP-1 [Sidman *et al.*, 1986], lyn [Chan *et al.*, 1997]) lead to increased numbers of B-1 cells. Lam and Rajewsky (1999) showed in gene-targeted mice that not only specificity but also surface density of BCR determines B-1 versus B-2 cell development. Third, mice expressing Ig transgenes commonly expressed by B-1 cells (*e.g.*, V_H12-V_k4 or V_H11-V9 encoding for antiphosphatidylcholine antibodies) have high numbers of transgene-expressing B cells, which predominantly have a B-1 cell phenotype (Arnold *et al.*,

1994; Chumley *et al.*, 2000). Conversely, transgenic expression of V_H genes often expressed by B-2 cells results in B-2 cell development (Lam and Rajewsky, 1999).

POSITIVE SELECTION IN B-1 CELLS

BCR signaling by self-antigens during early development seems to have differential effects in B-1 and B-2 cells. BCR signaling of immature B-2 cells during B cell development by self-antigens results in negative selection leading to clonal deletion or anergy, while B-2 cells that are not self-reactive persist. In contrast, there is evidence that B-1 cells undergo positive selection by self-antigens, during their development. B cells producing antibodies specific for the autoantigen phosphatidylcholine (PtC) are typically found in the B-1a subset. Mice transgenic for both Ig V_H12 heavy chain and V_k4 light chain genes or V_H11 and V_k9 (both resulting in PtC-specific antibodies) produce high numbers of transgene-expressing B-1a cells in spleen and peritoneal cavity (Arnold *et al.*, 1994; Chumley *et al.*, 2000). Several other examples show that B-1 cells are subjected to positive selection. It has long been known that the T15 idiotype ($V_HS107/V\kappa22$) recognizing phosphorylcholine is mainly expressed by B-1 cells, even in germfree mice (Sigal *et al.*, 1975). This antibody is instrumental in protecting against infections with *Streptococous pneumoniae* (Briles *et al.*, 1982). Recent experiments show that the T-15 idiotype can also recognize neodeterminants on oxidation products of low-density lipoproteins (LDLs) that are found in atherosclerotic lesions and on apoptotic cells (Shaw *et al.*, 2000). This suggests that even under germfree conditions, positive selection of this specificity within the B-1 cell pool contributes to a physiological clearance of cells and lipoproteins that have undergone oxidative changes. Another example comes from studies by Hayakawa *et al.* (1999 and 2003). The self-antigen CD90/Thy-1 antigen (antithymocyte autoantibody, ATA) is expressed by thymocytes and a fraction of the mature T cells. Autoantibodies specific for an ATA carbohydrate epitope are encoded by V_H3609 heavy chains and V_k21C-J_k2 light chains. Mice transgenic for V_H3609 heavy chains have high titers for ATA in the serum, and ATA B cells generated through pairing of transgenic V_H3609 heavy chains and endogenous V_k21C-J_k2 light chains accumulated in the peritoneal B-1 cell compartment. Whether stimulation of the Thy-1 antigen on T cells by the transgenic Ig results in extra T cell help for the autoantibody-producing B-1 cells is unclear. Most splenic B-2 cells also expressed the transgenic heavy chain but produced different light chains, resulting in antibodies that cannot bind to the Thy-1 self-antigen. When the V_H3609 transgenic B cells developed in the absence of the Thy-1 self-antigen (by the crossing of V_H3609 transgenic mice with Thy-1 deficient mice), high ATA titers and enrichment of peritoneal ATA B-1 cells were not seen. It remains to be shown whether all B-1 cells are the result of positive selection and whether (immature) B-2 cells can be subjected to positive selection.

THE PERITONEAL CAVITY AS A UNIQUE ENVIRONMENT

In mice, B-1 cells are clearly enriched in the peritoneal and pleural cavities. The chemokine CXCL13, which is mainly produced by cells of the omentum and peritoneal macrophages, is involved in preferential homing of B-1 cells to the body cavities (Ansel *et al.*, 2002). Differences in signaling properties could also be of functional advantage for B-1 cells within the peritoneal cavity. Prevention of activation of B-1 cells by their location in privileged sites such as the peritoneal cavity might protect them from deletion, as was suggested from studies by Honjo and colleagues in which autoreactive, transgenic antierythrocyte (RBC) B cells were deleted from spleen but not from the peritoneal cavity (Murakami *et al.*, 1992). Development of B-1 cells within the peritoneal cavity in such Tg mice seems to be partly dependent on T cells, since crossing with RAG-2 KO mice resulted in a decrease in B-1 cells. B-1 activation and differentiation into auto-antibody-producing cells in the anti-RBC Tg mice seem to be dependent on IL-5 and IL-10 production, for instance, by peritoneal macrophages after oral administration of LPS or after the breeding environment is changed from germfree to conventional conditions (Nisitani *et al.*, 1998; Sakiyama *et al.*, 1999).

The peritoneal cavity also contains factors that influence intracellular signaling in B cells. In the Vh12-Vk9 transgenic mice, splenic B-1 cells resemble phenotypically peritoneal B-1 cells, but they do not show the same intracellular signaling upon IgM crosslinking as that seen in peritoneal B-1 cells. Transfer of such Tg splenic B-1 cells into the peritoneal cavity resulted in conversion of splenic B-1 type to peritoneal B-1 cell type intracellular signaling patterns (Chumley *et al.*, 2002).

Experiments with congenic asplenic mice (*Hox11*-null mice) revealed that the spleen is indispensable for the generation and maintenance of the B-1 cell pool (Wardemann *et al.*, 2002). Which elements of the spleen are critical for this development is unknown.

CONTRIBUTION OF B-1 CELLS TO MUCOSAL IGA PRODUCTION

There is now general consensus that B-1 cells can, along with B-2 cells, contribute to mucosal IgA production. The contribution of B-1 and B-2 cells to IgA production in physiologically normal animals with intact immune systems is still an open question. In **Table 33.1** we give an overview of the different experimental settings that were used to examine the contribution of B-1 cells to IgA production. The different experimental systems, which all have their own bias, show a wide variety in the observed contribution to IgA production by B-1 cells.

Our own initial experiments used reconstitution of irradiated animals with mixtures of peritoneal B cells as the source of B-1 cells and Ig–congenically different bone marrow as a source for B-2 cells and showed that B-1 cells can contribute

up to 50% of the IgA production of the small intestine (Kroese *et al.*, 1989). Similarly, Ly5.1 congenic PeC cells were injected into sublethally irradiated B6 mice, and in their system about 14% of the surface-IgA-positive cells in the lamina propria were donor-derived (Kang *et al.*, 2002). Macpherson *et al.* used a comparable system in TCR βδ knockout (KO) mice, except that this time FACS-sorted B-1 cells were used. In these experiments the numbers of IgA-producing cells were low (approximately 10% of the IgA present in immunocompetent mice), but all IgA-producing cells appear to be derived from the injected B-1 cells (Macpherson *et al.*, 2000). The apparent T cell independence of B-1 cells to switch to IgA in TCR βδ–KO mice is discussed separately below.

In irradiated chimeric mice, the irradiation can seriously damage the gut epithelium, and the IgA plasma cells that persist after irradiation in the lamina propria could disturb the outcome. Therefore, neonatal chimeric mice were generated by temporal suppression of normal B cell (B-1 and B-2) development by administration of anti-IgM antibodies specific for the recipient IgM allotype and simultaneous injection of allotypically different peritoneal B cells. This resulted in about 30% to 40% of the IgA-producing cells in the gut lamina propria (LP) that have the B-1 cell allotype (Kroese *et al.*, 1989). In the previously mentioned experimental settings, B-2 cells must develop from bone marrow precursors, while B-1 cells are functionally active directly after injection. When such chimeric mice are raised under conventional conditions, the functionally active B-1 cells can respond immediately with IgA production, in contrast to the still developing B-2 cells.

To avoid direct IgA induction, we produced Ig-allotype neonatal chimeric mice under germfree conditions, and after establishment of the chimerism, the mice were monoassociated with different commensal bacterial species. In this system there was only a minimal contribution (1%–10%) of B-1 cells to the induced IgA production (Thurnheer *et al.*, 2003). It could be argued, however, that monoassociation of adult mice with one commensal bacterial strain is not comparable to natural colonization after birth where gradually different species are introduced under a shield of maternal IgA. Therefore, obtainment of neonatal Ig-allotype chimerical mice also was attempted under conventional conditions, without suppression of the normal B cell pool. The resulting contribution of donor B-1 cells to IgA production in these conventionally reared mice was also minimal (1%) (Thurnheer *et al.*, 2003). The level of chimerism among the B-1 cells in the latter experiments was low, however, and therefore much IgA production by endogenous B-1 cells could have been unnoticed.

In another model, mixtures of peritoneal (B-1) cells and Peyer's patch (B-2) cells were injected into conventionally reared severe combined immunodeficient (SCID) mice. The contribution of peritoneal (B-1) cells to production of IgA-positive cells within the small intestine was 40% to 60% (Bos *et al.*, 2000). When germfree SCID mice where reconstituted with mixtures of FACS-sorted B-1 cells and bone marrow cells and thereafter associated with different commensal bacteria, the percentage of B-1-cell-derived IgA varied between 10% and 38%, depending on the inducing bacteria (Jiang, Bos, and Cebra, unpublished results). Using SCID mice as a model for the physiological contribution of B-1 cells to IgA production has a disadvantage in that SCID mice lack development of a proper microenvironment for B-2 cells to switch to IgA, such as in Peyer's patches.

In all of the experiments described previously, Ig-allotype was used as a marker for the B-1 cells because other markers that can discriminate between B-1 and B-2 cells are missing on surface-IgA-positive cells and IgA plasma cells. In some experiments, however a low expression level of B220 (CD45) on IgA-positive cells within the LP was used to define B-1-derived IgA-producing cells. With use of this marker the contribution of B-1-cell-derived IgA-producing cells is estimated to be 85% to 90% (Hiroi *et al.*, 1999; Hiroi *et al.*, 2000). The expression of B220 (CD45), however, is downregulated on all B cells, irrespective of their origin, when they differentiate into plasma blasts and plasma cells, and therefore it is probably not a good marker for B-1-cell-derived IgA plasma blasts. It was argued that low B220 expression could be correlated with another B-1 cell marker, Mac-1 (CD11b) expression on these cells (Hiroi *et al.*, 2000). This observation is even more surprising in light of the finding that B-1 cells outside the peritoneal cavity appear to lack Mac-1 (CD11b) (Hardy and Hayakawa, 2001).

In conclusion, the observed contributions of B-1 cells to intestinal IgA production depend on the experimental systems, and the final answer on the physiological contribution still awaits genetic markers that are uniquely expressed on B-1 cells during all stages of development up to the IgA plasma cells within the LP of the gut. It is clear, however, that the antigens (*e.g.*, commensal bacteria) and factors that induce B-1 cells to switch to IgA can influence the level of B-1-cell-derived IgA.

ANTIGEN-SPECIFIC VERSUS POLYCLONAL ACTIVATION OF B-1 CELLS

B-1 cells can contribute significantly to rapid serum IgM antibody responses against many bacteria and viruses (Baumgarth *et al.*, 2000; Ochsenbein *et al.*, 1999). Evaluation of Ag-specific stimulation or involvement in immune responses of either B-1 or B-2 cells must always be judged against the baseline of the total amount of IgM or IgA produced in these animals. This becomes critical in animals kept under gnotobiological conditions in which background levels of IgG and IgA are severely reduced.

The involvement of BCR-mediated specific and selective antigen stimulation of B-1 cells during immune responses is not well known. B-1 cells are very sensitive to stimulation by T-cell-independent-1 (TI-1) antigens such as LPS through Toll-like receptors (TLRs), but this usually results in polyclonal stimulation. Su *et al.* (1991) showed that splenic B-1 cells can make antigen-specific antibody responses to the O/core region of LPS. Transferred peritoneal B cells respond in vivo to the TI-2 antigen α1-3 dextran but not to NP-CG (TD) or to NP-Ficoll (TI-2) (Forster and Rajewsky, 1987). In TI-2 antigen responses against bacterial-associated antigens, for example, phosphoryl-choline (PC)-containing heat-killed *S. pneumoniae*, both peritoneal B-1 and splenic marginal zone (MZ) B cells participate in a rapid IgM plasmablast response against PC (Martin *et al.*, 2001). The relative contribution of these two B cell subpopulations to this early IgM response seems to be dependent on the dose and route of antigen administration.

For T-dependent responses the evidence is even slimmer. Taki *et al.* (1992) showed a T-15 id⁺ B-1 cell IgM response after immunization with PC-KLH, but in this case PC-KLH on alum was combined with *Bordetella pertussis* as adjuvant. Vogel *et al.* (1995) showed that transferred B-1 cells can produce a T-dependent IgG1 immune response against hen egg-white lysozyme.

The involvement of B-1 cells in antigen-driven mucosal immune responses is also still unclear. Although Macpherson *et al.* (2000) noted an antigen-specific mucosal IgA response after introducing new antigens on commensal bacteria, they noted no antigen specificity in their B-1-cell-derived IgA samples. After rotavirus infection, both humoral and cellular immune responses are involved in resolving the infection and protection against reinfection. Although both B-1 and B-2 cells produced IgA after rotavirus infection, only B-2 cells produced rotavirus-specific IgA that is effective in resolving the infection (Kushnir *et al.*, 2001). Early after rotavirus infection, there is an increase of activated B cells in PP and MLN, even in TCR βδ KO mice, suggesting possible T-independent stimulation of B-2 cells (Blutt *et al.*, 2002). The efficiency of such T-independent rotavirus-specific IgA is limited, since only 5% of the amount of IgA that is produced in T-cell-competent mice can be found after rotavirus infection in TCR βδ KO mice and full resolution of the virus requires T cells (VanCott *et al.*, 2001).

ROLE OF T CELLS IN B-1-CELL-DERIVED ANTIBODY PRODUCTION AND ISOTYPE SWITCHING

There is some evidence that B-1 cells require at least some T-cell help (Taki *et al.*, 1992). B-1 cells seem to depend on IL-5 but not on IL-6 for isotype switching, whereas B-2 cells are dependent on IL-6 to switch to IgA (Beagley *et al.*, 1995; Erickson *et al.*, 2001; Wetzel, 1989). If switching to IgA already occurs within the peritoneal cavity, peritoneal T cells might provide these cytokines. A relatively high proportion of peritoneal T cells (50%–70%) have an "activated" phenotype (among others, they express high levels of CD11a and CD44). Furthermore, within the TCRαβ⁺, CD4⁺ T cell subset, there are 10 times more cells producing IFN-γ, IL-4, IL-5, and IL-10 and 2.5 to 5 times more IL-2- and IL-6-producing cells in the peritoneal cavity than in the spleen **(Fig. 33.1)** (F.G.M. Kroese, M.N. Hylkema, N. Baumgarth, and L.A. Herzenberg, unpublished results).

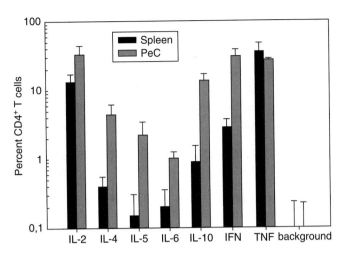

Fig. 33-1. The percentages of cytokine-producing TCR αβ CD4⁺ T cells were determined by 10-color, 12-parameter flow cytometry among peritoneal cavity (PeC) and spleen cells (F.G.M. Kroese, M.N. Hylkema, N. Baumgarth, and L.A. Herzenberg, unpublished results).

Recently, IL-15 was shown to stimulate proliferation of B-1 cells better than B-2 cells (Hiroi *et al.*, 2000). Also, IL-15 stimulates IgA⁺, B220^low cells more efficiently toward plasma cell differentiation than IgA⁺, B220^high cells (Hiroi *et al.*, 2000). Since B220^high, IgA⁺ cells within the LP are likely the immediate precursors of B220^low, IgA⁺ cells on their way to becoming IgA plasma cells and IL-15 can be produced by intestinal epithelial cells (Fehniger and Caligiuri, 2001), IL-15 can be regarded as an important local differentiation factor for all IgA plasma cells, independent of their B-1- or B-2-cell origin (Fagarasan *et al.*, 2001; Fagarasan and Honjo, 2003).

There is some intestinal IgA production in mice that are T-cell deficient or lack costimulation. Mice that are lacking MHC II still produce normal amounts of IgA, but when they were crossed with Xid mice that lack B-1 cells, the IgA production was severely reduced (Snider *et al.*, 1999). Also, transfer of sorted B-1 cells derived from BALB/c mice into TCR β, γ KO mice suggests that this T-cell-independent IgA might be derived from B-1 cells (Macpherson *et al.*, 2000). Conversely, we were unable to detect IgA production in the gut after transfer of purified B-1 cells into SCID mice (Bos *et al.*, 2001; Kushnir *et al.*, 2001). In transfer experiments with sorted B-1 cells, it is extremely important to check for accidental expansion of contaminating T cells, since we observed a very good correlation between (accidental) T cell outgrowth and IgA production by B-1 cells. When only minimal numbers of T cells were added to the purified B-1 cells, the IgA production increased dramatically (Jiang, Bos and Cebra, manuscript in preparation). This suggests that additional T cell help is also very important for B-1 cells to differentiate to IgA-secreting cells. The factors that are responsible for the T-cell-independent IgA production as seen in TCR β,γ KO mice are currently not known.

PP B cells switch to IgA efficiently after coculture with CD4 T cells, and CD40–CD40L interactions seem to be involved in this stimulation (Kang *et al.*, 2002). Human dendritic cells can induce class-switch to IgA in a CD40-independent way by interaction of BLyS (B lymphocyte stimulation protein, also called BAFF, TALL-1, THANK, and zTNF4) and/or APRIL (a proliferation-inducing ligand) with their receptors on human IgD⁺ B cells such as TACI (transmembrane activator and calcium modulator and cyclophylin ligand interactor), BCMA (B cell maturation antigen) and BAFF-R (Litinskiy *et al.*, 2002). This can also explain the IgA production as seen in CD40L-deficient mice (Renshaw *et al.*, 1994). BLyS and APRIL are upregulated on antigen-presenting cells (APCs) by IFN-α and IFN-γ that can be produced by APCs themselves in response to viral double-stranded RNA (dsRNA) or bacterial products (*e.g.*, CpG or LPS) (Litinskiy *et al.*, 2002). Whether B-1 or B-2 cells are more sensitive to this CD40-independent pathway is unknown.

In conclusion, B-1 cells seem to be able to produce some intestinal IgA in the absence of T cell help, probably by interactions with other immunoregulatory cells such as APCs and/or epithelial cells. On the other hand, IgA production by B-1 cells is greatly enhanced in the presence of T cells. In this interaction, cognate interaction between B-1 and T cells seems to be less important than T-cell-derived cytokines.

SITES OF SWITCHING TO IgA

Peritoneal B-1 cells may switch *in situ*, as indicated by the presence of germline IgA transcripts in peritoneal B-1 cells (B-1b subset) (Waard *et al.*, 1998; Hiroi *et al.*, 2000). Such germline transcripts are also observed among B220⁺, IgM⁺, and B220⁺ IgA⁺ cells in the LP or solitary follicles (Hiroi *et al.*, 2000). Other markers for class-switch recombination (CSR) are expression of activation-induced cytidine deaminase (AID) and the circle transcripts (aCT) that are looped out during CSR. In normal mice, the signs of active CSR to IgA were mostly found in IgM⁺, B220⁺ cells and IgA⁺, B220⁺ cells within the LP (LP proper and/or the isolated lymphoid follicles [ILF] therein; see next paragraph), while B220⁻, IgA⁺ cells in the LP still contain germline transcripts for IgA but are negative for AID and aCT (Fagarasan *et al.*, 2001). In AID-/-mice there is an accumulation of B220⁺, IgM⁺ cells within the LP that express active signs of CSR, such as aCT and germline transcripts (GLTs) for IgA, but that fail to switch because of the lack of AID (Fagarasan *et al.*, 2002). These data suggest active switching within the lamina propria in normal mice. However, it is unclear where these IgM-expressing B cells originate and where they were induced to start CSR. The LP IgM⁺, B220⁺ cells are more sensitive to factors produced by LP stromal cells such as IL-5, IL-6, and TGF-β stimulation to switch to IgA in vitro than are similar cells isolated from the PP (Fagarasan *et al.*, 2001). This suggests that the LP cells are in a different activation stage than PP cells. Signals such as LTβR on stromal lamina propria cells are required for IgA production, and migration of peritoneal cavity cells seems to be more affected in LTβR-/-mice than WT mice (Kang *et al.*, 2002). Taken together, these data show that there is active CSR within the LP, but the B-1 or B-2 cell origin of these IgA-committed cells remains elusive.

The site within the LP where these IgM cells accumulate could be the ILF (Hamada *et al.*, 2002), since AID–/–mice show great expansion of ILF over time (Fagarasan *et al.*, 2002). Recently, it was found that the chemokines CCL25 and CCL28 act as attractants into the gut for IgA-antibody-secreting cells expressing CCR9 and/or CCR10 (Bowman *et al.*, 2002; Kunkel *et al.*, 2003).

In conclusion, it is clear that Peyer's patches can be complemented in the induction of IgA production since appreciable CSR events from IgM to IgA can take place within the LP, including the ILF, but also within the peritoneal cavity. The B-1 or B-2 origin of the IgM cells committed to IgA switching is still unclear, however. B-1 cell migration to the LP seems to be more dependent on LT-induced factors than B-2 cells.

B-1 CELL FUNCTION

IgM antibodies

B-1 cells are thought to provide most of the natural (innate) (IgM) antibodies in the serum of normal mice (Hayakawa and Hardy, 2000). These antibodies are usually polyreactive and can bind with low affinity to autoantigens and microorganism coat antigens. Typical B-1-associated natural IgM antibodies include antibodies recognizing phosphorylcholine, phosphatidylcholine, thymocyte antigen, α1-3 dextran, and LPS. Baumgarth *et al.* (2000) showed that both B-1- and B-2-derived IgM antibodies can bind to influenza virus. In contrast to B-2-derived antibodies, the B-1-derived natural antivirus IgM titers do not increase, and cells that make it do not switch expression of Ig isotype in response to virus infection. Furthermore, these authors showed that both IgM types (natural and virus-induced) are required for the induction of virus-specific IgG antibodies (Baumgarth *et al.*, 2000). B-1-derived natural antibodies could play a role in efficient immune responses by preventing dissemination of pathogens and by enhanced antigen-trapping in lymphoid organs (Ochsenbein *et al.*, 1999). Rapid IgM responses that occur within 1 day, possibly derived from B-1 cells, are important in complement-mediated activation of T cells (Tsuji *et al.*, 2002). X-linked immunodeficient (Xid) mice have a point mutation in the pleckstrin homology domain of the Burton's tyrosine kinase gene (Btk) that results in severe depletion of the B-1 cell pool. Immunity against parasites is altered in Xid mice. Part of this vunerability to parasite infection can be explained by defective signaling of the Btk gene within T cells, macrophages, or granulocytes (Mukhopadhyay *et al.*, 2002).

Sometimes this defect results in decreased susceptibility to primary infections, as shown for *Leishmania major* (Hoerauf *et al.*, 1994) and *Trypanosoma cruzi* (Minoprio *et al.*, 1991), and sometimes in increased susceptibility to primary infections with, for instance, *Schistosoma mansoni* (Correa-Oliveira and Sher, 1985), *Strongyloides stercoralis* (Herbert *et al.*, 2002), and *Giardia muris* (Skea and Underdown, 1991). Immunization of Xid mice with the latter groups of parasites did not result in an increase of protective antigen-specific IgM responses, suggesting that B-1 cells in normal mice are responsible for the increase in antigen-specific IgM responses upon immunization. These experiments suggest that next to the production of natural IgM, B-1 cells are also important in early IgM immune responses.

IgA antibodies

As discussed above, both B-1 and B-2 cells can contribute to mucosal IgA production. Mucosal IgA production is clearly induced by colonization with commensal organisms. Evidence of GCR in PP has supported the T-cell dependence of at least part of the mucosal IgA response (Kramer and Cebra, 1995; Shroff *et al.*, 1995; Talham *et al.*, 1999; Weinstein and Cebra, 1991). In chimeric mice, we have shown that monoassociation with each of three different commensal gut organisms resulted in a clear GC response, and only a minor contribution of B-1 cells to the induced IgA production was evident (Thurnheer *et al.*, 2003). There was a regional and time-dependent IgA production difference between the various microorganisms (Thurnheer *et al.*, 2003). The presence of IgA in the gut can also influence the behavior of commensal organisms, as shown in the study by Jiang *et al.* (2001). Lack of either maternal IgA or neonatally derived IgA altered the distribution of segmented filamentous bacteria (SFB) in the intestinal tract. In the absence of IgA, SFB remained present in high numbers in the small intestine, whereas in immunocompetent animals the SFB retracted to the cecum and large intestine, as also seen under conventional conditions (Jiang *et al.*, 2001).

The specificity of such IgA interactions with the normal gut flora is still unknown. In conventionally reared animals the majority of intestinal bacteria are coated with IgA in vivo. Furthermore, after injection of PeC B cells into SCID mice, up to 90% of the intestinal bacteria became coated with IgA (Kroese *et al.*, 1995). Different mouse models interfering with production of S-IgA have become available, such as mice lacking IgA genes (IgA –/– mice) (Harriman *et al.*, 1999); mice lacking the J chain (J chain –/– mice), which is necessary for dimerization of IgA (Lycke *et al.*, 1999); and mice that are unable to transport IgA across the gut epithelium by deletion of the poly-Ig receptor (poly-IgR –/– mice) (Johansen *et al.*, 1999). No differences were seen in the bacterial populations of the terminal ileum between poly-IgR –/– mice and their normal controls (Sait *et al.*, 2003)

Also, in IgA–/– mice, no major changes were observed between the fecal bacterial populations from the KO mice and those from their normal controls (Harriman *et al.*, 1999). This could mean either that sIgA has no impact on the composition of the normal gut microbiota or that current quantitation methods to estimate the composition of the gut microbiota are not sensitive and discriminating enough to observe possible changes and shifts in conventionally reared mice. Development of gnotobiological models with a better controlled and less complex gut microbiota, in combination with more sensitive methods, should yield more definitive answers.

Poly-IgR –/– mice have elevated numbers of IgA plasma cells in the gut and do have some IgM, IgG, and IgA within their gut by passive leakage. It will be interesting to determine the effect of these alternative Ig molecules on the composition of the gut flora in the different compartments of the gut. Also, vaccine-induced protection against different mucosal pathogens such as influenza virus (Mbawuike et al., 1999), HSV-2, rotavirus (O'Neal et al., 2000), and *Helicobacter pylori* (Blanchard et al., 1999) seems to be unaffected in IgA–/– mice. However, J chain –/– mice seem to be more vulnerable to the toxic effects of cholera toxin (Lycke et al., 1999). Xid mice are more sensitive to salmonella infections (O'Brien et al., 1979), and the mucosal IgA response against *Salmonella typhimurium* can be restored by transfer of B-1 cells (Pecquet et al., 1992).

Macpherson et al. (2000) showed that T-independent IgA production is also induced by commensal bacteria. Furthermore, antigen-specific responses can be seen after introducing new members into an existing flora, even in TCR β,δ KO mice. Therefore, they argued that all mucosal IgA production is induced in a specific way and "natural" IgA does not exist. However, next to this antigen-specific response, we have shown that, depending on the nature of the stimulating commensal bacteria, most IgA does not seem to be antigen-specific and therefore should be considered to be "natural" or "bystander" IgA (Bos et al., 2001). Gut commensal bacteria can be considered part of the natural environment and obviously induce a lot of IgA production.

The functional relevance of this (possibly B-1-cell-derived) "natural" IgA is still open to speculation. We speculated that B-1-cell-derived IgA and B-2-cell-derived IgA may exert different functions, depending on their specificities and affinities (Bos et al., 2000). B-1-cell-derived IgA might play a role in maintaining a "balanced" intestinal microflora (homeostasis), whereas B-2-derived IgA might primarily be involved in immunoexclusion of (pathogenic) bacteria from the gut.

Recently, much attention has been given to cells that may switch within the LP from IgM to IgA production. The relevance of IgM or IgA in controlling the normal gut flora becomes obvious in mice lacking the AID gene. These mice are unable to switch to IgA or to exhibit somatic hypermutation (SHM) and show a strong increase in IgM plasma cells within the LP. This IgM response, however, seems to be inadequate to control the gut flora, since AID –/– mice seem to have a higher bacterial load of anaerobic bacteria, despite a significant expansion of the number and sizes of ILF (Fagarasan et al., 2002). When the bacterial load was decreased in the AID–/– mice with antibiotics, the number and size of the ILF decreased. Also, in other mucosal secretions such as saliva and tears, much IgA is secreted both in humans as well as in animal models. Much of this IgA is also regarded as "natural IgA," reacting with target antigens similar to those of "natural IgM" (Quan et al., 1997). The presence of IgA antibodies in tears of children that are reactive with conserved epitopes of *Toxoplasma gondii* that show epitope specificities different from those of *T. gondii* IgA antibodies after vaccination also suggests the presence of natural IgA antibodies in human tears that could be relevant as a first line of defense (Meek et al., 2002).

Production of IgA in human saliva is highly influenced by physiological stress and is regarded as a general measurement of "immune health status" (Klentrou et al., 2002). Similarly, an increase in serum natural IgM antibodies was seen in physically active rats. Although relatively much is known about both positive and negative selection of B-1 cells at the IgM level (see previous discussion), the repertoire of IgA-producing cells derived from either B-1 or B-2 cells is still largely unknown.

It is still unclear how important antigen-driven selection is for IgA-producing cells. Spectratype analysis of CDR3 lengths of IgA plasma cells suggests a very restricted repertoire for both B-1- and B-2-cell-derived IgA in the normal mouse intestine (Stoel et al., submitted for publication). Also in humans there is evidence that clonally expanded B cells are widely disseminated along the intestinal tract (Holtmeier et al., 2000; Dunn-Walters et al., 1997b). Analysis of involved V_H genes in the mouse intestine suggest that the precursors of most IgA plasma cells might be selected in another way than the antigen selection seen within the peripheral immune system (Stoel et al., submitted for publication). Selection, over evolutionary time, for expression of certain germline-encoded genes could provide a first-line protection against the most threatening pathogens in the natural environment. A relatively broad-specificity stimulation or even polyclonal stimulation would be expected to generate an effective, competent type of V(D)J rearrangement that may not require N-addition or somatic hypermutations to yield an effective antibody. However, analysis of the use of a particular set of V_H genes that are used by human IgA-producing cells within the LP shows very high numbers of somatic mutations (Dunn-Walters et al., 1997a). Such high numbers of somatic mutations were not seen in the same set of human V_H genes in human B cells derived from the peritoneal cavity, suggesting other selection criteria for peritoneal B cells and LP B cells in humans (Boursier et al., 2002).

B-1 CELLS AS REGULATORY CELLS

The ability of PeC B cells (B-1 cells) to present antigen to a T cell clone is better than that of splenic B cells (primarily B-2 cells) and comparable to splenic APCs that are commonly used in these types of assays **(Fig. 33.2)** (K.E. Shroff and J.J. Cebra, unpublished results). This can be partly explained by the constitutive expression of CD80 and CD86 on B-1 cells (Mohan et al., 1998). Despite this difference, B-2 cells can also act efficiently as APCs. Parenteral immunization in the footpad with rotavirus can induce a protective mucosal IgA response, and B-2 cells derived from the draining lymph nodes are responsible for transfer of such a protection response (Coffin et al., 1999). Surprisingly, the transferred B-2 cells themselves are not responsible for this protective IgA production, but they migrate to the gut and act as APCs for locally induced IgA production by the recipient (Coffin et al., 1999).

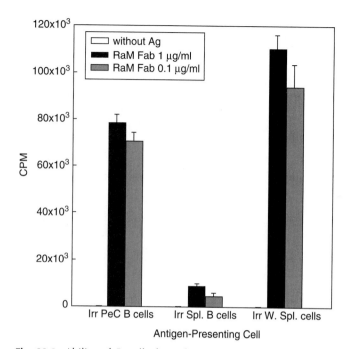

Fig. 33-2. Ability of B cells from the peritoneal cavity (PeC) and spleen (Spl) to present Ag, compared to unfractionated spleen cells that are commonly used as antigen-presenting cells. Th2 cell-line CDC35 cells (10^5), specific for rabbit Fab, were cultured along with 2×10^4 irradiated B cells from PeC or spleen or irradiated (2×10^4) unfractionated whole spleen (W. Spl.) cells and pulsed with either 1 μg/ml or 0.1 μg/ml of rabbit-anti-mouse $F(ab)_2$. Stimulation of T cells was measured by [^{3}H]thymidine incorporation (K.E. Shroff and J.J. Cebra, unpublished results).

B-1 cells are also a major source of IL-10 production, especially after LPS stimulation, and possibly they can skew T cell responses toward a Th-2 profile (O'Garra *et al.*, 1992). IL-10 expression in the mucosal environment is critical in resistance against inflammatory bowel disease (IBD), and a regulatory role for IL-10-producing B cells in IBD has been suggested (Mizoguchi *et al.*, 2000; Mizoguchi *et al.*, 2002). Disruption of the Gαi2 gene leads to a relative depletion of IL-10-producing B-1 cells and MZ B cells and to susceptibility for IBD, suggesting a possible regulatory role for B-1 cells in suppression of IBD under normal conditions (Dalwadi *et al.*, 2003).

CONCLUDING REMARKS

Although there is still much controversy in the literature about the developmental origin of B-1 cells (lineage model versus induced differentiation model), there is accumulating evidence that B-1-cell-derived antibodies play an essential role in the production of natural (innate) IgM and IgA antibodies. B-1 cells may be part of a "natural immune memory" and provide an important first line of humoral protection against infections with viruses and bacteria. Self-antigens play a critical role in establishing the B-1 cell IgM

immunoglobulin repertoire. Whether the IgA and IgM repertoires are selected in a similar way is still largely unknown. Elucidating B-1 cell development, activity, and function within the mucosal immune system is therefore of critical importance to understanding humoral immune protection against microorganisms and in maintaining a stable intestinal microflora.

ACKNOWLEDGMENTS

The authors thank Drs. Jiang, Shroff, Baumgarth, Hylkema, Herzenberg, and Stoel for use of their unpublished data.

REFERENCES

Ahearn, J. M., Fischer, M. B., Croix, D., Goerg, S., Ma, M., Xia, J., Zhou, X., Howard, R. G., Rothstein, T. L., and Carroll, M. C. (1996). Disruption of the Cr2 locus results in a reduction in B-1a cells and in an impaired B cell response to T-dependent antigen. *Immunity* 4, 251–262.

Ansel, K. M., Harris, R. B., and Cyster, J. G. (2002). CXCL13 is required for B1 cell homing, natural antibody production, and body cavity immunity. *Immunity* 16, 67–76.

Arnold, L. W., Pennell, C. A., McCray, S. K., and Clarke, S. H. (1994). Development of B-1 cells: segregation of phosphatidyl choline-specific B cells to the B-1 population occurs after immunoglobulin gene expression. *J. Exp. Med.* 179, 1585–1595.

Baumgarth, N., Herman, O. C., Jager, G. C., Brown, L. E., Herzenberg, L. A., and Chen, J. (2000). B-1 and B-2 cell-derived immunoglobulin M antibodies are nonredundant components of the protective response to influenza virus infection. *J. Exp. Med.* 192, 271–280.

Beagley, K. W., Bao, S., Ramsay, A. J., Eldridge, J. H., and Husband, A. J. (1995). IgA production by peritoneal cavity B cells is IL-6 independent: implications for intestinal IgA responses. *Eur. J. Immunol.* 25, 2123–2126.

Berland, R. and Wortis, H. H. (2002). Origins and functions of B-1 cells with notes on the role of CD5. *Annu. Rev. Immunol.* 20, 253–300.

Blanchard, T. G., Czinn, S. J., Redline, R. W., Sigmund, N., Harriman, G., and Nedrud, J. G. (1999). Antibody-independent protective mucosal immunity to gastric helicobacter infection in mice. *Cell. Immunol.* 191, 74–80.

Blutt, S. E., Warfield, K. L., Lewis, D. E., and Conner, M. E. (2002). Early response to rotavirus infection involves massive B cell activation. *J. Immunol.* 168, 5716–5721.

Bos, N. A., Cebra, J. J., and Kroese, F. G. (2000). B-1 cells and the intestinal microflora. *Curr. Top. Microbiol. Immunol.* 252, 211–220.

Bos, N. A., Jiang, H. Q., and Cebra, J. J. (2001). T cell control of the gut IgA response against commensal bacteria. *Gut* 48, 762–764.

Boursier, L., Farstad, I. N., Mellembakken, J. R., Brandtzaeg, P., and Spencer, J. (2002). IgVH gene analysis suggests that peritoneal B cells do not contribute to the gut immune system in man. *Eur. J. Immunol.* 32, 2427–2436.

Bowman, E. P., Kuklin, N. A., Youngman, K. R., Lazarus, N. H., Kunkel, E. J., Pan, J., Greenberg, H. B., and Butcher, E. C. (2002). The intestinal chemokine thymus-expressed chemokine (CCL25) attracts IgA antibody-secreting cells. *J. Exp. Med.* 195, 269–275.

Briles, D. E., Forman, C., Hudak, S., and Claflin, J. L. (1982). Anti-phosphorylcholine antibodies of the T15 idiotype are optimally protective against *Streptococcus pneumoniae*. *J. Exp. Med.* 156, 1177–1185.

Chan, V. W., Meng, F., Soriano, P., DeFranco, A. L., and Lowell, C. A. (1997). Characterization of the B lymphocyte populations in Lyn-deficient mice and the role of Lyn in signal initiation and down-regulation. *Immunity* 7, 69–81.

Chumley, M. J., Dal Porto, J. M., and Cambier, J. C. (2002). The unique antigen receptor signaling phenotype of B-1 cells is influenced by locale but induced by antigen. *J. Immunol.* 169, 1735–1743.

Chumley, M. J., Dal Porto, J. M., Kawaguchi, S., Cambier, J. C., Nemazee, D., and Hardy, R. R. (2000). A VH11V kappa 9 B cell antigen receptor drives generation of CD5⁺ B cells both *in vivo* and *in vitro*. *J. Immunol.* 164, 4586–4593.

Coffin, S. E., Clark, S. L., Bos, N. A., Brubaker, J. O., and Offit, P. A. (1999). Migration of antigen-presenting B cells from peripheral to mucosal lymphoid tissues may induce intestinal antigen-specific IgA following parenteral immunization. *J. Immunol.* 163, 3064–3070.

Correa-Oliveira, R. and Sher, A. (1985). Defective immunoglobulin M responses to vaccination or infection with Schistosoma mansoni in xid mice. *Infect. Immun.* 50, 409–414.

Dalwadi, H., Wei, B., Schrage, M., Spicher, K., Su, T. T., Birnbaumer, L., Rawlings, D. J., and Braun, J. (2003). B cell developmental requirement for the G alpha i2 gene. *J. Immunol.* 170, 1707–1715.

Dunn-Walters, D. K., Boursier, L., and Spencer, J. (1997a). Hypermutation, diversity and dissemination of human intestinal lamina propria plasma cells. *Eur. J. Immunol.* 27, 2959–2964.

Dunn-Walters, D. K., Isaacson, P. G., and Spencer, J. (1997b). Sequence analysis of human IgVH genes indicates that ileal lamina propria plasma cells are derived from Peyer's patches. *Eur. J. Immunol.* 27, 463–467.

Erickson, L. D., Foy, T. M., and Waldschmidt, T. J. (2001). Murine B1 B cells require IL-5 for optimal T cell-dependent activation. *J. Immunol.* 166, 1531–1539.

Fagarasan, S. and Honjo, T. (2003). Intestinal IgA synthesis: regulation of front-line body defences. *Nat. Rev. Immunol.* 3, 63–72.

Fagarasan, S., Kinoshita, K., Muramatsu, M., Ikuta, K., and Honjo, T. (2001). In situ class switching and differentiation to IgA-producing cells in the gut lamina propria. *Nature* 413, 639–643.

Fagarasan, S., Muramatsu, M., Suzuki, K., Nagaoka, H., Hiai, H., and Honjo, T. (2002). Critical roles of activation-induced cytidine deaminase in the homeostasis of gut flora. *Science* 298, 1424–1427.

Fehniger, T. A. and Caligiuri, M. A. (2001). Interleukin 15: biology and relevance to human disease. *Blood* 97, 14–32.

Forster, I. and Rajewsky, K. (1987). Expansion and functional activity of Ly-1+ B cells upon transfer of peritoneal cells into allotype-congenic, newborn mice. *Eur. J. Immunol.* 17, 521–528.

Hamada, H., Hiroi, T., Nishiyama, Y., Takahashi, H., Masunaga, Y., Hachimura, S., Kaminogawa, S., Takahashi-Iwanaga, H., Iwanaga, T., Kiyono, H., Yamamoto, H., and Ishikawa, H. (2002). Identification of multiple isolated lymphoid follicles on the antimesenteric wall of the mouse small intestine. *J. Immunol.* 168, 57–64.

Hao, Z. and Rajewsky, K. (2001). Homeostasis of peripheral B cells in the absence of B cell influx from the bone marrow. *J. Exp. Med.* 194, 1151–1164.

Hardy, R. R. and Hayakawa, K. (2001). B cell development pathways. *Annu. Rev. Immunol.* 19, 595–621.

Harriman, G. R., Bogue, M., Rogers, P., Finegold, M., Pacheco, S., Bradley, A., Zhang, Y., and Mbawuike, I. N. (1999). Targeted deletion of the IgA constant region in mice leads to IgA deficiency with alterations in expression of other Ig isotypes. *J. Immunol.* 162, 2521–2529.

Hayakawa, K., Asano, M., Shinton, S. A., Gui, M., Allman, D., Stewart, C. L., Silver, J., and Hardy, R. R. (1999). Positive selection of natural autoreactive B cells. *Science* 285, 113–116.

Hayakawa, K., Asano, M., Shinton, S. A., Gui, M., Wen, L. J., Dashoff, J., and Hardy, R. R. (2003). Positive selection of anti-thy-1 autoreactive B-1 cells and natural serum autoantibody production independent from bone marrow B cell development. *J. Exp. Med.* 197, 87–99.

Hayakawa, K. and Hardy, R. R. (2000). Development and function of B-1 cells. *Curr. Opin. Immunol.* 12, 346–353.

Herbert, D. R., Nolan, T. J., Schad, G. A., and Abraham, D. (2002). The role of B cells in immunity against larval Strongyloides stercoralis in mice. *Parasite Immunol.* 24, 95–101.

Herzenberg, L. A. (2000). B-1 cells: the lineage question revisited. *Immunol. Rev.* 175, 9–22.

Hiroi, T., Yanagita, M., Iijima, H., Iwatani, K., Yoshida, T., Takatsu, K., and Kiyono, H. (1999). Deficiency of IL-5 receptor alpha-chain selectively influences the development of the common mucosal immune system independent IgA-producing B-1 cell in mucosa-associated tissues. *J. Immunol.* 162, 821–828.

Hiroi, T., Yanagita, M., Ohta, N., Sakaue, G., and Kiyono, H. (2000). IL-15 and IL-15 receptor selectively regulate differentiation of common mucosal immune system-independent B-1 cells for IgA responses. *J. Immunol.* 165, 4329–4337.

Hoerauf, A., Solbach, W., Lohoff, M., and Rollinghoff, M. (1994). The Xid defect determines an improved clinical course of murine leishmaniasis in susceptible mice. *Int. Immunol.* 6, 1117–1124.

Holtmeier, W., Hennemann, A., and Caspary, W. F. (2000). IgA and IgM V(H) repertoires in human colon: evidence for clonally expanded B cells that are widely disseminated. *Gastroenterology* 119, 1253–1266.

Humbert, P. O. and Corcoran, L. M. (1997). oct-2 gene disruption eliminates the peritoneal B-1 lymphocyte lineage and attenuates B-2 cell maturation and function. *J. Immunol.* 159, 5273–5284.

Inaoki, M., Sato, S., Weintraub, B. C., Goodnow, C. C., and Tedder, T. F. (1997). CD19-regulated signaling thresholds control peripheral tolerance and autoantibody production in B lymphocytes. *J. Exp. Med.* 186, 1923–1931.

Jiang, H. Q., Bos, N. A., and Cebra, J. J. (2001). Timing, localization, and persistence of colonization by segmented filamentous bacteria in the neonatal mouse gut depend on immune status of mothers and pups. *Infect. Immun.* 69, 3611–3617.

Johansen, F. E., Pekna, M., Norderhaug, I. N., Haneberg, B., Hietala, M. A., Krajci, P., Betsholtz, C., and Brandtzaeg, P. (1999). Absence of epithelial immunoglobulin A transport, with increased mucosal leakiness, in polymeric immunoglobulin receptor/secretory component-deficient mice. *J. Exp. Med.* 190, 915–921.

Kang, H. S., Chin, R. K., Wang, Y., Yu, P., Wang, J., Newell, K. A., and Fu, Y. X. (2002). Signaling via LTbetaR on the lamina propria stromal cells of the gut is required for IgA production. *Nat. Immunol.* 3, 576–582.

Khan, W. N., Alt, F. W., Gerstein, R. M., Malynn, B. A., Larsson, I., Rathbun, G., Davidson, L., Muller, S., Kantor, A. B., and Herzenberg, L. A. (1995). Defective B cell development and function in Btk-deficient mice. *Immunity* 3, 283–299.

Klentrou, P., Cieslak, T., MacNeil, M., Vintinner, A., and Plyley, M. (2002). Effect of moderate exercise on salivary immunoglobulin A and infection risk in humans. *Eur. J. Appl. Physiol.* 87, 153–158.

Kramer, D. R. and Cebra, J. J. (1995). Early appearance of "natural" mucosal IgA responses and germinal centers in suckling mice developing in the absence of maternal antibodies. *J. Immunol.* 154, 2051–2062.

Kroese, F. G., Butcher, E. C., Stall, A. M., Lalor, P. A., Adams, S., and Herzenberg, L. A. (1989). Many of the IgA producing plasma cells in murine gut are derived from self-replenishing precursors in the peritoneal cavity. *Int. Immunol.* 1, 75–84.

Kroese, F. G., Ammerlaan, W. A., and Kantor, A. B. (1993). Evidence that intestinal IgA plasma cells in mu, kappa transgenic mice are derived from B-1 (Ly-1B) cells. *Int. Immunol.* 5, 1317–1327.

Kroese, F. G. M., Cebra, J. J., van der Cammen, M. J. F., Kantor, A. B., and Bos, N. A. (1995). Contribution of B1 cells to intestinal IgA production in the mouse. *Methods: A Companion to Methods in Enzymology* 8, 37–43.

Kunkel, E. J., Kim, C. H., Lazarus, N. H., Vierra, M. A., Soler, D., Bowman, E. P., and Butcher, E. C. (2003). CCR10 expression is a common feature of circulating and mucosal epithelial tissue IgA Ab secreting cells. *J. Clin. Invest.* 111, 1001–1010.

Kushnir, N., Bos, N. A., Zuercher, A. W., Coffin, S. E., Moser, C. A., Offit, P. A., and Cebra, J. J. (2001). B2 but not B1 cells can contribute to CD4+ T-cell-mediated clearance of rotavirus in SCID mice. *J. Virol.* 75, 5482–5490.

Lam, K. P. and Rajewsky, K. (1999). B cell antigen receptor specificity and surface density together determine B-1 versus B-2 cell development. *J. Exp. Med.* 190, 471–477.

Litinskiy, M. B., Nardelli, B., Hilbert, D. M., He, B., Schaffer, A., Casali, P., and Cerutti, A. (2002). DCs induce CD40-independent immunoglobulin class switching through BLyS and APRIL. *Nat. Immunol.* 3, 822–829.

Lu, L. S., Tung, J., Baumgarth, N., Herman, O., Gleimer, M., Herzenberg, L. A., and Herzenberg, L. A. (2002). Identification of a germ-line pro-B cell subset that distinguishes the fetal/neonatal from the adult B cell development pathway. *Proc. Natl. Acad. Sci. USA* 99, 3007–3012.

Lycke, N., Erlandsson, L., Ekman, L., Schon, K., and Leanderson, T. (1999). Lack of J chain inhibits the transport of gut IgA and abrogates the development of intestinal antitoxic protection. *J. Immunol.* 163, 913–919.

Macpherson, A. J., Gatto, D., Sainsbury, E., Harriman, G. R., Hengartner, H., and Zinkernagel, R. M. (2000). A primitive T cell-independent mechanism of intestinal mucosal IgA responses to commensal bacteria. *Science* 288, 2222–2226.

Macpherson, A. J., Lamarre, A., McCoy, K., Harriman, G. R., Odermatt, B., Dougan, G., Hengartner, H., and Zinkernagel, R. M. (2001). IgA production without mu or delta chain expression in developing B cells. *Nat. Immunol.* 2, 625–631.

Martin, F., Oliver, A. M., and Kearney, J. F. (2001). Marginal zone and B1 B cells unite in the early response against T-independent blood-borne particulate antigens. *Immunity* 14, 617–629.

Mbawuike, I. N., Pacheco, S., Acuna, C. L., Switzer, K. C., Zhang, Y., and Harriman, G. R. (1999). Mucosal immunity to influenza without IgA: an IgA knockout mouse model. *J. Immunol.* 162, 2530–2537.

Meek, B., Back, J. W., Klaren, V. N., Speijer, D., and Peek, R. (2002). Conserved regions of protein disulfide isomerase are targeted by natural IgA antibodies in humans. *Int. Immunol.* 14, 1291–1301.

Minoprio, P., Coutinho, A., Spinella, S., and Hontebeyrie-Joskowicz, M. (1991). Xid immunodeficiency imparts increased parasite clearance and resistance to pathology in experimental Chagas' disease. *Int. Immunol.* 3, 427–433.

Mizoguchi, A., Mizoguchi, E., Takedatsu, H., Blumberg, R. S., and Bhan, A. K. (2002). Chronic intestinal inflammatory condition generates IL-10-producing regulatory B cell subset characterized by CD1d upregulation. *Immunity* 16, 219–230.

Mizoguchi, E., Mizoguchi, A., Preffer, F. I., and Bhan, A. K. (2000). Regulatory role of mature B cells in a murine model of inflammatory bowel disease. *Int. Immunol* 12, 597–605.

Mohan, C., Morel, L., Yang, P., and Wakeland, E. K. (1998). Accumulation of splenic B1a cells with potent antigen-presenting capability in NZM2410 lupus-prone mice. *Arthritis Rheum.* 41, 1652–1662.

Mukhopadhyay, S., Mohanty, M., Mangla, A., George, A., Bal, V., Rath, S., and Ravindran, B. (2002). Macrophage effector functions controlled by Bruton's tyrosine kinase are more crucial than the cytokine balance of T cell responses for microfilarial clearance. *J. Immunol.* 168, 2914–2921.

Murakami, M., Tsubata, T., Okamoto, M., Shimizu, A., Kumagai, S., Imura, H., and Honjo, T. (1992). Antigen-induced apoptotic death of Ly-1 B cells responsible for autoimmune disease in transgenic mice. *Nature* 357, 77–80.

Nisitani, S., Sakiyama, T., and Honjo, T. (1998). Involvement of IL-10 in induction of autoimmune hemolytic anemia in anti-erythrocyte Ig transgenic mice. *Int. Immunol.* 10, 1039–1047.

O'Brien, A. D., Scher, I., Campbell, G. H., MacDermott, R. P., and Formal, S. B. (1979). Susceptibility of CBA/N mice to infection with Salmonella typhimurium: influence of the X-linked gene controlling B lymphocyte function. *J. Immunol.* 123, 720–724.

O'Garra, A., Chang, R., Go, N., Hastings, R., Haughton, G., and Howard, M. (1992). Ly-1 B (B-1) cells are the main source of B cell-derived interleukin 10. *Eur. J. Immunol.* 22, 711–717.

O'Neal, C. M., Harriman, G. R., and Conner, M. E. (2000). Protection of the villus epithelial cells of the small intestine from rotavirus infection does not require immunoglobulin A. *J. Virol.* 74, 4102–4109.

Ochsenbein, A. F., Fehr, T., Lutz, C., Suter, M., Brombacher, F., Hengartner, H., and Zinkernagel, R. M. (1999). Control of early viral and bacterial distribution and disease by natural antibodies. *Science* 286, 2156–2159.

Pecquet, S. S., Ehrat, C., and Ernst, P. B. (1992). Enhancement of mucosal antibody responses to Salmonella typhimurium and the microbial hapten phosphorylcholine in mice with X-linked immunodeficiency by B-cell precursors from the peritoneal cavity. *Infect. Immun.* 60, 503–509.

Quan, C. P., Berneman, A., Pires, R., Avrameas, S., and Bouvet, J. P. (1997). Natural polyreactive secretory immunoglobulin A autoantibodies as a possible barrier to infection in humans. *Infect. Immun.* 65, 3997–4004.

Renshaw, B. R., Fanslow, W. C., III, Armitage, R. J., Campbell, K. A., Liggitt, D., Wright, B., Davison, B. L., and Maliszewski, C. R. (1994). Humoral immune responses in CD40 ligand-deficient mice. *J. Exp. Med.* 180, 1889–1900.

Sait, L., Galic, M., Strugnell, R. A., and Janssen, P. H. (2003). Secretory antibodies do not affect the composition of the bacterial microbiota in the terminal ileum of 10-week-old mice. *Appl. Environ. Microbiol.* 69, 2100–2109.

Sakiyama, T., Ikuta, K., Nisitani, S., Takatsu, K., and Honjo, T. (1999). Requirement of IL-5 for induction of autoimmune hemolytic anemia in anti-red blood cell autoantibody transgenic mice. *Int. Immunol.* 11, 995–1000.

Sato, S., Ono, N., Steeber, D. A., Pisetsky, D. S., and Tedder, T. F. (1996). CD19 regulates B lymphocyte signaling thresholds critical for the development of B-1 lineage cells and autoimmunity. *J. Immunol.* 157, 4371–4378.

Shaw, P. X., Horkko, S., Chang, M. K., Curtiss, L. K., Palinski, W., Silverman, G. J., and Witztum, J. L. (2000). Natural antibodies with the T15 idiotype may act in atherosclerosis, apoptotic clearance, and protective immunity. *J. Clin. Invest.* 105, 1731–1740.

Shroff, K. E., Meslin, K., and Cebra, J. J. (1995). Commensal enteric bacteria engender a self-limiting humoral mucosal immune response while permanently colonizing the gut. *Infect. Immun.* 63, 3904–3913.

Sidman, C. L., Shultz, L. D., Hardy, R. R., Hayakawa, K., and Herzenberg, L. A. (1986). Production of immunoglobulin isotypes by Ly-1+ B cells in viable motheaten and normal mice. *Science* 232, 1423–1425.

Sigal, N. H., Gearhart, P. J., and Klinman, N. R. (1975). The frequency of phosphorylcholine-specific B cells in conventional and germfree BALB/C mice. *J. Immunol.* 114, 1354–1358.

Skea, D. L. and Underdown, B. J. (1991). Acquired resistance to Giardia muris in X-linked immunodeficient mice. *Infect. Immun.* 59, 1733–1738.

Snider, D. P., Liang, H., Switzer, I., and Underdown, B. J. (1999). IgA production in MHC class II-deficient mice is primarily a function of B-1a cells. *Int. Immunol.* 11, 191–198.

Solvason, N., Lehuen, A., and Kearney, J. F. (1991). An embryonic source of Ly1 but not conventional B cells. *Int. Immunol.* 3, 543–550.

Su, S. D., Ward, M. M., Apicella, M. A., and Ward, R. E. (1991). The primary B cell response to the O/core region of bacterial lipopolysaccharide is restricted to the Ly-1 lineage. *J. Immunol.* 146, 327–331.

Taki, S., Schmitt, M., Tarlinton, D., Forster, I., and Rajewsky, K. (1992). T cell-dependent antibody production by Ly-1 B cells. *Ann. N.Y. Acad. Sci.* 651, 328–335.

Talham, G. L., Jiang, H. Q., Bos, N. A., and Cebra, J. J. (1999). Segmented filamentous bacteria are potent stimuli of a physiologically normal state of the murine gut mucosal immune system. *Infect. Immun.* 67, 1992–2000.

Tarakhovsky, A., Turner, M., Schaal, S., Mee, P. J., Duddy, L. P., Rajewsky, K., and Tybulewicz, V. L. (1995). Defective antigen receptor-mediated proliferation of B and T cells in the absence of Vav. *Nature* 374, 467–470.

Thurnheer, M. C., Zuercher, A. W., Cebra, J. J., and Bos, N. A. (2003). B1 cells contribute to serum IgM, but not to intestinal IgA production in gnotobiotic Ig allotype chimeric mice. *J. Immunol.* 170, 4564–4571.

Tsuji, R. F., Szczepanik, M., Kawikova, I., Paliwal, V., Campos, R. A., Itakura, A., Akahira-Azuma, M., Baumgarth, N., Herzenberg, L. A., and Askenase, P. W. (2002). B cell-dependent T cell responses: IgM antibodies are required to elicit contact sensitivity. *J. Exp. Med.* 196, 1277–1290.

VanCott, J. L., McNeal, M. M., Flint, J., Bailey, S. A., Choi, A. H., and Ward, R. L. (2001). Role for T cell-independent B cell activity in the resolution of primary rotavirus infection in mice. *Eur. J. Immunol.* 31, 3380–3387.

Vogel, L. A., Sercarz, E. E., and Metzger, D. W. (1995). Antibody response of murine B1 cells to hen eggwhite lysozyme. *Cell. Immunol.* 161, 88–97.

de Waard, R., Dammers, P. M., Tung, J. W., Kantor, A. B., Wilshire, J. A., Bos, N. A., Herzenberg, L. A., and Kroese, F. G. (1998). Presence of germline and full-length IgA RNA transcripts among peritoneal B-1 cells. *Dev. Immunol.* 6, 81–87.

Wardemann, H., Boehm, T., Dear, N., and Carsetti, R. (2002). B-1a B cells that link the innate and adaptive immune responses are lacking in the absence of the spleen. *J. Exp. Med.* 195, 771–780.

Weinstein, P. D. and Cebra, J. J. (1991). The preference for switching to IgA expression by Peyer's patch germinal center B cells is likely due to the intrinsic influence of their microenvironment. *J. Immunol.* 147, 4126–4135.

Wetzel, G. D. (1989). Interleukin 5 regulation of peritoneal Ly-1 B lymphocyte proliferation, differentiation and autoantibody secretion. *Eur. J. Immunol.* 19, 1701–1707.

Wortis, H. H. and Berland, R. (2001). Cutting edge commentary: origins of B-1 cells. *J. Immunol.* 166, 2163–2166.

Zhang, R., Alt, F. W., Davidson, L., Orkin, S. H., and Swat, W. (1995). Defective signalling through the T- and B-cell antigen receptors in lymphoid cells lacking the vav proto-oncogene. *Nature* 374, 470–473.

Lymphocyte Homing: Chemokines and Adhesion Molecules in T cell and IgA Plasma Cell Localization in the Mucosal Immune System

Chapter 34

Kenneth R. Youngman, Nicole H. Lazarus, and Eugene C. Butcher

Laboratory of Immunology and Vascular Biology, Department of Pathology, Stanford University School of Medicine, Stanford, California; and the Center for Molecular Biology and Medicine, The Veterans Affairs Palo Alto Health Care System, Palo Alto, California

Leukocytes develop with characteristic inflammation- and/or tissue-selective trafficking properties. Lymphocytic components of the innate immune system such as γδ T-cell subsets, as well as specialized lymphoid dendritic populations, appear to be preprogrammed with particular tissue or inflammation tropisms during their development in primary lymphoid organs. Regulatory T cells and natural killer–like T cells display heterogeneous patterns of trafficking receptors, which may correlate with specialization of these phenotypically defined populations in cytokine production, tolerance, and bridging innate and adaptive immune responses. Within the adaptive immune system, comprising the bulk of αβ receptor-expressing T cells and of B cells in the adult animal, initial homing properties—a pronounced tropism for secondary lymphoid organs, including lymph nodes (LNs), Peyer's patches (PPs), and spleen—are also determined developmentally, prior to or in association with emigration from the thymus or bone marrow. Antigen-dependent stimulation and differentiation redirect homing properties, inducing or selecting for memory and effector cells displaying enhanced capacity to migrate to extralymphoid tissues and sites of inflammation, often with selective tropisms for intestines, skin, or other specific epithelial surfaces or organs in the body **(Fig. 34.1)**. For example, many antigen-reactive B and T memory and effector cells induced in response to intestinal immunization travel preferentially into the intestinal wall and/or into the intestine-associated lymphoid organs, and tissue-selective homing mechanisms target IgA antibody–secreting cells to mucosal surfaces. Tissue-selective targeting of antigen-reactive populations is thought to contribute to the efficiency of immune responses and to orchestrate and restrict the systemic competition between immunocytes that underlies the homeostatic regulation of memory and immune reactivity. From the perspective of mucosal physiology and pathology, selective trafficking also provides a mechanism for segregating the specialized immune response modalities characteristic of intestinal vs. systemic immune responses. This chapter provides a brief overview of tissue-selective lymphocyte trafficking, reviews some of the major homing receptors involved in intestinal lymphocyte recruitment, and highlights the recently defined role of tissue-specific lymphoid and epithelial chemokines and their receptors in targeting T cells and antibody secreting cells to and within the mucosal immune system.

CHEMOKINES AND ADHESION RECEPTORS MEDIATE LYMPHOCYTE–ENDOTHELIAL CELL RECOGNITION AND LYMPHOCYTE RECRUITMENT FROM THE BLOOD

The recruitment of circulating lymphocytes from the blood into intestinal tissues, as elsewhere, begins with their interaction with the vascular endothelium, principally within specialized postcapillary venules. In the mucosal lymphoid

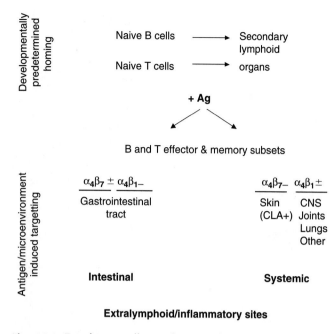

Naive B cells $\longrightarrow$ Secondary lymphoid

Naive T cells $\longrightarrow$ organs

+ Ag

B and T effector & memory subsets

Antigen/microenvironment induced targetting

$\alpha_4\beta_7 \pm \alpha_4\beta_1-$
Gastrointestinal tract

$\alpha_4\beta_7-$ $\alpha_4\beta_1\pm$
Skin CNS
(CLA+) Joints
Lungs
Other

Intestinal   **Systemic**

Extralymphoid/inflammatory sites

Fig. 34.1. Developmentally predetermined vs. directed homing properties of lymphoid mediators of adaptive immunity. Developmentally preprogrammed trafficking properties, controlling selectivity of recruitment from the blood, characterize naive B- and T-cell components of the adaptive immune system. In contrast, the homing of memory and effector cells is redirected as a function of microenvironmental characteristics at sites of antigenic stimulation.

organs, the PPs, appendix, and mesenteric lymph nodes (MLNs), these venules are lined by metabolically active, plump (or "high") endothelium and are defined as high endothelial venules (HEVs). In the intestinal lamina propria, postcapillary endothelium involved in lymphocyte recruit-

ment is less pronounced histologically, but here too, the endothelial cells are highly specialized for supporting interactions with circulating cells. Lymphocytes can recognize and differentially adhere to endothelium in different sites in the body, an ability that helps determine their trafficking patterns *in vivo*.

Multiple molecules and steps are required for engagement, arrest, and recruitment of circulating lymphocytes. Blood-borne lymphocytes flow with remarkable speed in relation to their size, requiring specialized mechanisms for interaction with postcapillary venule endothelium **(Fig. 34.2)** (reviewed in Johnston and Butcher, 2002). In the first step, microvillous processes deploying constitutively active adhesion receptors make contact with the specialized endothelium, initiating rolling of the lymphocyte along the vascular lumen. Many of the adhesion receptors mediating initial rolling are selectins, but in some instances additional rolling receptors can be required to slow rolling sufficiently for subsequent events to occur (most notably, the requirement of the α4β7 integrin to slow rolling of naïve lymphocytes in the intestinal PPs) (Bargatze *et al.*, 1995; Berlin *et al.*, 1995). Rolling delays the transit of lymphocytes dramatically, allowing "sampling" of the local microenvironment for activating factors, which are thought to act primarily through chemokine receptors of the Gαi protein-linked chemoattractant receptor subfamily. In this second step, these chemokines trigger rapid intracellular signaling in the leukocyte, leading to rapid lateral mobility and affinity activation of preexisting cell surface integrins (and perhaps other cell surface receptors) (Campbell *et al.*, 1998; Gunn *et al.*, 1998; Laudanna *et al.*, 2002). The activated integrins mediate firm arrest of the cell on the vessel wall (step 3), rendering the cell resistant to continuing blood shear forces. Firm arrest is reversible, and the lymphocyte can resume rolling and return to the blood, unless additional signals lead to transendothelial migration (step 4).

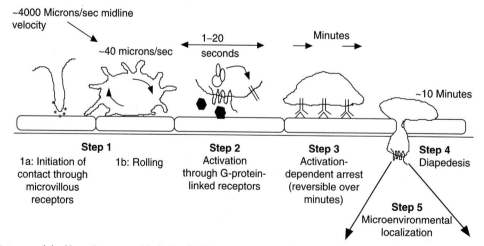

Fig. 34.2. The multistep model of lymphocyte–epithelial cell (EC) recognition and recruitment from the blood. The sequential requirement for multiple independently regulated receptor-ligand interactions allows combinatorial determination of the specificity of lymphocyte homing, implying that the specificity of the overall process can greatly exceed that of its component steps. Adapted with permission from Butcher and Picker (1996).

Chemokines or other chemoattractants are thought to provide such signals and selectively attract various lymphocyte subsets in *in vitro* assays (reviewed in Kunkel and Butcher, 2002). However, technical barriers have prevented identification of specific chemokine induction of diapedesis *in vivo*. Having entered the tissue, lymphocytes can segregate into specific areas, especially in secondary lymphoid organs (T cell zones or B-cell follicles), and chemokines clearly help control this microenvironmental organization (see Reif *et al.*, 2002). Thus chemokines and adhesion molecules work together in multistep processes that provide a combinatorial mechanism for the precise regulation of lymphocyte (and other leukocyte) recruitment, determined by the regional site, the developmental stage of the lymphocyte and of the tissue microenvironment, and the nature of any ongoing pathologic inflammation.

ADHESION/CHEMOKINE CASCADES IMPLICATED IN MUCOSAL LYMPHOCYTE HOMING

The current understanding of selectin, integrin, and chemokine participation in homing to mucosal sites is summarized in **Table 34.1**. Because of its importance to intestinal trafficking, we update the summary of MAdCAM-1 and its lymphocyte receptor α4β7 from the previous edition of this book. Involvement of β2 integrins and selectins in tissue-specific adhesion cascades has been previously reviewed (*e.g.*, Butcher *et al.*, 1999) and will be mentioned only briefly. We then focus on recent insights into the role of chemokines and their receptors in defining and targeting the mucosal immune response.

Table 34.1. Adhesion and Chemokine Receptors Regulate Lymphocyte Trafficking to Mucosal Tissues

Organ	Tethering and Rolling (Selectins and α4 Integrins)	Integrin Triggering and Diapedesis (Chemokines)	Activated Arrest (Integrins)
Peyer's patch (T cells)	L-selectin/PNAd α4β7/MAdCAM-1	CCR7/SLC	α4β7/MAdCAM-1 αLβ2/ICAMs
Peyer's patch (B cells)	L-selectin/:PNAd α4β7/MAdCAM-1	CCR7/SLC CXCR5/BCA-1 CXCR4/SDF-1	α4β7/MAdCAM-1 αLβ2/ICAMs
Peripheral lymph nodes (T cells)	L-selectin/PNAd	CCR7/SLC	αLβ2/ICAMs
Small intestine lamina propria (memory/effector T cells)	α4β7/MAdCAM-1	CCR9/TECK	αLβ2/ICAMs
Small intestine lamina propria (IgA plasmablasts)	α4β7/MAdCAM-1	CCR9/TECK CCR10/MEC	αLβ2/ICAMs
Large intestine lamina propria (IgA plasmablasts)	α4β7/MAdCAM-1	CCR10/MEC	αLβ2/ICAMs
Large intestine lamina propria (memory/effector T cells)	α4β7/MAdCAM-1 other?	Unknown	αLβ2/ICAMs
Bronchus-associated lymphoid tissues (naïve T/B)	L-selectin/PNAd	CCR7/SLC	αLβ2/ICAMs
Bronchus-associated lymphoid tissues (memory T cells)	L-selectin/PNAd α4β1/VCAM-1	Unknown	αLβ2/ICAMs
Bronchial wall (memory/effector T cells)	α4β1/VCAM-1	Unknown	αLβ2/ICAMs
Skin (memory/effector T cells in DTH)	CLA/E-selectin	CCR4/TARC CCR10/CTACK	αLβ2/ICAMs

Adhesion receptors, chemokines, and chemokine receptors implicated in selected homing events are presented. Note that we emphasize constitutive trafficking mechanisms, which may be supplemented by inflammatory chemokine pathways during infection or inflammation.

Adhesion molecules

MAdCAM-1, a mucosal vascular addressin involved in T and B cell homing to the gastrointestinal tract

As summarized in Table 34.1, in lymphocyte homing to the gut-associated lymphoid tissues and the small intestines, MAdCAM-1 acts as a key vascular "addressin," or address code molecule, for intestinal tissues (Butcher et al., 1999; Streeter et al., 1988a). It is an immunoglobulin family member related to other vascular adhesion molecules, such as vascular cell adhesion molecule-1 (VCAM-1) and intercellular adhesion molecules (ICAM-1 and ICAM-2), that each function as ligands for leukocyte integrins (Briskin et al., 1993). MAdCAM-1 is selectively though not exclusively expressed in postcapillary venules, defining sites of lymphocyte extravasation into intestinal lamina propria and into intestine-associated lymphoid tissues, especially the PPs and MLNs (Briskin et al., 1997; Streeter et al., 1988a). It also defines vessels involved in lymphocyte trafficking into the inflamed pancreas of NOD mice (Yang et al., 1997) and to the lactating mammary gland, where VCAM-1 is also expressed (Streeter et al., 1988a; van der Feltz et al., 2001). MAdCAM-1 is also expressed by vascular zone endothelium in the developing mouse placenta at the stage of active trophoblast invasion, where it appears to participate with P-selectin in recruiting a unique population of monocyte-related mononuclear cells (Kruse et al., 1999). Recent studies implicate MAdCAM-1 in hepatic inflammation (Grant et al., 2001; Hillan et al., 1999). It is interesting that MAdCAM-1 is also displayed by cells that help form the lining of the marginal sinus in the spleen (Kraal et al., 1995; Tanaka et al., 1996) and by choroid plexus epithelium in the central nervous system (Steffen et al., 1996), observations currently of undetermined significance. In contrast, although MAdCAM-1 can be upregulated in vitro by proinflammatory cytokines (Sikorski et al., 1993) in the adult animal, MAdCAM-1 is absent (or has been reported to be present at only very low levels, of uncertain physiologic significance) on venules in most nongastrointestinal sites of inflammation. Low levels of expression have been observed, for example, on inflamed peripheral lymph node (PLN) HEV, in inflamed bronchial tissues, and, under extraordinary circumstances, in inflamed joints (in murine Lyme disease models [Schaible et al., 1994]) and in the CNS (in chronic relapsing experimental allergic encephalomyelitis [O'Neill et al., 1991]). Other adhesion pathways dominate trafficking in these tissues, helping segregate intestinal from nonintestinal trafficking networks.

MAdCAM-1 and its lymphocyte receptor $\alpha 4\beta 7$ appear to play little or no role in lymphocyte homing to pulmonary or bronchial sites of inflammation. Similarly, the oral mucosa and tonsils lack significant histological expression of MAdCAM-1. Lymphocyte homing to these mucosal tissues also involves $\alpha 4$ integrins, but by interaction of $\alpha 4\beta 1$ with vascular VCAM-1, not $\alpha 4\beta 7$-MAdCAM-1. Memory T cell homing to bronchus-associated lymphoid tissues (BALT) and inflamed lung, for example, is mediated by $\alpha 4\beta 1$ and VCAM-1 in a manner analogous to the role of $\alpha 4\beta 7$-

MAdCAM-1 in PPs and gut lamina propria homing (Xu et al., 2003).

In addition to its expression by intestinal venules, MAdCAM-1 is also displayed by follicular dendritic cells (FDCs) in the mucosal lymphoid organs, especially within PPs and the appendix (Szabo et al., 1997). MAdCAM-1 decorates interlacing dendritic cells throughout PPs and appendix B cell follicles and is accentuated on FDCs of the germinal center light zone and on "junctional" dendritic cells overlapping the B zone border into the outer T zone and subepithelial dome region, sites associated with microenvironmental homing decisions and antigen presentation. In contrast, MAdCAM-1 is rarely displayed by FDCs in primary (resting) PLNs and is largely confined to the germinal center after lymph node immunization. Functional studies confirm that FDC-associated MAdCAM-1 plays an important and selective role in follicular binding of lymphocytes in PPs, when assayed in vitro on frozen tissue sections. Display of MAdCAM-1 by junctional and coronal FDCs in mucosal lymphoid organs may selectively support the development, retention, and function of lymphocytes expressing the mucosal homing receptor $\alpha 4\beta 7$, thus helping define and target intestinal memory and effector cells. It may also help influence the generation of intestinal homing properties ($\alpha 4\beta 7$ expression) during the antigen-specific generation of memory and effector B and T cells in PPs, working in conjunction with other local microenvironmental influences (i.e., cytokines) to determine the homing properties of lymphocytes responding to antigens presented in intestinal lymphoid organs. Indeed, these observations suggest that regional differences in the lymphoid stromal cells may help control the specialization of mucosal vs. nonmucosal immune responses.

The domain structure of human and mouse MAdCAM-1 is illustrated in **Figure 34.3** (Briskin et al., 1993, 1996). The two N-terminal Ig domains together confer optimal $\alpha 4\beta 7$-binding activity. The distal Ig domain contains a conserved LDTSL motif important to this interaction, but other elements in the first and second Ig loops contribute critically to the interaction and its specificity for $\alpha 4\beta 7$ (vs. $\alpha 4\beta 1$) as well (Briskin et al., 1996). A proximal mucinlike stalk, heavily O-glycosylated, may serve to extend the $\alpha 4\beta 7$-binding Ig domains away from the endothelial surface, facilitating adhesive interactions. This mucin domain can also serve as a site of presentation of L-selectin binding carbohydrates when MAdCAM-1 is expressed by HEV in MLNs and PPs (Berg et al., 1993). Modification of MAdCAM-1 by L-selectin binding carbohydrates does not appear to occur in venules in the normal mouse intestine. The mucin domain may also present chemokines to adherent gut homing lymphocytes. Thus, facultative display of L-selectin and potentially chemokine binding carbohydrates by MAdCAM-1 probably helps define the differential homing patterns of naive vs. memory/effector lymphocytes to mucosal lymphoid organs vs. the extralymphoid lamina propria (discussed later in the chapter).

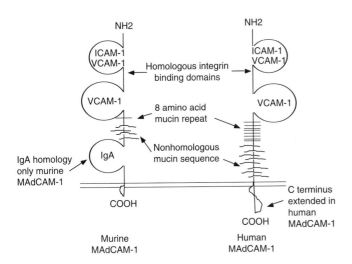

Fig. 34.3. Schematic diagram of the domain structure of mouse and human MAdCAM-1. Human and mouse MAdCAM-1 share strong homology in two N-terminal Ig domains, which together are required for efficient binding of α4β7 on lymphocytes. They also share prominent mucin domains, including an 8-amino-acid motif that is repeated several times in the human sequence. The mucin domain may serve as a stalk, facilitating presentation of the N-terminal integrin binding Ig domains; in addition, it can be modified by L-selectin-binding carbohydrates expressed in HEVs. Mouse but not human MAdCAM-1 also has a proximal Ig domain homologous to the Fc-binding region of IgA1: this domain is missing in an alternatively spliced mouse variant. Adapted with permission from Briskin et al. (1997).

The intestinal homing receptor, α4β7

α4β7 is a member of the heterodimeric integrin adhesion receptor family (reviewed in Hu et al., 1993). Leukocyte integrins, including α4β7, are displayed in relatively inactive or low avidity states on most resting and blood-borne lymphocytes but can be triggered to undergo dramatic functional activation in response to a variety of stimuli (reviewed in Hynes, 1992; Laudanna et al., 2002; Shimizu et al., 1992; Springer, 1995). In particular, chemoattractant receptors can trigger functional activation, assessed at the level of lymphocyte adhesion to integrin ligands, within seconds. This activation involves changes in receptor avidity through clustering, changes in receptor affinity through conformational alterations, and apparent rapid changes in the kinetics of integrin mobility that enhance encounters with dispersed vascular ligands (reviewed in Laudanna et al., 2002). Triggering of integrins by HEV or lamina propria venule–associated activating signals clearly plays an essential role in lymphocyte arrest (discussed later in the chapter). It is interesting, however, that α4 integrins display a significant if apparently low affinity/avidity activity even in the absence of stimulation. Moreover, circulating lymphocytes display these α4 integrins concentrated on the tips of microvilli (Berlin et al., 1995); for this reason, in some settings they can play an important role in activation-independent initial con-

tact formation or "tethering" (which depends on microvillous presentation) (von Andrian et al., 1995). In the absence of activation, α4 integrins, including α4β7, can also support reversible lymphocyte rolling (Berlin et al., 1995).

α4β7 binds MAdCAM-1 but also other ligands, including the CS1 peptide-containing splice variant of fibronectin, and VCAM-1 (reviewed in Ager, 1993; Imhof and Dunon, 1995; Kraal et al., 1995). These ligands may be important in gut-homing α4β7hi lymphocyte interactions within lymphoid tissues and within the lamina propria; however, there is as yet no evidence to support a significant role for α4β7 adhesion through VCAM-1 or fibronectin in the recruitment of lymphocytes from the blood. Indeed, at least on most circulating lymphocytes (including α4β7hi T cells, which tend to be α4β7low), binding to VCAM-1 is dominated by α4β1, with α4β7-VCAM-1 interaction being difficult to demonstrate except under artificial experimental conditions (Rott et al., 1996). Moreover, VCAM-1, although like MAdCAM-1 as an Ig family member that can be expressed by endothelium, is clearly distinguished from MAdCAM-1 by its patterns of expression. Although abundant in the stroma of PPs and the gastrointestinal lamina propria, VCAM-1 is largely excluded from expression by intestinal endothelium—even during chronic inflammation in, for example, inflammatory bowel disease (Salmi et al., 1994). Instead, VCAM-1 is induced on vessels involved in mononuclear cell recruitment in nonintestinal sites of inflammation: notably, the skin, heart, CNS, joints, and the lacrimal glands of autoimmune NOD mice, where inflammation is blocked by anti-VCAM-1 and anti-α4β1 antibodies but unaffected by MAdCAM-1 or α4β7 blockade (Mikulowska-Mennis et al., 2001). Thus, although it cannot be ruled out that activated α4β7 on, for example, immunoblasts may participate in VCAM-1-dependent extravasation in nonmucosal sites (Salmi et al., 1994), current data suggest that, in the context of leukocyte homing from the blood, α4β7-MAdCAM-1 and α4β1-VCAM-1 are largely independent homing receptor/vascular "addressin" interactions that play a major role in the differential trafficking of intestinal (α4β7+, α4β1low) vs. nonintestinal (α4β7−, α4β1+) memory and effector populations in vivo (see Fig. 34.1). Fibronectin has been implicated in α4β1-dependent lymphocyte adhesion to endothelium in vitro, but its ability to support physiologic α4β7-dependent adhesion and its importance to in vivo recruitment remain to be explored (Ager, 1993).

The expression of α4β7 by lymphocytes that embody intestinal immunity has been demonstrated in in vivo studies of rotavirus (RV) immunity in mice and humans. Rotavirus selectively infects the epithelium of the small intestines, providing a localized antigenic stimulus. In mice, B cell–mediated RV immunity is transferred to chronically infected immune-deficient (RAG−/−) mice only by α4β7+ memory B cells (Kuklin et al., 2001; Williams et al., 1998). Additionally, α4β7 expression is tightly regulated during development of RV-antigen-specific B cells; its expression correlates with the specific migration of memory and effector

B cells to intestinal tissues (Youngman et al., 2002). In the case of CD8[+] T cell–mediated immunity, studies in β7[-/-] mice reveal an α4β7 independent pathway; however, in normal mice, RV immunity is also found among α4β7[+] CD8[+] T cells (Kuklin et al., 2000; Rose et al., 1998). Finally, in humans, Gonzales et al. report that circulating RV-specific B cells are predominantly α4β7[+] (Gonzalez et al., 2003).

Other adhesion molecules involved in intestinal lymphocyte-endothelial interactions

L-selectin. The leukocyte L-selectin (CD62L) is a C-type calcium-dependent lectin of the selectin subfamily that binds a unique sulfated sialyl-Lewis X related carbohydrate structure found on many HEV glycoproteins (Hiraoka et al., 1999; Yeh et al., 2001). Together, the physiologically significant L-selectin ligand-presenting molecules comprise the PLN addressin (PNAd) (Rosen, 1999; Streeter et al., 1988b). A structure for the native HEV carbohydrate ligand for L-selectin has recently been derived (Yeh et al., 2001), and a sulfated L-selectin ligand found on two HEV-associated proteins (CD34 and podocalyxin-like protein) has been identified (Sassetti et al., 1998). L-selectin was originally identified as a PLN homing receptor, because L-selectin dominates the selectivity of lymphocyte recruitment to nonmucosal lymph nodes (Gallatin et al., 1983). HEVs in PLNs express extraordinarily high levels of L-selectin binding carbohydrates, much higher than those in PP-HEV (to be discussed below) (Streeter et al., 1988b; Warnock et al., 1998). Recently, a group of sulfotransferases critical to PNAd synthesis has been identified (Hemmerich and Rosen, 2000), several members of which are expressed in HEV, with one (designated GST-3) strongly and very selectively expressed in HEV (Bistrup et al., 1999; Hiraoka et al., 1999). While L-selectin appears critical to LN homing, L-selectin also plays an important if less dominant role in lymphocyte homing to PPs, where its principal but likely not exclusive HEV ligand is PNAd-decorated MAdCAM-1 (Fig. 34.3; Bargatze et al., 1995; Butcher and Picker, 1996).

αLβ2. αLβ2 (LFA-1, CD11a/CD18) is an integrin receptor for the widespread vascular and stromal cell ligands and is expressed by most circulating lymphocytes ICAM-1, ICAM-2, and ICAM-3 (Carlos and Harlan, 1994; Imhof and Dunon, 1995; Springer, 1995). Its affinity and mobility can be triggered by lymphocyte activation through chemoattractant receptors. Unlike the α4 integrins, however, LFA-1 is excluded from microvilli and is distributed instead to the planar cell body of leukocytes (Erlandsen et al., 1993). This topographic distribution may help explain the observation that LFA-1 plays no detectable role in initiating lymphocyte contact with high endothelium *in vivo* (Bargatze et al., 1995; Warnock et al., 1998) but is usually limited in its function to postactivation events, activation-triggered arrest, and subsequent transendothelial migration (although it can slow rolling of neutrophils in some settings).

αeβ7. The β7 integrin chain can be expressed as a heterodimer with αe as well as α4. αeβ7 is highly expressed by gut intraepithelial lymphocytes (IELs) and supports their interactions with intestinal epithelial cells by binding to epithelial or E-cadherin (reviewed in Shaw and Brenner, 1995). A small subset of circulating lymphocytes, especially CD8[+] (but also some CD4[+]) T cells, express αeβ7 and α4β7 together. The significance of this subset in the blood is unclear, as αeβ7 does not appear to participate in lymphocyte-EC interactions or extravasation *per se* (Strauch et al., 1994). αeβ7 is thought to help regulate and target IEL microenvironmental homing and interactions with the epithelium itself.

Vascular selectins and other potential adhesion molecules. Vascular E- and P-selectins (CD62E and CD62P) appear to play an insignificant role in lymphocyte trafficking to normal intestinal sites, either to intestinal lymphoid tissues or to the gut lamina propria. Neither selectin can be detected immunohistologically, for example, in the normal mouse small intestine or colon. This contrasts with important roles for vascular selectins in lymphocyte homing to certain extraintestinal sites. For example, E-selectin plays a critical role in cutaneous inflammation as a skin vascular "addressin," acting as a ligand for the cutaneous lymphocyte antigen on specialized skin homing memory T cells (reviewed in Butcher and Picker, 1996). However, E-selectin and likely P-selectin can be upregulated in nonintestinal mucosal tissues during inflammation, especially during acute inflammatory responses, during which they likely play important roles in facilitating neutrophil and monocyte recruitment from the blood.

Although not yet supported by *in vivo* studies, it is likely that additional molecules will prove to participate in lymphocyte trafficking to the gut, its associated lymphoid tissues, and other mucosal sites. An example is the vascular adhesion protein-1 (VAP-1), which may be involved in homing to the intestines, skin, inflamed joints, liver, and lungs (Lalor et al., 2002; Salmi et al., 1993; Salmi et al., 2001; Singh et al., 2003). VAP-1, an endothelial cell membrane–bound amine-oxidase, supports selectin independent adhesion and transmigration *in vitro* on hepatic sinusoidal endothelial cells (Lalor et al., 2002), perhaps by deamination of lymphocyte surface proteins, resulting in the formation of transient covalent bonds with the endothelium (Salmi et al., 2001).

CHEMOKINE AND CHEMOKINE RECEPTOR REGULATION OF LYMPHOCYTE HOMING

Chemokines and their receptors in rapid venular arrest and diapedesis of circulating lymphocytes

Gαi-linked receptors trigger the arrest of rolling lymphocytes on HEV in lymphoid tissues, and of granulocytes and monocytes in venules at sites of inflammation. Thus, it is likely that chemoattractant activation is required for arrest of rolling memory and effector T and B cells in sites of inflammation, as well. (Preactivated lymphocytes such as immunoblasts, which are among the most efficient subsets at homing to extralymphoid tissues, may express high levels of active integrins upon entering the blood and thus may potentially bypass the requirement for venule-associated adhesion triggering factors, although they will still required chemoattractants for localization within the tissue microenvironment.) Several members of the chemoattractant cytokine (chemokine) family (*i.e.*, SDF-1/CXCL12, MIP-3α/CCL20, MIP-3β/CCL19, and SLC/CCL21) trigger robust adhesion of blood lymphocytes to ICAM-1 (Campbell *et al.*, 1998). Moreover, triggered adhesion is extremely rapid, occurring within a second in *in vitro* flow assays. MIP-3β/CCL20, SLC/CCL21, and SDF-1/CXCL12 induce rapid binding of the majority of circulating CD4$^+$ T cells, including naive cells; MIP-3α/CCL19 triggers adhesion of memory but not naive CD4$^+$ T cells. Such adhesion-triggering chemokines are proving critical in controlling lymphocyte subset trafficking *in vivo* (see following discussion).

Lymphocyte subset recruitment into mucosal tissues is undoubtedly also regulated at the level of diapedesis and migration in the tissue parenchyma. Chemoattractants, especially members of the expanding chemokine family, are likely to be important in this regard as well, but as yet the molecular events involved remain incompletely understood. Early studies of Lamm and Czinn suggested the existence of chemoattractants that can selectively recruit IgA$^+$ immunoblasts, reinforcing the need for further molecular studies in this arena (Czinn and Lamm, 1986). Indeed, recent studies (summarized in the next section) point to a critical role for mucosal epithelial chemokines in mucosal lymphocyte and IgA plasma cell localization.

Homeostatic epithelial chemokines and the specialization of mucosal immunity

The mammalian immune system has developed intricate mechanisms to provide defense at epithelial surfaces and control potentially harmful responses to normal symbiotic flora. These mechanisms include numerous specialized T- and B-lymphocyte populations providing both cell-mediated and humoral immunity. At mucosal epithelial surfaces in particular, the local production and transepithelial transport of polymeric IgA secreted by resident plasma cells plays an important role in pathogen and toxin neutralization (Brandtzaeg *et al.*, 1999b; Kato *et al.*, 2001; Offit, 2001). The development of IgA antibody–secreting cells occurs primarily in secondary lymphoid tissues including PPs (Brandtzaeg *et al.*, 1999b), although recent data have suggested that *in situ* class-switching to IgA may also occur within the murine small intestine (Fagarasan *et al.*, 2001). Early IgA plasma cells, or plasmablasts, travel from lymphoid tissues through the blood to mucosal epithelial tissues, where they localize, secrete IgA, and terminally differentiate into plasma cells. It is interesting that local mucosal immunization leads to antigen-specific IgA production at distant mucosal sites in both humans (Czerkinsky *et al.*, 1991; Johansson *et al.*, 2001) and mice (McDermott and Bienenstock, 1979; Weisz-Carrington *et al.*, 1979), likely through the migration of IgA–secreting B cells (Brandtzaeg *et al.*, 1999a). These findings suggest that a simple nasal or oral vaccination may be effective at inducing IgA-dependent pathogen protection at multiple mucosal sites, in addition to systemic cell-mediated immunity (Kato *et al.*, 2001; Mestecky, 1987; Russell *et al.*, 1999; van Ginkel *et al.*, 2000). Understanding the mechanisms of mucosal immune T cell and IgA-secreting B cell trafficking to different distant mucosal sites may prove important to development of efficient vaccines capable of generating disseminated mucosal immunity.

Chemokines in lymphocyte homing to Peyer's patches

Peyer's patches are the first-line lymphoid organs of the intestinal tract. Here, antigens from the intestinal lumen are collected by the M cells of the dome epithelium, where dendritic cells, recruited in part by local production of the epithelial chemokine MIP1-α/CCL20, are thought to process antigen for presentation to memory and naïve lymphocytes that recirculate through the organ (Iwasaki and Kelsall, 2000). Naïve and subsets of α4β7$^+$ memory and effector lymphocytes recirculate through PP HEVs. Although B and T cells share use of L-selectin and α4β7 in initial contact and in slowing rolling, and LFA-1 in arrest, the sites of T and B cell firm arrest are segregated within PPs (Warnock *et al.*, 2000). HEVs supporting B cell accumulation are concentrated in or near follicles, the target domain of most B- cells entering PPs, whereas T cells preferentially accumulate in interfollicular HEVs **(Fig. 34.4)**. The HEV-expressed chemokine SLC/CCL21 triggers T cell arrest on HEV in the T cell zone through CCR7 on the T cell surface. In contrast, although B cells can also use CCR7, many B cells are triggered to bind to HEV segments upstream of the T zone HEV in vessel segments within or adjacent to B-cell follicles (Fig. 34.4). In this case, arrest can be triggered by any of several chemokines, including SDF-1/CXCL12 and BLC/CXCL13, as well as SLC/CCL21 (Okada *et al.*, 2002). This unexpected level of specialization of HEV may allow differential, segmental control of lymphocyte subset recruitment into functionally distinct lymphoid microenvironments *in vivo*, especially in the PPs.

Chemokines in lymphocyte homing to mucosal surfaces

Epithelial cell chemokines are emerging as important players in the homeostatic trafficking of lymphocyte subsets, including antibody-secreting cells and memory T cells (Kunkel and Butcher, 2002; Butcher and Kunkel, 2003). For instance, epithelial cells in the small intestine secrete the chemokine TECK/CCL25 (Kunkel *et al.*, 2000; Wurbel *et al.*, 2000), a ligand for the chemokine receptor CCR9, expressed on virtually all small intestinal T cells and on a subset of circulating mucosal (α4β7$^+$) memory T cells (Kunkel and Butcher, 2002; Zabel *et al.*, 1999). Moreover, TECK/CCL25 blockade reduces the efficiency of homing of CD8αα$^+$CD3$^+$ T cells to the IEL compartment and CD8αβ$^+$ CD3$^+$ T cells to

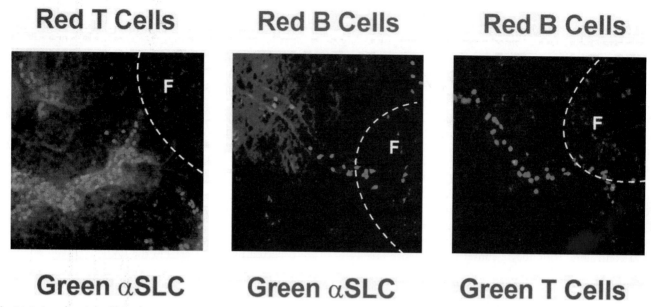

Fig. 34.4. Localization of lymphocytes in PP-HEV. Immunohistology of accumulated lymphocyte subpopulations in PPs. *Left,* T cells accumulated in SLC+ interfollicular segments of HEV; *middle,* B cells in SLC[low] HEV segments associated with primary follicles; *right,* segregation of sites of preferential T and B cell accumulation in relation to follicles. TRITC-labeled T cells (*left*) or B cells (*middle and right*) and CMFDA-labeled T cells (*right*) were observed in HEVs of normal animals. Adapted with permission from Warnock *et al.* (2000).

the small intestinal mucosa (Marsal *et al.*, 2002; Svensson *et al.*, 2002). Because CCR9+ lymphocytes are rare in the colon and virtually absent in other epithelial tissues (Kunkel *et al.*, 2000; Papadakis *et al.*, 2000), CCR9 and TECK/CCL25 may serve to segregate and compartmentalize the small-intestinal immune response. An analogous situation is the expression of the related chemokine CTACK/CCL27 by keratinocytes, the epithelial cells of the skin (Morales *et al.*, 1999). CCR10, the receptor for CTACK, is expressed on circulating CLA+ skin–homing memory lymphocytes (Hudak *et al.*, 2002; Morales *et al.*, 1999), and together with CCR4 and TARC/CCL17 and skin-selective adhesion receptors, it determines the selectivity of skin lymphocyte trafficking (Campbell *et al.*, 1999).

Intestinal epithelial expression of TECK thus appears to recruit a unique population of small-intestinal T cells, which may play a specialized role in small-intestinal immunity through specificity for local antigens, mediation of specialized immune properties, or both. It remains to be determined whether other homeostatic chemokines and G-protein-coupled receptors play an analogous specific role in recruiting T cell subsets to the large intestines, stomach, and other mucosal sites.

Most T cells in the gut wall, as in other extralymphoid tissues, also express receptors for inflammatory chemokines, in particular, CXCR3 and CCR5 for MIG/CXCL9 and RANTES /CCL5, respectively. The role of these chemokines and their receptors in the recruitment to or retention in the gut wall versus microenvironmental positioning, cell-to-cell

interactions, or other functions, remains to be determined. While skin lymphocytes also express CXCR3 and CCR5 and their ligands are induced in skin inflammation, homing of skin effector/memory cells to sites of delayed-type-hypersensitivity reactions in the mouse ear requires the receptor CCR4 for TARC/CCL17 or CCR10 for CTACK/CCL27, as blockade of these homeostatic skin-associated chemokine pathways is sufficient to inhibit T cell recruitment (Reiss *et al.*, 2001). Thus the role of inflammatory chemokines may lie in recruitment of more actively dividing cells or in other aspects of tissue inflammation.

Epithelial chemokines in the localization of IgA antibody–secreting cells

In addition to its role as a T-cell attractant to the small intestines, TECK/CCL25 is also a chemoattractant for splenic and small-intestinal IgA antibody–secreting cells that express CCR9 (Bowman *et al.*, 2002; Pabst *et al.*, 2004). Moreover, a related CCR10 ligand, the chemokine mucosal epithelial chemokine MEC/CCL28, is expressed by epithelial cells in a variety of mucosal tissues, including the salivary gland, mammary gland, small and large intestines, and trachea (Pan *et al.*, 2000; Wang *et al.*, 2000). Like CTACK/CCL27, MEC is also chemotactic for circulating CLA+ lymphocytes by virtue of being a CCR10 ligand (Pan *et al.*, 2000; Wang *et al.*, 2000), but CLA+ lymphocytes are virtually never found in gastrointestinal tissues because they do not express the α4β7 integrin, which is required for trafficking into these organs (via interaction with vascular MAdCAM-1 in intestinal sites)

(Jarmin *et al.*, 2000). Indeed, CCR10⁺ T cells are exceedingly rare in the gut lamina propria and other mucosal sites (Kunkel *et al.*, 2003).

In mucosal tissues, including the human gastrointestinal tract (*i.e.*, stomach, small intestine, and colon), salivary gland, and mucosa-associated lymphoid tissues (*i.e.*, tonsil and appendix), CCR10 is selectively expressed on IgA antibody–secreting cells (Kunkel *et al.*, 2003). Tonsillar IgA plasmablasts expressing CCR10 chemotax to MEC/CCL28 and ~70% of circulating IgA plasmablasts express CCR10, suggesting that blood IgA plasmablasts can home to and localize within MEC-expressing mucosal epithelial sites via CCR10 (Kunkel *et al.*, 2003). As mentioned previously, CCR9 is also expressed on a subset of circulating IgA plasmablasts and on IgA plasma cells within the small intestine (most of which also express CCR10) (Kunkel *et al.*, 2003). Together these results suggest a specialized involvement for CCR9 and TECK/CCL25 in small-intestinal IgA immunity and a broader role for CCR10 and MEC/CCL28 in unifying the localization of IgA plasma cells to the other disperse organs of the secretory IgA immune system (**Fig. 34.5**). It is likely that induction of CCR10 on pathogen-specific-IgA-secreting B cells may be an important factor for the successful dissemination of IgA-dependent protection following local mucosal infection or vaccination. In addition to upregulation of CCR9 and CCR10 on IgA ASCs, circulating and tissue-resident IgA (and IgG) plasmablasts downregulate their expression of CCR6, the receptor for MIP-3α/CCL20, expressed by naïve and memory B cells (Power *et al.*, 1997). This critical transition in chemokine receptor expression during ASC differentiation appears to determine IgA plasmablast localization to epithelial tissues.

While mucosal epithelial tissues also contain IgG plasma cells, these cells are usually less than 3% to 5% of the total

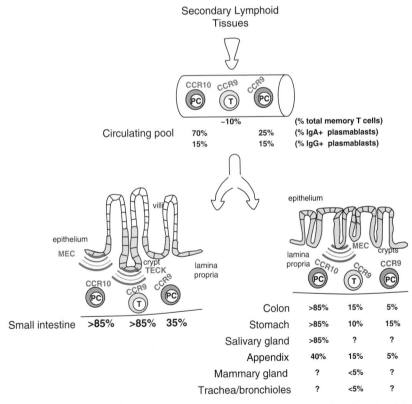

Fig. 34.5. MEC and CCR10 unify the epithelial IgA immune system. After development in secondary lymphoid tissues, IgA plasma cells (PCs) expressing CCR10 or CCR9 enter the circulation. By virtue of the expression of both MEC and TECK in the small intestine, both CCR10⁺ and CCR9⁺ PCs can enter this tissue (although CCR10⁺ PCs predominate). In other tissues where MEC expression predominates (*i.e.*, the colon and stomach), CCR10⁺ PCs predominate and CCR9⁺ PCs are less frequent. Other epithelial sites where MEC is expressed (*i.e.*, the mammary gland and trachea/bronchioles) and IgA is secreted may also contain CCR10⁺ PCs. CCR9⁺ T cells predominate in the small intestine where TECK is expressed and are found at lower levels in closely associated tissues such as the stomach and colon. This separate T lymphocyte localization pathway for the small intestine (via CCR9/TECK) allows functional compartmentalization of this organ, while physically dispersed organs that all share the function of pathogen neutralization by IgA are unified by CCR10/MEC. Adapted with permission from Kunkel *et al.* (2003).

plasma cell population. Many more IgG plasma cells are found in the spleen and bone marrow (McHeyzer-Williams and Ahmed, 1999). Few IgG plasma cells within MEC-expressing epithelial tissues express CCR10, and those that do so appear to express lower levels. Similarly, in the blood, the CD19^{int} large lymphocytes that express sIgG also contain few CCR10$^+$ cells. In the murine system, IgG antibody–secreting cells maintain high responsiveness to the chemokine SDF-1α/CXCL12 and become responsive to the CXCR3 ligands MIG/CXCL9 and IP-10/CXCL10 (Hauser *et al.*, 2002). The ability of murine IgG ASC to respond to SDF-1αCXCL12 may help in localization to the bone marrow (Hargreaves *et al.*, 2001), while responsiveness to MIG/CXCL9 or IP-10/CXCL10 may promote migration into inflammatory sites such as rheumatoid synovium. Few murine IgG ASCs (even from PPs or MLNs, two intestine-associated lymphoid tissues) respond to TECK/CCL25 or MEC/CCL28 (Bowman *et al.*, 2002; Lazarus *et al.*, 2003). Thus, it seems likely that, rather than homeostatic chemokines, inflammatory chemokines (particularly CXCR3 ligands) may play a dominant role in the localization of circulating IgG plasmablasts to epithelial (and other) tissues, allowing IgG plasmablast recruitment during tissue inflammation. Experimental confirmation of this hypothesis is needed.

It is interesting that in patients with selective IgA deficiency, the mucosal compartments of the upper aerodigestive tract commonly contain large numbers of IgD$^+$, IgM$^+$, and IgG$^+$ plasma cells, while the intestinal mucosal compartments largely contain IgG$^+$ and IgM$^+$ plasma cells (Brandtzaeg *et al.*, 1999b). It is unclear at this point whether CCR10 and MEC/CCL28 are involved in the mucosal migration of plasmablasts expressing other Ig isotypes, but in the absence of CCR10$^+$ IgA plasmablasts, it is very likely that CCR10$^+$ IgG and IgM antibody–secreting cells (which are only a small fraction of the total IgG and IgM plasmablast population in normal individuals) would have little competition for mucosal compartments and would therefore be able to fill these compartments. In fact, preliminary studies suggest that early in the human antirotavirus humoral response, rotavirus-specific plasmablasts expressing IgM or IgG can express CCR9 and/or CCR10 (M.C. Jaimes, E.J. Kunkel, H.B. Greenberg, and E.C. Butcher, unpublished data).

CONCLUSION

Homeostatic chemokines and leukocyte and vascular adhesion molecules operate in combination to control the trafficking of B and T cells responsible for mucosal immunity. CCR7 and its ligands, expressed constitutively in lymphoid tissues, help mediate the recirculation of naïve and memory lymphocytes through spleen, lymph nodes, and mucosal lymphoid tissues. Selectivity of recirculation through PPs (*i.e.*, for gut memory T cells), is permitted by differential expression of α4β7, the homing receptor for MAdCAM-1 on PP HEV, and high expression of α4β7 is characteristic of memory and immunoblasts that home to the gut wall. However, whereas most lymphocyte types use a common α4β7/MAdCAM-1 mechanism to home to the gastrointestinal tract, each differentiated population (*i.e.*, B vs. T or memory cell vs. plasmablast) seems to employ a distinct chemokine receptor or receptor combinations, thus allowing refined control of the types of immune cells recruited. For example, while naïve and memory B cells express CCR6, CXCR5, and variable CCR7, circulating and tissue IgA plasmablasts and plasma cells express CCR9 and CCR10, receptors for mucosal epithelial chemokines. This of course contrasts with IgG plasmablasts, which express CXCR3 and respond to inflammatory chemokines. Constitutive, tissue-specific expression of epithelial chemokines implies a surprising potential for local or tissue type–selective specialization in immune responses and modalities in the mucosal immune system. CCR9 is associated with IgA ASCs that localize to the TECK/CCL25-expressing small intestines, while CCR10, in conjunction with mucosal epithelial cell–derived MEC/CCL28, contributes to the broader localization of IgA ASCs to the physically dispersed organs of the secretory IgA immune system (**Fig. 34.6**). It should be noted that while CCR9 and TECK/CCL25 apparently play an equivalent role in memory T cell homing to the small intestine, chemoattractants regulating specific homing to colon, lung, and other mucosal tissues remain to be identified. These observations suggest a common chemoattractant mechanism for the dissemination of IgA-dependent immunity following local mucosal stimulation or vaccination but also indicate that unique combinatorial profiles of CCR9, CCR10, selectin, and integrin expression may result in selective trafficking of IgA ASCs or effector T cell subsets arising in response to mucosal immunization through nasal, lower airway, oral, colonic, or genitourinary tract sites. Refinement of our understanding of these processes will facilitate the design of effective vaccines against mucosal pathogens and treatment of mucosal inflammatory disease.

ACKNOWLEDGMENTS

The authors thank the many laboratory members who contributed to the work embodied in this review and especially E. Kunkel for discussion of unpublished studies on IgA ASCs and for assistance and input on the manuscript. Studies in the authors' laboratory were supported in part by grants from the National Institutes of Health, by an award from the U.S. Department of Veterans Affairs, and by the FACS Core Facility of the Stanford Digestive Disease Center.

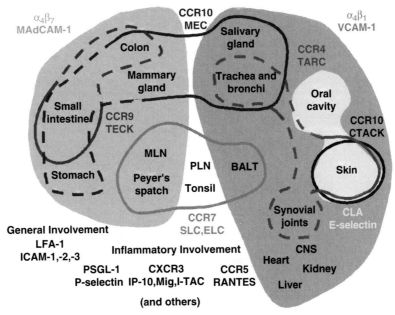

Fig. 34.6. Tissue-selective chemokine expression in the systemic organization of the immune system. In this model, tissue-selective chemokines and adhesion pathways control lymphocyte homing, while the selectivity of lymphocyte recruitment reflects the combination of vascular adhesion molecules and chemokines expressed in a given tissue site. This diagram groups body tissues according to the predominant constitutive tissue-selective lymphocyte-endothelial adhesion molecules that participate in lymphocyte recruitment (*solid colors*) and then further groups them by the homeostatic endothelial or epithelial chemokines (and their lymphocyte receptors) associated with each tissue (*solid lines; dashed lines* show sites where the chemokine is expressed at low levels in comparison with other grouped tissues and/or the receptor is only on a subset of lymphocytes). Thus, (1) the lymphoid tissue chemokines SLC/CCL21 and ELC/CCL19 and lymphocyte CCR7, in conjunction with L-selectin (not shown), help control lymphocyte entry into secondary lymphoid tissues; (2) endothelial TARC/CCL17 and its receptor CCR4 (expressed at high levels by T cells in skin and at lower levels in the lung and joints), along with CTACK/CCL27 and CCR10 (skin and perhaps oral cavity), in conjunction with CLA and E-selectin (skin and oral cavity) and $\alpha 4\beta 1$ and VCAM-1 (nonintestinal sites), control homing of cutaneous memory T cells to skin; (3) epithelial TECK/CCL25 (predominantly small intestine), in conjunction with $\alpha 4\beta 7$ and MAdCAM-1 (colon, mammary gland, and small intestine), is implicated in selective trafficking to the small intestine; and (4) MEC/CCL28 (colon, salivary gland, bronchi, and mammary gland), acting either with $\alpha 4\beta 1$ and VCAM-1 (nonintestinal sites) or with $\alpha 4\beta 7$ and MAdCAM-1 (mammary gland and intestines), is proposed to mediate lymphocyte subset recruitment to many mucosal tissues. Some adhesion molecules such as LFA-1 ($\alpha L\beta 2$) and its ligands (ICAM-1,-2,-3) are involved in lymphocyte homing to most tissues, and inflammation induces the expression of many other chemokines and adhesion molecules (*e.g.*, P-selectin and ligands for chemokine receptors such as CXCR3 and CCR5) that can complement the homeostatic tissue-selective recruitment mechanisms emphasized here. Adapted with permission from Kunkel and Butcher (2002).

REFERENCES

Ager, A. (1993). Lymphocyte-vascular endothelial cell interactions in the immune response. *Clin. Exp. Immunol.* 93(Suppl 1), 5–6.

Bargatze, R. F., Jutila, M. A., and Butcher, E. C. (1995). Distinct roles of L-selectin and integrins $\alpha 4\beta 7$ and LFA-1 in lymphocyte homing to Peyer's patch–HEV in situ: the multistep model confirmed and refined. *Immunity* 3, 99–108.

Berg, E. L., McEvoy, L. M., Berlin, C., Bargatze, R. F., and Butcher, E. C. (1993). L-selectin-mediated lymphocyte rolling on MAdCAM-1. *Nature* 366, 695–8.

Berlin, C., Bargatze, R. F., Campbell, J. J., von Andrian, U. H., Szabo, M. C., Hasslen, S. R., Nelson, R. D., Berg, E. L., Erlandsen, S. L., and Butcher, E. C. (1995). $\alpha 4$ integrins mediate lymphocyte attachment and rolling under physiologic flow. *Cell* 80, 413–22.

Bistrup, A., Bhakta, S., Lee, J. K., Belov, Y. Y., Gunn, M. D., Zuo, F. R., Huang, C. C., Kannagi, R., Rosen, S. D., and Hemmerich, S. (1999). Sulfotransferases of two specificities function in the reconstitution of high endothelial cell ligands for L-selectin. *J. Cell Biol.* 145, 899–910.

Bowman, E. P., Kuklin, N. A., Youngman, K. R., Lazarus, N. H., Kunkel, E. J., Pan, J., Greenberg, H. B., and Butcher, E. C. (2002). The intestinal chemokine thymus-expressed chemokine (CCL25) attracts IgA antibody–secreting cells. *J. Exp. Med.* 195, 269–75.

Brandtzaeg, P., Farstad, I. N., and Haraldsen, G. (1999a). Regional specialization in the mucosal immune system: primed cells do not always home along the same track. *Immunol. Today* 20, 267–77.

Brandtzaeg, P., Farstad, I. N., Johansen, F. E., Morton, H. C., Norderhaug, I. N., and Yamanaka, T. (1999b). The B-cell system of human mucosae and exocrine glands. *Immunol. Rev.* 171, 45–87.

Briskin, M., Winsor-Hines, D., Shyjan, A., Cochran, N., Bloom, S., Wilson, J., McEvoy, L. M., Butcher, E. C., Kassam, N., Mackay, C. R., Newman, W., and Ringler, D. J. (1997). Human mucosal addressin cell adhesion molecule-1 is preferentially expressed in intestinal tract and associated lymphoid tissue. *Am. J. Pathol.* 151, 97–110.

Briskin, M. J., McEvoy, L. M., and Butcher, E. C. (1993). MAdCAM-1 has homology to immunoglobulin and mucin-like adhesion receptors and to IgA1. *Nature* 363, 461–4.

Briskin, M. J., Rott, L., and Butcher, E. C. (1996). Structural requirements for mucosal vascular addressin binding to its lymphocyte receptor α4β7. Common themes among integrin-Ig family interactions. *J. Immunol.* 156, 719–26.

Butcher, E. C., and Picker, L. J. (1996). Lymphocyte homing and homeostasis. *Science* 272, 60–6.

Butcher, E. C., Williams, M., Youngman, K., Rott, L., and Briskin, M. (1999). Lymphocyte trafficking and regional immunity. *Adv. Immunol.* 72, 209–53.

Campbell, J. J., Haraldsen, G., Pan, J., Rottman, J., Qin, S., Ponath, P., Andrew, D. P., Warnke, R., Ruffing, N., Kassam, N., Wu, L., and Butcher, E. C. (1999). The chemokine receptor CCR4 in vascular recognition by cutaneous but not intestinal memory T cells. *Nature* 400, 776–80.

Campbell, J. J., Hedrick, J., Zlotnik, A., Siani, M. A., Thompson, D. A., and Butcher, E. C. (1998). Chemokines and the arrest of lymphocytes rolling under flow conditions. *Science* 279, 381–4.

Carlos, T. M., and Harlan, J. M. (1994). Leukocyte–endothelial adhesion molecules. *Blood* 84, 2068–101.

Czerkinsky, C., Svennerholm, A. M., Quiding, M., Jonsson, R., and Holmgren, J. (1991). Antibody-producing cells in peripheral blood and salivary glands after oral cholera vaccination of humans. *Infect. Immun.* 59, 996–1001.

Czinn, S. J., and Lamm, M. E. (1986). Selective chemotaxis of subsets of B lymphocytes from gut-associated lymphoid tissue and its implications for the recruitment of mucosal plasma cells. *J. Immunol.* 136, 3607–3611.

Erlandsen, S. L., Hasslen, S. R., and Nelson, R. D. (1993). Detection and spatial distribution of the β2 integrin (Mac-1) and L-selectin (LECAM-1) adherence receptors on human neutrophils by high-resolution field emission SEM. *J. Histochem. Cytochem.* 41, 327–33.

Fagarasan, S., Kinoshita, K., Muramatsu, M., Ikuta, K., and Honjo, T. (2001). In situ class switching and differentiation to IgA-producing cells in the gut lamina propria. *Nature* 413, 639–43.

Gallatin, W. M., Weissman, I. L., and Butcher, E. C. (1983). A cell-surface molecule involved in organ-specific homing of lymphocytes. *Nature* 304, 30–4.

Gonzalez, A. M., Jaimes, M. C., Cajiao, I., Rojas, O. L., Cohen, J., Pothier, P., Kohli, E., Butcher, E. C., Greenberg, H. B., Angel, J., and Franco, M. A. (2003). Rotavirus-specific B cells induced by recent infection in adults and children predominantly express the intestinal homing receptor α4β7. *Virology* 305, 93–105.

Grant, A. J., Lalor, P. F., Hubscher, S. G., Briskin, M., and Adams, D. H. (2001). MAdCAM-1 expressed in chronic inflammatory liver disease supports mucosal lymphocyte adhesion to hepatic endothelium (MAdCAM-1 in chronic inflammatory liver disease). *Hepatology* 33, 1065–72.

Gunn, M. D., Tangemann, K., Tam, C., Cyster, J. G., Rosen, S. D., and Williams, L. T. (1998). A chemokine expressed in lymphoid high endothelial venules promotes the adhesion and chemotaxis of naive T lymphocytes. *Proc. Natl. Acad. Sci. USA* 95, 258–63.

Hargreaves, D. C., Hyman, P. L., Lu, T. T., Ngo, V. N., Bidgol, A., Suzuki, G., Zou, Y. R., Littman, D. R., and Cyster, J. G. (2001). A coordinated change in chemokine responsiveness guides plasma cell movements. *J. Exp. Med.* 194, 45–56.

Hauser, A. E., Debes, G. F., Arce, S., Cassese, G., Hamann, A., Radbruch, A., and Manz, R. A. (2002). Chemotactic responsiveness toward ligands for CXCR3 and CXCR4 is regulated on plasma blasts during the time course of a memory immune response. *J. Immunol.* 169, 1277–82.

Hemmerich, S., and Rosen, S. D. (2000). Carbohydrate sulfotransferases in lymphocyte homing. *Glycobiology* 10, 849–56.

Hillan, K. J., Hagler, K. E., MacSween, R. N., Ryan, A. M., Renz, M. E., Chiu, H. H., Ferrier, R. K., Bird, G. L., Dhillon, A. P., Ferrell, L. D., and Fong, S. (1999). Expression of the mucosal vascular addressin, MAdCAM-1, in inflammatory liver disease. *Liver* 19, 509–18.

Hiraoka, N., Petryniak, B., Nakayama, J., Tsuboi, S., Suzuki, M., Yeh, J. C., Izawa, D., Tanaka, T., Miyasaka, M., Lowe, J. B., and Fukuda, M. (1999). A novel, high endothelial venule–specific sulfotransferase expresses 6-sulfo sialyl Lewis(x), an L-selectin ligand displayed by CD34. *Immunity* 11, 79–89.

Hu, M. C., Holzmann, B., Crowe, D. T., Neuhaus, H., and Weissman, I. L. (1993). The Peyer's patch homing receptor. *Curr. Top. Microbiol. Immunol.* 184, 125–38.

Hudak, S., Hagen, M., Liu, Y., Catron, D., Oldham, E., McEvoy, L. M., and Bowman, E. P. (2002). Immune surveillance and effector functions of CCR10(+) skin homing T cells. *J. Immunol.* 169, 1189–96.

Hynes, R. O. (1992). Integrins: versatility, modulation, and signaling in cell adhesion. *Cell* 69, 11–25.

Imhof, B. A., and Dunon, D. (1995). Leukocyte migration and adhesion. *Adv. Immunol.* 58, 345–416.

Iwasaki, A., and Kelsall, B. L. (2000). Localization of distinct Peyer's patch dendritic cell subsets and their recruitment by chemokines macrophage inflammatory protein (MIP)-3α, MIP-3β, and secondary lymphoid organ chemokine. *J. Exp. Med.* 191, 1381–94.

Jarmin, D. I., Rits, M., Bota, D., Gerard, N. P., Graham, G. J., Clark-Lewis, I., and Gerard, C. (2000). Cutting edge: identification of the orphan receptor G-protein-coupled receptor 2 as CCR10, a specific receptor for the chemokine ESkine. *J. Immunol.* 164, 3460–4.

Johansson, E. L., Wassen, L., Holmgren, J., Jertborn, M., and Rudin, A. (2001). Nasal and vaginal vaccinations have differential effects on antibody responses in vaginal and cervical secretions in humans. *Infect. Immun.* 69, 7481–6.

Johnston, B., and Butcher, E. C. (2002). Chemokines in rapid leukocyte adhesion triggering and migration. *Semin. Immunol.* 14, 83–92.

Kato, H., Kato, R., Fujihashi, K., and McGhee, J. R. (2001). Role of mucosal antibodies in viral infections. *Curr. Top. Microbiol. Immunol.* 260, 201–28.

Kraal, G., Schornagel, K., Streeter, P. R., Holzmann, B., and Butcher, E. C. (1995). Expression of the mucosal vascular addressin, MAdCAM-1, on sinus-lining cells in the spleen. *Am. J. Pathol.* 147, 763–71.

Kruse, A., Merchant, M. J., Hallmann, R., and Butcher, E. C. (1999). Evidence of specialized leukocyte-vascular homing interactions at the maternal/fetal interface. *Eur. J. Immunol.* 29, 1116–26.

Kuklin, N. A., Rott, L., Darling, J., Campbell, J. J., Franco, M., Feng, N., Muller, W., Wagner, N., Altman, J., Butcher, E. C., and Greenberg, H. B. (2000). α(4)β(7) independent pathway for CD8(+) T cell–mediated intestinal immunity to rotavirus. *J. Clin. Invest.* 106, 1541–52.

Kuklin, N. A., Rott, L., Feng, N., Conner, M. E., Wagner, N., Muller, W., and Greenberg, H. B. (2001). Protective intestinal anti-rotavirus B cell immunity is dependent on α4β7 integrin expression but does not require IgA antibody production. *J. Immunol.* 166, 1894–902.

Kunkel, E. J., and Butcher, E. C. (2002). Chemokines and the tissue-specific migration of lymphocytes. *Immunity* 16, 1–4.

Kunkel, E. J., and Butcher, E. C. (2003). Plasma-cell homing. *Nat. Rev. Immunol.* 3, 822–829.

Kunkel, E. J., Campbell, J. J., Haraldsen, G., Pan, J., Boisvert, J., Roberts, A. I., Ebert, E. C., Vierra, M. A., Goodman, S. B., Genovese, M. C., Wardlaw, A. J., Greenberg, H. B., Parker, C. M., Butcher, E. C., Andrew, D. P., and Agace, W. W. (2000). Lymphocyte CC chemokine receptor 9 and epithelial thymus-expressed chemokine (TECK) expression distinguish the small intestinal immune compartment: Epithelial expression of tissue-specific chemokines as an organizing principle in regional immunity. *J. Exp. Med.* 192, 761–8.

Kunkel, E. J., Kim, C. H., Lazarus, N. H., Vierra, M. A., Soler, D., Bowman, E. P., and Butcher, E. C. (2003). CCR10 expression is a common feature of circulating and mucosal epithelial tissue IgA Ab-secreting cells. *J. Clin. Invest.* 111, 1001–10.

Lalor, P. F., Edwards, S., McNab, G., Salmi, M., Jalkanen, S., and Adams, D. H. (2002). Vascular adhesion protein–1 mediates adhesion and transmigration of lymphocytes on human hepatic endothelial cells. *J. Immunol.* 169, 983–92.

Laudanna, C., Kim, J. Y., Constantin, G., and Butcher, E. (2002). Rapid leukocyte integrin activation by chemokines. *Immunol. Rev.* 186, 37–46.

Lazarus, N. H., Kunkel, E. J., Johnston, B., Wilson, E., Youngman, K. R., and Butcher, E. C. (2003). A common mucosal chemokine (mucosae-associated epithelial chemokine/ccl28) selectively attracts IgA plasmablasts. *J. Immunol.* 170, 3799–805.

Marsal, J., Svensson, M., Ericsson, A., Iranpour, A. H., Carramolino, L., Marquez, G., and Agace, W. W. (2002). Involvement of CCL25 (TECK) in the generation of the murine small-intestinal CD8α α+CD3+ intraepithelial lymphocyte compartment. *Eur. J. Immunol.* 32, 3488–97.

McDermott, M. R., and Bienenstock, J. (1979). Evidence for a common mucosal immunologic system. I. Migration of B immunoblasts into intestinal, respiratory, and genital tissues. *J. Immunol.* 122, 1892–8.

McHeyzer-Williams, M. G., and Ahmed, R. (1999). B cell memory and the long-lived plasma cell. *Curr. Opin. Immunol.* 11, 172–9.

Mestecky, J. (1987). The common mucosal immune system and current strategies for induction of immune responses in external secretions. *J. Clin. Immunol.* 7, 265–76.

Mikulowska-Mennis, A., Xu, B., Berberian, J. M., and Michie, S. A. (2001). Lymphocyte migration to inflamed lacrimal glands is mediated by vascular cell adhesion molecule-1/α(4)β(1) integrin, peripheral node addressin/l-selectin, and lymphocyte function–associated antigen-1 adhesion pathways. *Am. J. Pathol.* 159, 671–81.

Morales, J., Homey, B., Vicari, A. P., Hudak, S., Oldham, E., Hedrick, J., Orozco, R., Copeland, N. G., Jenkins, N. A., McEvoy, L. M., and Zlotnik, A. (1999). CTACK, a skin-associated chemokine that preferentially attracts skin-homing memory T cells. *Proc. Natl. Acad. Sci. USA* 96, 14470–5.

O'Neill, J. K., Butter, C., Baker, D., Gschmeissner, S. E., Kraal, G., Butcher, E. C., and Turk, J. L. (1991). Expression of vascular addressins and ICAM-1 by endothelial cells in the spinal cord during chronic relapsing experimental allergic encephalomyelitis in the Biozzi AB/H mouse. *Immunology* 72, 520–5.

Offit, P. A. (2001). Correlates of protection against rotavirus infection and disease. *Novartis Found. Symp.* 238, 106–13; discussion 114–24.

Okada, T., Ngo, V. N., Ekland, E. H., Forster, R., Lipp, M., Littman, D. R., and Cyster, J. G. (2002). Chemokine requirements for B cell entry to lymph nodes and Peyer's patches. *J. Exp. Med.* 196, 65–75.

Pabst, O., Ohl, L., Wendland, M., Wurbel, M. A., Kremmer, E., Malissen, B., Forster, R. (2004). Chemokine receptor CCR9 contributes to the localization of plasma cells to the small intestine. *J. Exp. Med.* 199, 411–416.

Pan, J., Kunkel, E. J., Gosslar, U., Lazarus, N., Langdon, P., Broadwell, K., Vierra, M. A., Genovese, M. C., Butcher, E. C., and Soler, D. (2000). A novel chemokine ligand for CCR10 and CCR3 expressed by epithelial cells in mucosal tissues. *J. Immunol.* 165, 2943–9.

Papadakis, K. A., Prehn, J., Nelson, V., Cheng, L., Binder, S. W., Ponath, P. D., Andrew, D. P., and Targan, S. R. (2000). The role of thymus-expressed chemokine and its receptor CCR9 on lymphocytes in the regional specialization of the mucosal immune system. *J. Immunol.* 165, 5069–76.

Power, C. A., Church, D. J., Meyer, A., Alouani, S., Proudfoot, A. E., Clark-Lewis, I., Sozzani, S., Mantovani, A., and Wells, T. N. (1997). Cloning and characterization of a specific receptor for the novel CC chemokine MIP-3α from lung dendritic cells. *J. Exp. Med.* 186, 825–35.

Reif, K., Ekland, E. H., Ohl, L., Nakano, H., Lipp, M., Forster, R., and Cyster, J. G. (2002). Balanced responsiveness to chemoattractants from adjacent zones determines B-cell position. *Nature* 416, 94–9.

Reiss, Y., Proudfoot, A. E., Power, C. A., Campbell, J. J., and Butcher, E. C. (2001). CC chemokine receptor (CCR)4 and the CCR10 ligand cutaneous T cell–attracting chemokine (CTACK) in lymphocyte trafficking to inflamed skin. *J. Exp. Med.* 194, 1541–7.

Rose, J. R., Williams, M. B., Rott, L. S., Butcher, E. C., and Greenberg, H. B. (1998). Expression of the mucosal homing receptor α4β7 correlates with the ability of CD8+ memory T cells to clear rotavirus infection. *J. Virol.* 72, 726–30.

Rosen, S. D. (1999). Endothelial ligands for L-selectin: from lymphocyte recirculation to allograft rejection. *Am. J. Pathol.* 155, 1013–20.

Rott, L. S., Briskin, M. J., Andrew, D. P., Berg, E. L., and Butcher, E. C. (1996). A fundamental subdivision of circulating lymphocytes defined by adhesion to mucosal addressin cell adhesion

molecule-1. Comparison with vascular cell adhesion molecule-1 and correlation with β7 integrins and memory differentiation. *J. Immunol.* 156, 3727–36.

Russell, M. W., Hedges, S. R., Wu, H. Y., Hook, E. W., 3rd, and Mestecky, J. (1999). Mucosal immunity in the genital tract: prospects for vaccines against sexually transmitted diseases: a review. *Am. J. Reprod. Immunol.* 42, 58–63.

Salmi, M., Granfors, K., MacDermott, R., and Jalkanen, S. (1994). Aberrant binding of lamina propria lymphocytes to vascular endothelium in inflammatory bowel diseases. *Gastroenterology* 106, 596–605.

Salmi, M., Kalimo, K., and Jalkanen, S. (1993). Induction and function of vascular adhesion protein-1 at sites of inflammation. *J. Exp. Med.* 178, 2255–60.

Salmi, M., Yegutkin, G. G., Lehvonen, R., Koskinen, K., Salminen, T., and Jalkanen, S. (2001). A cell surface amine oxidase directly controls lymphocyte migration. *Immunity* 14, 265–76.

Sassetti, C., Tangemann, K., Singer, M. S., Kershaw, D. B., and Rosen, S. D. (1998). Identification of podocalyxin-like protein as a high endothelial venule ligand for L-selectin: parallels to CD34. *J. Exp. Med.* 187, 1965–75.

Schaible, U. E., Vestweber, D., Butcher, E. C., Stehle, T., and Simon, M. M. (1994). Expression of endothelial cell adhesion molecules in joints and heart during *Borrelia burgdorferi* infection of mice. *Cell Adhes. Commun.* 2, 465–79.

Shaw, S. K., and Brenner, M. B. (1995). The β7 integrins in mucosal homing and retention. *Semin. Immunol.* 7, 335–42.

Shimizu, Y., Newman, W., Tanaka, Y., and Shaw, S. (1992). Lymphocyte interactions with endothelial cells. *Immunol. Today* 13, 106–12.

Sikorski, E. E., Hallmann, R., Berg, E. L., and Butcher, E. C. (1993). The Peyer's patch high endothelial receptor for lymphocytes, the mucosal vascular addressin, is induced on a murine endothelial cell line by tumor necrosis factor–α and IL-1. *J. Immunol.* 151, 5239–50.

Singh, B., Tschernig, T., Van Griensven, M., Fieguth, A., and Pabst, R. (2003). Expression of vascular adhesion protein-1 in normal and inflamed mice lungs and normal human lungs. *Virchows Arch.* 17, 17.

Springer, T. A. (1995). Traffic signals on endothelium for lymphocyte recirculation and leukocyte emigration. *Annu. Rev. Physiol.* 57, 827–72.

Steffen, B. J., Breier, G., Butcher, E. C., Schulz, M., and Engelhardt, B. (1996). ICAM-1, VCAM-1, and MAdCAM-1 are expressed on choroid plexus epithelium but not endothelium and mediate binding of lymphocytes in vitro. *Am. J. Pathol.* 148, 1819–38.

Strauch, U. G., Lifka, A., Gosslar, U., Kilshaw, P. J., Clements, J., and Holzmann, B. (1994). Distinct binding specificities of integrins α4β7 (LPAM-1), α4β1 (VLA-4), and αIELβ7. *Int. Immunol.* 6, 263–75.

Streeter, P. R., Berg, E. L., Rouse, B. T., Bargatze, R. F., and Butcher, E. C. (1988a). A tissue-specific endothelial cell molecule involved in lymphocyte homing. *Nature* 331, 41–6.

Streeter, P. R., Rouse, B. T., and Butcher, E. C. (1988b). Immunohistologic and functional characterization of a vascular addressin involved in lymphocyte homing into peripheral lymph nodes. *J. Cell. Biol.* 107, 1853–62.

Svensson, M., Marsal, J., Ericsson, A., Carramolino, L., Broden, T., Marquez, G., and Agace, W. W. (2002). CCL25 mediates the localization of recently activated CD8αβ(+) lymphocytes to the small-intestinal mucosa. *J. Clin. Invest.* 110, 1113–21.

Szabo, M. C., Butcher, E. C., and McEvoy, L. M. (1997). Specialization of mucosal follicular dendritic cells revealed by mucosal addressin–cell adhesion molecule-1 display. *J. Immunol.* 158, 5584–8.

Tanaka, H., Hataba, Y., Saito, S., Fukushima, O., and Miyasaka, M. (1996). Phenotypic characteristics and significance of reticular meshwork surrounding splenic white pulp of mice. *J. Electron Microsc. (Tokyo)* 45, 407–16.

van der Feltz, M. J., de Groot, N., Bayley, J. P., Lee, S. H., Verbeet, M. P., and de Boer, H. A. (2001). Lymphocyte homing and Ig secretion in the murine mammary gland. *Scand. J. Immunol.* 54, 292–300.

van Ginkel, F. W., Jackson, R. J., Yuki, Y., and McGhee, J. R. (2000). Cutting edge: the mucosal adjuvant cholera toxin redirects vaccine proteins into olfactory tissues. *J. Immunol.* 165, 4778–82.

von Andrian, U. H., Hasslen, S. R., Nelson, R. D., Erlandsen, S. L., and Butcher, E. C. (1995). A central role for microvillous receptor presentation in leukocyte adhesion under flow. *Cell* 82, 989–99.

Wang, W., Soto, H., Oldham, E. R., Buchanan, M. E., Homey, B., Catron, D., Jenkins, N., Copeland, N. G., Gilbert, D. J., Nguyen, N., Abrams, J., Kershenovich, D., Smith, K., McClanahan, T., Vicari, A. P., and Zlotnik, A. (2000). Identification of a novel chemokine (CCL28), which binds CCR10 (GPR2). *J. Biol. Chem.* 275, 22313–23.

Warnock, R. A., Askari, S., Butcher, E. C., and von Andrian, U. H. (1998). Molecular mechanisms of lymphocyte homing to peripheral lymph nodes. *J. Exp. Med.* 187, 205–16.

Warnock, R. A., Campbell, J. J., Dorf, M. E., Matsuzawa, A., McEvoy, L. M., and Butcher, E. C. (2000). The role of chemokines in the microenvironmental control of T versus B cell arrest in Peyer's patch high endothelial venules. *J. Exp. Med.* 191, 77–88.

Weisz-Carrington, P., Roux, M. E., McWilliams, M., Phillips-Quagliata, J. M., and Lamm, M. E. (1979). Organ and isotype distribution of plasma cells producing specific antibody after oral immunization: evidence for a generalized secretory immune system. *J. Immunol.* 123, 1705–8.

Williams, M. B., Rose, J. R., Rott, L. S., Franco, M. A., Greenberg, H. B., and Butcher, E. C. (1998). The memory B cell subset responsible for the secretory IgA response and protective humoral immunity to rotavirus expresses the intestinal homing receptor, α4β7. *J. Immunol.* 161, 4227–4235.

Wurbel, M. A., Philippe, J. M., Nguyen, C., Victorero, G., Freeman, T., Wooding, P., Miazek, A., Mattei, M. G., Malissen, M., Jordan, B. R., Malissen, B., Carrier, A., and Naquet, P. (2000). The chemokine TECK is expressed by thymic and intestinal epithelial cells and attracts double- and single-positive thymocytes expressing the TECK receptor CCR9. *Eur. J. Immunol.* 30, 262–71.

Xu, B., Wagner, N., Pham, L. N., V., M., Shan, Z., Butcher, E. C., and Michie, S. A. (2003). Lymphocyte homing to bronchus-associated lymphoid tissue (BALT) is mediated by l-selectin/PNAd, α4β1 integrin/VCAM-1, and LFA-1 adhesion pathways. *J. Exp. Med.* 197, 1255–1267.

Yang, X. D., Sytwu, H. K., McDevitt, H. O., and Michie, S. A. (1997). Involvement of β7 integrin and mucosal addressin cell adhesion molecule-1 (MAdCAM-1) in the development of diabetes in obese diabetic mice. *Diabetes* 46, 1542–7.

Yeh, J. C., Hiraoka, N., Petryniak, B., Nakayama, J., Ellies, L. G., Rabuka, D., Hindsgaul, O., Marth, J. D., Lowe, J. B., and Fukuda, M. (2001). Novel sulfated lymphocyte homing receptors and their control by a Core1 extension β 1,3-N-acetylglucosaminyltransferase. *Cell* 105, 957–69.

Youngman, K. R., Franco, M. A., Kuklin, N. A., Rott, L. S., Butcher, E. C., and Greenberg, H. B. (2002). Correlation of tissue distribution, developmental phenotype, and intestinal homing receptor expression of antigen-specific B cells during the murine anti-rotavirus immune response. *J. Immunol.* 168, 2173–81.

Zabel, B. A., Agace, W. W., Campbell, J. J., Heath, H. M., Parent, D., Roberts, A. I., Ebert, E. C., Kassam, N., Qin, S., Zovko, M., LaRosa, G. J., Yang, L. L., Soler, D., Butcher, E. C., Ponath, P. D., Parker, C. M., and Andrew, D. P. (1999). Human G protein-coupled receptor GPR-9-6/CC chemokine receptor 9 is selectively expressed on intestinal homing T lymphocytes, mucosal lymphocytes, and thymocytes and is required for thymus-expressed chemokine-mediated chemotaxis. *J. Exp. Med.* 190, 1241–56.

Proinflammatory Cytokines and Signaling Pathways in Intestinal Innate Immune Cells

Chapter 35

R. Balfour Sartor

Departments of Medicine and Microbiology & Immunology and Multidisciplinary Center for IBD Research and Treatment, University of North Carolina, Chapel Hill, North Carolina

Frank Hoentjen

Postdoctoral Research Fellow, University of North Carolina, Chapel Hill, North Carolina, and Free University Medical Center, Amsterdam, The Netherlands

Activated innate immune cells mediate a variety of protective and proinflammatory mucosal immune responses, with key roles in clearance of microbial pathogens, recruitment of effector cells into the inflammatory focus, tissue destruction and remodeling, and antigen presentation. These activities are relevant to both acute and chronic inflammatory processes at mucosal surfaces, including inflammatory bowel diseases (IBD), infection, asthma, periodontal disease, bronchitis and cystic fibrosis. Inflammatory cytokines, most notably interleukin-1 (IL-1), tumor necrosis factor (TNF), IL-6, and multiple chemokines, are secreted by a variety of activated innate immune cells of hematologic, mesenchymal, epithelial, and endothelial origin **(Table 35.1)**. In contrast, the Th1 polarizing cytokines IL-12, IL-18, and IL-23 are more selectively secreted by antigen-presenting cells (APCs), such as dendritic cells, macrophages, and in the case of IL-18, epithelial cells.

Many microbial products and proinflammatory molecules activate innate immune responses, culminating in increased transcription and secretion of proinflammatory cytokines. Microbial products stimulate cells through a family of pattern-recognition receptors that induce signals through NF-κB and mitogen-activated protein kinases (MAPK). In addition, innate immune cells can be activated by proinflammatory cytokines (IL-1 and TNF), reactive oxygen metabolites, and products of the coagulation and complement cascades.

Maintenance of mucosal homeostasis depends on the ability of activated innate immune cells to appropriately downregulate the inflammatory response to microbial and inflammatory signals through secreted and cytoplasmic regulatory molecules **(Table 35.2)**. Mechanisms of inhibition include suppression of responses to inflammatory signals by downregulation of membrane receptors, *i.e.*, CD14 and toll-like receptors (TLRs), which promotes unresponsiveness to ubiquitous stimuli by emigrating monocytes and maturing epithelial cells, as well as upregulation of suppressive molecules, including PPARγ, prostaglandins, suppressor of cytokine signaling (SOCS), and A20.

This chapter describes the biologic activities, signaling pathways, and regulatory mechanisms of the most common proinflammatory cytokines. The reader is referred to other chapters in this section for a more detailed description of bone marrow–derived APCs (Chapter 26), chemokines (Chapters 26 and 34), epithelial cells (Chapters 24 and 25), mast cells (Chapter 36), and eosinophils (Chapter 37) and to previous reviews on this topic (Sartor, 2003; Cominelli *et al.*, 2004).

PROFILE OF CYTOKINES SECRETED BY INNATE IMMUNE CELLS

Bone marrow–derived, epithelial, mesenchymal, and endothelial innate immune cells each secrete a unique characteristic profile of cytokines, inflammatory mediators, and antimicrobial peptides when stimulated with a variety of microbial products (Table 35.1). Because of conserved signaling pathways, proinflammatory cytokines induce expression of identical molecules in different cells, thereby amplifying the inflammatory response in cells not exposed to the original inciting agent and also broadening the repertoire of activating signals. Moreover, members of cytokine families

Table 35.1. Secretion of Proinflammatory Cytokines by Mucosal Innate Immune Cells

Cell Type	Function	Primary Cytokine Profile
Bone marrow–derived		
Macrophage	Effector, phagocytic, APC	IL-1, IL-6, IL-12, IL-18, IL-23, TNF, IFNα, GM-CSF, M-CSF, IL-1RA, chemokines
Dendritic cells[a]	APC	IL-10, IL-12, IL-18, IL-23, T cell chemokines
Neutrophil	Phagocytic, effector	IL-1, IL-6, TNF
Eosinophil	Effector, phagocytic	IL-1, TNF
Mast cell	Effector	IL-1, IL-6, TNF
Natural killer cell	Effector	IFN-γ
Epithelial origin		
Epithelial	Effector, barrier function APC	Chemokines, IL-18, IL-1RA
Paneth cell	Effector	
Mesenchymal origin		
Smooth muscle, fibroblast, myofibroblast	Motility, matrix secretion, tissue remodeling, effector	IL-1, IL-6, TNF, chemokines
Endothelial cell	Adhesion molecules, effector	IL-1, IL-6, TNF, chemokines

[a]Dendritic cell subsets: myeloid, lymphoid, plasmacytoid.

are usually stimulated or suppressed in concert via redundant transcriptional regulatory pathways.

Epithelial cells

Mucosal epithelial cells act as sensors of microbial invasion and secreted toxins by liberating chemokines and, to a lesser degree, proinflammatory molecules (see Chapter 25). These molecules activate protective mucosal inflammatory and immune responses by stimulating the emigration and activation of a variety of effector cells to respond to the inciting stimulus. Expression of chemotactic signals is temporally and spatially coordinated, leading to the emigration of first neutrophils, then monocytes, and finally lymphocytes. Furthermore, chemokines recruiting a single class of effector cells can be biphasic, so that the emigration of these cells can be prolonged. For example, *Salmonella* invasion of cultured colonic epithelial cell monolayers induces maximal expression of IL-8, which selectively recruits and activates neu-

Table 35.2. Regulatory Molecules Induced by Proinflammatory Cytokines

Molecule	Function	Primarily induced by
Secreted		
IL-10	Inhibits macrophage and APC activation, induces SOCS 3	IL-1, TNF, IFN-γ, CD40L
IL-1 receptor antagonist	Competitively inhibits IL-1α and IL-1β binding	IL-1, TNF
PGE$_2$, PGI$_2$, PGJ$_2$	Inhibits macrophage activation	IL-1, TNF
Corticosteroids	Blocks NF-κB, chemotaxis	IL-1, TNF, IL-6
IL-1RII	Binds IL-1 without signaling	IL-4
TNF RI (p55)	Binds TNF, LTα without signaling	IFN-α
Cytoplasmic		
A20	Inhibits TNF signaling	TNF
IκBα	Inhibits NF-κB activation	IL-1, TNF, bacterial products (NF-κB activation)
PPARγ	Inhibits NF-κB activation	Bacterial products (NF-κB activation)
COX 2	Inhibits macrophage activation	IL-1, TNF, IL-6, bacterial products (NF-κB activation)
iNOS	Inhibits NF-κB activation	IL-1, TNF, IL-6, bacterial products

trophils, at 4–6 hours, while epithelial neutrophil activating protein-78 (ENA-78) is maximally expressed 18–24 hours after bacterial invasion (Yang *et al.*, 1997; Dwinell *et al.*, 2001). IL-6 secreted by epithelial cells can promote the transition from acute to chronic inflammation by altering chemokine profiles to favor monocyte recruitment (Kaplanski *et al.*, 2003).

This sequential activation of chemokines leads to progressive recruitment of effector cells with distinct functions and also prolongs chemotactic signals to ensure efficient protective innate and acquired immune responses. In addition to chemotactic signals, activated NF-κB and MAP kinases in epithelial cells stimulate expression of adhesion molecules, including ICAM-1, class II major histocompatibility complex (MHC) molecules, cyclooxygenase-2 (COX-2), CARD15/NOD2, and certain proinflammatory cytokines, including IL-6 (Jung *et al.*, 1995; Jobin and Sartor, 2000; Rosenstiel *et al.*, 2003; Hisamatsu *et al.*, 2003). These molecules expand the immunologic function of mucosal epithelial cells beyond merely sensors of injury to active participants in the inflammatory response (Kagnoff and Eckmann, 1997; Jobin and Sartor, 2000). Mucosal defenses are further mediated by epithelial cell secretion of antimicrobial peptides, including α and β defensins (Chapter 6) and bacterial permeability–inducing peptide, lysozyme, and mucins. Proinflammatory cytokines stimulate expression of β defensins and secretion of mucus (O'Neil *et al.*, 1999).

Macrophages

Resident mucosal macrophages, which account for 8%–15% of intestinal lamina propria mononuclear cells, are less responsive to bacterial adjuvants and inflammatory signals than are newly recruited monocytes, because of low membrane expression of CD14 (LPS binding cofactor), CD11b (complement receptor 3), and CD16 (FcγIII receptor) (Rogler *et al.*, 1997; Pizarro *et al.*, 1999; Mahida, 2000; Smith *et al.*, 2001) (see Chapter 26). This relative nonresponsiveness prevents pathogenic responses to luminal commensal bacteria, and accounts for the observation that the majority of cytokines produced in active IBD are derived from freshly emigrated immature macrophages (Pizarro *et al.*, 1999). Chemotactic signals that selectively stimulate monocyte migration include MIP-1α and β, MCP-1, and MCP-2 (Papadakis and Targan, 2000). Macrophages are scattered throughout the lamina propria and are preferentially positioned under the subepithelial basement membrane, where they can easily respond to invading pathogens and translocating microbial products. Bacterial components primarily induce expression of proinflammatory molecules (IL-1, TNF, IL-6) and chemokines. In addition, mucosal macrophages secrete abundant IL-10 in response to bacterial stimulants and proinflammatory molecules, serving to downregulate the inflammatory response. The importance in macrophages and neutrophils in inducing and maintaining intestinal inflammation is demonstrated by therapeutic responses in patients with ulcerative colitis to granulocyte and monocyte aphoresis (Saniabadi *et al.*, 2003; Tsukada *et*

al., 2002), leading to decreased mucosal production of TNF, IL-1, IL-6, and IL-8. In addition, elimination of mucosal macrophages with rectal microspheres attenuates experimental colitis (Watanabe *et al.*, 2003).

Dendritic cells

Dendritic cells are efficient mucosal APCs because of their avid uptake of soluble antigens, efficient antigen processing and presentation, full complement of costimulatory molecules, and secretion of IL-12, IL-18, and IL-23 upon exposure to microbial adjuvants (see Chapter 26). Different types of dendritic cells (myeloid, lymphoid, and plasmacytoid) occupy various regions of organized mucosal lymphoid follicles (Kelsall and Strober, 1997) in the resting state, while myeloid dendritic cells are dramatically increased during mucosal inflammation (Stagg *et al.*, 2003). Migration of these cells to inflamed mucosal surfaces is governed by CCL 20 (MIP-3α) and CCL 9 (MIP-1γ), the expression of which is upregulated during inflammation, and perhaps β7 integrin (Zhao *et al.*, 2003; Stagg AJ *et al.*, 2003). M-DC8⁺ monocyte precursors are preferentially located in subepithelial areas of Peyer's patches and secrete large amounts of TNF; these are increased in Crohn's disease and decreased by corticosteroids (de Baey *et al.*, 2003). Maturation of dendritic cells is stimulated by exposure to bacterial microbial adjuvants, which signal through TLR membrane receptors, NOD intracellular receptors, and NF-κB, while MHC II expression is stimulated by IFN-γ exposure as well as by NF-κB activation by bacterial adjuvants, IL-1, or TNF. Costimulatory molecules in mucosal APCs are also upregulated by IL-1, TNF, and microbial adjuvants (Murtaugh and Foss, 2002).

Mast cells

Mast cells account for 2%–5% of intestinal lamina propria mononuclear cells and are located in all layers of the intestine and stomach (see Chapter 37). Mucosal mast cells are preferentially located adjacent to neuronal synapses (Stead *et al.*, 1989) and are activated by substance P, other neuropeptides, IgE binding to the IgE Fc receptor, activated complement, IL-3, and stem cell factor (C-kit) (Arizono *et al.*, 1993). Stimulated mast cells primarily secrete preformed granule constituents, such as histamine, serotonin, and proteases, but also produce proinflammatory cytokines and arachidonic acid metabolites. Distinctive mucosal and connective tissue mast cell subsets in rats arise from common precursors but secrete different products (see Chapter 36).

Eosinophils

Mucosal eosinophils primarily secrete arachidonic acid metabolites and preformed biologically active molecules stored in granules, including eosinophilic cationic protein, major basic protein, and peroxidase, but also can produce proinflammatory cytokines (see Chapter 37). These cells are activated by exposure to IgE and, to a lesser extent, IgA and IgG and are attracted to mucosal surfaces by eotaxin, MCP-3, and IL-8. The C-C chemokine eotaxin is selectively upregulated in intestinal epithelial cells by IL-4 but not by

IFNγ (Winsor *et al.*, 2000), and IL-5 contributes to this upregulation (Vallance *et al.*, 1998). In addition, ENA-78/CXCL5, IL-8/CXCL8, and TNF production by eosinophils is induced by TNF but decreased by IFN-γ (Persson *et al.*, 2003). Eosinophils contribute to clearance of helminths, gastrointestinal injury, and nerve damage in Th2-mediated hypersensitivity reactions (Hogan *et al.*, 2001).

Natural killer (NK) cells

NK cells are large granular lymphocytes that can express CD2 and αα homochimeric CD8, respond to IL-2, and produce IFN-γ, but they do not express T cell receptors or surface immunoglobulin. Instead, they can coexpress myeloid markers such as CD11b and CD11c, CD14, and the Fc receptor for IgG. Cytotoxic effects are largely independent of proinflammatory cytokine activity.

Mesenchymal cells

In addition to secretion of matrix components such as collagen and fibronectin that mediate fibrosis and secretion of matrix metalloproteases that are involved in tissue remodeling and activation of latent TGF-β, mucosal fibroblasts, myofibroblasts, and smooth-muscle cells are active participants in innate immune responses. These cells can be activated by proinflammatory cytokines, bacterial products, and TGF-β to proliferate, migrate, and secrete IL-1, TNF, IL-6, IL-8, M-CSF, GM-CSF, and metalloproteases and to express bioactive CD40 and adhesion molecules (Mifflin

et al., 2002; Pucilowska *et al.*, 2000; Powell *et al.*, 1999; Rogler *et al.*, 2001; Strong *et al.*, 1998). Secretion of IL-8, M-CSF, and GM-CSF by colonic myofibroblasts is NF-κB-dependent (Rogler *et al.*, 2001).

Endothelial cells

Likewise, endothelial cells respond to proinflammatory molecules and bacterial products by expressing adhesion molecules (such as ICAM-1 and ECAM-1) involved in the initial phase of cellular recruitment into an inflammatory focus, but they also actively participate in inflammation by expressing proinflammatory cytokines, including IL-1, IL-6, and TNF, and chemokines (Nilsen *et al.*, 1998).

MECHANISMS OF STIMULATING CYTOKINE EXPRESSION

Innate immune cells can be activated by a variety of mechanisms, including bacterial products and inflammatory mediators, such as IL-1, TNF, IL-6, neuropeptides, and reactive oxygen metabolites. However, these diverse stimuli induce cytokine transcription through two dominant intracellular kinase–signaling cascades, NF-κB and MAP kinases, thereby activating similar patterns of cytokine expression (**Fig. 35.1**). Different bacterial components selectively bind to various pattern-recognition receptors to trigger NF-κB and MAPK (Kobayashi *et al.*, 2003). Bacterial peptidoglycan, mycobac-

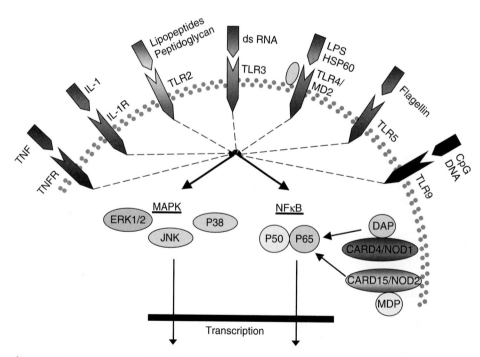

Fig. 35.1. Activation of innate immune responses via ligation of pattern recognition receptors. A wide range of microbial adjuvants selectively bind to homologous membrane-bound toll-like receptors (TLRs) or to intracellular CARD/NOD receptors. These pattern-recognition receptors, the IL-1 receptor (IL-1R), and tumor necrosis factor receptor (TNFR) signal through the central NF-κB and MAPK pathways to activate transcription of a large number of proinflammatory and protective molecules.

terial lipoarabinomannan, *Mycoplasma* lipopeptides, and heat shock protein 60 (HSP 60) bind to TLR2, which can complex with TLR3 or TLR6: viral DNA binds TLR3; LPS selectively ligates TLR4; flagellin binds to TLR5; and the bacterial DNA motif CpG ligates TLR9. Intracellular bacterial recognition is accomplished by CARD 4/NOD 1 (which ligates diaminopimelic acid), which is constitutively expressed in most intestinal cells, including epithelial cells, and by CARD 15/NOD-2 (which binds muramyl dipeptide), which is constitutively expressed in monocytes, dendritic cells, and Paneth cells and is induced in intestinal epithelial cells by IFNγ and TNF (Girardin *et al.*, 2003a; Girardin *et al.*, 2003b; Chamaillard *et al.*, 2003; Girardin *et al.*, 2003c).

The complexity of this system is increased by the ability of various TLR moieties to interact and by the ability of proinflammatory cytokines to affect expression of TLR and NOD molecules. For example, TLR2 complexes with homologous TLR1 to bind mycobacterial lipoarabinomannan and *Mycoplasma* triacylated lipopeptides, while *Mycoplasma* diacylated lipopeptides bind to TLR2/TLR6 complexes (Tapping and Tobias, 2003; Takeda *et al.*, 2002). These combinatorial repertoires are postulated to enhance the ability of the host to discriminate diverse bacterial products (Ozinsky *et al.*, 2000). In addition, efficacy of LPS binding to TLR4 is markedly enhanced by coligation of LPS binding protein and CD14. As mentioned in the section on macrophages, intestinal macrophages have lower expression of CD14 than do monocytes, providing a mechanism for relative nonresponsiveness to LPS produced by commensal enteric bacteria. Likewise, TLR and CARD15/NOD2 expression by native intestinal epithelial cells is relatively low, although Haller *et al.*, 2002, 2003) have demonstrated that *Bacteroides vulgatus* can stimulate expression of IL-6 and activate NF-κB in colonic epithelial cells after in vivo luminal colonization via LPS binding to TLR4. Similarly, feeding DNA from probiotic bacteria or *E. coli* can prevent and treat experimental colitis through interaction with TLR9 (Rachmilewitz *et al.*, 2004). TLR 2 is expressed in human alveolar type II epithelial cells and macrophages (Droemann *et al.*, 2003). IFN-γ upregulates expression, with resultant enhanced function, of CARD 4/NOD1 and the TLR4/MD-2 complex on intestinal epithelial cells (Hisamatsu *et al.*, 2003; Suzuki *et al.*, 2003), while TNF stimulates CARD15/NOD2 expression in epithelial cells (Rosenstiel *et al.*, 2003; Hisamatsu *et al.*, 2003).

Once ligation of various TLR molecules and bacterial products occurs, signaling converges on central pathways that are shared proximally by the IL-1/IL-1 receptor (IL-1R) and more distally by the CARD/NOD and TNF signaling pathways **(Fig. 35.2)**. The TLR and IL-1 signaling pathways require activation of toll-IL-1-1R (TIR) domain adaptor proteins, including MyD88, TIRAP, and TRIF. Although transcription of most proinflammatory cytokines requires MyD88, ligation of TLR3 and TLR4 can proceed through a MyD88-independent pathway mediated by TRIF. A TRIF-related adapter protein (TRAM) is required for TLR4-specific induction of IFNβ but not TLR3-stimulated responses (Yamamoto *et al.*, 2003). MyD88-dependent and -independent TLR, IL-1β,

TNF, and CARD/NOD pathways activate NF-κB through activation of the IKK complex to phosphorylate IκBα, which is ubiquinated and degraded by the 700-kDa proteasome complex (Jobin and Sartor, 2000), thereby freeing the previously complexed NF-κB heterodimer to be phosphorylated and translocate to the nucleus. Once NF-κB has homed to the nucleus, it stimulates transcription of multiple cytokines by binding to κB regulatory elements on the promoter region of the cytokine genes (Fig. 35.1). In addition to transcriptional regulation by NF-κB and other relevant transcription factors (Fig. 35.1), production and secretion of proinflammatory cytokines are dependent on stabilization of mRNA, protein translation, posttranslational modification, and in some cases such as IL-1 and IL-18, processing by precursor molecules.

TNF receptor ligation will also activate NF-κB but uses a different set of postreceptor scaffolding proteins (including TRAF6 [Fig. 35.2]). Similarly, CARD 4/NOD1 and CARD 15/NOD2, which selectively bind a diaminopimelic acid tripeptide from Gram-negative bacteria and muramyl dipeptide, respectively (Girardin *et al.*, 2003), activate NF-κB through the intermediate kinase Rip2 (RICK/CARDIAK), which appears to contribute to TLR, IL-1, and IL-18 signaling as well (Kobayashi *et al.*, 2002). Of considerable interest to the pathogenesis of Crohn's disease, the three most common polymorphisms of CARD 15/NOD 2, which are in the leucin-rich repeat region that binds bacterial cell wall peptides, diminish NF-κB activation (Bonen DK *et al.*, 2003).

IL-1, TNF, and TLRs activate parallel pathways in addition to NF-κB. A complex cascade of kinases leads to phosphorylation of c-jun NH2 terminal kinase (JNK) and p38 MAPK **(Fig. 35.3)**. These kinases activate c-fos and c-jun, the heterodimers of the AP-1 transcription factor complex. AP-1 transcriptionally regulates most proinflammatory cytokines, many in conjunction with NF-κB. Of considerable relevance to bacterial homeostasis, response to infection, and treatment of inflammation, selective blockade of JNK and p38 MAPK can have different effects, as suggested by their independent activation, function, and regulation. p38 MAPK, JNK, and ERK 1/2 are phosphorylated in active IBD (Hommes DW *et al.*, 2003; Waetzig GH *et al.*, 2002), and an uncontrolled study with an inhibitor of both p38 MAPK and JNK impressively inhibits active Crohn's disease (Hommes *et al.*, 2002). However, low-dose LPS administration to volunteers selectively activated p38 MAPK but not JNK in PBMNCs (Hommes *et al.*, 2003). Furthermore, a selective p38 MAPK inhibitor caused increased weight loss and higher levels of colonic cell TNF production in a TNBS model of colitis, although it decreased TNF production (S. van Deventer, unpublished observations). Thus, these pathways must be considered separately in mucosal inflammation.

Additional signaling pathways parallel to NF-κB include the inositol triphosphate (IP3) and phosphokinase B/AKT pathway, the NF IL-6 transcription factor, and ERK 1/2. The IP3/AKT system is activated by IL-1, IL-18, and LPS through the myD88/IRAK-1/TRAF6 complex (Neumann *et al.*, 2002), with both inflammatory and protective consequences. IP3/AKT stimulates intracellular calcium fluxes but also

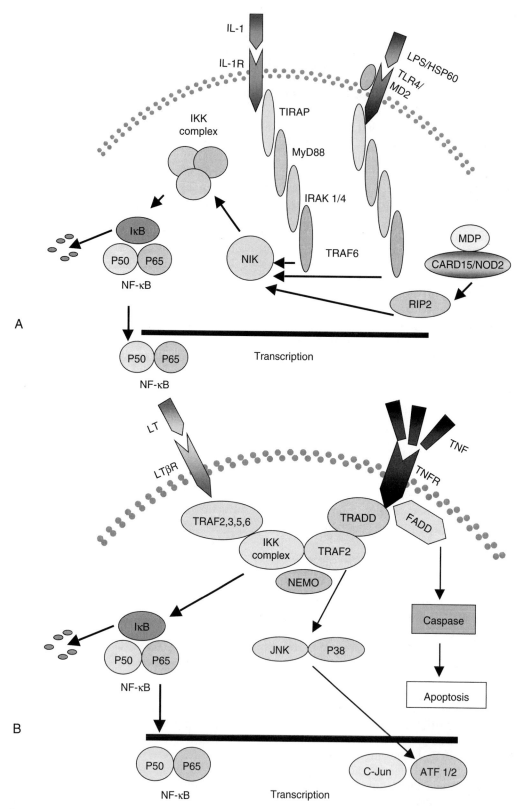

Fig. 35.2. Intracellular signal cascades activated by IL-1 receptor, TNF receptor, CARD15/NOD2 or TLR ligation. A, Parallel signaling mechanisms of the IL-1R and TLR pathways. Ligation of IL-1 or LPS to IL-1R and TLR4, respectively, activates signals through parallel signaling pathways involving a series of adaptor and scaffolding proteins and kinases. Activated kinases ultimately lead to the phosphorylation and degradation of IκBα. This releases NF-κB, which is phosphorylated and translocates to the nucleus, where it initiates transcription of a number of effector and regulatory molecules. **B,** Activation of multiple signaling and apoptotic pathways by TNF family member ligands. TNF (TNF-α) or lymphotoxin (TNF-β) bind to specific receptors that can activate either the NF-κB or MAPK signaling cascades through a series of specific adaptor molecules. In addition, TNF can initiate apoptosis through death domain adaptor molecules and caspases.

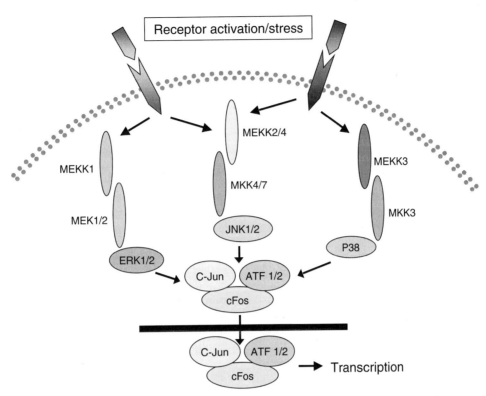

Fig. 35.3. Activation of mitogen-activated protein (MAP) kinases by multiple stimuli. A variety of stimuli, including growth factors, hormones, and proinflammatory cytokines (TNF, IL-1, etc) can activate a series of kinases that lead to liberation of transcription factors that operate in parallel with NF-κB. The MAPK effector molecules c jun and c fos can heterodimerize to form AP-1, or these molecules and ATF 1/2 can bind to DNA regulatory elements alone or in various combinations to regulate gene transcription.

mediates calcium/calmodulin-dependent protein kinase suppression of IL-1 and TLR signaling by uncoupling IRAK-1 and myD88 activity (Chan, 2002). In addition, TNF inhibits AKT phosphorylation, which is decreased in portal hypertensive gastropathy. Inhibition of AKT is postulated to contribute to gastric epithelial injury, since AKT stimulates epithelial cell proliferation, migration, and survival. Anti-TNF treatment restored gastric AKT levels and induced healing (Tsugawa *et al.*, 2003). IL-1, TNF, and IL-6 activate NF IL-6, a transcription factor binding along with NF-κB and AP-1 to the promoters of IL-6 and IL-8 to positively regulate transcription of these cytokines (Akira and Kishimoto, 1992). Finally, IL-1β can stimulate the extracellular signal-regulated protein kinase (ERK) 1/2 and AKT pathways via the association of phosphorylated SHPS and SHP-2 (MacGillivray *et al.*, 2003). LPS or LPS plus IFN-γ stimulation of dendritic cells increases ERK and p38 MAPK while stimulating IL-10 and IL-12. Blockade of ERK selectively decreases IL-10 and enhances IL-12 production, suggesting that ERK selectively induces IL-10, an endogenous inhibitor of IL-12 (Xia and Kao, 2003).

The regulation of these interacting pathways is extremely complex and has been evaluated predominantly in isolated cell lines and in peripheral blood mononuclear cells (PBMCs). It remains to be determined whether mucosal innate immune cells follow these paradigms or whether they exhibit unique regulatory features.

MECHANISMS OF INHIBITING PROINFLAMMATORY CYTOKINE EXPRESSION AND FUNCTION

Regulation of the expression and activity of proinflammatory cytokines is a key component of maintaining mucosal homeostasis and preventing excessive tissue injury after an inflammatory event. In addition, therapeutic blockade of innate immune responses is vital to treating mucosal inflammation.

Endogenous inhibitory mechanisms
Activation of signaling pathways by inflammatory cytokines or bacterial products stimulates a number of overlapping protective pathways that inhibit proinflammatory cytokine production by innate immune cells (Table 35.2). Many of these protective mechanisms can be induced by multiple cytokines, while others are selectively induced by a single stimulant. For example, IL-1, TNF, and IL-6 activate the hypothalamic/ pituitary/adrenal (HPA) axis, culminating in the release of immunosuppressive corticosteroids. The importance of this protective pathway is illustrated by the increased intensity and prolongation of experimental inflammation, accompanied by increased IL-1 and TNF levels in adrenalectomized rats or following pharmacologic blockade of corticotrophin-releasing hormone (Pothoulakis and LaMont, 2001). In addition to the more widely recognized proinflammatory

molecules induced by IL-1, TNF, and bacterial molecules, NF-κB activation leads to increased expression of multiple *protective* genes, including IκBα, cyclooxygenase-2 (COX-2), inducible nitric oxide synthetase (iNOS), and PPARγ. Production of IκBα is important in deactivating NF-κB by complexing nuclear p65/p50 heterodimers, interrupting gene transcription and transporting this complex back to the cytoplasm where it exists in an inactive complexed form. Although PGE$_2$, PGI$_2$, and other prostaglandins released during inflammation enhance epithelial chloride secretion, increase vascular permeability, and stimulate smooth-muscle contractions, thereby causing diarrhea, edema, and hypermotility, these products also inhibit proinflammatory cytokine production (Kunkel *et al.*, 1986) and stimulate mucosal healing (Cohn *et al.*, 1997). PGJ$_2$ may mediate protective effects through PPARγ activation. The importance of prostaglandin production in mucosal homeostasis, resolution of inflammation, and downregulation of inflammatory cytokines is illustrated by small intestinal and colonic inflammation following two injections of indomethacin in susceptible rat strains (Yamada *et al.*, 1993), piroxicam-triggering colitis in IL-10$^{-/-}$ mice on a resistant (C57BL/6) background (Berg *et al.*, 2002), potentiation of DSS-induced colitis in COX-2 deficient mice (Morteau *et al.*, 2000), and inhibition of DSS-induced colitis by ligation of EP4, the PGE$_2$ receptor (Nitta *et al.*, 2002). In each of these models, mucosal IL-1 and TNF are increased. Similarly, nitric oxide produced as a consequence of proinflammatory cytokine stimulation of iNOS has important protective properties. Nitric oxide inhibits NF-κB activation by blocking the IRAK/TRAF-6 interaction (Xiong *et al.*, 2004) and inhibits caspase 1/IL-1β converting enzyme (ICE) activity by 5-nitrosylation (Kim *et al.*, 1998).

IL-10 is induced by a number of agents, including IL-1, TNF, IL-6, IL-12, IFN-γ, and bacterial products. Of interest, the induction of IL-10 by bacterial products lags behind that of proinflammatory cytokines. Incubating unfractionated mesenteric lymph node (MLN) cells or splenocytes with LPS induces maximum TNF production by 4 hours, IL-1 by 6–8 hours, and IL-12 by 24 hours, but IL-10 secretion reaches maximal concentrations only after 72 hours of stimulation (Kim *et al.*, 2001). This progressive induction of first proinflammatory and then protective cytokines suggests a compensatory regulatory mechanism to downregulate responses to an inflammatory stimulus. The importance of endogenous IL-10 in host protection to the aggressive luminal environment is dramatically illustrated by spontaneous colitis in IL-10$^{-/-}$ mice raised in the presence of commensal bacteria (Sellon *et al.*, 1998; Kuhn *et al.*, 1993), and strikingly elevated IL-1β, TNF, IL-12, and IFN-γ secretion by LPS or cecal bacterial lysates stimulated MLN cells in IL-10$^{-/-}$ versus wild-type mice (Kim *et al.*, 2001). Secretion of soluble receptors by activated cells can bind IL-1 and TNF, thereby neutalizing their biologic effects. Finally, a number of inflammatory stimuli, including IL-1β, can stimulate expression of IL-1 receptor antagonist (IL-1RA), which competitively inhibits IL-1 receptor binding and down-

stream signaling (Dinarello, 2000). Of interest, IL-10 selectively inhibits IL-1β to a greater extent than IL-1RA in splenocytes exposed to LPS, profoundly altering the IL-1RA/IL-1 ratio to a less inflammatory profile.

Proinflammatory cytokines can selectively stimulate inhibitors that provide negative feedback on the inflammatory response. For example, TNF stimulates intracellular A20, which inhibits TNF signaling (Lee *et al.*, 2000). The importance of A20 in mucosal protection is evident by the colitis that develops in A20-deficient mice (Lee *et al.*, 2000). Although not selective, an inflammatory pathway stimulating production of an inhibitor that suppresses functions of the inductive stimulus is well documented; IL-1 stimulating IL-1RA and NF-κB increasing expression of IκBα are two obvious examples (Dinarello, 2000; Jobin and Sartor, 2000).

Mechanisms by which endogenous inhibitory molecules exert their protective effects are still not entirely clear. Many immunosuppressive molecules have multiple modes of action and target central signaling pathways. For example, corticosteroids inhibit phospholipase A2, thereby blocking arachidonic acid liberation; block NF-κB activity; suppress transcription by binding to the glucocorticoid regulatory element and the promoter of many proinflammatory molecules; prevent transcription factor binding to promoters by histone deacotylation; stabilize lysomal membranes; and inhibit adhesion of effector cells to endothelial cells (Barnes, 2001). Similarly, IL-10 inhibits NF-κB by multiple mechanisms yet to be fully understood. IL-10 transiently delays IκBα degradation after an inflammatory stimulus, but its probable mode of action is to inhibit p65 binding to DNA, although it does not block NF-κB p65/p50 nuclear transmigration (Schottelius *et al.*, 1999). In addition, IL-10 phosphorylates STAT 3 and stimulates production of the inhibitory molecule suppressor of cytokine synthesis (SOCS) 3 (Niemand *et al.*, 2003; Yasukawa *et al.*, 2003). TGF-β regulates aggressive T cell function by suppressing lymphocyte proliferation and activation but also stimulates IL-10 expression (Fuss *et al.*, 2002), perhaps explaining some of its diverse biologic activities. TGF-β phosphorylates SMAD 2 and SMAD 3, leading to activation of SMAD 4. Phosphorylation of SMAD 2 in colonic epithelial cells is evident 7 days after selective colonization of germ-free rats with *Bacteroides vulgatus*, which is temporally related to downregulation of in vitro epithelial NF-κB stimulation and IL-6 production (Haller *et al.*, 2003). In vitro studies showed that endogenous TGF-β could suppress LPS-induced IL-6 secretion by cultured colonic epithelial cells and affect NF-κB activation by blocking histone H3 acetylation (Haller *et al.*, 2003).

Exogenous compounds inhibiting proinflammatory cytokines

Although beyond the scope of this chapter, multiple clinically relevant pharmacologic agents, including traditional clinical therapies as well as biologic agents, have proven abilities to suppress proinflammatory cytokine transcription and biologic activity **(Table 35.3)**. Therapeutic effects of these

Table 35.3. Therapeutic Approaches to Blocking Inflammatory Cytokines Produced by Activated Innate Immune Cells

Approach	Target	Mechanism
Corticosteroids	IL-1, IL-6, IL-12, TNF, chemokines	Inhibits NF-κB, cytokine transcription
IL-10 (recombinant bacteria, transfected T cells)	APC, IL-12, IL-1, TNF, IL-6, chemokines	Inhibits NF-κB, APC activation
Block TNF – monoclonal antibodies, binding proteins, receptors	TNF	Inactivate secreted TNF, induce apoptosis of cells with membrane–bound TNF
Thalidomide analogues	TNF, IL-1	Inhibit synthesis
Pentoxifylline	TNF, IL-1	Inhibit synthesis
NF-κB – p65 antisense oligo-nucleotides, proteosome inhibitor	IL-1, TNF, IL-6, IL-12, chemokines	Block transcription
MAPK inhibitors – p38 MAPK, JNK	IL-1, IL-6, IL-12, TNF, chemokines	Block transcription

compounds, particularly those selectively active for individual cytokines, in clinical and experimental intestinal inflammation confirm the key contribution of proinflammatory cytokines in acute and chronic mucosal inflammation. Examples of the beneficial activities of compounds with selective activities are provided in the sections describing individual cytokines and signaling pathways.

STRUCTURE AND FUNCTION OF INDIVIDUAL PROINFLAMMATORY CYTOKINES

Consistent with their shared signaling pathways and receptors, many proinflammatory cytokines and chemokines have overlapping functions, yet each retains a unique pattern of responses. For example, IL-1 and TNF receptor ligation both stimulate NF-κB, MAP kinases, and AKT, yet TNF has a greater ability to activate Th1 lymphocyte responses and has an independent effect on apoptosis. Many chemokines share common heterodimeric molecules and receptors yet recruit different cell populations. These differential properties may be due to selective production by different cells or the differential kinetics of production. Many cytokine responses are either autocrine or paracrine in nature, such that biologic activity depends on the local cellular milieu. In addition, the activation state of a target cell can profoundly affect its response to a given stimulus as a result of upregulation or downregulation of membrane receptors, induction of endogenous protective molecules, or the degree of phosphorylation or dephosphorylation of signaling molecules.

Because of shared inductive mechanisms, in large part via NF-κB and AP-1 signaling pathways, proinflammatory cytokines tend to be expressed in tandem. For example, IL-1β, TNF, IL-6, and various chemokines are all induced in active IBD (Isaacs *et al.*, 1992; Sartor, 1994; Cominelli *et al.*, 2004), while a characteristic profile of cytokines is induced by IL-1, TNF, or invasive bacteria in cultured colonic epithelial cells (Jung *et al.*, 1995). Thus, it is physiologically and

pathophysiologically important to consider interactive, additive, and synergistic activities of cytokines rather than isolated expression and activities. However, the present discussion artificially considers the biologic effects of individual cytokines. Although many of the examples supporting physiologic and pathophysiologic effects of these cytokines are related to intestinal inflammation because of the wealth of investigations in this field and the particular expertise of the author, similar activities are found at other mucosal sites.

IL-1 family (IL-1α, IL-1β, IL-1RA and IL-1β converting enzyme)

Structure and secretion

IL-1 occurs in two forms, IL-1α and IL-1β, which share similar receptor-binding properties and hence have overlapping functions. IL-1α is membrane-bound or intracellular and therefore mediates its effects by cell contact or following liberation after cell lysis. Pro IL-1α (31 kDa) is cleaved by calpain or by extracellular proteases to a 17-dDa form. In contrast, IL-1β is an 18-kDa precursor that lacks a leader sequence and therefore remains in an intracellular cytoplasmic location unless activated by cleavage of ICE (caspase 1) (Siegmund, 2002). ICE itself is constitutively expressed as a 45-kDa inactive precursor that is cleaved at two locations to form an active heterodimer. ICE is cleaved by various caspases, including ICE itself, following cellular activation by bacterial products, proinflammatory cytokines, or CD40 ligation, but caspase activity is inhibited by nitric oxide. Following cleavage, biologically active IL-1β is secreted. IL-1RA is also present in two forms. A 22-kDa secreted form competitively inhibits IL-1 bioactivity by competitively binding to the two IL-1 receptor isoforms. A second splice variant form lacking a leader sequence remains in an intracellular cytoplasmic location (Watson *et al.*, 1995).

Expression

IL-1α and IL-1β are induced by multiple proinflammatory signals and are expressed in a variety of cell types. Levels are low in the normal intestine but are dramatically increased during active inflammation (Cominelli *et al.*, 1992; McCall *et al.*, 1994; Andus *et al.*, 1997; Isaacs *et al.*, 1992; Evgenikos *et al.*, 2002; McAlindon *et al.*, 1998). Tissue staining and cell extraction demonstrate that lamina propria macrophages, particularly newly immigrated cells with monocyte features, account for the majority of IL-1 production, although mesenchymal cells, endothelial cells, and to a lesser extent epithelial cells express mRNA and produce protein (McAlindon *et al.*, 1998; Mahida, 2000; Youngman *et al.*, 1993). IL-1RA is constitutively expressed in the normal intestine and in increased amounts following inflammation. Intracellular IL-1RA is constitutively expressed in intestinal epithelial cells, with mRNA expression in the crypt and accumulation of protein with cellular maturation (Bocker *et al.*, 1998). ICE is constitutively expressed, with expression but not cleavage upregulated by IFN-γ.

Signaling

IL-1α and IL-1β bind to two receptor isoforms that are selectively expressed on different cell types relevant to mucosal tissues. IL-1RI is present on intestinal epithelial cells, endothelial cells, mesenchymal cells, and T lymphocytes, while IL-1RII is expressed on monocytes/macrophages, neutrophils and B cells. IL-1RII binds IL-1 but does not transduce signals, raising the concept of a secreted "decoy" receptor that can inhibit responses (Colotta *et al.*, 1993). Ligation of either receptor transduces signals through a complex of kinases and scaffolding proteins (IRAK-1, TRAF-6, TAK1/TAB, and Rip 2) to activate the NF-κB pathways (Fig. 35.2). A comprehensive study by Mifflin *et al.* (2002) shows that IL-1α stimulates COX-2 mRNA transcription in intestinal myofibroblasts by activating the NF-κB, ERK, and protein kinase C (PKC) pathways. In parallel, IL-1α-stimulated p38 MAPK stabilizes COX-2 mRNA.

Function

Activation of NF-κB, MAPK, and AKT by ligation of the IL-1 receptors by IL-1α or IL-1β increases expression of a number of molecules involved in the inflammatory response (Fig. 35.1). Induction of IL-1, TNF, IL-6, IL-12, and chemokines by lamina propria innate immune cells and mesenchymal cells amplifies the inflammatory response, while stimulation of chemokine secretion and expression of adhesion molecules on mucosal epithelial cells leads to the emigration, transmigration, and excretion of effector cells (Sartor, 1994). IL-1 stimulates expression of costimulatory molecules on APC and upregulates IL-12 secretion, thereby enhancing T cell activation. Induction of metalloproteases results in matrix destruction, ulceration, and possibly fistula formation. Finally, enhanced expression of COX-2 leads to rapid production of eicosanoids that mediate epithelial chloride secretion and block sodium absorption, leading to diarrhea and bronchial secretion; smooth-muscle contractions resulting in cramps, airway spasm, and diarrhea; and increased vascular permeability.

Induction of iNOS, with resultant nitric oxide synthesis, enhances intracellular killing of phagocytosed microbial

agents; inhibits smooth-muscle contractions, possibly leading to ileus associated with intestinal inflammation; and regulates mucosal blood flow. Finally, IL-1 mediates anorexia associated with experimental colitis through induction of 5-HT in the hypothalamus (El-Haj *et al.*, 2002). In addition to its proinflammatory effects, IL-1 stimulates production of anti-inflammatory molecules such as prostaglandins, nitric oxide, and IL-1RA that inhibit inflammation (see previous section on endogenous inhibitory mechanisms). For example, IL-1β stimulates production of PGE2, 6-keto PGI2, and thromboxane B2 in the rabbit colon (Cominelli *et al.*, 1989), and administration of IL-1β 24 hours before administration of formalin and immune complexes in rabbits attenuates colitis through stimulation of endogenous prostaglandins (Cominelli *et al.*, 1990).

The net proinflammatory properties of endogenous IL-1 are documented by the ability of recombinant IL-1RA to attenuate experimental colitis in a number of models (Cominelli *et al.*, 1992; Cominelli and Pizarro, 1997; McCall *et al.*, 1994). Administration of IL-1RA not only decreases inflammation but also inhibits expression of a number of proinflammatory cytokines by the inflamed colon (McCall *et al.*, 1994). A trial of subcutaneous rIL-1RA in ulcerative colitis was not completed. Local mucosal administration via engineered bacteria may prove to be a better approach than systemic administration. Colonization of IL-2$^{-/-}$ mice with IL-1RA-secreting *Streptococcus gordonii* enhanced weight gain, although the colon was not examined (Ricci *et al.*, 2003). Attenuation of acute and chronic colitis in ICE-deficient mice (Siegmund *et al.*, 2001) and the ability to predict relapse of inactive Crohn's disease by the secretion of IL-1 (Arnott *et al.*, 2001) provide additional evidence of the pathogenic role of IL-1 (and IL-18).

Bioactivity of IL-1α and IL-1β is dependent on ligation of either IL-1RI or RII. Thus, the balance of IL-1 and IL-1RA determines receptor activation, although the levels of IL-1RA are increased and the IL-1/IL-1RA ratio is decreased during intestinal inflammation because of a greater increase in IL-1 than of IL-1RA (Casini-Raggi *et al.*, 1995; Isaacs *et al.*, 1992; McCall *et al.*, 1994; Andus *et al.*, 1997). This abnormal ratio may be a secondary phenomenon, since the ratio correlated with disease activity of IBD and was also decreased in nonspecific mucosal inflammation (Casini-Raggi *et al.*, 1995; McCall *et al.*, 1994). However, the association of polymorphisms in allele 2 of IL-1RA with ulcerative colitis and pouchitis suggests an etiologic role for defective IL-IRA activity, according to some authors (Mansfield *et al.*, 1994; Hacker *et al.*, 1997; Jostock *et al.*, 2001; Craggs *et al.*, 2001).

TNF and lymphotoxin
Structure and secretion

TNF (TNF-α, cachexin) is a 17-kDa protein that is produced as a 26-kDa precursor (pro-TNF). Pro-TNF is cleaved by TNFα cleavage enzyme (TACE or ADAM-17) or ADAM-10, which both are zinc-binding metalloprotease disintegrin members of the adamalysin family (Black *et al.*, 2003;

Mohan *et al.*, 2002). Secreted TNF forms trimeric complexes that optimally bind receptors. Structurally related lymphotoxin (TNF-β, LT-α) is also secreted as a trimer but can also complex with LT-β to form a membrane-bound heterodimer that has distinct functions. The TNF family of ligands and receptors comprise a complex and rapidly evolving group of immunologically relevant proteins and costimulatory molecules that include TNF, LT-α, LT-α/β, LIGHT, FasL, CD40L, TRAIL, RANKL, 4-1BBL, OC40L, GITRL, and BAFF (Mackay and Kalled, 2002) (Fig. 35.2).

Expression

Numerous cells in the inflamed mucosa produce TNF, including macrophages, Th1 lymphocytes, mast cells, mesenchymal cells, endothelial cells, and even epithelial cells, with activated macrophages being the primary source. Constitutive expression in the noninflamed gut is low but is dramatically increased during infection or inflammation in response to NF-κB and MAPK activation by bacterial products and IL-1. Tissue levels of TNF mRNA and protein in IBD have been somewhat controversial, with some investigators showing increases in Crohn's disease tissue and stool that correlates with disease activity and others finding no consistent elevation (Breese *et al.*, 1994; Isaacs *et al.*, 1992; Andus *et al.*, 1993; Dionne *et al.*, 2003). One reason for these inconsistent results is the relative instability of TNF mRNA, which is dependent on the Au-rich elements (ARE) in the 3′ untranslated region of the gene. Deletion of this ARE region leads to increased circulating and intestinal levels of TNF (Kontoyiannis *et al.*, 1999). TNF is primarily produced by lamina propria macrophages but is also expressed in subepithelial dendritic cell precursors and activated Th1 cells (Breese *et al.*, 1994; de Baey *et al.*, 2003).

LT-α is expressed in the same cell populations as TNF and is also increased in inflamed mucosal tissues. LT-α secretion by colonic biopsy explants is increased in Crohn's disease relative to ulcerative colitis (Noguchi *et al.*, 2001). LT-β is more selectively expressed by lymphoid cells.

Signaling

TNF binds to two membrane-bound receptors, TNFRI (p55) and TNFRII (p75), that are expressed in epithelial, bone marrow–derived, mesenchymal, and endothelial cells at mucosal surfaces (Bazzoni and Beutler, 1996). Expression of TNFRII is increased in colonic epithelial cells during experimental colitis and active IBD (Mizoguchi *et al.*, 2002). Ligation of TNFRII by TNF or LT-α trimers results in activation of proinflammatory effects mediated by stimulation of NF-κB, MAPK, PKC, and AKT (Fig. 35.2). Ligation of TNFRI by TNF or LT-α selectively induces apoptosis through a series of death domains (Fas-activated death domain, FADD, etc.). The TNF receptor–associated death domain (TRADD) is common to both pathways, which then diverge along two pathways regulated by TNF receptor–associated factor (TRAF) isoforms. TRAF 1 and 2 stimulate NF-κB and MAPK, while FADD mediates apoptotic signals through caspases. The α/β complex and Light bind to the LTβR.

Function

TNF both stimulates inflammatory responses in a variety of mucosal cell populations and induces apoptosis of epithelial cells. The ability of TNF to induce apoptosis is augmented by synergistic activities with IFN-γ (Targan *et al.*, 1991; Abreu-Martin *et al.*, 1995). The inflammatory effects are quite similar to those of IL-1, since both molecules activate NF-κB, MAPK, and AKT (Fig. 35.1), although cellular targets may vary because of differential expression of IL-1 and TNF receptors on different cell populations. The expression of TNFRII on epithelial cells may relate to mechanisms of mucosal hyperplasia during inflammation (Mizoguchi *et al.*, 2002). Transfer of CD4+ CD45RBhi T cells from wild-type and TNF−/− mice into wild-type or TNF−/− RAG2−/− mice demonstrates the importance of TNF production by non-T cells (Corazza *et al.*, 1999).

Like IL-1, TNF stimulates production of a variety of proinflammatory cytokines, chemokines, adhesion molecules, costimulatory molecules, COX-2, iNOS, and secreted matrix metalloproteases. In addition, TNF activates osteoclasts and inhibits osteoblast function, leading to bone resorption. Furthermore, TNF stimulates activity of lipoprotein lipase and (? leptin) decreases appetite at the hypothalamic level, leading to weight loss, hence its original name *cachexin*. Systemic injection of TNF induces mid-small-bowel inflammation and necrosis, possibly mediated through induction of platelet activating factor (Hsueh *et al.*, 2003), and Δ ARE transgenic mice overexpressing TNF spontaneously develop ileal inflammation, arthritis, and eventually multiorgan failure (Kontoyiannis *et al.*, 1999). Ileal inflammation in this model depends on the presence of both TNFRI and II, CD8+ T cells, IFN-γ, and IL-12 and is mediated by either myeloid or T cell–derived TNF (Kontoyiannis *et al.*, 2002). TNF neutralization attenuates inflammation in a variety of experimental colitis models (Neurath *et al.*, 1997; Zhang *et al.*, 2003; Rennick *et al.*, 1997) as well as ileal disease in the SAMP 1/Yit T cell transfer model (Kosiewicz *et al.*, 2001). However, in these models blockade of endogenous TNF was not as effective as inhibition of IL-12 in preventing or reversing intestinal inflammation. However, a chimeric IgG1 antibody to TNF (infliximab) has dramatic results in Crohn's disease, inducing responses in 65% of patients with luminal inflammation (Targan *et al.*, 1997) and 68% of patients with fistulae (Present *et al.*, 1999). However, these impressive results appear to be due to induction of apoptosis of activated T cells and monocytes bearing membrane-bound TNF rather than neutralizing free TNF since etanercept, a fusion protein of the extracellular domain of the p75 TNF receptor and the Fc portion of IgG, is not effective in Crohn's disease, despite equal binding affinity to TNF as infliximab (Lugering *et al.*, 2001; Sandborn, 2003; Van den Brande *et al.*, 2003). Whether the decreased efficacy of other more fully humanized anti-TNF antibodies in Crohn's disease relates to decreased induction of apoptosis remains to be established (Sandborn *et al.*, 2001) and will determine the effectiveness of PEGylated antibodies undergoing trials in Crohn's disease.

Finally, thalidomide, a TNF synthesis inhibitor, is effective in Crohn's disease, but well documented toxicities preclude its widespread use (Ehrenpreis et al., 1999; Vasiliauskas et al., 1999). The effectiveness of infliximab in ulcerative colitis is being evaluated by a large trial to resolve divergent early results (Sands et al., 2001; Probert et al., 2003). TNF is an important mediator of intracellular bacterial killing through upregulation of iNOS. Blockade of TNF is associated with increased bacterial infections (abscesses, sepsis) as well as reactivation and dissemination of mycobacterial infections (Sandborn, 2003; Sandborn et al., 2004). In an intestinal xenograft model of amebic colitis, TNF blockade was more effective than IL-1R blockade in decreasing explant inflammation, although *Entamoeba histolytica* invasion was unchanged (Zhang et al., 2003).

Animal models demonstrate an important function of LTα/β in mucosal immune development and inflammation. LTα/β, with IL-7, regulates lymphoid tissue development, notably in Peyer's patches and mesenteric lymph nodes, during embryogenesis and maintains secondary lymphoid structure in adults (Tumanov et al., 2003). In addition, LTβR signaling is required for formation and maintenance of follicular dendritic cell networks. More vigorous colitis in mice deficient in organized lymphoid tissue following neonatal blockade of LTβR suggests that cells in these tissues are protective (Spahn et al., 2002). In contrast, inhibition of LT-α/β and Light activity by soluble LTβR Ig fusion protein attenuated T cell–mediated colitis as effectively as anti-TNF antibody (Mackay et al., 1998). The latter results suggest that both LT-α/β and TNF mediate chronic colitis.

IL-6 soluble IL-6 receptor (IL-6R and gp130)
Structure and secretion

IL-6 is secreted without processing. Its receptor complex consists of two distinct membrane-bound glycoproteins: an 80-kDa cognate receptor (IL-6R) and a 130-kDa signal transducing element (gp130). Membrane-bound IL-6R can be shed after proteolytic cleavage by bacteria-derived metalloproteases and a not-yet fully-defined mammalian metalloprotease distinct from TACE (Jones et al., 2001). An alternative mechanism is differential mRNA splicing, leading to an isoform that lacks membrane-spanning and cytoplasmic domains (Jones et al., 2001).

Expression

IL-6 is produced by a variety of cells at mucosal surfaces, including macrophages, epithelial cells, mesenchymal cells, and endothelial cells. The normal intestine has detectible amounts of IL-6, which is dramatically upregulated in the inflamed intestine of patients with Crohn's disease, ulcerative colitis, and nonspecific inflammation, as well as during experimental colitis, with tissue levels correlating with the degree of inflammation (Gross et al., 1992; Hyams et al., 1993; Reinecker et al., 1993; Herfarth et al., 1996; Rath et al., 1996; Ito, 2003). Similarly, circulating levels of IL-6 and sIL-6R correspond with the activity of intestinal inflammation and have been proposed as indicators of disease activity

(Mitsuyama et al., 1995; Brown et al., 2002). IL-6 expression is induced by IL-1, TNF (through NF-κB and MAPK), IFN-γ (through STAT-1), LPS (through NF-κB), TGFβ, heat shock proteins, and prostaglandins (Haller et al., 2003; McGee et al., 1993; McLoughlin et al., 2003). IL-1β induces expression of IL-6 through transient activation of NF-κB; this is potentiated by IFN-γ through prolongation of NF-κB activation (McLoughlin et al., 2003). Polymorphisms of the IL-6 gene are not associated with Crohn's disease (Koss et al., 2000).

Glycoprotein 130 is constitutively expressed on most cells, while membrane-bound IL-6R is selectively expressed on monocytes, neutrophils, T and B lymphocytes, and hepatocytes. sIL-6R shedding by monocytic cell lines is enhanced by exposure to phorbol esters and certain bacterial toxins but not IL-1β, TNF, IFN-γ, IL-4, IL-6, IL-10, chemokines, or growth factors (Jones et al., 1998). However, neutrophils shed sIL-6R when exposed to C-reactive protein (CRP) through ligation of the FcγRIIa (Jones et al., 1999).

Signaling

IL-6 can transduce signals in two ways **(Fig. 35.4)** (Jones et al., 2001). IL-6 ligation of membrane-bound IL-6R induces homodimerization of membrane-bound gp130. Stimulation of this complex activates gp130-associated cytoplasmic tyrosine kinases (JAK-1, JAK-2, and Tyk 2), which phosphorylate STAT3. An alternative mechanism of activating cells that express only gp130 is trans-signaling, which is mediated by ligation of sIL-6R–IL-6 complexes with membrane-bound gp130 (Atreya et al., 2000). Trans-signaling then causes homodimerization of membrane gp130 and identical intracellular phosphorylation of STAT3. In parallel, either mechanism of signaling activates AP-1 and NF-IL-6 through the Ras/Raf pathway. A mechanism of regulating this pathology is provided by secretion of soluble gp130, which when bound to IL-6/sIL-6R prevents trans-signaling. IL-11 also transduces signals through gp130.

Function

IL-6 has pleiotropic effects on many cells, with both proinflammatory and anti-inflammatory properties. IL-6 can promote mucosal inflammation by inducing proliferation, activation, and prevention of apoptosis of T lymphocytes, differentiation of B cells, and stimulation of immunoglobulin production. At the same time, this molecule promotes neutrophil clearance from inflammatory foci (McLoughlin et al., 2003), decreases neutrophil chemokine production, activates the acute-phase response (hepatic synthesis of CRP, serum amyloid A, and haploglobulin), and induces expression of IL-1RA and the soluble p55 TNFR (Jones et al., 2001). IL-6 mediates IFN-γ–induced neutrophil clearance by decreasing KC production and enhancing PMN apoptosis through induction of caspase 3 (McLoughlin et al., 2003). IL-6 also promotes the transition from acute to chronic inflammation by recruitment of monocytes via alteration of chemokine profiles (Kaplanski et al., 2003).

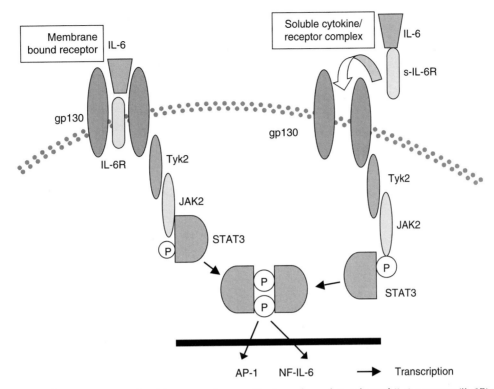

Fig. 35.4. IL-6 signaling pathways. IL-6 can signal by two pathways. Ligation of membrane-bound IL-6 receptor (IL-6R) causes homodimerization of membrane-bound gp130. This complex activates tyrosine kinases that phosphorylate STAT3, which homodimerizes to activate AP-1 or NF-IL-6. These transcription factors activate expression of a number of proinflammatory genes. An alternative transsignaling pathway is mediated by the complexing of secreted IL-6 with soluble IL-6 receptor (sIL-6R), which then binds to membrane-bound gp130. Subsequent signaling mechanisms are identical to ligation of membrane-bound receptor.

In contrast, transactivation of T cells through ligation of the sIL-6R/IL-6 complex with membrane gp130 *inhibits* apoptosis of activated T cells from patients with Crohn's disease and mice with Th1-mediated colitis through induction of the antiapoptotic genes bcl-2 and bcl-xl (Atreya *et al.*, 2000; Jostock *et al.*, 2001). A net proinflammatory effect of the transactivating properties of experimental Th1-mediated colitis is demonstrated by attenuation of disease by the blocking of sIL-1R-mediated signaling by anti-IL-6R antibodies or a gp 130–Fc fusion protein (Atreya *et al.*, 2000; Ito *et al.*, 2002; Yamamoto *et al.*, 2000; Mudter *et al.*, 2002). However, IL-6$^{-/-}$ mice exhibit increased expression of TNF, IFN-γ, GM-CSF, and MIP-2, as well as neutrophilia during acute inflammation (Xing *et al.*, 1998). Thus, it is probable that IL-6 stimulates both protective and inflammatory pathways in intestinal inflammation, perhaps by downregulating acute innate-mediated effects and stimulating T cell–mediated events. A primary role for circulating IL-6 in bone resorption is suggested by antibody blockade experiments using serum from patients with active Crohn's disease (Sylvester *et al.*, 2002).

IL-12 and IL-23

These immunoregulatory cytokines that polarize Th1 immune responses are briefly mentioned because they are produced by activated innate immune cells in response to many of the same stimuli that activate proinflammatory cytokines. This topic is covered in more detail in Chapter 28.

Structure

IL-12 is a homodimeric 70-kDa protein composed of p40 and p35 subsets. IL-12 p40 also can engage p19 to form IL-23, which has many functions overlapping with IL-12.

Expression

IL-12 is produced primarily by activated APCs, especially dendritic cells, as well as activated macrophages. Although noninflamed CD8$^+$ lymphoid dendritic cells produce IL-12 in preference to IL-10 and CD11b$^+$ myeloid dendritic cells produce very little IL-12 but have high levels of IL-10 in the normal intestine (Strober and Fuss, 2003), IL-12 production by mucosal CD11c$^+$ dendritic cells and CD11b$^+$ cells (macrophages and myeloid dendritic cells) is dramatically increased during Th1-mediated colitis in myeloid STAT3 conditional knockout mice (Kobayashi *et al.*, 2003). Likewise, IL-10-deficient myeloid dendritic cells stimulated with LPS or cecal bacterial lysate secrete high concentrations of IL-12 p40 (Albright *et al.*, 2002). These results indicate that endogenous IL-10 regulates IL-12 and IL-23 expression and that dendritic cells producing IL-12 are expanded during Th1-driven responses. TGF-β also inhibits IL-12 responses by downregulating IL-12, IL-12Rβ2, and IL-12Rβ2 subunits (Kitani *et al.*,

2000). Mucosal expression of IL-12 in the normal intestinal mucosa is very low, but it is substantially increased in experimental Th1-mediated colitis and human Crohn's disease. IL-12 expression is stimulated by NF-κB signaling in response to bacterial products (via TLR), TNF, and IL-1β, as well as IFNγ and CD40–CD40L ligation (Cong et al., 2000).

Signaling

IL-12 binds to a high-affinity complex of two receptors, β1 and β2. IL-12 and IL-23 signals are mediated by JAK2 and Tyk 2, which phosphorylate STAT4 (Mudter and Neurath, 2003). Accordingly, IL-12 stimulation of IFN-γ, Th1 responses, and NK cells are absent in STAT4$^{-/-}$ mice (Thierfelder et al., 1996).

Function

IL-12 and IL-23 polarize Th1 responses by inducing IFN-γ and TNF. In addition, IL-12 activates NK cells and stimulates cytotoxic T cells. IL-12 p40 expression—and hence IL-12 and IL-23 activity—is markedly increased in Th1-mediated intestinal inflammation, including experimental colitis and Crohn's disease (Sellon et al., 1998; Davidson et al., 1998; Neurath et al., 1995b; Monteleone et al., 1999; Fuss et al., 1996). A key role of IL-12 in the pathogenesis of intestinal inflammation is documented by potentiation of colitis by administration of recombinant IL-12 or the combination of rIL-12/IL-18 (Hans et al., 2000; Nakamura et al., 2000) and by near complete prevention and treatment of Th1-mediated colitis by anti-IL-12 antibody (Neurath et al., 1995b; Davidson et al., 1998). Fuss et al. (1999) demonstrated that this pronounced protection was accompanied by apoptosis of Th1 lymphocytes. Studies of tissue IL-12 expression and antibody blockade demonstrate that IL-12 mediates the early phase but not the late stage of colitis in IL-10$^{-/-}$ mice on a resistant C57BL/6 background (Spencer et al., 2002). A multicenter blinded study demonstrates therapeutic benefit of anti-IL-12 monoclonal antibody in the treatment of Crohn's disease (Mannon et al., 2004). Moreover, IL-12 and IL-18 can break oral tolerance in animal models, providing an additional mechanism to induce chronic inflammation (Neurath et al., 1996a; Eaton et al., 2003).

IL-18

This Th1 polarizing cytokine has structural and signaling similarities to IL-1β and functional overlap with IL-12.

Structure and secretion

IL-18 is an 18-kDa single peptide chain produced as a 24-kDa precursor protein that is activated by ICE (caspase 1) as well as proteinase 3, the same enzymes that secrete mature IL-1β (Nakanishi et al., 2001; Siegmund, 2002). Like IL-1β, IL-18 lacks a leader sequence and accumulates in the cytoplasm prior to activation. Secretion of mature IL-18 is stimulated by Fas ligand.

Expression

IL-18 is produced in the intestine by epithelial cells, lamina propria macrophages, and dendritic cells (Pizarro et al.,

1999). Expression of this cytokine is increased in active Crohn's disease but not in ulcerative colitis (Pizarro et al., 1999; Monteleone et al., 1999). Moreover, lamina propria mononuclear cells express IL-18 receptors (Kanai et al., 2001). LPMNCs from patients with Crohn's disease proliferate to a greater degree than do those from healthy persons when stimulated with IL-18. IL-18 gene expression is upregulated by IFN-γ, IFNα/β, or LPS through IFN consensus sequence-binding protein (ICSBP) and Pu.1 binding to regulatory elements on the two IL-18 promoters (Nakanishi et al., 2001).

Signaling

The IL-18 receptor is a heterodimer consisting of a ligand-binding subunit, IL-18Rα, which is identical to IL-1R-related protein, and a signaling subunit, IL-18Rβ, which is homologous to IL-1 RAcP. IL-18 binding protein (IL-18BP) is a soluble decoy receptor that can block binding of mature IL-18 with IL-18R, thereby inhibiting its biologic activity. Signaling proceeds through the IL-1R pathway involving the adapter protein MyD88, IRAK, and TRAF6 (Fig. 35.2). Stimulation of this complex activates the NF-κB and MAPK/AP-1 pathways. IL-18 activation of Th1 cells involves protein tyrosine kinase and the Src kinase LCK.

Function

IL-18 and IL-12 synergistically induce expression of IFN-γ through induction of NF-κB, AP-1 (IL-18), and STAT 4 (IL-12). By itself, IL-18 has minor effects, but the combination of IL-12 and IL-18 induces far more IFN-γ in T cells than either stimulus alone. These synergistic activities are evident in vivo, with no intestinal inflammation induced by injection of IL-18 alone and mild disease with IL-12 alone, but severe colitis, weight loss, and increased mortality occur with both IL-12 and IL-18 (Nakamura et al., 2000). This intestinal inflammation is IFNγ-dependent (Chikano et al., 2000). In addition, IL-18 stimulates production of TNF, IL-1β, C-C, and C-X-C chemokines by PBMCs and production of Fas-L and TNF by T cells and NK cells (Puren et al., 1998; Nakanishi et al., 2001). The contribution of IL-18 to intestinal inflammation is demonstrated by consistent attenuation of experimental colitis in multiple T cell–mediated and innate immune cell models (DSS, TNBS, T cell transfer to SCID mice) by a variety of IL-18-inhibitory strategies (antibody neutralization, IL-18BP binding, and antisense mRNA) (Siegmund et al., 2001; Kanai et al., 2001; ten Hove et al., 2001; Wirtz et al., 2002; Sivakumar et al., 2002). Furthermore, IL-18-transgenic mice are more susceptible to low-dose DSS-induced colitis, although macrophages appear to be more activated and more numerous than T lymphocytes (Ishikura et al., 2003). Of interest, IL-18BP expression and IL-18/IL-18BP complexes are increased in Crohn's disease, perhaps as a compensatory protective mechanism, although free (noncomplexed) IL-18 is found at the same time (Corbaz et al., 2002). As mentioned, IL-18 can break oral tolerance in mice (Eaton et al., 2003).

Other cytokines

Cytokines produced by both innate and cognate immune cells are being discovered at a rapid pace. This chapter emphasizes those molecules produced by innate immune cells that have been studied in the intestine; therefore, additional molecules are mentioned only briefly.

Chemokines

The rapidly expanding family of C-C and CXC chemokines is thoroughly covered in Chapter 34 and other comprehensive reviews (Papadakis and Targan, 2000) and is not emphasized in this discussion.

IFN-α, IFN-β

These molecules structurally related to IFN-γ are primarily secreted by activated macrophages. IFN-α has some antiinflammatory effects, including induction of IL-1RA and sTNFRI (p55) as well as inhibition of IL-5 and IL-13. Although an uncontrolled study showed a beneficial effect of IFN-α in ulcerative colitis (Sumer and Palabiyikoglu, 1995), a controlled study showed no benefit (Tilg *et al.*, 2003). IFN-β also has net antiinflammatory effects, with suppression of IFN-γ and TNF expression and stimulation of IL-10 expression and T cell–suppressor activity. Small open-label and controlled studies with IFN-β inhibited ulcerative colitis activity (Musch *et al.*, 2002; Nikolaus *et al.*, 2003).

M-CSF and GM-CSF

These growth factors have cytokine-like properties, including increasing the number and activation state of monocytes, macrophages, myeloid dendritic cells, and neutrophils (GM-CSF). G-CSF and CM-CSF production by LPMNCs is increased in active IBD (Pullman *et al.*, 1992; Noguchi *et al.*, 2001). A protective role for GM-CSF in Crohn's disease is supported by responses to recombinant protein in an open-label study (Dieckgraefe and Korzenik, 2002). The authors suggest that the beneficial effects of GM-CSF are mediated through stimulation of bacterial killing by mucosal phagocytic cells.

CONCLUSIONS

Proinflammatory cytokines induced by activated innate immune cells have an essential role in clearing enteric pathogens, mediating acute and chronic intestinal inflammation, and stimulating the effector T cell responses. Expansion of these cytokines is dependent on central transcription factors (NF-κB, AP-1, NF IL-6, JAK/STAT) that also serve to signal responses after receptor ligation by these same gene products. This conservation of redundant signaling pathways, together with widespread expression of cytokine receptors in many mucosal cell types and recruitment of additional effector cells through chemokines, leads to amplification of the inflammatory responses. This amplification is necessary to effectively clear invading pathogens, yet it can lead to irreversible tissue injury if not appropriately curtailed

once the inciting stimulus is resolved. The inflammatory response is efficiently suppressed in normal hosts by redundant inhibitory molecules that are induced by proinflammatory cytokines, bacterial products, and immunosuppressive molecules liberated by regulatory T-cell subsets, thus restoring immunologic tolerance and homeostasis with the commensal mucosally associated microflora.

Genetically susceptible individuals who are unable to mount appropriate suppressive signals develop chronic inflammation driven by overly aggressive innate and acquired immune responses to commensal bacteria. Most of the currently available therapies effective in IBD suppress proinflammatory cytokine transcription or function by inhibiting central signaling pathways or inducing apoptosis of key effector cells. Improved understanding of the regulation of expression and mode of action of these cytokines will lead to the development of new pharmacologic inhibitors that selectively block these key inducers of mucosal inflammatory responses.

REFERENCES

Abreu-Martin, M.T., Vidrich, A., Lynch, D.H., and Targan, S.R. (1995). Divergent induction of apoptosis and IL-8 secretion in HT-29 cells in response to TNF-alpha and ligation of Fas antigen. *J. Immunol.* 155, 4147–4154.

Akira, S., and Kishimoto, T. (1992). IL-6 and NF-IL6 in acute-phase response and viral infection. *Immunol. Rev.* 127, 25–50.

Albright, C., Tonkonogy, S.L., and Sartor, R.B. (2002). Endogenous IL-10 inhibits APC stimulation of T lymphocyte responses to luminal bacteria. *Gastroenterol.* 122, A270(Abstract)

Andus, T., Daig, R., Vogl, D., Aschenbrenner, E., Lock, G., Hollerbach, S., Kollinger, M., Scholmerich, J., and Gross, V. (1997). Imbalance of the interleukin 1 system in colonic mucosa–association with intestinal inflammation and interleukin 1 receptor agonist genotype 2. *Gut* 41, 651–657.

Andus, T., Targan, S.R., Deem, R., and Toyoda, H. (1993). Measurement of tumor necrosis factor alpha mRNA in small numbers of cells by quantitative polymerase chain reaction. *Reg. Immunol.* 5, 11–17.

Arizono, N., Kasugai, T., Yamada, M., Okada, M., Morimoto, M., Tei, H., Newlands, G.F., Miller, H.R., and Kitamura, Y. (1993). Infection of *Nippostrongylus brasiliensis* induces development of mucosal-type but not connective tissue-type mast cells in genetically mast cell-deficient Ws/Ws rats. *Blood* 81, 2572–2578.

Arnott, I.D., Drummond, H.E., and Ghosh, S. (2001). Gut mucosal secretion of interleukin 1beta and interleukin-8 predicts relapse in clinically inactive Crohn's disease. *Dig. Dis. Sci.* 46, 402–409.

Atreya, R., Mudter, J., Finotto, S., Mullberg, J., Jostock, T., Wirtz, S., Schutz, M., Bartsch, B., Holtmann, M., Becker, C., Strand, D., Czaja, J., Schlaak, J.F., Lehr, H.A., Autschbach, F., Schurmann, G., Nishimoto, N., Yoshizaki, K., Ito, H., Kishimoto, T., Galle, P.R., Rose-John, S., and Neurath, M.F. (2000). Blockade of interleukin 6 trans signaling suppresses T-cell resistance against apoptosis in chronic intestinal inflammation: evidence in Crohn's disease and experimental colitis in vivo. *Nat. Med.* 6, 583–588.

Barnes, P.J. (2001). Molecular mechanisms of corticosteroids in allergic diseases. *Allergy* 56, 928–936.

Bazzoni, F., and Beutler, B. (1996). The tumor necrosis factor ligand and receptor families. *N. Engl. J. Med.* 334, 1717–1725.

Berg, D.J., Zhang, J., Weinstock, J.V., Ismail, H.F., Earle, K.A., Alila, H., Pamkcu, R., Moore, S., and Lynch, R.G. (2002). Rapid development of colitis in NSAID-treated IL-10-deficient mice. *Gastroenterology* 123, 1527–1542.

Black, R.A., Doedens, J.R., Mahimkar, R., Johnson, R., Guo, L., Wallace, A., Virca, D., Eisenman, J., Slack, J., Castner, B., Sunnarborg, S.W., Lee, D.C., Cowling, R., Jin, G., Charrier, K., Peschon, J.J., and Paxton, R. (2003). Substrate specificity and inducibility of TACE (tumour necrosis factor alpha-converting enzyme) revisited: the Ala-Val preference, and induced intrinsic activity. *Biochem. Soc. Symp.* 39–52.

Bocker, U., Damiao, A., Holt, L., Han, D.S., Jobin, C., Panja, A., Mayer, L., and Sartor, R.B. (1998). Differential expression of interleukin 1 receptor antagonist isoforms in human intestinal epithelial cells. *Gastroenterology* 115, 1426–1438.

Bonen, D.K., Ogura, Y., Nicolae, D.L., Inohara, N., Saab, L., Tanabe, T., Chen, F.F., Foster, S.J., Duerr, R.H., Brant, S.R., Cho, J.H., and Nunez, G. (2003). Crohn's disease-associated NOD2 variants share a signaling defect in response to lipopolysaccharide and peptidoglycan. *Gastroenterology* 124, 140–146.

Breese, E.J., Michie, C.A., Nicholls, S.W., Murch, S.H., Williams, C.B., Domizio, P., Walker-Smith, J.A., and MacDonald, T.T. (1994). Tumor necrosis factor alpha-producing cells in the intestinal mucosa of children with inflammatory bowel disease. *Gastroenterology* 106, 1455–1466.

Brown, K.A., Back, S.J., Ruchelli, E.D., Markowitz, J.F., Mascarenhas, M., Verma, R., Piccoli, D.A., and Baldassano, R.N. (2002). Lamina propria and circulating interleukin-6 in newly diagnosed pediatric inflammatory bowel disease patients. *Am. J. Gastroenterol.* 97, 2603–2608.

Casini-Raggi, V., Kam, L., Chong, Y.J., Fiocchi, C., Pizarro, T.T., and Cominelli, F. (1995). Mucosal imbalance of IL-1 and IL-1 receptor antagonist in inflammatory bowel disease. A novel mechanism of chronic intestinal inflammation. *J. Immunol.* 154, 2434–2440.

Chamaillard, M., Hashimoto, M., Horie, Y., Masumoto, J., Qiu, S., Saab, L., Ogura, Y., Kawasaki, A., Fukase, K., Kusumoto, S., Valvano, M.A., Foster, S.J., Mak, T.W., Nunez, G., and Inohara, N. (2003). An essential role for NOD1 in host recognition of bacterial peptidoglycan containing diaminopimelic acid. *Nat. Immunol.* 4, 702–707.

Chikano, S., Sawada, K., Shimoyama, T., Kashiwamura, S.I., Sugihara, A., Sekikawa, K., Terada, N., Nakanishi, K., and Okamura, H. (2000). IL-18 and IL-12 induce intestinal inflammation and fatty liver in mice in an IFN-gamma dependent manner. *Gut* 47, 779–786.

Cohn, S.M., Schloemann, S., Tessner, T., Seibert, K., and Stenson, W.F. (1997). Crypt stem cell survival in the mouse intestinal epithelium is regulated by prostaglandins synthesized through cyclooxygenase-1. *J. Clin. Invest.* 99, 1367–1379.

Colotta, F., Re, F., Muzio, M., Bertini, R., Polentarutti, N., Sironi, M., Giri, J.G., Dower, S.K., Sims, J.E., and Mantovani, A. (1993). Interleukin-1 type II receptor: a decoy target for IL-1 that is regulated by IL-4. *Science* 261, 472–475.

Colombel, J.F., Loftus, E.V., Tremaine, W.J., Egan, L.J., Harmsen, W.S., Schleck, C.D., Zinsmeister, A.R., Sandborn, W.J. (2004). The safety profile of infliximab in patients with Crohn's disease: The Mayo Clinic experience in 500 patients. *Gastroenterol.* 126, 19–31.

Cominelli, F., Arseneau, K.A., and Pizarro, T.T. (2004). Cytokines and inflammatory mediators. *Kirsner's Inflammatory Bowel Diseases* (eds. Sartor RB and Sandborn WJ). Baltimore: WB Saunders: 179–198.

Cominelli, F., Nast, C.C., Dinarello, C.A., Gentilini, P., and Zipser, R.D. (1989). Regulation of eicosanoid production in rabbit colon by interleukin-1. *Gastroenterology* 97, 1400–1405.

Cominelli, F., Nast, C.C., Duchini, A., and Lee, M. (1992). Recombinant interleukin-1 receptor antagonist blocks the proinflammatory activity of endogenous interleukin-1 in rabbit immune colitis. *Gastroenterology* 103, 65–71.

Cominelli, F., Nast, C.C., Llerena, R., Dinarello, C.A., and Zipser, R.D. (1990). Interleukin 1 suppresses inflammation in rabbit colitis. Mediation by endogenous prostaglandins. *J. Clin. Invest.* 85, 582–586.

Cominelli, F., and Pizarro, T.T. (1997). Interleukin-1 receptor antagonist: a "novel" acute phase protein with antiinflammatory activities. *J. Clin. Invest.* 99, 2813

Cong, Y., Weaver, C.T., Lazenby, A., and Elson, C.O. (2000). Colitis induced by enteric bacterial antigen-specific CD4+ T cells

requires CD40-CD40 ligand interactions for a sustained increase in mucosal IL-12. *J. Immunol.* 165, 2173–2182.

Corazza, N., Eichenberger, S., Eugster, H.P., and Mueller, C. (1999). Nonlymphocyte-derived tumor necrosis factor is required for induction of colitis in recombination activating gene (RAG)2(–/–) mice upon transfer of CD4(+)CD45RB(hi) T cells. *J. Exp. Med.* 190, 1479–1492.

Corbaz, A., ten Hove, T., Herren, S., Graber, P., Schwartsburd, B., Belzer, I., Harrison, J., Plitz, T., Kosco-Vilbois, M.H., Kim, S.H., Dinarello, C.A., Novick, D., Van Deventer, S., and Chvatchko, Y. (2002). IL-18-binding protein expression by endothelial cells and macrophages is up-regulated during active Crohn's disease. *J. Immunol.* 168, 3608–3616.

Craggs, A., West, S., Curtis, A., Welfare, M., Hudson, M., Donaldson, P., and Mansfield, J. (2001). Absence of a genetic association between IL-1RN and IL-1B gene polymorphisms in ulcerative colitis and Crohn disease in multiple populations from northeast England. *Scand. J. Gastroenterol.* 36, 1173–1178.

Davidson, N.J., Hudak, S.A., Lesley, R.E., Menon, S., Leach, M.W., and Rennick, D.M. (1998). IL-12, but not IFN-gamma, plays a major role in sustaining the chronic phase of colitis in IL-10 deficient mice. *J. Immunol.* 161, 3143–3149.

de Baey, A., Mende, I., Baretton, G., Greiner, A., Hartl, W.H., Baeuerle, P.A., and Diepolder, H.M. (2003). A subset of human dendritic cells in the T cell area of mucosa-associated lymphoid tissue with a high potential to produce TNF-alpha. *J. Immunol.* 170, 5089–5094.

Dieckgraefe, B.K., and Korzenik, J.R. (2002). Treatment of active Crohn's disease with recombinant human granulocyte-macrophage colony-stimulating factor. *Lancet* 360, 1478–1480.

Dinarello, C.A. (2000). The role of the interleukin-1-receptor antagonist in blocking inflammation mediated by interleukin-1. *N. Engl. J. Med.* 343, 732–734.

Dionne, S., Laberge, S., Deslandres, C., and Seidman, E.G. (2003). Modulation of cytokine release from colonic explants by bacterial antigens in inflammatory bowel disease. *Clin. Exp. Immunol.* 133, 108–114.

Droemann, D., Goldmann, T., Branscheid, D., Clark, R., Dalhoff, K., Zabel, P., and Vollmer, E. (2003). Toll-like receptor 2 is expressed by alveolar epithelial cells type II and macrophages in the human lung. *Histochem. Cell. Biol.* 119, 103–108.

Dwinell, M.B., Lugering, N., Eckmann, L., and Kagnoff, M.F. (2001). Regulated production of interferon-inducible T-cell chemoattractants by human intestinal epithelial cells. *Gastroenterology* 120, 49–59.

Eaton, A.D., Xu, D., and Garside, P. (2003). Administration of exogenous interleukin-18 and interleukin-12 prevents the induction of oral tolerance. *Immunology* 108, 196–203.

Ehrenpreis, E.D., Kane, S.V., Cohen, L.B., Cohen, R.D., and Hanauer, S.B. (1999). Thalidomide therapy for patients with refractory Crohn's disease: an open-label trial. *Gastroenterology* 117, 1271–1277.

El-Haj, T., Poole, S., Farthing, M.J., and Ballinger, A.B. (2002). Anorexia in a rat model of colitis: interaction of interleukin-1 and hypothalamic serotonin. *Brain Res.* 927, 1–7.

Evgenikos, N., Bartolo, D.C., Hamer-Hodges, D.W., and Ghosh, S. (2002). Assessment of ileoanal pouch inflammation by interleukin 1 beta and interleukin 8 concentrations in the gut lumen. *Dis. Colon. Rectum.* 45, 249–255.

Fuss, I.J., Boirivant, M., Lacy, B., and Strober, W. (2002). The interrelated roles of TGF-beta and IL-10 in the regulation of experimental colitis. *J. Immunol.* 168, 900–908.

Fuss, I.J., Marth, T., Neurath, M.F., Pearlstein, G.R., Jain, A., and Strober, W. (1999). Anti-interleukin 12 treatment regulates apoptosis of Th1 T cells in experimental colitis in mice. *Gastroenterology* 117, 1078–1088.

Fuss, I.J., Neurath, M., Boirivant, M., Klein, J.S., de la, Matte, C. Strong, S.A., Fiocchi, C., and Strober, W. (1996). Disparate CD4+ lamina propria (LP) lymphokine secretion profiles in inflammatory bowel disease. Crohn's disease LP cells manifest increased secretion of IFN-gamma, whereas ulcerative colitis LP cells manifest increased secretion of IL-5. *J. Immunol.* 157, 1261–1270.

Girardin, S.E., Boneca, I.G., Carneiro, L.A., Antignac, A., Jehanno, M., Viala, J., Tedin, K., Taha, M.K., Labigne, A., Zahringer, U., Coyle, A.J., DiStefano, P.S., Bertin, J., Sansonetti, P.J., and Philpott, D.J. (2003a) Nod1 detects a unique neuropeptide from gram-negative bacterial peptidoglycan. *Science* 300, 1584–1587.

Girardin, S.E., Boneca, I.G., Viala, J., Chamaillard, M., Labigne, A., Thomas, G., Philpott, D.J., and Sansonetti, P.J. (2003b). Nod2 is a general sensor of peptidoglycan through muramyl dipeptide (MDP) detection. *J. Biol. Chem.* 278, 8869–8872.

Girardin, S.E., Travassos, L.H., Herve, M., Blanot, D., Boneca, I.G., Philpott, D.J., Sansonetti, P.J., and Mengin-Lecreulx, D. (2003c) Peptidoglycan molecular requirements allowing detection by Nod1 and Nod2. *J. Biol. Chem.* (in press).

Gross, V., Andus, T., Caesar, I., Roth, M., and Scholmerich, J. (1992). Evidence for continuous stimulation of interleukin-6 production in Crohn's disease. *Gastroenterology* 102, 514–519.

Hacker, U.T., Gomolka, M., Keller, E., Eigler, A., Folwaczny, C., Fricke, H., Albert, E., Loeschke, K., and Endres, S. (1997). Lack of association between an interleukin-1 receptor antagonist gene polymorphism and ulcerative colitis. *Gut* 40, 623–627.

Haller, D., Holt, L., Schwabe, R.F., Sartor, R.B., and Jobin, C. (2003). Transforming growth factor-β 1 inhibits non-pathogenic gram-negative bacteria-induced NF-κB recruitment to the interleukin-6 gene promoter in intestinal epithelial cells through modulation of histone acetylation. *J. Biol. Chem.* 278, 23851–23860.

Haller, D., Russo, M.P., Sartor, R.B., and Jobin, C. (2002). IKK beta and phosphatidylinositol 3-kinase/Akt participate in non-pathogenic Gram-negative enteric bacteria-induced RelA phosphorylation and NF-kappa B activation in both primary and intestinal epithelial cell lines. *J. Biol. Chem.* 277, 38168–38178.

Hans, W., Scholmerich, J., Gross, V., and Falk, W. (2000). Interleukin-12 induced interferon-gamma increases inflammation in acute dextran sulfate sodium induced colitis in mice. *Eur. Cytokine Netw.* 11, 67–74.

Herfarth, H.H., Mohanty, S.P., Rath, H.C., Tonkonogy, S., and Sartor, R.B. (1996). Interleukin 10 suppresses experimental chronic, granulomatous inflammation induced by bacterial cell wall polymers. *Gut* 39, 836–845.

Hisamatsu, T., Suzuki, M., and Podolsky, D.K. (2003). Interferon-gamma augments CARD4/NOD1 gene and protein expression through interferon regulatory factor-1 in intestinal epithelial cells. *J. Biol. Chem.* 278, 32962–32968.

Hisamatsu, T., Suzuki, M., Reinecker, H.C., Nadeau, W., *et al.* (2003). CARD15/NOD2 functions as an anti-bacterial factor in human intestinal epithelial cells. *Gastroenterology* 124, 993–1000.

Hogan, S.P., Mishra, A., Brandt, E.B., Royalty, M.P., Pope, S.M., Zimmermann, N., Foster, P.S., and Rothenberg, M.E. (2001). A pathological function for eotaxin and eosinophils in eosinophilic gastrointestinal inflammation. *Nat. Immunol.* 2, 353–360.

Hommes, D., van den Blink, B., Plasse, T., Bartelsman, J., Xu, C., Macpherson, B., Tytgat, G., Peppelenbosch, M.P., and Van Deventer, S. (2002). Inhibition of stress-activated MAP kinases induces clinical improvement in moderate to severe Crohn's disease. *Gastroenterology* 122, 7–14.

Hommes, D.W., Peppelenbosch, M.P., and van Deventer, S.J. (2003). Mitogen activated protein (MAP) kinase signal transduction pathways and novel anti-inflammatory targets. *Gut* 52, 144–151.

Hsueh, W., Caplan, M.S., Qu, X.W., Tan, X.D., De Plaen, I.G., and Gonzalez-Crussi, F. (2003). Neonatal necrotizing enterocolitis: clinical considerations and pathogenetic concepts. *Pediatr. Dev. Pathol.* 6, 6–23.

Hyams, J.S., Fitzgerald, J.E., Treem, W.R., Wyzga, N., and Kreutzer, D.L. (1993). Relationship of functional and antigenic interleukin 6 to disease activity in inflammatory bowel disease. *Gastroenterology* 104, 1285–1292.

Isaacs, K.L., Sartor, R.B., and Haskill, S. (1992). Cytokine messenger RNA profiles in inflammatory bowel disease mucosa detected by polymerase chain reaction amplification. *Gastroenterology* 103, 1587–1595.

Ishikura, T., Kanai, T., Uraushihara, K., Iiyama, R., Makita, S., Totsuka, T., Yamazaki, M., Sawada, T., Nakamura, T., Miyata, T., Kitahora, T., Hibi, T., Hoshino, T., and Watanabe, M. (2003).

Interleukin-18 overproduction exacerbates the development of colitis with markedly infiltrated macrophages in interleukin-18 transgenic mice. *J. Gastroenterol. Hepatol.* 18, 960–969.

Ito, H. (2003). IL-6 and Crohn's disease. *Curr. Drug. Targets. Inflamm. Allergy* 2, 125–130.

Ito, H., Hirotani, T., Yamamoto, M., Ogawa, H., and Kishimoto, T. (2002). Anti-IL-6 receptor monoclonal antibody inhibits leukocyte recruitment and promotes T-cell apoptosis in a murine model of Crohn's disease. *J. Gastroenterol.* 37, 56–61.

Jobin, C., and Sartor, R.B. (2000). The I kappa B/NF-kappa B system: a key determinant of mucosal inflammation and protection. *Am. J. Physiol. Cell Physiol.* 278, C451–C462

Jones, S.A., Horiuchi, S., Topley, N., Yamamoto, N., and Fuller, G.M. (2001). The soluble interleukin 6 receptor: mechanisms of production and implications in disease. *FASEB J.* 15, 43–58.

Jones, S.A., Horiuchi, S., Novick, D., Yamamoto, N., and Fuller, G.M. (1998). Shedding of the soluble IL-6 receptor is triggered by Ca2+ mobilization, while basal release is predominantly the product of differential mRNA splicing in THP-1 cells. *Eur. J. Immunol.* 28, 3514–3522.

Jones, S.A., Novick, D., Horiuchi, S., Yamamoto, N., Szalai, A.J., and Fuller, G.M. (1999). C-reactive protein: a physiological activator of interleukin 6 receptor shedding. *J. Exp. Med.* 189, 599–604.

Jostock, T., Mullberg, J., Ozbek, S., Atreya, R., Blinn, G., Voltz, N., Fischer, M., Neurath, M.F., and Rose-John, S. (2001). Soluble gp130 is the natural inhibitor of soluble interleukin-6 receptor transsignaling responses. *Eur. J. Biochem.* 268, 160–167.

Jung, H.C., Eckmann, L., Yang, S.K., Panja, A., Fierer, J., Morzycka-Wroblewska, E., and Kagnoff, M.F. (1995). A distinct array of proinflammatory cytokines is expressed in human colon epithelial cells in response to bacterial invasion. *J. Clin. Invest.* 95, 55–65.

Kagnoff, M.F., and Eckmann, L. (1997). Epithelial cells as sensors for microbial infection. *J. Clin. Invest.* 100, 6–10.

Kanai, T., Watanabe, M., Okazawa, A., Sato, T., Yamazaki, M., Okamoto, S., Ishii, H., Totsuka, T., Iiyama, R., Okamoto, R., Ikeda, M., Kurimoto, M., Takeda, K., Akira, S., and Hibi, T. (2001). Macrophage-derived IL-18-mediated intestinal inflammation in the murine model of Crohn's disease. *Gastroenterology* 121, 875–888.

Kaplanski, G., Marin, V., Montero-Julian, F., Mantovani, A., and Farnarier, C. (2003). IL-6: a regulator of the transition from neutrophil to monocyte recruitment during inflammation. *Trends Immunol.* 24, 25–29.

Kelsall, B.L., and Strober, W. (1997). Peyer's patch dendritic cells and the induction of mucosal immune responses. *Res. Immunol.* 148, 490–498.

Kim, S.C., Tonkonogy, S.L., and Sartor, R.B. (2001). Role of endogenous IL-10 in downregulating proinflammatory cytokine expression *Gastroenterology* 120, A183 [abstract].

Kim, Y.M., Talanian, R.V., Li, J., and Billiar, T.R. (1998). Nitric oxide prevents IL-1beta and IFN-gamma-inducing factor (IL-18) release from macrophages by inhibiting caspase-1 (IL-1 beta-converting enzyme). *J. Immunol.* 161, 4122–4128.

Kitani, A., Fuss, I.J., Nakamura, K., Schwartz, O.M., Usui, T., and Strober, W. (2000). Treatment of experimental (Trinitrobenzene sulfonic acid) colitis by intranasal administration of transforming growth factor (TGF)-beta1 plasmid: TGF-beta1-mediated suppression of T helper cell type 1 response occurs by interleukin (IL)-10 induction and IL-12 receptor beta2 chain downregulation. *J. Exp. Med.* 192, 41–52.

Kobayashi, K., Inohara, N., Hernandez, L.D., Galan, J.E., Nunez, G., Janeway, C.A., Medzhitov, R., and Flavell, R.A. (2002). RICK/Rip2/CARDIAK mediates signalling for receptors of the innate and adaptive immune systems. *Nature* 416, 194–199.

Kobayashi, K.S., Eynon, E.E., and Flavell, R.A. (2003). Intracellular debugging. *Nat. Immunol.* 4, 652–654.

Kobayashi, M., Kweon, M.N., Kuwata, H., Schreiber, R.D., Kiyono, H., Takeda, K., and Akira, S. (2003). Toll-like receptor-dependent production of IL-12p40 causes chronic enterocolitis in myeloid cell-specific Stat3-deficient mice. *J. Clin. Invest.* 111, 1297–1308.

Kontoyiannis, D., Boulougouris, G., Manoloukos, M., Armaka, M., Apostolaki, M., Pizarro, T., Kotlyarov, A., Forster, I., Flavell, R., Gaestel, M., Tsichlis, P., Cominelli, F., and Kollias, G. (2002).

Genetic dissection of the cellular pathways and signaling mechanisms in modeled tumor necrosis factor-induced Crohn's-like inflammatory bowel disease. *J. Exp. Med.* 196, 1563–1574.

Kontoyiannis, D., Pasparakis, M., Pizarro, T.T., Cominelli, F., and Kollias, G. (1999). Impaired on/off regulation of TNF biosynthesis in mice lacking TNF AU-rich elements: implications for joint and gut-associated immunopathologies. *Immunity* 10, 387–398.

Kosiewicz, M.M., Nast, C.C., Krishnan, A., Rivera-Nieves, J., Moskaluk, C.A., Matsumoto, S., Kozaiwa, K., and Cominelli, F. (2001). Th1-type responses mediate spontaneous ileitis in a novel murine model of Crohn's disease. *J. Clin. Invest.* 107, 695–702.

Koss, K., Satsangi, J., Welsh, K.I., and Jewell, D.P. (2000). Is interleukin-6 important in inflammatory bowel disease? *Genes Immun.* 1, 207–212.

Kuhn, R., Lohler, J., Rennick, D., Rajewsky, K., and Muller, W. (1993). Interleukin-10-deficient mice develop chronic enterocolitis. *Cell* 75, 263–274.

Kunkel, S.L., Chensue, S.W., and Phan, S.H. (1986). Prostaglandins as endogenous mediators of interleukin 1 production. *J. Immunol.* 136, 186–192.

Lee, E.G., Boone, D.L., Chai, S., Libby, S.L., Chien, M., Lodolce, J.P., and Ma, A. (2000). Failure to regulate TNF-induced NF-kappaB and cell death responses in A20-deficient mice. *Science* 289, 2350–2354.

Lugering, A., Schmidt, M., Lugering, N., Pauels, H.G., Domschke, W., and Kucharzik, T. (2001). Infliximab induces apoptosis in monocytes from patients with chronic active Crohn's disease by using a caspase-dependent pathway. *Gastroenterology* 121, 1145–1157.

MacGillivray, M., Herrera-Abreu, M.T., Chow, C.W., Shek, C., Wang, Q., Vachon, E., Feng, G.S., Siminovitch, K.A., McCulloch, C.A., and Downey, G.P. (2003). The protein tyrosine phosphatase SHP-2 regulates interleukin-1-induced ERK activation in fibroblasts. *J. Biol. Chem.* 278, 27190–27198.

Mackay, F., Browning, J.L., Lawton, P., Shah, S.A., Comiskey, M., Bhan, A.K., Mizoguchi, E., Terhorst, C., and Simpson, S.J. (1998). Both the lymphotoxin and tumor necrosis factor pathways are involved in experimental murine models of colitis. *Gastroenterology* 115, 1464–1475.

Mackay, F. and Kalled, S.L. (2002). TNF ligands and receptors in autoimmunity: an update. *Curr. Opin. Immunol.* 14, 783–790.

Mahida, Y.R. (2000). The key role of macrophages in the immunopathogenesis of inflammatory bowel disease. *Inflamm. Bowel Dis.* 6, 21–33.

Mannon, P., Fuss, I., Mayer, L., Elson, C.O., Sandborn, W.J., Orlin, B., Goodman, N., Groden, C., Hornung, R., Sulfold, J., Veldman, G.M., Schwertschalg, U., Strober, W. (2004). Anti-interleukin-12 treats active Crohn's disease. *Gastroenterol.* 126, A22 (abstract).

Mansfield, J.C., Holden, H., Tarlow, J.K., Di Giovine, F.S., McDowell, T.L., Wilson, A.G., Holdsworth, C.D., and Duff, G.W. (1994). Novel genetic association between ulcerative colitis and the anti-inflammatory cytokine interleukin-1 receptor antagonist. *Gastroenterology* 106, 637–642.

McAlindon, M.E., Hawkey, C.J., and Mahida, Y.R. (1998). Expression of interleukin 1 beta and interleukin 1 beta converting enzyme by intestinal macrophages in health and inflammatory bowel disease. *Gut* 42, 214–219.

McCall, R.D., Haskill, S., Zimmermann, E.M., Lund, P.K., Thompson, R.C., and Sartor, R.B. (1994). Tissue interleukin 1 and interleukin-1 receptor antagonist expression in enterocolitis in resistant and susceptible rats. *Gastroenterology* 106, 960–972.

McGee, D.W., Beagley, K.W., Aicher, W.K., McGhee, J.R. (1993). Transforming growth factor-beta and IL-1 beta act in synergy to enhance IL-6 secretion by the intestinal epithelial cell line, IEC-6. *J. Immunol.* 151, 970–978.

McLoughlin, R.M., Witowski, J., Robson, R.L., Wilkinson, T.S., Hurst, S.M., Williams, A.S., Williams, J.D., Rose-John, S., Jones, S.A., and Topley, N. (2003). Interplay between IFN-gamma and IL-6 signaling governs neutrophil trafficking and apoptosis during acute inflammation. *J. Clin. Invest.* 112, 598–607.

Mifflin, R.C., Saada, J.I., Di Mari, J.F., Adegboyega, P.A., Valentich, J.D., and Powell, D.W. (2002). Regulation of COX-2 expression in human intestinal myofibroblasts: mechanisms of IL-1-mediated induction. *Am. J. Physiol. Cell. Physiol.* 282, C824–C834.

Mitsuyama, K., Toyonaga, A., Sasaki, E., Ishida, O., Ikeda, H., Tsuruta, O., Harada, K., Tateishi, H., Nishiyama, T., and Tanikawa, K. (1995). Soluble interleukin-6 receptors in inflammatory bowel disease: relation to circulating interleukin-6. *Gut* 36, 45–49.

Mizoguchi, E., Mizoguchi, A., Takedatsu, H., Cario, E., de Jong, Y.P., Ooi, C.J., Xavier, R.J., Terhorst, C., Podolsky, D.K., and Bhan, A.K. (2002). Role of tumor necrosis factor receptor 2 (TNFR2) in colonic epithelial hyperplasia and chronic intestinal inflammation in mice. *Gastroenterology* 122, 134–144.

Mohan, M.J., Seaton, T., Mitchell, J., Howe, A., Blackburn, K., Burkhart, W., Moyer, M., Patel, I., Waitt, G.M., Becherer, J.D., Moss, M.L., and Milla, M.E. (2002). The tumor necrosis factor-alpha converting enzyme (TACE): a unique metalloproteinase with highly defined substrate selectivity. *Biochemistry* 41, 9462–9469.

Monteleone, G., MacDonald, T.T., Wathen, N.C., Pallone, F., and Pender, S.L. (1999). Enhancing lamina propria Th1 cell responses with interleukin 12 produces severe tissue injury. *Gastroenterology* 117, 1069–1077.

Monteleone, G., Trapasso, F., Parrello, T., Biancone, L., Stella, A., Iuliano, R., Luzza, F., Fusco, A., and Pallone, F. (1999). Bioactive IL-18 expression is up-regulated in Crohn's disease. *J. Immunol.* 163, 143–147.

Morteau, O., Morham, S.G., Sellon, R., Dieleman, L.A., Langenbach, R., Smithies, O., and Sartor, R.B. (2000). Impaired mucosal defense to acute colonic injury in mice lacking cyclooxygenase-1 or cyclooxygenase-2. *J. Clin. Invest.* 105, 469–478.

Mudter, J., and Neurath, M.F. (2003). The role of signal transducers and activators of transcription in T inflammatory bowel diseases. *Inflamm. Bowel. Dis.* 9, 332–337.

Mudter, J., Wirtz, S., Galle, P.R., and Neurath, M.F. (2002). A new model of chronic colitis in SCID mice induced by adoptive transfer of CD62L+ CD4+ T cells: insights into the regulatory role of interleukin-6 on apoptosis. *Pathobiology* 70, 170–176.

Murtaugh, M.P., and Foss, D.L. (2002). Inflammatory cytokines and antigen presenting cell activation. *Vet. Immunol. Immunopathol.* 87, 109–121.

Musch, E., Andus, T., and Malek, M. (2002). Induction and maintenance of clinical remission by interferon-beta in patients with steroid-refractory active ulcerative colitis-an open long-term pilot trial. *Aliment. Pharmacol. Ther.* 16, 1233–1239.

Nakamura, S., Otani, T., Ijiri, Y., Motoda, R., Kurimoto, M., and Orita, K. (2000). IFN-gamma-dependent and -independent mechanisms in adverse effects caused by concomitant administration of IL-18 and IL-12. *J. Immunol.* 164, 3330–3336.

Nakanishi, K., Yoshimoto, T., Tsutsui, H., and Okamura, H. (2001). Interleukin-18 is a unique cytokine that stimulates both Th1 and Th2 responses depending on its cytokine milieu. *Cytokine Growth Factor Rev.* 12, 53–72.

Neumann, D., Lienenklaus, S., Rosati, O., and Martin, M.U. (2002). IL-1beta-induced phosphorylation of PKB/Akt depends on the presence of IRAK-1. *Eur. J. Immunol.* 32, 3689–3698.

Neurath, M.F., Fuss, I., Kelsall, B.L., Presky, D.H., Waegell, W., and Strober, W. (1996) Experimental granulomatous colitis in mice is abrogated by induction of TGF-beta-mediated oral tolerance. *J. Exp. Med.* 183, 2605–2616.

Neurath, M.F., Fuss, I., Kelsall, B.L., Stuber, E., and Strober, W. (1995) Antibodies to interleukin 12 abrogate established experimental colitis in mice. *J. Exp. Med.* 182, 1281–1290.

Neurath, M.F., Fuss, I., Pasparakis, M., Alexopoulou, L., Haralambous, S., Meyer zum Buschenfelde, K.H., Strober, W., and Kollias, G. (1997). Predominant pathogenic role of tumor necrosis factor in experimental colitis in mice. *Eur. J. Immunol.* 27, 1743–1750.

Niemand, C., Nimmesgern, A., Haan, S., Fischer, P., Schaper, F., Rossaint, R., Heinrich, P.C., and Muller-Newen, G. (2003). Activation of STAT3 by IL-6 and IL-10 in primary human macrophages is differentially modulated by suppressor of cytokine signaling 3. *J. Immunol.* 170, 3263–3272.

Nikolaus, S., Rutgeerts, P., Fedorak, R., Steinhart, A.H., Wild, G.E., Theuer, D., Mohrle, J., and Schreiber, S. (2003). Interferon beta-

1a in ulcerative colitis: a placebo controlled, randomised, dose escalating study. *Gut* 52, 1286–1290.

Nilsen, E.M., Johansen, F.E., Jahnsen, F.L., Lundin, K.E., Scholz, T., Brandtzaeg, P., and Haraldsen, G. (1998). Cytokine profiles of cultured microvascular endothelial cells from the human intestine. *Gut* 42, 635–642.

Nitta, M., Hirata, I., Toshina, K., Murano, M., Maemura, K., Hamamoto, N., Sasaki, S., Yamauchi, H., and Katsu, K. (2002). Expression of the EP4 prostaglandin E2 receptor subtype with rat dextran sodium sulphate colitis: colitis suppression by a selective agonist, ONO-AE1-329. *Scand. J. Immunol.* 56, 66–75.

Noguchi, M., Hiwatashi, N., Liu, Z.X., and Toyota, T. (2001). Increased secretion of granulocyte-macrophage colony-stimulating factor in mucosal lesions of inflammatory bowel disease. *Digestion* 63 Suppl 1, 32–36.

O'Neil, D.A., Porter, E.M., Elewaut, D., Anderson, G.M., Eckmann, L., Ganz, T., and Kagnoff, M.F. (1999). Expression and regulation of the human beta-defensins hBD-1 and hBD-2 in intestinal epithelium. *J. Immunol.* 163, 6718–6724.

Ozinsky, A., Underhill, D.M., Fontenot, J.D., Hajjar, A.M., Smith, K.D., Wilson, C.B., Schroeder, L., and Aderem, A. (2000). The repertoire for pattern recognition of pathogens by the innate immune system is defined by cooperation between toll-like receptors. *Proc. Natl. Acad. Sci. USA* 97, 13766–13771.

Papadakis, K.A., and Targan, S.R. (2000). Role of cytokines in the pathogenesis of inflammatory bowel disease. *Annu. Rev. Med.* 51, 289–298.

Persson, T., Monsef, N., Andersson, P., Bjartell, A., Malm, J., Calafat, J., and Egesten, A. (2003). Expression of the neutrophil-activating CXC chemokine ENA-78/CXCL5 by human eosinophils. *Clin. Exp. Allergy* 33, 531–537.

Pizarro, T.T., Michie, M.H., Bentz, M., Woraratanadharm, J., Smith, M.F. Jr., Foley, E., Moskaluk, C.A., Bickston, S.J., and Cominelli, F. (1999). IL-18, a novel immunoregulatory cytokine, is up-regulated in Crohn's disease: expression and localization in intestinal mucosal cells. *J. Immunol.* 162, 6829–6835.

Pothoulakis, C., and LaMont, J.T. (2001). Microbes and microbial toxins: paradigms for microbial-mucosal interactions II. The integrated response of the intestine to *Clostridium difficile* toxins. *Am. J. Physiol. Gastrointest. Liver Physiol.* 280, G178–G183.

Powell, D.W., Mifflin, R.C., Valentich, J.D., Crowe, S.E., Saada, J.I., and West, A.B. (1999). Myofibroblasts. II. Intestinal subepithelial myofibroblasts. *Am. J. Physiol.* 277, C183–C201.

Present, D.H., Rutgeerts, P., Targan, S., Hanauer, S.B., Mayer, L., Van Hogezand, R.A., Podolsky, D.K., Sands, B.E., Braakman, T., DeWoody, K.L., Schaible, T.F., and van Deventer, S.J. (1999). Infliximab for the treatment of fistulas in patients with Crohn's disease. *N. Engl. J. Med.* 340, 1398–1405.

Probert, C.S., Hearing, S.D., Schreiber, S., Kuhbacher, T., Ghosh, S., Arnott, I.D., and Forbes, A. (2003). Infliximab in moderately severe glucocorticoid resistant ulcerative colitis: a randomised controlled trial. *Gut* 52, 998–1002.

Pucilowska, J.B., Williams, K.L., and Lund, P.K. (2000). Fibrogenesis. IV. Fibrosis and inflammatory bowel disease: cellular mediators and animal models. *Am. J. Physiol. Gastrointest. Liver Physiol.* 279, G653–G659.

Pullman, W.E., Elsbury, S., Kobayashi, M., Hapel, A.J., and Doe, W.F. (1992). Enhanced mucosal cytokine production in inflammatory bowel disease. *Gastroenterology* 102, 529–537.

Puren, A.J., Fantuzzi, G., Gu, Y., Su, M.S., and Dinarello, C.A. (1998). Interleukin-18 (IFNgamma-inducing factor) induces IL-8 and IL-1beta via TNFalpha production from non-CD14+ human blood mononuclear cells. *J. Clin. Invest.* 101, 711–721.

Rachmilewitz, D., Katakura, K., Karmeli, F., Hayashi, T., Reinus, C., Rudensky, B., Akira, S., Takeda, K., Lee, J., Takabayashi, K., and Raz, E. (2004). Toll-like receptor 9 signaling mediates the anti-inflammatory effects of probiotics in murine experimental colitis. *Gastroenterology* 126, 520–528.

Rath, H.C., Herfarth, H.H., Ikeda, J.S., Grenther, W.B., Hamm, T.E. Jr., Balish, E., Taurog, J.D., Hammer, R.E., Wilson, K.H., and Sartor, R.B. (1996). Normal luminal bacteria, especially *Bacteroides species* mediate chronic colitis, gastritis, and arthritis in HLA-B27/human beta2 microglobulin transgenic rats. *J. Clin. Invest.* 98, 945–953.

Reinecker, H.C., Steffen, M., Witthoeft, T., Pflueger, I., Schreiber, S., MacDermott, R.P., and Raedler, A. (1993). Enhanced secretion of tumour necrosis factor-alpha, IL-6, and IL-1 beta by isolated lamina propria mononuclear cells from patients with ulcerative colitis and Crohn's disease. *Clin. Exp. Immunol.* 94, 174–181.

Rennick, D.M., Fort, M.M., and Davidson, N.J. (1997). Studies with IL-10-/-mice: an overview. *J. Leukocyte. Biol.* 61, 389–396.

Ricci, S., Macchia, G., Ruggiero, P., Maggi, T., Bossu, P., Xu, L., Medaglini, D., Tagliabue, A., Hammarstrom, L., Pozzi, G., and Boraschi, D. (2003). In vivo mucosal delivery of bioactive human interleukin 1 receptor antagonist produced by *Streptococcus gordonii*. *BMC Biotechnol.* 3, 15.

Rogler, G., Andus, T., Aschenbrenner, E., Vogl, D., Falk, W., Scholmerich, J., and Gross, V. (1997). Alterations of the phenotype of colonic macrophages in inflammatory bowel disease. *Eur. J. Gastroenterol. Hepatol.* 9, 893–899.

Rogler, G., Gelbmann, C.M., Vogl, D., Brunner, M., Scholmerich, J., Falk, W., Andus, T., and Brand, K. (2001). Differential activation of cytokine secretion in primary human colonic fibroblast/myofibroblast cultures. *Scand. J. Gastroenterol.* 36, 389–398.

Rosenstiel, P., Fantini, M., Brautigam, K., Kuhbacher, T., Waetzig, G.H., Seegert, D., and Schreiber, S. (2003). TNF-alpha and IFN-gamma regulate the expression of the NOD2 (CARD15) gene in human intestinal epithelial cells. *Gastroenterology* 124, 1001–1009.

Sandborn, W.J. (2003). Strategies for targeting tumour necrosis factor in IBD. *Best Pract. Res. Clin. Gastroenterol.* 17, 105–117.

Sandborn, W.J., Feagan, B.G., Hanauer, S.B., Present, D.H., Sutherland, L.R., Kamm, M.A., Wolf, D.C., Baker, J.P., Hawkey, C., Archambault, A., Bernstein, C.N., Novak, C., Heath, P.K., and Targan, S.R.: CDP57/Crohn's Study Group. (2001). An engineered human antibody to TNF (CDP571) for active Crohn's disease: a randomized double-blind placebo-controlled trial. *Gastroenterology* 120, 1330–1338.

Sands, B.E., Tremaine, W.J., Sandborn, W.J., Rutgeerts, P.J., Hanauer, S.B., Mayer, L., Targan, S.R., and Podolsky, D.K. (2001). Infliximab in the treatment of severe, steroid-refractory ulcerative colitis: a pilot study. *Inflamm. Bowel. Dis.* 7, 83–88.

Saniabadi, A.R., Hanai, H., Takeuchi, K., Umemura, K., Nakashima, M., Adachi, T., Shima, C., Bjarnason, I., and Lofberg, R. (2003). Adacolumn, an adsorptive carrier based granulocyte and monocyte apheresis device for the treatment of inflammatory and refractory diseases associated with leukocytes. *Ther. Apher. Dial.* 7, 48–59.

Sartor, R.B. (2003). Innate immunity in the pathogenesis and therapy of IBD. *J. Gastroenterol.* 38, 43–47.

Sartor, R.B. (1994). Cytokines in intestinal inflammation: pathophysiological and clinical considerations. *Gastroenterology* 106, 533–539.

Schottelius, A.J., Mayo, M.W., Sartor, R.B., and Baldwin, A.S.J. (1999). Interleukin-10 signaling blocks inhibitor of kappaB kinase activity and nuclear factor kappaB DNA binding. *J. Biol. Chem.* 274, 31868–31874.

Sellon, R.K., Tonkonogy, S., Schultz, M., Dieleman, L.A., Grenther, W., Balish, E., Rennick, D.M., and Sartor, R.B. (1998). Resident enteric bacteria are necessary for development of spontaneous colitis and immune system activation in interleukin-10-deficient mice. *Infect. Immun.* 66, 5224–5231.

Siegmund, B. (2002). Interleukin-1beta converting enzyme (caspase-1) in intestinal inflammation. *Biochem. Pharmacol.* 64, 1–8.

Siegmund, B., Lehr, H.A., Fantuzzi, G., and Dinarello, C.A. (2001). IL-1 beta-converting enzyme (caspase-1) in intestinal inflammation. *Proc. Natl. Acad. Sci. USA* 98, 13249–13254.

Sivakumar, P.V., Westrich, G.M., Kanaly, S., Garka, K., Born, T.L., Derry, J.M., and Viney, J.L. (2002). Interleukin 18 is a primary mediator of the inflammation associated with dextran sulphate sodium induced colitis: blocking interleukin 18 attenuates intestinal damage. *Gut* 50, 812–820.

Smith, P.D., Smythies, L.E., Mosteller-Barnum, M., Sibley, D.A., Russell, M.W., Merger, M., Sellers, M.T., Orenstein, J.M., Shimada, T., Graham, M.F., and Kubagawa, H. (2001). Intestinal macrophages lack CD14 and CD89 and consequently are down-regulated for LPS- and IgA-mediated activities. *J. Immunol.* 167, 2651–2656.

Spahn, T.W., Herbst, H., Rennert, P.D., Lugering, N., Maaser, C., Kraft, M., Fontana, A., Weiner, H.L., Domschke, W., and Kucharzik, T. (2002). Induction of colitis in mice deficient of Peyer's patches and mesenteric lymph nodes is associated with increased disease severity and formation of colonic lymphoid patches. *Am. J. Pathol.* 161, 2273–2282.

Spencer, D.M., Veldman, G.M., Banerjee, S., Willis, J., and Levine, A.D. (2002). Distinct inflammatory mechanisms mediate early versus late colitis in mice. *Gastroenterology* 122, 94–105.

Stagg, A.J., Hart, A.L., Knight, S.C., and Kamm, M.A. (2003). The dendritic cell: its role in intestinal inflammation and relationship with gut bacteria. *Gut* 52, 1522–1529.

Stead, R.H., Dixon, M.F., Bramwell, N.H., Riddell, R.H., and Bienenstock, J. (1989). Mast cells are closely apposed to nerves in the human gastrointestinal mucosa. *Gastroenterology* 97, 575–585.

Strober, W., and Fuss, I.J. (2004). The regulation of mucosal homeostasis and its relation to inflammatory bowel diseases. *Kirsner's Inflammatory Bowel Diseases* (eds. Sartor R.B., and Sandborn, W.J.) Baltimore: WB Saunders, 60–79.

Strong, S.A., Pizarro, T.T., Klein, J.S., Cominelli, F., and Fiocchi, C. (1998). Proinflammatory cytokines differentially modulate their own expression in human intestinal mucosal mesenchymal cells. *Gastroenterol.* 114, 1244–1256.

Sumer, N., and Palabiyikoglu, M. (1995). Induction of remission by interferon-alpha in patients with chronic active ulcerative colitis. *Eur. J. Gastroenterol. Hepatol.* 7, 597–602.

Suzuki, M., Hisamatsu, T., and Podolsky, D.K. (2003). Gamma interferon augments the intracellular pathway for lipopolysaccharide (LPS) recognition in human intestinal epithelial cells through coordinated up-regulation of LPS uptake and expression of the intracellular Toll-like receptor 4-MD-2 complex. *Infect. Immun.* 71, 3503–3511.

Sylvester, F.A., Wyzga, N., Hyams, J.S., and Gronowicz, G.A. (2002). Effect of Crohn's disease on bone metabolism in vitro: a role for interleukin-6. *J. Bone Miner. Res.* 17, 695–702.

Takeda, K., Takeuchi, O., and Akira, S. (2002). Recognition of lipopeptides by Toll-like receptors. *J. Endotoxin Res.* 8, 459–463.

Tapping, R.I., and Tobias, P.S. (2003). Mycobacterial lipoarabinomannan mediates physical interactions between TLR1 and TLR2 to induce signaling. *J. Endotoxin Res.* 9, 264–268.

Targan, S.R., Deem, R.L., and Shanahan, F. (1991). Role of mucosal T-cell-generated cytokines in epithelial cell injury. *Immunol. Res.* 10, 472–478.

Targan, S.R., Hanauer, S.B., van Deventer, S.J., Mayer, L., Present, D.H., Braakman, T., DeWoody, K.L., Schaible, T.F., and Rutgeerts, P.J. (1997). A short-term study of chimeric monoclonal antibody cA2 to tumor necrosis factor alpha for Crohn's disease. Crohn's Disease cA2 Study Group. *N. Engl. J. Med.* 337, 1029–1035.

ten Hove, T., Corbaz, A., Amitai, H., Aloni, S., Belzer, I., Graber, P., Drillenburg, P., van Deventer, S.J., Chvatchko, Y., and Te Velde, A.A. (2001). Blockade of endogenous IL-18 ameliorates TNBS-induced colitis by decreasing local TNF-alpha production in mice. *Gastroenterology* 121, 1372–1379.

Thierfelder, W.E., van Deursen, J.M., Yamamoto, K., Tripp, R.A., Sarawar, S.R., Carson, R.T., Sangster, M.Y., Vignali, D.A., Doherty, P.C., Grosveld, G.C., and Ihle, J.N. (1996). Requirement for Stat4 in interleukin-12-mediated responses of natural killer and T cells. *Nature* 382, 171–174.

Tilg, H., Vogelsang, H., Ludwiczek, O., Lochs, H., Kaser, A., Colombel, J.F., Ulmer, H., Rutgeerts, P., Kruger, S., Cortot, A., D'Haens, G., Harrer, M., Gasche, C., Wrba, F., Kuhn, I., and Reinisch, W. (2003). A randomised placebo controlled trial of pegylated interferon alpha in active ulcerative colitis. *Gut* 52, 1728–1733.

Tsugawa, K., Jones, M.K., Akahoshi, T., Moon, W.S., Maehara, Y., Hashizume, M., Sarfeh, I.J., and Tarnawski, A.S. (2003). Abnormal PTEN expression in portal hypertensive gastric mucosa: A key to impaired PI 3-kinase/Akt activation and delayed injury healing? *FASEB J.* 17, 2316–2318.

Tsukada, Y., Nakamura, T., Iimura, M., Iizuka, B. E., and Hayashi, N. (2002). Cytokine profile in colonic mucosa of ulcerative colitis correlates with disease activity and response to granulocyta-pheresis. *Am. J. Gastroenterol.* 97, 2820–2828.

Tumanov, A.V., Kuprash, D.V., and Nedospasov, S.A. (2003). The role of lymphotoxin in development and maintenance of secondary lymphoid tissues. *Cytokine Growth Factor Rev.* 14, 275–288.

Vallance, B.A., Blennerhassett, P.A., Deng, Y., Matthaei, K.I., Young, I.G., and Collins, S.M. (1998). IL-5 contributes to worm expulsion and muscle hypercontractility in a primary *T. spiralis* infection. *Am. J. Physiol.* 277, G400–G408.

Van den Brande, J.M., Braat, H., Van den Brink, G.R., Versteeg, H.H., Bauer, C.A., Hoedemaeker, I., van Montfrans, C., Hommes, D.W., Peppelenbosch, M.P., and van Deventer, S.J. (2003). Infliximab but not etanercept induces apoptosis in lamina propria T-lymphocytes from patients with Crohn's disease. *Gastroenterology* 124, 1774–1785.

Vasiliauskas, E.A., Kam, L.Y., Abreu-Martin, M.T., Hassard, P.V., Papadakis, K.A., Yang, H., Zeldis, J.B., and Targan, S.R. (1999). An open-label pilot study of low-dose thalidomide in chronically active, steroid-dependent Crohn's disease. *Gastroenterology* 117, 1278–1287.

Waetzig, G.H., Seegert, D., Rosenstiel, P., Nikolaus, S., and Schreiber, S. (2002). p38 mitogen-activated protein kinase is activated and linked to TNF-alpha signaling in inflammatory bowel disease. *J. Immunol.* 168, 5342–5351.

Watanabe, N., Ikuta, K., Okazaki, K., Nakase, H., Tabata, Y., Matsuura, M., Tamaki, H., Kawanami, C., Honjo, T., Chiba, T. (2003). Elimination of local macrophages in intestine prevents chronic colitis in interleukin-10-deficient mice. *Dig. Dis. Sci.* 48, 408–414.

Watson, J.M., Lofquist, A.K., Rinehart, C.A., Olsen, J.C., Makarov, S.S., Kaufman, D.G., and Haskill, J.S. (1995). The intracellular IL-1 receptor antagonist alters IL-1-inducible gene expression without blocking exogenous signaling by IL-1 beta. *J. Immunol.* 155, 4467–4475.

Winsor, G.L., Waterhouse, C.C., MacLellan, R.L., and Stadnyk, A.W. (2000). Interleukin-4 and IFN-gamma differentially stimulate macrophage chemoattractant protein-1 (MCP-1) and eotaxin production by intestinal epithelial cells. *J. Interferon Cytokine. Res.* 20, 299–308.

Wirtz, S., Becker, C., Blumberg, R.S., Galle, P.R., and Neurath, M.F. (2002). Treatment of T cell-dependent experimental colitis in SCID mice by local administration of an adenovirus expressing IL-18 antisense mRNA. *J. Immunol.* 168, 411–420.

Xia, C.Q., and Kao, K.J. (2003). Suppression of interleukin-12 production through endogenously secreted interleukin-10 in activated dendritic cells: involvement of activation of extracellular signal-regulated protein kinase. *Scand. J. Immunol.* 58, 23–32.

Xing, Z., Gauldie, J., Cox, G., Baumann, H., Jordana, M., Lei, X.F., and Achong, M.K. (1998). IL-6 is an antiinflammatory cytokine required for controlling local or systemic acute inflammatory responses. *J. Clin. Invest.* 101, 311–320.

Xiong, H., Zhu, C., Li, F., Hegazi, R., He, K., Babyatsky, M., Bauer, A.J., and Plevy, S.E. (2004). Inhibition of interleukin-12 p40 transcription and NFkB activation by nitric oxide in murine macrophages and dendritic cells. *J. Biol. Chem.* 279, 10776–10783.

Yamada, T., Deitch, E., Specian, R.D., Perry, M.A., Sartor, R.B., and Grisham, M.B. (1993). Mechanisms of acute and chronic intestinal inflammation induced by indomethacin. *Inflammation* 17, 641–662.

Yamamoto, M., Sato, S., Hemmi, H., Uematsu, S., Hoshino, K., Kaisho, T., Takeuchi, O., Takeda, K., and Akira, S. (2003). TRAM is specifically involved in the Toll-like receptor 4-mediated MyD88-independent signaling pathway. *Nat. Immunol.* 4, 1144–1150.

Yamamoto, M., Yoshizaki, K., Kishimoto, T., and Ito, H. (2000). IL-6 is required for the development of Th1 cell-mediated murine colitis. *J. Immunol.* 164, 4878–4882.

Yang, S.K., Eckmann, L., Panja, A., and Kagnoff, M.F. (1997). Differential and regulated expression of C-X-C, C-C, and C-chemokines by human colon epithelial cells. *Gastroenterology* 113, 1214–1223.

Yasukawa, H., Ohishi, M., Mori, H., Murakami, M., Chinen, T., Aki, D., Hanada, T., Takeda, K., Akira, S., Hoshijima, M., Hirano, T., Chien, K.R., and Yoshimura, A. (2003). IL-6 induces an anti-inflammatory response in the absence of SOCS3 in macrophages. *Nat. Immunol.* 4, 551–556.

Youngman, K.R., Simon, P.L., West, G.A., Cominelli, F., Rachmilewitz, D., Klein, J.S., and Fiocchi, C. (1993). Localization of intestinal interleukin 1 activity and protein and gene expression to lamina propria cells. *Gastroenterology* 104, 749–758.

Zhang, Z., Mahajan, S., Zhang, X., and Stanley, S.L., Jr. (2003). Tumor necrosis factor alpha is a key mediator of gut inflammation seen in amebic colitis in human intestine in the SCID mouse-human intestinal xenograft model of disease. *Infect. Immun.* 71, 5355–5359.

Zhao, X., Sato, A., Dela Cruz, C.S., Linehan, M., Luegering, A., Kucharzik, T., Shirakawa, A.K., Marquez, G., Farber, J.M., Williams, I., and Iwasaki, A. (2003). CCL9 is secreted by the follicle-associated epithelium and recruits dome region Peyer's patch CD11b+ dendritic cells. *J. Immunol.* 171, 2797–2803.

Mast Cells In Mucosal Defenses and Pathogenesis

Tong-Jun Lin

Department of Microbiology and Immunology and Department of Pediatrics, Dalhousie University, Halifax, Nova Scotia, Canada

A. Dean Befus

Pulmonary Research Group, Department of Medicine, Faculty of Medicine, University of Alberta, Edmonton, Alberta, Canada

In 1878 Ehrlich identified mast cells through the metachromatic staining of their cytoplasmic granules. Mast cells have long been recognized as major effector cells of the allergic reactions through secretion of granule-associated and newly synthesized mediators. They are distributed widely in the body and are especially abundant in skin or mucosa, where they can interact with foreign materials such as allergens and pathogens. Mast cells are heterogeneous in their phenotypic and biologic features. Marked progress has been made recently in mast cell biology, especially the recent recognition of their importance in innate immunity. This review outlines knowledge on mast cell ontogeny, heterogeneity, and functions in allergy and immunity. The reader should also consult other reviews (*e.g.*, Metcalfe *et al.*, 1997; Williams and Galli, 2000; Féger *et al.*, 2002; Stassen *et al.*, 2002; Boyce, 2003; Befus and Denburg, 2004).

MAST CELL ONTOGENY

Basic characteristics of mast cells

Mature mast cells reside in tissues and are round, oval, spindle, or spiderlike in shape (Schwartz and Huff, 1993). They contain numerous cytoplasmic granules that may be homogeneously electron-dense or exhibit membrane or complex scroll-like patterns, highly organized crystalline structures, or combinations of these. Numerous biologically active products are synthesized and stored in these granules.

Origin of mast cells

Mast cells originate from pluripotential hematopoietic cells in bone marrow, undergo part of their differentiation in this site, and then enter the circulation and complete their differentiation in mucosal or connective tissues (Kitamura *et al.*, 1979; Befus and Denburg, 2004). In the bone marrow, the number of mast cell precursors in mice is estimated at 10 to 68 precursors per 10^5 bone marrow cells (Sonoda *et al.*, 1982; Thompson *et al.*, 1990). Mast cell progenitors are CD34+, but no mast cell–specific lineage marker has been described.

In normal mouse blood there are 1 to 2 mast cell precursors per 10^5 nucleated cells (Nakano *et al.*, 1987), and in the blood of fetal (day 15.5) mice these precursors are about 1/40 of the CD45+ leukocyte fraction (Rodewald *et al.*, 1996). The number of circulating mast cell precursors increases in diseases such as asthma (Mwamtemi *et al.*, 2001) and in infections (Sorden and Castleman, 1995). Although mast cells cannot be morphologically identified in the circulation normally (Nakano *et al.*, 1987), mast cell progenitors in peripheral blood are CD34+ mononuclear cells that differ from monocytes by their surface expression of kit (CD117) (Agis *et al.*, 1993; Rodewald *et al.*, 1996). CD117-negative mast cell precursors have also been reported to be present in peripheral blood (Welker *et al.*, 2000b). In mice, mast cell progenitors in blood are Thy-1^{lo}, CD117^{hi} and contain cytoplasmic granules and mRNA encoding mast cell–associated proteinases (Rodewald *et al.*, 1996). In humans, circulating mast cell progenitors are CD117+, CD34+, ly⁻, CD14⁻, CD17⁻ colony-forming cells (Agis *et al.*, 1993).

In tissues mast cells mature under the influence of microenvironmental factors. Mature mast cells express high levels of FcεRI (10^5 to 10^6 receptors per cell [Conrad *et al.*, 1975]) and CD117 on their surface. FcεRI has high affinity for IgE (10^9 to 10^{12} mol/l) and a low dissociation rate (Rossi *et al.*, 1977), resulting in retention of monomeric IgE on mast cells for long periods. Exposure to IgE upregulates surface expression of FcεRI on mast cells (Yamaguchi *et al.*, 1997), and there is a strong correlation between IgE levels and expression of FcεR1 on mast cells and basophils

(Kawakami and Galli, 2002). FcεRI-mediated activation contributes to many biological activities of mast cells. In addition, the stem cell factor (SCF) receptor CD117 has a leading role in mast cell maturation. Although other cell types also express CD117 or Fcε RI, these two receptors are used as markers of mature mast cells. Mature mouse mast cells express CD34 (Drew et al., 2002), but CD34 is undetectable on mature human mast cells (Agis et al., 1996).

Mast cell localization in mucosal and other tissues
The mechanisms by which mast cell progenitors localize in tissues are not well understood. Adhesion molecules on mast cell precursors and chemoattractants in the microenvironments are key factors influencing mast cell migration.

Mast cell chemoattractants
Several cytokines, chemokines, and growth factors are chemoattractants for mast cells **(Table 36.1)**. Both CC and CXC chemokines are chemoattractants for murine mast cells, including CCL2 (MCP-1), CCL3 (MIP-1α), CCL5 (RANTES), CCL11 (eotaxin), and CXCL4 (platelet factor-4) (Taub et al., 1995). CX3CL1 (fractalkine) also induces mouse mast cell migration but not degranulation (Papadopoulos et al., 2000). Some angiogenic factors such as platelet-derived growth factor-AB (PDGF-AB), vascular

Table 36.1. Mast Cell Chemoattractants and Their Receptors

Mast Cell Chemoattractants	Receptor(s)	Mast Cell (MC) Type	References
CC Chemokines			
CCL2 (MCP-1/MCAF)	CCR2	Mouse BMMC	(Taub et al., 1995)
CCL3 (MIP-1α/LD78α)	CCR1, CCR5	Mouse BMMC	(Taub et al., 1995)
CCL5 (RANTES)	CCR1, CCR3, CCR5	Human CBMC and mouse BMMC	(Juremalm et al., 2002; Taub et al., 1995)
CCL11 (eotaxin)	CCR3	Rat RBL 2H3 cell line	(Woo et al., 2002)
CXC chemokines			
CXCL1 (GROα)	CXCR2, CXCR1	HMC-1, CBMC	(Nilsson et al., 1999)
CXCL4 (platelet factor-4)	unknown	Human CBMC, HMC-1 and mouse BMMC	(Nilsson et al., 1999; Taub et al., 1995)
CXCL8 (IL-8)	CXCR1, CXCR3	Human CBMC	(Inamura et al., 2002; Nilsson et al., 1999)
CXCL12 (SDF-1)	CXCR4	Human CBMC, HMC-1	(Lin et al., 2000)
CX₃C chemokine			
CX₃CL1 (fractalkine)	CX3CR1	Mouse BMMC	(Papadopoulos et al., 2000)
Growth factors			
Nerve growth factor (NGF)	NGFR	Rat peritoneal MC	(Sawada et al., 2000)
Stem cell factor (SCF)	SCFR (kit)	Mouse peritoneal MC, BMMC, and HMC-1	(Meininger et al., 1992; Nilsson et al., 1994)
IL-3	IL-3R	Mouse peritoneal MC	(Matsuura and Zetter, 1989)
TGF-β	TGFR	Mouse BMMC, rat peritoneal MC, human CBMC and HMC-1	(Gruber et al., 1994) (Olsson et al., 2000a)
Other chemoattractants			
C3a	CD11b	Human CBMC and HMC-1	(Hartmann et al., 1997; Nilsson et al., 1996)
C5a	CD88	Human CBMC and HMC-1	(Hartmann et al., 1997; Nilsson et al., 1996)
Platelet-activating factor (PAF)	PAF-R	HMC-1	(Nilsson et al., 2000)
β-Defensin-2	CCR6	Rat peritoneal mast cell	(Niyonsaba et al., 2002a)
Cathelicidin-derived peptide LL-37	Unknown	Rat peritoneal mast cell	(Niyonsaba et al., 2002b)

endothelial cell growth factor (VEGF), and basic fibroblast growth factor (bFGF) cause directed migration of murine mast cells at picomolar concentrations (Gruber *et al.*, 1995). Nerve growth factor (NGF) (Sawada *et al.*, 2000), SCF (Meininger *et al.*, 1992), transforming growth factor-β (TGF-β) (Gruber *et al.*, 1994), and IL-3 (Matsuura and Zetter, 1989) exert chemotactic effects on rodent mast cells (Taub *et al.*, 1995). In addition, β-defensin-2 (Niyonsaba *et al.*, 2002a) and a cathelicidin family member of human antibacterial peptides, LL-37 (Niyonsaba *et al.*, 2002b), are mast cell chemoattractants. However, many of these factors, including CCL2, -3, -4, -7, and -8, IL-3, TGF-β, and NGF, have been reported to be ineffective on human mast cells (Nilsson *et al.*, 1994; Hartmann *et al.*, 1997). A recent study demonstrated that after sensitization with antigen-specific IgE, mouse mast cells migrate toward antigen (Ishizuka *et al.*, 2001), suggesting that Fcε RI functions not only in activation but also in mast cell migration.

In humans, a limited number of factors have been reported as chemoattractants for mast cells. These include CXCL8 (Inamura *et al.*, 2002), SCF (Nilsson *et al.*, 1994), complement components C3a and C5a (Hartmann *et al.*, 1997; Olsson *et al.*, 2000b), TGF-β (Olsson *et al.*, 2000a; Olsson *et al.*, 2000b), and stromal cell–derived factor-1α (SDF-1α, CXCL12) (Lin *et al.*, 2000). Most of the studies to test mast cell migration investigated extracellular matrix proteins such as laminin, fibronectin, vitronectin, or collagens. Unlike other leukocytes, the mechanism of mast cell migration across endothelium is less well understood. CXCL12 is the only factor reported to induce mast cell transmigration across endothelial monolayers (Lin *et al.*, 2000).

Expression of adhesion molecules on mast cells

Mast cells and their precursors express various adhesion molecules that are essential for the migration and localization of mast cells and their precursors in tissues. The β1 integrins α4β1 and α5β1 are expressed on mast cells from uterus (Guo *et al.*, 1992), lung (Sperr *et al.*, 1992), and skin (Columbo *et al.*, 1995). The human mast cell line HMC-1 expresses a different pattern of β1 integrins, including α2β1, α3β1, α6β1, and αVβ1 (Kruger-Krasagakes *et al.*, 1996). In human cord blood–derived mast cells (CBMCs) (Tachimoto *et al.*, 2001; Boyce *et al.*, 2002;) and human intestinal mucosal mast cells (Lorentz *et al.*, 2002), a number of β1 integrins are found, including α2β1, α3β1, α4β1, α5β1, and αVβ1. Human CBMCs also express several β2 integrins such as αMβ2 and αXβ2, as well as β3 integrin αVβ3 (Tachimoto *et al.*, 2001). ICAM-1, -2, and -3, VCAM-1, and selectins have also been found on mast cells (*e.g.*, Boyce *et al.*, 2002). Adhesion of human intestinal mucosal mast cells is preferentially mediated by β1 integrins (Lorentz *et al.*, 2002). Since the expression of adhesion molecules on mature mast cells differs from that on mast cell progenitors (Saeland *et al.*, 1992; Dercksen *et al.*, 1995), it is likely that expression of adhesion molecules is regulated during mast cell differentiation and maturation.

In mice, integrin α4β7 has an important role in tissue-specific homing of mast cells to the small intestine but not to other tissues such as lung (Gurish *et al.*, 2001). This integrin is also involved in parasite-induced intestinal mast cell hyperplasia (Issekutz *et al.*, 2001). Homing of mast cells to the peritoneum and skin involves αMβ2 (Rosenkranz *et al.*, 1998).

Expression of adhesion molecules and adhesion of mast cells to the extracellular matrix (ECM) are regulated by SCF, TGF-β, IL-4, IFN-γ, and nitric oxide (NO) (Wills *et al.*, 1999; Lorentz *et al.*, 2002; Rosbottom *et al.*, 2002). It is interesting that a cysteine protease, calpain, is involved in NO-mediated inhibition of mast cell adhesion, suggesting that calpain is involved in integrin clustering in mast cells (Forsythe and Befus, 2003). The change of adhesion molecule expression at different phases of mast cell development may facilitate emigration from the bone marrow into the circulation and contribute to tissue localization (Tachimoto *et al.*, 2001).

Mast cell growth factors

Growth factors are crucial for mast cell survival and development. The CD117 molecule (c-kit) is the receptor for SCF and is expressed on mast cells throughout their development. SCF plays a key role in mast cell development, especially in humans. SCF-dependent maturation of human mast cells can also be influenced by cofactors such as thrombopoietin (Sawai *et al.*, 1999), NGF (Welker *et al.*, 2000a), IL-6, and PGE$_2$ (Saito *et al.*, 1996). By contrast, mouse bone marrow cells can develop into relatively mature mast cells in the presence of IL-3 alone (Gurish *et al.*, 1992; Rottem *et al.*, 1992). Other cofactors involved in mouse mast cell development include SCF, IL-4, IL-9, IL-10, and eotaxin (Lantz and Huff, 1995; Rennick *et al.*, 1995; Quackenbush *et al.*, 1998).

Control of mast cell numbers in tissues

The number of mature mast cells increases in local tissues in various diseases such as asthma, rhinitis, rheumatoid arthritis, and cancer. The following mechanisms are involved in controlling mast cell numbers.

Migration of mature mast cells

Mature mast cells are generally considered to be relatively immobile. However, the rapid increase of mature mast cells (within hours) in the airway after antigen challenge suggests that mature mast cells may be mobile *in vivo* (Turner *et al.*, 1988). Recruited mast cells could have originated from adjacent tissues or from different organs. Several interesting studies have demonstrated potential "long-distance" migration of mature mast cells. Administration of antigen to sensitized skin induced a decrease in local mast cell density by ~50%, concurrent with a fivefold increase in mast cell numbers in draining lymph node (Wang *et al.*, 1998). Others have also demonstrated that when mature mast cells from the peritoneum are injected intravenously they cross the blood–brain barrier into brain tissues (Silverman *et al.*, 2000). In helminth-infected mice, senescent mast cells traffic from the jejunum to the spleen (Friend *et al.*, 2000). Thus, mature mast cells migrate from organ to organ *in vivo*, leading to a rapid increase of mast cell numbers in local tissues in response to physiological or pathological stimuli.

Recruitment of mast cell progenitors into tissues; subsequent proliferation and maturation

In animals (Sorden and Castleman, 1995) and a variety of human disorders, especially asthma (Mwamtemi et al., 2001), allergy (Otsuka et al., 1986), and drug reactions (Li et al., 1998), increased numbers of mast cells in local tissue are associated with increased progenitors in blood. It is likely that an allergen- or pathogen-induced increase in mast cell progenitors in the circulation is also associated with their enhanced transendothelial migration (Boyce et al., 2002). Chemokines, cytokines, or growth factors produced in local tissue not only will serve as chemoattractants for mast cells and their progenitors but also will stimulate adhesion molecule expression on endothelium, which enhances recruitment of mast cell precursors into local tissues. In dove brain it has been shown that immature mast cells infiltrate the central nervous system and undergo *in situ* differentiation within the neuropil (Zhuang et al., 1999). Thus, the recruitment of mast cell precursors and their subsequent local differentiation, proliferation, and maturation represent some of the mechanisms of mast cell increases in tissues.

MAST CELL APOPTOSIS

Apoptosis is an important homeostatic mechanism that regulates mast cell numbers and functions. Normally, mast cells are considered long-lived (up to months) and maintain relatively constant numbers in tissues. However, this can be altered. The bcl-2 family of proteins is a major class of intracellular regulators that include death agonists (bax, bak, bcl-X_s, bad, bid, and bik) and antagonists (bcl-2, bcl-X_L, bcl-w, mcl-1, and A1/bfl1) (Raff, 1998). Human and rodent mast cells express members of the bcl-2 family. Through a balance between death agonists and antagonists, cytokines and growth factors modulate mast cell survival or death. For example, in cultured human mast cells, SCF induces expression of bcl-2 and bcl-X_L and maintains mast cell survival (Mekori et al., 2001). In HMC-1 cells that are SCF-independent, death antagonists bcl-2 and bcl-X_L are expressed at high levels (Mekori et al., 2001). Similarly in rodents, SCF, NGF, IL-3, or IL-15 increases bcl-2 or bcl-X_L expression and promotes mast cell survival (Bullock and Johnson, 1996; Masuda et al., 2001). In contrast, a decrease in bcl-2 or bcl-X_L by Th2 cytokines IL-4 and IL-10 (Yeatman et al., 2000) or induction of death agonists such as bad (Yang et al., 2000) induces mast cell apoptosis. Bcl-2 proteins likely function at a critical point immediately upstream of an irreversible commitment to death in mast cells.

Two interesting recent studies demonstrated that binding of monomeric IgE to FcεRI enhances resistance of mast cells to growth factor depletion–induced apoptosis (Asai et al., 2001; Kalesnikoff et al., 2001). The survival-enhancing effect of IgE requires an interaction between IgE and FcεRI but not FcεRI cross-linking. This effect of IgE parallels its ability to enhance surface expression of FcεRI (Asai et al., 2001). Since the concentration of IgE that promotes mast cell survival (0.1–1.0 µg/ml) is present in mouse and human sera, IgE may be one of the factors that increases mast cell numbers in allergy or parasitic infections.

Upon activation by FcεRI cross-linking, mast cells withstand the exhaustive degranulation process and recover regranulation and can degranulate upon subsequent stimuli. One bcl-2 family member, the death antagonist A1, is essential for mast cell survival in this process (Xiang et al., 2001). Thus, bcl-2 family members may be potential targets for the treatment of allergic diseases. Indeed, chimeric proteins containing the Fc portion of IgE and a death agonist bcl-2 member bak or bax (Fcε-bak/bax) have been used to selectively eliminate FcεRI-bearing mast cells and basophils (Belostotsky and Lorberboum-Galski, 2001).

MAST CELL HETEROGENEITY

Human and rodent mast cells from different tissues vary in phenotype and function. Rodent mast cells are broadly divided into connective tissue–type mast cells (CTMCs) or mucosal-type mast cells (MMCs), based upon their location and characteristics. Human mast cells are divided into MC^T (containing tryptase only), MC^{TC} (containing both tryptase and chymase), or MC^C (containing chymase only) subpopulations. These different mast cells are most likely derived from a common precursor and individually tailored by their microenvironment to acquire selected phenotypes (Befus et al., 1988). Genetic background may also contribute to mast cell heterogeneity, as demonstrated in inbred strains of mice (Stevens et al., 1994).

The heterogeneity of mast cells involves differences in morphology, histochemical characteristics, mediator content, responsiveness to growth factors, and sensitivity to drugs and secretagogues. Histochemical heterogeneity was initially noted in rat tissues (Enerback, 1966) and relates to differences in expression of proteoglycans. CTMCs express heparin as the predominant proteoglycan, and MMCs mainly express chondroitin sulfates.

Many different proteinases in human, mouse, rat, dog, sheep, and cow mast cells (Miller and Pemberton, 2002) have been described. Like in humans, rodent mast cells from different tissues also express different proteinases. For example, mouse mast cell proteinase 1 (mMCP-1) is expressed by MMCs but not by CTMCs. In rat, MMCs express rat (r)MCP-2 but not rMCP-1, while CTMCs contain rMCP-1 but not rMCP-2. Given that some proteinases such as mMCP-1, rMCP-2, and human tryptase are soluble, they can be detected in the blood when released from mast cell granules. Levels of rMCP-2 and mMCP-1 in the blood of parasite-infected rats or mice can reach 5–10 µg/ml and have been used as an effective means of determining MMC activation *in vivo*.

Mast cells are also heterogeneous in their mediator content and responsiveness to secretagogues and antiallergic drugs, a subject extensively reviewed elsewhere (*e.g.*, Befus *et al.*, 1988). For example, MMCs metabolize arachidonic acid (AA) by both cyclo-oxygenase (COX) and lipoxygenase pathways to produce prostaglandin D_2 (PGD_2, 4.7 ng/10^6 cells) and leukotrienes (LTs) B_4 (12 ng/10^6 cells) and C_4 (29 ng/10^6 cells) (Heavey *et al.*, 1988), whereas CTMCs employ only the COX pathway to produce PGD_2 (50–260 ng/10^6 cells) (Murakami *et al.*, 1997). Thus, MMCs and CTMCs secrete a different profile of lipid mediators upon activation. Mast cell heterogeneity has been extended to cytokine and chemokine content. In human bronchial biopsies, MC^T express IL-4, IL-5, IL-6, and TNF, whereas MC^{TC} in the same tissue express only IL-4 (Bradding *et al.*, 1995). This difference likely contributes to the functional heterogeneity of mast cells.

MAST CELL ACTIVATION AND FUNCTIONAL REGULATION

Mast cell activation

Mast cells can be activated by the ligation of surface receptors such as FcεRI, CD117, and many others or by activation of specific intracellular signaling molecules such as calcium ionophore (calcium mobilization), compound 48/80 (activation of G proteins), or phorbol esters (activation of protein kinase C) (Stassen *et al.*, 2002). We will focus on FcεRI because it plays an essential role in allergic responses (**Fig. 36.1**).

FcεRI-mediated mast cell activation contributes to many mast cell–mediated responses and is central to the induction and maintenance of allergic reactions (Turner and Kinet, 1999). Allergen-specific IgE binds to high-affinity FcεRI and gives long-lasting sensitization of mast cells. Cross-linking of FcεRI by allergen binding to IgE initiates mast cell degranulation, production of eicosanoids and cytokines, and changes in gene expression and activity.

FcεRI is expressed on mast cells as a heterotetramer consisting of a single IgE-binding α-subunit, a β-subunit, and two disulfide-linked γ-subunits. The β- and γ-subunits each contain a conserved immunoreceptor tyrosine-based activation motif (ITAM) in their cytoplasmic tails and are rapidly phosphorylated on tyrosine after FcεRI cross-linking (Beaven and Baumgartner, 1996; Turner and Kinet, 1999). Tyrosine phosphorylation of the ITAMs in β and γ subunits is mediated by the src kinase Lyn in concert with cross-talk with another src, Fyn (Parravicini *et al.*, 2002). FcεRI cross-linking activates Syk through these src kinases. Lyn-deficient mast cells exhibit no β- or γ-subunit phosphorylation (Nishizumi and Yamamoto, 1997) but exhibit enhanced Fyn-dependent signals (Parravicini *et al.*, 2002). Syk-deficient mast cells fail to degranulate, synthesize leukotrienes, and secrete cytokines after FcεRI stimulation (Costello *et al.*, 1996), although they appear to respond normally to adenosine-mediated (G-protein-coupled) activation (Mocsai *et al.*, 2003). Aerosolized antisense to Syk inhibits allergic inflammation in the airways (Stenton *et al.*, 2002).

Activation of Lyn and Syk drives several intracellular signaling cascades, including phospholipase Cγ1 pathway—which leads to calcium mobilization by inositol (1,4,5)P_3 and PKC activation by diacylglycerol—and Ras/Raf-1/MEK/Erk pathway, as well as PI-3 kinase and Bruton's tyrosine kinase–related pathways. For details of FcεRI-mediated signaling mechanisms, see several excellent reviews (Beaven and Baumgartner, 1996; Turner and Kinet, 1999; Nadler *et al.*, 2000; Rivera, 2002).

Mast cell mediators and mediator secretion

Numerous presynthesized mediators are stored in mast cell granules, and upon activation mast cells secrete mediators by degranulation. Anaphylactic degranulation occurs in seconds to minutes and can be extensive, whereas piecemeal degranulation is less obvious morphologically and may occur over

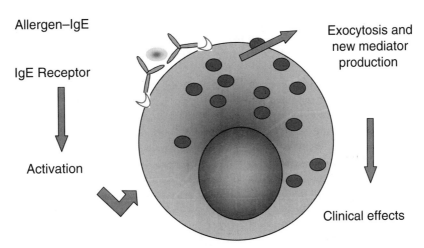

Fig. 36.1. Mast cells are major effector cells of allergic reactions mediated by allergen-induced cross-linking of high-affinity IgE receptors. This IgE-dependent activation induces release of stored mediators and the synthesis and secretion of other mediators that collectively produce the spectrum of clinical effects seen in allergies.

several days. When mast cells undergo anaphylactic degranulation, the granules appear to swell and fuse to form interconnecting channels that ultimately fuse with the plasma membrane to allow release of the contents (Dvorak, 1988). After degranulation, mast cells are able to recover and to degranulate again.

By contrast, in piecemeal degranulation, granule membranes do not fuse with each other or with the plasma membrane. Instead, it is postulated that vesicles containing granule contents bud off the granules and are transported to the cell surface. These exocytotic vesicles fuse with the plasma membrane and discharge their contents to the extracellular space (Dvorak, 1988). Piecemeal degranulation has been noted in Crohn's disease (Dvorak et al., 1980) and bullous pemphigoid (Dvorak et al., 1982) and is likely associated with secretion of selected mediators.

Granule-associated preformed mediators

Degranulation releases various granule-associated mediators. One well-known mediator is histamine, which can induce various reactions due to the widespread expression of H_1, H_2, H_3, and H_4 receptors (Repka-Ramirez, 2003). Histamine antagonists remain a major strategical component in the treatment of allergic reactions (e.g., rhinitis) in several target organs. Two proteoglycans, heparin (3–8 pg/cell) and chondroitin sulfates, are found in human mast cells. Proteoglycans function as storage matrices for other preformed mediators and they bind histamine, neutral proteinases, and acid hydrolases at acidic pH inside mast cell granules. Mast cells are the major source of heparin in the body (Zehnder and Galli, 1999). Two recent studies showed that mast cells in mice that are unable to synthesize sulphated heparin also lack metachromatic granules and have reduced amounts of histamine and mast-cell proteases (Forsberg et al., 1999; Humphries et al., 1999). When mast cells are activated, proteoglycans are secreted along with other granule mediators and are critical for the preservation of tryptase activity (e.g., Lindstedt et al., 1998).

Neutral proteases are the dominant protein components of secretory granules in mast cells, representing at least 20% to 50% of total cellular proteins (Schwartz and Huff, 1993). Over 50 mast cell–derived proteases have been identified in 11 species (Bairoch and Apweiler, 2000; Miller and Pemberton, 2002). These include tryptases, chymases, cathepsin G, and carboxypeptidase. In humans, several tetrameric tryptases with different specificities have been identified in mast cells, but only one chymase has been characterized (Miller and Pemberton, 2002). In other species, a larger family of chymases has been identified (e.g., Huang et al., 1998). Many of these proteases are specifically expressed in mast cells or in mast cell subpopulations, such as mMCP-1 (uniquely expressed in mouse MMC [Scudamore et al., 1997]) or rMCP 8 to 10 (expressed in rat MMC [Lutzelschwab et al., 1998]). Thus, these proteases serve as selective markers that distinguish mast cells from other cell types, including basophils, and different mast cell subpopulations from one another (Miller and Pemberton,

2002). Mast cell proteases have various natural substrates such as fibrinogen, fibronectin, substance P, proteinase-activated receptor-2, and many others (e.g., Huang et al., 2001), and thus they likely have diverse biological activities. Tryptase and chymase contribute to vascular permeability, tissue remodeling, and allergic reactivity during inflammation (Miller and Pemberton, 2002). The inhibition of inflammatory responses to allergen by pretreatment of animals with tryptase inhibitors suggests an important role of this protease in allergic inflammation (Clark et al., 1995; Oh et al., 2002).

Newly synthesized mediators

Upon activation, mast cells also secrete a range of *de novo* synthesized mediators such as lipid metabolites (leukotriene-C_4, -D_4, PGE_2, etc.), NO, and various cytokines and chemokines. Using techniques that define gene expression, investigators have reported on thousands of genes in human, mouse, and rat mast cells (Chen et al., 1998; Kuramasu et al., 2001; Nakajima et al., 2002). Many of them are specifically induced by FcεRI activation. However, because of the abundant sources of many of these mediators *in vivo*, the biological role of specific mast cell–derived mediators requires further study. Mast cell–derived TNF, leukotriene C_4, and proteinases have been implicated in neutrophil recruitment in IgE- and bacteria-induced inflammation *in vivo* (Echtenacher et al., 1996; Wershil et al., 1996; Malaviya and Abraham, 2000; Huang et al., 2001).

Mast cell inhibitory receptors

Mast cells express several surface receptors that inhibit activation (Ott and Cambier, 2000; Katz, 2002). Many of these receptors share a cytoplasmic consensus sequence, namely, the immunoreceptor tyrosine–based inhibitory motif (ITIM, $YxxLx_{6-8}YxxL$), that recruits and activates distinct SH2 domain–containing protein-tyrosine phosphatase (SHP)-1 and/or SHP-2 or SH2 domain–containing inositol polyphosphate 5′-phosphatase (SHIP)1 and/or SHIP2. Inhibitory receptors include FcγRIIB; gp49B1; paired Ig-like receptor (PIR)-B; signal regulatory protein (SIRP); mast cell function–associated antigen (MAFA); CD81; sialic acid–binding, Ig-like lectins (Siglec); and platelet endothelial cell adhesion molecule-1 (PECAM-1, CD31). *In vitro*, activation of these receptors by their natural ligands or specific antibodies inhibits mast cell activation. Animals deficient in some of these receptors have been generated, including FcγRIIB (Takai et al., 1996), gp49B1 (Daheshia et al., 2001), PIR-B (Ujike et al., 2002), and PECAM-1 (Wong et al., 2002). As anticipated, increased allergic susceptibility and severity are observed in these animals. Thus, these inhibitory receptors may be important therapeutic targets for mast cell–mediated allergic responses.

MAST CELLS AND HOST DEFENSE

Host defense against microbial pathogens involves innate and acquired immune responses. Innate immunity is not specific to the invading pathogen and does not generate immunologic memory (Medzhitov and Janeway, 2000). Toll-like receptors (TLRs) are a part of this innate immune defense as pattern recognition receptors (PRRs) that recognize common microbial structures (Takeuchi *et al.*, 1999; Medzhitov and Janeway, 2000; Krutzik *et al.*, 2001). By contrast, the acquired immune response is characterized by clonal selection of antigen-specific lymphocytes, which can give rise to long-lasting protection against pathogens. Increasing evidence suggests that mast cells and their mediators have major roles in both innate and acquired immunity **(Fig. 36.2)**.

Mast cells in innate immunity
Mast cells respond to many bacteria and their products
A critical role of mast cells in innate immunity against bacterial infection has been elegantly demonstrated in several studies using mast cell–deficient mice (W/W^v mice). In comparison with W/W^v mice reconstituted with normal mast cells, W/W^v mice had greater mortality rates associated with peritonitis and *Klebsiella pneumoniae* lung infection (Echtenacher *et al.*, 1996; Malaviya *et al.*, 1996a; Prodeus *et al.*, 1997). During bacterial infection, mast cells produce mediators including TNF, tryptase, and leukotrienes to recruit neutrophils to mount antibacterial host defenses (Echtenacher *et al.*, 1996; Malaviya *et al.*, 1996a; Malaviya and Abraham, 2000; Huang *et al.*, 2001). It is interesting that mast cell–dependent neutrophil infiltration has also been demonstrated in many other animal models of inflammation, such as immune complex–induced peritonitis (Zhang *et al.*, 1992), IgE-dependent gastric responses (Wershil *et al.*,

1996), skin reactions (Wershil *et al.*, 1991), implanted biomaterial–induced joint inflammation (Tang *et al.*, 1998), and experimental bullous pemphigoid (Chen *et al.*, 2002). Furthermore, survival of mice with acute bacterial peritonitis can be greatly enhanced by treatment with SCF, in part because of its effects on mast cell numbers and function (Maurer *et al.*, 1998).

In vitro studies show that human and rodent mast cells respond in various ways to many bacteria and their products, including secreted toxins, bacterial wall components, and nuclear DNA (*e.g.*, Leal-Berumen *et al.*, 1996; Abraham and Malaviya, 1997; Arock *et al.*, 1998; Zhu and Marshall, 2001; Supajatura *et al.*, 2002a, b). However, little is known about the components on mast cells that recognize bacterial pathogens or their products. Complement activation (Prodeus *et al.*, 1997), CD48 (Malaviya *et al.*, 1999), and caveoli (Shin *et al.*, 2000) have been implicated, and recent studies suggest that TLRs on mast cells play an important role **(Table 36.2)**.

Mast cells express multiple TLRs
The first human TLR (TLR1) was identified in 1996 (Taguchi *et al.*, 1996), and to date, 10 different TLRs have been identified (TLR1–10) (Lien and Ingalls, 2002). TLRs recognize pathogen-associated molecular patterns (PAMPs). Different TLRs play distinct roles in the activation of the immune and inflammatory responses to different microbial components. Several TLRs have been identified in mast cells (Table 36.2), including TLR1, TLR2, TLR4, TLR6, and TLR8 (McCurdy *et al.*, 2001; Supajatura *et al.*, 2001; Applequist *et al.*, 2002; Supajatura *et al.*, 2002a). In addition,

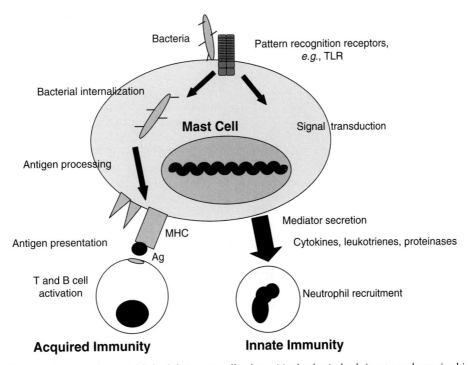

Fig. 36.2. Recent advances have established that mast cells play critical roles in both innate and acquired immunity.

Table 36.2 Toll-Like Receptors Expressed on Mast Cells and Their Microbial Ligands[a]

TLR	Mast Cell Expression	Selected Ligand(s)[b]
TLR1	Human CBMC, mouse mast cells	Lipopeptide (Pam3Cys)
TLR2	Human CBMC, mouse mast cells	Peptidoglycans, zymosan
TLR3	Undetectable (mouse mast cells)	Double-stranded RNA
TLR4	Human CBMC, mouse mast cells	Lipopolysaccharide, lipoteichoic acid, RSV F protein
TLR5	Undetectable (mouse mast cells)	Flagellin
TLR6	Human CBMC, mouse mast cells	Peptidoglycan, zymosan
TLR7	Undetectable (mouse mast cells)	Imidazoquinoline compounds
TLR8	Mouse mast cells	Unknown ligands
TLR9	Undetectable (mouse mast cells)	Bacterial DNA, CpG DNA
TLR10	Not studied	Unknown ligands

[a]For references, see McCurdy et al., 2001; Applequist et al., 2002; Supajatura et al., 2001, 2002a.
[b]For details, see review by Lien and Ingalls, 2002.

a TLR accessory protein, MD2, and a TLR signaling adaptor protein, MyD88, have also been found in mast cells (McCurdy et al., 2001; Applequist et al., 2002). However, mRNA for TLR3, TLR5, TLR7, and TLR9 was undetectable in murine mast cells (McCurdy et al., 2001; Supajatura et al., 2001; Applequist et al., 2002). In some cases, ligands for specific TLRs have been identified (Table 36.2; see Lien and Ingalls, 2002), and this assists in speculation about potential functions of TLRs in mast cell biology. However, several important issues regarding mast cell TLRs remain to be clarified: evidence of TLR expression in mast cells is limited to the mRNA level or to the ligand involved, but little is known about the proteins; there is no information about regulation of expression of TLRs on mast cells; although mast cells are heterogeneous, it is not clear whether different mast cell populations express distinct or similar TLR patterns; there is little information about TLR signaling in mast cells; and the clinical relevance of mast cell TLRs in humans has not been explored.

Regulation of mast cell function by TLRs
Using specific TLR ligands, investigators have studied the roles of TLR2 and TLR4. Activation of TLR2 on mouse bone marrow–derived mast cells by peptidoglycan from *Staphylococcus aureus* induced TNF, IL-4, IL-5, IL-6, and IL-13 but not IL-1β (McCurdy et al., 2001; Supajatura et al., 2002). In contrast, activation of mast cell TLR4 by lipopolysaccharide from *Escherichia coli* induced TNF, IL-1β, IL-6, and IL-13 but not IL-4 or IL-5 (McCurdy et al., 2001; Supajatura et al., 2001; 2002a). Moreover, mast cell degranulation and calcium mobilization were induced by TLR2-dependent but not by TLR4-dependent activation (Supajatura et al., 2002a). These data suggest that TLR2 and TLR4 have different roles in mast cell function. As demonstrated *in vivo*, mast cell TLR4 but not mast cell TLR2 is required for the full expression of innate immunity in a mast

cell–dependent sepsis model (Supajatura et al., 2002a), whereas TLR2-mediated activation of skin mast cells causes acute and late reactions following peptidoglycan application (Supajatura et al., 2002a).

TLR and FcεRI interaction in mast cells
Activation of mast cell TLR4 also synergistically enhanced IgE-dependent production of Th2-associated cytokines such as IL-5, IL-10, and IL-13 (Masuda et al., 2002). These findings may represent one of the mechanisms of how certain microbial infections can worsen asthma.

Mast cells in acquired immunity
There is growing evidence that mast cells can initiate acquired immunity against bacterial infection (Galli et al., 1999; Henz et al., 2001). Mast cells can phagocytose gram-positive and gram-negative bacteria (Sher et al., 1979; Malaviya et al., 1994; Lin et al., 2002) and process bacterial antigens (Malaviya et al., 1996b). Expression of receptor molecules on mast cells such as MHC-I, MHC-II, CD40L, ICAM-1 and ICAM-3, CD43, CD80, and CD86 allows them to interact with T and B lymphocytes (Gauchat et al., 1993; Agis et al., 1996; Raposo et al., 1997; Mekori and Metcalfe, 1999) and to present bacterial antigen to these cells (Malaviya et al., 1996b). MHC-I molecules mainly bind peptides derived from cytosolic antigens, for example, antigens derived from bacteria that escape from the phagosome to the cytosol (Harding et al., 2003). Antigens from a number of enterobacteria such as *Salmonella typhimurium* and *E. coli* are processed by mouse mast cells for MHC-I presentation to T cells (Malaviya et al., 1996b).

MHC-II molecules present antigens derived from phagocytic organelles (endosome/lysosome) (Harding et al., 2003). Both rodent and human mast cells can present antigen through MHC-II pathway (Frandji et al., 1993; Poncet et al., 1999). Thus, mast cells have antigen-processing and antigen-presentation functions using MHC-I and –II pathways. This evidence reinforces the concept that mast cells act as sentinels in host defense and not only initiate innate immunity but also are important players in acquired immunity by presenting bacterial antigens to lymphocytes to combat infection (Fig. 36.2).

REFERENCES

Abraham, S. N., and Malaviya, R. (1997). Mast cells in infection and immunity. *Infect. Immun.* 65, 3501–3508.

Agis, H., Willheim, M., Sperr, W. R., Wilfing, A., Kromer, E., Kabrna, E., Spanblochl, E., Strobl, H., Geissler, K., Spittler, A., Boltz-Nitulescu, G., Majdic, O., Lechner, K., and Valent, P. (1993). Monocytes do not make mast cells when cultured in the presence of SCF. Characterization of the circulating mast cell progenitor as a c-kit+, CD34+, Ly−, CD14−, CD17−, colony-forming cell. *J. Immunol.* 151, 4221–4227.

Agis, H., Fureder, W., Bankl, H. C., Kundi, M., Sperr, W. R., Willheim, M., Boltz-Nitulescu, G., Butterfield, J. H., Kishi, K., Lechner, K., and Valent, P. (1996). Comparative immunophenotypic analysis of human mast cells, blood basophils and monocytes. *Immunology* 87, 535–543.

Applequist, S. E., Wallin, R. P., and Ljunggren, H. G. (2002). Variable expression of Toll-like receptor in murine innate and adaptive immune cell lines. *Int. Immunol.* 14, 1065–1074.

Arock, M., Ross, E., Lai-Kuen, R., Averlant, G., Gao, Z., and Abraham, S. N. (1998). Phagocytic and tumor necrosis factor alpha response of human mast cells following exposure to gram-negative and gram-positive bacteria. *Infect. Immun.* 66, 6030–6034.

Asai, K., Kitaura, J., Kawakami, Y., Yamagata, N., Tsai, M., Carbone, D. P., Liu, F. T., Galli, S. J., and Kawakami, T. (2001). Regulation of mast cell survival by IgE. *Immunity* 14, 791–800.

Bairoch, A., and Apweiler, R. (2000). The SWISS-PROT protein sequence database and its supplement TrEMBL in 2000. *Nucleic Acids Res.* 28, 45–48.

Beaven, M. A., and Baumgartner, R. A. (1996). Downstream signals initiated in mast cells by Fc epsilon RI and other receptors. *Curr. Opin. Immunol.* 8, 766–772.

Befus, A. D. and Denburg, J. A. (2004). Basophilic leukocytes: Mast cells and basophils. In *Wintrobe's Clinical Hematology, 11th Edition* (eds. J. P. Greer, J. Foerster, J. Lukens, G. M. Rodgers, F. Paraskevas, and T. B. Glader). Baltimore: Williams & Wilkins. (pp. 335–348).

Befus, D., Fujimaki, H., Lee, T. D., and Swieter, M. (1988). Mast cell polymorphisms. Present concepts, future directions. *Dig. Dis. Sci.* 33, 16S–24S.

Belostotsky, R., and Lorberboum-Galski, H. (2001). Apoptosis-inducing human-origin Fc-epsilon-Bak chimeric proteins for targeted elimination of mast cells and basophils: a new approach for allergy treatment. *J. Immunol.* 167, 4719–4728.

Boyce, J. A. (2003). Mast cells: beyond IgE. *J. Allergy Clin. Immunol.* 111, 24–32.

Boyce, J. A., Mellor, E. A., Perkins, B., Lim, Y. C., and Luscinskas, F. W. (2002). Human mast cell progenitors use alpha4-integrin, VCAM-1, and PSGL-1 E-selectin for adhesive interactions with human vascular endothelium under flow conditions. *Blood* 99, 2890–2896.

Bradding, P., Okayama, Y., Howarth, P. H., Church, M. K., and Holgate, S. T. (1995). Heterogeneity of human mast cells based on cytokine content. *J. Immunol.* 155, 297–307.

Bullock, E. D., and Johnson, E. M., Jr. (1996). Nerve growth factor induces the expression of certain cytokine genes and bcl-2 in mast cells. Potential role in survival promotion. *J. Biol. Chem.* 271, 27500–27508.

Chen, H., Centola, M., Altschul, S. F., and Metzger, H. (1998). Characterization of gene expression in resting and activated mast cells. *J. Exp. Med.* 188, 1657–1668.

Chen, R., Fairley, J. A., Zhao, M. L., Giudice, G. J., Zillikens, D., Diaz, L. A., and Liu, Z. (2002). Macrophages, but not T and B lymphocytes, are critical for subepidermal blister formation in experimental bullous pemphigoid: macrophage-mediated neutrophil infiltration depends on mast cell activation. *J. Immunol.* 169, 3987–3992.

Clark, J. M., Abraham, W. M., Fishman, C. E., Forteza, R., Ahmed, A., Cortes, A., Warne, R. L., Moore, W. R., and Tanaka, R. D. (1995). Tryptase inhibitors block allergen-induced airway and inflammatory responses in allergic sheep. *Am. J. Respir. Crit. Care Med.* 152, 2076–2083.

Columbo, M., Bochner, B. S., and Marone, G. (1995). Human skin mast cells express functional beta 1 integrins that mediate adhesion to extracellular matrix proteins. *J. Immunol.* 154, 6058–6064.

Conrad, D. H., Bazin, H., Sehon, A. H., and Froese, A. (1975). Binding parameters of the interaction between rat IgE and rat mast cell receptors. *J. Immunol.* 114, 1688–1691.

Costello, P. S., Turner, M., Walters, A. E., Cunningham, C. N., Bauer, P. H., Downward, J., and Tybulewicz, V. L. (1996). Critical role for the tyrosine kinase Syk in signalling through the high affinity IgE receptor of mast cells. *Oncogene* 13, 2595–2605.

Daheshia, M., Friend, D. S., Grusby, M. J., Austen, K. F., and Katz, H. R. (2001). Increased severity of local and systemic anaphylactic reactions in gp49B1-deficient mice. *J. Exp. Med.* 194, 227–234.

Dercksen, M. W., Gerritsen, W. R., Rodenhuis, S., Dirkson, M. K., Slaper-Cortenbach, I. C., Schaasberg, W. P., Pinedo, H. M., von dem Borne, A. E., and van der Schoot, C. E. (1995). Expression of adhesion molecules on CD34+ cells: CD34+ L-selectin+ cells predict a rapid platelet recovery after peripheral blood stem cell transplantation. *Blood* 85, 3313–3319.

Drew, E., Merkens, H., Chelliah, S., Doyonnas, R., and McNagny, K. M. (2002). CD34 is a specific marker of mature murine mast cells. *Exp. Hematol.* 30, 1211–1218.

Dvorak, A. M. (1988). The fine structure of human basophils and mast cells. In *Mast Cells, Mediators and Disease* (ed. S. T. Holgate), 29–97. San Diego: Academic Publishers.

Echtenacher, B., Mannel, D. N., and Hultner, L. (1996). Critical protective role of mast cells in a model of acute septic peritonitis. *Nature* 381, 75–77.

Dvorak, A. M., Monahan, R. A., Osage, J. E., and Dickersin, G. R. (1980). Crohn's disease: transmission electron microscopic studies. II. Immunologic inflammatory response. Alterations of mast cells, basophils, eosinophils, and the microvasculature. *Hum. Pathol.* 11, 606–619.

Dvorak, A. M., Mihm, M. C., Jr., Osage, J. E., Kwan, T. H., Austen, K. F., and Wintroub, B. U. (1982). Bullous pemphigoid, an ultrastructural study of the inflammatory response: eosinophil, basophil and mast cell granule changes in multiple biopsies from one patient. *J. Invest. Dermatol.* 78, 91–101.

Enerback, L. (1966). Mast cells in rat gastrointestinal mucosa. 2. Dye-binding and metachromatic properties. *Acta Pathol. Microbiol. Scand.* 66, 303–312.

Féger, F., Varadaradjalou, S., Gao, Z., Abraham, S. N., and Arock, M. (2002). The role of mast cells in host defense and their subversion by bacterial pathogens. *TRENDS Immunol.* 23, 151–158.

Forsberg, E., Pejler, G., Ringvall, M., Lunderius, C., Tomasini-Johansson, B., Kusche-Gullberg, M., Eriksson, I., Ledin, J., Hellman, L., and Kjellen, L. (1999). Abnormal mast cells in mice deficient in a heparin-synthesizing enzyme. *Nature* 400, 773–776.

Forsythe, P., and Befus, A. D. (2003). Inhibition of calpain is a component of nitric oxide–induced down-regulation of human mast cell adhesion. *J. Immunol.* 170, 287–293.

Frandji, P., Oskeritzian, C., Cacaraci, F., Lapeyre, J., Peronet, R., David, B., Guillet, J. G., and Mecheri, S. (1993). Antigen-dependent stimulation by bone marrow–derived mast cells of MHC class II–restricted T cell hybridoma. *J. Immunol.* 151, 6318–6328.

Friend, D. S., Gurish, M. F., Austen, K. F., Hunt, J., and Stevens, R. L. (2000). Senescent jejunal mast cells and eosinophils in the mouse preferentially translocate to the spleen and draining lymph node, respectively, during the recovery phase of helminth infection. *J. Immunol.* 165, 344–352.

Galli, S. J., and Wershil, B. K. (1996). The two faces of the mast cell. *Nature 381*, 21–22.

Galli, S. J., Maurer, M., and Lantz, C. S. (1999). Mast cells as sentinels of innate immunity. *Curr. Opin. Immunol.* 11, 53–59.

Gauchat, J. F., Henchoz, S., Mazzei, G., Aubry, J. P., Brunner, T., Blasey, H., Life, P., Talabot, D., Flores-Romo, L., Thompson, J., Kishi, K., Butterfield, J., Dahinden, C., and Bonnefoy, J. Y. (1993). Induction of human IgE synthesis in B cells by mast cells and basophils. *Nature 365*, 340–343.

Gruber, B. L., Marchese, M. J., and Kew, R. R. (1994). Transforming growth factor-beta 1 mediates mast cell chemotaxis. *J. Immunol.* 152, 5860–5867.

Gruber, B. L., Marchese, M. J., and Kew, R. (1995). Angiogenic factors stimulate mast-cell migration. *Blood* 86, 2488–2493.

Guo, C. B., Kagey-Sobotka, A., Lichtenstein, L. M., and Bochner, B. S. (1992). Immunophenotyping and functional analysis of purified human uterine mast cells. *Blood* 79, 708–712.

Gurish, M. F., Ghildyal, N., McNeil, H. P., Austen, K. F., Gillis, S., and Stevens, R. L. (1992). Differential expression of secretory granule proteases in mouse mast cells exposed to interleukin 3 and c-kit ligand. *J. Exp. Med.* 175, 1003–1012.

Gurish, M. F., Tao, H., Abonia, J. P., Arya, A., Friend, D. S., Parker, C. M., and Austen, K. F. (2001). Intestinal mast cell progenitors require CD49dbeta7 (alpha4beta7 integrin) for tissue-specific homing. *J. Exp. Med.* 194, 1243–1252.

Harding, C. V., Ramachandra, L., and Wick, M. J. (2003). Interaction of bacteria with antigen presenting cells: influences on antigen presentation and antibacterial immunity. *Curr. Opin. Immunol.* 15, 112–119.

Hartmann, K., Henz, B. M., Kruger-Krasagakes, S., Kohl, J., Burger, R., Guhl, S., Haase, I., Lippert, U., and Zuberbier, T. (1997). C3a and C5a stimulate chemotaxis of human mast cells. *Blood* 89, 2863–2870.

Heavey, D. J., Ernst, P. B., Stevens, R. L., Befus, A. D., Bienenstock, J., and Austen, K. F. (1988). Generation of leukotriene C4, leukotriene B4, and prostaglandin D2 by immunologically activated rat intestinal mucosa mast cells. *J. Immunol.* 140, 1953–1957.

Henz, B. M., Maurer, M., Lippert, U., Worm, M., and Babina, M. (2001). Mast cells as initiators of immunity and host defense. *Exp. Dermatol.* 10, 1–10.

Huang, C., Sali, A., and Stevens, R. L. (1998). Regulation and function of mast cell proteases in inflammation. *J. Clin. Immunol.* 18, 169–183.

Huang, C., De Sanctis, G. T., O'Brien, P. J., Mizgerd, J. P., Friend, D. S., Drazen, J. M., Brass, L. F., and Stevens, R. L. (2001). Evaluation of the substrate specificity of human mast cell tryptase beta I and demonstration of its importance in bacterial infections of the lung. *J. Biol. Chem.* 276, 26276–26284.

Humphries, D. E., Wong, G. W., Friend, D. S., Gurish, M. F., Qiu, W. T., Huang, C., Sharpe, A. H., and Stevens, R. L. (1999). Heparin is essential for the storage of specific granule proteases in mast cells. *Nature 400*, 769–772.

Inamura, H., Kurosawa, M., Okano, A., Kayaba, H., and Majima, M. (2002). Expression of the interleukin-8 receptors CXCR1 and CXCR2 on cord-blood-derived cultured human mast cells. *Int. Arch. Allergy Immunol.* 128, 142–150.

Ishizuka, T., Okajima, F., Ishiwara, M., Iizuka, K., Ichimonji, I., Kawata, T., Tsukagoshi, H., Dobashi, K., Nakazawa, T., and Mori, M. (2001). Sensitized mast cells migrate toward the antigen: a response regulated by p38 mitogen–activated protein kinase and Rho-associated coiled-coil-forming protein kinase. *J. Immunol.* 167, 2298–2304.

Issekutz, T. B., Palecanda, A., Kadela-Stolarz, U., and Marshall, J. S. (2001). Blockade of either alpha-4 or beta-7 integrins selectively inhibits intestinal mast cell hyperplasia and worm expulsion in response to Nippostrongylus brasiliensis infection. *Eur. J. Immunol.* 31, 860–868.

Juremalm, M., Olsson, N., and Nilsson, G. (2002). Selective CCL5/RANTES-induced mast cell migration through interactions with chemokine receptors CCR1 and CCR4. *Biochem. Biophys. Res. Commun.* 297, 480–485.

Kalesnikoff, J., Huber, M., Lam, V., Damen, J. E., Zhang, J., Siraganian, R. P., and Krystal, G. (2001). Monomeric IgE stimulates signaling pathways in mast cells that lead to cytokine production and cell survival. *Immunity* 14, 801–811.

Katz, H. R. (2002). Inhibitory receptors and allergy. *Curr. Opin. Immunol.* 14, 698–704.

Kawakami, T., and Galli, S. J. (2002). Regulation of mast-cell and basophil function and survival by IgE. *Nat. Rev. Immunol.* 2, 773–786.

Kitamura, Y., Matsuda, H., and Hatanaka, K. (1979). Clonal nature of mast-cell clusters formed in W/Wv mice after bone marrow transplantation. *Nature 281*, 154–155.

Kruger-Krasagakes, S., Grutzkau, A., Baghramian, R., and Henz, B. M. (1996). Interactions of immature human mast cells with extracellular matrix: expression of specific adhesion receptors and their role in cell binding to matrix proteins. *J. Invest. Dermatol.* 106, 538–543.

Krutzik, S. R., Sieling, P. A., and Modlin, R. L. (2001). The role of Toll-like receptors in host defense against microbial infection. *Curr. Opin. Immunol.* 13, 104–108.

Kuramasu, A., Kubota, Y., Matsumoto, K., Nakajima, T., Sun, X. M., Watanabe, T., Saito, H., and Ohtsu, H. (2001). Identification of novel mast cell genes by serial analysis of gene expression in cord blood–derived mast cells. *FEBS Lett.* 498, 37–41.

Lantz, C. S., and Huff, T. F. (1995). Differential responsiveness of purified mouse c-kit+ mast cells and their progenitors to IL-3 and stem cell factor. *J. Immunol.* 155, 4024–4029.

Leal-Berumen, I., Snider, D. P., Barajas-Lopez, C., and Marshall, J. S. (1996). Cholera toxin increases IL-6 synthesis and decreases TNF-alpha production by rat peritoneal mast cells. *J. Immunol.* 156, 316–321.

Li, L., Li, Y., Reddel, S. W., Cherrian, M., Friend, D. S., Stevens, R. L., and Krilis, S. A. (1998). Identification of basophilic cells that express mast cell granule proteases in the peripheral blood of asthma, allergy, and drug-reactive patients. *J. Immunol.* 161, 5079–5086.

Lien, E., and Ingalls, R. R. (2002). Toll-like receptors. *Crit. Care Med.* 30, S1–S11.

Lin, T. J., Issekutz, T. B., and Marshall, J. S. (2000). Human mast cells transmigrate through human umbilical vein endothelial monolayers and selectively produce IL-8 in response to stromal cell–derived factor-1 alpha. *J. Immunol.* 165, 211–220.

Lin, T. J., Garduno, R., Boudreau, R. T., and Issekutz, A. C. (2002). Pseudomonas aeruginosa activates human mast cells to induce neutrophil transendothelial migration via mast cell–derived IL-1 alpha and beta. *J. Immunol.* 169, 4522–4530.

Lindstedt, K. A., Kokkonen, J. O., and Kovanen, P. T. (1998). Regulation of the activity of secreted human lung mast cell tryptase by mast cell proteoglycans. *Biochim. Biophys. Acta* 1425, 617–627.

Lorentz, A., Schuppan, D., Gebert, A., Manns, M. P., and Bischoff, S. C. (2002). Regulatory effects of stem cell factor and interleukin-4 on adhesion of human mast cells to extracellular matrix proteins. *Blood* 99, 966–972.

Lutzelschwab, C., Lunderius, C., Enerback, L., Hellman, L. (1998) A kinetic analysis of the expression of mast cell protease mRNA in the intestines of *Nippostrongylus brasiliensis*–infected rats. *Eur. J. Immunol.* 28, 3730–3737.

Malaviya, R., and Abraham, S. N. (2000). Role of mast cell leukotrienes in neutrophil recruitment and bacterial clearance in infectious peritonitis. *J. Leukoc. Biol.* 67, 841–846.

Malaviya, R., Ross, E. A., MacGregor, J. I., Ikeda, T., Little, J. R., Jakschik, B. A., and Abraham, S. N. (1994). Mast cell phagocytosis of FimH-expressing enterobacteria. *J. Immunol.* 152, 1907–1914.

Malaviya, R., Ikeda, T., Ross, E., and Abraham, S. N. (1996a). Mast cell modulation of neutrophil influx and bacterial clearance at sites of infection through TNF-alpha. *Nature 381*, 77–80.

Malaviya, R., Twesten, N. J., Ross, E. A., Abraham, S. N., and Pfeifer, J. D. (1996b). Mast cells process bacterial Ags through a phagocytic route for class I MHC presentation to T cells. *J. Immunol.* 156, 1490–1496.

Malaviya, R., Gao, Z., Thankavel, K., van der Merwe, P. A., and Abraham, S. N. (1999). The mast cell tumor necrosis factor alpha response to FimH-expressing *Escherichia coli* is mediated by the glycosylphosphatidylinositol-anchored molecule CD48. *Proc. Natl. Acad. Sci. USA* 96, 8110–8115.

Masuda, A., Matsuguchi, T., Yamaki, K., Hayakawa, T., and Yoshikai, Y. (2001). Interleukin-15 prevents mouse mast cell apoptosis through STAT6-mediated Bcl-xL expression. *J. Biol. Chem.* 276, 26107–26113.

Masuda, A., Yoshikai, Y., Aiba, K., and Matsuguchi, T. (2002). Th2 cytokine production from mast cells is directly induced by lipopolysaccharide and distinctly regulated by c-Jun N-terminal kinase and p38 pathways. *J. Immunol.* 169, 3801–3810.

Matsuura, N., and Zetter, B. R. (1989). Stimulation of mast cell chemotaxis by interleukin 3. *J. Exp. Med.* 170, 1421–1426.

Maurer, M., Echtenacher, B., Hultner, L., Kollias, G., Mannel, D. N., Langley, K. E., and Galli, S. J. (1998). The c-kit ligand, stem cell factor, can enhance innate immunity through effects on mast cells. *J. Exp. Med.* 188, 2343–2348.

McCurdy, J. D., Lin, T. J., and Marshall, J. S. (2001). Toll-like receptor 4-mediated activation of murine mast cells. *J. Leukoc. Biol.* 70, 977–984.

Medzhitov, R., and Janeway, C. A., Jr. (1997). Innate immunity: the virtues of a nonclonal system of recognition. *Cell* 91, 295–298.

Medzhitov, R., and Janeway, C., Jr. (2000). Innate immunity. *N. Engl. J. Med.* 343, 338–344.

Meininger, C. J., Yano, H., Rottapel, R., Bernstein, A., Zsebo, K. M., and Zetter, B. R. (1992). The c-kit receptor ligand functions as a mast cell chemoattractant. *Blood* 79, 958–963.

Mekori, Y. A., and Metcalfe, D. D. (1999). Mast cell–T cell interactions. *J. Allergy Clin. Immunol.* 104, 517–523.

Mekori, Y. A., Gilfillan, A. M., Akin, C., Hartmann, K., and Metcalfe, D. D. (2001). Human mast cell apoptosis is regulated through Bcl-2 and Bcl-XL. *J. Clin. Immunol.* 21, 171–174.

Metcalfe, D. D., Baram, D., and Mekori, Y. A. (1997). Mast cells. *Physiol. Rev.* 77, 1033–1079.

Miller, H. R., and Pemberton, A. D. (2002). Tissue-specific expression of mast cell granule serine proteinases and their role in inflammation in the lung and gut. *Immunology* 105, 375–390.

Mocsai, A., Zhang, H., Jakus, Z., Kitaura, J., Kawakami, T., Lowell, C. A. (2003). G-protein-coupled receptor signaling in Syk-deficient neutrophils and mast cells. *Blood* 101, 4155–4163.

Murakami, M., Tada, K., Nakajima, K., and Kudo, I. (1997). Cyclooxygenase-2-dependent delayed prostaglandin D2 generation is initiated by nerve growth factor in rat peritoneal mast cells: its augmentation by extracellular type II secretory phospholipase A2. *J. Immunol.* 159, 439–446.

Mwamtemi, H. H., Koike, K., Kinoshita, T., Ito, S., Ishida, S., Nakazawa, Y., Kurokawa, Y., Shinozaki, K., Sakashita, K., Takeuchi, K., Shiohara, M., Kamijo, T., Yasui, Y., Ishiguoi, A., Kawano, Y., Kitano, K., Miyazaki, H., Kato, T., Sakuma, S., and Komiyama, A. (2001). An increase in circulating mast cell colony–forming cells in asthma. *J. Immunol.* 166, 4672–4677.

Nadler, M. J., Matthews, S. A., Turner, H., and Kinet, J. P. (2000). Signal transduction by the high-affinity immunoglobulin E receptor Fc epsilon RI: coupling form to function. *Adv Immunol.* 76, 325–355.

Nakajima, T., Inagaki, N., Tanaka, H., Tanaka, A., Yoshikawa, M., Tamari, M., Hasegawa, K., Matsumoto, K., Tachimoto, H., Ebisawa, M., Tsujimoto, G., Matsudo, H., Nagai, H., and Saito, H. (2002). Marked increase in CC chemokine gene expression in both human and mouse mast cell transcriptomes following Fc epsilon receptor I cross-linking: an interspecies comparison. *Blood* 100, 3861–3868.

Nakano, T., Kanakura, Y., Nakahata, T., Matsuda, H., and Kitamura, Y. (1987). Genetically mast cell–deficient W/Wv mice as a tool for studies of differentiation and function of mast cells. *Fed. Proc.* 46, 1920–1923.

Nilsson, G., Butterfield, J. H., Nilsson, K., and Siegbahn, A. (1994). Stem cell factor is a chemotactic factor for human mast cells. *J. Immunol.* 153, 3717–3723.

Nilsson, G., Johnell, M., Hammer, C. H., Tiffany, H. L., Nilsson, K., Metcalfe, D. D., Siegbahn, A., and Murphy, P. M. (1996). C3a and C5a are chemotaxins for human mast cells and act through

distinct receptors via a pertussis toxin–sensitive signal transduction pathway. *J. Immunol.* 157, 1693–1698.

Nilsson, G., Mikovits, J. A., Metcalfe, D. D., and Taub, D. D. (1999). Mast cell migratory response to interleukin-8 is mediated through interaction with chemokine receptor CXCR2/interleukin-8RB. *Blood* 93, 2791–2797.

Nilsson, G., Metcalfe, D. D., and Taub, D. D. (2000). Demonstration that platelet-activating factor is capable of activating mast cells and inducing a chemotactic response. *Immunology* 99, 314–319.

Nishizumi, H., and Yamamoto, T. (1997). Impaired tyrosine phosphorylation and Ca2+ mobilization, but not degranulation, in lyn-deficient bone marrow–derived mast cells. *J. Immunol.* 158, 2350–2355.

Niyonsaba, F., Iwabuchi, K., Matsuda, H., Ogawa, H., and Nagaoka, I. (2002a). Epithelial cell–derived human beta-defensin-2 acts as a chemotaxin for mast cells through a pertussis toxin–sensitive and phospholipase C–dependent pathway. *Int. Immunol.* 14, 421–426.

Niyonsaba, F., Iwabuchi, K., Someya, A., Hirata, M., Matsuda, H., Ogawa, H., and Nagaoka, I. (2002b). A cathelicidin family of human antibacterial peptide LL-37 induces mast cell chemotaxis. *Immunology* 106, 20–26.

Oh, S. W., Pae, C. I., Lee, D. K., Jones, F., Ciang, G. K., Kim, H. O., Moon, S. H., Cao, B., Ogbu C., Jeong, K. W., Kozu, G., Nakanishi, H., Kahn, M., Chi, E. Y., and Henderson, W. R. Jr. (2002). Tryptase inhibition blocks airway inflammation in a mouse asthma model. *J. Immunol.* 168, 1992–2000.

Olsson, N., Piek, E., ten Dijke, P., and Nilsson, G. (2000). Human mast cell migration in response to members of the transforming growth factor-beta family. *J. Leukoc. Biol.* 67, 350–356.

Olsson, N., Rak, S., and Nilsson, G. (2000a). Demonstration of mast cell chemotactic activity in bronchoalveolar lavage fluid collected from asthmatic patients before and during pollen season. *J. Allergy Clin. Immunol.* 105, 455–461.

Otsuka, H., Dolovich, J., Befus, A. D., Telizyn, S., Bienenstock, J., and Denburg, J. A. (1986). Basophilic cell progenitors, nasal metachromatic cells, and peripheral blood basophils in ragweed-allergic patients. *J. Allergy Clin. Immunol.* 78, 365–371.

Ott, V. L., and Cambier, J. C. (2000). Activating and inhibitory signaling in mast cells: new opportunities for therapeutic intervention? *J. Allergy Clin. Immunol.* 106, 429–440.

Papadopoulos, E. J., Fitzhugh, D. J., Tkaczyk, C., Gilfillan, A. M., Sassetti, C., Metcalfe, D. D., and Hwang, S. T. (2000). Mast cells migrate, but do not degranulate, in response to fractalkine, a membrane-bound chemokine expressed constitutively in diverse cells of the skin. *Eur. J. Immunol.* 30, 2355–2361.

Parravicini, V., Gadina, M., Kovarova, M., Odom, S., Gonzalez-Espinosa, C., Furumoto, Y., Saitoh, S., Samelson, L. E., O'Shea, J. J., and Rivera, J. (2002). Fyn kinase initiates complementary signals required for IgE-dependent mast cell degranulation. *Nat. Immunol.* 3, 741–748.

Poncet, P., Arock, M., and David, B. (1999). MHC class II–dependent activation of CD4+ T cell hybridomas by human mast cells through superantigen presentation. *J. Leukoc. Biol.* 66, 105–112.

Prodeus, A. P., Zhou, X., Maurer, M., Galli, S. J., and Carroll, M. C. (1997). Impaired mast cell–dependent natural immunity in complement C3–deficient mice. *Nature* 390, 172–175.

Quackenbush, E. J., Wershil, B. K., Aguirre, V., and Gutierrez-Ramos, J. C. (1998). Eotaxin modulates myelopoiesis and mast cell development from embryonic hematopoietic progenitors. *Blood* 92, 1887–1897.

Raff, M. (1998). Cell suicide for beginners. *Nature* 396, 119–122.

Raposo, G., Tenza, D., Mecheri, S., Peronet, R., Bonnerot, C., and Desaymard, C. (1997). Accumulation of major histocompatibility complex class II molecules in mast cell secretory granules and their release upon degranulation. *Mol. Biol. Cell.* 8, 2631–2645.

Rennick, D., Hunte, B., Holland, G., and Thompson-Snipes, L. (1995). Cofactors are essential for stem cell factor–dependent growth and maturation of mast cell progenitors: comparative effects of interleukin-3 (IL-3), IL-4, IL-10, and fibroblasts. *Blood* 85, 57–65.

Repka-Ramirez, M. S. (2003). New concepts of histamine receptors and actions. *Curr. Allergy Asthma Rep.* 3, 227–231.

Rivera, J. (2002). Molecular adapters in Fc(epsilon)RI signaling and the allergic response. *Curr. Opin. Immunol.* 14, 688–693.

Rodewald, H. R., Dessing, M., Dvorak, A. M., and Galli, S. J. (1996). Identification of a committed precursor for the mast cell lineage. *Science* 271, 818–822.

Rosbottom, A., Scudamore, C. L., von der Mark, H., Thornton, E. M., Wright, S. H., and Miller, H. R. (2002). TGF-beta 1 regulates adhesion of mucosal mast cell homologues to laminin-1 through expression of integrin alpha 7. *J. Immunol.* 169, 5689–5695.

Rosenkranz, A. R., Coxon, A., Maurer, M., Gurish, M. F., Austen, K. F., Friend, D. S., Galli, S. J., and Mayadas, T. N. (1998). Impaired mast cell development and innate immunity in Mac-1 (CD11b/CD18, CR3)–deficient mice. *J. Immunol.* 161, 6463–6467.

Rossi, G., Newman, S. A., and Metzger, H. (1977). Assay and partial characterization of the solubilized cell surface receptor for immunoglobulin E. *J. Biol. Chem.* 252, 704–711.

Rottem, M., Barbieri, S., Kinet, J. P., and Metcalfe, D. D. (1992). Kinetics of the appearance of Fc epsilon RI–bearing cells in interleukin-3–dependent mouse bone marrow cultures: correlation with histamine content and mast cell maturation. *Blood* 79, 972–980.

Saeland, S., Duvert, V., Caux, C., Pandrau, D., Favre, C., Valle, A., Durand, I., Charbord, P., de Vries, J., and Bancherau, J. (1992). Distribution of surface-membrane molecules on bone marrow and cord blood CD34+ hematopoietic cells. *Exp. Hematol.* 20, 24–33.

Saito, H., Ebisawa, M., Tachimoto, H., Shichijo, M., Fukagawa, K., Matsumoto, K., Iikura, Y., Awaji, T., Tsujimoto, G., Yanagida, M., Uzumaki, H., Takahashi, G., Tsuji, K., and Nakahata, T. (1996). Selective growth of human mast cells induced by Steel factor, IL-6, and prostaglandin E2 from cord blood mononuclear cells. *J. Immunol.* 157, 343–350.

Sawada, J., Itakura, A., Tanaka, A., Furusaka, T., and Matsuda, H. (2000). Nerve growth factor functions as a chemoattractant for mast cells through both mitogen-activated protein kinase and phosphatidylinositol 3–kinase signaling pathways. *Blood* 95, 2052–2058.

Sawai, N., Koike, K., Mwamtemi, H. H., Kinoshita, T., Kurokawa, Y., Sakashita, K., Higuchi, T., Takeuchi, K., Shiohara, M., Kamijo, T., Ito, S., Kato, T., Miyazaki, H., Yamashita, T. and Komiyama, A. (1999). Thrombopoietin augments stem cell factor–dependent growth of human mast cells from bone marrow multipotential hematopoietic progenitors. *Blood* 93, 3703–3712.

Schwartz, L., and Huff, T. (1993). Biology of mast cells and basophils. In *Allergy: Principles and Practice* (eds. E. J. Middleton, C. E. Reed, E. F. Ellis, N. F. Adkinson, J. W. Yuninger, and W. W. Busse), 135–168. St. Louis: Mosby–Year Book, Inc.

Scudamore, C. L., McMillan, L., Thornton, E. M., Wright, S. H., Newlands, G. F., and Miller, H. R. (1997). Mast cell heterogeneity in the gastrointestinal tract: variable expression of mouse mast cell protease-1 (mMCP-1) in intraepithelial mucosal mast cells in nematode-infected and normal BALB/c mice. *Am. J. Pathol.* 150, 1661–1672.

Sher, A., Hein, A., Moser, G., and Caulfield, J. P. (1979). Complement receptors promote the phagocytosis of bacteria by rat peritoneal mast cells. *Lab. Invest.* 41, 490–499.

Shin, J. S., Gao, Z., and Abraham, S. N. (2000). Involvement of cellular caveolae in bacterial entry into mast cells. *Science* 289, 785–788.

Silverman, A. J., Sutherland, A. K., Wilhelm, M., and Silver, R. (2000). Mast cells migrate from blood to brain. *J. Neurosci.* 20, 401–408.

Sonoda, T., Ohno, T., and Kitamura, Y. (1982). Concentration of mast-cell progenitors in bone marrow, spleen, and blood of mice determined by limiting dilution analysis. *J. Cell Physiol.* 112, 136–140.

Sorden, S. D., and Castleman, W. L. (1995). Virus-induced increases in bronchiolar mast cells in Brown Norway rats are associated with both local mast cell proliferation and increases in blood mast cell precursors. *Lab. Invest.* 73, 197–204.

Sperr, W. R., Agis, H., Czerwenka, K., Klepetko, W., Kubista, E., Boltz-Nitulescu, G., Lechner, K., and Valent, P. (1992). Differential expression of cell surface integrins on human mast cells and human basophils. *Ann. Hematol.* 65, 10–16.

Stassen, M., Hültner, L. and Schmitt, E. (2002). Classical and alternative pathways of mast cell activation. *Crit. Rev. Immunol.* 22, 115–140.

Stenton, G. R., Ulanova, M., Dery, R. E., Merani, S., Kim, M. K., Gilchrist, M., Puttagunta, L., Musat-Marcu, S., James, D., Schreiber, A. D., and Befus, A. D. (2002). Inhibition of allergic inflammation in the airways using aerosolized antisense to Syk kinase. *J. Immunol.* 169, 1028–1036.

Stevens, R. L., Friend, D. S., McNeil, H. P., Schiller, V., Ghildyal, N., and Austen, K. F. (1994). Strain-specific and tissue-specific expression of mouse mast cell secretory granule proteases. *Proc. Natl. Acad. Sci. USA* 91, 128–132.

Supajatura, V., Ushio, H., Nakao, A., Okumura, K., Ra, C., and Ogawa, H. (2001). Protective roles of mast cells against enterobacterial infection are mediated by Toll-like receptor 4. *J. Immunol.* 167, 2250–2256.

Supajatura, V., Ushio, H., Nakao, A., Akira, S., Okumura, K., Ra, C., and Ogawa, H. (2002a). Differential responses of mast cell Toll-like receptors 2 and 4 in allergy and innate immunity. *J. Clin. Invest.* 109, 1351–1359.

Supajatura, V., Ushio, H., Wada, A., Yahiro, K., Okumura, K., Ogawa, H., Hirayama, T., and Ra, C. (2002b). Cutting edge: VacA, a vacuolating cytotoxin of *Helicobacter pylori*, directly activates mast cells for migration and production of proinflammatory cytokines. *J. Immunol.* 168, 2603–2607.

Tachimoto, H., Hudson, S. A., and Bochner, B. S. (2001). Acquisition and alteration of adhesion molecules during cultured human mast cell differentiation. *J. Allergy Clin. Immunol.* 107, 302–309.

Taguchi, T., Mitcham, J. L., Dower, S. K., Sims, J. E., and Testa, J. R. (1996). Chromosomal localization of TIL, a gene encoding a protein related to the Drosophila transmembrane receptor Toll, to human chromosome 4p14. *Genomics* 32, 486–488.

Takai, T., Ono, M., Hikida, M., Ohmori, H., and Ravetch, J. V. (1996). Augmented humoral and anaphylactic responses in Fc gamma RII–deficient mice. *Nature* 379, 346–349.

Takeuchi, O., Hoshino, K., Kawai, T., Sanjo, H., Takada, H., Ogawa, T., Takeda, K., and Akira, S. (1999). Differential roles of TLR2 and TLR4 in recognition of gram-negative and gram-positive bacterial cell wall components. *Immunity* 11, 443–451.

Tang, L., Jennings, T. A., and Eaton, J. W. (1998). Mast cells mediate acute inflammatory responses to implanted biomaterials. *Proc. Natl. Acad. Sci. USA* 95, 8841–8846.

Taub, D., Dastych, J., Inamura, N., Upton, J., Kelvin, D., Metcalfe, D., and Oppenheim, J. (1995). Bone marrow–derived murine mast cells migrate, but do not degranulate, in response to chemokines. *J. Immunol.* 154, 2393–2402.

Thompson, H. L., Metcalfe, D. D., and Kinet, J. P. (1990). Early expression of high-affinity receptor for immunoglobulin E (Fc epsilon RI) during differentiation of mouse mast cells and human basophils. *J. Clin. Invest.* 85, 1227–1233.

Turner, C. R., Kolbe, J., and Spannhake, E. W. (1988). Rapid increase in mast cell numbers in canine central and peripheral airways. *J. Appl. Physiol.* 65, 445–451.

Turner, H., and Kinet, J. P. (1999). Signalling through the high-affinity IgE receptor Fc epsilonRI. *Nature* 402, B24–30.

Ujike, A., Takeda, K., Nakamura, A., Ebihara, S., Akiyama, K., and Takai, T. (2002). Impaired dendritic cell maturation and increased T(H)2 responses in PIR-B(–/–) mice. *Nat. Immunol.* 3, 542–548.

Wang, H. W., Tedla, N., Lloyd, A. R., Wakefield, D., and McNeil, P. H. (1998). Mast cell activation and migration to lymph nodes during induction of an immune response in mice. *J. Clin. Invest.* 102, 1617–1626.

Welker, P., Grabbe, J., Gibbs, B., Zuberbier, T., and Henz, B. M. (2000a). Nerve growth factor–beta induces mast-cell marker expression during *in vitro* culture of human umbilical cord blood cells. *Immunology* 99, 418–426.

Welker, P., Grabbe, J., Zuberbier, T., Guhl, S., and Henz, B. M. (2000b). Mast cell and myeloid marker expression during early *in vitro* mast cell differentiation from human peripheral blood mononuclear cells. *J. Invest. Dermatol.* 114, 44–50.

Wershil, B. K., Wang, Z. S., Gordon, J. R., and Galli, S. J. (1991). Recruitment of neutrophils during IgE-dependent cutaneous late phase reactions in the mouse is mast cell–dependent. Partial inhibition of the reaction with antiserum against tumor necrosis factor-alpha. *J. Clin. Invest.* 87, 446–453.

Wershil, B. K., Furuta, G. T., Wang, Z. S., and Galli, S. J. (1996). Mast cell–dependent neutrophil and mononuclear cell recruitment in immunoglobulin E–induced gastric reactions in mice. *Gastroenterology* 110, 1482–1490.

Williams, C. M. and Galli, S. J. (2000). The diverse potential effector and immunoregulatory roles of mast cells in allergic disease. *J. Allergy Clin. Immunol.* 105, 847–859.

Wills, F. L., Gilchrist, M., and Befus, A. D. (1999). Interferon-gamma regulates the interaction of RBL-2H3 cells with fibronectin through production of nitric oxide. *Immunology* 97, 481–489.

Wong, M. X., Roberts, D., Bartley, P. A., and Jackson, D. E. (2002). Absence of platelet endothelial cell adhesion molecule-1 (CD31) leads to increased severity of local and systemic IgE-mediated anaphylaxis and modulation of mast cell activation. *J. Immunol.* 168, 6455–6462.

Woo, C. H., Jeong, D. T., Yoon, S. B., Kim, K. S., Chung, I. Y., Saeki, T., and Kim, J. H. (2002). Eotaxin induces migration of RBL-2H3 mast cells via a Rac-ERK-dependent pathway. *Biochem. Biophys. Res. Commun.* 298, 392–397.

Xiang, Z., Ahmed, A. A., Moller, C., Nakayama, K., Hatakeyama, S., and Nilsson, G. (2001). Essential role of the prosurvival bcl-2 homologue A1 in mast cell survival after allergic activation. *J. Exp. Med.* 194, 1561–1569.

Yamaguchi, M., Lantz, C. S., Oettgen, H. C., Katona, I. M., Fleming, T., Miyajima, I., Kinet, J. P., and Galli, S. J. (1997). IgE enhances mouse mast cell Fc(epsilon)RI expression *in vitro* and *in vivo*: evidence for a novel amplification mechanism in IgE-dependent reactions. *J. Exp. Med.* 185, 663–672.

Yang, F. C., Kapur, R., King, A. J., Tao, W., Kim, C., Borneo, J., Breese, R., Marshall, M., Dinauer, M. C., and Williams, D. A. (2000). Rac2 stimulates Akt activation affecting BAD/Bcl-XL expression while mediating survival and actin function in primary mast cells. *Immunity* 12, 557–568.

Yeatman, C. F., 2nd, Jacobs-Helber, S. M., Mirmonsef, P., Gillespie, S. R., Bouton, L. A., Collins, H. A., Sawyer, S. T., Shelburne, C. P., and Ryan, J. J. (2000). Combined stimulation with the T helper cell type 2 cytokines interleukin (IL)-4 and IL-10 induces mouse mast cell apoptosis. *J. Exp. Med.* 192, 1093–1103.

Zehnder, J. L., and Galli, S. J. (1999). Mast-cell heparin demystified. *Nature* 400, 714–715.

Zhang, Y., Ramos, B. F., and Jakschik, B. A. (1992). Neutrophil recruitment by tumor necrosis factor from mast cells in immune complex peritonitis. *Science* 258, 1957–1959.

Zhu, F. G., and Marshall, J. S. (2001). CpG-containing oligodeoxynucleotides induce TNF-alpha and IL-6 production but not degranulation from murine bone marrow–derived mast cells. *J. Leukoc. Biol.* 69, 253–262.

Zhuang, X., Silverman, A. J., and Silver, R. (1999). Distribution and local differentiation of mast cells in the parenchyma of the forebrain. *J. Comp. Neurol.* 408, 477–488.

Eosinophils

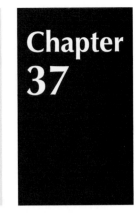

Chapter 37

Marc E. Rothenberg

Division of Allergy and Immunology, Department of Pediatrics, Cincinnati Children's Hospital Medical Center, Cincinnati, Ohio

Eosinophils are multifunctional proinflammatory leukocytes implicated in the pathogenesis of numerous diseases, especially allergic disorders, parasitic infections, malignancies, and a series of primary hypereosinophilic disorders (Gleich and Adolphson, 1986; Rothenberg, 1998; Weller, 1991). In healthy states, eosinophils normally represent only a small percentage of white blood cells in the bone marrow and blood (1%–3%), and low levels of eosinophils are present in several tissues. When a large series of biopsy and autopsy specimens were analyzed, the only organs that contained tissue eosinophils (at substantial levels) were the gastrointestinal tract, spleen, lymph nodes, and thymus (Kato *et al.*, 1998). Eosinophil infiltrations were associated with eosinophil degranulation only in the gastrointestinal tract. Similar to findings in human tissues, murine eosinophils also predominantly reside in the hematopoietic organs, gastrointestinal tract, and thymus (Matthews *et al.*, 1998). The lamina propria of the stomach, small intestine, cecum, and colon contains the main reservoir of eosinophils in the body. Notably, the baseline level of gastrointestinal eosinophils (comparable to that seen in adults) is achieved prior to birth and appears to be independent of endogenous flora (Mishra *et al.*, 1999). This strongly contrasts with the homing patterns of most other leukocytes (conventional lymphocytes and mast cells) (Ferguson and Parrott, 1972a; Ferguson and Parrott, 1972b; Watkins *et al.*, 1976; Woodbury and Neurath, 1978). For example, germfree mice, which have never come in contact with viable bacteria, have decreased levels of lymphocytes in the lamina propria (Ferguson, 1976) but normal levels of eosinophils (Mishra *et al.*, 2000). Thus, eosinophil homing into the gastrointestinal tract occurs prenatally, is independent of the presence of viable bacterial flora, and appears to be regulated by mechanisms distinct from those regulating other gastrointestinal leukocytes (*e.g.*, mast cells and lymphocytes). Indeed, important studies have elucidated that constitutively expressed chemokines (eotaxins) critically regulate the tissue distribution of eosinophils, providing a molecular mechanism to regulate the tissue distribution of eosinophils.

REGULATION OF EOSINOPHILS

Eosinophil development (hematopoiesis)

Eosinophils are produced in the bone marrow from pluripotential stem cells under the regulation of the transcription factor GATA-1 (Du *et al.*, 2002; Yu *et al.*, 2002). The eosinophil lineage is thought to be shared with the basophil lineage, on the basis of the identification of immature cells that coexpress eosinophilic and basophilic staining characteristics, the presence of shared molecules in these cell types (*e.g.*, the eotaxin receptor CCR3 and the βc hematopoietin receptor), and the utilization of common growth factors by these cells (*e.g.*, IL-3) (Boyce *et al.*, 1995). IL-3, IL-5, and GM-CSF are particularly important in regulating eosinophil expansion. These three growth factors, also known as eosinophilopoietins, bind to a heterodimeric receptor (R) that contains a common subunit (βc) and a unique chain (*e.g.*, IL-3Rα, IL-5Rα, GM-CSF Rα). IL-5, primarily derived from T cells, especially of the Th2 phenotype, is the most specific to the eosinophil lineage and is responsible for the selective differentiation of eosinophils (Sanderson, 1992) and their release from the bone marrow into the peripheral circulation (Collins *et al.*, 1995).

The critical role of IL-5 in the production of eosinophils is best demonstrated by genetic manipulation of mice. Overproduction of IL-5 by a variety of approaches, including transgenic overexpression in enterocytes, results in profound eosinophilia, and deletion of the IL-5 gene causes a marked reduction of eosinophils in the blood, lungs, and gastrointestinal tract after allergen challenge (Dent *et al.*, 1990; Foster *et al.*, 1996; Lee *et al.*, 1997b; Mishra *et al.*, 2001; Mishra *et al.*, 1999). Based on these results, a humanized anti-IL5-drug has been developed and tested in asthmatic individuals. Although this drug lowers circulating eosinophils by 80%, it reduces lung tissue levels by only ~55% (Flood-Page *et al.*, 2003b). Early results with anti-IL-5 have not shown improvements in airway function (*e.g.*, FEV1) (Leckie *et al.*, 2000), but it appears to induce significant improvements in markers of remodeling (associated with decreases in transforming growth factor beta (TGF-β) levels) (Flood-Page *et al.*, 2002; Flood-Page *et al.*, 2003a; Phipps *et al.*, 2003). This suggests the importance of other molecules involved in eosinophil tissue accumulation (*e.g.*, eotaxins) and an important role for eosinophils in the inflammatory changes associated with chronic remodeling.

Eosinophil adhesion

Eosinophil adhesion to blood vessel and tissue elements is regulated by a diverse set of mechanisms **(Fig. 37.1)**. Reversible interactions between eosinophils and endothelial cells are primarily mediated by selectins; eosinophils express the ligands (*e.g.*, sialylated Lewis-X antigen) for E- and P-selectins. The integrins expressed by eosinophils include members of the β1 (*e.g.*, very late antigen (VLA)-4), β2 (*e.g.*, CD18 family of molecules), and β7 families (*e.g.*, αβ7 molecule) (Bochner and Schleimer, 1994). The CD18 family of molecules includes lymphocyte function antigen (LFA)-1 and Mac-1, which both interact with endothelial cells via intercellular adhesion molecules (ICAMs); the VLA-4 integrin binds to vascular cell adhesion molecule (VCAM)-1. These adhesion interactions have been shown to be important for eosinophil recruitment into the lung and skin, but their role in eosinophil recruitment to the gastrointestinal tract has not been extensively evaluated (Broide and Sriramarao, 2001; Resnick and Weller, 1993; Tachimoto *et al.*, 2002). The αβ7 molecule, which is coexpressed on lymphocytes and eosinophils, may be the most important integrin for gastrointestinal eosinophils. This integrin binds to mucosal addressin cell adhesion molecule-1 (MAdCAM-1), a major adhesion molecule expressed on high endothelial venules in the intestinal lamina propria, lymph nodes, and Peyer's patches (Butcher *et al.*, 1999; Shaw and Brenner, 1995). Extensive studies focused on inhibiting the β7/MAdCAM-1 interaction with neutralizing antibodies or with β7 gene–targeted mice have supported a central role for this pathway in regulating lymphocyte and mast

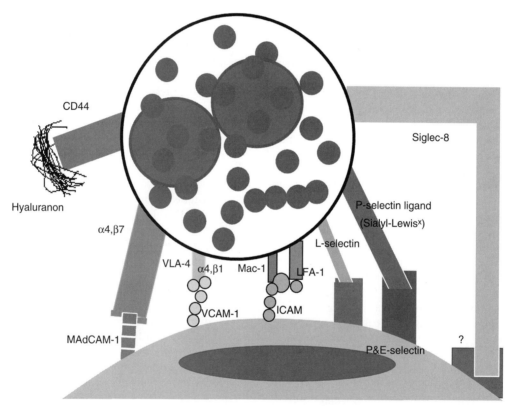

Fig. 37.1. Schematic diagram of eosinophil adhesion molecules and their ligands. Eosinophils express several classes of adhesion molecules, including members of the selectin and integrin families (more extensively reviewed in other publications [Bochner and Schleimer, 1994]). Depicted are eosinophil ligands (*e.g.*, sialylated Lewis-X antigen) for E- and P-selectins, which mediate reversible interactions between eosinophils and endothelial cells. In addition, eosinophils express L-selectin, but its exact ligand on endothelial cells is not known. Eosinophils have recently been demonstrated to selectively express a sialic acid–binding immunoglobulin-like lectin designated Siglec-8. The ligand for Siglec-8 has not yet been identified, but other members of the Siglec family of adhesion molecules have been shown to be important signaling receptors, employing immunomodulatory inhibitory motifs to interact with tyrosine phosphatases (*e.g.*, SHP-1). The integrins expressed by eosinophils include members of the β1 (*e.g.*, very late antigen [VLA]-4), β2 (*e.g.*, CD18 family of molecules), and β7 (*e.g.*, α4β7) families of molecules. The CD18 group of receptors includes lymphocyte function antigen (LFA)-1 and Mac-1, which both interact with endothelial cells via intercellular adhesion molecule (ICAM); the VLA-4 integrin (which is not expressed by neutrophils) binds to vascular cell adhesion molecule (VCAM)-1. The α4β7 molecule, which is coexpressed on lymphocytes and eosinophils, binds to mucosal addressin cell adhesion molecule-1 (MAdCAM-1), a major adhesion molecule expressed on high endothelial venules in the intestinal lamina propria, lymph nodes, and Peyer's patches. Eosinophils also express CD44, which is a receptor that recognizes multiple ligands, especially molecules that are part of the extracellular matrix such as hyaluronan and fibronectin. This figure has been adapted from Rothenberg *et al.* (2001b) with permission.

cell–progenitor cell homing into the intestine (Gurish *et al.*, 2001; Sandborn and Targan, 2002; von Andrian and Engelhardt, 2003). The findings that eotaxin-1-induced eosinophil recruitment to the lung and eotaxin-1-mediated chemoattraction *in vitro* are dependent upon VLA-4 (α4β1) (Kitayama *et al.*, 1997) suggest that the other α4-associated integrins on eosinophils (*e.g.*, α4β7) may also be involved in eotaxin-mediated events. Consistent with this, there is delayed intestinal hypersensitivity (including lymphocyte and eosinophil infiltrations) in response to intestinal infection with *Trichinella spiralis* in β7-deficient animals (Artis *et al.*, 2000). Additionally, the effect of the eotaxin-1 intestine transgene is dependent upon the β7 integrin (Mishra *et al.*, 2002b). In addition to expressing integrins, eosinophils have recently been demonstrated to selectively express a sialic acid–binding immunoglobulin-like lectin designated Siglec-8 (Floyd *et al.*, 2000; Kikly *et al.*, 2000). The ligand for Siglec-8 has not yet been identified, but other members of the Siglec family of adhesion molecules have been shown to be important signaling receptors, employing immunomodulatory inhibitory motifs to interact with tyrosine phosphatases (*e.g.*, SHP-1). In addition, eosinophils express adhesion molecules for extracellular matrix components, such as the hyaluronan receptor CD44 (Rothenberg, 2003); this molecule not only promotes eosinophil adhesion but also induces eosinophil activation and survival (Ohkawara *et al.*, 2000).

Eosinophil chemoattraction

The findings that eosinophils normally account for only a small percentage of circulating or tissue-dwelling cells and that their numbers markedly and selectively increase under specific disease states indicate the existence of molecular mechanisms that regulate the selective generation and accumulation of these leukocytes. The pathological role of eosinophils primarily is in tissues; therefore, a major focus of scientific investigation on eosinophils has been to elucidate the processes involved in eosinophil tissue recruitment. Numerous mediators have been identified as eosinophil chemoattractants, including diverse molecules such as lipid mediators (platelet activating factor, leukotrienes), bacterial products (fMLP), and recently chemokines such as RANTES and macrophage inflammatory protein (MIP)-1α (Resnick and Weller, 1993). However, none of these mediators selectively promote eosinophil recruitment. In contrast, a group of human chemokines—designated eotaxins—with eosinophil-selective chemoattractant activity has been identified.

Eotaxin was initially discovered with a biological assay in guinea pigs designed to identify the molecules responsible for allergen-induced eosinophil accumulation in the lungs. Using an *in vivo* chemotaxis assay in guinea pig skin, Jose *et al.* (1994) determined the partial amino acid sequence for the protein responsible for eosinophil chemoattraction in the bronchoalveolar lavage fluid in allergen-challenged guinea pigs. Subsequently, this sequence facilitated the genetic cloning of the genes and cDNA for guinea pig, murine, and human eotaxin, which led to the identification of eotaxin as a member of the CC chemokine family most homologous to the MCP subfamily (Garcia-Zepeda *et al.*, 1996; Ponath *et al.*, 1996b; Rothenberg *et al.* 1995a; Rothenberg *et al.*, 1995b). This subfamily of eotaxin and MCP chemokines is clustered on human chromosome 17q11, a region that also contains other CC chemokines (such as MIP-1α, I-309, RANTES, and HCC-1/2) (Luster and Rothenberg, 1997). An interesting finding is that this region has been linked to asthma susceptibility (Nickel *et al.*, 1999a; Nickel *et al.*, 1999b). With genomic analyses rather than biological assays, two additional chemokines have been identified in the human genome that encode for CC chemokines with eosinophil-selective chemoattractant activity and have hence been designated eotaxin-2 and eotaxin-3 (Forssmann *et al.*, 1997; Kitaura *et al.*, 1999; Patel *et al.*, 1997; Shinkai *et al.*, 1999; Zimmermann *et al.*, 2000). Eotaxin-2 and eotaxin-3 are only distantly related to eotaxin-1 since they are only ~30% identical in sequence and are located in a different chromosomal position (human 7q11.23) (Kitaura *et al.*, 1999; Nomiyama *et al.*, 1998; Zimmermann *et al.*, 2000). The specific activity of all eotaxins is mediated by the selective expression of the eotaxin receptor, CCR3, a seven-transmembrane spanning GPCR, primarily expressed on eosinophils (Combadiere, Ahuja and Murphy, 1995; Daugherty *et al.*, 1996; Ponath *et al.*, 1996a). CCR3 is a genetically polymorphic receptor that undergoes ligand-induced internalization, a process that is required for eotaxin-induced cellular activation (Zimmermann, Bernstein and Rothenberg, 1998; Zimmermann, Conkright and Rothenberg, 1999; Zimmermann and Rothenberg, 2003). CCR3 is a promiscuous receptor; it interacts with multiple ligands, including MCP-2, -3, -4, RANTES, and HCC-2 (MIP-5, leukotactin); however, the only ligands that signal exclusively through this receptor are the eotaxin chemokines, accounting for the cellular selectivity of eotaxins (Bertrand and Ponath, 2000; Zimmermann *et al.*, 2003). CCR3 appears to be the dominant eosinophil chemokine receptor, as suggested by the relatively high level of this receptor on eosinophils and the ability of an anti-CCR3 reagent to block the activity of RANTES, a chemokine that could signal through CCR1 or CCR3 (Heath *et al.*, 1997). Specific activities that have been associated with the human eotaxin chemokines *in vitro* include strong chemoattraction (eosinophils, basophils), cellular activation (such as induction of cytokine and leukotriene release from eosinophils and basophils), induction of basophil histamine release, and calcium transients (eosinophils, basophils, Th2 cells, dendritic cells) (Gutierrez-Ramos, Lloyd and Gonzalo, 1999).

When the eotaxin-1 cDNA from guinea pigs, mice, and humans was identified, the mRNA for this chemokine was noted to be constitutively expressed in a variety of tissues (Garcia-Zepeda *et al.*, 1996; Rothenberg, Luster and Leder, 1995; Rothenberg *et al.*, 1995). A finding in all species was that the intestine expressed relatively high levels of eotaxin-1 mRNA. Examination of multiple segments of the gastrointestinal tract of mice for expression of eotaxin-1 mRNA indicated that this chemokine was ubiquitously expressed, at variable levels, in all segments from the tongue to the colon.

Notably, the constitutive expression of eotaxin-1 was distinct from the expression of related chemokines (MCP-1, MCP-2, MCP-3, MIP-1α), which were not readily detectable. Only RANTES and eotaxin-2 were detectable, but they were not ubiquitously expressed (Mishra *et al.*, 1999; Zimmermann *et al.*, 2000).

The expression patterns of eosinophil-active chemokines at baseline indicated that eotaxin may be involved in the selective regulation of eosinophil homing in the gastrointestinal tract. Furthermore, eotaxin-1 mRNA expression in the small intestine is localized to mononuclear cells that reside in the lamina propria, the region where most gastrointestinal eosinophils reside (Matthews *et al.*, 1998). Indeed, the number of eosinophils in the gastrointestinal tract of mice deficient in eotaxin-1 (through gene targeting) (Rothenberg *et al.*, 1997) is significantly lower than in wild-type mice (Matthews *et al.*, 1998).

A variety of approaches have been used to determine the biological role of the eotaxin chemokines. *In vivo* administration studies involving guinea pigs and rodents have shown that the eotaxin chemokines are relatively potent and specific eosinophil chemoattractants (Gonzalo *et al.*, 1996; Jose *et al.*, 1994; Rothenberg *et al.*, 1996). Notably, the eotaxin chemokines cooperate with IL-5, the eosinophil growth and differentiation cytokine, in the induction of tissue eosinophilia (Collins *et al.*, 1995; Mould *et al.*, 1997; Mould *et al.*, 2000; Rothenberg *et al.*, 1996). For example, administration of eotaxin-1 into the lungs of IL-5 transgenic mice induces rapid (3-hour), specific lung eosinophilia; this activity is enhanced in comparison with that in administration studies in wild-type mice (Rothenberg *et al.*, 1996). Eotaxin-1 null mice and anti-eotaxin-1 neutralizing antibodies have definitively associated eotaxin-1 with the temporal and regional distribution of eosinophils in the lung and with the development of airway hyperreactivity in an allergen-induced model of asthma (Gonzalo *et al.*, 1998) (Campbell *et al.*, 1998). In addition to having a role in the respiratory tract, the eotaxin chemokines are involved in regulating eosinophils in other tissues. Under baseline conditions, eotaxin-1 and eotaxin-2 are constitutively expressed in a variety of tissues, with especially high levels in the gastrointestinal tract and thymus (Garcia-Zepeda *et al.*, 1996; Mishra *et al.*, 1999; Rothenberg *et al.*, 1995; Zimmermann *et al.*, 2000). Analysis of eotaxin-1-deficient mice has revealed that the constitutive expression of this chemokine is critically involved in regulating the baseline homing of eosinophils, especially in the intestine, the main reservoir of eosinophils (Matthews *et al.*, 1998; Mishra *et al.*, 1999). Additionally, induction of experimental gastrointestinal allergy in eotaxin-1-deficient mice has revealed an essential role for eotaxin-1 in regulating eosinophil-associated gastrointestinal pathology (Hogan *et al.*, 2000; Hogan *et al.*, 2001). Eotaxin-1 is also temporally induced in the developing mammary gland during puberty, and in the absence of eotaxin-1, there is a temporal deficiency in mammary gland eosinophils (Gouon-Evans, Rothenberg and Pollard, 2000). Finally, eotaxin-1-deficient mice, especially in conjunction

with IL-5 deficiency, have impaired eosinophil-associated antitumor immunity (Mattes *et al.*, 2003). Recently, CCR3-gene-targeted mice have been developed and have been analyzed at baseline and following induction of experimental asthma and experimental *T. spiralis* infection (Gurish *et al.*, 2002; Humbles *et al.*, 2002; Ma *et al.*, 2002). Consistent with the critical role of eotaxin-1 in regulating baseline and allergen-driven eosinophil homing into the gastrointestinal tract, CCR3−/− mice have decreased levels of intestinal eosinophils at baseline and following *T. spiralis* infection (Gurish *et al.*, 2002; Humbles *et al.*, 2002). Following a standard ovalbumin-induced model of experimental asthma, CCR3−/− mice have decreased eosinophil accumulation in the airway (Humbles *et al.*, 2002). It is interesting that eosinophils were found trapped in the subendothelial space, suggesting that CCR3-deficient eosinophils are capable of rolling, adhering, and transmigrating through endothelial cells but not crossing the elastic tissue into the lung parenchyma (Humbles *et al.*, 2002). Paradoxically, these mice exhibited increased allergen-induced mast cell hyperplasia in the lung and airway hyperreactivity, supporting a role for CCR3 in mast cell responses, but by an unclear mechanism. However, when CCR3-deficient mice were sensitized epicutaneously with ovalbumin, there was a marked deficiency of lung and biological fluid eosinophils and an impairment in the development of airway hyperresponsiveness (but no changes in mast cells) (Ma *et al.*, 2002). These apparently conflicting results may be related to the sensitization protocol. Collectively, these studies highlight the critical role of eotaxin/CCR3 in regulating eosinophil responses in experimental asthma.

There is now substantial preclinical evidence supporting a role for eotaxin chemokines in human allergic disease (Zimmermann *et al.*, 2003). Experimental induction of cutaneous and pulmonary late-phase responses in humans has revealed that the eotaxin chemokines are produced by tissue resident cells (*e.g.*, respiratory epithelial cells and skin fibroblasts) and allergen-induced infiltrative cells (*e.g.*, macrophages and eosinophils). Several studies have reported baseline increases in eotaxin-1 levels in the bronchoalveolar lavage fluid of asthmatics in comparison with control individuals (Lamkhioued *et al.*, 1997; Lilly *et al.*, 2001). Following allergen challenge, eotaxin-1 is induced early (within 6 hours) and correlates with early eosinophil recruitment; in contrast, eotaxin-2 correlates with eosinophil accumulation at 24 hours (Ying *et al.*, 1999a; Ying *et al.*, 1999b). In another study, eotaxin-1 and eotaxin-2 mRNA levels were found to be higher in patients with asthma than in normal controls; however, there was no further increase following allergen challenge (Berkman *et al.*, 2001). In contrast, eotaxin-3 mRNA was dramatically enhanced 24 hours after allergen challenge (Berkman *et al.*, 2001). The chemoattractant activity of the bronchoalveolar lavage fluid from patients with asthma is partially inhibited (~50%) by antibodies against RANTES, MCP-3, MCP-4, and eotaxin-1 (Lamkhioued *et al.*, 1997).

Further support for an important role of eotaxin-1 in human asthma is derived from analysis of a single nucleotide polymorphism (SNP) in the eotaxin-1 gene. A naturally occurring mutation encoding for a change in the last amino acid in signal peptide (alanine→threonine) results in less effective cellular secretion of eotaxin-1 *in vitro* and *in vivo* (Nakamura *et al.*, 2001). Notably, this SNP is associated with reduced levels of circulating eotaxin-1 and eosinophils and improved lung function (*e.g.*, FEV1) (Nakamura *et al.*, 2001). Recently, the activity of eotaxin-1 and eotaxin-2 in humans has been investigated by injection of these chemokines into the skin of humans; both eotaxin-1 and eotaxin-2 were able to induce an immediate wheal-and-flare response associated with mast cell degranulation and subsequent infiltrations by eosinophils, basophils, and neutrophils (Menzies-Gow *et al.*, 2002). The infiltration by neutrophils is likely to be mediated indirectly by mast cell degranulation. These results provide substantial evidence that the biological activities attributed to eotaxins in animals are conserved in humans.

Collectively, these studies have provided the impetus for the development of therapeutic agents aimed at blocking the action of eotaxins and/or CCR3. Indeed, small molecule inhibitors of CCR3 and a humanized anti–human eotaxin-1 antibody have been developed (Bertrand and Ponath, 2000;

Sabroe *et al.*, 2000; Zimmermann *et al.*, 2003). Early results in a phase I trial of humanized anti-eotaxin-1 in patients with allergic rhinitis have shown no serious adverse responses when this drug is administered by intravenous or intranasal routes (Pereira *et al.*, 2003; Salib *et al.*, 2003). Notably, anti-eotaxin-1 has been shown to markedly lower levels of eosinophils in nasal washes and nasal biopsy specimens and to improve nasal patency (Pereira *et al.*, 2003; Salib *et al.*, 2003). These early results have substantiated a role for eotaxin-1 in human allergic disease.

EOSINOPHIL PRODUCTS

Eosinophils express numerous receptors (for cytokines, immunoglobulins, complement proteins, and Toll-like receptor ligands) that when engaged lead to eosinophil activation, resulting in several processes, including the release of toxic secondary granule proteins (Rothenberg, 1998) **(Fig. 37.2)**. The secondary granule contains a crystalloid core composed of major basic protein (MBP)-1 and MBP-2 and a granule matrix that is mainly composed of eosinophil cationic protein (ECP), eosinophil neurotoxin (EDN), and eosinophil

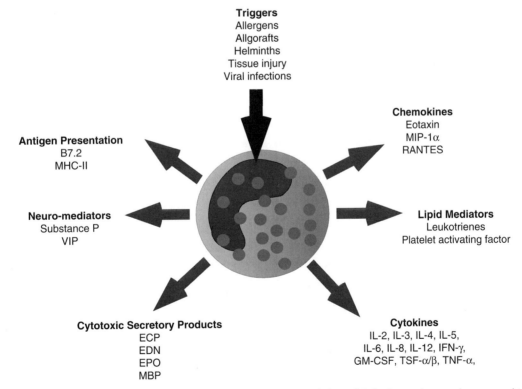

Fig. 37.2. Schematic diagram of an eosinophil and its diverse properties. Eosinophils are bilobed granulocytes that respond to diverse stimuli including allergens, helminths, viral infections, allografts, and nonspecific tissue injury. The secondary granules contain four primary cationic proteins, designated eosinophil peroxidase (EPO), major basic protein (MBP), eosinophil cationic protein (ECP), and eosinophil-derived neurotoxin (EDN). All four proteins are cytotoxic molecules; in addition, ECP and EDN are ribonucleases. In addition to releasing their preformed cationic proteins, eosinophils can also release a variety of cytokines (*e.g.*, IL-2, IL-3, IL-4, IL-5, IL-6, IL-8, IL-12, TSF-αβ, GM-CSF, TNF-α, and IFN-γ), chemokines (*e.g.*, eotaxin, RANTES, and MIP-1α), and neuromediators (vasoactive intestinal peptide [VIP] and substance P), and they can generate large amounts of leukotriene (LT)C$_4$. Last, eosinophils can be induced to express MHC class II and costimulatory (*e.g.*, B7.2) molecules and may be involved in propagating immune responses by presenting antigen to T cells. This figure has been adapted from Rothenberg *et al.* (2001b) with permission.

peroxidase (EPO). These proteins elicit potent cytotoxic effects on a variety of host tissues at concentrations similar to those found in biological fluid from patients with eosinophilia. The cytotoxic effects of eosinophils may be elicited through multiple mechanisms, including degrading cellular ribonucleic acid, since ECP and EDN have substantial functional and structural homology to a large family of ribonuclease genes (Rosenberg et al., 1995; Slifman et al., 1986). Notably, the coding sequences of ECP and EDN are the most divergent open reading frames in the entire human genome, even though their ribonuclease activity is preserved (Lander et al., 2001; Venter et al., 2001). The strong positive pressure for divergence of these enzymes suggests an important role for these molecules and eosinophils in degrading RNA; recent studies have suggested this response may be important in the immunity against single-strand RNA containing viruses such as respiratory syncytial virus (RSV) (Rosenberg and Domachowske, 2001). ECP also inserts ion-nonselective pores into the membranes of target cells, which may allow the entry of the cytotoxic proteins (Young et al., 1986). Further proinflammatory damage is caused by the generation of unstable oxygen radicals formed by the respiratory burst oxidase apparatus and EPO. Furthermore, direct degranulation of mast cells and basophils is triggered by MBP. In addition to being cytotoxic, MBP directly increases smooth-muscle reactivity by causing dysfunction of vagal muscarinic M2 receptors (Jacoby, Gleich and Fryer, 1993). Activation of eosinophils also leads to the generation of large amounts of LTC_4, which induces increased vascular permeability, mucous secretion, and smooth-muscle constriction (Lewis, Austen and Soberman, 1990). Additionally, activated eosinophils generate a wide range of cytokines, including IL-1, -3, -4, -5, -13, GM-CSF, TGF-α-β, TNF-α, RANTES, MIP-1α, and eotaxin-1, indicating that they have the potential to sustain or augment multiple aspects of the immune response, inflammatory reaction, and tissue repair process (Kita, 1996). Eosinophils also produce neuroactive mediators (e.g., substance P and vasoactive intestinal peptide [VIP]) (Metwali et al., 1994). Specimens from patients with eosinophilic gastroenteritis often display eosinophils undergoing marked degranulation near nerves, suggesting that they may indeed be involved in promoting inflammatory changes to neurons (Dvorak et al., 1993; Stead, 1992). The gastric dysmotility during experimental oral antigen-induced gastrointestinal inflammation is associated with eosinophils in the proximity of damaged nerves, suggesting a causal role for eosinophils in nerve dysfunction (Hogan et al., 2001). Additionally, experimental eosinophil accumulation in the gastrointestinal tract is associated with the development of weight loss, which is attenuated in eotaxin-deficient mice (Hogan et al., 2001). Finally, eosinophils have the capacity to initiate antigen-specific immune responses by acting as antigen-presenting cells (Mattes et al., 2002). Consistent with this, eosinophils express relevant costimulatory molecules (CD40, CD28, CD86, B7) (Ohkawara et al., 1996; Woerly et al., 1999), secrete cytokines capable of inducing T cell proliferation and maturation (IL-2, IL-4, IL-6, IL-10, IL-12)

(Kita, 1996; Lacy et al., 1998; Lucey, Nicholson and Weller, 1989), and can be induced to express MHC class-II molecules (Lucey, Nicholson and Weller, 1989). Experimental adoptive transfer of antigen-pulsed eosinophils induces antigen-specific T cell responses in vivo (Shi et al., 2000).

BENEFICIAL ROLE OF EOSINOPHILS

Antihelminth immunity

The beneficial function of eosinophils has been primarily attributed to their ability to defend the host against parasitic helminths. This is based on several lines of evidence, including the ability of eosinophils to mediate antibody-dependent (or complement-dependent) cellular toxicity against helminths in vitro (Butterworth, 1977; Butterworth, 1984); the observation that eosinophil levels increase during helminth infections and that eosinophils aggregate and degranulate in the local vicinity of damaged parasites in vivo; and the results obtained in parasite-infected mice that have been depleted of eosinophils by IL-5 neutralization and/or gene targeting (Behm and Ovington, 2000). However, it should be noted that murine studies are particularly problematic since mice are not the natural hosts of many of the experimental parasites. Nevertheless, in some primary infection models, a role for IL-5 (and hence eosinophils) in protective immunity has been suggested following infection with *Strongyloides venezuelensis*, *Strongyloides ratti*, *Nippostrongyloides brasiliensis*, and *Heligmosomoides polygyrus* (Behm and Ovington, 2000; Korenaga et al., 1991). Most recently, a role for eosinophils in the encystment of larvae in *T. spiralis* infection has been demonstrated (Gurish et al., 2002). In this study, a markedly lower level of gastrointestinal eosinophils was found in *T. spiralis*–infected CCR3 gene–targeted mice than in control infected mice that contained abundant degranulating eosinophils. The reduced level of eosinophils correlated with a greater number of intact encysted larvae. Thus, although the debate continues, it seems likely that eosinophils participate in protective immunity against selected helminths.

Immunoregulation

The localization of gastrointestinal eosinophils in juxtaposition with lymphocytes (e.g., lamina propria and Peyer's patches) suggests a functional interaction between these two leukocytes (Rothenberg et al., 2001b). While most studies have focused on the role of T cells in the regulation of eosinophils (e.g., through IL-5), it is likely that eosinophils may also regulate lymphocytes. Consistent with this possibility is that eosinophils are known to express the necessary cellular machinery for antigen presentation such as H-2 class II and costimulatory molecules (e.g., B7) (Lucey, Nicholson and Weller, 1989; Tamura et al., 1996; Woerly et al., 1999). Eosinophils are also known to express a variety of cytokines that can induce the proliferation and/or maturation of T cells (e.g., IL-2, IL-4, IL-12). Furthermore, preliminary investigations with human eosinophils in vitro have shown that eosinophils have the capacity to present antigen to T cells

(Lucey, Nicholson and Weller, 1989; Tamura *et al.*, 1996). Recent studies have shown that eosinophils isolated from the mouse lung can present antigen to T cells when adoptively transferred to naïve animals (Shi *et al.*, 2000). In addition, it has been proposed that lymph node eosinophils in patients with Hodgkin's disease may provide cellular ligands for TNF superfamily receptors and CD30, thereby transducing proliferation and antiapoptotic signals (Pinto *et al.*, 1996; Pinto *et al.*, 1997). Additional support for an interaction between eosinophils and T cells has recently been derived from analysis of thymic eosinophils. As mentioned earlier, the thymus is a primary site for eosinophils under healthy conditions. In young mice, thymic eosinophils are primarily located in the corticomedullary region, express IL-4 and IL-13, and are CD11b- and CD11c-positive (similar to dendritic cells) (Throsby *et al.*, 2000). In adult mice, eosinophils traffic to the medulla under the regulation of eotaxin (Matthews *et al.*, 1998). During experimental induction of tolerance, the level of thymic eosinophils increases and their location correlates with areas of active T cell apoptosis. Taken together, these studies indicate that regulation of T cell responses is one of the physiological functions of eosinophils.

Developmental biology

The finding that eosinophils home in the gastrointestinal tract during gestational development (Mishra *et al.*, 1999) suggests that eosinophils may have a role in tissue or organ development. A role for eosinophils in developmental processes in the gastrointestinal tract has not yet been identified. However, a physiological function for eosinophils in postnatal mammary gland development has been recently proposed (Gouon-Evans, Rothenberg and Pollard, 2000). In this investigation, F4/80-positive leukocytes were identified to be present in the developing mammary gland, primarily in the region of the terminal end buds. Surprisingly, on close histologic examination, the F4/80-positive cells were identified as macrophages and eosinophils. The important role for leukocytes in mammary gland development was demonstrated by depleting hematopoietic precursors by whole-body γ-irradiation. Following γ-irradiation, ductal outgrowth was impaired, and this abnormality was reversed by bone marrow transplantation. Interestingly, the level of eotaxin and eosinophils in the mammary gland was shown to increase with the development of the mammary gland during puberty. Furthermore, eotaxin-1-deficient mice had a near complete loss of mammary gland eosinophils, and this was associated with a decreased number of ductal branches and a defect in terminal end bud formation. Taken together, these data establish that eosinophils are critically involved in the branching morphogenesis of the mammary gland. The presence of constitutive eotaxin-1 and eosinophils in other endocrine organs (*e.g.*, uterus) (Hornung *et al.*, 2000; Salamonsen and Lathbury, 2000; Zhang, Lathbury and Salamonsen, 2000), as well as in the gastrointestinal tract, suggests that the involvement of tissue eosinophils in developmental processes is not likely to be restricted to the mammary gland. Indeed, eosinophils

cycle through the uterus by an estrogen-regulated mechanism that depends upon eotaxin-1 expression (Gouon-Evans and Pollard, 2001).

DETRIMENTAL ROLE OF EOSINOPHILS IN INFLAMMATORY DISEASE STATES

Eosinophils in inflammatory lung diseases

Eosinophils accumulate in numerous inflammatory lung diseases, including asthma, hypersensitivity pneumonitis, tropical pulmonary eosinophilia, Churg-Strauss syndrome, and both acute and chronic forms of eosinophilic pneumonia. A complete review of eosinophil-associated lung disorders is beyond the scope of this chapter; rather, the focus is on the involvement of eosinophils in allergic lung inflammation (primarily asthma), since a great deal of research has been dedicated to understanding this subject.

Asthma is a disease defined by reversible airflow obstruction and increased lung responsiveness to a variety of antigen-specific triggers (allergens) and antigen-nonspecific triggers (*e.g.*, cold air, cigarette smoke), strongly associated with atopy (IgE production) (Elias *et al.*, 2003). Asthma currently affects a large segment of the population in the western world (~8%), and its incidence is on the rise. Histologically, the asthmatic lung is characterized by an eosinophil-rich inflammation and by a variety of chronic changes that induce lung remodeling (including mucus production, smooth muscle hyperplasia, and deposition of extracellular matrix components) (Busse and Lemanske, 2001). Notably, recent studies have suggested that eosinophils are intimately linked with the development of these remodeling processes, at least in part (Flood-Page *et al.*, 2003a; Phipps *et al.*, 2003; Phipps, Ying and Kay, 2002; Phipps *et al.*, 2002).

Experimentation in the allergy field has largely focused on analysis of the cellular and molecular events induced by allergen exposure in sensitized animals (primarily mice) and humans (Busse and Lemanske, 2001; Leong and Huston, 2001). In patient studies, naturally sensitized individuals are challenged by exposure to allergen (*i.e.*, segmental antigen challenge) for analysis of asthmatic responses (Makker, Montefort, and Holgate, 1993). In the animal models, mice are typically subjected to sensitization with antigen (*e.g.*, ovalbumin) in the presence of adjuvant (*e.g.*, alum) by intraperitoneal injection (Hamelmann *et al.*, 1997b; Leong and Huston, 2001). Subsequently, mice are challenged by exposure to mucosal allergen (via intratracheal, intranasal, nebulized, or cutaneous routes), and pathological responses are monitored. While the use of an adjuvant is not necessary, it enhances the magnitude of the IgG1, IgE, and cellular responses. In other animal models, unsensitized mice are repeatedly exposed to allergens (*e.g.*, extracts of *Aspergillus fumigatus*) via mucosal or cutaneous routes, and the development of experimental allergy is monitored (Kurup *et al.*, 1992; Mishra *et al.*, 2001). Although no animal model adequately mimics human disease, experimentation in animals has provided an experimental framework to identify and dissect key cells and molecules involved in the pathogenesis of allergic responses.

Mechanism of eosinophilia in asthma

Animal and human experimental systems have demonstrated that allergic inflammatory responses are often biphasic and that eosinophils are associated with the second phase of allergic responses. For example, asthma is characterized by a biphasic bronchospasm response, consisting of an early phase asthmatic response (EAR) and a late-phase asthmatic response (LAR) (Bochner, Undem and Lichtenstein, 1994; Broide, 2001). The EAR phase is characterized by immediate bronchoconstriction in the absence of pronounced airway inflammation or morphological changes in the airway tissue. The EAR phase has been shown to directly involve IgE mast cell–mediated release of spasmogens (histamine, prostaglandin-D2, and cysteinyl-peptide leukotrienes [LTC_4, LTD_4, LTE_4], which are potent mediators of bronchoconstriction) (Drazen, Arm and Austen, 1996; Holgate *et al.*, 2003). Following the immediate response, individuals with asthma often experience an LAR, which is characterized by more persistent bronchoconstriction associated with extensive airway inflammation and its associated morphological changes (De Monchy *et al.*, 1985; Lam *et al.*, 1987). Clinical investigations have demonstrated that the LAR is associated with increased levels of inflammatory cells, in particular activated T lymphocytes and eosinophils. The elevated levels of T lymphocytes and eosinophils correlate with increased levels of eosinophilic constituents in the bronchoalveolar lavage fluid, the degree of airway epithelial cell damage, enhanced bronchial responsiveness to inhaled spasmogens, and disease severity (Foster *et al.*, 1996; Gleich, 2000; Hogan *et al.*, 1998a; Jarjour *et al.*, 1997). Th2 cells are thought to induce asthma through the secretion of an array of cytokines (*e.g.*, IL-4, IL-5, IL-9, IL-13, IL-25) that activate inflammatory and residential effector pathways both directly and indirectly (Bhathena *et al.*, 2000; Ray and Cohn, 1999). In particular, IL-4 and IL-13 are produced at elevated levels in allergic tissue and are thought to be central regulators of many of the hallmark features of the disease (Wills-Karp, 2001). However, in addition to Th2 cells, inflammatory cells (*e.g.*, eosinophils, basophils, and mast cells) within the allergic tissue also produce IL-4, IL-13, and a variety of other cytokines (Kita, 1996; Rothenberg, 1998). Notably, recent studies have found that eosinophils are a primary source of early IL-4, independent of T cells, following helminth infection (Shinkai, Mohrs, and Locksley, 2002). IL-4 promotes Th2 cell differentiation, IgE production, tissue eosinophilia, and in the case of asthma, morphological changes to the respiratory epithelium (Brusselle *et al.*, 1994; Rankin *et al.*, 1996). IL-13 induces mucus hypersecretion, eosinophil recruitment and survival, airway hyperresponsiveness, expression of adhesion molecules and chemokines (such as eotaxin-1), IgE production, and expression of CD23 and IgE (the last properties are observed in humans but not mice) (Bochner *et al.*, 1995; Wills-Karp, 2001; Zhu *et al.*, 1999). **Figure 37.3** summarizes the basic events that

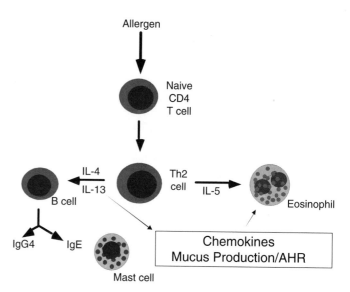

Fig. 37.3. Association of eosinophilia with a Th2 immune response. Allergens are presented to naive T cells, resulting in the generation of T cell polarization into the Th2 phenotype. Th2 cells produce a myriad of cytokines, including IL-4, IL-5, and IL-13. IL-4 and IL-13 promote IgE synthesis (leading to mast cell sensitization and their subsequent ability to recognize allergen). In addition, IL-4 and IL-13 directly activate tissue resident cells, including airway epithelium and smooth muscle, to produce mucus airway hyperresponsiveness (AHR) and chemokines (especially the eotaxin and MCP subfamily of chemokines). IL-5 promotes eosinophil expansion in the bone marrow and eosinophil release from the bone marrow into the circulation and primes eosinophils to respond to chemoattractants.

take place in a Th2-associated immune response that leads to eosinophilia.

Role of eosinophils in asthma

Elevated levels of eosinophil granule proteins (*e.g.*, MBP) have been found in biological fluid from patients with asthma; these concentrations are sufficient to induce cytotoxicity of a variety of host tissue, including respiratory epithelial cells, *in vitro* (Rothenberg, 1998). Direct degranulation of mast cells and basophils, triggered by MBP, is thought to also be involved in disease pathogenesis (Rothenberg, 1998). In addition to being cytotoxic, MBP directly increases smooth-muscle reactivity by causing dysfunction of vagal muscarinic M2 receptors, which is thought to contribute to the development of airway hyperreactivity, a cardinal feature of asthma (Jacoby, Gleich and Fryer, 1993). Additionally, eosinophils generate large amounts of the cysteinyl leukotrienes (Bandeira-Melo, Bozza and Weller, 2002; Lewis, Austen and Soberman, 1990). These mediators lead to increased vascular permeability and mucus secretion and are potent smooth-muscle constrictors. Indeed, inhibitors of cysteinyl leukotrienes are effective therapeutic agents for the treatment of allergic airway disease.

Multiple studies employing experimental models of asthma (primarily in mice, guinea pigs, and monkeys) have demonstrated that neutralization of IL-5, the major eosinophil growth factor, can block various aspects of asthma (Foster *et al.*, 1996; Hamelmann and Gelfand, 2001; Hamelmann *et al.*, 1997a). Although extensive investigations have implicated the eosinophil as a central effector cell in asthma and an important clinical target for the resolution of this disease, the role of this granulocyte in the development and exacerbation of asthma pathogenesis remains highly controversial. This controversy stems in part from distinctions between human asthma and experimental murine models of asthma. For example, in contrast to human asthma, mice with eosinophilic lung disease triggered by allergens or helminthic infection have variable levels of eosinophil degranulation (Denzler *et al.*, 2000; Shinkai, Mohrs and Locksley, 2002). In experimental models, inhibition of the actions of IL-5 consistently suppresses pulmonary eosinophilia in response to antigen inhalation; however, this effect does not always correlate with a reduction of airway hyperreactivity (Corry *et al.*, 1996; Foster *et al.*, 1996; Hamelmann *et al.*, 1997a; Hogan *et al.*, 1998a; Iwama *et al.*, 1992; Iwama *et al.*, 1993; Mauser *et al.*, 1993; Nagai *et al.*, 1993). This dichotomy is highlighted by findings in allergic IL-5-deficient (IL-5$^{-/-}$) mice of the C57BL/6 strain (Foster *et al.*, 1996) that do not develop antigen-induced airway hyperreactivity, while IL-5$^{-/-}$ BALB/c mice develop enhanced reactivity independently of this factor (Hogan *et al.*, 1998a).

Although eosinophil trafficking to the allergic lung is profoundly attenuated in IL-5$^{-/-}$ mice or those treated with anti-IL-5 antibodies in comparison with wild-type responses (Foster *et al.*, 2001; Hogan *et al.*, 1998b; Mattes *et al.*, 2002), a marked residual tissue eosinophilia can persist in these mice after allergen inhalation (Corry *et al.*, 1996; Foster *et al.*, 1996; Hamelmann *et al.*, 1997a; Hogan *et al.*, 1998a; Nagai *et al.*, 1993). Furthermore, the degree of residual tissue eosinophilia is under genetic regulation, as lung eosinophilia was 10-fold to 100-fold greater in the BALB/c strain, where airway hyperreactivity persists, than in the C57BL/6 strain, where airway hyperreactivity is abolished in the absence of IL-5 (Foster *et al.*, 1996; Hogan *et al.*, 1998a).

Studies with transgenic mice overexpressing IL-5 (in T cells, lung epithelial cells, or enterocytes) have demonstrated that high levels of IL-5 are sufficient for the development of eosinophilia (Dent *et al.*, 1990; Lee *et al.*, 1997a; Lee *et al.*, 1997b; Mishra *et al.*, 2002b; Tominaga *et al.*, 1991); however, elevated levels of eosinophils are not universally associated with the development of asthma-like changes in the lung. Since IL-5 receptors are also expressed by other cell types (including murine B cells, human basophils, and possibly human respiratory smooth-muscle cells) (Bischoff *et al.*, 1990; Hakonarson *et al.*, 1999; Sanderson, 1990; Sanderson, 1992), eosinophils may not be the only cells that are affected by manipulation of IL-5. A recent study has taken a new approach to deplete eosinophils in mice (administration of complement-fixing antibodies against CCR3) and demonstrated an important role for eosinophils in the development of asthma-associated airway hyperreactivity (Justice *et al.*, 2003); a role for other CCR3$^+$ cells was not ruled out, but there was no evidence of CCR3 expression by

noneosinophils (Justice *et al.*, 2003). Accordingly, a humanized antibody against IL-5 has been developed and was recently tested in phase I/II trials for asthma (Leckie *et al.*, 2000). In the early studies with this reagent, levels of circulating and sputum eosinophils in patients with mild to moderate asthma were shown to drop by more than fivefold (Leckie *et al.*, 2000). However, no clinical benefit (*e.g.*, improvement in FEV1) was demonstrated. This result prompted some investigators to conclude that eosinophils were not effector cells in human asthma (Leckie *et al.*, 2000); however, the anti-IL-5 study was not properly designed to fully address the efficacy of this drug (O'Byrne P, Inman, and Parameswaran, 2001).

With the discovery of the eotaxins and the finding that IL-5 cooperates with eotaxin-1 in regulating eosinophil tissue recruitment, it became critical to determine if the apparent lack of efficacy of anti-IL-5 in humans was related to the inability of this drug to block eosinophil tissue recruitment or the noneffector role of eosinophils. Along these lines, a very recent study has demonstrated that anti-IL-5 in humans blocks lung eosinophil recruitment by only 55% (Flood-Page *et al.*, 2003b), providing evidence that accessory molecules (in addition to IL-5) regulate lung eosinophilia. Thus, anti-IL-5 treatment does not completely resolve tissue eosinophilia in the allergic lung, and this cell may therefore still contribute to disease pathogenesis even in the presence of IL-5 neutralization. One possibility is that local chemokine systems (eotaxins) can operate independently of IL-5 to recruit eosinophils into the allergic lung. Studies with eotaxin-1 gene–targeted mice (–/–), IL-5$^{-/-}$, and eotaxin-1/IL-5 double –/– mice have revealed an independent and synergistic role for both of these molecules in regulating the tissue level of eosinophils in the asthmatic lung and in the induction of airway hyperreactivity (Mattes *et al.*, 2002). While early studies with anti-IL-5 in human asthma have continued to find no improvement in FEV1 measurements, pathological markers of chronic airway remodeling (*e.g.*, deposition of tenascin, procollagen III, and lumican) were improved by anti-IL-5 (Flood-Page *et al.*, 2002; Flood-Page *et al.*, 2003a; Phipps *et al.*, 2003). Decreased levels of TGF-β in the biological fluid following anti-IL-5 treatment have been found, suggesting that eosinophil-derived TGF-β regulates lung remodeling (Flood-Page *et al.*, 2002; Flood-Page *et al.*, 2003a; Phipps *et al.*, 2003).

In support for a role of eosinophils in the pathogenesis of human asthma, a very recent study has demonstrated improved clinical outcome when asthma treatment decisions are based on monitoring sputum eosinophil counts rather than conventional guidelines from the British Thoracic Society (Green *et al.*, 2002).

Eosinophils in gastrointestinal inflammatory disorders

The accumulation of eosinophils in the gastrointestinal tract is a common feature of numerous disorders, such as drug reactions (Rothenberg, 1998; Rothenberg *et al.*, 2001a); helminth infections (Behm and Ovington, 2000); idiopathic hypereosinophilic syndrome (Assa'ad *et al.*,

2000; Bauer *et al.*, 1996; Weller, 1994); eosinophilic esophagitis (Kelly, 2000; Rothenberg *et al.*, 2001c); eosinophilic gastroenteritis (Katz *et al.*, 1984; Keshavarzian *et al.*, 1985; Torpier *et al.*, 1988); allergic colitis (Hill and Milla, 1990; Odze *et al.*, 1995; Sherman and Cox, 1982); inflammatory bowel disease (Dvorak, 1980; Sarin *et al.*, 1978; Walsh and Gaginella, 1991); and gastroesophageal reflux (Brown, Goldman and Antonioli, 1984; Liacouras *et al.*, 1998; Winter *et al.*, 1982). A subset of these diseases, referred to as primary eosinophil-associated gastrointestinal disorders (EGIDs) (Hogan, Foster and Rothenberg, 2002), appear to have hypersensitivity disorders that lie in the middle of a spectrum ranging from anaphylaxis to celiac disease (Moon and Kleinman, 1995; Saavedra-Delgado and Metcalfe, 1985; Sampson, 1999) **(Fig. 37.4)**. EGID encompasses multiple disease entities, including eosinophilic esophagitis, eosinophilic gastritis, eosinophilic enteritis, eosinophilic colitis, and eosinophilic gastroenteritis (representing a combination of involved gastrointestinal segments) (Guajardo *et al.*, 2002). EGID occurs independently of peripheral blood eosinophilia ~50% of the time, indicating the potential significance of gastrointestinal-specific mechanisms for regulating eosinophil levels. In eosinophilic colitis, eosinophil accumulation occurs in the first few months of life and is a frequent cause of bloody diarrhea (Hill and Milla, 1990; Odze *et al.*, 1995; Sherman and Cox, 1982). In these patients, eosinophils predominantly accumulate in the colon in the presence or absence of peripheral blood eosinophilia. The eosinophil infiltration appears to be triggered by cow's milk protein hypersensitivity and improves upon withdrawal of the allergic triggers from the diet (Hill and Milla, 1990; Maluenda *et al.*, 1984; Saavedra-Delgado and Metcalfe, 1985). Eosinophil accumulation in the esophagus occurs in numerous diseases, including gastroesophageal reflux disease, as well as primary eosinophilic

esophagitis, and is part of the diagnostic criteria for gastroesophageal reflux disease (Brown, Goldman and Antonioli, 1984; Fox, Nurko and Furuta, 2002; Rothenberg *et al.*, 2001c). In gastroesophageal reflux disease, the magnitude of esophageal eosinophilia has been proposed to be a negative prognostic indicator (Liacouras *et al.*, 1998; Winter *et al.*, 1982) and adversely predicts response to conventional antigastroesophageal reflux medication (Ruchelli *et al.*, 1999). In at least a subset of refractory patients, the severity of the gastroesophageal inflammation is reversed by institution of an allergen-free diet (Kelly *et al.*, 1995). Eosinophilic esophagitis is distinguished from gastroesophageal reflux disease on the basis of several important differences, including the relatively higher prevalence of atopy, dysphagia, male gender, familial inheritance, degree of proximal esophagitis, and intensity of esophageal pathology (*e.g.*, epithelial hyperplasia and eosinophil density [generally >24 eosinophils/high-power field]) (Fox, Nurko, and Furuta, 2002; Rothenberg *et al.*, 2001c). Last, patients with inflammatory bowel disease also have an accumulation of eosinophils in the gastrointestinal tract. Both forms of inflammatory bowel disease, Crohn's disease and ulcerative colitis, are characterized by gastrointestinal eosinophilia; however, eosinophils usually represent only a small percentage of the infiltrating leukocytes (Desreumaux, Nutten and Colombel, 1999; Walsh and Gaginella, 1991). It is interesting that both diseases are associated with overproduction of eotaxin-1; however, there is controversy concerning whether IL-5 is overproduced in both disorders (Fuss *et al.*, 1996; Hankard *et al.*, 1997). Crohn's disease is thought to be a predominantly Th1 and tumor necrosis factor-α–associated response, whereas ulcerative colitis is predominantly a Th2-associated process accompanied by IL-5 overproduction. The level of eosinophils in inflammatory bowel disease lesions has been proposed to be a negative

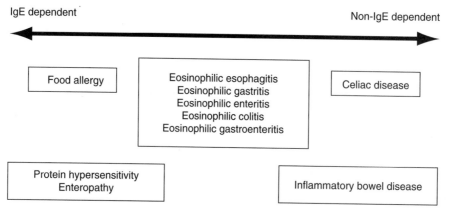

Fig. 37.4. The spectrum of inflammatory disorders of the gastrointestinal tract associated with eosinophil accumulation. Increased levels of eosinophils in the gastrointestinal tract occur in a wide variety of primary gastrointestinal disorders. These diseases vary in spectrum from strong dependence on IgE (*e.g.*, food anaphylaxis) to low dependence on IgE (*e.g.*, celiac disease). Diseases in the intermediate spectrum are characterized by specific organ inflammation, primarily associated with eosinophil accumulation (*e.g.*, eosinophilic esophagitis, eosinophilic gastritis, eosinophilic enteritis, eosinophilic colitis, and eosinophilic gastroenteritis) and are referred to as primary eosinophil-associated gastrointestinal diseases (EGIDs). In EGID, increased levels of IgE have been associated with the disorders in a subset of patients, but the etiological role of IgE is not clear. Diseases containing overlapping features with EGID include protein hypersensitivity enteropathy and inflammatory bowel disease.

prognostic indicator (Desreumaux, Nutten and Colombel, 1999; Nishitani *et al.*, 1998).

Mechanisms of eosinophil-associated damage in the gastrointestinal tract. In vitro studies have shown that eosinophil granule constituents are toxic to a variety of tissues, including intestinal epithelium (Tai *et al.*, 1984; Venge *et al.*, 1980; Frigas, Loegering and Gleich, 1980; Gleich *et al.*, 1979). Clinical investigations have demonstrated extracellular deposition of MBP and ECP in the small bowel of patients with eosinophilic gastroenteritis (Dvorak, 1980; Keshavarzian *et al.*, 1985; Tajima and Katagiri, 1996; Talley *et al.*, 1990; Torpier *et al.*, 1988) and have shown a correlation between the level of eosinophils and disease severity (Desreumaux *et al.*, 1996; Talley *et al.*, 1990). Electron microscopy studies have revealed ultrastructural changes in the secondary granules (indicative of eosinophil degranulation and mediator release) in duodenal samples from patients with eosinophilic gastroenteritis (Torpier *et al.*, 1988). Furthermore, Charcot-Leyden crystals, remnants of eosinophil degranulation, are commonly found on microscopic examination of stools obtained from patients with eosinophilic gastroenteritis (Cello, 1979; Klein *et al.*, 1970).

Experimental dissection of eosinophil-associated gastrointestinal disorders. Despite these clinical findings, there is currently only a limited understanding of the biological and pathological significance of eosinophils in the gastrointestinal tract. Most studies of eosinophils *in vivo* have concentrated on trafficking and activation of these cells in the lung. It remains to be determined if the mechanisms involved in the regulation of eosinophil recruitment in the lung are conserved in the gastrointestinal tract. Recent studies with experimental models of gastrointestinal allergy, especially oral antigen (in the form of enteric coated beads)–induced models of eosinophilic gastroenteritis, have revealed classic Th2-associated immunity, with prominent generation of IL-4, IL-5, and the eotaxin chemokines (Hogan *et al.*, 2000; Hogan *et al.*, 2001). Notably, eotaxin-1 gene–targeted mice do not develop intestinal eosinophilia (even though they develop peripheral blood eosinophilia) and are protected from antigen-induced gastromegaly and cachexia, strongly implicating eosinophils as effector cells in disease pathology (Hogan *et al.*, 2001). It is interesting that IL-5 gene–targeted mice fail to develop circulating eosinophilia but develop intestinal eosinophilia (Hogan *et al.*, 2000). Collectively, these studies indicate that intestinal eosinophilia can occur independently of IL-5 and that the relative balance between IL-5 and eotaxin-1 production can profoundly affect the tissue distribution of eosinophils (Rothenberg *et al.*, 2001b).

In a murine model of antigen-induced eosinophilic colitis associated with diarrhea, a dramatic infiltration of eosinophils, mast cells, and CD4[+] Th2 cells into the large but not small intestine was observed. Similar experimental analysis in mice showed that the targeted deletion of signal transducers and activators of transcription (STAT)6 completely eliminated the colonic eosinophils and the diarrhea (Kweon *et al.*, 2000). Adoptive transfer experiments showed that systemically primed splenic CD4[+] T cells were prefer-

entially recruited to the large but not small intestine upon oral allergen challenge. These results indicate that eosinophil-associated inflammation of the large intestine appears to be critically regulated by Th2 cells that specifically home to the colon. Recently, with use of a modified experimental regime, oral allergen–induced diarrhea has been shown to be accompanied by massive mast-cell degranulation and to be blocked by anti-IgE therapy or mast-cell depletion, strongly implicating mast cells with this cardinal feature of eosinophilic gastrointestinal diseases (Brandt *et al.*, 2003).

Recent advances have also taken place that further our understanding of the pathogenesis of eosinophil-associated esophagitis. The murine and human esophagus, in contrast to the more distal gastrointestinal segments, is devoid of resident eosinophils at baseline (Kato *et al.*, 1998; Mishra *et al.*, 1999). In an effort to understand the mechanisms and significance of eosinophil accumulation in the esophagus in diseased states, a murine model for antigen-induced esophagitis has been developed (Mishra *et al.*, 2001). Mice were repeatedly challenged with intranasal or intratracheal *Aspergillus fumigatus* allergen (under conditions which promote allergic airway inflammation) and were found to develop an increase of ~100– to 125-fold in their levels of esophageal eosinophils and epithelial hyperplasia (but had no changes in the gastrointestinal tract distal to the gastroesophageal junction). In contrast, exposure to repeated doses of oral or intragastric soluble allergen did not promote esophageal inflammation. Allergen challenge of IL-5 gene–targeted mice resulted in the complete loss of eosinophil recruitment to the esophagus and the onset of epithelial hyperplasia (Mishra *et al.*, 2001; Mishra *et al.*, 2002a). Consistent with the important role of Th2 cells and their cytokines, a clinical study of patients with eosinophilic esophagitis has demonstrated elevated levels of IL-4-secreting T cells in esophageal lesions (Nicholson *et al.*, 1997). These findings have several implications: they implicate aeroallergens and eosinophils in the etiology of eosinophilic esophagitis; they suggest that esophageal eosinophilic inflammation is mechanistically associated with pulmonary inflammation; and they suggest that targeting IL-5 (*e.g.*, with the humanized anti-IL-5) may be a useful strategy for patients with eosinophilic esophagitis and/or refractory gastroesophageal reflux. In addition, they suggest that distinct mechanisms regulate eosinophil accumulation in the esophagus versus other components of the gastrointestinal tract, such as the small intestine.

SUMMARY AND CONCLUDING REMARKS

Eosinophils are well known as proinflammatory leukocytes that account for a small subset of circulating blood cells. Under baseline (healthy) conditions, gastrointestinal eosinophils predominantly reside in the lamina propria in the stomach and intestine, and their numbers in these organs are substantially higher than in hematopoietic tissues. Eosinophils migrate to the gastrointestinal tract during embryonic development, and their concentrations in perinatal mice are comparable to those in adults, indicating that eosinophil homing occurs independent of intestinal flora. The chemokine eotaxin-1, an eosinophil-selective chemoattractant, is constitutively expressed throughout all segments of the gastrointestinal tract and is required for eosinophil homing to the lamina propria. During inflammatory conditions, eosinophils accumulate in their normal locations and in numerous other tissues, including the respiratory tract (nose and lung) and secondary lymphoid organs (Peyer's patches and lymph nodes). In the lung, the α4, β1, and β2 integrins are critically important for eosinophil homing, whereas in the gastrointestinal tract the α4 and β7 integrins appear to be important, suggesting that future therapeutics may include inhibitors of these integrins. The processes associated with eosinophil accumula-

tion in the gastrointestinal tract during inflammatory conditions are summarized in **Fig. 37.5**. Most eosinophil-associated diseases are characterized by Th2-associated immune responses, which provide a mechanism to explain eosinophilia. In particular, Th2 cell–derived IL-5 promotes eosinophil hematopoiesis and primes eosinophils to respond to chemoattractants. At the same time, Th2 cell–derived IL-4 and IL-13 induce eosinophil adhesion molecules (*e.g.*, ICAM-1 and VCAM-1) and eosinophil-selective chemokines (*e.g.*, eotaxins). In addition to being associated with Th2 immune responses, eosinophilia can develop as a consequence of aberrant somatic genetic events. In particular, a subset of patients with hypereosinophilic syndromes have a chromosome 4 microdeletion that results in the generation of an activated tyrosine kinase (Cools *et al.*, 2003). This tyrosine kinase is highly sensitive to imatinib, a recently approved drug for the treatment of

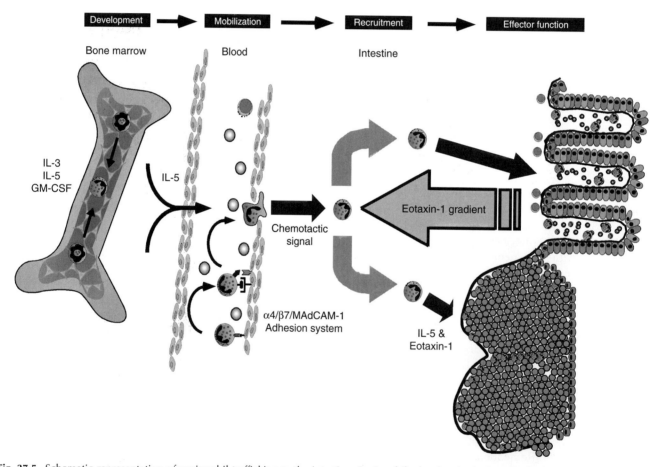

Fig. 37.5. Schematic representation of eosinophil trafficking to the intestine. Eosinophils develop in the bone marrow, where they differentiate from hematopoietic progenitor cells into mature eosinophils. Factors that control this process have not been fully defined; however, IL-3, IL-5, and GM-CSF are important in eosinophil expansion during conditions of hypereosinophilia. Eosinophil migration out of the bone marrow into the circulation is primarily regulated by IL-5. Circulating eosinophils subsequently interact with the endothelium by processes involving rolling, adhesion, and diapedesis. In the gastrointestinal tract, the adhesion α4β7 ligand on eosinophils interacts with the endothelial receptor mucosal vascular addressin MAdCAM-1. Eosinophils are mobilized into the lamina propria in response to a chemotactic gradient primarily established by the chemokine eotaxin-1, liberated from mononuclear cells in the crypts. Additionally, eosinophils are mobilized into the interfollicular and paracortical regions of Peyer's patches. The chemotactic response is enhanced by IL-5, an important eosinophil cytokine for eosinophil priming and survival. Depending upon the chemokine concentration gradient, gastrointestinal eosinophils can also migrate into the villi, residing in proximity to lymphocytes, and have the potential to degranulate, resulting in tissue damage. This figure has been adapted from Rothenberg *et al.* (2001b) with permission.

select malignancies. Regardless of the mechanism of disease induction, activated eosinophils have the capacity to participate in multiple aspects of disease, including the promotion of proinflammatory damage (through the secretion of cytotoxic granule proteins), tissue remodeling (through the secretion of pleiotropic cytokines such as TGF), sustenance of the immune response (by activating T cells via antigen presentation and by regulating T-cell cytokine production), and causing end-organ dysfunction (*e.g.*, antagonism of muscarinic receptors or elicitation of cardiomyopathy). Multiple therapeutic approaches are capable of interfering with eosinophils directly or indirectly. In particular, glucocorticoids promote eosinophil apoptosis and inhibit the production of eosinophil-directed cytokines (*e.g.*, IL-5 and eotaxins), and interferon-alpha inhibits eosinophilia, presumably by blocking Th2-cell cytokine production (Rothenberg, 1998). In select patients, imatinib therapy may also be a promising option. Early studies with humanized anti-IL-5 have demonstrated the potency of this agent in reducing circulating levels of eosinophils; the utility of this approach in various disease states is currently being pursued. In conclusion, eosinophils are resident cells of the mucosal immune system, their levels are increased by antigen exposure under Th2-associated conditions, and eotaxin and IL-5 differentially regulate their trafficking in a tissue-specific manner. We propose that eosinophils are integral members of the mucosal immune system (especially the gut-associated lymphoid tissue [GALT]) and are likely to be important in innate, regulatory, and inflammatory immune responses.

ACKNOWLEDGMENTS

Dr. Rothenberg was supported in part by National Institutes of Health grants R01 AI42242, R01 AI45898, and AI53479; the Human Frontier Science Program; the International Life Sciences Institute; and the Burroughs Wellcome Fund. The author thanks Dr. Nives Zimmermann and Andrea Lippelman for their editorial assistance as well as the numerous colleagues and trainees that contributed to the work presented in this chapter.

REFERENCES

Artis, D., Humphreys, N. E., Potten, C. S., Wagner, N., Muller, W., McDermott, J. R., Grencis, R. K., and Else, K. J. (2000). β7 integrin-deficient mice: delayed leukocyte recruitment and attenuated protective immunity in the small intestine during enteric helminthic infection. *Eur. J. Immunol.* 30, 1656–1664.

Assa'ad, A. H., Spicer, R. L., Nelson, D. P., Zimmermann, N., and Rothenberg, M. E. (2000). Hypereosinophilic syndromes. *Chem. Immunol.* 76, 208–229.

Bandeira-Melo, C., Bozza, P. T., and Weller, P. F. (2002). The cellular biology of eosinophil eicosanoid formation and function. *J. Allergy Clin. Immunol.* 109, 393–400.

Bauer, S., Schaub, N., Dommann-Scherrer, C. C., Zimmermann, D. R., Simon, H. U., and Wegmann, W. (1996). Long-term outcome of idiopathic hypereosinophilic syndrome: transition to eosinophilic gastroenteritis and clonal expansion of T-cells. *Eur. J. Gastroenterol. Hepatol.* 8, 181–185.

Behm, C. A., and Ovington, K. S. (2000). The role of eosinophils in parasitic helminth infections: insights from genetically modified mice. *Parasitol. Today* 16, 202–209.

Berkman, N., Ohnona, S., Chung, F. K., and Breuer, R. (2001). Eotaxin-3 but not eotaxin gene expression is upregulated in asthmatics 24 hours after allergen challenge. *Am. J. Respir. Cell Mol. Biol.* 24, 682–687.

Bertrand, C. P., and Ponath, P. D. (2000). CCR3 blockade as a new therapy for asthma. *Expert. Opin. Investig. Drugs* 9, 43–52.

Bhathena, P. R., Comhair, S. A., Holroyd, K. J., and Erzurum, S. C. (2000). Interleukin-9 receptor expression in asthmatic airways *In vivo. Lung* 178, 149–160.

Bischoff, S. C., Brunner, T., De Weck, A. L., and Dahinden, C. A. (1990). Interleukin 5 modifies histamine release and leukotriene generation by human basophils in response to diverse agonists. *J. Exp. Med.* 172, 1577–1582.

Bochner, B. S., Klunk, D. A., Sterbinsky, S. A., Coffman, R. L., and Schleimer, R. P. (1995). IL-13 selectively induces vascular cell adhesion molecule-1 expression in human endothelial cells. *J. Immunol.* 154, 799–803.

Bochner, B. S., and Schleimer, R. P. (1994). The role of adhesion molecules in human eosinophil and basophil recruitment. *J. Allergy Clin. Immunol.* 94, 427–438.

Bochner, B. S., Undem, B. J., and Lichtenstein, L. M. (1994). Immunological aspects of allergic asthma. *Annu. Rev. Immunol.* 12, 295–335.

Boyce, J. A., Friend, D., Matsumoto, R., Austen, K. F., and Owen, W. F. (1995). Differentiation *in vitro* of hybrid eosinophil/basophil granulocytes: autocrine function of an eosinophil developmental intermediate. *J. Exp. Med.* 182, 49–57.

Brandt, E. B., Strait, R. T., Hersko, D., Wang, Q., Muntel, E. E., Scribner, T. A., Zimmermann, N., Finkelman, F. D., and Rothenberg, M. E. (2003). Mast cells are required for experimental oral allergen-induced diarrhea. *J. Clin. Invest.* 112, 666–667.

Broide, D., and Sriramarao, P. (2001). Eosinophil trafficking to sites of allergic inflammation. *Immunol. Rev.* 179, 163–172.

Broide, D. H. (2001). Molecular and cellular mechanisms of allergic disease. *J. Allergy Clin. Immunol.* 108, S65–71.

Brown, L. F., Goldman, H., and Antonioli, D. A. (1984). Intraepithelial eosinophils in endoscopic biopsies of adults with reflux esophagitis. *Am. J. Surg. Pathol.* 8, 899–905.

Brusselle, G. G., Kips, J. C., Tavernier, J. H., van der Heyden, J. G., Cuvelier, C. A., Pauwels, R. A., and Bluethmann, H. (1994). Attenuation of allergic airway inflammation in IL-4 deficient mice. *Clin. Exper. Allergy* 24, 73–80.

Busse, W. W., and Lemanske, R. F., Jr. (2001). Asthma. *N. Engl. J. Med.* 344, 350–362.

Butcher, E. C., Williams, M., Youngman, K., Rott, L., and Briskin, M. (1999). Lymphocyte trafficking and regional immunity. *Adv. Immunol.* 72, 209–253.

Butterworth, A. E. (1977). The eosinophil and its role in immunity to helminth infection. *Curr. Top. Microbiol. Immunol.* 77, 127–168.

Butterworth, A. E. (1984). Cell-mediated damage to helminths. *Adv. Parasitol.* 23, 143–235.

Campbell, E. M., Kunkel, S. L., Strieter, R. M., and Lukacs, N. W. (1998). Temporal role of chemokines in a murine model of cockroach allergen–induced airway hyperreactivity and eosinophilia. *J. Immunol.* 161, 7047–7053.

Cello, J. P. (1979). Eosinophilic gastroenteritis: A complex disease entity. *Am. J. Med.* 67, 1097–1114.

Collins, P. D., Marleau, S., Griffiths-Johnson, D. A., Jose, P. J., and Williams, T. J. (1995). Cooperation between interleukin-5 and the chemokine eotaxin to induce eosinophil accumulation *in vivo. J. Exp. Med.* 182, 1169–1174.

Combadiere, C., Ahuja, S. K., and Murphy, P. M. (1995). Cloning and functional expression of a human eosinophil CC chemokine receptor. *J. Biol. Chem.* 270, 16491–16494.

Cools, J., DeAngelo, D. J., Gotlib, J., Stover, E. H., Legare, R. D., Cortes, J., Kutok, J., Clark, J., Galinsky, I., Griffin, J. D., Cross, N. C., Tefferi, A., Malone, J., Alam, R., Schrier, S. L., Schmid, J., Rose, M., Vandenberghe, P., Verhoef, G., Boogaerts, M.,

Wlodarska, I., Kantarjian, H., Marynen, P., Coutre, S. E., Stone, R., and Gilliland, D. G. (2003). A tyrosine kinase created by fusion of the PDGFRA and FIP1L1 genes as a therapeutic target of imatinib in idiopathic hypereosinophilic syndrome. *N. Engl. J. Med.* 348, 1201–1214.

Corry, D. B., Folkesson, M. L., Warnock, D. J., Erle, D. J., Matthay, M. A., Wiener-Kronish, J. P., and Locksley, R. C. (1996). Interleukin 4, but not interleukin 5 or eosinophils, is required in a murine model of acute airway hyperreactivity. *J. Exp. Med.* 183, 109–117.

Daugherty, B. L., Siciliano, S. J., DeMartino, J. A., Malkowitz, L., Sirotina, A., and Springer, M. S. (1996). Cloning, expression, and characterization of the human eosinophil eotaxin receptor. *J. Exp. Med.* 183, 2349–2354.

De Monchy, J. G., Kauffman, H. F., Venge, P., Koeter, G. H., Jansen, H. M., Sluiter, H. J., and De Vries, K. (1985). Bronchoalveolar eosinophilia during allergen-induced late asthmatic reactions. *Am. Rev. Respir. Dis.* 131, 373–376.

Dent, L. A., Strath, M., Mellor, A. L., and Sanderson, C. J. (1990). Eosinophilia in transgenic mice expressing interleukin 5. *J. Exp. Med.* 172, 1425–1431.

Denzler, K. L., Farmer, S. C., Crosby, J. R., Borchers, M., Cieslewicz, G., Larson, K. A., Cormier-Regard, S., Lee, N. A., and Lee, J. J. (2000). Eosinophil major basic protein-1 does not contribute to allergen-induced airway pathologies in mouse models of asthma. *J. Immunol.* 165, 5509–5517.

Desreumaux, P., Bloget, F., Seguy, D., Capron, M., Cortot, A., Colombel, J. F., and Janin, A. (1996). Interleukin 3, granulocyte-macrophage colony-stimulating factor, and interleukin 5 in eosinophilic gastroenteritis. *Gastroenterology* 110, 768–774.

Desreumaux, P., Nutten, S., and Colombel, J. F. (1999). Activated eosinophils in inflammatory bowel disease: do they matter? *Am. J. Gastroenterol.* 94, 3396–3398.

Drazen, J. M., Arm, J. P., and Austen, K. F. (1996). Sorting out the cytokines of asthma. *J. Exp. Med.* 183, 1–5.

Du, J., Stankiewicz, M. J., Liu, Y., Xi, Q., Schmitz, J. E., Lekstrom-Himes, J. A., and Ackerman, S. J. (2002). Novel combinatorial interactions of GATA-1, PU.1, and C/EBPepsilon isoforms regulate transcription of the gene encoding eosinophil granule major basic protein. *J. Biol. Chem.* 277, 43481–43494.

Dvorak, A. M. (1980). Ultrastructural evidence for release of major basic protein-containing crystalline cores of eosinophil granules *in vivo*: cytotoxic potential in Crohn's disease. *J. Immunol.* 125, 460–462.

Dvorak, A. M., Onderdonk, A. B., McLeod, R. S., Monahan-Earley, R. A., Antonioli, D. A., Cullen, J., Blair, J. E., Cisneros, R., Letourneau, L., and Morgan, E. (1993). Ultrastructural identification of exocytosis of granules from human gut eosinophils *in vivo*. *Int. Arch. Allergy Immunol.* 102, 33–45.

Elias, J. A., Lee, C. G., Zheng, T., Ma, B., Homer, R. J., and Zhu, Z. (2003). New insights into the pathogenesis of asthma. *J. Clin. Invest.* 111, 291–297.

Ferguson, A. (1976). Models of intestinal hypersensitivity. *Clin. Gastroenterol.* 5, 271–288.

Ferguson, A., and Parrott, D. M. (1972a). The effect of antigen deprivation on thymus-dependent and thymus-independent lymphocytes in the small intestine of the mouse. *Clin. Exp. Immunol.* 12, 477–488.

Ferguson, A., and Parrott, D. M. (1972b). Growth and development of "antigen-free" grafts of foetal mouse intestine. *J. Pathol.* 106, 95–101.

Flood-Page, P., Menzies-Gow, A., Phipps, S., Compton, C., Walls, C., Barnes, N., Robinson, D. S., and Kay, A. B. (2002). Reduction of tissue eosinophils in mild atopic asthmatics by an anti-IL-5 monoclonal antibody (mepolizumab) is associated with inhibition of tenascin deposition within the bronchial epithelium basement membrane. *Am. J. Respir. Crit. Care Med.* 109, 165.

Flood-Page, P., Phipps, S., Menzies-Gow, A., Ong, Y. E., and Kay, A. B. (2003a). Effect of intravenous administration of an anti-IL-5 (mepolizumab) on allergen-induced tissue eosinophilia, the late-phase allergic reaction and the expression of a marker of repair/remodeling in human atopic subjects. *J. Allergy Clin. Immunol.* 111, S261.

Flood-Page, P. T., Menzies-Gow, A. N., Kay, A. B., and Robinson, D. S. (2003b). Eosinophil's role remains uncertain as anti-interleukin-5 only partially depletes numbers in asthmatic airway. *Am. J. Respir. Crit. Care Med.* 167, 199–204.

Floyd, H., Ni, J., Cornish, A. L., Zeng, Z., Liu, D., Carter, K. C., Steel, J., and Crocker, P. R. (2000). Siglec-8. A novel eosinophil-specific member of the immunoglobulin superfamily. *J. Biol. Chem.* 275, 861–866.

Forssmann, U., Uguccioni, M., Loetscher, P., Dahinden, C. A., Langen, H., Thelen, M., and Baggiolini, M. (1997). Eotaxin-2, a novel CC chemokine that is selective for the chemokine receptor CCR3, and acts like eotaxin on human eosinophil and basophil leukocytes. *J. Exp. Med.* 185, 2171–2176.

Foster, P. S., Hogan, S. P., Ramsay, A. J., Matthaei, K. I., and Young, I. G. (1996). Interleukin 5 deficiency abolishes eosinophilia, airways hyperreactivity, and lung damage in a mouse asthma model. *J. Exp. Med.* 183, 195–201.

Foster, P. S., Mould, A. W., Yang, M., Mackenzie, J., Mattes, J., Hogan, S. P., Mahalingam, S., McKenzie, A. N., Rothenberg, M. E., Young, I. G., Matthaei, K. I., and Webb, D. C. (2001). Elemental signals regulating eosinophil accumulation in the lung. *Immunol. Rev.* 179, 173–181.

Fox, V. L., Nurko, S., and Furuta, G. T. (2002). Eosinophilic esophagitis: It's not just kid's stuff. *Gastrointest. Endosc.* 56, 260–270.

Frigas, E., Loegering, D. A., and Gleich, G. J. (1980). Cytotoxic effects of the guinea pig eosinophil major basic protein on tracheal epithelium. *Lab. Invest.* 42, 35–43.

Fuss, I. J., Neurath, M., Boirivant, M., Klein, J. S., de la Motte, C., Strong, S. A., Fiocchi, C., and Strober, W. (1996). Disparate CD4+ lamina propria (LP) lymphokine secretion profiles in inflammatory bowel disease. Crohn's disease LP cells manifest increased secretion of IFN-gamma, whereas ulcerative colitis LP cells manifest increased secretion of IL-5. *J. Immunol.* 157, 1261–1270.

Garcia-Zepeda, E. A., Rothenberg, M. E., Ownbey, R. T., Celestin, J., Leder, P., and Luster, A. D. (1996). Human eotaxin is a specific chemoattractant for eosinophil cells and provides a new mechanism to explain tissue eosinophilia. *Nat. Med.* 2, 449–456.

Gleich, G. J. (2000). Mechanisms of eosinophil-associated inflammation. *J. Allergy Clin. Immunol.* 105, 651–663.

Gleich, G. J., and Adolphson, C. R. (1986). The eosinophilic leukocyte: structure and function. *Adv. Immunol.* 39, 177–253.

Gleich, G. J., Frigas, E., Loegering, D. A., Wassom, D. L., and Steinmuller, D. (1979). Cytotoxic properties of the eosinophil major basic protein. *J. Immunol.* 123, 2925–2927.

Gonzalo, J.-A., Jia, G.-Q., Aquirre, V., Friend, D., Coyle, A. J., Jenkins, N. A., Lin, G.-S., Katz, H., Lichtman, A., Copeland, N., Kopf, M., and Gutierrez-Ramos, J.-C. (1996). Mouse eotaxin expression parallels eosinophil accumulation during lung allergic inflammation but is not restricted to a Th2-type response. *Immunity* 4, 1–14.

Gonzalo, J. A., Lloyd, C. M., Wen, D., Albar, J. P., Wells, T. N., Proudfoot, A., Martinez, A. C., Dorf, M., Bjerke, T., Coyle, A. J., and Gutierrez-Ramos, J. C. (1998). The coordinated action of CC chemokines in the lung orchestrates allergic inflammation and airway hyperresponsiveness. *J. Exp. Med.* 188, 157–167.

Gouon-Evans, V., and Pollard, J. W. (2001). Eotaxin is required for eosinophil homing into the stroma of the pubertal and cycling uterus. *Endocrinology* 142, 4515–4521.

Gouon-Evans, V., Rothenberg, M. E., and Pollard, J. W. (2000). Postnatal mammary gland development requires macrophages and eosinophils. *Development* 127, 2269–2282.

Green, R. H., Brightling, C. E., McKenna, S., Hargadon, B., Parker, D., Bradding, P., Wardlaw, A. J., and Pavord, I. D. (2002). Asthma exacerbations and sputum eosinophil counts: a randomised controlled trial. *Lancet* 360, 1715–1721.

Guajardo, J. R., Plotnick, L. M., Fende, J. M., Collins, M. H., Putnam, P. E., and Rothenberg, M. E. (2002). Eosinophil-associated gastrointestinal disorders: A world-wide-web based registry. *J. Pediatr.* 141, 576–581.

Gurish, M. F., Humbles, A., Tao, H., Finkelstein, S., Boyce, J. A., Gerard, C., Friend, D. S., and Austen, K. F. (2002). CCR3 is required for tissue eosinophilia and larval cytotoxicity after infection with *Trichinella spiralis*. *J. Immunol.* 168, 5730–5736.

Gurish, M. F., Tao, H., Abonia, J. P., Arya, A., Friend, D. S., Parker, C. M., and Austen, K. F. (2001). Intestinal mast cell progenitors require CD49β7 (α4β7 integrin) for tissue-specific homing. *J. Exp. Med.* 194, 1243–1252.

Gutierrez-Ramos, J. C., Lloyd, C., and Gonzalo, J. A. (1999). Eotaxin: from an eosinophilic chemokine to a major regulator of allergic reactions. *Immunol. Today* 20, 500–504.

Hakonarson, H., Maskeri, N., Carter, C., Chuang, S., and Grunstein, M. M. (1999). Autocrine interaction between IL-5 and IL-1beta mediates altered responsiveness of atopic asthmatic sensitized airway smooth muscle. *J. Clin. Invest.* 104, 657–667.

Hamelmann, E., and Gelfand, E. W. (2001). IL-5-induced airway eosinophilia: the key to asthma? *Immunol. Rev.* 179, 182–191.

Hamelmann, E., Oshiba, A., Loader, J., Larsen, G. L., Gleich, G., Lee, J., and Gelfand, E. W. (1997a). Antiinterleukin-5 antibody prevents airway hyperresponsiveness in a murine model of airway sensitization. *Am. J. Respir. Crit. Care Med.* 155, 819–825.

Hamelmann, E., Schwarze, J., Takeda, K., Oshiba, A., Larsen, G. L., Irvin, C. G., and Gelfand, E. W. (1997b). Noninvasive measurement of airway responsiveness in allergic mice using barometric plethysmography. *Am. J. Respir. Crit. Care Med.* 156, 766–775.

Hankard, G. F., Brousse, N., Cezard, J. P., Emilie, D., and Peuchmaur, M. (1997). In situ interleukin 5 gene expression in pediatric Crohn's disease. *J. Pediatr. Gastroenterol. Nutr.* 24, 568–572.

Heath, H., Qin, S. X., Rao, P., Wu, L. J., Larosa, G., Kassam, N., Ponath, P. D., and Mackay, C. R. (1997). Chemokine receptor usage by human eosinophils: the importance of CCR3 demonstrated using an antagonistic monoclonal antibody. *J. Clin. Invest.* 99, 178–184.

Hill, S. M., and Milla, P. J. (1990). Colitis caused by food allergy in infants. *Arch. Dis. Child.* 65, 132–133.

Hogan, S. P., Foster, P. S., and Rothenberg, M. E. (2002). Experimental analysis of eosinophil-associated gastrointestinal diseases. *Curr. Opin. Allergy Clin. Immunol.* 2, 239–248.

Hogan, S. P., Koskinen, A., Matthaei, K. I., Young, I. G., and Foster, P. S. (1998a). Interleukin-5-producing CD4+ T cells play a pivotal role in aeroallergen-induced eosinophilia, bronchial hyperreactivity, and lung damage in mice. *Am. J. Respir. Crit. Care Med.* 157, 210–218.

Hogan, S. P., Mishra, A., Brandt, E. B., Foster, P. S., and Rothenberg, M. E. (2000). A critical role for eotaxin in experimental oral antigen-induced eosinophilic gastrointestinal allergy. *Proc. Natl. Acad. Sci. USA* 97, 6681–6686.

Hogan, S. P., Mishra, A., Brandt, E. B., Royalty, M. P., Pope, S. M., Zimmermann, N., Foster, P. S., and Rothenberg, M. E. (2001). A pathological function for eotaxin and eosinophils in eosinophilic gastrointestinal inflammation. *Nat. Immunol.* 2, 353–360.

Hogan, S. P., Mould, A. W., Young, J. M., Rothenberg, M. E., Ramsay, A. J., Matthaei, K., Young, I. G., and Foster, P. S. (1998b). Cellular and molecular regulation of eosinophil trafficking to the lung. *Immunol. Cell Biol.* 76, 454–460.

Holgate, S. T., Peters-Golden, M., Panettieri, R. A., and Henderson, W. R., Jr. (2003). Roles of cysteinyl leukotrienes in airway inflammation, smooth muscle function, and remodeling. *J. Allergy Clin. Immunol.* 111, S18–S36.

Hornung, D., Dohrn, K., Sotlar, K., Greb, R. R., Wallwiener, D., Kiesel, L., and Taylor, R. N. (2000). Localization in tissues and secretion of eotaxin by cells from normal endometrium and endometriosis. *J. Clin. Endocrinol. Metab.* 85, 2604–2608.

Humbles, A. A., Lu, B., Friend, D. S., Okinaga, S., Lora, J., Al-Garawi, A., Martin, T. R., Gerard, N. P., and Gerard, C. (2002). The murine CCR3 receptor regulates both the role of eosinophils and mast cells in allergen-induced airway inflammation and hyperresponsiveness. *Proc. Natl. Acad. Sci. USA* 99, 1479–1484.

Iwama, T., Nagai, H., Suda, H., Tsuruoka, N., and Koda, A. (1992). Effect of murine recombinant interleukin-5 on the cell population in guinea-pig airways. *Brit. J. Pharmacol.* 105, 19–22.

Iwama, T., Nagai, H., Tsuruoka, N., and Koda, A. (1993). Effect of murine recombinant interleukin-5 on bronchial reactivity in guinea-pigs. *Clin. Exp. Allergy* 23, 32–38.

Jacoby, D. B., Gleich, G. J., and Fryer, A. D. (1993). Human eosinophil major basic protein is an endogenous allosteric antagonist at the inhibitory muscarinic M2 receptor. *J. Clin. Invest.* 91, 1314–1318.

Jarjour, N. N., Calhoun, W. J., Kelly, E. A., Gleich, G. J., Schwartz, L. B., and Busse, W. W. (1997). The immediate and late allergic response to segmental bronchopulmonary provocation in asthma. *Am. J. Respir. Crit. Care Med.* 155, 1515–1521.

Jose, P. J., Griffiths-Johnson, D. A., Collins, P. D., Walsh, D. T., Moqbel, R., Totty, N. F., Truong, O., Hsuan, J. J., and Williams, T. J. (1994). Eotaxin: a potent eosinophil chemoattractant cytokine detected in a guinea pig model of allergic airways inflammation. *J. Exp. Med.* 179, 881–887.

Justice, J. P., Borchers, M. T., Crosby, J. R., Hines, E. M., Shen, H. H., Ochkur, S. I., McGarry, M. P., Lee, N. A., and Lee, J. J. (2003). Ablation of eosinophils leads to a reduction of allergen-induced pulmonary pathology. *Am. J. Physiol. Lung Cell Mol. Physiol.* 284, L169–178.

Kato, M., Kephart, G. M., Talley, N. J., Wagner, J. M., Sarr, M. G., Bonno, M., McGovern, T. W., and Gleich, G. J. (1998). Eosinophil infiltration and degranulation in normal human tissue. *Anat. Rec.* 252, 418–425.

Katz, A. J., Twarog, F. J., Zeiger, R. S., and Falchuk, Z. M. (1984). Milk-sensitive and eosinophilic gastroenteropathy: similar clinical features with contrasting mechanisms and clinical course. *J. Allergy Clin. Immunol.* 74, 72–78.

Kelly, K. J. (2000). Eosinophilic gastroenteritis. *J. Pediatr. Gastroenterol. Nutr.* 30, S28–35.

Kelly, K. J., Lazenby, A. J., Rowe, P. C., Yardley, J. H., Perman, J. A., and Sampson, H. A. (1995). Eosinophilic esophagitis attributed to gastroesophageal reflux: improvement with an amino acid–based formula. *Gastroenterology* 109, 1503–1512.

Keshavarzian, A., Saverymuttu, S. H., Tai, P. C., Thompson, M., Barter, S., Spry, C. J., and Chadwick, V. S. (1985). Activated eosinophils in familial eosinophilic gastroenteritis. *Gastroenterology* 88, 1041–1049.

Kikly, K. K., Bochner, B. S., Freeman, S. D., Tan, K. B., Gallagher, K. T., D'Alessio K, J., Holmes, S. D., Abrahamson, J. A., Erickson-Miller, C. L., Murdock, P. R., Tachimoto, H., Schleimer, R. P., and White, J. R. (2000). Identification of SAF-2, a novel siglec expressed on eosinophils, mast cells, and basophils. *J. Allergy Clin. Immunol.* 105, 1093–1100.

Kita, H. (1996). The eosinophil: a cytokine-producing cell? *J. Allergy Clin. Immunol.* 97, 889–892.

Kitaura, M., Suzuki, N., Imai, T., Takagi, S., Suzuki, R., Nakajima, T., Hirai, K., Nomiyama, H., and Yoshie, O. (1999). Molecular cloning of a novel human CC chemokine (Eotaxin-3) that is a functional ligand of CC chemokine receptor 3. *J. Biol. Chem.* 274, 27975–27980.

Kitayama, J., Fuhlbrigge, R. C., Puri, K. D., and Springer, T. A. (1997). P-selectin, L-selectin, and alpha 4 integrin have distinct roles in eosinophil tethering and arrest on vascular endothelial cells under physiological flow conditions. *J. Immunol.* 159, 3929–3939.

Klein, N. C., Hargrove, R. L., Sleisenger, M. H., and Jeffries, G. H. (1970). Eosinophilic gastroenteritis. *Medicine* 49, 299–319.

Korenaga, M., Hitoshi, Y., Yamaguchi, N., Sato, Y., Takatsu, K., and Tada, I. (1991). The role of interleukin-5 in protective immunity to *Strongyloides venezuelensis* infection in mice. *Immunology* 72, 502–507.

Kurup, V. P., Mauze, S., Choi, H., Seymour, B. W., and Coffman, R. L. (1992). A murine model of allergic bronchopulmonary aspergillosis with elevated eosinophils and IgE. *J. Immunol.* 148, 3783–3788.

Kweon, M. N., Yamamoto, M., Kajiki, M., Takahashi, I., and Kiyono, H. (2000). Systemically derived large intestinal CD4(+) Th2 cells play a central role in STAT6-mediated allergic diarrhea. *J. Clin. Invest.* 106, 199–206.

Lacy, P., Levi-Schaffer, F., Mahmudi-Azer, S., Bablitz, B., Hagen, S. C., Velazquez, J., Kay, A. B., and Moqbel, R. (1998). Intracellular localization of interleukin-6 in eosinophils from atopic asthmatics and effects of interferon gamma. *Blood* 91, 2508–2516.

Lam, S., LeRiche, J., Phillips, D., and Chan-Yeung, M. (1987). Cellular and protein changes in bronchial lavage fluid after late asthmatic reaction in patients with red cedar asthma. *J. Allergy Clin. Immunol.* 80, 44–50.

Lamkhioued, B., Renzi, P. M., Abi-Younes, S., Garcia-Zepeda, E. A., Allakhverdi, Z., Ghaffar, O., Rothenberg, M. E., Luster, A. D., and Hamid, Q. (1997). Increased expression of eotaxin in bronchoalveolar lavage and airways of asthmatics contributes to the chemotaxis of eosinophils to the site of inflammation. *J. Immunol.* 159, 4593–4601.

Lander, E. S., Linton, L. M., Birren, B., Nusbaum, C., Zody, M. C., Baldwin, J., Devon, K., Dewar, K., Doyle, M., FitzHugh, W., Funke, R., Gage, D., Harris, K., Heaford, A., Howland, J., Kann, L., Lehoczky, J., LeVine, R., McEwan, P., McKernan, K., Meldrim, J., Mesirov, J. P., Miranda, C., Morris, W., Naylor, J., Raymond, C., Rosetti, M., Santos, R., Sheridan, A., Sougnez, C., Stange-Thomann, N., Stojanovic, N., Subramanian, A., Wyman, D., Rogers, J., Sulston, J., Ainscough, R., Beck, S., Bentley, D., Burton, J., Clee, C., Carter, N., Coulson, A., Deadman, R., Deloukas, P., Dunham, A., Dunham, I., Durbin, R., French, L., Grafham, D., Gregory, S., Hubbard, T., Humphray, S., Hunt, A., Jones, M., Lloyd, C., McMurray, A., Matthews, L., Mercer, S., Milne, S., Mullikin, J. C., Mungall, A., Plumb, R., Ross, M., Shownkeen, R., Sims, S., Waterston, R. H., Wilson, R. K., Hillier, L. W., McPherson, J. D., Marra, M. A., Mardis, E. R., Fulton, L. A., Chinwalla, A. T., Pepin, K. H., Gish, W. R., Chissoe, S. L., Wendl, M. C., Delehaunty, K. D., Miner, T. L., Delehaunty, A., Kramer, J. B., Cook, L. L., Fulton, R. S., Johnson, D. L., Minx, P. J., Clifton, S. W., Hawkins, T., Branscomb, E., Predki, P., Richardson, P., Wenning, S., Slezak, T., Doggett, N., Cheng, J. F., Olsen, A., Lucas, S., Elkin, C., Uberbacher, E., Frazier, M. (2001). Initial sequencing and analysis of the human genome. *Nature* 409, 860–921.

Leckie, M. J., ten Brinke, A., Khan, J., Diamant, Z., O'Connor, B. J., Walls, C. M., Mathur, A. K., Cowley, H. C., Chung, K. F., Djukanovic, R., Hansel, T. T., Holgate, S. T., Sterk, P. J., and Barnes, P. J. (2000). Effects of an interleukin-5 blocking monoclonal antibody on eosinophils, airway hyper-responsiveness, and the late asthmatic response. *Lancet* 356, 2144–2148.

Lee, J. J., McGarry, M. P., Farmer, S. C., Denzler, K. L., Larson, K. A., Carrigan, P. E., Brenneise, I. E., Horton, M. A., Haczku, A., Gelfand, E. W., Leikauf, G. D., and Lee, N. A. (1997a). Interleukin-5 expression in the lung epithelium of transgenic mice leads to pulmonary changes pathognomonic of asthma. *J. Exp. Med.* 185, 2143–2156.

Lee, N. A., McGarry, M. P., Larson, K. A., Horton, M. A., Kristensen, A. B., and Lee, J. J. (1997b). Expression of IL-5 in thymocytes/T cells leads to the development of a massive eosinophilia, extramedullary eosinophilopoiesis, and unique histopathologies. *J. Immunol.* 158, 1332–1344.

Leong, K. P., and Huston, D. P. (2001). Understanding the pathogenesis of allergic asthma using mouse models. *Ann. Allergy Asthma Immunol.* 87, 96–109.

Lewis, R. A., Austen, K. F., and Soberman, R. J. (1990). Leukotrienes and other products of the 5-lipoxygenase pathway. Biochemistry and relation to pathobiology in human diseases. *N. Engl. J. Med.* 323, 645–655.

Liacouras, C. A., Wenner, W. J., Brown, K., and Ruchelli, E. (1998). Primary eosinophilic esophagitis in children: successful treatment with oral corticosteroids. *J. Pediatr. Gastroenterol. Nutr.* 26, 380–385.

Lilly, C. M., Nakamura, H., Belostotsky, O. I., Haley, K. J., Garcia-Zepeda, E. A., Luster, A. D., and Israel, E. (2001). Eotaxin expression after segmental allergen challenge in subjects with atopic asthma. *Am. J. Respir. Crit. Care Med.* 163, 1669–1675.

Lucey, D. R., Nicholson, W. A., and Weller, P. F. (1989). Mature human eosinophils have the capacity to express HLA-DR. *Proc. Natl. Acad. Sci. USA* 86, 1348–1351.

Luster, A. D., and Rothenberg, M. E. (1997). Role of monocyte chemoattractant protein and eotaxin subfamily of chemokines in allergic inflammation. *J. Leukoc. Biol.* 62, 620–633.

Ma, W., Bryce, P. J., Humbles, A. A., Laouini, D., Yalcindag, A., Alenius, H., Friend, D. S., Oettgen, H. C., Gerard, C., and Geha, R. S.

(2002). CCR3 is essential for skin eosinophilia and airway hyper-responsiveness in a murine model of allergic skin inflammation. *J. Clin. Invest.* 109, 621–628.

Makker, H. K., Montefort, S., and Holgate, S. (1993). Investigative use of fibreoptic bronchoscopy for local airway challenge in asthma. *Eur. Respir. J.* 6, 1402–1408.

Maluenda, C., Phillips, A. D., Briddon, A., and Walker-Smith, J. A. (1984). Quantitative analysis of small intestinal mucosa in cow's milk–sensitive enteropathy. *J. Pediatr. Gastroenterol. Nutr.* 3, 349–356.

Mattes, J., Hulett, M., Xie, W., Hogan, S., Rothenberg, M. E., Foster, P., and Parish, C. (2003). Immunotherapy of cytotoxic T cell–resistant tumors by T helper 2 cells: An eotaxin and STAT6-dependent process. *J. Exp. Med.* 197, 387–393.

Mattes, J., Yang, M., Mahalingam, S., Kuehr, J., Webb, D. C., Simson, L., Hogan, S. P., Koskinen, A., McKenzie, A. N., Dent, L. A., Rothenberg, M. E., Matthaei, K. I., Young, I. G., and Foster, P. S. (2002). Intrinsic defect in T cell production of interleukin (IL)-13 in the absence of both IL-5 and eotaxin precludes the development of eosinophilia and airways hyperreactivity in experimental asthma. *J. Exp. Med.* 195, 1433–1444.

Matthews, A. N., Friend, D. S., Zimmermann, N., Sarafi, M. N., Luster, A. D., Pearlman, E., Wert, S. E., and Rothenberg, M. E. (1998). Eotaxin is required for the baseline level of tissue eosinophils. *Proc. Natl. Acad. Sci. USA* 95, 6273–6278.

Mauser, P. J., Pitman, A., Witt, A., Fernandez, X., Zurcher, J., Kung, T., Jones, H., Watnick, A. S., Egan, R. W., Kreutner, W., et al. (1993). Inhibitory effect of the TRFK-5 anti-IL-5 antibody in a guinea pig model of asthma. *Am. Rev. Respir. Dis.* 148:1623–1627.

Menzies-Gow, A., Ying, S., Sabroe, I., Stubbs, V. L., Soler, D., Williams, T. J., and Kay, A. B. (2002). Eotaxin (CCL11) and eotaxin-2 (CCL24) induce recruitment of eosinophils, basophils, neutrophils, and macrophages as well as features of early- and late-phase allergic reactions following cutaneous injection in human atopic and nonatopic volunteers. *J. Immunol.* 169, 2712–2718.

Metwali, A., Blum, A. M., Ferraris, L., Klein, J. S., Fiocchi, C., and Weinstock, J. V. (1994). Eosinophils within the healthy or inflamed human intestine produce substance P and vasoactive intestinal peptide. *J. Neuroimmunol.* 52, 69–78.

Mishra, A., Hogan, S. P., Brandt, E. B., and Rothenberg, M. E. (2000). Peyer's patch eosinophils: identification, characterization, and regulation by mucosal allergen exposure, interleukin-5, and eotaxin. *Blood* 96, 1538–1544.

Mishra, A., Hogan, S. P., Brandt, E. B., and Rothenberg, M. E. (2001). An etiological role for aeroallergens and eosinophils in experimental esophagitis. *J. Clin. Invest.* 107, 83–90.

Mishra, A., Hogan, S. P., Brandt, E. B., and Rothenberg, M. E. (2002a). IL-5 promotes eosinophil trafficking to the esophagus. *J. Immunol.* 168, 2464–2469.

Mishra, A., Hogan, S. P., Brandt, E. B., Wagner, N., Crossman, M. W., Foster, P. S., and Rothenberg, M. E. (2002b). Enterocyte expression of the eotaxin and interleukin-5 transgenes induces compartmentalized dysregulation of eosinophil trafficking. *J. Biol. Chem.* 277, 4406–4412.

Mishra, A., Hogan, S. P., Lee, J. J., Foster, P. S., and Rothenberg, M. E. (1999). Fundamental signals regulate eosinophil homing to the gastrointestinal tract. *J. Clin. Invest.* 103, 1719–1727.

Moon, A., and Kleinman, R. E. (1995). Allergic gastroenteropathy in children. *Ann. Allergy Asthma Immunol.* 74, 5–12.

Mould, A. W., Matthaei, K. I., Young, I. G., and Foster, P. S. (1997). Relationship between interleukin-5 and eotaxin in regulating blood and tissue eosinophilia in mice. *J. Clin. Invest.* 99, 1064–1071.

Mould, A. W., Ramsay, A. J., Matthaei, K. I., Young, I. G., Rothenberg, M. E., and Foster, P. S. (2000). The effect of IL-5 and eotaxin expression in the lung on eosinophil trafficking and degranulation and the induction of bronchial hyperreactivity. *J. Immunol.* 164, 2142–2150.

Nagai, H., Yamaguchi, S., Inagaki, N., Tsuruoka, N., Hitoshi, Y., and Takatsu, K. (1993). Effect of anti-IL-5 monoclonal antibody on allergic bronchial eosinophilia and airway hyperresponsiveness in mice. *Life Sci.* 53, L243–247.

Nakamura, H., Luster, A. D., Nakamura, T., In, K. H., Sonna, L. A., Deykin, A., Israel, E., Drazen, J. M., and Lilly, C. M. (2001). Variant eotaxin: its effects on the asthma phenotype. *J. Allergy Clin. Immunol.* 108, 946–953.

Nicholson, A. G., Li, D., Pastorino, U., Goldstraw, P., and Jeffery, P. K. (1997). Full thickness eosinophilia in oesophageal leiomyomatosis and idiopathic eosinophilic oesophagitis. A common allergic inflammatory profile? *J. Pathol.* 183, 233–236.

Nickel, R., Barnes, K. C., Sengler, C. A., Casolaro, V., Freidhoff, L. R., Weber, P., Naidu, R. P., Caraballo, L., Ehrlich, E., Plitt, J., Schleimer, R. P., Huang, S. K., and Beaty, T. (1999a). Evidence for linkage of chemokine polymorphisms to asthma in populations of African descent. *J. Allergy Clin. Immunol.* 103 (No. 1 Pt 2), S174.

Nickel, R. G., Saitta, F. P., Freidhoff, L. R., Yu, X.Y., Ehrlich, E., Barnes, K. C., Beaty, T., and Huang, S. K. (1999b). Positional candidate gene approach and functional genomics strategy in atopy gene discovery. *Int. Arch. Allergy Immunol.* 118, 282–284.

Nishitani, H., Okabayashi, M., Satomi, M., Shimoyama, T., and Dohi, Y. (1998). Infiltration of peroxidase-producing eosinophils into the lamina propria of patients with ulcerative colitis. *J. Gastroenterol.* 33, 189–195.

Nomiyama, H., Osborne, L. R., Imai, T., Kusuda, J., Miura, R., Tsui, L. C., and Yoshie, O. (1998). Assignment of the human CC chemokine MPIF-2/eotaxin-2 (SCYA24) to chromosome 7q11.23. *Genomics* 49, 339–340.

O'Byrne P, M., Inman, M. D., and Parameswaran, K. (2001). The trials and tribulations of IL-5, eosinophils, and allergic asthma. *J. Allergy Clin. Immunol.* 108, 503–508.

Odze, R. D., Wershil, B. K., Leichtner, A. M., and Antonioli, D. A. (1995). Allergic colitis in infants. *J. Pediatr.* 126, 163–170.

Ohkawara, Y., Lim, K. G., Xing, Z., Glibetic, M., Nakano, K., Dolovich, J., Croitoru, K., Weller, P. F., and Jordana, M. (1996). CD40 expression by human peripheral blood eosinophils. *J. Clin. Invest.* 97, 1761–1766.

Ohkawara, Y., Tamura, G., Iwasaki, T., Tanaka, A., Kikuchi, T., and Shirato, K. (2000). Activation and transforming growth factor-beta production in eosinophils by hyaluronan. *Am. J. Respir. Cell Mol. Biol.* 23, 444–451.

Patel, V. P., Kreider, B. L., Li, Y., Li, H., Leung, K., Salcedo, T., Nardelli, B., Pippalla, V., Gentz, S., Thotakura, R., Parmelee, D., Gentz, R., and Garotta, G. (1997). Molecular and functional characterization of two novel human C-C chemokines as inhibitors of two distinct classes of myeloid progenitors. *J. Exp. Med.* 185, 1163–1172.

Pereira, S., Taylor-Clark, T., Darby, Y., Powell, J., Howarth, P., and Scadding, G. (2003). Effects of anti-eotaxin monoclonal antibody CAT-213 on allergen-induced rhinitis. *J. Allergy Clin. Immunol.* 111, S268.

Phipps, S., Flood-Page, P., Menzies-Gow, A., Wangoo, A., Barnes, N. C., Barkans, J., Robinson, D. S., and Kay, A. B. (2003). Anti-IL-5 (mepolizumab) reduces the expression of tenascin, procollagen and lumican in the reticular basement membrane of human atopic asthmatics. *J. Allergy Clin. Immunol.* 111, S278.

Phipps, S., Ying, S., and Kay, A. B. (2002). The relationship of infiltrating eosinophils to markers of repair and resolution (myofibroblasts, TGF-β and tenascin) in allergen-induced late phase reactions in human skin. *J. Allergy Clin. Immunol.* 109, S169.

Phipps, S., Ying, S., Wangoo, A., Ong, Y. E., Levi-Schaffer, F., and Kay, A. B. (2002). The relationship between allergen-induced tissue eosinophilia and markers of repair and remodeling in human atopic skin. *J. Immunol.* 169, 4604–4612.

Pinto, A., Aldinucci, D., Gloghini, A., Zagonel, V., Degan, M., Improta, S., Juzbasic, S., Todesco, M., Perin, V., Gattei, V., Herrmann, F., Gruss, H. J., and Carbone, A. (1996). Human eosinophils express functional CD30 ligand and stimulate proliferation of a Hodgkin's disease cell line. *Blood* 88, 3299–3305.

Pinto, A., Aldinucci, D., Gloghini, A., Zagonel, V., Degan, M., Perin, V., Todesco, M., De Iuliis, A., Improta, S., Sacco, C., Gattei, V., Gruss, H. J., and Carbone, A. (1997). The role of eosinophils in the pathobiology of Hodgkin's disease. *Ann. Oncol.* 8, 89–96.

Ponath, P. D., Qin, S., Post, T. W., Wang, J., Wu, L., Gerard, N. P., Newman, W., Gerard, C., and Mackay, C. R. (1996). Molecular cloning and characterization of a human eotaxin receptor expressed selectively on eosinophils. *J. Exp. Med.* 183, 2437–2448.

Ponath, P. D., Qin, S. X., Ringler, D. J., Clark-Lewis, I., Wang, J., Kassam, N., Smith, H., Shi, X. J., Gonzalo, J. A., Newman, W., Gutierrez-Ramos, J. C., and Mackay, C. R. (1996). Cloning of the human eosinophil chemoattractant, eotaxin. Expression, receptor binding, and functional properties suggest a mechanism for the selective recruitment of eosinophils. *J. Clin. Invest.* 97, 604–612.

Rankin, J. A., Picarella, D. E., Geba, G. P., Temann, U.-A., Prasad, B., DiCosmo, B., Tarallo, A., Stripp, B., Whitsett, J., and Flavell, R. A. (1996). Phenotypic and physiologic characterization of transgenic mice expressing interleukin 4 in the lung: lymphocytic and eosinophilic inflammation without airway hyperreactivity. *Proc. Natl. Acad. Sci. USA* 93, 7821–7825.

Ray, A., and Cohn, L. (1999). Th2 cells and GATA-3 in asthma: new insights into the regulation of airway inflammation. *J. Clin. Invest.* 104, 985–993.

Resnick, M. B., and Weller, P. F. (1993). Mechanisms of eosinophil recruitment. *Am. J. Respir. Cell. Mol. Biol.* 8, 349–355.

Rosenberg, H. F., and Domachowske, J. B. (2001). Eosinophils, eosinophil ribonucleases, and their role in host defense against respiratory virus pathogens. *J. Leukoc. Biol.* 70, 691–698.

Rosenberg, H. F., Dyer, K. D., Tiffany, H. L., and Gonzalez, M. (1995). Rapid evolution of a unique family of primate ribonuclease genes. *Nat. Genet.* 10, 219–223.

Rothenberg, M. E. (1998). Eosinophilia. *N. Engl. J. Med.* 338, 1592–1600.

Rothenberg, M. E. (2003). CD44: a sticky target for asthma. *J. Clin. Invest.* 111, 1460–1462.

Rothenberg, M. E., Luster, A. D., and Leder, P. (1995a). Murine eotaxin: an eosinophil chemoattractant inducible in endothelial cells and in interleukin 4–induced tumor suppression. *Proc. Natl. Acad. Sci. USA* 92, 8960–8964.

Rothenberg, M. E., Luster, A. D., Lilly, C. M., Drazen, J. M., and Leder, P. (1995b). Constitutive and allergen-induced expression of eotaxin mRNA in the guinea pig lung. *J. Exp. Med.* 181, 1211–1216.

Rothenberg, M. E., MacLean, J. A., Pearlman, E., Luster, A. D., and Leder, P. (1997). Targeted disruption of the chemokine eotaxin partially reduces antigen-induced tissue eosinophilia. *J. Exp. Med.* 185, 785–790.

Rothenberg, M. E., Mishra, A., Brandt, E. B., and Hogan, S. P. (2001a). Gastrointestinal eosinophils. *Immunol. Rev.* 179, 139–155.

Rothenberg, M. E., Mishra, A., Brandt, E. B., and Hogan, S. P. (2001b). Gastrointestinal eosinophils in health and disease. *Adv. Immunol.* 78, 291–328.

Rothenberg, M. E., Mishra, A., Collins, M. H., and Putnam, P. E. (2001c). Pathogenesis and clinical features of eosinophilic esophagitis. *J. Allergy Clin. Immunol.* 108, 891–894.

Rothenberg, M. E., Ownbey, R., Mehlhop, P. D., Loiselle, P. M., Van de Rijn, M., Bonventre, J. V., Oettgen, H. C., Leder, P., and Luster, A. D. (1996). Eotaxin triggers eosinophil-selective chemotaxis and calcium flux via a distinct receptor and induces pulmonary eosinophilia in the presence of interleukin 5 in mice. *Molec. Med.* 2, 334–348.

Ruchelli, E., Wenner, W., Voytek, T., Brown, K., and Liacouras, C. (1999). Severity of esophageal eosinophilia predicts response to conventional gastroesophageal reflux therapy. *Pediatr. Dev. Pathol.* 2, 15–18.

Saavedra-Delgado, A. M., and Metcalfe, D. D. (1985). Interactions between food antigens and the immune system in the pathogenesis of gastrointestinal diseases. *Ann. Allergy* 55, 694–702.

Sabroe, I., Peck, M. J., Van Keulen, B. J., Jorritsma, A., Simmons, G., Clapham, P. R., Williams, T. J., and Pease, J. E. (2000). A small molecule antagonist of chemokine receptors CCR1 and CCR3. Potent inhibition of eosinophil function and CCR3-mediated HIV-1 entry. *J. Biol. Chem.* 275, 25985–25992.

Salamonsen, L. A., and Lathbury, L. J. (2000). Endometrial leukocytes and menstruation. *Hum. Reprod. Update* 6, 16–27.

Salib, R., Salagean, M., Lau, L., DiGiovanna, I., Brennan, N., Scadding, G., and Howarth, P. (2003). The anti-inflammatory response of anti-eotaxin monoclonal antibody CAT-213 on nasal allergen-induced cell infiltration and activation. *J. Allergy Clin. Immunol.* 111, S347.

Sampson, H. A. (1999). Food allergy. Part 1: immunopathogenesis and clinical disorders. *J. Allergy Clin. Immunol.* 103, 717–728.

Sandborn, W. J., and Targan, S. R. (2002). Biologic therapy of inflammatory bowel disease. *Gastroenterology* 122, 1592–1608.

Sanderson, C. J. (1990). The biological role of interleukin 5. *Int. J. Cell Cloning* 8, 147–153; discussion 153–144.

Sanderson, C. J. (1992). Interleukin-5, eosinophils, and disease. *Blood* 79, 3101–3109.

Sarin, S. K., Malhotra, V., Sen Gupta, S., Karol, A., Gaur, S. K., and Anand, B. S. (1978). Significance of eosinophil and mast cell counts in rectal mucosa in ulcerative colitis. A prospective controlled study. *Dig. Dis. Sci.* 32, 363–367.

Shaw, S. K., and Brenner, M. B. (1995). The beta 7 integrins in mucosal homing and retention. *Semin. Immunol.* 7, 335–342.

Sherman, M. P., and Cox, K. L. (1982). Neonatal eosinophilic colitis. *J. Pediatr.* 100, 587–589.

Shi, H. Z., Humbles, A., Gerard, C., Jin, Z., and Weller, P. F. (2000). Lymph node trafficking and antigen presentation by endobronchial eosinophils. *J. Clin. Invest.* 105, 945–953.

Shinkai, A., Yoshisue, H., Koike, M., Shoji, E., Nakagawa, S., Saito, A., Takeda, T., Imabeppu, S., Kato, Y., Hanai, N., Anazawa, H., Kuga, T., and Nishi, T. (1999). A novel human CC chemokine, eotaxin-3, which is expressed in IL-4-stimulated vascular endothelial cells, exhibits potent activity toward eosinophils. *J. Immunol.* 163, 1602–1610.

Shinkai, K., Mohrs, M., and Locksley, R. M. (2002). Helper T cells regulate type-2 innate immunity *in vivo*. *Nature* 420, 825–829.

Slifman, N. R., Loegering, D. A., McKean, D. J., and Gleich, G. J. (1986). Ribonuclease activity associated with human eosinophil–derived neurotoxin and eosinophil cationic protein. *J. Immunol.* 137, 2913–2917.

Stead, R. H. (1992). Innervation of mucosal immune cells in the gastrointestinal tract. *Reg. Immunol.* 4, 91–99.

Tachimoto, H., Ebisawa, M., and Bochner, B. S. (2002). Cross-talk between integrins and chemokines that influences eosinophil adhesion and migration. *Int. Arch. Allergy Immunol.* 128, 18–20.

Tai, P. C., Holt, M. E., Denny, P., Gibbs, A. R., Williams, B. D., and Spry, C. J. (1984). Deposition of eosinophil cationic protein in granulomas in allergic granulomatosis and vasculitis: the Churg–Strauss syndrome. *Br. Med. J.* 289, 400–402.

Tajima, K., and Katagiri, T. (1996). Deposits of eosinophil granule proteins in eosinophilic cholecystitis and eosinophilic colitis associated with hypereosinophilic syndrome. *Dig. Dis. Sci.* 41, 282–288.

Talley, N. J., Shorter, R. G., Phillips, S. F., and Zinsmeister, A. R. (1990). Eosinophilic gastroenteritis: a clinicopathological study of patients with disease of the mucosa, muscle layer, and subserosal tissues. *Gut* 31, 54–58.

Tamura, N., Ishii, N., Nakazawa, M., Nagoya, M., Yoshinari, M., Amano, T., Nakazima, H., and Minami, M. (1996). Requirement of CD80 and CD86 molecules for antigen presentation by eosinophils. *Scand. J. Immunol.* 44, 229–238.

Throsby, M., Herbelin, A., Pleau, J. M., and Dardenne, M. (2000). CD11c+ eosinophils in the murine thymus: developmental regulation and recruitment upon MHC class I–restricted thymocyte deletion. *J. Immunol.* 165, 1965–1975.

Tominaga, A., Takaki, S., Koyama, N., Katoh, S., Matsumoto, R., Migita, M., Hitoshi, Y., Hosoya, Y., Yamauchi, S., Kanai, Y., *et al.* (1991). Transgenic mice expressing a B cell growth and differentiation factor gene (interleukin 5) develop eosinophilia and autoantibody production. *J. Exp. Med.* 173, 429–437.

Torpier, G., Colombel, J. F., Mathieu-Chandelier, C., Capron, M., Dessaint, J. P., Cortot, A., Paris, J. C., and Capron, A. (1988). Eosinophilic gastroenteritis: ultrastructural evidence for a selective release of eosinophil major basic protein. *Clin. Exp. Immunol.* 74, 404–408.

Venge, P., Dahl, R., Hallgren, R., and Olsson, I. (1980). Cationic proteins of human eosinophils and their role in the inflammatory reaction. In *The Eosinophil in Health and Disease* (eds. A.A.F

Mahmoud and K.F. Austin), 1131–1142. New York: Grune & Stratton.

Venter, J. C., Adams, M. D., Myers, E. W., Li, P. W., Mural, R. J., Sutton, G. G., Smith, H. O., Yandell, M., Evans, C. A., Holt, R. A., Gocayne, J. D., Amanatides, P., Ballew, R. M., Huson, D. H., Wortman, J. R., Zhang, Q., Kodira, C. D., Zheng, X. H., Chen, L., Skupski, M., Subramanian, G., Thomas, P. D., Zhang, J., Gabor Miklos, G. L., Nelson, C., Broder, S., Clark, A. G., Nadeau, J., McKusick, V. A., Zinder, N., Levine, A. J., Roberts, R. J., Simon, M., Slayman, C., Hunkapiller, M., Bolanos, R., Delcher, A., Dew, I., Fasulo, D., Flanigan, M., Florea, L., Halpern, A., Hannenhalli, S., Kravitz, S., Levy, S., Mobarry, C., Reinert, K., Remington, K., Abu-Threideh, J., Beasley, E., Biddick, K., Bonazzi, V., Brandon, R., Cargill, M., Chandramouliswaran, I., Charlab, R., Chaturvedi, K., Deng, Z., Di Francesco, V., Dunn, P., Eilbeck, K., Evangelista, C., Gabrielian, A. E., Gan, W., Ge, W., Gong, F., Gu, Z., Guan, P., Heiman, T. J., Higgins, M. E., Ji, R. R., Ke, Z., Ketchum, K. A., Lai, Z., Lei, Y., Li, Z., Li, J., Liang, Y., Lin, X., Lu, F., Merkulov, G. V., Milshina, N., Moore, H. M., Naik, A. K., Narayan, V. A., Neelam, B., Nusskern, D., Rusch, D. B., Salzberg, S., Shao, W., Shue, B., Sun, J., Wang, Z., Wang, A., Wang, X., Wang, J., Wei, M., Wides, R., Xiao, C., Yan, C. (2001). The sequence of the human genome. *Science* 291, 1304–1351.

von Andrian, U. H., and Engelhardt, B. (2003). Alpha4 integrins as therapeutic targets in autoimmune disease. *N. Engl. J. Med.* 348, 68–72.

Walsh, R. E., and Gaginella, T. S. (1991). The eosinophil in inflammatory bowel disease. *Scand. J. Gastroenterol.* 26, 1217–1224.

Watkins, S. G., Dearin, J. L., Young, L. C., and Wilhelm, D. I. (1976). Association of mastopoiesis with haemopoietic tissues in the neonatal rat. *Experientia* 32, 1339–1340.

Weller, P. F. (1991). The immunobiology of eosinophils. *N. Engl. J. Med.* 324, 1110–1118.

Weller, P. F. (1994). The idiopathic hypereosinophilic syndrome. *Blood* 83, 2759–2779.

Wills-Karp, M. (2001). IL-12/IL-13 axis in allergic asthma. *J. Allergy Clin. Immunol.* 107, 9–18.

Winter, H. S., Madara, J. L., Stafford, R. J., Grand, R. J., Quinlan, J. E., and Goldman, H. (1982). Intraepithelial eosinophils: a new diagnostic criterion for reflux esophagitis. *Gastroenterology* 83, 818–823.

Woerly, G., Roger, N., Loiseau, S., Dombrowicz, D., Capron, A., and Capron, M. (1999). Expression of CD28 and CD86 by human eosinophils and role in the secretion of type 1 cytokines (interleukin 2 and interferon gamma). Inhibition by immunoglobulin A complexes. *J. Exp. Med.* 190, 487–496.

Woodbury, R. G., and Neurath, H. (1978). Purification of an atypical mast cell protease and its levels in developing rats. *Biochemistry* 17, 4298–4304.

Ying, S., Meng, Q., Zeibecoglou, K., Robinson, D. S., Macfarlane, A., Humbert, M., and Kay, A. B. (1999a). Eosinophil chemotactic chemokines (eotaxin, eotaxin-2, RANTES, monocyte chemoattractant protein-3 (MCP-3), and MCP-4), and C-C chemokine receptor 3 expression in bronchial biopsies from atopic and nonatopic (intrinsic) asthmatics. *J. Immunol.* 163, 6321–6329.

Ying, S., Robinson, D. S., Meng, Q., Barata, L. T., McEuen, A. R., Buckley, M. G., Walls, A. F., Askenase, P. W., and Kay, A. B. (1999b). C-C chemokines in allergen-induced late-phase cutaneous responses in atopic subjects: association of eotaxin with early 6-hour eosinophils, and of eotaxin-2 and monocyte chemoattractant protein-4 with the later 24-hour tissue eosinophilia, and relationship to basophils and other C-C chemokines (monocyte chemoattractant protein-3 and RANTES). *J. Immunol.* 163, 3976–3984.

Young, J. D., Peterson, C. G., Venge, P., and Cohn, Z. A. (1986). Mechanism of membrane damage mediated by human eosinophil cationic protein. *Nature* 321, 613–616.

Yu, C., Cantor, A. B., Yang, H., Browne, C., Wells, R. A., Fujiwara, Y., and Orkin, S. H. (2002). Targeted deletion of a high-affinity GATA-binding site in the GATA-1 promoter leads to selective loss of the eosinophil lineage *in vivo*. *J. Exp. Med.* 195, 1387–1395.

Zhang, J., Lathbury, L. J., and Salamonsen, L. A. (2000). Expression of the chemokine eotaxin and its receptor, CCR3, in human endometrium. *Biol. Reprod.* 62, 404–411.

Zhu, Z., Homer, R. J., Wang, Z., Chen, Q., Geba, G. P., Wang, J., Zhang, Y., and Elias, J. A. (1999). Pulmonary expression of interleukin-13 causes inflammation, mucus hypersecretion, subepithelial fibrosis, physiologic abnormalities, and eotaxin production. *J. Clin. Invest.* 103, 779–788.

Zimmermann, N., Bernstein, J. A., and Rothenberg, M. E. (1998). Polymorphisms in the human CC chemokine receptor-3 gene. *Biochim. Biophys. Acta* 1442, 170–176.

Zimmermann, N., Conkright, J. J., and Rothenberg, M. E. (1999). CC chemokine receptor-3 undergoes prolonged ligand-induced internalization. *J. Biol. Chem.* 274, 12611–12618.

Zimmermann, N., Hershey, G. K., Foster, P. S., and Rothenberg, M. E. (2003). Chemokines in asthma: Cooperative interaction between chemokines and IL-13. *J. Allergy Clin. Immunol.* 111, 227–242.

Zimmermann, N., Hogan, S. P., Mishra, A., Brandt, E. B., Bodette, T. R., Pope, S. M., Finkelman, F. D., and Rothenberg, M. E. (2000). Murine eotaxin-2: A constitutive eosinophil chemokine induced by allergen challenge and IL-4 overexpression. *J. Immunol.* 165, 5839–5846.

Zimmermann, N., and Rothenberg, M. E. (2003). Receptor internalization is required for eotaxin-induced responses in human eosinophils. *J. Allergy Clin. Immunol.* 111, 97–105.

Neuropeptides for Mucosal Immunity

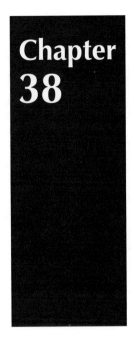

David W. Pascual

Veterinary Molecular Biology, Montana State University, Bozeman, Montana

Kenneth L. Bost

Department of Biology, University of North Carolina at Charlotte, Charlotte, North Carolina

Immune regulation is mediated via a cascade of events requiring cell–cell interactions and subsequent release of their soluble products, *e.g.*, cytokines, antibodies, and receptor molecules, to regulate these responses. In an attempt to describe immune regulation and give it order, there is the tendency to segregate the various immune functions into organized pathways. One unfortunate consequence of this tendency is to restrict such pathways and confine leukocyte function or their mediators. Similarly, the function of neurotransmitters, neuropeptides, and neuroendocrine hormones are often confined to neural pathways from which they originated. This chapter is an attempt to overcome such barriers and introduce a new dimension to immune regulation. We describe how the nervous system can interplay with the immune system and address the mutual expression of receptors and usage of soluble molecules that were originally derived from these two dissimilar systems. The relevance of neural intervention has no greater impact than at mucosal sites or mucosa-associated lymphoreticular tissue (MALT), where these neural mediators have been shown to concentrate. Thus, the focus of this chapter is to relate the significance of the sensory neurons, particularly the contents of the peripheral nerve fibers (peptidergic fibers) containing the neuropeptides (stored in secretory vesicles), for immunity. Specifically, this chapter describes the functions of the neuropeptides substance P and vasoactive intestinal peptide (VIP).

When considering cross-communication between the nervous and immune systems, one must examine the intrinsic properties of their mediators. Neuropeptides will most likely affect a localized area as opposed to inducing a systemic effect. This property complements leukocytes' inherent mobility and enhances the opportunity for neural-immune interactions. This suggests that leukocytes may be transiently innervated, especially in light of the ultrastructural studies with rat spleens demonstrating synaptic-like contacts between sympathetic nerve fibers and lymphocytes (Felten *et al.*, 1987).

Furthermore, the close approximation between lymphoid sites and nerve fibers (Felten *et al.*, 1985; Ottaway *et al.*, 1987; Stead *et al.*, 1987), in particular in mucosal sites of the gastrointestinal (GI) tract, poses the unique question as to whether mediators of one system can induce functional alterations of another system. This is particularly evident in those studies, suggesting that elements from the immune and nervous systems are shared—*e.g.*, neurotransmitters, neuropeptides, and neuroendocrine hormones—and can affect lymphoid function; conversely, cytokines can affect neural function. Obviously, for such effects to have validity, it is essential that a mode of uptake of such neuroimmune modifiers by the cells in question be demonstrated.

In this regard, an intriguing aspect of this neuroimmune network is the expression of neuropeptide and neuroendocrine hormone receptors on leukocytes. Neuropeptide receptors have been identified on both normal mononuclear and polymorphonuclear leukocytes and tumor cell lines **(Table 38.1)**. The expression and regulation of these receptors by leukocytes are energy demanding; therefore, we must assume that their expression is important and not the result of indiscriminate mRNA transcription and that these events are regulated. The expression of these receptors by various subpopulations of leukocytes on their cell surfaces provides the means to receive neuronal signals that can potentially alter immune function.

SUBSTANCE P AND VASOACTIVE INTESTINAL PEPTIDE ARE MUCOSAL NEUROPEPTIDES

Substance P and tachykinins

The CNS-derived, 11-amino-acid neuropeptide *substance P* (SP) is a product of the sensory ganglion cells, and it is

Table 38.1. Neuropeptide Receptor Expression by Mononuclear Cells

Neuropeptide Receptor[a]	Cell	Kd (nM)	Receptor Number	Reference
NK1-R	Guinea pig macrophages	19	ND[b]	Hartung et al., 1986
NK1-R	IM-9 B lymphocytes	0.65	22,641	Payan et al., 1984a
NK1-R	CH12.LX.C4.4F10 B lymphoma	0.69	632	Pascual et al., 1991a
NK1-R	CH12.LX.C4.5F5 B lymphoma	0.69	540	Pascual et al., 1991a
NK1-R	Murine Peyer's patch B cells	0.92	975	Stanisz et al., 1987
NK1-R	Murine splenic B cells	0.64	190	Stanisz et al., 1987
NK1-R	Murine Peyer's patch T cells	0.50	647	Stanisz et al., 1987
NK1-R	Murine splenic T cells	0.62	195	Stanisz et al., 1987
VIP-R	Murine Peyer's patch lymphocytes	0.24	490	Ottaway and Greenberg, 1984
VIP-R	Murine splenic lymphocytes	0.22	880	Ottaway and Greenberg, 1984
VIP-R	Murine lymph node T cells	0.19	3770	Ottaway and Greenberg, 1984
VIP-R	Molt 4b lymphoblasts	7.3	15,000	Beed et al., 1983

[a]NK1-R = neurokinin 1 receptor; VIP-R = vasoactive intestinal peptide receptor.
[b]ND = not determined.

transported to peripheral sites, where it is stored and released on noxious stimulation (Pernow, 1983). Classically, SP is recognized for its ability to induce contraction of smooth-muscle cells of the ileum and to act as a pain signal neurotransmitter (Pernow, 1983; Hokfelt et al., 2001). The amino acid sequence of SP is conserved among mammals (bovine, human, mouse, and rat sequences) and belongs to a family of related peptides called tachykinins, each of which bears a common C-terminus amino acid sequence, Phe-X-Gly-Leu-Met-NH$_2$, where X is a branched aliphatic or aromatic amino acid (**Table 38.2**). An additional feature intrinsic to many of the enteric neuropeptides is the amidation of its C-terminal residue. The two mammalian tachykinin genes encode preprotachykinin A (PPT-A), which generates SP and substance K (SK; neurokinin A), and preprotachykinin B (PPT-B), which produces neurokinin B (neuromedin K). Alternate RNA splicing of the PPT-A gene has the possibility of producing as many as four distinct SP-encoding mRNAs, designated α, β, γ, and δ forms of PPT-A. Recently, an additional tachykinin gene, preprotachykinin

Table 38.2. Sensory Neuropeptide Sequences

Gene	Translated Products	Amino Acid Sequences
Preprotachykinin A	Substance P (SP)	Arg-Pro-Lys-Pro-Gln-Gln-*Phe*-Phe-*Gly-Leu-Met-NH*$_2$
	Substance K (SK)	His-Lys-Thr-Asp-Ser-*Phe*-Val-*Gly-Leu-Met-NH*$_2$
Preprotachykinin B	Neurokinin B (NKB)	Asp-Met-His-*Phe*-Val-*Gly-Leu-Met-NH*$_2$
Preprotachykinin C	Hemokinin (HK)	Arg-Ser-Arg-Thr-Arg-Gln-*Phe*-Tyr-*Gly-Leu-Met-NH*$_2$
Vasoactive intestinal polypeptide	Vasoactive intestinal peptide (VIP)	His-Ser-Asp-Ala-Val-Phe-Thr-Asp-Asn-Tyr-Thr-Arg-Leu-Arg-Lys-Gln-Met-Ala-Val-Lys-Lys-Tyr-Leu-Asn-Ser-Ile-Leu-Asn-NH$_2$
	Peptide histidine isoleucine amide (PH1)	His-Ala-Asp-Gly-Val-Phe-Thr-Ser-Asp-Phe-Ser-Arg-Leu-Leu-Leu-Gly-Gln-Leu-Ser-Ala-Lys-Lys-Tyr-Leu-Glu-Ser-Leu-Ile-NH$_2$
	Peptide histidine methonine (PM1	Position 1-27 identical with PH1 ——Ser-Leu-Met-NH$_2$
Pituitary adenylate cyclase activating polypeptide (PACAP-38)	PACAP-38	His-Ser-Asp-Gly-Ile-Phe-Thr-Asp-Ser-Tyr-Ser-Arg-Tyr-Arg-Lys-Gln-Met-Ala-Val-Lys-Lys-Tyr-Leu-Ala-Ala-Val-Leu-Gly-Lys-Arg-Tyr-Lys-Gln-Arg-Val-Lys-Asn-Lys-NH$_2$

C (PPT-C), has been identified that encodes a novel tachykinin-designated hemokinin (Zhang *et al.*, 2000; Kurtz *et al.*, 2002).

The tachykinin or neurokinin receptor (NK-R) family is composed of three closely related G-protein-coupled, seven-transmembrane receptors sharing sequence homology but differing in ligand specificity (Maggi, 1995; Hokfelt *et al.*, 2001). The neuronal SP or NK1 receptor (NK1-R), which has the greatest affinity for SP (Maggi, 1995; Hokfelt *et al.*, 2001) and hemokinin (Bellucci *et al.*, 2002; Camarda *et al.*, 2002), is identical to the NK1-R expressed by leukocytes. In fact, a variety of methods have been used to demonstrate the presence of tachykinin receptors on leukocytes, including radiolabeled ligand–binding studies, expression of tachykinin receptor mRNA, and detection of NK1-R proteins with use of monospecific antibodies. It is surprising that macrophages (Hartung *et al.*, 1986; Lucey *et al.*, 1994; Kincy-Cain and Bost, 1996; Ho *et al.*, 1997; Goode *et al.*, 1998; Marriott and Bost, 2000), dendritic cells (Marriott and Bost, 2000, 2001), T lymphocytes (Cook *et al.*, 1994; McCormack *et al.*, 1996; Blum *et al.*, 2001; Qian *et al.*, 2001a; Guo *et al.*, 2002; Tripp *et al.*, 2002; Blum *et al.*, 2003), and B lymphocytes (Payan *et al.*, 1984; Pascual *et al.*, 1991a; Pascual *et al.*, 1991b; Bost and Pascual, 1992; Pascual *et al.*, 1992, 1995; van Ginkel and Pascual, 1996) each have the potential to express NK1-R.

Vasoactive intestinal peptide

First identified for its potent vasodilatory properties, vasoactive intestinal polypeptide (VIP) is a 28-amino-acid peptide with C-terminal amidated asparagine (Table 38.2). No deviation among bovine, rat, human, canine, and porcine sequences was evident, but variations were seen in guinea pig and chicken sequences. VIP is cotranslated from a 1.8-kb to 2.1-kb mature mRNA that encodes another C-terminal amidated peptide, designated PHI (peptide histidine isoleucine amide), and in humans, PHM (peptide histidine methionine amide), as a VIP-PHI/PHM preprohormone of 170 amino acids in length. The preprohormone is processed into a prohormone of 18 kDa. Further processing generates both VIP and PHI/PHM. Another VIP agonist is pituitary adenylate cyclase activating polypeptide 38 (PACAP38; Table 38.2), originally discovered in ovine hypothalami (Miyata *et al.*, 1989). It has been shown to cause the secretion of neuroendocrine hormones, growth hormone, prolactin, ACTH, and luteinizing hormone.

VIP is found in the central nervous system and in peripheral nerves, particularly in the peptidergic nerves (Ekblad *et al.*, 1987; Makhlouf, 1990; Schultzberg *et al.*, 1980). These types of nerve fibers are abundant in mucosal tissues: the GI tract, male and female genital tract, lungs, upper respiratory and nasal mucosa, and salivary glands (Polak and Bloom, 1982; Kaltreider *et al.*, 1997). In the GI tract, VIP-containing nerve fibers are present in both the small and large intestines, with extensive innervations in all tissue layers (Ekblad *et al.*, 1988; Ekblad *et al.*, 1987). VIP can also be found coexisting with SP in similar enteric neurons of the myenteric plexus and sub-

mucosal plexus (Makhlouf, 1990), and they have been found in lymphoid tissues, including the thymus, spleen, and Peyer's patches (Felten *et al.*, 1985; Ottaway *et al.*, 1987). In addition, lymphocytes have been shown to produce VIP (Gomariz *et al.*, 1990), particularly CD4+ Th2 cells (Delgado and Ganea, 2001a) upon their activation (Martinez *et al.*, 1999).

Three receptors for VIP ligands belong to the family of G-protein-coupled, seven-transmembrane receptors, and each acts through the adenylate cyclase pathway. The first cloned VIP-R was the VIP/PACAP type I receptor (VPAC$_1$; Ishihara *et al.*, 1992), and rank order displacement studies revealed that PACAP inhibited radiolabeled VIP binding slightly better than VIP. The second class of cloned VIP-R (referred to as VPAC$_2$) shared only a 50% amino acid homology with VPAC$_1$ (Lutz *et al.*, 1993). VPAC$_2$ showed equivalent affinity for the VIP ligands and exhibited a different tissue distribution than VPAC$_1$. The third class of VIP-R was called the PACAP receptor (PAC$_1$) and showed preferential binding for PACAP that was 1,000-fold greater than for VIP (Hashimoto *et al.*, 1993). T lymphocytes expressed both VPAC$_1$ and VPAC$_2$ (Delgado *et al.*, 1996), while macrophages expressed both VPAC$_1$ and PAC$_1$ (Delgado *et al.*, 1999a).

Earlier studies relied upon radiolabeled binding assays to detect the presence of VIP-R on leukocytes (Table 38.1). From these studies, VIP-R has been shown to be present on human MOLT-4b T lymphoblasts and is expressed as a single class of VIP-R with an apparent MW of 47,000 daltons (Wood and O'Dorisio, 1985), which correlates closely with VIP-R found on liver and pancreatic acinar cells. The VIP-R on the MOLT-4b T cells appears to activate cAMP via a stimulatory guanine nucleotide binding protein (O'Dorisio *et al.*, 1985). Normal mouse lymphocytes also have been shown to express VIP-R, and these receptors were primarily found on T cells (Ottaway and Greenberg, 1984). VIP-R density was greatest, in descending order, on lymphocytes isolated from subcutaneous lymph nodes, mesenteric lymph nodes, spleen, and Peyer's patches. Analysis at the mRNA level showed that both VIP receptors are expressed on CD4+ and CD8+ T cells (Delgado *et al.*, 1996). Radiolabeled binding studies were unrevealing as to the class of VIP-R that are present on lymphocytes, but RT-PCR demonstrated that VPAC$_1$ is constitutively expressed and that VPAC$_2$ is induced upon T-cell activation (Delgado *et al.*, 1996). Likewise, VPAC$_1$ is constitutively expressed on human CD4+ T cells (Lara-Marquez *et al.*, 2001). Freshly isolated intraepithelial and lamina propria T cells from small and large intestine also showed constitutive expression of VPAC$_1$, as suggested by mRNA analysis (Qian *et al.*, 2001b); however, only small-intestinal intraepithelial CD8+ T cells showed VPAC$_2$ mRNA.

CYTOKINE-LIKE POTENTIATION OF MUCOSAL IMMUNITY BY TACHYKININS AND VIP

The tantalizing question that remains for the subject of neuroimmunology is why neuropeptide receptors are expressed on the surfaces of mononuclear cells. Thus far, we have described the presence of peptidergic nerve fibers in close approximation with lymphocytes. This evidence suggests that, indeed, mononuclear cells are modified by neuropeptides, and the presence of neuropeptide receptors on lymphoid cell surfaces corroborates this point. To address the function of these neuropeptides on antigen-driven immune responses and the role of these neuropeptide receptors' expression on lymphocytes and macrophages, the following section is devoted to descriptions of those studies that show definitive immune effects on B cells, T cells, and antigen-presenting cells.

For neuropeptides to participate in mucosal immune responses, these mediators must be present in such tissues during host responses. Of particular interest to the mucosal immunologist is the observation that such neuropeptides can be found in high concentrations at mucosal sites. For example, outside the brain, SP is found in greatest concentrations in the GI tract (Pernow, 1983; Hokfelt et al., 2001), and this neuropeptide can be found in high levels in the lungs (Joos et al., 2001). Consequently, the presence of SP at nanomolar concentrations is suggestive of an SP contribution to the regulation of immune function in gut-associated lymphoreticular tissue (GALT) and bronchus-associated lymphoreticular tissue (BALT). Anatomical data have provided direct evidence of interactions between gut mast cells and nerve fibers containing SP (Stead et al., 1987; Stead, 1992). In Peyer's patches, some evidence suggests that SP-containing nerve fibers infiltrate T-cell zones and associate with macrophages, a result that contrasts with what is observed in the GI tract lamina propria. Here, IgA plasma cells can be found in densely innervated areas, suggesting that these cells may be more likely to be influenced by neuropeptides (Stead et al., 1987; Ichikawa et al., 1994; Kulkarni-Narla et al., 1999). In the mesenteric lymph nodes, SP innervation was sparse and found to be associated with 5% to 10% of the arterioles and venules in the medulla adjoining the T-cell region and in the capsule (Popper et al., 1988). In the same study, SP receptor binding sites were examined by quantitative receptor autoradiography. Between 25% and 35% of the germinal centers expressed SP binding sites, whereas limited binding sites were found on arterioles and venules in the T-cell region and internodular region near the capsule. SP-containing fibers are also found in the BALT. In the rat BALT, SP-containing fibers were localized to the subepithelial zone (Inoue et al., 1990). SP-containing fibers in human tonsils were primarily seen in the perivascular plexus, with low-level expression in the interfollicular areas and adjacent to T cells and macrophages (Weihe and Krekel, 1991). The association of SP-containing neurons with lymphoid organs is phylogenetically conserved, since the bursa of Fabricus in birds contains SP fibers that contact B lymphocytes (Zentel and Weihe, 1991).

Various studies have reported increased expression of neuronally associated SP following inflammation. For example, in patients with ulcerative colitis, SP-containing neurons are increased (Keranen et al., 1995; Vento et al., 2001), suggesting that neuronally derived SP contributes to the pathophys-

iology of this disease. The use of SP antagonists (Di Sebastiano et al., 1999) or the selective degradation of SP (Sturiale et al., 1999) significantly reduced colitis in these animal models.

However, neuronally derived SP may not be the only source of this neuropeptide during immune responses. Following activation, varieties of leukocytes have the potential to express neuropeptides. PPT-A mRNA expression has been detected in cultured macrophages (Bost et al., 1992; Ho et al., 1997; Killingsworth et al., 1997; Lai et al., 1998; Ho et al., 2002), dendritic cells (Lambrecht et al., 1999), lymphocytes (Lai et al., 1998; Qian et al., 2001a), and neutrophils (Metwali et al., 1994) following stimulation. In addition, PPT-C mRNA expression has been reported in B lymphocytes (Zhang et al., 2000). Fewer reports have quantified the levels of SP peptide that can be derived from macrophages (Pascual and Bost, 1990; Ho et al., 1997; Li et al., 2000), dendritic cells (Lambrecht et al., 1999), lymphocytes (Lai et al., 1998), and neutrophils (Metwali et al., 1994). Collectively, these studies clearly demonstrate that stimulated leukocytes can express PPT mRNA and the products of PPT genes, albeit at concentrations that are significantly less than those reported for neuronally derived tachykinins.

It is not altogether clear why leukocytes might express tachykinins, since neuronally derived peptides appear to be a significant source of these peptides and since SP-containing neurons have been localized to many lymphoid tissues. One may speculate and offer several possible explanations for the importance of leukocyte-derived tachykinins. First, it is highly likely that the stimuli that induce neuronal production and secretion of tachykinins will be significantly different from those stimuli that would evoke SP secretion by leukocytes. Therefore, the ability of leukocytes to produce SP during immune responses may reflect a need to respond to a diverse array of stimuli. Second, it is likely that leukocyte-derived neuropeptide production would allow such peptides to be produced in areas of limited innervation by peptidergic neurons. This would permit tachykinins to contribute to the development of immune responses in the absence of neuronally derived peptide.

Tachykinins and VIP as B-cell differentiation factors

The newly described tachykinin, hemokinin, is a selective NK1 receptor agonist (Bellucci et al., 2002; Camarda et al., 2002), and high concentrations of this neuropeptide stimulate the proliferation of IL-7-expanded B lymphocytes (Zhang et al., 2000). In fact, it has been suggested that hemokinin is an autocrine factor that contributes to the survival of B-cell precursors in the bone marrow (Zhang et al., 2000).

SP has also been shown to affect the ability of mature B lymphocytes to secrete Ig. In early *in vitro* studies describing SP function on lymphocytes, it was shown that addition of SP to concanavalin A–stimulated mononuclear cell fractions from the murine spleen, mesenteric lymph nodes, and Peyer's patches resulted in 70%, 40%, and 300% increases, respectively, in IgA production (Stanisz et al., 1986). To a lesser extent, IgM levels were altered significantly, by 20% to 40%; however, IgG levels were not affected. Such observations suggest that SP may preferentially stimulate IgA secretion or, alternatively, may indicate that SP is an IgA switching factor. A recent study using human T- and B-lymphocyte co-cultures suggested that tachykinins could augment Ig secretion in cytokine-stimulated cultures (Braun et al., 1999). This result was especially true for IgA synthesis. Together, these in vitro co-culture studies suggested that B lymphocytes could be stimulated by SP but required the presence of additional leukocyte populations that could potentially express NK1-R. Therefore, it was difficult to assess whether increased Ig synthesis was due to a direct or indirect action on B lymphocytes.

In an attempt to delineate the mechanisms of how SP behaves as a B-cell differentiation factor (Pascual et al., 1991b; Bost and Pascual, 1992; Pascual et al., 1992) and to assess the direct effect of SP, cloned B lymphoma cell lines were employed. To substantiate the ability of SP to stimulate B cells, particularly cloned B cells, it was important to demonstrate the presence of NK1-R. From radiolabeled binding experiments, it was shown that these CH12.LX subclones do bear NK1-R (between 500 and 600 receptors/cell). These experiments substantiated what was known about NK1-R expression on lymphocytes at that time, and the level of NK1-R expression and binding affinities (kD ~ 0.69 nM) were similar to those found on normal B lymphocytes (Stanisz et al., 1987) and IM-9 B lymphoblasts (Payan et al., 1984). On direct SP stimulation of CH12.LX.C4.4F10 cells, IgA production could be modestly enhanced at subnanomolar concentrations, whereas similar stimulation on CH12.LX.C4.5F5 cells resulted in no significant change in IgM produced. SP had no effect on cell proliferation when ascertained by ^{3}H-thymidine uptake.

The biological impact on the expression of NK1-R on B lymphocytes was evidenced by the ability of SP to augment Ig synthesis in the presence of a second signal. The addition of LPS to varying concentrations of SP to CH12.LX.C4.5F5 cells resulted in optimal IgM production (172% increase) at subnanomolar SP concentrations, whereas elevated doses of SP (100 nM) were not as effective. Modest increases in IgA production were obtained for CH12.LX.C4.4F10 cells when stimulated in a similar fashion, and again subnanomolar concentrations of SP were most effective for the enhancement of IgA production. These events were NK1-R-mediated, since the addition of excess SP antagonist to SP-treated cultures specifically inhibited the SP induction of IgM and IgA antibody production.

In the context of normal B cells, similar studies were performed with purified B cells isolated from the spleen (Pascual et al., 1991b) and Peyer's patches (Pascual et al., 1995). B lymphocytes (>99% sIg⁺) isolated from mouse spleens or Peyer's patches, when cultured with varying concentrations of SP (0.1 pM to 100 nM), showed no differences in Ig production. The addition of 10 µg/ml of LPS to these cultures resulted in optimal costimulation by subnanomolar concentrations of SP in IgM and IgG3 produc-

tion, with as much as 500% and 1,000% increases, respectively (Pascual et al., 1991b). Production of IgA in Peyer's patches was also enhanced when IL-6 was used as a costimulator (Pascual et al., 1995). Again, subnanomolar concentrations of SP induced three-fold increases in IL-6-induced production of IgA and IgG in Peyer's patch cell cultures.

The significance of these studies is twofold. First, SP could stimulate B cells directly in the absence of accessory cells. Second, physiologically relevant concentrations of SP could enhance Ig synthesis by purified B cells. This observation is in agreement with what has been previously reported (Stanisz et al., 1986) about the ability of SP to modify Ig synthesis. These increases in Ig synthesis were not the result of enhanced B cell proliferation by SP. In fact, at the doses optimal for Ig production, SP in the presence of LPS was antiproliferative and showed greater inhibitory activity at the higher SP concentrations (Pascual et al., 1991b).

VIP was shown to enhance IgM production (by 70%) while preferentially diminishing IgA production (by 70%) by Con A–stimulated Peyer's patch mononuclear cells (Stanisz et al., 1986). In contrast, VIP was shown to promote IgA production by human costimulated tonsillar B cells (Kimata and Fujimoto, 1994). When purified resting tonsillar B cells were isolated and stimulated with an anti-CD40 antibody, elevations in IgA1 and IgA2 production were obtained. The differences in these studies may be attributed to differences in cell populations tested, i.e., total mononuclear cells versus purified B cells. In the former study, VIP may have been exerting its effects indirectly upon B cells by activating T cells/macrophages, whereas in the latter study VIP was shown to affect B cells directly. Thus, depending upon the source of lymphocytes and the retention of organized lymphoid structures, i.e., disruption during inflammation, VIP may have selective effects upon VIP-R⁺ lymphocytes.

Regardless, it is clear from these studies that like SP, VIP stimulation of lymphocytes requires a costimulatory signal, and the observed induction of IgA antibody production was not the result of proliferating sIgA⁺ B cells; rather, resting sIgM⁺ B cells were stimulated (Kimata and Fujimoto, 1994), suggesting that VIP may be involved in IgA switching. Similar results were obtained with SP and murine B cells, whereby increased levels of α transcripts were found after costimulation of PP B cells with SP (unpublished results). These findings suggest that SP and VIP can stimulate B-cell differentiation. The requisite for a costimulatory signal implies that under resting conditions SP has minimal effects upon B cells. This is further supported by the observation that SP-containing nerve fibers fail to infiltrate into the PP B cell zones, suggesting that repeated or direct stimulation of PP B cell subsets can be avoided. This aversion may also represent an additional means of regulating B-cell activation, and possibly, during an inflammatory response, innervations into the B cell zones may occur, resulting in their activation. Alternatively, SP may also direct its action on T cells and accessory cells (see next section).

Thus far, we have discussed the potential in vivo significance of neuropeptides as neuroimmune modulators using various *in vitro* systems. The *in vivo* relevance of SP upon antibody production has been demonstrated (Helme *et al.*, 1987). In this study, peripheral stores of SP (and other neuropeptides) were depleted by treating neonatal rats with the neurotoxin capsaicin, which destroys unmyelinated sensory neurons present in peripheral tissues (Buck and Burks, 1986). The experimental paradigm was such that neonatally capsaicin-treated rats were allowed to mature and were then subjected to antigen (SRBC) challenge. This treatment resulted in a >80% reduction in IgM and IgG antibody-forming cell (AFC) responses by popliteal lymph nodes in comparison with AFC responses in untreated SRBC-challenged rats. Clearly, these results show the significance of neuronal input and particularly the presence of neuropeptides in the development of antibody responses.

This lack of antigen responsiveness or suppression exhibited by capsaicin-pretreated rats was reversible by coadministration of SP with SRBC. In a subsequent study (Eglezos *et al.*, 1990), a similar magnitude of inhibition in antibody responses was obtained with rats treated with the SP antagonist spantide during antigen priming. While these studies address the contribution of endogenous SP in mucosal immunity, the *in vivo* infusion of SP during immunization suggests that SP can act as an adjuvant. Mice were infused with SP for 1 week via miniosmotic pumps and simultaneously immunized with ultraviolet-inactivated rotavirus (Ijaz *et al.*, 1990). Increased levels of antirotavirus antibody in the milk of lactating females, as well as in the serum, were shown.

More recently, *in vivo* studies also have supported a role for SP in the development of antibody responses. Weinstock and colleagues demonstrated that schistosome granulomas that form in the presence of an NK1-R antagonist produce limited amounts of IgM in comparison with normal lesions (Blum *et al.*, 1996). The authors suggested that SP was an important factor in B-cell maturation at a terminal stage of differentiation. In related studies, NK1-R-deficient (NK1-R$^{-/-}$) mice were found to produce less IgG2a and IgE when challenged with *Schistosoma mansoni* (Blum *et al.*, 1999). Collectively, these studies suggest that, in each case, despite the differences in experimental conditions, SP required a coactivation signal to achieve an augmentation in Ig production. Furthermore, these *in vivo* and *in vitro* studies demonstrate an important role for tachykinins in the development of B lymphocytes and the ensuing antibody response.

Tachykinins and VIP as costimulation factors for T lymphocytes

Early studies showed that SP supports T-cell proliferation (Payan *et al.*, 1983; Stanisz *et al.*, 1986), suggesting that T lymphocytes can express NK1-R. In support of this possibility, recent investigations by several laboratories have demonstrated in vitro and in vivo expression of NK1-R by T lymphocytes. NK1-R mRNA expression by cultured murine (McCormack *et al.*, 1996) and human T cells (Li *et al.*, 2000) or T-cell lines has been reported. In addition, the functionality of NK1-R expression by T lymphocytes has been demonstrated in co-cultures with SP-producing dendritic cells

(Lambrecht *et al.*, 1999). It is interesting that NK1-R mRNA expression was observed in intraepithelial and lamina propria T lymphocytes but not in splenic T cells (Qian *et al.*, 2001a). During the host response against respiratory syncytial virus, NK1-R expression was markedly increased in CD4$^+$ T lymphocytes (Tripp *et al.*, 2002).

However, the most compelling evidence to date for the importance of NK1-R expression on T lymphocytes comes from studies by Weinstock and colleagues, using a murine model of schistosomiasis. Using NK1-R$^{-/-}$ mice, they observed significant reductions in the size of schistosome-induced granulomas in comparison with disease in wild-type mice (Blum *et al.*, 1999). The limited IFN-γ production by infected NK1-R$^{-/-}$ mice suggested that T cells may be an important target for SP during schistosomiasis. Additional studies clearly demonstrated that the presence of NK1-R on T lymphocytes was largely responsible for schistosome antigen–induced IFN-γ production (Blum *et al.*, 2003). Mechanistic studies demonstrated that schistosome antigen, as well as IL-12, could induce expression of NK1-R during murine schistosomiasis (Blum *et al.*, 2001). Collectively, these studies clearly demonstrate the importance of NK1-R expression and activity during the host response to a parasitic infection.

To further address the role of SP contribution to S-IgA responses, NK1-R$^{-/-}$ mice were orally immunized with an attenuated *Salmonella* construct expressing colonization factor antigen I (CFA/I). This vaccine construct has been shown to elicit a biphasic Th cell response (Pascual *et al.*, 1999) supported by early robust IL-4- and IL-5-producing CD4$^+$ T cells. When such a construct was used to orally immunize NK1-R$^{-/-}$ mice, a significant increase in antigen-specific S-IgA antibody titers was obtained (Trunkle *et al.*, 2003). Surprisingly, no significant differences in IFN-γ production were observed between NK1-R$^{+/+}$ and NK1-R$^{-/-}$ mice, but increased production to IL-6 was obtained. This evidence suggests, minimally, that some intracellular infections are resolvable in the absence of NK1-R function, perhaps via increases in S-IgA antibody responses.

VIP-containing nerve fibers also extend into the T-cell regions of the Peyer's patches (Ottaway *et al.*, 1987) to affect the CD4$^+$ T cells, whereby stimulation of CD4$^+$ T cells by SP or VIP can affect Ig synthesis. While SP has been shown to exert stimulatory effects upon T cells, VIP has the opposite effect and will inhibit mitogen-induced T-cell proliferation (Stanisz *et al.*, 1986; Ottaway and Greenberg, 1984). This effect apparently occurs through a reduction of IL-2 synthesis (Ottaway, 1987; Metawali *et al.*, 1993) and an inhibition of IL-4 in anti-CD3-stimulated T cells incubated with VIP (Wang *et al.*, 1996). These early studies suggested that VIP exhibited anti-inflammatory properties, but this was not confirmed until recently. As stated earlier, VPAC$_1$ is constitutively expressed, whereas VPAC$_2$ is inducible when T cells are stimulated with anti-CD3 antibody (Delgado *et al.*, 1996). Upon stimulation, VPAC$_1$ levels decrease, while VPAC$_2$ levels are induced. This evidence suggests that VIP action on CD4$^+$ T cells is via the effect of VPAC$_2$ acting specifically upon Th2 cells. To begin to address the regulation of $VPAC_1$ and $VPAC_2$, a mouse deficient in $VPAC_2$ was derived and exhibited enhanced delayed-type hypersensitivity (DTH) responses supported by increased IFN-γ production (Goetzl et al., 2001). To exacerbate Th2 cell function, a transgenic mouse was derived in which $CD4^+$ T cells express the human $VPAC_2$ (Voice et al., 2001). These mice showed increased serum IgE and IgG1 but not IgA antibodies. This Th2 cell bias was evidenced as enhanced susceptibility to TNP-induced cutaneous anaphylaxis and depressed DTH responses. Studies have yet to determine whether $VPAC_1$ and $VPAC_2$ are regulated in a similar fashion by Peyer's patch Th cells, in a manner analogous to that seen with splenic Th cells.

Tachykinins and VIP-mediated modulation of macrophage and dendritic cell function

While numerous investigations have focused on the ability of neuropeptides to significantly modulate antigen-specific T- and B-lymphocyte responses, a growing body of work suggests that the innate immune response can also be influenced by neuropeptides, particularly macrophages and dendritic cells. Of particular importance has been the demonstration of functional receptors for tachykinins on myeloid progenitors (Rameshwar and Gascon, 1997), macrophages (Hartung et al., 1986; Lotz et al., 1988; Kincy-Cain and Bost, 1996; Ho et al., 1997; Kincy-Cain and Bost, 1997; Marriott and Bost, 1998, 2000; Marriott et al., 2000), and dendritic cells (Marriott et al., 2000; Marriott and Bost, 2001). Upregulation of macrophage NK1-R expression can occur following stimulation of macrophages with a variety of agents, including morphine (Li et al., 2000), HIV or gp120 (Ho et al., 2002); IL-4; or IFN-γ (Marriott and Bost, 2000).

In vivo studies have suggested an important role for NK1-R expression by macrophages and dendritic cells in the initiation of the host response against bacterial and viral pathogens that invade mucosal surfaces. Salmonella enter through the gut mucosa where the bacterium survives as an intracellular pathogen of macrophages. Successful clearance of this pathogen requires IL-12-induced IFN-γ production, which amplifies macrophage activation, resulting in destruction of the pathogen. A murine model of salmonellosis was recently used to investigate the importance of SP-mediated macrophage activation following infection (Kincy-Cain and Bost, 1996). The rationale for hypothesizing that SP may play an important role in macrophage activation and destruction of this intracellular pathogen was based upon in vitro studies of the effect of SP on macrophage function and from the demonstration of inducible NK1-R expression by these cells (Hartung et al., 1986; Lotz et al., 1988; Kincy-Cain and Bost, 1996; Ho et al., 1997; Kincy-Cain and Bost, 1997; Marriott and Bost, 1998, 2000; Marriott et al., 2000). Cultured macrophages exposed to Salmonella were found to rapidly upregulate expression of NK1-R (Kincy-Cain and Bost, 1996). Such a response had added significance since it was already established that SP could augment the production of reactive oxygen intermediates by these cells (Hartung

et al., 1986). Thus, upregulation of NK1-R expression by Salmonella may significantly increase the SP-mediated macrophage response, directly killing the bacteria. In addition, SP can enhance IL-1, IL-6, and TNF-α secretion by macrophages (Lotz et al., 1988), which would augment the inflammatory response against this pathogen. Of particular interest is the recent finding that SP could synergize with LPS in the production of bioactive IL-12p70 (Kincy-Cain and Bost, 1997). Since the presence of IL-12 in vivo is an important step in resistance against salmonellosis (Kincy-Cain et al., 1996), SP-induced production of this monokine would have a significant impact on the cell-mediated immune response against this pathogen.

Collectively, these in vitro studies suggested mechanisms by which SP might augment the ability of macrophages to kill Salmonella, as well as mechanisms which would enhance the cell-mediated immune response via production of monokines. However, such a possibility depends upon expression of SP and its receptor at the site of the mucosal immune response against Salmonella, and more recent evidence suggests that the contribution by SP is impacted during the inductive phase of the host response (Trunkle et al., 2003).

In vivo studies show the relevance of SP and its receptor in mucosal immune responses against Salmonella. Surprisingly, after oral inoculation with Salmonella, a rapid and dramatic upregulation of the mRNAs encoding SP (Bost, 1995) and its receptor (Kincy-Cain and Bost, 1996) was observed in mucosal tissues. This result suggested that SP and its receptor were involved in the initiation of the response against this pathogen. To directly address this possibility, mice were pretreated with the potent SP antagonist spantide II prior to oral challenge with Salmonella. Mice pretreated with this SP antagonist could not resist the bacterial infection as well as control mice pretreated with an irrelevant peptide (Kincy-Cain and Bost, 1996). Treatment with the antagonist caused no apparent alterations in function of the GI tract, aside from a reduction in IL-12p40 mRNA expression in vivo following oral inoculation with Salmonella. Therefore, in vivo antagonism of SP/NK1-R interactions resulted in surprising and dramatic reductions in the resistance against the intracellular pathogen, Salmonella.

Mice deficient in NK1-R expression have also been used to investigate the importance of this neuropeptide receptor in the host response against pathogens. The significance of NK1-R expression during schistosomiasis has been discussed earlier (Blum et al., 1999). Recently, $NK1-R^{-/-}$ mice were used to investigate the host response following intranasal infection with murine γ-herpesvirus-68 (Elsawa and Bost, 2003), a $γ_2$-herpesvirus (Efstathiou et al., 1990b) that shares sequence homology and pathological similarities with Epstein-Barr virus (Efstathiou et al., 1990a) and human herpesvirus-8 (Sunil-Chandra et al., 1992b; Virgin et al., 1997). Nasal (Sunil-Chandra et al., 1992a) or gastric (Peacock and Bost, 2000) inoculation with murine γ-herpesvirus-68 results in an acute productive infection of lung or intestinal epithelial cells, respectively, followed by the dissemination of the virus to peripheral organs (Sunil-Chandra *et al.*, 1992a). B lymphocytes (Sunil-Chandra *et al.*, 1992b; Cardin *et al.*, 1996; Usherwood *et al.*, 1996b), macrophages (Weck *et al.*, 1999), and possibly dendritic cells (Flano *et al.*, 2000) become latently infected soon after inoculation. Levels of latent virus in the spleens of infected animals peak around 15 days postinfection, coinciding with marked splenomegaly (Sunil-Chandra *et al.*, 1992a; Cardin *et al.*, 1996; Usherwood *et al.*, 1996a) due to an unregulated expansion of leukocyte populations (Cardin *et al.*, 1996; Tripp *et al.*, 1997). The CTL response (Ehtisham *et al.*, 1993; Stevenson and Doherty, 1998; Usherwood *et al.*, 2000; Belz and Doherty, 2001), which develops during the primary infection, and possibly late-developing antiviral antibodies (Sangster *et al.*, 2000) are thought to limit secondary disease caused by the emergence of murine γ-herpesvirus-68 from latency.

Following nasal inoculation with this γ-herpesvirus, expression of SP and its receptor was increased in mucosal and peripheral lymphoid organs in wild-type strains of mice (Elsawa and Bost, 2003). Of particular interest was the finding that transcriptional activation of the NK1-R gene locus in response to viral infection was associated with marginal zone macrophages. Increased tachykinin and NK1-R mRNA expression suggested that these molecules were important components of the host response against this viral infection. To directly address such a possibility, murine γ-herpesvirus was used to infect mice genetically deficient in NK1-R expression. Surprisingly, these genetically deficient mice showed significant increases in latent viral burden in comparison with syngeneic C57BL/6 mice. Furthermore, NK1-R$^{-/-}$ mice showed a reduced CTL response against murine γ-herpesvirus 68, suggesting one possible mechanism that might help to explain this increased viral burden. Such limitations in the antigen-specific CTL response in NK1-R$^{-/-}$ mice could result from lowered expression of IL-12 during viral infection. Consistent with this hypothesis, increases in mRNA-encoding IL-12 and secretion of this cytokine into sera of infected wild-type animals were markedly reduced in NK1-R$^{-/-}$ mice.

Perhaps the most surprising result from these three well-studied models of microbial pathogenesis (i.e., schistosomiasis, salmonellosis, and γ-herpesvirus infection) is the magnitude of effects observed following the deletion (Blum *et al.*, 1999) (Elsawa and Bost, 2003) or antagonism of NK1-R (Kincy-Cain and Bost, 1996). Further surprises have been revealed as the mechanisms for SP-mediated modulation of the host response have been dissected. For schistosomiasis, NK1-R expression by T lymphocytes and its role in inducing IFN-γ production are key players in this immune response (Blum *et al.*, 2003). For salmonella infection, the importance of SP in the initiation of macrophage-derived IL-12 seems central to the protective host response (Kincy-Cain and Bost, 1996; Kincy-Cain *et al.*, 1996; Kincy-Cain and Bost, 1997). The role that NK1-R expression plays in the host response against murine γ-herpesvirus 68 (Elsawa and Bost, 2003) has only begun to be studied but may include NK1-R-mediated effects on macrophages, dendritic cells, CD4$^+$ T

lymphocytes, and CTLs. Whether such effects will be direct or indirect is not clear.

As for the ability of VIP to stimulate the anti-inflammatory arm for T cells, its anti-inflammatory properties are more pronounced on macrophages. While SP was shown to stimulate IL-12, VIP has an opposing effect and suppresses IL-12 production in response to endotoxin challenge (Delgado *et al.*, 1999a). In addition, VIP can inhibit TNF-α (Delgado *et al.*, 1999b) and IL-6 (Martinez *et al.*, 1998); its ability to suppress these proinflammatory cytokines is linked to VIP-induced production of IL-10 (Delgado *et al.*, 1999c) and IL-1R antagonist (Delgado *et al.*, 2001). In the same vein, VIP also exerts suppression of the proinflammatory chemokines, MIP-2, KC, MIP-1α, MIP-1β, RANTES, and MCP-1, by activated macrophages (Delgado and Ganea, 2001b). This suppression of proinflammatory chemokines appears to be associated with the induction of MDC (Jiang *et al.*, 2002).

BIDIRECTIONAL COMMUNICATION BETWEEN THE NERVOUS AND IMMUNE SYSTEMS: IS IT REAL?

We have provided here the experimental evidence of the existence of a communication system between the nervous and immune systems. Now that we have determined that various neuropeptides and neurotransmitters do play a role in modulation of the function in various arms of the cellular and humoral immune network, establishing the intracellular mechanisms involved becomes increasingly important. Furthermore, the shared expression of neuropeptide and cytokine receptors by elements of the immune and nervous systems, as well as the ability to respond to these diametric molecules, supports the existence of such a neuroimmune circuit. In view of these observations, efforts were put forth to investigate the possibility that neuropeptides were generated by cells other than those of neuronal origin. Consequently, leukocytes were shown to synthesize SP (Pascual and Bost, 1990) and VIP (Gomariz *et al.*, 1990; Matthew *et al.*, 1992; Martinez *et al.*, 1999; Delgado and Ganea, 2001a). These findings have led some researchers to speculate that the neuroimmune network is functionally bidirectional. If the neuroimmune network were bidirectional as proposed, this would imply that leukocyte-derived neuropeptides could act at neuronal or endocrine sites, even those at distant sites, in a systemic fashion; however, there exists no *in vivo* evidence to support this hypothesis. In fact, even if leukocyte-derived neuropeptides could reach their respective neuronal receptors, the concentration of leukocyte-derived neuropeptides generally has been found to be 1,000-fold less than neuronal concentrations. Thus, at these concentrations, leukocyte-derived neuropeptides seem unlikely to compete effectively with neuronal production and release.

One aspect of the studies addressing leukocyte-derived neuropeptides that has failed to attract consideration is why these neuropeptides are produced by leukocytes. While intricate studies have shown the production of neuropeptides by leukocytes, studies entailing the purpose of such production have been minimal. One possibility for their production is that low-level production of neuropeptides may represent a mechanism for maintaining the expression of their respective receptors on the leukocyte cell surface. In the case of macrophage-derived SP (Pascual and Bost, 1990), the proponents offered that macrophages produced SP in a paracrine/autocrine fashion to regulate cytokine production. Thus, if leukocyte-synthesized neuropeptides can affect their own function, then we must consider them functionally similar to cytokines. It may be important for them not to function at neuronal or endocrine sites; instead, they may exhibit properties not previously considered. Consequently, leukocyte-derived neuropeptides introduce a novel regulatory circuit to immune regulation. Such an additional regulatory pathway may also have its own mode of neuropeptide release. Previous studies have shown the sensitivity of neural elements to cytokine stimulation to induce the release of neuropeptides (Hart *et al.*, 1991; Jonakait and Schotland, 1990), but these same cytokines may not affect leukocyte-derived neuropeptide release.

There is still much to learn about the mechanisms utilized by the nervous system to regulate immune function in the MALT. We are beginning to learn about the ability of lymphocytes and macrophages to respond to neuropeptides. Subsequent studies should provide insight into the modulation of neuropeptide receptors on leukocytes and particularly lead to an understanding of the regulatory mechanisms and events responsible for the expression of neuropeptide receptors. This can be especially significant in mucosal tissues, where the presence of neuropeptides is greatly associated with leukocytes.

The consequence of understanding the relationship between the nervous system and the immune system is that it will provide a basis for future treatment of mucosal inflammatory bowel diseases (Crohn's disease and ulcerative colitis) and autoimmune diseases (arthritis and multiple sclerosis [myelin basic protein]), and will also serve as a basis for the development of new vaccines to mucosal pathogens. In general, this new field offers additional therapeutic strategies in the manipulation of immunity in various pathological states. When immune regulation in the MALT is considered, the importance of assessing the neuronal component will become more prevalent. Thus, with the development of cDNA probes and monoclonal antibodies to neuropeptide receptors, the regulation of these receptors on lymphoid cells and macrophages can be addressed readily, providing a functional understanding of the neural-immune network.

REFERENCES

Beed, E.A., O'Dorisio, M.S., O'Dorisio, T.M., and Gaginella, T.S. (1983). Demonstration of a functional receptor for vasoactive intestinal polypeptide on Molt 4b T lymphoblasts. *Regul. Pept.* 6, 1–12.

Bellucci, F., Carini, F., Catalani, C., Cucchi, P., Lecci, A., Meini, S., Patacchini, R., Quartara, L., Ricci, R., Tramontana, M., Giuliani, S., and Maggi, C.A. (2002). Pharmacological profile of the novel mammalian tachykinin, hemokinin 1. *Br. J. Pharmacol.* 135, 266–274.

Belz, G.T., and Doherty, P.C. (2001). Virus-specific and bystander CD8+ T-cell proliferation in the acute and persistent phases of a γ-herpesvirus infection. *J. Virol.* 75, 4435–4438.

Blum, A., Metwali, A., Elliott, D., Sandor, M., Lynch, R., and Weinstock, J.V. (1996). Substance P receptor antagonist inhibits murine IgM expression in developing schistosome granulomas by blocking the terminal differentiation of intragranuloma B cells. *J. Neuroimmunol.* 66, 1–10.

Blum, A.M., Metwali, A., Kim-Miller, M., Li, J., Qadir, K., Elliott, D.E., Lu, B., Fabry, Z., Gerard, N., and Weinstock, J.V. (1999). The substance P receptor is necessary for a normal granulomatous response in murine schistosomiasis mansoni. *J. Immunol.* 162, 6080–6085.

Blum, A.M., Metwali, A., Crawford, C., Li, J., Qadir, K., Elliott, D.E., and Weinstock, J.V. (2001). Interleukin 12 and antigen independently induce substance P receptor expression in T cells in murine schistosomiasis mansoni. *FASEB J.* 15, 950–957.

Blum, A.M., Metwali, A., Elliott, D.E., and Weinstock, J.V. (2003). T cell substance P receptor governs antigen-elicited IFN-γ production. *Am. J. Physiol. Gastrointest. Liver Physiol.* 284, G197–204.

Bost, K.L., and Pascual, D.W. (1992). Substance P: a late-acting B lymphocyte differentiation co-factor. *Am. J. Physiol.* 262, C537–C545.

Bost, K.L. (1995). Inducible preprotachykinin mRNA expression in mucosal lymphoid organs following oral immunization with *Salmonella. J. Neuroimmunol.* 62, 59–67.

Braun, A., Wiebe, P., Pfeufer, A., Gessner, R., and Renz, H. (1999). Differential modulation of human immunoglobulin isotype production by the neuropeptides substance P, NKA and NKB. *J. Neuroimmunol.* 97, 43–50.

Buck, S.H., and Burks, T.F. (1986). The neuropharmacology of capsaicin: review of some recent observations. *Pharmacol. Rev.* 38, 179–226.

Calvo, J.R., Guerrero, J.M., Lopez-Gonzalez, M.A., Osuna, C., and Segura, J.J. (1994). Characteristics of receptors for VIP in rat peritoneal macrophage membranes. *Peptides* 15, 309–315.

Camarda, V., Rizzi, A., Calo, G., Guerrini, R., Salvadori, S., and Regoli, D. (2002). Pharmacological profile of hemokinin 1: a novel member of the tachykinin family. *Life Sci.* 71, 363–370.

Cardin, R.D., Brooks, J.W., Sarawar, S.R., and Doherty, P.C. (1996). Progressive loss of CD8+ T cell-mediated control of a γ-herpesvirus in the absence of CD4+ T cells. *J. Exp. Med.* 184, 863–871.

Cook, G.A., Elliott, D., Metwali, A., Blum, A.M., Sandor, M., Lynch, R., and Weinstock, J.V. (1994). Molecular evidence that granuloma T lymphocytes in murine *Schistosomiasis mansoni* express an authentic substance P (NK-1) receptor. *J. Immunol.* 152, 1830–1835.

Delgado, M., Martinez, C., Johnson, M.C., Gomariz, R.P., and Ganea, D. (1996). Differential expression of vasoactive intestinal peptide receptors 1 and 2 (VIP-R1 and VIP-R2) mRNA in murine lymphocytes. *J. Neuroimmunol.* 68, 27–38.

Delgado, M., Muñoz-Elias, E.J., Gomariz, R.P., and Ganea, D. (1999a). VIP and PACAP inhibit IL-12 production in LPS-stimulated macrophages. Subsequent effect on IFN-γ synthesis by T cells. *J. Neuroimmunol.* 96, 167–181.

Delgado, M., Pozo, D., Martinez, C., Laceta, J., Calvo, J.R., Ganea, D., and Gomariz, R.P. (1999b). Vasoactive intestinal peptide and pituitary adenylate cyclase-activating polypeptide inhibit endotoxin-induced TNF-α production by macrophages: in vitro and in vivo studies. *J. Immunol.* 162, 2358–2367.

Delgado, M., Muñoz-Elias, E.J., Gomariz, R.P., and Ganea, D. (1999c). Vasoactive intestinal peptide and pituitary adenylate cyclase-activating polypeptide enhance IL-10 production by murine macrophages: in vitro and in vivo studies. *J. Immunol.* 162, 1707–1716.

Delgado, M., and Ganea, D. (2001a). Cutting edge: is vasoactive intestinal peptide a type 2 cytokine? *J. Immunol.* 166, 2907–2912.

Delgado, M., and Ganea, D. (2001b). Inhibition of endotoxin-induced macrophage chemokine production by vasoactive intestinal peptide and pituitary adenylate cyclase-activating polypeptide in vitro and in vivo. *J. Immunol.* 167, 966–975.

Delgado, M., Abad, C., Martinez, C., Leceta, J., and Gomariz, R.P. (2001). Vasoactive intestinal peptide prevents experimental arthritis by downregulating both autoimmune and inflammatory components of the disease. *Nat. Med.* 7, 563–568.

Di Sebastiano, P., Grossi, L., Di Mola, F.F., Angelucci, D., Friess, H., Marzio, L., Innocenti, P., and Buchler, M.W. (1999). SR140333, a substance P receptor antagonist, influences morphological and motor changes in rat experimental colitis. *Dig. Dis. Sci.* 44, 439–444.

Efstathiou, S., Ho, Y.M., Hall, S., Styles, C.J., Scott, S.D., and Gompels, U.A. (1990a). Murine herpesvirus 68 is genetically related to the γ-herpesviruses Epstein-Barr virus and herpesvirus saimiri. *J. Gen. Virol.* 71, 1365–1372.

Efstathiou, S., Ho, Y.M., and Minson, A.C. (1990b). Cloning and molecular characterization of the murine herpesvirus 68 genome. *J. Gen. Virol.* 71, 1355–1364.

Eglezos, A., Andrews, P.V., Boyd, R.L., and Helme, R.D. (1990). Effects of capsaicin treatment on immunoglobulin secretion in the rat: further evidence for involvement of tachykinin-containing afferent nerves. *J. Neuroimmunol.* 26, 131–138.

Ehtisham, S., Sunil-Chandra, N.P., and Nash, A.A. (1993). Pathogenesis of murine γ-herpesvirus infection in mice deficient in CD4 and CD8 T cells. *J. Virol.* 67, 5247–5252.

Ekblad, E., Winther, C., Ekman, R., Hakanson, R., and Sundler, F. (1987). Projections of peptide-containing neurons in rat small intestine. *Neuroscience* 20, 169–188.

Ekblad, E., Ekman, R., Håkanson, R., and Sundler, F. (1988). Projections of peptide-containing neurons in rat colon. *Neuroscience* 27, 655–674.

Elsawa, S.F., Taylor, W., Petty, C.C., Marriott, I., Weinstock, J.V., and Bost, K.L. (2003). Reduced CTL response and increased viral burden in substance P receptor-deficient mice infected with murine γ-herpesvirus 68. *J. Immunol.* 170, 2605–2612.

Felten, D.L., Felten, S.Y., Carlson, S.L., Olschowka, J.A., and Livnat, S. (1985). Noradrenergic and peptidergic innervation of lymphoid tissue. *J. Immunol.* 135, 755s–765s.

Felten, D.L., Felten, S.Y., Bellinger, D.L., Carlson, S.L., Ackerman, K.D., Madden, K.S., Olschowki, J.A., and Livnat, S. (1987). Noradrenergic sympathetic neural interactions with the immune system: structure and function. *Immunol. Rev.* 100, 225–260.

Flano, E., Husain, S.M., Sample, J.T., Woodland, D.L., and Blackman, M.A. (2000). Latent murine γ-herpesvirus infection is established in activated B cells, dendritic cells, and macrophages. *J. Immunol.* 165, 1074–1081.

Goetzl, E.J., Voice, J.K., Shen, S., Dorsam, G., Kong, Y., West, K.M., Morrison, C.F., and Harmar, A.J. (2001). Enhanced delayed-type hypersensitivity and diminished immediate-type hypersensitivity in mice lacking the inducible VPAC(2) receptor for vasoactive intestinal peptide. *Proc. Natl. Acad. Sci. USA* 98, 13854–13859.

Gomariz, R.P., Lorenzo, M.J., Cacicedo, L., Vicente, A., and Zapata, A.G. (1990). Demonstration of immunoreactive vasoactive intestinal peptide (IR-VIP) and somatostatin (IR-SOM) in rat thymus. *Brain Behav. Immun.* 4, 151–161.

Goode, T., O'Connell, J., Sternini, C., Anton, P., Wong, H., O'Sullivan, G.C., Collins, J.K., and Shanahan, F. (1998). Substance P (neurokinin-1) receptor is a marker of human mucosal but not peripheral mononuclear cells: molecular quantitation and localization. *J. Immunol.* 161, 2232–2240.

Guo, C.J., Lai, J.P., Luo, H.M., Douglas, S.D., and Ho, W.Z. (2002). Substance P up-regulates macrophage inflammatory protein-1β expression in human T lymphocytes. *J. Neuroimmunol.* 131, 160–167.

Hart, R.P., Shadiack, A.M., and Jonakait, G.M. (1991). Substance P gene expression is regulated by interleukin-1 in cultured sympathetic ganglia. *J. Neurosci. Res.* 29, 282–291.

Hartung, H.P., Wolters, K., and Toyka, K.V. (1986). Substance P: binding properties and studies on cellular responses in guinea pig macrophages. *J. Immunol.* 136, 3856–3863.

Hashimoto, H., Ishihara, T., Shigemoto, R., Mori, K., and Nagata, S. (1993). Molecular cloning and tissue distribution of a receptor for pituitary adenylate cyclase-activating polypeptide. *Neuron* 11, 333–342.

Helme, R.D., Eglezos, A., Dandie, G.W., Andrews, P.V., and Boyd, R.L. (1987). The effect of substance P on the regional lymph node antibody response to antigenic stimulation in capsaicin-pretreated rats. *J. Immunol.* 139, 3470–3473.

Ho, W.Z., Lai, J.P., Zhu, X.H., Uvaydova, M., and Douglas, S.D. (1997). Human monocytes and macrophages express substance P and neurokinin-1 receptor. *J. Immunol.* 159, 5654–5660.

Ho, W.Z., Lai, J.P., Li, Y., and Douglas, S.D. (2002). HIV enhances substance P expression in human immune cells. *FASEB J.* 16, 616–618.

Hokfelt, T., Johansson, O., Ljungdahl, A., Lundberg, J.M., and Schultzbert, M. (1980). Peptidergic neurons. *Nature* 284, 515–521.

Hokfelt, T., Pernow, B., and Wahren, J. (2001). Substance P: a pioneer amongst neuropeptides. *J. Intern. Med.* 249, 27–40.

Ichikawa, S., Sreedharan, S.P., Goetzl, E.J., and Owen, R.L. (1994). Immunohistochemical localization of peptidergic nerve fibers and neuropeptide receptors in Peyer's patches of the cat ileum. *Regul. Pept.* 54, 385–395.

Ijaz, M.K., Dent, D., and Babiuk, L.A. (1990). Neuroimmunomodulation of *in vivo* anti-rotavirus humoral immune response. *J. Neuroimmunol.* 26, 159–171.

Inoue, N., Magari, S., and Sakanaka, M. (1990). Distribution of peptidergic nerve fibers in rat bronchus-associated lymphoid tissue: light microscopic observations. *Lymphology* 23, 155–160.

Ishihara, T., Shigemoto, R., Mori, K., Takahashi, K., and Nagata, S. (1992). Functional expression and tissue distribution of a novel receptor for vasoactive intestinal polypeptide. *Neuron* 8, 811–819.

Jiang, X., Jing, H., and Ganea, D. (2002). VIP and PACAP down-regulate CXCL10 (IP-10) and upregulate CCL22 (MDC) in spleen cells. *J. Neuroimmunol.* 133, 81–94.

Jonakait, G.M., and Schotland, S. (1990). Conditioned medium from activated splenocytes increases substance P in sympathetic ganglia. *J. Neurosci. Res.* 26, 24–30.

Joos, G.F., De Swert, K.O., and Pauwels, R.A. (2001). Airway inflammation and tachykinins: prospects for the development of tachykinin receptor antagonists. *Eur. J. Pharmacol.* 429, 239–250.

Kaltreider, H.B., Ichidawa, S., Byrd, P.K., Ingram, D.A., Kashiyama, J.L., Sreedharan, S.P., Warnock, M.L., Beck, J.M., and Goetzl, E.J. (1997). Upregulation of neuropeptides and neuropeptide receptors in a murine model of immune inflammation in lung parenchyma. *Am. J. Respir. Cell Mol. Biol.* 16, 133–144.

Keranen, U., Kiviluoto, T., Jarvinen, H., Back, N., Kivilaakso, E., and Soinila, S. (1995). Changes in substance P-immunoreactive innervation of human colon associated with ulcerative colitis. *Dig. Dis. Sci.* 40, 2250–2258.

Killingsworth, C.R., Shore, S.A., Alessandrini, F., Dey, R.D., and Paulauskis, J.D. (1997). Rat alveolar macrophages express preprotachykinin gene-I mRNA-encoding tachykinins. *Am. J. Physiol.* 273, L1073–1081.

Kimata, H., and Fujimoto, M. (1994). Vasoactive intestinal peptide specifically induces human IgA1 and IgA2 production. *Eur. J. Immunol.* 24, 2262–2265.

Kincy-Cain, T., and Bost, K.L. (1996). Increased susceptibility of mice to *Salmonella* infection following in vivo treatment with the substance P antagonist, spantide II. *J. Immunol.* 157, 255–264.

Kincy-Cain, T., Clements, J.D., and Bost, K.L. (1996). Endogenous and exogenous interleukin-12 augment the protective immune response in mice orally challenged with *Salmonella dublin*. *Infect. Immun.* 64, 1437–1440.

Kincy-Cain, T., and Bost, K.L. (1997). Substance P-induced IL-12 production by murine macrophages. *J. Immunol.* 158, 2334–2339.

Kulkarni-Narla, A., Beitz, A.J., and Brown, D.R. (1999). Catecholaminergic, cholinergic and peptidergic innervation of gut-associated lymphoid tissue in porcine jejunum and ileum. *Cell. Tissue Res.* 298, 275–286.

Kurtz, M., Wang, R., Clements, M., Cascieri, M., Austin, C., Cunningham, B., Chicchi, G., and Liu, Q. (2002). Identification, localization and receptor characterization of novel mammalian substance P-like peptides. *Gene* 296, 205.

Lai, J.P., Douglas, S.D., Rappaport, E., Wu, J.M., and Ho, W.Z. (1998). Identification of a delta isoform of preprotachykinin mRNA in human mononuclear phagocytes and lymphocytes. *J. Neuroimmunol.* 91, 121–128.

Lambrecht, B.N., Germonpre, P.R., Everaert, E.G., Carro-Muino, I., DeVeerman, M., de Felipe, C., Hunt, S.P., Thielemans, K., Joos, G.F., and Pauwels, R.A. (1999). Endogenously produced substance P contributes to lymphocyte proliferation induced by dendritic cells and direct TCR ligation. *Eur. J. Immunol.* 29, 3815–3825.

Lara-Marquez, M., O'Dorisio, M., O'Dorisio, T., Shah, M., and Karacay, B. (2001). Selective gene expression and activation-dependent regulation of vasoactive intestinal peptide receptor type 1 and type 2 in human T cells. *J. Immunol.* 166, 2522–2530.

Li, Y., Tian, S., Douglas, S.D., and Ho, W.Z. (2000). Morphine Up-regulates expression of substance P and its receptor in human blood mononuclear phagocytes and lymphocytes. *Cell. Immunol.* 205, 120–127.

Lotz, M., Vaughan, J.H., and Carson, D.A. (1988). Effect of neuropeptides on production of inflammatory cytokines by human monocytes. *Science* 241, 1218–1221.

Lucey, D.R., Novak, J.M., Polonis, V.R., Liu, Y., and Gartner, S. (1994). Characterization of substance P binding to human monocytes/macrophages. *Clin. Diagn. Lab. Immunol.* 1, 330–335.

Lutz, E.M., Sheward, W.J., West, K.M., Morrow, J.A., Fink, G., and Harmar, A.J. (1993). The VIP2 receptor: molecular characterization of a cDNA encoding a novel receptor for vasoactive intestinal polypeptide. *FEBS Lett.* 334, 3–8.

Maggi, C.A. (1995). The mammalian tachykinin receptors. *Gen. Pharmacol.* 26, 911–944.

Makhlouf, G.M. (1990). Neural and hormonal regulation of function in the gut. *Hosp. Pract.* 25, 79–98.

Marriott, I., and Bost, K.L. (1998). Substance P diminishes lipopolysaccharide and IFN-γ-induced TGF-β1 production by cultured murine macrophages. *Cell. Immunol.* 183, 113–120.

Marriott, I., and Bost, K.L. (2000). IL-4 and IFN-γ up-regulate substance P receptor expression in murine peritoneal macrophages. *J. Immunol.* 165, 182–191.

Marriott, I., Mason, M.J., Elhofy, A., and Bost, K.L. (2000). Substance P activates NF-kappaB independent of elevations in intracellular calcium in murine macrophages and dendritic cells. *J. Neuroimmunol.* 102, 163–171.

Marriott, I., and Bost, K.L. (2001). Expression of authentic substance P receptors in murine and human dendritic cells. *J. Neuroimmunol.* 114, 131–141.

Martinez, C., Delgado, M., Pozo, D., Leceta, J., Calvo, J.R., Ganea, D., and Gomariz, R.P. (1998). Vasoactive intestinal peptide and pituitary adenylate cyclase-activating polypeptide modulate endotoxin-induced IL-6 production by murine peritoneal macrophages. *J. Leukoc. Biol.* 63, 591–601.

Martinez, C., Delgado, M., Abad, C., Gomariz, R.P., Ganea, D., and Leceta, J. (1999). Regulation of VIP production and secretion by murine lymphocytes. *J. Neuroimmunol.* 93, 126–138.

Mathew, R.C., Cook, G.A., Blum, A.M., Metwali, A., Felman, R., and Weinstock, J.V. (1992). Vasoactive intestinal peptide stimulates T lymphocytes to release IL-5 in murine schistosomiasis mansoni infection. *J. Immunol.* 148, 3572–3577.

McCormack, R.J., Hart, R.P., and Ganea, D. (1996). Expression of NK-1 receptor mRNA in murine T lymphocytes. *Neuroimmunomodulation* 3, 35–46.

Metwali, A., Blum, A., Mathew, R., Sandor, M., Lynch, R.G., and Weinstock, J.V. (1993). Modulation of T lymphocyte proliferation in mice infected with *Schistosoma mansoni*: VIP suppresses mitogen- and antigen-induced T cell proliferation possibly by inhibiting IL-2 production. *Cell. Immunol.* 149, 11–23.

Metwali, A., Blum, A.M., Ferraris, L., Klein, J.S., Fiocchi, C., and Weinstock, J.V. (1994). Eosinophils within the healthy or inflamed human intestine produce substance P and vasoactive intestinal peptide. *J. Neuroimmunol.* 52, 69–78.

Miyata, A., Arimura, A., Dahl, R.R., Minamino, N., Uehara, A., Jiang, L., Culler, M.D., and Coy, D.H. (1989). Isolation of a novel 38 residue-hypothalamic polypeptide which stimulates adenylate

cyclase in pituitary cells. *Biochem. Biophys. Res. Commun.* 164, 567–574.

Ottaway, C.A., and Greenberg, G.R. (1984). Interaction of vasoactive intestinal peptide with mouse lymphocytes: specific binding and the modulation of mitogen responses. *J. Immunol.* 132, 417–423.

Ottaway, C.A. (1987). Selective effects of vasoactive intestinal peptide on mitogenic response of murine T cells. *Immunology* 62, 291–297.

Ottaway, C.A., Lewis, D.L., and Asa, S.L. (1987). Vasoactive intestinal peptide-containing nerves in Peyer's patches. *Brain Behav. Immun.* 1, 148–158.

Pascual, D.W., and Bost, K.L. (1990). Substance P production by P388D1 macrophages: a possible autocrine function for this neuropeptide. *Immunology* 71, 52–56.

Pascual, D.W., Xu-Amano, J.C., Kiyono, H., McGhee, J.R., and Bost, K.L. (1991a). Substance P acts directly upon cloned B lymphoma cells to enhance IgA and IgM production. *J. Immunol.* 146, 2130–2136.

Pascual, D.W., McGhee, J.R., Kiyono, H., and Bost, K.L. (1991b). Neuroimmune modulation of lymphocyte function: I. Substance P enhances immunoglobulin synthesis in lipopolysaccharide activated murine splenic B cell culture. *Int. Immunol.* 3, 1223–1229.

Pascual, D.W., Bost, K.L., Xu-Amano, J., Kiyono, H., and McGhee, J.R. (1992). The cytokine-like action of substance P upon B cell differentiation. *Reg. Immunol.* 4, 100–104.

Pascual, D.W., Beagley, K.W., Kiyono, H., and McGhee, J.R. (1995). Substance P promotes Peyer's patch and splenic B cell differentiation. *Adv. Exp. Med. Biol.* 371A, 55–59.

Pascual, D.W., Hone, D.M., Hall, S., van Ginkel, F.W., Yamamoto, M., Walters, N., Fujihashi, K., Powell, R.I., Wu, S., VanCott, J.L., Kiyono, H., and McGhee, J.R. (1999). Expression of recombinant enterotoxigenic *Escherichia coli* colonization factor antigen I by *Salmonella typhimurium* elicits a biphasic T helper cell response. *Infect. Immun.* 67, 6249–6256.

Payan, D.G., Brewster, D.R., and Goetzl, E.J. (1983). Specific stimulation of human T lymphocytes by substance P. *J. Immunol.* 131, 1613–1615.

Payan, D.G., Brewster, D.R., and Goetzl, E.J. (1984a). Stereospecific receptors for substance P on cultured human IM-9 lymphoblasts. *J. Immunol.* 133, 3260–3265.

Payan, D.G., Hess, C.A., and Goetzl, E.J. (1984b). Inhibition by somatostatin of the proliferation of T-lymphocytes and Molt-4 lymphoblasts. *Cell. Immunol.* 84, 433–438.

Peacock, J.W., and Bost, K.L. (2000). Infection of intestinal epithelial cells and development of systemic disease following gastric instillation of murine γ-herpesvirus-68. *J. Gen. Virol.* 81, 421–429.

Pernow, B. (1983). Substance P. *Pharmacol. Rev.* 35, 85–140.

Polak, J.M., and Bloom, S.R. (1982). Distribution and tissue localization of VIP in the central nervous system and seven peripheral organs. In *Vasoactive Intestinal Peptide* (ed. S.I. Said), New York: Raven Press, 107.

Popper, P., Mantyh, C.R., Vigna, S.R., Maggio, J.E., and Mantyh, P.W. (1988). The localization of sensory nerve fibers and receptor binding sites for sensory neuropeptides in canine mesenteric lymph nodes. *Peptides* 9, 257–267.

Qian, B.F., Zhou, G.Q., Hammarström, M.L., and Danielsson, Å. (2001a). Both substance P and its receptor are expressed in mouse intestinal T lymphocytes. *Neuroendocrinology* 73, 358–368.

Qian, B.F., Hammarström, M.L., and Danielsson, Å. (2001b). Differential expression of vasoactive intestinal polypeptide receptor 1 and 2 mRNA in murine intestinal T lymphocyte subtypes. *J. Neuroendocrinol.* 13, 818–825.

Rameshwar, P., and Gascon, P. (1997). Hematopoietic modulation by the tachykinins. *Acta Haematol.* 98, 59–64.

Rasley, A., Bost, K.L., Olson, J.K., Miller, S.D., and Marriott, I. (2002). Expression of functional NK-1 receptors in murine microglia. *Glia* 37, 258–267.

Sangster, M.Y., Topham, D.J., D'Costa, S., Cardin, R.D., Marion, T.N., Myers, L.K., and Doherty, P.C. (2000). Analysis of the virus-specific and nonspecific B cell response to a persistent B-lymphotropic γherpesvirus. *J. Immunol.* 164, 1820–1828.

Schultzberg, M., Hokfelt, T., Nilsson, G., Terenius, L., Rehfeld, J.F., Brown, M., Elde, R., Goldstein, M., and Said, S. (1980). Distribution of peptide- and catecholamine-containing neurons in the gastro-intestinal tract of rat and guinea pig: immunohisto-chemical studies with antisera to substance P, vasoactive intestinal polypeptide, enkephalins, somatostatin, gastrin/cholecystokinin, neurotensin, and dopamine ß-hydroxylase. *Neuroscience* 5, 689–744.

Stanisz, A.M., Befus, D., and Bienenstock, J. (1986). Differential effects of vasoactive intestinal peptide, substance P, and somatostatin on immunoglobulin synthesis and proliferations by lymphocytes from Peyer's patches, mesenteric lymph nodes, and spleen. *J. Immunol.* 136, 152–156.

Stanisz, A.M., Scicchitano, R., Dazin, P., Bienenstock, J., and Payan, D.G. (1987). Distribution of substance P receptors on murine spleen and Peyer's patch T and B cells. *J. Immunol.* 139, 749–754.

Stead, R.H., Tomioka, M., Quinonez, G., Simon, G.T., Felten, S.Y., and Bienenstock, J. (1987). Intestinal mucosal mast cells in normal and nematode-infected rat intestines are in intimate contact with peptidergic nerves. *Proc. Natl. Acad. Sci. USA* 84, 2975–2979.

Stead, R.H. (1992). Innervation of mucosal immune cells in the gastrointestinal tract. *Reg. Immunol.* 4, 91–99.

Stevenson, P.G., and Doherty, P.C. (1998). Kinetic analysis of the specific host response to a murine γ herpesvirus. *J. Virol.* 72, 943–949.

Sturiale, S., Barbara, G., Qiu, B., Figini, M., Geppetti, P., Gerard, N., Gerard, C., Grady, E.F., Bunnett, N.W., and Collins, S.M. (1999). Neutral endopeptidase (EC 3.4.24.11) terminates colitis by degrading substance P. *Proc. Natl. Acad. Sci. USA* 96, 11653–11658.

Sunil-Chandra, N.P., Efstathiou, S., Arno, J., and Nash, A.A. (1992a). Virological and pathological features of mice infected with murine γ-herpesvirus 68. *J. Gen. Virol.* 73, 2347–2356.

Sunil-Chandra, N.P., Efstathiou, S., and Nash, A.A. (1992b). Murine γ-herpesvirus 68 establishes a latent infection in mouse B lymphocytes in vivo. *J. Gen. Virol.* 73, 3275–3279.

Tripp, R.A., Hamilton-Easton, A.M., Cardin, R.D., Nguyen, P., Behm, F.G., Woodland, D.L., Doherty, P.C., and Blackman, M.A. (1997). Pathogenesis of an infectious mononucleosis-like disease induced by a murine γ-herpesvirus: role for a viral superantigen? *J. Exp. Med.* 185, 1641–1650.

Tripp, R.A., Barskey, A., Goss, L., and Anderson, L.J. (2002). Substance P receptor expression on lymphocytes is associated with the immune response to respiratory syncytial virus infection. *J. Neuroimmunol.* 129, 141–153.

Trunkle, T., Walters, N., and Pascual, D.W. (2003). Substance P (SP) receptor-deficient (NK1R$^{-/-}$) mice show elevated secretory (S)-IgA responses to oral *Salmonella* vaccines and increased resistance to wild-type *Salmonella* challenge. *FASE B J* 17:C27, 32.18

Usherwood, E.J., Ross, A.J., Allen, D.J., and Nash, A.A. (1996a). Murine γ-herpesvirus-induced splenomegaly: a critical role for CD4 T cells. *J. Gen. Virol.* 77, 627–630.

Usherwood, E.J., Stewart, J.P., Robertson, K., Allen, D.J., and Nash, A.A. (1996b). Absence of splenic latency in murine γ-herpesvirus 68-infected B cell-deficient mice. *J. Gen. Virol.* 77, 2819–2825.

Usherwood, E.J., Roy, D.J., Ward, K., Surman, S.L., Dutia, B.M., Blackman, M.A., Stewart, J.P., and Woodland, D.L. (2000). Control of γ-herpesvirus latency by latent antigen-specific CD8^{+} T cells. *J. Exp. Med.* 192, 943–952.

van Ginkel, F.W., and Pascual, D.W. (1996). Recognition of neurokinin-1 receptor (NK1-R): an antibody to a peptide sequence from the third extracellular region binds to brain NK1-R. *J. Neuroimmunol.* 67, 49–58.

Vento, P., Kiviluoto, T., Keranen, U., Jarvinen, H.J., Kivilaakso, E., and Soinila, S. (2001). Quantitative comparison of growth-associated protein-43 and substance P in ulcerative colitis. *J. Histochem. Cytochem.* 49, 749–758.

Virgin, H.W. IV., Latreille, P., Wamsley, P., Hallsworth, K., Weck, K.E., Dal Canto, A.J., and Speck, S.H. (1997). Complete sequence and genomic analysis of murine γ-herpesvirus 68. *J. Virol.* 71, 5894–5904.

Voice, J.K., Dorsam, G., Lee, H., Kong, Y., and Goetzl, E.J. (2001). Allergic diathesis in transgenic mice with constitutive T cell expression of inducible vasoactive intestinal peptide receptor. *FASEB J.* 15, 2489–2496.

Wang, H.Y., Xin, Z., Tang, H., and Ganea, D. (1996). Vasoactive intestinal peptide inhibits IL-4 production in murine T cells by a post-transcriptional mechanism. *J. Immunol.* 156, 3243–3253.

Weck, K.E., Kim, S.S., Virgin, H.W. IV., and Speck, S.H. (1999). Macrophages are the major reservoir of latent murine γ-herpesvirus 68 in peritoneal cells. *J. Virol.* 73, 3273–3283.

Weihe, E., and Krekel, J. (1991). The neuroimmune connection in human tonsils. *Brain Behav. Immun.* 5, 41–54.

Wood, C.L., and O'Dorisio, M.S. (1985). Covalent cross-linking of vasoactive intestinal polypeptide to its receptors on intact human lymphoblasts. *J. Biol. Chem.* 260, 1243–1247.

Zentel, H.J., and Weihe, E. (1991). The neuro-B cell link of peptidergic innervation in the bursa fabricii. *Brain Behav. Immun.* 5, 132–147.

Zhang, Y., Lu, L., Furlonger, C., Wu, G.E., and Paige, C.J. (2000). Hemokinin is a hematopoietic-specific tachykinin that regulates B lymphopoiesis. *Nat. Immunol.* 1, 392–397.

Section C

Mucosal Immunity and Infection

Mucosal Immunity and Infection: An Overview

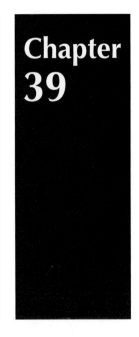

Chapter 39

Michael E. Lamm

Department of Pathology, Case Western Reserve University, Cleveland, Ohio

John Bienenstock

Departments of Medicine & Pathology and Molecular Medicine, McMaster University, Hamilton, Ontario, Canada

Section C deals with the manner in which the mucosal immune system interacts with microbes, including its ability to discriminate between pathogens and commensals—an especially important consideration because of the normal, abundant microbial flora in the intestinal tract. In fact, the normal flora of the intestinal and upper respiratory tracts greatly exceed potential pathogens in number and variety. Many of these commensal organisms themselves produce substances that may interfere with microbial well-being and might even be microbicidal. In turn, the flora and their products interact with mucosal epithelium in a variety of ways, promoting the secretion of mucus and other products. Normal peristalsis in the intestine, ciliary action in the respiratory tract, and urine flow in the urinary tract propel microorganisms and lessen their ability to adhere to the epithelium. Secretory products such as acid, enzymes, biliary constituents, lactoferrin, mucus, surfactant, and the complement system are all involved in homeostasis and defense against potentially pathogenic microorganisms.

Mucosal epithelium used to be thought of almost entirely as a physical barrier to the luminal contents, including microbes. Indeed, the tight junctions between epithelial cells help preserve the barrier function. The epithelium, however, also makes many pro- and anti-inflammatory substances constitutively, including products of arachidonic acid metabolism, potent microbicidal agents like defensins, and a gamut of cytokines and chemokines. These factors communicate not only with intraepithelial lymphocytes, dendritic cells, NK cells, mast cells, macrophages, eosinophils, and subsets of T lymphocytes, but also with different types of enteric nerves. Given that most cells in the body express receptors for neurotransmitters, enteric nerves are important regulators of physiological and inflammatory responses. Thus, an activated mucosal defense system comprises an integrated set of complex interactions, both specific and nonspecific, which, taken together, are usually beneficial for the host.

The chapters in Section C describe the kinds of surface structures and molecules that microbial pathogens use to adhere to and invade mucosal epithelium and to evade host defenses, as well as the cell surface receptors of the host with which they interact. These interactions trigger both the innate and adaptive arms of the mucosal immune system, which respond in ways that are designed to resist infection without provoking undue inflammation. In this context the chapters consider the kinds of effector and regulatory cells, antibodies, and mediator systems that come into play in mucosal defense against infection and how these both resemble and differ from their systemic counterparts.

The kinds of innate and adaptive host defense mechanisms that can be stimulated by pathogenic microbes are, of course, germane to strategies for preventing and treating infections. For dealing with mucosal infections, the most productive methods and strategies for prevention and treatment may well vary among different microbes, even within the same class of agent. In some cases, the most effective or practical ways to immunize against infections, or to treat them with passive antibody, will emphasize systemic routes, whereas for others, local mucosal routes will likely prove optimal. These issues are also considered.

Both common and distinctive properties of the different categories of infectious agents are delineated in Section C, which embraces bacteria, viruses, and parasites. Extensive new information is available with respect to bacterial and viral pathogens in the context of mucosal immunity. Unfortunately, comparatively little is known with regard to mucosal immunity to parasites, which are markedly heterogeneous and of particular significance in the economically disadvantaged parts of the world. For effective dealing with parasites, much needs to be accomplished.

Bacterial Interactions with Mucosal Epithelial Cells

Carlos J. Orihuela

Department of Infectious Diseases, St. Jude Children's Research Hospital, Memphis, Tennessee

George Fogg

Department of Pediatrics and Communicable Diseases, University of Michigan Medical School, Ann Arbor, Michigan

Victor J. DiRita

Department of Microbiology and Immunology, University of Michigan Medical School, Ann Arbor, Michigan

Elaine Tuomanen

Department of Infectious Diseases, St. Jude Children's Research Hospital, Memphis, Tennessee

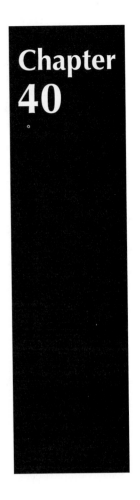

BACTERIAL INTERACTIONS WITH MUCOSAL EPITHELIAL CELLS IN THE RESPIRATORY TRACT

The human respiratory tract (RT) can be divided into two regions: the nasopharynx, the most common site for bacterial colonization, and the lungs, which are sterile. Epidemiological studies have demonstrated that while many bacteria are capable of infecting the lower RT, only few species do so commonly (Mandell, 1995). These pathogens cause two distinct types of disease. Infection limited to the airways is exemplified by that due to *Bordetella pertussis*, the cause of whooping cough (Locht, 1999; Coote, 2001). Infection of the alveoli produces pneumonia. In developed countries the most common agents of community-acquired pneumonia are *Streptococcus pneumoniae*, *Haemophilus influenzae*, *Moraxella catarrhalis*, and *Mycoplasma pneumoniae*. *S. pneumoniae* alone accounts for 8% to 46% of pneumonias.

Most respiratory pathogens initially colonize the nasopharynx and subsequently are aspirated into the lungs. All healthy children and adults are colonized repetitively and usually asymptomatically. Colonization progresses to disease more commonly in individuals who are immunocompromised, have underlying conditions (*e.g.*, cystic fibrosis, asthma, chronic pulmonary disease), or have habits or lifestyles that impair the normal functioning of the innate defense of the lung (*e.g.*, smoking or alcoholism) (Mandell, 1995; Ruiz *et al.*, 1999). While this chapter will focus on the interaction of pathogens with the lower RT, one must remember that pathogenic bacteria are only a small fraction of the total bacteria that colonize the upper RT. Like those in the gastrointestinal tract, most bacteria in the nasopharynx are commensal and exist in balance with the host. The presence of these bacteria is also most likely beneficial, if simply to occupy a niche and prevent colonization by more pathogenic strains.

The signature characteristic of bacteria that cause lower RT infection is the ability to adhere to and invade mucosal epithelial cells (MECs), either ciliated cells of the airways or type I and II alveolar cells in the terminal air sacs. To gain access to MECs, pathogens must overcome the gauntlet of innate and specific defenses present in mucosal secretions. These defenses routinely protect the host from the onslaught of commensal and pathogenic bacteria introduced into the RT daily. This section focuses on the mechanisms by which respiratory pathogens circumvent the innate immune system and cause pulmonary disease. While general concepts of microbial adhesion are discussed elsewhere (see Chapter 3), here bacterial adhesion in the context of invasive disease and lung damage is reviewed. It is our aim that the reader will gain an appreciation for the conserved mechanisms that distinct pathogens have developed to cause pneumonia. These mechanisms are striking examples of convergent evolution and provide important insight into the principal paradigms characterizing the bacteria–host interaction.

CILIA AND THE MUCIN LAYER

Mucus is the primary innate defense protecting mucosal epithelial cells from microorganisms and serves as a physical barrier to infection (Knowles *et al.*, 2002). Beating of cilia of epithelial cells transports mucus and entrapped particles to the mouth, where they can be swallowed and killed in the stomach. Mucin is a complex mixture of very diverse, high-molecular-weight, glycosylated macromolecules that, by virtue of carbohydrate diversity, is capable of binding almost any particle that lands on the airway surface (Klein *et al.*, 2000). Bacteria evade mucin entrapment by reducing the number of receptors on their surfaces or by enzymatic digestion of mucin by glycohydrolases (Gottschalk, 1960). Digestion of mucin reduces the viscosity of the mucus, enabling bacteria to penetrate to the epithelial surface. These enzymes also serve to cleave terminal carbohydrate structures from the surfaces of MECs, exposing previously cryptic antigens that then function as receptors for the bacteria (Tong *et al.*, 2000). For example, removal of sialic acid from glycans on host cells by neuraminidases is a strategy used by all respiratory pathogens, even viruses.

The most direct mechanism for protecting the host from bacteria is to kill microbes prior to their contact with MECs. Accordingly, the mucus layer, in addition to being a physical barrier, is a chemical shield exposing bacteria to an extensive array of antimicrobial peptides and inhibitory proteins. Antimicrobial factors present in mucus include complement, C-reactive protein, cathepsin G, elastase, defensins, surfactant, collectins, lysozyme, and lactoferrin (Brogden 2000). Mammals and even insects have evolved an extensive array of antimicrobial peptides or defensins to kill microbes in mucosal secretions. Defensins are secreted by epithelial cells and damage the bacterial cell membrane, causing blebs or lytic pores (Lehrer *et al.*, 1991). Bacterial strategies against defensins focus at either neutralizing the peptides or evading them (Brogden, 2000). Strategies include altering receptors for defensins (such as outer-membrane proteins, lipopolysaccharide [LPS] and teichoic acid), adsorbing charged molecules that repel the peptides, or actively transporting the defensins away from the bacterial surface.

Another important antimicrobial factor present in RT secretions is complement. LPS on gram-negative bacteria activates the alternative pathway by binding C3b and C5b, which then serve as a nucleus for the formation of the membrane attack complex (MAC) (Downey *et al.*, 1997). Alternatively, other components such as IgG and C-reactive protein (CRP), once bound, activate the classical comple-

ment pathway. Bound complement opsonizes bacteria for phagocytosis, while soluble C3a and C5a serve as potent chemotactic molecules for neutrophils and macrophages (Erdei *et al.*, 1997). Some gram-negative bacteria circumvent complement by attaching sialic acid to their surface. Sialic acid binds serum protein H, which in turn binds protein I. Protein I degrades C3b, thus preventing the formation of the C5 convertase (C462A3B) (Rautemaa *et al.*, 1999). This sialic acid–based defense is a common strategy with many variations. *Neisseria gonorrhoeae* binds sialic acid to the LPS O-antigen, while *Neisseria meningitidis* displays sialic acid as a major capsular component (Ram *et al.*, 1999). Alternatively, gram-negative bacteria can increase the length of the LPS O-antigen side chain in order to push MACs too far from the surface to have a bactericidal effect. Similarly, gram-positive bacteria are naturally resistant to MAC-killing, as the thick peptidoglycan cell wall prevents MAC access to the membrane (Fernie-King *et al.*, 2001).

Surfactant protein (SP)-A and SP-D also opsonize bacteria for phagocytosis and enhance superoxide production by alveolar macrophages. SP-A and SP-D are collectins, a subgroup of the mammalian protein family of C-type lectins that bind carbohydrates (Sastry *et al.*, 1993; LeVine *et al.*, 1999). Produced in the lungs by type II cells, nonciliated bronchial cells, and tracheobronchial glands, SP-A and SP-D form multimeric structures on the surfaces of the bacteria similar to the complement protein C1q (Sastry *et al.*, 1993). Phagocytes then bind to these multimeric structures via specific cell surface receptors, including the C1q receptor, and subsequently phagocytose the bacteria (LeVine *et al.*, 1999).

Although it is not possible to review all of the innate defense mechanisms, it should be emphasized that the majority of respiratory disease occurs only when the innate defense is hampered. In humans, a striking example of such susceptibility is cystic fibrosis. Cystic fibrosis (CF) is an autosomal recessive disorder in which the transporting of chloride across mucosal membranes is impossible, resulting in excessively viscid secretions. Respiratory manifestations are the result of impaired mucus clearance, resulting in obstruction of the airways and infection. The principal agents of morbidity and mortality among patients with CF are *Pseudomonas aeruginosa* and *Burkholderia cepacia* (Cant *et al.*, 2002). Colonization of the CF-affected lung by *P. aeruginosa* is associated with formation of biofilms on mucin plaques, a capability of the mucoid phenotype of *P. aeruginosa*. The mucoid phenotype expresses genes encoding for synthesis of a thick mucopolysaccharide surface layer and secretion of the major exoprotease elastase and a metalloproteinase (Firoved *et al.*, 2003). Similarly, *B. cepacia* also produces an elaborate array of virulence determinants, including a protease, lipase, hemolysin, and cytotoxin; in addition, some isolates produce a mucoid exopolysaccharide (Cant *et al.*, 2002).

A critical element making the mucous trap for bacteria effective is the expulsion of secretions from the lower RT by the ciliary escalator. Thus, it is not surprising that pathogens secrete toxins that can stop ciliary beating. The most specific of these toxins, tracheal cytotoxin, is derived from the cell wall of *B. pertussis* and is exquisitely potent and specific at killing ciliated cells (Wilson *et al.*, 1991). Other more general toxins, such as the pore-forming toxin, pneumolysin, can kill any cell in the RT, including ciliated cells (Feldman *et al.*, 1990).

NASOPHARYNGEAL COLONIZATION

RT pathogens regulate gene expression in response to signals present at each anatomical location (Stock *et al.*, 2000). This phase switching is under genetic control and serves to fine-tune the bacterial side of the bacterial/host cell interface. Switching between phases for *B. pertussis* allows for a phenotype adapted to transmission from person to person (nonadherent) or a phenotype adapted to high-level adherence to RT cells during infection (Cotter *et al.*, 1998). Phase switching for pneumococcus adapts the bacterial surface for mucosal adherence or survival in the bloodstream (Weiser 1998). In both cases, the bacteria use two-component signal transduction systems to enable the switch. These systems consist of a sensor kinase that detects environmental signals and autophosphorylates and a response regulator that then accepts the activated phosphate and binds to DNA to change gene transcription (Stock *et al.*, 2000). This mechanism of phase-switching in the RT was first understood in detail for the Bvg system in *B. pertussis*, a regulon that controls expression of adhesins and several toxins (Roy *et al.*, 1989).

Efficient colonization of the mucosa by pneumococci is controlled by the Cia system, which regulates expression of the serine protease HtrA, and other unknown genes (Sebert *et al.*, 2002) Another unknown genetic regulator controls the opaque-to-transparent-phase switch. Loss of CiaR/H results in a 1,000-fold decrease in the amount of bacteria colonizing the nasopharynx and a 25-fold decrease in expression of HtrA versus wild type. Mutants deficient in HtrA alone demonstrate a 100-fold reduction in virulence, indicating that other factors regulated by CiaR/H also contribute to nasopharyngeal colonization (Sebert *et al.*, 2002).

Prolonged colonization of the nasopharynx affords an opportunity for bacteria to enter the bloodstream without passing through the lower RT. One route of entry is via the polymeric immunoglobulin receptor (pIgR), an integral membrane protein produced by nasopharyngeal epithelial cells for transcytosis of IgA and IgM from the basolateral cell surface to the apical surface **(Fig. 40.1)** (Kaetzel, 2001). The pIgR-IgA dimer complex moves through a series of endosomal compartments to be secreted at the apex. Exported pIgR is cleaved, releasing secretory component (SC; the extracellular domain of pIgR) bound to the IgA dimer (S-IgA). *S. pneumoniae* binds to human SC (hSC) and human pIgR via a conserved hexapeptide motif in its major adhesin, CbpA (Zhang *et al.*, 2000). The interaction of CbpA with pIgR allows the bacteria to "co-opt" the pIgR translocation machinery and move across the epithelial cell from the apical to basolateral surface (Fig. 40.1). pIgR is not expressed in lung cells, and therefore CbpA-pIgR interactions repre-

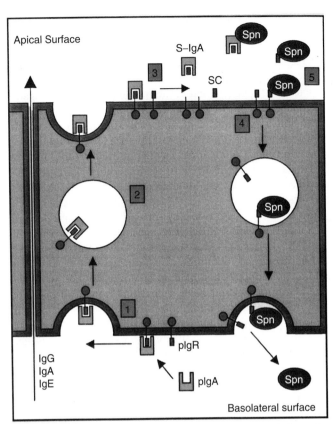

Fig. 40.1. Pneumococcal transcytosis. **(See page 10 of the color plates.)** (1) The polymeric immunoglobulin receptor (pIgR) on the basolateral surface of epithelial cells binds to polymeric IgA (pIgA) or IgM and is endocytosed. (2) During transcytosis pIgR, pIgR-pIgA is sorted into vesicles for transport to the apical surface. (3) On the apical surface a protease cleaves pIgR, releasing S-IgA or free secretory component (SC). (4) Uncleaved pIgR can be internalized and subsequently recycled to the apical surface or transcytosed to the basolateral side. (5) *Streptococcus pneumoniae* that binds to uncleaved pIgR can take advantage of the recycling of pIgR and along with pIgR transcytose across the epithelial cell to the basolateral surface.

sent a mechanism by which the pneumococcus crosses into the bloodstream without lower RT involvement.

WHOOPING COUGH VS. PNEUMONIA

The ability to invade MECs promotes infection in two ways. Most obvious is that it serves as a step for extracellular pathogens crossing epithelial cell barriers to gain access to the bloodstream. It also allows immune evasion, such as for the intracellular pathogen *Chlamydia pneumoniae* (Jones *et al.*, 2000). Pneumococci will be used as a prototype for bacteria that cause severe, invasive disease in the lower RT, since a third of all cases of pneumococcal pneumonia have bacteria detectable in the bloodstream (Mandell, 1995). In contrast, disease limited to the airways will be discussed in the setting of whooping cough, which involves bacterial attachment to RT cells but without translocation into the blood.

In the initial stages of infection, RT pathogens bind to carbohydrates located on the surfaces of lung cells. Pathogens such as *P. aeruginosa*, *H. influenzae*, *S. pneumoniae*, *Klebsiella pneumoniae*, *B. pertussis*, *S. aureus*, and *Escherichia coli* bind to the carbohydrate determinant N-acetylgalactosamine β1-3 galactose, commonly found in various lung cell glycoconjugates (Krivan *et al.*, 1988; Cundell *et al.*, 1994). Neuraminidases promote bacterial colonization by removing terminal sialic acid residues from the host cell surface, thereby exposing cryptic antigens such as N-acetylgalactosamine β1-3 galactose (Howie *et al.*, 1985; Tong *et al.*, 2000). Viral infections are also capable of enhancing bacterial adherence, in part because several respiratory viruses encode their own neuraminidase. Experiments in mice have demonstrated that viral infection with influenza primes the lungs for development of pneumococcal pneumonia by stripping sialic acid from the mucosa and consequently exposing pneumococcal receptors (McCullers *et al.*, 2003). To this end, dramatic increases in mortality are observed only when influenza infection precedes pneumococcal challenge and not the other way around.

For bacteria that never invade the bloodstream, the initial binding of bacteria to a carbohydrate does not induce translocation across the epithelium. *B. pertussis* binds to ciliated cells by an interaction of filamentous hemagglutinin with lactosylceramide (Tuomanen *et al.*, 1985; Prasad *et al.*, 1993). This interaction securely anchors the bacteria to the epithelial cell, and the production of toxins from that site eventually stops ciliary beating and kills the cell. *B. pertussis* infection remains localized to the airways without any alveolar or bloodstream invasion.

In contrast to pertussis, pneumococci bypass the airways and cause disease in the alveoli that commonly progresses to invasion of the bloodstream. After initial binding to host cell carbohydrates, upregulation of receptors for translocation to the bloodstream occurs as a result of inflammation. Components released by adherent bacteria activate the underlying epithelial cell, induce production of cytokines that in turn activate nearby cells, and eventually result in expression of neoreceptors. In the lower RT, bacterial invasion is commonly dependent on the upregulation of expression of platelet activating factor receptor (PAFr) (Cundell *et al.*, 1996; Swords *et al.*, 2001). Resting epithelial cells do not express high levels of PAFr. However, PAFr levels are enhanced on airway tissues during inflammation, such as with asthma (Nagase *et al.*, 2002) or smoking. Pathogens bind to PAFr in the same manner as the chemokine PAF, *i.e.*, by phosphorylcholine (ChoP) residues located on their surfaces. The surface expression of ChoP is a feature shared by the dominant respiratory pathogens, including *S. pneumoniae*, *H. influenzae*, *Mycoplasma pneumoniae*, *N. meningitidis*, *P. aeruginosa*, oral bacteria, and other pathogens such as nematodes (Kolberg *et al.*, 1997; Weiser *et al.*, 1998; Weiser *et al.*, 1998) **(Fig. 40.2)**. In most instances, ChoP is covalently bound to bacterial glycans or glycolipids (*e.g.*, teichoic acid, lipotechoic acid, lipooligosaccharides). One exception is *N. meningitidis*, which expresses ChoP on pili (Kolberg *et al.*, 1997). Bound bacteria are endocytosed in a PAFr-dependent manner and are translocated to the basolateral cell surface

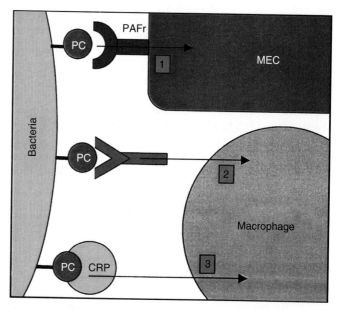

Fig. 40.2. Binding events mediated by phosphorylcholine. **(See page 10 of the color plates.)** Phosphorylcholine (PC) residues on bacteria allow the bacteria to (1) adhere to and invade mucosal epithelial cells expressing PAFr. Expression of PC on the bacterial surface allows opsonization of the bacteria either by (2) antibodies to PC or (3) CRP. Both activate complement deposition and subsequently further opsonize the bacteria for phagocytosis.

(Fig. 40.3). Bacteria not entering cells via PAFr presumably die in lysosomes (Ring *et al.*, 1998).

Although surface exposure of ChoP allows bacteria to adhere to PAFr, ChoP residues are also recognized by the host innate immune system and can be used to clear bacteria from the RT (Gould *et al.*, 2001) (Fig. 40.2). CRP, an acute-phase protein produced by the liver and MECs, binds ChoP and opsonizes bacteria for phagocytosis. Bound CRP also activates the classical complement cascade in an antibody-independent manner, resulting in formation of the MAC and further opsonization. By masking bacterial ChoP, CRP competitively inhibits bacterial binding to PAFr. Similarly, high levels of free ChoP in pulmonary surfactant competitively inhibit bacterial binding (Gould *et al.*, 2002).

Given the broad use of ChoP amongst respiratory pathogens and its role in innate defense, it is not surprising that bacteria have developed the ability to vary expression of the ChoP epitope on the bacterial surface (Weiser, 1998; Weiser *et al.*, 1998a; Weiser *et al.*, 1998b). Such phenotypic variation creates intrastrain variation among the infecting bacteria, such that some bacteria express more ChoP, allowing them to adhere to the mucosa, while others express less ChoP to avoid the bactericidal activity of CRP, especially in blood (Rosenow *et al.*, 1997; Weiser, 1998).

INFLAMMATION AND EPITHELIAL DAMAGE

The ability of the host to respond to bacterial products is dependent on a family of membrane proteins termed Toll-

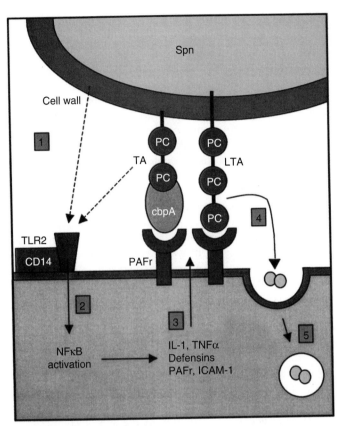

Fig. 40.3 PAFr-dependent adhesion and invasion. **(See page 10 of the color plates.)** (1) Gram-positive cell wall components such as peptidoglycan and teichoic acid bind their cognate pattern recognition protein (CD14/TLR2). (2) The CD14:cell wall complex binds to TLR2, initiating intracellular signaling that ultimately results in NF-κB activation. (3) NF-κB activation results in transcription and *de novo* production of inflammatory cytokines such as IL-1, TNFα, defensins, and surface receptors such as PAFr. (4) Enhanced expression of PAFr allows bacteria with phosphorylcholine to bind the PAFr. (5) In some bacteria such as the pneumococcus, binding of PAFr potentiates cell invasion in a cbpA-dependent manner.

like receptors (TLRs) (Medzhitov *et al.*, 1997). TLRs activate signaling pathways that initiate the innate response to infection and begin the process of adaptive immunity. These receptors play a major role in phagocytic cells such as alveolar macrophages and neutrophils but also dictate responsiveness of lung epithelial cells (Wang *et al.*, 2002). Conserved repetitive motifs on bacterial macromolecules (e.g., peptidoglycan, DNA, or LPS) are bound by soluble binding proteins (*e.g.*, LBP, sCD14) which then transfer the bacterial ligand to a corresponding TLR (Kopp *et al.*, 1999; Grassme *et al.*, 2000). TLR responses are tailored for the class of the infectious agent (Kopp *et al.*, 1999). For example, TLR4 recognizes LPS and as such is activated by gram-negative bacteria. TLR2 recognizes components of gram-positive bacteria such as peptidoglycan and teichoic acid. TLR9 recognizes nucleic acid motifs. Activation of TLRs triggers intracellular signaling, leading to induction of the innate response (defensins, cytokines, the expression of PAFr and ICAM) and recruitment of neutrophils and effector cells to clear the infection.

During the invasion process, several mucosal pathogens trigger apoptosis. Among the best studied are the gastrointestinal pathogens *Listeria monocytogenes*, *Shigella flexneri*, and *Salmonella typhimurium*. Although fewer RT bacteria have been implicated as causes of apoptosis, two of the most virulent, *P. aeruginosa* (Hauser *et al.*, 1999; Grassme *et al.*, 2000) and *S. pneumoniae* (Braun *et al.*, 2001; Braun *et al.*, 2002), appear to have this capability. *P. aeruginosa* has been shown to induce apoptosis in macrophages and certain lung epithelial cell lines. The process is mediated by a type III secretion system that injects ExoU, a cytotoxin, and an as-yet-unidentified protein into the host cells (Hauser *et al.*, 1999). Pneumolysin and hydrogen peroxide produced by pneumococci cause dramatic epithelial cell damage (Feldman *et al.*, 1990; Feldman *et al.*, 2002). Overall, cell death either by apoptosis or necrosis allows pathogens to avoid phagocytes and other immune modulators (Hauser *et al.*, 1999; Dockrell *et al.*, 2001) and damages the mucosa so as to facilitate bacterial entry into the bloodstream.

ANTHRAX: RESPIRATORY PATHOGENS AS BIOLOGICAL WARFARE AGENTS

Among RT pathogens, *Bacillus anthracis* is an effective biological warfare agent (Lew, 2000). Anthrax spores are suitable for such use because of their high potency, accessibility, ease of delivery, and capacity for storage. One millionth of a gram constitutes a lethal inhaled dose, whereas a kilogram has the potential to kill hundreds of thousands and render an area uninhabitable. Respiratory anthrax begins with inhalation and germination of the spores in the lower RT. The spores germinate into bacilli, which extend to regional lymph nodes, pleura, and subsequently the bowel. Survival is rare, with the first 3 days of infection marked by malaise, low-grade fever, and cough, followed by a sudden worsening of the condition, onset of sepsis, and death. The virulence of *B. anthracis* is due to a proteinaceous capsule that prevents phagocytosis of the bacilli (Koehler, 2002) and anthrax toxin, which suppresses macrophage function and causes epithelial cell necrosis (O'Brien *et al.*, 1985; Koehler, 2002). Experiments in animals suggest that spores deposited in the respiratory tract germinate and produce the toxin resulting in local lesions. Formation of these necrotic lesions then allows dissemination of the bacteria, resulting in systemic symptoms and toxicity (Lew, 2000).

BACTERIAL INTERACTIONS WITH THE GASTROINTESTINAL TRACT

The human gastrointestinal tract is the site of the most intensive interactions between the human host and the microbial world. The intestinal epithelium covers approximately 200 square meters and is colonized by bacteria that can reach densities of 10^{11} bacteria per milliliter in regions of the large intestine (Savage, 1977). Most of these microorganisms exist in a commensal relationship with the human host and under normal circumstances do not cause disease. A small subset of enteric bacteria, however, have developed virulence determinants that allow them to damage or even breach the intestinal epithelial barrier that separates the host tissues from this densely populated bacterial milieu. In the human gastrointestinal tract, pathogenic bacteria face a multitude of nonspecific host defenses such as the acidic environment of the stomach, interactions with mucins and IgA (discussed in the respiratory section), and soluble host factors such as lysozyme, proteases, lipases, antimicrobial peptides, and bile salts (Ouellette, 1997; Hecht, 1999). This section focuses on the virulence mechanisms that enteric pathogens use to overcome the host defenses at the mucosal epithelial cell (MEC) barrier. The different strategies employed by noninvasive and invasive enteric pathogens are discussed.

Noninvasive pathogens: toxin-mediated damage to the MEC

An indirect strategy employed by several enteric pathogens involves colonization of the digestive tract, with subsequent elaboration of enterotoxins that facilitate subsequent spread to other hosts. Classic members of this group of enteric pathogens include *Vibrio cholerae* and enterotoxigenic *Escherichia coli* (ETEC). The first step in the pathogenesis of these bacteria involves the coordinated expression of surface adhesion molecules that mediate colonization of the MEC **(Fig. 40.4)**. In the case of *V. cholerae*, an adhesin named the

"toxin coregulated pilus" (composed of subunits of TcpA protein) causes the bacteria to form microcolonies, which result in the colonization of the mucosal surface of the small intestine (Taylor *et al.*, 1987; Sharma *et al.*, 1989). The transcription of *tcpA* is under the control of the ToxR/TcpP/ToxT regulon, which also activates the transcription of the cholera toxin gene (*ctx*) (Herrington *et al.*, 1988; Krukonis *et al.*, 2000). Cholera toxin is composed of an enzymatically active A subunit and five B subunits that bind to GM1 ganglioside, the MEC cholera toxin surface receptor (Sixma *et al.*, 1991). The A subunit is internalized and causes a cAMP-mediated Cl⁻ secretion in the MEC (Betley *et al.*, 1986). The resulting voluminous secretory diarrhea carries the *V. cholerae* bacteria out of the host body, where they can colonize additional human hosts. Environmental signals in the small intestine activate the ToxR/TcpP/ToxT regulon, which restricts the expression of both the *tcpA* and ctx genes only to the region of the gastrointestinal tract, where they are required for virulence (Skorupski *et al.*, 1997; Lee *et al.*, 1999; Schuhmacher *et al.*, 1999).

Infections by ETEC follow a similar scenario in which adhesion is mediated by colonization factor antigen (Cfa) and enterotoxins (LT and ST toxins) are released (Levine, 1987; Gaastra *et al.*, 1996). For both *V. cholerae* and ETEC, the mucosal cell barrier remains intact and there is no evidence of invasion by the bacteria. Furthermore, although the toxins are potent mucosal immunogens and adjuvants, there is very little active inflammation at the site of colonization (Zhang *et al.*, 2003). Therefore, the pathogenic mechanism of disease seems to require only local colonization and enterotoxin production. The relationship between the bacterium and the host MEC remains a relatively indirect one that is mediated through the activity of a secreted toxin. A second major group of noninvasive enteric pathogens has developed a more intimate strategy of interacting with the host MEC.

Noninvasive pathogens: enteroadherent interactions with the MEC

Enteropathogenic *E. coli* (EPEC) and enterohemorrhagic *E. coli* (EHEC; O157:H7) remain extracellular but can subvert the normal function of the MEC through a mechanism that requires intimate attachment and major rearrangement of the host cell cytoskeleton. EPEC is a major cause of infantile diarrhea in the developing world, and EHEC is an important cause of sporadic foodborne outbreaks of bloody diarrhea (Nataro *et al.*, 1998). The characteristic pathological finding with infection of both of these bacteria is the attaching and effacing (A/E) lesion (Moon *et al.*, 1983). The multistep process involved in formation of the A/E lesion has been elucidated through a series of elegant studies (reviewed in De Vinney *et al.*, 1999; **Fig. 40.5**).

In the first step, the bacterium colonizes the MEC via a pilus called the bundle-forming pilus (BFP) (Giron *et al.*, 1991; Donnenberg *et al.*, 1992). This attachment is "nonintimate" and resembles the localized adherence by *V. cholerae*, described previously. This initial contact induces the formation of a syringe-like transfer apparatus, called a type III

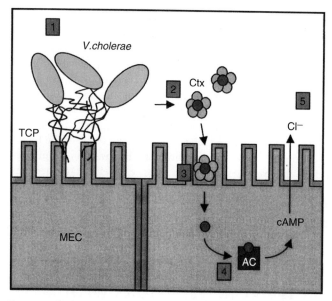

Fig. 40.4 Cholera toxin. **(See page 11 of the color plates.)** (1) *Vibrio cholerae* initially forms microcolonies and associates with the apical surface of the mucosal epithelial cell (MEC) through a type IV pilus called the toxin coregulated pilus (TCP). (2) Cholera toxin (Ctx), which is composed of one enzymatic A subunit (*red circles*) and five B subunits (*orange circles*), is coordinately expressed with TCP and secreted. (3) After the B subunits bind to the GM1 gangliosides on the MEC surface, the A subunit is translocated inside the cell. (4) Through the ADP-ribosylation activity, the A subunit constitutively activates adenylate cyclase (AC). (5) The resulting increase in intracellular cAMP causes efflux of chloride ions and secretory diarrhea.

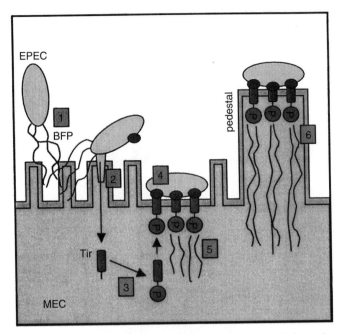

EPEC

BFP

pedestal

Tir

MEC

Fig. 40.5 EPEC formation of pedestals. **(See page 11 of the color plates.)** (1) Enteropathogenic *Escherichia coli* (EPEC) associates with the apical surface of MEC using a pilus called the bundle-forming pilus (BFP). (2) Using a type III secretion system (TTSS), the EPEC-derived protein Tir is injected into the MEC cytosol. Tir is a receptor for the EPEC outer-membrane protein intimin (*blue circles*). (3) Once inside the cytosol, Tir is phosphorylated by MEC kinases and inserted into the apical membrane. (4) Intimin on the bacteria binds tightly with Tir on the MEC to form "intimate attachment." (5) The cytosolic domains of Tir interact with host actin nucleation complexes after binding to intimin. The resulting actin polymerization causes the formation of protruding structures called pedestals and the subsequent effacement of the surrounding membrane surface.

secretion system (TTSS), to form a conduit through which bacterial proteins can be transferred into the host cell (Jarvis *et al.*, 1995). Type III secretion systems have been identified in several bacterial pathogens and are used by bacteria to efficiently deliver bacterial effector proteins to eukaryotic cells (reviewed in Hueck, 1998). EPEC and EHEC use their type III secretion apparatus to translocate the translocated intimin receptor (Tir) protein and other EPEC-secreted proteins (ESPs) into the host cell (Kenny *et al.*, 1997; Frankel *et al.*, 1998). Once inside the host cell, the EPEC-derived Tir is tyrosine-phosphorylated and inserted into the apical membrane (Kenny *et al.*, 1997). This membrane-bound form of Tir binds tightly to intimin, a bacterial outer-membrane protein, enabling what is termed "intimate attachment" (Kenny *et al.*, 1997). Thus, EPEC mediates intimate attachment to the host cell by delivering its own receptor to the host cell membrane.

Shortly after the intimin–Tir complex is formed, the intracellular domains of Tir initiate a profound accumulation of filamentous actin directly beneath the bacterial attachment site to form actin pedestals that can extend up to 10 μm above the host cell surface (Moon *et al.*, 1983; Kenny *et al.*, 1997). The formation of these structures also causes efface-

ment of the host cell microvilli along the apical brush border (Moon *et al.*, 1983). The exact mechanism by which these A/E lesions lead to diarrhea remains unclear.

There are some differences in the processes by which EPEC and EHEC establish their respective niches. For EHEC, the large intestine is the target organ, while EPEC infects the small bowel (Nataro *et al.*, 1998). In addition, the EHEC Tir protein is not phosphorylated inside of the host (DeVinney *et al.*, 2001). Although the mechanism of formation of the A/E lesions is similar to that of EPEC lesions, EHEC causes severe damage to the MEC because it also secretes a cytotoxin called shiga-like toxin, which inhibits host cell protein synthesis and has been associated with the development of hemorrhagic colitis (O'Brien *et al.*, 1987).

Another less characterized subgroup of noninvasive bacterial pathogens includes the enteroaggregative *E. coli* (EAEC). EAEC is responsible for chronic diarrhea in poorly nourished children and in HIV-infected patients (Bhan *et al.*, 1989; Mayer *et al.*, 1995). Like the other enteric pathogens described in this section, EAEC is noninvasive but adheres to the MEC in an aggregative pattern often described as a "stacked brick" formation (Nataro *et al.*, 1987). Several potential virulence factors involved in adhesion and toxin production have been identified, but none has been convincingly linked to the pathogenic phenotype of diarrheal disease (Okeke *et al.*, 2001).

Invasive pathogens: superficial mucosal invasion

An alternative strategy utilized by several enteric pathogens is to pursue an invasive lifestyle that allows bacteria access to deeper tissues in the host. Invasion provides many advantages to the bacteria, including evasion of the surface effectors of innate and adaptive immunity, access to nutrients, and the ability to travel to distant sites within the host. This strategy, however, presents multiple challenges to bacteria, since invasion also exposes them to more sophisticated arms of the immune response such as professional phagocytes, complement, and circulating immunoglobulins. This group of pathogens can be subdivided on the basis of the extent of dissemination they typically achieve during an infection.

The first subgroup of invasive enteric pathogens is represented by *Shigella* and the enteroinvasive *E. coli* (EIEC), both of which invade only the epithelial layer of the intestine. *Shigella* infection is characterized by dysentery, and histopathology of the colon usually shows extensive erosions of the mucosa and infiltration by large numbers of neutrophils (Wassef *et al.*, 1989; Mathan *et al.*, 1991). The mechanism of *Shigella* invasion explains how these extensive albeit superficial lesions are formed **(Fig. 40.6)**. *Shigella* cannot invade the MECs from their apical surface but efficiently enter via the basolateral surfaces (Perdomo *et al.*, 1994; Perdomo *et al.*, 1994).

In order to bypass the epithelial barrier presented by the MECs, the bacterium takes advantage of the M cell, a specialized cell type whose function is to sample luminal antigens and deliver them to the gut-associated lymphoid tissue

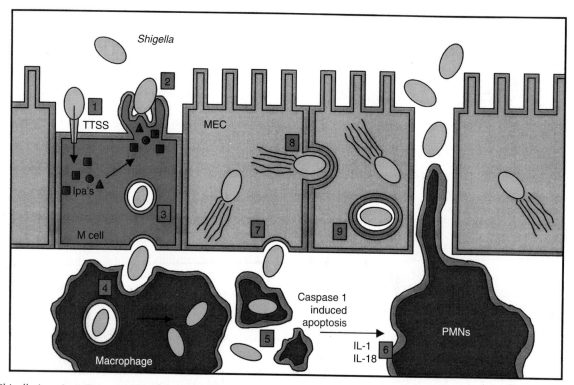

Fig. 40.6 Shigella invasion. **(See page 11 of the color plates.)** (1) *Shigella* interacts with M cells and injects the Ipa effector proteins into the cytosol through a TTSS. (2) The Ipa effectors stimulate membrane ruffling at the apical surface, and the bacterium is engulfed. (3) Once inside, the M cell translocates the membrane-bound bacteria to the lamina propria. (4) Resident macrophages engulf the *Shigella* and (5) are induced to undergo apoptosis through activation of caspase 1. (6) This also causes the release of inflammatory cytokines that recruit polymorphonuclear cells (PMNs) into the area. This inflammation creates a breach in the MEC barrier that allows more bacteria to infiltrate. (7) Shigella can efficiently infect the MEC from their basolateral surfaces. (8) Intracellular bacteria exit their vacuoles and propel themselves around the cytosol, using an actin-based motility. (9) Some bacteria are capable of moving into adjacent cells and are enclosed in a double membrane that is quickly destroyed by the bacterium.

(GALT) on their basolateral side. Normally, M cells overlie aggregations of lymphoid cells known as Peyer's patches. Luminal contents are collected by pinocytosis, and after transcytosis, they are delivered to antigen-presenting cells in the GALT (Hathaway et al. 2000). *Shigella* entry is targeted preferentially to the M cell. Once in contact with the M cell, a plasmid-encoded type III secretion system translocates the effector proteins IpaA, IpaC, and IpaD into the cell (Hale, 1991; Blocker *et al.*, 1999). These effector proteins interact with the M cell signal transduction pathways and cytoskeletal components to trigger engulfment of the bacterium (Tran Van Nhieu *et al.*, 1997; Tran Van Nhieu *et al.*, 1999; Niebuhr *et al.*, 2000). Shigellae transcytose across the M cell cytoplasm and are delivered to macrophages residing in the underlying GALT. Infected macrophages undergo apoptotic lysis mediated by interaction of IpaB with tripeptidyl peptidase II to activate caspase I (Chen *et al.*, 1996; Hilbi *et al.*, 1998; Hilbi *et al.*, 2000). Concurrently, IL-1β and IL-18 are released and lead to an inflammatory response with neutrophil recruitment (Sansonetti *et al.*, 2000).

This neutrophilic infiltration disrupts the MEC barrier, thereby providing an avenue for large-scale invasion of shigellae into the lamina propria layer of the gut wall. Despite this breach of the epithelial layer, shigellae rarely invade into deeper tissues but rather spread laterally. Internalized shigellae quickly escape from their endocytic vacuoles to gain access to the host cell cytoplasm (Sansonetti *et al.*, 1986). Motility within the cytoplasm is achieved by expressing IcsA, a bacterial outer-membrane protein, at one pole of the rod-shaped bacterium (Bernardini *et al.*, 1989).

IcsA interacts with and activates neural Wiskott-Aldrich syndrome protein (N-WASP) within the host cell (Egile *et al.*, 1999). Activation of N-WASP subsequently triggers actin nucleation and polymerization through interaction with the actin-related protein 2/3 (ARP 2/3) complex (Egile *et al.*, 1999). Actin polymerization generates sufficient force to move the bacterium through the host cell cytoplasm; photomicrographs of this process capture images of bacteria with filamentous actin at one pole forming structures termed "comet tails" (Goldberg *et al.*, 1995).

The gram-positive enteric pathogen *Listeria monocytogenes* uses a similar mechanism of cytoplasmic propulsion; however, its polar outer-membrane protein, termed ActA, interacts directly with the ARP 2/3 complex without the use of N-WASP (Portnoy *et al.*, 2002). Lateral spread of the shigellae to adjacent epithelial cells is mediated by active endocytosis of protrusions containing bacteria by the adjacent epithelial cells (Monack *et al.*, 2001). These bacteria are enclosed in a vacuole with two membrane layers that are quickly lysed by IpaB and IpaC proteins (Page *et al.*, 1999; Schuch *et al.*, 1999; Rathman *et al.*, 2000). Thus, *Shigella* exploits the transcytotic properties of the M cell for initial invasion, and the lateral cell-to-cell spreading strategy effectively maintains the bacterium in an intracellular compartment through the rest of the infection cycle. This strategy protects *Shigella* from resident submucosal macrophages, infiltrating neutrophils, and extracellular components of the immune system.

Invasive pathogens: regional submucosal invasion

Yersinia enterocolitica and *Yersinia pseudotuberculosis* are gram-negative enteric pathogens that cause disease characterized by invasion through the host cell epithelial barrier via M cells in the Peyer's patches and subsequent spread to the regional enteric lymphoid tissues **(Fig. 40.7)**. The major invasion factor is invasin, an outer-membrane protein that binds to the

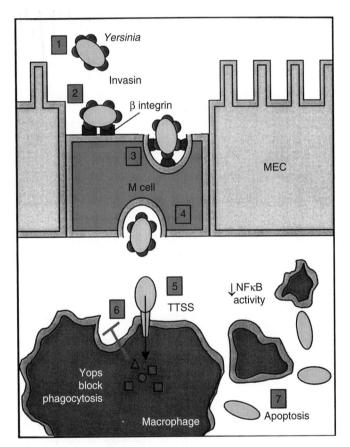

Fig. 40.7 *Yersinia* invasion. **(See page 12 of the color plates.)** (1) *Yersinia* has an outer-membrane protein called invasin. (2) Invasin can bind to β1-integrins on the surface of M cells. (3) Through a zippering mechanism, the bacteria are engulfed by the M cell. (4) The bacteria are translocated across the M cell and delivered to the lamina propria. (5) Plasmid-encoded effector proteins called *Yops* are transferred to the resident macrophage via a TTSS. (6) Through interference with host cell signaling cascades and interactions with the cytoskeleton, the Yops block phagocytosis. (7) In addition, another Yop inhibits NF-κB activity, which leads to apoptosis and allows the bacteria to remain extracellular and spread to the regional lymph nodes.

β-integrins on the apical surface of M cells by a mechanism that does not require an RGD sequence (Miller *et al.*, 1988; Van Nhieu *et al.*, 1991; Clark *et al.*, 1998; Schulte *et al.*, 2000).

Mutants deficient in invasin can cross the epithelium at greatly reduced efficiency, suggesting that *Yersinia* poses other, less efficient virulence factors that also mediate the internalization into M cells (Marra *et al.*, 1997; Schulte *et al.*, 2000). Internalization of *Yersinia* proceeds by a tightly adhering envelopment of the bacterium, as invasin and β1-integrin molecules engage each other throughout the process (Sansonetti, 2002). After engulfment, the bacteria are translocated across the MEC barrier by the M cells to the lamina propria submucosal tissues, where plasmid-encoded virulence factors disable host cell macrophages.

The interaction between *Yersinia* and macrophages has been intensively studied, and these studies demonstrate the complex interplay that has developed between the host and pathogen during evolution. *Yersinia* actively inhibits macrophage phagocytosis by injecting effector proteins called Yops (*Yersinia* outer proteins) into the macrophage through a type III secretion system (reviewed in Cornelis 2002). Three of these proteins—YopH, YopT, and YopE—disrupt effective cytoskeletal organization required for phagocytosis. YopH dephosphorylates proteins necessary for focal adhesion mediated by Fc-receptors and complement (Zhang *et al.*, 1992; Black *et al.*, 2000). YopT is a cysteine protease that cleaves Rho-dependent GTPases, which leads to actin depolymerization (Zumbihl *et al.*, 1999; Shao *et al.*, 2003). YopE functions as a Rho-GTPase activating protein to inactivate Rac, Rho, and CDC42 GTPases, which stabilize actin filaments (Black *et al.*, 2000). In addition to blocking phagocytosis, *Yersinia* also secretes Yops that disrupt host cell signaling pathways that upregulate inflammation. In *Yersinia enterocolitica*, YopP (the homolog of YopJ in *Yersinia pseudotuberculosis*) interferes with the proinflammatory transcription factor NF-κB by preventing its cytosolic inhibitor, IκB, from being degraded (Orth *et al.*, 2000). Mitogen-activated protein kinases (MAPKs) are also rendered nonfunctional by YopP (Orth *et al.*, 1999).

The result of all of this signal transduction interference is impaired expression of cytokines such as TNF, interleukin-1, and interleukin-8 (Schesser *et al.*, 1998). Moreover, decreased transcription of NF-κB anti-apoptosis genes also contributes to macrophage apoptosis (Ruckdeschel *et al.*, 2001). Finally, YopH has recently been shown to block elements of the phosphatidylinositol 3-kinase pathway to prevent the macrophage recruitment factor MCP-1 (Sauvonnet *et al.*, 2002). Therefore, *Yersinia* is capable of invading into deeper tissues to cause regional lymphadenitis.

Invasive pathogens: systemic dissemination

Salmonella is a diverse group of gram-negative enteric pathogens that cause diseases as mild as self-limited gastroenteritis to enteric (typhoid) fever, characterized by widespread dissemination throughout the host. Enteric fever is caused by *Salmonella typhi* and *Salmonella paratyphi*, which are serovars that are limited to humans as their only host (Ohl *et al.*, 2001). This infection is characterized by an initial asymptomatic invasion of bacteria from the small bowel to the liver, spleen, and bone marrow. Once established at these sites, the bacteria replicate and eventually cause prolonged bacteremia, which results in systemic spread to the gallbladder and kidneys and reinfection of the gut (Ohl *et al.*, 2001). In the course of this infectious cycle, *Salmonella* recapitulates many of the pathogenic themes used by other organisms as discussed earlier. Since the typhoid strains of *Salmonella* infect only humans, most of our knowledge of *Salmonella* pathogenesis has been gained from a mouse model using *S. typhimurium*, a *Salmonella* serovar that causes a disease similar to enteric fever in certain strains of mice.

Comparable to *Shigella*, *Salmonella* crosses the MEC barrier by inducing cells to take up extracellular bacteria in a process that involves apical membrane ruffling to endocytose the bacterium **(Fig. 40.8)**. The murine model of enteric fever suggests that M cells are the primary portal of entry for *Salmonella* into the deeper tissues (Clark *et al.*, 1996). However, most of the work to elucidate the cell biology of *Salmonella* invasion has been done in cultured human epithelial cells (reviewed in Zhou *et al.*, 2001). *Salmonella* use the Inv-Spa type III secretion system encoded within the *Salmonella* pathogenicity island-1 (SPI-1) to translocate several effector proteins that cause rearrangement of the host cytoskeleton (Galan *et al.*, 1989). These include SopE1 and SopE2, which are GDP/GTP exchange factors that activate the actin nucleation complex of N-WASP and ARP 2/3 via the Rho GTPases (Galan *et al.*, 2000). SipC, a structural component of the type III secretion system, also seems to be capable of promoting actin polymerization by itself (Hayward *et al.*, 1999).

After salmonellae are internalized, they reverse the effects on the cytoskeleton by secreting another effector protein, SptP, that has a Rho-GTPase activating protein activity (Fu *et al.*, 1999). Mutants deficient in many of these invasion proteins can still reach the spleen of mice after oral inoculation (Galan *et al.*, 1989). This *in vivo* finding implies that there are M cell–independent pathways for translocating *Salmonella* across the MEC barrier. In a bovine model of salmonella infection, both M cells and enterocytes demonstrated bacterial uptake in ligated ileal loops (Frost *et al.*, 1997). Recent studies in mice have demonstrated that mucosal dendritic cells that extend dendrites between the intestinal epithelial cells to sample the luminal contents may also support the internalization of bacteria (Vazquez-Torres *et al.*, 1999; Rescigno *et al.*, 2001; Rescigno *et al.*, 2001).

Once *Salmonella* invades below the epithelial layer, it must contend with the resident macrophages. Unlike the strategies pursued by *Shigella* or *Yersinia*, *Salmonella* does not avoid phagocytosis by these cells but is internalized and then embarks on a strategy of intracellular survival. In contrast to *Shigella*, *Salmonella* does not attempt to escape into the cytosol but instead manipulates its own vacuole called the *Salmonella*-containing vacuole (SCV) to divert it from normal cellular trafficking pathways that would deliver it to late endosomes and lysozomes (Uchiya *et al.*, 1999; Garvis *et al.*, 2001).

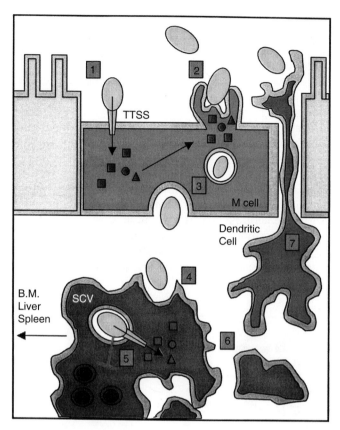

Fig. 40.8 *Salmonella* invasion. **(See page 12 of the color plates.)** (1) *Salmonella* interacts with the apical membrane of M cells and injects bacterial effector proteins into the M cells via the Inv-Spa TTSS. (2) These effectors induce membrane ruffling, and the bacterium is engulfed. (3) The M cell translocates the bacterium to the lamina propria. (4) Resident macrophages phagocytose the bacteria, where they are retained in a special compartment called the *Salmonella* containing vacuole (SCV). (5) From inside the SCV, *Salmonella* secretes another set of effector proteins into the macrophage cytosol, via the SPI-2 TTSS, that modulates expression of a large set of virulence genes controlled by the PhoP/PhoQ regulon and blocks the trafficking of the SCV to the endosome and lysosome. Retained bacteria replicate within the macrophage and are transported to the organs of the reticuloendothelial cell system. (6) Another fate of the resident macrophages is death shortly after infection, mediated by a caspase 1 pathway, or late-onset death after migration to distant sites through genes encoded by the SPI-2. (7) Uptake may also be mediated via dendritic cells, which sample luminal contents by sending dendrites between epithelial cells.

There are several advantages to staying within the macrophage. Among them is the fact that bacteria are shielded from complement and elements of the humoral immune response. Furthermore, macrophages facilitate dissemination throughout the host reticuloendothelial system, since these cells naturally migrate throughout the body. On the other hand, a maturing phagosome of a macrophage presents a hostile environment to *Salmonella* because of the potential for reactive oxidative species, antimicrobial peptides, and lysosomal enzymes to enter this space. To overcome these killing pathways, *Salmonella* uses genes regulated by the PhoP/PhoQ two-component regulatory system and a type III secretion system encoded by the *Salmonella* SPI-2. The PhoP/PhoQ regulon has more than 40 genes that are coordinately activated or repressed in response to low magnesium and calcium levels in the SCV (Miller *et al.*, 1989; Garcia Vescovi *et al.*, 1996). Activation of this regulon results in changes to the LPS and proteins in the *Salmonella* outer and inner membranes that make them more resistant to antimicrobial peptides (Fields *et al.*, 1989; Groisman *et al.*, 1992; Groisman, 1994; Guo *et al.*, 1998). Poorly characterized elements of the PhoP/PhoQ regulon also play an integral role in preventing the SCV from proceeding to the late endosome compartments (Garvis *et al.*, 2001). The SPI-2 type III secretion system also plays an important role in blocking maturation of the SCV (including attenuating the oxidative burst by preventing insertion of NADPH oxidase into the SCV membrane) (Vazquez-Torres *et al.*, 2000) and altering cellular trafficking of the SCV away from the degradative pathways (Garvis *et al.*, 2001; Yu *et al.*, 2002). However, the effector proteins involved in these functions have not been well established.

Salmonella is also capable of directly killing the macrophage. In a killing pathway that occurs early in infection, the SPI-1 effector protein, SipB, activates caspase 1 to cause macrophage lysis by a process that resembles cellular necrosis (Brennan *et al.*, 2000; Monack *et al.*, 2000). During a second, delayed killing pathway that requires elements of the SPI-2 genes, macrophages are induced to undergo apoptosis (van der Velden *et al.*, 2000). This pathway is likely important for the escape of *Salmonella* after the macrophage has migrated to distant sites, since it occurs late in infection. Thus, the interplay between *Salmonella* and macrophage demonstrates the sophisticated virulence factors bacteria have evolved to survive within the host organism.

SUMMARY

Gastrointestinal pathogens are capable of causing disease, such as diarrhea, in healthy individuals. In contrast, the majority of respiratory pathogens cause universal colonization of the nasopharynx without disease, two powerful exceptions being *B. pertussis and B. anthracis*, which infect even healthy airways. Overall, pneumonia can be considered more opportunistic in nature than gastrointestinal infection. This review has highlighted the conserved mechanisms shared by pathogens. In many instances these mechanisms are fascinating examples of convergent evolution and moreover provide important insight into the key interaction between host and pathogen.

REFERENCES

Bernardini, M.L., Mounier, J., d'Hauteville, H., Coquis-Rondon, M., and Sansonetti, P.J. (1989). Identification of icsA, a plasmid locus of Shigella flexneri that governs bacterial intra- and intercellular spread through interaction with F-actin. *Proc. Natl. Acad. Sci. USA*. 86(10):3867–3871.

Betley, M.J., Miller, V.L., and Mekalanos, J.J. (1986). Genetics of bacterial enterotoxins. *Annu. Rev. Microbiol*. 40:577–605.

Bhan, M.K., Raj, P., Levine, M.M., Kaper, J.B., Bhandari, N., Srivastava, R., Kumar, R., and Sazawal, S. (1989). Enteroaggregative *Escherichia coli* associated with persistent diarrhea in a cohort of rural children in India. *J. Infect. Dis*. 159(6):1061–1064.

Black, D.S., and Bliska, J.B. (2000). The RhoGAP activity of the *Yersinia pseudotuberculosis* cytotoxin YopE is required for antiphagocytic function and virulence. *Mol. Microbiol*. 37(3):515–527.

Black, D.S., Marie-Cardine, A., Schraven, B., and Bliska, J.B. (2000). The *Yersinia* tyrosine phosphatase YopH targets a novel adhesion-regulated signalling complex in macrophages. *Cell. Microbiol*. 2(5):401–414.

Blocker, A., Gounon, P., Larquet, E., Niebuhr, K., Cabiaux, V., Parsot, C., and Sansonetti, P. (1999). The tripartite type III secreton of *Shigella flexneri* inserts IpaB and IpaC into host membranes. *J. Cell. Biol*. 147(3):683–693.

Braun, J.S., Novak, R., Murray, P.J., Eischen, C.M., Susin, S.A., Kroemer, G., Halle, A., Weber, J.R., Tuomanen, E.I., and Cleveland, J.L. (2001). Apoptosis-inducing factor mediates microglial and neuronal apoptosis caused by pneumococcus. *J. Infect. Dis*. 184(10):1300–1309.

Braun, J.S., Sublett, J.E., Freyer, D., Mitchell, T.J., Cleveland, J.L., Tuomanen, E.I., and Weber, J.R. (2002). Pneumococcal pneumolysin and H(2)O(2) mediate brain cell apoptosis during meningitis. *J. Clin. Invest*. 109(1):19–27.

Brennan, M.A., and Cookson, B.T. (2000). *Salmonella* induces macrophage death by caspase-1-dependent necrosis. *Mol. Microbiol*. 38(1):31–40.

Brogden, K.A. (2000). Bacterial evasion of host-derived antimicrobial peptides on mucosal surfaces. *Virulence Mechanisms of Bacterial Pathogens* (ed. M.J. Wannemuehler). Washington, DC: ASM Press; 19–40.

Cant, A.J., Gordon, S.B., Read, R.C., Hart, C.A., and Winstanley, C. (2002). Respiratory infections. *J. Med. Microbiol*. 51(11): 903–914.

Chen, Y., Smith, M.R., Thirumalai, K., and Zychlinsky, A. (1996). A bacterial invasin induces macrophage apoptosis by binding directly to ICE. *Embo. J*. 15(15):3853–3860.

Clark, M.A., Hirst, B.H., and Jepson, M.A. (1998). M-cell surface β1 integrin expression and invasin-mediated targeting of *Yersinia pseudotuberculosis* to mouse Peyer's patch M cells. *Infect. Immun*. 66(3):1237–1243.

Clark, M.A., Reed, K.A., Lodge, J., Stephen, J., Hirst, B.H., and Jepson, M.A. (1996). Invasion of murine intestinal M cells by *Salmonella typhimurium* inv mutants severely deficient for invasion of cultured cells. *Infect. Immun*. 64(10):4363–4368.

Coote, J.G. (2001). Environmental sensing mechanisms in *Bordetella*. *Adv. Microb. Physiol*. 44:141–181.

Cornelis, G.R. (2002). *Yersinia* type III secretion: send in the effectors. *J. Cell. Biol*. 158(3):401–408.

Cotter, P.A., and Miller, J.F. (1998). In vivo and ex vivo regulation of bacterial virulence gene expression. *Curr. Opin. Microbiol*. 1(1):17–26.

Cundell, D.R., Gerard, C., Idanpaan-Heikkila, I., Tuomanen, E.I., and Gerard, N.P. (1996). PAf receptor anchors *Streptococcus pneumoniae* to activated human endothelial cells. *Adv. Exp. Med. Biol*. 416:89–94.

Cundell, D.R., and Tuomanen, E.I. (1994). Receptor specificity of adherence of *Streptococcus pneumoniae* to human type-II pneumocytes and vascular endothelial cells in vitro. *Microb. Pathog*. 17(6):361–374.

DeVinney, R., Knoechel, D.G., and Finlay, B.B. (1999). Enteropathogenic *Escherichia coli*: cellular harassment. *Curr. Opin. Microbiol*. 2(1): 83–88.

DeVinney, R., Puente, J.L., Gauthier, A., Goosney, D., and Finlay, B.B. (2001). Enterohaemorrhagic and enteropathogenic *Escherichia coli* use a different Tir-based mechanism for pedestal formation. *Mol. Microbiol*. 41(6):1445–1458.

Dockrell, D.H., Lee, M., Lynch, D.H., and Read, R.C. (2001). Immune-mediated phagocytosis and killing of *Streptococcus pneumoniae* are associated with direct and bystander macrophage apoptosis. *J. Infect. Dis*. 184(6):713–722.

Donnenberg, M.S., Giron, J.A., Nataro, J.P., and Kaper, J.B. (1992). A plasmid-encoded type IV fimbrial gene of enteropathogenic *Escherichia coli* associated with localized adherence. *Mol. Microbiol.* 6(22):3427–3437.

Downey, G.P., and Granton, J.T. (1997). Mechanisms of acute lung injury. *Curr. Opin. Pulm. Med.* 3(3):234–241.

Egile, C., Loisel, T.P., Laurent, V., Li, R., Pantaloni, D., Sansonetti, P.J., and Carlier, M.F. (1999). Activation of the CDC42 effector N-WASP by the *Shigella flexneri* IcsA protein promotes actin nucleation by Arp2/3 complex and bacterial actin-based motility. *J. Cell. Biol.* 146(6): 1319–1332.

Erdei, A., Kerekes, K., and Pecht, I. (1997). Role of C3a and C5a in the activation of mast cells. *Exp. Clin. Immunogenet.* 14(1):16–18.

Feldman, C., Anderson, R., Cockeran, R., Mitchell, T., Cole, P., and Wilson, R. (2002). The effects of pneumolysin and hydrogen peroxide, alone and in combination, on human ciliated epithelium in vitro. *Respir. Med.* 96(8):580–585.

Feldman, C., Mitchell, T.J., Andrew, P.W., Boulnois, G.J., Read, R.C., Todd, H.C., Cole, P.J., and Wilson, R. (1990). The effect of *Streptococcus pneumoniae* pneumolysin on human respiratory epithelium in vitro. *Microb. Pathog.* 9(4):275–284.

Fernie-King, B.A., Seilly, D.J., Willers, C., Wurzner, R., Davies, A., and Lachmann, P.J. (2001). Streptococcal inhibitor of complement (SIC) inhibits the membrane attack complex by preventing uptake of C567 onto cell membranes. *Immunology* 103(3):390–398.

Fields, P.I., Groisman, E.A., and Heffron, F. (1989). A *Salmonella* locus that controls resistance to microbicidal proteins from phagocytic cells. *Science* 243(4894 Pt 1):1059–1062.

Firoved, A.M., and Deretic, V. (2003). Microarray Analysis of Global Gene Expression in Mucoid *Pseudomonas aeruginosa. J. Bacteriol.* 185(3):1071–1081.

Frankel, G., Phillips, A.D., Rosenshine, I., Dougan, G., Kaper, J.B., and Knutton, S. (1998). Enteropathogenic and enterohaemorrhagic *Escherichia coli*: more subversive elements. *Mol. Microbiol.* 30(5):911–921.

Frost, A.J., Bland, A.P., and Wallis, T.S. (1997). The early dynamic response of the calf ileal epithelium to *Salmonella typhimurium. Vet. Pathol.* 34(5):369–386.

Fu, Y., and Galan, J.E. (1999). A salmonella protein antagonizes Rac-1 and Cdc42 to mediate host-cell recovery after bacterial invasion. *Nature* 401(6750):293–297.

Gaastra, W., and Svennerholm, A.M. (1996). Colonization factors of human enterotoxigenic *Escherichia coli* (ETEC). *Trends Microbiol.* 4(11):444–452.

Galan, J.E., and Curtiss, R., 3rd (1989). Cloning and molecular characterization of genes whose products allow *Salmonella typhimurium* to penetrate tissue culture cells. *Proc. Natl. Acad. Sci. USA.* 86(16):6383–6387.

Galan, J.E., and Zhou, D. (2000). Striking a balance: modulation of the actin cytoskeleton by *Salmonella. Proc. Natl. Acad. Sci. USA.* 97(16):8754–8761.

Garcia Vescovi, E., Soncini, F.C., and Groisman, E.A. (1996). Mg2+ as an extracellular signal: environmental regulation of *Salmonella* virulence. *Cell* 84(1):165–174.

Garvis, S.G., Beuzon, C.R., and Holden, D.W. (2001). A role for the PhoP/Q regulon in inhibition of fusion between lysosomes and *Salmonella*-containing vacuoles in macrophages. *Cell. Microbiol.* 3(11):731–744.

Giron, J.A., Ho, A.S., and Schoolnik, G.K. (1991). An inducible bundle-forming pilus of enteropathogenic *Escherichia coli. Science* 254(5032):710–713.

Goldberg, M.B., and Theriot, J.A. (1995). *Shigella flexneri* surface protein IcsA is sufficient to direct actin-based motility. *Proc. Natl. Acad. Sci. USA* 92(14):6572–6576.

Gottschalk, A. (1960). Correlation between composition, structure, shape, and function of a salivary mucoprotein. *Nature* 186:949–951.

Gould, J.M., and Weiser, J.N. (2001). Expression of C-reactive protein in the human respiratory tract. *Infect. Immun.* 69(3):1747–1754.

Gould, J.M., and Weiser, J.N. (2002). The inhibitory effect of C-reactive protein on bacterial phosphorylcholine platelet-activating factor receptor-mediated adherence is blocked by surfactant. *J. Infect. Dis.* 186(3):361–371.

Grassme, H.S., Kirschnek, S., Riethmueller, J., Riehle, A., von Kurthy, G., Lang, F., Weller, M., and Gulbins, E. (2000). CD95/CD95 ligand interactions on epithelial cells in host defense to *Pseudomonas aeruginosa. Science* 290(5491):527–530.

Groisman, E.A. (1994). How bacteria resist killing by host-defense peptides. *Trends Microbiol.* 2(11):444–449.

Groisman, E.A., Parra-Lopez, C., Salcedo, M., Lipps, C.J., and Heffron, F. (1992). Resistance to host antimicrobial peptides is necessary for *Salmonella* virulence. *Proc. Natl. Acad. Sci. USA.* 89(24):11939–11943.

Guo, L., Lim, K.B., Poduje, C.M., Daniel, M., Gunn, J.S., Hackett, M., and Miller, S.I. (1998). Lipid A acylation and bacterial resistance against vertebrate antimicrobial peptides. *Cell* 95(2):189–198.

Hale, T.L. (1991). Genetic basis of virulence in *Shigella* species. *Microbiol. Rev.* 55(2):206–224.

Hathaway, L.J., and Kraehenbuhl, J.P. (2000). The role of M cells in mucosal immunity. *Cell. Mol. Life Sci.* 57(2):323–332.

Hauser, A.R., and Engel, J.N. (1999). *Pseudomonas aeruginosa* induces type-III-secretion-mediated apoptosis of macrophages and epithelial cells. *Infect. Immun.* 67(10):5530–5537.

Hayward, R.D., and Koronakis, V. (1999). Direct nucleation and bundling of actin by the SipC protein of invasive *Salmonella. Embo. J.* 18(18):4926–4934.

Hecht, G. (1999). Innate mechanisms of epithelial host defense: spotlight on intestine. *Am. J. Physiol.* 277(3 Pt 1):C351–358.

Herrington, D.A., Hall, R.H., Losonsky, G., Mekalanos, J.J., Taylor, R.K., and Levine, M.M. (1988). Toxin, toxin-coregulated pili, and the toxR regulon are essential for *Vibrio cholerae* pathogenesis in humans. *J. Exp. Med.* 168(4):1487–1492.

Hilbi, H., Moss, J.E., Hersh, D., Chen, Y., Arondel, J., Banerjee, S., Flavell, R.A., Yuan, J., Sansonetti, P.J., and Zychlinsky, A. (1998). *Shigella*-induced apoptosis is dependent on caspase-1 which binds to IpaB. *J. Biol. Chem.* 273(49):32895–32900.

Hilbi, H., Puro, R.J., and Zychlinsky, A. (2000). Tripeptidyl peptidase II promotes maturation of caspase-1 in *Shigella flexneri*-induced macrophage apoptosis. *Infect. Immun.* 68(10):5502–5508.

Howie, A.J., and Brown, G. (1985). Effect of neuraminidase on the expression of the 3-fucosyl-N-acetyllactosamine antigen in human tissues. *J. Clin. Pathol.* 38(4):409–416.

Hueck, C.J. (1998). Type III protein secretion systems in bacterial pathogens of animals and plants. *Microbiol. Mol. Biol. Rev.* 62(2):379–433.

Jarvis, K.G., Giron, J.A., Jerse, A.E., McDaniel, T.K., Donnenberg, M.S., and Kaper, J.B. (1995). Enteropathogenic *Escherichia coli* contains a putative type III secretion system necessary for the export of proteins involved in attaching and effacing lesion formation. *Proc. Natl. Acad. Sci. USA.* 92(17):7996–8000.

Jones, R.B., and Batteiger, B.E. (2000). Chlamydial diseases. In *Mandell, Douglas, and Bennett's Principles and Practice of Infectious Diseases* (ed. R. Dolin). Philadelphia: Churchill Livingstone, 1986–1988.

Kaetzel, C.S. (2001). Polymeric Ig receptor: defender of the fort or Trojan horse? *Curr. Biol.* 11(1):R35–38.

Kenny, B., DeVinney, R., Stein, M., Reinscheid, D.J., Frey, E.A., and Finlay, B.B. (1997). Enteropathogenic *E. coli* (EPEC) transfers its receptor for intimate adherence into mammalian cells. *Cell* 91(4):511–520.

Klein, A., Strecker, G., Lamblin, G., and Roussel, P. (2000). Structural analysis of mucin-type O-linked oligosaccharides. *Methods Mol. Biol.* 125:191–209.

Knowles, M.R., and Boucher, R.C. (2002). Mucus clearance as a primary innate defense mechanism for mammalian airways. *J. Clin. Invest.* 109(5):571–577.

Koehler, T.M. (2002). Bacillus anthracis genetics and virulence gene regulation. *Curr. Top. Microbiol. Immunol.* 271:143–164.

Kolberg, J., Hoiby, E.A., and Jantzen, E. (1997). Detection of the phosphorylcholine epitope in streptococci, *Haemophilus* and pathogenic *Neisseriae* by immunoblotting. *Microb. Pathog.* 22(6):321–329.

Kopp, E.B., and Medzhitov, R. (1999). The Toll-receptor family and control of innate immunity. *Curr. Opin. Immunol.* 11(1):13–18.

Krivan, H.C., Roberts, D.D., and Ginsburg, V. (1988). Many pulmonary pathogenic bacteria bind specifically to the carbohydrate sequence GalNAc beta 1-4Gal found in some glycolipids. *Proc. Natl. Acad. Sci. USA* 85(16):6157–6161.

Krukonis, E.S., Yu, R.R., and DiRita, V.J. (2000). The *Vibrio cholerae* ToxR/TcpP/ToxT virulence cascade: distinct roles for two membrane-localized transcriptional activators on a single promoter. *Mol. Microbiol.* 38(1):67–84.

Lee, S.H., Hava, D.L., Waldor, M.K., and Camilli, A. (1999). Regulation and temporal expression patterns of *Vibrio cholerae* virulence genes during infection. *Cell* 99(6):625–634.

Lehrer, R.I., Ganz, T., and Selsted, M.E. (1991). Defensins: endogenous antibiotic peptides of animal cells. *Cell* 64(2):229–230.

LeVine, A.M., Kurak, K.E., Wright, J.R., Watford, W.T., Bruno, M.D., Ross, G.F., Whitsett, J.A., and Korfhagen, T.R. (1999). Surfactant protein-A binds group B streptococcus enhancing phagocytosis and clearance from lungs of surfactant protein-A-deficient mice. *Am. J. Respir. Cell Mol. Biol.* 20(2):279–286.

Levine, M.M. (1987). *Escherichia coli* that cause diarrhea: enterotoxigenic, enteropathogenic, enteroinvasive, enterohemorrhagic, and enteroadherent. *J. Infect. Dis.* 155(3):377–389.

Lew, D.P. (2000). Bacillus anthracis (anthrax). In *Mandell, Douglas, and Bennett's Principles and Practice of Infectious Diseases.* (ed. R. Dolin). Philadelphia: Churchill Livingstone, 2215–2220.

Locht, C. (1999). Molecular aspects of *Bordetella pertussis* pathogenesis. *Int. Microbiol.* 2(3):137–144.

Mandell, L.A. (1995). Community-acquired pneumonia: etiology, epidemiology, and treatment. *Chest* 108(2 Suppl):35S–42S.

Marra, A., and Isberg, R.R. (1997). Invasin-dependent and invasin-independent pathways for translocation of *Yersinia pseudotuberculosis* across the Peyer's patch intestinal epithelium. *Infect. Immun.* 65(8):3412–3421.

Mathan, V.I., and Mathan, M.M. (1991). Intestinal manifestations of invasive diarrheas and their diagnosis. *Rev. Infect. Dis.* 13(Suppl 4):S311–313.

Mayer, H.B., and Wanke, C.A. (1995). Enteroaggregative *Escherichia coli* as a possible cause of diarrhea in an HIV-infected patient. *N. Engl. J. Med.* 332(4):273–274.

McCullers, J.A., and Bartmess, K.C. (2003). Role of neuraminidase in lethal synergism between influenza virus and *Streptococcus pneumoniae*. *J. Infect. Dis.*

Medzhitov, R., Preston-Hurlburt, P., and Janeway, C.A., Jr. (1997). A human homologue of the *Drosophila* Toll protein signals activation of adaptive immunity. *Nature* 388(6640):394–397.

Miller, S.I., Kukral, A.M., and Mekalanos, J.J. (1989). A two-component regulatory system (phoP phoQ) controls *Salmonella typhimurium* virulence. *Proc. Natl. Acad. Sci. USA* 86(13):5054–5058.

Miller, V.L., and Falkow, S. (1988). Evidence for two genetic loci in *Yersinia enterocolitica* that can promote invasion of epithelial cells. *Infect. Immun.* 56(5):1242–1248.

Monack, D.M., Hersh, D., Ghori, N., Bouley, D., Zychlinsky, A., and Falkow, S. (2000). *Salmonella* exploits caspase-1 to colonize Peyer's patches in a murine typhoid model. *J. Exp. Med.* 192(2):249–258.

Monack, D.M., and Theriot, J.A. (2001). Actin-based motility is sufficient for bacterial membrane protrusion formation and host cell uptake. *Cell Microbiol.* 3(9):633–647.

Moon, H.W., Whipp, S.C., Argenzio, R.A., Levine, M.M., and Giannella, R.A. (1983). Attaching and effacing activities of rabbit and human enteropathogenic *Escherichia coli* in pig and rabbit intestines. *Infect. Immun.* 41(3):1340–1351.

Nagase, T., Ishii, S., Shindou, H., Ouchi, Y., and Shimizu, T. (2002). Airway hyperresponsiveness in transgenic mice overexpressing platelet activating factor receptor is mediated by an atropine-sensitive pathway. *Am. J. Respir. Crit. Care Med.* 165(2):200–205.

Nataro, J.P., and Kaper, J.B. (1998). Diarrheagenic *Escherichia coli*. *Clin. Microbiol. Rev.* 11(1):142–201.

Nataro, J.P., Kaper, J.B., Robins-Browne, R., Prado, V., Vial, P., and Levine, M.M. (1987). Patterns of adherence of diarrheagenic *Escherichia coli* to HEp-2 cells. *Pediatr. Infect. Dis. J.* 6(9):829–831.

Niebuhr, K., Jouihri, N., Allaoui, A., Gounon, P., Sansonetti, P.J., and Parsot, C. (2000). IpgD, a protein secreted by the type III secretion machinery of *Shigella flexneri*, is chaperoned by IpgE and implicated in entry focus formation. *Mol. Microbiol.* 38(1):8–19.

O'Brien, A.D., and Holmes, R.K. (1987). *Shiga* and *Shiga*-like toxins. *Microbiol. Rev.* 51(2):206–220.

O'Brien, J., Friedlander, A., Dreier, T., Ezzell, J., and Leppla, S. (1985). Effects of anthrax toxin components on human neutrophils. *Infect. Immun.* 47(1):306–310.

Ohl, M.E., and Miller, S.I. (2001). *Salmonella*: a model for bacterial pathogenesis. *Annu. Rev. Med.* 52:259–274.

Okeke, I.N., and Nataro, J.P. (2001). Enteroaggregative *Escherichia coli*. *Lancet. Infect. Dis.* 1(5):304–313.

Orth, K., Palmer, L.E., Bao, Z.Q., Stewart, S., Rudolph, A.E., Bliska, J.B., and Dixon, J.E. (1999). Inhibition of the mitogen-activated protein kinase kinase superfamily by a *Yersinia* effector. *Science* 285(5435):1920–1923.

Orth, K., Xu, Z., Mudgett, M.B., Bao, Z.Q., Palmer, L.E., Bliska, J.B., Mangel, W.F., Staskawicz, B., and Dixon, J.E. (2000). Disruption of signaling by *Yersinia* effector YopJ, a ubiquitin-like protein protease. *Science* 290(5496):1594–1597.

Ouellette, A.J. (1997). Paneth cells and innate immunity in the crypt microenvironment. *Gastroenterology* 113(5):1779–1784.

Page, A.L., Ohayon, H., Sansonetti, P.J., and Parsot, C. (1999). The secreted IpaB and IpaC invasins and their cytoplasmic chaperone IpgC are required for intercellular dissemination of *Shigella flexneri*. *Cell Microbiol.* 1(2):183–193.

Perdomo, J.J., Gounon, P., and Sansonetti, P.J. (1994). Polymorphonuclear leukocyte transmigration promotes invasion of coloni epithelial monolayer by *Shigella flexneri*. *J. Clin. Invest.* 93(2):633–643.

Perdomo, O.J., Cavaillon, J.M., Huerre, M., Ohayon, H., Gounon, P., and Sansonetti, P.J. (1994). Acute inflammation causes epithelial invasion and mucosal destruction in experimental shigellosis. *J. Exp. Med.* 180(4):1307–1319.

Portnoy, D.A., Auerbuch, V., and Glomski, I.J. (2002). The cell biology of *Listeria monocytogenes* infection: the intersection of bacterial pathogenesis and cell-mediated immunity. *J. Cell. Biol.* 158(3):409–414.

Prasad, S.M., Yin, Y., Rodzinski, E., Tuomanen, E.I., and Masure, H.R. (1993). Identification of a carbohydrate recognition domain in filamentous hemagglutinin from *Bordetella. pertussis*. *Infect. Immun.* 61(7):2780–2785.

Ram, S., Mackinnon, F.G., Gulati, S., McQuillen, D.P., Vogel, U., Frosch, M., Elkins, C., Guttormsen, H.K., Wetzler, L.M., Oppermann, M., Pangburn, M.K., and Rice, P.A. (1999). The contrasting mechanisms of serum resistance of *Neisseria gonorrhoeae* and group B *Neisseria. meningitidis*. *Mol. Immunol.* 36(13–14):915–928.

Rathman, M., Jouihri, N., Allaoui, A., Sansonetti, P., Parsot, C., and Tran Van Nhieu, G. (2000). The development of a FACS-based strategy for the isolation of *Shigella flexneri* mutants that are deficient in intercellular spread. *Mol. Microbiol.* 35(5):974–990.

Rautemaa, R., and Meri, S. (1999). Complement-resistance mechanisms of bacteria. *Microbes. Infect.* 1(10):785–794.

Rescigno, M., Rotta, G., Valzasina, B., and Ricciardi-Castagnoli, P. (2001). Dendritic cells shuttle microbes across gut epithelial monolayers. *Immunobiology* 204(5):572–581.

Rescigno, M., Urbano, M., Valzasina, B., Francolini, M., Rotta, G., Bonasio, R., Granucci, F., Kraehenbuhl, J.P., and Ricciardi-Castagnoli, P. (2001). Dendritic cells express tight junction proteins and penetrate gut epithelial monolayers to sample bacteria. *Nat. Immunol.* 2(4):361–367.

Ring, A., Weiser, J.N., and Tuomanen, E.I. (1998). Pneumococcal trafficking across the blood-brain barrier: molecular analysis of a novel bidirectional pathway. *J. Clin. Invest.* 102(2):347–360.

Rosenow, C., Ryan, P., Weiser, J.N., Johnson, S., Fontan, P., Ortqvist, A., and Masure, H.R. (1997). Contribution of novel choline-binding proteins to adherence, colonization and immunogenicity of *Streptococcus pneumoniae*. *Mol. Microbiol.* 25(5):819–829.

Roy, C.R., Miller, J.F., and Falkow, S. (1989). The bvgA gene of *Bordetella pertussis* encodes a transcriptional activator required for coordinate regulation of several virulence genes. *J. Bacteriol.* 171(11):6338–6344.

Ruckdeschel, K., Mannel, O., Richter, K., Jacobi, C.A., Trulzsch, K., Rouot, B., and Heesemann, J. (2001). *Yersinia* outer protein P or *Yersinia enterocolitica* simultaneously blocks the nuclear factor-κB pathway and exploits lipopolysaccharide signaling to trigger apoptosis in macrophages. *J. Immunol.* 166(3):1823–1831.

Ruiz, M., Ewig, S., Torres, A., Arancibia, F., Marco, F., Mensa, J., Sanchez, M., and Martinez, J.A. (1999). Severe community-acquired pneumonia: risk factors and follow-up epidemiology. *Am. J. Respir. Crit. Care. Med.* 160(3):923–929.

Sansonetti, P. (2002). Host-pathogen interactions: the seduction of molecular cross talk. *Gut* 50 Suppl 3:III2–8.

Sansonetti, P. J., Phalipon, A., Arondel, J., Thirumalai, K., Banerjee, S., Akira, S., Takeda, K., and Zychlinsky, A. (2000). Caspase-1 activation of IL-1beta and IL-18 are essential for *Shigella flexneri*–induced inflammation. *Immunity.* 12(5):581–590.

Sansonetti, P.J., Ryter, A., Clerc, P., Maurelli, A.T., and Mounier, J. (1986). Multiplication of *Shigella flexneri* within HeLa cells: lysis of the phagocytic vacuole and plasmid-mediated contact hemolysis. *Infect. Immun.* 51(2):461–469.

Sastry, K., and Ezekowitz, R.A. (1993). Collectins: pattern recognition molecules involved in first line host defense. *Curr. Opin. Immunol.* 5(1):59–66.

Sauvonnet, N., Lambermont, I., van der Bruggen, P., and Cornelis, G.R. (2002). YopH prevents monocyte chemoattractant protein 1 expression in macrophages and T-cell proliferation through inactivation of the phosphatidylinositol 3-kinase pathway. *Mol. Microbiol.* 45(3):805–815.

Savage, D.C. (1977). Microbial ecology of the gastrointestinal tract. *Annu. Rev. Microbiol.* 31:107–133.

Schesser, K., Spiik, A.K., Dukuzumuremyi, J.M., Neurath, M.F. Pettersson, S., and Wolf-Watz, H. (1998). The yopJ locus is required for *Yersinia*-mediated inhibition of NF-κB activation and cytokine expression: YopJ contains a eukaryotic SH2-like domain that is essential for its repressive activity. *Mol. Microbiol.* 28(6):1067–1079.

Schuch, R., Sandlin, R.C., and Maurelli, A.T. (1999). A system for identifying post-invasion functions of invasion genes: requirements for the Mxi-Spa type III secretion pathway of *Shigella flexneri* in intercellular dissemination. *Mol. Microbiol.* 34(4):675–689.

Schuhmacher, D.A., and Klose, K.E. (1999). Environmental signals modulate ToxT-dependent virulence factor expression in *Vibrio cholerae*. *J Bacteriol.* 181(5):1508–1514.

Schulte, R., Kerneis, S., Klinke, S., Bartels, H., Preger, S., Kraehenbuhl, J.P., Pringault, E., and Autenrieth, I.B. (2000). Translocation of *Yersinia enterocolitica* across reconstituted intestinal epithelial monolayers is triggered by *Yersinia* invasin binding to beta1 integrins apically expressed on M-like cells. *Cell Microbiol.* 2(2):173–185.

Sebert, M.E., Palmer, L.M., Rosenberg, M., and Weiser, J.N. (2002). Microarray-based identification of htrA, a *Streptococcus pneumoniae* gene that is regulated by the CiaRH two-component system and contributes to nasopharyngeal colonization. *Infect. Immun.* 70(8):4059–4067.

Shao, F., Vacratsis, P.O., Bao, Z., Bowers, K.E., Fierke, C.A., and Dixon, J.E. (2003). Biochemical characterization of the *Yersinia* Yop T protease: cleavage site and recognition elements in Rho GTPases. *Proc. Natl. Acad. Sci. USA.* 100(3):904–909.

Sharma, D.P., Stroeher, U.H., Thomas, C.J., Manning, P.A., and Attridge, S.R. (1989). The toxin-coregulated pilus (TCP) of *Vibrio cholerae*: molecular cloning of genes involved in pilus biosynthesis and evaluation of TCP as a protective antigen in the infant mouse model. *Microb. Pathog.* 7(6):437–448.

Sixma, T.K., Pronk, S.E., Kalk, K.H., Wartna, E.S., van Zanten, B.A., Witholt, B., and Hol, W.G. (1991). Crystal structure of a cholera toxin-related heat-labile enterotoxin from *E. coli.* *Nature* 351(6325):371–377.

Skorupski, K., and Taylor, R.K. (1997). Control of the ToxR virulence regulon in *Vibrio cholerae* by environmental stimuli. *Mol. Microbiol.* 25(6):1003–1009.

Stock, A.M., Robinson, V.L., and Goudreau, P.N. (2000). Two-component signal transduction. *Annu. Rev. Biochem.* 69:183–215.

Swords, W.E., Ketterer, M.R., Shao, J., Campbell, C.A., Weiser, J.N., and Apicella, M.A. (2001). Binding of the non-typeable *Haemophilus influenzae* lipooligosaccharide to the PAF receptor initiates host cell signalling. *Cell Microbiol.* 3(8):525–536.

Taylor, R.K., Miller, V.L., Furlong, D.B., and Mekalanos, J.J. (1987). Use of phoA gene fusions to identify a pilus colonization factor coordinately regulated with cholera toxin. *Proc. Natl. Acad. Sci. USA.* 84(9):2833–2837.

Tong, H.H., Blue, L.E., James, M.A., and DeMaria, T.F. (2000). Evaluation of the virulence of a *Streptococcus pneumoniae* neuraminidase-deficient mutant in nasopharyngeal colonization and development of otitis media in the chinchilla model. *Infect. Immun.* 68(2):921–924.

Tran Van Nhieu, G., Ben-Ze'ev, A., and Sansonetti, P.J. (1997). Modulation of bacterial entry into epithelial cells by association between vinculin and the *Shigella* IpaA invasin. *Embo. J.* 16(10):2717–2729.

Tran Van Nhieu, G., Caron, E., Hall, A., and Sansonetti, P.J. (1999) IpaC induces actin polymerization and filopodia formation during *Shigella* entry into epithelial cells. *Embo. J.* 18(12):3249–3262.

Tuomanen, E., and Weiss, A. (1985). Characterization of two adhesins of *Bordetella pertussis* for human ciliated respiratory-epithelial cells. *J. Infect. Dis.* 152(1):118–125.

Uchiya, K., Barbieri, M.A., Funato, K., Shah, A.H., Stahl, P.D., and Groisman, E.A. (1999). A *Salmonella* virulence protein that inhibits cellular trafficking. *Embo. J.* 18(14):3924–3933.

van der Velden, A.W., Lindgren, S.W., Worley, M.J., and Heffron, F. (2000). *Salmonella* pathogenicity island 1-independent induction of apoptosis in infected macrophages by *Salmonella enterica* serotype *typhimurium*. *Infect. Immun.* 68(10):5702–5709.

Van Nhieu, G.T., and Isberg, R.R. (1991). The *Yersinia pseudotuberculosis* invasin protein and human fibronectin bind to mutually exclusive sites on the alpha 5 beta 1 integrin receptor. *J. Biol. Chem.* 266(36):24367–24375.

Vazquez-Torres, A., Jones-Carson, J., Baumler, A.J., Falkow, S., Valdivia, R., Brown, W., Le, M., Berggren, R., Parks, W.T., and Fang, F.C. (1999). Extraintestinal dissemination of *Salmonella* by CD18-expressing phagocytes. *Nature* 401(6755):804–808.

Vazquez-Torres, A., Xu, Y., Jones-Carson, J., Holden, D.W., Lucia, S.M., Dinauer, M.C., Mastroeni, P., and Fang, F.C. (2000). *Salmonella* pathogenicity island 2-dependent evasion of the phagocyte NADPH oxidase. *Science* 287(5458):1655–1658.

Wang, X., Moser, C., Louboutin, J.P., Lysenko, E.S., Weiner, D.J., Weiser, J.N., and Wilson, J.M. (2002). Toll-like receptor 4 mediates innate immune responses to *Haemophilus influenzae* infection in mouse lung. *J. Immunol.* 168(2):810–815.

Wassef, J.S., Keren, D.F., and Mailloux, J.L. (1989). Role of M cells in initial antigen uptake and in ulcer formation in the rabbit intestinal loop model of shigellosis. *Infect. Immun.* 57(3):858–863.

Weiser, J.N. (1998). Phase variation in colony opacity by *Streptococcus pneumoniae*. *Microb. Drug. Resist.* 4(2):129–135.

Weiser, J.N., Goldberg, J.B., Pan, N., Wilson, L., and Virji, M. (1998a). The phosphorylcholine epitope undergoes phase variation on a 43-kilodalton protein in *Pseudomonas aeruginosa* and on pili of *Neisseria meningitidis* and *Neisseria gonorrhoeae*. *Infect. Immun.* 66(9):4263–4267.

Weiser, J.N., Pan, N., McGowan, K.L., Musher, D., Martin, A., and Richards, J. (1998b). Phosphorylcholine on the lipopolysaccharide of *Haemophilus influenzae* contributes to persistence in the respiratory tract and sensitivity to serum killing mediated by C-reactive protein. *J. Exp. Med.* 187(4):631–640.

Wilson, R., Read, R., Thomas, M., Rutman, A., Harrison, K., Lund, V., Cookson, B., Goldman, W., Lambert, H., and Cole, P. (1991). Effects of *Bordetella pertussis* infection on human respiratory epithelium in vivo and in vitro. *Infect. Immun.* 59(1):337–345.

Yu, X.J., Ruiz-Albert, J., Unsworth, K.E., Garvis, S., Liu, M., and Holden, D.W., (2002). SpiC is required for secretion of *Salmonella* pathogenicity island 2 type III secretion system proteins. *Cell Microbiol.* 4(8):531–540.

Zhang, D., Xu, Z., Sun, W., and Karaolis, D.K. (2003). The *Vibrio* pathogenicity island–encoded mop protein modulates the pathogenesis and reactogenicity of epidemic vibrio cholerae. *Infect. Immun.* 71(1):510–515.

Zhang, J.R., Mostov, K.E., Lamm, M.E., Nanno, M., Shimida, S., Ohwaki, M., and Tuomanen, E. (2000). The polymeric immunoglobulin receptor translocates pneumococci across human nasopharyngeal epithelial cells. *Cell* 102(6):827–837.

Zhang, Z.Y., Clemens, J.C., Schubert, H.L., Stuckey, J.A., Fischer, M.W., Hume, D.M., Saper, M.A., and Dixon, J.E. (1992). Expression, purification, and physicochemical characterization of a recombinant *Yersinia* protein tyrosine phosphatase. *J. Biol. Chem.* 267(33):23759–23766.

Zhou, D., and Galan, J. (2001). *Salmonella* entry into host cells: the work in concert of type III secreted effector proteins. *Microbes. Infect.* 3(14–15):1293–1298.

Zumbihl, R., Aepfelbacher, M., Andor, A., Jacobi, C.A., Ruckdeschel, K., Rouot, B., and Heesemann, J. (1999). The cytotoxin YopT of *Yersinia enterocolitica* induces modification and cellular redistribution of the small GTP-binding protein RhoA. *J. Biol. Chem.* 274(41):29289–29293.

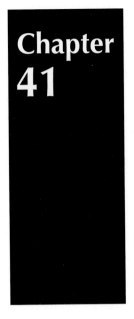

Virus Infection of Epithelial Cells

Chapter 41

Richard W. Compans

Department of Microbiology and Immunology, Emory University School of Medicine, Atlanta, Georgia

Georg Herrler

Institut für Virologie, Tierärztliche Hochschule Hannover, Hannover, Germany

VIRUS LIFE CYCLE

Viruses contain a genome consisting of either DNA or RNA, which is surrounded by a protein coat that is usually assembled in either an icosahedral or helical configuration. In many viruses the core is enclosed in a lipid-containing membrane called the viral envelope, which consists of a lipid bilayer containing one or more virus-coded surface glycoproteins. The structural properties of virus particles (virions) provide the basis for their classification into families. Important features that distinguish each family are the size and type of nucleic acid, the size and symmetry of the nucleocapsid, and the presence or absence of an envelope. Based on these and a few other characteristics, animal viruses have been classified into families, each of which has a characteristic virion structure and a common replication strategy.

The viral replication cycle is initiated by adsorption of the virion to host cell receptors, which are described in more detail in the next section. Following adsorption, enveloped viruses enter cells by a process of membrane fusion, which may be either low pH–dependent or pH-independent (White, 1992), and is mediated by specific viral glycoproteins. The pH-independent fusion occurs directly with the cellular plasma membrane; such fusion has been well documented for paramyxoviruses and certain retroviruses. In contrast, many other enveloped viruses enter cells by endocytosis. They subsequently are localized in endosomes, and the low pH of the endosome triggers a conformational change in the viral glycoprotein that activates their membrane fusion activity. The viral envelope then fuses with the surrounding endosomal membrane. The best-studied example of this fusion mechanism is with influenza virus, for which the molecular structure of the fusion protein (hemagglutinin) has been determined in

both its neutral pH form (Wilson *et al.*, 1981) and its low pH form (Bullough *et al.*, 1994), demonstrating that exposure to low pH triggers a dramatic conformational change that activates fusion activity. Most nonenveloped viruses also enter cells by endocytosis, but the exact process by which their genomes subsequently are released into cells is not well understood.

All viruses share two processes that are fundamental to their replication: synthesis of proteins encoded by the viral genome and replication of the viral nucleic acid. The replication of most RNA viruses is restricted to the cytoplasm, whereas the replication of DNA viruses usually takes place in the nucleus. During replication, the biosynthetic machinery of the infected cell is diverted to synthesis of viral components. Icosahedral viruses form by a process of self-assembly; the protein subunits form a symmetrical shell (capsid) containing the viral nucleic acid. The assembly and release of enveloped viruses occurs by budding at a cellular membrane **(Table 41.1)**. Viral membrane glycoproteins are synthesized in the rough endoplasmic reticulum and are transported through the exocytic pathway. For many enveloped viruses, assembly occurs by budding at the cell surface, and the completed virions are released immediately from the cell. However, some families of enveloped viruses are assembled by budding at intracellular membranes, as described in more detail below.

Many viruses initiate their infection processes by interaction with epithelial cells at mucosal surfaces. The cell biology of this virus–cell interaction is one of the important factors that play a role as a determinant of viral pathogenesis. In this chapter, we discuss the alternative routes of entry of viruses into mucosal epithelial cells, which are primarily determined by the distribution of viral receptors on cell surfaces. We also describe the process of viral release, which typically occurs in a polarized fashion in epithelial cells and tissues.

Table 41.1. Cellular Sites of Replication and Assembly of Selected Virus Families

Virus Family	Envelope	Site of Replication and Neocapsid Assembly	Site of Budding (for enveloped viruses)
RNA viruses			
Arenavirus	+	Cytoplasm	Plasma membrane
Bunyavirus	+	Cytoplasm	Golgi complex
Coronavirus	+	Cytoplasm	Rough endoplasmic reticulum
Orthomyxovirus	+	Nucleus and cytoplasm	Plasma membrane
Paramyxovirus	+	Cytoplasm	Plasma membrane
Picornavirus	−		
Calicivirus	−	Cytoplasm	
Astrovirus	−	Cytoplasm	
Reovirus	−	Cytoplasm	
Retrovirus	+	Nucleus and cytoplasm	Plasma membrane
Rhabdovirus	+	Cytoplasm	Plasma membrane
Filovirus	+	Cytoplasm	Plasma membrane
Togavirus	+	Cytoplasm	Plasma membrane
Flavivirus	+	Cytoplasm	Endoplasmic reticulum
DNA viruses			
Adenovirus	−	Nucleus	
Herpesvirus	+	Nucleus	Nuclear envelope
Hepadnavirus	+	Nucleus	Endoplasmic reticulum
Papillomavirus	−	Nucleus	
Parvovirus	−	Nucleus	
Polyomavirus	−	Nucleus	
Poxvirus	+	Cytoplasm/plasma membrame	Cytoplasm

VIRAL RECEPTORS

Definition of virus receptors

The initial event in the viral life cycle is the interaction of one or more viral surface proteins with specific components present on the cell surface. The macromolecules on the plasma membrane that are essential for the virus to initiate the infectious cycle are designated as virus receptors. Either cell surface proteins or surface lipids may serve as receptors for specific viruses. The presence or absence of suitable receptors is an important factor for determining whether a cell is sensitive or resistant to infection by a specific virus. Therefore, the tropism of a virus, *e.g.*, for neural, respiratory, or intestinal cells, is often determined by the level of expression of virus receptors in such tissues. Multiple noncovalent interactions between viral proteins and cell surface components are required to mediate the specific binding of a virus to a cell. The residues of the viral proteins that are involved in this interaction are designated as the receptor binding site. In the case of enveloped viruses, they usually are part of an individual protein, *e.g.*, in the influenza hemagglutinin, where they are arranged in the form of a pocket at the tip of the glycoprotein molecule. The residues of the receptor binding site may, however, belong to more than one viral polypeptide, as in the case of the nonenveloped polioviruses, where they are part of a canyon-like depression in the capsid structure. The portion of the receptor that is actu-

ally interacting with the virus, the receptor determinant, may be composed of a number of amino acids, as in the case of CD4, the receptor for human immunodeficiency virus (HIV), or intercellular adhesion molecule 1 (ICAM-I), the receptor for most strains of rhinoviruses.

Influenza viruses and several other viruses specifically recognize sialic acid residues. For these viruses, sialic acid functions as a receptor determinant. It should be noted that it is not appropriate to designate sialic acid as the receptor, because free sialic acid is bound very weakly by virions and, more important, is unable to mediate the infection of cells. It is functional only when present as a constituent of a glycoprotein or glycolipid. Therefore, cell surface sialoglycoconjugates are the receptors for the viruses that recognize sialic acids.

Cellular receptors for virus attachment

To identify a specific surface protein as a virus receptor, an approach involving the following two criteria has been most successful: a monoclonal antibody directed against this protein prevents virus infection; and receptor-negative cells become sensitive to virus infection after transfection with the receptor-encoding gene from receptor-positive cells. By these approaches, receptors for a number of viruses have been identified and their functions have been verified by additional evidence such as tissue distribution and in vitro binding studies (**Table 41.2**). However, the initiation of virus

Table 41.2.   Viruses that Recognize Defined Proteins as Virus Receptors

Virus	Receptor	Reference
Retroviruses		
HIV	CD4	Maddon et al., 1996
Murine leukemia viruses		
ecotropic (murine cells)	Cationic amino acid	Albritton et al., 1989
amphotropic (murine and other cells)	Phosphate transporter (GLVR2)	Miller et al., 1994; Zeijl et al., 1994
Gibbon ape leukemia virus	Phosphate transporter (GLVR1)	O'Hara et al., 1990
Feline leukemia virus, avian leukosis	Phosphate transporter (GLVR1)	Takeuchi et al., 1992
sarcoma virus		
Subgroup A	ALSV-A receptor	Bates et al., 1993
Subgroups B and D	Cytopathic ALSV receptor (CAR1)	Brojatsch et al., 1996
Bovine leukemia virus	BLV receptor	Ban et al., 1993
Picornaviruses		
Poliovirus	Poliovirus receptor	Mendelsohn et al., 1989
Rhinovirus, major serogroup	Intercellular adhesion molecule (ICAM-1)	Greve et al., 1989; Staunton et al., 1989
Rhinovirus, minor serogroup	Low-density lipoprotein receptor	Hofer et al., 1994
Echoviruses 1 and 8	Integrin (VLA-2)	Bergelson et al., 1992
Echovirus 7	Decay-accelerating factor (DAF; CD55)	Bergelson et al., 1992; Ward et al., 1994
Coxsackievirus B	Coxsackievirus-adenovirus receptor (CAR)	Bergelson et al., 1997
Hepatitis A virus	HAVcr-1	Kaplan et al., 1996; Huber et al., 1994
Encephalomyocarditis virus	Vascular cell adhesion molecule (VACM-1)	
Togaviruses		
Sindbis virus	Laminin receptor	Wang et al., 1992
Coronaviruses		
TGEV, FIPV, CCoV, HCoV-229E	Aminopeptidase N	Delmas et al., 1992; Yeager et al., 1992
Mouse hepatitis virus	Biliary glycoprotein (MHVR)	Dveksler et al., 1991
SARS-CoV	Angiotensin-converting enzyme 2	Li et al., 2003
Paramyxovirus		
Measles virus	Membrane cofactor protein (MCP, CD46), signaling leukocyte activation molecule (SLAM)	Naniche et al., 1993; Dorig et al., 1993; Tatsuo et al., 2000
Adenoviruses		
Adenovirus 2	Coxsackievirus-adenovirus receptor (CAR)	Bergelson et al., 1997
Herpesviruses		
Herpes simplex virus 1 and 2	Nectin-1, nectin-2	Geraghty et al., 1998
Pseudorabies virus	Tumor necrosis factor receptor family	Montgomery et al., 1996
Epstein-Barr virus	Complement receptor 2 (CD21)	Frade et al., 1985; Nemerow et al., 1985

infection may be more complex than a simple interaction of the virus with a single receptor. For example, viruses may use alternative surface constituents for attachment to cells. HIV has been reported to attach not only to CD4 (Dalgleish *et al.*, 1984) but also to galactosyl ceramide (Bhat *et al.*, 1991), although with lower affinity. It also requires an interaction with specific coreceptors, CXCR4 or CCR5, to initiate infection (see the following section).

The criteria for receptor identification mentioned previously apply only to defined protein receptors. A large number of viruses recognize determinants that may be present on multiple surface components (**Table 41.3**). Herpes simplex viruses use glycosaminoglycan chains of surface proteoglycans for attachment to cells (WuDunn and Spear, 1989). Influenza viruses and several members of the paramyxoviruses and coronaviruses are known to recognize sialic acids (a designation for all derivatives of neuraminic acid). The importance of this acidic sugar for virus binding can be demonstrated by the inactivation of receptors after treatment with sialidase (neuraminidase) and by the regeneration of receptors by enzymatic resialylation of cells. In this way it has been shown that these viruses may have a strict preference for a certain type of sialic acid. While influenza A and B viruses have a preference for N-acetyl-neuraminic acid (Rogers and Paulson, 1983), influenza C virus recognizes only N-acetyl-9-O-acetylneuraminic acid as a receptor determinant (Herrler *et al.*, 1985). Furthermore, virus binding may be restricted to sialic acids

that are connected to the adjacent sugar in a defined linkage type.

Human influenza viruses, for example, have a clear preference for N-acetylneuraminic acid attached to galactose in an α-2,6-linkage (Rogers and Paulson, 1983). This example already shows that it is not appropriate to designate sialic acid as the receptor, because only those surface glycoconjugates that contain the correct type of sialic acid in the correct linkage may serve as receptors for these viruses. Another restriction in the recognition of sialic acid–containing receptors is imposed by the fact that the interaction between individual sialic acid residues and the influenza hemagglutinin is rather weak. Therefore, an efficient binding of influenza viruses to the cell surface requires a multivalent interaction between the virus and its cellular receptors, and the number of sialic acid residues and their spatial orientation are important factors for a receptor for influenza viruses. Mucin-type glycoproteins that are highly glycosylated and contain clusters of O-linked oligosaccharides are expected to be suitable receptors. Among the surface proteins of Madin-Darby canine kidney (MDCK) cells, influenza C virus was found to bind primarily to a mucin-type glycoprotein designated gp40 (Zimmer *et al.*, 1995). Therefore, this sialoglycoprotein is a potential receptor for the infection of MDCK cells by influenza C virus. Sialic acid may serve as a receptor determinant not only on glycoproteins but also on glycolipids. The potential role of specific gangliosides as receptors has been demonstrated for Sendai virus, a member of the paramyxovirus family (Markwell *et al.*,

Table 41.3. Viruses that Recognize the Carbohydrate Portion of Glycoproteins as Receptor Determinants

Viruses	Receptors	Receptor Determinant	Reference
Influenza A and B	Sialoglycoconjugates	Neu5Ac	Carrol and Paulson, 1983
Influenza C	Sialoglycoconjugates (gp40)	Neu5,9Ac$_2$	Herrler and Klenk, 1987
Paramyxoviruses	Sialoglycoconjugates (gangliosides)	Neu5Ac	Markwell *et al.*, 1981
Coronaviruses BCoV, HCoV-OC43	Sialoglycoconjugates (gp40)	Neu5,9Ac$_2$	Schultze *et al.*, 1996
Reoviruses	Sialoglycoconjugates	Sialic acid	Paul *et al.*, 1989
Rotaviruses	Sialoglycoconjugates	Sialic acid	Yolken *et al.*, 1987
Polyomaviruses	Sialoglycoconjugates (gp40–42)	Sialic acid	Fried *et al.*, 1981
Canine parvovirus	—	Sialic acid	Basak *et al.*, 1994
Herpes simplex virus	Proteoglycans	Glycosaminoglycans	WuDunn and Spear, 1989
Pseudorabies virus	Proteoglycans	Glycosaminoglycans	Mettenleiter *et al.*, 1990
Respiratory syncytial virus	Proteoglycans	Glycosaminoglycans	Krusat and Streckert, 1997
Theiler's murine encephalomyelitis virus	Sialoglycoconjugates Proteoglycans	Sialic acid Glycosaminoglycans	Zhou *et al.*, 1997 Reddi and Lipton, 2002
Porcine reproductive and respiratory syndrome virus	Proteoglycans	Glycosaminoglycans	Jusa *et al.*, 1997
Adeno-associated virus-2	Proteoglycans	Glycosaminoglycans	Summerford and Samulski, 1998
HIV	Galactosyl ceramide		Bhat *et al.*, 1991
Parvovirus B19	P antigen (globoside)		Brown *et al.*, 1993

1981). Irrespective of the binding to a glycoprotein or to a glycolipid, for the reasons given earlier, only a subset of the surface sialoglycoconjugates are expected to be suitable receptors for viruses that use sialic acid as a receptor determinant.

Viruses may also attach to the cell surface and initiate infection without involving their own receptor-binding activity. HIV has been shown to incorporate cell surface components such as ICAM-1 and cyclophilin A into the viral membrane (Fortin *et al.*, 1997; Saphire *et al.*, 1999); the binding activities of these molecules allow HIV to attach to cells by interacting with lymphocyte function–associated molecule 1 (LFA-1) and surface-bound heparin sulfate structures, respectively. Virus attachment may also be mediated by cellular C-type lectin receptors that recognize the mannose-rich oligosaccharide side chains on the surface protein gp120 of HIV (Curtis *et al.*, 1992). Some of these binding activities may be used in a concerted action and enable the virus to attach to cells that express only a low level of CD4. Cells containing receptors for immunoglobulins may be infected by viruses that are complexed with nonneutralizing antibodies (Porterfield, 1986). This mechanism of virus entry has been described for several viruses, *e.g.*, HIV and dengue virus. Overall, the availability of alternative binding strategies may broaden the spectrum of cells that are susceptible to infection.

Cellular receptors for virus entry

Virus entry is best understood in the case of viruses with a lipid envelope (see first section of text), which introduce their genome into the cell by a fusion event between the viral and the cellular membrane. Whether fusion occurs by a low-pH-dependent or a pH-independent process, it usually requires a conformational change of the viral fusion protein just prior to the fusion reaction. In this process a fusion-active domain is exposed and thus is able to interact with the target membrane. With paramyxoviruses, in which the receptor-binding activity and the fusion activity are located on different surface proteins, fusion occurs at the plasma membrane. The receptor binding protein (HN) interacts with the fusion protein (F). Binding to sialic acid residues of cell surface receptors is thought to trigger a conformational change in the HN protein that induces the F protein to adapt the fusion-active form (Lamb, 1993).

Cellular proteins may also be involved in the virus-induced fusion reaction. In the case of HIV, binding to CD4 results in attachment to cells but not in virus entry. Chemokine receptors have been shown to be required for the fusion of the viral membrane with the host cell membrane (Weiss and Clapham, 1996). It has been suggested that binding of the viral protein gp120 to CD4 results in a conformational change in gp120, and this in turn results in the creation of a new recognition site for a chemokine receptor. The interaction of gp120 with the chemokine receptor is thought to trigger the fusion activity of the transmembrane protein gp41 and is an important determinant of the viral tropism.

Macrophage-tropic strains that predominate in the early stage of an HIV infection use a different type of receptor

(CC-CCR5) than do T-cell tropic strains that are more prominent in later stages of infection, which use the receptor CXCR-4. This finding shows that there is a high degree of flexibility in the interaction of the viral surface proteins with cellular receptors. Some strains of HIV have been reported to use chemokine receptors even to infect CD4-negative cells. A role for cellular proteins in mediating the fusion reaction after virus attachment has also been reported for herpes simplex virus. Following primary attachment via the surface glycoproteins gC and gB to glycosaminoglycans on surface proteoglycans (WuDunn and Spear, 1989), another surface protein, gD, binds to a specific receptor of the nectin family of surface proteins (Krummenacher *et al.*, 1998). This interaction enables HSV—in a reaction that also involves the additional viral glycoproteins gB, gH, and gL—to initiate the fusion between the viral and the cellular membrane.

There is no generally accepted designation for cellular proteins involved in the process of virus entry following the attachment to the plasma membrane, but designations such as entry mediators, coreceptors, or entry cofactors have been used to distinguish them from attachment receptors. However, in some cases it may be difficult or impossible to differentiate between the proteins involved in attachment and those involved in virus entry, because some variants or strains of viruses may have evolved to use the latter cellular proteins also for virus attachment.

VIRUS ENTRY INTO EPITHELIAL CELLS

Virus receptors on epithelial cells

The presence or absence of suitable surface receptors is a critical determinant for the sensitivity or resistance, respectively, of cells to virus infection. The plasma membrane of epithelial cells is divided into an apical domain and a basolateral domain that differ from each other in their composition. As a consequence, virus receptors may be present on one domain of the cell surface and absent from the other. A polarized distribution of virus receptors is expected to have important implications for virus infections. If a virus receptor is restricted to the apical surface, virus infection is possible only through this membrane domain and, in the context of an organism, only via the lumen of the body cavity that is lined by the respective epithelium **(Table 41.4)**. An example of an apical virus receptor is aminopeptidase N, which serves as a receptor for porcine transmissible gastroenteritis virus (TGEV) and related human, canine, and feline coronaviruses (Delmas *et al.*, 1992). These viruses enter the organism via the respiratory or gastrointestinal tract, causing localized infections of the respective epithelium, and therefore require virus receptors only on the apical surfaces of epithelial cells. The surface distribution of aminopeptidase N is consistent with the role of this protein as a coronavirus receptor. Apical surface receptors are also required for infections by human influenza viruses.

Sialic acid, the receptor determinant recognized by these viruses, is abundantly present on both the apical and

Table 41.4. Sites of Entry and Release of Selected Viruses in Polarized Epithelial Cells

Virus (family, species)	Cell Type	Site of Entry	Site of Release	References
Bunyavirus				
Punta Toro	Vero C1008	ND	Basolateral	Chen et al., 1991
Black Creek Canal	Vero C1008	Apical	Apical	Ravkov et al., 1997
Coronavirus				
Transmissible gastroenteritis	LLCPK1	Apical	Apical	Rossen et al., 1994
Bovine coronavirus	MDCK	Apical	Apical	Schultz et al., 1996
Mouse hepatitis	Murine kidney	Apical	Basolateral	Rossen et al., 1995
Orthomyxovirus				
Influenza	MDCK	Nonpolar	Apical	Rodriguez-Boulan and Sabatini, 1978; Fuller et al., 1984
Paramyxovirus				
Measles	Caco-2, Vero C1008	Apical	Apical	Blau and Compans, 1995
Sendai wild type	MDCK	ND	Apical	Rodriguez-Boulan and Sabatini, 1978
Sendai F1-R mutant	MDCK		Bidirectional	Tashiro et al., 1990
Retrovirus				
HIV-1	Vero C1008	ND	Basolateral	Owens et al., 1991
Rhabdovirus				
Vesicular stomatitis	MDCK	Basolateral	Basolateral	Rodriguez-Boulan and Sabatini, 1978; Fuller et al., 1984

ND, not determined

basolateral surfaces of most epithelial cells. As mentioned in the preceding section, there are several restrictions in the recognition of sialic acids. Therefore, only a limited number of surface sialoglycoconjugates are expected to fulfill the requirements for an influenza virus receptor. Suitable receptors appear not to be present on all epithelial cells of the respiratory tract. Within the tracheal epithelium, human influenza A viruses were found to bind to ciliated cells but not to nonciliated cells, suggesting that functional receptors are expressed on the surface of the former cells (Couceiro et al., 1993). A further limitation in the use of sialoglycoconjugates as receptors is imposed by the requirement of influenza viruses for endocytotic uptake. In this context it is interesting to note that glycoprotein gp40, a potential receptor for influenza C virus, is subject to endocytosis at a rate that is similar to the kinetics of virus internalization (Zimmer et al., 1995). Localization on the apical surface of epithelial cells is also characteristic of proteins that are membrane-anchored by glycosol phosphatidyl inositol residues. Decay accelerating factor, which belongs to this group of proteins, is a receptor for some members of the picornavirus family (Ward et al., 1994).

Virus receptors on the basolateral plasma membrane domain are required for viruses that approach epithelial cells from the serosal side, e.g., after spread via the blood stream. Both CD4 and galactosyl ceramide, an alternative attachment receptor for HIV, have been reported to be localized on the basolateral side of epithelial cells (Yahi et al., 1992), and this may explain the intestinal tropism of HIV. Canine parvovirus has also been shown to infect epithelial cells via the basolateral domain (Basak and Compans, 1989). This entry site is consistent with the basolateral location of the transferrin receptor, which has been identified as a receptor for canine and feline parvoviruses (Parker et al., 2001). The viruses for which receptor expression is restricted to the basolateral domain may nevertheless enter through the lumen of the intestine and be transported to the basolateral surface by binding to M cells, followed by transcytosis. Several viruses, including reoviruses, poliovirus, and HIV, have been reported to be transported efficiently across the M cells by transcytosis (Amerongen et al., 1991), after which they could initiate a retrograde infection of the epithelial cell layer.

Membrane cofactor protein (CD46), a regulatory protein of the complement system, has been identified as a receptor for measles virus (Naniche et al., 1993). With several epithelial cells, CD46 has been shown in vivo and in vitro to be a basolateral protein (Maisner et al., 1996). This distribution is consistent with the infection of epithelial cells in the late stage of a measles virus infection, when the virus spreads from the bloodstream to different epithelial tissues. In CaCo-2 cells, CD46 has been shown to be localized predominantly on the apical surface (Blau and Compans, 1995). An apical localization of CD46 would be consistent with the initial stage of the measles virus infection, when the virus enters the organism via the respiratory tract. However, CD46 serves as a receptor only for vaccine strains that are applied by injection and do not enter the organism via respiratory infection.

Signaling leukocyte activation molecule (SLAM) has been shown to function as a high-affinity receptor for wild-type measles virus (Tatsuo et al., 2000). This protein is present on various types of lymphocytes and activated macrophages but absent from epithelial, endothelial, and neuronal cells. SLAM-negative cells are infected with low efficiency, possibly by using a so far unidentified low-affinity-receptor (Hashimoto et al., 2002). Such a receptor may also be involved in the apical infection of the respiratory epithelium in the initial stage of the measles virus infection. Alternatively, measles virus may cross the epithelial barrier through sites where the integrity of the epithelial sheath is damaged or by intercellular passage of infected macrophages.

Some viruses make use of the asialoglycoprotein receptor or the immunoglobulin receptor to initiate infection. Both proteins are localized on the basolateral surface of epithelial cells. The asialoglycoprotein receptor has been reported to be a potential receptor for Marburg virus (Becker et al., 1995), and its presence on hepatocytes may explain the hepatotropism of this virus, although different receptors may be required to infect other tissues. The receptor for polymeric IgA has been reported to mediate the entry of antibody-complexed Epstein-Barr virus into an established human epithelial cell line (Sixbey and Yao, 1992). While CD21 is used by this virus to infect B lymphocytes and several epithelial cells, the antibody-dependent route is an alternative way to enter epithelial cells. To what extent this mechanism contributes to the infection of the nasopharyngeal epithelium remains to be established.

Polarity of virus entry

The examples presented in the preceding section show how the surface distribution of receptors affects the way in which a virus enters an epithelial cell. At present, our knowledge about this aspect of virology is very limited because the identity of the majority of virus receptors has not yet been elucidated. In addition, several cellular proteins, acting either as alternative receptors or in a consecutive way, may be involved in the initial stage of virus infection. The polarized distribution of any of these cell surface constituents, whether it is required for the attachment or for the entry step, may restrict the uptake of a virus to a specific domain of the plasma membrane. For some viruses, polarity of virus entry (see Table 41.4) has been demonstrated, although their receptors have not yet been identified. In the case of SV40, a nonenveloped virus, attachment to the cell surface and infection have been detected only via the apical membrane domain of epithelial cells (Clayson and Compans, 1988). On the other hand,

vesicular stomatitis virus and vaccinia virus, two enveloped viruses, infect epithelial cells predominantly via the basolateral domain (Fuller et al., 1984; Rodriguez et al., 1991). The cellular receptors for these viruses appear to be restricted to the respective segment of the plasma membrane.

Virus entry is not polarized for all viruses. The receptor for poliovirus, which is a structural homolog of the nectin family of adhesion molecules, is present mainly on the basolateral surface of epithelial cells (Tucker et al., 1993a). Nevertheless, a significant fraction of it was detected on the apical membrane domain. Recognition of the 65-kD protein by poliovirus is so efficient that virus infection is possible from both the serosal and the luminal side (Tucker et al., 1993a). However, the poliovirus receptor is present also on M cells and germinal centers within Peyer's patches (Iwasaki et al., 2002). Therefore, poliovirus enters the organism not necessarily via the apical surface of the intestinal epithelium. In contrast to the poliovirus receptor, the mucin-like glycoprotein gp40 is localized predominantly on the apical surface of the MDCK-1 cells, with only a minor fraction detectable on the basolateral side (Zimmer et al.,1995). This glycoprotein is the major surface protein of MDCK-1 cells recognized by influenza C virus and bovine coronavirus. Despite this similarity, bidirectional entry was found for the influenza C virus, as has been shown also for influenza A viruses (Fuller et al.,1984; Schultze et al., 1996). On the other hand, coronavirus was able to infect only via the apical surface (Schultze et al. 1996). It remains to be shown whether bovine coronavirus is unable to recognize the low amount of gp40 present on the basolateral surface or whether it requires an additional cellular surface protein that is present only on the apical membrane domain.

A complex picture has been described for the entry of herpes simplex virus into MDCK cells. While wild-type virus can initiate infection via both domains of the plasma membrane, mutants lacking either of the viral surface glycoproteins gC or gG are restricted in virus entry to the basolateral side (Tran et al., 2000). The exact function of gG is unclear, but it appears to be involved in a postattachment step of virus entry. The viral glycoprotein gC mediates the binding to glycosaminoglycans on surface proteoglycans (see later discussion). Such glycan structures are present on both surfaces of MDCK cells, consistent with the bidirectional entry of wild-type HSV. As mentioned earlier in this chapter, entry of herpes simplex viruses or pseudorabies virus requires the interaction of glycoprotein gD with a member of the nectin family of adherence proteins. This cellular receptor for herpesvirus colocalizes with adherence junctions and may explain infection via the basolateral membrane by viruses spreading from neurons to epithelial cells. However, the cellular localization of nectins does not provide a straightforward explanation of infection via the apical membrane. Disruption of tight junctions results in redistribution of nectins from the junction sites to the whole cell surface, with a concomitant increase in susceptibility to infection by herpes simplex virus (Yoon and Spear, 2002). Thus, virus approaching the epithelium from the apical side may enter the organism by infection of cells that have lost their polarized organization or by using a receptor different from nectin in the adherence junction, possibly with the help of glycoprotein gG.

Colocalization with cellular junction complexes is not unique to herpesvirus receptors. Both the receptor for several coxsackieviruses and adenoviruses, CAR (Bergelson et al., 1997), and the junction adhesion molecule, a reovirus receptor (Barton et al., 2001), are integral tight-junction proteins. This location is consistent with the inefficiency of these viruses to infect epithelial cells via the apical plasma membrane (Rubin, 1987; Walters et al., 1999). As far as adenoviruses are concerned, major histocompatibility complex (MHC)-I-α-2 protein, a potential alternative attachment receptor, and integrins $\alpha_v\beta_{3/5}$, which facilitate virus entry, are also basolateral proteins and not available for apical infection. Therefore, these viruses are efficient in entering epithelial cells from the basolateral side. For initial infection of an organism, they depend on other entry strategies: they may infect the epithelium at sites where the polarized organization of the cells is disturbed; they may use receptors that have not yet been identified; they may be taken up by a nonspecific mechanism (pinocytosis); and they may be transcytosed by M cells, as has been reported for reoviruses. These examples not only illustrate the complexity of virus–receptor interactions in the infection of epithelial cells but also demonstrate the importance of the identification of additional virus receptors to understand this process.

Accessory factors affecting virus entry into epithelial cells

The fusion activity of many viral surface glycoproteins depends on a posttranslational proteolytic cleavage event. At the cleavage site, most of the fusion proteins contain a motif of several basic amino acids that is recognized by furin-like proteases. Such proteases are encountered by the viral glycoproteins during passage through the secretory pathway of most cells. The hemagglutinin of human influenza viruses, however, contains a single arginine at the cleavage site, requiring a trypsin-like protease for the activation process. Such a protease, tryptase clara, is secreted by Clara cells that are part of the respiratory epithelium (Kido et al., 1992). Influenza viruses that are released into the lumen of the respiratory tract can be converted by this protease into the infectious, fusogenic form. The availability of an enzyme for proteolytic activation is one factor that restricts the infection by human influenza viruses to the respiratory epithelium. Proteolytic activation events also are known to be important for the initiation of infection by rotaviruses and reoviruses, which encounter the appropriate enzymes in the lumen of the intestinal tract. Thus, epithelial cells may provide conditions that favor the infection by certain viruses.

On the other hand, the environmental conditions of some epithelia may exclude the infection by certain viruses. In order to infect an organism in the intestinal epithelium via the oral route, viruses have to survive the harsh conditions encountered within the gastrointestinal tract: low pH, proteolytic enzymes, and bile salts. The detergent-like action of bile salts is expected to be especially detrimental for

enveloped viruses and explains why intestinal infections are caused mainly by nonenveloped viruses, e.g., rotaviruses, caliciviruses, and enteroviruses.

Coronaviruses are exceptional among viruses with an intestinal tropism, because they contain a lipid envelope. Porcine TGEV is an enteropathogenic coronavirus. As mentioned earlier, TGEV uses aminopeptidase N as a receptor to infect cells of the intestinal epithelium. In addition, it has a sialic acid binding activity. This binding activity is dispensable for infection of cultured cells. However, loss of the sialic acid binding activity, e.g., by a point mutation, results in the loss of enteropathogenicity (Krempl et al., 1997). It has been proposed that the ability of TGEV to recognize sialic acid results in the binding of sialoglycoconjugates to the viral surface. Sialylated cellular components such as intestinal mucins that are bound to the viral surface glycoprotein may increase virus stability and help it to survive the detrimental action of bile salts. In addition, binding to sialoglycoproteins may enable TGEV to attach to and penetrate through the glycocalix covering the apical membrane of intestinal cells (Schwegmann-Wessels et al., 2002). The glycocalix has been shown to prevent apical infection of epithelial cells by adenovirus, even when the CAR receptor was redirected to the apical membrane (Pickles et al., 2000), and treatment of cells with neuraminidase abolished this inhibitory effect. Therefore, the viral receptor–destroying enzymes of influenza viruses, paramyxoviruses, and coronaviruses (neuraminidases or acetylesterases) may be required not only for release from the infected cell but also for penetration through the glycocalix. A hydrolytic enzyme activity that acts on mucins has also been ascribed to the sigma1 protein of reoviruses (Bisaillon et al., 1999). This enzyme facilitates the penetration through the protective barrier of the mucus layer covering the intestinal epithelium. Thus, infection of mucosal surfaces may require viruses to evolve protective mechanisms to survive under specific environmental conditions.

POLARIZED RELEASE OF VIRUSES FROM EPITHELIAL CELLS

Virus assembly at the plasma membrane

Early studies of the release of influenza virus from polarized cells by Murphy and Bang (1952) reported that influenza virus is assembled and released by budding from the surface of the chorioallantoic membrane of embryonated eggs. They also observed that the release of the virus was polarized, occurring exclusively at the free apical surface. Rodriguez-Boulan and Sabatini (1978) reported the directional budding of enveloped viruses from polarized MDCK cells; vesicular stomatitis virus (VSV) was released predominantly from the basolateral plasma membrane, whereas influenza and Sendai virions were released from the apical domain. Subsequent studies with many viruses have revealed that viruses which assemble by budding at the plasma membrane are usually released from epithelial cells in a polarized fashion and that such directional release also occurs with some nonenveloped viruses.

The glycoproteins of enveloped viruses accumulate at the site of virus assembly, and association of viral core proteins with the viral glycoproteins leads to virus release by a process of budding, or outfolding, of the membrane. The glycoproteins of a number of enveloped viruses that assemble at the plasma membrane were found to be directionally transported to the same surface from which virus buds, even when expressed from recombinant vectors in the absence of other virus-specific proteins (Roth et al., 1983; Jones et al., 1985; Stephens et al., 1986). These observations led to the hypothesis that the site of plasma membrane accumulation of the envelope glycoprotein(s) determines the site of viral assembly. Studies of the assembly and release of HIV particles in polarized epithelial cells supported this hypothesis (Owens et al., 1991). Expression of the HIV core (Gag) protein in epithelial cells in the absence of the envelope glycoprotein resulted in the assembly and release of HIV-like particles in approximately equivalent amounts from both the apical and basolateral surfaces. In contrast to this nondirectional pattern of release, coexpression of the Gag and envelope proteins resulted in directional release of viral particles at the basolateral domain. The HIV envelope glycoprotein, when expressed from a recombinant vector, is almost exclusively found at the basolateral surface (Owens and Compans, 1989), indicating that its interaction with the core proteins determines the site of viral assembly and release.

In contrast to these observations, recent studies have provided evidence that factors other than the glycoproteins of some enveloped viruses can play a key role in determining the site of virus release. Measles virus was released from the apical surface of polarized epithelial cells, although its surface glycoproteins H and F were expressed at high levels on the basolateral membranes (Maisner et al., 1998). The glycoprotein (GP) of Marburg virus, a filovirus, was transported preferentially to the apical surfaces of polarized MDCK cells, whereas the release of infectious progeny virus occurs at the basolateral surface (Sanger et al., 2001). A VSV mutant was also constructed in which the glycoprotein lacked a basolateral targeting signal and was expressed in a nonpolarized fashion; however, release of the virus still occurred mainly at the basolateral surface (Zimmer et al., 2001). All of these viruses possess a matrix protein that is believed to play a major role in virus assembly and could be responsible for determining the site of viral assembly and release. Such a role for the matrix protein has been demonstrated in the case of measles virus (Naim et al., 2000).

Virus assembly at intracellular membranes

Bunyaviruses and coronaviruses are two families of enveloped RNA viruses that are assembled by budding at intracellular membranes. Assembly of most bunyaviruses occurs by budding at smooth-surfaced membranes in the Golgi complex (Murphy et al., 1973; Smith and Pifat, 1982). Punta Toro virus, a member of the sandfly fever group of bunyaviruses, was assembled in the Golgi complex and sub-

sequently released almost exclusively from the basolateral surfaces of polarized epithelial cells (Chen et al., 1991). Immunoelectron microscopic analysis of hepatocytes infected with another bunyavirus, Rift Valley fever virus, also indicated preferential release from the basolateral domain (Anderson and Smith, 1987). However, Rift Valley fever virus budding at the basolateral plasma membrane was also sometimes observed, indicating that at least one of the viral components contains the appropriate signals to direct vectorial transport of the viral proteins to the basolateral surface. The available evidence indicates that the viruses which assemble at intracellular membranes are transported to the cell surface by vesicular transport, thus resembling secretory proteins. The polarized release of enveloped virions may therefore be analogous to the directional release of endogenous secretory proteins from polarized cells. A possible mechanism for such polarized secretion involves a specific interaction with a membrane-bound receptor, which is targeted to a specific plasma membrane domain. In the case of some viruses, it is possible that the polarized transport of the viral receptor itself could play a role in such targeting. However, in other viruses, entry and release occur at opposite sides of epithelial cell layers, and other mechanisms must be involved in the release process. Release of certain viruses could occur by a default pathway for secretion, which may be directional or nondirectional, depending on the cell type examined.

Nonenveloped viruses

The assembly and release of nonenveloped viruses in epithelial cells has only been investigated to a limited extent, and the mechanism of release of such viruses is not well understood. However, studies with SV40 and poliovirus have indicated that nonenveloped viruses may also be targeted for release at a particular plasma membrane domain. SV40 is a nonenveloped DNA virus that is assembled in the nucleus of infected cells, and virions were found to be almost exclusively released from the apical surfaces of polarized monkey kidney epithelial cells (Clayson et al., 1989). It was also found that treatment of infected cells with the sodium ionophore monensin, which is known to be an effective inhibitor of vesicular transport, resulted in the inhibition of SV40 release but had no inhibitory effect upon viral protein synthesis or the intracellular assembly of infectious virus. High levels of SV40 release were observed prior to detectable cell lysis, and numerous virions were found to be enclosed within membrane-bound cytoplasmic vesicles during the period of maximal viral release (Clayson et al., 1989). These results suggested that the vectorial transport and release of SV40 may be mediated by a vesicular transport mechanism. Since the SV40 receptor is expressed on apical surfaces (Clayson and Compans, 1988), targeting of progeny virions to this domain might be mediated by their association with membrane-bound viral receptor molecules within transport vesicles.

Poliovirus is a nonenveloped RNA virus that replicates and is assembled in the cytoplasm, and progeny virions are observed free within the cytoplasm or within membrane-enclosed vesicular bodies (Dales *et al.*, 1965; Suhy *et al.*, 2000). Poliovirus was found to be released predominantly from the apical surfaces of infected human Caco-2 intestinal cells (Tucker *et al.*, 1993a). Although the mechanism of vectorial release is unclear, the targeting of poliovirus-containing vesicles or cytoplasmic aggregates to the apical plasma membrane may be involved.

Adenovirus was found to be released preferentially from basolateral surfaces of human airway epithelial cells (Walter *et al*, 2002). Subsequent to release, the integrity of the epithelial cell layers was disrupted in a process mediated by binding of the viral fiber protein to its receptor, CAR, allowing the virus to be released by paracellular passage to the apical surface. Further work is needed to unravel the process by which such nonenveloped viruses are directionally released from cells.

POLARIZED ENTRY AND RELEASE AS DETERMINANTS OF VIRAL PATHOGENESIS

The finding of polarized entry and release of viruses in epithelial cells has led to increasing interest in the importance of such processes within the infected organism. There are several alternative mechanisms by which viruses may traverse epithelial cell layers, and the cell biology of virus infection could play a role in this process. If a viral receptor molecule is localized exclusively on basolateral surfaces, the barrier to virus entry at epithelial tissues is more substantial than if the receptor is expressed on the apical surface or is nonpolarized. Free virus or infected cells could traverse the epithelial or endothelial barrier by paracellular passage through junctional complexes. Alternatively, virus could penetrate epithelial cell layers by transcytosis, a process that has been observed following interaction of several viruses (including HIV) with M cells, which cover mucosal lymphoid tissues (Wolf *et al.*, 1981; Amerongen *et al.*, 1991). Another mechanism could involve infection via the apical surface and subsequent release of progeny virions at the opposite surface. Finally, the epithelial cell layers could be disrupted as a result of the infection process, enabling the virus to traverse the barrier.

The release of a virus from the apical surface of an epithelial cell results in shedding into the lumen and away from underlying tissues, and such infections may have an increased likelihood of remaining localized at the epithelial surface. Conversely, basolateral release might be expected to favor the establishment of a systemic infection. Although these simple generalizations are probably not applicable to many virus infections, in some cases correlations of these types have been observed. Sendai virus, a murine parainfluenza virus, is found to be exclusively pneumotropic, whereas a Sendai mutant designated F1-R results in a systemic infection (Tashiro *et al.*, 1990). The wild-type virus was released by budding at the apical surfaces of the bronchial epithelium, whereas the F1-R mutant virions were observed to be released by budding in a bipolar manner at both the apical and basolateral surfaces. The bidirectional budding of the F1-R mutant was shown to be correlated with the distribution of viral glycoproteins on both plasma membrane domains (Tashiro *et al.*, 1990). Based on these observations, it was concluded that the site of budding of Sendai virus from the bronchial epithelium is a primary determinant of organ tropism in mice.

Viruses in the family *Coronaviridae* exhibit interesting differences in their patterns of entry and release in epithelial cells. TGEV causes a localized infection in the epithelial cells of the intestinal tract of pigs, and viral entry as well as virus release occur preferentially at the apical plasma membrane (Rossen *et al.*, 1994). The infectious process is therefore likely to involve shedding of virus into the gut lumen, with spread to adjacent epithelial cells. In contrast to TGEV, murine hepatitis virus (MHV) initially infects nasal epithelial cells but subsequently establishes a systemic infection. In epithelial cell cultures, MHV was found to infect cells at the apical surface, but progeny virions were preferentially released at the basolateral surface (Rossen *et al.*, 1995), suggesting that differences in the sites of release between the two viruses could play a role in the different disease patterns that they induce.

The *Bunyaviridae* represent another virus family in which interesting differences have been observed in the pattern of virus entry and release. Most members of this family are transmitted to humans by an insect vector and result in a systemic infection. They are assembled intracellularly by budding into the lumen of the Golgi cisternae. Their glycoproteins are localized in the Golgi complex, presumably because of specific Golgi retention signals. After budding intracellularly, virions are transported by vesicular transport to the basolateral plasma membrane, where virus release occurs (Chen and Compans, 1991). Recently, a novel group of New World hantaviruses has been discovered that are transmitted by aerosol and cause an acute pulmonary syndrome with high mortality. Unlike other members of the *Bunyaviridae*, the New World hantaviruses were found to be released exclusively at the apical plasma membrane, and virus entry was also restricted to the apical surface (Ravkov *et al.*, 1997). The glycoproteins of New World hantaviruses were found to be expressed at high levels on the apical cell surfaces, and assembly of virions by budding was observed at the apical plasma membranes of infected cells (Goldsmith *et al.*, 1995; Ravkov *et al.*, 1997). This site of entry and release is consistent with the tropism of these viruses for the respiratory tract. Hantaviruses are excreted in the urine of their rodent hosts, and the apical release of virus from kidney cells may also be relevant to this process.

EXAMPLES OF VIRAL INFECTION OF EPITHELIAL TISSUES

Gastrointestinal tract

The infectious process of reoviruses provides a model for the pathogenesis of viral infections associated with the gastrointestinal tract (Sharpe and Fields, 1985). Following ingestion, the reovirus particle undergoes proteolytic cleavage mediated by a host protease in the lumen of the gastrointestinal tract (Bodkin et al., 1989). The infection is subsequently established in epithelial cells, predominantly in the ileum in the case of reovirus type 1, or throughout the small intestine and colon in the case of reovirus type 3 (Rubin et al., 1986). Following oral inoculation of mice, binding of virus to the apical surface of M cells was observed, followed by transcytosis to the basolateral surface (Wolf et al., 1981). Once released from the basolateral surface, the virus establishes an infection in the adjacent epithelial cells and subsequently spreads to other sites, probably via the lymphatic system and bloodstream (Kauffman et al., 1983). Infection of the enterocytes adjacent to the M cells is thought to be mediated by virus binding to their basolateral surface; preferential binding to the basolateral surfaces of intestinal epithelial cells has been demonstrated in a cell culture system (Rubin, 1987).

Poliovirus is one of the most important enteroviruses that infects humans. Shortly after ingestion, virus can be recovered from lymphoid tissues, suggesting that these are the sites of primary replication. Within 4 days of ingestion, the highest titers of virus were found to be associated with the tonsils and Peyer's patches (Bodian, 1959). Occasionally, infection with poliovirus results in invasion of the central nervous system, probably via the blood (Bodian, 1959). Infection of neurons leads to transport to the anterior horn of the spinal cord and is associated with significant pathological lesions. In the later stages of infection, virus may be recovered from the feces, which is the predominant means by which dissemination occurs. Poliovirus infection of the gastrointestinal epithelium results in lesions of the Peyer's patches, and evidence suggests that poliovirus is endocytosed by M cells of human Peyer's patches (Sicinski et al., 1990). A likely scenario for the infection process is as follows: ingested poliovirus binds to the surface of M cells, which are subsequently infected and/or transport the virus by transcytosis to the underlying lymphoid tissue. A localized infection of cells in the Peyer's patch is initiated, followed by a viremia leading to infection of other target organs and tissues such as the central nervous system, brown fat, and somatic lymph nodes (Bodian, 1959). Release of virus into the feces may be mediated by the movement of infected lymphocytes from lymphoid tissues into the lumen of the gut (Bodian, 1959) and/or infection of nonlymphoid gut epithelial cells (Sabin, 1956), resulting in vectorial transport and preferential release of virions from their apical surface into the gut lumen (Tucker et al., 1993b).

Respiratory tract

Influenza virus is one of the most important causes of morbidity and mortality in humans. Influenza A viruses preferentially establish an infection in the ciliated epithelial cells of the respiratory tract. The infected cells are destroyed, leaving a layer of basal cells overlying the basement membrane, with gaps between cells that allow passage of fluids into the lumen (Small, 1990). Following this early destruction phase, the remaining epithelial cells of the basal layer begin to divide and regenerate the epithelia. Although damage is generally confined to the epithelium lining the upper respiratory tract, in some cases severe pathological changes can also occur in the epithelia of the lower respiratory tract, resulting in viral pneumonia. Influenza infections of humans do not usually result in extensive viremia (Louria et al., 1959). Influenza virus entry and release are likely to be largely restricted to the apical surfaces of epithelial cells, as observed in epithelial cell culture systems. Such a restriction is consistent with the establishment of the type of localized infection observed during influenza infection of humans.

The primary site of replication of rhinoviruses is the epithelial surface of the nasal mucosa (Douglas, 1975). Immunolocalization studies have demonstrated a tropism for columnar epithelial cells in this region (Turner et al., 1982). The cellular receptor for rhinoviruses has been identified as the ICAM-1 (Greve et al., 1989), which is restricted to the luminal surface of the lung epithelium (Albelda, 1991). Since ICAM-1 is widely distributed in other tissues, it is unlikely to have an important role as a determinant of tissue tropism. The receptor is expressed on the apical surface, so transepithelial transport is not required for infection, suggesting there is little selective pressure for the virus to further invade the mucosal surface. Virus is shed into nasal secretions, and the titers of progeny virus in secretions are correlated with the extent of mucosal infection and the severity of illness. There are several potential reasons for restriction of the infection to the upper respiratory tract (Couch, 1996). Because of the sensitivity of rhinoviruses to reduced pH, they are unable to survive passage through the gastrointestinal tract. However, direct inoculation of rhinoviruses into the small intestine of volunteers also failed to result in the establishment of infection, indicating that the low pH sensitivity of the virus is not the sole cause of the failure of these viruses to infect the intestinal tract. The optimal growth temperature of these viruses is 33°C, as found in the upper respiratory tract, and this may play a major role in restricting the site of infection.

IMPLICATIONS FOR EFFECTIVE VACCINES

Viruses exhibit a diverse pattern of interactions with epithelial cells. The site of virus entry is determined by the distribution of specific cellular receptors, whereas the site of release is determined primarily by sorting signals present in the viral proteins and their interaction with cellular transport pathways. The restriction of entry and release of some types of viruses to apical surfaces is consistent with a pattern of localized infection of epithelial cell surfaces by these agents. Other types of viruses are released at basolateral plasma membrane domains after infection of epithelial cells or are transported across epithelia by transcytosis and are thus more readily able to spread to other tissues. In both types of infection, immune responses in mucosal secretions represent the first line of defense against the initial interaction of a virus with apical cell surfaces. Therefore, development of vaccines that induce such responses is an important objective for prevention of virus infection at mucosal surfaces. For viruses that cause localized infections at epithelial surfaces, mucosal immune responses are also likely to be the most important mechanism for preventing spread of the infection process. Viruses that are able to traverse epithelial cell layers are subsequently also accessible to systemic immune responses, which play a role in preventing the spread of infection to other sites. In addition, following the initial infection of epithelial cells, the infected cells also can serve as targets for cytotoxic T lymphocytes by presentation of processed viral antigens in association with MHC molecules on their basolateral surfaces. It is believed that such responses play an important role in the clearance of virus from infected tissues.

REFERENCES

Albelda, S. M. (1991). Endothelial and epithelial cell adhesion molecules. *Am. J. Respir. Cell. Mol. Biol.* 4, 195–203.

Amerongen, H. M., Weltzin, R., Mack, J. A., Winner III, L. S., Michetti, P., Apter, F. M., Kraehenbuhl, J.-P., and Neutra, M. R. (1991). M cell-mediated antigen transport and monoclonal IgA antibodies for mucosal immune protection. *Ann. N.Y. Acad. Sci.* 622, 18–26.

Anderson, G. W. J., and Smith, J. F. (1987). Immunoelectron microscopy of rift valley fever viral morphogenesis in primary rat hepatocytes. *Virology* 161, 91–100.

Barton, E. S., Forrest, J. C., Connolly, J. L., Chappell, J. D., Liu, Y., Schnell, F. J., Nusrat, A., Parkos, C. A., and Dermody, T. S. (2001). Junction adhesion molecule is a receptor for reovirus. *Cell* 104, 441–451.

Basak, S., and Compans, R. W. (1989). Polarized entry of canine parvovirus in an epithelial cell line. *J. Virol.* 63, 3164–3167.

Becker, S., Spiess, M., and Klenk, H. D. (1995). The asialoglycoprotein receptor is a potential liver-specific receptor for Marburg virus. *J. Gen. Virol.* 76, 393–399.

Bergelson, J. M., Cunningham, J. A., Droguett, G., Kurt-Jones, E. A., Krithivas, A., Hong, J. S., Horwitz, M. S., Crowell, R. L., and Finberg, R. W. (1997). Isolation of a common receptor for Coxsackie B viruses and adenoviruses 2 and 5. *Science* 275, 1320–1323.

Bhat, S., Spitalnik, S., Gonzalez-Scarano, F., and Silberberg, D. (1991). Galactosyl ceramide or a derivative is an essential component of the neural receptor for human immunodeficiency virus type 1 envelope glycoprotein gp120. *Proc. Natl. Acad. Sci.* 88, 7131–7134.

Bisaillon, M., Senechal, S., Bernier, L., and Lemay, G. (1999). A glycosyl hydrolase activity of mammalian reovirus sigma1 protein can contribute to viral infection through a mucus layer. *J. Molec. Biol.* 286, 759–773.

Blau, D. M., and Compans, R. W. (1995). Measles virus entry and release are polarized in epithelial cells. *Virology* 210, 91–99.

Bodian, D. (1959). Poliomyelitis: pathogenesis and histopathology. In *Viral and Rickettsial Infections of Man* (eds. F.L. Horsfell, Jr., and I. Tamm) 3rd ed. Philadelphia: JB Lippincott.

Bodkin, D. K., Nibert, M. L., and Fields, B. N. (1989). Proteolytic digestion of reovirus in the intestinal lumens of neonatal mice. *J. Virol.* 63, 4676–4681.

Bullough, P. A., Hughson, F. M., Skehel, J. J., and Wiley, D. C. (1994). Structure of influenza haemagglutinin at the pH of membrane fusion. *Nature (London)* 371, 37–43.

Chen, S.-Y., and Compans, R. W. (1991). Oligomerization, transport and Golgi retention of Punta Toro virus glycoproteins. *J. Virol.* 65, 5902–5909.

Chen, S.-Y., Matsuoka, Y., and Compans, R. W. (1991). Assembly and polarized release of Punta Toro virus and the effects of brefeldin A. *J. Virol.* 65, 1427–1439.

Clayson, E. T., Brando, L. V. J., and Compans, R. W. (1989). Release of SV40 virions from epithelial cells is polarized and occurs without cell lysis. *J. Virol.* 63, 2278–2288.

Clayson, E. T., and Compans, R. W. (1988). Entry of SV40 is restricted to apical surfaces of polarized epithelial cells. *Mol. Cell Biol.* 8, 3391–3396.

Couceiro, J. N., Paulson, J. C., and Baum, L. G. (1993). Influenza virus strains selectively recognize sialyloligosaccharides on human respiratory epithelium; the role of the host cell in selection of hemagglutinin receptor specificity. *Virus Res.* 29, 155–165.

Couch, R. B. (1996). Rhinoviruses. In *Fields Virology*, 3rd ed. (eds. B. N. Fields, D. M. Knipe, and P. M. Howley), 713–734. Philadelphia: Lippincott.

Curtis, B. M., Scharnowske, S., and Watson, A. J. (1992). Sequence and expression of a membrane-associated C-type lectin that exhibits CD4-independent binding of human immunodeficiency virus envelope glycoprotein gp120. *Proc. Natl. Acad. Sci. USA* 89, 8356–8360.

Dales, S., Eggers, H. J., Tamm, I., and Palade, G. E. (1965). Electron microscopic study of the formation of poliovirus. *Virology* 26, 379–389.

Dalgleish, A. G., Beverley, P. C., Clapham, P. R., Crawford, D. H., Greaves, M. F., and Weiss, R. A. (1984). The CD4 (T4) antigen is an essential component of the receptor for the AIDS retrovirus. *Nature* 312, 763–767.

Delmas, B., Gelfi, J., L'Haridon, R., Vogel, L., Sjostrom, H., Noren, O., and Laude, H. (1992). Aminopeptidase N is a major receptor for the entero-pathogenic coronavirus TGEV. *Nature* 357, 417–420.

Douglas, R. G. J. (1975). In *The Influenza Virus and Influenza* (ed. E. D. Kilbourne), 395–447. Orlando: Academic Press.

Fortin, J. F., Cantin, R., Lamontagne, G., and Tremblay, M. (1997). Host-derived ICAM-1 glycoproteins incorporated on human immunodeficiency virus type 1 are biologically active and enhance viral infectivity. *J. Virol.* 71, 3588–3596.

Fuller, S. D., von Bonsdorff, C.-H., and Simons, K. (1984). Vesicular stomatitis virus infects and matures only through the basolateral surface of the polarized epithelial cell line, MDCK. *Cell* 38, 65–77.

Goldsmith, C. S., Elliott, L. H., Peters, C. J., and Zaki, S. R. (1995). Ultrastructural characteristics of Sin Nombre virus, causative agent of hantavirus pulmonary syndrome. *Arch. Virol.* 140, 2107–2122.

Greve, J. M., Davis, G., Meyer, A. M., Forte, C. P., Yost, S. C., Marlor, C. W., Kamarck, M. E., and McClelland, A. (1989). The major human rhinovirus receptor is ICAM-1. *Cell* 56, 839–847.

Hashimoto, K., Ono, N., Tatsuo, H., Minagawa, H., Takeda, M., Takeuchi, K., and Yanagi, Y. (2002). SLAM (CD150)-independent measles virus entry as revealed by recombinant virus expressing green fluorescent protein. *J. Virol.* 76, 6743–6749.

Herrler, G., Rott, R., Klenk, H. D., Muller, H. P., Shukla, A. K., and Schauer, R. (1985). The receptor-destroying enzyme of influenza C virus is neuraminate-O-acetylesterase. *EMBO J.* 4, 1503–1506.

Iwasaki, A., Welker, R., Mueller, S., Linehan, M., Nomoto, A., and Wimmer, E. (2002). Immunofluorescence analysis of poliovirus receptor expression in Peyer's patches of humans, primates, and CD155 transgenic mice: implications for poliovirus infection. *J. Infect. Dis.* 186, 585–592.

Jones, L. V., Compans, R. W., Davis, A. R., Bos, T. J., and Nayak, D. P. (1985). Surface expression of the influenza neuraminidase, an amino-terminally anchored viral membrane glycoprotein, in polarized epithelial cells. *Mol. Cell Biol.* 5, 2181–2189.

Kauffman, R. S., Wolf, J. L., Finberg, R., Trier, J. S., and Fields, B. N. (1983). The sigma 1 protein determines the extent of spread of reovirus from the gastrointestinal tract of mice. *Virology* 124, 403–410.

Kido, H., Yokogoshi, Y., Sakai, K., Tashiro, M., Kishino, Y., Fukutomi, A., and Katunuma, N. (1992). Isolation and characterization of a novel trypsin-like protease found in rat bronchiolar epithelial

Clara cells. A possible activator of the viral fusion glycoprotein. *J. Biol. Chem.* 267, 13573–13579.

Krempl, C., Schultze, B., Laude, H., and Herrler, G. (1997). Point mutations in the S protein connect the sialic acid binding activity with the enteropathogenicity of transmissible gastroenteritis coronavirus. *J. Virol.* 71, 3285–3287.

Krummenacher, C., Nicola, A. V., Whitbeck, J. C., Lou, H., Hou, W., Lambris, J. D., Geraghty, R. J., Spear, P. G., Cohen, G. H., and Eisenberg, R. J. (1998). Herpes simplex virus glycoprotein D can bind to poliovirus receptor-related protein 1 or herpesvirus entry mediator, two structurally unrelated mediators of virus entry. *J. Virol.* 72, 7064–7074.

Lamb, R. A. (1993). Paramyxovirus fusion: a hypothesis for changes. *Virology* 197, 1–11.

Louria, D. B., Blumenfeld, H. L., Ellis, J. T., Kilbourne, E. D., and Rogers, D. E. (1959). Studies on influenza in the pandemic of 1957–1958. II. Pulmonary complications of influenza. *J. Clin. Invest.* 38, 213–265.

Maisner, A., Klenk, H.-D., and Herrler, G. (1998). Polarized budding of measles virus is not determined by viral surface glycoproteins. *J. Virol.* 72, 5276–5278.

Maisner, A., M.K., L., Atkinson, J. P., Schwartz-Albiez, R., and Herrler, G. (1996). Two different cytoplasmic tails direct isoforms of the membrane cofactor protein (CD46) to the basolateral surface of Madin-Darby canine kidney cells. *J. Biol. Chem.* 271, 18853–18858.

Markwell, M. A. K., Svennerholm, L., and Paulson, J. C. (1981). Specific gangliosides function as host cell receptors for Sendai virus. *Proc. Natl. Acad. Sci. USA* 78, 5406–5410.

Murphy, F. A., Harrison, A. K., and Whitfield, S. G. (1973). Bunyaviridae: Morphologic and morphogenetic similarities of Bunyamwera serologic supergroup viruses and several other arthropod-borne viruses. *Intervirology* 1, 297–316.

Murphy, J. S., and Bang, F. B. (1952). Observations with the electron microscope on cells of the chick chorion-allantoic membrane infected with influenza virus. *J. Exp. Med.* 95, 259.

Naim, H. Y., Ehler, E., and Billeter, M. A. (2000). Measles virus matrix protein specifies apical virus release and glycoprotein sorting in epithelial cells. *EMBO J.* 19, 3576–3585.

Naniche, D., Varior-Krishman, G., Cervoni, F., Wild, T. F., Rossi, B., Rabourdin-Combe, C., and Gerlier, D. (1993). Human membrane co-factor protein (CD46) acts as a cellular receptor for measles virus. *J. Virol.* 67, 6025–6032.

Owens, R. J., and Compans, R. W. (1989). Expression of the HIV envelope glycoprotein is restricted to basolateral surfaces of polarized epithelial cells. *J. Virol.* 63, 978–982.

Owens, R. J., Dubay, J., Hunter, E., and Compans, R. W. (1991). The human immunodeficiency virus envelope protein determines the site of virus release in polarized epithelial cells. *Proc. Natl. Acad. Sci.* 88, 3987–3991.

Parker, J. S., Murphy, W. J., Wang, D., O'Brien, S. J., and Parrish, C. R. (2001). Canine and feline parvoviruses can use human or feline transferrin receptors to bind, enter, and infect cells. *J. Virol.* 75, 3896–3902.

Pickles, R. J., Fahrner, J. A., Petrella, J. M., Boucher, R. C., and Bergelson, J. M. (2000). Retargeting the coxsackievirus and adenovirus receptor to the apical surface of polarized epithelial cells reveals the glycocalyx as a barrier to adenovirus-mediated gene transfer. *J. Virol.* 74, 6050–6057.

Porterfield, J. S. (1986). Antibody-dependent enhancement of viral infectivity. *Adv. Virus Res.* 31, 335–355.

Ravkov, E. V., Nichol, S. T., and Compans, R. W. (1997). Polarized entry and release in epithelial cells of Black Creek Canal virus, a New World hantavirus. *J. Virol.* 71(2), 1147–1154.

Rodriguez, D., Rodriguez, J. R., Ojakian, G. K., and Esteban, M. (1991). Vaccinia virus preferentially enters polarized epithelial cells through the basolateral surface. *J. Virol.* 65, 494–498.

Rodriguez-Boulan, E., and Sabatini, D. D. (1978). Asymmetric budding of viruses in epithelial monolayers: a model system for study of epithelial polarity. *Proc. Natl. Acad. Sci.* 75, 5071–5075.

Rogers, G. N., and Paulson, J. C. (1983). Receptor determinants of human and animal influenza virus isolates: differences in recep-

tor specificity of the H3 hemagglutinin based on species of origin. *Virology* 127, 361–373.

Rossen, J. W., Bekker, C. P., Voorhout, W. F., Strous, G. J., van der Ende, A., and Rottier, P. J. (1994). Entry and release of transmissible gastroenteritis coronavirus are restricted to apical surfaces of polarized epithelial cells. *J. Virol.* 68, 7966–7973.

Rossen, J. W., Voorhout, W. F., Horzinek, M. C., van der Ende, A., Strous, G. J., and Rottier, P. J. (1995). MHV-A59 enters polarized murine epithelial cells through the apical surface but is released basolaterally. *Virology* 210, 54–66.

Roth, M. G., Compans, R. W., Giusti, L., Davis, A. R., Nayak, D. P., Gething, M. J., and Sambrook, J. (1983). Influenza virus hemagglutinin expression is polarized in cells infected with recombinant SV40 viruses carrying cloned hemagglutinin DNA. *Cell* 33, 435–442.

Rubin, D. H. (1987). Reovirus serotype 1 binds to the basolateral membrane of intestinal epithelial cells. *Microb. Pathog.* 3, 215–219.

Rubin, D. H., Eaton, M. A., and Anderson, A. O. (1986). Reovirus infection in adult mice: the virus hemagglutinin determines the site of intestinal disease. *Microb. Pathog.* 1, 79–87.

Sabin, A. B. (1956). Pathogenesis of poliomyelitis; (reappraisal in light of new data). *Science* 123, 1151–1156.

Sanger, C., Muhlberger, E., Ryabchikova, E., Kolesnikova, L. V., Klenk, H. D., and Becker, S. (2001). Sorting of Marburg virus surface protein and virus release take place at opposite surfaces of infected polarized epithelial cells. *J. Virol.* 75, 1274–1283.

Saphire, A. C., Bobardt, M. D., and Gallay, P. A. (1999). Host cyclophilin A mediates HIV-1 attachment to target cells via heparins. *EMBO J.* 18, 6771–6785.

Schultze, B., Zimmer, G., and Herrler, G. (1996). Virus entry into a polarized epithelial cell line (MDCK): similarities and dissimilarities between influenza C virus and bovine coronavirus. *J. Gen. Virol.* 77, 2507–2514.

Schwegmann-Wessels, C., Zimmer, G., Laude, H., Enjuanes, L., and Herrler, G. (2002). Binding of transmissible gastroenteritis coronavirus to cell surface sialoglycoproteins. *J. Virol.* 76, 6037–6043.

Sharpe, A. H., and Fields, B. N. (1985). Pathogenesis of viral infections. Basic concepts derived from the reovirus model. *N. Engl. J. Med.* 312, 486–497.

Sicinski, P., Rowinski, J., Warchol, J. B., Jarzabek, Z., Gut, W., Szcygiel, B., Bielecki, K., and Koch, G. (1990). Poliovirus type 1 enters the human host through intestinal M cells. *Gastroenterology* 98, 56–58.

Sixbey, J. W., and Yao, Q. Y. (1992). Immunoglobulin A-induced shift of Epstein-Barr virus tissue tropism. *Science* 255, 1578–1580.

Small, P. A., Jr. (1990). Influenza: pathogenesis and host defense. *Hosp. Pract.* Nov. 15, 51–62.

Smith, J. F., and Pifat, D. Y. (1982). Morphogenesis of sandfly fever viruses (*Bunyaviridae* family). *Virology* 121, 61–81.

Stephens, E. B., Compans, R. W., Earl, P., and Moss, B. (1986). Surface expression of viral glycoproteins in polarized epithelial cells using vaccinia virus vectors. *EMBO J.* 5, 237–245.

Suhy, D. A., Giddings, T. H., Jr., and Kirkegaard, K. (2000). Remodeling the endoplasmic reticulum by poliovirus infection and by individual viral proteins: an autophagy-like origin for virus-induced vesicles. *J. Virol.* 74, 8953–8965.

Tashiro, M., Yamakawa, M., Tobita, K., Seto, J. T., Klenk, H.-D., and Rott, R. (1990). Altered budding site of a pantropic mutant of sendai virus, F1-R, in polarized epithelial cells. *J. Virol.* 64, 4672–4677.

Tatsuo, H., Ono, N., Tanaka, K., and Yanagi, Y. (2000). SLAM (CDw150) is a cellular receptor for measles virus. *Nature* 406, 893–897.

Tran, L. C., Kissner, J. M., Westerman, L. E., and Sears, A. E. (2000). A herpes simplex virus 1 recombinant lacking the glycoprotein G coding sequences is defective in entry through apical surfaces of polarized epithelial cells in culture and in vivo. *Proc. Natl. Acad. Sci. USA* 97, 1818–1822.

Tucker, S. P., Thornton, C. L., Wimmer, E., and Compans, R. W. (1993a). Bi-directional entry of poliovirus into polarized epithelial cells. *J. Virol.* 67(1), 29–38.

Tucker, S. P., Thornton, C. L., Wimmer, E., and Compans, R. W. (1993b). The vectorial release of the poliovirus from polarized human intestinal epithelial cells and the effect of Brefeldin A. *J. Virol.* 67, 4274–4282.

Turner, R. B., Hendley, J. O., and Gwaltney, J. M. J. (1982). Shedding of infected ciliated epithelial cells in rhinovirus cold. *J. Infect. Dis.* 145, 849–853.

Walters, R. W., Grunst, T., Bergelson, J. M., Finberg, R. W., Welsh, M. J., and Zabner, J. (1999). Basolateral localization of fiber receptors limits adenovirus infection from the apical surface of airway epithelia. *J. Biol. Chem.* 274, 10219–10226.

Ward, T., Pipkin, P. A., Clarkson, N. A., Stone, D. M., Minor, P. D., and Almond, J. W. (1994). Decay-accelerating factor CD55 is identified as the receptor for echovirus 7 using CELICS, a rapid immuno-focal cloning method. *EMBO J.* 13, 5070–5074.

Weiss, R. A., and Clapham, P. R. (1996). Hot fusion of HIV. *Nature* 381, 647–648.

White, J. M. (1992). Membrane fusion. *Science* 258, 917–924.

Wilson, I. A., Skehel, J. J., and Wiley, D. C. (1981). Structure of the hemagglutinin membrane glycoprotein of influenza virus at 3 A resolution. *Nature (London)* 289, 366–373.

Wolf, J. L., Rubin, D. H., Finberg, R., Dambrauskas, R., and Trier, J. S. (1981). Intestinal M cells: a pathway for entry of retrovirus into the host. *Science* 212, 471–472.

WuDunn, D., and Spear, P. G. (1989). Initial interaction of herpes simplex virus with cells is binding to heparan sulfate. *J. Virol.* 63, 52–58.

Yahi, N., Baghdiguian, S., Moreau, H., and Fantini, J. (1992). Galactosyl ceramide (or a closely related molecule) is the receptor for human immunodeficiency virus type 1 on human colon epithelial HT-29 cells. *J. Virol.* 66, 4848–4854.

Yoon, M., and Spear, P., G. (2002). Disruption of adherens junctions liberates nectin-1 to serve as receptor for herpes simplex virus and pseudorabies virus entry. *J. Virol.* 76, 7203–7208.

Zimmer, G., Klenk, H. D., and Herrler, G. (1995). Identification of a 40-kDa cell surface sialoglycoprotein with the characteristics of a major influenza C virus receptor in a Madin-Darby canine kidney cell line. *J. Biol. Chem.* 270, 17815–17822.

Zimmer, G., Trotz, I., and Herrler, G. (2001). N-glycans of F protein differentially affect fusion activity of human respiratory syncytial virus. *J. Virol.* 75, 4744–4751.

Mucosal Immunity to Bacteria

Jan Holmgren and Ann-Mari Svennerholm

Department of Medical Microbiology and Immunology, and Göteborg University Vaccine Research Institute, Göteborg University, Göteborg, Sweden

The mucosal surfaces of especially the oropharynx, the large intestine, and the female genital tract are colonized with various commensal bacteria, or normal microflora; there are at least 100 bacteria for each human epithelial cell in a normal human subject. These commensals normally do not cause any harm, and in some cases they may be directly beneficial for the host. In addition, the mucosal surfaces are frequently exposed to a large number of food and environmental antigens to which it could be wasteful and potentially even harmful to respond immunologically.

At the same time, it is clear that the ability to mount mucosal immune responses protecting against bacterial pathogens is of critical importance for our health. The mucosal surfaces represent a very large area, and most mammals, including humans, live in a pathogen-rich environment. In the absence of efficient nonspecific and specific immune defense mechanisms, we would rapidly succumb to bacterial pathogens. An important feature of the mucosal immune system is therefore to be able to specifically recognize and react to exposure to pathogens, while avoiding reacting with or at least not responding with inflammation against the normal flora or against ingested or inhaled harmless food or environmental antigens.

However, even in the presence of normally effective mucosal immune mechanisms, bacterial infections in the gastrointestinal, respiratory, and urogenital mucosae represent a major global health problem and are important targets for vaccine development. Thus, enteric and acute respiratory tract infections are among the leading causes of illness and death globally, especially in infants and preschool children in developing countries. Although effective mucosal vaccines have recently been developed against a few of these infections, such as cholera and rotavirus diarrhea, there remains a great need for vaccine development against many of the most important gastrointestinal, respiratory, and urogenital pathogens.

Bacteria colonizing or invading mucosal tissues may also, either directly or via their interaction with the mucosal epithelium, induce production of several potent proinflammatory and immunomodulating cytokines and chemokines, which may recruit both acute and chronic inflammatory cells to the site of infection. For example, there is substantial evidence to suggest a link between inflammatory bowel disease (IBD), bacteria, and a disturbed mucosal response, although the precise role of bacteria and their products in starting and perpetuating IBD remains to be defined. Likewise, it has also been suggested that various gram-negative bacteria contribute to the development of some chronic inflammatory diseases believed to be of autoimmune origin, such as insulin-dependent diabetes, rheumatoid arthritis, and multiple sclerosis.

This presumed association presents several challenges with regard to vaccine development against certain pathogens. For instance, it cannot be excluded that there is a risk that vaccination with bacterial antigens might induce or aggravate inflammation, *e.g.*, pelvic inflammation in response to chlamydia vaccination, IBD after *Salmonella*, *Campylobacter*, or *Yersinia* vaccination, or gastritis after *Helicobacter pylori* vaccination. On the other hand, the phenomenon of oral tolerance might be exploited to construct immunomodulating vaccines that could suppress harmful immune reactions, both in relation to infectious agents and perhaps also more broadly against chronic tissue-destroying autoimmune reactions such as rheumatoid arthritis or multiple sclerosis.

Similar to the situation for genital human papilloma virus infections and cervical cancer, it has recently become clear that there is also a direct link between a specific bacterial mucosal pathogen and gastrointestinal cancer. Thus, infection with *H. pylori* is now recognized as the leading cause of stomach cancer, and it has been estimated that the infection results in approximately half a million new cases of adenocarcinoma each year (Peek and Blaser, 2002). The fact that stomach cancer is normally preceded by chronic atrophic gastritis suggests that the mucosal immune system plays a role in the outcome of *H. pylori* infection, *i.e.*, in determining whether the infection will remain asymptomatic, which is the case in about 85% of those infected, or give rise to peptic ulcer or even stomach cancer. Thus, if effective vaccines can be developed against *H. pylori* and possibly against certain other as yet unidentified bacterial pathogens that may be associated with cancer development, these vaccines may serve also as anticancer vaccines.

In this chapter we discuss interactions between bacteria and bacterial components and the mucosal immune system. A special emphasis is given to those innate and adaptive mucosal immune responses that may be protective, immunopathogenic, or tolerogenic and thus are of special relevance for both current and future development of vaccines against mucosal bacterial infections.

COMMENSAL BACTERIA AND MUCOSAL IMMUNITY

Influence of commensal bacteria on mucosal immune responses

The normal microflora colonizes the whole intestine from the stomach to the rectum. The proximal part of the intestine harbors various *Lactobacillus* and *Streptococcus* species, and the bacterial load then increases progressively toward the distal part, the large bulk of bacteria being dominated by different anaerobes in the colon. The resident normal microflora is stable over several years and may have both beneficial and detrimental effects on the host. This has been exemplified both in experimental studies and in humans when studying the effect of the intestinal normal flora on several important intestinal functions with use of modern genetic techniques. Thus, when germ-free mice were colonized with *Bacteroides thetaiotaomicron*, a prominent component of the normal mouse and human intestinal microflora, it was found with DNA microarrays as well as laser-capture microdissection methods that this bacterium modulates the expression of host gut genes involved in such diverse functions as, *e.g.*, mucosal barrier formation, angiogenesis, and postnatal intestinal maturation (Hooper and Gordon, 2001). These findings provide novel perspectives on the essential nature and breadth of the interactions between resident microorganisms and their hosts.

An important positive effect of the commensals is that they may prevent colonization of enteric pathogens. For instance, anaerobic bifidobacteria have been reported to have protective effects against various intestinal pathogens such as enterohemorrhagic *Escherichia coli* O157:H7, *Salmonella typhimurium*, and rotavirus in experimental animals. It was suggested that the protective effect of the bacteria was dependent on their modulatory effect on the intestinal immune responses against pathogens, since oral administration of *Bifidobacterium bifidum* has been described to augment both total IgA production in the intestine and specific IgA antibody responses against enteropathogens and also to increase systemic antibody responses (Park *et al.*, 2002). Consistent with this, *B. bifidum* has been shown to nonspecifically enhance antibody synthesis by B lymphocytes *in vitro* and to increase the total number of IgA-secreting cells in cultures of mesenteric lymph nodes as well as spleen cells (Park *et al.*, 2002). On the other hand, other commensals such as *Clostridium difficile* may become enteropathogens and cause severe disease if allowed to proliferate as a result of antibiotic killing of the competing normal microflora.

Various Enterobacteriaceae, for example, *E. coli* expressing type 1 pili or *Proteus*-like (P) fimbriae that do not cause problems when part of the normal intestinal flora, are potential pathogens if they reach the urinary tract, where they can cause cystitis (type-1 pili) or pyelonephritis (P-fimbriae) (Agace and Svanborg, 1996). In immunocompromised individuals or neonates, Enterobacteriaceae can also cause septicemia and meningitis after translocation of the bacteria through a defective mucosal barrier (Van Camp *et al.*, 1994).

Although the mammalian gut must be sufficiently permeable to support efficient absorption of nutrients, it must avoid potentially damaging immune responses to dietary proteins and commensals. Innate defense mechanisms, such as epithelial production of α-defensins and mucins and the "nonspecific" binding of several types of bacteria through the sugar moieties of secretory IgA (S-IgA), help to prevent bacteria from crossing the mucosal barrier (Hooper and Gordon, 2001). The mucosal immune system also has developed an ingenious way of allowing the induction of antigen-specific IgA responses to commensal bacteria without risk of inducing concomitant inflammation. Thus, in contrast to the S-IgA responses to pathogen-derived epitopes that require costimulation by antigen-specific T cells, induction of S-IgA against antigens on commensal bacteria has been found to be largely T cell–independent in mice (Macpherson *et al.*, 2000). This presumably allows the host to respond to shifts in the commensal flora without eliciting a deleterious immune response.

There is mounting evidence that commensals acquired during the early postnatal period are required for the development of normal immunologic tolerance not only to themselves but also to other luminal antigens. For example, Sudo *et al.* (1997) reported that T helper 2 (Th2)-mediated immune responses to ovalbumin were not susceptible to oral tolerance induction in germ-free mice, but susceptibility was restored after the introduction in neonates of a single component of the preweaning microflora. The increasing prevalence of atopy in Western industrialized societies has led to the hypothesis that an overly hygienic lifestyle has altered the normal pattern of intestinal colonization during infancy and produced a lack of tolerance to otherwise harmless food proteins and inhaled antigens (Wold, 1998).

Commensal bacteria and break of normal tolerance in IBD

Since commensals are located in close proximity to the intestinal lymphoid tissue, induction of a state of immunological tolerance against these bacteria may be required to avoid the development of inflammation (Mowat and Viney, 1997), even though, as mentioned, there are also other escapes from inflammation (Macpherson *et al.*, 2000). The pathogenesis of IBD appears to involve an "inappropriate" activation of the mucosal immune system, and this activation has been linked to a loss of tolerance to gut commensals (Duchmann *et al.*, 1996). The spontaneous colitis that develops in human leukocyte antigen B27/β2-microgloblin-transgenic rats and in knockout (KO) mice that lack IL-2 or T-cell receptors is abrogated when animals are raised under germ-free conditions. What is not clear is whether the inflammatory responses in IBD, both within the gut and at extraintestinal sites, are elicited in response to a specific subset of intestinal microbes or whether tolerance to commensals is affected generally. An interesting question is whether the normal epithelial barrier function is first compromised by "intrinsic" defects in epithelial integrity, by infection with enteropathogens, or by loss of commensal-dependent signals necessary to maintain the physical integrity of the epithelium and the normal hyporesponsiveness of the mucosal immune system. Part of this question may be answered when human IBD susceptibility genes are identified. Normal tolerance is clearly antigen-specific, since human intestinal lamina propria and peripheral blood lymphocytes proliferated in response to commensal bacteria from another individual but not to the subject's own intestinal microflora (Duchmann et al., 1996). However, lamina propria lymphocytes isolated from inflamed but not uninflamed areas of the intestine of IBD patients strongly proliferated to the patient's own intestinal bacteria. Local and systemic tolerance against the intestinal bacteria was also broken in a murine model of chronic intestinal inflammation. Interestingly, tolerance to the autologous strain was restored and colitis was abrogated in mice systemically treated with IL-10 or antibodies to IL-12 (Duchmann et al., 1996). There is a breakdown of tolerance also with respect to antibody production in IBD patients. Thus, IgG is produced in high quantities locally in the intestine, and these antibodies have been shown to be directed against commensal bacteria (Macpherson et al., 1996).

At the same time, many bacterial enteropathogens, particularly those invading the mucosal lymphoid tissues such as *Shigella*, *Salmonella*, *Campylobacter*, and *Yersinia*, usually give rise to vigorous inflammation and immune responses. Still, infections with these organisms normally resolve and do not result in subsequent IBD. This indicates that the previously cited break of tolerance to commensal bacteria in IBD patients may result from rather than be a primary cause of IBD. A complex set of host factors is likely to regulate the outcome of an active immune response in the gut, as indicated by the many genetically defined KO mice that have recently been found to be associated with IBD (Elson et al., 1995). In each of these animal models of IBD, an abnormal immunological reaction with primarily pathogenic or commensal bacteria triggers disease.

Commensal bacteria as therapeutic agents

The adaptations of commensals in nutritionally advantageous host niches provide a rationale for using these organisms as therapeutic agents. Components of the normal flora are given as live biological supplements (probiotics) that confer some host benefit. For example, giving *Lactobacillus* species to IL-10-deficient mice has resulted in attenuation of their colitis (Madsen, 2001). Probiotic preparations containing *Bifidobacterium*, *Lactobacillus*, and *Streptococcus* species have been beneficial in treating chronic "pouchitis," a complication following surgical intervention for ulcerative colitis (Gionchetti et al., 2002). In addition, the administration of nonpathogenic *E. coli* has provided effective probiotic ther-

apy in a randomized double-blind trial of patients with active ulcerative colitis (Rembachen et al., 1999).

Recently genetically engineered commensals have also been used for delivering drugs, antimicrobial agents, and even vaccines to defined host niches. For example, a strain of *Lactococcus lactis* programmed to produce IL-10 provided therapeutic benefits in two mouse models of IBD (Steidler et al., 2000), and oral inoculation of lactobacilli-expressing tetanus toxin fragment C induced local and systemic immune responses to the expressed antigen (Shaw et al., 2000).

PATHOGENIC MECHANISMS IN BACTERIAL MUCOSAL INFECTIONS

Adherence and colonization

The first critical step for the bacterial pathogen in establishing an infection at or from a mucosal surface is to colonize the mucosal epithelium. Adherence is a complex process dependent on receptor–ligand interactions, which may be specific for the species, host, and tissue. All bacterial mucosal pathogens presumably possess distinct colonization factors (CFs). These are often referred to as adhesins, and they may be expressed as fimbrial or fibrillar proteins or as bacterial surface proteins (Gaastra and Svennerholm, 1996; Klemm and Schembri, 2000). The host receptors, on the other hand, often consist of complex sugar moieties present in glycolipids and/or glycoproteins on the epithelial cell surface or in mucin-type glycoproteins in the mucus layer associated with the mucosal epithelium (Karlsson, 1989; Francis et al., 1998).

Binding of fimbriated bacteria to specific receptors on the epithelial cells may induce strong epithelial cytokine and chemokine responses that in turn lead to recruitment of inflammatory cells to the site of infection, as exemplified by urinary tract infections (Agace et al., 1996). Colonization by uropathogenic P-fimbriated *E. coli* bacteria represents one of the best-examined examples of such ligand-receptor interactions important for subsequent pathogenicity. Both the tip adhesin, PapG, on the P fimbriae and the $Gal\alpha1$-$4Gal\beta$-containing glycolipid receptor, including the membrane-anchoring ceramides in the lipid bilayer, have been well characterized (Bock et al., 1985; Lund et al., 1987; Dodson et al., 2001). In several cases the bacterial adhesins have also been identified. Examples among gastrointestinal pathogens include the toxin coregulated pilus (TCP) of pathogenic (toxigenic) *Vibrio cholerae* (Taylor et al., 1987), more than 20 different colonization factors (CFs) on different types of enterotoxigenic *E. coli* (ETEC) (Gaastra and Svennerholm, 1996), and the Lewis[b] binding antigen, BabA, of *H. pylori* (Ilver et al., 1998). Among respiratory bacterial pathogens are the Hap adhesin of *Haemophilus influenzae* (Cutter et al., 2002) and the filamentous hemagglutinin of *Bordetella pertussis*. In some cases, the binding structures for these adhesins were identified, sometimes even before the bacterial adhesin could be identified. For example, the Lewis[b] blood group antigen was recognized as a likely receptor for *H. pylori* in the stomach epithelium (Borén et al., 1993).

In addition to these classic adhesin-receptor interactions, mucosal colonization may be facilitated by the interaction of mucosal cells and specific molecules on pathogens called pathogen-associated molecular patterns (PAMPs). PAMPs are recognized by so-called pattern recognition receptors (PRRs) that are found on many cells of the innate immune system, including epithelial cells, macrophages/monocytes, granulocytes, mast cells, and dendritic cells, both inside and on mucosal tissues. The family of Toll-like receptors (TLRs) plays a pivotal role in the recognition of PAMPs by the innate immune system (Rock *et al.*, 1998). TLRs are an evolutionarily conserved set of proteins found in plants, insects, and mammals. It was earlier demonstrated that TLRs control important antimicrobial responses against bacteria in the *Drosophila* fly (Lemaitre *et al.*, 1996). At least 10 mammalian TLRs have been identified and several have been implicated in cellular responses to bacterial pathogens (Underhill and Ozinsky, 2002). TLR2 binds lipopeptides, lipoproteins, lipoarabinomannan, and peptidoglycan, making it a broad recognition receptor for many different gram-positive bacteria; TLR3 binds double-stranded RNA; TLR4 binds LPS and heat shock protein 60 (HSP60), thus making it a broad recognition receptor for mainly gram-negative bacteria but also other pathogens that may express HSP60; TLR5 is activated by bacterial flagellin (Hyashi *et al.*, 2000); and TLR9 is a receptor for so-called CpG motifs in bacterial DNA (Hemmi *et al.*, 2000). The rapid induction of proinflammatory mediators in epithelial cells exposed to bacteria may be due to a large extent to the interaction of PAMPs and corresponding TLRs. Thus, it was recently shown that type 1 pili–positive *E. coli* bind to and activate bladder epithelial cells by the binding of bacterial surface lipopolysaccharide (LPS) to CD14 and TLR-4, resulting in production of IL-6 and IL-8 (Schilling *et al.*, 2003). P fimbriae on uropathogenic *E. coli* also depend on TLR-4 for activation (Svanborg *et al.*, 2001). Thus, P fimbriae use the glycosphingolipids Galα1-4 Galβ as the primary receptor for binding to epithelial cells and then recruit TLR-4 as a co-receptor for LPS-mediated signal transduction and cell activation. On the other hand, it was recently shown that the epithelium in the stomach mucosa (Bäckhed *et al.*, 2003) as well as the human cervicovaginal epithelium (Fichorova *et al.*, 2002) do not express TLR-4 and thus could not respond to protein-free preparations of *H. pylori* and *N. gonorrhoeae*, respectively.

Triggering of disease

Several mechanisms have been described by which bacterial mucosal pathogens can cause disease. These can be classified primarily as production of exotoxins, induction of inflammation, and/or tissue-destroying invasion. Disease is commonly caused or at least influenced by a combination of two or more of these factors. Bacterial gastrointestinal infections illustrate each of these disease mechanisms.

Enterotoxins

In the group of diarrheal diseases known as enterotoxin-induced, the so-called enterotoxic enteropathies, the coloniz-ing bacteria do not invade the intestinal epithelium but produce one or more protein enterotoxins. After binding to specific receptors, these toxins produce diarrhea, leading sometimes to life-threatening dehydration. Cholera, the feared diarrheal disease caused by *V. cholerae* of the O1 serogroup and, since 1992, also by the O139 serogroup, is the prototype for this type of pathogenic mechanism, while diarrhea caused by ETEC is the most frequent toxin-mediated illness (Holmgren and Svennerholm, 1992). Both cholera toxin (CT) and the closely related heat-labile enterotoxin (LT) of ETEC bacteria consist of two different types of subunits responsible, respectively, for cell-binding (B subunit) and toxic activities (A subunit) (Holmgren, 1981). After binding to specific cell surface receptors through the B subunits, the toxins are internalized and their toxic-active A subunit is released to mediate its cellular action. In the case of CT and LT, the A subunit, through an enzymatic reaction, adenosine diphosphate (ADP)–ribosylates adenylate cyclase in a manner leading to increased production of cyclic adenosine monophosphate (cAMP). This results in a dramatic net secretion of electrolytes and water, causing the profuse diarrhea and fluid loss characteristic of cholera and other enterotoxic enteropathies. Indeed, the specific binding of the CTB to the GM1 ganglioside receptor on intestinal and other cells was not only the first-ever-described chemically defined biologic ligand–receptor interaction but also remains the best studied and the most extensively practically exploited such specific binding system. Although these events may occur without any structural damage to the intestinal epithelium or macroscopic signs of inflammation, it has recently been shown in biopsies of intestinal specimens from patients infected with *V. cholerae* O1 that the mucosa is mildly to moderately inflamed, with an influx of inflammatory cells that might contribute to the diarrheal process (Qadri *et al.*, 2002). In addition to *V. cholerae* and ETEC, a number of other gram-negative bacteria have also been found to produce enterotoxins or cytotoxins, for example, *Vibrio parahaemolyticus*, enterohemorrhagic *E. coli* (EHEC), *Salmonella*, *Campylobacter*, and *Shigella*. However, as discussed in the next section, invasiveness and inflammation are more prominent pathogenic mechanisms of the latter bacteria than of their enterotoxin production (Holmgren and Svennerholm, 1992, Willshaw *et al.*, 1997).

Invasion and inflammation

The other main pathogenic mechanism involves invasion of the pathogen into or across the intestinal epithelium, resulting in inflammation. Invasive microorganisms such as *Shigella* and enteroinvasive *E. coli* directly damage the intestinal epithelium, with ulceration and microscopic blood loss (Phalipon and Sansonetti, 1999). These bacteria appear to lack specific attachment or colonization factors for the intestinal epithelium but can easily be taken up by M cells of Peyer's patches. This uptake is important for the host to initiate a protective immune response, but it also allows the pathogens to have several days to enter the enterocytes from the basolateral side, multiply intracellularly, cause intense inflammation, and spread from cell to cell laterally with tissue destruction, bleeding, and often death as the result before a protective immune response has developed. Non-*typhi Salmonella*, *Campylobacter jejuni*, and *Yersinia enterocolitica*, on the other hand, which are also capable of invading the intestinal mucosa, usually do not cause much direct damage to the epithelium, but instead they evoke severe inflammatory responses in the lamina propria and Peyer's patches. The invasive property of all these microorganisms is determined by large plasmids, which encode a set of incompletely defined proteins that mediate cell attachment and uptake; however, in addition there may be an important contribution by soluble protein toxins in the disease process evoked by these invasive organisms (Kopecko *et al.*, 1989; Phalipon and Sansonetti, 1999).

Epithelial cells appear to have important roles in regulating inflammation in response to bacterial antigens. This is largely explained by the fact that many mucosal epithelial cells express TLRs that can recognize and respond to different PAMPs on mucosal pathogens. There appear, however, to be significant differences in the way epithelial cells from the nonsterile intestine and from normally sterile environments, such as the urinary bladder, respond to adhesion at the apical surface. As discussed above, the intestine contains commensals that can adhere to the epithelial cells without signaling any danger to the cell, and intestinal epithelial cells seem to be tolerant to the presence of microbes and LPS at their apical surfaces (Kagnoff and Eckman, 1997). In "sterile" sites, epithelial cells are able to respond to adhesion and the presence of LPS because of the presence of TLRs, CD14, and other PRRs; for instance, the adherence of *E. coli* to uroepithelial cells efficiently triggers the secretion of chemokines by the epithelial cells (Godaly *et al.*, 1998). However, once in contact with the basolateral side of the intestinal epithelial cells, a number of enteroinvasive bacteria, *e.g.*, salmonellae, have been found to stimulate production of proinflammatory cytokines and chemokines (Kagnoff and Eckman, 1997; Eckman and Kagnoff, 2001), including several members of the CXC family of chemokines, such as IL-8, GROα, and ENA-78, that may attract and activate polymorphonuclear leukocytes (PMNs). A mucosal influx of PMNs is a hallmark of the initial inflammatory response that results after infection of the intestinal tract with pathogenic bacteria (Kagnoff and Eckman, 1997). The activated epithelial cells may also secrete a range of C-C chemokines, such as macrophage chemoattractant protein (MCP)-1, major intrinsic protein (MIP)-1β, and RANTES (regulated upon activation, normal T cell expressed and secreted), which can act as chemoattractants of monocytes and eosinophils, and IP-H-10 (CXCL10) and I-TAC (CXCL11), which can attract subpopulations of T cells. All of these recruited cell types are important components of inflammatory responses after infection with enteric bacterial pathogens and play a role in both innate and acquired host defense against *Salmonellae*. Thus, the epithelial chemokine responses can provide a mechanistic explanation for the trafficking of different leukocyte subsets to the subepithelial regions after salmonella infection (Eckman and

Kagnoff, 2001). In addition to the release of chemokines, bacteria-activated intestinal epithelium may also release other cytokines that can activate phagocytic cells, *e.g.*, granulocyte- (G-) and granulocyte-macrophage-(GM-) colony stimulating factor (CSF), and induce the production of other proin-flammatory factors such as IL-1β, IL-6, and tumor necrosis factor (TNF)α from these cells. Infection with enteroinvasive bacteria may also regulate epithelial cell responses to cytokine and chemokine stimulation by upregulating cytokine and chemokine receptors (Dwinell *et al.*, 1999).

Salmonella infection is also associated with rapid upregulation of interferon (IFN)γ expression in the intestinal mucosa, Peyer's patches, and mesenteric lymph nodes. In an experimental mouse model it was shown that neutralization of IFN-γ with specific antibodies increased bacterial numbers and decreased survival in the host (Bao *et al.*, 2000). Similarly, specifically gene-targeted IFN-γ KO mice have readily succumbed to salmonella infection. These findings suggest that IFN-γ plays a central role in controlling salmonella infection, most likely by activating the ability of macrophages to kill salmonellae (Eckman and Kagnoff, 2001). The cells that produce IFN-γ, *i.e.*, T cells and natural killer (NK) cells, have little direct contact with the salmonellae during the course of infection but may be stimulated through communication with other cells that have such contact, *e.g.*, macrophages that produce IL-12 and IL-18, which have strong IFN-γ-inducing properties. It has also been shown that neutralization of these two cytokines results in increased bacterial load and decreased host survival in *Salmonella*-infected mice (Dybing *et al.*, 1999).

H. pylori *infection and disease*

The infection caused by *H. pylori* appears to present an exceptionally complex set of interactions between pathogen and host mucosa. The host mucosa characteristically either produces a sufficiently strong proinflammatory innate and adaptive immune response to control the extent of bacterial multiplication, albeit at the risk of inducing both acute and chronic mucosal inflammation (gastritis), or it downregulates the inflammatory response at the cost of more extensive bacterial colonization and risk of necrotizing tissue damage (duodenal ulcer). When *H. pylori* bacteria bind to gastric epithelial cells, they induce cytokine and chemokine production, in particular IL-8. This chemokine, together with several proinflammatory cytokines, *e.g.*, IL-1β, IL-6, and TNFα, is found in significantly higher levels in the gastric epithelium of the *H. pylori*–infected versus -noninfected gastric mucosa (Crabtree *et al.*, 1994; Lindholm *et al.*, 1998). In particular, *H. pylori* strains that express the virulence-associated factor CagA have been shown to induce more IL-8 than strains lacking CagA, indicating an important role of this factor in the induction of gastric inflammation (Crabtree *et al.*, 1994). *H. pylori*, as well as several other mucosal bacterial pathogens, has also been shown to upregulate the expression of MHC class II as well as the costimulatory molecules B7-1 and B7-2 on gastric epithelial cells (Archimandritis *et al.*, 2000; Lundin *et al.*, 2003), suggesting that the epithelial cells may also function as antigen-presenting cells (APCs) in the *H. pylori*–infected mucosa.

Epithelial production or expression of different cytokines and chemokines may be important for the outcome of *H. pylori* infection. Although the staining for several cytokines and chemokines (Lindholm *et al.*, 1998) as well as the bacterial density of mucosal biopsy specimens from the stomachs of patients with duodenal ulcers (DUs) and asymptomatic carriers are comparable, there are marked differences between these groups in the duodenal mucosa, which is the site of most *H. pylori*–induced ulcers. On average, 20-fold higher numbers of *H. pylori* are found in the duodenum of DU patients than in asymptomatic carriers (Hamlet *et al.*, 1999). This is associated with—and we believe also partly explained by—significantly decreased expression of IL-1β, IL-6, and IL-8 and also decreased staining for IFN-γ; the latter apparently is due to the higher production of the IFN-γR by duodenal epithelial cells in DU patients than in noninfected subjects or asymptomatic carriers (Strömberg *et al.*, 2003). Since *H. pylori* causes a chronic infection with constant influx of PMNs, these cytokines and chemokines may play an important role in the inflammatory and protective immune response during infection.

The decreased production of IL-8 in the duodenal epithelium of DU patients might result in impaired neutrophil transmigration across the epithelium. This may in turn result in neutrophil entrapment within the lamina propria of the duodenal mucosa and, subsequently, accumulation of harmful reactive metabolites and enzymes that may destroy the mucosa rather than eliminate the bacteria from the epithelial surface. The resulting high bacterial load on the epithelial surface in the duodenum of DU patients may result in increased production of bacterial toxins and enzymes that may cause further tissue destruction. The epithelial expression of the anti-inflammatory cytokine TGFβ has also been shown to be lower in the duodenal mucosa of DU patients than in asymptomatic or noninfected subjects (Strömberg *et al.*, 2003). This circumstance and the observed increased number of regulatory T cells (Treg) that may suppress T-cell responses in the mucosa of DU patients in comparison with asymptomatic carriers could be important factors in the deficient control of infection in DU patients (Lundgren *et al.*, 2003; Lundgren *et al.*, 2004). Considering the importance of TGFβ in ulcer healing, decreased expression of this cytokine might impair the wound healing process in the damaged duodenal mucosa of DU patients.

Other examples

As mentioned above, and different from the intestinal epithelium, the urinary tract mucosa can respond directly to apical surface contact by pathogens with cytokine production. In urinary tract infections it has been observed that binding of noninvasive type 1 fimbriated *E. coli* to bladder epithelium and uropathogenic *E. coli* to renal epithelial cells resulted in rapid production of several inflammatory mediators such as IL-6 and IL-8 (Svanborg *et al.*, 1999; Schilling *et al.*, 2003). This stimulation of proinflammatory cytokines and chemo-

kines induces migration of neutrophils through the urinary tract epithelial barrier into the lumen, where they may phagocytose and kill the colonizing bacteria (Svanborg *et al.*, 1999). It has been speculated that recurrent urinary tract infections may be due to a defect in the receptor for IL-8, and recently, lesser expression of CXC receptors on neutrophils was observed in children with recurrent infections or acute pyelonephritis than on neutrophils of age-matched controls without urinary tract infections (Frendéus *et al.*, 2000).

Another class of mucosal bacterial pathogens appears to adhere only to the intestinal microvillus membrane, which becomes locally disrupted, but otherwise there is no gross structural damage to the epithelium. Examples include enteropathogenic *E. coli* (EPEC) and *Cryptosporidium* (Donnenberg *et al.*, 1997). These organisms, however, may also produce cytotoxins or enterotoxins that contribute to epithelial damage.

In a few important respiratory tract infections caused by bacteria, the production of exotoxin can explain most or all of the disease manifestations. Diphtheria and whooping cough are typical examples of such diseases (Rappouli, 1997). However, in most bacterial respiratory infections, disease is due to a combination of severe inflammation and tissue destruction following invasion of the bacterial pathogen into or across the lining epithelium. Pneumococci, meningococci, and *H. influenzae* cause infections in which severe local inflammation and tissue destruction may be accompanied by bacteremic spread of organisms, a process promoted by the fact that these bacteria have polysaccharide capsules that prevent phagocytosis.

In some mucosal infections, *e.g.*, genital infections caused by *C. trachomatis*, the infection itself usually results in only mild symptoms. However, severe disease may occur as a result of inflammation owing to delayed-type-hypersensitivity (Stephens, 1992). In women in whom chlamydia infection reaches the Fallopian tubes, the inflammation may lead to tissue scarring and permanent occlusion of the tubes, resulting in sterility.

IMMUNE MECHANISMS

Nonimmunological defense mechanisms

The mucosal surfaces are protected by a complex set of both nonspecific and specific immune mechanisms that function in conjunction with other nonimmunological chemical and mechanical mechanisms to protect the host. Important roles of these factors are to prevent excessive growth of bacterial pathogens on the mucosal surfaces, block the entry of pathogens across the mucosa, and avoid tissue-damaging inflammation.

A number of mechanical cleansing mechanisms are important in preventing infection of mucosal surfaces. One such example is the combined effect of respiratory mucus entrapment with retrograde movement of microorganisms by the ciliated respiratory epithelium and the cough reflex to protect the deeper respiratory tissues against inhaled microorganisms, including bacteria. Examples in the small intestine are peristaltic movement, mucus discharge from goblet cells, and even diarrheal fluid production that can counteract the colonization and growth of organisms. An example in the urinary tract is urine flow, which normally keeps the mucosa sterile. Major disturbances in any of these functions increase the susceptibility to bacterial infection.

Likewise, a number of chemical factors contribute to non-specific mucosal defense, such as lysozyme in tear fluid and nasal secretions, which is capable of attacking gram-positive bacteria, and acid produced by the gastric mucosa, which can kill a large variety of swallowed bacteria. *H. pylori* can colonize the gastric mucosa by inhibiting mucus secretion by goblet cells (Sidebotham *et al.*, 1991) and by producing urease capable of raising the pH around the bacteria during passage through the stomach, before the bacteria reach the epithelial surface where pH is neutral. In the intestine, lactoferrin and lactoperoxidase remove iron or act in concert with immune factors such as IgA to limit the growth of pathogens. Likewise, antibiotic peptides and the presence of a normal flora producing colicins and other factors limit the establishment and overgrowth of pathogens (Selsted *et al.*, 1992; Bals, 2000).

The best characterized antibiotic peptides produced by epithelial cells are the so-called human α-defensins 5 and 6 (HD-5 and HD-6) produced by Paneth cells in the small intestine and by epithelial cells of the female urogenital tract; α-defensin 1 (HD-1), expressed constitutively in urinary and respiratory epithelial cells; and α-defensin 2 (HD-2), the expression of which is induced in a broad range of epithelial cells by infectious and inflammatory stimuli. Defensins and other antimicrobial peptides have a broad spectrum of activity against gram-positive and gram-negative bacteria, fungi, and enveloped viruses. Defensins can bind to LPS and inactivate its biological activity. In addition to their antimicrobial activity, antimicrobial peptides can partake in the regulation of both innate and adaptive immune responses (Basset *et al.*, 2003).

Pathogens have evolved mechanisms to avoid the antimicrobial effects of defensins and other peptides, and three mechanisms have been defined: modification of LPS and other bacterial cellular components (Starner *et al.*, 2002); activation of an efflux pump (Bengoechea and Skurnik, 2000); and release of dermatan sulfate, a molecule that inhibits defensins by the action of extracellular proteinases of several common pathogenic bacteria (Schmidtchen *et al.*, 2001).

The innate immune system

In addition to the important barrier function combined with the mechanical cleansing mechanisms and different chemical antimicrobial factors provided by the lining epithelium of different mucosal tissues, the mucosa also contains a number of other essential cells of the innate immune system: phagocytic neutrophils and macrophages, dendritic cells (DCs), NK cells, and mast cells. As excellently reviewed by Basset *et al.* (2003), these cell types provide important contributions to the immune defense against pathogens. Phagocytic cells are essential effector cells of innate immunity by eliminating pathogenic invaders before they can spread and, in the case of

resident macrophages, by initiating adaptive immune responses through antigen presentation to T cells. An even more important link between the innate and adaptive immune systems is provided by the DCs, which are widely distributed in the body in both lymphoid and nonlymphoid tissues, including the mucosal tissues. DCs have on their surface different TLRs and can therefore recognize and respond to PAMPs, and they have the ability to stimulate immune responses from both naïve and memory T-cells. During the initial phases of host–pathogen interaction, DCs are recruited to the local areas along with NK cells. The latter cells contain two sets of potent killing mechanisms for target cells: first, the molecules perforin and granzyme are released during cell-to-cell contact and can kill virus-infected or tumor cells, and second, the cells have the ability to kill via the fas/fasL apoptotic pathway. Unlike cytotoxic T cells, NK cells do not recognize specific antigens but instead have killer Ig-like receptors (KIRs) that recognize class I MHC molecules, with different NK cells recognizing different human leukocyte antigens (HLAs). If engaged by the HLA proteins, the KIRs signal to inhibit the release of perforins, which means that cells lacking HLA proteins, such as tumor and virus-infected cells, cannot signal via the KIR and thus the NK cell releases its killing agents. NKT cells, an intermediate cell-type, are mainly CD4+ cells but possess some cell surface receptors normally found on NK cells. They have a restricted T-cell receptor repertoire that recognizes glycolipid antigens presented by CD1d molecules on APCs and can secrete both IFN-γ and IL-4, thereby augmenting either or both cell-mediated and antibody-mediated responses (Basset *et al.*, 2003). Finally, mast cells reside in the mucosal connective tissues of the respiratory and gastrointestinal tracts. In addition to the classic activation of mast cells by allergens and other antigens binding to IgE bound to Fcε receptors on the cell surface, mast cells also express TLR1, TLR2, and TLR6 and thereby can recognize and react with *e.g.*, a variety of gram-positive bacteria and mycoplasma-associated antigens.

As evident from the above, the recognition of different PAMPs by TLRs is a key event in activating the innate immune response in many mucosal bacterial infections. On engagement of these receptors, a series of intracellular signaling events occurs. Usually the signaling takes place through the association of the cytoplasmic tail of the ligand-engaged TLR with an adaptor molecule called MyD88, followed by a cascade of signals which ultimately leads to the activation of NFκB, which in turn can bind to specific DNA regions in the nucleus and upregulate a number of proinflammatory genes involved in host defense (Kopp and Medzhitov, 2003). Other enzymes that are part of the innate response are cyclo-oxygenase-2 (COX-2) and inducible nitric oxide synthetase (iNOS), which contribute to defense against invading pathogens (Kim *et al.*, 2003; Ejima *et al.*, 2003; Tanigawa *et al.*, 2003). An important aspect of the innate response is also the augmentation of the acquired immune response by the combined effects of processing and presentation of microbial antigens and the upregulation of costimulatory molecules on APCs. The stimulation of maturation of APCs provides the key link between the innate and acquired immune system, the former instructing the latter to respond to the pathogens and potentially also directing the type of response, depending on the initial type of PAMP-TLR interaction.

Not surprisingly, microbes can affect these signaling pathways in many ways in order to avoid the host's immune attack (see Basset *et al.*, 2003). In some cases, NFκB is activated by pathogens such as *Shigella*, inducing a proinflammatory response, which is believed to assist in dissemination of the organism. In the case of intracellular pathogens such as *Chlamydia*, the activation of NFκB prevents apoptosis of the infected cell and thus allows the bacterium to replicate. However, commonly, activation of NFκB is inhibited. For instance, *Yersinia* bacteria inject proteins into the host cell cytoplasm by a type III secretion system that inhibits NFκB activation, and similar effects on NFκB can also be induced by *E. coli* and *Salmonella* bacteria (Neish *et al.*, 2000).

Secretory IgA (S-IgA) and other antibodies

The adaptive humoral response on mucosal surfaces is to a significant extent mediated by S-IgA, which is the major Ig isotype in mucosal secretions. The resistance of S-IgA to normal intestinal proteases makes antibodies of this isotype uniquely well suited for host defense at mucosal surfaces, particularly in the gastrointestinal tract **(Table 42.1)**. Furthermore, the secretory component ensures the appropriate tissue colonization of S-IgA by anchoring the antibodies to the mucus lining of the epithelial surfaces (Phalipon *et al.*, 2002). This influences the localization of S-IgA, and the secretory component is thus directly involved in S-IgA function *in vivo*. Mucosal defense against pathogens requires that the microorganisms are hindered from colonizing the mucosal lumen, *e.g.*, by specific S-IgA antibodies that prevent the attachment to and possible invasion of mucosal epithelium. S-IgA antibodies might even exert positive influences on the inductive phases of mucosal immunity by facilitating antigen uptake by Peyer's patches (Weltzin *et al.*, 1989). An IgA-mediated excretory pathway has also been shown to occur *in vivo* to eliminate antigens present in tissues via binding to IgA and subsequent polymeric Ig receptor (pIgR)–mediated transport of the resulting immune complexes through the epithelial cells (Robinson *et al.*, 2001). As IgA acts mainly by blocking the binding of microorganisms to the epithelium, it does not elicit an inflammatory response since it has little, if any, capacity to activate complement or inflammatory cells (Kraehenbuhl and Neutra, 2000). Indeed, by preventing the uptake and competing for contact of antigens with other immunoglobulins, IgA can be regarded as an antiphlogistic component of the mucosal immune system (see Table 42.1).

In noninvasive enteric infections, such as those caused by *V. cholerae* and ETEC, S-IgA appears to be the main—although perhaps not the only—protective molecule (Holmgren and Svennerholm, 1992). In both of these infections, protective IgA antibodies have been demonstrated to be directed against the bacteria and their specific adhesins as

Table 42.1. Properties of S-IgA and Functions in Mucosal Immune Defense

> Excessive production: >50 mg per kg body weight per 24 hours
> Specific transport into mucosal secretions
> Resistant to host proteases
> Inhibits:
>   Bacterial adhesion
>   Macromolecule absorption
>   Inflammatory effects of other immunoglobulins
> Neutralizes bacterial toxins (and viruses)
> Enhances nonspecific defense mechanisms:
>   Lactoperoxidase
>   Lactoferrin
> Eliminates antigens in tissue via binding to IgA and subsequent poly Ig receptor–mediated transport of immune complexes through epithelial cells

well as against the diarrhea-inducing enterotoxins. Indeed, when present together in the intestine, these types of antibody specificities have been shown to have a synergistic rather than simply additive protective effect. This is the basis for the development of an effective, widely licensed oral vaccine against cholera (Dukoral; SBL Vaccines, Sweden) containing inactivated whole bacterial cells together with cholera toxin B subunit (CTB) (Holmgren and Bergquist, 2004). It is also the basis for the development of oral ETEC vaccines comprising a combination of colonizing factors either expressed on whole inactivated bacteria or as purified proteins; these components are given together with heat-labile toxin B subunit (LTB) or, as has been practically used to date, the closely related, cross-reactive, and large-scale recombinantly produced CTB (Holmgren and Svennerholm, 1998).

The relative significance of IgA antibodies in protection against invasive enteric bacterial infections, such as those caused by *Shigella*, *Salmonella*, and *Campylobacter*, is less well defined. The same holds true for the role of IgA in respiratory and urogenital bacterial infections. In all of these infections there appears to be a potential complementary or alternative role for both cell-mediated immune mechanisms and antibodies of other isotypes, particularly IgG, which may be of either local or systemic (transudation) origin. In invasive enteric infections, the bacteria may be directly accessible for systemic antibodies once they have been taken up through M cells and reached the deeper mucosal tissues. This may explain the significant protection against shigella and salmonella infections obtained by injectable vaccines stimulating mainly IgG and IgM LPS serum antibodies (Robbins *et al.*, 1997, Cohen *et al.*, 1997).

In experimental systems, S-IgA has also been observed to induce phagocytic cell responses by engaging CD89 expressed on myeloid cells (Van Egmond *et al.*, 2001) and to interfere with the utilization of necessary growth factors for bacterial pathogens in the intestinal environment, such as iron.

In genital infections, both the mucosal and systemic immune responses against different bacterial pathogens, such as those causing uncomplicated gonorrhea, chlamydia urethritis, or chancroid (*Hemophilus ducreyi*), are usually weak, whether they are measured as IgA or IgG antibodies in genital secretions or as cellular immune response cytokines (Russell and Mestecky, 2002). This has been suggested to at least in part reflect the limited ability of the female genital tract to respond to foreign antigens. Both the female and male genital tracts lack organized lymphoid follicles and thus inductive sites capable of disseminating antigen-specific B cells and T cells to remote sites of the mucosal immune system. Furthermore, the female genital tract appears to have limited capacity to generate local mucosal immune responses, although there are certain sites where IgA plasma cells are located near pIgR-expressing epithelium and IgA is transported into the epithelium. As compared with most other mucosal secretions, the proportion of polymeric IgA versus monomeric IgA is considerably lower, with only about 70% S-IgA in cervical secretions and approximately equal proportions of polymeric and monomeric IgA in vaginal secretions. With regard to Ig-producing cells, IgA- and IgG-secreting cells are dominant in the uterine mucosa.

Secretion of S-IgA takes place at certain sites in the genital tract, e.g., in females primarily in the cervix and to a lesser extent in the uterus. The uterine expression of S-IgA is under control of hormones; e.g., estradiol results in elevation, and progesterone partially suppresses the expression (Wira *et al.*, 1999). The mechanism by which IgG, normally the major isotype both in male and female genital secretions, reaches the lumen is unclear. Some IgG seems to originate from serum through transudation, but a significant portion originates from plasma cells in genital mucosa (Russell and Mestecky, 2002).

In the respiratory mucosa, which, similar to the genital mucosa, is substantially more permeable and less protease-rich than the intestinal mucosa, transudated serum-derived IgG can also contribute significantly to the specific antibody levels on the mucosal surface. In humans, the surfaces of the lower respiratory tract seem to be considerably more permissive for transudation of serum IgG than the nasal mucosa. The mucosa of the upper respiratory tract contain similar proportions of IgA- and IgG-producing cells, and specific IgG of local origin can be found together with S-IgA in nasal secretions after intranasal vaccination (Rudin *et al.* 1998).

T-cell immunity

Although as discussed earlier the innate immune system is the primary line of defense against invasive bacteria, the acquired immune system is usually needed for clearing infection as well as for providing effective protection against subsequent infection with homologous or related strains (Hughes and Galan, 2002).

For protection against mucosal invasive infections such as those caused by *Salmonella*, cell-mediated immune responses seem to play the major role in clearing an already established infection, whereas mucosal and/or systemic antibodies would be most important for preventing infection.

Adaptive cellular anti-infectious immune responses are mediated by either or both of CD8+ cytotoxic T cells (CTLs) and CD4+ CD25− T-helper (Th) cells. The Th cells can be divided into two major subsets based on the cytokines they secrete, *i.e.*, Th1 cells that secrete IFNγ, TNFα, and IL-2 and that activate cellular immunity and inflammation, and Th2 cells that produce IL-4, IL-5, and IL-13 and induce B cell activation and differentiation. In most cases CD4+ T cells and more specifically Th1 cells have been shown to be more important than CD8+ T cells for protection against salmonellae (Hess *et al.*, 1996; Mastroeni *et al.*, 1998). However, it is not known when T cells first encounter APCs presenting *Salmonella* antigens together with MHC antigens, but DCs in Peyer's patches and other lymphoid follicles in the intestine are the most likely candidates for antigen sampling (Yrlid *et al.*, 2001).

In *H. pylori* infections, cell-mediated immune responses also seem to be of prime importance for protection (for an overview, see Svennerholm, 2002). *H. pylori* induces both CD4+ and CD8+ T-cell responses systemically as well as locally in the mucosa. Recently, activation of CD4+ rather than CD8+ T cells was observed after infection with *H. pylori* (Lundgren *et al.*, 2003). However, CD8+ T cells produce high levels of IFN-γ after stimulation with *H. pylori* antigens (Quiding-Järbrink *et al.*, 2001), and large numbers of CD8+ T cells are present in the gastric mucosa, suggesting that CTLs contribute to the T-cell response against *H. pylori*.

The local cytokine milieu in *H. pylori*–infected mucosa, largely due to macrophages producing IL-12, will preferentially activate a Th1 response. Thus, increased production of IFN-γ but little or no increase in IL-4 or IL-5 have been found in the *H. pylori*–infected mucosa of asymptomatic carriers as well as duodenal ulcer patients (Bamford *et al.*, 1998, Lindholm *et al.*, 1998).

IFN-γ–producing T cells and NK cells in the gut mucosa might be especially important in intestinal immune defense. These cells are present in large numbers in the human duodenal mucosa and may undergo significant expansion after intestinal antigenic exposure (Quiding *et al.*, 1991). IFN-γ enhances IgA production, increases MHC antigen expression, and probably allows antigen presentation by different mucosal cells, including enterocytes. It also increases the expression of pIgR on the enterocyte surface, which facilitates S-IgA transport. Furthermore, IFN-γ has been found to interfere with tight junction permeability between intestinal epithelial cells as well as with active electrolyte secretion by enterocytes *in vitro* (Madara *et al.*, 1989; Holmgren *et al.*, 1989). In addition, IFN-γ may interfere with the receptivity of epithelial cells for invasive enteric pathogens such as *Shigella* (Hess *et al.*, 1990), and IFN-γ also stimulates infected epithelial cells as well as macrophages to produce nitric oxide, which is strongly bactericidal (Nussler and Billiar, 1993).

Recent findings have also shed new light on the role of cell-mediated immunity (CMI) in genital infections, such as those caused by *C. trachomatis* (Morrison and Caldwell, 2002). It was previously known that disease manifestations associated with chronic inflammation are largely, if not exclusively, mediated by CMI reactions associated with delayed-type hypersensitivity (DTH), while it was assumed that protection is mediated mainly by antibodies directed against major outer membrane protein (MOMP) antigens. A protective role of mucosal antibodies, especially locally produced IgA, in preventing initial infection or recurrence of infection is likely, since B-cell-deficient KO mice had a higher incidence of reinfection than control mice (Su *et al.*, 1997). However, in mice the clearance of an already established infection is due mainly, if not exclusively, to CMI. Results of adoptive transfer experiments and monoclonal antibody–mediated *in vivo* cell depletions have identified a protective role for CD4⁺ T cells in resolution of chlamydia genital infection (Su and Caldwell, 1995). Cain and Rank (1995) demonstrated that local Th1-like responses are induced in mice by intravaginal infection with *C. trachomatis*, and recent work by several groups has provided direct support for the notion that, at least in mouse models of female genital tract infection, mucosal immunity to *C. trachomatis* is mediated predominantly by Th1-type cells (Yang *et al.*, 1996; Perry *et al.*, 1997; Johansson *et al.*, 1997). Clearance of *C. trachomatis* from the genital mucosa appears to be mediated by an IL-12-dependent, IFN-γ-independent mechanism, while in contrast, the prevention of disseminated disease requires IFN-γ (Perry *et al.*, 1997). The nature of Th1 control over mucosal infections remains to be defined but could involve T-cell mediated cytotoxicity induction of Fas-mediated apoptosis (Yagita *et al.*, 1995) as well as IFN-γ-induced activation of macrophages via the IFN-γ-iNOS pathway (Igietseme, 1996). A potential contribution of CD8⁺ cytotoxic T cells has also been proposed on the basis of both *in vitro* cytotoxicity studies (Stambach, 1995) and *in vivo* protection obtained with specific T-cell clones (Igietseme *et al.*, 1994). However, recent work with gene KO mice has failed to support a role for class I MHC–restricted cytotoxicity in protection against *C. trachomatis* (Morrison *et al.*, 1995). This might suggest that the observed protective function of CD8⁺ T cells may be as a source of cytokines to drive protective CD4⁺ Th1 cells rather than by a direct cytotoxic function. Likewise, within the limitations of the mouse model, data have so far failed to support a significant contribution of Th2 cells, γδT cells, or serum antibodies in immune-mediated clearance of *C. trachomatis* (Perry *et al.*, 1997).

There is also evidence of an important role for Th1 immune responses in bacterial clearance of *B. pertussis* in a murine respiratory infection model (Mills *et al.*, 1993). Nude mice, which are deficient in T cells, developed a persistent infection and could not clear the bacteria after aerosol challenge, in contrast to normal adult mice. Adoptive transfer of immune spleen cells into nude or sublethally irradiated normal mice before challenge restored the ability to clear the infection. Furthermore, transfer of enriched T cells or purified CD4⁺ T cells but not CD8⁺ T cells from immune mice conferred a high level of protection. Recently, respiratory infection of B-cell-deficient mice resulted in persistent infection and failure to clear the bacteria after aerosol inocula-

tion, indicating that both CD4⁺ T cells and B cells are required for complete elimination of *B. pertussis* from the lungs (Mahon *et al.*, 1997).

Regulatory T cells

Several types of differentiated CD4⁺ T-cell populations have been described that inhibit the activation of other T cells. Tr1 cells can be generated by repetitive stimulation of naive CD4⁺ T cells *in vitro* in the presence of exogenous IL-10. Following antigen stimulation, these cells produce high levels of IL-10 and are able to inhibit both Th1 and Th2 responses *in vivo* (Groux *et al.*, 1997). Th3 is another population of T cells that exhibits regulatory activity. These cells are induced following oral or nasal administration of antigen and secrete predominantly TGFβ, a potent immunosuppressive cytokine, but also a switch factor for IgA production (Inobe *et al.*, 1998). A third, naturally occurring type of regulatory T cell is CD4⁺CD25 T cells that constitutively express IL-2R and intracellular CTLA-4 (Suri-Payer *et al.*, 1998). While all of these regulatory T cells have been extensively studied in relation to their ability to inhibit immunopathology in a number of animal models of autoimmune disease and colitis, only recently has a picture begun to emerge of an important anti-inflammatory function of regulatory T cells (Tregs) in infections. Investigators recently described a role for CD4⁺ CD25⁺ Tregs in immune responses to pathogens in mouse models of infection with *Leishmania major* and *Pneumocystis carinii* (Hori *et al.*, 2002; Aseffa *et al.*, 2002). Depletion of CD4⁺ CD25⁺ Treg resulted in a reduced infection load but at the cost of more severe pathology. Furthermore, McGuirch *et al.* (2002; Ref 125 Sukanya) have shown that persistent infection with *B. pertussis* results in the generation of Tr1 clones in the lungs of mice specific for filamentous hemagglutinin and pertactin. These Tr1 clones produced high levels of IL-10 and suppressed Th1 responses to *B. pertussis*. This was proposed by the authors to represent a novel strategy for evasion of protective Th1 responses by *B. pertussis* (McGuirk *et al.*, 2002). A significant role for CD4⁺ CD25⁺ Treg has also recently been found in a mouse model of *H. pylori* infection (Raghaven *et al.*, 2003, 2004). The absence of CD4⁺ CD25⁺ Tregs was found to be associated with a loss of regulation leading to increased pathology (gastritis), even though the absence of such Tregs also led to significant reduction in the bacterial load. Conversely, adoptive transfer of CD4⁺ CD25⁺ Tregs to mice infected with *H. pylori* resulted in suppression of the gastritis and an increased bacterial load. The results indicate that CD4⁺ CD25⁺ Treg can significantly modulate *H. pylori* infection by inhibiting both the protective anti-infectious and immunopathological activities of CD4⁺ effector T (Th1) cells (Raghavan *et al.*, 2003).

IMPLICATIONS FOR MUCOSAL VACCINE DEVELOPMENT

It would be beyond the scope of this chapter to provide a comprehensive review of current strategies to develop vaccines against the many bacteria that cause mucosal infections. Here, we focus on only a few principles that have been utilized to date. First, it is important to identify those infections in which a mucosal vaccine would be critical for inducing protection versus those against which protection may also be achieved by parenteral immunization. In this regard there is a difference between infections in the small intestine and those in the respiratory or female genital tract mucosae. The intestinal mucosa is normally relatively tight for macromolecules, and if serum antibodies transudate into the gut lumen they would rapidly be degraded by the strong proteases present in the gut. In the respiratory and female genital tract mucosae, on the other hand, transudation of IgG from the circulation is considerably more prominent and transuded IgG is less subject to enzymatic degradation.

The depth of bacterial infection or toxin action is also important. If neither the bacteria nor their toxins pass across or even into the epithelial cells, as occurs, for example, in *V. cholerae* and ETEC infections, only antibodies appearing on the mucosal surface and in secretions can interfere with the infectious process. Since disease caused by these infections is strictly limited to the small intestinal mucosa, cholera and ETEC vaccines are probably the most typical examples of vaccines that should be administered mucosally to induce S-IgA in order to protect effectively (Holmgren and Svennerholm, 1998). In contrast, some pathogens can clearly also be attacked by systemic IgG and IgM antibodies in addition to being blocked from initial colonization by locally produced IgA antibodies. This is the case in infections like those caused by salmonellae reaching deeply into the mucosal lymphoid and even more in severe cases reaching the bloodstream or penetrating and spreading through the epithelium after being taken up by M cells, as described for shigellae. Consistent with this, protection against these infections may be achieved by oral as well as injectable vaccines (Robbins *et al.*, 1997).

In the development of vaccines against mucosal infections, it is important to determine the relative contribution of antibody-mediated and cell-mediated immune mechanisms and identify the target antigens for such responses. The disease-inducing mechanisms in invasive infections normally involve severe inflammation and/or intraepithelial bacterial multiplication, associated with cell death and epithelial destruction. In noninvasive infections, disease is instead predominantly mediated by toxins and/or more subtle cell-to-cell contacts between bacteria and epithelial cells. A common feature of mucosal infection is the initial adhesion of the microorganisms to epithelial cells. Thus, logical steps in the development of bacterial vaccines include the stimulation of protective immune responses against both bacterial surface and fimbrial antigens involved in epithelial adherence and against toxins and other extracellular factors that are involved in disease induction. The recently developed oral cholera and ETEC diarrhea vaccines (Holmgren and Svennerholm, 1998) are examples of mucosal vaccines designed to interfere with such defined pathogenic events.

Mucosal infections in which CMI may be involved in both protection and immunopathological events is a challenge for future vaccine development. This applies to, for example, *C. trachomatis* infections in the genital tract, *H. pylori* infection of the gastric mucosa, and shigella and salmonella infections. The design of vaccines to protect against *Chlamydia*-induced disease should probably aim at three different objectives simultaneously: stimulation of mucosal antibodies capable of preventing primary infection of the genital mucosa as well as ascending infection; stimulation of protective CD4+ Th1 cells while at the same time avoiding activation of immunopathologic CD4+ Th1 cells; and possibly also active tolerization of the latter cells that are responsible for immunopathology. Since *H. pylori*, shigella infections, and salmonella infections, similar to chlamydia infections, also involve a combination of analogous protective and immunopathologic immune response components, optimal vaccine development against these infections might use similar guidelines.

Different species of bacteria, including both attenuated pathogens and commensals, have also attracted much interest as orally administered vectors for various foreign antigens (**Table 42.2**). These antigens are inserted as plasmids or genetic constructs and are expected to be expressed during bacterial multiplication *in vivo*. Such organisms include, for example, genetically modified attenuated bacille Calmette-Guerin (BCG), *Salmonella, Shigella,* and *V. cholerae* bacteria as well as nonpathogenic bacteria such as *E. coli, Lactobacillus,* and *Streptococcus gordonii* (Hormaeche and Khan, 1997; Medaglini *et al.*, 1997). Also, attenuated *B. pertussis* and *Salmonella* organisms have been constructed as vectors for nasal use (Mielcarek *et al.*, 1998). All of these organisms have, with varying degree of efficiency, been able to stimulate antibody production and/or T-cell responses to a wide variety of foreign antigens incorporated for *in vivo* expression by the vector organisms. An advantage of this approach to vaccine development, apart from potentially inexpensive vaccine production, is that the live nature of the delivery system and the "danger signals" thereby provided may render normally weak or tolerogenic antigens more immunogenic (Matzinger, 1994). The dominant immunogenicity of the host organism may also help to steer the immune response in the preferred direction, for example, when antigen is presented by BCG to yield mainly a Th1-driven CMI response, as compared with a predominantly Th2-driven antibody response when *V. cholerae* or *B. pertussis* is used as a vector. In model systems, it has been possible to also insert genes allowing for expression of immunomodulating cytokines, such as IFN-γ, IL-5, and IL-6, to further stimulate and direct the immune response (Ramshaw *et al.*, 1992).

However, despite these promising features, each of these vector systems has a long way to go before it can be used in practice in humans. To date, none of the attenuated vector strains have a sufficient margin of safety, particularly considering the risks of using them as vaccine vectors in immunocompromised individuals. The nonpathogenic species, on the other hand, have so far failed to give sufficiently strong immune responses to the expressed foreign antigens to be truly promising in their present form. None of the bacterial

Table 42.2. Examples of Bacteria Used as Oral Live Vectors for Delivery of Heterologous Bacterial Antigens and Shown to Induce Protection in Animal Models[a]

Vector Organism	Expressed Foreign Antigen	Immune Response
S. typhimurium (various *aro* mutations)	*C. tetani* C fragment	Ab+; Protection (P)+
	B. pertussis pertactin	Ab−; CMI+; P+
	E. coli K1	Ab−; P+
	E. coli K88	Ab+; P+
	S. pyogenes M protein	Ab+, P+
	Y. pseudotuberculosis invasin	Ab+; P+
	Y. pestis F1 capsular antigen	Ab+; CMI+; P+
S. typhimurium cya crp asd	*F. tularensis* 17 kDa	Ab+; P+
S. typhi Ty21a (*gale-*)	*S. flexneri* O antigen	Ab+; P+
BCG	*B. burgdorferi* OspA	Ab+; P+
	S. pneumoniae PspA	Ab+; P+
Vibrio cholerae ctx	Shiga-like toxin I	Ab+; P(+)

[a]Adapted from Chatfield and Dougan, 1997; Fennelly *et al.*, 1997; Butterton and Calderwood, 1997.

vector candidates have as yet been tested in humans for their ability to stimulate immune responses to an expressed foreign antigen without inducing adverse reactions.

REFERENCES

Agace, W.W., and Svanborg, C. (1996). Mucosal immunity in the urinary system. In *Mucosal Vaccines* (eds. H. Kiyono, P.L. Ogra, and J.R. McGhee), 389-402. London: Academic Press.

Archimandritis, A., Sougioultzis, S., Foukas, P. G., Tzivras, M., Davaris, P., and Moutsopoulos, H. M. (2000). Expression of HLA-DR, costimulatory molecules B7-1, B7-2, intercellular adhesion molecule-1 (ICAM-1) and Fas ligand (FasL) on gastric epithelial cells in *Helicobacter pylori* gastritis: influence of *H. pylori* eradication. *Clin. Exp. Immunol.* 119, 464–471.

Aseffa, A., Gumy, A., Launois, P., MacDonald, H.R., Louis, J.A., and Tacchini-Cottier, F. (2002). The early IL-4 response to Leishmania major and the resulting Th2 cell maturation steering progressive disease in BALB/c mice are subject to the control of regulatory CD4+CD25+ T cells. *J. Immunol.* 169, 3232–41.

Bäckhed F., Rokbi B., Torstensson E., Zhao Y., Nilsson C., Seguin D., Normark S., Buchan AM and Richter-Dahlfors A. (2003). Gastric mucosal recognition of *Helicobacter pylori* is independent of toll-like receptor 4. *J. Infect. Dis.* 187, 829–836.

Bals, R. (2000). Epithelial anti-microbial peptides in host defence against infection. *Respir. Res.* 1:141–150.

Bao, S., Beagley, K. W., France, M. P., Shen, J., and Husband, A. J. (2000). Interferon-gamma plays a critical role in intestinal immunity against *Salmonella typhimurium* infection. *Immunology* 99, 464–472.

Basset, C., Holton, J., O'Mahony, R., and Roitt, I. (2003). Innate immunity and pathogen-host interaction. *Vaccine* 21:12–23.

Bengoechea, J.A., and Skurnik, M. (2000). Temperature-regulated efflux pump/potassium antiporter system mediates resistance to cationic anti-microbial peptides in *Yersinia. Mol. Microbiol.* 37, 67–80.

Bock, K., Breimer, M.E., Brignole, A., Hansson, G.C., Karlsson, K.A., Larson, G., Leffler, H., Samuelsson, B.E., Strömberg, N., Svanborg-Edén, C., and Thurin, J. (1985). Specificity of binding of a strain of uropathogenic *Escherichia coli* to Galα1→4Gal-containing glycosphingolipids. *J. Biol. Chem.* 260, 8545–8551.

Borén, T., Falk, P., Roth, K. A., Larsson, G., and Normark, S. (1993). Attachment of *Helicobacter pylori* to human gastric epithelium mediated by blood group antigens. *Science* 262 (5141), 1892–1895.

Borody T., Ren Z., Pang G., and Clancy R. (2002). Impaired host immunity contributes to *Helicobacter pylori* eradication failure. *Am. J. Gastroenterol.* 97, 3032–3037.

Cain, T.K., and Rank, R.G. (1995). Local Th1-like responses are induced by intravaginal infection of mice with the mouse pneumonitis biovar of *Chlamydia trachomatis. Infect. Immun.* 63, 1784–1789.

Cohen D, Ashkenazi S., Green M.S., Gdalevich M., Robin G., Slepon R., Yavzori M., Orr N., Block C., Ashkenazi I., Shemer J., Taylor D.N., Hale T.L., Sadoff J.C., Pavliakova D., Schneerson R., and Robbins J.B. (1997). Double-blind vaccine-controlled randomised efficacy trial of an investigational Shigella sonnei conjugate vaccine in young adults. *Lancet* 349, 155–159.

Cong Y., Weaver C.T, Lazenby A., and Elson C.O. (2002). Bacterial-reactive T regulatory cells inhibit pathogenic immune responses to the enteric flora. *J. Immunol.* 169, 6112–6119.

Crabtree, J. E., Farmery, S. M., Lindley, I. J., Figura, N., Peichl, P., and Tompkins, D. S. (1994). CagA/cytotoxic strains of *Helicobacter pylori* and interleukin-8 in gastric epithelial cell lines. *J. Clin. Pathol.* 47, 945–950.

Cutter D., Mason K.W., Howell A.P., Fink D.L., Green B.A., and St Geme J.W. 3rd. (2002). Immunization with Haemophilus influenzae Hap adhesin protects against nasopharyngeal colonization in experimental mice. *J. Infect. Dis.* 186, 1115–1121.

Donnenberg, M.S., Kaper, J.B., and Finlay, B.B. (1997). Interactions between enteropathogenic *Escherichia coli* and host epithelial cells. *Trends Microbiol.* 5 (3), 109–114.

Dodson, K. W., Pinkner, J. S., Rose, T., Magnusson, G., Hultgren, S. J., and Waksman, G. (2001) Structural basis of the interaction of the pyelonephritic *E. coli* adhesion to its human kidney receptor. *Cell* 105, 733–743.

Duchmann, R., Schmitt, E., Knolle, P., Meyer zum Büschenfelde K.-H., and Neurath, M. (1996). Tolerance towards resident intestinal flora in mice is abrogated in experimental colitis and restored by treatment with interleukin-10 or antibodies to interleukin-12. *Eur. J. Immunol.* 26, 934–938.

Dwinell, M.B., Eckmann, L., Leopard, J.D., Varki, N.M., and Kagnoff, M.F. (1999). Chemokine receptor expression by human intestinal epithelial cells. *Gastroenterology* 117, 359–367.

Dybing, J. K., Walters, N., and Pascual, D. W. (1999) Role of endogenous interleukin-18 in resolving wild-type and attenuated *Salmonella typhimurium* infections *Infect. Immun.* 67, 6242–6248.

Eckmann L., and Kagnoff M.F. (2001). Cytokines in host defense against *Salmonella*. *Microbes Infect*. 3, 1191–1200.

Ejima, K., Layne, M.D., Carvajal, I.M., Kritek, P.A., Baron, R.M., Chen, Y.H., Vom Saal, J., Levy, B.D., Yet, S.F., and Perrella, M.A. (2003). Cyclooxygenase-2-deficient mice are resistant to endotoxin-induced inflammation and death. *FASEB J*. 17, 1325–1327.

Elewaut D., DiDonato J.A., Kim J.M., Truong F., Eckmann L and Kagnoff M.F. (1999). NF-kappa B is a central regulator of the intestinal epithelial cell innate immune response induced by infection with enteroinvasive bacteria. *J. Immunol*. 163, 1457–1466.

Elson, C.O., Sartor, R.B., Tennyson, G.S., and Riddell R.H. (1995). Experimental models of inflammatory bowel disease. *Gastroenterology* 109, 1344–1367.

Ernst P.B., and Pappo J. (2001). T-cell-mediated mucosal immunity in the absence of antibody: lessons from *Helicobacter pylori* infection. *Acta Odontol. Scand*. 59, 216–221.

Fichorova R.N., Cronin A.O., Lien E., Anderson D.J., and Ingalls R.R. (2002). Response to *Neisseria gonorrhoeae* by cervicovaginal epithelial cells occurs in the absence of toll-like receptor 4-mediated signaling. *J. Immunol*. 168, 2424–2432.

Francis D.H., Grange P.A., Zeman D.H., Baker D.R., Sun R., and Erickson A.K. (1998). Expression of mucin-type glycoprotein K88 receptors strongly correlates with piglet susceptibility to K88+ enterotoxigenic *Escherichia coli*, but adhesion of this bacterium to brush borders does not. *Infect. Immun*. 66, 4050–4055.

Frendéus B., Godaly G., Hang L., Karpman D., Lundstedt A.C., and Svanborg C. (2000). Interleukin 8 receptor deficiency confers susceptibility to acute experimental pyelonephritis and may have a human counterpart. *J. Exp. Med*. 192, 881–890.

Gaastra, W., and Svennerholm, A.-M. (1996). Colonization factors of human enterotoxigenic *Escherichia coli*: (ETEC). *Trends Microbiol*. 4, 444–452.

Gionchetti, P., Amadini, C., Rizzello, F., Venturi, A., Palmonari, V., Morselli, C., Romagnoli, R., and Campieri, M. (2002). Probiotics–role in inflammatory bowel disease. *Dig. Liver Dis*. 34, S58–S62.

Groux, H., O'Garra, A., Bigler, M., Rouleau, M., Antonenko, S., de Vries, J.E., and Roncarolo, M.G. (1997). A CD4+ T-cell subset inhibits antigen-specific T-cell responses and prevents colitis. *Nature* 389, 737–42.

Hamlet A., Thoreson A-C., Nilsson O., Svennerholm A-M., and Olbe L. (1999). Duodenal *Helicobacter pylori* infection differs in cagA genotype between asymptomatic subjects and patients with duodenal ulcers. *Gastroenterology* 116, 259–268.

Hayashi F., Smith K.D., Ozinsky A., Hawn T.R., and Yi E.C. (2001). The innate immune response to bacterial flagellin is mediated by Toll-like receptor 5. *Nature* 410, 1099–1103.

Hemmi H., Kaisho T., Takeda K., and Akira S. (2003). The roles of Toll-like receptor 9, MyD88, and DNA-dependent protein kinase catalytic subunit in the effects of two distinct CpG DNAs on dendritic cell subsets. *J. Immunol*. 170, 3059–3064.

Hess, C. B., Niesel, D. W., Holmgren, J. Jonson, G., and Klimpel, G. R. (1990). Interferon production by *Shigella flexneri*-infected fibroblasts depends upon intracellular bacterial metabolism. *Infect. Immun*. 58, 399–405.

Holmgren, J. (1981). Actions of cholera toxin and the prevention and treatment of cholera. *Nature* 292, 413.

Holmgren, J., Fryklund, J., and Larsson, H. (1989). Gamma-interferon-mediated down-regulation of electrolyte secretion by intestinal epithelial cells: A local immune mechanism? *Scand. J. Immunol*. 30, 499–503.

Holmgren, J., and Svennerholm, A-M. (1992). Bacterial enteric infections and vaccine development. In *Mucosal Immunology* (eds. RP McDermott and CO Elson). *Gastroenterology Clinics of North America*. Baltimore: WB Saunders, 283–302.

Holmgren, J., and Svennerholm, A.-M. (1998). Vaccines against diarrheal diseases. In *Handbook of Experimental Pharmacology*, vol. 133, *Vaccines* (eds. Perlmann and H. Wigzell). Berlin-Heidelberg-New York: Springer-Verlag, 291–328.

Holmgren, J., and Bergquist, C. (2004). Oral B subunit-killed whole cell cholera vaccine. In *New Generation Vaccines*, Levine, M.M., Kaper, J., Rappuoli, R., Liu, M.A., and Good, M.F. (eds.). New York: Marcel Dekker, 499–509.

Hooper, L. V., and Gordon, J. I. (2001). Commensal host-bacterial relationships in the gut. *Science* 292, 1115–1118.

Hori, S., Carvalho, T.L., and Demengeot, J. (2002). CD25+CD4+ regulatory T cells suppress CD4+ T cell-mediated pulmonary hyperinflammation driven by Pneumocystis carinii in immunodeficient mice. *Eur. J. Immunol*. 32, 1282–1291.

Hughes E.A., and Galan J.E. (2002). Immune response to *Salmonella*: location, location, location? *Immunity* 16, 325–328.

Igietseme, J.U. (1996). Molecular mechanism of T-cell control of *Chlamydia* in mice: role of nitric oxide *in vivo*. *Immunology* 88, 1–5.

Igietseme, J.U., Magee, D.M., Williams, D.M., and Rank, R.G. (1994). Role for CD8+ T cells in antichlamydial immunity defined by *Chlamydia*-specific T-lymphocyte clones. *Infect. Immun*. 62, 5195–5197.

Ilver, D., Arnqvist, A., Ogren, J., Frick, I. M., Kersulyte, D, Incecik, E. T., Berg, D. E., Covacci, A., Engstrand, L., and Boren, T. (1998). *Helicobacter pylori* adhesin binding fucosylated histo-blood group antigens revealed by retagging. *Science* 279, 373–377.

Inobe, J., Slavin A.J., Komagata, Y., Chen, Y., Liu, L., and Weiner, H.L. (1998). IL-4 is a differentiation factor for transforming growth factor-beta secreting Th3 cells and oral administration of IL-4 enhances oral tolerance in experimental allergic encephalomyelitis. *Eur. J. Immunol*. 28, 2780–2790.

Johansson, T., Schön, K., Ward, M., and Lycke, N. (1997). Genital tract infection with *Chlamydia trachomatis* fails to induce protective immunity in gamma interferon receptor-deficient mice despite a strong local immunoglobulin A response. *Infect. Immun*. 65, 1032–1044.

Kagnoff M.F., and Eckmann L. (1997). Epithelial cells as sensors for microbial infection. *J. Clin. Invest*. 100, 6–10.

Karlsson, K.-A. (1989). Animal glycosphingolipids as membrane attachment sites for bacteria. *Ann. Rev. Biochem*. 58, 309–350.

Kim, J.M., Kim, J.S., Jung, H.C., Oh, Y.K., Chung, H.Y., Lee, C.H., Song, I.S. (2003). Helicobacter pylori infection activates the NF-κB signal pathway to induce iNOS and protect human gastric epithelia cells from apoptosis. *Am. J. Physiol. Gastrointest. Liver Physiol*. 285, G1171–G1180.

Klemm, P., Schembri, M.A. (2000) Bacterial adhesins: function and structure. *Int. J. Med. Microbiol*. 290:27–35.

Kopecko, D.J., Venkatesan, M., and Buysse, J.M. (1989). Basic mechanisms and genetic control of bacterial invasion. In *Enteric Infection: Mechanisms, Manifestation and Management* (eds. M.J.G. Farthing and G.T. Keusch), 41–63. London: Chapman and Hall.

Kopp, E., and Medzhitov, R. (2003). Recognition of microbial infection by Toll-like receptors. *Curr. Opin. Immunol*. 15:396–401.

Kraehenbuhl J.P., and Neutra M.R. (2000). Epithelial M cells: differentiation and function. *Cell. Dev. Biol*. 16, 301–332.

Lemaitre, B. (1996). The dorsoventral regulatory gene cassette spatzle/Toll/cactus controls the potent antifungal response in *Drosophila* adults. *Cell* 86, 973–983.

Lindholm, C., Quiding-Järbrink, M, Lönroth, H., Hamlet, A., and Svennerholm, A.-M. (1998). Local cytokine response in *Helicobacter pylori*-infected subjects. *Infect. Immun*. 66, 5964–5971.

Lund, B., Lindberg, F., Marklund, B.-I., and Normark, S. (1987). The PapG protein is the α-D-galactopyranosyl-(1,4)-β-D-galactopyranose-binding adhesin of uropathogenic *Escherichia coli*. *Proc. Natl. Acad. Sci. USA* 84, 5898–5902.

Lundgren, A., Suri-Payer, E., Enarsson, K., Svennerholm, A.-M., and Lundin, B. S. (2003). *Helicobacter pylori*-specific CD4+CD25high regulatory T cells suppress memory T-cell responses to *H. pylori* in infected individuals. *Infect. Immun*. 71, 1755–1762.

Lundgren, A., Strömberg, E., Sjöling, Å., Lindholm, C., Enarsson, K., Edebo, A., Johnsson, E., Suri-Payer, E., Larsson, P., Rudin, A., Svennerholm, A-M., Lundin, B.S. (2004). Mucosal *FOXP3*-expressing CD4+CD23high regulatory T cells in *Helicobacter pylori*-infected patients. *Infect. Immun*. (in press).

Macpherson, A., Khoo, U. Y, Forgacs, I., Philpott-Howard, J., and Bjarnason, I. (1996). Mucosal antibodies in inflammatory bowel disease are directed against intestinal bacteria. *Gut* 38, 365–375.

Macpherson, A. J., Gatto, D., Sainsbury, E., Harriman, G. R., Hengartner, H., and Zinkernagel, R. M. (2000). A primitive

T cell-independent mechanism of intestinal mucosal IgA responses to commensal bacteria. *Science* 23, 2222–2226.

Madara, J. L., and Stafford, J. (1989). Interferon-γ directly affects barrier function of cultured intestinal epithelial monolayers. *J. Clin. Invest.* 83, 724–727.

Madsen, K. L. (2001). Inflammatory bowel disease: lessons from the IL-10 gene-deficient mouse. *Clin. Invest. Med.* 24, 250–257.

Mahon, B. P., Sheahan, B. J., Griffin, F., Murphy, G., and Mills, K. H. G. (1997). Atypical disease after *Bordetella pertussis* respiratory infection of mice with targeted disruptions of interferon-γ receptor or immunoglobulin μ chain genes. *J. Exp. Med.* 186, 1843–1851.

Mastroeni, P., Harrison, J. A., Robinson, J. H., Clare, S., Khan, S., Maskell, D. J., Dougan, G., and Hormaeche, C. E. (1998). Interleukin-12 is required for control of the growth of attenuated aromatic-compound-dependent salmonellae in BALB/c mice: role of gamma interferon and macrophage activation. *Infect. Immun.* 66, 4767–4776.

Matzinger, P. (1994). Tolerance, danger and the extended family. *Ann. Rev. Immunol.* 12, 809–838.

McGuirk, P., McCann, C., and Mills, K. H. (2002). Pathogen-specific T regulatory 1 cells induced in the respiratory tract by a bacterial molecule that stimulates interleukin-10 production dendritic cells: a novel strategy for evasion of protective T helper type 1 responses by *Bordetella pertussis. J. Exp. Med.* 195, 221–231

McSorley, S.J., Asch, S., Costalonga, M., Reinhardt, R.L., and Jenkins, M.K. (2002). Tracking salmonella-specific CD4 T cells in vivo reveals a local mucosal response to a disseminated infection. *Immunity* 16, 365–377.

Medaglini, D., Oggioni, M. R., and Pozzi, G. (1997). Vaginal immunization with recombinant gram-positive bacteria. *Am. J. Reprod. Immunol.* 39, 199–208.

Mielcarek, N., Riveau, G., Remoué, F., Antoine, R., Capron, A., and Locht, C. (1998). Homologous and heterologous protection after single intranasal administration of live attenuated recombinant *Bordetella pertussis. Nature Biotechnol.* 5, 454–457.

Mills, K.H.G., Barnard, A., Watkins, J., and Redhead, K. (1993). Cell mediated immunity to *Bordetella pertussis*: role of Th1 cells in bacterial clearance in a murine respiratory infection model. *Infect. Immun.* 61, 399–410.

Mohammadi, M.S., Czinn, S., Redline, R, and Nedrud, J. (1996). *Helicobacter*-specific cell-mediated immune responses display a predominant TH1 phenotype and promote a delayed-type response in the stomachs of mice. *J. Immunol.* 156, 4729–4738.

Morrison, R.P. Feilzer, K., and Tumas, D.M. (1995). Gene knockout mice establish a primary protective role for major histocompatibility complex class II-restricted responses in *Chlamydia trachomatis* genital tract infection. *Infect. Immun.* 63, 4661–4668.

Mowat, A.McI., and Viney, J.L. (1997). The anatomical basis of intestinal immunity. *Immunol. Rev.* 156, 145–166.

Neish A.S., Gewirtz A.T., Zeng H., Young A.N., Hobert M.E., Karmali V., Rao A.S., and Madara J.L. (2000). Prokaryotic regulation of epithelial responses by inhibition of IkappaB-alpha ubiquitination. *Science* 289, 1560–1563.

Nussler, A. K., and Billiar, T. R. (1993). Inflammation, immunoregulation, and inducible nitric oxide synthase. *J. Leuk. Biol.* 54, 171.

Park J.-H., Um J.-I., Jin Lee B.-J., Goh J.-S., Park S.-Y., Kim W.-S., and Kim P.-H. (2002). Encapsulated *Bifidobacterium bifidum* potentiates intestinal IgA production. *Cell Immunol.* 219, 22–27.

Peek, R. M., and Blaser, M. J. (2002). *Helicobacter pylori* and gastrointestinal tract adenocarcinomas. *Nat. Rev. Cancer* 2, 28–37.

Perry, L.L., Feilzer, K., and Caldwell, H.D. (1997). Immunity to *Chlamydia trachomatis* is mediated by T helper 1 cells through IFN-γ-dependent and -independent pathways. *J. Immunol.* 158, 3344–3352.

Phalipon A., and Sansonetti P.J. (1999). Microbial-host interactions at mucosal sites. Host response to pathogenic bacteria at mucosal sites. *Curr. Top. Microbiol. Immunol.* 236, 163–189.

Phalipon A., Cardona A., Kraehenbuhl J-P., Edelman L., Sansonetti P.J., and Corthésy B. (2002). Secretory component: A new role in secretory IgA-mediated immune exclusion in vivo. *Immun.* 17, 107–115.

Purvén, M., and Lagergård, T. (1992). *Haemophilus ducreyi*, a cytotoxin-producing bacterium. *Infect. Immun.* 60, 1156–1162.

Qadri F., Raqib R., Ahmed F., Rahman T., Wenneras C., Das S.K., Alam N.H., Mathan M.M., and Svennerholm A-M. (2002). Increased levels of inflammatory mediators in children and adults infected with *Vibrio cholerae* O1 and O139. *Clin. Diagn. Lab. Immunol.* 9, 221–229.

Raghavan, S., Fredriksson, M., Svennerholm, A-M., Holmgren, J., and Suri-Payer, E. (2003). Absence of CD4⁺CD25⁺ regulatory T cells is associated with a loss of regulation leading to increased pathology in *Helicobacter pylori*-infected mice. *Clin. Exp. Immunol.* 132:393–400.

Raghavan, S., Suri-Payer, E., and Holmgren, J. (2004). Antigen-specific in vitro suppression of murine *Helicobacter pylori*–reactive immunopathological T cells by CDC4CD25 regulatory T cells. *Scand. J. Immunol.* 60, 82–88.

Ramshaw, I.A., Ruby, J., Ramsay, A.J., Ada, G.L., and Karupiah, G. (1992). Expression of cytokines by recombinant vaccinia viruses: A model for studying cytokines in virus infections *in vivo. Immunol. Rev.* 127, 157–182.

Rappuoli, R. (1997). New and improved vaccines against diphtheria and tetanus. In *New Generation Vaccines* (eds. M. M. Levine, G. C. Woodrow, J. B. Kaper, and G. S. Cobon), 417–436. New York: Marcel Dekker.

Raupach, B., and Kaufmann, S. H. (2001). Bacterial virulence, proinflammatory cytokines and host immunity: how to choose the appropriate *Salmonella* vaccine strain? *Microbes Infect.* 3, 1261–1269.

Rembacken, B.J., Snelling, A.M., Hawkey, P.M., Chalmers, D.M., and Axon, A.T. (1999). Non-pathogenic *Escherichia coli* versus mesalazine for the treatment of ulcerative colitis: a randomized trial. *Lancet* 354, 635–639.

Robbins, J.B., Schneerson, R., and Szu, S.C. (1997). O-specific polysaccharide-protein conjugates for prevention of enteric bacterial diseases. In *New Generation Vaccines* (eds. M.M. Levine, G.C. Woodrow, J.B. Kaper, and G.S. Cobon), 803–815.

Robinson, J.K., Blanchard, T.G., Levine, A.D., Emancipator, S.N., and Lamm, M.E. (2001). A mucosal IgA-mediated excretory immune system in vivo. *J. Immunol.* 166, 3688–3692.

Rudin, A., Johansson, E.-L., Bergquist, C., and Holmgren, J. (1998). Differential kinetics and distribution of antibodies in serum, and nasal and vaginal secretions after nasal and oral vaccination of humans. *Infect. Immun.* 66, 3390–3396.

Rudin, A., Riise, G., Berg, M., and Holmgren, J. (1999). Antibody responses in lower respiratory and urinary tract after nasal and oral vaccination of humans with cholera toxin B-subunit. *Infect. Immun.* 67, 2884–2890.

Russell M.W., and Mestecky J. (2002). Humoral immune responses to microbial infections in the genital tract. *Microbes Infect.* 4, 667–677.

Sansonetti, P.J. (1991). Genetic and molecular basis of epithelial cell invasion by *Shigella* species. *Rev. Infect. Dis.* 13, 285–292.

Schilling J.D., Martin S.M., Hunstad D.A., Patel K.P., Mulvey M.A., Justice S.S., Lorenz R.G., and Hultgren S.J. (2003). CD-14- and toll-like receptor-dependent activation of bladder epithelial cells by lipopolysaccharide and type 1 piliated *Escherichia coli. Infect. Immun.* 71, 1470–1480.

Schmidtchen, A., Frick, I.M., and Bjorck, L. (2001). Dermatan sulphate is released by proteinases of common pathogenic bacteria and inactivates anti-bacterial α-defensin. *Mol. Microbiol.* 39:708–713.

Selsted M.E., Miller S.I., Henschen A.H., and Quellette A.J. (1992). Enteric defensins: Antibiotic peptide components of intestinal host defense. *J. Cell. Biol.* 118:929–936.

Shaw, D. M., Gaerthe, B., Leer, R. J., van der Stap, J. G., Smittenaar, C., Heijne den Bak-Glashouwer, M., Thole, J. E., Tielen, F. J., Pouwels, P. H., and Havenith, C. E. (2000). Engineering the microflora to vaccinate the mucosa: serum immuno-globulin G responses and activated draining cervical lymph nodes following mucosal application of tetanus toxin fragment C-expressing lactobacilli. *Immunology* 100, 510–518.

Sidebotham, R.L., Batten, J.J., Karim, Q.N., Spencer, J., and Baron, J.H. (1991). Breakdown of gastric mucus in presence of *Helicobacter pylori.* J. Clin. Pathol. 44:52–57.

Stambach, M.N. (1995). Murine cytotoxic T lymphocytes induced following *Chlamydia trachomatis* intraperitoneal or genital tract infection respond to cells infected with multiple serovars. *Infect. Immun.* 63, 3527.

Starner, T.D., Swords, W.E., Apicella, M.A., and McCray, Jr. P.B. (2002). Susceptibility of non-typeable *Haemophilus influenzae* to human β defensins is influenced by lipooligosaccharide acylation. *Infect. Immunol.* 70:5287–5289.

Stephens, R.S. (1992). Challenge of *Chlamydia* research. *Infect. Agents Dis.* 1, 279–293.

Strömberg E., Edebo A., Svennerholm A-M., and Lindholm C. (2003). Decreased epithelial cytokine responses in the duodenal mucosa of *Helicobacter pylori*-infected duodenal ulcer patients. *Clin. Diagn. Lab. Immunol.* 10, 116–124.

Su, H., and Caldwell, H. D. (1995). CD4+ T cells play a significant role in adoptive immunity to *Chlamydia trachomatis* infection of the mouse genital tract. *Infect. Immun.* 63, 3302–3308.

Su, H., Feilzer, K., Caldwell, H. D., and Morrison, R. P. (1997). *Chlamydia trachomatis* genital tract infection of antibody-deficient gene knockout mice. *Infect. Immun.* 65, 1993–1999.

Sudo, N., Sawamura, S., Tanaka, K., Aiba, Y., Kubo, C., and Koga, Y. (1997). The requirement of intestinal bacterial flora for the development of an IgE production system fully susceptible to oral tolerance induction. *J. Immunol.* 159, 1739–1745.

Suri-Payer, E., Amar, A.Z., Thornton, A.M., Shevach, E.M. (1998). CD4+CD25+ T cells inhibit both the induction and effector function of autoreactive T cells and represent a unique lineage of immunoregulatory cells. *J. Immunol.* 160:1212–1218.

Steidler, L., Hans, W., Schotte, L., Neirynck, S., Obermeier, F., Falk, W., Fiers, W., and Remaut, E. (2000). Treatment of murine colitis by *Lactococcus lactis* secreting interleukin-10. *Science* 289, 1352–1355.

Svanborg C., Godaly G., and Hedlund M. (1999). Cytokine responses during mucosal infections: role in disease pathogenesis and host defence. *Curr. Opin. Microbiol.* 2, 99–105.

Svanborg C., Frendéus B, Godaly G., Hang L., Hedlund M., and Wachtler C. (2001). Toll-like receptor signalling and chemokine receptor expression influence the severity of urinary tract infection. *J. Infect. Dis.* 183, 61–65.

Tagliabue, A., Nencioni, L. Villa, Z., Keren, D. F., Lowell, G. H., and Braaschi, D. (1983). Antibody-dependent cell-mediated antibacterial activity of intestinal lymphocytes with secretory IgA. *Nature* 306, 184–186.

Tanigawa, T., Watanabe, T., Hamaguchi, M., Sasaki, E., Tominaga, K., Fujiwara, Y., Oshitani, N., Matsumoto, T., Higuchi, K., and Arakawa, T. (2003). Anti-inflammatory effect of two isoforms of cyclooxygenase in *Helicobacter pylori*-induced gastritis in mice: possible involvement of prostaglandin E2. *Am. J. Physiol. Gastrointest. Liver Physiol.*, 286, G148–G156.

Taylor, R. K., Miller, V. L., Furlong, D. B., and Mekalanos, J. J. (1987). Use of *phoA* gene fusions to identify a pilus colonization factor coordinately regulated with cholera toxin. *Proc. Natl. Acad. Sci. USA* 84, 2833–2837.

Tullus, K., Kuhn, I., Orskov, I., Orskov, F., and Möllby, R. (1992). The importance of P- and type 1-fimbriae for the persistence of *Escherichia coli* in the human gut. *Epidemiol. Infect.* 108, 415–421.

Underhill, D.M., Ozinsky, A. (2002). Toll-like receptors: key mediators of microbe detection. *Curr. Opin. Immunol.* 14, 103–110.

Wallin R. P.A., Lundqvist A., Moré S.H., von Bonin A., Kiessling R., and Ljunggren H-G. (2002). Heat-shock proteins as activators of the innate immune system. *Trends Immunol.* 23, 130–135.

Van Camp, J. M., Tomaselli, V., and Coran, A. G., (1994). Bacterial translocation in the neonate. *Curr. Opin. Pediatr.* 6, 327–333.

Weltzin, R.A., Lucia Jandris, P., Michetti, P., Fields, B.N., Kraehenbuhl, J.P., and Neutra, M.R. (1989). Binding and transepithelial transport of immunoglobulin by intestinal M cells. Demonstration using monoclonal IgA antibodies against enteric viral proteins. *J. Cell. Biol.* 108, 1673–1685.

Willshaw, G. A., Scotland, S. M., and Rowe, B. (1997). Vero-cytotoxin-producing *Escherichia coli*. In *Escherichia coli: Mechanisms of Virulence* (ed. M. Sussman), 421–448. Cambridge: Cambridge University Press.

Wira, C.R., Roche, M.A., and Rossoll, R.M. (2002). Antigen presentation by vaginal cells: role of TGFbeta as a mediator of estradiol inhibition of antigen presentation. *Endocrinology* 143, 2872–2879.

Wold, A.E. (1998). The hygiene hypothesis revised: is the rising frequency of allergy due to changes in the intestinal flora? *Allergy* 53, 20–25.

Yagita, H., Hanabuchi, S., Asano, Y., Tamura, T., Nariuchi, H., and Okumura, K. (1995). Fas-mediated cytotoxicit—a new immunoregulatory and pathogenic function of Th1 CD4+ T cells. *Immunol. Rev.* 146, 223.

Yang, X., HayGlass, K.T., and Brunham, R.C. (1996). Genetically determined differences in IL-10 and IFN-γ responses correlate with clearance of *Chlamydia trachomatis* mouse pneumonitis infection. *J. Immunol.* 156, 4338.

Yrlid, U., Svensson, M., Kirby, A., and Wick, M.J. (2001). Antigen-presenting cells and anti-Salmonella immunity. *Microbes Infect* 3, 1239–1248.

Mucosal Immunity to Viruses

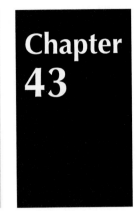

Brian R. Murphy

Respiratory Viruses Section, Laboratory of Infectious Diseases, National Institute of Allergy and Infectious Disease, National Institutes of Health, Bethesda, Maryland

The mucosal surfaces of the body, including primarily the respiratory and gastrointestinal tracts, are readily infected with a wide variety of DNA and RNA viruses. Important viral pathogens of mucosal surfaces such as influenza viruses, adenoviruses, paramyxoviruses (respiratory syncytial virus and the parainfluenza viruses), and rotaviruses cause serious disease upon first infection, often requiring hospitalization. Other viruses such as caliciviruses and rhinoviruses cause less severe disease in the gut or respiratory tract, respectively, but since these two virus groups contain multiple serotypes, frequent infection results in significant overall morbidity. Mucosal immunity induced by infection with some of these highly infectious viruses can be short-lived following first infection (especially if the first infection occurs early in infancy), and reinfection one or more times by such mucosal pathogens is common. Disease often occurs during reinfection but is usually less severe than that experienced during first infection. Infection with several viruses such as measles virus and polioviruses, which initiate replication on mucosal surfaces and then spread to systemic sites where they cause disease, can induce lifelong immunity against the systemic disease, but previous infection with these viruses does not necessarily protect against reinfection of the mucosal tissues.

Several general observations can be made about the ability of the mucosal immune system to reduce disease resulting from viral infection: in the absence of immunity resulting from prior infection, immunization, or acquisition of maternal antibodies, severe disease can ensue, with mucosal immunity primarily involved in clearance of the primary infection; in the presence of low to moderate levels of immunity, reinfection results in a milder illness; in the presence of intermediate to high levels of immunity, an asymptomatic infection occurs; and in the presence of high levels of antibody, infection can be prevented (Ogra and Karzon, 1969a). Because it is difficult to maintain a very high level of mucosal immunity, the major function of the mucosal immune system appears to be that of converting a severe infection to one that is mild or asymptomatic. The large volume, the rapid transit time of mucosal fluids, and the hostile environment of the respiratory and gastrointestinal tracts most likely contribute to the inability to maintain high levels of mucosal antibodies, which are major mediators of immunity. Further

complicating the story, levels of mucosal immunity that are effective against a low dose of virus can be overcome by exposure to a higher dose.

In this quantitative race between virus replication and host response, the host calls upon innate immunity and the cellular and humoral components of adaptive immunity to limit the extent of virus replication, to clear virus, and to prevent reinfection. Immunity to mucosal viruses is very complex and, most important, it is functionally very redundant. As outlined below, independent contributions to immunity can be identified for CD8[+] cytotoxic T cells (TCs), CD4[+] helper T (Th) cells, IgG (both IgG Fc–dependent and independent contributions), IgM, and IgA antibodies. The cellular and humoral immune responses are each composites of individual responses to multiple viral proteins and epitopes within these proteins. These cellular and humoral effectors can be in the form of highly activated effector cells or preformed antibodies, or, alternatively, these active T cells or antibodies can be generated from memory lymphocytes resident in mucosal tissues following reinfection. Antibodies exhibit multiple antiviral functions against virus in extracellular spaces, against virus-infected cells, and against virus transiting through or replicating intracellularly (especially IgA antibodies). With this complex and multifaceted array of immune mediators, it is not surprising that it is often not possible to identify a single correlate of immunity to viruses that replicate primarily on mucosal surfaces, whereas titer of serum neutralizing antibodies is often highly correlated with resistance to viruses that spread via the bloodstream. Although the innate antiviral effectors (interferons, natural killer [NK] cells, and phagocytic cells) make important contributions to defense against mucosal viruses, only the role of the adaptive cellular and humoral immune systems will be considered further in this chapter.

CELLULAR ANTIVIRAL IMMUNE MECHANISMS OPERATIVE ON MUCOSAL SURFACES

Major histocompatibility complex (MHC) class I–restricted TCs and MHC class II–restricted CD4[+] Th cells can each function as antiviral effector cells against viruses that infect mucosal surfaces (Doherty *et al.*, 1997).

TC response

TCs are the major T-cell effector in the restriction of virus replication and direct their antiviral activity against virus-infected cells (Dharakul, Rott, and Greenberg, 1990; Kast *et al.*, 1986; Munoz *et al.*, 1991; Offit and Dudzik, 1990; Taylor and Askonas, 1986; Yap, Ada, and McKensie, 1978). The receptor on TCs recognizes a short peptide processed from an endogenously expressed viral protein in the context of the MHC-class I, β2-microglobulin heterodimer expressed on the surface of an infected cell (Madden *et al.*, 1991). Since the MHC class I restriction elements are present on almost all cells except neurons, TCs can exert their antiviral effects against almost all infected cells present on mucosal surfaces. Since viral infection of a cell is generally required to provide the intracellular proteins for antigen presentation by the MHC class I β2-microglobulin heterodimer, it is clear that TCs cannot function to prevent infection. Instead, these lymphocytes function to lyse cells that are already infected or, alternatively, to secrete cytokines that restrict virus replication in the infected cells (Guidotti *et al.*, 1996; Kagi *et al.*, 1995). The net effect of TC activity is to decrease the amount of virus released by an infected cell and thereby to prevent further spread of virus. Passive transfer of TC clones or TC populations to mice results in restriction of virus replication and clearance of virus in mucosal epithelium, demonstrating the functional capabilities of this T-cell subset (Cannon, Openshaw, and Askonas, 1988; Mackenzie and Taylor, 1989; McDermott *et al.*, 1987; Munoz *et al.*, 1991). The antiviral activity of TCs is optimally mediated by recently activated lymphocytes (Cerwenka, Morgan, and Dutton, 1999). Animals lacking TCs can clear primary viral infection, indicating that the immune response is functionally redundant regarding clearance (Eichelberger *et al.*, 1991a; Eichelberger *et al.*, 1991b; Lightman *et al.*, 1987; Scherle, Palladino, and Gerhard, 1992). However, clearance can be delayed in such TC-deficient animals, highlighting the important role that the TC arm of the immune system plays in resolving viral infection (Franco and Greenberg, 1999; Taylor *et al.*, 1995). Disease enhancement can occur after passive transfer of large numbers of cloned virus-specific TCs capable of clearing virus infection (Cannon, Openshaw, and Askonas, 1988), suggesting that in some circumstances TCs might mediate some of the pathology that develops during primary viral infection of mucosal surfaces.

The time course of TC activation in Peyer's patches and nasal associated lymphoid tissue (NALT) (Zuercher *et al.*, 2002a) during primary viral infection is consistent with a predominant role in clearance of infection. The cytotoxic activity of primary (also called direct) pulmonary TCs peaks early during a paramyxovirus infection (day 7). CD8+ T cells can also be quantified by the more sensitive techniques of tetramer staining or Elispot analysis (Hogan *et al.*, 2001), but the kinetics of the TC response measured in this manner is similar to that seen for cytotoxic T cells. TC cytotoxic activ-

ity declines to barely detectable levels by day 12 and is associated temporally with the elimination of virus infection (Anderson *et al.*, 1990). Thus, restriction of virus replication in mucosal tissues mediated by TCs is active early during the acute stage of the virus infection, but this activity wanes rapidly by day 28 (Connors *et al.*, 1991; Gaddum *et al.*, 1996; Gerhard, 2001). These observations suggest that the TC component of the immune response is primarily operative during the early phase of infection, from the time just before peak titer of virus is reached to the time virus-infected cells are cleared. Later, TCs persist in a less active (or memory) state (Connors *et al.*, 1991; Nicholas *et al.*, 1991). TCs traffic preferentially to the mucosal sites at which virus replication occurred, e.g., TCs induced by rotavirus infection of the gut traffic back to the intestines and TCs induced by a respiratory virus preferentially track to the respiratory tract. This is achieved by the expression of specific homing and chemokine receptors on the surface of the TCs (Kuklin *et al.*, 2000; Kunkel and Butcher, 2002), and such TCs can persist in the lamina propria of mucosa and in alveolar tissues following recovery from virus infection, but their numbers decline with time (Hogan *et al.*, 2002; Hogan *et al.*, 2001). TCs capable of clearing rotavirus infection in immunodeficient mice reside both in a subset expressing a high level of the lymphocyte homing receptor, the α4β7 integrin (Rose *et al.*, 1998), and in an α4β7 integrin–independent subset (Kuklin *et al.*, 2000).

The role of TC receptors directing effector TCs to respiratory tract tissues remains to be defined. For influenza viruses and paramyxoviruses that replicate rapidly on mucosal surfaces, the recruitment of memory TCs and their proliferation at the site of virus replication is often not sufficiently rapid to alter the peak titer of virus achieved in the respiratory tract (Bot *et al.*, 1996; Endo *et al.*, 1991; McMichael *et al.*, 1983; Webster *et al.*, 1991). TCs induced by prior infection can, in some (Flynn *et al.*, 1998; Franco and Greenberg, 1999) but not all (Lawson *et al.*, 1994) instances, restrict replication of virus during reinfection. However, restriction of virus replication by TCs during reinfection is generally less effective than that mediated by antibodies (Gerhard, 2001). Since clinical illness occurs often at the time that peak titer of virus is achieved, it is not surprising that immunization with antigens that induce predominantly TC activity in the absence of antibody is much less successful in restricting replication of challenge virus and preventing illness than immunization that induces a sustained antibody response (Gerhard, 2001). Therefore, in contrast to the immune system's functional redundancy in clearing primary viral infection, it relies heavily on the humoral arm of the immune response to prevent or modify reinfection (Franco and Greenberg, 1999; Gerhard, 2001).

The mechanisms by which TCs exert their antiviral effects *in vivo* are diverse, involving lysis of infected cells via a perforin- or Fas-dependent pathway as well as by release of antiviral cytokines (Aung, Rutigliano, and Graham, 2001; Doherty *et al.*, 1997; Franco and Greenberg, 1999; Topham, Tripp, and Doherty, 1997). This indicates that there is considerable functional redundancy in the mechanisms by which TCs mediate their antiviral response.

Th cell response

Th cells are known to provide help to B cells, thereby augmenting antibody responses (Gerhard, 2001), and they can also provide help to TCs, especially to their maintenance following acute infection (Belz *et al.*, 2002; Riberdy *et al.*, 2000). Th cells themselves can have antiviral activities *in vivo* (McDermott *et al.*, 1987; McNeal *et al.*, 2002; Plotnicky-Gilquin *et al.*, 2002; Taylor, Esquivel, and Askonas, 1990; Zhong, Roberts, and Woodland, 2001). The ability of Th cells to mediate this antiviral effect can require γ-interferon (Plotnicky-Gilquin *et al.*, 2002). In some instances, cooperation between both TCs and Th cells are required for an antiviral effect in the absence of antiviral antibodies (Benton *et al.*, 2001; Crowe, Firestone, and Murphy, 2001; McNeal *et al.*, 2002; Zhong, Roberts, and Woodland, 2001). The contribution made by the direct antiviral activity of Th cells to the overall immunity that is induced appears to be less than the contribution of TCs. This is consistent with the more limited distribution of its restricting element, *i.e.*, the MHC class II, α,β heterodimer that is present predominantly on B lymphocytes and antigen-presenting cells such as macrophages. In addition to having antiviral activity, Th cells can mediate immunopathology (Leung and Ada, 1980; Simeckova-Rosenberg *et al.*, 1995; Taylor, Esquivel, and Askonas, 1990; Varga and Braciale, 2002).

IgG ANTIBODIES ON MUCOSAL SURFACES

IgG antibodies present in the blood can gain access to mucosal surfaces by passive diffusion across the epithelium. Much of the IgG antibody present on mucosal surfaces is derived from serum, as indicated by three observations: there is a linear relationship between the titer of serum and nasal wash influenza virus–specific IgG antibodies (Wagner *et al.*, 1987); the ratio of IgG1/IgG3 influenza virus–specific antibody titer is similar in serum and nasal washes (Wagner *et al.*, 1987); and the specific activity (*i.e.*, the ratio of isotype-specific virus antibody titer to the total concentration of the Ig isotype tested) of IgA and IgM antibodies in mucosal secretions is greater than that in serum, indicating active transport of these immunoglobulins, whereas the specific activity of IgG is less than or equal to that in serum, indicating passive transport (Murphy *et al.*, 1982). Although most IgG present in mucosal secretions is derived primarily by transudation from serum, virus-specific IgG antibodies produced by mucosal B cells in the lamina propria can also contribute to total antiviral activity in mucosal secretions (Belec *et al.*, 1996; Haan *et al.*, 2001; Heinen *et al.*, 2000; Johnson *et al.*, 1986; McBride and Ward, 1987; Ogra *et al.*, 1974). Some IgG antibodies that are synthesized locally in submucosal tissues might gain access to the lumenal surface via simultaneous binding of mucosal IgA and IgG to a multivalent viral antigen that is then transported across epithelial cells by the polymeric Ig receptor–mediated transport system (Kaetzel, Robinson, and Lamm, 1994).

The antiviral activity of IgG antibodies against viruses that replicate on mucosal surfaces has been documented following transudation of antibodies that are derived from three different sources: antibodies produced by the host in response to prior infection or immunization (Clements *et al.*, 1986); maternally derived antibodies (Lepow *et al.*, 1961; Puck *et al.*, 1980; Reuman, Ayoub, and Small, 1987; Reuman *et al.*, 1983); and passively transferred polyclonal or monoclonal antibodies (Besser *et al.*, 1988; Bodian and Nathanson, 1960; Offit, Shaw, and Greenberg, 1986; Prince, Horswood, and Chanock, 1985; Ramphal *et al.*, 1979). The IgG antiviral antibodies can prevent infection (Lepow *et al.*, 1961); decrease virus replication (Bodian and Nathanson, 1960; Clements *et al.*, 1986; Lepow *et al.*, 1961; Prince, Horswood, and Chanock, 1985); clear virus infection (Gerhard, 2001); and eliminate or lessen the severity of disease (Puck *et al.*, 1980). The ability of IgG antibodies to exert antiviral activity on mucosal surfaces is the basis for the licensure of a neutralizing IgG monoclonal antibody administered parenterally to prevent respiratory syncytial virus infection in infants (Sanchez, 2002). In the case of respiratory viruses, passively transferred serum IgG antibodies restrict virus replication in the lung more effectively than in the trachea or nose (Prince, Horswood, and Chanock, 1985; Ramphal *et al.*, 1979). Furthermore, passively transferred IgG antibodies restrict the replication of poliovirus to a greater extent in the throat than in the lower intestinal tract (Bodian and Nathanson, 1960). Considered together, these data demonstrate that a gradient exists regarding the ability of serum-derived IgG antibodies to restrict virus replication on mucosal surfaces; this gradient is lung > nasopharynx > lower intestinal tract (Johnson *et al.*, 1988; Kimman *et al.*, 1987; Kimman, Westenbrink, and Straver, 1989; Murphy *et al.*, 1986a; Murphy *et al.*, 1989; Murphy *et al.*, 1986b; Murphy *et al.*, 1988; Reuman *et al.*, 1983; Sabin *et al.*, 1963a; Sabin *et al.*, 1963b). An explanation for the existence of this gradient is that serum antibodies can more readily diffuse across alveolar walls than across the mucosa of the upper respiratory tract and that the hostile environment of the gastrointestinal tract and the dilution of the IgG antibodies with intestinal secretions further limit the effectiveness of passively derived IgG antibodies at this site. The antiviral activity of IgG antibodies *in vivo* involves direct neutralization of viral infectivity, as evidenced by the restriction of respiratory syncytial virus replication in the lungs of passively immunized rodents depleted of complement and by the finding that parenterally or mucosally administered $F(ab')_2$ fragments of IgG can restrict pulmonary virus replication as effectively as whole IgG molecules from which they were derived (Palladino *et al.*, 1995; Prince *et al.*, 1990). Thus, complement-dependent immune cytolysis and antibody-dependent cell cytotoxicity are not required for the antiviral activity of IgG antibodies (Palladino *et al.*, 1995; Prince *et al.*, 1990). However, complement has been reported to be necessary for the efficient clearance of influenza A virus infection in mice (Hicks *et al.*, 1978), and a role for the Fc fragment of IgG in resistance to influenza A virus infection has been confirmed in FcRγ-KO mice (Huber *et al.*, 2001). These findings underscore the functional redundancy of the mucosal immune system.

Many viruses infect mucosal surfaces during the first 6 months of life, despite the presence of maternal IgG antibodies in serum. In addition, infants are immunized with live poliovirus vaccine when passively acquired maternal antibodies are present. For these reasons, there has been interest in studying the effect of passively derived IgG antibodies on the development of immunity to mucosal viral infections. It has been repeatedly demonstrated that passively acquired IgG antibodies can significantly reduce the mucosal and systemic antibody response to virus infection, despite a high level of virus replication in the mucosal epithelium (Galletti, Beauverger, and Wild, 1995; Kimman *et al.*, 1987; Murphy *et al.*, 1986a; Sabin *et al.*, 1963a; Yamazaki *et al.*, 1994). However, individuals whose primary immune response had apparently been completely suppressed by passively acquired serum IgG antibodies can nevertheless experience a normal secondary immune response following rechallenge with virus or viral antigens (Reuman *et al.*, 1983; Sabin *et al.*, 1963b). Despite the reduction in magnitude of the primary antibody response to initial infection in such subjects, partial resistance to subsequent challenge is evident (Murphy *et al.*, 1989; Reuman *et al.*, 1983; Sabin *et al.*, 1963a). The immunosuppressive effect of passively acquired IgG antibody is greater when viral antigen is administered parenterally rather than mucosally (Murphy *et al.*, 1989). A secretory IgA response can still develop in individuals whose IgG antibody response is suppressed by passively derived serum IgG antibodies, suggesting that the mucosal IgA antibody response is less easily suppressed by passive IgG antibodies than is the systemic IgG response (Jayashree *et al.*, 1988; Kimman and Westenbrink, 1990; Tsutsumi *et al.*, 1995). This finding is a partial explanation for the development of mucosal resistance to infection in the presence of high levels of maternally derived antibodies.

A second way in which passively derived IgG antibodies can modify the antibody response to virus is by altering the functional activity (*i.e.*, quality) of the antiviral antibodies that are induced (Murphy *et al.*, 1988). The neutralizing activity of a given amount of virus-specific antibody is markedly decreased when the immunizing viral infection occurred in the presence of passively derived IgG antibodies (Murphy *et al.*, 1988). The mechanisms by which passively acquired IgG antibodies mediate their effects on the magnitude and quality of the antibody response remain to be defined.

THE MUCOSAL IgA AND IgM ANTIBODY RESPONSE

Although passively transferred IgG antibodies and Th and TC effector cells contribute to mucosal immunity, the major

mediators of resistance to reinfection with mucosal viruses are polymeric IgA antibodies, with a lesser role played by IgM antibodies. IgA antiviral antibodies also play a major role in clearance of viral infections where they work in concert with TCs to combat the infection.

Viral antigens recognized by IgA or IgM antibodies

The major viral antigens that induce a protective antibody response are the surface glycoproteins of viruses that contain lipid envelopes or the proteins present on the surface of icosahedral viruses. IgA antibodies recognize the same viral proteins as IgG antibodies. For instance, polyclonal IgA antibodies, like polyclonal IgG antibodies, recognize the hemagglutinin of influenza virus (Clements *et al.*, 1986; Murphy *et al.*, 1982); the gp70 (fusion) and gp90 (attachment glycoprotein) of respiratory syncytial virus (Murphy *et al.*, 1986c); the gp340 of Epstein-Barr virus (Yao *et al.*, 1991); the viral protein (VP)1, VP2, and VP3 of polioviruses (Zhaori *et al.*, 1989); and the VP4 or VP7 of rotaviruses (Conner *et al.*, 1991; Richardson and Bishop, 1990; Shaw *et al.*, 1991). In general, the specificity of the neutralizing activity of IgA and IgG antibodies for antigenically related variant viruses appears similar (Buscho *et al.*, 1972; Richman *et al.*, 1974), *i.e.*, the mucosal IgA antibody response does not appear to be more broad than that of the systemic IgG antibody response. However, cryptic epitopes on the surface proteins of some enteric viruses can be exposed by proteolytic enzymes in the gut. Thus, the immunogenicity of a virus that replicates in the intestinal tract can differ from that of a parenterally administered inactivated vaccine produced from tissue culture–grown virus. For example, the mucosal IgA response to the poliovirus VP3, which is cleaved by intestinal enzymes following oral administration of live virus, thereby exposing unique epitopes on the protein, is more broad than that following immunization with inactivated virus given parenterally (Zhaori *et al.*, 1989). This is so despite the finding that the antibody responses to VP1 and VP2 were comparable between the two groups. The IgA antibody response to rotavirus antigens also appears to be influenced by the route of immunization (Giammarioli *et al.*, 1996).

The IgA antibody response to the attachment and fusion glycoprotein antigens of respiratory syncytial virus is depressed in infants infected in the presence of maternal antibodies (Murphy *et al.*, 1986a; Wright *et al.*, 2000). Furthermore, the magnitude of the response to the fusion protein correlates with the age of the subject, and the magnitude of the response to the G glycoprotein is inversely related to the level of maternally derived antibodies (Murphy *et al.*, 1986a). Thus, factors influencing IgA responses to viral glycoproteins are complex, with protein structure, age of host, presence of passively acquired IgG antibody, and route of immunization each influencing the magnitude and quality of the response.

IgA monoclonal antibodies to viruses that infect mucosal surfaces have been produced to further define the epitopes on the virus proteins that are seen by IgA antibodies (Lyn *et al.*, 1991; Maoliang, 1986; Weltzin *et al.*, 1989). The same epitopes appear to be recognized by IgG and IgA mono-clonal antibodies (Buttinelli *et al.*, 2001). Neutralization-resistant viral mutants selected with neutralizing IgA and IgG monoclonal antibodies have been shown to have identical reactivity patterns against a panel of monoclonal antibodies (Maoliang, 1986) or to have identical amino acid substitutions (Lyn *et al.*, 1991). Some epitopes of the HN glycoprotein of Sendai virus are recognized by IgA antibodies but not by IgG antibodies; however, a very large panel of IgG and IgA monoclonal antibodies would need to be independently generated and analyzed to determine if any epitope or antigenic site on a viral protein is seen exclusively by IgA antibodies (Buttinelli *et al.*, 2001; Lyn *et al.*, 1991). The mechanism of heavy chain switching in which the antibody-binding regions are maintained but constant regions of the heavy chains are exchanged is compatible with the observations outlined above; namely, IgG and IgA in general have similar specificities for viral antigens and their epitopes. Very little is known about the epitopes recognized by IgM antibodies induced by mucosal virus infection.

The time course of the mucosal IgA response to viral infection

Mucosal immune responses are initiated at inductive sites in mucosa-associated lymphoid tissues (MALT); activated antigen-presenting cells (APCs) traffic to the lymph nodes, where maturation of the T and B cell response ensues; virus-specific T and B cells enter the blood; and finally they make their way back to the lamina propria of mucosal tissues, where they act as effectors (IgA-producing B cells or TCs) or reside as memory cells. The time course of an idealized mucosal IgA response is shown in **Figure 43.1**, and it reflects the pattern of lymphocyte maturation and trafficking. The mucosal IgA response to a primary viral infection is rapid following first infection and can be detected as early as the third day following infection (Blandford and Heath, 1972; Rubin, Anderson, and Lucis, 1983). The primary response peaks within the first 6 weeks and can decrease to a low, often barely detectable, level by 3 months (Bishop *et al.*, 1990; Buscho *et al.*, 1972; Coulson *et al.*, 1990; Friedman, 1982; Friedman, Phillip, and Dagan, 1989; Kaul *et al.*, 1981; Nishio *et al.*, 1990; Sonza and Holmes, 1980). The short duration of the primary mucosal antibody response partially explains the susceptibility of the host to

disease following reinfection, a common observation for viruses that infect mucosal surfaces. This susceptibility to reinfection also reflects the progressive decline in the number of memory IgA antibody-secreting cells (ASCs) in mucosal tissues following primary infection (Liang, Hyland, and Hou, 2001; Yuan and Saif, 2002). Reinfection or boosting with antigen results in a secondary antibody response that is characterized by a more rapid rise in IgA antibody titer; a rise to a higher peak titer; and maintenance of detectable levels of IgA antibody and IgA ASCs over a longer period of time (Asanuma *et al.*, 1998; Bishop *et al.*, 1990; Buscho *et al.*, 1972; Coulson *et al.*, 1990; Kaul *et al.*, 1981; Merriman *et al.*, 1984; Wright *et al.*, 1983; Yamaguchi *et al.*, 1985; Yuan and Saif, 2002).

In addition to a mucosal IgA response, a serum IgA response occurs following mucosal viral infection. A correlation between the magnitude of the serum and mucosal IgA antiviral antibody responses has been observed in some instances, suggesting that some of the serum IgA antibody is produced at mucosal sites and, after escaping the polymeric Ig receptor (pIgR)-mediated transport, reaches the blood via the lymphatics (Burlington *et al.*, 1983). The polymeric structure of postinfection antiviral serum IgA antibodies is consistent with a mucosal origin of the B cells that secrete the antibody, since serum IgA antibodies are generally monomeric (Brown *et al.*, 1985; Ponzi *et al.*, 1985). A correlation also exists between the magnitude of rotavirus-specific IgA ASCs in both blood and small intestinal lamina propria following acute rotavirus infection in humans (Brown *et al.*, 2000). Following recent rotavirus infection of children, rotavirus-specific IgM ASCs that bear intestine-specific integrins (see next section) are present in the blood, indicating that both IgM and IgA cells induced in the intestine can be identified as they circulate in the blood (Gonzalez *et al.*, 2003).

Polymeric IgA serum antibodies and IgA ASCs can be readily induced by parenteral immunization of persons who had previously experienced a wild-type or attenuated virus infection (Brown *et al.*, 1987; Herremans *et al.*, 1999) but can be induced only with difficulty in immunologically naive hosts. This suggests that IgA memory B cells of mucosal origin not only return to local sites of induction but also seed systemic sites following infection and that antigenic stimulation of such peripherally located B cells can yield IgA antibodies whose polymeric nature and subclass are characteristic of mucosal IgA antibodies. In this context, it is important to reiterate that parenteral immunization with viral antigens is very inefficient at inducing IgA antibodies or IgA ASCs at mucosal sites (Clements and Murphy, 1986; Coffin, Klinek, and Offit, 1995; Takao *et al.*, 1997), even in hosts with prior experience with related antigens (Clements and Murphy, 1986).

The number of virus-specific IgG-, IgA-, or IgM-secreting B cells at mucosal sites of virus replication has been studied in nasal tissues, lungs, and the small intestine following infection with enteric or respiratory virus (Coffin, Klinek, and Offit, 1995; Jones and Ada, 1986; Merchant *et al.*, 1991; Tamura *et al.*, 1998; Yuan and Saif, 2002; Yuan *et al.*, 1996).

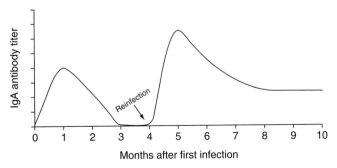

Fig. 43.1. Time course of mucosal IgA response to viral infection.

An IgG B-cell response predominated in the lungs, as is expected since IgG antibody is the predominant immunoglobulin isotype in the secretions of the lower respiratory tract (Jones and Ada, 1986). Also as expected, an IgA B-cell response predominated in the intestine (Merchant *et al.*, 1991; Yuan and Saif, 2002).

The local nature of the mucosal IgA antibody response

Evidence of the existence of a common mucosal immune system comes from the observation that immunization of a mucosal site often leads to detectable immune responses at distant mucosal sites (Mestecky, 1987). This seeding of distal mucosal sites is likely due to the trafficking of locally stimulated mucosal B-lymphocytes to distant sites, where they reside as IgA plasma cells actively producing antibody or as memory B cells (Czerkinsky *et al.*, 1987; Mestecky, 1987; Rudzik *et al.*, 1975). Specifically, immunization of the gastrointestinal tract mucosa or the respiratory tract mucosa can give rise to an IgA antibody response at distal sites, including the mucosa of the genital tract (Chen, Burlington, and Quinnan, 1987; Haneberg *et al.*, 1994; Hirabayashi *et al.*, 1990; Staats, Nichols, and Palker, 1996; Waldman *et al.*, 1986). Although this common mucosal system exists, it does not appear to be very efficient in protecting the sites that are not directly stimulated with antigen (Nedrud *et al.*, 1987a; Ogra and Karzon, 1969a; Smith *et al.*, 1970). Oral immunization with live adenovirus vaccine enclosed in enteric coated tablets selectively infects the lower intestinal tract and induces a fecal IgA and serum IgG antiviral antibody response that is protective against disease, but it fails to induce a detectable nasal wash IgA antibody response (Scott *et al.*, 1972; Smith *et al.*, 1970). In this case, the serum IgG antibodies induced by the intestinal infection protected against illness in the upper respiratory tract rather than locally produced respiratory tract IgA antibodies. Intestinal infection of mice with reovirus yields similar findings (Zuercher *et al.*, 2002b). In contrast, live adenovirus vaccine administered to the upper respiratory tract induces a vigorous nasal wash IgA antibody response (Smith *et al.*, 1970). In a similar study, selective infection of the colon of infants with live poliovirus virus vaccine by administration of virus directly into the orifice of a colostomy resulted in a vigorous neutralizing IgA antibody response in the colon but not in the nasopharynx (Ogra and Karzon, 1969a). When the upper respiratory tract and the colon of these infants were challenged with poliovirus vaccine, vaccine virus replicated to high titer in the pharynx but not the colon (Ogra and Karzon, 1969a). Similar studies with rotavirus infection in infants and children demonstrated that the IgA antiviral response in the duodenum, which is the major site of viral replication, was greater than in saliva, a representative distant mucosal site not known to support rotavirus replication (Grimwood *et al.*, 1988). During experimental studies in rodents, immunization of the gut with an inactivated parainfluenza virus vaccine plus adjuvant was less protective of the respiratory tract than

intranasally administered vaccine (Nedrud *et al.*, 1987a). In some instances, a protective response at a distal mucosal site can be achieved (Chen, Burlington, and Quinnan, 1987). Despite the occasional exception, these studies in humans and animals suggest that induction of a highly protective mucosal IgA response at a site distant to the site of immunization will be difficult to achieve.

The local nature of the mucosal antibody response even within the respiratory tract was observed in two studies. In the first study, the quantity of mucosal antibody in sputum or nasal secretions of volunteers given an inactivated influenza A virus vaccine by aerosol was a function of the size of the aerosolized particles (Waldman *et al.*, 1970). The adult volunteers vaccinated with an aerosol containing small particles of a size that is predominantly deposited in the lung developed high sputum but low nasal secretory antibody titers, whereas individuals immunized with larger particles that are predominantly deposited in the nose developed high nasal but low sputum antibody titers. In the second study, intranasal administration of inactivated influenza A virus vaccine induced a greater nasal wash neutralizing antibody response than a salivary antibody response, indicating that a greater mucosal response developed at the site of antigenic stimulation, *i.e.*, the nasal passages, than at the distant site, *i.e.*, the salivary glands (Waldman *et al.*, 1968). These observations demonstrate that mucosal antibody responses are more localized than systemic responses since IgG antibodies, in the latter case, are disseminated widely via the circulatory system.

A partial explanation for the local nature of the mucosal responses comes from the finding that the concentration of virus-specific IgA producing B cells at the site of antigenic stimulation is much higher than at more distant sites (Dharakul *et al.*, 1988). The molecular basis of the preferential production of IgA antibodies at the site of induction is beginning to be defined. Rotavirus-specific IgA B cells that home to the lamina propria of the small intestine express the $\alpha 4\beta 7$ integrin that specifically recognizes the MAdCAM-1 addressin expressed on venules in the lamina propria of the small intestine (Butcher *et al.*, 1999; Youngman *et al.*, 2002). In addition, small intestine epithelial cells secrete a chemokine designated TECK or CCl25 that serves as a specific attractant for IgA ASCs which bear the TECK receptor CCR9 (Bowman *et al.*, 2002). In this way, virus-specific IgA ASCs return from the lymph nodes to the lamina propria at sites of induction (*i.e.*, sites of virus replication), guided by the combined effect of integrin-addressin and specific chemokine-receptor interactions. The specific homing mechanisms for IgA ASCs bound for the lamina propria of the respiratory tract remain to be defined. Thus, although B cells track between mucosal sites, it appears that, as a result of site-specific homing mechanisms, the levels of antiviral antibody and resistance to infection achieved at distant sites are much less than at sites of direct antigenic stimulation. Mucosal immunization is thus most successfully achieved by antigenic stimulation at sites directly involved in viral replication.

IgA and IgM antibodies are associated with clearance of primary infection and resistance to reinfection

It has long been recognized that immunization by a mucosal route could induce greater resistance to virus infection than systemic immunization and that resistance correlated with the level of mucosal antibodies (De St. Groth and Donnelley, 1950). The appearance of IgA antibodies in mucosal secretions correlates with the cessation of virus shedding during mucosal viral infection in animals and humans in both the respiratory and gastrointestinal tracts **(Fig. 43.2)** (Corthier and Vannier, 1983; Keller and Dwyer, 1968; McIntosh *et al.*, 1978; McIntosh, McQuillin, and Gardner, 1979; Ogra, 1970; Valtanen *et al.*, 2000). The appearance of virus-IgA or virus-IgM immune complexes at the time of virus clearance is consistent with the role of these isotypes in resolution of virus infection (Tamura *et al.*, 1998). As mentioned earlier, animals rendered deficient in their TC or Th responses are able to clear virus infection similarly to their fully immunocompetent counterparts, but with a slight delay (Eichelberger *et al.*, 1991a; Eichelberger *et al.*, 1991b; Gerhard, 2001; Lightman *et al.*, 1987; Nguyen *et al.*, 2001). This suggests that antibodies participate in clearance of virus-infected cells from mucosal surfaces and that they can even be sufficient in this regard (Gerhard, 2001). Furthermore, the presence of virus-specific IgA antibody at the time of reinfection correlates with resistance **(Table 43.1)**, and the number of IgA ASCs present has also been associated with resistance to reinfection (Tamura *et al.*, 1998; Yuan and Saif, 2002). A quantitative inverse relationship exists between the level of mucosal IgA antibodies and the extent of virus replication (Ogra and Karzon, 1969a), indicating that the level of protection is a function of the quantity of antibody present at the time of challenge. One study even demonstrated that local IgA memory to bovine respiratory syncytial virus in the absence of detectable IgA antibodies was associated with resistance to reinfection with virus (Kimman, Westenbrink, and Straver, 1989). In this instance, it appeared that a local IgA response to reinfection was sufficiently rapid to limit the extent of virus replication, or alternatively, undetectable levels of antibody were present that modified the infection. In sum, these results clearly indicate that mucosal IgA antibodies participate in resolution of primary viral infection and that they also play a major role in resistance to reinfection. IgM antibodies can make independent contributions to resistance to mucosal viral infections (Baumgarth *et al.*, 2000; Kopf, Brombacher, and Bachmann, 2002; O'Neal, Harriman, and Conner, 2000).

How do IgA antibodies clear viral infections and prevent reinfection? Certain viral proteins can induce highly protective immune responses, whereas other proteins induce antibodies that are less protective; e.g., for influenza viruses, the hemagglutinin (HA) induces highly protective antibodies, whereas the neuraminidase (NA) and M2 proteins induce weaker, less protective, antibodies (Gerhard, 2001). In general, the antiviral activity of the highly protective mucosal antibodies resides in their ability to neutralize viral infectivity, as measured by an *in vitro* neutralization assay; e.g., for influenza viruses, HA but not NA or M2 induces neutralizing antibodies (Gerhard, 2001). For rotaviruses, neutralizing antibodies to the VP4 and VP7 protective antigens are more protective than the nonneutralizing antibodies induced by VP6 (Coste *et al.*, 2000; Yuan and Saif, 2002). The mechanisms by which antiviral antibodies against mucosal viruses exert their antiviral effect are diverse, but they primarily include prevention of attachment (Burton, 2002; Klasse and Sattentau, 2002; Knossow *et al.*, 2002), inhibition of fusion of the viral membrane with the cell membrane (Outlaw and Dimmock, 1991), and prevention of the disassembly of non-lipid-containing virions (e.g., for rotaviruses) required for initiation of transcription (Ludert *et al.*, 2002). These antiviral mechanisms are collectively referred to as immune exclusion, in which IgA or other mucosal antibodies interact with virus in the lumen of the respiratory or gastrointestinal tract and prevent infection of the epithelial cells by neutralization. Although IgA antibodies to influenza appear to be slightly more efficient than IgG antibodies at preventing attachment of virus to infected cells in tissue culture (Outlaw and Dimmock, 1991), direct comparisons *in vivo* indicate a comparable level of antiviral activity (Fisher *et al.*, 1999; Mazanec *et al.*, 1992b).

The main difference between the abilities of IgA/IgM and IgG antibodies to protect mucosal surfaces is the preferential

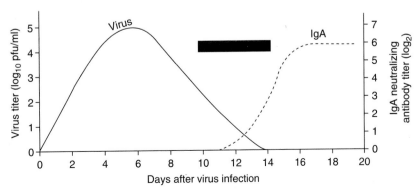

Fig. 43.2. An idealized viral infection of a mucosal surface, in which clearance of infectious virus is associated with the appearance of neutralizing IgA antibodies. The black bar indicates the time at which IgA–virus immune complexes are likely to be present.

Table 43.1. Association of Mucosal Antibodies with Resistance to Viral Infections

Studies in Humans or Animals	Virus	Resistance Observed		References
		Reduced Infection or Disease	Prevented Infection	
Humans				
	RSV	+		Mills *et al.*, 1971; Watt *et al.*, 1990
	PIV	+	+	Smith *et al.*, 1966
	Influenza	+		Clements *et al.*, 1986; Reuman, Keely, and Schiff, 1990
	Influenza		+	Clements *et al.*, 1983; Johnson *et al.*, 1986
	Influenza	+	+	Murphy *et al.*, 1973
	Rhinovirus		+	Perkins *et al.*, 1969
	Rotavirus	+		Hjelt *et al.*, 1987; Ward *et al.*, 1989
	Rotavirus	+	+	Feng *et al.*, 1997; Matson *et al.*, 1993; Ward *et al.*, 1990
	Poliovirus	+		Ogra and Karzon, 1969b; Onorato et al., 1991
	Poliovirus	+	+	Ogra and Karzon, 1969a
Animals				
Mice	Influenza	+	+	De St. Groth and Donnelley, 1950
Mice	Influenza		+	Liew *et al.*, 1984
Mice	PIV	+		Liang, Lamm, and Nedrud, 1988; Nedrud *et al.*, 1987b; Takao *et al.*, 1997
Hamsters	PIV	+	+	Ray *et al.*, 1988
Bovines	RSV	+		Kimman and Westenbrink, 1990

RSV, respiratory syncytial virus; PIV, parainfluenza virus.

secretion of J-chain containing polymeric IgA/IgM antibodies via the pIgR that enables IgA/IgM antibodies to achieve much higher levels on the lumenal surface than IgG antibodies. For example, systemically administered neutralizing polymeric monoclonal IgA antibody to influenza A virus hemagglutinin, but not IgG antibody, was able to restrict the replication of influenza virus in the upper respiratory tract of the mouse (Renegar and Small, 1991). Thus, the main advantage of IgA antibodies in protecting mucosal surfaces of the respiratory tract appears to be their ability to be selectively transported across mucosal surfaces on which they can reach high titers rather than their inherently greater antiviral activity. The second major advantage of IgA (or IgM) versus IgG antibodies is their ability to exert antiviral activity inside an epithelial cell during pIgR-mediated transcytosis from the basolateral to apical surface of the cell. This is a mode of *in vivo* neutralization that is not reproduced in typical *in vitro* neutralization assays.

A diverse set of neutralizing and nonneutralizing antiviral IgA, but not IgG, antibodies directed at different virion proteins, including virion surface proteins and nucleocapsid proteins, can exert an antiviral effect intracellularly via a diverse set of mechanisms (Bomsel *et al.*, 1998; Feng *et al.*, 2002; Fujioka *et al.*, 1998; Mazanec, Coudret, and Fletcher, 1995; Mazanec *et al.*, 1992a; Ruggeri *et al.*, 1998; Yan *et al.*,

2002). The mechanisms by which this antiviral effect can be achieved include an action against virus following its entry into the cell but before its replication, as well as during its replication and assembly. Some viruses such as HIV do not infect epithelial cells but instead traverse the cells on their way to infect lymphocytes and other cells in the lamina propria. Anti-HIV IgA or IgM antibodies that are present intracellularly can disrupt the safe passage of such viruses (Bomsel *et al.*, 1998). Nonneutralizing rotavirus VP6 IgA antibodies can bind intracellularly to partially decapsidated virions and prevent primary transcription (Feng *et al.*, 2002). Other neutralizing and nonneutralizing antibodies can colocalize with viral proteins present intracellularly and prevent efficient replication or assembly (Fujioka *et al.*, 1998; Yan *et al.*, 2002). IgA antibodies can have other effects such as promoting clearance of viral antigens present in the subepithelial space, by a process referred to as immune excretion in which an IgA antibody in the lamina propria binds a protein, and the complex is then transported via pIgR-mediated transcytosis to the lumen, where it is degraded or excreted. IgA antibodies to different virus proteins can exert different levels of immune excretion, e.g., the IgA antibodies to the fusion protein of measles virus were more efficient at immune excretion than IgA hemagglutinin antibodies (Yan *et al.*, 2002). IgA antibodies can promote uptake of viral antigens present in lumenal spaces via immunoglobulin receptors present on the specialized absorptive epithelial M cells, which would facilitate antigen presentation (Weltzin *et al.*, 1989).

Specific evidence demonstrating the role of antiviral IgA antibodies in mucosal immunity

The ability of IgA antibodies to exert antiviral activity against mucosal viruses has been demonstrated by passive transfer studies in which IgA antibodies that are administered parenterally (Renegar and Small, 1991) or directly onto a mucosal surface (Mazanec, Nedrud, and Lamm, 1987; Tamura *et al.*, 1990) or that are secreted by hybridoma cells (or other B cells) (Burns *et al.*, 1996; Kuklin *et al.*, 2001) decrease the replication of the virus on the mucosal surface. The efficacy of virus-specific IgA and IgG antibodies was comparable when the antibodies were directly applied to the mucosal surface, whereas polymeric IgA antibodies are more efficacious than IgG antibodies when the antibodies or ASCs are administered systemically, reflecting the specific transport of IgA antibodies as described earlier. However, it is important to emphasize that IgA antibodies are not essential in clearance and that other immunoglobulins such as IgM or IgG, under certain experimental conditions, can mediate clearance in the absence of IgA (Kuklin *et al.*, 2001).

The role of IgA antibodies in mucosal immunity to viral infections in previously infected or immunized animals has also been examined by instillation of an antibody to IgA or IgG into the upper respiratory tract prior to virus challenge in an attempt to specifically ablate the IgA or IgG component of mucosal immunity, leaving all other induced responses active. The antibody to IgA or IgG binds to the respective immunoglobulin in the lumen and inhibits its antiviral activity. A major role of IgA, but not IgG, in providing resistance to the upper respiratory tract was observed with this approach (Renegar and Small, 1991; Takao *et al.*, 1997).

Studies with KO mice deficient in total Ig, IgA, IgM, J-chain, or pIgR have clearly defined an important contribution of antibody in general, and IgA and IgM in particular, in clearance of virus following primary infection or in resistance to reinfection (Arulanandam *et al.*, 2001; Asahi *et al.*, 2002; Ruggeri *et al.*, 1998; Schwartz-Cornil *et al.*, 2002; Silvey *et al.*, 2001). This is experimentally challenging since the mucosal immune system is so functionally redundant that dissection of the relative contribution of individual components of the immune system is not always easy to achieve (O'Neal, Harriman, and Conner, 2000; Schwartz-Cornil *et al.*, 2002; Silvey *et al.*, 2001).

In conclusion, both the cellular and humoral immune systems participate actively in the resolution of first and subsequent mucosal viral infections. Specifically, TCs and IgA/IgM antibodies each make important contributions during resolution of primary infection, while IgA antibodies induced by prior infection or immunization offer the most effective resistance to reinfection. IgG antibodies are less effective at accessing the lumenal surfaces but are an important component of long-term immunity, especially in the lung. TCs and Th memory cells take time to expand and activate following reinfection and make a smaller contribution than IgA antibodies to inhibition of viral replication during reinfection.

REFERENCES

Anderson, J. J., Norden, J., Saunders, D., Toms, G. L., and Scott, R. (1990). Analysis of the local and systemic immune responses induced in BALB/c mice by experimental respiratory syncytial virus infection. *J. Gen. Virol.* 71, 1561–1570.

Arulanandam, B. P., Raeder, R. H., Nedrud, J. G., Bucher, D. J., Le, J., and Metzger, D. W. (2001). IgA immunodeficiency leads to inadequate Th cell priming and increased susceptibility to influenza virus infection. *J. Immunol.* 166(1), 226–231.

Asahi, Y., Yoshikawa, T., Watanabe, I., Iwasaki, T., Hasegawa, H., Sato, Y., Shimada, S., Nanno, M., Matsuoka, Y., Ohwaki, M., Iwakura, Y., Suzuki, Y., Aizawa, C., Sata, T., Kurata, T., and Tamura, S. (2002). Protection against influenza virus infection in polymeric Ig receptor knockout mice immunized intranasally with adjuvant-combined vaccines. *J. Immunol.* 168(6), 2930–2938.

Asanuma, H., Aizawa, C., Kurata, T., and Tamura, S. (1998). IgA antibody-forming cell responses in the nasal-associated lymphoid tissue of mice vaccinated by intranasal, intravenous and/or subcutaneous administration. *Vaccine* 16(13), 1257–1262.

Aung, S., Rutigliano, J. A., and Graham, B. S. (2001). Alternative mechanisms of respiratory syncytial virus clearance in perforin knockout mice lead to enhanced disease. *J. Virol.* 75(20), 9918–9924.

Baumgarth, N., Herman, O. C., Jager, G. C., Brown, L. E., Herzenberg, L. A., and Chen, J. (2000). B-1 and B-2 cell-derived immunoglobulin M antibodies are nonredundant components of the protective response to influenza virus infection. *J. Exp. Med.* 192(2), 271–280.

Belec, L., Tevi-Benissan, C., Dupre, T., Mohamed, A. S., Prazuck, T., Gilquin, J., Kanga, J. M., and Pillot, J. (1996). Comparison of cervicovaginal humoral immunity in clinically asymptomatic (CDC A1 and A2 category) patients with HIV-1 and HIV-2 infection. *J. Clin. Immunol.* 16(1), 12–20.

Belz, G. T., Wodarz, D., Diaz, G., Nowak, M. A., and Doherty, P. C. (2002). Compromised influenza virus-specific CD8$^{(+)}$-T-cell memory in CD4$^{(+)}$-T-cell-deficient mice. *J. Virol.* 76(23), 12388–12393.

Benton, K. A., Misplon, J. A., Lo, C. Y., Brutkiewicz, R. R., Prasad, S. A., and Epstein, S. L. (2001). Heterosubtypic immunity to influenza A virus in mice lacking IgA, all Ig, NKT cells, or gamma delta T cells. *J. Immunol.* 166(12), 7437–7445.

Besser, T. E., Gay, C. C., McGuire, T. C., and Evermann, J. F. (1988). Passive immunity to bovine rotavirus infections associated with transfer of serum antibody into the intestinal lumen. *J. Virol.* 62, 2238–2242.

Bishop, R., Lund, J., Cipriani, E., Unicomb, L., and Barnes, G. (1990). Clinical serological and intestinal immune responses to rotavirus infection of humans. In *Medical Virology 9* (eds. L. M. de la Maza and E. M. Peterson). New York: Plenum Press.

Blandford, G., and Heath, R. B. (1972). Studies on the immune response and pathogenesis of Sendai virus infection of mice. I. The fate of viral antigens. *Immunology* 22(4), 637–649.

Bodian, D., and Nathanson, N. (1960). Inhibitory effects of passive antibody on virulent poliovirus excretion and on immune response in chimpanzees. *Bull. Johns Hopkins Hosp.* 107, 143–162.

Bomsel, M., Heyman, M., Hocini, H., Lagaye, S., Belec, L., Dupont, C., and Desgranges, C. (1998). Intracellular neutralization of HIV transcytosis across tight epithelial barriers by anti-HIV envelope protein dIgA or IgM. *Immunity* 9(2), 277–287.

Bot, A., Reichlin, A., Isobe, H., Bot, S., Schulman, J., Yokoyama, W. M., and Bona, C. A. (1996). Cellular mechanisms involved in protection and recovery from influenza virus infection in immunodeficient mice. *J. Virol.* 70(8), 5668–5672.

Bowman, E. P., Kuklin, N. A., Youngman, K. R., Lazarus, N. H., Kunkel, E. J., Pan, J., Greenberg, H. B., and Butcher, E. C.

(2002). The intestinal chemokine thymus-expressed chemokine (CCL25) attracts IgA antibody-secreting cells. *J. Exp. Med.* 195(2), 269–275.

Brown, K. A., Kriss, J. A., Moser, C. A., Wenner, W. J., and Offit, P. A. (2000). Circulating rotavirus-specific antibody-secreting cells (ASCs) predict the presence of rotavirus-specific ASCs in the human small intestinal lamina propria. *J. Infect. Dis.* 182(4), 1039–1043.

Brown, T. A., Clements, M. L., Murphy, B. R., Radl, J., Haaijman, J. J., and Mestecky, J. (1987). Molecular form and subclass distribution of IgA antibodies after immunization with live and inactivated influenza A vaccines. *Adv. Exp. Med. Biol.* 216B, 1691–1700.

Brown, T. A., Murphy, B. R., Radl, J., Haaijman, J. J., and Mestecky, J. (1985). Subclass distribution and molecular form of immunoglobulin A hemagglutinin antibodies in sera and nasal secretions after experimental secondary infection with influenza A virus in humans. *J. Clin. Microbiol.* 22, 259–264.

Burlington, D. B., Clements, M. L., Meiklejohn, G., Phelan, M., and Murphy, B. R. (1983). Hemagglutinin specific antibody responses in the IgG, IgA and IgM isotypes as measured by ELISA after primary or secondary infection of man with influenza A virus. *Infect. Immunol.* 41, 540–545.

Burns, J. W., Siadat-Pajouh, M., Krishnaney, A. A., and Greenberg, H. B. (1996). Protective effect of rotavirus VP6-specific IgA monoclonal antibodies that lack neutralizing activity. *Science* 272(5258), 104–107.

Burton, D. R. (2002). Antibodies, viruses and vaccines. *Nat. Rev. Immunol.* 2(9), 706–713.

Buscho, R. F., Perkins, J. C., Knopf, J. L. S., Kapikian, A. Z., and Chanock, R. (1972). Further characterization of the local respiratory tract antibody response induced by intranasal instillation of inactivated rhinovirus 13 vaccine. *J. Immunol.* 108, 169–177.

Butcher, E. C., Williams, M., Youngman, K., Rott, L., and Briskin, M. (1999). Lymphocyte trafficking and regional immunity. *Adv. Immunol.* 72, 209–253.

Buttinelli, G., Ruggeri, F. M., Marturano, J., Novello, F., Donati, V., and Fiore, L. (2001). Antigenic sites of poliovirus type 3 eliciting IgA monoclonal antibodies in orally immunized mice. *Virology* 281(2), 265–271.

Cannon, M. J., Openshaw, P. J., and Askonas, B. A. (1988). Cytotoxic T cells clear virus but augment lung pathology in mice infected with respiratory syncytial virus. *J. Exp. Med.* 168, 1163–1168.

Cerwenka, A., Morgan, T. M., and Dutton, R. W. (1999). Naive, effector, and memory CD8 T cells in protection against pulmonary influenza virus infection: homing properties rather than initial frequencies are crucial. *J. Immunol.* 163(10), 5535–5543.

Chen, K. S., Burlington, D. B., and Quinnan, G. V. (1987). Active synthesis of hemagglutinin-specific immunoglobulin A by lung cells of mice that were immunized intragastrically with inactivated influenza virus vaccine. *J. Virol.* 61, 2150–2154.

Clements, M. L., Betts, R. F., Tierney, E. L., and Murphy, B. R. (1986). Serum and nasal wash antibodies associated with resistance to experimental challenge with influenza A wild-type virus. *J. Clin. Microbiol.* 24, 157–160.

Clements, M. L., and Murphy, B. R. (1986). Development and persistence of local and systemic antibody responses in adults given live attenuated or inactivated influenza A virus vaccine. *J. Clin. Microbiol.* 23, 66–72.

Clements, M. L., O'Donnell, S., Levine, M. M., Chanock, R. M., and Murphy, B. R. (1983). Dose response of A/Alaska/6/77 (H3N2) cold-adapted reassortant vaccine virus in adult volunteers: role of local antibody in resistance to infection with vaccine virus. *Infect. Immun.* 40, 1044–1051.

Coffin, S. E., Klinek, M., and Offit, P. A. (1995). Induction of virus-specific antibody production by lamina propria lymphocytes following intramuscular inoculation with rotavirus. *J. Infect. Dis.* 172, 874–878.

Conner, M. E., Gilger, M. A., Estes, M. K., and Graham, D. Y. (1991). Serologic and mucosal immune response to rotavirus infection in the rabbit model. *J. Virol.* 65, 2562–2571.

Connors, M., Collins, P. L., Firestone, C. Y., and Murphy, B. R. (1991). Respiratory syncytial virus (RSV) F, G, M2 (22K), and N pro-

teins each induce resistance to RSV challenge, but resistance induced by M2 and N proteins is relatively short-lived. *J. Virol.* 65(3), 1634–1637.

Corthier, G., and Vannier, P. (1983). Production of coproantibodies and immune complexes in piglets infected with rotavirus. *J. Infect. Dis.* 147, 293–296.

Coste, A., Sirard, J. C., Johansen, K., Cohen, J., and Kraehenbuhl, J. P. (2000). Nasal immunization of mice with virus-like particles protects offspring against rotavirus diarrhea. *J. Virol.* 74(19), 8966–8971.

Coulson, B. S., Grimwood, K., Masendycz, P. J., Lund, J. S., Mermelstein, N., Bishop, R. F., and Barnes, G. L. (1990). Comparison of rotavirus immunoglobulin A coproconversion with other indices of rotavirus infection in a longitudinal study in childhood. *J. Clin. Microbiol.* 28, 1367–1374.

Crowe, J. E., Jr., Firestone, C. Y., and Murphy, B. R. (2001). Passively acquired antibodies suppress humoral but not cell-mediated immunity in mice immunized with live attenuated respiratory syncytial virus vaccines. *J. Immunol.* 167(7), 3910–3918.

Czerkinsky, C., Prince, S. J., Michalek, S. M., Jackson, S., Russell, M. W., Moldoveanu, Z., McGhee, J. R., and Mestecky, J. (1987). IgA antibody-producing cells in peripheral blood after antigen ingestion: Evidence for a common mucosal immune system in humans. *Proc. Natl. Acad. Sci. USA* 84, 2449–2453.

De St. Groth, S. F., and Donnelley, M. (1950). Studies in experimental immunology of influenza. IV. The protective value of active immunization. *Aust. J. Exp. Bio. Med. Sci.* 28, 61–75.

Dharakul, T., Riepenhoff-Talty, M., Albini, B., and Ogra, P. L. (1988). Distribution of rotavirus antigen in intestinal lymphoid tissues: Potential role in development of the mucosal immune response to rotavirus. *Clin. Exper. Immunol.* 74, 14–19.

Dharakul, T., Rott, L., and Greenberg, H. B. (1990). Recovery from chronic rotavirus infection in mice with severe combined immunodeficiency: virus clearance mediated by adoptive transfer of immune CD8+ T lymphocytes. *J. Virol.* 64(9), 4375–4382.

Doherty, P. C., Topham, D. J., Tripp, R. A., Cardin, R. D., Brooks, J. W., and Stevenson, P. G. (1997). Effector CD4+ and CD8+ T-cell mechanisms in the control of respiratory virus infections. *Immunol. Rev.* 159, 105–117.

Eichelberger, M., Allan, W., Zijlstra, M., Jaenisch, R., and Doherty, P. C. (1991a). Clearance of influenza virus respiratory infection in mice lacking class 1 major histocompatibility complex-restricted CD8+ T cells. *J. Exp. Med.* 174, 875–880.

Eichelberger, M. C., Wang, M., Allan, W., Webster, R. G., and Doherty, P. C. (1991b). Influenza virus RNA in the lung and lymphoid tissue of immunologically intact and CD4-depleted mice. *J. Gen. Virol.* 72, 1695–1698.

Endo, A., Itamura, S., Iinuma, H., Funahashi, S.-L., Shida, H., Koide, F., Nerome, K., and Oya, A. (1991). Homotypic and heterotypic protection against influenza virus infection in mice by recombinant vaccinia virus expressing the haemagglutinin or nucleoprotein gene of influenza virus. *J. Gen. Virol.* 72, 699–703.

Feng, N., Lawton, J. A., Gilbert, J., Kuklin, N., Vo, P., Prasad, B. V., and Greenberg, H. B. (2002). Inhibition of rotavirus replication by a non-neutralizing, rotavirus VP6-specific IgA mAb. *J. Clin. Invest.* 109(9), 1203–1213.

Feng, N., Vo, P. T., Chung, D., Vo, T.-V. P., Hoshino, Y., and Greenberg, H. B. (1997). Heterotypic protection following oral immunization with live heterologous rotaviruses in a mouse model. *J. Infect. Dis.* 175, 330–341.

Fisher, R. G., Crowe, J. E., Jr., Johnson, T. R., Tang, Y. W., and Graham, B. S. (1999). Passive IgA monoclonal antibody is no more effective than IgG at protecting mice from mucosal challenge with respiratory syncytial virus. *J. Infect. Dis.* 180(4), 1324–1327.

Flynn, K. J., Belz, G. T., Altman, J. D., Ahmed, R., Woodland, D. L., and Doherty, P. C. (1998). Virus-specific CD8+ T cells in primary and secondary influenza pneumonia. *Immunity* 8(6), 683–691.

Franco, M. A., and Greenberg, H. B. (1999). Immunity to rotavirus infection in mice. *J. Infect. Dis.* 179 Suppl 3, S466–S469.

Friedman, M. G. (1982). Radioimmunoassay for the detection of virus-specific IgA antibodies in saliva. *J. Imunol. Meth.* 54, 203–211.

Friedman, M. G., Phillip, M., and Dagan, R. (1989). Virus-specific IgA in serum, saliva, and tears of children with measles. *Clin. Exp. Immunol.* 75, 58–63.

Fujioka, H., Emancipator, S. N., Aikawa, M., Huang, D. S., Blatnik, F., Karban, T., DeFife, K., and Mazanec, M. B. (1998). Immunocytochemical colocalization of specific immunoglobulin A with sendai virus protein in infected polarized epithelium. *J. Exp. Med.* 188(7), 1223–1229.

Gaddum, R. M., Cook, R. S., Wyld, S. G., Lopez, J. A., Bustos, R., Melero, J. A., and Taylor, G. (1996). Mutant forms of the F protein of human respiratory syncytial (RS) virus induce a cytotoxic T lymphocyte response but not a neutralizing antibody response and only transient resistance to RS virus infection. *J. Gen. Virol.* 77, 1239–1248.

Galletti, R., Beauverger, P., and Wild, T. F. (1995). Passively administered antibody suppresses the induction of measles virus antibodies by vaccinia-measles recombinant viruses. *Vaccine* 13, 197–201.

Gerhard, W. (2001). The role of the antibody response in influenza virus infection. *Curr. Top. Microbiol. Immunol.* 260, 171–190.

Giammarioli, A. M., Mackow, E. R., Fiore, L., Greenberg, H. B., and Ruggeri, F. M. (1996). Production and characterization of murine IgA monoclonal antibodies to the surface antigens of rhesus rotavirus. *Virology* 225, 97–110.

Gonzalez, A. M., Jaimes, M. C., Cajiao, I., Rojas, O. L., Cohen, J., Pothier, P., Kohli, E., Butcher, E. C., Greenberg, H. B., Angel, J., and Franco, M. A. (2003). Rotavirus-specific B cells induced by recent infection in adults and children predominantly express the intestinal homing receptor α4β7. *Virology* 305(1), 93–105.

Grimwood, K., Lund, J. C. S., Coulson, B. S., Hudson, I. L., Bishop, R. F., and Barnes, G. L. (1988). Comparison of serum and mucosal antibody responses following severe acute rotavirus gastroenteritis in young children. *J. Clin. Microbiol.* 26, 732–738.

Guidotti, L. G., Ishikawa, T., Hobbs, M. V., Matzke, B., Schreiber, R., and Chisari, F. V. (1996). Intracellular inactivation of the hepatitis B virus by cytotoxic T lymphocytes. *Immunity* 4(1), 25–36.

Haan, L., Verweij, W. R., Holtrop, M., Brands, R., van Scharrenburg, G. J., Palache, A. M., Agsteribbe, E., and Wilschut, J. (2001). Nasal or intramuscular immunization of mice with influenza subunit antigen and the B subunit of Escherichia coli heat-labile toxin induces IgA- or IgG-mediated protective mucosal immunity. *Vaccine* 19(20–22), 2898–2907.

Haneberg, B., Kendall, D., Amerongen, H. M., Apter, F. M., Kraehenbuhl, J. P., and Neutra, M. R. (1994). Induction of specific immunoglobulin A in the small intestine, colon-rectum, and vagina measured by a new method for collection of secretions from local mucosal surfaces. *Infect. Immun.* 62, 15–23.

Heinen, P. P., van Nieuwstadt, A. P., Pol, J. M., de Boer-Luijtze, E. A., van Oirschot, J. T., and Bianchi, A. T. (2000). Systemic and mucosal isotype-specific antibody responses in pigs to experimental influenza virus infection. *Viral Immunol.* 13(2), 237–247.

Herremans, T. M., Reimerink, J. H., Buisman, A. M., Kimman, T. G., and Koopmans, M. P. (1999). Induction of mucosal immunity by inactivated poliovirus vaccine is dependent on previous mucosal contact with live virus. *J. Immunol.* 162(8), 5011–5018.

Hicks, J. T., Ennis, F. A., Kim, E., and Verbonitz, M. (1978). The importance of an intact complement pathway in recovery from a primary viral infection: Influenza in decomplemented and in C5-deficient mice. *J. Immunol.* 121, 1437–1445.

Hirabayashi, Y., Kurata, H., Funato, H., Nagamine, T., Aizawa, C., Tamura, S.-I., Shimada, K., and Kurata, T. (1990). Comparison of intranasal inoculation of influenza HA vaccine combined with cholera toxin B subunit with oral or parenteral vaccination. *Vaccine* 8, 243–249.

Hjelt, K., Grauballe, P. C., Paerregaard, A., Nielsen, O. H., and Krasilnikoff, P. A. (1987). Protective effect of preexisting rotavirus-specific immunoglobulin A against naturally acquired rotavirus infection in children. *J. Med. Virol.* 21, 39–47.

Hogan, R. J., Cauley, L. S., Ely, K. H., Cookenham, T., Roberts, A. D., Brennan, J. W., Monard, S., and Woodland, D. L. (2002). Long-term maintenance of virus-specific effector memory CD8+ T cells in the lung airways depends on proliferation. *J. Immunol.* 169(9), 4976–4981.

Hogan, R. J., Usherwood, E. J., Zhong, W., Roberts, A. A., Dutton, R. W., Harmsen, A. G., and Woodland, D. L. (2001). Activated antigen-specific CD8+ T cells persist in the lungs following recovery from respiratory virus infections. *J. Immunol.* 166(3), 1813–1822.

Huber, V. C., Lynch, J. M., Bucher, D. J., Le, J., and Metzger, D. W. (2001). Fc receptor-mediated phagocytosis makes a significant contribution to clearance of influenza virus infections. *J. Immunol.* 166(12), 7381–7388.

Jayashree, S., Bhan, M. K., Kumar, R., Raj, P., Glass, R., and Bhandari, N. (1988). Serum and salivary antibodies as indicators of rotavirus infection in neonates. *J. Infect. Dis.* 158, 1117–1119.

Johnson, M. P., Meitin, C. A., Bender, B. S., and Small, P. A. (1988). Passive immune serum inhibits antibody response to recombinant vaccinia virus. In *Vaccines 88: Modern Approaches to New Vaccines, Including Prevention of AIDS* (eds. R. M. Chanock, R. A. Lerner, F. Brown, and H. Ginsberg). Cold Spring Harbor, NY: Cold Spring Harbor Laboratory Press.

Johnson, P. R., Feldman, S., Thompson, J. M., Mahoney, J. D., and Wright, P. F. (1986). Immunity to influenza A virus infection in young children: a comparison of natural infection, live cold-adapted vaccine, and inactivated vaccine. *J. Infect. Dis.* 154(1), 121–127.

Jones, P. D., and Ada, G. L. (1986). Influenza virus-specific antibody-secreting cells in the murine lung during primary influenza virus infection. *J. Virol.* 60, 614–619.

Kaetzel, C. S., Robinson, J. K., and Lamm, M. E. (1994). Epithelial transcytosis of monomeric IgA and IgG cross-linked through antigen to polymeric IgA. A role for monomeric antibodies in the mucosal immune system. *J. Immunol.* 152(1), 72–76.

Kagi, D., Seiler, P., Pavlovic, J., Ledermann, B., Burki, K., Zinkernagel, R. M., and Hengartner, H. (1995). The roles of perforin- and Fas-dependent cytotoxicity in protection against cytopathic and noncytopathic viruses. *Eur. J. Immunol.* 25(12), 3256–3262.

Kast, W. M., Bronkhorst, A. M., de Waal, L. P., and Melief, C. J. (1986). Cooperation between cytotoxic and helper T lymphocytes in protection against lethal Sendai virus infection. Protection by T cells is MHC-restricted and MHC-regulated; a model for MHC-disease associations. *J. Exp. Med.* 164(3), 723–738.

Kaul, T. N., Welliver, R. C., Wong, D. T., Udwadia, R. A., Riddlesberger, K., and Ogra, P. L. (1981). Secretory antibody response to respiratory syncytial virus infection. *Am. J. Dis. Child.* 135, 1013–1016.

Keller, R., and Dwyer, J. E. (1968). Neutralization of poliovirus by IgA coproantibodies. *J. Immunol.* 101, 192–202.

Kimman, T. G., and Westenbrink, F. (1990). Immunity to human and bovine respiratory syncytial virus. *Arch. Virol.* 112, 1–25.

Kimman, T. G., Westenbrink, F., Schreuder, B. E., and Straver, P. J. (1987). Local and systemic antibody response to bovine respiratory syncytial virus infection and reinfection in calves with and without maternal antibodies. *J. Clin. Microbiol.* 25(6), 1097–1106.

Kimman, T. G., Westenbrink, F., and Straver, P. J. (1989). Priming for local and systemic antibody memory responses to bovine respiratory syncytial virus: effect of amount of virus, virus replication, route of administration and maternal antibodies. *Vet. Immunol. Immunopathol.* 22(2), 145–160.

Klasse, P. J., and Sattentau, Q. J. (2002). Occupancy and mechanism in antibody-mediated neutralization of animal viruses. *J. Gen. Virol.* 83(Pt 9), 2091–2108.

Knossow, M., Gaudier, M., Douglas, A., Barrere, B., Bizebard, T., Barbey, C., Gigant, B., and Skehel, J. J. (2002). Mechanism of neutralization of influenza virus infectivity by antibodies. *Virology* 302(2), 294–298.

Kopf, M., Brombacher, F., and Bachmann, M. F. (2002). Role of IgM antibodies versus B cells in influenza virus-specific immunity. *Eur. J. Immunol.* 32(8), 2229–2236.

Kuklin, N. A., Rott, L., Darling, J., Campbell, J. J., Franco, M., Feng, N., Muller, W., Wagner, N., Altman, J., Butcher, E. C., and Greenberg, H. B. (2000). alpha(4)beta(7) independent pathway for CD8(+) T cell-mediated intestinal immunity to rotavirus. *J. Clin. Invest.* 106(12), 1541–1552.

Kuklin, N. A., Rott, L., Feng, N., Conner, M. E., Wagner, N., Muller, W., and Greenberg, H. B. (2001). Protective intestinal anti-rotavirus B cell immunity is dependent on alpha 4 beta 7 integrin expression but does not require IgA antibody production. *J. Immunol.* 166(3), 1894–1902.

Kunkel, E. J., and Butcher, E. C. (2002). Chemokines and the tissue-specific migration of lymphocytes. *Immunity* 16(1), 1–4.

Lawson, C. M., Bennink, J. R., Restifo, N. P., Yewdell, J. W., and Murphy, B. R. (1994). Primary pulmonary cytotoxic T lympho-cytes induced by immunization with a vaccinia virus recombi-nant expressing influenza A virus nucleoprotein peptide do not protect mice against challenge. *J. Virol.* 68(6), 3505–3511.

Lepow, M. L., Warren, R. J., Gray, N., Ingram, V. G., and Robbins, F. C. (1961). Effect of Sabin type 1 poliomyelitis vaccine administered by mouth to newborn infants. *N. Engl. J. Med.* 264, 1071–1078.

Leung, K. N., and Ada, G. L. (1980). Cells mediating delayed-type hypersensitivity in the lungs of mice infected with an influenza A virus. *Scandinavian Journal of Immunology* 12, 393–400.

Liang, B., Hyland, L., and Hou, S. (2001). Nasal-associated lymphoid tissue is a site of long-term virus-specific antibody production following respiratory virus infection of mice. *J. Virol.* 75(11), 5416–5420.

Liang, X. P., Lamm, M. E., and Nedrud, J. G. (1988). Oral administra-tion of cholera toxin-Sendai virus conjugate potentiates gut and respiratory immunity against Sendai virus. *J. Immunol.* 141(5), 1495–1501.

Liew, F. Y., Russell, S. M., Appleyard, G., Brand, C. M., and Beale, J. (1984). Cross-protection in mice infected with influenza A virus by the respiratory route is correlated with local IgA anti-body rather that serum antibody or cytoxic T cell reactivity. *Eur. J. Immunol.* 14, 350–356.

Lightman, S., Cobbold, S., Waldmann, H., and Askonas, B. A. (1987). Do L3T4+ T cells act as effector cells in protection against influenza virus infection? *Immunology* 62(1), 139–144.

Ludert, J. E., Ruiz, M. C., Hidalgo, C., and Liprandi, F. (2002). Antibodies to rotavirus outer capsid glycoprotein VP7 neutralize infectivity by inhibiting virion decapsidation. *J. Virol.* 76(13), 6643–6651.

Lyn, D., Mazanec, M. B., Nedrud, J. G., and Portner, A. (1991). Location of amino acid residues important for the structure and biological function of the haemagglutinin-neuraminidase glyco-protein of Sendai virus by analysis of escape mutants. *J. Gen. Virol.* 72, 817–824.

Mackenzie, C. D., and Taylor, P. M. (1989). Rapid recovery of lung his-tology correlates with clearance of influenza virus by specific CD8+ cytotoxic T cells. *Immunology* 67, 375–381.

Madden, D. R., Gorga, J. C., Strominger, J. L., and Wiley, D. C. (1991). The structure of HLA-B27 reveals nonamer self-peptides bound in an extended conformation. *Nature* 353, 321–325.

Maoliang, W. (1986). Production of IgA monoclonal antibodies against influenza A virus. *J. Virol. Method* 13, 21–26.

Matson, D. O., O'Ryan, M. L., Herrera, I., Pickering, L. K., and Estes, M. K. (1993). Fecal antibody responses to symptomatic and asymptomatic rotavirus infections. *J. Infect. Dis.* 167, 577–583.

Mazanec, M. B., Coudret, C. L., and Fletcher, D. R. (1995). Intracellular neutralization of influenza virus by immunoglobulin A anti-hemagglutinin monoclonal antibodies. *J. Virol.* 69(2), 1339–1343.

Mazanec, M. B., Kaetzel, C. S., Lamm, M. E., Fletcher, D., and Nedrud, J. G. (1992a). Intracellular neutralization of virus by immunoglobulin A antibodies. *Proc. Natl. Acad. Sci. USA* 89(15), 6901–6905.

Mazanec, M. B., Lamm, M. E., Lyn, D., Portner, A., and Nedrud, J. G. (1992b). Comparison of IgA versus IgG monoclonal antibodies for passive immunization of the murine respiratory tract. *Virus Res.* 23(1–2), 1–12.

Mazanec, M. B., Nedrud, J. G., and Lamm, M. E. (1987). Immunoglobulin A monoclonal antibodies protect against Sendai virus. *J. Virol.* 61(8), 2624–2626.

McBride, B. W., and Ward, K. A. (1987). Herpes simplex-specific IgG subclass response in herpetic keratitis. *J. Med. Virol.* 21, 179–189.

McDermott, M. R., Lukacher, A. E., Braciale, V. L., Braciale, T. J., and Bienenstock, J. (1987). Characterization and in vivo distribution

of influenza-virus-specific T-lymphocytes in the murine respira-tory tract. *Am. Rev. Respir. Dis.* 135(1), 245–249.

McIntosh, K., Masters, H. B., Orr, I., Chao, R. K., and Barkin, R. M. (1978). The immunologic response to infection with respiratory syncytial virus in infants. *J. Infect. Dis.* 138(1), 24–32.

McIntosh, K., McQuillin, J., and Gardner, P. S. (1979). Cell-free and cell-bound antibody in nasal secretions from infants with respi-ratory syncytial virus infection. *Infect. Immun.* 23(2), 276–281.

McMichael, A. J., Gotch, F. M., Noble, G. R., and Beare, P. A. S. (1983). Cytotoxic T-cell immunity to influenza. *N. Engl. J. Med.* 309, 13–17.

McNeal, M. M., VanCott, J. L., Choi, A. H., Basu, M., Flint, J. A., Stone, S. C., Clements, J. D., and Ward, R. L. (2002). CD4 T cells are the only lymphocytes needed to protect mice against rotavirus shedding after intranasal immunization with a chimeric VP6 protein and the adjuvant LT(R192G). *J. Virol.* 76(2), 560–568.

Merchant, A. A., Groene, W. S., Cheng, E. H., and Shaw, R. D. (1991). Murine intestinal antibody response to heterologous rotavirus infection. *J. Clin. Microbiol.* 29, 1693–1701.

Merriman, H., Woods, S., Winter, C., Fahnlander, A., and Corey, L. (1984). Secretory IgA antibody in cervicovaginal secretions from women with genital infection due to herpes simplex virus. *J. Infect. Dis.* 149, 505–510.

Mestecky, J. (1987). The common mucosal immune system and current strategies for induction of immune responses in external secre-tions. *J. Clin. Immunol.* 7, 265–276.

Mills, J., Van Kirk, J. E., Wright, P. F., and Chanock, R. M. (1971). Experimental respiratory syncytial virus infection of adults. Possible mechanisms of resistance to infection and illness. *J. Immunol.* 107(1), 123–130.

Munoz, J. L., McCarthy, C. A., Clark, M. E., and Hall, C. B. (1991). Respiratory syncytial virus infection in C57BL/6 mice: clearance of virus from the lungs with virus-specific cytotoxic T cells. *J. Virol.* 65(8), 4494–4497.

Murphy, B. R., Alling, D. W., Snyder, M. H., Walsh, E. E., Prince, G. A., Chanock, R. M., Hemming, V. G., Rodriguez, W. J., Kim, H. W., and Graham, B. S. (1986a). Effect of age and preexisting anti-body on serum antibody response of infants and children to the F and G glycoproteins during respiratory syncytial virus infec-tion. *J. Clin. Microbiol.* 24(5), 894–898.

Murphy, B. R., Chalhub, E. G., Nusinoff, S. R., Kasel, J., and Chanock, R. M. (1973). Temperature-sensitive mutants of influenza virus. III. Further characterization of the ts-1(E) influenza A recombi-nant (H3N2) virus in man. *J. Infect. Dis.* 128(4), 479–487.

Murphy, B. R., Collins, P. L., Lawrence, L., Zubak, J., Chanock, R. M., and Prince, G. A. (1989). Immunosuppression of the antibody response to respiratory syncytial virus (RSV) by pre-existing serum antibodies: partial prevention by topical infection of the respiratory tract with vaccinia virus-RSV recombinants. *J. Gen. Virol.* 70, 2185–2190.

Murphy, B. R., Graham, B. S., Prince, G. A., Walsh, E. E., Chanock, R. M., Karzon, D. T., and Wright, P. F. (1986b). Serum and nasal-wash immunoglobulin G and A antibody response of infants and children to respiratory syncytial virus F and G gly-coproteins following primary infection. *J. Clin. Microbiol.* 23(6), 1009–1014.

Murphy, B. R., Nelson, D. L., Wright, P. F., Tierney, E. L., Phelan, M. A., and Chanock, R. M. (1982). Secretory and systemic immunological response in children infected with live attenu-ated influenza A virus vaccines. *Infect. Immun.* 36(3), 1102–1108.

Murphy, B. R., Olmsted, R. A., Collins, P. L., Chanock, R. M., and Prince, G. A. (1988). Passive transfer of respiratory syncytial virus (RSV) antiserum suppresses the immune response to the RSV fusion (F) and large (G) glycoproteins expressed by recom-binant vaccinia viruses. *J. Virol.* 62(10), 3907–3910.

Murphy, B. R., Prince, G. A., Walsh, E. E., Kim, H. W., Parrott, R. H., Hemming, V. G., Rodriguez, W. J., and Chanock, R. M. (1986c). Dissociation between serum neutralizing and glycoprotein anti-body responses of infants and children who received inactivated respiratory syncytial virus vaccine. *J. Clin. Microbiol.* 24(2), 197–202.

Nedrud, J. G., Liang, X. P., Hague, N., and Lamm, M. E. (1987a). Combined oral/nasal immunization protects mice from Sendai virus infection. *J. Immunol.* 139(10), 3484–3492.

Nedrud, J. G., Mazanec, M. B., Liang, X., Hague, N., and Lamm, M. E. (1987b). Induction and expression of respiratory IgA immunity against Sendai virus in mice. *Adv. Exp. Med. Biol.* 216B, 1847–1854.

Nguyen, H. H., van Ginkel, F. W., Vu, H. L., McGhee, J. R., and Mestecky, J. (2001). Heterosubtypic immunity to influenza A virus infection requires B cells but not CD8[+] cytotoxic T lymphocytes. *J. Infect. Dis.* 183(3), 368–376.

Nicholas, J. A., Rubino, K. L., Levely, M. E., Meyer, A. L., and Collins, P. L. (1991). Cytotoxic T cell activity against the 22-kDa protein of human respiratory syncytial virus (RSV) is associated with a significant reduction in pulmonary RSV replication. *Virology* 182(2), 664–672.

Nishio, O., Sumi, J., Sakae, K., Ishihara, Y., Isomura, S., and Inouye, S. (1990). Fecal IgA antibody responses after oral poliovirus vaccination in infants and elder children. *Microbiol. Immunol.* 34, 683–689.

O'Neal, C. M., Harriman, G. R., and Conner, M. E. (2000). Protection of the villus epithelial cells of the small intestine from rotavirus infection does not require immunoglobulin A. *J. Virol.* 74(9), 4102–4109.

Offit, P. A., and Dudzik, K. I. (1990). Rotavirus-specific cytotoxic T lymphocytes passively protect against gastroenteritis in suckling mice. *J. Virol.* 64, 6325–6328.

Offit, P. A., Shaw, R. D., and Greenberg, H. B. (1986). Passive protection against rotavirus-induced diarrhea by monoclonal antibodies to surface proteins VP3 and VP7. *J. Virol.* 58, 700–703.

Ogra, P. L. (1970). Distribution of echovirus antibody in serum nasopharynx, rectum, and spinal fluid after natural infection with echovirus type 6. *Infect. Immun.* 2, 150–155.

Ogra, P. L., Coppola, P. R., MacGillivray, M. H., and Dzierba, J. L. (1974). Mechanism of mucosal immunity to viral infections in A immunoglobulin-deficiency syndromes. *Proc. Soc. Exp. Biol. Med.* 145, 811–816.

Ogra, P. L., and Karzon, D. T. (1969a). Distribution of poliovirus antibody in serum, nasopharynx and alimentary tract following segmental immunization of lower alimentary tract with poliovaccine. *J. Immunol.* 102, 1423–1430.

Ogra, P. L., and Karzon, D. T. (1969b). Polivirus antibody response in serum and nasal secretions following intranasal inoculation with inactivated poliovaccine. *J. Immunol.* 102, 15–23.

Onorato, I. M., Modlin, J. F., McBean, A. M., Thomas, M. L., Losonsky, G. A., and Bernier, R. H. (1991). Mucosal immunity induced by enhanced-potency inactivated and oral polio vaccines. *J. Infect. Dis.* 163, 1–6.

Outlaw, M. C., and Dimmock, N. J. (1991). Insights into neutralization of animal viruses gained from study of influenza virus. *Epidemiol. Infect.* 106, 205–220.

Palladino, G., Mozdzanowska, K., Washko, G., and Gerhard, W. (1995). Virus-neutralizing antibodies of immunoglobulin G (IgG) but not of IgM or IgA isotypes can cure influenza virus pneumonia in SCID mice. *J. Virol.* 69(4), 2075–2081.

Perkins, J. C., Tucker, D. N., Knopf, H. L. S., Wenzel, R. P., Kapikian, A. Z., and Chanock, R. M. (1969). Comparison of protective effect of neutralizing antibody in serum and nasal secretions in experimental rhinovirus type 13 illness. *Am. J. Epidemiol.* 90, 519–526.

Plotnicky-Gilquin, H., Cyblat-Chanal, D., Aubry, J. P., Champion, T., Beck, A., Nguyen, T., Bonnefoy, J. Y., and Corvaia, N. (2002). Gamma interferon-dependent protection of the mouse upper respiratory tract following parenteral immunization with a respiratory syncytial virus G protein fragment. *J. Virol.* 76(20), 10203–10210.

Ponzi, A. N., Merlino, C., Angeretti, A., and Penna, R. (1985). Virus-specific polymeric immunoglobulin A antibodies in serum from patients with rubella, measles, varicella, and herpes zoster virus infections. *J. Clin. Microbiol.* 22, 505–509.

Prince, G. A., Hemming, V. G., Horswood, R. L., Baron, P. A., Murphy, B. R., and Chanock, R. M. (1990). Mechanism of antibody-mediated viral clearance in immunotherapy of respiratory syncytial virus infection of cotton rats. *J. Virol.* 64(6), 3091–3092.

Prince, G. A., Horswood, R. L., and Chanock, R. M. (1985). Quantitative aspects of passive immunity to respiratory syncytial virus infection in infant cotton rats. *J. Virol.* 55(3), 517–520.

Puck, J. M., Glezen, W. P., Frank, A. L., and Six, H. R. (1980). Protection of infants from infection with influenza A virus by transplacentally acquired antibody. *J. Infect. Dis.* 142, 844–849.

Ramphal, R., Cogliano, R. C., Shands, J. W., and Small, P. A. (1979). Serum antibody prevents lethal murine influenza pneumonitis but not tracheitis. *Infect. Immun.* 25, 992–997.

Ray, R., Glaze, B. J., Moldoveanu, Z., and Compans, R. W. (1988). Intranasal immunization of hamsters with envelope glycoproteins of human parainfluenza virus type 3. *J. Infect. Dis.* 157(4), 648–654.

Renegar, K. B., and Small, P. A. (1991). Passive transfer of local immunity to influenza virus infection by IgA antibody. *J. Immunol.* 146, 1972–1978.

Reuman, P. D., Ayoub, E. M., and Small, P. A. (1987). Effect of passive maternal antibody on influenza illness in children: A prospective study of influenza A in mother-infant pairs. *Pediatr. Infect. Dis. J.* 6, 398–403.

Reuman, P. D., Keely, S. P., and Schiff, G. M. (1990). Rapid recovery in mice after combined nasal/oral immunization with killed respiratory syncytial virus. *J. Med. Virol.* 32(1), 67–72.

Reuman, P. D., Paganini, C. M. A., Ayoub, E. M., and Small, P. A. (1983). Maternal-infant transfer of influenza-specific immunity in the mouse. *J. Immunol.* 130, 932–936.

Riberdy, J. M., Christensen, J. P., Branum, K., and Doherty, P. C. (2000). Diminished primary and secondary influenza virus-specific CD8(+) T-cell responses in CD4-depleted Ig(–/–) mice. *J. Virol.* 74(20), 9762–9765.

Richardson, S. C., and Bishop, R. F. (1990). Homotypic serum antibody responses to rotavirus proteins following primary infection of young children with serotype 1 rotavirus. *J. Clin. Microbiol.* 28, 1891–1897.

Richman, D. D., Murphy, B. R., Tierney, E. L., and Chanock, R. M. (1974). Specificity of the local secretory antibody to influenza A virus infection. *J. Immunol.* 113(5), 1654–1656.

Rose, J. R., Williams, M. B., Rott, L. S., Butcher, E. C., and Greenberg, H. B. (1998). Expression of the mucosal homing receptor alpha4beta7 correlates with the ability of CD8[+] memory T cells to clear rotavirus infection. *J. Virol.* 72(1), 726–730.

Rubin, D. H., Anderson, A. O., and Lucis, D. (1983). Potentiation of the secretory IgA response by oral and enteric administration of CP 20,961. *Ann. NY Acad. Sci.* 409, 866–870.

Rudzik, R., Clancy, R. L., Perey, D. Y. E., Day, R. P., and Bienenstock, J. (1975). Repopulation with IgA-containing cells of bronchial and intestinal lamina propria after transfer of homologous Peyer's patch and bronchial lymphocytes. *J. Immunol.* 114, 1599–1604.

Ruggeri, F. M., Johansen, K., Basile, G., Kraehenbuhl, J. P., and Svensson, L. (1998). Antirotavirus immunoglobulin A neutralizes virus in vitro after transcytosis through epithelial cells and protects infant mice from diarrhea. *J. Virol.* 72(4), 2708–2714.

Sabin, A. B., Michaels, R. H., Krugman, S., Eiger, M. E., Berman, P. H., and Warren, J. (1963a). Effect of oral poliovirus vaccine in newborn children. I. Excretion of virus after ingestion of large doses of type I or of mixture of all three types, in relation to level of placentally transmitted antibody. *Pediatrics* 31, 623–640.

Sabin, A. B., Michaels, R. H., Ziring, P., Krugman, S., and Warren, J. (1963b). Effect of oral poliovirus vaccine in newborn children. II. Intestinal resistance and antibody response at 6 months in children fed type I vaccine at birth. *Pediatrics* 31, 641–654.

Sanchez, P. J. (2002). Immunoprophylaxis for respiratory syncytial virus. *Pediatr. Infect. Dis. J.* 21(5), 473–478.

Scherle, P. A., Palladino, G., and Gerhard, W. (1992). Mice can recover from pulmonary influenza virus infection in the absence of class I-restricted cytotoxic T cells. *J. Immunol.* 148(1), 212–217.

Schwartz-Cornil, I., Benureau, Y., Greenberg, H., Hendrickson, B. A., and Cohen, J. (2002). Heterologous protection induced by the inner capsid proteins of rotavirus requires transcytosis of mucosal immunoglobulins. *J. Virol.* 76(16), 8110–8117.

Scott, R. M., Dudding, B. A., Romano, S. V., and Russell, P. K. (1972). Enteric immunization with live adenovirus type 21 vaccine. II.

Systemic and local immune responses following immunization. *Infect. Immun.* 5, 300–304.

Shaw, R. D., Groene, W. S., Mackow, E. R., Merchant, A. A., and Cheng, E. H. (1991). VP4-specific intestinal antibody response to rotavirus in a murine model of heterotypic infection. *J. Virol.* 65, 3052–3059.

Silvey, K. J., Hutchings, A. B., Vajdy, M., Petzke, M. M., and Neutra, M. R. (2001). Role of immunoglobulin A in protection against reovirus entry into Murine Peyer's patches. *J. Virol.* 75(22), 10870–10879.

Simeckova-Rosenberg, J., Yun, Z., Wyde, P. R., and Atassi, M. Z. (1995). Protection of mice against lethal viral infection by synthetic peptides corresponding to B- and T-cell recognition sites of influenza A hemagglutinin. *Vaccine* 13(10), 927–932.

Smith, C. B., Purcell, R. H., Bellanti, J. A., and Chanock, R. M. (1966). Protective effect of antibody to parainfluenza type 1 virus. *N. Engl. J. Med.* 275(21), 1145–1152.

Smith, T. J., Buescher, E. L., Top, F. H., Altemeier, W. A., and McCown, J. M. (1970). Experimental respiratory infection with type 4 adenovirus vaccine in volunteers: Clinical and immunological responses. *J. Infect. Dis.* 122, 239–248.

Sonza, S., and Holmes, I. H. (1980). Coproantibody response to rotavirus infection. *Med. J. Aust.* 2, 496–499.

Staats, H. F., Nichols, W. G., and Palker, T. J. (1996). Mucosal immunity to HIV-1: systemic and vaginal antibody responses after intranasal immunization with the HIV-1 C4/V3 peptide T1SP10 MN(A). *J. Immunol.* 157(1), 462–472.

Takao, S. I., Kiyotani, K., Sakaguchi, T., Fujii, Y., Seno, M., and Yoshida, T. (1997). Protection of mice from respiratory Sendai virus infections by recombinant vaccinia viruses. *J. Virol.* 71(1), 832–838.

Tamura, S., Iwasaki, T., Thompson, A. H., Asanuma, H., Chen, Z., Suzuki, Y., Aizawa, C., and Kurata, T. (1998). Antibody-forming cells in the nasal-associated lymphoid tissue during primary influenza virus infection. *J. Gen. Virol.* 79 (Pt 2), 291–299.

Tamura, S.-I., Funato, H., Hirabayashi, Y., Kikuta, K., Suzuki, Y., Nagamine, T., Aizawa, C., Nakagawa, M., and Kurata, T. (1990). Functional role of respiratory tract haemagglutinin-specific IgA antibodies in protection against influenza. *Vaccine* 8, 479–485.

Taylor, G., Thomas, L. H., Wyld, S. G., Furze, J., Sopp, P., and Howard, C. J. (1995). Role of T-lymphocyte subsets in recovery from respiratory syncytial virus infection in calves. *J. Virol.* 69(11), 6658–6664.

Taylor, P. M., and Askonas, B. A. (1986). Influenza nucleoprotein-specific cytotoxic T-cell clones are protective *in vivo*. *Immunology* 58, 417–420.

Taylor, P. M., Esquivel, F., and Askonas, B. A. (1990). Murine CD4+ T cell clones vary in function in vitro and in influenza infection in vivo. *Int. Immunol.* 2(4), 323–328.

Topham, D. J., Tripp, R. A., and Doherty, P. C. (1997). CD8+ T cells clear influenza virus by perforin or Fas-dependent processes. *J. Immunol.* 159(11), 5197–5200.

Tsutsumi, H., Matsuda, K., Yamazaki, H., Ogra, P. L., and Chiba, S. (1995). Different kinetics of antibody responses between IgA and IgG classes in nasopharyngeal secretion in infants and children during primary respiratory syncytial virus infection. *Acta Paediatr. Jpn.* 37(4), 464–468.

Valtanen, S., Roivainen, M., Piirainen, L., Stenvik, M., and Hovi, T. (2000). Poliovirus-specific intestinal antibody responses coincide with decline of poliovirus excretion. *J. Infect. Dis.* 182(1), 1–5.

Varga, S. M., and Braciale, T. J. (2002). RSV-induced immunopathology: dynamic interplay between the virus and host immune response. *Virology* 295(2), 203–207.

Wagner, D. K., Clements, M. L., Reimer, C. B., Snyder, M., Nelson, D. L., and Murphy, B. R. (1987). Analysis of immunoglobulin G antibody responses after administration of live and inactivated influenza A vaccine indicates that nasal wash immunoglobulin G is a transudate from serum. *J. Clin. Microbiol.* 25(3), 559–562.

Waldman, R. H., Kasel, J. A., Fulk, R. V., Togo, Y., Hornick, R. B., Heiner, G. G., Dawkins, A. T., and Mann, J. J. (1968). Influenza antibody in human respiratory secretions after subcutaneous or respiratory immunization with inactivated virus. *Nature* 218, 594–595.

Waldman, R. H., Stone, J., Bergmann, K. C., Khakoo, R., Lazzell, V., Jacknowitz, A., Waldman, E. R., and Howard, S. (1986). Secretory antibody following oral influenza immunization. *Am. J. Med. Sci.* 292, 367–371.

Waldman, R. H., Wood, S. H., Torres, E. J., and Small, P. A. (1970). Influenza antibody response following aerosol administration of inactivated virus. *Am. J. Epidemiol.* 91, 575–584.

Ward, R. L., Bernstein, D. I., Shukla, R., McNeal, M. M., Sherwood, J. R., Young, E. C., and Schiff, G. M. (1990). Protection of adults rechallenged with a human rotavirus. *J. Infect. Dis.* 161, 440–445.

Ward, R. L., Bernstein, D. I., Shukla, R., Young, E. C., Sherwood, J. R., McNeal, M. M., Walker, M. C., and Schiff, G. M. (1989). Effects of antibody to rotavirus on protection of adults challenged with a human rotavirus. *J. Infect. Dis.* 159, 79–88.

Watt, P. J., Robinson, B. S., Pringle, C. R., and Tyrrell, D. A. (1990). Determinants of susceptibility to challenge and the antibody response of adult volunteers given experimental respiratory syncytial virus vaccines. *Vaccine* 8(3), 231–236.

Webster, R. G., Kawaoka, Y., Taylor, J., Weinberg, R., and Paoletti, E. (1991). Efficacy of nucleoprotein and haemagglutinin antigens expressed in fowlpox virus as vaccine for influenza in chickens. *Vaccine* 9, 303–308.

Weltzin, R., Lucia-Jandris, P., Michetti, P., Fields, B. N., Kraehenbuhl, J. P., and Neutra, M. R. (1989). Binding and transepithelial transport of immunoglobulins by intestinal M cells: Demonstration using monoclonal IgA antibodies against enteric viral proteins. *J. Cell Biol.* 108, 1673–1685.

Wright, P. F., Karron, R. A., Belshe, R. B., Thompson, J., Crowe Jr, J. E., Boyce, T. G., Halburnt, L. L., Reed, G. W., Whitehead, S. S., Anderson, E. L., Wittek, A. E., Casey, R., Eichelberger, M., Thumar, B., Randolph, V. B., Udem, S. A., Chanock, R. M., and Murphy, B. R. (2000). Evaluation of a live, cold-passaged, temperature-sensitive, respiratory syncytial virus vaccine candidate in infancy. *J. Infect. Dis.* 182(5), 1331–1342.

Wright, P. F., Murphy, B. R., Kervina, M., Lawrence, E. M., Phelan, M. A., and Karzon, D. T. (1983). Secretory immunological response after intranasal inactivated influenza A virus vaccinations: evidence for immunoglobulin A memory. *Infect. Immun.* 40(3), 1092–1095.

Yamaguchi, H., Inouye, S., Yamauchi, M., Morishima, T., Matsuno, S., Isomura, S., and Suzuki, S. (1985). Anamnestic response in fecal IgA antibody production after rotaviral infection of infants. *J. Infect. Dis.* 152, 398–400.

Yamazaki, H., Tsutsumi, H., Matsuda, K., Nagai, K., Ogra, P. L., and Chiba, S. (1994). Effect of maternal antibody on IgA antibody response in nasopharyngeal secretion in infants and children during primary respiratory syncytial virus infection. *J. Gen. Virol.* 75(Pt 8), 2115–2119.

Yan, H., Lamm, M. E., Bjorling, E., and Huang, Y. T. (2002). Multiple functions of immunoglobulin A in mucosal defense against viruses: an in vitro measles virus model. *J. Virol.* 76(21), 10972–10979.

Yao, Q. Y., Rowe, M., Morgan, A. J., Sam, C. K., Prasad, U., Dang, H., Zeng, Y., and Rickinson, A. B. (1991). Salivary and serum IgA antibodies to the Epstein-Barr virus glycoprotein gp340: Incidence and potential for virus neutralization. *Int. J. Cancer* 48, 45–50.

Yap, K. L., Ada, G. L., and McKensie, I. F. C. (1978). Transfer of specific cytotoxic T lymphocytes protects mice inoculated with influenza virus. *Nature* 273, 238–239.

Youngman, K. R., Franco, M. A., Kuklin, N. A., Rott, L. S., Butcher, E. C., and Greenberg, H. B. (2002). Correlation of tissue distribution, developmental phenotype, and intestinal homing receptor expression of antigen-specific B cells during the murine anti-rotavirus immune response. *J. Immunol.* 168(5), 2173–2181.

Yuan, L., and Saif, L. J. (2002). Induction of mucosal immune responses and protection against enteric viruses: rotavirus infection of gnotobiotic pigs as a model. *Vet. Immunol. Immunopathol.* 87(3–4), 147–160.

Yuan, L., Ward, L. A., Rosen, B. I., To, T. L., and Saif, L. J. (1996). Systemic and intestinal antibody-secreting cell responses and correlates of protective immunity to human rotavirus in a gnotobiotic pig model of disease. *J. Virol.* 70(5), 3075–3083.

Zhaori, G., Sun, M., Faden, H. S., and Ogra, P. L. (1989). Nasopharyngeal secretory antibody response to poliovirus type 3 virion proteins exhibit different specificities after immunization with live or inactivated poliovirus vaccines. *J. Infect. Dis.* 159, 1018–1024.

Zhong, W., Roberts, A. D., and Woodland, D. L. (2001). Antibody-independent antiviral function of memory CD4+ T cells in vivo requires regulatory signals from CD8+ effector T cells. *J. Immunol.* 167(3), 1379–1386.

Zuercher, A. W., Coffin, S. E., Thurnheer, M. C., Fundova, P., and Cebra, J. J. (2002a). Nasal-associated lymphoid tissue is a mucosal inductive site for virus-specific humoral and cellular immune responses. *J. Immunol.* 168(4), 1796–1803.

Zuercher, A. W., Jiang, H. Q., Thurnheer, M. C., Cuff, C. F., and Cebra, J. J. (2002b). Distinct mechanisms for cross-protection of the upper versus lower respiratory tract through intestinal priming. *J. Immunol.* 169(7), 3920–3925.

Mucosal Immune Response to Parasitic Infections

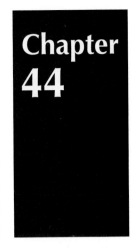

Chapter 44

Mohamed D. Abd-Alla and Jonathan I. Ravdin

Department of Medicine, University of Minnesota, Minneapolis, Minnesota

Mucosal immune responses to parasitic infestations are a sequel of direct contact between the parasite and the host mucosa, the outcome of which is both host and parasite dependent. A competent host immune system, antigenicity of parasite constituents, and duration of contact are factors contributing to development of mucosal immunity. The spectrum of mucosal antiparasitic immune responses is broad, and knowledge is still developing in most parasitic infections.

Parasites live on or in another organism during some aspect of their life cycle to draw nourishment from the host. More than half the population of the world harbors parasites, often without demonstrable injury to the host. The intensity of the infection, the nature of the parasite, and specific host–parasite interactions determine the degree of tissue injury and manifestations of disease.

There is a complex interplay between parasite and host; many parasites have sophisticated mechanisms for evading human immune responses. In some instances, parasites hide within host cells or modulate their surface antigen expression. The success of a parasite may also depend on its achieving the right location within the host. Host factors like nutritional condition, genetic susceptibility, and immune status may influence the outcome of the infection.

Many parasites interact with the mucosal immune system (Weinstock, 1996), including protozoans such as *Entamoeba histolytica* and *Giardia lamblia*, nematodes like *Ascaris lumbricoides*, trematodes such as *Clonorchis sinensis* (biliary fluke), and cestodes like *Taenia saginata* (beef tapeworm). The success of their parasitism depends on establishing a tranquil relationship with host mucosal defenses. Parasites inhabit distinct regions of the intestines, establishing unique immunological relationships. The objective of this chapter is to review our current understanding of the host mucosal immune response to intestinal parasites.

PROTOZOAL INFECTIONS

Parasitic protozoa are a major cause of global infection. The most commonly encountered intestinal protozoa producing gastrointestinal manifestations are *E. histolytica*, *G. lamblia* and *Cryptosporidium parvum*. Diseases associated with immunodeficiency predispose to severe intestinal infections by *Isospora belli* and microsporidia. These protozoans are extracellular parasites. A critical step in their host interaction is the evasion of the innate immune system. There are many other intestinal protozoa such as *Entamoeba coli*, *Endolimax nana*, and *Entamoeba polichi* that are harmless commensals.

Amebiasis

General comments

Human amebiasis is caused by *E. histolytica* and *Entamoeba dispar*, which are separate but morphologically identical species. *E. dispar* infection is always asymptomatic and noninvasive. *E. histolytica* causes both invasive and asymptomatic infection. Each is a unicellular protozoan parasite with a two-stage life cycle involving cyst and trophozoite forms. The parasites are transmitted by consumption of food or water contaminated with amebic cysts or by the direct fecal-oral route. In the small intestine excystation occurs, resulting in four trophozoites, which go on to colonize in the colon and multiply by binary fission. Trophozoites have the ability to either adhere to colonic mucosa, producing an established infection, or encyst and recycle back into the environment with excreta. Amebic infection is almost always associated with lack of proper sanitation, poor hygiene, or oral–anal sexual practices. The highest infection rates are in developing countries. In developed countries, high-risk groups for amebic infection include inhabitants of prisons and mental institutions, travelers to endemic regions, and sexually promiscuous homosexual men.

Infection in the host's colon is mediated by the amebic galactose-inhibitable adherence lectin, allowing trophozoites to adhere to colonic mucins. A Ca^{++} mediated lethal hit produced by *E. histolytica* trophozoites kills host cells. Disease syndromes produced by *E. histolytica* include colitis and liver abscess, and both symptomatic and asymptomatic *E. histolytica* infection is associated with pathological changes in the colonic mucosa. Clearance of *E. histolytica* is directly related to development of the host's mucosal and humoral immune response. Infection with *E. dispar* trophozoites is not associated with pathological changes in the colon. Clearance of *E. dispar* may also be related to the development of a mucosal immune response. Continuous availability of amebic cysts in different environments in endemic areas makes parasite recycling among the population unavoidable.

Amebiasis is the third leading parasite cause of death worldwide, after malaria and schistosomiasis, resulting from over 40 million cases of severe colitis or liver abscess annually. The diagnosis of intestinal amebiasis rests mostly on microscopic demonstration of either cysts or trophozoites in the stool or mucosal biopsies. Serological tests are most helpful in the diagnosis of amebic liver abscess. Trials for detection of fecal amebic ribosomal DNA by polymerase chain reaction (PCR) (Blessmann *et al.*, 2002) and amebic surface adherence lectin protein by enzyme-linked immunosorbent assay (ELISA) (Abd-Alla *et al.*, 1993; Haque *et al.*, 2000) are promising. Patients harboring *E. histolytica* require treatment of both tissue and luminal phases.

Host immunity

Colonic mucins are the first protective barrier against intestinal pathogens, and adhesion of *E. histolytica* to mucins and depletion of mucins occur prior to parasite invasion (Petri *et al.*, 2002). Amebic trophozoites resist mechanical washout with intestinal contents and peristalsis by interaction between the ameba's galactose-inhibitable lectin and colonic mucins (Petri *et al.*, 1987). Secreted proteases, Ca^{++} mediated lethal hits, and phagocyte activities of amebic trophozoites may follow adhesion and lead to invasion. The breakdown of colonic epithelium by trophozoites leads to the formation of a flask-shaped ulcer, resulting in direct contact of the parasite with systemic and mucosal immune cells. Humans cured of prior invasive amebiasis are immune to new or recurrent infection for at least 18 months.

The mucosal antiamebic antibody response to *E. histolytica* differs from that to *E. dispar*. Contact time with the colonic mucosa may be for up to 1 year for *E. dispar* and up to 3 months for *E. histolytica* before eliciting a mucosal immune response. After a primary mucosal immune response, reinfection with *E. dispar* does not boost the local immune system (adaptive immunity). Re-infection with *E. histolytica* usually succeeds in boosting mucosal immunity. A protective mucosal immune response occurs in *E. histolytica* infection and is associated with an antilectin IgA antibody response (Haque *et al.*, 2002).

Persistence of the mucosal immune response is dependent on the clinical presentation. Patients cured of amebic liver abscess have a protective fecal antiamebic IgA antibody response that lasts for more than 18 months (Ravdin *et al.*, 2003). Patients cured of acute amebic colitis demonstrated high titers of protective fecal antiamebic IgA antibodies for more than 12 months (Ramos *et al.*, 1997). Asymptomatic amebic infections produce a protective mucosal antiamebic IgA antibody response for few weeks in children (Haque *et al.*, 2001) and for over 12 months in adults (Ravdin *et al.*, 2003).

Recognition of unique lectin epitopes by IgA antibodies has been reported (Haque *et al.*, 2002; Abd-Alla *et al.*, 2004).

Assays of mucosal antiamebic IgA antibodies in stool and saliva were demonstrated in several studies to have utility in diagnosis of amebic infection. Salivary and fecal antilectin IgA antibodies can be used to diagnose *E. histolytica* infection in amebic liver abscess, acute amebic colitis, and asymptomatic carriers. Extra-intestinal infections, as in amebic liver abscess, give rise to higher titers of both fecal and salivary IgA antibodies compared to acute amebic colitis and asymptomatic infection (Kelsall *et al.*, 1994; Abou El-Magd *et al.*, 1995; Abd-Alla *et al.*, 2000).

Experimentally, mucosal antiamebic IgA antibodies inhibit adherence of *E. histolytica* to Chinese hamster ovary (CHO) cells (Beving *et al.*, 1996), and blocking adherence of amebic trophozoites to colonic mucins and mucosa is the goal of a mucosal-immunity mediated-vaccine against amebic infection. In this regard more research is required before evaluating the efficacy of the available recombinant protein fragments for use as a vaccine.

The reported resistance of *E. histolytica* trophozoites to low levels of human secretory IgA antibodies by Ravdin and Kelsall (1994) might explain the ability of the parasite to overcome low-titer IgA responses. Most cases of amebic liver abscess result in high-titer fecal antiamebic IgA antibody and are followed by negative cultures for *E. histolytica*. This might indicate why high levels of mucosal immune response in acute invasive amebiasis are considered more effective in providing immunity to recurrent infection (Ravdin *et al.*, 2003). Nonimmune factors such as competition with gut flora, host hormonal status (estrogens and progesterone), and dominance of certain alleles among certain populations are expected to play a considerable role in whether persistence or clearance of amebic trophozoites from the host colon occurs.

Studies using human leukocytes and animal models have explored the importance of cell-mediated immunity in resistance to invasive amebiasis. T cells from patients with invasive amebiasis or from animals immunized with *E. histolytica* lysates can proliferate in response to soluble amebic antigens and kill trophozoites *in vitro* (Salata *et al.*, 1986). Impairment of T-cell–mediated immunity in humans or in animal models promotes the severity of invasive amebiasis.

Attachment of trophozoites to epithelial and stromal cells induces expression of chemoattractant and proinflammatory cytokines like interleukin (IL)-8 and granulocyte-macrophage colony stimulating factor (GM-CSF) (Eckmann *et al.*, 1995). This may be one mechanism by which the host initiates an acute inflammatory response to the parasite. Macrophage-mediated effector mechanisms are considered important in host defense against this parasite. Naive macrophages can kill trophozoites if activated with recombinant interferon (rIFN)-γ, lipopolysaccharide (LPS), recombinant tumor necrosis factor (rTNF)-α, or other factors. The galactose-inhibitable adherence surface lectin of *E. histolytica* can directly stimulate macrophages to make TNF-α (Seguin *et al.*, 1995) and reactive oxygen radicals. Animal studies suggest that NO, with O_2 and H_2O_2 serving as cofactors, is the macrophage product responsible for this cytotoxicity (Lin and Chadee, 1992).

The parasite can modulate immune responses to allow for its survival in the host. Trophozoites activate the alternative pathway of complement during invasion of the colon but are resistant to killing by the complement complexes deposited on their plasma membranes. Human blood cells, such as polymorphonuclear white blood cells, express CD59, which is a membrane-bound inhibitor of the complement C5b-9 complex. *E. histolytica* expresses a surface adhesin that shares sequence similarity with CD59 and confers resistance to the C5b-9 complex (Braga *et al.*, 1992). Moreover, it is proposed that trophozoites release factors that can downregulate macrophage functions. For instance, soluble parasite antigens inhibit macrophage Ia expression through stimulating production of prostaglandin (PG)E2 and thus may impede antigen presentation (Wang and Chadee, 1995).

Giardiasis

General comments

Giardia intestinalis (also called *G. lamblia*) is the infectious agent responsible for giardiasis. The infection begins when the host ingests *Giardia* cysts present in contaminated water or food. In the proximal small intestine, the cysts release freely mobile trophozoites, which burrow into the mucus layer and attach to the surface epithelium. The trophozoites remain in the proximal small bowel, where they reproduce by binary fission. Some of the trophozoites encyst and leave the host in the stool, allowing continuation of the life cycle. The cysts survive well in the external environment, particularly when exposed to cool and moist conditions. Some wild and domestic animals can act as reservoirs of human infection. Cysts can contaminate natural and domestic freshwater supplies and are relatively resistant to chlorination. Swimming pools can also be a source of infection. The disease occurs worldwide, in both temperate and tropical climates. Regional prevalence rates vary from 2% to 30%, with industrialized societies having the lowest frequency. Some groups are at higher risk of infection; these include infants and young children, campers, travelers to regions with high prevalence, immunodeficient individuals, and people with poor hygiene or who are institutionalized.

Giardiasis can present in several different ways. Most people acutely infected with *Giardia* have few or no symptoms but may develop a carrier state. Others have acute but self-limiting, nonbloody diarrhea lasting from 2 to 6 weeks. Still others develop chronic diarrhea with malabsorption and weight loss. Children may suffer impairment of growth and development. Parasite strain variations or undefined host factors may play an important role in determining the clinical presentation. The diagnosis can be made by microscopic identification of cysts or trophozoites in the stool, duodenal biopsy specimens, or duodenal aspirates or with an immunological test that detects specific *Giardia* antigens in feces.

Several medications are effective against *G. intestinalis*, but there are treatment failures.

Host immunity

Giardia trophozoites reside in the proximal small intestine close to the apical surface of the epithelium and do not invade. Microscopic examination of duodenal or jejunal biopsies may reveal partial villous atrophy with a mild lymphocytic infiltrate or no abnormalities. It is unknown exactly how this parasite induces epithelial injury and diarrhea. Symptoms may result from release of parasite-derived cytopathic factors, direct contact injury, stimulation of the host's own immunological mechanisms, deconjugation of bile salts, or inhibition of luminal enzyme activity.

The immunological mechanisms required for parasite clearance or protective immunity have not been determined. Some immunodeficiency states predispose to chronic giardiasis and its associated diarrhea. This condition is reported most frequently in patients having common variable immunodeficiency syndrome with hypogammaglobulinemia. Yet, giardiasis is not a major clinical problem for patients with acquired immunodeficiency syndrome (AIDS). *Giardia* induced some degree of proliferation and IFN-γ production by CD4+ T lymphocytes in intestine and blood but did not trigger cytotoxicity or migration (Ebert, 1999). A T-cell–dependent mechanism is essential for controlling acute giardia infection, which is independent of antibody or B cells (Singer and Nash, 2000).

Infection results in an antibody response against the trophozoite, which includes serum antibodies (IgG, IgM, IgA) and intestinal secretory IgA (Char *et al.*, 1993). Salivary IgA antibodies to membrane-rich protein fraction were detected in patients with giardiasis; they may be important in protection or in diagnosis (Rosales-Borjas *et al.*, 1998). Prior *Giardia* infection may afford some protective immunity. Exposure of cysts to cyst-specific antibodies or wheat germ agglutinin can inhibit excystation *in vitro* (Meng *et al.*, 1996). Clinical and experimental studies indicate that B cell–dependent host defense mechanisms, particularly IgA, are important for controlling and clearing infection (Eckman and Gillin, 2001). However, it is undetermined whether the antibody response to the parasite promotes parasite elimination or prevents recolonization.

Giardia can undergo surface antigenic variation by modulating expression of different variant-specific surface proteins (VSPs), perhaps permitting immune evasion (Byrd *et al.*, 1994; Lujan *et al.*, 1995). The large number of VSP genes in *G. lamblia* may allow the parasite to infect different hosts, and the antigenic variation could be a mechanism to expand the parasite's host range (Singer *et al.*, 2001). Milk anti-VSP IgA antibodies from mice have a giardicidal effect both *in vitro* and *in vivo* (Stager *et al.*, 1998). A fragment of VSP protein subtype H7, consisting of 12 amino acids, stimulates a strong intestinal immune response (Bienz *et al.*, 2001).

Excretory–secretory product (ESP) is a heat-stable and protease-sensitive glycoprotein located on the outer surface of *Giardia*. Serum antibodies from patients with *G. lamblia* infection recognized the purified ESP protein (Kaur *et al.*, 2001). Immunization of mice with ESP protein stimulates local immunity, evidenced by enhancement of T helper (Th)/inducer activity and an increase in IgA-bearing cells (Kaur *et al.*, 1999).

There are experimental hosts for *Giardia* infection, including a *G. muris* mouse model, *G. intestinalis* weanling mouse model, *G. intestinalis* adult-mouse model, and the *G. intestinalis* gerbil model. Clearance of the rodent parasite *G. muris* requires $CD4^+$ but not $CD8^+$ T lymphocytes (Heyworth *et al.*, 1997). Ingestion of antitrophozoite antibodies affords some protection against infection and decreases the intensity of colonization, possibly by impeding parasite attachment. It is unlikely that natural killer (NK) cells, luminal macrophages, or complement have any role in parasite destruction (Heyworth, 1992). Trophozoites undergo antigenic variation when colonizing immunocompetent mice but not animals with severe combined immunodeficiency (Byrd *et al.*, 1994), suggesting that it is adaptive pressure on the trophozoite that results in altered antigen expression.

Cryptosporidiosis
General comments

Cryptosporidium parvum has been recognized as a zoonotic parasite of veterinary and human medical importance. Immunocompetent hosts are known to develop parasite-specific immune responses that prevent or terminate *C. parvum* infection. In immunocompetent hosts, a self-limited infection occurs that is localized to the intestinal tract, followed by relative resistance to reinfection and clinical disease (Riggs, 1997). However, *C. parvum* is the most important parasitic cause of prolonged diarrhea (>2 weeks) in children in the developing world.

This organism can cause life-threatening diarrhea in immunocompromised individuals such as patients with AIDS. Susceptible hosts usually acquire the disease when they drink water containing *C. parvum* oocysts. The oocysts release sporozoites that attach to intestinal epithelial cells and mature into trophozoites. The trophozoites can enter the epithelial cells and develop into merozoites, which undergo sexual reproduction and form new oocysts. These oocysts exit the body with the stool. *C. parvum* is resistant to chlorine, and contamination of municipal water supplies has resulted in large outbreaks of cryptosporidiosis. People consuming deep-well water are less liable to catch infection than are surface-water consumers (Isaac-Renton *et al.*, 1999). The organism is also transmissible among family members. *C. parvum* causes disease in cattle and other animals, which serve as reservoirs. In patients with AIDS, *C. parvum* can colonize the biliary and pancreatic ducts, causing stenosis of the papilla of Vater, sclerosing cholangitis, acalculous cholecystitis, and pancreatitis. The disease is diagnosed through visual identification of *C. parvum* organisms in intestinal tissue or stool or by immunoassay of stool for *C. parvum* antigens. In severe disease, intravenous hydration and electrolyte management may prove critical for survival. In AIDS patients with chronic cryptosporidiosis, administration of enriched colostral immunoglobulin fraction from cows immunized with whole *C. parvum* decreases the frequency of diarrhea and stool weight but does not eliminate infection (Greenberg and Cello, 1996). These findings suggest an important role for mucosal immunity in prevention and eradication of *C. parvum* infection.

Host immunity

Effective mucosal and systemic immunity is expected, as the disease is self-limiting in immunocompetent individuals. Even in symptomatic patients with diarrhea, resolution of symptoms and elimination of infection coincide with the appearance of serum and mucosal antibodies. Decreased severity of infection may also be attributed to mucosal and humoral antibody responses (Riggs, 1997; Crabb, 1998; Chappell *et al.*, 1999; Moss *et al.*, 1998).

There is a high degree of antigenic conservation between the sexual and asexual stages of *C. parvum* (Riggs, 1997)., Human sera recognize at least eight different antigens; six are glycoproteins and include CSL1300, GP900, CP47, and GP60/40/15. The other two antigens are the Gal/GalNAc lectin and the thromboprotein-related anonymous protein of *C. parvum* (TRAP-Cp). These antigens are involved in motility, attachment, invasion, and intracellular development of the parasite (Riggs, 2002). Monoclonal antibodies against other parasite antigens such as GP25-200, P23, and CP15/60 are available. Immunization with monoclonal antibodies provides up to 40% protection against new infection and up to 93% reduction of infectious burden in experimental animals (Schaefer *et al.*, 2000). Parenterally administered anti-P23 dimeric IgA monoclonal antibodies migrate to the hepatobiliary system, and study of their protective role has been initiated.

In humans infected with *C. parvum*, a prominent role of mucosal IFN-γ has been identified. In immunocompetent patients, mucosal IFN-γ was detected during infection but not in AIDS cases. A mucosal IFN-γ response correlates with prior exposure to *C. parvum* and enables the host to control oocyst production (White *et al.*, 2000). In contrast, IL-15 is found only in primary *C. parvum* infection in previously unexposed humans (Robinson *et al.*, 2001).

Mice are useful models for studying *C. parvum* infection. Treatment of immunocompetent or immunodeficient mice with systemic rIL-12 prevents establishment of infection. Data also suggest that endogenously produced IL-12 limits *C. parvum* infection by promoting IFN-γ production (Urban *et al.*, 1996). SCID mice are deficient in both T and B cells but remain resistant to *C. parvum* infection unless treated with neutralizing anti-IFN-γ antibody (Chen *et al.*, 1993). This suggests that IFN-γ can control *C. parvum* infection through T- and B-cell-independent mechanisms. IFN-γ makes intestinal epithelial cells more resistant to *C. parvum* penetration. Rapid elimination of established *C. parvum* infection in SCID mice requires both IFN-γ and $CD4^+$ but not $CD8^+$ T cells (Chen *et al.*, 1993; McDonald *et al.*, 1994). The relative importance of $CD4^+$ versus $CD8^+$ T cells is also illustrated by the greater susceptibility of mice to infection when they are deficient in major histocompatibility complex (MHC) class II but not MHC class I molecules (Aguirre *et al.*, 1994). Experiments using αβ or γδ T-cell-deficient animals suggest that αβT cells are more critical (Waters and Harp, 1996). The composition of the intestinal flora also may be a determinant.

HELMINTHIC INFECTIONS

Helminths are elaborate multicellular worms with complex organs. There are two groups of helminths that colonize the human intestine: nematodes (nonsegmented roundworms) and platyhelminths (flatworms). Perhaps more than one third of the population of the world harbors one or more of these organisms at any time.

Common nematodes that reside in the human gut are *Ascaris lumbricoides*, *Trichuris trichiura* (whipworm), *Ancylostoma duodenale* and *Necator americanus* (hookworms), *Enterobius vermicularis* (pinworm), *Strongyloides stercoralis*, and *Capillaria philippinensis*. *Trichinella spiralis* is a nematode with a short intestinal phase.

The platyhelminths include trematodes and cestodes. The most common adult trematodes that live in the human intestines are *Fasciolopsis*, *Echinostoma*, and *Heterophyes* species. Those most frequently living in the biliary system include *Clonorchis sinensis*, *Opisthorchis viverrini* and *O. felineus*, and *Fasciola hepatica*. *Schistosoma* lives in the venous system, but several species chronically affect the gut by the passage of eggs through the intestinal wall. The cestodes are tapeworms. Adult cestodes commonly infecting humans are *Diphyllobothrium* species (fish tapeworm), *Taenia saginata* (beef tapeworm), *Taenia solium* (pork tapeworm), and *Hymenolepis nana* (dwarf tapeworm).

Little is known about the human immune response to most intestinal helminthic infections. Most of the information derives from the study of rodent parasites. Trichuris is one of the few intestinal roundworm infections that has a species, *Trichuris muris* (mouse whipworm), that can infect laboratory mice. *Trichinella spiralis* also can infect rodents, allowing study of the gut immune response to the intestinal phase of this organism. A frequently studied murine roundworm is *Nippostrongylus brasiliensis*.

Nematodes
Trichinosis
Trichinella is a parasite mostly of temperate regions. The main repositories for human disease are domestic pigs, wild boar, and bears. Trichinosis results from eating undercooked meat containing cysts of *T. spiralis*. The cysts release larvae, which penetrate the epithelial lining of the small intestine and mature into adult worms. During this initial phase, the host experiences nausea, abdominal pain, fever, and diarrhea. Within 7 days, newborn larvae pass through the lymphatic system or directly into the bloodstream to encyst in striated muscle. This initiates a strong local, eosinophilic inflammatory response associated with muscle tenderness,

swelling, fever, and eosinophilia. Larvae may migrate to the brain or myocardium, causing serious complications. Symptoms peak in about 6 weeks and gradually decline over the next several months as the larvae encyst and the intestines expel the worms. Larvae remain alive in the cysts for years, releasing antigens that can induce continuous eosinophilia. Antihelminthics can eradicate the intestinal worms, and corticosteroids are used to treat the muscle stage when symptoms are severe.

Both mice and rats can host *T. spiralis*. In response to infection, susceptible animals mount a strong eosinophil-rich intestinal inflammation associated with IgE and mastocytosis, resulting in worm expulsion. This immune response not only limits the duration of the intestinal phase of the initial infection but also curtails development of subsequent infections. Treatment of *Trichinella*-infected mice with anti-IL-5 monoclonal antibody substantially depletes circulating and tissue eosinophils but still allows an inflammatory response to the parasite. Eosinophil depletion does not affect muscle-stage juvenile worm recovery, intestinal worm expulsion, or reinfection resistance (Hemdon and Kayes, 1992). Although the eosinophil frequently is regarded as an antihelminth effector cell, it does not have an essential role in the host immune response to this nematode. However, mast cell–deficient mice do show a delay in worm expulsion. Moreover, recombinant IL-3 treatment increases circulating IgE concentrations, enhances tissue mastocytosis, and promotes worm elimination (Korenaga *et al.*, 1996).

Transfer of IgE can protect if given with antigen-sensitized, CD4+ CD45RC− T cells. These observations suggest that IgE and mast cells may have an important role in worm clearance. Most of the IgE produced as a result of infection is transported from the gut wall into the lumen, with little entering the serum. Thus, serum IgE levels do not reflect the magnitude of the response (Negrao-Correa *et al.*, 1996).

Onset of the peak of the contractile muscle response, as well as the magnitude of a sustained response, contributes to parasite eviction from the gut (Vallance *et al.*, 1998). The addition of CD4 T cells is required to induce intestinal muscle pathophysiology (Vallance *et al.*, 1999). IgE antibodies produced by the intestinal mucosa or associated lymphoid organs might contribute independently from mast cell degranulation to worm elimination (Negrao-Corea, 2001). Experiments with immunodeficient mice have shown that both antitrichinella IgE and IgG1 independently can induce a fatal anaphylactic response (Bruschi *et al.*, 1999). In addition, worm burdens are inversely proportional to intestinal histamine-forming capacity (Hegazy, 1998).

In rats, parasite expulsion requires CD4+ T cells of the CD45RC− phenotype, which appear in the intestines and thoracic duct lymph during infection (Korenaga *et al.*, 1996). When injected into naive rats, they home to the intestines and provide protective immunity. Integrin α4 assists lymphocyte adherence to vascular endothelium and lymphocyte migration into Peyer's patches, mesenteric lymph nodes, and possibly intestinal mucosa. Blocking of integrin α4 can markedly impair the normal development and expression of immunity to this nematode (Bell and Issekutz, 1993). The protective CD4+ CD45RC− T cell subset responds to *T. spiralis* recall antigens *in vitro* with the production of IL-4 and IL-5. Also generated is an antigen-responsive CD4+ CD45RC+ T cell that produces Th1 cytokines like IFN-γ and TNF-α. This cell also homes to the gut but does not transfer immunity. Analysis of cytokine concentrations in intestinal lymph shows increased levels of IL-4, IL-5, and IFN-γ. Worm expulsion is associated with the maximal increase in IL-4 and IL-5 levels, which also are accentuated by adoptive transfer of protective CD4+ CD45RC− cells (Ramaswamy et al., 1996). This suggests that Th2 rather than Th1-type cytokines are protective. In summary, the adult worm is expelled by mast cell–dependent mechanisms and the larvae are killed by eosinophils (Gurish *et al.*, 2002).

The results of experimental manipulation of cytokines reflect their key functions. IL-18 was found to be a negative regulator in *T. spiralis* infection. IL-18 knockout mice are resistant to infection. The inhibitory effect of IL-18 on mastocytosis and Th2 cytokine secretion is independent of IFN-γ (Helmby and Grencis, 2002). Ad5IL-12-treated mice experience prolonged worm survival, and the intestinal hypercontractility and goblet cell hyperplasia normally associated with infection are markedly reduced. IL-12 upregulates INF-γ and downregulates IL-13 (Khan *et al.*, 2001). Neutrophil infiltration of the small intestinal epithelium contributes to stimulation of epithelial cell cytokine production. Anti-CD18 monoclonal antibodies block neutrophil infiltration and reduce epithelial cytokine mRNA (Stadnyk *et al.*, 2000). Following ketotifen treatment there is a reduction in IL-5, eosinophilia, and IgA antibody responses, affecting both the size and number of worms present (Doligalska and Laskowska, 2000). The changes in smooth muscle contractility are T-cell-dependent, whereas alterations in myenteric nerve function are T-cell-independent. Cytokine-induced effects in the myenteric plexus may not require the local influx of inflammatory cells.

In human trichinosis, peripheral blood mononuclear cells produce IL-2, IL-5, IL-10, and IFN-γ in response to trichinella antigen. There is a high degree of association between cytokine mRNA expression and protein production (Morales *et al.*, 2002). During the course of an infection by *T. spiralis*, antibodies to the muscle-larval excretory-secretory protein provide an immunoevasive mechanism by newborn larvae for avoidance of host antibody effector mechanisms (Venturiello *et al.*, 2000). ELISA is used to detect early IgA antibodies to newborn *T. spiralis* larva group (TSL)-1 and the phosphorylcholine antigens. Further evaluation of this test is required before application to diagnosis and epidemiological surveys of *T. spiralis* infection (Mendez-Loredo, 2001).

Trichuriasis (whipworm)

Trichuris trichiura infects over a billion people worldwide and is the causative agent for trichuriasis, with highest prevalence in the tropics. Ingestion of eggs present in soil initiates infection. The eggs release larvae that penetrate the cecal epithelium. Within 90 days, the larvae mature into adult worms.

which produce eggs that pass with the feces. The worms remain partly embedded in the cecal epithelium and live 1 to 3 years. Most people who have this parasite are infected lightly and remain asymptomatic. The parasite does not replicate within the host because the ova require a soil phase to embryonate. Heavy infection leads to more extensive involvement of the gastrointestinal tract, and patients can develop trichuris dysentery. Some people have chronic diarrhea and minimal histological changes on colonic mucosal biopsy. Others develop colitis associated with bloody diarrhea, anemia, and occasionally rectal prolapse.

Identification of the characteristic eggs on stool examination confirms the diagnosis. Adult worms about 4 cm long are readily evident on colonoscopic inspection. There are highly effective therapeutic agents. Upon rechallenge, some individuals expel the worms, whereas others are prone to high-level reinfection. This is in part related to the immune profile and nutritional status of the host. A low dietary level of iron can change the location and increase the worm burden. Vitamin A deficiency leads to earlier worm loss and a decreased fecal excretion of eggs. In children chronically infected by *T. trichiura*, the host reaction in the mucosa is characterized by a high concentration of IgE, many degranulating mast cells, and release of histamine. Circulating IgE is also elevated.

Extensively studied is the mouse whipworm, *T. muris* (Grenis, 1993). Measurable levels of IgG1, IgG4, IgA, and IgE antibodies against *T. muris* antigen are detected in humans, reflecting a degree of conserved antigenicity between both species (Turner *et al.*, 2002). Protective immunity to this murine intestinal nematode is CD4+ T-cell-dependent and strongly influenced by host genetics. Mouse strains that expel worms readily mount a strong Th2 response (IL4), whereas those that retain worms produce a Th1 pattern of inflammation (IFN-γ). As with other nematodes, worm expulsion does not appear to depend on the associated intestinal eosinophilia or the mucosal mastocytosis. IL-4 may have a critical role in worm expulsion, since treatment with anti-IL-4 or anti-IL-4 receptor monoclonal antibody can convert strains that normally expel the parasite into animals that accept chronic infection (Else *et al.*, 1994). However, this observation is now in question since recent studies suggest that IL-4 mutant mice expel worms normally. Treatment of mice that normally harbor chronic infection with anti-IFN-γ converts them to the responder phenotype, resulting in parasite expulsion (Bancroft *et al.*, 1994). The mechanisms that permit some mouse strains to produce the desirable Th2-dominated immune response are unknown. Antigen load is one possibly important factor. A moderate level of infection in BALB/c mice results in a strong Th2 response and expulsion of the worms. Yet, a light infection in the same strain favors development of a Th1 response and worm retention (Bancroft *et al.*, 1994).

T. muris–infected IL-10-deficient mice fail to expel the parasite and have intense inflammation, loss of Paneth cells, and absence of mucus in the cecum. In contrast, IL-10/IL-12-deficient mice are completely resistant to infection and mount a high-level Th2 cytokine response, indicating that susceptibility of IL-10-deficient mice to infection is dependent on IL-12 (Schopf et al., 2002). A protective function of immunoglobulins is demonstrated by resistance to *T. muris* infection when deficient mice are administered parasite-specific IgG1 antibodies and sensitized B cells (Blackwell and Else, 2001). *In vivo* neutralization of IL-13 prevents expulsion of *T. muris* while its addition markedly reduces the worm burden (Bancroft et al. 2000). Immunization of *T. muris*-resistant mice with anti-IL-9 antibodies results in their being susceptible to prolonged infection (Richard et al., 2000). Resistance to *T. muris* infection is dependent on IL-4 and IL-13. *In vivo* blockade of TNF-α in normally resistant mice does not alter IL-4, IL-5, or IL-13 production but delays worm expulsion. IL-13-mediated worm expulsion in IL-4-deficient mice is TNF-α dependent (Artis et al., 1999). Driving Th1 responses by IL-12 in *T. muris*-resistant mice causes chronic infection and elevated levels of IgG2a antibodies (Bancroft et al. 1997). Mucosal mast cells are not required for protection against *T. muris* infection in mice (Koyama and Ito, 2000).

Strongyloidiasis

Human strongyloidiasis is caused by *Strongyloides stercoralis*. Internal autoinfection is a major characteristic of this disease. Exposure to the free-living infective larvae in soil is the mode of transmission. Larvae enter the skin and the worms reach the gastrointestinal tract by poorly defined pathways. Mature females remain embedded in the small bowel mucosa and produce eggs, which hatch into rhabditiform larvae that migrate into the lumen and are excreted in the stool. In the host, rhabditiform larvae can mature into infective filariform larvae and reenter host tissue (internal autoinfection). Thus, a unique feature of this nematode is its potential for endogenous replication within the host. Strongyloidiasis is endemic to tropical and some temperate regions. Frequently, infection with *S. stercoralis* is clinically inapparent. Corticosteroid therapy can activate asymptomatic *S. stercoralis* infection, resulting in a hyperinfective syndrome. This condition can manifest by nausea, diarrhea, abdominal pain, wheezing, and cough. The organism can also migrate to other organs when there is heavy infection.

Antibody responses to *S. stercoralis* have been studied in humans. Total IgE antibodies persist for years after elimination of infection and resolution of eosinophilia (Poirriez, 2001). Detection of serum IgG antibodies against frozen sections of *S. stercoralis* and *S. ratti* larvae demonstrated more than 90% sensitivity and specificity in an immunofluorescence-based test (Costa-Cruz et al., 1997). An immediate hypersensitivity skin reaction to filariform larvae was successful in diagnosing 82% to 100% of *S. stercoralis* infections with use of a crude or secretory/excretory parasite antigen but demonstrated cross-reactivity with filarial infection (Neva et al., 2001). Western blots of human immune sera against *S. stercoralis* crude antigen identified eight antigens with molecular weights ranging from 26 to 96 kDa (Siddiqui et al., 1997). *S. stercoralis* infection in human T-cell leukemia virus

(HTLV)-1–positive patients with decreased IL-5 and IgE antibodies (switching from a Th2 to a Th1 immune response) is controlled by different mechanisms (Porto et al., 2001).

Mice have been well studied as an experimental model for immunity to *S. stercoralis*. Third larval antigenic protein (L3) is a target for the murine immune system. In mice vaccinated with the L3 protein, administration of anti-IL-4 and IL-5 monoclonal antibodies reduces the protective efficacy. Conversion of a Th2 to a Th1 response by IL-12 in immunized mice reduces the eosinophil number, eosinophil peroxidase level, and parasite-specific IgG1 antibody while increasing parasite-specific IgG2a antibodies. Inactivation of eosinophils by anti-IL5 monoclonal antibodies abolishes the protective immunity mediated by L3 vaccination (Rotman et al., 1996, 1997). Passive immunization with purified anti-L3 IgG polyclonal antibodies produced in mice yields up to 83% protection in animals challenged with infective larvae (Herbert et al., 2002).

Ascariasis

The intestinal nematode *Ascaris lumbricoides* is the cause of human ascariasis, one of the world's most prevalent parasite infestations. The host acquires *A. lumbricoides* by ingestion of eggs present in contaminated soil. The eggs survive gastric acidity and hatch into larvae within the intestines. The released larvae penetrate the colonic wall and migrate through the portal venous system and eventually to the lung. They leave the venous system and ascend the bronchial tree to the pharynx and are swallowed. The worms reach adult stature in the small intestine, achieving a length of 20 to 30 cm, and produce eggs, exiting with stool to complete the life cycle. Although 25% of the world's population harbors this parasite, the majority are asymptomatic. Migrating worms or a high parasite burden produces symptoms. Worms migrating into the pancreatic or biliary ducts can induce pancreatitis or ascending cholangitis. Heavy infection may result in intestinal obstruction, especially in children. Larvae migrating through the lung can induce an allergic pneumonitis and asthma-type symptoms.

Little is known about immunity in ascariasis. The intensity of the parasitic burden plays an important role in stimulating production of nonspecific polyclonal IgE antibodies, which diminish the effectiveness of the parasite-specific response to the infection. Nutritional deficiency downregulates mucosal immunity and increases production of polyclonal IgE antibodies (Ortize et al., 2000). An IgG4 antibody response to the *A. lumbricoides* secretory/excretory antigen (AI IIIb) was detected in 100% of ascariasis patients by ELISA without any cross-reactivity with other helminths (Chatterjee et al., 1996). In ascariasis, the peripheral eosinophil count is increased, but the eosinophil count in the nasal mucosal is normal. Nasal itching in ascariasis is differentiated from that of atopic allergy by the normal eosinophil count in nasal mucosa (Yazicio et al., 1996). Contact with a low dose of *A. lumbricoides* antigen is associated with both specific and increased total IgE antibody responses (Dol et al., 1998). There is an increased production of IL-4 and IL-5 by human sensitized peripheral blood mononuclear cells on exposure to ascaris antigen. The ratio of Th2 to Th1 type responses is increased (Cooper *et al.*, 2000).

Hookworm

Two major species infect humans, *Necator americanus* and *Ancylostoma duodenale*. *Ancylostoma caninum*, the dog hookworm, can also inhabit humans, causing diarrhea, abdominal pain, and severe eosinophilic gastroenteritis. Hookworm infections are important because as many as a billion subjects throughout the world harbor these parasites. The eggs release their larvae into the soil, and the host usually acquires hookworm infection through penetration of the skin. In the host, the larvae pass through the lungs, are swallowed, and mature in the small intestine. Infection causes chronic gastrointestinal blood loss and iron-deficiency anemia, which may impede childhood development. *A. duodenale* can also be transmitted through the oral route.

Adult hookworm infection is associated with an antibody response dominated by IgE, IgG1, and IgG4, which are controlled by Th2 cytokines. These antibodies are detected by immunoprecipitation around the parasite's oral opening or by ELISA and Western blotting with use of somatic or excretory/secretory antigens. Anti–stage 3 larvae (L3) antibodies recognize the surface antigen of ensheathed larvae but not exsheathed L3. Antibodies detected in exsheathing fluid reflect antigens that divert the immune response. IgE antibody responses to the parasite's L3 antigen are highly specific and sensitive for diagnosing infection with little if any cross-reactivity. The rapid resistance to L3 developed in mice is attributed to increasing levels of IgM, IgG1, and IgE antibodies, despite the incomplete life cycle (Loukas and Prociv, 2001).

The leukocytic response to adult hookworm infection is dominated by eosinophils, and the number of eosinophils in peripheral blood reflects the burden of infection. The small initial increase in the eosinophil count, followed by a sharp rise just before ova appear in the stool, is attributed to larval hypobiosis and reactivation of *A. duodenale* infection. Exposure to L3 protein in subjects with a history of *Necator* infection induces a rapid rise in the blood eosinophil level. Tissue eosinophilia is predominant in L3 infection. Eosinophils from subjects infected with *Necator* are activated and secrete superoxide. Little is known about T cell reactivity and cytokine secretion in hookworm infection. In necator infection, peripheral blood T cells react strongly to mitogens and weakly to hookworm antigen (Loukas and Prociv, 2001).

Pinworm

Enterobius vermicularis is a very common parasitic infection, especially among children. This white nematode inhabits the cecum and adjacent gut. The gravid females migrate at night through the large intestine and up to the anal and perineal area for oviposition. It is rare to find their eggs in feces. The most reliable method of diagnosis is by examination with adhesive cellophane tape pressed against the perianal region early in the morning. Pinworm is very contagious, and its mode of transmission is fecal–oral. External autoinfection is common. The eggs do not require a soil phase and ingested eggs release larvae, which mature in the colon. Most infections are asymptomatic. The clinical manifestations are related to perianal and perineal pruritus. The infection may cause right iliac cavity discomfort, diarrhea, and rarely appendicitis. Migration from anus to vagina may cause vaginitis, leukorrhea, and even urinary tract infection.

Nearly nothing is known about the immune response to this parasite. In uncomplicated enterobiasis, pinworms remain in the lumen and rarely cause any hematological changes. Cases of eosinophilia with gastroenteritis, salpingitis, epididymitis, and cystitis have been reported. Peripheral blood eosinophilia occurs whenever pinworms leave the intestine and migrate to extraintestinal organs. Durmaz *et al.* (1998) focused on increases in total serum IgE levels in children infected with *E. vermicularis*, which returned to normal 2 weeks after treatment.

Trematodes
Schistosomiasis

Schistosoma are parasitic blood flukes that cause schistosomiasis (bilharziasis). More than 200 million people in tropical and subtropical regions harbor schistosome flukes. The climatic requirements of the snail intermediate host determine the geographic distribution of the disease. The three most common species infecting humans are *Schistosoma mansoni*, *S. haematobium*, and *S. japonicum*.

Schistosoma species have complex life cycles. Schistosome eggs leave the host with the stool (*S. mansoni, S. japonicum*) or urine (*S. haematobium*). The eggs hatch, releasing miracidia that infect appropriate freshwater snail species, whose habitat is restricted to a subtropical or tropical climate. In the snail, the parasite produces sporocysts which mature into cercariae, which are released into the water to infect humans or other mammalian species, usually through skin penetration. The parasites migrate through the lungs and settle in the mesenteric veins, which collect blood returning from the intestines (*S. mansoni, S. japonicum*) or vesical veins, which drain the urinary bladder (*S. haematobium*). Here they mature into adult worms, which produce large numbers of eggs. Many of the eggs move through the intestinal (*S. mansoni, S. japonicum*) or bladder wall (*S. haematobium*) and pass with the stool or urinary stream back into the freshwater environment. Also, the venous blood sweeps eggs into the liver and other organs where they lodge. The intestinal and bladder walls capture some as well. The worms evade the immune system of the host, inducing no apparent immune response. Yet, the eggs that do not exit the host release antigens and toxic substances that incite a vigorous, eosinophilic granulomatous response that produces Th2-type cytokines.

Patients frequently remain asymptomatic, but many ultimately die of the disease. In heavy infection, the intestinal inflammation can result in bloody diarrhea, intestinal fibrosis, and obstruction. Bladder involvement (*S. haematobium*) may induce dysuria, hematuria, ureteral obstruction, and bladder cancer. Many years of infection can lead to hepatic fibrosis, portal hypertension, ascites, and variceal bleeding. Involvement of other organs causes additional complications that are correspondingly severe. The usual method of diagnosis is visualization of eggs in tissue biopsies, stool, or urine. There are medications that effectively eradicate the worms. Concomitant immunity limits the survival rate of newly infecting cercariae in a host already bearing adult worms, yet individuals cured of schistosomiasis can readily acquire a new infection. It is uncertain whether previous infection leads to partial immunity. Some people appear more susceptible to heavy infection or liver fibrosis because of undefined, inherited susceptibility factors.

Periportal hepatic fibrosis induced by the granulomatous reaction to *S. mansoni* eggs compromises liver function and enhances complications from viral infection. Higher rates of hepatitis B and C viral markers are found in hepatosplenic schistosomiasis patients. Impaired generation of hepatitis virus–specific CD$^{(+)}$Th1 T cells might explain the delayed clearance of virus and the increased severity of infection in hepatosplenic schistosomiasis (Aquino *et al.*, 2000; Kamal *et al.*, 2001).

Adults similarly exposed to *Schistosoma mansoni* may be either resistant or susceptible to new infection; some remain susceptible to infection despite repeated treatment (Karanja *et al.*, 2002). The infective burden and clinical outcome of prolonged infection are defined to a major extent by the host cytokine response. IFN-γ reduces the parasite load and inhibits periportal fibrosis. TNF-α aggravates periportal fibrosis (Henri *et al.*, 2002). In some cases the cytokine response correlates with the clinical presentation of schistosomiasis. TNF-α is elevated in patients with abdominal pain, and IFN-γ levels in peripheral blood mononuclear cells are higher in acute than in chronic disease. IL-5 levels are high in chronic infection and are associated with weight loss. A marked drop in the C3 level is a characteristic of chronic schistosomiasis (de-Jesus *et al.*, 2002; el-Shakawy *et al.*, 2002). Immunologic responses to *Schistosoma* infection often reflect the extent of pathology. Antisoluble egg antigen IgG4 antibodies are detected only in patients with periportal fibrosis (Silvera *et al.*, 2002).

Murine schistosomiasis mimics human disease and is an important experimental model for studying the immune response to *S. mansoni* and *S. japonicum* infection. Evidence from murine *S. mansoni* suggests that the Th2-type granulomatous inflammatory response to schistosome ova protects the host from antigens and other toxins released from the eggs. Although schistosome antigens are highly immunogenic, the chronically infected human host shows no systemic signs of allergic disease. However, some patients develop chronic glomerulonephropathy as a result of deposition of immune complexes within the kidneys. Also, it is probable that the eggs require intestinal inflammation to successfully breach the intestinal wall (Amiri *et al.*, 1992).

Eggs that lodge in tissue can survive for several weeks, even under a vigorous immune attack. They are quickly enveloped in a collagen network containing eosinophils, mature macrophages, T and B lymphocytes, and mast cells. Eventually, the inflammation kills and removes the surrounded egg. The focal inflammatory response resolves, leaving little or no scarring. Yet, the schistosome worm deposits hundreds of new eggs daily, which evoke repeated injury. There are no data regarding the circuits controlling intestinal fibrosis in schistosomiasis.

Undefined local tissue and systemic factors influence granuloma formation diversely in various organs. The cellular composition of liver granulomas is about 50% eosinophils, 30% macrophages, 10% T cells, and 5% B cells. Intestinal granulomas are smaller than those in the liver and have a somewhat different cell composition and morphology. There are even substantial differences between the granulomas that form in response to schistosome ova lodged in the ileum and colon (Weinstock and Boros, 1983).

T cells are critical for the development of schistosome granulomas in the intestines and other organs. Animals deficient in T cells or depleted of CD4$^+$ T lymphocytes produce a minimal inflammatory response to ova (Mathew and Boros, 1986). Much less critical are CD8$^+$ and γδ$^+$ T cells (Iacomini *et al.*, 1995). Granulomas have B cells that secrete IgM, IgG1, IgA, and IgE. Also, the intact intestinal mucosa secretes IgA and other antibody classes when challenged with schistosome egg antigen. Large Th2-type granulomas form in mice treated with anti-IL-5 to deplete eosinophils (Sher *et al.*, 1990). Depletion of various cellular elements alters granuloma morphology and function; however, CD4$^+$ T cells are most important for induction and maintenance of the inflammation.

The schistosome granuloma is a strong Th2-type inflammation rich in eosinophils and mast cells and constitutively produces large amounts of IL-4, IL-5, IgG1, and IgE. Serum IgE concentrations also are high. The granulomas make little IFN-γ or IgG2a, and macrophages express Ia antigen and Fcγ3 receptors only at low density. Moreover, dispersed granuloma cells, splenocytes, or mucosal inflammatory cells challenged with egg antigens secrete predominantly Th2-type cytokines. Within the granulomas, T cells make IL-5 and IFN-γ but are not likely the major source of IL-4.

As with other nematodes, IL-4 is critically important in establishing the Th2 nature of the inflammation. Transgenic mice lacking IL-4 produce granulomas with no mast cells and fewer eosinophils among other cellular alterations. In addition, there are substantial reductions in IL-5 and IgG1 production and no detectable IgE. Yet, the resulting vigorous inflammation is not a Th1 response. Thus, IL-4 production is not the critical factor limiting secretion of IFN-γ and expression of other aspects of Th1 type inflammation (Metawali *et al.*, 1996). The IL-4-deficient state also is not detrimental to the host, at least over the short term.

Cytokines like IL-12, IL-10, and TGF-β can regulate IFN-γ secretion. The granulomas produce these molecules. Dispersed granuloma cells from IL-4-deficient mice cultured *in vitro* in the presence of rIL-12, anti-IL-10, or anti-TGF-β monoclonal antibody produce substantially more IFN-γ. Cells from wild-type mice do likewise, but to a much lesser degree. Thus, these cytokines and the circuits that regulate them probably play a role in modulating IFN-γ production during the ongoing inflammatory response in wild-type animals and more so in IL4-deficient animals. Yet, wild-type mice treated with rIL-12 or animals deficient in IL-10 still develop predominantly Th2-type granulomatous inflammation in the liver and probably in the intestines during natural infection.

Early interaction of schistosome antigens with the innate immune system stimulates chemokines favorably for induction of the Th2-type response (Chensue et al., 1996). After cercarial infection, both type 1–associated and type 2–associated chemokines were elevated in the liver of mice presensitized with eggs and recombinant IL-12, a regimen that diminished pathology. Neutralization of IL-12 or IFN-γ during egg deposition led to formation of large granulomas, persistently elevated levels of the thymus-derived chemotactic-3 protein, eotaxin, and macrophage inflammatory protein 1α, and reduction in type 1–associated chemokines, despite a dominant Th1-type cytokine response in draining lymph nodes. This new relationship between chemokines and immune response suggests that end organ inflammation might be altered by chemokine blockade without necessarily reversing the phenotype of the majority of differentiated T cells (Park et al., 2001).

Granuloma inflammatory cells in murine S. mansoni make neurokines like substance P (SP), somatostatin (SOM), and vasoactive intestinal peptide (VIP). Intestinal nerves and neuroendocrine cells also produce these substances. Granuloma CD4+ T lymphocytes and other cellular elements express authentic neurokine receptors. Functioning through these authentic receptors, SP stimulates whereas SOM inhibits Th1 cells' secretion of IFN-γ. The mucosal immune system is under constant immune stimulation from the parasite ova and luminal factors. This immune response must be controlled tightly to avoid needless organ damage. It is likely that SP and SOM help maintain the mucosal balance between Th1 and Th2 and help control the intensity of the inflammation (Weinstock and Elliot, 1997).

Experimental downregulation of IL-4 and IL-13 effectively arrests granuloma formation. Both IL-4 and IL-13 are implicated in the in vivo production of IgE antibodies. Mast cells are not needed to form Th2-type granulomas, but they influence the release of IL-4 from different cells in granulomas. Th2 granuloma development in schistosomiasis is partly dependent on IL-4-producing CD4+ T cells (Jakubzick et al., 2002; Cetre et al., 2000; Metwali et al., 2002).

In murine S. mansoni infection, cross-reactive idiotypes (CRIs) are evident early on. CRIs are regulatory and possibly determine subsequent morbidity (Montesano et al., 2002). Sensitization of macrophages with soluble egg antigen (SEA) enhances their phagocytic activity via increasing expression of the macrophage adhesion molecule 1 (Mac-1). This leads to rapid destruction of the ova, a decreased inflammatory response to infection, and amelioration of the hepatic pathology (El-Ahwany et al., 2000).

Prevention of schistosomiasis by vaccination is receiving a great deal of attention, and field trials are going on in different places worldwide. Immune reactivity of human T and B cells to recombinant schistosome glyceraldehyde 3-phosphate dehydrogenase enzyme correlates with resistance to reinfection (El-Ridi et al., 2001). Active immunization of mice with anticercarial monoclonal antibody NP30 provides a degree of protection against infection with S. japonicum cercariae (Feng et al., 2002). The S. mansoni antigen paramyosin-3 induces production of IL-5, which significantly lowers levels of infection (de Jesus et al., 2000).

Intestinal and biliary flukes

Fasciolopsis, Echinostoma, and Heterophyes species are the trematodes that inhabit the human intestines. The biliary system is home to Clonorchis sinensis, Opisthorchis viverrini and O. felineus, and Fasciola hepatica. Their life cycles are akin to that of Schistosoma except that their cercariae need to encyst in a second intermediate host before they can infect the primary host. Depending on the species of fluke, specific types of freshwater vegetables, fish, or crustaceans serve as secondary hosts. Human infection results from ingestion of raw or poorly cooked food harboring cysts, and most of these infections are endemic to Asia. O. felineus is encountered in eastern and central Europe, whereas Fasciola is found in sheep- and cattle-raising areas worldwide. Biliary flukes can cause gallstones, biliary strictures, cholecystitis, ascending cholangitis, and cholangiocarcinoma. Intestinal flukes may induce nausea, abdominal pain, and focal intestinal eosinophilic inflammation. Essentially nothing is known about host immunity.

CESTODES

Taenia saginata (beef tapeworm), T. solium (pork tapeworm), Hymenolepis nana (dwarf tapeworm), and Diphyllobothrium species (fish tapeworm) are the cestodes that most often infect humans. They live in the small intestine. The natural definitive host of both T. solium and T. saginata adults is humans. Ingestion of raw or poorly cooked beef (T. saginata) or pork (T. solium) containing cysticerci causes taeniasis. The adult tapeworm produces eggs, which are shed with the feces. Eggs infect the appropriate intermediate host and hatch to release hexacanth larvae, which migrate and encyst in muscle. Cattle are the intermediate host for T. saginata and pigs for T. solium. Cysticercosis occurs only in T. solium infection as a result of egg hatching and extraintestinal migration of larvae in the definitive host (internal autoinfection). Infection with adult worms is asymptomatic in most cases. The circulating larvae in cysticercosis, on reaching the brain, eyes, and other organs, produce serious complications.

A dwarf tapeworm named H. nana, the most common human cestode, causes hymenolepiasis. Fecal-oral transmission of eggs is the route of transmission. The ingested eggs hatch, producing oncospheres, which penetrate the small intestinal mucosa. Oncospheres develop into cysticercoid larvae, which reenter the intestinal lumen and grow into adult worms. Thus, a secondary host is not required and eggs do not need soil for maturation. Internal autoinfection results from hatching of eggs in a current infection. The disease is asymptomatic and self-limiting.

Diphyllobothrium cysticerci ingestion in poorly cooked fish causes diphyllobothriasis. The life cycle of *Diphyllobothrium* species requires a crustacean as a second intermediate host. Anemia from vitamin B12 deficiency is the most common clinical presentation.

Cysticercosis occurring as a consequence of *T. solium* infection has a major clinical impact. Research efforts have been directed mainly toward the humoral immune response for diagnosis and vaccination purposes in both definitive and intermediate hosts. Immunologic diagnosis with use of both crude and recombinant antigens in antibody detection has acceptable levels of specificity and sensitivity. Whole crude antigen from *T. crassiceps* and *T. solium* are successfully used in detecting IgG and IgA antibodies in cerebrospinal fluid (CSF) and sera from patients with neurocysticercosis (Bueno *et al.*, 2000). A low-molecular-weight *T. solium* cysticercus antigen (18 kDa) was recognized by CSF and serum IgG antibodies from patients with neurocysticercosis in immunoblotting (Rossi *et al.*, 2000). Glycosylation increased the antigenicity of low-molecular-weight antigen (Obregon-Henao *et al.*, 2001). Sera from patients with cysticercosis identify the carboxyl end of *T. cysticercus* paramyosin, an immunodominant antigen. Cell-mediated immunity did not show any reaction to this antigen (Vazquez-Talavera *et al.* 2001). Recombinant antigens of *T. solium* species, including NC-3, TS14, Ag1V1, and Ag1V2, were used successfully to detect specific antibodies in neurocysticercosis (Greene *et al.*, 2000; Hubert *et al.*, 1999; Sako *et al.*, 2000). Serologic diagnosis of the intermediate host (pigs) has an important role in prevention. Excretory-secretory antigen from cysticerci helps to diagnose most cases of pig infection (D'Souza and Hafeez, 1999). Passive transfer of anticysticercal antibodies to piglets occurs solely via colostrum (Gonzalez *et al.*, 1999). Vaccination of pigs with recombinant DNA (Cai *et al.*, 2001) and synthetic peptide (Huetra *et al.*, 2001) significantly reduced infection burden and induced protection. A Th1 profile response has been identified in mice vaccinated with full-length recombinant paramyosin (Vazquez-Talavera *et al.*, 2001) and KETc1 (Toledo *et al.*, 2001) antigens.

H. nana can infect mice. *In vivo* suppression of T-cell immunity by tacrolimus (FK506) is related to complete inhibition of IL-2 and IFN-γ mRNA expression in mesenteric CD4$^+$ cells that were induced by *H. nana* infection. Egg infection induces a rapid increase in INF-γ. The Th2 immune response is predominant during luminal infection (IL-4 and Il-5), whereas a Th1 response is apparent during the tissue phase (Asano *et al.*, 1996). An extract from oncospheres of *H. nana* induces eosinophilic chemotactic activity *in vitro* and in mice. Intestinal mucosa from challenged mice shows a markedly higher number of eosinophils than in primary infection. Intestinal eosinophils may be a major contributor to oxygen radical production (Niwa and Miyazota, 1996 a,b).

As in humans, the larval form lives in the intestinal tissue, whereas adults reside in the lumen. Strong immunity to reinfection develops, limiting the tissue phase, which leads to gradual clearance of the adult worms. Infection initiates a mononuclear and neutrophilic cellular infiltrate, with subsequent appearance of eosinophils and mastocytosis. The process peaks 20 days after initiation of the infection and then declines coincidentally with worm expulsion. The mice develop resistance to reinfection. T-cell–deficient mice cannot clear the infection. Also, T cells from mesenteric lymph nodes of immune mice adoptively transferred into naive neonatal or T cell–deficient recipients afford nearly complete protection. Thus, it appears that T lymphocytes are essential for an effective immune response against this organism (Asano and Okamoto, 1991; Bortoletti *et al.*, 1992). The parasite also elicits an antibody response of unknown significance.

Parasites and conditioning of the immune response

An ongoing Th2-type response to a particular parasite can modulate the immune response to other concomitant parasitic, bacterial, and viral infections. Data suggest that humans with schistosomiasis are more resistant to infection with *Ascaris* and *Trichuris*. Mice naturally susceptible to infection with the intestinal nematode *T. muris* acquire resistance when coinfected with *S. mansoni*. Intraperitoneal injection of schistosome ova into uninfected mice affords similar protection. Markers of Th1 and Th2 responses *in vivo* are production of IgG2a and IgG1. Levels of IgG2a are high in mice infected with *T. muris* alone, yet no IgG2a is detectable in coinfected animals, although the level of total IgG remains unchanged (Curry *et al.*, 1995).

Mice injected with *Mycobacterium avium* develop chronic infection associated with a strong Th1 response and granulomas in the lungs and liver. Splenocytes and granuloma cells from these infected animals normally produce large amounts of IgG2a and IFN-γ but no IL-4 or IL-5. Mice infected with *S. mansoni* following establishment of an *M. avium* infection produce mycobacterial granulomas containing eosinophils. Also, in coinfected mice, splenocytes and granuloma cells secrete more IgG but much less IgG2a.

There are other examples of parasitic infection altering immune responses. Infection of mice with *S. mansoni* delays clearance of vaccinia virus and alters responsiveness to sperm whale myoglobin (Kullberg *et al.*, 1992). Mice also develop a Th2 response when infected with the microfilaria *Brugia malayi* or immunized with a soluble filarial extract from this parasite. The ongoing Th2 response to this helminth antigen modulates the Th1 response to mycobacterial antigen (Pearlman *et al.*, 1993). Moreover, *N. brasiliensis*, a murine intestinal nematode, stimulates Th2 activity, and *Nippostrongylus* infection delays kidney graft rejection in rats. Cross-regulatory suppression of Th1 activity probably is the mechanism (Ledingham *et al.*, 1996).

These findings have important implications. Persons harboring helminths possibly are more apt to mount a diminished Th1 response when challenged with other antigens. This could render them more susceptible to infection with mycobacteria, chronic hepatitis viruses, and other infections controlled by the Th1 response. However, helminth infections may afford protection against infectious agents controlled by Th2-type inflammation.

Perhaps more than half the population of the world have had a helminthic infection at some time. These infections are most frequent in childhood. In the past, humans have always harbored parasites; now this is not the case. Individuals living in increasingly hygienic temperate climates acquire helminths less frequently. Within this population subset, there appears to be an increasing prevalence of autoimmunity-related afflictions and Crohn's disease. In general, parasites often provide some benefit to the host. Perhaps the failure to acquire these infections and to experience Th2 conditioning predisposes humans to aberrant inflammatory illnesses.

REFERENCES

Asano K., Taki M., Matsuo S., Yamada K. (1996). Mode of action of FK-506 on protective immunity to *Hymenolepis nana* in mice. *In vivo* 10, 537–545.

Abd-Alla, M.D., Jackson, T.F.H.G., Gathiram, V., El-Hawey, A.M., and Ravdin, J.I. (1993). Differentiation of pathogenic *Entamoeba histolytica* infection from nonpathogenic infection by detection of galactose inhibitable adherence protein antigen in sera and feces. *J. Clin. Microbiol.* 31, 2845–2850.

Abd-Alla, M.D., Jackson, T.F.H.G., Reddy, S., Ravdin, J.I. (2000). Diagnosis of invasive amebiasis by ELISA of saliva to detect amebic lectin antigen and anti-lectin IgG antibodies. *J. Clin. Microbiol.* 38, 2344–2347.

Abd-Alla, M.D., Jackson, T.F., Soong, G.C., Mazanec, M., Ravdin, J.I. (2004). Identification of the *Entamoeba histolytica* galactose-inhibitable lectin epitopes recognized by human immunoglobulin A antibodies following cure of amebic liver abscess. *Infect. Immun.* 72, 3974–3980.

Abo-El-Maged, I., Soong, G., El-Hawey, A., and Ravdin, J. (1996). Humoral and mucosal IgA antibody response to a recombinant 52-kDa cysteine-rich portion of the *Entamoeba histolytica* galactose-inhibitable lectin correlates with detection of native 170-kDa antigen in serum patients with amebic colitis. *J. Infect. Dis.* 174, 157–162.

Aguirre, S.A., Mason, P.H., and Perryman, L.E. (1994). Susceptibility of major histocompatibility complex MHQ class I- and MHC class II deficient mice to *Cryptosporidium panum* infection. *Infect. Immun.* 62, 697–699.

Amiri, P., Locksley, R.M., Parslow, T.G., Sadick, M., Rector, E., Ritter, D., and McKerrow, J.H. (1992). Tumor necrosis factor α restores granulomas and induces parasite egg-laying in schistosome-infected SCID mice. *Nature* 356, 604–607.

Aquino, R.T., Chieffi, P.P., Catunda, S.M., Araujo, M.F., Riberiro, M.C., Taddeo, E.F., Rolim, E.G. (2000). Hepatitis B and C virus markers among patients with hepatosplenic mansinic schistosomiasis. *Revista do Instatuto de Medicina tropical de Sao Paulo.* 42, 313–320.

Artis D., Humphreys, N.E., Bancroft, A.J., Rothwell, N.J., Potten, C.S., Grencis, R.K. (1999). Tumor necrosis factor alpha is a critical component of interleukin 13-mediated protective T helper cell type 2 responses during helminth infection. *J. Exper. Med.* 190, 953–962.

Asano, K., and Okamoto, K. (199 1). Transfer of T-cell mediated immunity to *Hymenolepis nana* from mother mice to their neonates. *Experientia.* 48, 67–71.

Bancroft, A.J., Else, K.J., and Grencis, R.K. (1994). Low-level infection with *Trichuris muris* significantly affects the polarization of the CD4 response. *J. Immunol.* 24, 3113–3118.

Bancroft, A.J., Artis, D., Donaldson, D.D., Sypek, J.P., Grencis, R.K. (2000). Gastrointestinal nematode expulsion in IL-4 knockout mice is IL-13 dependent. *Eur. J. Immunol.* 30, 2083–2091.

Bancroft, A.J., Else, K.J., Sypek, J.P., Grencis, R.K. (1997). Interleukin-12 promotes a chronic intestinal nematode infection. *Eur. J. Immunol.* 27, 866–870.

Bell, R.G., and Issekutz, T. (1993). Expression of a protective intestinal immune response can be inhibited at three distinct sites by treatment with anti-ot4 integrin. *J. Immunol.* 151(9), 4790–4802.

Beving, D.E, Soong, C.J, Ravdin, J.I. (1996). Oral immunization with a recombinant cysteine-rich section of *Entamoeba histolytica* galactose-inhibitable lectin elicits an intestinal secretory immunoglobulin A response that has *in vitro* adherence inhibition activity. *Infect. Immun.* 64(4), 1473–1476.

Bienz, M., Wittwer, P., Zimmermann, V., Muller N. (2001). Molecular characterization of a predominant antigen region of *Giardia lamblia* variant surface protein H7. *Intl. J. Parasitol.* 31, 827–832.

Blackwell, N.M., Else, K.J. (2001). B cells and antibodies are required for resistance to parasitic gastrointestinal nematode *Trichuris muris. Infect. Immunity* 69, 3860–3868.

Blessman, J., Buss, H., Antonnu, P., Thi, H.D., Abd Alla, M.D., Jackson, T.F.H.G., Ravdin, J.R., Tannich, E. Real time PCR Detection and Differentiation of *Entamoeba histolytica* and *Entamoeba dispar* in fecal samples (2002). *J. Clin. Microbiol.* 40(12), 4413–4417.

Bortoletti, G., Gabriele, F., and Palmas, C. (1992). Mechanisms of protective immunity in *Hymenolepis nana*/mouse model. *Parasitologia* 34, 17–22.

Braga, L.L., Ninomiya, H., McCoy, J.J., Eacker, S., Wiedmer, T., Pham, C., Wood, S., Sims, P.J., and Petri, W. A., Jr. (1992). Inhibition of the complement membrane attack complex by the galactose-specific adhesin of *Entamoeba histolytica. J. Clin. Invest.* 90, 1131–1137.

Bruschi, F., Pozio, E., Watanabe, N., Gomez-Morales, M.A., Ito, M., Huang, Y., Binaghi, R. (1999). Anaphylactic response to parasite antigens: IgE and IgG1 independently induced death in Trichinella-infected mice. *International Archives of Allergy and Immunology* 119, 291–296.

Bueno, E.C., Vaz, A.J., Machado, L.D., Livramento, J.A. (2000). Neurocysticercosis: detection of IgG, IgA and IgE antibodies in cerebrospinal fluid, serum and saliva samples by ELISA with *T. solium* and *T. crassiceps* antigen. *Arquivos de Neeuro-Psiquiatria* 58, 18–24.

Byrd, L.G., Conrad, J.T., and Nash, T.E. (1994). *Giardia lamblia* infections in adult mice. *Infect. Immun.* 62(8), 3583–3585.

Cai, X., Chia, Z., Jing, Z., Wang, P., Luo, X., Chen, J., Dou, Y., Feng, S., Su, C., Jin, J. (20001). Studies on the development of DNA vaccine against *Cysticercus cellulosae* infection and its efficacy. *Southeast Asian J. Trop. Med. Public Health.* 32, 105–110.

Cetre, C., Pierrot, C., Maire, E., Capron, M., Capron, A., Khalife, J. (2000). Interleukin-13 and IgE antibodies in experimental schistosomiasis. *European Cytokine Network* 11, 241–249.

Chappell, C.L., Okhuysen, P.C, Sterling, C.R., Wang, C., Jakubowski, W., DuPont, H.L. (1999). Infectivity of *Cryptosporidium parvum* in healthy adults with pre-existing anti-*C. parvum* serum immunoglobulin G. *Am. J. Trop. Med. Hyg.* 60, 157–164.

Char, S., Cevallos, A.M., Yarnson, P., Sullivan, P.B., Neale, G., and Farthing, M.J.G. (1993). Impaired IgA response to *Giardia* heat shock antigen in children with persistent diarrhea and giardiasis. *Gut* 34, 38–40.

Chatterjee, B.P., Santra, A., Kamakar, P.R., Mazumder, D.N. (1996). Evaluation of IgG4 response in ascariasis by ELISA for serodiagnosis. *Trop. Med. Intl. Health* 1, 633–639.

Chen, W., Harp, J.A., and Harmsen, A.G. (1993). Requirements for CD4+ cells and γ interferon in resolution of established *Cryptosporidium parvum* infection in mice. *Infect. Immun.* 61(9), 3928–3932.

Chensue, S.W., Warmington, K.S., Ruth, J.H., Sanghi, P.S., Lincoln, P., and Kunkel, S.L. (1996). Role of monocyte chemoattractant protein 1 (MCP-1) in Th1 (mycobacterial) and Th2 (schistosomal) antigen induced granuloma formation: Relationship to local inflammation, Th cell expression, and IL-12 production. *J. Immunol.* 157, 4602–4608.

Cooper, P.J., Chico, M.E., Sandovel, C., Espinel, I,. Gyevara, A., Kennedy, M.W., Urban, J.F., Griffin, G.E., Nutman, T.B. (2000). Human infection with *Ascaris lumbricoides* is associated with a polarized cytokine response. *J. Infect. Dis.* 182, 1207–1213.

Costa-Cruz, J.M., Bullamah, C.B., Goncalves-Pires, R., Campos, D.M., Vieira, M.A. (1997). Cryo-microtome section of coproculture larvae of *Strongyloides stercoralis* and *Strongyloides ratti* as antigen source for immune diagnosis of human strongyloidiasis. *Revista do Instatuto de Medicina de Sao Paulo.* 39, 313–317.

Crabb, J.H. (1998). Antibody-based immunotherapy of cryptosporidiosis. *Adv. Parasitol.* 40, 121–149.

Curry, A.J., Else, K.J., Jones, F., Bancroft, A., Grencis, R.K., and Dunne, D.W. (1995). Evidence that cytokine-mediated immune interaction induced by *Schistosoma mansoni* alters disease outcome in mice concurrently infected with *Trichuris muris*. *J. Exp. Med.* 181, 769–774.

D'Souza, P.E., Hafeez, M. (1999). Detection of *Taenia solium* cysticercosis in pigs by ELISA with an excretory-secretory antigen. *Vet. Res. Comm.* 23, 293–298.

de Jesus, A.R., Silva, A., Santana, L.B., Magalhaes, A., de Jesus, A.A., De Almeida, R.P., Rego, M.A., Burattini, M.N. Pearce E.J. Carvalho E.M. (2002). Clinical and immunologic evaluation of 31 patients with acute schistosomiasis mansoni. *J. Infect. Dis.* 185, 98–105.

Dol, S., Heinrich, J, Wichmann, H.E., Wjst, M. (1998). Ascaris-specific IgE and allergic sensitization in a cohort of school children in former East Germany. *J. Allergy Clin. Immunol.* 102, 414–420.

Doligalska, M., Laskowska, M. (2000). Inhibition of protective IgA response by ketotifen is related to inflammatory reaction in the peritoneal cavity and intestinal mucosa of BALB/c mice infected with *Trichinella spiralis*. *Parasitol. Res.* 86, 480–485.

Durmaz, B., Yakinic, C., Koro, L.M., Durmaz, R. (1998). Concentration of total serum IgE in parasitized children and the effect of the antiparasitic therapy on IgE levels. *J. Trop. Ped.* 44, 121.

Ebert, E.C. (1999). Giardia induces proliferation and IFNγ production by intestinal lymphocytes. *Gut* 44, 342–346

Eckmann, L., Reed, S.L., Smith, J.R., and Kagnoff, M.F. (1995). *Entamoeba histolytica* trophozoites induced in inflammatory cytokine response by cultured human cells through the paracrine action of cytolytically released interleukin-la. *J. Clin. Invest.* 96, 1269–1279.

Eckmann, L., Gillin, F.D. (2001). Microbes and microbial toxins: paradigms for microbial–mucosal interactions I. Pathophysiological aspects of enteric infection with the lumen-dwelling protozoan pathogen *Giardia lamblia*. *Am. J. Physiol. Gastrointest. Liver Physiol.* 280, 1–6.

El Ridi, R., Shoemaker, C.B., Farouk, F., El Sherif, N.H., Afifi, A. (2001). Human T-and B-cell responses to *Schistosoma mansoni* recombinant glyceraldehyde 3-phosphate dehydrogenase correlate with resistance to reinfection with *S. mansoni* or *Schistosoma haematobium* after chemotherapy. *Infect. Immun.* 69, 237–244.

El-Ahwany, E.G., Hanallah, S.B., Zada, S.E.L, Ghorab, N.M., Badir, B., Badawy, A., Sharmy, R., Hassanein, H.I. (2000). Immunolocalization of macrophage adhesion molecule-1 and macrophage inflammatory protein-1 in schistosomal soluble egg antigen-induced granulomatous hyporesponsiveness. *Intl. J. Parasitol.* 30, 837–842.

El-Sarkawy, I.M., Ibrahim, A.A., el-Bassuoni, M.A. (2002). Neutrophil apoptosis in acute and chronic *Schistosoma mansoni* infection. *J. Egypt Soc. Parasitol.* 32, 507–516.

Else, K.J., Finkelman, F.D., Maliszewski, C.R., and Grencis, R.K. (1994). Cytokine-mediated regulation of chronic intestinal helminth infection. *J. Exp. Med.* 179, 347–351.

Feng, Z., Qui, Z., Li, Y., Zhu, C., Xue, W., Guan, X. (2002). Protective immunity induced by anti-idiotypic monoclonal antibody NP30 of *Schistosoma japonicum*. *Chin. Med. J.* 115, 576–579.

Gonzalez, A.E., Verastegui, M., Noh, J.C., Gavidia, C., Falcon, N., Bernal, T., Garcia, H.H., Tasang, V.C., Gilman R.H., Wilkins, P.P. (1999). Persistence of passively transferred antibodies in procine *Taenia solium* cysticercosis. Cysticercosis working group in Peru. *Vet. Parasitol.* 86, 113–118.

Green, R.M., Hancock, K., Wilkins, P.P., Tsang, V. C. (2000). *Taenia solium:* molecular cloning and serologic evaluation of 14- and 18-kDa related, diagnostic antigens. *J. Parasitol.* 86, 1001–1007.

Greenberg, P.D., Cello, J.P. (1996). Treatment of severe diarrhea caused by *Cryptosporidium parvum* with oral bovine immunoglobulin concentrate in patient with aids. *J. AIDS* 13, 348–354.

Grenis, R.K. (1993). Cytokine-mediated regulation of intestinal helminth infections: The *Trichuris* muris model. *Ann. Trop. Med. Parasitol.* 87(16), 643–647.

Gurish, M.F., Humbles, A., Tao, H., Finkelstein, S., Boyce, J.A., Gerard, C., Fried, D.S., Austen, K.F. (2002). CCR3 is required for tissue eosinophilia and larval cytotoxicity after infection with *Trichinella spiralis*. *J. Immunol.* 11, 5730–5736.

Haque, R., Ali, I. M., Sack, R.B., Farr, B.M., Ramakrishnan, G., Petri, W.A. (2001). Amebiasis and mucosal IgA antibody against *Entamoeba histolytica* adherence lectin in Bangladeshi children. *J. Infect. Dis.* 183, 1787–1793.

Haque, R., Mollah, N.U., Ali, I.K.M., *et al.* (2000) Diagnosis of amebic liver abscess and intestinal infection with the TechLab *Entamoeba histolytica* II antigen detection and antibody tests. *J. Clin. Microbiol.* 38, 3235–3239.

Haque, R., Duggal, P., Ali, I.M., *et al.* (2002) Innate and acquired resistance to amebiasis in Bangladeshi children. *J. Infect. Dis.* 86(4), 547–552.

Hebert, D.R., Nalon, T.J., Schad, G.A., Lustigman, S., Abraham, D. (2002). Immunoaffinity-isolated antigens induce protective immunity against larval *Strongyloides stercoralis* in mice. *Exper. Parasitol.* 100, 112–120.

Hegazy, I.H. (1998). Function correlation between histamine metabolism and worm expulsion in *Trichinella spiralis*. *J. Egypt Soc. Parasitol.* 28, 247–256.

Helmby, H., Grencis, R.K. (2002). IL-18 regulates intestinal mastocytosis and Th2 cytokine production independently of INF-γ during *Trichinella spiralis* infection. *J. Immunol.* 196, 2553–2560.

Hemdon, F.J., and Kayes, S.G. (1992). Depletion of eosinophils by anti-IL-5 monoclonal antibody treatment of mice infected with *Trichinella spiralis* does not alter parasite burden of immunologic resistance to reinfection. *J. Immunol.* 149(11), 3642–3647.

Henri, S., Chevillard, C., Mergani, A., Paris, P., Gaudart, J., Camilla, C., Dessein, H., Montero, F., Elwili, N.E., Saeed, O.K., Magzoub, M., Dessein, A.J. (2002). Cytokine regulation of periportal fibrosis in humans infected with *Schistosoma mansoni*: IFN-γ is associated with protection against fibrosis and TNF-alpha with aggravation of disease. *J. Immunol.* 169, 929–936.

Heyworth, M. (1992). Immunology of giardia and cryptosporidium infections. *J. Infect. Dis.* 166, 465–472.

Heyworth, M.F., Carlson, J.R., and Ermak, T.H. (1997). Clearance of *Giardia muris* infection requires helper/inducer T lymphocytes. *J. Exp. Med.* 165, 1743–1748.

Hubert, K., Andriantsimahavandy, A., Michault, A., Frosch, M., Muhlschlegel, F.A. (1999). Serological diagnosis of human cysticercosis by use of recombinant antigens from *Taenia solium* cysticerci. *Clin. Diagn. Lab. Immunol.* 6, 479–482.

Huerta, M., de Aluja, A.S., Fragoso, G., Toledo, A., Villalobos, N., Hernandez, M., *et al.* (2001). Synthetic peptide vaccine against *Taenia solium* pig cysticercosis: successful vaccination in controlled field trial in rural Mexico. *Vaccine* 20, 262–266.

Isaac-Renton, J., Blatherwick, J., Bowie, W.R., Fyfe, M., Khan, M., Li, A., King, A., MacLean, M., Medd, L., Moorehead, W., Ong, C.S., Robertson, W. (1999). Epidemic and endemic prevalence of antibodies to cryptosporidiosis and *Giardia* in residents of three communities with different drinking water supplies. *Am. J. Trop. Med. Hyg.* 60, 578–583.

Jakubzick, C., Kunkel, S.L., Joshi, B.H., Puri, R.K., Hogaboam, C.M. (2002). Interleukin-13 fusion cytotoxin arrests *Schistosoma mansoni* egg-induced pulmonary granuloma formation in mice. *Am. J. Pathol.* 161, 1283–1297.

Kamal, S.M., Bianchi, L., Al Tawil, A., Koziel, M., El Sayed Khalifa K., Peter, T., Rasenack, J.W. (2001). Specific cellular immune response and cytokine patterns in patients coinfected with hepatitis C virus and *Schistosoma mansoni*. *J. Infect. Dis.* 184, 972–982.

Karanja, D.M., Hightower, A.W., Colley, D.G., Mwinzi, P.N., Galil, K., Andove, J., Secor, W.E. (2002). Resistance to reinfection with *Schistosoma mansoni* in occupationally exposed adults and effect of HIV-1 co-infection on susceptibility to schistosomiasis: a longitudinal study. *Lancet.* 360, 592–596.

Kaur, H., Ghosh, S., Samra, H., Vinayak, V.K., Ganguly, N.K. (2001). Identification and characterization of an excretory-secretory producer from *Giardia lamblia. Parasitology* 123, 347–356.

Kaur, H., Samra, H., Vinayak, V.K., Ganguly, N.K. (1999). Immune effector response of an excretory-secretory product of *Giardia lamblia. FEMS Immunol. Med. Microbiol.* 23, 93–105.

Kelsall, B.L., Jackson, T.F.H.G.V., Pearson, R.D, and Ravdin, J.I. (1994). Secretory immunoglobulin A antibodies to the galactose inhibitable adherence protein in the saliva of patients with amebic liver abscess. *Am. J. Trop. Med. Hyg.* 83, 454–459.

Khan, W.I., Blennerhassett, P.A., Deng, Y., Gauldie, J., Vallance, B.A., Collins, S.M. (2001). IL-12 gene transfer alters gut physiology and host immunity and nematode-infected mice. *Am. J. Physiol. Gastrointest. Liver Physiol.* 281, 102–110.

Korenaga, M., Watanabe, N., Abe, T., and Hashiguchi, Y. (1996). Acceleration of IgE responses by treatment with recombinant interleukin-3 prior to infection with *Trichinella spiralis* in mice. *Immunology.* 87, 642–646.

Koyama, K., Ito, Y. (2000). Mucosal mast cell responses are not required for protection against infection with the murine nematode parasite *Trichuris muris. Parasite Immunol.* 22, 13–20.

Kullberg, M.C., Pearce, E.J., Hieny, S.E., Sher, A., and Berzofsky, J.A. (1992). Infection with *Schistosoma mansoni* alters Th1/Th2 cytokine responses to a non-parasite antigen. *Immunology* 148(10), 3264–3270.

Lacomini, J., Ricklan, D.E., and Stadecker, M.J. (1995). T cells expressing the γδ T cell receptor are not required for egg granuloma formation in schistosomiasis. *J. Immunol.* 25, 884–888.

Ledingham, D.L., McAlister V.C., Ehigiator, H.N., Giacomantonio, C., Theal, M., and Lee, T.D.G. (1996). Prolongation of rat kidney allograft survival by nematodes. *Transplantation* 61(2), 184–188.

Lin, J.Y., and Chadee, K. (1992). Macrophage cytotoxicity against *Entamoeba histolytica* trophozoites is mediated by nitric oxide from L-arginine. *J. Immunol.* 148(12), 3999–4005.

Loukas, A., Prociv, P. (2001). Immune response in hookworm infections. *Clin. Microbiol. Rev.* 14, 689–703.

Lujan, H.D., Mowatt, M.R., Wit, J-J., Lu, Y., Lees, A., Chance, M.R., and Nash, T.E. (1995). Purification of a variant specific surface protein of *Giardia lamblia* and characterization of its metal-binding properties. *J. Biol. Chem.* 270(23), 13807–13813.

Mathew, R.C., and Boros, D.L. (1986). Anti-L3T4 antibody treatment suppresses hepatic granuloma formation and abrogates antigen-induced interleukin-2 production in *Schistosoma mansoni* infection. *Infect. Immunol.* 54(3), 820–826.

McDonald, V., Robinson, H.A., Kelly, J.P., and Bancroft, G.J. (1994). *Cryptosporidium muris* in adult mice: Adoptive transfer of immunity and protective roles of CD4 versus CD8 cells. *Infect. Immun.* 62(6), 2289–2294.

Mendez-Loredo, B., Martinez, Y., Zamora, R., Chapa-ruiz, R., Ortiga-Pierres, G., Salinas-Tobon, R. (2001). The stage-specificity of the IgA response to newborn larva and TSL-1 antigens of *Trichinella spiralis* in humans infected with the parasite. *Parasite* 8, S158–S162.

Meng, T.C., Hetsko, M.L., and Gillin, F.D. (1996). Inhibition of *Giardia lamblia* excystation by antibodies against cyst walls and by wheat germ agglutinin. *Infect. Immun.* 64(6), 2151–2157.

Metawali, A., Elliott, D., Blum A.M., Li, J., Sandor, M., Lynch, R., Noben Trauth, N., and Weinstock, J.V. (1996). The granulomatous response in murine schistosomiasis mansoni does not switch to Th1 in IL-4 deficient C57BL/6 mice. *J. Immunol.* 157, 4546–4553.

Metwali, A., de Andres, B., Blum, A., Elliott, D., Li, J., Qadir, K., Sandor, M., Weinstock, J. (2002). Th2-type granuloma development in acute schistosomiasis is partly dependent on CD4⁺ T cells as the source of IL-4. *Eur. J. Immunol.* 32, 1242–1252.

Montesano, M.A., Colley, D.G., Willard, M.T., Freeman, G.L. Jr., Secor, W.E. (2002). Idiotype expressed early in experimental *Schistosoma mansoni* infections predicts clinical outcomes of chronic disease. *J. Exp. Med.* 195, 1223–1228.

Morales, M.A., Mele, R., Sanchez, M., Sacchini D., De Giacomo, M., Pozio, E. (2002). Increased CD8(⁺)-T-cell expression and type 2 cytokine pattern during the muscular phase of trichinella infection in humans. *Infect. Immun.* 70, 233–239.

Moss, D.M., Chappell, C.L., Okhuysen, P.C, DuPont, H.L, Arrowood, M.J., Hightower, A.W., Lammie, P.J. (1999). The antibody response to 27-, 17-, and 15-kDa *Cryptosporidium* antigens following experimental infection in humans. *J. Infect. Dis.* 178, 827–833.

Negra-Correa, D., Adams, L.S., and Bell, R.G. (1996). Intestinal transport and catabolism of IgE: A major blood-independent pathway of IgE dissemination during a *Trichinella spiralis* infection of rats. *J. Immunol.* 157, 4037–4044.

Negreo-Corea, D. (2001). Importance of immunoglobulin E (IgE) in the protective mechanism against gastrointestinal nematode infection: looking at intestinal mucosa. *Revista do Instituto de Medicina Tropical de Sao Paulo.* 43, 291–299.

Neva, F.A., Gam, A.A., Maxwell, C., Pelletier, L.L. (2001). Skin test antigens for immediate hypersensitivity prepared from infective larvae of *Strongyloides stercoralis. Am. J. Trop. Med. Hyg.* 65, 567–572.

Niwa, A, Miyazato, T. (1996a). Enhancement of intestinal eosinophilia during *Hymenolepis nana* infection in mice. *J. Helmenth.* 70, 33–41.

Niwa, A, Miyazato, T. (1996b). Reactive oxygen intermediates from eosinophils in mice infected with *Hymenolepis nana. Parasite Immunology.* 18, 285–295.

Obregon-Henao, A., Gil, D.L., Gomez, D.I., Sanzon, F., Teale, J.M., Restrepo, B.I. (2001). The role of N-linked carbohydrates in the antigenicity of *Taenia solium* metacestode glycoproteins of 12, 16 and 18 KD. *Molec. Biochem. Parasitol.* 114, 209–215.

Ortiz, D., Afonso, C., Hagel, I., Rodriguez, O, Ortiz, C., Palenque, M., Lynch, N.R. (2000). Influence of helminthic infection and nutritional status in immune response in Venezuelan children. *Pan Am. J. Public Health* 8, 156–163.

Park, M.K., Hoffmann, K.F., Cheever, A.W., Amichay, D., Wynn, T.A., Farber, J.M. (2001). Pattern of cytokine expression in models of *Schistosoma mansoni* inflammation and infection reveal relationships between type 1 and type 2 response and chemokines *in vivo. Infect. Immunity* 69, 6755–6768.

Pearlman, E., Kazura, J.W., Hazlett, F.E., Jr., and Boom, W.H. (1993). Modulation of urine cytokine responses to mycobacterial antigen. b) helminth-induced T helper 2 cell responses. *J. Immunol.* 151(9), 4857–4864.

Petri, W.A. Jr, Haque, R., Mann, B.J. (2002) The bittersweet interface of parasite and host: Lectin-carbohydrate interactions during human invasion by the parasite *Entamoeba histolytica. Annu. Rev. Microbiol.* 56, 39–64.

Petri, W., Smith, R., Schlesinger, P., and Ravdin, J. (1987) Isolation of galactose-binding lectin which mediates the *in vitro* adherence of *Entamoeba histolytica. J. Clin. Invest.* 80, 1238–1244.

Poirriez, J. (2001). A three year follow-up of total serum IgE levels in three patients treated for strongyloidiasis. *Parasite* 8, 359–362.

Porto, A.F., Neva, F.A., Bittencourt, H., Lisbeo, W., Tompson, R., Alcantara, L., Carvalho, E.M. (2001). HTLV-1 decreased Th2 type of immune response in patients with strongyloidiasis. *Parasite Immunology* 23, 503–507.

Ramaswamy, K., Negrao-Correa, D., and Bell, R. (1996). Local intestinal immune responses to infection with *Trichinella spiralis*: Real-time, continuous assay of cytokines in the intestine (afferent) and efferent thoracic duct lymph of rats. *J. Immunol.* 156, 4328–4337.

Ramos, F., Valenzuela, A., Moran, P., Gonzalez, E., Ramiro, M., Cidello, R., Martinez, M.D.C., Melendro, E.I., and Ximenez, C. 1997. Anti-*E. histolytica* IgA antibodies in saliva of *E. histolytica* and *E. dispar* infected individuals: longitudinal study of cohorts. *Arch. Med. Res.* 28, S327–S239.

Ravdin, J.I., and Kelsall, B.L. (1994). Role of mucosal secretory immunity in the development of an amebiasis vaccine. *Am. J. Trop. Med. Hyg.* 50(5), 36–41.

Ravdin, J.I., Abd-Alla, M.D., Welles, S.L., Reddy, S., Jackson, T.F. (2003). Intestinal antilectin immunoglobulin A antibody response and immunity to *Entamoeba dispar* infection following cure of amebic liver abscess. *Infect. Immun.* 71, 6899–6905.

Richard, M., Grencis, R.K., Humphreys, N.E., Renauld, J.C., Van Snick, J. (2000). Anti-IL-9 vaccination prevents worm expulsion and blood eosinophilia in *Trichuris muris* infected mice. *Proc. Natl. Acad. Sci. USA* 97, 767–772.

Riggs, M.W. (2002). Recent advances in cryptosporidiosis: the immune response. *Microb. Infect.* 4, 1067–1080.

Riggs, M.W., (1997). *Cryptosporidium and Cryptosporidiosis*. Boca Raton, Florida: CRC Press, 129–161.

Robinson, P., Okhuysen, P.C., Chappell, C.L, Lewise, D.E., Shahab, I., White, A.C. (2001). Expression of IL-15 and IL-4 in IFNγ dependent control of experimental human *Cryptosporidium parvum* infection. *Cytokine* 15, 39–46.

Rosales-Borjas, D.M., Diaz-Rivadeneyra, J., Dona-Leyva, A., Zambrno-Villa, S.A., Mascaro, C., Osuna, A., Ortiz-Ortiz, L. (1998). Secretory immune response to membrane antigen during *Giardia lamblia* infection in humans. *Infect. Immun.* 66, 756–759.

Rossi, N., Rivas, I., Hernands, M., Urdaneta, H. (2000). Immunodiagnosis of neurocysticercosis: comparative study of antigen extract from *Cysticercus cellulosae* and *Taenia crassiceps*. *Revista Cubana de Medicina Tropical.* 52, 157–164.

Rotman, H.L., Schnyder-Candrian, S., Scott, P., Nolan, T.J., Schad, G.A., Abraham, D. (1997). IL-12 eliminates the Th-2 dependent protective immune response of mice to larval *Strongyloides stercoralis*. *Parasite Immunology* 19, 20–39.

Rotman, H.L., Yutanawiboonchai, W., Bigandi, R.A., Leon, O., Gleich, G.J., Nolan, T.J., Schad, G.A., Abraham D. (1996). *Strongyloides stercoralis*: Eosinophil-dependent immune-mediated killing of third stage larvae in BALB/cByJ mice. *Exp. Parasitol.* 82, 267–278.

Sako, Y., Nakao, M., Ikejima, T., Piao, X.Z., Nakaya, K., Ito., A. (2000). Molecular characterization and diagnostic value of *Taenia solium* low-molecular-weight antigen genes. *J. Clin. Microbiol.* 38, 4439–4444.

Salata, R.A., Martinez-Palomo, A., Murphy, C.F., Conales, L., Segovia, E., Trevino, R., Murray, H.W., Ravdin, J.I. (1986). Patients treated for amebic liver abscess develop a cell-mediated immune response effective *in vitro* against *Entamoeba histolytica*. *J. Immunol.* 136, 2633–2639.

Schaefer, D.A., Auerbach-Dixon, B.A., Riggs, M.W. (2000). Characterization and formulation of multiple epitope-specific neutralizing monoclonal antibodies for passive immunization against cryptosporidiosis. *Infect. Immun.* 68, 2608–2616.

Schopf, L.R., Hoffmann, K.F., Cheever, A.W., Urban, J.F., Jr., Wynn, T.A. (2002). Il-10 is critical for host resistance and survival during gastrointestinal helminth infection. *J. Immunol.* 168, 2383–2392.

Seguin, A., Mann, B.J., Keller, K., and Chadee, K. (1995). Identification of the galactose lectin epitopes of *Entamoeba histolytica* that stimulate tumor necrosis factor-α production by macrophages. *Proc. Natl. Acad. Sci. USA* 92, 12175–12179.

Sher, A., Coffman, R.L., Hiery, S., Scott, P., and Cheever, A.W. (1990). Interleukin 5 is required for the blood and tissue eosinophilia but not granuloma formation induced by infection with *Schistosoma mansoni*. *Proc. Natl. Acad. Sci. USA* 87, 61–67.

Siddiqui, A.A. Koenig, N.M., Sinensky, M., Berk, S.L. (1997). *Strongyloides stercoralis*: identification of antigens in natural human infections from endemic areas of the United States. *Parasitology Research.* 83, 655–658.

Silveira, A.M., Bethony, J., Gazzinelli, A., Kloos, H., Fraga, L.A., Alvares, M.C., Prata, A., Guerra, H.L. Loverde P.T., Correa-Olivera, R., Gazzinelli, G. (2002). High levels of IgG4 to *Schistosoma mansoni* egg antigens in individuals with periportal fibrosis. *Am. J. Trop. Med. Hyg.* 66, 542–549.

Singer, S.M., Elmendof, H.G., Conrad, J.T., Nash, T.E. (2001). Biological selection of variant-specific surface proteins in *Giardia lamblia*. *J. Infect. Dis.* 183, 119–124.

Singer, S.M., Nash, T.E. (2000). T-cell-dependent control of acute *Giardia lamblia* infection in mice. *Infect. Immun.* 68, 170–175.

Stadnyk, A.W., Dollard, C.D., Isskutz, A.C. (2000). Neutrophil mitogens stimulates intestinal epithelial cell cytokine expression during helminth infection. *J. Leukoc. Biol.* 68, 821–827.

Stager, S., Gottstein, B., Sager, H., Jungi, T.W., Muller, N. (1998). Influence of antibodies in mother's milk on antigenic variation of *Giardia lamblia* in the murine mother-offspring model of infection. *Infect. Immun.* 66, 1287–1292.

Toledo, A., Fragoso, G., Hernandez, M., Gevorkian, G., Lopez-Casillas, F., Hernandez, B., *et al.* (2001). Two epitopes shared by *Taenia crassiceps* and *Taenia solium* confer protection against murine *T. crassiceps* cysticercosis along with a prominent T1 response. *Infect. Immun.* 69, 1766–1773.

Turner, J., Faulkner, H., Kamgno, J., Else, K., Boussinesq, M., Bradley, J. E. (2002). A comparison of cellular and humoral immune responses to trichurid antigen in human trichuriasis. *Parasite Immunol.* 24, 83–93.

Urban, J.F., Jr., Fayer, R., Chen, S-J, Gause, W.C., Gately, M.K., and Finkelman, F.D. (1996). IL-12 protects immunocompetent and immunodeficient neonatal mice against infection with *Cryptosporidium parvum*. *J. Immunol.* 156, 263–268.

Vallance, B.A., Croitoru, K., Collins, S.M. (1998). T lymphocyte-dependent and -independent intestinal smooth muscle dysfunction in the *T. spiralis*-infected mouse. *Am. J. Physiol.* 275, 1157–1165.

Vallance, B.A., Caleazzi, F., Collins, S.M., Snider, D.P. (1999). CD4 T cells and major histocompatibility complex class II expression influence worm expulsion and increased intestinal muscle contraction during *Trichinella spiralis* infection. *Infect. Immun.* 67, 6090–6097.

Vazquez-Talavera, J., Solis, C.F., Medina-Escutia, E., Lopez, Z.M., Proano, J., Correa, D., Laclette, J.P. (2001). Human T and B cell epitope mapping of *T. solium* paramyosin. *Parasite Immunol.* 23, 575–579.

Vazquez-Talavera, J., Solis, C.F., Terrazas, L.I., Laclette, J.P. (2001). Characterization and protective potential of the immune response to *Taenia solium* paramyosin in a murine mode of cysticercosis. *Infect Immun.* 69, 5412–5416.

Venturiello, S.M., Malmassari, S.L., Costantino, S.N., Nunez, G.G. (2000). Cytotoxicity-blocking antibodies in human chronic trichinellosis. *Parasitol Res.* 86, 762–767.

Wang, W., and Chadee, K. (1995). *Entamoeba histolytica* suppresses γ interferon-induced macrophage class II major histocompatibility complex Ia molecule and I-Aβ mRNA expression by a prostaglandin E2 dependent mechanism. *Infect. Immun.* 63(3), 1089–1094.

Waters, W.R., and Harp, J.A. (1996). *Cryptosporidium parvum* infection in T-cell receptor (TCR)-α- and TCR-β-deficient mice. *Infect. Immun.* 64(5a), 1854–1857.

Weinstock, J.V. (1996). Parasitic diseases of the liver and intestine. *Clin. Gastroenterol.* 25(3).

Weinstock, J.V., and Boros, D.L. (1983). Organ-dependent differences in composition and function observed in hepatic and intestinal granulomas isolated from mice with *Schistosoma mansoni*. *J. Immunol.* 130, 418–422.

Weinstock, J., and Elliott, D. (1998). The substance P and somatostatin interferon-γ immunoregulatory circuit. *Ann. N.Y. Acad. Sci.* 840, 532–539.

White, A.C., Robinson, P., Okhuysen, P.C., Lewise, D.E., Shahab, I., Lahoti, S., DuPont, H.L., Chappell, C.L. (2000). IFNγ-expression in jejunal biopsies in experimental human cryptosporidiosis correlates with prior sensitization and control of oocyst excretion. *J. Infect. Dis.* 181, 701–709.

Yazicio Lu, M., One, U., Yalcin, I. (1996). Peripheral and nasal eosinophilia and serum total immunoglobulin E levels in children with ascariasis. *Turkish J. Pediatr.* 38, 477–484.

Parenteral Immunization Induces Mucosal Protection: A Challenge to the Mucosal Immunity Paradigm

Chapter 45

Brian J. Underdown

Department of Pathology, Faculty of Health Sciences, McMaster University, Hamilton, Ontario, Canada

Development of vaccines for administration via mucosal routes (*e.g.*, oral, nasal) has been a major goal of academic and industrial-based researchers for the past few decades. Mucosally administered vaccines are of particular interest for application against infectious agents that cause disease at mucosal sites and may also have application against systemic infection and disease. While mucosally administered vaccines have advanced closer to the clinic, there may still be a place for achieving both systemic and mucosal protection with vaccines administered parenterally.

Review of the evidence obtained from human clinical trials suggests that parenteral immunization may provide significant protection at mucosal surfaces, as well as against systemic disease. The purpose of this chapter is to review the data from human trials that describe the mucosal immune response to parenteral immunization and, in particular, the evidence that parenteral immunization affects clinical outcome at mucosal sites.

PARENTERAL IMMUNIZATION AND MUCOSAL IMMUNITY

To some extent, the ability of parenteral immunization to provide effective immunity at mucosal surfaces may depend on the type of immune effector functions required and the location of the infection. For example, where antibody is implicated in protective immunity, generation of high levels of serum IgG antibody via parenteral immunization may offer a ready source of functional antibody, provided the IgG antibody can reach the mucosal surface. In this regard, the secretions of the lower respiratory tract and female repro-

ductive tract contain as much IgG as IgA. The relatively high concentrations of IgG seen at these particular mucosal sites may reflect combinations of constitutive transcellular/paracellular transport from the systemic compartment and specific transport mechanisms. In addition, inflammatory processes that may be triggered early during an infection would be expected to promote transudation of IgG from the systemic compartment to the mucosal secretion. It follows that some of the protective effects observed in the respiratory and genitourinary tracts following parenteral immunization may result from the IgG antibody in serum that subsequently finds its way to the mucosae.

IgG antibody in mucosal secretions would be expected to function by limiting multiplication and entry of mucosal pathogens, as has been postulated for IgA antibody. It is also possible that IgG antibodies may promote bactericidal mechanisms involving inflammatory cells and/or complement at mucosal sites, particularly in the lamina propria of the mucosa, but few experimental data exist to support this hypothesis.

Since parenteral immunization is less effective in inducing IgA responses than IgG responses, it might be expected to be less effective at the gastrointestinal tract and nasal surface, where IgA is the predominant isotype. Thus, the need to induce IgA antibodies for infections of the lower respiratory tract and female reproductive tract may have been overemphasized. However, to the extent that IgA antibodies might be beneficial, parenteral immunization has been reported to induce a polymeric IgA response in serum early after immunization (Tarkowski *et al.*, 1990) and some of this antibody may find its way from the vasculature to the mucosal secretion (Renegar and Small, 1991).

The generation of specific antibody following immunization provides protection as long as sufficient levels can be maintained. Over time, the benefit of immunization accrues from the presence of memory cells that can be recalled at the time of infectious challenge. Parenteral immunization has also been reported to stimulate IgA antibody-secreting cells (ASCs) in the systemic circulation, with a concomitant appearance of IgA in saliva (Nieminen *et al.*, 1999; Engstrom *et al.*, 2002). Interestingly, in the latter study specific IgA2 antibody responses were higher in parotid saliva than in whole saliva, suggesting an emigration of IgA ASCs to the parotid gland. The importance of previous mucosal priming was demonstrated in a study of Herremans *et al.* (1999) in which subjects immunized with parenteral polio vaccine produced strong IgA memory responses and circulating α4β7 B cells capable of homing to mucosal surfaces (Butcher and Picker, 1996). However, this response was observed only in subjects previously vaccinated with oral polio vaccine. It should be noted that the early work of McDermott and Bienenstock (1979) indicated that while cells generated at the mucosae home best to mucosal sites, peripherally generated immune cells also localize to the mucosae, albeit less efficiently. In summary, parenteral immunization can induce both IgG and IgA antibodies, which in turn can provide antibody-mediated protection at the mucosae.

Cell-mediated immunity (CMI) is also thought to be a potential component of protective responses at mucosal surfaces (Woodland, 2003). A recent study with a human papillomavirus vaccine demonstrated cellular immune responses in peripheral blood. The ability of these effector cells to migrate to the cervical mucosa and to contribute to the pro-tection observed was not studied (Pinto *et al.*, 2003). Whether parenteral immunization can generate effective CMI at mucosal surfaces is not clear, and experimentally, it is difficult to determine in humans. It is possible that the dependence on specific mucosal homing receptors may be different for cell-mediated immune responses in comparison with antibody-mediated immunity. If this is true, it is possible that parenteral immunization might be less effective in generating protective mucosal immunity against infectious agents that are largely intracellular.

Examples of situations in which parenteral immunization appears to provide significant protective immunity in humans **(Table 45.1)** are described below.

THE POLIO PARADIGM

Both parenteral inactivated polio vaccine (IPV) and live-attenuated orally administered polio vaccine (OPV) prevent paralytic polio. One of the most cited examples of the advantages offered by mucosal immunization came from the elegant studies of Ogra and associates, who compared in humans the relative efficacy of IPV and OPV to induce mucosal antibody responses, believed to be important for reducing virus excretion and subsequent transmission to uninfected hosts. The results of these studies indicated that in general, OPV was superior to IPV in inducing mucosal antibody responses. Upon challenge of immunized subjects with a dose of OPV, OPV-immunized subjects excreted less virus than did subjects immunized with the parenteral IPV preparation. In addition, since IPV administered nasally was

Table 45.1. Mucosal Immunity Induced by Parenteral Immunization

| Vaccine[a] | Degree of Efficacy | | | |
	Prevents Disease	Disease Site	Prevents Mucosal Replication	Promotes Herd Immunity
IPV (inactivated polio)	≅ 95%	Systemic (CNS)	++ (respiratory tract), + (gastrointestinal)	Yes
Hib	≅ 95%	Systemic (CNS)	65% (respiratory tract)	Yes
Pertussis	≅ 85–95%[b]	Mucosae (respiratory)	? (respiratory tract)	Yes
Meningococcal polysaccharide	≅ 85%	Systemic (CNS)	50% (respiratory tract)	Possibly
Pneumococcal polysaccharide	≅ 60%	Mucosae-systemic	+ (respiratory tract)	Yes (adults)
Influenza subunit	≅ 65%[c]	Mucosae-systemic	90% with respect to influenza (respiratory tract)	?
Cholera	≅ 50%	Mucosae	? (GI tract)	Possibly
Typhoid	≅ 50–75%	Mucosae-systemic	? (GI tract)	?
Shigella	≅ 74%[d]	Mucosae	? (GI tract)	?

[a]See text for details.
[b]With whole-cell vaccines most potent.
[c]Depends on age group and relatedness of the vaccine and challenge strains.
[d]Based on one small study

also superior to IPV administered parenterally in inducing mucosal antibody responses, the route of immunization seemed to be a critical factor for optimal induction of mucosal responses (Ogra, 1995).

Nevertheless, the killed parenteral vaccine, used exclusively in Scandinavia and the Netherlands, resulted in considerable reduction in virus transmission among the population as well as prevention of poliomyelitis in vaccinated subjects (reviewed in Murdin et al., 1996). Small outbreaks that did occur were due to importation of virus into small clusters of unvaccinated subjects. The IPV used in these countries was generally of higher potency than the IPV preparations used initially in North America, but in the United States too, evidence of diminished spread of wild-type virus in children vaccinated with IPV was reported (Marine et al., 1962). Subsequent studies comparing an enhanced formulation of the parenteral preparation (E-IPV) indicated that both E-IPV and OPV induced comparable mucosal responses in the nasopharyngeal tract, although OPV was still superior to E-IPV with respect to the induction of mucosal immunity and prevention of shedding from the gastrointestinal tract (Onorato et al., 1991). It appears that a key factor in the success of IPV in preventing community spread of infection is the fact that nasopharyngeal shedding of wild-type virus is thought to be more significant than fecal shedding for polio virus transmission (Salk and Salk, 1977), and in this respect, IPV and OPV appear equally efficacious in attenuating multiplication of virus in the nasopharynx (reviewed in Murdin et al., 1996).

The ability of IPV to prevent multiplication of virus in the mucosae could be related to the generation of levels of antibody in the systemic compartment sufficient to overflow into the mucosal secretions. Transudation of serum IgG antibody into saliva and nasopharyngeal secretions is likely greater than that observed for the gastrointestinal tract. In addition to providing high levels of systemic antibody for transudation to the nasopharyngeal surface, it is likely that parenteral immunization with IPV resulted in the priming of mucosal immune tissue in vaccinees that could be recalled upon subsequent booster immunizations, especially following exposure to wild-type virus. Indeed, experimental evidence exists to support this hypothesis (reviewed in Murdin et al., 1996). The recent introduction of a combined (IPV-OPV) approach offers the potential to obtain the maximum protection against paralytic disease and community spread of wild-type virus (Plotkin, 1997).

RESPIRATORY INFECTIONS

Bacterial infections

Development of polysaccharide–protein conjugate vaccines has been key to the development of improved bacterial vaccines, particularly for respiratory infections (Robbins et al., 1996; Makela and Kayhty, 2002). Induction of T cell–dependent immune responses is seen as critical to the effectiveness of conjugate vaccines, particularly as it relates to

induction of memory responses and the subsequent attenuation of carriage of bacteria in the secretions, with a concomitant induction of herd immunity and reduction of community spread of infections. However, recent data have indicated that conjugate vaccines that have been successful in attenuating carriage and community spread in the general population at risk are not as effective in communities where the general health status is low. A number of factors could contribute to this observation, including overcrowding (with greater chance of transmission) and low general health status due to poor nutrition (O'Brien, 2001). In addition, the generation of conjugate vaccines that do not include the majority, if not all, of the polysaccharide antigens associated with pathogenic phenotypes may result in the replacement of one set of persisting pathogenic organisms for another set (Obaro and Adegbola, 2002).

Haemophilus influenzae type b

The recent introduction of a protein–polysaccharide conjugate vaccine for the prevention of meningitis associated with Haemophilus influenzae type b infection has resulted in the virtual elimination of this disease in developed countries where the vaccine has been widely adopted (Petola et al., 1992; Makela and Kayhty, 2002). In addition to preventing infection, a decrease in mucosal carriage of H. influenzae type b was also observed in vaccinees versus case-controls. This effect was extended to unvaccinated siblings of vaccinees (reviewed in Barbour et al., 1996). Overall, it appears that the efficacy of the conjugate H. influenzae type b vaccine (Hib vaccine) in reducing the prevalence of carriage is approximately 60% to 65%, while the efficacy of preventing meningitis is 90% or greater. These data, taken together, suggest that parenteral immunization with the conjugate Hib vaccine generates herd immunity within the population in addition to preventing disease associated with infection.

There are substantial data to indicate that the protective effects of conjugate Hib vaccines arise from the induction of antibody. For example, conjugate Hib vaccine induces high levels of serum IgG anti–polyribosylribitol phosphate (PRP) antibody in serum and IgG and IgA antibody in saliva (Pichichero and Insel, 1983; Kauppi et al., 1995). In the study of Kauppi et al., some subjects had detectable salivary IgA antibodies in the absence of detectable IgA antibodies in serum. This finding suggested that parenteral immunization (two times) gave rise to local IgA antibody synthesis. Secretory component was associated with the salivary IgA antibody, consistent with the notion that the salivary IgA antibody was locally derived. The induction of salivary IgA antibodies following parenteral immunization could be envisioned to take place by a number of mechanisms: dispersion of antigen from the parenteral site to mucosal sites and subsequent stimulation of the mucosal immune system; migration of antigen-stimulated B cells to distant mucosal sites, with or without subsequent boosting by natural infection; and transudation of IgG and IgA synthesized in the periphery from the blood space to the interstitial fluid bathing the epithelia, followed by subsequent transcytosis by epithelial cells. The relative role of IgG and IgA in the secretions in mediating protection is also not known. It appears that if antibody in secretions is to prevent carriage, it must precede infection. For example, immunization of *H. influenzae* type b carriers with the conjugate Hib vaccine did not cause a reduction of *H. influenzae* type b carriage (Barbour *et al.*, 1995). A study by Siber *et al.* (1992) supported the hypothesis that protection could be mediated by serum antibody, since passive immunization with serum immune globulin reduced the risk of *H. influenzae* type b–associated meningitis and, by extension, infection. Other studies have argued that in addition to antibody, cell-mediated immunity may be involved in generating protective immunity to *H. influenzae* type b. Whatever the mechanism, the fact that parenteral Hib vaccine reduces carriage and interrupts transmission to unvaccinated hosts seems indisputable (Barbour *et al.*, 1995; Barbour, 1996). However, the extent to which Hib conjugate vaccines protect the community depends on a variety of factors that in disadvantaged populations conspire to provide less protection against spread than in advantaged populations. For example, American Indian and Alaskan native children are more prone to infection and carriage than the general population (Millar *et al.*, 2000; Lucher *et al.*, 2002). In addition, other factors such as immunization schedule and the inclusion of other components in combination vaccines containing Hib vaccine may affect the efficacy of the latter (McVernon *et al.*, 2003; Preston, 2003).

Pertussis

Infection of the respiratory mucosae by *Bordetella pertussis* is the cause of whooping cough. Parenteral immunization was reported to prevent both infection and whooping cough (Blackwelder *et al.*, 1991). There appears to be general agreement that protection against systemic disease is mediated by antibody, although there is some dispute over the antibody specificities that correlate with protection. Immunity induced by acellular vaccines appears to correlate with IgG serum antibodies to pertussis toxin, pertactin, and fimbriae (Olin *et al.*, 2001). Protection against disease may be primarily mediated by antibody to pertussis toxin. Supporting this notion is the observation that passive transfer of immune globulin containing high levels of antibodies to pertussis toxin, the etiologic agent of whooping cough, provided protection against disease (Granstrom *et al.*, 1991).

Transmission of pertussis infection occurs primarily via household contacts (Deen *et al.*, 1995). Early studies indicated that in addition to preventing disease, acellular and whole cell vaccines induced "herd immunity" (Nielsen and 1994; Olin *et al.*, 2003). Surprisingly, a study of a parenteral vaccine consisting of pertussis toxoid compounded with diphtheria and tetanus toxoids produced 70% to 75% efficacy not only against disease but also against carriage. This protection could be correlated with levels of anti–pertussis toxin antibody (Taranger *et al.*, 2001).

Meningococcus

Neisseria meningitidis is a major cause of bacterial meningitis, especially in those below 20 years of age. The major route of transmission is via excretion from the nasopharyngeal secretions, although only a small proportion of infected individuals develop systemic disease. Protection against invasive disease caused by two of the major serotypes (A and C) is associated with antibodies (Goldschneider *et al.*, 1969). Parenteral vaccines based on the isolated capsular polysaccharides from serotypes A and C have been demonstrated to be approximately 85% effective, although protection, especially against serotype C, was believed to be less effective in children. As with all polysaccharide vaccines, protection is not long-lived (Reingold *et al.*, 1985).

More recently, meningococcal C conjugate vaccines have been developed and have been reported to reduce infection by as much as 87% in vaccinees, with a concomitant decrease in deaths due to invasive disease (Balmer *et al.*, 2002; Ruggeberg and Heath, 2003; Bose *et al.*, 2003). Studies of the immune responses following vaccination with the conjugate as well as the polysaccharide vaccines indicate that parenteral immunization with both these vaccine types induces both serum and salivary antibodies, although such responses were more robust in adolescents than in infants (Zhang *et al.*, 2000, 2001, 2002).

Studies of carriage and/or transmission with the new conjugate meningococcus vaccine are incomplete. However, earlier studies with a prototype type C polysaccharide vaccine administered parenterally indicated that in addition to prevention of disease, acquisition of infection was also reduced by 50% in comparison with controls (Gotschlich *et al.*, 1969; Artenstein *et al.*, 1970). Similar results were also reported by Balmer *et al.* (2002) for meningococcal conjugate vaccines. Both the polysaccharide and conjugate vaccines induced antibody in saliva, which may reflect the ability of these vaccines to induce herd immunity (Balmer *et al.*, 2002).

Pneumococcus

Streptococcus pneumoniae is a major cause of middle ear infection (otitis media) and can also be responsible for invasive diseases such as pneumonia, meningitis, and bacteremia. Pathology associated with pneumococcal infection can be classified as primarily mucosal (otitis media and pneumonia) or systemic (meningitis and bacteremia). Recently, a heptavalent pneumococcal conjugate vaccine has been developed that provides approximately 97% protection against systemic disease by pneumococcal strains represented in the vaccine (Black and Shinefield, 2002; Darkes and Plosker 2002). This vaccine was also shown to have a small but distinct effect on the occurrence of otitis media in vaccinees in comparison with controls (7% to 9% reduction); the vaccine was up to 23% effective in preventing frequent otitis media (Giebink, 2001). Additional studies have indicated that parenteral pneumococcal vaccines (polysaccharide only and conjugate vaccine) induce antibody in mucosal secretions and that the conjugate vaccine reduced nasopharyngeal carriage of vaccine strains (Dagan *et al.*, 1996, 2000; Mbelle *et al.*, 1999; Millar *et al.*, 2002; Palmu *et al.*, 2002). There is a need to increase the number of polysaccharide serotypes in the currently licensed conjugate vaccine, since there is evidence that elimination of one set of pathogenic pneumococci via vaccination leaves the population vulnerable to other pathogenic strains not covered by the current vaccine (O'Brien, 2001).

Viral infections

Influenza

Numerous studies have indicated that current parenteral vaccines against influenza are effective in reducing morbidity and mortality associated with infection in the elderly (Nichol *et al.*, 1994; Nordin *et al.*, 2001). Moreover, challenge studies in healthy adults have demonstrated the efficacy of parenteral influenza immunization against infection (Couch *et al.*, 1981), and there is evidence that vaccination of healthy working-age adults may also be cost-effective (Nichol *et al.*, 1995).

While current parenteral influenza vaccines are licensed on the basis of their ability to stimulate serum neutralizing antibodies, experimental studies in humans and animals suggest that mucosal antibody and local cellular responses may also play a role in mediating protection (Renegar and Small, 1991; Powers *et al.*, 1996; Clements *et al.*, 1986). The extent to which parenteral influenza vaccines induce immune responses at the mucosae is unclear. While parenteral immunization with conventional inactivated influenza vaccine has been reported to produce antibody responses in mucosal secretions (Brokstad *et al.*, 1995; Moldoveanu *et al.*, 1995), such antibody may be serum-derived. In this regard, Brokstad *et al.* (2002) reported that no significant increase in anti-flu antibody-secreting cells was observed in the nasal mucosae of human subjects immunized with the parenteral influenza vaccine.

It should be pointed out that some studies indicate that a combination of parenteral immunization with the current split subunit vaccine, together with a live-attenuated nasal vaccine, may provide better mucosal immune responses than either vaccine, although no determination of correlation with efficacy was undertaken in these studies (Gorse *et al.*, 1996). There appears to be a need to increase the efficacy of influenza vaccination with respect to reducing the incidence of clinical disease associated with influenza (Demicheli *et al.*, 2001). Nasally administered influenza vaccines have matured in recent years, with a live attenuated vaccine reaching the markets and several nasal subunit vaccines in clinical development. Such vaccines have the potential for increased efficacy and ease of use.

Respiratory syncytial virus (RSV)

While a licensed vaccine against RSV has not yet been developed, it is interesting that passive immunization with high-titered RSV immune globulin is effective in preventing RSV disease and infection of the lower respiratory tract in infants (Groothuis *et al.*, 1993). This is not surprising since, as described above, the lower respiratory tract is well endowed with IgG. Additional transudation of antibody from serum early after the infectious challenge might also amplify the role of IgG antibody in neutralizing the virus and preventing its entry and/or replication in the respiratory tract. Passive immunization is believed to be useful in providing protection only for short periods in infants at high risk, such as those about to undergo cardiac surgery or infants born prematurely. These findings suggest that a parenteral vaccine that induces high levels of serum neutralizing antibody should also be sufficient to prevent RSV infection in individuals at risk, such as infants and children and possibly the elderly. As mentioned previously, parenteral immunization may induce local IgA antibody as well as IgG antibody, but it is not clear to what extent secretory IgA (S-IgA) antibodies are required for optimal protection against RSV. In the case of RSV, the choice of parenteral versus mucosal vaccine for infants will also take into account the potential of each to induce enhanced disease following natural infection, as was observed with an experimental vaccine evaluated in the 1960s (Kim *et al.*, 1969).

Cytomegalovirus (CMV)

Postnatal infection of infants and/or mothers with cytomegalovirus is thought to occur via the nasal/oral route. While both cell-mediated and humoral immunity are important for immunity to CMV, efforts to develop a parenteral vaccine have been stimulated by the fact that naturally acquired maternal antibody appears to be protective against damaging congenital infection (Fowler *et al.*, 1992), and passive immunization of renal transplant patients with immune globulin also reduced the severity of disease caused by CMV (Snydman *et al.*, 1990). A study of individuals immunized with either of two candidate vaccines provided further support for the notion that parenteral immunization can generate antibody responses in mucosal secretions. Both live attenuated (Towne strain) and an adjuvanted subunit (gB protein in MF59) candidate vaccine induced antibody responses in mucosal secretions as well as in serum. The greatest responses were observed in individuals who had received two immunizations of the adjuvanted subunit vaccine. The quantity of IgG and IgA antibody measured in parotid saliva and nasal wash correlated positively with the quantity of antibody measured for each respective isotype in serum, suggesting that in this case, transudation from serum to these mucosal secretions could account for the appearance of IgG and IgA antibody following parenteral immunization (Wang *et al.*, 1996). In the case of CMV, parenteral immunization might be expected to prevent disease caused by systemically disseminated virus and possibly by preventing infection at the mucosae. Clinical trials will be required to establish these points.

Rubella

Rubella virus infection is transmitted via the nasopharynx, where it replicates. Approximately 2 weeks following infection, a prolonged viremia develops. Protection against disease is thought to be mediated by serum antibody (Davis *et al.*, 1971; Matter *et al.*, 1997). Following natural infection, reinfection may occur if a seropositive individual is exposed to rubella, its incidence depending on the size of the challenge, the level of serum antibody, and probably the presence of secretory antibody, as discussed below.

Studies of a live attenuated rubella vaccine (strain RA27/3), which is capable of replicating in the nasopharynx, indicated that protective immunity could be induced whether the vaccine was given by the nasal route or by the parenteral route. In these studies, protection was scored by the lack of a secondary antibody response following challenge with wild-type virus (Ogra et al., 1971; Fogel et al., 1978). In contrast, another rubella vaccine (HPV-77) did not prevent reinfection. Analysis of the antibody responses induced by these two vaccines indicated that the RA27/3 strain induced both serum and nasal antibody, while the HPV-77 strain induced only serum antibody (Banatvala et al., 1979). These data suggested that resistance to reinfection correlated, in part, with the presence of mucosal antibody responses, and these could be induced by both parenteral and intranasal administration (Plotkin et al., 1973).

GASTROINTESTINAL INFECTIONS

Cholera

One of the best studied mucosal infections is that caused by Vibrio cholerae. Studies of acquired immunity following natural infection or immunization indicate that the best correlate of acquired immunity is serum vibriocidal antibody (Levine and Kaper, 1993). While IgM vibriocidal antibody was first thought to be the primary correlate of resistance, later studies indicated that serum IgG vibriocidal antibodies were a better correlate of resistance (Losonsky et al., 1996). The findings of these studies are consistent with those of early studies in animals and support a role for serum antibody in mediating cholera immunity (Ahmed et al., 1970).

It is not clear how serum antibody could mediate protection to what is, in essence, a noninvasive mucosal infection. Robbins has argued that transudation of IgG onto the intestinal surface may provide protection in cholera (Robbins et al., 1995). Since the contribution of IgG to the antibody content of the intestinal secretions is quite small, an alternative explanation is that serum IgG vibriocidal antibody is merely a correlate of an as yet undefined immune element that is critical in mediating immunity to cholera infection. Since IgG antibodies have been associated with T helper 2 (Th2)-type cytokines, Losonsky et al. (1996) suggested that the latter may be an important effector of immunity to cholera. In addition, studies in experimental animals have also suggested that IgA antibody can act as an effector of immunity to cholera by neutralizing cholera toxin (Winner et al., 1991).

The cumulative experience with killed cholera vaccines administered parenterally indicates an overall efficacy of approximately 50% (Sack, 1994). It has been argued that the relatively poor efficacy of parenteral immunization to cholera is due to the fact that killed vaccines preferentially induce an IgM antibody response and that a synthetic conjugate of a carrier protein coupled to the O-specific polysaccharide of V. cholerae may improve the efficacy of the parenteral approach (Gupta et al., 1998).

Most effort at developing vaccines against cholera has focused on the development of safe and effective vaccines for oral administration (Ledon et al., 2003; Liang et al., 2003). Earlier work with either killed whole cell or live attenuated V. cholerae showed that killed whole cell vaccines administered orally were approximately 50% effective, similar to the efficacy observed previously with parenteral administration. However, protection lasted for up to 1 year in infants and up to 3 years in older children and adults, and the vaccine was judged to be safer than previously studied parenteral whole cell killed cholera vaccines. Orally administered live attenuated vaccines, in nonrandomized control studies, appear to be as safe as orally administered killed vaccines but produce greater efficacy. These vaccines produce both vibriocidal IgG serum antibody as well as local immune responses, and in both experimental and field challenge studies they have been shown to be up to 80% to 85% effective. Larger field studies will be required to establish more accurate estimates of efficacy (Ryan and Claderwood, 2000; Cohen et al., 2002). The live attenuated approach should also produce herd immunity, observed previously with earlier oral cholera vaccines (Clements, 1990).

Typhoid

Typhoid fever, caused by Salmonella typhi, begins as an infection of the intestinal tract, but the principal disease caused by the organism is the result of passage of bacteria to the mesenteric lymph nodes and from there into the circulation. Disease is associated with symptoms of sepsis and spread to the liver, spleen, and meninges. Among the antigens of the organism is a capsular polysaccharide, termed Vi, that appears to be present on nearly all S. typhi that gain access to the bloodstream (Felix and Pitt, 1934). Antibodies against Vi are thought to mediate protection against systemic disease (Landy, 1964).

A vaccine consisting of Vi capsular polysaccharide conjugated to the nontoxic recombinant aeruginosa exotoxin A was recently reported to be over 90% efficacious against systemic disease and was associated with high levels of IgG antibodies in serum (Lin et al., 2001; Lanh et al., 2003a,b). This is consistent with findings in studies of parenteral vaccines consisting either of whole killed bacteria or of the purified Vi polysaccharide, which induced good serum antibody responses and were found to be approximately 50% to 75% effective against typhoid fever in earlier vaccine trials (reviewed in Plotkin and Bouveret-LeCam, 1995). To date, there has been little study of the ability of parenteral Vi conjugate vaccines to induce mucosal immune responses or to interrupt transmission of infection in the population. Nevertheless, it possible that IgA and other mucosal responses may be induced.

There is also considerable interest in the development of an orally administered live attenuated Salmonella vaccine based on the hypothesis that improved protection against systemic disease as well as decreased mucosal infection and transmission might be achieved (Salerno et al., 2003).

Shigella

Members of the Shigella genus are the major cause of bacillary dysentery worldwide. The infection is transmitted via the fecal–oral route, and in most individuals infection is self-limiting (Dupont, 1990). In some individuals infection of the colonic epithelium, including M cells, also occurs (Sansonetti, 2002). Intracellular spread and ulceration of the epithelium are believed to occur following escape of the *Shigella* bacteria from the phagolysosome, with resulting ulceration of the colonic mucosa. During this process, bacteria are inevitably exposed to the systemic immune system.

A double-blind vaccine-controlled study of a candidate *Shigella sonnei* polysaccharide conjugate vaccine administered parenterally generated efficacy of 74%. A subgroup analysis of one of the vaccinated groups indicated that protection correlated with serum IgG and IgA antibody responses to the lipopolysaccharide, with greater statistical significance attributed to serum IgG antibody (Cohen *et al.*, 1997). This finding was consistent with previous studies that indicated a correlation of pre-existing serum anti-lipopolysaccharide (LPS) antibody and resistance to infection (Cohen *et al.*, 1991). It is not clear to what extent parenteral immunization can contribute to mucosal antibody responses following shigella infection, but the early exposure of invading bacteria to the subepithelial space may afford serum-derived IgG antibody the opportunity to contribute to protection against disease.

GENITOURINARY INFECTIONS

Human papillomavirus

Human papillomavirus (HPV) is associated with the development of cervical and anogenital cancers in a small proportion of infected individuals (Nobbenhuis *et al.*, 1999). Recent development of a parenterally administered virus-like particle elicited 90% to 100% efficacy against infection and preinvasive disease in previously uninfected individuals (Koutsky *et al.*, 2002). While 50% of cervical cancers are associated with HPV-16, this study indicated that extension of this approach to the other main serotypes associated with cervical and anogenital cancers could result in their prevention. The mechanism of protection is not known but could be associated with antibody as well as cellular immune responses (Pinto *et al.*, 2003).

Herpes simplex virus (HSV)

Candidate vaccines against genital herpes have also been developed and tested in human clinical trials (Stanberry *et al.*, 2002). A subunit vaccine consisting of glycoprotein-D derived from HSV-2 was found to be approximately 74% effective in preventing infection in women but not men, who were both HSV-2- and HSV-1-negative.

CONCLUSION

We have attempted in this chapter to summarize the evidence obtained from human trials that parenteral immunization produces clinically significant protection against infections that begin at the mucosal surface and cause mucosal and/or systemic disease. The data available come primarily from trials directed toward infections of the respiratory and gastrointestinal tracts. Few human data are available for other sites such as the genitourinary tract, with emerging evidence that the parenteral approach can be effective in reducing infection and disease in the genitourinary tract.

In our view, the evidence that parenteral immunization induces substantial protection against infection as well as disease in the respiratory tract is quite convincing. With respect to enteric infection, in some cases such as hepatitis A, the gastrointestinal tract is merely a portal of entry, and little disease ensues within the gastrointestinal tract. In this case, systemic immunity induced by parenteral immunity is clearly sufficient (Stapleton *et al.*, 1991; Andre, 1995). For other gastrointestinal infections such as typhoid in which there is both systemic and mucosal infection, the evidence indicates that parenteral immunization can be effective in providing systemic immunity as well as protection at the mucosae.

Analysis of current efforts to develop a rotavirus vaccine provides interesting examples of some of the issues surrounding the development of the mucosal versus parenteral approach. A subunit vaccine was hampered by the difficulties in maintaining epitope integrity (Conner *et al.*, 1994), despite studies in experimental animals that indicated that parenteral immunization provided adequate protection even against this largely luminal infection (Conner *et al.*, 1996). For rotavirus infections, it might be concluded that the relative importance of local immunity versus systemic immunity is likely to be greater, since this infection is largely restricted to the surface and lumen of the intestine. Efforts to develop a live attenuated rotavirus vaccine have been stymied by the occurrence of intussusception, a relatively rare but serious adverse event (Myers *et al.*, 2002). The results reviewed here indicating that parenteral immunization, in many cases, provides adequate protection against mucosal infection and disease do not imply that a mucosal approach, if successfully developed, would not be desirable. Clearly, administration of vaccines via the oral route is particularly suited for mass vaccination, as demonstrated by the success of live oral polio vaccine. Where a live, attenuated approach is technically feasible, development of mucosal delivery may be viable. Where purified subunit vaccines are required, the major obstacle to mucosal vaccine development has been the development of safe and effective adjuvants and delivery systems that can function via the mucosal route. A number of promising subunit approaches for nasally administered vaccines are in clinical trial for respiratory infection.

The need for a delivery system for oral administration stems from the fact that doses of subunit vaccines normally used parenterally are subjected to substantial dilution by the large volume of the gastrointestinal tract, which also contains proteases and bile salts likely to inactivate the immunogen. Moreover, effective mucosal responses require uptake of immunogen by M cells, which also requires the immunogen to be in a particulate form. For this reason, particulate delivery systems that protect the vaccine and promote uptake by

M cells will likely be required before oral immunization becomes a generally available strategy, at least for subunit vaccines. Recently, considerable interest has been expressed in exploiting the nasal route for the induction of protective immune responses for mucosal infection and disease.

REFERENCES

Ahmed, A., Bhattacharjee, A.K., and Mosley, W.J. (1970). Characteristics of the serum vibriocidal and agglutinating antibodies in cholera cases and in normal residents of the endemic and nonendemic cholera areas. *J. Immunol.* 105, 431–441.

Andre, F.E. (1995). Approaches to a vaccine against hepatitis A: Development and manufacture of inactivated vaccine. *J. Infect. Dis.* 171 Suppl, S33–39.

Artenstein, M.S., Gold, R., Zimmerly, J.G., Wyle, F.A., Schneider, H., and Harkins. C. (1970). Prevention of meningococcal disease by group C polysaccharide vaccine. *N. Engl. J. Med.* 282, 417–420.

Balmer, P., Borrow, R and Miller, E. (2002). Impact of meningococcal C conjugate vaccine in the UK. *J. Med. Microbiol.* 51, 717–722.

Banatvala, J.E., Best, J.M., O'Shea, S., and Waldman, R.H. (1979). Rubella immunity gap: is intranasal vaccination the answer? *Lancet* 1, 970.

Barbour, M.L., Mayon-White, R.T., Coles, C., and Crook D.W.M. (1995) The impact of conjugate vaccine on carriage of haemophilus influenzae type b. *J. Infect. Dis.* 171, 93–98.

Barbour, M.L. (1996). Conjugate vaccines and the carriage of *Haemophilus influenzae* type b. *Emerg. Infect. Dis.* 2, 176–182.

Black, S., and Shinefield, H. (2002) Safety and efficacy of the seven-valent pneumococcal conjugate vaccine: evidence from Northern California. *Eur. J. Pediatr.* 161: Suppl 2, S127–S131.

Blackwelder, W.C., Storsaeter, J., Olin, P., and Hallander, H.O. (1991) Acellular pertussis vaccines. Efficacy and evaluation of clinical case definitions. *Am. J. Dis. Child.* 145, 1285–1289.

Borrow, R., Fox, A.J., Cartwright, K., Begg, N.E., and Jones, D.M. (1999). Salivary antibodies following parenteral immunization of infant with a meningococcal serogroup A and C conjugated vaccine. *Epidemiol. Infect.* 123, 201–208.

Bose, A., Coen, P., Tully, T., Viner, R., and Booy, R (2003). Effectiveness of meningococcal C conjugate vaccine in teenagers in England. *Lancet.* 391, 675–676.

Brokstad, K.A., Cox, R.J., Olofsson, J., Jonsson, R., and Haaheim, L.R. (1995). Parenteral influenza vaccination induces a rapid systemic and local immune response. *J. Infect. Dis.* 171, 198–203.

Brokstad, K.A., Eriksson, J.C., Cox, R.J. Tynning, T., Ollofsson, J., Jonsson, R., and Davidson, A. (2002). Parenteral vaccination against influenza does not induce a local antigen-specific immune response in the nasal mucosae. *J. Infect. Dis.* 185, 878–884.

Butcher, E.C., and Picker, L.J. (1996). Lymphocyte homing and homeostasis. *Science* 272, 60–66.

Clements, M.L., Betts, R.F., Tierney, E.L., and Murphy, B.R. (1986). Serum and nasal wash antibodies associated with resistance to experimental challenge with influenza A wild-type virus. *J. Clin. Microbiol.* 24, 157–160.

Cohen, D., Green, M.S., Block, C., Slepon, R., and Ofek, I. (1991). A prospective study on the association between serum antibodies to lipopolysaccharide and attack rate of shigellosis. *Clin. Microbiol.* 29, 386–389.

Cohen, D., Ashkenazi, S., Green, M.S., Gdalevich, M., Robin, G., Slepon, R., Yavzori, M., Orr, N. Block, C., Ashkenazi, I., Shemer, J., Taylor, D.N., Hale, T.L., Sadoff, J.C., Pavilakova, D., Schneerson, R., and Robbins, J.B. (1997). Double-blind vaccine-controlled randomized efficacy trial of an investigational *Shigella sonnei* conjugate vaccine in young adults. *Lancet* 349, 155–159.

Cohen, M.B., Giannella R.A., Bean, J., Taylor, D.N., Parker, S., Hoeper, A., Wowk, S., Hawkins, J., Kochi, S.K., Schiff, G., and Killeen, K.P. (2002). Randomized, controlled human challenge study of

the safety, immunogenicity, and protective efficacy of a single dose of Peru-15, a live attenuated oral cholera vaccine. *Infect. Immun.* 70(4), 1965–1970.

Conner, M.E., Crawford, S.E., Barone, C., O'Neal, C., Zhou, Y.J., Fernandez, F., Parwani, A., Saif, J., Cohen, J., and Estes, M.K., (1996). Rotavirus subunit vaccines. *Arch. Virol.* 12(suppl.), 199–206.

Conner, M.E., Matson, D.O., and Estes, M.K. (1994). Rotavirus vaccines and vaccination potential. In *Rotaviruses* (ed. R. Ramig), 286–337. Berlin: Springer-Verlag.

Couch, R.B., Kasel, J.A., Six, H.R., and Cate, T.R. (1981). The basis for immunity to influenza in man. In *Genetics Variation among Influenza Viruses. ICN-UCLA Symposia on Molecular and Cellular Biology* xxi (eds. Nayak, D., and Fox, C.F.), 535. New York: Academic Press.

Dagan, R., Melamed, R., Muallem, M., Piglansky, L., Greenberg, D., Abramson, O., Mendelman, P.M., Hohidar, N., and Yagupsky P. (1996). Reduction of nasopharyngeal carriage of pneumococci during the second year of life by a heptavalent conjugate pneumococcal vaccine. *J. Infect. Dis.* 174, 1271–1278.

Dagan, R., Fraser D. (2000). Conjugate pneumonococcal vaccine and antibiotic-resistant *Streptococcus pneumoniae:* herd immunity and reduction of otitis morbidity. *Pediatr. Infect. Dis. J.* Suppl 19, S79–S87.

Darkes, M.J., and Plosker, G.L. (2002). Pneumococcal conjugate vaccine (Prevnar, PNCRM7): a review of its use in the prevention of *Streptococcus pneumoniae* infection. *Paediatr. Drugs* 4, 609–630.

Davis, W.J. Larson, H.E., Simsarian, J.P., Parkman, P.D., and Meyer, H.M. (1971). A study of rubella immunity and resistance to infection. *JAMA* 215, 600–608.

Deen, J.L., Mink, C.M., Cherry, J.D., Christenson, P.D., Pineda, E.F., Lewis, K., Blumberg, D.A., and Ross, L.A. (1995). Household contact study of Bordetella pertussis infections. *Clin. Infect. Dis.* 21, 1211–1219.

Demicheli, V., Rivetti, D., Deeks, J.J., and Jefferson, T.O. (2001). Vaccines for preventing influenza in healthy adults. *Cochrane Database Syst Rev.* 4, CD001269.

Dupont, H.L. (1990). *Shigella* species: bacillary dysentery. In *Principles and Practice of Infectious Disease* (eds. G.L. Mandell, R. G. Douglas, Jr., and J. E. Bennett), 1716–1722. London: Churchill-Livingstone.

El-Madhun, A.S., Cox, R.J., Soreide, A., Oloffson, J., and Haaheim, L.R. (1998). Systemic and mucosal immune responses in young children and adults after parenteral influenza vaccination. *J. Infect. Dis.* 178, 933–939.

Engstrom, P.E., Gustafson, Granberg, M., and Engstron, G.N. (2002). Specific IgA subclass responses in serum and saliva: a 12-month follow-up study after parenteral booster immunization with tetanus toxoid. *Acta Odontol. Scand.* 60, 198–202.

Felix, P., and Pitt, R. (1934). A new antigen of *B. typhosus,* its relation to virulence and in active and passive immunization. *Lancet* 2, 186–191.

Fogel, A., Gerichter, C., Barnea, B., Handsher, R., and Heeger, E. (1978). Response to experimental challenge in persons immunized with different rubella vaccines. *J. Pediatrics* 92, 26–29.

Fowler, K.B., Stagno, S., Pass, R.F., Britt, W.J., Bell, T.J., and Alford, C.A. (1992). The outcome of congenital cytomegalovirus infection in relation to maternal antibody status. *N. Engl. J. Med.* 326, 663–667.

Giebink, G.C. (2001). The prevention of pneumococcal disease in children. *N. Engl. J. Med.* 345, 1177–1183.

Goldschneider, I. Gotschlich, E.C., and Artenstein, M.S. (1969). Human immunity to the meningococcus-I. The role of humoral antibodies. *J. Exp. Med.* 129, 1307–1326.

Gorse, G.J., Otto, E.E., Powers, D.C., Chambers, G.W., Eickhoff, C.S., and Newman, F.K. (1996). Induction of mucosal antibodies by live attenuated and inactivated influenza virus vaccines in the chronically ill elderly. *J. Infect. Dis.* 173, 285–290.

Gotschlich, E.C., Goldschneider, I., and Artenstein, M.S. (1969). Human immunity to the meningococcus-V. The effect of immunization with meningococcal group C polysaccharide vaccine. *J. Exp. Med.* 129, 1385–1395.

Granstrom, M., Olinder-Nielsen, A.M., Holmbad, P., Marks, A., and Hanngren, K. (1991). Specific immunoglobulin for treatment of whooping cough. *Lancet* 33, 1230–1232.

Groothuis, J.R., Simoes, E.A.F., Levin, M.J., Hall, C.B., Long, C.E., Rodriguez, W.J., Arrobio, J., Meissner, H.C., Fulton, D.R., Welliver, R.C., Tristram, D.A., Siber, G.R., Prince, G.A., Van Raden, M., and Hemming, V.G. (1993). Prophylactic administration of respiratory syncytial virus immune globulin to high-risk infants and young children. *N. Engl. J. Med.* 329, 1524–1527.

Gupta, R.K., Taylor, D.N., Bryla, D.A., Robbins, J.B., and Szu, S.C. (1998). Phase 1 evaluation of *Vibrio cholerae* O1, serotype Inaba, polysaccharide-cholera toxin conjugates in adult volunteers. *Infect. Immun.* 66(7), 3095–3099.

Herremans, T.D., Reimerink, J.H., Buisman, A.M., Kimman T.G., and Loopmans, M.P. (1999). Induction of mucosal immunity by inactivated poliovirus vaccine is dependent on previous mucosal contact with live virus. *J. Immunol.* 162, 5011–5018.

Kauppi, M., Eskola, J., Kayhty, H. (1995). Anti-capsular polysaccharide antibody concentrations in saliva after immunization with *Haemophilus influenzae* type b conjugate vaccines. *Pediatr. Infect. Dis. J.* 14, 286–294.

Keren, D.F., McDonald, R.A., and Carey, J.L. (1988). Combined parenteral and oral immunization results in an enhanced mucosal immunoglobulin A response to *Shigella flexneri*. *Infect. Immun.* 56, 910–915.

Kim, H.W., Canchola, J.G., Brandt, C.D., Pyles, G., Chanock, R.M., Jensen, K., and Parrot, R.H. (1969). Respiratory syncytial virus disease in infants despite prior administration of antigenic inactivated vaccine. *Am. J. Epidemiol.* 89, 422–434.

Koutsky, L.A., Ault, K.A., Wheeler, C. M., Brown, D.R., Barr, E., Alvarez, F.B., Chiacchierini, L.S., and Jansen, K.U. (2002). A controlled trial of a human papillomavirus type 16 vaccine. *N. Engl. J. Med.* 347, 1645–1651.

Landy, M. (1964). Studies on Vi antigen: Immunization of human beings with purified Vi Antigen. *Am. J. Hygiene* 60, 62.

Lahn, M.N., Phan, V.B., Vo, A.H., Tran, C.T., Lin, F.Y., Bryla, D.A., Chu, C., Schiloach, J., Robbins, J.B., Schneerson, R., and Szu, S.C. (2003). Persistent efficacy of Vi conjugate vaccine against typhoid fever in young children. *N. Engl. J. Med.* 239, 1390–1391.

Ledon, T., Valle, E., Valmaseda, T., Cedre, B., Campos, J., Rodriguex, B.D., M, K., Garcia, H., Carcia, L., and Fando, R. (2003). Construction and characterisation of O139 cholera vaccine candidates. *Vaccine* 21, 1282–1291.

Levine, M.M., and Kapper, J. (1993). Live vaccines against cholera: an update. *Vaccine* 11, 207–212.

Liang, W., Wang, S., Y, F., Zhang, L., Qi, G., Liu, Y., Gao, S., and Kan, B. (2003). Construction and evaluation of a safe, live, oral *Vibrio cholerae* vaccine candidate, IEM108. *Infect. Immun.* 71, 5498–5504.

Lin, Feng Ying C., Ho, V.A., Khiem, H.B., Trach, D.D., Bay, Ph.Vn., Thanh, T.C., Kozzaczka, Z., Bryla, D.A., Shiloach, J., Robbins, J.B., Schneerson and Szu, S.C., (2001). The efficacy of a *Salmonella typhi* vi conjugate vaccine in two-five-year old children. *N. Engl. J. Med.* 344, 1263–1269.

Losonsky, G.A., Yunyongying, J., Lim, V., Reymann, M., Lim, Y.L., Wasserman, S.S., and Levine, M.M. (1996). Factors influencing secondary vibriocidal immune responses: Relevance for understanding immunity to cholera. *Infect. Immun.* 64, 10–15.

Luchner, L.A., Reeves, M., Hennessy, T., Levine, O.S., Popovic, T., Rosenstein, N., and Parkinson (2002). *J. Infect. Dis.* 186, 958–965.

Makela, P.H., and Kayhty, H. (2002) Evolution of conjugate vaccines. *Expert Rev. Vaccines* 1, 399–410.

Marine, W.M., Chin, T.D.Y., and Gravelle, C.R. (1962). Limitation of fecal and pharyngeal poliovirus excretion in salk-vaccinated children. *Am. J. Hyg.* 76, 173–195.

Matter, L., Kogelschatz, K., and Germann, D. (1997). Serum levels of rubella virus antibodies indicating immunity: Response to vaccination of subjects with low or undetectable antibody concentrations. *J. Infect. Dis.* 175, 749–755.

Mbelle, N., Huebner, R.E., Wasas, A.D., Kimura, A., Chang, I., and Klugman, O.P. (1999). Immunogenicity and impact on nasopha-

ryngeal carriage of a nonvalent pneumococcal conjugate vaccine. *J. Infect Dis.* 180, 1171–1176.

McDermott, M.R., and Bienenstock, J. (1979). Evidence for a common mucosal immunologic system. I. Migration of B immunoblasts into intestinal, respiratory and genital tissues. *J. Immunol.* 122, 1892–1898.

McVernon, J., Andrews, N., Slack, M.P.E., Ramsay, M.E. (2003). Risk of vaccine failure after *Haemophilus influenzae* type b(Hib) combination vaccines with acellular pertussis. *Lancet* 361, 1521–1523.

Millar, E.V., O'Brian, K.L., Levine, O.S., Kvamme, S., Reid, R., and Santosham, M. (2000). Carriage disease among high risk American Indian children. *Am. J. Public Health* 90, 1550–1554.

Millar, E.V., O'Brien, K.L., Watt, J.P., et al. (2002). Duration of protection against pneumococcal nasopharyngeal carriage by 7-valent pneumococcal conjugate vaccine (pNCRM7) in Navajo and Apache children. In *Abstracts of ISPPD-2202, the 3rd International Symposium on Pneumococci and Pneumococcal diseases, Anchorage, Alaska.*

Moldoveanu, Z., Clement, M.L., Primie, S.J., Murphy, B.R., Mestecky J. (1995). Human immune responses to influenza virus vaccines administered by systemic or mucosal routes. *Vaccine* 13, 1006–1012.

Murdin, A.D., Barreto, L., and Plotkin, S. (1996). Inactivated poliovirus vaccine: past and present experience. *Vaccine* 14, 735–746.

Myers, P.G. (2002) Intussusception, rotavirus and oral vaccines: summary of a workshop. *Pediatrics* 110, e17.

Neilsen, A., and Larsen, S.O. (1994). Epidemiology of pertussis in Denmark: the impact of herd immunity. *Int. J. Epidemiol.* 23, 1300–1307.

Nichol, K.L., Lind, A., and Margolis, K.L. (1995). The effectiveness of vaccination against influenza in healthy working adults. *N. Engl. J. Med.* 333, 889–893.

Nobbenhuis M.A., Walboomers, J.M., Helmerhorst, T.J., Rozendaal, L., Remmink, A.J., Risse, E.K., van der Linden, H.C., Voorhorst, F.J., Kenemans, P., and Meijer, C.J. (1999). Relation of human papillomavirus status to cervical lesions and consequences for cervical-cancer screening: a prospective study. *Lancet* 354, 20–25.

Nieminen, T., Kayhty, H., Leroy, O., and Eskola, J. (1999). Pneumococcal conjugate vaccination in toddlers: mucosal antibody response measured as circulating antibody-secreting cells and as salivary antibodies. *Pediatr. Infect Dis. J.* 18, 764–772.

Nordin, J., Mullooley, J., Pobledte, S., Strikas, R., Petrucci, R., Wei, F., Rush, B., Safirstein, B., Wheeler, D., and Nichol, L.D. (2001). Influenza vaccine effectiveness in preventing hospitalizations and deaths in persons 65 years or older in Minnesota, New York and Oregon: data from 3 healthy plans. *J. Infect. Dis.* 184, 665–670.

Obaro, S., and Adegbola, R. (2002). The pneumococcus: carriage, disease and conjugate vaccines. *J. Microbiol.* 51, 98–104.

O'Brien, K. (2001). Disease transmission, routes, contributing factors and herd immunity. *IJCP Suppl.* 118, 5–7.

Ogra, P. L., Kerr-Grant, D., Umana, G., Dzierba, J., and Weintraub, D. (1971). Antibody response in serum and nasopharynx after naturally acquired and vaccine-induced infection with rubella virus. *N. Engl. J. Med.* 285, 1333–1339.

Ogra, P.L. (1995). Comparative evaluation of immunization with live attenuated and inactivated poliovirus vaccines. *Ann. N.Y. Acad. Sci.* 754, 97–107.

Olin, P., (1993). Defining surrogate serologic tests with respect to predicting protective vaccine efficacy: pertussis vaccination. *Ann. N.Y. Acad. Sci.* 754, 273–277.

Olin, P., Hallander, H.O., Gustafsson, L., Reizenstein, E., and Storsaeter, J. (2001). How to make sense of pertussis immunogenicity data. *Clin. Infect. Dis.* 33 Suppl 4, S288–S291.

Olin, P., Gustafsson, L., Barreto, L., Hessel, L., Mast, T.C., Rie, A.V., Bogaerts, H., and Storsaeter, J. (2003). Declining pertussis incidence in Sweden following the introduction of acellular pertussis vaccine. *Vaccine* 21, 17–18.

Onorato, I.M., Modlin, J.F., McBean, A.M., Thoms, M.L., Losonsky, G.A., and Bernier, R.H. (1991). Mucosal immunity induced by enhanced-potency inactivated and oral polio vaccines. *J. Infect. Dis.* 163, 1–6.

Palmu, A.A., Kaijalainen, T., Verho, J., Herva, E., Makela, P.H., and Kilpi, T.M. (2002). Long-term efficacy of the sevenvalent PncCRN vaccine on nasopharyngeal carriage. In *Abstracts of ISPPD-2002, the 3rd International Symposium on Pneumococci and Pneumococcal Diseases, Anchorage, Alaska.*

Petola, H., Kilpi, T., and Anttila, M. (1992). Rapid disappearance of *Haemophilus influenzae* type b meningitis after routine childhood immunization with conjugate vaccines. *Lancet* 340, 592–594.

Pichichero, M.E., and Insel, R.A. (1983). Mucosal antibody response to parenteral vaccination with *Haemophilus influenzae* type b capsule. *J. Allergy Clin. Immunol.* 72, 481–486.

Pinto, LA., Edwards, J., Castle, P.E., Harro, C.D., Lowy, D.R., Schiller, J.T., Wallace D., Kopp, W., Adesberger, J.W., Baseler, M.W., Berzofsky, J.A., and Hildesheim, A. (2003). Cellular immune responses to human papillomavirus (HPV)-16 L1 in healthy volunteers immunized with recombinant HPV-16 L1 virus-like particles. *J. Infect. Dis.* 188, 327–338.

Plotkin, S.A., and Bouveret-LeCam, N. (1995). A new typhoid vaccine composed of the Vi capsular polysaccharide. *Arch. Intern. Med.* 155, 2293–2299.

Plotkin, S. A., Farquhar, J.D., and Ogra, P. L. (1973). Immunologic properties of RA27/3 rubella virus vaccine. *JAMA* 225, 585–590.

Plotkin, S.A. (1997). Developed countries should use inactivated polio vaccine for the prevention of poliomyelitis. *Rev. Med. Virol.* 7, 75–81.

Powers, D.C., Gorse, G.J., Otto, E.E., Chambers, G.W., Eichoff, C.S., and Newman, F.K. (1996). Induction of mucosal antibodies by live attenuated and inactivated influenza virus vaccines in the chronically ill elderly. *J. Infect. Dis.* 173, 285–290.

Preston, N.W. (2003). Why the rise in *Haemophilus Influenza* type b infections? *Lancet* 362, 330–331.

Reingold, A.L., Hightower A.W., Bolan, G.A., Jones, E.E., Tiendrebeogo, H., Broome, C.V., Ajello, G.W., Adamsbaum, C., Phillips, C., and Yada, A. (1985). Age specific differences in duration of clinical protection after vaccination with meningococcal polysaccharide A vaccine. *Lancet* 20, 114–118.

Renegar, K.B., and Small, P.A. Jr. (1991) Passive transfer of local immunity to influenza virus infection by IgA antibody. *J. Immunol.* 146, 1972–1978.

Robbins, J.B., Schneerson, R., Anderson, P., and Smith, D.H. (1996). The 1996 Albert Lasker Medical Research Awards. Prevention of systemic infections, especially meningitis, caused by *Haemophilus influenzae* type b. Impact on public health and implications for other polysaccharide-based vaccines. *JAMA* 276, 1181–1185.

Robbins, J.B., Schneerson, R., Szu, S.C., and Yang, Y.H. (1986). Prospects for polysaccharide-protein conjugate vaccines. *Ann. Sclavo. Collano. Monogr.* 3, 213–232.

Robbins, J.B., Schneerson, R., and Szu, S.C. (1995). Perspective: Hypothesis: Serum IgG antibody is sufficient to confer protection against infectious diseases by inactivating the inoculum. *J. Infect. Dis.* 171, 1387–1398.

Ruggeberg, J., and Heath, P.T. (2003). Safety and efficacy of meningococcal group C conjugate vaccine. *Expert Opin. Drug Saf.* 2, 7–19.

Ryan, E.T and Calgerwood, S.B. (2000). Cholera vaccines. *Clin. Infect. Dis.* 31(2), 561–565.

Sack, D.A. (1994). Cholera control. *Lancet* 344, 616–617.

Salerno-Goncalves, R., Wyant, T.L., Pasetti, M.F., Fernandez-Vina, M., Tacket, C.O., Levine, M.M., and Sztein, M.B. (2003). *J. Immunol.* 170, 2734–2741.

Salk, J., and Salk, D. (1977). Control of influenza and poliomyelitis with killed virus vaccines. *Science* 195, 834–847.

Sansonetti, P. (2002). Host-pathogen interactions: the seduction of molecular cross tal. *Gut* 50 Suppl 3, 1112–1118.

Siber, G.R., Thompson, C., Reid, G.R., Almeido-Hill, J., Zacher, B., Wolff, M., and Santosham, M. (1992). Evaluation of bacterial polysaccharide immune globulin for the treatment or prevention of *Haemophilus influenzae* type b and pneumococcal disease. *J. Infect. Dis.* 165, Suppl 1, S129–133.

Silfverdal, S.A., Bodin, L., and Olcén, P. (2003). Why the rise in *Haemophilus influenzae* type b infections? *Lancet* 362, 331.

Stapleton, J.T., Lange, D.K., LeDuc, J.W., Binn, L.N., Jansen, R.W., and Lemon, S.M. (1991). The role of secretory immunity in hepatitis A virus infection. *J. Infect. Dis.* 163, 7–11.

Snydman, D.R., Werner, B.G., Heinze-Lacey B., Berardi V.P., Tilney, N.L., Kirkman, R.L., Milford, E.L., Cho S.I., Bush, H.L.Jr., Levey, A.S. (1987). Use of cytomegalovirus immune globulin to prevent cytomegalovirus disease in renal-transplant recipients. *N. Engl. J. Med.* 317, 1049–1054.

Snydman, D.R. (1990). Cytomegalovirus immunoglobulins in the prevention and treatment of cytomegalovirus disease. *Rev. Infect. Dis.* 12 suppl 7. S839–S848.

Stanberry, L.R., Spruance, Sp. L., Cunningham, A.L., Bernstein, D.I., Mindal, A., Sacks, S., Tyring, S., Aoki, F.Y., Slaoui M., Denis, M., Vanderpapeliere, P., and Dubin, G. For the GlaxoSmithKline Herpes Vaccine Efficacy Study Group. (2002). Glycoprotein-D-adjuvant vaccine to prevent genital herpes. *N. Engl. J. Med.* 347, 1652–1661.

Taranger J., Trollfors, B., Bergfors, E., Knutsson, N., Lagergard, T., Schneerson, R., and Robbins, J.B. (2001). Immunologic and epidemiologic experience of vaccination with monocomponent pertussis toxoid vaccine. *Pediatrics* 108, E115.

Tarkowski, A., Lue, C., Moldoveanu, Z., Kiyono, H., McGhee, J.R., and Mestecky, J. (1990). Immunization of humans with polysaccharide vaccines induces systemic, predominantly polymeric IgA2-subclass antibody responses. *J. Immunol.* 144, 3770–3778.

Wang, J.B., Adler, S.P., Hempfling, S., Burke, R.L., Duliege, A.M., Starr, S.E., and Plotkin, S.A. (1996). Mucosal antibodies to human cytomegalovirus glycoprotein B occur following both natural infection and immunization with human cytomegalovirus. *J. Infect. Dis.* 174, 387–392.

Winner, L. 3rd., Mach, J., Weltzin, R., Mekalanos, J.J., Kraehenbuhl, J.P., and Neutra, M.R. (1991). New model for analysis of mucosal immunity: intestinal secretion of specific monoclonal immunoglobulin A from hybridoma tumors protects against *Vibrio cholerae* infection. *Infect. Immun.* 59(3), 977–982.

Woodland, D.L. (2003). Cell-mediated immunity to respiratory virus infections. *Curr. Opin. Immunol.* 15, 430–435.

Zhang, Q., Choo, S., Everard, J., Jennings, R., and Finn, A. (2000). Mucosal immune responses to meningococcal group C conjugate and group A and C polysaccharide vaccines in adolescents. *Infect. Immun.* 68, 2692–2697.

Zhang, Q., Lakshman, R., Burkinshaw, R., Choo, S., Everard J., Akhtar, S and Fi, A (2001). Primary and booster mucosal immune responses to meningococcal group A and C conjugate and polysaccharide vaccines administered to university students in the United Kingdom. *Infect. Immun.* 69, 4337–4341.

Zhang, Q., Pettitt, E., Burkinshaw, R., Race, G., Shaw, L., and Finn, A. (2002). Mucosal immune responses to meningococcal conjugate polysaccharide vaccines in infants. *Pediatr. Infect. Dis. J.* 21, 209–213.

Passive Immunization: Systemic and Mucosal

Kathryn B. Renegar

Department of Pediatric Infectious Diseases, Vanderbilt University, Nashville, Tennessee

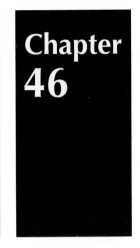

The passive transfer of maternal immunity is responsible for keeping all mammalian species alive. The process of evolution developed effective mechanisms for the passive transfer of both systemic and mucosal immunity from the mother to her offspring. Experimental passive transfer of systemic immunity via serum antibody is well established, but the experimental passive transfer of mucosal immunity has only recently been accomplished. This chapter addresses the contributions of both natural and experimental mechanisms to the study of passive immunization.

NATURAL PASSIVE IMMUNIZATION

Systemic immunity

The transfer of systemic immunity (IgG) from mother to offspring occurs prenatally via the placenta or yolk sac and after birth via the colostrum. Species vary in the contribution each route makes to the transfer of immunity (Waldman and Strober, 1969) and can be grouped into three categories: prenatal transfer only, combined prenatal and postnatal transfer, and postnatal transfer only.

Prenatal transfer only

This group includes primates, rabbits, and guinea pigs. Transport of IgG in primates occurs almost exclusively through the placenta. IgG transfer occurs via a receptor-mediated transcytosis across the syncytiotrophoblast and a transcellular pathway through the fetal endothelium (Leach *et al.,* 1990). Human placental transfer of protective IgG antibodies to a number of pathogens, including hepatitis B (Hockel and Kaufman, 1986), measles (Lennon and Black, 1986), and group B streptococcus (Baker *et al.,* 1988), has been reported. This process suggests an effective method of neonatal immunization, *i.e.,* immunization of the pregnant mother in order to protect the neonate. Prenatal transfer of IgG in the rabbit occurs via the yolk sac, and in the guinea pig, via both the yolk sac and fetal gut (Waldman and Strober, 1969).

Combined prenatal and postnatal transfer

This group includes rats, mice, cats, and dogs. Prenatal transmission occurs via the yolk sac/placenta and the fetal gut in the rat (Waldman and Strober, 1969). IgG is bound rapidly to receptors on the surface of the yolk sac membrane (Mucchielli *et al.,* 1983), is endocytosed in clathrin-coated vesicles, and, early in gestation, is stored in subapical vacuoles. By late gestation, the antibody has been hydrolyzed or transferred to fetal capillaries (Jollie, 1985). Prenatal transmission in mice occurs by a similar mechanism (Gardner, 1976).

Although placental transfer occurs, studies in rodents have shown that most transport of antibody occurs postnatally from colostrum or milk (Arango-Jaramillo *et al.,* 1988; Barthold *et al.,* 1988; Heiman and Weisman, 1989; Kohl and Loo, 1984; Nejamkis *et al.,* 1975; Oda *et al.,* 1983) over a period of 10 to 21 days, depending on the species. There is a gradual decrease in transmission over the last 3 days (Waldman and Strober, 1969), and transmission is limited to antibodies of the IgG class (Appleby and Catty, 1983; Hammerberg *et al.,* 1977). Transport is a receptor-mediated process (Simister and Rees, 1983). In rats, the receptor (FcRn) is found in enterocytes of the proximal intestine during the early postnatal period but is absent after weaning (Jakoi *et al.,* 1985). FcRn is specific for IgG and its Fc fragment and consists of two similar polypeptides of 48,000 to 52,000 daltons (p51) in association with β2 microglobulin (Jakoi *et al.,* 1985; Simister and Mostov, 1989). The Fc binding subunit (p51) has three extracellular domains and a transmembrane region that are all homologous to the corresponding domains of class I major histocompatibility complex (MHC) antigens (Simister and Mostov, 1989). Junghans and Anderson (1996) have shown that disruption of the FcRn in knockout mice also destroys the receptor (FcRp) necessary for the prolonged half-life of serum IgG in adults, suggesting that the same receptor protein that mediates transient IgG transport across the neonatal gut functions as the FcRp throughout life.

Postnatal transfer only

This group includes ruminants (cattle, sheep, goats), horses, and pigs (reviewed in Tizzard, 1987). Transport of colostral proteins from the lumen of the ileum in ruminants is largely nonspecific, but in the horse and the pig, IgG and IgM are preferentially absorbed. Proteins are actively taken up by epithelial cells through pinocytosis and passed through these cells into the lacteals and intestinal capillaries (Tizzard, 1987). Intestinal absorption occurs for only the first 24 to 48 hours after birth. Following this, the "open gut" closes down, and no further transfer from milk or colostrum occurs (Ellis *et al.*, 1986; Francis and Black, 1984; Tizzard, 1987; Waldman and Strober, 1969). Newborn piglets have also been shown to absorb colostral lymphoid cells during this period (Tuboly *et al.*, 1988). It is unclear whether these cells are fully functional and capable of immune processes such as the transfer of delayed-type hypersensitivity (DTH).

Absorption of colostral immunoglobulin is normally extremely effective, supplying the newborn with serum immunoglobulin (particularly IgG) at a level approaching that found in adults (Tizzard, 1987); however, failure of passive transfer (FPT) can occur and, when it does, can pose a considerable problem in animal husbandry. About 25% of newborn foals fail to obtain sufficient quantities of immunoglobulin (McGuire *et al.*, 1975; Tizzard, 1987). In the McGuire study (1975), two of nine foals affected by FPT died of infections within a few days of birth, and five of the remaining seven developed nonfatal respiratory infections between 2 and 5 weeks of age. McGuire *et al.* (1976) also reported FPT in calves, finding that 85% of calves less than 3 weeks old dying from infectious diseases have significant hypogammaglobulinemia. Although adequate methods to diagnose and treat FPT are available (Bertone *et al.*, 1988; Tizzard, 1987), the phenomenon remains a significant veterinary problem.

Mucosal immunity

Mother's milk provides passive protection of the mucosal surfaces it contacts. This protection may be mediated either by specific immunity or by nonspecific factors found in milk, such as lactoferrin, lysozyme, fatty acids, and complement (reviewed in Goldman *et al.*, 1985). The antibody composition of milk differs from that of colostrum (Tizzard, 1987), and the class of protective antibody in milk varies with the species and the route of immunization of the mother. With the exception of IgG in rodents, these protective antibodies are not systemically absorbed by the suckling offspring, but exert their protective effect locally by neutralizing viruses or virulence factors and by binding to microbial pathogens and preventing their attachment to the mucosal surface (Goldman *et al.*, 1985). Secretory IgA (S-IgA) is especially suited to this protective role, because secretory component enhances its resistance to proteolytic enzymes and gastric acid (Kenny *et al.*, 1967; Lindh, 1975; Tomasi, 1970; Zikan *et al.*, 1972), providing extra antibody stability in mucosal secretions.

Milk antibody in rodents

Rodents have been a popular model for the study of passive transfer of maternal immunity via milk; however, this class of animals has a major drawback as a model for passive *mucosal* immunity. Both rats and mice can actively transport IgG from the gut into the serum for approximately 2 weeks (see Combined Prenatal and Postnatal Transfer earlier in this chapter); thus, observed protection could be due either to antibody in the milk bathing the mucosal surfaces or to maternal antibody being transported into the serum and secretions of the offspring. This caveat should be kept in mind during evaluation of the many reports of milk-borne protection in these species. Three rodent models in which protection of mucosal surfaces is due to milk-borne, not serum-derived, antibody are described next.

The predominant immunoglobulin in mouse milk is IgG, although significant levels of IgA can also be present (Ijaz *et al.*, 1987). Protection of infant mice from colonization with *Campylobacter jejuni* can be achieved by the consumption of immune milk at and after the time of bacterial challenge. Infant mice were not protected by prior consumption of colostrum, showing that milk antibody was required in the gut lumen for protection to be observed (Abmiku and Dolby, 1987). A similar requirement for antibodies active at the intestinal cell surface in immunity to primate rotavirus SA-11 was reported by Offit and Clark (1985).

Protection of rats against dental caries by milk can be due to either IgG or S-IgA antibodies, depending on the route of maternal immunization. Rat dams immunized intravenously with heat-killed *Streptococcus mutans* developed IgG antibodies in their colostrum, milk, and serum. Their offspring demonstrated significant protection against *S. mutans*–induced caries formation. Rat dams locally injected in the region of the mammary gland with heat-killed *S. mutans* or fed formalin-killed *S. mutans* developed S-IgA antibodies in their colostrum and milk. Their offspring were also protected against caries formation (Michalek and McGhee, 1977). Caries protection in suckling rats could theoretically be due to bathing of mucosal surfaces and/or leakage of antibody into the saliva from the serum. Nonimmune adult rats can be protected from *S. mutans*–induced caries by feeding on lyophilized immune bovine milk or on immune bovine whey containing specific IgG (Michalek *et al.*, 1978a; Michalek *et al.*, 1987). Since adult rats are unable to transport orally administered IgG into their serum, protection must be from milk-derived antibodies bathing the oral cavity.

Milk antibody in ungulates

In ruminants (sheep, cattle, goats), the predominant antibody in both colostrum and milk is IgG. The predominant antibody in the colostrum of pigs and horses is also IgG, but as lactation progresses and colostrum becomes milk, IgA predominates (Tizzard, 1987). Protection can be mediated by either antibody class. While bathing of the mucosal surfaces by milk-derived antibodies can provide passive immunity to some pathogens, the high rate of infections in FPT foals and calves shows that milk (mucosal immunity) alone cannot provide complete protection to neonates.

In cattle and pigs, passive immunity against enteric infections with viruses such as rotaviruses and coronaviruses (transmissible gastroenteritis, or TGE) is dependent on the continual presence in the gut lumen of a protective level of specific antibodies (Crouch, 1985). Passive immunity against intestinal infection with the TGE virus is generally more complete in piglets ingesting IgA antibodies than in those ingesting IgG antibodies, although both classes of antibody are protective. The class of antibody present in the sow's milk depends on the route of immunization (Bohl and Saif, 1975). In cattle, passive immunity in calf scours (neonatal bovine colibacillosis caused by *Escherichia coli*) correlates with the level of specific IgA antibody in the mother's milk (Wilson and Jutila, 1976).

Milk antibody in primates
In primates, IgA is the predominant immunoglobulin in both colostrum and milk (Tizzard, 1987). Both lysozyme and S-IgA in human milk remain functional in the digestive tract of the early infant (Eschenburg et al., 1990). Human milk has been shown to contain S-IgA antibodies to at least five viral and nine bacterial pathogens, as well as to fungi, parasites, and food antigens (Goldman et al., 1985). Mucosal immunity to rotavirus, for example, was shown to be transferred to the infant by the S-IgA in milk; there was a positive correlation between titers of secretory component (SC) in the mother's milk and the infant's feces vs. virus-specific IgA in the infant's fecal samples (Rahman et al., 1987). In addition to providing passive mucosal immunity, human breast milk also stimulates the early local production of S-IgA in the urinary and gastrointestinal tracts, thereby accelerating the development of an active local host defense in the infant (Koutras and Vigorita, 1989; Prentice, 1987).

EXPERIMENTAL PASSIVE IMMUNIZATION

Since the original demonstration of transfer of immunity by the injection of serum (von Behring and Kitasato, 1890), passive transfer of humoral immunity has been intensively investigated. The use of specific serum antibody (IgG) to transfer protection to nonimmune individuals is now standard medical practice in, for example, the postexposure prophylaxis for rabies and tetanus and the treatment of snakebite (Arnold, 1982; Centers for Disease Control, 1991a, 1991b), while intravenous immunoglobulin (IVIg) treatment has been shown to lower the incidence of pneumonia in patients with common variable immunodeficiency (Busse et al., 2002).

Local immunity has been correlated with the level of IgA antibody in various secretions (reviewed in Renegar and Small, 1993); however, direct demonstration of the mediation of local immunity by injected IgA could not occur until specific transport of passively administered IgA had been confirmed.

Transport of passively administered IgA to mucosal surfaces
Gastrointestinal tract
In rabbits, rats, and mice, polymeric IgA (pIgA) is efficiently transported from the circulation into the bile via the liver (Delacroix et al., 1985; Koertge and Butler, 1986a; Mestecky and McGhee, 1987; Orlans et al., 1978, 1983). These species express pIg receptor (pIgR) on their hepatocytes (Socken et al., 1979) and, in addition, have pIgA as the primary molecular form in their serum (Heremans, 1974; Vaerman, 1973). Serum IgA is also efficiently transported into bile in cattle (Butler et al., 1986). In fact, most IgA in ruminant bile may be of serum origin.

Transport of serum IgA into bile in humans has been reported (Delacroix et al., 1982; Dooley et al., 1982), although IgA transport is about 50-fold less efficient than in rats and rabbits. The human biliary IgA level is approximately 20% of the human serum IgA level and, under physiologic conditions, only 50% of human biliary IgA is derived from the serum (Vaerman and Delacroix, 1984). Even though transport is possible, passively administered IgA does not reach high levels in human bile. In one study, less than 3% of intravenously injected radiolabeled pIgA was found in human bile at 24 hours (Vaerman and Delacroix, 1984).

Saliva
Serum pIgA can be transported into saliva in dogs (Montgomery et al., 1977), monkeys (Challacombe et al., 1978), mice (Falero-Diaz et al., 2000), and humans (Delacroix et al., 1982; Kubagawa et al., 1987). In humans the amount of IgA acquired from the plasma is low (only 2%) compared with the amount acquired from local production (Delacroix et al., 1982). Transfer of pIgA from the plasma into canine or murine saliva is a selective process requiring the pIgR (Montgomery et al., 1987; Falero-Diaz et al., 2000), while transport into oral fluids in monkeys appears to be by leakage from the plasma into the crevicular spaces surrounding the deciduous molars (Challacombe et al., 1978).

Milk
In sheep, active transport of IgA from the circulation into milk seems likely (Sheldrake et al., 1984); however, studies on the transport of IgA into murine milk have produced conflicting results. Using radiolabeled IgA, Halsey et al. (1983) demonstrated that in the mouse, IgA can be transported from the circulation into milk during early lactation. Other investigators (Koertge and Butler, 1986b; Russell et al., 1982), using assays based on antibody-binding activity, were unable to show transport of IgA into murine milk. Using radiolabeled IgA, Koertge and Butler (1986b) were able to show that the IgA present in milk was degraded and suggested that the previous study (Halsey et al., 1983) detected only IgA fragments that had been transudated into the milk from the serum and not specifically transported IgA. Passively administered IgA is not transported into the milk of rats (Dahlgren et al., 1981; Koertge and Butler, 1986b).

Respiratory tract

Only a limited number of studies on the transport of antibodies into respiratory secretions have been reported, but the results have shown that selective transport of passively administered serum IgA into the respiratory tract is possible in sheep and mice. Because of their importance as background to the experiments demonstrating the passive transfer of local immunity by IgA, these respiratory transport studies will be addressed in more detail.

Sheep. Using the intravenous injection of radioiodinated ovine immunoglobulin, Scicchitano et al. (1984) showed that 35% of the IgA in the mediastinal lymph of sheep is plasma-derived. It was further demonstrated (Scicchitano et al., 1986) by the simultaneous intravenous injection of radiolabeled IgA and radiolabeled IgG_1 or IgG_2 that IgA is selectively transported into ovine respiratory secretions. Transport of IgA was approximately 4.5 times greater than transport of IgG, and the transported IgA was intact in the secretions. Biological activity of the transported IgA was not determined.

Mice. Mazanec et al. (1989) found that 4 to 5 hours after the intravenous injection of radiolabeled monomeric or polymeric IgA anti-Sendai virus monoclonal antibodies into mice, transport of pIgA into nasal secretions was three to seven times more efficient than transport of monomeric IgA (mIgA), while pIgA transport into bronchoalveolar lavages was only one to three times more efficient. This difference may reflect an increased contribution of serum antibody due to the transudation of IgG into alveolar fluids. Transport of pIgA into the gut was four to five times more efficient than the transport of mIgA, as expected. The agreement of the nasal secretion and gut transport indices suggests that transport at these two sites could occur by a similar mechanism. The investigators were unable to demonstrate the presence of functionally intact pIgA in the upper respiratory tract.

The pIgA transported into murine nasal secretions in the studies reported by Renegar and Small (1991a) was, in contrast, functionally intact. To avoid problems associated with the quantification of intact vs. degraded radiolabeled IgA in secretions (described by Koertge and Butler, 1986b), this study used an anti-influenza enzyme-linked immunosorbent assay (ELISA) to evaluate the transport of monomeric or polymeric IgA or IgG_1 monoclonal anti-influenza antibodies into the nasal secretions of mice. Nonimmune mice were injected intravenously with influenza-specific mIgA, pIgA, or IgG_1, and sacrificed at varying times between 2 and 24 hours postinjection. The peak nasal wash pIgA titer was reached 4 hours after antibody injection and was approximately 35 times greater than the nasal wash titer of either monomeric immunoglobulin.

To determine whether pIgA was selectively transported relative to IgG_1, the investigators injected a mixture of the two monoclonals intravenously into nonimmune mice and calculated a selective transport index for nasal antibody for each mouse. Twenty-nine of the 31 mice studied showed selective transport of IgA relative to IgG. Using a similar model, Steinmetz et al. (1994) determined that passively

administered monoclonal pIgA isotype-switch variants, generated from IgG hybridomas producing antibodies specific for bacterial respiratory tract pathogens, were selectively transported relative to IgG into both the upper and lower respiratory tract secretions of mice. In agreement with the results of Renegar and Small (1991a), Falero-Diaz et al. (2000) showed that, in mice, parenterally administered (either intravenously or by "backpack" tumor growth) monoclonal pIgA acquired SC as it was transported from the serum into nasal or vaginal secretions or into the bile, while similarly administered IgG did not, suggesting specific transport of the IgA but not the IgG. In contrast to Steinmetz et al. (1994) but in agreement with Mazanec et al. (1989), the Falero-Diaz group found efficient transmission of IgG but not of pIgA into the lungs of mice. In fact, they found that topical administration under light anesthesia of IgA as nosedrops was a more effective method for the delivery of IgA into the lungs than either parenteral method.

Thus, transport of serum IgA into nasal secretions is possible in some species. The relevance of this transport to the passive transfer of local immunity will be addressed in the following section.

Protection of mucosal surfaces by passively administered antibodies

Studies of the passive transfer of local immunity can be classified into two categories. In the first are those studies in which the antibody is introduced into the local secretions exogenously or mixed with the target pathogen prior to host challenge. The second category includes those studies in which systemically administered pIgA must be physiologically transported by a pIgR-mediated mechanism to its site of activity.

Exogenously administered antibody

The studies in this category have investigated the role of IgA in mucosal immunity by feeding antibody or instilling it intranasally or intravaginally and then challenging, or by administering antibody-pathogen mixtures intranasally.

Oral antibody. Offit and Clark (1985) demonstrated the ability of milk-derived IgG and IgA to protect the murine intestine from infection with primate rotavirus SA-11. Suckling mice were protected by milk from dams that had been orally immunized with SA-11 virus. This protective activity was detected in both the IgG and IgA fractions, but the IgA fraction was more potent *in vivo* than the IgG fraction. In newborn mice from immune dams foster-nursed on seronegative dams, the presence of circulating systemic antirotavirus antibodies in high titer did not protect against SA-11 viral infection. Thus, the specific antibody had to be present in the gut lumen to protect the intestinal cell surface from viral infection, and S-IgA could mediate this protection.

Enriquez and Riggs (1998) developed a series of dimeric IgA monoclonal antibodies directed toward the sporozoite antigen P23 of *Cryptosporidium parvum*, an important diarrhea-causing protozoan parasite. When administered orally prior to parasitic challenge, these antibodies were able to reduce the number of intestinal parasites in infected neonatal mice by up to 70%. These results extend the work of Albert *et al.* (1994), who successfully treated cryptosporidiosis in nude mice by the oral administration of rat bile containing *C. parvum*–specific IgA, while Czinn *et al.* (1993) protected germ-free mice from infection by *Helicobacter felis* by incubating the bacteria with specific IgA antibody prior to oral administration. The protective antibody was later shown to be directed against urease (Blanchard *et al.*, 1995).

A significant number of systemic infections in the human neonate originate from the gastrointestinal tract, especially in premature infants with immature gut barriers. Maxson *et al.* (1996) fed rabbit pups human S-IgA via intragastric gavage, then challenged them with *E. coli* K100. IgA-treated pups had significantly fewer bacteria translocated from the gut to the liver, spleen, and mesenteric lymph nodes. This neonatal rabbit model provides the first demonstration of control of bacterial translocation by IgA and suggests that oral supplementation with IgA may be beneficial for patients at risk for gut-origin sepsis.

Intranasal antibody. A number of studies have shown that exogenously administered IgA can protect against intranasal challenge with a pathogen. Bessen and Fischetti (1988) showed that S-IgA given by the intranasal route protected mice against streptococcal infection. Live streptococci were mixed with affinity-purified human salivary S-IgA or serum IgG antibodies directed toward the streptococcal M6 protein. The mixture was administered intranasally to mice. The S-IgA antibody protected against streptococcal infection, while the serum antibody had no effect. This study suggested that S-IgA alone is capable of protecting the mucosa against bacterial invasion.

Mazanec *et al.* (1987) demonstrated that IgA can protect mucosal surfaces against viral infection. Ascites containing IgA anti-Sendai virus monoclonal antibody was administered intranasally to lightly anesthetized mice before and after the mice were challenged intranasally with live virus. Three days later, mice were sacrificed and lung viral titers were determined. Animals treated with the specific monoclonal antibody were protected against viral infection. Further work from the same laboratory showed that local immunity to Sendai virus can also be mediated by intranasally administered IgG (Mazanec *et al.*, 1990). Tamura *et al.* (1991) purified anti-influenza S-IgA antibodies from the respiratory tracts of mice immunized with influenza hemagglutinin molecules. This IgA, when given intranasally, protected nonimmune mice from influenza infection. Protection was observed up to 3 days after antibody administration, was proportional to the amount of IgA administered, and was observed at IgA doses equivalent to naturally occurring antibody titers.

Intravaginal antibody. Zeitlin *et al.* (1998) were able to protect the mouse vagina from infection with herpes simplex virus 2 (HSV-2) by the topical administration of either IgG or IgA monoclonal antibody directed against glycoprotein D of HSV-2.

These studies show that topically administered local IgA or IgG can protect against viral or bacterial infection of the mucosa. They do not show that physiologically transported (secretory) IgA or serum-derived IgG actually does so. For that demonstration, antibody must be administered parenterally and transported into the mucosal secretions by a physiologic mechanism. The studies presented in the next section satisfy that criterion.

Systemically administered antibody

The definitive studies in this category have involved the respiratory and gastrointestinal tracts, although passive transfer of uterine immunity by pIgA has also been observed (Renegar and Small, 1993; Cotter *et al.* 1995; Pal *et al.* 1997), and Leher *et al.* (1999) demonstrated the protection of Chinese hamsters and pigs against *Acanthamoeba castellanii*–mediated keratitis by intraperitoneally administered antigen-specific monoclonal IgA. Work with the respiratory and gastrointestinal tracts will be presented in more detail.

Respiratory tract. The respiratory tract can be separated into an upper region (nose and trachea) and a lower region (lungs and bronchi) with immunity at each site involving different elements of the immune system. Numerous studies have shown that passively administered serum anti-influenza antibody (IgG) can prevent lethal viral pneumonia (Barber and Small, 1978; Kris *et al.*, 1988; Loosli *et al.*, 1953; Ramphal *et al.*, 1979; Palladino *et al.*, 1995). Serum antibody, however, does not prevent influenza infection of the upper respiratory tract (Barber and Small, 1978; Kris *et al.*, 1988; Ramphal *et al.*, 1979). Protection of the nose correlates with an increased nasal secretion IgA antibody level (reviewed in Renegar and Small, 1993), making influenza an excellent model in which to investigate the hypothesis that nasal immunity is mediated by S-IgA.

The first demonstration of the passive transfer of local immunity by physiologically transported S-IgA was reported by Renegar and Small (1991a) in the murine influenza model. They showed, as described above, that intravenously administered pIgA is transported into nasal secretions. To determine whether intravenously administered pIgA anti-influenza monoclonal antibody could mediate protection against local influenza virus challenge, passively immunized mice were challenged intranasally while awake with influenza virus. Twenty-four hours later the mice were sacrificed and the amount of virus shed in their nasal secretions was determined. Of the 24 saline-injected control mice, 23 shed virus into the nasal secretions, while only 5 of the 25 pIgA injected mice shed virus, and those 5 that did shed virus had a low titer. The observed protection was significant ($p < 0.001$). Passive immunization with influenza-specific pIgA therefore conferred complete protection against viral infection in 80% of the mice and partial protection in the remaining 20%. Serum IgG was found to confer only limited protection against nasal influenza infection (minimal reduction in viral shedding [$p < 0.02$], with only one of eight mice intravenously injected with influenza-specific IgG not shedding virus [$p < 0.5$]).

The passive protection studies showed that IgA *can* mediate local immunity. To confirm that IgA *is* the mediator of local immunity, mice passively immunized with pIgA were given nose drops of anti-IgA antibody 10 minutes before and 6 hours after they were challenged intranasally with influenza virus suspended in anti-IgA antiserum. Anti-IgA treatment abrogated IgA-mediated protection in the passively immunized mice (Renegar and Small, 1991a). To show that the passive transfer of local immunity by IgA was a reflection of the natural situation, the abrogation technique was extended to mice convalescent from influenza infection (Renegar and Small, 1991b). Nonimmune mice and convalescent mice, *i.e.,* mice that had recovered from an influenza virus infection 4 to 6 weeks earlier and were therefore naturally immune, were treated intranasally with antiserum to IgA or IgG or with a mixture of antisera to IgG and IgM and then challenged while awake with influenza virus mixed with antiserum. Intranasal administration of antiserum was continued at intervals for 24 hours. One day after viral challenge, the mice were killed and their nasal washes were assayed for virus shedding. Nonimmune mice all became infected, regardless of whether the virus was administered in saline, normal rabbit serum, or anti-immunoglobulin antiserum. Convalescent mice, as expected, were protected from viral infection. Administration of influenza virus in either anti-IgG or a mixture of anti-IgG and anti-IgM antisera did not affect protection, *i.e.,* the convalescent mice were still immune. Administration of virus in anti-IgA antiserum, however, abrogated convalescent immunity. These results demonstrate that IgA is a major mediator of murine nasal immunity and suggest that passive immunization mimics the role S-IgA plays in natural immunity. These observations were extended by the work of Philipon *et al.* (1995). Using the backpack method of monoclonal antibody administration, they demonstrated that monoclonal IgA antibody directed against *Shigella flexneri* serotype 5a lipopolysaccharide protects mice against intranasal challenge with *S. flexneri.*

Mbawuicke *et al.* (1999), however, have used the IgA knockout mouse model to challenge these findings. Mice unable to produce IgA antibodies were able to generate a protective anti-influenza response and to transport passively administered anti-influenza antibodies into both the upper and lower respiratory tracts. Knockout mice, however, may not be the best model in which to study the role of IgA in nasal immunity, because, with the congenital loss of IgA, production of other classes of antibody such as IgG may be increased as a compensatory mechanism. The data of Mbawuicke *et al.* suggest that this may be the case, as influenza-specific IgG levels were higher in immune knockout mice than in normal mice, and an altered IgG subclass distribution in response to influenza infection was observed (Harriman *et al.,* 1999; Zhang *et al.,* 2002). Furthermore, perturbation of mucosal IgA transport in the pIgR knockout mouse (Johansen *et al.,* 1999) led to increased mucosal leakiness and increased serum total IgG levels, indicating a defect in the mucosal barriers. It is known (Renegar *et al.,* 2004) that at a dose high enough to give a serum titer seven times the normal anti-influenza IgG titer of convalescent mice, intravenously administered influenza-specific IgG can

lower or eliminate the nasal secretion viral load; however, scanning electron microscopy has revealed that even this high IgG dose does not prevent infection of the nasal epithelium. Thus, the lowered nasal secretion viral titers reported in IgG-protected mice may be due to neutralization of newly replicated virus by serum antibody leaking through the virally damaged epithelium. Furthermore, the serum anti-influenza IgG antibody titer has to be several times higher than that normally observed for the IgG effect to be observed, because serum antibody at a level comparable to that of normal convalescent mice neither depresses viral shedding nor prevents viral pathology in the nasal epithelium.

Since the publication of the IgA knockout mouse work, a model has been reported in which mucosal IgA levels are depressed in genetically normal mice while serum IgG remains unaffected (Renegar *et al.,* 2001a, 2001b). In mice, total parenteral nutrition (TPN) depressed nasal mucosal immunity to influenza virus, resulting in increased viral shedding from the noses of TPN-fed immune mice (**Fig. 46.1A**). In these mice, nasal influenza–specific IgA was severely depressed (**Fig. 46.1B**), while the serum anti-influenza IgG titer was unaffected (**Fig. 46.1C**). Thus, in genetically normal ICR mice, serum IgG alone is not capable of preventing viral infection of the nose. Protection could be restored by the intravenous administration of influenza-specific pIgA monoclonal antibody (**Fig. 46.1D**). This work strongly suggests that IgA is required for the prevention of influenza virus infection in the noses of normal mice.

Gastrointestinal tract. Additional evidence that S-IgA is the mediator of local immunity comes from studies of the gastrointestinal tract. Polymeric IgA hybridomas against *Vibrio cholerae* were generated and the resulting monoclonal antibodies were used to determine whether IgA can mediate immunity toward a bacterial pathogen in the gut (Winner *et al.,* 1991). The investigators selected a clone that produced dimeric monoclonal IgA antibodies directed against an Ogawa-specific lipopolysaccharide carbohydrate antigen exposed on the bacterial surface. These antibodies were able to cross-link bacterial organisms *in vitro,* suggesting that they might be effective in preventing mucosal colonization by the pathogen *in vivo.* To provide continuous physiologic (*i.e.,* secretory-component–mediated) transport of specific antibody into the gut, hybridoma cells were injected subcutaneously into the backs of adult BALB/c mice.

These "backpack" tumors released monoclonal IgA into the circulation, and the plasma IgA was transported into the gut lumen. Neonatal mice bearing these backpack tumors survived challenge with *V. cholerae,* while neonatal mice bearing backpack tumors of unrelated IgA hybridomas and non-tumor-bearing neonatal mice died. This ingenious model provided the first evidence that S-IgA alone can mediate mucosal immunity to a bacterial pathogen. Michetti *et al.* (1992) have since demonstrated that pathogen-specific monoclonal S-IgA can protect mice from infection by *Salmonella typhimurium* following oral challenge.

The backpack model has also been used to treat rotavirus infections of the gastrointestinal tract of mice (Burns *et al.,*

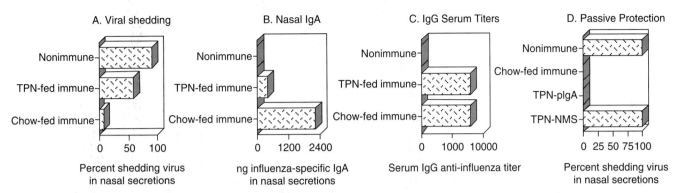

Fig. 46.1. Influenza immunity in total parenteral nutrition (TPN)–fed mice. **A,** Viral shedding: Following the surgical placement of intravenous catheters, influenza immune mice were fed mouse chow or intravenous TPN solution (IV-TPN). Nonimmune mice were fed chow. Following 5 days on their respective protocols, mice were challenged intranasally while awake (i.n.) with influenza virus and were assayed 42 hours later for the shedding of virus in their nasal secretions. This figure represents the pooled data from 17 experiments. Nonparametric statistical analysis: chow-fed immune vs. IV-TPN–fed immune, $p < 0.0001$; chow-fed immune vs. nonimmune, $p < 0.0001$. **B,** Nasal IgA: Fifteen mice were infected i.n. while awake with PR8 (H1N1) influenza virus. Three weeks later, they underwent surgical instrumentation and were randomized to IV TPN feeding ($n = 8$) or chow feeding ($n = 7$). Following 5 days on protocol, the mice were sacrificed. Levels of influenza-specific IgA in nasal secretions were determined by ELISA and normalized to ng-specific IgA/100 µg nasal protein (chow vs IV TPN, $P < 0.05$, ANOVA). Influenza-specific IgA was undetectable in nonimmune mice. **C,** Influenza-specific serum IgG titers: Immune mice ($n = 11$) underwent instrumentation and were randomized to IV TPN feeding ($n = 6$) or chow feeding ($n = 5$). Following 5 days on protocol, mice were sacrificed and serum IgG anti-influenza titers and nasal viral shedding were determined. Antibody titers were the serum dilution with an ELISA absorbance reading of 0.200 or greater. The IgG titers were comparable in chow-fed and TPN-fed immune mice. All of the TPN-fed mice shed virus in their nasal secretions, while none of the chow-fed mice did so. **D,** Passive protection: Immune mice were fed on mouse chow or IV-TPN. Following 5 days on their respective protocols, the IV-TPN mice were divided into two groups. Nonimmune controls, ($n = 5$), the chow-fed immune mice ($n = 5$), and one of the IV-TPN groups (TPN-NMS, $n = 4$) received 400µl ascites fluid containing MOPC 315 (does not recognize influenza) pIgA monoclonal Ab IV. The second IV-TPN group (TPN-pIgA, $n = 4$) received 400 µl ascites fluid containing pIgA anti-influenza monoclonal Ab. Four hours later, all mice were challenged i.n. with PR8 influenza virus. After 48 hours, the mice were euthanized and their nasal secretions assayed for viral shedding. Nonparametric statistical analysis: nonimmune vs. TPN-NMS, $p = $ NS; immune vs. TPN-pIgA, $p = $ NS; nonimmune vs. immune chow-fed, $p < 0.0001$; nonimmune vs. TPN-pIgA, $p < 0.0001$. Panels **A–C** modified from Renegar et al., 2001b. Panel **D** from Renegar et al., 2001a)

1996). Non-neutralizing monoclonal IgA antibodies directed against VP6, a major inner capsid viral protein, were capable of both preventing primary and resolving chronic murine rotavirus infections. These findings are consistent with the hypothesis that *in vivo* intracellular viral inactivation by pIgA during transcytosis is a mechanism of host defense against rotavirus infection.

CLINICAL APPLICATIONS

The general approach of passive parenteral transfer of mucosal immunity has proven to be a useful research tool for determining the role of S-IgA in protection against various mucosal pathogens. The possibility of therapy by passively administered IgA antibody is more problematic. Passive protection by injection is highly speculative because of both the questionable efficiency of transport to the targeted mucosal surface and the potential adverse effects of intravenous IgA antibody. Serum IgA has been associated with both decreased complement activation (Russell et al., 1989) and decreased immune lysis (Griffiss and Goroff, 1983). Systematically administered pIgA may also be suppressive of both specific humoral and cellular responses (Renger and Small, unpublished observations). A more thorough knowledge of the role IgA can play in regulating the immune response is needed before intravenous passive mucosal immunization can

become an acceptable means of therapy in man; however, the direct oral or respiratory application of antibodies to the mucosal surfaces is both practical and acceptable.

Control of dental carries is a feasible target for topical IgA administration. One study is particularly intriguing. Ma et al. (1998) generated a monoclonal secretory antibody in transgenic plants and showed that it survived up to 3 days in the human oral cavity; furthermore, this antibody afforded specific protection against oral streptococcal colonization for at least 4 months.

The literature contains a number of reports of the passive transfer of immunity against gastrointestinal pathogens in humans (reviewed in Bogstedt et al., 1996, and in Hammarström et al. 1994). This immunity has been provided by the oral administration of purified human IgG or serum IgA and has been used as both a prophylactic and a therapeutic measure against rotavirus infection in children (Barnes et al. 1982; Guarino et al., 1994) and as a therapeutic measure against bacterial diarrheas (Tjellstrom et al., 1993; Hammarström et al., 1993). Oral administration of bovine antibodies has also been used successfully in the prophylaxis of bacterial and rotaviral diarrheas in man and in the treatment of human rotavirus infections (Bogstedt et al., 1996; Mitra et al., 1995). Chicken egg yolk antibody (IgY) protects calves against bovine rotavirus (Kuroki et al., 1994).

Provision of passive immunity by the intranasal administration of antibodies has been reported in both human and nonhuman primate models. Human gamma globulin administered intranasally showed promise in challenge experiments with influenza or coxsackie A-21 viruses (Fruchtman *et al.*, 1972; Buthala *et al.*, 1970). IgA antibodies (IgAbulin), given as a nasal spray to the Swedish ski team during the Albertville Winter Olympic Games, significantly reduced the level of upper respiratory tract infections (Hammarström *et al.*, 1994); however, IgAbulin treatment had no effect on the frequency of upper respiratory tract symptoms in elite canoeists studied during hard and moderate training regimens (Lindberg and Berglund, 1996). IgAbulin nosedrop treatment of variable immunodeficiency patients who were chronic nasopharyngeal carriers of nonencapsulated *Haemophilus influenzae* eliminated the carrier state in 2 of 5 patients and alleviated coughing in all 5 (Lindberg *et al.*, 1993). Heikkinen *et al.* (1998) treated 40 children aged 1 to 4 years intranasally with IgA or a placebo and found a 42% reduction in rhinitis in the IgA-treated group. Thus, intranasal instillation of antibodies is feasible and may prove to be effective in the management of immunosuppressed patients.

Intranasal administration of specific antibodies may prove to be even more exciting. Weltzin *et al.* (1996) treated rhesus monkeys with nose drops containing mouse monoclonal IgA antibody against respiratory syncytial virus (RSV). Treated monkeys had reduced viral shedding in the nose, throat, and lungs and developed neutralizing serum antibody to RSV, even in the absence of detectable viral replication. RSV is a major cause of lower respiratory tract disease in infants and young children, producing severe disease in children with underlying conditions of the heart or lungs. These results suggest that prophylactic administration of monoclonal antibody nose drops could provide effective protection against RSV infection in at-risk human infants.

REFERENCES

Abimiku, A.G., and Dolby, J.M. (1987). The mechanism of protection of infant mice from intestinal colonization with *Campylobacter jejuni*. *J. Med. Microbiol.* 23, 339–344.

Albert, M.M., Rusnak, J., Luther, M.F., and Graybill, J.R. (1994). Treatment of murine cryptosporidiosis with anticryptosporidial immune rat bile. *Am. J. Trop. Med. Hyg.* 50, 112–119.

Appleby, P., and Catty, D. (1983). Transmission of immunoglobulin to foetal and neonatal mice. *J. Reprod. Immunol.* 5, 203–213.

Arango-Jaramillo, S., Wisseman, C.L., Jr., and Azad, A.F. (1988). Newborn rats in the murine typhus enzootic infection cycle: studies on transplacental infection and passively acquired maternal antirickettsial antibodies. *Am. J. Trop. Med. Hyg.* 39, 391–397.

Arnold, R.E. (1982). Treatment of rattlesnake bites. In *Rattlesnake Venoms: Their Actions and Treatment* (ed. A.T. Tu), 315–338. New York: Marcel Dekker.

Baker, C.J., Rench, M.A., Edwards, M.S., Carpenter, R.J., Hays, B.M., and Kasper, D.L. (1988). Immunization of pregnant women with a polysaccharide vaccine of group B streptococcus. *N. Engl. J. Med.* 319, 1180–1185.

Barber, W.H., and Small, P.A., Jr. (1978). Local and systemic immunity to influenza infections in ferrets. *Infect. Immun.* 21, 221–228.

Barnes, G.L., Hewson, P.H., McLellan, J.A., Doyle, L.W., Knoches, A.M.L., Kitchen, W.H., and Bishop, R.F. (1982). A randomized trial of oral gammaglobulin in low-birth weight infants infected with rotavirus. *Lancet* 1, 1371–1373.

Barthold, S.W., Beck, D.S., and Smith, A.L. (1988). Mouse hepatitis virus and host determinants of vertical transmission and maternally-derived passive immunity in mice. *Arch. Virol.* 100, 171–183.

Bertone, J.J., Jones, R.L., and Curtis, C.R. (1988). Evaluation of a test kit for determination of serum immunoglobulin G concentration in foals. *J. Vet. Intern. Med.* 2, 181–183.

Bessen, D., and Fischetti, V.A. (1988). Passive acquired mucosal immunity to group A streptococci by secretory immunoglobulin A. *J. Exp. Med.* 167, 1945–1950.

Blanchard, T.G., Czinn, S.J., Maurer, R., Thomas, W.D., Soman, G., and Nedrud, J.G. (1995). Urease-specific monoclonal antibodies prevent *Helicobacter felis* infection in mice. *Infect. Immun.* 63, 1394–1399.

Bogstedt, A.K., Johansen, K., Hatta, H., Kim, M., Casswall, T., Svensson, L., and Hammarström, L. (1996). Passive immunity against diarrhoea. *Acta Paediatr.* 85, 125–128.

Bohl, E.H., and Saif, L.J. (1975). Passive immunity in transmissible gastroenteritis of swine: immunoglobulin characteristics of antibodies in milk after inoculating virus by different routes. *Infect. Immun.* 11, 23–32.

Burns, J.W., Siadat-Pajouh, M., Krishnaney, A.A., and Greenberg, H.B. (1996). Protective effect of rotavirus VP6-specific IgA monoclonal antibodies that lack neutralizing activity. *Science* 272, 104–107.

Busse, P.J., Razvi, S., and Cunningham-Rundles, C. (2002). Efficacy of intravenous immunoglobulin in the prevention of pneumonia in patients with common variable immunodeficiency. *J. Allergy Clin. Immunol.* 109, 1001–1004.

Buthala, D.A., and Damiano, B.S. (1970). Studies on Coxackie A-21 (COE) virus-infected volunteers: Effect of local therapy with gamma globulin. *Ann. N.Y. Acad. Sci.* 173, 794.

Butler, J.E., Frenyo, V.L., Whipp, S.C., Wilson, R.A., and Koertge, T.E. (1986). The metabolism and transport of bovine serum SIgA. *Comp. Immunol. Microbiol. Infect. Dis.* 9, 303–315.

Centers for Disease Control. (1991a). Rabies prevention–United States: recommendations of the Immunization Practices Advisory Committee (ACIP). *MMWR Morb. Mortal. Wkly. Rep.* 40 (RR-3), 7–8.

Centers for Disease Control (1991b). Diphtheria, tetanus, and pertussis.: recommendations for vaccine use and other preventative measures: recommendations of the Immunization Practices Advisory Committee (ACIP). *MMWR Morb. Mortal. Wkly. Rep.* 40 (RR-10), 21–22.

Challacombe, S.J., Russell, M.W., Hawkes, J.E., Bergmeier, L.A., and Lehner, T. (1978). Passage of immunoglobulins from plasma to the oral cavity in rhesus monkeys. *Immunology* 35, 923–931.

Cotter, T.W., Meng, Q., Shen, Z.L., Zhang, Y.X., Su, H., and Caldwell, H.D. (1995). Protective efficacy of major outer membrane protein-specific immunoglobulin A (IgA) and IgG monoclonal antibodies in a murine model of *Chlamydia trachomatis* genital tract infection. *Infect. Immun.* 63, 4704–4714.

Crouch, C.F. (1985). Vaccination against enteric rota and coronaviruses in cattle and pigs: enhancement of lactogenic immunity. *Vaccine* 3, 284–291.

Czinn, S.J., Cai, A., and Nedrud, J.G. (1993). Protection of germ-free mice from infection by *Helicobacter felis* after active oral or passive IgA immunization. *Vaccine* 11, 637–642.

Dahlgren, U., Ahlstedt, S., Hedman, L., Wadsworth, C., and Hanson, L.Å. (1981). Dimeric IgA in the rat is transferred from serum into bile but not into milk. *Scand. J. Immunol.* 14, 95–98.

Delacroix, D.L., Hodgson, H.J., McPherson, A., Dive, C., and Vaerman, J.P. (1982). Selective transport of polymeric immunoglobulin A in bile. Quantitative relationships of monomeric and polymeric immunoglobulin A., immunoglobulin M, and other proteins in serum, bile, and saliva. *J. Clin. Invest.* 70, 230–241.

Delacroix, D.L., Malburny, G.N., and Vaerman, J.P. (1985). Hepatobiliary transport of plasma IgA in the mouse: contribution to the clearance of intravascular IgA. *Eur. J. Immunol.* 15, 893–899.

Dooley, J.S., Potter, B.J., Thomas, H.C., and Sherlock, S. (1982). A comparative study of the biliary secretion of human dimeric and monomeric IgA in the rat and in man. *Hepatology* 2, 323–327.

Ellis, T.M., Carman, H., Robinson, W.F., and Wilcox, G.E. (1986). The effect of colostrum-derived antibody on neonatal transmission of caprine arthritis-encephalitis virus infection. *Aust. Vet. J.* 63, 242–245.

Enriquez, F.J., and Riggs, M.W. (1998). Role of immunoglobulin A monoclonal antibodies against P23 in controlling murine *Cryptosporidium parvum* infection. *Infect. Immun.* 66, 4469–4473.

Eschenburg, G., Heine, W., and Peters, E. (1990). [Fecal sIgA and lysozyme excretion in breast feeding and formula feeding]. *Kinderarztl. Prax.* 58, 255–260.

Falero-Diaz, G., Challacombe, S., Rahman, D., Mistry, M., Douce, G., Dougan, G., Acosta, A., and Ivany, J. (2000). Transmission of IgA and IgG monoclonal antibodies to mucosal fluids following intranasal or parenteral delivery. *Int. Arch. Allergy Immunol.* 122, 143–150.

Francis, M.J., and Black, L. (1984). The effect of vaccination regimen on the transfer of foot and mouth disease antibodies from the sow to her piglets. *J. Hyg. Lond.* 93, 123–131.

Fruchtman, M.H., Mauceri, A.A., Migley, F.M., and Waldman, R.H. (1972). Aerosol administration of human gamma globulin as prophylaxis against influenza virus challenge. *Clin. Med.* 79, 17.

Gardner, M.M. (1976). Localization of rabbit gamma globulins in the mouse visceral yolk sac placenta. *Anat. Rec.* 184, 665–677.

Goldman, A.S., Ham-Pong, A.J., and Goldblum, R.M. (1985). Host defenses: development and maternal contributions. *Adv. Pediatr.* 32, 71–100.

Griffiss, J.M., and Goroff, D.K. (1983). IgA blocks IgM and IgG-initiated immune lysis by separate molecular mechanisms. *J. Immunol.* 130, 2882–2885.

Guarino, A., Cabani, R.B., Russo, S., Albano, F., Canani, M.B., Ruggeri, F.M., Donelli, G., and Rubino, A. (1994). Oral immuoglobulins for treatment of acute rotaviral gastroenteritis. *Pediatrics* 93, 12–16.

Halsey, J.F., Mitchell, C.S., and McKenzie, S.J. (1983). The origin of secretory IgA in milk: a shift during lactation from a serum origin to local synthesis in the mammary gland. *Ann. N.Y. Acac. Sci.* 409, 452–459.

Hammerberg, B., Musoke, A.J., Williams, J.F., and Leid, R.W. (1977). Uptake of colostral immunoglobulins by the suckling rat. *Lab. Anim. Sci.* 27, 50–53.

Hammarström, L., Gardulf, A., Hammarström, V., Janson, A., Lindberg, K., and Edvard Smith, C.I. (1994). Systemic and topical immunoglobulin treatment in immunocompromised patients. *Immun. Rev.* 139, 43–70.

Hammarström, V., Smith, C.I.E., and Hammarström, L. (1993). Oral immunoglobulin treatment in *Campylobacter jejuni* enteritis. *Lancet* 341, 1036.

Harriman, G.R., Bogue, M., Rogers, P., Finegold, M., Pacheco, S., Bradley, A., Zhang, Y., and Mbawuike, I.N. (1999). Targeted deletion of the IgA constant region in mice leads to IgA deficiency with alterations in expression of other Ig isotypes. *J. Immunol.* 162, 2521–2529.

Heikkinen, T., Ruohola, A., Ruskanen, O., Wari, S.M., Uhari, M., and Hammarstrom, L. (1998). Intranasally administered immunoglobulin for the prevention of rhinitis in children. *Pediatr. Infect. Dis. J.* 17, 367–372.

Heiman, H.S., and Weisman, L.E. (1989). Transplacental or enteral transfer of maternal immunization-induced antibody protects suckling rats from type III group B streptococcal infection. *Pediatr. Res.* 26, 629–632.

Heremans, J.F. (1974). Immunoglobulin A. In *The Antigens*. Vol. 2. (ed. M. Sela), 365–522. London: Academic Press.

Hjelt, K., Grauballe, P.C., Nielsen, O.H., Schiotz, P.O., and Krasilnikoff, P.A. (1985). Rotavirus antibodies in the mother and her breast-fed infant. *J. Pediatr. Gastroenterol. Nutr.* 4, 414–420.

Hockel, M., and Kaufmann, R. (1986). Placental transfer of class G immunoglobulins treated with beta-propiolactone (beta-PL) for intravenous application—a case report. *J. Perinat. Med.* 14, 205–208.

Ijaz, M.K., Sabara, M.I., Frenchick, P.J., and Babiuk, L.A. (1987). Effect of different routes of immunization with bovine rotavirus on lactogenic antibody response in mice. *Antiviral Res.* 8, 283–297.

Jakoi, E.R., Cambier, J., and Saslow, S. (1985). Transepithelial transport of maternal antibody: purification of IgG receptor from newborn rat intestine. *J. Immunol.* 135, 3360–3364.

Johansen, F.-E., Pekna, M., Norderhaug, I.N., Haneberg, B., Hietala, M.A., Krajci, P., Betsholtz, C., and Brandzaeg, P. (1999). Absence of epithelial immunoglobulin A transport, with increased mucosal leakiness, in polymeric immunoglobulin receptor/secretory component-deficient mice. *J. Exp. Med.* 190, 915–922.

Jollie, W.P. (1985). Immunocytochemical localization of antibody during placental transmission of immunity in rats. *J. Reprod. Immunol.* 7, 261–274.

Junghans, R.P., and Anderson, C.L. (1996). The protection receptor for IgG catabolism is the beta2-microglobulin-containing neonatal intestinal transport receptor. *Proc. Natl. Acad. Sci. U.S.A.* 93, 5512–5516.

Kenny, J.F., Boesman, M.I., and Michaels, R.H. (1967). Bacterial and viral coproantibodies in breast-fed infants. *Pediatrics* 39, 202–213.

Koertge, T.E., and Butler, J.E. (1986a). Dimeric mouse IgA is transported into rat bile five times more rapidly than into mouse bile. *Scand. J. Immunol.* 24, 567–574.

Koertge, T.E., and Butler, J.E. (1986b). Dimeric M315 is transported into mouse and rat milk in a degraded form. *Mol. Immunol.* 23, 839–845.

Kohl, S., and Loo, L.S. (1984). The relative role of transplacental and milk immune transfer in protection against lethal neonatal herpes simplex virus infection in mice. *J. Infect. Dis.* 149, 38–42.

Koutras, A.K., and Vigorita, V.J. (1989). Fecal secretory immunoglobulin A in breast milk versus formula feeding in early infancy. *J. Pediatr. Gastroenterol. Nutr.* 9, 58–61.

Kris, R.M., Yetter, R.A., Cogliano, R., Ramphal, R., and Small, P.A., Jr. (1988). Passive serum antibody causes temporary recovery from influenza virus infection of the nose, trachea, and lung of nude mice. *Immunology* 63, 349–353.

Kubagawa, H., Bertoli, L.F., Barton, J.C., Koopman, W.J., Mestecky, J., and Cooper, M.D. (1987). Analysis of paraprotein transport into the saliva by using anti-idiotype antibodies. *J. Immunol.* 138, 435–439.

Kuroki, M., Ohta, M., Ikemori, Y., Peralta, R.C., Yokoyama, H., and Kodama, Y. (1994). Passive protection against bovine rotavirus in calves by specific immunoglobulins from chicken egg yolk. *Arch. Virol.* 138, 143–148.

Leach, L., Eaton, B.M., Firth, J.A., and Contractor, S.F. (1990). Uptake and intracellular routing of peroxidase-conjugated immunoglobulin-G by the perfused human placenta. *Cell Tissue Res.* 261, 383–388.

Leher, H., Zaragoza, F., Taherzadeh, S., Alizad eh, H., and Niederkorn, J. Y. (1999). Monoclonal IgA antibodies protect against *Acanthamoeba* keratitis. *Exp. Eye Res.* 69, 75–84.

Lennon, J.L., and Black, F.L. (1986). Maternally derived measles immunity in era of vaccine-protected mothers. *J. Pediatr.* 108, 671–676.

Lindberg, K., and Berglund, B. (1996). Effect of treatment with nasal IgA on the incidence of infectious disease in world-class canoeists. *Int. J. Sports Med.* 17, 235–238.

Lindberg, K., Samuelson, A., Rynnel-Dagöö, B., Smith, C.I.E., and Hammarström, L. (1993). Nasal administration of IgA to individuals with hypogamma-globulinemia. *Scand. J. Infect. Dis.* 25, 395.

Lindh, E. (1975). Increased resistance of immunoglobulin dimers to proteolytic degradation after binding of secretory component. *J. Immunol.* 114, 284–286.

Loosli, C.G., Hamre, D., and Berlin, B.S. (1953). Airborne influenza virus A infections in immunized animals. *Trans. Assoc. Am. Phys.* 66, 222–230.

Ma, J. K., Hikmat, B. Y., Wycoff, K., Vine, N. D., Chargelegue, D., Yu, L., Hein, M. I., and Lehner, T. (1998). Characterization of a recombinant plant monoclonal secretory antibody and preventive immunotherapy in humans. *Nat. Med.* 4, 601–606.

Maxson, R.T., Johnson, D.D., Jackson, R.J., and Smith, S.D. (1996). The protective role of enteral IgA supplementation in neonatal gut-origin sepsis. *Ann. N. Y. Acad. Sci.* 778, 405–407.

Mazanec, M.B., Lamm, M.E., Lyn, D., Portner, A., and Nedrud, J.G. (1987). Comparison of IgA versus IgG monoclonal antibodies for passive immunization of the murine respiratory tract. *J. Virol.* 61, 2624–2626

Mazanec, M.B., Nedrud, J.G., and Lamm, M.E. (1987). Immunoglobulin A monoclonal antibodies protect against Sendai virus. *J. Virol.* 61, 2624–2626.

Mazanec, M.B., Nedrud, J.G., Liang, X., and Lamm, M.E. (1989). Transport of serum IgA into murine respiratory secretions and its implications for immunization strategies. *J. Immunol.* 142, 4275–4281.

Mbawuike, I. N., Pacheco, Acuna, C. L., Switzer, K. C., Zhang, Y., and Harriman, G. R. (1999). Mucosal immunity to influenza without IgA: an IgA knockout mouse model. *J. Immunol.* 162, 2530–2537.

McGuire, T.C., Poppie, M.J., and Banks, K.L. (1975). Hypogammaglobulinemia predisposing to infection in foals. *J. Am. Vet. Med. Assoc.* 166, 71–75.

McGuire, T.C., Pfeiffer, N.E., Weikel, J.M., and Bartsch, R.C. (1976). Failure of colostral immunoglobulin transfer in calves dying from infectious disease. *J. Am. Vet. Med. Assoc.* 169, 713–718.

Mestecky, J., and McGhee, J.R. (1987). Immunoglobulin A (IgA): molecular and cellular interactions involved in IgA biosynthesis and immune response. *Adv. Immunol.* 40, 153–245.

Michalek, S.M., and McGhee, J.R. (1977). Effective immunity to dental caries: passive transfer to rats of antibodies to *Streptococcus mutans* elicits protection. *Infect. Immun.* 17, 644–650.

Michalek, S.M., Gregory, R.L., Harmon, C.C., Katz, J., Richardson, G.J., Hilton, T., Filler, S.J., and McGhee, J.R. (1987). Protection of gnotobiotic rats against dental caries by passive immunization with bovine milk antibodies to *Streptococcus mutans*. *Infect. Immun.* 55, 2341–2347.

Michetti, P., Mahan, M.J., Slauch, J.M., Mekalanos, J.J., and Neutra, M.R. (1992). Monoclonal secretory IgA protects mice against oral challenge with the invasive pathogen *Salmonella typhimurium*. *Infect. Immun.* 60, 1786–1792.

Mitra, A.K., Mahalanabis, D., Ashraf, H., Uicomb, L., Eeckels, R., and Tzipori, S. (1995). Hyperimmune cow colostrum reduces diarrhoea due to rotavirus: a double-blind, controlled clinical trial. *Acta Paediatr.* 84, 996–1001.

Montgomery, P.C., Khaleel, S.A., Goudswaard, J., and Virella, G. (1977). Selective transport of an oligomeric IgA into canine saliva. *Immunol. Commun.* 6, 633–642.

Mucchielli, A., Laliberte, F., and Laliberte, M.F. (1983). A new experimental method for the dynamic study of the antibody transfer mechanism from mother to fetus in the rat. *Placenta* 4, 175–183.

Nejamkis, M.R., Nota, N.R., Weissenbacher, M.C., Guerrero, L.B., and Giovanniello, O.A. (1975). Passive immunity against Junin virus in mice. *Acta Virol. Praha.* 19, 237–244.

Oda, M., Izumiya, K., Sato, Y., and Hirayama, M. (1983). Transplacental and transcolostral immunity to pertussis in a mouse model using acellular pertussis vaccine. *J. Infect. Dis.* 148, 138–145.

Offit, P.A., Clark, H.F., Kornstein, M.J., and Plotkin, S.A. (1984). A murine model of oral infection with a primate rotavirus (simian SA-11). *J. Virol.* 51, 233–236.

Orlans, E., Peppard, J., Reynolds, J., and Hall, J. (1978). Rapid active transport of immunoglobulin A from blood to bile. *J. Exp. Med.* 147, 588–592.

Orlans, E., Peppard, J.V., Payne, A.W., Fitzharris, B.M., Mullock, B.M., Hinton, R.H., and Hall, J.G. (1983). Comparative aspects of the hepatobiliary transport of IgA. *Ann. N. Y. Acad. Sci.* 409, 411–427.

Pal, S., Theodor, I., Peterson, E. M., and de la Maza, L. M. (1997). Monoclonal immunoglobulin A antibody to the major outer membrane protein of the *Chlamydia trachomatis* mouse pneumonitis biovar protects mice against a chlamydial genital challenge. *Vaccine* 15, 575–582.

Palladino, G., Mozdzanowska, K., Washko, G., and Gerhard, W. (1995). Virus-neutralizing antibodies of immunoglobulin G (IgG) but not of IgM or IgA isotypes can cure influenza virus pneumonia in SCID mice. *J. Virol.* 69, 2075–2081.

Phalipon, A., Kaufman, M., Michetti, P., Cavaillon, J.M., Huerre, M., Sansonetti, P., and Kraehenbuhl, J.P. (1995). Monoclonal immunoglobulin A antibody directed against serotype-specific epitope of *Shigella flexnerii* lipopolysaccharide protects against murine experimental shigellosis. *J. Exp. Med.* 182, 769–778.

Prentice, A. (1987). Breast feeding increases concentrations of IgA in infants' urine. *Arch. Dis. Child.* 62, 792–795.

Rahman, M.M., Yamauchi, M., Hanada, N., Nishikawa, K., and Morishima, T. (1987). Local production of rotavirus specific IgA in breast tissue and transfer to neonates. *Arch. Dis. Child.* 62, 401–405.

Ramphal, R., Cogliano, R.C., Shands, J.W., Jr., and Small, P.A., Jr., (1979). Serum antibody prevents lethal murine influenza pneumonitis but not tracheitis. *Infect. Immun.* 25, 992–997.

Renegar, K.B., and Small, P.A., Jr. (1991a). Passive transfer of local immunity to influenza virus infection by IgA antibody. *J. Immunol.* 146, 1972–1978.

Renegar, K.B., and Small, P.A., Jr. (1991b). Immunoglobulin A mediation of murine nasal anti-influenza virus immunity. *J. Virol.* 65, 2146–2148.

Renegar, K. B., Kudsk, K. A., Dewitt, R. C., and King, B. K. (2001a). Impairment of mucosal immunity by parenteral nutrition: depressed nasotracheal influenza-specific secretory IgA levels and transport in parenterally fed mice. *Ann. Surg.* 233, 134–138.

Renegar, K. B., Johnson, C. D., Dewitt, R. C., King, B. K., Li, J., Fukatsu, K., and Kudsk, K. A. (2001b). Impairment of mucosal immunity by total parenteral nutrition: requirement for IgA in murine nasotracheal anti-influenza immunity. *J. Immunol.* 166, 819–825.

Renegar, K.B., Small, P.A., Jr., Boykins, L., and Wright, P. (2004). Role of IgA vs. IgG in the control of influenza viral infection in the murine respiratory tract. *J. Immunol* 173, 1978–1986.

Renegar, K.B., Menge, A.C., Small, P.A., Jr., and Mestecky, J. Influenza infection of the murine uterus: A model for the study of mucosal immunity in the female reproductive tract. Manuscript in preparation.

Russell, M.W., Brown, T.A., and Mestecky, J. (1982). Preferential transport of IgA and IgA-immune complexes into bile compared with other external secretions. *Mol. Immunol.* 19, 677–682.

Russell, M.W., Reinholdt, J., and Kilian, M. (1989). Anti-inflammatory activity of human IgA antibodies and their Fab alpha fragments: inhibition of IgG-mediated complement activation. *Eur. J. Immunol.* 19, 2243–2249.

Scicchitano, R., Husband, A.J., and Cripps, A.W. (1984). Immunoglobulin-containing cells and the origin of immunoglobulins in the respiratory tract of sheep. *Immunol.* 52, 529–537.

Scicchitano, R., Sheldrake, R.F., and Husband, A.J. (1986). Origin of immunoglobulins in respiratory tract secretion and saliva of sheep. *Immunol.* 58, 315–321.

Sheldrake, R.F., Husband, A.J., Watson, D.L., and Cripps, A.W. (1984). Selective transport of serum-derived IgA into mucosal secretions. *J. Immunol.* 132, 363–368.

Simister, N.E., and Mostov, K.E. (1989). An Fc receptor structurally related to MHC class I antigens. *Nature* 337, 184–187.

Simister, N., and Rees, A.R. (1983). Properties of immunoglobulin G-Fc receptors from neonatal rat intestinal brush borders. *Ciba Found. Symp.* 95, 273–286.

Socken, D.J., Jeejeebhoy, K.N., Bazin, H., and Underdown, B.J. (1979). Identification of secretory component as an IgA receptor on rat hepatocytes. *J. Exp. Med.* 150, 1538–1548.

Steinmetz, I., Albrecht, F., Haussler, S., and Brenneke, B. (1994). Monoclonal IgA class-switch variants against bacterial surface antigens: molecular forms and transport into murine respiratory secretions. *Eur. J. Immunol.* 24, 2855–2862.

Tamura, S., Funato, H., Hirabayashi, Y., Suzuki, Y., Nagamine, T., Aizawa, C., and Kurata, T. (1991). Cross-protection against influenza A virus infection by passively transferred respiratory tract IgA antibodies to different hemagglutinin molecules. *Eur. J. Immunol.* 21, 1337–1344.

Tizzard, I. (1987). Immunity in the fetus and newborn. In *Veterinary Immunology—An Introduction* (ed. I. Tizzard), 3rd ed., 171–184. Philadelphia: WB Saunders.

Tjellström, B., Stenhammar, L., Ericksson, S, and Magnusson, K.-E. (1993). Oral immunoglobulin A supplement in treatment of *Clostridium difficile* enteritis. *Lancet* 341, 701–702.

Tomasi, T.B., Jr. (1970). The structure and function of mucosal antibodies. *Ann. Rev. Med.* 21, 281–298.

Tsunemitsu, H., Shimizu, M., Hirai, T., Yonemichi, H., Kudo, T., Mori, K., and Onoe, S. (1989). Protection against bovine rotaviruses in newborn calves by continuous feeding of immune colostrum. *Nippon Juigaku Zasshi* 51, 300–308.

Tuboly, S., Bernath, S., Glavits, R., and Medveczky, I. (1988). Intestinal absorption of colostral lymphoid cells in newborn piglets. *Vet. Immunol. Immunopathol.* 20, 75–85.

Vaerman, J.P. (1973). Comparative immunochemistry of IgA. *Res. Immunochem. Immunobiol.* 3, 91.

Vaerman, J.P., and Delacroix, D.L. (1984). Role of the liver in the immunobiology of IgA in animals and humans. *Contrib. Nephrol.* 40, 17–31.

von Behring and Kitasato (1890). On the acquisition of immunity against diphtheria and tetanus in animals. *Detsch. Med. Wochenschr.* 16, 1113–1114.

Waldman, T.A., and Strober, W. (1969). Metabolism of immunoglobulins. *Progr. Allergy* 13, 1–110.

Weltzin, R., Hsu, S.A., Mittler, E.S., Georgakopoulos, K., and Monath, T.P. (1994). Intranasal monoclonal immunoglobulin A against respiratory syncytial virus protects against upper and lower res-piratory tract infections in mice. *Antimicrob. Agents Chemother.* 38, 2785–2791.

Weltzin, R., Traina-Dorge, V., Soike, K., Zhang, J.-Y., Mack, P., Soman, G., Drabik, G., and Monath, T.P. (1996). Intranasal monoclonal IgA antibody to respiratory syncytial virus protects rhesus monkeys against upper and lower respiratory tract infections. *J. Infect. Dis.* 174, 256–261.

Wilson, R.A., and Jutila, J.W. (1976). Experimental neonatal colibacillosis in cows: immunoglobulin classes involved in protection. *Infect. Immun.* 13, 100–107.

Winner, L., III, Mack, J., Weltzin, R., Mekalanos, J.J., Kraehenbuhl, J.-P., and Neutra, M.R. (1991). New model for analysis of mucosal immunity: intestinal secretion of specific monoclonal immunoglobulin A from hybridoma tumors protects against *Vibrio cholerae* infection. *Infect. Immun.* 59, 977–982.

Zeitlin, L., Castle, P. E., Whaley, K. J., Moench, T. R., and Cone, R. A. (1998). Comparison of an anti-HSV-2 monoclonal IgG and its IgA switch variant for topical immunoprotection of the mouse vagina. *J. Reprod. Immunol.* 40, 93–101.

Zhang, Y., Pacheco, S., Acuna, C. L., Switzer, K. C., Wang, Y., Gilmore, X., Harriman, G. R., and Mbawuike, I. N. (2002). Immunoglobulin A-deficient mice exhibit altered T helper 1-type immune responses but retain mucosal immunity to influenza virus. *Immunology* 105, 286–294.

Zikan, J., Mestecky, J., Schrohenloher, R.E., Tomana, M., and Kulhavy, R. (1972). Studies on human secretory immunoglobulin A. V. Trypsin hydrolysis at elevated temperatures. *Immunochemistry* 9, 1185–1193.

Section D

Mucosal Vaccines

Mucosal Vaccines: An Overview

Chapter 47

Prosper N. Boyaka

Department of Microbiology, University of Alabama at Birmingham, Birmingham, Alabama

Jerry R. McGhee

Department of Microbiology, University of Alabama at Birmingham, Birmingham, Alabama

Cecil Czerkinsky

Faculte de Medecine-Pasteur, Universite de Nice, Nice, France

Jiri Mestecky

Departments of Microbiology and Medicine, University of Alabama at Birmingham, Birmingham, Alabama

The exposure of mucosal tissues to antigens (Ags) results in the induction of local and disseminated responses in the mucosal compartment as well as systemic immune responses manifested by the presence of Ag-specific antibodies (Abs) in external secretions and plasma, and T cells of various subsets in both mucosal and systemic lymphoid tissues. Thus, both mucosal and systemic immune compartments respond, under normal conditions, to a vast spectrum of environmental antigens of mainly food and microbial origin. As described in preceding chapters, this enormous antigenic load has resulted in a strategic distribution of cells involved in the uptake, processing, and presentation of Ags, the production of Abs, and cell-mediated immune (CMI) T-cell defenses at the front line of mucosal tissues.

For almost 100 years, researchers have attempted to design vaccines to be administered by a variety of mucosal routes rather than by conventional parenteral injections (see the Historical Introduction at the beginning of this book). Mucosal vaccination has many attractive features, including easy and painless administration, potential for mass immunization in case of emergencies, and reduced cost of production, storage, and delivery. More important, only mucosal vaccines consistently promote immune responses at the most common sites of entry of infectious agents. These desirable features immediately prompt a question: why do we have so few mucosal vaccines? As will become obvious from the ensuing chapters in this section, the optimal doses of Ag for mucosal vaccination are difficult to establish because of the low and unpredictable absorption from intestinal surfaces and the interference with quantitatively superior antigens in the gastrointestinal (GI) tract. Therefore, a need to develop methodologies that would mediate the preferential absorption of desired Ags is obvious. Furthermore, because of the presence of proteolytic enzymes in external secretions, most Ags need to be protected from digestion (see Chapter 1). To enhance the magnitude or quality of immune responses, many mucosal adjuvants have been extensively tested in experimental animals and to a very limited degree in humans (see Chapter 54). Although many of these substances displayed desired effects, their acceptance in humans is restricted because of their potential toxicity (*e.g.*, cholera toxin [CT] and the heat-labile toxin [LT] of *E. coli*) and low adjuvanticity in humans as opposed to animals (*e.g.*, QS-21); however, some mucosal adjuvants have not been adequately evaluated in humans.

Although the stimulation of protective immune responses to mucosal infectious agents is the ultimate criterion for a vaccine's performance, the possibility of induction of a state of systemic unresponsiveness to mucosally administered antigen—mucosal tolerance—has been frequently considered to be a negative factor in acceptance of mucosal vaccines. Mucosal tolerance is indeed a fundamental feature of the mucosal immune system and a critical functional component that efficiently prevents and suppresses otherwise unavoidable overstimulation of the entire immune system by environmental Ags. Thus, the enhancement of protective mucosal immune responses to infectious agents that is sought by vaccinologists and the suppression of systemic responses may seem paradoxical. As discussed next, such outcomes are not mutually exclusive because of a hierarchy in the quality of immune responses.

INDUCTIVE AND EFFECTOR SITES AND THE COMMON MUCOSAL IMMUNE SYSTEM

Extensive studies concerning the origin of B- and T-lymphocytes that ultimately populate mucosal tissues and secretory glands and of immunization routes effective in the induction of mucosal immune responses indicated that the common mucosal immune system (CMIS) can be divided into two functionally distinct compartments, namely, inductive versus effector sites. This network is highly integrated and finely regulated, and the outcome of mucosal tissue encounters with foreign Ags and pathogens can range from mucosal and plasma Abs, T-cell CMI, and cytotoxic T-lymphocyte (CTL) responses, on the one hand, to systemic anergy or mucosal tolerance on the other. This physiological division is of paramount importance in the design of vaccines effective for the induction of protective immunity within the mucosal immune system and, in particular, its humoral branch. Experiments performed in animal models revealed that the inductive sites present in certain locations, such as gut-associated or in some species bronchus-associated lymphoepithelial tissues (GALT, represented by Peyer's patches, and BALT, respectively), function as primary sources of precursor cells which migrate through the lymphatics and blood and after directed extravasation populate remote mucosal tissues and glands (Phillips-Quagliata and Lamm, 1988; Scicchitano et al., 1988). More recent studies suggest that such inductive sites are not necessarily restricted to Peyer's patches found mainly in the small intestine and the BALT in bronchi. Additional sites have been identified in nasal mucosa; palatine tonsils and other organized lymphoid tissues of Waldeyer's ring in the nasopharynx (Kuper et al., 1992; Kiyono, 1997); the large intestine, especially the rectum; and the genital tract.

Numbers and types of cells involved in immune responses and their products, primarily Abs and mediators (cytokines, chemokines), are remarkably different in the mucosal and systemic compartments of the immune system. Thus, secretory IgA (S-IgA) differs from plasma IgA not only in terms of specific Ab activity but also in the proportions of polymeric versus monomeric forms and of origin in secretory tissues versus bone marrow plasma cells. The ontogenies of the mucosal and systemic IgA compartments display characteristic and apparently independent patterns of maturation. Adult levels of IgA are reached in external secretions considerably earlier (1 month to 2 years) than in the blood plasma (adolescence) (Allansmith et al., 1968; Mellander et al.,

1984). Experiments addressing the origin of mucosal Abs have led to the clear conclusion that an overwhelming proportion of such Abs are produced locally in mucosal tissues and that only a minor fraction derive from the circulation in most species, including humans (Brandtzaeg, 1984; Mestecky and McGhee, 1987; Mestecky et al., 1997).

Inductive sites of the gastrointestinal tract

Inductive sites for mucosal immune responses were initially described in mucosal locations such as small intestinal Peyer's patches of the GALT (Phillips-Quagliata and Lamm, 1988). Earlier studies have shown that surgical removal of Peyer's patches from the intestine of rats does not affect the total number of IgA-containing cells in the lamina propria or the development of a normal antibody response to intestinal immunization (Heatley et al., 1981). More recently, mice lacking Peyer's patches by in utero treatment with a lympho-toxin-β receptor-Ig molecule fusion protein developed normal mucosal and systemic immunity to oral immunization (Yamamoto et al., 2000) suggesting that alternative inductive sites for mucosal immunity are present in the GALT. In fact, other lymphoid follicles, termed "isolated lymphoid follicles (ILFs)" or "solitary lymphoid follicles," were reported in the intestinal wall of rabbits (Keren et al., 1978), guinea pigs (Rosner and Keren, 1984), and humans (Moghaddami et al., 1998; Neutra et al., 2001). These structures have now been demonstrated in mice (Hamada et al., 2002; Fagarasan et al., 2003; Lorenz et al., 2003), where their number and maturation appear to be triggered by lumenal stimuli such as the bacterial flora (Fagarasan et al., 2003; Lorenz et al., 2003).

Pharyngeal and nasal lymphoepithelial tissues

Organized lymphoid tissues, including palatine, lingual, and nasopharyngeal tonsils (Waldeyer's ring), are strategically positioned at the beginning of the digestive and respiratory tracts and are continuously exposed to ingested and inhaled antigens. These nasopharyngeal-associated lymphoepithelial tissues (NALT) possess structural features similar to both lymph nodes and Peyer's patches of the GALT (Brandtzaeg, 1984; Ogra, 1971; see Chapter 83). For example, tonsillar crypts possess a lymphoepithelium which contains M cells for selective antigen uptake as well as B and T cells, plasma cells, and antigen-presenting cells (APCs). The distribution of IgA1- and IgA2-producing cells in the nasal and gastric mucosa and in lacrymal and salivary glands is similar to the distribution in tonsils, suggesting that tonsils may serve as a source for precursors of IgA plasma cells found in the upper respiratory and digestive tracts. Furthermore, tonsillectomized children display lower levels of S-IgA antibodies to the oral poliovirus vaccine than children with intact tonsils (Ogra, 1971). Others have shown that direct unilateral injection of antigens (cholera toxin B subunit [CT-B] and tetanus toxoid [TT]) into the tonsil of human volunteers resulted in the induction of mainly mucosal immune responses, manifested by the appearance of antigen-specific IgG and, to a lesser degree, IgA-forming cells (AFCs) in the injected tonsil (Quiding-Järbrink *et al.*, 1995a). Recent studies confirm the prevalence of IgG antibodies in tonsils and demonstrated that these structures display features of both mucosal inductive and effector sites (Boyaka *et al.*, 2000). Therefore, the tonsils may serve as an inductive site analogous to GALT in some species. Organized BALT were also noted at airway branches of experimental animals, although these structures rarely occur in humans (Pabst, 1992).

Several studies have emphasized the importance of inductive sites in the nasal cavity for the generation of mucosal and systemic immune responses that may exceed in magnitude those induced by oral immunization (Bergquist *et al.*, 1997; Di Tommaso *et al.*, 1996; Gallichan and Rosenthal, 1995; Lubeck *et al.*, 1994; Pal *et al.*, 1996; Russell *et al.*, 1996; Staats *et al.*, 1996). When introduced into the nasal cavity, usually along with mucosal adjuvants such as CT and/or CT-B, viral and bacterial antigens induce superior immune responses in external secretions such as saliva and, surprisingly, in female genital tract secretions of rodents, rhesus monkeys, chimpanzees, and humans (Quiding-Järbrink *et al.*, 1995b; Russell and Mestecky, 2002). Whether such antibody responses are also induced in the male genital tract remains to be determined. Nevertheless, this finding may have important implications for the design of vaccines effective in the induction of immune responses in the genital tract (Russell and Mestecky, 2002; see Chapter 95). Although analogous studies with bacterial antigens have not been performed in humans, induction of genital tract immune responses by nasal immunization would have profound implications for the prevention of sexually transmitted diseases, including AIDS (see Chapter 52). Thus, different mucosal immunization routes (nasal and oral) can induce generalized mucosal immune responses, although the relative representation of dominant antibody isotypes may vary. Circulating IgA AFCs induced after nasal vaccination express a more promiscuous profile of homing receptors than their corresponding counterparts raised after oral or rectal immunization (Quiding-Järbrink *et al.*, 1997; Kantele *et al.*, 1998). This could explain the fact that nasal immunization appears to induce S-IgA immunity in a broader range of mucosal tissues than oral vaccination.

Lymphoepithelial tissues in the large intestine and rectal immunization

Although most investigations of GALT mucosal IgA inductive sites have primarily centered on Peyer's patches and the appendix, analogous follicular structures are also found in the large intestine, with especially pronounced accumulations in the rectum (Langman and Rowland, 1986; O'Leary and Sweeney, 1986). The potential importance of rectal lymphoid tissues as an IgA inductive site and as a source of IgA plasma cell precursors is suggested by several studies. The predominance of IgA2 cells over IgA1 cells in the lamina propria of the large intestine clearly diverges from the relative apportioning of the IgA subclass distribution in other mucosal tissues (Crago *et al.*, 1984; Kett *et al.*, 1986). That this is also the case in the female genital mucosal tissues

(uterus, cervix, fallopian tubes, and vagina) (Kutteh *et al.*, 1988) suggests that rectal lymphoid tissues may be an important source of IgA precursors destined for the genital tract. The potential importance of rectal lymphoid tissues as an inductive site is suggested from several studies performed with humans, nonhuman primates (NHPs), and mice. Rectal immunization of humans with a microbial vaccine (*e.g.*, *Salmonella typhi* Ty21a) or various viruses induced specific antibodies not only at the site of immunization but also in saliva and other secretions (Forrest *et al.*, 1990; Kozlowski *et al.*, 1997, 2002; Russell and Mestecky, 2002; see Chapters 94 and 95). The rectal route of immunization has also been evaluated in animal experimentation. Rhesus macaques immunized rectally with simian immunodeficiency virus (SIV) displayed both T- and B-cell-mediated immune responses, including the induction of anti-SIV antibodies (Lehner *et al.*, 1992, 1993). Mice immunized rectally with CT or recombinant vaccinia virus expressing gp120 of SIV also generated humoral immune responses in genital tract secretions as well as in serum; this immunization route was frequently superior to either the gastric or vaginal route (Moldoveanu *et al.*, 1995; Haneberg *et al.*, 1994). Therefore, the rectal immunization route appears to be effective in the induction of not only local but also generalized mucosal immune responses because of the presence of inductive site tissue. However, there are pronounced species differences with respect to the magnitude of the immune response induced: mice display a more vigorous response than humans. The type and dose of antigen, as well as the frequency of immunization, may be partially responsible for such observed differences. Further studies will be necessary to validate limited results obtained thus far, and males will be included in future immunization attempts to determine whether specific immune responses are generated in male genital tract secretions.

MUCOSAL HOMING AND COMPARTMENTALIZATION OF MUCOSAL IMMUNE RESPONSES

Early evidence of selective mucosal homing was revealed by the finding that rabbit Peyer's patch B cells repopulated the gut and became IgA plasma cells (Craig and Cebra, 1971, 1975). Further, the mesenteric lymph nodes of orally immunized experimental animals were found to contain antigen-specific precursors of IgA plasma cells, which repopulated the lamina propria of the gut and mammary, lacrymal, and salivary glands (McDermott and Bienenstock, 1979; McWilliams *et al.*, 1975, 1977; Roux *et al.*, 1977). Other evidence of the existence of the CMIS in humans was provided by the finding of specific S-IgA antibodies in secretions of the intestinal, respiratory, and genital tracts, as well as in tears, saliva, and milk, and by the observation of IgA-secreting cells in peripheral blood following oral immunization (Czerkinsky *et al.*, 1987; Kantele, 1990; Mestecky, 1987; McGhee *et al.*, 1992). Of importance for vaccine development, as mentioned earlier, is that immunization at certain inductive sites can give rise to a humoral immune response preferentially manifested at certain effector sites and resulting in further subcompartmentalization of the CMIS. For example, repeated nasal immunization may induce elevated mucosal immune responses not only in nasal secretions but also in saliva. On the other hand, rectal vaccination may induce preferential immune responses at the site of immunization and in some instances in the female genital tract.

A number of studies have now established that the mucosal addressin cell adhesion molecule-1 (MAdCAM-1) is the major homing receptor ligand in the GALT (Berlin et al., 1993; Holzmann et al., 1989; Bell and Issekutz, 1993; Hamann et al., 1994; Rott et al., 1996; see Chapter 34). In addition, pairing of α4 with β7 represents the major integrin molecule responsible for lymphocyte binding to MAdCAM-1 expressed on high endothelial venules (HEVs) in Peyer's patches (Holzmann et al., 1989). In contrast to the GALT, L-selectin and peripheral lymph node addressins play predominant roles in the binding of naive lymphocytes to NALT HEVs (Csencsits et al., 1999, 2001). Additional studies showed expression of L-selectin by most effector B cells induced by systemic immunization, with only a small proportion expressing α4β7, while the opposite was seen after enteric (oral or rectal) immunization (Quiding-Jabrink et al., 1995b, 1997). Interestingly, effector B cells induced by nasal immunization displayed a more promiscuous pattern of adhesion molecules, with a large majority of these cells expressing both L-selectin and α4β7 (Quiding-Jabrink et al., 1997).

It is now clear that chemokines are directly involved in mucosal homing of effector B and T cells. For example, loss of secondary lymphoid tissue chemokine (SLC) results in lack of naive T-cell or dendritic cell (DC) migration into spleen or Peyer's patches (Gunn et al., 1999). Further, thymus-expressed chemokine (TECK) mediated human memory T cell migration into the small intestinal lamina propria of the GI tract. In fact, gut homing α4β7^hi T-cell expression of the TECK receptor CCR-9 (Zabel et al., 1999) and reduction in levels of total intraepithelial lymphocytes (IELs) occur in the small intestine of CCR9^−/− mice (Wurbel et al., 2001). In addition to its chemoattractant activity on T cells, TECK efficiently recruits IgA-producing but not IgG- or IgM-producing cells from spleen, Peyer's patches, and the mesenteric lymph nodes (Bowman et al., 2002). While all CD4+ and CD8+ T lymphocytes in the small intestine express high levels of CCR9, only a small subset of lymphocytes in the colon are CCR9+ (Kunkel et al., 2000). Lymphocytes from other tissues, including tonsils, lung, inflamed liver, normal or inflamed skin, inflamed synovium and synovial fluid, breast milk, and seminal fluid, do not express CCR9 (Kunkel et al., 2000). Consistent with CCR9 expression, TECK expression is also restricted to the small intestine (Kunkel et al., 2000). These findings imply a restricted role for lymphocyte CCR9 and its ligand TECK in the small intestine and add support to the functional compartmentalization of

immune responses in different segments of the gastrointestinal (GI) tract and the CMIS in general.

Recent studies have shown that CCR10, a receptor for the mucosa-associated epithelial chemokine MEC (CCL28), is selectively expressed by IgA+CD38^hiCD19^int/−CD20− IgA antibody-secreting cells, including circulating IgA+ plasmablasts and almost all IgA+ plasma cells in the salivary gland, the small and large intestines, the appendix, and the tonsils (Kunkel et al., 2003; Lazarus et al., 2003). Further, MEC attracts IgA-producing but not IgG- or IgM-producing AFCs from the intestines, lungs, and lymph nodes draining the bronchopulmonary tree and oral cavity (Lazarus et al., 2003). Interestingly, T cells from mucosal sites fail to respond to MEC, suggesting that distinct chemokine signaling is needed for mucosal homing of B versus T cells. This concept is further supported by the fact that CCR9, whose ligand TECK/CCL25 is predominantly restricted to the small intestine and thymus, is expressed by a fraction of IgA antibody–AFCs and almost all T cells in the small intestine but by only a small percentage of plasma cells in other sites (Kunkel et al., 2003; Lazarus et al., 2003).

ROUTES OF IMMUNIZATION FOR PROTECTION OF MUCOSAL SURFACES

Mucosal immunization

Mucosal routes remain the preferred ones for vaccine delivery for induction of mucosal immunity. However, application of antigens to mucosal areas that lack inductive sites such as intestinal Peyer's patches is usually inefficient in the generation of disseminated mucosal and systemic immune responses. For example, the administration of nonreplicating antigens in the conjunctival sac, vagina, or intestinal loops, without Peyer's patches, results in a local, low immune response (for review see Mestecky, 1987; Mestecky and McGhee, 1987). Similarly, injection of antigens into the lactating mammary or salivary glands induces S-IgA and high IgG antibody responses in milk and saliva collected from immunized glands but not in secretions of other mucosal sites (for review see Mestecky, 1987). A concomitant IgG response in plasma suggests that injection of antigens into effector sites should be considered as systemic rather than mucosal immunization. This also seems to be the case when antigens are injected in the vicinity of regional lymph nodes draining certain mucosal sites.

Systemic immunization

Systemic immunization generally elicits weak humoral responses in external secretions and cellular responses in mucosal tissues. However, external secretions of the female and male genital tracts (cervical mucus and vaginal wash, and pre-ejaculate and ejaculate) contain approximately equal levels of IgA and IgG of mostly circulatory origin (see Chapter 96). Therefore, systemic immunization may be of considerable importance in the induction of protective responses in the genital tract secretions. Furthermore, systemic immunization with conjugated polysaccharide (*Haemophilus influenzae* or *Streptococcus pneumoniae*)–protein tetanus toxoid (TT) or diphtheria toxoid (DT) vaccine induce both IgA and IgG responses in plasma and secretions and predominantly IgA-secreting cells in the peripheral blood of systemically immunized volunteers (Lue *et al.*, 1990; Fattom *et al.*, 1990). Until the recent approval of the cold-adapted live attenuated influenza virus nasal vaccine (FluMist; MedImmune Vaccines, Inc., Gaithersburg, MD) in June 2003, systemic immunization with inactivated or split influenza virus has been and may continue to be the vaccine of choice. Thus, systemic immunization can be used as an effective route of antigen administration and ensuing protection in several mucosally contracted diseases (see Chapter 91).

Another important aspect of systemic immunization concerns its primary effects on subsequent mucosal immunization. Many previous studies indicate that single and even repeated immunization at the same mucosal site is not a particularly effective mode of induction of vigorous immune responses. Instead, empirical experience convincingly demonstrates that a combination of mucosal immunization routes (*e.g.*, oral and rectal) elicits better responses. Of upmost importance for induction of responses to HIV-1 is the need for the stimulation of both mucosal and systemic immunity. This goal may not be easily attainable by strictly mucosal (*e.g.*, oral or nasal) immunization. However, the combination of systemic priming and mucosal boosting will most likely lead to the desired outcome. Previous experiments (Moldoveanu *et al.*, 1993) have shown that systemic priming, even with minute doses of antigens (in this case the influenza virus) followed by mucosal boosting, elicited better mucosal and systemic immune responses than did mucosal immunization only. Furthermore, systemic priming does not preclude humoral and CMI responses induced by mucosal boosting (Belyakov *et al.*, 1999)—a distinct advantage of this sequence of immunization. The reversed order of immunizations—mucosal priming and systemic boosting—may create some undesirable complications (Czerkinsky *et al.*, 1999). In a recent phase II clinical trial, intramuscular immunization with a live recombinant canarypox HIV-1 vaccine could induce CTL responses in both the systemic and mucosal compartments (Musey *et al.*, 2003). The study also showed that CD8$^+$ CTL clones established from rectal and systemic cells of one vaccine recipient exhibited similar Env-specific responses and major histocompatibility complex (MHC) restriction (Musey *et al.*, 2003). This result suggests that parenteral vaccination can induce HIV-1-specific CTLs that localize to sites of HIV-1 infection.

Transdermal immunization

Immune responses have been induced through transdermal (skin) immunization by scarification such as in smallpox inoculation (Benenson *et al.*, 1977). More recently, the skin emerged as an attractive target for vaccine delivery. For example, depilatory agents (Tang *et al.*, 1997) and epidermal powder delivery system were shown to promote both mucosal and systemic immunity (Chen *et al.*, 2001). More interestingly, several studies in humans (Glenn *et al.*, 2000) and animal models

(Glenn *et al.*, 1998; Sharton-Kerten *et al.*, 2000; Beignon *et al.*, 2001; Anjuere *et al.*, 2003; Guebre-Xabier *et al.*, 2003) suggest that, in addition to systemic immunity, mucosal immunity can be achieved by topical application to intact skin of a vaccine antigen and the appropriate adjuvant. Adjuvants including CT, CT-B, LT, nontoxic mutants of LT, CpG, and cytokines promoted immunity to cutaneous vaccines (Scharton-Kersten *et al.*, 2000; Beignon *et al.*, 2001; Chen *et al.*, 2001; Anjuere *et al.*, 2003), suggesting that enhancement of the immune response to topical vaccines is not restricted to native enterotoxins. Epidermal dendritic cells (DCs) or Langerhans cells appear to play a major role in the immune responses to transcutaneous immunization (Baca-Estrada *et al.*, 2002). External factors such as vitamin D or ultraviolet radiation B were also reported to regulate systemic and mucosal immunity to transcutaneous vaccines (Enioutina *et al.*, 2002). However, the mechanisms underlying the induction of mucosal immunity by transcutaneous vaccines remain elusive.

PROTECTIVE MECHANISMS INDUCED BY MUCOSAL VACCINES

S-IgA antibodies

Most if not all current vaccines exert their protective effect through the induction of specific Abs. Mucosal Abs, which are predominantly IgA and to a lesser degree IgG, exhibit their protective function by mechanisms that are distinct from specific antibodies present in the plasma (see Chapter 14). Inhibition of microbial adherence is a critical initial step for the protection of the host and is mediated by both specific and nonspecific mechanisms. For instance, the agglutinating ability of S-IgA specific to capsular polysaccharide of *H. influenzae* seems to be crucial for preventing colonization by *H. influenzae* (Kauppi-Korkeila *et al.*, 1996). Furthermore, another nonspecific mechanism that inhibits microbial adherence is due to the presence of carbohydrate chains on the S-IgA molecule that bind to bacteria or other antigens (Davin *et al.*, 1991; Wold *et al.*, 1990). S-IgA antibodies have been shown to be effective in neutralizing viruses at different steps in the infectious process. In particular, S-IgA specific to influenza hemagglutinin can interfere with the initial binding of influenza virus to target cells or with the internalization and the intracellular replication of the virus (Armstrong and Dimmock, 1992). The S-IgA can neutralize the catalytic activity of many enzymes of microbial origin (such as neuraminidase, hyaluronidase, glycosyltransferase, and IgA-specific protease) as well as the toxic activity of bacterial enterotoxins (CT and the related LT of *E. coli*). *In vitro* experiments employing murine polarized epithelial cells have demonstrated that antibodies specific for rotavirus and hepatitis virus can neutralize the respective viruses inside the epithelial cells (Mazanec *et al.*, 1992, 1995), and evidence has been provided that similar mechanisms occur *in vivo* (Burns *et al.*, 1996). Similarly, it has been shown that transcytosis of primary HIV isolates is blocked by polymeric IgA specific to HIV envelope proteins (Bomsel *et al.*, 1998). It should be mentioned that S-IgA antibodies appear to be important in limiting inflammatory responses at mucosal surfaces. In fact, IgA antibodies are unable to activate complement and interfere with IgM- and IgG-mediated complement activation (Griffiss and Goroff, 1983; Russell and Mansa, 1989). Furthermore, IgA can downregulate the synthesis of TNF-α and IL-6 as well as enhance the production of IL-1R antagonists by LPS-activated human monocytes (Wolf *et al.*, 1994, 1996). An additional anti-inflammatory mechanism of S-IgA-mediated protection has been recently suggested. Thus, S-IgA can colocalize with LPS in the apical recycling endosome compartment, preventing LPS-induced NF-κB translocation and a subsequent proinflammatory response (Fernandez *et al.*, 2003).

Mucosal CTLs

There is a clear demarcation between inductive sites, which harbor precursor CTLs (pCTLs), and effector sites, which include lamina propria and the epithelial cells where activated CD8[+] CTLs function. It is now established that administration of virus into the GI tract results in a higher frequency of pCTL in Peyer's patches (Offit *et al.*, 1991; London *et al.*, 1987). For example, reovirus localizes to T-cell regions and is clearly associated with increased CD8[+] pCTLs and memory B cell responses (London *et al.*, 1990). Oral administration of *Vaccinia* to rats resulted in the induction of virus-specific CTLs in Peyer's patches and mesenteric lymph nodes (Issekutz, 1984). Virus-specific CTLs are also generated in mucosa-associated tissues by oral immunization with reovirus and rotavirus (Offit *et al.*, 1991; London *et al.*, 1987), and a high frequency of virus-specific CTLs are present in the Peyer's patches as early as 6 days after oral immunization. These studies suggest that oral immunization with live virus can induce antigen-specific CTLs in both mucosal inductive and effector tissues for mucosal responses and in systemic lymphoid tissues as well.

The vaginal and gastrointestinal models of NHP infection with SIV have been useful to demonstrate that successful vaccine protection against SIV/HIV may require CTL responses in the mucosa. It has been shown that vaginal inoculation of NHPs with a low dose of pathogenic SIV induces CTLs, which could develop in the absence of detectable antibodies (McChesney *et al.*, 1998) and protect or delay the onset of disease upon challenge (Wilson *et al.*, 2000). Other studies have shown CTL responses in GI mucosal tissues of chronically SIVmac-infected NHPs, which contained levels of CTLs comparable to those found in the peripheral blood and lymph nodes (Schmitz *et al.*, 2001). Finally, while high CTL responses develop at a similar rate and magnitude in both peripheral and mucosal lymphoid tissues in primary SIV infection, mucosal CTL responses may predominate later in the course of the disease (Veazey *et al.*, 2003).

Cytokines/chemokines in mucosal immunity

The role of T helper (Th) cell–derived cytokines for antibody and CMI responses is now well established. Thus, interleukin (IL)-12, IL-18, and IFN-γ trigger Th0 cells to differentiate along the Th1 pathway (Kobayashi *et al.*, 1989; Chan *et al.*, 1991; Micaleef *et al.*, 1996; Okamura *et al.*, 1998). Mature

Th1 cells produce IL-2, IFN-γ, and lymphotoxin-α (LT-α, also known as TNF-β), LT-β, and TNF-α (Mosmann and Coffman, 1989) and mediate Th1-type responses that are associated with CMI and the IgG2a antibody subclass in the mouse system (Snapper and Paul, 1987). On the other hand, IL-4 promotes differentiation of Th2 cells that produce IL-4, IL-5, IL-6, IL-9, IL-10, and IL-13 (Mosmann and Coffman, 1989) and provide effective help for IgG1, IgG2b, and IgE antibody responses (Coffman *et al.*, 1988; Finkelman *et al.*, 1990; Esser and Radbruch, 1990). Both Th1 and Th2 cells are quite sensitive to cross-regulation. Thus, IFN-γ inhibits both Th2 cell proliferation and B-cell isotype switching stimulated by IL-4 (Gajewski and Fitch, 1988). Likewise, IL-10 inhibits IFN-γ secretion by Th1 cells, allowing the development of Th2-type cells. Further, the Th2 cell subset is an effective helper phenotype for supporting the IgA isotype in addition to IgG1, IgG2b, and IgE responses in the mouse system.

Earlier studies established a major role for IL-5 and IL-6, two Th2-type cytokines, for inducing sIgA[+] B cells to differentiate into IgA-producing plasma cells in both mice (Beagley *et al.*, 1988, 1989, 1991) and humans (Fujihashi *et al.*, 1991). Thus, IL-10 has also been shown to play an important role in the induction of IgA synthesis, especially in humans (Briere *et al.*, 1994; Defrance *et al.*, 1992). Finally, high frequencies of Th2 cells producing IL-5, IL-6, and IL-10 were shown in mucosal effector sites (*e.g.*, the intestinal lamina propria and the salivary glands) where IgA responses occur (Mega *et al.*, 1992; Taguchi *et al.*, 1990). More recent studies with a number of mucosal adjuvants and vaccine delivery systems have now shown that Th1-type cytokines are also important for mucosal S-IgA (Van Cott *et al.*, 1996; Marinaro *et al.*, 1997; Arulanandam *et al.*, 1999; Boyaka *et al.*, 1999). This finding underlines the importance of S-IgA for protection of host mucosal surfaces against both soluble toxins and allergens as well as intracellular pathogens that require complement-fixing antibodies and CMI.

It is now clear that Th1- and Th2-type cells express distinct patterns of chemokine receptors (Bonnecchi *et al.*, 1998; Sallusto *et al.*, 1998; Kim *et al.*, 2003). For example, CCR5 and the CXC chemokine receptors CxCR3 and CxCR5 are preferentially expressed by human Th1 cell clones, while Th2 cells express CCR4 and to a lesser extent CCR3 (Sallusto *et al.*, 1998; Imai *et al.*, 1999). It has also been shown that mouse Th1 cells but not Th2 cells express CCR7 (Randolph *et al.*, 1999). Interestingly, only CCR7- Th2 cells localize in the periphery of the T-cell zones, from where they can provide help to nearby B cells in B-cell follicles (Randolph *et al.*, 1999). To what extent such dichotomy between localization of Th1 and Th2 cells occurs in mucosal inductive and effector tissues remains to be determined.

MUCOSAL IMMUNE RESPONSES TO VACCINES

Almost all viral and bacterial pathogens to which vaccines would be desirable, invade mucosal tissues where cell-mediated and antibody-mediated immunity would be most effective. It is therefore striking that very few of the current vaccines were given by a mucosal route until the recent approval of the nasal FluMist influenza vaccine **(Table 47.1)**. As indicated earlier in this chapter, mucosal delivery of vaccines has to overcome a number of problems, including vaccine stability and optimal antigen dosing in mucosal inductive sites. The most effective mucosal adjuvants are enterotoxins (*i.e.*, CT and LT) and, as such, are unsuitable for use in humans (see Chapter 54). Until recently, their mechanisms of action were poorly understood, and this has hampered the development of safe mucosal vaccines. However, the interest in mucosal vaccine development has increased significantly in the scientific community and has led to over 2,000 publications on adjuvants and delivery systems for mucosal vaccines during the last 5 years **(Figure 47.1)**. Studies over the past decade have now identified the sites of actions and several mechanisms that contribute to the mucosal adjuvanticity. Thus, mucosal adjuvants can act through pattern recognition such as Toll-like receptors (TLRs) on epithelial cells **(Figure 47.2)**. They can also improve antigen delivery in mucosal inductive sites by increasing the permeability of the epithelial layer or by targeting M cells (Figure 47.2). More recently, studies have established that APCs are key players in the development of mucosal immunity. In fact, adjuvants including enterotoxins and cytokines upregulate costimulatory and MHC class II molecule expression by macrophages (MØ) and DCs and thus favor their interaction with effector B and T cells (Cong *et al.*, 1997; Yamomoto *et al.*, 1999; Gagliardi *et al.*, 2000; Staats *et al.*, 2001) (Figure 47.2). In addition, cytokines secreted by APCs, including IL-1, IL-12, and IL-18, act as adjuvants for induction of antibody and CMI responses (Staats *et al.*, 2001; Bradney *et al.*, 2003). Cytokines such as Flt3 ligand (Flt3 L) or GM-CSF, which increase the number of DCs and stimulate their maturation (Williamson *et al.*, 1999; Dauer *et al.*, 2003), also promote

immunity to mucosal vaccines. Mucosal adjuvants can stimulate maturation and differentiation of effector B cells and trigger B-cell switching for production of S-IgA antibodies (Figure 47.2). They may also influence the development of targeted Th1-type responses for protection against intracellular pathogens or Th2-type responses required for protection against soluble antigens, allergens, and toxins (Figure 47.2). As described below, CT and LT virtually employ all the mechanisms listed earlier to enhance mucosal immunity, confirming these enterotoxins as the preferred model systems for studying regulation of mucosal immunity by mucosal adjuvants **(Table 47.2)**.

Enterotoxins and nontoxic derivatives as mucosal adjuvants

The major enterotoxins produced by *Vibrio cholerae* and *Escherichia coli*, CT and LT, respectively, have continued to be the most studied mucosal adjuvants (see Chapter 54) and account for nearly 40% of all the publications on mucosal vaccines during the last 5 years (Figure 47.1). The B subunits of these molecules bind to cell surface gangliosides and thus could target vaccines to mucosal epithelial cells. CT and LT could also enhance immune responses by increasing the permeability of epithelial membranes. Studies in the 1980s and early 1990s showed the role of CT for B-cell switching and S-IgA antibody production. It has also become clear over the past few years that mucosal adjuvants play a major role in the differentiation of CD4+ T cells and subsequent Th1- or Th2-type responses for protection against intracellular pathogens or toxins. In this regard, the mucosal adjuvant activity of CT after oral immunization of mice with protein antigen and CT as adjuvant involves IL-4 and Th2-type responses (Xu-Amano *et al.*, 1993; Marinaro *et al.*, 1995; Vajdy *et al.*, 1995). On the other hand, oral immunization with LT resulted in mixed CD4+ Th1- and Th2-type responses that included IFN-γ, IL-5, IL-6, and IL-10

Table 47.1. Mucosal Vaccines for Humans

Vaccine	Route	Comments
Polio vaccine of Sabin	Oral	Used to eradicate polio (no longer used in the United States)
Flu-Mist Trivalent: cold-adapted live influenza vaccine (MedImmune Vaccines, Inc)	Nasal	Approved in the United States since June 2003
Salmonella typhi Ty21A: Live typhoid vaccine (Vivotif Berna vaccine, Berna Biotech ag)	Oral	Licensed in the United States (not available in the United States)
CT-B / Killed whole-cell cholera vaccine (Dukoral, Chiron)	Oral	Approved in 18 countries including Canada; awaiting approval in Europe
CVD 103-HgR: Single-dose cholera vaccine (Orochol or Mutacol, Berna Biotech ag)	Oral	Pending registration in the United States
Nonliving nasal influenza HA plus *E. coli* LT adjuvant (Berna Biotech ag)	Nasal	Off market; associated with cases of Bell's palsy
Rhesus reassortant rotavirus vaccine (Rotashield, Wyeth-Lederle Vaccine)	Oral	Withdrawn from the market in 2000; cases of intussusception

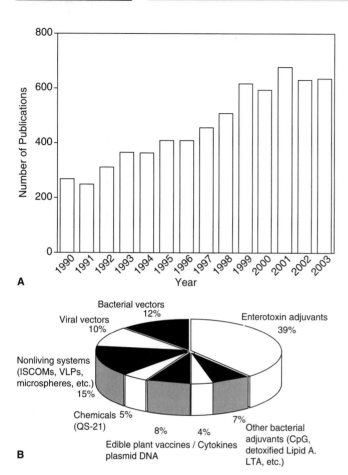

Fig. 47.1. A, Numbers of publications since 1990 on the subject of mucosal vaccine or mucosal immunization, taken from MEDLINE and additional life science journals (PubMed, U.S. National Library of Medicine). By mid November in 2003 alone, 561 manuscripts had been published. **B,** The percentage of publications for each major category of mucosal adjuvants and delivery systems, since 1999.

production (Takahashi *et al.*, 1996). Studies with chimeras of CT and LT have shown that the nature of the subunits of these enterotoxins, but not the ADP ribosyltransferase activity, direct the type of CD4+ T-cell responses (Bowman and Clements, 2001; Kweon *et al.*, 2002; Boyaka *et al.*, 2003). It has now been established that enterotoxins upregulate costimulatory and MHC class II molecule expression by MØ and DCs and thus favor their interaction with effector B and T cells (Cong *et al.*, 1997; Yamamoto *et al.*, 1999; Gagliardi *et al.*, 2000). Further, CT induces IL-1 secretion by APCs, and this cytokine has now been shown to promote mucosal immunity by mechanisms resembling those mediated by CT (Staats *et al.*, 1999). The mutants of CT and LT (mCTs and mLTs) generated by amino acid substitution are generally poor adjuvants when given by the oral route (see Chapter 54). Since safety issues are associated with the use of enterotoxins as nasal adjuvants (see next section), the next important challenge for mucosal vaccinologists will be to devise

enzymatically inactive mCTs and mLTs capable of acting as mucosal adjuvant for oral vaccines.

Immunostimulatory DNA sequences

It is now clear that stimulation via pattern recognition such as TLRs favor the development of mucosal immunity. Bacterial but not eukaryotic DNA contain immunostimulatory sequences consisting of short palindromic nucleotides centered around a CpG dinucleotide core, *e.g.*, 5′-purine-purine-CG-pyrimidine-pyrimidine-3′ or CpG motifs (Krieg, 2002; see Chapter 53). It is now clear that CpG motifs can induce B-cell proliferation and Ig synthesis as well as secretion of cytokines (*i.e.*, IL-6, IFN-α, IFN-β, IFN-γ, IL-12, and IL-18) by a variety of immune cells (Tighe *et al.*, 1998). Since CpG motifs create a cytokine microenvironment favoring Th1-type responses, they can be used as adjuvants to stimulate antigen-specific Th1-type responses or to redirect harmful allergic or Th2-dominated autoimmune responses. Indeed, coinjection of bacterial DNA or CpG motifs with a DNA vaccine or with a protein antigen promotes Th1-type responses even in mice with a pre-existing Th2-type of immunity (Roman *et al.*, 1997; Klinman *et al.*, 1996). More important for this chapter, CpG motifs can enhance systemic as well as mucosal immune responses when given to mice by the nasal route (McCluskie and Davis, 1998; Moldoveanu *et al.*, 1998; Gallichan *et al.*, 2001) or oral route (McCluskie *et al.*, 2000). A recent study provided evidence that CpG oligodeoxynucleotides (ODNs) could also induce innate immune protection of the female genital tract (Harandi *et al.*, 2003). In fact, vaginal administration of CpG ODNs rapidly induced IFN-γ, IL-12, IL-18, and RANTES production in the genital tract mucosa (Harandi *et al.*, 2003). The vaginal CpG ODN treatment protected mice against vaginal challenge with otherwise lethal doses of herpes simplex virus type 2, demonstrating the induction of innate immunity (Harandi *et al.*, 2003). It is interesting that two of the innate molecules induced by CpG (*i.e.*, IL-12 and RANTES) were reported to bridge the mucosal innate with the adaptive immune system (see next section).

Zonula occludens toxin

Zonula occludens toxin (Zot) is produced by toxigenic strains of *Vibrio cholerae* and has the ability to reversibly alter intestinal epithelial tight junctions, allowing the passage of macromolecules through the mucosal barrier. Nasal immunization of mice with a protein antigen and recombinant Zot, either alone or fused to the maltose-binding protein (MBP-Zot), induced high antigen-specific IgA antibody titers in plasma, as well as in vaginal and intestinal secretions (Marinaro *et al.*, 1999a). Moreover, Zot as adjuvant induced antigen-specific IgG subclasses that consisted of IgG1, IgG2a, and IgG2b antibodies and resembled the pattern induced by LT (Marinaro *et al.*, 1999). Zot was recently shown to also act as adjuvant for rectal immunization (Marinaro *et al.*, 2003). These studies illustrate the importance of increasing the permeability of mucosal tissues for induction of mucosal immunity to vaccines.

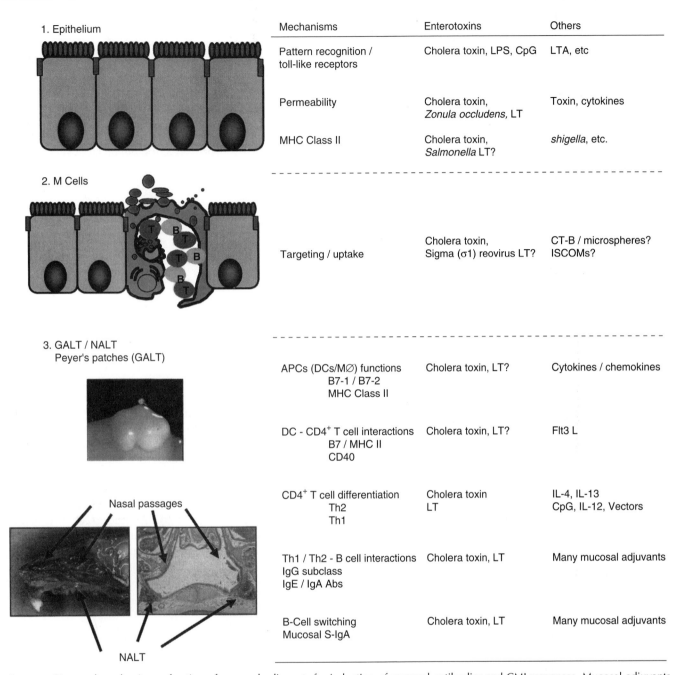

1. Epithelium

2. M Cells

3. GALT / NALT
Peyer's patches (GALT)

Nasal passages

NALT

Mechanisms	Enterotoxins	Others
Pattern recognition / toll-like receptors	Cholera toxin, LPS, CpG	LTA, etc
Permeability	Cholera toxin, *Zonula occludens*, LT	Toxin, cytokines
MHC Class II	Cholera toxin, *Salmonella* LT?	*shigella*, etc.
Targeting / uptake	Cholera toxin, Sigma (σ1) reovirus LT?	CT-B / microspheres? ISCOMs?
APCs (DCs/MØ) functions B7-1 / B7-2 MHC Class II	Cholera toxin, LT?	Cytokines / chemokines
DC - CD4$^+$ T cell interactions B7 / MHC II CD40	Cholera toxin, LT?	Flt3 L
CD4$^+$ T cell differentiation Th2 Th1	Cholera toxin LT	IL-4, IL-13 CpG, IL-12, Vectors
Th1 / Th2 - B cell interactions IgG subclass IgE / IgA Abs	Cholera toxin, LT	Many mucosal adjuvants
B-Cell switching Mucosal S-IgA	Cholera toxin, LT	Many mucosal adjuvants

Fig. 47.2. Sites and mechanisms of action of mucosal adjuvants for induction of mucosal antibodies and CMI responses. Mucosal adjuvants promote mucosal immunity by a variety of mechanisms, including stimulation of epithelial cells, targeting/enhancing Ag uptake, activation of mucosal APCs, and stimulation of effector B and T cells.

Cytokines and chemokines as adjuvants for mucosal Abs and CMI

The use of cytokines and chemokines to enhance immune responses to mucosal vaccines is an attractive strategy for at least two reasons. First, cytokines and chemokines act by often known mechanisms through specific interactions with corresponding receptors. Further, mucosal delivery of cytokines could help avoid the toxicity that is often associated with the large and repeated parenteral cytokine doses generally needed (Marinaro *et al.*, 1997, 1999b; Huber *et al.*, 2003). Finally, cytokines/chemokines that influence the development of Th cell subsets can help promote targeted Th1-type responses for protection against intracellular pathogens or Th2-type responses required for protection against soluble antigens, allergens, and toxins.

Table 47.2. Mucosal Adjuvants in Common Experimental Use

Bacterial Products	Viral Products	Others
Native enterotoxins	Reovirus protein sigma one (pσ1)	Cytokines
CT, LT		IL-1, IL-12, GM-CSF, Flt3 L
CT-B, LT-B		
CT-A, LT-A		Chemokines
		RANTES, Lymphotactin, MIP-1β
Enterotoxin derivatives		
Mutant CTs		Saponins (QS-21)
Mutants LTs		
Chimera of CT-LT		
LPS and derivatives		
Zonula occludens toxin		
CpG ODNs		

Cytokines as mucosal adjuvants

Consistent with the fact that CT induces IL-1 secretion by APCs and epithelial cells (Bromander et al., 1991, 1993), IL-1 has been shown to enhance mucosal immune responses to coadministered antigens and to promote a pattern of plasma IgG subclasses similar to the Th2-type response inducer CT (Staats et al., 1999). Both CMI and CTL responses could also be induced when IL-1 was nasally administered in combination with the Th1-type inducing cytokines IL-12, IL-18, or IL-12 plus GM-CSF (Bradney et al., 2002). CT has also been shown to induce IL-6 secretion by epithelial cells (McGee et al., 1993). However, in contrast to IL-1, nasal delivery of IL-6 together with a protein antigen promoted antigen-specific systemic immunity but failed to induce mucosal S-IgA antibody responses (Boyaka et al., 1999). Thus, not all cytokines induced by CT can provide signals for mucosal S-IgA antibody responses. IL-12 is a major cytokine produced by APCs in response to a variety of stimuli. This cytokine has been shown to induce antibodies to nasally coadministered protein vaccines in both the systemic compartment and mucosal tissues (Aralandandam et al., 1999; Boyaka et al., 1999) via mechanisms involving CD4+ Th1 cells (Boyaka et al., 1999). In addition, nasal (Marinaro et al., 1999b; Belyakov et al., 2000) or oral (Marinaro et al., 1999b) coadministration of IL-12 and CT redirected CT-induced Th2-type responses toward a Th1-type and optimized the induction of CTLs by a mucosal HIV peptide vaccine (Belyakov et al., 2000). A single intratracheal dose of Flt3 L was recently reported to increase the number of DCs and T cells in rat lung tissues and to enhance mucosal antibody responses to a protein antigen delivered thereafter (Pabst et al., 2003). Along the same line, nasal coadministration of a protein antigen and a plasmid DNA expressing Flt3 L (pFlt3 L) promoted antigen-specific mucosal and systemic antibody responses (Kataoka et al., 2004). Interestingly, unlike CpG ODNs, which stimulate Th1-type responses, pFlt3 L promoted Th2-type responses (Kataoka et al., 2004).

Induction of mucosal immunity by chemokines as adjuvant

Innate molecules secreted in mucosal epithelia have also been tested to determine their potential to provide signals to bridge the innate with the adaptive mucosal immune systems. Lymphotactin (Lptn) is a C chemokine produced predominantly by NK and CD8+ T cells, including γδ TCR+ IELs. Nasal coadministration of Lptn and a protein antigen enhanced antigen-specific antibody responses both in blood plasma and in mucosal secretions (Lillard et al., 1999). Lptn as adjuvant induced antigen-specific CD4+ Th1- and Th2-type cells and IgG1>IgG2a=IgG2b=IgG3 antibody subclasses (Lillard et al., 1999). Another CC chemokine, RANTES, also displayed mucosal adjuvant activity for nasally coadministered protein antigen (Lillard et al., 2001). RANTES as adjuvant promoted antigen-specific CD4+Th1-type cytokine responses and supported Th1-associated plasma IgG subclass responses (Lillard et al., 2001). As was discussed for CT and LT above, similar chemokines may have different effects on mucosal antibody and CMI responses. For example, MIP-1α and MIP-1β are distinct but highly homologous CC chemokines that share affinity for CCR5. MIP-1α also binds CCR1 as well as CCR3 in the mouse, while MIP-1β is a ligand for CCR8. A recent study has shown that nasally delivered MIP-1α promotes strong plasma IgG antibodies as well as mucosal and systemic CMI responses to coadministered antigen (Lillard et al., 2003). On the other hand, MIP-1β was a less effective adjuvant for plasma IgG antibodies and failed to induce CMI responses. However, MIP-1β supported higher levels of mucosal S-IgA antibodies (Lillard et al., 2003).

Saponin derivatives

QS-21 is a highly purified complex triterpene glycoside isolated from the bark of the *Quillaja saponaria* Molina tree (Kensil and Kramer, 1998). This molecule promotes both humoral and CMI responses when added to systemic vaccine formulations and has now been tested in several parenteral vaccine formulations (Livingston *et al.*, 1997; Kensil and Kramer, 1998). QS-21 was reported to promote both systemic and mucosal immunity to a nasal DNA vaccine (Sasaki *et al.*, 1998). Others have shown that QS-21 also acts as adjuvant when given to mice by the oral route (Boyaka *et al.*, 2001). Interestingly, low oral QS-21 doses promoted mucosal S-IgA Ab responses, while no S-IgA antibodies were induced by high oral QS-21 (Boyaka *et al.*, 2001). On the other hand, stronger Th1-type responses were seen after immunization with high oral QS-21 doses (Boyaka *et al.*, 2001). It is possible that the mild detergent activity of QS-21 and related saponin derivatives such as QS-7 (Kensil and Kramer, 1998) may enhance immune responses by facilitating antigen uptake. This point and mechanisms by which saponin derivatives promote mucosal immunity and control CD4$^+$Th cell subset differentiation remain to be determined.

Mucosal vaccine delivery systems

Empirical experience with mucosal immunization has resulted in the commonly held view that repeated administration of high doses of antigen is required to achieve the levels of immune response induced by systemic immunization. This conclusion is physiologically justifiable since the primary function of the mucosal immune system is to prevent overstimulation of the entire immune system. It does so by eliminating mucosally applied antigens with denaturing acids, degradative enzymes, and other factors of innate immunity or through intestinal peristalsis and ciliary movement on epithelia in the respiratory tract. As a result of the concerted interactions of such factors, little antigen remains to be absorbed and thereby to stimulate inductive sites for mucosal and systemic immune responses. Mucosal vaccinologists have devised delivery systems which circumvent such obstacles. The comparative advantages and disadvantages of mucosal antigen delivery will be dealt with here, and the details are covered in ensuing chapters. Furthermore, it should be emphasized that most results obtained have been generalized in animal models rather than in humans, with all unavoidable limitations.

M cell targeting delivery systems

The ability of some viral outer capsid proteins to bind to M cells covering mucosal inductive sites has recently been exploited to devise a delivery systems protein, DNA, and possibly polysaccharide vaccines (see Chapter 7). In this regard, reoviruses are nonenveloped, double-stranded RNA icosahedral viruses composed of three serotypes (Schiff and Fields, 1990). The most widely studied serotypes, 1 and 3, enter the host via M cells in the FAE. Binding to M cells is mediated via the C-terminus of the minor outer capsid protein sigma one (pσ1) (Mah *et al.*, 1990). The pσ1 subunit is 45 kDa and polymerizes via its N-terminus to form a stable tetramer (Bassel-Duby *et al.*, 1987). Incorporation of pσ1 into liposomes was shown to allow their binding to mouse L cells and rat Peyer's patches (Rubas *et al.*, 1990). Likewise, the pσ1 can bind to NALT M cells (Wu *et al.*,

2000, 2001). Of major interest for mucosal vaccine development, immunization with DNA complexed to pσ1 could overcome the low immunogenicity of naked DNA and promote elevated S-IgA and plasma IgG antibody responses (Wu *et al.*, 2001). Protein and polysaccharide vaccine antigens could be linked to pσ1 for optimal targeting of M cells and mucosal inductive sites. However, extrapolation of this strategy for human vaccination will first require that we determine the serotype of reovirus with the best affinity for human M cells.

Inert vaccine delivery systems

Since Ags are more immunogenic in particulate form than in solutions and are vulnerable to antigen-degrading enzymes and acids, they have often been incorporated into vehicles that are by themselves nontoxic and nonimmunogenic but which protect vaccine material from degradation, enhance their uptake from mucosal surfaces, and may exhibit some adjuvant effect (see Chapter 55). A few examples are discussed next.

Gelatin capsules

Gelatin capsules coated with substances (*e.g.*, cellulose acetate phthalate) that dissolve at alkaline pH in the intestine but not at acid pH in the stomach have been used for oral delivery of bacterial and viral vaccines in several studies performed in humans. Although vaccines given in enteric-coated capsules have not been rigorously shown to be more effective than free antigens, influenza virus exposed to acid pH is lowly immunogenic, while it remains intact when the virus is placed in enteric-coated gelatin capsules, where the drop in pH is greatly diminished (Moldoveanu *et al.*, 1993).

Mucoadhesive polymers

Mucoadhesive polymers that adhere to mucosal surfaces extend the time of the exposure of vaccines and thus facilitate the induction of immune responses. Compounds such as highly viscous inert polysaccharide eldexomer and carboxymethyl cellulose were used for oral, nasal, or vaginal delivery of antigens such as influenza virus or CT-B and could promote both local mucosal and systemic immune responses. Other compounds that have been considered are carbapol, polycarbophil, sodium alginate, and hydroxypropyl cellulose, which are used in medicine for delivery of drugs to combat diarrhea and constipation and to promote wound healing.

ISCOMs

Immunostimulating complexes (ISCOMs) are cage-like particles generated after addition of cholesterol to the Quil A from the bark of the *Quillaja saponaria* Molina tree. ISCOMs are effective oral delivery systems that promote mucosal and systemic immunity. More recently, ISCOMs containing a fusion protein comprising the OVA (323–339) peptide epitope linked to CTA1-DD were highly immunogenic when given in nanogram doses by the oral or nasal routes (Mowat *et al.*, 2001). Interestingly, ISCOMs containing the enzymatically inactive CTA1-R7K-DD mutant protein were much less effective, suggesting that at least part of the activity of the combined vector requires the ADP-ribosylating property of CTA1 (Mowat *et al.*, 2001).

Biodegradable microspheres

Biodegradable microspheres composed of antigens incorporated into polymers of lactic and glycolic acid have been used far more extensively in mucosal vaccinology than any other mucosal delivery system (Mestecky *et al.*, 1997). Soluble proteins, viral and bacterial glycoproteins, and viruses (*e.g.*, influenza and SIV) have been given as microencapsulated vaccines orally or intratracheally to humans, monkeys, and rodents in many studies. Microspheres are to be preferred to most of the other delivery systems because of their stability, which allows them to protect incorporated antigens from acids and enzymes; the ease with which their size and rapidity of biodegradation can be modified during the fabrication process; their nontoxicity and resulting unparalleled record of safety; and their biodegradability.

Transgenic plants

Novel molecular methods have allowed the production of subunit vaccines in transgenic plants (see Chapters 58 and 59). Plants can be engineered to synthesize and assemble an adjuvant and one or more antigens which retain both T and B-cell epitopes (Haq *et al.*, 1995; Tacket *et al.*, 1998; Yu and Langride, 2001). The feeding of transgenic potato tubers was shown to induce systemic and mucosal immune responses in mice (Haq *et al.*, 1995) and in humans (Tacket *et al.*, 1998). In order to circumvent potential denaturation of antigen during cooking, recombinant plants that do not require cooking such as bananas and tomatoes are being developed.

Live recombinant vaccine delivery systems

Many bacterial and viral vectors (*Salmonella, E. coli*, mycobacteria, lactobacilli, polio-, adeno-, rhino-mengo-, influenza, vaccinia, and canarypox viruses) have been used with variable success in animal models (see Chapters 56 and 57). A recombinant bacterial vector (*i.e.*, *Salmonella typhi* Ty21A) is licensed in the United States for use as an oral vaccine (Table 47.1). In June 2003, a cold-adapted live influenza vaccine (*i.e.*, FluMist) was approved as a nasal vaccine for humans (Table 47.1). Despite these significant advances, further studies will be required to determine optimal mucosal immunization protocols and to enhance the expression of future live recombinant vaccines while diminishing responses to the vector to prevent its elimination by immune mechanisms. In fact, vectored delivery has been limited to former pathogens that have been subjected to attenuating mutations or genomic deletions. Nonpathogenic strains of bacteria such as lactobacilli are being evaluated as vaccine delivery systems. In most instances, host immune responses develop both to recombinant vectors and to the transgenes. The use of different recombinant vectors for priming and boosting could help reduce potential immunity to the vectors.

IMMUNE RESPONSE VERSUS MUCOSAL TOLERANCE

Extensive experiments performed in animals clearly indicate that oral or nasal exposure to certain antigens (*e.g.*, myelin basic protein, ovalbumin, cartilage type II collagen) induces a state of unresponsiveness in the systemic compartment upon systemic immunization (see Chapter 27). Recently, the existence of this phenomenon was documented in humans immunized orally (Husby *et al.*, 1994; Kraus *et al.*, 2004) or nasally (Waldo *et al.*, 1994) with keyhole limpet hemocyanin (KLH). Subsequent systemic immunization with the same antigen clearly demonstrated boostable mucosal and systemic humoral immune responses but suppressed T-cell proliferation and delayed-type hypersensitivity (DTH) reactions (so called split tolerance). Consequently, it is unlikely that orally or nasally applied vaccines would induce the state of unresponsiveness in the humoral arm of the immune response. Considering the fact that all vaccines used so far in human medicine exhibit their protective effect through the induction of specific antibodies rather than CTLs, the possibility of inducing tolerance by mucosal exposure is minimal. Nevertheless, the suppression of Th1 and perhaps Th2 responses would be counterproductive in immunization strategies whose aim is to induce protective T cell–mediated responses (*e.g.*, to HIV). However, it should be emphasized that the suppression of T cell–mediated responses occurs only when the same antigen is administered by the mucosal route to the previously naïve animal. In sharp contrast, initial systemic priming and ensuing B- and T-cell responses cannot be suppressed by subsequent mucosal immunization. This fact of basic impact is unfortunately often disregarded. Therefore, it has been assumed that ongoing systemic immune responses, particularly of autoimmune character, can be suppressed by mucosal exposure to antigens that elicited preceding systemic responses. Contrary to this assumption, Chase (1946) dramatically demonstrated that the cell-mediated responses induced by systemic immunization of animals with a hapten-carrier cannot be suppressed by oral administration of the same antigen. In the same vein, DTH reactions to poison ivy or poison oak cannot be suppressed by oral administrations of dried leaves or their various extract in humans (for reviews see Stevens, 1945; Klingman, 1958). More recent studies have clearly demonstrated that ongoing vigorous responses induced by systemic immunization with autoantigens are refractory to suppression by nasal or oral administration of the same antigen (for review see Czerkinsky, 1999). These studies were recently extended to humans and indicated that ongoing humoral and cellular responses induced by systemic immunization with KLH cannot be suppressed by subsequent extended ingestion of large doses of KLH (Elson, C.O., University of Alabama at Birmingham, personal communication).

In summary, the sequence of systemic priming followed by mucosal boosting provides vigorous humoral and cellular immune responses in both mucosal and systemic compartments, with minimal danger of inducing tolerance in the cell-mediated arm of the immune response.

Mucosal therapeutic vaccines against autoimmune and inflammatory infectious diseases

It is now well established that adjuvants are required for effective induction of mucosal immunity. Less appreciated is the fact that delivery systems and/or adjuvants are also needed to enhance mucosal tolerance for effective immunotherapeutic applications. Thus far, the most promising vehicle for inducing mucosal tolerance is CT-B. Thus, mucosal delivery of CT-B chemically linked or genetically fused to various autoantigens is generally a more effective method for inducing tolerance than mucosal administration of autoantigen alone. For example, oral or nasal treatment with low-dose CT-B chemically conjugated or genetically linked (fusion proteins) to myelin basic protein (Sun *et al.*, 2000), insulin (Bergerot *et al.*, 1997), or collagen II (Tarkowski *et al.*, 1999) and/or selected peptides derived from these antigens could totally or markedly suppress the development of experimental autoimmune encephalitis (EAE), type I diabetes, or collagen-induced arthritis, respectively. In addition, prolonged oral treatment with low doses of allergen conjugated to CT-B markedly suppressed IgE antibody responses and allergic reactions in sensitized mice (Rask *et al.*, 2000). More recently, mucosally induced uveitis could be prevented in rat by oral administration of CT-B linked with the uveitogenic peptide (aa 336-351) derived from human heat-shock protein (HSP) 60 (Phipps *et al.*, 2003).

The mechanisms underlying the enhancement of oral tolerance by CT-B-Ag conjugates are probably complex and only partially understood. As for induction of mucosal immunity, DCs appear to also play a critical role in mucosal tolerance (Viney *et al.*, 1998). Thus, priming of DCs may constitute a major step in the induction of immune responses to mucosally delivered antigens. The development of active adaptive responses versus tolerance could then be dictated by additional stimuli including cytokines and costimulatory molecules.

For example, treatment with different CT-B-Ag conjugates or fusion proteins was reported to promote actively tolerogenic APCs and TGF-β-secreting suppressive–regulatory T cells in mucosal tissues and draining lymph nodes (Sun *et al.*, 2000). Oral feeding of CT-B was shown to both prevent and cure Th1-driven experimental colitis in mice, through reduction of IL-12 production within the large intestine (Boirivant *et al.*, 2001). Furthermore, tolerization was also shown to downregulate chemokines, including RANTES (Sun *et al.*, 2000), a chemokine that stimulates adaptive immunity (Lillard *et al.*, 1999).

SAFETY OF MUCOSAL VACCINES, ADJUVANTS, AND DELIVERY SYSTEMS

The watery diarrhea induced by native enterotoxin is the major safety concern identified thus far for oral vaccines. As seen above, nontoxic mutant has been developed to overcome this toxicity. Unfortunately, nontoxic enterotoxin mutants are generally poor adjuvants for oral vaccines, although they often retain their adjuvanticity for nasally coadministered vaccine antigens. While reviewing the safety, immunogenicity, and efficacy of oral rhesus–human reassortant vaccine candidates, a Rotavirus Working Group of the Advisory Committee on Immunization Practices (ACIP) of the Centers for Diseases Control and Prevention (CDC) noted 5 cases of intussusception among 10,054 vaccinees, 3 of which occurred during the first week postvaccination, and 1 case among 4,633 placebo recipients (Margaret *et al.*, 2000). While none of these cases had been judged by the clinical study investigators to be directly attributable to the vaccine, the product was withdrawn from the market. Thus, better methods are needed to analyze and predict potential toxicity of oral vaccines.

The nasal cavity is anatomically close to the olfactory nerves/epithelium (ON/E) and olfactory bulbs (OBs). Recent studies examined whether, in addition to NALT, CT as adjuvant could target these tissues of the central nervous system. Both CT and its B subunit (CT-B) entered the ON/E and OB and persisted for 6 days, although neither molecule was present in NALT beyond 24 hours after nasal delivery (van Ginkel *et al.*, 1999). This uptake into olfactory regions was monosialoganglioside (GM1)-dependent. Nasal vaccination with ^{125}I-TT together with unlabeled CT as adjuvant resulted in uptake into the ON/E but not the OB, whereas ^{125}I-TT alone did not penetrate into the CNS. This study suggested that GM1-binding molecules like CT target the ON/E and are retrograde-transported into the OB and may promote uptake of vaccine proteins into olfactory neurons. This raises concerns about the role of GM1-binding molecules that target neuronal tissues in mucosal immunity (van Ginkel *et al.*, 1999). The targeting of CNS tissues by nasally administered bacterial enterotoxins is possibly related to a higher incidence of Bell's palsy (facial paresis) among volunteers of a nasal vaccination trial with native LT as mucosal adjuvant. Thus, of the serious adverse events reported for approximately 3,600 subjects participating in a clinical (safety) trial for a nonliving nasal flu vaccine (Nasalflu) in 2000, there were 9 cases of Bell's palsy and 1 of trigeminal neuralgia that developed into facial paresis. Furthermore, five cases of Bell's palsy were spontaneously reported from among approximately 90,000 recipients of Nasalflu, and the vaccine was withdrawn from the market (www.niaid.nih.gov/dmid/enteric/intranasal.htm; Table 47.1). The recent approval of the trivalent FluMist cold-adapted live influenza vaccine demonstrates that the nasal route remains a viable choice for delivery of carefully devised mucosal vaccines.

SUMMARY AND PERSPECTIVES

Like HIV and AIDS some 20 years ago, the recent worldwide outbreak of severe acute respiratory syndrome (SARS) dramatically reminded us that infectious diseases remain a major global threat that is no longer restricted to developing countries or selected populations. The newly discovered coronavirus responsible for SARS (Kuiken *et al.*, 2003) infects the host via mucosal tissues of the respiratory tract, where both mucosal antibodies and CMI responses could provide the host with lifesaving protection. The cases of inhalational anthrax related to a bioterrorism attack in the United States during October and November 2001 (Jernigan *et al.*, 2001; Guarner *et al.*, 2003) further demonstrated the importance of mucosal tissues as portals for entry of pathogenic agents used as bioterrorism agents. In this regard, transmission of all the Category A bioterrorist agents/diseases listed by the CDC occurs by either inhalation or ingestion. Our understanding of mechanisms by which adjuvants control mucosal antibody and CMI responses has greatly improved over the past decade. In fact, we now know that pattern recognitions, together with innate factors such as cytokines and chemokines and the APC function of DCs, are crucial for initiation of mucosal immunity. New and improved delivery systems will be critical for use with new mucosal vaccines such as the nasal FluMist vaccine. The ADP ribosyltransferase activity of bacterial enterotoxins has been the only potential toxicity investigated in mucosal vaccines. The recent knowledge that nasal vaccines can potentially bind to neurons has fostered research on the safety of mucosal vaccines and should help in the design of safer vaccines to be administered by the nasal or other mucosal routes. The recently approved FluMist vaccine could then be the first of a long list of new-generation mucosal vaccines.

REFERENCES

Allansmith, M., McClellan, B.H., Butterworth, M., and Maloney, J.R. (1968). The development of immunoglobulin levels in man. *J. Pediatr.* 72, 276–290.

Anjuere, F., George-Chandy, A., Audant, F., Rousseau, D., Holmgren, J., and Czerkinsky, C. (2003). Transcutaneous immunization with cholera toxin B subunit adjuvant suppresses IgE antibody responses via selective induction of Th1 immune responses. *J. Immunol.* 170, 1586–1592.

Armstrong, S.J., and Dimmock, N.J. (1992). Neutralization of influenza virus by low concentrations of hemagglutinin-specific polymeric immunoglobulin A inhibits viral fusion activity, but activation of the ribonucleoprotein is also inhibited. *J. Virol.* 66, 3823–3832.

Arulanandam, B.P., O'Toole, M., and Metzger, D.W. (1999). Intranasal interleukin-12 is a powerful adjuvant for protective mucosal immunity. *J. Infect. Dis.* 180, 940–949.

Baca-Estrada, M.E., Ewen, C., Mahony, D., Babiuk, L.A., Wilkie, D., and Foldvari, M. (2002). The haemopoietic growth factor, Flt3L, alters the immune response induced by transcutaneous immunization. *Immunology* 107, 69–76.

Bassel-Duby, R., Nibert, M.L., Homcy, C.J., Fields, B.N., and Sawutz, D.G. (1987). Evidence that the sigma 1 protein of reovirus serotype 3 is a multimer. *J.Virol.* 61, 1834–1841.

Beagley, K.W., Eldridge, J.H., Kiyono, H., Everson, M.P., Koopman, W.J., Honjo, T. and McGhee, J.R. (1988). Recombinant murine IL-5 induces high rate IgA synthesis in cycling IgA-positive Peyer's patch B cells. *J. Immunol.* 141, 2035–2042.

Beagley, K.W., Eldridge, J.H., Lee, F., Kiyono, H., Everson, M.P., Koopman, W.J., Hirano, T., Kishimoto, T., and McGhee, J.R. (1989). Interleukins and IgA synthesis. Human and murine interleukin 6 induce high rate IgA secretion in IgA-committed B cells. *J. Exp. Med.* 169, 2133–2148.

Beagley, K.W., Eldridge, J.H., Aicher, W.K., Mestecky, J., Di Fabio, S., Kiyono, H., and McGhee, J.R. (1991). Peyer's patch B cells with

memory cell characteristics undergo terminal differentiation within 24 hours in response to interleukin-6. *Cytokine* 3, 107–116.

Beignon, A.S., Briand, J.P., Muller, S,., and Partidos, C.D. (2001). Immunization onto bare skin with heat-labile enterotoxin of *Escherichia coli* enhances immune responses to coadministered protein and peptide antigens and protects mice against lethal toxin challenge. *Immunology* 102, 344–351.

Bell, R.G., and Issekutz, T. (1993). Expression of a protective intestinal immune response can be inhibited at three distinct sites by treatment with anti-alpha 4 integrin. *J. Immunol.* 151, 4790–4802.

Belyakov, I.M., Moss, B., Strober, W., and Berzofsky, J.A. (1999). Mucosal vaccination overcomes the barrier to recombinant vaccinia immunization caused by preexisting poxvirus immunity. *Proc. Natl. Acad. Sci. (USA)* 96, 4512–4517.

Belyakov I.M., Ahlers J.D., Clements J.D., Strober W., Berzofsky J.A. (2000). Interplay of cytokines and adjuvants in the regulation of mucosal and systemic HIV-specific CTL. *J. Immunol.* 165, 6454–6462.

Benenson, A.S., Cherry, J.D., McIntosh. K., Connor. J.D., Alling, D.W., Nakano, J., Rolfe, U.T., Schanberger, J.E., Todd, W.A., DeCastro, F., Horvath, F.L, Bairan, A., Phillips, I.A., Galasso, G.J., and Matthels, M.J. (1977). Clinical and serologic study of four smallpox vaccines comparing variations of dose and route of administration. Basic study and laboratory standardization. *J. Infect. Dis.* 135, 135–144.

Bergerot, I., Ploix, C., and Petersen, J. (1997). A cholera toxoid–insulin conjugate as an oral vaccine against spontaneous autoimmune diabetes. *Proc. Natl. Acad. Sci. USA* 94, 4610–4614.

Bergquist, C., Johansson, E.-L., Lagergard, T., Holmgren, J., and Rudin, A. (1997). Intranasal vaccination of humans with recombinant cholera toxin B subunit induces systemic and local antibody responses in the upper respiratory tract and the vagina. *Infect. Immun.* 65, 2676–2684

Berlin, C., Berg, E.L., Briskin, M.J., Andrew, D.P., Kilshaw, P.J., Holzmann, B., Weissman, I.L., Hamann, A., and Butcher, E.C. (1993). Alpha 4 beta 7 integrin mediates lymphocyte binding to the mucosal vascular addressin MAdCAM-1. *Cell* 74, 185–195.

Boirivant, M., Fuss, I.J., Ferroni, L., De Pascale, M., and Strober, W. (2001). Oral administration of recombinant cholera toxin subunit B inhibits IL-12-mediated murine experimental (trinitrobenzene sulfonic acid) colitis. *J. Immunol.* 166, 3522–3532.

Bomsel, M., Heyman, M., Hocini, H., Lagaye, S., Belec, L., Dupont, C., and Desgranges, C. (1998). Intracellular neutralization of HIV transcytosis across tight epithelial barriers by anti-HIV envelope protein dIgA or IgM. *Immunity* 9, 277–287.

Bonecchi, R., Bianchi, G., Bordignon, P.P., D'Ambrosio, D., Lang, R., Borsatti, A., Sozzani, S., Allavena, P., Gray, P.A., Mantovani, A. and Sinigaglia, F. (1998). Differential expression of chemokine receptors and chemotactic responsiveness of type 1 T helper cells (Th1s) and Th2s. *J. Exp. Med.* 187, 129–134.

Boyaka, P.N., Marinaro, M., Jackson, R.J., Menon, S., Kiyono, H., Jirillo, E. and McGhee, J.R. (1999). IL-12 is an effective adjuvant for induction of mucosal immunity. *J. Immunol.* 162, 122–128.

Boyaka, P.N., Wright. P.F., Marinaro. M., Kiyono, H., Johnson, J.E., Gonzales, R.A., Ikizler, M.R., Werkhaven, J.A., Jackson, R.J., Fujihashi, K., Di Fabio, S., Staats, H.F., and McGhee, J.R. (2000). Human nasopharyngeal-associated lymphoreticular tissues. Functional analysis of subepithelial and intraepithelial B and T cells from adenoids and tonsils. *Am. J. Pathol.* 157, 2023–2035.

Boyaka, P.N., Marinaro, M., Jackson, R.J., van Ginkel, F.W., Cornet-Boyaka, E., Kirk, K.L. Kensil, C.R., and McGhee, J.R. (2001). Oral QS-21 requires early IL-4 help for induction of mucosal and systemic immunity. *J. Immunol.* 166, 2283–2290.

Boyaka, P.N., Ohmura, M., Fujihashi, K., Koga, T., Yamamoto, M., Kweon, M.N., Takeda, Y., Jackson, R.J., Kiyono, H., Yuki, Y., and McGhee, J.R. (2003). Chimeras of labile toxin one and cholera toxin retain mucosal adjuvanticity and direct Th cell subsets via their B subunit. *J. Immunol.* 170, 454–462.

Bowman, C.C., and Clements, J.D. (2001). Differential biological and adjuvant activities of cholera toxin and *Escherichia coli* heat-labile enterotoxin hybrids. *Infect. Immun.* 69, 1528–1535

Bowman, E.P, Kuklin, N.A., Youngman, K.R., Lazarus, N.H., Kunkel, E.J., Pan, J., Greenberg, H.B., and Butcher, E.C. (2002). The intestinal chemokine thymus-expressed chemokine (CCL25) attracts IgA antibody-secreting cells. *J. Exp. Med.* 195, 269–275.

Bradney, C.P., Sempowski, G.D., Liao, H.X., Haynes, B.F., and Staats, H.F. (2002). Cytokines as adjuvants for the induction of anti-human immunodeficiency virus peptide immunoglobulin G (IgG) and IgA antibodies in serum and mucosal secretions after nasal immunization. *J. Virol.* 76, 517–524.

Brandtzaeg, P. (1984). Immune functions of human nasal mucosa and tonsils in health. In *Immunology of the Lung and Upper Respiratory Tract* (ed. J. Bienenstock), 28–95. New York: McGraw-Hill.

Briere, F., Bridon, J.M., Chevet, D., Souillet, G., Bienvenu, F., Guret, C., Martinez-Valdez, H., and Bancherau, J. (1994). Interleukin 10 induces B lymphocytes from IgA-deficient patients to secrete IgA. *J. Clin. Invest.* 94, 97–104.

Bromander, A., Holmgren, J., and Lycke, N. (1991). Cholera toxin stimulates IL-1 production and enhances antigen presentation by macrophages *in vitro. J. Immunol.* 146, 2908–2914.

Bromander, A., Kjerrulf, M., Holmgren, J., and Lycke, N. (1993). Cholera toxin enhances alloantigen presentation by cultured intestinal epithelial cells. *Scand. J. Immunol.* 37, 452–458.

Burns, J.W., Siadat-Pajouh, M., Krishnaney, A.A., and Greenberg, H.B. (1996). Protective effect of rotavirus VP6-specific IgA monoclonal antibodies that lack neutralizing activity. *Science* 272, 104–107.

Chase, M.V. (1946). Inhibition of experimental drug allergy by prior feeding of the sensitizing agent. *Proc. Soc. Exp. Biol. Med.* 61, 257–259.

Chan, S.H., Perussia, B., Gupta, J.W., Kobayashi, M., Pospisil, M., Young, H.A., Wolf, S.F., Young, D., Clark, S.C., and Trinchieri, G. (1991). Induction of interferon gamma production by natural killer cell stimulatory factor: characterization of the responder cells and synergy with other inducers. *J. Exp. Med.* 173, 869–879.

Chen, D., Periwal, S.B., Larrivee, K., Zuleger, C., Erickson, C.A., Endres, R.L., and Payne, L.G. (2001). Serum and mucosal immune responses to an inactivated influenza virus vaccine induced by epidermal powder immunization. *J. Virol.* 75, 7956–7965.

Coffman, R.L., Seymour, B.W., Lebman, D.A., Hiraki, D.D., Christiansen, J.A., Shrader, B., Cherwinski, H.M., Savelkoul, H.F., Finkelman, F.D., and Bond, M.W. (1988). The role of helper T cell products in mouse B cell differentiation and isotype regulation. *Immunol. Rev.* 102, 5–28.

Cong, Y., Weaver, C.T. and Elson, C.O. (1997). The mucosal adjuvanticity of cholera toxin involves enhancement of costimulatory activity by selective up-regulation of B7.2 expression. *J. Immunol.* 159, 5301–5308.

Crago, S.S., Kutteh, W.H., Moro, I., Allansmith, M.R., Radl, J., Haaijman, J. J., and Mestecky, J. (1984). Distribution of IgA1-, IgA2-, and J chain-containing cells in human tissues. *J. Immunol.* 132, 16–18.

Craig, S.W., and Cebra, J.J. (1971). Peyer's patches: an enriched source of precursors for IgA-producing immunocytes in the rabbit. *J. Exp. Med.* 134, 188–200.

Craig, S.W., and Cebra, J.J. (1975). Rabbit Peyer's patches, appendix, and popliteal lymph node B lymphocytes: a comparative analysis of their membrane immunoglobulin components and plasma cell precursor potential. *J. Immunol.* 114, 492–502.

Crowley-Nowick, P.A., Bell, M.C., Brockwell, R., Edwards, R.P., Chen, S., Partridge, E.E., and Mestecky, J. (1997). Rectal immunization for induction of specific antibody in the genital tract of women. *J. Clin. Immunol.* 17, 370–379.

Csencsits, K.L., Jutila, M.A., and Pascual, D.W. (1999). Nasal-associated lymphoid tissue: phenotypic and functional evidence for the primary role of peripheral node addressin in naive lymphocyte adhesion to high endothelial venules in a mucosal site. *J. Immunol.* 163, 1382–1389.

Csencsits, K.L., Walters, N., and Pascual, D.W. (2001). Cutting edge: dichotomy of homing receptor dependence by mucosal effector B cells: alpha(E) versus L-selectin. *J. Immunol.* 167, 2441–2445.

Czerkinsky, C., Prince, S.J., Michalek, S.M., Jackson, S., Russell, M.W., Moldoveanu, Z., McGhee, J.R., and Mestecky, J. (1987). IgA antibody-producing cells in peripheral blood after antigen ingestion: evidence for a common mucosal immune system in humans. *Proc. Natl. Acad. Sci. USA* 84, 2449–2453.

Czerkinsky, C., Anjuere, F., McGhee, J.R., George-Chandy, A., Holmgren, J., Kieny, M.P., Fujihashi, K., Mestecky, J.F., Pierrefite-Carle, V., Rask, C., and Sun, J.B. (1999). Mucosal immunity and tolerance: relevance to vaccine development. *Immunol. Rev.* 170, 197–222.

Dauer, M., Obermaier, B., Herten, J., Haerle, C., Pohl, K., Rothenfusser, S., Schnurr, M., Endres, S., and Eigler, A. (2003). Mature dendritic cells derived from human monocytes within 48 hours: a novel strategy for dendritic cell differentiation from blood precursors. *J. Immunol.* 170, 4069–4076.

Davin, J.C., Senterre, J., and Mahieu. P.R. (1991). The high lectin-binding capacity of human secretory IgA protects nonspecifically mucosae against environmental antigens. *Biol. Neonate* 59, 121–125.

Defrance, T., B. Vanbervliet, F. Briere, I. Durand, F. Rousset, and J. Bancherau. (1992). Interleukin 10 and transforming growth factor beta cooperate to induce anti-CD40-activated naive human B cells to secrete immunoglobulin A. *J. Exp. Med.* 175, 671–682.

Di Tommaso, A., Saletti, G., Pizza, M., Rappuoli, R., Dougan, G., Abrignani, S., Douce, G., and De Magistris, M.T. (1996). Induction of antigen-specific antibodies in vaginal secretions by using a nontoxic mutant of heat-labile enterotoxin as a mucosal adjuvant. *Infect. Immun.* 64, 974–979.

Enioutina, E.Y., Visic, D.M., and Daynes, R.A. (2002). The induction of systemic and mucosal immunity to protein vaccines delivered through skin sites exposed to UVB. *Vaccine* 20, 2116–2130.

Esser, C., and Radbruch, A. (1990). Immunoglobulin class switching: molecular and cellular analysis. *Annu. Rev. Immunol.* 8, 717–735.

Fagarasan, S., and Honjo, T. (2003). Intestinal IgA synthesis: regulation of front-line body defences. *Nat. Rev. Immunol.* 3, 63–72.

Fattom, A., Lue, C., Szu, S.C., Mestecky, J., Schiffman, G., Bryla, D., Vann, W.F., Watson, D., Kimzey, L.M., Robbins, J.B., and Schneerson, R. (1990). Serum antibody response in adult volunteers elicited by injection of *Streptococcus pneumoniae* type 12F polysaccharide alone or conjugated to diphtheria toxoid. *Infect. Immun.* 58, 2309–2312.

Fernandez, M.I., Pedron ,T., Tournebize, R., Olivo-Marin, J.C., Sansonetti, P.J., and Phalipon, A. (2003). Anti-inflammatory role for intracellular dimeric immunoglobulin a by neutralization of lipopolysaccharide in epithelial cells. *Immunity* 18, 739–749.

Finkelman, F.D., Holmes, J., Katona, I.M., Urban, Jr., J.F., Beckmann, M.P., Park, L.S., Schooley, K.A., Coffman, R.L., Mosmann, T.R., and Paul, W.E. (1990). Lymphokine control of *in vivo* immunoglobulin isotype selection. *Annu. Rev. Immunol.* 8, 303–333.

Forrest, B.D., Shearman, D.J., and LaBrooy, J.T. (1990). Specific immune response in humans following rectal delivery of live typhoid vaccine. *Vaccine* 8, 209–212.

Fujihashi, K., McGhee, J.R., Lue, C., Beagley, K.W., Taga, T., Hirano, T., Kishimoto, T., Mestecky, J., and Kiyono, H. (1991). Human appendix B cells naturally express receptors for and respond to interleukin 6 with selective IgA1 and IgA2 synthesis. *J. Clin. Invest.* 88, 248–252.

Gagliardi, M.C., Sallusto, F., Marinaro, M., Langenkamp, A., Lanzavecchia, A., and De Magistris, M.T. (2000). Cholera toxin induces maturation of human dendritic cells and licences them for Th2 priming. *Eur. J. Immunol.* 30, 2394–2403.

Gallichan, W.S., and Rosenthal, K.L. (1995). Specific secretory immune responses in the female genital tract following intranasal immunization with a recombinant adenovirus expressing glycoprotein B of herpes simplex virus. *Vaccine* 13, 1589–1595.

Gallichan, W.S., Woolstencroft, R.N., Guarasci, T., McCluskie, M.J., Davis, H.L., and Rosenthal, K.L. (2001). Intranasal immunization with CpG oligodeoxynucleotides as an adjuvant dramatically increases IgA and protection against herpes simplex virus-2 in the genital tract. *J Immunol.* 166, 3451–3457.

Gajewski, T.F., and Fitch, F.W. (1988). Anti-proliferative effect of IFN-gamma in immune regulation. I. IFN-gamma inhibits the proliferation of Th2 but not Th1 murine helper T lymphocyte clones. *J. Immunol.* 140, 4245–4252.

van Ginkel, F.W., Jackson, R.J., Yuki Y., and McGhee, J.R. (2000). Cutting edge: the mucosal adjuvant cholera toxin redirects vaccine proteins into olfactory tissues. *J. Immunol.* 165, 4778–4782.

Glenn, G.M., Rao, M., Matyas, G.R., and Alving, C.R. (1998). Skin immunization made possible by cholera toxin. *Nature* 391, 851–851.

Glenn, G.M., Taylor, D.N., Li, X., Frankel, S., Montemarano, A., and Alving C.R. (2000). Transcutaneous immunization: a human vaccine delivery strategy using a patch. *Nat. Med.* 6, 1403–1406.

Griffiss, J.M., and Goroff, D.K. (1983). IgA blocks IgM and IgG-initiated immune lysis by separate molecular mechanisms. *J. Immunol.* 130, 2882–2885.

Guarner, J., Jernigan, J.A., Shieh, W.J., Tatti, K., Flannagan, L.M., Stephens, D.S., Popovic, T., Ashford, D.A., Perkins, B.A., Zaki, S.R., and Inhalational Anthrax Pathology Working Group. (2003). Pathology and pathogenesis of bioterrorism-related inhalational anthrax. *Am. J. Pathol.* 163, 701–709.

Guebre-Xabier, M., Hammond, S.A., Epperson, D.E., Yu, J., Ellingsworth, L., and Glenn, G.M. (2003). Immunostimulant patch containing heat-labile enterotoxin from *Escherichia coli* enhances immune responses to injected influenza virus vaccine through activation of skin dendritic cells. *J. Virol.* 77, 5218–5225.

Gunn, M.D., Kyuwa, S., Tam, C., Kakiuchi, T., Matsuzawa, A., Williams, L.T., and Nakano, H. (1999). Mice lacking expression of secondary lymphoid organ chemokine have defects in lymphocyte homing and dendritic cell localization. *J. Exp. Med.* 189, 451–460.

Haq, T.A., Mason, H.S., Clements, J.D., and Arntzen, C.J. (1995). Oral immunization with a recombinant bacterial antigen produced in transgenic plants. *Science* 268, 714–716.

Hamada, H., Hiroi, T., Nishiyama, Y., Takahashi, H., Masunaga, Y., Hachimura, S., Kaminogawa, S., Takahashi-Iwanaga, H., Iwanaga, T., Kiyono, H., Yamamoto, H., and Ishikawa, H. (2002). Identification of multiple isolated lymphoid follicles on the antimesenteric wall of the mouse small intestine. *J. Immunol.* 168, 57–64.

Hamann, A., Andrew, D.P., Jablonski-Westrich, D., Holzmann, B., and Butcher, E.C. (1994). Role of alpha 4-integrins in lymphocyte homing to mucosal tissues *in vivo. J. Immunol.* 152, 3282–3293.

Haneberg, B., Kendall, D., Amerongen, H.M., Apter, F.M., Kraehenbuhl, J.-P., and Neutra, M.R. (1994). Induction of specific immunoglobulin A in the small intestine, colon-rectum, and vagina measured by a new method for collection of secretions from local mucosal surfaces. *Infect. Immun.* 62, 15–23.

Harandi, A.M., Eriksson, K., and Holmgren J. (2003). A protective role of locally administered immunostimulatory CpG oligodeoxynucleotide in a mouse model of genital herpes infection. *J. Virol.* 77, 953–962.

Heatley, E.V., Stark, J.M., Horsewood, P., Bandouvas, E., Cole, F., and Bienenstock, J. (1981). The effects of surgical removal of Peyer's patches in rat on systemic antibody responses to intestinal antigen. *Immunology* 44, 543–548.

Holzmann, B., McIntyre, B.W., and Weissman, I.L. (1989). Identification of a murine Peyer's patch–specific lymphocyte homing receptor as an integrin molecule with an alpha chain homologous to human VLA-4 alpha. *Cell* 56, 37–46.

Huber, V.C., Arulanandam. B.P., Arnaboldi, P.M., Elmore, M.K., Sheehan, C.E., Kallakury, B.V., and Metzger, D.W. (2003). Delivery of IL-12 intranasally leads to reduced IL-12-mediated toxicity. *Int. Immunopharmacol.* 3, 801–809.

Husby, S., Mestecky, J., Moldoveanu, Z., Holland, S., and Elson, C.O. (1994). Oral tolerance in humans. T cell but not B cell tolerance after antigen feeding. *J. Immunol.* 152, 4663–4670.

Imai, T., Nagira, M., Takagi, S., Kakizaki, M., Nishimura, M., Wang, J., Gray, P.W., Matsushima, K., and Yoshie, O. (1999). Selective recruitment of CCR4-bearing Th2 cells toward antigen-presenting cells by the CC chemokines thymus and activation-regulated chemokine and macrophage-derived chemokine. *Int. Immunol.* 11, 81–88.

Issekutz, T.B. (1984). The response of gut-associated T lymphocytes to intestinal viral immunization. *J. Immunol.* 133, 2955–2960.

Jernigan, J.A., Stephens, D.S., Ashford, D.A., Omenaca, C., Topiel, M.S., Galbraith, M., Tapper, M., Fisk, T.L., Zaki, S., Popovic, T., Meyer, R.F., Quinn, C.P., Harper, S.A., Fridkin, S.K., Sejvar, J.J., Shepard, C.W., McConnell, M., Guarner, J., Shieh, W.J., Malecki, J.M., Gerberding, J.L., Hughes, J.M., Perkins, B.A., and Anthrax Bioterrorism Investigation Team. (2001). Bioterrorism-related inhalational anthrax: the first 10 cases reported in the United States. *Emerg. Infect. Dis.* 7, 933–944.

Kantele, A. (1990). Antibody-secreting cells in the evaluation of the immunogenicity of an oral vaccine. *Vaccine* 8, 321–326.

Kantele, A., Hakkinen, M., Moldoveanu, Z., Lu, A., Savilahti, E., Alvarez, R.D., Michalek. S., and Mestecky, J. (1998). Differences in immune responses induced by oral and rectal immunizations with *Salmonella typhi* Ty21a: evidence for compartmentalization within the common mucosal immune system in humans. *Infect. Immun.* 66, 5630–5635.

Kataoka, K., McGhee, J. R., Kobayashi, R., Fujihashi, K., Shizukuishi, S., and Fujihashi, K. (2004). Nasal Flt3 ligand cDNA elicits CD11c⁺ CD8⁺ dendritic cells for enhanced mucosal immunity. *J. Immunol.* 172, 3612–3619.

Kauppi-Korkeila, M., van Alphen, L., Madore, D., Saarinen, L., and Kayhty. H. (1996). Mechanism of antibody-mediated reduction of nasopharyngeal colonization by *Haemophilus influenzae* type b studied in an infant rat model. *J. Infect. Dis.* 174, 1337–1340.

Kett, K., Brandtzaeg, P., Radl, J., and Haaijman, J.F. (1986). Different subclass distribution of IgA-producing cells in human lymphoid organs and various secretory tissues. *J. Immunol.* 136, 3631–3635.

Kensil, C.R., and Kammer, R. (1998). QS-21: A water-soluble triterpene glycoside adjuvant. *Expert Opinion Invest. Drugs* 7, 1475–1482.

Keren, D.F., Holt, P.S., Collins, H.H., Gemski, P., and Formal, S.B. (1978). The role of Peyer's patches in the local immune response of rabbit ileum to live bacteria. *J. Immunol.* 120, 1892–1896.

Kim, C.H., Nagata, K., and Butcher, E.C. (2003). Dendritic cells support sequential reprogramming of chemoattractant receptor profiles during naive to effector T cell differentiation. *J. Immunol.* 171, 152–158.

Kiyono, H. (1997). Nasal-associated lymphoid tissue (NALT). *Mucosal Immunol. Update* 5, 1–20.

Klingman, A.M. (1958). Poison ivy (*Rhus*) dermatitis. *Arch. Dermatol.* 77, 149–180.

Klinman, D.M., Yi, A.K., Beaucage, S.L., Conover, J. and Krieg, A.M. (1996). CpG motifs present in bacteria DNA rapidly induce lymphocytes to secrete interleukin 6, interleukin 12, and interferon gamma. *Proc. Natl. Acad. Sci. USA* 93, 2879–2883.

Kobayashi, M., Fitz, L., Ryan, M., Hewick, R.M., Clark, S.C., Chan, S.C, Loudon, R., Sherman, F., Perussia, B., and Trinchieri, G. (1989). Identification and purification of natural killer cell stimulatory factor (NKSF), a cytokine with multiple biologic effects on human lymphocytes. *J. Exp. Med.* 170, 827–845.

Kozlowski, P.A., Cu-Uvin, S., Neutra, M.R., and Flanigan, T.P. (1997). Comparison of the oral, rectal, and vaginal immunization routes for induction of antibodies in rectal and genital tract secretions of women. *Infect. Immun.* 65, 1387–1394.

Kozlowski, P.A., Williams, S.B., Lynch, R.M., Flanigan, T.P., Patterson, R.R., Cu-Uvin, S., and Neutra, M.R. (2002). Differential induction of mucosal and systemic antibody responses in women after nasal, rectal, or vaginal immunization: influence of the menstrual cycle. *J. Immunol.* 169, 566–574.

Kraus, T.A., Toy, L., Chan, L., Childs, J., Cheisetz, A., and Mayer, L. (2004). Oral tolerance failure in Crohn's disease and ulcerative colitis patients. *Ann. N.Y. Acad. Sci.* (in press).

Krieg, A.M. (2002). CpG motifs in bacterial DNA and their immune effects. *Annu. Rev. Immunol.* 20, 709–760.

Kuiken, T., Fouchier, R.A., Schutten, M., Rimmelzwaan, G.F., van Amerongen, G., van Riel, D., Laman, J.D., de Jong, T., van Doornum, G., Lim, W., Ling, A.E., Chan, P.K., Tam, J.S., Zambon, M.C., Gopal, R., Drosten, C., van der Werf, S., Escriou, N., Manuguerra, J.C., Stohr, K., Peiris, J.S., and Osterhaus, A.D. (2003). Newly discovered coronavirus as the primary cause of severe acute respiratory syndrome. *Lancet* 362, 263–270.

Kunkel, E.J., Campbell, J.J., Haraldsen, G., Pan, J., Boisvert, J., Roberts, A.I., Ebert, E.C., Vierra. M.A., Goodman, S.B., Genovese, M.C., Wardlaw, A.J., Greenberg, H.B., Parker, C.M., Butcher, E.C., Andrew, D.P., and Agace, W.W. (2000). Lymphocyte CC chemokine receptor 9 and epithelial thymus-expressed chemokine (TECK) expression distinguish the small intestinal immune compartment: Epithelial expression of tissue-specific chemokines as an organizing principle in regional immunity. *J. Exp. Med.* 192, 761–768.

Kunkel, E.J., Kim, C.H., Lazarus, N.H., Vierra, M.A., Soler, D., Bowman, E.P., and Butcher, E.C. (2003). CCR10 expression is a common feature of circulating and mucosal epithelial tissue IgA Ab-secreting cells. *J. Clin. Invest.* 111, 1001–1010.

Kuper, C.F., Koornstra, P.J., Hameleers, D.M., Biewenga, J., Spit, B.J., Duijvestijn, A.M., van Breda Vriesman, P.J., and Sminia, T. (1992). The role of nasopharyngeal lymphoid tissue. *Immunol. Today* 13, 219–224.

Kutteh, W.H., Hatch, K.D., Blackwell, R.E., and Mestecky, J. (1988). Secretory immune system of the female reproductive tract: I. Immunoglobulin and secretory component-containing cells. *Obstet. Gynecol.* 71, 56–60.

Kweon, M.N., Yamamoto, M., Watanabe, F., Tamura, S., van Ginkel, F.W., Miyauchi, A., Takagi, H., Takeda, Y., Hamabata, T., Fujihashi, K., McGhee, J.R., and Kiyono, H. (2002). A nontoxic chimeric enterotoxin adjuvant induces protective immunity in both mucosal and systemic compartments with reduced IgE antibodies. *J. Infect. Dis.* 186, 1261–1269.

Langman, J.M., and Rowland, R. (1986). The number and distribution of lymphoid follicles in the human large intestine. *J. Anat.* 149, 189–194.

Lazarus, N.H., Kunkel, E.J., Johnston, B., Wilson, E., Youngman, K.R., and Butcher. E.C. (2003). A common mucosal chemokine (mucosae-associated epithelial chemokine/CCL28) selectively attracts IgA plasmablasts. *J. Immunol.* 170, 3799–805.

Lehner, T., Panagiotidi, C., Bergmeier, L.A., Ping, T., Brooks, R., and Adams, S.E. (1992). A comparison of the immune response following oral, vaginal, or rectal route of immunization with SIV antigens in non-human primates. *Vaccine Res.* 1, 319–330.

Lehner, T., Brookes, R., Panagiotidi, C., Tao, L., Klavinskis, L.S., Walker, J., Walker, P., Ward, R., Hussain, L., Gearing, A.J., Adams, S.E., and Bergmeier, L.A. (1993). T- and B-cell functions and epitope expression in nonhuman primates immunized with simian immunodeficiency virus antigen by the rectal route. *Proc. Natl. Acad. Sci. USA* 90, 8638–8642.

Lillard, J.W., Jr., Boyaka, P.N., Hedrick, J.A., Zlotnik, A., and McGhee, J.R. (1999). Lymphotactin acts as an innate mucosal adjuvant. *J. Immunol.* 162, 1959–1965.

Lillard, J.W., Boyaka, P.N., Taub, D.D. and McGhee, J.R. (2001). RANTES potentiates antigen-specific mucosal immune responses. *J. Immunol.* 166, 162–169.

Lillard, J.W. Jr., Singh, U.P., Boyaka, P.N., Singh, S., Taub, D.D., and McGhee, J.R. (2003). MIP-1alpha and MIP-1beta differentially mediate mucosal and systemic adaptive immunity. *Blood* 101, 807–814.

Livingston, P., Zhang, S., Adluri, S., Yao, T.J., Graeber, L., Ragupathi, G., Helling, F., and Fleisher, M. (1997). Tumor cell reactivity mediated by IgM antibodies in sera from melanoma patients vaccinated with GM2 ganglioside covalently linked to KLH is increased by IgG antibodies. *Cancer Immunol. Immunother.* 43, 324–330.

London, S.D., Rubin, D.H. and Cebra, J.J. (1987). Gut mucosal immunization with reovirus serotype 1/L stimulates virus-specific cytotoxic T cell precursors as well as IgA memory cells in Peyer's patches. *J. Exp. Med.* 165, 830–847.

London, S.D., Cebra-Thomas, J.A., Rubin, D.H., and Cebra, J.J. (1990). CD8 lymphocyte subpopulations in Peyer's patches induced by reovirus serotype 1 infection. *J. Immunol.* 144, 3187–3194.

Lorenz, R.G., Chaplin, D.D., McDonald, K.G., McDonough, J.S., and Newberry, R.D. (2003). Isolated lymphoid follicle formation is inducible and dependent upon lymphotoxin-sufficient B lymphocytes, lymphotoxin receptor, and TNF receptor I function. *J. Immunol.* 170, 5475–5482.

Lubeck, M.D. Natuk, R.J., Chengalvala, M., Chanda, P.K., Murthy, K.K., Murthy, S., Mizutani, S., Lee, S.-G., Wade, M.S., Bhat, B.M.,

Bhat, R., Kheer, S.K., Eichberg, J.W., Davis, A.R., and Hung, P.P. (1994). Immunogenicity of recombinant adenovirus-human immunodeficiency virus vaccines in chimpanzees following intranasal administration. *AIDS Res. Hum. Retroviruses* 10, 1443–1449.

Lue, C., Prince, S.J., Fattom, A., Schneerson, R., Robbins, J.B., and Mestecky, J. (1990). Antibody-secreting peripheral blood lymphocytes induced by immunization with a conjugate consisting of *Streptococcus pneumoniae* type 12F polysaccharide and diphtheria toxoid. *Infect. Immun.* 58, 2547–2554.

Mah, D.C., Leone, G., Jankowski, J.M., and Lee, P.W. (1990). The N-terminal quarter of reovirus cell attachment protein sigma 1 possesses intrinsic virion-anchoring function. *Virology* 179, 95–103.

Margaret, B., and Rennels, M.D. (2000). The rotavirus vaccine story: A clinical investigator's view. *Pediatrics* 106, 123–125.

Marinaro, M., Staats, H.F., Hiroi, T., Jackson, R.J., Coste, M., Boyaka, P.N., Okahashi, N., Yamamoto, M., Kiyono, H., Bluethmann, H., Fujihashi, K., and McGhee, J.R. (1995). Mucosal adjuvant effect of cholera toxin in mice results from induction of T helper 2 (Th2) cells and IL-4. *J. Immunol.* 155, 4621–4629.

Marinaro, M., Boyaka, P.N., Finkelman, F.D., Kiyono, H., Jackson, R.J., Jirillo, E., and McGhee, J.R. (1997). Oral but not parenteral interleukin (IL)-12 redirects T helper 2 (Th2)-type responses to an oral vaccine without altering mucosal IgA responses. *J. Exp. Med.* 185, 415–427.

Marinaro, M., Di Tommaso, A., Uzzau, S., Fasano, A., and De Magistris, M.T. (1999a). Zonula occludens toxin is a powerful mucosal adjuvant for intranasally delivered antigens. *Infect. Immun.* 67, 1287–1291.

Marinaro, M., Boyaka, P.N., Jackson, R.J., Finkelman, F.D., Kiyono, H., Jirillo, E. and McGhee, J.R. (1999b). Use of intranasal IL-12 to target predominantly Th1 responses to nasal and Th2 responses to oral vaccines given with cholera toxin. *J. Immunol.* 162, 114–1121.

Marinaro, M., Fasano, A. and De Magistris, M.T. (2003). Zonula occludens toxin acts as an adjuvant through different mucosal routes and induces protective immune responses. *Infect. Immun.* 71, 1897–1902.

Mazanec, M.B., Kaetzel, C.S., Lamm, M.E., Fletcher, D., and Nedrud, J.G. (1992). Intracellular neutralization of virus by immunoglobulin A antibodies. *Proc. Natl. Acad. Sci. USA* 89, 6901–6905.

Mazanec, M.B., Coudret, C.L. and Fletcher, D.R. (1995). Intracellular neutralization of influenza virus by immunoglobulin A anti-hemagglutinin monoclonal antibodies. *J. Virol.* 69, 1339–1343.

McCluskie, M.J., and Davis, H.L. (1998). CpG DNA is a potent enhancer of systemic and mucosal immune responses against hepatitis B surface antigen with intranasal administration to mice. *J. Immunol.* 161, 4463–4466.

McCluskie, M.J., Weeratna, R.D., Krieg, A.M., and Davis, H.L. (2000). CpG DNA is an effective oral adjuvant to protein antigens in mice. *Vaccine* 19, 950–957.

McChesney, M.B., Collins, J.R., Lu, D., Lu, X., Torten, J., Ashley, R.L., Cloyd, M.W., and Miller, C.J. (1998). Occult systemic infection and persistent simian immunodeficiency virus (SIV)-specific CD4+ T-cell proliferative responses in rhesus macaques that were transiently viremic after intravaginal inoculation of SIV. *J. Virol.* 72, 10029–10035.

McDermott, M.R., and Bienenstock, J. (1979). Evidence for a common mucosal immunologic system. I. Migration of B immunoblasts into intestinal, respiratory, and genital tissues. *J. Immunol.* 122, 1892–1898.

McGee, D.W., Elson, C.O., and McGhee, J.R. (1993). Enhancing effect of cholera toxin on interleukin-6 secretion by IEC-6 intestinal epithelial cells: mode of action and augmenting effect of inflammatory cytokines. *Infect. Immun.* 61, 4637–4644.

McGhee, J.R., Mestecky, J., Dertzbaugh, M.T., Eldridge, J.H., Hirasawa, M., and Kiyono, H. (1992). The mucosal immune system: from fundamental concepts to vaccine development. *Vaccine* 10, 75–88.

McWilliams, M., Phillips-Quagliata, J.M., and Lamm, M.E. (1975). Characteristics of mesenteric lymph node cells homing to gut-associated lymphoid tissue in syngeneic mice. *J. Immunol.* 115, 54–58.

McWilliams, M., Phillips-Quagliata, J.M., and Lamm, M.E. (1977). Mesenteric lymph node B lymphoblasts which home to the small intestine are precommitted to IgA synthesis. *J. Exp. Med.* 145, 866–875.

Mega, J., McGhee, J.R. and Kiyono, H. (1992). Cytokine- and Ig-producing T cells in mucosal effector tissues: analysis of IL-5- and IFN-gamma-producing T cells, T cell receptor expression, and IgA plasma cells from mouse salivary gland-associated tissues. *J. Immunol.* 148, 2030–2039.

Mellander, L., Carlsson, B., and Hanson, L.A. (1984). Appearance of secretory IgM and IgA antibodies to *Escherichia coli* in saliva during early infancy and childhood. *J. Pediatr.* 104, 564–568.

Mestecky J. (1987). The common mucosal immune system and current strategies for induction of immune responses in external secretions. *J. Clin. Immunol.* 7, 265–276.

Mestecky, J., and McGhee, J.R. (1987). Immunoglobulin A (IgA): molecular and cellular interactions involved in IgA biosynthesis and immune response. *Adv. Immunol.* 40, 153–245.

Mestecky, J., Moldoveanu, Z, Michalek, S.M., Morrow, C., Compans, R.W., Schafer, D.P., and Russell, M.W. (1997). Current options for vaccine delivery systems by mucosal routes. *J. Control. Rel.* 48, 243–257.

Micallef, M.J., Ohtsuki, T., Kohno, K., Tanabe, F., Ushio, S., Namba, M., Tanimoto, T., Torigoe, K., Fujii, M., Ikeda, M., Fukuda, S., and Kurimoto, M. (1996). Interferon-gamma-inducing factor enhances T helper 1 cytokine production by stimulated human T cells: synergism with interleukin-12 for interferon-gamma production. *Eur. J. Immunol.* 26, 1647–1651.

Moghaddami, M., Cummins, A., and Mayrhofer, G. (1998). Lymphocyte-filled villi: comparison with other lymphoid aggregations in the mucosa of the human small intestine. *Gastroenterology* 115, 1414–1425.

Moldoveanu, Z., Novak, M., Huang, W.-Q., Gilley, R.M., Staas, J.K., Schafer, D., Compans, R.W., and Mestecky, J. (1993). Oral immunization with influenza virus in biodegradable microspheres. *J. Infect. Dis.* 167, 84–90.

Moldoveanu, Z., Porter, D.C., Lu, A., McPherson, S., and Morrow, C.D. (1995). Immune responses induced by administration of encapsidated poliovirus replicons which express HIV-1 gag and envelope proteins. *Vaccine* 13, 1013–1022.

Moldoveanu, Z., Love-Homan, L., Huang, W.Q., and Krieg, A.M. (1998). CpG DNA, a novel immune enhancer for systemic and mucosal immunization with influenza virus. *Vaccine* 16, 1216–1224.

Mosmann, T.R., and Coffman, R.L. (1989). Th1 and Th2 cells: different patterns of lymphokine secretion lead to different functional properties. *Annu. Rev. Immunol.* 7, 145–173.

Mowat, A.M., Donachie, A.M., Jagewall, S., Schon, K., Lowenadler, B., Dalsgaard, K., Kaastrup, P., and Lycke, N. (2001). CTA1-DD-immune stimulating complexes: a novel, rationally designed combined mucosal vaccine adjuvant effective with nanogram doses of antigen. *J. Immunol.* 167, 3398–3405.

Musey, L., Ding, Y., Elizaga, M., Ha, R., Celum, C., and McElrath, M.J. (2003). HIV-1 vaccination administered intramuscularly can induce both systemic and mucosal T cell immunity in HIV-1-uninfected individuals. *J. Immunol.* 171, 1094–1101.

Neutra, M.R., Mantis, N.J., and Kraehenbuhl, J-P. (2001). Collaboration of epithelial cells with organized mucosal lymphoid tissues. *Nat. Immunol.* 2, 1004–1009.

Offit, P.A., Cunningham, S.L., and Dudzik, K.I. (1991). Memory and distribution of virus-specific cytotoxic T lymphocytes (CTLs) and CTL precursors after rotavirus infection. *J. Virol.* 65, 1318–1324.

O'Leary, A.D., and Sweeney, E.C. (1986). Lymphoglandular complexes of the colon: structure and distribution. *Histopathol.* 10, 267–283.

Ogra, P.L. (1971). Effect of tonsillectomy and adenoidectomy on nasopharyngeal antibody response to poliovirus. *N. Engl. J. Med.* 284, 59–64.

Okamura, H., Kashiwamura, S., Tsutsui, H., Yoshimoto, T., and Nakanishi, K. (1998). Regulation of interferon-gamma production by IL-12 and IL-18. *Curr. Opin. Immunol.* 10, 259–264.

Pal, S., Peterson, E.M., and de la Maza, L.M. (1996). Intranasal immunization induces long-term protection in mice against a *Chlamydia trachomatis* genital challenge. *Infect. Immun.* 64, 5341–5348.

Pabst, R. (1992). Is BALT a major component of the human lung immune system ? *Immunol. Today* 13, 119–122.

Pabst, R., Luhrmann, A., Steinmetz, I., and Tschernig, T. (2003). A single intratracheal dose of the growth factor Fms-like tyrosine kinase receptor-3 ligand induces a rapid differential increase of dendritic cells and lymphocyte subsets in lung tissue and bronchoalveolar lavage, resulting in an increased local antibody production. *J. Immunol.* 171, 325–330.

Phillips-Quagliata, J.M., and Lamm, M.E. (1988). Migration of lymphocytes in the mucosal immune system. In *Migration and Homing of Lymphoid Cells* (ed. A. J. Husband), 53–75. Boca Raton, Florida: CRC Press.

Phipps, P.A., Stanford, M.R., Sun, J.B., Xiao, B.G., Holmgren, J., Shinnick, T., Hasan, A., Mizushima, Y., and Lehner, T. (2003). Prevention of mucosally induced uveitis with a HSP60-derived peptide linked to cholera toxin B subunit. *Eur. J. Immunol.* 33, 224–232.

Quiding-Järbrink, M., Granström, G., Nordström, I., Holmgren, J., and Czerkinsky, C. (1995a). Induction of compartmentalized B-cell responses in human tonsils. *Infect. Immun.* 63, 853–857.

Quiding-Järbrink, M., Lakew, M., Nordström, I., Banchereau, J., Butcher, E., Holmgren, J., and Czerkinsky, C. (1995b). Human circulating specific antibody-forming cells after systemic and mucosal immunizations: differential homing commitments and cell surface differentiation markers. *Eur. J. Immunol.* 25, 322–327.

Quiding-Järbrink, M., Nordström, I., Granström, G., Kilander, A., Jertborn, M., Butcher, E. C., Lazarovits, A. I., Holmgren, J., and Czerkinsky, C. (1997). Differential expression of tissue-specific adhesion molecules on human circulating antibody-forming cells after systemic, enteric and nasal immunizations. A molecular basis for the compartmentalization of effector B cell responses. *J. Clin. Invest.* 99, 1281–1286.

Randolph, D.A., Huang, G., Carruthers, C.J., Bromley, L.E., and Chaplin, D.D. (1999). The role of CCR7 in Th1 and Th2 cell localization and delivery of B cell help *in vivo*. *Science* 286, 2159–2162.

Rask, C., Holmgren, J., Fredriksson, M., Lindblad, M., Nordstrom, I., Sun, J.B., and Czerkinsky, C. (2000). Prolonged oral treatment with low doses of allergen conjugated to cholera toxin B subunit suppresses immunoglobulin E antibody responses in sensitized mice. *Clin. Exp. Allergy* 30, 1024–1032.

Roman, M., Martin-Orozco, E., Goodman, J.S., Nguyen, M.D., Sato, Y., Ronaghy, A., Kornbluth, R.S., Richman, D.D., Carson, D.A., and Raz, E. (1997). Immunostimulatory DNA sequences function as T helper-1-promoting adjuvants. *Nat. Med.* 3, 849–854.

Rosner, A.J., and Keren, D.F. (1984). Demonstration of M cells in the specialized follicle-associated epithelium overlying isolated lymphoid follicles in the gut. *J. Leukoc. Biol.* 35, 397–404.

Rott, L.S., Briskin, M.J., Andrew, D.P., Berg, E.L., and Butcher, E.C. (1996). A fundamental subdivision of circulating lymphocytes defined by adhesion to mucosal addressin cell adhesion molecule-1. Comparison with vascular cell adhesion molecule-1 and correlation with beta 7 integrins and memory differentiation. *J. Immunol.* 156, 3727–3736.

Roux, M.E., McWilliams, M., Phillips-Quagliata, J.M., Weisz-Carrington. P. and Lamm. M.E. (1977). Origin of IgA-secreting plasma cells in the mammary gland. *J. Exp. Med.* 146, 1311–1322.

Rubas, W., Banerjea, A.C., Gallati, H., Speiser, P.P., and Joklik, W.K. (1990). Incorporation of the reovirus M cell attachment protein into small unilamellar vesicles: incorporation efficiency and binding capability to L929 cells *in vitro*. *J. Microencapsul.* 7, 385–395.

Russell, M.W., and Mansa, B. (1989). Complement-fixing properties of human IgA antibodies. Alternative pathway complement activation by plastic-bound, but not specific antigen-bound, IgA. *Scand. J. Immunol.* 30, 175–183.

Russell, M. W., Moldoveanu, Z., White, P. L., Sibert, G. J., Mestecky, J., and Michalek, S. M. (1996). Salivary, nasal, genital, and systemic antibody responses in monkeys immunized intranasally with a bacterial protein antigen and the cholera toxin B subunit. *Infect. Immun.* 64, 1272–1283.

Russell, M. W., and Mestecky, J. (2002). Humoral immune responses to microbial infections in the genital tract. *Microbes Infect.* 4, 667–677.

Sallusto, F., Lenig, D., Mackay, C. R., and Lanzavecchia, A. (1998). Flexible programs of chemokine receptor expression on human polarized T helper 1 and 2 lymphocytes. *J. Exp. Med.* 187, 875–883.

Sasaki, S., Sumino, K., Hamajima, K., Fukushima, J., Ishii, N., Kawamoto, S., Mohri, H., Kensil, C. R., and Okuda, K. (1998). Induction of systemic and mucosal immune responses to human immunodeficiency virus type 1 by a DNA vaccine formulated with QS-21 saponin adjuvant via intramuscular and intranasal routes. *J. Virol.* 72, 4931–4939.

Schiff, L. A., and Fields, B. N. (1990). Reoviruses and their replication. In *Virology* (eds. Fields, B. N., and Knipe, D. M.), 1275–1306. New York: Raven Press.

Scicchitano, R., Stanisz, A., Ernst, P. B., and Bienenstock, J. (1988). A common mucosal immune system revisited. In *Migration and Homing of Lymphoid Cells* (ed. A. J. Husband), 1–34. Boca Raton, Florida: CRC Press.

Scharton-Kersten, T., Yu, J., Vassell, R., O'Hagan, D., Alving, C. R., and Glenn, G. M. (2000). Transcutaneous immunization with bacterial ADP-ribosylating exotoxins, subunits, and unrelated adjuvants. *Infect. Immun.* 68, 5306–5313.

Schmitz, J. E., Veazey, R. S., Kuroda, M. J., Levy, D. B., Seth, A., Mansfield, K. G., Nickerson, C. E., Lifton, M. A., Alvarez, X., Lackner, A. A., and Letvin, N. L. (2001). Simian immunodeficiency virus (SIV)-specific cytotoxic T lymphocytes in gastrointestinal tissues of chronically SIV-infected rhesus monkeys. *Blood* 98, 3757–3761.

Snapper, C. M., and Paul, W. E. (1987). Interferon-gamma and B cell stimulatory factor-1 reciprocally regulate Ig isotype production. *Science* 236, 944–947.

Spangler, B. D. (1992). Structure and function of cholera toxin and the related *Escherichia coli* heat-labile enterotoxin. *Microbiol. Rev.* 56, 622–647.

Staats, H. F., Nichols, W. G., and Palker, T. J. (1996). Mucosal immunity to HIV-1: Systemic and vaginal antibody response after intranasal immunization with the HIV-1 C4/V3 peptide T1SP10 MN(A). *J. Immunol.* 157, 462–472.

Staats, H. F., and Ennis, Jr., F. A. (1999). IL-1 is an effective adjuvant for mucosal and systemic immune responses when coadministered with protein immunogens. *J. Immunol.* 162, 6141–6147.

Staats, H. F., Bradney, C. P., Gwinn, W. M., Jackson, S. S., Sempowski, G. D., Liao, H. X., Letvin, N. L., and Haynes, B. F. (2001). Cytokine requirements for induction of systemic and mucosal CTL after nasal immunization. *J. Immunol.* 167, 5386–5394.

Stevens, F. A. (1945). Council on pharmacy and chemistry. Report of the council: status of poison ivy extracts. *J. Am. Med. Assoc.* 127, 912–921.

Sun, J.-B., Xiao, B.-G., Lindblad, M., Li, B.L., Link, H., Czerkinsky, C., and Holmgren, J. (2000). Oral administration of cholera toxin B subunit conjugated to myelin basic protein protects against experimental autoimmune encephalomyelitis by inducing transforming growth factor-β-secreting cells and suppressing chemokine expression. *Int. Immunol.* 12, 1449–1457.

Tacket, C. O., Mason, H. S., Losonsky, G., Clements, J. D., Levine, M. M., and Arntzen, C. J. (1998). Immunogenicity in humans of a recombinant bacterial antigen delivered in a transgenic potato. *Nat. Med.* 4, 607–609.

Taguchi, T., McGhee, J. R., Coffman, R. L., Beagley, K. W., Eldridge, J. H., Takatsu, K., and Kiyono, H. (1990). Analysis of Th1 and Th2 cells in murine gut-associated tissues. Frequencies of CD4+ and CD8+ T cells that secrete IFN-gamma and IL-5. *J. Immunol.* 145, 68–77.

Takahashi, I., Marinaro, M., Kiyono, H., Jackson, R.J., Nakagawa, I., Fujihashi, K., Hamada, S. Clements, J.D., Bost, K.L., and

McGhee, J.R. (1996). Mechanisms for mucosal immunogenicity and adjuvancy of *Escherichia coli* labile enterotoxin. *J. Infect. Dis.* 173, 627–35.

Tang, D.C., Shi, Z., and Curiel, D.T. (1997). Vaccination onto bare skin. *Nature* 388, 729–730.

Tarkowski, A., Sun, J.-B., Holmdahl, R., Holmgren, J., and Czerkinsky, C. (1999). Treatment of experimental autoimmune arthritis by nasal administration of a type II collagen–cholera toxoid conjugate vaccine. *Arthritis Rheum.* 42,1628–1634.

Tighe, H., Corr, M., Roman, M. and Raz, E. (1998). Gene vaccination: plasmid DNA is more than just a blueprint. *Immunol. Today* 19, 89–97.

Vajdy, M., Kosco-Vilbois, M.H., Kopf, M., Kohler, G., and Lycke, N. (1995). Impaired mucosal immune responses in interleukin 4-targeted mice. *J. Exp. Med.* 181, 41–53.

VanCott, J.L., Staats, H.F., Pascual, D.W., Roberts, M., Chatfield, S.N., Yamamoto, M., Coste, M., Carter, P.B., Kiyono, H. and McGhee, J.R. (1996). Regulation of mucosal and systemic antibody responses by T helper cell subsets, macrophages, and derived cytokines following oral immunization with live recombinant *Salmonella*. *J. Immunol.* 156, 1504–1514.

Veazey, R.S., Lifson, J.D., Schmitz, J.E., Kuroda, M.J., Piatak, M. Jr., Pandrea, I., Purcell, J., Bohm, R., Blanchard, J., Williams, K.C., and Lackner, A.A. (2003). Dynamics of Simian immunodeficiency virus-specific cytotoxic T-cell responses in tissues. *J. Med. Primatol.* 32, 194–200.

Viney, J.L., Mowat, A.M., O'Malley, J.M., Williamson, E., and Fanger, N.A. (1998). Expanding dendritic cells *in vivo* enhances the induction of oral tolerance. *J. Immunol.* 160, 5815–5825

Waldo, F.B., van den Wall Bake, A.W., Mestecky, J., and Husby, S. (1994). Suppression of the immune response by nasal immunization. *Clin. Immunol. Immunopathol.* 72, 30–34

Williamson, E., Westrich, G.M., and Viney, J.L. (1999). Modulating dendritic cells to optimize mucosal immunization protocols. *J. Immunol.* 163, 3668–3675.

Wilson, L.A., Murphey-Corb, M., Martin, L.N., Harrison, R.M., Ratterree, M.S., and Bohm, R.P. (2000). Identification of SIV env-specific CTL in the jejunal mucosa in vaginally exposed, seronegative rhesus macaques (Macaca mulatta). *J. Med. Primatol.* 29, 173–181.

Wold, A.E., Mestecky, J., Tomana, M., Kobata, A., Ohbayashi, H., Endo, T., and Eden, C.S. (1990). Secretory immunoglobulin A carries oligosaccharide receptors for *Escherichia coli* type 1 fimbrial. *Infect. Immun.* 58, 3073–3077.

Wolf, H.M., Fischer, M.B., Puhringer, H., Samstag, A., Vogel, E., and Eibl, M.M. (1994). Human serum IgA downregulates the release of inflammatory cytokines (tumor necrosis factor-alpha, interleukin-6) in human monocytes. *Blood* 83, 1278–1288.

Wolf, H.M., Hauber, I., Gulle, H., Samstag, A., Fischer, M.B., Ahmad, R.U., and Eibl, M.M. (1996). Anti-inflammatory properties of human serum IgA: induction of IL-1 receptor antagonist and Fc alpha R (CD89)-mediated down-regulation of tumour necrosis factor-alpha (TNF-alpha) and IL-6 in human monocytes. *Clin. Exp. Immunol.* 105, 537–543.

Wu, Y., Boysun, M.J., Csencsits, K.L., and Pascual, D.W. (2000). Gene transfer facilitated by a cellular targeting molecule, reovirus protein sigma1. *Gene Ther.* 7, 61–69.

Wu, Y., Wang, X., Csencsits, K.L., Haddad, A., Walters, N., and Pascual, D.W. (2001). M cell-targeted DNA vaccination. *Proc. Natl. Acad. Sci. USA* 98, 9318–9323.

Wurbel, M.A., Malissen, M., Guy-Grand, D., Meffre, E., Nussenzweig, M.C., Richelme, M., Carrier, A., and Malissen, B. (2001). Mice lacking the CCR9 CC-chemokine receptor show a mild impairment of early T- and B-cell development and a reduction in T-cell receptor gamma delta(+) gut intraepithelial lymphocytes. *Blood* 98, 2626–2632.

Xu-Amano, J., Kiyono, H., Jackson, R.J., Staats, H.F., Fujihashi, K., Burrows, P.D., Elson, C.O., Pillai, S., and McGhee, J.R. (1993). Helper T cell subsets for immunoglobulin A responses: Oral immunization with tetanus toxoid and cholera toxin as adjuvant selectively induces Th2 cells in mucosa associated tissues. *J. Exp. Med.* 178, 1309–1320.

Yamamoto, M., Kiyono, H. ,Yamamoto, S., Batanero, E., Kweon, M.N., Otake, S., Azuma, M. Takeda, Y., and McGhee, J.R. (1999). Direct effects on antigen-presenting cells and T lymphocytes explain the adjuvanticity of a nontoxic cholera toxin mutant. *J. Immunol.* 162, 7015–7021.

Yamamoto, M., Rennert, P., McGhee, J.R., Kweon, M.N., Yamamoto, S., Dohi, T., Otake, S., Bluethmann, H., Fujihashi, K., and Kiyono, H. (2000). Alternate mucosal immune system: organized Peyer's patches are not required for IgA responses in the gastrointestinal tract. *J. Immunol.* 164, 5184–5191.

Yu, J., and Langridge, W.H. (2001). A plant-based multicomponent vaccine protects mice from enteric diseases. *Nat. Biotechnol.* 19, 548–552.

Zabel, B.A., Agace, W.W., Campbell, J.J., Heath, H.M., Parent, D., Roberts, A.I., Ebert, E.C., Kassam, N., Qin, S., Zovko, M., LaRosa, G.J., Yang, L.L., Soler, D., Butcher, E.C., Ponath, P.D., Parker, C.M., and Andrew, D.P. (1999). Human G protein-coupled receptor GPR-9-6/CC chemokine receptor 9 is selectively expressed on intestinal homing T lymphocytes, mucosal lymphocytes, and thymocytes and is required for thymus-expressed chemokine-mediated chemotaxis. *J. Exp. Med.* 190, 1241–1256.

Enteric Bacterial Vaccines: *Salmonella, Shigella, Vibrio cholerae, Escherichia coli*

Chapter 48

James P. Nataro

Center for Vaccine Development, University of Maryland School of Medicine, Baltimore, Maryland

Jan R. Holmgren

Department of Medical Microbiology and Immunology, and Göteborg University Vaccine Research Institute, Göteborg University, Göteborg, Sweden

Myron M. Levine

Center for Vaccine Development, University of Maryland School of Medicine, Baltimore, Maryland

Enteric bacterial infections remain among the most important infectious diseases. Estimates of diarrheal disease mortality suggest that at least 2 million persons succumb annually to diarrhea, and in countless others, the infections aggravate malnutrition and its attendant ills. Prevention of enteric illness by virtue of improved hygiene and provision of sanitation and water treatment is impractical in most developing countries, where enteric disease–related morbidity and mortality are highest. For this reason, development of vaccines against the most important gastrointestinal (GI) tract infections has been pursued aggressively. Here, we discuss the current status of vaccine efforts against four of the most important species causing gastrointestinal infection.

SALMONELLA VACCINES

Typhoid fever remains a major cause of morbidity and mortality in much of the developing world. Typhoid is maintained in developing populations via fecal contamination of food and water, due in part to the presence of active cases but also to the presence of long-term asymptomatic carriers. The high mortality of untreated typhoid, coupled with the difficulty in controlling this disease at the population level, has mandated a high priority for the development of typhoid vaccines.

Parenteral typhoid vaccines have been available for over 100 years. The killed whole-cell vaccines, as initially developed by Pfeiffer and Kolle and by Wright and Semple, demonstrated acceptable efficacy, but at the cost of significant reactogenicity, unacceptable by today's standards. The recently introduced purified Vi vaccine is about 70% efficacious over 10 years of follow-up, with a low rate of adverse reactions. However, parenteral vaccines can be difficult to administer in developing populations, providing impetus to the development of oral vaccines.

Live attenuated *Salmonella* vaccines

The affinity of *Salmonella typhi* for the gut-associated lymphoreticular tissue (GALT) makes it an ideal candidate for attenuation as a strategy in vaccine development. In the 1970s, Germanier and Furer derived an effective attenuated *S. typhi* vaccine (designated Ty21a) by nonspecific chemical mutagenesis of parent strain Ty2 (Germanier and Fuer, 1975). Ty21a harbors a galactose epimerase mutation, does not express the Vi (virulence) capsular polysaccharide, and exhibits many additional mutations that collectively contribute to its attenuation. When given in three to four doses on alternate days, the vaccine provides >70% efficacy against typhoid fever, with a very low incidence of adverse reactions (Levine *et al.*, 1990). However, the need for multiple doses limits the utility of this vaccine as a public health tool.

The advent of genetic engineering provides an opportunity to develop improved *Salmonella* vaccines by introducing defined mutations. Several such engineered vaccines have shown promise in humans. These include Ty800 (attenuated by virtue of mutation in the two-component regulatory system PhoPQ) (Hohmann *et al.*, 1996); x4372 (inactivated in the CRP transcriptional regulator and the *cdt* locus) (Tacket *et al.*, 1992a); CVD 908-*htrA* (inactivated in aromatic biosynthesis pathway and production of a stress protease) (Tacket *et al.*, 2000b); and ZH9 (inactivated in the aromatic biosynthesis pathway and the *Salmonella* pathogenicity island–2 type III secretion system secreton) (Hindle *et al.*, 2002).

The most advanced in terms of development is CVD 908-*htrA*, derived from a prior construct called CVD 908 (Hone *et al.*, 1991). Both of these vaccines are attenuated by virtue of two nonreverting deletion mutations within the chromosomal *aroC* and *aroD* genes. *AroC* and *aroD* encode enzymes critical in the biosynthetic pathway, leading to synthesis of chorismate, the key precursor required for synthesis of the aromatic amino acids (Hoiseth and Stocker, 1981); chorismate is further required for the synthesis of *p*-aminobenzoic acid, which is ultimately converted to the purine nucleotides ATP and GTP. In multiple studies, volunteers immunized with CVD 908 developed excellent immune responses with few and mild adverse reactions (Tacket *et al.*, 1992b). However, a silent vaccinemia was detected in 100% of volunteers who ingested 5×10^8 colony-forming units (cfu), wherein vaccine organisms were recovered from blood cultures collected between days 4 and 8 after vaccination (Levine *et al.*, 1996, 1997). Accordingly, further attenuation to obviate vaccinemias was pursued.

CVD 908 was therefore attenuated further by the introduction of a defined deletion mutation in the *htrA* gene, which encodes a heat shock–induced serine protease responsible for degradation of misfolded periplasmic proteins (Pallen and Wren, 1997). As expected, CVD 908-*htrA* was well tolerated at doses up to 5×10^9 and did not result in vaccinemias (Tacket *et al.*, 1997b). Volunteers ingesting CVD 908-*htrA* manifested a broad immune response to *S. typhi* antigens, including both cellular and humoral responses, which included both intestinal secretory IgA (S-IgA) and serum IgG.

Curtiss and colleagues have constructed *S. typhi* strains attenuated by deletion of adenylate cyclase (*cya*) and cyclic AMP (cAMP) receptor genes (*crp*). The gene products of *cya* and *crp* have multiple effects on bacterial transport and regulation of both housekeeping and virulence-related genes. Since the introduction of these two mutations alone was insufficiently attenuating in *S. typhi* strain Ty2 (Tacket *et al.*, 1992a), an additional mutation was introduced in the *cdt* locus, implicated in the ability of the bacterium to invade host tissue (Nardelli-Haefliger *et al.*, 1996; Tacket *et al.*, 1997a). When given in three doses of up to 10^9 cfu, the vaccine was well-tolerated and acceptably immunogenic.

Ty800 is a derivative of *S. typhi* Ty2, attenuated by deletion of the PhoPQ two-component regulatory system. The PhoPQ regulon includes a number of unlinked virulence-associated genes implicated in resistance to host defenses (Miller *et al.*, 1993). In escalating single-dose volunteer trials, Ty800 induced fever and diarrhea at a dose of 4×10^{10} cfu. Lower doses were less immunogenic but were better tolerated. A dose of 6×10^8 cfu was well-tolerated and elicited a mean number of anti–*S. typhi* lipopolysaccharide (LPS) antibody-forming cells (AFCs) of 833 per 10^6 peripheral blood mononuclear cells (PBMCs). This vaccine is undergoing further development, including its use as a vaccine vector.

A recent approach to the attenuation of specific virulence genes is the construction of strain ZH9, which consists of Ty2 attenuated in the SPI-2 pathogenicity island, as well as *aro C* (Hindle *et al.*, 2002; Khan *et al.*, 2003). SPI-2 products are required for survival of *S. typhi* within the phagosomal vacuole. In an escalating single-dose trial, ZH9 was well tolerated at doses as high as 10^9 cfu. Anti-LPS AFCs were observed at all doses, with a mean of 21 AFCs/10^6 PBMCs (Hindle *et al.*, 2002). Immunogenicity was not dose-related.

The versatility of *S. typhi* as a vector to deliver foreign antigens has been well documented. Volunteers receiving two doses of *S. typhi* CVD 908 expressing the *Plasmodium falciparum* circumsporozoite protein (CSP) developed CTLs to CSP-transfected target cells (Gonzalez *et al.*, 1994). In another study, 21 healthy adult volunteers received a single dose of CVD 908*htrA* carrying plasmid-encoded tetanus toxin fragment C under the control of one or two different *in vivo*–expressed promoters (p*nirB* and p*lpp*) (Tacket *et al.*, 2000a). Neither vaccine induced fever or vaccinemia. Of three seronegative volunteers who received a 10^9 cfu dose of CVD 908*htrA* (pTET*lpp*), a single oral dose of the live vector expressing fragment C seroconverted one of the three and elicited a rise in serum tetanus antitoxin 43 times above the protective level.

McKenzie and colleagues fed CVD 908-*htrA* expressing *H. pylori* urease to healthy volunteers at doses up to ~ 5×10^9 cfu (McKenzie *et al.*, 2002); the vaccine was well tolerated and induced urease-specific IgA and IgG AFCs in 25% and 88% of the vaccinated subjects.

With the ability of *S. typhi* to deliver foreign antigens established, attention has turned to improving the technical aspects of heterologous gene expression (Galen and Levine, 2001). Accordingly, genetic tools have been developed to express heterologous antigens from strong *in vivo*–induced promoters; ensure recombinant plasmid replication in the absence of antibiotic selection (Galen *et al.*, 1999); and enable secretion of foreign antigens to the extracellular milieu. With experience and expertise accumulating rapidly, the future of *Salmonella* as a live attenuated vector vaccine appears bright.

SHIGELLA VACCINES

Shigella species remain important enteric pathogens in many parts of the world. A recent analysis of the global burden of *Shigella* infections estimated 164 million episodes of such infection per year worldwide, with a resultant 1.1 million deaths annually (Kotloff *et al.*, 1999). Greater than 99% of this disease occurs in developing countries, where it is most severe in young children, with 69% of all episodes and 61% of all deaths occurring in children under 5 years of age. *Shigella* infects humans with doses as low as 100 organisms or even less, complicating control by affordable hygienic interventions. The shigellae cause diarrhea that is frequently persistent and/or severe, encompassing loss of fluid, electrolytes, and protein. Thus, vaccine development for *Shigella* continues to be a high global priority.

Four species of *Shigella* cause significant disease in humans: *S. dysenteriae*, *S. flexneri*, *S. sonnei*, and *S. boydii*. All *Shigella* species invade the colonic epithelium through M cells and then proceed to spread from cell to cell (Sansonetti, 2001a, b). Invasion is accompanied by inflammation of the mucosa, a clinical hallmark of the disease. The ability of *Shigella* to invade and spread through the epithelium is mediated by specialized factors encoded on a high-molecular-weight virulence plasmid. *S. dysenteriae* 1, the most virulent *Shigella* serotype, also elaborates Shiga toxin, which inhibits protein synthesis in eukaryotic cells and leads to severe systemic complications.

Epidemiologic and volunteer studies suggest that protective immunity to *Shigella* is directed to the somatic-O antigen and is type-specific (Ferreccio *et al.*, 1991). Although the four species of *Shigella* are divided into more than 47 serotypes, some serotypes are more common than others (Kotloff *et al.*, 1999).

Live attenuated vaccines
The potential of live attenuated *Shigella* vaccines was demonstrated in the 1960s independently by Mel (Mel *et al.*, 1971; Mel *et al.*, 1968) and Formal (Formal *et al.*, 1966). Mel *et al.* tested two different attenuated strains, including a streptomycin-dependent (SmD) mutant and a serially passaged *Shigella* strain (Istrati T_{32}) (Mel *et al.*, 1968, 1971). Though both vaccines were only mildly immunogenic (requiring multiple high doses), each provided respectable efficacy and elicited few adverse reactions. Formal published a report of similar success with a *Shigella/E. coli* chromosomal hybrid strain (Formal *et al.*, 1966).

As with *Salmonella* vaccines, the advent of genetic engineering technology has brought vigorous efforts to prepare more immunogenic *Shigella* vaccines by precise mutagenesis. These efforts have focused either on introducing metabolic auxotrophies that will result in global attenuation of the organism or on specific virulence-related traits.

In this regard, one group constructed SFL124, a *Shigella flexneri* Y strain mutated at the *aroA* locus (Lindberg *et al.*, 1990). The SFL124 was generally well tolerated and immunogenic in volunteers. One or three doses of 2×10^9 cfu elicited *Shigella*-specific anti-LPS antibody responses in serum and stool and AFCs in peripheral blood (Li *et al.*, 1992). In field studies of SFL124 on Vietnamese adults and children, the vaccine was found to be safe and immunogenic (Li *et al.*, 1993, 1994). In a second similar construct, an *aroD* mutation was introduced into *S. flexneri* 2a strain SFL1070. This strain produced mild adverse reactions in volunteers in

a dose-dependent fashion; the most severe symptoms of abdominal pain, fever, or watery diarrhea were experienced by approximately half of the volunteers ingesting 10^9 cfu (Karnell *et al.*, 1995). Experience with these vaccines demonstrates that a single mutation strategy may not yield identical results in all host strains, a theme that will be seen again. Nevertheless, these early live, attenuated vaccine candidates demonstrated the feasibility and promise of using an auxotrophic mutant as an enteric vaccine but indicated that achieving the correct balance between immunogenicity and lack of reactogenicity is a challenge.

In a different strategy, Sansonetti and coworkers made a series of strains with mutations in the *icsA (virG)* gene, which is involved in cell-to-cell spread of *Shigella* within the intestinal epithelium (Bernardini *et al.*, 1989). This approach was predicated on the assumption that if the *Shigella* strain could colonize the intestine and enter the epithelial cells, it would elicit an immune response, but the inability of the bacterium to spread through the epithelium would preclude enteric symptoms. Coupling this strategy with either additional virulence-related mutations or with metabolic auxotrophies, Sansonetti and coworkers have produced the strain *S. flexneri* 5a, containing mutations in *virG* and *ompB* or *virG* and *iuc*, the last encoding the iron-scavenging molecule aerobactin (Sansonetti *et al.*, 1991). In animal studies, the *ompB*, *virG* strain was well tolerated but only mildly immunogenic (Sansonetti *et al.*, 1991), whereas the *virG*, *iuc* strain was 100% protective but reactogenic (Sansonetti and Arondel, 1989). Subsequently, an *S. flexneri* 2a vaccine was constructed including *virG* and *iuc* mutations (SC602). In clinical trials, ingestion of 10^6 or 10^8 cfu caused symptoms of mild shigellosis in most volunteers, while a dose of 10^4 caused only mild symptoms in a few volunteers (Coster *et al.*, 1999). In subsequent challenge studies, volunteers ingesting a single dose of 10^4 SC602 were protected against challenge with wild-type *S. flexneri* 2a. Further studies on this vaccine candidate are under way.

Whereas a *virG* mutation alone is not sufficiently attenuating in *S. flexneri*, a *virG* mutant of *S. sonnei*, designated WRSS1, is only mildly reactogenic. In phase 1 clinical trials, a single dose of 10^3, 10^4, 10^5, or 10^6 cfu caused low-grade fever or mild diarrhea in 22% of recipients (Kotloff *et al.*, 2002). Moreover, the vaccine was highly immunogenic, generating strong serum anti-LPS and anti-LPS IgA AFC responses.

Noriega and coworkers constructed an *S. flexneri* 2a strain with mutations in *aroA* and *virG* (Noriega *et al.*, 1994), designated CVD 1203. Doses of 10^8 or 10^9 cfu of CVD 1203 elicited short-lived, dose-related adverse reactions, including fever, diarrhea, and/or mild dysentery (Kotloff *et al.*, 1996). Importantly, however, a single dose of 10^6 cfu was immunogenic and well tolerated by all subjects. Following this positive start, but with a desire to further attenuate the organism, Noriega and coworkers constructed *S. flexneri* 2a CVD 1204, harboring a deletion in the *guaBA* operon. This mutation renders the bacterium auxotrophic for guanine, which is not available in human tissues or the lumen of the gastrointestinal tract. Two further derivatives of CVD 1204 carried additional mutations in one or both of two *Shigella* entero-toxins: ShET1, encoded by the *set* genes, and ShET2, encoded by the *sen* gene. Human studies of these vaccine candidates are under way.

Non-*Shigella* vector vaccines

The principal protective antigen in *Shigella* infection appears to be the LPS-associated O antigen, which determines the serogroup of the strain. Presentation of *Shigella* LPS in the context of a non-*Shigella* vaccine vector has been accomplished by a number of investigators. As early as 1981, Formal and colleagues expressed the O antigen of *S. sonnei* in *S. typhi* vaccine strain Ty21A (see previous section) (Formal *et al.*, 1981) to create strain 5076-1C. Initial trials showed the strain to be well tolerated and protective against challenge, but these results were not consistently reproducible, varying by lot tested (Black *et al.*, 1987a; Herrington *et al.*, 1990; Tramont *et al.*, 1984). An *E. coli/S. flexneri* chromosomal hybrid strain, *EcSf*2a-2, was constructed by classical genetic techniques and comprised an *aroD*-deleted enteroinvasive *E. coli* strain expressing the LPS of *S. flexneri* 2a (Newland *et al.*, 1992). Strain *EcSf*2a-2 was subject to several volunteer studies and field studies. Volunteer studies showed the vaccine to be generally well tolerated but insufficiently immunogenic (Kotloff *et al.*, 1992a, 1995).

Parenteral *Shigella* vaccines

Robbins and coworkers have produced parenteral conjugate vaccines consisting of purified *Shigella* LPS conjugated to a protein carrier (Robbins, 1992). Three conjugate vaccines have been tested, including *S. dysenteriae* 1 LPS conjugated to tetanus toxoid, *S. flexneri* 2a LPS conjugated to recombinant *Pseudomonas* exoprotein A, and *S. sonnei* LPS conjugated to exoprotein A. These three candidates were immunogenic and protective against shigellosis in field trials with the Israeli Defense Force (Chu *et al.*, 1991; Cohen *et al.*, 1996; Taylor *et al.*, 1993). Further refinements of these vaccines are under way (Passwell *et al.*, 2001). Such parenteral vaccines may be useful for travelers but are impractical for use in developing countries. In addition, the many serogroups within the genus *Shigella* constitute a daunting obstacle to LPS-based vaccination strategies.

VACCINES AGAINST CHOLERA

Cholera continues to be responsible for substantial morbidity and economic disruption in endemic regions of the developing world. *Vibrio cholerae* is a noninvasive organism that colonizes the lining epithelium of the GI tract after penetrating the mucus layer. It affects the small intestine through its secreted cholera toxin (CT) that is composed of five receptor-binding B subunits surrounding one toxic-active A subunit. For its toxic action, CT is dependent on a specific receptor, the monosialosyl ganglioside GM1. Binding of CT increases the intestinal levels of cAMP by increasing the adenylate cyclase activity, and it results in secretion of chloride and bicarbonate into the small intestine. As a result, water is drawn from the intravascular and extracellular spaces of the body and is rapidly lost into the GI tract lumen.

Protective immunity in cholera is mediated mainly by antibodies produced locally in the intestinal mucosa and secreted onto the gut mucosal surface. These antibodies are directed against bacterial components including, as the main protective antigens, cell-surface LPS O-antigen and CT, and they protect by inhibiting bacterial colonization and multiplication and by blocking toxin action.

Whereas aggressive oral rehydration therapy is effective for mild and moderate cases of cholera, severe cases require intravenous rehydration, which represents a problem for cases that do not have ready access to medical care. For this reason, and to protect certain travelers to endemic and epidemic regions, the development of a safe and effective cholera vaccine is a priority. Two oral cholera vaccines, one live attenuated and one inactivated, have been licensed in many countries.

Live attenuated *Vibrio cholerae* vaccines

Given that the principal virulence factor of *V. cholerae* is CT itself, development of a live vaccine deleted for CT was an obvious first approach. Unfortunately, several such constructs have proven to retain reactogenicity in human trials. Additional attenuating mutations have therefore been introduced, giving rise to a series of attenuated cholera vaccines with substantial promise.

CVD 103-HgR (*ctxA⁻*, *hly⁻*, classical Inaba strain 569B) was the first recombinant live attenuated cholera vaccine that proved to be well tolerated, immunogenic, and protective, and it is the only such vaccine currently licensed for human use. CVD 103-HgR is derived from *V. cholerae* O1 classic Inaba strain 569B, which shows a mild defect in its ability to colonize the mouse and human intestine (Levine *et al.*, 1988). In addition to deletions in the catalytic A subunit of CT, CVD 103-HgR also harbors mutations in the putative virulence factor Hly (which is not expressed by classical biotype strains). CVD 103-HgR has been administered to more than 6,000 individuals in a series of placebo-controlled phase 1 and phase 2 trials (Acheson *et al.*, 1996; Cookson *et al.*, 1997; Cryz *et al.*, 1990, 1992, 1995; Gotuzzo *et al.*, 1993; Kaper *et al.*, 1994; Kotloff *et al.*, 1992b; Lagos *et al.*, 1995, 1999a,b; Levine *et al.*, 1988; Losonsky *et al.*, 1993; Migasena *et al.*, 1989; Perry *et al.*, 1998; Richie *et al.*, 2000; Simanjuntak *et al.*, 1993; Su-Arehawaratana *et al.*, 1992; Suharyono *et al.*, 1992; Tacket *et al.*, 1992c, 1999; Taylor *et al.*, 1997, 1999). In all studies, neither diarrhea nor any other adverse reaction occurred significantly more often in vaccinees than in placebo recipients. CVD 103-HgR is highly immunogenic and protective against wild-type challenge in a single dose. In a randomized, double-blind, placebo-controlled multicenter trial, a single dose of this strain conferred 91% protective efficacy against moderate or severe diarrhea after challenge with toxigenic El Tor *V. cholerae* (Tacket *et al.*, 1999). Protection is observed as early as 8 days after vaccination and lasts for at least 6 months, the longest interval tested (Tacket *et al.*, 1992c). These data strongly support the utility of CVD 103-HgR as a vaccine for travelers to areas of endemicity.

The ability of CVD 103-HgR to provide long-term protection against natural cholera infection among populations living in areas of endemicity has been more difficult to prove. In a 4-year prospective study in Indonesia, only 14% overall efficacy was observed (Richie *et al.*, 2000). However, during the first 6 months of this trial (when protection should be strongest), few cases of cholera occurred in the study cohort; protection was observed during this period, but the number of cases was too small to reach statistical significance. In postlicensure evaluation conducted during a cholera outbreak in Micronesia, the vaccine provided 79% effectiveness against clinical cholera (Claire-Lise Chaignat, World Health Organization, personal communication), an observation more consistent with volunteer studies.

Several nonmotile derivatives have been evaluated as cholera vaccines. The most promising of these vaccines is Peru-15, derived by deleting the CT genetic element, introducing the gene encoding CT B subunit (CT-B) into *recA*, and screening for nonmotility in a *V. cholerae* O1 El Tor Inaba strain (Cohen *et al.*, 2002; Sack *et al.*, 1997). In a recent trial, 59 volunteers were randomly allocated to groups to receive either a single dose of 2×10^8 cfu of Peru-15 or placebo; 3 months later, 36 of these volunteers were challenged with approximately 10^5 cfu of virulent *V. cholerae* O1 El Tor Inaba strain N16961(Cohen *et al.*, 2002). Five (42%) of the 12 placebo recipients and none (0%) of the 24 vaccinees developed moderate or severe diarrhea on challenge ($P = 0.002$; protective efficacy, 100%). A total of 7 (58%) of the 12 placebo recipients and 1 (4%) of the 24 vaccinees had any diarrhea ($P < 0.001$; protective efficacy, 93%). Peru-15 is a promising vaccine candidate that is undergoing further clinical development.

Several other live attenuated cholera vaccine candidates have been tested in early clinical trials, and some offer promise (Benitez *et al.*, 1999; Liu *et al.*, 1995; Taylor *et al.*, 1997, 1999; Yamamoto, 2000). Moreover, work done in this area has illuminated important scientific concepts in live attenuated vaccine science.

Killed whole-cell cholera vaccine

An oral cholera vaccine consisting of the nontoxic, highly immunogenic CTB protein, in combination with heat- and formalin-killed *V. cholerae* O1 classical and El Tor vibrios, has been developed in Sweden. This CT-B-whole-cell (B-WC) vaccine, which is given together with a bicarbonate buffer to preserve the B subunit pentameric structure, has been tested extensively in clinical trials, including large field studies, and has proved to be safe and protective against cholera and also, to a lesser extent, against diarrhea caused by enterotoxigenic *E. coli* (ETEC) producing CT-like heat-labile enterotoxin (LT) (Holmgren *et al.*, 1994; Jertborn *et al.*, 1994; van Loon *et al.*, 1996). This vaccine is licensed in over 20 countries world-wide. Another oral killed whole-cell vaccine modeled on the Swedish vaccine, but which does not include CT-B,

has been developed and produced in Vietnam (Trach *et al.*, 1997, 2002), and analogous locally produced, whole-cell vaccines are also under development in Indonesia, China, and India.

The B-WC vaccine was designed to evoke antitoxic as well as antibacterial intestinal immunity, since in animal studies these types of immunity have been shown to provide synergistic cooperative protection (Svennerholm and Holmgren, 1976). Phase 1 and phase 2 clinical studies established that the B-WC vaccine does not cause any detectable side effects and that, after either two or three doses, it stimulates a GI tract mucosal IgA antitoxic and antibacterial immune response (including memory) comparable to that induced by cholera disease itself (Jertborn *et al.*, 1992, 1994; Svennerholm *et al.*, 1984). Furthermore, immunization with the complete B-WC vaccine was found to protect American volunteers against challenge with a dose of live cholera vibrios (biotype El Tor) that caused disease in 100% of concurrently tested unvaccinated controls; oral vaccination with the WC component alone induced protection against challenge, which was only marginally less than that afforded by the B-WC vaccine (Black *et al.*, 1987b). On this basis, a large, double-blind placebo-controlled field trial with more than 90,000 participants was undertaken in rural Bangladesh with a prototype B-WC vaccine. The results established that both the B-WC vaccine and the WC component alone protect against cholera of either classic or El Tor biotype. The B-WC vaccine had a higher initial efficacy level than the WC vaccine (85% versus 58% for the initial 4- to 6-month period) (Clemens *et al.*, 1986). The B-WC continued to be significantly more protective than the WC-alone vaccine for the first 8 months after vaccination. Thereafter, the efficacy was similar: approximately 60% for both vaccines over a 2-year follow-up period, as estimated for a vaccinated population older than 2 years (Clemens *et al.*, 1990). Still higher (about 70%) long-term protective efficacy was seen in those over age 5 years when vaccinated. A secondary subgroup analysis suggested that protection was of similar magnitude after two or three doses of vaccine (Clemens *et al.*, 1990).

Three field trials of efficacy were undertaken with a definitive commercial formulation of the B-WC vaccine. The first study was a randomized, placebo-controlled efficacy field trial among Peruvian military personnel in 1992, soon after cholera first appeared in Peru (Sanchez *et al.*, 1994). This trial differed in many respects from the Bangladesh trial: for example, only two doses of vaccine were used, the vaccine contained recombinant rather than native B subunit, all cholera was caused by the El Tor biotype (apparently due to a common-source outbreak that occurred several weeks after vaccination), and the attack rate in the placebo group was very high. The protective efficacy (PE) observed during the 5-month follow-up period was strikingly similar to the efficacy during the same follow-up period in Bangladesh (PE = 85%; 95% confidence interval [CI], 36–97%; $P = 0.004$ for comparison with the placebo group).

A large field trial involving civilian adults and children was also conducted in Peru (Taylor *et al.*, 2000). In this study, two primary vaccinations were given to all subjects, regardless of age, followed by a third booster dose after 1 year. The analysis of this study was the subject of some debate (Clemens *et al.*, 2001). No protection (0% efficacy) was seen during the first year of surveillance, when very few patients with cholera sought treatment at a hospital and the cholera cases recorded were identified by active surveillance. However, during the second year, following a third booster dose and when there were more hospitalized patients, there was 60% protection against cholera (78% protection against cases necessitating hospitalization).

Through its B subunit component, the B-WC vaccine also has been shown to provide substantial short-term protection against diarrhea caused by LT-producing ETEC (Clemens *et al.*, 1988; Peltola *et al.*, 1991; Scerpella *et al.*, 1995). In the cholera vaccine trial in Bangladesh, the protection against disease caused by ETEC producing LT or LT together with heat-stable toxin (ST) was about 67% for the first 3 months after vaccination. The protection was more pronounced against ETEC diarrhea associated with severe life-threatening dehydration (86% efficacy) than against milder disease (56% efficacy) (Clemens *et al.*, 1988).

Two randomized, placebo-controlled studies have also evaluated protection by the B-WC cholera vaccine against ETEC diarrhea in travelers. The first study involved Finnish travelers going to Morocco (Peltola *et al.*, 1991), among whom a protective efficacy of 60% was seen against LT-producing ETEC. A second travel study involved U.S. students going to Mexico (Scerpella *et al.*, 1995). In contrast to the Finnish tourists, who were vaccinated before departure, the U.S. students in this study were vaccinated immediately upon arrival in Mexico. This was unfortunate, since the majority of diarrhea cases occurred during the first 2 weeks after arrival, when the vaccine could not be expected to protect. When only cases occurring more than 7 days after the second vaccination were considered, there was 50% (CI, 14–71%) protection against all ETEC diarrhea.

In Vietnam, a whole-cell vaccine modeled on the Swedish WC vaccine has been developed and locally produced for an estimated cost of U.S. $0.20 per dose. This vaccine was evaluated in a large-scale field trial conducted in more than 22,000 households in the central coastal city of Hue. Persons aged over 1 year were allocated in alternate households to receive two doses of vaccine or no vaccine (67,000 persons in each group). During an outbreak of El Tor cholera that occurred 8 to 10 months after vaccination, 66% protection was noted among the persons who received the two-dose vaccine regimen, and protection was similar for children aged 1 to 5 years (68%) and for older persons (66%) (Trach *et al.*, 1997). Recently, a second generation of this vaccine, comprising O139 vibrios in addition to the O1 whole-cell component, has been prepared and tested with good results in a phase 2 trial in Vietnam (Trach *et al.*, 2002). These findings clearly lend encouragement to the notion that an inexpensive, locally produced, effective oral cholera vaccine may

be within reach of the limited health care budget of poor countries with endemic cholera (Svennerholm and Holmgren, 1976). Work is in progress to produce similar oral whole-cell cholera vaccines for local use also in Indonesia, China, and India.

DIARRHEAGENIC *ESCHERICHIA COLI* VACCINES

Escherichia coli is the most abundant facultative anaerobic bacterium in the human intestine. As such, the mucosal immune system is highly tolerant of this organism and does not mount a significant ongoing immune response to *E. coli* antigens. However, at least six distinct pathotypes of *E. coli* have evolved the capacity to induce enteric disease (reviewed in Nataro and Kaper, 1998). The two most important of these pathotypes, from a public health perspective, are Shiga toxin–producing *E. coli* (STEC, also known as Vero-toxin producing and enterohemorrhagic *E. coli* [EHEC]) and enterotoxigenic *E. coli* (ETEC), a major cause of both traveler's diarrhea and weanling diarrhea in developing countries. STEC commonly colonizes bovine herds in the United States and other industrialized countries. It causes disease in humans following ingestion of a very small infectious dose, and its eradication from the food supply is a formidable task. Therefore, there is considerable interest in vaccine development for high-risk human or bovine populations. The infectious dose of ETEC is a great deal higher than that of STEC, yet its substantial contribution to diarrhea in developing countries renders it an important target of vaccine development efforts. ETEC vaccine development is driven by the financial incentive of preventing traveler's diarrhea, yet an effective vaccine may also make an impact on pediatric diarrhea in tropical countries.

Shiga-toxin-producing *E. coli*

STEC derive their name from their carriage of the phage encoding Shiga toxin (Stx), first characterized in *Shigella dysenteriae* (Sandvig, 2001; Kaper, 1998; Tarr and Neill, 2001). STEC colonize the colonic mucosa and induce local damage without significant invasion. Infection is accompanied by watery diarrhea, frequently progressing to frank hemorrhagic colitis (Tarr and Neill, 2001). Systemic absorption of Stx leads to serious sequelae, including hemolytic uremic syndrome (HUS), which develops in up to 20% of pediatric patients. Other potentially fatal complications include intestinal perforation and cerebrovascular accident. Epidemiologically and clinically, the most important STEC clone belongs to serotype O157:H7. In addition to Stx, this bacterium expresses an impressive array of virulence-related factors, including adherence factors and secreted host-damaging proteins (reviewed in Tarr and Neill, 2001).

Shiga toxin toxoids

Stx is comprised of a single catalytic A subunit of 32 kDa and five B subunits of 7.7 kDa each (reviewed in Sandvig,

2001). The B subunit mediates binding to the cell via the glycolipid globotriaosylceramide (Gb3). The A subunit is an N-glycosidase that catalyzes the depurination of a single site in the 28S eukaryotic rRNA, thereby inhibiting protein synthesis and leading to the death of the target cell. The Stx family comprises two subgroups, Stx1 and Stx2, sharing 55% amino acid identity with little immunologic cross-reactivity. Most cases of HUS are attributable to Stx2.

Antibodies against the Stx B subunit will prevent binding of the toxin to target cells (Marcato et al., 2001). However, the A–B complex is considerably more immunogenic than the B subunit alone, and thus both B and A–B toxoids have drawn attention as vaccine candidates. The B subunit mediates the binding of Stx to the eukaryotic cell, but it may itself elicit some response on the part of the cell (Marcato et al., 2002); therefore, use of StxB as a vaccine may require some degree of inactivation.

Keusch and colleagues have demonstrated that parenteral administration of Stx2 inactivated with formalin-lysine provided 100% protection to mice subsequently challenged intraperitoneally with 1000 LD_{50} Stx2 (Keusch et al., 1998). Whereas it is unlikely that parenteral immunization will be accepted as a vaccine strategy for STEC infection, such a vaccine may have application in management of epidemics of *S. dysenteriae* infection.

Mucosal immunization is likely to be a more acceptable route for Stx administration. Byun et al. and coworkers (2001) immunized mice nasally with purified recombinant Stx1B, accompanied by a cholera toxin adjuvant. Brisk serum IgG and mucosal IgA antibody responses and the serum antibody binding of Stx to its receptor were observed.

O-specific polysaccharide conjugate vaccines

Parenteral administration of the O157 polysaccharide may engender systemic IgG antibodies that transudate into the GI tract, potentially reducing colonization by O157:H7. However, although an *E. coli* O157 polysaccharide–albumin conjugate elicited a strong serum antibody response in mice, the vaccine did not protect the mice from intestinal colonization by *E. coli* O157 (Conlan et al., 1999a). Similarly, mice orally vaccinated with a glycoconjugate vaccine containing the O157 antigen mixed with CT as adjuvant were not protected from colonization with O157:H7 (Conlan et al., 2000). It is also important to note that non-O157 serogroups are an important cause of diarrhea and HUS, especially outside of the United States (Nataro and Kaper, 1998). Therefore, reliance on anti-O157 immunity will not provide complete protection against STEC disease.

Live attenuated STEC vaccine candidates

Most efforts at developing live attenuated STEC vaccines have focused on the expression of Stx in live attenuated bacterial vectors. Stx2 has been coexpressed along with the STEC outer membrane protein adhesin intimin in an attenuated *V. cholerae* vector, Peru2 (Butterton et al., 1997). This construct was tested in a rabbit model and found to elicit antibodies to StxB; one of two rabbits responded to the

intimin protein. An *E. coli* hemolysin–based system has been adapted to facilitate secretion of STx2B across the outer membrane of an *S. typhimurium aroA* auxotrophic vaccine vector (Tzschaschel et al., 1996a,b). This construct exports StxB efficiently but has yet to be proven effective in humans.

Conlan et al. have found that orally administered *S. landau*, a *Salmonella* strain that naturally expresses the O157 antigen, is able to elicit protection of mice from colonization by *E. coli* O157 (Conlan et al., 1999b). These results suggest that mucosal exposure to the O157 antigen may induce resistance when delivered by *Salmonella*, although humans exposed to STEC do not generate highly protective O157 responses after natural infection. Perhaps the ability of *Salmonella* to target antigens to the mucosa-associated immune system may increase the response to the antigen. This vaccine and its associated concept are undergoing further examination.

Enterotoxigenic *E. coli*

ETEC infection in susceptible hosts is characterized by profuse watery diarrhea lasting several days. Infection is usually self-limited but may lead to dehydration, especially in infants and young children (Nataro and Kaper, 1998). ETEC causes disease following ingestion of contaminated food or water by attachment to the small bowel mucosa, followed by elaboration of heat labile toxin (LT) and/or heat stabile toxin (ST). Intestinal colonization is mediated by a large array of antigenically diverse adherence fimbriae called *coli* surface antigens (CSs) or colonization factor antigens (CFAs) (Cassels and Wolf, 1995); individual ETEC strains typically express one to three of the many CFAs described. More than 20 types of ETEC fimbriae have been identified on human isolates, with seven types occurring most frequently, including CFA/I and CS1 through CS6. Immune responses against these fimbriae appear to be at least partially protective in volunteers (Tacket et al., 1994).

Immunity to ETEC LT toxin may also contribute to protection. The LT holotoxin, similar to CT, is composed of a single catalytic A subunit and five identical B subunits, which mediate binding to eukaryotic cells. Anti-LT responses are elicited in most people who have had diarrhea due to ETEC (Stoll et al., 1986; Wennerås et al., 1999), and as noted above, CT-based vaccines provide some cross-protection against ETEC (Peltola et al., 1991). In contrast to LT, ST is not immunogenic and is not considered a candidate vaccine antigen.

Whole-cell CFA plus B subunit killed vaccine

The most advanced ETEC vaccine candidate consists of a killed whole-cell formulation plus recombinant cholera toxin B subunit (rCT-B). The vaccine comprises five strains of formalin-killed ETEC, which collectively express the most prevalent fimbriae: CFA/I and CS1 through CS6 (Holmgren and Svennerholm, 1998). This vaccine has been found to be safe and immunogenic in adult volunteers as well as in children between 2 and 12 years of age (Ahrén et al., 1998; Jertborn *et al.*, 1998; Savarino *et al.*, 1998). Immune responses, as measured by intestinal lavage and antibody, were elicited against rCT-B as well as each fimbrial type (Jertborn *et al.*, 1998). In addition, this vaccine has been found to be immunogenic when tested in endemic areas, including adults and children in Bangladesh and Egypt (Qadri *et al.*, 2000; Savarino *et al.*, 1998, 1999).

Live ETEC vaccines

Investigators at Acambis Ltd. in the United Kingdom have developed two live attenuated nontoxigenic ETEC prototype vaccine candidates, mutated at the *aroC* and *ompR* genes, or the *aroC, ompC,* and *ompF* genes. The common parent strain of both vaccines, E1392-75-2A1, expresses CS1 and CS3 (components of CFA/II) and would be expected to protect against organisms expressing one or both of these factors. Both vaccine candidates were fairly well tolerated by volunteers at doses of 10^7 to 10^9 cfu in a phase 1 study (Turner *et al.*, 2001). Immune responses to the fimbrial components were observed in volunteers ingesting the highest dose, although in this group 15% of volunteers developed mild diarrhea. Interestingly, this result is similar to that observed with the wild-type parent strain (Levine, 1984).

An alternative strategy being pursued by investigators at the University of Maryland Center for Vaccine Development involves presenting the ETEC fimbrial antigens in a live attenuated *Shigella* vaccine strain. Preclinical animal studies have shown candidate vaccine formulations to be immunogenic, eliciting serum and mucosal immune responses to both the *Shigella* vector and the ETEC antigens (Barry *et al.*, 2003). Such a vaccine may stimulate immunity against two diseases common in populations at risk.

ETEC subunit vaccines

Since inhibition of adherence by anti-pilus antibodies is an obvious strategy for ETEC vaccine development, direct administration of ETEC fimbriae has been attempted via multiple routes. However, oral administration of purified unprotected fimbriae results in degradation and denaturation in the acid pH of the stomach (Levine, 1986). Several strategies have been pursued to provide protection against degradation. Encapsulation of CFA/II components in polylactide–polyglycolide microspheres resulted in modest antifimbrial antibody responses but poor levels of protection against homologous challenge (Tacket *et al.*, 1994).

An alternative approach to stimulation of antipilus immunity is to bypass the stomach completely. Purified CS6 has been coadministered with LT (as both adjuvant and immunogen) via transcutaneous patch (Guerena-Burgueno *et al.*, 2002; Yu *et al.*, 2002). In one study, subjects received patches containing 250, 500, 1000, or 2000 µg of CS6 alone or with 500 µg of LT, dosed at 0, 1, and 3 months. In the absence of LT, there were no demonstrable immune responses to the CS6 antigen; however, when CS6 was given with LT, 68% and 53% had anti-CS6 IgG and IgA antibodies, respectively, and 100% and 90% had anti-LT IgG and IgA antibodies, respectively. Fourteen (74%) of 19 volunteers developed mild delayed-type hypersensitivity (DTH) skin reactions after the second or third dose, but no other adverse events were reported.

Several additional strategies have been employed to present ETEC antigens to the human immune system. One creative approach is expression of foreign proteins in edible plants (Tacket *et al.*, 1998; Yu and Langridge, 2001). Expression of LT in transgenic potatoes resulted in induction of anti-LT antibodies in rabbits and humans. DNA vaccines have also been adapted to deliver ETEC fimbrial antigens. Alves *et al.* immunized mice with DNA encoding the CFA/I fimbrial subunit and derived antibodies capable of blocking fimbrial adhesion (Alves *et al.*, 2000).

SUMMARY AND CONCLUDING REMARKS

Despite the implementation of oral rehydration therapy and the availability of powerful antibiotics, enteric diseases remain a high public health priority for much of the world's population. Improvement of sanitation and hygiene would have a favorable impact on this problem, but resources are not available to effect these interventions worldwide. Thus, vaccines against some diarrheal diseases are needed urgently. There has been much success in this arena, but much more needs to be done. Solutions will depend upon both new and old technologies and on continued dedication of human and financial resources to address problems of global significance.

REFERENCES

Acheson, D.W., Levine, M.M., Kaper, J.B., and Keusch, G.T. (1996). Protective immunity to Shiga-like toxin I following oral immunization with Shiga-like toxin I B-subunit-producing *Vibrio cholerae* CVD 103-HgR. *Infect. Immun.* 64, 355–357.

Ahren, C., Jertborn, M., and Svennerholm, A.M. (1998). Intestinal immune responses to an inactivated oral enterotoxigenic *Escherichia coli* vaccine and associated immunoglobulin A responses in blood. *Infect. Immun.* 66, 3311–3316.

Alves, A.M., Lasaro, M.O., Almeida, D.F., and Ferreira, L.C. (2000). DNA immunisation against the CFA/I fimbriae of enterotoxigenic *Escherichia coli* (ETEC). *Vaccine* 19, 788–795.

Barry, E.M., Altboum, Z., Losonsky, G., and Levine, M.M. (2003). Immune responses elicited against multiple enterotoxigenic *Escherichia coli* fimbriae and mutant LT expressed in attenuated *Shigella* vaccine strains. *Vaccine* 21, 333–340.

Benitez, J.A., Garcia, L., Silva, A., Garcia, H., Fando, R., Cedre, B., Perez, A., Campos, J., Rodriguez, B.L., Perez, J.L., Valmaseda T., Perez, O., Perez, A., Ramirez, M., Ledon, T., Jidy, M.D., Lastre, M., Bravo, L., and Sierra, G. (1999). Preliminary assessment of the safety and immunogenicity of a new CTXPhi-negative, hemagglutinin/protease-defective El T or strain as a cholera vaccine candidate. *Infect. Immun.* 67, 539–545.

Bernardini, M.L., Mounier, J., d'Hauteville, H., Coquis-Randon, M., and Sansonetti, P.J. (1989). Identification of icsA, a plasmid locus of *Shigella flexneri* that governs bacterial intra- and intercellular spread through interaction with F-actin. *Proc. Natl. Acad. Sci. USA* 86, 3867–3871.

Black, R.E., Levine, M.M., Clements, M.L., Losonsky, G., Herrington, D., Berman, S., and Formal, S.B. (1987a). Prevention of shigellosis by a *Salmonella typhi-Shigella sonnei* bivalent vaccine. *J. Infect. Dis.* 155, 1260–1265.

Black, R.E., Levine, M.M., Clements, M.L.,Young, C.R., Svennerholm, A.M., and Holmgren, J. (1987b). Protective efficacy in humans of killed whole-vibrio oral cholera vaccine with and without the B subunit of cholera toxin. *Infect. Immun.* 55, 1116–1120.

Butterton, J.R., Ryan, E.T., Acheson, D.W., and Calderwood, S.B. (1997). Coexpression of the B subunit of Shiga toxin 1 and EaeA from enterohemorrhagic *Escherichia coli* in *Vibrio cholerae* vaccine strains. *Infect. Immun.* 65, 2127–2135.

Byun, Y., Ohmura, M., Fujihashi, K., Yamamoto, S., McGhee, J.R., Udaka, S., Kiyono, H., Takeda, Y., Kohsaka, T., and Yuki, Y. (2001). Nasal immunization with *E. coli* verotoxin 1 (VT1)-B subunit and a nontoxic mutant of cholera toxin elicits serum neutralizing antibodies. *Vaccine* 19, 2061–2070.

Cassels, F.J., and Wolf, M.K. (1995). Colonization factors of diarrheagenic *E. coli* and their intestinal receptors. *J. Ind. Microbiol.* 15, 214–226.

Chu, C.Y., Liu, B.K., Watson, D., Szu, S.S., Bryla, D., Shiloach, J., Schneerson, R., and Robbins, J.B. (1991). Preparation, characterization, and immunogenicity of conjugates composed of the O-specific polysaccharide of *Shigella dysenteriae* type 1 (Shiga's bacillus) bound to tetanus toxoid. *Infect. Immun.* 59, 4450–4458.

Clemens, J.D., Jertborn, M., Sack, D., Stanton, B., Holmgren, J., Khan, M.R., and Huda, S.. (1986). Effect of neutralization of gastric acid on immune responses to an oral B subunit, killed whole-cell cholera vaccine. *J. Infect. Dis.* 154, 175–178.

Clemens, J.D., Harris, J.R., Sack, D.A., Chakraborty, J., Ahmed, F., Stanton B.F., Khan, M.U., Kay, B.A., Huda, N., and Khan, M.R. (1988). Field trial of oral cholera vaccines in Bangladesh: results of one year of follow-up. *J. Infect. Dis.* 158, 60–69.

Clemens, J.D., Sack, D.A., Harris, J.R., Van Loon, F., Chakraborty, J., Ahmed, F., Rao, M.R., Khan, M.R., Yunu, M., and Huda, N. (1990). Field trial of oral cholera vaccines in Bangladesh: results from three-year follow-up. *Lancet* 335, 270–273.

Clemens, J.D., Sack, D.A., and Ivanoff, B. (2001). Misleading negative findings in a field trial of killed, oral cholera vaccine in Peru. *J. Infect. Dis.* 183, 1306–1309.

Cohen, D., Ashkenazi, S., Green, M., Lerman,Y., Slepon, R., Robin, G., Orr, N., Taylor, D.N., Sadoff, J.C., Chu, C., Shiloach, J., Schneerson, R., and Robbins, J.B. (1996). Safety and immunogenicity of investigational *Shigella* conjugate vaccines in Israeli volunteers. *Infect. Immun.* 64, 4074–4077.

Cohen, M.B., Giannella, R.A., Bean, J., Taylor, D.N., Parker, S., Hoeper, A., Wowk, S., Hawkins, J., Kochi, S.K., Schiff, G., and Killeen, K.P. (2002). Randomized, controlled human challenge study of the safety, immunogenicity, and protective efficacy of a single dose of Peru-15, a live attenuated oral cholera vaccine. *Infect. Immun.* 70, 1965–1970.

Conlan, J.W., Cox, A.D., KuoLee, R., Webb, A., and Perry, M.B. (1999a). Parenteral immunization with a glycoconjugate vaccine containing the O157 antigen of *Escherichia coli* O157:H7 elicits a systemic humoral immune response in mice, but fails to prevent colonization by the pathogen. *Can. J. Microbiol.* 45, 279–286.

Conlan, J.W., KuoLee, R., Webb, A., and Perry, M.B. (1999b). *Salmonella landau* as a live vaccine against *Escherichia coli* O157:H7 investigated in a mouse model of intestinal colonization. *Can. J. Microbiol.* 45, 723–731.

Conlan, J.W., KuoLee, R., Webb, A., Cox, A.D., and Perry, M.B. (2000). Oral immunization of mice with a glycoconjugate vaccine containing the O157 antigen of *Escherichia coli* O157:H7 admixed with cholera toxin fails to elicit protection against subsequent colonization by the pathogen. *Can. J. Microbiol.* 46, 283–290.

Cookson, S.T., Stamboulian, D., Demonte, J., Quero, L., Martinez de Arquiza, C., Aleman, A., Lepetic, A., and Levine, M.M. (1997). A cost-benefit analysis of programmatic use of CVD 103-HgR live oral cholera vaccine in a high-risk population. *Int. J. Epidemiol.* 26, 212–219.

Coster, T.S., Hoge, C.W., VanDeVerg, L.L., Hartman, A.B., Oaks, E.V., Venkatesan, M.M., Cohen, D., Robin, G., Fontaine-Thompson, A., Sansonetti, P.J., and Hale, T.L. (1999). Vaccination against shigellosis with attenuated *Shigella flexneri* 2a strain SC602. *Infect. Immun.* 67, 3437–3443.

Cryz, S.J., Jr., Levine, M.M., Kaper, J.B., Furer, E., and Althaus, B. (1990). Randomized double-blind placebo controlled trial to evaluate the safety and immunogenicity of the live oral cholera vaccine strain CVD 103-HgR in Swiss adults. *Vaccine* 8, 577–580.

Cryz, S.J., Jr., Levine, M.M., Losonsky, G., Kaper, J.B., and Althaus, B. (1992). Safety and immunogenicity of a booster dose of *Vibrio cholerae* CVD 103-HgR live oral cholera vaccine in Swiss adults. *Infect. Immun.* 60, 3916–3917.

Cryz, S.J., Jr., Que, J.U., Levine, M.M., Wiedermann, G., and Kollaritsch, H. (1995). Safety and immunogenicity of a live oral bivalent typhoid fever (*Salmonella typhi* Ty21a)-cholera (*Vibrio cholerae* CVD 103-HgR) vaccine in healthy adults. *Infect. Immun.* 63, 1336–1339.

Ferreccio, C., Prado, V., Ojeda, A., Cayyazo, M., Abrego, P., Guers, L., and Levine, M.M. (1991). Epidemiologic patterns of acute diarrhea and endemic *Shigella* infections in children in a poor periurban setting in Santiago, Chile. *Am. J. Epidemiol.* 134, 614–627.

Formal, S.B., Kent, T.H., May, H.C., Palmer, A., Falkow, S., and LaBrec, E.H. (1966). Protection of monkeys against experimental shigellosis with a living attenuated oral polyvalent dysentery vaccine. *J. Bacteriol.* 92, 17–22.

Formal, S.B., Baron, L.S., Kopecko, D.J., Washington, O., Powell, C., and Life, C.A. (1981). Construction of a potential bivalent vaccine strain: introduction of *Shigella sonnei* form I antigen genes into the *galE Salmonella* typhi Ty21a typhoid vaccine strain. *Infect. Immun.* 34, 746–750.

Galen, J.E., Nair, J., Wang, J.Y., Wasserman, S.S., Taner, M.K., Sztein, M.B., and Levine, M.M. (1999). Optimization of plasmid maintenance in the attenuated live vector vaccine strain *Salmonella* typhi CVD 908-htrA. *Infect. Immun.* 67, 6424–6433.

Galen, J.E., and Levine, M.M. (2001). Can a 'flawless' live vector vaccine strain be engineered? *Trends Microbiol.* 9, 372–376.

Germanier, R., and Fuer, E. (1975). Isolation and characterization of Gal E mutant Ty 21a of *Salmonella typhi*: a candidate strain for a live, oral typhoid vaccine. *J. Infect. Dis.* 131, 553–558.

Gonzalez, C., Hone, D., Noriega, F.R., Tacket, C.O., Davis, J.R., Losonsky, G., Nataro, J.P., Hoffman, S., Malik, A., and Nardin, E. (1994). *Salmonella typhi* vaccine strain CVD 908 expressing the circumsporozoite protein of *Plasmodium falciparum*: strain construction and safety and immunogenicity in humans. *J. Infect. Dis.* 169, 927–931.

Gotuzzo, E., Butron, B., Seas, C., Penny, M., Ruiz, R., Losonsky, G., Lanata, C.F., Wasserman, S.S., Salazar, E., and Kaper, J.B. (1993). Safety, immunogenicity, and excretion pattern of single-dose live oral cholera vaccine CVD 103-HgR in Peruvian adults of high and low socioeconomic levels. *Infect. Immun.* 61, 3994–3997.

Guerena-Burgueno, F., Hall, E.R., Taylor, D.N., Cassels, F.J., Scott, D.A., Wolf, M.K., Roberts, Z.J., Nesterova, G.V., Alving, C.R., and Glenn, G.M. (2002). Safety and immunogenicity of a prototype enterotoxigenic *Escherichia coli* vaccine administered transcutaneously. *Infect. Immun.* 70, 1874–1880.

Herrington, D.A., Van de Verg, L., Formal, S.B., Hale, T.L., Tall, B.D., Cryz, S.J., Tramont, E.C., and Levine, M.M. (1990). Studies in volunteers to evaluate candidate Shigella vaccines: further experience with a bivalent *Salmonella* typhi-*Shigella sonnei* vaccine and protection conferred by previous *Shigella sonnei* disease. *Vaccine* 8, 353–357.

Hindle, Z., Chatfield, S.N., Phillimore, J., Bentley, M., Johnson, J., Cosgrove, C.A., Ghaem-Maghami, M., Sexton, A., Khan, M., Brennan, F.R., Everest, P., Wu, T., Pickard, D., Holden, D.W., Dougan, G., Griffin, G.E., House, D., Santangelo, J.D., Khan, S.A., Shea, J.E., Feldman, R.G., and Lewis, D.J. (2002). Characterization of *Salmonella enterica* derivatives harboring defined aro C and *Salmonella* pathogenicity island 2 type III secretion system (ssaV) mutations by immunization of healthy volunteers. *Infect. Immun.* 70, 3457–3467.

Hohmann, E.L., Oletta, C.A., Killeen, K.P., and Miller, S.I. (1996). phoP/phoQ-deleted *Salmonella typhi* (Ty800) is a safe and immunogenic single-dose typhoid fever vaccine in volunteers. *J. Infect. Dis.* 173, 1408–1414.

Hoiseth, S.K., and Stocker, B.A. (1981). Aromatic-dependent *Salmonella typhimurium* are non-virulent and effective as live vaccines. *Nature* 291, 238–239.

Holmgren, J., Czerkinsky, C., Lycke, N., and Svennerholm, A.M. (1994). Strategies for the induction of immune responses at mucosal surfaces making use of cholera toxin B subunit as immunogen, carrier, and adjuvant. *Am. J. Trop. Med. Hyg.* 50, 42–54.

Holmgren, J., and Svennerholm, A. (1998). Vaccines against diarrheal diseases. In *Handbook of Experimental Pharmacology*. Vol. 133. (eds. Perlman, P., and Wigzell, H.), 291–328. Berlin-Heidelberg-New York: Springer-Verlag.

Hone, D.M., Harris, A.M., Chatfield, S., Dougan, G., and Levine, M.M. (1991). Construction of genetically defined double aro mutants of *Salmonella typhi*. *Vaccine* 9, 810–816.

Jertborn, M., Svennerholm, A.M., and Holmgren, J. (1992). Safety and immunogenicity of an oral recombinant cholera B subunit-whole cell vaccine in Swedish volunteers. *Vaccine* 10, 130–132.

Jertborn, M., Svennerholm, A.M., and Holmgren, J. (1994). Immunological memory after immunization with oral cholera B subunit whole-cell vaccine in Swedish volunteers. *Vaccine* 12, 1078–1082.

Jertborn, M., Ahren, C., Holmgren, J., and Svennerholm, A.M. (1998). Safety and immunogenicity of an oral inactivated enterotoxigenic *Escherichia coli* vaccine. *Vaccine* 16, 255–260.

Kaper, J.B., Michalski, J., Ketley, J.M., and Levine, M.M. (1994). Potential for reacquisition of cholera enterotoxin genes by attenuated *Vibrio cholerae* vaccine strain CVD 103-HgR. *Infect. Immun.* 62, 1480–1483.

Kaper, J.B. (1998). Enterohemorrhagic *Escherichia coli*. *Curr. Opin. Microbiol.* 1, 103–108.

Karnell, A., Li, A., Zhao, C.R., Karlsson, K., Nguyen, B.M., and Lindberg, A.A. (1995). Safety and immunogenicity study of the auxotrophic *Shigella flexneri* 2a vaccine SFL1070 with a deleted aroD gene in adult Swedish volunteers. *Vaccine* 13, 88–99.

Keusch, G., Acheson, D., Marchant, C., and McIver, J. (1998). Toxoid-based active and passive immunization to prevent and/or modulate hemolytic-uremic syndrome due to Shiga toxin-producing *Escherichia coli*. In *Escherichia coli O157:H7 and Other Shiga Toxin—Producing E. coli Strains* (eds. Kaper, J., and O'Brien, A.), 409–418. Washington, DC: American Society for Microbiology.

Khan, S.A., Stratford, R., Wu, T., Mckelvie, N., Bellaby, T., Hindle, Z., Sinha, K.A., Eltze, S., Mastroeni, P., Pickard, D., Dougan, G., Chatfield, S.N., and Btrennan, F.R. (2003). *Salmonella typhi* and *S. typhimurium* derivatives harbouring deletions in aromatic biosynthesis and *Salmonella* Pathogenicity Island-2 (SPI-2) genes as vaccines and vectors. *Vaccine* 21, 538–548.

Kotloff, K.L., Herrington, D.A., Hale, T.L., Newland, J.W., Van De Verg, L., Cogan, J.P., Snoy, P.J., Sadoff, J.C., Formal, S.B., and Levine, M.M. (1992a). Safety, immunogenicity, and efficacy in monkeys and humans of invasive *Escherichia coli* K-12 hybrid vaccine candidates expressing *Shigella flexneri* 2a somatic antigen. *Infect. Immun.* 60, 2218–2224.

Kotloff, K.L., Wasserman, S.S., O'Donnell, S., Losonsky, G.A., Cryz, S.J., and Levine, M.M. (1992b). Safety and immunogenicity in North Americans of a single dose of live oral cholera vaccine CVD 103-HgR: results of a randomized, placebo-controlled, double-blind crossover trial. *Infect. Immun.* 60, 4430–4432.

Kotloff, K.L., Losonsky, G.A., Nataro, J.P., Wasserman, S.S., Hale, T.L., Taylor, D.N., Newland, J.W., Sadoff, J.C., Formal, S.B., and Levine, M.M. (1995). Evaluation of the safety, immunogenicity, and efficacy in healthy adults of four doses of live oral hybrid *Escherichia coli-Shigella flexneri* 2a vaccine strain EcSf2a-2. *Vaccine* 13, 495–502.

Kotloff, K.L., Noriega, F., Losonsky, G.A., Sztein, M.B., Wasserman, S.S., Nataro, J.P., and Levine, M.M. (1996). Safety, immunogenicity, and transmissibility in humans of CVD 1203, a live oral *Shigella flexneri* 2a vaccine candidate attenuated by deletions in aro A and vir G. *Infect. Immun.* 64, 4542–4548.

Kotloff, K.L., Winickoff, J.P., Ivanoff, B., Clemens, J.D., Swerdlow, D.L., Sansonetti, P.J., Adak, G.L., and Levine, M.M. (1999). Global burden of *Shigella* infections: implications for vaccine development and implementation of control strategies. *Bull. World Health Organ.* 77, 651–666.

Kotloff, K.L., Taylor, D.N., Sztein, M.B., Wasserman, S.S., Losonsky, G.A., Nataro, J.P., Venkatesan, M., Hartman, A., Picking, W.D., Katz,

D.E., Campbell, J.D., Levine, M.M., and Hale, T.L. (2002). Phase I evaluation of delta virG *Shigella sonnei* live, attenuated, oral vaccine strain WRSS1 in healthy adults. *Infect. Immun.* 70, 2016–2021.

Lagos, R., Avendano, A., Prado, V., Horwitz, I., Wasserman, S., Losonsky, G., Cryz, S., Jr., Kaper, J.B., and Levine, M.M. (1995). Attenuated live cholera vaccine strain CVD 103-HgR elicits significantly higher serum vibriocidal antibody titers in persons of blood group O. *Infect. Immun.* 63, 707–709.

Lagos, R., Fasano, A., Wasserman, S.S., Prado, V., San Martin, O., Abrego, P., Losonsky, G.A., Alegria, S., and Levine, M.M. (1999a). Effect of small bowel bacterial overgrowth on the immunogenicity of single-dose live oral cholera vaccine CVD 103-HgR. *J. Infect. Dis.* 180, 1709–1712.

Lagos, R., San Martin, O., Wasserman, S.S., Prado, V., Losonsky, G.A., Bustamante, C. and Levine, M.M. (1999b). Palatability, reactogenicity and immunogenicity of engineered live oral cholera vaccine CVD 103-HgR in Chilean infants and toddlers. *Pediatr. Infect. Dis. J.* 18, 624–630.

Levine, M., Black, R.E., Clements, M.L., Young, C.R., Cheney, C.P., Schad, P., Collins, H., and Boedeker, E.C. (1984). Prevention of enterotoxigenic *Escherichia coli* diarrheal infection by vaccines that stimulate antiadhesion (antipili) immunity. In *Attachment of Organisms to the Gut Mucosa* (ed. Boedeker, E.C.), 223–244. Boca Raton, Florida: CRC Press.

Levine, M.M. (1986). Clinical and field trials to assess the efficacy of vaccines against bacterial enteric infections. *Ann. Sclavo. Collana. Monogr.* 3, 41–50.

Levine, M.M., Kaper, J.B., Herrington, D., Ketley, J., Losonsky, G., Tacket, C.O., Tall, B., and Cryz, S. (1988). Safety, immunogenicity, and efficacy of recombinant live oral cholera vaccines, CVD 103 and CVD 103-HgR. *Lancet* 2, 467–470.

Levine, M.M., Ferreccio, C., Cryz, S., and Ortiz, E. (1990). Comparison of enteric-coated capsules and liquid formulation of Ty21a typhoid vaccine in randomised controlled field trial. *Lancet* 336, 891–894.

Levine, M.M., Galen, J., Barry, E., Noriega, F., Chatfield, S., Sztein, M., Dougan, G., and Tacket, C. (1996). Attenuated *Salmonella* as live oral vaccines against typhoid fever and as live vectors. *J. Biotechnol.* 44, 193–196.

Levine, M.M., Galen, J., Barry, E., Noriega, F., Tacket, C., Sztein, M., Chatfield, S., Dougan, G., Losonky, G., and Kotloff, K. (1997). Attenuated *Salmonella typhi* and *Shigella* as live oral vaccines and as live vectors. *Behring Inst. Mitt.* 120–123.

Li, A., Pal, T., Forsum, U., and Lindberg, A.A. (1992). Safety and immunogenicity of the live oral auxotrophic *Shigella flexneri* SFL124 in volunteers. *Vaccine* 10, 395–404.

Li, A., Karnell, A., Huan, P.T., Dac Cam, P., Binh Minh, N., Ngoc, Tram, L., Phu Qiu, N., Duc Trach, D., Karlsson, K., Lindberg, G., and Lindberg, A.A. (1993). Safety and immunogenicity of the live oral auxotrophic *Shigella flexneri* SFL124 in adult Vietnamese volunteers. *Vaccine* 11, 180–189.

Li, A., Cam, P.D., Islam, D., Minh, N.B., Huan, P.T., Rong, Z.C., Karlsson, K., Lindberg, G., and Lindberg, A.A. (1994). Immune responses in Vietnamese children after a single dose of the auxotrophic, live *Shigella flexneri* Y vaccine strain SFL124. *J. Infect.* 28, 11–23.

Lindberg, A.A., Karnell, A., Pal, T., Sweiha, H., Hultenby, K., and Stocker, B.A. (1990). Construction of an auxotrophic *Shigella flexneri* strain for use as a live vaccine. *Microb. Pathog.* 8, 433–440.

Liu, Y.Q., Qi, G.M., Wang, S.X., Yu, Y.M., Duan, G.C., Zhang, L.J., and Gao, S.Y. (1995). A natural vaccine candidate strain against cholera. *Biomed. Environ. Sci.* 8, 350–358.

Losonsky, G.A., Tacket, C.O., Wasserman, S.S., Kaper, J.B., and Levine, M.M. (1993). Secondary *Vibrio cholerae*-specific cellular antibody responses following wild-type homologous challenge in people vaccinated with CVD 103-HgR live oral cholera vaccine: changes with time and lack of correlation with protection. *Infect. Immun.* 61, 729–733.

Marcato, P., Mulvey, G., Read, R.J., Vander Helm, K., Nation, P.N., and Armstrong, G.D. (2001). Immunoprophylactic potential of cloned Shiga toxin 2 B subunit. *J. Infect. Dis.* 183, 435–443.

Marcato, P., Mulvey, G., and Armstrong, G.D. (2002). Cloned Shiga toxin 2 B subunit induces apoptosis in Ramos Burkitt's lymphoma B cells. *Infect. Immun.* 70, 1279–1286.

McKenzie, R., Baqar, S., Forbes, E. (2002). A Phase 1 study of the safety and immunogenicity of two attenuated *Salmonella typhi* vectors expressing the urease vaccine antigen of *H. pylori*. In *Proceedings of the 102nd General Meeting of the American Society for Microbiology, Salt Lake City, UT*, E-45. Washington, DC: American Society for Microbiology.

Mel, D., Gangarosa, E.J., Radovanovic, M.L., Arsic, B.L., and Litvinjenko, S. (1971). Studies on vaccination against bacillary dysentery. 6. Protection of children by oral immunization with streptomycin-dependent *Shigella* strains. *Bull. World Health Organ.* 45, 457–464.

Mel, D.M., Arsic, B.L., Nikolic, B.D., and Radovanic, M.L. (1968). Studies on vaccination against bacillary dysentery. 4. Oral immunization with live monotypic and combined vaccines. *Bull. World Health Organ.* 39, 375–380.

Migasena, S., Pitisuttitham, P., Prayurahong, B., Suntharasamai, P., Suntharasamai, P., Supanaranond, W., Desakorn, V., Gongsthongsri, U., Tall, B., Ketley, J., and Losonsky, G. (1989). Preliminary assessment of the safety and immunogenicity of live oral cholera vaccine strain CVD 103-HgR in healthy Thai adults. *Infect. Immun.* 57, 3261–3264.

Miller, S.I., Loomis, W.P., Alpuche-Aranda, C., Behlau, I., and Hohmann, E. (1993). The PhoP virulence regulon and live oral *Salmonella* vaccines. *Vaccine* 11, 122–125.

Nardelli-Haefliger, D., Kraehenbuhl, J.P., Curtiss, R., 3rd, Schodel, F., Potts, A., Kelly, S., and De Grandi, P. (1996). Oral and rectal immunization of adult female volunteers with a recombinant attenuated *Salmonella typhi* vaccine strain. *Infect. Immun.* 64, 5219–5224.

Nataro, J.P., and Kaper, J.B. (1998). Diarrheagenic *Escherichia coli*. *Clin. Microbiol. Rev.* 11, 142–201.

Newland, J.W., Hale, T.L., and Formal, S.B. (1992). Genotypic and phenotypic characterization of an aroD deletion-attenuated *Escherichia coli* K12-*Shigella flexneri* hybrid vaccine expressing S. flexneri 2a somatic antigen. *Vaccine* 10, 766–776.

Noriega, F.R., Wang, J.Y., Losonsky, G., Maneval, D.R., Hone, D.M., and Levine, M.M. (1994). Construction and characterization of attenuated delta aroA delta virG *Shigella flexneri* 2a strain CVD 1203, a prototype live oral vaccine. *Infect. Immun.* 62, 5168–5172.

Pallen, M.J., and Wren, B.W. (1997). The HtrA family of serine proteases. *Mol. Microbiol.* 26, 209–221.

Passwell, J.H., Harlev, E., Ashkenazi, S., Chu, C., Miron, D., Ramon, R., Farzan, N., Shiloach, J., Bryla, D.A., Majadly, F., Roberson, R., Robbins, J.B., and Schneerson, R. (2001). Safety and immunogenicity of improved *Shigella* O-specific polysaccharide-protein conjugate vaccines in adults in Israel. *Infect. Immun.* 69, 1351–1357.

Peltola, H., Siitonen, A., Kyronseppa, H., Simula, I., Mattila, L., Oksanen, P., Kataja, M.J., and Cadoz, M. (1991). Prevention of travellers' diarrhoea by oral B-subunit/whole-cell cholera vaccine. *Lancet* 338, 1285–1289.

Perry, R.T., Plowe, C.V., Koumare, B., Bougoudogo, F., Kotloff, K.L., Losonsky, G.A., Wasserman, S.S., and Levine, M.M. (1998). A single dose of live oral cholera vaccine CVD 103-HgR is safe and immunogenic in HIV-infected and HIV-noninfected adults in Mali. *Bull. World Health Organ.* 76, 63–71.

Qadri, F., Wenneras, C., Ahmed, F., Asaduzzaman, M., Saha, D., Albert, M.J., Sack, R.B., and Svennerholm, A. (2000). Safety and immunogenicity of an oral, inactivated enterotoxigenic *Escherichia coli* plus cholera toxin B subunit vaccine in Bangladeshi adults and children. *Vaccine* 18, 2704–2712.

Richie, E.E., Punjabi, N.H., Sidharta, Y.Y., Peetosutan, K.K., Sukandar, M.M., Wasserman, S.S., Lesmana, M.M., Wangsasaputra, F.F., Pandam, S.S., Levine, M.M., O'Hanley, P.P., Cryz, S.J., and Simanjuntak, C.H. (2000). Efficacy trial of single-dose live oral cholera vaccine CVD 103-HgR in North Jakarta, Indonesia, a cholera-endemic area. *Vaccine* 18, 2399–2410.

Robbins, J.B., Chu, C., and Schneerson, R. (1992). Hypothesis for vaccine development: protective immunity to enteric diseases caused by nontyphoidal *Salmonellae* and *Shigellae* may be conferred by serum IgG antibodies to the O-specific polysaccharide of their lipopolysaccharides. *Clin. Infect. Dis.* 15, 346–361.

Sack, D.A., Sack, R.B., Shimko, J., Gomes, G., O'Sullivan, D., Metcalfe, K., and Spriggs, D. (1997). Evaluation of Peru-15, a new live oral vaccine for cholera, in volunteers. *J. Infect. Dis.* 176, 201–205.

Sanchez, J.L., Vasquez, B., Begue, R.E., Meza, R., Castellares, G., Cabezas, C., Watts, D.M., Svennerholm, A.M., Sadoff, J.C., and Taylor, D.N. (1994). Protective efficacy of oral whole-cell/recombinant-B-subunit cholera vaccine in Peruvian military recruits. *Lancet* 344, 1273–1276.

Sandvig, K. (2001). Shiga toxins. *Toxicon* 39, 1629–1635.

Sansonetti, P.J., and Arondel, J. (1989). Construction and evaluation of a double mutant of *Shigella flexneri* as a candidate for oral vaccination against shigellosis. *Vaccine* 7, 443–450.

Sansonetti, P.J., Arondel, J., Fontaine, A., d'Hauteville, H., and Bernardini, M.L. (1991). OmpB (osmo-regulation) and icsA (cell-to-cell spread) mutants of *Shigella flexneri*: vaccine candidates and probes to study the pathogenesis of shigellosis. *Vaccine* 9, 416–422.

Sansonetti, P.J. (2001a). Rupture, invasion and inflammatory destruction of the intestinal barrier by *Shigella*, making sense of prokaryote-eukaryote cross-talks. *FEMS Microbiol. Rev.* 25, 3–14.

Sansonetti, P.J. (2001b). Microbes and microbial toxins: paradigms for microbial-mucosal interactions III. Shigellosis: from symptoms to molecular pathogenesis. *Am. J. Physiol. Gastrointest. Liver Physiol.* 280, G319–323.

Savarino, S.J., Brown, F.M., Hall, E., Bassily, S., Youssef, F., Wierzba, T., Peruski, L., El-Masry, N.A., Safwat, M., Rao, M., Jertbron, M., Svennerholm, A.M., Lee, Y.J., and Clemens, J.D. (1998). Safety and immunogenicity of an oral, killed enterotoxigenic *Escherichia coli*-cholera toxin B subunit vaccine in Egyptian adults. *J. Infect. Dis.* 177, 796–799.

Savarino, S.J., Hall, E.R., Bassily, S., Brown, F.M., Youssef, F., Wierzba, T.F., Peruski, L., El-Masry, N.A., Safwat, M., Rao, M., El Mohamady, H., Abu-Elyazeed, R., Naficy, A., Svennerholm, A.M., Jertborn, M., Lee, Y.J., and Clemens, J.D. (1999). Oral, inactivated, whole cell enterotoxigenic *Escherichia coli* plus cholera toxin B subunit vaccine: results of the initial evaluation in children. PRIDE Study Group. *J. Infect. Dis.* 179, 107–114.

Scerpella, E.G., Sanchez, J.L., Mathewson, I.J., Mathewson, J.J., III, Torres-Cordero, J.V., Sadoff, J.C., Svennerholm, A.M., DuPont, H.L., Taylor, D.N., and Ericsson, C.D. (1995). Safety, immunogenicity, and protective efficacy of the whole-cell/recombinant B subunit (WC/rBS) oral cholera vaccine against travelers' diarrhea. *J. Travel Med.* 2, 22–27.

Simanjuntak, C.H., O'Hanley, P., Punjabi, N.H., Noriega, F. Pazzoglia, G., Dykstra, P., Kay, B., Budiarso, A., and Rifai, A.R. (1993). Safety, immunogenicity, and transmissibility of single-dose live oral cholera vaccine strain CVD 103-HgR in 24- to 59-month-old Indonesian children. *J. Infect. Dis.* 168, 1169–1176.

Stoll, B.J., Svennerholm, A.M., Gothefors, L., Barua, D., Huda, S., and Holmgreen, J. (1986). Local and systemic antibody responses to naturally acquired enterotoxigenic *Escherichia coli* diarrhea in an endemic area. *J. Infect. Dis.* 153, 527–534.

Su-Arehawaratana, P., Singharaj, P., Taylor, D.N., Hoge, C., Trofa, A., Kuvanont, K., Migasena, S., Pitisuttitham, P., Lim, Y.L., and Losonsky, G. (1992). Safety and immunogenicity of different immunization regimens of CVD 103-HgR live oral cholera vaccine in soldiers and civilians in Thailand. *J. Infect. Dis.* 165, 1042–1048.

Suharyono, Simanjuntak, C., Witham, N., Punjabi, N., Heppner, D.G., Losonsky, G., Totosudirjo, H., Rifai, A.R., Clemens, J., and Lim, Y.L. (1992). Safety and immunogenicity of single-dose live oral cholera vaccine CVD 103-HgR in 5–9-year-old Indonesian children. *Lancet* 340, 689–694.

Svennerholm, A.M., and Holmgren, J. (1976). Synergistic protective effect in rabbits of immunization with *Vibrio cholerae* lipopolysaccharide and toxin/toxoid. *Infect. Immun.* 13, 735–740.

Svennerholm, A.M., Jertborn, M., Gothefors, L., Karim, A.M., Sack, D.A., and Holmgren, J. (1984). Mucosal antitoxic and antibacterial immunity after cholera disease and after immunization with a combined B subunit-whole cell vaccine. *J. Infect. Dis.* 149, 884–893.

Tacket, C.O., Hone, D.M., Curtiss, R., 3rd, Kelly, S.M., Losonsky, G., Guers, L., Harris, A.M., Edelman, R., and Levine, M.M.

(1992a). Comparison of the safety and immunogenicity of delta aroC delta aroD and delta cya delta crp *Salmonella typhi* strains in adult volunteers. *Infect. Immun.* 60, 536–541.

Tacket, C.O., Hone, D.M., Losonsky, G.A., Guers, L., Edelman, R., and Levine, M.M. (1992b). Clinical acceptability and immunogenicity of CVD 908 *Salmonella typhi* vaccine strain. *Vaccine* 10, 443–446.

Tacket, C.O., Losonsky, G., Nataro, J.P., Cryz, S.J., Edelman, R., Kaper, J.B., and Levine, M.M. (1992c). Onset and duration of protective immunity in challenged volunteers after vaccination with live oral cholera vaccine CVD 103-HgR. *J. Infect. Dis.* 166, 837–841.

Tacket, C.O., Reid, R.H., Boedeker, E.C., Losonsky, G., Nataro, J.P., Bhagat, H., and Edelman, R. (1994). Enteral immunization and challenge of volunteers given enterotoxigenic *E. coli* CFA/II encapsulated in biodegradable microspheres. *Vaccine* 12, 1270–1274.

Tacket, C.O., Kelly, S.M., Schodel, F., Losonsky, G., Nataro, J.P., Edelman, R., Levine, M.M., and Curtiss, R., III. (1997a). Safety and immunogenicity in humans of an attenuated *Salmonella typhi* vaccine vector strain expressing plasmid-encoded hepatitis B antigens stabilized by the Asd-balanced lethal vector system. *Infect. Immun.* 65, 3381–3385.

Tacket, C.O., Sztein, M.B., Losonsky, G.A., Wasserman, S.S., Nataro, J.P., Edelman, R., Pickard, D., Dougan, G., Chatfield, S.N., and Levine, M.M. (1997b). Safety of live oral *Salmonella typhi* vaccine strains with deletions in htrA and aroC aroD and immune response in humans. *Infect. Immun.* 65, 452–456.

Tacket, C.O., Mason, H.S., Losonsky, G., Clements, J.D., Levine, M.M., and Artzen, C.J. (1998). Immunogenicity in humans of a recombinant bacterial antigen delivered in a transgenic potato. *Nat. Med.* 4, 607–609.

Tacket, C.O., Cohen, M.B., Wasserman, S.S., Losonsky, G., Livio, S., Kotloff, K., Edelman, R., Kaper, J.B., Cryz, S.J., Giannella, R.A., Schiff, G., and Levine, M.M. (1999). Randomized, double-blind, placebo-controlled, multicentered trial of the efficacy of a single dose of live oral cholera vaccine CVD 103-HgR in preventing cholera following challenge with *Vibrio cholerae* O1 El tor inaba three months after vaccination. *Infect. Immun.* 67, 6341–6345.

Tacket, C.O., Galen, J., Sztein, M.B., Losonsky, G., Wyant, T.L., Nataro, J., Wasserman, S.S., Edelman, R., Chatfield, S., Dougan, G., and Levine, M.M. (2000a). Safety and immune responses to attenuated *Salmonella enterica* serovar *typhi* oral live vector vaccines expressing tetanus toxin fragment C. *Clin. Immunol.* 97, 146–153.

Tacket, C.O., Sztein, M.B., Wasserman, S.S., Losonsky, G., Kotloff, K.L., Wyant, T.L., Naaro, J.P., Edelman, R., Perry, J., Bedford, P., Brown, D., Chatfield, S., Dougan, G., and Levine, M.M. (2000b). Phase 2 clinical trial of attenuated *Salmonella enterica* serovar *typhi* oral live vector vaccine CVD 908-htrA in U.S. volunteers. *Infect. Immun.* 68, 1196–1201.

Tarr, P.I., and Neill, M.A. (2001). *Escherichia coli* O157:H7. *Gastroenterol. Clin. North Am.* 30, 735–751.

Taylor, D.N., Trofa, A.C., Sadoff, J., Chu, C., Bryla, D., Shiloach, J., Cohen, D., Ashkenazi, S., Lerman, Y., and Egan, W. (1993). Synthesis, characterization, and clinical evaluation of conjugate vaccines composed of the O-specific polysaccharides of *Shigella dysenteriae* type 1, *Shigella flexneri* type 2a, and *Shigella sonnei* (*Plesiomonas shigelloides*) bound to bacterial toxoids. *Infect. Immun.* 61, 3678–3687.

Taylor, D.N., Tacket, C.O., Losonsky, G., Castro, O., Gutierrez, J., Meza, R., Nataro, J.P., Kaper, J.B., Wasserman, S.S., Edelman, R., Levine, M.M., and Cryz, S.J. (1997). Evaluation of a bivalent (CVD 103-HgR/CVD 111) live oral cholera vaccine in adult volunteers from the United States and Peru. *Infect. Immun.* 65, 3852–3856.

Taylor, D.N., Sanchez, J.L., Castro, J.M., Lebron, C., Parrado, C.M., Johnson, D.E., Tacket, C.O., Losonsky, G.A., Wasserman, S.S., Levine, M.M., and Cryz, S.J. (1999). Expanded safety and immunogenicity of a bivalent, oral, attenuated cholera vaccine, CVD 103-HgR plus CVD 111, in United States military personnel stationed in Panama. *Infect. Immun.* 67, 2030–2034.

Taylor, D.N., Cardenas, V., Sanchez, J.L., Begue, R.E., Gilman, R., Bautista, C., Perez, J., Puga, R., Gaillour, A., Mza, R., Echeverria, P., and Sadoff, J. (2000). Two-year study of the protective efficacy of the oral whole cell plus recombinant B subunit cholera vaccine in Peru. *J. Infect. Dis.* 181, 1667–1673.

Trach, D.D., Clemens, J.D., Ke, N.T., Thuy, H.T., Son, N.D., Canh, D.G., Hang, P.V. and Rao, M.R. (1997). Field trial of a locally produced, killed, oral cholera vaccine in Vietnam. *Lancet* 349, 231–235.

Trach, D.D., Cam, P.D., Ke, N.T., Rao, M.R., Dinh, D., Hang, P.V., Hung, N.V., Canh, D.G., Thiem, V.D., Naficy, A., Ivanoff, B., Svennerholm, A.M., Holmgren, J., and Clemens, J.D. (2002). Investigations into the safety and immunogenicity of a killed oral cholera vaccine developed in Viet Nam. *Bull. World Health Organ.* 80, 2–8.

Tramont, E.C., Chung, R., Berman, S., Keren, D., Kapfer, C., and Formal, S.B. (1984). Safety and antigenicity of typhoid-*Shigella sonnei* vaccine (strain 5076-1C). *J. Infect. Dis.* 149, 133–136.

Turner, A.K., Terry, T.D., Sack, D.A., Londono-Arcila, P., and Darsley, M.J. (2001). Construction and characterization of genetically defined aro omp mutants of enterotoxigenic *Escherichia coli* and preliminary studies of safety and immunogenicity in humans. *Infect. Immun.* 69, 4969–4979.

Tzschaschel, B.D., Guzman, C.A., Timmis, K.N., and de Lorenzo, V. (1996a). An *Escherichia coli* hemolysin transport system-based vector for the export of polypeptides: export of Shiga-like toxin IIeB subunit by *Salmonella typhimurium* aro A. *Nat. Biotechnol.* 14, 765–769.

Tzschaschel, B.D., Klee, S.R., de Lorenzo, V., Timmis, K.N., and Guzman, C.A. (1996b). Towards a vaccine candidate against *Shigella dysenteriae* 1: expression of the Shiga toxin B-subunit in an attenuated *Shigella flexneri* aroD carrier strain. *Microb. Pathog.* 21, 277–288.

van Loon, F.P., Clemens, J.D., Chakraborty, J., Rao, M.R., Kay, B.A., Sack, D.A., Yunus, M., Ali, M., Svennerholm, A.M., and Holmgren, J. (1996). Field trial of inactivated oral cholera vaccines in Bangladesh: results from 5 years of follow-up. *Vaccine* 14, 162–166.

Wenneras, C., Qadri, F., Bardhan, P.K., Sack, R.B., and Svennerholm, A.M. (1999). Intestinal immune responses in patients infected with enterotoxigenic *Escherichia coli* and in vaccinees. *Infect. Immun.* 67, 6234–6241.

Yamamoto, T. (2000). Current status of cholera and rise of novel mucosal vaccine. *Jpn. J. Infect. Dis.* 53, 181–188.

Yu, J., and Langridge, W.H. (2001). A plant-based multicomponent vaccine protects mice from enteric diseases. *Nat. Biotechnol.* 19, 548–552.

Yu, J., Cassels, F., Scharton-Kersten, T., Hammond, S.A., Hartman, A., Angov, E., Corthesy, B., Alving, C., and Glenn, G. (2002). Transcutaneous immunization using colonization factor and heat-labile enterotoxin induces correlates of protective immunity for enterotoxigenic *Escherichia coli*. *Infect. Immun.* 70, 1056–1068.

Viral Gastroenteritis Vaccines

Chapter 49

Richard L. Ward

Division of Infectious Diseases, Children's Hospital Medical Center, University of Cincinnati, Cincinnati, Ohio

Harry B. Greenberg

Department of Microbiology and Immunology, Veterans Affairs Hospital, Stanford University, Palo Alto, California

Mary K. Estes

Department of Molecular Virology and Microbiology, Baylor College of Medicine, Houston, Texas

The gastrointestinal tract is one of the most common portals of entry for pathogens, and viruses are frequently spread by fecal–oral routes. The first successful vaccine against an enteric viral infection was the parenteral inactivated poliovirus vaccine, which was subsequently followed by live attenuated oral poliovirus vaccines. Poliovirus vaccines have been extremely effective and have been used as models in the development of vaccines against other enteric viral infections. In fact, no cases of wild-type poliovirus have been reported in the Americas since 1989, and worldwide eradication of poliovirus is now being pursued. Although poliovirus enters the host via the gastrointestinal tract, levels of serum neutralizing antibody induced by these vaccines are clear correlates of protection. Thus, poliovirus vaccines protect against systemic paralytic disease by inducing serum neutralizing antibodies that prevent extraintestinal virus spread. This mechanism of action is not clearly associated with protective immunity in other enteric virus infections.

This chapter reviews three enteric viral infections of humans in which the primary or sole site of viral replication and the underlying mechanisms of pathogenesis result from local infections in the cells of the gastrointestinal tract. Rotaviruses, human caliciviruses, and astroviruses are considered, with emphasis on rotaviruses because of their significant clinical impact in children and because rotavirus vaccines are in phase III trials and the furthest toward licensure. Immunity for these enteric viruses is complex, but studies on immunization and vaccine development involving these viruses are clearly useful as models for probing virus–cell interactions in the gastrointestinal tract and for learning how to induce mucosal immunity to prevent local infections.

ROTAVIRUSES

Introduction

Rotaviruses are the single most important cause of severe infantile gastroenteritis. In the United States alone, these viruses are estimated to cause 50,000 to 100,000 hospitalizations in young children each year and approximately 20 to 40 deaths. On a world scale, rotaviruses are estimated to be responsible for nearly 1 million deaths annually (Kapikian et al., 2001). Cost estimates for hospitalizations due to rotavirus infections in the United States are greater than $300 million each year, and this does not account for the cost of doctors' visits and home care associated with 2 million less severe rotavirus illnesses. For these reasons, rotaviruses have received a high priority as a target for vaccine development.

Rotavirus transmission occurs by the fecal–oral route, providing a highly efficient mechanism for universal exposure that has circumvented differences in regional and national cultural practices and public health standards. The symptoms associated with rotavirus disease are typically diarrhea and vomiting, accompanied by fever, nausea, anorexia, cramping, and malaise, which can be mild and of short duration or produce severe dehydration. Severe disease occurs primarily in young children, most commonly between 6 and 24 months of age. Approximately 90% of children in both developed and developing countries experience a rotavirus infection by 3 years of age. Rotavirus infection normally provides short-term protection and immunity against subsequent severe illnesses but does not provide life-long immunity, and there are numerous reports of sequential illnesses. Neonates can also experience rotavirus infections, and these occur endemically in some settings but are typically asymptomatic. These neonatal infections have been reported to reduce the morbidity associated with a subsequent rotavirus infection (Bishop *et al.*, 1983; Bhan *et al.*, 1993). Rotavirus illnesses also occur in adults and the elderly, but the symptoms generally have been believed to be mild. A recent study conducted in Japan, however, suggests that rotaviruses are a major cause of hospitalization of adults due to acute diarrhea (Nakajima *et al.*, 2001).

Because of the frequency of rotavirus infections and the reduced severity of illness typically associated with sequential infections, a realistic goal for a rotavirus vaccine may be to protect against severe disease. Several vaccine candidates have been developed and evaluated in infants, with promising results. Incorporation of an effective rotavirus vaccine into the infant immunization schedule in developed countries could reduce hospitalizations due to dehydrating diarrhea in young children by 40% to 60%. More important, worldwide usage of such a vaccine could decrease total diarrheal deaths by approximately 10% to 20%. Until an effective vaccine is available, control of rotavirus disease is limited to nonspecific methods, particularly rehydration therapy for replacement of body fluids and electrolytes.

History

Particles approximately 100 nm in diameter with a wheel-like appearance, later associated with rotaviruses, were first observed by electron microscopy in 1963 in specimens from mice (Adams and Kraft, 1963) and monkeys (Malherbe *et al.*, 1963). The correlation between these viruses and human diarrheal disease was first reported by Bishop *et al.* (1973). Within a short time, these and other investigators confirmed the association between the presence of rotavirus in feces and acute gastroenteritis. In addition to their distinctive morphology, these human viruses along with their animal rotavirus counterparts were later shown to share a group antigen and have been classified as members of the *Rotavirus* genus within the Reoviridae family. In 1980, particles that were morphologically indistinguishable from established rotavirus strains but lacked the common group antigen were discovered in pigs (Bridger, 1980; Saif *et al.*, 1980). This observation subsequently lead to the identification of rotaviruses belonging to six additional groups (B–G) based on a common group antigen, with the original rotavirus strains classified as group A. Rotaviruses in different groups have restricted nucleic acid sequence similarity and do not appear to undergo gene reassortment following coinfection. Only groups A–C are associated with human diseases, and most known cases of rotavirus gastroenteritis are caused by group A strains. However, non–group A rotaviruses have been associated with outbreaks of disease in China, India, and Japan, which suggests that they could become major pathogens in the future.

Properties of the virus

Rotaviruses are complex, relatively large (100 nm), nonenveloped, icosahedral viruses. The capsid consists of three concentric protein layers **(Fig. 49.1)** (Prasad and Chiu,

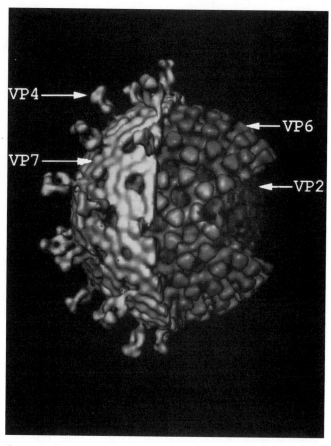

Fig. 49.1. Computer-generated image of the triple-layered rotavirus particle obtained by cryoelectron microscopy. The cut-away diagram shows the outer capsid, composed of VP4 spikes and a VP7 shell, an intermediate VP6 layer, and an inner VP2 layer surrounding the core containing the 11 double-stranded RNA segments and VP1 and VP3. (Photograph courtesy of B.V.V. Prasad, Baylor College of Medicine, Houston, Texas.)

1994). The outer layer is composed of two structural proteins, VP4 and VP7. VP4 forms a spike that radiates from the intermediate capsid layer composed of the major structural protein VP6. The inner layer is composed of VP2, and it surrounds the viral genome and two additional structural proteins, VP1 and VP3, the viral transcriptase and capping enzyme, respectively.

The genome of rotavirus is composed of 11 segments of double-stranded RNA that encode the six structural proteins, VP1–VP4, VP6, and VP7, and six nonstructural proteins designated NSP1–NSP6 **(Table 49.1)**. Each segment except segment 11, which appears to be bicistronic (Mattion *et al.*, 1991), encodes one known rotavirus protein whose functions have been investigated but in some cases remain poorly defined. The genome segments have sizes ranging from approximately 660 to 3300 bp, and their encoded proteins have molecular weights of approximately 12,000 to 125,000 Da. These genome segments of rotavirus can be extracted from viral particles and separated by polyacrylamide gel electrophoresis into 11 distinct bands. Each

Table 49.1. Sizes of Rotavirus Gene Segments and Properties of Encoded Proteins

RNA Segment	No. of Base Pairs	Encoded Protein	Molecular Weight of Protein ($\times 10^{-4}$)	Properties of Protein
1	3300	VP1	12.5	Inner core protein, RNA binding, RNA transcriptase
2	2700	VP2	10.2	Inner capsid protein, RNA binding
3	2600	VP3	9.8	Inner core protein, guanyl transferase
4	2360	VP4	8.7	Outer capsid protein, HA, NP, sialic acid binding, fusogenic protein
5	1600	NSP1	5.9	Nonstructural protein, RNA binding, contains zinc fingers, host range determinant (?)
6	1360	VP6	4.5	Intermediate capsid protein, group and subgroup antigen
7	1100	NSP3	3.5	Nonstructural protein, RNA binding, translational control
8	1060	NSP2	3.7	Nonstructural protein, RNA binding, NTPase
9	1060	VP7	3.7	Outer capsid glycoprotein, NP
10	750	NSP4	2.0	Nonstructural glycoprotein, transmembrane protein, enterotoxin
11	660	NSP5	2.2	Nonstructural protein, phosphorylated, O-glycosylated
		NSP6	1.2	Nonstructural protein, interacts with NSP5

rotavirus strain has a characteristic RNA profile or electropherotype, a property employed extensively in epidemiological studies of these viruses. Electropherotypes have also been used to identify reassortants of human and animal rotavirus strains having the desired combination of segments from each parental virus for use as vaccine candidates (see later discussion).

Serotypes

Both outer capsid proteins of rotavirus, VP4 and VP7, contain neutralization epitopes, and both are thereby involved in serotype determination. Because these are neutralization proteins, they are targeted for antibody responses following vaccination. Rotavirus serotypes based on VP4 and VP7 are classified as P and G types to describe the protease sensitivity and glycosylated structure of these two proteins, respectively (Estes and Cohen, 1989). Although the numbers continue to grow, 14 G types and 21 P types have been identified to date. Human rotaviruses belonging to 10 G serotypes have been isolated, but until very recently, the vast majority have been identified as G1, G2, G3, or G4. Likewise, nine P genotypes have been found in humans, but most illnesses have been associated with P genotypes 4 and 8. However, other G and P types, particularly G9 strains, have been the most frequently isolated from ill children in some settings, such as India, Brazil, and several African nations (Griffin *et al.*, 2002).

Growth restrictions and mechanisms of pathogenesis

Rotaviruses have an extremely wide host range, but natural cross-species infections appear to be rare. A number of human isolates appear to originate from animal strains or to be animal–human rotavirus reassortants, but their importance in human disease may be limited. It has been suggested but not yet demonstrated that once adapted to replication in humans, such strains may become important human pathogens (Nakagomi and Nakagomi, 1993). Host restriction has been utilized extensively to develop rotavirus vaccine candidates for humans by using naturally attenuated bovine and simian rotaviruses. Oral immunization of infants with these experimental live virus vaccines has resulted in low levels of intestinal replication and partial protection against human rotavirus illnesses. Thus, the barrier of host restriction can be sufficiently bypassed under these controlled conditions to permit the development of protective immune responses in a heterologous host.

There are also age restrictions associated with rotavirus disease. In the animals examined, rotavirus illness is limited to the first weeks of life. In contrast, severe human rotavirus disease is most common between 6 and 24 months of age, but milder rotavirus illnesses occur throughout life (Kapikian *et al.*, 2001). Neonatal rotavirus infections, which are usually asymptomatic in humans, are common and in some newborn nurseries appear to be endemic. Causes for the reduced severity of rotavirus disease during the first few months after birth and after the first years of life are subjects of intense investigation. Possibly, nonimmunological age-dependent changes occur within the intestine that can account for this effect in young infants. Likewise, protection may be at least partially due to transplacental antibody that persists for the first months of life. Mechanisms by which transplacental maternal antibody might protect against intestinal infection are unclear. Passive transfer of neutralizing antibody to the intestine of both humans and animals is associated with protection, but passively acquired circulating rotavirus IgG was found to confer little protection in animals (Snodgrass and Wells, 1978; Offit and Clark, 1985). Possibly, maternal IgG in humans is transferred into the intestine, where it neutralizes rotaviruses prior to infection. Regardless of why rotavirus infection of neonates is typically asymptomatic, these infections have been found to reduce the severity of rotavirus illnesses in older infants (Bishop et al., 1983; Bhan et al., 1993). For these reasons, several rotavirus strains obtained from neonates have been developed as vaccine candidates.

The reduced severity of rotavirus disease in older children and adults is probably due primarily to immune responses stimulated by previous rotavirus infections. Protection against rotavirus infection and disease in adults has been correlated with titers of both circulating and intestinal rotavirus antibody (Ward et al., 1989). Although these antibodies have not been established as the effectors of protection, their presence is indicative of a natural infection that has elicited a protective immune response.

The mechanisms by which rotaviruses induce gastrointestinal illnesses is also an area of intense investigation. In commercially important domestic animals and humans, rotavirus infection appears to be primarily restricted to the mature enterocytes on the tips of the intestinal villi, where extensive destruction is readily visualized **(Fig. 49.2)**. It has been suggested that this destruction results in malabsorption of nutrients, electrolyte imbalance, and diarrhea. The villus stunting that occurs in large mammals is very limited in mice, even though neonatal mice can experience severe rotavirus diarrhea for up to 15 days of life (Wolf et al., 1981). For these reasons, Osborne et al. (1988) suggested that rotavirus diarrhea in mice was due to vascular damage rather than to enterocyte destruction.

Recent studies of mice suggested other mechanisms for rotavirus diarrhea due, at least in part, to enterotoxin-like properties of viral proteins. Shaw et al. (1995) reported that inoculation of neonatal mice with very large quantities of purified inactivated rhesus rotavirus produced moderate to severe diarrhea in most animals. This indicated that mere attachment or uptake of rotavirus particles was sufficient to induce diarrhea. Subsequently, Ball et al. (1996) reported that purified preparations of the nonstructural protein NSP4, or a synthetic peptide from this protein from the simian rotavirus SA11, induced diarrhea in neonatal mice and rats. Further studies have shown that this protein functions as an enterotoxin by activation of a calcium-dependent signaling pathway that results in chloride secretion using a channel that is not CFTR (Ball et al., 1996; Dong et al., 1997; Morris et al., 1999). Antibody to NSP4 protects neonatal mice from virus-induced diarrhea, suggesting NSP4 is another vaccine candidate (Ball et al., 1996; Yo and Langridge, 2001). The importance of NSP4 in naturally acquired rotavirus disease in animals and humans remains to be determined, but children do make antibodies to NSP4 (Johansen et al., 1999).

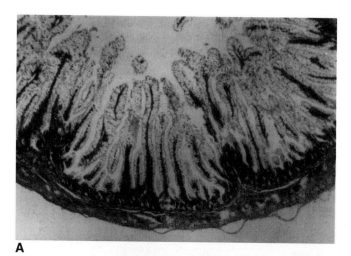

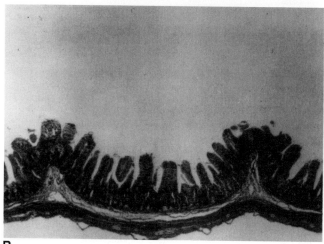

Fig. 49.2. A, Normal histologic appearance of ileum from an 8-day-old gnotobiotic pig. Normal mature vacuolate absorptive cells cover the villi. Hematoxylin and eosin stain. **B,** Ileum from an 8-day-old gnotobiotic pig after oral inoculation with virulent human rotavirus (Wa strain). Severe villous atrophy and early crypt hyperplasia are evident. Hematoxylin and eosin stain. (Photomicrographs courtesy of L.A. Ward, Ohio Agricultural Research and Development Center, Ohio State University, Wooster, Ohio.)

Further studies to identify the protein(s) responsible for rotavirus illness have been conducted with animals inoculated with reassortants composed of various gene combinations from pathogenic and nonpathogenic rotaviruses. Initial studies of mice suggested that virulence of rotavirus was associated with VP4 (Offit et al., 1986). Later studies, however, provided evidence that neither VP4 nor the outer capsid protein, VP7, was primarily responsible for virulence in mice (Broome et al., 1993). In that study, the protein most significantly associated with virulence was NSP1, encoded by segment 5 ($P < 0.008$). Another study conducted with human (DS-1) and porcine (SB-1A) reassortants linked virulence in piglets to the presence of four rotavirus proteins (VP3, VP4, VP7, and NSP4), any one of which was absolutely and exclusively required (Hoshino et al., 1995).

Thus, it is unclear whether specific rotavirus proteins are responsible for virulence or whether virulence is multigenic, resulting from a combined effect of the interactive properties of some or all of the 11 rotavirus proteins. It is likely that the genetic determinants of virulence are dependent, as well, on the specific phenotype of the parental strain used for reassortant analysis.

Immunity

In immunocompetent children, rotavirus disease is normally resolved within days, resulting in at least partial protection against subsequent rotavirus illness. Resolution of acute rotavirus disease can be prolonged in immunocompromised children, however, leading to chronic shedding and gastrointestinal symptoms. Thus, immune mechanisms are involved in both the resolution of rotavirus disease and the prevention of subsequent rotavirus illnesses.

The immunological effectors that prevent rotavirus disease have been partially identified, particularly through studies with animal models, but those in humans remain poorly understood. Because rotaviruses replicate in intestinal enterocytes, resulting in the associated gastrointestinal symptoms, it is generally assumed that effector mechanisms must be active at the intestinal mucosa. The most obvious immunological effector is secretory IgA (S-IgA). Following infection of mice with a high dose of heterologous rotavirus, up to 50% of all IgA-producing plasma cells in the lamina propria of the intestine can be rotavirus-specific (Shaw et al., 1993). Furthermore, protection against rotavirus infection in orally immunized mice correlates with levels of intestinal (stool) and serum rotavirus IgA but not serum rotavirus IgG (McNeal et al., 1994; Feng et al., 1994). Similarly, piglets orally immunized with a virulent human rotavirus (strain Wa) develop significantly greater numbers of cells that secrete rotavirus IgA (but not IgG) in their intestines and blood than piglets vaccinated with an avirulent Wa strain (Yuan et al., 1996, 2001a). When subsequently challenged with virulent Wa, the numbers of rotavirus IgA-secreting cells present in the intestines of these piglets correlate with protection from disease. In humans, titers of serum rotavirus IgG and IgA as well as intestinal rotavirus S-IgA correlate with protection following natural infection (Ward et al., 1989; Clemens et al., 1992; Coulson et al., 1992; Matson et al., 1993; O'Ryan et al., 1994, Velazquez et al., 2000). However, the titer of any isotype of rotavirus-specific antibody could not be consistently correlated with protection after either natural infection or vaccination. Thus, the possibility remains that rotavirus antibody is merely an indicator of protection and not the actual effector.

The most obvious mechanism of protection by antibody is by virus neutralization. Passive protection has been definitively linked with the consumption of neutralization antibody in both animal and human studies. Evidence that active immunity induced by oral immunization with live rotavirus or natural rotavirus infection is due to neutralizing antibody is varied. In an early report of a study on sequential rotavirus illnesses with the same serotype conducted at a Japanese orphanage, a close association was found between the titers of serotype-specific neutralizing antibody and protection (Chiba et al., 1986). Further support for neutralization as the mechanism of protection was found in a study on piglets where protection was dependent on oral immunization with rotaviruses containing genes for either VP4 or VP7 of the same serotype as the challenge strain (Hoshino et al., 1988). Rotaviruses containing only heterotypic genes for these proteins elicited some protection but less than that induced by homotypic immunization.

In contrast, a large case-control study with children in Bangladesh found protection following natural infection correlated with rotavirus antibody titers, but the best correlations were found with heterotypic neutralizing antibody (Ward et al., 1992). Initial vaccine trials with both bovine and simian rotaviruses suggested that protection developed in the absence of neutralizing antibody to the circulating human rotavirus strains. Protection was inconsistent, however, and subsequent vaccine trials with a rhesus rotavirus (RRV, simian) strain suggested that protection may be serotype-specific (Flores et al., 1987; Santosham et al., 1991). These results led to the development of bovine and simian rotavirus vaccine strains containing genes for human rotavirus neutralization proteins, which have been or are currently being evaluated in infants. Even in the most recent trials with simian rotavirus reassortants, however, the relationship between serum neutralizing antibody titers and protection is inconsistent, and protection is seen in infants that failed to develop serotype-specific neutralizing antibody responses to the circulating human rotavirus strains (Ward et al., 1997).

Most data from animal studies indicate that classical neutralization is not the only mechanism of protection. The most immunogenic protein is VP6, which does not appear to stimulate neutralizing antibody responses. Evidence, however, suggests that IgA antibodies directed at VP6 are protective by mechanisms that are not yet completely understood (Burns et al., 1996; Feng et al., 2002). Vaccination with either virus-like particles (VLPs) that lack the outer capsid proteins, and thus do not induce neutralizing antibody, or a chimeric VP6 can also elicit protective immunity against infection in adult mice (O'Neal et al., 1997; Choi et al., 1999). Passive protection against murine rotavirus disease in neonatal mice has also been produced by adoptive transfer of CD8+ T cells from spleens of mice previously infected (orally) with either homologous or heterologous rotavirus strains (Offit and Dudzik, 1990). Similarly, CD8+ splenic or intraepithelial lymphocytes from rotavirus-infected mice can eliminate chronic rotavirus shedding in mice with severe combined immunodeficiency (SCID) (Dharakul et al., 1990). Thus, at least passive protection against rotavirus disease and resolution of rotavirus shedding can be promulgated with cytotoxic T cells.

An adult mouse model of rotavirus infection has been particularly useful in examining the mechanisms of active immunity against rotavirus in mice (Ward et al., 1990). Since adult mice become infected with rotavirus but do not develop disease, this model uses protection against infection as its endpoint. According to this model, protection against live oral murine rotavirus infection is not correlated with either serum or intestinal neutralizing antibody titers against the challenge virus. However, it is correlated with total serum and stool rotavirus IgA titers (McNeal *et al.*, 1994; Feng *et al.*, 1994, 1997), as well as high titers of rotavirus-specific IgA at the intestinal mucosal surface (Moser *et al.*, 1998). Subsequently, the use of B-cell-deficient mice that cannot produce antibody has shown that long-term protection against rotavirus infection depends primarily on antibody (Franco and Greenberg, 1995; McNeal *et al.*, 1995). Even after parenteral immunization, migration of antigen-presenting cells (APCs) from the peripheral lymphoid tissues to the gut-associated lymphoid tissues (GALT) may contribute to mucosal S-IgA responses and protection (Coffin *et al.*, 1999). Although protection in this model is typically associated with rotavirus IgA, genetically modified mice that cannot produce IgA are also protected after live virus immunization, presumably due to increased titers of rotavirus IgG (O'Neal *et al.*, 2000). Recent studies have also demonstrated the importance of integrin-mediated B cell homing to the intestine for their antirotaviral effectiveness (Kuklin *et al.*, 2001).

Resolution of rotavirus shedding and protection against subsequent rotavirus infection of mice has also been associated with rotavirus-specific CD8+ T cells. Depletion of CD8+ T cells in B cell–deficient mice prior to oral inoculation with live murine rotavirus prevents resolution of the initial infection (Franco and Greenberg, 1995; McNeal *et al.*, 1995). Thus, cytotoxic T cells appear to be critical for the initial resolution of virus shedding when antibody is not present. In fully immunocompetent mice, however, CD8+ T cell depletion merely delays the resolution of shedding, which occurs with the appearance of antibody. Therefore, CD8+ T cells appear to be the normal primary effectors of rotavirus resolution, but long-term protection appears to be primarily dependent on antibody in this mouse model. Subsequently, it was shown that immune CD8+ T cells actively restricted but did not completely eliminate rotavirus replication on rechallenge for several weeks after immunization (Franco *et al.*, 1997a). Mechanistic studies indicate that CD8+ T cells do not mediate their protective effects via perforin-, Fas-, or IFN-γ-dependent pathways (Franco *et al.*, 1997b). More recently it was shown that nasal or oral inoculation of mice with a chimeric VP6 protein, or even a 14–amino acid peptide of VP6, along with an effective adjuvant, consistently elicited >95% reductions in rotavirus shedding after challenge (Choi *et al.*, 1999, 2000). CD4+ T cells were subsequently found to be the only lymphocytes required to elicit this protection, *i.e.*, B-cell-deficient mice that were depleted of CD8+ T cells were completely protected against rotavirus challenge, while depletion of CD4+ from these mice resulted in complete loss of protection (McNeal *et al.*, 2002). However, Schwartz-Cornil *et al.* (2002) reported that J-chain-deficient mice that were unable to mediate IgA and IgM transcytosis were only marginally protected against rotavirus shedding when immunized nasally with VLPs plus adjuvant and subsequently challenged with murine rotavirus.

This result suggested a role for antibody in rotavirus clearance in mice under these conditions. Therefore, B, CD8+, and CD4+ T cells have all been identified as effectors of protection against rotavirus shedding in mice, and the relative importance of each appears to be dependent on the immunogen and the method of immunization. A summary of the major findings on immune mechanisms in this adult mouse model are listed in **Table 49.2**.

Most studies on rotavirus immunity in both animals and humans have focused on oral immunization with live rotaviruses. Early studies on passive immunization in animals indicated that intestinal and not circulating rotavirus antibody was protective (Snodgrass and Wells, 1978; Offit and Clark, 1985). More recent reports in mice and rabbits, however, suggest that parenteral immunization with a variety of rotavirus antigens (*e.g.*, live virus, inactivated virus, VLPs, individual viral proteins encoded by DNA) of both homologous and heterologous origin can elicit at least partial protection against infection with homologous rotavirus strains (McNeal *et al.*, 1992; Conner *et al.*, 1993; Herrmann *et al.*, 1996; Coffin and Offit, 1998). Where examined, immunization by parenteral routes elicits little or no serum or intestinal rotavirus IgA responses, leading to the possibility that protection is due to rotavirus IgG, cytotoxic T-lymphocytes (CTLs), or the antiviral activity of cytokines (Bass, 1997).

In contrast to the results found in mice and rabbits, parenteral immunization of gnotobiotic piglets with an inactivated human rotavirus and adjuvant provided no protection against shedding or diarrhea following challenge with the same strain of rotavirus (To *et al.*, 1998). Furthermore, gnotobiotic piglets have also been generally less protected than mice after oral immunization with live attenuated rotaviruses or nasally with VLPs and adjuvant (Yuan *et al.*, 2000, 2001b). The reasons for the differences are unclear, and the relevance of these findings to human immunization has generated polarized views, ranging from suggestions that piglets are much more similar to humans than are mice to questions regarding the authenticity of gnotobiotic animals for studies on intestinal immunity. Resolution of the actual reasons for the wide range of results found with the different animal models will be critical for vaccine development and will probably be fully resolved only when the studies are conducted in humans.

Vaccines

Based upon the belief that protection from rotavirus is best achieved by inducing mucosal intestinal immune responses and the finding that natural rotavirus infections induce at least partial protection against subsequent rotavirus disease, vaccine efforts have been primarily directed at the development of live attenuated orally deliverable rotavirus vaccines. Most of these efforts have concentrated on the use of animal rotavirus strains that are naturally attenuated for humans and stimulate largely heterotypic immune responses. More recently, human rotavirus genes have been introduced into these animal strains by creating reassortant viruses to increase their serotypic relatedness to

Table 49.2. Effector Mechanisms of Resolution and Protection Identified in the Adult Mouse Model

Mouse Strain	Immunization	Outcome	Reference
BALB/c (normal)	Oral, several live homologous and heterologous rotaviruses	Protection correlates with serum rotavirus IgA	McNeal et al., 1994
BALB/c	Oral, live RRV, EDIM	Protection correlates with intestinal rotavirus IgA	Feng et al., 1994; Moser et al., 1998
$J_H D$ (B-cell-deficient)	Oral, live murine rotaviruses	Resolution dependent on CD8$^+$ cells; protection primarily dependent on antibody	Franco and Greenberg, 1995; McNeal et al., 1995
$J_H D$	Oral, live murine rotavirus	Partial protection related to CD8$^+$ cells	Franco et al., 1997a
BALB/c	Intramuscular with live murine rotavirus	Intestinal IgA production after parenteral immunization	Coffin et al., 1999
IgA$^{-/-}$	Oral, live murine rotavirus	Intestinal IgG associated with protection	O'Neal et al., 2000
$\beta 7^{-/-}$	Adoptive transfer of immune B or CD8$^+$ T cells into chronically shedding Rag-2-deficient mice	B but not CD8$^+$ T cells require $\alpha_4 \beta_7$ homing receptor	Kuklin et al., 2000, 2001
$J_H D$	Nasal immunization with VP6	CD4$^+$ cells are only lymphocytes required for protection	McNeal et al., 2002
J chain$^{-/-}$	Nasal immunization with 2/6 VLPs	Marginal protection in absence of transcytosed IgA, IgM	Schwartz-Cornil et al., 2002

human rotaviruses. Human rotaviruses have also been developed as vaccine candidates. Most are neonatal strains that may be naturally attenuated. However, the most extensively evaluated human rotavirus vaccine candidate is strain 89-12, a G1[P8] obtained from the stool of a symptomatic child and attenuated by multiple cell culture passages. One of the challenges in producing a live attenuated vaccine candidate for a pathogen that replicates in the gastrointestinal tract is finding the appropriate level of attenuation and immunogenicity, both of which are probably in some way related to the replication properties of the virus. Several vaccine candidates have been tested only for safety and immunogenicity; others have been tested in major vaccine efficacy trials **(Table 49.3)**.

The initial rotavirus vaccine trials were with RIT4237, a bovine rotavirus. These were followed by trials with a simian strain (RRV or MMU 18006), another bovine rotavirus (WC3), and reassortants of RRV, WC3, and a third bovine strain, UK. Less extensive studies have been performed with neonatal human strains M37, RV3, 116E, and I321, which are believed to be naturally attenuated human rotavirus strains. Human rotavirus strain 89–12 (attenuated by multiple passages in tissue culture) is presently one of the two candidate vaccines under extensive investigation in multiple countries throughout the world, the other being the WC3 reassortant strains. Finally, a lamb rotavirus has been developed in China and administered to large numbers of subjects locally.

The initial studies with the RIT vaccine produced excellent results in Finland, providing a protective efficacy of about 50% against all disease and >80% protection against severe disease (Vesikari, 1993). Later studies in developing countries and on a Navajo reservation in Arizona (Santosham et al., 1991), however, were disappointing, showing little or no efficacy. It should be noted that the RIT vaccine was efficacious in Finland, despite the fact that it was serotypically unrelated to the circulating human rotavirus strains.

The WC3 bovine rotavirus vaccine also appeared to be free of side effects, but like the RIT vaccine, belonged to serotype G6 and stimulated little or no neutralizing antibody to human strains. Although it replicates poorly in humans, infants developed some neutralizing antibody to WC3 and both rotavirus-specific IgA and IgG. The initial studies with WC3 conducted in Philadelphia, Pennsylvania (USA), appeared very promising (Clark et al., 1988), but later trials in Cincinnati, Ohio (USA) (Bernstein et al., 1990), and in less developed countries did not show significant protection.

Numerous trials were performed to evaluate RRV as a vaccine candidate. RRV replicates better in humans than the bovine vaccine strains but also produces mild side effects, including low-grade fever and mild diarrhea, especially when given to older children. RRV induces serum rotavirus IgG and IgA, intestinal rotavirus IgA, and serotype-specific neutralizing antibody to RRV and other serotype G3 strains.

Table 49.3. Selected Vaccine Studies

Vaccine	Country	Number of Subjects	Number of Doses	Percentage[a] Protection (Overall/Severe Disease)
RTT 4237	Finland	178	1	50/58
	Finland	328	2	58/82
	Rwanda	245	3	0/0
	Gambia	185	3	0/37
	Peru	391	3	40/75
WC3	USA (Philadelphia, PA)	104	1	43/89
	USA (Cincinnati, OH)	206	1	17/41
	Central African Republic	472	2	0/36
RRV	USA (Rochester, NY)	176	1	0/0
	Venezuela	247	1	68/100
	Finland	200	1	38/67
	Venezuela	320	1	64/90
	USA (Rochester, NY)	223	1	66/ND
	USA (Indian Reservation)	321	1	0/ND
RRV reassortants				
RRV G1	Finland	359	1	67/ND
RRV G2				66/ND
RRV G1	USA (Rochester, NY)	223	1	77/ND
RRV G1	USA	898	3	69/73
RRV TV				64/82
RRV G1	USA	1187	3	54/69
RRV TV				49/80
RRV TV	Finland	2273	3	66/91
RRV TV	Venezuela	2207	3	48/88
WC3 reassortants				
WC3 G1	USA (Rochester, NY)	325	3	64/87
WC3 TV	USA	417	3	73/73
89-12	USA	215	2	89/100

[a] Measured in the first year after vaccination
ND, not determined.

Protection with this vaccine has been inconsistent, ranging from >50%, even in developing countries, to nonexistent. Although there is some evidence suggesting that protection was predominantly against G3 strains (Flores *et al.*, 1987; Santosham *et al.*, 1991), this evidence is not conclusive, and the RRV vaccine has clearly demonstrated efficacy against serotypes other than G3 human strains in some trials.

Because of the belief that immunity to human rotavirus neutralization antigens may increase the magnitude and consistency of protection seen with the animal strains, reassortant rotaviruses were made that contained VP7 (RRV–human rotavirus reassortants) or VP7 and VP4 (WC3–human rotavirus reassortants) neutralization proteins of human rotavirus strains on parental animal rotavirus backgrounds. Although vaccine preparations containing between one and three RRV reassortants have been tested, the vaccine candidate prepared for licensure contained four viruses, each with a different VP7 protein gene (G1–G4) representative of the major G serotypes

of human rotaviruses. Vaccination with the tetravalent RRV vaccine stimulated serum rotavirus IgG and IgA responses, but neutralizing antibodies produced were predominantly to RRV rather than to the human rotavirus serotypes (Ward *et al.*, 1997). Because no greater titers of neutralizing antibody developed against the human G3 strain than against the G1, G2, and G4 human strains used in the laboratory analyses, the immune responses to RRV were primarily directed against its VP4, which is serotypically unrelated to the VP4 proteins found in the human strains used in the analyses.

Extensive evaluations of the reassortant RRV vaccine were performed. In two large trials conducted at centers across the United States (Bernstein *et al.*, 1995; Rennels *et al.*, 1996), the tetravalent vaccine was shown to be safe, although a slight increase in fever may be seen after the first dose. The efficacy of the vaccine against rotavirus disease for the first year was 49% to 64%, and it was 57% over 2 years. Protection was increased against more severe disease, to a level of about 80% for very severe illness. In a large trial carried out in Finland, the tetravalent RRV vaccine was even more protective (68% against all rotavirus disease and 100% against severe disease requiring hospitalization) (Joensuu et al., 1997). These results are consistent with findings in two less developed settings, including Venezuela (Perez-Schael et al., 1997) and a Navajo reservation in Arizona (USA) (Santosham et al., 1997).

Although this vaccine has consistently elicited good protection, the relationship between its ability to stimulate serotype-specific neutralizing antibody responses and to protect against rotavirus disease was not clearly established (Ward et al., 1997). The tetravalent RRV vaccine became the first and only licensed rotavirus vaccine when it was approved in the USA in 1998. However, within less than 1 year, the vaccine was withdrawn because of an increased risk of intussusception in the week following administration of the first dose of vaccine, thus again leaving the world without an approved rotavirus vaccine (Murphy et al., 2001).

A quadrivalent WC3-based reassortant vaccine has also been evaluated that consists of both VP7 and VP4 human rotavirus gene substitutions (G1, G2, G3, or P8) on a WC3 background. In a study conducted at multiple centers in the United States, it was shown to be safe, with only a slight increase in diarrhea after the first dose (Clark et al., 1995). The vaccine was 73% effective against all cases of rotavirus gastroenteritis and 73% effective against more severe cases, efficacy rates similar to those found with the tetravalent RRV vaccine. A fifth reassortant strain (G4) has since been added to this vaccine candidate, and the new quintavalent WC3-based vaccine is being evaluated in multiple sites around the world. It is one of two rotavirus vaccine candidates presently being seriously considered for international use.

Other approaches to rotavirus vaccines, including use of attenuated human viruses, are also being evaluated. The initial evaluation of M37, a strain isolated from an asymptomatic newborn, showed reduced immunogenicity and a lack of efficacy (Vesikari et al., 1991), while evaluations of another neonatal strain (RV3) are continuing, but so far few subjects have been given this candidate vaccine (Barnes et al., 2002). A phase 2 trial of human strain 89–12, which was protective after natural infection and attenuated by multiple tissue-culture passages, showed excellent protection in a small trial in the United States against the circulating G1 strains, the same G serotype as this single-strain vaccine candidate. Safety, immunogenicity, and efficacy trials of this vaccine are now being conducted worldwide, and this is the second rotavirus vaccine candidate presently being considered for international use.

Subunit and DNA vaccines, various expression vectors, synthetic peptides, and virus-like particles (VLPs) produced from baculovirus-expressed rotavirus capsid proteins are also being considered as alternative vaccine candidates. In every animal model of active and passive immunity examined, VLPs have been shown to be nonreplicating particles that are safe, highly immunogenic, and capable of inducing protective immunity (O'Neal et al., 1997; Cialet et al., 1998; Yuan et al., 2001b; Coste et al., 2000). VLPs are scheduled to begin to be tested

as vaccine candidates in humans. Nasal or oral inoculation of a chimeric VP6 along with a mucosal adjuvant has also been shown to provide excellent protection against rotavirus shedding in the adult mouse model (Choi et al., 1999).

On the basis of the finding that sequential illnesses with even the same serotypes of rotaviruses are not uncommon, it is difficult to envision how any live virus vaccine delivered orally can, by itself, stimulate complete and lasting protection against all rotavirus illnesses. Therefore, a reasonable goal for present vaccine candidates is to eliminate severe rotavirus disease in children during their most vulnerable period, between 6 months and 2 years of age. To do this, the vaccine must be delivered at an early age, a time when maternal components such as transplacental antibody and possibly innate resistance factors may limit immune responses to it, and when the immune system is immature. To overcome possible age-dependent inhibitory factors and stimulate more durable immune responses, parenteral rotavirus vaccines are receiving serious consideration. Studies in animals suggest that this route of immunization may provide excellent protection, either alone or in combination with oral immunization. Novel and less invasive means of vaccine delivery by the parenteral route are being investigated, and these may enhance the feasibility of this approach and help overcome a general resistance toward the development of additional parenteral childhood vaccines. Therefore, even though a rotavirus vaccine was licensed and then withdrawn, development of future rotavirus vaccines remains a fertile area for investigation. An important goal that remains is to establish a clear correlate of protection. If this could be achieved for children, it would greatly simplify future evaluations of new rotavirus vaccine candidates.

ENTERIC HUMAN CALICIVIRUSES

Introduction

Caliciviruses consist of a family of viruses that infect humans and animals. Animal caliciviruses cause a spectrum of diseases, including respiratory illness, hemorrhagic liver disease, abortions, skin lesions, glossitis, and gastroenteritis. Human caliciviruses have been associated only with gastrointestinal disease; this section considers these human viruses briefly, as well as the need and prospects for development of a vaccine to prevent such infections.

History and clinical significance

The Norwalk virus (NV) represents the prototype human calicivirus that causes epidemic gastroenteritis in humans. This virus is named for the location of an outbreak of gastroenteritis in Norwalk, Ohio, that began in October 1968. During a 2-day period, acute gastrointestinal illness developed in 50% of 232 students and teachers at an elementary school, and a secondary attack rate of 32% was observed among family contacts of primary cases. The disease lasted about 24 hours and had an incubation period of approximately 48 hours. Although some patients had diarrhea, the predominant clinical manifestations were vomiting and nausea (Adler and Zickl, 1969). Subsequent transmission of this disease to adult volunteers given bacteria-free fecal filtrates proved that a virus could cause gastroenteritis. The virus was not visualized until several years later, when a new method of immune electron microscopy was used to aggregate virus particles in fecal material from the Norwalk outbreak by coating them with convalescent serum (Kapikian et al., 1972). Subsequent studies in the 1970s and 1980s showed that NV and similar agents are the major cause of epidemic nonbacterial gastroenteritis, a disease that occurs in family and community-wide outbreaks and predominantly affects school-aged children and adults. Outbreaks occur in many settings, including recreational camps, cruise and military ships, communities, hospitals, schools, nursing homes, and families. This illness is transmitted by the fecal–oral route and is often food- or water-borne.

The genome of NV was characterized by cloning and sequence analysis, and it was found to be an RNA virus belonging to the family Caliciviridae (Jiang et al., 1990, 1993b; Matsui et al., 1991; Lambden et al., 1993). Following this breakthrough, our understanding of the epidemiology of infections with NV and related viruses began to change with the use of new, more sensitive diagnostic assays for detecting the viral genome, the capsid protein, and antibody responses to the viral proteins. Studies using new diagnostic assays developed with recombinant NV (rNV) VLPs have shown that the epidemiological significance of NV infections was previously greatly underestimated. For example, antibody prevalence studies indicate that NV infections occur in young children in developed countries (Green et al., 1993; Dimitrov et al., 1997; Estes et al., 1997). In addition, NV caused illness among Desert Storm troops in Kuwait and has resulted in significant debilitating illness during military maneuvers in Somalia, on aircraft carriers, and on pleasure cruise ships (Hyams et al., 1993; Sharp et al., 1995).

Growth properties, clinical illness, and mechanisms of pathogenesis

NV is an enteric virus whose host range is restricted to humans. Attempts to cultivate this virus and other noroviruses in cell culture and in animals have failed. NV is now recognized as the prototype strain of a large group of viruses that are classified in the genus *Norovirus* in the family Caliciviridae. These viruses are the most common cause of outbreaks of nonbacterial gastroenteritis in the United States, Europe, and Japan, with 60% to >90% of the outbreaks being associated with noroviruses (Fankhauser et al., 1998; Vinje and Koopmans, 1996; Inouye et al., 2000). Noroviruses are also being detected as causes of significant disease in the elderly and in young children (Green et al., 2002; Sakai et al., 2001). Human caliciviruses in a second genus, *Sapovirus*, of the Caliciviridae are also associated with gastroenteritis, but the disease they cause appears to be less common and less severe. Noroviruses are spread by food and

water and from person to person (Kapikian et al., 1996). Oral ingestion of infectious particles typically results in acute gastroenteritis.

The clinical manifestations of NV infections include sudden onset of vomiting and/or diarrhea after a 24- to 48-hour incubation period; symptoms typically last 12 to 24 hours. Only occasionally do infected individuals require intravenous fluid therapy.

The histopathology of NV and Hawaii virus illness was studied in detail during volunteer studies in the 1970s. Proximal intestinal biopsies from ill volunteers were obtained. The intestinal villi were broadened and blunted, crypt cells were hyperplastic, and there was polymorphonuclear and mononuclear cell infiltration into the lamina propria. The mucosa remained intact. Small intestinal brush-border enzymatic activities were decreased, resulting in fat and carbohydrate malabsorption (Agus et al., 1973; Schreiber et al., 1974).

An unexplained observation in the volunteer studies was that a subset of individuals were resistant to infection, and a genetic control of susceptibility and/or resistance was proposed (Parrino et al., 1977). Recent studies have found that ABO histo-blood group type is a partial explanation for this resistance (Hutson et al., 2002a), and the ability of virus to bind to intestinal cells may also be affected by an individual's secretor status (Marionneau et al., 2002). The H antigen has been discovered to be a carbohydrate that initially binds to NV (Marionneau et al., 2002; Hutson et al., 2002b).

Volunteer studies

The volunteer challenge model was used to reevaluate the clinical, virological, and immunological responses to NV challenge in volunteers, with use of highly sensitive diagnostic assays such as enzyme-linked immunosorbent assays (ELISAs) with rNV antigen for antibody detection and reverse transcriptase polymerase chain reaction (RT-PCR) for detecting the viral genome (Graham et al., 1994). A higher infection rate, more subclinical infections, and longer virus excretion following NV inoculations were found than in the earlier volunteer studies. Of 50 volunteers challenged with NV, 41 (82%) became infected; of these infections, 68% were symptomatic and 32% were asymptomatic. The peak of virus shedding was between 25 and 72 hours, and virus first appeared in stool 15 hours after inoculation. Surprisingly, stool specimens collected 7 days after inoculation remained ELISA-positive for individuals with both symptomatic and asymptomatic infections. The high rate of asymptomatic infection and the prolonged shedding in volunteers have clarified the public health significance of NV, since these characteristics contribute to increased transmission of this virus.

Immunity to NV

The inability to cultivate NV and other enteric human caliciviruses has hampered studies on viral immunity because *in vitro* neutralization assays are not available. Studies on NV immunity have involved measuring antibody in volunteers and naturally infected individuals and attempting to correlate serum responses with clinical outcomes. Epidemiological and volunteer rechallenge studies have indicated that at least short-term protective immunity is induced by infection (Kapikian *et al.*, 1996), and other studies indicate that multiple exposures lead to immunity that correlates with levels of antibody (Johnson *et al.*,1990). In other studies, a relationship between antibody and protection has been unclear for adults infected with NV. This may be because previous assays were measuring both antibody and secreted H antigen in serum that binds to virus but would not be involved in the acquired immune response. A correlation between serum antibody and protective immunity has been reported for young children infected with a different strain (HuCV Sapporo) of human caliciviruses (Nakata *et al.*, 1985a, b).

NV vaccines

Because our understanding of protective immunity to NV and other HuCVs is incomplete, it remains unclear whether vaccination will be able to prevent such illnesses. However, vaccines should prove effective if the evidence of short-term protection in adults and long-term protection in children is correct. It is clearly important to determine the number of serotypes of HuCVs and whether cross-protection among serotypes can be induced. The discovery that expression of the capsid protein leads to high yields of spontaneously folded VLPs lacking nucleic acid makes a subunit vaccine available. Such rNV VLPs are produced in high concentrations (22 mg of purified particles from 2×10^8 infected cells), and characterization of these particles has shown that they have desirable properties for use as a subunit vaccine. Specifically, these particles are stable following lyophilization and when exposed to acid (pH, 2.5); highly immunogenic when injected parenterally into animals (Jiang *et al.*, 1992, 1995b); immunogenic when given orally or nasally to mice in the absence of adjuvant (Ball *et al.*, 1998; Guerrero *et al.*, 2001); and safe and immunogenic when given orally to antibody-positive adult volunteers (Ball *et al.*, 1999; Tacket *et al.*, 2000). NV particles can also be expressed in plants (Mason *et al.*, 1996), and particles delivered in transgenic potatoes are immunogenic in volunteers (Tacket *et al.*, 2000). Although challenge efficacy studies remain to be performed, these results suggest that rNV VLPs could be used to immunize against NV.

VLPs of many strains of HuCVs have now been produced (Jiang *et al.*, 1992, 1995a; Dingle *et al.*, 1995; Numata *et al.*, 1997; Leite *et al.*, 1996), and it remains to be determined if a single type of VLP will be able to induce broadly cross-reactive protective immunity against infections with multiple types of HuCVs or if immunization with multiple types of VLPs will be necessary. Initial targets for such a vaccine would likely be the military and travelers. The unique structure of the single capsid protein in these particles suggests they also may be useful as a carrier for delivering other vaccine antigens (Prasad *et al.*, 1994; Prasad and Estes, 1997). A second NV candidate vaccine has been made by using a

Venezuelan equine encephalitis virus replicons (Harrington *et al.*, 2002).

ASTROVIRUSES

Introduction

The Astroviridae is a virus family containing viruses that infect several mammalian and avian species and usually cause diarrheal disease in these infected animals (Monroe *et al.*, 1995). Astroviruses are small, nonenveloped viruses that display a characteristic starlike appearance when visualized by negative-stain electron microscopy. Recent advances in astrovirus research, including cloning and sequencing of the plus-sense RNA genome, isolation of an "infectious" cDNA clone, development of cell culture systems, and availability of sensitive diagnostic reagents, have led to a better understanding of these emerging pathogens. We are becoming increasingly aware of their clinical importance in children and adults but still lack knowledge concerning the basic determinants of pathogenesis and immunity.

History and clinical significance

Astroviruses were first described in 1975 (Madeley and Cosgrove, 1975; Appleton and Higgins, 1975). Initially, astroviruses could be identified only when they displayed their typical starlike morphology on observation by electron microscopy (EM) in fecal specimens. Following the detection of astroviruses in fecal specimens from young children with gastroenteritis, similar particles were observed in stool specimens from a wide variety of animals. It was not until the cultivation of human astroviruses and the development of sensitive second-generation solid-phase immunoassays that a clear-cut picture of the epidemiology and clinical significance of astroviruses began to emerge (Lee and Kurtz, 1981; Herrmann *et al.*, 1990).

Human astrovirus infection appears to be very common and to occur early in life. In one study that detected antibody by an immunofluorescence assay, three-quarters of the children tested had antibody to astroviruses by the age of 10 years (Kurtz and Lee, 1978). Astrovirus antibodies have been identified in serum specimens from all parts of the world and in commercial preparations of IgG.

Astroviruses have been identified as pathogens in four general groups of people: normal infants and toddlers, the elderly, immunocompromised patients, and school-aged children and adults exposed to contaminated water or food sources. Although astroviruses have been clearly identified as etiological agents in each of these circumstances, with the exception of disease in infants and toddlers, it has been hard to determine the relative importance of astroviruses as etiological agents of diarrheal disease.

Properties of the virus

Astroviruses are icosahedral structures between 30 and 40 nm in diameter. They have a buoyant density of 1.37 g/ml in cesium chloride and 1.32 g/ml in tartrate–glycerol (Matsui *et al.*, 1993; Ashley and Caul, 1982). The astrovirus genome is a 6800-nucleotide-long, plus-sense RNA with a poly A tract at the 3′ terminus (Lewis *et al.*, 1994; Willcocks *et al.*, 1994; Jiang *et al.*, 1993a). In infected cells, a subgenomic RNA of approximately 2300 bases is found (Monroe *et al.*, 1993). Infectious RNA transcribed *in vitro* from a genome-length cDNA clone of human astrovirus serotype 1 has been described (Geigenmüller *et al.*, 1997). The genome is composed of three long open reading frames (ORFs) called ORF1a, ORF1b, and ORF2. Sequence analysis indicates that ORFs 1a and 1b probably encode the viral serine protease and RNA-dependent RNA polymerase, respectively. ORF1a also contains a functional nuclear localization signal of unknown biologic significance (Willcocks *et al.*, 1999). The intracellular processing of the ORF1a product, msPla, has recently been characterized (Geigenmüller *et al.*, 2002). Analysis of the coding sequences in ORF1a and 1b and *in vitro* transcription and translation studies indicate that astroviruses regulate the translation of ORF1b by a (−1) ribosomal frame-shifting mechanism (Jiang *et al.*, 1993a; Lewis and Matsui, 1994).

ORF2 is located at the 3′ end of the plus strand and is found in both genomic and subgenomic RNA species. This ORF encodes a 90-kDa protein that appears to be cleaved posttranslationally into at least three capsid proteins that make up the virion (Monroe *et al.*, 1991; Sanchez-Fauquier, 1994, Mendez, *et al.*, 2002). Neutralizing antibody is directed at the capsid structure, but the precise location of neutralization domains has not yet been determined.

Viral serotypes and detection

Eight serotypes of human astrovirus have been identified to date. It appears that serotype 1 viruses are most commonly encountered, with the other types accounting for 10% or less of isolates. Although it is reasonable to assume that immunity to astroviruses is type-specific, proof of this hypothesis is not yet available and the role of viral serotypes in the epidemiology of infection remains to be demonstrated.

Astrovirus infection can be diagnosed with use of several assay systems. Virus can now be efficiently cultivated from fecal specimens with use of CaCo-2 cells (Pinto *et al.*, 1994). Cultivation permits serotypic analysis of the isolate but is obviously labor-intensive and costly. Viral antigen can be detected in stool by EM, immune electron microscopy (IEM), and enzyme immunoassay (EIA). The latter assay is clearly the most efficient and sensitive and is currently the assay of choice. More recently, RT-PCR-based assays have also been developed, and these tests correlate well with EIA, although they appear to be somewhat more sensitive (Mitchell *et al.*, 1995; Matsui *et al.*, 1994). RT-PCR assays can determine viral serotype as well (Guix *et al.*, 2002).

Epidemiology and pathogenesis

Astrovirus infection generally causes acute self-limited gastroenteritis characterized by diarrhea, vomiting, fever, anorexia, and a variety of constitutional symptoms. The illness usually lasts 4 days or less and is indistinguishable from rotavirus infection except that it tends to be less severe, at least in young children. Volunteer studies and epidemiological analysis indicate that the incubation period for astrovirus-associated illness is 24 to 36 hours (Kurtz *et al.*, 1979).

Multiple studies have attempted to determine the role of astroviruses in acute gastroenteritis in young children under the age of 5 years (Mitchell *et al.*, 1995; Cruz *et al.*, 1992; Kotloff *et al.*, 1992; Lew *et al.*, 1991, Guix *et al.*, 2002; Marie-Cardine *et al.*, 2002). These studies have generally, but not exclusively, been outpatient-based and have occurred in both rural and urban settings. In most cases, astroviruses were isolated with a substantially greater frequency from ill subjects than from controls. The percentage of diarrheal cases associated with astrovirus shedding ranged from 2.3% to 13%. It seems likely, on the basis of these studies, that astroviruses are a common cause of mild to severe diarrheal disease in young children but less important than rotaviruses (Rodriguez-Baez *et al.*, 2002; Dennehy *et al.*, 2001).

Symptomatic astrovirus infections have been reported in the elderly, although the importance of this agent in the geriatric population remains to be fully examined (Matsui *et al.*, 1994). The role of astroviruses in immunocompromised patients has been studied in the setting of bone marrow transplantation and human immunodeficiency virus (HIV) infection (Grohmann *et al.*, 1993; Cox *et al.*, 1994; Cubbitt *et al.*, 1999). In each case, astroviruses appeared to play a significant but modest role as a cause of gastroenteritis. Finally, astrovirus infection has been associated with several food- or water-borne epidemics of gastroenteritis, primarily in Japan. Some of these epidemics were quite large, involving several thousand people. The existence of large epidemics of astrovirus infection in populations of older children and adults presumably indicates that immunity to astroviruses is not complete or lifelong. Knowledge concerning the pathogenesis of human astrovirus infection is very limited. In one report, astroviruses were detected in intestinal epithelial cells (Phillips *et al.*, 1982). In studies on a variety of mammalian species, it appears that astrovirus replication occurs primarily in mature villus enterocytes. Presumably, diarrhea results from the lytic destruction of these absorptive cells. In cell culture, astroviruses appear to be able to infect both the apical and basolateral sides of polarized epithelial monolayers (Willcocks *et al.*, 1990). Viral entry appears to be mediated via an endocytic pathway (Donelli *et al.*, 1992).

Immunity and treatment

Very little is known about immunity to astroviruses. Clearly, young children appear to be more susceptible to illness than adults, indicating that immunity probably plays some role in preventing illness. In volunteer studies with adults, susceptibility to illness was rare and appeared to correlate with lower levels of serum antibody to astrovirus (Kurtz *et al.*, 1979; Midthun *et al.*, 1993). The role of astrovirus serotype in immunity has not been studied, nor is it clear which arm of the immune system (antibody or cell-mediated immunity [CMI]/delayed-type hypersensitivity [DTH]) is involved.

Astrovirus illness is, in virtually all cases, self-limited. Hence, general supportive measures and oral rehydration, if necessary, are normally the only treatment required.

The need for vaccination against astroviruses is not clear. Clarification will require additional epidemiological data concerning the role of the pathogen in various settings. It is also not clear what form of immunity an effective vaccine would be required to induce. However, given the restriction of astroviruses to the intestine, it is likely that local immune effector mechanisms, such as S-IgA, will be most important.

SUMMARY AND CONCLUSIONS

In spite of major advances in public health practices in developed countries and worldwide usage of vaccines, morbidity and mortality due to diarrheal diseases continue to be a major health problem throughout the world. Much has been learned about viral diarrheal agents in the past 3 decades, but this knowledge has yet to have an impact on prevention of the diseases for which these pathogens are responsible, since there are no licensed vaccines for these agents. Although treatment is limited to nonspecific supportive practices, the oral rehydration therapy used worldwide has saved innumerable lives. The future goal will be to prevent viral diarrheal diseases through vaccine development. Rotavirus has been established as the major cause of severe infantile gastroenteritis, and the first rotavirus vaccine was licensed in the United States in 1998. Because of an unexpected side effect, it was withdrawn from the market the next year. Other rotavirus vaccine candidates are under development, and two are in phase 3 trials. The primary goal of these vaccines is to prevent severe rotavirus gastroenteritis, a goal that may require more effective second-generation vaccines to be fully realized. Whether these vaccines will be broadly used or will significantly reduce the global burden of viral diarrhea remains to be determined.

Other viral agents responsible for diarrhea have also been identified and characterized within the past 25 years. Included in this group are astroviruses and caliciviruses. The former is an established cause of gastroenteritis in young children, but the severity of astrovirus diarrhea is probably less than that typically caused by rotavirus. The importance of astroviruses, however, is only beginning to be realized. Caliciviruses also cause infantile diarrhea and are an important cause of juvenile and adult diarrhea. As with astroviruses, their overall contribution to human gastrointestinal illnesses and deaths remains to be determined. Development of vaccines against these agents is under way, and new epidemiological data will help focus target groups for these vaccines.

REFERENCES

Adams, W.R., and Kraft, L.M. (1963). Epizootic diarrhea of infant mice: Identification of the etiologic agent. *Science* 141, 359–360.

Adler, I., and Zickl, R. (1969). Winter vomiting disease. J. *Infect. Dis.* 119, 668–673.

Agus, S.G., Dolin, R., Wyatt, R.G., Tousimis, A.J., and Northrup, R.S. (1973). Acute infectious nonbacterial gastroenteritis: intestinal histopathology. Histologic and enzymatic alterations during illness produced by the Norwalk agent in man. *Ann. Intern. Med.* 79, 18–25.

Appleton, H., and Higgins, P.G. (1975). Viruses and gastroenteritis in infants. *Lancet* 1, 1297.

Ashley, C.R., and Caul, E.O. (1982). Potassium tartrate-glycerol as a density gradient substrate for separation of small, round viruses from human feces. *J. Clin. Microbiol.* 16, 377–381.

Ball, J.M., Graham, D.Y., Opekun, A.R., Gilger, M.A., Guerroro, R.A., and Estes, M.K. (1999). Recombinant Norwalk virus-like particles given orally to volunteers: phase I study. *Gastroenterology* 117, 40–48.

Ball, J. M., Hardy, M. E., Atmar, R. L., Conner, M. E., and Estes, M. K. (1998). Oral immunization with recombinant Norwalk virus-like particles induces a systemic and mucosal immune response in mice. *J. Virol.* 72, 1345–1353.

Ball, J.M., Tian, P., Zeng, C.Q., Morris, A.P., and Estes, M.K. (1996). Age-dependent diarrhea induced by a rotaviral nonstructural glycoprotein. *Science* 272, 101–104.

Barnes, G.L., Lund, J.S., Mitchell, S.V., De Bruyn, L., Piggford, L., Smith, A.L., Furmedge, J., Masendycz, P.J., Bugg, H.C., Bogdanovic-Sakran, N., Carlin, J.B., and Bishop, R.F. (2002). Early phase II trial of human rotavirus vaccine candidate RV3. *Vaccine* 20, 2950–2956.

Bass, D.M. (1997). Interferon gamma and interleukin 1, but not interferon alfa, inhibit rotavirus entry into human intestinal cell lines. *Gastroenterology* 113, 81–89.

Bernstein, D.I., Glass, R.I., Rodgers, G., Davidson, B.L., and Sack, D.A. (1995). Evaluation of rhesus rotavirus monovalent and tetravalent reassortant vaccines in US children. US Rotavirus Vaccine Efficacy Group. *JAMA* 273, 1191–1196.

Bernstein, D.I., Smith, V.E., Sander, D.S., Pax, K.A., Schiff, G.M., and Ward, R.L. (1990). Evaluation of WC3 rotavirus vaccine and correlates of protection in healthy infants. *J. Infect. Dis.* 162, 1055–1062.

Bhan, M.K., Lew, J.F., Sazawal, S., Das, B.K., Gentsch, J.R., and Glass, R.I. (1993). Protection conferred by neonatal rotavirus infection against subsequent rotavirus diarrhea. *J. Infect. Dis.* 168, 282–287.

Bishop, R.F., Barnes, G.L., Cipriani, E., and Lund, J.S. (1983). Clinical immunity after neonatal rotavirus infection. A prospective longitudinal study in young children. *N. Engl. J. Med.* 309, 72–76.

Bishop, R.F., Davidson, G.P., Holmes, I.H., and Ruck, B.J. (1973). Virus particles in epithelial cells of duodenal mucosa from children with acute non-bacterial gastroenteritis. *Lancet* 2, 1281–1283.

Bridger, J.C. (1980). Detection by electron microscopy of caliciviruses, astroviruses and rotavirus-like particles in the faeces of piglets with diarrhoea. *Vet. Rec.* 107, 532–533.

Broome, R.L., Vo, P.T., Ward, R.L., Clark, H.F., and Greenberg, H.B. (1993). Murine rotavirus genes encoding outer capsid proteins VP4 and VP7 are not major determinants of host range restriction and virulence. *J. Virol.* 67, 2448–2455.

Burns, J.W., Siadat-Pajouh, M., Krishnaney, A.A., and Greenberg, H.B. (1996). Protective effect of rotavirus VP6-specific IgA monoclonal antibodies that lack neutralizing activity. *Science* 272, 104–107.

Chiba, S., Yokoyama, T., Nakata, S., Morita, Y., Urasawa, T., Taniguchi, K., Urasawa, S., and Nakao, T. (1986). Protective effect of naturally acquired homotypic and heterotypic rotavirus antibodies. *Lancet.* 2, 417–421.

Choi, A.H., Basu, M., McNeal, M.M., Clements, J.D., and Ward, R.L. (1999). Antibody-independent protection against rotavirus infection of mice stimulated by intranasal immunization with chimeric VP4 or VP6 protein. *J. Virol.* 73, 7574–7581.

Choi A.H., Basu, M., McNeal, M.M., Flint, J., VanCott, J.L., Clements, J.D., and Ward, R.L. (2000). Functional mapping of protective domains and epitopes in the rotavirus VP6 protein. *J. Virol.* 74, 11574–11580.

Ciarlet, M., Crawford, S.E., Barone, C., Bertolotti-Ciarlet, A., Ramig, R.F., Estes, M.K., and Conner, M.E. (1998). Subunit rotavirus vaccine administered parenterally to rabbits induces active protective immunity. *J. Virol.* 72, 9233–9246.

Clark, H.F., Borian, F.E., Bell, L.M., Modesto, K., Gouvea, V., and Plotkin, S.A. (1988). Protective effect of WC3 vaccine against rotavirus diarrhea in infants during a predominantly serotype 1 rotavirus season. *J. Infect. Dis.* 158, 570–587.

Clark, H.F., White, C.J., Offit, P.A., Stinson, D., Eiden, J., Weaver, S., Cho, I., Shaw, A., Krah, D., Ellis, R., and the QHBRV Study Group (1995). Preliminary evaluation of safety and efficacy of quadrivalent human-bovine reassortant rotavirus vaccine (QHBRV). Abstract 1016. *Pediatr. Res.* 37, 172A.

Clemens, J.D., Ward, R.L., Rao, M.R., Sack, D.A., Knowlton, D.R., van Loon, F.P., Huda, S., McNeal, M., Ahmed, F., and Schiff, G. (1992). Seroepidemiologic evaluation of antibodies to rotavirus as correlates of the risk of clinically significant rotavirus diarrhea in rural Bangladesh. *J. Infect. Dis.* 165, 161–165.

Coffin, S.E., and Offit, P.A. (1998). Induction of mucosal B-cell memory by intramuscular inoculation of mice with rotavirus. *J. Virol.* 72, 3479–3483.

Coffin, S.E., Clark, S.L., Bos, N.A., Brubaker, J.O., and Offit, P.A. (1999). Migration of antigen-presenting B cells from peripheral to mucosal lymphoid tissues may induce intestinal antigen-specific IgA following parental immunization. *J. Immunol.* 163, 3064–3070.

Conner, M.E., Crawford, S.E., Barone, C., and Estes, M.K. (1993). Rotavirus vaccine administered parenterally induces protective immunity. *J. Virol.* 67, 6633–6641.

Coste, A., Sirard, J.C., Johansen, K., Cohen, J., and Kraehenbuhl, J.P. (2000). Nasal immunization of mice with virus-like particles protects offspring against rotavirus diarrhea. *J. Virol.* 74(19), 8966–8971.

Coulson, B.S., Grimwood, K., Hudson, I.L., Barnes, G.L., and Bishop, R.F. (1992). Role of coproantibody in clinical protection of children during reinfection with rotavirus. *J. Clin. Microbiol.* 30, 1678–1684.

Cox, G.J., Matsui, S.M., Lo, R.S., Hinds, M., Bowden, R.A., Hackman, R.C., Meyer, W.G., Mori, M., Tarr, P.I., and Oshiro, L.S. (1994). Etiology and outcome of diarrhea after marrow transplantation: a prospective study. *Gastroenterology* 107, 1398–1407.

Cruz, J.R., Bartlett, A.V., Herrmann, J.E., Caceres, P., Blacklow, N.R., and Cano, F. (1992). Astrovirus-associated diarrhea among Guatemalan ambulatory rural children. *J. Clin. Microbiol.* 30, 1140–1144.

Cubitt, W.D., Mitchell, D.K., Carter, M.J., Willcocks, M.M., and Holzel, H. (1999). Application of electron microscopy, enzyme immunoassay, and RT-PCR to monitor an outbreak of astrovirus type 1 in a paediatric bone marrow transplant unit. *J. Med. Virol.* 57, 313–321.

Dennehy, P.H., Nelson, S.M., Spangenberger, S., Noel, J.S., Monroe, S.S., and Glass, R.I. (2001). A prospective case-control study of the role of astrovirus in acute diarrhea among hospitalized young children. *J. Infect Dis.* 184, 10–15.

Dharakul, T., Rott, L., and Greenberg, H.B. (1990). Recovery from chronic rotavirus infection in mice with severe combined immunodeficiency: virus clearance mediated by adoptive transfer of immune CD8 + T lymphocytes. *J. Virol.* 64, 4375–4382.

Dimitrov, D. H., Dashti, S.A., Ball, J.M., Bishbishi, E., Alsaeid, K., Jiang, X., and Estes, M. K. (1997). Prevalence of antibodies to human caliciviruses in Kuwait established by ELISA using baculovirus-expressed capsid antigens representing two genogroups of HuCVs. *J. Med. Virol.* 51, 115–118.

Dingle, K.E., Lambden, P.R., Caul, E.O., and Clarke, I.N. (1995). Human enteric Caliciviridae: the complete genome sequence and expression of virus-like particles from a genetic group II small round structured virus. *J. Gen. Virol.* 76, 2349–2355.

Donelli, G., Superti, F., Tinari, A., and Marziano, M.L. (1992). Mechanism of astrovirus entry into Graham 293 cells. *J. Med. Virol.* 38, 271–277.

Dong, Y., Zeng, C., Q., Ball, J.M., Estes, M.K., and Morris, A.P. (1997). The rotavirus enterotoxin NSP4 mobilized intracellular calcium in human intestinal cells by stimulating phospholipase C-mediated inositol 1,4,5-triphosphate production. *Proc. Natl. Acad. Sci. USA* 94, 3960–3965.

Estes, M.K., and Cohen, J. (1989). Rotavirus gene structure and function. *Microbiol. Rev.* 53, 410–449.

Estes, M.K., Atmar, R.L., and Hardy, M.E. (1997). Norwalk and related diarrhea viruses. In *Clinical Virology* (eds. D.D. Richman, R.J. Whitley, and F.G. Hayden), 1073–1095. New York: Churchill Livingstone.

Fankhauser, R.L., Monroe, S.S., Noel, J.S., Humphrey, C.D., Bresee, J.S., Parashar, U.D., Ando, T., and Glass, R.I. (2002). Epidemiologic and molecular trends of "Norwalk-like viruses" associated with outbreaks of gastroenteritis in the United States. *J. Infect. Dis.* 186, 1–7.

Feng, N., Burns, J.W., Bracy, L., and Greenberg, H.B. (1994). Comparison of mucosal and systemic humoral immune responses and subsequent protection in mice orally inoculated with a homologous or a heterologous rotavirus. *J. Virol.* 68, 7766–7773.

Feng, N., Vo, P.T., Chung, D., Vo, T.V., Hoshino, Y., and Greenberg, H.B. (1997). Heterotypic protection following oral immunization with live heterologous rotaviruses in a mouse model. *J. Infect. Dis.* 175, 330–341.

Feng, N., Lawton, J.A., Gilbert, J., Kuklin, N., Vo, P., Prasad, B.V., and Greenberg, H.B. (2002). Inhibition of rotavirus replication by a non-neutralizing, rotavirus VP6-specific IgA mAb. *J. Clin. Invest.* 109, 1203–1213.

Flores, J., Perez-Schael, I., Gonzalez, M., Garcia, D., Perez, M., Daoud, N., Cunto, W., Chanock, R.M., and Kapikian, A.Z. (1987). Protection against severe rotavirus diarrhoea by rhesus rotavirus vaccine in Venezuelan infants. *Lancet.* 1, 882–884.

Franco, M.A., and Greenberg, H.B. (1995). Role of B cells and cytotoxic T lymphocytes in clearance of and immunity to rotavirus infection in mice. *J. Virol.* 69, 7800–7806.

Franco, M.A., Tin, C., and Greenberg, H.B. (1997). CD8 + T cells can mediate almost complete short-term and partial long-term immunity to rotavirus in mice. *J. Virol.* 71, 4165–4170.

Franco, M.A., Tin, C., Rott, L.S., VanCott, J.L., McGhee, J.R., and Greenberg, H.B. (1997). Evidence for CD8 + T-cell immunity to murine rotavirus in the absence of perforin, fas, and gamma interferon. *J. Virol.* 71, 479–486.

Geigenmüller, U., Ginzton, N.H., and Matsui, S.M. (1997). Construction of a genome-length cDNA clone for human astrovirus serotype 1 and synthesis of infectious RNA transcripts. *J. Virol.* 71, 1713–1717.

Geigenmüller, U., Chew, T., Ginzton, N.H., and Matsui, S.M. (2002). Processing of nonstructural protein 1a of human astrovirus. *J. Virol.* 76, 2003–2008.

Graham, D.Y., Jiang, X., Tanaka, T., Opekun, A.R., Madore, H.P., and Estes, M.K. (1994). Norwalk virus infection of volunteers: new insights based on improved assays. *J. Infect. Dis.* 170, 34–43.

Green, K.Y., Lew, J.F., Jiang, X., Kapikian, A.Z., and Estes, M.K. (1993). Comparison of the reactivities of baculovirus-expressed recombinant Norwalk virus capsid antigen with those of the native Norwalk virus antigen in serologic assays and some epidemiologic observations. *J. Clin. Microbiol.* 31, 2185–2191.

Green, K.Y., Belliot, G., Taylor, J.L., Valdesuso, J., Lew, J.F., Kapikian, A.Z., and Lin, F.Y. (2002). A predominant role for Norwalk-like viruses as agents of epidemic gastroenteritis in Maryland nursing homes for the elderly. *J. Infect. Dis.* 185(2), 133–146.

Griffin, D.D., Nakagomi, T., Hoshino, Y., Nakagomi, O., Kirkwood, C.D., Parashar, U.D., Glass, R.I., and Gentsch, J.R. (2002). Characterization of nontypeable rotavirus strains from the United States: identification of a new rotavirus reassortant (P2A[6],G12) and rare P3[9] strains related to bovine rotaviruses. *Virology* 294, 256–269.

Grohmann, G.S., Glass, R.I., Pereira, H.G., Monroe, S.S., Hightower, A.W., Weber, R., and Bryan, R.T. (1993). Enteric viruses and diarrhea in HIV-infected patients. Enteric Opportunistic Infections Working Group. *N. Engl. J. Med.* 329, 14–20.

Guerrero, R.A., Ball, J.M., Krater, S.S., Pacheco, S.E., Clements, J.D., and Estes, M.K. (2001). Recombinant Norwalk virus-like particles administered intranasally to mice induce systemic and mucosal (fecal and vaginal) immune responses. *J. Virol.* 75, 9713–9722.

Guix S., Caballero, S., Villena, C., Bartolome, R., Latorre, C., Rabella, N., Simo, M., Bosch, A., and Pinto, R.M. (2002). Molecular epidemiology of astrovirus infection in Barcelona, Spain. *J. Clin. Microbiol.* 40, 133–139.

Harrington, P.R., Yount, B., Johnston, R.E., Davis, N., Moe, C., and Baric, R.S. (2002). Systemic, mucosal, and heterotypic immune induction in mice inoculated with Venezuelan equine encephalitis replicons expressing Norwalk virus-like particles. *J. Virol.* 76, 730–742.

Herrmann, J.E., Chen, S.C., Fynan, E.F., Santoro, J.C., Greenberg, H.B., Wang, S., and Robinson, H.L. (1996). Protection against rotavirus infections by DNA vaccination. *J. Infect. Dis.* 174 (suppl. 1), S93–S97.

Herrmann, J.E., Nowak, N.A., Perron-Henry, D.M., Hudson, R.W., Cubitt, W.D., and Blacklow, N.R. (1990). Diagnosis of astrovirus gastroenteritis by antigen detection with monoclonal antibodies. *J. Infect. Dis.* 161, 226–229.

Hoshino, Y., Saif, L.J., Kang, S.-Y., Sereno, M.M., Chen, W.-K., and Kapikian, A.Z. (1995). Identification of group A rotavirus genes associated with virulence of a porcine rotavirus and host range restriction of a human rotavirus in the gnotobiotic piglet model. *Virology* 209, 274–280.

Hoshino, Y., Saif, L.J., Sereno, M.M., Chanock, R.M., and Kapikian, A.Z. (1988). Infection immunity of piglets to either VP3 or VP7 outer capsid protein confers resistance to challenge with a virulent rotavirus bearing the corresponding antigen. *J. Virol.* 62, 744–748.

Hutson, A.M., Atmar, R.L., Graham, D.Y., and Estes, M.K. (2002). Norwalk virus infection and disease is associated with ABO histo-blood group type. *J. Infect. Dis.* 185(9), 1335–1337.

Hutson, A.M., Atmar, R.L., Marcus, D.M., and Estes, M.K. (2003). Norwalk virus-like particle hemagglutination by binding to h histo-blood group antigens. *J. Virol.* 77, 405–415.

Hyams, K.C., Malone, J.D., Kapikian, A.Z., Estes, M.K., Xi, J., Bourgeois, A.L., Paparello, S., Hawkins, R.E., and Green, K.Y. (1993). Norwalk virus infection among Desert Storm troops. *J. Infect. Dis.* 167, 986–987.

Inouye, S., Yamashita, K., Yamadera, S., Yoshikawa, M., Kato, N., and Okabe, N. (2000). Surveillance of viral gastroenteritis in Japan: pediatric cases and outbreak incidents. *J. Infect. Dis.* 181 Suppl 2, S270–274.

Jiang, X., Graham, D.Y., Wang, K.N., and Estes, M.K. (1990). Norwalk virus genome cloning and characterization. *Science* 250, 1580–1583.

Jiang, X., Matson, D.O., Ruiz-Palacios, G.M., Hu, J., Treanor, J., and Pickering, L.K. (1995). Expression, self-assembly, and antigenicity of a snow mountain agent-like calicivirus capsid protein. *J. Clin. Microbiol.* 33, 1452–1455.

Jiang, B., Monroe, S.S., Koonin, E.V., Stine, S.E., and Glass, R.I. (1993). RNA sequence of astrovirus: distinctive genomic organization and a putative retrovirus-like ribosomal frameshifting signal that directs the viral replicase synthesis. *Proc. Natl. Acad. Sci. USA* 90, 10539–10543.

Jiang, X., Wang, J., and Estes, M.K. (1995). Characterization of SRSVs using RT-PCR and a new antigen ELISA. *Arch. Virol.* 140, 363–374.

Jiang, X., Wang, M., Graham, D.Y., and Estes, M.K. (1992). Expression, self-assembly, and antigenicity of the Norwalk virus capsid protein. *J. Virol.* 66, 6527–6532.

Jiang, X., Wang, M., Wang, K., and Estes, M.K. (1993). Sequence and genomic organization of Norwalk virus. *Virology* 195, 51–61.

Joensuu, J., Koskenniemi, E., Pang, X.-L., and Vesikari, T. (1997). Randomised placebo-controlled trial of rhesus-human reassortant rotavirus vaccine for prevention of severe rotavirus gastroenteritis. *Lancet* 350, 1205–1209.

Johansen, K., Hinkula, J., Espinoza, F., Levi, M., Zeng, C., Vesikari, T., Estes, M.K., and Svensson, L. (1999). Humoral and cell-mediated immune responses in humans to the NSP4 enterotoxin of rotavirus. *J. Med. Virol.* 59, 369–377.

Johnson, P.C., Mathewson, J.J., DuPont, H.L., and Greenberg, H.B. (1990). Multiple-challenge study of host susceptibility to Norwalk gastroenteritis in U.S. adults. *J. Infect. Dis.* 161, 18–21.

Kapikian, A.Z., Hoshino, Y., and Chanock, R.M. (2001). Rotaviruses. In *Fields Virology* (eds. D.M. Knipe, P.M. Howley, D.E. Griffin, R.A. Lamb, M.A. Martin, B. Roizman, and S.E. Strauss), 4th ed., 1787–1833. Philadelphia: Lippincott Williams & Wilkins.

Kapikian, A.Z., Estes, M.K., and Chanock, R.M. (1996). Norwalk group of viruses. In *Virology* (eds. B.N. Fields, D.M. Knipe, and P.M. Howley), 3rd ed., 783–810. New York: Lippincott-Raven.

Kapikian, A.Z., Wyatt, R.G., Dolin, R., Thornhill, T.S., Kalica, A.R., and Chanock, R.M. (1972). Visualization by immune electron microscopy of a 27-nm particle associated with acute infectious nonbacterial gastroenteritis. *J. Virol.* 10, 1075–1081.

Kotloff, K.L., Herrmann, J.E., Blacklow, N.R., Hudson, R.W., Wasserman, S.S., Morris, J.G., Jr., and Levine, M.M. (1992). The frequency of astrovirus as a cause of diarrhea in Baltimore children. *Pediatr. Infect. Dis. J.* 11, 587–589.

Kuklin, N.A., Rott, L., Darling, J., Campbell J.J., Franco, M., Feng, N., Muller, W., Wagner, N., Altman, J., Butcher, E.C., and Greenberg, H.B. (2000). $\alpha_4\beta_7$ independent pathway for CD8⁺T cell-mediated intestinal immunity to rotavirus. *J. Clin. Invest.* 106, 1541–1552.

Kuklin, N.A., Rott, L., Feng, N., Conner, M.E., Wagner, N., Muller, W., and Greenberg, H.B. (2001). Protective intestinal anti-rotavirus B cell immunity is dependent on $\alpha_4\beta_7$ integrin expression but does not require IgA antibody production. *J. Immunol.* 166, 1894–1902.

Kurtz, J., and Lee, T. (1978). Astrovirus gastroenteritis age distribution of antibody. *Med. Microbiol. Immunol.* 166, 227–230.

Kurtz, J.B., Lee, T.W., Craig, J.W., and Reed, S.E. (1979). Astrovirus infection in volunteers. *J. Med. Virol.* 3, 221–230.

Lambden, P.R., Caul, E.O., Ashley, C.R., and Clarke, I.N. (1993). Sequence and genome organization of a human small round-structured (Norwalk-like) virus. *Science* 259, 516–519.

Lee, T.W., and Kurtz, J.B. (1981). Serial propagation of astrovirus in tissue culture with the aid of trypsin. *J. Gen. Virol.* 57, 421–424.

Leite, J.P., Ando, T., Noel, J.S., Jiang, B., Humphrey, C.D., Lew, J.F., Green, K.Y., Glass, R.I., and Monroe, S.S. (1996). Characterization of Toronto virus capsid protein expressed in baculovirus. *Arch. Virol.* 141, 865–875.

Lew, J.F., Moe, C.L., Monroe, S.S., Allen, J.R., Harrison, B.M., Forrester, B.D., Stine, S.E., Woods, P.A., Hierholzer, J.C., Herrmann, J.E., Blacklow, N.R., Barlett, A.V., and Glass, R.I. (1991). Astrovirus and adenovirus associated with diarrhea in children in day care settings. *J. Infect. Dis.* 164, 673–678.

Lewis, T.L., and Matsui, S.M. (1995). An astrovirus frameshift signal induces ribosomal frameshifting *in vitro. Arch. Virol.* 140, 1127–1135.

Lewis, T.L., Greenberg, H.B., Herrmann, J.E., Smith, L.S., and Matsui, S.M. (1994). Analysis of astrovirus serotype 1 RNA, identification of the viral RNA-dependent RNA polymerase motif, and expression of a viral structural protein. *J. Virol.* 68, 77–83.

Madeley, C.R., and Cosgrove, B.P. (1975). Viruses in infantile gastroenteritis. *Lancet* 2, 124.

Malherbe, H.H., Harwin, R., and Ulrich, M. (1963). The cytopathic effect of vervet monkey viruses. *S. Afr. Med. J.* 37, 407–411.

Marie-Cardine, A., Gourlain, K., Mouterde, O., Castignolles, N., Hellot, M.F., Mallet, E., and Buffet-Janvresse, C. (2002). Epidemiology of acute viral gastroenteritis in children hospitalized in Rouen, France. *Clin. Infect. Dis.* 34, 1170–1178.

Marionneau, S., Ruvoen, N., Le Moullac-Vaidye, B., Clement, M., Cailleau-Thomas, A., Ruiz-Palacios, G., Huang, P., Jiang, X., and Le Pendu, J. (2002). Norwalk virus binds to histo-blood group antigens present on gastroduodenal epithelial cells of secretor individuals. *Gastroenterology* 122, 1967–1977.

Mason, H.S., Ball, J.M., Shi, J-J., Jiang, X., Estes, M.K., and Arntzen, C.J. (1996). Expression of Norwalk virus capsid protein in transgenic tobacco and potato and its oral immunogenicity in mice. *Proc. Natl. Acad. Sci. USA* 93(11), 5335–5340.

Matson, D.O., O'Ryan, M.L., Herrera, I., Pickering, L.K., and Estes, M.K. (1993). Fecal antibody responses to symptomatic and asymptomatic rotavirus infections. *J. Infect. Dis.* 167, 577–583.

Matsui, S.M., Kim, J.P., Greenberg, H.B., Su, W., Sun, Q., Johnson, P.C., DuPont, H.L., Oshiro, L.S., and Reyes, G.R. (1991). The isolation and characterization of a Norwalk virus-specific cDNA. *J. Clin. Invest.* 87, 1456–1461.

Matsui, S.M., Kim, J.P., Greenberg, H.B., Young, L.M., Smith, L.S., Lewis, T.L., Herrmann, J.E., Blacklow, N.R., Dupuis, K., and Reyes, G.R. (1993). Cloning and characterization of human astrovirus immunoreactive epitopes. *J. Virol.* 67, 1712–1715.

Matsui, S.M., Lewis, T.L., Chiu, E., Smith, L.S., Dupuis, K., Cahill, C.K., and Oshiro, L.S. (1994). An outbreak of astrovirus gastroenteritis in a nursing home and molecular characterization of the virus. *Gastroenterology* 106, A730.

Mattion, N.M., Mitchell, D.B., Both, G.W., and Estes, M.K. (1991). Expression of rotavirus proteins encoded by alternative open reading frames of genome segment 11. *Virology* 181, 295–304.

McNeal, M.M., Barone, K.S., Rae, M.N., and Ward, R.L. (1995). Effector functions of antibody and CD8 + cells in resolution of rotavirus infection and protection against reinfection in mice. *Virology* 214, 387–397.

McNeal, M.M., Broome, R.L., and Ward, R.L. (1994). Active immunity against rotavirus infection in mice is correlated with viral replication and titers of serum rotavirus IgA following vaccination. *Virology* 204, 642–650.

McNeal, M.M., Sheridan, J.F., and Ward, R.L. (1992). Active protection against rotavirus infection of mice following intraperitoneal immunization. *Virology* 191, 150–157.

McNeal, M.M., VanCott, J.L., Choi, A.H., Basu, M., Flint, J.A., and Stone, S.C., Clements, J.D., and Ward R.L. (2002). CD4 T cells are the only lymphocytes needed to protect mice against rotavirus shedding after intranasal immunization with a chimeric VP6 protein and the adjuvant LT(R192G). *J. Virol.* 76, 560–568.

Mendez, E., Fernandez-Luna, T., Lopez, S., Mendez-Toss, M., and Arias, C.F. (2002). Proteolytic processing of a serotype 8 human astrovirus ORF2 polyprotein. *J. Virol.* 76, 7996–8002.

Midthun, K., Greenberg, H.B., Kurtz, J.B., Gary, G.W., Lin, F.-Y. and Kapi Kian, A.Z. (1993). Characterization and seroepidemiology of a type 5 astrovirus associated with an outbreak of gastroenteritis in Marin County, California. *J. Clin. Microbiol.* 31, 955–962.

Mitchell, D.K., Monroe, S.S., Jiang, X., Matson, D.O., Glass, R.I., and Pickering, L.K. (1995). Virologic features of an astrovirus diarrhea outbreak in a day care center revealed by reverse transcriptase-polymerase chain reaction. *J. Infect. Dis.* 172, 1437–1444.

Monroe, S.S., Carter, M.J., Herrmann, J.E., Kurtz, J.B., and Matsui, S.M. (1995). Family Astroviridae. In *Classification and Nomenclature of Viruses. Sixth Report of the International Committee on Taxonomy of Viruses* (eds. F.A. Murphy, D.H.L. Bishop, *et al.*), 364–384. Berlin: Springer-Verlag.

Monroe, S.S., Jiang, B., Stine, S.E., Koopmans, M., and Glass, R.I. (1993). Subgenomic RNA sequence of human astrovirus supports classification of Astroviridae as a new family of RNA viruses. *J. Virol.* 67, 3611–3614.

Monroe, S.S., Stine, S.E., Gorelkin, L., Herrmann, J.E., Blacklow, N.R., and Glass, R.I. (1991). Temporal synthesis of proteins and RNAs during human astrovirus infection of cultured cells. *J. Virol.* 65, 641–648.

Morris, A.P., Scott, J.K., Ball, J.M., Zeng, C.Q., O'Neal, W.K., and Estes, M.K. (1999). NSP4 elicits age-dependent diarrhea and Ca(2+)-mediated I(−) influx into intestinal crypts of CF mice. *Am. J. Physiol.* 277, G431–G444.

Moser, C.A., Cookinham, S, Coffin, S.E., Clark, H.F., and Offit, P.A. (1998). Relative importance of rotavirus-specific effector and memory B cells in protection against challenge. *J. Virol.* 72, 1108–1114.

Murphy, T.V., Gargiullo, P.M., Massoudi, M.S., Nelson, D.B., Jumaan, A.O., Okoro, C.A., Zanardi, L.R., Setia, S., Fair, E., LeBaron, C.W., Wharton, M., Livengood, J.R., and Livingood, J.R. (2001). Intussusception among infants given an oral rotavirus vaccine. *N. Engl. J. Med.* 344, 564–572.

Nakajima, H., Nakagomi, T., Kamisawa, T., Sakaki, N., Muramoto, K., Mikami, T., Nara, H., and Nakagomi, O. (2001). Winter seasonality and rotavirus diarrhoea in adults. *Lancet* 357, 1950.

Nakagomi, O., and Nakagomi, T. (1993). Interspecies transmission of rotaviruses studied from the perspective of genogroup. *Microbiol. Immunol.* 37, 337–348.

Nakata, S., Chiba, S., Terashima, H., and Nakao, T. (1985). Prevalence of antibody to human calicivirus in Japan and Southeast Asia determined by radioimmunoassay. *J. Clin. Microbiol.* 22, 519–521.

Nakata, S., Chiba, S., Terashima, H., Yokoyama, T., and Nakao, T. (1985). Humoral immunity in infants with gastroenteritis caused by human calicivirus. *J. Infect. Dis.* 152, 274–279.

Numata, K., Hardy, M.E., Nakata, S., Chiba, S., and Estes, M. K. (1997). Molecular characterization of morphologically typical human calicivirus Sapporo. *Arch. Virol.* 142, 1537–1552.

O'Neal, C.M., Crawford, S.E., Estes, M.K., and Conner, M.E. (1997). Rotavirus virus-like particles administered mucosally induce protective immunity. *J. Virol.* 71, 8707–8717.

O'Neal, C.M., Harriman, G.R., and Conner, M.E. (2000). Protection of the villus epithelial cells of the small intestine from rotavirus infection does not require immunoglobulin A. *J. Virol.* 74, 4102–4109.

Offit, P.A., and Clark, H.F. (1985). Protection against rotavirus-induced gastroenteritis in a murine model by passively acquired gastrointestinal but not circulating antibodies. *J. Virol.* 54, 58–64.

Offit, P.A., and Dudzik, K.I. (1990). Rotavirus-specific cytotoxic T lymphocytes passively protect against gastroenteritis in suckling mice. *J. Virol.* 64, 6325–6328.

Offit, P.A., Blavat, G., Greenberg, H.B., and Clark, H.F. (1986). Molecular basis of rotavirus virulence: role of gene segment 4. *J. Virol.* 57, 46–49.

O'Ryan, M.L., Matson, D.O., Estes, M.K., and Pickering, L.K. (1994). Anti-rotavirus G type-specific and isotype-specific antibodies in children with natural rotavirus infections. *J. Infect. Dis.* 169, 504–511.

Osborne, M.P., Haddon, S.J., Spencer, A.J., Collins, J., Starkey, W.G., Wallis, T.S., Clarke, G.J., Worton, K.J., Candy, D.C., and Stephen, J. (1988). An electron microscopic investigation of time-related changes in the intestine of neonatal mice infected with murine rotavirus. *J. Pediatr. Gastroenterol. Nutr.* 7, 236–248.

Parrino, T.A., Schreiber, D.S., Trier, J.S., Kapikian, A. Z., and Blacklow, N.R. (1977). Clinical immunity in acute gastroenteritis caused by Norwalk agent. *N. Engl. J. Med.* 297, 86–89.

Perez-Schael, I., Guntinas, M.J., Perex, M., Pagone, V., Rojas, A.M., Gonzalez, R., Cunto, W., Hoshino, Y., and Kapikian, A.Z. (1997). Efficacy of the rhesus rotavirus-based quadrivalent vaccine in infants and young children in Venezuela. *N. Engl. J. Med.* 337, 1181–1187.

Phillips, A.D., Rice, S.J., and Walker-Smith, J.A. (1982). Astrovirus within human small intestinal mucosa. *Gut* 23, A923–A924.

Pinto, R.M., Diez, J.M., and Bosch, A. (1994). Use of the colonic carcinoma cell line CaCo-2 for *in vivo* amplification and detection of enteric viruses, *J. Med. Virol.* 44, 310–315.

Prasad, B.V., and Chiu, W. (1994). Structure of rotavirus. *Curr. Top. Microbiol. Immunol.* 185, 9–29.

Prasad, B.V.V., and Estes, M.K. (1997). Molecular basis of rotavirus replication: structure-function correlations. In *Structural Biology of Viruses* (eds. W. Chiu, R.M. Burnett, and R. Garcea), 239–268. Oxford, UK: Oxford University Press.

Prasad, B.V., Rothnagel, R., Jiang, X., and Estes, M.K. (1994). Three-dimensional structure of baculovirus-expressed Norwalk virus capsids. *J. Virol.* 68, 5117–5125.

Rennels, M.B., Glass, R.I., Dennehy, P.H., Bernstein, D.I., Pichichero, M.E., Zito, E.T., Mack, M.E., Davidson, B.L., and Kapikian, A.Z. (1996). Safety and efficacy of high-dose rhesus-human reassortant rotavirus vaccines—report of the National Multicenter Trial. United States Rotavirus Vaccine Efficacy Group. *Pediatrics* 97, 7–13.

Rodriguez-Baez, N., O'Brien, R., Qiu, S.Q., and Bass, D.M. (2002). Astrovirus, adenovirus, and rotavirus in hospitalized children: prevalence and association with gastroenteritis. *J. Pediatr. Gastroenterol. Nutr.* 35, 64–68.

Saif, L.J., Bohl, E.H., Theil, K.W., Cross, R.F., and House, J.A. (1980). Rotavirus-like, calicivirus-like, and 23-nm virus-like particles associated with diarrhea in young pigs. *J. Clin. Microbiol.* 12, 105–111.

Sakai, Y., Nakata, S., Honma, S., Tatsumi, M., Numata-Kinoshita, K., and Chiba, S. (2001). Clinical severity of Norwalk virus and

Sapporo virus gastroenteritis in children in Hokkaido, Japan. *Pediatr. Infect. Dis. J.* 20, 849–853.

Sanchez-Fauquier, A., Carrascosa, A.L., Carrascosa, J.L., Otero, A., Glass, R.I., Lopez, J.A., San Martin, C., and Melero, J.A. (1994). Characterization of a human astrovirus serotype 2 structural protein (VP26) that contains an epitope involved in virus neutralization. *Virology* 201, 312–320.

Santosham, M., Letson, G.W., Wolff, M., Reid, R., Gahagan, S., Adams, R., Callahan, C., Sack, R.B., and Kapi Kian, A.Z. (1991). A field study of the safety and efficacy of two candidate rotavirus vaccines in a Native American population. *J. Infect. Dis.* 163, 483–487.

Santosham, M., Moulton, L.H., Reid, R., Croll, J., Weatherholt, R., Ward, R., Forro, J., Zito, E., Mack, M., Brenneman, G., and Davidson, B.L. (1997). Efficacy and safety of high-dose rhesus-human reassortant rotavirus vaccine in Native American populations. *J. Pediatrics* 131, 632–638.

Schreiber, D.S., Blacklow, N.R., and Trier, J.S. (1974). The small intestinal lesion induced by Hawaii agent acute infectious nonbacterial gastroenteritis. *J. Infect. Dis.* 129, 705–708.

Schwartz-Cornil, I., Benureau, Y., Greenberg, H., Hendrickson, B.A., and Cohen, J. (2002). Heterologous protection induced by the inner capsid proteins of rotavirus requires transcytosis of mucosal immunoglobulins. *J. Virol.* 76, 8110–8117.

Sharp, T.W., Hyams, K.C., Watts, D., Trofa, A.F., Martin, G.J., Kapikian, A.Z., Green, K.Y., Jiang, X., Estes, M.K., and Waack, M. (1995). Epidemiology of Norwalk virus during an outbreak of acute gastroenteritis aboard a US aircraft carrier. *J. Med. Virol.* 45, 61–67.

Shaw, R.D., Hempson, S.J., and Mackow, E.R. (1995). Rotavirus diarrhea is caused by nonreplicating viral particles. *J. Virol.* 69, 5946–5950.

Shaw, R.D., Merchant, A.A., Groene, W.S., and Cheng, E.H. (1993). Persistence of intestinal antibody response to heterologous rotavirus infection in a murine model beyond 1 year. *J. Clin. Microbiol.* 31, 188–191.

Snodgrass, D.R., and Wells, P.W. (1978). Passive immunity in rotaviral infections. *J. Am. Vet. Med. Assoc.* 173, 565–568.

Tacket, C.O., Mason, H.S., Losonsky, G., Estes, M.K., Levine, M.M., and Arntzen C.J. (2000). Human immune responses to a novel Norwalk virus vaccine delivered in transgenic potatoes. *J. Infect. Dis.* 182(1), 302–305.

To, T.L., Ward, L.A., Yuan, L. and Saif, L.J. (1998). Serum and intestinal isotype antibody responses and correlates of protective immunity to human rotavirus in a gnotobiotic pig model of disease. *J. Gen. Virol.* 79, 2661–2672.

Velazquez, F.R., Matson, D.O., Guerrero, M.L., Shults, J., Calva, J.J., Morrow, A.L., Glass, R.I., Pickering, L.K., and Ruiz-Palacios, G.M. (2000). Serum antibody as a marker of protection against natural rotavirus infection and disease. *J. Infect. Dis.* 182, 1602–1609.

Vesikari, T. (1993). Clinical trials of live oral rotavirus vaccines: The Finnish experience. *Vaccine.* 11, 255–261.

Vesikari, T., Ruuska, T., Koivu, H.-P., Green, K.Y., Flores, J., and Kapikian, A.Z. (1991). Evaluation of the M37 human rotavirus vaccine in 2- to 6-month-old infants. *Pediatr. Infect. Dis. J.* 10, 912–917.

Vinje, J., and Koopmans, M.P. (1996). Molecular detection and epidemiology of small round-structured viruses in outbreaks of gastroenteritis in the Netherlands. *J Infect. Dis.* 174, 610–615.

Ward, R.L., Bernstein, D.I., Shukla, R., Young, E.C., Sherwood, J.R., McNeal, M.M., Walker, M.C., and Schiff, G.M. (1989). Effects of antibody to rotavirus on protection of adults challenged with a human rotavirus. *J. Infect. Dis.* 159, 79–88.

Ward, R.L., Clemens, J.D., Knowlton, D.R., Rao, M.R., van Loon, F.P., Huda, N., Ahmed, F., Schiff, G.M., and Sack, D.A. (1992). Evidence that protection against rotavirus diarrhea after natural infection is not dependent on serotype-specific neutralizing antibody. *J. Infect. Dis.* 166, 1251–1257.

Ward, R.L., Knowlton, D.R., Zito, E.T., Davidson, B.L., Rappaport, R., and Mack, M.E. (1997). Serological correlates of immunity in a tetravalent reassortant rotavirus vaccine trial. US Rotavirus Vaccine Efficacy Group. *J. Infect. Dis.,* 176, 570–577.

Ward, R.L., McNeal, M.M., and Sheridan, J.F. (1990). Development of an adult mouse model for studies on protection against rotavirus. *J. Virol.* 64, 5070–5075.

Willcocks, M.M., Brown, T.D., Madeley, C.R., and Carter, M.J. (1994). The complete sequence of a human astrovirus. *J. Gen. Virol.* 75, 1785–1788.

Willcocks, M.M., Carter, M.J., Laidler, F.R., and Madeley, C.R. (1990). Growth and characterisation of human faecal astrovirus in a continuous cell line. *Arch. Virol.* 113, 73–81.

Willcocks, M.M., Boxall, A.S., and Carter, M.J. (1999). Processing and intracellular location of human astrovirus non-structural proteins. *J. Gen. Virol.* 80, 2607–2611.

Wolf, J.L., Cukor, G., Blacklow, N.R., Dambrauskas, R., and Trier, J.S. (1981). Susceptibility of mice to rotavirus infection: effects of age and administration of corticosteroids. *Infect. Immun.* 33, 565–574.

Yu, J., and Langridge, W.H. (2001). A plant-based multicomponent vaccine protects mice from enteric diseases. *Nat. Biotechnol.* 19, 548–552.

Yuan, L., Ward, L.A., Rosen, B.I., To, T.L., and Saif, L.J. (1996). Systemic and intestinal antibody-secreting cell responses and correlates of protective immunity to human rotavirus in a gnotobiotic pig model of disease. *J. Virol.* 70, 3075–3083.

Yuan, L., Geyer, A., Hodgins, D.C., Fan, Z., Qian, Y., Chang, K.O., Crawford, S.E., Parreno, V., Ward, L.A., Estes, M.K., Conner, M.W., and Saif, L.J. (2000). Intranasal administration of 2/6-rotavirus-like particles with mutant *Escherichia coli* heat-labile toxin (LT-R192G) induces antibody-secreting cell responses but not protective immunity in gnotobiotic pigs. *J. Virol.* 74, 8843–8853.

Yuan, L., Geyer, A., and Saif, L.J. (2001). Short-term immunoglobulin A B-cell memory resides in intestinal lymphoid tissues but not in bone marrow of gnotobiotic pigs inoculated with Wa human rotavirus. *Immunology* 103, 188–198.

Yuan, L., Iosef, C., Azevedo, M.S., Kim, Y., Qian, Y., Geyer, A., Nguyen, T.V., Chang, K.O., and Saif, L.J. (2001). Protective immunity and antibody-secreting cell responses elicited by combined oral attenuated Wa human rotavirus and intranasal Wa 2/6-VLPs with mutant *Escherichia coli* heat-labile toxin in gnotobiotic pigs. *J. Virol.* 75, 9229–9238.

Respiratory Bacterial Vaccines

Chapter 50

Edward N. Janoff

Mucosal and Vaccine Research Center and Infectious Disease Section, Veterans Affairs Medical Center, University of Minnesota School of Medicine, Minneapolis, Minnesota

David E. Briles

Department of Microbiology, University of Alabama at Birmingham, Birmingham, Alabama

Jeffrey B. Rubins

Mucosal and Vaccine Research Center and Pulmonary Section, Veterans Affairs Medical Center, University of Minnesota School of Medicine, Minneapolis, Minnesota

Successful mucosal colonization with bacterial respiratory pathogens is typically asymptomatic and represents a balance of bacterial factors and host defenses. Pathogen-associated disease arises in uniquely susceptible hosts or when specific bacterial virulence factors overwhelm or subvert host immune mechanisms. Clinical illness may result from release of bacterial toxins, contiguous spread of bacteria through the respiratory tract, or invasion and dissemination of the bacteria through the blood. In industrialized countries, bacterial infections localized to the upper respiratory tract (e.g., otitis media, sinusitis, bronchitis) are associated with substantial morbidity, with appreciable social and economic consequences. Although less common, invasive bacterial infections of the lower respiratory tract cause significant mortality, especially among patients immunocompromised by the extremes of age or by underlying medical illnesses. An even greater disease burden is present in developing countries, where respiratory bacterial infections vie with gastrointestinal infections as the leading causes of death among infants and children (3–4 million per year each) (Murray and Lopez, 1997).

Discovery of the virulence factors expressed by these respiratory mucosal pathogens has led to the development of effective vaccines that prevent severe clinical illness and in many instances inhibit asymptomatic colonization. In this chapter, we review the currently available vaccines against four prominent and prototypical respiratory mucosal bacteria—*Corynebacterium diphtheriae*, *Bordetella pertussis*, *Haemophilus influenzae*, and *Streptococcus pneumoniae*—and highlight the virulence mechanisms involved in mucosal infection that form the basis for these immunogenic and clinically efficacious vaccines **(Table 50.1)**.

DIPHTHERIA VACCINE

Pathogenesis of clinical infection

The development of an effective vaccine against *Corynebacterium diphtheriae* transformed diphtheria from among the most common and fatal diseases in the United States at the beginning of this century to a rarity that few contemporary American physicians have ever seen. This unprecedented control of *C. diphtheriae* infection has closely paralleled advances in microbiology and immunology over the last century. Indeed, prominent in the earliest work on mechanisms of immunity were examinations of systemic responses to mucosal infection, particularly diphtheria. Despite these advances, diphtheria remains a serious problem in areas of social and political turmoil and where cost and accessibility limit use of the vaccine (Centers for Disease Control, 1993).

C. diphtheriae, a gram-positive bacillus that primarily infects humans, is spread person-to-person by respiratory droplets, highlighting the importance of mucosal colonization in transmission and initiation of disease. Asymptomatic pharyngeal colonization was first described by Loeffler, who also observed that the organism remained confined to the mucosa, even during severe infection with peripheral manifestations (MacGregor, 1995).

In 1826, Bretonneau characterized the signs and natural history of throat "distemper," differentiating it from other pharyngeal infections by the presence of the inflammatory false membrane ("diphthera" is Greek for skin or hide). On the upper respiratory tract epithelia of tonsils, oropharynx, and contiguous sites, infection is associated with local tissue injury and cell death in nonimmune hosts. Suffocation on

Table 50.1. Characteristics of Vaccine-Preventable Respiratory Bacterial Pathogens

Organism	Gram Stain	Encapsulated	Invasive	Vaccine Target(s)	Intracellular Viability in Respiratory Epithelium
Corynebacterium diphtheriae	Positive	No	No	Exotoxin	Unknown
Bordetella pertussis	Negative	No	No	Exotoxin, adhesins	Yes
Haemophilus influenzae	Negative	Invasive strains[a]	Yes	Capsule	Yes
Streptococcus pneumoniae	Positive	Yes	Yes	Capsule	Some strains

[a]Most invasive strains in children and approximately half of invasive strains in adults.

the detached membrane is a common cause of death, particularly among children. The bacteria, however, do not invade deeper into local tissues or the blood. Although Klebs observed the organism in stains of smears from the adherent membrane in 1883 and Loeffler grew the organism and induced disease in animals in 1884, it remained for Roux and Yersin in 1888 to confirm that a soluble heat-labile exotoxin in culture supernatants produced systemic disease in animals (Willett, 1992).

By this secondary mechanism, the localized mucosal infection is able to induce necrosis and dramatic pathologic effects in organs distant from the primary pharyngeal bacterial focus. Although diphtheria toxin (DT) can affect any cell, cardiac toxicity is a prominent complication. Severe myocarditis may result in congestive heart failure, electrical conduction defects, and death. However, cardiac abnormalities, peripheral and cranial neuropathies (including pharyngeal paralysis), and renal effects are typically self-limited. The frequency and gravity of these distant effects are related to the intensity and duration of the local upper respiratory tract process and, presumably, the amount of DT produced and absorbed.

Virulence factors

The DT induces most of the local and systemic pathogenicity of the infection. A lysogenic β-phage carrying the toxin gene (tox+) may infect the bacteria, integrate into the bacterial genome, replicate, and lyse a subset of bacteria upon appropriate stimulation. That DT production is locally regulated by environmental factors such as low iron (Pappenheimer, 1982) may suggest a potential role for the toxin in maintaining growth of the organism on the mucosa. All virulent *C. diphtheriae* strains produce identical forms of the 61-kDa DT, composed of two components, of which the B fragment (40 kDa) is responsible for membrane binding and transport of the disulfide-bound active A fragment (21 kDa) into the target cell cytoplasm. Once released, the A subunit catalyzes inactivation of only one specific eukaryotic enzyme, "elongation factor 2," which uncouples the interaction of tRNA from mRNA (Willett, 1992; Pappenheimer,

1982). As little as one molecule of fragment A introduced into the cytoplasm inhibits its protein synthesis and kills the cell (Yamaizumi et al., 1978). In addition to its inhibition of protein synthesis, a DT-associated apoptosis-like nuclease activity, which is inhibitable by specific antitoxin, has been described (Chang et al., 1989) but remains controversial.

The presence of secondary virulence factors in addition to toxin was suggested by molecular epidemiologic data showing clustering of isolates, all tox+, causing epidemic and severe cases of *C. diphtheriae* infection in Sweden (Rappuoli et al., 1988). Although those factors were not identified, local pathogenicity of *C. diphtheriae* strains, independent of toxin production, has been ascribed to strain-specific surface protein K antigens, responses to which may confer antibacterial immunity, and to a glycolipid core factor that inhibits mitochondrial function in murine cells (Willett, 1992).

Protective immune responses

The presence of serum antibody to DT appears to be the most predictive marker of protective immunity. Critical support for the central role of toxins in the pathogenesis of infectious diseases and of humoral immunity in defense against these diseases was provided in 1890 by von Behring and Kitasato, who demonstrated that antibodies provide protection against the secreted toxins of both diphtheria and tetanus (Silverstein, 1989).

The B fragment is the immunogenic moiety of DT, and antibodies to this subunit protect against disease. Although genetic factors influence antibody responses to DT, six immunodominant region sequences, all peptides of the receptor binding and transmembrane components of the toxin's B fragment, are recognized by CD4+ T cells from immune adults, independent of their human leukocyte antigen haplotype (Raju et al., 1995). Moreover, antitoxin neutralizes only toxin binding, with no effect on previously infected cells (Mortimer, 1994). This conclusion is supported by data from two studies showing that mortality was lower (1.5%–4.2 %) when antitoxin was given on the first day of illness than when given 7 or more days later (15%–20%) (Mortimer, 1994). Levels of antitoxin in serum correlate with protection against disease. Epidemic investigations confirm that most symptomatic cases of diphtheria involve persons with <0.01 IU of antitoxin/mL, whereas >90% of asymptomatic carriers had levels >0.1 IU/mL (Björkholm et al., 1986).

Although symptomatic infection does not reliably elicit antibodies to the toxin, pharyngeal colonization and skin infection induce protective immunity. Prior to immunization, children are at greatest risk of illness (English, 1985), and the prevalence of antitoxin antibodies increases with age while rates of colonization with toxigenic strains decrease. Natural immunity to diphtheria may therefore relate to protection against the effects of the toxin and to strain-specific antibacterial immunity (e.g., to surface K antigens). The immunizing potential of cutaneous diphtheria is suggested by the low rates of diphtherial disease and of pharyngeal colonization with toxigenic strains in areas with high rates of C. diphtheriae skin lesions, such as Uganda (Bezjak and Farsey, 1970). In addition, rates of systemic protection against the toxin, as detected by a negative Schick test, are often high in poorly vaccinated children in these areas.

Although no studies have correlated mucosal responses to diphtheria antigens with protection against colonization or disease, it is clear that DT-specific antibodies in serum are sufficient to protect against serious mucosal infection and death. The demonstration by Roux in 1894 that immunized horses produced functional antitoxin and that treatment with this equine antiserum reduced mortality among patients with diphtheria by half (51% to 24%) provided the impetus to develop toxin-based preventive vaccines. Subsequent demonstrations that serum antitoxin levels of 0.01–0.1 IU /mL were protective provided a tangible surrogate marker for vaccine efficacy.

The DT vaccine
Early efforts to develop a diphtheria vaccine were hindered by practical difficulties in inactivating the toxin antigen. Attempts by Von Pirquet and Schick in 1906 and Smith in 1909 to neutralize DT in toxin-antitoxin combinations and to induce protection in humans were successful but were complicated by the risk of serum sickness from the equine serum. The development of the intradermal Schick test in 1913 to predict protective immunity facilitated evaluation of vaccine efficacy. Formalin treatment of DT, used to this day as "toxoid" with an alum adjuvant, eliminated the toxicity of DT while retaining the immunogenicity of the native form.

Although no randomized placebo-controlled double-blinded trial of efficacy of diphtheria vaccine has been performed, the clinical and epidemiologic data supporting its effectiveness are compelling. One unblinded trial involving almost 500 patients in the late 19th century showed a reduction in mortality from 12.2% to 3.3% (Mortimer, 1994). Moreover, as with earlier passive immunization with antitoxin, active immunization has consistently resulted in dramatic decreases in the rates and severity of disease as well as case-fatality rates during epidemics and in the general population (Mortimer, 1994; Brooks et al., 1974).

The reasons for the protective efficacy of specific immunity solely to DT are intriguing. Clearly, neutralization of toxin limits tissue damage and its associated morbidity and mortality during infection. However, immunization with toxoid also decreases rates of carriage of toxin-producing strains but not of nonvirulent strains (Pappenheimer, 1982). Conceivably, the toxin confers a survival benefit to the phage and bacterium, and phage production may be energy-inefficient for the bacterium if the toxin is ineffective in an immune host. Nontoxigenic strains likely employ other virulence mechanisms. Lower carriage rates in a population may account for the low rates of disease in the United States that persist despite waning immunity in 20%–50% of adults, particularly women and the elderly. These observations are consistent with the presence of herd immunity (Karzon and Edwards, 1988).

The reactogenicity (side-effect profile) of the current DT preparation is low, but the need to give three to four intramuscular doses to provide durable protective levels has directed attention to producing a more purified, epitope-selective preparation. Nevertheless, the consistent immunogenicity of DT makes it and its congeners popular, effective adjuvants for other vaccines. Purely synthetic peptides and anti-idiotypes have also been shown to elicit toxin-neutralizing activity. Little attention has been directed to developing vaccines based on other potential virulence factors (e.g., those necessary for adherence, colonization, or evasion of host defenses) because of the striking and consistent protective efficacy of parenteral immunization with DT against this strictly mucosal bacterial respiratory infection.

However, diphtheria toxoid, particularly the genetically inactivated mutant diphtheria toxin CRM197 (cross-reacting material), is currently in use as a protein conjugate to enhance the immunogenicity and T-cell dependence of capsular polysaccharides from H. influenzae type b and S. pneumoniae given parenterally (see relevant sections, further in text). Recent data also suggest that nasal immunization with diphtheria toxoid (Aggerbeck et al., 1997) or CRM197 (the latter particularly with the bioadhesive polycationic polysaccharide chitosan; Mills et al., 2003) can induce specific systemic antibody responses comparable to or greater than those achieved with parenteral immunization. Moreover, nasal IgA responses accompany the mucosal exposure but not parenteral immunization. Thus, nasal immunization with CRM197 or a range of other antigen-adjuvant combinations may be a promising approach to providing effective local and systemic immunity.

Summary
The development of an effective vaccine against C. diphtheriae infections was a direct consequence of novel microbiologic insights into the pathogenic mechanisms of the organism (e.g., the central role of the exotoxin in inducing local and distant injury) and of original immunologic discoveries of the immunogenicity of the protein and the ability of humoral factors (particularly serum antibody) to arrest its effects. The initial high frequency of this severe infection,

isolation of a specific pathogenic mechanism, and identification of predictive surrogate markers of susceptibility and protection all greatly facilitated vaccine development and utilization. Of particular note, systemic immunity alone, both active and passive, provided clear protection against both mucosal and systemic disease. However, novel approaches to the use of diphtheria toxoid and CRM197 as nasal vaccines have expanded the potential of this protein to facilitate the generation of protective mucosal and systemic responses against other pathogen-derived antigens.

PERTUSSIS VACCINE

Pathogenesis of clinical infection

Bordetella pertussis causes the clinical syndromes of whooping cough, which is associated with substantial morbidity in children, and can progress to lethal pneumonia in infants. Prior to the development and use of effective vaccines, pertussis accounted for an estimated 600,000 deaths annually worldwide. Although it is considered primarily a pediatric disease, serologic studies have indicated that pertussis may also be endemic in young adults, among whom the organism may be an occult etiology for chronic cough (Nennig *et al.*, 1996).

Similar to *C. diphtheriae*, *B. pertussis* remains confined to the respiratory tract throughout the course of the disease and does not invade beyond the epithelial layer in normal hosts. Also, as with diphtheria, lethal systemic disease is generally the consequence of release of cytotoxins and only rarely is from disseminated infection. However, *B. pertussis* can invade and survive within epithelial cells and macrophages, possibly as a means of evading the host immune response (Saukkonen *et al.*, 1991). Consequently, a protective immune response may require both a humoral response to pertussis virulence factors and a cellular response to eliminate intracellular organisms.

Virulence factors

All known virulence factors for *B. pertussis* infection are involved in attachment of the organism to the respiratory epithelium. Expression of each of these adhesins and toxins necessary for adherence is controlled at a single gene locus (*bvg*), which simultaneously activates their translation while suppressing the expression of motility factors, which are required only during nutrient depletion (Yuk *et al.*, 1996). The prominent *B. pertussis* virulence factors, including pertussis toxin (PT), filamentous hemagglutinin (FHA), pertactin (PRN), and fimbrial proteins (FIMs), have been fully characterized and incorporated into recently approved acellular pertussis vaccines (see the Vaccine section) (Patel and Wagstaff, 1996). PT disrupts cellular signaling by ADP-ribosylating the catalytic subunit of eukaryotic membrane G proteins and preventing normal processing of G-protein-transduced signals. Although PT disrupts immune cell function, its precise action in facilitating successful *B. pertussis* colonization of human respiratory epithelium is not completely defined.

FHA and PRN are loosely associated surface components of *B. pertussis* that share structural similarities and mediate bacterial adherence to eukaryotic cells. FHA, a 220-kDa surface protein that can be recovered from *B. pertussis* culture media, binds predominantly to sulfated glycosaminoglycans on cell-surface proteoglycans (Brennan and Shahin, 1996). Deletion of the FHA gene in mutant *B. pertussis* strains decreases bacterial adherence to epithelial cells by 70% (Menozzi *et al.*, 1994), confirming its role in the pathogenesis of *B. pertussis* colonization of the respiratory tract. As with FHA, *B. pertussis* mutant strains deficient in PRN expression also show decreased adherence to epithelial cells (Brennan and Shahin, 1996), although the cellular binding site for this adhesin has not been characterized. However, both FHA and PRN contain the ARG-GLY-ASP peptide sequence motif, which characterizes eukaryotic proteins that interact with integrins (Brennan and Shahin, 1996), and soluble peptides containing the ARG-GLY-ASP motif inhibit adherence, epithelial cell invasion, and intracellular survival of *B. pertussis* (Leininger *et al.*, 1991; Saukkonen *et al.*, 1991; Relman *et al.*, 1990).

Protective immune responses

The potential of these virulence factors to abrogate *B. pertussis* infection was suggested by their ability to stimulate systemic and mucosal immunity and to mediate protection against colonization of the upper respiratory tract in animals. For FHA and PRN, both active systemic immunization and passive immunization with monoclonal antibodies protected mice against subsequent aerosol challenge with *B. pertussis* (Shahin *et al.*, 1992; Kimura *et al.*, 1990). Systemic immunization of mice with FHA in solution or in biodegradable poly (lactide-co-glycolide) microspheres generated substantial serum IgG antibodies but minimal concentrations of IgA antibodies in lung and nasal lavage. In contrast, nasal immunization of mice with FHA produced strong systemic IgG responses and measurable anti-FHA IgA and IgG in lung lavages (Cahill *et al.*, 1995). Although both systemic and mucosal immunization produced antibodies that blocked adherence of *B. pertussis* to epithelial cells *in vitro* and provided protection against subsequent aerosol challenge with *B. pertussis*, mice immunized nasally cleared bacteria slightly faster than those immunized systemically (Cahill *et al.*, 1995). Mucosal (nasal) immunization of mice with a combination of PT, FHA, and PRN in biodegradable microspheres similarly produced serum IgG and lavage IgA responses to the individual component antigens and provided better protection against subsequent respiratory challenge with *B. pertussis* than any single antigen (Shahin *et al.*, 1995). In addition, stimulation of mucosal immunity by oral immunization of mice with *B. pertussis* FIMs encapsulated in microspheres not only produced systemic antigen-specific IgG comparable to that with intraperitoneal injection but also generated mucosal IgA and IgG antibodies to FIMs that were not detected after systemic immunization (Jones *et al.*, 1996). Furthermore, mucosal immunity to FIMs was protective against subsequent respiratory challenge of mice with *B. pertussis* (Jones *et al.*, 1996).

The pertussis vaccine

The immunogenicity and efficacy of these virulence factors to prevent mucosal infection in murine models identified PT, FHA, PRN, and FIMs as ideal immunogens when acellular pertussis vaccines were formulated to replace earlier whole-cell vaccines. The original whole-cell vaccine composed of inactivated *B. pertussis* bacteria was protective in pediatric immunization programs world-wide, most often in combination with diphtheria and tetanus toxoids (Centers for Disease Control and Prevention, 1994). However, the frequent incidence of minor adverse effects (fever, protracted crying, and local erythematous reactions) and concerns regarding rare reports of serious neurologic effects caused a decline in its acceptance and use (Baraff *et al.*, 1984). Indeed, pertussis vaccine was not included in the formal pediatric immunization schedules in Sweden and Japan, and declines in its use in Italy and Germany were associated with subsequent rises in the incidence of pertussis in these countries (Patel and Wagstaff, 1996). Although follow-up studies have failed to confirm any evidence of serious or permanent neurologic damage from the whole-cell vaccine (AAPCID, 1996; Patel and Wagstaff, 1996), acellular pertussis vaccines were formulated to improve tolerability and acceptance.

Currently available acellular pertussis vaccines incorporating PT and one to three of the other virulence factors (FHA, PRN, FIMs) involved in respiratory mucosal adherence and infection are consistently associated with decreased adverse effects (Gustafsson *et al.*, 1996; Patel and Wagstaff, 1996, Jefferson *et al.*, 2002). Serum IgG antibody responses to these virulence factors are consistently higher after systemic immunization with the acellular vaccine than with the whole-cell vaccine (Patel and Wagstaff, 1996; Jefferson *et al.*, 2002). However, because serum antibody responses are not highly correlated with protection from infection, a number of large, placebo-controlled clinical studies have directly compared the efficacy of acellular vaccines with whole-cell pertussis vaccines.

Several large clinical trials have demonstrated that the overall clinical efficacy of acellular vaccines is approximately 85%, with effectiveness increasing in proportion to the number of virulence factors included in the vaccine (**Table 50.2**). For studies of clinical efficacy, pertussis infection has been uniformly defined as 21 or more days of paroxysmal cough, with *B. pertussis* infection confirmed by culture or serologic testing, and efficacy is prevention of infections for 30 days after the third primary immunization. Systematic reviews have shown that three- and five-component acellular vaccines are as effective or more effective than whole-cell vaccines against pertussis, which in turn are more effective than two-component acellular vaccines (Jefferson *et al.*, 2003). Thus, systemic immunization with acellular pertussis vaccines incorporating virulence factors involved in adherence and mucosal infection have clinical efficacy against *B. pertussis* infection comparable or superior to that provided by the killed whole-cell vaccine.

Clinical trials of the acellular pertussis vaccines have also demonstrated a role for a cell-mediated immune response to *B. pertussis* infection. Murine studies indicated that *B. pertussis* infection or systemic immunization with the whole-cell vaccine stimulated macrophages to produce IL-12 and stimulated T helper type 1 (Th1) proliferative lymphocyte responses (Mahon *et al.*, 1996). In contrast, acellular vaccines preferentially stimulated Th2-type T-cell responses in mice (Barnard *et al.*, 1996; Mahon *et al.*, 1996). However, in clinical trials involving infants, the tricomponent acellular vaccine stimulated T-cell proliferative responses against all three vaccine components, and antigen-stimulated T cells produced IL-2 and IFN-γ, indicative of a preferential Th1 cell pattern (Zepp *et al.*, 1996). T-cell responses were durable in children for up to 12 months after primary immunization and did not correlate with serum specific IgG levels. Despite these discrepancies in the patterns of T-cell responses between animal and clinical trials, the common findings of these studies indicate that *B. pertussis* virulence factors stimulate T-cell-mediated immunity, which may be protective against pertussis infection. A cell-mediated immune response may explain the protective efficacy of acellular vaccines, which does not correlate with humoral immune responses. Also, cell-mediated immunity would be an essential component of the host response to *B. pertussis* infection if the recently demonstrated ability of the organism to invade

Table 50.2. Clinical Studies of Pertussis Vaccine Efficacy

Vaccine Components	Population	Percent Efficacy (95% CI)	References
Whole-cell	Household contacts	48.3 (37–58)	Gustafsson *et al.*, 1996
		85.0 (46–95)	Preziosi and Halloran, 2003
	Children <2 years old	36 (14–52)	Greco *et al.*, 1996
PT	Children <2 years old	71 (63–78)	Trollfors *et al.*, 1995
PT + FHA	Household contacts	58.9 (51–66)	Gustafsson *et al.*, 1996
PT + FHA + PRN	Children <2 years old	84 (76–90)	Greco *et al.*, 1996
	Household contacts	88.7 (76–95)	Schmitt *et al.*, 1996

FHA, filamentous hemagglutinin; PRN, pertactin; PT, pertussis toxin.

and survive intracellularly is fundamental to the pathogenesis of pertussis infection.

Summary

B. pertussis is a noninvasive respiratory mucosal pathogen with well-characterized virulence factors that mediate adherence to host tissues. The function and immunogenicity of these factors form the basis for clinically efficacious immunization against this serious infection. Recent revelations regarding intracellular invasion and survival of *B. pertussis* and about the cell-mediated immune response to this bacterium may lead to further improvements in pertussis vaccines. In addition, the potential of mucosal immunization against *B. pertussis*, which has been demonstrated in murine models, has yet to be explored in immunization of children.

HAEMOPHILUS INFLUENZAE VACCINE

Pathogenesis of clinical infection

Mucosal respiratory infections, including otitis media, sinusitis, conjunctivitis, bronchitis, and pneumonia, account for the majority of *H. influenzae*–related morbidity. However, *H. influenzae*, particularly encapsulated type b, has dramatic potential to cause bacteremia and meningitis in specific high-risk groups. Among children less than 5 years of age the rates of *H. influenzae* bacteremia (38–145 per 100,000 person-years) are 100-fold higher than among adults, and the risk for children less than 1 year of age is twofold to threefold higher still (Shapiro and Ward, 1991). In addition to young age, genetic factors may contribute to the strikingly higher rates of invasive *H. influenzae* infection among Native American children (214–601 per 100,000 person-years for children less than 5 years old and up to 1700 per 100,000 person-years for infants less than 1 year old), rates that are among the highest in the world (Shapiro and Ward, 1991).

Virulence factors

In contrast to *C. diphtheriae* and *B. pertussis*, the greater invasive potential of *H. influenzae* is related to its polysaccharide capsule, which the other pathogens lack. Of the six structurally and antigenically distinct capsular polysaccharides (serotypes a through f), serotype b (Hib) has a unique polyribosylribitol phosphate (PRP) polysaccharide that prevents direct complement-mediated lysis. Accordingly, Hib causes 90% of cases of invasive *H. influenzae* infection and meningitis (Robbins *et al.*, 1996). In contrast, infections from nonencapsulated and therefore nontypeable *H. influenzae* (NTHi) are usually localized to the respiratory tract, with invasive infections occurring primarily in immunocompromised persons (neonates, elderly, children in developing countries) (Shapiro and Ward, 1991). Nevertheless, unencapsulated *H. influenzae* accounts for approximately half of invasive cases in adults.

Although the polysaccharide capsule is the major virulence factor in invasive disease, a number of *H. influenzae* adhesins are involved in bacterial attachment to the respiratory epithelium and in colonization (St. Geme, 1996; Hakansson

et al., 1996). Surface pili enhance Hib adherence to human nasopharyngeal and nasal tissue in organ culture and augment nasopharyngeal colonization in primates (St. Geme, 1996). During infection, expression of pili is regulated at the transcriptional level: nasopharyngeal Hib isolates are usually piliated, whereas invasive Hib isolates are almost always nonpiliated (St. Geme, 1996). In nonpiliated *H. influenzae*, adherence to human nasopharyngeal organ culture and to the primate nasopharynx is mediated by surface fibrils, which can be distinguished from pili by transmission electron microscopy (St. Geme, 1996). The fibril Hsf protein is regulated by a defined genetic *hsf* locus and is ubiquitous among geographically and evolutionarily diverse *H. influenzae* isolates (St. Geme, 1996). In addition to structurally defined pili and fibrils, colony opacity factor protein in the outer Hib membrane produces a spontaneous, reversible variation in colony opacity from transparent colonies on agar plates to intermediate or opaque colonies. Transparent strains are efficient colonizers of the infant rat nasopharynx, whereas opaque and intermediate strains are rapidly cleared in this model (Weiser, 1993). Expression of these adhesins in Hib may be coordinately regulated with expression of the polysaccharide capsule, which actually interferes with bacterial adherence of Hib to respiratory epithelial cells and mucins (St.Geme, 1996; Hakansson *et al.*, 1996).

Consistent with the negative effects of the bacterial capsule on colonization, NTHi strains are relatively more efficient colonizers of the respiratory mucosa and attach more avidly to epithelial cells and respiratory mucins (Hakansson *et al.*, 1996). NTHi strains possess a different complement of adhesins than do Hib strains. Only 35% of NTHi isolates express pili and agglutinate erythrocytes, and none is known to express fibrils. However, NTHi isolates express *H. influenzae* adhesins (Hia), which are structurally and functionally homologous with fibrils and efficiently mediate adherence to epithelial cells (St. Geme, 1996). NTHi isolates also express high-molecular-weight adhesins (HMW 1 and 2), which share amino acid sequence and antigenic similarity with *B. pertussis* FHA and, through distinct cellular binding specificities, enhance adherence of *H. influenzae* to epithelial cells (van Schilfgaarde, 2000).

Like *B. pertussis*, *H. influenzae* is generally considered an extracellular pathogen but appears capable of invading and surviving within cultured human epithelial cells and macrophages (St. Geme and Falkow, 1990; Craig, 2001). Viable intracellular *H. influenzae* isolates have also been recovered from resected adenoid tissue in children, particularly within the reticular crypt epithelium, and in tissue macrophages (Forsgren *et al.*, 1994). Intracellular *H. influenzae* was found more frequently in bronchial biopsies of patients with chronic bronchitis than from healthy subjects, suggesting that intracellular *H. influenzae* has a role in the pathogenesis of this disease (Bandi *et al.*, 2001).

Protective immune responses

Although colonization of respiratory mucosa is as essential to the pathogenesis of *H. influenzae* infection as it is for

B. pertussis and *C. diphtheriae* infections, immunity to the Hib capsular polysaccharide is the basis for natural and vaccine-induced immunity against this invasive disease. Antibodies to Hib polysaccharide activate complement, are bactericidal, and protect animals from lethal challenge (Shapiro and Ward, 1991). Accordingly, the highest incidence of invasive infection in humans corresponds to periods of deficient natural immunity to Hib polysaccharide. Newborns are protected for the first 2–3 months of life by antibodies transferred from the maternal circulation, and by the age of 6 years children have acquired protective immunity to Hib polysaccharide from responses to cross-reactive respiratory and intestinal bacterial polysaccharide (including *Streptococcus pneumoniae* type 6 and *Escherichia coli* K100) (Robbins *et al.*, 1996) and, presumably, from asymptomatic colonization and noninvasive mucosal infections. Thus, the goal of vaccination against *H. influenzae* has been to induce protective immunity in children between 3 months and 6 years of age.

The Hib vaccine

The major obstacles to formulating an effective vaccine against *H. influenzae* capsular polysaccharide relate to the inherently poor immunogenicity of relatively T-cell-independent polysaccharide antigens (TI type 2). Primary antibody responses to polysaccharide are age-related, and minimal immunity is generated in infants during the first 18 months of life, the precise age of highest risk for invasive *H. influenzae* infection. In addition, T-cell-independent antigens typically do not induce a booster or anamnestic immune response with repeated exposures; thus, immunity gradually declines from the time of primary immunization.

Despite these obstacles, a pure Hib polysaccharide vaccine was shown to have 90% protective efficacy (95% confidence interval, 56%–96%) in children between 18 and 71 months of age in Finland, and consequently it was licensed in the

United States in 1985 and recommended for children more than 18 months old (Shapiro and Ward, 1991; Peltola *et al.*, 1984). However, concerns about the protective efficacy of the Hib polysaccharide vaccine were raised after licensure. The vaccine was ineffective for infants, who have the highest attack rate of invasive Hib infection, and even in older children it produced protective antibodies that lasted on average only 1 year (Robbins *et al.*, 1996). In addition, some postlicensure case-control studies suggested that rates of invasive disease actually increased in the immediate postimmunization period (Shapiro and Ward, 1991; Osterholm *et al.*, 1988). Consequently, more immunogenic and durably efficacious vaccines were sought.

Conjugate Hib vaccines provided such an enhanced potency product by covalently linking PRP to immunogenic protein carriers, thereby generating T-cell-dependent responses to the Hib polysaccharide. Such Hib conjugate vaccines stimulate appreciable antibody levels to PRP, even in infants less than 12 months old, as well as booster responses. In addition, prior or concurrent administration of the linked protein antigen produces heightened antibody responses to PRP by "carrier priming" (Robbins *et al.*, 1996). On the other hand, preexisting passively acquired maternal antibodies to the carrier antigen may decrease immune responses to conjugate in infants during the first 2–3 months of life, therefore limiting the application of these vaccines to very young infants (Barington *et al.*, 1994; Robbins *et al.*, 1996).

The structural properties of different Hib conjugates produce vaccines with differing immunogenicities and efficacies in specific populations at risk **(Tables 50.3 and 50.4)**. The first Hib conjugate vaccine, PRP linked to DT (PRP-D), generated moderately increased immunogenicity for infants and only fair durability of immunity over 12 months following vaccination. Accordingly, PRP-D was shown to

Table 50.3. Formulations of *Haemophilus influenzae* Conjugate Vaccines

Vaccine	Carrier Antigen	Linkage	Polysaccharide Size	First-Dose Response in Infants	Third-Dose Response in Infants[a]	Durability at 3–12 Months
PRP-D	Diphtheria toxoid	6-carbon spacer	Medium	Minimal	<50%	Decrease in antibody
HbOC	CRM$_{197}$ diphtheria toxoid	None	Short	Minimal	>95%	Continues >12 months
PRP-OMP	Outer-membrane protein from group B *Neisseria meningitidis*	Bigeneric spacer	Medium	High	90%	Decreases over 12 months
PRP-T	Tetanus toxoid	6-carbon spacer	Large	Intermediate	>99%	Stable

[a]Percentage with PRP antibody concentrations >1.0 μg/ml.

Table 50.4. Efficacy of *Haemophilus influenzae* Conjugate Vaccines

Vaccine[a]	Study Site/Population	Population Age (months)	Percent Efficacy (95% CI)	References
PRP-D	Minnesota	15–60	96 (65–99)	Osterholm *et al.*, 1990
	Los Angeles	15–60	87 (62–95)	Greenberg *et al.*, 1991
	Centers for Disease Control	15–60	82 (46–95)	Wenger *et al.*, 1990
	Connecticut/ Pennsylvania	15–60	96 (77–99)	Shapiro and Wald, 1990
	Finland	<12	89 (70–96)	Eskola *et al.*, 1990a
	Native Alaskan	<12	35 (57–73)	Ward *et al.*, 1990
HbOC	Finland	<12	100 (68–100)	Eskola *et al.*, 1990b
	Northern California	<12	100 (65–100)	Black *et al.*, 1991
PRP-OMP	Navajo Indian	<12	95 (73–99)	Santosham *et al.*, 1991

[a]Randomized clinical trials using PRP-T were discontinued prior to completion, when efficacy of other Hib conjugate vaccines was proven.

be effective at preventing invasive disease in children from 15 to 60 months of age but was less effective in infants, particularly among native Alaskans. Subsequent formulation of shorter PRP molecules linked to a genetically engineered DT (HbOC) had markedly improved and sustained immunogenicity as well as efficacy for infants (Madore *et al.*, 1990; Bulkov *et al.*, 1993). However, vaccine failures after the first or second dose of either the PRP-D or HbOC vaccine (Black *et al.*, 1992) provided the impetus to conjugate medium-length PRP molecules with the outer membrane proteins of group B *Neisseria meningitidis* (PRP-OMP), producing a vaccine with significantly higher immune responses after the initial immunization in infants (Schlesinger *et al.*, 1992). Unfortunately, serum antibodies to PRP after immunization with PRP-OMP were lower in avidity and in bacteriolytic activity than with other formulations, and immunity following the third dose of vaccine waned appreciably over time (Schlesinger *et al.*, 1992). In contrast, PRP-tetanus toxoid (PRP-T) vaccine produced protective immunity after the initial dose and was highly immunogenic in nearly 100% of infants after three doses, with stable vaccine-specific antibody levels over the ensuing 12 months (Decker *et al.*, 1992; Capeding *et al.*, 1996). PRP-T was capable of inducing protective immunity even in immunocompromised infants, such as those with sickle cell disease (Goldblatt *et al.*, 1996), and its effectiveness was established in developing countries, including the Gambia, Chile, and The Philippines (Lagos *et al.*, 1996; Capeding *et al.*, 1996; Robbins *et al.*, 1996). Of note, none of the Hib conjugate vaccines has achieved greater than a 37% immune response in HIV-infected children after a single dose, regardless of the type of conjugate (Peters and Sood, 1994).

In addition to protecting from invasive *H. influenzae* disease, Hib conjugate vaccines appear to substantially reduce asymptomatic colonization in immunized populations and induce herd immunity. The mechanism(s) by which antibodies specific for the *H. influenzae* capsule polysaccharide can block colonization, which is presumably mediated by the distinct adhesins, are not completely understood. Conceivably, a Quellung-type reaction induced by specific antibodies to the *H. influenzae* capsular polysaccharide may sterically hinder surface adhesins from binding to epithelial cells or, alternatively, may alter signaling for bacterial growth and viability by blocking influx of essential nutrients or chemokines (van Alphen *et al.*, 1996). In animal models, colonization of infant rats with Hib but not NTHi strains was specifically inhibited by nasal or intraperitoneal administration of human secretory IgA (S-IgA) or serum IgG specific for Hib polysaccharide (Kauppi *et al.*, 1993) and by nasal injection of anti-Hib polysaccharide monoclonal IgG (Kauppi-Korkeila *et al.*, 1996). *In vitro* studies confirmed that antibodies to Hib polysaccharide but not to adhesins or *H. influenzae* lipopolysaccharide inhibit adherence of *H. influenzae* to oropharyngeal epithelial cells (van Alphen *et al.*, 1996). Whereas the concentrations of Hib polysaccharide antibodies required to inhibit adherence in these assays were much higher than those achieved in human sera or breast milk, Hib growth *in vitro* was inhibited by tenfold lower concentrations (1 μg/mL) of anti-Hib polysaccharide (van Alphen *et al.*, 1996), suggesting that antipolysaccharide antibodies may decrease colonization preferentially through their effects on bacterial growth rather than on adherence per se.

Clinical studies have confirmed that immunization against PRP can decrease carriage and transmission of Hib. Immunization of children with the PRP-D conjugate in Finland reduced Hib carriage (from 3.5% to 0%), whereas carriage of NTHi (19%) and *S. pneumoniae* (18%) were not affected (Takala *et al.*, 1991). In subsequent studies, immunization of infants with PRP-T decreased carriage from 3.8% to 0% at 6 months and from 5.6% to 0.5% at

12 months (Barbour *et al.*, 1995). Similarly, Hib conjugate vaccines decreased carriage rates after immunization of native American children (Takala *et al.*, 1993) and children in day-care settings, despite direct exposure to index cases of Hib (Murphy *et al.*, 1993). Reductions in nasopharyngeal carriage after HiB vaccination appears to correlate with serum antibody levels of ≥5 μg/mL, levels substantially higher than those thought to provide protection against invasive Hib disease (1 μg/mL) (Fernandez, 2000).

In addition to reducing carriage in vaccinated children, immunization with Hib conjugate vaccines also decreased Hib carriage in unvaccinated siblings, from 12% to 3.3%, compared with a control population at 12 months (Barbour *et al.*, 1995). Such herd immunity likely has contributed to the decline in the incidence of *H. influenzae* meningitis and other systemic infections in both immunized and nonimmunized children in the United States and Europe since the introduction of Hib vaccines (Muhlemann *et al.*, 1996; Robbins *et al.*, 1996).

Mucosal vaccination with Hib may prove even more effective at reducing nasopharyngeal carriage and transmission of disease. Although current Hib vaccines induce some degree of mucosal immunity, the use of mucosal adjuvants, such as synthetic oligodeoxynucleotide containing immunostimulatory sequences, which powerfully stimulate type 1 immune responses, significantly improved mucosal IgA and systemic IgG responses after mucosal immunization of mice with a conjugate vaccine of Hib and cross-reacting material from diphtheria toxin (Mariotti, 2002).

Despite these successes against Hib infection, alternative strategies are needed for prevention of invasive Hib infection in the subset of young infants who lack sufficient maternal antibodies, for prevention of disease in uniquely susceptible populations within the United States and globally and for prevention of respiratory tract disease caused by NTHi strains. Recent studies suggest that immunization of mothers with conjugate Hib vaccines during the third trimester protected young infants against invasive Hib infection by dramatically increasing concentrations of PRP antibodies transferred from their mothers (Englund *et al.*, 1995). Thus, maternal immunization with Hib conjugate vaccines early in the third trimester may prove an effective strategy to decrease invasive Hib infection among young infants in high-risk populations.

Within the United States, infants and young children in rural Alaska continue to have high rates of invasive Hib disease and nasopharyngeal carriage, despite availability of Hib vaccines (Singleton, 2000). Although rates of invasive Hib disease among native Alaskan children less than 5 years old fell dramatically after introduction of Hib vaccines (from 332 per 100,000 between 1980 and 1991 to 11 cases per 100,000 children after 1991), rates of invasive disease continue to be unacceptably high among native Alaskan children living in rural areas (approximately 66 per 100,000). It is interesting that the change in type of Hib vaccine used, from PRP-OMP in 1992–1995 to HbOC in 1996–1997, was associated with a dramatic rise in invasive Hib disease in this population

(Singleton, 2000). Subsequent use of an initial immunization with PRP-OMP followed by HbOC resulted in a decline in these rates, but nasopharyngeal carriage rates continued to remain high. The study of the interplay of unique host characteristics with vaccination programs in this United States population may provide strategies for elimination of Hib disease in the global community, where the availability of safe and efficacious vaccines has reduced the burden of Hib disease only by an estimated 2% (Peltola, 2000).

In contrast to Hib, vaccines against the nonencapsulated NTHi strains must be directed against alternative virulence factors. Two surface lipoproteins, lipoprotein D and P6, each widely distributed and antigenically conserved among Hib and NTHi strains, elicit protective immunity in animals. Immunization of rats with the 42-kDa membrane-derived lipoprotein D elicited specific serum antibodies that were bactericidal *in vitro* against homologous and heterologous NTHi strains (Akkoyunlu *et al.*, 1996). Lipoprotein D is naturally immunogenic in humans, and concentrations of specific serum IgG against this antigen increase during the first 20 years of life. However, thus far human antibodies against lipoprotein D have not had detectable bactericidal activity against NTHi strains when assayed *in vitro*. The potential for lipoprotein D as a component of vaccines against NTHi will depend upon identifying the mechanism of protection afforded by specific antibodies.

Systemic immunization with the 16-kDa surface peptidoglycan-associated lipoprotein P6 induces high titers of bactericidal serum IgG against P6 in chinchillas (Demaria *et al.*, 1996). In this model, there were trends towards decreased incidence and duration of middle ear infection in immunized animals, but these did not achieve statistical significance (Demaria *et al.*, 1996). Furthermore, systemic immunization with P6 did not affect nasopharyngeal colonization in the chinchilla model (Demaria *et al.*, 1996). On the other hand, mucosal immunization of rats with direct injection of purified P6 into intestinal Peyer's patches, followed by tracheal instillation of P6 at 14 days, provided protection against subsequent pulmonary challenge with both Hib and NTHi strains (Kyd *et al.*, 1995). Also, mucosal (nasal) immunization of mice with recombinant P6 combined with cholera toxin stimulated P6-specific mucosal IgA and systemic IgG responses and enhanced clearance of NTHi from the nasopharynx and middle ear (Hotomi *et al.*, 2002; Sabirov *et al.*, 2001). Thus, these data suggest that the design of future NTHi vaccines should be directed toward mucosal immunization with *H. influenzae* surface lipoproteins and possibly other NTHi antigens.

Summary

Protective immunization against Hib has incorporated the immunologic principles of conjugating polysaccharide to carrier proteins to increase immune responses at younger ages and to provide durable and anamnestic responses to subsequent antigen challenge. Hib conjugate vaccines not only have been effective at preventing invasive Hib infection but also have decreased carriage rates and elicited herd immunity, demonstrating that antibodies against capsular polysaccharide, which are not directly involved in bacterial adherence to respiratory mucosa, can nevertheless decrease colonization and transmission of *H. influenzae* infection. The remaining challenges of preventing invasive Hib infection in young infants and in decreasing disease from NTHi strains may be met by maternal immunization and mucosal immunization strategies, respectively.

PNEUMOCOCCAL VACCINE

Pathogenesis of clinical infection

Although *S. pneumoniae* was discovered more than a century ago, this well-studied encapsulated gram-positive mucosal organism remains the preeminent respiratory bacterial pathogen in the world today. The versatility of *S. pneumoniae* is highlighted by its ability to colonize the nasopharynx asymptomatically or to cause localized mucosal infections (e.g., otitis media, sinusitis, bronchitis, or pneumonia), while retaining the potential to cause devastating invasive infections (e.g., necrotizing pneumonia, bacteremia, and meningitis). Localized infections are much more common; invasive infections are more often fatal.

The impact of pneumococcal disease is tremendous. Respiratory diseases, among which pneumococcal infections are prominent in all age groups, are the leading cause of childhood mortality worldwide (over 4 million deaths per year) (Murray *et al.*, 1997) and the sixth leading cause of death among Americans. Annually in the United States, approximately 6 million cases of otitis media in children occur and 1 in 5000 adults experiences pneumococcal bacteremia. Rates of invasive infection increase with age, are threefold higher among black Americans than among whites (Bennett *et al.*, 1992), and are fivefold to 10-fold higher in geographically diverse native American adults (Davidson *et al.*, 1994). Young children are also particularly susceptible to invasive pneumococcal disease, with rates 10 times greater than those among matched adults (Bennett *et al.*, 1992; Dagan *et al.*, 1992; Davidson *et al.*, 1994).

Virulence factors

Compared with the respiratory bacterial pathogens discussed previously, a greater variety of virulence factors have been identified for *S. pneumoniae* (**Table 50.5**), particularly those involved in bacterial invasion and multiplication in tissues, such as the polysaccharide capsule, cell wall, autolysin, pneumolysin, and the pneumococcal surface protein A (PspA). The pneumococcal polysaccharide capsule, the major determinant of virulence, was the first nonprotein antigen described and provided the first convincing evidence that polysaccharides would induce antibody responses. Currently, more than 90 antigenically distinct pneumococcal capsular serotypes have been identified. Noninflammatory and not directly toxic to any cell, the pneumococcal capsule provides relative resistance to direct complement activation and to opsonophagocytosis and killing. The capsule accomplishes this role by stearic hindrance, its net negative charge,

Table 50.5. *Streptococcus pneumoniae* Virulence Factors

Factor	Proposed Mechanism
With known virulence functions	
Capsular polysaccharide	Reduces opsonophagocytosis
Cell wall polysaccharide	Pro-inflammatory
	Directly cytotoxic to endothelial cells
Pneumolysin	Disrupts tissue barriers
	Inhibits immune responses
	Consumes complement in local environment
Surface protein, PspA	Interferes with complement deposition
	Interferes with killing by lactoferrin
With possible virulence functions	
Autolysin	Release of inflammatory cell wall and cytoplasmic factors
Neuraminidase	May unmask cell-surface binding receptors
Hyaluronidase	May enhance disruption of cell-matrix barriers
IgA1 protease	Enhances adherence of encapsulated *S. pneumoniae* to epithelial cells *in vitro*
	May inhibit complement-killing of *S. pneumoniae* by phagocytes
	May prevent IgA-mediated immune exclusion; IgA F(ab) fragments may prevent IgG binding

Data are from Paton *et al.*, 1993; Briles *et al.*, 2001; Weiser *et al.*, 2003.

and its hydrophilicity (Bayer and Bayer, 1994). Capsule formation is regulated in response to environmental factors, with strains generally producing less capsule during colonization than during invasion.

In contrast to the bacterial capsule, the peptidoglycan cell wall is readily immunogenic and highly proinflammatory. Cell wall components may promote disease by stimulating inflammation and tissue injury in the middle ear, lung, and meninges (Tuomanen *et al.*, 1995). Although antibody and complement components bind to cell wall antigens, the pneumococcal capsule may hinder access of phagocytes to opsonized cell wall in the intact bacteria. However, disruption of the cell wall by autolysin, a 36-kDa *N*-acetylmuramic acid, ι-alanine amidase in the cell envelope, releases free cell wall components (Holtje and Tomasz, 1976) and cytoplasmic toxins.

Pneumolysin is the principal pneumococcal cytotoxin released by pneumococci. Pneumolysin can be released by autolysin but can also be released through a nonlytic process (Rubins and Janoff, 1998; Balachandran *et al.*, 2001). Pneumolysin abrogates ciliary clearance mechanisms of the bronchial epithelium and disrupts the alveolar-capillary barrier within the lung, thus facilitating bacterial invasion and dissemination (Rayner *et al.*, 1995; Rubins *et al.*, 1993). Pneumolysin also promotes bacterial multiplication by subverting complement-mediated clearance mechanisms and by directly inhibiting phagocyte functions (Paton *et al.*, 1993; Rubins *et al.*, 1996).

Despite the variety of known and suspected pneumococcal virulence factors, the *S. pneumoniae* adhesins involved in respiratory mucosal colonization have not been characterized, although cellular binding sites have been identified. A glycoconjugate binding site (containing the disaccharide GlcNAcα 1-3Gal) has been identified for pneumococci on human pharyngeal epithelial cells (Andersson *et al.*, 1983), and selected domains of fibronectin may also serve as a binding substrate (van der Flier *et al.*, 1995). Bacterial binding to epithelial cells may be significantly increased during inflammation. Local cytokines may induce the expression of epithelial membrane receptors, including induced platelet-activating factor receptors, which bind to pneumococcal phosphorylcholine (Tuomanen *et al.*, 1995). Perturbation of epithelial cells by pneumolysin or by viral respiratory infections (e.g., adenovirus or influenza) also appears to enhance pneumococcal adherence. In addition, pneumococcal neuraminidase may enhance bacterial attachment by exposing cellular binding sites. Finally, pneumococcal IgA1 protease, which cleaves the effector Fc portion of IgA1 from its pathogen-binding component, has been reported to facilitate pneumococcal colonization by inhibiting functional bacterial opsonization by mucosal IgA antibodies. This modulation of charge provides exposure of phosphorylcholine to its epithelial cell receptors (Kilian *et al.*, 1988; Weiser *et al.*, 2003).

Putative pneumococcal adhesins include cell wall components, such as phosphorylcholine. PsaA is necessary for manganese transport, which is, in turn, responsible for unknown changes required for *in vivo* colonization and bacterial adherence *in vitro* (Tuomanen *et al.*, 1995; Paton *et al.*,

1993). However, PspA itself is not likely to serve directly as an adhesin. As discussed previously with regard to *H. influenzae*, pneumococci also undergo spontaneous, reversible variation in colony opacity on agar plates, from transparent colonies, which efficiently colonize the nasopharynx, to intermediate or opaque colonies, which are rapidly cleared from the respiratory mucosa (Weiser, 1998; Tuomanen *et al.*, 1995). As yet, the pneumococcal homolog to the *H. influenzae* colony opacity factor protein has not been identified.

Pneumococci also have the potential to invade and survive within respiratory epithelial cells (Talbot *et al.*, 1996), similar to *B. pertussis* and *H. influenzae*. Invasion of the epithelium may allow pneumococci to evade mucosal clearance mechanisms during colonization. Of note, the pneumococcal capsule interfered with the ability of different pneumococcal strains to invade respiratory epithelial cells (Talbot *et al.*, 1996).

Protective immune responses

Most children and adults do not experience serious pneumococcal infections. Such exemption from disease is likely related to an array of host factors, such as intact anatomic defenses (mucus, bronchial ciliary movement, epithelial cell integrity) and soluble nonimmune factors (e.g., lactoferrin, lysozyme, and lactoperoxidase), in concert with systemic and mucosal immune mechanisms. Host immune factors important in protection against systemic infection include inflammation, complement, phagocytes, and cytokines. Prominent among the immune factors that can play a role in protection against systemic infection is capsule-specific serum antibody. Most often present in older children and adults in the absence of overt infection or immunization, natural antibodies to the pneumococcal capsule may be induced by structurally similar or cross-reactive antigens (e.g., antibodies to *H. influenzae* type b and *E. coli* K100 cross-react with *S. pneumoniae* type 6B). Alternatively, they may be polyreactive antibodies produced by the CD5+ subset of B cells or may be produced in response to asymptomatic colonization (Musher *et al.*, 1997). These initial responses to polysaccharides appear to occur in specific immunologic venues, such as the marginal zones of splenic germinal centers (Martin *et al.*, 2001) in association with dendritic cells (Colino *et al.*, 2002; Balazs *et al.*, 2002) and in the context of specific activation requirements (Wu *et al.*, 1999; Wu *et al.*, 2000).

Pneumococcal capsular polysaccharides mediate resistance to phagocytosis. Opsonization of the organism by capsule-specific IgG, IgM, or polymeric IgA greatly facilitates efficient complement-dependent binding, phagocytosis, and killing of the organism (Janoff *et al.*, 1999; Finn *et al.*, 2002). Opsonophagocytic activity *in vitro* correlates reasonably well with serum concentrations of capsule-specific antibodies. Accordingly, low serum concentrations of these antibodies have been invoked as a major risk factor for increased rates of invasive pneumococcal disease among young children, patients with hypogammaglobulinemia, and patients infected with HIV-1 (Janoff and Rubins, 1998).

In addition to capsular polysaccharide, other pneumococcal virulence factors, including cell wall, pneumolysin, IgA1 protease, PspA, and PsaA, induce antibody responses in clinical and animal studies (Paton *et al.*, 1993; Briles *et al.*, 2000b). Although partially protective against respiratory challenge in animal studies, none of these antibody responses has been shown to provide protection against pneumococcal infection in humans (Musher *et al.*, 1997). However, levels of human antibodies elicited to an experimental PspA vaccine and human antibodies to pneumolysin as a result of natural infection correlate with their ability to protect mice from otherwise fatal pneumococcal infections (Briles *et al.*, 2000a; Briles *et al.*, 2000b; Musher *et al.*, 2001).

The pneumoccal vaccine

Diphtheria, pertussis, and invasive *H. influenzae* disease can be potentially controlled with adequate utilization of safe and effective vaccines in appropriate populations. However, until recently, the goals for a pneumococcal vaccine have been more modest and its efficacy has been more limited, in a narrower age range of patients (primarily adults). Now, as the populations at risk increase (especially socially disadvantaged children, the elderly, and immunocompromised patients) and as rates of antimicrobial resistance rise, focused efforts must be made to develop innovative strategies to prevent pneumococcal infections with cost-effective vaccines.

In 1945, MacLeod *et al.* reported the protective efficacy of a capsular polysaccharide vaccine in 17,000 military personnel during an outbreak of pneumococcal pneumonia in a training facility. Immunization with purified capsular polysaccharide represented a major medical advance, because vaccine reactogenicity (e.g., local abscess formation) was significantly less than with the previously used inactivated whole bacteria and because the isolated polysaccharides were more stable and more reliably standardized. Use of this vaccine also supported the concept that a single specific virulence factor could be targeted, isolated, purified, and ultimately effective in preventing disease. Protection afforded by immunization with the polysaccharide vaccine was specific for the four serotypes included in the vaccine, with little impact on nonvaccine serotypes in this population of healthy men with high underlying rates of disease. In addition, the vaccine was also thought to have decreased rates of pneumococcal infection with vaccine serotypes in the nonvaccinees, perhaps due to induction of herd immunity by decreasing rates of carriage and transmission (MacLeod *et al.*, 1945).

This initial study, along with those by Austrian *et al.* (1976) and others among South African gold miners and adults in the New Guinea Highlands (Riley *et al.*, 1977), confirmed the efficacy of parenteral immunization with purified capsular polysaccharide in preventing pneumococcal disease, particularly that due to vaccine serotypes, in immunocompetent adults in high-incidence settings. Subsequently, a thoughtful and rigorous meta-analysis by Fine in 1994 of the properly randomized, controlled trials of

pneumococcal vaccine efficacy examined its effect on definite and presumptive pneumococcal pneumonia, pneumococcal disease overall, pneumonia, bronchitis, and all-cause and pneumococcal disease–specific mortality. In these studies, the vaccine produced a statistically significant reduction in numbers of cases of definitive (bacteremic) pneumococcal pneumonia caused by vaccine serotypes alone, as well as that related to all serotypes, in healthy young men in high-risk situations. Also, there were statistical trends toward reduction of presumptive pneumococcal pneumonia cases involving vaccinated subjects.

However, the vaccine did not significantly reduce rates of overall pneumococcal disease in patients considered "high risk" for pneumococcal infection, e.g., patients >55 years of age and those with chronic underlying medical conditions or immunosuppression (Fine *et al.*, 1994). The efficacy of pneumococcal vaccines primarily against invasive disease is supported by a series of retrospective case-control studies showing 47%–81% protection in high-risk patients, as defined earlier, against bacteremic infection (Fedson and Musher, 1994). The lack of protection against pneumococcal pneumonia or all-cause pneumonia in older adults was confirmed in a recent prospective randomized trial (Ortqvist *et al.*, 1998) and a large, retrospective cohort study of more than 47,000 patients (Jackson *et al.*, 2003).

Although prevention of the lethal complications of invasive pneumococcal infection in adults is an important goal of immunization, the major burden of *S. pneumoniae* disease is mucosal, not invasive, and occurs in children as well as in adults (Murray and Lopez, 1997). The high risk of pneumococcal infection for young children appears related to their inability to produce antibodies to polysaccharide antigens. This humoral defect, likely under T-cell control, may derive in part from compromised production of the IgG2 subclass, which comprises an appreciable proportion of capsule-specific IgG (Chudwin *et al.*, 1987). The enhanced ability of capsular polysaccharide to stimulate specific IgG when conjugated to protein antigens was the basis for the outstanding clinical efficacy of newer *H. influenzae* vaccines (see previous discussion). Field trials of similarly conjugated pneumococcal vaccines have demonstrated the immunogenicity of these vaccines in Western and African infants (Leach *et al.*, 1996).

Subsequent randomized controlled trials have demonstrated that a protein-polysaccharide pneumococcal conjugate vaccine containing CRM197 and seven common pediatric serotypes (4, 6B, 9V, 14, 18C, 19F, and 23F) (Prevnar, Wyeth Lederle Vaccines), which represent 86% of invasive pneumococcal strains in children (directly or by cross-reactivity), provided greater than 90% protection against invasive pneumococcal disease in children in northern California (Black *et al.*, 2000). Office visits for otitis media, only a fraction of which are caused by *S. pneumoniae*, were reduced by almost 8% (Fireman *et al.*, 2003). Episodes of pneumonia were reduced by 4%–32%, with the higher rates of protection earlier in life and against more severe cases (Black *et al.*, 2002). On the basis of these data, the vaccine is recommended for children less than 5 years of age

(Centers for Disease Control and Prevention, 2000). Since introduction of the vaccine in early 2000, rates of invasive pneumococcal disease have declined for children <2 years old by 78% and 50% for vaccine serotypes and vaccine-related serotypes, respectively, and by 32% for adults of peak child-bearing ages (20–39 years) (Whitney et al., 2003). This vaccine and related vaccines also decrease rates of colonization with vaccine serotypes but may increase colonization with nonvaccine serotypes (reviewed in Pelton et al., 2002).

Work is in progress to broaden the distribution and accessibility of the vaccine to high-risk children around the world. Alternative strategies (which avoid the four-dose regimen and high cost of the vaccine) to protect infants, among whom rates of pneumococcal disease are highest, include maternal immunization with the 23-valent polysaccharide vaccine. Protection may be afforded by passive transfer of antibodies through cord blood and breast milk. Indeed, recent data show that capsule-specific S-IgA antibodies are present in breast milk of immunized mothers and support complement-dependent killing of the organism by neutrophils (Finn et al., 2002). The efficacy of this strategy against the development of otitis media is under evaluation.

Summary

S. pneumoniae is currently the single most common cause of potentially preventable respiratory bacterial disease in children and adults worldwide, with tremendous medical, social, and economic impact. Although the current capsular polysaccharide vaccine has efficacy against invasive disease in adults, an optimal vaccine should provide greater documented efficacy in elderly and compromised patients, particularly against pneumonia and other mucosal manifestations. To date, the conjugates include fewer serotypes and do not appear to provide significantly greater immunogenicity in adults, including high-risk patients with HIV-1 infection, than the 23-valent vaccine does (Shelly et al., 1997). However, the newly introduced protein-polysaccharide vaccine is remarkably effective against invasive infections in children, with more modest effects on pneumonia and otitis media. Some of these limitations result from the variable proportion of these infections caused by S. pneumoniae and likely in part from the difficulty of introducing effective mucosal responses with parenteral vaccines. Promising alternative approaches are directed toward identifying and integrating other pneumococcal virulence factors into vaccines as primary antigens or as additional protein conjugates to provide protection against a broader array of capsular serotypes. These factors, which are implicated in the early events of pneumococcal infection at mucosal surfaces, include pneumolysin, PspA, and PsaA (Briles et al., 2001).

Whether to prevent invasive or mucosal pneumococcal disease and whether systemic immunity will be sufficient to achieve both goals with this serotypically diverse organism are critical questions to address at this juncture. Clearly, systemic immunization is effective in preventing localized respiratory bacterial infections with C. diphtheriae and B. pertussis and both invasive infections and colonization with

H. influenzae. Diphtheria vaccine is directed toward a single but pivotal disease-related toxin; pertussis vaccine integrates the bacteria's toxin in conjunction with clearly identified factors required for mucosal adherence and colonization; and H. influenzae vaccine is directed toward a single prominent virulence mechanism, the polysaccharide capsule, but toward only one capsule (type b) on a complement-lysis-sensitive gram-negative organism. In contrast, S. pneumoniae has no preeminent single disease-determining toxin, adherence mechanisms are not as yet well characterized, and efficient killing of this gram-positive complement-lysis-resistant organism requires the combination of complement, phagocytic cells, and specific antibody to many capsular polysaccharides.

A serious challenge for the microbiologist, vaccinologist, and mucosal immunologist is to eschew prior bias and objectively determine the contribution of systemic and mucosal immune responses to protection against pneumococcal infection. The quality and relevance of these responses should be characterized and judged on the basis of their impact on antigens of defined structure and function. This done, the most reasonable and promising approaches to elicit such responses, whether with parenteral, nasal, or oral formulations in liposomes, microspheres, live vectors, or other innovative vehicles, will become more readily apparent. What is abundantly clear, however, is that the wealth and depth of creative investigation related to the pathogenesis of S. pneumoniae infections at this time should be integrated with a clear goal of producing a vaccine capable of controlling both mucosal and systemic infections in adults and children in the West and worldwide.

REFERENCES

Aggerbeck, H., Gizurarson, S., Wantzin, J., and Heron, I. (1997). Intranasal booster vaccination against diphtheria and tetanus in man. Vaccine 15, 307–316.

Akkoyunlu, M., Janson, H., Ruan, M., and Forsgren, A. (1996). Biological activity of serum antibodies to a nonacylated form of lipoprotein D of Haemophilus influenzae. Infect. Immun. 64, 4586–4592.

American Academy of Pediatrics Committee on Infectious Diseases (AAPCID). The relationship between pertussis vaccine and central nervous system sequelae: continuing assessment. (1996). Pediatrics 97, 279–281.

Andersson, B., Dahmén, J., Frejd, T., Leffler, H., Magnusson, G., Noori, G., and Edén, C.S. (1983). Identification of an active disaccharide unit of a glycoconjugate receptor for pneumococci attaching to human pharyngeal epithelial cells. J. Exp. Med. 158, 559–570.

Austrian, R., Douglas, R.M., Schiffman, G., Coetzee, A.M., Koornhof, H.J., Hayden-Smith, S., and Reid, R.D. (1976). Prevention of pneumococcal pneumonia by vaccination. Trans. Assoc. Am. Physicians 89, 184–194.

Balachandran, P., Hollingshead, S.K., Paton, J.C., and Briles, D.E. (2001). The autolytic enzyme LytA of Streptococcus pneumoniae is not responsible for releasing pneumolysin. J. Bacteriol. 183, 3108–3116.

Balazs, M., Martin, F., Zhou, T., and Kearney, J. (2002). Blood dendritic cells interact with splenic marginal zone B cells to initiate T-independent immune responses. Immunity 17, 341–352.

Bandi, V., Apicella, M.A., Mason, E., Murphy, T.F., Siddiqi, A., Atmar, R.L., and Greenberg, S.B. (2001). Nontypeable Haemophilus *influenzae* in the lower respiratory tract of patients with chronic bronchitis. *Am. J. Respir. Crit. Care Med.* 164, 2114–2119.

Baraff, L.J., Cody, C.L., and Cherry, J.D. (1984). DTP-associated reactions: an analysis by injection site, manufacturer, prior reactions, and dose. *Pediatrics* 73, 31–36.

Barbour, M.L., Mayon-White, R.T., Coles, C., Crook, D.W., and Moxon, E.R. (1995). The impact of conjugate vaccine on carriage of *Haemophilus influenzae* type b. *J. Infect. Dis.* 171, 93–98.

Barington, T., Gyhrs, A., Kristensen, K., and Heilmann, C. (1994). Opposite effects of actively and passively acquired immunity to the carrier on responses of human infants to a *Haemophilus influenzae* type b conjugate vaccine. *Infect. Immun.* 62, 9–14.

Barnard, A., Mahon, B.P., Watkins, J., Redhead, K., and Mills, K.H. (1996). Th1/Th2 cell dichotomy in acquired immunity to *Bordetella pertussis*: variables in the *in vivo* priming and *in vitro* cytokine detection techniques affect the classification of T-cell subsets as Th1, Th2 or Th0. *Immunology* 87, 372–380.

Bayer, M.E, and Bayer, M.H. (1994). Biophysical and structural aspects of the bacterial capsule. *ASM News* 60, 192–198.

Bennett, N.M., Buffington, J., and LaForce, F.M. (1992). Pneumococcal bacteremia in Monroe County, New York. *Am. J. Public Health* 82, 1513–1516.

Bezjak, V, and Farsey, S.J. (1970). *Corynebacterium diphtheriae* in skin lesions in Ugandan children. *Bull. World Health Organ.* 43, 643–650.

Björkholm, B., Böttiger, M., Christenson, B., and Hagberg, L. (1986). Antitoxin antibody levels and the outcome of illness during an outbreak of diphtheria among alcoholics. *Scand. J. Infect. Dis.* 18, 235–239.

Black, S.B., Shinefield, H.R., Fireman, B., Hiatt, R., Polen, M., and Vittinghoff, E. (1991). Efficacy in infancy of oligosaccharide conjugate *Haemophilus influenzae* type b (HbOC) vaccine in a United States population of 61,080 children. The Northern California Kaiser Permanente Vaccine Study Center Pediatrics Group. *Pediatr. Infect. Dis. J.* 10, 97–104.

Black, S.B., Shinefield, H.R., Fireman, B., and Hiatt, R. (1992). Safety, immunogenicity, and efficacy in infancy of oligosaccharide conjugate *Haemophilus influenzae* type b vaccine in a United States population: possible implications for optimal use. *J. Infect. Dis.* 165 (Suppl 1), S139–S143.

Black, S., Shinefield, H., Fireman, B., Lewis, E., Ray, P., Hansen, J.R., Elvin, L., Ensor, K.M., Hackell, J., Siber, G., Malinoski, F., Madore, D., Chang, I., Kohberger, R., Watson, W., Austrian, R., and Edwards, K. (2000). Efficacy, safety and immunogenicity of heptavalent pneumococcal conjugate vaccine in children. Northern California Kaiser Permanente Vaccine Study Center Group. *Pediatr. Infect. Dis. J.* 19, 187–195.

Black, S.B., Shinefield, H.R., Ling, S., Hansen, J., Fireman, B., Spring, D., Noyes, J., Lewis, E., Ray, P., Lee, J., and Hackell, J. (2002). Effectiveness of heptavalent pneumococcal conjugate vaccine in children younger than five years of age for prevention of pneumonia. *Pediatr. Infect. Dis. J.* 21, 810–815.

Brennan, M.J, and Shahin, R.D. (1996). Pertussis antigens that abrogate bacterial adherence and elicit immunity. *Am. J. Respir. Crit. Care Med.* 154, S145–S149.

Briles, D.E., Hollingshead, S.K., King, J., Swift, A., Braun, P.A., Park, M.K., Ferguson, L.M., Nahm, M.H., and Nabors, G.S. (2000a). Immunization of humans with rPspA elicits antibodies that passively protect mice from fatal infection with *Streptococcus pneumoniae* bearing heterologous PspA. *J. Infect. Dis.* 182, 1694–1701.

Briles, D.E., Paton, J.C., Nahm, M.H., and Swiatio E. (2000b). Immunity to *Streptococcus pneumoniae*. In *Effect of Microbes on the Immune System* (eds. M. Cunningham, R. S. Fujinami). Philadelphia: Lippincott-Raven, 263–280.

Briles, D.E., Hollingshead, S., Nabors, G.S., Paton, J.C., and Brooks-Walter, A. (2000). The potential for using protein vaccines to protect against otitis media caused by *Streptococcus pneumoniae*. *Vaccine* 19, (Suppl. 1) S87–S95.

Brooks, G.F., Bennett, J.V., and Feldman, R.A. (1974). Diphtheria in the United States, 1959–1970. *J. Infect. Dis.* 129, 172–8.

Bulkow, L.R., Wainwright, R.B., Letson, G.W., Chang, S.J., and Ward, J.I. (1993). Comparative immunogenicity of four *Haemophilus*

influenzae type b conjugate vaccines in Alaska Native infants. *Pediatr. Infect. Dis. J.* 12, 484–492.

Cahill, E.S., O'Hagan, D.T., Illum, L., Barnard, A., Mills, K.H., and Redhead, K. (1995). Immune responses and protection against *Bordetella pertussis* infection after intranasal immunization of mice with filamentous haemagglutinin in solution or incorporated in biodegradable microparticles. *Vaccine* 13, 455–462.

Capeding, M.R., Nohynek, H., Pascual, L.G., Kayhty, H., Sombrero, L.T., Eskola, J., and Ruutu, P. (1996). The immunogenicity of three *Haemophilus influenzae* type B conjugate vaccines after a primary vaccination series in Philippine infants. *Am. J. Trop. Med. Hyg.* 55, 516–520.

Centers for Disease Control and Prevention. (1993). Diphtheria outbreak: Russian Federation, 1990–1993. *MMWR Morb. Mortal. Wkly. Rep.* 42, 840–847.

Centers for Disease Control and Prevention. General recommendations on immunization. Recommendations of the Advisory Committee on Immunization Practices (ACIP). (1994). *MMWR Morb. Mortal. Wkly. Rep.* 43, 1–38.

Centers for Disease Control and Prevention. Preventing pneumococcal disease among infants and young children. (2000). Recommendations of the Advisory Committee on Immunization Practices (ACIP). *MMWR Morb. Mortal. Wkly. Rep.* 49, 1–35.

Chang, M.P., Baldwin, R.L., Bruce, C., and Wisnieski, B.J. (1989). Second cytotoxic pathway of diphtheria toxin suggested by nuclease activity. *Science* 246, 1165–1168.

Chudwin, D.S., Artrip, S.G., and Schiffman, G. (1987). Immunoglobulin G class and subclass antibodies to pneumococcal capsular polysaccharides. *Clin. Immunol. Immunopathol.* 44, 114–121.

Colino, J., Shen, Y., and Snapper, C.M. (2002). Dendritic cells pulsed with intact *Streptococcus pneumoniae* elicit both protein- and polysaccharide-specific immunoglobulin isotype responses in vivo through distinct mechanisms. *J. Exp. Med.* 195, 1–13.

Craig, J.E., Cliffe, A., Garnett, K., and High, N.J. (2001). Survival of nontypeable *Haemophilus influenzae* in macrophages. *FEMS Microbiol. Lett.* 203, 55–61.

Dagan, R., Engelhard, D., Piccard, E, and Englehard, D. (1992). Epidemiology of invasive childhood pneumococcal infections in Israel. The Israeli Pediatric Bacteremia and Meningitis group. *JAMA* 268, 3328–3332.

Davidson, M., Parkinson, A.J., Bulkow, L.R., Fitzgerald, M.A., Peters, H.V., and Parks, D.J. (1994). The epidemiology of invasive pneumococcal disease in Alaska, 1986–1990: ethnic differences and opportunities for prevention. *J. Infect. Dis.* 170, 368–376.

Decker, M.D., Edwards, K.M., Bradley, R., and Palmer, P. (1992). Comparative trial in infants of four conjugate *Haemophilus influenzae* type b vaccines. *J. Pediatr.* 120, 184–189.

Demaria, T.F., Murwin, D.M., and Leake, E.R. (1996). Immunization with outer membrane protein P6 from nontypeable *Haemophilus influenzae* induces bactericidal antibody and affords protection in the chinchilla model of otitis media. *Infect. Immun.* 64, 5187–5192.

English, P.C. (1985). Diphtheria and theories of infectious disease: centennial appreciation of the critical role of diphtheria in the history of medicine. *Pediatrics* 76, 1–9.

Englund, J.A., Glezen, W.P., Turner, C., Harvey, J., Thompson, C., and Siber, G.R. (1995). Transplacental antibody transfer following maternal immunization with polysaccharide and conjugate *Haemophilus influenzae* type b vaccines. *J. Infect. Dis.* 171, 99–105.

Eskola, J., Käyhty, H., Takala, A.K., Peltola, H., Rönnberg, P-R., Kela, E., Pekkanen, E., McVerry, P.H., and Mäkelä, P.H. (1990a). A randomized, prospective field trial of a conjugate vaccine in the protection of infants and young children against invasive *Haemophilus influenzae* type b disease. *N. Engl. J. Med.* 323, 1381–1387.

Eskola, J., Peltola, H., and Takala, A. (1990b). Protective efficacy of the *Haemophilus influenzae* type b conjugate vaccine HbOC in Finnish infants. In *Program and Abstracts of the 30th Interscience Conference on Antimicrobial Agents and Chemotherapy* [Atlanta; abstract no. 60]. Washington, DC: American Society for Microbiology.

Fedson, D.S, and Musher, D.M. (1994). Pneumococcal vaccine. In *Vaccines* (eds. Plotkin, S.A., Mortimer, E.A., Jr.). Philadelphia: WB Saunders, 517–564.

Fernandez, J., Levine, O.S., Sanchez, J., Balter, S., LaClaire, L., Feris, J., and Romero-Steiner, S. (2000). Prevention of *Haemophilus influenzae* type b colonization by vaccination: correlation with serum anti-capsular IgG concentration. *J. Infect. Dis.* 182, 1553–1556.

Fine, M.J., Smith, M.A., Carson, C.A., Meffe, F., Sankey, S.S., Weissfeld, L.A., Detsky, A.S., and Kapoor, W.N. (1994). Efficacy of pneumococcal vaccination in adults: a meta-analysis of randomized controlled trials. *Arch. Intern. Med.* 154, 2666–2677.

Finn, A., Zhang, Q., Seymour, L., Fasching, C., Pettitt, E., and Janoff, E.N. (2002). Induction of functional secretory IgA responses in breast milk, by pneumococcal capsular polysaccharides. *J. Infect. Dis.* 186, 1422–1429.

Fireman, B., Black, S.B., Shinefield, H.R., Lee, J., Lewis, E., and Ray, P. (2003). Impact of the pneumococcal conjugate vaccine on otitis media. *Pediatr. Infect. Dis. J.* 22, 10–16.

Forsgren, J., Samuelson, A., Ahlin, A., Jonasson, J., Rynnel-Dagoo, B., and Lindberg, A. (1994). *Haemophilus influenzae* resides and multiplies intracellularly in human adenoid tissue as demonstrated by *in situ* hybridization and bacterial viability assay. *Infect. Immun.* 62, 673–679.

Goldblatt, D., Johnson, M., and Evans, J. (1996). Antibody response to *Haemophilus influenzae* type b conjugate vaccine in sickle cell disease. *Arch. Dis. Child* 75, 159–161.

Greco, D., Salmaso, S., Mastrantonio, P., Giuliano, M., Tozzi, A.E., Anemona, A., Ciofi degli Atti, M.L., Giammanco, A., Panei, P., Blackwelder, W.C., Klein, D.L., and Wassilak, S.G. (1996). A controlled trial of two acellular vaccines and one whole-cell vaccine against pertussis. Progetto Pertosse Working Group. *N. Engl. J. Med.* 334, 341–348.

Greenberg, D.P., Vadheim, C.M., Bordenave, N., Ziontz, L., Christenson, P., Waterman, S.H., and Ward, J.I. (1991). Protective efficacy of *Haemophilus influenzae* type b polysaccharide and conjugate vaccines in children 18 months of age and older. *JAMA* 265, 987–992.

Gustafsson, L., Hallander, H.O., Olin, P., Reizenstein, E., and Storsaeter, J. (1996). A controlled trial of a two-component acellular, a five-component acellular, and a whole-cell pertussis vaccine. *N. Engl. J. Med.* 334, 349–355.

Hakansson, A., Carlstedt, I., Davies, J., Mossberg, A.K., Sabharwal, H., and Svanborg, C. (1996). Aspects on the interaction of *Streptococcus pneumoniae* and *Haemophilus influenzae* with human respiratory tract mucosa. *Am. J. Respir. Crit. Care Med.* 154, S187–S191.

Holtje, J.V, and Tomasz, A. (1976). Purification of the pneumococcal N-acetylmuramyl-L-alanine amidase to biochemical homogeneity. *J. Biol. Chem.* 251, 4199–4207.

Hotomi, M., Yamanaka, N., Shimada, J., Suzumoto, M., Ikeda, Y., Sakai, A., Arai, J., and Green, B. (2002). Intranasal immunization with recombinant outer membrane protein P6 induces specific immune responses against nontypeable *Haemophilus influenzae*. *Int. J. Pediatr. Otorhinolaryngol.* 65, 109–116.

Jackson, L.A., Neuzil, K.M., Yu, O., Benson, P., Barlow, W.E., Adams, A.L., Hanson, C.A., Mahoney, L.D., Shay, D.K., and Thompson, W.W. (2003). Vaccine Safety Datalink. Effectiveness of pneumococcal polysaccharide vaccine in older adults. *N. Engl. J. Med.* 348, 1747–1755.

Janoff, E.N., and Rubins, J.B. (1998) Invasive pneumococcal disease in immunocompromised patients. In *Streptococcus pneumoniae* (ed. A. Tomasz). Larchmont, NY: Mary Ann Liebert, Inc.

Janoff, E.N., Fasching, C., Orenstein, J.M., Rubins, J.B., Opstad, N.L., and Dalmasso, A.P. (1999). Killing of *Streptococcus pneumoniae* by capsular polysaccharide-specific polymeric IgA, complement, and phagocytes. *J. Clin. Invest.* 104, 1139–1147.

Jefferson, T., Rudin, M., and DiPietrantonj, C. (2003). Systematic review of the effects of pertussis vaccines in children. *Vaccine* 21, 2012–2023.

Jones, D.H., McBride, B.W., Thornton, C., O'Hagan, D.T., Robinson, A., and Farrar, G.H. (1996). Orally administered microencapsu-

lated *Bordetella pertussis* fimbriae protect mice from *B. pertussis* respiratory infection. *Infect. Immun.* 64, 489–494.

Karzon, D.T, and Edwards, K.M. (1988). Diphtheria outbreaks in immunized populations. *N. Engl. J. Med.* 318, 41–43.

Kauppi, M., Saarinen, L., and Kayhty, H. (1993). Anti-capsular polysaccharide antibodies reduce nasopharyngeal colonization by *Haemophilus influenzae* type b in infant rats. *J. Infect. Dis.* 167, 365–371.

Kauppi-Korkeila, M., van Alphen, L., Madore, D., Saarinen, L., and Kayhty, H. (1996). Mechanism of antibody-mediated reduction of nasopharyngeal colonization by *Haemophilus influenzae* type b studied in an infant rat model. *J. Infect. Dis.* 174, 1337–1340.

Kilian, M., Mestecky, J., and Russell, M.W. (1988). Defense mechanisms involving Fc-dependent functions of immunoglobulin A and their subversion by bacterial immunoglobulin A proteases. *Microbiol. Rev.* 52, 296–303.

Kimura, A., Mountzouros, K.T., Relman, D.A., Falkow, S., and Cowell, J.L. (1990). *Bordetella pertussis* filamentous hemagglutinin: evaluation as a protective antigen and colonization factor in a mouse respiratory infection model. *Infect. Immun.* 58, 7–16.

Kyd, J.M., Dunkley, M.L., and Cripps, A.W. (1995). Enhanced respiratory clearance of nontypeable *Haemophilus influenzae* following mucosal immunization with P6 in a rat model. *Infect. Immun.* 63, 2931–2940.

Lagos, R., Horwitz, I., Toro, J., San Martin, O., Abrego, P., Bustamante, C., Wasserman, S.S., Levine, O.S., and Levine, M.M. (1996). Large scale, postlicensure, selective vaccination of Chilean infants with PRP-T conjugate vaccine: practicality and effectiveness in preventing invasive *Haemophilus influenzae* type b infections. *Pediatr. Infect. Dis. J.* 15, 216–222.

Leach, A., Ceesay, S.J., Banya, W.A., and Greenwood, B.M. (1996). Pilot trial of a pentavalent pneumococcal polysaccharide/protein conjugate vaccine in Gambian infants. *Pediatr. Infect. Dis. J.* 15, 333–339.

Leininger, E., Roberts, M., Kenimer, J.G., Charles, I.G., Fairweather, N., Novotny, P., and Brennan, M.J. (1991). Pertactin, an Arg-Gly-Asp-containing *Bordetella pertussis* surface protein that promotes adherence of mammalian cells. *Proc. Natl. Acad. Sci. USA* 88, 345–349.

MacGregor, R.R. (1995). *Corynebacterium diphtheriae*. In *Principles and Practice of Infectious Diseases*, 4th ed. (eds. Mandell, G.L., Bennet, J.E., Dolin, R.) New York: Churchill-Livingston, 1865–1872.

MacLeod, C.M., Hodges, R.G., Heidelberger, M., and Bernhard, W.G. (1945). Prevention of pneumococcal pneumonia by immunization with specific capsular polysaccharides. *J. Exp. Med.* 82, 445–465.

Madore, D.V., Johnson, C.L., Phipps, D.C., Popejoy, L.A., Eby, R., and Smith, D.H. (1990). Safety and immunologic response to *Haemophilus influenzae* type b oligosaccharide-CRM$_{197}$ conjugate vaccine in 1- to 6-month-old infants. *Pediatrics* 85, 331–337.

Mahon, B.P., Ryan, M.S., Griffin, F., and Mills, K.H. (1996). Interleukin-12 is produced by macrophages in response to live or killed *Bordetella pertussis* and enhances the efficacy of an acellular pertussis vaccine by promoting induction of Th1 cells. *Infect. Immun.* 64, 5295–5301.

Mariotti, S., Teloni, R., von Hunolstein, C., Romagnoli, G., Orefici, G., and Nisini, R. (2002). Immunogenicity of anti–*Haemophilus influenzae* type b CRM197 conjugate following mucosal vaccination with oligodeoxynucleotide containing immunostimulatory sequences as adjuvant. *Vaccine* 20, 2229–2239.

Martin, F., Oliver, A.M., and Kearney, J.F. (2001). Marginal zone and B1 cells unite in the early response against T-independent blood-borne particulate antigens. *Immunity* 14, 617–629.

Menozzi, F.D., Mutombo, R., Renauld, G., Gantiez, C., Hannah, J.H., Leininger, E., Brennan, M.J., and Locht, C. (1994). Heparin-inhibitable lectin activity of the filamentous hemagglutinin adhesin of *Bordetella pertussis*. *Infect. Immun.* 62, 769–778.

Mills, K.H., Cosgrove, C., McNeela, E.A., Sexton, A., Giemza, R., Jabbal-Gill, I., Church, A., Lin, W., Illum, L., Podda, A., Rappuoli, R., Pizza, M., Griffin, G.E., and Lewis, D.J. (2003). Protective levels of diphtheria-neutralizing antibody induced in healthy volunteers by unilateral priming-boosting intranasal immunization associated with restricted ipsilateral mucosal secretory immunoglobulin a. *Infect. Immun.* 71, 726–732.

Mortimer, E.A., Jr. (1994). Diphtheria toxoid. In *Vaccines*, 2nd ed. (eds. Plotkin, S.A., Mortimer, Jr., E.A.) Philadelphia: WB Saunders, 41–56.

Muhlemann, K., Alexander, E.R., Pepe, M., Weiss, N.S., and Schopfer, K. (1996). Invasive *Haemophilus influenzae* disease and epiglottitis among Swiss children from 1980 to 1993: evidence for herd immunity among older age groups. The Swiss *Haemophilus influenzae* Study Group. *Scand. J. Infect. Dis.* 28, 265–268.

Murphy, T.V., Pastor, P., Medley, F., Osterholm, M.T., and Granoff, D.M. (1993). Decreased *Haemophilus* colonization in children vaccinated with *Haemophilus influenzae* type b conjugate vaccine. *J. Pediatr.* 122, 517–523.

Murray, C.J, and Lopez, A.D. (1997). Mortality by cause for eight regions of the world: Global Burden of Disease Study. *Lancet* 349, 1269–1276.

Musher, D.M., Groover, J.E., Reichler, M.R., Riedo, F.X., Schwartz, B., Watson, D.A., Baughn, R.E., and Breiman, R.F. (1997). Emergence of antibody to capsular polysaccharides of *Streptococcus pneumoniae* during outbreaks of pneumonia: association with nasopharyngeal colonization. *Clin. Infect. Dis.* 24, 441–446.

Musher, D.M., Phan, H.M., and Baughn, R.E. (2001). Protection against bacteremic pneumococcal infection by antibody to pneumolysin. *J. Infect. Dis.* 183, 827–830.

Nennig, M.E., Shinefield, H.R., Edwards, K.M., Black, S.B., and Fireman, B.H. (1996). Prevalence and incidence of adult pertussis in an urban population. *JAMA* 275, 1672–1674.

Örtqvist, A., Hedlund, J., Burman, L.A., Elbel, E., Höfer, M., Leinonen, M., Lindblad, I., Sundelöf, B., and Kalin, M. (1998). Randomised trial of 23-valent pneumococcal capsular polysaccharide vaccine in prevention of pneumonia in middle-aged and elderly people. Swedish Pneumococcal Vaccination Study Group. *Lancet* 351, 399–403.

Osterholm, M.T., Rambeck, J.H., White, K.E., Jacobs, J.L., Pierson, L.M., Neaton, J.D., Hedberg, C.W., MacDonald, K.L., and Granoff, D.M. (1988). Lack of efficacy of *Haemophilus* b polysaccharide vaccine in Minnesota. *JAMA* 260, 1423–1428.

Osterholm, M.T., Jacobs, J.L., and White, K.E. (1990). Efficacy of *Haemophilus influenzae* b plain polysaccharide (PRP) vaccine and conjugate vaccine (PRP-D) in Minnesota. In *Program and Abstracts of the 30th Interscience Conference on Antimicrobial Agents and Chemotherapy* [Atlanta; abstract no. 449A]. Washington, DC: American Society for Microbiology.

Pappenheimer, A.M., Jr. (1980-81). Diphtheria: studies on the biology of an infectious disease. *Harvey Lect.* 76, 45–73.

Patel, S.S, and Wagstaff, A.J. (1996). A cellular pertussis vaccine (Infanrix-DTPa; SB-3). A review of its immunogenicity, protective efficacy and tolerability in the prevention of *Bordetella pertussis* infection. *Drugs* 52, 254–275.

Paton, J.C., Andrew, P.W., Boulnois, G.J., and Mitchell, T.J. (1993). Molecular analysis of the pathogenicity of *Streptococcus pneumoniae*: the role of pneumococcal proteins. *Annu. Rev. Microbiol.* 47, 89–115.

Peltola, H., Kayhty, H., Virtanen, M., and Makela, P.H. (1984). Prevention of *Haemophilus influenzae* type b bacteremic infections with the capsular polysaccharide vaccine. *N. Engl. J. Med.* 310, 1561–1566.

Peltola H. (2000). Worldwide *Haemophilus influenzae* type b disease at the beginning of the 21st century: global analysis of the disease burden 25 years after the use of the polysaccharide vaccine and a decade after the advent of conjugates. *Clin. Microbiol. Rev.* 13, 302–317.

Pelton, S.I., Dagan, R., Gaines, B.M., Klugman, K.P., Laufer, D., O'Brien, K., and Schmitt, H-J. (2003). Pneumococcal conjugate vaccines: proceedings from an Interactive Symposium at the 41st Interscience Conference on Antimicrobial Agents and Chemotherapy. *Vaccine* 21, 1562–1571.

Préziosi, M-P, and Halloran, M.E. (2003). Effects of pertussis vaccination on transmission: vaccine efficacy for infectiousness. *Vaccine* 21, 1853–1861.

Peters, V.B, and Sood, S.K. (1994). Immunity to *Haemophilus influenzae* type b polysaccharide capsule in children with human immunodeficiency virus infection immunized with a single dose of *Haemophilus* vaccine. *J. Pediatr.* 125, 74–77.

Raju, R., Navaneetham, D., Okita, D., Diethelm-Okita, B., McCormick, D., and Conti-Fine, B.M. (1995). Epitopes for human CD4+ cells on diphtheria toxin: structural features of sequence segments forming epitopes recognized by most subjects. *Eur. J. Immunol.* 25, 3207–3214.

Rappuoli, R., Perugini, M, and Falsen, E. (1988). Molecular epidemiology of the 1984–1986 outbreak of diphtheria in Sweden. *N. Engl. J. Med.* 318, 12–14.

Rayner, C.F., Jackson, A.D., Rutman, A., Dewar, A., Mitchell, T.J., Andrew, P.W., Cole, P.J., and Wilson, R. (1995). Interaction of pneumolysin-sufficient and -deficient isogenic variants of *Streptococcus pneumoniae* with human respiratory mucosa. *Infect. Immun.* 63, 442–447.

Relman, D., Tuomanen, E., Falkow, S., Golenbock, D.T., Saukkonen, K., and Wright, S.D. (1990). Recognition of a bacterial adhesion by an integrin: macrophage CR3 (αMβ2,CD11b/CD18) binds filamentous hemagglutinin of *Bordetella pertussis*. *Cell* 61, 1375–1382.

Riley, I.D., Tarr, P.I., Andrews, M., Pfeiffer, M., Howard, R., Challands, P., and Jennison, G. (1977). Immunization with a polyvalent pneumococcal vaccine. Reduction of adult respiratory mortality in a New Guinea Highlands community. *Lancet* 1, 1338–41.

Robbins, J.B., Schneerson, R., Anderson, P., and Smith, D.H. (1996). The 1996 Albert Lasker Medical Research Awards. Prevention of systemic infections, especially meningitis, caused by *Haemophilus influenzae* type b. Impact on public health and implications for other polysaccharide-based vaccines. *JAMA* 276, 1181–1185.

Rubins, J.B., Duane, P.G., Clawson, D., Charboneau, D., Young, J., and Niewoehner, D.E. (1993). Toxicity of pneumolysin to pulmonary alveolar epithelial cells. *Infect. Immun.* 61, 1352–1358.

Rubins, J.B, and Janoff, E.N. (1998). Pneumolysin: a multifunctional pneumococcal virulence factor. *J. Lab. Clin. Med.* 131, 21–27.

Sabirov, A., Kodama, S., Hirano, T., Suzuki, M., and Mogi, G. (2001). Intranasal immunization enhances clearance of nontypeable *Haemophilus influenzae* and reduces stimulation of tumor necrosis factor alpha production in the murine model of otitis media. *Infect. Immun.* 69, 2964–2971.

Santosham, M., Wolff, M., Reid, R., Hohenboken, M., Bateman, M., Goepp, J., Cortese, M., Sack, D., Hill, J., and Newcomer, W., et al. (1991). The efficacy in Navajo infants of a conjugate vaccine consisting of *Haemophilus influenzae* type b polysaccharide and *Neisseria meningitidis* outer-membrane protein complex. *N. Engl. J. Med.* 324, 1767–1772.

Saukkonen, K., Cabellos, C., Burroughs, M., Prasad, S., and Tuomanen, E. (1991). Integrin-mediated localization of *Bordetella pertussis* within macrophages: role in pulmonary colonization. *J. Exp. Med.* 173, 1143–1149.

Schlesinger, Y, and Granoff, D.M., (1992). Avidity and bactericidal activity of antibody elicited by different *Haemophilus influenzae* type b conjugate vaccines. The Vaccine Study Group. *JAMA* 267, 1489–1494.

Schmitt, H.J., von Konig, C.H., Neiss, A., Bogaerts, H., Bock, H.L., Schulte-Wissermann, H., Gahr, M., Schult, R., Folkens, J.U., Rauh, W., and Clemens, R. (1996). Efficacy of acellular pertussis vaccine in early childhood after household exposure. *JAMA* 275, 37–41.

Shahin, R., Leef, M., Eldridge, J., Hudson, M., and Gilley, R. (1995). Adjuvanticity and protective immunity elicited by *Bordetella pertussis* antigens encapsulated in poly (DL-lactide-co-glycolide) microspheres. *Infect. Immun.* 63, 1195–2000.

Shahin, R.D., Amsbaugh, D.F., and Leef, M.F. (1992). Mucosal immunization with filamentous hemagglutinin protects against *Bordetella pertussis* respiratory infection. *Infect. Immun.* 60, 1482–1488.

Shapiro, E.D, and Wald, E.R. (1990). Protective efficacy of PRP-D conjugate vaccine against *Haemophilus influenzae* type b. In *Program and Abstracts of the 30th Interscience Conference on Antimicrobial Agents and Chemotherapy* [Atlanta; abstract no. 604]. Washington, DC: American Society for Microbiology.

Shapiro, E.D, and Ward, J.I. (1991). The epidemiology and prevention of disease caused by *Haemophilus influenzae* type b. *Epidemiol. Rev.* 13, 113–142.

Shelly, M.A., Jacoby, H., Riley, G.J., Graves, B.T., Pichichero, M., and Treanor, J.J. (1997). Comparison of pneumococcal polysaccharide and CRM$_{197}$-conjugated pneumococcal oligosaccharide vaccines in young and elderly adults. *Infect. Immun.* 65, 242–247.

Silverstein, A.M. (1989). *History of Immunology*. San Diego: Academic Press.

Singleton, R., Bulkow, L.R., Levine, O.S., Butler, J.C., Hennessy, T.W., and Parkinson, A. (2000). Experience with the prevention of invasive *Haemophilus influenzae* type b disease by vaccination in Alaska: the impact of persistent oropharyngeal carriage. *J. Pediatr.* 137, 313–320.

St. Geme, J.W., 3rd, and Falkow, S. (1990). *Haemophilus influenzae* adheres to and enters cultured human epithelial cells. *Infect. Immun.* 58, 4036–4044.

St. Geme, J.W., 3rd. (1996). Molecular determinants of the interaction between *Haemophilus influenzae* and human cells. *Am. J. Respir. Crit. Care Med.* 154, S192–S196.

Takala, A.K., Eskola, J., Leinonen, M., Kayhty, H., Nissinen, A., Pekkanen, E., and Makela, P.H. (1991). Reduction of oropharyngeal carriage of *Haemophilus influenzae* type b (Hib) in children immunized with an Hib conjugate vaccine. *J. Infect. Dis.* 164, 982–986.

Takala, A.K., Santosham, M., Almeido-Hill, J., Wolff, M., Newcomer, W., Reid, R., Kayhty, H., Esko, E., and Makela, P.H. (1993). Vaccination with *Haemophilus influenzae* type b meningococcal protein conjugate vaccine reduces oropharyngeal carriage of *Haemophilus influenzae* type b among American Indian children. *Pediatr. Infect. Dis. J.* 12, 593–599.

Talbot, U.M., Paton, A.W., and Paton, J.C. (1996). Uptake of *Streptococcus pneumoniae* by respiratory epithelial cells. *Infect. Immun.* 64, 3772–3777.

Trollfors, B., Taranger, J., Lagergard, T., Lind, L., Sundh, V., Zackrisson, G., Lowe, C.U., Blackwelder, W., and Robbins, J.B. (1995). A placebo-controlled trial of a pertussis-toxoid vaccine. *N. Engl. J. Med.* 333, 1045–1050.

Tuomanen, E.I., Austrian, R., and Masure, H.R. (1995). Pathogenesis of pneumococcal infection. *N. Engl. J. Med.* 332, 1280–1284.

van Alphen, L., Eijk, P., Kayhty, H., van Marle, J., and Dankert, J. (1996). Antibodies to *Haemophilus influenzae* type b polysaccharide affect bacterial adherence and multiplication. *Infect. Immun.* 64, 995–1001.

van der Flier, M., Chhun, N., Wizemann, T.M., Min, J., McCarthy, J.B., and Tuomanen, E.I. (1995). Adherence of *Streptococcus pneumoniae* to immobilized fibronectin. *Infect. Immun.* 63, 4317–4322.

van Schilfgaarde, M., van Ulsen, P., Eijk, P., Brand, M., Stam, M., Kouame, J., van Alphen, L., and Dankert, J. (2000). Characterization of adherence of nontypeable *Haemophilis influenzae* to human epithelial cells. *Infect. Immun.* 68, 4658–4665.

Ward, J., Brenneman, G., Letson, G.W., and Heyward, W.L. (1990). Limited efficacy of a *Haemophilus influenzae* type b conjugate vaccine in Alaska Native infants. The Alaska *H. Influenzae* Vaccine Study Group. *N. Engl. J. Med.* 323, 1393–1401.

Weiser, J.N. (1993). Relationship between colony morphology and the life cycle of *Haemophilus influenzae*: the contribution of lipopolysaccharide phase variation to pathogenesis. *J. Infect. Dis.* 168, 672–680.

Weiser, J.N. (1998). Phase variation in colony opacity by *Streptococcus pneumoniae*. *Microb. Drug. Resist.* 4, 129–135.

Weiser, J.N., Bae, D., Fasching, C., Scamurra, R.W., Ratner, A.J., and Janoff, E.N. (2003) Antibody-enhanced pneumococcal adherence requires IgA1 protease. *Proc. Natl. Acad. Sci. USA* 100, 4215–4220.

Wenger, J.D., Plikaytis B., and Pierce, R. Protective efficacy of *Haemophilus influenzae* type b (Hib) conjugate (CNJ) and polysaccharide (PRP) vaccines in children 18 months and older. (1990) In *Program and Abstracts of the 30th Interscience Conference on Antimicrobial Agents and Chemotherapy* [Atlanta; abstract no. 607]. Washington, DC: American Society for Microbiology.

Whitney, C.G., Farley, M.M., Hadler, J., Harrison, L.H., Bennett, N.M., Lynfield, R., Reingold, A., Cieslak, P.R., Pilishvili, T., Jackson, D., Facklam, R.R., Jorgensen, J.H., and Schuchat, A., for Active Bacterial Core Surveillance of the Emerging Infections Program Network. (2003). Decline in invasive pneumococcal disease after the introduction of protein-polysaccharide conjugate vaccine. *N. Engl. J. Med.* 348, 1737–1746.

Willett, H.P. (1992) *Corynebacterium*. In *Zinsser Microbiology*, 20th ed. (eds. Joklik, W.H., Willett, H.P., Amos, D.B., Wilfert, C.M.). East Norwalk, CT: Appleton and Lange, 487–496.

Wu, Z.Q., Vos, Q., Shen, Y., Lees, A., Wilson, S.R., Briles, D.E., Gause, W.C., Mond, J.J., and Snapper, C.M. (1999). *In vivo* polysaccharide-specific IgG isotype responses to intact *Streptococcus pneumoniae* are T cell dependent and require CD40- and B7-ligand interactions. *J. Immunol.* 163, 659–667.

Wu, Z.Q., Khan, A.Q., Shen, Y., Schartman, J., Peach, R., Lees, A., Mond, J.J., Gause, W.C., and Snapper, C.M. (2000). B7 requirements for primary and secondary protein- and polysaccharide-specific Ig isotype responses to *Streptococcus pneumoniae*. *J. Immunol.* 165, 6840–6848.

Yamaizumi, M., Mekada, E., Uchida, T., and Okada, Y. (1978). One molecule of diphtheria toxin fragment A. introduced into a cell can kill the cell. *Cell* 15, 245–250.

Yuk, M.H., Cotter, P.A., Miller, J.F. (1996). Genetic regulation of airway colonization by *Bordetella* species. *Am. J. Respir. Crit. Care Med.* 154, S150–S154.

Zepp, F., Knuf, M., Habermehl, P., Schmitt, J.H., Rebsch, C., Schidtke, P., Clemens, R., and Slaoui, M. (1996). Pertussis-specific cell-mediated immunity in infants after vaccination with a tricomponent acellular pertussis vaccine. *Infect. Immun.* 64, 4078–4084.

Respiratory Viral Vaccines

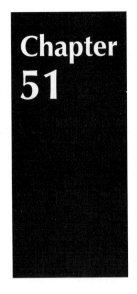

D. Scott Schmid

Viral Immunology Section, Centers for Disease Control and Prevention, Atlanta, Georgia

Barry T. Rouse

Department of Microbiology, The University of Tennessee at Knoxville, Knoxville, Tennessee

The respiratory mucosa is vulnerable to invasion by a number of important human pathogens, including a variety of viruses. Proficient mucosal, antigen-specific immune responses are essential to prevent the disruption of critical functions that may be substantially impaired in the course of respiratory virus infection. Unfortunately, the most severe respiratory complications tend to occur on first exposure in very young children and among the elderly in whom immunocompetence has begun to erode. As such, vaccines that effectively target those populations are needed to provide protection where it is most urgently needed. Passive transfer of specific immunoglobulin is generally not protective against respiratory virus infections. Only two vaccines for respiratory viruses, influenza and adenovirus, have been licensed for use; neither vaccine is highly effective and neither is recommended for use in children less than 2 years of age. The difficulty in designing beneficial mucosal vaccines is compounded by the fact that the mucosal immune system appears to be prone to polarizing toward either T helper (Th) type 1 (Th1) or Th2 dominance, the latter of which can actually lead to immune-mediated airway obstructive disease. A more complete understanding of the mechanisms underlying this polarization could well lead to superior strategies for priming the mucosal immune system against respiratory pathogens. The importance for doing so is manifest, since these viral agents are a leading cause of morbidity among adults and of mortality among the very young and the elderly. Notably, more persons in the 20th century perished in the 1918 influenza pandemic than perished in both world wars.

What follows is a summary of the salient features of the pathogenesis of respiratory viruses responsible for the greatest public health impact, together with current and anticipated progress in vaccine development, including the use of adjuvants and other biological modifiers to enhance vaccine performance. The pathogens causing the largest burden of respiratory disease in humans include influenza (flu) virus, respiratory syncytial virus (RSV), parainfluenza viruses (PIVs), rhinoviruses, coronaviruses, and adenoviruses.

INFLUENZA VIRUS

Viral pathogenesis

Influenza is a single-stranded negative-sense RNA virus belonging to the Orthomyxovirus family and is classified as influenza viruses A, B, and C. The influenza virus genome is divided into seven (influenza C) or eight (influenza A and B) segments that encode a variable number of gene products. All influenza viruses share the property of binding to mucus (to sialic acid–bearing cell surface receptors), and the three types are distinguished on the basis of antigenic differences in the nucleocapsid and matrix proteins (Wright and Webster, 1996). Influenza A viruses are most commonly responsible for severe respiratory illness in humans, followed by influenza B. Influenza C is only rarely responsible for lower respiratory disease in humans. Influenza A viruses are distinguished by their rapid antigen variation, which is accomplished through two mechanisms, antigenic shift and antigenic drift. Antigenic shift results from recombination in the hemagglutinin (HA) and neuraminidase (NA) genes between parent strains, a process believed to involve intermediate animal hosts, particularly migratory waterfowl and pigs. Fifteen HA and nine NA subtypes have been identified. Antigenic drift results from continuous mutational changes in the HA and NA proteins. Shift variants emerge constantly against which previously induced antibodies have reduced avidity, and these are responsible for annual epidemics of influenza. The periodic emergence of shift variants, for which large numbers of people in the population have no history of exposure, can lead to influenza pandemics. Both types of variation pose considerable problems for influenza vaccination strategy and currently make annual vaccination with updated vaccine formulations essential for the control of influenza disease.

Influenza viruses replicate rapidly, are highly infectious, and spread principally by aerosol. Influenza is an infection of primarily the upper respiratory tract. During the course of infection the virus spreads to the lower respiratory tract, where it can cause viral pneumonia or enhance susceptibility to bacterial infections. Virus replication peaks within 48 hours after exposure and then slowly declines for approximately 1 week (Wright and Webster, 2001). Upon recovery, the patient is permanently immune to reinfection to the identical strain but may be fully susceptible to shift variants. Protection from symptomatic infection with drift variants usually persists for several years (Frank et al., 1987).

Influenza infection is a major cause of morbidity and mortality in most areas of the world, resulting in at least 20,000 deaths and 114,000 hospitalizations annually in the United States (Centers for Disease Control and Prevention [CDC], 2000). Infections occur most frequently in children and adults, but the elderly are regarded as the highest risk group for life-threatening disease (Webster, 2000). Very young children and persons of all ages with chronic lung disorders are also at high risk for serious complications and death from influenza infection (Betts and Treanor, 2000).

The relative importance of innate, humoral, cellular, and mucosal immunity for the control of and protection from influenza virus infection remains poorly understood. High levels of proinflammatory cytokines such as IL-6 and interferon (IFN)-α are induced by influenza infection, usually peaking by day 2 (Hayden et al., 1998; Kaiser et al., 2001). These cytokines are believed to play a direct role in impairing viral infection and in driving the immune response toward a CD4$^+$Th1 cytokine pattern. A transient infiltration of natural killer (NK) cells has also been observed during influenza infection and has been suggested as an important early defense mechanism (Skoner et al., 1996). Neutrophils also play an important role in clearance of virus from the lung. Mice irradiated to reduce the number of peripheral polymorphonuclear leukocytes have increased viral titers after influenza infection of the lung (Wright and Webster, 2001). In addition, deficiency in the C3 component of complement, which has well-described opsonin activities, also results in impaired ability to clear influenza (Wright and Webster, 2001). However, enthusiasm for nonspecific defenses must be tempered by the observation that they function poorly against shift variants, particularly in the populations at greatest risk. Thus, innate defenses would seem inadequate alone to prevent and control influenza infections. Moreover, influenza virus directly impairs neutrophil function, which appears to be responsible for a reduced capacity to clear bacterial infections in complicating pneumonias (Ruben and Cate, 1987; LeVine et al., 2001)

The presence of antibodies specific for HA and NA are an absolute requirement for prevention of influenza infection (Webster, 2000). Mucosal IgA antibody in nasal and bronchial secretions appears particularly effective for the neutralization of influenza virus and may also play an important role in viral clearance (Tamura et al., 1998). Humoral IgG antibodies to HA and NA are also produced in response to influenza, and these enhance resistance to influenza virus infection in both humans and animal models (Wright and Webster, 2001).

Neutralizing antibodies against influenza are directed to the surface glycoproteins HA and NA and thus against the specific influenza subtype (i.e., they are homosubtypic). T cell responses, in contrast, are predominantly directed to epitopes on invariant proteins such as NP and matrix protein and are thus influenza type–specific (heterosubtypic). The results of studies comparing mucosal and systemic immunization suggest that the former induces an effective memory response, while the latter does not (Gorse and Belshe, 1990; Clover et al., 1991; Brühl et al., 2001).

The role of T cells in prevention of influenza infection, especially in humans, is not well defined. However, since CD8$^+$T cell responses are directed mainly against the shared proteins among A strains, protection would be expected to be highly cross-reactive. In fact, in humans, cross-protection occurs only among drift variants and is more effective when levels of cross-reactivity detected by antibodies are high (Wright and Webster, 2001). The relevance of cross-reactive CD8$^+$ T cell immunity to influenza has been studied in mice in circumstances where antibody-mediated cross-reactivity to HA or NA epitopes is avoided. In such studies, effective cross-protection occurs for a month or so and appears to principally involve "effector memory" CD8$^+$ cytotoxic T lymphocytes (CTLs) present in alveolar spaces and interstitial tissues of the respiratory tract (Woodland, 2003; Hogan et al., 2001). Although similar cells may be present in the draining lymphoid tissues, these cells seem not to participate in the protective response. After a few months post–primary infection, the mucosal effector memory CD8$^+$ T cells have largely disappeared and no longer participate directly in immunity to reinfection. In these circumstances, if they lack cross-reactive antibody, the CD8$^+$ T cell–primed animals become susceptible to clinical disease upon challenge, although the syndrome may be shorter and of milder severity than occurs in challenged naïve animals (Woodland, 2003). Accordingly, CD8$^+$ T cells would seem to play at best a minor role in effecting resistance to secondary infection, except in the immediate post–primary infection period.

Less is known about the function of CD4$^+$ T cells in mediating protection against reinfection. However, it is also believed that CD4$^+$ T cells (in mice at least) play little or no role in mediating protection to secondary infection. Nevertheless, the CD4$^+$ T cell response is required for optimal antibody responses to influenza proteins and may also be needed for robust CD8$^+$ T cell responses (Epstein et al., 1998).

The function of T cells in immunity is mainly required to effect recovery from infection. In primary infections, this is chiefly a function of CD8$^+$ T cells and may largely involve both cytotoxicity and cytokine production (Cerwenka et al., 1999; Sarawar et al., 1994). In the mouse, the CD8$^+$ T cell response becomes evident around 7 days after primary infection and peaks at day 10, a time that corresponds with viral clearance (Eichelberger *et al.*, 1991; Flynn *et al.*, 1998; Riberdy *et al.*, 2000). The induction of CD8+ T cell responses occurs both in the nasal associated lymphoreticular tissue (NALT) and in draining lymph nodes. However, the effector CD8+ T cells responsible for viral clearance from the lung likely derive largely from the mucosal lymphoid site.

The crucial outcome of primary infection is the establishment of immunological memory. In the mouse, T cell memory cells are found in both nonlymphoid and lymphoid sites. The memory in nonlymphoid sites, which includes the respiratory tract itself, is of shorter duration than lymphoid memory (Hogan *et al.*, 2002). Recall from both sites takes at least 4–5 days, a circumstance explaining why T cells are not readily available to contain infection in the early stages of infection. However, once the T cells are recruited and activated into effectors, both CD8+ and CD4+ T cells participate in viral clearance (Doherty *et al.*, 1992). CD4+ T cells function by producing type 1 cytokines, particularly IFN-γ.

The recent understanding of immunity to murine influenza may have implications with regard to vaccine design. Thus, it would seem that mucosal memory is an important goal for vaccines against influenza. Moreover, it is suspected that different types of vaccines may variably stimulate long-term mucosal and systemic memory. The immune response to influenza is thus complex, and crafting effective vaccination strategies requires accounting for a variety of factors, including route of inoculation, vaccine composition and type, and strain variation.

Vaccine development

The inactivated influenza vaccine in current use in the United States comprises three split influenza strains; these strains are selected on the basis of the previous year's surveillance data on the most prevalent subtypes, and vaccine composition may vary from year to year, particularly the influenza A component. In contrast to natural infection, intramuscular inoculation of inactivated trivalent influenza vaccine induces the production of serum antibodies but is not effective at inducing mucosal or cell-mediated immune responses. Some influenza-specific systemic antibody transudates to the lung and is credited with this vaccine formulation's observed reduction of severe lower respiratory tract disease. Nonetheless, the immunity elicited by inactivated, parenterally administered vaccine is strain-specific and of short duration, making annual revaccination necessary. In addition, the protection rate varies by age group and is especially low in the populations most susceptible to disease complications and death: the elderly, infants, and persons with chronic pulmonary conditions (Wright and Webster, 2001). The basis for the reduced efficacy of vaccine in the elderly is not well understood; studies have variously implicated heterogeneity in the response to the component strains and in the type of adaptive immune response that is generated (Webster, 2000; Remarque, 1999; Treanor and Falsey, 1999; Bernstein *et al.*, 1999).

Since respiratory infection by influenza induces both humoral and mucosal antibody as well as cross-reactive cell-mediated immunity (CMI), it is widely believed, although not proven, that vaccine efficacy will be improved through nasal administration. A number of nasal vaccine strategies are under investigation, including the use of live attenuated strains (Bradshaw and Wright, 2002; Belshe, 1999; Gruber *et al.*, 1996; Murphy, 1993); recombinant (Berglund *et al.*, 1999; Ferko *et al.*, 1998; Watanabe *et al.*, 2002), virosomal (Cusi *et al.*, 2000), DNA (Ljungberg *et al.*, 2002; Ban *et al.*, 1997), peptide (Matsuki *et al.*, 1999; Yedidia *et al.*, 1998; Jeon and Arnon, 2002), and purified subunit vaccines (Barchfield *et al.*, 1999; Asanuma *et al.*, 2001; Saurwein-Teissl *et al.*, 1998); and immune-stimulating complexes (ISCOMs) (Sjölander *et al.*, 2001; Sjölander *et al.*, 1997).

Nasally administered, live, attenuated, cold-adapted, trivalent influenza-virus vaccine (ca vaccine) may represent a convenient and effective approach to the prevention of influenza in children. The segmented genome characteristic of influenza facilitates reassortment between two strains dually infecting individual cells. By exploiting this phenomenon, the vaccine antigens can be updated annually, substituting genes encoding the HA and NA antigens from contemporary influenza A and B viruses for those present in established master attenuated strains (Bradshaw and Wright, 2002). Ca vaccine will be administered with a spray device that delivers an aerosol of large particles to the upper respiratory tract.

The vaccine has been extensively field-tested in subjects ranging from 6 months to 65 years of age and is well tolerated, immunogenic, and protective, particularly in young children (Belshe *et al.*, 1998; Belshe *et al.*, 2000; Edwards *et al.*, 1994; Treanor *et al.*, 2000; Boyce *et al.*, 2000; Gruber *et al.*, 1996; Murphy, 1993). In one field trial of seronegative children, the individual viruses present in the vaccine induced fourfold or greater increases in titer in 61% to 96% of recipients (Belshe *et al.*, 1998). A clinical trial involving 4000 participants of all ages revealed that, while the inactivated vaccine induced higher levels of serum antibody than the live vaccine, the latter induced much higher levels of mucosal immunity (Edwards *et al.*, 1994). The vaccine has been shown to induce strain-specific mucosal IgA in the majority of children after two doses (Boyce *et al.*, 2000). In a challenge study of 103 adult volunteers, the protective efficacy of ca vaccine was estimated at 85%, compared with 71% for the currently available inactivated vaccine (Treanor *et al.*, 2000). In a separate study of children aged 1 to 6, the vaccine was determined to be 92% effective at preventing culture-confirmed influenza A and B infection (Belshe *et al.*, 2000). One early study of influenza vaccine in children suggests that risk for acquiring influenza infections in all age groups could be reduced substantially if community-wide coverage levels of 70% were achieved in young children (Monto and Kioumehr, 1975). This is considered an achievable goal with ca vaccine, in large part because the nasal route of administration is more readily accepted than subcutaneous or intramuscular injection, particularly for children.

Ca vaccine has been associated with some side effects, generally mild. Recipients have been found to be at slightly elevated risk for rhinorrhea and low-grade fever (Belshe et al., 1998). Elevated fever is also observed in a comparable fraction of inactivated influenza vaccine recipients, and ca vaccine has not been associated with Guillain-Barré syndrome, which is observed at very low incidence in inactivated-vaccine recipients (Lasky et al., 1998).

While the live, attenuated vaccine appears to be less efficacious in the elderly, one study suggested that conventional inactivated trivalent vaccine given in combination with nasal ca vaccine may enhance protection in elderly recipients (Treanor and Betts, 1998). The live, attenuated intranasal vaccine was licensed for use in late 2003. However, the Advisory Committee on Immunization Practices has recommended its use only in persons between the ages of 5 and 49. Thus, the vaccine is not yet available for the age groups at highest risk for life-threatening disease (Harper et al., 2004).

A nasal virosomal vaccine consisting of purified HA and NA encapsulated in lecithin has also been evaluated in clinical trials in Europe. Study populations included children (6–12 years old), adults, and the elderly (>60 years old); the vaccine induced both influenza-specific systemic IgG and mucosal IgA and was estimated to be 85% efficacious in all adults and had 89% efficacy in children. The highest immunogenicity was seen when the vaccine was coadministered with the adjuvant LT (heat-labile toxin of *Escherichia coli*) (Cusi et al., 2000). Unfortunately, this vaccine was associated with an increased incidence of Bell's Palsy or facial paralysis, and it has been taken off the market. The Semliki Forest virus (SFV) recombinant vaccines expressing HA and NA have been shown to induce protective, strain-specific secretory IgA (S-IgA) antibody responses in mice, and SFV recombinant vaccine expressing influenza NP elicited antigen-specific CTLs that protected mice from infectious challenge (Berglund et al., 1999). ISCOMs, including influenza HA and NA, administered nasally induced protective immunity in mice, with measurable antigen-specific mucosal and systemic antibody and CMI (T helper and cytotoxic activity) (Sjölander et al., 1997). Both the cytokine profile and localization of the T cell response induced by ISCOMs was shown in a separate study to depend upon the type of adjuvant used (Sjölander et al., 2001).

It has been suggested that plasmid DNA vaccines have an advantage over recombinant viral vectors such as SFV because no immune response is generated against the vector itself. As such, it should be possible to revaccinate indefinitely without a reduction in the expression of the target proteins. A nasal plasmid DNA vaccine expressing influenza HA has been evaluated in mice but, disappointingly, failed to elicit detectable antibody in the respiratory tract (Ban et al., 1997). A similar vaccine given parenterally was able to induce a CMI response (Ljungberg et al., 2002). However, DNA vaccines in general are more effective in mice than in humans. In fact, one must conclude that currently there is little enthusiasm for a DNA vaccine against human influenza.

Other strategies are also under investigation for vaccination against influenza. For example, there is interest in exploiting the common mucosal immune system to induce respiratory immunity by delivering vaccines at other mucosal sites. Trials with an oral vaccine thought to engage the intestinal Peyer's patches by means of particle formations of inert microspheres containing protein antigens represent one such approach under investigation (Clancy et al., 1995). Another approach that is under study is the use of epidermal powder immunization, in which trivalent split vaccine is administered to mice with a compressed-air injector. An initial study demonstrated both systemic and mucosal antibody, as well as enhanced protection from infectious challenge (Chen et al., 2001). Coadministration of almost every candidate vaccine with various antigens is also being actively explored, as is the tactic of using both intranasal and parenteral vaccine to induce maximal immunity.

Given the intensive level of activity in this field, it seems very likely that new alternatives to the currently used vaccine will be available within a relatively short period.

RESPIRATORY SYNCYTIAL VIRUS

Viral pathogenesis

Respiratory syncytial virus (RSV) is the most important cause of serious lower respiratory tract illness among infants and children in the United States, particularly before the age of 2 years. In the United States alone, RSV infections account for between 85,000 and 144,000 hospitalizations and thousands of deaths each year, and health care costs have been estimated at several million dollars annually (Shay et al., 1999; Institute of Medicine, 1985). Together with parainfluenza virus 3, these two viruses are responsible for nearly one-third of all cases of respiratory tract disease necessitating hospitalization of children. Most hospitalizations resulting from RSV infection are of newborn infants with no prior exposure to RSV and, in general, hospitalized infants carry no recognized risk factors for severe disease in comparison with other infants of the same age. In developed countries throughout the world, RSV is the leading cause of morbidity and mortality among infants and young children (Crowe et al., 1997). Respiratory virus infections are estimated to cause about 4 million deaths each year in children less than 5 years of age, and RSV is the leading contributor to those deaths. RSV is also a significant cause of severe respiratory tract illness in elderly and immunocompromised persons (Nicholson et al., 1997; Walsh et al., 1999). Infants born prematurely and persons with underlying heart or lung disease (notably, bronchopulmonary dysplasia) are at heightened risk for developing severe RSV disease (Hall et al., 1986; MacDonald et al., 1982; Groothius et al., 1988). RSV disease displays seasonality, with most community outbreaks occurring during the winter months. There is currently no effective treatment for RSV disease, although prophylactic administration of RSV antibody is approved for high-risk infants and appears to offer protection against severe disease.

RSV (as with most other respiratory viruses) has been implicated as a predisposing factor for the development of otitis media, leading to speculation that an effective vaccine could also reduce the morbidity associated with that disease (Anderson, 2001). RSV spreads very efficiently among infants and young children; most have primary infection by age 2 years.

RSV is a nonsegmented negative-strand RNA virus, a member of Paramyxoviridae. The virus codes for 11 proteins, including three transmembrane surface proteins (G, F, and SH), the virion matrix protein (M), the nucleocapsid and polymerase proteins (N, P, M2-1, and L), the putative transcription-replication regulatory factor (M2-2), and two nonstructural proteins (NS1 and NS2). The genome consists of 15,222 nucleotides. Two antigenically distinct subgroups of RSV have been characterized on the basis of both antigenic and sequence variability: RSV A and RSV B. Subgroup A has been most frequently isolated in community outbreaks and appears to be associated more frequently with severe disease. The attachment glycoprotein (G) contains most of the observed variability between subgroups. Strains of RSV within a subgroup display a high level of antigenic similarity, but the antigenic diversity between subgroup A and B strains can be as high as 95% for G and as high as 50% for the fusion protein (F) (Collins et al., 2001).

RSV establishes infection in the upper respiratory tract, replicating initially in the nasopharynx. Symptoms manifest after 4 to 5 days. If virus spreads to the lower tract, which often happens in the most susceptible 2- to 7-month-old age group, severe bronchiolitis and pneumonia develop within 1–2 days. Symptoms persist for 2–3 weeks, with continual viral shedding. Except in immunocompromised individuals, virus rarely spreads beyond the superficial epithelium. Lung lesions in severe disease are likely a consequence of direct virus-induced tissue damage along with an immunopathological reaction (Collins et al., 2001).

Animal models have played an important role in acquiring information about the pathogenesis of RSV (Brandenburg et al., 2001). The mouse model has been especially useful, permitting robust studies, for example, aimed at defining the underlying mechanisms responsible for the failure of formalin-inactivated RSV vaccine. Other animals, such as the cotton rat and nonhuman primates such as the African green monkey, bonnet monkey, and chimpanzee have also provided useful insights into RSV disease. Such models, as for all infectious agents, have serious limitations, however. Mice, for instance, are not fully permissive for RSV infection, and challenge doses do not cause death. Cotton rats are more susceptible to infection, but the range of immunological reagents available for mouse studies is not available for the rat, and the high body temperature of this animal complicates the assessment of the attenuation of temperature-sensitive strains developed as vaccine candidates. Nonhuman primate models have permitted essential preclinical studies of vaccine tolerance and virulence, but these animals are still less permissive than humans for RSV infection. As such, the critical assessments of candidate RSV vaccines will need to be performed in human subjects and ultimately will involve assess-

ment in the youngest, most vulnerable population, to whom an RSV vaccine will need to be targeted.

The immunological response to RSV is complex and dependent on multiple factors, including the age of the patient, level of immunological maturity, and presence of maternal, passively transferred antibodies. The antigenic diversity of RSV allows both subgroups to circulate in a community at the same time. While exposure to an RSV of one subgroup confers short-lived resistance to disease by subsequent infection with the alternative subgroup, protection against the homotypic subgroup is superior. Since antibodies to G and F are considered to be principally responsible for resistance to reinfection, and since the intertypic variation is greatest in these same proteins, there is the possibility that a bivalent RSV vaccine will be required to achieve optimal effectiveness.

The humoral response to RSV is directed almost exclusively against the F and G surface glycoproteins, and these proteins are the major neutralization targets for mucosal and serum antibody. While several components of the immune system have been implicated in the control and resolution of RSV infection, the increased resistance to reinfection observed in persons previously infected seems to be mediated primarily by RSV-specific secretory and serum antibodies (Mills et al., 1971; Prince et al., 1985). Serum IgG antibodies protect the lower but not the upper respiratory tract; the role of protecting the latter is largely the province of S-IgA antibodies. Although antibodies confer protection against severe disease, the protection is incomplete, and multiple reinfection, even by the same strain, can take place despite high circulating titers of neutralizing antibody. A recent study of antibodies cloned from natural responses to RSV revealed that the virus engineers an evasive tactic by presenting the F antigen in multiple forms during an immune response, skewing the antibody response toward the production of nonneutralizing antibodies (Sakurai et al., 1999). The study also revealed that the neutralizing power of an antibody was more important than its isotype, showing in a mouse model that an IgG monoclonal antibody (mAb) with high neutralizing titer was more protective than an IgA antibody with lower neutralizing titer.

RSV-specific CMI can lead to both advantageous and immunopathologic endpoints during acute infection. Resolving acute infection appears to require the presence of CTLs, the peak activation levels of which coincide with virus clearance (Collins et al., 2001). The period of RSV shedding is prolonged in animals or patients that lack functional T cells (Cannon et al., 1987; Bangham et al., 1986). CD8+ CTLs are present in the circulation of persons who have had a known primary exposure, and both CD4+ and CD8+ T cells can eliminate RSV from infected animals. While CTLs play an important role in viral clearance, they are not believed to contribute substantially to the prevention of reinfection, largely because the response is very short-lived.

There are two curious aspects of immunity to RSV. First, natural infection fails to result in resistance to reinfection. In fact, repeated infections can occur throughout life (Hall et al.,

1991). Second, pulmonary disease following infection appears to result mainly from a host immune inflammatory response (Varga and Braciale, 2002). This situation was exaggerated following the use of a formalin-inactivated vaccine in children. Many vaccine recipients developed severe disease, several of which were lethal following natural infection with RSV (Kapikian et al., 1969). The explanation for the ineffective and untoward immune response to RSV remains obscure. Thus, infection induces neutralizing antibody production as well as CD4+ and CD8+ T-cell responses to peptides from most viral proteins. For unknown reasons, infection can occur in the presence of neutralizing antibody and T-cell immunity. The latter form of immunity, however, is of brief duration, especially in the respiratory tract (Varga and Braciale, 2002). Solutions to these immune mysteries are likely to emerge from ongoing studies in animal model systems.

As mentioned previously, several animal models are available to study RSV immunopathology, none of which is ideal. Most recent progress has come from studies in the BALB/c mouse strain. In such animals, it is possible to simulate vaccine-induced pulmonary disease. For example, if RSV G protein–specific Th2 CD4+ T cells are transferred into mice that were subsequently RSV-infected, then a pulmonary disease reminiscent of that in vaccinated children occurred (Alwan et al., 1994). Other approaches have since confirmed that memory CD4+ T cell responses to the G protein are responsible for pulmonary immunopathology. Surprisingly, in BALB/c mice a single peptide of the G protein is the recognized epitope, and the memory T cells involved are highly oligoclonal (Varga et al., 2000). The cells that recognize the peptide can be of either Th1 or Th2 effector phenotype, but the Th2 cells, although the minor population, are responsible for lesions (Varga et al., 2000).

CD8+ T cells also play a role in immunopathology since they serve to influence the phenotype of the G protein–specific CD4+ T cells involved. Thus, in the adoptive transfer model described previously, the cotransfer of M2 protein–specific CD8+ T cells along with G-specific CD4+ T cells resulted in diminished pathology (Alwan et al., 1994). Moreover, incorporation of the M2 MHC class I–restricted epitope into G protein constructs used to prime for injury-provoking memory CD4+ T cells reduced pulmonary disease expression (Srikiatkhachorn and Braciale, 1997). Thus the CD8+ T-cell response is protective, a lesson for future vaccine design. Unfortunately, the environment of the lung, or perhaps exposure to one or more RSV proteins, appears to impair the function of CD8+ T cells. In addition, such cells persist only briefly in the lungs. Residence of CD8+ T cells in the lung impairs their antigen-induced cytokine production, compromising their protective efficacy (Chang and Braciale, 2002). The exact mechanism of CD8+ T cell functional damage is not understood, but its mechanistic resolution could lead to the design of effective vaccines against RSV.

In recent years, evidence has mounted that both infectious RSV and individual RSV proteins are capable of modulating the innate and antigen-specific host immune responses. The F protein has been implicated in the contact-mediated impairment of peripheral blood lymphocyte (PBL) proliferation (Schlender et al., 2002). PBLs exposed to RSV-infected cells or to cells expressing F protein in the absence of infectious RSV were arrested in G_0G_1 phase. Activation marker could still be induced on the surface of these cells with use of T-cell mitogens. The RSV nonstructural proteins NS1 and NS2 were shown in a separate study to coordinately antagonize the antiviral effect of type 1 IFN (Schlender et al., 2000). Both of these effects were observed for both human and bovine RSV and to function most effectively when cells of the homologous species were used. The F protein was also shown to augment innate immunity through the receptors CD14 and Toll-like receptor 4 (TLR4) by inducing the proinflammatory cytokine IL-6 (Kurt-Jones et al., 2000). Recently, the CX3C chemokine receptor 1 (CX3CR1) has been shown to facilitate RSV infection. The G glycoprotein binds to CX3CR1, and a short region of G has been shown to have moderate amino acid homology to fractaline, the only CX3C chemokine identified thus far (Tripp et al., 2001). More recent studies indicate that glycoprotein G has CX3C chemokine activity that can be blocked by anti-G antibody and that the G glycoprotein is responsible for generating the enhanced disease caused by inactivated RSV (Tripp, personal communication). Finally, a study of CD8+ T cells infiltrating the lung parenchyma in BALB/c mice showed they are impaired in both cytolytic activity and cytokine secretion (Chang and Brachiale, 2002). This impairment appears to be attributable to a T-cell-receptor signaling defect that is in turn dependent upon pulmonary infection by RSV. Thus, it seems clear that RSV has developed a number of mechanisms for altering or curtailing the host immune response.

Vaccine development

The preceding section documents some of the difficulties associated with developing safe and effective vaccines for RSV. One- to 2-month-old infants are the population most likely to develop RSV infections requiring hospitalization, and as such they constitute a critical target group for RSV vaccine. Live virus vaccines tend to be more immunogenic than other types of vaccine at this age, when maternal antibody and immunologic maturity can render the immune system refractory to antigenic stimulation (Crowe, 2001). Unfortunately, live virus vaccines also pose a potential risk, since an insufficiently attenuated virus may actually cause disease in young infants. In addition, candidate RSV vaccines must induce a robust circulating titer of neutralizing antibody, since they have been shown to play an instrumental role in protection against reinfection. Finally, any candidate vaccine for RSV will need to be carefully evaluated to ensure that it does not cause the disease enhancement on primary exposure to wild-type virus that was associated with formalin-inactivated vaccine (Kapikian et al., 1969). Although there is no vaccine currently licensed for RSV, a variety of vaccine development strategies have been assessed, including those involving peptide (Jiang et al., 2002), subunit (Simoes et al., 2002; Goetsch et al., 2001; Power et al., 2001; Prince et al.,

2000), virus vector (Dollenmaier *et al.*, 2001; Schmidt *et al.*, 2002), plasmid DNA/RNA (Andersson *et al.*, 2000; Fleeton *et al.*, 2001), and live attenuated vaccines (Collins and Murphy, 2002; Crowe *et al.*, 1999; Wright *et al.*, 2000).

While subunit and peptide vaccines provide a higher level of safety than vectored or live virus vaccines, they generally have the disadvantage of failing to induce protective levels of neutralizing antibody. This is primarily due to the fact that most of the neutralizing antibodies to RSV are directed against the mature, membrane-bound/virion-associated form of F, and subunit and peptide vaccines present the immature form of F. At least two subunit/peptide RSV vaccines are being actively pursued. One is a purified preparation of the F glycoprotein and the other is a glycoprotein G specific peptide conjugated to the albumin-binding site of the streptococcus G protein, which serves a carrier function. Neither appears to be sufficiently immunogenic in young infants, and both are being targeted for use in older children and the elderly. Efforts are being made to address the need to induce adequate levels of neutralizing antibody by expressing F glycoprotein in a suitable vector. In one study, for example, the immunogenicity of a human rhinovirus replicon expressing the RSV F protein was evaluated in mice; while the majority of the F protein produced was of the immature form, a fraction was expressed as the mature form, and titers of neutralizing antibody were readily measurable in immunized animals (Dollenmaier *et al.*, 2001). Similar observations have been made for RSV glycoproteins expressed in vaccinia and bovine parainfluenza virus (Crowe 2002; Schmidt *et al.*, 2001). Plasmid DNA vaccines are transfected into cells on administration, leading to a transient expression of the immunogenic antigens. The approach has been demonstrated to be effective in mice with use of recombinant constructs containing either RSV F or G protein in an SFV expression system (Fleeton *et al.*, 2001). However, there is scant evidence that such an approach will prove sufficiently immunogenic in humans. The pursuit of live attenuated RSV vaccines has begun to yield promising results. One potential advantage to a live attenuated RSV vaccine (also possibly applicable for plasmid DNA or vectored vaccines) is the possibility of intranasal administration. This immunization strategy has been demonstrated to mimic a natural RSV infection, inducing a neutralizing antibody response in both the nasopharyngeal mucosum and in serum, as well as cell-mediated immunity (Crowe, 2002).

Initially, live candidate RSV vaccines were derived in the conventional fashion, by passaging the virus repeatedly in culture at low temperature, leading to a strain of RSV that was attenuated in chimps as well as seropositive adults and children (Crowe, 2002). This virus was further mutagenized chemically to produce a series of temperature-sensitive mutants that, while clearly more attenuated, remained capable of causing transient respiratory illness in infants when administered intranasally. Furthermore, some of these mutations have been shown capable of reverting during replication in vivo (McIntosh *et al.*, 1974). However, extensive sequencing data have provided a catalog of specific temper-

ature-sensitive mutations for RSV, and the next generation of candidate RSV vaccines is being created with use of site-directed mutation (Collins and Murphy, 2002). With use of the best current generation of attenuated strains as a starting point, a cDNA copy of the virus is produced, and various characterized mutations are introduced, whereupon the cDNA copy can be transfected into cells to produce infectious virions of the new vaccine strain. By this approach, multiple attenuating mutations (point mutations, gene insertions, deletions) can be introduced into RSV and evaluated independently and in combination for immunogenicity, pathogenicity, and stability in test animals and humans. The possibility of introducing immunomodulatory genes, such as IL-2 or IL-12, into an RSV live virus vaccine is also being explored as a means for driving the anti-RSV toward the Th1 cytokine profile and, concomitantly, to reduce the risk of causing vaccine-enhanced illness.

PARAINFLUENZA

Viral pathogenesis

Parainfluenza viruses (PIVs) are single-stranded, negative-sense RNA viruses belonging to the family Paramyxoviridae. The envelopes of these viruses display two glycoproteins, hemagglutinin-neuraminidase (HN) and fusion (F) proteins, against which the major antibody response is generated. Four distinct serological types have been identified, termed PIV-1 through PIV-4. Human PIVs are a major cause of acute respiratory infections, particularly in infants and young children (Chanock *et al.*, 2001). PIV-1 is responsible for the majority of cases of croup, and PIV-3 is the second most frequent etiologic agent, after RSV, in pediatric lower respiratory disease. More recently, PIVs, predominantly PIV-3, have been shown to cause acute pneumonia, persistent infection, and death in immunocompromised patients. It is estimated that in the United States, PIV-1, -2, and -3 are responsible for about 20% of cases of pediatric respiratory disease requiring hospitalization (Murphy *et al.*, 1988).

PIV subtypes exhibit clear differences in epidemiology. PIV-1, -2, and to a lesser extent PIV-4 occur most commonly in the fall and winter months, whereas PIV-3 infections occur year-round, with peak infection in the spring and summer (Laurichess *et al.*, 1999). PIV-1 and PIV-2 are effectively controlled by maternal antibody in infants, which delays the onset of disease caused by these subtypes until the preschool years. PIV-3 infection is unimpaired by maternal antibody, so that half of all children seroconvert to this subtype during the first year of life (Glezen *et al.*, 1984).

In common with influenza and RSV, reinfection by the homologous subtype occurs, even in the presence of virus-specific antibody. In general, reinfection is restricted to the upper respiratory tract, probably because serum IgG, which is present in the lungs, endures longer than secretory IgA in the upper respiratory tract. The predominant humoral immune response is directed against HN and F, which are involved in virus attachment and fusion, respectively

(Chanock *et al.*, 2001). Both serum IgG and S-IgA antibodies are produced in response to PIV infection, but their contribution to viral clearance is uncertain. T-cell immunity is thought to play an important role in recovery from PIV infection, since disseminated disease, including spread to the brain, can occur in T-cell–immunosuppressed patients (Fishout *et al.*, 1980). Virus shedding also tends to be more prolonged in persons with impaired cell-mediated immune responses (Rabella *et al.*, 1999). Additional support for the participation of cell-mediated immunity in PIV recovery comes from studies in mice, where the participation of CD8[+] CTLs can effect virus clearance in the absence of other cell types (Hou *et al.*, 1992). Conversely, patients with PIV-3-induced bronchiolitis display elevated levels of PIV-3-specific lymphocyte transformation, suggesting that immunopathogenic responses to PIV-3 may occur (Chanock *et al.*, 2001). Maternally acquired anti-PIV antibody appears to protect infants from severe PIV-3-associated lower respiratory tract disease in infants, suggesting an important role for humoral immunity. However, nasal wash IgA produced by infants during primary infection with PIV-1 or PIV-2 is usually unable to neutralize virus (Chanock *et al.*, 2001).

In adults, PIV illnesses spread only in rare instances to the lower respiratory tract. Nonetheless, PIV has been increasingly identified as the causative agent in serious respiratory illness in elderly care facilities. Rates of pneumonia in this population have been reported to be as high as 29%, and deaths due to PIV have also been confirmed. PIVs have also been shown to exacerbate chronic obstructive pulmonary disease in the elderly (Chanock *et al.*, 2001).

PIV vaccine development

Given the complex and variable pathology of PIVs, compounded by uncertainties about the relative contribution of various facets of immunity in controlling infection, vaccine development for these viruses is somewhat problematic. No vaccine has been licensed to date; nonetheless, several approaches to PIV vaccine development are currently under investigation. Early candidate vaccines were formalin-inactivated but failed to provide any protection against PIV infection or disease. Fortunately, in contrast to the experience with inactivated RSV vaccine, enhanced PIV disease in infants was not a consequence of vaccination with formalin-inactivated PIV vaccine (Chin *et al.*, 1969). Two PIV-3 vaccine candidates, a live chimeric vaccine (HN and F of human PIV-3 recombined into bovine PIV-3) (Schmidt *et al.*, 2001b) and a cold-adapted vaccine strain (cp45) (Karron *et al.*, 1995), have undergone clinical trials and were determined to be both safe and immunogenic in seronegative infants ≥6 months of age.

A number of attempts have been made to develop a live-attenuated intranasal vaccine with temperature-sensitive, cold-adapted PIV. However, attenuated PIV strains were discovered to retain the capacity to infect central neurons in the nasal cavity, and as such they had the potential for causing adverse events in the central nervous system (Mori *et al.*, 1996). Thus, the strategy of oral immunization with this vaccine was investigated in mice as an alternative approach to establishing anti-PIV mucosal immunity, and this strategy was found to provide protection. This has not yet been attempted in primates or human subjects. In addition, purified HN and F and viral vectors expressing these proteins are immunogenic in various animal models but have yet to be evaluated in primates and humans (Chanock *et al.*, 2001).

Hamsters, cotton rats, mice, and ferrets have been useful small animal models for the evaluation of candidate PIV vaccines. Chimpanzees have also been employed, and recent evidence suggests that African green monkeys provide a superior animal model for the assessment of live PIV vaccines (Durbin *et al.*, 2000).

It seems that we are on the brink of developing acceptable PIV vaccines. Recent efforts to apply the technique of reverse genetics with PIV3 could lead to the development of vaccine strains that lack neurotropism and would thus be suitable for nasal administration. The payoff from such powerful new techniques has yet to materialize, but the prospects appear promising.

ADENOVIRUSES

Viral pathogenesis and vaccine development

The human adenoviruses are a large family of double-stranded DNA viruses comprising more than 50 serotypes, divided into six subgroups (A–F). A small number of serotypes in subgroups B and C are estimated to cause between 5% and 15% of all respiratory diseases in children and about 3% of respiratory illnesses in adults. In children, adenovirus infections can cause severe interstitial pneumonia that results rarely in death. Symptomatic respiratory infections are usually febrile and are often accompanied by conjunctivitis. Under conditions in which persons are housed in close quarters, such as military barracks, dormitories, and long-term-care facilities, adenoviruses can cause large-scale epidemics of acute respiratory disease. Subgroup A viruses such as Ad31 have also been associated with pneumonia in immunocompromised patients. Neutralizing antibodies directed against the capsid proteins (hexon and fiber proteins) are considered to be primarily responsible for the prevention of reinfection by adenovirus. While these viruses cause both upper and lower respiratory disease, only serum antibodies appear to have a role in protective immunity (Horwitz, 2001). A highly effective live virus vaccine against serotypes 4 and 7 was administered to military recruits until 1998. This vaccine was administered orally in enteric coated capsules; the virus, which was not attenuated in the nasopharyngeal cavity, could replicate in the gastrointestinal tract without causing disease, generating a protective response in both the upper and lower respiratory tract (Howell *et al.*, 1998). The vaccine went out of production in 1996, and supplies have now unfortunately been exhausted. The loss of this vaccine has already precipitated respiratory disease epidemics among military recruits, and adenovirus has now reemerged as the leading cause of febrile respiratory disease in this population. A similarly constructed quadrivalent vaccine for serotypes 1, 2, 3, and 5 should be developed and assessed for use in children, since those serotypes cause more than 80% of adenovirus-associated respiratory disease in young children (Schmidt *et al.*, 2001a).

Since recombinant adenoviruses efficiently transfer foreign genes into host cells in vivo, a great deal of attention has been focused on the use of these viruses as vectors to express recombinant genes for gene therapy (Carroll *et al.*, 2001). This is achieved by deleting the E1 region from the wild-type viral genome. The adenoviruses used for gene therapy have extensive gene deletions and thus cannot replicate in normal cells. The primary interest in adenovirus vectors is for use in correcting gene defects such as cystic fibrosis and to make certain cancers more immunogenic. Similarly, the well-characterized immune modulatory effects of these viruses are being explored as a means for controlling autoimmune disease and transplant rejection.

RHINOVIRUSES

The human rhinoviruses (HRVs) are nonenveloped, positive-strand RNA viruses of the family Picornaviridae. More than 100 antigenically distinct serotypes have been identified. HRVs are the etiologic agents responsible for more than 50% of common colds. HRVs are highly infectious and replicate rapidly in the epithelium and adjacent lymphoid tissues of the upper respiratory tract, causing symptoms in 1–4 days. Usually lesions are confined to the upper respiratory tract, mostly the nose, and only very rarely does pneumonia occur. Recovery occurs quickly and appears to depend mainly on innate defense mechanisms, especially IFNs. Characteristically, nasal and serum antibodies appear late after infection and can be delayed until 21 days in primary disease. Titers may continue to rise until 4–5 weeks after infection, and immunity, once developed, is stable and long-lasting (2–4 years). However, it remains uncertain whether serum IgG transudate, nasal IgA, or both defend against reinfection (Couch, 2001). Because so many antigenically distinct serotypes occur in nature and no infection is homotypic, vaccine development for the prevention of HRV infection is theoretically possible but probably not practical.

CORONAVIRUSES

First isolated in 1965, human coronaviruses are enveloped, positive-strand, RNA viruses with a large (30,000-nucleotide) genome. The viruses are classified as two serotypes (designated simply 1 and 2), represented respectively by the strains 229E and OC43. Coronaviruses are estimated to cause between 15% and 30% of common colds. The disease has a longer incubation and shorter course than disease due to rhinoviruses. Occasionally coronaviruses cause severe lower respiratory tract disease in infants and small children. Recovery from infection leaves patients immune, but the duration of immunity is shorter than that for rhinoviruses (Holmes, 2001). The mechanism of immunity is not understood, and no attempts have been made to develop a vaccine against human coronavirus infection.

This situation may be about to change. By April 2003, the world had suddenly become aware of coronaviruses as human pathogens. Around November 2002, new coronavirus strains appeared in Southern China that represent major respiratory pathogens. The syndrome has been termed *SARS*, for severe acute respiratory syndrome (Ksiazek *et al.*, 2003; Drosten *et al.*, 2003). Unlike previously described coronavirus strains, which usually cause mild upper respiratory tract lesions, the SARS strains affect the lower tract, markedly damage alveolar epithelial cells, and may become viremic. Furthermore, infection results in death, and in some communities the mortality rate may be as high as 5%. Modern travel is rapidly disseminating the virus around the world, and given the high mortality and the lack of effective antiviral therapy or vaccines, this is causing considerable alarm. The origin of the new virus remains unknown, but its genomic structure suggests it is a zoonosis, or a recombination of animal and human strains. The National Institutes of Health (NIH) and the governments of other countries are in the process of significantly funding coronavirus research to find improved means of diagnosis, treatment, and control. As mentioned above, vaccines are not available for human coronavirus, but some animal coronaviruses are controlled by vaccines, the efficacy of which is not well established (Ladman *et al.*, 2002). It appears likely that vaccines against the SARS strains will represent a high priority issue for the future.

THE MUCOSAL IMMUNE SYSTEM AND VIRAL VACCINES

Obstacles and possible strategies

The example of formalin-inactivated RSV vaccine illustrates the potential hazards of immunizing humans with the aim of inducing protective immunity at a mucosal surface. Because mucosal surfaces are continuously visited with a large variety of foreign, albeit mostly harmless antigens, the local immune system is predisposed to be hyporesponsive to most of these materials. The perturbations caused by invading microbes, such as bacteria and viruses, are thought to arm the mucosal surface to a state of responsiveness. Consequently, nasally administered vaccine viruses, which have been carefully designed to exhibit limited virulence, may insufficiently disturb the mucosal surface to generate an effective immune response. In addition, even when preparations are sufficiently immunogenic, resident antigen-presenting cells in concert with T lymphocytes can direct individual responses toward Th1 or Th2 dominance (Neurath *et al.*, 2002). The cytokine profile secreted by activated Th1 cells promotes the development of antigen-specific cytotoxic T lymphocytes, and Th2 cells promote the activation of B cells to produce specific antibodies, including S-IgA antibodies. Both responses make important contributions to the resolution of respiratory infections, but overproduction of STAT6 and GATA-3 can polarize the immune response toward Th2 cell hyperactivity, leading to allergic responses such as asthma (Neurath *et al.*, 2002). Similarly, activation of the transcription factor T-bet can lead to Th1 hyperresponsiveness, leading to immunopathologic responses such as that seen with Crohn's disease (Ouyang *et al.*, 2000). Thus, respiratory viral vaccines (including materials coadministered to enhance immunogenicity) must be carefully evaluated to ensure that they lack the capacity to induce harmful immune responses in recipients.

A variety of experimental adjuvants have been evaluated for their ability to improve the immunogenicity of mucosal vaccines. The two most widely investigated adjuvants are the heat-labile enterotoxin of *Escherichia coli* (LT) and cholera toxin (CT) (Pizza *et al.*, 2001). Normal LT has been shown to have too much toxicity to be used as an adjuvant; however, studies of nasal immunization in mice have demonstrated that the mutated LT (which lacks the toxic ADP-ribosylation activity) provides an adjuvant effect comparable to that of the intact heterodimer. Likewise, CT has been shown to cause both inflammation and enhanced production of IgE antibody, which will likely preclude its use as an adjuvant in humans, but selected mutations of CT have resulted in reduced toxicity variants that retain adjuvancy. Another adjuvant that shows promise for nasal immunization is CpG oligodeoxynucleotide (ODN). Unmethylated CpG oligonucleotide motifs occur commonly in bacterial DNA and trigger immune responsiveness in mammals. Studies of nasal immunization using CpG ODN as an adjuvant showed that the material enhanced both humoral and cell-mediated responses and was well tolerated (McCluskie and Davis, 2001; Moldoveanu *et al.*, 1998).

Another pair of experimental adjuvants under investigation for nasal administration, proteosomes and emulsomes, were shown in animal studies to polarize immunity toward a Th1- or Th2/3-type cytokine profile. Proteosomes, a complex of neisserial membrane proteins with lipopolysaccharide from *Shigella flexneri* or *Plesiomonas shigelloides*, induced Th1-type cytokines in mice in response to nasally coadministered influenza HA (Jones *et al.*, 2002). Emulsomes are lipoidal particulate vehicles comprising a hydrophobic solid fat core surrounded and stabilized by one or more phospholipid bilayers. Emulsomes have been shown in mice to enhance nasal immunogenicity, polarizing the response toward the Th2/3 cytokine profile (Lowell *et al.*, 1997).

The coadministration of nasal influenza vaccine with the cytokine IL-12 has also been evaluated in mice and was found to substantially enhance protective antibody responses over those obtained with vaccine alone (Arulanandam *et al.*, 1999).

One significant drawback to vaccination strategies for viruses such as influenza that induce homotypic and usually transient immunity is that continual revaccination is required. T-cell immunity, which is primarily directed against nonvariant internal antigens of these viruses (heterotypic immunity), has the potential to provide cross-protection against recurrent disease. Unfortunately, CD8+ CMI responses to respiratory viruses appear to decline rather rapidly (Woodland, 2003). Recent studies in mice have revealed that long-term CD8+ CMI responses can be generated, particularly with use of DNA vaccination. These studies, while still relatively early, may eventually lead to vaccine strategies that target the induction of long-term, cross-reactive T-cell immunity that could reduce the requirement for revaccination. The complexities of the mucosal immune system thus present daunting challenges for vaccinologists. Many of the strategies under study have enormous promise, but they must be examined with great care to guard against the equally great capacity for inadvertent harm.

SUMMARY AND CONCLUSIONS

Respiratory virus infections are a major cause of human disease. None is satisfactorily controlled by vaccines, and for most infections licensed vaccines do not exist. The reasons for this situation are likely multiple. They include the fact that some are antigenically mobile or exist as multiple serotypes. Moreover, none persists beyond a usually brief infection/disease episode. Hence, there is no continual source of antigen, which some investigators maintain is necessary to sustain functional long-term memory (Ahmed and Gray, 1996). In addition, it has been evident since the pioneering work of Tomasi and Ogra that the biology of immunity at mucosal surfaces differs from central systemic immunity (Tomasi *et al.*, 1965; Ogra and Karzon, 1969). Initially, the focus was on the types of antibodies involved. Thus, S-IgA is usually the principal Ig isotype at mucosal sites, and this is mainly produced by lymphoid tissue associated with mucosal surfaces (Tomasi *et al.*, 1965). It seems that the half-life for IgA is less than that for IgG which dominates systemic immunity. The long-term presence of Ig requires that cells continue to produce it. Some have argued that IgG-producing plasma cells can exist for long periods at least in the bone marrow (Slifka and Ahmed, 1996). It is not clear if similar long-term IgA-producing plasma cells also exist in mucosa-associated lymphoreticular tissue (MALT). Should they be absent, this could account for the loss of protective IgA at mucosal surfaces.

Contemporary research has focused on T-cell immunity, especially immunological memory, the basis for protective vaccines. As discussed previously, T cells, especially CD8+ T cells, do participate in immunity to respiratory virus infections. However, unlike neutralizing antibody, they do not function to impede infection. Instead T cells serve to effect recovery from infection, a process that involves cytotoxicity and cytokine production. Following infection, effector-memory cells are induced in lung tissues, and these are responsible mainly for the control of infection. The cells exert direct protective effects and maintain this function in nonlymphoid parenchymal tissues of the lung for some time. However, after a few months, effector memory cell activity is barely detectible. At this stage, self-renewing memory cells are present in central lymphoid tissue, and these may persist for years, seemingly without the need for antigen restimulation to sustain them (Sprent and Tough, 2001; Wherry *et al.*, 2003). This issue, however, remains debatable (Hogan *et al.*, 2002). In addition, it is not clear if mucosal lymphoid and nonlymphoid sites similarly act as repositories of memory cells. However, some have suggested that mucosal memory is of shorter duration than central memory (Hogan *et al.*, 2001). Wherever noneffector memory cells exist, it takes 4–5 days for their recruitment as effector memory cells in lung tissues. Meanwhile, a rapidly replicating respiratory virus could be well established and be in the process of causing lesions.

Another unresolved issue is the location of cells that are recruited and activated following reinfection to become lung effector memory cells. Conceivably, it cannot be mucosal lymphoid sites if such cells do indeed disappear quickly after antigen exposure. Experiments have shown that the central lymphoid organs can provide a source of protective T cells long after initial infection (Wherry *et al.*, 2003). It could be that some forms of antigen reexposure might preferentially recruit this source of cells. Additionally, it is conceivable that certain forms of vaccination may induce a readily recruitable form of memory cells from lymphoid tissues. Novel adjustments might serve to influence such events. It is anticipated that ongoing fundamental research on mucosal and central memory should reveal clues that are exploitable to improve the efficacy of respiratory viral vaccines. We hope that any future rewrite of this review will be able to report positive progress on these issues.

REFERENCES

Ahmed, R., and Gray, D. (1996). Immunological memory and protective immunity: understanding their relation. *Science* 272, 54–60.

Alwan, W.H., Kozlowska, W.J., and Openshaw, P.J. (1994). Distinct types of lung disease caused by functional subsets of antiviral T cells. *J. Exp. Med.* 179, 81–89.

Arulanandam, B.P., O'Toole, M., and Metzger, D.W. (1999). Intranasal interleukin-12 is a powerful adjuvant for protective mucosal immunity. *J. Infect. Dis.* 180, 940–949.

Anderson, L.J. (2000). Respiratory syncytial virus vaccines for otitis media. *Vaccine* 19, S59–S65.

Andersson, C., Liljestrom, P., Stahl, S., and Power, U.F. (2000). Protection against respiratory syncytial virus (RSV) elicited in mice by plasmid DNA immunization encoding a secreted RSV G protein–derived antigen. *FEMS Immun. Med. Microbiol.* 29, 247–253.

Asanuma, H., Hirokawa, K., Uchiyama, M., Suzuki, Y., Aizawa, C., Kurata, T., Sata, T., and Tamura, S. (2001). Immune responses and protection in different strains of aged mice immunized intranasally with an adjuvant-combined influenza vaccine. *Vaccine* 19, 3981–3989.

Ban, E.M., van Ginkel, F.W., Simecka, J.W., Kiyono, H., Robinson, H.L., and McGhee, J.R. (1997). Mucosal immunization with DNA encoding influenza hemagglutinin. *Vaccine* 15, 811–813.

Bangham, C.R., Openshaw, P.J., Ball, L.A., King, A.M., Wertz, G.W., and Askonas, B.A. (1986). Human and murine cytotoxic T cells specific to respiratory syncytial virus recognize the viral nucleoprotein (N), but not the major glycoprotein (G), expressed by vaccinia virus recombinants. *J. Immunol.* 137, 3973–3977.

Barchfeld, G.L., Hessler, A.L., Chen, M., Pizza, M., Rappuoli, R., and Van Nest, G.A. (1999). The adjuvants MF59 and LT-K63 enhance the mucosal and systemic immunogenicity of subunit influenza vaccine administered intranasally in mice. *Vaccine* 17, 695–704.

Belshe, R.B. (1999). Influenza prevention and treatment: current practices and new horizons. *Ann. Intern. Med.* 131, 621–623.

Belshe, R.B., Gruber, W.C., Mendelman, P.M., Mehta, H.B., Mahmood, K., Reisinger, K., Treanor, J., Zangwill, K., Hayden, F.G., Bernstein, D.I., Kotloff, K., King, J., Piedra, P.A., block, S.L., Yan, L., and Wolff, M. (2000). Correlates of immune protection induced by live, attenuated, cold-adapted, trivalent, intranasal influenza virus vaccine. *J. Infect. Dis.* 181, 1133–1137.

Belshe, R.B., Mendelman, P.M., Treanor, J., King, J., Gruber, W.C., Piedra, P., Bernstein, D.I., Hayden, F.G., Kotloff, K., Zangwill, K., Iacuzio, D., and Wolff, M. (1998). The efficacy of live attenuated, cold-adapted, trivalent, intranasal influenzavirus vaccine in children. *N. Engl. J. Med.* 338, 1405–1412.

Ben-Yedidia, T., Abel, L., Arnon, R., and Globerson, A. (1998). Efficacy of anti-influenza peptide vaccine in aged mice. *Mech. Ageing Dev.* 104, 11–23.

Berglund, P., Fleeton, M.N., Smerdou, C., and Liljeström, P. (1999) Immunization with recombinant Semliki Forest virus induces protection against influenza challenge in mice. *Vaccine* 17, 497–507.

Bernstein, E., Kaye, D., Abrutyn, E., Gross, P., Dorfman, M., and Murasko, D.M. (1999). Immune response to influenza vaccination in a large healthy elderly population. *Vaccine* 17, 82–94.

Betts, R.F., and Treanor, J.J. (2000). Approaches to improved influenza vaccination. *Vaccine* 18, 1690–1695.

Boyce, T.G., Gruber, W.C., Coleman-Dockery, S.D., Sannella, E.C., Reed, G.W., Wolff, M., and Wright, P.F. (2000). Mucosal immune response to trivalent live attenuated intranasal influenza vaccine in children. *Vaccine* 18, 82–88.

Bradshaw, J., and Wright, P.F. (2002). Cold-adapted influenza vaccines. *Curr. Opin. Pediatr.* 14, 95–98.

Brühl, P., Kerschbaum, A., Kistner, O., Barrett, N., Dorner, F., and Gerencer, M. (2000). Humoral and cell-mediated immunity to vero cell–derived influenza vaccine. *Vaccine* 19, 1149–1158.

Cannon, M.J., Stott, E.J., Taylor, G. and Askonas, B.A. (1987). Clearance of persistent respiratory syncytial virus infections in immunodeficient mice following transfer of primed T cells. *Immunology* 62, 133–138.

Carroll, M.W., Wilkinson, G.W., and Lundstrom, K. (2001). Mammalian expression systems and vaccination. In *Genetically Engineered Viruses* (eds. C.J.A. Ring and E.D. Blair), Oxford: Bios Scientific Publishers, 107–157.

Centers for Disease Control and Prevention. (2000). Prevention and control of influenza: recommendations of the Advisory Committee on Immunization Practices (ACIP). *MMWR Morb. Mortal. Wkly. Rep.* 49(27), 619–622.

Cerwenka, A, Morgan, T.M., Harmsen, A.G., and Dutton, R.W. (1999). Migration kinetics and final destination type 1 and type 2 CD8 effector cells predict protection against pulmonary virus infection. *J. Exp. Med.* 189, 423–434.

Chang, J., and Braciale, T.J. (2002). Respiratory syncytial virus infection suppresses lung CD8+ T-cell effector activity and peripheral CD8+ T-cell memory in the respiratory tract. *Nat. Med.* 8, 54–60.

Chanock, R.M., Murphy, B.R., and Collins, P.L. (2001). Parainfluenza viruses. In *Field's Virology I* (eds. D.M. Knipe and P.M. Howley), Philadelphia: Lippincott-Raven, 1341–1379.

Chen, D., Periwal, S.B., Larrivee, K., Zuleger, C., Erickson, C.A., Endres, R.L., and Payne, L.G. (2001). Serum and mucosal immune responses to an inactivated influenza virus vaccine induced by epidermal powder immunization. *J. Virol.* 75, 7956–7965.

Chin, J., Magoffin, R.L., Shearer, L.A., Schieble, J.H., Lennette, E.H. (1969). Field evaluation of a respiratory syncytial virus vaccine and a trivalent parainfluenza virus vaccine in a pediatric population. *Am. J. Epidemiol.* 89, 449–463.

Clancy, R.L. (1995). Mucosal vaccines for the prevention of influenza. *Drugs* 50, 587–594.

Clover, R.D., Crawford, S., Glezen, W.P., Taber, L.H., Matson, C.C., and Couch, R.B. (1991). Comparison of heterotypic protection against influenza A/Taiwan/86 (H1N1) by attenuated and inactivated vaccines to A/Chile/83-like viruses. *J. Infect. Dis.* 163, 300–304.

Collins, P.L., Chanock, R.M., and Murphy, B.R. (2001). Respiratory syncytial virus. In *Field's Virology I* (eds. D.M. Knipe and P.M. Howley). Philadelphia: Lippincott-Raven, pp. 1443–1485.

Collins, P.L., and Murphy, B.R. (2002). Respiratory syncytial virus: reverse genetics and vaccine strategies. *Virology* 296, 204–211.

Crowe, J.E., Jr. (2001) Respiratory syncytial virus vaccine development. *Vaccine* 20, S32–S37.

Crowe, J.E., Jr. (2001) Influence of maternal antibodies on neonatal immunization against respiratory viruses. *Clin. Infect. Dis.* 33, 1720–1727.

Crowe, J.E., Jr., Collins, P.L., Chanock, R.M., and Murphy, B.R. (1997). Vaccines against respiratory syncytial virus and parainfluenza virus type 3. In *New Generation Vaccines* (eds. M.M. Levine, G.C. Woodrow, J.B. Kaper, and G.S. Cobon), 2nd ed. New York: Marcel Dekker, pp. 711–725.

Crowe, J.E., Jr., Randolph, V., and Murphy, B.R. (1999). The live attenuated subgroup B respiratory syncytial virus vaccine candidate RSV 2B33F is attenuated and immunogenic in chimpanzees, but exhibits partial loss of the *ts* phenotype following replication in vivo. *Virus Res.* 59, 13–22.

Couch, R.B. (2001). Rhinoviruses. In *Field's Virology I* (eds. D.M. Knipe and P.M. Howley). Philadelphia: Lippincott-Raven, 777–798.

Cusi, M.G., Lomagistro, M.M., Valassina, M., Valensin, P.E., and Glück, R. (2000). Immunopotentiating of mucosal and systemic antibody responses in mice by intranasal immunization with HLT-combined influenza virosomal vaccine. *Vaccine* 18, 2838–2842.

Doherty, P.C., Allan, W., Eichelberger, M., and Carding, S.R. (1992). Roles of α/β and γ/δ T cell subsets in viral immunity. *Annu. Rev. Immunol.* 10, 123–151.

Dollenmaier, G., Mosier, S.M., Scholle, F., Sharma, N. McKnight, K.L., and Lemon, S.M. (2001). Membrane-associated respiratory syncytial virus F protein expressed from a human rhinovirus type 14 vector is immunogenic. *Virology* 281, 216–230.

Drosden, C., Gunther, S., Preiser, W., van der Werf, S., Brodt, H.-R., Becker, S., Rabenau, H., Panning, M., Kolesnikova, L., Fouchier, R.A.M., Berger, A., Burgiere, A.-M., Cinatl, J., Eickmann, M., Escriou, N., Grywna, K., Kramme, S., Manuguerra, C., Muller, S., Rikerts, V., Sturmer, M., Vieth, S., Klenk, H.-D., Osterhaus, A.D.M.E, Schmitz, H., and Doerr, H.W. (2003). Identification of a novel coronavirus in patients with severe acute respiratory syndrome. *N. Engl. J. Med.* (Online Publication, April 18).

Durbin, A.P., Elkins, W.R., and Murphy, B.R. (2000). African green monkeys provide a useful nonhuman primate model for the study of human parainfluenza virus types -1, -2, and -3 infection. *Vaccine* 18, 2462–2469.

Edwards, K.M., Dupont, W.D., Westrich, M.K., Plummer, W.D. Jr., Palmer, P.S., and Wright, P.F. (1994). A randomized controlled trial of cold-adapted and inactivated vaccines for the prevention of influenza A disease. *J. Infect. Dis.* 169, 68–76.

Eichelberger, M., Allan, W., Zijlstra, M., Jaenisch, R., and Doherty, P.C. (1991). Clearance of influenza virus respiratory infection in mice lacking class I major histocompatibility complex–restricted CD8+ T cells. *J. Exp. Med.* 174, 875–880.

Epstein, S.L., Lo, C.Y., Misplon, J.A., and Bennink, J.R. (1998). Mechanism of protective immunity against influenza virus infection in mice without antibodies. *J. Immunol.* 160, 322–327.

Ferko, B., Katinger, D., Grassauer, A., Egorov, A., Romanova, J., Niebler, B., Katinger, H., and Muster, T. (1998). Chimeric influenza virus replicating predominantly in the murine upper respiratory tract induces local immune responses against human immunodeficiency virus type 1 in the genital tract. *J. Infect. Dis.* 178, 1359–1368.

Fishaut, M., Tubergen, D., and McIntosh, K. (1980). Cellular response to respiratory viruses with particular reference to children with disorders of cell-mediated immunity. *J. Pediatr.* 96, 179–186.

Flynn, K.J., Belz, G.T., Altman, J.D., Ahmed, R., Woodland, D.L., and Doherty, P.C. (1998). Virus-specific CD8+ T cells in primary and secondary influenza pneumonia. *Immunity* 8, 683–691.

Frank, A.L., Taber, L.H., and Porter, C.M. (1987). Influenza B virus reinfection. *Am. J. Epidemiol.* 89, 576–586.

Glezen, W.P., Frank, A.L., Taber, L.H., and Kasel, J.A. (1984). Parainfluenza virus type 3: seasonality and risk of infection and reinfection in young children. *J. Infect. Dis.* 150, 851–857.

Goetsch, L., Plotnicky-Gilquin, H., Aubry, J.P., De-Lys, P., Haeuw, J.F., Bonnefoy, J.Y., Nguyen, N.T., Corvaia, N., and Velin, D. (2001). BBG2Na an RSV subunit vaccine candidate intramuscularly injected to human confers protection against viral challenge after nasal immunization in mice. *Vaccine* 19, 4036–4042.

Gorse, G.J., and Belshe, R.B. (1990). Enhancement of anti-influenza A virus cytotoxicity following influenza A virus vaccination in older, chronically ill adults. *J. Clin. Microbiol.* 28, 2539–2550.

Groothuis, J.R., Gutierrez, K.M., and Lauer, B.A. (1988). Respiratory syncytial virus infection in children with bronchopulmonary dysplasia. *Pediatrics* 82, 199–203.

Gruber, W.C., Belshe, R.B., King, J.C., Treanor, J.J., Piedra, P.A., Wright, P.F., Reed, G.W., Anderson, E., and Newman, F. (1996). Evaluation of live attenuated influenza vaccines in children 6–18 months of age: safety, immunogenicity, and efficacy. National Institute of Allergy and Infections Diseases Vaccine and Treatment Evaluation Program and the Wyeth-Ayerst ca Influenza Vaccine Investigators Group. *J. Infect. Dis.* 173, 1313–1319.

Hall, C.B., Powell, K.R., MacDonald, N.E., Gala, C.L., Menegus, M.E., Suffin, S.C., and Cohen, H.J. (1986). Respiratory syncytial viral infection in children with compromised immune function. *N. Engl. J. Med.* 315, 77–81.

Hall, C.B., Walsh, E.E., Long, C.E., and Schnabel, K.C. (1991). Immunity to and frequency of reinfection with respiratory syncytial virus. *J. Infect. Dis.* 163, 693–698.

Hayden, F.G., Fritz, R., Lobo, M.C., Alvord, W., Strober, W., and Straus, S.E. (1998). Local and systemic cytokine responses during experimental human influenza A virus infection. Relation to symptom formation and host defense. *J. Clin. Invest.* 101, 643–649.

Hogan, R.J., Cauley, L.S., Ely, K.H., Cookenham, T., Roberts, A.D., Brennan, J.W., Monard, S., and Woodland, D.L. (2002). Long-term maintenance of virus-specific effector memory CD8+ T cells in the lung airways depends on proliferation. *J. Immunol.* 169, 4976–4981.

Hogan, R.J., Usherwood, E.J., Zhong, W., Roberts, A.A., and Dutton, R.W., Harmsen, A.G., and Woodland, D.L. (2001). Activated antigen-specific CD8+ T cells persist in the lungs following recovery from respiratory virus infections. *J. Immunol.* 166, 1813–1822.

Holmes, K.V. (2001). Coronaviruses. In *Field's Virology I* (eds. D.M. Knipe and P.M. Howley). Philadelphia: Lippincott-Raven, 1443–1485.

Horwitz, M.S. (2001). Adenoviruses. In *Field's Virology I* (eds. D.M. Knipe and P.M. Howley). Philadelphia: Lippincott-Raven, 1443–1485.

Hou, S., Doherty, P.C., Zijlstra, M., Jaenisch, R., and Katz, J.M. (1992). Delayed clearance of Sendai virus in mice lacking class I MHC–restricted CD8+ T cells. *J. Immunol.* 149, 1319–1325.

Howell, M.R., Nang, R.N., Gaydos, C.A., and Gaydos, J.C. (1998) Prevention of adenoviral acute respiratory disease in Army recruits: cost-effectiveness of a military vaccination policy. *Am. J. Prev. Med.* 14, 168–175.

Institute of Medicine. (1985). Appendix N: prospects for immunizing against respiratory syncytial virus. In *New Vaccine Development: Establishing Priorities*, vol 1. Washington, DC: Institute of Medicine, 397–409.

Jeon, S.H., and Arnon, R. (2002) Immunization with influenza virus hemagglutinin globular region containing the receptor-binding pocket. *Viral Immunol.* 15, 165–176.

Jiang, S., Borthwick, N.J., Morrison, P., Gao, G.F., Steward, M.W. (2002). Virus-specific CTL responses induced by an H-2K^d-restricted, motif-negative 15-mer peptide from the fusion protein of respiratory syncytial virus. *J. Gen. Virol.* 83, 429–438.

Jones, T., Rioux, C., Plante, M., Allard, M., Gelinas, F., Tran, A, Cyr, S., Diamantakis, H., Bellerose, N., Lowell, N., and Burt, G. (2002). A novel mucosal adjuvant for induction of enhanced serum IgG, mucosal IgA and type 1 cytokine responses. In *11th International*

Congress of Mucosal Immunology. Mucosal Immunology Update. Orlando: Society for Mucosal Immunology, 2756.

Kaiser, L., Fritz, R.S., Straus, S.E, Gubareva, L., and Hayden, F.G. (2001). Symptom pathogenesis during acute influenza: interleukin-6 and other cytokine responses. *J. Med.Virol.* 64, 262–268.

Kapikian, A.Z., Mitchell, R.H., Chanock, R.M., Shvedoff, R.A., and Stewart C.E. (1969). An epidemiologic study of altered clinical reactivity to respiratory syncytial (RS) virus infection in children previously vaccinated with an inactivated RS virus vaccine. *Am. J. Epidemiol.* 89, 405–421.

Karron, R.A., Wright, P.F., Newman, F.K., Makhene, M., Thompson, J., Samorodin, R., Wilson, M.H., Anderson, E.L., Clements, M.L., Murphy, B.R., and Belshe, R.B. (1995). A live human parainfluenza type 3 virus vaccine is attenuated and immunogenic in healthy infants and children. *J. Infect. Dis.* 172, 1445–1450.

Ksiazek, T.G., Erdman, D., Goldsmith, C., Zaki, S.R., Peret, T., Emery, S., Tong, S., Urbani, C., Comer, J.A., Lim, W., Rollin, P.E., Dowell, S., Ling, A.-E., Humphrey, C., Shieh, W.-J., Guarner, J., Paddock, C.D., Rota, P., Fields, B., DeRisi, J., Yang, J.-Y., Cox, N., Hughes, J., LeDuc, J.W., Bellini, W., and Anderson, L.J. (2003). A novel coronavirus associated with severe acute respiratory syndrome. *N. Engl. J. Med.* (Online publication, April 18).

Kurt-Jones, E.A., Popova, L., Kwinn, L., Haynes, L.M., Jones, L.P., Tripp, R.A., Walsh, E.E., Freeman, M.W., Golenbock, D.T., Anderson, L.J., and Finberg, R.W. (2000). Pattern recognition receptors TLR4 and CD14 mediate response to respiratory syncytial virus. *Nat. Immunol.* 1, 398–401.

Ladman, B.S., Pope, C.R., Ziegler, A.F., Swieczkowski, T., Callahan, C.J., Davison, S., and Gelb, J. Jr. (2002). Protection of chickens after live and inactivated virus vaccination against challenge with nephropathogenic infectious bronchitis virus. *Avian Dis.* 46, 938–944.

Lasky, T., Terracciano, G.J., Magder, L., Koski, C.L., Ballesteros, M., Nash, D., Clark, S., Haber, P., Stolley, P.D., Schonberger, L.B., and Chen, R.T. (1998). The Guillain-Barre syndrome and the 1992–1993 and 1993–1994 influenza vaccines. *N. Engl. J. Med.* 339, 1797–1802.

LeVine, A.M., Koeningsknecht, V. and Stark, J.M. (2001). Decreased pulmonary clearance of *S. pneumoniae* following influenza A infection in mice. *J. Virol. Methods* 94, 173–186.

Ljungberg, K., Kolmskog, C., Wahren, B., van Amerongen, G., Baars, M., Osterhaus, A., Linde, A., and Rimmelzwaan, G. (2002). DNA vaccination of ferrets with chimeric influenza A virus hemagglutinin (H3) genes. *Vaccine* 20, 2045–2052.

Lowell, G.H., Kaminski, R.W., VanCott, T.C., Slike, B., Kersey, K., Zawoznik, E., Loomis-Price, L., Smith, G., Redfield, R.R., Amselem, S., and Birx, D.L. (1997). Proteosomes, emulsomes, and cholera toxin B provide nasal immunogenicity of human immunodeficiency virus gp160 in mice: induction of serum, intestinal, vaginal, and lung IgA and IgG. *J. Infect. Dis.* 175, 292–301.

MacDonald, N.E., Hall, C.B., Suffin, S.C., Alexson, C., Harris, P.J., and Manning, J.A. (1982). Respiratory syncytial viral infection in infants with congenital heart disease. *N. Engl. J. Med.* 307, 397–400.

Matsuki, N., Ogasawara, K., Takami, K., Namba, K., Takahashi, A., Fukui, Y., Sasazuki, T., Iwabuchi, K., Good, R.A., and Onoé, K.. (1999). Prevention of infection of influenza virus in DQ6 mice, a human model, by a peptide vaccine prepared according to the cassette theory. *Vaccine* 17, 1161–1168.

McIntosh, K., Arbeter, A.M., Stahl, M.K., Orr, I.A., Hodes, D.S., and Ellis, E.F. (1974). Attenuated respiratory syncytial virus vaccines in asthmatic children. *Pediatr. Res.* 8, 689–696.

McCluskie, M.J., and Davis. H.L. (2000). Oral, intrarectal, and intranasal immunizations using CpG and non-CpG oligodeoxynucleotides as adjuvants. *Vaccine* 19, 413–422.

Mills, J., 5th, van Kirk, J.E., Wright, P.F., and Chanock, R.M. (1971). Experimental respiratory syncytial virus infection of adults. Possible mechanisms of resistance to infection and illness. *J. Immunol.* 107, 123–130.

Moldoveanu, Z., Love-Homan, L., Huang, W.Q., and Krieg, A.M. (1998). CpG DNA, a novel immune enhancer for systemic and mucosal immunization with influenza virus. *Vaccine* 16, 1216–1224.

Monto, A.S., and Kioumehr, F. (1975). The Tecumseh Study of Respiratory Illness. IX. Occurrence of influenza in the community, 1966–1971. *Am. J. Epidemiol.* 102, 553–563.

Mori, I., Nakakuki, K, and Kimura, Y. (1996). Temperature-sensitive parainfluenza type 1 vaccine virus directly accesses the central nervous system by infecting olfactory neurons. *J. Gen.Virol.* 77, 2121–2124.

Murphy, B.R. (1993). Use of live attenuated cold-adapted influenza A reassortant virus vaccines in infants, children, young adults, and elderly adults. *Infect. Dis. Clin. Pract.* 2, 174–181.

Murphy, B.R., Prince, G.A., Collins, P.L., Van Wyke Coelingh, K., Olmsted, R.A., Spriggs, M.K., Parrott, R.H., Kim, H.W., Brandt, C.D., and Chanock, R.M. (1988). Current approaches to the development of vaccines effective against parainfluenza and respiratory syncytial viruses. *Virus Res.* 11, 1–15.

Neurath, M.F., Finotto, S., and Glimcher, L.H. (2002). The role of Th1/Th2 polarization in mucosal immunity. *Nat. Med.* 8, 567–573.

Nicholson, K.G., Kent, J., Hammersley, V, and Cancio, E. (1997). Acute viral infections of upper respiratory tract in elderly people living in the community: comparative, prospective, population-based study of disease burden. *BMJ* 315, 1060–1064.

Ogra, P., and Karzon, D. (1971). Formation and function of poliovirus antibody in different tissues. *Progr. Med. Virol.* 13, 156–193.

Ouyang, W., Lohning, M., Gao, Z., Assenmacher, M., Ranganath, S., Radbruch, A., and Murphy, K.M. (2000). Stat6-independent GATA-3 autoactivation directs IL-4 independent Th2 development and commitment. *Immunity* 12, 27–37.

Pizza, M., Giuliani, M.M., Fontana, M.R., Monaci, E., Douce, G., Dougan, G., Mills, K.H., Rappouli, R., and Del Giudice, G. (2001). Mucosal vaccines: nontoxic derivatives of LT and CT as mucosal adjuvants. *Vaccine* 19, 2534–2541.

Power, U.F., Nguyen, T.N., Rietveld, E., de Swart, R.L., Groen, J., Osterhaus, A.D., de Groot, R., Corvaia, N., Beck, A., Bouveret-le-Cam, N, and Bonnefoy, J-Y. (2001). Safety and immunogenicity of a novel recombinant subunit respiratory syncytial virus vaccine (BBG2Na) in healthy young adults. *J. Infect. Dis.* 184, 1456–1460.

Prince, G.A., Capiau, C., Deschamps, M., Fabry, L., Garcon, N., Gheysen, D., Prieels, J-P., Thiry, G., van Opstal, O., and Porter, D.D. (2000). Efficacy and safety studies of a recombinant chimeric respiratory syncytial virus FG glycoprotein vaccine in cotton rats. *J. Virol.* 74, 10287–10292.

Prince, G.A., Horswood, R.L., and Chanock, R.M. (1985). Quantitative aspects of passive immunity to respiratory syncytial virus infection in infant cotton rats. *J. Virol.* 55, 517–520.

Rabella, N., Rodriguez, P., Labeaga, R., Otegui, M., Mercader, M., Gurgui, M., and Prats, G. (1999). Conventional respiratory viruses recovered from immunocompromised patients: clinical considerations. *Clin. Infect. Dis.* 28, 1043–1048.

Remarque, E.J. (1999). Influenza vaccination in elderly people. *Exp. Gerontol.* 34, 445–452.

Riberdy, J.M., Christensen, J.P., Branum, K. and Doherty, P.C. (2000). Diminished primary and secondary influenza virus-specific CD8+ T-cell responses in CD4-depleted Ig-/- mice. *J. Virol.* 74, 9762–9765.

Ruben, F.L., and Cate, T.R. (1987). Influenza pneumonia. *Semin. Respir. Infect.* 2, 122–129.

Sakurai, H., Williamson, R.A., Crowe, J.E., Beeler, J.A., Poignard, P., Bastidas, R.B., Chanock, R.M., and Burton, D.R. (1999). Human antibody responses to mature and immature forms of viral envelope in respiratory syncytial virus infection: significance for subunit vaccines. *J. Virol.* 73, 2956–2962.

Sarawar, S.R., and Doherty, P.C. (1994). Concurrent production of interleukin-2, interleukin-10, and gamma interferon in the regional lymph nodes of mice with influenza pneumonia. *J. Virol.* 68, 3112–3119.

Saurwein-Teissl, M., Zisterer, K., Schmitt, T.L., Gluck, R., Cryz, S., and Grubeck-Loebenstein, B. (1998). Whole virus influenza vaccine activates dendritic cells (DC) and stimulates cytokine production by peripheral blood mononuclear cells (PBMC) while subunit vaccines support T cell proliferation. *Clin. Exp. Immunol.* 114, 271–276.

Schlender, J., Walliser, G., Fricke, J., and Conzelmann, K-K. (2002). Respiratory syncytial virus fusion protein mediates inhibition of mitogen-induced T-cell proliferation by contact. *J. Virol.* 76, 1163–1170.

Schmidt, A.C., Couch, R.B., Galasso, G.J., Hayden, F.G., Mills, J., Murphy, B.R., and Chanock, R.M. (2001a). Current Research on Respiratory Viral Infections: Third International Symposium. *Antiviral Res.* 50, 157–196.

Schmidt, A.C., McAuliffe, J.M., Murphy, B.R., and Collins, P.L. (2001b). Recombinant bovine/human parainfluenza virus type 3 (B/HPIV3) expressing the respiratory syncytial virus (RSV) G and F proteins can be used to achieve simultaneous mucosal immunization against RSV and HPIV3. *J. Virol.* 75, 4594–4603.

Schmidt, A.C., Wenzke, D.R., McAuliffe, J.M., St. Claire, M., Elkins, W.R., Murphy, B.R., and Collins, P.L. (2002). Mucosal immunization of rhesus monkeys against respiratory syncytial virus subgroups A and B and human parainfluenza virus type 3 by using a live cDNA-derived vaccine based on a host range-attenuated bovine parainfluenza virus type 3 vector backbone. *J. Virol.* 76, 1089–1099.

Shay, D.K., Holman, R.C., Newman, R.D., Liu, L.L, Stout, J.W., and Anderson, L.J. (1999) Bronchiolitis-associated hospitalizations among US children, 1980–1996. *JAMA* 282, 1440–1446.

Simoes, E.A., Tan, D.H., Ohlsson, A., Sales, V., and Wang, E.E. (2001). Respiratory syncytial virus vaccine: a systemic overview with emphasis on respiratory syncytial virus subunit vaccines. *Vaccine* 20, 954–960.

Sjölander, S., Drane, D, Davis, R., Beezum, L., Pearse, M., and Cox, J. (2001). Intranasal immunization with influenza-ISCOM induces strong mucosal as well as systemic antibody and cytotoxic T-lymphocyte responses. *Vaccine* 19, 4072–4080.

Skoner, D.P., Whiteside, T.L., Wilson, J.W., Doyle, W.J., Herberman, R.B., and Fireman, P. (1996). Effect of influenza A virus infection on natural and adaptive cellular immunity. *Clin. Immunol. Immunopathol.* 79, 294–302.

Slifka, M.K., and Ahmed, R. (1996). Long-term antibody production is sustained by antibody-secreting cells in the bone marrow following acute viral infection. *Ann. N.Y. Acad. Sci.* 797, 166–176.

Sprent, J., and Tough, D.F. (2001). T cell death and memory. *Science* 293, 245–248.

Srikiatkhachorn, A. and Braciale, T.J. (1997). Virus-specific CD8⁺ T lymphocytes downregulate T helper cell type 2 cytokine secretion and pulmonary eosinophilia during experimental murine respiratory syncytial virus infection. *J. Exp. Med.* 186, 421–432.

Tamura, S., Iwasaki, T., Thompson, A.H., Asanuma, H., Chen, Z., Suzuki, Y., Aizawa, C., and Kurata, T. (1998). Antibody-forming cells in the nasal-associated lymphoid tissue during primary influenza virus infection. *J. Gen. Virol.* 79, 291–299.

Tomasi, T.B., Jr., Tan, E.M., Solomon, A., and Prendergast, R.A. (1965). Characteristics of an immune system common to certain external secretions. *J. Exp. Med.* 121, 101–124.

Treanor, J.J., and Betts, R.F. (1998). Evaluation of live, cold-adapted influenza A and B virus vaccines in elderly and high-risk subjects. *Vaccine* 16, 1756–1760.

Treanor, J., and Falsey, A. (1999). Respiratory viral infections in the elderly. *Antiviral Res.* 44, 79–102.

Treanor, J.J., Kotloff, K., Betts, R.f., Belshe, R.B., Newman, F., Iacuzio, D., Wittes, J., Bryant, M. (2000). Evaluation of trivalent, live, cold-adapted (CAIV-T) and inactivated (TIV) influenza vaccines in prevention of virus infection and illness following challenge of adults with wild-type influenza A (H1N1), A (H3N2), and B viruses. *Vaccine* 18, 899–906.

Tripp, R.A., Jones, L.P., Haynes, L.M., Zheng, H., Murphy, P.M., and Anderson, L.J. (2001). CX3C chemokine mimicry by respiratory syncytial virus G glycoprotein. *Nat. Immunol.* 2, 732–738.

Varga, S.M., and Braciale, T.J. (2002). RSV-induced immunopathology: dynamic interplay between the virus and host immune response. *Virology* 295, 203–207.

Varga, S.M., Wissinger, E.L., and Braciale, T.J. (2000). The attachment (G) glycoprotein of respiratory syncytial virus contains a single immunodominant epitope that elicits both Th1 and Th2 CD4+ T cell responses. *J. Immunol.* 165, 6487–6495.

Walsh, E.E., Falsey, A.R., and Hennessey, P.A. (1999). Respiratory syncytial and other viral infections in persons with chronic cardiopulmonary disease. *Am. J. Respir. Crit. Care Med.* 160, 791–795.

Watanabe, T., Watanabe, S., Kida, H., and Kawaoka, Y. (2002). Influenza A virus with defective M2 ion channel activity as a live vaccine. *Virology* 299, 266–270.

Webster, R.G. (2000). Immunity to influenza in the elderly. *Vaccine* 18, 1686–1689.

Wherry, E.J., Teichgraber, V., Becker, T.C., Masopust, D., Kaech, S.M., Antia, R., Von Andrian, U.H., Ahmed, R. (2003). Lineage relationship and protective immunity of memory CD8 T cell subsets. *Nat. Immunol.* 4, 225–234.

Woodland, D.L. (2003). Cell-mediated immunity to respiratory virus infections. *Curr. Opin. Immunol.* 15, 336–342.

Wright, P.F., Karron, R.A., Belshe, R.B., Thompson, J., Crowe, J.E., Jr., Boyce, T.G., Halburnt, L.L., Reed, G.W., Whitehead, S.S., Anderson, E.L., Wittek, A.E., Casey, R., Eichelberger, M., Thumar, B., Randolph, V.B., Udem, S.A., Chanock, R.M., and Murphy, B.R. (2000). Evaluation of a live, cold-passaged, temperature-sensitive, respiratory syncytial virus vaccine candidate in infancy. *J. Infect. Dis.* 182, 1331–1342.

Wright, P.F., and Webster R.G. (2001). Orthomyxoviruses. In *Field's Virology I* (eds. D.M. Knipe and P.M. Howley). Philadelphia: Lippincott-Raven, 1443–1485.

Mucosal Immunity and Vaccines Against Simian Immunodeficiency Virus and Human Immunodeficiency Virus

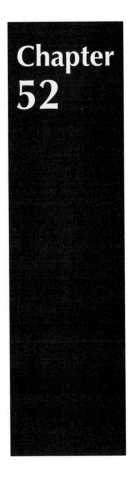

M. Juliana McElrath

Program in Infectious Diseases, Clinical Research Division, Fred Hutchinson Cancer Research Center, and Department of Medicine, University of Washington, Seattle, Washington

Christopher J. Miller

Center for Comparative Medicine and Department of Veterinary Pathology, Microbiology, and Immunology, School of Veterinary Medicine, and California National Primate Research Center, University of California at Davis, Davis, California

INTRODUCTION: THE GLOBAL HIV EPIDEMIC

The human immunodeficiency virus (HIV) pandemic grows unabated, with 38 million people living with HIV in 2003 (World Health Organization, Joint United Nations Program on HIV/AIDS). Approximately 14,000 new infections occur daily, and in adults, transmission occurs mainly through sexual contact. Nearly half of these new infections occur in women, and each of these women has the potential to transmit the virus to her children. Oral exposure is an important route for mother-to-child HIV-1 transmission (Gaillard *et al.*, 2000; Goedert *et al.*, 1991; Mandelbrot *et al.*, 1999). Thus, mucosal transmission accounts for the vast majority of HIV infections, and a vaccine capable of preventing HIV infection will need to induce mucosal anti-HIV immune responses at the mucosal sites of HIV entry.

Extensive efforts to prevent HIV transmission have focused on education and counseling, screening blood donors, use of condoms and other barriers, needle-exchange programs, and testing of topical microbicides. Clearly, these measures have led to reduction in frequencies of new infections in some populations at risk. In addition, the administration of antiretroviral agents to mothers during the peripartum period and more important to infants at birth

can markedly reduce vertical transmission. Despite ongoing implementation of these beneficial procedures, almost 5 million new infections occurred during 2003, and there is evidence that this trend will continue unless an effective vaccine becomes available. Clearly, the best long-term global strategy to control HIV infection is through the development and implementation of a safe and efficacious HIV-1 vaccine.

Development of an HIV-1 vaccine presents a challenge not previously encountered with an infectious disease. The hallmark of HIV-1 infection lies in its propensity to infect and consequently deplete CD4-positive (CD4+) T cells, either by direct or indirect mechanisms. This leads to the inevitable morbidity related to opportunistic infections and neoplasms and the host's eventual demise. Untreated HIV-1 infection, with rare exceptions, is lethal. Thus, a vaccine that will protect against disease must either strictly prevent infection or rapidly control replication. This requirement is unlike that for other vaccines against viral infections of public health importance. With other viral pathogens, the major strategy has been to protect against disease and not to prevent infection. There is no known example of a vaccine that elicits sterilizing immunity in humans, and it is unreasonable to expect that an HIV vaccine will impart sterilizing immunity. Moreover, there is general acceptance that even a partially effective vaccine that can control infection and prevent deterioration of the immune system can have a powerful effect on the epidemic.

One of the major difficulties in developing a global HIV-1 vaccine is the marked genetic variability of HIV-1. The lack of proofreading activity during reverse transcription leads to approximately one nucleotide substitution in each newly produced virion (Bebenek et al., 1989). Deletions, insertions, duplication, and recombination events also occur and with increased frequency in the setting of high viral loads and high rates of replication. Further diversity arises in response to immune pressure, either by HIV-1-specific antibodies or by CD8⁺ cytotoxic T lymphocytes (CTLs). Together, these events lead to approximately 10% genetic alteration in an infected individual over the course of infection (Korber et al., 2001). Twenty percent to 30% differences exist in the nucleotide sequences of HIV envelope genes in the HIV-1 subtypes that account for the global epidemic. Thus, the development of one global vaccine that can protect against all HIV-1 subtypes may not be feasible.

One goal of HIV vaccine development is to elicit immune responses that attack HIV-1 immediately after deposition onto the genital mucosa and prior to widespread systemic dissemination. To do this, an effective anti-HIV response must be present in the genital and gastrointestinal mucosa to combat HIV-1 as it enters the host. Knowledge of the nature of the transmitting virus, the cells first targeted for infection, the pathways of HIV-1 spread, and the immune response that can rapidly contain infection must be understood in order to develop a successful HIV-1 vaccine. These aspects will be discussed in detail later, and we will summarize information gained from humans with HIV-1 infection and from significant studies in the rhesus macaque (Macaca mulata) model of simian immunodeficiency virus (SIV) infection. We will then highlight investigations that are particularly noteworthy with respect to candidate HIV-1 vaccines that target the mucosal immune system.

HIV-1 TRANSMISSION

Epidemiology

Recent studies among discordant couples (one sexual partner HIV-infected, the other partner uninfected) in Uganda provide insight into the factors involved in HIV-1 transmission (Quinn et al., 2000; Gray et al., 2001). Rates of HIV-1 transmission from infected male to female versus infected female to male were similar (12.0 and 11.6 per 100 person-years, respectively). The major determinant in predicting risk of transmission was the plasma HIV RNA (vRNA) level in the infected partner. Transmission was rare when plasma vRNA levels were <1500 copies/mL (Quinn et al., 2000); the probability of HIV-1 transmission per coital heterosexual act was 0.0011 (95% confidence interval [CI], 0.0008–0.0015). Transmission rates per coital act were higher if the plasma vRNA levels were high in the infected partner or if either partner had genital ulcerative disease (Gray et al., 2001). Further HIV-1 acquisition was reduced among males cir-

cumcised before puberty, but this observation may be confounded by cultural and behavioral factors (Gray et al., 2001).

Transmission of HIV-1 also occurs through the oral mucosa of neonates by ingestion of amnionic fluid in utero or ingestion of fluids in the birth canal during delivery (Mandelbrot et al., 1999). In addition, infants can acquire infection during breastfeeding from their infected mothers (Embree et al., 2000). In one study, the overall frequency of HIV-1 transmission through breastfeeding was 16%, and the majority of infections were observed within the first 6 months of life. Higher levels of secretory leukocyte protease inhibitor in saliva are associated with reduced transmission of HIV-1 to infants through breast milk (Farquhar et al., 2002). Additional studies indicate that oral HIV-1 exposure may lead to systemic infection in adults as well as infants (Faruque et al., 1996; Wallace et al., 1997).

Host factors that influence vaginal HIV transmission

Epidemiologic studies suggest that the rate of male-to-female HIV transmission is higher in Africa and Asia than it is in the United States and Europe. Heterosexual HIV transmission is estimated to occur 5.6 times more frequently per exposure in Thailand than in the United States (Kunanusont et al., 1995). While differences in transmission efficiency may be due in part to viral factors (Kunanusont et al., 1995), host factors have a significant impact, and these include practices or conditions that damage the cervicovaginal epithelium or induce genital tract inflammation. Notably, the use of vaginal irritants or drying agents during sexual intercourse (reviewed in Strathdee et al., 1996), bacterial vaginosis (BV) (Sewankambo et al., 1997), and sexually transmitted diseases (STDs) (reviewed in Miller et al., 1993) can alter mucosal integrity and induce inflammation. Proinflammatory cytokines increase CCR5 expression in human peripheral blood mononuclear cells (PBMCs) and CD4⁺ T cells (Patterson, et al., 1999; Syrbe et al., 1999), and inflammation increases the expression of viral receptors and co-receptors on the resident target cells in mucosal surfaces (Kabashima et al., 2002). Oral contraceptive use also increases CCR5 expression on cervical T cells of healthy women (Prakash et al., 2002). In addition, genital tract inflammation increases the number of activated potential HIV target cells within the mucosa by recruitment and activation of immune cells from the circulation (reviewed in Douek et al., 2003). Furthermore, inflammation may lead to ulceration, eliminating the barrier effects of an intact epithelium and directly exposing the full range of lamina propria target cells to infectious virus.

In the United States, prior to the initiation of semen donor screening, donor insemination accounted for HIV transmission in up to 141 women (Wortley et al., 1998). In one study, four of eight women acquired HIV infection through insemination with cryopreserved semen from one asymptomatic HIV-infected donor (Stewart et al., 1985). Thus, HIV can be transmitted during an atraumatic clinical procedure, which strongly suggests that adequate numbers of HIV target cells are in the intact genital mucosal epithelium. In addition,

HIV was transmitted by vaginal intercourse to a woman who congenitally lacked a cervix and uterus (Kell *et al.*, 1992). In the primate model of AIDS, intravaginal SIV inoculation results in systemic infection (Miller *et al.*, 1989; Miller *et al.*, 1998; Miller *et al.*, 1994), and SIV is efficiently transmitted to hysterectomized female macaques by inoculation of cell-free virus into vaginal pouches (Miller *et al.*, 1992a; Miller *et al.*, 1993). Thus, the SIV monkey model data and human epidemiologic evidence suggest that HIV can enter through the intact mucosal epithelium of the cervix and vagina.

Characteristics of susceptible and permissive HIV target cells

HIV target cells must permit the fusion of the virus membrane and cell membrane by the sequential interaction of the virus envelope glycoproteins (gp120) with cell surface CD4 and one of two chemokine (CC) receptor molecules, CXCR4 or CCR5. Expression of these CC receptors can confer susceptibility *in vitro* to previously HIV-resistant CD4+ T cells (Alkhatib *et al.*, 1996; Deng *et al.*, 1996; Dragic *et al.*, 1996). The expression of CCR5 has been shown to be critical for HIV infection, and individuals expressing a homozygous deletion mutation in the CCR5 gene have a greatly reduced rate of HIV infection (Dean *et al.*, 1996; Liu *et al.*, 1996).

Productive HIV infection occurs in macrophages, T cells, and dendritic cells (DCs). In addition, DCs can bind HIV to their cell surface without becoming infected and can maintain or even enhance viral infectivity in T cell cocultures. This ability is linked to expression of the C-type lectin receptor DC-SIGN (DC-specific intercellular adhesion molecule [ICAM]–grabbing nonintegrin) by mature human dendritic cells (Geijtenbeek *et al.*, 2000; Pohlmann *et al.*, 2001). It is becoming clear that DC-SIGN is one of a number of C-type lectin receptors that are capable of binding HIV to human DCs (Turville *et al.*, 2001). DC-SIGN plays no discernable role in the ability of macaque DCs to capture and transmit lentivirus infection (Wu *et al.*, 2002). Thus, the ability of HIV to effectively use DCs in virus transmission without becoming directly infected may be dependent upon a range of cell-surface receptors in addition to DC-SIGN.

Epithelial barriers of mucosal surfaces

The mucosa of the oral cavity, esophagus, oropharynx, anus, vagina, and ectocervix consists of a stratified squamous epithelium resting on an indistinct lamina propria and an underlying vascular submucosa **(Fig. 52.1)**. This multilayered structure can be 20–45 cells thick and comprises four zones: the basal, squamous, granular and cornified layers (Robboy *et al.*, 1992). Intercellular desmosomes and amorphous lipoidal material within the cornified and granular layers restrict passive diffusion of molecules into the deeper layers of the epithelium (King, 1983; Shattock *et al.*, 2000). As they migrate upward from the dividing cells of the germinal basal layer, epithelial cells become flattened and keratinized with small pyknotic nuclei. The rectum, colon, and endocervix consist of a mucus-secreting, simple columnar epithelium covering a vascular lamina propria. Mucus may act as a barrier to infected cells, and it contains proteins with anti-HIV-1 activity, including secretory leukocyte protease inhibitors (Moriyama *et al.*, 1999) and, potentially, anti-HIV antibodies.

Organization of immune cells in the female reproductive tract

The mucosal immune system in the lower female genital tract consists of a resident population of DCs, monocytes/macrophages, T cells, and B cells in the lamina propria of the vagina and cervix. Collections of lymphocytes are occasionally found in the lamina propria, and CD20+ B cells are relatively common in these nodules (Ma *et al.*, 2001; Miller *et al.*, 1992b), forming a mucosa-associated lymphoreticular tissue (MALT). CD8+ T cells comprise over 60% of the total T cells in the cervicovaginal mucosa and are common in the deep layers of the vaginal epithelium or in the superficial lamina propria (Edwards and Morris, 1985; Fawcett, 1986; Ma *et al.*, 2001; Miller *et al.*, 1992b). Detailed studies of immune cell distribution in monkeys demonstrated that the density of T cells and Langerhans cells (LCs) but not B cells is higher in the distal vagina than in the ectocervix and that the immune cell populations of the lower genital tract remain stable through the menstrual cycle (Ma *et al.*, 2001).

Because of the difficulty in obtaining human samples, similarly detailed studies in normal-cycling women have not been undertaken. LCs are abundant in the epithelial layer of the vaginal and ectocervical mucosa of women (Bjercke *et al.*, 1983; Morris *et al.*, 1983) and rhesus macaques (Ma *et al.*, 2001; Miller *et al.*, 1992b), and they are especially frequent in the vulva. Cervicovaginal T cells are predominantly TCR αβ+, CD45RO+, CD69+, CD28+, CD29+, CD44+, and CD62L−, and more CD8+ T cells (63%) than CD4+ T cells (32%) express CD103 (Hladik *et al.*, 1999b). The frequencies of various lymphocyte subsets are stable at all stages of the menstrual cycle (Ma *et al.*, 2001; Patton *et al.*, 2000).

The antigen-presenting cells (APCs) of the genital mucosa include the intraepithelial CD1a+, MHC class II+, fascin-bundling protein (p55)+, CD11c+, CD123−, DC-SIGN−, CD4+ LCs and the CD1a−, MHC II+, p55+, DC-SIGN+, CD4+ DCs in the lamina propria of the mucosa. In addition, MHC II+/CD4+ macrophages (MØs) and MHC II+ B cells are present in the vaginal mucosa and probably act as APCs (Ma *et al.*, 2001). In the rectum, there are numerous DC-SIGN+ cells at all levels of the mucosa (Jameson *et al.*, 2002), including directly beneath epithelial cells.

In general, T cells, MØs, DCs, and LCs can express CXCR4 and CCR5 (Lee *et al.*, 1999; Rubbert *et al.*, 1998; Weissman *et al.*, 1997; Zaitseva *et al.*, 1997; Zoeteweij and Blauvelt, 1998); however, expression levels are dependent upon the localized cytokine milieu and cellular differentiation. Studies using immunohistochemical techniques have shown that CCR5 and CXCR4 expression levels are very low in women without genital tract inflammation, with positive cells predominantly localized to the lamina propria (Rottman *et al.*, 1997; Zhang *et al.*, 1998). However, CCR5

A. Epithelial barriers that HIV must cross to reach mucosal target cells

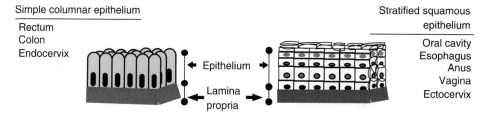

Simple columnar epithelium

Rectum
Colon
Endocervix

← Epithelium →

← Lamina propria →

Stratified squamous
epithelium

Oral cavity
Esophagus
Anus
Vagina
Ectocervix

B. Routes used by HIV to traverse the epithelial barriers

Simple columnar epithelium

Epithelial disruption
Trauma
Inflammation
M cell transfer
Epithelial cell transcytosis
DC/IEL infection

Stratified squamous epithelium

Epithelial disruption
Trauma
Inflammation
DC infection

C. Mucosal HIV target cells

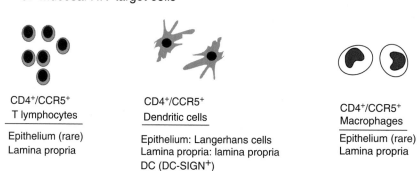

CD4⁺/CCR5⁺
T lymphocytes

Epithelium (rare)
Lamina propria

CD4⁺/CCR5⁺
Dendritic cells

Epithelium: Langerhans cells
Lamina propria: lamina propria
DC (DC-SIGN⁺)

CD4⁺/CCR5⁺
Macrophages

Epithelium (rare)
Lamina propria

Fig. 52.1. Mucosal epithelial barriers and target cells in HIV transmission. To enter the host and infect target cells expressing the appropriate viral receptors, HIV must penetrate mucosal surfaces that are covered by either simple columnar or stratified squamous epithelia. If the epithelia are intact, then intraepithelial dendritic cells (DCs) sampling luminal contents can become infected and carry the infection to lamina propria lymphoid nodules and draining lymph nodes where large numbers of HIV target cells reside. Once HIV is in lymphoid tissues, viral replication ensues. If the epithelia are compromised, virus has direct access to target cells in the lamina propria; these include HIV-infected migratory DCs that can carry the virus to lymphoid nodules and draining lymph nodes.

expression on T cells, MØs, and DCs is likely to be increased in women with vaginitis (Rottman *et al.*, 1997). Furthermore, studies using flow cytometric methods showed that CCR5⁺ CD4⁺ T cells were commonly found in the cervicovaginal tissue of women without genital tract inflammation (Hladik *et al.*, 1999a, b). Thus, mucosal inflammation may be key in recruiting additional target cells for HIV-1 and rendering the local cell population susceptible to HIV infection. The other mucosal surfaces that HIV crosses to gain access to the body have a population of immune cells and thus of HIV target cells that is similar to that of the female genital tract (Fig. 52.1), although the level of organization and the density of the immune cells can vary widely from one anatomic site to another, as described in detail elsewhere in this textbook.

In vitro studies of mucosal HIV transmission
CD4⁺ T cells and macrophages support HIV replication *in vitro*. Activated CD4⁺ T cells are susceptible to HIV iso-

lates that use CXCR4 (X4), CCR5 (R5), or both (dual tropic), but macrophages are predominantly susceptible to CCR5-utilizing virus. HIV can also infect DCs (Patterson and Knight, 1987) and LCs (Kawamura *et al.*, 2000), which permit much higher levels of virus replication *in vitro* than T cells without the usual cytopathic effects associated with HIV infection (Blauvelt *et al.*, 1997; Langhoff *et al.*, 1991; Macdonald *et al.*, 2002). Furthermore, others demonstrated that DCs derived from the noninflamed cervicovaginal mucosa support replication of both X4 and R5 HIV-1 variants (Hladik *et al.*, 1999a). After *in vitro* infection of cells emigrated from vaginal mucosa, HIV-1 particles were found budding from DC cytoplasmic membranes, and some DCs had intracellular inclusions typical of HIV-1 replication by electron microscopy (Hladik *et al.*, 1999a) **(Fig. 52.2)**. In contrast, mature DCs appear refractory to HIV infection, but they efficiently capture infectious HIV via surface receptors, including DC-SIGN, leading to robust HIV replication in T cell–DC conjugates (Geijtenbeek *et al.*, 2000). Thus, all

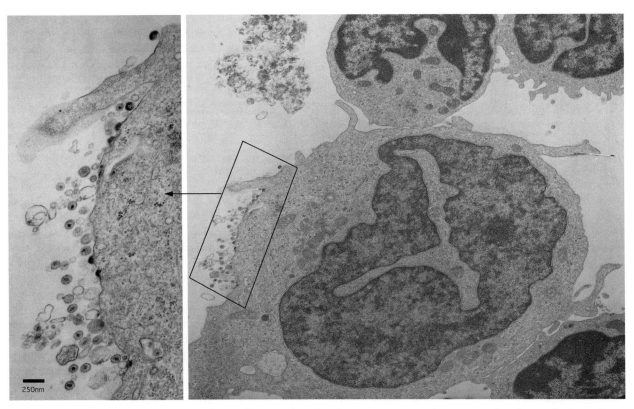

Fig. 52.2. Electron micrograph of a genital dendritic cell (DC) infected with HIV-1Ba-L. Vaginal tissue was placed in media for 36 hours, and emigrated mononuclear cells were infected with HIV-1Ba-L at a multiplicity of infection (MOI) of 0.5. After 4 additional days of culture, cells were processed for electron microscopy. The picture shows a conjugate of one DC with two lymphocytes demonstrating productive HIV-1 infection of the DC (X5000). Inset: higher magnification of a portion of the DC shows assembly and budding of retroviral particles in the productively infected DC (X40,000). Note the characteristic morphology of the lentiviral particles (photomicrograph courtesy of F. Hladik, University of Washington, Seattle).

of the CD4$^+$ cell types found in mucosal surfaces can either directly support HIV replication *in vitro* or efficiently transfer infectious virus to susceptible partners.

Although early studies suggested that CD4-negative vaginal and cervical epithelial cells were targets of HIV (Phillips and Bourinbaiar, 1992), more recent studies employing primary cervical and vaginal epithelial cells have failed to demonstrate their susceptibility to infection. In addition, infectious virions are unable to transcytose through these primary genital epithelial cells (Dezzutti *et al.*, 2001; Greenhead *et al.*, 2000) but in recent models this capacity appears intact (Hladik *et al.*, unpublished). HIV can transcytose from the apical to basolateral surface of human intestinal and endometrial cell lines (Hocini and Bomsel, 1999). Using CXCR4 and galactosyl cerebroside (GalCer) receptors on the apical surface of M cells, R4 HIV strains cross Caco-2 M cell monolayers and infect underlying CD4$^+$ T cells. The Caco-2 M cells must be transfected with the CCR5 co-receptor gene to permit passage of R5 HIV variants (Fotopoulos *et al.*, 2002). *In vivo*, CCR5 and GalCer, but not CXCR4, are expressed on the luminal side of human follicular-associated epithelium enterocytes (FAEs) and M cells (Fotopoulos *et al.*, 2002). Thus, rectal or duodenal HIV transmission may involve

transepithelial transport of virus by M cells. Primary human jejunal epithelial cells express CCR5 and these cells transfer R5 HIV to the basolateral surface, probably through endocytic uptake and transcytosis of HIV (Meng *et al.*, 2002). Thus, transcytosis of virus by epithelial cells may have a role to play in transmission of HIV across the gastrointestinal mucosa, but the process is less clear across the female reproductive tract or the upper gastrointestinal (GI) tract.

Ex vivo (explant) studies of mucosal HIV transmission

Human skin has been utilized as an *in vitro* model for the movement of HIV across the genital tract epithelium and into the lamina propria (Kawamura *et al.*, 2000; Reece *et al.*, 1998). In this system, HIV productively infects LCs within 4–6 days of virus inoculation onto an intact cornified layer of the epidermis. Cervical explant culture systems (Collins *et al.*, 2000; Greenhead *et al.*, 2000) using biopsy or postoperative cervical tissue from healthy premenopausal women become infected upon addition of cell-free or cell-associated X4 or R5 HIV strains. There is no evidence of migration of donor-labeled or infected cells into the epithelium of these systems, as has been reported to occur in progesterone-treated mice (Ibata *et al.*, 1997; Zacharopoulos *et al.*, 1997). Subepithelial T cells and MØs are the predominant cell types productively infected in these explant systems at 6–7 days postinoculation. HIV-infected epithelial cells or DCs are not seen, nor is there any evidence that epithelial transcytosis is a mechanism of HIV transfer across genital epithelia, which is consistent with findings of some *in vitro* studies using primary epithelial cells. Immune activation (e.g., stimulation with PHA and IL-2) dramatically increased the replication of primary and T-cell tropic strains (Greenhead *et al.*, 2000), while others found that 20%–30% of cervical samples were resistant to infection (Collins *et al.*, 2000). These data suggest that infection of cervical tissue is critically influenced by the activation state of resident immune cells.

Animal studies of mucosal HIV transmission

To initiate an infection, HIV must cross the epithelial barrier of the genital tract. The first site of HIV infection in the female genital tract is presumed to be the vagina and/or cervix. Target cells in the vaginal mucosa are the only known requirement for SIV transmission, as removal of the cervix and upper genital tract does not alter susceptibility of monkeys to atraumatic vaginal SIV inoculation (Miller *et al.*, 1992a). Exogenous estrogen administration decreases the efficiency of SIV transmission after intravaginal inoculation (Smith *et al.*, 2000), and chronic exogenous progesterone administration increases transmission efficiency (Marx *et al.*, 1996). These effects have been attributed to the hormone-dependent changes in epithelial thickness. However, these hormones also have profound effects on innate and adaptive immune function in women (Lu, submitted for publication) and rhesus macaques (Lu *et al.*, 2002) that may influence transmission.

Intravaginal transmission of SIV to macaques is efficient when cell-free virus is used as the inoculum, but inoculation of SIV-infected cells rarely produces systemic infection. Intravaginal inoculation with 10^5 infected cells produced systemic infection in only one of two monkeys, and all monkeys resisted infection after inoculation with less than 10^5 infected cells (Sodora *et al.*, 1998; Miller, unpublished). The relatively low infectivity of SIV-infected cells parallels observations from *ex vivo* studies using human cervical tissue, suggesting that HIV-infected cells merely provide a transient source for production of infectious virions within the cervicovaginal lumen (Collins *et al.*, 2000; Greenhead *et al.*, 2000). Dual-tropic or T-cell tropic SIV isolates (Greenier *et al.*, 2001) and R5- or X4-using simian HIV (SHIV) (Harouse *et al.*, 2001) cause systemic infection after vaginal inoculation of rhesus monkeys. In fact, the only virologic measure that predicts intravaginal infectivity is the relative ability of viruses to replicate *in vivo* after intravenous inoculation (*in vivo* replication capacity). Viruses with a high *in vivo* replication capacity are more efficient at producing systemic infection after intravaginal inoculation than are viruses with low replication capacity (Miller *et al.*, 1998).

Several investigators have attempted to define the early events in vaginal SIV infections. Within 48 hours, SIV-infected cells are present in the lamina propria of the cervicovaginal mucosa (Spira *et al.*, 1996). In this study, putative DCs were similarly located in adjacent tissue sections, suggesting that DCs were early target cells in vaginal SIV transmission. Others demonstrated that SIV enters the vaginal mucosa of rhesus macaques within 60 minutes of intravaginal exposure and SIV-infected cells are found in the vaginal epithelium and lamina propria within 18 hours (Hu *et al.*, 2000). SIV-infected cells in the lamina propria are predominantly CD3+ T cells with both activated and quiescent phenotypes and less common CD68+ MØs (Hu *et al.*, 2000; Zhang *et al.*, 1998). In the epithelium, 50%–90% of the SIV-infected cells are LCs (Hu *et al.*, 2000). These SIV-infected cells (presumably LCs) are present in the subcapsular sinus of the genital tract lymph nodes at 18 and 24 hours (Hu *et al.*, 2000). Furthermore, in a mouse model, HIV-1 is transported by LCs to the draining lymph nodes within 24 hours after intravaginal inoculation (Masurier *et al.*, 1998). Taken together, these findings provide one clear explanation of how HIV crosses the intact stratified squamous epithelial barrier of the lower female genital tract. Of course, if breaks in the epithelial barrier occur, then the virus will have direct access to T cells, DCs, and MØs in the lamina propria, which may explain the productive infection of lamina propria T cells and MØs within 18 hours of SIV inoculation (Hu *et al.*, 2000). In fact, there was a correlation between the level of inflammation, the number of histologically detectable breaks/10 µm of vaginal epithelium, and the ability to detect SIV DNA in genital and systemic tissues in the initial hours and days after vaginal SIV inoculation (C.J. Miller and A. Haase, unpublished).

After rectal inoculation of macaques, SIV replication was first observed in T cells and macrophages in the paracolic lymph nodes prior to systemic dissemination (Couedel-Courteille *et al.*, 1999). This stepwise dissemination pattern following intrarectal infection was distinct from intravenous infection, in which the infection spread simultaneously to all lymph nodes (Couedel-Courteille *et al.*, 1999). Similarly, after tonsillar inoculation, SIV first infects T cells and MØs in the subepithelial lymphoid aggregates of the mucosa (Stahl-Hennig *et al.*, 1999).

Findings in mucosal tissues from HIV-infected patients

HIV-infected MØs, T cells, and DCs can be detected in the female genital tract during chronic infection (Nuovo *et al.*, 1993; Pomerantz *et al.*, 1988). HIV-infected LCs are found in the vaginal mucosa of asymptomatic women infected with HIV-1 subtype E (Bhoopat *et al.*, 2001) and in the oral mucosa of infected patients (Chou *et al.*, 2000). As yet there has been no definitive demonstration *in vivo* of HIV-infected genital tract epithelial cells. Both infectious HIV and viral DNA can be detected in the rectal mucosa of HIV-infected patients, indicating ongoing viral replication, which is associated with higher levels of proinflammatory cytokines than in the rectal mucosa of healthy controls (Di Stefano *et al.*, 2001).

Summary of biology of mucosal HIV transmission

The events following mucosal HIV-1 exposure that lead to systemic infection require the interaction of both host and viral factors. HIV transmission, as defined by virus crossing the epithelial barrier and productively infecting a permissive target cell, may occur through several nonexclusive mechanisms (Fig. 52.1 and **Fig. 52.3**). Vaginal tears in the epithelium can be detected histologically in >60% of women following consensual sexual intercourse (Novell *et al.*, 1984). Presumably, the extent of trauma to the simple columnar epithelium of the rectum during anal intercourse is much greater than to the stratified squamous epithelium of the vagina. Where microscopic or macroscopic defects in the mucosal epithelium occur, HIV has direct access to susceptible T cells, DCs, and MØs in the lamina propria. This may permit HIV to establish a local infection and/or may permit uptake of infectious virions by migratory DCs, followed by rapid dissemination (Fig. 52.3 and **Fig. 52.4**). In the vaginal mucosa of HIV-infected women and SIV-infected monkeys, LCs comprise the majority of infected cells in the epithelium

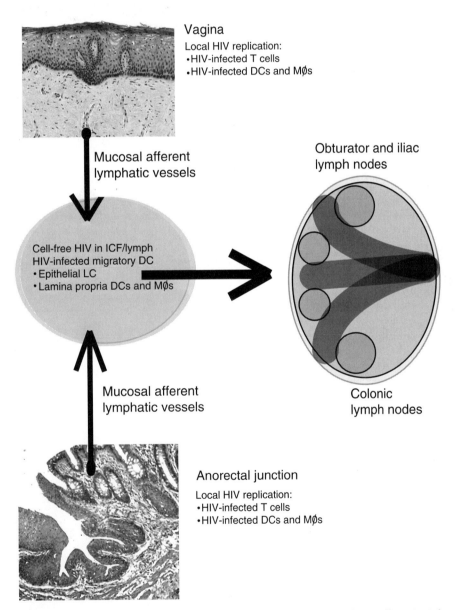

Fig. 52.3. HIV replication and initial dissemination from mucosal surfaces. Either migratory dendritic cells (DCs) infected by the initial inoculum or cell-free virus and infected cells produced by replication after an infection are established in the lamina propria, enter mucosal lymphatic vessels, and are carried to the draining lymph nodes. Migratory DCs and lymphocytes move to the T-cell-rich paracortex of the lymph node, where the infection spreads and expands. The fate of cell-free virus in the first few days postexposure is less certain, as there is no antigen-trapping of immune complex–bound virions by follicular DCs prior to the development of an antiviral antibody response at 10–14 days postinfection. However, it is likely that virions are carried by the flow of lymph through the paracortex toward the lymph node medulla.

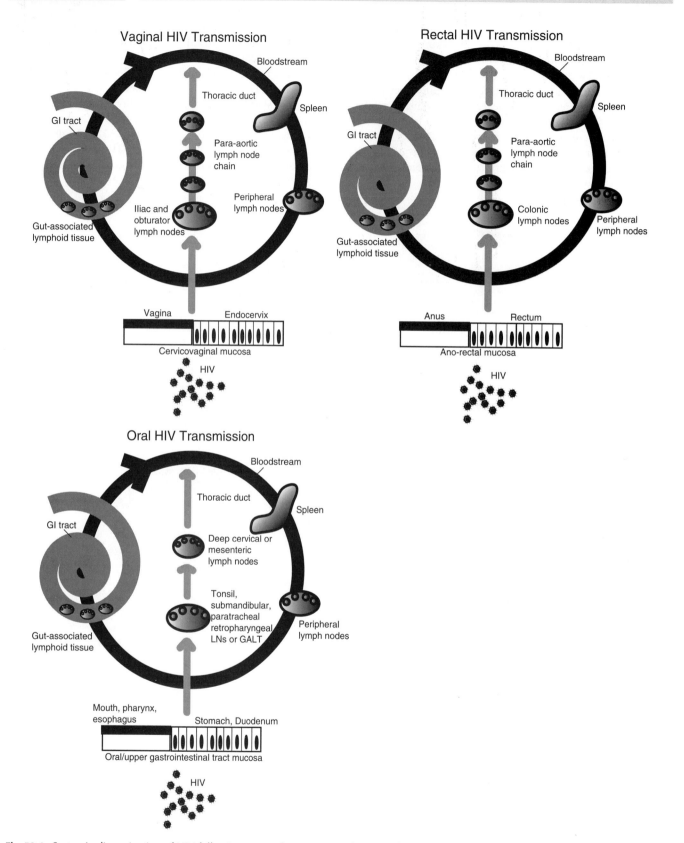

Fig. 52.4. Systemic dissemination of HIV following mucosal exposure. With HIV replication occurring in the mucosal site of transmission and draining lymph nodes, HIV-infected cells and virions move with the flow of lymph through a chain of lymph nodes to the thoracic duct where lymph enters the systemic circulation. Once in the bloodstream, HIV is rapidly disseminated to all lymphoid tissues, including the systemic lymphoid tissues and MALT.

and DCs represent 50% of the infected cells in the lamina propria (Bhoopat *et al.*, 2001; Hu *et al.*, 2000; Hu *et al.*, 1998). These findings strongly suggest that LCs play a part in HIV transmission across an intact genital mucosa. However, as sexual HIV transmission frequently occurs in the setting of an inflamed and friable mucosa, the extent of the role of LC in infection of the human genital tract requires further characterization.

Inflammation and immune activation play a critical role in HIV disease and transmission. The level of T cell activation in blood correlates with the decline in peripheral CD4$^+$ T cells as well as (and perhaps to an even greater extent than) plasma HIV RNA copy number (Leng *et al.*, 2001). The ability of HIV to replicate robustly in the first few hours after mucosal exposure is likely the single most important factor in determining if an exposure will result in systemic infection. Induction of high levels of proinflammatory cytokines occurs with mucosal infections. For example, TNF-α, IL-10, and IL-1β levels increase with BV and nonulcerative genital tract infections (Cohen *et al.*, 1999; Sturm-Ramirez *et al.*, 2000) and may be associated with amplification of local HIV replication in the first few hours after exposure. In addition, mucosal inflammation stimulates the production of chemokines that can recruit (Kabashima *et al.*, 2002) and activate HIV target cells (reviewed in Douek *et al.*, 2003) in the mucosa. Thus, inflammation-induced changes in the mucosa increase the interactions between HIV and target cells, increasing the susceptibility of the individual to HIV infection. This hypothesis is supported by epidemiological evidence linking STD prevalence with HIV seroconversion in adults (Grosskurth *et al.*, 1995) and the association between oral thrush and acquisition of HIV in infants (Embree *et al.*, 2000). Once infection commences, viral replication induces cytokine and CC expression by infected cells, including DCs (Izmailova *et al.*, 2003), leading to local inflammation in lymphoid tissues and recruitment of more target cells for replication to these tissues (Reinhart *et al.*, 2002). Thus, the goal of vaccination is to elicit specific antiviral immunity on mucosal surfaces yet avoid excessive concurrent inflammation that may be detrimental.

IMMUNE RESPONSES TO HIV/SIV INFECTION AT MUCOSAL SURFACES

Anti-HIV and anti-SIV antibodies in mucosal secretions

Numerous investigators have sought to understand the potential role of IgG and IgA antibodies in containing local HIV-1 replication. Overall, different profiles of HIV-specific antibodies occur within the GI and reproductive tracts among infected patients. Although differences are not surprising, discrepancies may be attributed to the methodologies for collection of specimens and detection of antibodies. Measurement of S-IgA in saliva has been hampered by its binding to components of culture supernatants containing HIV-recombinant proteins used in enzyme-linked immuno-

sorbent assay (ELISA) determinations (Jackson *et al.*, 2000). Thus, the technical challenges in measuring HIV-specific antibodies in human secretions should be considered when reviewing the relevant literature.

Gastrointestinal tract secretions

Anti-HIV antibodies are present in the GI tract secretions of HIV-infected patients (Mathewson *et al.*, 1994; Janoff *et al.*, 1989; Janoff *et al.*, 1994; Raux *et al.*, 1999), and large numbers of anti-HIV antibody-forming cells (AFCs), both IgG and IgA, are present in the duodenum and rectum of HIV-infected individuals (Eriksson *et al.*, 1995; Eriksson *et al.*, 1998; Schneider *et al.*, 1997; Schneider *et al.*, 1998). One blinded study of HIV-1 anti-Env antibody in rectal washes from 16 infected and 14 uninfected donors at six laboratories revealed that HIV-1-specific IgA antibodies were absent in most samples (Wright *et al.*, 2002). Despite a 10-fold lower level of total IgG than IgA, HIV-1-specific IgG rather than IgA was more commonly detected in infected individuals.

Saliva and breast milk

A number of studies have shown that anti-HIV antibodies are present in saliva of HIV-infected people, and although some anti-HIV S-IgA antibodies are present, IgG antibodies are the predominant immunoglobulin isotype of the HIV-specific antibodies in saliva (Jackson *et al.*, 2000; Artenstein *et al.*, 1997; Moja *et al.*, 2000; Raux *et al.*, 1999; Skott *et al.*, 1999; Archibald *et al.*, 1987). Anti-HIV S-IgA is present in the breast milk of about 60% of infected women, but there is no association between the presence of these antibodies and the rates of HIV transmission to nursing infants (Belec *et al.*, 1990; Duprat *et al.*, 1994).

Cervicovaginal secretions

Both mucosally produced and plasma-derived antibodies contribute to the pool of immunoglobulin in female genital tract secretions to varying degrees (Kutteh *et al.*, 1996; Miller *et al.*, 1996). IgG plasma cells are abundant in the female genital tract of primates (Crowley-Nowick *et al.*, 1995; Eriksson *et al.*, 1998; Lu *et al.*, 2002; Ma *et al.*, 2001). Anti-HIV antibodies have been found in the cervicovaginal secretions (CVSs) (Archibald *et al.*, 1987; Belec *et al.*, 1990; Belec *et al.*, 1995; Belec *et al.*, 1996; Lü *et al.*, 1991; Lü *et al.*, 1993) of seropositive individuals. Anti-HIV IgG predominates in CVSs of HIV-infected women (Belec *et al.*, 1995; Lü *et al.*, 1993; Williams *et al.*, 2002) and SIV-infected rhesus macaques (Miller *et al.*, 1996; Miller *et al.*, 1997). The IgG antibodies in secretions are thought to be both locally produced and serum-derived (Kozlowski *et al.*, 1997; Kozlowski *et al.*, 2002; Quesnel *et al.*, 1997; Lü *et al.*, 2002). Anti-SIV antibodies are present in the vaginal secretions of SIV-infected, hysterectomized rhesus macaques with intact ovaries (Miller *et al.*, 1996), although the levels of both anti-SIV IgG and IgA antibodies were lower than in SIV-infected female macaques with intact uteri. As in intact animals, the levels of total and anti-SIV serum IgG were much higher than those of serum anti-SIV IgA. Thus, the bulk of the anti-SIV

IgG in vaginal secretions either is produced in or transudes through the mucosa of the upper genital tract (cervix, uterus). That anti-SIV IgA levels are less affected then anti-SIV IgG levels by the absence of the upper genital tract is more likely explained by significant local production of secreted IgA in the vaginal mucosa, but it can also be attributed to preferential transport of serum IgA into the vaginal secretions of the hysterectomized animals.

Sex steroid hormones are important in regulating both the systemic and secretory immune system (reviewed in Grossman, 1984). *In vitro*, estrogens enhance nonspecific differentiation of APCs (Paavonen *et al.*, 1981; Sthoeger *et al.*, 1988), and this estrogen-mediated enhancement is thought to be due to inhibition of suppressor T cells (Paavonen *et al.*, 1981). In rhesus macaques and women, immunoglobulin isotype and antibody levels in cervical mucus and vaginal fluid are relatively low around the time of ovulation (Jalanti and Isliker, 1977; Kutteh *et al.*, 1996; Lü *et al.*, 1999; Schumacher and Yang, 1977) and are relatively high during menstruation and the luteal phase. This fluctuation in antibody levels is not associated with shifts in mucosal immune cell populations, as the number of B cells in the cervicovaginal mucosa remains constant during the menstrual cycle (Ma *et al.*, 2001; Patton *et al.*, 2000). However, the menstrual cycle dramatically affects the ability of B cells to secrete immunoglobulin, as evidenced by the cyclic changes in the frequency of spontaneous immunoglobulin-secreting cells (ISCs) in all lymphoid tissues of female monkeys (Lü *et al.*, 2002) and in the PBMCs of women (Lü *et al.*, submitted). The addition of progesterone to PBMC cultures decreases the number of spontaneous or pokeweed mitogen–induced ISCs, while addition of estrogen increases the number of ISCs in a dose-dependent manner and through a mechanism that requires the presence of CD8+ T cells (Lü *et al.*, 2002). The effects of the menstrual cycle on immunoglobulin secretion need to be considered when assessing immune responses to HIV and HIV vaccines. Furthermore, because women of reproductive age using long-acting progestins for birth control are a critical target population for HIV vaccination, the effects of ovarian hormones on vaccine-induced immune responses may need to be considered in HIV vaccine design.

Several groups have reported HIV-specific IgA in the genital tract secretions of HIV-1-resistant female commercial sex workers and discordant partners of HIV-infected individuals, apparently occurring independently of HIV-specific T-helper lymphocyte responses (Kaul *et al.*, 1999; Mazzoli *et al.*, 1997). However, the presence of genital anti-HIV-specific antibodies in highly exposed seronegative sex workers has not been confirmed in other reports (Belec *et al.*, 1989; Buchacz *et al.*, 2001; Dorrell *et al.*, 2000; Skurnick *et al.*, 2002). As the assays to detect anti-HIV IgA are known to be problematic (Jackson *et al.*, 2000), it is possible that the differences in the methodologies used to detect mucosal antibodies account for the contradictory results of these studies. This conclusion is indirectly supported by studies in a macaque model with virologic and immunologic features of HIV-exposed seronegative sex workers. In this model, multiple vaginal wash samples from 10 monkeys with occult systemic SIV infections were examined for IgG and IgA antibodies to SIV (McChesney *et al.*, 1998). Occult SIV infections are characterized by a brief period in which SIV-infected PBMCs can be detected soon after inoculation (Miller *et al.*, 1994). However, this brief period of transient viremia is followed by a complete inability to detect SIV-infected PBMCs, the lack of serum anti-SIV antibodies (despite regular monthly to yearly assessments), and the presence of SIV-specific T cell proliferative responses (McChesney *et al.*, 1998). Although the clinical presentation of these animals is indistinguishable from "highly exposed HIV-resistant" sex workers, all these macaques lacked detectable anti-SIV antibodies in cervicovaginal secretions (McChesney *et al.*, 1998). This finding argues against mucosal antiviral antibody production in occult SIV-infected (persistently seronegative, transiently viremic) monkeys inoculated intravaginally with SIV and suggests that inconsistencies in the measurements of these responses in HIV-exposed seronegative women may account for the discrepancies in the aforementioned findings.

HIV- and SIV-specific cellular immune responses at mucosal surfaces

Numerous CD8+ T cells are present in the epithelium and lamina propria of the vagina and cervix of rhesus macaques and humans (Edwards and Morris, 1985; Ma *et al.*, 2001; Miller *et al.*, 1992b; Musey *et al.*, 1997b; Patton *et al.*, 2000; Roncalli *et al.*, 1988; Johansson *et al.*, 1999). Functional studies of CD8+ T cells isolated from the cervicovaginal mucosa of SIV-infected monkeys and HIV-infected women have shown that these cells include virus-specific CTLs (Lohman *et al.*, 1995; Musey *et al.*, 1997a; Shacklett *et al.*, 2000b). In addition, HIV-specific CTLs are present in the semen of HIV-infected patients (Musey *et al.*, 2003; Quayle *et al.*, 1998), and virus-specific CD8+ T cells are present in the gut of SIV-infected monkeys (Murphey-Corb *et al.*, 1999; Schmitz *et al.*, 2001) and HIV-infected patients (Musey *et al.*, 2003; Shacklett *et al.*, 2000a). HIV-1-specific CD8+ CTLs have been noted in the mucosa and PBMCs (Kaul *et al.*, 2000) of individuals repeatedly exposed to HIV-1 for years who do not have other evidence of systemic infection, and this has been interpreted as evidence that CTLs play a role in the control of HIV-1 replication.

The role of CTLs in conferring protection from HIV infection may be limited, as the role of the CTLs is to eliminate infected cells. Even in well-defined mouse models of CTL-mediated "viral clearance," CTLs cannot completely clear the viral infection (Ciurea *et al.*, 1999). There are no other known examples of infectious agents that can produce immune responses upon exposure but without infection of a host. Thus, the presence of anti-HIV CTLs in "exposed, uninfected" people is controversial. The most plausible explanation for these observations is that individuals with these responses are or have been HIV infected but that the level of infection and the site(s) of viral replication cannot be detected by means of standard clinical techniques and sporadically collected blood samples (Zhu et al., 2003).

HIV-1-specific CD8+ CTL lines and clones established from the blood, cervix, rectum, and semen were used to examine in vitro mechanisms of target cell lysis. These clones all demonstrated perforin-dependent lysis of HIV-1-expressing targets rather than Fas-FasL- or anti-TNF-mediated lysis (Musey et al., 2003). Clones from the mucosal sites and blood had similar epitope specificities and were frequently restricted by the same MHC class I molecules. Moreover, identical clonotypes were detected within the mucosal and systemic compartments of two patients, which indicates that the anti-HIV CTLs in the blood and mucosa can have a common origin and traffic between anatomically distinct compartments (Musey et al., 2003). Of note, HIV-1-specific CTLs were present in the mucosa regardless of whether or not plasma or mucosal HIV vRNA was detectable (Musey et al., 2003).

VACCINES TO ELICIT ANTI-HIV IMMUNITY AT MUCOSAL SURFACES

Is there a need for HIV vaccines to elicit mucosal immune responses?

As described previously in detail, HIV is a mucosally transmitted pathogen, and thus mucosal immune responses would seem to be beneficial for any HIV vaccine. Two studies in the SIV model found that systemically administered antisera (Joag et al., 1999) or attenuated SIV vaccines (Marthas et al., 1992) that protect monkeys from intravenous SIV challenge do not protect animals from mucosal SIV challenge. However, oral or subcutaneous immunization with an attenuated SHIV protects monkeys from vaginal challenge with pathogenic SHIV (Joag et al., 1998), and a large study found that there was no significant difference in the rates of protection from intravaginal SIV challenge between monkeys immunized with an attenuated SHIV vaccine by nasal or intravenous routes (Abel et al., 2003). It is interesting that monkeys immunized with this attenuated virus vaccine by the intravaginal route had delayed replication of the vaccine virus and the lowest rates of protection from subsequent intravaginal challenge with pathogenic SIV. It is important to note that "protection" in the previously mentioned studies is defined as inability to detect challenge virus and/or a reduction in plasma vRNA in vaccinated versus control monkeys (Abel et al., 2003). Plasma vRNA levels in monkeys and humans are highly predictive of clinical outcome (Hirsch et al., 1996; Mellors et al., 1995, 1996) and of the likelihood of mucosal HIV transmission to an uninfected partner (Mandelbrot et al., 1999; Quinn et al., 2000). Thus, if the observed reduction in plasma vRNA levels after vaccination in monkeys can be duplicated by immunization with an HIV vaccine in people, then the rates of HIV transmission would potentially decline and the pandemic would be significantly blunted. If this is the goal of HIV vaccination, then strong systemic anti-HIV immune responses may

be sufficient to elicit this level of protection, and specific strategies to elicit mucosal immune responses may not be necessary.

If the goal of vaccination is to prevent infection with HIV, then anti-HIV-specific immunity in the mucosa at the portal of entry will likely be critical to the success of the vaccine. As CD8+ T cells produce antiviral cytokines and chemokines that may reduce HIV replication, their central role is to recognize and lyse cells after they have become infected with HIV. Thus, innate antiviral immune responses in mucosal tissues or anti-HIV neutralizing antibodies in mucosal secretions and interstitial fluid offer the best defense in preventing HIV infection in mucosally exposed individuals (**Fig. 52.5**). Innate immune responses may render cells resistant to viral replication, and neutralizing antibodies may inhibit the interaction of HIV with receptors or block preintegration steps in the HIV replication cycle. Thus, S-IgA antibodies can neutralize virus within mucosal epithelial cells, in the mucosal interstitium, or in the lumen prior to binding to target cells (reviewed in Mazanec et al., 1993). In summary, induction of anti-HIV S-IgA, neutralizing anti-HIV envelope IgG, and innate antiviral effector molecules at the sites of mucosal transmission may be the most effective strategy to prevent HIV infection by vaccination.

Routes of immunization

In developing vaccines to prevent mucosal HIV transmission, it is worth noting that the anatomic site of the immune response to HIV vaccine antigens could be as critical as the immunogenicity of the HIV vaccine antigens. It is not known which routes are optimal to induce mucosal antibody responses to HIV-1, as few studies have addressed the induction of these responses in monkeys or humans. It has become increasingly clear that the well-described "common" mucosal immune system of mice that results in antigen-specific response at multiple mucosal sites remote from the site of mucosal immunization is not well developed in primates. In fact, the mucosal immune system of primates seems to be much more compartmentalized than in mice. In one study, oral immunization of rhesus monkeys with SIV subunit vaccine formulated with cholera toxin adjuvant induced rectal and systemic immune responses, but no antigen-specific antibodies were detected in cervicovaginal secretions (Kubota et al., 1997). In addition, intranasal immunization of rhesus monkeys with the same SIV subunit vaccine and adjuvant elicited higher antibody titers in the vagina than did oral immunization (Imaoka et al., 1998; Kubota et al., 1997). Vaccines containing killed vibrios and cholera toxin B subunit (CT-B) or CT-B alone have been used to compare the induction of antibodies by various mucosal immunization routes in women (Kozlowski et al., 1997; Kozlowski et al., 2002; Bergquist et al., 1997). Nasal immunization induces specific IgG and IgA antibody responses in serum, rectal secretions, and vaginal secretions (Bergquist et al., 1997; Kozlowski et al., 1997), while intravaginal and intrarectal immunization induced specific antibody in serum and secretions at the site of immunization

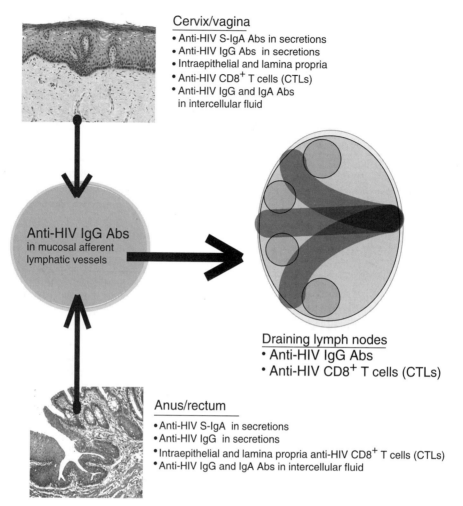

Cervix/vagina
- Anti-HIV S-IgA Abs in secretions
- Anti-HIV IgG Abs in secretions
- Intraepithelial and lamina propria
- Anti-HIV CD8$^+$ T cells (CTLs)
- Anti-HIV IgG and IgA Abs in intercellular fluid

Anti-HIV IgG Abs
in mucosal afferent
lymphatic vessels

Draining lymph nodes
- Anti-HIV IgG Abs
- Anti-HIV CD8$^+$ T cells (CTLs)

Anus/rectum
- Anti-HIV S-IgA in secretions
- Anti-HIV IgG in secretions
- Intraepithelial and lamina propria anti-HIV CD8$^+$ T cells (CTLs)
- Anti-HIV IgG and IgA Abs in intercellular fluid

Fig. 52.5. Potential vaccine-inducible immune barriers to mucosal HIV transmission and dissemination. HIV-specific S-IgA and IgG antibodies (Abs) in mucosal secretions binding to cell-free virus could prevent infection of initial target cells. Furthermore, HIV-specific IgG and IgA antibodies in the intercellular fluid (ICF) of the lamina propria can neutralize cell-free virus, and IgG in lymph can neutralize cell-free virus in the draining lymph node. In the mucosa and draining lymph nodes, antiviral IgG antibodies can also contribute to Ab-dependent cellular cytotoxicity and complement-mediated lysis of virions. After an infection is established in the mucosa, antiviral CD8$^+$ T cells in the mucosa and the draining lymph nodes can control viral replication by killing infected cells or releasing innate immune factors capable of inhibiting viral replication. Once HIV infection reaches the systemic lymphoid tissues and MALT distant to the site of initial virus transmission, both antibody- and T-cell-mediated, antiviral immune responses are expected to contribute to control HIV replication. The possible role of innate antiviral immune responses in vaccine-mediated protection from HIV infection is not shown.

(Kozlowski *et al.*, 1997). In fact, nasal immunization was as effective as direct vaginal inoculation at inducing cervical anti-CT-B IgA (Kozlowski *et al.*, 2002). However, very high antigen doses may be required to induce potent mucosal immune responses in the genital and rectal tissue, and the durability of these responses remains to be determined.

Systemic HIV-1 vaccination with virus vectors can elicit virus-specific CTLs at mucosal sites. Canarypox vectors containing HIV-1 gene inserts have undergone extensive testing in phase I and II trials. Notably, vCP205, containing HIV-1 genes encoding *env*, *gag*, and portions of *pol*, has induced cumulatively HIV-specific CD8$^+$ CTLs in the peripheral blood of 30% to 50% of HIV-seronegative vaccine recipients. Within a phase II clinical trial evaluating the safety and immunogenicity of vCP205 in low- and high-risk

HIV-seronegative volunteers (Belshe *et al.*, 2001; Salmon-Ceron *et al.*, 1999), a smaller study was undertaken to examine the induction of both systemic (PBMCs) and mucosal (cervical, rectal) CTLs in consenting volunteers (Musey *et al.*, 2003). Remarkably, intramuscular injection of recombinant canarypox vector containing HIV-1 gene inserts induced HIV-specific CD8$^+$ T cells that were cytolytic for targets expressing HIV-1 Gag, Env, or both, and in some cases were capable of secreting IFN-γ upon antigen stimulation. These results are consistent with those of recent vaccine studies in nonhuman primates, in which SIV-specific cells were identified in the intestinal and vaginal mucosa after systemic immunization (Baig *et al.*, 2002; Mitchell *et al.*, 1998). Thus, systemic immunization can induce antiviral CTLs in the rectal and genital mucosa of vaccine recipients, although direct mucosal immunization may improve these responses.

WHICH IMMUNE RESPONSES ARE MOST LIKELY TO PROTECT FROM HIV EXPOSURE?

One of the greatest challenges in HIV-1 vaccine development is to understand the components of immunity necessary to protect against infection. Their identification in humans can be done only in a large-scale vaccine efficacy trial, and to date only two such trials have been initiated (Francis *et al.*, 2003). Apart from humans, the only practical model that can be used to understand HIV transmission and pathogenesis is SIV infection in rhesus macaques (Desrosiers and Letvin, 1987). The amino acid sequences of envelope proteins of HIV-1 and SIV diverge significantly; thus, to improve understanding of antibody recognition of HIV-1 envelope in the context of preventive vaccines, a chimeric SHIV construct is frequently employed, which contains the SIV backbone but the HIV-1 envelope gene. However, the SHIV viruses have altered *in vivo* virulence in comparison with SIV and HIV, due to altered mechanisms of pathogenesis (Feinberg and Moore, 2002; Lifson and Martin, 2002; Zhang *et al.*, 2002). Furthermore, a number of approaches that have been unsuccessful in preventing SIV transmission seem to be effective against SHIV (McChesney *et al.*, 1999). Thus, the extent to which the SHIV constructs are useful models for HIV vaccine development is unclear.

The components of immunity that are presumed but not proven to correlate with vaccine-induced protection include the induction of broadly reactive neutralizing antibodies to HIV-1 and T cells, both helper and cytotoxic, that recognize HIV-1 epitopes in association with MHC molecules. HIV-1 avoids antibody-mediated neutralization by escape, and recent studies indicate that conformational masking enables HIV-1 to maintain receptor binding as it resists neutralization (Kwong *et al.*, 2002). Numerous studies attest to the critical role of class I MHC–restricted CD8$^+$ CTLs in controlling HIV-1 infection in humans and SIV or SHIV infection in macaques (Barouch *et al.*, 2000; Borrow *et al.*, 1994; Jin *et al.*, 1998; Koup, 1994; Musey *et al.*, 1997a). Thus, vaccine strategies that elicit neutralizing antibodies and/or T-cell responses have been pursued in the monkey preclinical models and in human clinical trials.

MUCOSAL CHALLENGE STUDIES IN MONKEYS

Results of vaccination studies

Recent vaccine studies have demonstrated an association between the induction of CD8$^+$ CTLs in macaques first immunized with SIV-, SHIV-, or HIV-2-based vaccines and subsequently challenged mucosally with more virulent SIV strains (Abel *et al.*, 2003; Almond *et al.*, 1997; Murphey-

Corb *et al.*, 1999; Miller *et al.*, 1997). These results suggest that mucosal CTLs contribute to control of initial viral replication; thus, if mucosal CTLs can be elicited by vaccination, they may provide immune surveillance upon exposure to HIV-1 by sexual contact. Vaccination of rhesus macaques with live, attenuated *nef*-deleted SIV provides protection against more pathogenic SIV challenge (Daniel *et al.*, 1992). Detailed investigations have revealed that vaccine induces a range of SIV-specific immune effector mechanisms, including relatively potent CTL and antibody responses. These responses either individually or together have correlated with protection, but the relative importance of each of these individually is not known (reviewed by Johnson, 2002). In a live-attenuated SHIV vaccine system, protection from vaginal SIV challenge was also associated with antiviral CTL responses and the ability of animals to produce IFN-α in the first few weeks postchallenge (Abel *et al.*, 2003).

A number of studies in monkeys have shown that mucosal anti-SIV immune responses can be induced in the relevant compartments and that monkeys can be protected from mucosal challenge with virus. Oral immunization with *Salmonella enterica* serovar *typhimurium* and serovar *typhi* expressing fragments of SIV Gag fused to the type III–secreted SopE protein elicited Gag-specific CTLs in both the blood and colon of rhesus macaques. However, this response was not sufficient to protect against subsequent rectal challenge with pathogenic SIV mac239 (Evans *et al.*, 2003). In another study, 48 hours after intrarectal challenge with SIVmac251, rhesus macaques that had been immunized with NYVAC/SIV containing Env, Gag, and Pol genes had SIV-specific CD8$^+$ CTLs that were confined mainly to mucosal tissues, regardless of whether the animals were immunized nasally, intramuscularly, or intrarectally (Stevceva *et al.*, 2002). A vaccine regimen that involved DNA priming and boosting with recombinant modified vaccinia Ankara (rMVA) was shown to successfully control an intrarectal challenge with SIV (Amara *et al.*, 2001).

Some of the most robust systemic SIV-specific immune responses have been induced with a replication-incompetent adenovirus type 5 vector expressing SIV Gag (Shiver *et al.*, 2002), used either as a single agent or following a Gag DNA vaccine prime. Upon intravenous challenge with SHIV, animals receiving the vaccine were better able to control viral replication, a circumstance indicating that vaccine-induced CD8$^+$ T cells recognizing HIV-1 Gag can attenuate infection and prevent HIV-1 disease. Not surprisingly, CTLs do not protect against infection but play a role in ameliorating disease progression.

Since HIV-1 infection is acquired primarily through mucosal routes, the presence of virus-specific CD8$^+$ CTLs at the site of viral entry may be critical in restricting viral dissemination to the lymphoid tissue and the blood. The presence of HIV-specific, activated effector T cells at mucosal surfaces may be critical in rapid control of viral infection after exposure. The success of vaccine candidates may best correlate with their ability to induce such responses mucosally, as has been reported in recent primate studies demonstrating that only animals with local HIV- or SIV-specific IgG, IgA, or CTLs were protected against challenge with a more virulent strain (Bagarazzi *et al.*, 1999; Haigwood, 1999; Heeney *et al.*, 1999; Murphey-Corb *et al.*, 1999; Nilsson *et al.*, 1998; Yoshino *et al.*, 2000).

Results of passive antibody transfer studies

A systemically administered cocktail of anti-HIV envelope monoclonal IgG antibodies can protect progesterone-treated monkeys from vaginal SHIV challenge (Mascola *et al.*, 2000; Parren *et al.*, 2001). However, intravaginal application of the same antibody cocktail does not protect monkeys from the same intravaginal SHIV challenge (J. Mascola, personal communication). Another study demonstrated that IgG monoclonal anti-HIV antibodies applied to the vaginal surface can prevent vaginal transmission of SHIV (Veazey *et al.*, 2003); thus, while vaccine-induced anti-HIV IgG in secretions could be effective at preventing HIV infection, the levels and specificities of the IgG antibodies may be critical. Protection from oral SIV or SHIV challenge has also been achieved with use of systemically administered hyperimmune serum (Van Rompay *et al.*, 1998) or anti-HIV envelope IgG monoclonal antibodies (mAbs) (Ferrantelli and Ruprecht, 2002). Thus, in the SHIV model, systemic passive administration of very high doses of anti-HIV envelope IgG antibodies can provide protection from at least two routes of mucosal transmission. Whether the levels of antibodies used in these studies can be induced and maintained through an active immunization protocol remains to be demonstrated.

A BRIEF OVERVIEW OF CLINICAL HIV VACCINE STUDIES

The initial HIV vaccine clinical trials in the 1990s focused on assessment of safety and immunogenicity of recombinant HIV-1 envelope glycoprotein subunit vaccines in several different adjuvant formulations. The evidence is overwhelming that HIV-1 rgp120 and other envelope subunit constructs have been safe thus far in human testing (Keefer *et al.*, 1994) but they have limited immunogenicity based on titer, breadth and function of the antibodies elicited (McElrath *et al.*, 2000). Envelope subunit vaccines do not reliably induce antiviral CTLs in macaques and humans, but do induce T helper cell responses (Evans and Desrosiers, 2001; McElrath *et al.*, 2000). Recombinant viral vectors administered alone elicit low-level antibody responses. Combining vectors with a subunit vaccine such as rgp160 or rgp120 in prime-boost protocols stimulates CD8+ CTLs and higher titers of neutralizing antibodies. Thus, the prime-boost approach has been tested in numerous trials and is currently the preferred approach to induce anti-HIV responses from both the humoral and cellular arms of immunity.

The first successful approach in eliciting anti-HIV CD8+ CTLs in uninfected individuals was with use of recombinant vaccinia virus vector containing HIV-1 *env* (Cooney *et al.*,

1993; Hammond *et al.*, 1992). Priming with recombinant vaccinia and boosting with envelope subunit protein induced both neutralizing antibodies and CTLs (McElrath *et al.*, 1997). Recent efforts have focused on using replication-defective poxviruses such as canarypox or modified vaccinia Ankara. Canarypox vectors (Aventis-Pasteur) encoding *env*, *gag*, protease (ALVAC-HIV vCP205), and *nef* (ALVAC vCP1452) have been administered with remarkable safety (Belshe *et al.*, 2001; Evans *et al.*, 1999; Gupta *et al.*, 2002; Corey *et al.*, 1998) and have induced CD8+ CTLs in more than one-third of vaccinees (Corey *et al.*, 1998). However, in a randomized, placebo-controlled phase II study involving volunteers at high risk for acquiring HIV infection, the vaccine did not meet predetermined minimum immunogenicity criteria for advancement to a larger efficacy trial. Thus, the overall safety of the canarypox vaccine is high, but some inconsistencies in immunogenicity have been noted. Nevertheless, a separately designed, smaller phase III trial to determine efficacy without relationship to laboratory correlates of immunity is underway in Thailand and involves the use of a clade E canarypox vector.

VACCINES IN THE PIPELINE

As described previously, it appears on the basis of preclinical studies that several new prime-boost regimens hold significant promise in eliciting virus-specific T cell immunity, and these are currently under evaluation in early clinical trials. Recombinant DNA with or without adjuvant and replication-defective adenovirus vectors delivered by the intramuscular route have been tested thus far in phase I clinical studies led by Merck Research Laboratories, and additional constructs are being evaluated by the NIH Vaccine Research Center and the HIV Vaccine Trials Network. Another strategy receiving attention following primate studies is the use of DNA and then modified vaccinia Ankara (MVA) (Hanke and McMichael, 1999; McMichael and Hanke, 1999). Clinical trials have commenced in Oxford and Nairobi, Kenya, of an HIV clade A DNA immunogen (HIVA), to be followed by an MVA boost. The role of vaccinia vectors in HIV-1 vaccine design may fall into disfavor, however, because of the recent smallpox immunization recommendations in response to potential bioterror attacks. Other recombinant viral vectors containing HIV-1 genes moving into clinical trials include Venezuelan equine encephalitis virus replicons (AlphaVax) (Caley *et al.*, 1999), attenuated vesicular stomatitis virus (Haglund *et al.*, 2002), herpes simplex virus, and Sindbis virus. These constructs have the potential for mucosal delivery, which may induce a more rapid response following HIV-1 exposure.

CONCLUSIONS

HIV is primarily transmitted across mucosal surfaces. Thus, a successful vaccine to prevent HIV transmission and infection may require induction of mucosal immune responses. It is known that anti-SIV/HIV antibodies are present in the vaginal secretions of infected individuals. IgG is the major isotype of anti-SIV/HIV antibodies in vaginal secretions. There is also clear evidence of antiviral CD8[+] T-cell effector function in mucosal tissues. Anti-SIV CTLs are present in the GI tract and vaginal epithelium of SIV-infected rhesus macaques, and anti-HIV CTLs are present in the GI tract and endocervix of HIV-infected patients. Future trials of anti-HIV vaccines should include an analysis of mucosal immune responses induced by the vaccine candidates. It is likely that a successful vaccine will be capable of rapidly inducing the full range of mucosal anti-HIV immune responses that occur during natural infection.

ACKNOWLEDGMENTS

The work cited from Dr. Miller's Laboratory was supported by National Institutes of Health (NIH) grants AI35545, HD 33169, HD 29125, RR14555, and RR00169 and by the Rockefeller Foundation. The work cited from Dr. McElrath's laboratory was supported by NIH grants AI35605 and A27757 and by the Burroughs Wellcome Foundation.

REFERENCES

Abel, K., L. Compton, T. Rourke, D. Montefiori, D. Lu, K. Rothaeusler, L. Fritts, K. Bost, and C. J. Miller (2003). Simian-human immunodeficiency virus SHIV89.6-induced protection against intravaginal challenge with pathogenic SIVmac239 is independent of the route of immunization and is associated with a combination of cytotoxic T-lymphocyte and alpha interferon responses. *J. Virol.* 77, 3099–3118.

Alkhatib, G., C. Combadiere, C. C. Broder, Y. Feng, P. E. Kennedy, P. M. Murphy, and E. A. Berger (1996). CC CKR5: a RANTES, MIP-1alpha, MIP-1beta receptor as a fusion cofactor for macrophage-tropic HIV-1. *Science* 272, 1955–1958.

Almond, N., J. Rose, R. Sangster, P. Silvera, R. Stebbings, B. Walker, and E. J. Stott (1997). Mechanisms of protection induced by attenuated simian immunodeficiency virus. I. Protection cannot be transferred with immune serum. *J. Gen. Virol.* 78 (Pt 8), 1919–1922.

Amara, R. R., F. Villinger, J. D. Altman, S. L. Lydy, S. P. O'Neil, S. I. Staprans, D. C. Montefiori, Y. Xu, J. G. Herndon, L. S. Wyatt, M. A. Candido, N. L. Kozyr, P. L. Earl, J. M. Smith, H. L. Ma, B. D. Grimm, M. L. Hulsey, J. Miller, H. M. McClure, J. M. McNicholl, B. Moss, and H. L. Robinson (2001). Control of a mucosal challenge and prevention of AIDS by a multiprotein DNA/MVA vaccine. *Science* 292, 69–74.

Archibald, D. W., D. J. Witt, D. E. Craven, M. W. Vogt, M. S. Hirsch, and M. Essex (1987). Antibodies to human immunodeficiency virus in cervical secretions from women at risk for AIDS. *J. Infect. Dis.* 156, 240–241.

Artenstein, A. W., T. C. VanCott, K. V. Sitz, M. L. Robb, K. F. Wagner, S. C. Veit, A. F. Rogers, R. P. Garner, J. W. Byron, P. R. Burnett, and D. L. Birx (1997). Mucosal immune responses in four distinct compartments of women infected with human immunodeficiency virus type 1: a comparison by site and correlation with clinical information. *J. Infect. Dis.* 175, 265–271.

Bagarazzi, M. L., J. D. Boyer, M. A. Javadian, M. A. Chattergoon, A. R. Shah, A. D. Cohen, M. K. Bennett, R. B. Ciccarelli, K. E. Ugen, and D. B. Weiner (1999). Systemic and mucosal immunity is elicited after both intramuscular and intravaginal delivery of human immunodeficiency virus type 1 DNA plasmid vaccines to pregnant chimpanzees. *J. Infect. Dis.* 180, 1351–1355.

Baig, J., D. B. Levy, P. F. McKay, J. E. Schmitz, S. Santra, R. A. Subbramanian, M. J. Kuroda, M. A. Lifton, D. A. Gorgone, L. S. Wyatt, B. Moss, Y. Huang, B. K. Chakrabarti, L. Xu, W. P. Kong, Z. Y. Yang, J. R. Mascola, G. J. Nabel, A. Carville, A. A. Lackner, R. S. Veazey, and N. L. Letvin (2002). Elicitation of simian immunodeficiency virus–specific cytotoxic T lymphocytes in mucosal compartments of rhesus monkeys by systemic vaccination. *J. Virol.* 76, 11484–11490.

Barouch, D. H., S. Santra, J. E. Schmitz, M. J. Kuroda, T. M. Fu, W. Wagner, M. Bilska, A. Craiu, X. X. Zheng, G. R. Krivulka, K. Beaudry, M. A. Lifton, C. E. Nickerson, W. L. Trigona, K. Punt, D. C. Freed, L. Guan, S. Dubey, D. Casimiro, A. Simon, M. E. Davies, M. Chastain, T. B. Strom, R. S. Gelman, D. C. Montefiori, M. G. Lewis, E. A. Emini, J. W. Shiver, and N. L. Letvin (2000). Control of viremia and prevention of clinical AIDS in rhesus monkeys by cytokine-augmented DNA vaccination. *Science* 290, 486–492.

Bebenek, K., J. Abbotts, J. D. Roberts, S. H. Wilson, and T. A. Kunkel (1989). Specificity and mechanism of error-prone replication by human immunodeficiency virus-1 reverse transcriptase. *J. Biol. Chem.* 264, 16948–16956.

Belec, L., J. C. Bouquety, A. J. Georges, M. R. Siopathis, and P. M. Martin (1990). Antibodies to human immunodeficiency virus in the breast milk of healthy, seropositive women. *Pediatrics* 85, 1022–1026.

Belec, L., T. Dupre, T. Prazuck, C. Tevi-Benissan, J. M. Kanga, O. Pathey, X. S. Lu, and J. Pillot (1995). Cervicovaginal overproduction of specific IgG to human immunodeficiency virus (HIV) contrasts with normal or impaired IgA local response in HIV infection. *J. Infect. Dis.* 172, 691–697.

Belec, L., A. J. Georges, G. Steenman, and P. M. Martin (1989). Antibodies to human immunodeficiency virus in vaginal secretions of heterosexual women. *J. Infect. Dis.* 160, 385–391.

Belec, L., C. Tevi-Benissan, T. Dupre, A. S. Mohamed, T. Prazuck, J. Gilquin, J. M. Kanga, and J. Pillot (1996). Comparison of cervicovaginal humoral immunity in clinically asymptomatic (CDC A1 and A2 category) patients with HIV-1 and HIV-2 infection. *J. Clin. Immunol.* 16, 12–20.

Belshe, R. B., C. Stevens, G. J. Gorse, S. Buchbinder, K. Weinhold, H. Sheppard, D. Stablein, S. Self, J. McNamara, S. Frey, J. Flores, J. L. Excler, M. Klein, R. E. Habib, A. M. Duliege, C. Harro, L. Corey, M. Keefer, M. Mulligan, P. Wright, C. Celum, F. Judson, K. Mayer, D. McKirnan, M. Marmor, and G. Woody (2001). Safety and immunogenicity of a canarypox-vectored human immunodeficiency virus Type 1 vaccine with or without gp120: a phase 2 study in higher- and lower-risk volunteers. *J. Infect. Dis.* 183, 1343–1352.

Bergquist, C., E. L. Johansson, T. Lagergard, J. Holmgren, and A. Rudin (1997). Intranasal vaccination of humans with recombinant cholera toxin B subunit induces systemic and local antibody responses in the upper respiratory tract and the vagina. *Infect. Immun.* 65, 2676–2684.

Bhoopat, L., L. Eiangleng, S. Rugpao, S. S. Frankel, D. Weissman, S. Lekawanvijit, S. Petchjom, P. Thorner, and T. Bhoopat (2001). In vivo identification of Langerhans and related dendritic cells infected with HIV-1 subtype E in vaginal mucosa of asymptomatic patients. *Mod. Pathol.* 14, 1263–1269.

Bjercke, S., H. Scott, L. R. Braathen, and E. Thorsby (1983). HLA-DR-expressing Langerhans-like cells in vaginal and cervical epithelium. *Acta Obstet. Gynecol. Scand.* 62, 585–589.

Blauvelt, A., H. Asada, M. W. Saville, V. Klaus-Kovuton, D. J. Altman, R. Yarchoan, and S. I. Katz (1997). Productive infection of dendritic cells by HIV-1 and their ability to capture virus are mediated through separate pathways. *J. Clin. Invest.* 100, 2043–2053.

Borrow, P., H. Lewicki, B. H. Hahn, G. M. Shaw, and M. B. Oldstone (1994). Virus-specific CD8+ cytotoxic T-lymphocyte activity associated with control of viremia in primary human immunodeficiency virus type 1 infection. *J. Virol.* 68, 6103–6110.

Buchacz, K., B. S. Parekh, N. S. Padian, A. van der Straten, S. Phillips, J. Jonte, and S. D. Holmberg (2001). HIV-specific IgG in cervicovaginal secretions of exposed HIV-uninfected female sexual partners of HIV-infected men. *AIDS Res. Hum. Retroviruses* 17, 1689–1693.

Caley, I. J., M. R. Betts, N. L. Davis, R. Swanstrom, J. A. Frelinger, and R. E. Johnston (1999). Venezuelan equine encephalitis virus vectors expressing HIV-1 proteins: vector design strategies for improved vaccine efficacy. *Vaccine* 17(23–24), 3124–3135.

Chou, L. L., J. Epstein, S. A. Cassol, D. M. West, W. He, and J. D. Firth (2000). Oral mucosal Langerhans' cells as target, effector and vector in HIV infection. *J. Oral Pathol. Med.* 29, 394–402.

Ciurea, A., P. Klenerman, L. Hunziker, E. Horvath, B. Odermatt, A. F. Ochsenbein, H. Hengartner, and R. M. Zinkernagel (1999). Persistence of lymphocytic choriomeningitis virus at very low levels in immune mice. *Proc. Natl. Acad. Sci. USA* 96, 11964–11969.

Cohen, C. R., F. A. Plummer, N. Mugo, I. Maclean, C. Shen, E. A. Bukusi, E. Irungu, S. Sinei, J. Bwayo, and R. C. Brunham (1999). Increased interleukin-10 in the endocervical secretions of women with non-ulcerative sexually transmitted diseases: a mechanism for enhanced HIV-1 transmission? *AIDS* 13, 327–332.

Collins, K. B., B. K. Patterson, G. J. Naus, D. V. Landers, and P. Gupta (2000). Development of an in vitro organ culture model to study transmission of HIV-1 in the female genital tract. *Nat. Med.* 6, 475–479.

Cooney, E. L., M. J. McElrath, L. Corey, S. L. Hu, A. C. Collier, D. Arditti, M. Hoffman, R. W. Coombs, G. E. Smith, and P. D. Greenberg (1993). Enhanced immunity to human immunodeficiency virus (HIV) envelope elicited by a combined vaccine regimen consisting of priming with a vaccinia recombinant expressing HIV envelope and boosting with gp160 protein. *Proc. Natl. Acad. Sci. USA* 90, 1882–1886.

Corey, L., M. J. McElrath, K. Weinhold, T. Matthews, D. Stablein, B. Graham, M. Keefer, D. Schwartz, and G. Gorse (1998). Cytotoxic T cell and neutralizing antibody responses to human immunodeficiency virus type 1 envelope with a combination vaccine regimen. AIDS Vaccine Evaluation Group. *J. Infect. Dis.* 177, 301–309.

Couedel-Courteille, A., C. Butor, V. Juillard, J. G. Guillet, and A. Venet (1999). Dissemination of SIV after rectal infection preferentially involves paracolic germinal centers. *Virology* 260, 277–294.

Crowley-Nowick, P. A., M. Bell, R. P. Edwards, D. McCallister, H. Gore, A. Kanbour-Shakir, J. Mestecky, and E. E. Partridge (1995). Normal uterine cervix: characterization of isolated lymphocyte phenotypes and immunoglobulin secretion. *Am. J. Reprod. Immunol.* 34(4), 241–247.

Daniel, M. D., F. Kirchhoff, S. C. Czajak, P. K. Sehgal, and R. C. Desrosiers (1992). Protective effects of a live attenuated SIV vaccine with a deletion in the nef gene. *Science* 258, 1938–1941.

Dean, M., M. Carrington, C. Winkler, G. A. Huttley, M. W. Smith, R. Allikmets, J. J. Goedert, S. P. Buchbinder, E. Vittinghoff, E. Gomperts, S. Donfield, D. Vlahov, R. Kaslow, A. Saah, C. Rinaldo, R. Detels, and S. J. O'Brien (1996). Genetic restriction of HIV-1 infection and progression to AIDS by a deletion allele of the CKR5 structural gene. Hemophilia Growth and Development Study, Multicenter AIDS Cohort Study, Multicenter Hemophilia Cohort Study, San Francisco Cohort, ALIVE Study. *Science* 273, 1856–1862.

Deng, H., R. Liu, W. Ellmeier, S. Choe, D. Unutmaz, M. Burkhart, P. Di Marzio, S. Marmon, R. E. Sutton, C. M. Hill, C. B. Davis, S. C. Peiper, T. J. Schall, D. R. Littman, and N. R. Landau (1996). Identification of a major co-receptor for primary isolates of HIV-1. *Nature* 381, 661–666.

Desrosiers, R. C., and N. L. Letvin (1987). Animal models for acquired immunodeficiency syndrome. *Rev. Infect. Dis.* 9, 438–446.

Dezzutti, C. S., P. C. Guenthner, J. E. Cummins, Jr., T. Cabrera, J. H. Marshall, A. Dillberger, and R. B. Lal (2001). Cervical and prostate primary epithelial cells are not productively infected but sequester human immunodeficiency virus type 1. *J. Infect. Dis.* 183, 1204–1213.

Di Stefano, M., A. Favia, L. Monno, P. Lopalco, O. Caputi, A. C. Scardigno, G. Pastore, J. R. Fiore, and G. Angarano (2001). Intracellular and cell-free (infectious) HIV-1 in rectal mucosa. *J. Med. Virol.* 65, 637–643.

Dorrell, L., A. J. Hessell, M. Wang, H. Whittle, S. Sabally, S. Rowland-Jones, D. R. Burton, and P. W. Parren (2000). Absence of specific mucosal antibody responses in HIV-exposed uninfected sex workers from the Gambia. *AIDS* 14, 1117–1122.

Douek, D. C., L. J. Picker, and R. A. Koup (2003). T cell dynamics in HIV-1 infection. *Annu. Rev. Immunol.* 21, 265–304.

Dragic, T., V. Litwin, G. P. Allaway, S. R. Martin, Y. Huang, K. A. Nagashima, C. Cayanan, P. J. Maddon, R. A. Koup, J. P. Moore, and W. A. Paxton (1996). HIV-1 entry into CD4+ cells is mediated by the chemokine receptor CC-CKR-5. *Nature* 381, 667–673.

Duprat, C., Z. Mohammed, P. Datta, W. Stackiw, J. O. Ndinya-Achola, J. K. Kreiss, K. K. Holmes, F. A. Plummer, and J. E. Embree (1994). Human immunodeficiency virus type 1 IgA antibody in breast milk and serum. *Pediatr. Infect. Dis. J.* 13, 603–608.

Edwards, J. N. and H. B. Morris (1985). Langerhans' cells and lymphocyte subsets in the female genital tract. *Br. J. Obstet. Gynaecol.* 92, 974–982.

Embree, J. E., S. Njenga, P. Datta, N. J. Nagelkerke, J. O. Ndinya-Achola, Z. Mohammed, S. Ramdahin, J. J. Bwayo, and F. A. Plummer (2000). Risk factors for postnatal mother-child transmission of HIV-1. *AIDS* 14, 2535–2541.

Eriksson, K., A. Kilander, L. Hagberg, G. Norkrans, J. Holmgren, and C. Czerkinsky (1995). Virus-specific antibody production and polyclonal B-cell activation in the intestinal mucosa of HIV-infected individuals. *AIDS* 9, 695–700.

Eriksson, K., M. Quiding-Jarbrink, J. Osek, A. Moller, S. Bjork, J. Holmgren, and C. Czerkinsky (1998). Specific-antibody-secreting cells in the rectums and genital tracts of nonhuman primates following vaccination. *Infect. Immun.* 66(12), 5889–5896.

Evans, D. T., L. M. Chen, J. Gillis, K. C. Lin, B. Harty, G. P. Mazzara, R. O. Donis, K. G. Mansfield, J. D. Lifson, R. C. Desrosiers, J. E. Galan, and R. P. Johnson (2003). Mucosal priming of simian immunodeficiency virus–specific cytotoxic T-lymphocyte responses in rhesus macaques by the *Salmonella* type III secretion antigen delivery system. *J. Virol.* 77, 2400–2409.

Evans, D. T., and R. C. Desrosiers (2001). Immune evasion strategies of the primate lentiviruses. *Immunol. Rev.* 183, 141–158.

Evans, T. G., M. C. Keefer, K. J. Weinhold, M. Wolff, D. Montefiori, G. J. Gorse, B. S. Graham, M. J. McElrath, M. L. Clements-Mann, M. J. Mulligan, P. Fast, M. C. Walker, J. L. Excler, A. M. Duliege, and J. Tartaglia (1999). A canarypox vaccine expressing multiple human immunodeficiency virus type 1 genes given alone or with rgp120 elicits broad and durable CD8+ cytotoxic T lymphocyte responses in seronegative volunteers. *J. Infect. Dis.* 180, 290–298.

Farquhar, C., T. C. VanCott, D. A. Mbori-Ngacha, L. Horani, R. K. Bosire, J. K. Kreiss, B. A. Richardson, and G. C. John-Stewart (2002). Salivary secretory leukocyte protease inhibitor is associated with reduced transmission of human immunodeficiency virus type 1 through breast milk. *J. Infect. Dis.* 186, 1173–1176.

Faruque, S., B. R. Edlin, C. B. McCoy, C. O. Word, S. A. Larsen, D. S. Schmid, J. C. Von Bargen, and Y. Serrano (1996). Crack cocaine smoking and oral sores in three inner-city neighborhoods. *J. Acquir. Immune Defic. Syndr. Hum. Retrovirol.* 13, 87–92.

Fawcett, D. W. (1986). *Bloom and Fawcett's Textbook of Histology.* Philadelphia: WB Saunders.

Feinberg, M. B., and J. P. Moore (2002). AIDS vaccine models: challenging challenge viruses. *Nat. Med.* 8, 207–210.

Ferrantelli, F., and R. M. Ruprecht (2002). Neutralizing antibodies against HIV: back in the major leagues? *Curr. Opin. Immunol.* 14(4), 495–502.

Fotopoulos, G., A. Harari, P. Michetti, D. Trono, G. Pantaleo and J. P. Kraehenbuhl (2002). Transepithelial transport of HIV-1 by M cells is receptor-mediated. *Proc. Natl. Acad. Sci. USA* 99, 9410–9414.

Francis, D. P., W. L. Heyward, V. Popovic, P. Orozco-Cronin, K. Orelind, C. Gee, A. Hirsch, T. Ippolito, A. Luck, M. Longhi, V. Gulati, N. Winslow, M. Gurwith, F. Sinangil, and P. W. Berman (2003). Candidate HIV/AIDS vaccines: lessons learned from the World's first phase III efficacy trials. *AIDS* 17, 147–156.

Gaillard, P., C. Verhofstede, F. Mwanyumba, P. Claeys, V. Chohan, K. Mandaliya, J. Bwayo, J. Plum, and M. Temmerman (2000).

Exposure to HIV-1 during delivery and mother-to-child transmission. *AIDS* 14(15), 2341–2348.

Geijtenbeek, T. B., D. S. Kwon, R. Torensma, S. J. van Vliet, G. C. van Duijnhoven, J. Middel, I. L. Cornelissen, H. S. Nottet, V. N. KewalRamani, D. R. Littman, C. G. Figdor, and Y. van Kooyk (2000). DC-SIGN, a dendritic cell-specific HIV-1-binding protein that enhances trans-infection of T cells. *Cell* 100, 587–597.

Goedert, J. J., A. M. Duliege, C. I. Amos, S. Felton, and R. J. Biggar (1991). High risk of HIV-1 infection for first-born twins. The International Registry of HIV-exposed Twins. *Lancet* 338, 1471–1475.

Gray, R. H., M. J. Wawer, R. Brookmeyer, N. K. Sewankambo, D. Serwadda, F. Wabwire-Mangen, T. Lutalo, X. Li, T. vanCott, and T. C. Quinn (2001). Probability of HIV-1 transmission per coital act in monogamous, heterosexual, HIV-1-discordant couples in Rakai, Uganda. *Lancet* 357, 1149–1153.

Greenhead, P., P. Hayes, P. S. Watts, K. G. Laing, G. E. Griffin, and R. J. Shattock (2000). Parameters of human immunodeficiency virus infection of human cervical tissue and inhibition by vaginal virucides. *J. Virol.* 74, 5577–5586.

Greenier, J. L., C. J. Miller, D. Lu, P. J. Dailey, F. X. Lu, K. J. Kunstman, S. M. Wolinsky, and M. L. Marthas (2001). Route of simian immunodeficiency virus inoculation determines the complexity but not the identity of viral variant populations that infect rhesus macaques. *J. Virol.* 75(8), 3753–3765.

Grosskurth, H., F. Mosha, J. Todd, E. Mwijarubi, A. Klokke, K. Senkoro, P. Mayaud, J. Changalucha, A. Nicoll, and G. ka-Gina. (1995). Impact of improved treatment of sexually transmitted diseases on HIV infection in rural Tanzania: randomised controlled trial. *Lancet* 346, 530–536.

Grossman, C. J. (1984). Regulation of the immune system by sex steroids. *Endocr. Rev.* 5, 435–455.

Gupta, K., M. Hudgens, L. Corey, M. J. McElrath, K. Weinhold, D. C. Montefiori, G. J. Gorse, S. E. Frey, M. C. Keefer, T. G. Evans, R. Dolin, D. H. Schwartz, C. Harro, B. Graham, P. W. Spearman, M. Mulligan, and P. Goepfert (2002). Safety and immunogenicity of a high-titered canarypox vaccine in combination with rgp120 in a diverse population of HIV-1-uninfected adults: AIDS Vaccine Evaluation Group Protocol 022A. *J. Acquir. Immune Defic. Syndr.* 29, 254–261.

Haglund, K., I. Leiner, K. Kerksiek, L. Buonocore, E. Pamer, and J. K. Rose (2002). Robust recall and long-term memory T-cell responses induced by prime-boost regimens with heterologous live viral vectors expressing human immunodeficiency virus type 1 Gag and Env proteins. *J. Virol.* 76, 7506–7517.

Haigwood, N. L. (1999). Progress and challenges in therapies for AIDS in nonhuman primate models. *J. Med. Primatol.* 28, 154–163.

Hammond, S. A., R. C. Bollinger, P. E. Stanhope, T. C. Quinn, D. Schwartz, M. L. Clements, and R. F. Siliciano (1992). Comparative clonal analysis of human immunodeficiency virus type 1 (HIV-1)-specific CD4+ and CD8+ cytolytic T lymphocytes isolated from seronegative humans immunized with candidate HIV-1 vaccines. *J. Exp. Med.* 176, 1531–1542.

Hanke, T., and A. McMichael (1999). Pre-clinical development of a multi-CTL epitope-based DNA prime MVA boost vaccine for AIDS. *Immunol. Lett.* 66, 177–181.

Harouse, J., A. Gettie, T. Eshetu, R. Fuller, J. Blanchard, and C. Cheng-Mayer (November 7–10, 2001). Co-transmission and growth of CCR5 and CxCR4 specific SHIVs after intravaginal or intravenous exposure. 19th Annual Symposium on Nonhuman Primate Models for AIDS, San Juan, Puerto Rico.

Heeney, J., L. Akerblom, S. Barnett, W. Bogers, D. Davis, D. Fuller, G. Koopman, T. Lehner, P. Mooij, B. Morein, C. de Giuli Morghen, B. Rosenwirth, E. Verschoor, R. Wagner, and H. Wolf (1999). HIV-1 vaccine–induced immune responses which correlate with protection from SHIV infection: compiled preclinical efficacy data from trials with ten different HIV-1 vaccine candidates. *Immunol. Lett.* 66, 189–195.

Hirsch, V. M., T. R. Fuerst, G. Sutter, M. W. Carroll, L. C. Yang, S. Goldstein, M. J. Piatak, W. R. Elkins, W. G. Alvord, D. C. Montefiori, B. Moss, and J. D. Lifson (1996). Patterns of viral replication correlate with outcome in simian immunodeficiency virus (SIV)–infected macaques: effect of prior immunization with a trivalent SIV vaccine in modified vaccinia virus Ankara. *J. Virol.* 70, 3741–3752.

Hladik, F., G. Lentz, R. E. Akridge, G. Peterson, H. Kelley, A. McElroy, and M. J. McElrath (1999a). Dendritic cell–T-cell interactions support coreceptor-independent human immunodeficiency virus type 1 transmission in the human genital tract. *J. Virol.* 73, 5833–5842.

Hladik, F., G. Lentz, E. Delpit, A. McElroy, and M. J. McElrath (1999b). Coexpression of CCR5 and IL-2 in human genital but not blood T cells: implications for the ontogeny of the CCR5+ Th1 phenotype. *J. Immunol.* 163, 2306–2313.

Hocini, H., and M. Bomsel (1999). Infectious human immunodeficiency virus can rapidly penetrate a tight human epithelial barrier by transcytosis in a process impaired by mucosal immunoglobulins. *J. Infect. Dis.* 179 Suppl 3, S448–453.

Hu, J., M. B. Gardner, and C. J. Miller (2000). Simian immunodeficiency virus rapidly penetrates the cervicovaginal mucosa after intravaginal inoculation and infects intraepithelial dendritic cells. *J. Virol.* 74, 6087–6095.

Hu, J., M. Pope, C. Brown, U. O'Doherty, and C. J. Miller (1998). Immunophenotypic characterization of SIV-infected dendritic cells in the cervix, vagina and draining lymph nodes of rhesus monkeys. *Lab. Invest.* 78, 435–451.

Ibata, B., E. L. Parr, N. J. King, and M. B. Parr (1997). Migration of foreign lymphocytes from the mouse vagina into the cervicovaginal mucosa and to the iliac lymph nodes. *Biol. Reprod.* 56, 537–543.

Imaoka, K., C. J. Miller, M. Kubota, M. B. McChesney, B. Lohman, M. Yamamoto, K. Fujihashi, K. Someya, M. Honda, J. R. McGhee, and H. Kiyono (1998). Nasal immunization of nonhuman primates with simian immunodeficiency virus p55gag and cholera toxin adjuvant induces Th1/Th2 help for virus-specific immune responses in reproductive tissues. *J. Immunol.* 161(11), 5952–5958.

Izmailova, E., F. M. Bertley, Q. Huang, N. Makori, C. J. Miller, R. A. Young, and A. Aldovini (2003). HIV-1 Tat reprograms immature dendritic cells to express chemoattractants for activated T cells and macrophages. *Nat. Med.* 9, 191–197.

Jackson, S., S. Prince, R. Kulhavy, and J. Mestecky (2000). False positivity of enzyme-linked immunosorbent assay for measurement of secretory IgA antibodies directed at HIV type 1 antigens. *AIDS Res. Hum. Retroviruses* 16, 595–602.

Jalanti, R., and H. Isliker (1977). Immunoglobulins in human cervicovaginal secretions. *Int. Arch. Allergy Appl. Immunol.* 53, 402–408.

Jameson, B., F. Baribaud, S. Pohlmann, D. Ghavimi, F. Mortari, R. W. Doms, and A. Iwasaki (2002). Expression of DC-SIGN by dendritic cells of intestinal and genital mucosae in humans and rhesus macaques. *J. Virol.* 76, 1866–1875.

Janoff, E., S. Wahl, and P. Smith (1989). Antibodies to human immunodeficiency virus-1 (HIV) in the small intestine are primarily IgG, not IgA (abstract). *Gastroenterology* 96, 236A.

Janoff, E. N., S. Jackson, S. M. Wahl, K. Thomas, J. H. Peterman, and P. D. Smith (1994). Intestinal mucosal immunoglobulins during human immunodeficiency virus type 1 infection. *J. Infect. Dis.* 170, 299–307.

Jin, X., C. G. Roberts, D. F. Nixon, Y. Cao, D. D. Ho, B. D. Walker, M. Muldoon, B. T. Korber, and R. A. Koup (1998). Longitudinal and cross-sectional analysis of cytotoxic T lymphocyte responses and their relationship to vertical human immunodeficiency virus transmission. ARIEL Project Investigators. *J. Infect. Dis.* 178, 1317–1326.

Joag, S. V., Z. Li, C. Wang, L. Foresman, F. Jia, E. B. Stephens, W. Zhuge, and O. Narayan (1999). Passively administered neutralizing serum that protected macaques against infection with parenterally inoculated pathogenic simian-human immunodeficiency virus failed to protect against mucosally inoculated virus. *AIDS Res. Hum. Retroviruses* 15, 391–394.

Joag, S. V., Z. Q. Liu, E. B. Stephens, M. S. Smith, A. Kumar, Z. Li, C. Wang, D. Sheffer, F. Jia, L. Foresman, I. Adany, J. Lifson, H. M. McClure, and O. Narayan (1998). Oral immunization of macaques with attenuated vaccine virus induces protection against vaginally transmitted AIDS. *J. Virol.* 72, 9069–9078.

Johansson, E. L., A. Rudin, L. Wassen, and J. Holmgren (1999). Distribution of lymphocytes and adhesion molecules in human cervix and vagina. *Immunology* 96, 272–277.

Johnson, R. P. (2002). Mechanisms of protection against simian immuno-deficiency virus infection. *Vaccine* 20, 1985–1987.

Kabashima, H., M. Yoneda, K. Nagata, T. Hirofuji, and K. Maeda (2002). The presence of chemokine (MCP-1, MIP-1alpha, MIP-1beta, IP-10, RANTES)-positive cells and chemokine receptor (CCR5,CXCR3)–positive cells in inflamed human gingival tissues. *Cytokine* 20, 70–77.

Kaul, R., F. A. Plummer, J. Kimani, T. Dong, P. Kiama, T. Rostron, E. Njagi, K. S. MacDonald, J. J. Bwayo, A. J. McMichael, and S. L. Rowland-Jones (2000). HIV-1-specific mucosal CD8+ lymphocyte responses in the cervix of HIV-1-resistant prostitutes in Nairobi. *J. Immunol.* 164, 1602–1611.

Kaul, R., D. Trabattoni, J. J. Bwayo, D. Arienti, A. Zagliani, F. M. Mwangi, C. Kariuki, E. N. Ngugi, K. S. MacDonald, T. B. Ball, M. Clerici, and F. A. Plummer (1999). HIV-1-specific mucosal IgA in a cohort of HIV-1-resistant Kenyan sex workers. *AIDS* 13, 23–29.

Kawamura, T., S. S. Cohen, D. L. Borris, E. A. Aquilino, S. Glushakova, L. B. Margolis, J. M. Orenstein, R. E. Offord, A. R. Neurath, and A. Blauvelt (2000). Candidate microbicides block HIV-1 infection of human immature Langerhans cells within epithelial tissue explants. *J. Exp. Med.* 192, 1491–1500.

Keefer, M. C., B. S. Graham, R. B. Belshe, D. Schwartz, L. Corey, D. P. Bolognesi, D. M. Stablein, D. C. Montefiori, M. J. McElrath, and M. L. Clements (1994). Studies of high doses of a human immunodeficiency virus type 1 recombinant glycoprotein 160 candidate vaccine in HIV type 1–seronegative humans. The AIDS Vaccine Clinical Trials Network. *AIDS Res. Hum. Retroviruses* 10, 1713–1723.

Kell, P. D., S. E. Barton, D. K. Edmonds, and F. C. Boag (1992). HIV infection in a patient with Meyer-Rokitansky-Kuster-Hauser syndrome. *J. R. Soc. Med.* 85, 706–707.

King, B. F. (1983). The permeability of nonhuman primate vaginal epithelium: a freeze-fracture and tracer-perfusion study. *J. Ultrastruct. Res.* 83(1), 99–110.

Korber, B., B. Gaschen, K. Yusim, R. Thakallapally, C. Kesmir, and V. Detours (2001). Evolutionary and immunological implications of contemporary HIV-1 variation. *Br. Med. Bull.* 58, 19–42.

Koup, R. A. (1994). Virus escape from CTL recognition. *J. Exp. Med.* 180, 779–782.

Kozlowski, P. A., S. Cu-Uvin, M. R. Neutra, and T. P. Flanigan (1997). Comparison of the oral, rectal, and vaginal immunization routes for induction of antibodies in rectal and genital tract secretions of women. *Infect. Immun.* 65, 1387–1394.

Kozlowski, P. A., S. B. Williams, R. M. Lynch, T. P. Flanigan, R. R. Patterson, S. Cu-Uvin, and M. R. Neutra (2002). Differential induction of mucosal and systemic antibody responses in women after nasal, rectal, or vaginal immunization: influence of the menstrual cycle. *J. Immunol.* 169, 566–574.

Kubota, M., C. J. Miller, K. Imaoka, S. Kawabata, K. Fujihashi, J. R. McGhee, and H. Kiyono (1997). Oral immunization with simian immunodeficiency virus p55 gag and cholera toxin elicits both mucosal IgA and systemic IgG immune responses in nonhuman primates. *J. Immunol.* 158, 5321–5329.

Kunanusont, C., H. M. Foy, J. K. Kreiss, S. Rerks-Ngarm, P. Phanuphak, S. Raktham, C. P. Pau, and N. L. Young (1995). HIV-1 subtypes and male-to-female transmission in Thailand. *Lancet* 345, 1078–1083.

Kutteh, W. H., S. J. Prince, K. R. Hammond, C. C. Kutteh, and J. Mestecky (1996). Variations in immunoglobulins and IgA subclasses of human uterine cervical secretions around the time of ovulation. *Clin. Exp. Immunol.* 104, 538–542.

Kwong, P. D., M. L. Doyle, D. J. Casper, C. Cicala, S. A. Leavitt, S. Majeed, T. D. Steenbeke, M. Venturi, I. Chaiken, M. Fung, H. Katinger, P. W. Parren, J. Robinson, D. Van Ryk, L. Wang, D. R. Burton, E. Freire, R. Wyatt, J. Sodroski, W. A. Hendrickson, and J. Arthos (2002). HIV-1 evades antibody-mediated neutralization through conformational masking of receptor-binding sites. *Nature* 420, 678–682.

Langhoff, E., E. F. Terwilliger, H. J. Bos, K. H. Kalland, M. C. Poznansky, O. M. Bacon, and W. A. Haseltine (1991). Replication of human immunodeficiency virus type 1 in primary dendritic cell cultures. *Proc. Natl. Acad. Sci. USA* 88, 7998–8002.

Lee, B., M. Sharron, L. J. Montaner, D. Weissman, and R. W. Doms (1999). Quantification of CD4, CCR5, and CXCR4 levels on lymphocyte subsets, dendritic cells, and differentially conditioned monocyte-derived macrophages. *Proc. Natl. Acad. Sci. USA* 96, 5215–5220.

Leng, Q., G. Borkow, Z. Weisman, M. Stein, A. Kalinkovich, and Z. Bentwich (2001). Immune activation correlates better than HIV plasma viral load with CD4 T-cell decline during HIV infection. *J. Acquir. Immune Defic. Syndr.* 27, 389–397.

Lifson, J. D., and M. A. Martin (2002). One step forwards, one step back. *Nature* 415, 272–273.

Liu, R., W. A. Paxton, S. Choe, D. Ceradini, S. R. Martin, R. Horuk, M. E. MacDonald, H. Stuhlmann, R. A. Koup, and N. R. Landau (1996). Homozygous defect in HIV-1 coreceptor accounts for resistance of some multiply-exposed individuals to HIV-1 infection. *Cell* 86, 367–377.

Lohman, B. L., C. J. Miller, and M. B. McChesney (1995). Antiviral cytotoxic T lymphocytes in vaginal mucosa of simian immunodeficiency virus–infected rhesus macaques. *J. Immunol.* 155, 5855–5860.

Lü, F. X., K. Abel, Z. Ma, T. Rourke, D. Lu, J. Torten, M. McChesney, and C. J. Miller (2002). The strength of B cell immunity in female rhesus macaques is controlled by CD8+ T cells under the influence of ovarian steroid hormones. *Clin. Exp. Immunol.* 128, 10–20.

Lü, F. X., Z. Ma, T. Rourke, S. Srinivasan, M. McChesney, and C. J. Miller (1999). Immunoglobulin concentrations and antigen-specific antibody levels in cervicovaginal lavages of rhesus macaques are influenced by the stage of the menstrual cycle. *Infect. Immun.* 67, 6321–6328.

Lu, N.S., L. Belec, P. M. Martin, and J. Pillot (1991). Enhanced local immunity in vaginal secretions of HIV-infected women. *Lancet* 338, 323–324.

Lu, X. S., L. Belec, and J. Pillot (1993). Anti-gp160 IgG and IgA antibodies associated with a large increase in total IgG in cervicovaginal secretions from human immunodeficiency virus type 1-infected women. *J. Infect. Dis.* 167, 1189–1192.

Ma, Z., F. X. Lu, M. Torten, and C. J. Miller (2001). The number and distribution of immune cells in the cervicovaginal mucosa remain constant throughout the menstrual cycle of rhesus macaques. *Clin. Immunol.* 100, 240–249.

MacDougall, T. H., R. J. Shattock, C. Madsen, B. M. Chain, and D. R. Katz (2002). Regulation of primary HIV-1 isolate replication in dendritic cells. *Clin. Exp. Immunol.* 127, 66–71.

Mandelbrot, L., M. Burgard, J. P. Teglas, J. L. Benifla, C. Khan, P. Blot, E. Vilmer, S. Matheron, G. Firtion, S. Blanche, M. J. Mayaux, and C. Rouzioux (1999). Frequent detection of HIV-1 in the gastric aspirates of neonates born to HIV-infected mothers. *AIDS* 13, 2143–2149.

Marthas, M., S. Sutjipto, C. Miller, J. Higgins, J. Torten, R. Unger, H. Kiyono, J. McGhee, P. Marx, and N. Pedersen (1992). Efficacy of live-attenuated and whole-inactivated simian immunodeficiency virus vaccines against intravenous and intravaginal challenge. In *Vaccines 1992* (eds. F. Brown, R. M. Chanock, H. S. Ginsberg, and R. A. Lerner), Cold Spring Harbor, NY: Cold Spring Harbor Laboratory Press, 117–122.

Marx, P. A., A. I. Spira, A. Gettie, P. J. Dailey, R. S. Veazey, A. A. Lackner, C. J. Mahoney, C. J. Miller, L. E. Claypool, D. D. Ho, and N. J. Alexander (1996). Progesterone implants enhance SIV vaginal transmission and early virus load. *Nat. Med.* 2, 1084–1089.

Mascola, J. R., G. Stiegler, T. C. VanCott, H. Katinger, C. B. Carpenter, C. E. Hanson, H. Beary, D. Hayes, S. S. Frankel, D. L. Birx, and M. G. Lewis (2000). Protection of macaques against vaginal transmission of a pathogenic HIV-1/SIV chimeric virus by passive infusion of neutralizing antibodies. *Nat. Med.* 6(2), 207–210.

Masurier, C., B. Salomon, N. Guettari, C. Pioche, F. Lachapelle, M. Guigon, and D. Klatzmann (1998). Dendritic cells route human immunodeficiency virus to lymph nodes after vaginal or intravenous administration to mice. *J. Virol.* 72(10), 7822–7829.

Mathewson, J. J., Z. D. Jiang, H. L. DuPont, C. Chintu, N. Luo, and A. Zumla (1994). Intestinal secretory IgA immune response against human immunodeficiency virus among infected patients with acute and chronic diarrhea. *J. Infect. Dis.* 169, 614–617.

Mazanec, M. B., J. G. Nedrud, C. S. Kaetzel, and M. E. Lamm (1993). A three-tiered view of the role of IgA in mucosal defense. *Immunol. Today* 14, 430–435.

Mazzoli, S., D. Trabattoni, S. Lo Caputo, S. Piconi, C. Ble, F. Meacci, S. Ruzzante, A. Salvi, F. Semplici, R. Longhi, M. L. Fusi, N. Tofani, M. Biasin, M. L. Villa, F. Mazzotta, and M. Clerici (1997). HIV-specific mucosal and cellular immunity in HIV-seronegative partners of HIV-seropositive individuals. *Nat. Med.* 3, 1250–1257.

McChesney, M., E. Sawaii, and C. J. Miller (1999). Simian immunodeficiency virus. In *Persistent Viral Infections* (eds. R. Ahmed and I. Chen). West Sussex, England: John Wiley and Sons, 321–346.

McChesney, M. B., J. R. Collins, D. Lu, X. Lü, J. Torten, R. L. Ashley, M. W. Cloyd, and C. J. Miller (1998). Occult systemic infection and persistent SIV-specific CD4+ T-cell-proliferative responses in rhesus macaques that were transiently viremic after intravaginal inoculation of SIV. *J. Virol.* 72, 10029–10035.

McElrath, M. J., L. Corey, D. Montefiori, M. Wolff, D. Schwartz, M. Keefer, R. Belshe, B. S. Graham, T. Matthews, P. Wright, G. Gorse, R. Dolin, P. Berman, D. Francis, A. M. Duliege, D. Bolognesi, D. Stablein, N. Ketter, and P. Fast (2000). A phase II study of two HIV type 1 envelope vaccines, comparing their immunogenicity in populations at risk for acquiring HIV type 1 infection. AIDS Vaccine Evaluation Group. *AIDS Res. Hum. Retroviruses* 16, 907–919.

McElrath, M. J., R. F. Siliciano, and K. J. Weinhold (1997). HIV type 1 vaccine-induced cytotoxic T cell responses in phase I clinical trials: detection, characterization, and quantitation. *AIDS Res. Hum. Retroviruses* 13, 211–216.

McMichael, A. J., and T. Hanke (1999). Is an HIV vaccine possible? *Nat. Med.* 5, 612–614.

Mellors, J. W., L. A. Kingsley, C. R. Rinaldo, Jr., J. A. Todd, B. S. Hoo, R. P. Kokka, and P. Gupta (1995). Quantitation of HIV-1 RNA in plasma predicts outcome after seroconversion. *Ann. Intern. Med.* 122, 573–579.

Mellors, J. W., C. R. Jr. Rinaldo, P. Gupta, R. M. White, J. A. Todd, and L. A. Kingsley (1996). Prognosis in HIV-1 infection predicted by the quantity of virus in plasma. *Science* 272, 1167–1170.

Meng, G., X. Wei, X. Wu, M. T. Sellers, J. M. Decker, Z. Moldoveanu, J. M. Orenstein, M. F. Graham, J. C. Kappes, J. Mestecky, G. M. Shaw, and P. D. Smith (2002). Primary intestinal epithelial cells selectively transfer R5 HIV-1 to CCR5+ cells. *Nat. Med.* 8, 150–156.

Miller, C. J., N. J. Alexander, S. Sutjipto, A. A. Lackner, A. Gettie, A. G. Hendrickx, L. J. Lowenstine, M. Jennings, and P. A. Marx (1989). Genital mucosal transmission of simian immunodeficiency virus: animal model for heterosexual transmission of human immunodeficiency virus. *J. Virol.* 63, 4277–4284.

Miller, C. J., N. J. Alexander, P. Vogel, J. Anderson, and P. A. Marx (1992a). Mechanism of genital transmission of SIV: a hypothesis based on transmission studies and the location of SIV in the genital tract of chronically infected female rhesus macaques. *J. Med. Primatol.* 21, 64–68.

Miller, C. J., M. Marthas, J. Greenier, D. Lu, P. J. Dailey, and Y. Lu (1998). *In vivo* replication capacity rather than *in vitro* macrophage tropism predicts efficiency of vaginal transmission of simian immunodeficiency virus or simian/human immunodeficiency virus in rhesus macaques. *J. Virol.* 72, 3248–3258.

Miller, C. J., M. Marthas, J. Torten, N. J. Alexander, J. P. Moore, G. F. Doncel, and A. G. Hendrickx (1994). Intravaginal inoculation of rhesus macaques with cell-free simian immunodeficiency virus results in persistent or transient viremia. *J. Virol.* 68, 6391–6400.

Miller, C. J., M. McChesney, and P. F. Moore (1992b). Langerhans' cells, macrophages and lymphocyte subsets in the cervix and vagina of rhesus macaques. *Lab. Invest.* 67, 628–634.

Miller, C. J., M. B. McChesney, and X. S. Lu (1996). Mucosal immune responses to SIV infection. *Semin. Virol.* 7, 139–145.

Miller, C. J., M. B. McChesney, X. Lü, P. J. Dailey, C. Chutkowski, D. Lu, P. Brosio, B. Roberts, and Y. Lu (1997). Rhesus macaques previously infected with SHIV are protected from vaginal challenge with pathogenic SIVmac239. *J. Virol.* 71, 1911–1921.

Miller, C. J., J. R. McGhee, and M. B. Gardner (1993). Mucosal Immunity, HIV transmission and AIDS. *Lab. Invest.* 68, 129–145.

Mitchell, E. A., L. A. Bergmeier, C. Doyle, R. Brookes, L. A. Hussain, Y. Wang, and T. Lehner (1998). Homing of mononuclear cells from iliac lymph nodes to the genital and rectal mucosa in non-human primates. *Eur J. Immunol.* 28(10), 3066–3074.

Moja, P., C. Tranchat, I. Tchou, B. Pozzetto, F. Lucht, C. Desgranges, and C. Genin (2000). Neutralization of human immunodeficiency virus type 1 (HIV-1) mediated by parotid IgA of HIV-1-infected patients. *J. Infect. Dis.* 181, 1607–1613.

Moriyama, A., K. Shimoya, I. Ogata, T. Kimura, T. Nakamura, H. Wada, K. Ohashi, C. Azuma, F. Saji, and Y. Murata (1999). Secretory leukocyte protease inhibitor (SLPI) concentrations in cervical mucus of women with normal menstrual cycle. *Mol. Hum. Reprod.* 5, 656–661.

Morris, H. H., K. C. Gatter, H. Stein, and D. Y. Mason (1983). Langerhans' cells in human cervical epithelium: an immunohistologic, immunohistological study. *Br. J. Obstet. Gynaecol.* 90, 400–411.

Murphey-Corb, M., L. A. Wilson, A. M. Trichel, D. E. Roberts, K. Xu, S. Ohkawa, B. Woodson, R. Bohm, and J. Blanchard (1999). Selective induction of protective MHC class I–restricted CTL in the intestinal lamina propria of rhesus monkeys by transient SIV infection of the colonic mucosa. *J. Immunol.* 162, 540–549.

Musey, L., Y. Ding, M. Elizaga, R. Ha, C. Celum, and M. J. Mc Elrath. (2003). HIV-1 vaccination administered intramuscularly can induce both systemic and mucosal T-cell immunity in HIV-1 infected individuals. *J. Immunol.* 171, 1094–1101.

Musey, L., Y. Ding, J. Cao, J. Lee, C. Galloway, A. Yuen, K. R. Jerome, and M. J. McElrath (2003). Ontogeny and specificities of mucosal and blood human immunodeficiency virus type 1–specific CD8(+) cytotoxic T lymphocytes. *J. Virol.* 77, 291–300.

Musey, L., Y. Hu, L. Eckert, M. Christensen, T. Karchmer, and M. J. McElrath (1997a). HIV-1 induces cytotoxic T lymphocytes in the cervix of infected women. *J. Exp. Med.* 185, 293–303.

Musey, L., J. Hughes, T. Schacker, T. Shea, L. Corey, and M. J. McElrath (1997b). Cytotoxic-T-cell responses, viral load, and disease progression in early human immunodeficiency virus type 1 infection. *N. Engl. J. Med.* 337, 1267–1274.

Nilsson, C., B. Makitalo, R. Thorstensson, S. Norley, D. Binninger-Schinzel, M. Cranage, E. Rud, G. Biberfeld, and P. Putkonen (1998). Live attenuated simian immunodeficiency virus (SIV)mac in macaques can induce protection against mucosal infection with SIVsm. *AIDS* 12(17), 2261–2270.

Novell, M. K., G. I. Benrudi, and R. J. Thompson (1984). Investigation of microtrauma after sexual intercourse. *J. Reprod. Med.* 29, 269–271.

Nuovo, G. J., A. Forde, P. MacConnell, and R. Fahrenwald (1993). In situ detection of PCR-amplified HIV-1 nucleic acids and tumor necrosis factor cDNA in cervical tissues. *Am. J. Pathol.* 143, 40–48.

Paavonen, T., L. C. Andersson, and H. Adlercreutz (1981). Sex hormone regulation of in vitro immune response. Estradiol enhances human B cell maturation via inhibition of suppressor T cells in pokeweed mitogen–stimulated cultures. *J. Exp. Med.* 154(6), 1935–1945.

Parren, P. W., P. A. Marx, A. J. Hessell, A. Luckay, J. Harouse, C. Cheng-Mayer, J. P. Moore, and D. R. Burton (2001). Antibody protects macaques against vaginal challenge with a pathogenic R5 simian/human immunodeficiency virus at serum levels giving complete neutralization *in vitro*. *J. Virol.* 75, 8340–8347.

Patterson, B. K., M. Czerniewski, J. Andersson, Y. Sullivan, F. Su, D. Jiyamapa, Z. Burki, and A. Landay (1999). Regulation of CCR5 and CXCR4 expression by type 1 and type 2 cytokines: CCR5 expression is downregulated by IL-10 in CD4-positive lymphocytes. *Clin. Immunol.* 91, 254–262.

Patterson, S., and S. C. Knight (1987). Susceptibility of human peripheral blood dendritic cells to infection by human immunodeficiency virus. *J. Gen. Virol.* 68, 1177–1181.

Patton, D. L., S. S. Thwin, A. Meier, T. M. Hooton, A. E. Stapleton, and D. A. Eschenbach (2000). Epithelial cell layer thickness and immune cell populations in the normal human vagina at different stages of the menstrual cycle. *Am. J. Obstet. Gynecol.* 183, 967–973.

Phillips, D. M., and A. S. Bourinbaiar (1992). Mechanism of HIV spread from lymphocytes to epithelia. *Virology* 186, 261–273.

Pohlmann, S., F. Baribaud, and R. W. Doms (2001). DC-SIGN and DC-SIGNR: helping hands for HIV. *Trends Immunol.* 22, 643–646.

Pomerantz, R. J., S. M. de la Monte, S. P. Donegan, T. R. Rota, M. W. Vogt, D. E. Craven, and M. S. Hirsch (1988). Human immunodeficiency virus (HIV) infection of the uterine cervix. *Ann. Intern. Med.* 108, 321–327.

Prakash, M., M. S. Kapembwa, F. Gotch, and S. Patterson (2002). Oral contraceptive use induces upregulation of the CCR5 chemokine receptor on CD4(+) T cells in the cervical epithelium of healthy women. *J. Reprod. Immunol.* 54, 117–131.

Quayle, A. J., W. M. Coston, A. K. Trocha, S. A. Kalams, K. H. Mayer, and D. J. Anderson (1998). Detection of HIV-1-specific CTLs in the semen of HIV-infected individuals. *J. Immunol.* 161, 4406–4410.

Quesnel, A., S. Cu-Uvin, D. Murphy, R. L. Ashley, T. Flanigan, and M. R. Neutra (1997). Comparative analysis of methods for collection and measurement of immunoglobulins in cervical and vaginal secretions of women. *J. Immunol. Methods* 202, 153–161.

Quinn, T. C., M. J. Wawer, N. Sewankambo, D. Serwadda, C. Li, F. Wabwire-Mangen, M. O. Meehan, T. Lutalo, and R. H. Gray (2000). Viral load and heterosexual transmission of human immunodeficiency virus type 1. Rakai Project Study Group. *N. Engl. J. Med.* 342, 921–929.

Raux, M., L. Finkielsztejn, D. Salmon-Ceron, H. Bouchez, J. L. Excler, E. Dulioust, J. M. Grouin, D. Sicard, and C. Blondeau (1999). Comparison of the distribution of IgG and IgA antibodies in serum and various mucosal fluids of HIV type 1–infected subjects. *AIDS Res. Hum. Retroviruses* 15, 1365–1376.

Reece, J. C., A. J. Handley, E. J. Anstee, W. A. Morrison, S. M. Crowe, and P. U. Cameron (1998). HIV-1 selection by epidermal dendritic cells during transmission across human skin. *J. Exp. Med.* 187, 1623–1631.

Reinhart, T. A., B. A. Fallert, M. E. Pfeifer, S. Sanghavi, S. Capuano, 3rd, P. Rajakumar, M. Murphey-Corb, R. Day, C. L. Fuller, and T. M. Schaefer (2002). Increased expression of the inflammatory chemokine CXC chemokine ligand 9/monokine induced by interferon-gamma in lymphoid tissues of rhesus macaques during simian immunodeficiency virus infection and acquired immunodeficiency syndrome. *Blood* 99, 3119–3128.

Robboy, S. J., M. Prade, and G. Cunha (1992). Vagina. In *Histology for Pathologists* (ed. S. S. Sternberg). North Holland, NY: Raven Press, 881–892.

Roncalli, M., M. Sideri, P. Gie, and E. Servida (1988). Immunophenotypic analysis of the transformation zone of human cervix. *Lab. Invest.* 58, 141–149.

Rottman, J. B., K. P. Ganley, K. Williams, L. Wu, C. R. Mackay, and D. J. Ringler (1997). Cellular localization of the chemokine receptor CCR5. Correlation to cellular targets of HIV-1 infection. *Am. J. Pathol.* 151, 1341–1351.

Rubbert, A., C. Combadiere, M. Ostrowski, J. Arthos, M. Dybul, E. Machado, M. A. Cohn, J. A. Hoxie, P. M. Murphy, A. S. Fauci, and D. Weissman (1998). Dendritic cells express multiple chemokine receptors used as coreceptors for HIV entry. *J. Immunol.* 160, 3933–3941.

Salmon-Ceron, D., J. L. Excler, L. Finkielsztejn, B. Autran, J. C. Gluckman, D. Sicard, T. J. Matthews, B. Meignier, C. Valentin, R. El Habib, C. Blondeau, M. Raux, C. Moog, J. Tartaglia, P. Chong, M. Klein, B. Milcamps, F. Heshmati, and S. Plotkin (1999). Safety and immunogenicity of a live recombinant canarypox virus expressing HIV type 1 gp120 MN MN tm/gag/protease LAI (ALVAC-HIV, vCP205) followed by a p24E-V3 MN synthetic peptide (CLTB-36) administered in healthy volunteers at low risk for HIV infection. AGIS Group and L'Agence Nationale de Recherches sur Le Sida. *AIDS Res. Hum. Retroviruses* 15, 633–645.

Schmitz, J. E., R. S. Veazey, M. J. Kuroda, D. B. Levy, A. Seth, K. G. Mansfield, C. E. Nickerson, M. A. Lifton, X. Alvarez, A. A. Lackner, and N. L. Letvin (2001). Simian immunodeficiency virus (SIV)–specific cytotoxic T lymphocytes in gastrointestinal tissues of chronically SIV-infected rhesus monkeys. *Blood* 98, 3757–3761.

Schneider, T., T. Zippel, W. Schmidt, G. Pauli, W. Heise, U. Wahnschaffe, E. O. Riecken, M. Zeitz, and R. Ullrich (1997). Abnormal predominance of IgG in HIV-specific antibodies produced by short-term cultured duodenal biopsy specimens from HIV-infected patients. *J. Acquir. Immune Defic. Syndr. Hum. Retrovirol.* 16, 333–339.

Schneider, T., T. Zippel, W. Schmidt, G. Pauli, U. Wahnschaffe, S. Chakravarti, W. Heise, E. O. Riecken, M. Zeitz, and R. Ullrich (1998). Increased immunoglobulin G production by short term cultured duodenal biopsy samples from HIV infected patients. *Gut* 42, 357–361.

Schumacher, G. F. B., and S. L. Yang (1977). Cyclic changes of immunoglobulins and specific antibodies in human and rhesus monkey cervical mucus. In *The Uterine Cervix in Reproduction* (eds V. Insler and G. Bettendorf). Stuttgart: Georg Thieme Verlag, 187–203.

Sewankambo, N., R. H. Gray, M. J. Wawer, L. Paxton, D. McNaim, F. Wabwire-Mangen, D. Serwadda, C. Li, N. Kiwanuka, S. L. Hillier, L. Rabe, C. A. Gaydos, T. C. Quinn, and J. Konde-Lule (1997). HIV-1 infection associated with abnormal vaginal flora morphology and bacterial vaginosis. *Lancet* 350, 546–550.

Shacklett, B. L., T. J. Beadle, P. A. Pacheco, J. H. Grendell, P. A. Haslett, A. S. King, G. S. Ogg, P. M. Basuk, and D. F. Nixon (2000a). Characterization of HIV-1-specific cytotoxic T lymphocytes expressing the mucosal lymphocyte integrin CD103 in rectal and duodenal lymphoid tissue of HIV-1-infected subjects. *Virology* 270, 317–327.

Shacklett, B. L., S. Cu-Uvin, T. J. Beadle, C. A. Pace, N. M. Fast, S. M. Donahue, A. M. Caliendo, T. P. Flanigan, C. C. Carpenter, and D. F. Nixon (2000b). Quantification of HIV-1-specific T-cell responses at the mucosal cervicovaginal surface. *AIDS* 14, 1911–1915.

Shattock, R. J., G. E. Griffin, and G. I. Gorodeski (2000). In vitro models of mucosal HIV transmission. *Nat. Med.* 6, 607–608.

Shiver, J. W., T. M. Fu, L. Chen, D. R. Casimiro, M. E. Davies, R. K. Evans, Z. Q. Zhang, A. J. Simon, W. L. Trigona, S. A. Dubey, L. Huang, V. A. Harris, R. S. Long, X. Liang, L. Handt, W. A. Schleif, L. Zhu, D. C. Freed, N. V. Persaud, L. Guan, K. S. Punt, A. Tang, M. Chen, K. A. Wilson, K. B. Collins, G. J. Heidecker, V. R. Fernandez, H. C. Perry, J. G. Joyce, K. M. Grimm, J. C. Cook, P. M. Keller, D. S. Kresock, H. Mach, R. D. Troutman, L. A. Isopi, D. M. Williams, Z. Xu, K. E. Bohannon, D. B. Volkin, D. C. Montefiori, A. Miura, G. R. Krivulka, M. A. Lifton, M. J. Kuroda, J. E. Schmitz, N. L. Letvin, M. J. Caulfield, A. J. Bett, R. Youil, D. C. Kaslow, and E. A. Emini (2002). Replication-incompetent adenoviral vaccine vector elicits effective anti-immunodeficiency-virus immunity. *Nature* 415, 331–335.

Skott, P., E. Lucht, I. Julander, J. Dillner, and E. Bjorling (1999). Salivary sIgA response in HIV-1 infection. *J. Acquir. Immune Defic. Syndr.* 21, 73–80.

Skurnick, J. H., P. Palumbo, A. DeVico, B. L. Shacklett, F. T. Valentine, M. Merges, R. Kamin-Lewis, J. Mestecky, T. Denny, G. K. Lewis, J. Lloyd, R. Praschunus, A. Baker, D. F. Nixon, S. Stranford, R. Gallo, S. H. Vermund, and D. B. Louria (2002). Correlates of nontransmission in US women at high risk of human immunodeficiency virus type 1 infection through sexual exposure. *J. Infect. Dis.* 185, 428–438.

Smith, S. M., G. B. Baskin, and P. A. Marx (2000). Estrogen protects against vaginal transmission of simian immunodeficiency virus. *J. Infect. Dis.* 182(3), 708–715.

Sodora, D. L., A. Gettie, C. J. Miller, and P. A. Marx (1998). Vaginal transmission of SIV: assessing infectivity and hormonal influences in macaques inoculated with cell-free and cell-associated viral stocks. *AIDS Res. Hum. Retroviruses* 14 Suppl 1, S119–123.

Spira, A. I., P. A. Marx, B. K. Patterson, J. Mahoney, R. A. Koup, S. M. Wolinsky, and D. D. Ho (1996). Cellular targets of infection and route of viral dissemination after an intravaginal inoculation of simian immunodeficiency virus into rhesus macaques. *J. Exp. Med.* 183, 215–225.

Stahl-Hennig, C., R. M. Steinman, K. Tenner-Racz, M. Pope, N. Stolte, K. Matz-Rensing, G. Grobschupff, B. Raschdorff, G. Hunsmann, and P. Racz (1999). Rapid infection of oral mucosal-associated lymphoid tissue with simian immunodeficiency virus. *Science* 285, 1261–1265.

Stevceva, L., B. Kelsall, J. Nacsa, M. Moniuszko, Z. Hel, E. Tryniszewska, and G. Franchini (2002). Cervicovaginal lamina propria lymphocytes: phenotypic characterization and their importance in cytotoxic T-lymphocyte responses to simian immunodeficiency virus SIVmac251. *J. Virol.* 76, 9–18.

Stewart, G. J., J. P. Tyler, A. L. Cunningham, J. A. Barr, G. L. Driscoll, J. Gold, and B. J. Lamont (1985). Transmission of human T-cell lymphotropic virus type III (HTLV-III) by artificial insemination by donor. *Lancet* 2, 581–585.

Sthoeger, Z. M., N. Chiorazzi, and R. G. Lahita (1988). Regulation of the immune response by sex hormones. I. In vitro effects of estradiol and testosterone on pokeweed mitogen–induced human B cell differentiation. *J. Immunol.* 141, 91–98.

Strathdee, S. A., R. S. Hogg, M. V. O'Shaughnessy, J. S. Montaner, and M. T. Schechter (1996). A decade of research on the natural history of HIV infection: Part 2. Cofactors. *Clin. Invest. Med.* 19, 121–130.

Sturm-Ramirez, K., A. Gaye-Diallo, G. Eisen, S. Mboup, and P. J. Kanki (2000). High levels of tumor necrosis factor–alpha and interleukin–1beta in bacterial vaginosis may increase susceptibility to human immunodeficiency virus. *J. Infect. Dis.* 182, 467–473.

Syrbe, U., J. Siveke, and A. Hamann (1999). Th1/Th2 subsets: distinct differences in homing and chemokine receptor expression? *Springer Semin. Immunopathol.* 21, 263–285.

Turville, S. G., J. Arthos, K. M. Donald, G. Lynch, H. Naif, G. Clark, D. Hart, and A. L. Cunningham (2001). HIV gp120 receptors on human dendritic cells. *Blood* 98, 2482–2488.

Van Rompay, K. K., C. J. Berardi, S. Dillard-Telm, R. P. Tarara, D. R. Canfield, C. R. Valverde, D. C. Montefiori, K. S. Cole, R. C. Montelaro, C. J. Miller, and M. L. Marthas (1998). Passive immunization of newborn rhesus macaques prevents oral simian immunodeficiency virus infection. *J. Infect. Dis.* 177, 1247–1259.

Veazey, R. S., R. J. Shattock, M. Pope, J. C. Kirijan, J. Jones, Q. Hu, T. Ketas, P. A. Marx, P. J. Klasse, D. R. Burton, and J. P. Moore (2003). Prevention of virus transmission to macaque monkeys by a vaginally applied monoclonal antibody to HIV-1 gp120. *Nat. Med.* 9, 343–346.

Wallace, J. I., J. Porter, A. Weiner, and A. Steinberg (1997). Oral sex, crack smoking, and HIV infection among female sex workers who do not inject drugs. *Am. J. Public Health* 87, 470.

Weissman, D., A. Rubbert, C. Combadiere, P. M. Murphy, and A. S. Fauci (1997). Dendritic cells express and use multiple HIV coreceptors. *Adv. Exp. Med. Biol.* 417, 401–406.

Williams, S. B., T. P. Flanigan, S. Cu-Uvin, K. Mayer, P. Williams, C. A. Ettore, A. W. Artenstein, A. Duerr, and T. C. VanCott (2002).

Human immunodeficiency virus (HIV)–specific antibody in cervicovaginal lavage specimens obtained from women infected with HIV type 1. *Clin. Infect. Dis.* 35, 611–617.

Wortley, P. M., T. A. Hammett, and P. L. Fleming (1998). Donor insemination and human immunodeficiency virus transmission. *Obstet. Gynecol.* 91, 515–518.

Wright, P. F., P. A. Kozlowski, G. K. Rybczyk, P. Goepfert, H. F. Staats, T. C. VanCott, D. Trabattoni, E. Sannella, and J. Mestecky (2002). Detection of mucosal antibodies in HIV type 1–infected individuals. *AIDS Res. Hum. Retroviruses* 18, 1291–1300.

Wu, L., A. A. Bashirova, T. D. Martin, L. Villamide, E. Mehlhop, A. O. Chertov, D. Unutmaz, M. Pope, M. Carrington, and V. N. KewalRamani (2002). Rhesus macaque dendritic cells efficiently transmit primate lentiviruses independently of DC-SIGN. *Proc. Natl. Acad. Sci. USA* 99, 1568–1573.

Yoshino, N., Y. Ami, K. Someya, S. Ando, K. Shinohara, F. Tashiro, Y. Lu, and M. Honda (2000). Protective immune responses induced by a non-pathogenic simian/human immunodeficiency virus (SHIV) against a challenge of a pathogenic SHIV in monkeys. *Microbiol. Immunol.* 44, 363–372.

Zacharopoulos, V. R., M. E. Perotti, and D. M. Phillips (1997). A role for cell migration in the sexual transmission of HIV-1? *Curr. Biol.* 7, 534–537.

Zaitseva, M., A. Blauvelt, S. Lee, C. K. Lapham, V. Klaus-Kovtun, H. Mostowski, J. Manischewitz, and H. Golding (1997). Expression and function of CCR5 and CXCR4 on human Langerhans cells and macrophages: implications for HIV primary infection. *Nat. Med.* 3, 1369–1375.

Zhang, L., T. He, A. Talal, G. Wang, S. S. Frankel, and D. D. Ho (1998). In vivo distribution of the human immunodeficiency virus/simian immunodeficiency virus coreceptors: CXCR4, CCR3, and CCR5. *J. Virol.* 72, 5035–5045.

Zhang, Z. Q., T. M. Fu, D. R. Casimiro, M. E. Davies, X. Liang, W. A. Schleif, L. Handt, L. Tussey, M. Chen, A. Tang, K. A. Wilson, W. L. Trigona, D. C. Freed, C. Y. Tan, M. Horton, E. A. Emini, and J. W. Shiver (2002). Mamu-A*01 allele-mediated attenuation of disease progression in simian-human immunodeficiency virus infection. *J. Virol.* 76, 12845–12854.

Zhu, T., L. Corey, Y. Hwangbo, J. Lee, G. H. Learn, J. I. Mullins, and M. J. McElrath. (2003). Persistence of extraordinarily low levels of genetically homogenous HW-1 in exposed seronegative individuals. *J. Virol.* 77, 6108–6116.

Zoeteweij, J. P., and A. Blauvelt (1998). HIV-dendritic cell interactions promote efficient viral infection of T cells. *J. Biomed. Sci.* 5, 253–259.

CpG Oligodeoxynucleotides for Mucosal Vaccines

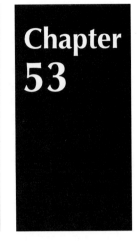

Chapter 53

Arthur M. Krieg

Coley Pharmaceutical Group, Wellesley, Massachusetts

THE ROLE OF TOLL-LIKE RECEPTORS IN THE IMMUNE RECOGNITION OF CpG MOTIFS

Several generations of immunologists have recognized the potent adjuvant activity of bacterial extracts. An emulsion of killed bacteria, complete Freund's adjuvant (CFA), has long been the "gold standard" experimental injected vaccine adjuvant for immunologists, but it is generally considered to be too toxic for use in humans. Recent discoveries in immunology have revealed the mechanism through which bacterial extracts activate the immune system. To detect the presence of infectious agents, the immune system appears to have evolved one or more families of "pattern recognition receptors" (PRRs). The best characterized family of PRRs are the Toll-like receptors, or TLRs, of which 10 members have been identified in humans (Janeway *et al.*, 2002). TLRs are expressed on certain innate immune cells such as dendritic cell (DC) subsets, macrophages, monocytes, and neutrophils and trigger cell activation when they bind their ligands. Different TLRs bind different conserved microbial-specific molecules, such as peptidoglycans, zymosan, lipopolysaccharides (LPSs), and certain unmethylated CpG dinucleotides (Janeway *et al.*, 2002).

Several of these microbial molecules likely contribute to the immune activity of CFA, bacille Calmette-Guerin (BCG), and other bacterial extracts. Studies to identify the component responsible for the antitumor properties of BCG revealed this to be the bacterial DNA; little or no antitumor activity could be detected in the protein, RNA, lipid, or carbohydrate fractions of BCG (Tokunaga *et al.*, 1999). Treatment of CFA or other microbial extracts with nuclease severely reduces their immune stimulating activity (Brown *et al.*, 1998; Ronaghy *et al.*, 2002), further supporting the identification of bacterial DNA as a key active ingredient of bacterial extracts. It is now realized that these immune stimulatory effects of bacterial DNA are a consequence of the presence of unmethylated CpG dinucleotides in particular base contexts, termed "CpG motifs" (Krieg *et al.*, 1995).

CpG motifs are common in bacterial DNA but are underrepresented and methylated in vertebrate DNA (Krieg, 2002).

TLR9 is the receptor used by the innate immune system for detecting CpG motifs, as mice lacking TLR9 fail to respond to CpG stimulation (Hemmi *et al.*, 2000). In humans TLR9 is expressed only in B cells and in plasmacytoid dendritic cells (pDCs), which are known as the cells that produce most of the type I interferon (IFN) that is made in response to viral infection (Bauer *et al.*, 2001; Hornung *et al.*, 2002; Kadowaki *et al.*, 2001; Krug *et al.*, 2001). Since no other known immune activator has this specificity, TLR9 is the most selective TLR pathway for inducing IFN-α expression. IFN-α triggers strong adaptive Th1 T-cell responses (Biron *et al.*, 2002), so the possibility of triggering endogenous IFN-α production through deliberate activation of the TLR9 pathway is of considerable interest for vaccination. TLR9 activation for adjuvant vaccines is easily accomplished through the use of synthetic oligodeoxynucleotides (ODNs) of about 8 to 30 bases in length that contain a nuclease-resistant phosphorothioate backbone and the appropriate CpG motifs for the species to be treated. There are species-specific differences with regard to the optimal CpG motif. For example, the optimal immune stimulatory ODN CpG motif is GACGTT for mice (Krieg *et al.*, 1995; Rankin *et al.*, 2001; Yi *et al.*, 1998) but GTCGTT for humans (Hartmann *et al.*, 2000) and many other vertebrate species, including cow, sheep, cat, dog, goat, horse, pig, and chicken (Brown *et al.*, 1998; Rankin *et al.*, 2001). The immune stimulatory activity of an ODN is determined not only by the activity of a given hexamer CpG motif but also by several other factors, including the number of CpG motifs in an ODN, where 2 or 3 are optimal; the spacing of the CpG motifs, which are best separated by at least two intervening bases, preferably Ts; the presence of poly G sequences or other flanking sequences in the ODN; and the ODN backbone, where a nuclease-resistant phosphorothioate backbone is best for *in vivo* use (Ballas *et al.*, 1996; Hartmann *et al.*, 2000; Hartmann *et al.*, 2000; Krieg *et al.*, 1995; Pisetsky *et al.*, 1998; Yi *et al.*, 1998). In addition, the immune stimulatory effects of the ODNs are enhanced if it has a TpC dinucleotide on the 5′ end and is pyrimidine rich on the 3′ side (Hartmann et al., 2000; Hartmann et al., 2000; Yi et al., 1998). Mice and humans also differ in the types of immune cells that express TLR9 and therefore are able to respond to CpG. In contrast to humans, where only the pDCs and B cells are known to express the TLR9 receptor (Kadowaki et al., 2001; Krug et al., 2001), TLR9 expression in mice is broader, including the mouse myeloid DC and monocyte/macrophages. These interspecies differences cause obvious difficulties in extrapolating from mouse models to predict results in humans.

The immune effects of activating TLR9-expressing cells with CpG ODNs are Th1-like and may be considered in two stages: an early innate immune activation and a later enhancement of adaptive immune responses. Within minutes of exposure of B cells or pDCs to CpG, the ODNs appear to enter an endosomal compartment where they interact with TLR9, leading to the activation of cell-signaling pathways that culminate in the expression of costimulatory molecules, resistance to apoptosis, upregulation of the chemokine receptor CCR7 that causes cell trafficking to the T cell zone of the lymph nodes, and secretion of Th1-promoting-like chemokines and cytokines such as MIP-1, IP-10, and other IFN-inducible genes (Krieg, 2002). PDCs secrete type I IFN and mature to highly effective antigen-presenting cells (Krug et al., 2001). These CpG-induced type I IFN, cytokines, and chemokines trigger within hours a wide range of secondary effects, such as natural killer (NK) cell activation and enhanced polymorphonuclear (PMN) cell migration in response to inflammatory signals. The innate immune activation and pDC maturation are followed by the generation of adaptive immune responses. B cells are strongly constimulated if they bind specific antigen at the same time as TLR9 stimulation (Krieg et al., 1995). This selectively enhances the development of antigen-specific antibodies, especially of the isotype associated with Th1-like immune responses (e.g., IgG2a in mice). Following CpG stimulation, both B cells and pDCs can present antigen to T cells. CpG-induced antigen presentation occurs in a Th1-like cytokine milieu, stimulating the development of Th1 cells, and can result in primary effector CTL (Sparwasser et al., 2000). Moreover, the enhancement of IL-12 production by CpG establishes strong memory T-cell responses. In vivo administration of CpG ODNs by subcutaneous injection or intradermally or nasally creates a Th1-like milieu and lymphadenopathy in the draining lymph node (LN) that peaks at 7–10 days (Kobayashi et al., 1999; Lipford et al., 2000). DCs increase in number and exhibit a mature phenotype with increased expression of costimulatory molecules. This Th1-like environment appears to be sustained for several weeks, since CpG-primed mice respond to an antigen injection with a Th1-biased response and CTL even 5 weeks later (Kobayashi et al., 1999; Lipford et al., 2000).

We have identified three main families of CpG ODNs with distinct structural and biological characteristics. The A class is a potent activator of NK cells and IFN-α secretion from DCs but is a poor stimulator of B cells. The B class is a strong B-cell stimulator but is weaker for induction of NK activity or IFN-α. Otherwise, both classes induce Th1-type cytokines (Krieg, 2002). The most recently discovered C class has properties of both the A and B classes (Vollmer et al., 2004). Since virtually all published studies to date using CpG ODNs as a vaccine adjuvant have been carried out with B class CpG ODNs, the following sections refer to "CpG ODN" generically, but this is actually referring to the B class. All three ODN classes require the presence of TLR9, as they have no immune stimulatory effects in mice deficient in TLR9 (Vollmer et al., 2004).

CpG ODN AS A VACCINE ADJUVANT

The utility of CpG ODN as a vaccine adjuvant for inducing antigen-specific humoral and cellular responses has been confirmed in studies using a wide variety of antigens, including peptide or protein antigens, live or killed viruses, DC vaccines, autologous cellular vaccines, and polysaccharide conjugates. CpG ODNs do not appear to be effective adjuvants for most pure polysaccharide antigens but are quite effective if a protein carrier is conjugated to the polysaccharide (Chu et al., 2000; Kovarik et al., 2001; von Hunolstein et al., 2000). Conjugation of CpG ODN directly to the antigen has been used to enhance antigen uptake and reduce antigen requirements (Cho et al., 2000; Tighe et al., 2000). The adjuvant effects of CpG ODN are not limited to mice but have also been shown to enhance antibody responses in Aotus monkeys against peptide sequences derived from the circumsporozoite protein from Plasmodium falciparum in a mineral oil emulsion (Jones et al., 1999) and for a hepatitis B vaccine in chimpanzees (Hartmann et al., 2000). Orangutans are hyporesponders to the commercial HBV vaccine (Davis 1999), but addition of a CpG ODN increased their seroconversion rates after two doses to 100%, with much higher antibody titers (Davis, 1999). A CpG ODN has been tested in two human trials in combination with Engerix-B (GlaxoSmithKline), a commercial HBV vaccine that contains HBsAg adsorbed to alum. A double-blind phase I clinical trial in healthy human volunteers showed that addition of a clinical grade CpG ODN optimized for interaction with the human TLR9, called CpG 7909, at a dose of 125 µg, 500 µg, or 1 mg to Engerix-B given at 0, 1, and 6 months by intramuscular injection dramatically accelerated seroconversion, with most of the subjects achieving protective levels of IgG antibodies in just 2 weeks (Cooper et al., 2004). The experimental and control vaccines were well tolerated, both locally and systemically.

The adjuvant activity of CpG has also been seen in a clinical trial in immunocompromised HIV-infected patients. This study was designed to evaluate the immunogenicity of Engerix-B vaccine plus CpG 7909 and included 38 HIV-seropositive adults aged 18–55 years, half of whom had no prior hepatitis B vaccination and half of whom had been vaccinated previously with at least three doses of the regular vaccine but did not have protective antibody titers. Patients receiving CpG 7909 with their hepatitis B vaccine produced protective antibodies more rapidly than patients receiving the vaccine alone (Krieg, 2002). By 8 weeks, only 42% of patients receiving vaccine alone had protective titers (≥10 mIU/mL), compared with 89% of CpG subjects. In addition to these increased rates of seroconversion, patients receiving CpG 7909 also had significantly higher antibody titers. For example, after two doses, geometric mean antibody titers were 18 for controls versus 252 for CpG 7909 recipients, and after three doses they were 119 for controls versus 1594 for CpG recipients (Cooper *et al.*, manuscript submitted).

Comparisons of different adjuvants in mouse models have demonstrated CpG ODNs to be stronger Th1-promoting adjuvants than any other agent, even including CFA, as measured by the ability of CpG ODNs to drive the differentiation of CTL and IFN-γ-secreting T cells (Chu *et al.*, 1997; Kim *et al.*, 1999; Lipford *et al.*, 1997; Roman *et al.*, 1997). Moreover, CpG ODNs accomplish this level of antigen-specific activation without inducing the harsh local inflammatory effects seen with CFA. Nevertheless, the adjuvant efficacy of CpG ODN can be further enhanced by coadministration with other adjuvants, especially adjuvants that may provide some depot function, such as alum or various lipid emulsions and nanoparticles or microparticles (Davis, 2000). Such formulations are especially important when the antigen is relatively weak. Combinations of CpG ODNs with QS21, Titermax, and MPL also have shown synergistically increased activity in mice (Kim *et al.*, 2000).

The vaccine adjuvant activity of CpG ODNs appears to result from several mechanisms. First, purified B cells are synergistically activated when stimulated by CpG ODNs in the presence of antigen, indicating cross-talk between the B-cell receptor and CpG signaling pathways (Krieg *et al.*, 1995). Although CpG DNA can activate essentially any B cell without regard to its antigen specificity, the synergy observed in B-cell activation through CpG and the BCR suggests that antigen-specific B cells will be preferentially activated. Second, the induction of increased costimulatory molecule expression on B cells and other APCs suggests that these should be more effective at promoting antigen-specific immune responses. Third, CpG ODNs inhibit B-cell apoptosis, contributing to a more sustained immune response (Yi *et al.*, 1996; Yi *et al.*, 1998). Fourth, the CpG-induced activation of DCs creates a Th1-like cytokine and chemokine environment in the secondary lymphoid organs (Lipford *et al.*, 2000; Sparwasser *et al.*, 2000). CpG ODNs promote cross-presentation with strong cytolytic T-cell and antibody responses to peptides and protein antigens independently of T-cell help (Lipford *et al.*, 1997; Roman *et al.*, 1997; Sparwasser *et al.*, 2000; Vabulas *et al.*, 2000; Wild *et al.*, 1999).

Inducing immunity during the neonatal period or in elderly or immune-compromised hosts is extremely important from the public health standpoint but generally is difficult to accomplish efficiently. Even with repeated vaccination, immune responses are generally modest in neonatal or aged mice or humans. Moreover, the neonatal immune system

tends to be skewed more toward the generation of Th2 responses rather than the more desirable Th1 responses. It is therefore noteworthy that CpG ODNs have proven to be highly effective Th1 adjuvants in neonatal and aged mice (Kovarik *et al.*, 1999).

GMP production of CpG ODNs is well established and highly economical. ODNs are produced in bulk (Kg scale) by a solid-phase synthesis. Stability of the bulk product appears to be at least several years when it is stored frozen; other ODNs have been reported to be stable for at least 2 years, even at room temperature. Aqueous solubility is excellent, and the ODNs are relatively nonreactive and nonpyrogenic.

MUCOSAL ADJUVANT ACTIVITY OF CpG ODNs

Because most pathogens enter the body through one of the vast mucosal surfaces, there is a great deal of interest in identifying adjuvants for achieving effective mucosal immunization. Although systemic vaccination can induce mucosal immune responses, most investigators have found that vaccination through the mucosal route provides superior humoral and cellular immune responses. Cholera toxin (CT) and heat-labile enterotoxin (LT) have been demonstrated to be effective mucosal adjuvants in animal models but are considered too toxic for general human use. The addition of CpG oligos to mucosal vaccines significantly enhances both systemic and mucosal fecal, serum, and bronchoalveolar lavage IgA and T-cell responses, including CTLs (Horner *et al.*, 1998; McCluskie *et al.*, 1998; Moldoveanu *et al.*, 1998). In addition to enhancing these humoral and cellular responses, CpG increases the induction of antigen-specific β-chemokine production against HIV vaccines (Dumais *et al.*, 2002; Horner *et al.*, 2001). A particularly potent method to induce very strong mucosal immunity was to prime systemically (intramuscularly) and boost mucosally (nasally) or vice versa; this yielded even higher IgA levels than both priming and boosting nasally (McCluskie *et al.*, 2002). The CpG oligos are noteworthy for enhancing the Th1 character of the systemic and mucosal immune response after mucosal vaccination, including directing antibody production toward the IgG2a isotype and stimulating the development of IFN-γ-secreting T cells in the spleen (McCluskie *et al.*, 1998). Human clinical trials with CpG ODNs as mucosal vaccine adjuvants have not yet been performed.

CpG ODNs have compared well to other mucosal vaccine adjuvants. For inducing both local and distant mucosal IgA responses, CpG ODNs have been shown to be similar in efficacy to cholera toxin (CT) and the *E. coli* labile toscin LT but are much better tolerated (Horner *et al.*, 1998; McCluskie *et al.*, 1998; McCluskie *et al.*, 2000a; McCluskie *et al.*, 2000b; McCluskie *et al.*, 2001a; McCluskie *et al.*, 2001b; Moldoveanu *et al.*, 1998). The combination of the detoxified LTR72 plus CpG given through the nasal route is as good as wild-type LT for enhancing the local and systemic humoral and cellular responses to mucosal vaccination to peptide

(Olszewska *et al.*, 2000). In addition, the inclusion of CpG in the vaccine changes the response from the Th2 response that is normally promoted by LTR72 to a Th1 response.

The volume used for nasal mucosal vaccination in mouse models is very important. Larger vaccine volumes, which presumably target not only the nasal mucosa but also parts of the lower respiratory tract, induce stronger immune responses to the CpG-adjuvanted vaccine (McCluskie *et al.*, 2000). This is also true when the CpG is used in combination with CT or LT. A surprising observation in these studies has been that although the Th1-effective mucosal vaccination requires the CpG motif, non-CpG control ODNs with a phosphorothioate backbone also have adjuvant activity in mucosal vaccination, but these responses were more Th2-like than those achieved with CpG ODN (Joseph *et al.*, 2002; McCluskie *et al.*, 2000). Almost all of the mucosal vaccination studies with CpG ODNs have used the nuclease-resistant phosphorothioate backbone. However, native bacterial DNA also is effective for nasal vaccination (Moldoveanu *et al.*, 1998) and one report also demonstrated that ODNs with a native phosphodiester backbone can be used for oral CpG vaccination (Eastcott *et al.*, 2001).

Comparison of different routes for mucosal vaccination with tetanus toxoid show that the intrarectal route is generally the weakest for inducing generalized mucosal or systemic immune responses (McCluskie *et al.*, 2000). Both the nasal and oral routes show similar ability to enhance systemic immune responses, but the nasal route appears to be more consistently successful at inducing optimal local and distant mucosal IgA responses (McCluskie *et al.*, 2000). Similarly, the nasal route is superior to gastric vaccination with *Helicobacter felis* (Jiang *et al.*, 2003).

CpG ODNs have been used as mucosal adjuvants for multiple different types of vaccines. They have enhanced the generation of systemic and mucosal immune responses to peptide antigens (Gierynska *et al.*, 2002; Olszewska *et al.*, 2000); proteins (Choi *et al.*, 2002; Gallichan *et al.*, 2001; Horner *et al.*, 1998; McCluskie *et al.*, 1998; McCluskie *et al.*, 2000); a polysaccharide conjugate (Mariotti *et al.*, 2002); immune complexes (McCluskie *et al.*, 1998); live attenuated BCG (Freidag *et al.*, 2000); viruslike particles (Gerber *et al.*, 2001; Kang *et al.*, 2003); and inactivated flu virus (Moldoveanu *et al.*, 1998). Formulation of the vaccine such as with liposomes can further improve the adjuvant activity of the CpG ODNs, providing superior mucosal and systemic humoral and cellular immune responses with either intramuscular or nasal vaccination (Davis, 2000; Joseph *et al.*, 2002). In general, coformulation of the CpG ODNs with the antigen yields the best responses.

In addition to enhancing the generation of immune responses, mucosal vaccination with CpG oligos has also provided superior protection against pathogen challenges. In a mouse rotavirus model, the use of CpG as a vaccine adjuvant reduced viral shedding almost as well as did CT or LT (Choi *et al.*, 2002). A liposomal formulation with HN was as good or better than CT for reducing viral titers in mice after intranasal flu challenge (Joseph *et al.*, 2002). Mice given an

aerosol challenge with virulent *Mycobacterium tuberculosis* had decreased colony-forming units in the lungs if they had been vaccinated with BCG plus CpG through the systemic route or especially through the nasal route (Freidag *et al.*, 2000). In an *H. felis* model, nasal CpG alone did not induce protective responses to a vaccine, but when used in combination with CT it showed synergy for immune enhancement, including providing sterilizing immunity against pathogen challenge (Jiang *et al.*, 2003).

Furthermore, mucosal vaccination with nasal CpG can protect against challenge at a different mucosal site. Mice immunized nasally with CpG and an HIV antigen preparation showed a >1-log decrease in ovarian viral titers in comparison with control mice following an intravaginal challenge with recombinant vaccinia virus expressing an HIV-1 gag protein (Dumais *et al.*, 2002). Likewise, mice vaccinated nasally with a recombinant HSV-1 glycoprotein had a 1-log decrease in viral titer after intravaginal challenge with HSV-2 in comparison with mice vaccinated without the CpG (Gallichan *et al.*, 2001). Moreover, these investigators demonstrated that nasal vaccination with CpG provided continuously high vaginal IgA titers throughout the estrous cycle, whereas mice vaccinated without CpG had very low vaginal IgA titers, especially during the diestrus phase of the estrous cycle (Gallichan *et al.*, 2001).

CpG ODNs AS ADJUVANTS FOR ALLERGY VACCINES

Allergic diseases result from Th2-type immune responses against otherwise harmless environmental antigens. Such responses lead to the generation of Th2 T cells that produce IL-4 and IL-5 and promote the differentiation of B cells into IgE-secreting cells. This IgE binds to the high-affinity IgE Fc receptor on the surface of mast cells and basophils. Subsequent exposure of these cells to an allergen results in the binding of the allergen by surface IgE, crosslinking of the IgE Fc receptors, and activation and degranulation of the mast cells or basophils. These cells release a variety of preformed proinflammatory and vasoactive compounds, including histamine, prostaglandins, leukotrienes, and cytokines. This results in an immediate inflammatory response (within 15 minutes), followed by a secondary late-phase reaction several hours later.

Considering the well-described Th1 immune effects of CpG ODNs and the inhibitory effects of Th1 responses on allergic Th2 responses, it is not surprising that their potential applications in the treatment of Th2-mediated allergic disease have attracted much interest. Several investigators have demonstrated the efficacy of systemic CpG ODN therapy in preventing or reversing allergic disease in mouse models (reviewed in Kline, 2000). In addition, mucosal coadministration of allergen and CpG oligos prevents the development of allergic responses (Shirota *et al.*, 2000). In a mouse model of allergic conjunctivitis, established disease was effectively treated by mucosal administration of CpG oligos (Magone *et* al., 2000). Conjugation of the CpG ODNs to the allergen can reduce the CpG dose required for immunotherapy. A recent study demonstrated that nasal immunotherapy with such a CpG conjugate is superior to intradermal immunotherapy for treating allergic disease in sensitized mice (Takabayashi *et al.*, 2003).

SUMMARY

CpG ODNs are a new class of Th1-type immune stimulant that, by stimulating the TLR9 receptor, have proven to be a highly effective adjuvant for mucosal vaccines against infectious diseases and allergies in mice. Mucosal vaccination with CpG ODNs provides enhanced systemic and mucosal humoral and cellular immune responses and enhanced protection against pathogen challenge, even when the challenge is at a different mucosal site. For infectious diseases, this may allow the induction of protective immune responses with fewer and lower doses of antigen, even in neonates and hyporesponders. Finally, the Th1 effects and the ability of CpG to reduce the adverse effects of preexisting Th2 responses make them ideal for mucosal allergy vaccines. Although human clinical trials indicate that CpG ODNs enhance seroconversion and antibody titers and are generally well tolerated for injectable vaccines, further studies will be needed to determine their efficacy and safety as a human mucosal adjuvant.

REFERENCES

Ballas, Z.K., Rasmussen, W.L., and Krieg, A.M. (1996). Induction of NK activity in murine and human cells by CpG motifs in oligodeoxynucleotides and bacterial DNA. *J. Immunol.* 157, 1840–1845.

Bauer, S., Kirschning, C.J., Hacker, H., Redecke, V., Hausmann, S., Akira, S., Wagner, H., and Lipford, G.B. (2001). Human TLR9 confers responsiveness to bacterial DNA via species-specific CpG motif recognition. *Proc. Natl. Acad. Sci. USA* 98, 9237–9242.

Biron, C.A., Nguyen, K.B., and Pien, G.C. (2002). Innate immune responses to LCMV infections: natural killer cells and cytokines. *Curr. Top. Microbiol. Immunol.* 263, 7–27.

Brown, W.C., Estes, D.M., Chantler, S.E., Kegerreis, K.A., and Suarez, C.E. (1998). DNA and a CpG oligoncleotide derived from *Babesia bovis* are mitogenic for bovine B cells. *Infect. Immun.* 66, 5423–5432.

Cho, H.J., Takabayashi, K., Cheng, P.M., Nguyen, M.D., Corr, M., Tuck, S., and Raz, E. (2000). Immunostimulatory DNA-based vaccines induce cytotoxic lymphocyte activity by a T-helper cell-independent mechanism. *Nat. Biotechnol.* 18, 509–514.

Choi, A.H., McNeal, M.M., Flint, J.A., Basu, M., Lycke, N.Y., Clements, J.D., Bean, J.A., Davis, H.L., McCluskie, M.J., VanCott, J.L., and Ward, R.L. (2002). The level of protection against rotavirus shedding in mice following immunization with a chimeric VP6 protein is dependent on the route and the coadministered adjuvant. *Vaccine* 20, 1733–1740.

Chu, R.S., Targoni, O.S., Krieg, A.M., Lehmann, P.V., and Harding, C.V. (1997). CpG oligodeoxynucleotides act as adjuvants that switch on T helper 1 (Th1) immunity. *J. Exp. Med.* 186, 1623–1631.

Chu, R.S., McCool, T., Greenspan, N.S., Schreiber, J.R., and Harding, C.V. (2000). CpG oligodeoxynucleotides act as adjuvants for pneumococcal polysaccharide-protein conjugate vaccines and enhance antipolysaccharide immunoglobulin G2a (IgG2a) and IgG3 antibodies. *Infect. Immun.* 68, 1450–1456.

Cooper, C. L., Davis, H. L., Morris, M. L., Efler, S. M., Al-Adhani, M., Kreig, A. M., Cameron, D. W., and Heathcote, J. (2004). CpG 7909, on immunostimulatory T1 agonist oligodeoxynucleotide, as adjuvant to Engerix-B® HBV vaccine in healthy adults: a double-blind phase I/II study. *J. Clin. Immunol.*, In press.

Davis, H.L. (1999). DNA vaccines for prophylactic or therapeutic immunization against hepatitis B virus. *Mt. Sinai. J. Med.* 66, 84–90.

Davis, H.L. (2000). Use of CpG DNA for enhancing specific immune responses. *Curr. Top. Microbiol. Immunol.* 247, 171–183.

Dumais, N., Patrick, A., Moss, R.B., Davis, H.L., and Rosenthal, K.L. (2002). Mucosal immunization with inactivated human immuno-deficiency virus plus CpG oligodeoxynucleotides induces genital immune responses and protection against intravaginal challenge. *J. Infect. Dis.* 186, 1098–1105.

Eastcott, J.W., Holmberg, C.J., Dewhirst, F.E., Esch, T.R., Smith, D.J., and Taubman, M.A. (2001). Oligonucleotide containing CpG motifs enhances immune response to mucosally or systemically administered tetanus toxoid. *Vaccine* 19, 1636–1642.

Freidag, B.L., Melton, G.B., Collins, F., Klinman, D.M., Cheever, A., Stobie, L., Suen, W., and Seder, R.A. (2000). CpG oligodeoxynucleotides and interleukin-12 improve the efficacy of *Mycobacterium bovis* BCG vaccination in mice challenged with *M. tuberculosis. Infect. Immun.* 68, 2948–2953.

Gallichan, W.S., Woolstencroft, R.N., Guarasci, T., McCluskie, M.J., Davis, H.L., and Rosenthal, K.L. (2001). Intranasal immunization with CpG oligodeoxynucleotides as an adjuvant dramatically increases IgA and protection against herpes simplex virus-2 in the genital tract. *J. Immunol.* 166, 3451–3457.

Gerber, S., Lane, C., Brown, D.M., Lord, E., DiLorenzo, M., Clements, J.D., Rybicki, E., Williamson, A.L., and Rose, R.C. (2001). Human papillomavirus virus-like particles are efficient oral immunogens when coadministered with *Escherichia coli* heat-labile enterotoxin mutant R192G or CpG DNA. *J. Virol.* 75, 4752–4560.

Gierynska, M., Kumaraguru, U., Eo, S.K., Lee, S., Krieg, A., and Rouse, B.T. (2002). Induction of CD8 T-cell-specific systemic and mucosal immunity against herpes simplex virus with CpG-peptide complexes. *J. Virol.* 76, 6568–6576.

Hartmann, G. and Krieg, A.M. (2000). Mechanism and function of a newly identified CpG DNA motif in human primary B cells. *J. Immunol.* 164, 944–953.

Hartmann, G., Weeratna, R.D., Ballas, Z.K., Payette, P., Blackwell, S., Suparto, I., Rasmussen, W.L., Waldschmidt, M., Sajuthi, D., Purcell, R.H., Davis, H.L., and Krieg, A.M. (2000). Delineation of a CpG phosphorothioate oligodeoxynucleotide for activating primate immune responses *in vitro* and *in vivo. J. Immunol.* 164, 1617–1624.

Hemmi, H., Takeuchi, O., Kawai, T., Kaisho, T., Sato, S., Sanjo, H., Matsumoto, M., Hoshino, K., Wagner, H., Takeda, K., and Akira, S. (2000). A Toll-like receptor recognizes bacterial DNA. *Nature* 408, 740–745.

Horner, A.A., Ronaghy, A., Cheng, P.M., Nguyen, M.D., Cho, H.J., Broide, D., and Raz, E. (1998). Immunostimulatory DNA is a potent mucosal adjuvant. *Cell Immunol.* 190, 77–82.

Horner, A.A., Datta, S.K., Takabayashi, K., Belyakov, I.M., Hayashi, T., Cinman, N., Nguyen, M.D., Van Uden, J.H., Berzofsky, J.A., Richman, D.D., and Raz, E. (2001). Immunostimulatory DNA-based vaccines elicit multifaceted immune responses against HIV at systemic and mucosal sites. *J. Immunol.* 167, 1584–1591.

Hornung, V., Rothenfusser, S., Britsch, S., Krug, A., Jahrsdorfer, B., Giese, T., Endres, S., and Hartmann, G. (2002). Quantitative expression of toll-like receptor 1-10 mRNA in cellular subsets of human peripheral blood mononuclear cells and sensitivity to CpG oligodeoxynucleotides. *J. Immunol.* 168, 4531–4537.

Janeway, C.A., Jr. and Medzhitov, R. (2002). Innate immune recognition. *Annu. Rev. Immunol.* 20, 197–216.

Jiang, W., Baker, H.J., and Smith, B.F. (2003). Mucosal immunization with *Helicobacter*, CpG DNA, and cholera toxin is protective. *Infect. Immun.* 71, 40–46.

Jones, T.R., Obaldia, N., III, Gramzinski, R.A., Charoenvit, Y., Kolodny, N., Kitov, S., Davis, H.L., Krieg, A.M., and Hoffman, S.L. (1999). Synthetic oligodeoxynucleotides containing CpG motifs enhance immunogenicity of a peptide malaria vaccine in Aotus monkeys. *Vaccine* 17, 3065–3071.

Joseph, A., Louria-Hayon, I., Plis-Finarov, A., Zeira, E., Zakay-Rones, Z., Raz, E., Hayashi, T., Takabayashi, K., Barenholz, Y., and Kedar, E. (2002). Liposomal immunostimulatory DNA sequence (ISS-ODN): an efficient parenteral and mucosal adjuvant for influenza and hepatitis B vaccines. *Vaccine* 20, 3342–3354.

Kadowaki, N., Ho, S., Antonenko, S., de Waal, M.R., Kastelein, R.A., Bazan, F., and Liu, Y.J. (2001). Subsets of human dendritic cell precursors express different toll-like receptors and respond to different microbial antigens. *J Exp. Med.* 194, 863–870.

Kang, S.M. and Compans, R.W. (2003). Enhancement of mucosal immunization with virus-like particles of simian immunodeficiency virus. *J Virol.* 77, 3615–3623.

Kim, S.K., Ragupathi, G., Musselli, C., Choi, S.J., Park, Y.S., and Livingston, P.O. (1999). Comparison of the effect of different immunological adjuvants on the antibody and T-cell response to immunization with MUC1-KLH and GD3-KLH conjugate cancer vaccines. *Vaccine* 18, 597–603.

Kim, S.K., Ragupathi, G., Cappello, S., Kagan, E., and Livingston, P.O. (2000). Effect of immunological adjuvant combinations on the antibody and T-cell response to vaccination with MUC1-KLH and GD3-KLH conjugates. *Vaccine* 19, 530–537.

Kline, J.N. (2000). Effects of CpG DNA on Th1/Th2 balance in asthma. *Curr. Top. Microbiol. Immunol.* 247, 211–225.

Kobayashi, H., Horner, A.A., Takabayashi, K., Nguyen, M.D., Huang, E., Cinman, N., and Raz, E. (1999). Immunostimulatory DNA pre-priming: a novel approach for prolonged Th1-biased immunity. *Cell Immunol.* 198, 69–75.

Kovarik, J., Bozzotti, P., Love-Homan, L., Pihlgren, M., Davis, H.L., Lambert, P.H., Krieg, A.M., and Siegrist, C.A. (1999). CpG oligodeoxynucleotides can circumvent the Th2 polarization of neonatal responses to vaccines but may fail to fully redirect Th2 responses established by neonatal priming. *J. Immunol.* 162, 1611–1617.

Kovarik, J., Bozzotti, P., Tougne, C., Davis, H.L., Lambert, P.H., Krieg, A.M., and Siegrist, C.A. (2001). Adjuvant effects of CpG oligodeoxynucleotides on responses against T-independent type 2 antigens. *Immunology* 102, 67–76.

Krieg, A.M., Yi, A.K., Matson, S., Waldschmidt, T.J., Bishop, G.A., Teasdale, R., Koretzky, G.A., and Klinman, D.M. (1995). CpG motifs in bacterial DNA trigger direct B-cell activation. *Nature* 374, 546–549.

Krieg, A.M. (2002). From A to Z on CpG. *Trends Immunol.* 23, 64–65.

Krieg, A.M. (2002). CpG motifs in bacterial DNA and their immune effects. *Annu. Rev. Immunol.* 20, 709–760.

Krug, A., Rothenfusser, S., Hornung, V., Jahrsdorfer, B., Blackwell, S., Ballas, Z.K., Endres, S., Krieg, A.M., and Hartmann, G. (2001). Identification of CpG oligonucleotide sequences with high induction of IFN-alpha/beta in plasmacytoid dendritic cells. *Eur. J. Immunol.* 31, 2154–2163.

Krug, A., Towarowski, A., Britsch, S., Rothenfusser, S., Hornung, V., Bals, R., Giese, T., Engelmann, H., Endres, S., Krieg, A.M., and Hartmann, G. (2001). Toll-like receptor expression reveals CpG DNA as a unique microbial stimulus for plasmacytoid dendritic cells which synergizes with CD40 ligand to induce high amounts of IL-12. *Eur. J. Immunol.* 31, 3026–3037.

Lipford, G.B., Bauer, M., Blank, C., Reiter, R., Wagner, H., and Heeg, K. (1997). CpG-containing synthetic oligonucleotides promote B and cytotoxic T cell responses to protein antigen: a new class of vaccine adjuvants. *Eur. J. Immunol.* 27, 2340–2344.

Lipford, G.B., Sparwasser, T., Zimmermann, S., Heeg, K., and Wagner, H. (2000). CpG-DNA-mediated transient lymphadenopathy is associated with a state of Th1 predisposition to antigen-driven responses. *J. Immunol.* 165, 1228–1235.

Magone, M.T., Chan, C.C., Beck, L., Whitcup, S.M., and Raz, E. (2000). Systemic or mucosal administration of immunostimulatory DNA inhibits early and late phases of murine allergic conjunctivitis. *Eur. J. Immunol.* 30, 1841–1850.

Mariotti, S., Teloni, R., von Hunolstein, C., Romagnoli, G., Orefici, G., and Nisini, R. (2002). Immunogenicity of anti-Haemophilus influenzae type b CRM197 conjugate following mucosal vaccination with oligodeoxynucleotide containing immunostimulatory sequences as adjuvant. *Vaccine* 20, 2229–2239.

McCluskie, M.J. and Davis, H.L. (1998). CpG DNA is a potent enhancer of systemic and mucosal immune responses against hepatitis B surface antigen with intranasal administration to mice. *J. Immunol.* 161, 4463–4466.

McCluskie, M.J., Wen, Y.M., Di, Q., and Davis, H.L. (1998). Immunization against hepatitis B virus by mucosal administration of antigen-antibody complexes. *Viral Immunol.* 11, 245–252.

McCluskie, M.J., Weeratna, R.D., Krieg, A.M., and Davis, H.L. (2000a). CpG DNA is an effective oral adjuvant to protein antigens in mice. *Vaccine* 19, 950–957.

McCluskie, M.J., Weeratna, R.D., and Davis, H.L. (2000b). Intranasal immunization of mice with CpG DNA induces strong systemic and mucosal responses that are influenced by other mucosal adjuvants and antigen distribution. *Mol. Med.* 6, 867–877.

McCluskie, M.J. and Davis, H.L. (2000). Oral, intrarectal and intranasal immunizations using CpG and non-CpG oligodeoxynucleotides as adjuvants. *Vaccine* 19, 413–422.

McCluskie, M.J., Weeratna, R.D., Clements, J.D., and Davis, H.L. (2001a). Mucosal immunization of mice using CpG DNA and/or mutants of the heat-labile enterotoxin of *Escherichia coli* as adjuvants. *Vaccine* 19, 3759–3768.

McCluskie, M.J., Weeratna, R.D., and Davis, H.L. (2001b). The potential of oligodeoxynucleotides as mucosal and parenteral adjuvants. *Vaccine* 19, 2657–2660.

McCluskie, M.J., Weeratna, R.D., Payette, P.J., and Davis, H.L. (2002). Parenteral and mucosal prime-boost immunization strategies in mice with hepatitis B surface antigen and CpG DNA. *FEMS Immunol. Med. Microbiol.* 32, 179–185.

Moldoveanu, Z., Love-Homan, L., Huang, W.Q., and Krieg, A.M. (1998). CpG DNA, a novel immune enhancer for systemic and mucosal immunization with influenza virus. *Vaccine* 16, 1216–1224.

Olszewska, W., Partidos, C.D., and Steward, M.W. (2000). Antipeptide antibody responses following intranasal immunization: effectiveness of mucosal adjuvants. *Infect. Immun.* 68, 4923–4929.

Pisetsky, D.S. and Reich, C.F., III. (1998). The influence of base sequence on the immunological properties of defined oligonucleotides. *Immunopharmacology* 40, 199–208.

Rankin, R., Pontarollo, R., Ioannou, X., Krieg, A.M., Hecker, R., Babiuk, L.A., and van Drunen Littel-van den Hurk. (2001). CpG motif identification for veterinary and laboratory species demonstrates that sequence recognition is highly conserved. *Antisense Nucleic Acid Drug Dev.* 11, 333–340.

Roman, M., Martin-Orozco, E., Goodman, J.S., Nguyen, M.D., Sato, Y., Ronaghy, A., Kornbluth, R.S., Richman, D.D., Carson, D.A., and Raz, E. (1997). Immunostimulatory DNA sequences function as T helper-1-promoting adjuvants [see comments]. *Nat. Med.* 3, 849–854.

Ronaghy, A., Prakken, B.J., Takabayashi, K., Firestein, G.S., Boyle, D., Zvailfler, N.J., Roord, S.T., Albani, S., Carson, D.A., and Raz, E. (2002). Immunostimulatory DNA sequences influence the course of adjuvant arthritis. *J. Immunol.* 168, 51–56.

Shirota, H., Sano, K., Kikuchi, T., Tamura, G., and Shirato, K. (2000). Regulation of T-helper type 2 cell and airway eosinophilia by transmucosal coadministration of antigen and oligodeoxynucleotides containing CpG motifs. *Am. J. Respir. Cell Mol. Biol.* 22, 176–182.

Sparwasser, T., Vabulas, R.M., Villmow, B., Lipford, G.B., and Wagner, H. (2000). Bacterial CpG-DNA activates dendritic cells in vivo: T helper cell-independent cytotoxic T cell responses to soluble proteins. *Eur. J. Immunol.* 30, 3591–3597.

Takabayashi, K., Libet, L., Chisholm, D., Zubeldia, J., and Homer, A.A. (2003). Intranasal immunotherapy is more effective than intradermal immunotherapy for the induction of airway allergen tolerance in Th2-sensitized. *J. Immunol.* 170, 3898–3907.

Tighe, H., Takabayashi, K., Schwartz, D., Marsden, R., Beck, L., Corbeil, J., Richman, D.D., Eiden, J.J., Jr., Spiegelberg, H.L., and Raz, E. (2000). Conjugation of protein to immunostimulatory

DNA results in a rapid, long-lasting and potent induction of cell-mediated and humoral immunity. *Eur. J. Immunol.* 30, 1939–1947.

Tokunaga, T., Yamamoto, T., and Yamamoto, S. (1999). How BCG led to the discovery of immunostimulatory DNA. *Jpn. J. Infect. Dis.* 52, 1–11.

Vabulas, R.M., Pircher, H., Lipford, G.B., Hacker, H., and Wagner, H. (2000). CpG-DNA activates in vivo T cell epitope presenting dendritic cells to trigger protective antiviral cytotoxic T cell responses. *J. Immunol.* 164, 2372–2378.

Vollmer, J., Weeratna, R. W., Payette, P., Jurk, M., Schetter, C., Laucht, M., Wader, T., Tluk, S., Liu, M., Davis, H. L., and Kreig, A. M. (2004). Characterization of the three CpG oligodeoxynucleotide classes with distinct immunostimulatory activities. *Eur. J. Immunol.* 34, 251–262.

von Hunolstein, C., Teloni, R., Mariotti, S., Recchia, S., Orefici, G., and Nisini, R. (2000). Synthetic oligodeoxynucleotide containing CpG motif induces an anti-polysaccharide type 1-like immune response after immunization of mice with Haemophilus influenzae type b conjugate vaccine. *Int. Immunol.* 12, 295-303.

Wild, J., Grusby, M.J., Schirmbeck, R., and Reimann, J. (1999). Priming MHC-I-restricted cytotoxic T lymphocyte responses to exogenous hepatitis B surface antigen is CD4+ T cell dependent. *J. Immunol.* 163, 1880–1887.

Yi, A.K., Hornbeck, P., Lafrenz, D.E., and Krieg, A.M. (1996). CpG DNA rescue of murine B lymphoma cells from anti-IgM-induced growth arrest and programmed cell death is associated with increased expression of c-myc and bcl-xL. *J. Immunol.* 157, 4918–4925.

Yi, A.K., Chang, M., Peckham, D.W., Krieg, A.M., and Ashman, R.F. (1998). CpG oligodeoxyribonucleotides rescue mature spleen B cells from spontaneous apoptosis and promote cell cycle entry [erratum appears in *J. Immunol.* 1999; 163(2):1093]. *J. Immunol.* 160, 5898–5906.

Mucosal Adjuvants

Charles O. Elson

Division of Gastroenterology and Hepatology, Department of Medicine, University of Alabama at Birmingham, Birmingham, Alabama

Mark T. Dertzbaugh

United States Army Medical Research Institute of Infectious Disease, Fort Detrick, Maryland

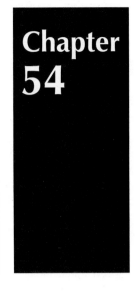

Adjuvants are substances that enhance immune responses; that is, they stimulate an immune response of greater magnitude than that which occurs when the antigen is given alone. Many if not most antigens yield only weak or poor immune responses when given by themselves. The need for strong, reliable adjuvants has been accentuated by modern molecular techniques that generate weakly immunogenic recombinant proteins or peptides from pathogens for use in vaccines. This has led to a renewed interest in vaccine adjuvants, particularly those that can be used in humans (Hooper, 1991). Adjuvants affect virtually every measurable aspect of antibody responses, including the kinetics, duration, quantity, isotype, avidity, and generation of neutralizing activity. Adjuvants have been shown to affect the specificity of antibody responses as well, in that they alter the selection of epitopes of complex antigens to which antibody is directed (Hui *et al.*, 1991). Adjuvants can also enhance the development of cell-mediated immunity (CMI), both delayed-type hypersensitivity (DTH) mediated by CD4 T cells and cytotoxic T lymphocyte (CTL) responses mediated by CD8 T cells. However, adjuvants that stimulate CMI responses tend to be fewer in number than those that stimulate antibody formation.

Most protein antigens are poor immunogens when given mucosally and may induce immunological tolerance instead. Thus, mucosal adjuvants are needed to overcome this potential outcome of mucosal antigen exposure. (The reader is referred to other chapters in this volume that cover in detail the mucosal immune system, oral immunization, and oral tolerance.) An important concept for this discussion is that of the common mucosal immune system, in which immunization of one mucosal surface also sensitizes other, remote mucosal surfaces. This paradigm has formed the basis for a strategy of oral immunization in which the antigen is delivered into the intestine, which has the greatest amount of mucosal lymphoid tissue, to prime the entire mucosal immune system; such priming is then followed by either local mucosal or systemic boosting. The intestine is a very harsh environment for most

antigens because of its intrinsic properties as a digestive organ. This has generated interest in modification of this paradigm to utilize other mucosal sites for mucosal immunization, particularly the nasal mucosa. The latter mucosal surface requires smaller amounts of antigen and adjuvant, and administration would be easy. However, enthusiasm for the nasal route has been dampened by the recognition that the cholera-like toxin adjuvants are taken up into the olfactory nerve and central nervous system (van Ginkel *et al.*, 2000; Alisky *et al.*, 2002). Because different mucosal surfaces have different microenvironments, mucosal adjuvants may well have different effects at different mucosal sites, a point that needs to be kept in mind as we review different mucosal adjuvants.

Adjuvants have been used empirically by immunologists for many years, without much insight as to how they work. It has long been known that most adjuvants are of microbial origin and that most induce or mimic inflammation. These elements can now be linked by the discovery of a family of molecules that recognize and bind selected microbial products on the basis of their molecular patterns. The discovery of this family of receptors, particularly the Toll-like receptors (TLRs), represents an important advance in our understanding about how the immune system senses and responds to microbes and their products. Most adjuvants are ligands for Toll-like receptors. The signaling pathways that follow the binding of a ligand to a TLR eventuate in the activation of the transcription factor NF-κB. NF-κB translocates to the nucleus, where it activates a host of genes. When this sequence of events occurs in dendritic cells, they become activated and mature, express high amounts of costimulatory molecules, and secrete costimulatory cytokines, the effect of which is to render them extremely potent antigen-presenting cells. The activation of dendritic cells by adjuvants acting through TLRs is likely essential for the induction of immune responses, but effects on other cell types, including T cells and B cells also occur and may explain how adjuvants modulate virtually every aspect of immune response, as mentioned above.

CHOLERA-LIKE TOXINS

Cholera toxin (CT) is the most potent mucosal immunogen yet identified and is also an effective mucosal adjuvant, i.e., CT can enhance the immunogenicity of relatively poor mucosal immunogens when mixed or conjugated with them and given orally (Elson and Ealding, 1984a). The receptor for CT on cells is not a pattern recognition receptor like the Toll-like receptors. Instead, it binds to GM1 ganglioside which is on the surface of all nucleated cells, including the brush border of intestinal epithelial cells. Once bound, CT is endocytosed by many cells, including intestinal epithelial cells, antigen presenting cells, and lymphocytes. The A subunit of CT then activates the stimulatory G protein of adenylate cyclase and increases intracellular cyclic AMP. In contrast to other bacterial products that act as adjuvants, CT does not induce inflammation or activate NF-κB. Nevertheless, CT does activate antigen-presenting cells (APCs), similar in many ways to the activation induced by bacterial ligands for the TLRs, and this is probably crucial for the adjuvant properties of CT, as will be discussed later.

Enterotoxigenic strains of *Escherichia coli* produce several types of heat-labile toxins (LTs), of which one, LT-I, is highly homologous to CT. A second genetic locus, LT-II, encodes toxins as well, but these differ in their protein sequence and carbohydrate binding specificities (Jobling and Holmes, 1991, 1992). LT-I toxin of *E. coli* has a crystal structure virtually identical to that of CT. It binds to GM1 ganglioside on cells also, but it can bind other gangliosides and glycoproteins as well. LT-I has been used with success as a mucosal adjuvant (Clements *et al.*, 1988), but less is known about its mucosal immunogenicity and adjuvanticity than is known about CT; thus, the following discussion focuses mainly on the effects of CT, but the similarities and differences between adjuvant effects of CT and LT also are discussed.

CT as a mucosal immunogen
CT is the most potent mucosal immunogen yet identified, inducing strong intestinal S-IgA responses and plasma IgG responses after oral administration (Elson and Ealding, 1984b). It has been estimated that at the peak of the response in rodents, up to 5% of all the plasma cells in the intestine produce antibody to it (Pierce and Cray, 1982). Contrary to most protein antigens, feeding CT does not induce oral tolerance for antibody responses (Elson and Ealding, 1984a); rather, it induces extended memory responses in the mucosa (Lycke and Holmgren, 1986a). Although generalized mucosal immunity occurs after mucosal application of CT, the local mucosal response is greatest at the mucosal site directly exposed to CT (Pierce and Cray, 1982). Despite these remarkable properties as a mucosal immunogen, the mucosal response to CT follows the "rules" applicable to more conventional protein antigens in that the response is CD4+ T cell–dependent (Hornquist *et al.*, 1991) and requires antigen presentation via major histocompatibility complex (MHC) class II molecules (Elson and Ealding, 1987). In mice, the response to CT after intestinal immunization is predominately a Th2 response (Xu-Amano *et al.*, 1993). These properties of CT as an oral immunogen are summarized here in **Table 54.1** because the same properties seem to extend to antigens for which CT acts as a mucosal adjuvant.

Most of the work done with CT has focused on the antibody response, and much less is known about the CMI or delayed type hypersensitivity (DTH) response to CT. Kay and Ferguson (1989a,b) found that feeding CT or its toxoid prior to systemic immunization induced oral tolerance for DTH but not for the antibody response. Experiments with cell transfer indicated that this oral tolerance for DTH involved the induction of suppressor cells that were not further characterized. Thus, the B cell and T cell response to CT can be regulated independently.

The bulk of the data concerning CT as a mucosal immunogen comes from studies in rodents. In humans, CT-B is immunogenic and well tolerated (Czerkinsky *et al.*, 1991; Quiding *et al.*, 1991). Contrary to the situation in mice, where CT is consistently much more immunogenic than CT-B, in humans CT-B can induce levels of serum antibody in volunteers comparable to those found following clinical cholera (Svennerholm *et al.*, 1984). Extended memory responses after immunization with a CT-B-containing oral vaccine can persist for years (Jertborn *et al.*, 1988). Antigen-specific T cells can be demonstrated in the peripheral blood of humans after oral immunization for up to 1 year after immunization with CT-B (Lewis *et al.*, 1993; Castello-Branco *et al.*, 1994), consistent with the induction of a prolonged T-cell memory response as well. Many of these results parallel those found in rodents. More detailed studies are needed concerning the immune response to oral immunization with CT-B, particularly with regard to whether it can serve as a mucosal adjuvant in humans.

CT as a mucosal adjuvant: general characteristics
The initial demonstration of the adjuvant effects of CT came from studies on whether the feeding of CT resulted in oral tolerance (Elson and Ealding, 1984a). CT was fed to mice either alone or with the unrelated protein antigen, keyhole limpet hemocyanin (KLH). CT did not induce oral tolerance to itself, and when both proteins were fed together, it abrogated oral tolerance to KLH. At the same time CT also induced an intestinal S-IgA response to KLH that did not

Table 54.1. Key Properties of Cholera Toxin (CT) as a Mucosal Immunogen

> Stimulates S-IgA and serum IgG response
> Does not include oral tolerance for antibody responses
> Induces extended memory in mucosal tissues
> Local response best at mucosal site in contact with CT
> Restricted by I-A subregion of H-2 MHC
> CD4+ T-cell-dependent
> Induces a predominant Th2 response after oral immunization

occur when KLH alone was fed. The ability of CT to act as a mucosal adjuvant has since been confirmed by many investigators with a variety of antigens **(Table 54.2)**. Although many of these are protein antigens, CT has been effective as a mucosal adjuvant for both lipid and carbohydrate types of antigens, as well as for whole viruses, bacteria, *Candida*, and protozoa. Thus, although the mucosal adjuvant effects of CT may not apply to all antigens, it has shown efficacy with a remarkably broad array of antigen types.

A number of important parameters of the mucosal adjuvanticity of CT are listed in **Table 54.3**. In order to induce immunity to the target antigen, CT has to be administered simultaneously with the antigen, and both the antigen and CT must be administered by the same route, namely,

Table 54.2. Antigens with which Cholera Toxin (CT) or CT-B Has Been Effective as an Adjuvant

Antigen (adjuvant)	Route	Reference
Proteins		
Keyhole limpet hemocyanin (CT)	IG	Elson and Ealding, 1984a
Horseradish peroxidase (CT-B)	IG	McKenzie and Halsey, 1984
Ovalbumin (CT)	IG	Van der Heijden *et al.*, 1991
Tetanus toxoid (CT)	IG	Jackson *et al.*, 1993
M protein epitope of group		
A streptococci (CT-B)	IN	Bessen and Fischetti, 1988
Antigen I/II of *S. mutans* (CT/CT-B)	IG	Czerkinsky *et al.*, 1989; Wu and Russell, 1993
Protein antigen of *S. mutans* (CT-B)	IN	Takahashi *et al.*, 1990b
Hemagglutinin of influenza virus (CT/CT-B)	IG, IN	Tamura, *et al.*, 1988
Respiratory syncytial virus FG glycoprotein (CT/CT-B)	IN	Walsh, 1993
Streptococcus mutans		
GtfB.1::PhoA fusion protein (CT)	IG	Tomasi *et al.*, 1997
Polysaccharides		
Shigella lipopolysaccharide (CT-B)	IG	Orr *et al.*, 1994
Dextran-CT-B conjugate (CT)	IG, IN	Bergquist *et al.*, 1995
Pseudomonas aeruginosa polysaccharide (CT)	IG	Abraham and Robinson, 1991
Viruses		
Whole influenza virus (CT)	IG	Chen and Strober, 1990
Sendai virus (CT)	IG, IN	Nedrud *et al.*, 1987
Measles virus (CT-B)	IN	Muller *et al.*, 1995
Respiratory syncytial virus (CT)	IN	Reuman *et al.*, 1991
Rotavirus (CT, LT)	IN	O'Neal *et al.*, 1998
HIV macromolecular peptide (CT)	IG	Bukawa *et al.*, 1995
SIVp55 gag (CT)	IN	Imaoka *et al.*, 1998
Bacteria/fungi		
Helicobacter pylori (CT)	IG	Czinn and Nedrud, 1991
Helicobacter felis (CT-B + CT)	IG	Lee and Chen, 1994
Group B streptococci (CT)	Colon	Hordness *et al.*, 1995
Candida (CT)	IN	DeBarnardis *et al.*, 2002
Protozoa		
Toxoplasma gondii (CT)	IG	Bourguin *et al.*, 1991
Pneumococcus (CT)	IN	Malley *et al.*, 2001
Entamoeba histolytica		
peptide-CT-B fusion protein	IG	Zhang *et al.*, 1995

IG, intragastric; IN, intranasal.

Table 54.3. Important Features of Mucosal Adjuvanticity of Cholera Toxin (CT)

Dose: usually in micrograms
Route: must be mucosal
Timing: must be simultaneous with antigen
Genetics: works best in high responders to CT
Memory: long term
Class of antigen: many types of antigens
Antigen form: mixtures, covalent conjugates, molecular chimeras

mucosally (Lycke and Holmgren, 1986b). Giving CT by a route different from that of the antigen is not effective. These features are consistent with a requirement for CT to bind to and activate the same APCs that take up the antigen that is delivered with the CT. It is interesting that CT does not induce antibody responses to food antigens that would be expected to be present in the intestine at the time of its administration (Nedrud and Sigmund, 1991), nor does it stimulate polyclonal B-cell responses (Jackson et al., 1993). The dose of CT required in mice for mucosal adjuvanticity ranges between 1 and 10 µg (Lycke and Holmgren, 1986b; Kusnecov et al., 1992) and may vary depending on the antigen involved; i.e., although very small amounts of CT suffice to potentiate the immune response to CT-B, much larger amounts have been used to enhance mucosal responses to viruses. CT induces long-term mucosal and systemic memory B- and T-cell responses to antigens coadministered with it (Vajdy and Lycke, 1993). Although most studies have measured simple enhancement of antibody titers, CT as a mucosal adjuvant has been found to provide protection against pathogenic challenge in several different systems, e.g., sendai virus (Nedrud et al., 1987), influenza virus (Tamura et al., 1991), tetanus toxin (TT) (Jackson et al., 1993), and measles virus (Muller et al., 1995).

Although the induction of antibody responses by CT is well established, less is known about the induction of cellular immune responses or DTH by CT. As mentioned earlier, CT feeding in mice has been found to induce oral tolerance for DTH reactions to CT (Kay and Ferguson, 1989a,b). Nevertheless, there are reports of enhanced priming of DTH reactions by CT as a mucosal adjuvant (Kusnecov et al., 1992; Tamura et al., 1995), as well as by CT-B containing small amounts of CT (Tamura et al., 1996). Nasal administration of inactivated respiratory syncytial virus (RSV) plus CT yielded an IgG2a response, a subclass representative of Th1 responses in mice (Reuman et al., 1991). Indeed, some workers have found priming of both Th1 and Th2 cytokines on antigen restimulation in vitro after antigen plus CT was given mucosally (Wilson et al., 1991; Vajdy and Lycke, 1993), although others have found only the priming of Th2 cytokines (Xu-Amano et al., 1993). Last, priming of cytotoxic T-cell responses after the feeding of ovalbumin plus CT and/or LT as adjuvant has been reported (Bowen et al.,

1994; Simmons et al., 1999). However, a cytokine mixture of nasal IL-1α, IL-12, IL-18, and GM-CSF was able to substitute for CT in the generation of CTL in mice. These cytokines were not shown to be secreted locally after CT was used as an adjuvant, and CT is an inhibitor of IL-12 in both mouse (Cong, et al., 2001) and human (Braun et al., 1999). However, these results are consistent with induction of cellular immune responses by mucosal CT adjuvant. The duration of this cellular response is unknown.

The adjuvanticity of CT appears to be related to and dependent on its immunogenicity; e.g., the response of mice to KLH given together with CT orally was significantly higher in H-2 congenic mouse strains that are high responders to CT than in strains that are low responders to CT (Elson, 1992). In addition, mutant CT molecules lacking immunogenicity also lack adjuvanticity, and vice versa, as will be discussed later. Although CT generates a strong mucosal and systemic response to itself when coadministered as an adjuvant, preexisting mucosal immunity to CT does not impair its mucosal adjuvanticity (Tamura et al., 1989; Wu and Russell, 1994).

CT has been effective as a mucosal adjuvant in mice, rats, rabbits, and ferrets but did not work in one study in chickens (Hoshi et al., 1995). Because CT induces significant diarrhea in humans (Levine et al., 1983), the holotoxin itself cannot be tested orally, and it remains unknown whether CT-B or a nontoxic CT mutant has mucosal adjuvanticity in humans. It is thus reassuring that nasal application of Streptococcus mutans antigen I/II plus CT-B to monkeys resulted in IgA antibody responses at multiple mucosal sites, including the female genital tract (Russell et al., 1996). CT-B containing a trace amount of CT (0.1%–5%) has shown mucosal adjuvanticity equivalent to that of the holotoxin in mice, whether given orally (Wilson et al., 1990; Lee and Chen, 1994a) or nasally (Tamura et al., 1994b). This combination is attractive as a method for reducing the toxicity enough to allow use in humans, particularly with a nasal route of administration. The incorporation of CT within the lipid particles of multiple emulsions has been found to preserve adjuvanticity while markedly decreasing toxicity and is another possible strategy for translation to humans (Tomasi et al., 1994).

Site of adjuvant activity

The effects of CT might differ at various mucosal surfaces with very distinct microenvironments, e.g., the nasal versus the intestinal mucosa. Nasal immunization with CT or CT-B has been the focus of a number of studies (Table 54.2), from which a number of general conclusions are evident. Most combinations of antigen plus CT or CT-B as adjuvant that immunize when introduced into the intestine also do so when given nasally. In some instances, antigen plus CT-B as adjuvant is effective nasally even though the same combination is ineffective when introduced into the intestine. The distribution of the response systemically and at various mucosal sites is roughly equivalent when antigen plus adjuvant is given either nasally or orally to mice (Wu and Russell, 1993). Because the dose of CT or CT-B used intranasally is frequently equivalent to that used in the intestine, the ratio of dose to mucosal surface area is much greater with nasal administration. Second, many antigen preparations, particularly recombinant-derived antigens, contain bacterial lipopolysaccharide (LPS) and other TLR ligands that have adjuvant activity. This may partly explain some of the previously mentioned differences as well as the apparent lack of genetic restriction of the adjuvant effect when the nasal route is used (Hirabayashi *et al.*, 1991), a restriction that is apparent after gastric administration (Elson, 1992). The nasal mucosa contains organized lymphoid tissue, nasal-associated lymphoreticular tissue (NALT) (Kuper *et al.*, 1992), which is analogous to GALT in the intestine, but the exact site of the adjuvant effect of CT or CT-B in nasal mucosa is not clear.

With regard to the intestine, our current understanding is that the induction of mucosal immune responses occurs in GALT and requires the transport of antigen by specialized M cells into the underlying lymphoid follicles where antigen is processed and presented to antigen-specific T and B cells. Thus, the adjuvant effect of CT presumably occurs in GALT. There is evidence from some studies that this is at least one site of CT adjuvanticity. CT is an effective adjuvant when inserted with antigen into the lipid particles of multiple emulsions and delivered into the gut (Tomasi *et al.*, 1994). Such multiple emulsion particles enter the lymphoid follicles but not the epithelium or lamina propria of the intestine (Hearn, 1995). CT induced the migration of microparticle-containing DCs from the subepithelial dome region of Peyer's patches into B-cell follicles and T-cell zones (Schreedhar *et al.*, 2003). In addition, the major cell type responsible for CT adjuvant effects in nasal mucosa was identified as DC in nasal-associated lymphoid tissue (Porgador *et al.*, 1998).

Gut epithelial cells can act as antigen-presenting cells *in vitro*, although the functional effect of this presentation has been suppression (Bland and Warren, 1986; Mayer *et al.*, 1988). T cells in the epithelium have a greatly restricted T-cell receptor (TCR) repertoire, making this site an unlikely location for induction of primary immune responses. Gut epithelial cells bind the great majority of CT, and in an immunohistochemical light microscopy study, CT was present within epithelial cells as well as within mononuclear cells in the underlying lamina propria (Hansson *et al.*, 1984), indicating that it can traverse the epithelial layer. These mononuclear cells taking up CT may be DCs that sit just below the epithelial layer and under some circumstances can extend processes into the lumen to sample lumenal antigen (Rescigno 2001). These DCs can then migrate into draining lymph nodes. Overall, DCs in the Peyer's patches, the subepithelial area of the intestine, and in NALT appear to be the primary site of adjuvanticity of CT.

Cellular targets of adjuvanticity
Antigen-presenting cells
Details about the mechanisms of antigen presentation in GALT remain sketchy. CT and CT-B do not alter macrophage APC antigen uptake or processing *in vitro* (Woogen *et al.*, 1987) or affect macrophage MHC class II

expression (Bromander *et al.*, 1991). However, CT has been shown to stimulate the production of IL-1 *in vitro*, an effect that may enhance antigen presentation (Lycke *et al.*, 1989). CT increases CD86 expression and functional activity on macrophages in vitro (Cong *et al.*, 1997), and blocking CD86 with monoclonal antibodies (mAbs) reduces the mucosal adjuvanticity of CT *in vivo*. CT stimulates IL-1β, IL-6, and IL-10 by bone-marrow-derived macrophages and DCs, but it inhibits TNF-α, IL-12, and nitric oxide synthase (NOS) production *in vitro* (Cong *et al.*, 2001). Thus, enhancement of APC costimulation via surface molecules and cytokines by CT is likely a major factor in its adjuvanticity. Consistent with this idea, increased T-cell priming in mucosal tissues after delivery of antigen plus CT has been demonstrated *in vivo*. Thus, an enhancement of antigen presentation through increased costimulatory activity seems to be a major mechanism—if not *the* major mechanism—by which CT acts as a mucosal adjuvant.

Other cells in the intestine might also act as APCs, such as dendritic cells, B cells, and epithelial cells. There is little or no information available on the first two with regard to the adjuvant effects of CT. Epithelial cells are now recognized as an active and important component of the mucosal immune system. They express both MHC class I and class II molecules, produce certain cytokines, and respond to an even wider array of cytokines. CT stimulates the production of IL-6 by the IEC-6 epithelial cell line *in vitro*, and such stimulation is synergistically enhanced by the presence of TGF-β, TNF-α, or IL-1β in the cultures (McGee *et al.*, 1993a, b). The IEC-17 epithelial cell line showed enhanced alloantigen presentation *in vitro* after treatment with CT, an effect that seemed to be related to increased IL-1 and IL-6 production (Bromander *et al.*, 1993). Although there is no direct evidence that epithelial cells present antigen *in vivo*, they may influence the process by secreting such cytokines.

Other cellular targets
T cells
Restimulation of T cells with KLH *in vitro* from mice previously fed KLH plus CT as an adjuvant has been shown to cause substantial proliferative responses in Peyer's patches, gut lamina propria, mesenteric lymph node, and spleen (Clarke *et al.*, 1991; Hornquist and Lycke, 1993). Similar responses did not occur in mice fed KLH alone. In addition, T cells from these same tissues produced a variety of cytokines when restimulated with KLH, including IL-2, IFN-γ, IL-4, IL-5, and IL-6, although their relative quantity varied among these tissues (Wilson *et al.*, 1990; Clarke *et al.*, 1991; Hornquist and Lycke, 1993). Thus, CT as a mucosal adjuvant induced antigen-specific T-cell activation and expansion in both mucosal and systemic lymphoid tissues. The T cells responding in these cultures were predominately CD4+ (Hornquist and Lycke, 1993), and the mucosal adjuvanticity of CT was not evident in CD4−/− mice lacking CD4+ T cells; thus, this subset is clearly an essential target for CT mucosal adjuvanticity (Hornquist *et al.*, 1996). Because the direct effect of CT on T cells *in vitro* is very inhibitory, as

discussed later, this T-cell priming *in vivo* is not likely to be due to direct effects of CT on T cells but rather to indirect effects, e.g., through enhanced APC function and/or down-regulation of cells producing inhibitory cytokines.

Murine CD4$^+$ T cells have been further subdivided into Th1 and Th2 subtypes on the basis of the pattern of cytokines they secrete (Mosmann and Coffman, 1989). In mice the IgG2a subclass antibody response is Th1-dependent, whereas IgG1 and IgE antibody responses are Th2-dependent (Finkelman *et al.*, 1990); the amounts of IgG1 and IgG2a antibodies produced during a given immune response can be used as a rough estimate of the proportion of the response that is Th1 versus Th2, although this is not a substitute for direct measurement of the relevant cytokines. There appear to be multiple factors determining whether a given antigen triggers a Th1- or Th2-dominated response, one of which is that certain antigens seem to preferentially induce one pathway or the other. Another factor is the adjuvant used. As mentioned previously, early after immunization with KLH and CT, both Th1 and Th2 cytokines are detectable in restimulation assays; however, these cytokine phenotypes take time to develop fully, and the previously mentioned studies were short-term. CT as a mucosal adjuvant seems to preferentially enhance Th2-type responses, e.g., the feeding of ovalbumin plus CT to mice primed for or induced IgE responses (Snider *et al.*, 1994; Tamura *et al.*, 1994a), the latter being sufficient to result in anaphylaxis after intraperitoneal challenge with ovalbumin. The feeding of TT plus CT generated TT-specific lamina propria T cells producing Th2 but not Th1 cytokines (Xu-Amano *et al.*, 1993). Last, IL-6 and IL-10 were detected in intestinal secretions of ligated loops in mice after CT exposure, although the cellular source of these cytokines was not identified (Klimpel *et al.*, 1995). It is still possible that the antigens used in these studies themselves triggered a Th2 response that CT simply amplified, because CT appears able to enhance a Th1 response to some antigens. For example, inactivated RSV (Reuman *et al.*, 1991) and TT fragment C (Roberts *et al.*, 1995) plus CT as adjuvant given nasally induced a substantial or a predominant IgG2a response, respectively. The feeding of ovalbumin plus a mixture of CT-B and CT induced MHC class I restricted CTL responses to an ovalbumin-transfected cell line (Bowen *et al.*, 1994). A wider variety of antigens needs to be tested in order to settle this question, particularly for those that preferentially induce Th1 responses.

The feeding of most protein antigens (other than CT) results in a state of immunological unresponsiveness or oral tolerance, one mechanism of which is the induction of regulatory cells producing suppressive cytokines (Weiner *et al.*, 1994). CT is able to abrogate the induction of oral tolerance to other antigens, but it does not "break" tolerance that is already established (Grdic *et al.*, 1998). This would argue that the adjuvant effect of CT is exerted mainly on the APCs rather than on T cells. However, CT and CT-B are able to directly inhibit both CD4$^+$ and CD8$^+$ T cells *in vitro* (Woogen *et al.*, 1987, 1993; Elson *et al.*, 1995a), a mechanism which is associated with downregulation of IL-2 and

the IL-2 receptor expression. This may have relevance *in vivo* in that CT introduced into the mouse intestine caused a marked depletion of intraepithelial lymphocytes in the small intestine as well as in the cells in the dome epithelium over the Peyer's patches (Elson *et al.*, 1995a). Coincident with these effects, CT inhibited the generation of suppressor cells that mediate oral tolerance: in an adoptive transfer system, the feeding of KLH to mice generated suppressor T cells that inhibited both the S-IgA and the plasma IgG response to KLH, but the feeding of both KLH and CT together eliminated this suppression (Elson *et al.*, 1995a). The data are inconclusive as to whether direct perturbation of T cells is involved in the mucosal immunogenicity or adjuvanticity of CT.

B cells

There are many stages of B-cell development that must be traversed before reaching the antibody-secreting plasma cell. The major steps of B-cell development, including isotype commitment or switching, clonal expansion, and terminal differentiation, are all dependent on and regulated by cytokines, which act on B cells at defined stages of development. For example, the IgE and IgG1 isotypes are preferentially enhanced by IL-4 (Snapper and Paul, 1987), and the IgA isotype by IL-5 (Murray *et al.*, 1987). CT can affect any one or more of these steps.

CT may drive B cells toward IgA-committed precursors. Lebman *et al.* (1988) have shown that CT given intraduodenally can change the isotype pattern displayed by Peyer's patch B cells primed for an unrelated hapten from IgM to IgG and IgA after antigen-dependent clonal expansion *in vitro*. CT appeared to nonspecifically alter the responsiveness of Peyer's patch B cells to isotype switching signals present in *in vitro* cultures. This might be due to a direct effect on B cells or could be attributed to the effect CT had on cytokine-mediated signals within the Peyer's patch. CT has direct effects on B-cell isotype differentiation *in vitro* by enhancing the effect of both IL-4 and IL-5 on purified B cells stimulated by LPS (Lycke and Strober, 1989). In the presence of CT, IL-4 enhanced IgG1-producing B cells threefold to fourfold, and IL-5 had a similar effect on IgA-producing B cells. This effect of CT was on sIgM$^+$ B cells, which is consistent with CT inducing isotype switching in synergy with IL-4. Subsequent analysis demonstrated that CT plus IL-4 increased the expression of germline γ-1 RNA transcripts, providing direct support for this idea (Lycke *et al.*, 1990). It is interesting that CT plus IL-4 did not have a similar effect on IgA heavy-chain gene transcription. Two mechanisms appear to be involved: an increase in cAMP that causes the increase in the germline IgH gene RNA transcripts and an enhancement of B-cell differentiation due to CT-B binding to its ligand, GM1 ganglioside, on the cell surface (Lycke, 1993).

Similar to its effects on T cells, CT inhibits B-cell proliferation *in vitro* even though it seems to be predominantly stimulatory *in vivo*. Woogen *et al.* (1987) found that CT inhibited proliferation of purified B cells *in vitro* when they were polyclonally stimulated either by anti-IgM or by LPS; CT-B inhibited B cells stimulated by anti-IgM but not by LPS. The inhibition of B-cell proliferation is accompanied by enhancement of differentiation as manifested by an increase in MHC class II expression (Francis *et al.*, 1992). Lycke *et al.* (1989) also found that CT inhibited the B-cell proliferative response to LPS but observed a mild stimulatory effect on B-cell proliferation relative to the control when the culture period was prolonged to 6 days and low doses of CT were used, although the former condition may not be physiologically relevant. CT can stimulate the proliferation of anti-IgM prestimulated human B cells, an effect mediated through increased cAMP (Anastassiou *et al.*, 1992). The effects of CT on B-cell proliferation *in vivo*, particularly after the brief exposures expected there, remain to be determined but seem predominantly stimulatory. Certainly the large number of plasma cells producing anti-CT in the lamina propria following oral immunization with CT, which has been estimated to be up to 5% of the total IgA plasma cells at the peak of the response, indicates that clonal expansion occurs and is vigorous *in vivo*. Just as with T cells, this may well be an indirect effect resulting from the stimulation of cytokines by other cell types.

Epithelial cells or M cells
Can the mucosal adjuvanticity of CT or CT-B be explained by an increased delivery of antigen into intestinal follicles, perhaps related to their ability to bind to mucosa and thus persist in the intestine? Although it is difficult to perceive how this would be a mechanism when antigens are simply mixed with CT or CT-B, this idea has appeal as a mechanism by which CT might potentiate the immune response to fusion chimeras or to antigens to which it is chemically conjugated. There are no firm data pro or con. The form and size of the resulting antigen might be important variables, in that 28-nm colloidal gold particles to which CT-B had been conjugated selectively localized to the M cells of the follicle-associated epithelium of the rabbit intestine (Frey *et al.*, 1996), whereas soluble CT was bound diffusely to the microvillus surface of all enterocytes. Larger coated particles 1 μm in size did not bind to either M cells or enterocytes, presumably because they were not able to get through the glycocalyx. Therefore, selective uptake of antigen by coupling to CT or CT-B may apply only to antigens of a certain size or form.

Toward a nontoxic toxin adjuvant
The molecular structure of CT has been characterized extensively (Betley *et al.*, 1986). It is composed of A and B subunits **(Fig. 54.1)**. The toxinogenic A subunit (CT-A) is a 28-kDa protein that ADP-ribosylates the stimulatory Gs protein of adenylate cyclase. The A subunit is cleaved post-translationally into A1 and A2 peptides, which remain connected via a disulfide bond, and it is the A1 peptide that has enzymatic activity. Crystallographic data on CT and on the closely related *E. coli* heat-labile toxin (LT) indicate that in both these enterotoxins the A2 peptide forms an α helix connecting the A1 peptide with the binding subunit (Sixma *et al.*, 1991). The B subunit of cholera toxin (CT-B) is a

homopentamer composed of noncovalently associated subunits (each 11.6 kDa) that form a ringlike structure with a central pore through which the A2 subunit projects (Hol *et al.*, 1995). This structure, which is common to both CT and *E. coli* LT, has been likened to a "ring on a finger" (van Heyningen, 1991). CT-B binds to the monosialoganglioside GM1 (Cuatrecasas, 1973), which is present on all nucleated cells, including the surface of intestinal epithelial cells. CT is endocytosed at the apical border of the enterocyte, and in a multistep process the toxin-containing endosomal vesicles transcytose to the basolateral membrane where adenylate cyclase is located (Lencer *et al.*, 1993). The exact cellular location of the interaction between A1 peptide and Gs is unknown. Binding of the B subunit to the cell membrane is required for endocytosis, but whether other parts of the molecule participate is not yet known.

Role of CT subunits in mucosal adjuvanticity and genetically engineered mutant toxins
The role that A and B subunits play in the mucosal immunogenicity and adjuvanticity of CT has been a subject of continuing interest. McKenzie and Halsey (1984) reported first that horseradish peroxidase (HRP) chemically conjugated to CT-B elicited higher antibody levels in the gut and serum than those observed after feeding either HRP alone or an unconjugated mixture of HRP and CT-B. Since then, the use of CT-B as a vaccine adjuvant has been examined by others, with mixed results. In one study, mixtures of KLH and CT-B were unable to stimulate immunity to KLH unless very small doses (<50 ng) of holotoxin were added (Lycke and Holmgren, 1986b); however, KLH conjugated to CT-B was not tested. The use of CT-B conjugates has been reported to be effective in some cases (Bessen and Fischetti, 1988; Tamura *et al.*, 1988) but not in others (Czerkinsky *et al.*, 1989; Liang *et al.*, 1989b). The poor responses observed with CT-B conjugates in some cases may be due to the coupling procedure. The degree of cross-linking and the coupling procedure used can significantly affect the immunogenicity of protein conjugates (Verheul *et al.*, 1989). The mucosal route used could be another important variable, in that CT-B has been more effective as a mucosal adjuvant when used for nasal immunization (Wu and Russell, 1993; Muller *et al.*, 1995), a route discussed in the next section.

Fusion of peptides to CT-B by recombinant gene technology has generated chimeric neoantigens (Sanchez *et al.*, 1988; Dertzbaugh *et al.*, 1990; Oien *et al.*, 1994). This approach has been used to determine whether CT-B has intrinsic adjuvant activity in comparison with that of a control bacterial protein. Thus, the same immunogenic peptide of *S. mutans* glucosyltransferase B was fused to either CT-B or to *E. coli* alkaline phosphatase, and each purified chimeric protein was fed to mice (Dertzbaugh and Elson, 1993a). These studies demonstrated that CT-B has intrinsic adjuvant activity, but this activity was much less potent than that found with the holotoxin. The size of the peptide that can be fused to CT-B is effectively restricted to about 20–25 residues. Peptides or proteins larger than this impair the

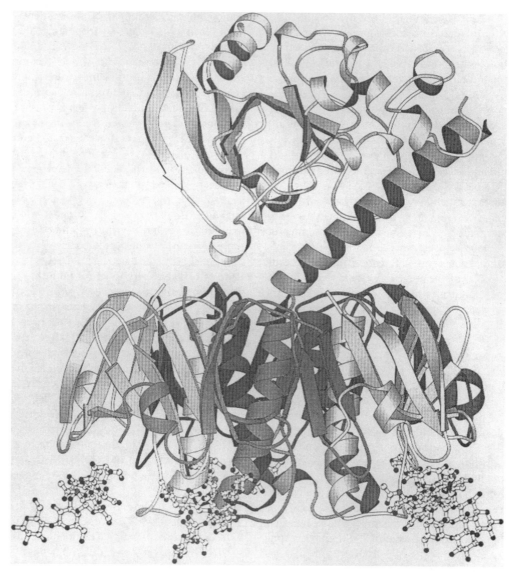

Fig. 54.1. Composite model for AB$_5$ holotoxin bound to the saccharide moieties of five receptor molecules. This model was derived from the x-ray structures of the complete *E. coli* LT bound to the simple sugar galactose (Merritt *et al.*, 1994b) and of the CT-B pentamer bound to the GM1 pentasaccharide (Merritt *et al.*, 1994a). The secondary and tertiary structures of the two toxins are essentially identical, with the possible exception that the C-terminal portion of the A subunit extends into or through the central pore of the B pentamer (figure courtesy of E. Merritt and W. Hol).

ability of CT-B to fold properly, to bind to GM1 ganglioside, and to form pentamers, thus abolishing its activity (Dertzbaugh and Elson, 1993b). A solution to this problem is suggested by the crystallographic structure of CT and LT (Fig. 54.1), namely, the substitution of an antigen for the A1 subunit of CT. This approach was shown to be feasible (Jobling and Holmes, 1992), and the resulting fusion protein containing A2 subunit reassembled with B monomers to form holotoxin-like chimeras. Such a chimera containing a streptococcal protein adhesin induced strong S-IgA and serum IgG responses when fed to mice (Hajishengallis *et al.*, 1995), which persisted at substantial levels for almost 1 year (Hajishengallis *et al.*, 1996). This result is again compatible

with the notion that the B subunit has intrinsic adjuvant activity. It is interesting that the adjuvant activity of CT-B may be qualitatively different from that of CT, in that antigen–CT-B conjugates have been found to be potent inducers of tolerance for DTH responses, even when given in very small amounts (Sun *et al.*, 1994, 1996). This tolerance does not occur if even trace amounts of CT holotoxin are present.

Information on the role of the A subunit has been conflicting. In mice the consistently higher potency of holotoxin than of the B subunit for both immunogenicity and adjuvanticity argues for an important role for the A subunit. Liang *et al.* (1989a) concluded that GM1 binding but not toxic activity was necessary for the mucosal adjuvanticity of

CT–Sendai virus conjugates, on the basis of studies with glutaraldehyde-treated CT. However, very small amounts of residual A subunit may be sufficient, and this study does not provide a definitive answer. The opposite conclusion, that the ADP-ribosyltransferase activity of the A subunit was crucial to CT mucosal adjuvanticity, was reached in another study, showing deficient mucosal adjuvanticity by recombinant CT-B and by a mutant *E. coli* LT in which a single amino acid substitution inactivated its enzymatic activity (Lycke *et al.*, 1992). Again, this is not a definitive result.

In order to define the role of the A and B subunits in the immunogenicity and adjuvanticity of CT, mutants of both A and B subunits that lacked enzymatic and binding ability, respectively, were generated by site-directed mutagenesis. Holotoxins containing only an A mutant, only a B mutant, or both A and B mutants were compared to wild-type CT for immunogenicity and adjuvanticity in mouse intestine. Each was fed to mice along with TT. Mice receiving wild-type CT had strong responses to both CT and TT. Mice receiving the A mutant or CT-B alone had moderate and weak anti-CT responses, respectively, but no TT response. Mice given the B mutant or the double A and B mutant had no response to either CT or TT (Elson *et al.*, 1995b). These results show clearly that both a functional A subunit and a functional B subunit are required for optimal immunogenicity and adjuvanticity of CT in the intestine. They also illustrate that the intestinal adjuvanticity of CT appears to be linked to its immunogenicity.

The contributions of the two subunits might vary at different mucosal surfaces. For example, a nontoxic mutant, LTK7, of *E. coli* LT with a single amino acid substitution in its A subunit was effective as a mucosal adjuvant when administered nasally (Douce *et al.*, 1995). However, this mutant LT was ineffective as a mucosal adjuvant when given orally. These results are similar to those mentioned earlier in which CT-B or LT-B was effective nasally but much less or not at all effective when given orally.

A variety of genetically engineered mutant toxins have been generated in a search for a nontoxic mucosal adjuvant. In all cases the mutations involved the A subunit. For cholera toxin, mutant toxins have included CT (S61F), CT (E112K) (Yamamoto *et al.*, 2001), and CT (E29H) (Periwal *et al.*, 2003). Mutants have also been developed for *E. coli* LT, including LT (S63Y), LT (del 110/112) (Park *et al.*, 2000), and LT (R192G) (Lu *et al.*, 2002). All of these mutants have shown some adjuvant activity after nasal delivery. Chimeric mutant toxins have also been produced, for example, a combination of a nontoxic mutant A subunit of CT(E112K) with the B subunit of LT (Kweon *et al.*, 2002). As mentioned above, all of these mutant toxins able to bind GM1 ganglioside will be taken up into the olfactory nerve and CNS after nasal delivery; thus, translation of these mutants to human use is problematic.

An alternative but related strategy for a nontoxic toxin adjuvant has been the creation of a fusion protein of the A1 subunit of CT coupled to the Ig-binding fragment D of *Staphylococcus aureus*. The latter targets the fusion protein to B cells. This construct has shown adjuvant activity when administered systemically or mucosally (in ISCOMs) to mice, without detectable toxicity (Lycke, 2001; Mowat *et al.*, 2001).

Comparison of the effects of *E. coli* LT and CT

Given the close relationship between CT and *E. coli* LT, it is not surprising that LT is not only a good mucosal immunogen but also an effective mucosal adjuvant. These molecules are not identical, however, and it is possible there may be some properties that are not shared. The clinical syndrome induced by toxigenic *E. coli* is more benign than that caused by *Vibrio cholerae*, which might suggest that LT is less toxic in humans. However, this difference is more likely due to secretion of CT but not of LT by their respective bacteria *in vivo* than to any difference in their intrinsic ability to induce intestinal secretion. Indeed, a trial involving oral immunization in humans with LT as adjuvant resulted in diarrhea in two-thirds of the volunteers (Michetti *et al.*, 1999). There are differences in MHC class II restrictions between CT-B and LT-B (Nashar and Hirst, 1995), probably related to primary sequence differences that alter the major T-cell epitope (Cong *et al.*, 1996), but this difference is unlikely to have a major effect on their mucosal adjuvanticity. In two inbred strains of mice, LT induced a mixed Th1 and Th2 response (Takahashi *et al.*, 1996), whereas in other studies by the same group, CT consistently induced a predominant Th2 response (Xu-Amano *et al.*, 1993).

Because CT stimulates predominant Th2 responses but LT stimulates predominant Th1 responses, chimeras of CT-A with LT-B and LT-A with CT-B were generated to determine their relative contribution to Th2 subset responses. Interestingly, it was found that the different effects on Th1 or Th2 responses were due to the B subunits rather than the A subunits (Boyaka *et al.*, 2003). The detailed molecular signaling pathway used by the B subunits was not defined in this study. However, a mutant LT-B subunit, EtxB(H47S), has been generated that is able to bind to Gm1 ganglioside on cells and to be internalized but is unable to provide immunomodulatory signals to lymphoid cells (Fraser *et al.*, 2003). These results reinforce the importance of both subunits in the adjuvant effects of these toxins.

Much remains to be learned about the mechanism of both the immunogenicity and adjuvanticity of CT, particularly the importance *in vivo* of the multiple effects of CT found *in vitro*. The properties of CT as a mucosal immunogen appear to extend to antigens delivered with it to mucosal surfaces. The mucosal adjuvanticity of CT appears to be related to its immunogenicity, and both its subunits are required. CT has been effective as a mucosal adjuvant with a wide variety of antigen types. The dose, timing, route, antigen type, and genetic background of the host are all important variables. There are indications that the mechanism of CT adjuvanticity involves multiple aspects of immune induction in the mucosa, but particularly the upregulation of costimulatory cytokines and cell surface molecules by APCs **(Fig. 54.2)**. Other mechanisms include enhancement of T-cell priming; perturbations of regulatory T cells; stimulation of B-cell switching to IgA

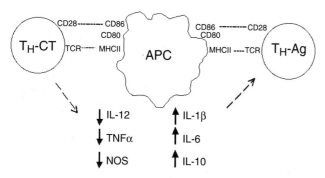

Fig. 54.2. Proposed mechanism of cholera toxin (CT) adjuvanticity. CT binds to antigen-presenting cells (APCs) and alters their expression of costimulatory molecules, upregulating CD86, but perhaps other molecules as well. At the same time CT inhibits the production of certain cytokines such as IL-12 and tumor necrosis factor (TNF)-α and of nitric oxide synthase (NOS), while increasing the production of IL-1, IL-6, and IL-10. T cells reactive to CT as an antigen (Th-CT) are stimulated by these APCs through their T cell receptor (TCR) and, in turn, further upregulate costimulatory cytokines and surface molecules by the APCs. T cells reactive to the exogenous antigen (Th-Ag) coadministered with CT are stimulated by this activated APC and begin to clonally expand, initiating an active immune response.

and IgG; and possibly enhancement of B-cell clonal expansion. Different components of these multiple effects may be of more importance for some antigens than for others. Similar mechanisms likely apply to LT. CT and LT, or their derivatives, remain attractive as adjuvants for mucosal vaccines.

OTHER BACTERIALLY DERIVED MUCOSAL ADJUVANTS

In contrast to the information available on CT and LT, the literature on the use of other agents as mucosal adjuvants is sparse. More recently, interest in the development of effective mucosal vaccines has increased activity in this field. As the following discussion attests, a number of new agents have been evaluated as mucosal adjuvants. However, none has equaled the potency of CT and LT. Rigorous, careful study of more candidates is needed.

Historically, some of the most effective adjuvants used in vaccines have been derived from bacterial components. These agents are now recognized as ligands for TLRs that serve to detect pathogen-associated molecular patterns (PAMPs) and activate innate immune cells. Ten TLRs have now been identified, each recognizing different microbial molecules.

Lipopolysaccharide

The adjuvant activity of LPS was first demonstrated in 1956 (Johnson *et al.* 1956). An unusual feature of its adjuvanticity, relative to that of other agents, is that it can be delivered at a different site and at a different time than antigen (Ulrich *et al.*, 1991). LPS activates the immune system by binding to TLR4, resulting in stimulation of macrophages to produce cytokines such as IL-1 and colony stimulating factors

(CSFs), stimulation of B cell proliferation, alteration of MHC class II expression on APCs, and stimulation of IFN-γ production and of DTH (Ohta *et al.*, 1982; Warren *et al.*, 1986). Despite its potent adjuvant effects, LPS has been used only as an experimental adjuvant because of its toxicity. The lipid A component of LPS is its active moiety and can mimic all the toxic and biological effects of LPS (Chiller *et al.*, 1973).

Many studies have been performed with use of chemically modified forms of lipid A in an effort to find a less toxic but still immunostimulatory compound (Takayama *et al.*, 1981; Takada and Kotani, 1989). Multiple forms of lipid A have been produced and tested as nontoxic alternatives. One of these, monophosphorylipid A, has been shown to possess many of the adjuvant effects of LPS itself. It stimulates macrophages to release IL-1, TNF-α, and CSF, increases production of IFN-γ *in vivo*, and can increase the nonspecific resistance of mice to bacterial infection (Ulrich *et al.*, 1991). This material can be combined with other adjuvants, and its safety has been evaluated in humans.

These studies suggest that lipid A may be an effective adjuvant for mucosal immunization, but its effects on the immune system are complex. LPS increased serum antibody to inhaled bovine serum albumin (BSA) or ovalbumin when it was included in the inhalant (Mizoguchi *et al.*, 1986) and enhanced the antibody response to BSA after oral administration of BSA in liposomes (Ogawa *et al.*, 1986). Studies of rodents suggest that LPS depresses the response to certain antigens such as sheep red blood cells given orally. The administration of LPS to germ-free mice induced oral tolerance to sheep red blood cells subsequently fed to the same mice (Michalek *et al.*, 1983). Administration of LPS or lipid A orally with myelin basic protein (MBP) to rats enhanced the generation of oral tolerance to this antigen; in contrast, LPS given subcutaneously at the time of antigen feeding abrogated oral tolerance to MBP (Khoury *et al.*, 1990). Others have reported that intravenous administration of LPS to mice abrogates orally induced humoral (IgG) but not cellular (DTH) tolerance to ovalbumin (Mowat *et al.*, 1986). These studies illustrate that the effects of LPS or lipid A at mucosal surfaces are complex.

The effect of LPS on different forms of antigen and at various mucosal surfaces, including those not normally bathed in bacterial endotoxin, must be defined. Because antigen and LPS do not need to be given by the same route, combined parenteral and mucosal administration may be effective in stimulating mucosal responses, as has been found in studies with *Shigella* LPS (Keren *et al.*, 1988). Last, lipid A derivatives can be combined with other adjuvants, and such combinations may have much greater efficacy than lipid A alone. The availability of nontoxic lipid A derivatives for human use makes a reexamination of their mucosal adjuvant effects a worthwhile endeavor.

Pertussigen

Killed *Bordetella pertussis* has been used experimentally as a parenteral adjuvant. This material is a complex mixture, including LPS as well as variable amounts of pertussis toxin. The latter has many biological effects, probably related to its ability to bind to signal-transducing G proteins in a diverse number of cell types. Purified pertussigen has been found to exert adjuvant activity. In particular, it enhances the cell-mediated immunity (CMI) response, as measured by delayed skin test responses to soluble antigens and increased inflammatory responses such as footpad swelling after the injection of Freund's complete adjuvant. *Bordetella* and pertussigen both increase IgG and IgE responses to antigens and have been reported to abrogate humoral tolerance (Herzenberg and Tokuhisa, 1982) and cell-mediated tolerance (Tamura *et al.*, 1985) to antigens in some systems, an effect of some interest for mucosal immunity because of the propensity for tolerance induction by antigen feeding. Like LPS, pertussigen can be given by a different route and at a different time than the antigen and still exert its adjuvant effects.

Data on the mucosal adjuvanticity of pertussigen are emerging. One can induce IgE antibody responses in rats fed ovalbumin by administering pertussigen intradermally, intraperitoneally, or orally (Bazin and Platteau, 1976; Jarrett *et al.*, 1976). The IgE isotype is not one that vaccines are usually intended to induce; thus, the value of this antibody response is questionable. Perhaps related to its ability to induce IgE responses or, alternatively, to induce DTH, immunization with nematode worm antigens plus pertussigen stimulated resistance to two different intestinal nematodes in rodents (Murray *et al.*, 1979; Mitchell and Munoz, 1983). A genetically detoxified derivative of pertussis toxin, PT-9K/129G, has been generated that has mucosal adjuvanticity when administered with antigen nasally. When TT plus PT-9K/129G was administered nasally to mice, IgG$_1$ and IgA but not IgE anti-TT were induced, and the mice were protected from TT challenge (Roberts *et al.*, 1995). This is an exciting and promising observation that might make the use of this agent as a mucosal adjuvant feasible if these results are confirmed in humans.

The propensity of pertussigen to produce adverse effects is a concern. Pertussis vaccine has been associated with severe reactions in humans, including encephalitis (Cavanagh *et al.*, 1981). These potential toxicities may be lessened by employing a mucosal route of administration. However, pertussigen has induced intestinal hypersecretory responses to some inflammatory mediators and neurotransmitters, and this responsiveness may be prolonged by oral immunization (Crowe *et al.*, 1990). These and other potential adverse reactions with pertussigen may limit its usefulness as a mucosal adjuvant except for experimental use.

Muramyl dipeptide

Muramyl dipeptide (MDP; *N*-acetyl-muramyl-L-alanyl-D-isoglutamine) is derived from the cell wall of mycobacteria. It is the smallest structural component of the cell wall that still retains adjuvant activity and is one of the active components in Freund's complete adjuvant. MDP is one of the ligands for TLR2. MDP has been used parenterally for experimental vaccines and immunotherapy, but data on the use of MDP as a mucosal adjuvant are limited.

MDP has been used as an adjuvant for intravaginal immunization in mice (Thapar *et al.*, 1990). Multiple large doses of horse ferritin were combined with aluminum hydroxide, MDP, monophosphoryl lipid A, or CT. Although MDP was not the most effective adjuvant for this route, it was shown to potentiate the secretory immune response to horse ferritin. Depending on the route of immunization chosen, the level and isotype of antibody to horse ferritin varied (Thapar *et al.*, 1990). Pelvic immunization induced greater IgA and IgG responses in the vagina than did intravaginal immunization.

MDP has also been used as an adjuvant for oral immunization (Thapar *et al.*, 1990). Trinitrophenyl (TNP)-haptenated whole cells or cell wall from the cariogenic bacterium *S. mutans* was combined with MDP and administered intragastrically to mice. MDP boosted anti-TNP IgA responses in LPS-responsive C3H/HeN mice but not in LPS-unresponsive C3H/HeJ mice. The salivary immune response to *S. mutans* whole cells or cell walls in gnotobiotic rats was augmented more than twofold when they were administered orally with MDP. The use of MDP in combination with *S. mutans* resulted in a significant reduction in bacterial colonization of tooth surfaces and in the number of carious lesions produced (Morasaki *et al.*, 1983). MDP augmented the mucosal immune response to *Neisseria gonorrhoeae* major outer-membrane protein when given intraduodenally or injected directly into Peyer's patches (Jeurissen *et al.*, 1987). Lipophilic derivatives of MDP have been synthesized and tested for their mucosal adjuvanticity. Some derivatives enhanced the mucosal response of rats to soluble BSA administered in saline, whereas others were active only when incorporated with antigen in liposomes (Ogawa *et al.*, 1986).

The preceding observations suggest that MDP can be presented to the mucosal lymphoid tissue and can stimulate both secretory and systemic immunity to antigens administered with it. The mechanism of action at these sites is unknown but probably involves, at least in part, the ability of MDP to induce IL-1 production and increase processing and presentation of antigen by macrophages.

Lipopeptides and proteosomes

Lipopeptides, derived from bacterial lipoproteins, which are the ligand for TLRs 2 and 6, have been shown to be potent adjuvants for parenteral immunization. They have also been used as carriers for haptens, resulting in elicitation of hapten-specific antibody responses. The structure of certain lipopeptides has been characterized, and some can be produced synthetically. One synthetically produced lipopeptide, P3CSK4, has been shown to be an effective adjuvant for oral immunization (Heinevetter *et al.*, 1995). This compound has been observed to stimulate murine lymphocytes from Peyer's patches in a dose-dependent manner without any apparent toxicity.

Proteosomes are multimolecular preparations of meningococcal outer-membrane proteins (Lowell *et al.*, 1988). The ability of proteosomes to act as B-cell mitogens suggested that they may be useful as vaccine adjuvants. Nasal or intramuscular immunization of mice and intramuscular immunization of rabbits with formalinized staphylococcal enterotoxin B (SEB) toxoid in saline elicited higher anti-SEB serum IgG titers when the toxoid was formulated with proteosomes (Lowell *et al.*, 1996). In addition, nasal immunization of mice with this proteosome–toxoid vaccine combination elicited high levels of anti-SEB IgA in lung and intestinal secretions, whereas the toxoid without proteosomes did not. Furthermore, proteosome–toxoid delivered nasally in saline afforded significant protection against challenge by a lethal aerosol exposure to SEB. Efficacy correlated with the induction of high serum levels of anti-SEB IgG. Nasal immunization with toxoid in saline without proteosomes was not significantly protective.

Bacterial DNA

Bacterial-derived DNA sequences are the ligand for TLR9. Bacterial DNA has immunostimulatory properties (Tokunaga *et al.*, 1984; see Chapter 54), including production of interferon and IL-12 (Sato *et al.*, 1996) and stimulation of B-cell proliferation and production of IL-6 (Cowdery *et al.*, 1996). Natural killer (NK) cell activity was also reportedly enhanced by the addition of specific DNA sequences (Yamamoto *et al.*, 1992). This activity is associated with specific palandromic DNA sequences that can be encoded by single-stranded oligonucleotides (Klinman *et al.*, 1996). The ability to synthesize these oligonucleotides on a large scale makes their use as vaccine adjuvants attractive. The CpG oligodeoxynucleotides were effective as a mucosal adjuvant for viruslike particles of simian immunodeficiency virus when coadministered with antigen to the nasal mucosa of mice (Kang *et al.*, 2003). CpG oligodeoxynucleotides were effective at inducing immune responses to hepatitis B surface antigen and could act synergistically with cholera toxin (McCluskie *et al.*, 1998).

SYNTHETIC ADJUVANTS

Synthetic adjuvants are based on the concept that antigen can be packaged into particles composed of emulsions or detergents. Particle size appears to be crucial for efficient uptake by GALT. The particles also appear to protect antigen against the harsh environment of the gastrointestinal tract, ensuring that a greater amount of intact antigen reaches GALT. Although a limited number of these agents have been evaluated as mucosal adjuvants, some appear to be quite promising, as described in the following sections.

Saponin-based adjuvants

Quil A

Quil A is a component of saponin, a detergent derived from the plant *Quillaja saponaria Molina*, that has been shown to have adjuvant activity (Dalsgaard, 1974). Quil A is one of the biologically active components of immunostimulating

complexes (ISCOMs), but it has also been employed alone as an adjuvant. The usefulness of Quil A as an adjuvant has been hampered by its apparent toxicity, which has been observed in small animals after parenteral immunization with this adjuvant, and such toxicity may well limit its usefulness. However, nontoxic immunostimulatory fractions of Quil A have been identified that may reduce or eliminate this problem (Kensil *et al.*, 1991). While Quil A by itself does not appear to be highly effective as a mucosal adjuvant, its use as one of the components of ISCOMs appears to be critical for the effectiveness of this system, which is described next.

Immunostimulating complexes (ISCOMs)

The term *ISCOM* was coined by Morein to describe 40-nm cagelike particles that form spontaneously when cholesterol is mixed with Quil A (Morein, 1987; Morein *et al.*, 1990). Protein antigens can be incorporated into such particles, with Quil A serving as a built-in adjuvant. The incorporation of antigens into ISCOMs occurs via hydrophobic interactions, which could potentially limit the utility of this adjuvant for protein antigens. However, modification of proteins by either palmitification or acidification (followed by the addition of phosphatidylcholine) permits a greater variety of proteins to be incorporated into ISCOMs (Morein *et al.*, 1990; Mowat *et al.*, 1991). Much smaller amounts of antigen can be employed in ISCOMs than in oil-based adjuvants, which makes them useful as adjuvants in cases where the quantity of antigen is limiting (Nagy *et al.*, 1990). ISCOMs have been effectively used as adjuvants for parenteral vaccines in a variety of species, including mice, cats, sheep, cattle, and monkeys (Morein *et al.*, 1990).

ISCOMs stimulate a strong response for all immunoglobulin classes (Lovgren, 1988). They also stimulate CMI, as measured by proliferative T-cell responses and DTH (Fossum *et al.*, 1990). Perhaps a unique feature of ISCOMs is their ability to induce CD8+ CTL responses. A single subcutaneous immunization of mice with ISCOMs containing either purified human immunodeficiency virus (HIV) gp160 or influenza hemagglutinin resulted in priming of antigen-specific CD8+ MHC class I–restricted CTLs (Takahashi *et al.*, 1990a). This suggests that ISCOMs cause exogenous proteins to enter the endogenous pathway of antigen processing. It appears that the Quil A component is essential for this effect since it did not occur with simple liposomes or with free palmitified antigen (Mowat *et al.*, 1991). The ability of ISCOMs to redirect exogenous antigens into the class I pathway may be unique among adjuvants.

Intranasal administration of ISCOMs containing influenza virus resulted in high levels of virus-specific antibody and protected mice against challenge with influenza virus (Lovgren, 1988). These results were equivalent to those obtained by subcutaneous immunization with virus alone. Oral administration of ovalbumin in ISCOMs to mice orally tolerized to ovalbumin resulted in the production of ovalbumin-specific serum antibody (Mowat *et al.*, 1991). After repeated feeding of ovalbumin in ISCOMs, ovalbumin-specific CTLs were elicited (Mowat *et al.*, 1991). After several oral feedings, strong S-IgA antibody responses to ovalbumin were detected in intestinal washings. Thus, the oral administration of ovalbumin in ISCOMs generated a wide spectrum of humoral and cellular immune responses. Last, parenteral immunization of mice in the pelvic pre-sacral space with sheep erythrocyte membrane proteins in ISCOMs generated significant IgA titers against this antigen in vaginal fluid (Thapar *et al.*, 1991). Administration of ISCOMs by a mucosal route of immunization may help to avoid some of the toxicity issues raised by the use of Quil A in parenteral vaccines.

Multiple emulsions

Multiple emulsions have been used for decades for parenteral immunization but only recently for mucosal immunization. Water-in-oil-in-water emulsions utilizing a biodegradable squalene as the lipid and nonionic block copolymers as emulsifiers have been tested for their ability to induce an immune response to antigen incorporated, with or without adjuvant, in the inner water phase. The response to antigen plus CT as adjuvant in multiple emulsions has been found to induce strong intestinal S-IgA and plasma IgG responses to the antigen. Moreover, this delivery system not only protected the antigen from the intestinal bile and proteases but also sequestered the CT and protected the mucosa from the secretory effects of CT (Tomasi *et al.*, 1997).

Whether such multiple emulsions represent a delivery system or an adjuvant remains unclear. Nonionic block copolymers are both powerful systemic adjuvants and effective stabilizers of water-in-oil-in-water multiple emulsions. Block copolymers are composed of hydrophilic polyoxyethylene (POE) and hydrophobic polyoxypropylene (POP) that differ in molecular weight, percentage of POE, and mode of linkage of POP to POE (Zigterman *et al.*, 1987). Block copolymers, such as Titermax, have been used extensively as adjuvants for parenteral immunization (Brey, 1995) and can elicit both CMI and humoral immunity as well as modulate the antibody isotype produced (Hunter *et al.*, 1994). The copolymers appear to adhere to lipids, thereby promoting retention of protein antigen in local tissue and facilitating the uptake of antigen by APCs.

One of the intriguing results of the studies on the use of multiple emulsions for oral immunization is that incorporation of antigen alone induced oral tolerance (Elson *et al.*, 1996). This occurred after delivery of three different antigens, including a recombinant bacterial protein derived from *E. coli*. The same preparation given parenterally induced strong humoral responses. These results support the idea that mucosal tolerance can be enhanced by adjuvants. Another example of this effect is the strong induction of tolerance following mucosal application of antigen-rCT-B complexes (Sun *et al.*, 1994; Sun *et al.*, 1996). Oral tolerance has been used in the treatment of a number of experimental autoimmune diseases but requires the feeding of large quantities of antigen on a daily basis. Although adjuvants are not generally thought of in relation to enhancement of tolerance, such adjuvants will likely be necessary if oral tolerance is to become an effective treatment for human disorders.

CYTOKINES AND OTHER IMMUNOMODULATORS

It is probable that stimulation of cytokine production is central to adjuvant activity. This understanding, combined with the availability of recombinant cytokines, has stimulated interest in using cytokines themselves as adjuvants. It is hoped that this approach will prove less toxic and might allow the resulting immune response to be directed into specific pathways of immunity that are beneficial to the host. cytokine are unlikely to be practical via the oral route, but their application to other mucosal surfaces, such as nasal mucosa, may be effective.

Cytokines

Certain cytokines have been associated with the production of IgA. Thus, these cytokines are prime candidates for use in mucosal vaccines, including IL-4, IL-5, and IL-6, which are produced primarily by Th2 cells. Th2 responses appear to be the dominant helper cell type elicited by mucosal vaccination with protein antigens plus CT. IL-6 given intranasally along with TT antigen stimulated serum IgG but not S-IgA responses (Boyaka *et al.*, 1999). Deletion of the IL-6 gene in mice markedly reduced mucosal IgA in one study (Ramsay *et al.*, 1994) but had no effect on the production of IgA in another (Bromander *et al.*, 1996). In the case of IL-4, results have been conflicting also; complete ablation of IgA responses was achieved in one study (Vajdy *et al.*, 1995) but only partial ablation was achieved in another (Okahashi, *et al.*, 1996). This may be related partly to the overlapping effects of many cytokines, the housing environment, and the genetic background of the strains used. Certain cytokines appear to act as "master switches" controlling the balance between Th1 and Th2 responses. Other cytokines might modulate DCs, such as in a study in which flt3L and IL-1α given parenterally activated DCs, resulting in an active immune response to fed antigen in the absence of a traditional mucosal adjuvant (Williamson *et al.*, 1999). The following discussion describes some preliminary studies that used such cytokines to influence the type of immune response elicited to orally administered antigens.

Interleukin-12

Interleukin-12 has been used experimentally in mice to alter the response elicited by orally administered antigens. Systemic administration of recombinant murine IL-12 to C56B1/6 mice orally immunized with TT plus CT shifted the Th2 responses normally produced by these antigens to a mixed Th1/Th2 response (Marinaro *et al.*, 1996). This change was associated with an increase in DTH and a shift in IgG subclass to IgG2a and IgG3. Serum IgE and mucosal IgA antibody responses were both depressed by systemic

IL-12 treatment. Mucosally delivered IL-12 stimulated both IgG and S-IgA responses to TT (Boyaka *et al.*, 1999) and could modulate the mucosal adjuvanticity of CT intranasally, enhancing Th1 responses to TT (Marinaro *et al.*, 1999). IL-12 may be useful for the generation of a Th1 response to orally administered antigens, which is critical for protection against many types of intracellular pathogens.

Interleukin-13

The importance of IL-13 in the development of mucosal and systemic antibody responses was demonstrated by the ability of high-affinity polyclonal antibody to IL-13 to block the response normally elicited by oral immunization with the B subunit of *E. coli* LT (LT-B) (Bost *et al.*, 1995). Mice treated with antibody to IL-13 prior to oral immunization with a single dose of LT-B had significantly lower intestinal IgA and serum IgG responses than did untreated mice. Inhibition of IL-13 also affected the production of antibody to subsequent immunizations with LT-B. *In vitro* restimulation of lymphocytes isolated from the mesenteric lymph nodes and spleens of antibody-treated mice depressed Th2 responses, but Th1 responses were unaffected by the treatment. This study suggests that IL-13 may be able to enhance Th2 responses to mucosally administered vaccines, but this hypothesis remains to be tested.

OTHER CANDIDATE ADJUVANTS

A number of agents have been tested for their ability to serve as mucosal adjuvants, but there are insufficient data to draw firm conclusions. These include *Clostridium difficile* toxins (Thomas *et al.*, 1995), dehydroepiandrosterone (DHEA) (Araneo *et al.*, 1995a), vitamin D3 (Araneo *et al.*, 1995b), and Avridine (Bergmann and Waldman, 1988).

REFERENCES

Abraham, E., and Robinson, A. (1991). Oral immunization with bacterial polysaccharide and adjuvant enhances antigen-specific pulmonary secretory antibody response and resistance to pneumonia. *Vaccine* 9, 757–764.

Alisky, J.M., van de Wetering, C.I., and Davidson, B.L. (2002). Widespread dispersal of cholera toxin subunit B to brain and spinal cord neurons following systemic delivery. *Exp. Neurol.* 178, 13–46.

Anastassiou, E.D., Yamada, H., Boumpas, D.T., Tsokos, G.C., Thyphronitis, G., Balow, J., and Mond, J.J. (1992). Cholera toxin promotes the proliferation of anti-mu antibody-prestimulated human B cells. *Cell. Immunol.* 140, 237–247.

Araneo, B., Dowell, T., Woods, M.L., Daynes, R., Judd, M., and Evans, T. (1995a). DHEAS as an effective vaccine adjuvant in elderly humans: Proof-of-principle studies. *Ann. N.Y. Acad. Sci.* 774, 232–248.

Araneo, B., Kreisel, J., Ricigliano, J., and Norton, S. (1995b). Vitamin D3-enhanced protection in two murine models of viral infection: influenza and herpes simplex 2. *Clin. Immunol. Immunopathol.* 76, S122, A718.

Bazin, H., and Platteau, B. (1976). Production of circulating reaginic (IgE) antibodies by oral administration of ovalbumin to rats. *Immunology* 30, 679–684.

Bergmann, K.C., Waldman, R.H. (1988). Enhanced murine respiratory tract IgA antibody response to oral influenza vaccine when combined with a lipoidal amine (Avridine). *Int. Arch. Allergy. Appl. Immunol.* 87, 334–335.

Bergquist, C., Lagergard, T., Lindblad, M., and Holmgren, J. (1995). Local and systemic antibody responses to dextran-cholera toxin B subunit conjugates. *Infect. Immun.* 63, 2021–2025.

Bessen, D., and Fischetti, V.A. (1988). Influence of intranasal immunization with synthetic peptides corresponding to conserved epitopes of M protein on mucosal colonization by group A streptococci. *Infect. Immun.* 56, 2666–2672.

Betley, M., Miller, V., and Mekalanos, J. (1986). Genetics of bacterial enterotoxins. *Annu. Rev. Microbiol.* 40, 577–605.

Bland, P.W., and Warren, L.G. (1986). Antigen presentation by epithelial cells of the rat small intestine. II. Selective induction of suppressor cells. *Immunology* 58, 9–14.

Bost, K.L., Holton, R.H. and Clements, J.D. (1995). In vivo treatment with antibodies against IL-13 dramatically inhibits mucosal and systemic humoral responses in mice orally immunized with the B subunit of *E. coli* heat labile enterotoxin. *Clin. Immunol. Immunopathol.* 76, S122, A719.

Bourguin, I., Chardes, T., Mevelec, M.N., Woodman, J.P., and Bout, D. (1991). Amplification of the secretory IgA response to *Toxoplasma gondii* using cholera toxin. *FEMS Microbiol. Lett.* 65, 265–271.

Bowen, J.C., Nair, S.K., Reddy, R., and Rouse, B.T. (1994). Cholera toxin acts as a potent adjuvant for the induction of cytotoxic T-lymphocyte responses with nonreplicating antigens. *Immunology* 81, 338–342.

Boyaka, P.N., Marinaro, M., Jackson, R.J., Menon, S., Kiyono, H., Jirillo, E., and McGhee, J.R. (1999). IL-12 is an effective adjuvant for induction of mucosal immunity. *J. Immunol.* 162, 122–128.

Boyaka, P.N., Ohmura, M., Fujihashi, K., Koga, T., Yamamoto, M., Kweon, M.N., Takeda, Y., Jackson, R.J., Kiyono, H., Yuki, Y., and McGhee, J.R. (2003). Chimeras of labile toxin one and cholera toxin retain mucosal adjuvanticity and direct Th cell subsets via their B subunit. *J. Immunol.* 170, 454–462.

Braun, M.C., He, J., Wu, C.Y., and Kelsall, B.L. (1999). Cholera toxin suppresses interleukin (IL)-12 production and IL-12 receptor a1 and a2 chain expression. *J. Exp. Med.* 189, 541–552.

Brey, R.N. (1995). Development of vaccines based on formulations containing nonionic block copolymers. *Pharm. Biotechnol.* 6, 297–311.

Bromander, A., Holmgren, J., and Lycke, N. (1991). Cholera toxin stimulates IL-1 production and enhances antigen presentation by macrophages in vitro. *J. Immunol.* 146, 2908–2914.

Bromander, A.K., Ekman, L., Kopf, M., Nedrud, J.G., and Lycke, N.Y. (1996). IL-6-deficient mice exhibit normal mucosal IgA responses to local immunizations and *Helicobacter felis* infection. *J. Immunol.* 156, 4290–4297.

Bromander, A.K., Kjerrulf, M., Holmgren, J., and Lycke, N. (1993). Cholera toxin enhances alloantigen presentation by cultured intestinal epithelial cells. *Scand. J. Immunol.* 37, 452–458.

Bukawa, H., Sekigawa, K., Hamajima, K., Fukushima, J., Yamada, Y., Kiyono, H., and Okuda, K. (1995). Neutralization of HIV-1 by secretory IgA induced by oral immunization with a new macromolecular multicomponent peptide vaccine candidate. *Nature Med.* 1, 681–685.

Castello-Branco, L.R., Griffin, G.E., Poulton, T.A., Dougan, G., and Lewis, D.J. (1994). Characterization of the circulating T-cell response after oral immunization of human volunteers with cholera toxin B subunit. *Vaccine* 12, 65–72.

Cavanagh, N.P., Brett, E.M., Marshall, W.C., and Wilson, J. (1981). The possible adjuvant role of *Bordetella pertussis* and pertussis vaccine in causing severe encephalopathic illness: A presentation of three case histories. *Neuropediatrics* 12, 374–381.

Chen, K.S., and Strober, W. (1990). Cholera holotoxin and its B subunit enhance Peyer's patch B cell responses induced by orally administered influenza virus: Disproportionate cholera toxin enhancement of the IgA B cell response. *Eur. J. Immunol.* 20, 433–436.

Chiller, J.M., Skidmore, B.J., Morrison, D.C., and Weigle, W.O. (1973). Relationship of the structure of bacterial lipopolysaccharides to its function in mitogenesis and adjuvanticity. *Proc. Natl. Acad. Sci. USA* 70, 2129–2135.

Clarke, C.J., Wilson, A.D., Williams, N.A., and Stokes, C.R. (1991). Mucosal priming of T-lymphocyte responses to fed protein antigens using cholera toxin as an adjuvant. *Immunology* 72, 323–328.

Clements, J.D., Hartzog, N.M., and Lyon, F.L. (1988). Adjuvant activity of *Escherichia coli* heat-labile enterotoxin and effect on the induction of oral tolerance in mice to unrelated protein antigens. *Vaccine* 6, 269–277.

Cong, Y., Bowdon, H.R., and Elson, C.O. (1996). Identification of an immunodominant T cell epitope on cholera toxin. *Eur. J. Immunol.* 26, 2587–2594.

Cong, Y., Weaver, C.T., and Elson, C.O. (1977). The mucosal adjuvanticity of cholera toxin involves enhancement of costimulatory activity by selective up-regulation of B7.2 expression. *J. Immunol.* 159, 5301–5308.

Cong, Y., Oliver, A.O., and Elson, C.O. (2001). Effects of cholera toxin on macrophage production of co-stimulatory cytokines. *Eur. J. Immunol.* 31, 64–71.

Cowdery, J.S., Chace, J.H., Yi, A.K., and Krieg, A.M. (1996). Bacterial DNA induces NK cells to produce IFN-γ in vivo and increases the toxicity of lipopolysaccharides. *J. Immunol.* 156, 4570–4575.

Crowe, S.E., Sestini, P., and Perdue, M.H. (1990). Allergic reactions of rat jejunal mucosa: Ion transport responses to luminal antigen and inflammatory mediators. *Gastroenterology* 99, 74–82.

Cuatrecasas, P. (1973). Gangliosides and membrane receptors for cholera toxin. *Biochemistry* 12, 3558–3556.

Czerkinsky, C., Russell, M.W., Lycke, N., Lindblad, M., and Holmgren, J. (1989). Oral administration of a streptococcal antigen coupled to cholera toxin B subunit evokes strong antibody responses in salivary glands and extramucosal tissues. *Infect. Immun.* 57, 1072–1077.

Czerkinsky, C., Svennerholm, A.M., Quiding, M., Jonsson, R., and Holmgren, J. (1991). Antibody-producing cells in peripheral blood and salivary glands after oral cholera vaccination of humans. *Infect. Immun.* 59, 996–1001.

Czinn, S.J., and Nedrud, J.G. (1991). Oral immunization against *Helicobacter pylori*. *Infect. Immun.* 59, 2359–2363.

Dalsgaard, K. (1974). Saponin adjuvants. 3. Isolation of a substance from *Quillaja saponaria Molina* with adjuvant activity in foot-and-mouth disease vaccines. *Arch. Gesamte. Virusforsch.* 44, 243–254.

Daynes, R.A., Enioutina, E.Y., Butler, S., Mu, H.H., McGee, Z.A., and Araneo, B.A. (1996). Induction of common mucosal immunity by hormonally immunomodulated peripheral immunization. *Infect. Immun.* 64, 1100–1109.

De Bernardis, F., Boccanera, M., Adriani, D., Girolamo, A., and Cassone, A. (2002). Intravaginal and intranasal immunizations are equally effective in inducing vaginal antibodies and conferring protection against vaginal candidiasis. *Infect. Immun.* 70, 2725–2729.

Dertzbaugh, M.T., and Elson, C.O. (1991). Cholera toxin as a mucosal adjuvant. In *Topics in Vaccine Adjuvant Research* (eds. D.R. Spriggs and W.C. Koff). Boca Raton, FL: CRC Press, 119–131.

Dertzbaugh, M.T., and Elson, C.O. (1993a). Comparative effectiveness of the cholera toxin B subunit and alkaline phosphatase as carriers for oral vaccines. *Infect. Immun.* 61, 48–55.

Dertzbaugh, M.T., and Elson, C.O. (1993b). Reduction in oral immunogenicity of cholera toxin B subunit by N-terminal peptide addition. *Infect. Immun.* 61, 384–390.

Dertzbaugh, M.T., Peterson, D.L., and Macrina, F.L. (1990). Cholera toxin B subunit gene fusion: Structural and functional analysis of the chimera protein. *Infect. Immun.* 58, 70–79.

Douce, G., Turcotte, C., Cropley, I., Roberts, M., Pizza, M., Domenghini, M., Rappuoli, R., and Dougan, G. (1995). Mutants of *Escherichia coli* heat-labile toxin lacking ADP-ribosyl-transferase activity act as non-toxic, mucosal adjuvants. *Proc. Natl. Acad. Sci. USA* 92, 1644–1648.

Elson, C.O. (1992). Cholera toxin as a mucosal adjuvant: Effects of H-2 major histocompatibility complex and *lps* genes. *Infect. Immun.* 60, 2874–2879.

Elson, C.O., and Ealding, W. (1984a). Cholera toxin feeding did not induce oral tolerance in mice and abrogated oral tolerance to an unrelated protein antigen. *J. Immunol.* 133, 2892–2897.

Elson, C.O., and Ealding, W. (1984b). Generalized systemic and mucosal immunity in mice after mucosal stimulation with cholera toxin. *J. Immunol.* 132, 2736–2742.

Elson, C.O., and Ealding, W. (1987). Ir gene control of the murine secretory IgA response to cholera toxin. *Eur. J. Immunol.* 17, 425–428.

Elson, C.O., Holland, S.P., Dertzbaugh, M.T., Cuff, C.F., and Anderson, A.O. (1995a). Morphologic and functional alterations of mucosal T cells by cholera toxin and its B subunit. *J. Immunol.* 154, 1032–1040.

Elson, C.O., Tomasi, M., Chang, T.-T., Jobling, M.G., and Holmes, R.K. (1995b). Immunogenicity and adjuvanticity of mutant cholera toxin (CT) molecules. *FASEB J.* 9, A290.

Elson, C.O., Tomasi, M., Dertzbaugh, M.T., Thaggard, G., Hunter, R., and Weaver, C. (1996). Oral-antigen delivery by way of a multiple emulsion system enhances oral tolerance. *Ann. N.Y. Acad. Sci.* 778, 156–162.

Finkelman, F.D., Holmes, J., Katona, I.M., Urban, J.F.J., Beckmann, M.P., Park, L.S., Schooley, K.A., Coffman, R.L., Mosmann, T.R., and Paul, W.E. (1990). Lymphokine control of in vivo immunoglobulin isotype selection. *Annu. Rev. Immunol.* 8, 303–333.

Fossum, C., Bergstrom, M., Lovgren, K., Watson, D.L., and Morein, B. (1990). Effect of ISCOMs and their adjuvant moiety (matrix) on the initial proliferation and IL-2 responses: Comparison of spleen cells from mice inoculated with ISCOMs and/or matrix. *Cell. Immunol.* 129, 414–425.

Francis, M.L., Ryan, J., Jobling, M.G., Holmes, R.K., Moss, J., and Mond, J.J. (1992). Cyclic AMP-independent effects of cholera toxin on B cell activation. II. Binding of ganglioside GM1 induces B cell activation. *J. Immunol.* 148, 1999–2005.

Fraser, S.A., de Haan, L., Hearn, A.R., Bone, H.K., Salmond, R.J., Rivett, A.J., Williams, N.A., and Hirst, T.R. (2003). Mutant *Escherichia coli* heat-labile toxin B subunit that separates toxoid-mediated signaling and immunomodulatory action from trafficking and delivery functions. *Infect. Immun.* 71, 1527–1537.

Frey, A., Giannasca, K.T., Weltzin, R., Giannasca, P.J., Reggio, H., Lencer, W.I., and Neutra, M.R. (1996). Role of the glycocalyx in regulating access of microparticles to apical plasma membranes of intestinal epithelial cells: Implications for microbial attachment and oral vaccine targeting. *J. Exp. Med.* 184, 1045–1059.

Gizurarson, S., Tamura, S., Aizawa, C., and Kurata, T. (1992). Stimulation of the transepithelial flux of influenza HA vaccine by cholera toxin B subunit. *Vaccine* 10, 101–106.

Grdic, D., Hornquist, E., Kjerrulf, M., and Lycke, N.Y. (1998). Lack of local suppression in orally tolerant CD8-deficient mice reveals a critical regulatory role of CD8+ T cells in the normal gut mucosa. *J. Immunol.* 160, 754–762.

Hajishengallis, G., Hollingshead, S.K., Koga, T., and Russell, M.W. (1995). Mucosal immunization with a bacterial protein antigen genetically coupled to cholera toxin A2/B subunits. *J. Immunol.* 154, 4322–4332.

Hajishengallis, G., Michalek, S.M., and Russell, M.W. (1996). Persistence of serum and salivary antibody responses after oral immunization with a bacterial protein antigen genetically linked to the A2/B subunits of cholera toxin. *Infect. Immun.* 64, 665–667.

Hansson, H.A., Lange, S., and Lonnroth, I. (1984). Internalization in vivo of cholera toxin in the small intestinal epithelium of the rat. *Acta Pathol. Microbiol. Immunol. Scand. [A]* 92, 15–21.

Hearn, T.I. (1995). *Murine Mucosal and Systemic Immune Responses to Antigens Delivered by Oral Infusion in Water-in-Oil-in-Water Emulsions Containing Block Copolymer P1005*. Ph.D. thesis. Atlanta: Emory University.

Heinevetter, L., Baier, W., Wiesmuller, H.H., Jung, G., and Bessler, W.G. (1995). Synthetic lipopeptides as adjuvants in oral immunization. *Clin. Immunol. Immunopathol.* 76, S18.

Herzenberg, L.A., and Tokuhisa, T. (1982). Epitope-specific regulation I. Carrier-specific induction of suppression for IgG anti-hapten antibody responses. *J. Exp. Med.* 155, 1730–1740.

Hirabayashi, Y., Tamura, S.I., Suzuki, Y., Nagamine, T., Aizawa, C., Shimada, K. and Kurata, T. (1991). H-2-unrestricted adjuvant effect of cholera toxin B subunit on murine antibody responses to influenza virus haemagglutinin. *Immunology* 72, 329–335.

Hol, W.G.J., Sixma, T.K., and Meritt, E.A. (1995). Structure and function of *E. coli* heat-labile enterotoxin and cholera toxin B pentamer. In *Bacterial Toxins and Virulence Factors in Disease* (eds. J. Moss, B. Iglewski, M. Vaughan and A.T. Tu). New York: Marcel Dekker, 185–223.

Hooper, C. (1991). The new age of vaccine adjuvants. *J. NIH Res.* 3, 21–23.

Hordnes, K., Digranes, A., Haugen, I.L., Helland, D.E., Ulstein, M., Jonsson, R., and Haneberg, B. (1995). Systemic and mucosal antibody responses to group B streptococci following immunization of the colonic rectal mucosa. *J. Reprod. Immunol.* 28, 247–262.

Hornquist, E., and Lycke, N. (1993). Cholera toxin adjuvant greatly promotes antigen priming of T cells. *Eur. J. Immunol.* 23, 2136–2143.

Hornquist, E., Goldschmidt, T.J., Holmdahl, R., and Lycke, N. (1991). Host defense against cholera toxin is strongly CD4$^+$ T cell dependent. *Infect. Immun.* 59, 3630–3638.

Hornquist, E., Grdic, D., Mak, T., and Lycke, N. (1996). CD8-deficient mice exhibit augmented mucosal immune responses and intact adjuvant effects to cholera toxin. *Immunology* 87, 220–229.

Hoshi, S., Nakamura, T., Nunoya, T., and Ueda, S. (1995). Induction of protective immunity in chickens orally immunized with inactivated infectious bursal disease virus. *Vaccine* 13, 245–252.

Hui, G.S.N., Chang, S.P., Gibson, H., Hashimoto, A., Hashiro, C., Barr, P.J., and Kotani, S. (1991). Influence of adjuvants on the antibody specificity to the *Plasmodium falciparum* major merozoite surface protein, gp195. *J. Immunol.* 147, 3935–3941.

Hunter, R.L., McNicholl, J. and Lal, A.A. (1994). Mechanisms of action of nonionic block copolymer adjuvants. *AIDS Res. Hum. Retroviruses* 10, S95–S98.

Imaoka, K., Miller, C.J., Kubota, M., McChesney, M.B., Lohman, B., Yamamoto, M., Fuhihashi, K., Someya, K., Honda, M., McGhee, J.R., and Kiyono, H. (1998). Nasal immunization of nonhuman primates with simian immunodeficiency virus P55gag and cholera toxin adjuvant induces Th1/Th2 help for virus-specific immune responses in reproductive tissues. *J. Immunol.* 161, 5952–5958.

Jackson, R.J., Fujihashi, K., Xu-Amano, J., Kiyono, H., Elson, C.O., and McGhee, J.R. (1993). Optimizing oral vaccines: Induction of systemic and mucosal B-cell and antibody responses to tetanus toxoid by use of cholera toxin as an adjuvant. *Infect. Immun.* 61, 4272–4279.

Jarrett, E.E., Haig, D.M., McDougall, W., and McNulty, E. (1976). Rat IgE production. II. Primary and booster reaginic antibody responses following intradermal or oral immunization. *Immunology* 30, 671–677.

Jertborn, M., Svennerholm, A.M., and Holmgren, J. (1988). Five-year immunologic memory in Swedish volunteers after oral cholera vaccination. *J. Infect. Dis.* 157, 374–377.

Jeurissen, S.H., Sminia, T., and Beuvery, E.C. (1987). Induction of mucosal immunoglobulin A immune response by preparations of *Neisseria gonorrhoeae* porin proteins. *Infect. Immun.* 55, 253–257.

Jobling, M.G., and Holmes, R.K. (1991). Analysis of structure and function of the B subunit of cholera toxin by the use of site-directed mutagenesis. *Mol. Microbiol.* 5, 1755–1767.

Jobling, M.G., and Holmes, R.K. (1992). Fusion proteins containing the A2 domain of cholera toxin assemble with B polypeptides of cholera toxin to form immunoreactive and functional holotoxin-like chimeras. *Infect. Immun.* 60, 4915–4924.

Johnson, A.J., Gaines, S., and Landy, M. (1956). Studies on the O antigen of *Salmonella typhosa*. V. Enhancement of the antibody response to protein antigens by the purified lipopolysaccharide. *J. Exp. Med.* 103, 225–233.

Justewicz, D.M., Morin, M.J., Robinson, H.L., and Webster, R.G. (1995). Antibody-forming cell response to virus challenge in mice immunized with DNA encoding the influenza virus hemagglutinin. *J. Virol.* 69, 7712–7717.

Kang, S.M., and Compans, R.W. (2003). Enhancement of immunization with virus-like particles of simian immunodeficiency virus. *J. Virol.* 77, 3615–3623.

Kay, R.A., and Ferguson, A. (1989a). The immunological consequences of feeding cholera toxin. I. Feeding cholera toxin suppresses the induction of systemic delayed-type hypersensitivity but not humoral immunity. *Immunology* 66, 410–415.

Kay, R.A., and Ferguson, A. (1989b). The immunological consequences of feeding cholera toxin. II. Mechanisms responsible for the induction of oral tolerance for DTH. *Immunology* 66, 416–421.

Kensil, C.R., Patel, U., Lennick, M., and Marciani, D. (1991). Separation and characterization of saponins with adjuvant activity from *Quillaja saponaria Molina* cortex. *J. Immunol.* 146, 431–437.

Keren, D.F., McDonald, R.A., and Carey, J.L. (1988). Combined parenteral and oral immunization results in an enhanced mucosal immunoglobulin A response to *Shigella flexneri*. *Infect. Immun.* 56, 910–915.

Khoury, S.J., Lider, O., Al-Sabbagh, A., and Weiner, H.L. (1990). Suppression of experimental autoimmune encephalomyelitis by oral administration of myelin basic protein. III. Synergistic effect of lipopolysaccharide. *Cell. Immunol.* 131, 302–310.

Klimpel, G.R., Asuncion, M., Haithcoat, J., and Niesel, D.W. (1995). Cholera toxin and *Salmonella typhimurium* induce different cytokine profiles in the gastrointestinal tract. *Infect. Immun.* 63, 1134–1137.

Klinman, D.M., Yi, A.K., Beaucage, S.L., Conover, J., and Krieg, A.M. (1996). CpG motifs present in bacteria DNA rapidly induce lymphocytes to secrete interleukin 6, interleukin 12, and interferon-α. *Proc. Natl. Acad. Sci. USA* 93, 2879–2883.

Kuper, C.F., Koornstra, P.J., Hameleers, D.M., Biewenga, J., Spit, B.J., Duijvestijn, A.M., van Breda Vriesman, P.J.C., and Sminia, T. (1992). The role of nasopharyngeal lymphoid tissue. *Immunol. Today* 13, 219–224.

Kuznecov, A.W., Cohen, N., and Moynihan, J. (1992). Adjuvant effects of freely ingested cholera toxin on systemic antibody and DTH responses to protein antigen. *Reg. Immunol.* 4, 153–161.

Kweon, M.N., Yamamoto, M., Watanabe, F., Tamura, S., Van Ginkel, F. W., Miyauchi, A., Takagi, H., Takeda, Y., Hamabata, T., Fujihashi, K., McGhee, J. R., and Kiyono, H. (2002). A nontoxic chimeric enterotoxin adjuvant induces protective immunity in both mucosal and systemic compartments with reduced IgE antibodies. *J. Infect. Dis.* 186, 1261–1269.

Lebman, D.A., Fuhrman, J.A., and Cebra, J.J. (1988). Intraduodenal application of cholera holotoxin increases the potential of clones from Peyer's patch B cells of relevant and unrelated specificities to secrete IgG and IgA. *Reg. Immunol.* 1, 32–40.

Lee, A., and Chen, M. (1994). Successful immunization against gastric infection with *Helicobacter* species: use of a cholera toxin B-subunit-whole-cell vaccine. *Infect. Immun.* 62, 3594–3597.

Lencer, W.I., de Almeida, J.B., Moe, S., Stow, J.L., Ausiello, D.A., and Madara, J.L. (1993). Entry of cholera toxin into polarized human intestinal epithelial cells: Identification of an early brefeldin A sensitive event required for A1-peptide generation. *J. Clin. Invest.* 92, 2941–2951.

Levine, M.M., Kaper, J.B., Black, R.E., and Clements, M.L. (1983). New knowledge on pathogenesis of bacterial enteric infections as applied to vaccine development. *Microbiol. Rev.* 47, 510–550.

Lewis, D.J., Castello, B.L.R., Novotny, P., Dougan, G., Poulton, T.A., and Griffin, G.E. (1993). Circulating cellular immune response to oral immunization of humans with cholera toxin B-subunit. *Vaccine* 11, 119–121.

Liang, X., Lamm, M.E., and Nedrud, J.G. (1989a). Cholera toxin as a mucosal adjuvant: Glutaraldehyde treatment dissociates adjuvanticity from toxicity. *J. Immunol.* 143, 484–490.

Liang, X.P., Lamm, M.E., and Nedrud, J.G. (1989b). Cholera toxin as a mucosal adjuvant for respiratory antibody responses in mice. *Reg. Immunol.* 2, 244–248.

Lovgren, K. (1988). The serum antibody response distributed in subclasses and isotypes after intranasal and subcutaneous immunization with influenza virus immunostimulating complexes. *Scand. J. Immunol.* 27, 241–245.

Lowell, G.H., Ballou, W.R., Smith, L.F., Wirtz, R.A., Zollinger, W.D., and Hockmeyer, W.T. (1988). Proteosome-lipopeptide vaccines: enhancement of immunogenicity for malaria. CS peptides. *Science* 240, 800–803.

Lowell, G.H., Kaminski, R.W., Grate, S., Hunt, R.E., Charney, C., Zimmer, S., and Colleton, C. (1996). Intranasal and intramuscular proteasome-staphylococcal enterotoxin B (SEB) toxoid vaccines: Immunogenicity and efficacy against lethal SEB intoxication in mice. *Infect. Immun.* 64, 1706–1713.

Lu, X., Clements, J.D., and Katz, J.M. (2002). Mutant *Escherichia coli*-heat-labile enterotoxin [LT(R192G)] enhances protective humoral and cellular immune responses to orally administered inactivated influenza vaccine. *Vaccine* 20, 7–8.

Lycke, N., Bromander, A.K., Ekman, L., Karlsson, U., and Holmgren, J. (1989). Cellular basis of immunomodulation by cholera toxin *in vitro* with possible association to the adjuvant function *in vivo*. *J. Immunol.* 142, 20–27.

Lycke, N., Hellstrom, U., and Holmgren, J. (1987). Circulating cholera antitoxin memory cells in the blood one year after oral cholera vaccination in humans. *Scand. J. Immunol.* 26, 207–211.

Lycke, N., and Holmgren, J. (1986a). Intestinal mucosal memory and presence of memory cells in lamina propria and Peyer's patches in mice 2 years after oral immunization with cholera toxin. *Scand. J. Immunol.* 23, 611–616.

Lycke, N., and Holmgren, J. (1986b). Strong adjuvant properties of cholera toxin on gut mucosal immune responses to orally presented antigens. *Immunology* 59, 301–308.

Lycke, N., and Holmgren, J. (1987). Long-term cholera antitoxin memory in the gut can be triggered to antibody formation associated with protection within hours of an oral challenge immunization. *Scand. J. Immunol.* 25, 407–407.

Lycke, N., Karlsson, U., Sjolander, A., and Magnusson, K.E. (1991). The adjuvant action of cholera toxin is associated with an increased intestinal permeability for luminal antigens. *Scand. J. Immunol.* 33, 691–698.

Lycke, N., Severinson, E., and Strober, W. (1990). Cholera toxin acts synergistically with IL-4 to promote IgG_1 switch differentiation. *J. Immunol.* 145, 3316–3316.

Lycke, N., and Strober, W. (1989). Cholera toxin promotes B cell isotype differentiation. *J. Immunol.* 142, 3781–3787.

Lycke, N., Tsuji, T., and Holmgren, J. (1992). The adjuvant effect of *Vibrio cholerae* and *Escherichia coli* heat-labile enterotoxins is linked to their ADP-ribosyltransferase activity. *Eur. J. Immunol.* 22, 2277–2281.

Lycke, N.Y. (1993). Cholera toxin promotes B cell isotype switching by two different mechanisms: cAMP induction augments germ-line Ig H-chain RNA transcripts whereas membrane ganglioside GM1-receptor binding enhances later events in differentiation. *J. Immunol.* 150, 4810–4821.

Lycke, N. (2001). The B-cell targeted CTA1-DD vaccine adjuvant is highly effective at enhancing antibody as well as CTL responses. (2001). *Curr. Opin. Mol. Ther.* 3, 37–44.

Malley, R., Lipsitch, M., Stack, A., Saladino, R., Fleisher, G., Pelton, S., Thompson, C., Briles, D., and Anderson, P. (2001). Intranasal immunization with killed unencapsulated whole cells prevents colonization and invasive disease by capsulated pneumococci. *Infect. Immun.* 69, 4870–4873.

Marinaro, M., Boyaka, P.N., Jackson, R.J., Finkelman, F.D., Kiyono, H., and McGhee, J.R. (1996). Interleukin-12 alters helper T-cell subsets and antibody profiles induced by the mucosal adjuvant cholera toxin. *Ann. N.Y. Acad. Sci.* 795, 361–365.

Marinaro, M., Boyaka, P.N., Jackson, R.J., Finkelman, F.D., Kiyono, H., Jirillo, E., and McGhee, J.R. (1999). Use of intranasal IL-12 to target predominantly Th1 responses to nasal and Th2 responses to oral vaccines given with cholera toxin. *J. Immunol.* 162, 114–121.

Matousek, M.P., Nedrud, J.G., and Harding, C.V. (1996). Distinct effects of recombinant cholera toxin B subunit and holotoxin on different stages of class II MHC antigen processing and presentation by macrophages. *J. Immunol.* 156, 4137–4145.

Mayer, L., Eisenhardt, D., and Shlien, R. (1988). Selective induction of antigen nonspecific suppressor cells with normal gut epithelium as accessory cells. *Monogr. Allergy* 24, 78–80.

McCluskie, M.J., Weeratna, R.d., Payette, P.J., and Davis, H.L. (2002). Parenteral and mucosal prime-boost immunization strategies in mice with hepatitis B surface antigen and CpG DNA. *FEMS Immunol. Med. Microbiol.* 32, 179–185.

McGee, D.W., Beagley, K.W., Aicher, W.K., and McGhee, J.R. (1993a). Transforming growth factor-β and IL-1β act in synergy to enhance IL-6 secretion by the intestinal epithelial cell line, IEC-6. *J. Immunol.* 151, 970–978.

McGee, D.W., Elson, C.O., and McGhee, J.R. (1993b). Enhancing effect of cholera toxin on interleukin-6 secretion by IEC-6 intestinal epithelial cells: Mode of action and augmenting effect of inflammatory cytokines. *Infect. Immun.* 61, 4637–4644.

McKenzie, S.J., and Halsey, J.F. (1984). Cholera toxin B subunit as a carrier protein to stimulate a mucosal immune response. *J. Immunol.* 133, 1818–1824.

Merritt, E.A., Sarfaty, S., van den Akker, F., L'Hoir, C., Martial, J.A., and Hol, W.G. (1994a). Crystal structure of cholera toxin B-pentamer bound to receptor GM1 pentasaccharide. *Protein Sci.* 3, 166–175.

Merritt, E.A., Sixma, T.K., Kalk, K.H., Van Zanten, B.A.M., and Hol, W.G.J. (1994b). Galactose binding site in *E. coli* heat-labile enterotoxin (LT) and cholera toxin (CT). *Mol. Microbiol.* 13, 745–753.

Michalek, S.M., McGhee, J.R., Kiyono, H., Colwell, D.E., Eldridge, J.H., Wannemuehler, M.J., and Koopman, W.J. (1983). The IgA response: Inductive aspects, regulatory cells, and effector functions. *Ann. N.Y. Acad. Sci.* 409, 48–69.

Michel, F.B., Dussourd, D.H.L., Bousquet, J., Pinel, A.M., and Normier, G. (1978). Immuno-stimulation by a ribosomal vaccine associated with a bacterial cell wall adjuvant in humans. *Infect. Immun.* 20, 760–769.

Michetti, P., Kreiss, C., Kotloff, K., Porta, N., Blanco, J.L., Bachmann, D., Saldinger, P.F., Corthesy-Theulaz, I., Losonsky, G., and Nichols, R. Herranz, M., et al. (1999). Oral immunization with urease and *Escherichia coli* heat-labile endotoxin is safe and immunogenic in *Helicobacter pylori*-infected adults. *Gastroenterology* 116, 804–812.

Mitchell, G.F., and Munoz, J.J. (1983). Vaccination of genetically susceptible mice against chronic infection with *Nematospiroides dubius* using pertussigen as adjuvant. *Aust. J. Exp. Biol. Med. Sci.* 61, 425–434.

Mizoguchi, K., Nakashima, I., Hasegawa, Y., Isobe, K., Nagase, F., Kawashima, K., Shimokata, K., and Kato, N. (1986). Augmentation of antibody responses of mice to inhaled protein antigens by simultaneously inhaled bacterial lipopolysaccharides. *Immunobiology* 173, 63–71.

Morasaki, I., Michalek, S.M., Harmon, C.C., Torii, M., Hamada, S., and McGhee, J.R. (1983). Effective immunity to dental caries: Enhancement of salivary anti-*Streptococcus mutans* antibody responses with oral adjuvants. *Infect. Immun.* 40, 577–591.

Morein, B. (1987). Potentiation of the immune response by immunization with antigens in defined multimeric physical forms. *Vet. Immunol. Immunopathol.* 17, 153–159.

Morein, B., Fossum, C., Lovgren, K., and Hoglund, S. (1990). The ISCOM—A modern approach to vaccines. *Virology* 1, 49–55.

Mosmann, T.R., and Coffman, R.L. (1989). Th1 and Th2 cells: Different patterns of lymphokine secretion lead to different functional properties. *Annu. Rev. Immunol.* 7, 145–147.

Mowat, A.M., Donachie, A.M., Reid, G., and Jarrett, O. (1991). Immune-stimulating complexes containing Quil A and protein antigen prime class I MHC-restricted T lymphocytes in vivo and are immunogenic by the oral route. *Immunology* 72, 317–322.

Mowat, A.M., Thomas, M.J., MacKenzie, S., and Parrott, D.M. (1986). Divergent effects of bacterial lipopolysaccharide on immunity to orally administered protein and particulate antigens in mice. *Immunology* 58, 677–683.

Mowat, A.M., Donachie, A.M., Jagewall, S., Schon, K., Lowenadler, B., Dalsgaard, K., Kaastrup, P., and Lycke, N. (2001). CTA1-DD-immune stimulating complexes: a novel, rationally designed, combined mucosal vaccine adjuvant effective with nanogram doses of antigen. *J. Immunol.* 167, 3398–3405.

Muller, C.P., Beauverger, P., Schneider, F., Jung, G., and Brons, N.H. (1995). Cholera toxin B stimulates systemic neutralizing antibodies after intranasal coimmunization with measles virus. *J. Gen. Virol.* 76, 1371–1380.

Murray, M., Robinson, P.B., Grierson, C., and Crawford, R.A. (1979). Immunization against *Nippostrongylus brasiliensis* in the rat: A study on the use of antigen extracted from adult parasites and the parameters which influence the level of protection. *Acta Trop.* 36, 297–322.

Murray, P.D., McKenzie, D.T., Swain, S.L., and Kagnoff, M.F. (1987). Interleukin 5 and interleukin 4 produced by Peyer's patch T cells selectively enhance immunoglobulin A expression. *J. Immunol.* 139, 2669–2674.

Nagy, B., Hoglund, S., and Morein, B. (1990). ISCOM (immunostimulating complex) vaccines containing mono- or polyvalent pili of enterotoxigenic *E. coli*: Immune response of rabbit and swine. *Zentralbl. Veterinarmed. [B]* 37, 728–738.

Nashar, T.O., and Hirst, T.R. (1995). Immunoregulatory role of H-2 and intra-H-2 alleles on antibody responses to recombinant preparations of B-subunits of *Escherichia coli* heat-labile enterotoxin (rEtxB) and cholera toxin (rCtxB). *Vaccine* 13, 803–810.

Nedrud, J.G., and Sigmund, N. (1991). Cholera toxin as a mucosal adjuvant. III. Antibody responses to nontarget dietary antigens are not increased. *Reg. Immunol.* 3, 217–222.

Nedrud, J.G., Liang, X.P., Hague, N., and Lamm, M.E. (1987). Combined oral/nasal immunization protects mice from Sendai virus infection. *J. Immunol.* 139, 3484–3492.

Ogawa, T., Kotani, S., and Shimauchi, H. (1986). Enhancement of serum antibody production in mice by oral administration of lipophilic derivatives of muramyl peptides and bacterial lipopolysaccharides with bovine serum albumin. *Methods Find. Exp. Clin. Pharmacol.* 8, 19–26.

Ohta, M., Nakashima, I., and Kato, N. (1982). Adjuvant action of bacterial lipopolysaccharide in induction of delayed-type hypersensitivity to protein antigens. II. Relationships of intensity of the action to that of other immunological activities. *Immunobiology* 163, 460–466.

Oien, N.L., Brideau, R.J., Walsh, E.E., and Wathen, M.W. (1994). Induction of local and systemic immunity against human respiratory syncytial virus using a chimeric FG glycoprotein and cholera toxin B subunit. *Vaccine* 12, 731–735.

Okahashi, N., Yamamoto, M., Vancott, J.L., Chatfield, S.N., Roberts, M., Bluethmann, H., Hiroi, T., Kiyono, H., and McGhee, J.R. (1996). Oral immunization of interleukin-4 (IL-4) knockout mice with a recombinant *Salmonella* strain or cholera toxin reveals that CD4+ Th2 cells producing IL-6 and IL-10 are associated with mucosal immunoglobulin A responses. *Infect. Immun.* 64, 1516–1525.

Okutomi, T., Inagawa, H., Nishizawa, T., Oshima, H., Soma, G., and Mizuno, D. (1990). Priming effect of orally administered muramyl dipeptide on induction of exogenous tumor necrosis factor. *J. Biol. Resp. Med.* 9, 564–569.

O'Neal, C.M., Clements, J.D., Estes, M.K., and Conner, M.E. (1998). Rotavirus 2/6 virus-like particles administered intranasally with cholera toxin, *Escherichia coli* heat-labile toxin (LT), and LT-R192G induce protection from rotavirus challenge. *J. Virol.* 72, 3390–3393.

Orr, N., Arnon, R., Rubin, G., Cohen, D., Bercovier, H., and Lowell, G.H. (1994). Enhancement of anti-*Shigella* lipopolysaccharide (LPS) response by addition of the cholera toxin B subunit to oral and intranasal proteosome-*Shigella flexneri* 2a LPS vaccines. *Infect. Immun.* 62, 5198–5200.

Parant, M., Parant, F., and Chedid, L. (1978). Enhancement of the neonate's nonspecific immunity to *Klebsiella* infection by muramyl dipeptide, a synthetic immunoadjuvant. *Proc. Natl. Acad. Sci. USA* 75, 3395–3399.

Park, E.J., Chang, J.H., Kim, J.S., and Chung, S.I. (2000). The mucosal adjuvanticity of two nontoxic mutants of *Escherichia coli* heat-labile enterotoxin varies with immunization routes. *Exp. Mol. Med.* 32, 72–78.

Periwal, S.B., Kourie, K.R., Ramachandaran, N., Blakeney, S.J., DeBruin, S., Zhu, D., Zamb, T.J., Smith, L., Udem, S., Eldridge, J.H., Shroff, K.E., and Reilly, P.A. (2003). A modified cholera holotoxin CT-E29H enhances systemic and mucosal immune responses to recombinant Norwalk virus-virus like particle vaccine. *Vaccine* 21, 376–385.

Pierce, N.F., and Cray, W.C. (1982). Determinants of the localization, magnitude, and duration of a specific mucosal IgA plasma cell response in enterically immunized rats. *J. Immunol.* 128, 1311–1315.

Pierce, N.F., and Gowans, J.L. (1975). Cellular kinetics of the intestinal immune response to cholera toxoid in rats. *J. Exp. Med.* 142, 1550–1563.

Porgador, A., Staats, H.F., Itoh, Y., and Kelsall, B.L. (1998). Intranasal immunization with cytotoxic T-lymphocyte epitope peptide and mucosal adjuvant cholera toxin: selective augmentation of peptide-presenting dendritic cells in nasal mucosa-associated lymphoid tissue. *Infect. Immun.* 66, 5876–5881.

Quiding, M., Nordstrom, I., Kilander, A., Andersson, G., Hanson, L.A., Holmgren, J., and Czerkinsky, C. (1991). Intestinal immune responses in humans: Oral cholera vaccination induces strong intestinal antibody responses and interferon-γ production and evokes local immunological memory. *J. Clin. Invest.* 88, 143–148.

Ramsay, A.J., Husband, A.J., Ramshaw, I.A., Bao, S., Matthaei, K.I., Koehler, G., and Kopf, M. (1994). The role of interleukin-6 in mucosal IgA antibody responses in vivo. *Science* 264, 561–563.

Rehmani, S.F., and Spradbrow, P.B. (1995). The influence of adjuvants on oral vaccination of chickens against Newcastle disease. *Vet. Microbiol.* 46, 63–68.

Rescigno, M., Urbano, M., Valzasina, B., Francolini, M., Rotta, G., Bonasio, R., Granucci, F., Kraehenbuhl, J.P., and Ricciardi-Castagnoli, P. (2001). Dendritic cells express tight junction proteins and penetrate gut epithelial monolayers to sample bacteria. *Nat. Immunol.* 2, 361–367.

Reuman, P.D., Keely, S.P., and Schiff, G.M. (1991). Similar subclass antibody responses after intranasal immunization with UV-inactivated RSV mixed with cholera toxin or live RSV. *J. Med. Virol.* 35, 192–197.

Robert, D., Quillon, J.P., Ivanoff, B., Beaudry, Y., Fontanges, R., Normier, G., Pinel, A.M., and D'Hinterland, L.D. (1979). Role of interferon in mice in protection against influenza A virus by bacterial ribosomes together with membranal glycoproteins of *Klebsiella pneumoniae* as adjuvant. *Infect. Immun.* 26, 515–519.

Roberts, M., Bacon, A., Rappuoli, R., Pizza, M., Cropley, I., Douce, G., Dougan, G., Marinaro, M., McGhee, J., and Chatfield, S. (1995). A mutant pertussis toxin molecule that lacks ADP-ribosyltransferase activity, PT-9K/129G, is an effective mucosal adjuvant for intranasally delivered proteins. *Infect. Immun.* 63, 2100–2108.

Russell, M.W., Moldoveanu, Z., White, P.L., Sibert, G.J., Mestecky, J., and Michalek, S.M. (1996). Salivary, nasal, genital, and systemic antibody responses in monkeys immunized intranasally with a bacterial protein antigen and the cholera toxin B subunit. *Infect. Immun.* 64, 1272–1283.

Sanchez, J., Svennerholm, A.M., and Holmgren, J. (1988). Genetic fusion of a nontoxic heat-stable enterotoxin-related decapeptide antigen to cholera toxin B-subunit. *FEBS Lett.* 241, 110–114.

Sato, Y., Roman, M., Tighe, H., Lee, D., Corr, M., Nguyen, M., Silverman, G.J., Lotz, M., Carson, D.A., and Raz, E. (1996). Immunostimulatory DNA sequences necessary for effective intradermal gene immunization. *Science* 273, 352–354.

Shreedhar, V.K., Kelsall, B.L., and Neutra, M.R. (2003). Cholera toxin induces migration of dendritic cells from the subepithelial dome region to T- and B-cell areas of Peyer's patches. *Infect. Immun.* 71, 504–509.

Simmons, C.P., Mastroeni, P., Fowler, R., Ghaem-maghami, M., Lycke, N., Pizza, M., Rappuoli, R., and Dougan, G. (1999). MHC class I-restricted cytotoxic lymphocyte responses induced by enterotoxin-based mucosal adjuvants. *J. Immunol.* 163, 6502–6510.

Sixma, T.K., Pronk, S.E., Kalk, K.H., Wartna, E.S., van Zanten, B.A.M., Witholt, B., and Hol, W.G. (1991). Crystal structure of a cholera toxin-related heat-labile enterotoxin from *E. coli*. *Nature* 351, 371–377.

Snapper, C.M., and Paul, W.E. (1987). Interferon-γ and B cell stimulatory factor-1 reciprocally regulate Ig isotype production. *Science* 236, 944–947.

Snider, D.P., Marshall, J.S., Perdue, M.H., and Liang, H. (1994). Production of IgE antibody and allergic sensitization of intestinal and peripheral tissues after oral immunization with protein Ag and cholera toxin. *J. Immunol.* 153, 647–657.

Spriggs, D.R., and Koff, W.C., Ed. (1991). *Topics in Vaccine Adjuvant Research*. Boca Raton, FL: CRC Press.

Suckow, M.A., Keren, D.F., Brown, J.E., and Keusch, G.T. (1994). Stimulation of gastrointestinal antibody to Shiga toxin by orogastric immunization in mice. *Immunol. Cell. Biol.* 72, 69–74.

Sun, J.B., Holmgren, J., and Czerkinsky, C. (1994). Cholera toxin B subunit: an efficient transmucosal carrier-delivery system for induction of peripheral immunological tolerance, *Proc. Natl. Acad. Sci. USA* 91, 10795–10799.

Sun, J.B., Rask, C., Olsson, T., Holmgren, J., and Czerkinsky, C. (1996). Treatment of experimental autoimmune encephalomyelitis by feeding myelin basic protein conjugated to cholera toxin B subunit. *Proc. Natl. Acad. Sci. USA* 93, 7196–7201.

Svennerholm, A.M., Jertborn, M., Gothefors, L., Karim, A.M.M.M., Sack, D.A., and Holmgren, J. (1984). Mucosal antitoxic and antibacterial immunity after cholera disease and after immunization with a combined B subunit-whole cell vaccine. *J. Infect. Dis.* 149, 884–893.

Takada, H., and Kotani, S. (1989). Structural requirements of lipid A for endotoxicity and other biological activities. *Crit. Rev. Microbiol.* 16, 477–523.

Takahashi, H., Takeshita, T., Morein, B., Putney, S., Germain, R. N., and Berzofsky, J. A. (1990a). Induction of CD8+ cytotoxic T cells by immunization with purified HIV-1 envelope protein in ISCOMs. *Nature* 344, 873–875.

Takahashi, I., Marinaro, M., Kiyono, H., Jackson, R. J., Nakagawa, I., Fujihashi, K., Hamada, S., Clements, J. D., Bost, K. L., and McGhee, J. R. (1996). Mechanisms for mucosal immunogenicity and adjuvanticity of *Escherichia coli* labile enterotoxin. *J. Infect. Dis.* 173, 627–635.

Takahashi, I., Okahashi, N., Kanamoto, T., Asakawa, H., and Koga, T. (1990b). Intranasal immunization of mice with recombinant protein antigen of serotype c *Streptococcus mutans* and cholera toxin B subunit. *Arch. Oral. Biol.* 35, 475–477.

Takayama, K., Ribi, E., and Cantrell, J. L. (1981). Isolation of a nontoxic lipid A fraction containing tumor regression activity. *Cancer Res.* 41, 2654–2660.

Tamura, S., Funato, H., Hirabayashi, Y., Suzuki, Y., Nagamine, T., Aizawa, C., and Kurata, T. (1991). Cross-protection against influenza A virus infection by passively transferred respiratory tract IgA antibodies to different hemagglutinin molecules. *Eur. J. Immunol.* 21, 1337–1344.

Tamura, S., Funato, H., Nagamine, T., Aizawa, C., and Kurata, T. (1989). Effectiveness of cholera toxin B subunit as an adjuvant for nasal influenza vaccination despite pre-existing immunity to CTB. *Vaccine* 7, 503–505.

Tamura, S., Ishihara, K., Miyata, K., Aizawa, C., and Kurata, T. (1995). Mechanism of enhancement of the immune responses to influenza vaccine with cholera toxin B subunit and a trace amount of holotoxin. *Vaccine* 13, 339–341.

Tamura, S., Miyata, K., Matsuo, K., Asanuma, H., Takahashi, H., Nakajima, K., Suzuki, Y., Aizawa, C., and Kurata, T. (1996). Acceleration of influenza virus clearance by Th1 cells in the nasal site of mice immunized intranasally with adjuvant-combined recombinant nucleoprotein. *J. Immunol.* 156, 3892–3900.

Tamura, S., Samegai, Y., Kurata, H., Nagamine, T., Aizawa, C., and Kurata, T. (1988). Protection against influenza virus infection by vaccine inoculated intranasally with cholera toxin B subunit. *Vaccine* 6, 409–413.

Tamura, S., Shoji, Y., Hasiguchi, K., Aizawa, C., and Kurata, T. (1994a). Effects of cholera toxin adjuvant on IgE antibody response to orally or nasally administered ovalbumin. *Vaccine* 12, 1238–1240.

Tamura, S., Yamanaka, A., Shimohara, M., Tomita, T., Komase, K., Tsuda, Y., Suzuki, Y., Nagamine, T., Kawahara, K., and Danbara, H. (1994b). Synergistic action of cholera toxin B subunit (and *Escherichia coli* heat-labile toxin B subunit) and a trace amount of cholera whole toxin as an adjuvant for nasal influenza vaccine. *Vaccine* 12, 419–426.

Tamura, S.I., Tanaka, H., Takayama, R., Sato, H., Sato, Y., and Uchida, N. (1985). Break of unresponsiveness of delayed-type hypersensitivity to sheep red blood cells by pertussis toxin. *Cell. Immunol.* 92, 376–382.

Thapar, M.A., Parr, E.L., Bozzola, J.J., and Parr, M.B. (1991). Secretory immune responses in the mouse vagina after parenteral or intravaginal immunization with an immunostimulating complex (ISCOM). *Vaccine* 9, 129–133.

Thapar, M.A., Parr, E.L., and Parr, M.B. (1990). The effect of adjuvants on antibody titers in mouse vaginal fluid after intravaginal immunization. *J. Reprod. Immunol.* 17, 207.

Thomas, W.D., Zhang, Z., Lei, W., Torres, J.F., and Monath, T.P. (1995). New mucosal adjuvants for *Helicobacter pylori* vaccines. *Clin. Immunol. Immunopathol.* 76, S94.

Tokunaga, T., Yamamoto, H., Shimada, S., Abe, H., Fukuda, T., Fujisawa, Y., Furutani, Y., Yano, O., Kataoka, T., and Sudo, T. (1984). Antitumor activity of deoxyribonucleic acid fraction from *Mycobacterium bovis* BCG. I. Isolation, physicochemical characterization, and antitumor activity. *J. Natl. Cancer Inst.* 72, 955–962.

Tomasi, M., Dertzbaugh, M., Hunter, H., and Elson, C. (1994). Use of multiple emulsions containing cholera toxin (CT) for mucosal immunization. *FASEB J.* 8, A283.

Tomasi, M., Dertzbaugh, M.T., Hearn, T.I., Hunter, R.L., and Elson, C.O. (1997). Strong mucosal adjuvanticity of cholera toxin within lipid particles of a new multiple emulsion delivery system for oral immunization. *Eur. J. Immunol.* 27, 2720–2725.

Ulrich, J.T., Cantrell, J.L., Gustafson, G.L., K.R., M., Rudbach, J.A., and Hiernaux, J.R. (1991). The adjuvant activity of monophosphoryl lipid A. In *Topics in Vaccine Adjuvant Research*. Boca Raton, FL: CRC Press, 133–143.

Vajdy, M.m and Lycke, N. (1993). Stimulation of antigen-specific T- and B-cell memory in local as well as systemic lymphoid tissues following oral immunization with cholera toxin adjuvant. *Immunology* 80, 197–203.

Vajdy, M., Kosco-Vilbois, M.H., Kopf, M., Kohler, G., and Lycke, N. (1995). Impaired mucosal immune responses in interleukin 4-targeted mice. *J. Exp. Med.* 181, 41–53.

Van der Heijden, P.J., Bianchi, A.T., Dol, M., Pals, J.W., Stok, W., and Bokhout, B.A. (1991). Manipulation of intestinal immune responses against ovalbumin by cholera toxin and its B subunit in mice. *Immunology* 72, 89–93.

van Ginkel, F.W., Jackson, R.J., Yuki, Y., and McGhee, J.W. (2000). Cutting edge: the mucosal adjuvant cholera toxin redirects vaccine proteins into olfactory tissues. *J. Immunol.* 165, 4778–4782.

van Heyningen, S. (1991). The ring on a finger. *Nature* 351, 351.

Verheul, A.F.M., Versteeg, A., DeReuver, M.J., Jansze, M., and Snippe, H. (1989). Modulation of the immune response to pneumococcal type 14 capsular polysaccharide-protein conjugates by the adjuvant Quil A depends on the properties of the conjugates. *Infect. Immun.* 57, 1078–1083.

Waksman, B.H. (1979). Adjuvants and immune regulation by lymphoid cells. *Springer Sem. Immunopathol.* 2, 5–33.

Walsh, E.E. (1993). Mucosal immunization with a subunit respiratory syncytial virus vaccine in mice. *Vaccine* 11, 1135–1138.

Warren, H.S., Vogel, F.R., and Chedid, L.A. (1986). Current status of immunological adjuvants. *Annu. Rev. Immunol.* 4, 369–388.

Weiner, H.L., Friedman, A., Miller, A., Khoury, S.J., al-Sabbagh, A., Santos, L., Sayegh, M., Nussenblatt, R.B., Trentham, D.E., and Hafler, D.A. (1994). Oral tolerance: Immunologic mechanisms and treatment of animal and human organ-specific autoimmune diseases by oral administration of autoantigens. *Annu. Rev. Immunol.* 12, 809–837.

Williamson, E., Westrich, G.M., and Viney, J.L. (1999). Modulating dendritic cells to optimize mucosal immunization protocols. *J. Immunol.* 163, 3668–3675.

Wilson, A.D., Bailey, M., Williams, N.A., and Stokes, C.R. (1991). The in vitro production of cytokines by mucosal lymphocytes immunized by oral administration of keyhole limpet hemocyanin using cholera toxin as an adjuvant. *Eur. J. Immunol.* 21, 2333–2339.

Wilson, A.D., Clarke, C.J., and Stokes, C.R. (1990). Whole cholera toxin and B subunit act synergistically as an adjuvant for the mucosal immune response of mice to keyhole limpet haemocyanin. *Scand. J. Immunol.* 31, 443–451.

Woogen, S.D., Ealding, W., and Elson, C.O. (1987). Inhibition of murine lymphocyte proliferation by the B subunit of cholera toxin. *J. Immunol.* 139, 3764–3770.

Woogen, S.D., Turo, K., Dieleman, L.A., Beagley, K.W., and Elson, C.O. (1993). Inhibition of murine T cell activation by cholera toxin B subunit is not mediated through the phosphatidylinositol second messenger system. *J. Immunol.* 150, 3274–3283.

Wu, H.Y., and Russell, M.W. (1993). Induction of mucosal immunity by intranasal application of a streptococcal surface protein antigen with the cholera toxin B subunit. *Infect. Immun.* 61, 314–322.

Wu, H.Y., and Russell, M.W. (1994). Comparison of systemic and mucosal priming for mucosal immune responses to a bacterial protein antigen given with or coupled to cholera toxin (CT) B subunit, and effects of pre-existing anti-CT immunity. *Vaccine* 12, 215–222.

Xu-Amano, J., Jackson, R.J., Staats, H.F., Fujihashi, K., Kiyono, H., Burrows, P.D., Elson, C.O., Pillai, S., and McGhee, J.R. (1993). Helper T cell subsets for IgA responses: Oral immunization with tetanus toxoid and cholera toxin as adjuvant selectively induces Th2 cells in mucosa-associated tissues. *J. Exp. Med.* 178, 1309–1320.

Yamamoto, S., Yamamoto, T., Shimada, S., Kuramoto, E., Yano, O., Kataoka, T., and Tokunaga, T. (1992). DNA from bacteria, but not from vertebrates, induces interferons, activates natural killer cells and inhibits tumor growth. *Microbiol. Immunol.* 36, 983–997.

Yamamoto, M., McGhee, J.R., Hagiwara, Y., Otake, S., and Kiyono, H. (2001). Genetically manipulated bacterial toxin as a new generation mucosal adjuvant. *Scand. J. Immunol.* 53, 211–217.

Zhang, T., Li, E., and Stanley, S.L., Jr. (1995). Oral immunization with the dodecapeptide repeat of the serine-rich *Entamoeba histolytica* protein (SREHP) fused to the cholera toxin B subunit induces a mucosal and systemic anti-SREHP antibody response. *Infect. Immun.* 63, 1349–1355.

Zigterman, G.J., Snippe, H., Jansze, M., and Willers, J.M. (1987). Adjuvant effects of nonionic block polymer surfactants on liposome-induced humoral immune response. *J. Immunol.* 138, 220–225.

Antigen Delivery Systems I: Nonliving Microparticles, Liposomes, and Immune Stimulating Complexes (ISCOMs)

Suzanne M. Michalek

Department of Microbiology, University of Alabama at Birmingham, Birmingham, Alabama

Derek T. O'Hagan

Chiron Corporation, Emeryville, California

Noel K. Childers

Department of Oral Biology, University of Alabama at Birmingham, Birmingham, Alabama

Albert D.M.E. Osterhaus

Department of Virology, Erasmus University, Rotterdam, The Netherlands

Guus F. Rimmelzwaan

Department of Virology, Erasmus University, Rotterdam, The Netherlands

In designing a vaccine, several issues that need to be considered are its safety for use in animals and humans, the convenience and cost of reproducibly generating the vaccine in large quantities, and its effectiveness in inducing the desired host response. Particulate antigens have been shown to be more effective mucosal immunogens than soluble antigens in inducing local and generalized secretory and systemic immune responses. There are several reasons for this. First, the size of macromolecular complexes may allow them to more effectively survive the mucosal environment, such as the low pH, bile salts, and proteolytic enzymes of the stomach and gastrointestinal tract. Second, at least some particulates are adsorbed through the M cells into the IgA inductive sites, such as the Peyer's patches, with greater efficiency than soluble molecules, thus providing a higher local antigen concentration within this mucosal immune inductive site. Third, particulates may act as a depot for the slow release of antigen, and fourth, the major portion of an ingested soluble protein antigen crosses the epithelial barrier of the gut in the form of amino acids and low-molecular-weight peptides, which could result in systemic tolerance.

This information and the availability of modern technology have facilitated the development of delivery systems for most antigens that render them particulate-like and that exhibit immunopotentiating activity for the induction of protective mucosal and systemic immune responses against microbial pathogens. This chapter reviews nonreplicating antigen delivery systems, including microparticles (D. O'Hagan), liposomes (S. Michalek and N. Childers), and immunostimulating complexes (ISCOMs) (A. Osterhaus and G. Rimmelzwaan), which have received considerable attention for their use in vaccine development.

MICROPARTICLES

Alternative routes of immunization

There are several alternative routes available for mucosal immunization, including oral, nasal, pulmonary, vaginal, and rectal. The most attractive route is oral because of the ease and acceptability of oral administration. However, because of the presence of the low pH in the stomach, an extensive range of digestive enzymes in the intestine, and a protective coating of mucus that limits access to the mucosal epithelium, oral immunization has proven extremely difficult, particularly with nonliving antigens. Yet novel delivery systems, including a range of microparticles, may be used to significantly enhance responses following oral immunization.

In addition, the nasal route is attractive for several reasons. The nose, like the mouth, is a practical site for easy self-administration, with use of commercially available delivery devices. In contrast, delivery of vaccines to the lower lung is much more difficult, requiring sophisticated technologies, and causes heightened concerns in relation to potential toxicity at this site, since the consequences of adverse effects are potentially life-threatening. Nevertheless, the lungs are exposed to a diverse range of noxious materials on a daily basis because of environmental contamination, and they seem to deal with such insults reasonably well.

Although the oral route is much preferred, nasal immunization generally requires much lower doses of antigen, which has important implications for many recombinant antigens that are often costly to produce. Lower doses are possible by this route mainly because nasal immunization does not expose antigens to low pH and secreted enzymes. A particularly attractive feature of nasal immunization is that this route has been shown to induce potent immune responses both in the respiratory and the genital tracts, as a consequence of the common mucosal immune system (McGhee *et al.*, 1999). In contrast to immunization of the genital tract, nasal immunization is more convenient and acceptable. In addition, it has been shown to induce more potent local and systemic responses (Gallichan and Rosenthal, 1995; Johansson *et al.*, 1998; Staats *et al.*, 1997; Wu *et al.*, 2000). Finally, compared with rectal immunization, the nasal route is more readily accessible and culturally more acceptable. Nevertheless, the optimal route of immunization for each vaccine needs to be defined by extensive studies in discriminating animal models, preferably involving challenge with the relevant or closely related pathogens.

Poly (lactide coglycolide) microparticles for vaccine delivery

In recent years, the principal polymers used for the preparation of microencapsulated vaccines have been the aliphatic polyesters, the poly (lactide coglycolide) microparticles, abbreviated as PLG. PLG are the primary candidates for the development of microencapsulated vaccines because they are biodegradable and biocompatible and have been used in humans for many years as suture material and as controlled-release drug delivery systems (Anderson and Shive, 1997). PLG polymers have also been extensively evaluated for the development of controlled-release single-dose vaccines, an area which has recently been reviewed (O'Hagan *et al.*, 1998). However, one of the limitations of PLG in relation to vaccine development is that these polymers are soluble in only a limited range of organic solvents and are insoluble in water. Hence, the most commonly used solvent for PLG is dichloromethane (DCM), although ethyl acetate and others may also be used. In addition, the methods used for the preparation of microencapsulated vaccines usually involve the emulsification of aqueous solutions of antigens into organic solvents containing the polymer and extraction or evaporation of the solvent to form microparticles. The preparation methods commonly employed for the encapsulation of vaccines into PLG polymers have been described in detail (O'Hagan, 1998). A significant problem with PLG microencapsulation is the possibility of antigen denaturation as a consequence of exposure to organic solvents, high shear, aqueous/organic interfaces, and localized elevated temperatures. Nevertheless, despite these significant problems, a number of proteins have been successfully entrapped in PLG microparticles with full maintenance of structural and immunologic integrity (O'Hagan, 1997). Moreover, some proteins have also induced neutralizing antibodies and protective immunity following microencapsulation in PLG microparticles and mucosal delivery (O'Hagan, 1998; O'Hagan *et al.*, 1998).

Despite the problems with this technology, the use of polymeric microparticles offers significant potential for the development of mucosally administered vaccines. The main advantage of microparticles is that they can be designed to protect entrapped vaccines against degradation and to target vaccines for uptake into the mucosal-associated lymphoreticular tissue (MALT). Moreover, microparticles can be prepared from a range of different polymers, including bioadhesive polymers, which can be designed to retain microparticles and associated antigens at mucosal sites.

Mucosal immunization with protein antigens in PLG microparticles

In mice, oral immunization with PLG microparticles has been shown to induce potent mucosal and systemic immunity (Challacombe *et al.*, 1992; Eldridge *et al.*, 1990; Murillo *et al.*, 2001; O'Hagan, 1994). In addition, mucosal immunization with microparticles induced protection against challenge with *Bordetella pertussis* (Cahill *et al.*, 1995; Conway *et al.*, 2001; Jones *et al.*, 1996; Shahin *et al.*, 1995), *Chlamydia trachomatis* (Whittum-Hudson *et al.*, 1996), *Yersinia pestis* (Eyles *et al.*, 2000), *Brucella ovis* (Murillo *et al.*, 2001), and *Salmonella typhimurium* (Allaoui-Attarki *et al.*, 1997). Oral or intratracheal immunization with microparticles containing entrapped simian immunodeficiency virus (SIV) induced protective immunity in systemically primed macaques against repeated intravaginal challenge with SIV (Marx *et al.*, 1993). In contrast, systemic or oral immunization alone did not provide protection, and a parenteral prime was needed prior to mucosal immunization. In a separate nonhuman primate study, intratracheal immunization following systemic priming induced optimal protection in rhesus monkeys (4/4) against aerosol challenge with staphylococcal enterotoxin B (Tseng *et al.*, 1995). Again, a systemic prime was needed to induce optimal protection, since intratracheal immunization alone (2/4) and oral immunization alone (1/4) protected only limited numbers of monkeys (Tseng *et al.*, 1995). The term *IN* (or intranasal) immunization has often been used inaccurately in the literature to describe intranasal administration of vaccines to anesthetized mice, since anesthesia results in the delivery of the bulk of the vaccine into the lung. This results in relatively easy access of the vaccine to the systemic lymphoid tissue and the induction of potent immune responses. However, this cannot accurately reflect the likely immune responses that would be induced in humans following nasal immunization, unless the vaccine is delivered efficiently to the lungs. In some studies, the term *intratracheal* immunization has been used, but this normally involves a process in which the trachea is surgically opened and the vaccine is directly introduced, under anesthesia (Malone *et al.*, 1997). Following nasal immunization of anesthetized mice, Eyles *et al.* (1999) found that if 10 µl of a vaccine formulation was applied through the nose, most of it remained in the nasal passages. However, if 50 µl was administered, almost half was found in the lung. Moreover, only the 50-µl volume resulted in immune responses in lung lavage (Eyles *et al.*, 1999). Hence, the term nasal immunization in mice should be restricted to vaccine administration in small volumes (<20 µl), preferably in the complete absence of anesthesia.

We recently compared the potency of PLG microparticles with various alternative adjuvants and delivery systems for the induction of antibody responses against gD2 from herpes simplex virus following nasal immunization (Ugozzoli *et al.*, 1998). In these studies, gD2 was administered in the water-in-oil emulsion, MF59, entrapped in PLG microparticles, associated with ISCOMs, or mixed with LTK63, a genetically detoxified mutant of heat-labile enterotoxin (LT). We demonstrated that gD2 entrapped in PLG induced the highest specific IgA titers in mucosal secretions (**Fig. 55.1**). In addition, gD2 entrapped in PLG also induced strong serum IgG titers, but LTK63 was more potent (**Fig. 55.2**). In fact, LTK63 and gD2, when given by the nasal route, induced comparable serum antibody responses to intramuscular immunization with MF59, a potent emulsion-based adjuvant (Ugozzoli *et al.*, 1998). These data show that nasal immunization with protein antigens entrapped in PLG microparticles is one of the most effective means of enhancing specific antibody responses in various mucosal secretions, while also inducing strong systemic antibody responses.

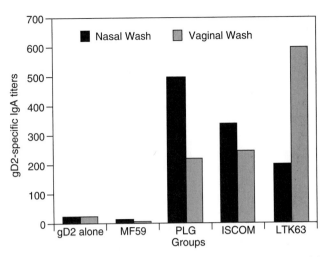

Fig. 55.1. Specific IgA responses in mucosal secretions 2 weeks following nasal immunization with 10 µg HSV gD2 in combination with MF59 emulsion, PLG microparticles, ISCOMs, or LTK63 adjuvants.

Nasal immunization in mice with microencapsulated antigens has also been shown to induce protective immunity against pathogen challenge. For example, several antigens from *B. pertussis* were entrapped in microparticles and, following nasal immunization, induced protective immunity against aerosol challenge (Cahill *et al.*, 1995; Shahin *et al.*, 1995). Optimal protection was achieved when more than one antigen was administered simultaneously (Shahin *et al.*, 1995). Nasal immunization of mice with ricin toxoid in microparticles also induced long-lasting protection against aerosol challenge with the toxin (Yan *et al.*, 1996). Furthermore, nasal immunization with protein-linked phosphorylcholine protected mice against a lethal challenge with *Streptococcus pneumoniae* (Trolle *et al.*, 2000). The nasal-associated lymphoreticular tissue (NALT), which has been well

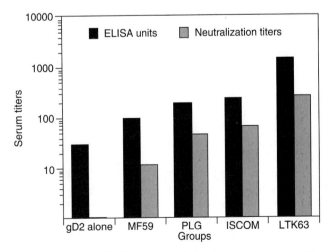

Fig. 55.2. Serum antibody responses following nasal immunization with HSV gD2 in combination with MF59 emulsion, PLG microparticles, ISCOMs, or LTK63 adjuvants. The results are presented as gD2-specific serum ELISA units and neutralization titers.

defined in mice (Kuper *et al.*, 1992), has been assumed to be the site of uptake of microparticles from the nasal cavity. However, in humans, the organized lymphoid tissue of the upper respiratory tract is represented by the tonsils and the Waldeyer's rings of the trachea (Boyaka *et al.*, 2000). Hence, although it has been claimed that the mouse is a good model to predict the likely outcome of nasal immunization in humans (Kuper *et al.*, 1992), this seems unlikely.

Although most studies on the induction of immune responses through nasal immunization have involved induction of humoral immunity, nasal immunization can also result in induction of strong cell-mediated immunity. Mora and coworkers (1998) reported that nasal immunization of anesthetized mice with a lipidated HIV-1 gp120 peptide entrapped in PLG particles induced gp120-specific cytotoxic T-lymphocyte (CTL) and antibody responses. Previously, we had reported that nasal immunization with HIV-1 gp120 entrapped in microparticles induced systemic CTL responses and mucosal antibodies in mice (Moore *et al.*, 1995). We also reported that ovalbumin entrapped in PLG microparticles induced CTL responses following oral immunization, but this approach was less potent than ISCOMs (Maloy *et al.*, 1994).

The vagina is considered to be a component of the common mucosal immune system, and oral immunization of mice with microparticles has been shown to induce a vaginal antibody response (Challacombe *et al.*, 1997). In addition, nasal immunization with microparticles also induced antibodies in the lower genital tract of mice (Ugozzoli *et al.*, 1998). However, intravaginal (IVAG) immunization protocols in small animal models have not normally met with great success, despite the use of novel delivery systems and adjuvants (O'Hagan *et al.*, 1992; O'Hagan *et al.*, 1993; Thaparr *et al.*, 1991). Moreover, the local immune response in the vagina is subject to significant hormonal regulation, with major changes in local antibodies at different stages of the menstrual cycle (Wira *et al.*, 1994). A recent study in mice showed that the nasal route of immunization was more effective than the IVAG route for the induction of immune responses in the vagina (Di Tommaso *et al.*, 1996). Consequently, the vaginal route of immunization appears unlikely to be easily exploited for the development of novel vaccines. A more successful strategy for the induction of immunity in the lower genital tract is likely to involve oral, nasal, or rectal immunization (Di Tommaso *et al.*, 1996; Haneberg *et al.*, 1994; Ugozzoli *et al.*, 1998). A recent study has confirmed that the nasal route of immunization may be exploited for the induction of genital tract antibody responses in female humans (Bergquist *et al.*, 1997). While microparticles have significant potential for mucosal delivery of vaccines, their potency may be improved by their use in combination with additional adjuvants. This is likely to be a prerequisite for the development of effective oral vaccines, since the challenges should not be underestimated. Accumulated experimental evidence suggests that simple encapsulation of vaccines into microparticles is unlikely to result in the successful development of oral vaccines, and

improvements in the current technology are clearly needed (Brayden, 2001). Nevertheless, data from small animal models suggest that microparticles may have significant potential for delivery of vaccines involving nasal immunization.

Mucosal immunization with DNA and PLG microparticles

Although vaccines normally comprise bacterial toxoids, live attenuated viruses, killed bacteria, or recombinant proteins, much attention has recently been focused on DNA vaccines. Immunization with DNA has several advantages over immunization with proteins, including the induction of potent CTL responses in nonhuman primates (Donnelly *et al.*, 1995; Donnelly *et al.*, 1997). The ruggedness and simplicity of DNA offer the potential for improved vaccine stability and reduced costs for vaccine production. Moreover, compared with attenuated viruses, plasmid DNA offers a safe alternative. Clinical trials involving intramuscular immunization with DNA vaccines have already been performed, and the approach appears to be safe and well tolerated (Roy *et al.*, 2000; Wang *et al.*, 1998). However, although DNA vaccines have proven potent in small animal models, the potency in larger primates, including humans, has been disappointing. Consequently, there is a clear need to improve the potency of DNA vaccines for human immunization.

We recently described the development of novel cationic PLG microparticles with adsorbed DNA, which were used to induce enhanced immune responses following intramuscular immunization (Singh *et al.*, 2000). Previously, the use of PLG microparticles with entrapped DNA for oral immunization was described by Jones *et al.* (1997). In a subsequent publication, the ability of orally administered microencapsulated DNA to offer protection against challenge with rotavirus was described (Chen *et al.*, 1998). Nevertheless, although PLG microparticles appear to have significant potential for delivery of DNA, the formulations previously described had significant limitations. For example, it has been reported that microencapsulation of DNA results in a significant reduction in the amount of supercoiled DNA, with only 10% to 20% of the encapsulated material retaining super-coiled structure (Ando *et al.*, 1999). Moreover, encapsulation efficiency is low, with only 20% to 50% of DNA successfully encapsulated (Ando *et al.*, 1999). To overcome these and other significant problems, we developed the novel approach of adsorbing DNA onto the surface of microparticles. Adsorption of DNA to cationic microparticles results in maintenance of super-coiled DNA and allows high efficiency of DNA association with the microparticles (Singh *et al.*, 2000).

Recently, we explored the potential of cationic PLG microparticles to induce local and systemic immunity following intranasal immunization with DNA encoding HIV-1 gag. We found that cationic PLG microparticles with adsorbed DNA induced enhanced local (**Table 55.1**) and systemic (**Fig. 55.3**) cell-mediated as well as humoral (**Fig. 55.4**) immunity against HIV-1 gag. Thus, nasal immunizations with DNA adsorbed onto cationic microparticles

Table 55.1. Induction of CMI Responses Following Nasal Immunization with DNA Vaccines

Vaccine Formulation	Cervical Lymph Nodes	Spleen
PLG-CTAB/DNA	247 + 31	480 + 74
Naked DNA	0	157 + 60

Mucosal and systemic immune responses induced by DNA encoding HIV-1 gag adsorbed onto cationic PLG microparticles compared to naked DNA was measured by an IFN-γ ELISPOT assay. The data show the number of gag-specific IFN-γ secreting cells per 10 million mononuclear cells + one SD of a minimum of three wells from pools of five mice per group.

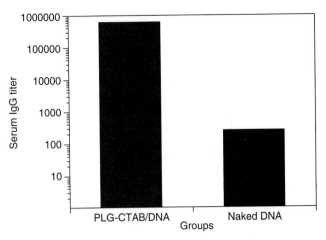

Fig. 55.4. Induction of systemic humoral immune responses following nasal immunization with DNA encoding HIV-1 gag adsorbed onto cationic PLG microparticles, as compared with naked plasmid DNA as measured by ELISA.

appeared to be a novel approach for the induction of enhanced local and systemic cell-mediated as well as humoral immune responses.

To investigate a possible mechanism for the enhanced immune responses induced following nasal immunizations with PLG/DNA, we localized and phenotypically identified the cells that expressed gag protein in local and systemic lymphoid tissues. Following a single nasal immunization with PLG-DNA expressing HIV-1 gag, we localized and identified the cells that expressed the encoded gene by immunofluorescent staining (Singh *et al.*, 2002). The majority of gag-expressing cells were CD11b+, suggesting that this population is responsible for uptake and expression of DNA following nasal immunization with PLG/DNA. Although

CD11b is expressed by many cell populations, it is primarily considered a marker for tissue macrophages (MØs) and dendritic cells (DCs), which are both professional antigen-presenting cells (APCs). However, compared with MØs, DCs are more potent APCs. Our previous *in vitro* data showed that bone marrow–derived DCs can take up PLG/DNA encoding HIV-1 gag and present it to a gag-specific T cell hybridoma (Denis-Mize *et al.*, 2000).

The prolonged expression of DNA following nasal immunizations with PLG/DNA may be due in part to protection of DNA from damage by tissue DNAse, which has previously been reported *in vitro* (Singh *et al.*, 2000). In addition, the presence of the cationic surfactant CTAB on the surface of PLG microparticles may contribute to disruption of endosomes and subsequent release of DNA into the cytoplasm, to enhance the response.

Alternative microencapsulation approaches for mucosal immunization

Encapsulation of antigens into particulate delivery systems, including liposomes, microparticles, and ISCOMs, has been extensively evaluated for mucosal delivery of vaccines. However, all of these approaches share some serious limitations. Uptake of the delivery system into the MALT is often very inefficient, resulting in most of the formulation not reaching the intended site of action. This problem is most apparent following oral delivery, necessitating high doses for oral immunization, but it is also a problem following nasal immunization. In addition, many of the particulate delivery systems used do not have sufficient stability to withstand the challenging environment in the gut, including low pH, gastric enzymes, and bile salts. Nevertheless, polymeric microparticles can be specifically designed to survive the low pH of the stomach and to release the entrapped antigen within the vicinity of the local lymphoid tissue. Hence, so-called enteric-coated formulations have some attributes of a desirable

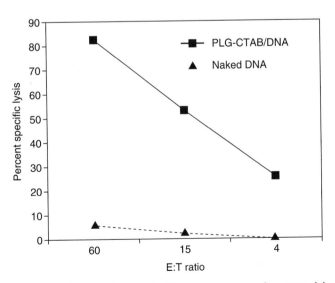

Fig. 55.3. Induction of systemic CTL responses in splenocytes following intranasal immunization with DNA encoding HIV-1 gag adsorbed onto cationic PLG-CTAB microparticles, as compared with naked DNA as measured by a 51Cr-release assay. E:T ratio, ratio of the number of effector cells to target cells.

formulation for oral delivery. The use of enteric-coated formulations can also overcome the problem of limited uptake of particulates into lymphoid tissue, since these formulations are not designed for uptake; rather, the antigen is released locally for direct uptake. However, most protein and DNA vaccines are unlikely to be sufficiently immunogenic to induce potent immune responses even in this situation, and additional formulation components may prove necessary to protect the antigens against degradation or to promote uptake. Nevertheless, more potent responses may be expected, if the antigen can directly bind to the epithelium as well as provide its own adjuvanticity (e.g., secreted bacterial toxins, particularly mutated enterotoxins like LT). Overall, the significant challenges to the development of effective oral vaccines using nonreplicating delivery systems should not be underestimated, and success in smaller animal models using high doses of antigen should not be overinterpreted.

Evidence of dissemination of antigen-specific, antibody-secreting cells from NALT to the cervical lymph nodes and spleen following intranasal immunizations has been provided by Heritage et al. (1998). These responses were generated by entrapment of human serum albumin (HSA) in polymer-grafted microparticles (3-(triethoxysilyl)-propyl-terminated polydimethylsiloxane [TS-PDMS]) with a size range of 1 μm to 100 μm. McDermott et al. (1998) also reported that polymer-grafted starch microparticles have been used as an alternative to PLG particles for oral or nasal immunizations and induced mucosal and systemic humoral responses. However, in comparison with PLG, these microparticles are poorly defined, and their biocompatibility has not been tested in humans. In another study, a single nasal or oral immunization with a Schistosoma mansoni antigen entrapped in PLG or polycaprolactone (PCL) microparticles resulted in sustained serum IgG responses (Baras et al., 1999). Interestingly, it was noted that only PLG-entrapped and not PCL-entrapped vaccine resulted in strong neutralizing antibody responses following either nasal or oral immunization. Moreover, the humoral responses were detectable earlier following PLG versus PCL immunizations, presumably because of the physicochemical differences between the two polymers and different rates of antigen release.

Nasal immunization of anesthetized mice with hemagglutinin from influenza virus entrapped in one of four microparticle resins (sodium polystyrene sulfonate, calcium polystyrene sulfinate, polystyrene benzyltrimethylammonium chloride, or polystyrene divinylbenzene) sized to 20–45 μm enhanced serum hemagglutinin-inhibiting antibodies and nasal wash IgA antibodies (Higaki et al., 1998). An important finding of this study was that immunization reduced viral burden in the lungs following nasal administration of virus. Debin et al. (2002) described an approach to nasal immunization using polymerized polysaccharide nanoparticles, with a coating of lipids. Using hepatitis B surface antigen (HbsAg) in mice, they reported the induction of potent antibody and CTL responses; the approach has also been evaluated in clinical trials involving human volunteers (von Hoegen, 2001).

An alternative approach to mucosal immunization with particles is represented by the use of virus-like particles (VLPs), which are nonreplicating viral proteins that naturally self-assemble into particulates when they are expressed in vitro (Boisgerault et al., 2002). On a number of occasions, VLPs have been shown to be potent immunogens following mucosal delivery, particularly by the nasal route (Guerrero et al., 2001). In addition, an alternative kind of VLP is represented by replicons, including those derived from Sindbis virus, which are designed to encode an antigen of interest but are capable of only a single cycle of replication in vivo. Potent immune responses and protection against challenge have been induced following mucosal delivery of Sindbis replicons (Vajdy et al., 2001).

Microparticles as delivery systems for immunization with mutants of LT

Genetically detoxified mutants of LT have been shown to be potent adjuvants for inducing mucosal and systemic immune responses. LT is toxic in its native state and induces accumulation of intestinal fluid and diarrhea in humans. In order to retain the adjuvanticity of these molecules but reduce their toxicity, several mutants have been generated by site-directed mutagenesis. Of these, two mutants of the enzymatic A subunit, LTK63 and LTR72, maintain a high degree of adjuvanticity (Barackman et al., 2001). LTK63 is the result of a substitution of serine 63 with a lysine in the A subunit, which renders it enzymatically inactive and nontoxic, while LTR72 is derived from a substitution of alanine 72 with an arginine in the A subunit and contains about 0.6% of the enzymatic activity of wild-type LT. LTR72 is 25 to 100 times less toxic than wild-type LT in the rabbit ileal loop assay (Giuliani et al., 1998).

Since LT mutants are potently immunogenic following mucosal immunization, there is a concern that immunity to LT might affect the potency of these molecules when used as adjuvants for several proteins consecutively. Nevertheless, we found that preexisting immunity to LTK63 did not affect its potency as an adjuvant, when used for nasal immunization with a second vaccine, soon after the first (Ugozzoli et al., 2001).

Moreover, in a recent study, we showed that hemagglutinin given nasally, together with LTK63, in a novel bioadhesive delivery system prepared from esterified hyaluronic acid microspheres (HYAFF), induced enhanced serum IgG as well as nasal IgA responses in mice and pigs (Singh et al., 2001) **(Figs. 55.5 and 55.6)**. Thus, combination of LT mutant adjuvants with a delivery system enhanced mucosal and systemic humoral immunity. Collectively, these data show that LT mutants are effective mucosal adjuvants in small and large animal models and can be used in combination with delivery systems to enhance their potency.

Conclusions about microparticles
The successful development of orally administered vaccines with nonreplicating approaches remains tremendously chal-

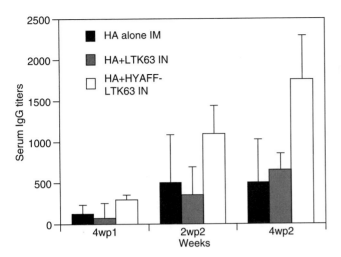

Fig. 55.5. Anti-hemagglutinin (HA) serum IgG titers in three groups of pigs immunized with either HA alone intramuscularly (IM), HA + LTK63 intranasally (IN), or HA + LTK63 + HYAFF (bioadhesive microspheres) intranasally (IN). The graphs represent the geometric mean titer ± one standard error of the mean for each group. 4wp1, 4 weeks post first immunization; 2wp2, 2 weeks post second immunization; 4wp2, 4 weeks post second immunization.

lenging, and no single approach currently looks very promising. In light of this, nasal immunization with protein or DNA encapsulated in or adsorbed onto PLG microparticles offers an attractive approach for enhancement of mucosal and systemic cell-mediated and humoral immune responses. The nasal route of immunization has several advantages over other routes of mucosal immunization, including the potential for induction of enhanced immunity in the genitourinary and respiratory tracts. Polymeric delivery systems can be designed to enhance the efficacy of mucosally administered vaccines in a

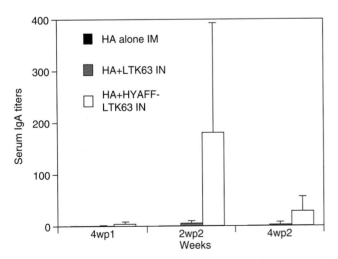

Fig. 55.6. Anti-hemagglutinin (HA) IgA titers in nasal secretions in three groups of pigs immunized with either HA alone intramuscularly (IM), HA + LTK63 intranasally (IN), or HA + LTK63 + HYAFF (bioadhesive microspheres) intranasally (IN). The graphs represent the geometric mean titer ± one standard error of the mean for each group. 4wp1, 4 weeks post first immunization; 2wp2, 2 weeks post second immunization, 4wp2, 4 weeks post second immunization.

number of ways: they can protect antigens from degradation, concentrate them in one area of the mucosal tissue for better uptake, extend their residence time in the body, and target them to specific sites of antigen uptake (e.g., NALT). Significant progress has been made recently with PLG, allowing the effective stabilization of proteins and DNA in or on microparticles during the preparation process. Thus, nasal delivery of entrapped or adsorbed antigens may prove to be a practical and feasible approach for vaccination. Developments in the aerosolization of PLG microparticles also offers the potential of delivery of vaccines to the lungs (Edwards *et al.*, 1997; Masinde and Hickey, 1993). The potential of targeting ligands to enhance particle uptake in larger animal models, including humans, is currently unknown, although in rodents, the extent of uptake of microparticles can be enhanced with use of targeting ligands. Nevertheless, the advantages of a highly complex system for mucosal administration involving a targeting agent need to be justified by a large increase in potency over nontargeted systems. Future research in the use of nonspecific bioadhesives to retain antigens in the nasal cavity for extended periods may prove beneficial, particularly if these agents are combined with potent mucosal adjuvants.

LIPOSOMES

Introduction

Bangham and coworkers (1965) were the first to demonstrate almost 40 years ago that the addition of water to a flask containing a film of phospholipids results in the appearance of microscopic closed vesicles. Since that time, liposomes have been extensively studied for use in targeted drug delivery and as vaccine delivery systems. These studies have resulted in the development of several injectable liposome-based formulations that have been licensed for use in humans (reviewed in Gregoriadis, 1995). A number of aspects pertaining to the usefulness of liposomes as vaccine delivery systems are similar to those described for PLG microparticles and ISCOMs.

In brief, liposomes can act as adjuvants in potentiating immune responses, and therefore the amount of antigen needed to induce a response is smaller when it is incorporated into liposomes than when given alone. Liposomes can also convert nonimmunogenic substances into immunogenic forms, e.g., by rendering soluble substances particulate in nature. A variety of substances can be incorporated into liposomes, including multiple antigens, adjuvants, cytokines, and substances such as antibodies to cell surface antigens for targeted delivery. Liposomes are taken up by macrophages (MØs) and by microfold (M) cells (i.e., the specialized epithelial cells covering Peyer's patches and other IgA inductive sites) for antigen processing and/or presentation to other lymphoid cells for the induction of immune responses. They can also directly present antigens to lymphoid cells for the induction of immune responses. Since liposomes can be composed of substances (*e.g.*, phospholipids) that make up host cells, they can represent nontoxic, safe, efficacious vaccine delivery systems for use in animals and humans. Liposomes can also mediate DNA or RNA transfection of cells and may represent a useful means for transfer of genetic material encoding vaccine antigens. For more detailed discussion of this subject, the reader is referred to other reviews (Alving, 1991, 1995; Chen and Langer, 1998; Childers and Michalek, 1994; Duzgunes and Shlomo, 1999; Gregoriadis, 1990, 1995; Gregoriadis *et al.*, 1999; Lasic, 1998; Michalek *et al.*, 1994).

Properties of liposomes

Liposomes are bilayered membranes consisting of amphipathic molecules (polar and nonpolar portions) such as phospholipids forming multilayered or unilayered (lamellar) vesicles. Multilamellar vesicles (MLVs) have several lipid bilayers separated by thin aqueous phases, whereas unilamellar vesicles (UVs) have a single bilayer membrane surrounding an aqueous core and are characterized as being either small (SUVs) or large (LUVs). Many of the phospholipids used to make liposomes are purified from food products (e.g., egg yolk); therefore, they are nontoxic and safe for human use. These vesicles form spontaneously when an aqueous solution is added to a dried film of the lipid components. The hydrophilic (water-soluble or polar head) portion of the lipid molecule is oriented toward the aqueous phase, and the hydrophobic (water-insoluble) portion is aligned inside the membrane. Thus, in preparing liposome vaccines, water-soluble substances can be incorporated into the enclosed aqueous space, whereas lipid-soluble molecules can be added to the solvent during vesicle formation and incorporated into the lipid bilayer.

Liposomes can be prepared that vary in membrane stability, fluidity, and permeability, depending on their lipid content and their charge. Net negative-charged liposomes can be prepared by using anionic phospholipids or by adding a negatively charged compound such as dicetyl phosphate. Positively charged or neutral liposomes can also be made, depending on the components used in production. A common formulation for production of negatively charged liposomes consists of dipalmitoyl phosphatidylcholine and dicetyl phosphate. Cholesterol is often added as a stabilizer and to increase membrane fluidity by interrupting the orderly interdigitation of the dipalmitoyl phosphatidylcholine molecules. These types of vesicles are likely to be stable in the gastrointestinal tract for long periods of time (Kokkona *et al.*, 2000). Each property of the vesicles influences how effective a liposome preparation will be as an antigen delivery system.

A commonly used method for producing liposomes has involved sonication of the aqueous phospholipid suspension. The liposomes generated are a mixture of small-diameter (0.1 μm) to large-diameter (>1.0 μm) vesicles that are mostly multilamellar. For use in vaccine delivery systems, it is necessary to use techniques that reproducibly generate liposome preparations of controlled size and composition. Methods used to produce homogenous unilamellar liposomes include microemulsification, ultracentrifugation, and membrane extrusion. Microemulsification involves the production of liposomes in a pressurized chamber under controlled pressure and cycling time. This procedure results in SUVs of a desired diameter and has been extensively used to generate liposomes containing antigens for use as oral vaccines (reviewed in Childers and Michalek, 1994; Michalek et al., 1994, 1995). To ensure the size and lamellar characteristics of liposomes, a commonly used procedure is electron microscopy. The size characteristics of liposomes can also be determined by dynamic light scatter analysis. Perhaps the most convenient method to qualitatively analyze liposomes would be to record laser light scatter of a suspension with flow cytometry, a technique available to most laboratories. Another method for preparing liposomes involves the generation of dehydrated-rehydrated vesicles (DRVs) (reviewed in Gregoriadis, 1990, 1992). This procedure has been shown to result in a high-yield entrapment of drugs and has been used to reproducibly incorporate various substances such as tetanus toxoid, influenza virus subunit peptides, recombinant hepatitis B surface antigen, *Leishmania major* antigens, and poliovirus. A method has also been developed for high-yield entrapment of solutes in SUVs (Zadi and Gregoriadis, 2000). Various liposome preparations need to be directly prepared in order to establish whether one type is more effective as a vaccine delivery system for the induction of protective immune responses.

Processing of liposome vaccines

Several explanations have been proposed by which liposomes can be effective delivery systems and adjuvants for the induction of immune responses (reviewed in Alving, 1991; Gregoriadis, 1990, 1992, 1995). Liposomes, regardless of their composition and size, can adsorb to most cells and release their incorporated substances, which can then act on the cell. Liposomes can also be taken up by MØs and other phagocytic cells in the blood, lymph, and various tissues (e.g., lymph nodes, liver, and spleen) with the subsequent release of antigen. The liver and spleen take up nearly all liposomes introduced by the intravenous route, whereas most liposomes injected via the subcutaneous or intramuscular route are retained at the site of injection (depot) and are taken up by infiltrating MØs. The ability of APCs to more efficiently take up and process antigens associated with liposomes for enhanced immune responses is another explanation of the immunoadjuvant property of liposomes. It has also been suggested that the liposomes may act directly in presenting antigen to lymphoid cells for the induction of responses.

Although liposomes have been extensively studied for their ability to augment immune responses when given systemically, some studies have shown that they can also serve as an immunoadjuvant for mucosal immunization (reviewed in Alving, 1995; Childers and Michalek, 1994; Michalek et al., 1994, 1995). Whether the adjuvant quality of liposomes is due to the more effective uptake by M cells of Peyer's patches and/or to their subsequent interaction with antigen-processing cells has not been established. However, liposomes have been found in endocytic vesicles of M cells in close proximity to lymphocytes following intestinal administration. Because liposomes are bilayered membrane vesicles, which mimic cell membranes, by enclosing the antigen in the lipid vesicle, the uptake and processing of antigen may be enhanced. Another proposed mechanism for the adjuvant properties of liposomes is their ability to protect the antigen from acids and proteolytic enzymes of the gastrointestinal system. Although they are not completely resistant to lipases and bile salts found in the small intestine, at least partial resistance has been found with use of cholesterol-containing liposomes. The use of polymerized liposomes (composed of modified phospholipids that are cross-linked via diene groups on the 1 or 2 carbons of the acyl chains) has also been shown to increase the stability of the vesicles while inside the gastrointestinal tract (Chen *et al.*, 1996a).

Liposome vaccines *in vivo*
During the past decade, numerous studies have been performed to establish the usefulness of the liposome vaccine delivery system for inducing protective immune responses against various infectious diseases. Studies with liposome-antigen or liposome-DNA vaccines have frequently involved systemic routes of administration, and a number of these are on the market or in clinical development (reviewed by Lasic, 1998). However, evidence is accumulating that liposomes can serve as carriers of antigens and as adjuvants for inducing enhanced mucosal immune responses. **Table 55.2** is a partial list of studies that have investigated liposomes as mucosal vaccine delivery systems. In these studies, mucosal and systemic immune responses to microbial and viral antigens were evaluated, and in some cases protection against the pathogen was assessed. In these studies and those involving systemic routes of liposome vaccine administration, the spatial arrangement of the antigens within liposomes and characteristics of the vesicles, such as size and number of lamellae, were not always determined. It is generally accepted that a physical association between the liposome membrane and antigen (as opposed to their simple mixing) is an important consideration in formulating a delivery system for inducing immune responses. Antigen can be incorporated into the aqueous phase of the vesicles, adsorbed onto their surface, partitioned into the bilayers (hydrophobic antigens), or covalently coupled to a membrane component. The specific formulation of liposome delivery systems may differ for the development of vaccines that are effective in inducing protective immunity against different infectious organisms.

Induction of mucosal responses by oral immunization with liposome vaccines
A number of studies have been done to determine the effectiveness of liposomes as mucosal vaccines (reviewed in Alving, 1995; Childers and Michalek, 1994; Michalek *et al.*, 1994, 1995). The use of liposomes containing antigen as oral vaccines was first investigated to determine their ability to augment protective salivary immune responses against the oral pathogen *Streptococcus mutans* in an experimental rat caries model. Initial investigations compared liposomal *S.*

mutans antigens to other vaccine preparations when given orally. Liposomal *S. mutans* antigens were found to enhance salivary antibody activity and protection against *S. mutans*–induced dental caries better than did control whole cell or antigen only. The dose of *S. mutans* antigen necessary to produce a mucosal immune response following oral administration was much lower when antigen was incorporated in liposomes. Responses induced with the liposomal antigens were comparable with those seen in animals given *S. mutans* antigens with other adjuvants such as peptidoglycan, muramyl dipeptide, monophosphoryl lipid A, and water-in-oil emulsion. However, the addition of muramyl dipeptide to liposomal antigen was shown to further augment the protective immune response to *S. mutans*. When the mucosal adjuvant CT was given in (or in addition to) the liposomal antigen preparation, no additional enhancement in the immune response was seen. This may be partially due to the fact that incorporating CT in liposomes may interfere with the binding of CT-B to GM1 ganglioside on the surface of host cells. However, when the CT-B was attached to the surface of liposomes, an enhanced mucosal response was observed to the antigen incorporated in the liposome following oral or intranasal immunization (Harokopakis *et al.*, 1998, unpublished results). These findings support the concept that CT-B present on lipid vesicles will target them to mucosal cells expressing surface GM1 (Lian and Ho, 1997). Furthermore, these studies and others confirm the potential usefulness of liposomal-antigen delivery systems for protection against *S. mutans*–induced dental caries (Wachsmann *et al.*, 1985, 1986; reviewed in Michalek *et al.*, 1994, 1995).

A challenge regarding the design of oral liposomal vaccines has been to determine the optimal characteristics of liposomes and the form of liposomal antigen used in the induction of immune responses. When various liposome preparations containing *S. mutans* glucosyltransferase (GTF) that differed in homogeneity and size of liposomes were evaluated for their ability to induce protective immune responses, all liposomal-GTF preparations induced immune responses that were more protective than that evoked by GTF alone (Childers *et al.*, 1996). It was also shown that smaller, more homogeneous (unilamellar) liposomal-GTF were more effective in inducing protective responses. Human studies utilizing oral liposomal–*S. mutans* antigen vaccines have provided preliminary data indicating their safety and immunogenicity (reviewed in Childers and Michalek, 1994, and Michalek *et al.*, 1995). Oral administration of liposomal–*S. mutans* cell wall carbohydrate antigen in enteric-coated capsules resulted in a transient salivary IgA anticarbohydrate response in comparison with preimmunization levels. A second immunization resulted in a more rapid response of higher magnitude. In this study, the liposome preparation was maintained in an aqueous phase that is difficult to package. Therefore, in a subsequent human study, a dehydrated liposomal–*S. mutans* GTF vaccine was tested (Childers *et al.*, 1994). Volunteers who swallowed capsules containing the liposome vaccine showed increased salivary IgA anti-GTF responses with a predominant salivary

Table 55.2. Mucosal Immunization Studies with Liposomal Vaccines Delivery Systems

Antigen/Adjuvant	Liposome Composition	Route of Administration	Host	Major Findings/References
Cholera toxin-lipoidal amine-lipid A	DPPC, Chol, DP (MLV)	Oral	Rats	Enhanced intestinal IgA response (Pierce and Sacci, 1984; Pierce et al., 1984)
Mutans streptococcal Anti-idiotypic antibodies Carbohydrate Carbohydrate-lipophilic MDP Peptide-CTB Protein-CTB Proteins Ribosomes	DPPC, Chol, DP (SUV)	Oral	Rats	Adjuvant effect—induction of salivary IgA antibodies; reduced infection by mutans streptococci (Childers et al., 1996; reviewed in Michalek et al., 1992, 1994, 1995)
Carbohydrate-protein conjugate		Oral	Rats	Adjuvant effect—induction of serum and salivary antibodies (Wachsmann et al., 1985, 1986)
Protein/MPL		Oral or N	Mice	Mucosal and systemic IgA responses 10-fold higher with N than oral immunization; augmented responses with MPL (Childers et al., 2000).
Streptococcus mutans Carbohydrate Protein	DPPC, Chol, DP	Oral	Humans (adults)	Adjuvant effect—induction of salivary and serum IgA antibodies (Childers et al., 1994; reviewed in Michalek et al., 1994, 1995)
Streptococcus mutans Protein	DPPC, Chol, DP	N or Tonsil	Humans (adults)	Induction of IgA response in nasal secretions, saliva, and serum; low response with tonsillar immunization (Childers et al., 1999; Childers et al., 2002)
Bacteroides gingivalis Fimbriae/L18-MDP or GM-53-MDP Influenza virus	DPPC, Chol	Oral or SubQ	Mice	Adjuvant effect—enhanced by GM-53-MDP > L18-MDP (salivary and serum antibodies) (reviewed in Michalek et al., 1994, 1995)
Glycoprotein	octyl-β-D-glucopyranoside	N	Mice	Induced local IgA and systemic antibody responses and protection from virus challenge (El Guink et al., 1989; reviewed in Michalek et al., 1994, 1995)
Subunit antigen	PC, Chol, DCP	N	Mice	Induced mucosal IgA and serum IgG antibody responses and protection against infection (de Haan et al., 1995a); induced S-IgA responses in vaginal and respiratory tract secretions and serum IgG (de Haan et al., 1995b)
Subunit vaccine	DSPC, Chol, BisHOP (DRV)	N, IM	Mice	Mucosal route less effective in inducing local or systemic responses and protection (Ben Ahmeida et al., 1993)
Antibody	PC, Chol, PS or PC, Chol, SA	N, IT or IV		Enhanced delivery of antibody to lung and protection against infection with negative charged liposomes (PC, Chol, PS) given by the N route (Wong et al., 1994)

(Continued)

Table 55.2. Mucosal Immunization Studies with Liposomal Vaccines Delivery Systems *(Continued)*

Antigen/Adjuvant	Liposome Composition	Route of Administration	Host	Major Findings/References
Ricin	DMPC, DMPG, Chol, lipid A	N, IM or IV	Mice	Elevated IgG and IgA responses in lung washes (N group only). All mice protected against N challenge with ricin (Matyas and Alving, 1996)
DNA/Adjuvant	**Composition**	**Administration**	**Host**	**Major Findings/References**
CMV promoter-env gp160 & rev genes-cytokines	DC-Chol, DOPE	N	Mice	Enhanced intestinal and vaginal IgA responses; with cytokines, induced high levels of HIV-specific CTLs (Okada *et al.*, 1997)

Chol, cholesterol; CT-B, cholera toxin B subunit; DC-Chol, 3β(N′, N′-dimethylaminoethane)carbamoyl) cholesterol; DMPC, dimyristoyl phosphatidylcholine; DOPE, dioleoylphosphatidylethanolamine; DP, dicethyl phosphate; DPPC, dipalmitoyl phosphatidylcholine; DMPG, dimyristoyl phosphatidylglycerol; MDP, muramyl dipeptide; MPL, monophosphorly lipid A; IM, intramuscular; IT, intratracheal; MLV, multilamellar vesicles; N, nasal; PC, phosphatidylcholine; SA, stearylamine; SubQ, subcutaneous; SUV, small unilamellar vesicles; DSPC, distearoyl phosphatidyl choline; BisHOP, 1,2-bis(hexadecyl-cycloxy-3-trimethyl amino propane); DRV, dehydrated-rehydrated vesicles.

IgA2 anti-GTF response. Since naturally occurring IgA anti–*S. mutans* protein responses are predominantly IgA1, it is possible that the presentation of the antigen in liposomes accounted for the shift in the subclass of the IgA response. In recognition of the fact that IgA1 proteases are produced by some bacteria colonizing the oral cavity (and teeth; e.g., *Streptococcus sanguis*), an IgA2 response could be more advantageous to the host because it would be resistant to degradation by this microbial protease.

The *in vivo* studies described thus far have concentrated on experimental data utilizing oral liposome vaccines containing antigens of *S. mutans* because of the number of investigations, the existence of an experimental animal model to study protection against *S. mutans*–induced dental caries, and the human studies that have been done. Collectively, these studies provide a strong basis for the use of this approach for the development of a caries vaccine for human use. Oral immunization studies with liposomes containing antigens of other pathogens have also been reported. Rhalem and coworkers (1988) reported that mice orally immunized with antigens from *Nippostrongylus brasiliensis* showed the greatest protection against infection with this helminth when the antigen was given in liposomes. Other microbial antigens used to investigate liposomes as mucosal vaccines were obtained from pathogens such as *Clostridium tetani*, *Vibrio cholerae*, *Porphyromonas gingivalis*, HIV, and *B. pertussis*. This research showed augmentation of mucosal and systemic immune responses in the various systems employed; however, protective responses were not assessed (reviewed in Alving, 1995; Michalek *et al.*, 1995).

Nasal immunization with liposome vaccines

Mucosal immunization with use of liposomes is not limited to oral administration. Abraham (1992) has tested nasal applica-

tion of large unilamellar liposomes containing bacterial polysaccharide antigens in BALB/c mice. This study revealed enhanced immune responses in pulmonary secretions in mice immunized with the liposomal antigen, in comparison with antigen alone. These responses were found to be much stronger than those following oral immunization (nasal immunization produced comparable antibody titers at 1/30 the oral dose). When liposomal *Pseudomonas aeruginosa* polysaccharide was administered nasally, mortality among the animals after challenge was decreased. Abraham and Shah (1992) also reported an improvement in immune responses when antigens were given in liposomes containing IL-2 (but not with liposomes containing IL-4). An 80-fold increase in pulmonary specific antibody-producing plasma cells was found.

A number of studies have also used the nasal route to immunize with liposomes containing influenza virus antigens. El Guink *et al.* (1989) immunized mice with proteoliposomes containing the envelope glycoprotein of the influenza virus by either the nasal or systemic route. The mice were anesthetized for nasal immunization. The results showed that mice immunized by the nasal route had higher levels of IgA in nasal washes and slightly lower serum antibody responses than the systemically immunized mice and were protected against influenza virus challenge. These results were not in agreement with those of Ben Ahmeida *et al.* (1993), who used live influenza A or subunit vaccine preparations as the immunogen. These investigators reported that nasal immunization of anesthetized mice with live virus or systemic immunization with the subunit vaccine preparation in ISCOMs resulted in higher mucosal and systemic immune responses and protection than observed with the liposome vaccine given by either route. In fact, the liposome-subunit vaccine prepared by the DRV method appeared to be less effective than the subunit vaccine alone in inducing immune responses.

Subsequent studies by de Haan and coworkers (1995a,b) showed that nasal immunization of mice with liposomes containing an influenza subunit preparation resulted in a serum IgG and lung and nasal cavity IgA response that persisted for about 5 months and was protective against infection (de Haan *et al.*, 1995a). Vaccines consisting of negatively charged but not zwitterionic liposomes were effective in inducing responses. Furthermore, these investigators indicated that systemic and mucosal responses were also induced when the liposomes were coadministered with the antigen. In another study in which the same liposome-antigen vaccine was used, it was shown that nasal immunization of anesthetized mice resulted not only in a systemic and mucosal immune response but also in a specific IgA response in vaginal secretions (de Haan *et al.*, 1995b). Vaginal and lung wash IgA responses were not detected in nonanesthetized mice immunized by the oral or nasal route. These results provide evidence that immunization with a liposome-antigen vaccine in the lower respiratory tract of mice resulted in both local and distal mucosal responses. These studies with influenza A virus vaccines have used liposomes to actively immunize the host, whereas studies by Wong *et al.* (1994) showed protection against influenza A infection following nasal administration of liposomes containing antiviral antibody to anesthetized mice. The protection seen in these animals was greater than that in mice given free antibody. The authors concluded that the greater protection seen with liposomes could be due to enhanced delivery and to the retention of antibodies in the lung.

Matyas and Alving (1996) reported that nasal immunization of anesthetized mice with liposomes containing ricin, a glycoprotein toxin from castor beans, resulted in IgG and IgA antiricin antibodies in lung secretions and in levels of serum IgG antibody similar to those seen in systemically immunized mice. Elevated levels of antibody were seen in lung washes and in serum of nasally immunized mice for 3 to 4 months. Since the systemically and mucosally immunized groups of mice were both protected against nasal challenge with ricin, the authors concluded that humoral immunity was mainly responsible for protection. The liposomes used in this study contained lipid A as an added adjuvant and have been extensively studied for their ability to augment responses to various antigens following systemic immunization (reviewed in Alvin 1991, 1995). However, little is known about the potential of this liposome formulation for enhancing mucosal immune responses.

Recent studies of humans in which liposomal–*S. mutans* GTF was compared with antigen alone showed that both were effective in inducing mucosal IgA responses following intranasal immunization (Childers *et al.*, 1999). Interestingly, it was noted that the levels of nasal wash IgA1 anti-GTF activity were higher in subjects immunized with the liposomal vaccine than in those immunized with antigen alone, thus suggesting that the form of the antigen affected the magnitude of the local mucosal response. The finding that the levels of IgA antibody activity in nasal wash secretions were higher than those seen in saliva suggests that nasal immu-

nization with the GTF vaccines was more effective in inducing a local than a disseminated immune response. In this study, serum antibodies were also induced, providing additional evidence that nasal immunization can result in the induction of both mucosal and systemic immune responses.

In a subsequent experiment, Childers *et al.* (2002) investigated the effectiveness of nasal versus tonsillar immunization with the GTF vaccines for inducing mucosal immune responses. Adult subjects immunized by the nasal route had higher levels of IgA antibody activity in saliva and nasal wash samples than individuals immunized via the tonsillar route. These results provide evidence that topical application of antigen to tonsils may not be an effective method for immunization of adults. However, these results cannot rule out the potential usefulness of this approach in children, whose tonsils are fully developed and are likely to be actively responding to antigens, in comparison with the atrophied tonsils in adults. Finally, the liposomal GTF vaccine induced higher responses than the soluble antigen following nasal immunization; however, the differences were not significant. Additional studies in humans are necessary to establish whether a liposomal vaccine will be more effective than a soluble vaccine in inducing mucosal (local versus disseminated) and systemic responses following nasal immunization.

Novel approaches of liposome vaccination

Other strategies to improve mucosal vaccines that use liposomes are being tested. One approach involves covalent linkage of antigens or ligands to the surface of liposomes. By using an antibody to a specific receptor or a ligand for the surface of a target cell, e.g., *Ulex europaeus* agglutinin I or wheat germ agglutinin (Chen *et al.*, 1996b), it is possible to specifically target vaccines to an antigen-processing cell or to M cells and thus provide a more efficient system for immunization. Other studies are exploring the effectiveness of conjugating antibodies to the surface of liposomes for use in passive immune protection (Robinson *et al.*, 1998). Another growing area of liposome research involves the packaging of RNA- and DNA-encoding antigens that could be inserted into antigen-processing cells or APCs to provide a renewable source of antigen for continuous immunization (Felgner *et al.*, 1987; Farhood *et al.*, 1994) and for gene therapy (Simoes *et al.* 1999a; Simoes *et al.*, 1999b). Cationic liposomes are used and complexed to negatively charged, naked DNA by simple mixing the two such that the complex has a net positive charge. Studies in this area have been very promising; however, much work is needed to develop new and improved liposome formulations for effective gene transfer and efficient methods for *in vivo* delivery.

ISCOMS

Introduction

The immune stimulating complex (ISCOM) is a highly versatile and effective antigen presentation system that has been extensively studied as an adjuvant system for a range of viral antigens. Furthermore, several bacterial, parasite, and other antigens have been presented in ISCOMs, and these studies have provided evidence of the usefulness of the ISCOM structure in inducing desired immune responses. The results of these studies have led to the application of ISCOM-based vaccines for commercial veterinary use and clinical trials involving humans.

ISCOM matrix and ISCOMs

The ISCOM structure was first described in 1984 (Morein et al., 1984) as a cagelike structure about 30 to 40 nm in diameter that is composed of glycosides present in the adjuvant Quil A, cholesterol, the antigenic component, and in most cases also a phospholipid such as phosphatidyl choline or phosphatidylethanolamine. Quil A is prepared from the bark of the tree *Quillaja saponaria,* and its adjuvant activity is based on the presence of a complex mixture of closely related triterpene glycosides. Quil A itself is widely used as an adjuvant in veterinary vaccines. The typical cagelike structure of ISCOMs is formed by hydrophobic interactions between the triterpene glycosides and cholesterol, interactions that are apparently so strong that the structure is extremely stable. For example, ISCOMs resist lyophilization procedures routinely used for vaccine formulation (Morein et al., 1984). Furthermore, the ISCOM matrix can be formed in the absence of the immunogenic component, and this structure can act as a potent adjuvant (Lövgren and Morein, 1988). However, evidence exists that for the efficient induction of HLA class I–restricted CTL responses, which is a hallmark of the potential of the ISCOM structure, physical incorporation of the immunogen is required (Van Binnendijk et al., 1992). Others, however, have provided data that conflict with these findings and have demonstrated that proteins mixed with empty matrix can also induce the activation of virus-specific CD8[+] T cells (Voeten et al., 2000).

The structure and morphology of ISCOMs are not significantly influenced by the incorporated immunogen. It has been shown that small amounts of phospholipid are necessary for the efficient incorporation of proteins into ISCOMs. This is probably related to the increase in flexibility of the structure that can be achieved, thus facilitating protein incorporation within the structure (Lövgren and Morein, 1988). Although a wide range of proteins can be incorporated into ISCOMs, until recently most experience was generated with membrane proteins of viruses since these immunogens induce virus-neutralizing (VN) antibodies and T cell responses. As a result of hydrophobic interactions, most viral membrane proteins are incorporated spontaneously into ISCOMs when present during their formation. For this reason, virus particles or cellular membranes expressing these proteins are usually solubilized by detergent treatment, which allows their exposure in a monomeric form. If required, the protein may first be purified before incorporation. Then, in the presence of cholesterol, Quil A components, and phospholipids, the ISCOMs containing the protein of interest are spontaneously formed when the

detergent is removed in a controlled way. Several methods have been used to achieve this goal.

The use of ultracentrifugation through sucrose gradients was the first method described (Morein et al., 1984). The use of dialyzable detergents like octylglucoside or Mega-10 allows their removal by dialysis. Chromatographic methods have also been employed. The introduction of proteins, which do not have membrane insertion or anchor sequences, may be more complicated, and several approaches allowing their incorporation into ISCOMs have been developed. The protein may be coupled to hydrophobic carriers such as palmatic acid (Mowat et al., 1991) or lipopolysaccharides (Weiss et al., 1990). Pretreatment of hydrophilic proteins by lowering the pH may expose hidden hydrophobic regions, which may then interact with the forming ISCOM matrix (Morein et al., 1990).

More recently, recombinant DNA technology has been used to attach hydrophobic regions to hydrophilic regions (Voeten et al., 2000; Andersson et al., 1999, 2000). The removal of cleavage sites between surface and transmembrane parts of proteins may also facilitate incorporation of the surface part into ISCOMs, as was shown for the membrane glycoproteins of certain lentiviruses (Rimmelzwaan et al., 1994; Hulskotte et al., 1995).

It should be realized that all these procedures may influence the antigenicity and immunogenicity of the incorporated immunogens. Changes in conformation-dependent B-cell epitopes may occur, depending on the procedures and proteins used. Therefore, a detailed analysis of these properties is usually required to determine the best method of incorporation. Actual formation of the desired ISCOMs may be confirmed by negative contrast electron microscopy, revealing the typical structures. This can be followed by confirmation of their physical characteristics, e.g., a well-defined sedimentation constant (19S), chemical composition, and antigenic properties measured by antibody recognition patterns. An important factor in the efficiency of ISCOM preparation is the relative concentrations of the respective components forming the ISCOM. A generally practiced rule of thumb is to use a cholesterol to protein solution to Quil A ratio of 1:1:5 (w/w/w), respectively.

Much effort has been made to characterize the essential components in the crude Quil A mix that are involved in the actual formation of ISCOMs, contribute to their immunity-enhancing properties, and do not induce toxic side effects. This has now resulted in a commercially available preparation containing purified Quil A components (Iscoprep 703, Iscotec AB, Uppsala, Sweden).

Immune-enhancing properties of ISCOMs

Since they were first described in 1984 (Morein et al., 1984), the immunity-enhancing properties of the ISCOM have been extensively studied in several systems. The induction of high-titer and biologically active antibodies, which persisted for long periods of time, was first described in a series of viral systems. Perhaps the most striking initial finding was that an inactivated measles virus preparation that failed to induce biologically active antibodies against the fusion protein of this virus did induce a response after it was incorporated into ISCOMs (Morein *et al.*, 1984). This was soon followed by a series of observations in other viral systems, including feline leukemia virus (Osterhaus *et al.*, 1985), lentiviruses (Osterhaus *et al.*, 1992; Siebelink *et al.*, 1995), and influenza viruses (Rimmelzwaan *et al.*, 1997, 1999, 2000). In some of these studies, it was shown that less antigen was required to induce a comparable antibody response when it was incorporated into ISCOMs than when soluble antigen was administered with the adjuvant Quil A. In most of these studies, it was shown that strong virus-neutralizing antibody responses were induced.

Another important finding was that when other vaccines or candidate vaccine preparations failed to induce protective antibody responses because of the presence of pre-existing neutralizing antibodies, the same antigens presented in ISCOMs were capable of inducing protective antibody. This was shown in the cynomolgus macaque model for measles (Van Binnendijk *et al.*, 1997). This may be an important issue, especially for measles and other morbillivirus infections, since the presence of maternal antibodies at the time of vaccination is considered one of the major problems interfering with the success of vaccination. Also, for other virus infections like influenza, preexisting, virus-specific antibodies may be a major stumbling block to successful vaccination.

The fact that ISCOM presentation results in a more potent, longer-lasting antibody response may be explained in part by the induction of a Th cell response that indirectly influences the subsequent B cell response via the release of a complex series of soluble factors. In several studies, it has been shown that a multimeric presentation alone, e.g., the presentation via protein micelles, results in enhanced antibody responses. The combination with a built-in adjuvant in the multimeric presentation form probably enhances this effect. The role of the multimeric presentation was elegantly shown in experiments in which different numbers of biotin molecules were coupled to preformed ISCOMs. The presence of three or more biotin molecules per ISCOM resulted in specific antibody responses 10 times higher than those obtained with ISCOMs in which only one biotin molecule had been incorporated (Lövgren *et al.*, 1987).

ISCOMs were shown to be potent inducers not only of antibody responses but also of T-cell responses. Besides the role of Th cells, the importance of CTLs has now been demonstrated in the protection from and the clearance of many infectious diseases. Therefore, effective vaccines should in many cases induce not only antibody and Th cell responses but also CTL responses against the proper antigens.

For the processing and presentation of antigens to either Th cells or CTLs, two different pathways exist. For presentation to $CD4^+$ T cells, antigens are taken up into the endosomes of APCs via the exogenous pathway, where they are degraded to peptides that associate with MHC class II molecules. For presentation to $CD8^+$ T cells, usually *de novo* synthesized proteins are degraded in the cytosol and the formed peptides are transported into the endoplasmic reticulum via the endogenous pathway to associate with MHC class I molecules. Consequently, vaccines that are not based on actively replicating antigen do not or only minimally activate specific $CD8^+$ T cells since no *de novo* synthesis of the antigen takes place. Therefore, the use of inactivated or subunit vaccines may be prohibited if their success depends on the elicitation of $CD8^+$ T cells. However, it has been shown that certain antigen presentation forms may still allow processing and presentation of such antigens via the endogenous pathway that stimulates $CD8^+$ T cells.

Probably the most effective in this respect is the ISCOM preparation form. In several studies, it was shown that antigen-specific $CD8^+$ CTLs were induced *in vivo* when the immunizing antigen was incorporated into the ISCOM matrix. These include studies with lentiviruses HIV-1 and SIV (Takahashi *et al.*, 1990; Hulskotte *et al.*, 1995), influenza viruses (Takahashi *et al.*, 1990; Rimmelzwaan *et al.*, 2000), and ovalbumin used as model antigen (Mowat *et al.*, 1991). Using human $CD4^+$ and $CD8^+$ T cell clones specific for the F protein of measles virus and HLA-matched APCs, we were able to show that only when this antigen was physically incorporated into the ISCOM matrix was it processed via the endogenous pathway, and the resulting peptides were presented in the context of HLA class I to stimulate the $CD8^+$ T cell clone. Nonincorporated F protein presented together with Quil A failed to stimulate the $CD8^+$ T cell clones but did stimulate the $CD4^+$ cell clones. Stimulation of both types of T cells by the F-ISCOM preparation proved to be insensitive to chloroquine activity, which blocks the exogenous pathway by raising the pH of the endosomes (Van Binnendijk *et al.*, 1992). Presentation of the F protein to the $CD8^+$ but not the $CD4^+$ T cell clones was absent in a transporter-protein-negative mutant of an APC line that presented this antigen to both types of clones (Van Binnendijk *et al.*, 1992). Collectively, these data show that presentation of nonreplicating antigens incorporated into or associated with the ISCOM matrix allows their processing and presentation via the endogenous and exogenous pathways, resulting in the stimulation of both $CD4^+$ and $CD8^+$ T cells.

Basis for ISCOM-mediated immune enhancement

The overall adjuvant activity of the Quil A moiety is probably retained in ISCOMs. Its mode of action is not fully understood, but retention time of the antigen at the site of injection and the selective uptake in lymphoid tissue are probably important factors. The progressive redistribution of antigens in ISCOMs to the spleen, where they are taken up by a distinct subset of MØs not involved in the uptake of free antigen (Claassen *et al.*, 1995), is another interesting phenomenon. As mentioned earlier, multimeric presentation of an antigen in the ISCOM structure was shown to lead to a major increase in antibody responses (Lövgren *et al.*, 1987). The extent to which this multimeric presentation is also important in the induction of T cell responses is not clear.

How ISCOM presentation leads to processing through the endogenous pathway and presentation via MHC class I to stimulate $CD8^+$ T cells is also not understood at present. It seems most likely that ISCOMs act as carriers, which allow the proteins to be transported into and subsequently through the plasma and endosomal membranes, directly resulting in introduction of the antigen into the respective proteolytic compartments of the APC. Furthermore, temporary introduction of the protein into the membranes may shield them from proteolysis by enzymes other than those of the cellular proteolytic compartments. It was shown that intact and partially degraded ISCOM structures were attached to cell membranes of MØs. In addition, they were shown to be present in phagosomal membranes. The hydrophobic nature of the ISCOM structure and the presence of saponins in this structure, which may intercalate into cholesterol-containing membranes, may form the basis for the capacity of ISCOMs to integrate into membranes and traffic their antigenic moieties over these membranes.

Induction of mucosal immunity after ISCOM vaccination

Parenteral immunization

It has been shown that parenteral immunization with ISCOMs containing sheep erythrocyte antigen results in an immune response in the female reproductive tract of mice. Immunization in the pelvic presacral space (which is an intramuscular site) stimulated significant anti-erythrocyte IgA titers in vaginal fluid that were higher than after intraperitoneal, subcutaneous, intravaginal, or intraperitoneal-intravaginal immunizations with the same vaccine. Specific IgG titers in vaginal washings were found to be less dependent on the route of immunization (Thapar et al., 1991), although the intravaginal route of administration resulted in lower IgG titers.

In a more recent study, it was shown that a genital mucosal Th1 response was induced against *Chlamydia trachomatis* upon intramuscular immunization with ISCOMs containing the major outer membrane protein of this microorganism. Upon transfer of T cells obtained from ISCOM-immunized mice, recipients were protected against an intravaginal challenge (Igietseme and Murdin, 2000). In addition, intradermally administered ISCOMs were efficacious in eliciting both systemic and mucosal IgG and IgA antibodies in sheep, pigs, and mice (Chin et al., 1996). Also, intramuscular immunization of mice with an influenza–ISCOM preparation resulted in the development of IgA and IgG antibodies in nasal washes, which conferred partial protection against a homologous challenge infection (Ben Ahmeida et al., 1993). Thus, parenteral immunization with an ISCOM-based vaccine can induce mucosal IgA and IgG antibodies.

Oral immunization

The first evidence that oral immunization with ISCOMs elicited mucosal and systemic immune responses was obtained with use of ovalbumin as a model antigen (Mowat et al., 1991a,b, 1993; Maloy et al., 1995). Oral immunization with ISCOMs containing ovalbumin induced not only serum antibodies but also mucosal IgA antibodies and MHC class I restricted CTL responses after repeated immunization, as well as Th1 and Th2 T-cell responses. For the induction of immune responses by oral immunization, higher doses of immunizing antigen are required than for parenteral immunization. This may be related to immunogen degradation in the gastrointestinal tract before ISCOMs reach immunocompetent cells of the lymphoid organs of the gut.

It has been shown that the modulation of antigen uptake and induction of local innate immune responses contribute to the mucosal adjuvant properties of ISCOMs. In mice that were fed ISCOMs containing ovalbumin, recruitment of dendritic cells (DCs), activation of MØs and lymphocytes in the mesenteric lymph nodes, and recruitment of MØs and B cells in the Peyer's patches were observed (Furrie et al., 2002). In addition, feeding ISCOMs prior to a tolerogenic dose of ovalbumin prevented the induction of tolerance, as measured by the development of delayed-type hypersensitivity and IgG responses upon transfer of serum of immunized mice to naïve recipients. The enhanced immunogenicity of ISCOMs is dependent on the induction of IL-12 but not other mediators of innate immunity such as IL-4, IL-6, NO, and IFN-γ (Mowat et al., 1999; Grdic et al., 1999; and Smith et al., 1999).

The potential of ISCOMs given by the oral route to induce protective immunity has been evaluated for a variety of microbial pathogens. Oral immunization of mice with influenza antigens induced virus-specific serum IgG and nasal wash IgG and IgA antibodies, although comparable doses of ISCOMs given by the intramuscular route were found to be more immunogenic (Ghazi et al., 1995). Mice given herpes simplex virus (HSV)-2 ISCOM preparations by the oral route developed serum IgG and nasal IgA antibodies (Mohamedi et al., 2001). In addition, virus-specific T-cell responses were induced, as measured by lymphoproliferative responses and IL-2, IL-4 and IFN-γ production in splenocyte cultures. When HSV-2 ISCOMs were given orally or subcutaneously to mice that had experienced a previous infection with HSV-2, these mice were protected against a lethal challenge with HSV-1. Furthermore, in mice primed by infection with a human rotavirus, strong local and systemic B-cell responses were induced upon vaccination with virus-like particles (VLPs) adhered to ISCOM matrix but not after vaccination with VLPs alone. The induced B cell responses correlated with protection against a challenge infection in these animals (Iosef et al., 2002). Finally, oral immunization of mice with ISCOMs containing the P27 *E. falciformis* sporozoite surface antigen induced systemic IgG, mucosal IgA, and cellular responses and provided partial protection against an oocyte challenge (Kazanji et al., 1994).

Nasal immunization

Upon nasal immunization with ISCOMs containing the major outer-membrane protein of *Chlamydia trachomatis*, mice developed genital Th1 responses; however, these were much lower than after intramuscular immunization (Igietseme and Murdin, 2000). Following a high dosing of influenza ISCOM, mice developed systemic IgG and IgA responses, IgA antibodies in nasal washes, and a systemic CTL response, comparable to the responses to a low dose of influenza ISCOMs given by the subcutaneous route (Lövgren *et al.*, 1990; Sjölander *et al.*, 2001). When a low dose (0.25 µg) of influenza ISCOM was used for nasal immunization of mice, no mucosal antibody response was observed (Ben Ahmeida *et al.*, 1993). In mice, nasal immunization with ISCOMs containing the membrane antigens of *Mycoplasma mycoides* subs. *mycoides* resulted in potent systemic and mucosal antibody responses, which were higher than those induced after subcutaneous or nasal immunization with whole-cell antigen (Abusugra and Morein, 1999). ISCOMs have also been found to be an efficient mucosal delivery system for the envelope proteins of respiratory syncytial virus (RSV), an important causative agent of viral respiratory tract infections. Nasal immunization of mice with an RSV ISCOM vaccine resulted in potent IgA antibody responses in the upper respiratory tract and the lungs, systemic antibody responses, CTL responses, and reduced virus titers upon challenge with RSV (Trudel *et al.*, 1992; Hu *et al.*, 1998). Nasal ISCOM immunization of cows also proved to be effective in protecting the animals from disease after infection with bovine herpesvirus 1 (BHV-1) and reduced virus shedding considerably (Trudel *et al.*, 1988).

The adjuvant activity of ISCOMs administered by the nasal or oral routes could be further enhanced by the addition of a fusion protein of the cholera toxin CTA1 subunit and a B cell targeting moiety D of the *Staphylococcus aureus* protein A (Mowat *et al.*, 2001). Furthermore, studies with ISCOMs that were targeted to receptors at mucosal sites and to which other antigens had been coupled showed the potential of ISCOMs as a vehicle for the directional delivery of several antigens to mucosal surfaces and for inducing local and systemic immune responses (Ekström *et al.*, 1999).

Toxicity issues of ISCOM-based vaccines: selection of the optimal saponin combination

The use of new generations of adjuvants or adjuvant systems in vaccines for human use can be considered only if no major mucosal or systemic side effects are associated with their use. When ISCOMs are considered for human use, it should probably first be noted that Quil A, as a crude extract of the bark of the *Q. saponaria Molina*, is and has been widely used as an adjuvant for veterinary vaccines at concentrations about 100- to 1000-fold higher than those used in ISCOM preparations. So far, only limited numbers of studies have been published on the *in vivo* toxicity of ISCOMs. An early study using crude Quil A as a basis for ISCOM formulation showed that only moderate inflammatory reactions were found in rats inoculated with an ISCOM dose into which about 60 µg of Quil A was incorporated (Speijers *et al.*, 1988). Furthermore, it was shown that the hemolytic activity of Quil A incorporated into ISCOMs was about 10 times lower that that of unincorporated Quil A.

Several groups have now attempted to define Quil A components that are not toxic but do exhibit the characteristic immunity-enhancing properties when incorporated into ISCOMs. By reverse-phase high-pressure liquid chromatography (HPLC), several fractions of Quil A have been identified that seem to fulfill these criteria. One fraction, called QS-7, was defined that was relative nontoxic for mice and had a high adjuvant activity, although it was not tested as an adjuvant moiety in the ISCOM matrix (Kensil *et al.*, 1991). Separation of several fractions and combinations of fractions of Quil A in basically the same way resulted in the identification of a number of purified or partly purified fractions of saponins that formed ISCOMs with immunogenic properties that could not be distinguished from those of unpurified Quil A–based ISCOMs (Kersten, 1991).

A mixture of well-defined, purified Quil A components that apparently fulfills all the previously mentioned criteria has become available (Iscoprep 703; see earlier discussion). It should also be noted that a commercial ISCOM-based equine influenza vaccine using crude Quil A as a source of saponins has been on the market for several years without causing any problems involving side effects. Furthermore, ongoing clinical trials involving humans and ISCOM-based candidate vaccines have not shown problems of this nature so far. Finally, it should be realized that if ISCOMs are used for mucosal and especially orally applied vaccines in the future, the toxicity issue will probably become even less relevant since saponins are widely accepted and used as food additives.

Conclusions about ISCOMs

The ISCOM matrix is a highly promising structure for use in vaccines, since it complies with basically all the requirements for a modern adjuvant system **(Table 55.3)**. ISCOM-based vaccines induce high titers of long-lasting biologically relevant antibodies, which also takes place in the presence of pre-existing specific antibodies. ISCOM-based vaccines induce potent specific cell-mediated immune responses,

Table 55.3. Advantages of ISCOMs as Antigen Presentation Systems

Induction of potent antibody responses
Biologically active (e.g., virus neutralizing), long lasting
Also in the presence of preexisting specific antibody
Induction of potent T-cell responses
MHC class II restricted CD4+ T cells
MHC class I restricted CD8+ cytotoxic T lymphocytes
Function in the presence of preexisting specific antibody
Induction of immunity after mucosal delivery
Mucosal immunity
Systemic immunity
Induction of protective immune responses
Absence of toxicity
Accepted for animal vaccines
Accepted for human vaccines—selected glycosides
Suitable for large-scale vaccine production
Well-defined production technology
Very stable vaccines (lyophilization possible)

including CD8[+] MHC class I restricted CTL responses, which also takes place in the presence of preexisting specific antibodies. Both mucosal and systemic immune responses can be elicited by administering ISCOM vaccines either by mucosal or parenteral routes. The induced immune responses have been shown to be protective for long periods of time in many viral, bacterial, and parasitic systems. To date, the mechanisms by which the ISCOM presentation form exerts its adjuvant activities are not fully understood, although several research groups are presently conducting studies to elucidate the basic mechanism underlying these activities. On the basis of present knowledge, it may be expected that ISCOM-based vaccines will contribute to the combat of infectious diseases for which no adequate vaccines are currently available.

ACKNOWLEDGMENTS

The author of the microparticles section (D. O'Hagan) thanks the members of the Vaccine Delivery group at Chiron for generating the data used in this chapter, particularly Manmohan Singh, Michael Vajdy, and Mildred Ugozzoli, and also thanks Nelle Cronen for editorial assistance. The studies described in this chapter, which were performed in the laboratories of the authors of the liposome section (S. Michalek and N. Childers) were supported in part by U.S. Public Health Service grants DE 08182, DE 09081, and DE 09846 from the National Institutes of Health, grants from the World Health Organization, and contracts from the U.S. Army Medical Research Acquisition Activity. The authors of the ISCOM section (G. Rimmelzwaan and A. Osterhaus) thank Conny Kruyssen for assistance in preparing the manuscript. The authors of this chapter thank Keli Broome for editorial assistance.

REFERENCES

Abraham, E. (1992). Intranasal immunization with bacterial polysaccharide containing liposomes enhances antigen-specific pulmonary secretory antibody response. *Vaccine* 10, 461–468.

Abraham, E., and Shah, S. (1992). Intranasal immunization with liposomes containing IL-2 enhances bacterial polysaccharide antigen–specific pulmonary secretory antibody response. *J. Immunol.* 149, 3719–3726.

Abusugra, I., and Morein B. (1999). ISCOM is an efficient mucosal delivery system for *Mycoplasma mycoides* subsp. *mycoides* (MmmSC) antigens inducing high mucosal and systemic antibody responses. *FEMS Immunol. Med. Microbiol.* 23, 5–12.

Allaoui-Attarki, K., Pecquet, S., Fattal, E., Trolle, S., Chachaty, E., Couvreur, P., and Andremont, A. (1997). Protective immunity against *Salmonella typhimurium* elicited in mice by oral vaccination with phosphorylcholine encapsulated in poly (DL-lactide-co-glycolide) microspheres. *Infect. Immun.* 65, 853–857.

Alving, C.R. (1991) Liposomes as carriers of antigens and adjuvants. *J. Immunol. Methods* 140, 1–13.

Alving, C.R. (1995) Liposomes as vehicles for vaccines: induction of humoral, cellular, and mucosal immunity. In *Bacterial Toxins and Virulence Factors in Disease* (eds. J. Moss, B. Iglewski, M. Vaughan, and A.T. Tu). New York: Marcel Dekker, 47–58.

Andersson, C., Sandberg, L., Wernerus, H., Johansson, M., Lövgren-Bengtsson, K., Stahl S. (2000). Improved systems for hydrophobic tagging of recombinant immunogens for efficient ISCOM incorporation. *J. Immunol. Methods* 238, 181–193.

Andersson, C., Sandberg, L., Murby, M., Sjölander, A., Lövgren-Bengtsson, K., and Stahl, S. (1999). General expression vectors for production of hydrophobically tagged immunogens for direct ISCOM incorporation. *J. Immunol. Methods* 222, 171–182.

Ando, S., Putnam, D., Pack, D. W., and Langer, R. (1999). PLGA microspheres containing plasmid DNA: Preservation of supercoiled DNA via cryopreparation and carbohydrate stabilization. *J. Pharm. Sci.* 88, 126–130.

Bangham, A.D., Standish, M.M., and Watkins, J.C. (1965). Diffusion of univalent ions across the lamellae of swollen phospholipids. *J. Mol. Biol.* 13, 238–252.

Barackman, J. D., Ott, G., Pine, S., and O'Hagan, D. T. (2001). Oral administration of influenza vaccine in combination with the adjuvants LT-K63 and LT-R72 induces potent immune responses comparable to or stronger than traditional intramuscular immunization. *Clin. Diagn. Lab. Immunol.* 8, 652–657.

Baras, B., Benoit, M. A., Dupre, L., Poulain-Godefroy, O., Schacht, A. M., Capron, A., Gillard, J., and Riveau, G., (1999). Single-dose mucosal immunization with biodegradable microparticles containing a *Schistosoma mansoni* antigen. *Infect. Immun.* 67, 2643–2648.

Ben Ahmeida, E.T., Gregoriadis, G., Potter, C.W., and Jennings, R. (1993). Immunopotentiation of local and systemic humoral immune responses by ISCOMs, liposomes and FCA: Role in protection against influenza A in mice. *Vaccine* 11, 1302–1309.

Bergquist, C., Johansson, E. L., Lagergard, T., Holmgren, J., and Rudin, A. (1997). Intranasal vaccination of humans with recombinant cholera toxin B subunit induces systemic and local antibody responses in the upper respiratory tract and the vagina. *Infect. Immun.* 65, 2676–2684.

Boisgerault, F., Moron, G., and Leclerc, C. (2002). Virus-like particles: a new family of delivery systems. *Expert Rev. Vaccines* 1, 101–109.

Boyaka, P. N., Wright, P. F., Marinaro, M., Kiyono, H., Johnson, J. E., Gonzales, R. A., Ikizler, M. R., Werkhaven, J. A., Jackson, R. J., Fujihashi, K., Di Fabio, S., Staats, H. F., and McGhee, J. R. (2000). Human nasopharyngeal-associated lymphoreticular tissues: functional analysis of subepithelial and intraepithelial B and T cells from adenoids and tonsils. *Am. J. Pathol.* 157, 2023–35.

Brayden, D. J. (2001). Oral vaccination in man using antigens in particles: current status. *Eur. J. Pharm. Sci.* 14, 183–189.

Cahill, E. S., O'Hagan, D. T., Illum, L., Barnard, A., Mills, K. H., and Redhead, K. (1995). Immune responses and protection against *Bordetella pertussis* infection after intranasal immunization of mice with filamentous haemagglutinin in solution or incorporated in biodegradable microparticles. *Vaccine* 13, 455–462.

Challacombe, S. J., Rahman, D., Jeffery, H., Davis, S. S., and O'Hagan, D. T. (1992). Enhanced secretory IgA and systemic IgG antibody responses after oral immunization with biodegradable microparticles containing antigen. *Immunology* 76, 164–168.

Challacombe, S. J., Rahman, D., and O'Hagan, D. T. (1997). Salivary, gut, vaginal and nasal antibody responses after oral immunization with biodegradable microparticles. *Vaccine* 15, 169–175.

Chen, H., and Langer, R. (1998). Oral particulate delivery: status and future trends. *Adv. Drug Deliv. Rev.* 34, 339–350.

Chen, H. Torchilin. V. and Langer, R. (1996a). Polymerized liposomes as potential oral vaccine carriers: stability and bioavailability. *J. Controlled Release* 42, 263–272.

Chen, H. Torchilin. V. and Langer, R. (1996). Lectin-bearing polymerized liposomes as potential oral vaccine carriers. *Pharm. Res.* 13, 1378–1383.

Chen, S. C., Jones, D. H., Fynan, E. F., Farrar, G. H., Clegg, J. C., Greenberg, H. B., and Herrmann, J. E. (1998). Protective immunity induced by oral immunization with a rotavirus DNA vaccine encapsulated in microparticles. *J. Virol.* 72, 5757–5761.

Childers, N.K., and Michalek, S.M. (1994). Liposomes. In *Novel Delivery Systems for Oral Vaccine Development* (ed. D.T. O'Hagan). Boca Raton, Florida: CRC Press, 241–254.

Childers, N.K., Miller, K.L., Tong, G., Llarena, J.C., Greenway, T., Ulrich, J.T., and Michalek, S.M. (2000). Adjuvant activity of monophosphoryl lipid A for nasal and oral immunization with soluble or liposome associated antigen. *Infect. Immun.* 68, 5509–5516.

Childers, N.K., Tong, G., Mitchell, S., Kirk, K., Russell, M.W., and Michalek, S.M. (1999). A controlled clinical study of the effect of nasal immunization with a *Streptococcus mutans* antigen alone or incorporated into liposomes on induction of immune responses. *Infect. Immun.* 67, 618–623.

Childers, N.K., Tong, G., Li, F., Dasanayake, A.P., Kirk, K., and Michalek, S.M. (2002). Humans immunized with *Streptococcus mutans* antigens by mucosal routes. *J. Dent. Res.* 81, 48–52.

Childers, N.K., Zhang, S.S., Harokopakis, E., Harmon, C.C., and Michalek, S.M. (1996). Properties of practical oral liposome–*Streptococcus mutans* glucosyltransferase vaccines for effective induction of caries protection. *Oral Microbiol. Immunol.* 11, 172–180.

Childers, N.K., Zhang, S.S., and Michalek, S.M. (1994). Oral immunization of humans with dehydrated liposomes containing *Streptococcus mutans* glucosyltransferase induces salivary IgA2 antibody responses. *Oral Microbiol. Immunol.* 9, 146–153.

Chin, J., San Gil, F., Novak, M., Eamens, G., Djordjevic, S., Simecka, J., Duncan, J., and Mullbacher, A. (1996). Manipulating systemic and mucosal immune responses with skin-deliverable adjuvants. *J. Biotechnol.* 44, 13–19.

Claassen, I.J., Osterhaus, A.D., and Claassen, E. (1995). Antigen detection in vivo after immunization with different presentation forms of rabies virus antigen: involvement of marginal metallophilic macrophages in the uptake of immune-stimulating complexes. *Eur. J. Immunol.* 25, 1446–1452.

Conway, M. A., Madrigal-Estebas, L., McClean, S., Brayden, D. J., and Mills, K. H. (2001). Protection against *Bordetella pertussis* infection following parenteral or oral immunization with antigens entrapped in biodegradable particles: Effect of formulation and route of immunization on induction of Th1 and Th2 cells. *Vaccine* 19, 1940–1950.

Debin, A., Kravtzoff, R., Santiago, J. V., Cazales, L., Sperandio, S., Melber, K., Janowicz, Z., Betbeder, D., and Moynier, M. (2002). Intranasal immunization with recombinant antigens associated with new cationic particles induces strong mucosal as well as systemic antibody and CTL responses. *Vaccine* 20, 2752–2763.

de Haan, A., Geerligs, H.J., Huchshorn, J.P., van Scharrenburg, G.J.M., Palache, A.M., and Wilschut, J. (1995). Mucosal immunoadjuvant activity of liposomes: Induction of systemic IgG and secretory IgA responses in mice by intranasal immunization with an influenza subunit vaccine and coadministered liposomes. *Vaccine* 13, 155–162.

de Haan, A., Renegar, K.B., Small, P.A., Jr., and Wilschut, J. (1995). Induction of a secretory IgA response in the murine female urogenital tract by immunization of the lungs with liposome-supplemented viral subunit antigen. *Vaccine* 13, 613–616.

Denis-Mize, K. S., Dupuis, M., MacKichan, M. L., Singh, M., Doe, B., O'Hagan, D., Ulmer, J. B., Donnelly, J. J., McDonald, D. M., and Ott, G. (2000). Plasmid DNA adsorbed onto cationic microparticles mediates target gene expression and antigen presentation by dendritic cells. *Gene Ther.* 7, 2105–2112.

Di Tommaso, A., Saletti, G., Pizza, M., Rappuoli, R., Dougan, G., Abrignani, S., Douce, G., and De Magistris, M. T. (1996). Induction of antigen-specific antibodies in vaginal secretions by using a nontoxic mutant of heat-labile enterotoxin as a mucosal adjuvant. *Infect. Immun.* 64, 974–979.

Donnelly, J.J., Ulmer, J. B., and Liu, M. A. (1997). DNA vaccines. *Life Sci.* 60, 163–172.

Donnelly, J. J., Friedman, A., Martinez, D., Montgomery, D. L., Shiver, J. W., Motzel, S. L., Ulmer, J. B., and Liu, M. A. (1995). Preclinical efficacy of a prototype DNA vaccine: enhanced protection against antigenic drift in influenza virus. *Nat. Med.* 1, 583–587.

Duzgunes, N., and Shlomo, N. (1999). Mechanisms and kinetics of liposome-cell interactions. *Adv. Drug Deliv. Rev.* 40, 3–18.

Edwards, D. A., Hanes, J., Caponetti, G., Hrkach, J., Ben Jebria, A., Eskew, M. L., Mintzes, J., Deaver, D., Lotan, N., and Langer, R.

(1997). Large porous particles for pulmonary drug delivery. *Science* 276, 1868–1871.

Ekström, J., Hu, K.F., Bengtsson, K.L., and Morein, B. (1999). ISCOM and ISCOM-matrix enhance by intranasal route the IgA responses to OVA and rCTB in local and remote mucosal secretions. *Vaccine* 17, 2690–2701.

Eldridge, J. H., Hammond, C. J., Meulbroek, J. A., Staas, J. K., Gilley, R. M., and Tice, T. R. (1990). Controlled vaccine release in the gut-associated lymphoid tissues. I. Orally administered biodegradable microspheres target the Peyer's patches. *J. Controlled Release* 11, 205–214.

el Guink, N., Kris, R.M., Goodman-Snitkoff, G., Small, P.A., Jr., and Mannino, R.J. (1989). Intranasal immunization with proteoliposomes protects against influenza. *Vaccine* 7, 147–151.

Eyles, J.E., Williamson, E.D., and Alpar, H. O. (1999). Immunological responses to nasal delivery of free and encapsulated tetanus toxoid: Studies on the effect of vehicle volume. *Int. J. Pharm.* 189, 75–79.

Eyles, J. E., Williamson, E. D., Spiers, I. D., and Alpar, H. O. (2000). Protection studies following bronchopulmonary and intramuscular immunisation with *Yersinia pestis* F1 and V subunit vaccines coencapsulated in biodegradable microspheres: A comparison of efficacy. *Vaccine* 18, 3266–71.

Farhood, H., Gao, X., Son, K., Yang, Y.-Y., Lazo, J.S., Huang, L., Barsoum, J., Bottega, R., and Epand, R.M. (1994). Cationic liposomes for direct gene transfer in therapy of cancer and other diseases. *Ann. N.Y. Acad. Sci.* 716, 23–34.

Felgner, P.L., Gadek, T.R., Holm, M., Roman, R., Chan, H.W., Wenz, M., Northrop, J.P., Ringold, G.M., and Danielsen, M. (1987). Lipofection: a highly efficient, lipid-mediated DNA-transfection procedure. *Proc. Natl. Acad. Sci. USA* 84, 7413–7417.

Furrie, E., Smith, R.E., Turner, M.W., Strobel, S. and Mowat, A.M. (2002). Induction of local innate immune responses and modulation of antigen uptake as mechanisms underlying the mucosal adjuvant properties of immune stimulating complexes (ISCOMs). *Vaccine* 20, 2254–2262.

Gallichan, W. S., and Rosenthal, K. L. (1995). Specific secretory immune responses in the female genital tract following intranasal immunization with a recombinant adenovirus expressing glycoprotein B of herpes simplex virus. *Vaccine* 13, 1589–1595.

Ghazi, H.O., Potter, C.W., Smith, T.L., and Jennings, R. (1995). Comparative antibody responses and protection in mice immunised by oral or parenteral routes with influenza virus subunit antigens in aqueous form or incorporated into ISCOMs. *J. Med. Microbiol.* 42, 53–61.

Giuliani, M. M., Del Giudice, G., Giannelli, V., Dougan, G., Douce, G., Rappuoli, R., and Pizza, M. (1998). Mucosal adjuvanticity and immunogenicity of LTR72, a novel mutant of *Escherichia coli* heat-labile enterotoxin with partial knockout of ADP-ribosyltransferase activity. *J. Exp. Med.* 187, 1123–1132.

Grdic, D., Smith, R., Donachie, A., Kjerrulf, M., Hörnquist, E., Mowat, A., and Lycke, N. (1999). The mucosal adjuvant effects of cholera toxin and immune-stimulating complexes differ in their requirement for IL-12, indicating different pathways of action. *Eur. J. Immunol.* 29, 1774–1784.

Gregoriadis, G. (1990). Immunological adjuvants: A role for liposomes. *Immunol. Today* 11, 89–97.

Gregoriadis, G. (1992). Liposomes as immunological adjuvants: approaches to immunopotentiation including ligand-mediated targeting to macrophages. *Res. Immunol.* 143, 178–185.

Gregoriadis, G. (1995). Engineering liposomes for drug delivery: progress and problems. *Trends Biotechnol.* 13, 527–537.

Gregoriadis, G., McCormack, B., Obrenovic, M., Saffie, R., Zadi, B., and Perrie, Y. (1999). Vaccine entrapment in liposomes. *Methods* 19, 156–162.

Guerrero, R. A., Ball, J. M., Krater, S. S., Pacheco, S. E., Clements, J. D., and Estes, M. K. (2001). Recombinant Norwalk virus–like particles administered intranasally to mice induce systemic and mucosal (fecal and vaginal) immune responses. *J. Virol.* 75, 9713–9722.

Haneberg, B., Kendall, D., Amerongen, H. M., Apter, F. M., Kraehenbuhl, J. P., and Neutra, M. R. (1994). Induction of specific immunoglobulin A in the small intestine, colon–rectum, and vagina measured by a new method for collection of secretions from local mucosal surfaces. *Infect. Immun.* 62, 15–23.

Harokopakis, E., Hajishengallis, G., and Michalek, S.M. (1998). Effectiveness of liposomes possessing surface-linked recombinant B subunit of cholera toxin as an oral antigen delivery system. *Infect. Immun.* 66, 4299–4304.

Heritage, P. L., Brook, M. A., Underdown, B. J., and McDermott, M. R. (1998). Intranasal immunization with polymer-grafted microparticles activates the nasal-associated lymphoid tissue and draining lymph nodes. *Immunology* 93, 249–256.

Higaki, M., Takase, T., Igarashi, R., Suzuki, Y., Aizawa, C., and Mizushima, Y. (1998). Enhancement of immune response to intranasal influenza HA vaccine by microparticle resin. *Vaccine* 16, 741–745.

Hu, K.F., Elvander, M., Merza, M., Akerblom, L., Brandenburg, A., and Morein, B. (1998). The immunostimulating complex (ISCOM) is an efficient mucosal delivery system for respiratory syncytial virus (RSV) envelope antigens inducing high local and systemic antibody responses. *Clin. Exp. Immunol.* 113, 235–243.

Hulskotte, E.G., Geretti, A.M., Siebelink, K.H., van Amerongen, G., Cranage, M.P., Rud, E.W., Norley, S.G., de Vries, P., and Osterhaus, A.D. (1995). Vaccine-induced virus-neutralizing antibodies and cytotoxic T cells do not protect macaques from experimental infection with simian immunodeficiency virus SIVmac32H (J5). *J. Virol.* 69, 6289–96.

Igietseme, J.U., and Murdin, A. (2000). Induction of protective immunity against *Chlamydia trachomatis* genital infection by a vaccine based on major outer membrane protein–lipophilic immune response–stimulating complexes. *Infect. Immun.* 68, 6798–6806.

Iosef, C., van Nguyen, T., Jeong, K., Bengtsson, K., Morein, B., Kim, Y., Chang, K.-O., Azevedo, M.S., Yuan, L., Nielsen, P., and Saif, L.J. (2002). Systemic and intestinal antibody secreting cell responses and protection in gnotobiotic pigs immunized orally with attenuated Wa human rotavirus and Wa 2/6-rotavirus-like particles associated with immunostimulating complexes. *Vaccine* 20, 1741–1753.

Johansson, E. L., Rask, C., Fredriksson, M., Eriksson, K., Czerkinsky, C., and Holmgren, J. (1998). Antibodies and antibody-secreting cells in the female genital tract after vaginal or intranasal immunization with cholera toxin B subunit or conjugates. *Infect. Immun.* 66, 514–520.

Jones, D. H., Corris, S., McDonald, S., Clegg, J. C., and Farrar, G. H. (1997). Poly(DL-lactide-co-glycolide)-encapsulated plasmid DNA elicits systemic and mucosal antibody responses to encoded protein after oral administration. *Vaccine* 15, 814–817.

Jones, D. H., McBride, B. W., Thornton, C., O'Hagan, D. T., Robinson, A., and Farrar, G. H. (1996). Orally administered microencapsulated *Bordetella pertussis* fimbriae protect mice from *B. pertussis* respiratory infection. *Infect. Immun.* 64, 489–494.

Kazanji, M., Laurent, F., and Pery, P. (1994). Immune responses and protective effect in mice vaccinated orally with surface sporozoite protein of *Eimeria falciformis* in ISCOMs. *Vaccine* 12, 798–804.

Kensil, C.R., Patel, U., Lennick, M., and Marciani, D. (1991). Separation and characterization of saponins with adjuvant activity from *Quillaja saponaria Molina* cortex. *J. Immunol.* 146, 431–437.

Kersten, G.F.A. (1991). Aspects of ISCOMs: analytical, pharmaceutical and adjuvant properties. Thesis. Utrecht, The Netherlands, State University.

Kokkona, M., Kallinteri, P., Fatouros, D., and Antimisiaris, S.G. (2000). Stability of SUV liposomes in the presence of cholate salts and pancreatic lipases: effect of lipid composition. *Eur. J. Pharm. Sci.* 9, 245–252.

Kuper, C. F., Koornstra, P. J., Hameleers, D. M., Biewenga, J., Spit, B. J., Duijvestijn, A. M., van Breda Vriesman, P. J., and Sminia, T. (1992). The role of nasopharyngeal lymphoid tissue [see comments]. *Immunol. Today* 13, 219–224.

Lasic, D.D. (1998). Novel applications of liposomes. *Trends Biotechnol.* 16, 307–321.

Lian, T., and Ho, R.J. (1997). Cholera toxin B–mediated targeting of lipid vesicles containing ganglioside GM1 to mucosal epithelial cells. *Pharm. Res.* 14, 1309–1315.

Lövgren, K., Lindmark, J., Pipkorn, R., and Morein, B. (1987). Antigenic presentation of small molecules and peptides conjugated to a preformed ISCOM as carrier. *J. Immunol. Methods* 98, 137–143.

Lövgren, K., and Morein, B. (1988). The requirement of lipids for the formation of immunostimulating complexes (ISCOMs). *Biotechnol. Appl. Biochem.* 10, 161–172.

Lövgren, K., Kaberg, H., and Morein, B. (1990). An experimental influenza subunit vaccine (ISCOMs): induction of protective immunity to challenge infection in mice after intranasal or subcutaneous administration. *Clin. Exp. Immunol.* 82, 435–439.

Malone, J. G., Bergland, P. J., Liljestrom, P., Rhodes, G. H., and Malone, R.W. (1997). Mucosal immune responses associated with polynucleotide vaccination. *Behring Inst. Mitt.* 98, 63–72.

Maloy, K.J., Donachie, A.M., and Mowat, A.M. (1995). Induction of Th1 and Th2 CD4+ T cell responses by oral or parenteral immunization with ISCOMs. *Eur. J. Immunol.* 25, 2835–2841.

Maloy, K. J., Donachie, A. M., O'Hagan, D. T., and Mowat, A. M. (1994). Induction of mucosal and systemic immune responses by immunization with ovalbumin entrapped in poly(lactide-co-glycolide) microparticles. *Immunology* 81, 661–667.

Marx, P. A., Compans, R. W., Gettie, A., Staas, J. K., Gilley, R. M., Mulligan, M. J., Yamshchikov, G. V., Chen, D., and Eldridge, J. H. (1993). Protection against vaginal SIV transmission with microencapsulated vaccine. *Science* 260, 1323–1327.

Masinde, L. E., and Hickey, A. J. (1993). Aerosolized suspensions of poly (L-lactic acid) microspheres. *Int. J. Pharm.* 100, 123–131.

Matyas, G.R., and Alving, C.R. (1996). Protective prophylactic immunity against intranasal ricin challenge induced by liposomal ricin A subunit. *Vaccine Res.* 5, 163–172.

McDermott, M. R., Heritage, P. L., Bartzoka, V., and Brook, M. A. (1998). Polymer-grafted starch microparticles for oral and nasal immunization. *Immunol. Cell Biol.* 76, 256–262.

McGhee, J. R., Lamm, M. E., and Strober, W. (1999). Mucosal immune responses. In *Mucosal Immunology* (eds. P. L. Ogra, J. Mestecky, M. E. Lamm, W. Strober, J. Bienenstock, and J. R. McGhee). San Diego: Academic Press, 485–506.

Michalek, S.M., Childers, N.K., Katz, J., Dertzbaugh, M., Zhang, S., Russell, M.W., Macrina, F.L., Jackson, S., and Mestecky, J. (1992). Liposomes and conjugate vaccines for antigen delivery and induction of mucosal immune responses. In *Genetically Engineered Vaccines: Prospects for Oral Disease Prevention* (eds. J. Ciardi, J. Keith, and J.R. McGhee). New York: Plenum Publishing Corporation, 191–198.

Michalek, S.M., Childers, N.K., and Dertzbaugh, M.T. (1995). Vaccination strategies for mucosal pathogens. In *Virulence Mechanisms of Bacterial Pathogens* (eds. J.A. Roth, C.A. Bolin, K.A. Brogden, F.C. Minion, and M.J. Wannemuehler), 2nd ed. Washington, DC: ASM Press, 269–302.

Michalek, S.M., Eldridge, J.H., Curtiss, R. III, and Rosenthal, K.L. (1994). Antigen delivery systems: new approach to mucosal immunization. In: *Handbook of Mucosal Immunology* (eds P.L. Ogra, J. Mestecky, M.E. Lamm, W. Strober, J. McGhee, and J. Bienenstock). San Diego: Academic Press, 373–386.

Mohamedi, S.A., Heath, A.W., and Jennings, R. (2001). A comparison of oral and parenteral routes for therapeutic vaccination with HSV-2 ISCOMs in mice; cytokine profiles, antibody responses and protection. *Antiviral Res.* 49, 83–99.

Moore, A., McGuirk, P., Adams, S., Jones, W. C., McGee, J. P., O'Hagan, D. T., and Mills, K. H. (1995). Immunization with a soluble recombinant HIV protein entrapped in biodegradable microparticles induces HIV-specific CD8+ cytotoxic T lymphocytes and CD4+ Th1 cells. *Vaccine* 13, 1741–1749.

Mora, A. L., and Tam, J. P. (1998). Controlled lipidation and encapsulation of peptides as a useful approach to mucosal immunizations. *J. Immunol.* 161, 3616–3623.

Morein, B., Sundquist, B., Hoglund, S., Dalsgaard, K., and Osterhaus, A.D. (1984). ISCOM, a novel structure for antigenic presentation of membrane proteins from enveloped viruses. *Nature* 308, 457–460.

Morein, B., Ekström, J., and Lövgren, K. (1990). Increased immunogenicity of a non-amphipathic protein (BSA) after inclusion into ISCOMS. *J. Immunol. Methods* 128, 177–181.

Mowat, A.M., Donachie, A.M., Jägewall, S., Schön, K., Löwenadler, B., Dalsgaard, K., Kaastrup, P., and Lycke, N. (2001). CTA1-DD-immune stimulating complexes: a novel, rationally designed combined mucosal vaccine adjuvant effective with nanogram doses of antigen. *J. Immunol.* 167, 3398–3405.

Mowat, A.M., Donachie, A.M., Reid, G., and Jarrett, O. (1991). Immune-stimulating complexes containing Quil A and protein antigen prime class I MHC-restricted T lymphocytes *in vivo* and are immunogenic by the oral route. *Immunology* 72, 317–322.

Mowat, A.M., Maloy, K.J., and Donachie, A.M. (1993). Immune-stimulating complexes as adjuvants for inducing local and systemic immunity after oral immunization with protein antigens. *Immunology* 80, 527–534.

Mowat, A.M., and Donachie, A.M. (1991). ISCOMs: a novel strategy for mucosal immunization? *Immunol. Today* 12, 383–385.

Mowat, A.M., Smith, R.E., Donachie, A.M., Furie, E., Grdic, D., and Lycke, N. (1999). Oral vaccination with immune stimulating complexes. *Immunol. Today* 65, 133–140.

Murillo, M., Grillo, M. J., Rene, J., Marin, C. M., Barberan, M., Goni, M. M., Blasco, J. M., Irache, J. M., and Gamazo, C. (2001). A *Brucella ovis* antigenic complex bearing poly-epsilon-caprolactone microparticles confer protection against experimental brucellosis in mice. *Vaccine* 19, 4099–4106.

O'Hagan, D. T. (1994). Microparticles as oral vaccines. In *Novel Delivery Systems for Oral Vaccines* (ed. D. T. O'Hagan). Boca Raton, Florida: CRC Press, 175–205.

O'Hagan, D. T. (1997). Prospects for the development of new and improved vaccines through the use of microencapsulation technology. In *New Generation Vaccines* (eds. M. M. Levine, G. C. Woodrow, J. B. Kaper, and G. S. Cobon). New York: Marcel Dekker, 215–228.

O'Hagan, D. T. (1998). Microparticles and polymers for the mucosal delivery of vaccines. *Adv. Drug Deliv. Rev.* 34, 305–320.

O'Hagan, D. T., Rafferty, D., McKeating, J. A., and Illum, L. (1992). Vaginal immunization of rats with a synthetic peptide from human immunodeficiency virus envelope glycoprotein. *J. Gen. Virol.* 73, 2141–2145.

O'Hagan, D. T., Rafferty, D., Wharton, S., and Illum, L. (1993). Intravaginal immunization in sheep using a bioadhesive microsphere antigen delivery system. *Vaccine* 11, 660–664.

Gupta, R. K., Singh, M., and O'Hagan, D. T. (1998). Poly(lactide-co-glycolide) microparticles for the development of single-dose controlled-release vaccines. *Adv. Drug Deliv. Rev.* 32, 225–246.

Okada, E., Sasaki, S., Ishii, N., Aoki, I., Yasuda, T., Nishioka, K., Fukushima, J., Miyazaki, J., Wahren, B., and Okuda, K. (1997). Intranasal immunization of a DNA vaccine with IL-12- and granulocyte-macrophage colony–stimulating factor (GM-CSF)-expressing plasmids in liposomes induces strong mucosal and cell-mediated immune responses against HIV-1 antigens. *J. Immunol.* 159, 3638–3647.

Osterhaus, A., de Vries, P., and Heeney, J. (1992). AIDS vaccine developments. *Nature* 355, 684–685.

Osterhaus, A., Weijer, K., Uytdehaag, F., Jarrett, O., Sundquist, B., and Morein, B. (1985). Induction of protective immune response in cats by vaccination with feline leukemia virus ISCOM. *J. Immunol.* 135, 591–596.

Pierce, N.F., and Sacci, J.B., Jr. (1984). Enhanced mucosal priming by cholera toxin and procholeragenoid with a lipoidal amine adjuvant (avridine) delivered in liposomes. *Infect. Immun.* 44, 469–473.

Pierce, N.F., Sacci, J.B., Jr., Alving, C.R., and Richardson, E.C. (1984). Enhancement by lipid A of mucosal immunogenicity of liposome-associated cholera toxin. *Rev. Infect. Dis.* 6, 563–566.

Rhalem, A., Bourdieu, C., Luffau, G., and Pery, P. (1988). Vaccination of mice with liposome-entrapped adult antigens of *Nippostrongylus brasiliensis. Ann. Inst. Pasteur Immunol.* 139, 157–166.

Rimmelzwaan, G.F., Nieuwkoop, N., Brandenburg, A., Sutter, G., Beyer, W.E., Maher, D., Bates, J., and Osterhaus, A.D. (2000). A randomized, double blind study in young healthy adults comparing cell mediated and humoral immune responses induced by influenza ISCOM vaccines and conventional vaccines. *Vaccine* 19, 1180–1187.

Rimmelzwaan, G.F., Claas, E.C., van Amerongen, G., de Jong, J.C., and Osterhaus, A.D. (1999). ISCOM vaccine induced protection against a lethal challenge with a human H5N1 influenza virus. *Vaccine* 17, 1355–1358.

Rimmelzwaan, G.F., Baars, M., van Beek, R., van Amerongen, G., Lövgren-Bengtsson, K., Claas, E.C., and Osterhaus, A.D. (1997). Induction of protective immunity against influenza virus in a macaque model: comparison of conventional and iscom vaccines. *J. Gen. Virol.* 78, 757–765.

Rimmelzwaan, G.F., Siebelink, K.H., Huisman, R.C., Moss, B., Francis, M.J., and Osterhaus, A.D. (1994). Removal of the cleavage site of recombinant feline immunodeficiency virus envelope protein facilitates incorporation of the surface glycoprotein in immune-stimulating complexes. *J. Gen. Virol.* 75, 2097–2102.

Robinson, A.M., Creeth, J.E., and Jones, M.N. (1998). The specificity and affinity of immunoliposome targeting to oral bacteria. *Biochim. Biophys. Acta* 1369, 278–286.

Roy, M. J., Wu, M. S., Barr, L. J., Fuller, J. T., Tussey, L. G., Speller, S., Culp, J., Burkholder, J. K., Swain, W. F., Dixon, R. M., Widera, G., Vessey, R., King, A., Ogg, G., Gallimore, A., Haynes, J. R., and Heydenburg Fuller, D. (2000). Induction of antigen-specific CD8+ T cells, T helper cells, and protective levels of antibody in humans by particle-mediated administration of a hepatitis B virus DNA vaccine. *Vaccine* 19, 764–778.

Shahin, R., Leef, M., Eldridge, J., Hudson, M., and Gilley, R. (1995). Adjuvanticity and protective immunity elicited by *Bordetella pertussis* antigens encapsulated in poly(DL-lactide-co-glycolide) microspheres. *Infect. Immun.* 63, 1195–1200.

Shive, M.S. and Anderson, J.M. (1997). Biodegradation and biocompatability of PLA and PLGA microspheres. *Adv. Drug Deliv. Rev.* 28, 5–24.

Siebelink, K.H., Tijhaar, E., Huisman, R.C., Huisman, W., de Ronde, A., Darby, I.H., Francis, M.J., Rimmelzwaan, G.F., and Osterhaus, A.D. (1995). Enhancement of feline immunodeficiency virus infection after immunization with envelope glycoprotein subunit vaccines. *J. Virol.* 69, 3704–3711.

Simoes, S., Pires, P., Duzgunes, N., and Pedroso de Lima, M.C. (1999). Cationic liposomes as gene transfer vectors: Barriers to successful application in gene therapy. *Curr. Opin. Mol. Ther.* 1, 147–157.

Simoes, S., Slepushkin, V., Pires, P., Gaspar, R., Pedroso de Lima, M.C., and Duzgunes, N. (1999). Mechanisms of gene transfer mediated by lipoplexes associated with targeting ligands or pH-sensitive peptides. *Gene Ther.* 6, 1798–1807.

Singh, M., Briones, M., and O'Hagan, D.T. (2001). A novel bioadhesive intranasal delivery system for inactivated influenza vaccines. *J. Controlled Release* 70, 267–276.

Singh, M., Briones, M., Ott, G., and O'Hagan, D. (2000). Cationic microparticles: A potent delivery system for DNA vaccines. *Proc. Natl. Acad. Sci. USA* 97, 811–816.

Singh, M., Vajdy, M., Gardner, J., Briones, M., and O'Hagan, D. (2001). Mucosal immunization with HIV-1 gag DNA on cationic microparticles prolongs gene expression and enhances local and systemic immunity. *Vaccine* 20, 594–602.

Sjölander, S., Drane, D., Davis, R., Beezum, L., Pearse, M., and Cox, J. (2001). Intranasal immunisation with influenza-ISCOM induces strong mucosal as well as systemic antibody and cytotoxic T-lymphocyte responses. *Vaccine* 19, 4072–4080.

Smith, R.E., Donachie, A.M., Grdic, D., Lycke, N., and Mowat, A.M. (1999). Immune-stimulating complexes induce an IL-12-dependent cascade of innate immune responses. *J. Immunol.* 162, 5536–5546.

Speijers, G.J., Danse, L.H., Beuvery, E.C., Strik, J.J., and Vos, J.G. (1988). Local reactions of the saponin Quil A and a Quil A containing ISCOM measles vaccine after intramuscular injection of rats: A comparison with the effect of DPT-polio vaccine. *Fundam. Appl. Toxicol.* 10, 425–430.

Staats, H. F., Montgomery, S. P., and Palker, T. J. (1997). Intranasal immunization is superior to vaginal, gastric, or rectal immunization for the induction of systemic and mucosal anti-HIV antibody responses. *AIDS Res. Hum. Retroviruses* 13, 945–952.

Takahashi, H., Takeshita, T., Morein, B., Putney, S., Germain, R.N., and Berzofsky, J.A. (1990). Induction of CD8+ cytotoxic T cells by immunization with purified HIV-1 envelope protein in ISCOMs. *Nature* 344, 873–875.

Thapar, M.A., Parr, E.L., Bozzola, J.J., and Parr, M.B. (1991). Secretory immune responses in the mouse vagina after parenteral or intravaginal immunization with an immunostimulating complex (ISCOM). *Vaccine* 9, 129–33.

Trolle, S., Chachaty, E., Kassis-Chikhani, N., Wang, C., Fattal, E., Couvreur, P., Diamond, B., Alonso, J., and Andremont, A. (2000). Intranasal immunization with protein-linked phosphorylcholine protects mice against a lethal intranasal challenge with *Streptococcus pneumoniae*. *Vaccine* 18, 2991–2998.

Trudel, M., Boulay, G., Sequin, C., Nadon, F., and Lussier, G. (1988). Control of infectious bovine rhinotracheitis in calves with a BHV-1 subunit-ISCOM vaccine. *Vaccine* 6, 525–529.

Trudel, M., Nadon, F., Seguin, C., Brault, S., Lusignan, Y., and Lemieux S. (1992). Initiation of cytotoxic T-cell response and protection of BALB/c mice by vaccination with an experimental ISCOMs respiratory syncytial virus subunit vaccine. *Vaccine* 10, 107–112.

Tseng, J., Komisar, J. L., Trout, R. N., Hunt, R. E., Chen, J.Y., Johnson, A. J., Pitt, L., and Ruble, D. L. (1995). Humoral immunity to aerosolized staphylococcal enterotoxin B (SEB), a superantigen, in monkeys vaccinated with SEB toxoid-containing microspheres. *Infect. Immun.* 63, 2880–2885.

Ugozzoli, M., O'Hagan, D. T., and Ott, G. S. (1998). Intranasal immunization of mice with herpes simplex virus type 2 recombinant gD2: the effect of adjuvants on mucosal and serum antibody responses. *Immunology* 93, 563–571.

Ugozzoli, M., Santos, G., Donnelly, J., and O'Hagan, D. T. (2001). Potency of a genetically detoxified mucosal adjuvant derived from the heat-labile enterotoxin of *E. coli* (LTK63) is not adversely affected by the presence of pre-existing immunity to the adjuvant. *J. Infect. Dis.* 183, 351–354.

Vajdy, M., Gardner, J., Neidleman, J., Cuadra, L., Greer, C., Perri, S., O'Hagan, D., and Polo, J. M. (2001). Human immunodeficiency virus type 1 Gag-specific vaginal immunity and protection after local immunizations with Sindbis virus–based replicon particles. *J. Infect. Dis.* 184, 1613–1616.

Van Binnendijk, R.S., Poelen, M.C., van Amerongen, G., de Vries, P., and Osterhaus, A.D. (1997). Protective immunity in macaques vaccinated with live attenuated, recombinant, and subunit measles vaccines in the presence of passively acquired antibodies. *J. Infect. Dis.* 175, 524–532.

Van Binnendijk, R.S., van Baalen, C.A., Poelen, M.C., de Vries, P., Boes, J., Cerundolo, V., Osterhaus, A.D., and UytdeHaag, F.G.C.M. (1992). Measles virus transmembrane fusion protein synthesized *de novo* or presented in immunostimulating complexes is endogenously processed for HLA class I– and class II–restricted cytotoxic T cell recognition. *J. Exp. Med.* 176, 119–128.

Voeten, J.T., Rimmelzwaan, G.F., Nieuwkoop, N.J., Lövgren-Bengtsson, K., Osterhaus, A.D. (2000). Introduction of the haemagglutinin transmembrane region in the influenza virus matrix protein facilitates its incorporation into ISCOM and activation of specific CD8(+) cytotoxic T lymphocytes. *Vaccine* 19, 514–522.

von Hoegen, P. (2001). Synthetic biomimetic supra molecular Biovector (SMBV) particles for nasal vaccine delivery. *Adv. Drug Deliv. Rev.* 51, 113–125.

Wachsmann, D., Klein, J.P., Scholler, M., and Frank, R.M. (1985). Local and systemic immune response to orally administered liposome-associated soluble *S. mutans* cell wall antigens. *Immunology* 54, 189–193.

Wachsmann, D., Klein, J.P., Scholler, M., Ogier, J., Ackermans, F., and Frank, R.M. (1986). Serum and salivary antibody responses in rats orally immunized with *Streptococcus mutans* carbohydrate protein conjugate associated with liposomes. *Infect. Immun.* 52, 408–413.

Wang, R., Doolan, D. L., Le, T. P., Hedstrom, R. C., Coonan, K. M., Charoenvit, Y., Jones, T. R., Hobart, P., Margalith, M., Ng, J., Weiss, W. R., Sedegah, M., de Taisne, C., Norman, J. A., and Hoffman, S. L. (1998). Induction of antigen-specific cytotoxic T lymphocytes in humans by a malaria DNA vaccine. *Science* 282, 476–480.

Weiss, H.P., Stitz, L., and Becht, H. (1990). Immunogenic properties of ISCOM prepared with influenza virus nucleoprotein. *Arch. Virol.* 114, 109–120.

Whittum-Hudson, J. A., An, L. L., Saltzman, W. M., Prendergast, R. A., and MacDonald, A. B. (1996). Oral immunization with an anti-idiotypic antibody to the exoglycolipid antigen protects against experimental *Chlamydia trachomatis* infection. *Nat. Med.* 2, 1116–1121.

Wira, C. R., Richardson, J., and Prabhala, R. (1994). Endocrine regulation of mucosal immunity: effect of sex hormones and cytokines on the afferent and efferent arms of the immune system in the female reproductive tract. In *Handbook of Mucosal Immunology* (eds. P. L. Ogra, M. E. Lamm, J. R. McGhee, J. Mestecky, W. Strober, and J. Bienenstock). San Diego: Academic Press, 705–718.

Wong, J.P., Stadnyk, L.L., and Saravolac, E.G. (1994). Enhanced protection against respiratory influenza A infection in mice by liposome-encapsulated antibody. *Immunology* 81, 280–284.

Wu, H.Y., Abdu, S., Stinson, D., and Russell, M.W. (2000). Generation of female genital tract antibody responses by local or central (Common) mucosal immunization. *Infect. Immun.* 68, 5539–5545.

Yan, C., Rill, W. L., Malli, R., Hewetson, J., Naseem, H., Tammariello, R., and Kende, M. (1996). Intranasal stimulation of long-lasting immunity against aerosol ricin challenge with ricin toxoid vaccine encapsulated in polymeric microspheres. *Vaccine* 14, 1031–1038.

Zadi, B., and Gregoriadis, G. (2000). A novel method for high-yield entrapment of solutes into small liposomes. *J. Liposome Res.* 10, 73–80.

Antigen Delivery Systems II: Development of Live Recombinant Attenuated Bacterial Antigen and DNA Vaccine Delivery Vector Vaccines

Roy Curtiss III

Biodesign Institute and School of Life Sciences, Arizona State University, Tempe, Arizona

Attenuated bacteria that colonize on or invade through mucosal surfaces and/or mucosa-associated lymphoreticular tissues (MALT) can be and have been used as antigen or DNA (nucleic acid) vaccine delivery vectors to induce mucosal, systemic, and cellular immunities to bacterial, viral, parasitic, and fungal pathogens. In general, live recombinant attenuated bacteria are most often successfully used to deliver protective antigens to induce immunities to bacterial pathogens. These attenuated bacterial antigen delivery vectors can also be successfully used to deliver linear T- and B-cell epitopes derived from protective antigens from any pathogen and also non-posttranslationally modified (nonglycosylated) protective antigens from viral, parasitic, and fungal pathogens (provided that they fold correctly upon synthesis in the bacterial vector).

Use of attenuated bacteria to synthesize protective antigens for many viral, parasitic, and fungal pathogens does not result in a vaccine capable of inducing protective immunity because these protective antigens, when synthesized in a eukaryotic host, are usually posttranslationally modified, often by glycosylation, and have specific requirements to cause correct disulfide bond-dependent folding. The use of DNA vaccines against infections caused by viral, parasitic, and fungal pathogens thus has the potential to induce relevant protective immunities, since the protective antigens encoded by the nucleic acid vaccines are synthesized and appropriately modified and folded in the eukaryotic host being immunized. It follows that the use of nucleic acid vaccines to encode bacterial protective antigens will very often not induce relevant immunities unless the amino acid sequence of the bacterial protective antigen lacks N- and O-glycosylation sites and also folds properly upon synthesis in the eukaryotic cytoplasm. Since there are significant economies in using attenuated bacteria to deliver DNA vaccines to immunized animal and human hosts in comparison with the use of DNA vaccines isolated from bacterial cultures, there has been considerable interest and some success in using attenuated bacteria to deliver such DNA vaccines to elicit relevant protective immune responses to viral, parasitic and fungal pathogens (Dietrich *et al.*, 2000).

The focus of this review chapter will be on the use of attenuated bacterial systems to deliver antigens or DNA vaccine vectors to induce protective immunity to microbial pathogens that colonize on or invade through a mucosal surface. In other words, the focus will be on systems for the induction of mucosal immunity that are delivered to a mucosal site, usually by nasal or oral immunization. I have therefore ignored, without prejudice, reports primarily focusing on induction of cellular immunities with use of attenuated bacteria to deliver antigens and/or DNA vaccine vectors, unless they contain teachings relevant to the development of vaccine constructions that would be effective in inducing mucosal immunities. I have also ignored reports describing results obtained when vaccines were delivered by needles unless induction of mucosal immunity was quantitated.

Earlier research accomplishments in this field have been the subject of numerous reviews (Roberts *et al.*, 1994; Schodel and Curtiss, 1995; Curtiss *et al.*, 1996; Doggett and Brown, 1996; Hantman *et al.*, 1999; Liljeqvist and Stahl, 1999; Oggioni *et al.*, 1999; Sirard *et al.*, 1999; Levine, 2000; Mastroeni *et al.*, 2001; Galen and Levine, 2001; Curtiss, 2001; Drabner and Guzman, 2001; Medina and Guzman, 2001; Mielcarek *et al.*, 2001; Ohara and Yamada, 2001; Curtiss, 2002).

BACTERIAL DELIVERY VECTOR SYSTEMS

Bacterial delivery vector systems can be divided into two main groups: those that colonize on and invade through a mucosal surface and those that are noninvasive colonizers in proximity to a mucosal surface. The first group contains strains of *Salmonella*, *Shigella*, *Listeria*, *Mycobacterium*, and *Brucella*. The noninvasive colonizers include strains of *Vibrio*, *Escherichia*, *Yersinia*, *Streptococcus*, and *Lactobacillus*. Some bacteria are being evaluated for antigen delivery that are invasive into tissues but not invasive into cells. Strains of *Bacillus anthracis* and some of the so-far poorly studied *Bordetella* and *Yersinia* vaccine delivery systems are in this category. Focused attention will be given to studies in which the invasive and noninvasive mucosal colonizers were used, since they are superior in eliciting mucosal immune responses.

DESIRED ATTRIBUTES OF RECOMBINANT ATTENUATED BACTERIAL VACCINE SYSTEMS

The design of attenuated bacterial systems for the delivery of recombinant antigens or nucleic acid vaccines is dependent on at least three bodies of information that need to be considered to achieve both safety and high efficacy in inducing protective immunity (Galen and Levine, 2001; Curtiss, 2002). First, it is necessary to understand as fully as possible the mechanism by which the bacterial pathogen selected for use gains entrance to the host, colonizes a mucosal surface, invades tissues (if relevant), and causes disease. This is because it is necessary that the mutational alteration(s) to attenuate the bacterial host preclude induction of disease symptoms on the one hand but does (do) not impair functions necessary for the attenuated bacterial strain expressing a recombinant antigen or delivering a nucleic acid vector to result in high immunogenicity and a protective immune response. Second, it is necessary to define and characterize antigens of bacterial, viral, parasitic, and fungal pathogens that will induce protective immune responses when expressed and delivered by the attenuated bacterial vector or when expressed in the immunized eukaryotic host after delivery of the nucleic acid vaccine by the attenuated bacterial vector. Third, it is important, insofar as possible, to understand the means by which the bacterial pathogen to be used as the attenuated delivery vector evades, suppresses, or otherwise circumvents induction of host defense/immune responses. This is of critical importance to avoid creating vaccines that establish a carrier state but instead induce a long-lasting protective immunity based on induction of immunological memory. Unfortunately, we know altogether too little about such aspects of pathogen–host interactions, and this persistent ignorance probably most compromises our abilities to achieve success in the development of safe, efficacious live recombinant attenuated vaccines. In spite of this limitation, the ideal live recombinant attenuated vaccine strain must be able to colonize host tissues efficiently and invade to reach and then persist in effector lymphoid tissues to induce a maximal immune response and yet be unable to induce disease symptoms or to establish a carrier state.

The first body of information to consider relates to the basic host–pathogen interactions governing the pathogenesis of the bacterial vector. (The second and third topics enumerated in the previous paragraph will be dealt with in later sections of this chapter). Successful vaccine design is dependent on understanding the means by which the selected bacterial pathogen to be used as the vaccine vector survives the stresses encountered in reaching the site for mucosal colonization; the means of access and adherence to mucosal surfaces; the mechanism of invasion through cell surfaces into tissues; and the mechanisms for survival and nonsurvival to host defenses and in various cell types likely encountered, especially in lymphoid tissues.

Most bacterial pathogens possess many sensors, often as two-component regulatory systems, to detect changes in the environment with ensuing regulatory cascades, enabling rapid differential gene expression to cope with these ever-changing environments and to succeed in survival, infection, pathogenesis, and transmission. Since there is a more complete body of information concerning the stress responses, colonizing ability, invasiveness, and survival capabilities of *Salmonella* than of other bacterial genera used as vaccine vectors and since attenuated strains of *Salmonella* have been prevalently used as antigen and DNA vaccine delivery vectors, I will discuss this body of knowledge and indicate both key known attributes and intellectual voids in knowledge concerning the other bacterial pathogens with significant potential as antigens and/or DNA vaccine vectors.

Many of the bacterial pathogens used as antigen or DNA vaccine vectors are frequently transmitted from contaminated food or water to infect warm-blooded animal and human hosts. No studies have investigated whether gene expression under ambient conditions found in such environments leads to synthesis of adhesins or other attributes that facilitate success of bacteria used as vaccine vectors in the initial infection of warm-blooded hosts; this does occur with regard to Agf (curli) and Tsh adhesins in avian pathogenic *E. coli* (APEC) strains (Provence and Curtiss, 1992, 1994; Dozois *et al.*, 2000). If so, design of vaccines for constitutive expression of such attributes might reduce the required dose of the vaccine vector to elicit protective immunity, which could also reduce the likelihood of undesirable side effects.

A corollary benefit would be the induction of a more protective immune response.

The doses of recombinant *Salmonella* vaccines to elicit maximal immune responses are lower for nasal immunization than they are for oral immunization (Hopkins *et al.*, 1995; Nardelli-Haefliger *et al.*, 1997). This may be due, in part, to killing of orally administered vaccines by the acid stress of the stomach (Giannella *et al.*, 1973), quickly followed by exposure to bile in the duodenum. We have determined that these two stresses in succession are more effective in causing bacterial cell death than the sum of killing by each stress alone. *Salmonella* possesses a large constellation of genes that confer acid tolerance and resistance to acid stress (Foster and Spector, 1995; Audia *et al.*, 2001), and inactivation of these genes or their inability to be expressed by induction reduces virulence (Wilmes-Riesenberg *et al.*, 1996). In this regard, the regulatory proteins RpoS (Lee *et al.*, 1995), Fur (Hall and Foster, 1996), PhoPQ (Bearson *et al.*, 1998), and OmpR (Bang *et al.*, 2000, 2002) are all necessary to confer resistance to acid stress and/or shock in *S. typhimurium*. Similarly, many genes are turned on in response to exposure to bile, and some of these gene products transiently repress invasion while bacteria reside in the intestinal lumen (van Velkinburgh and Gunn, 1999; Gunn, 2000; Prouty and Gunn, 2000). The exceedingly low dose of *Shigella* needed for oral infectivity correlates well with the innate expression of high resistance to acid stresses (Waterman and Small, 1996) and the presumed nonimportance of bile stress.

Since rough mutants of *Salmonella* lacking lipopolysaccharide (LPS) O-antigen side chains or portions of the core are avirulent and fail to colonize the intestinal tract (Stocker and Makela, 1978, 1986), it is likely that such mutants fail to invade into or through mucin covering the intestinal mucosa to enable adherence to cells prior to invasion. With complete sequencing of the genomes of many bacterial pathogens, it now becomes possible to conduct searches for fimbrial operons or other genes encoding potential nonfimbrial adhesins to commence a thorough investigation of the importance of these adhesins for colonization of mucosal cell surfaces. *S. typhimurium* possesses 12 fimbrial operons (McClelland *et al.*, 2001), but some of these fimbrial operons are either absent or inactivated by frame shift mutations in *S. typhi* (Townsend *et al.*, 2001). The Lpf fimbriae seem to facilitate attachment to M cells and thus colonization of the gut-associated lymphoreticular tissues (GALT; Peyer's patches) (Baumler *et al.*, 1996). However, absence of many of these fimbriae, due to mutation, does not seem to appreciably reduce infection of orally administered *Salmonella* in mice or chickens (Lockman and Curtiss 1992; Curtiss *et al.*, 1993; Navis *et al.*, 1998; van der Velden *et al.*, 1998). This may be due, in part, to the presence of the diversity of fimbrial adhesins, such that absence of some does not significantly impair attachment to cells sufficient to facilitate subsequent invasion.

In keeping with this speculation, expression of some of these fimbrial operons is enhanced in the intestinal tract (Humphries *et al.*, 2003). As *Salmonella* traverses the intestinal tract, there is an increase in osmolarity and a decrease in available oxygen, both of these environmental signals induce the expression of the *Salmonella* pathogenicity island 1 (SPI-1) genes necessary for cell invasion (Galan and Curtiss 1990; Ernst *et al.*, 1990; Lee and Falkow, 1990), as does the succession of low pH passage through the stomach, followed by the neutral pH of the ileal contents (Bajaj *et al.*, 1996). There are also likely stresses to ions, defensins, and other metabolites that might impair the ability of bacterial vaccine vectors, depending on the means of attenuation, to persist in the intestinal tract for sufficient time to enable cell attachment and invasion. In this regard, genes regulated by PhoPQ (van Velkinburgh and Gunn, 1999) and PmrAB (Gunn *et al.*, 2000; Wosten and Groisman, 1999; Wosten *et al.*, 2000) very much contribute to resistance to bile stress, defensins, and iron stress. Even though genes encoded on the *Salmonella* virulence plasmid present in *S. enterica* serovars typhimurium, dublin, enteritidis, and choleraesuis, including those dependent on RpoS (Fang *et al.*, 1992) for their transcription, are not necessary for colonization of Peyer's patches (Pardon *et al.*, 1986; Hackett *et al.*, 1986; Gulig and Curtiss, 1987), RpoS-deficient mutants of *S. typhimurium* are very much attenuated (Fang *et al.*, 1992) and very much impaired in their ability to colonize Peyer's patches (Coynault *et al.*, 1996; Nickerson and Curtiss, 1997). This implies that RpoS-regulated chromosomal genes are involved either in invasion of and/or persistence in M cells and/or other cells of the GALT (Nickerson and Curtiss, 1997). In accord with this observation, RpoS⁻ recombinant attenuated *S. typhimurium* vaccine strains expressing hepatitis B virus (HBV) epitopes are far less immunogenic in inducing antibody responses against *Salmonella* or HBV antigens than are their RpoS⁺ homologs (Zhang *et al.*, 2003). This is true for both nasal as well as oral immunization.

The previous discussion shows how important it is to have mutations contributing to attenuation or other beneficial vaccine attributes that do not impair the abilities of the vaccine to adjust to and/or withstand a diversity of stresses encountered at any location within the gastrointestinal tract (if administered orally) or in the respiratory tract (if administered nasally). Likewise, the vaccine strain should have wild-type abilities not compromised by attenuating or other mutations to penetrate through mucin, to attach to cells in the mucosal epithelium, and to invade those cells. I will discuss in the following section how some of the currently used attenuating strategies for *Salmonella* potentially compromise vaccine effectiveness.

Information concerning responses to stresses encountered in the respiratory or gastrointestinal tracts or of the genetic control of these stress responses is sparse with regard to *Shigella*, *Listeria*, *Mycobacterium*, and *Brucella* strains that have potential as invasive colonizing vaccine delivery systems.

Shigella is infectious at very low doses (DuPont *et al.*, 1989) and is thus likely tolerant of all stresses encountered in the gastrointestinal tract, including acid stress (Waterman and Small, 1996). Invasion is through M cells of the GALT to reach the basolateral pole of intestinal epithelial cells. Considerable information is known about the genetic control of these events and the means for harnessing host cell functions to achieve invasion, survival, and distribution in host tissues (Sansonetti and Egile, 1998; Adam, 2001; Goldberg, 2001).

Relevant information to facilitate oral infection/immunization with *Listeria monocytogenes* is only now being acquired. This is because most animal studies have used needle delivery routes of infection because of the very high cell numbers (~10^9 CFU) needed for oral infection. A bile salts hydrolase, Bsh, is necessary for bile resistance and liver colonization. The *bsh* gene is PrfA-regulated and is expressed optimally under the low-O_2-tension intestinal environment (Dussurget *et al.*, 2002). Internalin (InlA) and the InlB cell-surface proteins interact with E-cadherin and c-Met cell receptors, respectively (Pizarro-Cerda *et al.*, 2002; Schubert *et al.*, 2002), and cell-surface glycosaminoglycans are essential for InlB to facilitate entry into epithelial cells (Jonquieres *et al.*, 2001). Sortases, such as SrtA, are needed to anchor InlA to the *L. monocytogenes* cell surface, and their absence results in noninvasiveness (Bierne *et al.*, 2002). A lipoprotein like the PsaA adhesin of *Streptococcus pneumoniae*, termed LpeA, also facilitates invasion into epithelial cells but not macrophages (Reglier-Poupet *et al.*, 2003). Exit from the endosome/phagosome is dependent on listeriolysin O (LLO), encoded by the *hylA* gene, whereas movement in the cytoplasm for cell-to-cell spread requires the ActA protein (Gaillard *et al.*, 1987; Tilney and Portnoy, 1989; Mounier *et al.*, 1990). The ActA protein is also reported to facilitate invasion (Suarez *et al.*, 2001).

Since the proposed use of *Mycobacterium bovis* bacillus Calmette-Guerin (BCG) as a recombinant antigen delivery vector (Jacobs *et al.*, 1988), there has been little research investigating oral delivery for induction of mucosal immunity (Lagranderie *et al.*, 1993). Although BCG was initially administered orally as a vaccine, numerous instances of lymphadenitis led to discontinuation of oral immunization, to be replaced by intradermal vaccination. Consequentially, we have little or no information about genetic attributes of *M. bovis* or *Mycobacterium tuberculosis* that would facilitate development of safe vaccine vectors to be given orally to stimulate mucosal immunity.

Although we have some understanding of the means by which oral streptococci colonize in the oral cavity on teeth or gums (Kolenbrander, 2000) and a beginning genetic understanding (Duncan, 2003), we have less information about other colonizing noninvasive vaccine delivery systems derived from lactic acid bacteria, for example. Since these bacteria are nonpathogens, are noninvasive, are components of food, and are prevalent as normal flora, they are used as antigen delivery vectors without introducing attenuating mutations (Mielcarek *et al.*, 2001). Nevertheless, since they are genetically endowed with the ability to express protective antigens from other pathogens, their ability to survive, per-

sist, and exchange genetic information with other microbes deserves some level of scrutiny.

CONSEQUENCES OF ATTENUATING MUTATIONS ON VACCINE ATTRIBUTES

Vaccine strains that colonize mucosal surfaces and that are invasive must possess some mutational alteration that confers attenuation to preclude induction of disease symptoms. Although bacterial vaccine vectors that are nonpathogenic and noninvasive may not require attenuating mutations, they certainly should possess mutational alterations that restrict them to surviving only in the immunized animal or human host. In other words, these noninvasive bacterial vaccine vectors would benefit from possessing biological containment attributes. In attenuated bacterial vaccine vectors, it is preferable for the vaccine strain to possess multiple attenuating mutations as a safety feature. This may not be essential, however, if the attenuating mutation represents a defined deletion of genetic information. Although some individuals and regulatory agencies have expressed concern about potential gene transfer to eliminate a single attenuating mutation, this would require the presence of a high number (density) of wild-type bacteria of the same species and restriction-modification genotype/phenotype, a situation that already would kill or at least render severely ill the immunized individual. However, if the vaccine strain is shed into the environment with some potential for survival, gene transfer could theoretically occur and result in a wild-type strain expressing a recombinant cloned gene derived from a heterologous pathogen. Because of the likely inclusion of multiple mutations in vaccine strains to optimize their performance, these issues of probability of gene transfer have decreased importance.

It is best for the attenuating phenotype to be irreversible by diet constituents. Thus, reliance on mutations conferring auxotrophy as the sole means of attenuation are unlikely to be ethically justifiable for immunization of diverse human populations with highly varied food consumption practices. In this regard, reversibility of attenuation of auxotrophic mutants can be achieved by supplementation of diets or drinking water to cause induction of disease and sometimes death. It is also of critical importance to not use a means of attenuation to generate a vaccine strain that can be cleared only from immunized individuals whose host defense/immune system is fully functioning. This becomes important because of the increasing prevalence of individuals that are immunocompromised because of disease, health care practices, or age. Since it is not possible to anticipate the basis for all conceivable environmental and/or genetic factors that might lead to an adverse vaccine reaction in an immunized individual, it is imperative that the vaccine strain be sensitive to all antibiotics that might be useful in treating such a patient. In this regard, the sensitivities should be to antibiotics still used in the developing world, even though they are not used in the developed world.

Table 56.1 lists attenuating mutations included in bacterial vaccine vectors that have been used for antigen or nucleic acid vaccine delivery. There is quite an array of additional attenuating mutations that have been evaluated for rendering strains avirulent and immunogenic but without monitoring these attenuated mutants for induction of mucosal immunity or for expression of foreign protective antigens to induce mucosal, systemic, and cellular immunities. Some of these mutations are mentioned later in the text.

Salmonella

Attenuating mutations have been most fully investigated in *Salmonella*, commencing with the work of Bacon *et al.* (1950,

1951). The *galE* mutation was first used to attenuate and render *S. typhimurium* immunogenic in mice (Germanier and Furer, 1971). Germanier and Furer (1975) went on to construct an *S. typhi* Ty2 derivative possessing a *galE* mutation, although this Ty21a strain possesses other still unknown mutations induced by the nitrosoguanidine mutagenesis treatment. This strain is also RpoS⁻ (Robbe-Saule *et al.*, 1995), due to a mutation present in its parent Ty2 (Robbe-Saule and Norel, 1999). Although the *galE* mutation alone is insufficient to confer adequate attenuation to *S. typhi* for humans (Hone *et al.*, 1988a), the Ty21a vaccine is exceedingly safe and, after administration of multiple doses, induces protective immunity to at least two-thirds of the

Table 56.1. Attenuating Mutations Evaluated in Recombinant Attenuated Invasive Bacterial Antigen Delivery Systems and Their Limitations

Mutation	Basis of Attenuation	Limitations	Reference
Used in *Salmonella*			
Δ*galE*	Lacks UDP-Gal epimerase	Growth with galactose yields nonimmunogenic Galʳ mutants	Germanier and Furer, 1971, 1975
Δ*pmi*	Lacks phospho-mannose isomerase	Retains some virulence at high doses	Collins *et al.*, 1991
Δ*aro*	Blocks synthesis of pABA, dihydroxy benzoic acid, Vit K & Q and aromatic amino acids	Remedial nutrient requirement and lethal to some immuno-deficient mice	Hoiseth and Stocker, 1981
Δ*cya crp*	Eliminates adenylate cyclase and cAMP receptor protein	Continues to grow slowly and probably lethal to some immunodeficient mice	Curtiss and Kelly, 1987
Δ*phoPQ*	Eliminates two-component regulatory system essential for virulence	Diminished invasion and colonization of lymphoid tissues but safe and immunogenic	Galan and Curtiss, 1989
Used in *Shigella*			
Δ*virG* (*icsA*)	Blocks intercellular spread		d' Hauteville and Sansonetti, 1992
Δ*iuc*	Eliminates aerobactin system		Barzu *et al.*, 1996
Δ*sen* Δ*set*	Eliminates enterotoxins		Kotloff *et al.*, 2000
Δ*guaBA*	Blocks synthesis of guanine nucleotides	Likely remedial nutrient requirement	Noriega *et al.*, 1996a
Δ*asd*	Requirement for DAP	Hyperattenuated	Sizemore *et al.*, 1995
Used in *Listeria*			
hlyA	Eliminates or alters listeriolysin O	Remains in endosome	Gahan and Collins, 1995
mpl	Metalloprotease		Paglia *et al.*, 1997
actA	Eliminates intercellular spread movement		Domann *et al.*, 1992
plcB	Phospholipase		Brundage *et al.*, 1993
dal dat	Requires D-alanine for growth and survival	Hyperattenuated	Thompson *et al.*, 1998 Vasquez-Boland *et al.*, 1992

immunized population for at least 5 to 6 years following immunization (Levine et al., 1999). Unfortunately, vaccine strains with galE mutations must be grown in the presence of galactose to enable synthesis of UDP-galactose needed for synthesis of the LPS core and O-antigen (Fukasawa and Nikaido, 1961). This is necessary, since as stated above, rough strains of Salmonella are not only avirulent but also not immunogenic because of an inability to adequately invade and colonize lymphoid tissues. The problem with galE mutant strains arises from the fact that they are also sensitive to galactose (Adhya and Shapiro, 1969) and accumulate secondary mutations blocking either galactose uptake or its conversion via galactose kinase and UDP-Gal transferase to UDP-Gal. These galactose-resistant mutants are rough, avirulent, and therefore not immunogenic. This lessens the effectiveness of the Ty21a vaccine on a per-live-cell basis.

The pmi gene encodes phospho-mannose isomerase, which interconverts mannose-6-P and fructose-6-P (Rosen et al., 1965). Mannose, via conversion of mannose-6-P to GDP-Man, is incorporated into LPS O-antigen side chains (Makela and Stocker, 1969). Bacteria with a deletion (Δ) mutation in the pmi gene synthesize LPS O-antigen side chains only when grown in the presence of mannose. When such strains are inoculated into medium without mannose, LPS O-antigen side chain synthesis ceases and the strains gradually become rough, with absence of O-antigen side chains following 8 to 10 generations of growth. Since free nonphosphorylated mannose is unavailable in animal tissues, O-antigen side chain synthesis ceases when a Δpmi mutant resides in vivo; Δpmi mutants of S. typhimurium are significantly attenuated but cause some deaths in mice at oral doses of 10^8 to 10^9 CFU (Collins et al., 1991). Such strains are highly immunogenic, however, since all surviving mice acquire protective immunity. An important observation is that Δpmi mutants are not mannosal sensitive, and thus rough mutants do not arise during growth of pmi mutants in media with added mannose. In view of the retained virulence of ΔgalE S. typhi strains in humans, even though ΔgalE mutants of S. typhimurium are completely attenuated in mice, I infer that a Δpmi mutation would be even more inadequate to attenuate S. typhi for humans.

By far the most widely studied attenuating mutations, first evaluated by Hoiseth and Stocker (1981), are in aro genes, more specifically in the aroA, aroC, and aroD loci. These mutations, which block the aromatic pathway prior to chorismic acid, impose nutritional requirements for p-aminobenzoic acid (pABA), dihydroxy benzoate, vitamin K, vitamin Q, and the three aromatic amino acids tyrosine, phenylalanine, and tryptophan. Even though S. typhimurium strains with single aro mutations are totally avirulent and highly immunogenic in mice (Hoiseth and Stocker, 1981), S. typhi Ty2 strains (which possess an attenuating rpoS mutation) with ΔaroC ΔaroD (Hone et al., 1991) mutations caused some reactogenicity in human volunteers and resulted in bacteremia when administered at high doses (Tacket et al., 1992a, 1992b). An S. typhi ISP1820 ΔaroC ΔaroD strain (that is RpoS⁺ due to presence of the wild-type rpoS gene)

and a ΔaroA ΔaroD S. typhi CDC 10-80 strain (presumably RpoS⁺) were even more reactogenic and induced more frequent bacteremias in humans (Hone et al., 1992; Dilts et al., 2000).

In addition, S. typhimurium strains with Δaro mutations are able to grow very slowly but sufficiently to kill mice with some, but not all, knockout mutations for certain cytokines (Van Cott et al., 1998). It is therefore evident that the nutrients necessary to satisfy the growth requirements of aro mutants are present in the diet and can be absorbed to a sufficient extent to enable slow in vivo growth of such attenuated vaccine strains (Stocker, 2000). For these reasons, subsequent studies of S. typhi vaccine constructions in human volunteers have included the ΔhtrA mutation in addition to ΔaroC and ΔaroD mutations (Tacket et al., 1997a). The htrA gene encodes a periplasmic heat-shock protease, and a mutation in this gene is able to render S. typhimurium attenuated and immunogenic for mice (Chatfield et al., 1992b).

A more recently proposed added attenuation to ΔaroC S. typhimurium and S. typhi Ty2 strains has been the inclusion of the ΔssaV mutation that inactivates the SPI-2 encoded functions for systemic infection (Khan et al., 2003).

Deletion of the cya gene for adenylate cyclase and the crp gene for the cAMP receptor protein render S. typhimurium avirulent and highly immunogenic for mice (Curtiss and Kelly, 1987). Strains with the Δcya and Δcrp mutations grow more slowly than their wild-type parent, are defective in uptake and catabolism of peptides and carbohydrates, cease to synthesize some outer membrane proteins, and are deficient in synthesizing some fimbrial adhesins, including the type 1 fimbriae, and flagella and in display of motility (Botsford and Harman, 1992). Nevertheless, an S. typhi Ty2 strain with Δcya and Δcrp mutations was too reactogenic in human volunteers and caused bacteremia at even moderate doses (Tacket et al., 1992a). During the generation of Δcrp mutations by excision of Tn10, some mutants were recovered that still exhibited avirulence and immunogenicity when the crp mutation was complemented with the wild-type allele on a plasmid vector (Kelly et al., 1992; Zhang et al., 1997). Many of these deletions extended into the cysG gene to impose a nutritional requirement for cysteine. Since this crp-linked mutation enabled a wild-type level of colonization of the GALT but a decreased ability to colonize the spleen, we termed the attenuating mutation cdt for colonization of deep tissues (Kelly et al., 1992; Zhang et al., 1997).

A Δcya Δcrp-cdt mutant derivative of S. choleraesuis is completely attenuated and highly immunogenic in mice (Kelly et al., 1992) and in swine (Kennedy et al., 1999; Gibson et al., 1999; Charles et al., 1999). This strain is commercially marketed as a vaccine to control S. choleraesuis and S. typhimurium infections of pigs. The inclusion of the Δcrp-cdt mutation with the Δcya mutation in S. typhi Ty2 yielded a strain that was well tolerated and displayed immunogenicity in human volunteers (Tacket et al., 1997b) that was very similar to that displayed by the S. typhi Ty2 ΔaroC ΔaroD ΔhtrA strain (Tacket et al., 1997a). Because of the presence of the *rpoS* mutation in *S. typhi* Ty2 and the realization that such mutations decrease the immunogenicity of recombinant attenuated *S. typhimurium* strains for mice (Zhang *et al.*, 2003), a derivative of the RpoS⁺ *S. typhi* ISP1820 strain was constructed with defined Δ*cya* and Δ*crp-ctd* mutations. Even though the human trial with this vaccine construct unwisely made use of lyophilized vaccine inocula, all individuals mounting significant immune responses also developed bacteremias and often experienced other adverse reactions (Frey *et al.*, 2001).

During the course of these studies, we learned that the *crp-cdt* deletion mutations deleted the *pabA* gene. This discovery was slow in coming since Δ*pabA* mutants grow in the absence of any pABA supplementation on minimal agar and display reduced growth only when purified Noble agar is used. In any event, it is likely that this low-level pABA requirement is sufficient to give reduced avirulence and enhanced immunogenicity to the RpoS⁻ *S. typhi* Ty2 Δ*cya* Δ*crp-cdt* vaccine strain in human volunteers. Since we believe that the Δ*cya* Δ*crp* strains would continue to grow slowly *in vivo* in immunocompromised individuals (Van Cott *et al.*, 1998) and know that the pABA nutritional requirement imposed by the *cdt* mutation can be reversed by the diet, we have ceased to use this constellation of mutations for any vaccines except those used for investigational research with laboratory animals.

Fields *et al.* (1986) isolated *S. typhimurium* mutants by transposon mutagenesis and identified a class that was defective in survival in murine macrophages in culture. They later determined (Fields *et al.*, 1989) that some of these macrophage-sensitive mutants had mutations in the *phoP* gene previously identified as controlling acid phosphatase production (Kier *et al.*, 1979). In attempting to use the *phoP12* mutation isolated in these earlier studies (Kier *et al.*, 1979) to enable generation and use of PhoA fusions, my colleague and I discovered that *S. typhimurium* strains with this mutant allele (now known to be a frameshift mutation in the *phoQ* gene and thus designated *phoQ12*) were totally avirulent in mice and induced high-level protective immunity to subsequent challenge with wild-type *S. typhimurium* strains (Galan and Curtiss, 1989). These results were confirmed by Miller *et al.* (1989), who along with Groisman *et al.* (1989) demonstrated the existence of the *phoPQ* two-component regulatory system that governs many attributes important to *Salmonella* virulence.

In the course of these studies, it was demonstrated that phosphorylated PhoP activated transcription of genes termed *pag* and repressed transcription of other genes termed *prg* (Miller, 1991). Other studies demonstrated that the PhoQ sensor kinase was responsive to levels of Mg⁺⁺, which, via phospho-transfer from PhoQ-P to PhoP, regulated transcriptional expression of *pag* and *prg* genes (Garcia-Vescovi *et al.*, 1996). *S. typhimurium* mutants with Δ*phoP*, Δ*phoQ*, or Δ*phoPQ* mutations are all totally avirulent for mice and highly immunogenic in inducing protective immunity to challenge with virulent wild-type strains. This is surprising in that such mutants, although colonizing the GALT

to reasonable levels in spite of their increased sensitivity to acid stress, defensins, and bile (van Velkinburgh and Gunn, 1999), are found in the mesenteric lymph nodes and spleens of orally immunized mice at much reduced levels in comparison with titers in CFU observed after oral administration of either Δ*aro* or Δ*cya* Δ*crp* attenuated strains. These collective results demonstrate that Δ*phoPQ* mutants are totally avirulent and highly immunogenic but imply that some of the attenuation is due to a reduced ability to colonize lymphoid tissues. If so, delaying expression of the mutant phenotype, as described later in the text for the *fur* gene, might enhance the immunogenicity.

The first human trials to evaluate an *S. typhi* Ty2 strain with a Δ*phoPQ* mutation evaluated a double mutant that also possessed a Δ*aroA* mutation. This vaccine strain was well tolerated at oral doses of up to 10¹⁰ CFU but was hyperattenuated and induced disappointingly minimal immune responses (Hohmann *et al.*, 1996a). A subsequent trial with human volunteers (Hohmann *et al.*, 1996b) evaluated the *S. typhi* Ty800 strain with a defined Δ*phoPQ* mutation in comparison with equivalent oral doses of the already approved and widely used *S. typhi* Ty21a vaccine. The Ty800 strain was well tolerated at doses of up to 10¹⁰ CFU with but minor instances of diarrhea in some volunteers and, importantly, induced far superior immune responses (mucosal, systemic, and cellular) in comparison with the Ty21a vaccine.

Ty800 also possesses the attenuating *rpoS* frameshift mutation (present in *S. typhi* Ty2), which differs from the wild-type allele by only a single base-pair insertion capable of reversion. In addition, the defined Δ*phoPQ* mutation present in Ty800 is an internal DNA fragment that results in an in-frame fusion protein possessing the N-terminal portion of the PhoP protein, including the aspartate residue that is normally phosphorylated in the wild-type PhoP protein, and the C-terminal portion of PhoQ, which retains the histidine residue normally phosphorylated in the wild-type PhoQ protein under conditions of low Mg⁺⁺ (Hohmann *et al.*, 1996a). In hindsight, it would have been preferable to delete the entire *phoPQ* encoding gene sequence.

Other attenuating mutations introduced into *S. typhimurium* have led to strains evaluated in mice for immunogenicity/induction of protective immunity and sometimes in other animal species, but few if any of these attenuated strains have been investigated as potential live recombinant attenuated antigen delivery vectors. The genes investigated include *purA* (McFarland and Stocker, 1987) and *purE* (Everest *et al.*, 1997), *ompR* (Dorman *et al.*, 1989), *hemA* (Benjamin *et al.*, 1991), *recA* (Buchmeier *et al.*, 1993), *guaBA* (Noriega *et al.*, 1996a), *nuoG* (Zhang-Barber *et al.*, 1998), *fur* (Wilmes-Riesenberg *et al.*, 1996), *poxA* (Kaniga *et al.*, 1998), *dam* (Heithoff *et al.*, 1999), *surA* (Sydenham *et al.*, 2000), *clpXP*, and *lon* (Matsui *et al.*, 2003). Purine-requiring mutants tend to be hyperattenuated and strains in tissues for long periods. I am concerned about the genetic stability of strains with *recA* and *dam* mutations because of the potential for enhanced frequencies of chromosomal rearrangements and/or mutational changes leading to instability of avirulence and immunogenic phenotypes. The OmpR-EnvZ two-component system is responsive to changes in osmolarity, regulates expression of genes for the major outer membrane proteins OmpC and OmpF, controls functions in infection and virulence (Mills *et al.*, 1998), and also regulates genes encoded in SPI-2 involved in systemic infection (Feng *et al.*, 2003). The importance of these different functions to the development of a safe, efficacious recombinant attenuated bacterial antigen delivery system remains to be determined.

Strains with *fur* mutations constitutively express genes encoding iron-regulated outer membrane proteins (IROMPs) and other genes necessary for iron acquisition. The *fur* gene is autoregulated but is also regulated by Crp and OxyR in response to catabolic and oxidative stresses, respectively (Zheng *et al.*, 1999). The *fur* mutants are attenuated when administered orally (Wilmes-Riesenberg *et al.*, 1996) or intraperitoneally (Garcia-del Portillo *et al.*, 1993) but are not very immunogenic. This may be due to the fact that orally administered *fur* mutants do not survive well in the intestinal tract (*i.e.*, in the ileum), quite possibly because of iron toxicity leading to a reduced ability to colonize the GALT. Iron is present because of the poor absorption of dietary iron and is contributed in bile as a product of red cell degradation and processing in the liver. We have rectified these problems by deleting the entire *fur* promoter sequence, including recognition sequences for Fur, Crp, and OxyR, and substituting a transcription terminator (TT) *araC* P_{BAD} sequence linked to and regulating expression of the *fur* gene (Zhang *et al.*, 2002).

In this construction, *fur* gene expression is dependent on the presence of arabinose, which is present in Luria broth but is totally absent (in either a nonphosphorylated or noncomplex form) in animal tissues. An orally-administered, Luria broth–grown *S. typhimurium* strain with this ΔP_{fur}::TT *araC* P_{BAD} *fur* deletion–insertion mutation survives in the intestinal tract of mice and chickens to efficiently colonize the GALT and internal lymphoid tissues in which complete derepression occurs, leading to constitutive expression of all genes used for iron acquisition. Such a strain is totally avirulent and induces a very high level of protective immunity to challenge with virulent *S. typhimurium* strains (Zhang *et al.*, 2002). By analogy, and in view of the diminished colonizing ability of lymphoid tissues by strains with $\Delta phoPQ$ mutations, we are constructing an *S. typhimurium* strain with a ΔP_{phoPQ}::TT *araC* P_{BAD} *phoPQ* deletion–insertion mutation in anticipation of increasing colonizing ability and enhancing immunogenicity.

The means to genetically manipulate *Salmonella* to achieve lysis for release of DNA vaccines *in vivo* is considered below.

Shigella

The attenuating mutations (in addition to $\Delta aroA$) recently evaluated in strains of *Shigella flexneri* 2a or 5a that have been studied as antigen or nucleic acid vaccine delivery vectors are also listed in Table 56.1. *Shigella sonnei* with a $\Delta icsA$ ($\Delta virG$) mutation alone is attenuated and immunogenic but too reac-

togenic in human volunteers (Kotloff *et al.*, 2002). *S. flexneri* candidate vaccines have included $\Delta aroA$ (Noriega *et al.*, 1994), Δiuc (Coster *et al.*, 1999), and $\Delta guaBA$ (Kotloff *et al.*, 2000), in addition to the $\Delta icsA$ mutation. These strains are more attenuated, and undesired reactions are very minimal. The inclusion of mutations to eliminate toxin production (*i.e.*, Δsen Δset) further reduces potential for inducing disease symptoms. The use of the Δasd attenuating mutation to affect cell lysis for the release of DNA vaccines *in vivo* is more fully discussed later in the text.

Listeria monocytogenes

L. monocytogenes has begun to be investigated as an antigen and DNA vaccine delivery vector (Dietrich *et al.*, 2000; Medina and Guzman, 2001). Since mice possess an E-cadherin receptor that is incompatible with the InlA *L. monocytogenes* adhesin (Lecuit *et al.*, 2001), *L. monocytogenes* wild-type virulent strains can only be demonstrated to be nonspecifically invasive in mice by administration of very high (~10^9 CFU) oral doses. As a consequence, most recombinant attenuated *L. monocytogenes* vaccine candidates have been delivered to mice by needle primarily to evaluate induction of cellular immune responses and with little or no attention to their potential to induce mucosal immunity. Use of an animal model that shares with humans a compatible adhesin-receptor and invasion system is thus necessary to enable such studies (see later discussion).

Nevertheless, some important work has been initiated to evaluate different attenuating mutations that are listed in Table 56.1 to potentiate the use of *L. monocytogenes* as an antigen and DNA vaccine delivery vector. The inclusion of the Δact and $\Delta plcB$ mutations (Angelakopoulos *et al.*, 2002) engenders safety since both mutations decrease invasion into neurons (Dramsi *et al.*, 1998).

Mycobacterium

Mycobacterium species have the potential to be used as antigen and DNA vaccine delivery vectors to induce mucosal immunity, but this has yet to be investigated. Current work has focused on construction and evaluation of deletion mutants with auxotrophic requirements for leucine (Hondalus *et al.*, 2000), pantothenate (Sambandamurthy *et al.*, 2002), and lysine (Pavelka *et al.*, 2003) that are attenuating and immunogenic. Although some safety issues concerned with attenuation in immunodeficient mice have been addressed, the issue of attenuation relative to diet constituents has not.

ATTENUATION ATTRIBUTES OF NONINVASIVE MUCOSAL COLONIZING BACTERIAL ANTIGEN DELIVERY SYSTEMS

The strains of *Streptococcus gordonii* and *Lactobacillus* species that have been investigated for antigen delivery capabilities have generally not been genetically modified except with regard to delivery of foreign antigens. An exception is the recent success in engineering a *Lactococcus lactis* orally delivered strain to decrease its survival following excretion due to thymine-less death and to efficiently prevent transmission of recombinant information (Steidler *et al.*, 2003).

Attenuated nontoxigenic derivatives of *Vibrio cholerae* are currently being evaluated as antigen delivery vector systems. In that *V. cholerae* has specific mechanisms for adhering to the intestinal mucosa via TCP pili and other adhesins, they have the capacity to colonize on a mucosal surface with potential for delivery of protective antigens encoded by gene sequences from other pathogens to elicit mucosal, systemic, and cellular immunities. These attenuated *V. cholerae* strains all possess a deletion of the *ctxA* gene for cholera toxin (Kaper *et al.*, 1984). The strains sometimes also have the *zot* deletion to eliminate production of the zonula occludens toxin (Fasano *et al.*, 1991), a Δ*ace* mutation to eliminate the accessory cholera toxin (Trucksis *et al.*, 1993), and sometimes deletion of the attachment site for the converting phage that carries *ctx* genes in addition to the *ctx* and *zot* genes (Butterton *et al.*, 1995). Although prolonging colonization on the intestinal mucosa can cause inflammation leading to fluid loss, modification of the *hap* gene to retain mucinase activity to facilitate colonization while eliminating, if possible, the protease activity that normally disassociates *V. cholerae* from the intestinal mucosa (Benitez *et al.*, 2001) might prolong intestinal colonization and thus the period for antigen delivery.

Pathogenic strains of *E. coli* with the potential to colonize the intestinal mucosa have also been considered as antigen delivery vectors (Turner *et al.*, 2001). The systems would be analogous to using *V. cholerae* as an antigen delivery vector and would require genetic manipulation to eliminate their ability to produce toxins or cause adverse disease symptoms associated with their ability to colonize on the intestinal mucosa.

DESIRED ATTRIBUTES OF VECTOR COMPONENTS OF RECOMBINANT ATTENUATED BACTERIAL ANTIGEN DELIVERY SYSTEMS

The development of safe, efficacious recombinant attenuated bacterial antigen delivery systems requires attention to some desired attributes that are not as important/relevant when attempting to elicit protective immunity with an attenuated bacterial vaccine (Galen and Levine, 2001; Curtiss, 2002). Thus, vaccine design should be focused on enhancing immunogenicity and the magnitude and duration of the immune response to the expressed protective antigen and on diminishing the potentially competing immune responses to antigens of the attenuated bacterial antigen delivery vector. The latter objective gains importance with preservation of the ability to reuse an antigen delivery system for vaccines to prevent multiple infectious diseases. In this regard, the impact of prior exposure to a vaccine strain on the immune

response to a heterologous antigen delivered by a second vaccine strain of the same serotype is still unresolved (Bao and Clements, 1991; Whittle and Verma, 1997; Attridge *et al.*, 1997; Roberts *et al.*, 1999; Kohler *et al.*, 2000; Vindurampulle and Attridge, 2003).

Depending upon the disease to be prevented and the nature of the pathogen causing that disease, it may be necessary to make further genetic modifications of the antigen delivery system to maximize a Th2 response important for inducing mucosal and systemic antibody responses or, in other cases, a Th1 response to enhance cellular immunity. Last, it is undesirable to have individuals who do not elect or are not targeted for immunization to be immunized by exposure to surviving recombinant attenuated bacterial vaccines shed from immunized individuals into the environment. This becomes increasingly important when live recombinant attenuated vaccines are administered by aerosol spraying of farm animals in agricultural settings. There is also the potential concern if recombinant vaccine constructions survive in nature to transmit DNA sequences encoding virulence determinants from the vaccine strains to other microorganisms encountered in the environment. Thus, it is potentially desirable to introduce biological containment features into vaccines to prevent their survival and persistence in environments into which they might be introduced as a consequence of immunization.

The magnitude of protective immunity to an expressed protective antigen, at least in regard to mucosal and systemic antibody responses, is more or less dependent on the amount of protective antigen delivered to the immunized host. Much more success has therefore been achieved when the protective antigen is specified by a gene on a multicopy plasmid vector rather than residing in the chromosome (Schodel and Curtiss, 1995). This is not universally true, since, for example, synthesis and assembly of a fimbrial adhesin encoded by a fimbrial operon may result in toxicity if expressed from a plasmid vector. Such overexpression of a fimbrial operon might impair growth or, more important, diminish colonization of relevant lymphoid tissues. In such a case, chromosomal insertion (Hone *et al.*, 1988b; Strugnell *et al.*, 1990) of the fimbrial operon encoding a protective fimbrial adhesin might represent a more realistic vaccine design to achieve success. The selection of a plasmid vector copy number to use will depend to some extent on the tolerance of the host-vector system for synthesis and processing, if any, of the plasmid-encoded protective antigen. To ensure maximum immunogenicity, the recombinant attenuated bacterial vector should synthesize as much protective antigen as possible and yet be able to grow nearly as well as the vector control strain not expressing the protective antigen. More important, the recombinant vaccine strain should be able to colonize target lymphoid tissues within an animal as well as the vector control strain following, for example, oral immunization.

Synthesis of protective antigens encoded by plasmid vector genes has often made use of strong constitutive promoters such as P_{trc}, P_{tac}, P_{ompA}, and P_{lpp} that can intensify problems associated with protective antigen toxicity when expressed on high-copy-number plasmid vectors. These vectors contain a diversity of multiple cloning sites after the promoter and usually include a strong transcription terminator to block transcription into genes needed for plasmid maintenance and replication.

Maintenance of a multicopy plasmid vector by the vaccine strain following immunization of an animal or human can be ensured in several ways. This can be accomplished by using a balanced lethal host-vector system in which the chromosome of the vaccine strain possesses a deletion of an essential gene involved in the synthesis of a cell component that is totally absent from animal tissues (Nakayama *et al.*, 1988). In this case, the plasmid vector possesses the wild-type gene to complement the defect due to the chromosomal mutation and to enable the strain to multiply and survive *in vivo* in the absence of an exogenous supply of the required component necessitated by the chromosomal mutation; loss of the plasmid would lead to cell death. One widely used system employs a deletion of the chromosomal *asd* gene, which imposes a requirement for diaminopimelic acid (DAP), an essential constituent of the rigid layer of the bacterial cell wall that is not synthesized by nonprokaryotic organisms, with the wild-type *asd* gene placed on the plasmid vector to complement the chromosomal mutation (Galan *et al.*, 1990). Overexpression of the plasmid *asd* gene is actually detrimental to the bacterial host and contributes some attenuation due to interference by the excess Asd protein with the normal formation of an enzyme complex of aspartokinases with the β-aspartate semialdehyde dehydrogenase encoded by the *asd* gene. This problem has been rectified by deletion of the *asd* promoter on high-copy-number (pBR *ori* and pUC *ori*) plasmids with retention of the Shine-Dalgarno sequence preceding the *asd* structural gene (Kang *et al.*, 2002a). Some years ago, Gerdes and colleagues developed a plasmid maintenance system dependent upon the *hok* gene that specifies a small toxic polypeptide and the *sok* gene that encodes a very unstable antisense RNA that prevents translation of the *hok* gene mRNA (Gerdes *et al.*, 1997). Loss of plasmid with the *hok* and *sok* genes results in rapid absence of *sok* mRNA to cause expression of the *hok* gene whose product causes cytoplasmic membrane damage to result in cell killing.

This system has been used in the development of a host–vector system for recombinant attenuated bacterial vaccine systems and ensures that all recombinant vaccine cells within an immunized animal retain the plasmid vector encoding the protective antigen (Galen *et al.*, 1999). The use of this system requires the presence of a selectable plasmid marker to facilitate strain construction, which of course should not confer antibiotic resistance.

In some cases, the expression of a protective antigen is deleterious and it is not possible to engineer the antigen gene to reduce or eliminate toxicity of the product. In this case, an invertible promoter on the plasmid vector can be used so that expression of the gene encoding the protective antigen occurs in only some of the bacterial cells that now exhibit a decreased proliferative ability but nevertheless induce immune responses to the protective antigen. In the pro-

moter-off cell population, growth and proliferation in lymphoid tissues continue until such time as the invertible switch in some cells leads to synthesis of protective antigens. This system was well developed with use of the bacteriophage Mu Gin invertase (Tijhaar *et al.*, 1994).

Another approach to reduce impairment of the efficacy of recombinant attenuated bacterial vaccines due to consequences of protective antigen synthesis is to employ promoters that are *in vivo* inducible. Thus, Chatfield *et al.* (1992a) introduced the use of the *nirB* promoter that is more active anaerobically than aerobically, in accord with the more likely *in vivo* anaerobic environment. The *pagC* (Hohmann *et al.*, 1995), *htrA* (Roberts *et al.*, 1998), and *dmsA* (Orr *et al.*, 2001) promoters have also been used to enhance *in vivo* expression of genes for protective antigens, although the *pagC* promoter was used only with a chromosomal insertion for expression of the protective antigen. The P_{trc} promoter used in Asd$^+$ vectors (Kang *et al.*, 2002a), as well as P_{tac}, is constitutive under most environments but actually is more transcriptionally active both anaerobically and aerobically than the *nirB* promoter (see Chatfield *et al.*, 1992a, Fig. 1, lanes 2 and 5 vs. lanes 1 and 4). For this reason, we have generated *araC* P_{BAD} *lacI* constructions either inserted into chromosomal genes or present on low-copy compatible plasmids. Thus, vaccine strains grown in medium in the presence of arabinose synthesize the LacI repressor to repress transcription from P_{trc} on plasmid vectors until after immunization, when the vaccine strain is already colonizing internal lymphoid tissues. Actually, the derepression leading to expression of the protective antigen is gradual, since the LacI concentration decreases by half at each cell division. The P_{tac} promoter was found to be superior to the *in vivo*–inducible heat shock *htpG* and iron-inducible *irgA* promoters in recombinant attenuated *V. cholerae* in terms of murine serum IgG titers to CtxB (John *et al.*, 2000). It is evident that assessment of promoter efficacy needs to be related to the impact of constitutive versus *in vivo* inducible protective antigen synthesis on the ability of the recombinant attenuated bacterial antigen delivery strain to both colonize lymphoid tissues and induce relevant immune responses (John *et al.*, 2000).

Plasmid expression vectors have been designed to employ the type III secretion system (TTSS) of *Salmonella* (Russmann *et al.*, 1998; Evans *et al.*, 2003) and *Yersinia* (Russmann *et al.*, 2000) to deliver antigens to the cytoplasm for MHC class I presentation by antigen-processing cells to elicit CTL responses. More relevant for the induction of mucosal and systemic antibody responses are vector systems that preferentially enhance antigen processing by a Th2-dependent pathway. Initial efforts were directed at inserting B-cell epitopes derived from protective antigens by fusion into surface-exposed domains of outer membrane proteins such as LamB, MalE (Charbit *et al.*, 1997), OmpA (Stathopoulos *et al.*, 1996), and PhoE (Janssen and Tommassen, 1994), but the immune responses to these epitopes were generally quite modest. This might have been caused by masking due to surface LPS O-antigen side chains. This possibility could be alleviated by employing an attenuated *Salmonella* antigen display/delivery vector with a Δ*pmi* mutation that would cause a vaccine strain to gradually become rough *in vivo*, due to the absence of free mannose for continued synthesis of LPS O-antigen side chains.

B-cell epitopes derived from protective antigens have also been inserted in place of the variable region of flagellar antigens (Newton *et al.*, 1989; Pereira *et al.*, 2001) or into the principal subunit of fimbrial adhesins (Chen and Schifferli, 2000, 2001) to elicit rather good antibody responses, at least when the inserted epitopes did not severely compromise assembly of a wild-type level of flagella or fimbriae on the bacterial cell surface. These approaches have some limitations, however, since populations to be immunized are genetically diverse and not all individuals are able to mount immune responses to any given epitope derived from a protective antigen. Thus, the strategies for vaccine design would seem to mandate expression of multiple epitopes in multiple surface-exposed antigens in the recombinant attenuated bacterial antigen delivery vector.

Enhancement of a Th2-dependent response has also been achieved with use of the *E. coli* hemolysin secretion system (Welch, 1991; Thomas *et al.*, 1992) in *Salmonella* (Mollenkopf *et al.*, 2001) antigen delivery systems for cell surface placement and/or secretion. IgA proteases of *Neisseria* and *Haemophilus* are encoded by genes that specify proteins that cause autotransport and proteolytic release of the protease. The *Neisseria* IgA protease was engineered for use in attenuated *Salmonella*, but transport of fusion-protective antigens was complicated by improper protein folding (Klauser *et al.*, 1990). The discovery of a class of autotransporting proteases in the Enterobacteriaceae (Provence and Curtiss, 1994) might enable development of a system for protective antigen epitope export out of vaccine cells that would be operational in attenuated *Salmonella*, *Shigella*, *Vibrio*, and *Yersinia* antigen delivery vector systems (Dutta *et al.*, 2002). In this regard, the AIDA autotransporter has been successfully used to secrete *Y. enterocolitica* antigens from *S. typhimurium* (Kramer *et al.*, 2003). Use of this and related autotransporter systems to induce mucosal immunity has yet to be investigated.

Plasmid vectors have been constructed to enable fusions to the β-lactamase signal sequence to cause transport of α-helical protein domains from gram-positive pathogens by recombinant *Salmonella* (Kang *et al.*, 2002a). This led to some of the antigen being exported into the culture supernatant, some transported to the periplasm, and about half retained within the cytoplasm. Antigen retention in the cytoplasm might have been due to oversaturation of the Sec-dependent secretion system. These constructs generated antibody titers to a pneumococcal protective antigen that were in excess of antibody titers to *Salmonella* outer-membrane protein (OMP) or LPS antigens. Expression of this same pneumococcal protein antigen in the cytoplasm of recombinant attenuated *S. typhimurium* antigen delivery strains led to minimal and very inferior antibody titers relative to the induced antibody titers for *Salmonella* OMP and LPS antigens (Kang and Curtiss,

2003). The immune response to the pneumococcal antigen was a mixed Th1–Th2 response with enhancement in production of IgG1 antibodies following a booster immunization. In other studies, either deletion of genes for synthesis of type 1 fimbriae or introduction of mutations to constitutively overexpress type 1 fimbriae shifted the antibody responses from IgG2a to IgG1 (Kang et al, 2002b). These and other studies (Tzschaschel *et al.*, 1996; Gentschev *et al.*, 2000) reveal that protective antigen expression on the surface or by export out of the vaccine cell enhances induction of mucosal and systemic antibody responses by a predominately Th2 cell pathway.

The twin arginine transport (TAT) system causes export of proteins that fold into a mature form within the cytoplasm across the cytoplasmic membrane into the periplasm (Berks, 1996). It has recently been discovered that some virulence antigens are secreted with use of the TAT system (Ochsner *et al.*, 2002). It therefore follows that this system, which is becoming increasingly well characterized (Palmer and Berks, 2003), could be used to export protective antigens by recombinant attenuated bacterial antigen delivery strains.

ATTENUATED BACTERIAL DNA VACCINE DELIVERY SYSTEMS

Sizemore *et al.* (1995) used a *Shigella flexneri* 2a strain with a Δ*asd* mutation to deliver a DNA vaccine vector encoding β-galactosidase that resulted in β-galactosidase synthesis in eukaryotic cells in culture. The DNA vaccine vector was released since the Δ*asd* mutant strain underwent DAP-less death with lysis *in situ*. This strain was then used for immunization of mice, and antibody responses to β-galactosidase were elicited (Sizemore *et al.*, 1997), even though *Shigella* cannot cause infection or disease in mice but can be invasive in cells lining the intestinal tract (where DNA vaccine vector release must have occurred). A beneficial attribute of *Shigella* is that it invades cells and multiplies freely in the cytoplasm without being incorporated into an endosome. Thus, the DNA vaccine is released into the cytoplasm, where it can traverse to the nucleus and be transcribed with the mRNA trafficking to the cytoplasm for translation. The protein antigen synthesized can then be subjected to processing to elicit antibody and cellular immunities. Because of its invasion of cells on mucosal surfaces, *Shigella* would seem to be an ideal bacterial vector for delivery of DNA vaccines to elicit mucosal immunity. A Δ*dapA E. coli* mutant endowed with invasiveness by expression of the *Yersinia pseudotuberculosis inv* gene has been used to deliver plasmid DNA to eukaryotic cells (Grillot-Courvalin *et al.*, 1998) but has not yet been investigated further for inducing immune responses in animals. Attenuated *L. monocytogenes*, which also escapes the endosome to gain access to the cytoplasm of infected eukaryotic cells, has been used to deliver, by genetically engineered lysis, an antigen-encoding plasmid into the cytosol of macrophages (Spreng *et al.*, 2000).

Although *Salmonella* is encased within an endosome upon entry into epithelial cells and macrophages (Finlay and Falkow, 1990), attenuated *S. typhimurium* strains have been successfully used to deliver DNA vaccines into animal hosts (Dietrich *et al.*, 2000). In one study (Hess *et al.*, 2000a), the *S. typhimurium* was endowed with the ability to produce listeriolysin to facilitate breakdown of the endosome membrane so that the bacteria could release plasmid DNA into the cytoplasm of antigen-presenting cells. In other studies, the Δ*aroA S. typhimurium* strains possessed no added attributes that may cause lysis for escape from an endosome or phagosome and/or lysis for release of the DNA vaccine. Nevertheless, immune responses were elicited in mice but only after multiple immunizations. Since CTL responses were induced in these studies (Woo *et al.*, 2001; Cochlovius *et al.*, 2002), it can be argued that the attenuated *S. typhimurium* somehow occasionally delivered the DNA vaccine into the cytoplasm of invaded cells to have permitted synthesis of the antigen and its presentation in association with MHC class I molecules that is essential to generate a CTL immune response.

The DNA vaccine plasmids delivered by these attenuated bacterial vector systems have the bacterial promoter and multiple cloning site sequence deleted and replaced with a eukaryotic expression cassette. This cassette most often uses the cytomegalovirus (CMV) enhancer-promoter sequence followed by a Kozak sequence, a multiple cloning site, and a polyadenylation sequence often derived from the bovine growth hormone gene. Unfortunately, most of the DNA vectors used to investigate their delivery by attenuated bacterial DNA vaccine delivery hosts permit expression of the gene for the protective antigen in the bacterial host. (This is a consequence of transcription that occurs on high-copy-number plasmids in the absence of a prokaryotic promoter in proximity to a coding sequence) (Kang *et al.*, 2002a). This protective antigen expression can be precluded only by inclusion of strong transcription terminator sequences flanking the eukaryotic expression cassette. In the absence of this precaution, immune responses in immunized animals may often be due to or at least contributed to by potentially improperly processed antigen synthesized in the bacterial DNA vaccine delivery strain prior to the release of the DNA vaccine.

Using DNA vaccine vectors encoding resistance to ampicillin or kanamycin such that selective maintenance of the DNA vaccine within the attenuated bacterium cannot be ensured *in vivo* has further complicated the studies on DNA vaccine delivery by attenuated bacteria. In this regard, expression of ampicillin resistance on pUC *ori* plasmids, which are most often used in DNA vaccines, causes instability in attenuated *S. typhimurium* strains. This is due, in part, to overexpression of the β-lactamase gene and the difficulty in exporting all of this overexpressed β-lactamase across the cytoplasmic membrane to the periplasm. This problem can be eliminated by deleting the β-lactamase gene promoter, as was done for the *asd* gene promoter (Kang *et al.*, 2002a). We thus constructed a DNA vaccine vector with a promoter-less *asd*+ gene that has the added benefit of encoding an immune-enhancing CpG sequence that is absent from the kanamycin resistance gene.

We have recently constructed a host–vector system with regulatable delayed lysis for release of either antigens synthesized in the recombinant attenuated bacterial delivery cells or DNA vaccine vectors (Kong *et al.*, 2003 a, b). The host–vector system is based on regulated expression of the *murA* gene, which encodes the first enzyme in muramic acid synthesis, and the *asd* gene, which is essential for DAP synthesis. Both muramic acid and DAP are unique constituents of the rigid layer of the bacterial cell wall, with muramic acid required for the carbohydrate backbone and DAP needed for the amino acid cross-links. A series of plasmid vectors have been constructed with the same regulatory domain to confer regulated delayed lysis *in vivo* with either eukaryotic or prokaryotic expression systems to use as DNA vaccine vectors or as antigen delivery vectors, respectively. The *Salmonella* bacterial hosts for these systems possess a Δ*asd* mutation with an inserted *araC* P_{BAD} *c2* cassette that specifies synthesis of the bacteriophage P22 C2 repressor when the strain is grown in the presence of arabinose; a deletion of the *murA* promoter replaced with an *araC* P_{BAD} insertion so that synthesis of the *murA* gene product is dependent upon the continued presence of arabinose in growth media; a Δ(*gmd-fcl*) mutation to preclude colanic acid synthesis (Andiranopoulos *et al.*, 1998) as a stress response during the course of death by muramic acid and DAP starvation; a Δ*relA* mutation to uncouple the occurrence of cell wall–less death from dependence on protein synthesis; and a Δ*endA* mutation to reduce possible degradation of released DNA vaccine vectors by the periplasmic endonuclease I.

The plasmid vectors for this *S. typhimurium* host strain possess three cassettes. One cassette contains the genes that control regulated delayed lysis and includes an improved *araC* P_{BAD} fusion to the *murA* and *asd* genes in tandem (which both have GTG start codons to reduce translation efficiency) and a C2-repressible P22 P_R in the opposite orientation that causes synthesis of an antisense mRNA for the *asd* and *murA* genes. The second cassette contains the origin of plasmid replication: p15A *ori* or pBR *ori* for antigen delivery and pUC *ori* for DNA vaccine delivery. The third cassette contains a promoter with transcription initiation and translation-enhancing domains, a multiple cloning site, and the appropriate gene termination domain for either expression in eukaryotes or prokaryotes. The combination of one of these plasmids in the *Salmonella* mutant host generates an arabinose-dependent host–vector system that will undergo lysis as a function of cell divisions occurring in environments lacking arabinose, due to dilution by half in the amounts of the MurA and Asd enzymes and C2 repressor after each cell division. These events occur *in vivo* since there is no free arabinose present in animal tissues. The number of cell generations before onset of lysis has been further modulated by introducing chromosomal mutations that govern the uptake and breakdown of arabinose (Kong *et al.*, 2003 a, b). Oral immunization of mice with this host–vector combination can induce fever due to release of endotoxin during cell lysis, and this can be decreased by introducing mutations such as Δ*msbB* that detoxify lipid A (Hone *et al.*, 1998).

BIOLOGICAL CONTAINMENT FEATURES OF RECOMBINANT ATTENUATED BACTERIAL ANTIGEN AND DNA VACCINE DELIVERY SYSTEMS

The biological containment features of live attenuated bacterial vaccines are of little importance for the conduct of research to investigate the best means to achieve optimal desired immune responses. Nevertheless, the ultimate goal of this research is to design, construct, and clinically evaluate vaccines that will be used for immunization of animals and humans to protect against a diversity of infectious diseases causing substantial morbidity and/or mortality. It is in these latter instances that considerations need to be given to improve biological containment features of live bacterial vaccines. This is to prevent immunization of individuals who did not elect to be immunized and to diminish the potential for gene transfer to other bacteria of cloned genes that might represent virulence attributes in some instances. This importance was recognized when at the 2003 General Meeting of the American Society for Microbiology, data were presented demonstrating the persistence of a Δ*cya* Δ*crp S. typhimurium* vaccine at significant titers in soil for a period of 1 year (M. P. Doyle, personal communication). This same vaccine, used for aerosol immunization of broiler chickens, has also been recovered on carcasses following slaughter in processing plants (S. Kelly-Aihle, personal communication). It is likely that most attenuated bacterial vaccines have some potential for survival in soil, water, and other environments outside of an animal host, but these issues have been inadequately investigated. I surmise that auxotrophs, mutants with metabolic defects, mutants with diminished ability to respond to stresses, and rough mutants lacking cell-surface protective layers may be less able to survive in nature than wild-type strains. Molin *et al.* (1993) have considered some of these issues, but there is minimal information in the literature pertaining to enhancing the biological containment features of recombinant attenuated bacterial vaccines.

The system described in the previous section for regulated delayed lysis is arabinose-dependent, but an investigation of the presence of arabinose in soil, water, or other potential environments into which a bacterial vaccine may be shed has not been done.

In regard to decreasing the duration and therefore the numbers of vaccine cells shed, the inclusion of a *shdA* mutation into *Salmonella* vaccine strains should be beneficial (Kingsley *et al.*, 2000). It is also interesting that the *shdA* gene product has homology to the *Shigella icsA* gene product. Thus, the inclusion of the Δ*icsA* mutation in *Shigella* vaccine vectors may have the additional benefit of reducing duration

of intestinal colonization and decreasing the number of bacteria shed in feces.

IDENTIFICATION OF PROTECTIVE ANTIGENS

A diversity of means has been used to identify putative protective antigens of pathogens to express in recombinant attenuated bacterial antigen and DNA vaccine delivery systems (Roberts *et al.*, 1994; Mastroeni *et al.*, 2001; Curtiss, 2002). Presence of antibodies in an animal host surviving infection is one approach. However, the presence of antibodies to a specific antigen does not always correlate with protection. Purification of the antigen and demonstration that immunization with that antigen confers some protection to an animal or isolation of a monoclonal antibody (mAb) that can passively protect animals are observations validating the high likelihood that the antigen would induce protective immune responses. Phage display technology can be used to identify peptides recognized by lymphocytes isolated from animals possessing protective immunity (Warren *et al.*, 1990). Also, the identification of antigen-specific T cells whose passive transfer can confer protective immunity has also been used to identify protective antigens for vaccine evaluation. In cases in which an antigen is surface-localized on or secreted from a pathogen, evidence that a mutant unable to synthesize that antigen is avirulent is another useful means to identify potential protective antigens.

A word of caution is in order with regard to secreted antigens. Many pathogens such as *Salmonella*, *Shigella*, and *Yersinia* use a TTSS to secrete effector proteins into the cytoplasm of host cells for the benefit of the pathogen (Galan and Collmer, 1999). Although using a different mechanism, *Mycobacterium* species likely use a similar process to facilitate their entry into host cells. In any of these cases, the secreted protein antigens have been subjected to potential processing and presentation by MHC class I molecules that would be expected to induce CD8-dependent CTL responses that should theoretically be protective. Obviously, this would be detrimental to the success of the pathogen, and it is highly likely that pathogen antigens translocated into the cytoplasm of host cells have undergone selection during the course of evolution to eliminate epitopes that would induce such protective immunity.

Theoretically microbial pathogens (not viruses) can, under some environmental condition prior to infection, synthesize and assemble adhesins and/or invasins to facilitate their initial success in infecting an animal host, with complete shutdown of expression of genes for these antigens *in vivo*. This regulatory means of antigen nonexpression would likely not lead to significant immune responses against these antigens in an infected host, and such cell surface antigens should yield candidates that might represent protective antigens for inducing mucosal immune responses that should interfere with the initial phase of infection. On the other hand, many pathogen virulence attributes are displayed only after infection, and the genes for these antigens are usually silent under *in vitro* growth conditions, unless one is able to mimic *in vitro* an environmental stress encountered *in vivo* that is responsible for expression of these genes. Various means have been devised to identify genes expressed *in vivo*, including *in vivo* expression technology (IVET) (Mahan *et al.*, 1993), signature-tagged mutagenesis (STM) (Hensel *et al.*, 1995), and selective capture of transcribed sequences (SCOTS) (Graham and Clark-Curtiss, 1999; Daigle *et al.*, 2002). Although not replicating all the potentially diverse *in vivo* conditions encountered by a pathogen, intracellular gene expression studies using microarrays has some potential to reveal candidate antigens (Eriksson *et al.*, 2003). Proteins constitutively synthesized by recombinant clones containing genes uniquely expressed *in vivo* can then be used to recognize either antibodies or lymphocyte populations responding to that antigen or to induce immune responses that can be evaluated for protectiveness. Genomic analysis can also be useful in looking for homologs encoded in the genome of one pathogen of proteins from other related pathogens that have been demonstrated to induce protective immunity.

BIOTECHNOLOGICAL CONSIDERATIONS IN IMPROVING VACCINE EFFICACY

Once protective antigens have been identified, significant improvement in the efficacy of antigen delivery to stimulate immune responses can be achieved by technological manipulations of the host-vector system. These changes can result in recombinant attenuated strains that exhibit growth and colonizing potentials quite similar to those exhibited by the vector control strain. To date, most vaccine improvements have focused on selection of the promoter sequence used to drive expression of a plasmid-encoded protective antigen and occasionally on codon optimization to enhance the level of synthesis of protective antigens. Selection or regulated expression of a promoter to cause expression of protective antigens was discussed previously. Codon usage patterns have species-specific and expression level–specific differences. Thus, codons in genes specifying an antigen from a heterologous species often need to be optimized for high-level expression in the vaccine strain. If this is not done, pausing in translation because of low concentrations of required charged tRNA species can lead to translation termination and synthesis of truncated proteins. The enhanced stability of mRNA can be achieved by adding DNA sequences specifying 5′ (Emory *et al.*, 1992) and 3′ (McLaren *et al.*, 1991) untranslated mRNA sequences that create stem–loop structures. Also, removing potential targets within the coding mRNA sequences to minimize mRNA degradation by the mRNA degradosome (Liou *et al.*, 2001) can increase antigen yields with a decrease in expenditure of energy by the vaccine strain. This must be done, of course, without altering the amino acid sequence of the protective antigen. Deletion of the gene for

poly (A) polymerase I can also increase mRNA stability (O'Hara *et al.*, 1995) to possibly improve the productive fitness of the recombinant vaccine strain.

It is potentially beneficial to engineer stability of the synthesized antigen in the bacterial antigen delivery strain to preclude toxicity of breakdown products as well as to enhance induction of the desired type of immune response after delivery to the immunized host. Thus, T-cell antigens, which need to be degraded by the proteosome prior to antigen presentation, might benefit from changes that decrease their stability. Conversely, antigens to which a systemic immune response is desired should more likely be engineered for greater stability in the immunized host. Attention to the N-terminal rule for protein degradation (Varshavsky, 1996), the presence of PEST sequences (Rogers *et al.*, 1986), and other protease cleavage sites in the antigen are important in designing these modifications. If the protective antigen contains cysteine residues, the potential for anomalous protein-folding requires consideration. Such potential problems can be rectified by deleting Cys-encoding sequences, changing the environment of the antigen delivery strain with regard to Eh potential, including a chaperone for the expressed antigen, or modifying the *dsb* system for isomerization of proteins with disulfide bonds (Ritz and Beckwith, 2001). Other means to enhance immunogenicity of an expressed protective antigen might be to include sequences leading to lipidation since lipoproteins can be taken up more efficiently by antigen-presenting cells to induce an array of desired immune responses (Baier *et al.*, 2000; Hosmalin *et al.*, 2001; Wiesmuller *et al.*, 2001; Cote-Sierra *et al.*, 2002). Since expression of proteins with extensive hydrophobic domains very often results in toxicity to the antigen delivery vector, it is advantageous to delete these sequences since immune responses to them are seldom protective. Fusions can also be used to stabilize proteins or to enhance induction of immune responses with the fusion partner encoding a strong or universal epitope. Consideration can be given to the impact of coexpression of cytokines, many of which can be synthesized and secreted from recombinant attenuated bacterial antigen delivery strains (Saltzman *et al.*, 1996; Dunstan *et al.*, 1996; Xu *et al.*, 1998).

EVALUATION OF CANDIDATE VACCINES *IN VITRO* AND *IN VIVO*

It is essential to fully characterize candidate vaccine strains during the course of their construction. In using gram-negative attenuated bacterial delivery systems, a frequent mistake is selection of a rough variant during the introduction of the recombinant plasmid vector, resulting in a vaccine strain that is hyperattenuated and thus unlikely to induce the desired immune responses. It is thus necessary to verify the presence of LPS O-antigen side chains and conduct complete morphological and biochemical analyses of the candidate vaccine to verify the presence of all properties that will be important in conferring attenuation, biological containment, and immune-enhancing attributes. The candidate vaccine strains should exhibit good growth in relevant culture media, since this is correlated with ability to colonize host lymphoid tissues to levels needed to induce maximal immune responses. It is of critical importance that important properties be genetically stable over a considerable number of generations of growth.

In regard to *in vivo* evaluation of strains, Mastroeni *et al.* (2001) presented a complete list of types of studies that could be profitably undertaken. These studies with laboratory animals should include an evaluation of vaccine persistence in animal tissues and its potential for shedding into the environment. It should be emphasized that comparative vaccinology research is needed to maximize progress in this field. A comparison of single candidate vaccines versus the vector control in either laboratory animals or humans does not enable a meaningful evaluation. Only by comparison between candidate vaccines, often requiring collaborative endeavors, can we ever hope to succeed in selecting the best vaccines for use in disease-prevention programs (see Tacket *et al.*, 1992a; Dunstan *et al.*, 1998; Roberts *et al.*, 1998, 2000; Hohmann *et al.*, 1996b).

Another most difficult challenge concerns evaluation of candidate vaccines generated from human host–adapted pathogens. The use of surrogate systems is of considerable benefit, but, for example, the disease caused by *S. typhimurium* in mice is not exactly the same as that caused by *S. typhi* infection in humans. Furthermore, the mutations that attenuate *S. typhimurium* to be immunogenic in mice very often are insufficiently attenuating for *S. typhi* in humans (Hone *et al.*, 1988a; Tacket *et al.*, 1992a,b; Bumann *et al.*, 2000; Frey *et al.*, 2001). An additional concern is the fact that most research with *S. typhimurium* uses inbred strains of mice that possess unique susceptibility to infection, such that this system does not represent a likely scenario for immunizing genetically diverse human populations. Some of the mandated assays of attenuation of *S. typhi* generate misleading results. For example, inoculation of *S. typhi* intraperitoneally into outbred mice in the presence of iron-supplemented hog gastric mucin (Powell *et al.*, 1980) demonstrates the ability of *S. typhi* to grow in this medium rather than its attenuation. Thus, *S. typhi* Δ*phoPQ* mutants inoculated at low dose grow in this assay as well as wild-type bacteria to cause death by endotoxic shock (Baker *et al.*, 1997), whereas some virulent auxotrophic mutants fail to grow to incorrectly suggest their attenuation. Similar difficulties are encountered in evaluating in animals the attenuating attributes of mutant candidate vaccines derived from *Shigella* species, *V. cholerae*, *Mycobacterium* species, and *L. monocytogenes*. The recent generation of transgenic mice with a human E-cadherin receptor facilitating *L. monocytogenes* infection after oral inoculation (Lecuit *et al.*, 2001) could provide an improved model for developing recombinant attenuated *L. monocytogenes* vaccines for humans. The oral doses necessary to infect these transgenic mice still approximate 10^9 CFU, a dose that makes it difficult to genetically analyze virulence attributes and other genetic traits that might be useful in constructing improved vaccines. The recent demonstration (Peters and Paterson, 2003) that animal passage of attenuated *L. monocytogenes* strains

enhances their ability to infect mice and their resulting immunogenicity suggests a means for improving animal evaluations of recombinant attenuated *L. monocytogenes* vaccines. On the other hand, this potential nonstability of virulence/avirulence phenotypes will be troublesome for regulatory agencies. These considerations make it clear that successful design of recombinant attenuated bacterial antigen and DNA vaccine delivery systems will invariably require use of human volunteers to acquire basic information not now available as well as to conduct clinical trials to demonstrate the safety and efficacy of vaccine candidates judged to have significant merit.

As noted earlier, nasal immunization of mice with recombinant attenuated *S. typhimurium* antigen delivery strains is very effective in inducing immune responses with use of significantly lower doses of viable CFU than need to be administered orally to achieve equivalent immune responses. This difference is much more pronounced when recombinant attenuated *S. typhi* vaccines are administered nasally rather than orally (Pasetti *et al.*, 2000). This is the basis for the increasingly popular means of evaluating immunogenicity of recombinant attenuated *S. typhi* vaccines with use of nasal immunization of mice (Galen *et al.*, 1997, Pickett *et al.*, 2000).

However, because meningitis is a frequent occurrence associated with *S. typhi* infection in children (Denis *et al.*, 1977) and occasionally in adults (Karim and Islam, 2002), we were concerned that nasal delivery of attenuated *Salmonella* may enable *Salmonella* to reach the brain. This concern is due to the anatomy of the nasopharynx and the proximity of the cribriform plate of the ethmoid bone and the ascending olfactory nerve to the nasal cavity. Our findings (Bollen *et al.*, 2003) indicate that following nasal immunization (<10 μL doses) of unanesthetized mice, both attenuated and wild-type strains of *S. typhimurium* and *S. typhi* reach the brain with more rapid clearance of the non-host-adapted *S. typhi* strains than of the host-compatible *S. typhimurium* strains. These results would suggest against nasal immunization of humans with live bacterial vaccines until we learn means of attenuation or other genetic alterations to decrease the potential risk associated with nasal immunization.

These results indicate the need to investigate the possibility of brain colonization for any live bacterial vaccine candidate contemplated for delivery via the nasal route. This is particularly important for *L. monocytogenes*, which is neurotrophic (Dramsi *et al.*, 1998). The use of Δ*actA* Δ*pls* to attenuate vaccine candidates (Angelakopoulos *et al.*, 2002) is probably a wise choice since both mutations significantly decrease the ability of *L. monocytogenes* to invade neurons (Dramsi *et al.*, 1998).

RECOMBINANT ATTENUATED BACTERIAL ANTIGEN DELIVERY SYSTEMS

Table 56.2 lists the more recently published descriptions of the use of various attenuated bacterial species to deliver

Table 56.2. Recombinant Attenuated Bacterial Antigen Delivery Vaccines[a]

Pathogen	Protective Antigen	Host and Attenuation	Reference
Attenuated *S. enterica*			
Streptococcus sobrinus	SpaA	Stm *cya crp*	Redman *et al.*, 1996
S. mutans	AgI/II	Stm *aroA*	Huang *et al.*, 2000
Porphyromonas gingivalis	HagB	Stm *cya crp*	Kohler *et al.*, 1998
P. gingivalis	*HagA*	*Stm cya crp*	Kozarov *et al.*, 2000
Bordetella pertussis	S1 toxin	Sty *aroC aroD*	Barry *et al.*, 1996
B. pertussis	Pertactin	Stm *aroA aroD*	Anderson *et al.*, 1996
B. pertussis	S1, S2, S3, S4, S5 toxin subunits	Stm *aroA*	Dalla Pozza *et al.*, 1998
Streptococcus pneumoniae	PspA	Stm *cya crp*	Nayak *et al.*, 1998
S. pneumoniae	PspA	Stm *crp*	Kang *et al.*, 2002a
Yersinia pestis	F1-Vag fusion	Stm *aroA*	Leary *et al.*, 1997
Y. pestis	F1 antigen	Stm *aroA*	Bullifent *et al.*, 2000
Y. pestis	V antigen	Stm *aroA*	Garmory *et al.*, 2003
Myccobacterium bovis	30kDa antigen	Stm *aroA*	Hess *et al.*, 2000b
M. tuberculosis	ESAT-6	Stm *aroA*	Mollenkopf *et al.*, 2001
Helicobacter pylori	UreAB	Stm *aroA*	Gomez Duarte *et al.*, 1998
H. pylori	UreAB	Stm PhoP (*phoQ24*)	Corthesy-Theulaz *et al.*, 1998
H. pylori	UreAB	Sty *phoPQ*	DiPetrillo *et al.*, 2000
H. pylori	UreAB	Stm *aroA*	Koesling *et al.*, 2001
H. pylori	UreAB	Sty *aroC aroD* ±*htrA*	Londono-Arcila *et al.*, 2002
ETEC	CS3-ST and LT-B fusions	Stm *aroA*	Yakhchali & Manning, 1997
EHEC	O111 antigen	Stm *aroA*	Wang *et al.*, 1999
EPEC	BfpA pilus	Stm *aroA*	Schriefer *et al.*, 1999
ETEC	CFA/1 fimbriae	Stm *aroA*	Lasaro *et al.*, 1999
ETEC	CFA/1 fimbriae	Stm *aroA*	Pascual *et al.*, 1999
ETEC	Nontoxic ST	Stm *aroA*	Guillobel *et al.*, 2000
ETEC	987P fimbriae	Stm *aroA*	Chen and Schifferli, 2000
ETEC	CS3-ST and LT-B fusions	Stm *cya crp*	Xu *et al.*, 2002
ETEC	Flagellar-ST fusion	Stm *aroA*	Pereira *et al.*, 2001
Listeria monocytogenes	p60, Hly (LLO)	Stm *aroA*	Hess *et al.*, 1996
L. monocytogenes	Hly	Stm *aroA*	Hess *et al.*, 2000a
L. monocytogenes	Hly (LLO), p60	Stm *aroA*	Russmann *et al.*, 2001
Clostridium difficile	Toxin A	Stm *aroA*	Ward *et al.*, 1999
Corynebacterium diptheriae	CRM-197	Sty *aroC aroD htrA*	Orr *et al.*, 1999
Clostridum tetani	Toxin fragment C	Stm *aroA aroD*	Van Cott *et al.*, 1996
C. tetani	Toxin fragment C	Sty *guaBA*	Pasetti *et al.*, 1999
C. tetani	Toxin fragment C	Sty *aroC aroD htrA*	Tacket *et al.*, 2000
Measles	MV epitopes	Stm *aroA*	Spreng *et al.*, 2000
HBV	pre S1, S2	Stm *cya crp*	Schodel *et al.*, 1996
HBV	pre S1, S2	Sty *cya crp-cdt*	Nardelli-Haefliger *et al.*, 1996
HBV	pre S1, S2	Sty *cya crp-cdt*	Tacket *et al.*, 1997b
HBV	HBVcore	Stm *phoP, cya crp* & PhoP[c] (=*phoQ24*)	Nardelli-Haefliger *et al.*, 2001

(Continued)

Table 56.2. Recombinant attenuated bacterial antigen delivery vaccines[a] (Continued)

Pathogen	Protective antigen	Host and attenuation	Reference
HIV	gp120	Stm *aroA*	Wu *et al.*, 1997
SIV	Capsid p27	Stm *aroA*	Steger *et al.*, 1999
SIV	Gag epitopes	Sty *phoPQ* Stm *phoPQ*	Evans *et al.*, 2003
TGEV	Spike protein	Stm *cya crp*	Chen & Schifferli, 2001
HSV-1	gpD	Stm *cya crp*	Karem *et al.*, 1997
HSV-2	gpD	Stm *aroA*	Flo *et al.*, 2001
Papilloma	HBVc-E7 epitope fusion	Stm *aroA*	Londono *et al.*, 1996
Papilloma	L1 V-L particles	Stm PhoP[c] (*phoQ24*)	Nardelli-Haefliger *et al.*,1997
Papilloma	L1 V-L particles	Stm PhoP[c] (*phoQ24*)	Revaz *et al.*, 2001
Echinococcus granulosus	Tetanus toxin C-fatty acid binding protein fusion	Stm *aroA*	Chabalgoity *et al.*, 1997
Entamoeba histolytica	Serine-rich protein	Sty *cya crp-cdt*	Zhang and Stanley,1997
Leishmania major	gp63	Stm *aroA aroD*	McSorley *et al.*, 1997
L. major	gp63	Sty *araC aroD*	Gonzalez *et al.*, 1998
Plasmodium falciparum	MSP-1	Sty *aroC aroD*	Wu *et al.*, 2000
Schistosoma haematobium	Tetanus toxin C-glutathoione S-transferase fusion	Stm *galE*	Lee *et al.*, 2000
Attenuated *Shigella*			
C. tetani	Toxin fragment C	Sh fl 2a Δ*guaBA*	Anderson *et al.*, 2000
ETEC	CS3	Sh fl 2a Δ*aroA* Δ*virG (icsA)*	Noriega *et al.*, 1996b
ETEC	CFA/1 & LT-Tox⁻	Sh fl 2a Δ*guaBA*	Koprowski *et al.*, 2000
ETEC	CS2 & CS3 fimbriae	Sh fl 2a Δ*guaBA*	Altboum *et al.*, 2001
ETEC	CS4 fimbriae	Sh fl 2a Δ*guaBA*	Altboum *et al.*, 2003
ETEC	CFA/1, CS2, CS3, & CS4	Sh fl 2a Δ*guaBA*	Barry *et al.*, 2003
Attenuated *L. monocytogenes*			
Leishmania major	LACK protein	Lm Δ*actA*	Saklani-Jusforgues *et al.*, 2003
Attenuated *V. cholerae*			
Clostridium difficile	Toxin A-HlyA fusion	Vc 01 Δ*ctxAB*	Ryan *et al.*, 1997a
Entamoeba histolytica	ctxB–serine rich protein fusion	Vc Peru2 Δ*attRS1*	Ryan *et al.*, 1997b
EHEC	Shiga toxin B and EaeA	Vc Peru2 Δ*attRS1*	Butterton *et al.*, 1997
ETEC	Tox⁻ LT	Vc Peru2 Δ*attRS1* Δ*irgA*	Ryan *et al.*, 1999
ETEC	ctxB	Vc Peru2 Δ*attRS1*	Ryan *et al.*, 2000
ETEC	ctxB	Vc Peru2 Δ*attRS1*	John *et al.*, 2000
Vibrio cholerae	Tox⁻ CT	Vc E1 Tor Δ*ctxAB*	Fontana *et al.*, 2000

[a]Only articles published during or after 1996 are included.
Stm, *S. typhimurium*; Sty, *S. typhi*; Sh fl 2a, *S. flexneri* 2a; Vc, *V. cholerae*.

protective antigens from other pathogens to elicit primarily mucosal immune responses but also systemic and cellular immunities. Reports focusing on induction of cellular immunity or describing recombinant vaccine constructions not delivered to a mucosal tissue or not evaluating induction of mucosal immunity have been omitted from consideration. We also limit citations in the table to reports published since 1996, because earlier works have been described in numerous reviews (Curtiss, 1990; Roberts *et al.*, 1994; Schodel and Curtiss, 1995; Hantman *et al.*, 1999).

Since bacterial enteric pathogens are likely to represent the best systems with capabilities to induce mucosal immunity and since bacterial enteropathogens cause significant global morbidity and some 1.5 to 2 million deaths annually (World Bank), an important focus in developing recombinant attenuated bacterial antigen delivery systems should be the development of vaccines that would diminish the prevalence and/or severity of infections with *Salmonella enterica* serotypes, *Shigella* species, *V. cholerae*, *E. coli* (especially EPEC, ETEC, and EHEC strains), *C. jejuni*, and *L. monocytogenes*. In this regard, the best antigen delivery vectors are likely to be derived from the listed pathogens that have been successful in colonizing and/or invading tissues of the gastrointestinal system. These vector systems, especially those capable of delivering DNA vaccines, can also be used for immunization against other enteric pathogens such as rotavirus, Norwalk virus, *Giardia*, and *Entamoeba histolytica*.

The use of recombinant attenuated *S. typhi* vaccines in human volunteers has often been associated with episodes of diarrhea (10% to 30% of vaccinated individuals). This problem is even more prevalent in the use of recombinant attenuated *Shigella* vaccines and will likely be experienced with the use of attenuated *V. cholerae* strains for antigen delivery. Consideration therefore needs to be given to means to reduce these sequelae that will likely lessen the popularity of such vaccines. The question arises as to whether genetic modifications can be made to eliminate or greatly reduce induction of diarrhea without compromising and indeed while enhancing immunogenicity to expressed protective antigens. Inactivation of the master flagellar synthesis control gene *flhD* in *S. typhimurium* significantly reduces fluid secretion into ligated ileal loops of calves but also decreases the LD_{50} some 10-fold in orally infected mice (Schmitt *et al.*, 2001). The introduction of mutations into the *S. typhimurium sop* genes also reduces fluid secretion into ileal loops of calves (Zhang *et al.*, 2002, 2003), and these mutations may have the potential for modification of *S. typhi* strains to be used for humans.

Although comparative studies of *S. typhimurium* strains with different types of attenuating mutations have revealed that strains with *phoPQ* attenuation give enhanced Th1-type CD4- and CD8-dependent cellular immunities (Wick *et al.*, 1995; Svensson *et al.*, 1997) and strains with *aro*, *ompR*, *htrA*, and *cya crp* mutations a mixed Th1-Th2-type response more favorable to production of secretory mucosal and systemic antibody responses (Dunstan *et al.*, 1998), little or nothing is known about how to maximize mucosal and systemic antibody

responses with use of recombinant attenuated antigen delivery systems in humans. Both the deletion of genes for expression of type 1 fimbriae and the constitutive overexpression of type 1 fimbriae caused a shift from a Th1-type to a Th2-type immune response in a *S. typhimurium phoP* strain expressing the pneumococcal PspA antigen (Kang *et al.*, 2002b).

The use of recombinant attenuated bacterial antigen delivery systems to develop food-safety vaccines that would prevent and/or reduce infection of agriculturally important animals with bacterial enteropathogens such as *Salmonella*, *E. coli* pathovars, *C. jejuni*, *Enterococcus* species, and *L. monocytogenes* would lessen the likelihood for transmission of these pathogens through the food chain to humans. Since many of these human bacterial enteropathogens acquire antibiotic resistance due to use of antibiotics for promotion of growth and disease prevention in farm animals, these food safety vaccines would likely also reduce transmission of both pathogenic and nonpathogenic bacteria with drug-resistance traits through the food chain to humans. Examples of and success with nonrecombinant attenuated vaccines to prevent *Salmonella* infection in farm animals have recently been reviewed (Mastroeni *et al.*, 2001). There are reports (Pawelec *et al.*, 1997; Wyszyznska *et al.*, 2002) of expressing *C. jejuni*–protective antigens in attenuated *S. typhimurium* strains, but there is no information on induction of protective immunity of poultry to *C. jejuni* infection. A recombinant attenuated *S. typhimurium* vaccine expressing protective antigens from an avian pathogenic *E. coli* (APEC) strain has been constructed and shown to confer protective immunity to infection against APEC strains (Roland *et al.*, 1999). This may or may not be beneficial for humans, since although APEC and UPEC O1 K1 and O2 K2 strains have much in common, they also have numerous differences (Caya *et al.*, 1999).

Some of the most promising research in directly inducing protective immunity in humans to bacterial enteropathogens will likely derive from use of attenuated *S. flexneri* antigen delivery vectors such as CVD1207 (Kotloff *et al.*, 2000). This strain has Δ*guaBA* and Δ*icsA* attenuating mutations with the Δ*sen* and Δ*set* mutations to eliminate enterotoxin production (Table 56.1). Prior research in successfully delivering colonization antigens and detoxified LT and ST components specified by genes from ETEC and EPEC strains (Table 56.2) from *S. flexneri* strains not as well attenuated/contained as CVD1207 provides optimism for future success in preventing/reducing human diarrheal disease.

RECOMBINANT ATTENUATED BACTERIAL DNA VACCINE DELIVERY SYSTEMS

Table 56.3 lists examples in which strains of *Shigella*, *S. typhimurium*, and *L. monocytogenes* have been used to deliver DNA vaccines encoding protective antigens from other pathogens. Most research to date has focused more on inducing cellular immunity to tumors or to pathogens that require

Table 56.3. Recombinant Attenuated Bacterial DNA Vaccine Delivery Systems

Pathogen	Protective Antigen	Host and Attenuation	Reference
Delivered by *Salmonella*			
HBV	S antigen	Stm *aroA*	Woo *et al.*, 2001
HBV	S antigen	Stm *aroA*	Zheng *et al.*, 2002
Herpes simplex virus 2	gpD	Stm *aroA*	Flo *et al.*, 2001
HIV	Env gp120	Stm *aroA*	Hone *et al.*, 2002
ETEC HIV	CTA1 gp120	Stm *aroA*	Bagley *et al.*, 2003
Delivered by *Shigella*			
Measles	F, HA & NP antigens	Sh fl 2a Δ*asd*	Fennelly *et al.*, 1999
HIV	gp120	Sh fl 2a Δ*aroA* Δ*icsA*	Shata and Hone, 2001
HIV	gp120	Sh fl 2a Δ*asd*	Vecino *et al.*, 2002
HIV	Gag	Sh fl 2a *rfbF*	Xu *et al.*, 2003

Stm, *S. typhimurium*; Sh fl 2a, *S. flexneri* 2a.0

a cellular immune response to achieve protective immunity. Thus, research using these technologies to more specifically induce immunities effective at the mucosal cell surface is so far not prevalent. The technologies described earlier that have been used to achieve regulated delayed lysis of *S. typhimurium* for the release of DNA vaccines were developed to investigate induction of protective immunity against *Eimeria* species that colonize the intestinal tracts of poultry and cause coccidiosis (Kong *et al.*, 2003a). This DNA vaccine delivery system induces mucosal and systemic antibody responses, but evaluating the degree of protective immunity, which requires challenge studies, has not yet been done.

It is likely that technologies for the delivery of nucleic acid vaccines will improve if the highly cost-effective means for their delivery with use of attenuated bacterial systems can be perfected. As stated earlier, *Shigella* probably has the most ideal attributes as a nucleic acid vaccine delivery system to especially induce protective mucosal (and systemic) immune responses. Strains of *Shigella* genetically modified to enable regulated delayed release of nucleic acid vaccines are needed to more fully realize the potential of this delivery system.

In the development of nucleic acid vaccine delivery by strains of *Salmonella*, what is needed is a means by which *Salmonella* could escape the endosome prior to lysis with liberation of the nucleic acid vaccine. In the case of *L. monocytogenes*, strains that can be orally administered at much lower doses than now required are needed to make this delivery strategy competitive. In all cases, significant improvements can be made in enhancing the level of expression of genetic information for protective antigens after the nucleic acid vaccine is delivered by the attenuated bacterial strains. One can include sequences in the DNA vaccine vector that would enhance trafficking of the DNA to the nucleus for transcription (Suh *et al.*, 2003). Alternatively, the DNA vaccine vector could be designed to enable synthesis of mRNA templates either in bacteria prior to delivery or in eukaryotic cells after delivery to enable immediate mRNA translation in the cytoplasm of eukaryotic host cells.

CONCLUDING THOUGHTS

Improving health, nutrition, and economic well-being (the latter dependent on the first two) provides the best means to enhance the quality of life globally. Some 18 to 19 million of the total 54 million deaths globally each year are due to infectious diseases. Morbidity due to infectious diseases is an even more invidious curse on society, as chronic respiratory and diarrheal diseases in infancy, coupled with malnutrition, preclude the normal mental development necessary to achieve self-sufficiency by those that survive past age 5 years. The onset of parasitic infections exacerbates the problems and severely diminishes the ability of many to become productive citizens. The more universal use of existing vaccines and the development of improved vaccines that are safe, efficacious, and cost-effective can address these problems.

Live recombinant attenuated bacterial antigen and nucleic acid delivery vaccines can be manufactured, preserved by lyophilization, and reconstituted at the time of use for oral immunization. The cost for growth by fermentation, concentration, lyophilization, bottling, and labeling range from $0.001 to about $0.10 per dose of vaccine for poultry versus humans, respectively. Research to enhance the stability and resistance of such vaccines to temperature stress needs to be conducted. Although progress is being made in the development of these live recombinant vaccines, there is still much to learn to achieve success in developing these safe and efficacious vaccines. We thus know too little about how the successful bacterial pathogens we use evade, modulate, circumvent, and/or suppress host immune responses. We also do not understand very well how some of these pathogens are able to establish a carrier state. We have yet to fully understand how to harness and optimally recruit the innate immune system to enhance induction of acquired immunity with use of these recombinant live vaccine systems. We also have insufficient knowledge of how to modulate and/or enhance Th2- vs. Th1-dependent responses, and this is of critical importance in inducing mucosal immunity. In this regard, we know too little about how to induce antigen-specific memory responses to ensure prompt recall. Last, much more needs to be learned and done to ensure the safety of these live recombinant vaccines by precluding their access to certain host tissues and, by means of biological containment features, ensuring their inability to establish carrier states and survive in the environment.

ACKNOWLEDGMENTS

The author thanks Erika Arch, Vjollca Konjufca, Soo Young Wanda, Wendy Bollen, and Josephine Clark-Curtiss in the preparation of this review chapter.

REFERENCES

Adam, T. (2001). Exploitation of host factors for efficient infection by *Shigella. Int. J. Med. Microbiol.* 291, 287–298.

Adhya, S.L., and Shapiro, J.A. (1969). The galactose operon of *E. coli* K-12. I. Structural and pleiotropic mutations of the operon. *Genetics* 62, 231–247.

Altboum, Z., Barry, E.M., Losonsky, G., Galen, J.E., and Levine, M.M. (2001). Attenuated *Shigella flexneri* 2a ∆*guaBA* strain CVD 1204 expressing enterotoxigenic *Escherichia coli* (ETEC) CS2 and CS3 fimbriae as a live mucosal vaccine against *Shigella* and ETEC infection. *Infect. Immun.* 69, 3150–3158.

Altboum, Z., Levine, M.M., Galen, J.E., and Barry, E.M. (2003). Genetic characterization and immunogenicity of coli surface antigen 4 from enterotoxigenic *Escherichia coli* when it is expressed in a *Shigella* live-vector strain. *Infect. Immun.* 71, 1352–1360.

Anderson, R., Dougan, G., and Roberts, M. (1996). Delivery of the pertactin/P.69 polypeptide of *Bordetella pertussis* using an attenuated *Salmonella typhimurium* vaccine strain: expression levels and immune response. *Vaccine* 14, 1384–1390.

Anderson, R.J., Pasetti, M.F., Sztein, M.B., Levine, M.M., and Noriega, F.R. (2000). ∆*guaBA* attenuated *Shigella flexneri* 2a strain CVD 1204 as a *Shigella* vaccine and as a live mucosal delivery system for fragment C of tetanus toxin. *Vaccine* 18, 2193–2202.

Andrianopoulos, K., Wang, L., and Reeves, P.R. (1998). Identification of the fucose synthetase gene in the colanic acid gene cluster of *Escherichia coli* K-12. *J. Bacteriol.* 180, 998–1001.

Angelakopoulos, H., Loock, K., Sisul, D.M., Jensen, E.R., Miller, J.F., and Hohmann, E.L. (2002). Safety and shedding of an attenuated strain of *Listeria monocytogenes* with a deletion of *actA/plcB* in adult volunteers: a dose escalation study of oral inoculation. *Infect. Immun.* 70, 3592–3601.

Attridge, S.R., Davies, R., and LaBrooy, J.T. (1997). Oral delivery of foreign antigens by attenuated *Salmonella*: consequences of prior exposure to the vector strain. *Vaccine* 15, 155–162.

Audia, J.P., Webb, C.C., and Foster, J.W. (2001). Breaking through the acid barrier: an orchestrated response to proton stress by enteric bacteria. *Int. J. Med. Microbiol.* 291, 97–106.

Bacon, G.A., Burrows, T.W., and Yates, M. (1950). The effects of biochemical mutation on the virulence of *Bacterium typhosum*: the virulence of mutants. *Br. J. Exp. Pathol.* 37, 714–724.

Bacon, G.A., Burrows, T.W., and Yates, M. (1951). The effects of biochemical mutation on the virulence of *Bacterium typhosum*: the loss of virulence of certain mutants. *Br. J. Exp. Pathol.* 32, 85–96.

Bagley, K.C., Shata, M.T., Onyabe, D.Y., DeVico, A.L., Fouts, T.R., Lewis, G.K., and Hone, D.M. (2003). Immunogenicity of DNA vaccines that direct the coincident expression of the 120 kDa glycoprotein of human immunodeficiency virus and the catalytic domain of cholera toxin. *Vaccine* 21, 3335–3341.

Baier, W., Masihi, N., Huber, M., Hoffmann, P., and Bessler, W.G. (2000). Lipopeptides as immunoadjuvants and immunostimulants in mucosal immunization. *Immunobiology* 201, 391–405.

Bajaj, V., Lucas, R.L., Hwang, C., and Lee, C.A. (1996). Co-ordinate regulation of *Salmonella typhimurium* invasion genes by environmental and regulatory factors is mediated by control of *hilA* expression. *Mol. Microbiol.* 22, 703–714.

Baker, S.J., Daniels, C., and Morona, R. (1997). PhoP/Q regulated genes in *Salmonella typhi* identification of melittin sensitive mutants. *Microb. Pathog.* 22, 165–179.

Bang, I.S., Audia, J.P., Park, Y.K., and Foster, J.W. (2002). Autoinduction of the *ompR* response regulator by acid shock and control of the *Salmonella enterica* acid tolerance response. *Mol. Microbiol.* 44, 1235–1250.

Bang, I.S., Kim, B.H., Foster, J.W., and Park, Y.K. (2000). OmpR regulates the stationary-phase acid tolerance response of *Salmonella enterica* serovar Typhimurium. *J. Bacteriol.* 182, 2245–2252.

Bao, J.X., and Clements, J.D. (1991). Prior immunologic experience potentiates the subsequent antibody response when *Salmonella* strains are used as vaccine carriers. *Infect. Immun.* 59, 3841–3845.

Barry, E.M., Altboum, Z., Losonsky, G., and Levine, M.M. (2003). Immune responses elicited against multiple enterotoxigenic *Escherichia coli* fimbriae and mutant LT expressed in attenuated *Shigella* vaccine strains. *Vaccine* 21, 333–340.

Barry, E.M., Gomez-Duarte, O., Chatfield, S., Rappuoli, R., Pizza, M., Losonsky, G., Galen, J., and Levine, M.M. (1996). Expression and immunogenicity of pertussis toxin S1 subunit-tetanus toxin fragment C fusions in *Salmonella typhi* vaccine strain CVD 908. *Infect. Immun.* 64, 4172–4181.

Barzu, S., Fontaine, A., Sansonetti, P., and Phalipon, A. (1996). Induction of a local anti-IpaC antibody response in mice by use of a *Shigella flexneri* 2a vaccine candidate: implications for use of IpaC as a protein carrier. *Infect. Immun.* 64, 1190–1196.

Baumler, A.J., Tsolis, R.M., and Heffron, F. (1996). The *lpf* fimbrial operon mediates adhesion of *Salmonella typhimurium* to murine Peyer's patches. *Proc. Natl. Acad. Sci. USA.* 93, 279–283.

Bearson, B.L., Wilson, L., and Foster, J.W. (1998). A low pH-inducible, PhoPQ-dependent acid tolerance response protects *Salmonella typhimurium* against inorganic acid stress. *J. Bacteriol.* 180, 2409–2417.

Benitez, J.A., Silva, A.J., and Finkelstein, R.A. (2001). Environmental signals controlling production of hemagglutinin/protease in *Vibrio cholerae. Infect. Immun.* 69, 6549–6553.

Benjamin, W.H., Jr., Hall, P., and Briles, D.E. (1991). A *hemA* mutation renders *Salmonella typhimurium* avirulent in mice, yet capable of eliciting protection against intravenous infection with *S. typhimurium. Microb. Pathog.* 11, 289–295.

Berks, B.C. (1996). A common export pathway for proteins binding complex redox cofactors? *Mol. Microbiol.* 22, 393–404.

Bierne, H., Mazmanian, S.K., Trost, M., Pucciarelli, M.G., Liu, G., Dehoux, P., Jansch, L., Garcia-del Portillo, F., Schneewind, O., Cossart, P., and The European *Listeria* Genome Consortium (2002). Inactivation of the *srtA* gene in *Listeria monocytogenes* inhibits anchoring of surface proteins and affects virulence. *Mol. Microbiol.* 43, 869–881.

Bollen, W.S., Gunn, B., Lay, M., and Curtiss III, R. (2003). Colonization of the brain following intranasal inoculation with *Salmonella* [E-086]. Washington, DC: American Society for Microbiology, 103rd General Meeting, 265.

Botsford, J.L., and Harman, J.G. (1992). Cyclic AMP in prokaryotes. *Microbiol. Rev.* 56, 100–122.

Brundage, R.A., Smith, G.A., Camilli, A., Theriot, J.A., and Portnoy, D.A. (1993). Expression and phosphorylation of the *Listeria monocytogenes* ActA protein in mammalian cells. *Proc. Natl. Acad. Sci. U.S.A.* 90, 11890–11894.

Buchmeier, N.A., Lipps, C.J., So, M.Y., and Heffron, F. (1993). Recombination-deficient mutants of *Salmonella typhimurium* are avirulent and sensitive to the oxidative burst of macrophages. *Mol. Microbiol.* 7, 933–936.

Bullifent, H.L., Griffin, K.F., Jones, S.M., Yates, A., Harrington, L., and Titball, R.W. (2000). Antibody responses to *Yersinia pestis* F1-antigen expressed in *Salmonella typhimurium aroA* from in vivo-inducible promoters. *Vaccine* 18, 2668–2676.

Bumann, D., Hueck, C., Aebischer, T., and Meyer, T.F. (2000). Recombinant live *Salmonella* spp. for human vaccination against heterologous pathogens. *FEMS Immunol. Med. Microbiol.* 27, 357–364.

Butterton, J.R., Beattie, D.T., Gardel, C.L., Carroll, P.A., Hyman, T., Killeen, K.P., Mekalanos, J.J., and Calderwood, S.B. (1995). Heterologous antigen expression in *Vibrio cholerae* vector strains. *Infect. Immun.* 63, 2689–2696.

Butterton, J.R., Ryan, E.T., Acheson, D.W., and Calderwood, S.B. (1997). Coexpression of the B subunit of Shiga toxin 1 and EaeA from enterohemorrhagic *Escherichia coli* in *Vibrio cholerae* vaccine strains. *Infect. Immun.* 65, 2127–2135.

Caya, F., Fairbrother, J.M., Lessard, L., and Quessy, S. (1999). Characterization of the risk to human health of pathogenic *Escherichia coli* isolates from chicken carcasses. *J. Food Prot.* 62, 741–746.

Chabalgoity, J.A., Harrison, J.A., Esteves, A., Demarco de Hormaeche, R., Ehrlich, R., Khan, C.M., and Hormaeche, C.E. (1997). Expression and immunogenicity of an *Echinococcus granulosus* fatty acid–binding protein in live attenuated *Salmonella* vaccine strains. *Infect. Immun.* 65, 2402–2412.

Charbit, A., Newton, S.M., Klebba, P.E., Clement, J.M., Fayolle, C., Lo-Man, R., Leclerc, C., and Hofnung, M. (1997). Expression and immune response to foreign epitopes in bacteria. Perspectives for live vaccine development. *Behring Inst. Mitt.* 98, 135–142.

Charles, S., Trigo, E., Settje, T., Abraham, A., and Johnson, P. (1999). Evaluation of a Δ*cya* Δ(*crp-cdt*) *Salmonella choleraesuis* commercial vaccine to protect against clinical signs caused by and reduced shedding of *Salmonella typhimurium* in pigs. Proceedings of the 3rd International Symposium on the Epidemiology and Control of *Salmonella* in Pork, Washington D.C. (P.B. Bahnson, Ed.), pp. 293–295. Iowa State University, Extended and Continuing Education, Ames, IA.

Charles, S.D., Abraham, A.S., Trigo, E.T., Jones, G.F., and Settje, B.A. (2000). Reduced shedding and clinical signs of *Salmonella typhimurium* in nursery pigs vaccinated with a *Salmonella choleraesuis* vaccine. *Swine Health and Production* 8, 107–112.

Chatfield, S., Charles, I.G., Makoff, A.J., Oxer, M.D., Dougan, G., Pickard, D., Slater, D., and Fairweather, N.F. (1992a). Use of the *nirB* promoter to direct the stable expression of heterologous antigens in *Salmonella* oral vaccine strains: Development of a single-dose oral tetanus vaccine. *Biotechnology* 10, 888–892.

Chatfield, S.N., Strahan, K., Pickard, D., Charles, I.G., Hormaeche, C.E., and Dougan, G. (1992b). Evaluation of *Salmonella typhimurium* strains harbouring defined mutations in *htrA* and *aroA* in the murine salmonellosis model. *Microb. Pathog.* 12, 145–151.

Chen, H., and Schifferli, D.M. (2000). Mucosal and systemic immune responses to chimeric fimbriae expressed by *Salmonella enterica* serovar Typhimurium vaccine strains. *Infect. Immun.* 68, 3129–3139.

Chen, H., and Schifferli, D.M. (2001). Enhanced immune responses to viral epitopes by combining macrophage-inducible expression with multimeric display on a *Salmonella* vector. *Vaccine* 19, 3009–3018.

Cochlovius, B., Stassar, M.J., Schreurs, M.W., Benner, A., and Adema, G.J. (2002). Oral DNA vaccination: antigen uptake and presentation by dendritic cells elicits protective immunity. *Immunol. Lett.* 80, 89–96.

Collins, L.V., Attridge, S., and Hackett, J. (1991). Mutations at *rfc* or *pmi* attenuate *Salmonella typhimurium* virulence for mice. *Infect. Immun.* 59, 1079–1085.

Corthesy-Theulaz, I.E., Hopkins, S., Bachmann, D., Saldinger, P.F., Porta, N., Haas, R., Zheng-Xin, Y., Meyer, T., Bouzourene, H., Blum, A.L., and Kraehenbuhl, J.P. (1998). Mice are protected from *Helicobacter pylori* infection by nasal immunization with attenuated *Salmonella typhimurium phoP*^c expressing urease A and B subunits. *Infect. Immun.* 66, 581–586.

Coster, T.S., Hoge, C.W., VanDeVerg, L.L., Hartman, A.B., Oaks, E.V., Venkatesan, M.M., Cohen, D., Robin, G., Fontaine-Thompson, A., Sansonetti, P.J., and Hale, T.L. (1999). Vaccination against shigellosis with attenuated *Shigella flexneri* 2a strain SC602. *Infect. Immun.* 67, 3437–3443.

Cote-Sierra, J., Bredan, A., Toldos, C.M., Stijlemans, B., Brys, L., Cornelis, P., Segovia, M., de Baetselier, P., and Revets, H. (2002). Bacterial lipoprotein–based vaccines induce tumor necrosis factor–dependent type 1 protective immunity against *Leishmania major*. *Infect. Immun.* 70, 240–248.

Coynault, C., Robbe-Saul, V., and Norel, F. (1996). Virulence and vaccine potential of *Salmonella typhimurium* mutants deficient in the expression of the RpoS (σ^S) regulon. *Mol. Microbiol.* 22, 149–160.

Curtiss III, R. (1990). Attenuated *Salmonella* strains as live vectors for the expression of foreign antigens. In *New Generation Vaccines* (eds. G. C. Woodrow and M. M. Levine). New York: Marcel Dekker, 161–188.

Curtiss III, R. (2001). Vaccines and vaccine technology to prevent typhoid and *Salmonella* diarrheal diseases. In *Typhoid Fever and other Salmonellosis. Proceedings of the 4th International Symposium.* Taipei, Taiwan, ROC: Jeou-Chou Book Co., 1–24.

Curtiss III, R. (2002). Perspective: Bacterial infectious disease control by vaccine development. *J. Clin. Invest.* 110, 1061–1066.

Curtiss III, R., Doggett, T., Nayak, A., and Srinivasan, J. (1996). Strategies for the use of live recombinant avirulent bacterial vaccines for mucosal immunization. In *Essentials of Mucosal Immunology* (eds. H. Kiyono & M. F. Kagnoff). San Diego: Academic Press, 499–511.

Curtiss III, R., and Kelly, S.M. (1987). *Salmonella typhimurium* deletion mutants lacking adenylate cyclase and cyclic AMP receptor protein are avirulent and immunogenic. *Infect. Immun.* 55, 3035–3043.

Curtiss III, R., MacLeod, D.L., Lockman, H.A., Galan, J.E., Kelly, S.M., and Mahairas, G.G. (1993). Colonization and invasion of the intestinal tract by *Salmonella*. In *Biology of Salmonella* (ed. F. Cabello). New York: Plenum Press, 191–198.

d' Hauteville, H., and Sansonetti, P.J. (1992). Phosphorylation of IcsA by cAMP-dependent protein kinase and its effect on intracellular spread of *Shigella flexneri*. *Mol. Microbiol.* 6, 833–841.

Daigle, F., Hou, J.Y., and Clark-Curtiss, J.E. (2002). Microbial gene expression elucidated by selective capture of transcribed sequences (SCOTS). *Meth. Enz.* 358, 108–122.

Dalla Pozza, T., Yan, H., Meek, D., Guzman, C.A., and Walker, M.J. (1998). Construction and characterisation of *Salmonella typhimurium aroA* simultaneously expressing the five pertussis toxin subunits. *Vaccine* 16, 522–529.

Denis, F., Badiane, S., Chiron, J.P., Sow, A., and Mar, I.D. (1977). *Salmonella* meningitis in infants. *Lancet* 1, 910.

Dietrich, G., Spreng, S., Gentschev, I., and Goebel, W. (2000). Bacterial systems for the delivery of eukaryotic antigen expression vectors. *Antisense Nucleic Acid Drug Dev.* 10, 391–399.

Dilts, D.A., Riesenfeld-Orn, I., Fulginiti, J.P., Ekwall, E., Granert, C., Nonenmacher, J., Brey, R.N., Cryz, S.J., Karlsson, K., Bergman, K., Thompson, T., Hu, B., Bruckner, A.H., and Lindberg, A.A. (2000). Phase I clinical trials of *aroA aroD* and *aroA aroD htrA* attenuated *S. typhi* vaccines; effect of formulation on safety and immunogenicity. *Vaccine* 18, 1473–1484.

DiPetrillo, M.D., Tibbetts, T., Kleanthous, H., Killeen, K.P., and Hohmann, E.L. (2000). Safety and immunogenicity of *phoP/phoQ*-deleted *Salmonella typhi* expressing *Helicobacter pylori* urease in adult volunteers. *Vaccine* 18, 449–459.

Doggett, T., and Brown, P.K. (1996). Attenuated *Salmonella* as vectors for oral immunization. In *Mucosal Vaccines* (eds. H. Kiyono, P. L. Ogra, and J. R. McGhee). San Diego: Academic Press, 105–118.

Domann, E., Wehland, J., Rohde, M., Pistor, S., Hartl, M., Goebel, W., Leimeister-Wachter, M., Wuenscher, M., and Chakraborty, T.

(1992). A novel bacterial virulence gene in *Listeria monocytogenes* required for host cell microfilament interaction with homology to the proline-rich region of vinculin. *EMBO J.* 11, 1981–1990.

Dorman, C.J., Chatfield, S., Higgins, C.F., Hayward, C., and Dougan, G. (1989). Characterization of *porin* and *ompR* mutants of a virulent strain of *Salmonella typhimurium: ompR* mutants are attenuated *in vivo. Infect. Immun.* 57, 2136–2140.

Dozois, C.M., Dho-Moulin, M., Bree, A., Fairbrother, J.M., Desautels, C., and Curtiss III, R. (2000). Relationship between the Tsh autotransporter and pathogenicity of avian *Escherichia coli* and localization and analysis of the Tsh genetic region. *Infect. Immun.* 68, 4145–4154.

Drabner, B., and Guzman, C.A. (2001). Elicitation of predictable immune responses by using live bacterial vectors. *Biomolecular Engineering* 17, 75–82.

Dramsi, S., Levi, S., Triller, A., and Cossart, P. (1998). Entry of *Listeria monocytogenes* into neurons occurs by cell-to-cell spread: an in vitro study. *Infect. Immun.* 66, 4461–4468.

Duncan, M.J. (2003). Genomics of oral bacteria. *Crit. Rev. Oral Biol. Med.* 14, 175–187.

Dunstan, S.J., Ramsay, A.J., and Strugnell, R.A. (1996). Studies of immunity and bacterial invasiveness in mice given a recombinant *Salmonella* vector encoding murine interleukin-6. *Infect. Immun.* 64, 2730–2736.

Dunstan, S.J., Simmons, C.P., and Strugnell, R.A. (1998). Comparison of the abilities of different attenuated *Salmonella typhimurium* strains to elicit humoral immune responses against heterologous antigen. *Infect. Immun.* 66, 732–740.

DuPont, H.L., Levine, M.M., Hornick, R.B., and Formal, S.B. (1989). Inoculum size in shigellosis and implications for expected mode of transmission. *J. Infect. Dis.* 159, 1126–1128.

Dussurget, O., Cabanes, D., Dehoux, P., Lecuit, M., The European *Listeria* Genome Consortium, Buchrieser, C., Glaser, P., and Cossart, P. (2002). *Listeria monocytogenes* bile salt hydrolase is a PrfA-regulated virulence factor involved in the intestinal and hepatic phases of listeriosis. *Mol. Micobiol.* 45, 1095–1106.

Dutta, P.R., Cappello, R., Navarro-Garcia, F., and Nataro, J.P. (2002). Functional comparison of serine protease autotransporters of Enterobacteriaceae. *Infect. Immun.* 70, 7105–7113.

Emory, S.A., Bouvet, P., and Belasco, J.G. (1992). A 5′-terminal stem-loop structure can stabilize mRNA in *Escherichia coli. Genes Dev.* 6, 135–148.

Eriksson, S., Lucchini, S., Thompson, A., Rhen, M., and Hinton, J.C. (2003). Unravelling the biology of macrophage infection by gene expression profiling of intracellular *Salmonella enterica. Mol. Microbiol.* 47, 103–118.

Ernst, R.K., Dombroski, D.M., and Merrick, J.M. (1990). Anaerobiosis, type 1 fimbriae, and growth phase are factors that affect invasion of HEp-2 cells by *Salmonella typhimurium. Infect. Immun.* 58, 2014–2016.

Evans, D.T., Chen, L.M., Gillis, J., Lin, K.C., Harty, B., Mazzara, G.P., Donis, R.O., Mansfield, K.G., Lifson, J.D., Desrosiers, R.C., Galan, J.E., and Johnson, R.P. (2003). Mucosal priming of simian immunodeficiency virus–specific cytotoxic T-lymphocyte responses in rhesus macaques by the *Salmonella* type III secretion antigen delivery system. *J. Virol.* 77, 2400–2409.

Everest, P., Allen, J., Papakonstantinopoulou, A., Mastroeni, P., Roberts, M., and Dougan, G. (1997). *Salmonella typhimurium* infections in mice deficient in interleukin-4 production: role of IL-4 in infection-associated pathology. *J. Immunol.* 159, 1820–1827.

Fang, F.C., Libby, S.J., Buchmeier, N.A., Loewen, P.C., Switala, J., Harwood, J., and Guiney, D.G. (1992). The alternative sigma factor *katF* (*rpoS*) regulates *Salmonella* virulence. *Proc. Natl. Acad. Sci. USA.* 89, 11978–11982.

Fasano, A., Baudry, B., Pumplin, D.W., Wasserman, S.S., Tall, B.D., Ketley, J.M., and Kaper, J.B. (1991). *Vibrio cholerae* produces a second enterotoxin, which affects intestinal tight junctions. *Proc. Natl. Acad. Sci. USA.* 88, 5242–5246.

Feng, X., Oropeza, R., and Kenney, L.J. (2003). Dual regulation by phospho-OmpR of *ssrA/B* gene expression in *Salmonella* pathogenicity island 2. *Mol. Microbiol.* 48, 1131–1143.

Fennelly, G.J., Khan, S.A., Abadi, M.A., Wild, T.F., and Bloom, B.R. (1999). Mucosal DNA vaccine immunization against measles

with a highly attenuated *Shigella flexneri* vector. *J. Immunol.* 162, 1603–1610.

Fields, P.I., Groisman, E.A., and Heffron, F. (1989). A *Salmonella* locus that controls resistance to microbicidal proteins from phagocytic cells. *Science* 243, 1059–1062.

Fields, P.I., Swanson, R.V., Haidaris, C.G., and Heffron, F. (1986). Mutants of *Salmonella typhimurium* that cannot survive within the macrophage are avirulent. *Proc. Natl. Acad. Sci. USA.* 83, 5189–5193.

Finlay, B.B., and Falkow, S. (1990). *Salmonella* interactions with polarized human intestinal Caco-2 epithelial cells. *J. Infect. Dis.* 162, 1096–1106.

Flo, J., Tisminetzky, S., and Baralle, F. (2001). Oral transgene vaccination mediated by attenuated Salmonellae is an effective method to prevent herpes simplex virus–2 induced disease in mice. *Vaccine* 19, 1772–1782.

Fontana, M.R., Monaci, E., Yanqing, L., Guoming, Q., Duan, G., Rappuoli, R., and Pizza, M. (2000). IEM101, a naturally attenuated *Vibrio cholerae* strain as carrier for genetically detoxified derivatives of cholera toxin. *Vaccine* 19, 75–85.

Foster, J.W., and Spector, M.P. (1995). How *Salmonella* survive against the odds. *Annu. Rev. Microbiol.* 49, 145–174.

Frey, S.E., Bollen, W., Sizemore, D., Campbell, M., and Curtiss III, R. (2001). Bacteremia associated with live attenuated χ8110 *Salmonella enterica* serovar Typhi ISP1820 in healthy adult volunteers. *Clin. Immunol.* 101, 32–37.

Fukasawa, T., and Nikaido, H. (1961). Galactose mutants of *Salmonella typhimurium. Genetics* 46, 1295–1303.

Gahan, C.G.M., and Collins, J.K. (1995). Vaccination of mice with attenuated mutants of *Listeria monocytogenes*: requirement for induction of macrophage Ia expression. *Microb. Path.* 18, 417–422.

Gaillard, J.L., Berche, P., Mounier, J., Richard, S., and Sansonetti, P. (1987). In vitro model of penetration and intracellular growth of *Listeria monocytogenes* in the human enterocyte-like cell line Caco-2. *Infect. Immun.* 55, 2822–2829.

Galan, J.E., and Collmer, A. (1999). Type III secretion machines: bacterial devices for protein delivery into host cells. *Science* 284, 1322–1328.

Galan, J.E., and Curtiss III, R. (1989). Virulence and vaccine potential of *phoP* mutants of *Salmonella typhimurium. Microb. Pathog.* 6, 433–443.

Galan, J.E., and Curtiss III, R. (1990). Expression of *Salmonella typhimurium* genes required for invasion is regulated by changes in DNA supercoiling. *Infect. Immun.* 58, 1879–1885.

Galan, J.E., Nakayama, K., and Curtiss III, R. (1990). Cloning and characterization of the *asd* gene of *Salmonella typhimurium*: use in stable maintenance of recombinant plasmids in *Salmonella* vaccine strains. *Gene* 94, 29–35.

Galen, J.E., Gomez-Duarte, O.G., Losonsky, G.A., Halpern, J.L., Lauderbaugh, C.S., Kaintuck, S., Reymann, M.K., and Levine, M.M. (1997). A murine model of intranasal immunization to assess the immunogenicity of attenuated *Salmonella typhi* live vector vaccines in stimulating serum antibody response to expressed foreign antigens. *Vaccine* 15, 700–708.

Galen, J.E., and Levine, M.M. (2001). Can a 'flawless' live vector vaccine strain be engineered? *Trends Microbiol.* 9, 372–376.

Galen, J.E., Nair, J., Wang, J.Y., Wasserman, S.S., Tanner, M.K., Sztein, M.B., and Levine, M.M. (1999). Optimization of plasmid maintenance in the attenuated live vector vaccine strain *Salmonella typhi* CVD 908-*htrA. Infect. Immun.* 67, 6424–6433.

Garcia-del Portillo, F., Foster, J.W., and Finlay, B.B. (1993). Role of acid tolerance response genes in *Salmonella typhimurium* virulence. *Infect. Immun.* 61, 4489–4492.

Garcia-Vescovi, E., Soncini, F.C., and Groisman, E.A. (1996). Mg2+ as an extracellular signal: environmental regulation of *Salmonella* virulence. *Cell* 84, 165–174.

Garmory, H.S., Griffin, K.F., Brown, K.A., and Titball, R.W. (2003). Oral immunisation with live *aroA* attenuated *Salmonella enterica* serovar Typhimurium expressing the *Yersinia pestis* V antigen protects mice against plague. *Vaccine* 21, 3051–3057.

Gentschev, I., Dietrich, G., Spreng, S., Kolb-Maurer, A., Daniels, J., Hess, J., Kaufmann, S.H., and Goebel, W. (2000). Delivery of protein antigens and DNA by virulence-attenuated strains of *Salmonella typhimurium* and *Listeria monocytogenes*. *J. Biotechnol.* 83, 19–26.

Gerdes, K., Gultyaev, A.P., Franch, T., Pedersen, K., and Mikkelsen, N.D. (1997). Antisense RNA-regulated programmed cell death. *Annu. Rev. Genet.* 31, 1–31.

Germanier, R., and Furer, E. (1971). Immunity in experimental salmonellosis. II. Basis for the avirulence and protective capacity of *galE* mutants of *Salmonella typhimurium*. *Infect. Immun.* 4, 663–673.

Germanier, R., and Furer, E. (1975). Isolation and characterization of GalE mutant Ty 21a of *Salmonella typhi*: a candidate strain for a live, oral typhoid vaccine. *J. Infect. Dis.* 131, 553–558.

Giannella, R.A., Washington, O., Gemski, P., and Formal, S.B. (1973). Invasion of HeLa cells by *Salmonella typhimurium*: a model for study of invasiveness of *Salmonella*. *J. Infect. Dis.* 128, 69–75.

Gibson, K.J., Blaha, T., Frank, R.K., Charles, S.D., and Trigo, E. (1999). Investigation into the capability of a *Salmonella choleraesuis* live vaccine to reduce the shedding of *Salmonella tyhimurium* in swine. Proceedings of the 3rd International Symposium on the Epidemiology and Control of *Salmonella* in Pork, Washington D.C. (P.B. Bahnson, Ed.), pp. 302–304. Iowa State University, Extended and Continuing Education, Ames, IA.

Goldberg, M.B. (2001). Actin-based motility of intracellular microbial pathogens. *Microbiol. Mol. Biol. Rev.* 65, 595–626.

Gomez-Duarte, O.G., Lucas, B., Yan, Z.X., Panthel, K., Haas, R., and Meyer, T.F. (1998). Protection of mice against gastric colonization by *Helicobacter pylori* by single oral dose immunization with attenuated *Salmonella typhimurium* producing urease subunits A and B. *Vaccine* 16, 460–471.

Gonzalez, C.R., Noriega, F.R., Huerta, S., Santiago, A., Vega, M., Paniagua, J., Ortiz-Navarrete, V., Isibasi, A., and Levine, M.M. (1998). Immunogenicity of a *Salmonella typhi* CVD 908 candidate vaccine strain expressing the major surface protein gp63 of *Leishmania mexicana mexicana*. *Vaccine* 16, 1043–1052.

Graham, J.E., and Clark-Curtiss, J.E. (1999). Identification of *Mycobacterium tuberculosis* RNAs synthesized in response to phagocytosis by human macrophages by selective capture of transcribed sequences (SCOTS). *Proc. Natl. Acad. Sci. USA.* 96, 11554–11559.

Grillot-Courvalin, C., Goussard, S., Huetz, F., Ojcius, D.M., and Courvalin, P. (1998). Functional gene transfer from intracellular bacteria to mammalian cells. *Nat. Biotechnol.* 16, 862–866.

Groisman, E.A., Chiao, E., Lipps, C.J., and Heffron, F. (1989). *Salmonella typhimurium phoP* virulence gene is a transcriptional regulator. *Proc. Natl. Acad. Sci. USA.* 86, 7077–7081.

Guillobel, H.C., Carinhanha, J.I., Cardenas, L., Clements, J.D., de Almeida, D.F., and Ferreira, L.C. (2000). Adjuvant activity of a nontoxic mutant of *Escherichia coli* heat-labile enterotoxin on systemic and mucosal immune responses elicited against a heterologous antigen carried by a live *Salmonella enterica* serovar Typhimurium vaccine strain. *Infect. Immun.* 68, 4349–4353.

Gulig, P.A., and Curtiss III, R. (1987). Plasmid-associated virulence of *Salmonella typhimurium*. *Infect. Immun.* 55, 2891–2901.

Gunn, J.S. (2000). Mechanisms of bacterial resistance and response to bile. *Microbes Infect.* 2, 907–913.

Gunn, J.S., Ernst, R.K., McCoy, A.J., and Miller, S.I. (2000). Constitutive mutations of the *Salmonella enterica* serovar Typhimurium transcriptional virulence regulator *phoP*. *Infect. Immun.* 68, 3758–3762.

Hackett, J., Kotlarski, I., Mathan, V., Francki, K., and Rowley, D. (1986). The colonization of Peyer's patches by a strain of *Salmonella typhimurium* cured of the cryptic plasmid. *J. Infect. Dis.* 153, 1119–1125.

Hall, H.K., and Foster, J.W. (1996). The role of *fur* in the acid tolerance response of *Salmonella typhimurium* is physiologically and genetically separable from its role in iron acquisition. *J. Bacteriol.* 178, 5683–5691.

Hantman, M.J., Hohmann, E.L., Murphy, C.G., Knipe, D.M., and Miller, S.I. (1999). Antigen delivery systems: development of recombinant live vaccines using viral or bacterial vectors. In *Mucosal Immunology* (eds. P. L. Ogra, M. E. Lamm,

J. Bienenstock, J. Mestecky, W. Strober, and J. R. McGhee). San Diego: Academic Press, 779–791.

Heithoff, D.M., Sinsheimer, R.L., Low, D.A., and Mahan, M.J. (1999). An essential role for DNA adenine methylation in bacterial virulence. *Science* 284, 967–970.

Hensel, M., Shea, J.E., Gleeson, C., Jones, M.D., Dalton, E., and Holden, D.W. (1995). Simultaneous identification of bacterial virulence genes by negative selection. *Science* 269, 400–403.

Hess, J., Gentschev, I., Miko, D., Welzel, M., Ladel, C., Goebel, W., and Kaufmann, S.H. (1996). Superior efficacy of secreted over somatic antigen display in recombinant *Salmonella* vaccine induced protection against listeriosis. *Proc. Natl. Acad. Sci. USA.* 93, 1458–1463.

Hess, J., Grode, L., Gentschev, I., Fensterle, J., Dietrich, G., Goebel, W., and Kaufmann, S.H. (2000a). Secretion of different listeriolysin cognates by recombinant attenuated *Salmonella typhimurium*: superior efficacy of haemolytic over non-haemolytic constructs after oral vaccination. *Microbes Infect.* 2, 1799–1806.

Hess, J., Grode, L., Hellwig, J., Conradt, P., Gentschev, I., Goebel, W., Ladel, C., and Kaufmann, S.H. (2000b). Protection against murine tuberculosis by an attenuated recombinant *Salmonella typhimurium* vaccine strain that secretes the 30-kDa antigen of *Mycobacterium bovis* BCG. *FEMS Immunol. Med. Microbiol.* 27, 283–289.

Hohmann, E.L., Oletta, C.A., Killeen, K.P., and Miller, S.I. (1996b). *phoP/phoQ*-deleted *Salmonella typhi* (Ty800) is a safe and immunogenic single-dose typhoid fever vaccine in volunteers. *J. Infect. Dis.* 173, 1408–1414.

Hohmann, E.L., Oletta, C.A., Loomis, W.P., and Miller, S.I. (1995). Macrophage-inducible expression of a model antigen in *Salmonella typhimurium* enhances immunogenicity. *Proc. Natl. Acad. Sci. USA.* 92, 2904–2908.

Hohmann, E.L., Oletta, C.A., and Miller, S.I. (1996a). Evaluation of a *phoP/phoQ*-deleted, *aroA*-deleted live oral *Salmonella typhi* vaccine strain in human volunteers. *Vaccine* 14, 19–24.

Hoiseth, S.K., and Stocker, B.A. (1981). Aromatic-dependent *Salmonella typhimurium* are non-virulent and effective as live vaccines. *Nature* 291, 238–239.

Hondalus, M.K., Bardarov, S., Russell, R., Chan, J., Jacobs Jr., W.R., and Bloom, B.R. (2000). Attenuation of and protection induced by a leucine auxotroph of *Mycobacterium tuberculosis*. *Infect. Immun.* 68, 2888–2889.

Hone, D., Attridge, S., van den Bosch, L., and Hackett, J. (1988b). A chromosomal integration system for stabilization of heterologous genes in *Salmonella* based vaccine strains. *Microb. Pathog.* 5, 407–418.

Hone, D.M., Attridge, S.R., Forrest, B., Morona, R., Daniels, D., LaBrooy, J.T., Bartholomeusz, R.C., Shearman, D.J., and Hackett, J. (1988a). A *galE* via (Vi antigen–negative) mutant of *Salmonella* typhi Ty2 retains virulence in humans. *Infect. Immun.* 56, 1326–1333.

Hone, D.M., DeVico, A.L., Fouts, T.R., Onyabe, D.Y., Agwale, S.M., Wambebe, C.O., Blattner, W.A., Gallo, R.C., and Lewis, G.K. (2002). Development of vaccination strategies that elicit broadly neutralizing antibodies against human immunodeficiency virus type 1 in both the mucosal and systemic immune compartments. *J. Hum. Virol.* 5, 17–23.

Hone, D.M., Harris, A.M., Chatfield, S., Dougan, G., and Levine, M.M. (1991). Construction of genetically defined double *aro* mutants of *Salmonella typhi*. *Vaccine* 9, 810–816.

Hone, D.M., Powell, J., Crowley, R.W., Maneval, D., and Lewis, G.K. (1998). Lipopolysaccharide from an *Escherichia coli htrB msbB* mutant induces high levels of MIP-1 α and MIP-1 β secretion without inducing TNF-α and IL-1 β. *J. Hum. Virol.* 1, 251–256.

Hone, D.M., Tacket, C.O., Harris, A.M., Kay, B., Losonsky, G., and Levine, M.M. (1992). Evaluation in volunteers of a candidate live oral attenuated *Salmonella typhi* vector vaccine. *J. Clin. Invest.* 90, 412–420.

Hopkins, S., Kraehenbuhl, J.P., Schodel, F., Potts, A., Peterson, D., de Grandi, P., and Nardelli-Haefliger, D. (1995). A recombinant *Salmonella typhimurium* vaccine induces local immunity by four different routes of immunization. *Infect. Immun.* 63, 3279–3286.

Hosmalin, A., Andrieu, M., Loing, E., Desoutter, J.F., Hanau, D., Gras-Masse, H., Dautry-Varsat, A., and Guillet, J.G. (2001). Lipopeptide presentation pathway in dendritic cells. *Immunol. Lett.* 79, 97–100.

Huang, Y., Hajishengallis, G., and Michalek, S.M. (2000). Construction and characterization of a *Salmonella enterica* serovar Typhimurium clone expressing a salivary adhesin of *Streptococcus mutans* under control of the anaerobically inducible *nirB* promoter. *Infect. Immun.* 68, 1549–1556.

Humphries, A.D., Raffatellu, M., Winter, S., Weening, E.H., Kingsley, R.A., Droleskey, R., Zhang, S., Figueiredo, J., Khare, S., Nunes, J., Adams, L.G., Tsolis, R.M., and Baumler, A.J. (2003). The use of flow cytometry to detect expression of subunits encoded by 11 *Salmonella enterica* serotype Typhimurium fimbrial operons. *Mol. Microbiol.* 48, 1357–1376.

Jacobs, W.R., Jr., Snapper, S.B., and Bloom, B.R. (1988). Beyond BCG: developing recombinant BCG multivaccine vehicle. In *Molecular Biology and Infectious Diseases* (ed. M. Schwartz). New York: Elsevier, 207–212.

Janssen, R., and Tommassen, J. (1994). PhoE protein as a carrier for foreign epitopes. *Int. Rev. Immunol.* 11, 113–121.

John, M., Crean, T.I., Calderwood, S.B., and Ryan, E.T. (2000). In vitro and in vivo analyses of constitutive and in vivo–induced promoters in attenuated vaccine and vector strains of *Vibrio cholerae*. *Infect. Immun.* 68, 1171–1175.

Jonquieres, R., Pizarro-Cerda, and Cossart, P. (2001). Synergy between the N- and C-terminal domains of InlB for efficient invasion of non-phagocytic cells by *Listeria monocytogenes*. *Mol. Micobiol.* 42, 955–965.

Kang, H.Y., and Curtiss III, R. (2003). Immune responses dependent on antigen location in recombinant attenuated *Salmonella typhimurium* vaccines following oral immunization. *FEMS Immunol. Med. Microbiol.* 37, 99–104.

Kang, H.Y., Lee, T.H., Zhang, X., and Curtiss III, R. (2002b). Variation of the PspA immune responses induced by live PspA-*Salmonella* vaccines carrying different types of attenuations and surface adhesions [E-56]. In *American Society for Microbiology, 102nd General Meeting, Salt Lake City, Utah*. Washington, DC: American Society for Microbiology, 197.

Kang, H.Y., Srinivasan, J., and Curtiss III, R. (2002a). Immune responses to recombinant pneumococcal PspA antigen delivered by live attenuated *Salmonella enterica* serovar *typhimurium* vaccine. *Infect. Immun.* 70, 1739–1749.

Kaniga, K., Compton, M.S., Curtiss III, R., and Sundaram, P. (1998). Molecular and functional characterization of *Salmonella enterica* serovar *typhimurium poxA* gene: effect on attenuation of virulence and protection. *Infect. Immun.* 66, 5599–5606.

Kaper, J.B., Lockman, H., Baldini, M.M., and Levine, M.M. (1984). Recombinant nontoxinogenic *Vibrio cholerae* strains as attenuated cholera vaccine candidates. *Nature* 308, 655–658.

Karem, K.L., Bowen, J., Kuklin, N., and Rouse, B.T. (1997). Protective immunity against herpes simplex virus (HSV) type 1 following oral administration of recombinant *Salmonella typhimurium* vaccine strains expressing HSV antigens. *J. Gen. Virol.* 78, 427–434.

Karim, M., and Islam, N. (2002). *Salmonella meningitis*: report of three cases in adults and literature review. *Infection* 30, 104–108.

Kelly, S.M., Bosecker, B.A., and Curtiss III, R. (1992). Characterization and protective properties of attenuated mutants of *Salmonella choleraesuis*. *Infect. Immun.* 60, 4881–4890.

Kennedy, M.J., Yancey, R.J., Jr., Sanchez, M.S., Rzepkowski, R.A., Kelly, S.M., and Curtiss III, R. (1999). Attenuation and immunogenicity of Δ*cya* Δ*crp* derivatives of *Salmonella choleraesuis* in pigs. *Infect. Immun.* 67, 4628–4636.

Khan, S.A., Stratford, R., Wu, T., Mckelvie, N., Bellaby, T., Hindle, Z., Sinha, K.A., Eltze, S., Mastroeni, P., Pickard, D., Dougan, G., Chatfield, S., and Brennan, F.R. (2003). *Salmonella typhi* and *S. typhimurium* derivatives harbouring deletions in aromatic biosynthesis and *Salmonella* Pathogenicity Island-2 (SPI-2) genes as vaccines and vectors. *Vaccine* 21, 538–548.

Kier, L.D., Weppelman, R.M., and Ames, B.N. (1979). Regulation of nonspecific acid phosphatase in *Salmonella: phoN* and *phoP* genes. *J. Bacteriol.* 138, 155–161.

Kingsley, R.A., van Amsterdam, K., Kramer, N., and Baumler, A.J. (2000). The *shdA* gene is restricted to serotypes of *Salmonella enterica* subspecies I and contributes to efficient and prolonged fecal shedding. *Infect. Immun.* 68, 2720–2727.

Klauser, T., Pohlner, J., and Meyer, T.F. (1990). Extracellular transport of cholera toxin B subunit using *Neisseria* IgA protease β-domain: conformation-dependent outer membrane translocation. *EMBO J.* 9, 1991–1999.

Koesling, J., Lucas, B., Develioglou, L., Aebischer, T., and Meyer, T.F. (2001). Vaccination of mice with live recombinant *Salmonella typhimurium aroA* against *H. pylori*: parameters associated with prophylactic and therapeutic vaccine efficacy. *Vaccine* 20, 413–420.

Kohler, J.J., Pathangey, L.B., and Brown, T.A. (1998). Oral immunization with recombinant *Salmonella typhimurium* expressing a cloned *Porphyromonas gingivalis* hemagglutinin: effect of boosting on mucosal, systemic and immunoglobulin G subclass response. *Oral Microbiol. Immunol.* 13, 81–88.

Kohler, J.J., Pathangey, L.B., Gillespie, S.R., and Brown, T.A. (2000). Effect of preexisting immunity to *Salmonella* on the immune response to recombinant *Salmonella enterica* serovar Typhimurium expressing a *Porphyromonas gingivalis* hemagglutinin. *Infect. Immun.* 68, 3116–3120.

Kolenbrander, P.E. (2000). Oral microbial communities: biofilms, interactions, and genetic systems. *Annu. Rev. Microbiol.* 54, 413–437.

Kong, W., Wanda, S.Y., and Curtiss III, R. (2003a). Construction and application of hot-vector systems for DNA vaccine vector delivery [Z-016]. In *American Society for Microbiology, 103rd General Meeting, Washington, DC*. Washington, DC: American Society for Microbiology, 677.

Kong, W., Wanda, S.Y., and Curtiss III, R. (2003b). Regulated bacterial lysis for antigen release [E-031]. In *American Society for Microbiology, 103rd General Meeting, Washington, DC*. Washington, DC: American Society for Microbiology, 255.

Koprowski, H., 2nd, Levine, M.M., Anderson, R.J., Losonsky, G., Pizza, M., and Barry, E.M. (2000). Attenuated *Shigella flexneri* 2a vaccine strain CVD 1204 expressing colonization factor antigen I and mutant heat-labile enterotoxin of enterotoxigenic *Escherichia coli*. *Infect. Immun.* 68, 4884–4892.

Kotloff, K.L., Noriega, F.R., Samandari, T., Sztein, M.B., Losonsky, G.A., Nataro, J.P., Picking, W.D., Barry, E.M., and Levine, M.M. (2000). *Shigella flexneri* 2a strain CVD 1207, with specific deletions in *virG*, *sen*, *set*, and *guaBA*, is highly attenuated in humans. *Infect. Immun.* 68, 1034–1039.

Kotloff, K.L., Taylor, D.N., Sztein, M.B., Wasserman, S.S., Losonsky, G.A., Nataro, J.P., Venkatesan, M., Hartman, A., Picking, W.D., Katz, D.E., Campbell, J.D., Levine, M.M., and Hale, T.L. (2002). Phase I evaluation of Δ*virG Shigella sonnei* live, attenuated, oral vaccine strain WRSS1 in healthy adults. *Infect. Immun.* 70, 2016–2021.

Kozarov, E., Miyashita, N., Burks, J., Cerveny, K., Brown, T.A., McArthur, W.P., and Progulske-Fox, A. (2000). Expression and immunogenicity of hemagglutinin A from *Porphyromonas gingivalis* in an avirulent *Salmonella enterica* serovar Typhimurium vaccine strain. *Infect. Immun.* 68, 732–739.

Kramer, U., Konstantin, R., Apfel, H., Autenrieth, I.B., and Lattemann, C.T. (2003). Autodisplay: Development of an efficacious system for surface display of antigenic determinants in *Salmonella* vaccine strains. *Infect. Immun.* 71, 1944–1952.

Lagranderie, M., Murray, A., Gicquel, B., Leclerc, C., and Gheorghiu, M. (1993). Oral immunization with recombinant BCG induces cellular and humoral immune responses against the foreign antigen. *Vaccine* 11, 1283–1290.

Lasaro, M.O., Alves, A.M., Guillobel, H.C., Almeida, D.F., and Ferreira, L.C. (1999). New vaccine strategies against enterotoxigenic *Escherichia coli*. II: Enhanced systemic and secreted antibody responses against the CFA/I fimbriae by priming with DNA and boosting with a live recombinant *Salmonella* vaccine. *Braz. J. Med. Biol. Res.* 32, 241–246.

Leary, S.E., Griffin, K.F., Garmory, H.S., Williamson, E.D., and Titball, R.W. (1997). Expression of an F1/V fusion protein in attenuated *Salmonella typhimurium* and protection of mice against plague. *Microb. Pathog.* 23, 167–179.

Lecuit, M., Vandormael-Pournin, S., Lefort, J., Huerre, M., Gounon, P., Dupuy, C., Babinet, C., and Cossart, P. (2001). A transgenic model for listeriosis: role of internalin in crossing the intestinal barrier. *Science* 292, 1722–1725.

Lee, C.A., and Falkow, S. (1990). The ability of *Salmonella* to enter mammalian cells is affected by bacterial growth state. *Proc. Natl. Acad. Sci. USA.* 87, 4304–4308.

Lee, I.S., Lin, J., Hall, H.K., Bearson, B.L., and Foster, J.W. (1995). The stationary-phase sigma factor sigma S (RpoS) is required for a sustained acid tolerance response in virulent *Salmonella typhimurium*. *Mol. Micobiol.* 17, 155–167.

Lee, J.J., Sinha, K.A., Harrison, J.A., de Hormaeche, R.D., Riveau, G., Pierce, R.J., Capron, A., Wilson, R.A., and Khan, C.M. (2000). Tetanus toxin fragment C expressed in live *Salmonella* vaccines enhances antibody responses to its fusion partner *Schistosoma haematobium* glutathione *S*-transferase. *Infect. Immun.* 68, 2503–2512.

Levine, M.M. (2000). Immunization against bacterial diseases of the intestine. *J. Pediatr. Gastroenterol. Nutr.* 31, 336–355.

Levine, M.M., Ferreccio, C., Abrego, P., Martin, O.S., Ortiz, E., and Cryz, S. (1999). Duration of efficacy of Ty21a, attenuated *Salmonella typhi* live oral vaccine. *Vaccine* 17, S22–27.

Liljeqvist, S., and Stahl, S. (1999). Production of recombinant subunit vaccines: proteins immunogens, live delivery systems and nucleic acid vaccines. *J. Biotech.* 73, 1–33.

Liou, G.G., Jane, W.N., Cohen, S.N., Lin, N.S., and Lin-Chao, S. (2001). RNA degradosomes exist in vivo in *Escherichia coli* as multicomponent complexes associated with the cytoplasmic membrane via the N-terminal region of ribonuclease E. *Proc. Natl. Acad. Sci. USA.* 98, 63–68.

Lockman, H.A., and Curtiss III, R. (1992). Isolation and characterization of conditional adherent and non–type 1 fimbriated *Salmonella typhimurium* mutants. *Mol. Microbiol.* 6, 933–945.

Londono, L.P., Chatfield, S., Tindle, R.W., Herd, K., Gao, X.M., Frazer, I., and Dougan, G. (1996). Immunisation of mice using *Salmonella typhimurium* expressing human papillomavirus type 16 E7 epitopes inserted into hepatitis B virus core antigen. *Vaccine* 14, 545–552.

Londono-Arcila, P., Freeman, D., Kleanthous, H., O'Dowd, A.M., Lewis, S., Turner, A.K., Rees, E.L., Tibbitts, T.J., Greenwood, J., Monath, T.P., and Darsley, M.J. (2002). Attenuated *Salmonella enterica* serovar Typhi expressing urease effectively immunizes mice against *Helicobacter pylori* challenge as part of a heterologous mucosal priming-parenteral boosting vaccination regimen. *Infect. Immun.* 70, 5096–5106.

Mahan, M.J., Slauch, J.M., and Mekalanos, J.J. (1993). Selection of bacterial virulence genes that are specifically induced in host tissues. *Science* 259, 686–688.

Makela, P.H., and Stocker, B.A. (1969). How genes determine the structure of the *Salmonella* lipopolysaccharide. *J. Gen. Microbiol.* 57, vi.

Mastroeni, P., Chabalgoity, J.A., Dunstan, S.J., Maskell, D.J., and Dougan, G. (2001). *Salmonella*: immune responses and vaccines. *Vet. J.* 161, 132–164.

Matsui, H., Suzuki, M., Isshiki, Y., Kodama, C., Eguchi, M., Kikuchi, Y., Motokawa, K., Takaya, A., Tomoyasu, T., and Yamamoto, M. (2003). Oral immunization with ATP-dependent protease-deficient mutants protects mice against subsequent oral challenge with virulent *Salmonella enterica* serovar Typhimurium. *Infect. Immun.* 71, 30–39.

McClelland, M., Sanderson, K.E., Spieth, J., Clifton, S.W., Latreille, P., Courtney, L., Porwollik, S., Ali, J., Dante, M., Du, F., Hou, S., Layman, D., Leonard, S., Nguyen, C., Scott, K., Holmes, A., Grewal, N., Mulvaney, E., Ryan, E., Sun, H., Florea, L., Miller, W., Stoneking, T., Nhan, M., Waterston, R., and Wilson, R.K. (2001). Complete genome sequence of *Salmonella enterica* serovar Typhimurium LT2. *Nature* 413, 852–856.

McFarland, W.C., and Stocker, B.A. (1987). Effect of different purine auxotrophic mutations on mouse-virulence of a Vi-positive strain of *Salmonella dublin* and of two strains of *Salmonella typhimurium*. *Microb. Pathog.* 3, 129–141.

McLaren, R.S., Newbury, S.F., Dance, G.S., Causton, H.C., and Higgins, C.F. (1991). mRNA degradation by processive 3′–5′

exoribonucleases in vitro and the implications for prokaryotic mRNA decay in vivo. *J. Mol. Biol.* 221, 81–95.

McSorley, S.J., Xu, D., and Liew, F.Y. (1997). Vaccine efficacy of *Salmonella* strains expressing glycoprotein 63 with different promoters. *Infect. Immun.* 65, 171–178.

Medina, E., and Guzman, C.A. (2001). Use of live bacterial vectors for antigen delivery: potential and limitations. *Vaccine* 19, 1573–1580.

Mielcarek, N., Alonso, S., and Locht, C. (2001). Nasal vaccination using live bacterial vectors. *Advanced Drug Delivery Reviews* 51, 55–69.

Miller, S.I. (1991). *PhoP/PhoQ*: macrophage-specific modulators of *Salmonella* virulence? *Mol. Microbiol.* 5, 2073–2078.

Miller, S.I., Kukral, A.M., and Mekalanos, J.J. (1989). A two-component regulatory system (*phoP phoQ*) controls *Salmonella typhimurium* virulence. *Proc. Natl. Acad. Sci. USA.* 86, 5054–5058.

Mills, S.D., Ruschkowski, S.R., Stein, M.A., and Finlay, B.B. (1998). Trafficking of porin-deficient *Salmonella typhimurium* mutants inside HeLa cells: *ompR* and *envZ* mutants are defective for the formation of *Salmonella*-induced filaments. *Infect. Immun.* 66, 1806–1811.

Molin, S., Boe, L., Jensen, L.B., Kristensen, C.S., Givskov, M., Ramos, J.L., and Bej, A.K. (1993). Suicidal genetic elements and their use in biological containment of bacteria. *Annu. Rev. Microbiol.* 47, 139–166.

Mollenkopf, H.J., Groine-Triebkorn, D., Andersen, P., Hess, J., and Kaufmann, S.H. (2001). Protective efficacy against tuberculosis of ESAT-6 secreted by a live *Salmonella typhimurium* vaccine carrier strain and expressed by naked DNA. *Vaccine* 19, 4028–4035.

Mounier, J., Ryter, A., Coquis-Rondon, M., and Sansonetti, P.J. (1990). Intracellular and cell-to-cell spread of *Listeria monocytogenes* involves interaction with F-actin in the enterocytelike cell line Caco-2. *Infect. Immun.* 58, 1048–1058.

Nakayama, K., Kelly, S., and Curtiss III, R. (1988). Construction of Asd⁺ expression-cloning vector: Stable maintenance and high level expression of cloned genes in a *Salmonella* vaccine strain. *Bio/Tech.* 6, 693–697.

Nardelli-Haefliger, D., Benyacoub, J., Lemoine, R., Hopkins-Donaldson, S., Potts, A., Hartman, F., Kraehenbuhl, J.P., and De Grandi, P. (2001). Nasal vaccination with attenuated *Salmonella typhimurium* strains expressing the hepatitis B nucleocapsid: dose response analysis. *Vaccine* 19, 2854–2861.

Nardelli-Haefliger, D., Kraehenbuhl, J.P., Curtiss III, R., Schodel, F., Potts, A., Kelly, S., and De Grandi, P. (1996). Oral and rectal immunization of adult female volunteers with a recombinant attenuated *Salmonella typhi* vaccine strain. *Infect. Immun.* 64, 5219–5224.

Nardelli-Haefliger, D., Roden, R.B., Benyacoub, J., Sahli, R., Kraehenbuhl, J.P., Schiller, J.T., Lachat, P., Potts, A., and De Grandi, P. (1997). Human papillomavirus type 16 virus-like particles expressed in attenuated *Salmonella typhimurium* elicit mucosal and systemic neutralizing antibodies in mice. *Infect. Immun.* 65, 3328–3336.

Navis, C.J., Nickerson, C.A., Wilmes-Riesenberg, M.R., and Curtiss III, R. (1998). Construction of *Salmonella typhimurium* strains containing mutations in one or more adhesins and their effect on virulence [B-213]. In: *American Society for Microbiology, 98th General Meeting, Atlanta*. Washington, DC: American Society for Microbiology, 91.

Nayak, A.R., Tinge, S.A., Tart, R.C., McDaniel, L.S., Briles, D.E., and Curtiss III, R. (1998). A live recombinant avirulent oral *Salmonella* vaccine expressing pneumococcal surface protein A induces protective responses against *Streptococcus pneumoniae*. *Infect. Immun.* 66, 3744–3751.

Newton, S.M., Jacob, C.O., and Stocker, B.A. (1989). Immune response to cholera toxin epitope inserted in *Salmonella* flagellin. *Science* 244, 70–72.

Nickerson, C.A., and Curtiss III, R. (1997). Role of sigma factor RpoS in initial stages of *Salmonella typhimurium* infection. *Infect. Immun.* 65, 1814–1823.

Noriega, F.R., Losonsky, G., Lauderbaugh, C., Liao, F.M., Wang, J.Y., and Levine, M.M. (1996b). Engineered ΔaguaB-A ΔvirG *Shigella flexneri* 2a strain CVD 1205: construction, safety, immunogenicity, and potential efficacy as a mucosal vaccine. *Infect. Immun.* 64, 3055–3061.

Noriega, F.R., Losonsky, G., Wang, J.Y., Formal, S.B., and Levine, M.M. (1996a). Further characterization of Δ*aroA* Δ*virG Shigella flexneri* 2a strain CVD 1203 as a mucosal *Shigella* vaccine and as a live-vector vaccine for delivering antigens of enterotoxigenic *Escherichia coli*. *Infect. Immun.* 64, 23–27.

Noriega, F.R., Wang, J.Y., Losonsky, G., Maneval, D.R., Hone, D.M., and Levine, M.M. (1994). Construction and characterization of attenuated Δ*aroA* Δ*virG Shigella flexneri* 2a strain CVD 1203, a prototype live oral vaccine. *Infect. Immun.* 62, 5168–5172.

O'Hara, E.B., Chekanova, J.A., Ingle, C.A., Kushner, Z.R., Peters, E., and Kushner, S.R. (1995). Polyadenylylation helps regulate mRNA decay in *Escherichia coli*. *Proc Natl Acad Sci USA.* 92, 1807–1811.

Ochsner, U.A., Snyder, A., Vasil, A.I., and Vasil, M.L. (2002). Effects of the twin-arginine translocase on secretion of virulence factors, stress response, and pathogenesis. *Proc. Natl. Acad. Sci. USA.* 99, 8312–8317.

Oggioni, M.R., Medaglini, D., Maggi, T., and Pozzi, G. (1999). Engineering the gram-positive cell surface for construction of bacterial vaccine vectors. *Methods* 19, 163–173.

Ohara, N., and Yamada, T. (2001). Recombinant BCG vaccines. *Vaccine* 19, 4089–4098.

Orr, N., Galen, J.E., and Levine, M.M. (1999). Expression and immunogenicity of a mutant diphtheria toxin molecule, CRM(197), and its fragments in *Salmonella typhi* vaccine strain CVD 908-*htrA*. *Infect. Immun.* 67, 4290–4294.

Orr, N., Galen, J.E., and Levine, M.M. (2001). Novel use of anaerobically induced promoter, *dmsA*, for controlled expression of fragment C of tetanus toxin in live attenuated *Salmonella enterica* serovar Typhi strain CVC 908-*htrA*. *Vaccine* 19, 1694–1700.

Paglia, P., Aroli, I., Frahm, N., Chakraborty, T., Colombo, M.P., and Guzman, C.A. (1997). The defined attenuated *Listeria monocytogenes mpl2* mutant is an effective oral vaccine carrier to trigger a long-lasting immune response against a mouse fibrosarcoma. *Eur. J. Immunol.* 27, 1570–1576.

Palmer, T., and Berks, B.C. (2003). Moving folded proteins across the bacterial cell membrane. *Microbiology* 149, 547–556.

Pardon, P., Popoff, M.Y., Coynault, C., Marly, J., and Miras, I. (1986). Virulence-associated plasmids of *Salmonella* serotype Typhimurium in experimental murine infection. *Ann. Inst. Pasteur Microbiol.* 137B, 47–60.

Pascual, D.W., Hone, D.M., Hall, S., van Ginkel, F.W., Yamamoto, M., Walters, N., Fujihashi, K., Powell, R.J., Wu, S., Van Cott, J.L., Kiyono, H., and McGhee, J.R. (1999). Expression of recombinant enterotoxigenic *Escherichia coli* colonization factor antigen I by *Salmonella typhimurium* elicits a biphasic T helper cell response. *Infect. Immun.* 67, 6249–6256.

Pasetti, M.F., Anderson, R.J., Noriega, F.R., Levine, M.M., and Sztein, M.B. (1999). Attenuated Δ*guaBA Salmonella typhi* vaccine strain CVD 915 as a live vector utilizing prokaryotic or eukaryotic expression systems to deliver foreign antigens and elicit immune responses. *Clin Immunol* 92, 76–89.

Pasetti, M.F., Pickett, T.E., Levine, M.M., and Sztein, M.B. (2000). A comparison of immunogenicity and in vivo distribution of *Salmonella enterica* serovar Typhi and Typhimurium live vector vaccines delivered by mucosal routes in the murine model. *Vaccine* 18, 3208–3213.

Pavelka Jr., M.S., Chen, B., Kelley, C.L., Collins, F.M., and Jacobs Jr., W.R. (2003). Vaccine efficacy of a lysine auxotroph of *Mycobacterium tuberculosis*. *Infect. Immun.* 71, 4190–4192.

Pawelec, D., Rozynek, E., Popowski, J., and Jagusztyn-Krynicka, E.K. (1997). Cloning and characterization of a *Campylobacter jejuni* 72Dz/92 gene encoding a 30 kDa immunopositive protein, component of the ABC transport system; expression of the gene in avirulent *Salmonella typhimurium*. *FEMS Immunol. Med. Microbiol.* 19, 137–150.

Pereira, C.M., Guth, B.E., Sbrogio-Almeida, M.E., and Castilho, B.A. (2001). Antibody response against *Escherichia coli* heat-stable enterotoxin expressed as fusions to flagellin. *Microbiology* 147, 861–867.

Peters, C., and Paterson, Y. (2003). Enhancing the immunogenicity of bioengineered *Listeria monocytogenes* by passaging through live animal hosts. *Vaccine* 21, 1187–1194.

Pickett, T.E., Pasetti, M.F., Galen, J.E., Sztein, M.B., and Levine, M.M. (2000). In vivo characterization of the murine intranasal model for assessing the immunogenicity of attenuated *Salmonella enterica* serovar Typhi strains as live mucosal vaccines and as live vectors. *Infect. Immun.* 68, 205–213.

Pizarro-Cerda, J., Jonquieres, R., Gouin, E., Vandekerckhove, J., Garin, J., and Cossart, P. (2002). Distinct protein patterns associated with *Listeria monocytogenes* InlA- or InlB-phagosomes. *Cell Microbiol.* 4, 101–115.

Powell, C.J., Jr., DeSett, C.R., Lowenthal, J.P., and Berman, S. (1980). The effect of adding iron to mucin on the enhancement of virulence for mice of *Salmonella typhi* strain TY2. *J. Biol. Stand.* 8, 79–85.

Prouty, A.M., and Gunn, J.S. (2000). *Salmonella enterica* serovar Typhimurium invasion is repressed in the presence of bile. *Infect. Immun.* 68, 6763–6769.

Provence, D.L., and Curtiss III, R. (1992). Role of *crl* in avian pathogenic *Escherichia coli*: a knockout mutation of *crl* does not affect hemagglutination activity, fibronectin binding, or curli production. *Infect. Immun.* 60, 4460–4467.

Provence, D.L., and Curtiss III, R. (1994). Isolation and characterization of a gene involved in hemagglutination by an avian pathogenic *Escherichia coli* strain. *Infect. Immun.* 62, 1369–1380.

Redman, T.K., Harmon, C.C., and Michalek, S.M. (1996). Oral immunization with recombinant *Salmonella typhimurium* expressing surface protein antigen A (SpaA) of *Streptococcus sobrinus*: effects of the *Salmonella* virulence plasmid on the induction of protective and sustained humoral responses in rats. *Vaccine* 14, 868–878.

Reglier-Poupet, H., Pellegrini, E., Charbit, A., and Berche, P. (2003). Identification of LpeA, a PsaA-like membrane protein that promotes cell entry by *Listeria monocytogenes*. *Infect. Immun.* 71, 474–482.

Revaz, V., Benyacoub, J., Kast, W.M., Schiller, J.T., De Grandi, P., and Nardelli-Haefliger, D. (2001). Mucosal vaccination with a recombinant *Salmonella typhimurium* expressing human papillomavirus type 16 (HPV16) L1 virus-like particles (VLPs) or HPV16 VLPs purified from insect cells inhibits the growth of HPV16-expressing tumor cells in mice. *Virology* 279, 354–360.

Ritz, D., and Beckwith, J. (2001). Roles of thiol-redox pathways in bacteria. *Annu. Rev. Microbiol.* 55, 21–48.

Robbe-Saule, V., Coynault, C., and Norel, F. (1995). The live oral typhoid vaccine Ty21a is a *rpoS* mutant and is susceptible to various environmental stresses. *FEMS Microbiol. Lett.* 126, 171–176.

Robbe-Saule, V., and Norel, F. (1999). The *rpoS* mutant allele of *Salmonella typhi* Ty2 is identical to that of the live typhoid vaccine Ty21a. *FEMS Microbiol. Lett.* 170, 141–143.

Roberts, M., Bacon, A., Li, J., and Chatfield, S. (1999). Prior to homologous and heterologous *Salmonella* serotypes suppresses local and systemic anti-fragment C antibody responses and protection form tetanus toxin in mice immunized with *Salmonella* strains expressing fragment C. *Infect. Immun.* 67, 3810–3815.

Roberts, M., Chatfield, S., Pickard, D., Li, J., and Bacon, A. (2000). Comparison of abilities of *Salmonella enterica* serovar Typhimurium *aroA aroD* and *aroA htrA* mutants to act as live vectors. *Infect. Immun.* 68, 6041–6043.

Roberts, M., Chatfield, S.N., and Dougan, G. (1994). *Salmonella* as carriers of heterologous antigens. In *Novel Delivery Systems for Oral Vaccines* (ed. D. T. O'Hagan). Boca Raton, Florida: CRC Press, 27–58.

Roberts, M., Li, J., Bacon, A., and Chatfield, S. (1998). Oral vaccination against tetanus: Comparison of the immunogenicities of *Salmonella* strains expressing fragment C form the *nirB* and *htrA* promoters. *Infect. Immun.* 66, 3080–3087.

Rogers, S., Wells, R., and Rechsteiner, M. (1986). Amino acid sequences common to rapidly degraded proteins: the PEST hypothesis. *Science* 234, 364–368.

Roland, K., Curtiss III, R., and Sizemore, D. (1999). Construction and evaluation of a Δcya Δcrp *Salmonella typhimurium* strain expressing avian pathogenic *Escherichia coli* O78 LPS as a vaccine to prevent airsacculitis in chickens. *Avian Dis.* 43, 429–441.

Rosen, S.M., Zeleznick, L.D., Fraenkel, D., Wiener, I.M., Osborn, M.J., and Horecker, B.L. (1965). Characterization of the cell wall lipopolysaccharide of a mutant of *Salmonella typhimurium* lacking phosphomannose isomerase. *Biochem. Z.* 342, 375–386.

Russmann, H., Igwe, E.I., Sauer, J., Hardt, W.D., Bubert, A., and Geginat, G. (2001). Protection against murine listeriosis by oral vaccination with recombinant *Salmonella* expressing hybrid *Yersinia* type III proteins. *J. Immunol.* 167, 357–365.

Russmann, H., Shams, H., Poblete, F., Fu, Y., Galan, J.E., and Donis, R.O. (1998). Delivery of epitopes by the *Salmonella* type III secretion system for vaccine development. *Science* 281, 565–568.

Russmann, H., Weissmuller, A., Geginat, G., Igwe, E.I., Roggenkamp, A., Bubert, A., Goebel, W., Hof, H., and Heesemann, J. (2000). *Yersinia enterocolitica*–mediated translocation of defined fusion proteins to the cytosol of mammalian cells results in peptide-specific MHC class I-restricted antigen presentation. *Eur. J. Immunol.* 30, 1375–1384.

Ryan, E.T., Butterton, J.R., Smith, R.N., Carroll, P.A., Crean, T.I., and Calderwood, S.B. (1997a). Protective immunity against *Clostridium difficile* toxin A induced by oral immunization with a live, attenuated *Vibrio cholerae* vector strain. *Infect. Immun.* 65, 2941–2949.

Ryan, E.T., Butterton, J.R., Zhang, T., Baker, M.A., Stanley, S.L., Jr., and Calderwood, S.B. (1997b). Oral immunization with attenuated vaccine strains of *Vibrio cholerae* expressing a dodecapeptide repeat of the serine-rich *Entamoeba histolytica* protein fused to the cholera toxin B subunit induces systemic and mucosal antiamebic and anti–*V. cholerae* antibody responses in mice. *Infect. Immun.* 65, 3118–3125.

Ryan, E.T., Crean, T.I., John, M., Butterton, J.R., Clements, J.D., and Calderwood, S.B. (1999). In vivo expression and immunoadjuvancy of a mutant of heat-labile enterotoxin of *Escherichia coli* in vaccine and vector strains of *Vibrio cholerae*. *Infect. Immun.* 67, 1694–1701.

Ryan, E.T., Crean, T.I., Kochi, S.K., John, M., Luciano, A.A., Killeen, K.P., Klose, K.E., and Calderwood, S.B. (2000). Development of a ΔglnA balanced lethal plasmid system for expression of heterologous antigens by attenuated vaccine vector strains of *Vibrio cholerae*. *Infect. Immun.* 68, 221–226.

Saklani-Jusforgues, H., Fontan, E., Soussi, N., Milon, G., and Goossens, P.L. (2003). Enteral immunization with attenuated recombinant *Listeria monocytogenes* as a live vaccine vector: organ-dependent dynamics of CD4 T lymphocytes reactive to a *Leishmania major* tracer epitope. *Infect. Immun.* 71, 1083–1090.

Saltzman, D.A., Heise, C.P., Hasz, D.E., Zebede, M., Kelly, S.M., Curtiss III, R., Leonard, A.S., and Anderson, P.M. (1996). Attenuated *Salmonella typhimurium* containing interleukin-2 decreases MC-38 hepatic metastases: a novel anti-tumor agent. *Cancer Biother. Radiopharm.* 11, 145–153.

Sambandamurthy, V.K., Wang, X., Chen, B., Russell, R.G., Derrick, S., Collins, F.M., Morris, S.L., and Jacobs, W.R., Jr. (2002). A pantothenate auxotroph of *Mycobacterium tuberculosis* is highly attenuated and protects mice against tuberculosis. *Nat. Med.* 8, 1171–1174.

Sansonetti, P., and Egile, C. (1998). Molecular bases of epithelial cell invasion by *Shigella flexneri*. *Antonie Van Leeuwenhoek* 74, 191–197.

Schmitt, C.K., Ikeda, J.S., Darnell, S.C., Watson, P.R., Bispham, J., Wallis, T.S., Weinstein, D.L., Metcalf, E.S., and O'Brien, A.D. (2001). Absence of all components of the flagellar export and synthesis machinery differentially alters virulence of *Salmonella enterica* serovar Typhimurium in models of typhoid fever, survival in macrophages, tissue culture invasiveness, and calf enterocolitis. *Infect. Immun.* 69, 5619–5625.

Schodel, F., and Curtiss III, R. (1995). *Salmonella* as oral vaccine carriers. *Dev. Biol. Stand.* 84, 245–253.

Schodel, F., Kelly, S., Tinge, S., Hopkins, S., Peterson, D., Milich, D., and Curtiss III, R. (1996). Hybrid hepatitis B virus core antigen as a vaccine carrier moiety. II. Expression in avirulent *Salmonella* spp. for mucosal immunization. *Adv. Exp. Med. Biol.* 397, 15–21.

Schriefer, A., Maltez, J.R., Silva, N., Stoeckle, M.Y., Barral-Netto, M., and Riley, L.W. (1999). Expression of a pilin subunit BfpA of the bundle-forming pilus of enteropathogenic *Escherichia coli* in an *aroA* live *Salmonella* vaccine strain. *Vaccine* 17, 770–778.

Schubert, W.D., Urbanke, C., Ziehm, T., Beier, V., Machner, M.P., Domann, E., Wehland, J., Chakraborty, T., and Heinz, D.W. (2002). Structure of internalin, a major invasion protein of *Listeria monocytogenes*, in complex with its human receptor E-cadherin. *Cell* 111, 825–836.

Shata, M.T., and Hone, D.M. (2001). Vaccination with a *Shigella* DNA vaccine vector induces antigen-specific CD8(+) T cells and antiviral protective immunity. *J. Virol.* 75, 9665–9670.

Sirard, J.C., Niedergang, F., and Kraehenbuhl, J.P. (1999). Live attenuated *Salmonella*: a paradigm of mucosal vaccines. *Immunol. Rev.* 171, 5–26.

Sizemore, D.R., Branstrom, A.A., and Sadoff, J.C. (1995). Attenuated *Shigella* as a DNA delivery vehicle for DNA-mediated immunization. *Science* 270, 299–302.

Sizemore, D.R., Branstrom, A.A., and Sadoff, J.C. (1997). Attenuated bacteria as a DNA delivery vehicle for DNA-mediated immunization. *Vaccine* 15, 804–807.

Spreng, S., Gentschev, I., Goebel, W., Weidinger, G., ter Meulen, V., and Niewiesk, S. (2000). *Salmonella* vaccines secreting measles virus epitopes induce protective immune responses against measles virus encephalitis. *Microbes Infect.* 2, 1687–1692.

Stathopoulos, C., Georgiou, G., and Earhart, C.F. (1996). Characterization of *Escherichia coli* expressing an Lpp OmpA(46-159)-PhoA fusion protein localized in the outer membrane. *Appl. Microbiol. Biotechnol.* 45, 112–119.

Steger, K.K., Valentine, P.J., Heffron, F., So, M., and Pauza, C.D. (1999). Recombinant, attenuated *Salmonella typhimurium* stimulate lymphoproliferative responses to SIV capsid antigen in rhesus macaques. *Vaccine* 17, 923–932.

Steidler, L., Neirynck, S., Huyghebaert, N., Snoeck, V., Vermeire, A., Goddeeris, B., Cox, E., Remon, J.P., and Remaut, E. (2003). Biological containment of genetically modified *Lactococcus lactis* for intestinal delivery of human interleukin 10. *Nat. Biotechnol.* 21, 785–789.

Stocker, B.A. (2000). Aromatic-dependent *Salmonella* as anti-bacterial vaccines and as presenters of heterologous antigens or of DNA encoding them. *J. Biotech.* 83, 45–50.

Stocker, B.A., and Makela, P.H. (1978). Genetics of the (gram-negative) bacterial surface. *Proc. R. Soc. Lond. B Biol. Sci.* 202, 5–30.

Stocker, B.A., and Makela, P.H. (1986). Genetic determination of bacterial virulence, with special reference to *Salmonella*. *Curr. Top. Microbiol. Immunol.* 124, 149–172.

Strugnell, R.A., Maskell, D., Fairweather, N., Pickard, D., Cockayne, A., Penn, C., and Dougan, G. (1990). Stable expression of foreign antigens from the chromosome of *Salmonella typhimurium* vaccine strains. *Gene* 88, 57–63.

Suarez, M., Gonzalez-Zorn, B., Vega, Y., Chico-Calero, I., and Vazquez-Boland, J.A. (2001). A role for ActA in epithelial cell invasion by *Listeria monocytogenes*. *Cell Microbiol.* 3, 853–864.

Suh, J., Wirtz, D., and Hanes, J. (2003). Efficient active transport of gene nanocarriers to the cell nucleus. *Proc. Natl. Acad. Sci. USA.* 100, 3878–3882.

Svensson, M., Pfeifer, J., Stockinger, B., and Wick, M.J. (1997). Bacterial antigen delivery systems: phagocytic processing of bacterial antigens for MHC-I and MHC-II presentation to T cells. *Behring. Inst. Mitt.* 98, 197–211.

Sydenham, M., Douce, G., Bowe, F., Ahmed, S., Chatfield, S., and Dougan, G. (2000). *Salmonella enterica* serovar Typhimurium *surA* mutants are attenuated and effective live oral vaccines. *Infect. Immun.* 68, 1109–1115.

Tacket, C.O., Galen, J., Sztein, M.B., Losonsky, G., Wyant, T.L., Nataro, J., Wasserman, S.S., Edelman, R., Chatfield, S., Dougan, G., and Levine, M.M. (2000). Safety and immune responses to attenuated *Salmonella enterica* serovar Typhi oral live vector vaccines expressing tetanus toxin fragment C. *Clin. Immunol.* 97, 146–153.

Tacket, C.O., Hone, D.M., Curtiss III, R., Kelly, S.M., Losonsky, G., Guers, L., Harris, A.M., Edelman, R., and Levine, M.M. (1992a). Comparison of the safety and immunogenicity of ΔaroC ΔaroD and Δcya Δcrp Salmonella typhi strains in adult volunteers. Infect. Immun. 60, 536–541.

Tacket, C.O., Hone, D.M., Losonsky, G., Guers, L., Edelman, R., and Levine, M.M. (1992b). Clinical acceptability and immunogenicity of CVD 908 Salmonella typhi vaccine strain. Vaccine 10, 443–446.

Tacket, C.O., Kelly, S.M., Schodel, F., Losonsky, G., Nataro, J.P., Edelman, R., Levine, M.M., and Curtiss III, R. (1997b). Safety and immunogenicity in humans of an attenuated Salmonella typhi vaccine vector strain expressing plasmid-encoded hepatitis B antigens stabilized by the Asd-balanced lethal vector system. Infect. Immun. 65, 3381–3385.

Tacket, C.O., Sztein, M.B., Losonsky, G.A., Wasserman, S.S., Nataro, J.P., Edelman, R., Pickard, D., Dougan, G., Chatfield, S.N., and Levine, M.M. (1997a). Safety of live oral Salmonella typhi vaccine strains with deletions in htrA and aroC aroD and immune response in humans. Infect. Immun. 65, 452–456.

Thomas, W.D., Jr., Wagner, S.P., and Welch, R.A. (1992). A heterologous membrane protein domain fused to the C-terminal ATP-binding domain of HlyB can export Escherichia coli hemolysin. J. Bacteriol. 174, 6771–6779.

Thompson, R.J., Bouwer, H.G., Portnoy, D.A., and Frankel, F.R. (1998). Pathogenicity and immunogenicity of a Listeria monocytogenes strain that requires D-alanine for growth. Infect. Immun. 66, 3552–3561.

Tijhaar, E.J., Zheng-Xin, Y., Karlas, J.A., Meyer, T.F., Stukart, M.J., Osterhaus, A.D., and Mooi, F.R. (1994). Construction and evaluation of an expression vector allowing the stable expression of foreign antigens in a Salmonella typhimurium vaccine strain. Vaccine 12, 1004–1111.

Tilney, L.G., and Portnoy, D.A. (1989). Actin filaments and growth, movement, and spread of the intracellular bacterial parasite, Listeria monocytogenes. J. Cell Biol. 109, 1597–1608.

Townsend, S.M., Kramer, N.E., Edwards, R., Baker, S., Hamlin, N., Simmonds, M., Stevens, K., Maloy, S., Parkhill, J., Dougan, G., and Baumler, A.J. (2001). Salmonella enterica serovar Typhi possesses a unique repertoire of fimbrial gene sequences. Infect. Immun. 69, 2894–2901.

Trucksis, M., Galen, J.E., Michalski, J., Fasano, A., and Kaper, J.B. (1993). Accessory cholera enterotoxin (Ace), the third toxin of a Vibrio cholerae virulence cassette. Proc. Natl. Acad. Sci. USA. 90, 5267–5271.

Turner, A.K., Terry, T.D., Sack, D., Londono-Arcila, P., and Darsley, M.J. (2001). Construction and characterization of genetically defined aro omp mutants of enterotoxigenic Escherichia coli and preliminary studies of safety and immunogenicity in humans. Infect. Immun. 69, 4969–4979.

Tzschaschel, B.D., Guzman, C.A., Timmis, K.N., and de Lorenzo, V. (1996). An Escherichia coli hemolysin transport system-based vector for the export of polypeptides: export of Shiga-like toxin IIeB subunit by Salmonella typhimurium. Nat. Biotechnol. 14, 765–769.

Van Cott, J.L., Chatfield, S.N., Roberts, M., Hone, D.M., Hohmann, E.L., Pascual, D.W., Yamamoto, M., Kiyono, H., and McGhee, J.R. (1998). Regulation of host immune responses by modification of Salmonella virulence genes. Nat. Med. 4, 1247–1252.

Van Cott, J.L., Staats, H.F., Pascual, D.W., Roberts, M., Chatfield, S.N., Yamamoto, M., Coste, M., Carter, P.B., Kiyono, H., and McGhee, J.R. (1996). Regulation of mucosal and systemic antibody responses by T helper cell subsets, macrophages, and derived cytokines following oral immunization with live recombinant Salmonella. J. Immunol. 156, 1504–1514.

van der Velden, A.W., Baumler, A.J., Tsolis, R.M., and Heffron, F. (1998). Multiple fimbrial adhesins are required for full virulence of Salmonella typhimurium in mice. Infect. Immun. 66, 2803–2808.

van Velkinburgh, J.C., and Gunn, J.S. (1999). PhoP-PhoQ-regulated loci are required for enhanced bile resistance in Salmonella spp. Infect. Immun. 67, 1614–1622.

Varshavsky, A. (1996). The N-end rule: functions, mysteries, uses. Proc. Natl. Acad. Sci. USA. 93, 12142–12149.

Vasquez-Boland, J.A., Kocks, C., Dramsi, S., Ohayon, H., Geoffroy, C., Mengaud, J., and Cossart, P. (1992). Nucleotide sequence of the lecithinase operon of Listeria monocytogenes and possible role of lecithinase in cell-to-cell spread. Infect. Immun. 60, 219–230.

Vecino, W.H., Morin, P.M., Agha, R., Jacobs, W.R., Jr., and Fennelly, G.J. (2002). Mucosal DNA vaccination with highly attenuated Shigella is superior to attenuated Salmonella and comparable to intramuscular DNA vaccination for T cells against HIV. Immunol. Lett. 82, 197–204.

Vindurampulle, C.J., and Attridge, S.R. (2003). Impact of vector priming on the immunogenicity of recombinant Salmonella vaccines. Infect. Immun. 71, 287–297.

Wang, L., Curd, H., and Reeves, P.R. (1999). Immunization of mice with live oral vaccine based on a Salmonella enterica (sv Typhimurium) aroA strain expressing the Escherichia coli O111 O antigen. Microb. Pathog. 27, 55–59.

Ward, S.J., Douce, G., Figueiredo, D., Dougan, G., and Wren, B.W. (1999). Immunogenicity of a Salmonella typhimurium aroA aroD vaccine expressing a nontoxic domain of Clostridium difficile toxin A. Infect. Immun. 67, 2145–2152.

Warren, R.L., Lu, D., Sizemore, D.R., Baron, L.S., and Kopecko, D.J. (1990). Method for identifying microbial antigens that simulate specific lymphocyte responses: application to Salmonella. Proc. Natl. Acad. Sci. USA. 87, 9823–9827.

Waterman, S.R., and Small, P.L. (1996). Identification of sigma S-dependent genes associated with the stationary-phase acid-resistance phenotype of Shigella flexneri. Mol. Micobiol. 21, 925–940.

Welch, R.A. (1991). Pore-forming cytolysins of gram-negative bacteria. Mol. Microbiol. 5, 521–528.

Whittle, B.L., and Verma, N.K. (1997). The immune response to a B-cell epitope delivered by Salmonella is enhanced by prior immunological experience. Vaccine 15, 1737–1740.

Wick, M.J., Harding, C.V., Twesten, N.J., Normark, S.J., and Pfeifer, J.D. (1995). The phoP locus influences processing and presentation of Salmonella typhimurium antigens by activated macrophages. Mol. Microbiol. 16, 465–476.

Wiesmuller, K.H., Fleckenstein, B., and Jung, G. (2001). Peptide vaccines and peptide libraries. Biol. Chem. 382, 571–579.

Wilmes-Riesenberg, M.R., Bearson, B., Foster, J.W., and Curtiss III, R. (1996). The role of the acid tolerance response in the virulence of Salmonella typhimurium. Infect. Immun. 64, 1085–1092.

Woo, P.C., Wong, L.P., Zheng, B.J., and Yuen, K.Y. (2001). Unique immunogenicity of hepatitis B virus DNA vaccine presented by live-attenuated Salmonella typhimurium. Vaccine 19, 2945–2954.

World Bank. Communicable Diseases. www.worldbank.org/hnp.

Wosten, M.M., and Groisman, E.A. (1999). Molecular characterization of the PmrA regulon. J. Biol. Chem. 274, 27185–27190.

Wosten, M.M., Kox, L.F., Chamnongpol, S., Soncini, F.C., and Groisman, E.A. (2000). A signal transduction system that responds to extracellular iron. Cell 103, 113–125.

Wu, S., Beier, M., Sztein, M.B., Galen, J., Pickett, T., Holder, A.A., Gomez-Duarte, O.G., and Levine, M.M. (2000). Construction and immunogenicity in mice of attenuated Salmonella typhi expressing Plasmodium falciparum merozoite surface protein 1 (MSP-1) fused to tetanus toxin fragment C. J. Biotechnol. 83, 125–135.

Wu, S., Pascual, D.W., Lewis, G.K., and Hone, D.M. (1997). Induction of mucosal and systemic responses against human immunodeficiency virus type 1 glycoprotein 120 in mice after oral immunization with a single dose of a Salmonella-HIV vector. AIDS Res. Hum. Retroviruses 13, 1187–1194.

Wyszyznska, A., Pawelec, D.P., and Jagusztyn-Krynicka, E.K. (2002). Immunological characterization of the Campylobacter jejuni 72Dz/92 cjaD gene product and its fusion with B subunit of E. coli LT toxin. Acta Microbiol. Pol. 51, 313–326.

Xu, B., Zhang, Z.S., Li, S.Q., Shu, D., and Huang, C.F. (2002). Simultaneous expression of CS3 colonization factor antigen and LT-B/ST fusion enterotoxin antigen of enterotoxigenic Escherichia coli by attenuated Salmonella typhimurium. Yi Chuan Xue Bao 29, 370–376.

Xu, D., McSorley, S.J., Tetley, L., Chatfield, S., Dougan, G., Chan, W.L., Satoskar, A., David, J.R., and Liew, F.Y. (1998). Protective effect on *Leishmania major* infection of migration inhibitory factor, TNF-alpha and IFN-gamma administered orally via attenuated *Salmonella typhimurium*. *J. Immunol.* 160, 1285–1289.

Xu, F., Hong, M., and Ulmer, J.B. (2003). Immunogenicity of an HIV-1 *gag* DNA vaccine carried by attenuated *Shigella*. *Vaccine* 21, 644–648.

Yakhchali, B., and Manning, P.A. (1997). Epitope analysis of the CS3 fimbrial subunit of human enterotoxigenic *Escherichia coli* and the construction of novel CS3::ST and CS3::LT-B immunogens. *Behring Inst. Mitt.* 98, 124–134.

Zhang, S., Kingsley, R.A., Santos, R.L., Andrews-Polymenis, H., Raffatellu, M., Figueiredo, J., Nunes, J., Tsolis, R.M., Adams, L.G., and Baumler, A.J. (2003). Molecular pathogenesis of *Salmonella enterica* serotype *typhimurium*–induced diarrhea. *Infect. Immun.* 71, 1–12.

Zhang, S., Santos, R.L., Tsolis, R.M., Stender, S., Hardt, W.D., Baumler, A.J., and Adams, L.G. (2002). The *Salmonella enterica* serotype Typhimurium effector proteins SipA, SopA, SopB, SopD, and SopE2 act in concert to induce diarrhea in calves. *Infect. Immun.* 70, 3843–3855.

Zhang, T., and Stanley, S.L., Jr. (1997). Expression of the serine rich *Entamoeba histolytica* protein (SREHP) in the avirulent vaccine strain *Salmonella typhi* Ty2 χ4297 (Δcya Δcrp Δasd): safety and immunogenicity in mice. *Vaccine* 15, 1319–1322.

Zhang, X., Kang, H.Y., Bollen, W., and Curtiss III, R. (2002). *Salmonella typhimurium* UK-1 ΔPfur::araC P$_{BAD}$fur Δpmi mutants are highly

attenuated and induced protective immunity in BALB/c mice [Z-29]. In: *American Society for Microbiology, 102nd General Meeting, Salt Lake City, Utah*. Washington, DC: American Society for Microbiology, 512.

Zhang, X., Kelly, S.M., Bollen, W.S., and Curtiss III, R. (1997). Characterization and immunogenicity of *Salmonella typhimurium* SL1344 and UK-1 Δcrp and Δcdt deletion mutants. *Infect. Immun.* 65, 5381–5387.

Zhang, X., Nickerson, C.A., Bollen, W.S., and Curtiss III, R. (1997). Antibody responses induced in mice by attenuated *Salmonella*, with RpoS$^+$ phenotype expressing HBV hybrid core-pre-S protein [E-3]. In *American Society for Microbiology, 100th General Meeting, Los Angeles, California*. Washington, DC: American Society for Microbiology, 293.

Zhang-Barber, L., Turner, A.K., Dougan, G., and Barrow, P.A. (1998). Protection of chickens against experimental fowl typhoid using a *nuoG* mutant of *Salmonella* serotype *Gallinarum*. *Vaccine* 16, 899–903.

Zheng, B.J., Ng, M.H., Chan, K.W., Tam, S., Woo, P.C., Ng, S.P., and Yuen, K.Y. (2002). A single dose of oral DNA immunization delivered by attenuated *Salmonella typhimurium* down-regulates transgene expression in HBsAg transgenic mice. *Eur. J. Immunol.* 32, 3294–3304.

Zheng, M., Bernard, D., Schneider, T.D., and Storz, G. (1999). OxyR and SoxRS regulation of *fur*. *J. Bacteriol.* 181, 4639–4643.

Recombinant Live Viral Vectors as Vaccines for Mucosal Immunity

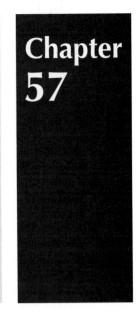

Kenneth L. Rosenthal

Centre for Gene Therapeutics, Department of Pathology & Molecular Medicine, McMaster University Health Sciences Centre, Hamilton, Ontario, Canada

As early as the 5th century in China, protection against smallpox involved collecting scabs from lesions and blowing a powder made from them into an infant's nose (Mazumdar, 2003). Thus, one of the earliest vaccines appears to have been delivered via a mucosal route. It is unfortunate, therefore, that the term *vaccination* has come to be associated with inoculation. Indeed, today most vaccines are delivered via inoculation, despite the fact that most infectious agents initiate infection at the extensive mucosal surfaces of the body.

In industrialized countries, widespread application of vaccines has successfully resulted in the disappearance of many epidemic infections, particularly acute infections in children (Ehreth, 2003b; Ehreth, 2003a). Together with clean water and antibiotics, vaccines have had remarkable success that has profoundly affected human society, not the least of which was the global eradication of smallpox in the late 1970s and the possibility of eradicating polio in the near future. Successful vaccines have been generated against viruses that tend to be relatively genetically stable and cause acute self-limiting infections followed by long-lasting immunity. These vaccines work by generating neutralizing antibodies of long enough duration for lasting protection (Zinkernagel, 2003). However, pathogens that cause chronic infections, such as human immunodeficiency virus (HIV-1), herpesviruses, hepatitis C virus (HCV), mycobacteria, and parasites, require new strategies to induce more effective immune responses for better control. This is due, in part, to the fact that these pathogens establish persistent or latent infections in the host and have evolved sophisticated mechanisms to evade both innate and adoptive immunity. Additionally, chronic infectious agents tend to be noncytopathic or weakly cytopathic and persist in extralymphoid tissues. Since T-cell-mediated immunity appears to be critical in controlling chronic viral infections, currently much emphasis is being placed on developing novel vaccines that can promote the generation of strong T-cell-mediated immunity (CMI).

To induce strong CMI responses, effective vaccines should mimic the processing and presentation seen during natural virus infection. Live attenuated viral vaccines achieve this very effectively, but for infectious agents that are able to establish persistent, often lifelong, infections, there are concerns about safety. Therefore, live recombinant viral vectors provide a novel and safer method to achieve this goal. Recombinant viral vectors can elicit both neutralizing antibodies and T-cell immunity. Additional advantages include relative ease of growth and delivery, including via the mucosal route; ability to naturally target cells or tissues of interest; and provision of a natural adjuvant effect mediated by the release of cytokines and chemokines due to host response to the vector itself.

Some concerns associated with live viral vectors are appropriate attenuation to limit vaccine-induced pathology, especially in immunocompromised individuals; preexisting or induction of immunity to the vector itself; and the capacity of the candidate vectors to accommodate large foreign gene inserts. A number of recombinant viral vectors have been evaluated in extensive preclinical studies in animal models, and several have moved into human clinical trials. Much of the impetus to advance recombinant viral vectors into clinical trials emanates from the urgent need for a safe and effective vaccine against HIV-1 (Voltan and Robert-Guroff, 2003). One must keep in mind that it is unlikely that a single vector system will be optimal in all respects. Furthermore, the generation of strong immune responses to the vector itself will allow only a limited number of applications for a specific vaccine vector in a given population.

Therefore, efforts to produce an ideal vector for all applications are likely to be unproductive. Rather, a strong case must be made for parallel development of multiple viral vaccine vectors, in order to take advantage of the unique properties of each for specific applications. Ultimately, selection of candidate vectors for clinical trials will have to rely on head-to-head comparative studies.

A number of recombinant viral vectors have the advantage of being based on viruses that are naturally transmitted via mucosal routes. Thus, they are tropic for mucosal tissues, and this feature can be exploited for induction of local mucosal immune responses. In order to prevent mucosally transmitted infections through vaccination, the administration route used for vaccine delivery is as critical as vaccine immunogenicity (Kozlowski and Neutra, 2003). We and others have demonstrated a clear dichotomy between mucosal immunization and systemic immunization, in that mucosal immunization is critical for induction and long-term maintenance of mucosal immune responses (Rosenthal and Gallichan, 1997; Stevceva et al., 2000). In contrast, systemic immunization does not effectively induce mucosal IgA or T-cell-mediated immunity.

This dichotomy likely reflects preferential homing of activated lymphocytes to sites of induction (Kantele et al., 1999). For example, administration of vaccines via parenteral routes results in activation of lymphocytes that express L-selectin or other adhesion molecules that preferentially target their migration to peripheral lymphoid tissues but not mucosal sites. On the other hand, entry of lymphocytes into the intestinal mucosa is promoted by expression of tissue-specific adhesion molecules, such as $\alpha4\beta7$, which promotes migration into intestinal lamina propria after interaction with the mucosal addressin MADCAM-1, expressed on high endothelial venules (Briskin et al., 1997; Butcher et al., 1999).

In this chapter we summarize features of some of the more promising recombinant viral vectors and focus on those that have potential utility for mucosal immunity.

RECOMBINANT DNA VIRUS VECTORS

Poxviruses

The orthopox family includes smallpox virus, vaccinia, and the avian poxviruses (canarypox and fowlpox). One of the greatest achievements in vaccinology was the successful eradication of smallpox, which was accomplished through a worldwide vaccination program employing vaccinia virus. Poxviruses are large and complex. The poxvirus genome is a double-stranded DNA molecule of approximately 130 to 300 kb for the mammalian and avian poxviruses, respectively. The genome has over 190 open reading frames (ORFs) and can accommodate large insertions of greater than 20 kb of foreign DNA. Heterologous sequences are usually inserted at sites encoding nonessential genes, such as the viral thymidine kinase. These viruses can be readily manipulated in the laboratory and have a wide host range

(Moss, 1996; Paoletti, 1996). Poxviruses replicate in the cytoplasm of infected cells, and since they have their own transcriptional system, viral promoters are necessary in the expression cassette for foreign genes. The natural promoters, P7.5 and H5, are relatively weak, so the use of a synthetic early/late promoter (Chakrabarti et al., 1997) is currently the most common choice for achieving high-level expression of biologically active proteins (Ourmanov et al., 2000; Nilsson et al., 2002; Sharpe et al., 2001). Vaccinia recombinants have been tested in phase I trials, and their use in nonimmune individuals is generally well tolerated, with limited side effects. But the use of replication-competent vaccinia is a safety concern, especially in immunocompromised individuals, where it may cause eczema, encephalitis, and disseminated infection. Additionally, prior vaccinia exposure may lead to failure of subsequent use of recombinant vaccinia vaccines. Today, this is especially important in light of renewal of smallpox vaccination programs to protect against the threat of bioterrorism. To address these concerns, several highly attenuated poxvirus vectors with limited pathogenic potential and host range were developed.

Modified vaccinia virus Ankara (MVA) was attenuated by extensive passage in chicken embryo fibroblasts (CEFs) (Mayr, 1975). This resulted in extensive deletions in the virus genome and a shift in host range (Meyer et al., 1991; Wyatt et al., 1998; Antoine et al., 1998). Although MVA replicates well in CEF cells, it is unable to replicate productively in mammalian cells. This is due to a block in virion formation that prevents generation of infectious progeny. Despite this defect, MVA is still able to infect cells normally and undergo DNA replication and protein expression, so expression of foreign genes in MVA recombinants is efficient (Sutter and Moss, 1992). An important observation is that some of the deleted viral genes encoded soluble receptors for interferon-γ, α/β-interferons, tumor necrosis factor (TNF), and CC-chemokines, which are normally secreted by poxvirus-infected cells to evade host immune responses (Blanchard et al., 1998). The lack of expression of these genes appears to contribute to the increased immunogenicity of MVA in comparison with vaccinia virus (Carroll et al., 1997; Blanchard et al., 1998). MVA was used as a vaccine in the final stages of the global smallpox eradication campaign in Germany and Turkey. Its use proved to be highly successful and showed no significant side effects. Indeed, at least 120,000 humans were inoculated with MVA without any adverse effects, confirming its safety in humans.

MVA has shown good success in many preclinical models of infectious diseases, including HIV, malaria, and tuberculosis. In nonhuman primates, immunization with MVA-SIVenv or gag-pol recombinants elicited simian immunodeficiency virus (SIV)-specific CD8[+] T cell responses (Seth et al., 1998), primed for neutralizing antibody in response to SIV challenge (Ourmanov et al., 2000), and reduced viral burden following challenge (Seth et al., 2000). The success of MVA recombinants in preclinical models of HIV has led to a number of phase I clinical trials involving HIV, including a trial based on the use of MVA encoding a consensus clade A HIV-1 gag gene plus a number of HIV-specific cytotoxic T lymphocyte (CTL) epitopes. As discussed later in the text, it was shown in prime-boost studies that priming with plasmid DNA followed by boosting with rMVA was able to protect against a virulent rectal challenge with simian–human immunodeficiency virus (SHIV)89.6 (Amara *et al.*, 2001; Hanke *et al.*, 1998; Hanke *et al.*, 1999). In light of these results, a number of DNA prime-MVA boost clinical trials against HIV-1 are under way (www.iavi.org; www.vrc.nih.gov; http://aidscience.com).

NYVAC is a vaccinia-based vaccine that was further attenuated by genetic engineering. It was derived from the Copenhagen strain of vaccinia virus by specific deletion of 18 viral genes that encoded virulence, pathogenicity, and host-range regulation of the virus (Tartaglia *et al.*, 1992). Like MVA, NYVAC is unable to productively replicate in human cells, but its replication is blocked at an early stage in the virus cycle. Nevertheless, NYVAC recombinants still express foreign genes and induce protective immune responses in immunized hosts. NYVAC-based vaccines have been successful in several veterinary applications (Paoletti, 1996), and a phase I trial of NYVAC encoding HIV gag, pol, nef, and env is under way in the United Kingdom and Switzerland.

ALVAC is a canarypox virus that is naturally restricted to replication in avian species. Although the virus can infect mammalian cells and express foreign recombinant genes, it undergoes an abortive infection that inhibits production of viral progeny. These features make ALVAC-based vectors safe and immunogenic in both normal and immunocompromised individuals. ALVAC was one of the first live recombinant viral vectors to advance to clinical trials. Indeed, a number of phase I trials have been conducted and phase II trials are under way. These clinical studies have shown good safety, but ALVAC by itself does not appear to be as immunogenic as some other vectors. Recently, a phase II trial of a prime-boost regimen with use of ALVAC-HIV recombinants for priming failed to elicit sufficiently high cellular immune responses in at least 30% of vaccinees (Check, 2002). This resulted in its failure to advance to a phase III trial in the United States. Nevertheless, a phase III trial of the approach was proposed to be conducted in Thailand. Human trials of DNA prime followed by ALVAC boost will be important to determine whether recombinant ALVAC can significantly boost immune responses against HIV.

Adenoviruses

Adenoviruses (Ads) are associated with the common cold and cause respiratory, intestinal, and eye infections in humans. More than 100 Ad serotypes have been isolated and characterized from humans and from most mammalian and avian species (Ishibashi, 1984). Of the human Ads, types 2 and 5 have been most extensively studied as recombinant viral vectors (Lai *et al.*, 2002; Babiuk and Tikoo, 2000). Since Ads are mucosally transmitted, they are attractive vectors for delivering vaccines to mucosal surfaces. Ads have well-defined molecular biology, can be grown to extremely high titers (10^{10} to 10^{11} pfu/mL), thus reducing the cost of vaccine production and delivery, and can infect a variety of cells and tissues. An important observation is that Ads can infect and be expressed in dendritic cells (DCs), the most potent antigen presenting cell (APC). Ads can also infect a variety of postmitotic cells. A number of effective Ad vaccines have been licensed for use in humans and animals, providing extensive experience with safety and efficacy. Indeed, millions of military recruits have been safely and effectively protected against acute respiratory disease following oral mucosal immunization with Ad4 and Ad7 vaccines in gelatin-coated capsules (Top *et al.*, 1971a; Top *et al.*, 1971b; Top, 1975).

Ads are nonenveloped viruses containing a linear double-stranded DNA genome that varies in size (30 to 45 kb), depending on the species from which they were isolated. Two main types of recombinant Ads have been developed: replication-competent and replication-defective. Replication-competent Ads are constructed by deleting the early 3 (E3) region genes, which modulate host immune responses to the virus but are not essential for replication. These vectors do not require complementing cells for growth *in vitro* and can be used at lower doses to induce immune responses *in vivo*. A disadvantage of replication-competent rAds is they can accept only 3 to 4 kb of foreign DNA. Replication-defective Ads lack the E1 region genes, which are essential for virus replication. Replication-defective Ads require a complementing cell line for growth *in vitro*. E1 and E1, E3–deleted Ads can accommodate up to 8.3 kb of foreign DNA inserted into either the E1 or E3 region. Replication-defective Ad vectors have been used to deliver vaccines in animal models and in the veterinary field (Babiuk and Tikoo, 2000). They have provided protection against challenge with rabies virus (Vos *et al.*, 2001; Tims *et al.*, 2000; Lees *et al.*, 2002); bovine herpesvirus (Reddy *et al.*, 2000; Gogev *et al.*, 2002); infectious bursal disease virus (Sheppard *et al.*, 1998); foot-and-mouth disease virus (Moraes *et al.*, 2002); measles virus (Sharpe *et al.*, 2002); Ebola virus (Sullivan *et al.*, 2000); SHIV (Shiver *et al.*, 2002); and HIV-1 (Yoshida *et al.*, 2001).

Recently, helper-dependent "gutless" (or perhaps, more appropriately, "gutted") Ads have been developed that lack all adenovirus structural genes (Kumar-Singh and Chamberlain, 1996; Kochanek *et al.*, 1996; Fisher *et al.*, 1996). These vectors contain only the inverted terminal repeats (ITRs) required for replication and the *cis*-acting Ad encapsidation signals necessary for packaging. The deletion of all the viral genes permits gutted Ad vectors even greater cloning capacity and addresses the problem of antivector immunity. However, these vectors are difficult to produce and require the use of a helper virus to provide all the viral proteins in *trans*. Since a helper virus is used to produce the gutted vector, one of the main problems associated with them is the final separation of helper and vector viruses during purification. However, recent improvements in the production of gutless Ad vectors has helped in the obtainment of purified vectors that contain 0.1% helper virus (Parks *et al.*, 1996). Although gutted Ad vectors have been tested in gene therapy, they have yet to be tested in vaccine studies.

Human Ad5 is the most commonly used vector for pre-clinical studies. A hurdle in extrapolating studies of human rAd5-based vectors from animal models to humans is the presence of anti-Ad5 neutralizing antibodies in humans. Humoral immune responses to Ad5 are strong and are found in up to 45% of adults in the United States. Depending on route of delivery, they have been shown to decrease the infection efficacy in animal models as well as humans. Strategies to bypass preexisting immunity include switching of Ad serotype (Morral *et al.*, 1999; Mastrangeli *et al.*, 1996; Kass-Eisler *et al.*, 1996) and the use of animal adenoviruses (Farina *et al.*, 2001; Hofmann *et al.*, 1999; Moffatt *et al.*, 2000). While an advantage of animal adenoviruses is that neutralizing antibodies are absent, the lack of knowledge regarding their biology—including tropism in humans—and the possibility of *in vivo* recombination with human types has so far limited their application. Therefore, extensive screening was conducted to identify human adenoviruses with low seroprevalence and Ad type 35 (Vogels *et al.*, 2003). Subsequently, replication-deficient human Ad35 vectors were constructed and were shown to bypass anti-Ad5 neutralizing antibodies and to have tropism similar to that of Ad5 (Vogels *et al.*, 2003).

We were among the first groups to explore recombinant human Ads as mucosal vaccines and have been strong proponents of its application against HIV. rAds have been described for a variety of animal viruses, including hepatitis B virus, hepatitis C virus, vesicular stomatitis virus (VSV), herpes simplex virus, rabies virus, parainfluenza virus, and HIV.

Today, studies of rAd vectors are generating much interest as vaccines against HIV (Voltan and Robert-Guroff, 2003). Most groups have pursued replication-defective Ad5/HIV and SIV recombinants. These have been found to have good immunogenicity. Recently, a study demonstrating that immunization with rAd/SIVgag, with or without prior priming with SIVgag DNA, elicited potent cellular immune responses and protected macaques against SHIV89.6 challenge. This has led to a phase I trial being conducted in the United States, evaluating DNA versus rAd prime, followed by rAd boost, and a phase II rAd/HIVgag evaluation is being conducted by the National Institute of Allergy and Infectious Diseases (NIAID) and Merck in a number of countries. Additionally, some groups have pursued use of replication-competent rAd vectors, using a strategy based on sequential immunization with rAd of different serotypes. Studies in nonhuman primates have shown induction of strong humoral, cellular, and mucosal immune responses.

Tuberculosis, caused by *Mycobacterium tuberculosis*, remains a global epidemic: one-third of the world's population is infected, and 8 million new cases and 2 to 2.5 million deaths occur annually (Wang and Xing, 2002; Dye *et al.*, 1999). Recently, a recombinant replication-defective Ad-based vaccine expressing *M. tuberculosis* Ag85A (AdAg85A) was engineered and evaluated for its potential to serve as a respiratory mucosal tuberculosis vaccine in a murine model of pulmonary tuberculosis (Wang *et al.*, submitted). A single nasal immunization with AdAg85A provided potent protection against airway *M. tuberculosis* challenge. Indeed, mice immunized mucosally with AdAg85A were much better protected than those immunized parenterally with AdAg85A or even with bacillus Calmette-Guerin (BCG) vaccine. Such superior protection following nasal AdAg85A was mediated by both CD4-positive (CD4$^+$) and CD8$^+$ T cells and was correlated with greater accumulation and retention of antigen-specific T cells in the lung. Thus, these results lend further support to the critical advantage of respiratory mucosal vaccination over other routes of vaccination in the fight against tuberculosis.

Herpesviruses

Herpes simplex virus type 1 (HSV-1), attenuated herpesviruses, and varicella-zoster virus (VZV) have been used to express foreign genes (Burton *et al.*, 2002). Herpesviruses are large enveloped viruses that contain a linear double-stranded DNA genome that can accommodate large amounts of foreign DNA. These viruses are being studied as vaccines against genital herpes, and since they target mucosal surfaces, they may be attractive vectors for use against HIV (Voltan and Robert-Guroff, 2003). Additionally, since herpesviruses establish persistent lifelong infections from which they can periodically reactivate, they may be useful to induce long-term immune responses. Indeed, strong humoral and cell-mediated immune responses can be easily detected for long periods of time (Whitley *et al.*, 1993). Studies of both attenuated, replication-competent (Meignier *et al.*, 1990; Spector *et al.*, 1998), and replication-defective HSV recombinants have shown partial protection against a virulent SIVmac239 challenge (Murphy *et al.*, 2000). Other investigators used HSV amplicons encoding HIV gp120 to elicit humoral and T-cell-mediated immune responses in mice that persisted for more than 5 months after a single immunization (Hocknell *et al.*, 2002). Since herpesviruses are ubiquitous, a concern has been the effect of prior host immunity on efficacy of the vector. Indeed, for both poxvirus (Flexner *et al.*, 1988; Etlinger and Altenburger, 1991) and adenovirus vectors (Schulick *et al.*, 1997; Papp *et al.*, 1999; Parr *et al.*, 1998), prior immunity has been shown to suppress efficacy of these vectors. Recently, it was shown in a mouse model that preexisting immunity to HSV did not diminish induction of antibody or T-cell-proliferative responses to a replication-defective HSV-derived vaccine vector (Brockman and Knipe, 2002). Some safety concerns with these viruses, though, are its ability to establish a latent infection and its use in immunocompromised individuals.

Adeno-Associated Viruses

Adeno-associated virus (AAV) is a small, nonenveloped, single-stranded DNA virus belonging to the Parvoviridae family (Hoggan, 1970; Berns, 1990). It is a defective virus dependent on the presence of a helper virus, usually Ad or herpesvirus, for replication (Buller *et al.*, 1981; Casto *et al.*, 1967). In the absence of these helper viruses, AAV establishes latency by integrating into human chromosome 19q.

Thus, its integration is site-specific. About 50% to 90% of the adult population is seropositive for AAV (Samulski *et al.*, 1991; Kotin *et al.*, 1990, 1992; Erles *et al.*, 1999; Chirmule *et al.*, 1999), and the virus has been detected in the human genital tract (Hermonat *et al.*, 1997). However, there is no evidence of association of AAV with any disease to date. Indeed, some studies have suggested that AAV may have a protective role against human papillomavirus-associated cervical cancer (Walz *et al.*, 2002; Meyers *et al.*, 2001).

Six AAV serotypes have been identified, and AAV-2 isolated from humans has been the most extensively characterized to date. The AAV genome is a 4.6-kb ssDNA molecule with inverted terminal repeat (ITR) sequences of 145 nucleotides at each end (Berns, 1990). The ITRs are the only *cis*-acting elements required for replication, packaging, and integration. Thus, rAAV vectors are generated by replacing the AAV genome with foreign sequences between the two ITRs, allowing packaging of 4.1 to 4.9 kb (Dong *et al.*, 1996). Ad helper genes (e.g., E1, E2a, E4) are provided in *trans* to produce titers of up to 10^{14} particles/mL. AAV has a broad host range, and expression of the inserted gene is long-lasting. Further, nonenveloped AAV vectors are stable and resistant to temperature, organic solvents, and extremes of pH (Hoggan *et al.*, 1966, Hoggan, 1970). Their insensitivity to acid makes them suitable for oral delivery to mucosal inductive sites in the intestine.

Persistence of rAAVs *in vivo* for months or years has been attributed to the limited cellular response elicited by this vector, which is devoid of all viral genes except the transgene product and the ITRs. Delivery of rAAV has been followed by a lack of inflammation (Xiao *et al.*, 1996; Conrad *et al.*, 1996), which may be due to poor transduction of APCs (Hernandez *et al.*, 1999; Jooss *et al.*, 1998). On the other hand, humoral responses to AAV virion capsid have been detected following rAAV delivery. Furthermore, the presence of neutralizing antibodies to AAV can reduce the success of vector readministration (Xiao *et al.*, 1999; Chirmule *et al.*, 2000). Another concern with AAV is its ability to integrate (Nakai *et al.*, 2001; Nakai *et al.*, 2000). This is a double-edged sword since integration is site-specific and permits long-term transgene expression, so it may be beneficial for sustaining immune responses.

AAV has been used extensively in gene therapy studies with considerable success (Monahan and Samulski, 2000; Lai *et al.*, 2002). With regard to its use as a vaccine, much of the work has focused on development rAAV for HIV (Voltan and Robert-Guroff, 2003). rAAV expressing HIV env, tat, and rev genes under a cytomegalovirus (CMV) promoter demonstrated induction of HIV-specific serum IgG for 10 months and fecal secretory IgA (S-IgA) antibodies and class I–restricted CTL activity following systemic immunization (Xin *et al.*, 2001). More recently, a single oral administration of rAAV expressing HIV-1 env stimulated strong HIV-specific humoral immunity and CTL (Xin *et al.*, 2002). This response significantly reduced viral load following rectal challenge with recombinant vaccinia virus expressing the HIV env gene. A novel approach to control of HIV employed

rAAV encoding the gene for the broadly cross-reactive neutralizing monoclonal antibody designated b12 to mouse muscle, a sort of genetic passive antibody transfer (Lewis *et al.*, 2002). A single administration of the vector led to long-term neutralizing antibody activity in the sera of mice for more than 6 months.

RECOMBINANT RNA VIRUS VECTORS

Alphaviruses

Alphaviruses are members of the Togaviridae family (Strauss and Strauss, 1994). Three alphaviruses, Semliki Forest virus (SFV) (Liljestrom and Garoff, 1991), Sindbis virus (SIN) (Xiong *et al.*, 1989), and Venezuelan equine encephalitis virus (VEE) (Davis *et al.*, 1989), have been engineered to serve as useful expression vectors (Lundstrom, 2002; Lundstrom, 2003). Alphavirus vectors demonstrate high expression of heterologous proteins in a broad range of host cells. This, coupled with their strong cytoplasmic replicon-driven RNA replication, has made them attractive vectors. The alphavirus genome consists of a single-stranded positive-sense RNA of between 11,000 and 12,000 nucleotides. Alphavirus vectors can be used for vaccine delivery as naked RNA, DNA plasmids, or recombinant replication-deficient viral particles. While SIN and SFV have been studied in small animal models (Vajdy *et al.*, 2001; Lemiale *et al.*, 2001; Nilsson *et al.*, 2001), VEE vector development has advanced to studies in macaques.

Alphaviruses, including VEE, are spread by mosquitoes and can cause fatal infections in humans during epizootic outbreaks among horses. Live VEE vaccines have been constructed to contain mutations that strongly attenuate the virus while maintaining its ability to induce mucosal and humoral immunity. Three features of VEE suggest it may be especially useful as a vaccine vector (Davis *et al.*, 1996). First, most humans are not already immune to VEE, so preexisting immunity would not limit expression of the heterologous antigen; second, VEE replicates in local lymphoid tissues, including Langerhans cells and follicular DCs, thus favoring induction of immune responses; and last, parenteral immunization of rodents and humans with live attenuated VEE vaccines results in protection against systemic as well as mucosal (nasal) aerosol challenges.

A variety of viral proteins have been expressed from alphavirus replicons, as recombinant viral particles, naked RNA molecules, or DNA plasmids. Subcutaneous immunization with VEE particles expressing influenza hemagglutinin have resulted in strong immune responses, including serum antihemagglutinin IgG and IgA, and protection against nasal challenge with influenza virus (Davis *et al.*, 1996). Thus, significant mucosal immune responses were elicited to restrict challenge virus replication in the lung and protect against signs of disease. An interesting observation is that immunization with SFV particles expressing the fusion (F) and glycoprotein (G) of respiratory syncytial virus (RSV) protected against RSV only following nasal immunization

(Chen *et al.*, 2002). It was recently shown that VEE replicons expressing the capsid protein gene of Norwalk virus were capable of self-assembly of Norwalk virus–like particles (VLPs) in baby hamster kidney cells (Harrington *et al.*, 2002). Subcutaneous inoculation of mice with VEE particles expressing Norwalk virus capsid proteins elicited systemic and mucosal immune responses to Norwalk VLPs. Protection against lethal challenges with Ebola virus was demonstrated after immunization of mice and guinea pigs with VEE vectors expressing the nucleoprotein (NP) and glycoprotein (G) (Wilson and Hart, 2001; Pushko *et al.*, 2000); however, these vectors failed to protect nonhuman primates against Ebola virus (Geisbert *et al.*, 2002).

Studies with use of attenuated VEE replicon vectors against SIV have been conducted in rhesus macaques (Davis *et al.*, 2000, 2002). Following three sequential subcutaneous immunizations of a cocktail of VEE replicons expressing SIV gag, gp160, and gp140, both humoral and cellular responses were induced. Although all animals challenged intrarectally became infected, reduced viral burdens and no CD4+ T cell loss were observed. In light of these results, a phase I trial of VEE replicons expressing HIV-1 gag from clade C is being conducted in South Africa.

Vesicular stomatitis virus

Interest in vesicular stomatitis virus (VSV) as a recombinant vector stems from its simplicity of structure, ease of manipulation, and very rapid growth to high titer in a variety of mammalian cells (Haglund *et al.*, 2002a; Roberts *et al.*, 1999; Rose *et al.*, 2001). VSV is the prototype of the family Rhabdoviridae and has a single negative-stranded RNA genome of 11 kb. It infects a broad range of animals, including cattle, horses, and swine. Although rarely fatal, VSV infection of livestock causes vesicular lesions around the mouth, hoofs, and teats, mimicking hoof-and-mouth disease in horses and cattle (Walton *et al.*, 1987). Viral replication occurs in the cytoplasm, thus avoiding any possibility of integration. It encodes five structural proteins, including the nucleoprotein (N), P and L polymerase subunits, matrix (M) protein, and the transmembrane glycoprotein (G) (Wagner, 1996). Cloning is relatively easy and expression is efficient (Schnell *et al.*, 1996; Lawson *et al.*, 1995; Haglund *et al.*, 2000; Kretzschmar *et al.*, 1997). VSV can accommodate at least 4.5 kb of foreign sequence and has a number of advantages as a live replication-competent vector (Haglund *et al.*, 2000). The virus replicates rapidly to high titers, so it can be easily prepared in large quantities. VSV efficiently shuts off host mRNA translation, so the level of gene expression is high, resulting in high-level production of recombinant protein. VSV recombinants can be administered via the mucosal route to elicit mucosal immune responses (Roberts *et al.*, 1999). Seroprevalence of anti-VSV antibodies within the general human population is extremely low, and its lack of serious pathogenicity in humans is an advantage for the potential use of VSV as a recombinant vector vaccine in humans. Also, a number of serotypes of VSV are available, thus permitting prime-boost vaccination strategies.

Early studies reported that nasal vaccination of mice with rVSV expressing influenza virus hemagglutinin protein (VSV/HA) completely protected mice from lethal nasal influenza virus challenge (Roberts *et al.*, 1998). Prior to challenge, mice had high levels of serum neutralizing antibodies against influenza virus. Subsequently, VSV vectors were further attenuated by truncations or complete deletion of the VSV glycoprotein. These attenuated VSV vectors were protective and nonpathogenic and did not induce neutralizing antibodies to the vector itself (Roberts *et al.*, 1999).

VSV was recently introduced as a potential vector for HIV vaccines (Voltan and Robert-Guroff, 2003). VSV recombinants based on different serotypes and expressing HIV env and SIV gag genes were evaluated in rhesus macaques for immunogenicity and protection against SHIV89.6 challenge (Rose *et al.*, 2001). Intramuscular immunizations followed by mucosal boost conferred protection against disease with low viral burden and with preservation of CD4 T cells. Decreases in antivector antibody responses after each immunization may have been due to T-cell-mediated immunity against the vector.

Studies in mice suggested that VSV/HIV recombinants induced more potent cellular immune responses than vaccinia recombinants expressing the same genes (Haglund *et al.*, 2002a). However, sequential VSV recombinant immunization followed by a vaccinia virus boost triggered significantly enhanced CTL responses (Haglund *et al.*, 2002b). Thus, the use of heterologous viruses in prime-boost strategies may provide stronger immune responses.

PRIME-BOOST VACCINATION

Most immunization strategies require booster immunizations to achieve maximal efficacy. Concerns that antivector immunity will limit the reapplication of a particular recombinant-based vector vaccine led to evaluation of heterologous prime-boost strategies employing different vectors (Plotkin, 2003; Excler and Plotkin, 1997). One of the earliest trials of the prime-boost concept concerned priming with avipox vectors containing HIV genes and boosting with inoculations of HIV envelope gp120 protein (Pialoux *et al.*, 1995). This resulted in significantly greater generation of both antibodies and cell-mediated immunity than with either vaccine alone in macaques.

Interest in enhancing T-cell-mediated immunity has focused largely on heterologous vaccination with use of plasmid DNA to prime and recombinant viruses to boost. Heterologous prime-boost has resulted in unprecedented immune responses in highly pathogenic models of SIV, tuberculosis, and malaria challenges, where other vaccine modalities have failed (McShane *et al.*, 2001; Sedegah *et al.*, 1998; Schneider *et al.*, 1998; Robinson *et al.*, 1999; Amara *et al.*, 2001). In an impressive study in nonhuman primates, monkeys primed with DNA coding for SIV Gag, Pol, Vif, Vpx, and Vpr and for HIV-1 Env, Tat, and Rev and boosted with rMVA expressing SIV Gag and Pol and HIV-1 Env controlled a rectal challenge with highly pathogenic SHIV-89.6P 7 months after the booster (Amara *et al.*, 2002). Containment of the viral challenge was associated with a burst of antiviral T cells. A number of human clinical trials of HIV vaccines based on DNA prime-recombinant rMVA boost are under way in Europe and Africa (www.iavi.org). Similarly, a phase I trial of DNA-rAd boost is under way in the United States following success in nonhuman primates (Shiver *et al.*, 2002).

The mechanism whereby heterologous prime-boost vaccination enhances immunization is poorly understood. Ramshaw and Ramsay (2000) have hypothesized that persistent low-level gene expression associated with plasmid DNA immunization results in induction of high-avidity T cells. The subsequent boost with virus provides a greater antigenic challenge than boosting with pDNA, causing greater expansion of the high-avidity cells and thus greater protection. Alternatively, Leitner *et al.* (1999) have suggested two other possibilities. This first is that the presence of viral vector antigens following priming may deviate the immune response away from the specific vaccine antigen. The second possibility is that the presence of immunosuppressive molecules encoded by the viral vector might impair the immune response.

An important study assessing prime-boost immunization strategies using a DNA vaccine encoding HSV glycoprotein B (gB DNA) and an attenuated recombinant vaccinia virus vector expressing HSVgB demonstrated that systemic prime-boost failed to induce detectable humoral or T-cell-mediated responses at mucosal surfaces (Eo *et al.*, 2001). However, such responses were induced if immunizations, particularly the priming dose, were administered mucosally. It is curious that whereas optimal immunity with systemic priming and boosting occurred when gB DNA was used to prime and rVacgB was used to boost, mucosal responses were optimal when animals were mucosally primed with rVacgB and boosted with gB DNA given mucosally. Furthermore, notable mucosal immune responses also occurred in animals that were mucosally primed with rVacgB and boosted systemically with gB DNA. These results suggest that the rules governing optimal prime-boost strategies may differ if one is seeking to optimize systemic versus mucosal immunity. Since the mucosal prime-boost immunization strategy also induced strong systemic immune responses, this approach may be useful to protect against infections for which both mucosal and systemic immunity are important.

Recently, we examined protection against intravaginal challenge with HSV-2 following various prime-boost combinations delivered mucosally, employing recombinant Ad vectors expressing HSVgB (AdgB) or recombinant HSV-2 gB protein plus CpG oligodeoxynucleotide (ODNs) as an adjuvant (Kwant, A., and Rosenthal, K.L., manuscript in preparation). Mice immunized nasally with AdgB followed by boost with rgB plus CpG ODNs provided the greatest protection against intravaginal HSV-2 challenge. Indeed, this prime-boost combination protected better than in mice given homologous prime-boost or primed with rgB plus

CpG and boosted with AdgB. The level of HSV-2 in vaginal washes of the AdgB-primed/rgB plus CpG–boosted group was also shown to be at least a log lower than nearly all of the other groups 2 days following intravaginal challenge. These results suggest that mucosal (nasal) priming with a recombinant viral vector and boosting with a recombinant subunit viral protein plus CpG is the most effective way of inducing a mucosal immune response and providing protection against a sexually transmitted virus. This approach should be of use when designing vaccination strategies for sexually transmitted pathogens, such as HSV or HIV.

MODIFICATIONS OF VIRAL VECTORS TO ENHANCE MUCOSAL IMMUNITY

In addition to the enhanced immune responses and protection following heterologous prime-boost delivery, an alternative strategy has been to insert various cytokine, chemokine, and costimulatory genes into viral vectors to enhance and/or redirect immune responses (Ahlers *et al.*, 2003; Berzofsky *et al.*, 2001; Bukreyev and Belyakov, 2002). It is well known that many vaccines require the use of adjuvants to induce optimal protective immune responses. Adjuvants achieve this, in part, by inducing relevant cytokines and chemokines and upregulating expression of costimulatory molecules on APCs. Inclusion of immunomodulating genes in live vectors mimics adjuvant-induced signals and results in local production of specific immunomodulatory factors in the context of encoded antigens to improve immunogenicity or qualitatively affect immune responses, such as polarizing them toward Th1- or Th2-type immunity. Furthermore, this approach may serve to eliminate the need to formulate the vaccine with particular adjuvants.

Recombinant vaccinia viruses engineered to express human IL-2 were among the earliest vectors to be examined for modulation of immunobiological properties (Flexner *et al.*, 1987; Ramshaw *et al.*, 1987). Following inoculation of immunodeficient athymic nude mice, wild-type vaccinia virus caused generalized infection and killed the mice, whereas vaccinia virus expressing IL-2 resulted in limited infection with significantly lower viral titers and greatly reduced mortality. Immunogenicity of this vector was examined by inclusion of the influenza hemagglutinin gene in vaccinia encoding IL-2 (Flexner *et al.*, 1987). The antibody response to the recombinant vector expressing hemagglutinin and IL-2 was equal to or significantly greater than that for the control virus expressing hemagglutinin alone. This study was also extended to primates, and despite lower levels of replication, the virus expressing hemagglutinin and IL-2 induced levels of antihemagglutinin antibodies equal to or higher than those induced by the control virus expressing hemagglutinin alone (Flexner *et al.*, 1990).

In a study in the macaque model (Benson *et al.*, 1998), NYVAC expressing SIV gag, pol, and env genes was mixed with a separate NYVAC vector expressing human IL-12 p35 and p40 subunits, as well as the IL-2 gene, and was delivered intramuscularly. The overall CTL response was greater, at the expense of proliferative and humoral responses, in animals that were immunized with both vectors versus those immunized with the NYVAC-SIV vaccine alone. An important observation was that five of 11 vaccinated monkeys exposed mucosally to SIVmac251 showed a transient peak of viremia at 1 week after challenge and then their infection appeared to clear. In contrast, all 12 animals inoculated intravenously became infected, but 5 to 6 months later, virus replication appeared to be under control in four animals, and the virus appeared to progress more slowly in these four.

Secretory IgA is a major effector molecule in protection against mucosal infections (Mazanec et al., 1993). Both IL-5 and IL-6 have been shown to enhance IgA production in vitro (Schoenbeck et al., 1989; Kunimoto et al., 1989; Beagley et al., 1988; Beagley et al., 1989). We examined in vivo effects of these two cytokines, using recombinant adenoviruses capable of expressing each of these cytokines (Braciak et al., 2000). Nasal immunization of mice with Ad expressing IL-5 or IL-6 increased Ad-specific IgA titers in lung lavage threefold, relative to control virus. Although Ad expressing IL-6 had the greatest impact, simultaneous expression of both IL-5 and IL-6 following coinoculation resulted in faster kinetic and greater-than-additive increases in anti-Ad IgA titers in the lung.

Similarly, in normal mice, infection with recombinant vaccinia virus expressing influenza virus hemagglutinin and IL-6 resulted in a fourfold increase in hemagglutinin-specific mucosal antibodies in comparison with the titers with control virus expressing hemagglutinin alone (Ramsay et al., 1994). In separate studies, infection with recombinant fowlpox virus expressing hemagglutinin and murine IL-6 resulted in an eightfold increase in mucosal IgG and 33-fold increases in IgA following secondary immunization, relative to immunization with vector expressing hemagglutinin alone (Leong et al., 1994, Ramsay et al., 1994). A significant increase in the number of mucosal IgG and IgA-secreting B cells was also observed following immunization with this recombinant vector expressing both hemagglutinin and IL-6. Thus, IL-6 is a promising cytokine candidate for coexpression by live recombinant vectors to promote mucosal humoral immune responses.

Costimulatory molecules have also been shown to enhance vaccine efficacy (Freund et al., 2000; Chamberlain et al., 1996). For example, a combination of IL-12 and B7-1 (CD80) was found to be synergistic in a recombinant viral vaccine (Rao et al., 1996). Last, expression of a triple combination of costimulatory molecules, including CD80, intercellular adhesion molecule 1 (ICAM-1; CD54), and lymphocyte function–associated protein 3 (LFA-3; CD58) has been found to be synergistic for the induction of CTL and antitumor immunity (Hodge et al., 1999). Indeed, these so-called TRICOM vectors were shown to make B cells into APCs as effective in vitro as DCs and to make DCs into "super APCs" (Zhu et al., 2001; Hodge et al., 1999).

In addition to amplifying immune responses, cytokines and chemokines can control the type of responses induced.

Indeed, codelivery of Th1 cytokines, including IL-2, IL-12, IL-15, and IL-18, enhanced survival and reduced pathology of herpetic lesions following intravaginal HSV-2 challenge. In contrast, coinoculation of Th2 cytokine genes increased morbidity and mortality among challenged mice.

Although inclusion of cytokine genes in recombinant viral vectors holds much promise, as with any new technology, it may also have negative effects. Notably, inclusion of certain cytokine genes can increase the level of viral pathogenicity of a live recombinant vector. For example, inclusion of interleukin 4 (IL-4) into a recombinant vaccinia virus suppressed antiviral CTL, reduced the number of CTL precursors, downregulated production of mRNA for IFN-γ, IL-12, and IL-2, and delayed clearance of infection in mice in comparison with control virus (Sharma et al., 1996). Since IL-4 tends to promote Th2 responses and suppress Th1 responses and vaccinia virus is controlled by Th1 responses, inclusion of this cytokine in the vector resulted in increased pathogenicity. This was more dramatically shown by studies demonstrating that inclusion of the murine IL-4 gene into recombinant ectromelia or mousepox virus resulted in dramatic suppression of natural killer (NK) and CTL activity in mice and high mortality (Jackson et al., 2001). Indeed, strains of mice normally resistant to ectromelia virus developed symptoms and died following infection with recombinant ectromelia expressing IL-4. Furthermore, since introduction of live virus vectors can result in serious illness in immunocompromised individuals, and since inclusion of immunomodulatory genes can affect the pathogenicity of live recombinant vectors, the safety of recombinant viruses expressing cytokines needs to be examined in immunocompromised individuals.

CONCLUSIONS

Since most infections are initiated mucosally, it will be important to develop immunization strategies that elicit strong mucosal as well as systemic immune responses. Recombinant viral vectors have proven very effective in eliciting strong immune responses. But because of the compartmentalization of our immune system and selective homing of lymphocytes, mucosal delivery of recombinant viral vaccines has been shown to be critical for induction and long-term durability of mucosal immune responses. Indeed, mucosal delivery of vaccines induces both mucosal and systemic immune responses, whereas parenteral immunization is not effective at generation of long-term mucosal immunity or protection. Many recombinant viral vectors have been shown to induce strong systemic and mucosal immune responses and protection against mucosal viral challenge in animal models and nonhuman primates.

Recent studies have clearly demonstrated the ability of heterologous prime-boost to strongly promote induction of immune responses and protection. Furthermore, the flexibility of recombinant viral vectors permits inclusion of cytokines, chemokines, and costimulatory molecules that can also enhance and direct the immunogenicity of these vectors. Although a number of the recombinant viral vectors reviewed here are currently in human clinical trials, they are being delivered via parenteral routes of immunization. In light of our current understanding of mucosal immune responses, it will be important that trials incorporating mucosal delivery of these recombinant viral vectors be investigated.

REFERENCES

Ahlers, J. D., Belyakov, I. M., and Berzofsky, J. A. (2003). Cytokine, chemokine and costimulatory molecule modulation to enhance efficacy of HIV vaccines. *Curr. Mol. Med.* 3, 285–301.

Amara, R. R., Villinger, F., Altman, J. D., Lydy, S. L., O'Neil, S. P., Staprans, S. I., Montefiori, D. C., Xu, Y., Herndon, J. G., Wyatt, L. S., Candido, M. A., Kozyr, N. L., Earl, P. L., Smith, J. M., Ma, H. L., Grimm, B. D., Hulsey, M. L., McClure, H. M., McNicholl, J. M., Moss, B., and Robinson, H. L. (2002). Control of a mucosal challenge and prevention of AIDS by a multiprotein DNA/MVA vaccine. *Vaccine* 20, 1949–1955.

Amara, R. R., Villinger, F., Altman, J. D., Lydy, S. L., O'Neil, S. P., Staprans, S. I., Montefiori, D. C., Xu, Y., Herndon, J. G., Wyatt, L. S., Candido, M. A., Kozyr, N. L., Earl, P. L., Smith, J. M., Ma, H. L., Grimm, B. D., Hulsey, M. L., Miller, J., McClure, H. M., McNicholl, J. M., Moss, B., and Robinson, H. L. (2001). Control of a mucosal challenge and prevention of AIDS by a multiprotein DNA / MVA vaccine. *Science* 292, 69–74.

Antoine, G., Scheiflinger, F., Dorner, F., and Falkner, F. G. (1998). The complete genomic sequence of the modified vaccinia Ankara strain: comparison with other orthopoxviruses. *Virology* 244, 365–396.

Babiuk, L. A., and Tikoo, S. K. (2000). Adenoviruses as vectors for delivering vaccines to mucosal surfaces. *J. Biotechnol.* 83, 105–113.

Beagley, K. W., Eldridge, J. H., Kiyono, H., Everson, M. P., Koopman, W. J., Honjo, T., and McGhee, J. R. (1988). Recombinant murine IL-5 induces high rate IgA synthesis in cycling IgA-positive Peyer's patch B cell. *J. Immunol.* 141, 2035–2042.

Beagley, K. W., Eldridge, J. H., Lee, F., Kiyono, H., Everson, M. P., Koopman, W. J., Hirano, T., Kishimoto, T., and McGhee, J. R. (1989). Interleukins and IgA synthesis. Human and murine interleukin 6 induce high rate IgA secretion in IgA-committed B cells. *J. Exp. Med.* 169, 2133–2148.

Benson, J., Chougnet, C., Robert-Guroff, M., Montefiori, D., Markham, P., Shearer, G., Gallo, R. C., Cranage, M., Paoletti, E., Limbach, K., Venzon, D., Tartaglia, J., and Franchini, G. (1998). Recombinant vaccine-induced protection against the highly pathogenic simian immunodeficiency virus SIV (mac251): dependence on route of challenge exposure. *J. Virol.* 72, 4170–4182.

Berns, K. I. (1990). Parvovirus replication. *Microbiol. Rev.* 54, 316–329.

Berzofsky, J. A., Ahlers, J. D., and Belyakov, I. M. (2001). Strategies for designing and optimizing new generation vaccines. *Nat. Rev. Immunol.* 1, 209–219.

Blanchard, T. J., Alcami, A., Andrea, P., and Smith, G. L. (1998). Modified vaccinia virus Ankara undergoes limited replication in human cells and lacks several immunomodulatory proteins: implications for use as a human vaccine. *J. Gen. Virol.* 79 (Pt 5), 1159–1167.

Braciak, T. A., Gallichan, W. S., Graham, F. L., Richards, C. D., Ramsay, A. J., Rosenthal, K. L., and Gauldie, J. (2000). Recombinant adenovirus vectors expressing interluekin-5 and -6 specifically enhance mucosal immunoglobulin A responses in the lung. *Immunology* 101, 388–396.

Briskin, M., Winsor-Hines, D., Shyjan, A., Cochran, N., Bloom, S., Wilson, J., McEvoy, L. M., Butcher, E. C., Kassam, N., Mackay, C. R., Newman, W., and Ringler, D. J. (1997). Human mucosal addressin cell adhesion molecule-1 is preferentially expressed in intestinal tract and associated lymphoid tissue. *Am. J. Pathol.* 151, 97–110.

Brockman, M. A., and Knipe, D. M. (2002). Herpes simplex virus vectors elicit durable immune responses in the presence of preexisting host immunity. *J. Virol.* 76, 3678–3687.

Bukreyev, A., and Belyakov, I. M. (2002). Expression of immunomodulating molecules by recombinant viruses: can the immunogenicity of live virus vaccines be improved? *Expert Rev. Vaccines* 1, 233–245.

Buller, R. M., Janik, J. E., Sebring, E. D., and Rose, J. A. (1981). Herpes simplex virus types 1 and 2 completely help adenovirus-associated virus replication. *J. Virol.* 40, 241–247.

Burton, E. A., Fink, D. J., and Glorioso, J. C. (2002). Gene delivery using herpes simplex virus vectors. *DNA Cell Biol.* 21, 915–936.

Butcher, E. C., Williams, M., Youngman, K., Rott, L., and Briskin, M. (1999). Lymphocyte trafficking and regional immunity. *Adv. Immunol.* 72, 209–253.

Carroll, M. W., Overwijk, W. W., Chamberlain, R. S., Rosenberg, S. A., Moss, B., and Restifo, N. P. (1997). Highly attenuated modified vaccinia virus Ankara (MVA) as an effective recombinant vector: a murine tumor model. *Vaccine* 15, 387–394.

Casto, B. C., Armstrong, J. A., Atchison, R. W., and Hammon, W. M. (1967). Studies in the relationship between adeno-associated virus type 1 (AAV-1) and adenoviruses. II. Inhibition of adenovirus plaques by AAV; its nature and specificity. *Virology* 33, 452–458.

Chakrabarti, S., Sisler, J. R., and Moss, B. (1997). Compact, synthetic, vaccinia virus early/late promoter for protein expression. *Biotechniques* 23, 1094–1097.

Chamberlain, R. S., Carroll, M. W., Bronte, V., Hwu, P., Warren, S., Yang, J. C., Nishimura, M., Moss, B., Rosenberg, S. A., and Restifo, N. P. (1996). Costimulation enhances the active immunotherapy effect of recombinant anticancer vaccines. *Cancer Res.* 56, 2832–2836.

Check, E. (2002). Army HIV vaccine to undergo clinical trial as rival is halted. *Nature* 416, 6.

Chen, M., Hu, K. F., Rozell, B., Orvell, C., Morein, B., and Liljestrom, P. (2002). Vaccination with recombinant alphavirus or immune-stimulating complex antigen against respiratory syncytial virus. *J. Immunol.* 169, 3208–3216.

Chirmule, N., Propert, K., Magosin, S., Qian, Y., Qian, R., and Wilson, J. (1999). Immune responses to adenovirus and adeno-associated virus in humans. *Gene Ther.* 6, 1574–1583.

Chirmule, N., Xiao, W., Truneh, A., Schnell, M. A., Hughes, J. V., Zoltick, P., and Wilson, J. M. (2000). Humoral immunity to adeno-associated virus type 2 vectors following administration to murine and nonhuman primate muscle. *J. Virol.* 74, 2420–2425.

Conrad, C. K., Allen, S. S., Afione, S. A., Reynolds, T. C., Beck, S. E., Fee-Maki, M., Barrazza-Ortiz, X., Adams, R., Askin, F. B., Carter, B. J., Guggino, W. B., and Flotte, T. R. (1996). Safety of single-dose administration of an adeno-associated virus (AAV)-CFTR vector in the primate lung. *Gene Ther.* 3, 658–668.

Davis, N. L., Brown, K. W., and Johnston, R. E. (1996). A viral vaccine vector that expresses foreign genes in lymph nodes and protects against mucosal challenge. *J. Virol.* 70, 3781–3787.

Davis, N. L., Caley, I. J., Brown, K. W., Betts, M. R., Irlbeck, D. M., McGrath, K. M., Connell, M. J., Montefiori, D. C., Frelinger, J. A., Swanstrom, R., Johnson, P. R., and Johnston, R. E. (2000). Vaccination of macaques against pathogenic simian immunodeficiency virus with Venezuelan equine encephalitis virus replicon particles. *J. Virol.* 74, 371–378.

Davis, N. L., West, A., Reap, E., MacDonald, G., Collier, M., Dryga, S., Maughan, M., Connell, M., Walker, C., McGrath, K., Cecil, C., Ping, L. H., Frelinger, J., Olmsted, R., Keith, P., Swanstrom, R., Williamson, C., Johnson, P., Montefiori, D., and Johnston, R. E. (2002). Vaccination of macaques against pathogenic simian immunodeficiency virus with Venezuelan equine encephalitis virus replicon particles. *IUBMB Life* 53, 209–211.

Davis, N. L., Willis, L. V., Smith, J. F., and Johnston, R. E. (1989). *In vitro* synthesis of infectious Venezuelan equine encephalitis virus RNA from a cDNA clone: analysis of a viable deletion mutant. *Virology* 171, 189–204.

Dong, J. Y., Fan, P. D., and Frizzell, R. A. (1996). Quantitative analysis of the packaging capacity of recombinant adeno-associated virus. *Hum. Gene Ther.* 7, 2101–2112.

Dye, C., Scheele, S., Dolin, P., Pathania, V., and Raviglione, M. C. (1999). Consensus statement. Global burden of tuberculosis: estimated incidence, prevalence, and mortality by country. WHO Global Surveillance and Monitoring Project. *JAMA* 282, 677–686.

Ehreth, J. (2003a). The global value of vaccination. *Vaccine* 21, 596–600.

Ehreth, J. (2003b). The value of vaccination: a global perspective. *Vaccine* 21, 4105–4117.

Eo, S. K., Gierynska, M., Kamar, A. A., and Rouse, B. T. (2001). Prime-boost immunization with DNA vaccine: mucosal route of administration changes the rules. *J. Immunol.* 166, 5473–5479.

Erles, K., Sebokova, P., and Schlehofer, J. R. (1999). Update on the prevalence of serum antibodies (IgG and IgM) to adeno-associated virus (AAV). *J. Med. Virol.* 59, 406–411.

Etlinger, H. M., and Altenburger, W. (1991). Overcoming inhibition of antibody responses to a malaria recombinant vaccinia virus caused by prior exposure to wild type virus. *Vaccine* 9, 470–472.

Excler, J. L., Plotkin, S. A. (1997). The prime-boost concept applied to HV preventive vaccines. *AIDS* 11, S127–S137.

Farina, S. F., Gao, G. P., Xiang, Z. Q., Rux, J. J., Burnett, R. M., Alvira, M. R., Marsh, J., Ertl, H. C., and Wilson, J. M. (2001). Replication-defective vector based on a chimpanzee adenovirus. *J. Virol.* 75, 11603–11613.

Fisher, K. J., Choi, H., Burda, J., Chen, S. J., and Wilson, J. M. (1996). Recombinant adenovirus deleted of all viral genes for gene therapy of cystic fibrosis. *Virology* 217, 11–22.

Flexner, C., Hugin, A., and Moss, B. (1987). Prevention of vaccinia virus infection in immunodeficient mice by vector-directed IL-2 expression. *Nature* 330, 259–262.

Flexner, C., Moss, B., London, W. T., and Murphy, B. R. (1990). Attenuation and immunogenicity in primates of vaccinia virus recombinants expressing human interleukin-2. *Vaccine* 8, 17–21.

Flexner, C., Murphy, B. R., Rooney, J. F., Wohlenberg, C., Yuferov, V., Notkins, A. L., and Moss, B. (1988). Successful vaccination with a polyvalent vector despite existing immunity to an expressed antigen. *Nature* 335, 259–262.

Freund, Y. R., Mirsalis, J. C., Fairchild, D. G., Brune, J., Hokama, L. A., Schindler-Horvat, J., Tomaszewski, J. E., Hodge, J. W., Schlom, J., Kantor, J. A., Tyson, C. A., and Donohue, S. J. (2000). Vaccination with a recombinant vaccinia vaccine containing the B7-1 co-stimulatory molecule causes no significant toxicity and enhances T cell-mediated cytotoxicity. *Int. J. Cancer* 85, 508–517.

Geisbert, T. W., Pushko, P., Anderson, K., Smith, J., Davis, K. J., and Jahrling, P. B. (2002). Evaluation in nonhuman primates of vaccines against Ebola virus. *Emerg. Infect. Dis.* 8, 503–507.

Gogev, S., Vanderheijden, N., Lemaire, M., Schynts, F., D'Offay, J., Deprez, I., Adam, M., Eloit, M., and Thiry, E. (2002). Induction of protective immunity to bovine herpesvirus type 1 in cattle by intranasal administration of replication-defective human adenovirus type 5 expressing glycoprotein gC or gD. *Vaccine* 20, 1451–1465.

Haglund, K., Forman, J., Krausslich, H. G., and Rose, J. K. (2000). Expression of human immunodeficiency virus type 1 Gag protein precursor and envelope proteins from a vesicular stomatitis virus recombinant: high-level production of virus-like particles containing HIV envelope. *Virology* 268, 112–121.

Haglund, K., Leiner, I., Kerksiek, K., Buonocore, L., Pamer, E., and Rose, J. K. (2002a). High-level primary CD8(+) T-cell response to human immunodeficiency virus type 1 gag and env generated by vaccination with recombinant vesicular stomatitis virus. *J. Virol.* 76, 2730–2738.

Haglund, K., Leiner, I., Kerksiek, K., Buonocore, L., Pamer, E., and Rose, J. K. (2002b). Robust recall and long-term memory T-cell responses induced by prime-boost regimens with heterologous live viral vectors expressing human immunodeficiency virus type 1 Gag and Env proteins. *J. Virol.* 76, 7506–7517.

Hanke, T., Blanchard, T. J., Schneider, J., Hannan, C. M., Becker, M., Gilbert, S. C., Hill, A. V., Smith, G. L., and McMichael, A. (1998). Enhancement of MHC class I-restricted peptide-specific T cell induction by a DNA prime/MVA boost vaccination regime. *Vaccine* 16, 439–445.

Hanke, T., Samuel, R. V., Blanchard, T. J., Neumann, V. C., Allen, T. M., Boyson, J. E., Sharpe, S. A., Cook, N., Smith, G. L., Watkins, D. I., Cranage, M. P., and McMichael, A. J. (1999). Effective induction of simian immunodeficiency virus-specific cytotoxic T lymphocytes in macaques by using a multiepitope gene and DNA prime-modified vaccinia virus Ankara boost vaccination regimen. *J. Virol.* 73, 7524–7532.

Harrington, P. R., Lindesmith, L., Yount, B., Moe, C. L., and Baric, R. S. (2002). Binding of Norwalk virus-like particles to ABH histo-blood group antigens is blocked by antisera from infected human volunteers or experimentally vaccinated mice. *J. Virol.* 76, 12335–12343.

Hermonat, P. L., Plott, R. T., Santin, A. D., Parham, G. P., and Flick, J. T. (1997). Adeno-associated virus Rep78 inhibits oncogenic transformation of primary human keratinocytes by a human papillomavirus type 16-ras chimeric. *Gynecol. Oncol.* 66, 487–494.

Hernandez, Y. J., Wang, J., Kearns, W. G., Loiler, S., Poirier, A., and Flotte, T. R. (1999). Latent adeno-associated virus infection elicits humoral but not cell-mediated immune responses in a non-human primate model. *J. Virol.* 73, 8549–8558.

Hocknell, P. K., Wiley, R. D., Wang, X., Evans, T. G., Bowers, W. J., Hanke, T., Federoff, H. J., and Dewhurst, S. (2002). Expression of human immunodeficiency virus type 1 gp120 from herpes simplex virus type 1-derived amplicons results in potent, specific and durable cellular and humoral immune responses. *J. Virol.* 76, 5565–5580.

Hodge, J. W., Sabzevari, H., Yafal, A. G., Gritz, L., Lorenz, M. G., and Schlom, J. (1999). A triad of costimulatory molecules synergize to amplify T-cell activation. *Cancer Res.* 59, 5800–5807.

Hofmann, C., Loser, P., Cichon, G., Arnold, W., Both, G. W., and Strauss, M. (1999). Ovine adenovirus vectors overcome preexisting humoral immunity against human adenoviruses *in vivo*. *J. Virol.* 73, 6930–6936.

Hoggan, M. D. (1970). Adenovirus associated viruses. *Prog. Med. Virol.* 12, 211–239.

Hoggan, M. D., Blacklow, N. R., and Rowe, W. P. (1966). Studies of small DNA viruses found in various adenovirus preparations: physical, biological, and immunological characteristics. *Proc. Natl. Acad. Sci. USA* 55, 1467–1474.

Ishibashi, M., Yasue, H., eds. (1984). *Adenoviruses of Animals*. New York: Plenum Press.

Jackson, R. J., Ramsay, A. J., Christensen, C. D., Beaton, S., Hall, D. F., and Ramshaw, I. A. (2001). Expression of mouse interleukin-4 by a recombinant ectromelia virus suppresses cytolytic lymphocyte responses and overcomes genetic resistance to mousepox. *J. Virol.* 75, 1205–1210.

Jooss, K., Yang, Y., Fisher, K. J., and Wilson, J. M. (1998). Transduction of dendritic cells by DNA viral vectors directs the immune response to transgene products in muscle fibers. *J. Virol.* 72, 4212–4223.

Kantele, A., Zivny, J., Hakkinen, M., Elson, C. O., and Mestecky, J. (1999). Differential homing commitments of antigen-specific T cells after oral or parenteral immunization in humans. *J. Immunol.* 162, 5173–5177.

Kass-Eisler, A., Leinwand, L., Gall, J., Bloom, B., and Falck-Pedersen, E. (1996). Circumventing the immune response to adenovirus-mediated gene therapy. *Gene Ther.* 3, 154–162.

Kochanek, S., Clemens, P. R., Mitani, K., Chen, H. H., Chan, S., and Caskey, C. T. (1996). A new adenoviral vector: replacement of all viral coding sequences with 28 kb of DNA independently expressing both full-length dystrophin and beta-galactosidase. *Proc. Natl. Acad. Sci. USA* 93, 5731–5736.

Kotin, R. M., Linden, R. M., and Berns, K. I. (1992). Characterization of a preferred site on human chromosome 19q for integration of adeno-associated virus DNA by non-homologous recombination. *EMBO J.* 11, 5071–5078.

Kotin, R. M., Siniscalco, M., Samulski, R. J., Zhu, X. D., Hunter, L., Laughlin, C. A., McLaughlin, S., Muzyczka, N., Rocchi, M., and Berns, K. I. (1990). Site-specific integration by adeno-associated virus. *Proc. Natl. Acad. Sci. USA* 87, 2211–2215.

Kozlowski, P. A., and Neutra, M. R. (2003). The role of mucosal immunity in prevention of HIV transmission. *Curr. Mol. Med.* 3, 217–228.

Kretzschmar, E., Buonocore, L., Schnell, M. J., and Rose, J. K. (1997). High-efficiency incorporation of functional influenza virus glycoproteins into recombinant vesicular stomatitis viruses. *J. Virol.* 71, 5982–5989.

Kumar-Singh, R., and Chamberlain, J. S. (1996). Encapsidated adenovirus minichromosomes allow delivery and expression of a 14 kb dystrophin cDNA to muscle cells. *Hum. Mol. Genet.* 5, 913–921.

Kunimoto, D. Y., Nordan, R. P., and Strober, W. (1989). IL-6 is a potent cofactor of IL-1 in IgM synthesis and of IL-5 in IgA synthesis. *J. Immunol.* 143, 2230–2235.

Lai, C. M., Lai, Y. K., and Rakoczy, P. E. (2002). Adenovirus and adeno-associated virus vectors. *DNA Cell Biol.* 21, 895–913.

Lawson, N. D., Stillman, E. A., Whitt, M. A., and Rose, J. K. (1995). Recombinant vesicular stomatitis viruses from DNA. *Proc. Natl. Acad. Sci. USA* 92, 4477–4481.

Lees, C. Y., Briggs, D. J., Wu, X., Davis, R. D., Moore, S. M., Gordon, C., Xiang, Z., Ertl, H. C., Tang de, C. C., and Fu, Z. F. (2002). Induction of protective immunity by topic application of a recombinant adenovirus expressing rabies virus glycoprotein. *Vet. Microbiol.* 85, 295–303.

Leitner, W. W., Ying, H., and Restifo, N. P. (1999). DNA- and RNA-based vaccines: principles, progress and prospects. *Vaccine* 18, 765–777.

Lemiale, F., Brand, D., Lebigot, S., Verrier, B., Buzelay, L., Brunet, S., and Barin, F. (2001). Immunogenicity of recombinant envelope glycoproteins derived from T-cell line-adapted isolates or primary HIV isolates: a comparative study using multivalent vaccine approaches. *J. Acquir. Immune Defic. Syndr.* 26, 413–422.

Leong, K. H., Ramsay, A. J., Boyle, D. B., and Ramshaw, I. A. (1994). Selective induction of immune responses by cytokines coexpressed in recombinant fowlpox virus. *J. Virol.* 68, 8125–8130.

Lewis, A. D., Chen, R., Montefiori, D. C., Johnson, P. R., and Clark, K. R. (2002). Generation of neutralizing activity against human immunodeficiency virus type 1 in serum by antibody gene transfer. *J. Virol.* 76, 8769–8775.

Liljestrom, P., and Garoff, H. (1991). A new generation of animal cell expression vectors based on the Semliki Forest virus replicon. *Biotechnology (NY)* 9, 1356–1361.

Lundstrom, K. (2002). Alphavirus-based vaccines. *Curr. Opin. Mol. Ther.* 4, 28–34.

Lundstrom, K. (2003). Alphavirus vectors for vaccine production and gene therapy. *Expert Rev. Vaccines* 2, 447–459.

Mastrangeli, A., Harvey, B. G., Yao, J., Wolff, G., Kovesdi, I., Crystal, R. G., and Falck-Pedersen, E. (1996). Sero-switch adenovirus-mediated *in vivo* gene transfer: circumvention of anti-adenovirus humoral immune defenses against repeat adenovirus vector administration by changing the adenovirus serotype. *Hum Gene Ther.* 7, 79–87.

Mayr, A., Hochstein-Mintzel, V., and Stickl, H. (1975). *Infection* 3, 6–14.

Mazanec, M. B., Nedrud, J. G., Kaetzel, C. S., and Lamm, M. E. (1993). A three-tiered view of the role of IgA in mucosal defense. *Immunol. Today* 14, 430–435.

Mazumdar, P. (2003) In *Fundamental Immunology* (ed. Paul, W. E.). Philadelphia: Lippincott Williams & Wilkins, 23–46.

McShane, H., Brookes, R., Gilbert, S. C., and Hill, A. V. (2001). Enhanced immunogenicity of CD4(+) T-cell responses and protective efficacy of a DNA-modified vaccinia virus Ankara prime-boost vaccination regimen for murine tuberculosis. *Infect. Immun.* 69, 681–686.

Meignier, B., Martin, B., Whitley, R. J., and Roizman, B. (1990). *In vivo* behavior of genetically engineered herpes simplex virus R7017 and R7020. II. Studies in immunocompetent and immunosuppressed owl monkeys (Aotus trivirgatus). *J. Infect. Dis.* 162, 313–321.

Meyer, H., Sutter, G., and Mayr, A. (1991). Mapping of deletions in the genome of the highly attenuated vaccinia virus MVA and their influence on virulence. *J. Gen. Virol.* 72 (Pt 5), 1031–1038.

Meyers, C., Alam, S., Mane, M., and Hermonat, P. L. (2001). Altered biology of adeno-associated virus type 2 and human papillomavirus during dual infection of natural host tissue. *Virology* 287, 30–39.

Moffatt, S., Hays, J., HogenEsch, H., and Mittal, S. K. (2000). Circumvention of vector-specific neutralizing antibody response by alternating use of a human and non-human adenoviruses: implications in gene therapy. *Virology* 272, 159–167.

Monahan, P. E., and Samulski, R. J. (2000). Adeno-associated virus vectors for gene therapy: more pros than cons? *Mol. Med. Today* 6, 433–440.

Moraes, M. P., Mayr, G. A., Mason, P. W., and Grubman, M. J. (2002). Early protection against homologous challenge after a single dose of replication-defective human adenovirus type 5 expressing capsid proteins of foot and mouth disease virus (FMDV) strain A24. *Vaccine* 20, 1631–1639.

Morral, N., O'Neal, W., Rice, K., Leland, M., Kaplan, J., Piedra, P. A., Zhou, H., Parks, R. J., Velji, R., Aguilar-Cordova, E., Wadsworth, S., Graham, F. L., Kochanek, S., Carey, K. D., and Beaudet, A. L. (1999). Administration of helper-dependent adenoviral vectors and sequential delivery of different vector serotype for long-term liver-directed gene transfer in baboons. *Proc. Natl. Acad. Sci. USA* 96, 12816–12821.

Moss, B. (1996). Genetically engineered poxviruses for recombinant gene expression, vaccination, and safety. *Proc. Natl. Acad. Sci. USA* 93, 11341–11348.

Murphy, C. G., Lucas, W. T., Means, R. E., Czajak, S., Hale, C. L., Lifson, J. D., Kaur, A., Johnson, R. P., Knipe, D. M., and Desrosiers, R. C. (2000). Vaccine protection against simian immunodeficiency virus by recombinant strains of herpes simplex virus. *J. Virol.* 74, 7745–7754.

Nakai, H., Storm, T. A., and Kay, M. A. (2000). Recruitment of single-stranded recombinant adeno-associated virus vector genomes and intermolecular recombinant are responses for stable transduction of liver *in vivo*. *J. Virol.* 74, 9451–9463.

Nakai, H., Yant, S. R., Storm, T. A., Fuess, S., Meuse, L., and Kay, M. A. (2001). Extrachromosomal recombinant adeno-associated virus vector genomes are primarily responsible for stable liver transduction *in vivo*. *J. Virol.* 75, 6969–6976.

Nilsson, C., Makitalo, B., Berglund, P., Bex, F., Liljestrom, P., Sutter, G., Erfle, V., ten Haaft, P., Heeney, J., Biberfeld, G., and Thorstensson, R. (2001). Enhanced simian immunodeficiency virus-specific immune responses in macaques induced by priming with recombinant Semliki Forest virus and boosting with modified vaccinia virus Ankara. *Vaccine* 19, 3526–3536.

Nilsson, C., Sutter, G., Walther-Jallow, L., ten Haaft, P., Akerblom, L., Heeney, J., Erfle, V., Bottiger, P., Biberfeld, G., and Thorstensson, R. (2002). Immunization with recombinant modified vaccinia virus Anakara can modify mucosal simian immunodeficiency virus infection and delay disease progression in macaques. *J. Gen. Virol.* 83, 807–818.

Ourmanov, I., Brown, C. R., Moss, B., Carroll, M., Wyatt, L., Pletneva, L., Goldstein, S., Venzon, D., and Hirsch, V. M. (2000). Comparative efficacy of recombinant modified vaccinia virus Ankara expressing simian immunodeficiency virus (SIV) Gag-Pol and/or Env in macaques challenged with pathogenic SIV. *J. Virol.* 74, 2740–2751.

Paoletti, E. (1996). Applications of pox virus vectors to vaccination: an update. *Proc. Natl. Acad. Sci. USA* 93, 11349–11353.

Papp, Z., Babiuk, L. A., and Baca-Estrada, M. E. (1999). The effect of pre-existing adenovirus-specific immunity on immune responses induced by recombinant adenovirus expressing glycoprotein D of bovine herpesvirus type 1. *Vaccine* 17, 933–943.

Parks, R. J., Chen, L., Anton, M., Sankar, U., Rudnicki, M. A., and Graham, F. L. (1996). A helper-dependent adenovirus vector system: removal of helper virus by Cre-mediated excision of the viral packaging signal. *Proc. Natl. Acad. Sci. USA* 93, 13565–13570.

Parr, M. J., Wen, P. Y., Schaub, M., Khoury, S. J., Sayegh, M. H., and Fine, H. A. (1998). Immune parameters affecting adenoviral vector gene therapy in the brain. *J. Neurovirol.* 4, 194–203.

Pialoux, G., Excler, J. L., Riviere, Y., Gonzalez-Canali, G., Feuillie, V., Coulaud, P., Gluckman, J. C., Matthews, T. J., Meignier, B., Kieny, M. P., and et al. (1995). A prime-boost approach to HIV preventive vaccine using a recombinant canarypox virus expressing glycoprotein 160 (MN) followed by a recombinant glycoprotein 160 (MN/LAI). The AGIS Group, and l'Agence Nationale de Recherche sur le SIDA. *AIDS Res. Hum. Retroviruses* 11, 373–381.

Plotkin, S. A. (2003). Vaccines, vaccination and vaccinology. *J. Infect. Dis.* 187, 1349–1359.

Pushko, P., Bray, M., Ludwig, G. V., Parker, M., Schmaljohn, A., Sanchez, A., Jahrling, P. B., and Smith, J. F. (2000). Recombinant RNA replicons derived from attenuated Venezuelan equine encephalitis virus protect guinea pigs and mice from Ebola hemorrhagic fever virus. *Vaccine* 19, 142–153.

Ramsay, A. J., Leong, K. H., Boyle, D., Ruby, J., and Ramshaw, I. A. (1994). Enhancement of mucosal IgA responses by interleukin 5 and 6 encoded in recombinant vaccine vectors. *Reprod. Fertil. Dev.* 6, 389–392.

Ramshaw, I. A., Andrew, M. E., Phillips, S. M., Boyle, D. B., and Coupar, B. E. (1987). Recovery of immunodeficient mice from vaccinia virus/IL-2 recombinant infection. *Nature* 329, 545–546.

Ramshaw, I. A., and Ramsay, A. J. (2000). The prime-boost strategy: exciting prospects for improved vaccination. *Immunol. Today* 21, 163–165.

Rao, J. B., Chamberlain, R. S., Bronte, V., Carroll, M. W., Irvine, K. R., Moss, B., Rosenberg, S. A., and Restifo, N. P. (1996). IL-12 is an effective adjuvant to recombinant vaccinia virus-based tumor vaccines: enhancement by simultaneous B7-1 expression. *J. Immunol.* 156, 3357–3365.

Reddy, P. S., Idamakanti, N., Pyne, C., Zakhartchouk, A. N., Godson, D. L., Papp, Z., Baca-Estrada, M. E., Babiuk, L. A., Mutwiri, G. K., and Tikoo, S. K. (2000). The immunogenicity and efficacy of replication-defective and replication-competent bovine adenovirus-3 expressing bovine herpesvirus-1 glycoprotein gD in cattle. *Vet. Immunol. Immunopathol.* 76, 257–268.

Roberts, A., Buonocore, L., Price, R., Forman, J., and Rose, J. K. (1999). Attenuated vesicular stomatitis viruses as vaccine vectors. *J. Virol.* 73, 3723–3732.

Roberts, A., Kretzschmar, E., Perkins, A. S., Forman, J., Price, R., Buonocore, L., Kawaoka, Y., and Rose, J. K. (1998). Vaccination with a recombinant vesicular stomatitis virus expressing an influenza virus hemagglutinin provides complete protection from influenza virus challenge. *J. Virol.* 72, 4704–4711.

Robinson, H. L., Montefiori, D. C., Johnson, R. P., Manson, K. H., Kalish, M. L., Lifson, J. D., Rizvi, T. A., Lu, S., Hu, S. L., Mazzara, G. P., Panicali, D. L., Herndon, J. G., Glickman, R., Candido, M. A., Lydy, S. L., Wyand, M. S., and McClure, H. M. (1999). Neutralizing antibody-independent containment of immunodeficiency virus challenges by DNA priming and recombinant pox virus booster immunizations. *Nat. Med.* 5, 526–534.

Rose, N. F., Marx, P. A., Luckay, A., Nixon, D. F., Moretto, W. J., Donahoe, S. M., Montefiori, D., Roberts, A., Buonocore, L., and Rose, J. K. (2001). An effective AIDS vaccine based on live attenuated vesicular stomatitis virus recombinants. *Cell* 106, 539–549.

Rosenthal, K. L., and Gallichan, W. S. (1997). Challenge for vaccination against sexually-transmitted diseases: induction and long-term maintenance of mucosal immune responses in the female genital tract. *Semin. Immunol.* 9, 303–314.

Samulski, R. J., Zhu, X., Xiao, X., Brook, J. D., Housman, D. E., Epstein, N., and Hunter, L. A. (1991). Targeted integration of adeno-associated virus (AAV) into human chromosome 19. *EMBO J.* 10, 3941–3950.

Schneider, J., Gilbert, S. C., Blanchard, T. J., Hanke, T., Robson, K. J., Hannan, C. M., Becker, M., Sinden, R., Smith, G. L., and Hill, A. V. (1998). Enhanced immunogenicity for CD8+ T cell induction and complete protective efficacy of malaria DNA vaccination by boosting with modified vaccinia virus Ankara. *Nat. Med.* 4, 397–402.

Schnell, M. J., Buonocore, L., Whitt, M. A., and Rose, J. K. (1996). The minimal conserved transcription stop-start signal promotes stable expression of a foreign gene in vesicular stomatitis virus. *J. Virol.* 70, 2318–2323.

Schoenbeck, S., McKenzie, D. T., and Kagnoff, M. F. (1989). Interleukin 5 is a differentiation factor for IgA B cells. *Eur. J. Immunol.* 19, 965–969.

Schulick, A. H., Vassalli, G., Dunn, P. F., Dong, G., Rade, J. J., Zamarron, C., and Dichek, D. A. (1997). Established immunity precludes adenovirus-mediated gene transfer in rate carotid arteries. Potential for immunosuppression and vector engineering to overcome barriers of immunity. *J. Clin. Invest.* 99, 209–219.

Sedegah, M., Jones, T. R., Kaur, M., Hedstrom, R., Hobart, P., Tine, J. A., and Hoffman, S. L. (1998). Boosting with recombinant vaccinia increases immunogenicity and protective efficacy of malaria DNA vaccine. *Proc. Natl. Acad. Sci. USA* 95, 7648–7653.

Seth, A., Ourmanov, I., Kuroda, M. J., Schmitz, J. E., Carroll, M. W., Wyatt, L. S., Moss, B., Forman, M. A., Hirsch, V. M., and Letvin, N. L. (1998). Recombinant modified vaccinia virus Ankara-simian immunodeficiency virus gag pol elicits cytotoxic T lymphocytes in rhesus monkeys detected by a major histocompatibility complex class I/peptide tetramer. *Proc. Natl. Acad. Sci. USA* 95, 10112–10116.

Seth, A., Ourmanov, I., Schmitz, J. E., Kuroda, M. J., Lifton, M. A., Nickerson, C. E., Wyatt, L., Carroll, M., Moss, B., Venzon, D., Letvin, N. L., and Hirsch, V. M. (2000). Immunization with a modified vaccinia virus expressing simian immunodeficiency virus (SIV) Gag-Pol primes for an anamnestic Gag-specific cytotoxic T-lymphocyte response and is associated with reduction of viremia after SIV challenge. *J. Virol.* 74, 2502–2509.

Sharma, D. P., Ramsay, A. J., Maguire, D. J., Rolph, M. S., and Ramshaw, I. A. (1996). Interleukin-4 mediates down regulation of antiviral cytokine expression and cytotoxic T-lymphocyte responses and exacerbates vaccinia virus infection *in vivo*. *J. Virol.* 70, 7103–7107.

Sharpe, S., Fooks, A., Lee, J., Hayes, K., Clegg, C., and Cranage, M. (2002). Single oral immunization with replication deficient recombinant adenovirus elicits long-lived transgene-specific cellular and humoral immune responses. *Virology* 293, 210–216.

Sharpe, S., Polyanskaya, N., Dennis, M., Sutter, G., Hanke, T., Erfle, V., Hirsch, V., and Cranage, M. (2001). Induction of simian immunodeficiency virus (SIV)-specific CTL in rhesus macaques by vaccination with modified vaccinia virus Ankara expressing SIV transgenes: influence of pre-existing anti-vector immunity. *J. Gen. Virol.* 82, 2215–2223.

Sheppard, M., Werner, W., Tsatas, E., McCoy, R., Prowse, S., and Johnson, M. (1998). Fowl adenovirus recombinant expressing VP2 of infectious bursal disease virus induces protective immunity against bursal disease. *Arch. Virol.* 143, 915–930.

Shiver, J. W., Fu, T. M., Chen, L., Casimiro, D. R., Davies, M. E., Evans, R. K., Zhang, Z. Q., Simon, A. J., Trigona, W. L., Dubey, S. A., Huang, L., Harris, V. A., Long, R. S., Liang, X., Handt, L., Schleif, W. A., Zhu, L., Freed, D. C., Persaud, N. V., Guan, L., Punt, K. S., Tang, A., Chen, M., Wilson, K. A., Collins, K. B., Heidecker, G. J., Fernandez, V. R., Perry, H. C., Joyce, J. G., Grimm, K. M., Cook, J. C., Keller, P. M., Kresock, D. S., Mach, H., Troutman, R. D., Isopi, L. A., Williams, D. M., Xu, Z., Bohannon, K. E., Volkin, D. B., Montefiori, D. C., Miura, A., Krivulka, G. R., Lifton, M. A., Kuroda, M. J., Schmitz, J. E., Letvin, N. L., Caulfield, M. J., Bett, A. J., Youil, R., Kaslow, D. C., and Emini, E. A. (2002). Replication-incompetent adenoviral vaccine vector elicits effective anti-immunodeficiency-virus immunity. *Nature* 415, 331–335.

Spector, F. C., Kern, E. R., Palmer, J., Kaiwar, R., Cha, T. A., Brown, P., and Spaete, R. R. (1998). Evaluation of a live attenuated recombinant virus RAV 9395 as a herpes simplex virus type 2 vaccine in guinea pigs. *J. Infect. Dis.* 177, 1143–1154.

Stevceva, L., Abimiku, A. G., and Franchini, G. (2000). Targeting the mucosa: genetically engineered vaccines and mucosal immune responses. *Genes Immun.* 1, 308–315.

Strauss, J. H., and Strauss, E. G. (1994). The alphaviruses: gene expression, replication and evolution. *Microbiol. Rev.* 58, 491–562.

Sullivan, N. J., Sanchez, A., Rollin, P. E., Yang, Z. Y., and Nabel, G. J. (2000). Development of a preventive vaccine for Ebola virus infection in primates. *Nature* 408, 605–609.

Sutter, G., and Moss, B. (1992). Nonreplicating vaccinia vector efficiently expresses recombinant genes. *Proc. Natl. Acad. Sci. USA* 89, 10847–10851.

Tartaglia, J., Perkus, M. E., Taylor, J., Norton, E. K., Audonnet, J. C., Cox, W. I., Davis, S. W., van der Hoeven, J., Meignier, B., Riviere, M., and et al. (1992). NYVAC: a highly attenuated strain of vaccinia virus. *Virology* 188, 217–232.

Tims, T., Briggs, D. J., Davis, R. D., Moore, S. M., Xiang, Z., Ertl, H. C., and Fu, Z. F. (2000). Adult dogs receiving a rabies booster dose with a recombinant adenovirus expressing rabies virus glycoprotein develop high titers of neutralizing antibodies. *Vaccine* 18, 2804–2807.

Top, F. H., Jr. (1975). Control of adenovirus acute respiratory disease in U.S. Army trainees. *Yale J. Biol. Med.* 48, 185–195.

Top, F. H., Jr., Buescher, E. L., Bancroft, W. H., and Russell, P. K. (1971a). Immunization with live types 7 and 4 adenovirus vaccines. II. Antibody response and protective effect against acute respiratory disease due to adenovirus type 7. *J. Infect. Dis.* 124, 155–160.

Top, F. H., Jr., Grossman, R. A., Bartelloni, P. J., Segal, H. E., Dudding, B. A., Russell, P. K., and Buescher, E. L. (1971b). Immunization with live types 7 and r adenovirus vaccines. I. Safety, infectivity, antigenicity, and potency of adenovirus type 7 vaccine in humans. *J. Infect. Dis.* 124, 148–154.

Vajdy, M., Gardner, J., Neidleman, J., Cuadra, L., Greer, C., Perri, S., O'Hagan, D., and Polo, J. M. (2001). Human immunodeficiency virus type 1 Gag-specific vaginal immunity and protection after local immunization with Sindbis virus-based replicon particles. *J. Infect. Dis.* 184, 1613–1616.

Vogels, R., Zuijdgeest, D., van Rijnsoever, R., Hartkoorn, E., Damen, I., de Bethune, M. P., Kostense, S., Penders, G., Helmus, N., Koudstaal, W., Cecchini, M., Wetterwald, A., Sprangers, M., Lemckert, A., Ophorst, O., Koel, B., van Meerendonk, M., Quax, P., Panitti, L., Grimbergen, J., Bout, A., Goudsmit, J., and Havenga, M. (2003). Replication-deficient human adenovirus type 35 vectors for gene transfer and vaccination: efficient human cell infection and bypass of preexisting adenovirus immunity. *J. Virol.* 77, 8263–8271.

Voltan, R., and Robert-Guroff, M. (2003). Live recombinant vectors for AIDS vaccine development. *Curr. Mol. Med.* 3, 273–284.

Vos, A., Neubert, A., Pommerening, E., Muller, T., Dohner, L., Neubert, L., and Hughes, K. (2001). Immunogenicity of an E1-deleted recombinant human adenovirus against rabies by different routes of administration. *J. Gen. Virol.* 82, 2191–2197.

Wagner, R. R., and Rose, J. K. (1996). In *Fields Virology* (eds. Fields, B. Knipe, D. M., Howley, P. M., Griffin, D. E., and Lamb, R. A.) New York: Lippincott-Raven, 1121–1136.

Walton, T. E., Webb, P. A., Kramer, W. L., Smith, G. C., Davis, T., Holbrook, F. R., Moore, C. G., Schiefer, T. J., Jones, R. H., and Janney, G. C. (1987). Epizootic vesicular stomatitis in Colorado, 1982: epidemiologic and entomologic studies. *Am. J. Trop. Med. Hyg.* 36, 166–176.

Walz, C. M., Correa-Ochoa, M. M., Muller, M., and Schlehofer, J. R. (2002). Adenoassociated virus type 2-induced inhibition of the human papillomavirus type 18 promoter in transgenic mice. *Virology* 293, 172–181.

Wang, J., and Xing, Z. (2002). Tuberculosis vaccines: the past, present and future. *Expert Rev. Vaccines* 1, 341–354.

Whitley, R. J., Kern, E. R., Chatterjee, S., Chou, J., and Roizman, B. (1993). Replication, establishment of latency, and induced reactivation of herpes simplex virus gamma 1 34.5 deletion mutants in rodent models. *J. Clin. Invest.* 91, 2837–2843.

Wilson, J. A., and Hart, M. K. (2001). Protection from Ebola virus mediated by cytotoxic T lymphocytes specific for the viral nucleoprotein. *J. Virol.* 75, 2660–2664.

Wyatt, L. S., Carroll, M. W., Czerny, C. P., Merchlinsky, M., Sisler, J. R., and Moss, B. (1998). Marker rescue of the host range restriction defects of modified vaccinia virus Ankara. *Virology* 251, 334–342.

Xiao, W., Chirmule, N., Berta, S. C., McCullough, B., Gao, G., and Wilson, J. M. (1999). Gene therapy vectors based on adeno-associated virus type 1. *J. Virol.* 73, 3994–4003.

Xiao, X., Li, J., and Samulski, R. J. (1996). Efficient long-term gene transfer into muscle tissue of immunocompetent mice by adeno-associated virus vector. *J. Virol.* 70, 8098–8108.

Xin, K. Q., Ooki, T., Mizukami, H., Hamajima, K., Okudela, K., Hashimoto, K., Kojima, Y., Jounai, N., Kumamoto, Y., Sasaki, S., Klinman, D., Ozawa, K., and Okuda, K. (2002). Oral administration of recombinant adeno-associated virus elicits human immunodeficiency virus-specific immune responses. *Hum. Gene Ther.* 13, 1571–1581.

Xin, K. Q., Urabe, M., Yang, J., Nomiyama, K., Mizukami, H., Hamajima, K., Nomiyama, H., Saito, T., Imai, M., Monahan, J., Okuda, K., and Ozawa, K. (2001). A novel recombinant adeno-associated virus vaccine induces a long-term humoral immune response to human immunodeficiency virus. *Hum. Gene Ther.* 12, 1047–1061.

Xiong, C., Levis, R., Shen, P., Schlesinger, S., Rice, C. M., and Huang, H. V. (1989). Sindbis virus: an efficient, broad host range vector for gene expression in animal cells. *Science* 243, 1188–1191.

Yoshida, T., Okuda, K., Xin, K. Q., Tadokoro, K., Fukushima, J., Toda, S., Hagiwara, E., Hamajima, K., Koshino, T., and Saito, T. (2001). Activation of HIV-1-specific immune responses to an HIV-1 vaccine constructed from a replication-defective adenovirus vector using various combinations of immunization protocols. *Clin. Exp. Immunol.* 124, 445–452.

Zhu, M., Terasawa, H., Gulley, J., Panicali, D., Arlen, P., Schlom, J., and Tsang, K. Y. (2001). Enhanced activation of human T cells via avipox-vector-mediated hyperexpression of a triad of costimulatory molecules in human dendritic cells. *Cancer Res.* 61, 3725–3734.

Zinkernagel, R. M. (2003). On natural and artificial vaccinations. *Annu. Rev. Immunol.* 21, 515–546.

Transgenic Plants for Mucosal Vaccines

Hugh S. Mason, Rachel Chikwamba, Luca Santi, Richard T. Mahoney, and Charles J. Arntzen

Arizona State University Biodesign Institute and School of Life Sciences, Tempe, Arizona

Modern biotechnology provides a huge potential for human health improvement by the development of new therapies and vaccines against infectious diseases. In the best cases, vaccines can provide great economic value with cost-benefit ratios of 1:10 (Centers for Disease Control and Prevention, 1998). However, the development and implementation of new vaccines often encounter substantial cost and logistical barriers that are difficult to overcome in many countries that are economically depressed. The use of transgenic plant-derived recombinant proteins is a promising strategy that combines the innovations in medical science and plant biology to create affordable vaccines. The potential benefits are low cost, heat stability, oral administration, and convenience of production in developing countries. A growing number of laboratories are investing in plant-derived protein pharmaceuticals, expanding on the seminal works that first proposed this idea (Curtis and Cardineau, 1990; Mason *et al.*, 1992). The subject of plant-derived vaccines has been reviewed several times in recent years (Koprowski and Yusibov, 2001; Mason *et al.*, 2002), and a nearly comprehensive list of vaccine antigens produced in plants has been provided (Daniell *et al.*, 2001). While much research is yet needed to optimize plant production of vaccines and to validate them in large-scale clinical trials, the results to date show a very promising technology that is on the brink of commercial development. Ingestion of transgenic plants expressing vaccine antigens can, via the gut lymphoid system, result in specific mucosal secretory IgA (S-IgA) and serum IgG antibody responses. Although protective efficacy of a plant-derived vaccine has yet to be determined in humans, some challenge studies in animals have shown promising results and are discussed later in the text. The previous chapter in this series (Palmer *et al.*, 1999) described plant expression systems and their use in vaccine studies in some detail. In this chapter, we examine the advances in the field of transgenic plant-derived mucosal vaccines, focusing on the results of human clinical trials and on orally delivered animal vaccines. Another chapter in this volume (Lomonossoff, G.P.; see Chapter 59) describes work involving plant viruses to produce vaccines.

PLANT-DERIVED VACCINES FOR HUMANS: CLINICAL TRIALS

Bacterial diarrhea: enterotoxigenic *Escherichia coli* (ETEC) and *Vibrio cholerae*

Diarrhea caused by bacterial and viral infections can cause severe dehydration, which is particularly dangerous in children and the elderly. Especially in developing countries, infectious diarrheal diseases are major causes of morbidity and mortality. It is estimated that diarrhea causes up to 2.5 million deaths yearly, mostly in the age group of less than 1 year. Several different bacteria can cause acute gastroenteritis by colonizing the gastrointestinal (GI) tract via contaminated water or food. Some of these are capable of systemic infection by crossing the mucosal epithelium (septicemic forms); others colonize the intestinal tract and secrete toxins that are absorbed by the enterocytes and cause diarrhea (enterotoxigenic forms). Two of the most widely spread and well studied of the latter are enterotoxigenic *E. coli* (ETEC) and *Vibrio cholerae*. The toxins they produce, labile toxins (LTs) and cholera toxins (CTs), respectively, are very similar in primary sequence, structure, and mechanism of action (Sixma *et al.*, 1991). The ring-shaped pentamer formed by the five identical noncovalently linked B subunits is responsible for binding to the G_{M1} ganglioside (both CTs and LTs) and to other gangliosides (LTs only) on the mucosal epithelial cells, while the toxic A subunit is translocated into the epithelial cells of the GI tract, where its ADP-ribosyl transferase activity promotes the efflux of water and electrolytes. Both LT-B and CT-B are among the most potent oral immunogens known, with oral delivery efficiently causing accumulation of specific serum (IgG, IgA) and mucosal S-IgA antibodies (Holmgren *et al.*, 1993). Both LT and CT also function as mucosal adjuvants, stimulating antibody production against codelivered antigens. The ganglioside-binding activity of the LT-B pentamer is required both for its mucosal immunogenicity and for the adjuvanticity of the holotoxin (Guidry *et al.*, 1997).

Plant systems have been used to express both LT-B and CT-B. For example, others reported the expression of ganglioside-binding pentameric LT-B in transgenic potato and tobacco plants (Haq *et al.*, 1995). Mice fed transgenic tubers showed production of serum and mucosal antibodies against LT-B. Later, a plant-optimized LT-B gene was synthesized with preferred codons and avoidance of spurious mRNA processing signals, ultimately resulting in increased expression in potatoes (Mason *et al.*, 1998). Mice were fed 5 g of these transgenic tubers, containing 50 µg of LT-B, at 4-day intervals over 3 weeks, and the titers of anti-LT-B serum IgG and fecal IgA antibodies were improved over those in the earlier experiment. These mice were partially protected from a 25-µg dose of LT, indicating the potential for efficacious use of the potato vaccine in humans. In a similar study, others found that LT-B expressed in corn and eaten as raw corn meal stimulated antibody responses in mice that were partially protective against toxin challenge (Streatfield *et al.*, 2001).

The preclinical studies with potatoes expressing LT-B led to the first trial of a transgenic plant-derived vaccine administered to humans (Tacket *et al.*, 1998). Fourteen volunteers ingested either 100 g of transgenic potato, 50 g of transgenic potato, or 50 g of nontransgenic potato. The LT-B content of the tubers varied between 3.7 and 15.7 µg per gram of tuber weight, and the doses were given on days 0, 7, and 21. Volunteers reported only a few instances of minor side effects (nausea, cramps, or diarrhea), and the raw potato was well-tolerated overall. Ten of 11 volunteers who ate the potatoes expressing LT-B (and none who ate placebo potatoes) developed at least fourfold increases in levels of toxin-neutralizing serum IgG antibodies against LT-B. Five of 10 volunteers showed at least fourfold rises in anti-LT-B IgA detected in stool samples. These data compared favorably with those from an earlier study in which volunteers were challenged with 10^9 ETEC cells (Tacket *et al.*, unpublished). This study was significant as the first ever to examine an edible plant vaccine in humans and showed great potential for this new strategy.

The CT-B molecule has also been expressed in transgenic potato tubers at up to 0.3% of TSP (Arakawa *et al.*,1997). The plant-produced CT-B assembled into the pentameric structure was shown to bind G_{M1} ganglioside and to react with specific anti-CT-B IgG antibody. Mice immunized by being fed raw potato tubers expressing CT-B developed specific serum and mucosal antibodies (Arakawa *et al.*, 1998). It is interesting that in previously immunized mice, the edible CT-B was able to trigger a significant boosting response. Moreover, the CT-B produced in plants was heat-resistant: transgenic potato tubers cooked until soft retained 50% of the ganglioside-binding activity.

Viral diarrhea: Norwalk virus

The Norwalk virus and related Norwalk-like viruses are responsible for 42% of outbreaks of acute epidemic gas-troenteritis in the United States. The Norwalk virus capsid protein (NVCP) was the antigen chosen to develop an oral edible vaccine, since when expressed in insect cells it assembled into 38-nm Norwalk virus–like particles (VLPs) and reacted with serum of infected humans (Jiang *et al.*, 1992). Tobacco and potato plants were transformed with constructs harboring the NVCP sequence; the plant recombinant protein assembled into VLPs identical to the insect cell–derived antigen (Mason *et al.*, 1996). Mice that were gavaged with partially purified VLPs from tobacco leaf or fed with transgenic tubers developed serum IgG and fecal IgA antibodies specific for NVCP.

A clinical trial was performed with the same potatoes used for the preclinical study (Tacket *et al.*, 2000). Of 20 adult volunteers, 10 received two doses (days 0 and 7) and 10 received three doses (days 0, 7, and 21) of 150 g of raw transgenic potato tubers containing NVCP at 215 to 750 µg/dose. It is important to note that tuber expression was quite variable, and at most only half of NVCP in these potatoes was assembled as VLP; thus, the effective dose of potato vaccine was ~325 µg/dose. Unassembled subunits are likely to be much less stable in the GI tract and thus less immunogenic. However, 19 of 20 subjects in the experimental group showed significant increases in the numbers of IgA antibody–forming cells (AFCs), ranging from 6 to 280 per 10^6 peripheral blood mononuclear cells (PBMCs), and 6 of 20 subjects in this group developed increases in IgG AFCs. Four volunteers showed increases in serum IgG anti-NVCP antibody titers, 4 had increased serum IgM, and 6 showed increased IgA in their stool samples (17-fold mean increase). Although the antibody responses were less impressive than those obtained with LT-B, the study showed that a plant-derived protein other than LT-B and CT-B can stimulate human immune responses after oral delivery. Insect cell–derived 250-µg doses of purified Norwalk VLP provided more effective seroconversion (Ball *et al.*, 1999); thus it is likely that part of the potato-delivered NVCP was unavailable for uptake in the GI tract. More recent studies in transgenic tomato fruits with a plant-optimized NVCP gene resulted in higher expression and more potent immune responses in mice fed freeze-dried tomatoes (X. Zhang and H.S. Mason, unpublished results). A clinical trial is planned in which dried tomato powder formulated in gelatin capsules will be used to evaluate safety and immunogenicity (D. Kirk, H.S. Mason, and C.J. Arntzen, trial investigators).

Hepatitis B virus

The World Health Organization (WHO) has estimated that there are approximately 350 million chronic carriers of hepatitis B virus (HBV). Infection with HBV leads to liver cancer resulting in as many as 1 million deaths annually. Transmission of HBV is primarily through blood and/or sexual contact, but there is also a high incidence of mother-child transmission during childbirth. Thus a vaccine that provides mucosal immune protection in addition to serum antibodies could be an improvement over the currently used intramuscularly injected hepatitis B surface antigen (HBsAg), produced in transgenic yeast cells (McAleer *et al.*, 1984). Two types of hepatitis B vaccine are licensed by the U.S. Food and Drug Administration (FDA) for human use, both purified for intramuscular injection. The first is based on HBsAg derived from human plasma; the second is a recombinant yeast-derived HBsAg. Beyond the potential for mucosal immunity, an orally administered plant-derived vaccine would be useful for several reasons: it could improve the success rate of full immunization because the vaccine could be taken without the requirement of returning to a facility that can provide injections; it would be heat stable and could thus reach children in more remote areas; and it would not require the use of needles that pose the risk of infection themselves. However, in light of the increasingly global use of yeast-derived hepatitis B vaccine in both developed and developing countries, any plant-derived vaccine would have to offer distinct advantages and not interfere with efforts to expand vaccination.

The report of expression of HBsAg in tobacco leaf was the first description of plant expression of vaccine immunogen (Mason *et al.*, 1992). The recombinant tobacco HBsAg was recovered as spherical particles of an average diameter of 22 nm, similar to the native subviral particle from blood of infected humans and similar to the yeast-derived vaccine (McAleer *et al.*, 1984). The tobacco-derived HBsAg stimulated immune responses in mice vaccinated intraperitoneally that were similar to those produced by the commercial vaccine, including production of all IgG subclasses and IgM (Thanavala *et al.*, 1995). In addition, T cells from the mice immunized with the plant-derived HBsAg proliferated in response to a yeast-derived HBsAg, indicating the fidelity of the T-cell epitopes on the plant-produced protein. Studies that followed aimed to improve the amount of antigen produced by the plant system by optimizing different constructs (Richter *et al.*, 2000; Sojikul *et al.*, 2003), as well as proving that orally delivered plant material could elicit an immune response (Kong *et al.*, 2001). A construct containing the unmodified HBsAg driven by the constitutive CaMV 35S promoter and terminated by the potato PinII polyadenylation signal yielded the highest expression of HBsAg in potato tubers (Richter *et al.*, 2000). Immuno-electron microscopy of sectioned potato leaf showed that spherical and filamentous subviral particles assembled *in vivo* and accumulated in endoplasmic reticulum (ER)-derived vesicles. Mice fed once a week for 3 weeks with 5 g of raw tubers (containing an average of 42 μg of HBsAg/dose) were compared with mice that were gavaged with the purified yeast recombinant HBsAg (Kong *et al.*, 2001). In either case, 10 μg CT per dose was given as a mucosal adjuvant. The potato-delivered HBsAg was a more potent immunogen when delivered orally: a primary serum IgG antibody response began after two feedings of the transgenic potatoes (containing a total of 84 μg of HBsAg), whereas no primary immune response was detected after two doses of yeast-derived HBsAg (containing a total of 300 μg of HBsAg). The authors suggested that the difference was due to enhanced stability of the antigen when it is retained in the plant cells. Serum IgG antibody levels in

the potato-primed mice declined after a few weeks but rebounded dramatically with high and lasting titers after a single intraperitoneal injection with a subimmunogenic dose of yeast recombinant vaccine. Furthermore, mice primed with a subimmunogenic intraperitoneal dose of the commercial vaccine and fed with HBsAg potatoes responded with a long-lasting secondary antibody response. The antibody titer decreased with time but remained above the estimated protection level (10 IU/L) up to 5 months after the challenge, when the experiment was terminated (Kong *et al.*, 2001). This result suggests that priming with a single injection followed by additional doses of orally delivered plant-derived vaccine could be used in humans. A change in immunization strategies would be especially useful in developing countries, where the injection delivery of multiple doses of vaccine is a significant problem for massive immunization.

There is one published report on the immunogenicity in humans of orally delivered HBsAg expressed in plants (Kapusta *et al.*, 1999). Two of three volunteers who ate two 150-g doses of transgenic lettuce (containing ~1 to 2 μg HBsAg per dose) developed a modest but protective (>10 IU/L) serum antibody titer after the second dose. The serum antibody titers declined rapidly after 4 weeks, probably because of the very low dosage; however, the study showed that presumably naïve subjects could be seroconverted by oral delivery of plant-expressed HBsAg. In the United States, others directed a clinical trial at the Roswell Park Cancer Institute (Buffalo, NY) to test the oral immunogenicity of recombinant potatoes expressing HBsAg (Kong *et al.*, 2001). Since chronic HBV infection can lead to liver cancer, the FDA was concerned that oral delivery of HBsAg could cause oral tolerance. Thus, the study was limited to volunteers who had previously been vaccinated and seroconverted with the standard injectable HBsAg. The experiment involved 33 volunteers who ate either two (days 0 and 28) or three (days 0, 14, and 28) 100-g doses of HBsAg potato tubers containing ~1 mg HBsAg per dose, as measured by the Auszyme monoclonal immunoassay (Abbott Laboratories, Abbott Park, IL). A group of 10 volunteers ate nontransgenic potatoes only. The potato HBsAg vaccine stimulated boosting of serum IgG antibody titers in more than half of the volunteers (Thanavala *et al.*, unpublished results, 2003), which suggests that oral ingestion of plant-produced HBsAg could be a viable delivery system for an HBV vaccine.

Rotavirus vaccines currently under study

Rotavirus is a common form of diarrhea and is estimated to cause approximately 600,000 deaths annually, primarily among children in developing countries. It is the most frequent cause of childhood diarrhea-related hospitalizations in the United States. Group A rotavirus (GAR) is one of the leading causes of acute infectious viral diarrhea in humans and livestock. The rotavirus major inner capsid protein (VP6) has been defined as a protective antigen (Choi *et al.*, 1999), and VP6 constitutes about 51% by weight of the virion protein and is well conserved in each virus serogroup (Kapikian *et al.*, 1990). In addition to the capsid proteins, a nonstructural protein, NSP4, and its 22–amino acid peptide, which functions as a viral enterotoxin, were also identified (Ball *et al.*, 1996). Induction of antibodies against the NSP4 22 amino acid peptide alone might confer protection from clinical disease, without the need for induction of antibodies against the structural proteins (O'Neal *et al.*, 1997). Others have shown that VP6 elicits protection against rotavirus shedding in a mouse model, and this protection was attributed to a CD4[+] T cell epitope in the protein. These attributes indicate that the VP6 protein has potential as a candidate subunit vaccine against rotavirus (Choi *et al.*, 1999).

Others have reported that expression of VP6 from bovine group A rotavirus in transgenic potato plants occurs at levels in leaf and tuber tissues of 0.006% and 0.002% of TSP, respectively (Matsumura *et al.*, 2002). Mice were vaccinated intraperitoneally with concentrated potato tuber extracts estimated to contain 750 ng of VP6, which resulted in anti-GAR antibodies detected by Western blotting. Expression of VP6 in potato tubers was boosted by using two tandem repeats of the 5′-upstream sequence of the CaMV 35S promoter and the 5′ untranslated region of tobacco mosaic virus, which yielded 0.1% VP6 of TSP in tubers, a 17-fold increase. Subsequent experiments will test oral immunization with tuber-produced VP6.

Adopting a different approach, others used a fusion protein approach with the NSP4 22–amino acid peptide and subunits of the cholera toxin (Yu and Langridge, 2001). This group reported the expression in potato tuber of a recombinant holotoxin in which the 22–amino acid immunodominant murine rotavirus enterotoxin NSP4 to the C-terminus of CT-B and an ETEC bacterial fimbrial protein (CF1) fused to the N-terminus of the A subunit. The recombinant A and B particles assemble into a holotoxin-like molecule. CD-1 mice orally immunized with five doses of tuber tissues containing 10 µg of fusion protein per dose showed serum and mucosal antibodies to NSP4, as well as high levels of IL-2 and IFN-γ, indicating a Th1-type immune response. Offspring born to dams orally immunized with CT-B-NSP4 fusion proteins were partially protected from challenge from live murine rotavirus. The success of this multiple fusion protein strategy shows the possibility of a plant-based multicomponent vaccine against several diarrheal pathogens.

PLANT-DERIVED VACCINES FOR ANIMALS

Swine transmissible gastroenteritis virus

Swine transmissible gastroenteritis (TGE) is an economically important herd health problem globally. It is a highly contagious viral diarrheal disease in neonatal pigs that can result in up to 100% mortality among severe cases (Saif and Wesley, 1992; see Chapter 61). Because of the rapid course of disease and the immaturity of their immune systems, newborn piglets are unable to develop their own protective immunity and depend upon the presence of S-IgA in mother's milk for protection against the virus. To date,

commercially available vaccines, either attenuated or inactivated, are unable to adequately protect piglets (Tuboly *et al.*, 2000). Swine TGE is caused by the transmissible gastroenteritis virus (TGEV), a coronavirus with an immunodominant spike (S) protein. The S protein can induce neutralizing antibodies against the virus, and protective immunity in the host is directed toward this protein, which contains four major antigenic sites in its N-terminal region (Jiminez *et al.*, 1986). The S protein has been expressed in many systems, including baculovirus (Tuboly *et al.*, 1994) and human adenovirus (Torres *et al.*, 1996).

Others have reported the expression of the TGEV S protein in transgenic *Arabidopsis thaliana*, a convenient plant model system (Gomez *et al.*, 1998). The level of S protein obtained in leaves was between 0.03% and 0.06% of TSP. Immunization of mice intramuscularly with crude plant extracts induced TGEV-specific antibodies, with a virus-neutralizing index of 2.2 to 3.5, in comparison with an index of 5 for rabbit sera, with anti-TGEV antibodies used as a positive control. The S protein has been expressed in tobacco leaves at 0.1% to 0.2% of TSP (Tuboly *et al.*, 2000). Transgenic leaf extracts given intraperitoneally to pigs stimulated TGEV-specific serum antibodies with low levels of virus-neutralizing activity. In this study, the N-terminal domain of the S protein was codon-optimized for tobacco cells, which resulted in expression levels that were 10 times higher than had been obtained previously (Gomez *et al.*, 1998). No data on mucosal immunization were described in either study report; however, the results indicate that the plant-expressed S protein presents virus-neutralizing epitopes and is thus a competent immunogen.

Perhaps the most promising study showing protection with a mucosally delivered plant-based vaccine involved TGEV S protein expressed in corn (Streatfield *et al.*, 2001; Lamphear *et al.*, 2002). This group reported on the oral immunization of 10-day-old, specific-pathogen-free, TGEV-seronegative piglets with transgenic corn meal expressing the S protein. Test animals were fed nontransgenic corn mixed with 50 g of transgenic corn containing 2 mg of the S protein in a medicated milk replacer daily over a 10-day period, and control groups were orally immunized with either a commercial modified live vaccine or nontransgenic corn. All piglets were then orally challenged with a virulent form of the virus, and clinical symptoms were evaluated. While 50% of the pigs vaccinated with transgenic corn developed diarrhea, 78% in the group immunized by the commercially available vaccine and 100% of those that were fed with nontransgenic corn became ill. These observations suggest that the corn-derived S protein generated an immune response adequate to confer partial protection from the virus. No specific antibody assays were reported for this study; however, animals vaccinated with the commercial vaccine appeared to recover much faster, an observation suggesting that the commercial vaccine generated a stronger cytotoxic T-cell (CTL) response that was boosted by infection. In subsequent experiments (Lamphear *et al.*, 2002), piglets orally immunized with the corn-expressed S protein had a memory immune response leading to rapid accumulation of virus-neutralizing antibodies when orally immunized piglets were exposed to enough TGEV to cause subclinical infection. A study of different dosage regimens (4, 8, or 16 consecutive days) with S protein corn or with the commercial vaccine showed animals on the S protein corn 4-day regimen had no morbidity, while 50% of animals fed nontransgenic corn displayed symptoms. The animals fed the transgenic corn on the 8- and 16-day dosage regimens showed 20% and 36% morbidity, respectively, indicating that the 4-day dosage regimen was more effective in protecting the pigs. The frequency of dosage is therefore critical for this vaccine. In the group immunized with the commercial vaccine the morbidity rate was 9%, in comparison with zero for the corn-derived-vaccine recipients on the 4-day dosage regimen, a result which suggests that the corn-derived S protein is marginally more effective. However, this work should be explored further with virus challenge titers that are relevant in the field, rather than just enough to cause subclinical infection.

These efforts indicate the feasibility of producing a plant-based TGEV vaccine in transgenic plants. The work on the corn-derived S protein is especially interesting in that corn is a main constituent of livestock diets and does not require extensive heating during processing. Furthermore, the stability of antigen in the corn kernel matrix has been established, and a dosage size of 2 mg of S protein in 50 g of corn meal (Streatfield et al., 2001) indicates reasonable expression levels were attained for this antigen in maize.

Foot-and-mouth disease

Foot-and-mouth disease virus (FMDV) is considered the most economically important veterinary pathogen because of its highly infectious nature, ability to cause persistent infections, and long-term effects on the condition and productivity of the many animal species it affects. Countries where FMDV infections are active face many trade restrictions (Knowles and Samuels, 2003). Once an outbreak of the disease occurs, formal quarantine approaches are generally employed to contain the disease. Vaccination of all susceptible hosts with inactivated virus is a viable strategy for control of the disease, but is not used in most countries because of the expense or the difficulty in distinguishing immunized from infected animals. FMD is caused by several strains of virus that belong to the genus *Aphthovirus*, of the Picornaviridae family. Critical epitopes resulting in the induction of neutralizing antibodies have been identified on the VP1 structural protein of FMDV (Brown, 1992).

One group reported the expression of the FMDV VP1 in transgenic *A. thaliana* plants (Carillo et al., 1998). In this study, BALB/c mice were immunized intraperitoneally with plant extracts in incomplete Freund's adjuvant, which stimulated serum antibodies that reacted strongly with intact FMDV particles. The mice were challenged intraperitoneally with a virulent virus and were protected, as determined by absence of viremia 48 hours postinoculation, while the control groups were not protected. Others reported the expression of VP1 protein in transgenic alfalfa; in this study, mice

fed 0.3 g of transgenic leaves on a fortnightly basis in three doses of 15 to 20 mg of total soluble protein each developed virus-neutralizing antibodies, and 66% to 75% of animals were protected from intraperitoneal challenge (Wigdorovitz et al., 1999).

A common problem in all FMDV studies has been the low level of expression of the VP1 protein, resulting in limited immunogenicity. For example, one group developed a methodology for rapidly screening transgene expression levels in large numbers of transgenic plants from independent transgenic events (Dus Santos et al., 2002). This methodology involved the fusion of FMDV peptides to the readily assayable *gus* reporter gene and yielded a high correlation between expression of GUS and a VP135–160 epitope to which it was fused (between 0.05% and 0.1% of TSP). Mice immunized intraperitoneally with crude extracts from selected transgenic plants readily developed strong and completely protective immune responses. At the observed levels of expression, this peptide vaccine resulted in higher antibody titers than those previously reported when the full VP1 protein was expressed in alfalfa (Carillo et al., 1998).

Rabies

Rabies is a viral disease of mammals and is most commonly transmitted through the bite of a rabid animal. This disease is unusual in that it affects humans, wildlife, and domestic animals and is readily transmitted between animals and humans. In the United States, most rabies cases reported to the Centers for Disease Control and Prevention each year occur in wild animals such as raccoons, skunks, bats, and foxes, and a few (less than 10%) have been reported to occur in domestic animals such as cats, cattle, and dogs. However, rabies remains a major threat to humans in the world today, with about 50,000 fatal cases reported by the WHO each year (Plotkin, 2000). Globally, an estimated 10 million people receive postexposure antiserum treatment each year, after being exposed to rabies-suspect animals (WHO Fact Sheet number 99, 2001). Modern vaccines for humans are expensive, especially for densely populated countries in Africa and Asia, where rabies is endemic and remains a major health problem. For example, it has been reported that in India, most individuals exposed to rabies receive a primitive brain tissue vaccine because the safer and more efficacious modern products are unaffordable (Koprowski and Yusibov, 2001).

The rabies virus infects the central nervous system, causing encephalopathy and inevitable death. The rabies virus glycoprotein (G protein) is the major viral protein responsible for the induction of a protective immune response, while the nucleoprotein (N protein) triggers T cell responses, facilitating the production of neutralizing antibodies and other immune functions (Tollis et al., 1991). Oral vaccination with the baculovirus-expressed G protein was shown to protect raccoons from lethal challenge with the virus, and boosting with the N protein enhanced the protective immune response (Fu et al., 1993). A plant-based edible rabies vaccine that is very low in cost and orally administered would be very useful in preexposure vaccination of children and older persons in developing countries where rabies is highly endemic.

It has been reported that the production in transgenic tomato fruit of the rabies virus G protein can be estimated at 0.001% of TSP (McGarvey et al., 1995). However no immunization studies were described with this protein. This group observed that the tomato-synthesized G protein was smaller than the mammalian protein and yet larger than the predicted size for the unglycosylated protein, indicating that the plant glycosylation occurred, but perhaps the absence of sialic acid in plant glycans results in the observed smaller molecule size. Chimeric plant viruses were used to express immunogenic rabies virus G protein B-cell epitope and a T-cell epitope from the N protein (Yusibov et al., 1997). This work suggests that optimized transgenic plant expression could produce a viable rabies vaccine.

Poultry vaccines

The poultry industry is a significant component of global agriculture, and its success depends on the ability to maintain healthy birds. Vaccination is one of the key strategies for disease management, and in many cases, birds are immunized with attenuated live vaccines. The use of edible vaccines for the poultry industry should result in significant cost savings by greatly simplifying the current vaccination strategies and avoiding the practice of immunization via live vaccines. Infectious bursal disease virus (IBDV) is a globally important poultry pathogen. The major antigen in this virus is the structural protein VP2.

One group is currently working on a USDA-funded project for the production of a recombinant VP2 protein in transgenic plants (Scissum-Gunn [Alabama State University] and colleagues). In this work, oral immunization and boosting of 3-week-old unvaccinated chicks, challenge with IBDV, and serum and bursal tissue examinations were planned. Preliminary results following oral vaccination with recombinant VP2 expressed in transgenic A. thaliana were encouraging, and future expression in alfalfa is planned (K. Scissum-Gunn, personal communication, 2003).

SUMMARY AND CONCLUSIONS

Based upon the results presented in this chapter, it is clear that plant-based vaccines hold great promise and will likely form an integral part of the future arsenal of antigen production systems for vaccination. Transgenic plant-derived vaccine antigens have been shown to be orally immunogenic in humans and several animals species, and partial protection from pathogen challenge was shown for TGEV and FMDV in mice. Several issues remain to be addressed, including potential risk factors associated with the production of these pharmaceuticals in transgenic plants. First, progress needs to be made in improving the yield of antigens, in ensuring uniformity of yield, in enhancing immunogenicity of orally administered vaccines, and in assessing the potential for development of immune tolerance. Second, there are several

regulatory issues. For materials produced in the field, interaction with biotic and abiotic factors in the environment could affect expression stability and potentially compromise the integrity of the product. Thus, it is important to ensure sufficient analysis of the plant-derived product to validate its uniformity and functionality. Potential risk to the environment and the associated public perception of risk must be carefully considered. To that end, the USDA recently proposed strict measures to minimize environmental risks, including physical containment and rigorous regulation of transportation, processing, and disposal of plant-made pharmaceuticals. Biological containment practices to minimize unintentional release include the use of male sterile lines to minimize transgene escape via pollen and tissue or organ-specific expression of recombinant protein. The choice of crop for production of vaccines has a direct bearing on the ability to contain transgenes, with pollen-shedding crops presenting a greater challenge than those like tomatoes or other self-pollinating species. Strategies for monitoring genes within the environment should be employed, such as use of dominant marker genes, high-resolution detection systems, and efficient production, processing, and monitoring systems.

Finally, active participation of the plant biotechnology industry is an important step in the development of plant-based vaccines. Dow AgroSciences, LLC (DAS; Indianapolis, IN) has invested substantial effort toward the development of plant-derived vaccines for animals (Butch Mercer, DAS, personal communication). Results of DAS-supported studies are encouraging and may lead to commercialization of this exciting new technology.

REFERENCES

Arakawa T., Chong, D.K., Merritt, J.L., and Langridge, W.H. (1997). Expression of cholera B subunits oligomers in transgenic potato plants. Transgenic Res. 6, 403–413.

Arakawa T., Chong, D.K. , and Langridge, W.H. (1998). Efficacy of food plant–based oral cholera toxin B subunit vaccine. Nat. Biotechnol. 16, 292–297.

Ball, J.M., Tian, P., Zeng, C.Q., Morris, A.P., and Estes, M.K. (1996). Age-dependent diarrhea induced by a rotavirus nonstructural glycoprotein. Science 272, 101–104.

Ball, J.M., Graham, D.Y., Opekun, A.R., Gilger, M.A., Guerrero, R.A., and Estes, M.K. (1999) Recombinant Norwalk virus–like particles given orally to volunteers: phase I study. Gastroenterology 117, 40–48.

Brown, F. (1992). New approaches to vaccination against foot-and-mouth disease. Vaccine 10, 1022–1026.

Carrillo, C., Wigdorovitz, A., Oliveros, J.C., Zamorano, P. I., Sadir, A.M., Gómez, N. Salinas, J. Escribano, J.M., and Borca M.V. (1998). Protective immune response to foot-and-mouth disease virus with VP1 expressed in transgenic plants. J. Virol. 72, 1688–1690.

Carrillo, C., Wigdorovitz, A., Trono, K., Dus Santos, M.J., Castanon, S., Sadir, A.M., Ordas, R., Escribano, J.M., and Borca, M.V. (2001). Induction of a virus-specific antibody response to foot and mouth disease virus using the structural protein VP1 expressed in transgenic potato plants. Viral Immunol. 14, 49–57.

Centers for Disease Control (1998). Preventing emerging infectious diseases: a strategy for the 21st century. MMWR Morb. Mortal.Wkly. Rep. 47, 1–4.

Choi, A.H., Basu, M., McNeal, M.M., Clements, J.D., and Ward, R.L. (1999). Antibody-independent protection against rotavirus infection of mice stimulated by intranasal immunization with chimeric VP4 or VP6 protein. *J. Virol.* 73, 7574–7581.

Curtiss, R.C., and Cardineau, G.A. (1990) Oral immunisation by transgenic plants. In *World Intellectual Property Organization PCT/US89/03799.* St. Louis: Washington University.

Daniell, H., Streatfield, S. J., and Wycoff, K. (2001) Medical molecular farming: production of antibodies, biopharmaceuticals and edible vaccines in plants. *Trends Plant Sci.* 6, 219–226.

Dus Santos, M.J., Wigdorovitz, A., Trono, K., Rios, R.D., Franzone, P.M., Gil, F., Moreno, J., Carrillo, C., Escribano, J.M., and Borca, M.V. (2002). A novel methodology to develop a foot and mouth disease virus (FMDV) peptide-based vaccine in transgenic plants. *Vaccine* 20, 1141–1147.

Fu, Z.F., Rupprecht, C.E., Dietzschold, B. Saikumar, P. Niu, H.S., Babka I., Wunner, W.H., and Koprowski, H. (1993). Oral vaccination of raccoons (*Procyon lotor*) with baculovirus-expressed rabies virus glycoprotein. *Vaccine* 11, 925–928.

Gómez, N., Carrillo, C., Salinas, J., Parra, F., Borca M.V., and Escribano, J.M. (1998). Expression of immunogenic glycoprotein S polypeptides from transmissible gastroenteritis coronavirus in transgenic plants. *Virology* 249, 352–358.

Guidry, J.J., Cardenas, L., Cheng, E., and Clements, J.D. (1997) Role of receptor binding in toxicity, immunogenicity, and adjuvanticity of *Escherichia coli* heat-labile enterotoxin. *Infect. Immun.* 65, 4943–4950.

Haq, T.A., Mason, H.S., Clements, J.D., and Arntzen, C.J. (1995) Oral immunization with a recombinant bacterial antigen produced in transgenic plants. *Science* 268, 714–716.

Holmgren, J., Lycke, N., and Czerkinsky, C. (1993). Cholera toxin and cholera B subunit as oral-mucosal adjuvant and antigen vector systems. *Vaccine* 11, 1179–1184.

Jiang, X., Wang, M., Graham, D.Y., and Estes, M.K. (1992) Expression, self-assembly, and antigenicity of the Norwalk virus capsid protein. *J. Virol.* 66, 6527–6532.

Jimenez, G., Correa, I., Melgosa, M.P., Bullido, M.J., and Enjuanes, L. (1986). Critical epitopes in transmissible gastroenteritis virus neutralization. *J. Virol.* 60, 131–139.

Johansen, K., Hinkula, J., Espinoza, F., Levi, M., Zeng, C., Ruden, U., Vesikari, T., and Estes, M., and Svensson, L. (1999). Humoral and cell-mediated immune responses in humans to the NSP4 enterotoxin of rotavirus *J Med. Virol.* 59, 369–377.

Kapikian, A.Z., and Chanock, R.M. (1990). Rotavirus. In *Virology* (eds. Fields, B.N., Knipe, D.M., Chanock, R.M., Hirsch, M.S., Melnick, J.L., Monath, T.P., Roizman, B.), 2nd ed. New York: Raven Press, 1353–1404.

Kapusta, J., Modelska, A., Figlerowicz, M., Pniewski, T., Letellier, M., Lisowa, O., Yusibov, V., Koprowski H., Plucienniczak, A., and Legocki, A. B. (1999). A plant-derived edible vaccine against hepatitis B virus. *FASEB J.* 13, 1796–1799.

Knowles N.J., and Samuel A.R., (2003). Molecular epidemiology of foot-and-mouth disease virus. *Virus Res.* 91, 65–80.

Kong, Q., Richter, L., Yang, Y. F., Arntzen, C. J., Mason, H.S and Thanavala, Y. (2001). Oral immunization with hepatitis B surface antigen expressed in transgenic plants. *Proc. Natl. Acad. Sci. USA* 98, 11539–11544.

Koprowski, H., and Yusibov, V. (2001). The green revolution: plants as heterologous expression vectors. *Vaccine* 19, 2735–2741.

Lamphear, B.J., Streatfield, S.J., Jilka, J.M., Brooks, C.A., Barker, D.K., Turner, D.D., Delaney, D.E., Garcia, M., Wiggins, B., Woodard, S.L., Hood, E.E, Tizard I.R., Lawhorn, B., and Howard, J.A. (2002). Delivery of subunit vaccines in maize seed. *J. Control Release* 85, 169–180.

Mason, H.S., Lam, D.M., and Arntzen, C.J. (1992). Expression of hepatitis B surface antigen in transgenic plants. *Proc. Natl. Acad. Sci. USA* 89, 11745–11749.

Mason, H. S., Ball J. M., Shi J. J., Jiang X., Estes M. K., and Arntzen C. J. (1996). Expression of Norwalk virus capsid protein in transgenic tobacco and potato and its oral immunogenicity in mice. *Proc Natl Acad Sci USA* 93, 5335–5340.

Mason, H.S., Haq, T.A., Clements, J.D., and Arntzen, C.J. (1998). Edible vaccine protects mice against *E. coli* heat-labile enterotoxin (LT): potatoes expressing a synthetic LT-B gene. *Vaccine* 16, 1336–1343.

Mason, H.S., Warzecha ,H., Mor, T., and Arntzen, C.J. (2002). Edible plant vaccines: applications for prophylactic and therapeutic molecular medicine. *Trends Mol. Med.* 8, 324–329.

Matsumura, T., Itchoda, N., and Tsunemitsu, H. (2002). Production of immunogenic VP6 protein of bovine group A rotavirus in transgenic potato plants. *Arch. Virol.* 147, 1263–1270.

McAleer, W.J. Buynak, E.B., Maigetter, R.Z., Wampler, D.E., Miller, W.J., and Hilleman, M.R. (1984). Human hepatitis B vaccine from recombinant yeast. *Nature* 307, 178–180.

McGarvey, P.B., Hammond, J., Dienelt, M.M., Hooper, D.C., Fu, Z.F., Dietzschold, B., Koprowski, H., Michaels, F.H. (1995). Expression of the rabies virus glycoprotein in transgenic tomatoes. *Biotechnology* 13, 1484–1487.

O'Neal, C.M., Crawford, S.E., Estes, M.K., and Conner, M.E. (1997). Rotavirus-like particles administered mucosally induce protective immunity. *J. Virol.* 71: 8707–8717.

Palmer, K.E., Arntzen, C.J., and Lomonossoff, G.P. (1999). Antigen delivery systems III. Transgenic plants and recombinant plant viruses. In *Mucosal Immunology*, 2nd ed. (eds. P.L. Ogra, J. Mestecky, M.E. Lamm, W. Strober, J. R. McGhee, J. Bienenstock). San Diego: Academic Press, 793–807.

Plotkin, S.A. (2000). Rabies. *Clin. Infect. Dis.* 30, 4–12.

Richter, L. J., Thanavala, Y., Arntzen, C., and Mason, H.S. (2000). Production of hepatitis B surface antigen in transgenic plants for oral immunization. *Nat. Biotechnol.* 18, 1167–1171.

Saif, L.J., and Wesley, R.D. (1992). Transmissible gastroenteritis. In *Disease of Swine* (eds. A.D. Leman, B.E. Straw, W.L. Mengeling, S. D'Allaire, and D.J. Taylor). Prescott, Arizona: Wolfe Publishing, Ltd., 362–386.

Sixma, T.K., Pronk, S.E., Kalk, K.H., Wartna, E.S., van Zanten, B.A., Witholt, B., and Hol, W.G. (1991). Crystal structure of a cholera toxin–related heat-labile enterotoxin from *E. coli. Nature* 351, 371–377.

Sojikul, P., Buehner, N., and Mason, H.S. (2003). A plant signal peptide–hepatitis B surface antigen fusion protein with enhanced stability and immunogenicity expressed in plant cells. *Proc. Natl. Acad. Sci. USA* 100, 2209–2214.

Streatfield, S. J., Jilka, J. M., Hood, E. E., Turner, D. D., Bailey, M. R., Mayor, J. M., Woodard, S. L., Beifuss, K. K., Horn, M. E., Delaney, D. E., Tizard, I. R., and Howard, J. A. (2001). Plant-based vaccines: unique advantages. *Vaccine* 19, 2742–2748.

Tacket, C.O., Mason, H.S., Losonsky, G., Clements, J.D., Levine, M.M., and Arntzen, C.J. (1998). Immunogenicity in humans of a recombinant bacterial antigen delivered in transgenic potato. *Nat. Med.* 4, 607–609.

Tacket, C.O., Mason, H. S., Losonsky, G., Estes M.K., Levine, M. M., and Arntzen, C. J. (2000). Human immune responses to a novel Norwalk virus vaccine delivered in transgenic potatoes. *J. Infect. Dis.* 182, 302–305.

Thanavala, Y., Yang, Y. F., Lyons, P., Mason, H.S., and Arntzen C. (1995). Immunogenicity of transgenic plant-derived hepatitis B surface antigen. *Proc Natl Acad Sci USA* 92, 3358–3361.

Tollis, M., Dietzschold, B., Volia, C.B., and Koprowski, H., (1991). Immunization of monkeys with rabies ribonucleoprotein (RNP) confers protective immunity against rabies. *Vaccine* 9, 134–136.

Torres, J.M, Alonso, C., Ortega, A., Mittal, S., Graham, F., and Enjuanes, L. (1996). Tropism of human adenovirus type 5–based vectors in swine and their ability to protect against transmissible gastroenteritis coronavirus. *J. Virol.* 70, 3770–3780.

Tuboly, T., Nagy, E., Dennis, J.R., and Derbyshire, J.B. (1994). Immunogenicity of the S protein of transmissible gastroenteritis virus expressed in baculovirus. *Arch. Virol.* 137, 55–67.

Tuboly, T., Yu, W., Bailey, S., Degrandis, S., Du, S., Erickson, L., and Nagy, E. (2000). Immunogenicity of porcine transmissible gastroenteritis virus spike protein expressed in plants. *Vaccine* 18, 2023–2028.

Wigdorovitz, A., Carrillo, C., Dus Santos, M.J., Trono, K., Peralta, A., Gomez, M.C., Rios, R.D., Franzone, P.M., Sadir, A.M., Escribano, J.M., and Borca, M.V. (1999). Induction of a protective antibody response to foot and mouth disease virus in mice following oral or parenteral immunization with alfalfa transgenic plants expressing the viral structural protein VP1. *Virology* 255, 347–353.

Yu, J., and Langridge W. H. (2001). A plant-based multicomponent vaccine protects mice from enteric diseases. *Nat. Biotechnol.* 19, 548–552.

Yusibov, V., Moldelska, A., Steplewski, K., Agadjanyan, M., Weiner, D., Hooper, D.C., and Koprowski, H. (1997). Antigens produced in plants by infection with chimeric plant viruses immunize against rabies virus and HIV-1. *Proc. Natl. Acad. Sci. USA* 94, 5784–5788.

Antigen Delivery Systems III: Use of Recombinant Plant Viruses

Chapter 59

George P. Lomonossoff

John Innes Centre, Norwich, United Kingdom

The most widely used approach to the expression of foreign proteins in plants is stable genetic transformation. This involves integration of heterologous genes into the chromosomes of a host plant and has been used successfully to express a number of immunologically active proteins (see Chapter 58). An alternative approach involves the use of plant virus–based vectors. One of the main attractions of this approach is that viral genomes multiply within infected cells, potentially leading to very high levels of protein expression. Additional advantages include the fact that viral genomes are very small and therefore relatively easy to manipulate and that the infection process is simpler than transformation/regeneration. There are, inevitably, disadvantages to the approach: the foreign gene is not heritable, there are limitations on the size and complexity of the sequences that can be expressed in a genetically stable manner, and there are concerns about the ability of modified viruses to spread in the environment. Nonetheless, the virus vector approach has been used to express a number of immunologically active proteins, and this article reviews the progress in the field and problems that remain to be solved.

TYPES OF VIRAL VECTOR

The first plant viruses to be investigated as potential gene vectors were those with DNA genomes. However, for a number of reasons, these proved difficult to develop into practical vectors for large-scale protein expression, and they have not been used for the production of immunologically active proteins. Details of the development and applications of DNA virus–based vectors are therefore outside the scope of the current chapter, and the reader is referred to Porta and Lomonossoff (1996, 2002) for a discussion of these systems.

Most plant viruses have genomes that consist of one or more strands of positive-sense RNA. These viruses can grow in a wide range of hosts, and some can reach extremely high titers. As with animal RNA viruses, they use a variety of strategies for gene expression, including the use of subgenomic promoters and polyprotein processing. The availability of infectious cDNA clones was prerequisite for the development of RNA virus–based vectors. Since their advent, members of several virus families have been developed as useful vectors (**Fig. 59.1**). Initial attempts at vector construction were based on gene replacement strategies in which a sequence encoding a non-essential viral function was replaced by a gene of interest. Though several of these early constructs could replicate in isolated plant cells, they generally could not systemically infect whole plants. A more successful approach has been the development of vectors based on gene addition. In these a foreign sequence is added to the complement of viral genes, rather than substituting for one. For reviews of the development of RNA virus-based vectors the reader is referred to Scholtof *et al.* (1996), and Porta and Lomonossoff (1998, 2002).

Two basic types of systems have been developed for the production of immunogenic peptides and proteins in plants. The first type, often termed epitope presentation, involves inserting a sequence encoding an antigenic peptide into the viral coat protein gene in such a manner that the peptide is expressed on the surface of assembled virus particles. The modified virions are often referred to as chimeras or chimeric virus particles. Such particles are attractive as potential novel vaccines, since the presentation of multiple copies of an antigenic peptide on the surface of a macromolecular assembly can significantly increase its immunogenicity (Lomonossoff and Johnson, 1996). With these systems it is generally anticipated that the modified particles will be at least partially purified prior to administration to animals. The second type, often referred to as polypeptide expression, involves introducing a whole gene into the viral genome in such a manner that it is efficiently expressed in infected cells, usually as an unfused polypeptide. Though purification of the expressed protein may be necessary or desirable, this type of system could be suitable for the production of

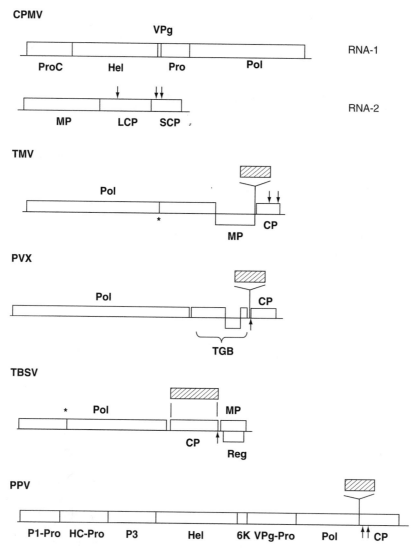

Fig. 59.1. Genome organization of viruses used to express heterologous peptides and proteins in plants. Positions where epitopes have been inserted into the coat proteins of the various viruses are shown by black arrows. The positions where foreign proteins (shown hatched) have been inserted into the viral genomes are also indicated. The functions of various virus genes are shown as follows: CP, coat protein; HC-Pro, helper component proteinase; Hel, helicase; MP, movement protein; LCP, large coat protein; Pol, RNA-dependent RNA polymerase; Pro, proteinase; ProC, proteinase cofactor; Reg, regulatory protein; TGB, triple gene block; VPg, virus protein genome-linked; P1-Pro, P1-proteinase; P3, protein P3; 6K, 6-kDa protein; SCP, small coat protein; and VPg-Pro, VPg-proteinase. The *asterisk* represents a leaky termination codon.

immunogens that can be supplied orally by direct feeding of plant material to animals.

EPITOPE PRESENTATION SYSTEMS

A number of viruses of various morphologies have been adapted for use as epitope presentation systems. The main prerequisites for such a use are that the presence of the foreign sequence does not interfere with ability of the modified coat protein to assemble into virions and that the peptide is displayed on the surface of assembled particles. Thus, attention to date has focused on those viruses for which there is at least some information available about the topology of the coat protein in the assembled virions. As more structural information accumulates, it is likely that additional plant viruses will be developed into epitope presentation systems.

Cowpea mosaic virus (CPMV)
Construction of CPMV chimeras
Cowpea mosaic virus (CPMV) was the first plant virus to be developed as an epitope presentation system (Usha *et al.*, 1993; Porta *et al.*, 1994, 1996). CPMV is a bipartite RNA virus (Fig. 59.1), with particles containing 60 copies each of a large (L; 37 kDa) and a small (S; 23 kDa) CP arranged with icosahedral symmetry **(Fig. 59.2)**. The virus

CPMV

TMV

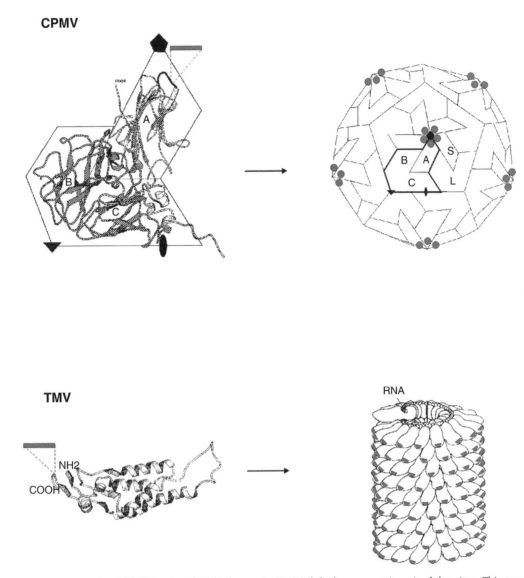

Fig. 59.2. Epitope presentation using CPMV (*top*) and TMV (*bottom*). CPMV: *left*, the assymetric unit of the virus. This consists of one copy each of the large (L; C and B domains) and small (S; A domain) coat proteins. The site most commonly used for the insertion of foreign peptides, the βB-βC loop of the S coat protein, is indicated. The icosahedral particles *(right)* contain 60 copies each of the S and L coat proteins, and the positions on assembled virus particles of an epitope inserted in the βB-βC loop of the S coat protein are shown as *grey dots*. TMV: *left,* the position on the coat protein subunit near the C-terminus where insertions have been made in most chimeras. The approximate positions of inserted epitopes are shown as *shaded dots* on a segment of an assembled virus particle *(right)*.

was an attractive candidate for development as an epitope presentation system because it grows to high titers and the detailed three-dimensional structure of the coat protein was known. This enabled a rational choice to be made regarding potential insertion sites (Lomonossoff and Johnson, 1995). Since the original reports describing the construction of chimeric virus particles, a large variety of epitopes have been expressed on the surface of CPMV particles (for examples, see Lomonossoff and Hamilton, 1999, and Porta *et al.*, 2003). In most cases, the foreign sequence has been inserted into the most exposed loop of the virus surface, the βB-βC loop of the S protein (Fig. 59.2). However, other sites, such as the βE-αB loop of the L protein and the βC'-βC'' loop of the S protein, have also been used successfully (Brennan *et al.*, 1999a; Taylor *et al.*, 2000; Chatterji *et al.*, 2002; Porta *et al.*, 2003). Generally, provided the inserted peptide is less than 40 amino acids and has a pI below 9.0 (Porta *et al.*, 2003), the yields of modified particles are similar to those obtained with wildtype CPMV (up to 1 mg of particles per gram of infected leaf tissue). In each case, the chimeric virus particles present 60 copies of the inserted peptide on the virus surface, though preliminary experiments indicate that it will be possible to utilize more than one insertion site simultaneously. Where appropriate antisera are available, detection of the inserted epitope on the modified coat protein subunits has proven to be straightforward (Usha *et al.*, 1993; Porta *et al.*, 1994, 1996).

Immunogenicity of CPMV chimeras

The first CPMV chimera and, indeed, the first modified plant virus particle to be assessed for the immunogenicity of a foreign peptide contained a 14–amino acid epitope (the NIm1A site) from human rhinovirus 14 (HRV-14). The modified particles proved capable of inducing specific antibodies against the insert when supplied parenterally to rabbits (Porta *et al.*, 1994). However, due to the nature of the expressed sequence, the antisera were nonneutralizing. Nonetheless, CPMV chimeras expressing this site have proven valuable in assessing the effect of mode of presentation of epitopes on their immunological structure. In particular, it allowed the effect of the proteolytic cleavage that occurs at or near the carboxy-terminus of the inserted sequence to be investigated (Lin *et al.*, 1996; Taylor *et al.*, 1999, 2000).

A number of CPMV-based chimeras have been subjected to detailed immunological analysis. The first to be analyzed in this regard was a chimera expressing a 22–amino acid epitope from gp41 (the "Kennedy epitope") of human immunodeficiency virus type 1 (CPMV-HIV/1; Porta *et al.*, 1994). Initial analysis of the immunogenicity of this chimera focused on the parenteral administration of purified particles to mice in the presence of alum adjuvant (McLain *et al.*, 1995). Sera obtained after boosting gave a strong ELISA response against the gp41 peptide. At a 1:100 dilution, antisera from all of the mice were found to be neutralizing against three strains of HIV-1, IIIB, RF, and SF2 (McLain *et al.*, 1995; 1996a). Further studies showed that neutralizing antibody production elicited by CPMV-HIV/1 did not have a narrow genetic restriction (McLain *et al.*, 1996b). An investigation into the effectiveness of five adjuvants at enhancing the immune response to CPMV-HIV/1 in mice showed that Quil A was the most effective of those tested (McInerney *et al.*, 1999). It was also the only one to stimulate an in vitro proliferative T-cell response. An additional, potentially significant finding from these experiments was that mice receiving chimeric particles in the absence of any adjuvant were also able to mount a secondary immune response. This indicates that the particles themselves can present antigens effectively to the immune system and may obviate the need to use adjuvants for at least some applications.

A curious feature of the immune response to CPMV-HIV/1 was that when the dose of particles was decreased from 100 µg to 1 µg there was a >230-fold decrease in the ELISA antibody titer while the neutralizing antibody titer dropped only twofold (McLain *et al.*, 1996a,b). The differential response of the ELISA and neutralizing antibody titers provided the first indication that mice make HIV-1-specific antibodies to two distinct epitopes present in the gp41 peptide, one neutralizing and one nonneutralizing. The presence of two such epitopes has subsequently been demonstrated (Buratti *et al.*, 1998). The nonneutralizing epitope is antigenically dominant, and deletion of this epitope results in a stronger neutralizing antibody response (Cleveland *et al.*,

2000a). The dissection of the "Kennedy epitope" through the use of CPMV-based chimeras has made a significant contribution to our understanding of the topology of gp41 from HIV-1 (Cleveland *et al.*, 2000b).

The key demonstration of the utility of plant virus–based vaccines, the ability to stimulate protective immunity, has been reported (Dalsgaard *et al.*, 1997) **(Table 59.1)**. This study involved a CPMV chimera (CPMV-PARVO1) that contained a 17–amino acid epitope from the N-terminal region of the VP2 capsid protein of canine parvovirus (CPV). This peptide is also found in VP2 of related parvoviruses, mink enteritis virus (MEV), and feline panleukopenia virus (FPV). CPMV-PARVO1 was administered subcutaneously to mink as a single dose of 100 µg or 1 mg with use of an alum/Quil A adjuvant, and 4 weeks' postvaccination the animals were challenged with MEV. Protection was afforded by either dose, and shedding of MEV was almost completely eliminated with the 1-mg dose. Subsequently, an ultraviolet light-inactivated form of CPMV-PARVO1 was shown to be capable of protecting dogs against a lethal challenge with CPV (Langeveld *et al.*, 2001). As in the case of the mink experiments, the chimera was mixed with an alum/Quil A adjuvant prior to inoculation, and a comparatively high dose (7.5 mg of purified particles per animal) was used. The levels of antibody response, protection, and virus shedding were similar to those obtained with the CPV peptide linked to keyhole limpet hemocyanin.

The work described above all concerned the properties of CPMV chimeras that express epitopes of viral origin. However, there have also been reports of immunological studies on chimeras expressing epitopes of bacterial origin. For example, the properties of a chimera expressing the 30–amino acid D2 domain of the fibronectin-binding protein (FnBP) from *Staphylococcus aureus* has been investigated (Brennan *et al.*, 1999b). The chimera was able to elicit antibodies in rats that completely inhibited the binding of fibronectin to immobilized FnBP and blocked the adherence of *S. aureus* to fibronectin. The construct was subsequently found to protect rats against endocarditis, and the serum from the rats protected mice against weight loss due to *S. aureus* bacteremia (Rennermalm *et al.*, 2001).

The construction of a chimera, CPMV-PAE5, which expressed a 34–amino acid sequence containing two epitopes (peptides 10 and 18) from the outer membrane (OM) protein F of *Pseudomonas aeruginosa* in tandem, has been described (Brennan *et al.*, (1999a). The antibodies induced in mice to this chimera, which were exclusively directed against the peptide 10 epitope, were able to recognize the F protein from all seven immunotypes of *P. aeruginosa*. Furthermore, immunized mice were protected against challenge by two different immunotypes of *P. aeruginosa* in a model of chronic pulmonary infection (Brennan *et al.*, 1999c; Table 59.1).

Tobacco mosaic virus

Construction of tobacco mosaic virus chimeras

Particles of tobacco mosaic virus (TMV) consist of a single molecule of genomic RNA (Fig. 59.1) encapsidated by 2130

Table 59.1. Protective Immunity Induced by the Administration of Peptides and Proteins Expressed in Plants with Use of Viral Vectors

Type of Virus Construct	Expressed Sequence	Species Protected	Immunization Route	Reference(s)
CPMV chimera	CPV VP2 epitope	Mink, dog	Parenteral	Dalsgaard et al. (1997); Langeveld et al. (2001)
CPMV chimera	P. aeruginosa OMF protein epitopes	Mouse	Parenteral	Brennan et al. (1999)
CPMV chimera	S. aureus D2 domain of FnBN	Rat	Parenteral	Rennermalm et al. (2001)
TMV chimera	MHV spike protein epitope	Mouse	Parenteral, nasal	Koo et al. (1999)
TMV chimera	P. aeruginosa OMF protein epitopes	Mouse	Parenteral	Stacek et al. (2000)
TMV/AlMV chimera	Rabies virus epitopes	Mouse	Parenteral, oral	Modelska et al. (1998)
TMV-expressed protein	FMDV VP1	Mouse	Parenteral	Wigdorovitz et al. (1999)
PPV-expressed protein	RHDV VP60	Rabbit	Parenteral	Fernandez-Fernandez et al. (2001)
PVX-expressed protein	HPV-16 E7	Mouse	Parenteral	Franconi et al. (2002)

copies of the 17.5-kDa coat protein arranged with helical symmetry. The first example of the presentation of foreign peptides on the TMV coat protein was reported in 1986 (Haynes et al., 1986). However, in this case the modified coat protein bearing an eight–amino acid poliovirus epitope at its C-terminus was expressed in *Escherichia coli* rather than in plants. The production of modified TMV particles in plants was first attempted in 1990 (Takamatsu et al., 1990). In these experiments, a sequence encoding Leu-enkephalin was fused to the C-terminus of the viral coat protein. However, the modified coat protein was not competent for virion assembly. This highlighted a problem with using TMV particles to express foreign peptides. The fact that TMV particles contain a large number of subunits, making the system potentially very attractive for peptide expression, is also a problem in that the subunits are very tightly packed, allowing little space on the virus surface for the expression of foreign sequences (Fig. 59.2).

To address the problem of steric hindrance, a TMV vector was developed that permitted the synthesis of both native and C-terminally modified versions of the coat protein from the same viral RNA (Hamamoto et al., 1993). This was achieved by engineering a leaky termination codon at the C-terminus of the coat protein gene. This system produced particles in plants in which up to 5% of the coat protein subunits were modified at their C-termini and has been used to express epitopes from several animal pathogens (Sugiyama et al., 1995; Turpen et al., 1995). As with CPMV-based chimeras, the inserted peptides could be detected on the surface of assembled virions. Subsequently, by modifying the site of peptide insertion, TMV-based systems were developed in which all the coat protein subunits could be modified to express foreign peptides without abolishing virus

viability (Turpen et al., 1995; Fitchen et al., 1995; Beachy et al., 1996). As a result, most TMV-based chimeras now contain inserts between amino acids 154 and 155, near but not at the C-terminus of the coat protein (Fig. 59.2). The size of inserts that can be tolerated even at this optimized position seems to be quite small, the largest reported to date being 23 amino acids in a chimera that grew substantially more slowly than wild-type TMV (Bendahmane et al., 1999).

Immunogenicity of TMV chimeras

The first analysis of the immunogenicity of a TMV chimera involved a construct expressing 13 amino acids from the glycoprotein ZP3 from the murine zona pellucida (Fitchen et al., 1995), a sequence previously shown to be capable of inducing antibody-mediated contraception. The modified virions were capable of eliciting antibodies in mice that bound to the zona pellucida, but the effectiveness of these antibodies in contraception could not be assessed.

Using the vector developed by Fitchen et al. (1995), Koo et al. (1999) expressed two sequences, of 10 and 15 amino acids, from the 5B19 epitope from the spike protein of the coronavirus, murine hepatitis virus (MHV). Counterintuitively, the construct harboring the 15–amino acid insert (TMV-5B19L) could be purified more readily than that with the smaller one (TMV-5B19), despite the latter sequence being entirely contained within the former. Mice immunized nasally (5B19L) or subcutaneously (5B19L or 5B19) with purified virions produced antibodies against the MHV epitope, and those with high antibody titers were protected from subsequent nasal challenge with the virus (Table 59.1).

In experiments similar to those reported previously with CPMV (Brennan, 1999a,c), Stacek et al. (2000) expressed an epitope (peptide 9) from the OM protein F of *P. aeruginosa* on the surface of TMV (Stacek *et al.*, 2000). As found with the CPMV construct expressing different epitopes (peptides 10 and 18), antibodies induced in mice to the TMV chimera recognized the F protein from all seven immunotypes of *P. aeruginosa*, and immune mice were protected against challenge with *P. aeruginosa* (Table 59.1). In an attempt to develop a combined vaccine in which several epitopes from protein F of *P. aeruginosa* are presented simultaneously, mice were immunized with a mixture of the TMV chimera expressing peptide 9 and a chimeric influenza virus containing peptide 10 (Gilleland *et al.*, 2000). The mice produced antibodies against both epitopes and were protected against challenge at a level similar to that found when the individual components were used.

To overcome the limitation on the size of peptide that can be fused to the TMV coat protein, others have developed an approach that combined the use of TMV as vector with the known ability of the coat protein of alfalfa mosaic virus (AlMV) to tolerate foreign peptides at its N–terminus (Yusibov *et al.*, 1997). In this system, an appropriately modified version of the AlMV coat protein is expressed from an additional copy of the TMV coat protein subgenomic promoter. Using this approach, a 40–amino acid sequence containing epitopes from the glycoprotein and nucleoprotein of rabies virus and a 47–amino acid sequence from gp120 from HIV-1 were fused to the AlMV coat protein and the fusion protein expressed in *Nicotiana benthamiana*. In infected leaf tissue, the modified AlMV CP subunits assembled into ellipsoid particles that expressed multiple copies of the antigenic insert. When purified and injected into mice, these particles elicited the production of appropriate virus-neutralizing antibodies, even in the absence of adjuvant. Particles expressing the rabies virus epitopes were subsequently shown to protect mice against a normally lethal challenge with the virus when supplied either intraperitoneally or orally (Modelska *et al.*, 1998; Table 59.1).

In a related epitope/polypeptide approach, others have expressed a fusion protein consisting of a potentially neutralizing epitope from hepatitis C virus (HCV) linked to the C-terminus of the cholera toxin B subunit (CT-B) (Nemchimov *et al.*, 2000). Plants infected with the recombinant TMV produced functionally active pentameric CT-B presenting the inserted epitope. Nasal administration of crude plant material to mice elicited the production of antibodies against both the HCV epitope and CT-B.

Other plant viruses
Tomato bushy stunt virus
Tomato bushy stunt virus (TBSV) is a monopartite virus (Fig. 59.1), particles of which contain 180 copies of a single type of coat protein arranged with icosahedral symmetry. Sequences derived from gp120 of HIV-1 have been fused to the C-terminus of the coat protein, and the ability of the modified virus to infect *N. benthamiana* has been examined (Joelson *et al.*, 1997). When a sequence encoding 162 amino

acids was expressed at this site, a large proportion of the inserted sequence was lost on serial passaging. By contrast, when a 13–amino acid sequence, corresponding to the V3 loop of gp41, was expressed at the same location, the construct was genetically stable and the inserted epitope could be detected immunologically. Though the modified virions stimulated only a weak response when injected into mice (Sjölander *et al.*, 1996), plates coated with particles could detect anti-V3 antibodies in HIV-positive individuals (Joelson *et al.*, 1997).

Plum pox virus
Plum pox virus (PPV) has flexuous rod-shaped particles consisting of more than 2000 copies of a single-coat protein encapsidating a single RNA molecule (Fig. 59.1). Though a detailed structure of PPV coat protein was not available, immunological analyses of related viruses suggested that both the N- and C-termini are surface-exposed. Furthermore, it had been shown that it was possible to fuse foreign sequences to the N-terminus of the coat protein of Johnsongrass mosaic virus (JGMV), a member of the same genus as PPV, without abolishing the ability of the coat protein molecules to assemble into viruslike particles in heterologous systems (Jagadish *et al.*, 1993). Making use of this information, one group fused a 15–amino acid epitope, equivalent to that used by Dalsgaard *et al.* (1997), from VP2 of CPV to a position near the N-terminus of the PPV coat protein, either as a single copy or as a tandem duplication (Fernandez-Fernandez *et al.*, 1998). Both constructs could be propagated in *N. clevelandii* and gave yields of virus particles similar to those obtained with wild-type PPV, and the inserted epitope could be detected on the virion surface. Antisera produced in either mice or rabbits with specificity for particles of either construct showed neutralizing activity in a monolayer-protection assay. The site of expression of peptides on the PPV coat protein has subsequently been refined (Fernandez-Fernandez *et al.*, 2002), raising the prospect that PPV may have general utility as an epitope-presentation system.

Potato virus X
Potato virus X (PVX) has filamentous particles consisting of approximately 1260 coat protein subunits encapsidating a single RNA molecule (Fig. 59.1). It has proven possible to express proteins at the surface–exposed N-terminus of either a proportion (Santa Cruz *et al.*, 1996) (see discussion of PVX in the section on Polypeptide Expression Systems) or all of the subunits (Marusic *et al.*, 2001). To assess whether peptides expressed in this way were immunogenic, one group fused a 38–amino acid sequence from the D2 domain of the fibronectin-binding protein (FnBP) from *Staphylococcus aureus* (Brennan *et al.*, 1999). The sequence was a C-terminally extended version of the 30–amino acid sequence from the epitope expressed on CPMV (see section on Immunogenicity of CPMV Chimeras). In the resulting chimeric particles it was estimated that about 10% of the subunits carried the inserted sequence. Though some of

the details varied, the immunogenicity of the PVX construct was generally similar to that of the equivalent CPMV one. Using a related approach, one group expressed a highly conserved hexapeptide epitope from gp41 of HIV-1 on all the PVX subunits (Marusic *et al.*, 2001). Mice immunized either intraperitoneally or nasally with the chimeric particles produced high levels of HIV-1-specific IgG and IgA antibodies. The potential human response to the chimera was assessed using immunodeficient mice reconstituted with human peripheral blood lymphocytes (hu–PBL-SCID mice). These mice made human primary antibody responses to the gp41 peptide, and the serum exerted an anti-HIV-1-neutralizing activity.

Alfalfa mosaic virus

Recently, an attempt to express the rabies epitopes described in the section on Immunogenicity of TMV Chimeras on the surface of AlMV particles using an AlMV rather than a TMV vector was reported (Fleysch *et al.*, 2001). The potential advantage of using AlMV itself rather than TMV is that the former can infect edible plants such as soybean. Though the initial experiments appeared promising, it has not been possible to reproduce them (Brodzik *et al.*, 2002).

POLYPEPTIDE EXPRESSION SYSTEMS

A number of RNA viruses, particularly but not exclusively those which produce rod-shaped or filamentous particles, have been adapted to act as vectors for the production of free foreign proteins in plants. The preference for these types of virus over those with isometric particles is mainly due to the absence of any absolute limit on the size of RNA that can be packaged in the particles.

Tobacco mosaic virus

The first virus to be used to express a whole protein (chloramphenicol acetyl transferase, or CAT) was TMV (Takamatsu *et al.*, 1987; Dawson *et al.*, 1989). Subsequently, TMV vectors were developed in which expression of an inserted sequence is driven by an additional copy of the coat protein subgenomic promoter (Donson *et al.*, 1991), with genetic stability being improved by the use of promoters from heterologous strains. These have been used to express high levels (up to 2% of soluble proteins) of several valuable proteins in plants. These include a eukaryotic ribosome-inactivating protein (RIP), α-trichosanthin (Kumagai *et al.*, 1993), and single-chain (ScFvs; McCormick *et al.*, 1999) or full-length monoclonal antibodies (Verch *et al.*, 1998). Furthermore, it has proven possible to synthesize glycosylated proteins with TMV vectors (Kumagai *et al.*, 2000; Dirnberger *et al.*, 2001).

There are a number of examples in which the TMV vector system has been used to produce immunogenic proteins. One group (Wigdorovitz *et al.*, 1999) expressed VP1 from FMDV in *N. benthamiana* using the vector developed by others (Donson *et al.*, 1991). This group detected significant quantities (50–150 µg per gram of leaf, fresh weight) of VP1 in leaves and used leaf extracts to inoculate mice intraperitoneally in the presence of Freund's complete adjuvant. All mice immunized in this manner developed significant antibody titers directed to a VP1 epitope. When challenged with FMDV, all immunized mice were protected in two separate experiments (Table 59.1). This was the first example in which a whole protein, rather than a peptide fusion, expressed in plants using a viral vector was shown to be capable of conferring protective immunity. Another group expressed a major birch pollen antigen (Betv1) in *N. benthamiana* and showed that the B-cell epitopes from natural Betv1 were preserved in the plant-expressed protein (Krebitz *et al.*, 2000). Mice immunized with crude leaf extracts from *N. benthamiana* expressing Betv1 generated immunological responses comparable to those induced by the protein expressed in *E. coli* or extracted from birch pollen.

Potato virus X

Potato virus X (PVX) has been used to express polypeptide immunogens in two different formats. The first uses duplicated subgenomic promoters (Chapman *et al.*, 1992) and is similar to that developed with TMV (see discussion on TMV in section on Polypeptide Expression Systems; Fig. 59.1). Such vectors have proven very useful in expression studies with a number of proteins such as ScFv antibodies (Hendy *et al.*, 1999; Franconi *et al.*, 1999; Ziegler *et al.*, 2000). In terms of immunogens, there are only two examples. One group expressed the major capsid protein, VP6, from a murine rotavirus and showed that although the protein retained its ability to form trimers, it tended to assemble into paracrystalline sheets and tubes rather than viruslike particles (VLPs) (O'Brien *et al.*, 2000). Another group used PVX to express the E7 protein human papillomavirus 16 (HPV-16), a virus implicated in the induction of cervical cancer, in *N. benthamiana* (Franconi *et al.*, 2002). Mice immunized with foliar extracts containing the E7 protein in the presence of Quil A as an adjuvant developed both antibody and cell-mediated immune responses. The isotypic profile of the IgG antibodies indicated that both Th1 and Th2 responses were present, and 40% of mice remained tumor-free after challenge with an E7-expressing tumor cell line. The tumors that did develop in mice vaccinated with the plant-expressed E7 were considerably smaller in volume than those that developed in untreated mice (Table 59.1). The results obtained in this study were particularly significant, as previous attempts to produce large amounts of unfused E7 in other expression systems had been unsuccessful.

The second type of PVX polypeptide expression system involves the fusion of the foreign protein to the N-terminus of the coat protein gene via the 2A catalytic peptide from FMDV. The 2A sequence promotes cotranslational cleavage between the foreign gene insert and the CP, although this is not 100% efficient, resulting in some CP subunits still bearing the inserted protein. These fusion proteins were found to retain their ability to be incorporated into virus capsids, resulting in particles that display the inserted polypeptide. By means of this approach it is possible, with the use of the same construct, to produce a protein of interest in both a free (unfused) state where cleavage by 2A has occurred and as a CP fusion where it is incorporated in PVX particles. The functionality of a foreign protein when incorporated into virions was demonstrated by the observation that an ScFv expressed as a CP fusion could still bind to its antigen, the herbicide Diuron (Smolenska *et al.*, 1998). When this system was used to express the rotavirus VP6 sequence, the uncleaved VP6-2A-CP assembled into PVX virions while the VP6-2A cleavage product formed typical VP6 VLPs (O'Brien *et al.*, 2000).

Plum pox virus

The PPV genomic RNA contains a single ORF that encodes a multifunctional polyprotein (Fig. 59.1). This is self-processed by proteinase domains within it to produce the mature viral proteins. To develop PPV as a polypeptide expression system, sequences encoding foreign proteins, initially marker genes, were inserted such that the free polypeptide would be released through the action of the VPg-proteinase (Fig. 59.1). This was achieved by flanking the inserted sequence with the appropriate proteinase recognition sites (Guo *et al.*, 1998). Subsequently, a PPV vector in which the foreign sequence was inserted between the polymerase (Pol) and coat protein (CP) genes (Fig. 59.1) was used to express the VP60 structural protein from the calicivirus, rabbit hemorrhagic disease virus (RHDV) in *N. clevelandii* (Fernandez-Fernandez *et al.*, 2001). Inoculation with a crude preparation from infected leaf tissue in the presence of adjuvant fully protected rabbits against subsequent challenge with a lethal dose of RHDV (Table 59.1). Taking into account the dose required to confer immunity and the time taken to grow the PPV-infected plants, Fernandez-Fernandez *et al.* (2001) estimated that 1 m² of greenhouse space and 21 days would be sufficient to obtain enough material to protect 50 rabbits against RHDV.

Tomato bushy stunt virus

To overcome the potential limitation on the size of insertion that could be tolerated in the isometric TBSV particles, one group exploited the fact that the TBSV coat protein is not essential for infectivity and produced constructs in which most of the region encoding the coat protein was replaced with marker genes (Fig. 59.1) (Scholtof *et al.*, 1993). A refined version of the vector was subsequently produced in which the coat protein gene was replaced with a polylinker (Scholtof, 1999). This, coupled with improvements to the infection process, permitted the facile expression of heterologous sequences in the inoculated leaves of plants. The approach has been used to express the nucleocapsid protein p24 from HIV-1 as a fusion with the 5′ terminal portion of the CP gene (Zhang *et al.*, 2000). The modified TBSV RNA was capable of replicating in both protoplasts and in the inoculated leaves of whole plants. Accumulation of the CP-p24 fusion protein could be detected in inoculated leaves but, as yet,

there has been no report concerning the immunological properties of the plant-expressed protein.

MUCOSAL IMMUNIZATION

One of the potential advantages of using plants to produce vaccines is that it may be possible to supply the immunological material to mucosal surfaces without a high degree of purification. However, to demonstrate the immunogenicity of plant-expressed material, initial investigations involved parenteral administration in the presence of adjuvant (Table 59.1). However, parenteral immunization does not generally elicit a mucosal immune response, and there have been a number of recent studies aimed at investigating the efficacy of supplying material by other routes.

To investigate whether purified particles of CPMV chimeras can elicit a mucosal immune response, one group administered CPMV-HIV/1 (see section on Immunogenicity of CPMV Chimeras) particles either nasally or orally in the presence of cholera toxin as an adjuvant (Durrani *et al.*, 1998). All the mice immunized nasally produced anti-HIV IgA in feces as well as serum IgG antibodies. Oral immunization was considerably less effective, with only serum antibody being stimulated in a minority of mice. Similar results were obtained when mice were immunized nasally or orally with a CPMV chimera expressing a 30–amino acid sequence from the *S. aureus* FnBP (Brennan *et al.*, 1999d). Detailed characterization of the immune responses in mice immunized nasally with CPMV chimeras expressing epitopes from CPV provided further support to the idea that it will be possible to stimulate mucosal immunity by this route (Nicholas *et al.*, 2002).

Evidence that it may, in fact, be possible to administer CPMV-based chimeras orally was provided by studies on the related virus, cowpea severe mosaic virus (CPSMV). When purified virus particles or crude extracts of CPSMV-infected cowpea leaves were used to immunize mice orally, anti-CPSMV IgG and IgA but not IgE antibodies were produced systemically (Florindo *et al.*, 2002). Significantly, no antibodies were produced in response to the leaf proteins from either healthy or CPSMV-infected cowpeas, and no pathogenic effects were noted in any of the mice. Though these results were obtained with a wild-type virus rather than a chimera, they indicate that purification of virus particles may not be required prior to oral immunization.

The most thorough study to date on the effectiveness of different modes of immunization on protective immunity was carried out by a group using chimeric AlMV viruslike particles carrying rabies virus epitopes (see section on Immunogenicity of TMV Chimeras) (Modelska *et al.*, 1998). The immunogen was supplied to mice in three different ways: intraperitoneally, by gastric intubation, or by feeding on virus-infected leaves. The first two routes involved supplying purified virus particles, while the third used spinach leaves containing the recombinant protein. Though less effective in affording protection than the intraperitoneal route, both forms of oral administration stimulated IgG and IgA antibody synthesis and ameliorated symptoms of a subsequent challenge with an attenuated strain of rabies virus. In similar experiments, others compared the efficacy of purified particles of TMV chimeras expressing an epitope from the spike protein of MHV (see section on Immunogenicity of TMV Chimeras) when supplied to mice either subcutaneously in the presence of adjuvant or nasally (Koo et al., 1999). Nasal administration induced the production of epitope-specific IgG and IgA antibodies, while subcutaneous administration led to the production of only IgG antibodies. In both cases, mice were protected from subsequent challenge with MHV, and there appeared to be some correlation between the degree of protection obtained and the IgA antibody titers.

REGULATORY ISSUES

There are two types of regulatory issues that will need to be addressed before plant-based vaccines using viral vectors can be used. The first type concerns the equivalence between plant-expressed proteins and those produced by more conventional means. These concerns apply generically to proteins expressed in plants whether they are produced transgenically, transiently, or through the use of viral vectors. The problems in demonstrating equivalence have been specifically reviewed elsewhere (Miele, 1997) and will not be further discussed here.

The second type of issue is specifically related to the use of virus-based vectors for foreign gene expression. These principally concern the genetic stability of the expressed sequences and the possibility of spread of the modified viruses in the environment. RNA viruses are particularly prone to the accumulation of mutations during multiple rounds of replication, as RNA-dependent RNA polymerases lack proofreading functions. It was anticipated that this could be a particular problem when expressing heterologous sequences, since their presence, far from conferring a selective advantage on the virus, tends to reduce the rate of virus replication. Thus, the inserted sequence tends to be subjected to both genetic drift and deletion. Indeed, when RNA viruses were first mooted as potential vectors, there was some debate as to whether they would be of any practical use for the expression of foreign proteins (van Vloten-Doting et al., 1985; Siegel, 1985). However, studies on the stability of both constructs containing either whole genes or expressing peptides indicate that these problems will be manageable, provided excessive passaging is not undertaken (Kearney et al., 1993, 1999; Porta et al., 1994).

The second concern involves the potential of modified viruses to spread in the environment. This could lead to the expression of immunologically active material in unwanted locations, and the presence of the foreign sequence could conceivably alter the host range and/or the transmissibility of the modified virus. Complete elimination of the ability of modified viruses to infect healthy host plants is clearly unde-sirable, as it is this property that makes viral vectors attractive in the first place. However, limitation of the ability to spread would be an advantage. At present this is most commonly achieved by growing infected plants under physically contained conditions, but this may not always be possible if large quantities of material are to be produced. In a pilot experiment to assess the potential spread of recombinant viruses in a field situation, adjacent rows of tobacco in a field were spray-inoculated with two different recombinant TMV constructs (Pogue et al., 2002). No cross-contamination between plants was found, despite the rows being only 18 inches apart. In addition, the fact that recombinants are at a disadvantage in terms of replication rate when compared with the wild-type virus leads to the deletion of the inserted sequence after multiple rounds of multiplication (Guo et al., 1998; Kearney et al., 1999; Rabindran and Dawson, 2001). This is likely to effectively prevent the widespread unwanted expression of foreign protein in the environment during propagation.

To address the problem of potential virus spread after material has been purified and/or administered to animals, one group carried out ultraviolet inactivation experiments on CPMV-PARVO1 (see section on Immunogenicity of CPMV Chimeras) (Langeveld et al., 2001). This group showed that it was possible to completely abolish the infectivity of chimera on plants without affecting either the structural integrity of the particles or their ability to stimulate protective immunity. Since ultraviolet irradiation is a U.S. Food and Drug Administration–approved method for virus inactivation, this method may be a generally useful pretreatment for purified preparations of chimeric virus particles.

The possibility that a modified virus may have its host range or transmission ability altered has been raised in the case of chimeric virus particles. Though there is no evidence that host range is determined directly by the sequence of the viral coat protein, transmission is known to be affected. Thus, it is conceivable that expression of a foreign peptide on the surface of virus particles may, by chance, change the ability of a virus to spread in the environment. To investigate this possibility, one group examined the host ranges and transmission characteristics of two CPMV chimeras, expressing epitopes from HRV-14 and HIV-1 (Porta et al., 2003). The host ranges of the chimeras were identical to that of wild-type CPMV, but they had a reduced ability to be transmitted by beetles, the natural insect vectors. Furthermore, the chimeras had not gained an ability to be transmitted by aphids or through seed. Though these experiments were inevitably somewhat limited in scope, they have provided further support to the idea that incorporation of foreign peptides on a virus surface if anything reduces the ability of the virus to spread in the environment.

SUMMARY AND FUTURE PROSPECTS

The past few years have seen significant progress in the use of plant virus vectors for the production of immunogens in plants. Particularly encouraging is the fact that it is now clear that peptides or proteins expressed in this manner can confer protective immunity against a number of diseases (Table 59.1), in some cases in the target animals (Dalsgaard *et al.*, 1997; Langeveld *et al.*, 2001; Fernandez-Fernandez *et al.*, 2001). In most of these cases, immunity was stimulated by parenteral immunization, but there are encouraging signs that mucosal immunization may be possible (Modelska *et al.*, 1998; Koo *et al.*, 1999; Durrani *et al.*, 1999). This raises the prospect that it may be possible to confer protective immunity by simply feeding with plant material infected with an appropriate virus construct. To achieve this, it will be necessary not only to express peptides or proteins that can stimulate mucosal immunity but also to express the material in edible plants. In this regard, the continued development of vectors that can infect edible plants such as those based on CPMV (Gopinath *et al.*, 2000), clover yellow vein virus (ClYVV; Masuta *et al.*, 2000), and pea early browning virus (PEBV; MacFarlane and Popovich, 2000), all of which infect legumes; wheat streak mosaic virus (WSMV; Choi *et al.*, 2000), which infects cereals; and zucchini yellow mosaic virus (ZYMV; Arazi *et al.*, 2001), which infects cucurbits, is likely to play a prominent role. In addition, the development of combined transgene/virus complementation systems, such as that described by others (Sanchez-Navarro *et al.*, 2001; Mori *et al.*, 2001), may allow the use of defective viral replicons for the expression of foreign sequences, thereby reducing the risk of environmental spread.

Even if direct feeding of plant material is shown to be efficacious, there will still be need to purify, at least partially, proteins and chimeric particles for certain applications. Though sufficient material for initial characterization can be obtained by laboratory-scale extractions, a substantial scale-up of procedures will be necessary for its widescale use. One group reported the results of experiments on the large-scale growth and purification of a TMV chimera expressing a 12–amino acid malarial peptide (Pogue *et al.*, 2002). The results indicate that although growth under field conditions gives a lower yield per gram (fresh weight) of tissue than growth in a greenhouse or growth chamber, in excess of 1 kg per acre (planted area) of purified particles could be obtained. It was shown that large quantities (up to 10 mg per gram, fresh weight) of wild-type CPMV could be extracted from fresh or frozen cowpea leaves by methods suitable for large-scale application (Nichols *et al.*, 2002). The development of methods for the industrial-scale production and/or purification of plant-derived vaccines will make an important contribution to the practical use of such material.

REFERENCES

Arazi, T., Slutsky S.G., Shiboleth, Y.M., Wang, Y., Rubinstein, M., Barak, S., Yang, J., and Gal-on, A. (2001). Engineering zucchini yellow mosaic polyvirus as a non-pathogenic vector for expression of heterologous proteins in cucurbits. (2001). *J. Biotechnol.* 87, 67–82.

Beachy, R.N., Fitchen, J.H., and Hein, M.B. (1996). Use of plant viruses for delivery of vaccine epitopes. *Ann. Acad. Sci.* 792, 43–49.

Bendahmane, M., Koo, M., Karrer, E., and Beachy, R.N. (1999). Display of epitopes on the surface of tobacco mosaic virus: impact of charge and isoelectric point of the epitope on virus-host interactions. *J. Mol. Biol.* 290, 9–20.

Brennan, F.R., Jones, T.D., Gilleland L.B., Bellaby, T., Xu, F., North, P.C., Thompson, A., Staczek, J., Lin, T., Johnson, J.E., Hamilton, W.D., and Gilleland, H.E., Jr. (1999a). Pseudomonas aeruginosa outer-membrane protein F epitopes are highly immunogenic in mice when expressed on a plant virus. *Microbiology* 145, 211–220.

Brennan, F.R., Jones, T.D., Longstaff, M., Chapman, S., Bellaby, T., Smith, H., Xu, F., Hamilton, W.D., and Flock, J.-I. (1999b). Immunogenicity of peptides derived from a fibronectin-binding protein of S. aureus expressed on two different plant viruses. *Vaccine* 17, 1846–1857.

Brennan, F.R., Gilleland L.B., Staczek, J., Bendig, M.M., Hamilton, W.D., and Gilleland, H.E., Jr. (1999c). A chimaeric plant virus vaccine protects mice against a bacterial infection. *Microbiology* 145, 2061–2067.

Brennan, F.R., Bellaby, T., Helliwell, S.M., Jones, T.D., Kamstrup, S., Dalsgaard, K, Flock, J-I., and Hamilton, W.D. (1999d). Chimeric plant virus particles administered nasally or orally induce systemic and mucosal immune responses in mice. *J. Virol.* 73, 930–938.

Brodzik, R., Deka, D., Karasev, A., and Koprowski, H. (2002). Pathogenesis of Alfalfa mosaic virus in soybean (Glycine max) and expression of chimeric rabies peptide in virus-infected soybean plants: a reexamination. *Phytopathology* 92, 1260–1261.

Buratti, E., McLain, L., Tisminetzky, S., Cleveland, S.M., Dimmock, N.J., and Baralle, F.E. (1998). The neutralizing antibody response against a conserved region of human immunodeficiency virus type 1 gp41 (amino acid residues 731-752) is uniquely directed against a conformational epitope. *J. Gen. Virol.* 79, 2709–2716.

Chapman, S., Kavanagh, T., and Baulcombe, D. (1992). Potato virus X as a vector for gene expression in plants. *Plant J.* 2, 549–557.

Chatterji, A., Burns, L.L., Taylor, S.S., Lomonossoff, G.P., Johnson, J.E., Lin, T., and Porta, C. (2002). Cowpea mosaic virus: from the presentation of antigenic peptides to the display of active biomaterials. *Intervirology* 45, 362–370.

Choi, I.R., Stenger, D.C., Morris, T.J., and French, R. (2000). A plant virus vector for systemic expression of foreign genes in cereals. *Plant J.* 23, 547–555.

Cleveland, S.M., Buratti, E., Jones, T.D., North, P., Baralle, F., McLain, L., McInerney, T., Durrani, Z., and Dimmock, N.J. (2000a). Immunogenic and antigenic dominance of a nonneutralizing epitope over a highly conserved neutralizing epitope in the gp41 envelope glycoprotein of human immunodeficiency virus type 1: its deletion leads to a strong neutralizing response. *Virology* 266, 66–78.

Cleveland, S.M., Jones, T.D., and Dimmock, N.J. (2000b). Properties of a neutralizing antibody that recognizes a conformational form of epitope ERDRD in the gp41 C-terminal tail of human immunodeficiency virus type 1. *J. Gen. Virol.* 81, 1251–1260.

Dalsgaard, K., Uttenthal, Å., Jones T.D., Xu F., Merryweather, A., Hamilton, W.D., Langeveld, J.P., Boshuizen, R.S., Kamstrup, S., Lomonossoff, G.P., Porta, C., Vela C., Casal, J.I., Meloen, R.H., and Rodgers P.B. (1997). Plant-derived vaccine protects target animals against a viral disease. *Nat. Biotechnol.* 15, 248–252.

Dawson, W.O., Lewandowski, D.J., Hilf, M.E., Bubrick, P., Raffo, A.J., Shaw, J.J., Grantham, G.L., and Desjardins, P.R. (1989). A tobacco mosaic virus-hybrid expresses and loses an added gene. *Virology* 172, 285–292.

Dirnberger, D., Steinkellner, H., Abdennebi, L., Remy, J-J., and van de Wiel, D. (2001). Secretion of biologically active glycoforms of bovine follicle stimulating hormone in plants. *Eur. J. Biochem.* 268, 4570–4579.

Donson, J., Kearney, C.M., Hilf, M.E., and Dawson, W.O. (1991). Systemic expression of a bacterial gene by a tobacco mosaic virus-based vector. *Proc. Natl. Acad. Sci. USA* 88, 7204–7208.

Durrani, Z., McInerney, T.L., McLain, L., Jones, T., Bellaby, T., Brennan, F.R., and Dimmock, N.J. (1998). Intranasal immunization with a plant virus expressing a peptide from HIV-1 gp41 stimulates better mucosal and systemic HIV-1-specific IgA and IgG than oral immunization. *J. Immunol. Methods* 220, 93–103.

Fernandez-Fernandez, M.R., Martinez-Torrecuadrada, J.L., Casal, J.I., and Garcia, J.A. (1998). Development of an antigen presentation system based on plum pox polyvirus. *FEBS Lett.* 427, 229–235.

Fernandez-Fernandez, M.R., Mourino, M., Rivera, J., Rodriguez, F., Plana-Duran, J., and Garcia, J.A. (2001). Protection of rabbits against rabbit hemorrhagic disease virus by immunization with the VP60 protein expressed in plants with a potyvirus-based vector. *Virology* 280, 283–291.

Fernandez-Fernandez, M.R., Martinez-Torrecuadrada, J.L., Roncal, F., Dominguez, E., and Garcia, J.A. (2002). Identification of immunogenic hot spots within plum pox potyvirus capsid protein for efficient antigen presentation. *J. Virol.* 76, 12646–12653.

Fitchen, J., Beachy, R.N., and Hein, M.B. (1995). Plant virus expressing hybrid coat protein with added murine epitope elicits autoantibody response. *Vaccine* 13, 1051–1057.

Fleysch, N., Deka, D., Drath, M., Koprowski, H., and Yusibov, V. (2001). Pathogenesis of Alfalfa mosaic virus in soybean (Glycine max) and expression of chimeric rabies peptide in virus-infected soybean plants. *Phytopathology* 91, 941–947.

Florindo, M.I., de Aragao, M.E., da Silva, A.C., Otoch, M.L., Melo, D.F., Lima, J.A., and Lima, M.G. (2002). Immune response induced in mice by oral immunization with Cowpea severe mosaic virus. *Braz. J. Med. Biol. Res.* 35, 827–835.

Franconi, A., Roggero, P., Pirazzi, P., Arias, F.J., Desiderio, A., Bitti, O., Pashkoulov, D., Mattei, B., Bracci, L., Masenga, V., Milne, R.G., and Benvenuto, E. (1999). Functional expression in bacteria and plants of an scFv antibody fragment against tospoviruses. *Immunotechnology* 4, 189–201.

Franconi, R., Di Bonito, P., Dibello, F., Accardi, L., Muller, A., Cirilli, A., Simeone, P., Dona, M.G., Venuti, A., and Giorgi, C. (2002). Plant derived-human papillomavirus 16 E7 oncoprotein induces immune response and specific tumour protection. *Cancer Res.* 62, 3654–3658.

Gilleland, H.E., Gilleland, L.B., Staczek, J., Harty, R.N., Garcia-Sastre. A., Palese, P., Brennan, F.R., Hamilton, W.D., Bendahmane, M., and Beachy, R.N. (2000). Chimeric animal and plant viruses expressing epitopes of outer membrane protein F as a combined vaccine against *Pseudomonas aeruginosa* lung infection. *FEMS Immunol. Med. Microbiol.* 27, 291–297.

Gopinath, K., Wellink, J., Porta, C., Taylor, K.M., Lomonossoff, G.P., and van Kammen, A. (2000). Engineering cowpea mosaic virus RNA-2 into a vector to express heterologous proteins in plants. *Virology* 267, 159–173.

Guo, H.S., Lopez-Moya, J.J., and Garcia, J.A. (1998). Susceptibility to recombination rearrangements of a chimeric plum pox potyvirus genome after insertion of a foreign gene. *Virus Res.* 57, 183–195.

Hamamoto, H., Sugiyama, Y., Nakagawa, N., Hashida, E., Matsunaga, Y., Takemoto, S., Watanabe, Y., and Okada, Y. (1993). A new tobacco mosaic virus vector and its use for the systemic production of angiotensin-I-converting enzyme inhibitor in transgenic tobacco and tomato. *Biotechnology* 11, 930–932.

Haynes, J.R., Cunningham, J., von Seefried, A., Lennick, M., Garvin, R.T., and Shen, S-H. (1986). Development of a genetically engineered, candidate polio vaccine employing the self-assembling properties of the tobacco mosaic virus coat protein. *Biotechnology* 4, 637–641.

Hendy, S., Chen, Z.C., Barker, H., Santa Cruz, S., Chapman, S., Torrance, L., Cockburn, W., and Whitelam, G.C. (1999) Rapid production of single-chain Fv fragments in plants using a potato virus X episomal vector. *J. Immunol. Methods* 231, 137–146.

Jagadish, M.N., Hamilton, R.C., Fernandez, C.S., Schoofs, P., Davern, K.M., Kalnins, H., Ward, C.W., and Nisbet, I.T. (1993). High level production of hybrid potyvirus-like particles carrying repetitive copies of foreign antigens in *Escherichia coli. Biotechnology* 11, 1166–1170.

Joelson, T., Åkerblom, L, Oxelfelt, P., Strandberg, B., Tomenius, K., and Morris, T.J. (1997). Presentation of a foreign peptide on the surface of tomato bushy stunt virus. *J. Gen. Virol.* 78, 1213–1217.

Kearney, C.M., Donson, J., Jones, G.E., and Dawson W.O. (1993). Low level of genetic drift in foreign sequences replicating in an RNA virus in plants. *Virology* 192, 11–17.

Kearney, C.M., Thomas, M.J., and Roland, K.E. (1999). Genome evolution of tobacco mosaic virus populations during long-term passaging in a diverse range of hosts. *Arch. Virol.* 144, 1513–1526.

Koo, M., Bendahmane, M., Lettieri, G.A., Paoletti, A.D., Lane, T.E., Fitchen, J.H., Buchmeier, M.J., and Beachy, R.N. (1999). Protective immunity against murine hepatitis virus (MHV) induced by intranasal or subcutaneous administration of hybrids of tobacco mosaic virus that carries an MHV epitope. *Proc. Natl. Acad. Sci. USA* 96, 7774–7779.

Krebitz, M., Wiedermann, U., Essl, D., Steinkellner, H., Wagner, B., Turpen, T.H., Ebner, C., Scheiner, O., and Breiteneder, H. (2000). Rapid production of the major birch pollen allergen Bet v 1 in Nicotiana benthamiana plants and its immunological in vitro and in vivo characterization. *FASEB J.* 14, 1279–1288

Kumagai, M.H., Turpen, T.H., Weinzettl, N., della-Cioppa, G., Turpen, A.M., Donson, J., Hilf, M.E., Grantham, G.L., Dawson, W.O., Chow, T.P., Piatak, M., and Grill, L.K. (1993). Rapid, high-level expression of biologically active alpha-trichosanthin in transfected plants by an RNA viral vector. *Proc. Natl. Acad. Sci. USA* 90, 427–430.

Kumagai, M.H., Donson, J., della-Cioppa, G., and Grill, L.K. (2000). Rapid, high-level expression of glycosylated rice alpha-amylase in transfected plants by an RNA viral vector. *Gene* 245, 169–174.

Langeveld, J.P., Brennan, F.R., Martinez-Torrecuadrada, J.L., Jones, T.D., Boshuizen, R.S., Vela, C., Casal, J.I., Kamstrup, S., Dalsgaard, K., Meloen, R.H., Bendig, M.M., and Hamilton, W.D. (2001). Inactivated recombinant plant virus protects dogs from a lethal challenge with canine parvovirus. *Vaccine* 19, 3661–3670.

Lin, T., Porta, C., Lomonossoff, G., and Johnson, J.E., (1996). Structure-based design of peptide presentation on a viral surface: the crystal structure of a plant/animal virus chimera at 2.8 Å resolution. *Fold Des.* 1, 179–187.

Lomonossoff, G.P., and Hamilton, W.D. (1999). Cowpea mosaic virus-based vaccines. *Curr. Top. Microbiol. Immunol.* 240, 177–189.

Lomonossoff, G.P., and Johnson, J.E. (1995). Eukaryotic viral expression systems for polypeptides. *Semin. Virol.* 6, 257–267.

Lomonossoff, G.P., and Johnson, J.E. (1996). Use of macromolecular assemblies as expression systems for peptides and synthetic vaccines. *Curr Opin. Struct. Biol.* 6, 176–182.

MacFarlane, S.A., and Popovich, A.H. (2000). Efficient expression of foreign proteins in roots from tobravirus vectors. *Virology* 267, 29–35.

Marusic, C., Rizza, P., Lattanzi, L., Mancini, C., Spada, M., Belardelli, F., Benvenuto, E., and Capone, I. (2001). Chimeric plant virus particles as immunogens for inducing murine and human immune responses against human immunodeficiency virus type 1. *J. Virol.* 75, 8434–8439.

Masuta, C., Yamana, T., Tacahashi, Y., Uyeda, I., Sato, M., Ueda, S., and Matsumura, T. (2000). Development of clover yellow vein virus as an efficient, stable gene-expression system for legume species. *Plant J.* 23, 539–546.

McCormick, A.A., Kumagai, M.H., Hanley, K., Turpen, T.H., Hakim, I., Grill, L.K., Tuse, D., Levy, S., and Levy, R. (1999). Rapid production of specific vaccines for lymphoma by expression of the tumor-derived single-chain Fv epitopes in tobacco plants. *Proc. Natl. Acad. Sci. USA* 96, 703–708.

McInerney, T.L., Brennan, F.R., Jones, T.D., and Dimmock, N.J. (1999). Analysis of the ability of five adjuvants to enhance immune responses to a chimeric plant virus displaying an HIV-1 peptide. *Vaccine* 17, 1359–1368.

McLain, L., Porta, C., Lomonossoff, G.P., Durrani, Z., and Dimmock, N.J. (1995). Human immunodeficiency virus type 1-neutralizing antibodies raised to a glycoprotein 41 peptide expressed on the surface of a plant virus. *AIDS Res. Hum. Retroviruses* 11, 327–334.

McLain, L., Durrani, Z., Wisniewski, L.A., Porta, C., Lomonossoff, G.P.,. and Dimmock, N.J. (1996a). Stimulation of neutralizing antibodies to human immunodeficiency virus type 1 in three strains of mice immunized with a 22 amino acid peptide of gp41 expressed on the surface of a plant virus. *Vaccine* 14, 799–810.

McLain , L., Durrani, Z., Dimmock, N.J., Wisniewski, L.A, Porta, C., and Lomonossoff, G.P. (1996b). A plant virus-HIV-1 chimaera stimulates antibody that neutralizes HIV-1. In *Vaccines 96* (eds. F. Brown, D.R. Burton, J. Collier, J. Mekalanos and E. Norrby). New York: Cold Spring Harbor Press, 311–316.

Miele, L. (1997). Plants as bioreactors for biopharmaceuticals: regulatory considerations. *Trends Biotechnol.* 15, 45–50.

Modelska A., Dietzschold, B., Sleysh, N., Fu, Z.F., Steplewski, K., Hooper, D.C., Koprowski, H., and Yusibov, V. (1998). Immunization against rabies with plant-derived antigen. *Proc. Natl. Acad. Sci. USA* 95, 2481–2485.

Mori, M., Fujihara, N., Mise, K., and Furusawa, I. (2001). Inducible high-level mRNA amplification system by viral replicase in transgenic plants. *Plant J.* 27, 79–86.

Nemchinov, L.G., Liang, T.J., Rifaat, M.M., Mazyad, H.M., Hadidi, A., and Keith, J.M. (2000). Development of a plant-derived subunit vaccine candidate against hepatitis C virus. *Arch. Virol.* 145, 2557–2573.

Nicholas, B.L., Brennan, F.R., Martinez-Torrecuadrada, J.L., Casal, J.I., Hamilton, W.D., and Wakelin, D. (2002). Characterization of the immune response to canine parvovirus induced by vaccination with chimaeric plant viruses. *Vaccine* 20, 2727–2734.

Nichols, M.E., Stanislaus, T., Keshavarz-Moore, E., and Young, H.A. (2002). Disruption of leaves and initial extraction of wild-type CPMV virus as a basis for producing vaccines from plants. *J. Biotechnol.* 92, 229–235.

O'Brien, G.J., Bryant, C.J., Voogd, C., Greenberg, H.B., Gardner, R.C., and Bellamy, A.R. (2000). Rotavirus VP6 expressed by PVX vectors in Nicotiana benthamiana coats PVX rods and also assembles into virus like particles. *Virology* 270, 444–453.

Pogue, G.P., Lindbo, J.A., Garger, S.J., and Fitzmaurice, W.P. (2002). Making an ally from an enemy: plant virology and the new agriculture. *Annu. Rev. Phytopathol.* 40, 45–74.

Porta, C., and Lomonossoff, G.P. (1996). Use of viral replicons for the expression of genes in plants. *Mol. Biotechnol.* 5, 209–221.

Porta, C., and Lomonossoff, G.P. (1998). Scope for using plant viruses to present epitopes from animal pathogens. *Rev. Med. Virol.* 8, 25–41.

Porta, C., and Lomonossoff, G.P. (2002). Viruses as vectors for the expression of foreign sequences in plants. *Biotechnol. Genet. Eng. Rev.* 19, 245–291.

Porta, C., Spall, V.E., Loveland, J., Johnson, J.E., Barker, P.J., and Lomonossoff, G.P. (1994). Development of cowpea mosaic virus as a high-yielding system for the presentation of foreign peptides. *Virology* 202, 949–955.

Porta, C., Spall, V.E., Lin, T., Johnson, J.E., and Lomonossoff, G.P. (1996). The development of cowpea mosaic virus as a potential source of novel vaccines. *Intervirology* 39, 79–84.

Porta, C., Spall, V.E., Findlay, K.C., Gergerich, R.C., Farrance, C.E., and Lomonossoff, G.P. (2003). Cowpea mosaic virus-based chimaeras: effects of inserted peptides on the phenotype, host-range and transmissibility of the modified viruses. *Virology* 310, 50–63.

Rabindran, S., and Dawson, W.O. (2001). Assessment of recombinants that arise from the use of a TMV-based transient expression vector. *Virology* 284, 182–189.

Rennermalm, A., Li, Y.H., Bohaufs, L., Jarstrand, C., Brauner, A., Brennan, F.R., and Flock, J.I. (2001). Antibodies against a truncated Staphylococcus aureus fibronectin-binding protein protect against dissemination of infection in the rat. *Vaccine* 19, 3376–3383.

Sanchez-Navarro, J., Miglino, R., Ragozzini, A., and Bol, J.F. (2001). Engineering of alfalfa mosaic virus RNA 3 into an expression vector. *Arch. Virol.* 146, 923–939.

Santa Cruz, S., Chapman, S., Roberts, A.G., Roberts, I.M., Prior, D.A., and Oparka, K.J. (1996). Assembly and movement of a plant virus carrying a green fluorescent protein overcoat. *Proc. Natl. Acad. Sci. USA* 93, 6286–6290.

Scholthof, H.B. (1999). Rapid delivery of foreign genes into plants by direct rub-inoculation with intact plasmid DNA of a tomato bushy stunt virus gene vector. *J. Virol.* 73, 7823–7829.

Scholthof, H.B., Morris, T.J., and Jackson, A.O. (1993). The capsid protein gene of tomato bushy stunt virus is dispensable for systemic movement and can be replaced for localized expression of foreign genes. *Mol. Plant-Microbe Interact.* 6, 309–322.

Scholthof, H.B., Scholthof, K.B., and Jackson, A.O. (1996). Plant virus gene vectors for transient expression of foreign proteins in plants. *Annu. Rev. Phytopathol.* 34, 299–323.

Siegel, A. (1985) Plant-virus-based vectors for gene transfer may be of considerable use despite a presumed high error frequency during RNA synthesis. *Plant Mol. Biol.* 4, 327–329.

Sjölander, S., Hansen, J.-E., Lövgren-Bengtsson, K., Åkerblom, L., and Morein, B. (1996). Induction of homologous virus neutralizing antibodies in guinea-pigs immunized with two human immunodeficiency virus type I glycoprotein gp120-iscom preparations. A comparison with other adjuvant systems. *Vaccine* 14, 344–352.

Smolenska, L., Roberts, I.M., Learmonth, D., Porter, A.J., Harris, W.J., Wilson, T.M., and Santa Cruz, S. (1998). Production of a functional single chain antibody attached to the surface of a plant virus. *FEBS Lett.* 441, 379–382.

Staczek, J., Bendahmane, M., Gilleland, L.B., Beachy, R.N., and Gilleland, H.E., Jr. (2000). Immunization with a chimeric tobacco mosaic virus containing an epitope of outer membrane protein F of Pseudomonas aeruginosa provides protection against challenge with P. aeruginosa. *Vaccine* 18, 2266–2274.

Sugiyama, Y., Hamamoto, H., Takemoto, S., Watanabe, Y., and Okada, Y. (1995). Systemic production of foreign peptides on the particle surface of tobacco mosaic virus. *FEBS Lett.* 359, 247–250.

Takamatsu, N., Ishikawa, M., Meshi, T., and Okada, Y. (1987) Expression of bacterial chloramphenicol acetyltransferase gene in tobacco plants mediated by TMV-RNA. *EMBO J.* 6, 307–311.

Takamatsu N, Watanabe Y, Yanagi H, Meshi T, Shiba T, and Okada Y. (1990). Production of enkephalin in tobacco protoplasts using tobacco mosaic virus RNA vector. *FEBS Lett.* 269, 73–76.

Taylor, K.M., Porta, C., Lin, T., Johnson, J.E., Barker, P.J., and Lomonossoff, G.P., (1999). Position-dependent processing of peptides presented on the surface of cowpea mosaic virus. *J. Biol. Chem.* 380, 387–392.

Taylor, K.M., Lin, T., Porta, C., Mosser, A.G., Giesing, H.A., Lomonossoff, G.P., and Johnson, J.E. (2000). Influence of three-dimensional structure on the immunogenicity of a peptide expressed on the surface of a plant virus. *J. Mol. Recognit.* 13, 71–82.

Turpen, T.H., Reinl, S.J., Charoenvit, Y., Hoffman, S.L., Fallarme, V., and Grill, L.K. (1995). Malarial epitopes expressed on the surface of recombinant tobacco mosaic virus. *Biotechnology* 13, 53–57.

Usha, R., Rohll, J.B., Spall, V.E., Shanks, M., Maule. A.J., Johnson, J.E., and Lomonossoff, G.P. (1993). Expression of an animal virus antigenic site on the surface of a plant virus particle. *Virology* 197, 366–374.

van Vloten-Doting, L., Bol, J.F., and Cornelissen, B. (1985). Plant virus-based vectors for gene transfer will be of limited use because of the high error frequency during viral RNA synthesis. *Plant Mol. Biol.* 4, 323–326.

Verch, T., Yusibov, V., and Koprowski, H. (1998). Expression and assembly of a full-length monoclonal antibody in plants using a plant virus vector. *J. Immunol. Methods* 220, 69–75.

Wigdorovitz, A., Perez Filgueira, D.M., Robertson, N., Carillo, C., Sadir, A.M., Morris, T.J., and Borca, M.V. (1999). Protection of mice against challenge with foot and mouth disease virus (FMDV) by immunization with foliar extracts from plants infected with recombinant tobacco mosaic virus expressing the FMDV structural protein VP1. *Virology* 264, 85–91.

Yusibov, V., Modelska, A., Steplewski, K., Agadjanyan, M., Weiner, D., Hooper, D.C., and Koprowski, H. (1997). Antigens produced in plants by infection with chimeric plant viruses immunize against rabies virus and HIV-1. *Proc. Natl. Acad. Sci. USA* 94, 5784–5788.

Zhang, G.C., Leung, C., Murdin, L., Rovinski, B., and White, K.A. (2000). In planta expression of HIV-1 p24 protein using an RNA plant virus-based expression vector. *Mol. Biotechnol.* 14, 99–107.

Ziegler, A., Cowan, G.H., Torrance, L., Ross, H.A., and Davies, H.V. (2000). Facile assessment of cDNA constructs for expression of functional antibodies in plants using the potato virus X vector. *Mol. Breeding* 6, 327–335.

DNA Vaccines for Mucosal Immunity to Infectious Diseases

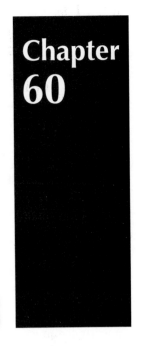

Chapter 60

John E. Herrmann

Division of Infectious Diseases and Immunology, University of Massachusetts Medical School, Worcester, Massachusetts

Harriet L. Robinson

Division of Microbiology and Immunology, Yerkes Primate Research Center of Emory University, Atlanta, Georgia

DNA vaccines are plasmid DNAs encoding specific proteins that can be expressed in cells of an inoculated host. The plasmids used are eukaryotic expression vectors, which contain the necessary elements for expression in eukaryotic cells. Plasmid DNAs encoding α-galactosidase, luciferase, or acetylcholine transferase expressed these enzymes in muscle cells after injection of the plasmid into the quadriceps of mice (Wolff *et al.*, 1990). Enzyme production in muscle tissue was detected up to 2 months after inoculation. Others have described production of antibodies to human growth hormone by gene gun immunization of DNA-coated gold microparticles, demonstrating that plasmid DNAs could be administered by this route and elicit antibody production (Tang *et al.*, 1992).

The first DNA vaccines that demonstrated protective immunity in animal models were described in 1993 for plasmids encoding influenza hemagglutinin (Robinson *et al.*, 1993; Fynan *et al.*, 1993) and influenza nucleoprotein (Ulmer *et al.*, 1993). Most studies to date have involved administration of DNA vaccines by intramuscular, intravenous, or intradermal injection or by gene-gun delivery of DNA-coated particles into the epidermis. Of these methods, gene-gun delivery requires the least amount of DNA to induce immune responses (Fynan *et al.*, 1993; Robinson *et al.*, 1997).

DNA vaccines have inherent advantages over traditional inactivated whole microbial vaccines and subunit vaccines. For one, they do not require the use of purified proteins or viral vectors. More important, vaccines that use inactivated microorganisms or their components do not provide endogenously synthesized proteins and generally do not elicit cytotoxic T lymphocyte (CTL) responses, which are important in controlling infection. The use of DNA vaccines encoding specific microbial proteins is an approach to subunit vaccines that allows for the expression of immunizing proteins by host cells that take up the inoculated DNA. Expression of the immunizing proteins in host cells results in the presentation of normally processed proteins to the immune system, which is important for inducing immune responses against the native forms of proteins (Webster *et al.*, 1994). Expression of the immunogen in host cells also results in the immunogen having access to class I major histocompatibility complex presentation, which is necessary for eliciting CD8+ CTL responses.

Inoculation of DNA has been shown to generate protective immunity for several viral, bacterial, and parasitic agents in animal models. A few examples of protective models for DNA vaccines for viruses include cytomegalovirus (Gonzalez-Armas *et al.*, 1996), influenza A viruses (Fynan *et al.*, 1993; Ulmer *et al.*, 1993), lymphocytic choriomeningitis virus (Martins *et al.*, 1995; Yokoyama *et al.*, 1995; Zarozinski *et al.*, 1995), hepatitis B virus (Prince *et al.*, 1997), herpes simplex virus (HSV) type 1 (Ghiasi *et al.*, 1995; Manickan *et al.*, 1995) and type 2 (Bourne *et al.*, 1996; Kriesel *et al.*, 1996; McClements *et al.*, 1996), human immunodeficiency virus (HIV) type 1 (Boyer *et al.*, 1997), infectious hematopoietic necrosis virus (Anderson *et al.*, 1996), papillomavirus (Donnelly *et al.*, 1996; Sundarum *et al.*, 1997), rabies virus (Xiang *et al.*, 1994, 1995), rotavirus (Herrmann *et al.*, 1996 a,b), and St. Louis encephalitis virus (Phillpotts *et al.*, 1996). Some examples of protective models for DNA vaccines against bacteria include those for *Borrelia burgdorferi* (Simon *et al.*, 1996; Zhong *et al.*, 1996; Luke *et al.*, 1997), *Mycoplasma pulmonis* (Barry *et al.*, 1995), and *Mycobacterium tuberculosis* (Huygen *et al.*, 1996; Tascon *et al.*, 1996). Examples of protective immune responses with DNA vaccines for parasitic infections include *Leishmania major* (Xu and Liew, 1996), *Plasmodium yoelii* (Sedegah *et al.*, 1994; Doolan *et al.*, 1996; Gramzinski *et al.*, 1996), and *Taenia ovis* (Rothel *et al.*, 1997).

Protective immune responses to many other infectious agents have been obtained with DNA vaccines, so it can be expected that DNA vaccine models will continue to be developed. We found in a current search (mid-2003) that more than 2500 articles on all aspects of DNA vaccines have been published, and a study in 1999 noted that more than 1000 different published reports were found concerning DNA vaccines for viral, bacterial, and parasitic agents (Lewis and Babiuk, 1999). The protection studies elicited by DNA vaccines cited above were done primarily in mice, but numerous other animal models have been described, including nonhuman primates. For example, protection elicited by DNA vaccination against influenza has been shown in ferrets, chickens, primates (Fynan *et al.* 1993; Robinson *et al.* 1993; Webster *et al.*, 1994; Donnelly *et al.*, 1995), and pigs (Macklin *et al.*, 1998). Protection against HSV-2 has been demonstrated in guinea pigs (Bourne *et al.*, 1996), protection against infectious hematopoietic necrosis virus in rainbow trout (Anderson *et al.*, 1996), and protection against hepatitis B virus and HIV-1 in chimpanzees (Boyer *et al.*, 1997; Prince *et al.*, 1997). Protection against rabies virus was obtained in cynomolgus monkeys (Lodmell *et al.*, 1998), and protection against vaccinia virus has been shown in rhesus monkeys (Hooper *et al.*, 2003). Turkeys were protected against *Chlamydia psittaci* by DNA vaccination (Vanrompay *et al.*, 1999). Sheep immunized with a DNA vaccine and boosted with a recombinant adenovirus vaccine against the cestode parasite *Taenia ovis* were protected against experimental challenge (Rothel *et al.*, 1997), and DNA vaccination protected pigs against *Taenia solium* (Wang *et al.*, 2003). In large animals, the route of immunization may influence the magnitude of the immune responses obtained (Babiuk *et al.*, 2003; De Rose *et al.*, 2002).

Studies concerning the clinical effectiveness of DNA vaccines with regard to protection induced by DNA vaccines or their therapeutic use are in progress. A DNA vaccine against HIV has been tested for safety and immunogenicity (MacGregor *et al.*, 1998), and malaria DNA vaccines have been found in volunteers to elicit CD8+ CTLs (Wang *et al.*, 1998; Wang *et al.*, 2001) and IFN-γ (Wang *et al.*, 2001) but not antibody (Le *et al.*, 2000; Epstein *et al.*, 2002). A hepatitis B viral DNA vaccine inoculated into volunteers by gene gun resulted in the induction of serum antibodies to hepatitis B virus surface antigen at concentrations considered to be protective, showing promise for the DNA vaccine approach (Roy *et al.*, 2000). One report that is encouraging for a therapeutic application of DNA vaccines involved a DNA vaccine against papillomavirus proteins. In a phase II clinical study designed to determine the effectiveness of the vaccine in treating papillomavirus-induced cervical dysplasia, it was found that the dysplasia resolved in 70% of women ≤25 years of age after treatment with the DNA vaccine (Garcia *et al.*, 2003).

To date, DNA vaccines have proven to be safe and well tolerated. Safety concerns for DNA vaccines include two major areas: possible integration of vaccine DNA into host cell genomes and generation of antibodies to vaccine DNA. Studies to date have not shown development of antivaccine DNA antibodies (Mor *et al.*, 1997). Integration of plasmid DNA with Ig gene transcription units into B cells (Xiong *et al.*, 1997) and of DNA delivered to macrophages with an attenuated *Listeria monocytogenes* (Dietrich *et al.*, 1998) has been shown, but this phenomenon has not been reported for saline or gene gun injections of conventional vaccine plasmids. For example, others did not detect integration of vaccine DNA after intramuscular injection of mice (Martin *et al.*, 1999), and on the basis of the amount of plasmid DNA that was associated with purified genomic DNA, it was not considered a potential safety threat. Others have also concluded that the risk of integration of DNA into the host cell genome is lower than that of naturally occurring mutations (Ledwith *et al.*, 2000).

Possible induction of tolerance has been another concern. It was reported that a DNA vaccine against the circumsporozoite protein of the malarial parasite that induced protection in adult mice induced tolerance when given to 2- to 6-day-old BALB/c mice (Mor *et al.*, 1996). However, tolerance in viral infections has not been demonstrated. Immunization of neonatal mice with plasmid DNA encoding rabies virus glycoprotein did not induce tolerance (Wang, Xiang *et al.*, 1997), and newborn mice immunized with plasmid DNA encoding influenza virus nucleoprotein or hemagglutinin developed protective immunity, as measured by reduction of virus lung titer after challenge (Bot *et al.*, 1996; Pertmer *et al.*, 1999).

In this chapter we discuss mucosal immunity primarily in the context of DNA vaccination against infectious agents. However, it should be noted that plasmid DNAs encoding various proteins are being used in applications such as prevention of autoimmune disorders (Waisman *et al.*, 1996), treatment of allergies (Hsu *et al.*, 1996; Raz *et al.*, 1996), and production of monoclonal and polyclonal antibodies (Barry *et al.*, 1994; Robinson *et al.*, 1996; Sundaram *et al.*, 1996) and as an approach to the control of cancer (Syrengelas *et al.*, 1996). These and other applications have been reviewed (Robinson and Torres, 1997; Manickan *et al.*, 1997; Gurunathan *et al.*, 2000).

MUCOSAL DELIVERY SYSTEMS FOR DNA VACCINES

Induction of mucosal immunity by direct immunization of mucosal surfaces has been considered for many vaccination approaches, including those involving DNA vaccines. The potential advantage of mucosal immunization with DNA vaccines would be the ability to target immune responses at the site of microbial entry while stimulating general systemic immunity. However, whereas techniques for mucosal immunization with antigens have been well developed over several years, techniques for targeting DNA vaccines to mucosal surfaces remain in the early stages of development. While some approaches for mucosal immunization with DNA vaccines share delivery systems with those used for antigen delivery, some reflect the uniqueness of DNA vaccination. An example of the latter is the use of biolistic (gene gun) methods.

Biolistic (gene gun) vaccination

The gene gun is a device designed to propel DNA-coated gold microparticles into the epidermis or other tissues. The gold particles generally are 1 to 3 μm in diameter. Gene gun immunization of the epidermis has resulted in immunity to pathogens that invade mucosal surfaces, and it may be that epidermal inoculation is as effective in inducing immunity at distal mucosal sites as that obtained by direct mucosal immunization. This possibility has been tested in several models. In a murine rotavirus model, protection obtained by gene gun delivery to perineal tissue was higher than that for the same DNA vaccine given by gene gun immunization of skin at the same dose (Chen et al., 1999). This suggested that direct mucosal immunization could be a more effective means to generate protective immunity against mucosal pathogens.

DNA vaccines have also been administered to the vaginal mucosa, on the premise that IgA can be produced locally in the cervix and vagina upon vaginal challenge. Rats inoculated by gene gun delivery of a plasmid DNA encoding human growth hormone to the vaginal epithelium expressed the hormone in vaginal tissues at levels comparable to those obtained with gene gun administration of the same plasmid DNA to skin (Livingston et al., 1995, 1998). In cattle, intravulvomucosal delivery of a plasmid encoding bovine herpesvirus 1 gB induced strong cellular immune responses, although the cattle were not protected against challenge (Loehr et al., 2000), and gene gun delivery to the vagina of cattle with a plasmid encoding bovine herpesvirus 1 gD induced immunity at other mucosal surfaces (nasal secretions) as well as in the vagina (Babiuk et al., 2003). Gene gun delivery to the Peyer's patches of rabbits with a plasmid encoding a portion of HIV-1 gp 160 yielded IgA antibody responses in both fecal and vaginal washes (Winchell et al., 1998). DNA vaccines encoding influenza hemagglutinins given by gene gun to the tongue of pigs resulted in more effective mucosal immunity than that obtained by gene gun delivery to the epidermis (Macklin et al., 1998; Larsen and Olsen, 2000).

Most studies utilizing gene gun delivery of DNA vaccines into the epidermis show that the predominant T-helper response is of a Th2 type. Mucosal inoculation by gene gun also elicits primarily Th2-type responses (Chen et al., 1999; McCluskie et al., 1999). This is in contrast to that generally found following saline injections of DNA, which elicit Th1-type responses **(Table 60.1)**. The mechanisms that determine the predominant Th cell response induced by different routes of plasmid DNA inoculation have not been established. When DNA vaccines are injected intramuscularly, it

has been postulated that the adjuvant effect of unmethylated CpG sequences in plasmid DNA acting through the Toll 9–like receptor selectively activates stimuli for Th1-type responses (for reviews see McCluskie et al., 2001; Krieg, 2002). It appears that the method, not the target site, of DNA inoculation is the more important factor in the type of response generated. In studies by others, it was found that saline-DNA injections into skin or muscle generated Th1-type responses, whereas gene gun delivery of the same DNA to skin or to muscle raised Th2-type responses (Feltquate et al., 1997).

Mucosal inoculation with naked DNA

Inoculation of mucosal surfaces with DNA vaccines has the potential for providing effective mucosal protection at proximal as well as distal sites. Direct application of naked DNA to mucosal sites has been attempted by several routes and methods. Direct injection of naked DNA vaginally generated mucosal immune responses in both mice and primates (Wang, Dang et al., 1997; Bagarazzi et al., 1997). Rectal immunization of mice with an HIV DNA vaccine also generated mucosal antibodies and CTL responses (Hamajima et al., 2002), and rectal immunization of rhesus monkeys with an SIV vaccine generated IgA antibodies and some protection if combined with intradermal administration (Wang et al., 2000). Application of plasmid DNA encoding herpesvirus glycoprotein B to ocular surfaces in mice generated protective immunity against challenge and generated mucosal antibody at ocular as well as vaginal and intestinal distal sites (Daheshia et al., 1998).

Needle-free jet delivery devices have been used to administer naked DNA to the epidermis of humans (Epstein et al., 2002) and animals (van Rooij et al., 1998). The use of a jet delivery device has also been used to apply naked DNA to a mucosal surface. A high-pressure jet injector used in dentistry was used to inject plasmid against HIV-1 into the buccal cavity of mice (Lundholm et al., 1999). This method generated overall higher IgA responses in lung lavages and intestinal washes than those obtained with DNA administered nasally, by injection of the tongue, or by gene gun delivery to the oral cavity. Another method of administering naked DNA mucosally has been mixing plasmid DNA with melted suppositories and administering them to the vagina of cattle (Loehr et al., 2001; Babiuk et al., 2003).

Nasal inoculation has been tested in many studies for both respiratory and nonrespiratory pathogens. Studies with influenza virus have shown that nasal immunization with DNA vaccines resulted in protection in mice, but the vaccines were not as effective with gene gun epidermal immunization (Fynan et al., 1993). The same influenza DNA vaccine given nasally has been compared with that given intramuscularly for induction of mucosal immunity, with and without cationic lipids or cholera toxin (CT). No influenza-specific serum antibodies were detected in these studies, but antihemagglutinin-secreting B cells were detected in spleen and lung cells when CT was codelivered with the DNA vaccine (Ban et al., 1997).

Table 60.1. Examples of Techniques Used for DNA Immunization and Their Characteristics in Murine Models

Method	Model	Predominant Serum Antibody Isotype	Subset of T-Helper Response	Comment	Reference(s)
Intramuscular injection	Influenza virus	IgG2a	Th1	Cell-associated form of antigen	Feltquate et al., 1997, and Torres et al., 1999
		IgG1	Th2	Secreted form of antigen	Mavickian et al., 1994
	Herpes simplex virus	IgG2a	Th1	Cell-associated form of antigen	Higgins et al., 2000
		IgG1	Th2	Secreted form of antigen	
Gene gun, epidermis	Influenza virus	IgG1	Th2	Requires 25–100 fold less DNA than i.m.	Feltquate et al., 1997, and Pertmer et al., 1996
Gene gun, perineum/ anal mucosa	Rotavirus	IgG1	Th2	Required 5-fold less DNA than gene gun to epidermis	Chen et al., 1999
Nasal	HIV-1	IgG2a	Th1	Similar profile found with oral jet injector	Lundholm et al., 1999
Nasal with cholera toxin	Herpes simplex virus	IgG1	Th2	Induced vaginal IgA	Kuklin et al., 1997
Nasal in *Shigella* vector	Measles virus	IgG2a	Th1	Responses equal to *Salmonella* vector i.m.	Fennelly et al., 1999
Nasal, liposome-mediated	Mumps virus	IgG2a	Th1	IL-10 level indicated Th2 as well	Cusi et al., 2000
Oral delivery in PLG microparticles	Rotavirus	IgG1	Th2	Induced intestinal IgA	Chen et al., 1998; Herrmann et al., unpublished data

The nasal route has also been compared with the intramuscular route for induction of mucosal immunity by DNA vaccination against herpes simplex virus (Kuklin et al., 1997). In this study, nasal administration of a DNA vaccine encoding glycoprotein B of herpes simplex type 1 resulted in a distal IgA response in vaginal secretions. Coadministration of CT enhanced the IgA responses. Results of antigen-specific cytokine ELISPOT analyses and the serum IgG1/IgG2a ratios obtained indicated that Th2-type responses were generated by nasal coadministration of the vaccine with CT. Thus, this inoculation protocol gave Th responses similar to those found in studies that have used gene gun immunization. The intramuscular route induced a strong IgG response in the serum and vagina but was less efficient in generating mucosal IgA responses. However, in protection studies, intramuscular injection (despite the inefficient generation of IgA) was more effective than nasal inoculation in protecting against a lethal vaginal challenge of herpes simplex virus, although neither inoculation route prevented virus infection of the mucosa.

In another study comparing routes of DNA vaccine immunization against herpes simplex viruses, both the intradermal and intramuscular routes produced mucosal immune responses comparable to those obtained by nasal inoculation of the vaccine (Shroff et al., 1999). HIV DNA vaccines given nasally also have resulted in mucosal immune responses (Asakura et al., 1997; Hinkula et al., 1997; Hamajima et al., 1998; Sasaki et al., 1998; Xin et al., 1999). In a comparison of nasal and intramuscular administration to mice of the same HIV DNA vaccine, it was found that both routes gave similar levels of cell-mediated immunity, but the intestinal IgA response was higher in mice that received the vaccine nasally (Sasaki et al., 1998). Studies utilizing nasal administration of DNA complexed with liposomes have also been reported (see the following section on liposomes).

A study investigating the absorption and biodistribution of DNA administered nasally showed that plasmid DNA appeared in the serum and in lymph nodes, which could explain in part the systemic immunogenicity obtained after inoculation of DNA by this route (Oh et al., 2001). It has also been found that nasal administration of DNA vaccines is associated with the expression of the encoded protein in dendritic cells and macrophages at the site of DNA delivery, as well as in the spleen and lymph nodes (Barnfield *et al.*, 2000).

It may be expected that naked DNA given orally would be degraded by nucleases before significant uptake could occur, but it has been shown that naked DNA can yield immune responses when given in this manner. A plasmid encoding luciferase induced antibody responses, although encapsulation in microparticles enhanced the responses (Jones, Clegg *et al.*, 1997). DNA encoding measles antigen given orally generated CTL responses to that antigen (Etchart *et al.*, 1997), and partial protection was obtained after oral administration of a naked rotavirus VP7 DNA vaccine, although encapsulation in microparticles enhanced the responses, as found with the luciferase plasmid cited above (Herrmann *et al.*, 1999). DNA has also induced mucosal immunity after being injected into the oral cavity of lambs *in utero* (Gerdts *et al.*, 2002).

Liposomes

Liposomes have been used for targeted drug delivery and have been studied as vaccine delivery systems for antigens. Liposomes have adjuvant activity that results in lesser amounts of antigen being required to generate an immune response. The liposomes are taken up by macrophages and M cells and thus are suitable for targeting antigens in mucosal immunization (Michalek *et al.*, 1994, 1999). Liposomes have been used to facilitate transfection of cells *in vitro* by DNA and RNA. They also have been used to mediate gene transfer to lung cells *in vivo* in mice (Wheeler *et al.*, 1996) and in rhesus monkeys (Fortunati *et al.*, 1996). A potentially effective means to deliver lipid-DNA complexes to lung tissue would be through the use of aerosols, and methods have been described for these types of deliveries (Eastman *et al.*, 1997).

Intramuscular immunization of mice with a plasmid DNA encoding the S region of hepatitis B antigen entrapped in cationic liposomes resulted in improved humoral and cell-mediated immune responses. Cationic liposome–entrapped DNA vaccines yielded 100-fold higher antibody titers and increased levels of both IFN-γ and IL-4 than either naked DNA or DNA complexed with preformed similar cationic liposomes (Gregoriadis *et al.*, 1997). In addition to adjuvant effects and possible protection of DNA from nucleases, injected DNA complexed with liposomes facilitates uptake of plasmid DNA by antigen-presenting cells (Perrie *et al.*, 2001; Gregoriadis *et al.*, 2002). The ability of liposomes to enhance the effectiveness of DNA vaccines may depend on the liposome composition (Gregoriadis *et al.*, 2002). The type of liposome used may also affect the type of T-helper response obtained by DNA vaccination (Jiao *et al.*, 2003).

Mucosal delivery of DNA-liposome complexes has been primarily by the nasal route. It has been shown that nasal administration of plasmid DNA encoding luciferase results in dissemination of the DNA in respiratory and gastrointestinal tracts, draining lymph nodes, and spleens and

enhances the expression of the encoded protein in the respiratory tract. Luciferase-specific IgA responses were detected in both vaginal and rectal fluids (Klavinskis *et al.*, 1999).

Nasal administration of DNA vaccines to infectious agents has been described for HIV (Mitchell *et al.*, 1995; Ishii *et al.*, 1997; Okada *et al.*, 1997), mumps virus (Cusi *et al.*, 2000), and influenza virus (Wong *et al.*, 2001). Mucosal immune responses have been obtained in all these studies, and in the influenza model, mice were protected against influenza virus challenge (Wong *et al.*, 2001).

Other mucosal routes have also been tested. Cationic lipoplexes of a DNA vaccine to influenza nucleoprotein instilled into salivary glands of rats generated systemic antibody responses to nucleoprotein and IgA responses to nucleoprotein in saliva (Sankar *et al.*, 2002). Oral delivery of plasmid DNA encoding hepatitis B surface antigen incorporated in liposomes resulted in higher antigen-specific IgA responses in mice than did oral administration of naked DNA (Perrie *et al.*, 2002).

Live bacterial vectors

The possibility of directing a plasmid DNA to mucosal sites by using bacterial vectors as delivery vehicles was first tested with use of an attenuated strain of *Shigella flexneri* (Sizemore *et al.*, 1995). The *S. flexneri* strain contained a eukaryotic expression vector with DNA encoding the enzyme β-galactosidase. The enzyme was able to be expressed in infected cell cultures. A potential advantage of this type of system is that it may enhance local immunity at the target site. A disadvantage of using live bacterial vectors is that the process involves cell invasion, with its subsequent reactogenicity (Sizemore *et al.*, 1995, 1997), and in the case of *Listeria monocytogenes*, it may lead to integration of the DNA (Dietrich *et al.*, 1998).

The use of live vectors for mucosal delivery of DNA vaccines against infectious agents has been described for both *Shigella* and *Salmonella* vectors. The primary route of administration has been nasal, and some have been given by the oral route. Nasal vaccination with a *Shigella*-HIV gp 120 DNA vaccine vector was found to elicit in mice a CD8+ T-cell response to gp 120 that was equivalent in magnitude to that developed by intramuscular inoculation of the gp 120 DNA vaccine (Shata and Hone, 2001). In another HIV study, nasal delivery of an HIV DNA vaccine contained in *S. flexneri* yielded higher levels of HIV-specific IgA antibodies in vaginal washings than obtained with intramuscular delivery of the DNA vaccine (Vecino *et al.*, 2002). Nasal immunization with a *S. flexneri* vaccine vector containing a measles virus DNA vaccine resulted in measles virus–specific CD8+ CTL responses (Fennelly *et al.*, 1999). Strains of both *S. enterica* and *S. flexneri* have been used to deliver DNA vaccines encoding measles virus hemagglutinin nasally to cotton rats. The vaccination schemes reduced the measles virus titers in lungs after the mice had been challenged with wild-type measles virus (Pasetti *et al.*, 2003).

S. typhimurium was used for oral delivery of a DNA vaccine encoding *L. monocytogenes* virulence factors, which protected immunized mice against subsequent challenge with *L. monocytogenes* (Darji *et al.*, 2000). Oral immunization with live *Shigella* and *Salmonella* containing HIV DNA vaccines is being developed as a prime-boost strategy as well (Devico *et al.*, 2002).

Polymeric microparticles

Administration of DNA vaccines by the oral route would provide a convenient means of delivery and would also target the vaccines to mucosal tissues. The use of antigens entrapped in biodegradable microparticles for use in oral immunization is an established experimental procedure (O'Hagen, 1994; Michalek *et al.*, 1999). Several polymers have been used to prepare encapsulated antigens for implantation or for subcutaneous, intraperitoneal, or intramuscular administration, such as polymethylmethacrylate, polyethylene-vinyl acetate, polyacryl-starch, and polylactide-co-glycolide (PLG) (reviewed by Michalek *et al.*, 1994). Antigens in PLG microspheres have also been given by the oral route. More recently, methods for encapsulation of plasmid DNA have been developed that permit the DNA to be orally administered. Plasmid DNA encoding β-galactosidase encapsulated in polymers of fumaric and sebacic acid was found to target the tissues of Peyer's patches (Mathiowitz *et al.*, 1997). It was not determined whether immune responses to β-galactosidase were obtained. Plasmid DNA encoding insect luciferase was encapsulated in PLG microparticles, and oral (or intraperitoneal) administration of these PLG microparticles stimulated serum IgG, IgA, and IgM antibodies to the expressed luciferase (Jones *et al.*, 1997). Luciferase-specific IgA was also detected in stool samples, indicating that a mucosal immune response had occurred. Plasmid DNA complexed with chitosan to form nanoparticles has been used for oral immunization of plasmid DNA encoding a peanut allergen, but as yet it has not been used for infectious disease antigens (Roy *et al.*, 1999).

The advantages of oral immunization with DNA in microparticles are similar to those considered for antigens in microparticles. Ease of administration is an important feature. There is evidence that microparticles are taken up into Peyer's patches, and in studies to date, encapsulated DNA vaccines appear to be protected from degradation in the gut, as evidenced by the immune responses obtained (Jones *et al.*, 1997; Mathiowitz *et al.*, 1997; Chen *et al.*, 1998, Herrmann *et al.*, 1999; Kaneko *et al.*, 2000; Fooks *et al.*, 2000 Wierzbicki *et al.*, 2002). Encapsulation also offers the possibility for more than one DNA vaccine to be encapsulated and administered simultaneously. Finally, the polymers that have been used for microencapsulation are nonimmunogenic and have a known record of safety. This has been shown in their use for other purposes, such as in drug delivery and in surgical suture materials.

The ability of PLG-encapsulated DNA vaccines to protect against virus challenge was demonstrated in a rotavirus model (Chen *et al.*, 1998). It was found that mice were protected against rotavirus challenge after PLG-encapsulated plasmid DNA encoding the rotavirus group antigen (VP6)

was given orally to the mice. In studies with live murine rotaviruses given orally to mice, protection against challenge was associated with rotavirus-specific intestinal IgA responses, and it was found that prior to challenge with live rotavirus, intestinal IgA antibodies were elicited in mice immunized with the rotavirus DNA vaccine. This did not occur in mice immunized by gene gun delivery of the same DNA vaccine (Herrmann *et al.*, 1996a,b), indicating that targeting of mucosal tissues may be advantageous for raising IgA antibodies. In additional studies, the use of DNA vaccines against the rotavirus neutralization antigens VP4 and VP7 also generated intestinal IgA responses and protected against rotavirus challenge (Herrmann *et al.*, 1999). Subsequent to these studies, it was found that oral immunization of a measles DNA vaccine encapsulated in PLG microparticles generated virus-specific serum IgG (Fooks *et al.*, 2000), and a PLG-encapsulated DNA vaccine to HIV gp 160 induced specific serum antibodies and an increased level of specific IgA in fecal washes (Kaneko *et al.*, 2000). The immunized mice were also more resistant to rectal challenge with an HIV recombinant vaccinia virus.

Another approach to enhancing mucosal immunity with use of microparticles has been to adsorb DNA onto cationic PLG microparticles that can be delivered mucosally as well as by other routes. Immunization of mice nasally with PLG-DNA encoding HIV gag protein generated CTL and both local and systemic antibody responses, whereas nasal immunization with naked DNA did not (Singh *et al.*, 2001).

Prime-boost immunization

Because DNA vaccines may not be sufficiently immunogenic when given alone, a strategy for improving their efficacy has evolved that involves priming with a DNA vaccine and boosting with a recombinant viral vector or proteins (for reviews see Schneider *et al.*, 1999; Ramshaw and Ramsay, 2000). It has been particularly effective in improving the efficacy of DNA vaccines for HIV (Robinson *et al.*, 1999; Amara *et al.*, 2002; Shiver *et al.*, 2002). Prime-boost immunization has also been done by priming with DNA and boosting with a live vaccine (Skinner *et al.*, 2003) or boosting with an oral plant-derived vaccine (Webster *et al.*, 2002). These approaches may result in immunity at mucosal sites, but it was found that giving a mucosal (nasal) priming dose of a DNA vaccine encoding herpes simplex virus glycoprotein B (gB), followed by boosting with a recombinant vaccinia virus expressing gB, enhanced mucosal antibody responses at distant sites, as measured by gB-specific IgA in vaginal lavages (Eo *et al.*, 2001). It was further found that nasal immunization with the recombinant vaccinia vector followed by intranasal boosting with the plasmid encoding gB yielded the optimal mucosal responses. Priming by gene gun delivery of a DNA vaccine against bovine herpesvirus glycoproteins B and D to mucosal tissue followed by a modified live virus vaccine enhanced T-cell responses (Loehr *et al.*, 2001), and mucosal gene gun delivery of a DNA vaccine against influenza hemagglutinin protein primed pigs for killed-virus vaccine boosting (Larsen *et al.*, 2001).

Prime-boost strategies that use priming by mucosal delivery of encapsulated DNA vaccines have also been developed to enhance responses to HIV or SIV. Oral immunization with a PLG-encapsulated DNA vaccine encoding HIV gp 160 followed by a recombinant vaccinia virus expressing gp 160 gave enhanced anti-gp-160 responses in systemic and mucosal tissues of immunized mice (Wierzbicki et al., 2002). Rectal delivery of a PLG-encapsulated DNA vaccine encoding a multi-CTL epitope gene primed an SIV-specific CTL response after boosting with a recombinant modified vaccinia Ankara vaccine (Sharpe et al., 2003).

Most of the studies examining immune responses to mucosal DNA immunization against infectious agents have not included challenge with the agent to determine protective immunity. Some of the ones that have shown protection are provided in **Table 60.2**. Although it may be assumed that induction of a mucosal IgA response by the various means outlined in this chapter would enhance protection, there may not be a direct correlation. As noted for the herpesvirus model (Kuklin et al., 1977) discussed earlier and cited in Table 60.2, the intramuscular route induced a strong IgG response in the serum and vagina but was less efficient than the nasal route in generating mucosal IgA responses in the vagina. However, in protection studies, the intramuscular route was found to be more effective in protecting against a lethal vaginal challenge of herpes simplex virus. More such studies are needed comparing the degree of protection obtained by mucosal DNA immunization versus systemic immunization with methods such as intramuscular injection, gene gun delivery, or other means that have been shown to give protective immunity.

CONCLUSIONS

The first reports on protective immunity elicited by DNA vaccination appeared in 1993 (Robinson et al., 1993; Fynan et al., 1993; Ulmer et al., 1993). On the basis of the expanding number of publications on the subject, it appears that the interest in DNA vaccines continues to grow. Applications for the control of human and veterinary diseases are still few and in the early phases of clinical trials, and selection and optimization of delivery methods will be important to DNA vaccine acceptance. The techniques discussed in this chapter all offer potential for stimulating improved immune responses with DNA vaccinations. Most are still in the early stages of development, and many of the techniques have not been widely applied to protection against infectious agents in model challenge systems. Plasmid DNAs have an advantage of being stable, in comparison with live attenuated vaccines,

Table 60.2. Protective Immune Responses Obtained by Mucosal DNA Vaccination

Method	Mucosal Tissue Targeted	Route	Infectious Agent	Animal Model	Reference
Naked DNA	Nasal tissue, lung	Nasal droplet	Influenza virus[a]	Mice	Fynan et al., 1993
			Herpes simplex virus[b]	Mice	Kuklin et al., 1997
			Pseudorabies virus[c]	Pigs	Van Rooij et al., 1998
			Chlamydia psittaci[c]	Turkeys	Vanrompay et al., 1999
	Intestinal tract	Oral	Rotavirus	Mice	Herrmann et al., 1999
		Rectal	SIV[d]	Monkeys	Wang et al., 2000
Gene gun	Oral mucosa	Tongue	Influenza virus	Pigs	Macklin et al., 1998; Larsen and Olsen, 2002
	Intestinal tract	Anal mucosa	Rotavirus	Mice	Chen et al., 1999
Liposome-mediated	Nasal tissue, lung	Nasal	Influenza virus	Mice	Wong et al., 2001
Bacterial vectors	Intestinal tract	Oral	Measles virus	Cotton rats	Pasetti et al., 2003
			Listeria monocytogenes	Mice	Darji et al., 2000
Polymeric microparticles	Intestinal tract	Oral	Rotavirus	Mice	Chen et al., 1998; Herrmann et al., 1999
Mucosal prime-boost	Oral mucosa	Tongue	Influenza virus	Pigs	Larsen et al., 2001

[a] Gene gun to epidermis and i.m. injections gave better protective immunity.
[b] Greater protection obtained by i.m. injection.
[c] The nasal route was combined with i.m. injection.
[d] Rectal injection was combined with intradermal injection.

but one area that will need more attention is the stability of various DNA vaccine formulations under different conditions of storage and transport.

The majority of studies of DNA vaccines have used intramuscular inoculation, a route that has been traditional for many vaccines. Some of the other routes of administration discussed here that target mucosal surfaces may prove to be more effective for some vaccine applications. The methods and routes of DNA vaccine administration that may ultimately find the widest acceptance are the ones that offer a combination of effective protection, convenience, and simplicity of administration.

ACKNOWLEDGMENTS

These studies were supported by grant R01 AI47393 (to J.E.H.) and grants P01 AI49364, P01 AI 43045, and R01 AI34946 (to H.L.R.) from the National Institutes of Health, Bethesda, Maryland.

REFERENCES

Amara, R.R., Villinger, F., Altman, J.D., Lydy, S.L., O'Neil, S.P., Staprans, S.I., Montefiori, D.C., Xu, Y., Herndon, J.G., Wyatt, L.S., Candido, M.A., Kozyr, N.L., Earl, P.L., Smith, J.M., Ma, H.L., Grimm, B.D., Hulsey, M.L., McClure, H.M., McNicholl, J.M., Moss, B., and Robinson, H.L. (2002). Control of a mucosal challenge and prevention of AIDS by a multiprotein DNA/MVA vaccine. *Vaccine* 20, 1949–1955.

Asakura, Y., Hinkula, J., Leandersson, A.C., Fukushima, J., Okuda, K., and Wahren, B. (1997). Induction of HIV-1 specific mucosal immune responses by DNA vaccination. *Scand. J. Immunol.* 46, 326–330.

Asakura, Y., Liu, L.J., Shono, N., Hinkula, J., Kjerrstrom, A., Aoki, I., Okuda, K., Wahren, B., and Fukushima, J. (2000). Th1-biased immune responses induced by DNA-based immunizations are mediated via action on professional antigen-presenting cells to up-regulate IL-12 production. *Clin. Exp. Immunol.* 119, 130–139.

Anderson, E.D., Mourich, D.V., Fahrenkrug, S.C., LaPatra, S., Shepherd, J., and Leong, J.A. (1996). Genetic immunization of rainbow trout (*Oncorhynchus mykiss*) against infectious hematopoietic necrosis virus. *Mol. Mar. Biol. Biotechnol.* 5, 114–122.

Babiuk, L.A., Pontarollo, R., Babiuk, S., Loehr, B., and van Drunen Littel-van den Hurk, S. (2003). Induction of immune responses by DNA vaccines in large animals. *Vaccine* 21, 649–658.

Bagarazzi, M.L., Boyer, J.D., Javadian, M.A., Chattergoon, M., Dang, K., Kim, G., Shah, J., Wang, B., Weiner, D.B. (1997). Safety and immunogenicity of intramuscular and intravaginal delivery of HIV-1 DNA constructs to infant chimpanzees. *J. Med. Primatol.* 26, 27–33.

Ban, E.M., van Ginkel, F.W., Simecka, J.W., Kiyono, H., Robinson, H.L., and McGhee, J.R. (1997). Mucosal immunization with DNA encoding influenza hemagglutinin. *Vaccine* 15, 811–813.

Barnfield, C., Brew, R., Tilling, R., Rae, A., Wheeler, C., and Klavinskis, L.S. (2000). The cellular basis of immune induction at mucosal surfaces by DNA vaccination. *Dev. Biol. (Basel)* 104, 159–164.

Barry, M.A., Barry, M.E., and Johnston, S.A. (1994). Production of monoclonal antibodies by genetic immunization. *BioTechniques* 16, 616–620.

Barry, M.A., Lai, W.C., and Johnston, S.A. (1995). Protection against mycoplasma infection using expression-library immunization. *Nature* 377, 632–635.

Bot, A., Bot, S., Garcia-Sastre A., and Bona, C. (1996). DNA immunization of newborn mice with a plasmid-expressing nucleoprotein of influenza virus. *Viral Immunol.* 9, 207–210.

Bourne, N., Milligan, G.N., Schleiss, M.R., Bernstein, D.I., and Stanberry, L.R. (1996). DNA immunization confers protective immunity on mice challenged intravaginally with herpes simplex virus type 2. *Vaccine* 14, 1230–1234.

Bourne, N., Stanberry, L.R., Bernstein, D.I., and Lew, D. (1996). DNA immunization against experimental genital herpes simplex virus infection. *J. Infect. Dis* 173, 800–807.

Boyer, J.D., Ugen, K.E., Wang, B., Agadjanyan, M., Gilbert, L., Bagarazzi, M.L., Chattergoon, M., Frost, P., Javadian, A., Williams, W.V., Refaeli, Y., Ciccarelli, R.B., McCallus, D., Coney, L., Weiner, D.B. (1997). Protection of chimpanzees from high-dose heterologous HIV-1 challenge by DNA vaccination. *Nat. Med.* 3, 526–532.

Chen, S.C., Fynan, E.F., Greenberg, H.B., and Herrmann, J.E. (1999). Immunity obtained by gene-gun inoculation of a rotavirus DNA vaccine to the abdominal epidermis or anorectal epithelium. *Vaccine* 17, 3171–3176.

Chen, S.C., Jones, D.H., Fynan, E.F., Farrar, G.H., Clegg, J.C., Greenberg, H.B. and Herrmann, J.E. (1998). Protective immunity induced by oral immunization with a rotavirus DNA vaccine encapsulated in microparticles. *J. Virol.* 72, 5757–5761.

Cusi, M.G., Zurbriggen, R., Valassina, M., Bianchi, S., Durrer, P., Valensin, P.E., Donati, M., and Gluck, R. (2000). Intranasal immunization with mumps virus DNA vaccine delivered by influenza virosomes elicits mucosal and systemic immunity. *Virology* 277, 111–118.

Daheshia, M., Kuklin, N., Manickan, E., Chun, S., and Rouse, B.T. (1998). Immune induction and modulation by topical ocular administration of plasmid DNA encoding antigens and cytokines. *Vaccine* 16, 1103–1110.

Darji, A., zur Lage, S., Garbe, A.I., Chakraborty, T., and Weiss, S. (2000). Oral delivery of DNA vaccines using attenuated *Salmonella typhimurium* as carrier. *FEMS Immunol. Med. Microbiol.* 27, 341–349.

De Rose, R., Tennent, J., McWaters, P., Chaplin, P.J., Wood, P.R., Kimpton, W., Cahill, R., and Scheerlinck, J.P. (2002). Efficacy of DNA vaccination by different routes of immunisation in sheep. *Vet. Immunol. Immunopathol.* 90, 55–63.

Devico, A.L., Fouts, T.R., Shata, M.T., Kamin-Lewis, R., Lewis, G.K., and Hone, D.M. (2002). Development of an oral prime-boost strategy to elicit broadly neutralizing antibodies against HIV-1. *Vaccine* 20, 1968–1974.

Dietrich, G., Bubert, A., Gentschev, I., Sokolovic, Z., Simm, A., Catic, A., Kaufmann, S.H., Hess, J., Szalay, A.A., and Goebel, W. (1998). Delivery of antigen-encoding plasmid DNA into the cytosol of macrophages by attenuated suicide *Listeria monocytogenes. Nat. Biotechnol.* 16, 181–185.

Donnelly, J.J., Friedman, A., Martinez, D., Montgomery, D.L., Shiver, J.W., Motzel, S.L., Ulmer, J.B., and Liu, M.A. (1995). Preclinical efficacy of a prototype DNA vaccine: enhanced protection against antigenic drift in influenza virus. *Nat. Med.* 1, 583–587.

Donnelly, J.J., Martinez, D., Jansen, K.U., Ellis, R.W., Montgomery, D.L., and Liu, M.A. (1996). Protection against papillomavirus with a polynucleotide vaccine. *J. Infect. Dis.* 713, 314–320.

Doolan, D.L., Sedegah, M., Hedstrom, R.C., Hobart, P., Charoenvit, Y., and Hoffman, S.L. (1996). Circumventing genetic restriction of protection against malaria with multigene DNA immunization : CD8+ cell-, interferon γ-, and nitric oxide–dependent immunity. *J. Exp. Med.* 183, 1739–1746.

Eastman, S.J., Lukason, M.J., Tousignant, J.D., Murray, H., Lane, M.D., St. George, J.A., Akita, G.Y., Cherry, M., Cheng, S.H., and Scheule, R.K. (1997). A concentrated and stable aerosol formulation of cationic lipid: DNA complexes giving high-level gene expression in mouse lung. *Hum. Gene. Ther.* 8, 765–773.

Eo, S.K., Gierynska, M., Kamar, A.A., and Rouse, B.T. (2001). Prime-boost immunization with DNA vaccine: mucosal route of administration changes the rules. *J. Immunol.* 166, 5473–5479.

Epstein, J.E., Gorak, E. J., Charoenvit, Y., Wang, R., Freydberg, N., Osinowo, O., Richie, T.L., Stoltz, E.L., Trespalacios, F., Nerges, J., Ng, J., Fallarme-Majam, V., Abot, E., Goh, L., Parker, S., Kumar, S., Hedstrom, R.C., Norman, J., Stout, R., and Hoffman, S.L. (2002). Safety, tolerability, and lack of antibody responses after administration of a PfCSP DNA malaria vaccine via needle or needle-free jet injection, and comparison of intramuscular and combination intramuscular/intradermal routes. *Hum. Gene Ther.* 13, 1551–1560.

Etchart, N., Buckland, R., Liu, M.A., Wild, T.F., and Kaiserlian, D. (1997). Class I–restricted CTL induction by mucosal immunization with naked DNA encoding measles virus haemagglutinin. *J. Gen. Virol.* 78, 1577–1580.

Feltquate, D.M., Heaney, S., Webster, R.G., and Robinson, H.L. (1997). Different T helper cell types and antibody isotypes generated by saline and gene gun DNA immunization. *J. Immunol.* 158, 2278–2284.

Fennelly, G.J., Khan, S.A., Abadi, M.A., Wild, T.F., and Bloom, B.R. (1999). Mucosal DNA vaccine immunization against measles with a highly attenuated *Shigella flexneri* vector. *J. Immunol.* 162, 1603–1610.

Fooks, A.R., Sharpe, S.A., Shallcross, J.A., Clegg, J.C., and Cranage, M.P. (2000). Induction of immunity using oral DNA vaccines expressing the measles virus nucleocapsid protein. *Dev. Biol. (Basel)* 104, 65–71.

Fortunati, E., Bout, A., Zanta, M.A., Valerio, D., and Scarpa, M. (1996). *In vitro* and *in vivo* gene transfer to pulmonary cells mediated by cationic liposomes. *Biochem. Biophys. Acta.* 1306, 55–62.

Fynan, E.F., Webster, R.G., Fuller, D.H., Haynes, J.R., Santoro, J.C., and Robinson, H.L. (1993). DNA vaccines: protective immunizations by parenteral, mucosal, and gene-gun inoculations. *Proc. Natl. Acad. Sci. USA* 90, 11478–11482.

Garcia, F., Petry, K.U., Muderspach, L., Gold, M.A., Braly, P., Crum, C.P., Magill, M., Silverman, M., Urban, R., Hedley, M.L., and Beach, K.J. (2004). ZYC101a for treatment of high-grade cervical intraepithelial neoplasia: a randomized controlled trial. *Obstet. Gynecol.* 103, 317–326.

Gerdts, V., Snider, M., Brownlie, R., Babiuk, L.A., and Griebel, P.J. (2002). Oral DNA vaccination in utero induces mucosal immunity and immune memory in the neonate. *J. Immunol.* 168, 1877–1885.

Ghiasi, H., Cai, S., Slanina, S., Nesburn, A.B., and Wechsler, S.L. (1995). Vaccination of mice with herpes simplex virus type 1 glycoprotein D DNA produces low levels of protection against lethal HSV-1 challenge. *Antiviral Res.* 28, 147–157.

Gonzalez Armas, J.C., Morello, C.S., Cranmer, L.D., and Spector, D.H. (1996). DNA immunization confers protection against murine cytomegalovirus infection. *J. Virol.* 70, 7921–7928.

Gramzinski, R.A., Maris, D.C., Obaldia, N., Rossan, R., Sedegah, M., Wang, R., Hobart, P., Margalith, M., and Hoffman, S. (1996). Optimization of antibody responses of a malaria DNA vaccine in *Aotus* monkeys. *Vaccine Res.* 5, 173–184.

Gregoriadis, G., Saffie, R., and de Souza, J.B. (1997). Liposome-mediated DNA vaccination. *FEBS Lett.* 402, 107–110.

Gregoriadis, G., Bacon, A., Caparros-Wanderley, W., and McCormack, B. (2002). A role for liposomes in genetic vaccination. *Vaccine* 20, Suppl 5:B1–B9.

Gurunathan, S., Klinman, D.M., and Seder, R.A. (2000). DNA vaccines: immunology, application, and optimization. *Annu. Rev. Immunol.* 18, 927–974.

Hamajima, K., Hoshino, Y., Xin, K.Q., Hayashi, F., Tadokoro, K., and Okuda, K. (2002). Systemic and mucosal immune responses in mice after rectal and vaginal immunization with HIV-DNA vaccine. *Clin. Immunol.* 102, 12–18.

Hamajima, K., Sasaki, S., Fukushima, J., Kaneko, T., Xin, K.Q., Kudoh, I., and Okuda, K. (1998). Intranasal administration of HIV-DNA vaccine formulated with a polymer, carboxymethylcellulose, augments mucosal antibody production and cell-mediated immune response. *Clin. Immunol. Immunopathol.* 88, 205–210.

Herrmann, J.E., Chen, S.C., Fynan, E.F., Santoro, J.C., Greenberg, H.B., Wang, S., and Robinson, H.L. (1996a). Protection against rotavirus infections by DNA vaccination. *J. Infect. Dis.* 174, (Suppl. 1) S93–97.

Herrmann, J.E., Chen, S.C., Fynan, E.F., Santoro, J.C., Greenberg, H.B., and Robinson, H.L. (1996b) DNA vaccines against rotavirus infections. *Arch. Virol. Suppl.* 12, 207–215.

Herrmann, J.E., Chen, S.C., Jones, D.H., Tinsley-Bown, A., Fynan, E.F., Greenberg, H.B., and Farrar G.H. (1999). Immune

responses and protection obtained by oral immunization with rotavirus VP4 and VP7 DNA vaccines encapsulated in microparticles. *Virology* 259, 148–153.

Higgins, T.J., Herold, K.M., Arnold, R.L., McElhiney, S.P., Shroff, K.E., and Pachuk, C.J. (2000). Plasmid DNA-expressed secreted and nonsecreted forms of herpes simplex virus glycoprotein D2 induce different types of immune responses. *J. Infect. Dis.* 182, 1311–1320.

Hinkula, J., Lundholm, P., and Wahren, B. (1997). Nucleic acid vaccination with HIV regulatory genes: a combination of HIV-1 genes in separate plasmids induces strong immune responses. *Vaccine* 15, 874–878.

Hooper, J.W., Custer, D.M., and Thompson, E. (2003). Four-gene-combination DNA vaccine protects mice against a lethal vaccinia virus challenge and elicits appropriate antibody responses in nonhuman primates. *Virology* 306, 181–195.

Hsu, C.H., Chua, K.Y., Tao, M.H. Lai, Y.L., Wu, H.D., Huang, S.K., and Hsieh, K.H. (1996). Immunoprophylaxis of allergen-induced immunoglobulin E synthesis and airway hyperresponsiveness in vivo by genetic immunization. *Nat. Med.* 2, 540–544.

Huygen, K., Content, J., Denis, O., Montgomery, D.L., Yawman, A.M., Deck, R.R., DeWitt, C.M., Orme, I.M., Baldwin, S., D'Souza, C., Drowart, A., Lozes, E., Vandenbussche, P., Van Vooren, J-P., Liu, M.A., and Ulmer, J.B. (1996). Immunogenicity and protective efficacy of a tuberculosis DNA vaccine. *Nat. Med.* 2, 893–898.

Ishii, N., Fukushima, J., Kaneko, T., Okada, E., Tani, K., Tanaka, S.I., Hamajima, K., Xin, K.Q., Kawamoto, S., Koff, W., Nishioka, K., Yasuda, T., and Okuda K. (1997). Cationic liposomes are a strong adjuvant for a DNA vaccine of human immunodeficiency virus type 1. *AIDS Res. Hum. Retroviruses* 13, 1421–1428.

Jiao, X., Wang, R.Y., Feng, Z., Alter, H.J., and Shih, J.W. (2003). Modulation of cellular immune response against hepatitis C virus nonstructural protein 3 by cationic liposome encapsulated DNA immunization. *Hepatology* 37, 452–460.

Jones, D.H., Corris, S., McDonald, S., Clegg, J.C., and Farrar, G.H. (1997). Poly (DL-lactide-co-glycolide)-encapsulated plasmid DNA elicits systemic and mucosal antibody responses to encoded protein after oral administration. *Vaccine* 15, 814–817.

Jones, D.H., Clegg, J.C., and Farrar, G.H. (1998). Oral delivery of micro-encapsulated DNA vaccines. *Dev. Biol. Stand.* 92, 149–155.

Kaneko, H., Bednarek, I., Wierzbicki, A., Kiszka, I., Dmochowski, M., Wasik, T.J., Kaneko, Y., and Kozbor, D. (2000). Oral DNA vaccination promotes mucosal and systemic immune responses to HIV envelope glycoprotein. *Virology* 267, 8–16.

Klavinskis, L.S., Barnfield, C., Gao, L., and Parker, S. (1999). Intranasal immunization with plasmid DNA-lipid complexes elicits mucosal immunity in the female genital and rectal tracts. *J. Immunol.* 162, 254–262.

Kriesel, J.D., Spruance, S.L., Daynes, R.A., and Araneo, B.A. (1996). Nucleic acid vaccine encoding gD2 protects mice from herpes simplex virus type 2 disease. *J. Infect. Dis.* 173, 536–541.

Kuklin, N., Daheshia, M., Karem, K., Manickan, E., and Rouse, B.T. (1997). Induction of mucosal immunity against herpes simplex virus by plasmid DNA immunization. *J. Virol.* 71, 3138–3145.

Larsen, D.L., Karasin, A., and Olsen, C.W. (2001). Immunization of pigs against influenza virus infection by DNA vaccine priming followed by killed-virus vaccine boosting. *Vaccine* 19, 2842–2853.

Larsen, D.L., and Olsen, C.W. (2002). Effects of DNA dose, route of vaccination, and coadministration of porcine interleukin-6 DNA on results of DNA vaccination against influenza virus infection in pigs. *Am. J. Vet. Res.* 63, 653–659.

Le, T.P., Coonan, K.M., Hedstrom, R.C., Charoenvit, Y., Sedegah, M., Epstein, J.E., Kumar, S., Wang, R., Doolan, D.L., Maguire, J.D., Parker, S.E., Hobart, P., Norman, J., and Hoffman, S.L. (2000). Safety, tolerability and humoral immune responses after intramuscular administration of a malaria DNA vaccine to healthy adult volunteers. *Vaccine* 18, 1893–1901.

Ledwith, B.J., Manam, S., Troilo, P.J., Barnum, A.B., Pauley, C.J., Griffiths, T.G. 2nd, Harper, L.B., Beare, C.M., Bagdon, W.J., and Nichols, W.W. (2000). Plasmid DNA vaccines: investigation of integration into host cellular DNA following intramuscular injection in mice. *Intervirology* 43, 258–272.

Krieg AM. (2002). CpG motifs in bacterial DNA and their immune effects. *Annu Rev Immunol.* 20:709–760.

Lewis, P.J., and Babiuk, L.A. (1999). DNA vaccines: a review. *Adv. Virus Res.* 54, 129–188.

Livingston, J.B., Lu, S., Robinson, H.L., and Anderson, D.J. (1995). The induction of mucosal immunity in the female genital tract using gene-gun technology. Part 1: Antigen expression. *Ann. N.Y. Acad. Sci.* 772, 265–267.

Livingston, J.B., Lu, S., Robinson, H., and Anderson, D.J. (1998). Immunization of the female genital tract with a DNA-based vaccine. *Infect. Immun.* 66, 322–329.

Lodmell, D.L., Ray, N.B., Parnell, M.J., Ewalt, L.C., Hanlon, C.A., Shaddock, J.H, Sanderlin, D.S., and Rupprecht, C. E. (1998). DNA immunization protects nonhuman primates against rabies virus. *Nat. Med.* 4, 949–952.

Loehr, B.I., Willson, P., Babiuk, L.A., and van Drunen Littel–van den Hurk, S. (2000). Gene gun–mediated DNA immunization primes development of mucosal immunity against bovine herpesvirus 1 in cattle. *J. Virol.* 74, 6077–6086.

Loehr, B.I., Pontarollo, R., Rankin, R., Latimer, L., Willson, P., Babiuk, L.A., and van Drunen Littel–van den Hurk, S. (2001). Priming by DNA immunization augments T-cell responses induced by modified live bovine herpesvirus vaccine. *J. Gen. Virol.* 82, 3035–3043.

Loehr, B.I., Rankin, R., Pontarollo, R., King, T., Willson, P., Babiuk, L.A., and van Drunen Littel–van den Hurk, S. (2001). Suppository-mediated DNA immunization induces mucosal immunity against bovine herpesvirus-1 in cattle. *Virology* 289, 327–333.

Lu, S., Arthos, J., Montefiori D.C., Yasutomi, Y., Manson, K., Mustafa, F., Johnson, E., Santoro, J.C., Wissink, J., Mullins, J.I., Haynes, J.R., Letvin, N.L., Wyand, M., Robinson, H.L. (1996). Simian immunodeficiency virus DNA vaccine trial in macaques. *J. Virol.* 70, 3978–3991.

Luke, C.J., Carner, K., Liang X., and Barbour, A.G. (1997). An OspA-based DNA vaccine protects mice against infection with *Borrelia burgdorferi*. *J. Infect. Dis.* 175, 91–97.

Lundholm, P., Asakura, Y., Hinkula, J., Lucht, E., and Wahren, B. (1999). Induction of mucosal IgA by a novel jet delivery technique for HIV-1 DNA. *Vaccine* 17, 2036–2042.

MacGregor, R.R., Boyer, J.D., Ugen, K.E., Lacy, K.E., Gluckman, S.J., Bagarazzi, M.L., Chattergoon, M.A., Baine, Y., Higgins, T.J., Ciccarelli, R.B., Coney, L.R., Ginsberg, R.S., and Weiner, D.B. (1998). First human trial of a DNA-based vaccine for treatment of human immunodeficiency virus type 1 infection: safety and host response. *J. Infect. Dis.* 178, 92–100.

Macklin, M.D., McCabe, D., McGregor, M.W., Neumann, V., Meyer, T., Callan, R., Hinshaw, V.S., and Swain, W.F. (1998). Immunization of pigs with a particle-mediated DNA vaccine to influenza A virus protects against challenge with homologous virus. *J. Virol.* 72, 1491–1496.

Manickan, E., Rouse, R.J., Yu, Z., Wire, W.S., and Rouse, B.T. (1995). Genetic immunization against herpes simplex virus. Protection is mediated by CD4+ T lymphocytes. *J. Immunol.* 155, 259–265.

Manickan, E., Karem. K.L., and Rouse, BT. (1997). DNA vaccines: a modern gimmick or a boon to vaccinology? *Crit. Rev. Immunol.* 17, 139–154.

Martin, T., Parker, S.E., Hedstrom, R., Le, T., Hoffman, S.L., Norman, J., Hobart, P., and Lew, D. (1999). Plasmid DNA malaria vaccine: the potential for genomic integration after intramuscular injection. *Hum. Gene Ther.* 10, 759–768.

Martins, L.P., Lau, L.L., Asano, M.S., and Ahmed R. (1995). DNA vaccination against persistent viral infection. *J. Virol.* 69, 2574–2582.

Mathiowitz, E., Jacob, J.S., Jong, Y.S., Carino, G.P., Chickering, D.E., Chaturvedi, P., Santos, C.A., Vijayaraghavan, K., Montgomery, S., Bassett, M., and Morrell, C. (1997). Biologically erodable microspheres as potential oral drug delivery systems. *Nature* 386, 410–414.

McClements, W.L., Armstrong, M.E., Keys, R.D., and Liu, M.A. (1996). Immunization with DNA vaccines encoding glycopro-

tein D or glycoprotein B, alone or in combination, induces protective immunity in animal models of herpes simplex virus-2 disease. *Proc. Natl. Acad. Sci. USA* 93, 11414–11420

McCluskie, M.J., Brazolot Millan, C.L., Gramzinski, R.A., Robinson, H.L., Santoro, J.C., Fuller, J.T., Widera, G., Haynes, J.R., Purcell, R.H., Davis, H.L. (1999). Route and method of delivery of DNA vaccine influence immune responses in mice and nonhuman primates. *Mol. Med.* 5, 287–300.

McCluskie, M.J., Weeratna, R.D., and Davis, H.L. (2001). The potential of oligodeoxynucleotides as mucosal and parenteral adjuvants. *Vaccine* 19, 2657–2660.

Michalek, S.M., Eldrige, J.H., Curtiss, R. III, and Rosenthal, K.L. (1994). Antigen delivery systems: New approaches to mucosal immunization. In *Handbook of Mucosal Immunology* (eds. P.L. Ogra, M.L. Lamm, J.R.McGhee, J. Mestecky, W. Strober, and J. Bienenstock). San Diego: Academic Press, 373–390.

Michalek, S.M., O'Hagen, D.T., Gould-Fogerite, S., Rimmelzwaan, G.F., and Osterhaus, A.D.M.E. (1999). Antigen delivery systems: nonliving microparticles, liposomes, cochleates, and ISCOMs. In *Mucosal Immunology*, 2nd ed. (eds. P.L. Ogra, J. Mestecky, M.L. Lamm, W. Strober, J.R.McGhee, and J. Bienenstock). San Diego: Academic Press, 759–778.

Mitchell, W.M., Rosenbloom, S.T., and Gabriel J. (1995). Induction of mucosal anti-HIV antibodies by facilitated transfection of airway epithelium with lipospermine/DNA complexes. *Immunotechnology* 1, 211–219.

Montgomery, D.L., Shiver, J.W., Leander, K.R., Perry, H.C., Friedman, A., Martinez, D., Ulmer, J.B., Donnelly, J.J., and Liu, M.A. (1993). Heterologous and homologous protection against influenza A by DNA vaccination: optimization of DNA vectors. *DNA Cell. Biol.* 12, 777–783.

Mor, G., Yamshchikov, G., Sedegah, M., Takeno, M., Wang, R., Houghten, R.A., Hoffman, S., and Klinman, D.M. (1996). Induction of neonatal tolerance by plasmid DNA vaccination of mice. *J. Clin. Invest.* 98, 2700–2705.

Mor, G., Singla, M., Steinberg, A.D., Hoffman, S.L., Okuda, K., and Klinman, D.M. (1997). Do DNA vaccines induce autoimmune disease? *Hum. Gene Ther.* 8, 293–300.

Nichols, W.W., Ledwith, B.J., Manam, S.V., and Troilo, P.J. (1995). Potential DNA vaccine integration into host cell genome. *Ann. N.Y. Acad. Sci.* 772, 30–39.

Oh, Y.K., Kim, J.P., Hwang, T.S., Ko, J.J., Kim, J.M., Yang, J.S., Kim, C.K. (2001). Nasal absorption and biodistribution of plasmid DNA: an alternative route of DNA vaccine delivery. *Vaccine* 19, 4519–4525.

O'Hagen, T. (1994). Microparticles as oral vaccines. In *Novel Delivery Systems for Oral Vaccines* (ed. D. T. O'Hagen). Boca Raton, Florida: CRC Press, 175–205.

Okada, E., Sasaki, S., Ishii, N., Aoki, I., Yasuda, T., Nishioka, K., Fukushima, J., Miyazaki, J., Wahren, B., and Okuda, K. (1997). Intranasal immunization of a DNA vaccine with IL-12- and granulocyte-macrophage colony-stimulating factor (GM-CSF)-expressing plasmids in liposomes induces strong mucosal and cell-mediated immune responses against HIV-1 antigens. *J. Immunol.* 159, 3638–3647.

Pasetti, M.F., Barry, E.M., Losonsky, G., Singh, M., Medina-Moreno, S.M., Polo, J.M., Ulmer, J., Robinson, H., Sztein, M.B., and Levine, M.M. (2003). Attenuated *Salmonella enterica* serovar typhi and *Shigella flexneri* 2a strains mucosally deliver DNA vaccines encoding measles virus hemagglutinin, inducing specific immune responses and protection in cotton rats. *J. Virol.* 77, 5209–5217.

Perrie, Y., Frederik, P.M., Gregoriadis, G. (2001). Liposome-mediated DNA vaccination: the effect of vesicle composition. *Vaccine* 19, 3301–3310.

Perrie, Y., Obrenovic, M., McCarthy, D., and Gregoriadis, G. (2002). Liposome (Lipodine)–mediated DNA vaccination by the oral route. *J. Liposome Res.* 12, 185–197.

Pertmer, T.M., Roberts, T.R., and Haynes, J.R. (1996). Influenza virus nucleoprotein–specific immunoglobulin G subclass and cytokine responses elicited by DNA vaccination are dependent on the route of vector DNA delivery. *J. Virol.* 70, 6119–6125.

Pertmer, T.M., and Robinson, H.L. (1999). Studies on antibody responses following neonatal immunization with influenza hemagglutinin DNA or protein. *Virology* 257, 406–414.

Phillpotts, R.J., Venugopal, K., and Brooks, T. (1996). Immunisation with DNA polynucleotides protects mice against lethal challenge with St. Louis encephalitis virus. *Arch. Virol.* 141,743–749.

Prince, A.M., Whalen, R., and Brotman, B. (1997). Successful nucleic acid based immunization of newborn chimpanzees against hepatitis B virus. *Vaccine* 15, 916–919.

Raz, E., Tighe, H., Sato, Y., Corr, M., Dudler, J.A., Roman, M., Swain, S.L., Spiegelberg, H.L., and Carson, D.A. (1996). Preferential induction of a Th1 immune response and inhibition of specific IgE antibody formation by plasmid DNA immunization. *Proc. Natl. Acad. Sci. USA* 93, 5141–5145.

Ramshaw, I.A., and Ramsay, A.J. (2000). The prime-boost strategy: exciting prospects for improved vaccination. *Immunol. Today* 21, 163–165.

Robinson, H.L., Hunt, L.A., and Webster, R.G. (1993). Protection against a lethal influenza virus challenge by immunization with a haemagglutinin-expressing plasmid DNA. *Vaccine* 11, 957–960.

Robinson, W.H., Prohaska, S.S., Santoro, J.C., Robinson, H.L., and Parnes, J.R. (1995). Identification of a mouse protein homologous to the human CD6 T cell surface protein and sequence of the corresponding cDNA. *J. Immunol.* 155, 4739–4748.

Robinson, H.L., Boyle, C.A., Feltquate, D.M., Morin, M.J., Santoro, J.C., and Webster, R.G. (1997). DNA immunization for influenza virus: studies using hemagglutinin- and nucleoprotein-expressing DNAs. *J. Infect. Dis.* 176, Suppl 1:S50–55.

Robinson, H.L., and Torres. C.A. (1997). DNA vaccines. *Semin. Immunol.* 9, 271–283.

Robinson, H.L., Montefiori, D.C., Johnson, R.P., Manson, K.H., Kalish, M.L., Lifson, J.D., Rizvi, T.A., Lu, S., Hu, S.L., Mazzara, G.P., Panicali, D.L., Herndon, J.G., Glickman, R., Candido, M.A., Lydy, S.L., Wyand, M.S., and McClure, H.M. (1999). Neutralizing antibody–independent containment of immunodeficiency virus challenges by DNA priming and recombinant pox virus booster immunizations. *Nat. Med.* 5, 526–534.

Rothel, J.S., Boyle, D.B., Both, G.W., Pye, A.D., Waterkeyn, J.G., Wood, P.R., and Lightowlers, M.W. (1997). Sequential nucleic acid and recombinant adenovirus vaccination induces host-protective immune responses against *Taenia ovis* infection in sheep. *Parasite Immunol.* 19, 221–227.

Roy, K., Mao, H.Q., Huang, S.K., Leong, K.W. (1999). Oral gene delivery with chitosan-DNA nanoparticles generates immunologic protection in a murine model of peanut allergy. *Nat. Med.* 5, 387–391.

Roy, M.J., Wu, M.S., Barr, L.J., Fuller, J.T., Tussey, L.G., Speller, S., Culp, J., Burkholder, J.K., Swain, W.F., Dixon, R.M., Widera, G., Vessey, R., King, A., Ogg, G., Gallimore, A., Haynes, J.R., and Heydenburg Fuller, D. (2000). Induction of antigen-specific CD8+ T cells, T helper cells, and protective levels of antibody in humans by particle-mediated administration of a hepatitis B virus DNA vaccine. *Vaccine* 19, 764–778.

Sankar, V., Baccaglini, L., Sawdey, M., Wheeler, C.J., Pillemer, S.R., Baum, B.J., and Atkinson, J.C. (2002). Salivary gland delivery of pDNA-cationic lipoplexes elicits systemic immune responses. *Oral Dis.* 8, 275–281.

Sasaki, S., Hamajima, K., Fukushima, J., Ihata, A., Ishii, N., Gorai, I., Hirahara, F., Mohri, H., and Okuda, K. (1998). Comparison of intranasal and intramuscular immunization against human immunodeficiency virus type 1 with a DNA-monophosphoryl lipid A adjuvant vaccine. *Infect. Immun.* 66, 823–826.

Schneider, J., Gilbert, S.C., Hannan, C.M., Degano, P., Prieur, E., Sheu, E.G., Plebanski, M., and Hill, A.V. (1999). Induction of CD8+ T cells using heterologous prime-boost immunisation strategies. *Immunol. Rev.* 170, 29–38.

Sedegah, M., Hedstrom, R., Hobart, P., and Hoffman, S.L. (1994). Protection against malaria by immunization with plasmid DNA encoding circumsporozoite protein. *Proc. Natl. Acad. Sci. USA* 91, 9866–9870.

Shata, M.T., and Hone, D.M. (2001). Vaccination with a Shigella DNA vaccine vector induces antigen-specific CD8 (+) T cells and antiviral protective immunity. *J. Virol.* 75, 9665–9670.

Sharpe, S., Hanke, T., Tinsley-Bown, A., Dennis, M., Dowall, S., McMichael, A., and Cranage, M. (2003). Mucosal immunization with PLGA-microencapsulated DNA primes a SIV-specific CTL response revealed by boosting with cognate recombinant modified vaccinia virus Ankara. *Virology* 313, 13–21.

Shiver, J.W., Fu, T.M., Chen, L, Casimiro, D.R., Davies, M.E., Evans, R.K., Zhang, Z.Q., Simon, A.J., Trigona, W.L., Dubey, S.A., Huang, L., Harris, V.A., Long, R.S., Liang, X., Handt, L., Schleif, W.A., Zhu, L., Freed, D.C., Persaud, N.V., Guan, L., Punt, K.S., Tang. A, Chen, M., Wilson, K.A., Collins, K.B., Heidecker, G.J., Fernandez, V.R., Perry, H.C., Joyce, J.G., Grimm, K.M., Cook, J.C., Keller, P.M., Kresock, D.S., Mach, H., Troutman, R.D., Isopi, L.A., Williams, D.M., Xu, Z., Bohannon, K.E., Volkin, D.B., Montefiori, D.C., Miura, A., Krivulka, G.R., Lifton, M.A., Kuroda, M.J., Schmitz, J.E., Letvin, N.L., Caulfield, M.J., Bett, A.J, Youil, R., Kaslow, D.C., and Emini, E.A. (2002). Replication-incompetent adenoviral vaccine vector elicits effective anti-immunodeficiency-virus immunity. *Nature* 415, 331–335.

Shroff, K.E., Marcucci-Borges, L.A., de Bruin, S.J., Winter, L.A., Tiberio, L., Pachuk, C., Snyder, L.A., Satishchandran, C., Ciccarelli, R.B., and Higgins, T.J. (1999). Induction of HSV-gD2 specific CD4+ cells in Peyer's patches and mucosal antibody responses in mice following DNA immunization by both parenteral and mucosal administration. *Vaccine* 18, 222–230.

Simon, M.M., Gern, L., Hauser, P., Zhong, W., Nielsen, P.J., Kramer, M.D., Brenner, C., and Wallich, R. (1996). Protective immunization with plasmid DNA containing the outer surface lipoprotein A gene of *Borrelia burgdorferi* is independent of an eukaryotic promoter. *Eur. J. Immunol.* 26, 2831–2840.

Singh, M., Vajdy, M., Gardner, J., Briones, M., and O'Hagan, D. (2001). Mucosal immunization with HIV-1 gag DNA on cationic microparticles prolongs gene expression and enhances local and systemic immunity. *Vaccine* 20, 594–602.

Sizemore, D.R., Branstrom, A.A., and Sadoff, J.C. (1995). Attenuated *Shigella* as a DNA delivery vehicle for DNA-mediated immunization. *Science* 270, 299–302.

Sizemore, D.R., Branstrom, A.A., and Sadoff, J.C. (1997). Attenuated bacteria as a DNA delivery vehicle for DNA-mediated immunization. *Vaccine* 15, 804–807.

Skinner, M.A., Ramsay, A.J., Buchan, G.S., Keen, D.L., Ranasinghe, C., Slobbe, L., Collins, D.M., de Lisle, G.W., and Buddle, B.M. (2003). A DNA prime-live vaccine boost strategy in mice can augment IFN-gamma responses to mycobacterial antigens but does not increase the protective efficacy of two attenuated strains of *Mycobacterium bovis* against bovine tuberculosis. *Immunology* 108, 548–555.

Sundaram, P., Xiao, W., and Brandsma, J.L. (1996). Particle-mediated delivery of recombinant expression vectors to rabbit skin induces high-titered polyclonal antisera (and circumvents purification of a protein immunogen). *Nucleic Acid. Res.* 24, 1375–1377.

Syrengelas, A.D., Chen, T.T., and Levy, R. (1996). DNA immunization induces protective immunity against B-cell lymphoma. *Nat. Med.* 2, 1038–1041.

Tang, D.C., DeVit, M., and Johnston, S.A. (1992). Genetic immunization is a simple method for eliciting an immune response. *Nature* 356,152–154.

Tascon, R.E., Colston, M.J., Ragno, S., Stavropoulos, E., Gregory, D., and Lowrie, D.B. (1996). Vaccination against tuberculosis by DNA injection. *Nat. Med.* 2, 888–892.

Torres, C.A., Yang, K., Mustafa, F., and Robinson H.L. (1999). DNA immunization: effect of secretion of DNA-expressed hemagglutinins on antibody responses. *Vaccine* 18, 805–814.

Ulmer, J.B., Donnelly, J.J., Parker, S.E., Rhodes, G.H., Felgner, P.L., Dwarki, V.J., Gromkowski, S.H., Deck, R.R., DeWitt, C.M., Friedman, A., Hawe, L.A., Leander, K.R., Martinez, D., Perry, H.C., Shiver, J.W., Montgomery, D.L., and Liu, M.A. (1993). Heterologous protection against influenza by injection of DNA encoding a viral protein. *Science* 259, 1745–1749.

Vanrompay, D., Cox, E., Volckaert, G., and Goddeeris, B. (1999). Turkeys are protected from infection with *Chlamydia psittaci* by plasmid DNA vaccination against the major outer membrane protein. *Clin. Exp. Immunol.* 118, 49–55.

van Rooij, E.M., Haagmans, B.L., de Visser, Y.E., de Bruin, M.G., Boersma, W., and Bianchi AT. (1998). Effect of vaccination route and composition of DNA vaccine on the induction of protective immunity against pseudorabies infection in pigs. *Vet. Immunol. Immunopathol.* 66, 113–126.

Vecino, W.H., Morin, P.M., Agha, R., Jacobs, W.R., Jr., and Fennelly GJ. (2002). Mucosal DNA vaccination with highly attenuated *Shigella* is superior to attenuated *Salmonella* and comparable to intramuscular DNA vaccination for T cells against HIV. *Immunol. Lett.* 82, 197–204.

Waisman, A., Ruiz, P.J., Hirschberg, D.L., Gelman, A., Oksenberg, J.R., Brocke, S., Mor, F., Cohen, I.R., and Steinman, L. (1996). Suppressive vaccination with DNA encoding available region gene of the T-cell receptor prevents autoimmune encephalomyelitis and activates Th2 immunity. *Nat. Med.* 2, 899–905.

Wang, B., Dang, K., Agadjanyan, M.G., Srikantan, V., Li, F., Ugen, K.E, Boyer, J., Merva, M., Williams, W.V., and Weiner, D.B. (1997). Mucosal immunization with a DNA vaccine induces immune responses against HIV-1 at a mucosal site. *Vaccine* 15, 821–825.

Wang, Y., Xiang, Z., Pasquini, S., and Ertl, H.C. (1997). Immune response to neonatal genetic immunization. *Virology* 228, 278–284.

Wang, R., Doolan, D.L., Le, T.P., Hedstrom, R.C., Coonan, K.M., Charoenvit, Y., Jones, T.R., Hobart, P., Margalith, M., Ng, J., Weiss, W.R., Sedegah, M., de Taisne, C., Norman, J.A., and Hoffman, S.L. (1998). Induction of antigen-specific cytotoxic T lymphocytes in humans by a malaria DNA vaccine. *Science* 282, 476–480.

Wang, S.W., Kozlowski, P.A., Schmelz, G., Manson, K., Wyand, M.S., Glickman, R., Montefiori, D., Lifson, J.D., Johnson, R.P., Neutra, M.R., and Aldovini, A. (2000). Effective induction of simian immunodeficiency virus–specific systemic and mucosal immune responses in primates by vaccination with proviral DNA producing intact but noninfectious virions. *J. Virol.* 74, 10514–10522.

Wang, R., Epstein, J., Baraceros, F.M., Gorak, E.J., Charoenvit, Y., Carucci, D.J., Hedstrom, R.C., Rahardjo, N., Gay, T., Hobart, P., Stout, R., Jones, T.R., Richie, T.L., Parker, S.E., Doolan, D.L., Norman, J., and Hoffman, S.L. (2001). Induction of CD4 (+) T cell–dependent CD8 (+) type 1 responses in humans by a malaria DNA vaccine. *Proc. Natl. Acad. Sci. USA* 98, 10817–10822.

Wang, Q., Sun, S., Hu, Z., Wu, D., and Wang, Z. (2003). Immune response and protection elicited by DNA immunisation against *Taenia cysticercosis*. *Vaccine* 21, 1672–1680.

Webster, D.E., Cooney, M.L., Huang, Z., Drew, D.R., Ramshaw, I.A., Dry, I.B., Strugnell, R.A., Martin, J.L., and Wesselingh, S.L. (2002). Successful boosting of a DNA measles immunization with an oral plant-derived measles virus vaccine. *J. Virol.* 76, 7910–7912.

Webster, R.G., Fynan, E.F., Santoro, J.C., and Robinson, H. (1994). Protection of ferrets against influenza challenge with a DNA vaccine to the haemagglutinin. *Vaccine* 12, 1495–1498.

Wheeler, C.J., Felgner, PL., Tsai, Y.J., Marshall, J., Sakhu, L., Doh, S.G., Hartikka, J., Nietupski, J., Manthorpe, M., Nichols, M., Plewe, M., Liang, X., Norman, J., Smith, A., and Cheng, S.H. (1996). A novel cationic lipid greatly enhances plasmid DNA delivery and expression in mouse lung. *Proc. Natl. Acad. Sci. USA* 93, 11454–11459.

Wierzbicki, A., Kiszka, I., Kaneko, H., Kmieciak, D., Wasik, T.J., Gzyl, J., Kaneko, Y., and Kozbor, D. (2002). Immunization strategies to augment oral vaccination with DNA and viral vectors expressing HIV envelope glycoprotein. *Vaccine* 20, 1295–1307.

Winchell, J.M., Routray, S., Betts, P.W., Van Kruiningen, H.J., and Silbart, L.K. (1998). Mucosal and systemic antibody responses to a C4/V3 construct following DNA vaccination of rabbits via the Peyer's patch. *J. Infect. Dis.* 178, 850–853.

Wolff, J.A., Malone, R.W., Williams, P., Chong, W., Acsadi, G., Jani, A., and Felgner, P.L. (1990). Direct gene transfer into mouse muscle in vivo. *Science* 247, 1465–1468.

Wong, J.P., Zabielski, M.A., Schmaltz, F.L., Brownlee, G.G., Bussey, L.A., Marshall, K., Borralho, T., and Nagata, L.P. (2001). DNA vaccination against respiratory influenza virus infection. *Vaccine* 19, 2461–2467.

Xiang, Z.Q., Spitalnik, S., Tran, M., Wunner, W.H., Cheng, J., and Ertl, H.C. (1994). Vaccination with a plasmid vector carrying the rabies virus glycoprotein gene induces protective immunity against rabies virus. *Virology* 199, 132–140.

Xiang, Z.Q., Spitalnik, S.L., Cheng, J., Erikson, J., Wojczyk, B., and Ertl, H.C. (1995). Immune responses to nucleic acid vaccines to rabies virus. *Virology* 209, 569–579.

Xin, K.Q., Hamajima, K., Sasaki, S., Tsuji, T., Watabe, S., Okada, E., and Okuda, K. (1999). IL-15 expression plasmid enhances cell-mediated immunity induced by an HIV-1 DNA vaccine. *Vaccine* 17, 858–866.

Xiong, S., Gerloni, M., and Zanetti, M. (1997). In vivo role of B lymphocytes in somatic transgene immunization. *Proc. Natl. Acad. Sci. USA* 94, 6352–6357.

Xu, D., and Liew, F.Y. (1994). Genetic vaccination against leishmaniasis. *Vaccine* 12, 1534–1536.

Yokoyama, M., Zhang, J., and Whitton, J.L. (1995). DNA immunization confers protection against lethal lymphocytic choriomeningitis virus infection. *J. Virol.* 69, 2684–2688.

Zarozinski, C.C., Fynan, E.F., Selin, L.K., Robinson, H.L., and Welsh, R.M. (1995). Protective CTL-dependent immunity and enhanced immunopathology in mice immunized by particle bombardment with DNA encoding an internal virion protein. *J. Immunol.* 154, 4010–4017.

Zhong, W., Wiesmuller, K.H., Kramer, M.D., Wallich, R., and Simon, M.M. (1996). Plasmid DNA and protein vaccination of mice to the outer surface protein A of *Borrelia burgdorferi* leads to induction of T helper cells with specificity for a major epitope and augmentation of protective IgG antibodies *in vivo*. *Eur. J. Immunol.* 26, 2749–2757.

Mucosal Veterinary Vaccines: Comparative Vaccinology

Douglas C. Hodgins

Department of Pathobiology, Ontario Veterinary College, University of Guelph, Guelph, Ontario, Canada

Lijuan Yuan

Food Animal Health Research Program, Ohio Agricultural Research and Development Center, The Ohio State University, Wooster, Ohio

Viviana Parreño

Institute of Virology, Center of Research in Veterinary Science, National Institute of Agricultural Technology, Buenos Aires, Argentina

Lynette B. Corbeil

Department of Pathology, UCSD Medical Center, University of California at San Diego, San Diego, California

Linda J. Saif

Food Animal Health Research Program, Ohio Agricultural Research and Development Center, The Ohio State University, Wooster, Ohio

Chapter 61

In spite of advances in nutrition, genetics, housing, and therapeutics, diseases of the respiratory, reproductive, and enteric tracts of domestic animals and poultry continue to be major causes of morbidity and mortality, with economic losses of billions of dollars a year (Whiteley *et al.*, 1992). Although vaccines have been developed and licensed for prevention of many of these diseases (summarized in **Tables 61.1** to **61.3**), there is a need for improvement in vaccine efficacy. Reasons for low vaccine efficacy include inappropriate antigens in vaccine preparations (*e.g.*, *in vitro* expressed antigens instead of *in vivo* expressed antigens), inappropriate immune responses (*e.g.*, systemic instead of mucosal or Th2-type instead of Th1-type), and inappropriate use of otherwise efficacious vaccines (*e.g.*, vaccination after onset of disease) (Tizard, 2000).

The majority of current poultry vaccines are attenuated agents delivered orally, nasally, or by other mucosal routes, for reasons of ease of administration, economy, and protective efficacy. Until relatively recently, however, few vaccines for domestic mammals have been delivered by mucosal routes. Management practices for mammals differ from those for poultry, and mass vaccination techniques for mucosal delivery have not been pursued as zealously.

Recently, however, a number of attenuated live vaccines for nasal administration have been developed for respiratory tract infections, especially of horses and pets, with use of traditional methodologies. Improved protective efficacy and rapid onset of immunity, in comparison with killed vaccine products, have led to their widespread acceptance. Attenuated live vaccines for enteric diseases have also been marketed, but in many cases efficacy has been disappointing. Better strategies for induction of immunity in the gastrointestinal tract are needed. In contrast, effective parenteral vaccines for the most common diseases of the reproductive tract in veterinary species have been available for years, and there has been little motivation to develop mucosal vaccines.

Many of the diseases of the respiratory and gastrointestinal tracts are most devastating in the neonatal period. For these diseases, active immunization may not provide protection before natural exposure to the pathogen. Maternal vaccination to enhance passive immunity has been widely used in veterinary medicine, especially for

Table 61.1. Commercial Veterinary Vaccines for Diseases of the Gastrointestinal, Respiratory, and Reproductive Tracts of Ruminants

Species	Agent[a]	Diseases	Vaccine Types[b,c]	Comments[d]
Bovine	Bovine coronavirus	Enteritis in neonates, winter dysentery in adults, Respiratory tract infections in feedlot calves	K,L	Maternal vaccination for passive immunity, and/or oral vaccination of newborns
	Bovine herpesvirus-1	Respiratory tract infection, reproductive tract infection	K,L	Also modified live nasal
	Bovine respiratory syncytial virus	Respiratory tract infection	K,L	
	Bovine rotavirus	Neonatal enteritis	K,L	Maternal vaccination for passive immunity and/or oral vaccination of newborns
	Bovine virus, diarrhea virus	"Mucosal disease," respiratory tract infection, abortion	K,L	
	Brucella abortus	Reproductive tract infection, abortion	L	
	Campylobacter fetus subsp. veneralis	Reproductive tract infection, abortion	K	
	Dictyocaulus viviparus	Parasitic bronchitis (lungworm)	L	Oral administration of third-stage infective larvae
	Escherichia coli	Neonatal enteritis	K	maternal vaccination for passive immunity
	Haemophilus somnus	Bronchopneumonia, reproductive tract infection, abortion	K	
	Leptospira spp.	Reproductive tract infection, abortion, nephritis	K	
	Mannheimia (Pasteurella) haemolytica	Bronchopneumonia	K,L,S	Some bacterins are prepared from cultures grown under iron-restricted conditions
	Parainfluenza virus-3	Respiratory tract infection	K,L	Some live vaccines given nasally
	Pasteurella multocida	Bronchopneumonia	K,L	
	Salmonella spp.	Enteritis	K	
	Tritrichomonas foetus	Reproductive tract infection, abortion	K	
Ovine	Campylobacter fetus spp. fetus Campylobacter jejuni	Abortion	K	
	Chlamydia psittaci	Abortion	K	
	Mannheimia haemolytica	Bronchopneumonia	K	Some bacterins are prepared from cultures grown under iron-restricted conditions
	Pasteurella trehalosi	Bronchopneumonia	K	Some bacterins are prepared from cultures grown under iron-restricted conditions
	Toxoplasma gondii	Early embryonic death, abortion	L	Live tachyzoites

[a] Agents and vaccines have been selected as representative of common disease concerns and current commercial vaccines. Tabulation of all mucosal pathogens and all licensed commercial vaccines in all jurisdictions has not been attempted.

[b] K indicates a killed (inactivated) vaccine; L indicates live (attenuated or nonattenuated) vaccine; S indicates a culture supernatant vaccine.

[c] Vaccine data have been collated from manufacturers' product monographs, including monographs published in Entriken (2001) and Glennon and Jeffs (2000).

[d] Vaccines are administered by the intramuscular or subcutaneous routes unless indicated otherwise. Inclusion of a vaccine in the table does not imply efficacy.

Table 61.2. Commercial Veterinary Vaccines for Diseases of the Gastrointestinal, Respiratory, and Reproductive Tracts of Pigs and Horses

Species	Agent[a]	Diseases	Vaccine Types[b,c]	Comments[d]
Porcine	Actinobacillus pleuropneumoniae	Pneumonia	K,L	Maternal vaccination for passive immunity, with or without vaccination (nasal or intramuscular) of newborns
	Bordetella bronchiseptica	Atrophic rhinitis	K,L	Maternal vaccination for passive immunity
	Escherichia coli	Neonatal enteritis	K	
	Haemophilus parasuis	Pneumonia	K	
	Swine influenza virus	Respiratory tract infections	K	
	Leptospira spp.	Abortion, stillbirths	K	
	Mycoplasma hyopneumoniae	Enzootic pneumonia	K	
	Porcine parvovirus	Abortion, mummified fetuses, stillbirths	K	
	Pasteurella multocida	Atrophic rhinitis, pneumonia	K	
	Porcine reproductive and respiratory syndrome virus	Abortion, stillbirths, neonatal respiratory tract Infection	K,L	
	Porcine rotavirus	Neonatal enteritis	K,L	Maternal vaccination for passive immunity, with or without vaccination (intraperitoneal, oral, or intramuscular) of newborns
	Pseudorabies virus	Abortion, mummification, stillbirths, Respiratory tract infection	L	
	Salmonella spp.	Enteritis	K,L	Some by oral or nasal routes
	Streptococcus suis	Pneumonia, arthritis, meningitis	K	Maternal vaccination for passive immunity and/or vaccination of newborns
	Transmissible gastroenteritis virus	Enteritis	K,L	Maternal vaccination (some vaccines by oral route) for passive immunity, with or without intraperitoneal or oral vaccination of newborns
Equine	Influenza virus	Respiratory tract infection	K,L	A cold adapted live vaccine is given nasally; an ISCOM vaccine has been marketed since 1987
	Equine herpesvirus-4	Equine viral rhinopneumonitis	K,L	
	Equine rotavirus	Neonatal enteritis	K	Maternal vaccination for passive immunity
	Streptococcus equi	Strangles	E,L	A live vaccine is marketed for nasal use

[a] Agents and vaccines have been selected as representative of common disease concerns and current commercial vaccines. Tabulation of all mucosal pathogens and all licensed commercial vaccines in all jurisdictions has not been attempted.
[b] E indicates an extract or subunit vaccine; K indicates a killed (inactivated) vaccine; L indicates live (attenuated or nonattenuated) vaccine.
[c] Vaccine data have been collated from manufacturers' product monographs, including monographs published in Entriken (2001) and Glennon and Jeffs (2000). Inclusion of a vaccine in the table does not imply efficacy.
[d] Vaccines are administered by the intramuscular or subcutaneous routes unless indicated otherwise.

Table 61.3. Commercial Veterinary Vaccines for Diseases of the Gastrointestinal, Respiratory, and Reproductive Tracts of Dogs, Cats, and Chickens

Species	Agent[a]	Diseases	Vaccine Types	Comments
Canine	*Bordetella bronchiseptica*	Tracheobronchitis ("kennel cough")	K,L,E	Some live vaccines by nasal route, in combination with parainfluenza virus, with or without CAV2
	Canine adenovirus-2	Tracheobronchitis ("kennel cough")	L	In combination with other agents of tracheobronchitis
	Canine parvovirus-2	Enteritis	K,L	Vaccination of young puppies: suppressive effects of maternal antibodies are problematic; some low-passage and/or high-virus-titer vaccines are marketed
	Leptospira spp.	Nephritis	K	
	Parainfluenza virus-2	Tracheobronchitis ("kennel cough")	L	In combination with other agents of tracheobronchitis
Feline	Feline calicivirus	Respiratory tract infections	K,L	Some by nasal or ocular routes
	Chlamydia psittaci	Respiratory tract infection, conjunctivitis	K,L	
	Feline herpesvirus-1	Rhinotracheitis, conjunctivitis, keratitis, stomatitis, abortion, pneumonia	K,L	Some by nasal or ocular routes
Chicken	Infectious bronchitis virus	Respiratory tract infection, reproductive tract infection	K,L	Ocular, aerosol, nasal, or drinking water administration; killed vaccines parenterally after priming with live vaccine by mucosal route
	Eimeria spp.	Coccidiosis (enteritis)	L	Live oocysts on feed or in water in first week of life, up to 8 species of *Eimeria* simultaneously
	Infectious laryngotracheitis virus	Respiratory tract infection	L	Vaccination via cloaca, ocular, nasal, feather follicle, and drinking water
	Avian influenza virus	Respiratory tract infection	L	Recombinant vaccine in fowl pox virus vector
	Mycoplasma spp.	Respiratory tract infection	K,L	Ocular, aerosol
	Newcastle disease virus	Respiratory tract infection, enteritis, neurological disease	K,L	Ocular, aerosol, nasal, drinking water; killed vaccines parenterally after priming with live vaccine by mucosal route
	Pasteurella multocida	Fowl cholera	K,L	Live vaccine is administered in drinking water

[a] Agents and vaccines have been selected as representative of common disease concerns and current commercial vaccines. Tabulation of all mucosal pathogens and all licensed commercial vaccines in all jurisdictions has not been attempted.

[b] E indicates an extract or subunit vaccine; K indicates a killed (inactivated) vaccine; L indicates live (attenuated or nonattenuated) vaccine.

[c] Vaccine data have been collated from manufacturers' product monographs, including monographs published in Entriken (2001) and Glennon and Jeffs (2000). Inclusion of a vaccine in the table does not imply efficacy.

[d] Vaccines are administered by the intramuscular or subcutaneous routes unless indicated otherwise.

control of enteric diseases. Severe practical difficulties arise, however, with diseases such as parvovirus enteritis in puppies, in which a smooth transition must be made from protection by passive maternal antibodies to protection by active immunity, without permitting a window of disease susceptibility to occur in between. This transition is difficult to achieve because induction of active immunity is commonly inhibited by maternal antibodies. Various strategies are used to address this problem, but improved adjuvants and antigen delivery systems would improve the reliability of neonatal immunization.

Although progress is being made in disease prevention in veterinary species, ever-changing management practices (*e.g.*, earlier weaning of piglets, larger dairy operations) appear to be generating new patterns of disease, requiring new control strategies. The emergence of new pathogens (*e.g.*, porcine reproductive and respiratory syndrome virus [PRRSV], porcine circovirus-2) also presents new challenges for vaccine research before some of the older challenges have been met. In this chapter, we focus on mucosal veterinary vaccines and vaccine concepts related to selected pathogens associated with economically important respiratory, reproductive, and enteric diseases, with an emphasis on livestock species. Our intent is to highlight progress, to review existing and future vaccination strategies, and to acknowledge the unique contributions of this research to our understanding of mucosal vaccines and immunology.

RESPIRATORY VACCINES

Respiratory tract infections are a major cause of morbidity and mortality among farm animals, poultry, and pets (Tables 61.1 to 61.3). In many cases, disease conditions are intensified by current management practices such as the mixing of recently weaned, stressed beef calves from multiple sources in auction barns. Certain disease conditions, such as atrophic rhinitis of pigs, result from the interplay of several pathogens, and multiple agents must be represented in vaccines. Some respiratory pathogens such as *Mycoplasma hyopneumoniae* in young pigs are causing new patterns of disease as management practices change (*e.g.*, weaning at an earlier age), requiring changes in vaccine strategies. Other pathogens such as PRRSV have only recently emerged, and improved vaccines await advances in understanding of the agent and of disease pathogenesis. A discussion of respiratory vaccines for even the major pathogens of veterinary species is beyond the scope of the present review. This section therefore focuses on selected pathogens of cattle and horses to illustrate general principles.

Bovine respiratory vaccines
Introduction and background
Respiratory tract disease has been a major problem for beef, veal, and dairy producers for decades. From the perspectives of both economic and animal welfare considerations, efficacious and practical means to reduce the burden of disease

are long overdue. Most attention has focused on pneumonic pasteurellosis, commonly termed "shipping fever," in recently weaned beef calves soon after entry to feedlots. Economic losses to the North American feedlot industry alone have been estimated at nearly $1 billion per year (Whiteley *et al.*, 1992). This does not include losses due to enzootic pneumonia in veal, dairy, or beef calves before weaning. Both bacteria and viruses have been implicated in the disease processes, and vaccines have been marketed for over 80 years (Mosier *et al.*, 1989). We have summarized the agents associated with respiratory disease in cattle and the vaccine preparations marketed for their control (Table 61.1). *Mannheimia haemolytica* is discussed in detail as an example of past, current, and future vaccine approaches.

Mannheimia haemolytica
M. haemolytica, classified until recently as *Pasteurella haemolytica* (Angen *et al.*, 1999), is a gram-negative, facultatively anaerobic bacterium. In experimental studies, it causes a fibrinous pneumonia comparable to that seen in cattle dying of pneumonic pasteurellosis (Friend *et al.*, 1977; Shoo, 1989), and it is considered the most important bacterial pathogen in bovine pneumonias (Mosier, 1997). The first 7 decades of vaccine history have been reviewed by Mosier *et al.* (1989). As a single agent, this bacterium induces pneumonia in experimental studies, but most field cases of pneumonia involve predisposing factors of stress (sudden shifts in weather conditions, change of feed, weaning, and commingling with other cattle) and interactions with viral pathogens (reviewed by Yates [1982] and by Hodgins *et al.* [2002]). To be effective, vaccination strategies against respiratory disease in feedlot cattle will therefore need to induce immunity to multiple pathogens.

M. haemolytica can be cultured intermittently from the nasopharynx of healthy cattle and is considered part of the normal flora (Babiuk and Acres, 1984; Frank, 1984). Under ill-defined conditions of stress, *M. haemolytica* serotype A1 populations increase rapidly in the nasopharynx (Frank and Smith, 1983). Invasion of the lower respiratory tract, facilitated in many cases by viral effects on clearance mechanisms of the tracheal and bronchial mucosa, leads to vascular damage, exudation of fibrin, and necrosis of lung parenchymal tissue (lesions reviewed by Rehmtulla and Thomson [1981]). Morbidity rates of 15% to 45% and mortality rates of 1% to 5% are common among weaned calves arriving at feedlots (Kelly and Janzen, 1986). Antibiotics are used extensively in treatment and prevention (Mechor *et al.*, 1988; Hoar *et al.*, 1998).

The earliest vaccines for "shipping fever" were bacterins of doubtful efficacy (Miller *et al.*, 1927) or causing detrimental effects (Farley, 1932; Friend *et al.*, 1977). The identification and characterization of a heat-labile exotoxin (leukotoxin) cytolytic for ruminant leukocytes, produced by *M. haemolytica* during logarithmic growth (Shewen and Wilkie, 1985), initiated an intensive search for other protective antigens of *M. haemolytica* that continues today. Other antigens suggested as playing a role in disease pathogenesis and of potential value in vaccine formulation include the capsular polysaccharide of *M. haemolytica* A1 (Brogden *et al.*, 1995), a sialoglycoprotease (Abdullah *et al.*, 1992; Lee *et al.*, 1994), a neuroaminidase (Straus and Purdy, 1994), outer membrane proteins (Gatewood *et al.*, 1994), fimbriae (Morck *et al.*, 1987, 1989), and iron-regulated proteins (Morck *et al.*, 1991; Potter *et al.*, 1999).

Most of the *M. haemolytica* vaccines now available commercially consist of culture supernatants or cell extracts (with or without leukotoxin) and are licensed for use by the intramuscular or subcutaneous routes. Significant protection in experimental challenge studies has been reported for a number of these products (Conlon *et al.*, 1991, 1995; Confer and Fulton, 1995). Investigations of vaccine efficacy are conducted almost exclusively in ruminants because the leukotoxin, the best documented of its virulence factors, is toxic only to ruminant leukocytes (Kaehler *et al.*, 1980; Shewen and Wilkie, 1982). Efficacy in field trials can be considerably lower than in controlled experiments because of suboptimal timing of vaccination, variation in exposure to pathogens other than *M. haemolytica*, and variation in immunity to *M. haemolytica* in nonvaccinated control calves (Thorlakson *et al.*, 1990).

In general, the proportion of IgG to IgA in respiratory tract secretions increases from the upper respiratory tract to the lower respiratory tract. It is unclear, however, what proportion of IgG detected in the bovine lung results from local secretion and how much is serum derived (Butler, 1983). The protection mediated by parenteral vaccination with nonreplicating vaccines suggests that serum antibodies have at least limited access to the lung compartment.

A number of attempts have been made to develop live *M. haemolytica* vaccines for parenteral (intradermal or intramuscular) administration. Efficacy studies have yielded variable results (Smith *et al.*, 1985; Purdy *et al.*, 1986; Mosier *et al.*, 1998). This approach has limitations for use in feedlot calves because the use of antibiotics prevents adequate replication of the live vaccine.

A major challenge in developing effective vaccines against *M. haemolytica* is to adapt vaccines to existing management practices or to adapt management practices to feasible vaccines. There are limited opportunities to vaccinate beef calves raised on open-range land before weaning. Conventional two-dose vaccination, with primary vaccination weeks before weaning, is labor intensive and increases stress for the calves. Delayed vaccination, with a single dose of vaccine at the time of feedlot arrival, can induce anamnestic responses in calves that have been primed by natural exposure (Conlon *et al.*, 1995), but it does not allow sufficient time for naïve (highly susceptible) calves to respond immunologically. One approach with merit is to vaccinate calves at about 3 months of age when they are being handled for branding (Harland *et al.*, 1992), followed by a booster dose at weaning (6 to 8 months of age).

Oral vaccination. Recent studies have shown that transgenic clover expressing a truncated form of the leukotoxin of *M. haemolytica* is a potential oral vaccine (Lee *et al.*, 2001). Oral administration of dried transgenic plant material would

be a low-labor, low-stress method of vaccination. It is doubtful whether plant-expressed antigens survive passage through the rumen (first stomach) in ruminant species, but the authors hypothesize that repeated exposure of the tonsils to antigen during rumination will induce mucosal immune responses. Immunogenicity trials of the recombinant plant antigen in calves have not been reported.

Others have reported that live, genetically modified *M. haemolytica* can be administered to recently weaned calves as a top dressing over pelleted feed (Briggs and Tatum, 1999). It is hypothesized that the vaccine strain of *M. haemolytica* could colonize the nasopharynx (without causing pneumonic disease) and induce mucosal immune responses. Mortality of high-risk feedlot calves was reduced from 16% to 0%. Significant increases in IgA antibodies were noted in nasal secretions by 3 days postvaccination. While these results are promising, continued studies are needed to confirm a lack of virulence under varied feedlot conditions. Environmental considerations, such as the potential for contamination of run-off water in feedlots vaccinating thousands of cattle, could also block licensing.

Another approach has involved microencapsulation of nonreplicating antigens for oral immunization of ruminants (Bowersock *et al.*, 1994a). The anatomy of ruminant digestive tracts, with prolonged passage times for materials lingering in the rumen, complicates vaccination by the oral route. Incorporation of microencapsulated antigen into macroparticles (5 mm in diameter) allows antigen to bypass the rumen (Bowersock *et al.*, 1999) and pass promptly into the reticulum (second stomach). An oral vaccine containing microencapsulated antigens of *M. haemolytica* has been shown to induce partial protection (Bowersock *et al.*, 1994b).

Nasal vaccination. Preliminary work by Rebelatto *et al.* (2001) indicates that vaccination by the nasal route using alginate microencapsulated antigen may be useful in cattle. Nasal (but not oral) vaccination led to high levels of IgG antibodies in serum and nasal secretions.

DNA-based vaccine strategies. Immunization of large animals with plasmid vaccines has proven to be more difficult than for mice (Braun *et al.*, 1999; Babiuk *et al.*, 2002). Doses of up to 1000 μg have been administered to cattle in attempts to optimize immune responses (Babiuk, *et al.*, 1999). Although long-lived immune responses can be induced (Braun *et al.*, 1999), antibody responses develop slowly (in comparison with those induced by protein-based vaccines), and revaccination may be necessary for detectable responses (Braun *et al.*, 1999). These attributes discourage the use of plasmid DNA technology by itself for vaccination against *M. haemolytica*, since frequency of vaccination and labor costs are key issues. Further advances in plasmid design and delivery (Babiuk *et al.*, 2002) or combination of plasmid vaccines with other vaccination approaches may make DNA vaccines feasible for use in cattle. Unmethylated CpG oligodeoxynucleotides have been investigated as potential adjuvants for veterinary vaccines (Rankin *et al.*, 2001) and may find a role in conventional protein-based vaccines or plasmid DNA vaccines.

Equine respiratory vaccines

Introduction and background

Respiratory tract disease affects virtually every aspect of equine husbandry, including working, pleasure, and race horses. Considerable efforts are expended to prevent epizootics of respiratory disease in stables, fairs, shows, and race tracks. We have summarized the major respiratory pathogens of horses and the vaccine preparations marketed for their control (Table 61.2). Equine influenza virus is discussed in detail as an example of past, current, and future vaccine approaches.

Equine influenza virus

Equine influenza virus causes epizootics of upper and lower respiratory tract disease almost worldwide. Infection can occur in horses of all ages, but epidemics often involve younger animals (van Maanen and Cullinane, 2002). Clinical signs include high fever, a persistent dry cough, nasal discharge, anorexia, and depression (Ardans, 1999). Secondary bacterial pneumonia may complicate the clinical picture (Timoney, 1996).

Equine influenza viruses are classified as type A influenza. Antigenic differences in the hemagglutinin (H) and neuraminidase (N) glycoproteins define the two recognized subtypes, A/equine/1 (H7N7) and A/equine/2 (H3N8) (Wilson, 1993). The A/equine/1 subtype has not been associated with outbreaks of equine influenza since 1980 (Timoney, 1996; van Maanen and Cullinane, 2002). Two lineages of A/equine/2, American and European, have been identified (Yates and Mumford, 2000). Multiple virus strains are included in vaccines since protection against heterologous strains is incomplete (Yates and Mumford, 2000). Antigenic drift is sufficient to require regular reappraisal of strains included in vaccines (Mumford and Wood, 1993).

Natural infection induces IgA antibodies in nasal secretions, IgGa and IgGb antibodies in serum (Hannant et al., 1989; Nelson et al., 1998), and circulating cytotoxic T lymphocytes (Hannant and Mumford, 1989). Protection against reinfection persists for at least a year (Hannant et al., 1988). Vaccination with inactivated virus vaccines induces serum IgG (T) antibodies without detectable IgA in nasal secretions (Nelson et al., 1998) and without cytotoxic T cell activity (van Maanen and Cullinane, 2002). Two or three doses of vaccine are typically administered in the primary series, with booster doses administered at least once a year thereafter. More frequent vaccination is advised for horses at high risk of infection (Wilson, 1993). Protection is typically incomplete and of limited duration (Morley et al., 1999). Improved adjuvants can enhance the level and duration of antibody responses to inactivated virus vaccines (Mumford et al., 1994c; van Maanen and Cullinane, 2002). Suppressive effects of maternal antibodies on responses to inactivated vaccines have led to recommendations not to vaccinate foals before 6 months of age (van Oirschot et al., 1991; van Maanen and Cullinane, 2002).

Immune stimulating complex (ISCOM) vaccines. A subunit equine influenza vaccine based on the ISCOM adjuvant technology has been licensed and marketed in Europe since 1987 (Newmark, 1988). Antibody responses to ISCOM-based vaccines typically are of higher titer and are more persistent than those stimulated by conventional inactivated vaccines (Mumford et al., 1994a; Brugmann et al., 1997). Protection has been demonstrated against experimental challenge, 15 months after a three-dose vaccination series (Mumford et al., 1994b). Protection may be due in part to the ability of ISCOM-adjuvanted vaccines to induce cytotoxic T lymphocytes (CTLs) (Morein et al., 1999). Although ISCOM-based vaccines can induce IgA antibody responses following nasal administration (Hu et al., 2001), the commercial influenza ISCOM vaccine is administered parenterally.

Nasal vaccination. Nasal administration of inactivated equine influenza with cholera toxin B subunit has been reported to induce mucosal IgA antibodies and protection against experimental challenge (Hannant et al., 1998). Recently, a cold-adapted, temperature-sensitive live vaccine for nasal administration was commercialized (Chambers et al., 2001). Protection against experimental challenge was demonstrated 6 months after a single vaccination (Townsend et al., 2001). This is a notable improvement in efficacy and practicality over conventional killed vaccines.

Plasmid DNA vaccines. Experimental plasmid vaccines encoding the hemagglutinin gene of equine influenza have been examined in horses. Three doses of plasmid administered to the skin and mucosal sites (tongue, conjunctiva, and third eyelid) induced protection against clinical disease and partial protection against viral shedding. Protection against clinical disease was reduced if plasmid was administered only to the skin (Lunn et al., 1999).

Pox virus vectored vaccines. Both canarypox (ALVAC strain) and attenuated vaccinia virus (NYVAC strain) have been used as vaccine vectors for expression of hemagglutinins of A1 and A2 subtypes of equine influenza virus. Intramuscular vaccination induced serum antibodies and partial protection was achieved following natural exposure to A2 influenza virus (Taylor et al., 1992).

Future needs

For some respiratory pathogens (e.g., M. hyopneumoniae in pigs), the critical antigens associated with protective immune responses have not been identified. For other pathogens (e.g., PRRSV) there is also a need to identify the appropriate immune response (Th1 or Th2 type) needed for protection. For some complex disease conditions (e.g., pneumonic pasteurellosis in cattle) there is continuing uncertainty about whether all of the relevant contributing pathogens have been identified. Although many parenteral vaccines are efficacious in reducing lower respiratory tract disease, there is a need to investigate whether induction of mucosal immunity in the upper airways, in combination with systemic immunity, can further reduce infection rates, transmission of pathogens, and economic losses. Finally, there is a need to devise and implement changes in management procedures to reduce disease exposure (by nonimmunological methods) and to optimize immune interventions by improving the timing of vaccinations.

VACCINES FOR GENITAL INFECTIONS

Vaccines to prevent reproductive tract disease have received much emphasis in veterinary medicine. This is especially true of food-producing animals because reproductive failure is an economic problem. Although vaccines to prevent reproduction are of interest for abandoned pets or deer in areas of over-population, this section deals only with vaccines designed to prevent infectious disease of the reproductive mucosa. We have outlined and summarized pathogens associated with reproductive tract disease in veterinary species and the vaccine preparations marketed for their control (Tables 61.1 to 61.3).

Infections causing adverse pregnancy outcome can be classified by route of infection: hematogenous or ascending. Several hematogenous infections have a predilection for the gravid uterus, resulting in early or late abortions (Corbeil *et al.*, 2001). These include leptospirosis, chlamydial infection, and brucellosis in several animal species, *Haemophilus somnus* infection in cattle and sheep, and *Neospora caninum* infection in cattle. Although vaccines are available for leptospirosis and hemophilosis, the vaccine for brucellosis, which has been available since the 1940s, is the prototype. Several *Brucella* species cause abortion or epididymitis/orchitis in the primary host (*B. abortus* in cattle, *B. suis* in swine, *B. melitensis* in goats, *B. ovis* in sheep, *B. canis* in dogs, and *B. marinum* [or *B. delphini*] in marine mammals). Infection may be acquired via the gut mucosa or the conjunctiva/upper respiratory mucosa, and the infection localizes in the reticuloendothelial system and endometrium/placenta by systemic spread. Thus, systemic vaccines are effective. A modified live *B. abortus* vaccine, along with a "test and slaughter" eradication program, has been successful in controlling bovine brucellosis in North America. The modified live vaccine (*B. abortus* strain 19) is very effective in stimulating cell-mediated immunity (CMI), which is critical for protection against this facultative intracellular pathogen. Strain 19 now has been largely replaced by the new attenuated strain RB51, which does not stimulate an antibody response known to interfere with diagnostic assays. There is considerable information on mechanisms of immunity to brucellosis, but since the focus of this volume is mucosal immunity, no more will be said on hematogenous infection of the genital tract.

Ascending, local infections of the reproductive tract are usually transmitted sexually. The two best examples of vaccines for sexually transmitted infections of animals are *Campylobacter fetus* subsp. *venerealis* (formerly *Vibrio fetus* subsp. *venerealis*) and *Tritrichomonas foetus*. Both are host-specific, bovine sexually transmitted disease (STD) pathogens that infect only the reproductive mucosa. Both are extracellular pathogens that do not invade the mucosa of the reproductive tract but may be found in the placenta and fetus. The localized nature of these infections and transmission limited to coitus suggest that mucosal immunity must be important. Because a vaccine has been available for *C. fetus* subsp. *venerealis* for several decades and its use has controlled the disease in developed countries, that vaccine will be described first.

Vibriosis

Vibriosis (or campylobacteriosis) is a chronic bacterial genital infection with no overt clinical signs other than reproductive failure (Corbeil *et al.*, 1981). After months of infection, the uterus is cleared first, followed by the vagina. Convalescent immunity is partially protective for a limited time. Antibody is effective in protection against this extracellular pathogen, as demonstrated by systemic passive immunization (Berg *et al.*, 1979). The antibody response to infection is primarily IgA in the vagina and IgG in the uterus (Corbeil *et al.*, 1981). Systemic immunization with a whole cell vaccine results in both IgG1 and IgG2 antibody responses to surface antigen in serum, uterine, and vaginal secretions (Corbeil *et al.*, 1981). This response prevents infection and can rapidly clear infected cows (Corbeil and Winter, 1978). That is, the vaccine can be used prophylactically and therapeutically. Immunization is efficacious even though surface antigenic variation occurs in the face of a local immune response (Corbeil and Winter, 1978). Presumably, immune clearance occurs when the dynamic interaction between protection and evasion is shifted in favor of the host. This appears to occur earlier when the response is primarily IgG than when IgA predominates (Corbeil *et al.*, 1981). This may be related to the ability of the IgG antibodies to mediate opsonization and intracellular killing of the bacterium, an ability that IgA antibodies lack (Corbeil and Winter, 1978). Although this work was done many years ago, it sets a precedent for systemic immunization for prophylaxis and therapy for reproductive mucosal infections.

Trichomoniasis

Trichomoniasis is a similar chronic genital mucosal infection of cattle. It is caused by the protozoan *T. foetus* and results in pregnancy loss. *T. vaginalis* causes a human STD also associated with adverse pregnancy outcome. Thus, bovine trichomoniasis serves as a model for immune prevention of a human reproductive mucosal infection. Because of the economic significance of bovine trichomoniasis and because no chemotherapy is used owing to toxicity, investigations have focused on immunoprophylaxis and therapy. Like *C. fetus* subsp. *venerealis*, *T. foetus* colonizes the vaginal and uterine or preputial surfaces for months. In fact, mature bulls are often infected for life, whereas young bulls may clear the infection with time. This is probably related to innate immunity. Trichomonads are anaerobic parasites and are found deep in uterine glands and epithelial crypts of the penis and prepuce (Rhyan *et al.*, 1999), where the oxygen tension is probably lowest. In order to elucidate protective acquired immune responses, monoclonal antibodies (mAbs) with putative protective functions were chosen for immunoaffinity purification of a highly glycosylated surface antigen (Corbeil *et al.*, 2001).

Analysis of many isolates of *T. foetus* indicated that the two mAbs recognized different epitopes of the same antigen, which was conserved in all isolates tested. This glycosylated surface antigen was later shown to be a lipophosphoglycan (LPG)/protein complex. Systemic immunization with the immunoaffinity-purified surface antigen, followed by vaginal challenge with *T. foetus*, resulted in statistically significantly earlier clearance of the parasite from vaccinated animals than from controls (Corbeil *et al.*, 2001). Even more important, clearance of immunized animals most often occurred before 7 weeks of infection. Mucosal convalescent immunity cleared controls much later. Others showed that significant inflammation accompanied by reproductive failure did not occur until after 7 weeks of infection, so the vaccine should protect against fetal loss (Parsonsen *et al.*, 1976). Analysis of antibody responses demonstrated predominantly IgG1 responses in the serum and IgA plus IgG1 antibodies in secretions.

This raised several questions. First, why is the systemic response skewed toward IgG1 (a Th2-type response in cattle) and not IgG2 (a Th1-type response)? This question is under investigation. Second, which is more protective: IgG or IgA antibody? And how can that Ig class be enriched to enhance protection? To address the latter questions, preliminary studies were done in mice to determine the best routes and adjuvants to enrich for IgG or IgA in genital secretions (Corbeil *et al.*, 2001). Subcutaneous priming with the immunoaffinity purified surface antigen (called TF1.17 antigen) in Quil A adjuvant and subcutaneous boosting with whole cells enriched for IgG anti-TF1.17 antibodies, whereas subcutaneous priming and vaginal boosting greatly enriched for IgA antibodies in genital secretions. When cattle immunized by these two methods were challenged vaginally with *T. foetus*, those with predominantly IgA or predominantly IgG1 anti-TF1.17 antibodies in genital secretions were equally protected. Later studies with similar nasal immunizations showed that stimulation of the common mucosal immune system yielded results similar to those of vaginal immunization (Corbeil *et al.*, 2001). This raised the question of inductive sites for local immune responses in the genital tract.

Others have suggested that the genital tract is not an inductive site because M cells and mucosa-associated lymphoreticular tissue (MALT) are not present. This is true of cattle as well as mice and humans. However, even though control cows did not have histologically demonstrable MALT in the uterus and vagina, cows experimentally infected with *T. foetus* did (Corbeil *et al.*, 2001). Similar lymphoid nodules and follicles under a modified epithelium were detected in preputial and penial surfaces of bulls infected with *T. foetus* (Rhyan *et al.*, 1999). Immunostaining of parallel sections with mAb to TF1.17 antigen indicated uptake of antigen by epithelial cells and large macrophage or dendritic type cells under the basement membrane near the lymphoid follicles (Rhyan *et al.*, 1999). Similar antigen uptake has been detected in the infected female uterine and vaginal mucosa (unpublished data, Rhyan, J.C., BonDurant, R.H., and Corbeil, L.B.). Thus, even though the parasite is noninvasive, released TF1.17 antigen appears to be taken up

by epithelial cells. Rat uterine epithelial cells can present antigen to Th cells (Wira and Rossol, 1995). Also, macrophage/dendritic type cells positive for antigen should be antigen-presenting cells (APCs). Detection of IgG1 and IgA antibodies to TF1.17 antigen in genital secretions of infected animals (Rhyan *et al.*, 1999) and cows (Corbeil *et al.*, 2001) and the histologic demonstration of follicles and putative APCs suggest that inductive sites in the genital tract are formed in response to antigen.

Like *C. fetus* subsp. *venerealis*, *T. foetus* has mechanisms for evasion of immune responses. These include coating of the surface with Ig nonspecifically (Corbeil *et al.*, 1991), epitope variation (Ikeda *et al.*, 1993), and cleavage of IgG1, IgG2, and complement component 3 by extracellular cysteine proteinase (Talbot *et al.*, 1991; Kania *et al.*, 2001). However, as with *C. fetus*, it is clear that the dynamic interaction between host and parasite can be made to favor the host by systemic or mucosal immunization. The usefulness of whole cell vaccines in preventing *T. foetus* in cows has been demonstrated in clinical trials (Kvasnicka *et al.*, 1992). Earlier, Clark *et al.* (1984) demonstrated efficacious immunization of bulls with whole *T. foetus* cells or crude membrane glycoproteins that probably contained TF1.17 antigen. First-generation whole cell vaccines are now commercially available for prevention of trichomoniasis in cows.

Summary

The above studies with *C. fetus* subsp. *venerealis* and *T. foetus* show that:

- STDs can be prevented or even cured by systemic vaccination of both males and females.
- At least for one STD, IgG and IgA of the same antigen specificity are equally protective at the mucosal surface.
- Inductive sites are formed in the mucosa of infected male and female genital tracts, even with noninvasive pathogens.
- Strong and appropriate immune responses will clear microbial infection from the genital tract even when the microbe has multiple immune evasive mechanisms.
- Protection against two STDs has been demonstrated in the natural outbred host (cattle) and thus has advantages over murine models of STD vaccines. In the latter, the human pathogen is usually inoculated into the abnormal murine host and the disease does not mimic the human infection. Furthermore, although inbred mice provide a homogenous experimental model, they do not represent the variation in immune responses seen in the human population. The work on bovine vibriosis and trichomoniasis demonstrates protection under field conditions for two STDs that cause adverse pregnancy outcome in an outbred host. This is an encouraging precedent for control of human STDs and related adverse pregnancy outcomes.

Future needs

Future needs include identification of the protective antigens for most STDs. For antibody-mediated protection of the genital mucosa, several questions have not yet been addressed. As alluded to earlier, it is not clear how IgG crosses the mucosal epithelium into the secretions since it lacks secretory component and a polymeric Ig receptor-mediated type of transport. To our knowledge, the role of IgE in the genital tract has been largely unstudied. Last, manipulating genital immune responses to enhance Th1- or Th2-type responses is an unexplored research area. This should be important in protection against intracellular or extracellular pathogens. The use of DNA or recombinant vaccines including genes for appropriate cytokines may be an approach to meet this need.

ENTERIC VACCINES

Enteric disease is a major cause of mortality and morbidity in animals. Agents causing diarrhea in animals include viruses (*e.g.*, adenoviruses, pestiviruses, caliciviruses, coronaviruses, parvoviruses, rotaviruses, toroviruses), bacteria (*e.g.*, *Campylobacter* spp., *Clostridium* spp., diarrheagenic *Escherichia coli*, *Salmonella* spp., *Yersinia* spp.), and parasites (*e.g.*, *Coccidia* spp., *Cryptosporidium parvum*). These infections occur most commonly in suckling animals or in poultry less than 3 weeks of age but may also be common postweaning or in susceptible seronegative or stressed adult animals (Saif and Jackwood, 1990). We have summarized veterinary vaccines marketed for prevention and control of diseases caused by mucosal pathogens (Tables 61.1 to 61.3). Because attachment, adhesion, colonization, replication, and invasion by enteric pathogens are largely localized to the gastrointestinal tract, immune effectors on intestinal surfaces, *e.g.*, secretory (S)-IgA antibodies, cytokines, and cytotoxic NK and T cells, play critical roles in protective immunity. Enteric pathogens have different characteristics related to their intestinal tropism and replication, requiring different vaccination strategies.

Enteric viruses have predilections for replication in distinct vertical and longitudinal regions of the small intestine or the large intestine (Saif, 1999a). They cause diarrhea of variable severity via mechanisms that differ from those of enteric bacteria, most of which cause secretory diarrhea mediated by enterotoxins (Bertschinger, 1999). Enteric viruses produce cytolytic infections of enterocytes, leading to varying degrees of villus loss and fusion, resulting in reduced absorptive capacity in the small intestine and malabsorptive, maldigestive diarrhea. A rotavirus nonstructural protein, NSP4, reportedly functions as a viral enterotoxin and plays a role in the pathogenesis of rotavirus diarrhea, according to the results of studies of mice (Estes *et al.*, 2001). The role of NSP4 in rotavirus diarrhea in other species has not been confirmed.

The enteric nervous system has been recognized as a critical component in regulating fluid secretion in the normal gut and a key element in the pathophysiology of rotavirus diarrhea in mice (Lundgren *et al.*, 2000). Neural reflex pathways increase fluid secretion by enterocytes in response to

infection with rotavirus and other enteric pathogens (reviewed by Jones and Blikslager [2002]).

Enteropathogenic viruses can be divided into three types according to their preferred site of replication in the intestine (reviewed by Saif, 1999a). Although viruses such as hepatitis viruses and picornaviruses, including human polioviruses and enteroviruses, are shed in feces, they do not replicate in enterocytes and they cause systemic and not gastrointestinal infections. Poliovirus vaccines (oral and parenteral) are often cited as quintessential enteric viral vaccines, but they induce systemic neutralizing antibodies that prevent extraintestinal viral spread and paralytic polio. The applicability of poliovirus as a model for immunity to localized enteric infections is thus limited. Type I viruses infect small intestinal villous enterocytes via the luminal surface and include canine coronavirus, porcine transmissible gastroenteritis coronavirus (TGEV), rotavirus, astrovirus, and calicivirus. TGEV infects and destroys the absorptive enterocytes of the entire villi throughout the small intestine, causing pronounced villous atrophy and often fatal diarrhea. Rotavirus and astrovirus infections are more restricted within the villi and occur mainly in the mid to distal small intestine, causing less severe villous atrophy and diarrhea. Enteric caliciviruses infect villous enterocytes of the proximal small intestine, inducing moderate villous atrophy and diarrhea. Type II viruses such as adenoviruses, bovine coronaviruses, toroviruses, and porcine epidemic diarrhea coronavirus (PEDV) infect villous and crypt enterocytes in the distal small intestine and the large intestine, inducing moderate to severe villous atrophy, crypt aplasia, and diarrhea. Type III viruses such as enteric parvoviruses infect crypt enterocytes basolaterally, causing crypt aplasia, severe villous atrophy, mucosal collapse, and severe hemorrhagic and often fatal diarrhea (Saif, 1999a). Thus, parvovirus infections can be prevented by systemic immunity, whereas prevention of localized enteric virus infections (types I and II) relies largely on intestinal immunity.

The enteropathogenicity of bacteria is determined by their virulence factors, including adhesion factors (fimbriae or pili) and enterotoxins; therefore, bacterial vaccines generally need to prevent attachment and toxin action within the intestine (Bertschinger, 1999).

In the following sections, we review vaccine strategies for types I, II, and III enteric infections. TGEV and rotavirus vaccines in pigs will be reviewed to illustrate findings concerning domestic outbred animals instead of inbred laboratory rodent models.

Vaccines to induce passive and active immunity in neonates to type I enteric viruses infecting villous enterocytes

Passive immunity

Prevention of localized intestinal infections requires the presence of sufficient levels of antibodies at the site of pathogen attachment, replication, and invasion (gut lumen). The need to provide neonatal immunity against enteric pathogens prompted studies of maternal vaccines to enhance passive lactogenic immunity (maternal antibodies in colostrum and milk). The notion that live oral vaccines could mimic natural routes of infection and were preferable to conventional inactivated parenteral vaccines for stimulating protective lactogenic immunity (Bohl *et al.*, 1972; Saif *et al.*, 1972) was put forth over 30 years ago. Studies showed that in TGEV-seronegative sows, only oral immunization with virulent TGEV induced high rates of protection in suckling neonates. Oral immunization with live TGEV induced high titers of S-IgA antibodies in colostrum and milk, whereas systemic immunization induced mainly IgG antibodies. The ability of sows to transmit a high degree of passive lactogenic immunity to their suckling progeny was more closely associated with S-IgA than IgG TGEV antibodies. Bohl and Saif were the first to elaborate the concept of a gut–mammary gland–S-IgA immunologic axis, and these pioneering studies formed part of the basic tenet for a common mucosal immune system. Oral immunization of pregnant sows with attenuated TGEV and rotavirus vaccines is still used to induce passive immunity (Table 61.2). However, it was subsequently shown that in seropositive, naturally infected pregnant swine or cattle, lactogenic antibodies (S-IgA in swine and IgG1 in cattle) could also be enhanced by parenteral vaccination with live or appropriate killed or subunit vaccines (reviewed by Saif and Wesley, 1999; Saif and Fernandez, 1996). These observations concerning vaccine effects in TGEV-seronegative versus -seropositive animals explain some of the vaccine inconsistencies seen in field studies. Killed and modified live vaccines administered orally or parenterally to the mother are used extensively to increase lactogenic immunity in livestock and will be discussed further in the passive immunity section.

Active immunity

Rotavirus is a major cause of dehydrating diarrhea in young livestock, infants, and poultry (Saif and Fernandez, 1996). Multiple rotavirus serogroups (A, B, C, and E) based upon common inner-capsid VP6 antigens and multiple G (VP7, glycoprotein) and P (VP4, protease-sensitive) serotypes based on neutralizing epitopes on VP7 and VP4 capsid proteins of group A rotaviruses have been detected in humans, sheep, swine, cattle, horses, and poultry (Kapikian *et al.*, 2001). Characteristics of rotaviruses applicable to human and animal rotaviruses are reviewed in Chapter 49 on viral gastroenteritis vaccines. Among the distinct rotavirus serogroups and serotypes, cross-protection is minimal or nonexistent. The antigenic divergence among different sero/genotypes of rotaviruses (and enteric caliciviruses) presents a challenge for design of vaccines capable of inducing heterotypic protection.

Commercial modified live and killed rotavirus vaccines for rotavirus diarrhea in livestock and poultry are limited to group A rotaviruses and a group C rotavirus for pigs (Saif and Fernandez, 1996). The first oral rotavirus vaccine for calves was developed in 1972 (1 year prior to the discovery of human rotavirus) with use of a cell-culture-adapted neonatal calf diarrhea rotavirus (NCDV) strain (Mebus *et al.*, 1972). Although a significant reduction in morbidity

and mortality was observed in a field trial among vaccinated calves in the majority of herds (in comparison with previous years), subsequent field studies revealed variable efficacy. Experimental studies suggested that maternal antibodies interfered with live vaccine replication and suppressed development of active immunity (Saif and Fernandez, 1996).

The neonatal gnotobiotic pig model of rotavirus infection and disease has been used to study correlates of active protective immunity and to evaluate approaches to improve the immunogenicity and protective efficacy of rotavirus vaccines for nearly 2 decades (Saif *et al.*, 1996; Saif *et al.*, 1997; Yuan and Saif, 2002). Gnotobiotic pigs are free of maternal antibodies (placental transfer of Ig does not occur in swine), but they are immunocompetent at birth. They are maintained aseptically and free of exposure to extraneous rotaviruses, ensuring that exposure to a single pathogen can be analyzed. Initial studies were conducted to mimic natural rotavirus infection (Bohl *et al.*, 1984) and to examine immune correlates of protection (Saif *et al.*, 1997). Gnotobiotic pigs orally inoculated with virulent or attenuated porcine rotaviruses or human rotavirus (HRV) were completely protected from homotypic but not heterotypic (distinct P and G type) rotavirus challenge (Hoshino *et al.*, 1988; Saif *et al.*, 1997). Pigs inoculated with virulent HRV developed significantly higher numbers of virus-specific IgA and IgG antibody-forming cells (AFCs) and memory B cells and higher lymphocyte proliferative responses in the intestinal lamina propria than did pigs inoculated with attenuated HRV (Ward *et al.*, 1996b; Yuan *et al.*, 1996). Pigs inoculated with two or three doses of attenuated HRV were moderately protected against virus shedding and diarrhea after homotypic challenge, similar to results of clinical trials of oral attenuated rotavirus vaccines in infants (Bresee *et al.*, 1999). The magnitude of the intestinal IgA AFC and lymphocyte proliferative responses correlated with the level of protection induced (Ward *et al.*, 1996b; Yuan *et al.*, 1996).

Immunogenicity and protective efficacy of various rotavirus vaccine formulations (attenuated replicating virus, inactivated virus, and recombinant baculovirus-expressed virus-like particles [VLPs]), administration routes, and adjuvants also have been evaluated in the gnotobiotic pig model (Saif *et al.*, 1997; Yuan and Saif, 2002). Inactivated oral or intramuscular HRV vaccines failed to protect against virulent HRV challenge, despite high IgG antibody responses induced in serum and systemic lymphoid tissues by the intramuscular vaccine. Rotavirus subunit vaccines consisting of double-layered VLPs composed of rotavirus inner capsid proteins VP2 and VP6 (2/6-VLPs) administered nasally or orally with mutant heat-labile toxin of *E. coli* (mLT) or ISCOMs as adjuvants (Iosef *et al.*, 2002; Yuan and Saif, 2002) induced IgG AFC responses in systemic lymphoid tissues and low or no IgA AFC responses in intestinal lymphoid tissues and also failed to mediate protection. The failure of intramuscularly administered inactivated HRV vaccines demonstrates that protective immunity against rotavirus requires the induction of IgA antibodies in the intestine, since systemic IgG antibodies alone were not effective. The failure of nasal or oral 2/6-VLP vaccines suggests that protective immunity to rotavirus diarrhea in neonatal pigs requires the presence of intestinal IgA neutralizing antibodies to the outer capsid rotavirus proteins VP4 and VP7.

However, when 2/6-VLPs adjuvanted with MLT or ISCOM were used as nasal or oral booster doses in pigs orally primed with attenuated HRV, the protective efficacy increased significantly, and the highest numbers of intestinal IgA AFC and serum and intestinal IgA antibody titers were induced by this sequential prime/boost regimen (AttHRV/2/6-VLP), among all the vaccines tested in the gnotobiotic pig model (Iosef et al., 2002; Yuan and Saif, 2002). An interesting finding was that priming with two doses of 2/6-VLP followed by live attenuated HRV was ineffective for inducing IgA antibodies or protection. Thus, the use of a replicating vaccine to prime lymphocytes in the major inductive site (gut-associated lymphoreticular tissue, or GALT), followed by boosting with a nonreplicating vaccine at a second mucosal inductive site (nasopharyngeal-associated lymphoreticular tissue, or NALT), was a highly effective approach to stimulating the mucosal immune system and to inducing active protective immunity against infection and diarrhea.

Using the TGEV model for evaluation of active protection against diarrhea in pigs, researchers also revealed new information about compartmentalization in the common mucosal immune system and its impact on mucosal vaccine strategies and protection (VanCott et al., 1993, 1994). The natural occurrence of a deletion mutant of TGEV with exclusive respiratory tropism, referred to as porcine respiratory coronavirus (PRCV), provided a unique opportunity to study AFC responses and protective immunity to two antigenically related porcine coronaviruses with enteric (TGEV) versus respiratory (PRCV) tropism. The investigators showed that oral immunization of pigs with TGEV induced high numbers of IgA AFCs in the intestine and provided complete protection against TGEV challenge, whereas nasal immunization of pigs with PRCV induced mainly systemic immune responses (IgG AFCs) and provided only partial protection against TGEV challenge. Thus, the nasal PRCV alone failed to elicit sufficient intestinal IgA AFCs to provide full protection against the enteric pathogen, TGEV. Findings from this study, in addition to the studies of rotavirus vaccines, suggest that use of multiple mucosal inductive sites in a prime/boost vaccination regimen may be an effective approach to overcoming the compartmentalization in the common mucosal immune system.

Vaccines to induce active immunity in neonates to type III enteric viruses infecting crypt enterocytes

Canine parvovirus (CPV) infects crypt enterocytes, causing hemorrhagic gastroenteritis in pups (Bridger, 1990). Since CPV is likely disseminated to the basolateral surface of crypts by the hematogenous route, serum neutralizing antibodies (derived maternally or actively produced) are protective against the disease. In 1982, it was demonstrated that pups with hemagglutination inhibition (HI) serum antibody

titers of >1:80 were immune to oronasal CPV type 2 challenge (Pollock and Carmichael, 1982). CPV is highly stable in the environment, and pups became susceptible to infection as soon as maternal antibodies declined to HI titers of 1:64 to 1:80. A maternal HI antibody titer as low as 1:20 severely affected the efficacy of a live CPV vaccine, however (Carmichael et al., 1983).

Others have compared the immunogenicity and protective efficacy of commercial vaccines and concluded that substantial differences existed in their ability to immunize and protect pups with maternal antibodies (Larson and Schultz 1997). During the past 4 decades of CPV vaccine development, modified live viruses have proved to be superior to inactivated intramuscular vaccines (Appel, 1999). A study by Pratelli et al., (2000) showed that a modified-live variant CPV-2b vaccine elicited protective immunity in 100% of pups whose maternal antibody titers were 1:10 to 1:40 and even in 60% of pups with antibody titers of 1:320.

Synthetic peptides (Casal et al., 1995), DNA plasmids expressing VP1 (Jiang et al., 1998), recombinant VLPs formed by baculovirus-expressed VP2 (Casal, 1999), and chimeric plant viruses expressing VP2 peptide (Langeveld et al., 2001) have been evaluated in dogs or mice without maternal antibodies and have demonstrated good immunogenicity and/or protective efficacy. Further efficacy tests in pups in the presence of maternal antibodies are needed to assess their commercial potential.

Vaccines to induce immunity against enteric bacterial infections in neonates

Oral vaccines for induction of active immunity against bacterial diarrhea are not commonly used in livestock, although E. coli diarrhea is an important problem in postweaning pigs. Fimbrial vaccines are routinely administered parenterally to pregnant cattle, sheep, and swine to protect their suckling neonates against enterotoxigenic E. coli (ETEC) infections (Moon and Bunn, 1993). Such vaccines are practical and effective because (1) fimbriae are required for the adhesion-colonization of bacteria early in the pathogenesis of the disease; (2) most fatal ETEC infections in farm animals occur in the neonatal period; and (3) more than 90% of the ETEC strains in farm animals belong to a small family of fimbrial antigen types. Moreover, the vaccine strategy used to induce lactogenic immunity, parenteral vaccination of field-exposed seropositive mothers, is the same as that shown to be effective for parenteral application of rotavirus vaccines in rotavirus-seropositive mothers (Saif and Fernandez, 1996; Saif and Jackwood, 1990).

Studies of live oral enteric vaccines in animals have clarified the mechanisms of induction of protective immunity against enteric disease and contributed to our understanding of the common mucosal immune system. However, commercial live oral vaccines have often shown inadequate or inconsistent efficacy under field conditions (Saif and Jackwood, 1990). Major obstacles to improved efficacy of oral vaccines include maternal antibodies in the intestine of neonates (mainly colostrum and milk antibodies), which interfere with live vaccine replication; inability of attenuated vaccine strains to adequately infect or stimulate S-IgA antibodies in the intestine (*i.e.*, less immunogenic than virulent field strains); use of inappropriate or unstable antigens for subunit vaccines; lack of oral delivery vehicles or mucosal adjuvants for subunit vaccines; and infection by pathogens prior to vaccination.

Differences in veterinary species and mouse models

Studies of adult mice and rabbits have shown that inactivated rotavirus vaccines and various formulations of VLPs (VP2/6, VP2/6/7, VP2/4/6/7), administered via intramuscular, oral, or nasal routes with or without adjuvants, induce complete or significant partial protection against rotavirus infection (Crawford *et al.*, 1999; O'Neal *et al.*, 1998; Siadat-Pajouh and Cai, 2001). However, only protection against infection, not against diarrhea, can be assessed in adult mouse or rabbit models, as these species are susceptible to rotavirus-induced diarrhea only during the first 2 weeks of life (Ciarlet *et al.*, 1998; Ward *et al.*, 1990). Studies in pigs indicate that protection rates against rotavirus diarrhea upon challenge correlate with the magnitude of IgA AFC and memory B cell responses in intestinal lymphoid tissues but not with such responses in systemic lymphoid tissues (Yuan and Saif, 2002). Thus, the capacity to induce sufficient levels of intestinal IgA AFCs or antibodies and sufficient memory B cell responses appears to be critical for the efficacy of rotavirus vaccines in large animals and likely in human infants (Coulson *et al.*, 1992).

The relative importance of B cells versus CD4$^+$ and CD8$^+$ T cells in protective immunity to rotavirus has been extensively studied in adult mice because inbred mouse strains, antibodies to CD4 and CD8 T cells, and gene knockout mice are available to facilitate such studies (Franco and Greenberg, 2000; McNeal *et al.*, 2002). In these studies neither CD4$^+$/CD8$^+$ T cells nor antibodies were essential for induction of protective immunity to rotavirus infection in adult mice, but usually one of these effectors (T or B cells) was necessary for elimination of primary rotavirus infection. The redundant nature of the immune responses to rotavirus in mice, the multiple immunologic and possibly nonimmunologic pathways to resolve rotavirus infections (Franco and Greenberg, 2000), the age factor (adult models) and host differences in the pathogenesis of rotavirus infection in mice and pigs (Conner and Ramig, 1997; Saif *et al.*, 1997), and the use of highly inbred mouse strains contribute to the discrepancies seen between the adult mouse and neonatal gnotobiotic pig models.

Future directions

To develop more effective vaccines against enteric pathogens, improved methods are needed to induce high levels of intestinal IgA antibodies against the appropriate microbial antigens. Vaccines should also induce heterotypic protection, active immunity in the presence of maternal antibodies, and if possible long-lasting immunological memory against enteric pathogens. In nature, such memory is pre-sumably maintained by frequent boosting by repeated environmental exposure to these common and stable enteric pathogens, most of which are endemic in animal and human populations. Novel vaccines (*e.g.*, transgenic plants), adjuvants (*e.g.*, MLT, ISCOM, CpG-oligodeoxynucleotides, 1α, 25-dihydroxyvitamin D3), and vaccine delivery systems (*e.g.*, recombinant plant or animal viruses, bacterial vectors, and microparticles) should be explored and evaluated in relevant animal models.

A recent study showed that intramuscular immunization with *E. coli* F4 fimbriae reduced F4$^+$-*E. coli* excretion in feces of suckling pigs upon challenge. Addition of 1α, 25(OH)$_2$D3 (a Th2 modulating adjuvant) reduced shedding significantly and was associated with secondary IgA antibody responses postchallenge. Addition of CpG (a Th1 modulating adjuvant) reduced diarrhea and was associated with enhanced lymphocyte proliferative responses (Van der Stede *et al.*, 2003).

A newly developed coronavirus expression system (Alonso *et al.*, 2002; Enjuanes *et al.*, 2001) has potential for use as a virus vector for delivery of mucosal vaccines. Since coronaviruses infect the mucosal surfaces of the respiratory and intestinal tracts, these vaccines can be targeted to mucosal inductive sites. Nonpathogenic coronaviruses infecting many species of interest are available for development of expression systems. The tissue and species tropism of coronaviruses may be manipulated by engineering the S gene, which is the tropism determinant, to target specific tissues in their individual hosts (Enjuanes *et al.*, 2001).

Attenuated *S. typhimurium* strains expressing heterologous antigens have been widely evaluated, mostly in mice, as vector vaccines for human mucosal pathogens (reviewed by Fooks, 2000). Recombinant *S. typhimurium* has been used as an antigen delivery system for oral immunization of chicks against the coccidian parasite *Eimeria tenella* (Pogonka *et al.*, 2003). Recombinant *Salmonella* vaccines have also been used to express antigens of TGEV and of bovine enterotoxigenic *E. coli* (ETEC) K99 fimbriae (Chen and Schifferli, 2001; Ascon *et al.*, 1998).

Transgenic plants expressing recombinant proteins from enteropathogens may provide inexpensive edible vaccines for induction of intestinal immunity. Plants expressing antigens of enteric viruses, such as the TGEV S protein (Tuboly *et al.*, 2000) or rotavirus NSP4-cholera toxin B and A2 subunit fusion protein (Yu and Langridge, 2001), induce antibody responses following parenteral immunization. Further research is necessary to improve immune responses and immunological memory following ingestion of transgenic plant vaccines.

PASSIVE IMMUNITY

The passive transfer of maternal immunity provides essential protection in newborn mammals. Although the neonatal immune system is competent to mount primary immune responses against antigens of many infectious agents, developing both humoral and cell-mediated immunity, in many cases primary (active) immune responses do not develop quickly enough to prevent disease and death. Maternal immunologic assistance thus can provide a critical (though temporary) aid to survival for neonates.

The enhancement of passive immunity through vaccination of the mother has been a successful disease prevention strategy in domesticated animals. Vaccinated mothers develop higher levels of specific antibodies in colostrum and milk and thereby increase levels of immunity in their offspring (Glezen, 2001; Saif and Fernandez, 1996; Tizard, 2000). Passive immunity can also be enhanced by oral administration of immune milk or heterologous antibody preparations (*e.g.*, chicken egg yolk IgY, [Ikemori, 1992; Kuroki, 1994] or monoclonal antibodies) or by parenteral administration of hyperimmune plasma (Becu *et al.*, 1997).

Unfortunately, passive antibodies often interfere with active immunization of young animals and birds. Various vaccination strategies have been developed to minimize the suppressive effects of maternal antibodies, but improved adjuvants and antigen delivery systems are needed to facilitate efficient and predictable induction of active immunity in the presence of maternal antibodies. This section will address past, current, and future approaches and considerations for using passive immunity in veterinary species.

Transfer of maternal immunity

The transfer of systemic passive immunity from the mother to her offspring can occur prenatally, via the placenta or yolk sac, or postnatally via ingestion of colostrum and milk, depending upon the species. The main Ig isotype transferred in most species is IgG. Mechanisms of transport of Ig from dam to offspring are described elsewhere in this volume. In mice and rats, transplacental transfer of Ig occurs in combination with prolonged (16 and 21 days, respectively) postnatal transfer by means of colostrum and milk (Pastoret, 1998). In dogs and cats, transfer of IgG occurs by a combination of prenatal and postnatal mechanisms, with 5% to 10% of total transfer occurring before birth (Tizard, 2000). In ruminants, horses, and pigs, offspring are born virtually agammaglobulinemic, and transmission of Ig occurs only via colostrum for a limited time after birth (Pastoret, 1998; Wagstrom *et al.*, 2000). After the transition from production of colostrum to milk, Ig are no longer absorbed from the intestines and act only locally.

Immunoglobulin absorption in neonates of large domestic species is facilitated by the presence of protease inhibitors in the colostrum (Westrom *et al.*, 1982), and its efficiency declines rapidly after birth, with maximal absorption occurring in the first 4 hours. The cessation of absorption of intact macromolecules is termed "gut closure" and occurs at different ages in different species. In calves and pigs closure normally occurs by 24 to 36 hours after birth.

Failure of passive transfer (FPT) in domestic large animals

Absorption of colostral Ig can be highly effective, supplying the newborn with serum antibodies at similar levels to those in the mother's circulation. Failure of passive transfer is a common problem, however, in newborn calves and foals

(Besser and Gay, 1994; Tyler-McGowan and Hodgson, 1997). Failure of passive transfer may occur because of the production of low quantities of colostrum, production of colostrum with inadequate levels of maternal antibodies (e.g., with mastitis or agalactia), ingestion of low quantities of colostrum, or inefficient absorption in the gut (Quigley and Drewry, 1998). Colostral supplements and replacers (Arthington *et al.*, 2000; Quigley and Drewry, 1998) as well as plasma products have been developed commercially to address this problem, with variable success. Since transfer of maternal antibodies in farm animals is dependent upon ingestion of colostrum, the benefits of vaccination of the dam for enhancing passive immunity are lost if absorption of colostral Ig is inefficient (Hodgins and Shewen, 1994).

Mechanisms of clearance of passively acquired IgG

The half-life of Ig varies considerably among species of domestic animals. Recent findings suggesting that the FcRn is involved in homeostasis of serum levels of IgG in general do not preclude distinct mechanisms functioning in neonates. Studies conducted by Besser *et al.* (1987, 1988b) indicate that the main route of clearance of passively acquired IgG1 in calves is transfer from the serum to the intestine. Approximately 70% of passively acquired IgG1 is eliminated by this route. If titers of passive circulating antibodies are high enough, the transfer of antibodies from the circulation to the intestinal lumen is sufficiently efficient to mediate at least short-term partial protection against rotavirus diarrhea (Besser *et al.*, 1988a). The same mechanism may be functional in piglets (reviewed by Saif and Wesley, 1999; Parreño *et al.*, 1999; Ward *et al.*, 1996a). The persistence of titers of circulating maternal antibodies is generally considered in the design of vaccination strategies for young animals because of suppressive effects of maternal antibodies on active immune responses. However, it is not always necessary to wait for titers of maternal antibodies to decline to the limit of detection before vaccination (Hodgins and Shewen, 1998), and in maternally immune piglets, induction of memory can occur even in the presence of detectable antibodies (Boersema *et al.*, 1998).

Passive immunity in the respiratory tract

Experiments in colostrum-deprived lambs (Jones *et al.*, 1989) and calves (Mosier *et al.*, 1995) have demonstrated the ability of parenterally administered immune antisera of appropriate specificity and high titer to mediate protection following experimental challenge with *M. haemolytica*. Although antisera prepared against *M. haemolytica* continue to be marketed in some countries for prevention of pneumonia in calves, lack of documentation of the specificity and antibody titer of these products makes their value questionable. Parenteral administration of hyperimmune plasma raised against *R. equi* has been shown to protect against pneumonia in young foals in experimental (Hooper-McGrevy *et al.*, 2001) and field studies (Becu *et al.*, 1997). Hyperimmune plasma is available commercially for prophylactic use in foals.

Prepartum vaccination of beef cows (Van Donkersgoed *et al.*, 1995) and dairy cows (Hodgins and Shewen, 1994; Hodgins and Shewen, 1996) has been demonstrated to increase titers of antibody to *M. haemolytica* in their colostrum and in the serum of their calves. Virtually all adult cattle have serum antibodies to *M. haemolytica*; vaccination therefore serves to trigger anamnestic responses.

Passive immunity in the gastrointestinal tract

Rodents have been a popular model for the study of passive protection by milk antibodies. However, rats and mice actively transport IgG from the gut into the circulation during the first 2 weeks of life. Thus, antibodies in ingested milk contribute to both local and systemic immunity in rodents, in contrast to the strictly local effects occurring in humans and most domestic animals. In pigs, horses, dogs, and cats, IgG is the most abundant Ig in colostrum, but IgA predominates in milk. Parenteral vaccination, by enhancing serum IgG antibody titers, contributes to IgG antibodies in colostrum but has limited effects on IgA antibodies in milk. Although Saif and Bohl (1983) and Salmon (1995) observed IgA antibody responses in sow's milk after the administration of live viruses into the mammary gland, this is not the usual mechanism for induction of IgA antibodies to enteric pathogens in milk of seronegative animals. Rather, in swine, Bohl and Saif (Bohl *et al.*, 1972; Saif *et al.*, 1972) showed that IgA antibodies in milk with specificity for enteric pathogens appear after sufficient antigenic stimulation (TGEV infection) of the intestine. On the basis of these observations, they first proposed trafficking of IgA lymphoblasts from the gut to the mammary gland in monogastrics. This proposed gut–mammary–S-IgA immunologic axis provided part of the initial basis for the concept of a common mucosal immune system. The trafficking of gut-origin IgA lymphoblasts to the mammary gland was confirmed experimentally in mice (Roux *et al.*, 1977) and subsequently verified in swine (Salmon *et al.*, 1984). In contrast, Sheldrake and Husband (1985) found little evidence of a gut–mammary gland axis in ruminants. Instead, in ruminants, IgG1 is the main isotype in both colostrum and milk (Butler, 1983), and it is selectively transported from serum primarily prepartum, but also postpartum, with a marked decrease in serum IgG1 prepartum (Butler, 1983). An IgG1-specific Fc receptor, probably the FcRn (Kacskovics *et al.*, 2000), expressed on the basolateral surface of mammary gland alveolar epithelial cells is responsible for this transport. It is interesting that both the expression of this IgG1 receptor in ruminants and the trafficking of IgA lymphoblasts to the mammary gland in monogastrics are regulated by pregnancy hormones (prolactin, estrogen, and progesterone) (Weisz-Carrington *et al.*, 1978; Barrington *et al.*, 2000).

Milk antibodies provide passive protection to the neonatal intestinal tract by immune exclusion, preventing the attachment of viruses, bacteria, and parasites, and by neutralizing enterotoxins, virulence factors, and viruses. S-IgA antibodies, presumably because of their resistance to cleavage by digestive enzymes and their higher levels in milk, appear to be more efficient in mediating protection in the gut of pigs and other monogastrics (Saif and Jackwood, 1990; Saif and Fernandez, 1996), but high persisting levels of passive IgG antibodies are also protective (reviewed in Saif and Wesley 1999; Ward *et al.*, 1996a; Parreño *et al.*, 1999). In ruminants, IgG1 antibodies, also relatively resistant to proteolytic enzymes (Brock *et al.*, 1977) and predominant in milk, may supplant the role of S-IgA.

Numerous vaccines are marketed for vaccination of cows and sows to provide lactogenic immunity to rotavirus, coronavirus, and *E. coli* in suckling offspring (Table 61.2). Vaccine efficacy has been variable and is influenced by numerous factors related to the host, the vaccine, and management. A discussion of key concepts follows, in which coronavirus and rotavirus enteric vaccines in swine and cattle serve as examples (reviewed by Saif and Jackwood, 1990; Saif and Fernandez, 1996; Saif and Wesley, 1999).

Ideally, suckling animals become subclinically infected with enteric pathogens while receiving adequate passive antibodies to prevent disease, and they develop active immunity (or are primed; Boersema *et al.*, 1998) to prevent subsequent diarrhea. This balance between passive immunity and disease has been disrupted in intensive animal production systems by exposing animals to high pathogen doses in confined, contaminated environments. In addition, earlier weaning practices, with feeding of supplements or milk replacers, curtail or dilute milk antibodies. Consequently, without maternal vaccines, antibody titers to enteric pathogens usually decrease to unprotective levels in milk.

Maternal enteric vaccines are commonly used in two populations of pregnant animals. To control epidemic infections (such as epidemic TGEV), they are targeted for use in naïve, seronegative animals to induce primary immune responses. To control endemic infections (such as with rotavirus and *E. coli*), booster vaccines are used in seropositive, field-exposed animals to stimulate anamnestic responses. Vaccine strategies for the latter vaccines generally have been more successful than for the former, reflecting a greater success in designing vaccines to boost rather than to prime for mucosal immunity to provide lactogenic immunity against enteric pathogens. To date, only virulent TGEV given to pregnant sows effectively stimulates high levels of IgA antibodies in milk and passive protection (reviewed by Saif and Jackwood, 1990; Saif and Wesley, 1999). Use of oral highly attenuated TGEV vaccines (safe for piglets but which replicate poorly in sows) induces lower IgA milk antibody titers and low or variable efficacy in the field (Moxley and Olsen, 1989). Parenteral killed TGEV vaccines induce only low milk IgG antibody titers and usually the lowest protection rates. Attempts to develop maternal TGEV recombinant subunit vaccines based on the surface TGEV spike (S) protein that induces neutralizing antibodies or live vector vaccines expressing the S protein have also been of limited success in TGEV-seronegative swine (reviewed by Saif and Wesley, 1999). However, prime/boost strategies such as intramuscular administration of TGEV S protein following oral/nasal priming with attenuated TGEV have shown promise as a means of enhancing milk IgA antibody titers (Park *et al.*, 1998). Epidemic TGEV outbreaks have also declined following the appearance of a respiratory variant of TGEV. This variant induces TGEV-neutralizing antibodies in milk and at least moderate protection against TGEV after repeated respiratory infections in sows, raising unresolved questions about bronchus-associated lymphoid tissue (BALT)–mammary gland lymphocyte trafficking (reviewed in Saif and Wesley, 1999).

Whereas TGEV is associated with both epidemic and endemic infections in swine, rotavirus and *E. coli* infections are endemic in swine and cattle. Booster vaccination strategies are required to enhance lactogenic immunity to such endemic enteric pathogens because antibody titers in milk decline dramatically during lactation. Although studies are limited, parenteral vaccination of TGEV- or rotavirus-seropositive (field-exposed) pregnant sows with attenuated vaccines effectively boosted both S-IgA and IgG antibodies in milk (Saif and Jackwood, 1990; Saif and Fernandez, 1996; Saif and Wesley, 1999). These findings concur with reports of increased breast milk IgA antibodies in women endemically exposed to cholera and parenterally boosted with a cholera vaccine (Svennerholm *et al.*, 1977). The finding that parenteral boosting is effective in increasing IgA antibodies in mucosal secretions of animals orally primed with a live pathogen is consistent with observations that after intestinal replication of rotavirus in pigs, IgA memory B cells initially reside in the ileal Peyer's patches but are subsequently also present in substantial numbers in spleen but not bone marrow (Yuan *et al.*, 2001). Thus, systemic stimulation of such IgA memory B cells by parenteral booster vaccines could yield IgA antibodies in serum for transport to mucosal secretions via the polymeric Ig receptor. These observations have led to mucosal prime/boost strategies for human and animal rotavirus vaccines that are currently being tested in gnotobiotic pigs (Yuan and Saif, 2002).

Under field conditions, antibodies to endemic intestinal pathogens are also common in bovine colostrum and milk, but without the boosting effect of highly immunogenic vaccines, antibody titers are often too low to protect calves (Besser and Gay, 1994; Saif *et al.*, 1983; Saif and Fernandez, 1996; Saif and Jackwood, 1990). Thus, vaccines are marketed for prepartum vaccination of cows against rotavirus, coronavirus, and *E. coli* to enhance passive immunity in their calves (Table 61.1), but the field efficacy of these viral vaccines has been questioned (Waltner-Toews *et al.*, 1985). A number of important variables may account for vaccine failures. These include vaccine titer and dose, inactivating agent, virus strain, adjuvant, inoculation route, and parity of the mother (reviewed by Saif and Fernandez, 1996). Because colostrum and milk of ruminants contain mainly serum-derived IgG1, parenteral (intramuscular, subcutaneous, or intramammary) inoculation of rotavirus seropositive cows with optimal live, inactivated, or subunit (VP 2/4/6/7 VLP) rotavirus vaccines effectively boosts both IgG1 and virus-neutralizing antibody titers in serum and milk.

A positive correlation has been shown between serum titers of rotavirus-neutralizing antibodies in neonatal beef calves and resistance to rotavirus diarrhea (Kohara and Tsunemitsu, 2000). Vaccination of pregnant dairy cows with modified live ($\geq 10^7$ plaque-forming units), binary ethyleneamine (but not β-propiolactone) inactivated rotavirus in incomplete Freund's adjuvant (IFA) (but not AlOH adjuvant) or recombinant 2/4/6/7 VLPs in IFA significantly increased titers of IgG1 and virus-neutralizing antibody to rotavirus in colostrum and milk (Saif *et al.*, 1983; Saif and Fernandez, 1996; Kim *et al.*, 2002). These colostral supplements mediated passive protection in calves against experimental oral rotavirus challenge (reviewed by Saif and Fernandez, 1996; Saif *et al.*, 1983).

Prepartum vaccination of cows and sows with bacterins prepared from enteropathogenic *E. coli* for prevention of diarrhea in their offspring is also commonly practiced (Table 61.2). Under modern farming practices, dairy and veal calves rarely are fed whole milk from their dams for more than 1 or 2 days. Thus, vaccine efficacy is based on antibodies absorbed from colostrum or retained temporarily in the gut, rather than on a continuing supply of immune milk. Besser *et al.* (1988a) demonstrated that transfer of passive IgG1 antibodies from the serum to the intestine in calves could mediate this short-term protection. Piglets, in contrast, continue to receive immune milk until weaning at 2 to 3 weeks of age. The importance of a continuous supply of passive antibodies for protection against TGEV has been demonstrated experimentally (Saif and Wesley, 1999).

Numerous commercial Ig preparations with antibody activity against specific enteric pathogens have been marketed over the past several decades. Products intended for prevention of *E. coli* enteritis in calves include dried bovine colostrum and whey, hyperimmune sera raised in horses, and mouse monoclonal antibodies to the K99 (F5) antigen of *E. coli*. These products are administered orally in the first 12 hours of life to prevent adhesion of enteropathogenic *E. coli*. Bovine Ig products containing antibodies to antigens of *E. coli* pathogenic for neonatal pigs have also been marketed for oral use in piglets. Orally administered bovine colostral whey containing rotavirus antibodies also passively protected piglets (in the absence of circulating antibodies) against rotavirus in a dose-dependent manner but did not interfere with induction of active serum antibody responses (Schaller *et al.*, 1992).

Oral administration of chicken egg yolk antibodies

Immunization of chickens shows promise as an efficient method of producing polyclonal antibodies for passive protection. Specific antibodies of the IgY isotype are induced by vaccination and are concentrated in egg yolk. Laying hens can produce about 20 g of IgY per year. Yolk antibodies with virus neutralizing activity provide partial protection against rotavirus (Kuroki *et al.*, 1994) and coronavirus diarrhea (Ikemori *et al.*, 1997). Yolk antibodies have also provided protection against enterotoxigenic *E. coli* in calves (Ikemori *et al.*, 1992) and piglets (Yokoyama *et al.*, 1997). Protective effects of yolk antibodies are dependent on antibody titers in the oral preparations (Marquardt, 2000). Thus, development of better means to protect yolk antibodies from digestive processes will improve both the efficacy and the economic viability of yolk antibodies for clinical applications (Mine and Kovacs-Nolan, 2002).

Induction of active immunity in the presence of maternal antibodies

For many diseases of newborns and neonates, passive immunity is the only practical means of providing timely protection. Unfortunately, it is well documented that maternal antibodies can suppress active immune responses following vaccination. This effect has been observed with both live and nonreplicating vaccines and for both systemic and mucosal immune responses (Siegrist *et al.*, 1998; Parreño *et al.*, 1999). Antibody responses especially are affected; recent evidence suggests that T-lymphocyte responses may not be suppressed (Siegrist *et al.*, 1998). Titers of maternal antibodies are maximal for most species of interest in the first week of life and then decline gradually over the next few months, but variability of titers among individuals is high. With many vaccines, a "window of disease susceptibility" of variable duration occurs when titers of maternal antibodies are too low to mediate protection but too high to permit effective vaccination.

A number of strategies are used to cope with this problem. Some veterinary vaccines for cattle are sold with the disclaimer that "animals vaccinated before 6 months of age should receive a booster dose of vaccine at 6 months of age." This provides little solace for the many diseases of cattle occurring in the first weeks or months of life. A common strategy for vaccines of dogs and cats is to administer a series of doses of vaccine from an early age (at which only a few individuals will be responsive) and to continue vaccinating until an age at which virtually all can respond to vaccination. This strategy has economic disadvantages for the pet owner. Some manufacturers produce low-passage, high-virus-titer vaccines especially for use in situations where high titers of maternal antibodies and high pathogen exposure are anticipated. This is similar to a strategy once (but no longer) approved by the World Health Organization for vaccination of children in developing countries against measles (Gellin and Katz, 1994). Preliminary evidence suggests that incorporation of vaccine antigens in highly structured ISCOMs or nasal application of vaccines can enhance immune responses in the presence of maternal antibodies (Van Binnendijk *et al.*, 1997; Brockmeier *et al.*, 1997).

Future needs

Maternal vaccination to enhance passive immunity is already widely used in veterinary medicine. Some of these vaccines, especially vaccines against enteric viruses, have limited efficacy; new approaches are needed to enhance immunogenicity in an economically viable manner. Commercial products have already been developed as supplements for newborns that have received inadequate amounts or quality of colostrum. Although some of these products contain guaranteed minimum titers of antibodies against specific organ-

isms, there is a need to expand this quality control to additional common pathogens of neonates.

There is an urgent need for development of adjuvants and delivery systems capable of reliably inducing active immunity in neonates in spite of the presence of maternal antibodies. The ability to provide continuity of immune protection from birth, by combining passive immunity with active immunization, would have a major impact on neonatal morbidity and mortality in animals and humans.

CONCLUSIONS

Research on mucosal veterinary vaccines has contributed new concepts to the field of mucosal immunity. Investigations of pathogen–host interactions in outbred animals have illustrated the complexity of these interactions and have encouraged rethinking of established paradigms. Early studies of an enteric coronavirus infection of swine (TGEV) led to the concept of the gut–mammary gland–S-IgA immunologic axis and provided part of the basic tenet for a common mucosal immune system (Bohl *et al.*, 1972; Saif *et al.*, 1972). Later studies of TGEV and a deletion mutant of TGEV with respiratory tropism (PRCV) revealed that functional compartmentalization exists within the common mucosal immune system whereby nasal inoculation of pigs with PRCV failed to elicit sufficient intestinal IgA antibody responses to fully protect against the enteric pathogen TGEV (Van Cott *et al.*, 1993, 1994). Subsequent studies have explored new prime/boost mucosal immunization strategies to elicit intestinal immunity to the enteric pathogen rotavirus in naïve pigs (Saif, 1999b; Yuan and Saif, 2002). In these studies, only oral priming with attenuated virus led to successful nasal booster responses with use of nonreplicating (VLP) vaccines combined with mucosal adjuvants such as ISCOM or mLT. Thus, use of a replicating vaccine to prime lymphocytes at a major mucosal inductive site (GALT), followed by boosting with a nonreplicating vaccine at a second inductive site (NALT), effectively stimulated intestinal IgA antibodies and induced active protection against rotavirus diarrhea.

Although there is progress in developing safe and effective nonreplicating vaccines to boost mucosal immune responses, including the use of parenteral booster vaccines in field-exposed animals (Saif and Fernandez, 1996), there is still a need to develop effective, safe vaccines to prime for mucosal immunity. Mucosal adjuvants (mLT, ISCOM, CpG, cytokines [Rankin *et al.*, 2001]) and new delivery systems (replicating vectors, microparticles [Bowersock *et al.*, 1994a]) have shown promise in animal studies reviewed in this chapter. However, their economical production and their final evaluation under field conditions, including in the presence of maternal antibodies (as relevant), are needed.

Considerable research effort has been devoted to development of vaccines for respiratory diseases of domestic animals. In some instances attenuated organisms delivered by mucosal routes have demonstrated improved efficacy over nonreplicating antigens given by systemic routes. For many respiratory diseases, however, further progress in development of mucosal vaccines will have to await advances in understanding of disease pathogenesis and identification of protective antigens. In contrast, studies of ascending infections of the reproductive tract in cattle have demonstrated the efficacy of systemic vaccination to clear established infections and highlight the possibility of therapeutic vaccines.

Finally, it is important to realize that there are species differences to consider in designing vaccines to elicit mucosal immunity. For example, the primary Ig in mammary secretions of ruminants is IgG1, which is actively transported to the mammary gland from serum and provides effective passive immunity to the nursing offspring against enteric pathogens. Thus, parenteral immunization of the mother is effective in stimulating passive immunity in ruminants against enteric pathogens. In contrast, in monogastrics, IgA predominates in milk and IgA lymphoblasts that traffic to the mammary gland originate in the intestine. Therefore, oral vaccines in monogastrics may provide a more effective vaccine strategy to induce IgA antibodies in milk against enteric pathogens (Saif and Fernandez, 1996). If the aforementioned vaccine concepts and ones reviewed in this chapter are applied with new and effective mucosal adjuvants, delivery systems, and bioengineered vectors expressing the appropriate microbial antigens, it is likely that a new generation of veterinary vaccines will emerge to better cope with existing and emerging mucosal pathogens.

REFERENCES

Abdullah K. M., Udoh E. A., Shewen P.E., and Mellors A. (1992). A neutral glycoprotease of *Pasteurella haemolytica* A1 specifically cleaves O-sialoglycoproteins. *Infect. Immun.* 60, 56–62.

Alonso, S., Sola, I., Teifke, J. P., Reimann, I., Izeta, A., Balasch, M., Plana-Duran, J., Moormann, R. J., and Enjuanes, L. (2002). In vitro and in vivo expression of foreign genes by transmissible gastroenteritis coronavirus-derived minigenomes. *J. Gen. Virol.* 83, 567–579.

Angen O., Mutters R., Caugant D. A., Olsen J.E., and Bisgaard M. (1999). Taxonomic relationships of the [*Pasteurella*] haemolytica complex as evaluated by DNA–DNA hybridizations and 16S rRNA sequencing with proposal of *Mannheimia haemolytica* gen. nov., comb. nov., *M. granulomatis* comb. nov., *M. glucosida* sp. nov., *M. ruminalis* sp. nov., and *M. varigena* sp. nov. *Int. J. Syst. Bacteriol.* 49, 67–86.

Appel, M. J. (1999). Forty years of canine vaccination. *Adv. Vet. Med.* 41, 309–324.

Ardans A. A. (1999). Orthomyxoviridae. In *Veterinary Microbiology* (eds. Hirsh D.C., Zee Y.C.). Malden, Massachusetts: Blackwell Science, 396–402.

Arthington, J. D., Cattell, M. B., Quigley, J. D. 3rd, McCoy, G. C., and Hurley, W. L. (2000). Passive immunoglobin transfer in newborn calves fed colostrum or spray-dried serum protein alone or as a supplement to colostrum of varying quality. *J. Dairy Sci.* 83, 2834–2838.

Ascon, M. A., Hone, D. M., Walters, N., and Pascual, D. W. (1998). Oral immunization with a *Salmonella typhimurium* vaccine vector expressing recombinant enterotoxigenic *Escherichia coli* K99 fimbriae elicits elevated antibody titers for protective immunity. *Infect. Immun.* 66, 5470–5476.

Babiuk, L. A., and Acres, S. D. (1984). Models for bovine respiratory disease. In *Bovine Respiratory Disease* (ed. Loan R.W.). College Station, Texas: Texas A&M Press.

Babiuk, L. A., van Drunen Littel–van den Hurk, S., and Babiuk, S. L. (1999). Immunization of animals: from DNA to the dinner plate. *Vet. Immunol. Immunopathol.* 72, 189–202.

Babiuk, S., Baca-Estrada, M.E., Foldvari, M., Storms, M., Rabussay, D., Widera, G., and Babiuk, L.A. (2002). Electroporation improves the efficacy of DNA vaccines in large animals. *Vaccine* 20, 3399–3408.

Barrington, G. M., McFadden, T. B., Huyler, M. T., and Besser, T. E. (2000). Regulation of colostrogenesis in cattle. *Livest. Prod. Sci.* 70, 95–104.

Becu, T., Polledo, G., and Gaskin, J.M. (1997). Immunoprophylaxis of *Rhodococcus equi* pneumonia in foals. *Vet. Microbiol.* 56, 193–204.

Berg, R. L., Firehammer, B. D., Border, M., and Myers, L. L. (1979). Effects of passively and actively acquired antibody on bovine campylobacteriosis (vibriosis). *Am. J. Vet. Res.* 40, 21–25.

Bertschinger, H. U, Fairbrother, J. M. (1999). *Escherichia coli* infections. In *Diseases of Swine* (eds. B. E. Straw, S. D'Allaire, W. L. Mengeling, and D. Taylor), 8th ed. Ames, Iowa: Iowa State University Press, 431–454.

Besser, T. E., and Gay, C. C. (1994). The importance of colostrum to the health of the neonatal calf. *Vet. Clin. North Am. Food Anim. Pract.* 10, 107–117.

Besser, T.E., McGuire, T.C., and Gay, C.C. (1987). The transfer of serum IgG1 antibody into the gastrointestinal tract in newborn calves. *Vet. Immunol. Immunopathol.* 17, 51–56.

Besser, T. E., Gay, C. C., McGuire, T. C., and Evermann, J. F. (1988a). Passive immunity to bovine rotavirus infection associated with transfer of serum antibody into the intestinal lumen. *J. Virol.* 62, 2238–2242.

Besser, T. E., McGuire, T. C., Gay, C. C., and Pritchett, L. C. (1988b). Transfer of functional immunoglobulin G (IgG) antibody into the gastrointestinal tract accounts for IgG clearance in calves. *J. Virol.* 62, 2234–2237.

Boersma, W. J., Van Rooij, E. M., Scholten, J–W., Zwart, R. J., Kimman, T. G., and Bianchi, A. (1998). Silent memory induction in maternal immune young animals. *Vet. Q.* 20, S89–92.

Bohl, E. H., Gupta, R. K., Olquin, M. V., and Saif, L. J. (1972). Antibody responses in serum, colostrum, and milk of swine after infection or vaccination with transmissible gastroenteritis virus. *Infect. Immun.* 6, 289–301.

Bohl, E. H., Theil, K. W., and Saif, L. J. (1984). Isolation and serotyping of porcine rotaviruses and antigenic comparison with other rotaviruses. *J. Clin. Microbiol.* 19, 105–111.

Bowersock, T. L., Shalaby, W. S. W., Levy, M., Blevins, W. E., White, M. R., Borie, D. L., and Park, K. (1994a). The potential use of poly(methacrylic acid) hydrogels for oral administration of drugs and vaccines to ruminants. *J. Contr. Rel.* 31, 245–254.

Bowersock, T. L., Shalaby, W. S., Levy, M., Samuels, M. L., Lallone, R., White, M. R., Borie, D. L., Lehmeyer, J., and Park, K. (1994b). Evaluation of an orally administered vaccine, using hydrogels containing bacterial exotoxins of *Pasteurella haemolytica*, in cattle. *Am. J. Vet. Res.* 55, 502–509.

Bowersock, T. L., HogenEsch, H., Suckow, M., Guimond, P., Martin, S., Borie, D., Torregrosa, S., Park, H., and Park, K. (1999). Oral vaccination of animals with antigens encapsulated in alginate microspheres. *Vaccine* 17, 1804–1811.

Braun, R. P., Babiuk, L.A., Loehr, B. I., and van Drunen Littel–van den Hurk, S. (1999). Particle-mediated DNA immunization of cattle confers long-lasting immunity against bovine herpesvirus-1. *Virology* 265, 46–56.

Bresee, J. S., Glass, R. I., Ivanoff, B., and Gentsch, J. R. (1999). Current status and future priorities for rotavirus vaccine development, evaluation and implementation in developing countries. *Vaccine* 17, 2207–2022.

Bridger, J. C. (1990). Small viruses associated with gastroenteritis in animals. In *Viral Diarrheas of Man and Animals* (eds. L. J. Saif and K. W. Theil). Boca Raton, Florida: CRC Press, 161–182.

Briggs, R.E., and Tatum, F.M. (1999). New mucosal vaccine in beef cattle imparts rapid resistance to pneumonic pasteurellosis after mass-medicating on feed. Presented at the U.S. Animal Health Assoc. Mtg., San Diego, CA.

Brock, J.H., Arzabe, F.R., Ortega, F., and Pineiro, A. (1977). The effect of limited proteolysis by trypsin and chymotrypsin on bovine colostral IgG1. *Immunology* 32, 215–219.

Brockmeier, S.I., Lager, K. M., and Mengeling, W. L. (1997). Successful pseudorabies vaccination in maternally immune piglets using recombinant vaccinia virus vaccines. *Res. Vet. Sci.* 62, 281–285.

Brogden, K. A., DeBey, B., Audibert, F., Lehmkuhl, H., and Chedid, L. (1995). Protection of ruminants by *Pasteurella haemolytica* A1 capsular polysaccharide vaccines containing muramyl dipeptide analogs. *Vaccine* 13, 1677–1684.

Brugmann, M., Drommer, W., Reichl, U., and Boge, A. (1997). [Iscom (immunostimulating complex) vaccine of equine influenza virus: transmission electron microscopic investigation and literature review]. *Dtsch. Tierarztl. Wochenschr.* 104, 196–202.

Butler, J. E. (1983). Bovine immunoglobulins: an augmented review. *Vet. Immunol. Immunopathol.* 4, 43–152.

Carmichael, L. E., Joubert, J. C., and Pollock, R. V. (1983). A modified live canine parvovirus vaccine. II. Immune response. *Cornell Vet.* 73, 13–29.

Casal, J. I., Langeveld, J. P., Cortes, E., Schaaper, W. W., van Dijk, E., Vela, C., Kamstrup, S., and Meloen, R. H. (1995). Peptide vaccine against canine parvovirus: identification of two neutralization subsites in the N terminus of VP2 and optimization of the amino acid sequence. *J. Virol.* 69, 7274–7277.

Casal, J. I. (1999). Use of parvovirus-like particles for vaccination and induction of multiple immune responses. *Biotechnol. Appl. Biochem.* 29, 141–150.

Chambers, T. M., Holland, R. E., Tudor, L. R., Townsend, H. G., Cook, A., Bogdan, J., Lunn, D. P., Hussey, S., Whitaker-Dowling, P., Youngner, J. S., Sebring, R. W., Penner, S. J., and Stiegler, G. L. (2001). A new modified live equine influenza virus vaccine: phenotypic stability, restricted spread and efficacy against heterologous virus challenge. *Equine Vet. J.* 33, 630–636.

Chen, H., and Schifferli, D. M. (2001). Enhanced immune responses to viral epitopes by combining macrophage-inducible expression with multimeric display on a *Salmonella* vector. *Vaccine* 19, 3009–3018.

Ciarlet, M., Gilger, M. A., Barone, C., McArthur, M., Estes, M. K., and Conner, M. E. (1998). Rotavirus disease, but not infection and development of intestinal histopathological lesions, is age restricted in rabbits. *Virology* 251, 343–360.

Clark, B. L., Emery, D. L., Dufty, J. H. (1984). Therapeutic immunization of bulls with the membranes and glycoproteins of *Tritrichomonas foetus* var. *brisbane. Aust. Vet. J.* 61, 65–66.

Confer, A. W., and Fulton, R. W. (1995). Evaluation of *Pasteurella* and *Haemophilus* vaccines. *The Bovine Proceedings* 27, 136–141.

Conlon J. A., Shewen P. E., and Lo R. Y. (1991). Efficacy of recombinant leukotoxin in protection against pneumonic challenge with live *Pasteurella haemolytica* A1. *Infect. Immun.* 59, 587–591.

Conlon, J. A., Gallo, G. F., Shewen, P. E., and Adlam, C. (1995). Comparison of protection of experimentally challenged cattle vaccinated once or twice with a *Pasteurella haemolytica* bacterial extract vaccine. *Can. J. Vet. Res.* 59, 179–182.

Conner, M. E., Ramig, A. Viral enteric diseases. (1997). In *Viral Pathogenesis* (eds. N. Nathanson and R. Ahmed). Philadelphia: Lippincott-Raven, 713–742.

Corbeil, L. B., and Winter, A. J. (1978). Animal model for the study of genital immune mechanisms: venereal vibrosis of cattle. In *Immunobiology of Neisseria gonorrhoeae.* (ed. G. F. Brooks). Washington, DC: American Society for Microbiology, 293–299.

Corbeil, L. B., Schurig, G. G., Duncan, J. R., Wilkie, B. N., Winter, A. J. (1981). Immunity in the female bovine reproductive tract based on the response to *Campylobacter fetus. Adv. Exp. Med. Biol.* 137, 729–743.

Corbeil, L. B., Hodgson, J. L., Widders, P. R. (1991). Immunoglobulin binding by *Tritrichomonas foetus. J. Clin. Microbiol.* 29, 2710–2714.

Corbeil, L. B., Munson, L., Campero, C., BonDurant, R.H. (2001). Bovine trichomoniasis as a model for development of vaccines against sexually-transmitted disease. *Am. J. Reprod. Immunol.* 45, 310–319.

Coulson, B. S., Grimwood, K., Hudson, I. L., Barnes, G. L., and Bishop, R. F. (1992). Role of coproantibody in clinical protection of children during reinfection with rotavirus. *J. Clin. Microbiol.* 30, 1678–1684.

Crawford, S. E., Estes, M. K., Ciarlet, M., Barone, C., O'Neal, C. M., Cohen, J., and Conner, M. E. (1999). Heterotypic protection and induction of a broad heterotypic neutralization response by rotavirus-like particles. *J. Virol.* 73, 4813–4822.

Enjuanes, L., Sola, I., Almazan, F., Ortego, J., Izeta, A., Gonzalez, J. M., Alonso, S., Sanchez, J. M., Escors, D., Calvo, E., Riquelme, C., and Sanchez, C. (2001). Coronavirus derived expression systems. *J. Biotechnol.* 88, 183–204.

Entriken, T. (2001). *Veterinary Pharmaceuticals and Biologicals.* Lenexa, KS: Veterinary Healthcare Communications.

Estes, M. K., Kang, G., Zeng, C. Q., Crawford, S. E., and Ciarlet, M. (2001). Pathogenesis of rotavirus gastroenteritis. *Novartis Found. Symp.* 238, 82–96.

Farley, H. (1932). An epizoological study of shipping fever in Kansas. *J. Am. Vet. Med. Assoc.* 52, 165–172.

Fooks, A. R. Development of oral vaccines for human use. (2000). *Curr. Opin. Mol. Ther.* 2, 80–86.

Franco, M. A., and Greenberg, H. B. (2000). Immunity to homologous rotavirus infection in adult mice. *Trends Microbiol.* 8, 50–52.

Frank, G. H. (1984). Bacteria as etiologic agents in bovine respiratory disease. In *Bovine Respiratory Disease.* (ed. R.W. Loan). College Station, Texas: Texas A & M Press.

Frank, G. H., and Smith, P. C. (1983). Prevalence of *Pasteurella haemolytica* in transported calves. *Am. J. Vet. Res.* 44, 981–985.

Friend, S. C., Wilkie, B. N., Thomson, R. G., and Barnum, D. A. (1977). Bovine pneumonic pasteurellosis: experimental induction in vaccinated and nonvaccinated calves. *Can. J. Comp. Med.* 41, 77–83.

Gatewood, D. M., Fenwick, B. W., and Chengappa, M. M. (1994). Growth-condition dependent expression of *Pasteurella haemolytica* A1 outer membrane proteins, capsule, and leukotoxin. *Vet. Microbiol.* 41, 221–233.

Gellin, B. G., and Katz, S. L. (1994). Measles: state of the art and future directions. *J. Infect. Dis.* 170 (Suppl. 1), S3–S14.

Glennon, A., and Jeffs, J. (2000). *NOAH Compendium of Data Sheets for Veterinary Products.* Enfield, Middlesex, UK: National Office of Animal Health, Ltd.

Glezen, W. P. (2001). Maternal vaccines. *Prim. Care* 28, 791–806.

Hannant, D., and Mumford, J. A. (1989). Cell mediated immune responses in ponies following infection with equine influenza virus (H3N8): the influence of induction culture conditions on the properties of cytotoxic effector cells. *Vet. Immunol. Immunopathol.* 21, 327–337.

Hannant, D., Mumford, J. A., and Jessett, D. M. (1988). Duration of circulating antibody and immunity following infection with equine influenza virus. *Vet. Rec.* 122, 125–128.

Hannant, D., Jessett, D. M., O'Neill, T., and Mumford, J. A. (1989). Antibody isotype responses in the serum and respiratory tract to primary and secondary infections with equine influenza virus (H3N8). *Vet. Microbiol.* 19, 293–303.

Hannant, D., Easeman, R., and Mumford, J. (1998). Equine mucosal immune system: intranasal vaccination with inactivated equine influenza virus protects from infection. In *Proceedings of the 8th International Conference on Equine Infectious Diseases* (ed. W. Plowright). Newmarket, UK: R&W Publications, 50–56.

Harland, R. J., McCartney, D. H., and Potter, A. P. (1992). Evaluation of *P. haemolytica* vaccination strategies in beef calves. In *Proceedings of the 73rd Conference on Research Work in Animal Diseases*, Chicago, Illinois.

Hoar, B. R., Jelinski, M. D., Ribble, C. S., Janzen, E. D., and Johnson, J. C. (1998). A comparison of the clinical field efficacy and safety of florfenicol and tilmicosin for the treatment of undifferentiated bovine respiratory disease of cattle in western Canada. *Can. Vet. J.* 39, 161–166.

Hodgins, D.C., and Shewen, P.E. (1994). Passive immunity to *Pasteurella haemolytica* A1 in dairy calves: effects of preparturient vaccination of the dams. *Can. J. Vet. Res.* 58, 31–35.

Hodgins, D. C., and Shewen, P. E. (1996). Preparturient vaccination to enhance passive immunity to the capsular polysaccharide of *Pasteurella haemolytica* A1. *Vet. Immunol. Immunopathol.* 50, 67–77.

Hodgins, D. C., and Shewen, P. E. (1998). Serologic responses of young colostrum fed dairy calves to antigens of *Pasteurella haemolytica* A1. *Vaccine* 16, 2018–2025.

Hodgins, D. C., Conlon, J. A., Shewen, P. E. (2002). Respiratory viruses and bacteria in cattle. In *Polymicrobial Diseases* (eds. K.A. Brogden and J.M. Guthmiller). Washington, DC: American Society for Microbiology Press, 213–229.

Hooper-McGrevy, K. E., Giguere, S., Wilkie, B. N., and Prescott, J. F. (2001). Evaluation of equine immunoglobulin specific for *Rhodococcus equi* virulence-associated proteins A and C for use in protecting foals against *Rhodococcus equi*–induced pneumonia. *Am. J. Vet. Res.* 62, 1307–1313.

Hoshino, Y., Saif, L. J., Sereno, M. M., Chanock, R. M., and Kapikian, A. Z. (1988). Infection immunity of piglets to either VP3 or VP7 outer capsid protein confers resistance to challenge with a virulent rotavirus bearing the corresponding antigen. *J. Virol.* 62, 744–748.

Hu, K. F., Lovgren-Bengtsson, K., and Morein, B. (2001). Immunostimulating complexes (ISCOMs) for nasal vaccination. *Adv. Drug Deliv. Rev.* 51, 149–159.

Ikeda, J. S., BonDurant, R. H., Campero, C. M., and Corbeil, L. B. (1993). Conservation of a protective surface antigen of *Tritrichomonas foetus*. *J. Clin. Microbiol.* 31, 3289–3295.

Ikemori, Y., Kuroki, M., Peralta, R. C., Yokoyama, H., and Kodama, Y. (1992). Protection of neonatal calves against fatal enteric colibacillosis by administration of egg yolk powder from hens immunized with K99-piliated enterotoxigenic *Escherichia coli*. *Am. J. Vet. Res.* 53, 2005–2008.

Ikemori, Y., Ohta, M., Umeda, K., Icatlo, F. C. Jr, Kuroki, M., Yokoyama, H., and Kodama, Y. (1997). Passive protection of neonatal calves against bovine coronavirus-induced diarrhea by administration of egg yolk or colostrum antibody powder. *Vet. Microbiol.* 58, 105–111.

Iosef, C., Van Nguyen, T., Jeong, K., Bengtsson, K., Morein, B., Kim, Y., Chang, K. O., Azevedo, M. S., Yuan, L., Nielsen, P., and Saif, L. J. (2002). Systemic and intestinal antibody secreting cell responses and protection in gnotobiotic pigs immunized orally with attenuated Wa human rotavirus and Wa 2/6-rotavirus-like particles associated with immunostimulating complexes. *Vaccine* 20, 1741–1753.

Jiang, W., Baker, H. J., Swango, L. J., Schorr, J., Self, M. J., and Smith, B. F. (1998). Nucleic acid immunization protects dogs against challenge with virulent canine parvovirus. *Vaccine* 16, 601–607.

Jones, G. E., Donachie, W., Sutherland, A. D., Knox, D. P., and Gilmour, J. S. (1989). Protection of lambs against experimental pneumonic pasteurellosis by transfer of immune serum. *Vet. Microbiol.* 20, 59–71.

Jones, S. L., and Blikslager, A. T. (2002). Role of the enteric nervous system in the pathophysiology of secretory diarrhea. *J. Vet. Intern. Med.* 16, 222–228.

Kacskovics, I., Wu, Z., Simister, N. E., Frenyo, L. V., and Hammarstrom, L. (2000). Cloning and characterization of the bovine MHC class I–like Fc receptor. *J. Immunol.* 164, 1889–1897.

Kaehler, K. L., Markham, R. J., Muscoplat, C. C., and Johnson, D. W. (1980). Evidence of species specificity in the cytocidal effects of *Pasteurella haemolytica*. *Infect. Immun.* 30, 615–616.

Kania, S. A., Reed, S. L., Thomford, J. W., BonDurant, R. H., Hirata, K., Corbeil, R. R., North, M. J., Corbeil, L. B. (2001). Degradation of bovine complement C3 by trichomonad extracellular proteinase. *Vet. Immunol. Immunopathol.* 78, 83–96.

Kapikian, A. Z., Hoshino, Y., and Chanock, R. M. Rotaviruses. (2001). In *Fields Virology*, 4th ed. (eds. D.M. Kinipe and P.M. Howley). Philadelphia: Lippincott-Raven, 1787–1834.

Kelly, A. P., and Janzen, E. D. (1986). A review of morbidity and mortality rates and disease occurrence in North American feedlot cattle. *Can. Vet. J.* 27, 496–500.

Kim, Y., Nielsen, P. R., Hodgins, D., Chang, K. O., and Saif, L. J. (2002). Lactogenic antibody responses in cows vaccinated with recombinant bovine rotavirus-like particles (VLPs) of two serotypes or inactivated bovine rotavirus vaccines. *Vaccine* 20, 1248–1258.

Kohara, J., Tsunemitsu, H. (2000). Correlation between maternal serum antibodies and protection against bovine rotavirus diarrhea in calves. *J. Vet. Med. Sci.* 62, 219–221.

Kuroki, M., Ohta, M., Ikemori, Y., Peralta, R. C., Yokoyama, H., and Kodama, Y. (1994). Passive protection against bovine rotavirus in calves by specific immunoglobulins from chicken egg yolk. *Arch. Virol.* 138, 143–148.

Kvasnicka, W. G., Hanks, D., Huang, J.-C., Hall, M. R., Sandblom, D., Chu, H. J., Chavez, L., Acree, W. M. (1992). Clinical evaluation of the efficacy of inoculating cattle with a vaccine containing *Tritrichomonas foetus*. *Am. J. Vet. Res.* 53, 2023–2027.

Langeveld, J. P., Brennan, F. R., Martinez-Torrecuadrada, J. L., Jones, T. D., Boshuizen, R. S., Vela, C., Casal, J. I., Kamstrup, S., Dalsgaard, K., Meloen, R. H., Bendig, M. M., and Hamilton, W. D. (2001). Inactivated recombinant plant virus protects dogs from a lethal challenge with canine parvovirus. *Vaccine* 19, 3661–3670.

Larson, L. J., and Schultz, R. D. (1997). Comparison of selected canine vaccines for their ability to induce protective immunity against canine parvovirus infection. *Am. J. Vet. Res.* 58, 360–363.

Lee, C. W., Shewen, P. E., Cladman, W. M., Conlon, J. A., Mellors, A., and Lo, R. Y. (1994). Sialoglycoprotease of *Pasteurella haemolytica* A1: detection of antisialoglycoprotease antibodies in sera of calves. *Can. J. Vet. Res.* 58, 93–98.

Lee, R. W., Strommer, J., Hodgins, D., Shewen, P. E., Niu, Y., and Lo, R. Y. (2001). Towards development of an edible vaccine against bovine pneumonic pasteurellosis using transgenic white clover expressing a *Mannheimia haemolytica* A1 leukotoxin 50 fusion protein. *Infect. Immun.* 69, 5786–5793.

Lundgren, O., Peregrin, A. T., Persson, K., Kordasti, S., Uhnoo, I., and Svensson, L. (2000). Role of the enteric nervous system in the fluid and electrolyte secretion of rotavirus diarrhea. *Science* 287, 491–495.

Lunn, D. P., Soboll, G., Schram, B. R., Quass, J., McGregor, M. W., Drape, R. J., Macklin, M. D., McCabe, D. E., Swain, W. F., and Olsen, C. W. (1999). Antibody responses to DNA vaccination of horses using the influenza virus hemagglutinin gene. *Vaccine* 17, 2245–2258.

Marquardt, R. R. (2000). Control of intestinal diseases in pigs by feeding specific chicken egg antibodies. In *Egg Nutrition and Biotechnology* (eds. J.S. Sim, S. Nakai and W. Guenter). Wallingford, Oxon, UK: CABI Publishing, 289–299.

McNeal, M. M., VanCott, J. L., Choi, A. H., Basu, M., Flint, J. A., Stone, S. C., Clements, J. D., and Ward, R. L. (2002). CD4 T cells are the only lymphocytes needed to protect mice against rotavirus shedding after intranasal immunization with a chimeric VP6 protein and the adjuvant LT(R192G). *J. Virol.* 76, 560–568.

Mebus, C. A., White, R. G., Stair, E. L., Rhodes, M. B., and Twiehaus, M. J. (1972). Neonatal calf diarrhea: results of a field trial using a reo-like virus vaccine. *Vet. Med. Small Anim. Clin.* 67, 173–174.

Mechor, G. D., Jim, G. K., and Janzen, E. D. (1988). Comparison of penicillin, oxytetracycline, and trimethoprim-sulfadoxine in the treatment of acute undifferentiated bovine respiratory disease. *Can. Vet. J.* 29, 438–443.

Miller, A. W., Howard, L. H., Bayard, E. S., Smith, R. W., Stanard, S.J., Jones, J. D., Hilton, G., Killham, B. J., and Truam, J. (1927). Report of committee on miscellaneous transmissible diseases. *J. Am. Vet. Med. Assoc.* 70, 952–955.

Mine, Y., and Kovacs-Nolan, J. (2002). Chicken egg yolk antibodies as therapeutics in enteric infectious disease: a review. *J. Med. Food* 5, 159–169.

Moon, H. W., and Bunn, T. O. (1993). Vaccines for preventing enterotoxigenic *Escherichia coli* infections in farm animals. *Vaccine* 11, 200–213.

Morck, D. W., Raybould, T. J., Acres, S. D., Babiuk, L. A., Nelligan, J., and Costerton, J. W. (1987). Electron microscopic description of glycocalyx and fimbriae on the surface of *Pasteurella haemolytica*-A1. *Can. J. Vet. Res.* 51, 83–88.

Morck, D. W., Olson, M. E., Acres, S. D., Daoust, P. Y., and Costerton, J. W. (1989). Presence of bacterial glycocalyx and fimbriae on *Pasteurella haemolytica* in feedlot cattle with pneumonic pasteurellosis. *Can. J. Vet. Res.* 53, 167–171.

Morck, D. W., Ellis, B. D., Domingue, P. A., Olson, M. E., and Costerton, J. W. (1991). *In vivo* expression of iron regulated outer-membrane proteins in *Pasteurella haemolytica*-A1. *Microb. Pathog.* 11, 373–378.

Morein, B., Villacres-Eriksson, M., Ekstrom, J., Hu, K., Behboudi, S., and Lovgren-Bengtsson, K. (1999). ISCOM: a delivery system for neonates and for mucosal administration. *Adv. Vet. Med.* 41, 405–413.

Morley, P. S., Townsend, H. G., Bogdan, J. R., and Haines, D. M. (1999). Efficacy of a commercial vaccine for preventing disease caused by influenza virus infection in horses. *J. Am. Vet. Med. Assoc.* 215, 61–66.

Mosier, D. A. (1997). Bacterial pneumonia. *Vet. Clin. North Am. Food Anim. Pract.* 13, 483–493.

Mosier, D. A., Confer, A. W., and Panciera, R. J. (1989). The evolution of vaccines for bovine pneumonic pasteurellosis. *Res. Vet. Sci.* 47, 1–10.

Mosier, D. A., Simons, K. R., and Vestweber, J. G. (1995). Passive protection of calves with *Pasteurella haemolytica* antiserum. *Am. J. Vet. Res.* 56, 1317–1321.

Mosier, D. A., Panciera, R. J., Rogers, D. P., Uhlich, G. A., Butine, M. D., Confer, A. W., and Basaraba, R. J. (1998). Comparison of serologic and protective responses induced by two *Pasteurella* vaccines. *Can. J. Vet. Res.* 62, 178–182.

Moxley, R. A., and Olson, L. D. (1989). Clinical evaluation of transmissible gastroenteritis virus vaccines and vaccination procedures for inducing lactogenic immunity in sows. *Am. J. Vet. Res.* 50, 111–118.

Mumford, J., and Wood, J. (1993). WHO/OIE meeting: consultation on newly emerging strains of equine influenza. 18–19 May 1992, Animal Health Trust, Newmarket, Suffolk, UK. *Vaccine* 11, 1172–1175.

Mumford, J. A., Jessett, D., Dunleavy, U., Wood, J., Hannant, D., Sundquist, B., and Cook, R. F. (1994a). Antigenicity and immunogenicity of experimental equine influenza ISCOM vaccines. *Vaccine* 12, 857–863.

Mumford, J. A., Jessett, D. M., Rollinson, E. A., Hannant, D., and Draper, M. E. (1994b). Duration of protective efficacy of equine influenza immunostimulating complex/tetanus vaccines. *Vet. Rec.* 134, 158–162.

Mumford, J. A., Wilson, H., Hannant, D., and Jessett, D. M. (1994c). Antigenicity and immunogenicity of equine influenza vaccines containing a Carbomer adjuvant. *Epidemiol. Infect.* 112, 421–437.

Nelson, K. M., Schram, B. R., McGregor, M. W., Sheoran, A. S., Olsen, C. W., and Lunn, D. P. (1998). Local and systemic isotype-specific antibody responses to equine influenza virus infection versus conventional vaccination. *Vaccine* 16, 1306–1313.

Newmark, P. (1988). Bark extract amplifies vaccine. *Biotechnology* 6, 23.

O'Neal, C. M., Clements, J. D., Estes, M. K., and Conner, M. E. (1998). Rotavirus 2/6 viruslike particles administered intranasally with cholera toxin, *Escherichia coli* heat-labile toxin (LT), and LT-R192G induce protection from rotavirus challenge. *J. Virol.* 72, 3390–3393.

Park, S., Sestak, K., Hodgins, D. C., Shoup, D. I., Ward, L. A., Jackwood, D. J., and Saif, L. J. (1998). Immune response of sows vaccinated with attenuated transmissible gastroenteritis virus (TGEV) and recombinant TGEV spike protein vaccines and protection of their suckling pigs against virulent TGEV challenge exposure. *Am. J. Vet. Res.* 59, 1002–1008.

Parreño, V., Hodgins, D. C., de Arriba, L., Kang, S. Y., Yuan, L., Ward, L. A., To, T. L., and Saif, L. J. (1999). Serum and intestinal isotype antibody responses to Wa human rotavirus in gnotobiotic pigs are modulated by maternal antibodies. *J. Gen. Virol.* 80, 1417–1428.

Parsonson, I. M., Clark, B. L., Dufty, J. H. (1976) Early pathogenesis and pathology of *Tritrichomonas foetus* infection in virgin heifers. *J. Comp. Pathol.* 86, 59–66.

Pastoret, P. P. (1998). Immunology of cattle. In *Handbook of Vertebrate Immunology* (ed. P.P. Pastoret). San Diego: Academic Press.

Pogonka, T., Klotz, C., Kovacs, F., and Lucius, R. (2003). A single dose of recombinant *Salmonella typhimurium* induces specific humoral immune responses against heterologous *Eimeria tenella* antigens in chicken. *Int. J. Parasitol.* 33, 81–88.

Pollock, R. V., and Carmichael, L. E. (1982). Maternally derived immunity to canine parvovirus infection: transfer, decline, and interference with vaccination. *J. Am. Vet. Med. Assoc.* 180, 37–42.

Potter, A. A., Schryvers, A. B., Ogunnariwo, J. A., Hutchins, W. A., Lo, R. Y., and Watts, T. (1999). Protective capacity of the *Pasteurella*

haemolytica transferrin-binding proteins TbpA and TbpB in cattle. *Microb. Pathog.* 27, 197–206.

Pratelli, A., Cavalli, A., Normanno, G., De Palma, M. G., Pastorelli, G., Martella, V., and Buonavoglia, C. (2000). Immunization of pups with maternally derived antibodies to canine parvovirus (CPV) using a modified-live variant (CPV-2b). *J. Vet. Med. B Infect. Dis. Vet. Public Health* 47, 273–276.

Purdy, C. W., Livingston, C. W., Jr., Frank, G. H., Cummins, J.M., Cole, N.A., and Loan, R.W. (1986). A live *Pasteurella haemolytica* vaccine efficacy trial. *J. Am. Vet. Med. Assoc.* 188, 589–591.

Quigley, J. D. 3rd, and Drewry, J. J. (1998). Nutrient and immunity transfer from cow to calf pre- and postcalving. *J. Dairy Sci.* 81, 2779–2790.

Rankin, R., Pontarollo, R., Ioannou, X., Krieg, A.M., Hecker, R., Babiuk, L.A., and van Drunen Littel–van den Hurk, S. (2001). CpG motif identification for veterinary and laboratory species demonstrates that sequence recognition is highly conserved. *Antisense Nucleic Acid Drug Dev.* 11, 333–340.

Rebelatto, M. C., Guimond, P., Bowersock, T. L., and HogenEsch, H. (2001). Induction of systemic and mucosal immune response in cattle by intranasal administration of pig serum albumin in alginate microparticles. *Vet. Immunol. Immunopathol.* 83, 93–105.

Rehmtulla, A. J., and Thomson, R. G. (1981). A review of the lesions in shipping fever of cattle. *Can. Vet. J.* 22, 1–8.

Rhyan, J. C., Wilson, K. L., Wagner, B., Anderson, M. L., BonDurant, R. H., Burgess, D. E., Mutwiri, G. K., and Corbeil, L. B. (1999). Demonstration of *Tritrichomonas foetus* in the external genitalia and of specific antibodies in preputial secretions of naturally infected bulls. *Vet. Pathol.* 36, 406–411.

Roux, M. E., McWilliams, M., Phillips-Quagliata, J. M., Weisz-Carrington, P., and Lamm, M. E. (1977). Origin of IgA-secreting plasma cells in the mammary gland. *J. Exp. Med.* 146, 1311–1322.

Saif, L., Yuan, L., Ward, L., and To, T. (1997). Comparative studies of the pathogenesis, antibody immune responses, and homologous protection to porcine and human rotaviruses in gnotobiotic piglets. *Adv. Exp. Med. Biol.* 412, 397–403.

Saif, L. J. (1999a). Comparative pathogenesis of enteric viral infections of swine. In *Mechanisms in the Pathogenesis of Enteric Diseases 2* (eds. P. Paul and D. Francis). New York: Kluwer Academic/Plenum Publishers, 47–59.

Saif, L. J. (1999b). Enteric viral infections of pigs and strategies for induction of mucosal immunity. *Adv. Vet. Med.* 41, 429–446.

Saif, L. J., and Bohl, E. H. (1983). Passive immunity to transmissible gastroenteritis virus: intramammary viral inoculation of sows. *Ann. N. Y. Acad. Sci.* 409, 708–723. Saif, L. J., and Fernandez, F. M. (1996). Group A rotavirus veterinary vaccines. *J. Infect. Dis.* 174 Suppl 1, S98–S106.

Saif, L. J., and Jackwood, D. J. (1990). Enteric virus vaccines: theoretical considerations, current status, and future approaches. In *Viral Diarrheas of Man and Animals* (eds. L. J. Saif and K. W. Theil). Boca Raton, Florida: CRC Press, 313–329.

Saif, L. J., and Wesley, R. D. Transmissible gastroenteritis and porcine respiratory coronavirus. (1999). In *Diseases of Swine* (eds. Straw, B. E., D'Allaire, S., Mengeling, W. L., and Taylor, D.), 8th ed. Ames, Iowa: Iowa State University Press, 295–325.

Saif, L. J., Bohl, E. H., and Gupta, R. K. (1972). Isolation of porcine immunoglobulins and determination of the immunoglobulin classes of transmissible gastroenteritis viral antibodies. *Infect. Immun.* 6, 600–609.

Saif, L. J., Redman, D. R., Smith, K. L., and Theil, K. W. (1983). Passive immunity to bovine rotavirus in newborn calves fed colostrum supplements from immunized or nonimmunized cows. *Infect. Immun.* 41, 1118–1131.

Saif, L. J., Ward, L. A., Yuan, L., Rosen, B. I., and To, T. L. (1996). The gnotobiotic piglet as a model for studies of disease pathogenesis and immunity to human rotaviruses. *Arch. Virol. Suppl.* 12, 153–161.

Salmon, H. (1995). Lactogenic immunity and vaccinal protection in swine. *Vet. Res.* 26:232–237.

Salmon, H. (2000). Mammary gland immunology and neonate protection in pigs. In *Biology of the Mammary Gland* (eds. Mol, J. A. and Clegg, R. A.). New York: Kluwer Academic/Plenum, pp. 279–287.

Schaller, J. P., Saif, L. J., Cordle, C. T., Candler, E. Jr., Winship, T. R., and Smith, K. L. (1992). Prevention of human rotavirus-induced diarrhea in gnotobiotic piglets using bovine antibody. *J. Infect. Dis.* 165, 623–630.

Sheldrake, R. F., Husband, A. J., and Watson, D.L. (1985). Specific antibody–containing cells in the mammary gland of non-lactating sheep after intraperitoneal and intramammary immunization. *Res. Vet. Sci.* 38, 312–316.

Shewen, P. E., and Wilkie, B. N. (1982). Cytotoxin of *Pasteurella haemolytica* acting on bovine leukocytes. *Infect. Immun.* 35, 91–94.

Shewen, P. E., and Wilkie, B. N. (1985). Evidence for the *Pasteurella haemolytica* cytotoxin as a product of actively growing bacteria. *Am. J. Vet. Res.* 46, 1212–1214.

Shoo, M. K. (1989). Experimental bovine pneumonic pasteurellosis: a review. *Vet. Rec.* 124, 141–144.

Siadat-Pajouh, M., and Cai, L. (2001). Protective efficacy of rotavirus 2/6-virus-like particles combined with CT-E29H, a detoxified cholera toxin adjuvant. *Viral Immunol.* 14, 31–47.

Siegrist, C.-A., Barrios, C., Martinez, X., Brandt, C., Berney, M., Córdova, M., Kovarik, J., and Lambert, P.-H. (1998). Influence of maternal antibodies on vaccine responses: inhibition of antibody but not T cell responses allows successful early prime-boost strategies in mice. *Eur. J. Immunol.* 28, 4138–4148.

Smith, C. K., Davidson, J. N., and Henry, C. W. (1985). Evaluating a live vaccine for *Pasteurella haemolytica* in dairy calves. *Vet. Med.* 80, 78–88.

Straus, D. C., and Purdy, C. W. (1994). In vivo production of neuraminidase by *Pasteurella haemolytica* A1 in goats after transthoracic challenge. *Infect. Immun.* 62, 4675–4678.

Svennerholm, A. M., Holmgren, J., Hanson, L. A., Lindblad, B. S., Quereshi, F., and Rahimtoola, R. J. (1977). Boosting of secretory IgA antibody responses in man by parenteral cholera vaccination. *Scand. J. Immunol.* 6:1345–9.

Talbot, J. A., Nielsen, K., Corbeil, L. B. (1991). Cleavage of proteins of reproductive secretions by extracellular proteinases of *Tritrichomonas foetus*. *Can. J. Microbiol.* 37, 384–390.

Taylor, J., Tartaglia, J., Moran, T., Webster, R., Bouquet, J.-F., Quimby, F., Holmes, D., Laplace, E., Mickle, T., Paoletti, E. (1992). The role of poxvirus vectors in influenza vaccine development. In *Proceedings of the 3rd International Symposium on Avian Influenza.* Madison, Wisconsin: University of Wisconsin, 311–335.

Thorlakson, B., Martin, W., and Peters, D. (1990). A field trial to evaluate the efficacy of a commercial *Pasteurella haemolytica* bacterial extract in preventing bovine respiratory disease. *Can. Vet. J.* 31, 573–579.

Timoney, P. J. (1996). Equine influenza. *Comp. Immunol. Microbiol. Infect. Dis.* 19, 205–211.

Tizard, I. R. (2000). *Veterinary Immunology: An Introduction*, 6th ed. Philadelphia: WB Saunders, 210–252.

Townsend, H. G., Penner, S. J., Watts, T. C., Cook, A., Bogdan, J., Haines, D. M., Griffin, S., Chambers, T., Holland, R. E., Whitaker-Dowling, P., Youngner, J. S., and Sebring, R. W. (2001). Efficacy of a cold-adapted, intranasal, equine influenza vaccine: challenge trials. *Equine Vet. J.* 33, 637–643.

Tuboly, T., Yu, W., Bailey, A., Degrandis, S., Du, S., Erickson, L., and Nagy, E. (2000). Immunogenicity of porcine transmissible gastroenteritis virus spike protein expressed in plants. *Vaccine* 18, 2023–8.

Tyler-McGowan, C. M., Hodgson, J. L., and Hodgson, D. R. (1997). Failure of passive transfer in foals: incidence and outcome on four studs in New South Wales. *Aust. Vet. J.* 75, 56–59.

Van Binnendijk, R. S., Poelen, M. C., van Amerongen, G., de Vries, P., and Osterhaus, A. D. (1997). Protective immunity in macaques vaccinated with live attenuated, recombinant, and subunit measles vaccines in the presence of passively acquired antibodies. *J. Infect. Dis.* 175, 524–532.

VanCott, J. L., Brim, T. A., Simkins, R. A., and Saif, L. J. (1993). Isotype-specific antibody-secreting cells to transmissible gastroenteritis virus and porcine respiratory coronavirus in gut- and bronchus-associated lymphoid tissues of suckling pigs. *J. Immunol.* 150, 3990–4000.

VanCott, J. L., Brim, T. A., Lunney, J. K., and Saif, L. J. (1994). Contribution of antibody-secreting cells induced in mucosal lymphoid tissues of pigs inoculated with respiratory or enteric strains of coronavirus to immunity against enteric coronavirus challenge. *J. Immunol.* 152, 3980–3990.

Van der Stede, Y., Cox, E., Verdonck, F., Vancaeneghem, S., and Goddeeris, B. M. (2003). Reduced faecal excretion of F4(+)-*E. coli* by the intramuscular immunisation of suckling piglets by the addition of 1alpha, 25-dihydroxyvitamin D(3) or CpG-oligodeoxynucleotides. *Vaccine* 21, 1023–1032.

Van Donkersgoed, J., Guenther, C., Evans, B. N., Potter, A. A., and Harland, R. J. (1995). Effects of various vaccination protocols on passive and active immunity to *Pasteurella haemolytica* and *Haemophilus somnus* in beef calves. *Can. Vet. J.* 36, 424–429.

Van Maanen, C., and Cullinane, A. (2002). Equine influenza virus infections: an update. *Vet. Q.* 24, 79–94.

Van Oirschot, J. T., Bruin, G., de Boer–Luytze, E., and Smolders, G. (1991). Maternal antibodies against equine influenza virus in foals and their interference with vaccination. *Zentralbl. Veterinarmed [B].* 38, 391–396.

Wagstrom, E. A., Yoon, K. J., and Zimmerman, J. J. (2000). Immune components in porcine mammary secretions. *Viral Immunol.* 13, 383–397.

Waltner-Toews, D., Martin, S. W., Meek, A. H., McMillan, I., and Crouch, C. F. (1985). A field trial to evaluate the efficacy of a combined rotavirus-coronavirus/*Escherichia coli* vaccine in dairy cattle. *Can. J. Comp. Med.* 49, 1–9.

Ward, L. A., Rich, E. D., and Besser, T. E. (1996a). Role of maternally derived circulating antibodies in protection of neonatal swine against porcine group A rotavirus. *J. Infect. Dis.* 174, 276–282.

Ward, L. A., Yuan, L., Rosen, B. I., To, T. L., and Saif, L .J. (1996b). Development of mucosal and systemic lymphoproliferative responses and protective immunity to human group A rotaviruses in a gnotobiotic pig model. *Clin. Diagn. Lab. Immunol.* 3, 342–350.

Ward, R. L., McNeal, M. M., and Sheridan, J. F. (1990). Development of an adult mouse model for studies on protection against rotavirus. *J. Virol.* 64, 5070–5075.

Weisz-Carrington, P., Roux, M.E., McWilliams, M., Phillips-Quagliata, J.M., and Lamm, M.E. (1978). Hormonal induction of the secretory immune system in the mammary gland. *Proc. Natl. Acad. Sci. USA* 75, 2928–2932.

Westrom, B. R., Karlsson, B. W., and Svendsen, J. (1982). Levels of serum protease inhibitors during fetal and postnatal development of the pig. *Biol. Neonate* 41, 22–31.

Whiteley, L. O., Maheswaran, S. K., Weiss, D. J., Ames, T. R., and Kannan, M. S. (1992). *Pasteurella haemolytica* A1 and bovine respiratory disease: pathogenesis. *J. Vet. Intern. Med.* 6, 11–22.

Wilson, W. D. (1993). Equine influenza. *Vet. Clin. North Am. Equine Pract.* 9, 257–282.

Wira, C. R., and Rossoll, R. M. (1995). Antigen-presenting cells in the female reproductive tract: influence of estrous cycle on antigen presentation by uterine epithelial and stromal cells. *Endocrinology* 136, 4526–4534.

Yates, P., and Mumford, J. A. (2000). Equine influenza vaccine efficacy: the significance of antigenic variation. *Vet. Microbiol.* 74, 173–177.

Yates, W. D. (1982). A review of infectious bovine rhinotracheitis, shipping fever pneumonia and viral-bacterial synergism in respiratory disease of cattle. *Can. J. Comp. Med.* 46, 225–263.

Yokohama, H., Hashi, T., Umeda, K., Icatlo, F. C. Jr, Kuroki, M., Ikemori, Y., and Kodama, Y. (1997). Effect of oral egg antibody in experimental F18+ *Escherichia coli* infection in weaned pigs. *J. Vet. Med. Sci.* 59, 917–921.

Yu, J., and Langridge, W. H. (2001). A plant-based multicomponent vaccine protects mice from enteric diseases. *Nat. Biotechnol.* 19, 548–552.

Yuan, L., and Saif, L. J. (2002). Induction of mucosal immune responses and protection against enteric viruses: rotavirus infection of gnotobiotic pigs as a model. *Vet. Immunol. Immunopathol.* 87, 147–160.

Yuan, L., Ward, L. A., Rosen, B. I., To, T. L., and Saif, L. J. (1996). Systematic and intestinal antibody-secreting cell responses and

correlates of protective immunity to human rotavirus in a gnotobiotic pig model of disease. *J. Virol.* 70, 3075–3083.

Yuan, L., Geyer, A., and Saif, L. J. (2001). Short-term immunoglobulin
A B-cell memory resides in intestinal lymphoid tissues but not in
bone marrow of gnotobiotic pigs inoculated with Wa human
rotavirus. *Immunology* 103, 188–198.

Mucosal Vaccines for Dental Diseases

Chapter
62

Martin A. Taubman
Department of Immunology, The Forsyth Institute, Boston, Massachusetts

Robert J. Genco
State University of New York, University at Buffalo, Buffalo, New York

Roy C. Page
Regional Clinical Dental Research Center, University of Washington, Seattle, Washington

Host mucosal immunity has been demonstrated to be of considerable importance in dental infection with cariogenic pathogens. The role of salivary antibodies in periodontal infections is less well-documented, with gingival crevice fluid antibody also having the potential to alter the nature of the pathogenic flora. Dental infections are virtually ubiquitous in the teenage population in the United States. Evidence indicates that antibody can modify the course of infection and disease caused by mutans streptococci. Target antigens for dental caries vaccines include surface adhesin proteins, glucosyltransferases (GTFs), glucan-binding proteins (GBPs), other surface antigens, and cell wall carbohydrate of mutans streptococci. Passive antibody administration has been effective in diminishing mutans streptococcal infection in several different species, including humans. Phase I trials of clinical vaccines have established GTF as a safe antigen, with the ability to elicit IgA antibody.

Infants are immunocompetent with respect to salivary IgA at 1 year of age or before, which appears to be the appropriate time to immunize before mutans streptococci colonize. Periodontal diseases are related to the presence of certain primary microorganisms, including *Actinobacillus actinomycetemcomitans*, *Porphyromonas gingivalis*, and *Bacteroides forsythus*. Host response to these microorganisms seems to occur during disease and may accompany infection. The role of antibody may be protective in that many studies in rodents and nonhuman primates suggest that parenteral immunization and host serum antibody can result in reductions in infecting organisms and at times reductions in periodontal bone loss. It has also been demonstrated that inflammatory T-cell functions may contribute to experimental periodontal diseases. Although some results of studies of a vaccine to interfere with periodontal infection appear promising, much research must be performed before confidence in such a vaccine is engendered.

ORAL MUCOSAL IMMUNITY

The intestine is the largest immunological organ in the body, with 70% to 80% of all immunoglobulin-producing cells (about 10% to 20% of which end up outside of the gut mucosa). The cells produce 50 to 100 mg/kg of immunoglobulin per day, considerably more than the remaining antibody-producing cells (McGhee and Mestecky, 1990; Holmgren, 1991). Secretory IgA (S-IgA) antibodies function at mucosal surfaces, including the oral cavity, to neutralize bacterial toxins and viruses and to inhibit attachment, adherence, and colonization of the mucosal and tooth surfaces. Very small amounts of antigen are required, and several excellent vehicles and adjuvants that target IgA B cells in Peyer's patches have been developed. Attenuated strains of bacteria such as *Salmonella* have been used as vectors for targeting delivery. *Salmonella typhimurium* carrying *Streptococcus mutans* antigen I/II or GTF and *Salmonella typhi* expressing lipopolysaccharide from another bacterium have been used for oral immunization in animals and humans, respectively. These induce serum as well as secretory antibodies and protection (Mestecky and Eldridge, 1991). Other bacterial antigens, including the M protein of streptococci, bacterial fimbriae, and GTF peptides, have also been expressed recombinantly in strains of *Salmonella* (Eastcott *et al.*, 2002). Liposomes, phospholipid membrane vesicles, microspheres of poly-DL-lactide-co-glycolide, and antigen linked to the B subunit of cholera toxin have also been successfully used as targeting vehicles (McGhee and Mestecky, 1990; Holmgren, 1991; Moldoveanu *et al.*, 1993; Smith *et al.*, 2000).

Mucosal humoral immunity in the oral cavity, particularly mediated by S-IgA antibody, can interfere with colonization of bacteria (Williams and Gibbons, 1972). In particular, results from microbiological studies involving humans indicate that the mouth (including various mucosal surfaces) may be a reservoir for gingival challenges with oral pathogens (Ebersole *et al.*, 1987b). S-IgA is a deterrent to colonization of oral surfaces, so the mucosal immune system may function by reducing the frequency or degree of challenge by pathogens or their products, without the associated host destructive effects of secondary mediators of immunity (Brandtzaeg and Tolo, 1977).

An oral vaccine designed to induce S-IgA in saliva could be effective in interfering with bacterial adherence and colonization of the oral mucosa and teeth by dental and periodontal pathogens without inducing significant nonmucosal humoral immunity, which may contribute to periodontal pathology. The bacteria of concern, however, are predominantly anaerobic or facultative and are found mostly in periodontal pockets, which are not necessarily accessible to salivary components. Thus, while salivary antibodies could interfere with initial mucosal colonization of periodontal disease–associated microflora, they might not have access to the bacteria in the subgingival flora. In contrast to saliva, gingival crevicular fluid (GCF) is mostly a blood-derived exudate containing serum immunoglobulins as well as immunoglobulins produced by plasma cells in the periodontal pocket wall. GCF traverses periodontal pockets, where it bathes the bacteria (in plaque and those free in the pocket) and exudes into the mouth. Thus, GCF is an ideal vehicle for transporting specific antibodies to the subgingival bacteria as well as to the supragingival region around the necks of the teeth. It is for these reasons that investigators working to develop periodontal vaccines have considered traditional injectable vaccines (to elicit specific IgG antibody in GCF) and mucosal vaccines as complementary approaches to inducing protective immunity (Taubman and Smith, 1993).

The concept of mucosal inductive sites giving rise to primed lymphoid cells that migrate has been elaborated (Mestecky and McGhee, 1987). Inductive sites usually are in close association with antigen-handling cells such as M cells, macrophages, and dendritic cells. Initial stimulation of mucosal Ig-producing B cells is suggested to occur in the organized mucosa-associated lymphoreticular tissue (MALT), particularly the Peyer's patches. Effector cells migrate from these inductive sites from the peripheral blood to exocrine tissues throughout the body. It has been suggested that there are preferential pathways for migration of effector cells from MALT (*e.g.*, cells stimulated in the nasal [tonsils and adenoids]–associated lymphoreticular tissue [NALT] may show a preference to populate proximal sites such as lacrimal, nasal, and salivary glands) as opposed to more distal sites of the mucosal immune system such as the urogenital tract (Brandtzaeg and Haneberg, 1997). Therefore, the homing mechanisms—for example,

for mucosal B cells—are both generalized and regionalized. These cells are directed by the gate-keeper function of epithelial cells (Parker *et al.*, 1992; Tanaka *et al.*, 1993).

Adhesion molecules are involved in leukocyte-endothelial recognition, directing naive lymphocytes to organized GALT structures and primed B and T cells (memory lymphocytes, lymphoblasts) to the intestinal lamina propria. High endothelial venules (HEVs) in GALT in the parafollicular zone express MAdCAM-1, which contains O-linked carbohydrates that bind L-selectin, an interaction that initiates emigration of naive lymphocytes into the inductive GALT locations. Unmodified MAdCAM-1 expressed by lamina propria venules is important for targeting primed lymphoid cells expressing $\alpha 4\beta 7$ from the blood to the mucosal effector site (Farstad *et al.*, 1997). The use of such a system to direct cells to periodontal tissues has not been explored. However, it is clear that the cervical lymph nodes (CLNs) drain this NALT and salivary-associated lymphoid tissue area (Russell and Wu, 1997). The mucosal immunity expressed by mature S-IgA effector cells via the saliva(s) is of primary significance in cariogenic infections. Although gingival and periodontal tissues can be considered as mucosal tissues, they are not part of the mucosal immune system because IgA effector cells are not directly involved in gingival/periodontal tissue immunity. IgG and effector T cells are primarily involved in subgingival periodontal immunity via these tissues and the GCF. However, mucosal immunity may also be quite relevant on a supragingival level at various stages of periodontal infections. Altough the cervical lymph nodes drain the NALT, the salivary associated lymphoid tissue area, and the gingival/periodontal tissues (Russell and Wu, 1997), there is currently little information elucidating the dynamics of effector cell migration to gingival/periodontal tissues. Recently, investigations have begun to explore the migration mechanisms of effector cells to gingival/periodontal tissues (Taubman *et al.*, 1994, 1997; Kawai *et al.*, 1999, 2000, 2001). These mechanisms will be discussed in the periodontal disease section. Theoretically, this information could lead to the ability to interfere with or to direct migration of appropriate effector cells to these tissues to prevent or alleviate the sequelae of periodontal infection.

The mucosal immune system in dental infections

The principle of caries vaccine immunization was first demonstrated by Bowen (1969), who showed that intravenously immunized monkeys infected with *S. mutans* developed little disease. This principle was extended to include mucosal immunity by Taubman (1973) and later by Taubman and Smith (1974) and also McGhee and colleagues (1975), who immunized conventional and gnotobiotic rats in the vicinity of the salivary gland with intact mutans streptococcal cells. The resulting induction of salivary IgA and serum antibody was related to reductions in the levels of experimental mutans streptococcal infection and subsequent disease. Michalek and coworkers (1976) were the first to show that induction of immunity by a different mucosal route (oral feeding of whole cells) was sufficient to elicit a protective salivary IgA immune response in rats. Intraductal (Stenson's duct) immunization of primates with intact cells also induced salivary antibody (Evans *et al.*, 1975) that was associated with significant reductions in dental caries caused by experimental infection with mutans streptococci (Emmings *et al.*, 1975).

Mestecky and coworkers (1978) then demonstrated that ingestion of intact mutans streptococcal cells in capsules could elicit salivary S-IgA antibody in humans. These experiments helped to initiate and establish the concept of a common mucosal immune system, since S-IgA antibody levels were also increased in tears. Thus, in dental caries where the mutans streptococci appear to be the major pathogen, these early studies indicated that under controlled conditions, the host immune response to *S. mutans* cells could interfere with the pathogenesis of the caries process. The association between the protective aspects of the mucosal immune response and protection against cariogenic bacterial infection has been strengthened considerably in subsequent years (Ma *et al.*, 1987; Taubman and Smith, 1989a; Michalek and Childers, 1990; Russell, 1992; Taubman and Smith, 1993a, 1997).

The mucosal immune system in periodontal infections

While initial studies suggested that salivary antibodies have potential for diagnostic or protective aspects of periodontal disease assessment (Taubman *et al.*, 1982a; Smith *et al.*, 1985), the parotid salivary IgA concentration and secretion rate appear to be mostly independent of periodontal inflammation. The effects of salivary IgA on periodontal disease manifestations in humans may be extremely complex. Salivary antibody to periodontal pathogens can be detected after infection (Smith *et al.*, 1985). It is quite clear that periodontopathic microorganisms can be vulnerable to the effect of S-IgA in saliva during their natural colonization progression. The earliest phases of colonization with putative periodontal pathogens have not been investigated extensively, and data are less than optimal to evaluate use of the mucosal immune system for interference with periodontal infections. However, perhaps the most compelling evidence for the association of microorganisms with disease is the strong relationship between organisms and gingival immune responses (Ebersole *et al.*, 1985; Ebersole *et al.*, 1987). These findings highlight the significance of GCF antibody (predominantly IgG) in periodontal infection (Ebersole *et al.*, 1985). Both protective and destructive gingival inflammation and immunity seem to be inextricably related in the host response to periodontal infection.

In considering the development of a strategy for producing a vaccine that would protect against periodontopathic bacteria, several choices can be made involving the use of a traditional injectable vaccine aimed at inducing high levels of serum IgG antibodies, or an oral vaccine targeting the GALT for production of S-IgA antibodies, and induction of mucosal immunity. While the two strategies differ greatly, each has advantages and disadvantages.

Systemic antibody has been shown to function in antibacterial immunity by a variety of mechanisms. These include the ability to aggregate the bacteria, inhibit adherence and colonization, enhance phagocytosis, lyse the bacteria, and detoxify endotoxins and exotoxins. Examinations of these functions in periodontal disease have generally attempted to relate the levels or presence of antibody activity to the severity of disease and examine the ability of antibodies to inhibit colonization and to inhibit or antagonize other proposed virulence components of the bacteria (Ebersole and Taubman, 1994).

DENTAL CARIES: INTRODUCTION TO THE DISEASE—MOLECULAR PATHOGENESIS

Dental caries is a disease that results from the dissolution of mineral in the enamel and dentin of the tooth by organic acids that are the metabolic byproducts secreted by certain dental plaque microbiota. Mutans streptococci have been most often associated as the primary etiologic agents of this disease (Hamada and Slade, 1980; Loesche, 1986). *S. mutans* is the species most commonly isolated from humans, with *Streptococcus sobrinus* colonizing a minority of subjects (Coykendall and Gustafson, 1986). These oral streptococci have the ability to produce very large amounts of lactic acid at a significant rate and can tolerate extremes in sugar concentration, ionic strength, and pH. Dental caries can be initiated and transmitted by infection with mutans streptococci, especially in the presence of carbohydrate-rich diets that favor their accumulation. Animal studies and clinical trials have demonstrated that caries incidence declines when mutans streptococcal challenge is modified, further implicating these microorganisms in the pathogenesis of dental caries (Loesche, 1986).

There appear to be three main phases to the molecular pathogenesis of mutans streptococci–associated dental caries. The first phase seems to involve attachment of the organism to dental pellicle. This is mediated by an adhesin of the mutans streptococci (*e.g.*, Ag I/II, PAc; Russell and Lehner, 1978; Russell, 1992). The mutans streptococci can bind to appropriate molecules in the pellicle, presumably by this surface protein adhesin molecule (Lamont *et al.*, 1991). The second phase of accumulation is dependent on the presence of sucrose, GTF enzymes, and glucan-binding protein(s) (GBPs) on the mutans streptococci. GTF will synthesize water-soluble or water-insoluble polyglucans from the glucose moieties of sucrose after cleaving sucrose into its component saccharides, glucose and fructose. These multivalent glucans give rise to the interactions with GBP and GTF on the surface of the mutans streptococcal cell. These multiple aggregation events, including binding to GTF (glucan binding domain) and bacterial multiplication, result in the accumulation of large masses of mutans streptococci. When these accumulations are of sufficient magnitude and the sugar substrates (including glucose) are available, large amounts of the metabolic end-product lactic acid are produced that can cause enamel dissolution, and carious lesions ensue.

Epidemiology of dental caries in the United States
Estimate of overall and age-specific incidence

Dental caries was such a severe health problem in World War II that the impact of this devastating disease on the lack of eligibility of United States youths for the draft resulted in the founding of the National Institute of Dental Research in 1948. However, as the subsequent use of fluoride and antibiotics increased in the United States (Loesche, 1986), the former vast extent of this health problem diminished, with an increase in the average number of permanent teeth (in 18- to 50-year-olds) without decay or fillings between the periods of 1971 to 1974 and 1988 to 1994 (National Center for Health Statistics, 1975, 1996). Nevertheless, dental caries is the most prevalent bacterial infectious disease occurring in areas where refined sugars are utilized. In 1986 to 1987 the mean number of decayed, missing, or filled surfaces (DMFS) in United States schoolchildren 10 years of age was 1.69, and increased in 17-year-olds to 8.04 (Hicks and Flaitz, 1993; see **Table 62.1**). The DMFS in the United States is about 1.4 in 9-year-olds, and there are high-risk groups within this population who are particularly susceptible to disease (*e.g.*, in North American Indians, the mean number of decayed, missing, or filled teeth [DMFT] is 11.8 among 17-year-olds). However, the occurrence of dental caries remains fairly ubiquitous, with approximately 80% of all 17-year-olds affected (Stamm, 1991; see Table 62.1). The most recent large-scale study data available indicate that the prevalence of dental caries (decayed and filled teeth) increases with age (NCHS, 1996; Table 62.1).

Children are at the greatest risk of dental caries, although in 1987 adults older than 55 years were experiencing caries rates similar to those of children aged 6–11 years (DePaola, 1992). The caries incidence in grade-school children (Stamm *et al.*, 1988) is indicated in **Table 62.2**, showing that in 1988 from 46% to 66% of children in grade 5 had had dental caries. Also, dental caries is present in 80% of 17-year-olds, and root caries is present in 56% of individuals over 51 years of age. A higher percentage of poor people than nonpoor people have at least one untreated, decayed tooth. There are approximately twofold more poor individuals than nonpoor ones with untreated, decayed teeth at all ages studied (ages 2–9, 5–17, and 18 years or older) (NCHS, 1996). Although more recent data are not available, it is clear that dental caries continues to be a significant infectious disease.

Incidence of clinical disease

The neonatal oral cavity, which is sterile, becomes rapidly colonized by the maternal flora (Berkowitz and Jones, 1985), which can preferentially colonize mucosal surfaces (van Houte, 1976). The primary early components of the young infant's flora are *Streptococcus salivarius*, which colonizes shortly after birth (Carlsson *et al.*, 1970), and *Streptococcus mitis*, which soon accounts for the majority of streptococci in the oral cavity prior to the eruption of dentition (Smith *et al.*, 1993a). The eruption of teeth into the oral cavity midway through the first year of life signals a significant change in the kind and distribution of microbiota that colonize the oral cavity (Carlsson *et al.*, 1975; Kononen *et al.*, 1994). Teeth provide sites for *Streptococcus sanguis* and mutans streptococcal colonization. *S. sanguis* can be detected in a majority of children by the end of the first year of life (Carlsson *et al.*, 1975; Smith *et al.*, 1993a). Mutans streptococci colonize in

Table 62.1. Incidence of Dental Caries (per National Institutes of Health Studies)

Study Category	Incidence (%)
United States, 1986–1987: One or more dental caries lesions[a]	
All children aged 5–8 years	53
American Indian–Alaskan Native aged 6–8 years	52
Primary dentition	92
Black children aged 6–8 years	61
All adolescents aged 15 years	78
American Indian–Alaskan Native aged 15 years	93
Root caries in general population using fluoride, aged 51–65 years[b]	56
At least one carious lesion or filling in coronal portion of primary or permanent teeth[c]	
Children aged 5–9 years	52
Seventeen-year-olds	78
Adults 18 years or older	85

[a] Data derived from U.S. Department of Health and Human Services (1989).
[b] Data derived from Burt *et al.*, 1986.
[c] Data derived from NCHS, NHANES III (1996).

Table 62.2. Incidence of Dental Caries in Grade-School Children, 1988[a]

Location	n	Grade	Age (years)	Incidence (%)
Aiken, South Carolina	1099	1	6–7	58
	967	5	10–11	66
Portland, Maine	1085	1	6–7	31
	965	5	10–11	46

[a]Data derived from Stamm *et al.* (1988).

childhood, as determined by bacteriocin typing (Berkowitz and Jordan, 1975) and plasmid detection (Caufield *et al.*, 1982). Culture studies (Smith *et al.*, 1998) and DNA finger-printing studies (Li and Caufield, 1995) have indicated a predominant maternal source of infection with mutans streptococci. The extent and frequency of infection of the child are often related to the level of mutans streptococcal colonization of the mother (Kohler *et al.*, 1983, 1984; Caufield *et al.*, 1993; Smith *et al*, 1998).

Initial mutans streptococcal colonization of the child generally occurs during a "window of infectivity" (Caufield *et al.*, 1993) between 18 and 36 months of age. Many children do not become infected during this period and may remain uninfected until the secondary dentition erupts. Thus, although an erupted primary dentition is necessary for colonization with mutans streptococci, it is not solely sufficient to ensure colonization. Other factors besides the infectious dose of mutans streptococci and the presence of teeth also play a role in the ultimate colonization of the child. These include the dietary presence of sucrose and the host immune response. Thus, it is conceivable that although multiple initial attachment encounters occur, these are not accompanied by sucrose-dependent accumulation events. Also, although children are quite competent to produce mucosal S-IgA antibody before 12 months of age (Smith and Taubman, 1992), there is little or no antibody to GTFs at that time (Gahnberg *et al.*, 1985). Thus, mutans streptococcal infection is primarily manifested as colonization of the oral cavity of individuals with teeth. In general, the extent of the infectious challenge (maternal or otherwise) is related to the extent of the infection that is established (Kohler *et al.*, 1983, 1984).

Mutans streptococci are not avid colonizers of the tooth surface, and other organisms that compete for tooth surface sites (*e.g.*, *S. sanguis*) appear to colonize at an earlier time (by 12 months of age; Carlsson *et al.*, 1975). The relatively feeble ability of mutans streptococci to establish colonization bodes well for attempts to actively interfere with the establishment of this microorganism on the tooth. Thus, it may be possible to actively immunize with a mutans streptococcal antigen, which is crucial in the molecular pathogenesis of dental caries at a time when children are immunologically competent with respect to mucosal immunity. Such an approach could delay or prevent the effective establishment

and colonization of the mutans streptococci. Such procedures could be assisted by minimizing the (maternal) infectious challenge prior to enhancing host immunity by immunization (Taubman and Smith, 1989).

Immunological competence and dental caries
Legler and coworkers (1981) showed that subjects with combined immunodeficiencies in the ability to produce S-IgA and S-IgM had significantly more disease than matched controls. Congenitally athymic rats have significantly more dental caries than their euthymic counterparts after experimental infection (Stack *et al.*, 1990). These studies suggested that the presence of a functioning immune system is critical to oral health.

Characteristics of immunity
Adaptive immunity has numerous expressions in the oral cavity. Mucosal and systemic immune systems function in the oral cavity and can be modified to interfere with mutans streptococcal colonization and pathogenicity. Systemic immune elements, including IgG, IgA, IgM, B- and T-lymphocytes, cytokines, and complement components, enter the oral cavity in the GCF. These elements may exert a protective effect, primarily on the cervical areas of the tooth surface, by "conventional" systemic mechanisms. Mucosal immune elements, chiefly mucosal S-IgA, and lower concentrations of IgM and IgG antibody are secreted into the oral cavity from major and minor salivary glands. Mucosal immunization at a variety of inductive sites, including GALT or NALT, with antigens derived from mutans streptococci results in the migration of antigen-specific IgA-producing cells into salivary glands, differentiation, maturation, and the eventual secretion of salivary IgA antibody from these mucosal effector tissues (McGhee *et al.*, 1992). Once in the oral cavity, antibody from each of these sources has the potential to modify the colonization of cariogenic microbiota on dental surfaces. Also, a T-cell response to mutans streptococci and to various antigens (GTF, antigen I/II) has been demonstrated in the peripheral blood lymphocytes of individuals with disease. The three major antigens to which S-IgA antibody has been demonstrated are GTFs (sucrose-dependent accumulation), antigen I/II (surface adhesin), and GBPs (accumulation), as described in **Table 62.3.**

Table 62.3. *Streptococcus mutans* Antigens Involved in the Molecular Pathogenesis of Dental Caries: Mode of Immunization and Use in Experimental Vaccines

Antigen	Function	Mode	Result	Reference
Antigen I/II (PAc)	Adhesin	Injected	Protection	Lehner *et al.*, 1981; Russell, 1992; Katz *et al.*, 1993; Ma *et al.*, 1987
Portion (N-terminal)	Adhesin	Intraoral?	Protection	Redman *et al.*, 1995
Glucosyltransferase	Glucan synthesis accumulation	Salivary gland vicinity	Protection	Taubman *et al.*, 1977; Smith *et al.*, 1979, 1982, 1987; Taubman, 1996
GTF + Antigen I/II	Glucan synthesis and adhesion	Oral	Increase in salivary IgA2 antibody	Childers *et al.*, 1994
GTF + Antigen I/II	Glucan synthesis and adhesion	Nasal	Increase in nasal/ salivary IgA1 & salivary IgA2 antibody	Childers *et al.*, 1999
Glucan-binding protein(s)	Surface receptor accumulation	Salivary (oral) gland vicinity	Protection	Smith and Taubman, 1996
3.8-kDa antigen	Uknown adhesin?	Topical gingival application	Protection	Lehner *et al.*, 1989b, 1994
Serotype carbohydrate	Steric blockage of surface function	Oral	Protection	Childers *et al.*, 1991; Russell, 1992

Characteristics of antigen elicitation of antibody

Mutans streptococci can elicit antibodies both in saliva (mucosal; predominantly IgA) and in serum (predominantly IgG). Between the ages of 1 and 5 years, salivary S-IgA antibody has been detected to antigens of *S. mutans*, *S. sobrinus*, and *Streptococcus rattus*, when this antibody appears to be crucial. Salivary S-IgA antibody to *S. mutans* GTF was detected in only 6% of 2- to 48-month-old children, although most adults demonstrate IgA antibody to *S. mutans* GTF (Smith and Taubman, 1992). The absence or low level of salivary antibody to specific mutans streptococcal antigens (including antigen I/II) prior to colonization may increase the risk of permanent infection (Smith and Taubman, 1992).

Others have concluded that low caries experience was positively correlated with elevated serum IgG antibody to a surface protein of *S. mutans* in young people and have suggested that serum immunity, manifested in the oral cavity via the GCF, could alter cariogenic mutans streptococcal colonization and disease (Challacombe *et al.*, 1984). With advancing age, however, serum antibody levels ultimately appear to reflect the cumulative antigenic challenge provided by infections that lead to disease (Kent *et al.*, 1991). The presence of gingival crevicular IgG antibody (Smith *et al.*, 1994d) or salivary S-IgA (Gregory *et al.*, 1985) antibody to *S. mutans* has been associated with short-term modifications of indigenous (Smith and Taubman, 1987) or implanted (Camling *et al.*, 1991) mutans streptococcal colonization of teeth. These and other studies (Legler *et al.*, 1981; Stack *et al.*, 1990) have suggested that the presence of a functioning immune system

is critical to oral health and that antibody of the appropriate specificity could influence the course of dental caries, especially if antibody was present at the initiation of cariogenic infectious challenge.

Pathways to immunological intervention with mutans streptococcal infection

Several lines of evidence indicate that antibody may modify the course of infection and disease with cariogenic mutans streptococci (Michalek and Childers, 1990). Antibody to mutans streptococcal antigens, particularly to GTF, when incubated *in vitro* with growing pure cultures of mutans streptococci, reduced the amount of plaque formed on hard surfaces (Taubman *et al.*, 1982b). Epidemiologic evidence is more problematic because of uncontrolled variables such as diet, fluoride levels, medication, and length of association with the cariogenic flora.

Theoretically, several phases of mutans streptococcal infection are amenable to immune intervention. Microorganisms can be cleared from the oral cavity by antibody-mediated aggregation while still in the salivary phase, prior to colonization. Antibody could also block the surface receptor molecules necessary for colonization or accumulation, inactivate enzymes responsible for glucan formation, or modify metabolically important functions.

At this stage of investigation, knowledge of the pathogenic mechanisms of dental caries infection and advances in vaccinology and information relating to the ontogeny of immune development in the oral cavity, coupled with understanding of the natural history of streptococcal colonization of the mouth, would suggest that an effective vaccine can alleviate considerable suffering and save the billions of dollars that are spent on restorative dentistry in the United States. (Total dental health expenditures in the United States were between $30 billion and $40 billion in 1992 and were $60 billion in 2000. This represented approximately 5% of the total United States health expenditure. The majority of this expense is for the diagnosis and treatment of dental caries.)

Vaccine development

There are several different types of vaccine currently in development. The specific type is based on the antigen being used to make up the vaccine (see Table 62.3).

Target antigens for dental caries vaccines. Several purified mutans streptococcal antigens have induced protective immunity in experimental dental caries models and form the basis for the development of a vaccine (Table 62.3). These include surface proteins. Administration of antigen I/II and GTF has demonstrated effects in humans that were observed as reductions in indigenous mutans streptococci.

Antigen I/II (Adhesin) Russell and Lehner (1978) described a protein designated antigen I/II (also known as PAc or P1), which was found both in the culture supernatant and the *S. mutans* cell surface. This 190-kDa adhesin has been cloned and sequenced (Lee *et al.*, 1988; Okahashi *et al.*, 1989). It is composed of a polypeptide chain of approximately 1600 residues containing two internal repeating regions (Table 62.2). One proline-rich region is in the center of the molecule, and an alanine-rich region is located in the N-terminal portion. Although the actual function of antigen I/II is not completely clear, several investigators have identified regions of the molecule that bind to human salivary proteins. Crowley and colleagues (1993) and Nakai *et al.* (1993) have each described a region in the vicinity of the alanine-rich segment that can bind to experimental tooth pellicles. Others (Lehner *et al.*, 1994) have suggested that the proline-rich protein region may contain an adhesin segment, on the basis of adhesin inhibition assays using recombinant fragments of antigen I/II. Similar adhesins have been found and defined in other mutans streptococci (*e.g.*, SpaA from *S. sobrinus*; Curtiss *et al.*, 1986). Significant sequence homology has been observed among these mutans streptococcal adhesins (Ogier *et al.*, 1990; Tokuda *et al.*, 1990; LaPolla *et al.*, 1991) as well as with at least one adhesin from *Streptococcus gordonii*, a noncariogenic oral strain (Demuth *et al.*, 1990). Furthermore, others (Lamont *et al.*, 1991) have indicated that *S. mutans* can also bind to saliva-coated early plaque bacteria via antigen I/II.

Antibody to the intact antigen I/II molecule or to its salivary-binding segment blocked adherence of *S. mutans* to saliva-coated hydroxyapatite (Hajishengallis *et al.*, 1992). Furthermore, a variety of immunization approaches have shown that active (Lehner *et al.*, 1981; Russell, 1992; Katz *et al.*, 1993) immunization with intact antigen I/II or passive (Ma *et al.*, 1987) immunization with monoclonal antibody to this component can protect rodents or primates from

experimental dental caries caused by *S. mutans*. Immunization of mice with synthetic peptides from the alanine-rich segment of antigen I/II suppressed tooth colonization with *S. mutans* (Takahashi *et al.*, 1991). Immunization with mutans streptococcal adhesins has recently included protection after immunization with *S. sobrinus* SpaA constructs (Redman *et al.*, 1995). Further studies of an adherence domain and a structural region of *S. mutans* antigen I/II indicated that both the regions produced protective immunity against dental caries when administered nasally (Hajishengallis *et. al.*, 1998). Protection is theoretically implemented by interference with initial colonization and/or antibody-mediated prevention of accumulation by clearance of the bacteria that display the adhesin.

Glucosyltransferases Glucosyltransferases from mutans streptococci are the second category of components that have been effective as antigens in experimental models for dental caries. Mutans streptococcal GTFs synthesize glucans having a variety of α1–3 and α1–6 linkages, as well as different solubilities in water. These enzymes contain approximately 1400 to 1600 amino acid residues and include significant sequence homology, despite the variety of products. Genes encoding GTFs that synthesize water-insoluble and water-soluble glucans from *S. mutans* (Aoki *et al.*, 1986; Pucci *et al.*, 1987; Shiroza *et al.*, 1987) and *S. sobrinus* (Russell *et al.*, 1987, 1988) have been cloned. Early studies with mutations in the GTF gene of *S. mutans* responsible for insoluble glucan synthesis indicated that these mutants were relatively noncariogenic (Tanzer *et al.*, 1974). More recent studies of insertionally inactivated *S. mutans* GTF genes to replace functional wild-type copies of the gene indicated that caries was markedly diminished when *gtf-b* and *gtf-c* genes that coded for GTFs synthesizing water-insoluble or water-soluble glucan were inactivated. Therefore, both water-insoluble and water-soluble glucans from GTFs are important in dental caries pathogenesis (Yamashita *et al.*, 1993).

The activity of GTF is mediated through both catalytic and glucan-binding functions. The catalytic activity of GTF appears to be associated with at least two primary sites in the N-terminal third of the molecule. One of these sites contains an aspartic acid (residues 453 [*S. downei* GTF-I] or 451 [*S. mutans gtf-b*]) that has been suggested by Mooser and colleagues (1991) to be the residue to which the glucosyl moiety of sucrose is covalently bound in the active site. A second catalytic site has been identified by Funane and coworkers (1993) in *Leuconostoc mesenteroides* GTF. This second site appears to retain catalytic activity even when the more C-terminal catalytic aspartate previously described in mutans streptococci (Mooser *et al.*, 1991) is chemically blocked (Funane *et al.*, 1993). The *L. mesenteroides* sequence surrounding the aspartate in this second site is quite similar to that found in mutans streptococcal GTF sequences, where it may also participate in catalytic events.

The C-terminal region of the GTF molecule contains a pattern of repeating sequences that have been identified in all GTFs from mutans streptococci (Ferretti *et al.*, 1988; Hanada and Kuramitsu, 1989; Abo *et al.*, 1991). This region is associated with glucan-binding function because C-terminal, tryptic fragments of GTF (Wong *et al.*, 1990; Mooser *et al.*, 1991) retain the ability to bind α-1,6 glucan, and recombinant products containing the C-terminal third of GTF-I of *S. downei* or *S. sobrinus* also can bind α-1,6 glucan (Ferretti *et al.*, 1987; Abo *et al.*, 1991). Amino acid deletions in this region remove glucan-binding activity, and also a GBP of *S. mutans* contains reiterated sequences that are very similar to those found in this region of GTF (Banas *et al.*, 1990). In addition, toxin A from *Clostridium difficile*, which has been postulated to bind carbohydrate on intestinal epithelial cells, contains repeating sequences that are similar to those of the *S. mutans* GBP (Wren *et al.*, 1991; Von Eichel-Streiber *et al.*, 1992). These sequences include structural redundancies that are shared among toxin A, GBP, and GTF. Repetition of such aromatic acid–based motifs may be important in protein-carbohydrate complex formation (Wren *et al.*, 1991; Von Eichel-Streiber *et al.*, 1992).

The use of GTF as an antigen has been shown to result in protection from experimental dental caries in rodents (Taubman and Smith, 1977; Smith *et al.*, 1979; Smith *et al.*, 1982) and in the induction of S-IgA antibody in humans, accompanied by interference with reaccumulation of indigenous mutans streptococci after dental prophylaxis (Smith and Taubman, 1990). Local injection, gastric intubation, oral administration, and topical application have each resulted in successful demonstration of a protective effect with use of this antigen. The GTF vaccine consists of a mixture of purified GTF enzymes responsible for synthesis of water-soluble and water-insoluble glucan synthesis derived from *S. sobrinus*. Only enzyme protein is present in the vaccine (Smith and Taubman, 1987).

Synthetic peptides, based on sequences thought to be associated with catalytic or glucan-binding domains, have also been shown to elicit antibody that can inhibit GTF activity (Smith *et al.*, 1993b; Smith *et al.*, 1994c; Taubman *et al.*, 1995, 2001). Peptides (Dertzbaugh and Macrina, 1990; Chia *et al.*, 1993) containing sequences near the catalytic domain(s) of GTF also have elicited GTF-inhibitory activity. Synthetic peptide vaccines based on the putative catalytic or glucan-binding epitopes of GTF have recently been reported to protect rats from experimental dental caries (Taubman *et al.*, 1995, 2001). Although the exact basis for experimental protection with such GTF-type vaccines is presently unknown, it appears likely that such protection can involve functional inhibition of the catalytic and/or glucan-binding activity of GTF (Taubman *et al.*, 1995).

In strong support of this suggestion is the recent demonstration that coimmunization with complementary glucosyltransferase peptides from the catalytic and glucan binding regions of GTF resulted in enhanced immunogenicity and protection against dental caries (Taubman *et al.*, 2000). Even more compelling is the demonstration that immunization of rats with a synthetic diepitopic multi-antigenic peptide (MAP) construct consisting of peptide epitopes from the catalytic and glucan-binding regions of GTF markedly enhanced immunogenicity, inhibitory reac-

tivity with GTF, and protection against dental caries (Taubman *et al.*, 2001).

Glucan-Binding Proteins   Although several mutans streptococcal products with catalytic activities (*e.g.*, GTFs and dextranases) can also bind glucans, a separate group of proteins are synthesized that seem to function as a glucan receptor. These GBPs participate in the formation of dental plaque by providing receptors on the mutans streptococcal cell surface for attachment of glucose polymers synthesized by GTFs. Several *S. mutans* and *S. sobrinus* GBPs have been described (Russell, 1979; Landale and McCabe, 1987; Wu-Yuan and Gill, 1992; Smith *et al.*, 1994a). All *S. mutans* strains tested synthesize at least two GBPs (Smith *et al.*, 1995). One of these has a molecular mass of 74 kDa (GBP74) in SDS PAGE and bears significant sequence homology with the glucan-binding domain of GTF (Banas *et al.*, 1990). An immunologically distinct *S. mutans* 59-kDa GBP (GBP59) is also synthesized and appears to induce salivary IgA antibody formation in many humans. Immunization of rats with *S. mutans* GBP59 can inhibit the subsequent colonization of *S. mutans* on molar surfaces (Smith *et al.*, 1996). Passive immunization with egg yolk antibody to *S. mutans* GBP resulted in significant reduction in dental caries induced by *S. mutans* infection (Smith *et al.*, 2001).

Lehner and coworkers (1985) have described a 3.8-kDa surface antigen presumed to be from the *S. mutans* surface, which they have shown to prevent the colonization of *S. mutans* and to inhibit the development of dental caries in primates. This protein, which has been partially sequenced, appears to have cross-reactive segments in common with the antigen I/II of *S. mutans*. Also, cyclized and linear peptides of varying lengths derived from the 3.8-kDa antigen have been synthesized (Lehner *et al.*, 1989a) and elicit antibody in GCF and saliva after topical gingival application (Table 62.3). This immunization regimen inhibited the colonization of animals on a carbohydrate-rich diet with *S. mutans* (Lehner *et al.*, 1994).

Cell wall carbohydrates   Cell wall carbohydrates of *S. mutans* have also received attention as potential vaccine antigens. The *c* serotype carbohydrates have been used in both animal and human immunization studies (Childers *et al.*, 1991). This carbohydrate contains a backbone of alternating 1,2- and 1,3-linked rhamnose units to which α-glucose residues are attached as side chains in the two position (Briand *et al.*, 1992). The *f* serotype carbohydrate has been suggested to participate in the adhesion of *S. mutans* to salivary glycoproteins (Klein and Scholler, 1988). A potential advantage of immunization with the serotype carbohydrate antigens is that their inherent specificity permits targeting of the immune response to the human pathogens, *S. mutans* and *S. sobrinus*. Since carbohydrates are T cell–independent antigens, they are, by themselves, unsuited to induce mucosal immune responses that typically have T cell–dependent characteristics. However, serum and salivary antibody can be elicited when serotype carbohydrates are orally administered in liposomes with or without additional adjuvants (Wachsmann *et al.*, 1985; Michalek *et al.*, 1992) or with peptide carriers or protein (Lett *et al.*, 1994). Introduction of liposomes to the conjugate for immunization led to salivary IgA antibody to both conjugate components (Lett *et al.*, 1995). Conjugation of either tetanus toxoid (Taubman *et al.*, 1998) or *S. sobrinus* GTF (Taubman *et al.*, 1999) to water-soluble glucans synthesized by GTF significantly enhanced levels of serum IgG and salivary IgA antibody to the glucan and the conjugated protein. Serum GTF inhibition was also enhanced by the conjugation, in comparison with GTF alone.

Since *S. mutans* infection occurs when children are minimally immunocompetent with respect to polysaccharide antigens, conjugate vaccines may have a very important role in enhancing levels of protection in immunized children. Michalek and coworkers (1992) have shown that oral immunization with liposomes containing *c* serotype *S. mutans* carbohydrate not only induced salivary IgA antibody to *S. mutans* but also resulted in reduced numbers of *S. mutans* in plaque and reduced the extent of dental caries caused by experimental infection of rats.

Passive Immunization Passive immunization techniques, in which antibody to injected intact mutans streptococcal cells entered the oral cavity via milk (Michalek and McGhee, 1977), dietary supplements (Michalek *et al.*, 1987), or topical application of monoclonal antibody (Lehner *et al.*, 1989b), all resulted in successful interference with infection and disease caused by experimental or natural infections with cariogenic streptococci (Michalek and McGhee, 1977; Michalek *et al.*, 1987; Lehner *et al.*, 1989b). Hamada and his colleagues (1991) found that they could interfere with dental caries passive immunization with hen yolk antibody to *S. mutans* GTF. In addition, passive immunization with egg yolk antibody to *S. mutans* GbpB resulted in significant reduction in dental caries induced by *S. mutans* infection (Smith *et al.*, 2001). Studies in humans with mouse monoclonal IgG antibody specific for antigen I/II (Ma *et al.*, 1990) deferred recolonization with mutans streptococci for 2 years after a 9-day treatment with chlorhexidine.

Studies in humans with mouse monoclonal IgG antibody specific for antigen I/II (Ma *et al.*, 1990) deferred recolonization with mutans streptococci for 2 years after a 9-day treatment with chlorhexidine. Ma and coworkers (1998) have developed a transgenic tobacco plant mucosal human monoclonal IgA antibody with specificity for antigen I/II. After chlorhexadine treatment and passive application of the antibody, subjects remained free of mutans streptococci for 4 months or more. The specific reason for the duration of interference with colonization has been suggested to involve removal of *S. mutans* colonization sites in the biofilm by competing microorganisms.

Progression of vaccine development

The GTF vaccine has progressed through phase I trials (Smith and Taubman, 1987). These clinical trials involved young adults, although it is now known that this is not the optimal target population (see later discussion for descrip-

tion). Orally administered GTF vaccine (with aluminum phosphate) was shown to elicit parotid salivary IgA antibody. After a thorough prophylaxis, indigenous mutans streptococci were reduced for a longer period of time in the immunized group than in the placebo group. No untoward effects of GTF administration were observed (Smith and Taubman, 1987).

Other vaccines described are in preclinical phases, with the exception of passive immunization.

Combination vaccines

The intact *S. sobrinus* GTF vaccine is not likely to be a part of a combination vaccine. However, a GTF peptide subunit vaccine would contain at least two epitopes: one each from a catalytic region and a glucan-binding region (Taubman *et al.*, 2001). A GTF peptide subunit vaccine could also contain epitopes from other functionally significant mutans streptococcal molecules such as adhesins (e.g., antigen I/II) (Smith *et al.*, 1994a; Smith and Taubman, 1996). Other antigens that could be included are portions of molecules that might enhance mucosal immune response (such as cholera toxin subunits). It would also be possible to include other childhood vaccine components such as tetanus toxoid.

Appropriate target population for a vaccine

Caufield and colleagues (1993) and others have shown that most children do not become colonized with mutans streptococci until after 18 months of age, although children undergo multiple infectious challenges with these microorganisms throughout early childhood. These events occur in a mucosal environment that appears to be immunologically responsive to infectious challenge (Smith and Taubman, 1992). For example, salivary S-IgA responses can be detected by 3 to 5 weeks of age to microorganisms that colonize the oral cavity during this time (*e.g.*, *S. mitis* and *S. salivarius*). Salivary S-IgA of these young infants appears to be substantially intact, despite often high proportions of an IgA1-protease-secreting microbiota found to colonize their oral cavity (Smith *et al.*, 1993a). By 12 months of age, both S-IgA1 and S-IgA2 antibodies appear to be present to an increasing number of antigens associated with these early colonizing streptococci. However, the secretion of S-IgA2 may be delayed in some infants (Smith *et al.*, 1993a).

Longitudinal studies during the first 5 years of life have revealed differences in the apparent extent of immune response to mutans streptococcal infectious challenge (Smith *et al.*, 1994b). Some children who became heavily infected with mutans streptococci had little salivary IgA antibody to mutans streptococcal antigens. Salivary IgA antibody to mutans antigens can be detected in other children who are apparently marginally colonized with mutans streptococci. Even within families where children are likely to be challenged with similar mutans streptococcal biotypes, different patterns of salivary IgA antibody to streptococcal antigens were observed. Thus, although mucosal immune responses to oral infections occur in most children, different response characteristics may occur after colonization of teeth.

During the past decade, considerable information has been obtained regarding the functionally important epitopes on virulence antigens of *S. mutans*. New methods of delivering and presenting these epitopes to achieve enhanced responses and knowledge of the ontogeny of mucosal immune responses to streptococci that colonize the oral cavity are leading to the development of effective vaccine approaches. The challenges for the next decade will be to identify the best assembly of epitopes with functional and adjuvant activity that will afford the longest protection by routes that are safe, convenient, and effective in the induction of antibody at the site of mutans streptococcal colonization. The multiplicity of experimental routes, vectors, and delivery systems under study should eventually allow us to tailor the vaccine to the abilities of a public health network available to the at-risk population. The frequency or necessity of booster immunizations remains unknown. Host immune responses (or nonresponses) to natural exposures to cariogenic streptococci, although not clearly understood, may reveal the capacity for natural boosting of mucosal immunity (Taubman and Smith, 1993).

INTRODUCTION TO PERIODONTAL DISEASES

Prevalence and progression

Periodontitis is a destructive chronic inflammatory disease of the connective tissues and bone housing the teeth and is a major cause of tooth loss in adults. These diseases have an infectious etiology, which may consist of several different pathogenic species. The prevalence of periodontal diseases in the American population is relatively high, with approximately 35% of the population aged 30–89 years affected (Albander *et al.*, 1999). Moderate to severe progressive periodontitis that may endanger the survival of the dentition affects about 13% of the population **(Table 62.4)**. In contrast, progressive periodontal destruction of a magnitude sufficient to endanger the survival of the dentition occurs in a smaller but significant proportion of the population (Brown and Löe, 1993). This is also true for populations in

Sri Lanka and Africa, where dental care traditionally has not been available (Löe *et al.*, 1986; Pilot *et al.*, 1986). Thus, a discrete but significant proportion of the general adult population (about 70%), as well as patients receiving adequate periodontal therapy, is considered to be at high risk for periodontitis (Axelsson *et al.*, 1991).

While the presence of bacteria is essential for the initiation and progression of periodontitis, bacteria alone are insufficient. A susceptible host is also necessary. Host susceptibility is determined in major part by genetic and other risk factors such as tobacco smoking (Page and Beck, 1997). Major factors that enhance risk for periodontitis have been identified (Genco and Löe, 1993; Grossi *et al.*, 1994, 1995; Kornman *et al.*, 1997; Michalowitcz *et al.*, 1999), and a Web-based tool for identification of individuals at high and low risk has been described (Page *et al.*, 2002).

Microbiology of periodontitis

Studies of the microbial progression from periodontal health through gingivitis to periodontitis have indicated a substantial increase in spirochetes and a change from a predominantly gram-positive flora to a gram-negative flora (Tanner *et al.*, 1979; Slots, 1986). In addition, the environment appears to become increasingly anaerobic as the severity of the disease increases. The association of some specific microbial species with periodontitis in humans and animals has been established, and approximately 32 participating species of putative periodontal pathogens have been identified (Tanner *et al.*, 1979; Slots, 1986; Loesche, 1988; Zambon *et al.*, 1988a,b). Species most strongly implicated in the disease include *Actinobacillus actinomycetemcomitans* (especially serotype b), *Porphyromonas gingivalis*, *Tannerella forsythensis*, *Treponema denticola*, and possibly *Prevotella intermedia*. Other less likely species include *Eikenella corrodens*, *Campylobacter rectus*, *Fusobacterium nucleatum*, and *Peptostreptococcus micros* (Haffajee and Socransky, 1994; Consensus Report, 1996; Socransky *et al.*, 1998). Recent evidence has suggested that, in addition to individual pathogenic bacterial species, complexes of bacteria are important in the development of a putative pathogenic flora (Socransky *et al.*, 1998). A large group of bacterial species compose the normal oral flora found in most individuals. It seems that an intermediary complex found in some individuals must form before the pathogenic species (also known as the red complex) can appear (Socransky *et al.*, 1998).

Humoral immune response in patients with periodontitis

Early detection of response

The initiation of a specific host response is reflected by alterations in the local cellular infiltrate in the tissues, by a systemic humoral immune response manifested by enhanced levels of serum antibody (Genco *et al.*, 1980), and by the local antibody response in the periodontium and GCF (Ebersole *et al.*, 1982b, 1984; Gmür, 1985). A serum antibody response to the bacteria can result from systemic dissemination of antigen to draining lymph nodes and the

Table 62.4. Prevalence (%) of Periodontal Disease with Pockets (one or more lesions) in Males

Age (years)	NIDR, 1985–1986[a]	Stoltenberg et al., 1993[b]
35–39	18.9	56.3
45–49	25.5	55.6
55–59	23.3	71.4

[a] Data derived from Miller *et al.* (1987).
[b] Data derived from Stoltenberg *et al.* (1993).

spleen, with recirculation of memory B lymphocytes sensitized in the local tissues, or the migration of macrophages with processed antigen. Although products from subgingival plaque bacteria can cross epithelial surfaces of the periodontium, it must be considered that the mass of organisms is still external to the host systemic immune responses. Therefore, just as there are low levels of serum antibody to bacteria colonizing the gastrointestinal tract (*e.g.*, *Escherichia coli* and *Bacteroides fragilis*), there are levels in serum of IgG antibody to a wide variety of prospective periodontal pathogens in normal subjects (Ebersole, 1990).

Early studies presented evidence of a specific immunological response in the disease showing precipitating antibodies to *A. actinomycetemcomitans* antigens in the sera of patients with local juvenile periodontitis (LJP; aggressive periodontitis) that were absent from normal subjects (Genco *et al.*, 1980). An enzyme-linked immunosorbent assay (ELISA; Ebersole *et al.*, 1980) was developed and utilized to describe the levels of serum antibody in periodontitis patients and normal subjects to a large number of periodontal disease–associated bacteria. As periodontitis is initiated and periodontal pockets form, epithelium of the pocket wall becomes ulcerated, and intact bacteria and bacterial components and products can have access to the underlying connective tissues and the circulation, resulting in serum antibody titers much higher than those generally seen in periodontally normal individuals.

Patients with periodontitis produce a humoral response

Numerous studies have demonstrated that many although not all patients with periodontitis produce a humoral response during the course of a periodontal infection (Mouton *et al.*, 1981; Ebersole *et al.*, 1982a,b; Taubman *et al.*, 1982a; Tew *et al.*, 1985; Ebersole *et al.*, 1986; Vincent *et al.*, 1987; Ishikawa *et al.*, 1988; Murayama *et al.*, 1988; Zambon *et al.*, 1988a,b; Ogawa *et al.*, 1990; Chen *et al.*, 1991b; Whitney *et al.*, 1992; Ling *et al.*, 1993). The role such antibodies may play in the onset and progression of the disease is not totally clear. Antibody variation in IgG subclass response may indicate the bacterial immunodominant antigens and could provide clues to the nature of host protection (Ebersole *et al.*, 1985, 1989). For example, the primary response to *A. actinomycetemcomitans* lipopolysaccharides to whole cell sonicates and to serotype antigen is primarily IgG2 (Page *et al.*, 1991; Wilson and Hamilton, 1992), an isotype which may provide a less than optimal protective capacity. Additionally, significant elevations in IgG4 immunoglobulin (Wilton *et al.*, 1993) have been associated with periodontitis and suggest a chronic antigenic stimulation lacking the induction of sufficient protective functions. For example, antibodies of the IgG2 subclass (followed by IgG3, IgG1, and IgG4) to antigens of *A. actinomycetemcomitans* and *P. gingivalis* often predominate in the sera of patients with LJP or rapidly progressive periodontitis (RPP), respectively (Whitney *et al.*, 1992; Ling *et al.*, 1993). IgG2 antibodies do not fix complement nor enhance opsonization and phagocytosis and killing by neutrophils as effectively as IgG1

(Roitt *et al.*, 1989). However, recent studies show that IgG2 antibodies in LJP are effective opsonins when used with phagocytes expressing the proper allotype of the low-affinity IgG (Fc) receptor (CD32; Wilson *et al.*, 1995).

Functions of humoral antibody to periodontal infection

Although serum antibody titers may be rather high in some patients, measures of antibody function (such as avidity and enhancement of killing) can sometimes be relatively low (Chen *et al.*, 1991a; Sjöstrom *et al.*, 1992, 1994). Indeed, in a study by Sjöstrom *et al.* (1992), low-titer sera from periodontally normal individuals were more effective at enhancing phagocytosis and killing than were low-titer sera from RPP patients, suggesting that immediately following infection, normal subjects may produce antibodies that are effective in clearing the organisms prior to clinical signs of infection; however, individuals who are susceptible to periodontitis may be unable to do so, and clinical disease can develop. Despite these observations, evidence of antibody-based protection has also been reported. Baker and Wilson (1989) found opsonic IgG antibodies in high-titered sera from LJP patients. Ranney *et al.* (1982) observed fewer affected teeth and less severe disease in young adults having high levels of precipitating serum antibodies to antigens of periodontopathic bacteria than in subjects with lower titers. Similarly, Gunsolley *et al.* (1987) found an inverse relationship between levels of serum antibodies reactive with antigens of *A. actinomycetemcomitans* and *P. gingivalis* and the number of teeth having attachment loss. In addition, a negative correlation between specific serum IgG antibody and the number of pockets deeper than 4 mm has been reported (Schenck and Michaelsen, 1987).

Effect of periodontal therapy on humoral immune response

Periodontal therapy appears to have a marked effect on humoral immune response to antigens of periodontopathic bacteria (Ebersole *et al.*, 1985; Vincent *et al.*, 1987; Murayama *et al.*, 1988). Treatment by scaling and root planing or by surgery significantly enhances serum antibody levels and avidities to antigens of *P. gingivalis* and induces seroconversion in seronegative patients (Ebersole *et al.*, 1985; Chen *et al.*, 1991a; Sjöstrom *et al.*, 1994). A statistically significant positive correlation was observed between titer to whole-cell sonicate of *P. gingivalis* and both mean pocket and mean bone loss, and a significant negative correlation exists between avidity to the whole-cell sonicate and mean bone loss and mean pocket depth (Chen *et al.*, 1991a). In another study, RPP patients treated only by scaling and root planing manifested significantly elevated serum antibody titers and avidities to antigens of *A. actinomycetemcomitans*, and at 12 months posttreatment, sera showed significantly enhanced chemiluminescence, phagocytosis, and killing relative to pretreatment sera (Sjöstrom *et al.*, 1994). Thus, conventional therapeutic approaches such as scaling and root planing, which are known to result in transient bacteremias, appear to elicit the production of antibodies that may be more protective than antibodies produced before treatment of the spontaneously occurring infection.

Antibody can influence periodontal microorganisms

Mechanisms of antibody protection against the onset and progression of periodontitis have not been well studied. However, some evidence does exist that antibody can influence periodontal microorganisms. Using ligature-induced periodontitis in *Macaca fascicularis* and a vaccine containing intact periodontopathic bacteria, Ebersole *et al.* (1999) demonstrated a reduction in some species of bacteria and enhancement in others in subgingival flora samples from the immunized animals. Using the same animal model and a vaccine containing formalinized *P. gingivalis* (monkey strain) as antigen, Persson *et al.* (1994) demonstrated a significant reduction in alveolar bone loss and significantly lower proportions of *P. gingivalis* in the subgingival flora of vaccinated animals having high titers of opsonic anti–*P. gingivalis* antibody. These observations suggest that one mechanism of immune protection may be enhanced opsonization, phagocytosis, and killing of *P. gingivalis*. In the same immunized animals, PGE2 levels in gingival crevicular fluid samples (and presumably in the inflamed gingival tissues) were significantly reduced and the extent of reduction was related to site-specific reduction in alveolar bone loss. Thus, reduction in PGE2 levels may be another mechanism whereby immunization may inhibit the onset and progression of periodontitis.

Immunization studies in rodents

Investigations of mucosal immunity, A. actinomycetemcomitans, *and T lymphocytes*

Rodent models, mostly rats and mice but also rabbits and hamsters, have been used extensively in periodontitis immunization and host response studies. Early studies of experimental periodontal disease **(Table 62.5)** most importantly indicated that immunization to stimulate the mucosal immune system could be protective in rodents and that delayed-type hypersensitivity might be accompanied by increases in bone loss (Crawford *et al.*, 1978). Other studies (Taubman *et al.*, 1983a, 1984) used a rat model to examine aspects of host immune responses in periodontal disease. A defined antigen, ovalbumin, was administered to gnotobiotic rats and elicited increased gingival lymphocytes, sensitized spleen cells, and increased bone loss (Taubman *et al.*, 1984). Animals presensitized with ovalbumin showed increased bone loss and high IgG antibody levels, suggesting that a mixed-type hypersensitivity may be contributing to the progression of disease (Taubman *et al.*, 1983a). In companion studies (Yamashita *et al.*, 1991; Yoshie *et al.*, 1985, 1987), the ability of adoptively transferred normal or *A. actinomycetemcomitans*–sensitized T lymphocytes to contribute to the disease process in rats was examined. T cells transferred into nude rats had the capacity to facilitate production of normal levels of immunoglobulins (and antibody) and protect against increased bone loss (Yoshie *et al.*, 1985). Specific *A. actinomycetemcomitans*–sensitized T cells transferred into rats exacer-

bated disease and increased delayed-type hypersensitivity (DTH) after *A. actinomycetemcomitans* infection (Yoshie *et al.*, 1987). These results further indicated that the disease in this model could be associated with hypersensitivity and that T lymphocytes were critical in regulating both T-cell and B-cell activity to maintain homeostasis in the periodontium. Further studies showed that immunization of rats with *A. actinomycetemcomitans* resulted in DTH reactions and antibody, with accompanying increased bone loss (Taubman *et al.*, 1983a). These studies supported the concept that T-cell functions and thymic regulation of immune responses can contribute to protective and/or destructive effects in periodontal disease. Therefore, the necessity of enhancing the protective aspects of the immune response and minimizing the detrimental aspects to modify the disease through a more complex understanding of the host immune response was emphasized.

Immune responses induced by active immunization with *Actinomyces viscosus* (now *naeslundii*) resulted in significant antibody titers and T-lymphocyte responses. Alveolar bone loss was greater in the immunized and infected animals than in rats that were only infected. It was suggested that these findings indicate a hypersensitivity reaction in the progression of disease (Burckhardt *et al.*, 1981). Parenteral immunization of rats with a whole bacterial sonicate elicited significantly elevated antibodies in a germ-free rat model system that developed alveolar bone loss following monoassociation with *E. corrodens* (Behling *et al.*, 1981). The immunized rats showed less bone loss than infected controls.

Investigations involving P. gingivalis

Some studies (Evans *et al.*, 1992a; Kusumoto *et al.*, 1993) have concentrated on the colonization and subsequent disease related to infection by *P. gingivalis*, with a focus on the ability of antibody to interfere with the function of fimbriae. The reports have indicated that murine antibody to the fimbriae inhibits colonization and the resulting clinical changes of periodontitis following infection with this pathogen. Studies of periodontal infections in rodents have included induction of alveolar bone loss by exposure to various putative periodontopathic bacteria or antigens (Baker *et al.*, 1994), induction of skin abscesses by injection of specific bacterial species or combinations of species (P.B. Chen *et al.*, 1987, 1991), implantation of subcutaneous chambers (Dahlen and Slots, 1989), and passive transfer of sensitized or nonsensitized lymphoid cells (Yoshie *et al.*, 1985; Yamashita *et al.*, 1991; Taubman *et al.*, 1994).

Rodent models used to demonstrate protection and to understand the function of antibody in periodontal diseases include germfree rats monoinfected with *P. gingivalis* (Klausen *et al.*, 1993), mice infected with *P. gingivalis* (Baker *et al.*, 1994), ligated hamster teeth (Okuda *et al.*, 1988), subcutaneous abscesses in mice (van Steenbergen *et al.*, 1982), and subcutaneous chamber models in mice and rabbits (Dahlen and Slots, 1989; Genco *et al.*, 1992). The subcutaneous abscess and chamber models are useful in investigations concerning virulence once bacteria have been introduced into the tissue. Factors such as colonization and

Table 62.5. Rodent Studies of Periodontal Disease Vaccines

Antigens	Mode	Result	Reference
Whole cells from *S. mutans*, *A. naeslundii, A. viscosus*	Local immunization to produce salivary and serum antibodies	High salivary antibodies to *S. mutans* or *A. naeslundii*, reduction in bone loss; DTH to *A. viscosus*, increased bone loss	Crawford *et al.*, 1978
Whole cells from *A. actinomycetemcomitans*	Parenteral immunization	Increased bone loss	Taubman *et al.*, 1983b
Whole cells from *A. viscosus*	Parenteral immunization	Increased T-cell responsiveness; increased bone loss	Burckhardt *et al.*, 1981
Sonicate from *E. corrodens*	Parenteral immunization	Decreased bone loss	Behling *et al.*, 1981
Whole cells from *P. gingivalis*	Parenteral immunization	Decreased bone loss ·	Klausen *et al.*, 1991, 1993; Evans *et al.*, 1992c
Crude fimbriae from *P. gingivalis*	Parenteral immunization	Decreased bone loss	Evans *et al.*, 1992a
Purified fimbriae and fimbril subunit from *P. gingivalis*	Parenteral immunization	Decreased bone loss	Evans *et al.*, 1992c
Hemagglutinin from *P. gingivalis* passive rabbit antibody	Passive polyclonal antibody	Reduced *P. gingivalis* recovered	Okuda *et al.*, 1988
Th2-type-specific T-cell clone anti–*A. actino-mycetemcomitans*	T-cell clone injected, help for antibody production	Decreased bone loss	Yamashita *et al.*, 1991; Eastcott *et al.*, 1994
P. gingivalis Arg-gingipain-A/Lys-gingipain peptides from the catalytic and adhesin hemagglutinin domain	Mouse abscess model	Protected against challenge with *P. gingivalis*	O'Brien-Simpson *et al.*, 2000a, 2000b; Rajapakse *et al.*, 2002
P. gingivalis Arg-gingipain-A DNA	Mouse abscess model	Protected against challenge with *P. gingivalis*	Yonezawa *et al.*, 2001
P. gingivalis Arg-gingipain-A/Lys-gingipain	Bone loss model; parenteral immunization in IFA	Inhibition of alveolar bone loss	Sunethra *et al.*, 2001
P. gingivalis whole cells	Bone loss model	SCID mice without T or B cells show significant bone loss but less than immuno-competent mice	Baker *et al.*, 1994
P. gingivalis Arg-gingipain-A/Lys-gingipain	Mouse chamber	Protected against infection	Genco *et al.*, 1998
Recombinant *P. gingivalis* Rhemagglutinin-B (rHag B) Gingipain R1	Rat bone loss model Parenteral immunization Bone loss model	Protected against alveolar bone loss	Katz *et al.*, 1999; Gibson & Genco, 2001
A. actinomycetemcomitans Omp 29, *A. actino-mycetemcomitans* LPS + Th1-omp29-specific clone cells	Bone loss model Omp 29, LPS intragingival cells in tail	Increased bone resorption if Th1 cells are injected	Kawai *et al.*, 2000

destruction of periodontal bone and ligament, of course, cannot be studied in these models. However, colonization and destruction of periodontal bone and ligament can be studied in the gnotobiotic rat model monoinfected with *P. gingivalis* (Klausen *et al.*, 1991; Evans *et al.*, 1992a,b,c) (Table 62.5) or infected with *P. gingivalis* or other periodontopathic organisms in the presence of a controlled flora (Chang *et al.*, 1988) and in mice infected with *P. gingivalis* (Baker *et al.*, 1994).

In general, studies conducted can be grouped into four areas: identification of potentially pathogenic periodontal bacteria or combinations of bacteria; assessment of their pathogenic potential; antigen testing and immune protection; and elucidation of mechanisms of protection and tissue destruction such as the roles of specific antibody, DTH responses, T-cell function, and Th1/Th2 responses.

Despite the obvious differences such as keratinization of the sulcular epithelium and the prominence of polymorphonucleocytes (PMNs), rats are similar to humans with respect to periodontal structure as well as pathogenesis of periodontal disease (Page and Schroeder, 1982; Klausen *et al.*, 1991) and in the cellular composition of periodontal lesions (Taubman *et al.*, 1984). In addition, rats have been established as reliable models for the assessment of periodontal bone loss (Klausen *et al.*, 1989). Although it is difficult to establish *P. gingivalis* in rats for more than a few weeks (Evans *et al.*, 1992c), several studies have shown that this infection time is sufficient to induce detectable periodontal bone loss without ligation (Klausen *et al.*, 1991; Evans *et al.*, 1992a,b,c). Recent studies have shown the importance of the bacterial pathogenic potential in establishing rodent periodontal infection and bone resorption (Schreiner *et al.*, 2003).

Studies of putative periodontopathic bacteria and their pathogenic potential

Rat abscess models have been used to study the pathogenic properties of various oral microorganisms (van Steenbergen *et al.*, 1982; Chen *et al.*, 1987; H.A. Chen *et al.*, 1991; Kesavalu *et al.*, 1991, 1992). *Porphyromonas gingivalis* initiates a spreading, phlegmonous abscess in mice (van Steenbergen *et al.*, 1982). Chen and coworkers (1987) immunized mice with heat-killed *P. gingivalis* strains A7A I-28 and 381 or *P. intermedia* ATCC 25261 to induce serum antibody. Following subcutaneous challenge with viable microorganisms, only the homologous immunization protected the mice from an invasive lesion and systemic infection. In contrast, immunization with LPS had no effect on lesion progression and lethality. These investigators have also demonstrated the ability of *A. actinomycetemcomitans* and *C. rectus* to initiate lesions in mice (P.B. Chen *et al.*, 1991). A further study showed that immune responses elicited to the capsular polysaccharides of *P. gingivalis* decreased tissue destruction initiated by an infectious challenge with *P. gingivalis* (Schifferle *et al.*, 1993).

Antigen testing and immune protection

Antigens of P. gingivalis. Various killed antigens *of P. gingivalis* have been used in immunization studies in the rat (for example, heat-killed whole cells [Klausen *et al.*, 1991; Evans *et al.*, 1992c]). Whole cells, either live (Chen *et al.*, 1987, 1990) or heat-killed (Chen *et al.*, 1987; Genco *et al.*, 1992; Kesavalu *et al.*, 1992), and formalin-treated whole cells (Kesavalu *et al.*, 1992) have been used in the mouse abscess or chamber model. Fimbrial antigens (crude preparations [Evans *et al.*, 1992c], the 43-kDa pure preparation [Evans *et al.*, 1992c], and the 20-mer synthetic peptide [Evans *et al.*, 1992c]) have been used (Table 62.5). The 75-kDa antigen obtained from the cell surface of *P. gingivalis* has also been studied (Evans *et al.*, 1992c). The 41-kDa fimbriae have also been used in the mouse (Ogawa *et al.*, 1989; Shimauchi *et al.*, 1991), as have a lithium diiodosalicylate (LIS) extract (Chen *et al.*, 1990), LPS (Kesavalu *et al.*, 1992), and outer-membrane vesicles (Chen *et al.*, 1990; Kesavalu *et al.*, 1992).

Whole bacteria and bacterial sonicates. Parenteral immunization of rats with a whole bacterial sonicate elicited significantly elevated antibodies in a germ-free rat model system that developed alveolar bone loss following monoassociation with *E. corrodens* (Behling *et al.*, 1981). The immunized rats showed less bone loss than infected controls. Other studies (Evans *et al.*, 1992a; Kusumoto *et al.*, 1993) have concentrated on the ability of antibody to interfere with the function of fimbriae in the colonization and subsequent disease related to infection by *P. gingivalis*. Reports have indicated that murine antibody to the fimbriae inhibits colonization and the resulting clinical changes in periodontitis following infection with this pathogen.

Many studies have demonstrated a protective effect of immunization with *P. gingivalis* antigens on *P. gingivalis*–induced pathology. For example, in subcutaneous models in mice, immunization with whole *P. gingivalis* cells generally reduces the size of the primary lesion, inhibits invasion of bacteria, and prevents subsequent death of the animals on challenge with *P. gingivalis* (Chen *et al.*, 1987,1990; Genco *et al.*, 1992; Kesavalu *et al.*, 1992). Immunization of rabbits led to elimination of *P. gingivalis* in a subcutaneous chamber (Dahlen and Slots, 1989). In ligated hamsters, subcutaneous immunization with killed *P. gingivalis* cells resulted in a reduction in the number of *P. gingivalis* isolates. A strong effect was also seen on reducing organisms recovered from hamsters after passive immunization with rabbit antisera to *P. gingivalis* (Okuda *et al.*, 1988) (Table 62.5). Marked protection from *P. gingivalis*–induced periodontal bone loss was found in monoinfected rats after immunization with whole cells of *P. gingivalis* (Klausen *et al.*, 1991; Evans *et al.*, 1992c). Immunization also reduced the activity of gingival collagenase and cysteine proteinases. The controls (sham-immunized *P. gingivalis*–infected rats) had significantly greater bone loss and high gingival enzyme activities (Klausen *et al.*, 1991; Evans *et al.*, 1992c).

Hemagglutinin, LPS, membrane extract, and outer-membrane vesicles. Several antigen extracts and purified antigens from *P. gingivalis* have also been applied in immunization studies (Table 62.5). Results varied; for example, immunization with purified hemagglutinin of *P. gingivalis* appeared as effective as immunization with whole cells in reducing the recovery of *P. gingivalis* in ligated teeth in hamsters (Okuda *et al.*, 1988). Passive immunization with rabbit antiserum against hemagglutinin also resulted in marked reduction of *P. gingivalis* cultivatable from ligated teeth (Okuda *et al.*, 1988). In the mouse abscess model, LPS, which was found to be a weak immunogen, did not interfere with the disease process. However, an extract (LIS) of membranes from *P. gingivalis* reduced the incidence of secondary lesions but could not prevent invasion of tissues in all animals in the abscess model (Chen *et al.*, 1990). In another mouse abscess study, immunization with LPS slightly decreased the size of lesions and reduced the lethality to 60% of the control level (Kesavalu *et al.*, 1992). Immunization with a preparation of outer-membrane vesicles of *P. gingivalis* resulted in reduced lethality and in a slight reduction in abscess size (Kesavalu *et al.*, 1992).

Fimbrial structures. Fimbrial structures, crucial for the adherence of *P. gingivalis* to oral tissues (Okuda *et al.*, 1981; Lee *et al.*, 1992), have been studied extensively in the *P. gingivalis*–monoinfected rat model. *P. gingivalis* fimbriae are highly immunogenic (Ogawa *et al.*, 1999; Klausen *et al.*, 1991; Shimauchi *et al.*, 1991) and biochemically well characterized (Yoshimura *et al.*, 1985; Lee *et al.*, 1991). The fimbrillin 43-kDa subunit has been cloned and sequenced (Dickinson *et al.*, 1988). Rats immunized with purified fimbriae and with the purified fimbrillin subunit were protected from *P. gingivalis*–induced periodontal destruction as efficiently as rats immunized with whole *P. gingivalis* and gingival collagenase, and cysteine proteinases were also reduced to control levels in the fimbriae-immunized rats (Evans *et al.*, 1992c). These immunized rats had both salivary and serum antibodies to purified fimbriae of *P. gingivalis* (Evans *et al.*, 1992c). Titers of salivary antibodies were elevated in the protected groups only in response to the *P. gingivalis* fimbrillin. Similar results were obtained with a synthetic 20-amino-acid peptide epitope based on the known structure of the fimbrial protein (Evans *et al.*, 1992a), suggesting the possible development of genetically engineered or synthetic fimbrial vaccines. Recombinant fimbriae have been shown to induce immunity (Evans *et al.*, 1992a). Protection induced by immunization with *P. gingivalis* fimbriae appears to be specific since rats immunized with a purified 75-kDa outer membrane protein did not exhibit protection from *P. gingivalis*–induced periodontal bone loss (Evans *et al.*, 1992c).

Fimbriae share many common antigenic determinants that may elicit protective immunity (Lee *et al.*, 1991; Brant *et al.*, 1995). While these determinants may be somewhat serotype-specific, immunization of rats with whole cells from five different strains of *P. gingivalis* consistently induced antibodies to a component in the 43-kDa region (Genco *et al.*, 1992). The mechanism of immunity to *P. gingivalis* fimbriae is unknown, although there are several possibilities: antibodies from the mucosal immune system, known to be induced in the *P. gingivalis*–immunized animal, may confer protection against initial colonization; serum antibodies or humoral cell-mediated immunity (CMI) may

reduce other activities of the fimbriae, such as stimulation of macrophage production of lytic enzymes and proinflammatory cytokines; or CMI to *P. gingivalis* may manifest protective aspects. In summary, *P. gingivalis* fimbriae, fimbrillin, and sequences from these proteins have properties indicating they may be good candidates for an anti–*P. gingivalis* vaccine. These antigens are present on the cell surfaces in very high concentrations and induce high levels of specific antibody.

Antifimbrial antibody is highly opsonic and enhances phagocytosis and killing of *P. gingivalis* by human phagocytes (Fan *et al.*, 2001). Nevertheless, fimbriae may not be the best candidate for an anti–*P. gingivalis* vaccine. Five different fimbrial types of *P. gingivalis* have been identified, and opsonic target sites do not appear to be shared among them (Fan *et al.*, 2001). Thus, immunization using one fimbrial type would likely be ineffective against *P. gingivalis* strains of the other fimbrial types.

Cysteine proteases. Recently the cysteine proteases, arginine-porphypain [gingipain] (RgpA) and lysine-porphypain [gingipain] (Kgp), from *P. gingivalis* have received considerable attention as potential antigens in anti–*P. gingivalis* vaccines. These enzymes are potent virulence factors, and they account for more than 85% of the proteolytic activity of this species. Furthermore, these enzymes are present in all naturally occurring strains studied. *P. gingivalis*–induced alveolar bone loss in rats can be inhibited by immunization with either killed *P. gingivalis* or a combination of RgpA-Kgp in incomplete Freund's adduvant (IFA) (Rajapakse *et al.*, 2002). In a chamber model, Genco *et al.* (1998) immunized with RgpA, Kgp, and a peptide from the N-terminal region of the catalytic domain and protected against *P. gingivalis* infection, while adhesin and hemagglutinin domain peptides did not protect. By contrast, Katz *et al.* (1999) demonstrated that rats infected with *P. gingivalis* manifesting alveolar bone loss were protected after immunization with a recombinant hemagglutinin B domain from *P. gingivalis* (rHagB) cysteine protease. Yonezawa *et al.* (2001) immunized mice using an RgpA DNA vaccine that protects against challenge with *P. gingivalis* in an abscess. These proteins and sequences derived from them hold great promise as antigens for anti–*P. gingivalis* vaccines. The key question here is whether an anti–*P. gingivalis* vaccine can interfere with disease associated with antigens of other bacteria or an infectious group of bacteria (red complex).

Mechanisms of immunologic protection and tissue destruction

Delayed-type hypersensitivity. Early studies conducted in rodents indicated a role for DTH in the pathobiology of periodontitis. Taubman *et al.*, (1983a;1984) used a gnotobiotic rat model and a defined antigen, ovalbumin (OVA), to examine aspects of host immune responses in periodontal disease. Administration of the antigen elicited increased numbers of lymphocytes in the gingiva, sensitized spleen cells, and increased bone loss. Animals presensitized with OVA showed increased bone loss and high IgG antibody levels, suggesting that a mixed-type hypersensitivity may contribute to the progression of disease (Taubman *et al.*, 1983a). In companion studies (Yamashita *et al.*, 1991; Yoshie *et al.*, 1985,1987), the ability of adoptively transferred normal or *A. actinomycetemcomitans*–sensitized T lymphocytes to contribute to the disease process in rats was examined. T cells transferred into nude rats had the capacity to facilitate production of normal levels of immunoglobulins (and antibody) and to protect against increased bone loss (Yoshie *et al.*, 1985). Specific *A. actinomycetemcomitans*–sensitized T cells transferred into rats exacerbated disease and increased DTH after *A. actinomycetemcomitans* infection (Yoshie *et al.*, 1987). These results indicated that the disease in this model could be associated with hypersensitivity and that T lymphocytes were critical in regulating both T- and B-cell activity to maintain homeostasis in the periodontium. Further studies showed that immunization of rats with *A. actinomycetemcomitans* resulted in DTH reactions and antibody, with accompanying increased bone loss (Taubman *et al.*, 1983a). These studies support the concept that T-cell functions and thymic regulation of immune responses can contribute to protective effects and/or more significantly to destructive effects in periodontal disease. Therefore, the necessity of enhancing the protective aspects of the immune response and minimizing the detrimental aspects to modify the disease through a more complex understanding of the host immune response was emphasized.

T lymphocytes. Immune responses induced by active immunization with *A. viscosus* (now *A. naeslundii*) resulted in significant antibody levels and T-lymphocyte responses. Alveolar bone loss was greater in the immunized and infected animals than in rats that were only infected. It was suggested that these findings indicated a hypersensitivity reaction in the progression of disease (Burckhardt *et al.*, 1981). T lymphocytes, which are abundant in periodontal disease tissues, can regulate many of the symptomatic effects of this disease (Taubman *et al.*, 1994). The combined responses involving cell and cytokine networks may account for many of the symptoms of periodontal disease, including soft-tissue collagen lysis and bone resorption (Taubman *et al.*, 1994, 1997).

T helper (Th) cells and clones can be divided into at least two subsets, which, in general, regulate expression of humoral or cellular immune response (Mosmann and Coffman, 1989). Classification of these cells as Th1 and Th2 is based on differences in the patterns of secretion of cytokines and helper functions (Mosmann *et al.*, 1986; Paul *et al.*, 1994). The type or antigen specificity of a Th-cell clone may affect the migration, retention, and T-cell–mediated immune regulation in gingival tissues. Bacterial antigen-specific T cells migrate to periodontal tissues, where retention can be related to the presence of antigen (Taubman *et al.*, 1994; Kawai *et al.*, 1998). Some of the functional attributes of these mature cells have been described (Seymour *et al.*, 1997). Further investigations have suggested that the transmigration of mature antigen–activated T lymphocytes into periodontal tissues may anergize these potentially destructive Th1-type cells and thus be a protective mechanism in periodontal disease (Taubman *et al.*, 1997).

Cytokines. Early studies of cytokines indicated that IL-2 message expression was detected in 12 of 20 unstimulated cultures of total cells from patient with periodontal disease (Seymour *et al.*, 1985). Fujihashi and coworkers (1993) detected abundant IFN-γ, IL-5, and/or IL-6 and little or no IL-2 or IL-4 RNA message expression from adult periodontitis gingival mononuclear cells (GMCs) by polymerase chain reaction (PCR). Further studies (Fujihashi *et al.*, 1996) indicated two cytokine mRNA expression patterns by CD4$^+$ T cells, both of which demonstrated prominent IFN-γ expression. It was suggested that there was coexistence of Th1- and Th2-type cells in this disease. Indications (Wassenaar *et al.*, 1995) that a majority of collagen-reactive CD4$^+$ T-cell clones isolated from diseased human periodontal tissues produced quantitatively more IL-4 than IFN-γ suggested that these were Th2-type T-cell clones. Bacteria-reactive CD4$^+$ and CD8$^+$ clones were considered Th0 type, and some CD4$^+$ and CD8$^+$ clones of unknown specificity were considered Th1 (Wassenaar *et al.*, 1995). It is interesting that still other investigators (Yamazaki *et al.*, 1994, 1995) have detected IL-4 immunologically in periodontal disease tissues but have been unable to detect IL-4 transcripts by *in situ* hybridization.

It was suggested that mRNA for IL-4 may be short-lived in gingival tissues (Yamazaki *et al.*, 1994). Fujihashi and coworkers (1993) and others (Lundqvist *et al.*, 1994) were also unable to detect IL-4 messages by reverse transcriptase polymerase chain reaction (RT-PCR) in diseased periodontal tissues and detected IFN-γ messages ubiquitously. In our investigations (Taubman *et al.*, 1994; Takeichi *et al.*, 2000), IFN-γ mRNA expression was also detected most frequently. Cytokine gene expression by GMC and gingival T lymphocytes (CD4$^+$ or CD8$^+$) obtained from adult periodontitis (AP) patients were analyzed (Taubman *et al.*, 1994). IFN-γ and, to a lesser extent, IL-2 mRNA were detected from gingival mononuclear cells and T lymphocytes by RT-PCR, whereas IL-5 or IL-6 transcripts were not detected. It was concluded that the prominent subset of T lymphocytes associated with periodontal infections was of the Th1 type and that some Th2-type cells were also found (Takeichi *et al.*, 2000). Thus, in this disease there is a clear input of host-destructive T cells. Therefore, immunization approaches are considerably more complex than for dental caries vaccines.

The existence of these dichotomous T-cell populations can account for the apparently dichotomous results involving bone loss in rodent experimental disease, and experiments have provided a rational basis for understanding these findings. *A. actinomycetemcomitans*–specific Th2 type cell clones were adoptively transferred to conventional (Yamashita *et al.*, 1991) or congenitally athymic animals (Eastcott *et al.*, 1994). In both cases, copious amounts of antibody were produced, and reductions in bone loss were observed in the animals receiving these specific helper T cells. Thus, the results of abundant specific Th2-type cells can be protective against bone loss in periodontal infection. Indeed, we have suggested that Th1-type T cells, conversely, should enhance production of bone loss. In fact, this effect has been confirmed by Kawai *et al.* (1999), who demonstrated that adoptive transfer of antigen-specific T clone cells resulted in increased bone loss. These findings facilitate our understanding of the roles of T lymphocytes in periodontal diseases, suggest significant targets for vaccine production, and provide methods of avoiding the potentially destructive effects of immunization.

Not only have we shown that Th1-type T-cell clones can contribute to experimental periodontal bone loss when the antigen (OMP29) and LPS are injected into the gingival area (Kawai *et al.*, 2000); recently a link between the T cells and bone resorption has been discovered (Kong *et al.*, 1999). Bone remodelling requires control of the rates of bone formation by osteoblasts and degradation by osteoclasts (Ducy *et al.*, 2000). RANKL, receptor activator of (NF)-kB ligand; its cellular receptor, receptor activator of NF-kB (RANK); and the decoy receptor, osteoprotegrin (OPG) have been identified as the molecular regulation system for bone remodelling (Kong *et al.*, 1999; Yasuda *et al.*, 1998). RANKL is the main stimulatory factor for the formation of mature osteoclasts and is essential for their survival (Lacey *et al.*, 1998). The effects of RANKL are counteracted by OPG, which prevents RANKL from binding to RANK on osteoclasts, suppressing osteoclastogenesis. Recently the link between immune cells and bone resorption has been elucidated (Kong *et al.*, 1999), with T cells and other immune cells expressing RANKL on their surface (Taubman and Kawai, 2001). Alveolar bone destruction seen in periodontal infection has been shown in part by triggered induction of RANKL expression on T cells (Teng *et al.*, 2000; Taubman and Kawai, 2001). Thus, while many studies have addressed protective effects of immunization with bacteria or bacterial antigens, T cells bearing RANKL can contribute to periodontal bone resorption through RANKL-mediated osteoclastogenesis. However, little is known about the methods to modulate the positive effects of immunization and to ensure that no negative effects are observed. However, the roles of immune cells, RANKL, and osteoclastogenesis must be considered in any vaccine study.

Immunization studies in nonhuman primates

Studies of immunization of primates with intact bacteria (P. gingivalis, P. intermedia, and B. fragilis)

Nonhuman primates offer many advantages to investigators developing periodontal vaccines. The anatomic structure of the periodontium, the periodontal microflora, host immune responses, and host defense mechanisms closely resemble those of humans. Many monkey species develop spontaneously occurring periodontitis as they age. Spontaneously occurring disease in monkeys is not useful for most aspects of vaccine development because the disease generally takes many years to develop and varies greatly from one animal to another in severity. This problem has been circumvented by placement of ligatures at the gingival sulcus that act as enhancers of plaque accumulation. Ligature-induced lesions manifest an inflammatory response very similar to that seen in human periodontitis that results in alveolar bone destruction.

Several immunization studies have been performed with nonhuman primates **(Table 62.6)**. McArthur and coworkers (1989) conducted a study in squirrel monkeys (*Saimiri scuireus*) using a vaccine containing 10^9 *P. gingivalis* I-372 and IFA aimed at determining whether immunization could affect black-pigmented *Bacteroides* (BPB) in the subgingival flora. Prior to immunization, the animals had no detectable black-pigmenting bacteria and manifested very low serum levels of anti–*P. gingivalis* IgG, IgM, and IgA antibodies. Teeth in the mandibular right quadrant (quadrant 4) were ligated with silk suture material previously soaked in *P. gingivalis*, and following ligation, 10^{10} viable *P. gingivalis* were applied to the gingival margin throughout the entire mouth relative to the sham-immunized group. The immunized animals developed high serum levels of IgG to antigens of the immunizing

Table 62.6. Nonhuman Primate Studies of Periodontal Disease Vaccines

Antigens	Mode	Result	Reference
Whole cells from *P. gingivalis*	Parenteral immunization	Decreased bone loss	McArthur *et al.*, 1989
Whole cells from *B. macacae*	Parenteral immunization	Decreased disease	Nisengard *et al.*, 1989
Whole cells from *P. intermedia*	Parenteral immunization	Reduced reemergence of indigenous *P. intermedia*	Clark *et al.*, 1991
Whole cells from *P. gingivalis*, *P. intermedia*, *B. fragilis*	Parenteral immunization	Enhanced bone loss in all immunized	Ebersole *et al.*, 1991
Whole cells from *P. gingivalis*	Parenteral immunization	Reduced *P. gingivalis*, less bone loss	Persson *et al.*, 1994
Passive anti–*P. gingivalis*	Passive, on teeth	Reduced recovery	Lehner, 1994; Booth *et al.*, 1996
P. gingivalis cysteine protease	Bone loss in *M. fascicularis*	Inhibition of alveolar bone loss	Moritz *et al.*, 1998, Page *et al.*, 2004
P. gingivalis Arg-gingipain-A/ Lys-gingipain	Bone loss in *M. fascicularis*	Inhibition of alveolar bone loss	Page *et al.* (unpublished)

microorganism. There was a trend toward reduction in the mean values for *P. gingivalis* in samples from the ligated and directly opposing quadrants, although statistically significant differences (at the *P* < 0.05 level) could not be demonstrated. Thus, immunization may have affected *P. gingivalis* in the subgingival flora, but not to a significant degree.

In an additional study on colonization by *P. intermedia*, 12 monkeys were enrolled in immunized and control groups and treated by prophylaxis combined with administration of tetracycline to eliminate BPB from the flora (Clark *et al.*, 1991). The animals were immunized with *P. intermedia* 1447 (monkey isolate) in IFA, and very high titers of antibody were induced. After repeated samplings demonstrated that the animals were essentially free of *P. intermedia*, teeth in the mandibular right quadrant were ligated with silk sutures. Over a period of 100 days, the percentage of immunized animals infected in the ligated quadrant remained significantly lower than in the sham-immunized group. Thus, immunization is associated with a reduction in the reemergence of indigenous *P. intermedia*.

Using intact *P. gingivalis* 3079.03, *P. intermedia* 6235.02, and *Bacteroides fragilis* ATCC 225285 in IFA, Ebersole and colleagues (1991) evaluated the effect of immunization on the subgingival flora and on alveolar bone loss using the ligature model in *Macaca fascicularis*. Groups of monkeys were immunized with each of the vaccines and a fourth group received placebo vaccine containing adjuvant but no bacteria. After immunization, three adjacent teeth in the mandibular left quadrant were ligated, and the contralateral teeth served as nonligated controls. Significant increases in serum antibody of all three isotypes were observed in the immunized animals and resulted in a significant decrease in *P. gingivalis* at both ligated and nonligated sites and also caused a significant reduction in *P. intermedia*. However, immunization with *P. gingivalis* and *B. fragilis* resulted in a significant overgrowth of *A. actinomycetemcomitans* at ligated sites. Immunization with these three species enhanced periodontitis assessed by alveolar bone loss, relative to the sham-immunized controls.

Persson and coworkers (1994) performed a study aimed at two questions: Can immunization clear *P. gingivalis* from the subgingival flora, and can immunization alter the progression of experimental periodontitis? They used *M. fascicularis* and a vaccine of formalin-killed *P. gingivalis* (monkey isolate) and Syntex adjuvant formulation M (SAF-M). High titers of anti–*P. gingivalis* antibody were induced. Following immunization, ligatures were placed around the second premolar and first and second molars in one mandibular quadrant and the contralateral maxillary quadrants. Over an experimental period of 36 weeks, subgingival plaque, GCF, and blood samples were collected from ligated and nonligated teeth, blood samples were harvested, and alveolar bone status was assessed by digital subtraction radiography. DNA probes specific for *P. gingivalis* were used to measure *P. gingivalis* in the subgingival flora. Immunization significantly reduced the levels but did not eliminate *P. gingivalis* from the flora. The control animals manifested twice the amount of alveolar

bone loss as the immunized animals at both 30 and 36 weeks. Superinfection of a subgroup of animals by application of a slurry of viable *P. gingivalis* to the teeth between week 36 and week 44 had no effect on bone status in the immunized animals, but it induced rapid bone loss in the controls. Thus, immunization in this primate model inhibits the onset and progression of periodontitis, as assessed by alveolar bone status.

Studies of immunization of primates with purified antigen

Moritz *et al.* (1998) conducted the first study in nonhuman primates using a purified antigen from *P. gingivalis*. One group of *M. fascicularis* was immunized with the cysteine protease prophypain-2 in IFA, and controls received vaccine containing only the adjuvant. Gingivitis was allowed to develop, and ligatures were placed on test teeth (week 12) and removed on week 25. The study ended at week 30. Samples of subgingival plaque and blood and radiographic and clinical measurements were taken. Immunization did not suppress the emergence of *P. gingivalis* in the flora, although gram-negative anaerobes appeared sooner and proportions were greater in the samples from control versus immunized animals. Alveolar bone loss was greater in the control animals than in the immunized animals, but the differences were not statistically significant (see Table 62.6).

With use of the model described above and a protocol almost identical to that of Persson *et al.* (1994), another study was conducted involving the use of cysteine protease (RgpA/Kgp, porphypain) purified from *P. gingivalis* (Cibrowski *et al.*, 1994) as antigen and SAF-M adjuvant (Page *et al.*, 2004). Five young adult monkeys were immunized over a period of 16 weeks with complete vaccine, while five control animals received adjuvant only. *P. gingivalis* and five additional plaque bacterial species were monitored with DNA probes. Immunization resulted in significantly reduced levels of *P. gingivalis* in plaque samples. In contrast to the report by Ebersole *et al.* (1994), the levels of the other five species of bacteria monitored were not significantly affected. Inhibition of alveolar bone loss in the immunized animals was at least as great as that observed when the whole-cell vaccine was used, and inhibition was surprisingly uniform among animals. Levels of prostaglandin E2 in GCF and presumably in the tissues were significantly reduced in the immunized animals, and site-specific amounts of bone loss were positively associated with the extent of prostaglandin inhibition. This study has been repeated with 20 animals, with essentially the same results (Page *et al.*, unpublished; see Table 62.6).

Prospects for a vaccine that interferes with periodontal infection

The observations described earlier and data obtained from recent rodent studies support the idea that development of a vaccine for control and prevention of periodontitis may be feasible. However, severe challenges are involved in the development of a safe and effective periodontal vaccine.

Periodontitis is a multifactorial disease in which host defense mechanisms and poorly understood genetic factors play a major role. The possibility exists that systemic or cellular aspects of immunity contribute to the pathogenic processes leading to tissue destruction. In that case, induction of mucosal immunity may be a safer approach. The presence of periodontopathic bacteria in the subgingival flora is essential but insufficient for periodontitis to occur. Of equal importance, several bacterial species appear to be involved (Haffajee and Socransky, 1994; Socransky et al., 1998), altough not all the implicated microbial species may be essential for the disease to occur. Notably, in an epidemiologic study of 1426 patients (Grossi et al., 1994, 1995), P. gingivalis and T. forsythensis were the only subgingival species that were significantly linked to adult periodontitis.

Second, species associated with disease may express shared antigenic epitopes. Most of the putative periodontal pathogens are gram-negative and therefore have LPS. Antigenic epitopes in LPS, especially in lipid A and to a lesser extent in core carbohydrates, are highly conserved and may be shared among gram-negative bacteria (Aydintug et al., 1989; DiPadova et al., 1993). Immunization of rabbits or M. fascicularis with P. gingivalis induces serum antibodies reactive with ·LPS of both P. gingivalis and B. forsythus (Persson et al., 1994; Vasel et al., 1996).

Finally, even if several species are essential to the etiology of periodontitis, a successful vaccine may still be possible. Characterization of the epitopes of pathogenic function of significant antigens of each species responsible for induction of protective immunity could result in determination of the peptide sequences containing the necessary epitopes, as described previously for GTF functional epitopes. With the use of known sequences and recombinant DNA technology, an appropriate antigenic sequence (or series of sequences) may be constructed to induce immunity to several of the important periodontal pathogens.

What we learned from vaccination studies in rodents
The vaccination studies in rodents (Table 62.5) have shown that protective immunity to specific periodontal pathogens, such as P. gingivalis, can usually be obtained by inducing an immune response to whole cells or various antigens of periodontopathic bacteria prior to inoculation of the animal with the specific pathogen. The mechanism of action of protective immunity is unclear, but in one study of ligated hamsters (Okuda et al., 1988), passively administered antibody conferred protection against P. gingivalis–induced pathology, suggesting that the antibody may be responsible for protection.

Summary of rat protection mechanisms
On the basis of rodent studies, potential mechanisms of protective immunity against periodontal pathogens include the following.

Mucosal immunity. In higher species, mucosal immunity consists almost exclusively of S-IgA, but in rodents some IgG in saliva, as well as S-IgA, may play a role. These antibodies mediate their effects by inhibiting initial colonization, hence

limiting infection by periodontal pathogens to the oral cavity and adjacent tissues. (Some evidence exists to support this role of mucosal IgA antibody in periodontal disease.)

Humoral immunity of mucosal tissues. The antibodies in the serum are found in the gingival tissue and may be effective in enhancing phagocytosis by neutrophils in the gingiva, gingival crevice, or periodontal pocket. In addition, humoral antibodies could exert their protective effects by neutralizing toxin-like activities of periodontopathic bacteria. Toxins such as the leukocyte-lethal leukotoxin of *Actinobacillus* have been shown to be neutralized by antibody. In the presence of opsonic antibody, *Actinobacillus* is opsonized and phagocytosed by neutrophils. There are other mechanisms by which antibodies may exert protective effects, such as neutralizing bacteria-derived host cell lytic enzymes (*e.g.*, the proteases produced by *P. gingivalis*) or by inhibiting factors that trigger host cells. LPS or fimbrial stimulation of macrophages results in the release of tissue-destructive factors and proinflammatory cytokines such as IL-1, which in turn could cause hard-tissue destruction. Antibodies could block this reaction by interfering with LPS, fimbriae, or other triggering agents.

Cellular immunity. This technique could result in enhanced phagocytosis and killing of the organism by macrophages, or antibody-dependent cellular cytotoxicity mechanisms could operate to protect against periodontal pathogen(s). Several cellular mechanisms involving enhancement of host-derived destructive-type cells producing bone resorptive cytokines have been described and theoretically attributed to CMI and Th1-type cells. Consistent with the theoretical notions of protective immunity mediated by antibody are the findings in rodent experiments indicating that adoptive transfer of Th2-type cells giving rise to high levels of antibody to the specific pathogen are protective. All these are possible mechanisms of action, as validated in the rodent experiments; definitive evidence as to which single mechanism or combination of mechanisms is operative is still needed.

One can propose that in developing a vaccine an attempt should be made to maximize the potential for mucosal immunity, since this could be intrinsically the safest method of immunization. Specific induction of mucosal immunity mediated by S-IgA in the absence of, or with low levels of, humoral or cellular immunity could provide protection without adverse immunopathological effects that could be exerted by humoral antibodies or by cellular immunity to the periodontal pathogens.

Selection of antigens for a periodontal vaccine
Polymicrobial infectious disease. There are several approaches to the selection of antigens. The most direct approach that has proven to be effective in the design of vaccines for dental caries has been to select antigens that are of the most significance in the molecular pathogenesis of the disease. In the case of periodontal diseases, antigen selection is much more complex. In contrast to most infectious diseases, periodontitis is a polymicrobial, chronic infectious disease, and having had the disease does not usually confer immunity. Furthermore, in

most cases, the disease is not detected and diagnosed until a widely variable period of time from the onset. In addition, a rather wide range of putative potent virulence factors from multiple bacterial species is known to exist. Among the most well characterized of these are structural components such as lipopolysaccharide (LPS), fimbriae, and other cell surface polysaccharide and protein components and relatively large numbers of hydrolytic enzymes such as the cysteine proteases.

Microbial focus on P. gingivalis. Prior to attemping to select the antigen/s most likely to be successful in an antiperiodontitis vaccine, limiting the search to one or at least a very few bacterial species is necessary. In this area, a wealth of data exists upon which choices can be based. There appears to be a consensus that *A. actinomycetemcomitans* is the primary infectious agent in aggressive periodontitis and that *P. gingivalis*, *T. forsythensis*, and *T. denticola* are the species most strongly documented as involved in causing chronic periodontitis (Socransky and Haffajee, 1994; Consensus Report, 1996; Socransky *et al.*, 1998). Since chronic periodontitis accounts, by far, for most cases of periodontitis, it seems reasonable to focus on that disease for vaccine development. Among the three remaining bacterial species, the strength of the data implicating *P. gingivalis* as a major pathogen relative to *T. forsythensis* and *T. denticola* is significant. For example, in a large epidemiological study conducted by Grossi *et al.* (1994), the only species that could be linked statisically to periodontitis were *P. gingivalis* and *T. forsythensis*.

Other epidemiological evidence associates *P. gingivitis* with the onset, progression, and recurrence of periodontitis in humans and animals and its absence with periodontal health and stability. While few virulence factors have been demonstrated for *T. forsythensis* and *T. denticola*, a large number have been documented for *P. gingivalis*. *P. gingivalis* may be unique among the putative pathogens in that it appears to have "stealth" properties. Acute inflammation is usually the first event in development of host defense against bacterial challenge. An early event in the acute inflammatory response is the induced expression of E-selectin by endothelial cells of the microcirculation and the production of IL-8. E-selectin expression initiates and facilitates the emigration of granulocytes from the circulation to the extracellular compartment, where chemotactic agents such as IL-8 guide the cells to move to the location of the infection. *P. gingivalis* can block expression of E-selectin by vascular endothelium and production of IL-8 by gingival epithelial cells and thereby block a first step in host defense (Darveau *et al.*, 1995; 1998). This property may permit *P. gingivalis* and other periodontopathic bacteria in the immediate environment to establish a foothold and grow in the virtual absence of host defense.

On the basis of the earlier observations, there seems little doubt that a strong case exists for focusing on *P. gingivalis* for vaccine development. The question remains whether successful immunization against *P. gingivalis* infection will prevent or aleviate chronic periodontitis. Some data concerning this question exist. The study of Persson *et al.* (1994), previously described, demonstrated that immunization of *M. fas-*

cicularis with a vaccine containing killed *P. gingivalis* as antigen inhibits alveolar bone loss by approximately 50%. The periodontal flora of this animal closely resembles that of humans, and oral innoculation and *P. gingivalis* infection may induce periodontitis in this animal. These data indicate that successful immunization with a single species of bacteria can inhibit periodontitis in a single bacterial infection system even though it is a polymicrobial disease.

Since a vaccine containing intact *P. gingivalis* provided protection in the animal model describe earlier, this model provides a convenient way to identify the antigen/s most likely to be successful in a periodontitis vaccine. *P. gingivalis* expresses a host of possible virulence factors and other candidate antigens, including LPS (endotoxin), fimbriae and associated proteins, and surface-located cysteine proteases. One can use the preimmune and postimmune sera from the monkeys that were protected to identify which *P. gingivalis* antigen(s) induce the highest titers of biologically effective antibody. Although the role of *P. gingivalis* LPS in the pathogenesis of periodontitis is well documented, its use as a potential vaccine antigen is ruled out by its inate toxicity. Other potential antigens can be ruled out on other grounds. For example, it is clear that many genetically unique clonal types of the species *P. gingivalis* exist (Ali *et al.*, 1997; Menard and Mouton, 1995).

Although there is evidence (Loos *et al.*, 1993; Teanpaisan *et al.*, 1996; Leyes *et al.*, 1999; Griffen *et al.*, 1999), we do not yet know which clones or how many are pathogenic participants in human periodontitis. Thus, a successful vaccine antigen should be expressed by all *P. gingivalis* clonal types. Although there is abundant evidence that *P. gingivalis* fimbriae and associated proteins are excellent antigens, this requirement appears to rule out the use of fimbriae, fimbrillin, and other proteins associated with fimbriae as well as peptide sequences derived from fimbriae. There are at least five fimbrial types of *P. gingivalis* (Lee *et al.*, 1991), five serotypes (Ebersole *et al.*, 1995; Nagata *et al.*, 1991), and seven types based on cell-surface polysaccharide K antigens (Schifferle *et al.*, 1989, 1998). The antigenic molecular determinants of these various types do not cross-react, or they cross-react poorly (Fan *et al.*, 2000, 2001; Sims *et al.*, 2001) and therefore are not good candidates for a vaccine antigen.

Cysteine proteases. Although their involvement in the molecular pathogenesis of periodontitis is unknown, cysteine proteases appear to have potential to meet some criteria needed for a successful antiperiodontitis vaccine antigen. In addition to the properties listed in Table 62.6, sera of protected monkeys have high titers of IgG antibody specific for these molecules, and use of cysteine proteases (prophypain) in the *M. fascicularis* model induced protection (assessed as attenuation of alveolar bone loss) at least equivalent to that induced by a whole-cell vaccine. Furthermore, 15 animals have now been immunized with the cysteine protease vaccines, and no local or systemic signs of toxicity have been observed; nor have abnormalities been found in blood and urine chemistries (Page, unpublished). These antigens have also been tested in rodents. Sunethra *et al.* (2002) demonstrated that *P. gingivalis*–induced alveolar bone loss in rats can be inhibited by immunization with RgpA and Kgp in IFA. In a chamber model, Genco *et al.* (1998) immunized with RgpA, Kgp, and a peptide from the N-terminal region of the catalytic domain and protected against *P. gingivalis* infection, while adhesin and hemagglutinin domain peptides did not protect. By contrast, Katz *et al.* (1999) demonstrated that rats infected with *P. gingivalis* manifesting alveolar bone loss were protected after immunization with a recombinant hemagglutinin B domain from *P. gingivalis* (rHagB) cysteine protease. Yonezawa *et al.* (2001) immunized mice using a RgpA DNA vaccine that protects against challenge with *P. gingivalis* in an abscess.

These proteins and sequences derived from them hold promise as antigens for anti–*P. gingivalis* vaccines. Additional work is needed to better define the minimal peptide domain from the cysteine proteases that has the most potential to be protective in a human antiperiodontitis vaccine. Some tools and animal models needed for these studies are available, but those are clearly concerns when the abscess is used.

Vaccination studies in primates

Intact bacteria. Although the protocols and details of immunization studies using nonhuman primates differed greatly, many of the observations have been consistent among studies (Table 62.6). Reasonably high levels of serum IgG antibodies reactive with the immunizing species were observed. In the study by Persson *et al.* (1994), levels in the least-responsive animals were not much greater than in control levels. In all studies, the antibody levels observed were not completely enduring. For example, levels returning to a baseline level by week 51 (Ebersole *et al.*, 1991; Persson *et al.*, 1994) and in mean titers at the end of the experiment (week 36) were less than half-peak values. Levels that are not long-lasting may pose problems for the development of a vaccine for use in humans, although humoral immune response in humans to highly purified antigen administered with appropriate adjuvant may differ greatly from those in other primates. Other possibilities may include a replicating antigen with the potential to produce a more extended response.

Purified antigens. Others noted that immunization with *P. gingivalis* resulted not only in reductions in the immunizing organism but also in reductions in *P. intermedia* levels and overgrowth of *A. actinomycetemcomitans* and to a lesser extent *E. corrodens* and *C. rectus* (Ebersole *et al.*, 1991). The diminution of *P. intermedia* could have resulted from the presence of antigenic epitopes shared with *P. gingivalis*, from changes in the subgingival environment, or from altered interspecies interactions that are known to occur. The possibility that shared antigenic epitopes may exist is supported by the fact that epitopes, especially those in the lipid A and core carbohydrate components of LPS of gram-negative bacteria, are highly conserved (Aydintug *et al.*, 1989; DiPadova *et al.*, 1993). It is also notable that in the study conducted by Persson *et al.* (1994), animals immunized with *P. gingivalis* manifested serum antibodies reactive not only with the immunizing species but also with

B. forsythus that were cross-reactive with antigens in LPS of the two species (Vasel *et al.*, 1996). The immunization study conducted by Page *et al.* (unpublished) used purified cysteine protease from *P. gingivalis* as antigen in the *M. fascicularis* model, and they monitored five bacterial species in addition to *P. gingivalis* using specific DNA probes. While significant reduction in levels of *P. gingivalis* were observed, no affects on any of the other monitored species were detected. The same results were observed in another study, involving 20 animals (Page *et al.*, unpublished). Thus, the use of purified antigens appears to limit the effects of immunization on subgingival plaque to the targeted microorganism.

Biological effects of immunization. The nonhuman primate studies demonstrate that immunization can reduce levels of targeted bacterial species (*P. gingivalis*) in the subgingival microflora (McArthur *et al.*, 1989; Clark *et al.*, 1991). However, immunization did not result in clearance of the immunizing species from the subgingival flora in any study. Clearance in these experiments would be unlikely regardless of the effectiveness of the immunization because of the presence of the ligatures, which serve as foreign bodies and entrap bacteria. The study by Clark *et al.* (1991) supports the idea but does not prove that immunization may have the potential to suppress recolonization or reemergence of pathogenic species that have been previously eliminated or greatly reduced.

SUMMARY AND CONCLUSIONS

Studies performed with humans and experimental animals support the hypothesis that the host immune system has significant potential for intervention or interference in periodontal infection. Many periodontitis patients exhibit a humoral immune response during the course of their spontaneous infection. Many of those who are seronegative convert to seropositivity following routine periodontal therapy. The antibodies, however, may have relatively low avidity and capacity to opsonize. Nevertheless, there is evidence of immune protection. Taken as a whole, immunization studies demonstrate that immunization can reduce pathogenic subgingival flora, even in the presence of ligatures, and high levels of specific antibody titers can alter the progression of periodontal tissue destruction. It has also been demonstrated that T-cell and B-cell osteoclastogenic functions may contribute to bone resorption and inflammation in experimental periodontal diseases. Systematic evaluation of both mucosal and systemic vaccines is necessary, and the role of systemic and mucosal immunity in preventing, exacerbating, or altering the course of periodontitis remains unknown **(Table 62.7)**.

ACKNOWLEDGMENTS

The research reported in this chapter was supported in part by grants DE 04733, DE 03420, DE 08555, DE 07063,

Table 62.7. Characteristics of an Ideal Antigen for a Putative Periodontal Disease Vaccine

Of major importance in the molecular pathogenesis of periodontal disease associated with a particular microorganism
Present in large quantities on the bacterial cell surface
Probably has some type of associated virulence properties (*e.g.*, adhesin, hemagglutinin, protease)
Obtainable in a highly purified (recombinant if possible) form in large quantities
Induces an enduring high level of biologically effective antibody, preferably of the IgG1 and IgG3 isotypes, or an appropriate cell response, preferably of the Th2 type
Does not elicit Th1 or destructive host response (particularly in gingival and periodontal tissues)
Present in all serotypes and ribotypes of the species
Strongly enhances opsonization, phagocytosis, and killing of the species in question
No toxic side effects
Stable in a vaccine formulation

DE 04898, and DE 08240 from the National Institute of Dental and Craniofacial Research.

REFERENCES

Abo, H., Masumura, T., Kodama, T., Ohta, H., Fukui, K., Kato, K., and Kagawa, H. (1991). Peptide sequences for sucrose splitting and glucan binding within *Streptococcus sobrinus* glucosyltransferase (water-insoluble glucan synthetase). *J. Bacteriol.* 173, 989–996.

Albander, J.M., Brunelle, J.A., and Kingman, A. (1999). Active periodontal disease in adults 30 years of age and older in the United States, 1988–1994. *J. Periodontol.* 70, 13–29.

Ali, R.W., Martin, L., Haffajee, A.D., and Socransky, S.S. (1997). Detection of identical ribotypes of *Porphyromonas gingivalis* in patients residing in USA, Sudan, Romania and Norway. *Oral Microbiol. Immunol.* 12, 106–111.

Allison, A.C., and Byars, N.E. (1986). An adjuvant formulation that selectively elicits the formation of antibodies of protective isotypes and cell-mediated immunity. *J. Immunol. Methods* 95, 157–168.

Aoki, H., Shiroza, T., Hayakawa, M., Sato, S., and Kuramitsu, H.K. (1986). Cloning of *Streptococcus mutans* glucosyltransferase gene coding for insoluble glucan synthesis. *Infect. Immun.* 53, 587–594.

Aydintug, M.K., Inzana, T.H., Letonja, T., Davis, W.E., and Corbeil, L.B. (1989). Cross-reactivity of monoclonal antibodies to *Escherichia coli* J5 with heterologous gram-negative bacteria and extracted lipopolysaccharides. *J. Infect. Dis.* 160, 846–857.

Axelsson P, Lindhe J., and Nystrom B. (1991). On the prevention of caries and periodontal disease. Results of a 15-years longitudinal study in adults. *J. Clin. Periodontol.* 18, 182–189.

Baker, P., and Wilson, M. (1989). Opsonic IgG antibody against *Actinobacillus actinomycetemcomitans* in localized juvenile periodontitis. *Oral Microbiol. Immunol.* 4, 98–105.

Baker, P.J., Evans, R.T., and Roopenian, D.C. (1994). Oral infection with *Porphyromonas gingivalis* and induced alveolar bone loss in immunocompetent and severe combined immunodeficient mice. *Arch. Oral Biol.* 39, 1035–1040.

Banas, J.A., Russell, R.R., and Ferretti, J.J. (1990). Sequence analysis of the gene for the glucan-binding protein of *S. mutans* Ingbritt. *Infect. Immun.* 58, 667–673.

Behling, U.H., Sallay, C., Sanavi, F., Pham, P.H., and Nowotny, A. (1981). Humoral immunity and reduced periodontal bone loss in *Eikenella corrodens*–monoassociated rats. *Infect. Immun.* 33, 801–805.

Berkowitz, R.J., and Jones, P. (1985). Mouth-to-mouth transmission of the bacterium *Streptococcus mutans* between mother and child. *Archs. Oral Biol.* 30, 377–379.

Berkowitz, R.J., and Jordan, H.V. (1975). Similarity of bacteriocins of *Streptococcus mutans* from mother and infant. *Archs. Oral Biol.* 20, 725–730.

Booth, V., Ashley, F. P., and Lehner, T. (1996). Passive immunization with monoclonal antibodies against *Porphyromonas gingivalis* in patients with periodontitis. *Infect. Immun.* 64, 422–427.

Bowen, W.H. (1969). A vaccine against dental caries. A pilot experiment in monkeys (*Macaca irus*). *Brit. Dent.* J. 126, 159–166.

Brandtzaeg, P., and Tolo, K. (1977). Mucosal penetrability enhanced by serum-derived antibodies. *Nature* 266, 262–263.

Brandtzaeg, P., and Haneberg, B. (1997). Role of nasal-associated lymphoid tissue in the human mucosal immune system. *Muc. Immunol. Update* 5, 4–8.

Brant, E. E., Sojar, H.T., Sharma, A., Bedi, G.S., Genco, R. J., and De Nardin, E. (1995). Identification of linear antigenic sites on the *Porphyromonas gingivalis* 43-kDa fimbrillin subunit. *Oral Microbiol. Immunol.* 10, 146–150.

Briand, J. P., Barin, C., Van Regenmortel, M. H., and Muller, S. (1992). Application and limitations of the multiple antigen peptide (MAP) system in the production and evaluation of anti-peptide and anti-protein antibodies. *J. Immunol. Methods* 156, 255–265.

Brown, L. J., and Löe, H. (1993). Prevalence, extent, severity, and progression of periodontal disease. *Periodontology 2000* 4, Chapter 6.

Burckhardt, J.J., Gaegauf-Zollinger, R., Schmid, R., and Guggenheim, B. (1981). Alveolar bone loss in rats after immunization with *Actinomyces viscosus. Infect. Immun.* 31, 971–977.

Burt, B.A., Ismail, A.I., and Eklund, S.A. (1986). Root caries in an optimally fluoridated and a high-fluoride community. *J. Dent. Res.* 65, 1154–1158.

Camling, E., Gahnberg. L., Emilson, C.G., and Lindquist, B. (1991). Crevicular IgG antibodies and recovery of *S. mutans* implanted by mouth rinsing. *Oral Microbiol. Immunol.* 6, 134–138.

Carlsson, J., Grahnen, H., Jonsson, G., and Wikner, S. (1970). Early establishment of *Streptococcus salivarius* in the mouths of infants. *J. Dent. Res.* 49, 1143–1148.

Carlsson, J., Grahnen, H., and Jonsson, G. (1975). Lactobacilli and streptococci in the mouths of children. *Caries Res.* 9, 333–339.

Caufield, P.W., Wannemuehler, Y. M., and Hansen, J. B. (1982). Familial clustering of the *Streptococcus mutans* cryptic plasmid in a dental clinic population. *Infect. Immun.* 38, 785–787.

Caufield, P. W., Cutter, G. R., and Dasanayake, A. P. (1993). Initial acquisition of mutans streptococci by infants: evidence for a discrete window of infectivity. *J. Dent. Res.* 72, 37–45.

Challacombe, S. J., Bergmeier, L. A., and Reis, A. S. (1984). Natural antibodies in man to a protein antigen from the bacterium *Streptococcus mutans* related to dental caries experience. *Archs. Oral Biol.* 29, 179–184.

Chang, K. M., Ramamurthy, N. S., McNamara, T. F., Genco, R. J., and Golub, L.M. (1988). Infection with a gram-negative organism stimulates gingival collagenase production in non-diabetic and diabetic germfree rats. *J. Periodontal Res.* 23, 239–244.

Chen, H. A., Johnson, B. D., Sims, T. J., Darveau, R. P., Moncla, B. J., Whitney, C. W., Engel, L. D., and Page, R. C. (1991a). Humoral immune responses to *P. gingivalis* before and following therapy in rapidly progressive periodontitis patients. *J. Periodontol.* 62, 781–791.

Chen, P.B., Neiders, M. E., Millar, S. J., Reynolds, H. S., and Zambon, J. J. (1987). Effect of immunization on experimental *Bacteroides gingivalis* infection in a murine model. *Infect. Immun.* 55, 2534–2537.

Chen, P. B, Davern, L. B., Schifferle, R., and Zambon, J. J. (1990). Protective immunization experimental *Bacteroides (Porphyromonas gingivalis)* infection. *Infect. Immun.* 58, 3394–3400.

Chen, P. B., Davern, L. B., Neiders, M. E., Reynolds, H. S., and Zambon, J. J. (1991b). Analysis of *in vitro* lymphoproliferative responses and antibody formation following subcutaneous infection of *Actinobacillus actinomycetemcomitans* and *Wolinella recta* in a murine model. *Oral Microbiol. Immunol.* 6, 12–16.

Chia, J. -S., Lin, R. -H., Lin, S. -W., Chen, J. -Y., and Yang, C. -S. (1993). Inhibition of glucosyltransferase activities of *Streptococcus mutans* by a monoclonal antibody to a subsequence peptide. *Infect. Immun.* 61, 4689–4695.

Childers, N. K., Michalek, S. M., Prichard, D. G., and McGhee, J. R. (1991). Mucosal and systemic responses to an oral liposome–*Streptococcus mutans* carbohydrate vaccine in humans. *Reg. Immunol.* 3, 289–296.

Childers, N. K., Tong, G., Mitchell, S., Kirk, K., Russell, M. W., Michalek, S.M. (1999). A controlled clinical study of the effect of nasal immunization with a *Streptococcus mutans* antigen alone or incorporated into liposomes on induction of immune responses. *Infect. Immun.* 67, 618–623.

Clark, W. B., Magnusson, I., Beem, J. E., Jung, J. M., Marks, R. G., and McArthur, W. P. (1991). Immune modulation of *Prevotella intermedia* colonization in squirrel monkeys. *Infect. Immun.* 59, 1927–1931.

Consensus Report. Periodontal diseases: pathogenesis and microbial factors. Workshop on Periodontology, Vol. 1. *Ann. Periodontol.* 1, 926–932.

Coykendall, A.L., and Gustafson K.B. (1986). Taxonomy of *Streptococcus mutans*. In *Molecular Microbiology and Immunobiology of Streptococcus mutans* (eds. S. Hamada, S. M. Michalek, H. Kiyono, K. Menaker, and J. R. McGhee). New York: Elsevier Science Publishers B.V., 21–28.

Crawford, J. M., Taubman, M. A., and Smith, D. J. (1978). The effects of local immunization with periodontopathic microorganisms on periodontal bone loss in gnotobiotic rats. *J. Periodontal Res.* 13, 445–459.

Crowley, P. J., Brady, L. J., Piacentini, D. A., and Bleiweis, A. S. (1993). Identification of a salivary agglutinin-binding domain within cell surface adhesin P1 of *Streptococcus mutans*. *Infect. Immun.* 61, 1547–1552.

Curtiss, R. I., Goldschmidt, R., Pastina, R., Lyons, M., Michalek, S. M., and Mestecky, J. (1986). Cloning virulence determinants from *Streptococcus mutans* and the use of recombinant clones to construct bivalent oral vaccine strains to confer protective immunity against *S. mutans* induced dental caries. In *Molecular Microbiology and Immunobiology of Streptococcus mutans* (eds. S. Hamada, S. M. Michalek, H. Kiyono, L. Menaker, and J. R. McGhee). Amsterdam: Elsevier Science Publishers, 173–180.

Dahlén, G., and Slots, J. (1989). Experimental infections by *Bacteroides gingivalis* in nonimmunized and immunized rabbits. *Oral Microbiol. Immunol.* 4, 6–11.

Darveau, R. P., Belton, C. M., Reifie, R. A., Lamont, R. J. (1998). Local chemokine paralysis: a novel pathogenic mechanism for *Porphyromonas gingivalis*. *Infect Immun* 66, 1660–1665.

Darveau, R. P., Cunningham, M. D., Bailey, T., Seachord, C., Ratcliffe, K., Bainbridge, B., Dietsch, M., Page, R.C., Aruffo, A. (1995). Relationship between bacteria associated with chronic inflammatory disease, endothelial cell E-selectin expression, and neutrophil adhesion. *Infect. Immun.* 63, 1311–1317.

Demuth, D. R., Lammey, M. S., Huck, M., Lally, E. T., and Malamud, D. (1990). Comparison of *Streptococcus mutans* and *Streptococcus sanguis* receptors for human salivary agglutinin. *Microbiol. Pathog.* 9, 199–211.

DePaola, P. (1992). Caries in our aging population: what are we learning? In *Cariology for the Nineties* (eds. W. Bowen and L. Tabak), New York: University of Rochester Press, 25–35.

Dertzbaugh, M. T., and Macrina, F. L. (1990). Inhibition of *Streptococcus mutans* glucosyltransferase activity by antiserum to a subsequence peptide. *Infect. Immun.* 58, 1509–1513.

Dickinson, D. P., Kubiniec, M. A., Yoshimura, F., and Genco, R. J. (1988). Molecular cloning and sequencing of the gene encoding the fimbrial subunit protein of *Bacteroides gingivalis*. *J. Bacteriol.* 170, 1658–1665.

DiPadova, F. E., Brade, H., Barclay, G. R., Poxton, I. R., Liehl, E., Schuetze, E., Kocher, H. P., Ramsay, F., Scheier, H., Brian, D., McClellan, L., and Rietschel, E. T. (1993). A broad cross-protective monoclonal antibody binding to *Escherichia coli* and *Salmonella* lipopolysaccharides. *Infect. Immun.* 61, 3863–3872.

Ducy, P., Schinke, T., Karsenty, G. (2000). The osteoblast: a sophisticated fibroblast under central surveillance. *Science* 289, 1501–1504.

Eastcott, J. W., Yamashita, K., Taubman, M. A., Harada, Y., and Smith, D. J. (1994). Adaptive transfer of cloned T helper cells ameliorates periodontal disease in nude rats. *Oral Microbiol. Immunol.* 9, 284–289.

Eastcott, J. W., Orr, N., Smith, D. J., Hayden, T. L., Taubman, M. A. (2002) Expression and delivery of GTF peptides in *Salmonella enterica*. *J. Dent. Res.* 281, 475.

Ebersole, J. L. (1990). Systemic humoral immune responses in periodontal disease. *Crit. Rev. Oral Biol. Med.* 1, 283–331.

Ebersole, J. L., Frey, D. E., Taubman, M. A., and Smith, D. J. (1980). An ELISA for measuring serum antibodies to *Actinobacillus actinomycetemcomitans*. *J. Periodontal Res.* 15, 621–632.

Ebersole, J. L., Taubman, M. A., Smith, D. J., Genco, R. J., and Frey, D. E. (1982a). Human immune responses to oral microorganisms. I. Association of localized juvenile periodontitis (LJP) with serum antibody responses to *Actinobacillus actinomycetemcomitans*. *Clin. Exp. Immunol.* 47, 43–52.

Ebersole, J. L., Taubman, M. A., Smith, D. J., and Socransky, S.S. (1982b). Humoral immune responses and diagnosis of human periodontal disease. *J. Periodontal Res.* 17, 478–480.

Ebersole, J. L., Taubman, M. A., Smith, D. J., and Goodson, J. M. (1984). Gingival crevicular fluid antibody to oral microorganisms. I. Method of collection and analysis of antibody. *J. Periodontal Res.* 19, 124–132.

Ebersole, J. L., Taubman, M. A., Smith, D. J., and Haffajee, A. D. (1985). Effect of subgingival scaling on systemic antibody responses to oral microorganisms. *Infect. Immun.* 48, 534–539.

Ebersole, J. L., Taubman, M. A., Smith, D. J., and Frey, D. E. (1986). Human immune responses to oral microorganisms: Patterns of systemic antibody levels to *Bacteroides* species. *Infect. Immun.* 51, 507–513.

Ebersole, J. S., Taubman, M. A., Smith, D. J., Frey, D. E., Haffajee, A. D., Socransky, S. S. (1987a). Human serum antibody responses to oral microorganisms. IV. Correlation with homologous infection. *Oral Microbiol. Immunol.* 2, 53–59.

Ebersole, J. L., Frey, D. E., Taubman, M. A., and Socransky, S. S. (1987b). Dynamics of systemic antibody responses in periodontal disease. *J. Periodontal Res.* 22, 184–186.

Ebersole, J. E., Steffen, M. J., Sandoval, M.-N. (1989). Quantitation of IgG subclass antibodies to periodontopathogens. *J. Dent. Res.* 68, 222.

Ebersole, J. L., Brunsvold, M., Steffensen, B., Wood, R., and Holt, S. C. (1991). Effects of immunization with *Porphyromonas gingivalis* and *Prevotella intermedia* on progression of ligature-induced periodontitis in the nonhuman primate *Macaca fascicularis*. *Infect. Immun.* 59, 3351–3359.

Ebersole, J. L., and Taubman, M. A. (1994). The protective nature of host responses in periodontal diseases. *Periodontology 2000* 5, 112–141.

Ebersole, J. L., and Steffen, M .J. (1995). Human antibody responses to outer envelope antigens of *Porphyromonas gingivalis* serotypes. *J Periodontal Res* 30, 1–14.

Emmings, F. G., Evans, R. T., and Genco, R. J. (1975). Antibody response in the parotid fluid and serum of irus monkeys (*Macaca fascicularis*) after local immunization with *Streptococcus mutans*. *Infect. Immun.* 12, 287–292.

Evans, R. T., Emmings, F. G., and Genco, R. J. (1975). Prevention of *Streptococcus mutans* infection of monkeys (*Macaca fascicularis*). *Infect. Immun.* 12, 293–302.

Evans, R. T., Klausen, B., and Genco, R. J. (1992a). Immunization with fimbrial protein and peptide protects against *Porphyromonas gingivalis*–induced periodontal tissue destruction. In *Genetically Engineered Vaccines: Prospects for Oral Disease Prevention* (eds. J. Keith and J. McGhee). New York: Plenum, 255–262.

Evans, R. T., Klausen, B., Ramamurthy, N. S., Golub, L. M., Sfintescu, C., and Genco, R.J. (1992b). Periodontopathic potential of two strains of *Porphyromonas gingivalis* in gnotobiotic rats. *Arch. Oral Biol.* 37, 813–819.

Evans, R. T., Klausen, B., Sojar, H. T., Bedi, G. S., Sfintescu, C., Ramamurthy, N. S., Golub, L. M., and Genco, R. J. (1992c). Immunization with *Porphyromonas (Bacteroides) gingivalis* fimbriae protects against periodontal destruction. *Infect. Immun.* 60, 2926–2935.

Fan, Q., Sims, T. J., Nakagawa, T., Page, R. C. (2000). Antigenic cross-reactivity among *Porphyromonas gingivalis* serotypes. *Oral Microbiol Immunol* 15, 158–165.

Fan, Q., Sims, T., Sojar, H., Genco, R., Page, R. C. (2001). Fimbriae of *Porphyromonas gingivalis* induce opsonic antibodies that significantly enhance phagocytosis and killing by human polymorphonuclear leukocytes. *Oral Microbiol. Immunol.* 16,144–152.

Earstad, I. N., Hastensen, T. S., Kule, D., Fausa, O., Brandtzaig, P. (1997). Topographic distribution of homing receptors on B and T cells in human gut-associated lymphoid tissues: relation of L-selectin and integrin α4 β7 to naive and memory phenotypes. *Am. J. Pathol.* 150, 188–199.

Ferretti, J. J, Gilpin, M. L, and Russell, R. R. B. (1987). Nucleotide sequence of a glucosyltransferase gene from *Streptococcus sobrinus* MFe28. *J. Bacteriol.* 169, 4271–4278.

Ferretti, J. J., Huang, T. T., and Russell, R. R. (1988). Sequence analysis of the GTF A gene (gtfA) from *S. mutans* Ingbritt. *Infect. Immun.* 56, 1585–1588.

Fujihashi, K., Beagley, K. W., Kono, Y., Aicher, W. K., Yamamoto, M., DiFabio, S. *et al.* (1993). Gingival mononuclear cells from chronic inflammatory periodontal tissues produce interleukin (IL)-5 and IL-6 but not IL-2 and IL-4. *Am. J. Pathol.* 142, 1239.

Fujihashi, K., Yamamoto, M., Hiroi, T., Bamberg, T. V., McGhee, J. R., and Kiyono, A. (1996). Selected Th1 and Th2 cytokine mRNA expression by CD4+ T cells isolated from inflamed human gingival tissues. *Clin. Exp. Immunol.* 103, 422–428.

Funane, K., Shiraiwa, M., Hashimoto, K., Ichishima, E., and Kobayashi, M. (1993). An active-site peptide containing the second essential carboxyl group of dextran sucrose from *Leuconostoc mesenteroides* by chemical modifications. *Biochem.* 32, 13696–13702.

Gahnberg, L., Smith, D. J., Taubman, M. A., and Ebersole J. L. (1985). Salivary IgA antibody to glucosyltransferase of oral microbial origin in children. *Arch. Oral Biol.* 301, 551–556.

Genco, C. A., Odusanya, B. M., Potempa, J., Mikolajczyk- Pawlinska, J., Travis, J. (1998). A peptide domain on gingipain R which confers immunity against *Porphyromonas gingivalis* infection in mice. *Infect Immun* 66, 4108–4114.

Genco, R. J., and Löe, H. (1993). The role of systemic conditions and disorders in periodontal disease. *Periodontology 2000* 2, 98–116.

Genco, R. J., Taichman, N. A., and Sadowski, C. A. (1980). Precipitating antibodies to *Actinobacillus actinomycetemcomitans* in localized juvenile periodontitis. *J. Dent. Res.* 59, 329–336.

Genco, R. J., Lee, J. -Y., Sojar, H. T., Bedi, G. S., Loos, B. G., and Dyer, D. W. (1991). Antigenic heterogeneity of periodontal pathogens. In *Periodontal Disease: Pathogens and Host Immune Responses* (eds. S. Hamada, S. C. Holt, and J. R. McGhee). Tokyo: Quintessence Publishing, 167–186.

Genco, R. J., Kapczynski, D. R., Cutler, C. W., Arko, R. J., and Arnold, R.R. (1992). Influence of immunization on *Porphyromonas gingivalis* colonization and invasion in the mouse chamber model. *Infect. Immun.* 60, 1447–1454.

Gibson, F.C. III, and Genco, C. A. (2001). Prevention of *Porphyromonas gingivalis*–induced bone loss following immunization with gingipain R1. *Infect. Immun.* 69, 7959–7963.

Gmür, R. (1985). Human serum antibodies against *Bacteroides intermedius*. Antigenic heterogeneity impairs the interpretation of the host response. *J. Periodontal Res.* 20, 492–496.

Gregory, R. L., Michalek, S. M., Filler, S. J., Mestecky, J., and McGhee, J.R. (1985). Prevention of *Streptococcus mutans* colonization by salivary IgA antibodies. *J. Clin. Immunol.* 5, 55–62.

Griffen, A. L., Lyons, S. R., Becker, M. R., Moeschberger, M. L., Leys, E.J. (1999). *Porphyromonas gingivalis* strain variability and periodontitis. *J. Clin. Microbiol.* 37, 4028–4033.

Grossi, S. G., Zambon, J. J., Ho, A. W., Koch, G., Dunford, R. G., Machtei, E.E., Norderyd, O.M., and Genco, R.J. (1994). Assessment of risk for periodontal disease. I. Risk indicators for attachment loss. *J. Periodontol.* 65, 260–267.

Grossi, S. G., Genco, R. J., Machtei, E. E., Ho, A. W., Koch, G., Dunford, R., Zambon, J. J., and Hausmann, R. (1995). Assessment of risk for periodontal disease. II. Risk indicators for alveolar bone loss. *J. Periodontol.* 66, 23–29.

Gunsolley, J. C., Burmeister, J. A., Tew, J. G., Best, A. M., and Ranney, R.R. (1987). Relationship of serum antibody to attachment level patterns in young adults with juvenile periodontitis or generalized severe periodontitis. *J. Periodontol.* 58, 314–320.

Haffajee, A.D., and Socransky, S.S. (1994). Microbial etiological agents of destructive periodontal disease. *Periodontology 2000* 5, 78–111.

Hajishengallis, G., Nikolova, E., and Russell, M.W. (1992). Inhibition of *Streptococcus mutans* adherence to saliva-coated hydroxyapatite by human secretory immunoglobulin A (SIgA) antibodies to cell surface protein antigen I/II: reversal by IgA1 protease cleavage. *Infect. Immun.* 60, 5057–5064.

Hajishengallis, G., Russell, M. W., Michalek, S. M. (1998). Comparison of an adherence domain and a structural region of *Streptococcus mutans* antigen I/II in protective immunity against dental caries in rats after intranasal immunization. *Infect. Immun.* 66, 1740–1743.

Hamada, S., and Slade, H. D. (1980). Biology, immunology, and cariogenicity of *Streptococcus mutans*. *Microbiol. Rev.* 44, 331–384.

Hamada, S., Horikoshi, T., Minami, T., Kawabata, S., Hiraoka, J., Fujiwara, T., Ooshima, T. (1991). Oral passive immunization against dental caries in rats by use of hen egg yolk antibodies specific for cell-associated glucosyltransferase of *Streptococcus mutans*. *Infect. Immun.* 59, 4161–4167.

Hanada, N., and Kuramitsu, H. K. (1989). Isolation and characterization of the *Streptococcus mutans* gtfD gene, coding for primer-dependent soluble glucan synthesis. *Infect. Immun.* 57, 2079–2085.

Hicks, J. M., and Flaitz, C. M. (1993). Epidemiology of dental caries in the pediatric and adolescent population: A review of past and current trends. *J. Clin. Ped. Den.* 18, 43–49.

Holmgren, J. (1991). Mucosal immunity and vaccination. *FEMS. Microbiol. Immunol.* 89, 1–10.

Ishikawa, I., Watanabe, H., Horibe, M., and Izumi, Y. (1988). Diversity of IgG antibody responses in patients with various types of periodontitis. *Adv. Dent. Res.* 2, 334–338.

Katz, J., Black, K. P., Michalek, M. (1999). Host responses to recombinant hemagglutinin B of *Porphyromonas gingivalis* in an experimental rat model. *Infect Immun* 67, 4352–4359.

Katz, J., Harmon, C. C., Buckner, G. P., Richardson, G. J., Russell, M.W., and Michalek, S.M. (1993). Protective salivary immunoglobulin A responses against *Streptococcus mutans* infection after intranasal immunization with *S. mutans* antigen I/II coupled to the B subunit of cholera toxin. *Infect. Immun.* 61, 1964–1971.

Kawai, T., Shimauchi, H., Eastcott, J. W., Smith, D. J., Taubman, M. A. (1998). Antigen direction of specific T-cell clones into gingival tissues. *Immunology* 93, 11–19.

Kawai, T., Seki, M., Hiromatsu, K., Eastcott, J. W., Watts, G. F. M. Smith, D. J., Sugai, M., Porcelli, S. A., Taubman, M.A. (1999). Selective diapedesis of T helper 1 cells induced by endothelial cell RANTES. *J. Immunol.* 163, 3269–3278.

Kawai, T., Seki, M., Watanabe, H., Eastcott, J.W., Smith, D. J., Taubman, M.A. (2000a). Th1 transmigration anergy; a new concept of endothelial cell–T cell regulatory interaction. *Int. Immunol.* 12, 937–948.

Kawai, T., Eisen-Lev, R., Seki, M., Eastcott, J. W., Wilson, M. E., Taubman, M. A. (2000b). Requirement of B7 costimulation for

Th1-mediated inflammatory bone resorption in experimental periodontal disease. *J. Immunol.* 164, 2102–2109.

Kent, R., Smith, D. J., Jashipura, K. (1991). Associations among serum IgG antibody specificities and clinical variables in a population at risk for root surface caries. *J. Dent. Res.* 70, 317–327.

Kesavalu, L., Holt, S. C., Crawley, R. R., Borinski, R., and Ebersole, J. L. (1991). Virulence of *Wolinella recta* in a murine abscess model. *Infect. Immun.* 59, 2806–2817.

Kesavalu, L., Ebersole, J. E., Machen, R. L., and Holt, S. C. (1992). *Porphyromonas gingivalis* virulence in mice. Induction immunity to bacterial components. *Infect. Immun.* 60, 1455–1464.

Klausen, B., Evans, R. T., and Sfintescu, C. (1989). Two complementary methods of assessing periodontal bone level in rats. *Scand. J. Dent. Res.* 97, 494–499.

Klausen, B., Evans, R. T., Ramamurthy, N. S., Golub, L. M., Sfintescu, C., Lee, J.-Y., Bedi, G., Zambon, J. J., and Genco, R. J. (1991). Periodontal bone level and gingival proteinase activity in gnotobiotic rats immunized with *Bacteroides gingivalis*. *Oral Microbiol. Immunol.* 6, 193–201.

Klausen, B., Evans, R. T., and Genco, R. J. (1993). Vaccination against *Porphyromonas gingivalis* in experimental animals. In *Biology of the Species Porphyromonas gingivalis* (eds. H. N. Shah, D. Mayrand, and R. J. Genco). Boca Raton, Florida: CRC Press.

Klein, J.-P., and Scholler, M. (1988). Recent advances in the development of a *Streptococcus mutans* vaccine. *Eur. J. Epidemiol.* 4, 419–425.

Kohler, B., Bratthall, D., and Krasse, B. (1983). Preventive measures in mothers influence the establishment of the bacterium *Streptococcus mutans* in their infants. *Archs. Oral Biol.* 28, 225–231.

Kohler, B., Andreen, I., and Jonsson, B. (1984). The effect of caries-preventive measures in mothers on dental caries and the oral presence of the bacteria *Streptococcus mutans* and lactobacilli in their children. *Archs. Oral Biol.* 29, 879–883.

Komatsuzawa, H., Asakawa, R., Kawai, T., Ochiai, K., Fujiwara, T., Taubman, M.A., Ohara, M., Kurihara, H., Sugai, M. (2002). Identification of six major outer membrane proteins from *Actinobacillus actinomycetemcomitans*. *Gene* 288,195–201.

Kong, Y.Y., Yoshida, H., Sarosi, I., Tan, H. L., Timms, E., Capparelli, C., Moron, S., Oliveira-dos-Santos, A. J., Van, G., Itie, A., Khoo, W., Wakeham, A., Dunsta, C. R., Lacey, D. L., Mak, T. W., Boyle, W. J., Penninger, J. M. (1999). OPGL is a key regulator of osteoclastogenesis, lymphocyte development and lymph-node organogenesis. *Nature* 397, 315–323.

Kononen, E., Asikainen, S., Saarela, M., Karjaiainen, J., and Jousimies-Somer, H. (1994). The oral gram-negative anaerobic microflora in young children: longitudinal changes from edentulous to dentate mouth. *Oral Microbiol. Immunol.* 9, 136–141.

Kornman, K. S., Crane, A., Wang, H. Y., Digiovine, F. S., Newman, M. G., Pirk, F. W., Wilson, T. G., Higginbottom, F. L., and Dugg, G. W. (1997). The interleukin-1 genotype as a severity factor in adult periodontal disease. *J. Clin. Periodontol.* 24, 72–77.

Kusumoto, Y., Ogawa, T., and Hamada, S. (1993). Generation of specific antibody–secreting cells in salivary glands of BALB/c mice following parenteral in oral immunization with *Porphyromonas gingivalis*. *Arch. Oral Biol.* 38, 361–367.

Lacey, D. L., Timms, E., Tan, H. L., Kelley, M. J., Dunstan, C. R., Burgess, T., Elliot, R., Colombero, A., Elliott, G., Scully, S., Hsu, H., Sullivan, J., Hawkins, N., Davy, E., Capparelli, C., Eli, A., Qian, Y. X., Kaufman, S., Sarosi, I., Shalhoub, V., Senaldi, G., Guo, J., Delaney, J., Boyle, W. J. (1998). Osteoprotegrin ligand is a cytokine that regulates osteoclast differentiation and activation. *Cell* 93, 165–176.

Lamont, R.J., Demuth, O. R., Davis, C. A., Malamud, D., and Rosan, B. (1991). Salivary-agglutinin-mediated adherence of Streptococcus mutans to early plaque bacteria. *Infect. Immun.* 59, 3446–3450.

Landale, E. C., and McCabe, M. M. (1987). Characterization by affinity electrophoresis of an α-1,6-glucan-binding protein from *Streptococcus sobrinus*. *Infect. Immun.* 55, 3011–3016.

LaPolla, R. J., Haron, J. A., Kelly, C. G., Taylor, W. R., Bohart, C., Hendricks, M., Pyati, J., Graff, R. T., Ma, J. K., and Lehner, T. (1991). Sequence and structural analysis of surface protein antigen I/II (SpaA) of *Streptococcus sobrinus*. *Infect. Immun.* 59, 2677–2685.

Lee, J.-Y., Sojar, H. T., Bedi, G. S., and Genco, R. J. (1991). *Porphyromonas (Bacteroides) gingivalis* fimbrillin: Size, amino-terminal sequence, and antigenic heterogeneity. *Infect. Immun.* 59, 383–385.

Lee, J.-Y., Sojar, H. T., Bedi, G. S., and Genco, R. J. (1992). Synthetic peptides analogous to the fimbrillin sequence inhibit adherence of *Porphyromonas gingivalis*. *Infect. Immun.* 60, 1662–1670.

Lee, S. F., Progulske-Fox, A., and Bleiweis, A. S. (1988). Molecular cloning and expression of a *Streptococcus mutans* major surface protein antigen P1 (I/II) in *Escherichia coli*. *Infect. Immun.* 56, 2114–2119.

Legler, D. W., McGhee, J. R., Lynch, D. P., Mestecky, J. F., Schaffer, M. E., Carson, J., and Bradley, E. L. (1981). Immunodeficiency disease and dental caries in man. *Arch. Oral Biol.* 26, 905–910.

Lehner, T., Russell, M. W., Caldwell, J., and Smith, R. (1981). Immunization with purified protein antigen from *Streptococcus mutans* against dental caries in rhesus monkeys. *Infect. Immun.* 34, 407–415.

Lehner, T., Caldwell, J., and Smith, R. (1985). Local passive immunization by monoclonal antibodies against streptococcal antigen I/II in the prevention of dental caries. *Infect. Immun.* 50, 796–799.

Lehner, T., Walker, P., Bergmeier, L. A., and Haron, J. A. (1989b). Immunogenicity of synthetic peptides derived from the sequences of a *S. mutans* cell surface antigen in nonhuman primates. *J. Immunol.* 143, 2699–2705.

Lehner, T., Ma, J. K.-C., Munro, G., Walker, P., Childerstone, A., Todryk, S., Kendal, H., and Kelly, C. G. (1994). T-cell and B-cell epitope mapping and construction of peptide vaccines. In *Molecular Pathogenesis of Periodontal Disease* (eds. R. J. Genco, S. Hamada, T. Lehner, J. R. McGhee, and S. Mergenhagen). Washington, DC: American Society for Microbiology Press, 279–292.

Lett, E., Gangloff, M., Zimmermann, D., Wachsmann, D., and Klein, J. P. (1994). Immunogenicity of polysaccharides conjugated to peptides containing T- and B-cell epitopes. *Infect. Immun.* 62, 785–792.

Lett, E., Klopfenstein, C., Klein, J. P., Scholler, M., Wachsmann, D. (1995). Mucosal immunogenicity of polysaccharides conjugated to a peptide or multiple-antigen peptide containing T- and B-cell epitopes. *Infect. Immun.* 63, 2645–2651.

Leyes, E. J., Smith, J. H., Lyons, S. R., Griffen, A. L. (1999). Identification of *Porphyromonas gingivalis* strains by heteroduplex analysis of a detection of multiple strains. *J Clin Microbiol* 37, 3906–3911.

Li, Y., and Caufield, P. W. (1995). The fidelity of initial acquisition of mutans streptococci by infants from their mothers. *J. Dent. Res.* 74, 681–685.

Ling, T.Y., Sims, T. J., Chen, H. A., Whitney, C., Moncla, B., Engel, L. D., and Page, R. C. (1993). Titer and subclass distribution of serum IgG antibody reactive with *Actinobacillus actinomycetemcomitans* in localized juvenile periodontitis. *J. Clin. Immunol.* 13, 100–112.

Löe, H., Anerud, A., Boysen, H., and Morrison, E. (1986). Natural history of periodontal disease in man. *J. Clin. Periodontol.* 13, 431–445.

Loesche, W. J. (1986). Role of *Streptococcus mutans* in human dental decay. *Microbiol. Rev.* 50, 353–380.

Loesche, W. J. (1988). The role of spirochetes in periodontal disease. *Adv. Dent. Res.* 2, 275–283.

Loos, B. G., Dyer, D. S., Whittam, T.S., Selander, R. K. (1993). Genetic structure of populations of *Porphyromonas gingivalis* associated with periodontitis and other oral infections. *Infect Immun* 61, 204–212.

Lundqvist, C., Baranov, V., Teglund, S., Hammerstrom, S., and Hammerstrom, M.-L. (1994). Cytokine profile and ultrastructure of intrepithelial γδ T cells in chronically inflamed human gingiva suggest a cytotoxic effector function. *J. Immunol.* 153, 2302–2312.

Ma, J. K.-C., Smith, R., and Lehner, T. (1987). Use of monoclonal antibodies in local passive immunization to prevent colonization of human teeth by *Streptococcus mutans*. *Infect. Immun.* 55, 1274–1278.

Ma, J. K., and Lehner, T. (1990). Prevention of colonization of *Streptococcus mutans* by topical application of monoclonal antibodies in human subjects. *Arch. Oral Biol.* 35 (Suppl.), 115S–122S.

McArthur, W. P., Magnusson, I., Marks, R. G., and Clark, W. B. (1989). Modulation of colonization by black-pigmented *Bacteroides* species in squirrel monkeys by immunization with *Bacteroides gingivalis*. *Infect. Immun.* 57, 2313–2317.

McGhee, J. R., and Mestecky, J. (1990). In defense of mucosal surfaces: development of novel vaccines for IgA responses protective of the portals of entry of microbial pathogens. *Infect. Dis. Clin. North Am.* 4, 315–341.

McGhee, J. R., Michalek, S. M., Webb, J., Navia, J. M., Rahman, A. F. R., and Legler, D. W. (1975). Effective immunity to dental caries: protection of gnotobiotic rats by local immunization with *Streptococcus mutans*. *J. Immunol.* 16, 300–305.

McGhee, J. R., Mestecky, J., Dertzbaugh, M. T., Eldridge, J. H., Hirasawa, M., and Kiyono, H. (1992). The mucosal immune system: from fundamental concepts to vaccine development. *Vaccine* 10, 75–88.

Menard, C., Mouton, C. (1995). Clonal diversity of the taxon *Porphyromonas gingivalis* assessed by random amplified polymorphic DNA fingerprinting. *Infect Immun* 63, 2522–2531.

Mestecky, M. T., McGhee, J. R., Arnold, R. R., Michalek, S. M., Prince, S. J., and Babb, J. L. (1978). Selective induction of an immune response in human external secretions by ingestion of bacterial antigen. *J. Clin. Invest.* 61, 731–737.

Mestecky, M. T. and McGhee, J. R. (1987). Immunoglobulin A (IgA): molecular and cellular interactions involved in IgA biosynthesis and immune response. *Adv. Immunol.* 40, 153–245.

Mestecky, J., and Eldridge, J. H. (1991). Targeting and controlled release of antigens for the effective induction of secretory antibody responses. *Curr. Opin. Immunol.* 3, 492–495.

Michalek, S. M., McGhee, J. R., Mestecky, J., Arnold, R. R., and Bozzo, L. (1976). Ingestion of *S. mutans* induces secretory IgA and caries immunity. *Science* 192, 1238–1240.

Michalek, S. M., and McGhee, J. R. (1977). Effective immunity to dental caries: passive transfer to rats of antibodies to *Streptococcus mutans* elicit protection. *Infect. Immun.* 17, 644–650.

Michalek, S. M., Gregory, R. L., Harmon, C. C., Katz, J., Richardson, G. J., Hilton, T., Filler, S. J., and McGhee, J. R. (1987). Protection of gnotobiotic rats against dental caries by passive immunization with bovine milk antibodies to *Streptococcus mutans*. *Infect. Immun.* 55, 2341–2347.

Michalek, S. M., and Childers, N. K. (1990). Development and outlook for a caries vaccine. *Crit. Rev. Biol. Med.* 1, 37–54.

Michalek, S. M., Childers, N. K., Katz, J., Dertzbaugh, M. T., Zhang, S., Russell, M. W., Macrina, F. L., Jackson, S., and Mestecky, J. (1992). Liposomes and conjugate vaccines for antigen delivery and induction of mucosal immune responses. In *Genetically Engineered Vaccines* (eds. J. E. Ciardi *et al.*). New York: Plenum, 191–198.

Michalowicz, B. S., Diehl, S. S. R., Gunsolley, J. C. *et al.* (2000). Evidence of a substantial genetic basis for risk of adult periodontitis. *J Periodontol.* 71, 1699–1707.

Miller, A. J., Brunelle, J. A., Carlos J. P., Brown, L. J., and Löe, H. (1987). Oral health of United States adults. U. S. Department Health Human Services, NIH Publication No. 87-2868. Bethesda, MD.

Moldoveanu, A., Novak, M., Huang, W. -Q., Gilley, R. M., Stass, J. K., Schafer, D., Compans, R. W., and Mestecky, J. (1993). Oral immunization with influenza virus in biodegradable microspheres. *J. Infect. Dis.* 167, 84–90.

Moore, S. (1989a). Local oral immunization with synthetic peptides induces a dual mucosal IgG and salivary IgA antibody response and prevents colonization of *S. mutans*. *Immunology* 67, 419–424.

Mooser, G., Hefta, S. A., Paxton, R. J., Shively, J. E., and Lee, T. (1991). Isolation and sequence of an active-site peptide containing a catalytic aspartic acid from two *Streptococcus sobrinus* glucosyltransferases. *J. Biol. Chem.* 266, 8916–8922.

Mosmann, T. R., and Coffman, R. L. (1989). Th1 and Th2 cells: different patterns of lymphokine secretion lead to different functional properties. *Annu. Rev. Immunol.* 7, 145–173.

Mosmann, T. R., Cherwinski, H., Bond, M. W., Giedlin, M. A., and Coffman, R. L. (1986). Two types of murine helper T cell clones. I. Definition according to profiles of lymphokine activities and secreted proteins. *J. Immunol.*, 136, 2348–2357.

Mouton, C., Hammond, P. G., Slots, J., and Genco, R. J. (1981). Serum antibodies to oral *Bacteroides asaccharolyticus* (*Bacteroides gingivalis*): Relationship to age and periodontal disease. *Infect. Immun.* 31, 182–192.

Murayama, Y., Nagai, A., Okamura, K., Kurihara, H., Nomura, Y., Kokeguchi, S., and Kato, K. (1988). Serum immunoglobulin G antibody to periodontal disease. *Adv. Dent. Res.* 2, 339–345.

National Center for Health Statistics (NCHS). (1975). *First National Health and Nutrition Examination Survey (NHANES I)*. Hyattsville, MD: NCHS, U.S. Department of Health and Human Services, Centers for Disease Control.

National Center for Health Statistics (NCHS). (1996). *Third National Health and Nutrition Examination Survey (NHANES III)*. Hyattsville, MD: NCHS, U.S. Department of Health and Human Services, Centers for Disease Control and Prevention.

Nagata, A., Man, Y.-T. Sato, M., Nakamura, R. (1991). Serological studies of *Porphyromonas* (*Bacteroides*) *gingivalis* and correlation with enzyme activity. *J Periodontal Res* 26, 184–190.

Nakai, M., Oskahashi, N., Ohta, H., and Koga, T. (1993). Saliva-binding region of *Streptococcus mutans* surface protein antigen. *Infect. Immun.* 61, 433–4349.

Nisengard, R., Blann D., Zelonis L., McHenry K., Reynolds H., Zambon J. (1989). Effects of immunization with *B. macacae* on induced periodontitis: preliminary findings. *Immunol. Invest.* 18, 225–237.

O'Brien-Simpson, N. M., Black, C. L., Bhogal, P. S., Cleal, S. M., Slakeski, N., Higgins, T. J., Reynolds, E.C. (2000a). Serum immunoglobulin G (IgG) and IgG subclass responses to the RgpA-Kgp proteinase-adhesin complex of *Porphyromonas gingivalis* in adult periodontitis. *Infect. Immun.* 68, 2704–2712.

O'Brien-Simpson, N. M., Paolini, R. A., Reynolds, E.C. (2000b). RgpA-Kgp peptide-based immunogens provide proection against *Porphyromonas gingivalis* challenge in a murine lesion model. *Infect. Immun.* 68, 4055–4063.

Ogawa, T., Shimauchi, H., and Hamada, S. (1989). Mucosal and systemic immune responses in BALB/c mice to *Bacteroides gingivalis* fimbriae administered orally. *Infect. Immun.* 57, 3466–3471.

Ogawa, T., Kusumoto, Y., Hamada, S., McGhee, J. R., and Kiyono, H. (1990). *Bacteroides gingivalis*–specific serum IgG and IgA subclass antibodies in periodontal diseases. *Clin. Exp. Immunol.* 82, 318–325.

Ogier, J. A., Scholler, M., Lepoivre, Y., Pini, A., Sommer, P., and Klein, J. P. (1990). Complete nucleotide sequence of the sr gene from *Streptococcus mutans* OMZ 175. *FEMS. Microbiol. Lett.* 68, 223–228.

Okahashi, N., Sasakawa, M., Yoshikawa, M., Hamada, S., and Koga, T. (1989). Molecular characterization of a surface protein antigen gene from serotype c *Streptococcus mutans* implicated in dental caries. *Mol. Microbiol.* 3, 673–678.

Okuda, K., Slots, J., and Genco, R. J. (1981). *Bacteroides gingivalis*, *Bacteroides asaccharolyticus*, and *Bacteroides melaninogenicus* subspecies: cell surface morphology and adherence to erythrocytes and human buccal epithelial cells. *Curr. Microbiol.* 6, 7–12.

Okuda, K., Kato, K., Naito, Y., Takazoe, I., Kikuchi, Y., Nakamura, T., Kiyoshige, T., and Sasaki, S. (1988). Protective efficacy of active and passive immunization against experimental infection with *Bacteroides gingivalis* in ligated hamster. *J. Dent. Res.* 67, 807–811.

Page, R. C., and Schroeder, H. E. (1982). *Periodontitis in Man and Other Animals: A Comparative Review*. Basel: Karger.

Page, R. C., Sims, T. J., Engel, L. D., Moncla, G. J., Bainbridge, B., Stray, J., and Darveau, R. P. (1991). The immunodominant outer membrane antigen of *Actinobacillus actinomycetemcomitans* is located in the serotype-specific high molecular mass carbohydrate moiety of lipopolysaccharide. *Infect. Immun.* 59, 3451–3462.

Page, R. C., Beck, J. D. (1997). Risk assessment for periodontal diseases. *Internatl. Dent.* J. 47, 61–87.

Page, R. C., Krall, E. A., Marin, J., Mancl, L. A., Garcia, R. I. (2002). Validity and accuracy of a risk calculator for future periodontal disease. *J. Am. Dent. Assoc.* 133, 569–576.

Parker, C. M., Cepek, K. L., Russell, G. J., Shaw, S. K., Posnett, D. N., Schwarting, R., Brenner, M. B. (1992). A family of β7 integrins on human mucosal lymphocytes. *Proc. Natl. Acad. Sci. USA* 89, 1924–1928.

Paul, A., Bagwell, C. B., and Irvin, G. I. (1994). Lymphocyte responses and cytokines. *Cell* 76, 241–251.

Persson, G. R., Engel, L. D., Whitney, C. W., Weinberg, A., Moncla, B. J., Darveau, R. P., Houston, L., Braham, P., and Page, R. C. (1994). *Macaca fascicularis* as a model in which to assess the safety and efficacy of a vaccine for periodontitis. *Oral Microbiol. Immunol.* 9, 104–111.

Pilot, T., Barmes, D. E., Leclercq, M. H., McCombie, B. J., and Infirri, J. S. (1986). Periodontal conditions in adults, 34–44 years of age: An overview of CPITN data in the WHO global oral data bank. *Commun. Dent. Oral Epidemiol.* 14, 310–312.

Pucci, M. J., Jones, K. R., Kuramitsu, H. K., and Macrina, F. L. (1987). Molecular cloning and characterization of the glucosyltransferase C gene (gtfC) from *Streptococcus mutans* LM7. *Infect. Immun.* 55, 2176–2182.

Rajapakse, P. S., O'Brien-Simpson, N. M., Slakeski, N., Hoffman, B., Reynolds, E.C. (2002). Immunization with the RgpA-Kgp proteinase-adhesin complexes of *Porphyromonas gingivalis* protects against periodontal bone loss in the rat periodontitis model. *Infect. Immun.* 70, 2480–2486.

Ranney, R. R., Yanni, N. R., Burmeister, J. A., and Tew, J. G. (1982). Relationship between attachment loss and precipitating serum antibody to *Actinobacillus actinomycetemcomitans* in adolescents and young adults having severe periodontal destruction. *J. Periodontol.* 53, 1–7.

Redman, T. K., Harmon, C. C., Lallone, R. L., and Michalek, S. M. (1995). Oral immunization with recombinant *Salmonella typhimurium* expressing surface protein antigen A of *Streptococcus sobrinus*: dose response and induction of protective humoral responses in rats. *Infect. Immun.* 63, 2004–2011.

Roitt, I., Brostoff, J., and Male, D. (1989). *Immunology*, 2nd ed. St. Louis, Missouri: Mosby, 75.

Russell, M. W. (1992). Immunization against dental caries. *Curr. Opin. Dent.* 2, 72–80.

Russell, M. W., and Lehner, T. (1978). Characterization of antigens extracted from cells and culture fluids of *Streptococcus mutans* serotype c. *Arch. Oral Biol.* 23, 7–15.

Russell, M. W., and Wu, H.-Y. (1997). Nasal-associated lymphoid tissue and mucosal vaccine development. *Muc. Immunol. Update* 5, 12–14.

Russell, R. R. B. (1979). Glucan-binding proteins of *Streptococcus mutans* serotype c. *J. Gen. Microbiol.* 112, 197–201.

Russell, R. R. B., Gilpin, M. L., Mukasa, H., and Dougan, G. (1987). Characterization of glucosyltransferase expressed from a *Streptococcus sobrinus* gene cloned in *Escherichia coli*. *J. Gen. Microbiol.* 133, 935–944.

Russell, R. R. B., Shiroza, T., Kuramitsu, H. K., and Ferretti, J. J. (1988). Homology of glucosyltransferase gene and protein sequences from *Streptococcus sobrinus* and *Streptococcus mutans*. *J. Dent. Res.* 67, 543–547.

Schenck, K., and Michaelsen, T. E. (1987). IgG subclass distribution of serum antibodies against lipopolysaccharide from *Bacteroides gingivalis* in periodontal health and disease. *Acta. Path. Microbiol. Scand.* 95, 41–46.

Schifferle, R. E., Chen, P. B., Davern, L. B., Aguirre, A., Genco, R. J., and Levine, M. J. (1993). Modification of experimental *Porphyromonas gingivalis* murine infection by immunization with a polysaccharide-protein conjugate. *Oral Microbiol. Immunol.* 8, 266–271.

Schifferle, R. E., Promsudthi, A., Elvebak, L., Wrona, C. T., Beanan, J.M. (1998). Isolation and characterization of K5 polysaccharide antigen of *Porphyromonas gingivalis* strain E20-1. *Int. J. Oral Biol.* 23, 173–180.

Schifferle, R. E., Reddy, M. S., Zambon, J. J., Genco, R. J., Levine, M. J. (1989). Characterization of a polysaccharide antigen from *Bacteroides gingivalis*. *J. Immunol.* 143, 3035–3042.

Schreiner, H. C., Sinatra K., Kaplan, J. B., Furgang, D., Kachlany, S. C., Planet, P. J., Perez, B. A., Figurski, D. H., Fine, D. H. (2003)

Tight-adherence genes of *Actinobacillus actinomycetecomitans* are required for virulence in a rat model. *Proc. Natl. Acad. Sci. USA* 100, 7295–7300.

Seymour GJ, Cole K. L., Powell R. N., Lewins E., Cripps A. W., Clancy R.L. (1985). Interleukin-2 production and bone-resorption activity *in vitro* by unstimulated lymphocytes extracted from chronically-inflamed human periodontal tissues. *Arch. Oral Biol.* 30, 481–484.

Seymour, G. J., Taubman, M. A., Eastcott, J. W., Gemmell, E., and Smith, D. J. (1997). CD29 expression on CD4+ gingival lymphocytes supports migration of activated memory T lymphocytes to diseased periodontal tissue. *Oral Microbiol. Immunol.* 12, 129–134.

Shimauchi, H., Ogawa, T., and Hamada, S. (1991). Immune response gene regulation of the humoral immune response to *Porphyromonas gingivalis* fimbriae in mice. *Immunology* 74, 362–364.

Shiroza, T., Ueda, S., and Kuramitsu, H. K. (1987). Sequence analysis of the gtfB gene from *Streptococcus mutans*. *J. Bacteriol.* 169, 4263–4270.

Sims, T. J., Schifferle, R. E., Ali, W., Skaug, N., Page, R. C. (2001). Immunoglobulin G response of periodontitis patients to *Porphyromonas gingivalis* capsular carbohydrate and lipopolysaccharide antigens. *Oral Microbiol. Immunol.* 16, 193–201.

Sjöstrom, K., Darveau, R., Page, R., Whitney, C., and Engel D. (1992). Opsonic antibody activity against *Actinobacillus actinomycetemcomitans* in patients with rapidly progressive periodontitis. *Infect. Immun.* 60, 4819–4825.

Sjöstrom, K., Ou, J., Whitney, C., Johnson, B., Darveau, R., Engel, D., and Page, R. (1994). Effect of treatment on titer, function, and antigen recognition of serum antibodies to *Actinobacillus actinomycetemcomitans* in patients with rapidly progressive periodontitis. *Infect. Immun.* 62, 145–151.

Slots, J. (1986). Bacterial specificity in adult periodontitis. A summary of recent work. *J. Clin. Periodontol.* 13, 912–917.

Smith, D. J., and Taubman, M. A. (1990). Effect of local deposition of antigen on salivary immune responses and reaccumulation of mutans streptococci. *J. Clin. Immunol.* 10, 273–281.

Smith, D. J., and Taubman, M. A. (1992). Ontogeny of immunity to oral microbiota in humans. *Crit. Rev. Oral Biol. Med.* 3, 109–133.

Smith, D. J., Taubman, M. A., and Ebersole, J. L. (1979). Effect of oral administration of glucosyltransferase antigens on experimental dental caries. *Infect. Immun.* 26, 82–89.

Smith, D. J., Taubman, M. A., and Ebersole, J. L. (1982). Effects of local immunization on colonization of hamsters by *Streptococcus mutans*. *Infect. Immun.* 37, 656–661.

Smith, D. J., Ebersole, J. L., Taubman, M. A., and Gadalla, L. (1985). Salivary IgA antibody to *Actinobacillus actinomycetemcomitans* in a young adult population. *J. Periodontal Res.* 20, 8–11.

Smith, D. J. and Taubman, M. A. (1987). Oral immunization of humans with *Streptococcus sobrinus* glucosyltransferase. *Infect. Immun.* 55, 2562–2569.

Smith, D. J., Anderson, J. M., King, W. F., van Houte, J., and Taubman, M. A. (1993a). Oral streptococcal colonization of infants. *Oral Microbiol. Immunol.* 8, 1–4.

Smith, D. J., Taubman, M. A., Holmberg, C. J., Eastcott, J., King, W. F., and Ali-Salaam, P. (1993b). Antigenicity and immunogenicity of a synthetic peptide derived from a glucan-binding domain of mutans streptococcal glucosyltransferase. *Infect. Immun.* 61, 2899–2905.

Smith, D. J., Akita, H., King, W. F., and Taubman, M. A. (1994a). Purification and antigenicity of a novel glucan binding protein of *S. mutans*. *Infect. Immun.* 62, 2545–2552.

Smith, D. J., King, W. F., Imelmann, C., Akita, H., and Taubman, M. A. (1994b). Longitudinal association of salivary IgA antibody and initial mutans streptococcal infection in children. *J. Dent. Res.* 73, 153.

Smith, D. J., Taubman, M. A., King, W. F., Eida, S., Powell, J. R., and Eastcott, J. (1994c). Immunological characteristics of a synthetic peptide associated with a catalytic domain of mutans streptococcal glucosyltransferase. *Infect. Immun.* 62, 5470–5476.

Smith, D. J., van Houte, J., Kent, R., and Taubman, M. A. (1994d). Effect of antibody in gingival crevicular fluid on early colonization of exposed root surfaces by mutans streptococci. *Oral Microbiol. Immunol.* 9, 65–69.

Smith, D. J., King, W. F., and Taubman, M. A. (1995). Synthesis, cellular distribution and immunogenicity of *S. mutans* glucan binding protein. *J. Dent. Res.* 74, 123.

Smith, D. J. and Taubman, M. A. (1996). Experimental immunization of rats with a *Streptococcus mutans* 59-kilodalton glucan-binding protein protects against dental caries. *Infect. Immun.* 64, 3069–3073.

Smith, D. J., King, W. F., Akita, H., Taubman, M. A. (1998). Association of salivary IgA antibody and initial mutans streptococcal infection. *Oral Microbiol. Immunol.* 13, 278–285.

Smith, D. J., Trantolo, D. J., King, W. F., Gusek, E. J., Fackler, P. H., Gresser, J. D., De Souza, V. L., Wise, D. L. (2000). Induction of secretory immunity with bioadhesive poly (D,L-lactide-co-glycolide) microparticles containing *Streptococcus sobrinus* glucosyltransferase. *Oral Microbiol. Immunol..* 15, 124–130.

Smith, D. J., King, W. F., Godiska R. (2001). Passive transfer of immunoglobulin Y antibody to *Streptococcus mutans* glucan binding protein B can confer protection against experimental dental caries. *Infect. Immun.* 69, 3135–3142.

Socransky, S. S., Haffajee, A. D., Cugini, M. A., *et al.* (1998). Microbial complexes in subgingival plaque. *J. Clin. Periodontol.* 25,134–144.

Stack, W. E., Taubman, M. A., Tsukuda, T., Smith, D. J., Ebersole, J. L., and Kent, R. (1990). Dental caries in congenitally athymic rats. *Oral Microbiol. Immunol.* 5, 309–314.

Stamm, J. W. (1991). The epidemiology of permanent tooth caries in the Americas. In *Risk Markers for Oral Diseases* (ed. N. W. Johnson), *Vol. 1, Dental Caries.* Cambridge, UK: Cambridge University Press, 132–155.

Stamm, J. W., Disney, J. A., Graves, R. C., Bohannan, H. M., and Abernathy, J. R. (1988). The University of North Carolina Caries Risk Assessment Study 1: Rationale and content. *J. Publ. Health Dent.* 48, 225–232.

Stoltenberg, J. L., Osborn, J. B., Pilstrom, B. C., Hardie, N. A., Aeppli, D. M., Huso, B. A., Babdash, M. B., and Fischer, G. E. (1993). Prevalence of periodontal disease in a health maintenance organization and comparisons to the national survey of oral health. *J. Periodontol.* 64, 853–858.

Takahashi, I., Okahashi, N., Matsushita, K., Tokuda, M., Kanamoto, T., Munekata, E., Russell, M. W., and Koga, T. (1991). Immunogenicity and protective effect against oral colonization by *Streptococcus mutans* of synthetic peptides of a streptococcal surface protein antigen. *J. Immunol.* 146, 332–336.

Takeichi, O., Haber, J., Kawai, T., Smith D. J., Moro, I., Taubman, M. A. (2000). Cytokine profiles of cells from gingival tissues with pathological pocketing. *J. Dent. Res.* 79, 1548–1555.

Tanaka, Y., Adams, D. H., Shaw, S. (1993). Proteoglycans on endothelial cells present adhesion-inducing cytokines to leukocytes. *Immunol. Today* 14, 111–115.

Tanner, A. C. R., Haffer, C., Brathall, G. T., Visconti, R. A., and Socransky, S. S. (1979). A study of the bacteria associated with advancing periodontitis in man. *J. Clin. Periodontol.* 6, 278–307.

Tanzer, J. M., Freedman, M. L., Fitzgerald, R. J., and Larson, R. H. (1974). Diminished virulence of glucan synthesis–defective mutants of *Streptococcus mutans*. *Infect. Immun.* 10, 197–203.

Taubman, M. A. (1973). Role of immunization in dental disease. In *Comparative Immunology of the Oral Cavity* (eds. S. E. Mergenhagen and H. W. Scherp). Washington, DC: U. S. Government Printing Office, 138–158.

Taubman, M. A., and Smith, D. J. (1974). Effects of local immunization with *Streptococcus mutans* on induction of salivary immunoglobulin A antibody experimental dental caries in rats. *Infect. Immun.* 9, 1079–1091.

Taubman, M. A., and Smith, D. J. (1977). Effects of local immunization with glucosyltransferase fractions from *Streptococcus mutans* on dental caries in rats and hamsters. *J. Immunol.* 118, 710–720.

Taubman, M. A., Ebersole, J. L., Smith, D. J. (1982a). Association between systemic and local antibody and periodontal diseases. In *Host–Parasite Interactions in Periodontal Diseases* (eds. R. J. Genco and S. E. Mergenhagen). Washington, DC: American Society for Microbiology, 283–298.

Taubman, M. A., Smith, D. J., Ebersole, J. L., and Hillman, J. D. (1982b). Immunological interference with accumulation of cariogenic microorganisms on tooth surfaces. In *Recent Advances in Mucosal Immunity* (eds. W. Strober, L. A. Hanson, and K. W. Sell). New York: Raven Press, 371–382.

Taubman, M. A., Buckelew, J. M., Ebersole, J. L., and Smith, D. J. (1983a). Periodontal bone loss in ovalbumin sensitized germfree rats fed antigen-free diet with ovalbumin. *J. Periodontal Res.* 18, 292–302.

Taubman, M. A., Yoshie, H., Wetherell, J. R., Jr., Ebersole, J. L., and Smith, D.J. (1983b). Host response in experimental periodontal disease. *J. Dent. Res.* 63, 455–460.

Taubman, M. A., Yoshie, H., Ebersole, J. L., Smith, D.J., and Olson, C. L. (1984). Host response in experimental periodontal disease. *J. Dent. Res.* 63, 455–460.

Taubman, M. A., and Smith, D. J. (1989a). A vaccine for intervention in dental infection. In *Contemporary Issues in Infectious Diseases* (eds. R.K. Root, K.S. Warren, J. McCleod Griffiss, and M.A. Sande), Vol. 8. New York: Churchill Livingstone, 99–112.

Taubman, M. A., and Smith, D. J. (1989b). Oral immunization for the prevention of dental disease. *Curr. Top. Microbiol. Immunol.* 146, 187–195.

Taubman, M. A., and Smith, D. J. (1993a). Vaccination: A cariostatic option?. In *Cariology for the Nineties* (eds. W.H. Bowen and L. A. Tabeck). Rochester, NY: University of Rochester Press, 441–457.

Taubman, M. A., and Smith, D. J. (1993b). Significance of salivary antibody in dental diseases. *Ann. N.Y. Acad. Sci.* 694, 202–215.

Taubman, M. A., Eastcott, J.W., Shimauchi, H., Takeichi, O., and Smith, D. J. (1994). Modulatory role of T lymphocytes in periodontal inflammation. In *Molecular Pathogenesis of Periodontal Disease* (eds. R. J. Genco, S. Hamada, T. Lehner, J. McGhee, and S. E. Mergenhagen). Washington, DC: American Society for Microbiology, 147–157.

Taubman, M. A., Holmberg, C. J., and Smith, D. J. (1995). Immunization of rats with synthetic peptide constructs from the glucan binding or catalytic regions of mutans streptococcal glucosyltransferase protects against dental caries. *Infect. Immun.* 63, 3088–3093.

Taubman, M. A., Kawai, T., Eastcott, J. W., Smith, D. J., Watanabe, H. (1997). Protective mechanism in periodontal diseases can be triggered by T-lymphocyte transmigration. In *Mucosal Solutions: Advances in Mucosal Immunology*, Vol. 1 (eds. A.J. Husband, K.W. Beagley, R.L. Clancy, A.M. Collins, A.W. Cripps, E.L. Emery). Sydney, Australia: University of Sydney, 205–218.

Taubman, M. A., Smith, D. J., Holmberg, C. J., Ma, B. -Y., Shafer, D., and Lees, A. (1998). Protein-polysaccharide conjugates as potential caries vaccines. *J. Dent. Res.* 77, 792.

Taubman, M.A., Smith, D.J., Holmberg, C.J., Lees, A. (1999). GTF–S. sobrinus polysaccharide conjugates as potential caries vaccines. *J. Dent. Res.* 78, 453.

Taubman, M. A., Smith, D. J., Holmberg, C. J., and Eastcott, J. W. (2000). Coimmunization with complementary glucosyltransferase peptides results in enhanced immunogenicity and protection against dental caries. *Infect. Immun.* 68, 2698–2703.

Taubman, M. A., Holmberg, C. J., and Smith, D. J. (2001). Diepitopic construct of functionally relevant complementary peptides enhances immunogenicity, reactivity with glucosyltransferase and protection against dental caries. *Infect. Immun.* 69, 4210–4216.

Taubman, M. A., Kawai, T. (2001). Involvement of T lymphocytes in periodontal disease and in direct and indirect induction of bone resorption. *Crit. Rev. Oral. Biol. Med.* 12, 125–135.

Teanpaisan, R., Douglas, C. W. I., Eley, A. R., Walsh, T. F. (1996). Clonality of *Porphyromonas gingivalis*, *Prevotella intermedia* and *Prevotella nigrescens* isolated from periodontally diseased and healthy sites. *J. Periodont. Res.* 31, 423–432.

Teng, Y. T., Nguyen, H., Gao, X., Kong, Y.Y., Gorczynski, R. M., Singh, B., Ellen, R.P., Penninger, J.M. (2000). Functional human T-cell immunity and osteoprotegerin ligand control alveolar bone destruction in periodontal infection. *J. Clin. Invest.* 106, R59–R67.

Tew, J. G., Marshall, D. R., Moore, W. E. C., Best, A. M., Palcanis, K. G., and Ranney, R. R. (1985). Serum antibody reactive with predominant organisms in the subgingival flora of young adults with generalized severe periodontitis. *Infect. Immun.* 48, 303–311.

Tokuda, M., Okahashi, I., Takahashi, M., Nakai, S., Nagoika, M., Kawagoe, M., and Koga, T. (1990). Complete nucleotide sequence of the gene for a surface protein antigen of *Streptococcus sobrinus. Infect. Immun.* 59, 3309–3312.

U.S. Department of Health and Human Services. (1989). *Oral Health of United States Children: National and Regional Findings, Public Health Service.* NIH publication no. 89-2247. Bethesda, Maryland: National Institutes of Health.

U.S. Department of Health and Human Services (2000). *Oral Health in America: A Report of the Surgeon General. Executive Summary.* Rockville, MD: U.S. Department of Health and Human Services, National Institute of Dental and Craniofacial Research, National Institutes of Health.

van Houte, J. (1976). Oral bacterial colonization: mechanisms and implications. *Microbiol. Abstr.* 1(special suppl), 3–32.

van Steenbergen, T. J. M., Kastelein, P., Touw, J. J. A., and de Graff, J. (1982). Virulence of black-pigmented *Bacteroides* strains from periodontal pockets and other sites in experimentally induced skin lesions in mice. *J. Periodontal Res.* 17, 41–49.

Vasel, D., Sims, T. J., Bainbridge, B., Houston, L., Darveau, R., and Page, R. C. (1996). Shared antigens of *Porphyromonas gingivalis* and *Bacteroides gingivalis. Oral Microbiol. Immunol.* 11, 226–235.

Vincent, J. W., Falker, W. A., Cornett, W. C., and Suzuki, J. B. (1987). Effect of periodontal therapy on specific antibody responses to suspected periodontopathogens. *J. Clin. Periodontol.* 14, 412–417.

Von Eichel–Streiber, C., Sauerborn, M., and Kuramitsu, H. K. (1992). Evidence for a modular structure of the homologous repetitive C-terminal carbohydrate-binding sites of *Clostridium difficile* toxins and *Streptococcus mutans* glucosyltransferases. *J. Bacteriol.* 174, 6707–6710.

Wachsmann, D., Klein, J. P., Scholler, M., and Frank, R. M. (1985). Local and systemic immune response to orally administered liposome-associated soluble *S. mutans* cell wall antigens. *Immunology* 54, 189–193.

Wassenaar, A., Reinhardus, C., Thepen, T., Abraham-Inpijn, L., and Kievits, F. (1995). Cloning, characterization and antigen specificity of T-lymphocyte subsets extracted from gingival tissue of chronic adult periodontitis patients. *Infect. Immun.* 63, 2147–2153.

Whitney, C., Ant, J., Moncla, B., Johnson, B., Page, R. C., and Engel, L. D. (1992). Serum immunoglobulin G antibody to *Porphyromonas gingivalis* in rapidly progressive periodontitis: titer, avidity, and subclass distribution. *Infect. Immun.* 60, 2194–2200.

Williams, R. C., and Gibbons, R. J. (1972). Inhibition of bacterial adherence by secretory immunoglobulin A: a mechanism of antigen disposal. *Science* 177, 697–9.

Wilson, M. E., and Hamilton, R. G. (1992). Immunoglobulin G subclass response of localized juvenile periodontitis patients to *Actinobacillus actinomycetemcomitans* Y4 lipopolysaccharide. *Infect. Immun.* 60, 1806–1812.

Wilson, M. E., Bronson, P. M., and Hamilton, R. G. (1995). Immunoglobulin G2 antibodies promote neutrophil killing of *Actinobacillus actinomycetemcomitans. Infect. Immun.* 63, 1070–1075.

Wilton, J. M. A., Bampton, J. L. M., Hurst, T. J., Caves, J., and Powell, J. R. (1993). Interleukin-1β and IgG subclass concentrations in

gingival crevicular fluid from patients with adult periodontitis. *Arch. Oral Biol.* 38, 55–60.

Wong, C., Hefta, S. A., Paxton, R. J., Shively, J. E., and Mooser, G. (1990). Size and subdomain architecture of the glucan-binding domain of sucrose: 3-α-D-glucosyltransferase from *Streptococcus sobrinus. Infect. Immun.* 58, 2165–2170.

Wren, B. W., Russell, R. R. B., and Tabaqchali, S. (1991). Antigenic cross-reactivity and functional inhibition by antibodies to *Clostridium difficile* toxin A, *Streptococcus mutans* glucan-binding protein, and a synthetic peptide. *Infect. Immun.* 59, 3151–3155.

Wu-Yuan, C. D, and Gill, R. E. (1992). An 87-kilodalton glucan-binding protein of *Streptococcus sobrinus* B13. *Infect. Immun.* 60, 5291–5293.

Yamashita, K., Eastcott, J. W., Taubman, M. A., Smith, D. J., and Cox, D. S. (1991). Effect of adoptive transfer of cloned *Actinobacillus actinomycetemcomitans*–specific T helper cells on periodontal disease. *Infect. Immun.* 59, 1529–1534.

Yamashita, Y., Bowen, W. H., Burne, R. A., and Kuramitsu, H. K. (1993). Role of the *Streptococcus mutans* gtf genes in caries induction in the specific-pathogen free rat model. *Infect. Immun.* 61, 3811–3817.

Yamazaki, K., Nakajima, T., Gemmell, E., Polak, B., Seymour, G. J., and Hara, K. (1994). IL-4 and IL-6-producing cells in human periodontal disease tissue. *J. Oral Pathol. Med.* 23, 347–353.

Yamazaki, K., Nakajima, T., and Hara, K. (1995). Immunohistological analysis of T cell functional subsets in chronic inflammatory periodontal diseases. *Clin. Exp. Immunol.* 99, 384–391.

Yasuda, H., Shima, N., Nakagawa, N., Yamaguchi, K., Kinosaki, M., Mochizuki, S., Tomoyasu, A., Yano, K., Goto, M., Murakami, A., Tsuda, E., Morinaga, T., Higashio, K., Udagawa, N., Takahashi, N., Suda, T. (1998). Osteoclast differentiation factor is a ligand for osteoprotegerin/osteoclastogenesis-inhibitory factor and is identical to TRANCE/RANKL. *Proc. Natl. Acad. Sci. USA* 95, 3597–3602.

Yonezawa, H., Ishihara, K., Okuda, K. (2001). Arg-gingipain A DNA vaccine induces protective immunity against infection by *Porphyromonas gingivalis* in a murine model. *Infect. Immun.* 69, 2858–2864.

Yoshie, H., Taubman, M. A., Ebersole, J. L., Smith, D. J., and Olson, C. L. (1985). Periodontal bone loss and immune characteristics of congenitally athymic and thymus cell–reconstituted athymic rats. *Infect. Immun.* 50, 403–408.

Yoshie, H., Taubman, M. A., Olson, C. L., Ebersole, J. L., and Smith, D. J. (1987). Periodontal bone loss and immune characteristics after adoptive transfer of *Actinobacillus*-sensitized T cell to rats. *J. Periodontal Res.* 22, 499–505.

Yoshimura, F., Takasawa, T., Yoneyama, M., Yamaguchi, T., Shiokawa, H., and Suzuki, T. (1985). Fimbriae from the oral anaerobe *Bacteroides gingivalis*: physical, chemical, and immunological properties. *J. Bacteriol.* 163, 730–734.

Zambon, J. J., Reynolds, H., Fisher, J. G., Shlossman, M., Dunford, R., and Genco, R. J. (1988a). Microbiological and immunological studies of adult periodontitis in patients with noninsulin-dependent diabetes mellitus. *J. Periodontol.* 59, 23–31.

Zambon, J. J., Umemoto, T., DeNardin, E., Nakazawa, F., Christersson, L. A., and Genco, R. J. (1988b). *Actinobacillus actinomycetemcomitans* in the pathogenesis of human periodontal disease. *Adv. Dent. Res.* 2, 269–274.

Abbreviations

Note: Additional abbreviations may be used and defined in the individual chapters.

A2m	IgA2 allotype marker
Ab	antibody
ADCC	antibody-dependent cell-mediated cytotoxicity
AFC	antibody-forming cell(s)
Ag	antigen
AIDS	acquired immune deficiency syndrome
APC	antigen-presenting cell(s)
ASC	antibody-secreting cell(s)
BALT	bronchus-associated lymphoid tissue
C region	constant region of Ig
CD	cluster of differentiation or Crohn's disease
cDNA	complementary DNA
CSF	colony-stimulating factor
CSR	class switch recombination
CTL	cytotoxic T lymphocyte(s)
CTLA	cytolytic T lymphocyte-associated antigen
D region	diversity region of Ig or T-cell receptor for antigen
Da	dalton(s)
DC	dendritic cell(s)
ELISA	enzyme-linked immunosorbent assay
ELISPOT	enzyme-linked immunospot
Fab	antigen-binding fragment
FACS	fluorescence-activated cell sorter
FAE	follicle-associated epithelium
FcR	Fc receptor(s)
FDC	follicular dendritic cell(s)
FITC	fluorescein isothiocyanate
GALT	gut-associated lymphoid tissue
GM-CSF	granulocyte-macrophage CSF
H chain	heavy chain
H&E	hematoxylin and eosin
HEV	high endothelial venule(s)
HIV	human immunodeficiency virus
HLA	human leukocyte antigen(s)
IBD	inflammatory bowel disease
ICAM	intercellular adhesion molecule
IEC	intestinal epithelial cell(s)
IEL	intraepithelial lymphocyte(s)
IFN	interferon
Ig	immunoglobulin
IgA1	IgA subclass 1
IgA2	IgA subclass 2

IgH	Ig heavy chain
IL	interleukin
im	intramuscular
in	intranasal
ip	intraperitoneal
J chain	joining chain of oligomeric Ig
kDa	kilodalton(s)
L chain	light chain
LFA	leukocyte (lymphocyte) function-associated antigen
LPL	lamina propria lymphocyte(s)
LPMC	lamina propria mononuclear cell(s)
LPS	lipopolysaccharide
M cell	microfold cell in mucosal epithelium
mAb	monoclonal antibody
MAdCAM	mucosal addressin-cell adhesion molecule
MALT	mucosa-associated lymphoid tissue
M-CSF	macrophage CSF
MHC	major histocompatibility complex
mIgA	monomeric IgA
MLN	mesenteric lymph node(s)
MLR	mixed leukocyte (lymphocyte) reaction
mRNA	messenger RNA
mw	molecular weight
NALT	nasopharyngeal-associated lymphoid tissue
NF	nuclear factor
NK cell	natural killer cell
p	probability
PAGE	polyacrylamide gel electrophoresis
PBL	peripheral blood lymphocyte(s) or leukocyte(s)
PBMC	peripheral blood mononuclear cell(s)
PCR	polymerase chain reaction
PE	phycoerythrin
PFU	plaque-forming unit
pIgA	polymeric IgA
pIgR	polymeric immunoglobulin receptor
PLN	peripheral lymph node(s)
PP	Peyer's patch(es)
RALT	rectal-associated lymphoid tissue
RBC	red blood cell(s)
RT-PCR	reverse transcriptase polymerase chain reaction
sc	subcutaneous

SC	secretory component	STAT	signal transducer and activator of transcription
SCID	severe combined immunodeficiency	STD	sexually transmitted disease(s)
SD	standard deviation	TCR	T-cell receptor for antigen
SDS	sodium dodecyl sulfate	TGF	transforming growth factor
SE	standard error	Th cell	T helper cell
SEM	standard error of the mean	TLR	toll-like receptor
sIg	surface Ig	TNF	tumor necrosis factor
S-IgA	secretory IgA	TNP	trinitrophenyl
S-IgM	secretory IgM	UC	ulcerative colitis
SIV	simian immunodeficiency virus	V region	variable region of Ig or T-cell receptor
SRBC	sheep red blood cell(s)	VCAM	vascular cell adhesion molecule

Index